Bronchial Asthma

Bronchial Asthma

Mechanisms and Therapeutics

Third Edition

Edited by

Earle B. Weiss, M.D.
Visiting Professor of Anesthesia, Faculty of Medicine, Harvard Medical School;
Senior Pulmonary Scientist, Department of Anesthesia Research, Brigham and
Women's Hospital, Boston

Myron Stein, M.D.
Clinical Professor of Medicine, University of California, Los Angeles, UCLA
School of Medicine, Los Angeles; Codirector, Department of Pulmonary
Medicine, Brotman Medical Center, Culver City, California

Little, Brown and Company
Boston/Toronto/London

Library of Congress Cataloging-in-Publication Data

Bronchial asthma : mechanisms and therapeutics / edited by Earle B.
    Weiss, Myron Stein.—3rd ed.
        p.   cm.
    Includes bibliographical references and index.
    ISBN 0-316-92899-2 (cloth)
    1. Asthma.   I. Weiss, Earle B., 1932–   II. Stein, Myron,
1925–
    [DNLM: 1. Asthma.   WF 553 B869]
    RC591.B75   1993
    616.2′38—dc20
    DNLM/DLC
    for Library of Congress   92-49468
                                                              CIP

Printed in the United States of America

MV-NY

Sponsoring Editor: Laurie Anello
Production Editor: Anne Holm
Copyeditors: Mary N. Babcock, Betty Notzon, and Debbie Corman
Indexer: Alexandra Nickerson
Production Supervisor: F. David Bell
Designer: F. David Bell
Cover Designer: Jill Haber

Contents

Contributing Authors   xi

Preface   xix

I. Mechanisms

1. Definition and Clinical Categorization   3
   Definition of Asthma
   J. G. Scadding
   Definition of Asthma
   Kenneth M. Moser

2. Epidemiology and Natural History   15
   Scott T. Weiss and Frank E. Speizer

3. Genetic Factors   26
   John W. Gerrard and Malcolm N. Blumenthal

4. Mechanisms of Airway Hyperresponsiveness   32
   Donald W. Cockcroft and Paul M. O'Byrne

5. Immunochemical Properties of Antigens That Cause Atopic
   Diseases   43
   Te Piao King

6. Overview of Immune-Mediated Disease: Structure,
   Function, and Regulation of the Immune Response   50
   Joseph A. Bellanti and Josef V. Kadlec

7. Advances in IgE Biology   57
   Sho Matsushita, Mark L. Richards, and David H. Katz

8. IgE Immediate Hypersensitivity   68
   Samuel C. Bukantz and Richard F. Lockey

9. Inflammation   80
   Peter J. Barnes

10. Biochemical Mediators: Histamine, 5-Hydroxytryptamine,
    Kinins, Peptide Chemotactic Factors, and
    Complement   95
    Wayne H. Anderson

11. Chemical Mediators: Leukotrienes and Eicosanoids   112
    Jonathan P. Arm and Tak H. Lee

12. Late Asthmatic Reactions   135
    Jean-Luc Malo and André Cartier

13. Immunoregulation: Role of Macrophages and
    T-Cells   147
    Dennis J. Beer and Ross E. Rocklin

14. Adrenergic Regulation   165
    Andor Szentivanyi

15. Cyclic Nucleotides   192
    Ralph P. Miech

16. Advances in Receptor Biochemistry   203
    M. Maureen Dale and Stuart J. Hirst

17. Neural Control of the Airways and Cholinergic
    Mechanisms   217
    *Ronald L. Sorkness, William J. Calhoun, and
    William W. Busse*

18. Nonadrenergic, Noncholinergic Nerves and
    Neuropeptides   232
    Peter J. Barnes

19. Role of Adenosine and Adenosine Receptors   253
    *Stephen T. Holgate, Riccardo Polosa, and
    Gerrard D. Phillips*

20. Eosinophil   258
    Andrew J. Wardlaw and A. Barry Kay

21. Mast Cell and Basophil   271
    David Lagunoff

22. Platelet-Activating Factor, Platelets, and Asthma   287
    Clive P. Page and John Morley

23. Role of Epithelium   296
    Lauri A. Laitinen, Annika Laitinen, and Carl G. A. Persson

24. Bronchoalveolar Lavage   309
    *Gianni Marone, Vincenzo Casolaro, Giuseppe Spadaro, and
    Arturo Genovese*

25. Airway Smooth Muscle: Physiology, Bronchomotor Tone,
    Pharmacology, and Relation to Asthma   314
    Newman L. Stephens and Chun Y. Seow

26. Physiology and Gas Exchange   333
    Adrian J. Williams

27. Control of Breathing   346
    David W. Hudgel

28. Pathology   352
    James C. Hogg

29. Bronchial Mucus   356
    *Maria Teresa Lopez-Vidriero, K. Ramakrishnan Bhaskar,
    and Lynne M. Reid*

30. Mucociliary Function   371
    Alejandro D. Chediak and Adam Wanner

31. Experimental Asthma in Animals   382
    Carol A. Hirshman and Hall Downes

32. Aerosols   405
    Joseph D. Brain and James D. Blanchard

33. Immune-Neuroendocrine Circuitry and Its Relation to Asthma   421
    Andor Szentivanyi

II. Diagnostics and Laboratory

34. Clinical Incitants   441
    Paul P. VanArsdel, Jr.

35. Clinical Evaluation   447
    M. Henry Williams, Jr., and Chang Shim

36. Methods of Assessing Bronchoreversibility: Site of Airway Obstruction and Bronchodilator Response   455
    Archie F. Wilson

37. Differential Diagnosis   459
    Kenneth F. MacDonnell and Henry D. Beauchamp

38. Laboratory Methods for Diagnosing Allergic Asthma   485
    Lawrence M. Du Buske, Doris S. Pennoyer, and Albert L. Sheffer

39. Bronchial Provocation Tests   501
    Sheldon L. Spector

40. Correlation Between History, Skin Test, and Inhalation Test Results in Allergic Asthma   517
    Valentin T. Popa

41. Upper Respiratory Tract   533
    Raymond G. Slavin

42. Inhalant Aerobiology and Antigens   545
    Robert W. Ausdenmoore, Michelle B. Lierl, and Thomas J. Fischer

43. Food Allergens   559
    Michael K. Farrell

44. Bacteria and Viruses in Etiology and Treatment   564
    William J. Hall and Caroline Breese Hall

45. Environmental Factors: Air Pollution, Weather, and Noxious Gases   577
    Jack D. Hackney and William S. Linn

46. Occupational Asthma   585
    Stuart M. Brooks

47. Exercise-Induced Asthma   612
    Ephraim Bar-Yishay and Simon Godfrey

48. Drug-Induced Asthma   621
    Loren W. Hunt, Jr., and Edward C. Rosenow III

49. Hypersensitivity Pneumonitis and Allergic Bronchopulmonary Aspergillosis   632
    Michael A. Ganz, Paul A. Greenberger, and Roy Patterson

50. Cough Variant Asthma   644
    Henry Milgrom

51. Wheezing   650
    Robert G. Loudon and Raymond L. H. Murphy, Jr.

52. Sputum   655
    Mauricio J. Dulfano and Sadamu Ishikawa

53. Radiography   664
    Murray L. Janower

III. Therapy and Patient Management

54. Staging Therapy to Severity   683
    L. Jack Faling and Gordon L. Snider

55. Beta-Adrenergic Agonists   700
    John W. Jenne and Donald P. Tashkin

56. Aerosol Delivery Systems   749
    Archie F. Wilson

57. Intravenous Sympathomimetic Drugs in Acute Severe Asthma   756
    Nils Svedmyr and Claes-Göran A. H. Löfdahl

58. Methylxanthines   764
    Miles M. Weinberger

59. Standards and Study Design for Asthma Drugs   784
    Richard A. Nicklas

60. Corticosteroids   800
    Kian Fan Chung, John Wiggins, and John Collins

61. Aerosol Corticosteroids   818
    John H. Toogood, Barbara H. Jennings, Jon C. Baskerville, and Neville M. Lefcoe

62. Hypothalamic-Pituitary-Adrenal Function in Asthma   842
    Roger Ellul-Micallef

63. Nonsteroidal Antiallergic Drugs   854
    Jonathan A. Bernstein and I. Leonard Bernstein

64. Anticholinergic Agents   876
    Nicholas J. Gross

65. Histamine Antagonists   884
    Richard Wood-Baker and Stephen T. Holgate

66. Lipoxygenase, Cyclooxygenase, Alternative Fatty Acids, PAF Inhibitors, Gold, Diuretics, and Alcohol   889
    Elliot Israel and Jeffrey M. Drazen

67. Troleandomycin in Corticosteroid Dependency   901
    Robert S. Zeiger and Stanley J. Szefler

68. Potent Antiinflammatory Agents   910
    Michael F. Mullarkey

69. Hydration, Humidification, and Mucokinetic Therapy   917
    Irwin Ziment

70. Immunotherapy   934
    David F. Graft and Martin D. Valentine

71. Calcium, Calcium Antagonists, and Oxyradicals   945
    Wayne H. Anderson, Francis M. Cuss, and Earle B. Weiss

72. Acute Asthma   972
    Christopher H. Fanta

73. Status Asthmaticus   985
    Nicholas S. Hill and Earle B. Weiss

74. Geriatric Considerations   1017
    James F. Morris

75. Gastroesophageal Reflux and Esophageal Dysfunction   1023
    Michael K. Farrell

76. Nocturnal Asthma   1030
Philip W. Ind, Colin T. Dollery, and Peter J. Barnes

77. Therapeutic Approaches in the Cardiac-Hypertensive-Diabetic Patient   1038
Kenneth R. Chapman and Anthony S. Rebuck

78. Cardiac Interactions, Arrhythmias, and Pathology   1045
Curtis N. Sessler, Stephen M. Ayres, and Frederick L. Glauser

79. Chronic Severe Asthma   1054
Harold S. Nelson

80. Childhood Asthma   1062
Gerard J. Canny, Desmond J. Bohn, John J. Reisman, and Henry Levison

81. Pregnancy and Menses   1085
Sin-Ming J. Chien and Sheldon Mintz

82. Preoperative and Postoperative Considerations   1099
Klaus K. Geiger and John Hedley-Whyte

83. Respiratory Therapy Modalities   1114
Steven E. Levy

84. Fiberoptic Bronchoscopy   1118
Ralph L. Kendall

85. Psychiatric Aspects   1121
Jonathan Brush and Aleksander A. Mathé

86. Exercise and Sex   1132
Stanley Sabin and Alfred I. Kaplan

87. Air Environmental Controls   1137
Thomas J. Fischer and Michelle B. Lierl

88. Inappropriate and Unusual Remedies   1145
Irwin Ziment and Myron Stein

89. Oral Hyposensitization   1152
Ralph P. Miech

90. Fatal Asthma   1154
Joseph N. Gaddy, William W. Busse, and Albert L. Sheffer

91. Complications   1167
Guy W. Soo Hoo and Silverio Santiago

92. Financial Considerations   1179
Robert N. Ross

93. Asthma and Alpha₁-Antitrypsin   1185
Charlotte R. Colp and Jack Lieberman

94. Prevention of Asthma: Education and Self-Management Programs   1188
Gustave A. Laurenzi

95. Current Overview and Unresolved Issues   1194
James E. Fish and Stephen P. Peters

Appendixes

A. Botanical Regions of the United States and Canada   1203

B. Incidence of Individual Molds in the United States   1210

C. Asthma Education Materials   1212

D. Professional and Nonprofessional Organizations for Resource Information and Educational Programs   1215

E. Summer Camps for Children   1217

F. Theophylline Toxicity: A Management Algorithm   1220

G. Guidelines for Intravenous Terbutaline Use in Status Asthmaticus   1221
Donald L. Uden

H. Guidelines for Methotrexate Use in Severe Bronchial Asthma   1222
Michael F. Mullarkey

I. Technique for Cytologic and Bacteriologic Microscopic Examination of Sputum   1223
Mauricio J. Dulfano

J. Medications Available for the Treatment of Asthma, by Class and Generic Name   1224
Steven Kozel and Mauricio J. Dulfano

Index   1235

Contributing Authors

Wayne H. Anderson, Ph.D.
Associate Director, Respiratory Clinical Research, Glaxo Inc. Research Institute, Research Triangle Park, North Carolina
10. Biochemical Mediators: Histamine, 5-Hydroxytryptamine, Kinins, Peptide Chemotactic Factors, and Complement, 71. Calcium, Calcium Antagonists, and Oxyradicals

Jonathan P. Arm, M.D.
Clinical Lecturer in Medicine, United Medical and Dental Schools of Guy's and St. Thomas's Hospitals (University of London); Honorary Senior Registrar, Department of Allergy, Guy's Hospital, London
11. Chemical Mediators: Leukotrienes and Eicosanoids

Robert W. Ausdenmoore, M.D.
Clinical Professor of Allergy and Immunology, University of Cincinnati College of Medicine; Attending Physician, Division of Allergy/Immunology, Children's Hospital Medical Center, Cincinnati
42. Inhalant Aerobiology and Antigens

Stephen M. Ayres, M.D.
Dean, School of Medicine, Medical College of Virginia, Virginia Commonwealth University, Richmond, Virginia
78. Cardiac Interactions, Arrhythmias, and Pathology

Peter J. Barnes, M.A., D.M., D.Sc., F.R.C.P.
Professor of Thoracic Medicine and Director, Department of Thoracic Medicine, National Heart and Lung Institute (University of London); Honorary Consultant Physician, Royal Brompton and National Heart Hospital, London
9. Inflammation, 18. Nonadrenergic, Noncholinergic Nerves and Neuropeptides, 76. Nocturnal Asthma

Ephraim Bar-Yishay, Ph.D.
Head, Pulmonary Function Laboratories, Hadassah University Hospitals, Jerusalem
47. Exercise-Induced Asthma

Jon C. Baskerville, Ph.D.
Manager, Statistics Laboratory, Department of Statistical and Actuarial Sciences, University of Western Ontario Faculty of Medicine, London, Ontario, Canada
61. Aerosol Corticosteroids

Henry D. Beauchamp, M.D.
Assistant Professor of Medicine, Tufts University School of Medicine; Assistant Director, Division of Pulmonary and Critical Care Medicine, St. Elizabeth's Hospital, Boston
37. Differential Diagnosis

Dennis J. Beer, M.D.
Associate Professor of Medicine, Boston University School of Medicine; Chief, Allergy Department, and Director, Medical Intensive Care Unit, The University Hospital, Boston
13. Immunoregulation: Role of Macrophages and T-Cells

Joseph A. Bellanti, M.D.
Professor of Pediatrics and Microbiology, Georgetown University School of Medicine; Director, International Center for Inter-Disciplinary Studies of Immunology, Georgetown University Hospital, Washington
6. Overview of Immune-Mediated Disease: Structure, Function, and Regulation of the Immune Response

I. Leonard Bernstein, M.D.
Clinical Professor of Medicine and Environmental Health Sciences, University of Cincinnati College of Medicine; Codirector, Allergy Research Lab and Training Program, University of Cincinnati Hospital, Cincinnati
63. Nonsteroidal Antiallergic Drugs

Jonathan A. Bernstein, M.D.
Instructor in Clinical Medicine, Division of Immunology, University of Cincinnati College of Medicine; Attending Physician, Division of Immunology, University of Cincinnati Hospital, Cincinnati
63. Nonsteroidal Antiallergic Drugs

K. Ramakrishnan Bhaskar, Ph.D.
Associate Research Professor, Department of Medicine, Boston University School of Medicine; Research Associate in Gastroenterology, The University Hospital, Boston
29. Bronchial Mucus

James D. Blanchard, M.D.
Respiratory Biology Program, Department of Environmental Health, Harvard School of Public Health, Boston
32. Aerosols

Malcolm N. Blumenthal, M.D.
Clinical Professor of Medicine/Allergy, University of Minnesota Medical School—Minneapolis; Director, Section of Allergy, The University of Minnesota Hospital and Clinic, Minneapolis
3. Genetic Factors

Desmond J. Bohn, M.B., B.Ch., F.R.C.P.(C)
Associate Professor of Anesthesiology and Pediatrics, University of Toronto Faculty of Medicine; Assistant Director, Department of Critical Care, The Hospital for Sick Children, Toronto
80. Childhood Asthma

Joseph D. Brain, S.D. in Hyg.
Drinker Professor of Environmental Physiology, Director, Respiratory Biology Program, and Chair, Department of Environmental Health, Harvard School of Public Health, Boston
32. Aerosols

Stuart M. Brooks, M.D.
Professor and Chairman, Department of Environmental and Occupational Health, University of South Florida College of Public Health, Tampa, Florida
46. Occupational Asthma

Jonathan Brush, Ph.D.
Instructor in Psychiatry, Boston University School of Medicine; Psychologist, Mental Health Department, Harvard Community Health Plan, Boston
85. Psychiatric Aspects

Samuel C. Bukantz, M.D.
Professor of Medicine and Director Emeritus, Department of Internal Medicine, Division of Allergy and Immunology, University of South Florida College of Medicine, Tampa, Florida
8. IgE Immediate Hypersensitivity

William W. Busse, M.D.
Professor of Medicine, University of Wisconsin Medical School; Head, Allergy/Clinical Immunology, University of Wisconsin Hospital and Clinics, Madison, Wisconsin
17. Neural Control of the Airways and Cholinergic Mechanisms, 90. Fatal Asthma

William J. Calhoun, M.D.
Associate Professor of Medicine, Division of Pulmonary and Critical Care Medicine, University of Pittsburgh School of Medicine; Attending Physician, Division of Pulmonary and Critical Care Medicine, Presbyterian-University Hospital, Pittsburgh
17. Neural Control of the Airways and Cholinergic Mechanisms

Gerard J. Canny, M.D., B.Ch., F.R.C.P.(C)
Associate Professor of Pediatrics, University of Toronto Faculty of Medicine; Pediatric Pulmonologist, The Hospital for Sick Children, Toronto
80. Childhood Asthma

André Cartier, M.D.
Professor of Medicine, Université de Montréal Faculty of Medicine; Chest Physician, Chest Department, Hôpital du Sacré-Coeur, Montreal
12. Late Asthmatic Reactions

Vincenzo Casolaro, M.D.
Doctoral Student, Division of Clinical Immunology and Allergy, University of Naples Federico II School of Medicine, Naples, Italy
24. Bronchoalveolar Lavage

Kenneth R. Chapman, M.D., M.Sc., F.R.C.P.(C)
Assistant Professor of Medicine, University of Toronto Faculty of Medicine; Director, Asthma Center, The Toronto Hospital, Toronto
77. Therapeutic Approaches in the Cardiac-Hypertensive-Diabetic Patient

Alejandro D. Chediak, M.D.
Assistant Professor of Medicine, Pulmonary Division, University of Miami School of Medicine, Miami; Associate Attending Physician, Pulmonary Division, Mount Sinai Medical Center, Miami Beach
30. Mucociliary Function

Sin-Ming J. Chien, M.D., Ph.D., F.R.C.P.(C)
Fellow, Division of Respirology, University of Toronto Faculty of Medicine, Toronto
81. Pregnancy and Menses

Kian Fan Chung, M.D., M.R.C.P.
Senior Lecturer in Thoracic Medicine, National Heart and Lung Institute (University of London); Honorary Consultant Physician, Royal Brompton and National Heart Hospital, London
60. Corticosteroids

Donald W. Cockcroft, M.D., F.R.C.P.(C)
Professor, Division of Respiratory Medicine, University of Saskatchewan College of Medicine; Active Staff, Division of Respiratory Medicine, Department of Medicine, Royal University Hospital, Saskatoon, Saskatchewan, Canada
4. Mechanisms of Airway Hyperresponsiveness

John Collins, M.D.
Honorary Senior Lecturer, National Heart and Lung Institute (University of London); Consultant Physician, Royal Brompton and National Heart Hospital and Westminster Hospital, London
60. Corticosteroids

Charlotte R. Colp, M.D.
Associate Clinical Professor of Medicine, Mount Sinai School of Medicine of the City University of New York; Associate Attending Physician in Medicine, Beth Israel Medical Center, New York
93. Asthma and Alpha₁-Antitrypsin

Francis M. Cuss, M.A., M.B., B.Chir., M.R.C.P.
Adjunct Associate Professor of Medicine, Jefferson Medical College of Thomas Jefferson University, Philadelphia; Vice President, Clinical Research, Schering-Plough Research Institute, Kenilworth, New Jersey
71. Calcium, Calcium Antagonists, and Oxyradicals

M. Maureen Dale, M.B., B.Ch., Ph.D.
Honorary Lecturer in Pharmacology, University College London, London
16. Advances in Receptor Biochemistry

Colin T. Dollery, F.R.C.P.
Dean, Royal Postgraduate Medical School, London
76. Nocturnal Asthma

Hall Downes, M.D., Ph.D.
Professor and Acting Chairman, Department of Pharmacology, and Associate Professor of Anesthesiology, Oregon Health Sciences University School of Medicine, Portland, Oregon
31. Experimental Asthma in Animals

Jeffrey M. Drazen, M.D.
Parker B. Francis Professor of Medicine, Harvard Medical School; Chief, Combined Program in Pulmonary/Critical Care Medicine, Beth Israel Hospital and Brigham and Women's Hospital, Boston
66. Lipoxygenase, Cyclooxygenase, Alternative Fatty Acids, PAF Inhibitors, Gold, Diuretics, and Alcohol

Lawrence M. Du Buske, M.D.
Clinical Instructor in Medicine, Harvard Medical School; Clinical Associate Attending Physician and Consultant in Allergy, Brigham and Women's Hospital, Boston
38. Laboratory Methods for Diagnosing Allergic Asthma

Mauricio J. Dulfano, M.D.
Associate Professor of Medicine, Tufts University School of Medicine; Attending Physician, Department of Medicine, St. Elizabeth's Hospital, Boston
52. Sputum, Appendix I. Technique for Cytologic and Bacteriologic Microscopic Examination of Sputum, Appendix J. Medications Available for the Treatment of Asthma, by Class and Generic Name

Roger Ellul-Micallef, M.D.(Malta), Ph.D.(Edin.), F.R.C.P.(Edin.)
Professor and Head, Department of Clinical Pharmacology and Therapeutics, University of Malta Medical School; Consultant and Clinical, Physiology Unit, St. Luke's Teaching Hospital, Msida, Malta
62. Hypothalamic-Pituitary-Adrenal Function in Asthma

L. Jack Faling, M.D.
Associate Professor of Medicine, Tufts University School of Medicine; Associate Chief of Medicine and Pulmonary Medicine, Veterans Affairs Medical Center, Boston
54. Staging Therapy to Severity

Christopher H. Fanta, M.D.
Associate Professor of Medicine, Harvard Medical School; Clinical Director, Pulmonary and Critical Care Division, Brigham and Women's Hospital, Boston
72. Acute Asthma

Michael K. Farrell, M.D.
Associate Professor of Pediatrics, University of Cincinnati College of Medicine; Associate Attending Physician, Department of Pediatrics, Children's Hospital Medical Center, Cincinnati
43. Food Allergens, 75. Gastroesophageal Reflux and Esophageal Dysfunction

Thomas J. Fischer, M.D.
Associate Professor of Pediatrics, University of Cincinnati College of Medicine; Associate Director, Division of Allergy/Immunology, Children's Hospital Medical Center, Cincinnati
42. Inhalant Aerobiology and Antigens, 87. Air Environmental Controls

James E. Fish, M.D.
Professor of Medicine, Jefferson Medical College of Thomas Jefferson University; Director, Division of Pulmonary Medicine and Critical Care, Thomas Jefferson University Hospital, Philadelphia
95. Current Overview and Unresolved Issues

Joseph N. Gaddy, M.D.
Former Assistant Professor of Medicine, Allergy Section, University of Wisconsin Medical School, Madison, Wisconsin; Private Practice, Brownsburg, Indiana
90. Fatal Asthma

Michael A. Ganz, M.D.
Attending Physician, Division of Allergy/Immunology, St. Mary's Medical Center, Racine, Wisconsin
49. Hypersensitivity Pneumonitis and Allergic Bronchopulmonary Aspergillosis

Klaus K. Geiger, M.D.
Professor of Anesthesiology, Albert-Ludwigs-Universitaet; Director, Anesthesia Department, University Hospital, Freiburg, Germany
82. Preoperative and Postoperative Considerations

Arturo Genovese, M.D.
Associate Professor of Medicine, University of Naples Federico II School of Medicine, Naples, Italy
24. Bronchoalveolar Lavage

John W. Gerrard, D.M., F.R.C.P.(L), F.R.C.P.(C)
Professor Emeritus of Paediatrics, University of Saskatchewan College of Medicine; Active Staff, Department of Paediatrics, Royal University Hospital, Saskatoon, Saskatchewan, Canada
3. Genetic Factors

Frederick L. Glauser, M.D.
Chief, Pulmonary and Critical Care Division, Medical College of Virginia and McGuire Veterans Administration Medical Center, Richmond, Virginia
78. Cardiac Interactions, Arrhythmias, and Pathology

Simon Godfrey, M.D., Ph.D., F.R.C.P.
Professor of Pediatrics, Hebrew University; Chairman, Institute of Pulmonology, Hadassah University Hospital, Jerusalem
47. Exercise-Induced Asthma

David F. Graft, M.D.
Clinical Assistant Professor of Pediatrics, University of Minnesota Medical School—Minneapolis; Chairman, Allergy Department, Park Nicollet Medical Center, Minneapolis
70. Immunotherapy

Paul A. Greenberger, M.D.
Professor of Medicine and Associate Chief, Division of Allergy-Immunology, Northwestern University Medical School; Attending Physician, Department of Medicine, Northwestern Memorial Hospital, Chicago
49. Hypersensitivity Pneumonitis and Allergic Bronchopulmonary Aspergillosis

Nicholas J. Gross, M.D., Ph.D., F.R.C.P.
Professor of Medicine and Molecular Biochemistry, Loyola University of Chicago Stritch School of Medicine, Maywood; Chief, Section of Pulmonary Diseases, Edward Hines Jr. Veterans Affairs Medical Center, Hines, Illinois
64. Anticholinergic Agents

Jack D. Hackney, M.D.
Professor of Medicine, University of Southern California School of Medicine, Los Angeles; Chief, Environmental Health Service, Rancho Los Amigos Medical Center, Downey, California
45. Environmental Factors: Air Pollution, Weather, and Noxious Gases

Caroline Breese Hall, M.D.
Professor of Pediatrics and Medicine, University of Rochester School of Medicine and Dentistry; Attending Physician, Department of Pediatrics, Strong Memorial Hospital, Rochester, New York
44. Bacteria and Viruses in Etiology and Treatment

William J. Hall, M.D.
Professor of Medicine and Pediatrics, University of Rochester School of Medicine and Dentistry; Chief, Department of Medicine, Rochester General Hospital, Rochester, New York
44. Bacteria and Viruses in Etiology and Treatment

John Hedley-Whyte, M.D.
David S. Sheridan Professor of Anaesthesia and Respiratory Therapy, Harvard Medical School, and Professor of Health Policy and Management, Harvard School of Public Health; Veterans Affairs Medical Center, Boston
82. Preoperative and Postoperative Considerations

Nicholas S. Hill, M.D.
Associate Professor of Medicine, Brown University Program in Medicine; Director, Respiratory Care Unit, Rhode Island Hospital, Providence, Rhode Island
73. Status Asthmaticus

Carol A. Hirshman, M.D.
Professor of Anesthesiology, Environmental Health Sciences, and Medicine, Johns Hopkins University School of Medicine; Attending Physician, Department of Anesthesiology, Johns Hopkins Hospital, Baltimore
31. Experimental Asthma in Animals

Stuart J. Hirst, Ph.D.
Research Fellow, Respiratory Research Laboratories, Department of Medicine, United Medical and Dental Schools of Guy's and St. Thomas's Hospitals (University of London), London
16. Advances in Receptor Biochemistry

James C. Hogg, M.D., Ph.D.
Professor of Pathology, University of British Columbia Faculty of Medicine; Director, Pulmonary Research Laboratory, St. Paul's Hospital, Vancouver, British Columbia, Canada
28. Pathology

Stephen T. Holgate, M.D., D.Sc., F.R.C.P.
MRC Clinical Professor of Immunopharmacology, University of Southampton Medical School; Honorary Consultant Physician, Southampton General Hospital, Southampton, Hampshire, England
19. Role of Adenosine and Adenosine Receptors, 65. Histamine Antagonists

David W. Hudgel, M.D.
Associate Professor of Medicine, Case Western Reserve University School of Medicine; Director, Pulmonary and Critical Care Medicine, MetroHealth Medical Center, Cleveland
27. Control of Breathing

Loren W. Hunt, Jr., M.D.
Assistant Professor of Medicine, Allergic Diseases and Internal Medicine, Mayo Medical School; Attending Physician, St. Mary's and Methodist Hospitals, Rochester, Minnesota
48. Drug-Induced Asthma

Philip W. Ind, M.A., F.R.C.P.
Senior Lecturer in Medicine, Royal Postgraduate Medical School; Consultant Physician, Respiratory Medicine, Hammersmith Hospital, London
76. Nocturnal Asthma

Sadamu Ishikawa, M.D.
Associate Professor of Medicine, Tufts University School of Medicine; Director, Pulmonary Laboratory, St. Elizabeth's Hospital, Boston
52. Sputum

Elliot Israel, M.D.
Assistant Professor of Medicine, Harvard Medical School; Medical Director, Pulmonary Function Laboratory, Division of Pulmonary and Critical Care Medicine, Beth Israel Hospital, Boston
66. Lipoxygenase, Cyclooxygenase, Alternative Fatty Acids, PAF Inhibitors, Gold, Diuretics, and Alcohol

Murray L. Janower, M.D.
Professor of Radiology, University of Massachusetts Medical School; Physician-in-Chief, Department of Radiology, St. Vincent Hospital, Inc., Worcester, Massachusetts
53. Radiography

John W. Jenne, M.D.
Professor of Medicine (Pulmonary), Loyola University of Chicago Stritch School of Medicine, Maywood; Medical Director, Department of Respiratory Therapy, Edward Hines Jr. Veterans Affairs Medical Center, Hines, Illinois
55. Beta-Adrenergic Agonists

Barbara H. Jennings, Ph.D.
Senior Clinical Research Scientist, Medical Department, Astra Pharma Inc., Mississauga, Ontario, Canada
61. Aerosol Corticosteroids

Josef V. Kadlec, M.D., Ph.D., S.J.
Associate Professor of Pediatrics and Microbiology, Immunology Center, Georgetown University School of Medicine, Washington
6. Overview of Immune-Mediated Disease: Structure, Function, and Regulation of the Immune Response

Alfred I. Kaplan, M.D., M.P.H.
Codirector, Department of Pulmonary Medicine, Metrowest Medical Center, Natick, Massachusetts
86. Exercise and Sex

David H. Katz, M.D.
President and Chief Executive Officer, Medical Biology Institute, La Jolla, California
7. Advances in IgE Biology

A. Barry Kay, M.D., Ph.D., F.R.C.P.
Professor and Director, Department of Allergy and Clinical Immunology, National Heart and Lung Institute; Honorary Consultant Physician, Royal Brompton and National Heart Hospital, London
20. Eosinophil

Ralph L. Kendall, M.D.
Assistant Professor of Medicine, University of Massachusetts Medical School, Worcester; Director, Respiratory Care Services, Veterans Affairs Medical Center, Northampton, Massachusetts
84. Fiberoptic Bronchoscopy

Te Piao King, Ph.D.
Associate Professor of Biochemistry, Rockefeller University, New York
5. Immunochemical Properties of Antigens That Cause Atopic Diseases

Steven R. Kozel, Pharm. D.
Department of Pharmacology, Brotman Medical Center, Culver City, California
Appendix J. Medications Available for the Treatment of Asthma, by Class and Generic Name

David Lagunoff, M.D.
Professor and Chairman, Department of Pathology, Saint Louis University School of Medicine; Acting Director of Laboratories, St. Louis University Hospital, St. Louis
21. Mast Cell and Basophil

Annika Laitinen, M.D.
Senior Lecturer, Department of Anatomy, University of Helsinki, Helsinki, Finland
23. Role of Epithelium

Lauri A. Laitinen, M.D., Ph.D.
Professor of Pulmonary Medicine, University of Helsinki; Head, Department of Pulmonary Medicine, University Central Hospital, Helsinki, Finland
23. Role of Epithelium

Gustave A. Laurenzi, M.D.
Clinical Professor of Medicine, Tufts University School of Medicine, Boston; Chief of Pulmonary Medicine, Newton-Wellesley Hospital, Newton Lower Falls, Massachusetts
94. Prevention of Asthma: Education and Self-Management Programs

Tak H. Lee, M.D., F.R.C.P., M.R.C.Path.
Professor of Allergy and Allied Respiratory Disorders, United Medical and Dental Schools of Guys's and St. Thomas's Hospitals, (University of London); Honorary Consultant in Allergy and Allied Respiratory Disorders, Guy's Hospital, London
11. Chemical Mediators: Leukotrienes and Eicosanoids

Neville M. Lefcoe, M.D., F.R.C.P.(C)
Professor of Medicine, University of Western Ontario Faculty of Medicine; Attending Staff, Department of Medicine, Victoria Hospital, London, Ontario, Canada
61. Aerosol Corticosteroids

Henry Levison, M.D., F.R.C.P.(C)
Professor of Pediatrics, University of Toronto Faculty of Medicine; Head, Chest Division, The Hospital for Sick Children, Toronto
80. Childhood Asthma

Steven E. Levy, M.D.
Clinical Professor of Medicine, University of California, Los Angeles, UCLA School of Medicine, Los Angeles; Codirector, Department of Pulmonary Medicine, Brotman Medical Center, Culver City, California
83. Respiratory Therapy Modalities

Jack Lieberman, M.D.
Professor of Medicine, University of California, Los Angeles, UCLA School of Medicine, Los Angeles; Director, Pulmonary Biochemistry, Department of Pulmonary and Critical Care Medicine, Veterans Affairs Medical Center, Sepulveda, California
93. Asthma and Alpha₁-Antitrypsin

Michelle B. Lierl, M.D.
Assistant Professor of Clinical Pediatrics, University of Cincinnati College of Medicine; Acting Director, Division of Allergy/Immunology, Children's Hospital Medical Center, Cincinnati
42. Inhalant Aerobiology and Antigens, 87. Air Environmental Controls

William S. Linn, M.A.
Senior Project Scientist, Environmental Health Service, Rancho Los Amigos Medical Center, Downey, California
45. Environmental Factors: Air Pollution, Weather, and Noxious Gases

Richard F. Lockey, M.D.
Professor of Medicine, Pediatrics, and Public Health, and Director, Division of Allergy and Immunology, Department of Internal Medicine, University of South Florida College of Medicine; Chief, Section of Allergy and Immunology, James A. Haley Veterans Affairs Hospital, Tampa, Florida
8. IgE Immediate Hypersensitivity

Claes-Göran A. H. Löfdahl, M.D.
Associate Professor of Pulmonary Medicine, University of Göteborg; Chief Physician, Division of Pulmonary Medicine, Renström Hospital, Göteborg, Sweden
57. Intravenous Sympathomimetic Drugs in Acute Severe Asthma

Maria Teresa Lopez-Vidriero, M.D., Ph.D.
Corporate Medical Department, Boehringer Ingelheim GmbH, Ingelheim, Rhein, Germany
29. Bronchial Mucus

Robert G. Loudon, M.B., Ch.D.
Professor of Medicine, University of Cincinnati College of Medicine; Director, Pulmonary and Critical Care Medicine, University of Cincinnati Medical Center, Cincinnati
51. Wheezing

Kenneth F. MacDonnell, M.D.
Maurice S. Segal Professor of Medicine, Tufts University School of Medicine; Chairman, Department of Medicine, St. Elizabeth's Hospital, Boston
37. Differential Diagnosis

Jean-Luc Malo, M.D.
Associate Professor of Medicine, Université de Montréal Faculty of Medicine; Chest Physician, Chest Department, Hôpital du Sacré-Coeur, Montreal
12. Late Asthmatic Reactions

Gianni Marone, M.D.
Professor of Clinical Immunology and Allergy, University of Naples Federico II School of Medicine, Naples, Italy
24. Bronchoalveolar Lavage

Aleksander A. Mathé, M.D., Ph.D.
Vice-Chair, Department of Psychiatry, Karolinska Institute; Associate to Chief Physician, St. Görans Hospital, Stockholm, Sweden
85. Psychiatric Aspects

Sho Matsushita, M.D., Ph.D.
Assistant Member, Division of Immunology, Medical Biology Institute, La Jolla, California
7. Advances in IgE Biology

Ralph P. Miech, M.D., Ph.D.
Associate Professor of Biology and Medicine, Brown University Program in Medicine, Providence; Emergency Medicine Physician, Emergency Medicine Department, Landmark Medical Center, Woonsocket, Rhode Island
15. Cyclic Nucleotides, 89. Oral Hyposensitization

Henry Milgrom, M.D.
Associate Professor of Pediatrics, University of Colorado School of Medicine; Staff Physician and Director, Ambulatory Pediatric Allergy Program, National Jewish Center for Immunology and Respiratory Medicine, Denver
50. Cough Variant Asthma

Sheldon Mintz, M.D., F.R.C.P.(C)
Associate Professor of Medicine, University of Toronto Faculty of Medicine; Chief, Respiratory Division, Women's College Hospital, Toronto
81. Pregnancy and Menses

John Morley, F.R.C.Path.
Preclinical Research and Development, Sandoz Pharmaceutical Ltd., Basel, Switzerland
22. Platelet-Activating Factor, Platelets, and Asthma

James F. Morris, M.D.
Professor of Medicine, Oregon Health Sciences University School of Medicine; Chief, Pulmonary Disease Section, Veterans Affairs Medical Center, Portland, Oregon
74. Geriatric Considerations

Kenneth M. Moser, M.D.
Professor of Medicine, University of California, San Diego, School of Medicine, La Jolla; Director, Pulmonary and Critical Care Division, University of California, San Diego, Medical Center, San Diego
1. Definition of Asthma

Michael F. Mullarkey, M.D.
Attending Physician, Department of Medicine, Swedish Hospital Medical Center, Seattle
68. Potent Antiinflammatory Agents, Appendix H. Guidelines for Methotrexate Use in Severe Bronchial Asthma

Raymond L. H. Murphy, Jr., M.D.
Professor of Medicine, Tufts University School of Medicine; Medical Director, Pulmonary Department, Faulkner and Lemuel Shattuck Hospitals, Boston
51. Wheezing

Harold S. Nelson, M.D.
Professor of Medicine, University of Colorado School of Medicine; Senior Staff Physician, Department of Medicine, National Jewish Center for Immunology and Respiratory Medicine, Denver
79. Chronic Severe Asthma

Richard A. Nicklas, M.D.
Clinical Professor of Medicine, George Washington University School of Medicine and Health Sciences, Washington; Associate Clinical Professor of Medicine, Uniformed Services University of Health Sciences, Bethesda, Maryland
59. Standards and Study Design for Asthma Drugs

Paul M. O'Byrne, M.B., F.R.C.P.(I), F.R.C.P.(C)
Associate Professor of Medicine, McMaster University School of Medicine; Head, Division of Respirology, Chedoke-McMaster Hospital, Hamilton, Ontario, Canada
4. Mechanisms of Airway Hyperresponsiveness

Clive P. Page, Ph.D.
Reader in Pharmacology, King's College, University of London, London
22. Platelet-Activating Factor, Platelets, and Asthma

Roy Patterson, M.D.
Ernest S. Bazely Professor of Medicine, Northwestern University Medical School; Chief, Division of Allergy/Immunology, Northwestern Memorial Hospital, Chicago
49. Hypersensitivity Pneumonitis and Allergic Bronchopulmonary Aspergillosis

Doris S. Pennoyer, M.D.
Attending in Internal Medicine; Maine Medical Center, Portland, Maine
38. Laboratory Methods for Diagnosing Allergic Asthma

Carl G. A. Persson, Ph.D.
Professor of Clinical Pharmacology, University of Lund, Lund, Sweden
23. Role of Epithelium

Stephen P. Peters, M.D., Ph.D.
Professor of Medicine, Jefferson Medical College of Thomas Jefferson University; Associate Director, Division of Pulmonary Medicine and Critical Care, Thomas Jefferson University Hospital, Philadelphia
95. Current Overview and Unresolved Issues

Gerrard D. Phillips
Senior Registrar in Thoracic Medicine, Royal Brompton and National Heart Hospital, and Senior Registrar in Internal Medicine, St. George's Hospital, London
19. Role of Adenosine and Adenosine Receptors

Riccardo Polosa, M.D.
Research Associate in Respiratory Medicine, University of Catania; Resident in General Medicine, Ospedale Tomaselli, Catania, Italy
19. Role of Adenosine and Adenosine Receptors

Valentin T. Popa, M.D.
Associate Clinical Professor of Medicine, University of California, Davis, School of Medicine, Sacramento, California
40. Correlation Between History, Skin Test, and Inhalation Test Results in Allergic Asthma

Anthony S. Rebuck, M.D., F.R.C.P.(C)
Professor of Medicine, University of Toronto Faculty of Medicine; Director, Asthma Centre of The Toronto Hospital, Toronto
77. Therapeutic Approaches in the Cardiac-Hypertensive-Diabetic Patient

Lynne M. Reid, M.D.
Wolbach Professor of Pathology, Harvard Medical School; Pathologist-in-Chief, Emeritus, Children's Hospital, Boston
29. Bronchial Mucus

John J. Reisman, M.D., F.R.C.P.(C)
Assistant Professor of Pediatrics, University of Toronto Faculty of Medicine; Pediatric Pulmonologist, The Hospital for Sick Children, Toronto
80. Childhood Asthma

Mark L. Richards, Ph.D.
Assistant Member, Division of Immunology, Medical Biology Institute, La Jolla, California
7. Advances in IgE Biology

Ross E. Rocklin, M.D.
Senior Associate Director of Clinical Research, Boehringer Ingelheim Pharma Inc., Ridgefield; Staff Physician, Division of Allergy, Yale-New Haven Hospital, New Haven, Connecticut
13. Immunoregulation: Role of Macrophages and T-Cells

Edward C. Rosenow III, M.D.
Arthur M. and Gladys D. Gray Professor of Medicine, Mayo Medical School; Chair, Division of Thoracic Diseases, The Mayo Clinic, Rochester, Minnesota
48. Drug-Induced Asthma

Robert N. Ross, Ph.D.
Robert N. Ross Medical/Science Writing, Brookline, Massachusetts
92. Financial Considerations

Stanley Sabin, M.D.
Assistant Clinical Professor of Medicine, Tufts University School of Medicine, Boston; Chief, Department of Pulmonary Medicine, Metrowest Medical Center, Natick, Massachusetts
86. Exercise and Sex

Silverio Santiago, M.D.
Adjunct Professor of Medicine, University of California, Los Angeles, UCLA School of Medicine; Attending Physician, Pulmonary Disease Section, Wadsworth Veterans Affairs Medical Center, Los Angeles
91. Complications

J. G. Scadding, M.D., F.R.C.P.
Emeritus Professor of Medicine, National Heart and Lung Institute (University of London); Honorary Consultant Physician, Royal Brompton and National Heart Hospital, London
1. Definition of Asthma

Chun Y. Seow, Ph.D.
Research Associate and Assistant Professor of Medicine, University of Chicago, Pritzker School of Medicine, Chicago
25. Airway Smooth Muscle: Physiology, Bronchomotor Tone, Pharmacology, and Relation to Asthma

Curtis N. Sessler, M.D.
Associate Professor of Medicine, Division of Pulmonary and Critical Care Medicine, Virginia Commonwealth University, Medical College of Virginia, School of Medicine; Director, Medical Respiratory Intensive Care Unit, Medical College of Virginia Hospitals, Richmond, Virginia
78. Cardiac Interactions, Arrhythmias, and Pathology

Albert L. Sheffer, M.D.
Clinical Professor of Medicine, Harvard Medical School; Director, Allergy Clinic, Brigham and Women's Hospital; Head, Allergy Section, New England Deaconess Hospital, Boston
38. Laboratory Methods for Diagnosing Allergic Asthma, 90. Fatal Asthma

Chang Shim, M.D.
Professor of Medicine, Albert Einstein College of Medicine of Yeshiva University; Attending Physician, Department of Medicine, Bronx Municipal Hospital Center, Bronx, New York
35. Clinical Evaluation

Raymond G. Slavin, M.D.
Professor of Internal Medicine and Microbiology, Saint Louis University School of Medicine; Director, Division of Allergy and Immunology, St. Louis University Hospital, St. Louis
41. Upper Respiratory Tract

Gordon L. Snider, M.D.
Maurice B. Strauss Professor of Medicine, Boston University School of Medicine and Tufts University School of Medicine; Chief, Medical Service, Veterans Affairs Medical Center, Boston
54. Staging Therapy to Severity

Guy W. Soo Hoo, M.D.
Assistant Clinical Professor of Medicine, University of California, Los Angeles, UCLA School of Medicine; Director, Medical Intensive Care Unit, Pulmonary and Critical Care Section, Veterans Affairs Medical Center, West Los Angeles
91. Complications

Ronald L. Sorkness, Ph.D.
Associate Scientist, Department of Medicine, University of Wisconsin Medical School, Madison, Wisconsin
17. Neural Control of the Airways and Cholinergic Mechanisms

Giuseppe Spadaro, M.D.
Clinical and Research Associate, Clinical Immunology, University of Naples Federico II School of Medicine, Naples, Italy
24. Bronchoalveolar Lavage

Sheldon L. Spector, M.D.
Clinical Associate Professor of Medicine, University of California, Los Angeles, UCLA School of Medicine; Director, Allergy Research Foundation, Los Angeles
39. Bronchial Provocation Tests

Frank E. Speizer, M.D.
Professor of Medicine, Harvard Medical School; Senior Physician; Department of Medicine, Brigham and Women's Hospital, Boston
2. Epidemiology and Natural History

Myron Stein, M.D.
Clinical Professor of Medicine, University of California, Los Angeles, UCLA School of Medicine, Los Angeles; Codirector, Department of Pulmonary Medicine, Brotman Medical Center, Culver City, California
88. Inappropriate and Unusual Remedies

Newman L. Stephens, M.D. F.R.C.P.(Eng.)
Professor of Physiology, University of Manitoba Faculty of Medicine, Winnipeg, Manitoba, Canada
25. Airway Smooth Muscle: Physiology, Bronchomotor Tone, Pharmacology, and Relation to Asthma

Nils Svedmyr, M.D., Ph.D.
Professor and Chairman of Clinical Pharmacology, Sahlgrenska University Hospital, Göteborg, Sweden
57. Intravenous Sympathomimetic Drugs in Acute Severe Asthma

Stanley J. Szefler, M.D.
Professor of Pediatrics and Pharmacology, University of Colorado School of Medicine; Director of Clinical Pharmacology, National Jewish Center for Immunology and Respiratory Medicine, Denver
67. Troleandomycin in Corticosteroid Dependency

Andor Szentivanyi, M.D., D.Sc.
Distinguished Professor of Internal Medicine, University of South Florida College of Medicine, Tampa, Florida
14. Adrenergic Regulation, 33. Immune-Neuroendocrine Circuitry and Its Relation to Asthma

Donald P. Tashkin, M.D.
Professor of Medicine, University of California, Los Angeles, UCLA School of Medicine; Attending Physician, Division of Pulmonary/Critical Care Medicine, UCLA Medical Center, Los Angeles
55. Beta-Adrenergic Agonists

John H. Toogood, M.D., F.R.C.P.
Professor of Medicine, University of Western Ontario Faculty of Medicine; Director, Allergy Clinic, Victoria Hospital, London, Ontario, Canada
61. Aerosol Corticosteroids

Donald L. Uden, Pharm.D.
Associate Professor of Pharmacy Practice, University of Minnesota Medical School—Minneapolis
G. Guidelines for Intravenous Terbutaline Use in Status Asthmaticus

Martin D. Valentine, M.D.
Professor of Medicine, Johns Hopkins University School of Medicine; Attending Physician, Department of Medicine, Johns Hopkins Hospital, Baltimore
70. Immunotherapy

Paul P. VanArsdel, Jr., M.D.
Professor of Medicine, University of Washington School of Medicine; Head, Section of Allergy, University of Washington Medical Center, Seattle
34. Clinical Incitants

Adam Wanner, M.D.
Professor of Medicine, University of Miami School of Medicine, Miami; Chief, Pulmonary Division, Mount Sinai Medical Center, Miami Beach
30. Mucociliary Function

Andrew J. Wardlaw, Ph.D., M.R.C.P.
Senior Lecturer, Department of Medicine, Leicester University Medical School; Consultant Physician, Department of Respiratory Medicine, Glenfield Hospital, Leicester, England
20. Eosinophil

Miles M. Weinberger, M.D.
Professor of Pediatrics, University of Iowa College of Medicine; Director, Allergy and Pulmonary Division, Department of Pediatrics, University of Iowa Hospitals and Clinics, Iowa City, Iowa
58. Methylxanthines

Earle B. Weiss, M.D.
Visiting Professor of Anesthesia, Faculty of Medicine, Harvard Medical School; Senior Pulmonary Scientist, Department of Anesthesia Research, Brigham and Women's Hospital, Boston
71. Calcium, Calcium Antagonists, and Oxyradicals, 73. Status Asthmaticus

Scott T. Weiss, M.D., M.S.
Associate Professor Medicine, Harvard Medical School; Associate Physician, Pulmonary and Critical Care Division, Beth Israel Hospital and Brigham and Women's Hospital, Boston
2. Epidemiology and Natural History

John Wiggins, M.D.
Senior Medical Registrar, Royal Brompton and National Heart Hospital, London
60. Corticosteroids

Adrian J. Williams, M.B., F.R.C.P.
Professor of Clinical Medicine, University of California, Los Angeles, UCLA School of Medicine; Chief, Pulmonary Division, Veterans Affairs Medical Center, West Los Angeles
26. Physiology and Gas Exchange

M. Henry Williams, Jr., M.D.
Professor of Medicine, Albert Einstein College of Medicine of Yeshiva University; Director, Pulmonary Division, Bronx Municipal Hospital Center and Weiler Hospital, Bronx, New York
35. Clinical Evaluation

Archie F. Wilson, M.D., Ph.D.
Professor of Medicine, University of California, Irvine, College of Medicine; Chief, Pulmonary and Critical Care Medicine, University of California, Irvine, Medical Center, Orange, California
36. Methods of Assessing Bronchoreversibility: Site of Airway Obstruction and Bronchodilator Response, 56. Aerosol Delivery Systems

Richard Wood-Baker, M.B., B.S.
Clinical Research Fellow, University of Southampton, Southampton, England; Attending Physician, Department of Respiratory Medicine, Sir Charles Gardner Hospital, Nedlands, Perth, Western Australia
65. Histamine Antagonists

Robert S. Zeiger, M.D., Ph.D.
Clinical Professor of Pediatrics, University of California, San Diego, School of Medicine; Chief, Department of Allergy, Kaiser Permanente Medical Center, San Diego
67. Troleandomycin in Corticosteroid Dependency

Irwin Ziment, M.D., F.R.C.P.
Professor of Medicine, University of California, Los Angeles, UCLA School of Medicine; Chief, Department of Medicine, Olive View Medical Center, Sylmar, California
69. Hydration, Humidification, and Mucokinetic Therapy, 88. Inappropriate and Unusual Remedies

Preface

Dum spiro, spero. While I breathe, I hope.

"The intensity of the conviction that a hypothesis is true has no bearing on whether it is true or not."—P. B. Medawar

Some 2200 years ago Hippocrates used the word *asthma* to describe episodic shortness of breath. Since this early characterization many aspects of the causation of asthma have been unraveled, and irrational or ineffective remedies have been abandoned. The considerable advances in basic scientific knowledge in concert with the applied disciplines have complemented more effective diagnostic approaches and therapeutic modalities. As a result, there are increased demands on the physician for greater knowledge and precision in diagnosis, prevention, and treatment—an awareness of which has guided the editors in the formulation of the third edition of *Bronchial Asthma.*

As we have previously stated, we believe that a sound acquisition of fundamental mechanisms is a prerequisite to a rational therapeutic approach. This edition expands on the exponentially increasing information base and is an entirely new book with original and completely revised chapters. The volume comprises a comprehensive presentation of fundamentals, pathophysiology, and diagnostics, an expansive therapy section, and a comprehensive bibliography in addition to other added material.

From its earlier, simpler conceptual origins asthma has emerged as an important model of the complex biochemical, immunologic, physiologic, pharmacologic, and clinical interrelationships characterizing a medical disorder. The developments in our knowledge and understanding of asthma have appropriately focused on the application of therapeutic strategies aimed at preventing, ameliorating, or reversing the process. However, the fundamental mechanism remains elusive. Perhaps of humbling importance has been the ability to ask the more incisive question. Nevertheless, the implications of current advances have become sufficiently immense that it is doubtful any single investigator or physician can master the technical background required to assimilate the multiple disparate disciplines encompassing the entire subject. Not only are the therapeutic approaches numerous and under continuous evaluation and change but the various strategic approaches based on evolving epidemiology, pharmacology, environmental control, immunotherapy, and so forth may limit one book's ability to solve the dilemma of total information and integration.

The prevalence, morbidity, mortality, and human and financial costs of asthma emphasize its continued and current importance. While precise data on incidence and mortality are difficult to obtain in the United States, the burdensome nature and economic sequelae of the illness are considerable. Further, the physician caring for the asthmatic patient has been confronted by continuously shifting concepts—for example, the issue of increased morbidity and mortality from standard beta-agonist aerosol therapy—necessitating a continued awareness and careful evaluation of information to apply in clinical practice.

As we have previously stressed, the physician caring for the patient with asthma must be a humanistic scientist, rendering clear communications and guidance to the patient and family. The physician must not only be mindful of the factual details but also be compassionate to the total needs of the patient through all phases of this frightening and potentially life-threatening disorder. It is our intent that these pages provide guidance toward a rational understanding and management of a process often unpredictable in its course and often difficult to control. Complacency has no role in our enhanced understanding of this disorder.

As editors, we have gained much from the distinguished expert colleagues who helped bring this edition to fruition. Each subject represents the professional opinion and experience of its contributing authors. We endeavored to blend each topic into an integrated whole as a balanced and accurate presentation of the current status of asthma. The book is particularly directed to pulmonologists, allergists, and advanced students; we hope it will also be of value to internists and anesthesiologists and others who are seriously interested in the problem. Given this rapidly evolving discipline, in which there is an ever-increasing reliance on factual data based on careful science, we must apologize for certain omissions or limitations in scope or subject matter, which is of necessity constrained by human and technical factors. We encourage our readers to communicate their comments to us.

In the interval since the second edition we note with sadness the passing of our coeditor and colleague Dr. Maurice S. Segal, Professor Emeritus at Tufts University School of Medicine, and contributor Dr. Peter Knapp, Professor Emeritus at Boston University School of Medicine and University Hospital.

The book is lengthy and the time frame for its completion has been long. Many individuals' contributions engendered significant commitments. The final text is a tribute to basic and clinical scientists as well as physicians who have contributed immensely to the conquest of this disorder. Publication invariably involved the effort and dedication of numerous individuals. In particular we acknowledge the valuable critiques and suggestions of the staff of Little, Brown and Company—notably, Laurie Anello, Karen Oberheim, and Anne Holm. We thank the Department of Anesthesia and Anesthesia Research Laboratories of Brigham and Women's Hospital and Harvard Medical School—notably, the late Professor and Chairman Dr. Benjamin Covino (1930–1991) for encouragement and support and Ellen Jacobson and Rachel Abrams for technical assistance. The support of the administration and medical staff of Brotman Medical Center is acknowledged. Educational grants from the following pharmaceutical firms are acknowledged: Fisons Pharmaceuticals, Rochester, New York; Lilly Research Laboratories, Eli Lilly and Company, Indianapolis, Indiana; Purdue Frederick Company, Norwalk, Connecticut; Glaxo Pharmaceuticals Inc., Research Triangle Park, North Carolina; and Ciba-Geigy Corp., Summit, New Jersey. Finally, major support was provided by the Foundation for Research in Bronchial Asthma and Related Diseases.

E.B.W.
M.S.

I   Mechanisms

Definition and Clinical Categorization

1

Definition of Asthma

J. G. Scadding

The word *asthma* has been used in the past to refer to almost any sort of difficulty in breathing, especially if it was paroxysmal or episodic. At one time the paroxysmal nocturnal dyspnea caused by incipient or actual pulmonary edema owing to left ventricular failure was called *cardiac asthma,* but this usage is obsolescent; in both medical and nonmedical discourse asthma is now generally understood to refer to a disorder of the respiratory system characterized by episodes of difficulty in breathing, usually with wheezing. These episodes can be shown to be attributable to increases in resistance to expiratory flow in intrapulmonary airways.

This brief statement is acceptable as descriptive of the necessary implications of the word *asthma* in current medical discourse, and several groups who have considered the problems of definition of chronic bronchopulmonary diseases have suggested definitions of *asthma* compatible with it. For instance, a Ciba Foundation Guest Symposium in 1958 [4] suggested:

Asthma refers to the condition of subjects with widespread narrowing of the bronchial airways, which changes in severity over short periods of time either spontaneously or under treatment, and is not due to cardiovascular disease. The clinical characteristics are abnormal breathlessness, which may be paroxysmal or persistent, wheezing, and in most cases relief by bronchodilator drugs (including corticosteroids).

The Committee on Diagnostic Standards of the American Thoracic Society [1] suggested in 1962:

Asthma is a disease characterized by an increased responsiveness of the trachea and bronchi to a variety of stimuli and manifested by widespread narrowing of the airways that changes in severity either spontaneously or as a result of therapy. The term "asthma" is not appropriate for the bronchial narrowing which results solely from widespread bronchial infection, e.g., acute or chronic bronchitis; from destructive disease of the lung e.g., pulmonary emphysema; or from cardiovascular disorders. Asthma, as here defined, may occur in subjects with other bronchopulmonary or cardiovascular diseases, but in these instances the airway obstruction is not causally related to these diseases.

Nevertheless, when such a definition was submitted for consideration to a Ciba Foundation Study Group in 1971 [5], it was rejected by some participants because they did not think it defined what they would accept as "a disease." And in 1980 Gross [10] suggested that attempts to define asthma should be abandoned, and that in research and publication this "handy shorthand label" should be replaced by ad hoc descriptions of the subjects studied.

It is evident that these difficulties are in part due to confusion about the concept "a disease." If a disease terminology is to be used in scientific discourse, its factual implications must be made manifest: The medical concept of a disease must be defined.

THE CONCEPT OF A DISEASE IN MEDICINE

Definitions are of two sorts, which Popper [22] designated *essentialist* and *methodologically nominalist.* Essentialist definitions, which seek to express intuitions about the nature of the definiendum, have no place in science, in which all necessary definitions are nominalist, being no more than statements about how words or other symbols are to be related to observable phenomena. The essentialist idea of diseases as active agents making people ill is implicit in colloquial discourse; medical education discourages but does not entirely dispel it [3]. It has been accepted uncritically by some writers on computer-assisted diagnosis, who regard differential diagnosis as the selection from "a set of possible causes (diseases)" that which is most likely to produce "an observed effect (symptom complex)" [16], or who propose to "talk of diseases as if they existed as real entities" [9].

In fact, the name of a disease may have factual implications of several different sorts. It may refer to no more than a consistent syndrome whose cause is not known or various, but whose recognition is important because study of previous cases permits prognosis, and may have discovered helpful therapeutic procedures. It may refer to the effects of a specified disorder of structure or function, correction or amelioration of which may be possible, even though its cause remains unknown. It may refer to the effects of a specified causal agent or process (etiology). Thus, the causal implications of a diagnosis in the current disease terminology vary greatly. This heterogeneity must be openly acknowledged; if it is, the names of diseases can be used in concise diagnostic statements that take causal explanation only as far as the available evidence allows, and do not carry unjustified implications [24–26, 28, 30].

This analysis leads to the following general statement: In medical discourse the name of a disease refers to the sum of the abnormal phenomena displayed by a group of living organisms in association with a specified common characteristic by which they differ from the norm for their species in a biologically disadvantageous way.

Acceptance of this general statement makes it possible to define a particular disease by specification of the common characteristic of the group of organisms ("patients" in human medicine) on the study of which its description is based. For brevity, this may be called its *defining characteristic.* The first step must be to decide, in the light of existing knowledge, from which field of study this characteristic can most usefully be drawn. Must we admit the impossibility of going beyond clinical description or syndrome? Can more precise criteria in terms of a disorder of structure or of function be adopted? Or is it possible to define in terms of causal factors? Whatever sort of criterion is adopted, definition should leave no doubt about the field of study from which the current defining characteristic of the disease is derived.

Since it cannot be assumed that a group of patients who were selected because they have a common characteristic in one field of study will be similarly distinguishable in others, a primary or simple diagnostic category should be defined in a single field of study. It is often useful to recognize categories defined in more than one field of study, constituting compound diagnostic categories. An obvious example is *pneumococcal pneumonia,* which is the intersection of two simple sets—*pneumonia* defined in morbid-anatomic terms and *pneumococcal infection* defined etiologically—and a subset of each.

AN APPROACH TO THE DEFINITION OF ASTHMA

The foregoing analysis suggests that the formulation of an acceptable and workable definition of asthma entails the following steps:

1. A survey of the sorts of patients to whom the diagnostic label asthma is customarily applied and review of established knowledge about them—clinical, functional, structural, and etiologic.
2. An attempt to discover features that are common to all these patients.
3. Selection of the most useful of these to form the basis of a formal definition.

In general a definition based on clinical description only is less useful than, and will be displaced by, one based on a specified structural abnormality or disturbance of function; and one based on etiology will tend to displace all others. If it proves convenient to define asthma as a simple diagnostic category in any field short of etiology, the possibility of recognizing within it one or more subgroups defined in other ways, especially etiologically—compound diagnostic categories—should be considered.

Survey of Patients and Review of Knowledge

To what sorts of patient is the diagnostic label asthma applied? The diagnosis of asthma would be accepted without controversy in patients who complain of feeling abnormally breathless, either in episodes with intervals of freedom or in varying degrees of severity, often with wheezing in more severe episodes, and in whom these changes can be shown to be correlated with corresponding variations in expiratory airflow resistance. In such patients a variety of stimuli, both nonspecific and specific, have been found to induce abnormal increases in airflow resistance, but the effective stimuli vary from patient to patient. Most, if not all, can be shown to respond with bronchoconstriction to various stimuli, pharmacologic, chemical, and physical, some of which have a small effect of the same sort in normal subjects. This phenomenon has been called nonspecific bronchial or airway hyperreactivity (see Chap. 4). The validity of the term *nonspecific* is doubtful, since levels of hyperreactivity to stimuli of different sorts in individual patients are poorly correlated; the stimulus to which hyperreactivity has been detected should always be specified. Hyperreactivity may be increased temporarily after acute asthmatic episodes and intercurrent respiratory infections.

More specific reactions to inhaled substances in concentrations having no effect in normal individuals can be demonstrated in some patients. Several sorts of antigen-antibody reactions that may underlie these have been identified:

1. In a large and well-recognized group the characteristic antibody is of the IgE class. In this group asthma starts typically in childhood, sometimes masquerading as bronchitis initially because the early episodes may be prolonged, and sometimes

following infantile eczema, which may persist. Many of these patients have paroxysmal rhinitis, either seasonal hay fever because of pollen hypersensitivity or perennial and attributable to hypersensitivity to other environmental dusts. Such patients belong to a group, perhaps 10 percent of the population, who have a special liability to become sensitized to a wide range of antigens as a result of the minor exposures that are inevitably encountered in everyday life and which do not affect other people. Since patients with this sort of asthma and the associated hay fever and infantile eczema frequently have family histories of similar illnesses, this liability is thought to be genetically determined and has been called *atopy.* The antibodies concerned in their asthma belong to a special class of immunoglobulin, IgE; they are present in the circulating blood and become attached to the surface of cells, where their reaction with antigen leads to release of pharmacologically active substances, causing immediate wheal-and-flare reactions in the skin tests and narrowing of lumen in the bronchi. They can be passively transferred to the skin of normal subjects (the Prausnitz-Küstner reaction). While IgE antibodies typically mediate both skin and airways reactions of rapid onset, which reach their peak in about 10 minutes and are of short duration, in some circumstances they can mediate late as well as early reactions [7, 31]; also, as noted below, they may be concerned with antibodies of other types in the pathogenesis of other later-developing reactions. Thus they may be involved in some patients whose symptoms appear at long intervals after exposure to allergens.

2. Short-term sensitizing antibody of the IgG class (STS IgG) [19] has been implicated in some individuals with specific hypersensitivities demonstrated by both skin tests and bronchial challenge [2, 21]. STS may be accompanied by IgE antibody or may be the only demonstrable antibody.

3. Several sorts of delayed reaction, in addition to that associated with IgE noted above, have been described in both bronchial challenge and skin tests in asthmatics. The most frequent of these is a dual reaction with an initial transient bronchoconstriction and wheal-and-flare skin reaction followed by a second bronchoconstrictor response starting 2 to 3 hours after challenge, reaching a maximum in about 6 hours and lasting about 24 hours, together with a skin reaction to intradermal injection consisting of an ill-defined erythematous swelling and having a similar time course. This sort of dual reaction may occur in response to certain fungal antigens, including those of *Aspergillus fumigatus,* avian proteins, and some chemical dusts and fumes. The reactions induced by *Aspergillus* antigens (see Chap. 49) have been intensively studied. The second, prolonged component seems to occur only after the initial immediate reaction. In those asthmatics sensitized to *Aspergillus* who show dual reactions, both IgE and low levels of precipitating IgG antibody are found in the serum. The immediate component of the reaction is presumably IgE mediated. The late component of the skin reaction has clinical and histologic features compatible with an immune complex–mediated Type III reaction, but immunofluorescence studies have given inconsistent results; the immunologic reaction underlying the late airway response remains undetermined. Bronchoconstrictor responses occurring 1 to 3 hours after bronchial challenge and resolving in 5 hours and others occurring at night, 12 or more hours after challenge and possibly recurring during several subsequent nights, have also been reported, but their immunologic basis, if any, has not been elucidated.

4. Exposure to certain chemical substances, ranging from thiocyanates to complex salts of platinum, may cause bronchoconstriction in some instances only or principally in persons who have been previously exposed and in whom specific bronchial hypersensitivity can be demonstrated. Several sorts of occupational asthma so caused have been described (see Chap. 46).

5. In some patients with variable breathlessness that can be correlated with changes in airflow resistance and bronchial hy-

perreactivity to nonspecific stimuli, none of the specific factors or their immunologic counterparts outlined above can be found. It may be, of course, that among them are a few in whom investigation had failed to reveal recognized factors; and it may be expected that with further study factors at present unrecognized will be discovered. If it is important to emphasize that full investigation has failed to reveal specific factors, this group of patients can be designated as having cryptogenic asthma. Among them a clinically important group can be recognized, characterized by the appearance of symptoms in adult life, many in middle age and some as late as the eighth decade; the tendency to persistence of asthma with only small variations in severity; a poor response to treatment except by corticosteroids, to which response may be striking; and in many cases considerable eosinophilia in blood and bronchial secretions.

6. Wheezy breathlessness after exercise is a common symptom in asthmatic patients. It is a prominent feature in a few, who may complain only of this symptom. This exercise-induced asthma has been extensively studied and appears to be a special example of bronchial hyperreactivity, the stimulus being cooling of the airways mainly by evaporation occasioned by the high minute volume of respiration during exercise (see Chap. 47). Patients in whom exercise induction is a prominent feature of their asthma form a heterogeneous group in other respects; the wide variations in airflow resistance to which they are liable without the special factor of exercise may or may not be attributable to identifiable antigen-antibody reactions.

7. Breathlessness owing to chronic expiratory airflow limitation is a frequent symptom, especially in populations with a high proportion of cigarette smokers and exposed to general air pollution. It is variably associated with hypersecretion of bronchial mucus (bronchial catarrh). The terminology of the resulting symptom complex is confused [30]; it is variously called chronic obstructive lung or airway disease, chronic obstructive bronchitis, or chronic bronchitis and emphysema. Fletcher and his co-workers [8] have shown in a prospective study that airflow limitation and bronchial catarrh are independent effects of smoking, and it is a reasonable assumption that a similar relation holds for general air pollution. In this symptom complex, airflow limitation may be caused by structural changes in small airways, destructive enlargement of air spaces in acini (emphysema), or combinations of these. In a few patients emphysema is the predominant or even the only demonstrable cause of airflow limitation; many of these have a genetically determined deficiency of alpha$_1$-antitrypsin, and those who are nonsmokers may have no excess of bronchial secretion. Patients of all these sorts generally show some variability in severity of airflow limitation. Such variability may be attributable to evident factors such as episodes of heavy air pollution, viral infections of the respiratory tract, or exacerbations of bacterial infection in those with bronchial catarrh. Nevertheless, a few show wide variations without evident precipitating factors. Differences of opinion may arise about whether such patients should be said to be suffering from asthma.

8. In the past, knowledge of the gross and microscopic pathology of asthma (see Chap. 28) has been gained from necropsy in patients dying in status asthmaticus, from cytology of sputum (see Chap. 52), and from bronchial biopsy studies. Frequent findings during life are eosinophilia, widely varying from patient to patient and with time, in blood and sputum, and desquamated ciliated epithelial cells, Charcot-Leyden crystals, and Curschmann's spirals in sputum. Necropsy findings in fatal status asthmaticus are striking, and similar whatever the immunologic findings during life: plugging of small airways with viscid secretion containing epithelial cells and eosinophils; extreme overinflation of the lung, involving most alveoli but with scattered groups of alveoli showing air-absorption collapse; mucous glands that are more prominent than usual; and bronchial smooth muscle that may appear hypertrophied.

More recently, bronchoalveolar lavage has provided the means of sampling cells of the immune system from airways and acini, and permitted study at the cellular level of the complex interactions between lymphocytes, polymorphonuclear cells, monocytes, and alveolar macrophages and their products leading to the release of factors mediating airway narrowing (see Chaps. 10, 11, and 13). The demonstration that cells of these sorts, which are commonly associated with inflammation, are concerned in the pathogenesis of asthma has led to the suggestion that "inflammation" should be regarded as an important feature of asthma (see Chap. 9).

Common Features

The foregoing discussion shows that the only features common to all patients to whom the term asthma is customarily applied are the clinical syndrome of episodic or variable difficulty in breathing with expiratory wheezing, and the wide variations in resistance to flow in intrapulmonary airways that can be demonstrated, both in relation to these symptoms and in response to a variety of chemical and physical stimuli.

In the past there has been a tendency to include in attempted definitions of asthma findings derived from whatever aspect of its study was attracting current interest. Thus, at one time definitions often included immunologic hypersensitivity as a necessary feature. This presented no difficulty with the sorts of patient described in the paragraphs numbered 1, 2, and 3 of the preceding section, but led to problems with those who had the clinical features of asthma but in whom attempts to demonstrate hypersensitivity failed. They could be said to be suffering from asthma only on the assumption that this failure was due either to ineffective application of tests for hypersensitivity or to deficiency in knowledge, expected to be remedied in due course, or they would have to be excluded from the category asthma, leading to the need to devise some other diagnosis for them.

When tests for bronchial hyperreactivity were first receiving attention, a tendency to introduce "nonspecific bronchial hyperreactivity" into definitions of asthma became apparent. The definition of this concept is at least as difficult as that of asthma, and in the final analysis is similarly dependent on some measure of expiratory airflow resistance; thus this amounted to no more than a proposal to substitute a long phrase for a commonly accepted word.

Although the pathologist can recognize pathognomonic changes in fatal cases of asthma, and histologic changes in the airways in less severe cases are becoming better defined, the demonstration of such changes could never be a clinically applicable defining feature. It may be suspected that the current suggestion that asthma should be regarded as an "inflammatory" disease is intended to emphasize the distinction between two sorts of therapeutic agents—pharmacologic bronchodilators acting through the autonomic nervous system and agents such as corticosteroids and cromolyn sodium whose action may be regarded as "antiinflammatory." While this may be a useful distinction in encouraging appropriate therapy, it is an undue simplification of the complex effects of these agents, and the introduction of "inflammation" as a defining characteristic of asthma would lead to the unnecessary complication that it would require the preliminary definition of "inflammation."

Selecting a Basis for Primary Definition

Thus it seems that clinical description and a specified disorder of function are the two possible bases for primary definition of asthma. As already noted, definition in clinical-descriptive or syndromal terms is generally superseded when a more objective and quantifiable basis becomes available. This is immediately evident in relation to asthma, since a clinical-descriptive definition would necessarily include as an essential feature variable or episodic dyspnea with expiratory wheezing; this could only be quantified in terms of some measure of resistance to gas flow in the airways and so would lead to this functional criterion as the most precise basis for primary definition of the nosologic category asthma.

A few examples of the way hypotheses about asthma are investigated, both clinically and experimentally, serve to show that the demonstration of wide variations in resistance to expiratory airflow is in practice accepted as the most convincing evidence of asthma. The methods required to demonstrate this can be quite simple. The clinician observing wide variations in the severity of wheezy dyspnea, associated with changes in the duration and intensity of expiratory wheeze, or diminution in severity of symptoms and signs after administration of a bronchodilator can properly deduce that there have been corresponding changes in airflow resistance, justifying a diagnosis of asthma. He or she can quantify the observations approximately by the simple procedure of measuring the forced expiratory time [14], and with simple instrumental aid by the Wright peak expiratory flow meter or by the forced expiratory spirogram. Only for special purposes are more elaborate procedures such as flow-volume loops and body plethysmography required. Exercise-induced asthma is detected by finding an increase in airway resistance after exercise. The clinical pharmacologist, investigating the effect of drugs in asthma, and the clinical immunologist, challenging the bronchi in an inhalation test with a suspected antigen, quantify their observations by some test of expiratory airflow. In the experimental study of immunologic mechanisms, of chemical mediators of hypersensitivity reactions in the bronchi, and of possible antagonists, changes either in the caliber of airways or in tissues that are concerned in determining their caliber are generally regarded as evidence of relevance to asthma. Thus both clinically and experimentally, the definition of asthma in terms of widely variable resistance to airflow is in accord with existing usage, convenient, and quantifiable in ways that are applicable to a variety of practical situations.

It remains to consider the terms of a formal statement of the definition.

PRIMARY DEFINITION OF ASTHMA

The definitions of asthma suggested at the Ciba Foundation Guest Symposium in 1958 [4] and by the American Thoracic Society [1] were principally in terms of a disorder of function. They can be simplified if the analysis of the general concept of disease suggested above is accepted, including that part relating to simple and compound diagnostic categories, and if phrases indicative of the ways in which the defining characteristics may be sought, which are not in principle part of the definition itself, are relegated to an explanatory paragraph. These considerations lead to the following primary definition of asthma as a disorder of airway function:

Asthma is a disease characterized by wide variations over short periods of time in resistance to flow in the airways of the lungs.
Hyperreactivity of the airways to bronchoconstrictor stimuli, including pharmacologic agents and a variety of nonspecific chemical and physical agents, can usually be demonstrated. In some cases, specific antigen-antibody reactions, usually to inhaled antigens, can be shown to lead to increases in airflow resistance. Diminution of increased resistance in response to bronchodilator drugs or to corticosteroids is usually demonstrable. Although asthma is characteristically episodic, it may become persistent with only minor variations; in such instances, diagnosis may be justified by indirect evidence that wide variability has been present in the past, and confirmed by later observation of the clinical course, including the response to treat-

ment, or by the finding of histologic changes known to be associated with this functional abnormality.

Those who cannot renounce essentialist ideas of diseases as causes of illness can delete "is a disease characterized by" from this definition, and replace it by "refers to the condition of individuals with symptoms arising from."

CLINICAL CATEGORIZATION OF ASTHMA

The definition of asthma as a disorder of airway function leaves open the possibility that within the category so defined, subgroups definable in other fields of study, especially etiologically, can usefully be defined and named, constituting compound diagnostic categories. Is knowledge about any of the types of patients described in the previous numbered paragraphs sufficient to lead to the definition and naming of any such categories?

To consider each of these:

1. In this group of patients, narrowing of airways is caused by antigen-antibody reactions, the antigen being encountered in the environment and usually inhaled. The external source of this causal factor can be indicated by the use of the word *extrinsic.* Those patients who belong to the atopic group, producing IgE antibody, can be categorized accurately and informatively as having *extrinsic atopic asthma.*

2. and 3. It has been suggested [20] that those patients who are not atopic and in whom asthma can be shown to be owing to reactions between environmental antigens and antibodies of types other than IgE should be categorized as having *extrinsic nonatopic asthma.* This seems a clear and unequivocal usage, provided that it is recognized to be an abbreviation of extrinsic allergic but nonatopic asthma.

4. Asthma attributable to an inhaled chemical substance should be specified as asthma due to the relevant substance.

Thus all patients of Types 1 to 4 can be placed in compound diagnostic categories referring to specified causal factors as well as to the common functional disorder, asthma. These categories are of course not mutually exclusive: There is no reason a priori why more than one causal factor should not be concerned in one patient. Where one allergen is thought especially important, it can be specified (e.g., pollen asthma).

5. Those patients who show the functional defining characteristics of asthma for which no environmental causal factor or recognized type of antigen-antibody reaction can be identified can be said to be suffering from *cryptogenic asthma.* It is likely that in a few of them investigation has failed to reveal recognized factors, but there is little reason to doubt that in most as yet unidentified pathogenetic factors are at work.

As previously mentioned briefly, a small but important group can be differentiated among patients with cryptogenic asthma on certain clinical criteria: nonseasonal incidence, possibility of onset at any age in persons who have had no previous serious respiratory symptoms, tendency to persistence with variations in severity rather than complete remission, high eosinophilia in blood and sputum (though, like eosinophilia in nearly all contexts, this is subject to wide temporal variations), and in many instances unsatisfactory response to bronchodilators but prompt response to adrenal corticosteroids. The term *intrinsic* has been used to designate this pattern of asthma. It should not be taken to imply a belief that no external precipitating agent is concerned but rather that no specific factor or antigen-antibody reaction of types currently known to be associated with asthma has been identified, together with the presumption that immunologic factors of some other sort, possibly peculiar to this group of asthmatics, will eventually be discovered. Several features suggest this possibility: These patients have eosinophilia; if they die, they show the same morbid anatomic and histopathologic changes as do patients dying with extrinsic atopic asthma, and they respond to corticosteroid treatment. Other features differentiate this group from other asthmatic patients. A few are hypersensitive to aspirin, some dangerously and some with other manifestations, such as nasal polyposis and urticaria. A higher proportion of them than of extrinsic atopic asthmatics or control groups show autoantibodies to smooth muscle [35] and among women thyroid and gastric antibodies and antinuclear factor [12]. A few patients with intrinsic asthma develop various sorts of systemic vasculitis [27], and the asthma that is prodromal to some cases of polyarteritis nodosa is of the intrinsic type [15]. Some patients with intrinsic asthma develop transient infiltrations in the lungs with high eosinophilia, pathologically an eosinophilic pneumonia but of unknown pathogenesis and radiographically often showing a curious peripheral distribution—in these respects quite different from the eosinophilic infiltrations observed in extrinsic asthmatics, which can nearly always be shown to be owing to well-defined specific reactions to the mold *Aspergillus fumigatus* [27]. These points both confirm the usefulness of delineating this group of patients on clinical-descriptive criteria and suggest that as yet unelucidated immunologic reactions may be concerned in their pathogenesis. It cannot be assumed, of course, that this group is etiologically homogeneous, but it may be hoped that with advancing knowledge one or more categories definable in terms of specific pathogenesis may be distinguishable within it.

Some patients with asthma, especially of the intrinsic group, date their liability to wheezy dyspnea from an apparent or confirmed respiratory infection of variable severity, ranging from symptoms suggestive of no more than an upper respiratory viral infection to those of a pneumonia. The role of this initial illness generally remains uncertain. Did it draw attention to asthma that had been gradually developing? Was the apparent respiratory infection really the initial phase of the patient's reaction to the unidentified factors that led to the development of asthma? If it was in fact an infection, did it in some way trigger a continuing reaction which resulted in asthma? These questions can rarely be answered with confidence, and the answers to them may not be the same for all patients; the available evidence suggests that there is no good reason to describe a separate category of "infective" asthma. In those patients who conform best to the description of intrinsic asthma, the striking response to corticosteroid treatment makes it very unlikely that infection plays any direct role in pathogenesis; although in many asthmatic patients intercurrent respiratory infections tend to be associated with exacerbations of asthma, this situation occurs in atopic and other extrinsic as well as cryptogenic groups and seems explicable most simply as a nonspecific lowering of threshold to the factors, known and unknown, causing the asthma.

6. If bronchoconstriction after exercise is an important feature in any case of asthma, the term *exercise-induced asthma* can be used if it is required to draw attention to this factor. Exercise-induced asthma alone should be taken to refer to all cases in which exercise is an important precipitating factor, without commitment to categorization in other respects. But these include some (probably the majority) that can be shown to belong to the extrinsic atopic group and some that have the features of other groups.

7. Discussion of the problems presented by the minority of patients with chronic bronchopulmonary disease with persistent airflow limitation (chronic obstructive lung disease) who show important variations in airflow resistance is facilitated by the acceptance of a methodologically nominalist approach to nosology [29]. Table 1-1 presents an outline of a scheme of diagnostic

Table 1-1. Nominalist terminology for diseases in which airflow limitation is a feature

	Defined in terms of:	*Established associations*	*Comments*
Primary categories			
{ Bronchial catarrh { Simple chronic bronchitis	Clinical description	Morbid anatomy: mucous gland hyperplasia	Pathophysiology: Gross tests show no defect, but refined tests may show increased resistance to flow in small airways
Airflow limitation, persistent	Pathophysiology	Morbid anatomy: changes in small airways and/or emphysema	Variable association with bronchial catarrh, probably from common causation by smoking and air pollution
{ Airflow limitation, variable { Asthma	Pathophysiology	Pathogenesis known in some cases. These can be placed in compound categories.	Asthma alone implies only widely variable airflow limitation. To refer particularly to cases in which, in spite of investigation, causation remains unknown, the term cryptogenic is appropriate
Emphysema	Morbid anatomy	Pathophysiology: airflow limitation, large lung volumes, defective gas transfer	Clinical: Dyspnea is leading symptom, with hypoxic, initially hypocapnic respiratory failure
Compound categories Chronic obstructive bronchitis	Components { Bronchial catarrh (clinical description) { Airflow limitation (pathophysiology)		With acceptable evidence of emphysema and/or of changes in small airways, these diagnostic terms should be used Without emphysema, leads to chronic hypercapnic respiratory failure
Alpha₁-antitrypsin–deficient emphysema	{ Emphysema (morbid anatomy) { Alpha₁-antitrypsin deficiency (biochemical genetics)		Emphysema is panacinar, affecting lower parts of lungs more than upper
Extrinsic atopic asthma Extrinsic nonatopic asthma Asthma owing to specified factor	{ Asthma (pathophysiology) { Immunology Above + specified causal factor		Morbid anatomy similar for all pathogenetic types: eosinophilia, desquamation of ciliated epithelial cells, hypertrophy of smooth muscle, mucus plugging of airways
Intrinsic asthma	{ Asthma (pathophysiology) { Exclusion of known immunologic factors { Clinical description		The term intrinsic has been applied to a special type of cryptogenic asthma characterized by certain clinical features and occasional association with cryptogenic eosinophilic pneumonia and with systemic vasculitis

Source: J. G. Scadding and G. Cumming (eds.), *Scientific Foundations of Respiratory Medicine*. London: William Heinemann Medical Books, 1981. Chap. 58. Reprinted with permission.

categories, defined according to these rules, for patients in whom airflow limitation, persistent or variable, is a feature.

Two groups may be difficult to categorize. One consists of a few patients who otherwise present the usual picture of chronic obstructive lung disease but in whom airflow limitation is found to vary rather widely without obvious cause (such as intercurrent infections or episodes of heavy air pollution) or who show an unusually good response to bronchodilators. If the observed variations attain the level chosen for the diagnosis of asthma, the additional diagnostic term asthma can be applied to such patients; the use of this term without amplification should imply no more than the observed variability in airflow resistance. It is in this context that difficulties over cases at the borderline of whatever quantitative terms are chosen for insertion into the definition most frequently arise; this problem is discussed later. In a few cases the observed variability can be attributed to specific IgE-mediated or other hypersensitivities; this results in an unequivocal additional diagnosis of extrinsic atopic or nonatopic asthma. More often the problem is whether the unknown factors underlying intrinsic asthma are contributing to airway obstruction in such patients. If a significant eosinophilia is found in the blood, the sputum, or both, and especially if, in addition, there is a considerable or even dramatic response to corticosteroid treatment, the additional diagnosis of intrinsic asthma may reasonably be made. Indeed, in some instances reassessment after such a response to treatment may lead to revision of the diagnosis.

Much less frequently a patient with bronchial hypersecretion and severe airflow limitation with little variation or response to bronchodilators or to corticosteroids is found to have blood eosinophilia as well as eosinophils and desquamated bronchiolar epithelial cells in the sputum and even at necropsy may be found to have changes in the lungs of the sorts commonly found in asthma. If there is a history of earlier episodes and the patient can be shown to be atopic, the diagnosis of extrinsic atopic asthma is generally acceptable. If there is no evidence of this sort, a diagnosis of asthma would imply that the as yet unelucidated causal factors underlying intrinsic asthma have caused the observed persistent changes in the airways; this may be thought plausible on the ground that it is a reasonable deduction that at some time the defining characteristics of asthma must have been present. Alternatively, doubt may be admitted by a descriptive label for the clinical syndrome—for example, persistent airway obstruction with bronchial hypersecretion and eosinophilia.

Both episodically in acute attacks and more persistently in chronic asthma, there may be excessive secretion of bronchial mucus (see Chaps. 29 and 52). In a population in which cigarette smoking is a socially accepted habit and which also is exposed to general air pollution, it is to be expected that asthmatic subjects will be at least as susceptible as others to the effects of these factors in causing chronic hypersecretion of bronchial mucus and/or persistent airflow limitation. It frequently happens, therefore, that in a patient with long-standing asthma who has persistent cough and expectoration, the question arises whether these symptoms are due to the same causes as the asthma, to the private and public air pollution that are recognized as the most important cause of chronic bronchial hypersecretion and persistent airflow limitation, or to both these sets of factors. In a few cases this question can be answered with some confidence. If the patient has never smoked, lives in an area of low pollution, has had no important episodes of bacterial infection, and produces mucoid sputum in which eosinophils are the predominant cells, there can be little doubt that the bronchial hypersecretion is related to the asthma. At the other extreme, if he is a heavy cigarette smoker, lives in a heavily polluted area, has had frequent episodes of bacterial infection leading to purulent sputum, and continues to have bronchitic symptoms at times when the

Table 1-2. Diagnostic features of clinical categories of asthma

	Extrinsic		Cryptogenic	
	Atopic	Nonatopic	Intrinsic	Unspecified
Resistance to flow in intrapulmonary airways				
Lability	+	+	+	+
Increased by				
Nonspecific factors	+	+	+	+
Exercise	+	+ ±	+	+ ±
Allergens	+	±	0	0
Other specific factors	0	±	0	0
Diminished by				
Bronchodilators	+	+	+ ±	+
Corticosteroids	+	+	+ ±	+
Family history (asthma, hay fever, eczema)	±	–	–	–
Associated diseases				
Eczema, especially infantile	±	–	–	–
Rhinitis, hay fever	±	–	±	–
Systemic vasculitis	0	0	±	0
Aspirin sensitivity	0	0	±	0
Eosinophilic lung infiltrations				
Owing to *Aspergillus* hypersensitivity	±	0	0	0
Of unknown cause	0	0	±	0
Skin tests to inhalant allergens				
Type I (immediate)	+	As part of dual reaction	0	0
Dual	–	±	0	0
Eosinophilia	+ ±	±	+ or + +	±
Antibodies				
IgE	+	±	0	0
STS IgG	±	?	0	0
Precipitating	–	±	0	0

+ + = prominent; + = present; ± = in some cases; – = may occur; 0 = not found; + ± = usually; ? = unknown.

asthma is well controlled, it is a reasonable inference that the bronchial hypersecretion is at least in large part attributable to causes other than those causing the asthma. Of course, most cases fall between these two extremes, and only a well-informed guess at the relative importance of these two groups of causal factors is possible.

Clinical and laboratory findings in the diagnostic categories of asthma discussed above are summarized in Table 1-2.

QUANTITATIVE TERMS IN THE DEFINITION OF ASTHMA

In the first instance the definition of any disease is in qualitative terms—a statement of the sort of deviation from the norm that characterizes a particular group of patients. When the defining characteristic has been agreed on, it is necessary to specify quantitative terms for practical application of the definition. It was largely the difficulty of obtaining agreement on a degree of variability of airway obstruction that could be accepted as characterizing asthma and on how this should be measured that led the Ciba Foundation Study Group in 1971 [5] to abandon the attempt to define asthma and instead to urge "all those who use the word 'asthma' in publications to provide as much detailed information as possible on symptoms and clinical signs . . . on tests of lung function . . . on precipitating factors, on evidence of immunological abnormalities, on bronchial hyperreactivity and, where appropriate, on anatomical changes." This sort of difficulty over quantitative factors arises no matter what qualitative characteristics are chosen to define a disease. Consideration of examples of diseases defined in terms of clinical description, anatomic abnormality, disorder of function, and etiology will illustrate this point.

The Medical Research Council definition of chronic bronchitis suggested in 1965 was in clinical-descriptive terms [18]. Definitions based on it have been widely used in epidemiologic studies. For this practical purpose quantitative terms must be inserted into the qualitative prototype. Such terms have been selected for their usefulness and convenience and should not be thought of in terms of true or false. Indeed in some studies quantitative factors differing from those originally suggested have been used; this complicates comparison of results but causes no confusion, provided the quantitative factors used in each study are clearly stated.

Aortic stenosis is defined anatomically as the disease characterized by narrowing of the aortic valve. For practical application of this definition, quantitative factors must be stated and should be chosen for their appropriateness to the context: A pathologist or a surgeon may use direct measurement of the size of the valve orifice, and the cardiologist hemodynamic measurements. No confusion should arise from the use in different studies of different quantitative factors, provided they are clearly stated and appropriate.

Hypothyroidism is defined in terms of depression of thyroid function. What magnitude of deviation from the norm of what measures of this function shall be adopted for the practical application of this definition? Quantitative factors varying in both these respects are adopted in different contexts.

Even for diseases defined etiologically, the need for similar decisions about quantitative terms to be inserted into the qualitative definition may arise. For instance, tuberculosis is defined as the disease caused by *Mycobacterium tuberculosis.* What objective findings are required for the diagnosis of a case of this disease? For various purposes different criteria may quite properly be chosen, ranging from no more than a positive tuberculin test (which itself is quantified in well-chosen but still disputable terms) for some epidemiologic studies, through this combined with radiologic evidence, up to demonstration of tubercle bacilli, again requiring specification of methods and quantitative factors.

No matter how carefully the quantitative terms to be used in the practical application of a definition are chosen, there are certain to be borderline cases about which the wise person will reserve judgment and the disputatious will argue. There are certain special difficulties in suggesting quantitative terms of general applicability in the definition of asthma.

1. The factors concerned in determining resistance to gas flow in the lungs are complex [17] (see Chap. 26). The generally available clinical tests are related to various combinations of these factors and in some circumstances may show little change, though functionally important changes have in fact occurred. For instance, during severe asthma, hyperinflation of the lungs may lead to a situation where changes in total lung capacity are a better measure of variation in expiratory airflow limitation than tests based on the forced expiratory spirogram, especially during recovery, which is reflected in diminished total lung capacity before any change in forced expiratory volumes is apparent [36, 37].

2. Airway resistance shows some variability both in normal subjects and in patients with bronchopulmonary diseases not associated with the sort of variations that characterize asthma.

For normal subjects some information is available, from studies of relatively small numbers, about the magnitude of variations in the commonly used measures of ventilatory function, including airway resistance in tests repeated after relatively long intervals [6, 33, 34], daily [11, 32], and at 4-hour intervals through the day [13]. The quantitative factors for the definition of asthma must be set at a level that exceeds the variability seen in normal subjects, but this should cause no difficulty, since these variations are relatively small.

The variations that occur in patients with bronchopulmonary disease [15] impose greater difficulty. In clinical practice the term asthma would not normally be applied unless such variations are large enough to be symptomatically or therapeutically important. It would be convenient to choose quantitative factors for use in formal studies that correlate with this clinical criterion. No confusion should arise over the use of the diagnostic term asthma in this context, provided the quantitative factors are clearly stated and it is understood that it implies no more than the observed variability unless qualified by such additional terms as extrinsic atopic, extrinsic nonatopic, and intrinsic. If it is important to emphasize that a case falls into none of these groups, the term cryptogenic is appropriate.

3. Specification of variability must refer both to magnitude of changes and to time course. A study designed to obtain information about both these aspects of variability in patients with airflow limitation, including asthma of all sorts, would be a major undertaking, requiring frequently repeated tests on a carefully constituted representative sample of a defined population. Such a study might suggest quantitative factors defining distinctive patterns of variation to correlate usefully with diagnostic categories; at present only the description "wide variations over short periods of time" can be used to specify the variability of asthma.

Because of these difficulties, it is not possible to suggest a standard procedure and set of quantitative factors appropriate to all practical applications of the qualitative definition of asthma. But this does not detract from the validity of a primary definition of asthma in terms of a disorder of function; similar difficulties over quantitative factors and over procedures by which the presence of defining characteristics can be demonstrated or inferred arise in relation to many other diseases. In scientific work the quantitative factors adopted for each study must of course be stated. In clinical practice the criterion that the variability of airflow resistance is symptomatically or therapeutically important is sufficient. If the clinician is doubtful, he or she should be content to state briefly the findings with only a tentative interpretation. They will rarely be required to do this with the large number of cases, including nearly all those classifiable as extrinsic atopic or nonatopic asthma and many of those classifiable as intrinsic, in which variations in resistance to flow in the airways of the lungs are so large and readily demonstrable that the correctness of their categorization as asthma is undoubted.

CLINICAL SEVERITY GRADING

The clinical categorization discussed above and summarized in Table 1-1 is concerned with analysis as far as possible by etiology. It is relevant to some important aspects of treatment; in those patients who can be placed in one of the extrinsic categories, avoidance of or, in rare instances, desensitization to those environmental antigens to which they have been shown to be hypersensitive may be expected to be helpful, whereas in others this approach is not applicable. The physician should be more ready to accept the need for the use of systemic corticosteroids in long-term management of intrinsic asthma, since the response is usually excellent and other forms of treatment are frequently

Table 1-3. Clinical severity of asthma

Mild	Controlled by bronchodilators and avoidance of known precipitating factors; does not interfere with normal activities
Moderate	Occasionally interferes with normal activities; requires use of systemic corticosteroids in treatment
Severe	Seriously interferes with normal activities; life-threatening episodes (status asthmaticus)

Table 1-4. Temporal course of asthma

Episodic	Episodes of wheezy dyspnea with symptom-free intervals; frequency and severity of episodes may be indicated
Persistent	Persistent symptoms with episodic exacerbations; severity both of persistent symptoms and of episodes may be indicated

Other forms of chronic bronchopulmonary disease may be present, notably bronchial hypersecretion, persistent airway obstruction, and emphysema and may be partly responsible for persistent symptoms; if so, additional diagnostic terms, as appropriate, should be added

unsatisfactory. He or she should be alerted to different sets of possible complications in extrinsic atopic and in intrinsic asthma.

All these categories are symptomatically similar and vary greatly both in severity and in time course, from rare isolated episodes to persistence with frequent exacerbations; and the management of individual episodes, from trivial wheezy attacks to life-threatening status asthmaticus, and to some extent of persistent chronic asthma is similar, whatever the etiologic category. It is therefore useful to add to the diagnostic terms set forth in Table 1-1 some reference to clinical severity and temporal course. Suitable terms are presented in Tables 1-3 and 1-4. They are descriptive, since the complex situations to which they refer cannot be summarized in any manageable set of rigid quantitative criteria. Severe asthma that persists in spite of nonintensive therapy is life-threatening and generally called status asthmaticus; quantitative criteria defining this emergency situation are discussed in Chapter 73.

REFERENCES

1. American Thoracic Society Committee on Diagnostic Standards. Definitions and classification of chronic bronchitis, asthma, and pulmonary emphysema. *Am. Rev. Respir. Dis.* 85:762, 1962.
2. Bryant, D. H., Burns, M. W., and Lazarus, L. New type of allergic asthma due to IgG reaginic antibody. *Br. Med. J.* 4:589, 1973.
3. Campbell, E. J. M., Scadding, J. G., and Roberts, R. S. The concept of disease. *Br. Med. J.* 2:757, 1979.
4. Ciba Foundation Guest Symposium. Terminology, definitions and classification of chronic pulmonary emphysema and related conditions. *Thorax* 14:286, 1959.
5. Ciba Foundation Study Group No. 38. *Identification of Asthma.* London: Churchill-Livingstone, 1971.
6. Dawson, A. Reproducibility of spirometric measurements in normal subjects. *Am. Rev. Respir. Dis.* 93:264, 1966.
7. Dolovich, J., et al. Late cutaneous allergic responses in isolated IgE-dependent reactions. *J. Allergy Clin. Immunol.* 52:38, 1973.
8. Fletcher, C. M., et al. *The Natural History of Chronic Bronchitis and Emphysema.* Oxford: Oxford University Press, 1976.
9. Good, I. J., and Card, W. I. The diagnostic process with special reference to errors. *Methods Inf. Med.* 10:176, 1971.
10. Gross, N. J. What is this thing called love?—or, defining asthma. *Am. Rev. Respir. Dis.* 121:203, 1980.
11. Guyatt, A. R., et al. Variability of plethysmographic measurements of airways resistance in man. *J. Appl. Physiol.* 22:383, 1967.
12. Hall, R., Turner-Warwick, M. T., and Doniach, D. Autoantibodies in iodide goitre and asthma. *Clin. Exp. Immunol.* 1:285, 1966.
13. Kerr, H. D. Diurnal variation of respiratory function independent of air quality. *Arch. Environ. Health.* 26:144, 1973.
14. Lal, S., Ferguson, A. D., and Campbell, E. J. M. Forced expiratory time: A simple test for airways obstruction. *Br. Med. J.* 1:814, 1964.
15. Lewinsohn, H. C., Capel, L. H., and Smart, J. Changes in forced expiratory volumes throughout the day. *Br. Med. J.* 1:462, 1960.
16. Lipkin, M. The Role of Data Processing in the Diagnostic Process. In J. A. Jacquez (ed.), *The Diagnostic Process.* Ann Arbor, Mich: Malloy Lithographing, 1964. P. 255.
17. Macklem, P. T. Airway obstruction and collateral ventilation. *Physiol. Rev.* 51:368, 1971.
18. Medical Research Council Committee on Aetiology of Chronic Bronchitis. Definition and classification of chronic bronchitis for clinical and epidemiological purposes. *Lancet.* 1:775, 1965.
19. Parish, W. E. Short-term anaphylactic antibodies in human serum. *Lancet.* 2:591, 1970.
20. Pepys, J. Hypersensitivity to inhaled organic antigens. *J. R. Coll. Physicians Lond.* 2:42, 1967.
21. Pepys, J., et al. Clinical correlations between long-term (IgE) and short-term (IgG) anaphylactic antibodies in atopic and "non-atopic" subjects with respiratory allergic disease. *Clin. Allergy.* 9:645, 1979.
22. Popper, K. R. *The Open Society and its Enemies.* London: Routledge and Kegan Paul, 1945. Vol. 2, Chap. 11.
23. Rose, G. A., and Spencer, H. Polyarteritis nodosa. *Q. J. Med.* 26:43, 1957.
24. Scadding, J. G. Principles of definition in medicine. *Lancet* 1:323, 1959.
25. Scadding, J. G. The meaning of diagnostic terms in bronchopulmonary disease. *Br. Med. J.* 2:1423, 1963.
26. Scadding, J. G. Diagnosis: The clinician and the computer. *Lancet.* 2:877, 1967.
27. Scadding, J. G. Eosinophilic infiltrations of the lungs in asthmatics. *Proc. R. Soc. Med.* 64:381, 1971.
28. Scadding, J. G. The semantics of medical diagnosis. *Biomed. Computing.* 3:83, 1972.
29. Scadding, J. G. Talking Clearly About Broncho-Pulmonary Disease. In J. G. Scadding and G. Cumming (eds.), *Scientific Foundations of Respiratory Medicine.* Philadelphia: Saunders, 1981. P. 727.
30. Scadding, J. G. Health and disease: What can medicine do for philosophy? *J. Med. Ethics.* 12:118, 1988.
31. Solley, G. O., et al. The late phase of the immediate wheal and flare skin reaction: Its dependence upon IgE antibodies. *J. Clin. Invest.* 58:408, 1967.
32. Spicer, W. S., Jr., and Kerr, H. D. Variation of respiratory function: Studies on patients and normal subjects. *Arch. Environ. Health.* 12:217, 1966.
33. Spicer, W. S., Jr., and Kerr, H. D. Effects of environment on respiratory function: III. Weekly studies on young male adults. *Arch. Environ. Health.* 21:635, 1970.
34. Spodnik, M. J., Jr., et al. Effects of environment on respiratory function: Weekly studies on young male adults. *Arch. Environ. Health.* 13:243, 1966.
35. Turner-Warwick, M., and Haslam, P. Smooth muscle antibody in bronchial asthma. *Clin. Exp. Immunol.* 7:31, 1970.
36. Woolcock, A. J., and Read, J. Lung volumes in exacerbations of asthma. *Am. J. Med.* 41:259, 1966.
37. Woolcock, A. J., et al. Lung volume changes in asthma measured concurrently by two methods. *Am. Rev. Respir. Dis.* 104:703, 1971.

Definition of Asthma

Kenneth M. Moser

Trying to develop adequate definitions in medicine is a somewhat hazardous undertaking. This is particularly true when the entity to be defined is asthma, where the importance of *perspective* (from the molecular biology laboratory to the bedside) is vital.

There is an obvious need for definitions. There must be some consensus as to what asthma is. Without such consensus—at least at one point in time—investigations are not possible. One must define what one is studying as precisely as possible. Without such characterization, no investigative report regarding asthma can be interpreted.

Yet, despite such needs, the definition of asthma presents significant difficulties. Several international conferences have considered the definition of asthma and have attempted to provide documents that express a consensus view [3–5]. The American Thoracic Society also has provided a definition [27]: "Asthma is a clinical syndrome characterized by increased responsiveness of the tracheobronchial tree to a variety of stimuli." That basic definition then is expanded to include major symptoms (variable paroxysms of dyspnea, wheezing, and cough), primary physiologic abnormalities (airway obstruction), and histologic changes (eosinophilic bronchitis).

Examination of these attempts by experts to define asthma focuses on the central obstacle that asthma is not a disease but a syndrome. Attempts to develop a unitary description acceptable to all are limited because a unitarian identification of a single pathogenetic mechanism or clinical picture that is applicable to all patients appears not possible. As Professor Scadding indicates in his section of this chapter, the matter of definition depends heavily on one's perspective. A review of his erudite commentary here and in his other writings [21–23] regarding medical definitions is recommended to readers who might undertake the task of definition. Asthma poses special definition challenges, but seekers after truth about "what asthma is" ultimately must face the reality that there are no absolutes; rather, there are a variety of truths.

This unfortunately ill-defined situation is simply a reflection of the one accepted fact about asthma; namely, that airway dysfunction appears to be the final expressive pathway of a number of inciting events—some recognized and some obscure, some persistent and some transient. The clinician recognizes this inevitable variability because it is obvious that airway dysfunction can arise in multiple contexts, as discussed in detail in this text: after exposure to defined allergens or irritants in the workplace or elsewhere [14]; following ingestion of certain drugs; after viral or other respiratory infections [7]; during exercise [9]; and as a component of other chronic lung diseases such as chronic bronchitis [16], emphysema, and interstitial pneumonitis. In each context, a genetic predisposition may or may not be present. The clinician also is aware of the widely varying presentations and courses that asthmatic patients can offer—from mild cough to life-threatening respiratory failure, from a brief self-limited episode to a chronic, lifetime problem that resists intensive therapy.

And lastly, the clinician recognizes the variable response to therapy, despite the steadily expanding options available. Immunotherapy has a long and controversial history [8]; the same is true for methylxanthines, whose therapeutic value, in the judgement of various authors, still ranges from advocacy to rejection [10] (see also Chaps. 58 and 95). Beta agonists, cromolyn, corticosteroids, and anticholinergics—all in a variety of formulations—are potential therapeutic agents. And in development are many new agents, targeted on a variety of putative mediators of airway dysfunction [1, 13, 26, 29]. The clinician deals with this welter of variables as well as he or she can, further recognizing that patient education may be as vital a component of successful management as is any therapeutic agent.

The clinician must also remain ever alert to the fact that the "classic" symptoms of asthma may actually represent the symptoms of multiple other disorders ranging from left ventricular failure through pulmonary vascular diseases to a number of systemic disorders that can cause cough, wheezing, and episodic dyspnea. These other diagnostic candidates, detailed in Chapter 37, must be carefully excluded before a "primary" problem (asthma) with airways emerges as the most appropriate classification. The potential for such diagnostic errors is substantial. Errors evoke diagnostic delay and inappropriate therapy. Mitral stenosis and lymphangitic carcinoma, for example, do not respond well to intensive asthma therapy; indeed, such therapy may be harmful. Thus, the physician must remain cautious, excluding many other bases for episodic breathlessness and wheezing before a definitive diagnosis is concluded.

Given these considerations, the clinician often enlists the assistance of the physiology laboratory in an effort to confirm the clinical diagnosis and optimize management. Here, again, variability confounds those involved. The modern pulmonary physiology laboratory offers a wide variety of studies. These include standard spirometry (before and after various bronchodilator maneuvers), exercise-related spirometry, methacholine challenges, challenges with putative allergens or occupational materials, arterial blood gas analysis, and such other tests as carbon monoxide transfer as detailed in subsequent sections of this text. Selecting the optimal test(s) and test protocols is not easy and requires close clinician-laboratory interaction, as well as reliance on a laboratory that has established careful quality control and standardization technique. A major contribution of the laboratory is to identify those patients whose airways are functioning *normally* (therefore, either the asthma is in remission or an alternative diagnosis should be sought) and those with coexistent lung disease (e.g., interstitial pneumonitis, emphysema).

The clinician may also enlist the assistance of the pathologist. In the past, pathology information was usually limited to autopsy and/or cytology data. Now, however, the clinician can opt for analyses of bronchial and lung biopsy specimens and bronchoalveolar lavage fluid [2] (see Chaps. 24 and 28). Such approaches are useful in ruling out competing diagnoses, but their ability to provide findings characteristic of asthma remains limited. The results of such studies are of great investigative interest, but their current value to the clinician (except in exclusion of other entities) remains uncertain.

However, despite these diagnostic and definition constraints, one major new theme about asthma has emerged clearly in recent years. In the past, reversible or episodic *bronchospasm* was central in the approach to asthma. Now, airway inflammation has achieved at least equal consideration [20] (see Chap. 9). Indeed, the medical emphasis appears to have swung to *airway inflammation* as the dominant concern, with bronchospasm a parallel process. Whatever the final consensus, it is clear that airway inflammation and bronchospasm always have been intrinsic to and interactive in the asthma process and, hence, therapeutic attention must be directed toward both factors.

The other prominent development in our efforts to understand and more adequately define asthma has been the identification of a growing list of inflammatory-bronchospastic mediators [28]. Previous concerns about histamine release have been essentially replaced by a focus on leukotrienes, platelet-activating factor, endothelin, and other substances which, by local release or by cell-cell communications that promote release of other agents, can result in airway inflammation and bronchospasm. The impressive growth of molecular cellular biology may not result in a "unitary theory" regarding asthma, but it is likely to identify different asthmatic subgroups and fundamental mechanisms for which new therapeutic approaches may be highly effective.

Currently, what is the position in our efforts to define and to diagnose asthma—and to select appropriate therapy? The first step, it would appear, is to assure specificity. Specifically, if airway inflammation and bronchospasm, the two asthma hallmarks, are present as determined by history and other data, other confounding entities should be excluded before a therapeutic trial is implemented. What is not pulmonary embolism, infectious lung disease, left-sided heart failure, and so on, may of clinical necessity be cautiously labeled asthma. The second step is an effort to identify an inciting cause, by careful history and laboratory tests if possible. The third step is patient education. The fourth step is judicious selection of appropriate therapy that will remit airway inflammation and bronchospasm.

As these sequences are followed, however, it should be recognized that the apparently rising incidence of asthma and mortality due to asthma [25, 30] (see Chap. 90) contain some elements that are more societal than medical [15]. Society must deal with the issues of workplace and environmental pollution as well as the issue of access to medical care. Such lack of access—with attendant delay of appropriate and prompt therapy—certainly has been identified as a major factor in asthma mortality. All physicians who deal with asthma recognize that the neglected patient is the one who most commonly presents in the emergency room, requires hospital admission, and is at highest risk of death [17, 19] (see Chap. 90).

RELATIONSHIP OF ASTHMA TO OTHER CHRONIC OBSTRUCTIVE PULMONARY DISEASES

As has been inferred above, one of the issues to be addressed in dealing with the asthmatic patient is whether another chronic obstructive pulmonary disease coexists. Among those disorders are not only chronic bronchitis and emphysema, but also small-airway disease and obliterative bronchiolitis. Further, even interstitial ("restrictive") lung diseases are often associated with hyperreactive airways.

Sorting out whether asthma alone exists or whether one of these other diseases is also present is sometimes a simple and sometimes a complex problem. The complexities are introduced by three considerations: (1) that lung biopsy is often the only definitive means for excluding these other entities, (2) that symptoms and physiologic findings of the coexisting diseases may be similar, and (3) that many patients have combinations of these disorders. It is now clear, for example, that instances of "pure" emphysema or "pure" chronic bronchitis are uncommon. The vast majority of patients with chronic obstructive airway disease share a common association: inhalation of tobacco smoke or other irritants. Not surprisingly, then, the alveolar fragmentation of emphysema and the mucosal inflammation of chronic bronchitis usually coexist. Small-airway disease also carries similar associations. Thus, while the precise pathogenetic mechanisms responsible for these entities may differ significantly, as may therapy beyond avoidance of the irritant, the fact is that the different anatomic lesions often coexist. Equally true, however, is that one of the lesions often dominates in a given patient. In any of these conditions, episodic exacerbations characterized by asthmatic hallmarks (increased airway inflammation and bronchospasm) may occur. This situation has spawned such terms as *asthmatic bronchitis*.

How important it is to define the precision of diagnosis and its severity in differentiation is of value to both the physician and the patient in establishing prognosis and reasonable expectations for the results of therapeutic intervention. "Pure" asthma is potentially subject to total reversion. With relief of airway inflammation and bronchospasm, the patient can return to a normal clinical and physiologic state. Chronic bronchitis is also theoretically reversible, though over a longer time frame than even severe asthma. The alveolar fragmentation of emphysema is not reversible and is reflected by persistent symptoms (e.g., effort dyspnea) and physiologic findings (e.g., increased lung compliance, loss of normal elastic recoil). Thus, if anatomic fragmentation is advanced, reversion to a normal state will not occur, regardless of the intensity of any current therapy.

Furthermore, such definition is critical in efforts to educate the patient about his or her disease. Patients with asthma can be assured that asthma does not cause emphysema and that with appropriate management, they are not faced with relentless progression of respiratory dysfunction. Patients with emphysema can be guided to programs which emphasize techniques that slow disease progression, avoid preventable exacerbations, and maximize their ability to cope with their dysfunction (e.g., rehabilitation programs).

SEVERITY OF ASTHMA

Gauging the severity of asthma in a given patient is an important issue in patient care and one that may be subject to error. The most common error is the failure to recognize that airway inflammation is a major feature of this disorder so that the focus is directed exclusively to bronchospasm. This misdirected focus is the primary reason for certain commonly observed sequences and misperceptions. For example, a patient comes to the emergency room, wheezing and dyspneic with an acute asthmatic attack. After administration of intravenous or inhaled bronchodilator, the wheezing subsides; the patient is less dyspneic and discharged. A few hours later, the patient returns with the same symptoms, much to the chagrin of the treating physician. In the hospital, a similar sequence often is observed.

There is a plethora of carefully documented data indicating that these clinical failures are due to neglect of the presence and severity of the existing airway inflammation, and nonrecognition of the fact that relief of this inflammation—and the extensive mucus production associated with it—takes a substantially longer period of time to resolve than does wheezing [11]. Obviously, the goal of therapy in asthma is not to relieve wheezing, but to revert the airways to as normal a state as possible. Such reversion requires time, persistent application of antiinflammatory therapy, and meticulous observations by the responsible physician.

How can the underestimation of the degree of airway inflammation be avoided? There are helpful historical, physical, and physiologic clues [6, 11]. Historically, the chief clues are the patient's past behavior during "attacks," the patient's therapy (if any) prior to this attack, and the duration of the attack prior to the patient's being seen. The patient who ordinarily requires modest maintenance therapy, whose attacks are rare and have responded quickly to minimal treatment, who has never been hospitalized for asthma, and whose symptoms began shortly (hours) before being seen usually has *mild* asthma. Airway inflammation and mucus production and plugging are likely to be modest. The patient with *moderate* asthma usually relates a different story. This patient's prior attacks were more frequent, he or she receives more substantial maintenance therapy, prior attacks required intensive therapy, the patient may have been hospitalized, and the symptoms began many hours to days prior to being seen (see Chap. 54). The patient with *severe* asthma gives a history similar to that of the patient with moderate asthma, often has been hospitalized, is on either *little* maintenance therapy or *extensive* therapy, and has been progressively less responsive to usual therapy over a period of some days.

Physical examination also can provide clues to severity. The patient with mild asthma has minimal tachycardia and a modest increase in respiratory rate and is not cyanotic. Pulmonary examination discloses good diaphragmatic motion despite diffuse wheezing. The patient with moderate asthma is more tachypneic and tachycardic, may be cyanotic, and has moderate diaphragmatic motion and diffuse wheezing. The hallmarks of severe asthma are marked tachycardia and tachypnea, cyanosis, an appearance of fatigue, inspiratory retraction of the supraclavicular fossae, poor diaphragmatic motion, and pulsus paradoxus [18]. The more silent the lungs become, the more severe the airway obstruction is, as the disappearance of wheezing indicates that diffuse mucus plugging (and perhaps diaphragmatic fatigue) has developed. In these severe patients, disappearance of wheezing is an ominous sign; its reappearance during therapy is an early indication of improvement.

Spirometry can reflect historical and physical features. With increasing disease severity, there is more severe reduction in both inspiratory and expiratory flow rates. Further, air trapping elevates the residual volume–total lung capacity (RV/TLC) ratio, which is often reflected by a chest x-ray showing significant hyperinflation. Spirometric testing may not be possible, of course, in emergent situations. However, arterial blood gas analysis is possible under virtually all circumstances and is a good indicator of severity [12]. In mild asthma, arterial oxygen tension (PaO_2) is normal or slightly reduced and arterial carbon dioxide tension ($PaCO_2$) is normal to slightly *decreased*. With more severe asthma, the PaO_2 declines and $PaCO_2$ falls. Finally, in severe asthma, the $PaCO_2$ rises to normal and in the most severe cases, hypercapnia appears. Hypercapnia is an ominous sign. Such patients require hospital admission and intensive therapy.

Thus, the combination of historical, physiologic, and physical findings should allow the physician to stratify asthmatic patients reasonably well. This assessment of severity also provides a reasonable guideline regarding the intensity and duration of therapy for a given patient. The more severe the manifestations are, the more advanced is the degree of airway inflammation and mucus plugging. Furthermore, serial pulmonary spirometric tests have shown that the greater the initial dysfunction, the more slowly the abnormalities will return to normal. This is the reason why abatement of wheezing is such an unreliable guide to judgments about emergency room dismissal or hospital discharge. Substantial flow obstruction persists for days to weeks after a significant

asthmatic episode. Until this resolves, one must maintain effective antiinflammatory and bronchodilator therapy. The desire on the part of the patient or physician to rapidly taper such therapy should be resisted, a resistance that can be achieved by following the patient by objective measurements of expiratory flow. Devices that allow such measurements by the patient can be almost useful adjunct in both patient education and compliance [24].

However, true to its hallmark of variability, asthma may not neatly follow such characterizations of severity. Some patients, fortunately relatively uncommonly, may progress to respiratory failure and even death within a period of hours [14]. The key to successful management of these patients—and all asthmatic patients—is an educated patient who has a good relationship with the physician. While definitions of asthma are likely to remain controversial, there is no controversy about the fundamentals of optimal management, which are reviewed in detail in the remainder of this text.

REFERENCES

1. Barnes, P. J., Cung, K. F., and Page, C. P. Inflammatory mediators and asthma. *Pharmacol. Rev.* 40:49, 1988.
2. Bousquet, J., Chanez, P., and Lacoste, J. Eosinophilic inflammation in asthma. *N. Engl. J. Med.* 323:1033, 1990.
3. Ciba Foundation Guest Symposium. Terminology, definitions and classification of chronic pulmonary emphysema and related conditions. *Thorax.* 14:286, 1959.
4. Ciba Foundation Study Group No. 38. *Identification of Asthma.* London: Churchill-Livingstone, 1971.
5. Fletcher, C. M., and Pride, N. B. Definitions of emphysema, chronic bronchitis, asthma and airflow obstruction: 25 years on from the Ciba Symposium. *Thorax.* 39:81, 1984.
6. Gold, W. M. Clinical and physiologic evaluation of asthma. *Chest.* 87:305, 1985.
7. Hahn, P. L., Dodge, R. W., and Golubjatnikov, R. Association of *Chlamydia pneumonia* (strain TWAR) infection with wheezing, asthmatic bronchitis and adult-onset asthma. *JAMA* 266:225, 1991.
8. Lichtenstein, C. M. A re-evaluation of immunotherapy in asthma. *Am. Rev. Respir. Dis.* 129:657, 1984.
9. McFadden, E. R. Exercise and asthma. *N. Engl. J. Med.* 317:502, 1987.
10. McFadden, E. R., Jr. Methylxanthines in the treatment of asthma: The rise, the fall, and the possible rise again. *Ann. Intern. Med.* 115:323, 1991.
11. McFadden, E. R., Jr., Kiser, R., and deGroot, W. J. Acute bronchial asthma: Relations between clinical and physiologic manifestations. *N. Engl. J. Med.* 288:221, 1973.
12. McFadden, E. R., Jr., and Lyons, H. A. Arterial-blood gas tension in asthma. *N. Engl. J. Med.* 278:1027, 1968.
13. Morrison, J. F. J., et al. Platelet activation in nocturnal asthma. *Thorax.* 46:197, 1991.
14. O'Hollaren, M. T., Yunginger, J. W., and Offord, G. Exposure to an aeroallergen as a possible precipitating factor in respiratory arrest in young patients with asthma. *N. Engl. J. Med.* 324:359, 1991.
15. Ozone: Too much in the wrong place (editorial). *Lancet.* 338:221, 1991.
16. Ramsdell, J. E., Nachtwey, F. J., and Moser, K. M. Bronchial hyperreactivity in chronic obstructive bronchitis. *Am. Rev. Respir. Dis.* 126:829, 1982.
17. Read, J. The reported increase in mortality from asthma: A clinico-functional analysis. *Med. J. Aust.* 1:879, 1968.
18. Rebuck, A. S., and Pengelly, L. D. Development of pulsus paradoxus in the presence of airways obstruction. *N. Engl. J. Med.* 288:66, 1973.
19. Rebuck, A. S., and Read, J. Assessment and management of severe asthma. *Am. J. Med.* 51:788, 1971.
20. Reed, C. E. Aerosol steroids as primary treatment of mild asthma. *N. Engl. J. Med.* 325:425, 1991.
21. Scadding, J. G. The meaning of diagnostic terms in bronchopulmonary disease. *Br. Med. J.* 2:1423, 1963.
22. Scadding, J. G. The semantics of medical diagnosis. *Biomed. Computing.* 3:83, 1972.
23. Scadding, J. G. Definition and Clinical Categorization. In E. B. Weiss, M. S. Segal, and M. Stein (eds.), *Bronchial Asthma* (2nd ed.). Boston: Little, Brown, 1985. P. 3.
24. Shim, C. S., and Williams, M. H., Jr. Evaluation of the severity of asthma: Patients versus physicians. *Am. J. Med.* 68:11, 1980.

25. Sly, R. M. Increases in deaths from asthma. *Ann. Allergy* 53:20, 1984.

26. Springall, P. R., et al. Endothelin immunoreactivity of airway epithelium in asthmatic patients. *Lancet.* 337:697, 1991.

27. Standards for the diagnosis and care of patients with chronic obstructive pulmonary disease (COPD) and asthma. *Am. Rev. Respir. Dis.* 136:225, 1987.

28. Symposium. The clinical importance of leukotrienes and platelet-activat-ing factor in allergic respiratory disease. *Am. Rev. Respir. Dis.* 143:585, 1991.

29. Taylor, I. K., et al. Effect of cysteinyl leukotriene receptor antagonist ICI 204,219 on allergen-induced bronchoconstriction and airway hyperreac-tivity in atopic subjects. *Lancet* 337:690, 1991.

30. Woolcock, A. J. Worldwide differences in asthma prevalence and mortal-ity. *Chest.* 90:409, 1986.

Epidemiology and Natural History

Scott T. Weiss
Frank E. Speizer

2

Recognizable clinical descriptions of asthma date from antiquity [2]. However, the clinician, physiologist, or epidemiologist who attempts to investigate this disease today is still hampered by disagreements about the definition of this disorder. Part of the problem relates to the lack of specificity of respiratory symptoms. Osler recognized part of the problem with his famous aphorism, "All that wheezes is not asthma." McFadden [57] and Corrao and colleagues [27] noted that cough, either with or without phlegm and with or without dyspnea, can be the only presenting symptom for patients with asthma.

The overlap of symptoms traditionally associated with both chronic obstructive lung disease and asthma seriously compromises identification of asthmatic subjects by symptoms alone. Furthermore, the relationship of cigarette smoking, the major cause of chronic obstructive lung disease, to asthma is unclear but is potentially important. Thus, the traditional clinical view that attaches the diagnostic label *asthma* to the young, atopic, wheezing patient and *chronic obstructive lung disease* to the middle-aged, smoking, coughing patient may obscure rather than enhance our understanding of the potential risk factors involved in the production of these unique diseases and the natural history of their development.

Epidemiologists have been hampered by a second methodologic concern that relates directly to the definition of asthma. The American Thoracic Society [26] has defined asthma as "a disease characterized by an increased responsiveness of the trachea and bronchi to a variety of stimuli and manifested by widespread narrowing of the airways that changes in severity either spontaneously or as a result of therapy." Although acceptable to most clinicians and investigators, this definition appears to be in need of modification based on more recent data from population studies. These studies have emphasized the importance of physiologic testing to determine the degree of bronchial responsiveness either with a nonspecific agent, such as histamine, methacholine, or subfreezing air, or with a specific environmental antigen. The reader is referred to Chapter 1 which deals with the definition of asthma.

Still, in the clinical setting, tests of bronchial responsiveness are rarely used to systematically investigate symptomatic patients. Thus, the diagnostic classification of patients with asthma-like symptoms and signs is significantly influenced by the training and experience of the practitioner.

Partly because of the above-mentioned methodologic issues, epidemiologists have relied primarily on historic or questionnaire sources to identify patients with asthma. Cases have been identified either by physicians or by surveys of population groups in which the definition of who is asthmatic has been left to the patients themselves, the parents of patients, or the report of the diagnosis having been made by the patient's physician. Each of these means of selecting asthma patients has inherent weaknesses. One must assume that some bias in reporting of cases is present in each group, and it is more likely that the biases in each method of gathering data are different. Clearly, comparisons among different countries, regions, and population groups, which may depend on different diagnostic criteria, must be tentative at best. Table 2-1 summarizes the advantages and disadvantages of clinical, questionnaire, and physiologic approaches to identifying persons with asthma.

What follows is an attempt to describe the epidemiology and natural history of bronchial asthma. We will first discuss the incidence and prevalence of the disease and then consider some of the potential risk factors noted in Table 2-2. Occupation, exercise, and drugs are discussed in Chapters 46, 47, and 48, respectively. Finally, we will assess available data about the prognosis of the condition.

PREVALENCE AND INCIDENCE OF ASTHMA: RELATIONSHIP TO AGE AND SEX

Asthma is a common disease affecting 9 to 12 million people in the United States. There are no definitive population-based figures that have used uniform diagnostic criteria to estimate the incidence or prevalence of asthma in the United States. One source of prevalence data is the U.S. National Center for Health Statistics. In 1970, as part of the Health Interview Survey, a national sample of 116,000 people in 37,000 randomly selected households in the United States were asked if they had seen a physician for asthma in the preceding 2 weeks [1]. The overall disease prevalence was 3 percent, with slightly higher rates reported for younger (<6 years) and older (>65 years) males. Some regional variation in the disease also was reported, with the southern (4.4%) and western (2.3%) parts of the country reporting slightly more asthma than the Northeast (2.0%) (Table 2-3).

Several investigators [32, 33, 64] used asthmatic clinic or hospital populations for identification of age of onset of the disease. A bias in selection may flaw these studies, and a preferable approach would be to study a total population. Broder and colleagues [12] collected such data for the community of Tecumseh, Michigan, where almost 50 percent of all subjects had onset before the age of 10 years. Males tend to predominate in this youngest age group, the sexes are equally represented from ages 12 to 14, and females predominate through the rest of the age range. In contrast, 25 percent of all subjects had their disease onset after age 40. Sex and age play an important role in modifying other known or potential risk factors and on disease prognosis. Age-specific incidence rates for asthma are available from the Tucson Epidemiologic Study of lung diseases [34]. Males have an incidence of 1.4 percent per year between birth and 4 years old. The incidence drops to 1 percent per year between the ages of 5 and 9 years and is stable at 0.2 percent per year over the rest of

Table 2-1. Approaches for indentifying persons with asthma

Method	Problems
Clinical evaluation	Nonstandardization of physician criteria for diagnosis; bias toward more severe cases; bias by access to physician
Questionnaire history of diagnosis	Same as above, plus recall bias subjects
Questionnaire history of symptoms	Possibly influenced by frequency of other symptoms; less specific than physician's diagnosis
Response to bronchodilator	May be influenced by level of FEV_1 correlation with bronchodilator; may lack sensitivity
Bronchoconstrictor response	Influenced by level of FEV_1; may be nonspecific

Source: Modified from J. Samet. Epidemiologic approaches for the identification of asthma. *Chest* 91:745, 1987.

Table 2-2. Potential risk factors for the development of asthma

Risk factors	Methods of assessment
Airway responsiveness	Bronchial challenge testing with methacholine, histamine, and cold air
Atopic allergy	Skin testing, serum IgE level, blood eosinophilia, bronchial challenge testing with antigen
Air pollution, air temperature	Urban verus rural, levels of SO_2 and particulates, home or personal monitoring, measurement of air temperature
Respiratory infection	History of croup, bronchiolitis, or acute bronchitis; measurement of bronchial responsiveness during viral illness
Familial or household and genetic	Household associations, twin studies, HLA typing
Occupation	Years of exposure, challenge testing with environmental antigens, skin testing with environmental antigens
Sex	Directly measured
Age	Directly measured
Exercise	Directly measured, exercise challenge testing
Drugs	History of sensitivity to aspirin, tartarizine, dye, nitrites, beta-blocking drugs; direct bronchial challenge with drug
Cigarette smoking	Directly measured

Table 2-3. Prevalence of asthma per 1,000 persons in the United States in 1970, as reported in health interviews by age, sex, and region

	Under age 6	6–16	17–44	45–64	65 and over	All ages
Males	36.8	38.1	24.6	29.3	42.3	31.7
Females	21.5	25.7	27.6	36.7	31.1	28.8
Northeast	22.1	29.9	22.4	25.2	26.5	25.1
North Central	26.6	24.0	22.7	29.4	34.3	25.9
South	36.8	36.7	39.5	42.8	43.8	35.9
West	30.4	39.3	30.8	34.1	39.1	34.1
Total	29.3	32.0	26.2	33.1	35.8	30.2

Source: Adapted from U.S. Dept. of Health and Human Services, PHS Resources Administration. Prevalence of selected chronic respiratory conditions, United States, 1970. *Vital Health Stat.* Series 10, No. 84, September 1973.

Table 2-4. Relationship of age of onset of asthma in Tecumseh, Michigan, to prospectively observed incidence of disease measured in Tucson, Arizona

	Tecumseh (%)			Tucson (incidence/100)		
Age	Males	Females	Ratio males-females	Males	Females	Ratio males-females
0–4	36.0	26.3	1.4	1.4	0.9	1.6
5–9	23.0	11.0	2.1	1.0	0.7	1.4
10–14	10.6	9.3	1.1	0.2	0.3	0.7
15–19	6.7	14.4	0.5	—	—	—
20–29	7.7	16.0	0.5	0.2	0.4	0.5
30–39	10.6	11.9	0.9	—	0.4	—
40–49	4.8	6.8	0.7	—	0.4	—
50–59	—	3.4	—	—	0.5	—
60+	—	0.8	—	0.3	0.8	0.4

Source: Adapted from I. Broder, et al. Epidemiology of asthma and allergic rhinitis in a total community: Tecumseh, Michigan: III. Second survey of the community. *J. Allergy Clin. Immunol.* 53:127, 1974; and from R. R. Dodge and B. Burrows. The prevalence and incidence of asthma and asthma-like symptoms in a general population sample. *Am. Rev. Respir. Dis.* 122:567, 1980.

the age range. Females have a slightly lower incidence in the youngest age group—0.9 percent per year. The incidence of disease decreases to 0.7 percent per year. The incidence of disease decreases to 0.7 percent per year between the ages of 5 and 9 years and fluctuates from 0.4 to 0.8 percent per year over the rest of the age range.

The age of onset data from Tecumseh [12] tend to confirm the prospective incidence data from Tucson, and both studies suggest that asthma in early life (< age 15) tends to be predominantly a male disease, while asthma in later life (> age 40) tends to be more common in females (Table 2-4). One conceivable explanation for the gender difference is lower absolute level of lung function in females relative to males. However, this will need to be explored further.

AIRWAY RESPONSIVENESS

The definition of asthma centers on the concept of abnormal bronchial responsiveness as noted above [26]. Available clinical data suggest that bronchomotor tone to constricting agents such as histamine, methacholine, and cold air shows greater variability in subjects with asthma than in normal subjects and in subjects with allergic rhinitis. Both Townley and colleagues [83] and Deal and colleagues [30] found a gradient of responsiveness using different challenge tests, with current asthmatics having the greatest decrease in forced expiratory volume in 1 second (FEV_1), normals having the least response, and hay fever sufferers being intermediate between the other two groups. These clinical and physiologic studies, although valuable, are limited. Population-based studies are needed to define the underlying distribution of responsiveness in an unselected population and to assess the relationship of responsiveness to disease.

Cockcroft and Berscheid [23] examined nonspecific bronchial responsiveness to inhaled histamine in a randomly selected cohort of college students aged 20 to 29 years. Bronchial responsiveness was distributed in a unimodal fashion, skewed in the direction of greater responsiveness. All subjects with current or past asthma responded at a concentration of inhaled histamine of 4 mg/ml or less. Using this criterion of a responder, fully 20 percent (58/300) of these subjects with no respiratory symptoms had increased levels of bronchial responsiveness.

Lorber and coworkers used a bronchodilator response to inhaled isoproterenol [51]. They found that 20 percent of their

Table 2-5. Prevalence of increased bronchial responsiveness in random population samples of asymptomatic children and adults

Study	Population	Criteria for positive response	Prevalence of increased bronchial responsiveness (%)	Prevalence of asymptomatic increased responsiveness	
				Total population (%)	All responsive subjects (%)
Weiss [90]	East Boston, MA, random population children, young adults (N = 213), age range 6–24 yr	$\Delta FEV_1/FVC > 9\%$ to cold air	22	11	51
Salome et al. [73]	Australia, random population children (N = 2,363), age range 8–11 yr	PD_{20} $FEV_1 \leq 7.8$ μmole histamine	17.9	6.7	37
Sears [75]	New Zealand, random population sample (N = 766), mean age 9 yr	PD_{20} $FEV_1 < 25$ mg/ml methacholine	22	8	30
Woolcock et al. [95]	Busselton, Australia, random population sample (N = 876), mean age 49 yr	PD_{20} $FEV_1 \leq 3.9$ μmole histamine	11	2	19
Rijcken et al. [71]	Netherlands, random population adults (N = 1,905), age range 14–64+ yr	PC_{10} $FEV_1 \leq 16$ mg/ml histamine	24.5	14	58.5
Sparrow et al. [80]	Boston, MA, adult males (N = 458), mean age 60 yr	PD_{20} $FEV_1 \leq 50$ μmole methacholine	29.9	—	—
Burney et al. [17]	England, random population adults (N = 511), age range 18–64 yr	PD_{20} $FEV_1 \leq 8$ μmole histamine	14	—	—

random sample population with normal pulmonary function and no prior or current physician's diagnosis of asthma demonstrated a significant change in pulmonary function below a single challenge dose. This would suggest a rough correlation between bronchoconstrictive stimuli and bronchodilators in assessing responsiveness in asymptomatic subjects.

A summary of population-based studies of adults and children is given in Table 2-5. Even a cursory examination of this table reveals that the prevalence of asthma in these populations is twofold to threefold lower than the prevalence of increased airway responsiveness. In addition, 20 to 50 percent of all subjects with increased airway responsiveness have no symptoms at the time they are tested (see Table 2-5). Although definitional issues for asthma, respiratory symptoms, and increased responsiveness may contribute to some of the between-study differences, there can be no doubt that increased bronchial responsiveness and asthma are not identical phenomena. Increased levels of bronchial responsiveness are a necessary but not sufficient condition for the development of clinical disease.

Although the relationship between increased airway responsiveness and asthma is unclear at the present time, the concept of airway inflammation seems central to asthma pathophysiology (see Chap. 9). The relationship between increased bronchial responsiveness and airway inflammation is thought to be key in understanding why some bronchial responsiveness is associated with clinical disease and some is not [6]. Even in the absence of clinical disease, increased airway responsiveness predicts accelerated decline in FEV_1 [66] and the subsequent development of disease [46].

Exposure to environmental agents may produce airway inflammation in that segment of the population who is susceptible by virtue of having increased airway responsiveness at baseline. A wide variety of common environmental events such as respiratory infections [41], atopy or allergy [24], air temperature and humidity [31], and exercise [58] are known to influence airway responsiveness. Whether these environmental factors are simply enhancers of an underlying physiologic trait or whether they are the agents responsible for the distribution of responsiveness in the population is unknown. The intuitively most appealing theory, depicted in Figure 2-1, is that there is a biologic distribution of responsiveness in the population that is dynamic and modifiable by environmental exposures. This distribution appears to

change with age. Environmental factors may enhance or depress bronchial responsiveness and thus may influence the development of a clinical illness. What characteristics or factors are directly associated with an increased risk of clinical asthma is only partially known.

ATOPIC ALLERGY

Allergy is characterized by increases in serum IgE in response to exposure to environmental antigens. Atopy can be assessed in clinical and epidemiologic studies by three methods: skin test reactivity, serum IgE levels, and blood eosinophilia (see Chaps. 7 and 38).

Skin test reactivity is highly age dependent. Barbee and colleagues [3–5] studied 3,101 subjects between the ages of 2 and 80 years in Tucson, Arizona, using a battery of five skin tests. With the criterion of any skin test reactivity greater than control being positive, 20 percent of children younger than age 4 and 52 percent of individuals aged 20 to 25 were considered atopic (Fig. 2-2). However, in adults skin test reactivity declines with age. Therefore, individuals over 60 years old have skin test positivity rates approximating the rates in very young children.

Skin test reactivity correlates closely with serum IgE level; thus, serum IgE follows a distribution by age similar to that of skin test reactivity [3, 4, 14]. Because cigarette smoking is a major determinant of serum IgE level, when cigarette-smoking habits are taken into account, differences in IgE levels between males and females disappear [17, 18, 44].

Blood eosinophilia, a third test of the atopic state, shows a good correlation with skin test reactivity and serum IgE level [19, 44].

The relationship between atopy as assessed by any of the three measures (skin test, IgE level, eosinophilia) and respiratory symptoms is clearly complicated by the association of cigarette smoking with both atopy and respiratory symptoms in both adults [12, 17–20] and children [89, 90]. Burrows and colleagues [18] examined the relationship of skin test reactivity to respiratory symptoms after controlling for cigarette-smoking status in adults. They found that asthma, wheeze, and a family history of allergy all were associated with atopy. Burrows and colleagues showed that of the various allergy markers, total serum IgE level

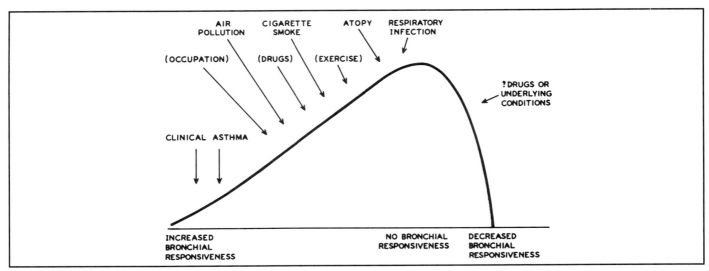

Fig. 2-1. *Hypothesized relationship between environmental and host factors responsible for clinical asthma. (Environmental factors in parentheses discussed in text.)*

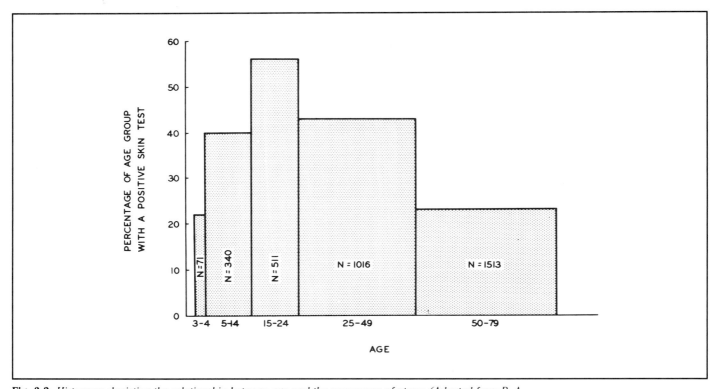

Fig. 2-2. *Histogram depicting the relationship between age and the occurrence of atopy. (Adapted from R. A. Barbee, et al. Immediate skin-test reactivity in a general population sample.* Ann. Intern. Med. *84:129, 1976.)*

correlates best with asthma while skin test reactivity correlates best with hay fever [21]. To date, no data are available combining the allergy markers and their relationship to asthma.

The prevalence of atopy in patients with asthma varies from 23 to 80 percent, depending on the age of the population and how asthma and atopy are defined. The strong association of atopy with early-life onset of disease is a feature of several large series [15, 59, 64]. Although several large cohort studies, notably those of Williams and McNichol [94] and Rackerman and Edwards [70], have found rates of atopy higher than those reported in the Tucson cohort, the relationship of atopy to asthma in these

studies may have depended to a large extent on bias in selection, definition of asthma, and unclear definitions of skin test reactivity. There seems little question that asthma in childhood that is associated with atopy is destined to be more severe than nonatopic disease. The current consensus is that in damp, temperate areas, exposure to antigens in the home (e.g., house dust, dust mites, dog and cat dander) provides the major environmental antigen burden and the relationship of these exposures to asthma still requires investigation in prospective studies.

To determine how the various definitions of atopy predict the onset of asthma requires prospective evaluation of population

Table 2-6. Relationship of atopic factors and cigarette smoking to the development of asthma in Tucson

	Developed asthma		Did not develop asthma		Ratio (of %)
	Number	%	Number	%	
Age <40	27		1,819		
Positive skin test		76.5		39.8	1.92
Eosinophilia 5%		30.0		8.0	3.75
Cigarette smoking		60.0		30.0	2.00
Age ≥40	22		1,564		
Positive skin test		27.3		26.5	1.03
Eosinophilia 5%		26.7		7.1	3.68
Cigarette smoking		45.5		30.5	1.49

Source: Adapted from R. R. Dodge and B. Burrows. The prevalence and incidence of asthma and asthma-like symptoms in a general population sample. *Am. Rev. Respir. Dis.* 122:567, 1980.

groups at risk of developing disease. Some of the best data come from Tucson where Dodge and Burrows [34] followed 3,860 subjects and examined the relationship of skin test reactivity and blood eosinophil levels to the subsequent development of asthma over a 3-year period (Table 2-6). In subjects less than 40 years old, positive skin test results were twice as common in subjects who developed asthma than in those who did not; eosinophilia greater than 5 percent was more than three times as common. Yet, cigarette smoking was also more common in subjects developing asthma than in those who did not. In subjects over the age of 40, positive skin test results were not more common in new asthmatic subjects when compared with nonasthmatic subjects. Eosinophilia and smoking were more common in new asthmatic than in nonasthmatic subjects.

RESPIRATORY INFECTION

Viral and bacterial respiratory infections in adults and children with asthma are often associated with clinical exacerbations. However, there are no conclusive epidemiologic data linking viral respiratory infection to the onset of asthma in previously normal individuals. Theoretically, infection has been linked to the development of asthma by directly inducing a change in bronchial responsiveness by a variety of physiologic mechanisms and by the induction of the atopic state (see Chap. 44). Empey and colleagues [35] studied bronchial responsiveness with histamine aerosols and citric acid aerosols in 16 normal subjects with colds (viral upper respiratory tract infection) and 11 healthy controls. Responsiveness was markedly increased in those subjects with colds. Atropine inhibition of this response suggested that airway epithelial damage by respiratory infections sensitizes airway receptors to be more responsive to environmental stimuli. Busse [22] noted a decrease in beta-adrenergic sensitivity of asthmatic patients with viral respiratory infections. An increase in mucosal permeability [45] (Chap. 23) may also be a physiologic factor in the increased levels of airway responsiveness seen in subjects with viral respiratory infections.

Although transient increases in airway responsiveness with viral respiratory illnesses are well documented, the relationship between a prior respiratory illness and the subsequent development of more permanent increased levels of responsiveness is unclear. In a retrospective cohort study, Zach and coworkers [96] followed 110 of 331 children who were hospitalized for croup 9 years after their initial episode: Twenty-one percent of these children had a bronchoresponsive response to inhaled histamine. Gurwitz and colleagues [41] reported on 8.5-year follow-up of 96 children from a similar group of 229 children hospitalized with croup: Thirty-five percent had increased bronchial responsiveness to inhaled methacholine. In a study of similar design, Gurwitz and colleagues [42] examined bronchial responsiveness to methacholine in a group of 48 children from a cohort of 145 hospitalized with bronchiolitis; bronchial responsiveness to methacholine was increased in 27 (56%).

However, several important biases flaw these clinical investigations. The hospital-based nature of these populations means that one can generalize these data only to other children who may have been hospitalized at the time of the study. One cannot be sure whether factors that determined need for hospitalization would be generally applicable to the population. Because only about one-third of the original group was subsequently evaluated, there is significant potential for bias in outcome with the previously mentioned studies. Sicker children are more likely to maintain contact with the hospital, and therefore for purposes of follow-up these children would be the most readily identified for further study.

Respiratory infections might produce or exacerbate asthma in other ways. Frick and associates [37] showed that viral respiratory infections commonly precede the development of the atopic state in children. However, Cogswell and coworkers [25] studying a larger cohort of children found no such association. Immunologic studies have documented transient increases in IgE levels following respiratory syncytial virus (RSV) infection in children [92]. If this correlates with other markers of the atopic state, viral respiratory infection could be an important environmental stimulant to the development of atopy.

Pullan and Hey [69] presented data on a cohort of 180 children admitted to a hospital during the first year of life with a documented RSV infection. One hundred and sixty-four were followed up 10 years later and compared with 110 control children of comparable age for a history of wheeze, a positive skin test result, and increases in bronchial responsiveness to inhaled histamine. Wheezing and abnormal bronchial responsiveness to histamine were more common in the RSV-infected group, and atopy was more common in the control group. However, parental cigarette smoking was more common in RSV-infected children in this investigation.

CIGARETTE SMOKING

Active Smoking

A number of cross-sectional, population-based epidemiologic studies have examined the relationship between chronic cigarette smoking and increased bronchial responsiveness (Table 2-7). Burney and coworkers [17] and Woolcock and associates [95] studied population-based random samples of adult subjects in England and Australia using histamine challenge. Both investigators found an increased occurrence of bronchial responsiveness among current smokers compared to former or never smokers: Total pack-years of smoking was not investigated in these studies. Similar results were obtained when methacholine [80] or cold air [93] was used as the bronchoconstrictive stimulus. In contrast to these results, Van der Lende and associates [86] observed no association between bronchial responsiveness to histamine and smoking status. Recently, Rijcken and coworkers [71] reexamined this question in a larger group of subjects from this population. Although no overall association was noted between bronchial responsiveness to histamine and current smoking status, within the group of current smokers bronchial responsiveness increased with both duration and amount smoked in a dose-response relationship. The total pack-year experience of subjects in this study was very low (<10 pack-years) and the mean age of the cohort was also the youngest of all studied populations.

Table 2-7. Relationship between chronic cigarette smoking and increased bronchial responsiveness

Study	Sample characteristics	Challenge type	Response measure	Findings
Woolcock et al. [95]	N = 876 random population sample, mean age 49 yr	Histamine	FEV_1	Smokers more responsive
Sparrow et al. [80]	N = 458 men participating in longitudinal study of aging, mean age 60 yr	Methacholine	FEV_1	Smokers more responsive
Rijcken et al. [71]	N = 1,905 random population sample, age range 14–64+ yr	Histamine	FEV_1, VC	No difference in "responder" rate; among smokers, weak positive association between responsiveness and cigarettes/day
Burney et al. [17]	N = 511 random population sample, mean age 41 yr	Histamine	FEV_1	Smokers more responsive
Pham et al. [68]	N = 1,109 male iron mine workers, mean age 46 yr	Acetylcholine	FEV_1	Smokers more responsive (borderline significance)
Van der Lende et al. [86]	N = 260 random population, mean age 38 yr	Histamine	FEV_1, VC	No difference between smokers and nonsmokers
Welty et al. [93]	N = 171 subsample from random population sample, median age 38 yr	Cold air hyperpnea	FEV_1	Smokers more responsive

Despite the apparent relationship between smoking and non-specific airway responsiveness, the presence of asthma in adults has generally appeared to be unrelated to smoking history in cross-sectional population samples [34]. However, these results may have been influenced by a bias toward diagnosing smokers with symptoms of wheeze and dyspnea as having chronic obstructive pulmonary disease rather than asthma. In addition, asthmatic subjects may tend not to become regular smokers or smoke less. A positive association between asthma and smoking in a cross-sectional sample of adults was reported by Kiviloog and associates [47]. Burrows and Dodge [34] observed a positive association between asthma and smoking among allergy skin test–negative subjects. They also reported longitudinal data indicating that the incidence of newly diagnosed asthma is greater among smoking than nonsmoking adults (see Table 2-4).

In addition to the issues of diagnostic bias, an important type of selection bias may be operating in the above-noted cross-sectional studies. Younger subjects with high degrees of bronchial responsiveness may be unable to smoke; thus, new-onset smokers come from the "hyporesponsive" end of the distribution. It is only after many years of heavy smoking that these initially unresponsive subjects develop increased bronchial responsiveness. Prospective data are currently lacking to directly test this hypothesis.

As noted earlier, induction of the atopic state might be another potential mechanism by which chronic cigarette smoking might be related to asthma. Burrows and colleagues [18, 34] noted a marked increase in serum IgE and eosinophilia in cigarette smokers. A nonspecific increase in bronchial permeability has been postulated by Hogg [45] as the mechanism by which cigarette smoke leads to an increase in serum IgE level. This nonspecific increase in permeability is consistent with the observation that the elevation in IgE level is nonspecific and that true "allergy" to tobacco smoke is extremely rare [38].

The epidemiologic data concerning the relationship of cigarette smoking to the development of asthma in adults are similarly sparse. Fletcher and coworkers [36], in their longitudinal study of workers in London, found 17 asthmatic adults, all but 2 of whom were current smokers or exsmokers. As previously discussed, Dodge and Burrows [34] found that in young adults (age 10–39) followed for 3 years, those who developed asthma were two times more likely to have smoked, relative to those who did not.

Passive Smoking

Only three investigations have addressed the question of passive smoking and its relationship to airway responsiveness in chil-

dren. Murray and Morrison [61] reported on a small number of asthmatic children drawn from a clinical population and noted that maternal cigarette smoke exposure was associated with a lower mean PD_{20} FEV_1 to histamine (a 20% decrease in FEV_1 from baseline with histamine provocation) than in non–smoke-exposed asthmatics. O'Connor and colleagues [63] confirmed these results in population-based samples using cold air as the challenge test. No effect of maternal smoking on airway responsiveness in nonasthmatic subjects could be determined in this investigation. Finally, Martinez and coworkers [56] studied the relationship of passive smoking to airway responsiveness in 166 children aged 9 years. Increased responsiveness was defined as a PD_{20} FEV_1 of 1,200 μg of carbachol or less. Overall, the odds ratio (OR) for having increased airway responsiveness if exposed to maternal cigarette smoke was 2.3. In addition, there was significant heterogeneity over the sex strata, with males (OR = 3.9) at much greater risk than females (OR = 1.4). These data are urgently in need of confirmation.

The relationship of parental smoking to wheezing symptoms and asthma episodes in children has been studied, with inconsistent results. O'Connell and Logan [62] identified 37 asthmatic children who were "bothered" by parental cigarette smoke. Parents of 20 of the children stopped smoking, and 18 (90%) of the 20 children had an improvement in symptoms. The control group consisted of 15 children (2 were not followed) whose parents did not stop smoking. Only 4 (27%) of these 15 children improved. In addition to possible bias in selection of cases and in reporting of symptoms by parents, subjective criteria for improvement and an unclear duration of follow-up flaw this study.

British workers, studying a birth cohort, demonstrated an increased incidence of wheezing over a 5-year period among nonasthmatic children who had two parents who smoked when compared to children who had two nonsmoking parents [11]. However, when examined by logistic regression, parental smoking was not a significant predictor of the occurrence of wheeze or the future occurrence of asthma.

In a subgroup of the cohort, 861 children of asymptomatic parents, Leeder and colleagues [50] were unable to show a significant trend in asthma-wheeze symptoms by increasing level of parental smoking over a 5-year period. In a study of 650 children aged 5 to 10 years, Weiss and colleagues [88] showed a significant trend in the reported prevalence of chronic wheezing with current parental smoking; the rates were 1.85 percent, 6.85 percent, and 11.8 percent for zero, one, and two smoking parents, respectively. Gortmaker and coworkers [39] studied two populations of children from birth to 17 years old. They found a significant association between parental reporting of children's asthma and maternal smoking. Maternal smoking alone accounted for approximately 20 percent of all asthma. The effect persisted when age and sex of the child, allergies, and family income and education were controlled for in the analysis. No control was attempted for the children's own smoking habits, and the potential of symptomatic parents being more apt to report symptoms in their children exists in these data.

These above-discussed data emphasize the potentially important relationship between cigarette smoking (both active and passive) and increased levels of airway responsiveness and the atopic status. Chronic smoking may directly influence airway responsiveness by causing bronchial mucosal inflammation and epithelial damage. Smoking also could lead to heightened nonspecific airway responsiveness indirectly by predisposing to allergy (as discussed above) or to an increased frequency of respiratory infection. In addition, by causing reduced levels of pulmonary function, smoking may be associated with heightened nonspecific airway responsiveness because of the association between decreased level of FEV_1 and increased bronchial responsiveness.

Evidence from population-based studies suggests that cigarette smoking causes heightened airway responsiveness in adults, but this relationship may be evident only among individuals with sufficiently high cumulative exposure in terms of pack-years. This may be true because smokers may be self-selected from the more hyporesponsive end of the responsiveness distribution. Cross-sectional studies, even those using random population-based samples, may underestimate the magnitude of the active cigarette smoking–airway responsiveness relationship because of a potential "healthy smoker effect." Longitudinal study designs would eliminate the selection bias seen in cross-sectional studies; such data, however, have not yet been reported. Finally, cigarette smoking may modify airway responsiveness by altering the responses to environmental antigens. The details of this mechanism, however, are currently unknown and likely to be complex.

FAMILIAL AGGREGATION OF ASTHMA

Familial aggregation of asthma has been documented in several investigations [29, 78, 85]. This finding is not, however, proof of a genetic basis for the disease, as common environmental factors (air pollution, smoking, and respiratory infection) as well as a relatively high prevalence of disease could possibly account for the finding. Whether familial aggregation of airway responsiveness exists is unknown because family studies with a physiologic test of airway responsiveness in all family members, using appropriate sampling and statistical techniques, have not been performed.

More is known concerning the genetics of atopic allergy (see Chap. 3). Although the IgE regulator gene has not been identified, a dominant inheritance for low IgE and a recessive model for

high IgE have been proposed [52]. In addition, there are some data from which one can postulate a linkage between the IgE regulating gene and the histocompatibility loci antigen (HLA) gene complex [53]. However, as noted earlier, environmental factors are also important determinants of the atopic allergic response, and a precise definition of the genetic factors influencing the atopic state will require much further investigation. Furthermore, since atopic allergy alone is not a sufficient condition for the development of asthma, the relationship of the familial aggregation of atopy itself to the pathogenesis of the disease is unknown.

WEATHER AND AIR POLLUTION

There is no question that weather can influence asthma symptoms [40] (see Chap. 45). Based on the physiologic theory of respiratory heat exchange proposed by Deal and colleagues [30, 31], one would expect that cold, dry climates would be associated with the greatest reporting of wheeze symptoms. However, there seems to be an imperfect correlation because other environmental conditions [40], most notably a change in weather, seem to better predict clinical disease.

There is also little argument for a differential effect of air pollution on the asthmatic subject when compared with the nonasthmatic subject. Asthma symptom severity and emergency room visits correlate with atmosphere pollution [9, 47]. Laboratory studies show significant changes in FEV_1 in a subset of asthmatics with exposure to sulfur dioxide as low as 0.5 ppm [76] and with even lower doses coupled with exercise [77]. Similar results have been demonstrated with acid sulfates [84]. What remains unclear is the relationship, if any, of specific air pollutants on lung development of asthma, and the role of chronic exposure to any such pollutants on lung development, or growth in pulmonary function that might affect the natural history of the disease.

NATURAL HISTORY OF ASTHMA

There are relatively few cohort studies that examine the natural history of asthma (Table 2-8). The bulk of the studies that have been performed have been conducted in children with follow-up into early adulthood. The methodologic problems presented by these investigations are relevant to their interpretation. All of these studies except for the McNichols and Williams study [59, 60, 94] were hospital or clinic based, thus leading to possible bias in selection of the more severely ill patients. Many were retrospective in design, thus raising important questions about loss to follow-up. No study incorporated a physiologic test of airway reactivity, although several examined the question of atopic allergy [14, 33, 49, 72]. No clear currently accepted definition of asthma was given in most of the studies. The criteria for skin test positivity were unclear in some, and none examined

---

Table 2-8. Prognosis in long-term follow-up studies of patients with asthma

Author(s) (year of publication)	Number of subjects	Years of observation	Improved or normal at follow-up	Asthma at follow-up	Deaths
Rackerman and Edwards (1952) [70]	688	20	388 (49.1%)	212 (30.8%)	10 (1.4%)
Kraepelien (1963) [49]	528	8–10	156 (29.6%)	370 (70%)	2 (0.4%)
Ryssing and Flensborg (1963) [72]	442	10–15	163 (36.8%)	279 (63.2%)	0 (0%)
Barr and Logan (1964) [7]	336	17–27	173 (51.5%)	160 (47.5%)	3 (1%)
Buffum and Settipane (1966) [15]	518	10	212 (41%)	301 (58.0%)	5 (1%)
Buffum (1963) [14]	136	20	75 (55.1%)	58 (42.7%)	3 (2.2%)
Ogilvie (1962) [64]	1,000	3–33	724 (72.4%)	276 (27.6%)	—
McNicol and Williams (1973) [60]	295	7	(48.0%)	(52%)	—
Blair (1979) [10]	244	20	123 (52.0%)	114 (48.0%)	3 (1.2%)

serum IgE levels. Perhaps most importantly, only one study utilized population-based controls. In connection with our earlier discussion of risk factors, only two studies examined the role of respiratory infection, and no study considered the potential role of cigarette smoking, either personal or parental. No study considered all risk factors, and none utilized multivariate techniques. In spite of these limitations, some conclusions about the natural history of asthma can be made, albeit tentative.

Children

Between 30 and 70 percent of children with asthma can expect to be markedly improved or become symptom free by early adulthood. On the other hand, significant disease will persist in approximately 30 percent of patients. Age of onset has a complicated relationship to disease prognosis. While children have a greater chance of remission than adults who develop the disease, within children an earlier age of onset carries a worse prognosis [60, 94]. Since skin test reactivity declines with age, there is a tendency to underdiagnose atopic allergy in individuals over the age of 40 years. Thus, it is impossible to assess the relationship of atopy to prognosis. Whether the presence of atopy increases disease severity after controlling for age is unknown. When Williams and McNicol [63] stratified their sample of children by age and examined their relationship of skin test reactivity to disease severity, they found atopy associated with increased severity of disease.

There are no reliable data that relate respiratory infection or cigarette smoking to prognosis.

There is little information on pulmonary function of asthma children followed for several years. Martin and coworkers [54, 55] followed a subgroup of the Williams and McNicol cohort and assessed their pulmonary function at age 21 years (14 years after study onset). Although statistically significant differences were found between the subjects when grouped by initial disease severity, the means for all groups were within the 80 to 120 percent of predicted range considered normal by clinicians and physiologists. For the most severely ill group, the mean was closer to 80 percent predicted than the 100+ percent predicted of the controls. This could have important implications for decline in adult life, as maximal attained level of function may be an important predictor of rate of decline [36]. Weiss and colleagues [91], performed an analysis of the effect of asthma on lung growth in a cohort of 5- to 9-year-old children from the population sample in East Boston over a 13-year period. The effect of asthma on lung growth was different for boys and girls. Boys with asthma had larger growth in vital capacity (VC) than boys without asthma. This projected over a 5-year period to be about an 8 percent larger vital capacity compared with that of nonasthmatic boys. Asthmatic girls, however, had reductions in FEV_1 and growth in forced expiratory flow in mid–expiratory phase ($FEF_{25\%-75\%}$) relative to nonasthmatic girls.

There are several plausible hypotheses to explain these data. Environmental events, for example, respiratory illness and cigarette smoke (vide supra), may explain the gender differences, at least in part. Alternatively, differences in pulmonary mechanics between males and females (e.g., muscle strength) may also be important.

Adults

Clinical studies of the relationship of airway responsiveness and its relationship to decline in FEV_1 may be biased by the selected nature of the patients and inadequate statistical methods [8]. Population-based data is preferred. There are only two population-based studies in which responsiveness has been related to decline in FEV_1. Taylor and colleagues [82] followed 227 men over 7.5 years and examined the relationship between nonspe-

cific airway responsiveness and rate of decline of FEV_1. Histamine airway responsiveness, expressed as $PC_{20} FEV_1$, was measured at the end of the follow-up period rather than at the beginning. There was a significant correlation between histamine responsiveness and the rate of decline of FEV_1, higher degrees of responsiveness being associated with more rapid decline in FEV_1. Because responsiveness was assessed at the end of follow-up, this report does not answer the question of whether heightened airway responsiveness was a cause or a consequence of the decline in FEV_1.

Pham and coauthors [68] reported the only prospective, longitudinal study of the relationship of nonspecific airway responsiveness to subsequent decline in pulmonary function. Spirometry and an acetylcholine challenge test were performed on 1,109 iron mine workers, and 820 of these subjects were available for reexamination 5 years later. A positive response to acetylcholine was defined as a 10 percent or greater decline in FEV_1 after inhaling acetylcholine aerosol for 3 minutes (an estimated delivered dose of 1,200 µg), and 19 percent of subjects had a positive response so defined. Subjects with a positive acetylcholine response experienced a significantly greater decline in the FEV_1/VC ratio during the subsequent 5 years than did nonresponders; a similar trend for FEV_1 was not statistically significant.

In both of the above-described studies, there was an inverse relationship between nonspecific airway responsiveness and level of pulmonary function, subjects with greater responsiveness having lower levels of function. However, the relationship between nonspecific airway responsiveness and rate of decline of pulmonary function was analyzed without adjustment for level of pulmonary function. Thus, the association of higher degrees of responsiveness with a more rapid rate of decline of pulmonary function may simply reflect the association of lower levels of function with a more rapid decline in function.

Based on the model of lung growth presented earlier in this chapter, it is unclear whether adjustment for level is or is not appropriate in examining the relationship of responsiveness to decline in pulmonary function: The extent to which bronchial responsiveness was present in childhood and influenced lung growth adjustment may be inappropriate; the extent to which responsiveness is a consequence of cigarette smoking and hence unrelated to maximal growth adjustment may be more relevant. These questions are even more complicated because so little is known about maximal lung growth. Until these issues are clearer, it seems prudent to present both adjusted and unadjusted analyses.

Longitudinal studies of adult subjects with asthma could provide insight into the question of whether increased levels of airway responsiveness are associated with an accelerated decline in lung function. Fletcher and associates [36] identified 17 men with a physician's diagnosis of asthma who were not treated and were followed for 8 years as part of a longitudinal study of decline in pulmonary function in a population of working men. The rate of decline in FEV_1 in milliliters per year adjusted for the mean value over the 8-year period was significantly more rapid (by 22 ml/yr) when compared with asymptomatic nonsmokers.

Schachter and coworkers [74] studied a rural white population of 1,303 subjects in Lebanon, Connecticut, over a 6-year period. Subjects were considered to have asthma if they responded affirmatively to the question "Have you ever had asthma?" Asthmatic adults experienced more rapid decline in FEV_1 than did nonasthmatics. Although these data were not adjusted for age, smoking, or initial level of FEV_1, the magnitude of the difference (18 ml/yr) was similar to that observed by Fletcher and colleagues [36].

Buist and Vollmer [16] studied a total of 35 asthmatic subjects drawn from a young working population and a health-screened older cohort. Subjects were considered to have asthma if a physician had ever informed them of that diagnosis. The results were presented as rate of decline of FEV_1 without adjustment for age or initial level but stratified by cohort of origin and smoking status. No consistent accelerated decline in FEV_1 was observed.

By far the largest set of data are those of Peat and coworkers [67], who analyzed results collected over an 18-year period in a random population sample in Busselton, Australia. Ninety-two asthmatic subjects, initially between the ages of 22 and 69 years, were compared with 186 normal subjects. Individual regressions of FEV_1/Ht^3 (height cubed) on age were used to compute FEV_1 slopes. Asthmatic subjects had greater rates of decline than did nonasthmatics, and the difference for males (15 ml/yr) was reasonably close to that observed by others. Although smoking asthmatics had the most rapid rate of decline, this did not reach statistical significance because of very small numbers. There was no adjustment for initial level of FEV_1 in this analysis.

Because relatively small numbers of asthmatic subjects have been studied to date, it is not clear to what extent conclusions from these data can be generalized to the larger number of nonasthmatic adults with relatively high levels of airway responsiveness. In addition, the potential importance of adjustment for level of FEV_1 complicates interpretation of these data. Only the analysis of Fletcher and colleagues [36] included adjustment for mean level of FEV_1. However, Fletcher's adjusted value is reasonably close to the unadjusted values observed by others. Finally, other potentially important factors such as smoking, age, sex, and diagnostic overlap with other conditions are not addressed in the existing data analyses. Thus, existing data on the decline of lung function in asthmatic adults are consistent with, but do not prove, the hypothesis that asthma is associated with an accelerated decline in lung function parameters cited above.

As noted in the follow-up studies (see Table 2-8), mortality from asthma is still a relatively rare event in the United States. Certain countries, namely Australia and New Zealand, have much higher rates. The reasons for these international differences are largely unknown and unexplored. Indeed, risk factors for mortality from asthma in any country are largely unknown. Black race and female gender are two epidemiologic characteristics that seem to be associated with increased mortality based on U.S. National Health Statistics data but the reasons for these associations are unknown and require further investigation. The only additional risk factor for mortality that has been identified is excessive sympathomimetic aerosol use, which was responsible for an epidemic of asthma-related deaths in England in the 1960s [81] and a recent epidemic in New Zealand [66] (see Chap. 90 for further discussion of this topic).

There is much controversy about whether asthma mortality is increasing in the United States. In the age group 5 to 34 years, the ages at which there are few other diseases that might be confused with asthma, there were 250 deaths in the year 1980, yielding a mortality rate of 2.6/100,000 persons. In 1984 there was a mortality rate of 3.2/100,000 persons aged 5 to 34. In older subjects where asthma and chronic obstructive pulmonary disease are often confused, the figure for 1986 is 6.7/100,000 [87, 89]. While the overall mortality rate for asthma has increased in the United States, the increase in the elderly may be due to changes in the coding of causes of death while in younger subjects the absolute increase is very small.

The following statements summarize the findings presented here:

1. Asthma affects 3 percent of the U.S. population. Below age 10, males are affected with asthma approximately 1.5 to 2.0 times as often as females. Above age 10, the onset of disease is slightly higher in females.
2. Airway responsiveness is the sine qua non of asthma; however, in isolation it does not define asthma. The distribution of responsiveness is unimodal and skewed toward a greater

reduction in FEV_1 following challenge testing in patients with asthma. A large number of responsive subjects are asymptomatic.
3. Atopy tends to enhance asthma severity. Both respiratory infection and cigarette smoking may be related to the development of the atopic state in those genetically susceptible. Males and females are equally affected.
4. Respiratory infections are common in asthmatic subjects. Whether these infections play an etiologic role or are linked by virtue of their relationship to the underlying inflammation in airways or more indirectly to cigarette smoking and atopy is unknown.
5. Cigarette smoking, both active and passive, has been linked to a number of the known or putative risk factors for asthma and needs much greater attention to clarify this important factor.
6. A variety of meteorologic conditions appear to worsen asthma severity. Laboratory investigations have suggested that at relatively low exposure levels, certain air pollutants (sulfur dioxide) can precipitate symptoms in some asthmatics. Whether chronic exposure to relatively high levels of specific pollutants increases the risk of asthma is unknown.
7. Because the disease frequency is high and the potential for incomplete penetrance may exist and there is no specific biologic marker of disease, the genetics of the disease have been difficult to establish. No knowledge is available about the inheritance of airway responsiveness. Atopy is at least in part genetically controlled.
8. The natural history of asthma is poorly understood. Childhood asthmatics have roughly a 50 percent chance of remission of their disease, although early age of onset and the atopic state argue for a poorer prognosis.
9. Mortality from asthma is a relatively rare event. However, because increased hospitalization for asthma, particularly among children and the poor, has been documented, greater concern about the availability of health care and the modes of therapy, particularly when that therapy may become complicated, is warranted.

REFERENCES

1. Adams, P. F., and Benson, V. Current estimates from the National Health Interview Survey 1989. National Center for Health Statistics. *Vital Health Stat.* Series 10, No. 176, 1990.
2. Aretaeus the Cappodocian. *The Extant Works of Aretaeus the Cappodocian,* edited and translated by Francis Adams. London: Syndenham Society, 1856. Quoted in M. Samter (ed.), *Excerpts from Classics in Allergy.* Columbus: Ross Laboratories, 1969.
3. Barbee, R. A., et al. Allergen skin-test reactivity in a community population sample: Correlation with age, histamine skin reactions and total serum immunoglobulin E. *J. Allergy Clin. Immunol.* 68:15, 1981.
4. Barbee, R. A., et al. Distribution of IgE in a community population sample: Correlations with age, sex, and allergen skin-test reactivity. *J. Allergy Clin. Immunol.* 68:106, 1981.
5. Barbee, R. A., et al. Immediate skin-test reactivity in a general population sample. *Ann. Intern. Med.* 84:129, 1976.
6. Barnes, P. J. A new approach to the treatment of asthma. *N. Engl. J. Med.* 321:161, 1989.
7. Barr, L. W., and Logan, G. B. Prognosis of children having asthma. *Pediatrics* 333:856, 1964.
8. Barter, C. E., and Campbell, A. H. Relationship of constitutional factors and cigarette smoking to decrease in 1-second forced expiratory volume. *Am. Rev. Respir. Dis.* 113:305, 1976.
9. Bates, D. V., and Sizto, R. Air pollution and hospital admission in Southern Ontario: The acid summer haze effect. *Environ. Res.* 48:317, 1987.
10. Blair, H. Natural history of wheezing in childhood. *J. R. Soc. Med.* 72:42, 1979.
11. Bland, M., et al. Effect of children's and parents' smoking on respiratory symptoms. *Arch. Dis. Child.* 53:100, 1978.

12. Broder, I., et al. Epidemiology of asthma and allergic rhinitis in a total community: Tecumseh, Michigan: III. Second survey of the community. *J. Allergy Clin. Immunol.* 53:127, 1974.
13. Brown, W. G., et al. The relationship of respiratory allergy, skin testing reactivity and serum IgE in a community sample. *J. Allergy Clin. Immunol.* 63:328, 1979.
14. Buffum, W. P. The prognosis of asthma in infancy. *Pediatrics* 32:453, 1963.
15. Buffum, W. P., and Settipane, G. A. Prognosis of asthma in childhood. *Am. J. Dis. Child.* 112:214, 1966.
16. Buist, A. S., and Vollmer, W. M. Prospective investigations in asthma. What have we learned from longitudinal studies about lung growth and senescence in asthma? *Chest* 91(Suppl.):119s, 1987.
17. Burney, P. G. J., et al. Descriptive epidemiology of bronchial reactivity in an adult population: Results from a community study. *Thorax* 42:38, 1987.
18. Burrows, B., et al. The relationship of serum immunoglobulin E, allergy skin tests, and smoking to respiratory disorders. *J. Allergy Clin. Immunol.* 70:199, 1982.
19. Burrows, B., et al. Epidemiologic observations on eosinophilia and its relationship to respiratory disorders. *Am. Rev. Respir. Dis.* 122:709, 1980.
20. Burrows, B., Lebowitz, M. D., and Barbee, R. A. Respiratory disorders and allergy skin test reactions. *Ann. Intern. Med.* 84:134, 1976.
21. Burrows, B., et al. The association of asthma with serum IgE levels and skin test reactivity to allergens. *N. Engl. J. Med.* 320:271, 1989.
22. Busse, W. W. Decreased granulocyte response to isoproterenol in asthma during upper respiratory infections. *Am. Rev. Respir. Dis.* 115:783, 1977.
23. Cockcroft, D. W., and Berscheid, B. A. Unimodal distribution of bronchial responsiveness to inhaled histamine in a random population. *Chest* 83:751, 1983.
24. Cockcroft, D. W., et al. Determinant of allergen-induced asthma: Dose of allergen, circulating IgE antibody concentration, and bronchial responsiveness to inhaled histamine. *Am. Rev. Respir. Dis.* 120:1053, 1979.
25. Cogswell, J. J., Halliday, D. F., and Alexander, J. R. Respiratory infections in the first year of life in children at risk of developing atopy. *Br. Med. J.* 284:1011, 1982.
26. Committee on Diagnostic Standards for Nontuberculosis Respiratory Diseases, American Thoracic Society. Chronic bronchitis, asthma, and pulmonary emphysema. *Am. Rev. Respir. Dis.* 85:762, 1962.
27. Corrao, W. M., Braman, S. S., and Irwin, R. S. Chronic cough as the sole presenting manifestation of bronchial asthma. *N. Engl. J. Med.* 300:633, 1979.
28. Crene, J., et al. Prescribed fenoterol and death from asthma in New Zealand, 1981–1983: Case-control study. *Lancet* 1:917, 1989.
29. Davis, J. B., and Bulpitt, C. J. Atopy and wheeze in children according to parental atopy and family size. *Thorax* 36:185, 1981.
30. Deal, E. C., Jr., et al. Airway responsiveness to cold air and hyperpnea in normal subjects and in those with hay fever and asthma. *Am. Rev. Respir. Dis.* 121:621, 1980.
31. Deal, E. C., Jr., et al. Hyperpnea and heat flux: Initial reaction sequence in exercise-induced asthma. *J. Appl. Physiol.* 46:47, 1979.
32. Dees, S. C. The asthmatic child: Development and course of asthma in children. *J. Dis. Child.* 93:228, 1957.
33. Derrick, E. H. The significance of the age of onset of asthma. *Med. J. Aust.* 1:1317, 1971.
34. Dodge, R. R., and Burrows, B. The prevalence and incidence of asthma and asthma-like symptoms in a general population sample. *Am. Rev. Respir. Dis.* 122:567, 1980.
35. Empey, D. W., et al. Mechanisms of bronchial hyperreactivity in normal subjects after upper respiratory tract infection. *Am. Rev. Respir. Dis.* 113:131, 1976.
36. Fletcher, C., et al. *The Natural History of Chronic Bronchitis and Emphysema: An Eight-Year Study of Early Chronic Obstructive Lung Disease in Working Men in London.* New York; Oxford University Press, 1976. P. 148.
37. Frick, A., German, D. F., and Mills, J. Development of allergy in children: I. Association with virus infections. *J. Allergy Clin. Immunol.* 63:228, 1979.
38. Gleich, G. J., et al. Allergy to tobacco, an occupational hazard. *N. Engl. J. Med.* 302:617, 1980.
39. Gortmaker, S. L., et al. Parental smoking and the risk of childhood asthma. *Am. J. Public Health* 72:574, 1982.
40. Greenberg, L., et al. Asthma and temperature change: II. 1964 and 1965 epidemiologic studies of emergency clinic visits for asthma in three large New York City hospitals. *Arch. Environ. Health* 12:561, 1966.
41. Gurwitz, D., Corey, M., and Levinson, H. Pulmonary function and bronchial reactivity in children after croup. *Am. Rev. Respir. Dis.* 122:95, 1980.
42. Gurwitz, D., Mindorff, C., and Levinson, H. Increased incidence of bronchial reactivity in children with a history of bronchiolitis. *J. Pediatr.* 98:551, 1981.
43. Hall, W. J., and Douglas, R. G. Pulmonary function during and after common respiratory infections. *Annu. Rev. Med.* 31:233, 1980.
44. Halonen, M., et al. An epidemiologic study of the interrelationships of total serum immunoglobulin E, allergy skin-test reactivity and eosinophilia. *J. Allergy Clin. Immunol.* 69:221, 1982.
45. Hcg, J. C. Bronchial mucosal permeability and its relationship to airways reactivity. *J. Allergy Clin. Immunol.* 67:421, 1981.
46. Hopp, R. J., et al. The presence of airway reactivity before the development of asthma. *Am. Rev. Respir. Dis.* 141:2, 1990.
47. Kiviloog, J., Irnell, L., and Eklund, G. The prevalence of bronchial asthma and chronic bronchitis in smokers and non-smokers in a representative local Swedish population. *Scand. J. Respir. Dis.* 55:262, 1974.
48. Korn, E. L., and Whittemore, A. S. Methods for analyzing panel studies of acute health effects of air pollution. *Biometrics* 35:795, 1979.
49. Kraepelien, S. Prognosis of asthma in childhood with special reference to pulmonary function and the failure of specific hyposensitization. *Acta Paediatr. Scand. Suppl.* 2:92, 1963.
50. Leeder, S. R., et al. Influence of family factors on asthma and wheezing during the first five years of life. *Br. J. Prev. Soc. Med.* 30:213, 1976.
51. Lorber, D. B., Kaltenborn, W., and Burrows, B. Responses to isoproterenol in a general population sample. *Am. Rev. Respir. Dis.* 118:855, 1978.
52. Marsh, D. G., Bias, W. B., and Ishizaka, K. Genetic control of basal serum immunoglobulin E level and its effect on specific reaginic sensitivity. *Proc. Natl. Acad. Sci. USA* 71:3588, 1974.
53. Marsh, D. G., Meyers, D. A., and Bias, W. B. The epidemiology and genetics of atopy allergy. *N. Engl. J. Med.* 305:1551, 1981.
54. Martin, A. J., Landau, K. I., and Phelan, P. H. Lung function in young adults who had asthma in childhood. *Am. Rev. Respir. Dis.* 122:609, 1980.
55. Martin, A. J., et al. The natural history of childhood asthma to adult life. *Br. Med. J.* 2:1939, 1980.
56. Martinez, F. D., et al. Parental smoking enhances bronchial responsiveness in nine-year-old children. *Am. Rev. Respir. Dis.* 138:518, 1988.
57. McFadden, E. R., Jr. Exertional dyspnea and cough as preludes to acute attacks of bronchial asthma. *N. Engl. J. Med.* 292:555, 1975.
58. McFadden, E. R., Jr., and Ingram, R. H., Jr. Exercise induced asthma: *N. Engl. J. Med.* 301:763, 1979.
59. McNicol, K. N., and Williams, H. B. Spectrum of asthma in children: I. Clinician physiological components. *Br. Med. J.* 4:7, 1973.
60. McNicol, K. N., and Williams, H. B. Spectrum of asthma in children: II. Allergic components. *Br. Med. J.* 4:12, 1973.
61. Murray, A. B., and Morrison, B. J. The effect of cigarette smoke from the mother on bronchial responsiveness and severity of symptoms in children with asthma. *J. Allergy Clin. Immunol.* 77:575, 1986.
62. O'Connell, E. J., and Logan, G. B. Parental smoking in childhood asthma. *Ann. Allergy* 32:142, 1974.
63. O'Connor, G. T., et al. The effect of passive smoking on pulmonary function and nonspecific bronchial responsiveness in a population-based sample of children and young adults. *Am. Rev. Respir. Dis.* 135:800, 1987.
64. Ogilvie, A. G. Asthma: A study in prognosis of 1,000 patients. *Thorax* 17:183, 1962.
65. Parker, D. R., et al. The relationship of nonspecific airway responsiveness and atopy to the rate of decline of lung function. *Am. Rev. Respir. Dis.* 141:589, 1990.
66. Pearce, N., et al. Case-control study of prescribed fenoterol and death from asthma in New Zealand 1977–81. *Thorax* 45:170, 1990.
67. Peat, J. K., Woolcock, A. J., and Cullen, K. Rate of decline of lung function in subjects with asthma. *Eur. J. Respir. Dis.* 70:171, 1987.
68. Pham, Q. T., et al. Prognostic value of acetylcholine challenge test: A prospective study. *Br. J. Ind. Med.* 41:267, 1984.
69. Pullan, C. R., and Hey, E. N. Wheezing, asthma and pulmonary dysfunction 10 years after infection with respiratory syncytial virus in infancy. *Br. Med. J.* 284:1665, 1982.
70. Rackerman, F. M., and Edwards, M. D. Asthma in children: A follow-up study of 688 patients after an interval of twenty years. *N. Engl. J. Med.* 246:815, 1952.
71. Rijcken, B., et al. The relationship of nonspecific bronchial responsiveness to respiratory symptoms in a random population sample. *Am. Rev. Respir. Dis.* 136:62, 1987.
72. Ryssing, E., and Flensborg, E. W. Prognosis after puberty for 442 asthmatic children examined and treated on specific allergologic principles. *Acta Paediatr. Scand.* 52:97, 1963.
73. Salome, C. M., et al. Bronchial hyperresponsiveness in two populations of

Australian schoolchildren. I. Relation to respiratory symptoms and diagnosed asthma. *Clin. Allergy* 17:271, 1987.

74. Schachter, E. N., Doyle, C. A., and Beck, G. J. A prospective study of asthma in a rural community. *Chest* 85:623, 1984.

75. Sears, W. R., et al. Relation between airway responsiveness and serum IgE in children with asthma and apparently normal children. *N. Engl. J. Med.* 325:1067, 1991.

76. Sheppard, D., et al. Exercise increases sulfur dioxide-induced bronchoconstriction in asthmatic subjects. *Am. Rev. Respir. Dis.* 123:486, 1981.

77. Sheppard, D., et al. Lower threshold and greater bronchomotor responsiveness of asthmatic subjects to sulfur dioxide. *Am. Rev. Respir. Dis.* 122:873, 1980.

78. Sibbald, B., Horn, M. E. C., and Grey, I. A family study of the genetic basis of asthma and wheezing bronchitis. *Arch. Dis. Child.* 35:354, 1980.

79. Sly, M. R. Mortality from asthma. *J. Allergy Clin. Immunol.* 84:421, 1989.

80. Sparrow, D., et al. The relationship of nonspecific bronchial responsiveness to the occurrence of respiratory symptoms and decreased levels of pulmonary function. The Normative Aging Study. *Am. Rev. Respir. Dis.* 135:1255, 1987.

81. Speizer, F. E., et al. Investigation into use of drugs preceding death from asthma. *Br. Med. J.* 1:339, 1968.

82. Taylor, R. G., et al. Bronchial reactivity to inhaled histamine and annual rate of decline in FEV_1 in male smokers and ex-smokers. *Thorax* 40:9, 1985.

83. Townley, R. G., et al. Bronchial sensitivity to methacholine in current and former asthmatic and allergic rhinitis patients and control subjects. *J. Allergy Clin. Immunol.* 56:429, 1975.

84. Utell, M. J., et al. Airway responses to sulfate and sulfuric acid aerosols in asthmatics. An exposure-response relationship. *Am. Rev. Respir. Dis.* 28:444, 1983.

85. Van Arsdel, P. P., Jr., and Motulsky, A. G. Frequency and heritability of asthma and allergic rhinitis in college students. *Acta. Genet.* 9:101, 1959.

86. Van der Lende, R., et al. Distribution of histamine threshold values in a random population. *Rev. Indust. Hyg. Mines.* 28:186, 1973.

87. Weiss, K. B., and Wagener, D. R. Changing patterns of asthma mortality, identifying target populations at high risk. *JAMA* 264:1683, 1990.

88. Weiss, S. T., et al. Persistent wheeze: Its relationship to respiratory illness, cigarette smoking, and level of pulmonary function in a population sample of children. *Am. Rev. Respir. Dis.* 122:697, 1980.

89. Weiss, S. T., et al. The relationship of respiratory infections in childhood to the occurrence of increased levels of airway responsiveness and atopy. *Am. Rev. Respir. Dis.* 131:573, 1985.

90. Weiss, S. T., et al. Airways responsiveness in a population sample of adults and children. *Am. Rev. Respir. Dis.* 129:898, 1984.

91. Weiss, S. T., et al. The effect of asthma on lung growth in children: a longitudinal study of male-female differences. *Amer. Rev. Respir. Dis.* 145:58, 1992.

92. Welliver, R. C., Kaul, T. N., and Ogra, P. L. The appearance of cell-bound IgE in respiratory-tract epithelium after respiratory syncytial-virus infection. *N. Engl. J. Med.* 303:1198, 1980.

93. Welty, C., et al. The relationship of airways responsiveness to cold air, cigarette smoking, and atopy to respiratory symptoms and pulmonary function in adults. *Am. Rev. Respir. Dis.* 130:198, 1984.

94. Williams, H., and McNicol, K. N. Prevalence, natural history and relationship of wheezy bronchitis and asthma in children: An epidemiological study. *Br. Med. J.* 4:321, 1969.

95. Woolcock, A. J., et al. Prevalence of bronchial hyperresponsiveness and asthma in a rural adult population. *Thorax* 41:283, 1986.

96. Zach, M., Erben, A., and Olinsky, A. Croup, recurrent croup, allergy, and airways hyperreactivity. *Arch. Dis. Child.* 56:336, 1981.

Genetic Factors

John W. Gerrard
Malcolm N. Blumenthal

FAMILIAL INCIDENCE OF ATOPIC DISEASE

It has been known for many years that diseases such as asthma, hay fever, and eczema tend to run in families. Cooke and Vander Veer in 1916 [20] undertook the first comprehensive study of the inheritance of allergy. They demonstrated that in many families asthma, hay fever, and urticaria occurred in successive generations, but they were unable to detect any consistent mode of inheritance. They were looking for a simple dominant or recessive mode of transmission. It is not surprising, in the light of our present knowledge, that no single, simple pattern emerged. Nevertheless, family histories are important, for they indicate to the physician whether the patient's symptoms are or are not likely to be allergic in origin. The importance of the family history was confirmed by Van Arsdel and Motulsky [75] who studied nearly 6,000 students at the University of Washington. They found that if both parents of the student were allergic, 58 percent of their offspring were allergic; if one parent was allergic, 20 percent of the offspring were allergic; and if no parent was allergic, only 6 percent of offspring were affected.

Meyers [60] noted that although the allergic status of the parent is important, the allergic status of siblings, who share both genetic and environmental factors with the child in question, also provides useful information. The importance of the subject's genetic constitution was underscored by Lubs' study [48] of 7,000 Swedish twin pairs. She found a greater concordance for asthma, hay fever, and eczema in monozygous (MZ) than in dizygous (DZ) twin pairs, though only the concordance for asthma was actually significant. Environmental factors were also found to be important, for more than half the MZ twin pairs with the same genetic makeup were in point of fact discordant for allergy. The risk factors that she [49] deduced for the development of allergy are indicated in Table 3-1.

In addition Gerrard and colleagues [31] showed that it is not only the susceptibility to develop allergic diseases that runs in families, but also their manifestation: Asthmatic parents are more likely to have children with asthma than children with hay fever or eczema, parents with hay fever are more likely to have children with hay fever than children with asthma or eczema, and parents with eczema are more likely to have children with eczema than children with asthma or hay fever. The localization of the atopic disorder in the respiratory tract, skin, or elsewhere is probably determined by genetic factors.

Cookson and colleagues [21] recently studied the transmission of atopy in 239 members of three extended and 40 nuclear families; in half the proband was atopic and in half it was not. Patients were labeled atopic if they had one or two of the following: one or more positive results on skin prick tests of common allergens, a total IgE that was more than 2 standard deviations above the population norm, and one or more positive results on radioallergosorbent tests (RASTs). They did not include symptoms such

as wheezing, for they were interested primarily in evidence of an immunologic IgE-mediated response. In the extended families, which were selected for their high incidence of atopy, atopy seemed to be transmitted in a dominant manner. In the nuclear families the evidence was not quite as convincing: The parents of two of the atopic asthmatic patients were not atopic. These investigators nevertheless concluded that atopy, defined as the propensity to produce IgE in response to common, usually inhalant antigens, is inherited in a simple autosomal dominant manner.

FACTORS, MAINLY NONGENETIC, INFLUENCING LEVELS OF IgE

Atopic State of the Patient

The term *atopy*, as originally introduced, meant "strange disease." Coca and Cooke [18] defined it as a type of hypersensitivity peculiar to humans, subject to hereditary influences, associated with circulating reaginic antibody, whealing-type reactions, and symptoms such as asthma and hay fever. The term as it is used today describes allergic diseases that involve the IgE system.

In westernized society, levels of IgE, apart from those in the rare patients with hyper-IgE syndrome and IgE myeloma, are closely related to atopy. IgE levels are highest in patients with asthma and eczema, being successively lower in those with asthma alone, eczema, hay fever, and allergic rhinitis [80]. Unfortunately, in the general population, levels of IgE do not segregate into clearly defined groups. Rather, IgE levels have a lognormal distribution, merging imperceptibly from the low to the intermediate to the high, with a few tailing off into the very high levels. There is no cutoff point below which it can be said that atopic disease does not occur (Fig. 3-1) [30].

Those individuals with the highest levels of IgE not only have the most extensive disease but also have the greatest variety of IgE antibodies, as was found when RASTs to a series of antigens were performed on sera from 42 atopic patients (J. W. Gerrard and C. Ko. Unpublished data, 1978). Two foods (cow's milk and egg), four animal danders (cat, dog, horse, and cow), seven pollens important locally (elm, maple, birch, timothy and Kentucky blue grass, Russian thistle, and lamb's quarters), and two mold spores (*Cladosporium* and *Alternaria*) were studied; ragweed is uncommon locally. Low levels of IgE were associated with a smaller proportion of positive results on RASTs; high levels were associated with a higher proportion.

Levels of IgE and/or Atopy

Although levels of IgE are closely linked in western societies to the development of atopic diseases, the environment as well as

Table 3-1. Risk of allergy in first-degree relatives of allergic individuals

Proband	Allergy	Normal population (%)	First-degree relatives (%)
Asthma	Asthma	3.8	9.2
	Hay fever	14.8	25.2
	Eczema	2.5	4.3
Hay fever	Asthma	3.8	6.0
	Hay fever	14.8	24.1
	Eczema	2.5	3.3
Eczema	Asthma	3.8	6.2
	Hay fever	14.8	24.1
	Eczema	2.5	7.7

Source: C. Cohen, Genetic aspects of allergy, *Med. Clin. North Am.* 58:25, 1974. Reprinted with permission.

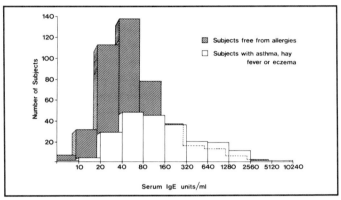

Fig. 3-1. *Histogram comparing serum IgE levels in those with asthma, hay fever, or eczema and in those free from allergies. (Reprinted with permission from J. W. Gerrard, et al. Serum IgE levels in white and metis communities in Saskatchewan.* Ann. Allergy *37:91, 1976.)*

host factors (genetic and nongenetic) play important roles in determining serum IgE levels and whether the patient will or will not develop atopy. Nongenetic factors include the age and sex of the host as well as environmental exposure to allergens, infections, and cigarette smoke.

If the incidence of allergy is to be reduced, and knowing the importance of the host and the environment in triggering atopic disorders, it is important to try and determine what it is that initiates sensitization.

Although the fetus can synthesize IgE, which has been identified in amniotic fluid as early as 13 weeks [70], the fetus seems to be protected in large measure from sensitization, for antenatal sensitization to foods is rare [83] and to inhalants is unknown. Antenatal sensitization to maternal parasitic infections with microfilaria has been documented [77]. Nevertheless, toward term, the fetus often makes IgE in measurable quantities; it is present in up to 82 percent of term infants [83], and levels of 0.9 U/ml or greater indicate that the fetus is potentially atopic, for 82 percent of such infants develop atopic disease by the age of 6 years [45].

Sensitization to Inhalant Allergens

The crucial role of inhalants in triggering atopic disease is indicated by the relative freedom from atopic disease in those still living in their pristine environments [46, 59]. In the western world, and probably in the world at large, the house dust mite allergen [26], followed by cat, dog, and cockroach allergens, are the most widespread and important of the domestic inhalant

allergens. Sensitization to these can occur in infancy, probably because the child is exposed to them on a daily basis. Exposure to cigarette smoke, particularly from the mother, accentuates the development of atopic disease, particularly in boys [65]. If children are to be shielded from the development of atopic disease, it is essential that these hazards be excluded from the home from before birth. It has been suggested that levels of house dust mite antigen (*Der p*) should be kept below 2 μg *Der p* I per gram of dust; this is equivalent to 100 mites per gram of dust [26].

Sensitization to Food Allergens

The most common manifestation of atopy in the first year of life is atopic dermatitis. Because atopic dermatitis is known to be often triggered by foods, studies have been carried out to determine the influence of feeding on its development. Modifying the mother's diet antenatally does not affect the incidence of atopic dermatitis in the baby, but breast-feeding does, provided the mother avoids common allergenic foods such as cow's milk, eggs, fish, and peanuts while she is breast-feeding her baby [16, 17]. Substituting a hydrolyzed casein formula, such as Nutramigen, also reduces the incidence of atopic dermatitis [17]. Early feeding with cow's milk is associated with an increase in atopy in babies with low levels of T-cells [44].

Antigenic Load

Although fewer breast-fed babies whose mothers avoid milk while breast-feeding have atopic dermatitis than formula-fed babies, they can develop severe IgE-mediated allergies to foods, with cow's milk, eggs, fish, and peanuts being the most common [27, 32]. In these instances they are usually asymptomatic until they are inadvertently given these foods (milk, egg, etc.), when they may develop anaphylactic reactions. Severe IgE-mediated reactions of this degree to cow's milk are never seen in formula-fed babies, indicating that low-dose sensitization—only traces of cow's milk appear in breast milk—leads to IgE sensitization. This is not surprising for if IgE antibody production is to play a role in the primary immune response, it must be triggered by trace amounts of the viral antigen in question. The antigenic load therefore plays a crucial role in determining sensitization. This applies not only to foods but also to inhalants, as indicated below. Confirmation that the amount of antigen to which the patient is exposed may be important in determining the response is suggested by the findings of Green and associates [35, 36] in the guinea pig. They noted that low levels of antigen stimulation (using Freund's adjuvant and bovine serum albumen [BSA]) provoked significant levels of BSA antibody in some strains of guinea pig but not in others. When antigenic exposure was increased, the differences between the strains disappeared. Atopic individuals may well be good responders to low antigen stimulation, and though this is a hazard to the atopic person in the modern world, it may well have been highly advantageous in primitive societies where survival depended on a brisk and early, as well as an effective, immune response to environmental pathogens.

Season of Birth

Settipane and Hagy [70] in the United States reported a significant increase in ragweed allergy in those born 3 months before the ragweed season. Bjorksten and Suoniemi [7] in Finland reported that babies born in the spring are more likely than those born at other times of the year to develop an allergy to birch and grass pollens, and that allergies are more likely to develop in seasons with a high pollen density [8], again indicating the importance of the dose of the allergen. It is tempting to speculate that there is a critical level below which there is no response, and that there may be another level above which the response is no longer IgE mediated.

Infections

Parasitic Infections

Although levels of IgE in the white population correlate closely with atopic disease, the biologic function of IgE is clearly not to cause allergic disease. In combination with other immune responses, its role is to play an integral part in the protection of the host against infection. The discovery of IgE and its relationship to the atopic state by Ishizakas and coworkers [40] and Johansson [42] was quickly followed by the finding that much higher levels were found in the developing world in heavily parasitized, preschool children [43]. The suggestion was made that the primary function of IgE was to protect the host from intestinal parasitism.

The highest levels of IgE in a normal population have been found in the Waorani Indians, living in the upper reaches of the Amazon [46]; their mean IgE level is 11,975 U/ml. They are heavily parasitized, but are otherwise healthy and are remarkably free from atopic disease. When the studies were undertaken, none had asthma. In another isolated community in the highlands of Papua New Guinea, whose first contact with civilization was in 1933, asthma was unknown. Even in 1974, 40 years later, only 0.2 to 0.3 percent of the adult population had developed asthma [2], but 10 years later, in 1985, after increasing westernization, its incidence had risen to 7.3 percent [25]. In less-sheltered but more westernized communities in Africa—the Gambia [34] and Rhodesia [59]—IgE levels are still high. They are higher, as might be expected, in rural areas, and have fallen in urban communities, presumably because of better hygiene. In the rural communities, even though IgE levels are high, there was no asthma in 1975 [34]. In the urban communities, with lower IgE levels, asthma had made its appearance.

It would seem that the introduction of hygiene is followed by a fall in parasitism and IgE levels, and the development of atopy. The fall in parasitism, it has been suggested, frees IgE-binding sites on mast cells, allowing them to accept antibodies directed against allergens [59], the most important of which may be the house dust mite [26]. There is some evidence, mainly anecdotal, that parasitism may predispose to the development of asthma, but surveys indicate that asthma is less common where intestinal parasitism is endemic, supporting the thesis that parasitism protects against the development of asthma [57]. Another possible explanation for the increase of atopic disorders would be the exposure of individuals, genetically tolerant to their pristine environment, to foreign allergens at the same time that their contact with parasites is decreased.

The introduction of the blanket in Papua New Guinea, by providing a home for the mite, probably played an important role in the genesis of asthma in that country [25]. If this is the case, the removal of parasitism opened the door to the mite and led to the emergence of asthma and other allergies. Even in Saskatchewan there is an inverse relationship between IgE levels in the white and North American Indian communities and the prevalence of asthma [30]. Asthma is twice as common in the white community as it is in the Indian, even though IgE levels are higher in the latter.

Viral Infections

In addition to IgE being involved in protection against parasites, there is evidence that it plays a role in combating viral infections [28, 66], infectious mononucleosis, and cytomegalovirus infections [3, 4]. In this capacity it contributes, with IgM and IgD, to the primary immune response; levels of specific antibodies fall as soon as the initial infection is over. Its postulated role in the primary response is that of a gate opener, the local release of histamine and leukotrienes leading to capillary dilatation, resulting in an increase in blood flow to the infected area, and increased capillary permeability, enabling macrophages and polymorphonuclear leukocytes to more readily enter the tissue spaces. The fact that IgE levels are high in childhood and decline at puberty may well be due in part to the fact that it is in childhood that many viral infections (measles, varicella, and poliomyelitis, for example) are encountered for the first time.

Bacterial and Fungal Infections

Certain bacteria such as *Staphylococcus aureus* or fungi such as *Candida albicans* will increase IgE levels in some patients with the hyper-IgE syndrome or atopic dermatitis.

Age, Sex, and Cigarette Smoke and Other Pollutants

IgE levels at birth are either undetectable or very low and then rise rapidly during the first 2 to 3 years of life, peaking at puberty [5, 30, 79]. IgE rises more rapidly and to much greater levels in the atopic subject, and atopy undoubtedly accounts for most of the increase in IgE levels. After puberty, levels in the nonatopic subject, already low, remain remarkably constant over the years; in the atopic subject they fall slowly, but tend to be higher in men than in women [5]. This is probably because in men, but not in women, smoking boosts levels of IgE, particularly in those with atopy. Barbee and colleagues [5] found that IgE levels in nonsmoking, nonatopic men and women are the same.

We do not know why smoking should boost levels of IgE [14, 29], particularly in the atopic male, but it has been suggested that smoking, by causing inflammation of the airways, facilitates the absorption of antigens, leading to sensitization and, in some instances, occupational asthma [84] (see also Chap. 2). It may also influence the immune response, for it depresses levels of IgG and IgM and possibly IgA [29]. It has been suggested that smoking potentiates sensitization. When studying risk factors in the development of allergic disease, Wittig and coworkers [80] found that in families in which there was smoking, atopic disease had an earlier onset and was accompanied by more positive results on skin tests of certain pollen antigens. Burrows and colleagues [15] found that smokers over the age of 54 who have high levels of IgE tend to have a form of chronic bronchitis that is very difficult to manage. Air pollution with particles and fumes have been reported to aggravate atopic disorders such as asthma [58, 63, 64, 73]. They may have a direct effect on the respiratory tract or have a synergistic effect with aeroallergens.

FACTORS, MAINLY GENETIC, INFLUENCING LEVELS OF IgE AND ATOPY

The genetic control of atopic disease is complex. It is probably polygenic, involving many genetic controls acting at several different stages involved in its development, for example, regulating the specific immune response to an allergen such as ragweed, the production of specific IgE antibodies, the ability of the IgE antibody to attach to cells and assist in the release of mediators, as well as the end-organ response to the mediators released. Others suggest that the atopic process in general is regulated by a major gene.

Regulation of the Specific Immune Response

The general expression of allergic disease has been known for many years to be familial and to have heritability. Recently the general expression of certain diseases was noted to be associated with the presence of extended HLA haplotypes [1, 24]. It is suggested that different extended haplotypes contain a different pattern of chromosomal deletions and insertions, some of which may influence the level of gene expression. As a result, certain combinations of alleles, especially of D/DR and complement loci, are seen to be highly associated with a disease. Blumenthal and associates [11] demonstrated that the frequencies of HLA-DR2 and the extended major histocompatibility complex (MHC) haplotype B7, SC31, DR2 were increased significantly in patients with asthma who had high titers of IgE anti-*Amb a* V. Conversely, these patients had decreased frequencies of HLA-DR3 and the extended haplotypes HLA-DR3 and HLA B8, SC01, DR3. These findings are consistent with a dominant MHC-linked gene or genes on HLA B7, SC31, DR2 controlling the IgE immune response to *Amb a* V and predisposing to asthma.

With complex allergens, such as ragweed *Amb* I, heritability can be demonstrated using family studies, as has been shown by Levine et al. [47], Blumenthal et al. [9], and Yoo et al. [82]. Wilcox and Marsh [78], in small multifamily studies, found no significant segregation.

Employing purified allergens, evidence that the immune response is associated with the MHC, specifically DR, has been demonstrated. Population studies demonstrating an association between the IgE response to *Amb a* V and HLA-DR2 and -Dw2 has been reported by Marsh et al. [53, 54] and confirmed by Blumenthal et al. [11] and Coulter et al. [23]. Additional studies by Marsh [52] showed that antibody responses to *Amb t* V, *Amb a* V, and *Amb p* V were associated with the HLA-DR2. The author concluded that the same immunoglobulin molecules associated with Dw2 participate in the immune recognition of structurally similar sites on all three *Amb a* V molecules. Studies [40] have also suggested that the presentation of ragweed *Amb a* V to the T-cell is determined by DR rather than DQ or DP. Other allergens that have shown HLA association include *Amb a* VI with DR5 and *Loi p* I, II, and III with DR3 [52].

The presence of an immunosuppressive gene linked to the HLA system was suggested by Sasazuki et al. [69] using streptococcal cell wall, cedar pollen, and schistosomal antigens. These authors regard susceptibility to cedar pollinosis as a recessive trait and resistance or suppression to be dominant. Their work has not been confirmed.

Regulation of IgE Levels

The regulation of IgE has been shown to be heritable; however, its exact mode of inheritance is not well established. Twin studies [13] have indicated a greater degree of concordance in IgE levels in MZ than in DZ twins; the degree of concordance is greatest in infancy and early childhood, diminishing with age due to the impact of environmental influences [6]. Studies of twins raised apart, maximizing the effect of environmental factors, indicate that in addition to the levels of IgE there is a greater degree of concordance for specific IgE antibodies, as indicated by RAST and skin tests, in MZ than in DZ twins [37]. Surprisingly, however, the clinical manifestations of atopy often differ markedly, suggesting not only that it is the level of specific antibody that determines the development of allergy, but also that other factors—for example, levels of IgG and IgA or alterations in the IgG/IgE ratio, as well as other host factors and environmental exposures—determine whether the subject will or will not manifest atopic disease.

Family studies have also been performed to study the relationship between high levels of IgE and genetic factors. Marsh and associates [55, 56] were the first to address this possibility. They studied 28 allergic families and concluded that high IgE levels were determined by a recessive factor. Gerrard and Rao and their colleagues [33, 67], using more sophisticated techniques and a larger population, came to the same conclusion. Blumenthal and coworkers [10], studying three large allergic pedigrees, also found heritability and demonstrated a major IgE-regulating locus, but found the overall results consistent with a dominant mode of

inheritance. Additional investigations by Meyers and colleagues [62], studying 23 large Amish and 533 members of Mormon pedigrees, and by Blumenthal and associates [13], demonstrated a great deal of genetic heterogeneity regarding regulation of serum IgE levels.

Cookson and coworkers [21, 22] more recently investigated a series of allergic families with asthma and allergic rhinitis. They looked at both total serum IgE levels and also at specific IgE responses to allergens as determined by skin testing and RAST. The data suggested that atopy, defined as the ability to produce an IgE response, using several parameters, is inherited as an autosomal dominant character, and that it is linked to chromosome 11q. This is probably not the final word; for Lympany and her colleagues [85], who studied nine families in which the index case had a history of atopy or asthma, and used the same criteria, as well as bronchial hyperresponsiveness, for atopy and asthma that Cookson had used, were unable to confirm his findings. Further studies are awaited.

Release of Mediators

The interaction of IgE with cells and their ability to release mediating substances has not been extensively investigated (see also Chap. 8). Histamine release has been noted in two studies to be influenced by genetic factors. Marone and coworkers [50, 51] investigated twins, studying the release of histamine from basophils in response to anti-IgE, f-met peptide, and Ca^{++} ionophore A 23187. They found the Ca^{++} ionophore– and anti-IgE–induced release of histamine to be under genetic control while f-met peptide–induced release was not. Furthermore, the IgE-mediated releasability was controlled by genetic factors that were independent of the genetics of serum IgE levels. Roitman-Johnson and colleagues [68], studying nuclear families, also demonstrated a heritability of histamine release that was independent of serum IgE levels.

Bronchial Hyperresponsiveness

Another factor associated with asthma is bronchial hyperresponsiveness (BHR) (see Chap. 4). Townley et al. [74] and Hopp et al. [38] studied the incidence of BHR in a large number of controls as well as in families in whom the proband had asthma. They found that the atopic member, when compared with normal family members, had increased BHR. They concluded that familial and possibly genetic factors influenced the development of clinical asthma, and that there was strong evidence that nonspecific BHR was found in certain individuals, and that its presence was likely determined by genetic factors. Cockcroft [19] reported that BHR is not present between seasons in seasonal asthmatics, suggesting that it is associated with but does not cause asthma. It would seem that although BHR is associated with asthma, particularly in those with late asthmatic responses, it does not exist in the atopic subject apart from asthma. The interrelationships between asthma and BHR and their genetics are not yet well defined.

INTRINSIC, NONATOPIC ASTHMA

So far only the genetic and environmental factors that play a part in the development of atopy and allergic asthma have been discussed. Atopy, asthma, and IgE levels are all the product of many factors, and only when their interrelationships are fully known will it be possible to explain why asthma develops only in certain susceptible individuals, and why it runs such varied courses, increasing in severity in some, running a relatively constant course in others, and diminishing in severity in still others.

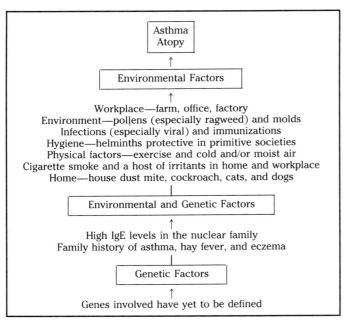

Asthma
Atopy
↑
Environmental Factors
↑
Workplace—farm, office, factory
Environment—pollens (especially ragweed) and molds
Infections (especially viral) and immunizations
Hygiene—helminths protective in primitive societies
Physical factors—exercise and cold and/or moist air
Cigarette smoke and a host of irritants in home and workplace
Home—house dust mite, cockroach, cats, and dogs
|
Environmental and Genetic Factors
↑
High IgE levels in the nuclear family
Family history of asthma, hay fever, and eczema
|
Genetic Factors
↑
Genes involved have yet to be defined

Fig. 3-2. *Although little is known about the genetic control of the many mechanisms involved in the development of asthma, probably the most important element is the patient's genetic constitution, HLA type, and chromosomal constitution. Asthma only develops when an individual comes in contact with and is sensitized to factors in the environment. The environment is therefore very important, and is the only factor that can be controlled. If the figure can be visualized as a tree, genetic factors are seen to form the roots, high IgE levels and the atopic state of close relatives (the result of their interaction with their environments) form the trunk, and the purely environmental factors form the branches.*

In this chapter we have only addressed the genetics of "extrinsic," "allergic," or "IgE"-mediated asthma. The factors that play a part in the development of intrinsic, nonallergic asthma have not been addressed. Sibbald [71] studied the familial incidence of these two types of asthma. She classified the extrinsic asthmatics as those we had evidence of atopy, either hay fever or atopic dermatitis, positive results on skin prick tests, and reactions to inhalants such as house dust, pollens, and animal danders. She found the incidence of the two types of asthma to be the same in the parents and offspring of both those with extrinsic and those with intrinsic asthma. This suggests that asthma, whether extrinsic or intrinsic, may have a common genetic origin. The prevalence of asthma in first-degree relatives was greater in the relatives of the subjects with extrinsic asthma than in those of subjects with intrinsic asthma, suggesting that separate factors may determine the development of atopy and asthma. Asthma can certainly be triggered by allergy, particularly in the young, but it can also be triggered by other, nonallergic factors. Only when we know the mechanisms involved will we be able to more fully understand the genetics of asthma.

In conclusion, asthma is a condition in which genetic factors have been shown to play a significant role in initiating specific immune responses to aeroallergens, in the production of IgE, in the release of mediators, and in the development of BHR, as well as in the clinical entity we call asthma. When the many genes involved in the development of allergic asthma, and the details of their interaction with environmental factors, have been identified, it should be possible to better define asthma, and to treat it in a more rational and less pragmatic manner. It may also enable us to provide more detailed genetic counseling with the possibility of genetic engineering (Fig. 3-2).

REFERENCES

1. Alpers, C. A., et al. Genetic prediction of non-response to hepatitis B vaccine. *N. Engl. J. Med.* 321:708, 1986.
2. Anderson, H. R. The epidemiological and allergic features of asthma in the New Guinea Highlands. *Clin. Allergy* 4:171, 1974.
3. Bahna, S. L., et al. IgE response in heterophil-positive infectious mononucleosis. *J. Allergy Clin. Immunol.* 62:167, 1978.
4. Bahna, S. L., Horwitz, C. A., and Heiner, D. C. IgE in cytomegalovirus mononucleosis (CMV mono). *J. Allergy Clin. Immunol.* 61:177, 1978.
5. Barbee, R. A., et al. A longitudinal study of serum IgE in a community cohort: Correlations with age, sex, smoking and atopic status. *J. Allergy Clin. Immunol.* 79:919, 1987.
6. Bazaral, M., Orgel, H. A., and Hamburger, R. N. Genetics of IgE and allergy: Serum IgE levels in twins. *J. Allergy Clin. Immunol.* 54:283, 1974.
7. Bjorksten, F., and Suoniemi, I. Dependence of immediate hypersensitivity on the month of birth. *Clin. Allergy* 6:165, 1976.
8. Bjorksten, F., and Suoniemi, I. Early Allergen Contacts, Adjuvant Factors and Subsequent Allergy. In J. W. Kerr and M. A. Gamderton (eds.), *Proceedings of the XIth International Congress of Allergology and Clinical Immunology.* London: Macmillan, 1983. Pp. 145–148.
9. Blumenthal, M. N., et al. Genetic mapping of the Ir locus in man: Linkage to second locus of HL-A. *Science* 184:1301, 1974.
10. Blumenthal, M. N., et al. Study of genetic transmission of serum IgE levels. *J. Allergy Clin. Immunol.* 63:169, 1979.
11. Blumenthal, M. N., et al. Ra5 immune responses, HLA antigens and complotypes. *J. Allergy Clin. Immunol.* 75:155, 1985.
12. Blumenthal, M. N., et al. Preventive allergy: Genetics of IgE mediated diseases. *J. Allergy Clin. Immunol.* 78:962, 1986.
13. Blumenthal, M. N., and Bonini, S. Immunogenetics of Specific Immune Responses to Allergens in Twins and Families. In D. Marsh, and M. N. Blumenthal (eds.), *The Genetic and Environmental Factors in Clinical Allergy.* Minneapolis: University of Minnesota Press, 1990 Pp. 132–142.
14. Burrows, B., et al. The relationship of serum immunoglobulin E to cigarette smoking. *Am. Rev. Respir. Dis.* 124:523, 1981.
15. Burrows, B., et al. The relationship of serum immunoglobulin E, allergy skin tests, and smoking to respiratory disorders. *J. Allergy Clin. Immunol.* 70:199, 1982.
16. Chandra, R. K., et al. Influence of maternal food allergy avoidance during pregnancy and lactation on incidence of atopic eczema in infants. *Clin. Allergy* 16:565, 1986.
17. Chandra, R. K., Puri, S., Hamed, A. Influence of maternal diet during lactation and use of formula feeds on development of atopic eczema in high risk infants. *Br. Med. J.* 299:228, 1989.
18. Coca, A. F., and Cooke, R. A. The classification of the phenomena of hypersensitivity. *J. Immunol.* 8:163, 1923.
19. Cockcroft, D. W., et al. Allergen-induced increase in non-allergic bronchial reactivity. *Clin. Allergy* 7:508, 1977.
20. Cooke, R. A., and Vander Veer, A. Human sensitization. *J. Immunol.* 1:201, 1916.
21. Cookson, W. O. C. M., and Hopkin, J. M. Dominant inheritance of atopic immunoglobulin-E responsiveness. *Lancet* 1:86, 1988.
22. Cookson, W. O. C. M., et al. Linkage between immunoglobulin-E responses underlying asthma and rhinitis and chromosome 11q. *Lancet* 1:1292, 1989.
23. Coulter, K. M., et al. Genetic Controls of IgE Antibody Responses in Human to Amb a V (Ra5) Model. In D. Marsh, and M. N. Blumenthal (eds.), *The Genetic and Environmental Factors in Clinical Allergy.* Minneapolis: University of Minnesota Press, 1990, Pp. 124–131.
24. Craven, D. E., et al. Non-responsiveness to hepatitis B vaccine in health care workers. Result of revaccination in genetic typing. *Ann Intern. Med.* 105:356, 1986.
25. Dowse, G. K., et al. The association between *Dermatophagoides* mites and the increasing prevalence of asthma in village communities within the Papua New Guinea highlands. *J. Allergy Clin. Immunol.* 75:83, 1985.
26. Dust mite allergens and asthma—a world wide problem. *J. Allergy Clin. Immunol.* 83:416, 1989.
27. Firer, M. A., Hosking, C. S., and Hill, D. J. Effect of antigen load on development of milk antibodies in infants allergic to milk. *Br. Med. J.* 283:693, 1981.
28. Frick, O. L., German, D. F., and Mills, J. Development of allergy in children: I. Association with virus infections. *J. Allergy Clin. Immunol.* 63:228, 1979.
29. Gerrard, J. W., et al. Immunoglobulin levels in smokers and nonsmokers. *Ann. Allergy* 44:261, 1980.
30. Gerrard, J. W., et al. Serum IgE levels in white and metis communities in Saskatchewan. *Ann. Allergy* 37:91, 1976.

31. Gerrard, J. W., et al. The familial incidence of allergic disease. *Ann. Allergy* 36:10, 1976.

32. Gerrard, J. W., and Perelmutter, L. IgE mediated allergy to peanut, cow's milk and egg in children with special reference of maternal diet. *Ann. Allergy* 56:351, 1986.

33. Gerrard, J. W., Rao, D. C., and Morton, N. E. A genetic study of immunoglobulin E. *Am. J. Hum. Genet.* 30:46, 1978.

34. Godfrey, R. C. Asthma and IgE levels in rural and urban communities in the Gambia. *Clin. Allergy* 5:201, 1975.

35. Green, I., and Benacerraf, B. Genetic control of immune responses to limiting doses of proteins and hapten protein conjugates in guinea pigs. *J. Immunol.* 107:374, 1971.

36. Green, I., Inman, J., and Benacerraf, B. Genetic control of the immune response of guinea pigs to limiting dose of bovine serum albumen. *Proc. Natl. Acad. Sci. USA* 66:1267, 1970.

37. Hanson, B., et al. Atopic disease and immunoglobulin E in twins reared apart and together. *Am. J. Hum. Genet.* 48:873, 1991.

38. Hopp, R., et al. Genetic Aspects of Bronchial Hyperreactivity. In D. Marsh, and M. N. Blumenthal (eds.), *The Genetic and Environmental Factors in Clinical Allergy*. Minneapolis: University of Minnesota Press, 1990. Pp. 143–152.

39. Huang, S. K., and Marsh, D. Genetic restriction of human T-cell clones to short ragweed allergen Amb a V. *Am. J. Hum. Genet.* 45:196, 1989.

40. Ishizaka, K., Ishizaka, T., and Hornbrook, M. M. Physiochemical properties of reaginic antibody; V. Correlation of reaginic activity with E-globulin antibody. *J. Immunol.* 97:840, 1966.

41. Jarret, E. E. E., and Basin, H. Elevation of total serum IgE in rats following helminth parasite infection. *Nature* 251:613, 1974.

42. Johansson, S. G. O. Raised levels of a new immunoglobulin class (IgND) in asthma. *Lancet* 2:951, 1967.

43. Johansson, S. G. O., Melbin, T., and Valquist, B. Immunoglobulin levels in Ethiopian school children with special reference to high concentrations of immunoglobulin E (IgND). *Lancet* 1:1118, 1968.

44. Juto, P. Elevated serum immunoglobulin E in T cell deficient infants fed cow's milk. *J. Allergy Clin. Immunol.* 66:402, 1980.

45. Kjellman, N-I. M., and Croner, S. Cord blood IgE determination for allergy prediction—A follow up to 7 years of age in 1651 children. *Ann. Allergy* 53:161, 1984.

46. Larrick, J. W., et al. Does hyperimmunoglobulin-E protect tropical populations from allergic disease? *J. Allergy Clin. Immunol.* 71:184, 1983.

47. Levine, B. B., Stember, R. H., and Fotino, M. Ragweed hay fever: Genetic control and linkage to HL-A haplotypes. *Science* 178:1201, 1972.

48. Lubs, M. L. E. Allergy in 7000 twin pairs. *Acta. Allergol.* 26:249, 1971.

49. Lubs, M. L. E. Empirical risks for genetic counselling in families with allergy. *J. Pediatr.* 80:26, 1972.

50. Marone, G., et al. Human basophil releasability. III. Genetic controls of the human basophil releasability. *J. Immunol.* 137:3588, 1986.

51. Marone, G., et al. The Role of Genetic and Environmental Factors in the Control of Basophil and Mast Cell Releasability. In D. Marsh, and M. N. Blumenthal (eds.), *The Genetic and Environmental Factors in Clinical Allergy*. Minneapolis: University of Minnesota Press, 1990. Pp. 153–160.

52. Marsh, D. Immunogenetic and Immunochemical Factors Determining Immune Responsiveness to Allergens: Studies in Unrelated Subjects. In D. Marsh, and M. N. Blumenthal (eds.), *The Genetic and Environmental Factors in Clinical Allergy*. Minneapolis: University of Minnesota Press, 1990. Pp. 97–123.

53. Marsh, D., Hsu, S. H., Roebber, M., et al. HLA-Dw2:A genetic marker for human immune response to short ragweed allergen Ra5 I response resulting primarily from natural antigenic exposure. *J. Exp. Med.* 155:1439, 1982.

54. Marsh, D., et al. HLA-Dw2:A genetic marker for human immune response to short ragweed allergen Ra5 II. Response after ragweed immunotherapy. *J. Exp. Med.* 155:1452, 1982.

55. Marsh, D. G., Bias, W. B., and Ishizaka, K. Genetic control of basal serum immunoglobulin E level, and its effect on specific reaginic sensitivity. *Proc. Natl. Acad. Sci. USA* 51:174, 1974.

56. Marsh, D. G., Meyers, D. A., and Bias, W. B. The epidemiology and genetics of atopic allergy. *N. Engl. J. Med.* 305:1551, 1981.

57. Masters, A., and Barret-Connor, E. Parasites and asthma—predictive or protective? *Epidemiol. Rev.* 1:49, 1985.

58. Matsumura, Y. The effects of ozone, nitrogen dioxide, and sulfur dioxide on the experimentally induced allergic respiratory disorders in Guinea pigs. *Am. Rev. Respir. Dis.* 102:430, 1970.

59. Merret, T. G., Merret, J., and Cookson, J. B. Allergy and parasites: The measurement of total and specific IgE levels in urban and rural communities in Rhodesia. *Clin. Allergy* 6:131, 1976.

60. Meyers, D. A. Family Analysis and Genetic Counselling for Allergic Diseases. In D. Marsh, and M. N. Blumenthal (eds.), *The Genetic and Environmental Factors in Clinical Allergy*. Minneapolis: University of Minnesota Press, 1990. Pp. 161–173.

61. Meyers, D. A., Bias, W. B., and Marsh, D. G. A genetic study of total IgE levels in the Amish. *Hum. Hered.* 32:15, 1982.

62. Meyers, D. A., et al. Total IgE levels in Mormon and Amish families (abstract). *J. Allergy Clin. Immunol.* 67:60, 1981.

63. Miyamoto, T., et al. Mechanism of asthmatic attack in bronchial asthma; 1. From the study of skin sensitizing antibody and hypersensitivity of respiratory tract. *Jpn. J. Allergy* 17:91, 1968.

64. Muranaka, M., et al. Adjuvant activity of diesel-exhaust particulates for the production of IgE antibody in mice. *J. Allergy Clin. Immunol.* 77:616, 1986.

65. Murray, A. B., and Morrison, B. J. Passive smoking by asthmatics: Its greater effect on boys than on girls and on older than on younger children. *Pediatrics* 84:451, 1989.

66. Perelmutter, L., Potvin, L., and Phipps, P. Immunoglobulin E responses during viral infections. *J. Allergy Clin. Immunol.* 64:127, 1979.

67. Rao, D. C., et al. Immunoglobulin E revisited. *Am. J. Hum. Genet.* 32:620, 1980.

68. Roitman-Johnson, B., and Blumenthal, N. M. Family analysis of histamine release (abstract). *J. Allergy Clin. Immunol.* 81:232, 1988.

69. Sasazuki, T., et al. MHC-link immune suppression genes and antigen specific T-cell in man. *Prog. Immunol.* 5:949, 1983.

70. Settipane, R. I., and Hagy, G. W. Effect of atmospheric pollen on the newborn. *Rhode Island Med. J.* 62:477, 1979.

71. Sibbald, B. Extrinsic and intrinsic asthma: Influence of classification on family history of asthma and allergic disease. *Clin. Allergy* 10:313, 1980.

72. Singer, A. D., et al. Evidence for secretory IgA and IgE in utero. *J. Allergy Clin. Immunol.* 53:94, 1974.

73. Takafuji, S., et al. Enhancing effect of suspended particulate matter on the IgE antibody production in mice. *Int. Arch. Allergy Appl. Immunol.* 90:1, 1989.

74. Townley, R. G., et al. Segregation analysis of bronchial response to methacholine inhalation challenge in families with and without asthma. *J. Allergy Clin. Immunol.* 77:101, 1986.

75. Van Arsdel, P. P., and Motulsky, A. G. Frequency and hereditability of asthma and allergic rhinitis in college students. *Acta. Genet. Stat. Med.* 9:104, 1959.

76. Venables, K. M., et al. Interaction of smoking and atopy in producing specific IgE antibody against a hapten protein conjugate. *Br. Med. J.* 290:201, 1985.

77. Weil, G. T., et al. Prenatal allergic sensitization to helminth antigens in offspring of parasitic infected mothers. *J. Clin. Invest.* 71:1124, 1983.

78. Wilcox, H., and Marsh, D. Genetic regulation of antibody heterogeneity. *Immunogenetics* 6:209, 1978.

79. Wittig, H. J., et al. Age related serum immunoglobulin E levels in healthy subjects and in patients with allergic disease. *J. Allergy Clin. Immunol.* 66:305, 1980.

80. Wittig, H. J., et al. Risk factors in the development of allergic disease: Analysis of 2,190 patient records. *Ann. Allergy* 41:84, 1978.

81. Wuthrich, B., et al. Total and specific IgE (RAST) in atopic twins. *Clin. Allergy* 11:147, 1981.

82. Yoo, T. J., et al. A family study of HLA antigen and immune response (Ir) gene linkage in ragweed and dust allergies. *J. Allergy Clin. Immunol.* 57:229, 1976.

83. Zeiger, R. S., et al. Effectiveness of dietary manipulation in the prevention of food allergy. *J. Allergy Clin. Immunol.* 78:224, 1986.

84. Zetterstrom, O., et al. Another smoking hazard: Raised serum IgE concentration and increased risk of occupational allergy. *Br. Med. J.* 283:1215, 1981.

85. Lympany, P., et al. Genetic analysis using DNA polymorphism of the linkage between chromosome 11q13 and atopy and bronchial hyperresponsiveness to methacholine. *J. Allergy Clin. Immunol.* 89:619, 1992.

Mechanisms of Airway Hyperresponsiveness

Donald W. Cockcroft
Paul M. O'Byrne

4

Airway hyperresponsiveness, the increased responsiveness of the airway to nonsensitizing physical or chemical stimuli, is a consistent feature of asthma, at least as it is currently defined [17, 27, 60] (see Chap. 1). Airway hyperresponsiveness has become part of more recent definitions of asthma [3]. Some experts are prepared to concede that airway hyperresponsiveness is virtually synonymous with asthma, whereas others believe that although not synonymous with asthma, airway hyperresponsiveness is at least very closely related to the clinical asthma syndrome [18]. Whatever the case, to better understand airway hyperresponsiveness, its measurement, its clinical significance, and its mechanisms is to better understand asthma. Unfortunately, the mechanisms surrounding the hyperresponsiveness of the airways in asthma remain obscure and somewhat controversial. This chapter will provide a broad overview of the various possible mechanisms responsible for airway hyperresponsiveness to nonsensitizing stimuli in asthma; many of these individual areas will be covered in greater detail in subsequent chapters. Airway responsiveness to sensitizing stimuli (e.g., allergen) will not be discussed except as it relates to airway hyperresponsiveness (to nonsensitizing stimuli).

AIRWAY HYPERRESPONSIVENESS: DEFINITION AND MEASUREMENT

Airway responsiveness is defined as the degree to which airways constrict in response to nonsensitizing physical or chemical stimuli [28]. The normal airway responsiveness probably serves a useful physiologic role, both in terms of helping to keep ventilation matched to perfusion [36] and to protect the pulmonary parenchyma from the detrimental effects of toxic inhalants.

Airway hyperresponsiveness, thus, is an increase above the normal responsiveness of the airways to these stimuli. When measured with histamine or methacholine, there is an increase both in the ease of airway narrowing (left shift of the dose-response curves) [30, 148] and in the magnitude of the airway constriction (elevation and eventual loss of the maximal response plateau) [148] (Fig. 4-1). Airway responsiveness is distributed continuously in a lognormal fashion in humans [24, 147] and animals [45, 127]. There is no sharp demarcation between normal responsiveness and hyperresponsiveness; the distinction is somewhat arbitrary and necessarily "gray" [27, 28].

Many stimuli can be used to measure airway responsiveness acting through different and often not completely understood mechanisms [28, 108]. Stimuli used to provoke airway narrowing include cholinergic agonists (methacholine, carbachol, acetylcholine), histamine, beta-adrenergic blockers, alpha-adrenergic agonists, serotonin, bradykinin, prostaglandins ($F_{2\alpha}$), leukotrienes (C_4, D_4, E_4), adenosine monophosphate (AMP), neuropeptides, as well as physical stimuli such as exercise, cold air, hyper-

ventilation, and nonisotonic aerosols [108] (see Chap. 39). Considering the different mechanisms and receptors involved in these different stimuli, it is surprising that there is as reasonable a correlation between different stimuli as there is. This is particularly true for histamine, methacholine, exercise, cold air, and probably arachidonic acid metabolites [1, 5, 49, 70, 104, 134]. It is, however, not surprising that correlations between different stimuli are not perfect.

Recently, the separation of bronchoconstrictor stimuli into direct (histamine, methacholine) and indirect (exercise, cold air, nonisotonic aerosols, propranolol, AMP, neurokinins, etc.) categories has been proposed [108]. Since bronchoconstriction under natural conditions in asthmatic subjects is likely to involve indirect mechanisms, it has been hypothesized that bronchoconstrictive responses to the indirect stimuli may correlate better with natural-occurring asthma [108]. While the sensitivity and specificity of these various stimuli with relevance to asthma have not been worked out and the "best agent" has not been clarified, some data support the hypothesis that the indirect stimuli differentiate asthma from chronic airflow limitation better than the direct stimuli.

Histamine and methacholine, both probably direct-acting stimuli, however, have been most widely used in the clinical and research assessment of airway responsiveness [17, 27, 28, 60]. Histamine and methacholine are generally administered by inhalation provocation tests, with doubling doses of agonist being given at fixed time intervals accompanied by appropriately timed measurements of airflow. Because of the continuous distribution of airway responsiveness [24, 45, 127, 147] (Fig. 4-2), and the gray or borderline area, careful regulation of all factors, both technical and nontechnical, surrounding inhalation provocation tests is necessary [61]. The results are usually expressed by a single number expressing the position of the dose-response curve. The provocation concentration (or dose) producing a 20 percent fall in forced expiration volume in 1 second (FEV_1), the PC_{20} (or PD_{20}), is most commonly used [61]. The plateau response [129, 148] has been addressed infrequently, at least in routine measurements of airway responsiveness.

Airway hyperresponsiveness correlates closely with other measures of variable airflow obstruction in subjects with [120, 149] and those without [58, 113] symptoms. Airway hyperresponsiveness also correlates with a number of indices of asthma severity [71, 94], but the overlap in such determinations makes this feature not routinely clinically useful. Airway hyperresponsiveness may simply be regarded as one objective way to demonstrate variable airflow obstruction [27], which remains the fundamental physiologic feature of current asthma definitions [3].

Subjects with perennial asthma have a relatively stable degree of chronic "baseline" airway hyperresponsiveness [72]. Superimposed on this, transient increases in airway responsiveness develop following exposure to a number of "inducers" [43]. Subjects

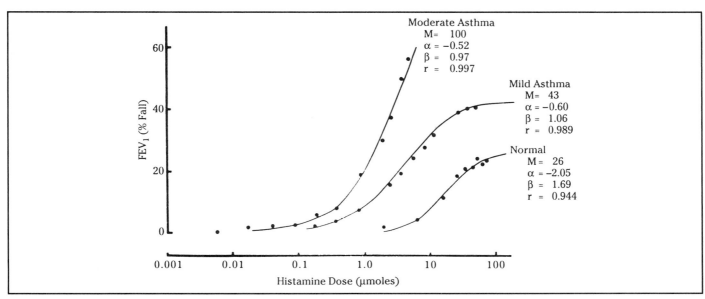

Fig. 4-1. *Histamine dose-response curves in a normal subject, a patient with mild asthma, and a patient with moderate asthma. (Reprinted with permission from A. J. Woolcock, C. M. Salome, and K. Yan. The shape of the dose-response curve to histamine in asthmatic and normal subjects. Am. Rev. Respir. Dis. 130:71, 1984.)*

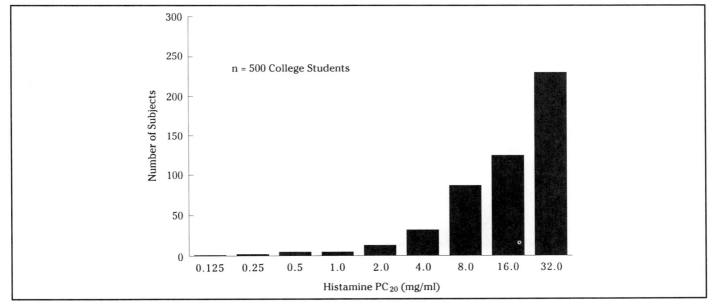

Fig. 4-2. *Unimodal continuous distribution of histamine PC_{20} values in 500 college students.*

with seasonal asthma may exhibit only this transient airway hyperresponsiveness [25, 30]. While the mechanisms of airway hyperresponsiveness remain uncertain, it is possible that several mechanisms may be involved and that the pathogenesis of transient airway hyperresponsiveness might be quantitatively or qualitatively different from the pathogenesis of the persistent airway responsiveness.

The numerous hypotheses to explain airway hyperresponsiveness are outlined below. These hypotheses are not mutually exclusive.

INFLAMMATION AND AIRWAY HYPERRESPONSIVENESS

The observation that even individuals with the mildest asthma have airway inflammation was recently emphasized [11, 79] (see

Chap. 9). This led to the hypothesis that asthma is primarily an inflammatory disease with airway hyperresponsiveness and subsequent symptoms of variable airflow obstruction are secondary features [43, 73, 75, 101, 115]. There are increasing data to link both persistent and transient airway responsiveness to airway inflammation. In individuals with mild stable asthma who have persistent airway hyperresponsiveness, inflammatory cells (eosinophils, metachromatic cells, lymphocytes) can be seen in bronchoalveolar lavage or bronchial biopsy material [40, 52, 56, 68, 77, 143] (see Chap. 24). Several studies have shown correlations between the numbers of metachromatic cells [56, 77, 143], eosinophils [52, 77, 143], neutrophils [40], lymphocytes [68], and alveolar macrophages [52] and the degree of airway responsiveness to histamine or methacholine. An example of these relationships is shown in Figure 4-3 [77]. Some studies have failed to find such a relationship [42].

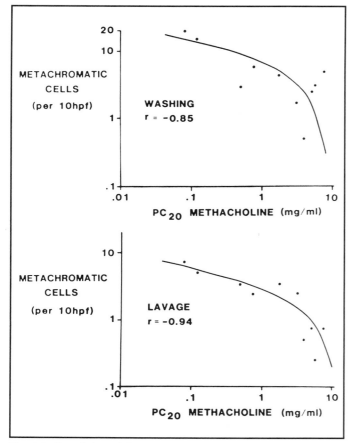

Fig. 4-3. *Correlation of the number of metachromatic cells (upper panel) and eosinophils (lower panel) and the degree of methacholine airway hyperresponsiveness in mild asthmatic subjects. The more airway hyperresponsiveness is present, the more inflammatory cells are in lavage fluid. (Reprinted with permission from J. C. Kirby. Bronchoalveolar cell profiles of asthmatic and nonasthmatic subjects. Am. Rev. Respir. Dis. 136:379, 1987.)*

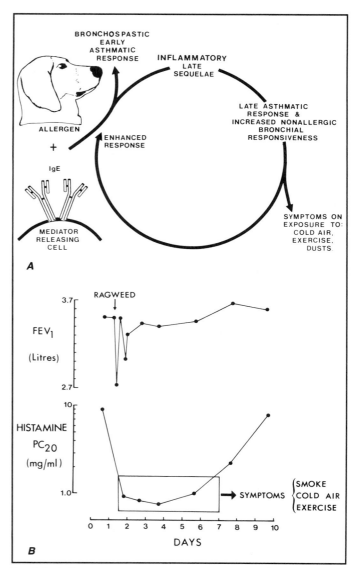

Fig. 4-4. *A. The inflammatory hypothesis explaining the development and maintenance of perennial (and seasonal) allergen-induced asthma. B. Allergen-induced increase in airway responsiveness to inhaled histamine in one subject. The top panel shows a spontaneously reversible dual asthmatic response. The bottom panel shows the associated increase in airway responsiveness to inhaled histamine lasting 1 week and associated with symptoms on exposure to bronchospastic triggers. (Reprinted with permission from D. W. Cockcroft. Mechanism of perennial allergic asthma. Lancet 2:253, 1983.)*

Transient airway hyperresponsiveness and transient airway inflammation occur in humans following exposure to allergen [21, 31, 41, 91], low-molecular-weight chemical sensitizers [51, 80, 81, 89], noxious gases such as ozone [128], and viral respiratory tract infections [50]. Although the airway hyperresponsiveness and airway inflammation have generally been demonstrated in separate studies, the temporal relationships and associations with late responses induced by allergen or chemical sensitizer strongly suggest that these go hand in hand. Allergen-induced increase in histamine or methacholine airway responsiveness [21, 31] and allergen-induced, predominantly eosinophilic airway inflammation [41, 91] occur primarily in conjunction with late asthmatic responses but not isolated early asthmatic responses, appear prior to the late response [47, 91], and persist for longer than 24 hours. Similar features have been observed for airway hyperresponsiveness and airway inflammation induced by low-molecular-weight chemical sensitizers such as plicatic acid [81, 128] or toluene diisocyanate [50, 89]. Animal models of allergen-induced airway hyperresponsiveness [93] and ozone airway hyperresponsiveness [105] have convincingly demonstrated the requirement for cells of the polymorphonuclear leukocyte series both for the appearance of late asthmatic responses, and of transient increases in airway responsiveness.

This evidence taken together provides strong support for the hypothesis that airway hyperresponsiveness, both transient and

persistent, is somehow caused by airway inflammation (Fig. 4-4) (see Chap. 9). However, this hypothesis does little to reduce the number of possible mechanisms underlying airway hyperresponsiveness. The theories outlined below for the most part are consistent with some feature of airway inflammation, and will be discussed in the context of the hypothesized importance of airway inflammation in the pathogenesis of airway hyperresponsiveness.

PHYSICAL OR STRUCTURAL ABNORMALITIES IN THE AIRWAYS

One school of thought surrounding airway hyperresponsiveness has been to attribute it to an artifact of some structural or physical abnormality caused by the asthmatic (inflammatory) airway abnormalities. It now seems unlikely that these features alone can explain the airway hyperresponsiveness in asthma. However, they are included both for the sake of completeness and because they may play some role either in true airway hyperresponsiveness or in apparent hyperresponsiveness by affecting the results of its measurement.

Reduced Airway Caliber

Reduction in baseline airway caliber has been suggested as a major determinant of hyperresponsiveness of the airways to inhaled chemical mediators [12]. This makes empirical sense for two reasons. First, the resistance to airflow in a tube is inversely proportional to the radius of the tube to either the fourth power (laminar flow) or the fifth power (turbulent flow) [46]. Therefore, a small reduction in radius would have a magnified effect on the resistance in a small tube when compared with a larger tube. The second reason is the (perhaps inappropriate) method of measuring responsiveness, in that most procedures look for a fixed percent reduction in lung function (e.g., 20% reduction in FEV_1) as an end point. Since a 20 percent reduction in FEV_1 in the presence of reduced airway caliber will indicate a smaller absolute fall in FEV_1, the airways may appear to be more sensitive. It is also possible, if not likely, that reduced airway caliber will alter the dose and deposition of the inhaled agonist, perhaps altering the measured responses in the opposite direction.

Now, many data suggest that reduced baseline airway caliber is not an important determinant of airway hyperresponsiveness in asthma. Studies between different individuals have shown that once asthma can be separated from chronic airflow limitation, unlike chronic airflow limitation there is either no correlation or a very small correlation between baseline FEV_1 and histamine or methacholine PC_{20} in asthmatics [30, 150]. Subjects with asthma and mild to moderate airway hyperresponsiveness, over a 10- to 20-fold range of PC_{20} values (0.5–10.0 mg/ml), do not have reduced airway caliber [120]. It is, however, studies within individuals that are most convincing. Moderate fluctuations in airway caliber in the absence of any other exacerbation of asthma have been shown not to influence airway responsiveness [119]. Induced airway hyperresponsiveness persists well beyond any measurable changes in even subtle measures of airway function [26, 31]. These studies suggest that in asthma, airway caliber alone is not an important determinant of airway responsiveness.

Airways of subjects with chronic airflow limitation but no asthma are also hyperresponsive to direct stimuli, namely histamine and methacholine. However, unlike asthma, this airway responsiveness is highly correlated with the degree of reduction in FEV_1 [48, 112, 114, 140] (Fig. 4-5). The airways in chronic airflow limitation are also less responsive for a given degree of airflow obstruction than those of asthmatic subjects [114] (see Fig. 4-5). Several other features differentiate this apparent airway hyperresponsiveness from that seen in asthma. It appears that despite the lower PC_{20}, the dose-response plateau is preserved in subjects with chronic airflow limitation [48]. Moreover, there are a number of stimuli that will provoke airway narrowing in asthma but do not appear to provoke airway narrowing in chronic airflow limitation despite the reduced histamine and methacholine PC_{20}. Subjects with chronic airflow limitation appear to be nonresponsive to cold air [112], beta-adrenergic blockers [146], and alpha-adrenergic stimulants [48]. These data would suggest that this "pseudo–airway hyperresponsiveness" seen in subjects with chronic airflow limitation is indeed an artifact created by the anatomic narrowing of the airways. Although probably not important in the pathogenesis of airway hyperresponsiveness in asthma, reduced airway caliber in asthmatic subjects may influence the result, at least when histamine and methacholine are used to measure airway responsiveness.

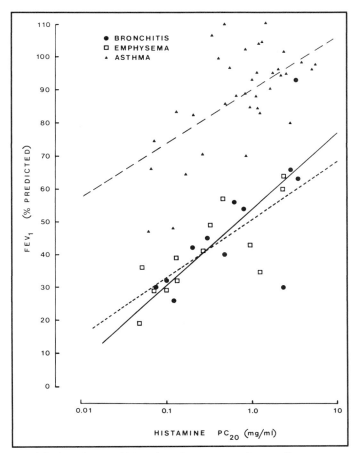

Fig. 4-5. *Correlation of histamine airway responsiveness (log histamine PC_{20}) with baseline airway caliber (FEV_1, % predicted) in subjects with emphysematous chronic airflow limitation (r = 0.79), nonemphysematous chronic airflow limitation or "bronchitis" (r = 0.73), and asthma (r < 0.50). There is no difference between the two chronic airflow limitation groups, whereas the asthmatic subjects are significantly more hyperresponsive. (Modified with permission from V. K. Verma, D. W. Cockcroft, and J. A. Dosman. Airway hyperresponsiveness to inhaled histamine in chronic obstructive airway disease. Chronic bronchitis vs. emphysema. Chest 94:457, 1988.)*

Airway Permeability

Ultrastructural observations in asthmatic airways have documented increased permeability due to a loss of tight junctions [64] (see Chap. 23). This provided a reasonable hypothesis for the development of airway hyperresponsiveness, namely that increased airway permeability would allow inhaled mediators (histamine, methacholine) easier access to the site of action, be it directly on the smooth muscle or on subepithelial nerves. This theory was supported by observations that transient airway hyperresponsiveness induced by allergen in monkeys was also associated with increased penetration of tritiated histamine into the systemic circulation [15]. Subsequent studies, however, have documented that airways of smokers with normal lung function were hyperpermeable to technetium 99m–labeled diethylenetriamine pentaacetate (^{99m}Tc-DTPA) but not hyperresponsive to histamine [100]. By contrast, the airways of subjects with stable asthma were hyperresponsive to histamine but not hyperpermeable to ^{99m}Tc-DTPA [100]. Thus, it appears that at least the stable airway hyperresponsiveness of asthmatics is not caused by or associated with hyperpermeability of the airway mucosa. The possibility that the transient inflammatory airway hyperresponsiveness could be at least in part associated with hyperpermeability remains.

Airway Wall Thickness

A recent hypothesis has emerged based on morphometric studies of asthmatic airways [67] and an elegant computer modeling of airway function [145]. The airways of asthmatics have increased cellularity and fluid. This increased volume or increased cross-sectional area of the airway wall may play a role in increasing airway responsiveness independent of neural, humoral, and muscular function. Computer modeling has suggested that increased airway wall thickness could have minimal effect on baseline airway resistance, and yet by virtue of its "space-occupying" nature contribute greatly to reduced cross-sectional airway caliber when the airway smooth muscle contracts and the inner airway wall "buckles" into the lumen [145]. This is in reality a more sophisticated "reduced airway caliber" hypothesis.

At the present time, such a hypothesis based on computer modeling is difficult either to prove or to disprove. However, the same observations suggesting that reduced airway caliber is unlikely to be the major mechanism of airway hyperresponsiveness in asthma apply at least to some extent to the hypothesis of increased airway wall thickness. Based on other observations (see below), it seems unlikely that increased airway wall thickness alone can account for airway hyperresponsiveness in asthma, although it may indeed play a role.

NEUROLOGIC ABNORMALITIES

The airways are richly innervated and many of the stimuli used to assess airway responsiveness act directly or indirectly through neural channels or neural receptors. It is therefore only natural that many investigators have turned to the nervous system and abnormalities therein in attempt to explain airway hyperresponsiveness and asthma. Attention initially was focused on the classic autonomic nervous system, giving rise to hypotheses of beta-adrenergic (sympathetic) blockade and cholinergic (parasympathetic) dominance. Recent description of additional components of the autonomic nervous system including a nonadrenergic noncholinergic (NANC) inhibitory system, NANC excitatory system, and various local axon reflexes has made understanding of the neural control of airways much more complex [8]. The precise role of the nervous system and abnormalities therein in the genesis of airway hyperresponsiveness remain uncertain. The reader is also referred to Chapters 17 and 18.

Beta-Adrenergic Blockade

Several years ago, a hypothesis for the pathogenesis of asthma and airway hyperresponsiveness based on partial beta-adrenergic blockade was presented [132]. Such a defect, probably of beta-adrenergic receptor function, would seem an attractive explanation for airway hyperresponsiveness, tipping the scales in the direction of enhanced cholinergic tone. The hypothesis has been supported by observations of reduced responses to beta-adrenergic agents in a number of nonairway tissues in asthmatics [34, 106].

However, it appears that beta-adrenergic receptor dysfunction alone cannot explain airway hyperresponsiveness and asthma. Although beta-adrenergic blockade increases airway responsiveness in asthmatic subjects [136], it does not produce airway hyperresponsiveness or asthma in normal subjects [117, 133, 151]. Impaired beta-adrenergic responsiveness in other tissues (and thus perhaps in the airway itself) may be secondary to treatment with beta agonists, since they can be reproduced by beta-agonist use in normal nonasthmatic subjects [33, 99].

The question of whether or not beta-adrenergic function is impaired has not been settled; this area has been reviewed recently in depth. Barnes concluded that even if beta-receptor function is abnormal in asthma, "such a defect is likely to be of little clinical significance" [8] (see also Chaps. 14 and 16).

Alpha-Adrenergic System

Alpha-adrenergic responsiveness may be increased in asthma [132]. Alpha agonists provoke bronchoconstriction [13] and alpha blockers are bronchodilators [110] and at least partial inhibitors of induced bronchoconstriction [8, 10, 107, 142]. However, it has been concluded that the role of alpha receptors in the pathogenesis of asthma is limited [8] and unlikely to explain airway hyperresponsiveness.

Cholinergic Overactivity

The cholinergic parasympathetic nerves regulate bronchomotor tone and airway secretions [96]. Many triggers of bronchoconstriction stimulate afferent vagal fibers and the induced bronchoconstriction can be at least partially blocked by atropine. The major hypothesized site of cholinergic overactivity is at the afferent irritant receptor where either exposure of the afferent nerve endings by inflammatory changes or irritation induced by inflammation might render them more easily stimulated [8, 50]. The possibility of efferent cholinergic overactivity either at the level of the ganglia or at the muscarinic receptor on the smooth muscle has also been considered [8].

Some triggers can be blocked at least in part by anticholinergic drugs [65, 97, 145], implying reflex vagal contribution to bronchoconstriction (or direct stimulation of muscarinic receptors as is the case for methacholine). By contrast, a number of other triggers are either unaffected or affected only slightly and often variably by anticholinergic drugs, in particular, bronchoconstriction induced by histamine [29], exercise [62], and antigens [32, 54]. Antigen-induced airway hyperresponsiveness to histamine is not inhibited any better by high-dose atropine than is the baseline airway responsiveness [16]. Although increased responsiveness to methacholine has led to the term *cholinergic hyperresponsiveness*, the airways are also hyperresponsive to several noncholinergic triggers [17, 27, 60, 108]. These data suggest that neither the transient nor the persistent asthmatic airway hyperresponsiveness is due to primary cholinergic overactivity.

Nonadrenergic Noncholinergic Inhibitory Nervous System

A NANC inhibitory nervous system was recently identified in human airways [7, 116] (see Chap. 18). This is analogous to the similar nervous system in the gut [20]. For the moment, the neurotransmitter remains uncertain although purines [20] and vasoactive intestinal peptide [121] have been suggested as possible mediators. The NANC inhibitory nervous system appears to be the sole bronchodilator innervation of the airways [8]. Its physiologic role in humans, both in health and in disease, however, is uncertain until such time as pharmacologic studies can be done; this will require definitive identification of the mediator. It has been postulated that a functional defect in this system could develop as a result of airway inflammation leading to uninhibited (or less inhibited) cholinergic tone [9].

Nonadrenergic Noncholinergic Excitatory Nerves

There is a component of electrically stimulated airway contraction that is not inhibited by atropine [4]. Substance P has been suggested as a possible neurotransmitter [8]. Although this has been demonstrated in animals, it is not easy to demonstrate in humans [83] and the relevance of a noncholinergic excitatory system in the airways of healthy or asthmatic humans is uncertain.

Local Axon Reflexes

Local axon reflexes may release tachykinins such as substance P, neurokinin, and calcitonin gene–related peptide. These have potent effects that mimic a number of the features of asthma. Increased axon reflex activity may be triggered by the inflammatory pathology involved in asthma [8]. Again, the precise role of these neuropeptides in the pathogenesis of airway hyperresponsiveness and asthma remains uncertain.

HUMORAL MEDIATORS

Many mediators have been implicated in causing airway hyperresponsiveness (Table 4-1). Those that have been most extensively studied have been the preformed mediators arising from mast cells, such as histamine; the newly formed lipid mediators, which arise from the action of phospholipases on cell membrane phospholipids causing the release of arachidonic acid; and those mediators known to be released from nerves, such as acetylcholine and the tachykinins. A great deal of interest has recently focused on the possibility that cytokines, released from a number of cells such as lymphocytes and mast cells, are important in the development of airway hyperresponsiveness. However, no direct evidence implicating these mediators yet exists, and they will not be reviewed in this chapter.

Humoral mediators are most easily considered in three groups, although some controversy exists as to the precise role of most of the mediators studied to date. These groups include the following:

1. Mediators that cause transient bronchoconstriction, such as histamine or acetylcholine, but that do not have any other action on airway function.
2. Mediators that cause influx of inflammatory cells and possibly activation of cells in the airways, such as platelet-activating factor (PAF) or leukotriene (LT) B_4.
3. Mediators that are released from inflammatory cells and cause airway hyperresponsiveness. For example, evidence for such mediators exists for thromboxane in dogs and tachykinins in guinea pigs.

Mediators Causing Transient Bronchoconstriction

These mediators are important in causing airway narrowing through airway smooth muscle constriction and/or effects on blood vessels causing vasodilation and airway edema. However, these effects are transient and do not appear to result in longer-term effects on airway function. This class of mediators has been the most extensively studied in asthma. The mediators that act in this way in humans include histamine [37], acetylcholine [135], the sulfidopeptide leukotrienes LTC_4 and LTD_4 [1] and probably thromboxane A_2 [122]. Each of these mediators has been implicated in causing exercise- [63, 87] and/or allergen-induced acute bronchoconstriction [85]. Current evidence suggests that the sulfidopeptide leukotrienes and histamine are together responsible for these acute bronchoconstrictor responses. However, none of these mediators has been convincingly demonstrated to cause either airway inflammation or airway hyperresponsiveness. Indeed, most of these mediators can cause the release of inhibitory prostaglandins in the airways, which inhibit the ability of the airway smooth muscle to develop further bronchoconstriction [84, 131].

Proinflammatory Mediators

It is likely that proinflammatory mediators are released in asthmatic airways and cause the chemotaxis and possibly activation of inflammatory cells into the airways, resulting in the development of airway hyperresponsiveness after the inhalation of stimuli such as allergens or occupational sensitizing agents [22, 31]. It is also possible, although much less extensively studied, that these mediators are involved in the pathogenesis of ongoing airway inflammation and hyperresponsiveness in patients with symptomatic asthma. The two mediators best studied in this regard are LTB_4 and PAF.

Inhaled LTB_4 has been demonstrated to cause both airway inflammation, with the predominant cellular infiltration being neutrophilic, and airway hyperresponsiveness in dogs [103]. The airway hyperresponsiveness lasted for up to 1 week. However, inhaled LTB_4 has not been demonstrated to cause airway hyperresponsiveness in humans [14]. By contrast, PAF has been shown to be released after allergen inhalation [98] and to cause both eosinophil influx and activation and airway hyperresponsiveness in a variety of animal models [23, 82] and in humans [38] (Fig. 4-6). As allergen inhalation also causes eosinophil infiltration into the airways [41, 91] and airway hyperresponsiveness [31], it is possible that allergen-induced PAF release may be the initiating stimulus for the airway events following allergen inhalation (see Chap. 22). However, preliminary evidence using potent and selective PAF antagonists has not demonstrated any inhibitory effects on allergen-induced responses in humans [57]. Therefore, the proinflammatory mediators that are important in causing airway inflammation in asthma are not yet known.

Mediators Causing Airway Hyperresponsiveness

The chemotaxis and activation of inflammatory cells in the airways of asthmatic subjects may cause the release of mediators

Table 4-1. Effects of inflammatory mediators implicated in asthma

Mediator	Bronchoconstriction	Airway secretion	Microvascular leakage	Chemotaxis	Bronchial hyperresponsiveness
Histamine	+	+	+	+	—
Prostaglandins D_2, $F_{2\alpha}$	+ +	+	?	?	+
Prostaglandin E_2	—	+	—	+	—
Thromboxane	+ +	?	—	±	+
Leukotriene B_4	—	—	±	+ +	±
Leukotrienes C_4, D_4, E_4	+ +	+ +	+ +	?	±
Platelet-activating factor	+ +	+	+ +	+ +	+ +
Bradykinin	+	+	+ +	—	—
Substance P	+	+ +	+ +	±	—
Complement fragments	+	+	+	+ +	—

+ + = pronounced effect; + = moderate effect; ± = uncertain effect; ? = information not available.
Source: K. F. Chung. Inflammatory Mediators in Asthma. In P. O'Byrne (ed.), *Asthma as an Inflammatory Disease.* New York: Marcel Dekker, 1990. P. 164. Reprinted by courtesy of Marcel Dekker, Inc.

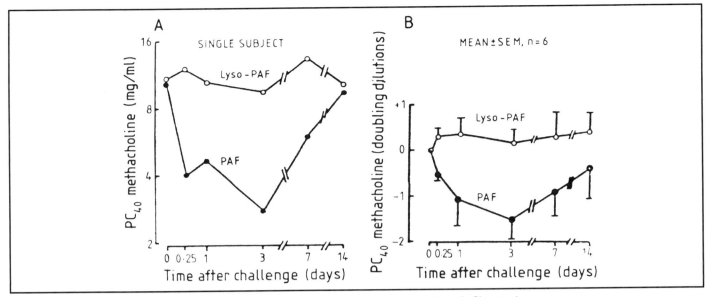

Fig. 4-6. *Platelet-activating factor (PAF)–induced airway hyperresponsiveness to methacholine. A. Changes in PC$_{40}$ methacholine in a single subject. B. Changes in mean PC$_{40}$ methacholine in six normal subjects after inhalation of PAF. There is a significant increase in airway responsiveness within 6 hours, an effect lasting up to 2 weeks. (Reprinted with permission from F. M. Cuss, C. M. S. Dixon, and P. J. Barnes. Effects of inhaled platelet activating factor on pulmonary function and bronchial responsiveness in man. Lancet 2:189, 1986.)*

that alter tissue responses or damage the airways, causing airway hyperresponsiveness. The best evidence to date for such events occurring comes from studies in dogs, which indicate that the proinflammatory mediator LTB$_4$ causes an influx of neutrophils into the airways and the release of thromboxane A$_2$ [103]. Inhibition of thromboxane production prevents the development of airway hyperresponsiveness in dogs [2, 103]. However, inhibition of thromboxane has not yet been successful in inhibiting induced airway hyperresponsiveness in humans [86].

Another interesting hypothesis to explain airway hyperresponsiveness suggests that toxic basic proteins released from activated eosinophils, such as major basic protein (MBP) or eosinophil cationic protein (ECP), cause epithelial damage and denudation in asthmatic airways [59]. This results in the loss of epithelium-derived relaxation factor (EpDRF), leading to airway hyperresponsiveness [137]. The evidence that these eosinophil products are released in asthmatic airways, particularly in those with more severe asthma, is convincing [143]. However, their precise role in causing airway hyperresponsiveness is not yet established (see also Chap. 20).

AIRWAY SMOOTH MUSCLE ABNORMALITIES

Since the airway smooth muscle is hyperresponsive to a number of different stimuli operating through many different mechanisms, it is attractive to speculate that the abnormality may lie in the final common pathway, namely the airway smooth muscle itself. This could be explained by some anatomic or physiologic change in the airway smooth muscle, or in its neurohumoral milieu. The rather predictable hyperresponsiveness to cholinergic muscarinic agonists suggests that such an abnormality would be at or distal to the muscarinic receptor.

A number of studies have addressed airway smooth muscle function in vitro. These studies have dealt with excised lung in subjects undergoing resection, usually for pulmonary nodules. In these studies, airway responsiveness in vivo and in vitro shows no correlation and in fact, it is difficult to demonstrate in vitro airway hyperresponsiveness in these specimens [6, 141]. How-

ever, it appears likely that many of these subjects undergoing resection for pulmonary nodules (suspected carcinoma) are in fact smokers with chronic airflow limitation who have the "pseudo–airway hyperresponsiveness" of reduced airway caliber. These data could be taken as support for the contention that the histamine and airway hyperresponsiveness seen in chronic airflow limitation is indeed an artifact created by the reduced airway caliber. By contrast, there are now preliminary reports that smooth muscle from subjects with bronchial asthma, when tested in vitro, is indeed hyperresponsive [39, 123]. Thus, it is possible that a defect, possibly acquired, possibly secondary to inflammatory mediators, could be present either chronically or intermittently in the airway smooth muscle itself. At the moment, the nature of such defect can only be speculated.

LOSS OF INHIBITORY MECHANISMS

The hypotheses outlined above, with the exception of a possible defect in the NANC inhibitory nervous system, attempt to explain why the airway smooth muscle contracts more easily and to a greater extent in asthmatic than in normal subjects. This is indeed the direction in which most attention has been focused. However, there are compelling reasons to consider the possibility that airway hyperresponsiveness is secondary to a loss of some potent protective inhibitory mechanism. Theoretically, isotonic contraction of airway smooth muscle has the potential to completely close the airways [145]. The fact that this does not occur suggests in part that airway smooth muscle may be contracting against a (presumably elastic) load [145]. An alternative explanation is that some other active protective mechanism prevents complete airway closure due to smooth muscle contraction. Such an inhibition in normal subjects is suggested by the shape of the dose-response curve, with a plateau above which increasing concentrations of agonist fail to produce any further bronchoconstriction [129, 130, 148]. This, along with the well-recognized bronchodilator effect of a deep inspiration (in normal subjects and in subjects who have mild asthma with induced bronchoconstriction) [53], suggests a powerful inhibitory system. Neither inspiration-induced bronchodilatation nor the maximal response plateau to methacholine are affected by beta-adrenergic blockade, (parasympathetic) ganglionic blockade, or indomethacin [130]. This suggests that neither adrenergic, cholinergic, nor NANC (ganglionically transmitted) inhibitory activity nor prostaglandins are likely to explain the abnormality [130].

A variety of studies have demonstrated that inhibitory mechanisms that attempt to limit bronchoconstriction exist in the airways, and these mechanisms depend on the release of inhibitory prostaglandins. For example, exercise refractoriness, which is progressively reduced bronchoconstriction with repeated exercise in asthmatic subjects, is prevented by pretreatment with indomethacin [90, 102]. Also, progressively reduced bronchoconstriction with repeated challenge with histamine occurs in subjects with mild, but not those with more severe asthma. Again, this effect is dependent on the release of inhibitory prostaglandins in the airways [84]. Lastly, a prostaglandin-mediated reduction in methacholine-induced bronchoconstriction occurs only in normal, but not asthmatic subjects [131]. These studies suggest that loss of this prostaglandin-mediated protective mechanism in the airways may be related to worsening asthma; however, this hypothesis has not yet been tested.

The other inhibitory influence that has been proposed to be important in limiting bronchoconstriction is the release of EpDRF from the airway epithelium [55]. EpDRF was described as the effect of intact airway epithelium to inhibit the magnitude of airway contraction caused by a variety of constrictor mediators, such as histamine and acetylcholine. Thus, loss of airway epithelium (and thereby EpDRF) in patients with asthma would potentially result in a greater contractile response to inhaled constrictor mediators [137]. However, studies in an animal model of airway hyperresponsiveness have not demonstrated any loss of EpDRF function in vitro when airway hyperresponsiveness is present in vivo [69]. Once again, the precise importance of this mechanism in human asthma is not known.

IATROGENIC FACTORS

Despite improved understanding of the pathophysiology of asthma and "improved" treatments, asthma-related morbidity and mortality have been rising throughout the industrialized world [19, 88, 118, 124, 126] (see Chap. 90). The reasons are uncertain; more accurate diagnosis, increasing prevalence of disease, and increasing severity have all been suggested. However, the possibility that increased morbidity and mortality from asthma are in whole or in part iatrogenic has been strongly suggested [118]. This could include indirect adverse effects (e.g., overreliance on potent symptomatic but non-antiinflammatory treatments), direct adverse effects, or both. Enhanced airway responsiveness might be one explanation for direct adverse effects.

Inhaled Beta$_2$ Agonists

Inhaled beta$_2$ agonists, particularly fenoterol, are a major concern, having been linked with both asthma morbidity [125] and mortality [35, 109]. There are now convincing data that regular frequent use of inhaled beta$_2$ agonists causes a significant modest increase in airway responsiveness in asthmatic subjects [74, 78, 125, 138, 139]. This was hypothesized as a possible cause of increasing asthma mortality [92] before the relationship of fenoterol to asthma morbidity [125] and mortality [35, 109] was observed. The mechanism of beta agonist–induced airway hyperresponsiveness is not clear; subsensitivity of beta receptors has been suggested [99] but in one study, appeared to be an unlikely explanation [92]. Although not the primary or major cause of airway hyperresponsiveness in asthmatics, this is one (possibly of several) modifying influence.

Allergen-Injection Therapy

Preseasonal allergen-injection therapy may partially inhibit seasonal airway hyperresponsiveness [111]. However, there are also data [95] and anecdotal observations [44] that allergen injections can lead to enhanced airway responsiveness. The mechanism is presumably through the genesis of inflammation such as that seen following inhaled allergen [21, 31, 41, 91].

In summary, much more information is necessary to unravel which of the mechanisms outlined above are responsible for the variable hyperresponsiveness of the airways seen in asthma. Most likely some links, be they humoral, neural, or both, between inflammatory cells and the airway smooth muscle will prove to be important. Reduced airway caliber, increased airway wall thickness, increased permeability, and iatrogenic effects likely play secondary or modifying roles in its pathogenesis. The reader is referred to a recent review on airway reactivity for further discussion of this subject [66].

REFERENCES

1. Adelroth, E., et al. Airway responsiveness to leukotrienes C$_4$ and D$_4$ and to methacholine in patients with asthma and normal controls. *N. Engl. J. Med.* 315:480, 1986.
2. Aizawa, H., et al. Significance of thromboxane generation in ozone-induced airway hyperresponsiveness in dogs. *J. Appl. Physiol.* 59:1918, 1985.
3. American Thoracic Society. Standards for the diagnosis and care of patients with chronic obstructive pulmonary disease (COPD) and asthma. *Am. Rev. Respir. Dis.* 136:225, 1987.
4. Andersson, R. G. G., and Grundstrom, N. The excitatory non-cholinergic, non-adrenergic nervous system of the guinea-pig airways. *Eur. J. Respir. Dis.* 64(Suppl. 131):141, 1983.
5. Anderton, R. C., et al. Bronchial responsiveness to inhaled histamine and exercise. *J. Allergy Clin. Immunol.* 63:315, 1979.
6. Armour, C. L., et al. A comparison of *in vivo* and *in vitro* human airway reactivity to histamine. *Am. Rev. Respir. Dis.* 129:907, 1984.
7. Barnes, P. J. The third nervous system in the lung: Physiology and clinical perspectives. *Thorax* 39:561, 1984.
8. Barnes, P. J. Neural control of human airways in health and disease. *Am. Rev. Respir. Dis.* 134:1289, 1986.
9. Barnes, P. J. Non-adrenergic non-cholinergic neural control of human airways. *Arch. Int. Pharmacodyn. Ther.* 280(Suppl.):208, 1986.
10. Barnes, P. J., Wilson, N. M., and Vickers, H. Prazosin, an alpha$_1$-adrenoceptor antagonist, partially inhibits exercise-induced asthma. *J. Allergy Clin. Immunol.* 68:411, 1981.
11. Beasley, R., et al. Cellular events in the bronchi in mild asthma and after bronchial provocation. *Am. Rev. Respir. Dis.* 139:806, 1989.
12. Benson, M. K. Bronchial hyperreactivity. *Br. J. Dis. Chest* 69:227, 1975.
13. Black, J. L., et al. Comparison between airways response to an alpha-adrenoreceptor agonist and histamine in asthmatic and nonasthmatic subjects. *Br. J. Clin. Pharmacol.* 14:464, 1982.
14. Black, P. N., et al. Effect of inhaled leukotriene B$_4$ alone and in combination with prostaglandin D$_2$ on bronchial responsiveness to histamine in normal subjects. *Thorax* 44:491, 1989.
15. Boucher, R. C., Pare, P. D., and Hogg, J. C. Relationship between airway hyperreactivity and hyperpermeability in *Ascaris*-sensitive monkeys. *J. Allergy Clin. Immunol.* 64:197, 1979.
16. Boulet, L. P., et al. The effect of atropine on allergen-induced increases in bronchial responsiveness to histamine. *Am. Rev. Respir. Dis.* 130:368, 1984.
17. Boushey, H. A., and Holtzman, M. J. Experimental airway inflammation and hyperreactivity. *Am. Rev. Respir. Dis.* 131:312, 1985.
18. Britton, J. Is hyperreactivity the same as asthma? *Eur. J. Respir. Dis.* 1: 478, 1988.
19. Buist, A. S. Asthma mortality: What have we learned? *J. Allergy Clin. Immunol.* 84:275, 1989.
20. Burnstock, G. Purinergic nerves. *Pharmacol. Rev.* 24:509, 1972.
21. Cartier, A., et al. Allergen-induced increase in bronchial responsiveness to histamine: Relationship to the late asthmatic response and change in airway caliber. *J. Allergy Clin. Immunol.* 70:170, 1982.
22. Chan-Yeung, M., and Lam, S. Occupational asthma: State of the art. *Am. Rev. Respir. Dis.* 133:686, 1986.

23. Chung, K. F., et al. Airway hyperresponsiveness induced by platelet-activating factor: Role of thromboxane generation. *J. Pharmacol. Exp. Ther.* 236:580, 1986.

24. Cockcroft, D. W., Berscheid, B. A., and Murdock, K. Y. Unimodal distribution of bronchial responsiveness to inhaled histamine in a random human population. *Chest* 83:751, 1983.

25. Cockcroft, D. W., et al. Sensitivity and specificity of histamine PC_{20} measurements in a random population. *J. Allergy Clin. Immunol.* 75:142(A), 1985.

26. Cockcroft, D. W., Cotton, D. J., and Mink, J. T. Nonspecific bronchial hyperreactivity after exposure to Western Red Cedar: A case report. *Am. Rev. Respir. Dis.* 119:505, 1979.

27. Cockcroft, D. W., and Hargreave, F. E. Airway hyperresponsiveness: Relevance of random population data to clinical usefulness (editorial). *Am. Rev. Respir. Dis.* 142:497, 1990.

28. Cockcroft, D. W., and Hargreave, F. E. Airway Hyperresponsiveness: Definition, Measurement and Clinical Relevance. In M. A. Kaliner, P. J. Barnes, and C. G. A. Persson (eds.), *Asthma: Its Pathology and Treatment.* New York: Marcel Dekker, 1991. Pp. 51–72.

29. Cockcroft, D. W., et al. Protective effect of drugs on histamine-induced asthma. *Thorax* 32:429, 1977.

30. Cockcroft, D. W., et al. Bronchial reactivity to inhaled histamine: A method and clinical survey. *Clin. Allergy* 7:235, 1977.

31. Cockcroft, D. W., et al. Allergen-induced increase in nonallergic bronchial reactivity. *Clin. Allergy* 7:503, 1977.

32. Cockcroft, D. W., Ruffin, R. E., and Hargreave, F. E. Effect of Sch 1000 in allergen-induced asthma. *Clin. Allergy* 8:361, 1978.

33. Conolly, M. E., and Greenacre, J. K. The lymphocyte beta-adrenoceptor in normal subjects and patients with bronchial asthma; the effect of different forms of treatment on receptor function. *J. Clin. Invest.* 58:1307, 1976.

34. Cookson, D. V., and Reed, C. E. A comparison of the effects of isoproterenol in normal and asthmatic subjects. *Am. Rev. Respir. Dis.* 88:636, 1963.

35. Crane, J., et al. Prescribed fenoterol and death from asthma in New Zealand, 1981–83: Case-control study. *Lancet* 1:917, 1989.

36. Crawford, A. B. H., Makowska, M., and Engel, L. A. Effect of bronchomotor tone on static mechanical properties of lung and ventilation distribution. *J. Appl. Physiol.* 63:2278, 1987.

37. Curry, J. J. The action of histamine on the respiratory tract in normal and asthmatic subjects. *J. Clin. Invest.* 25:785, 1946.

38. Cuss, F. M., Dixon, C. M. S., and Barnes, P. J. Effects of inhaled platelet activating factor on pulmonary function and bronchial responsiveness in man. *Lancet* 2:189, 1986.

39. de Jongste, J. C., et al. *In vitro* responses of airways from an asthmatic patient. *Eur. J. Respir. Dis.* 71:23, 1987.

40. de Jongste, J. C., et al. Comparison of human bronchiolar smooth muscle responsiveness in vitro with histological signs of inflammation. *Thorax* 42:870, 1987.

41. de Monchy, J. G. R., et al. Bronchoalveolar eosinophilia during allergen-induced late asthmatic reactions. *Am. Rev. Respir. Dis.* 131:373, 1985.

42. Djakanovic, R., et al. Quantitation of mast cells and eosinophils in the bronchial mucosa of symptomatic atopic asthmatics and healthy control subjects using immunohistochemistry. *Am. Rev. Respir. Dis.* 142:863, 1990.

43. Dolovich, J., and Hargreave, F. E. The asthma syndrome: Inciters, inducers, and host characteristics. *Thorax* 36:641, 1981.

44. Dolovich, J., Zimmerman, B., and Hargreave, F. E. Allergy in Asthma. In T. J. H. Clark and S. Godfrey (eds.), *Asthma.* London: Chapman and Hall, 1983. Pp. 132–157.

45. Douglas, J. S., Ridgway, P., and Brink, C. Airway responses to the guinea pig *in vivo* and *in vitro. J. Pharmacol. Exp. Ther.* 202:116, 1977.

46. Dubois, A. B. Resistance to Breathing. In W. O. Fenn and H. Rahn (eds.), *Handbook of Physiology,* Section 3: Respiration, Vol. I. Washington: American Physiologic Society, 1964. Pp. 451–462.

47. Durham, S. R., et al. Increases in airway responsiveness to histamine precede allergen-induced late asthmatic responses. *J. Allergy Clin. Immunol.* 82:764, 1988.

48. Du Toit, J. I., et al. Characteristics of bronchial responsiveness in smokers with chronic airflow limitation. *Am. Rev. Respir. Dis.* 134:498, 1986.

49. Eggleston, P. A. A comparison of the asthmatic response to methacholine and exercise. *J. Allergy Clin. Immunol.* 63:104, 1979.

50. Empey, D. W., et al. Mechanisms of bronchial hyperreactivity in normal subjects after upper respiratory tract infection. *Am. Rev. Respir. Dis.* 113:131, 1976.

51. Fabbri, L. M., et al. Bronchoalveolar neutrophilia during late asthmatic reactions induced by toluene diisocyanate. *Am. Rev. Respir. Dis.* 136:36, 1987.

52. Ferguson, A. C., and Wong, F. W. M. Bronchial hyperresponsiveness in asthmatic children: Correlation with macrophages and eosinophils in broncholavage fluid. *Chest* 96:988, 1989.

53. Fish, J. E., et al. Regulation of bronchomotor tone by lung inflation in asthmatic and nonasthmatic subjects. *J. Appl. Physiol. Respir. Environ. Exerc. Physiol.* 50:1079, 1981.

54. Fish, J. E., et al. The effect of atropine on acute antigen-mediated airway constriction in subjects with allergic asthma. *Am. Rev. Respir. Dis.* 115:371, 1977.

55. Flavahan, N. A., et al. Respiratory epithelium inhibits bronchial smooth muscle tone. *J. Appl. Physiol.* 58:834, 1985.

56. Flint, K. C., et al. Bronchoalveolar mast cells in extrinsic asthma: A mechanism for the initiation of antigen specific bronchoconstriction. *Br. Med. J.* 291:923, 1985.

57. Freitag, A., et al. The effect of treatment with an oral platelet activating factor antagonist (WEB 2086) on allergen-induced asthmatic responses. *Am. Rev. Respir. Dis.* In press.

58. Gibson, P. G., et al. Variable airflow obstruction in asymptomatic children with methacholine airway hyperresponsiveness. *Clin. Invest. Med.* 11:C105, 1988.

59. Gleich, G. J., et al. Cytotoxic properties of the eosinophil major basic protein. *J. Immunol.* 123:2925, 1979.

60. Hargreave, F. E., et al. Bronchial responsiveness to histamine or methacholine in asthma: Measurement and clinical significance. *J. Allergy Clin. Immunol.* 68:347, 1981.

61. Hargreave, F. E., and Woolcock, A. J. (eds.), *Airway Responsiveness: Measurement and Interpretation.* Astra Pharmaceuticals Canada, 1985. Pp. 22–28.

62. Hartley, J. P. R., and Davis, B. H. Cholinergic blockade in the prevention of exercise-induced asthma. *Thorax* 35:680, 1980.

63. Hartley, J. P. R., and Nogrady, S. G. Effect of an inhaled antihistamine on exercise-induced asthma. *Thorax* 35:675, 1980.

64. Hogg, J. C. Bronchial mucosal permeability and its relationship to airways hyperreactivity. *J. Allergy Clin. Immunol.* 67:421, 1981.

65. Holtzman, M. J., et al. Effect of ozone on bronchial reactivity in atopic and nonatopic subjects. *Am. Rev. Respir. Dis.* 120:1059, 1979.

66. International Symposium on Airway Reactivity. *Am. Rev. Respir. Dis.* 143(Pt 2):51, 1991.

67. James, A. L., Pare, P. D., and Hogg, J. C. The mechanics of airway narrowing in asthma. *Am. Rev. Respir. Dis.* 139:242, 1989.

68. Jeffery, P. K., et al. Bronchial biopsies in asthma: An ultrastructural quantitative study and correlation with hyperreactivity. *Am. Rev. Respir. Dis.* 140:1745, 1989.

69. Jones, G. L., Lane, C. G., and O'Byrne, P. M. Release of epithelium-derived relaxation factor (EpDRF) after ozone inhalation in dogs. *J. Appl. Physiol.* 65:1238, 1988.

70. Juniper, E. F., et al. Reproducibility and comparison of responses to inhaled histamine and methacholine. *Thorax* 33:705, 1978.

71. Juniper, E. F., Frith, P. A., and Hargreave, F. E. Airway responsiveness to histamine and methacholine: Relationship to minimum treatment to control symptoms of asthma. *Thorax* 36:575, 1981.

72. Juniper, E. F., Frith, P. A., and Hargreave, F. E. Long-term stability of bronchial responsiveness to histamine. *Thorax* 37:288, 1982.

73. Kaliner, M. Hypothesis on the contribution of late-phase allergic responses to the understanding and treatment of allergic diseases. *J. Allergy Clin. Immunol.* 73:311, 1984.

74. Kerribijn, K. F., van Essen-Zandvliet, E. E. M., and Neijens, H. J. Effects of long-term treatment with inhaled corticosteroids and beta-agonists on the bronchial responsiveness in children with asthma. *J. Allergy Clin. Immunol.* 79:653, 1987.

75. Kerribijn, W. F. Triggers of airway inflammation. *Eur. J. Respir. Dis.* 69(Suppl. 147):98, 1986.

76. Keyzer, J. J., et al. Urinary N^T-Methylhistamine During Early and Late Allergen-induced Bronchial Obstructive Reaction. In J. J. Keyzer (ed.), *Determinations of Histamine and Some of Its Metabolites and Their Clinical Applications* (1st ed.). Groningen: Drukkerij Van Denderen B. V., 1983. Pp. 100–109.

77. Kirby, J. C., et al. Bronchoalveolar cell profiles of asthmatic and nonasthmatic subjects. *Am. Rev. Respir. Dis.* 136:379, 1987.

78. Kraan, J., et al. Changes in bronchial hyperreactivity induced by 4 weeks of treatment with antiasthmatic drugs in patients with allergic asthma: A comparison between budesonide and terbutaline. *J. Allergy Clin. Immunol.* 76:628, 1985.

79. Laitinen, L. A., et al. Damage of the airway epithelium and bronchial reactivity in patients with asthma. *Am. Rev. Respir. Dis.* 131:599, 1985.

80. Lam, S. et al. Cellular and protein changes in bronchial lavage fluid after late asthmatic reaction in patients with red cedar asthma. *J. Allergy Clin. Immunol.* 80:44, 1987.

81. Lam, S., Wong, R., and Yeung, M. Nonspecific bronchial reactivity in occupational asthma. *J. Allergy Clin. Immunol.* 63:28, 1979.

82. Lellouch-Tubiana, A., et al. Eosinophil recruitment into guinea pig lungs after PAF-aceter and allergen administration. *Am. Rev. Respir. Dis.* 137:948, 1988.

83. Lundberg, J. M., Martling, C.-R., and Saria, A. Substance P and capsaicin-induced contraction of human bronchi. *Acta Physiol. Scand.* 119:49, 1983.

84. Manning, P. J., Jones, G. L., and O'Byrne, P. M. Tachyphylaxis to inhaled histamine in asthmatic subjects. *J. Appl. Physiol.* 63:1572, 1987.

85. Manning, P. J., et al. Urinary leukotriene E_4 levels during early and late asthmatic responses. *J. Allergy Clin. Immunol.* 86:211, 1990.

86. Manning, P. J., et al. The role of thromboxane in allergen-induced asthmatic responses. *Eur. J. Respir. Dis.* 4:667, 1991.

87. Manning, P. J., et al. Inhibition of exercise-induced bronchoconstriction by MK-571, a potent leukotriene D_4 receptor antagonist. *N. Engl. J. Med.* 323:1736, 1990.

88. Mao, Y., et al. Increased rates of illness and death from asthma in Canada. *Can. Med. Assoc. J.* 137:620, 1987.

89. Mapp, C. E., et al. Late, but not early, asthmatic reactions induced by toluene-diisocyanate are associated with increased airway responsiveness to methacholine. *Eur. J. Respir. Dis.* 69:276, 1986.

90. Margolskee, D. J., Bigby, B. G., and Boushey, H. A. Indomethacin blocks airway tolerance to repetitive exercise but not to eucapnic hyperpnea in asthmatic subjects. *Am. Rev. Respir. Dis.* 137:842, 1988.

91. Metzger, W. J., et al. Bronchoalveolar lavage of allergic asthmatic patients following allergen bronchoprovocation. *Chest* 89:477, 1986.

92. Mitchell, E. A. Is current treatment increasing asthma mortality and morbidity? *Thorax* 44:81, 1989.

93. Murphy, K. R., et al. The requirement for polymorphonuclear leukocytes in the late asthmatic response and heightened airways reactivity in an animal model. *Am. Rev. Respir. Dis.* 134:62, 1986.

94. Murray, A. B., Ferguson, A. C., and Morrison, B. Airway responsiveness to histamine as a test for overall severity of asthma in children. *J. Allergy Clin. Immunol.* 68:119, 1981.

95. Murray, A. B., Ferguson, A. C., and Morrison, B. J. Nonallergic bronchial hyperreactivity in asthmatic children decreases with age and increases with mite immunotherapy. *Ann. Allergy* 54:541, 1985.

96. Nadel, J. A. Autonomic Regulation of Airway Smooth Muscle. In C. Lenfant (ed.), *Physiology and Pharmacology of the Airways*, Vol. 15. Lung Biology in Health and Disease. New York: Marcel Dekker, 1980. Pp. 217–239.

97. Nadel, J. A., et al. Mechanism of bronchoconstriction during inhalation of sulfur dioxide. *J. Appl. Physiol.* 20:164, 1965.

98. Nakamura, T., et al. Platelet-activating factor in late asthmatic response. *Int. Arch. Allergy Appl. Immunol.* 82:57, 1987.

99. Nelson, H. S., et al. Subsensitivity to the bronchodilator action of albuterol produced by chronic administration. *Am. Rev. Respir. Dis.* 116:871, 1977.

100. O'Byrne, P. M., et al. Lung epithelial permeability: Relation to nonspecific airway responsiveness. *J. Appl. Physiol. Respir. Environ. Exerc. Physiol.* 57:77, 1984.

101. O'Byrne, P. M., Hargreave, F. E., and Kirby, J. G. Airway inflammation and hyperresponsiveness. *Am. Rev. Respir. Dis.* 136:S35, 1987.

102. O'Byrne, P. M., and Jones, G. L. The effect of indomethacin on exercise-induced bronchoconstriction and refractoriness after exercise. *Am. Rev. Respir. Dis.* 134:69, 1986.

103. O'Byrne, P. M., et al. Leukotriene B_4 induced airway hyperresponsiveness in dogs. *J. Appl. Physiol.* 59:1941, 1985.

104. O'Byrne, P. M., et al. Asthma induced by cold air and its relation to nonspecific bronchial responsiveness to methacholine. *Am. Rev. Respir. Dis.* 125:281, 1982.

105. O'Byrne, P. M., et al. Neutrophil depletion inhibits airway hyperresponsiveness induced by ozone exposure. *Am. Rev. Respir. Dis.* 130:214, 1984.

106. Parker, C. W., and Smith, J. W. Alterations in cyclic adenosine monophosphate metabolism in human bronchial asthma. *J. Clin. Invest.* 52:48, 1973.

107. Patel, K. R., and Kerr, I. W. Effect of alpha receptor blocking drug, thymoxamine, on allergen induced bronchoconstriction in extrinsic asthma. *Clin. Allergy* 5:311, 1975.

108. Pauwels, R., Joos, G., and van der Straeten, M. Bronchial hyperresponsiveness is not bronchial hyperresponsiveness is not bronchial asthma. *Clin. Allergy* 18:317, 1988.

109. Pearce, N., et al. Case-control study of prescribed fenoterol and death from asthma in New Zealand, 1977–81. *Thorax* 45:170, 1990.

110. Prime, F. J., et al. The effects on airways conductance of alpha-adrenergic stimulation and blocking. *Bull. Eur. Physiopathol. Respir.* 8:99, 1972.

111. Rak, S., Lowhagen, O., and Venge, P. The effect of immunotherapy on bronchial hyperresponsiveness and eosinophil cationic protein in pollen-allergic patients. *J. Allergy Clin. Immunol.* 82:470, 1988.

112. Ramsdale, E. H. et al. Bronchial responsiveness to methacholine in chronic bronchitis: Relationship to airflow obstruction and cold air responsiveness. *Thorax* 39:912, 1984.

113. Ramsdale, E. H., et al. Asymptomatic bronchial hyperresponsiveness in rhinitis. *J. Allergy Clin. Immunol.* 75:573, 1985.

114. Ramsdale, E. H., et al. Differences in responsiveness to hyperventilation and methacholine in asthma and chronic bronchitis. *Thorax* 40:422, 1985.

115. Reed, C. E. Basic mechanisms of asthma: Role of inflammation. *Chest* 94:175, 1988.

116. Richardson, J. B. Nonadrenergic inhibitory innervation of the lung. *Lung* 159:315, 1981.

117. Richardson, P. S., and Sterling, G. M. Effects of beta-adrenergic receptor blockade on airway conductance and lung volume in normal and asthmatic subjects. *Br. Med. J.* 3:143, 1969.

118. Robin, E. D. Deaths from bronchial asthma. *Chest* 93:614, 1988.

119. Rubinfeld, A. R., and Pain, M. C. F. Relationship between bronchial reactivity, airway calibre, and severity of asthma. *Am. Rev. Respir. Dis.* 115:381, 1977.

120. Ryan, G., et al. Bronchial responsiveness to histamine: Relationship to diurnal variation of peak flow rate, improvement after bronchodilator, and airway calibre. *Thorax* 37:423, 1982.

121. Said, S. I. Vasoactive intestinal polypeptide (VIP): Current status. *Peptides* 5:143, 1984.

122. Saroea, G., et al. The effect of an inhaled thromboxane mimetic (U46619) on airway function in human subjects. *Am. Rev. Respir. Dis.* 145:1270, 1992.

123. Schellenberg, R. R., and Foster, A. *In vitro* responses of human asthmatic airway and pulmonary vascular smooth muscle. *Int. Arch. Allergy Appl. Immunol.* 75:237, 1984.

124. Sears, M. R. Increasing asthma mortality—Fact or artifact? *J. Allergy Clin. Immunol.* 82:957, 1988.

125. Sears, M. R., et al. Regular inhaled beta-agonist treatment in bronchial asthma. *Lancet* 336:1391, 1990.

126. Sly, R. M. Mortality from asthma. *J. Allergy Clin. Immunol.* 84:421, 1989.

127. Snapper, J. R., et al. Distribution of pulmonary responsiveness to aerosol histamine in dogs. *J. Appl. Physiol.* 44:738, 1978.

128. Stelzer, J., et al. Ozone-induced changes in bronchial reactivity to methacholine and airway inflammation in humans. *J. Appl. Physiol.* 60:1321, 1986.

129. Sterk, P. J., et al. Limited bronchoconstriction to methacholine using partial flow-volume curves in nonasthmatics. *Am. Rev. Respir. Dis.* 133:272, 1985.

130. Sterk, P. J., et al. Limited maximal airway narrowing in nonasthmatic subjects: Role of neural control and prostaglandin release. *Am. Rev. Respir. Dis.* 132:865, 1985.

131. Stevens, W. H., Manning, P. J., and O'Byrne, P. M. Tachyphylaxis to inhaled methacholine in normal but not asthmatic subjects. *J. Appl. Physiol.* 69:875, 1990.

132. Szentivanyi, A. The beta adrenergic theory of the atopic abnormality in bronchial asthma. *J. Allergy* 42:203, 1968.

133. Tattersfield, A. E., Leaver, D. G., and Pride, N. B. Effect of beta-adrenergic blockade and stimulation on normal human airways. *J. Appl. Physiol.* 35:613, 1973.

134. Thomson, N. C., et al. Comparison of bronchial responses to prostaglandin F2 and methacholine. *J. Allergy Clin. Immunol.* 68:392, 1981.

135. Tiffeneau, R., and Beauvallet. Epreuve de bronchoconstriction et de bronchodilatation par aerosols. *Bull. Acad. Med.* 129:166, 1945.

136. Townley, R. C., McGeady, S., and Bewtra, A. The effect of beta adrenergic blockade on bronchial sensitivity to acetyl-beta-methacholine in normal and allergic rhinitis subjects. *J. Allergy Clin. Immunol.* 57:358, 1976.

137. Vahoutte, P. M. Airway epithelium and bronchial reactivity. *Can. J. Physiol. Pharmacol.* 65:448, 1987.

138. van Schayck, C. P., et al. Increased bronchial hyperresponsiveness after inhaling salbutamol during 1 year is not caused by subsensitization to salbutamol. *J. Allergy Clin. Immunol.* 86:793, 1990.

139. Vathenen, A. S., et al. Rebound increase in bronchial responsiveness after treatment with inhaled terbutaline. *Lancet* 1:554, 1988.

140. Verma, V. K., Cockcroft, D. W., and Dosman, J. A. Airway hyperresponsiveness to inhaled histamine in chronic obstructive airways disease. Chronic bronchitis vs. emphysema. *Chest* 94:457, 1988.

141. Vincenc, C. S., et al. Comparison of *in vivo* and *in vitro* responses to histamine in human airways. *Am. Rev. Respir. Dis.* 128:875, 1983.

142. Walden, S. M., et al. Effect of alpha-adrenergic blockade on exercise-induced asthma and conditioned cold air. *Am. Rev. Respir. Dis.* 130:357, 1984.

143. Wardlaw, A. J., et al. Eosinophils and mast cells in bronchoalveolar lavage in subjects with mild asthma. *Am. Rev. Respir. Dis.* 137:62, 1988.

144. Widdicombe, J. G., Kent, D. C., and Nadel, J. A. Mechanism of bronchoconstriction during inhalation of dust. *J. Appl. Physiol.* 17:613, 1962.

145. Wiggs, B., et al. A Model for the Mechanics of Airway Narrowing in Asthma. In M. A. Kaliner, P. J. Barnes, and C. G. A. Persson (eds.), *Asthma: Its Pathology and Treatment.* New York: Marcel Dekker, 1991. Pp. 51–72.

146. Woolcock, A. J., Cheung, W., and Salome, C. Relationship between bronchial responsiveness to propranolol and histamine. *Am. Rev. Respir. Dis.* 133:A177, 1986.

147. Woolcock, A. J., et al. Prevalence of bronchial hyperresponsiveness and asthma in a rural adult population. *Thorax* 42:361, 1987.

148. Woolcock, A. J., Salome, C. M., and Yan, K. The shape of the dose-response curve to histamine in asthmatic and normal subjects. *Am. Rev. Respir. Dis.* 130:71, 1984.

149. Woolcock, A. J., Yan, K., and Salome, C. M. Effect of therapy on bronchial hyperresponsiveness in the long-term management of asthma. *Clin. Allergy* 18:165, 1988.

150. Yan, K., Salome, C. M., and Woolcock, A. J. Prevalence and nature of bronchial hyperresponsiveness in subjects with chronic obstructive pulmonary disease. *Am. Rev. Respir. Dis.* 132:25, 1985.

151. Zaid, G., and Beall, G. N. Bronchial response to beta-adrenergic blockade. *N. Engl. J. Med.* 275:580, 1966.

Immunochemical Properties of Antigens That Cause Atopic Diseases

5

Te Piao King

All of us are exposed, by inhalation, ingestion, injection, or contact, to numerous antigens that are present in various sources in our environment. However, only certain genetically predisposed persons—about 10 percent of our population—become allergic under natural conditions of exposure to some of these antigens [12]. Antigens that induce allergic responses of the immediate type (atopy) are called *atopic allergens*. It is generally accepted that atopic allergy in people is primarily mediated by allergen-specific IgE antibodies [3, 29]. Some reports suggest that specific IgG4 antibodies may also be involved in atopic allergy [8, 79]. Also it is known that the synthesis of both IgE and IgG4 is stimulated by the lymphokine interleukin-4 (IL-4) and it is inhibited by the lymphokine interferon-gamma (IFN-γ) [28].

The common environmental sources of allergens include pollens from different weeds, grasses, and trees; molds; animal danders; insect venoms; mites, and foods: see Part II of this text. Reactive chemicals, such as some drugs or industrial substances, can also be allergens following their conjugation with body proteins or other macromolecules. Allergen extracts invariably contain many protein components that are immunogenic in experimental animals, yet not all of them are allergenic in humans. This difference is in part a consequence of different conditions of immunization. Under natural conditions of exposure, a person becomes sensitized on absorption of minute quantities of allergens. For example, the amount of proteins to which a person may be exposed in the course of a pollinating season [54] or by an insect sting [27] is measured in micrograms. By contrast, experimental animals such as rabbits are hyperimmunized with milligram amounts of proteins in the presence of a powerful adjuvant.

Each environmental source contains multiple allergens. On the basis of their relative allergenic activities, the allergens can be divided into major and minor ones. Major allergens are highly active in the majority of allergic individuals tested, while the minor ones are weakly active. However, minor allergens can be as active as or more active than major allergens in some selected individuals. The major allergens are usually proteins in the molecular weight range of 20,000 to 40,000, while the minor ones are more variable in weight from 3,000 to 70,000. Usually the major allergens are the most abundant ones in the allergen source.

Individuals may vary not only in their responses to different allergens but also in their responses to the different antigenic determinants (epitopes) of the same allergen molecule. For example, studies with chemically modified derivatives of the major bee venom allergen phospholipase suggest that persons who are allergic to bee venom produce IgE antibodies specific for distinct regions of phospholipase [41]. This variation in responses of individuals to different allergens or their determinants is believed to

be genetically determined; see also Chapter 3. It has been shown by Marsh and colleagues [54–56] and others that an individual's sensitivity to an allergen is correlated with their major histocompatibility complex (MHC) gene product.

BIOCHEMICAL STUDIES OF ALLERGENS

Table 5-1 lists some of the allergens that have been isolated and characterized. Most of these allergens were purified by standard techniques of gel filtration and ion-exchange chromatography, and in some cases by affinity chromatography on immunosorbents containing monoclonal antibodies [7]. The use of affinity chromatography can minimize the problem of proteolytic modification and/or degradation of allergens during isolation [35]. The most widely used in vitro tests are the radioallergosorbent test (RAST) [3] and crossed radioimmunoelectrophoresis (CRIE) [52] for measuring the reaction of allergens with their specific human IgE antibodies. A useful modification of RAST or CRIE is to substitute enzyme-labeled reagents for radiolabeled ones [71]. A recent advance is to immunoscreen the allergen(s) of interest in complementary DNA (cDNA) expression libraries with human IgE antibodies. This combined approach has the distinct advantage that the gene for the allergen can be obtained for sequence and expression studies [9, 77, 78, 84]. Chapter 38 further details these in vitro tests.

As given in Tables 5-1 and 5-2, some of the allergens have enzymatic activities but others have as yet unidentified biochemical functions. The amino acid sequences of nearly all the allergens in Table 5-1 are known and this is in large measure due to advances in the cloning and sequencing techniques of molecular biology in recent years. No common feature of the sequences of allergens is noted. But several of these allergens are found to have varying extents of sequence similarity with other proteins in our environment, as given in Table 5-2. Some of the sequence similarities in Table 5-2 are to be expected as they represent proteins of common biologic functions and they are from closely related sources. But some are surprising as they represent proteins from widely different sources. Two examples are given in Figures 5-1 and 5-2.

The sequence similarity of the bee venom allergen *Api m* I with phospholipases A₂ from bovine and human pancreas and from a lizard (Gila monster) venom is given in Figure 5-1. About two-thirds of the amino acid residues of the human and the bovine phospholipases are common to each other, while slightly less than one-fifth of the human and the bee enzymes are in common. About two-fifths of the bee and the lizard enzymes are in common, and their longest stretch of common sequences has seven amino residues at position 24-30.

The sequence similarity of the insect venom allergen *Dol m* V (form A and B) with proteins from tobacco and tomato leaves,

This research is supported in part by a grant from the United States Public Health Service, AI-17021.

Table 5-1. Properties of some purified allergens

Source	Allergens[a]			Molecular weight	Sequence data[b]	References
Pollens						
Short ragweed	*Amb*	*a*	I; antigen E	38,000	C	35, 75
(*Ambrosia artemisifolia*)	*Amb*	*a*	II; antigen K	38,000	C	32, 35
	Amb	*a*	III; Ra 3	11,000	C	42
	Amb	*a*	V; Ra 5	5,000	C	61
Rye grass	*Lol*	*p*	I; group I	30,000	C	54, 72
(*Lolium perenne*)	*Lol*	*p*	II; group II	11,000	C	1
	Lol	*p*	III; group III	11,000	C	1
Kentucky blue grass	*Poa*	*p*	Ia; group I	35,000	P	18, 48
(*Poa pratensis*)	*Poa*	*p*	Ib	33,000	P	48, 65
	Poa	*p*	IX	28,000	C	77
Birch tree	*Bet*	*v*	I	17,000	C	5
(*Betula verrucosa*)	*Bet*	*v*	II		C	85
Insect venoms						
Honey bee	*Api*	*m*	I; phospholipase A$_2$	16,000	C	24, 41, 43
(*Apis mellifera*)	*Api*	*m*	IV; melittin	3,000	C	24, 33, 41
White face hornet	*Dol*	*m*	I; phospholipase A$_1$	35,000	P	40
(*Dolichovespula maculata*)	*Dol*	*m*	V; antigen 5	23,000	C	38, 40
Foods						
Cod	*Gad*	*c*	I; allergen M	12,000	C	17
(*Gadus callarias*)						
Mustard seeds	*Sin*	*a*	I	14,000	C	59
(*Sinapis alba*)						
Others						
Cat saliva	*Fel*	*d*	I	38,000	C	64, 70
(*Felis domesticus*)						
Midges	*Chi*	*t*	I; hemoglobin	16,000	C	57, 73
(*Chironomus thummi thummi*)						
Mold						
(*Aspergillus fumigatus*)	*Asp*	*f*	I	18,000	C	2
(*Candida albicans*)	*Can*	*a*		40,000	C	25
Mites	*Der*	*p*	I; antigen P$_1$	24,000	C	10, 74
(*Dermatophagoides*	*Der*	*p*	II	16,000	C	9, 26
pteronyssinus)						
	Der	*p*	III	17,000	C	84
Mouse urine	*Mus*	*m*	I	19,000	no	51
(*Mus muscaris*)						

[a] The allergens are designated according to the recently adopted nomenclature system [55]; also given are their names used in the early literature.
[b] Allergens with known partial or complete sequence data are designated as P and C, respectively.

and a sperm-coating protein from rat epididymis is shown in Figure 5-2. Sequence alignments of *Dol m* VA and VB with tobacco or tomato leaf proteins and with rat epididymal protein show that about one-fifth and one-third of their amino acid residues are in common. The longest continuous stretch of sequence similarity is between *Dol m* V and the rat protein and it has seven amino acid residues at position 118-125 of rat protein. The biologic function of *Dol m* V is not known. The proteins from tobacco and tomato leaves are designated as pathogenesis-related proteins, as their synthesis is induced following infection or physical injury and they are present in the leaves of many plants [13, 53]. The protein from rat epididymis was shown to have a role in the process of fertilization [6].

The complete conformational structures of most proteins are not known since they can be determined only by x-ray crystallography and/or by nuclear magnetic resonance spectroscopy. In some cases they can be obtained from molecular modeling studies when the conformational structure of a closely related protein is known. Of the allergens listed in Table 5-1, the conformational structures are known only for bee venom phospholipase A$_2$, *Api m* I [76]; melittin, *Api m* IV [83]; and a chironomid hemoglobin, *Chi t* I [80].

Plate 1 shows the superimposed tracings of the Cα atoms of bee venom and bovine pancreatic phospholipase A$_2$. These two proteins of partial sequence similarity also have partial similarity of their three-dimensional backbones. The conserved catalytic

sites of these two enzymes are superimposable, and they are represented by the pink tracings of two antiparallel helices in the figure. One helix is represented by residue 45-57 of the bee and the bovine enzymes as given in Figure 5-1, and the other helix is represented by two separate regions of their linear sequences, residues 80-93 of the bee enzyme and 130-143 of the bovine enzyme. There is also partial similarity of the backbone regions for calcium ion binding of these two enzymes, residue 26-33. Just as is the case for the bovine enzymes, the human and the lizard enzymes in Figure 5-1 are likely to have conformational similarity with the bee enzyme.

IMMUNOLOGIC STUDIES OF ALLERGENS

A knowledge of the conformational structures of allergens is required for understanding their antibody-combining sites. These sites are also designated as B-cell epitopes since antibodies are the receptor molecules of B-lymphocytes. Most allergens listed in Table 5-1 show greatly reduced antibody-binding activities on denaturation, for example, ragweed allergens *Amb a* I, III, and V [22, 39]; group I mite allergen [50]; and bee venom phospholipase A$_2$ [41]. These results indicate that their B-cell epitopes are mainly of the topographic type consisting of discontinuous segments of the polypeptide chain [4]. But allergens also have B-cell epitopes of continuous segments of the polypeptide chain, for

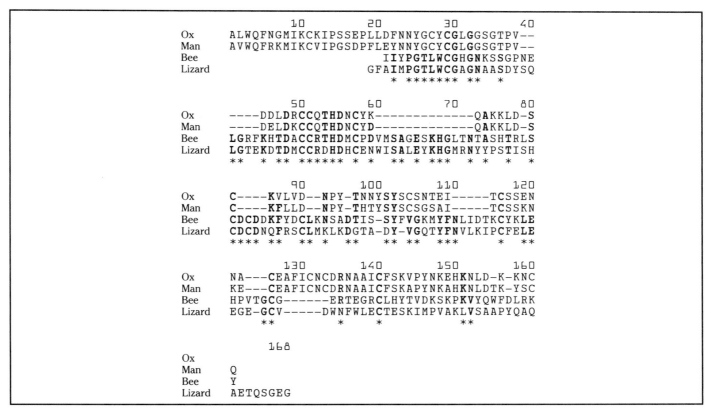

Fig. 5-1. *Amino acid sequences of phospholipases A₂ from bovine and human pancreas, and bee and lizard (Gila monster) venoms. The amino acid residues common to bee enzyme are in boldface and are indicated with stars. The hyphens indicate gaps introduced for maximal alignment of the sequences. Data are from [21, 43, 86].*

Table 5-2. Allergens having sequence similarity with other proteins

Allergen		Other proteins	References
Amb	a I	Pectate lyases	75
Api	m I	Phospholipases A₂ from bovine, porcine, and human pancreas, and Gila monster venom	21, 43, 86
Api	m IV[a]	Human complement C9	46
Asp	f I	Mitogillin family of cytoxins from other strains of *Aspergillus*	2
Bet	v I	Pea disease resistance response gene	5
Bet	v II	Actin-binding protein, profilin	85
Can	a 40 kd	Yeast alcohol dehydrogenase	25
Chi	t I	Human hemoglobin alpha chain	57, 73
Dol	m V	Pathogenesis-related proteins from tobacco and tomato leaves, and sperm-coating glycoprotein from rat epididymis	6, 13, 38, 53
Der	p I	Human cathepsin and other cysteine proteases	9
Fel	d I	Rabbit uteroglobin	64
Lol	p I[b]	Group I allergens of other grass pollens	18
Sin	a I	2S albumins from rapeseed, castor bean, and Brazil nuts	59

[a] *Api m* IV, melittin, probably also has sequence similarity with a calmodulin-binding protein [31] and with a mammalian phospholipase A₂ stimulatory protein [11], as these two proteins showed cross-reaction with melittin-specific antibodies.
[b] Comparisons are made with partial N-terminal sequence data.

example, the grass pollen group I allergens [18], the allergens from cod fish [16] and midge [57], and the bee venom allergen melittin [37]. Some allergens are glycoproteins, like bee venom phospholipase A₂, which has an oligosaccharide side chain of eight or nine monosaccharides attached to the asparagine residue at position 3. A recent report indicates that the oligosaccharide side chain of bee venom phospholipase A₂ is a B-cell epitope for IgE antibodies in bee venom allergic patients [88].

Melittin, a 26-residue peptide, has one major B-cell epitope which is in the C-terminal region of residue 20-26 [37]. This immunochemical property was shown to be related to its biophysical property of binding to cell membrane [19]. Melittin has a linear amphiphilic structure with 20 predominantly hydrophobic amino acids in the N-terminus and a cluster of six hydrophilic, including four cationic amino acids, in the C-terminus [24]. The distribution of polar and nonpolar amino acids in the N-terminus results in alpha-helical amphiphilicity. Melittin assumes the alpha-helical conformation in concentrated solutions, in crystals, or when associated with cell membrane [83, 87]. In the cell membrane, the hydrophobic N-terminus of melittin is inserted into the lipid bilayer and its hydrophilic and cationic C-terminus is exposed on the surface by charge interaction with the anionic head groups of phospholipid [87]. This model helps to explain why the major B-cell epitope of melittin is in its C-terminus.

Antigen- or allergen-specific IgE and IgG responses are known to require the collaboration of T- and B-lymphocytes [15, 29]; see also Chapters 7 and 13. T-cells are activated when their receptors bind processed antigens. The activated T-cells secrete lymphokines, which in turn stimulate antigen-activated B-cells to differentiate and secrete immunoglobulins; one of the lymphokines required for isotype switching and secretion of IgE is IL-4. In

```
Dol m VA   NNYCKIKCSR  GIHTLCKFGT  SMKPNCGSKI   30
Dol m VB   NNYCKIKCRK  GIHTLCKFGT  SMKPNCGRNV   30
Rat        DEW-----DR  DLENL----S  TTK-------   18

Dol m VA   VKVHGVSNDE  KNEIVNRHNQ  FRQKVAKGLE   60
Dol m VB   VKAYGLTNDE  KNEILKRHND  FRQNVAKGLE   60
Rat        -----LSVQE  --EIINKHNQ  LRRTVS----   37
Tobacco                            QNSQQD        6
Tomato                             QNSPQD        6

Dol m VA   TRGNPGPQPP  AKNMNVLVWN  DELAKIAQTW   90
Dol m VB   TRGKPGPQPP  AKNMNVLVWN  DELAKIAQTW   90
Rat        --------PS  GSDLLRVEWD  HDAYVNAQKW   59
Tobacco    YLDAHNTARA  DVGVEPLTWD  NGVAAYAQNY   36
Tomato     YLAVHNDARA  QVGVGPMSWD  ANLASRAQNY   36

Dol m VA   ANQCSFGHDQ  CRN-TEKYQV  GQNVAIASTT  119
Dol m VB   ANQCDFNHDD  CRN-TAKYQV  GQNIAISSTT  119
Rat        ANRCIYNHSP  LQHRTTLKC   GENLFMANYP   89
Tobacco    VSQLAADCNL  VHS-HGQY--  GENLA---QG   60
Tomato     ANSRAGDCNL  IHS--GA---  GENLA---KG   58

Dol m VA   GNSYATMSKL  IEMWENEVKD  FNPKKGTIGD  149
Dol m VB   ATQFDRPSKL  IKQWEDEVTE  FNYKVGLQNS  149
Rat        AS---WSS-V  IQDWYDESLD  FVFGFGPKKV  115
Tobacco    SGDFMTAAKA  VEMWVDEKQY  YDHDSNTCAQ   90
Tomato     GGDF-TGRAA  IQLWVSERPS  YNYATNQCVG   87

Dol m VA   NNFSKVGHYT  QMVWGKTKEI  GCGSVKYIEN  179
Dol m VB   N-FRKVGHYT  QMVWGKTKEI  GCGSIKYIED  178
Rat        G-V-KVGHYT  QVVWNSTFLV  ACGVAECPDQ  143
Tobacco    GQVC--GHYT  QVVWRNSVRV  GCARVKCNNG  118
Tomato     GKKC--RHYT  QVV-----RL  GCGRARCNNG  110

Dol m VA   NWHTHYLVCN  YGPAGNYMDQ  PIYERK      205
Dol m VB   NWYTHYLVCN  YGPGGNDFNQ  PIYERK      204
Rat        P-LKYFYVCH  YCPGGN-YVG  RLYSPY      167
Tobacco    G-YV--VSCN  YDPPGNVIGQ  SPY         138
Tomato     WWF----SCN  YDPVGNWIGQ  RPY         129
```

Fig. 5-2. *Amino acid sequences of* Dol m *VA and B, tobacco leaf protein PR-1b, tomato leaf protein p14, and a sperm-coating glycoprotein from rat epididymis. The hyphens indicate gaps introduced for maximal alignment of the sequences. Residues that are common to* Dol m *VA or B are enclosed in boxes. Data are from [6, 13, 38, 53].*

contrast to the B-cell epitopes that are dependent on the native conformation of an antigen, the T-cell epitopes are usually not and they contain linear segments of the polypeptide chain of about 8 to 15 amino acid residues. This is probably because T-cells do not bind native antigens. Antigens are first processed by antigen-presenting cells into small peptides; then the peptides are displayed on the cell surface together with the Class II MHC protein [62]. MHC proteins are highly polymorphic, and MHC proteins of different haplotypes can have different patterns of association with the processed antigen. Therefore T-cell epitopes of an antigen can vary with the haplotypes of the immunized hosts and this is one known mechanism for genetic control of immune response.

T-cell epitopes of several allergens have been studied. Mouse allergen *Mus m* I was studied in human T-cell lines, and one T-cell epitope was identified to have the same sequence as that of residue 80-108 of rat alpha$_2$-euglobulin [58]. Proliferation assays with human peripheral blood lymphocytes demonstrated that patients have varying patterns of recognition of T-cell peptides of *Chi t* I but one peptide, residue 98-111, was recognized by 9 of 13 patients tested [57]. Using mouse strains of different haplotypes, T-cell epitopes of the following allergens were mapped: ragweed allergen *Amb a* III [45], bee venom allergens phospholip-

ase *Api m* I [44] and melittin *Api m* III [19], and hornet venom allergen *Dol m* V [34]. Comparison of the sequence data of the T-cell epitopes of these allergens does not reveal any special features.

The B- and T-cell epitopes of an allergen may or may not represent separate regions of the molecule. For example, one of the B-cell epitopes of *Chi t* I is located in residue 91-101 and one of its T-cell epitopes is located in the overlapping region of residue 98-111 [57]. But the B- and T-cell epitopes of melittin do not occupy overlapping regions, as they are located in residues 11-19 and 19-26, respectively [19, 37]. Analogs of melittin, which differ only in the region of B-cell epitope [20], elicited analog-specific IgE and IgG responses in responder strains of mice, thus providing direct experimental support for the T-cell control of the B-cell response.

ARE ALLERGENS DIFFERENT FROM OTHER PROTEIN ANTIGENS?

Early animal model experiments have suggested that IgE antibody response to antigens is controlled by the dose, the adjuvant, and the genetic makeup of the host, and it does not depend on the chemical nature of antigens [47]. The known immunochemical properties of the allergens described above do not reveal any unusual features when their B- and T-cell epitopes are compared with those of other protein antigens. These data together with those of the animal model experiments would suggest that any antigen can be an allergen in susceptible persons under the proper immunizing conditions. However, the general observation is that some of the proteins present in various allergen extracts are more effective than others as allergens. Is this only a consequence of the specificity of the immunized host? Or are there other unknown factors in our environment [81] or in allergen extracts that may have an adjuvant role for IgE responses? Or is it that allergenic proteins have some intrinsic properties that can enhance their immunogenicity?

Sequence similarity of allergens with other proteins in our environment (see Table 5-2) may possibly represent one intrinsic property that can enhance the immunogenicity of a protein by antigenic cross-reactivity. Prior exposure to cross-reacting antigens primes a host for immune responses so that on subsequent exposures only trace amounts of allergens are sufficient to elicit antibody responses. The cross-reactivity can be at both T- and B-cell epitope levels, but it is more likely to be at the T-cell epitope level. As mentioned earlier, T-cell epitopes are less dependent on the native conformation of antigen and they are usually of short contiguous segments of the polypeptide chain.

Another possible intrinsic property of allergens is either specific or nonspecific interaction with the cell membrane, and this can result in prolonged antigenic stimulation. An example is the allergenicity of the 26-residue bee venom peptide melittin; the 18-residue bee venom peptide apamin has not been found to be an allergen [33, 41]. In responder strains of mice, melittin induced at least 10 times higher levels of antibodies than apamin did [14, 37]. Melittin differs from apamin in that it can bind to cell membrane tightly, as reflected by its lytic activity of red blood cells in micromolar concentration [20].

MODIFIED ALLERGENS AS IMMUNOTHERAPEUTIC REAGENTS

Chemically modified antigens usually have reduced allergenic activities. This is because they have a reduced number of antigenic determinants. Bridging of cell-bound specific IgE antibodies by multivalent antigens is known to be a necessary step for the release of cellular mediators of allergic symptoms [29]. Since the modified antigens cannot bridge IgE antibodies as well as the native antigens can, they have reduced allergenic activities. Such modified antigens, however, retain at least in part the immunogenicity of native antigens; therefore, they can be useful as immunotherapeutic agents in humans. The types of chemical modifications that have been investigated for this purpose include (1) polymerized antigen on treatment with formaldehyde [54] or glutaraldehyde [23, 63]; (2) antigen conjugates with nonimmunogenic polymers [36]; (3) denatured antigen [30]; and (4) antigen fragments obtained on protease digestion [49].

Polymerized antigens [23, 60, 67], antigen conjugates [68], as well as one denatured antigen [66] have been tested as immunotherapeutic reagents in humans. These modified antigens can be used safely in greater doses than the native antigens can. Patients treated with polymerized antigen or antigen conjugates demonstrated symptom reduction and gave IgE and IgG responses similar to those treated with native antigens. But patients treated with a denatured antigen, specifically the urea denatured antigen E (*Amb a* I) from ragweed pollen, did not show significant changes of their antigen E–specific IgE or IgG. In mice the denatured antigen E was poorly immunogenic for IgE and IgG antibody

responses and it partially suppressed ongoing antigen-specific IgE responses. This suppressive effect was suggested to be stimulation of antigen-specific suppressor T-cells [82]. However, in treatment of patients, it was not possible to attain the dosage levels used in mice. Another recent proposal on the mechanism of immunotherapy was suggested to be inactivation of allergen-specific T-cells [69].

REFERENCES

1. Ansari, A. A., Shenbagamurthi, P., and Marsh, D. G. Complete amino acid sequence of a Lolium perenne (perennial rye grass) allergen, Lol p III: Comparison with known Lol p I and II sequences. *Biochemistry* 28:8665, 1989.
2. Aruda, L. K., et al. Aspergillus fumigatus allergen I, a major IgE-binding protein, is a member of the mitogillin family of cytotoxins. *J. Exp. Med.* 172:1529, 1990.
3. Bennich, H., and Johansson, S. Structure and function of human IgE. *Adv. Immunol.* 13:1, 1971.
4. Berzofsky, J. Intrinsic and extrinsic factors in protein antigenic structure. *Science* 229:923, 1985.
5. Breiteneder, H., et al. The gene coding for the major birch pollen allergen Bet v I is highly homologous to a pea disease resistance response gene. *EMBO J.* 8:1935, 1989.
6. Brooks, D. E., et al. Molecular cloning of the cDNA for androgen-dependent sperm-coating glycoproteins secreted by the rat epididymis. *Eur. J. Biochem.* 161:13, 1986.
7. Chapman, M. D. Purification of allergens. *Curr. Opin. Immunol.* 1:647, 1989.
8. Chernokhvostova, E. V., et al. IgG4 antibodies in hay fever patients. Difference in IgG4 response to tree pollen and grass pollen allergens. *Int. Arch. Allergy Appl. Immunol.* 92:217, 1990.
9. Chua, K. Y., et al. Isolation of cDNA coding for the major mite allergen Der p II by IgE plaque immunoassay. *Int. Arch. Allergy Appl. Immunol.* 91:118, 1990.
10. Chua, K. Y., Stewart, G. A., and Thomas, W. R. Sequence analysis of cDNA encoding for a major house dust mite allergen, Der p I. *J. Exp. Med.* 167: 175, 1988.
11. Clark, M., et al. Identification and isolation of a mammalian protein which is antigenically and functionally related to the phospholipase A2 stimulatory peptide melittin. *J. Biol. Chem.* 262:4402, 1987.
12. Cooke, R. A. *Allergy in Theory and Practice.* Philadelphia: Saunders, 1947.
13. Cornelissen, B., et al. Molecular characterization of messenger RNAs for pathogenesis related proteins 1a, 1b and 1c produced by TMV infection of tobacco. *EMBO J.* 5:37, 1986.
14. Defendini, M., et al. H-2A linked control of T-cell and antibody responses to apamin. *Immunogenetics* 28:139, 1988.
15. Delespesse, G., Sarfati, M., and Heusser, C. IgE synthesis. *Curr. Opin. Immunol.* 2:506, 1990.
16. Elsayed, S., et al. The immunochemical reactivity of the three homologous repetitive tetrapeptides in the region 41-64 of allergen M from cod. *Scand. J. Immunol.* 16:77, 1982.
17. Elsayed, S., Von Bahr-Lindsrom, H., and Bennich, H. The primary structure of fragment TM2 of allergen M from cod. *Scand. J. Immunol.* 3:683, 1974.
18. Esch, R. E., and Klapper, D. G. Isolation and characterization of a major cross-reactive grass group I allergenic determinant. *Mol. Immunol.* 26:557, 1989.
19. Fehlner, P. F., et al. Murine T cell responses to melittin and its analogs. *J. Immunol.* 146:799, 1991.
20. Fehlner, P. F., Kochoumian, L., and King, T. P. Murine IgG and IgE responses to melittin and its analogs. *J. Immunol.* 146:2664, 1991.
21. Gomez, F., et al. Purification and characterization of five variants of phospholipase A2 and complete primary structure of the main phospholipase A2 variant in heloderma suspectum (gila monster) venom. *Eur. J. Biochem.* 186:23, 1989.
22. Goodfriend, L. Toward Structure-function Studies with Ragweed Allergens Ra3 and Ra5. In E. Mathov, T. Shindo, and P. Naranjo (eds.), *Allergy and Clinical Immunology.* Amsterdam: Excerpta Medica, 1977. Pp. 151–155.
23. Grammer, L., et al. A double-blind, placebo-controlled trial of polymerized whole ragweed for immunotherapy of ragweed allergy. *J. Allergy Clin. Immunol.* 69:494, 1982.
24. Habermann, E. Bee and wasp venoms. *Science* 177:314, 1972.
25. Han, S. H., Shen, H. D., and Choo, K. B. The 40 kd allergen of Candida

albicans is an alcohol dehydrogenase (abstract). *J. Allergy Clin. Immunol.* 87:327, 1991.

26. Heyman, P., et al. Antigenic and structural analysis of group II allergens (Der f II and Der p II) from house dust mites (Dermatophagoides spp). *J. Allergy Clin. Immunol.* 83:1055, 1989.

27. Hoffman, D. R., and Jackson, R. S. Allergens in hymenoptera venom. XIII. How much protein is in a sting? *Ann. Allergy* 52:276, 1984.

28. Ishizaka, A., et al. Regulation of IgE and IgG4 synthesis in patients with hyper IgE syndrome. *Immunology* 70:414, 1990.

29. Ishizaka, K. Basic mechanisms of IgE-mediated hypersensitivity. *Curr. Opin. Immunol.* 1:625, 1989.

30. Ishizaka, K., Okudaira, H., and King, T. P. Immunogenic properties of modified antigen E. II. Ability of urea-denatured antigen and alpha-polypeptide chain to prime T cells specific for antigen E. *J. Immunol.* 114:110, 1975.

31. Kaetzel, M., and Dedman, J. Affinity-purified melittin antibody recognized the calmodulin-binding domain on calmodulin target protein. *J. Biol. Chem.* 262:3726, 1987.

32. Keating, K. M., et al. Amb a I and Amb a II from short ragweed pollen are a multi-gene family of allergens (abstract). *J. Allergy Clin. Immunol.* 85:201, 1990.

33. Kemeny, D. M., et al. Antibodies to purified bee venom proteins and peptides. I. Development of a highly specific RAST for bee venom antigens and its application to bee sting allergy. *J. Allergy Clin. Immunol.* 71:505, 1983.

34. King, T. P. T cell epitopes of a vespid venom allergen Ag5 (abstract). *J. Allergy Clin. Immunol.* 85:213, 1990.

35. King, T. P., et al. Limited proteolysis of antigens E and K from ragweed pollen. *Arch. Biochem. Biophys.* 212:127, 1981.

36. King, T. P., Kochoumian, L., and Chiorazzi, N. Immunological properties of conjugates of ragweed antigen E with methoxypolyethylene glycol or a copolymer of D-glutamic acid and D-lysine. *J. Exp. Med.* 149:424, 1979.

37. King, T. P., Kochoumian, L., and Joslyn, A. Melittin-specific monoclonal and polyclonal IgE and IgG1 antibodies from mice. *J. Immunol.* 133:2668, 1984.

38. King, T. P., et al. Structural studies of a hornet venom allergen antigen 5, Dol m V and its sequence similarity with other proteins. *Protein Seq. Data Anal.* 3:263, 1990.

39. King, T. P., Norman, P., and Tao, N. Chemical modifications of the major allergen of ragweed pollen: Antigen E. *Immunochemistry* 11:83, 1974.

40. King, T. P., et al. Protein allergens of white-faced hornet, yellow hornet and yellowjacket venoms. *Biochemistry* 17:5165, 1978.

41. King, T. P., et al. Allergens of honeybee venom. *Arch. Biochem. Biophys.* 172:661, 1976.

42. Klapper, D., Goodfriend, L., and Capra, J. Amino acid sequence of ragweed allergen Ra3. *Biochemistry* 10:5729, 1980.

43. Kuchler, K., et al. Analysis of the cDNA for phospholipase A2 from honey bee venom glands: The deduced amino acid sequence reveals homology of the corresponding vertebrate enzymes. *Eur. J. Biochem.* 184:249, 1989.

44. Kuo, M., et al. Epitope mapping of T cell recognition of phospholipase A2 (abstract). *J. Allergy Clin. Immunol.* 83:251, 1989.

45. Kurisaki, J., Atassi, H., and Atassi, M. Z. T cell recognition of ragweed allergen Ra3: Localization of the full T cell recognition profile by synthetic overlapping peptides representing the entire protein chain. *Eur. J. Immunol.* 16:236, 1986.

46. Laine, R., and Esser, A. Identification of the discontinuous epitope in human complement C9 recognized by anti-melittin antibodies. *J. Immunol.* 143:553, 1989.

47. Levine, B., and Vaz, N. Effect of combinations of inbred strain, antigen and antigen dose on immune responsiveness and reagin production in the mouse. A potential mouse model for immune aspects of human atopic allergy. *Int. Arch. Allergy Appl. Immunol.* 39:156, 1970.

48. Lin, Z., et al. Isolation and characterization of Poa p I allergens of Kentucky bluegrass pollen with a murine monoclonal anti-Lol p I antibody. *Int. Arch. Allergy Appl. Immunol.* 87:294, 1988.

49. Litwin, A., Pesce, A. J., and Michael, J. G. Regulation of the immune response to allergens by immunosuppressive allergenic fragments. I. Peptic fragment of honey bee venom phospholipase A2. *Int. Arch. Allergy Appl. Immunol.* 87:361, 1988.

50. Lombardero, M., et al. Conformational stability of B cell epitopes on group I and group II Dermatophagoides spp. allergens: Effect of thermal and chemical denaturation on the binding of murine IgG and human IgE antibodies. *J. Immunol.* 144:1353, 1990.

51. LoRusso, J. R., Moffat, S., and Ohman, J. Immunologic and biochemical properties of the major mouse urinary allergen. *J. Allergy Clin. Immunol.* 78:928, 1986.

52. Lowenstein, H. Quantitative immunoelectrophoretic methods as a tool for the analysis and isolation of allergens. *Prog. Allergy* 25:1, 1978.

53. Lucas, J., et al. Amino acid sequence of the pathogenesis-related leaf protein p14 from viroid-infected tomato reveals a new type of structurally unfamiliar proteins. *EMBO J.* 4:2745, 1987.

54. Marsh, D. G. Allergens and the Genetics of Allergy. In M. Sela (ed.), *The Antigens,* Vol. III. New York: Academic, 1975. Pp. 271–359.

55. Marsh, D. G., et al. Allergen nomenclature. *J. Allergy Clin. Immunol.* 80:639, 1987.

56. Marsh, D. G., et al. Molecular studies of human response to allergens. *Cold Spring Harb. Symp. Quant. Biol.* 54:459, 1989.

57. Mazur, G., Baur, X., and Liebers, V. Hypersensitivity to hemoglobins of the Diptera family Cironomidae: Structural and functional studies of their immunogenic/allergenic sites. *Monogr. Allergy* 28:121, 1990.

58. McDonald, B., et al. A 29 amino acid peptide derived from rat alpha 2 euglobulin triggers murine allergen specific human T cells (abstract). *J. Allergy Clin. Immunol.* 83:251, 1988.

59. Menendez-Arias, L., et al. Epitope mapping of the major allergen from yellow mustard seeds, Sin a I. *Mol. Immunol.* 27:143, 1990.

60. Metzger, W., et al. Clinical and immunologic evaluation of glutaraldehyde-modified, tyrosine-adsorbed short ragweed extract: A double-blind, placebo-controlled trial. *J. Allergy Clin. Immunol.* 68:442, 1981.

61. Mole, L., et al. The amino acid sequence of ragweed pollen allergen Ra5. *Biochemistry* 14:1216, 1975.

62. Moller, G. Antigen processing. *Immunol. Rev.* 106:1, 1988.

63. Moran, D., et al. Chemical modification of crude timothy grass pollen extract. III. The effect of glutaraldehyde-induced aggregation on antigen and immunogenic properties. *Int. Arch. Allergy Appl. Immunol.* 54:315, 1977.

64. Morgenstern, J., et al. Determination of the amino acid sequence and cDNA cloning of the major allergen of domestic cat, Fel d I (abstract). *J. Allergy Clin. Immunol.* 87:327, 1991.

65. Nayak, B. N., and Kisil, F. T. NH2-terminal amino acid sequences of Poa p Ia and Ib allergens of Kentucky blue grass (abstract). *J. Allergy Clin. Immunol.* 87:325, 1991.

66. Norman, P., et al. Treatment of ragweed hay fever with urea-denatured antigen E. *J. Allergy Clin. Immunol.* 66:336, 1980.

67. Norman, P., et al. Controlled evaluation of allergoid in the immunotherapy of ragweed hay fever. *J. Allergy Clin. Immunol.* 70:248, 1982.

68. Norman, P. S., et al. Immunologic responses to conjugates of antigen E in patients with ragweed hay fever. *J. Allergy Clin. Immunol.* 73:787, 1984.

69. O'Hehir, R. E., et al. The specificity and T cell regulation of responsiveness to allergens. *Ann. Rev. Immunol.* 9:67, 1991.

70. Ohman, J. L., Lowell, F. C., and Block, K. I. Allergens of mammalian origin. V. Properties of extracts derived from the domestic cat. *Clin. Allergy* 6:419, 1976.

71. Peltre, G., Lapeyre, J., and David, B. Heterogeneity of grass pollen allergens (Dactyleis glomerata) recognized by IgE antibodies in human patient sera by a new nitrocellulose immunoprint technique. *Immunol. Lett.* 5:127, 1982.

72. Perez, M., et al. cDNA cloning and immunological characterization of the rye grass allergen Lol p I. *J. Biol. Chem.* 265:16210, 1990.

73. Pfletsinger, J., Plagenes, H., and Braunritzer, G. The primary structure of the monomeric hemoglobin component CTT IV of Chironomus thumus thumus. *Z. Naturforsch* 35:840, 1980.

74. Platts-Mills, T., and Chapman, M. Dust mites: Immunology, allergic disease and environmental control. *J. Allergy Clin. Immunol.* 80:755, 1987.

75. Rafnar, T., et al. Cloning of Amb a I (antigen E), the major allergen family of short ragweed pollen. *J. Biol. Chem.* 266:1229, 1991.

76. Scott, D. L., et al. Crystal structure of bee venom phospholipase A2 in a complex with a transition-state analogue. *Science* 250:1563, 1990.

77. Silvavovich, A., et al. Nucleotide sequence analysis of three cDNAs coding for Poa p IX isoallergen of Kentucky bluegrass pollen. *J. Biol. Chem.* 266:1204, 1991.

78. Singh, M., Smith, P. M., and Knox, R. B. Molecular biology of rye grass pollen allergens. *Monogr. Allergy* 28:101, 1990.

79. Stanworth, D. R. The molecular pathology of IgG4. *Monogr. Allergy* 19:227, 1986.

80. Steigemann, W., and Weber, E. Structure of erythrocruorin in different ligand status refined at 1.4 A resolution. *J. Mol. Biol.* 127:309, 1979.

81. Takafuji, S., et al. Enhancing effect of suspended particulate matter on the IgE antibody production in mice. *Int. Arch. Allergy Appl. Immunol.* 90:1, 1989.

82. Takatsu, K., Ishizaka, K., and King, T. P. Immunogenic properties of modified antigen E. III. Effect of repeated injections of modified antigen on

immunocompetent cells specific for native antigen. *J. Immunol.* 115:1469, 1975.

83. Terwilliger, T. C., and Eisenberg, D. The structure of melittin. II. Interpretation of the structure. *J. Biol. Chem.* 257:6016, 1982.

84. Tovey, E. R., et al. Cloning and sequencing of a cDNA expressing a recombinant house dust mite protein that binds human IgE and corresponds to an important low molecular weight allergen. *J. Exp. Med.* 170:1457, 1989.

85. Valenta, R., et al. A low molecular weight allergen of white birch (Betula vermicosa) is highly homologous with an ubiquitous cytoskeletal protein. *Int. Arch. Allergy Appl. Immunol.* 94:368, 1991.

86. Verheij, H., et al. The complete primary structure of phospholipase A2 from human pancreas. *Biochim. Biophys. Acta* 747:93, 1983.

87. Vogel, H., and Jahnig, F. The structure of melittin in membranes. *Biophys. J.* 50:573, 1986.

88. Weber, A., et al. Specific interaction of IgG antibodies with carbohydrate epitope of honey bee venom phospholipase A2. *Allergy* 42:464, 1989.

Overview of Immune-Mediated Disease: Structure, Function, and Regulation of the Immune Response

Joseph A. Bellanti
Josef V. Kadlec

One of the most fundamental properties of life is the conservation of self-identity and the distribution between "self" from "nonself" or foreignness. The immunologic system, the principal organ system involved in the recognition of foreignness, developed over the millennia in response to an ever-changing and potentially hostile environment. The immune response may be defined as all those physiologic mechanisms that enable the animal to recognize materials as foreign to itself and neutralize, eliminate, or metabolize them with or without injury to its own tissues [1].

This chapter provides an overview of the specific components of the immune response as a basis for more detailed descriptions of basic and clinical mechanisms of immunology and their applications to asthma, which will appear in subsequent chapters.

THE NATURE OF FOREIGNNESS

Broadly speaking, *foreignness* may be defined as those characteristics that are not recognized as "self." Those foreign substances that are formed have the capacity to evoke immunologic responses and are referred to as *antigens* or *immunogens* and all are recognized as foreign by the host. *Allergens* are a specialized class of immunogens which elicit the formation of IgE antibodies that trigger allergic reactions in certain genetically predisposed (i.e., atopic) individuals. Thus, all allergens are antigens but all antigens are not necessarily allergens.

THE RECOGNITION OF FOREIGNNESS

For ease of discussion we may speak of five components of the host's encounter with foreignness: (1) the environment, (2) the target cells, (3) the phagocytic cell, (4) the mediator cells and their products, and (5) the specific antigen recognition cells (B-lymphocytes and T-lymphocytes) and their products (Fig. 6-1).

The starting point in any discussion of the immunologic system is with the external environment, which includes the myriad of foreign substances ranging from simple low-molecular-weight chemicals to the most complex microbial agents that ultimately activate the immune processes as immunogens (antigens) or allergens. The introduction of an environmental agent into the host may have an adverse effect on a *target cell,* which may result in dysfunction or death of the target cell and subsequent disease. There are a variety of target cells; whether they are affected by a particular agent depends on their type, location, and portal of entry of the foreign substances (Table 6-1). The cells and cell products of the immune system therefore may be considered to be interacting in such a way as to protect the target cell from injury from the environmental agents.

The *phagocytic cells* are those cells that function in the initial process of engulfment and uptake of particles from the external environment and present a barrier between the environment and the target cell, protecting the target cell from subsequent injury (see Fig. 6-1). Phagocytosis is the process of uptake of foreign substances and, in the human, is carried out by three classes of phagocytic cells: (1) the mononuclear phagocytes (macrophages), (2) neutrophils, and (3) eosinophils. These cells, acting alone or in concert, are triggered by chemotactic factors generated from the complement system or from products derived from specific lymphocytes and can accumulate in areas of inflammation. The macrophages, in addition to their phagocytic function, are importantly involved in the processing and presentation of antigen to T- and B-lymphocytes [4]. Most of these activities are carried out by cell-surface receptors, which are formed on the membranes of these cells.

Certain other cells of the immune system, referred to as *mediator cells,* can amplify the effects of the phagocytic cells or may have a direct action on target cells (see Fig. 6-1). These cells function through their interaction with the environmental agent(s) and through the release of biologically active chemical substances referred to as *mediators.* These comprise a wide variety of low-molecular-weight and macromolecular mediators, shown in Table 6-2, and are described in greater detail in subsequent chapters. The release of these mediators from mediator cells may be triggered directly by interaction with the foreign antigen or by the interaction of antigen with specific antibodies (e.g., IgE) that bind to the surface of these cells through their Fc fragments. The release of these mediators is of extreme importance in the clinical expression of immediate hypersensitivity and is central to discussion of the immunologic reactions involved in the pathogenesis of bronchial asthma.

It is now recognized that IgE-mediated inflammation consists of a two-phase response: (1) an initial immediate effect on blood vessels, smooth muscles, and secretory glands triggered by the immediate release of mediators; and (2) a late-phase response that is mediated by cellular inflammatory responses (see Chap. 12). It is also now recognized that there are two types of surface receptors for IgE. Those found on the mast cells and basophils bear a surface Fcϵ RI or a high-affinity receptor. A second class of IgE receptors, found on eosinophils, monocytes (macrophages), lymphocytes, and platelets is referred to as *FcϵRII* or a *low-affinity receptor.* This receptor is expressed only when these cells are activated and plays no known role in the release of mediators or in IgE-mediated inflammation [9].

The specific antigen-recognition cells of the immune system include two universes of lymphocytes: the B-lymphocytes, which produce five classes of immunoglobulins (IgG, IgA, IgM, IgD, and IgE), and the T-lymphocytes, which are responsible for cell-mediated immune reactions (see Fig. 6-1). The interactions of the products of these two lymphocyte populations may be on the one hand beneficial to the host and be collectively referred to as *protective immune responses,* or at times may be detrimental

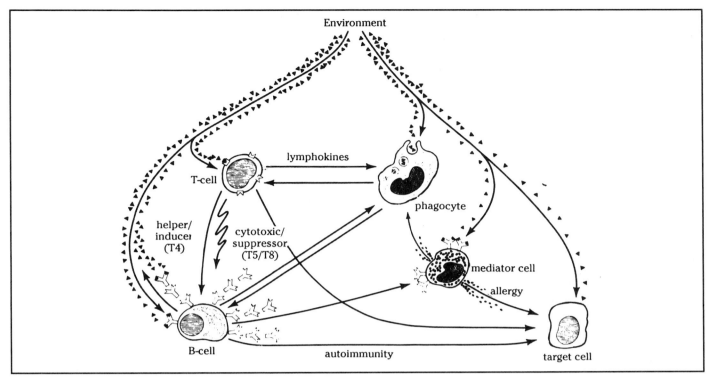

Fig. 6-1. *Total array of immunologic responses to the environment. (Reprinted with permission from J. A. Bellanti.* Immunology III. *Philadelphia: Saunders, 1985. P. 207).*

Table 6-1. Effects of the environment on target cells

Location of target cell	Example of effect	Result
Skin	Disruption of epidermal cells	Dermatitis
Gastrointestinal tract		
Mucosal cell	Destruction	Gastrointestinal bleeding
Smooth muscle	Increased contractility	Diarrhea, vomiting
Glandular cell	Increased secretion	Increased mucus production
Respiratory tract		
Smooth muscle	Increased contraction	Bronchospasm
Glandular cell	Increased secretion	Increased mucus production
Circulatory system		
Endothelial cell	Increased intercellular pore size	Edema
Formed elements	Destruction of erythrocytes	Anemia

Table 6-2. Mediators released in response to environmental agents

Low-molecular-weight mediators (<1,000)
    Histamine
    Serotonin
    Kinins
    Slow reactive substance of anaphylaxis (SRS-A) (now leukotrienes C_4, D_4, E_4)
    Arachidonic acid metabolites (i.e., prostaglandins, leukotrienes)
    Eosinophilic chemotactic factors of anaphylaxis (ECF-A)
    Platelet-activating factor (PAF)
Macromolecular mediators (>1,000)
    Lysosomal enzymes
    Cationic proteins of polymorphonuclear leukocytes
    Complement and coagulation components; neuropeptides

and give rise to adverse or harmful expressions of the immune response referred to as *hypersensitivity* or *allergic reactions.* The whole of the immune response is under genetic control, which has been implicated in the clinical expression of allergic diseases and specifically the atopic state.

THE MOLECULAR BASIS FOR ANTIGEN RECOGNITION

In recent years antigen recognition by cells of the immune system has been defined in molecular terms. It is now recognized that antigen specificity of every immune response is driven by three different systems of recognition structures: (1) the variable or V region of immunoglobulins expressed as free immunoglobulin molecules or bound on the surface of B-cells, (2) cluster of differentiation markers on lymphocytes that not only differentiate T- from B-lymphocytes but also perform important collaborative functions with other antigen-recognition structures, (3) the polymorphic regions (or V regions) of major histocompatibility complex (MHC) Class I and II molecules, and (4) the V regions of the T-cell receptor (TCR) chains (alpha, beta, gamma, delta).

The Immunoglobulins

As described above, immunoglobulins are glycoproteins produced by B-lymphocytes and comprise the humoral arm of immunity. Immunoglobulins have a symmetric four-chain structure composed of two identical heavy (H) and two identical light (L) chains joined together covalently by disulfide bridges. The four polypeptide chains are folded into globular regions (domains) by means of disulfide bonds. Each chain contains an amino-terminal portion, the V regions, and one or more carboxy-terminal portions, the constant (C) regions. Moreover, the V regions also contain three or four regions or "hot spots" where the amino acid sequence is even more variable and therefore these regions are referred to as the *hypervariable regions,* which form the antigen-binding sites of the immunoglobulin molecule. Thus, the immunoglobulins display an immense diversity of heterogeneity matched by the challenge of the heterogeneity of the vast array of foreign configurations present in our complex environment.

The five classes of immunoglobulins (IgG, IgA, IgM, IgD, and IgE) are defined by the antigenic differences in the C regions of their H chains. The IgC class of immunoglobulins can be further subdivided into four subclasses, referred to as IgG1, IgG2, IgG3, and IgG4, which are assuming increasing clinical importance in patients with asthma and other allergic states in which subclass deficiencies have been observed. In addition to the major structure of these molecules there are two types of light chains, referred to as kappa (κ) and lambda (λ) chains, which divide each major immunoglobulin class into kappa and lambda types.

Cluster of Differentiation Markers on Lymphocytes

By the late 1960s both the immunologic importance of the thymus and the existence of two major subsets of lymphocytes were clearly established. T- and B-lymphocytes, however, could not be distinguished by morphologic criteria alone and some major accomplishment was made when various cell-surface components on the lymphocytes became identifiable by the use of specific monoclonal antibodies, which allowed the differentiation of various surface markers on both B- and T-lymphocytes. These markers are referred to as *cluster of differentiation (CD) markers.* On the basis of these CD markers and antigen receptors, at least three distinct lineages of lymphocytes now have been identified: T-lymphocytes, B-lymphocytes, and natural killer (NK) cells. The T-cells recognize antigens by a membrane structure referred to as the CD3/T-cell antigen receptor (CD3/TCR) complex, described more fully below; the B-lymphocytes recognize antigens by surface immunoglobulin molecules. The nature of the antigen recognition structure of the NK cells has not been identified, but appears to be different from the TCR or the immunoglobulin structures. Table 6-3 lists commonly recognized CD structures on immune system cells and their postulated functions.

The Major Histocompatibility Complex Antigens

The second important recognition structure of the immune system consists of a group of molecules found on the surface of most nucleated cells, which are referred to as the *MHC antigens.* The human MHC is referred to as the *human leukocyte antigen (HLA) system.* The MHC is the most polymorphic complex known in the mammalian species and the molecules that are encoded by this region play a very important role in discrimination between "self" and "nonself" by the immune system. HLA molecules can be divided into three major classes: Class I, II, and III.

Class I and Class II molecules are cell-surface glycoproteins that can be distinguished according to their structure, function, and sites of tissue distribution. Class I molecules include the HLA-A, -B, and -C molecules and are found on the surface of all nucleated cells. Class II molecules include HLA-DR, -DQ and -DP molecules and are found on the surface of antigen-presenting cells. Class III molecules are responsible for the synthesis of certain components of the complement system (C2, C4, and Factor B).

Class I molecules (Fig. 6-2) consist of a beta-pleated sheet that forms a platform on which are found the coils of two alpha helices, thus forming the sides of a groove (i.e., the antigen-binding site). The structure of Class II molecules is postulated to be similar to that of Class I. Processed antigens fit into this groove and are presented to cells of the immunologic system (Fig. 6-3). The antigen-binding site varies from one HLA molecule to another, and one HLA molecule can bind only a limited number of specific peptide fragments. The foreign antigen is thus recognized only in the context of the antigen-presenting HLA molecules by the cells of the immune system.

This molecular recognition of the foreignness within the context of "self" also involves the interaction of HLA molecules that present "processed" foreign antigen to the T-cells via the TCR.

The T-Cell Receptor

The third recognition structure of the immune system consists of a TCR complex [4]. The TCR is a two-chain structure that

Table 6-3. Summary of major cluster of differentiation (CD) surface markers

Antigen*	Molecular weight	Distribution	Function
CD1 (T6)	45,000	Thymocytes, Langerhans' cells	—
CD2 (T11)	50,000	T-cells	E-rosette receptor
CD3 (T3)	20,000–26,000	T-cells	Part of T-cell receptor (TCR) complex
CD4 (T4)	60,000	Helper T-cells	Class II MHC interaction, HIV receptor
CD5 (T1)	67,000	T-cells, B-cells	?
CD6 (T12)	120,000	T-cells	?
CD7	40,000	T- and NK cells	IgM Fc receptor ?
CD8 (T8)	32,000	Cytotoxic/suppressor T-cells	Class I MHC interaction
CD10	100,000	Pre-B-cells (CALLA)	?
CD11a	180,000	Leukocytes	Alpha chain of LFA-1 (cellular adhesion)
CD11b	160,000	Myeloid and NK cells, T subset	Complement receptor (α-CR3)
CD11c	150,000	Myeloid and NK cells, T subset	Complement receptor (α-CR4)
CD16	50,000–60,000	Granulocytes, NK cells, T subset	FcR (low affinity) (IgG-Fc receptor type III)
CD18	95,000	Leukocytes	Beta subunit of CD11a, b, c
CD20	35,000	B-cells	?
CD21	140,000	B-cells	Complement receptor type 2
CD23α	45,000	Activated B-cells	Low-affinity IgE receptor, FcεRII
CD23β	45,000	B-cells, monocytes, eosinophils, T subsets	—
CD25	55,000	Activated T- and B-cells, macrophages	Low-affinity IL-2 receptor
CD35	220,000	Granulocytes, monocytes	Complement receptor type 1
CD45	180,000–220,000	Leukocyes	Leukocyte common antigen

NK = natural killer; CALLA = common acute lymphocytic leukemia antigen; HIV = human immunodeficiency virus; LFA-1 = lymphocyte function–associated antigen-1; FcR = Fc receptor; IL-2 = interleukin-2.
* Older nomenclature shown in parentheses.

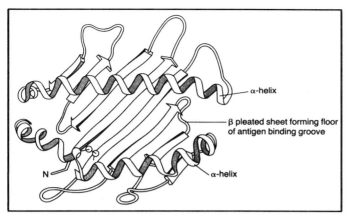

Fig. 6-2. *The structure of a Class I HLA molecule* (top view). *The molecule is shown as the T-cell receptor would see it. The antigen-binding site formed by the alpha helices* (ribbonlike structures) *and beta-pleated strands* (broad arrows) *is shown.* N = *the amino terminus. (Reprinted with permission from D. P. Stites and A. I. Terr (eds.).* Basic Human Immunology *(1st ed.). Norwalk: Appleton & Lange, 1991. P. 48.)*

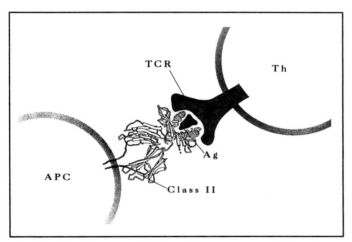

Fig. 6-3. *A T-cell receptor* (TCR) *attaches to an antigen* (Ag) *and a Class II HLA molecule, found on the cell surface.* Th = *helper T-cell;* APC = *antigen-presenting cell. (Courtesy of Drs. Carolyn K. Hurley and Kyung Wha Lee, The Lombardi Cancer Center, Georgetown University.)*

recognizes foreign antigens (i.e., processed antigen) bound to the major histocompatibility proteins either on the antigen-presenting cells (Class II) or on the target cells (Class I). This dual recognition requirement for antigen recognition is referred to as *HLA restriction.* The TCR functions in the context of a cluster of CD3 molecules, referred to as the *CD3/TCR complex* (Fig. 6-4).

One of the CD3-associated TCRs for antigen consists of a disulfide-linked heterodimer comprised of alpha and beta chains and is found on the majority of T-cells. Recently, another CD3-associated TCR heterodimer was described for a distinct T-cell subset composed of gamma and delta chains. All these chains are encoded by multiple rearranged genes. The precise role of this gamma-delta receptor is as yet unknown. The T-cells that bear the TCR can be further subdivided into the CD4$^+$8$^-$ (formerly T4, helper/inducer cells), which are involved in upregulation of cellular events, and CD4$^-$8$^+$ subsets (formerly the T8, suppressor or cytotoxic cells), which are involved in downregulation of cellular events or in cell-mediated destruction of target cells.

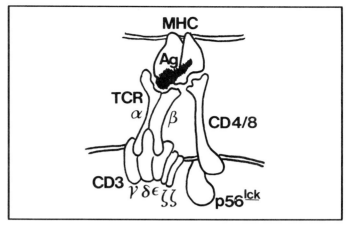

Fig. 6-4. *The aggregate formed by T-cell receptor* (TCR) *CD3, CD4, or CD8, major histocompatibility complex* (MHC), *antigen* (Ag), *and p56^{lck}. (Reprinted with permission from T. Mustelin and A. Altman. Do CD4 and CD8 control T-cell activation via a specific tyrosin protein kinase?* Immunol. Today *10:189, 1989.)*

THE IMMUNOGLOBULIN SUPERGENE FAMILY

Because of the structural similarities between the TCR, immunoglobulin, and MHC antigens, a unifying concept has been developed and is referred to as the *immunoglobulin supergene family* [3]. This represents a diverse collection of molecules found on immunoglobulins, TCRs, and the Class I and Class II of the MHC which represents repeating structures composed of similar V and C domains that appear to be derived from a common primordial cell-surface structure. It has been proposed that the immunoglobulin supergene family developed from a simple primordial surface receptor consisting of single V and C domains, and that during the course of evolution a number of more complex structures and configurations appeared and are now found on immunoglobulins, TCRs, and the MHC products as a result of gene duplications, genetic reassortments, and rearrangements of the V, diversity (D), joining (J), and C domains of a genetic locus. This ranges from a full array of V and C regions found on the L and H chains of immunoglobulins to the alpha and beta chains found on TCRs to the various domains found on the MHC. With continued selective pressures of evolution additional duplications of genetic elements encoding for the V and C regions appeared, providing additional information involved in lymphocyte gene rearrangement consisting of D and J gene segments. This hypothesis explains the great generation of the diversity characteristic of the immunoglobulin supergene family [3].

CYTOKINES

In the 1970s evidence accumulated that some of the active molecules produced by cells of the immune system other than immunoglobulins also were importantly involved in the communication network of intercellular communication. These substances are now referred to as *cytokines* rather than *lymphokines.* Cytokines produced by lymphocytes are now referred to as *lymphokines,* whereas products produced by monocytes or macrophages are referred to as *monokines.* Table 6-4 lists properties of commonly recognized cytokines.

There are now recognized 10 major classes of interleukins, each affecting a variety of target cells; three major classes of growth factors affecting granulocytes and monocytes; and three major classes of interferons. Tumor necrosis factor-alpha (TNF-α), which is involved in inflammation, has also been described.

Table 6-4. Characteristics of major cytokines

Cytokine	Molecular weight	Primary cell sources	Activity	Principal effects
IL-1	17,500	Macrophages, NK and B-cells	Immunoaugmentation	Inflammatory and hematopoietic
IL-2	15,500	T-lymphocytes and LGL	T- and B-cell growth factor	Activates T- and NK cells
IL-3	28,000	T-lymphocytes	Hematopoietic growth factor	Promotes growth of early myeloid progenitor cells
IL-4	20,000	TH cells	T- and B-cell growth factor; promotes IgE reactions	Promotes IgE switch and mast cell growth
IL-5	50,000–60,000	TH cells	Stimulates B-cells and eosinophils	Promotes IgA switch and eosinophilia
IL-6	25,000	Fibroblasts and others	Hybridoma growth factor; augments inflammation	Growth factor for B-cells and polyclonal immunoglobulin production
IL-7	25,000	Stromal cells	Lymphopoietin	Generates pre-B- and pre-T-cells and is lymphocyte growth factor
IL-8	8,800	Macrophages and others	Chemoattracts neutrophils and T-lymphocytes	Regulates lymphocyte homing and neutrophil infiltration
IL-9	30,000–40,000	Activated T-lymphocytes	T-cell growth factor; stimulation of hematopoiesis	Together with IL-2 increases fetal thymocyte proliferation; stimulates erythroid precursor cell proliferation
IL-10	18,000	B- and T-lymphocytes (TH2) and thymocytes	Effects on T-cells, B-cells, and mast cells; inhibition of cytokine synthesis by TH1 cells; IL-10 shows homology with EBV proteins	Proliferation of mature and immature thymocytes in presence of IL-2 and IL-4; stimulates mast cells only when combined with IL-3 and/or IL-4; interference with antigen presentation
IL-11	23,000	Bone marrow stromal cells	Functions as cofactor in hematopoiesis; B-cell growth factor; regulator of stem cell cycle	Stimulates megakaryocyte colony-forming units; stimulates Ig synthesis in the presence of T-cells
G-CSF	18,000–22,000	Monocytes and others	Myeloid growth factor	Generates neutrophils
M-CSF	18,000–26,000	Monocytes and others	Macrophage growth factor	Generates macrophages
GM-CSF	14,000–38,000	T-cells and others	Monomyelocytic growth factor	Myelopoiesis
IFN-α	18,000	Leukocytes	Antiviral, antiproliferative, and immunomodulating	Stimulates macrophages and NK cells; induces cell membrane antigens (e.g., MHC)
IFN-β	20,000	Fibroblasts		
IFN-γ	20,000–25,000	TH lymphocytes and NK cells		
TNF-α	17,000	Macrophages and others	Inflammatory, immunoenhancing, and tumoricidal	Vascular thromboses and tumor necrosis
LT-TNF-β	25,000	T-lymphocytes		
TGF-β	25,000	Platelets, bone, and others	Fibroplasia and immunosuppression	Wound healing and bone remodeling

IL = interleukin; G = granulocyte; CSF = colony-stimulating factor; M = monocyte; IFN = interferon; TNF = tumor necrosis factor; LT = lymphotoxin; TGF = transforming growth factor; NK = natural killer; LGL = large granular lymphocytes; TH = helper T-cell; EBV = Epstein-Barr virus.
Source: Adapted from Oppenheim, et al. Cytokines. In D. P. Stites and A. I. Terr (eds.), *Basic Human Immunology*. Norwalk: Appleton & Lange 1991. P. 79.

REGULATION OF THE IMMUNE SYSTEM

We can now construct a synthesizing framework to describe some of the more significant cellular interactions involved in the regulation system. There are three types of interactions: (1) macrophage–T-cell, (2) T-T, and (3) T-B.

Macrophage–T-Cell Interactions

When antigen is first encountered, it is metabolized by macrophages [8]. The product of this initial step leads to degraded peptide fragments called *processed antigen* and is presented to the helper/inducer T-cell population (CD4$^+$8$^-$) in the framework of the MHC Class II molecules, as described previously (see Fig. 6-3). In this process a number of interleukins are generated, for example, interleukin-1 (IL-1). The processed antigen is then presented to the helper T-cell subpopulation and is recognized by the CD3/TCR complex. This clone of T-cells then is induced to expand and to produce receptors specific for antigen and for IL-2 and is also stimulated to produce IL-2. IL-2 then can interact and expand a separate clone of antigen-sensitized T-cells, which can then synthesize other lymphokines such as interferon gamma. Interferon gamma can stimulate antigen-presenting cells (e.g., macrophages), to synthesize Class II molecules. Thus there exists a cascading system of intercellular communication of cellular interaction mediated through signals provided by macrophages, lymphocytes, and interleukins.

T-T Interactions

A second type of regulation involves the interactions of different subsets of T-cells. As described above, T-cells can communicate with other subpopulations of T-cells through IL-2 cytokine cascade (Fig. 6-5). CD4$^-$8$^+$ T-cells can also interact with target cells or with membrane-associated antigens on target cells in the context of Class I antigens, found on target cells, thus providing antigen presentation to the suppressor/cytotoxic (CD4$^-$8$^+$) T-cells. Recent evidence suggests that at least two subgroups of helper T-cells exist: Th1 and Th2. Different patterns of cytokine reactions have been identified with these helper T-cell subgroups, the Th1 mediating primarily delayed hypersensitivity reaction, and the Th2 mediating IgE synthesis and eosinophilia. Although the pattern of cytokine production in atopic asthma is unknown, a predominant Th2-like lymphocyte subpopulation has been found in bronchial biopsy specimens and bronchoalveolar lavage fluids of patients with bronchial asthma [11].

T-B Interactions

Another type of regulation occurs between T-lymphocytes and B-lymphocytes (see Fig. 6-1). Two major types of communication pathways between T-lymphocytes and B-lymphocytes are involved in regulation: upregulation and downregulation. T-lymphocytes involved in the upregulation of B-cell function are referred to as the *helper/inducer T-cell population* (CD4$^+$8$^-$).

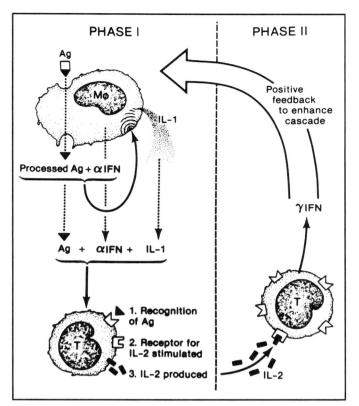

Fig. 6-5. *The role of the interferon* (IFN) *cascade in the normal immune response.* Ag = *antigen;* Mø = *macrophage;* IL = *interleukin. (Reprinted with permission from S. Skurkovich, B. Skurkovich, and J. A. Bellanti. A unifying model of the immunoregulatory role of the interferon system: Can interferon produce a disease in humans?* Clin. Immunol. Immunopathol. *43:362, 1987.)*

Another subset involved in the downregulation of B-cell function is referred to as *suppressor/cytotoxic* (CD4$^-$8$^+$) T-cells, which enhances B-cell differentiation and production of immunoglobulins. There are other interactions of interleukins involved in the synthesis of IgE such as IL-4, IL-5, and IL-6 and inhibitory responses seen with other lymphokines such as interferon gamma.

THE CONCEPT OF IMMUNOLOGICALLY MEDIATED DISEASE

The summation of the total immunologic capability of the host to foreign substances is shown schematically in Figure 6-6 [1]. There are three types of responses through which all foreign substances can proceed, the progression of which depends on either (1) the nature of the foreign substance or (2) the genetic constitution of the host. The first responses are referred to as *nonspecific responses,* the most primitive type, and consist of phagocytosis and inflammation. If the substance is completely eliminated at this stage, the host response terminates. Some substances are not completely eliminated at this stage and reflect antigen persistence, which proceeds to the second response.

The *specific responses* are more sophisticated and consist of two effector mechanisms: (1) the B-lymphocyte–mediated humoral immune responses with the elaboration of antibody of five major classes and (2) the T-lymphocyte–mediated responses.

If antigen continues to persist and is not eliminated, then the third type of response, the *tissue-damaging responses,* are called into play and reflect the breakdown of the above-described responses. If antigen persists, four types of immunologic interactions can be elicited—Types 1, 2, 3, and 4 (Table 6-5). The responses are no longer beneficial to the host and manifest as disease symptoms and immunologically mediated diseases. These responses may be temporary if the foreign substance can be eliminated or more permanent if it cannot. The allergic dis-

Fig. 6-6. *The total immunologic capability of the host based on the efficiency of the elimination of foreign matter.* Ag-Ab = *antigen-antibody. (Reprinted with permission from J. A. Bellanti.* Immunology III. *Philadelphia: Saunders, 1985. P. 347)*

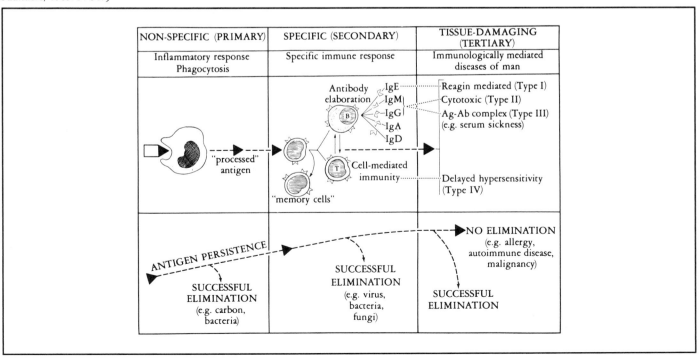

Table 6-5. Mechanisms of immunologically mediated diseases according to Gell and Coombs

Type	Target organs	Clinical manifestations	Mechanisms
I. Anaphylactic (cytotropic)	Gastrointestinal tract Skin Lungs	Gastrointestinal allergy, urticaria, atopic dermatitis, rhinitis, and asthma	IgE and other immunoglobulins
II. Cytolytic (cytotoxic)	Circulating blood elements (red cells, white cells, and platelets)	Hemolytic anemia, leukopenia, thrombocytopenia, hemolytic disease of newborn, and Goodpasture's disease	IgG, IgM, and phagocytes (opsonization) and mononuclear cells (ADCC) reactions, or antibody-mediated complement cytolysis
III. Arthus: immune complex (serum sickness)	Blood vessels of skin, joints, kidneys, and lungs	Serum sickness, systemic lupus erythematosus, nephrosis of quartan malaria, and chronic glomerulonephritis	Antigen-antibody complexes (IgG)
IV. Cell-mediated (delayed hypersensitivity)	Skin Lungs CNS Thyroid Other organs	Contact dermatitis Tuberculosis Allergic encephalitis Thyroiditis Primary homograft rejection	Sensitized T-lymphocytes
V. Mixed types I and II	—	Allergic bronchopulmonary aspergillosis	IgE and precipitating IgG antibodies
III and IV	—	Extrinsic allergic alveolitis	Antigen-antibody complexes and cell-mediated immunity

Source: P. G. H. Gell, R. R. A. Coombs, and P. J. Lachman. *Clinical Aspects of Immunology* (3rd ed.). Oxford: Blackwell, 1977.

eases, autoimmune diseases, and malignancy can be considered examples of a failure to eliminate the foreign configuration.

CLINICAL APPLICATIONS OF IMMUNOLOGIC REACTIONS

It is clear that the immunologic system is responsible for the recognition and elimination of foreignness and has direct applications for an understanding of the mechanisms and clinical expressions of the allergic diseases and asthma.

The terms *atopic* and *allergic* are frequently used interchangeably and are occasionally misunderstood or confused [5]. The term *allergy,* as originally advanced by von Pirquet in 1906, included both facets of the altered immunologic state including the beneficial and the deleterious aspects. The beneficial aspect was referred to as *immunity* and the harmful expressions, as *hypersensitivity* or *allergy* (altered reactivity). Today the terms are used interchangeably: *allergy* has become synonymous with the deleterious effects of hypersensitivity, and the broader responses to antigens are now encompassed by the term *immunity.* Allergy or hypersensitivity may be defined as a constellation of signs and symptoms in which the altered (Greek *allos*) immunologic reactions between foreign substances (antigens or allergens) and antibody or sensitized lymphocytes are thought to play a major role, resulting clinically in pathologic reactions referred to as the *allergic reactions.* The term *atopy* (Greek *a-topos,* out of place, strange), coined by Coca in 1931, was used to designate a group of allergic reactions that had a hereditary basis and a seasonal pattern and included seasonal and perennial allergic rhinitis, asthma, and atopic dermatitis, and in which specific sensitizing antibodies (atopic reagin, now recognized to be mainly IgE antibody) were found. Most allergists today include in the definition of the atopic state a complex of symptoms or disease-related constellations, such as dermatitis (eczema), asthma, allergic rhinitis, urticaria, or gastrointestinal allergy.

Rackemann [7] divided asthma into "intrinsic" and "extrinsic" forms. The extrinsic form was caused by exogenous antigens and mediated by IgE reactions and was found primarily in younger children and young adults. In contrast, intrinsic asthma was found mainly in adults in whom an exogenous antigen could not be identified and in whom IgE reactions were not thought to play a major role. Recent studies have disclosed that the distinction between these two forms of asthma may be less apparent and IgE is now thought to play a major role in both forms [2]. The common pathophysiologic pathway of asthma is related to the various stages and expressions of the inflammatory response.

The clinical diagnosis and management of the atopic and allergic states are now predicated on a firm understanding of the pathophysiology of these conditions, the identification of the genetically predisposed host, and the possibility of modifying the environment either through elimination of the offending antigens or by interference with their pathophysiologic expressions through the use of hyposensitization or pharmacologic therapy. In the case of bronchial asthma this will require a fuller understanding of the complex and rapidly emerging advances in immunology as well as a greater elucidation of the molecular basis of airway inflammation, which ultimately underlies the clinical patterns of this disorder [6].

REFERENCES

1. Bellanti, J. A. *Immunology III.* Philadelphia: Saunders, 1985. P. 7.
2. Burrows, B., et al. Association of asthma with serum IgE levels and skin-test reactivity to allergens. *N. Engl. J. Med.* 320:271, 1989.
3. Hood, L., Kronenberg, M., and Hunkapillar, T. T cell antigen receptors and the immunoglobulin supergene family. *Cell* 40:225, 1985.
4. Mustelin, T., and Altman, A. Do CD4 and CD8 control T-cell activation via a specific tyrosin protein kinase? *Immunol. Today* 10:189, 1989.
5. Nelson, H. S. The Bela Schick lecture for 1985. *Ann. Allergy* 55:441, 1985.
6. Plaut, M. Antigen-specific lymphokine secretory patterns in atopic disease. *J. Immunol.* 144:4497, 1990.
7. Rackemann, R. M. Intrinsic asthma. *J. Allergy* 11:147, 1940.
8. Skurkovich, S., Skurkovich, B., and Bellanti, J. A. A unifying model of the immunoregulatory role of the interferon system: Can interferon produce a disease in humans? *Clin. Immunol. Immunopathol.* 43:362, 1987.
9. Stites, D. P., and Terr, A. I., (eds.). *Basic Human Immunology* (1st ed.). Norwalk: Appleton & Lange, 1991. P. 137.
10. Möller, G., (ed.). *Immunological Reviews.* 125:37, 77, 1992.
11. Robinson, D. S., et al. Predominant TH2-like bronchoalveolar T-lymphocyte population in atopic asthma. *N. Engl. J. Med.* 326:298, 1992.

Advances in IgE Biology

Sho Matsushita
Mark L. Richards
David H. Katz

The discovery of IgE by Ishizaka and colleagues over 25 years ago [75] initiated the modern era of allergy research by providing a focus for the study of allergic phenomena. Indeed, IgE is primarily regarded as an agent of disease rather than a functionary in the immunologic network of disease prevention. However, with all the attention focused on the "adverse" effects of IgE, it should be mentioned that this class of immunoglobulins has been implicated in an immunologically beneficial role. Pathways that involve IgE have been demonstrated to be cytotoxic for parasites [18, 20, 76], and IgE was recently shown to be the central molecule in providing protective immunity against these infections [60].

In order to control the causes and manifestations of IgE-related diseases, it is imperative to gain an understanding of two fundamental and distinct aspects of IgE biology: (1) the factors and mechanisms that dictate the normal and aberrant processes that regulate IgE production, and (2) the role of IgE in effecting the initiation and perpetuation of an ongoing allergic response. The prevalence of allergic diseases has stimulated a vast outgrowth in the understanding of IgE system physiology. The complete structure of IgE is known at both the amino acid and gene levels, and the cellular receptors identified for IgE have been cloned and sequenced. Hence, the molecular groundwork is established for understanding the most important aspects of IgE activity. The cellular interactions involved in the synthesis of IgE have largely been elucidated and, to a certain extent, the lymphokines that regulate these interactions have been identified. Many of these lymphokines have also been cloned and sequenced. However, while studies have contributed greatly to our knowledge of the pathophysiology of IgE-mediated allergic diseases, much is still unknown. Technical advances such as genetic modulation using the transgenic mouse system or homologous recombinant stem cells promise to further accelerate our understanding of this complex system. Moreover, in attempting to understand the biology of the IgE system, it must be realized that its control is functionally integrated throughout. For example, lymphokines such as interleukin-4 (IL-4) and interferon gamma (IFN-γ), and, indeed, IgE itself regulate not only the production of IgE, but also the expression of IgE-specific receptors. Hence, the IgE system is best viewed as a whole, rather than focusing on its individual components.

PROPERTIES OF IgE

Kinetics

IgE exhibits several features that distinguish it from other immunoglobulins [122, 175]. The normal plasma IgE concentrations are in the *nanogram* range (50–300 ng/ml), as contrasted to other immunoglobulins which are present in *milligram* amounts. Immunization with an appropriate antigen causes levels of IgE to increase 3- to 12-fold, the majority of which is antigen specific. In contrast, IgG exhibits only a marginal increase in plasma level after antigen stimulation and only a fraction of that is antigen specific. Moreover, IgE levels decrease rapidly following antigen challenge because of a short serum half-life (2.5 days) and efficient epsilon-specific regulatory mechanisms. IgG concentrations are more stable owing to their 20- to 25-day half-life. These characteristics thus create a situation where the relative responsiveness of IgE to antigenic challenge is considerably exaggerated in comparison to other immunoglobulins.

Peptide Structure

The discovery of a rare IgE-secreting human myeloma ultimately resulted in the determination of the entire amino acid sequence of this protein [41]. Final delineation of its structure was provided by nucleotide sequencing of IgE complementary DNA (cDNA) and genomic DNA [81, 111]. Like other immunoglobulins and members of the immunoglobulin gene superfamily, IgE is composed of a tetrameric structure of two light chains (κ or λ) and two heavy chains (ϵ; this is diagrammed schematically in Fig. 7-1). The heavy chains are integrated into the IgE molecule as one variable region domain (Vϵ) and four constant region domains (Cϵ1–4). IgE is heavily glycosylated, with carbohydrate comprising 13 percent of its total mass, and six carbohydrate attachment sites have been identified on the IgE myeloma protein [41]. The total mass of IgE is 190 kd, which is comparable to monomeric IgM, and about 10 to 20 percent larger than other immunoglobulin isotypes [42, 122]. Much of this difference stems from the extent of IgE glycosylation, although the epsilon polypeptide chain is marginally the largest of the immunoglobulin heavy chains. The three-dimensional structure of IgE has been modeled on the basis of IgG crystallography data [128] and, although not entirely rigid, it is predicted to be a somewhat less flexible molecule than IgG [152].

Genomic Structure

Molecular biology studies have elucidated the structure of the immunoglobulin gene region [44, 151, 161] and the series of rearrangements that ultimately give rise to immunoglobulin gene expression [77, 136]. The constant region of the immunoglobulin heavy chain gene (C$_H$) locus spans about 200 kilobases (kb) and is found on human chromosome 14 just downstream of the variable (V) region gene [32]. Thus, the immunoglobulin heavy chain gene loci are arranged in tandem as follows: 5'-V region (variable [V]-diversity [D]-joining [J])-C region (Cμ-Cδ-Cγ3-Cγ1-Cα1-Cγ2-Cγ4-Cϵ-Cα2)-3'. Expression of an immunoglobulin is pre-

Support for the authors' contribution to the work described herein was provided by National Institutes of Health grants AI-24526, AI-19476, AI-19747, and AI-20958.

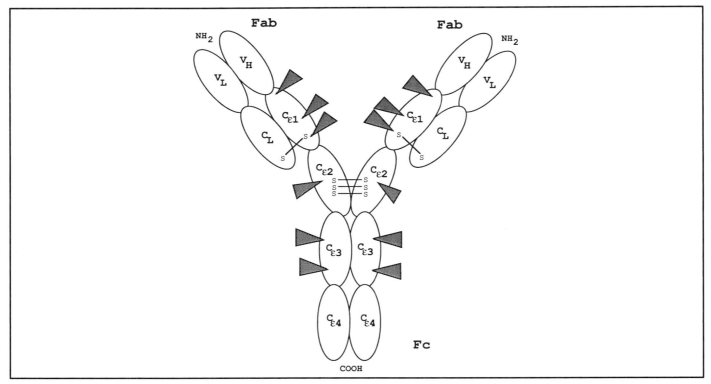

Fig. 7-1. *Structure of IgE. The organization of the constant (C) and variable (V) region domains of the heavy (H, ε) and light (L) chains of IgE is depicted. Shaded wedges indicate glycosylation sites on the Cε chain, and S—S denotes interchain disulfide bonds. Fab = antigen-binding domain; Fc = effector region.*

ceded by expression of the corresponding germline C_H gene [55]. B-lymphocytes first develop with surface IgM and, following activation, undergo somatic recombination to produce a new immunoglobulin isotype. This "switch" of immunoglobulin production is preceded by a juxtaposition of the V region to a new C_H locus [77, 136]. Somatic recombination occurs between highly homologous repetitive DNA sequences (switch regions) that are located in front of each C_H gene [137]. Thus, B-cells start with their V regions proximal to $C\mu$ (VDJ-$C\mu$), and during the process of class switching, the V region is placed proximal to $C\gamma$, $C\epsilon$, or any other downstream C_H. Moreover, B-lymphocytes that ultimately commit to IgE production can express any C_H upstream of the $C\epsilon$ locus prior to switching to $C\epsilon$ [137]. For example, B-cells might produce IgG1 prior to producing IgE [179], but once they produce IgE, they cannot switch to any upstream loci; that is, the only remaining class switch achievable is to $C\alpha2$. Hence, any immunoglobulin (except IgA2)-producing B-cell is potentially capable of switching to IgE production.

CELLULAR INTERACTIONS OF IgE

IgE Receptors and Other IgE-binding Proteins

A number of proteins capable of binding IgE have been identified. These include two distinct cellular receptors, the high-affinity (FcεRI) and the low-affinity (FcεRII or CD23) Fc receptors for IgE, and a variety of IgE-binding factors including epsilon-binding protein and the truncated soluble fragments of FcεRII.

FcεRI Receptor

The high-affinity IgE receptors are so named because the affinity of monomeric IgE for the FcεRI (association constant [kd] = 10^{-9}–10^{-10} M) is at least two orders of magnitude greater than

that for FcεRII (kd = 10^{-6}–10^{-7} M). FcεRI receptors are found on mast cells and basophils, and mediate the IgE antigen–dependent degranulation of these cells to release the various pharmacologic mediators of immediate hypersensitivity reactions [112, 134] (see Chaps. 8, 10, and 11). This process is so profound and so well characterized that it serves as a model system for the study of receptor aggregation and activation of second-messenger systems. The nucleotide sequence of FcεRI reveals it to be a member of the immunoglobulin gene superfamily, with a predicted tetrameric structure composed of one alpha, one beta, and two gamma subunits [9, 85, 86, 112]. The alpha chain is responsible for the molecular interaction with IgE, while the other three chains are required for transport and incorporation of FcεRI into the cell membrane [9]. The extracellular domain of FcεRI has a highly conserved nucleotide sequence, and some regions share substantial homology with IgG receptors [139]. The FcεRI interaction site on IgE has been localized to a 76-amino acid region that is predominantly on Cε3, with some overlap on Cε2 [2, 66, 123]. Hence, the actual Fc-terminal domain of IgE, Cε4, is not required for binding FcεRI. Efforts are currently underway to develop clinically useful peptides that are homologous with the FcεRI-binding region of IgE that will block the IgE-FcεRI interaction.

FcεRII Receptor

The low-affinity IgE receptor was first discovered on B-lymphocytes and macrophages [18, 93], and since has been found on eosinophils, platelets, T-cells, and Langerhans' cells [8, 20, 76, 177]. Although one of its functions on eosinophils, platelets, and macrophages has been reasonably well established as mediating IgE-dependent cytotoxicity, the role of FcεRII on lymphocytes remains a matter of considerable debate [142]. The FcεRII molecule is a single 45-kd glycopeptide [96, 132] and, as such, is distinguished from other Fc receptors, which are members of the immunoglobulin gene superfamily. Moreover, whereas other immunoglobulins and their cellular Fc receptors evolved from a common gene, thus permitting homotypic binding between each immunoglobulin and a corresponding receptor, the FcεRII gene is likely a hybrid of two primordial gene segments [143]. The distinct evolutionary origins of IgE and FcεRII probably account in part for their low binding affinity. cDNA cloning studies have predicted a unique Fc receptor protein that has an inverted membrane orientation (cytoplasmic amino-terminal) and an extracellular domain that is highly homologous with animal lectins [82, 90]. The lectin region of the FcεRII molecule is responsible for binding to IgE, but glycosylation of the IgE molecule is not required for the interaction to occur [7, 172]. This was a somewhat surprising finding because many of the features of the IgE-FcεRII interaction resemble the prototypical carbohydrate-lectin interaction [43, 141]. Indeed, based on its structure, FcεRII can be included among the selectin family of cellular adhesion proteins [156]. Moreover, its extensive α-helical coiled coil structure places FcεRII within a subfamily of the C-type lectin superfamily, which is characterized as dimeric or trimeric cell surface proteins with extracellular lectin "heads" [5a].

Two FcεRII subtypes have been identified, differing only in their cytoplasmic tails: FcεRIIa is expressed only on B-cells whereas FcεRIIb is expressed on B-cells, T-cells, macrophages, platelets, and eosinophils [124, 178]. Another interesting feature of this protein is its propensity to be proteolytically cleaved from the cell surface, yielding soluble FcεRII fragments that are also capable of binding IgE [96, 119]. These products can be detected in blood, particularly from patients with certain leukemias, but their function has not been definitively established [142]. Monoclonal antibody– and recombinant IgE–mapping studies have determined the Cε3 region of IgE as responsible for binding to FcεRII [29, 172]. This region of IgE overlaps with, but is distinct from, the segment that interacts with FcεRI. The higher affinity of Cε4-containing IgE peptides for FcεRII implies that dimerization of the IgE molecule promotes this interaction [172].

Other IgE-binding Proteins

In addition to cellular membrane receptors, several IgE-binding factors have been identified. Epsilon-binding protein was initially characterized because it adhered to an IgE-Sepharose column. Subsequent molecular studies revealed epsilon-binding protein to be a ubiquitous mammalian lectin that interacts with the carbohydrate moieties of IgE [98]. Both its function and the significance of its IgE binding are unknown. However, because of its extensive tissue distribution, sequence homology with Mac-2 [27], and multiple potential glycoligands, epsilon-binding protein probably has far more diverse functions than simply involvement in the IgE system. Indeed, recent evidence suggests that this lectin may act as a cell-adhesion protein on the surface of mast cells and macrophages [53a]. Molecular studies on another type of IgE-binding factor revealed striking structural homology with a highly conserved region of retroviral reverse transcriptase [114]. As for epsilon-binding protein, its role in the IgE system is unclear. Numerous other IgE-binding factors also have been reported, but either their structure has not been elucidated or they have been found to be one of the soluble truncated products of FcεRII [34, 73].

Cell Types That Interact with IgE

Mediators of IgE-dependent Cytotoxicity

One function that is shared by macrophages, eosinophils, and platelets is mediation of IgE-dependent inflammatory responses [18, 20, 76]. Binding of IgE-coated particles to the FcεRII of these cells results in their phagocytosis and release of potent cyto-

kines, such as leukotrienes [19] (Fig. 7-2). The complement receptor for C36i is required for both adherence of the IgE-coated particles and cytotoxicity [21]. The ability of these effector cells to act in this fashion is somewhat dependent on the level of FcεRII expression. Helminthic infestations and other factors that cause elevated IgE levels are associated with increased cellular density of FcεRII [20]. IL-4 enhances and dexamethasone suppresses FcεRII expression on macrophages, whereas the reported effects of interferons have been conflicting [78, 120, 121, 142, 165, 173].

In addition to their role in parasite cytotoxicity, recent evidence has shown that macrophages, eosinophils, and platelets contribute to IgE-dependent allergic/inflammatory responses. IgE-antigen complexes stimulate circulating monocytes to produce IL-1 and tumor necrosis factor-alpha (TNF-α), which, like leukotrienes, are potent effectors of inflammation [11]. These cells also have been implicated in precipitating the bronchial manifestations of allergy. This is suggested by the prevalence of macrophages in bronchial mucosa, and the accumulation of activated platelets in pulmonary vessels during anaphylaxis or bronchoconstriction in animal models [17, 138, 168]. Moreover, FcεRII expression is enhanced on macrophages and platelets of asthmatic patients [17], and cromoglycate directly inhibits IgE-dependent activation of macrophages, platelets, and eosinophils while having little effect on mast cell function [17, 169]. These results suggest the direct involvement of other cell types, in addition to mast cells and basophils, in forming the cellular basis for IgE-related allergic phenomena, particularly if bronchial manifestations exist.

B- and T-lymphocytes

The presence of FcεRII (CD23) on unstimulated T-cells has not been unequivocally established, although it is expressed following cytokine treatment, viral transformation, or allergen activation of T-lymphocytes [1, 125, 135, 142]. In contrast, about 8 to 10 percent of normal human peripheral blood B-lymphocytes and over half of murine splenic B-cells express FcεRII [35, 104, 142]. A high percentage of the B-cell phenotype that are IgM/IgD positive are also FcεRII positive, whereas the FcεRII is no longer expressed after isotype switching [83]. The dominant control of B-cell FcεRII expression seems to be exerted by the reciprocal effects of IL-4 (stimulatory) and IFN-γ (inhibitory) [33, 37, 83, 175a]. Corticosteroids and interferon alpha (IFN-α) also have been reported to downregulate FcεRII expression [33, 36, 37]. IgE enhances membrane FcεRII expression, but only by protecting it from the action of proteolytic enzymes [58, 78, 94, 121].

The primary function of the FcεRII on B-cells is a matter of considerable debate [142]. FcεRII has been implicated in mediating B-cell antigen presentation by IgE [79, 144], promotion of differentiation/maturation [140, 180], and regulation of B-cell IgE production [131, 146, 148] (see Fig. 7-2). IgE likely regulates its own production via a negative feedback process. IgE-antigen complexes suppress IgE production, and anti-FcεRII monoclonal antibodies inhibit IL-4–stimulated production of IgE [130, 146, 148]. Additionally, the truncated soluble fragments of FcεRII have been reported to enhance B-cell growth and IgE production, although these functions are controversial and by no means established [119, 146, 147, 170] (see Chap. 13).

Mast Cells and Basophils

The FcεRI of mast cells and basophils has long been associated with immediate hypersensitivity reactions. As illustrated in Figure 7-2, IgE-antigen complexes interact with the FcεRI of these cells, resulting in the release of histamine, leukotrienes, prostaglandins, IL-3, IL-4, IL-5, and IL-6 [14, 112, 134]. These cytokines act on secretory glands and smooth muscles (e.g., of blood vessels and bronchi) to give rise to the clinical manifestations of allergy. Inhibition of these responses can be achieved by adminis-

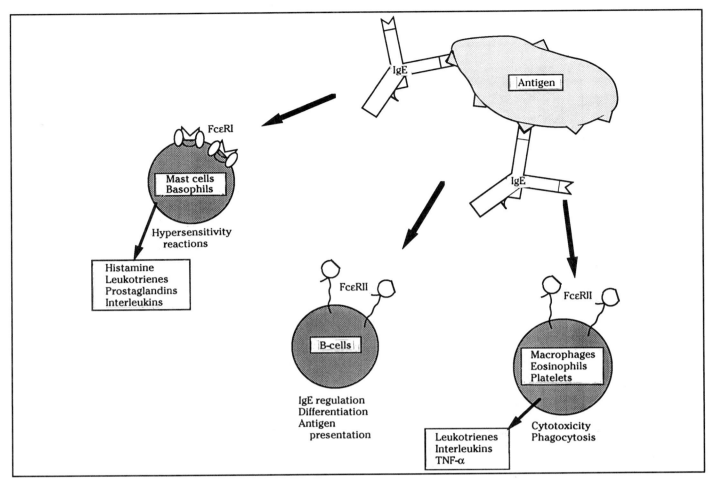

Fig. 7-2. *Cellular interactions of IgE. The cell types that interact with IgE-antigen complexes are illustrated together with the proposed sequelae. Cytokines that are released following this interaction are in boxes. TNF-α = tumor necrosis factor-alpha.*

tration of monoclonal antibodies directed to the FcεRI, thus documenting the participation of the IgE system in these processes [89]. The role of mast cells and basophils as effectors of allergy is discussed in more detail in Chapter 21. However, it should be reiterated that the cellular origins of allergic diseases are not limited to these cell types. Thus, the ability to control IgE production would permit artificial modulation of these aberrant inflammatory responses via two distinct receptor and cellular systems.

REGULATION OF IgE BIOSYNTHESIS

Basic Pathway

Soluble antigens (allergens), once exposed to immunocompetent cells, are trapped by particular cell populations such as macrophages, dendritic cells, and B-cells (see also Chap. 5). Four proposed mechanisms of antigen trapping have generally been accepted (Fig. 7-3). Macrophages take up antigens by phagocytosis of particles, which allow both primary and recall antigens to be internalized and processed. Dendritic cells and B-cells are incapable of phagocytosis but may use the more general process of pinocytosis [149]. B-cells also use antigen-specific surface immunoglobulin for antigen capture [91, 92], which is so efficient that the required antigen concentrations are 1,000 times less than

for pinocytosis [23, 91]. As noted earlier, B-cells can present antigen via an alternative pathway utilizing IgE and FcεRII. Antigens thus trapped by these cells are processed by intracellular proteolysis, and the peptide fragments are expressed back onto the cell surface together with the major histocompatibility complex (MHC) Class II molecules [16]. These cells then present antigens to T-cells by interaction of MHC Class II molecules and the T-cell receptor (TCR), with some help from adhesion molecules [156]. These cells are therefore designated antigen-presenting cells. In this process, IL-1, IL-6, and IL-7 produced by macrophages are essential for the activation of T-cells [54, 115]; that is, as "second signals" these molecules activate T-cells, which in turn will produce IL-2 and express IL-2 receptors to proliferate (Fig. 7-4). The activated T-cells will finally differentiate into helper T-cells (Th) or cytotoxic T-cells, which then produce lymphokines and express additional cell-surface molecules. These cells will play further important roles as immunocompetent T-cells or in activating B-cells independently. Th cells produce many lymphokines, such as IL-2, IL-4, IL-5, IL-6, and IFN-γ, which regulate B-cell proliferation and differentiation into immunoglobulin-producing cells, or plasma cells. Some of the lymphokines are characterized at the molecular level as "class-switch" factors, as described in the previous section. For instance, IL-4 induces IgG1 and IgE [31], and transforming growth factor-beta (TGF-β) induces IgA [30] on IgM-positive B-cells.

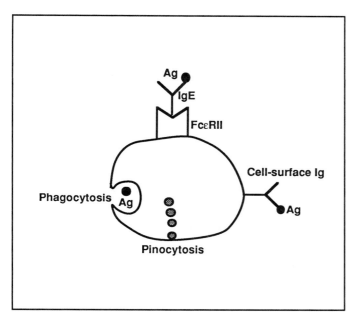

Fig. 7-3. *Four mechanisms of antigen (Ag) uptake. One cell is not able to use all four mechanisms; for example, macrophages use phagocytosis, while B-cells use pinocytosis, surface immunoglobulin, and FcεRII IgE.*

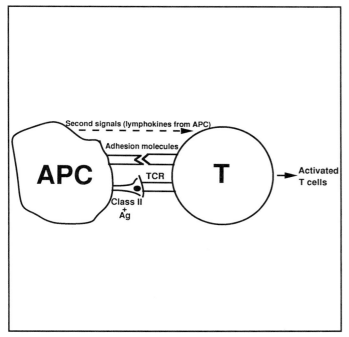

Fig. 7-4. *Interaction between antigen-presenting cells (APC) and T-cells. Many adhesion molecules and accessory molecules are involved. See [156] for details. TCR = T-cell receptor.*

Two Types of Helper T-cells

T-cells can be separated by surface markers and function into CD4$^+$ helper/suppressor inducer cells and CD8$^+$ cytotoxic/suppressor cells [40]. Long-term mouse Th cell clones, grown in vitro, can be further divided into two distinct groups (Th1 and Th2) (Table 7-1) based on their cytokine profile [28, 116]. Th1 clones secrete IL-2, IFN-γ, and lymphotoxin, whereas Th2 clones secrete IL-4, IL-5, IL-6, and IL-10 [28, 50, 70, 116, 159, 167]. Both

Table 7-1. Lymphokines produced by helper T-cell subsets

Th1	Th2	Both Th1 and Th2
Interferon gamma	Interleukin-4	Granulocyte-macrophage
Interleukin-2	Interleukin-5	colony-stimulating
Tumor necrosis	Interleukin-6	factor
factor-beta	Interleukin-10	Interleukin-3

types of cells express IL-3, granulocyte-macrophage colony-stimulating factor (GM-CSF), and tumor necrosis factor (TNF) [13, 28, 182]. Cell types with these two different cytokine patterns have very different functional capabilities. Both Th1 and Th2 clones can provide help for B-cells [157], but Th2 clones are more effective helpers, especially for IgE antibody responses, due to the production of IL-4 and IL-5 [10, 84]. Th1 clones can mediate a delayed-type hypersensitivity (DTH) reaction in an adoptive transfer system [26], in part via the production of IFN-γ [53], which results in the activation of macrophages [158]. Because IFN-γ suppresses IgE responses effectively, Th1 cells have suppressive function for IgE responses, which is reciprocal to Th2 (see the following sections for details). Alloreactive murine CD8$^+$ T-cell clones secrete the Th1 pattern of cytokines [52]. These two T-cell subsets not only produce different cytokines but also have different growth requirements; IL-1 has been reported to augment the proliferation of Th2, but not Th1 clones [59].

Although Th1 or Th2 cytokine patterns are expressed by the majority of long-term mouse Th cell clones, they are found infrequently among panels of human T-cell clones [102, 171]. Furthermore, recent studies demonstrated that a considerable percentage of mouse CD4$^+$ T-cells and a majority of human CD4$^+$ T-cells produce both IL-4 and IFN-γ [80, 129]. Some of these CD4$^+$ T-cells, which have combined characteristics of Th1 and Th2 cells and have been termed *Th0 cells* [51], may represent precursors of the Th1 or Th2 CD4$^+$ subpopulations. Although it is unclear whether CD4$^+$ T-cells with pure Th1 or Th2 secretory characteristics exist in vivo, it is clear that T-cell responses to different stimuli (or to the same stimulus in different mouse strains [118]) can have either a predominantly Th1 or Th2 character. This has proved to be of particular importance in murine leishmaniasis, in which a host response dominated by Th1 cells is associated with a self-limited infection, while a response dominated by Th2 cells is associated with a generalized and fatal infection [65]. Then, do Th2 clones explain all about the abnormalities of the atopic state? One intriguing possibility is that excess production of Th2-derived lymphokines could account for most of the manifestations of the atopic state [133], that is, induction of IgE production, basophil degranulation due to a unique IgE molecule (IgE$^+$ [101]), and abnormal responsiveness of airways and other tissues due to inflammatory responses such as IL-5–induced eosinophil activation [117].

Molecules Involved in Upregulation of IgE Biosynthesis

Many studies in recent years have suggested that IgE synthesis is regulated mainly by the reciprocal effects of IL-4 and IFN-γ, but several other factors also modulate this response. In this section, immunologic mechanisms and cell types involved in IgE regulation are discussed by focusing on each effector molecule.

Interleukin-4

Many lymphokines are not specific for B-cells and display more than one activity on the same cell. This phenomenon was observed for IL-4 (previously designated B-cell growth factor I [BCGFI] or B-cell stimulatory factor 1 [BSF1]), which possesses diverse pleiotropic effects. Briefly, IL-4 has been reported to be an activation factor of macrophages and resting B-cells (induction of Class II MHC molecules and FcεRII) and as a growth factor of B-cells. In mice, it has been shown that IL-4 can induce lipopolysaccharide-activated splenic B-cells to increase secretion of IgE and IgG1, and inhibit the secretion of IgG2a, IgG2b, and IgG3 without affecting IgA [155]. Studies in humans have shown that IL-4 induces IgE and IgG4 in vitro [99]; the latter resembles murine IgG1 in its inability to fix complement. In murine in vivo primary antibody responses to *Nippostrongylus brasiliensis* (Nb) and anti-IgD antibody, IgE, but not IgG1, synthesis is totally abrogated by anti–IL-4 antibody, indicating that IL-4 is required for the induction of primary polyclonal IgE, but not for IgG1 synthesis in vivo [49]. Anti–IL-4 antibody inhibited in vivo secondary antigen-specific IgE synthesis as well [47]. However, not all IgE responses appear to be totally dependent on the presence of IL-4. In the secondary in vivo IgE response to Nb, injection of anti–IL-4 antibody at the time of second Nb inoculation only partially inhibited IgE production, suggesting that the secondary Nb-specific IgE response has both IL-4–dependent and IL-4–independent components [47]. Similar findings have been made in secondary antigen-specific IgE responses in vitro [105]. Interestingly, IL-4–independent, secondary anti-Nb IgE responses can be inhibited when anti–IL-4 is present during the initial immunization. Further evidence for the IgE regulatory role of IL-4 in vivo has been demonstrated by studies with transgenic mice. Overexpression of IL-4 resulted in a marked increase in serum IgE and IgG1 levels [14a] and the appearance of an inflammatory ocular lesion with characteristic histopathologic features seen in allergic reactions [164].

Interleukin-5

IL-5 has been reported to have T-cell–replacing activity both by differentiating B-cells to produce antibody and stimulating B-cell growth, hence its previous nomenclature (T-cell–replacing factor [TRF] or B-cell growth factor II [BCGFII] [87]). Moreover, IL-5 drives differentiation of T-cells and eosinophils and supports growth of eosinophils. It also enhances IL-2 receptor expression on B-cells and acts together with IL-4 to preferentially enhance IgA synthesis by human and murine B-cells. In mice, IL-5 further enhances IL-4–induced IgE synthesis by lipopolysaccharide-activated B-cells. In humans, IL-4–induced IgE production as well as expression of FcεRII are enhanced by IL-5, whereas IL-5 alone has no effect [130, 160]. In some murine in vivo systems, however, there is no direct evidence that IL-5 contributes to the generation of IgE antibody responses [47].

Interleukin-6

IL-6 was previously known as interferon beta$_2$, B-cell stimulatory factor 2 (BSF2), 26-kd protein, hybridoma/plasmacytoma growth factor (HPGR or IL-HPI), hepatocyte-stimulating factor (HSF), and monocyte-granulocyte inducer type 2 (MGI-2). Molecular cloning studies have shown that all of these molecules are identical [150]. As is evident by the nomenclature, IL-6 acts on a wide range of tissues, exerting growth-inhibiting and differentiation-inducing effects, depending on the nature of the target cells, including induction of B- and T-cell differentiation and growth [67]. With regard to B-cell differentiation, IgE production obtained in the presence of suboptimal amounts of IL-4 was increased by IL-6 [130]. However, the role of IL-6 in modulating IgE responses in vivo has not been clarified.

Other Factors

As already mentioned in a previous section, there are several reports that soluble FcεRII fragments have B-cell growth–promoting activity. However, studies with recombinant soluble FcεRII have yielded conflicting results [170].

It was recently suggested that an interaction between T- and B-cells is necessary for IL-4–induced IgE synthesis by B-cells. Activated T-cells (not necessarily IL-4–producing T-cells) render B-cells responsive to IL-4. This stimulation is therefore required at the initiation of the culture for B-cells to make IgE. T-cell–B-cell contact via TCR MHC Class II is required for the activation of T-cells; however, once T-cells are activated, they can help B-cells respond to IL-4 without TCR-MHC interaction, that is, noncognate interaction will take place at a final stage. Activated T-cells can be substituted by lipopolysaccharide in the mouse system [31] and by Epstein-Barr virus [54a, 166], phorbol ester–activated thymoma cells [99], hydrocortisone [75a], and anti-CD40 antibody in the human system [3].

Included among the candidates to mediate this noncognate interaction are serine proteases. There have been several reports describing IgE-inducing activities of serine proteases, such as trypsin-like serine protease derived from *Schistosoma mansoni* [174], kallikrein-like glycosylation-enhancing factor [74], and epsilon receptor–modulating protein (εRMP) [107–109]. εRMP by itself can induce germline IgE heavy chain transcripts on B-cells [108a]. In this regard, FcεRII itself has been reported to have protease activity [97], which might explain the B-cell growth factor activity of FcεRII fragments. Recently, prostaglandin E$_2$ was reported to promote IL-4–induced IgE and IgG1 synthesis [145]. Relationship to serine proteases (such as kallikrein) awaits determination.

Finally, a newly discovered cytokine, IL-10, might be involved in the upregulation of IgE biosynthesis, because it is produced by Th2 cells and inhibits cytokine production by Th1 cells [159].

Molecules Involved in Downregulation of IgE Biosynthesis

Interferon Gamma and Alpha

In vitro murine studies have demonstrated that IFN-γ, which is produced by Th1 cells, can inhibit IL-4–induced IgG1 and IgE responses, and contribute to the generation of IgG2a responses at lower concentrations [153, 154]. IFN-α also has a similar effect in vitro [47]. In vivo studies with recombinant IFN-γ and IFN-α also showed similar results, and injections of anti–IFN-γ antibody had an effect opposite to that of IFN-γ [47]. Interestingly, IFN-α had less toxic effects on rodents [48], which is indicative of its potential for clinical application. The possible existence of an in vivo suppressive mechanism for IgE responses, distinct from IFN-γ, has been speculated based on studies of murine immune responses to *Brucella abortus*. *B. abortus*, which stimulates IFN-γ secretion, suppressed IgG1 and IgE, while enhancing IgG2a secretion. However, treatment of these mice with anti–IFN-γ did not reverse the suppressive effect of *B. abortus* on IgE secretion [48]. In another study using murine primary and secondary antigen-specific IgE antibody responses in vitro, antigen-stimulated secondary IgE responses were shown to be eightfold less sensitive than primary responses to the inhibitory effects of IFN-γ [105]. Furthermore, anti–IFN-γ antibody could not reverse the high-dose, antigen-dependent diminution of IgE production, thus indicating that IFN-γ is not the sole cause of high antigen dose–induced suppression of IgE biosynthesis [105]. The effect of IFN-γ among mouse strains is heterogeneous—that is, B-cell sensitivity to IgE-suppressive activity of IFN-γ is polymorphic and controlled by a non–H-2-linked gene [107a].

Interleukin-2

In some experiments, IL-2 and IL-4 have been shown to act in a synergistic manner [22, 157], whereas in other studies these seem to inhibit one another [153]. IL-2 inhibited the effect of IL-4 on lipopolysaccharide-stimulated IgE synthesis by B-cells of BALB/c or nude mice in vitro. In this system, only anti-IL-2, but not anti–IFN-γ antibody could neutralize the inhibitory action of IL-2 on the IL-4–induced IgE synthesis [113], suggesting that the inhibitory pathway of IL-2 is distinct from that of IFN-γ.

Suppressive Factor of Allergy

Another IgE-suppressive factor, designated suppressive factor of allergy (SFA), was first described as components in serum (or ascites fluids) obtained from mice that had been repeatedly injected with *Mycobacteria*-containing complete Freund's adjuvant, a poor adjuvant for eliciting IgE antibody responses. It was shown recently [109] that this activity is produced by CD4+ T-cells and is ascribed to a 30-kd protein, which suppresses lipopolysaccharide- and IL-4–induced IgE and IgG1 synthesis, but the effect is not blocked by anti–IFN-γ antibody. Thus, SFA is a lymphokine, distinct from IFN-γ, that is involved in suppressing IgE antibody synthesis.

Other Mechanisms of Downregulation

Hepatic accessory cells can function as antigen-presenting cells. However, although the liver is the major site for the clearance and degradation of foreign antigens from the portal circulation, antibody responses to orally or intraportally administered antigens are uncommon. For this reason, hepatic accessory cells have been shown to support the proliferation of Th1, but not Th2 clones [103]. Addition of hepatic accessory cells did not inhibit spleen cells from stimulating Th2 clones in the presence of antigen. Thus, inability of liver cells to stimulate the proliferation of Th2 cells appears to be secondary to an absence of either an unknown accessory cell cofactor or an accessory cell that preferentially presents antigen to Th2 cells. The selective activation of Th1, but not Th2 cells by hepatic accessory cells may result in suppression of IgE antibody responses to orally administered antigens [103].

Suppressor T-cells, as a functional subset of T-cells, have been under intensive investigation. Although the final effector function of suppressor T-cells is to suppress immune responses, their cell-surface markers and other characteristics suggest that they are functionally heterogeneous. The CD8+ suppressor T-cells relate to antigen-specific immune suppression, but the term *antigen specific* has been used for antigen-specific induction as well as for antigen-specific effector function of suppressor cells. There is a report that some suppressor T-cells can be induced by a specific antigenic stimulation, but become antigen nonspecific at a final effector stage [88, 110, 162]. Some "suppressor" T-cells such as Th1 cells or SFA-producing T-cells have CD4 as their marker. The Th1 population is indeed not a subset of suppressor T-cells, but it can be classified functionally as IgE (and IgG1) -specific suppressor T-cells by means of IFN-γ. Interestingly, these T-cell subsets have been described as irradiation-sensitive suppressor T-cells for IgE immune responses [4, 109]. Thus, it should be noted that CD8 (Leu-2, OKT8) -positive suppressor T-cells comprise just one of the T-cell populations with suppressive activity, especially with regard to immunoglobulin synthesis.

Antigen Specificity of IgE Biosynthesis

Another important feature of MHC(+antigen)-TCR interaction is the direct association with immune response gene phenomena, in which the degree of polymorphism of immune responsiveness to a particular antigen between individuals is genetically linked to MHC [6]. Molecular studies have demonstrated that with regard to a particular antigen, MHC Class II molecules (allelic products) have a wide spectrum in their ability to transduce signals to T-cells [69, 176]. This spectrum changes depending on the antigens presented. In other words, some MHC Class II molecules can transduce signals to T-cells in association with a particular antigen, whereas other Class II molecules cannot. This leads to a common observation that within the same environment, one individual can be allergic to mite but not to ragweed, whereas another is allergic to ragweed but not to mite [106, 110]. It should also be noted that some MHC Class II alleles may stimulate the induction of suppressor T-cells rather than helper cells in some human models such as cedar pollinosis [110], schistosomiasis [68], or bee venom allergy [100], probably through CD4+ suppressor-inducer T-cells.

BASIC ASPECTS OF HYPOSENSITIZATION

Hyposensitization, or specific immunotherapy, has been successfully used for the treatment of patients with severe pollinosis and other Type I allergies (see Chap. 70). Although the efficacy of this kind of therapy has been shown for many allergens, the underlying mechanisms are still a matter of controversy [12, 45]. Several physiologic responses, including blocking antibodies, modulation of specific IgE by restoration or by generation of suppressor T-cells [162], changes in cell sensitivity or activation [12, 45], and autoantiidiotypic antibodies [24, 25], are potentially important for immunotherapy to be successful. Among these mechanisms, the role of IgG4 antibodies in "blocking" allergic responses has received considerable attention. Experienced beekeepers can be stung several thousand times during bee season and develop an intense IgG4 antibody response after a few weeks with concurrent inhibition of any skin reactivity [181]. However, attempts to correlate clinical improvement with titers of IgG4 antibodies during immunotherapy demonstrated that a direct correlation of the two parameters could only be observed for parenteral allergies [46, 57]. IgG4 antibodies in Hymenoptera allergies were thereby considered to be "blocking antibodies" [95].

With regard to inhalant allergens, only a few authors have described positive correlation between clinical improvement and serum IgG levels [127]. Enhanced IgG levels and simultaneously decreased serum IgE levels have been observed [72], but no correlation with clinical improvement was found [56, 64, 163]. Thus, the concept of blocking antibodies directed against the allergen appears to remain controversial.

This raises questions about the physiologic role of the IgG4 response. The IgG4 isotype is the least abundant IgG subclass in humans, and represents approximately 4 percent of the total IgG in serum of adults. Nevertheless, the contribution of IgG4 antibodies to the total IgG response elicited by a particular antigen may sometimes exceed 90 percent of the IgG antibodies [63]. The association of IgG4 and IgE responses is especially important in conditions involving IL-4 production, because both isotypes are stimulated by IL-4 [99]. Moreover, basophil degranulation can be initiated not only by forming bridges between adjacent IgE molecules but also by bridging molecules of a subclass of IgG, thereby resulting in hypersensitivity reactions. This IgG was denoted for its ligand capacity: short-term sensitizing IgG (IgG S-TS). Anti-IgG4 antibody induces histamine release from leukocytes as anti-IgE does in some subjects, but additional studies aimed at demonstrating the presence of IgG4 on human basophil membranes were not conclusive. Another recent study indicated that human basophils might be activated by anti-IgG4 via two different mechanisms, depending on the antibody concentration: One is eosinophil dependent, and the other is eosinophil independent [5]. Further study is needed to reach a final consensus about the role of IgG4 in anaphylaxis [61, 62].

Parasitic infections have been one of the major causes of fatality for mammals throughout their evolution and generate specific as well as nonspecific IgE responses, which are also characteristics of mammals [39, 126]. Contrary to the adverse aspects of IgE responses as causes of allergic diseases, it has been suggested that immunologic pathways involving IgE can lead to damage to the developing parasite, and could have evolved as protection against helminth infections that might be largely dependent on IgE-dependent cytotoxicity with or without the involvement of Fcε receptors [15, 38]. Recent study in an area of endemic schistosomiasis has shown that reinfection is significantly less likely in those individuals possessing high levels of specific IgE antibody and more likely in those with high levels of IgG4 antibodies against either the worm or egg. This indicates that immunity to schistosomal infection may depend on pathways involving IgE, some of which might be blocked by high levels of IgG4 [60]. Although both IgE and IgG4 are enhanced by IL-4 and inhibited by IFN-γ as described above, low levels of IFN-γ can suppress only IgE, but not IgG4 [71]. Thus, segregation of IgE and IgG4 responses that might be dependent on the balance of IL-4 (produced by Th2) and IFN-γ (produced by Th1) could result in the loss of a protective role of IgE against parasitic infections on the one hand and the success of hyposensitization to allergens on the other.

In conclusion, this chapter has attempted to interweave many aspects of the IgE antibody system to create an overall perspective of the current state of knowledge about the biology of this fascinating antibody system. It is almost remarkable that the component of the immune system that produces quantities of molecules on orders of a magnitude less than those produced in other antibody systems has received such intense investigation in recent years. This reflects the enormous advances in cellular and molecular techniques used to identify the complexity of components that regulate and respond to IgE antibodies. Many interesting questions about the extent of the role of IgE molecules in a variety of physiologic and pathologic responses still need to be answered but it seems clear at this point that IgE involvement goes beyond allergic diseases and parasitic infections. It is also probable that additional, as yet undiscovered, lymphokines that interact with the IgE antibody system will eventually be recognized. Intensive study during the next 5 to 10 years should be most revealing in this respect.

REFERENCES

1. Armitage, R. J., Goff, L. K., and Beverley, P. C. Expression and functional role of CD23 on T cells. *Eur. J. Immunol.* 19:31, 1989.
2. Baird, B., et al. Interaction of IgE with its high affinity receptor. Structural basis and requirements for effective cross-linking. *Int. Arch. Allergy Appl. Immunol.* 88:23, 1989.
3. Banchereau, J., et al. Long-term human B cell lines dependent on interleukin-4 and antibody to CD40. *Science* 251:70, 1991.
4. Bass, H., Mosmann, T., and Strober, S. Evidence for mouse Th1- and Th2-like helper T cells in vivo: Selective reduction of Th1-like cells after total lymphoid irradiation. *J. Exp. Med.* 170:1495, 1989.
5. Beauvais, F., et al. Bimodal IgG4-mediated human basophil activation. *J. Immunol.* 144:3881, 1990.
5a. Beavil, A. J., et al. α-Helical coiled coil stalks in the low-affinity receptor for IgE (FcεRII/CD23) and related C-type lectins. *Proc. Natl. Acad. Sci. USA* 89:753, 1992.
6. Benacerraf, B., and McDevitt, H. O. Histocompatibility-linked immune response genes. *Science* 175:273, 1972.
7. Bettler, B., et al. Binding site for IgE of the human low affinity Fcε receptor (FcεRII/CD23) is confined to the domain homologous with animal lectins. *Proc. Natl. Acad. Sci. USA* 86:7118, 1989.
8. Bieber, T., et al. Induction of FcεR2/CD23 on human epidermal Langerhans' cells by recombinant interleukin 4 and γ-interferon. *J. Exp. Med.* 170:309, 1989.
9. Blank, U., et al. Complete structure and expression in transfected cells of high affinity IgE receptor. *Nature* 337:187, 1989.
10. Boom, W. H., Liano, D., and Abbas, A. K. Heterogeneity of helper/inducer T lymphocytes. II. Effects of interleukin 4- and interleukin 2-producing T cell clones on resting B lymphocytes. *J. Exp. Med.* 167:1352, 1988.
11. Borish, L., Mascali, J. J., and Rosenwasser, L. J. IgE-dependent cytokine production by human peripheral blood mononuclear phagocytes. *J. Immunol.* 146:63, 1991.
12. Bousquet, J., and Michel, F.-B. Specific immunotherapy. *Allergy* 43(Suppl. 8):16, 1988.
13. Brown, K. D., et al. A family of small inducible proteins secreted by leukocytes are members of a new superfamily that includes leukocyte and fibroblast-derived inflammatory agents, growth factors, and indicators of various activation processes. *J. Immunol.* 142:679, 1989.
14. Burd, P. R., et al. Interleukin 3-dependent and -independent mast cells stimulated with IgE and antigen express multiple cytokines. *J. Exp. Med.* 170:245, 1989.
14a. Burstein, H. J., et al. Humoral immune functions in IL-4 transgenic mice. *J. Immunol.* 147:2950, 1991.
15. Butterworth, A. E., et al. Antibody-dependent cell-mediated damage to schistosomula in vitro. *Nature* 252:503, 1974.
16. Buus, S., et al. Autologous peptides constitutively occupy the antigen binding site on Ia. *Science* 242:1045, 1988.
17. Capron, A., and Dessaint, J.-P. From protective immunity to allergy: The cellular partners of IgE. *Chem. Immunol.* 49:236, 1990.
18. Capron, A., et al. Specific IgE antibodies in immune adherence of normal macrophages to *Schistosoma mansoni* schistosomules. *Nature* 253:474, 1975.
19. Capron, A., et al. From parasites to allergy: The second receptor for IgE (FcεR2). *Immunol. Today* 7:15, 1986.
20. Capron, M., et al. Fc receptors for IgE on human and rat eosinophils. *J. Immunol.* 126:2087, 1981.
21. Capron, M., et al. Functional role of the α-chain of complement receptor type 3 in human eosinophil-dependent antibody-mediated cytotoxicity against schistosomes. *J. Immunol.* 139:2059, 1987.
22. Carding, S. R., and Bottomly, K. IL-4 (B cell stimulatory factor-1) exhibits thymocyte growth factor activity in the presence of IL-2. *J. Immunol.* 140:1519, 1988.
23. Casten, L. A., and Pierce, S. K. Receptor-mediated B cell antigen processing. *J. Immunol.* 140:404, 1988.
24. Castracane, J. M., and Rocklin, R. E. Detection of human auto-anti-idiotypic antibodies (Ab2). I. Isolation and characterization of Ab2 in the serum of a ragweed immunotherapy-treated patient. *Int. Arch. Allergy Appl. Immunol.* 86:288, 1988.
25. Castracane, J. M., and Rocklin, R. E. Detection of human auto-anti-idiotypic antibodies (Ab2). II. Generation of Ab2 in atopic patients undergoing allergen immunotherapy. *Int. Arch. Allergy Appl. Immunol.* 86:295, 1988.
26. Cher, D. J., and Mosmann, T. R. Two types of murine helper T cell clone. II. Delayed-type hyersensitivity is mediated by Th1 clones. *J. Immunol.* 138:3688, 1987.
27. Cherayil, B. J., Weiner, S. J., and Pillai, S. The Mac-2 antigen is a galactose-specific lectin that binds IgE. *J. Exp. Med.* 170:1959, 1989.
28. Cherwinski, H. M., et al. Two types of mouse helper T cell clone. III. Further differences in lymphokine synthesis between Th1 and Th2 clones revealed by RNA hybridization, functionally monospecific bioassays, and monoclonal antibodies. *J. Exp. Med.* 166:1229, 1987.
29. Chretien, I., et al. A monoclonal anti-IgE antibody against an epitope (amino acids 367-376) in the CH3 domain inhibits IgE binding to the low affinity IgE receptor (CD23). *J. Immunol.* 141:3128, 1988.
30. Coffman, R. L., Lebman, D. A., and Schrader, B. Transforming growth factor β specifically enhances IgA production by lipopolysaccharide-stimulated murine B lymphocytes. *J. Exp. Med.* 170:1039, 1989.
31. Coffman, R. L., et al. B cell stimulatory factor-1 enhances the IgE response of lipopolysaccharide-activated B cells. *J. Immunol.* 136:4538, 1986.
32. Croce, C. M., et al. Chromosomal location of the genes for human immunoglobulin heavy chains. *Proc. Natl. Acad. Sci. USA* 76:3416, 1979.
33. Defrance, T., et al. Human recombinant interleukin 4 induces Fcε receptors (CD23) on normal human B lymphocytes. *J. Exp. Med.* 165:1459, 1987.
34. Delespesse, G., and Sarfati, M. IgE-binding factors (soluble CD23) and IgE regulation. *Res. Immunol.* 141:75, 1990.
35. Delespesse, G., et al. IgE receptors on human lymphocytes. II. Detection of cells bearing IgE receptors on unstimulated mononuclear cells by means of a monoclonal antibody. *Eur. J. Immunol.* 16:815, 1986.
36. Delespesse, G., et al. IgE receptors on human lymphocytes. III. Expression of IgE receptors on mitogen-stimulated human mononuclear cells. *Eur. J. Immunol.* 16:1043, 1986.
37. Denoroy, M.-C., Yodoi, J., and Banchereau, J. Interleukin 4 and interferons α and γ regulate FcεRII/CD23 mRNA expression on normal human B cells. *Mol. Immunol.* 27:129, 1990.
38. Dessaint, J. P., and Capron, A. IgE and immune defense mechanism. *Clin. Rev. Allergy* 7:105, 1989.
39. Dessaint, J. P., et al. Quantitative determination of specific IgE antibodies

to schistosome antigens and serum IgE levels in patients with schistoso-miasis. *Clin. Exp. Immunol.* 20:427, 1975.

40. Dialynas, D. P., et al. Characterization of the murine antigenic determinant, designated L3T4a, recognized by monoclonal antibody GK1.5: Expression of L3T4a by functional T cell clones appears to correlate primarily with class II MHC antigen-restriction. *Immunol. Rev.* 74:29, 1983.

41. Dorrington, K. J., and Bennich, H. H. Structure-function relationships in human immunoglobulin E. *Immunol. Rev.* 41:3, 1978.

42. Dorrington, K. J., and Tanford, C. Molecular size and conformation of immunoglobulins. *Adv. Immunol.* 12:333, 1970.

43. Drickamer, K. Two distinct classes of carbohydrate recognition domains in animal lectins. *J. Biol. Chem.* 263:9557, 1988.

44. Early, P., et al. An immunoglobulin heavy chain variable region gene is generated from three segments of DNA: V_n, D and J_n. *Cell* 19:981, 1980.

45. Ewan, P. W. Allergen immunotherapy. *Curr. Opin. Immunol.* 1:672, 1989.

46. Ferrante, A., Mocatta, R., and Goh, D. H. B. Changes in IgG and IgE antibody levels during immunotherapy. *Int. Arch. Allergy Appl. Immunol.* 81:284, 1986.

47. Finkelman, F. D., et al. Lymphokine control of *in vivo* immunoglobulin isotype selection. *Annu. Rev. Immunol.* 8:303, 1990.

48. Finkelman, F. D., et al. Interferon-γ regulates the isotypes of immunoglobulin secreted during *in vivo* humoral immune responses. *J. Immunol.* 140:1022, 1988.

49. Finkelman, F. D., et al. Interleukin-4 is required to generate and sustain *in vivo* IgE responses. *J. Immunol.* 141:2335, 1988.

50. Fiorentino, D. F., Bond, M. W., and Mosmann, T. R. Two types of mouse helper T cells. IV. Th2 cells secrete a factor that inhibits cytokine production by Th1 clones. *J. Exp. Med.* 170:2081, 1989.

51. Firestein, G. S., et al. A new murine CD4$^+$ T cell subset with an unrestricted cytokine profile. *J. Immunol.* 143:518, 1989.

52. Fong, T. A. T., and Mosmann, T. R. Alloreactive murine CD8$^+$ T cell clones secrete the Th1 pattern of cytokines. *J. Immunol.* 144:1744, 1990.

53. Fong, T. A. T., and Mosmann, T. R. The role of IFN-γ in delayed-type hypersensitivity mediated by Th1 clones. *J. Immunol.* 143:2887, 1989.

53a. Frigeri, L. G., and Liu, F.-T. Surface expression of functional IgE binding protein, an endogenous lectin, on mast cells and macrophages. *J. Immunol.* 148:861, 1992.

54. Garmen, R. D., et al. B-cell stimulatory factor (beta 2 and interferon) functions as a second signal for interleukin 2 production by mature mutine T cells. *Proc. Natl. Acad. Sci. USA* 84:7629, 1987.

54a. Gauchat, J-F., et al. Regulation of germ-line ε transcription and induction of ε switching in cloned EBV-transformed and malignant human B cell lines by cytokines and CD4$^+$ T cells. *J. Immunol.* 148:2291, 1992.

55. Gerondakis, S. Structure and expression of murine germ-line immunoglobulin ε heavy chain transcripts induced by interleukin 4. *Proc. Natl. Acad. Sci. USA* 87:1581, 1990.

56. Gleich, G. J., et al. Effect of immunotherapy on immunoglobulin E and immunoglobulin G antibodies to ragweed antigens: A six-year prospective study. *J. Allergy Clin. Immunol.* 70:261, 1982.

57. Golden, D. B. K., et al. Clinical relevance of the venom-specific immunoglobulin G antibody level during immunotherapy. *J. Allergy Clin. Immunol.* 69:489, 1982.

58. Gollnick, S. O., et al. Isolation, characterization, and expression of cDNA clones encoding the mouse Fc receptor for IgE (FcεRII). *J. Immunol.* 144:1974, 1990.

59. Greenbaum, L. A., et al. Autocrine growth of CD4$^+$ T cells: Differential effects of IL-1 on helper and inflammatory T cells. *J. Immunol.* 140:1555, 1988.

60. Hagan, P., et al. Human IgE, IgG4 and resistance to re-infection with *Schistosoma haematobium*. *Nature* 349:243, 1991.

61. Halpern, G. M., and Scott, J. IgG4 antibody response in allergic patients during immunotherapy. *New England and Regional Allergy Proc.* 9:81, 1988.

62. Halpern, G. M. IgG4 antibodies and their role in asthmatic patients. *J. Asthma* 26:345, 1989.

63. Halpern, G. M. Nonreaginic anaphylactic and/or blocking antibodies. *Clin. Rev. Allergy* 1:179, 1983.

64. Hedlin, G., et al. Immunotherapy with cat- and dog-dander extracts. *J. Allergy Clin. Immunol.* 77:488, 1986.

65. Heinzel, F. P., et al. Reciprocal expression of interferon γ or interleukin 4 during the resolution or progression of murine leishmaniasis. Evidence for expansion of distinct helper T cell subsets. *J. Exp. Med.* 169:59, 1989.

66. Helm, B., et al. The mast cell binding site on human immunoglobulin E. *Nature* 331:180, 1988.

67. Hirano, T., et al. Biological and clinical aspects of interleukin 6. *Immunol. Today* 11:12, 1990.

68. Hirayama, K., et al. HLA-DQ is epistatic to HLA-DR in controlling the immune response to schistosomal antigen in humans. *Nature* 327:426, 1987.

69. Hochman, P. S., and Huber, B. T. A class II gene conversion event defines an antigen-specific Ir-gene epitope. *J. Exp. Med.* 160:1925, 1984.

70. Hodgkin, P. D., et al. Identification of IL-6 as a T cell-derived factor that enhances the proliferative response of thymocytes to IL-4 and phorbol myristate acetate. *J. Immunol.* 141:151, 1988.

71. Ishizaka, A., et al. The inductive effect of interleukin-4 on IgG4 and IgE synthesis in human peripheral blood lymphocytes. *Clin. Exp. Immunol.* 79:392, 1990.

72. Ishizaka, K. Cellular mechanisms of IgE antibody response. *Int. Arch. Allergy Appl. Immunol.* 49:255, 1975.

73. Ishizaka, K. IgE-binding factors and regulation of the IgE antibody response. *Annu. Rev. Immunol.* 6:513, 1988.

74. Ishizaka, K. Twenty years with IgE. *J. Immunol.* 135:i, 1985.

75. Ishizaka, K., Ishizaka, T., and Hornbrook, M. M. Physicochemical properties of human reaginic antibody. IV. Presence of a unique immunoglobulin as a carrier of reaginic activity. *J. Immunol.* 97:75, 1966.

75a. Jabara, H. H., et al. Hydrocortisone and IL-4 induce IgE isotype switching in human B cells. *J. Immunol.* 147:1557, 1991.

76. Joseph, M., et al. A new function for platelets: IgE-dependent killing of schistosomes. *Nature* 303:810, 1983.

77. Kataoka, T., et al. Rearrangement of immunoglobulin γ1-chain gene and mechanism for heavy-chain class switch. *Proc. Natl. Acad. Sci. USA* 77:919, 1980.

78. Kawabe, T., et al. Regulation of FcεR2/CD23 gene expression by cytokines and specific ligands (IgE and anti-FcεR2 monoclonal antibody). Variable regulation depending on the cell types. *J. Immunol.* 141:1376, 1988.

79. Kehry, M. R., and Yamashita, L. C. Fcε receptor II (CD23) function on mouse B cells: Role in IgE dependent antigen focusing. *Proc. Natl. Acad. Sci. USA* 86:7566, 1989.

80. Kelso, A., and Gough, N. M. Coexpression of granulocyte-macrophage colony-stimulating factor, γ-interferon, and interleukins 3 and 4 is random in murine alloreactive T-lymphocyte clones. *Proc. Natl. Acad. Sci. USA* 85:9189, 1988.

81. Kenten, J. H., et al. Cloning and sequence determination of the gene for the human immunoglobulin ε chain expressed in a myeloma cell line. *Proc. Natl. Acad. Sci. USA* 79:6661, 1982.

82. Kikutani, H., et al. Molecular structure of human lymphocyte receptor for immunoglobulin E. *Cell* 47:657, 1986.

83. Kikutani, H., et al. Fc receptor, a specific differentiation marker transiently expressed on mature B cells prior to isotype switching. *J. Exp. Med.* 164:1455, 1986.

84. Killar, L., et al. Cloned, Ia-restricted T cells that do not produce interleukin 4(IL 4)/B cell stimulatory factor 1 (BSF-1) fail to help antigen-specific B cells. *J. Immunol.* 138:1674, 1987.

85. Kinet, J.-P., et al. Isolation and characterization of cDNAs coding for the β subunit of the high-affinity receptor for immunoglobulin E. *Proc. Natl. Acad. Sci. USA* 85:6483, 1988.

86. Kinet, J.-P., et al. A cDNA presumptively coding for the α subunit of the receptor with high affinity for immunoglobulin E. *Biochemistry* 26:4605, 1987.

87. Kishimoto, T., and Hirano, T. Molecular regulation of B lymphocyte response. *Annu. Rev. Immunol.* 6:485, 1988.

88. Kishimoto, T., et al. Regulation of antibody response in different immunoglobulin classes. *J. Immunol.* 121:2106, 1978.

89. Kitani, S., et al. Inhibition of allergic reactions with monoclonal antibody to the high affinity IgE receptor. *J. Immunol.* 140:2585, 1988.

90. Koichi, I., et al. Human lymphocyte Fc receptor for IgE: Sequence homology of its cloned cDNA with animal lectins. *Proc. Natl. Acad. Sci. USA* 84:819, 1987.

91. Lanzavecchia, A. Antigen uptake and accumulation in antigen-specific B cells. *Immunol. Rev.* 99:39, 1987.

92. Lanzavecchia, A. Antigen-specific interaction between T and B cells. *Nature* 314:537, 1985.

93. Lawrence, D. A., Weigle, W. O., and Spiegelberg, H. L. Immunoglobulins cytophilic for human lymphocytes, monocytes, and neutrophils. *J. Clin. Invest.* 55:268, 1975.

94. Lee, W. T., Rao, M., and Conrad, D. H. The murine lymphocyte receptor for IgE. IV. The mechanisms of ligand-specific receptor upregulation on B cells. *J. Immunol.* 139:1191, 1987.

95. Lesourd, B., et al. Hymenoptera venom immunotherapy. I. Induction of

T cell-mediated immunity by honeybee venom immunotherapy: Relationships with specific antibody responses. *J. Allergy Clin. Immunol.* 83: 563, 1989.

96. Letellier, M., Nakajima, T., and Delespesse, G. IgE receptor on human lymphocytes. IV. Further analysis of its structure and of the role of N-linked carbohydrates. *J. Immunol.* 141:2374, 1988.

97. Letellier, M., et al. *J. Exp. Med.* 172:693, 1990.

98. Liu, F.-T. Molecular biology of IgE-binding protein, IgE-binding factors, and IgE receptors. *Crit. Rev. Immunol.* 10:289, 1990.

99. Lundgren, M., et al. Interleukin 4 induces synthesis of IgE and IgG4 in human B cells. *Eur. J. Immunol.* 19:1311, 1989.

100. Lympany, P., et al. An HLA-associated nonresponsiveness to melittin: A component of bee venom. *J. Allergy Clin. Immunol.* 86:160, 1990.

101. MacDonald, S. M., et al. Studies of IgE-dependent histamine releasing factors: Heterogeneity of IgE. *J. Immunol.* 139:506, 1987.

102. Maggi, E., et al. Profiles of lymphokine activities and helper function for IgE in human T cell clones. *Eur. J. Immunol.* 18:1045, 1988.

103. Magilavy, D. B., Fitch, F. W., and Gajewski, T. F. Murine hepatic accessory cells support the proliferation of Th1 but not Th2 helper T lymphocyte clones. *J. Exp. Med.* 170:985, 1989.

104. Marcelletti, J. F., and Katz, D. H. FcRε+ lymphocytes and regulation of the IgE antibody system. I. A new class of molecules, termed IgE-induced regulants (EIR), which modulate FcRε expression by lymphocytes. *J. Immunol.* 133:2821, 1984.

105. Marcelletti, J. F., and Katz, D. H. Antigen concentration determines helper T cell subset participation in IgE antibody responses. *Cell. Immunol.* In press.

106. Marsh, D. G., et al. HLA-Dw 2: A genetic marker for human immune response to short ragweed pollen allergen Ra 5. I. Response resulting primarily from natural antigenic exposure. *J. Exp. Med.* 155:1439, 1982.

107. Matsushita, S., and Katz, D. H. The murine CD23-modulating protein is a novel serine protease. *J. Allergy Clin. Immunol.* 87:244, 1991.

107a. Matsushita, S., and Katz, D. H. B cell sensitivity to IgE-suppressive activity of IFN-γ is polymorphic and controlled by a non-H-2-linked gene. *Cell. Immunol.* 143:212, 1992.

108. Matsushita, S., and Katz, D. H. The murine ε receptor modulating protein: A novel serine protease which modulates CD23 binding of IgE. *Cell. Immunol.* 137:252, 1991.

108a. Matsushita, S., and Katz, D. H. εRMP: A novel serine protease expressed on activated T-cell membranes enhances IL-4-induced IgE synthesis by B cells (abstract). *FASEB J.* 6:A1986, 1992.

109. Matsushita, S., et al. Purification of murine suppressive factor of allergy into distinct CD23-modulating and IgE-suppressive proteins. *Proc. Natl. Acad. Sci. USA* 88:4718, 1991.

110. Matsushita, S., et al. HLA-linked nonresponsiveness to Cryptomeria japonica pollen antigen. I. Nonresponsiveness is mediated by antigen-specific suppressor T cell. *J. Immunol.* 138:109, 1987.

111. Max, E. E., et al. Duplication and deletion in the human immunoglobulin ε genes. *Cell* 29:691, 1982.

112. Metzger, H., et al. The receptor with high affinity for immunoglobulin E. *Annu. Rev. Immunol.* 4:419, 1986.

113. Miyajima, H., et al. Suppression by IL-2 of IgE production by B cells stimulated by IL-4. *J. Immunol.* 146:457, 1991.

114. Moore, K. W., et al. Rodent IgE-binding factor genes are members of an endogenous, retrovirus-like gene family. *J. Immunol.* 136:4283, 1986.

115. Morrissey, P. J., et al. Recombinant interleukin 7, pre-B cell growth factor, has costimulatory activities on purified mature T cells. *J. Exp. Med.* 169: 707, 1989.

116. Mosmann, T. R., et al. Two types of murine helper T cell clone. I. Definition according to profiles of lymphokine activities and secreted proteins. *J. Immunol.* 136:2348, 1986.

117. Mosmann, T. R., and Coffman, R. L. Th1 and Th2 cells: Different patterns of lymphokine secretion lead to different functional properties. *Annu. Rev. Immunol.* 7:145, 1989.

118. Murray, J. S., et al. MHC control of CD4+ T cell subset activation. *J. Exp. Med.* 170:2135, 1989.

119. Nakajima, T., Sarfati, M., and Delespesse, G. Relationship between human IgE-binding factors and lymphocyte receptors for IgE. *J. Immunol.* 139: 848, 1987.

120. Naray-Fejes-toth, A., Cornwell, G. G., and Guyre, P. M. Glucocorticoids inhibit IgE receptor expression on the human monocyte cell line U937. *Immunology* 56:359, 1985.

121. Naray-Fejes-toth, A., and Guyre, P. M. Recombinant human immune interferon induces increased IgE receptor expression on the human monocyte cell line U937. *J. Immunol.* 133:1914, 1984.

122. Natvig, J. B., and Kunkel, H. G. Human immunoglobulins: Classes, subclasses, genetic variants, and idiotypes. *Adv. Immunol.* 10:106, 1969.

123. Nissim, A., Jouvin, M.-H., and Eshhar, Z. Mapping of the high affinity Fcε receptor binding site to the third constant region domain of IgE. *EMBO J.* 10:101, 1991.

124. Nonaka, M., et al. Cloning of cDNA coding for low-affinity Fc receptors for IgE on human T lymphocytes. *Int. Immunol.* 1:254, 1989.

125. Nutman, T. B., et al. IgE binding factors of T cell origin. I. Cloned and transformed T cells producing IgE-binding factors. *J. Immunol.* 139:4049, 1987.

126. Ogilivie, B. M. Reagin-like antibodies in animals immune to helminth parasites. *Nature* 204:91, 1964.

127. Ortolani, C., et al. Grass-pollen immunotherapy: A single-year, double-blind, placebo-controlled study in patients with grass pollen-induced asthma and rhinitis. *J. Allergy Clin. Immunol.* 73:283, 1984.

128. Padlan, E. A., and Davies, D. R. A model of the Fc immunoglobulin E. *Mol. Immunol.* 23:1063, 1986.

129. Palaird, X., et al. Simultaneous production of IL2, IL4, and IFNγ by activated human CD4+ and CD8+ T cell clones. *J. Immunol.* 141:849, 1988.

130. Péne, J. Regulatory role of cytokines and CD23 in the human IgE antibody synthesis. *Int. Arch. Allergy Appl. Immunol.* 90:32, 1989.

131. Péne, J., et al. IgE production by normal human lymphocytes is induced by interleukin 4 and suppressed by interferons γ, and α and prostaglandin E₂. *Proc. Natl. Acad. Sci. USA* 85:6880, 1988.

132. Peterson, L. H., and Conrad, D. H. Fine specificity, structure, and proteolytic susceptibility of the human lymphocyte receptor for IgE. *J. Immunol.* 135:2654, 1985.

133. Plaut, M. Antigen-specific lymphokine secretory patterns in atopic disease. *J. Immunol.* 144:4497, 1990.

134. Plaut, M., et al. Mast cell lines produce lymphokines in response to cross-linkage of FcεRI or to calcium ionophore. *Nature* 339:64, 1989.

135. Prinz, J. C., et al. Allergen-directed expression of Fc receptors for IgE (CD23) on human T lymphocytes is modulated by interleukin 4 and interferon-γ. *Eur. J. Immunol.* 20:1259, 1990.

136. Rabbitts, T. H., et al. The role of gene deletion in the immunoglobulin heavy chain switch. *Nature* 283:351, 1980.

137. Radbruch, A., et al. Control of immunoglobulin class switch recombination. *Immunol. Rev.* 89:69, 1986.

138. Rankin, J. A., et al. Human airway lining fluid (ALF): Cellular and protein constituents (abstract). *Am. Rev. Respir. Dis.* 137(Suppl.):5, 1988.

139. Ravetch, J. V., et al. Structural heterogeneity and functional domains of murine immunoglobulin G Fc receptors. *Science* 234:718, 1986.

140. Richards, M. L., and Katz, D. H. FcεRII and the activation of B lymphocytes. In J. Gordon (ed.), *Monographs in Allergy.* Basel: Karger, 1991. Pp. 124–134.

141. Richards, M. L., and Katz, D. H. The binding of IgE to murine FcεRII is calcium-dependent but not inhibited by carbohydrate. *J. Immunol.* 144: 2638, 1990.

142. Richards, M. L., and Katz, D. H. Biology and chemistry of the low affinity IgE receptor (FcεRII/CD23). *Crit. Rev. Immunol.* 11:65, 1991.

143. Richards, M. L., Katz, D. H., and Liu, F.-T. Complete genomic sequence of the murine low affinity Fc receptor for IgE (FcεRII): Demonstration of alternative transcripts and conserved sequence elements. *J. Immunol.* 147:1067, 1991.

144. Richards, M. L., Marcelletti, J. F., and Katz, D. H. IgE-antigen complexes enhance FcεR and Ia expression by murine B lymphocytes. *J. Exp. Med.* 168:571, 1988.

145. Roper, R. L., et al. Prostaglandin E₂ promotes IL-4-induced IgE and IgG1 synthesis. *J. Immunol.* 145:2644, 1990.

146. Sarfati, M., and Delespesse, G. Possible role of human lymphocyte receptor for IgE (CD23) or its soluble fragments in the *in vitro* synthesis of human IgE. *J. Immunol.* 141:2195, 1988.

147. Sarfati, M., et al. *In vitro* synthesis of IgE by human lymphocytes. III. IgE-potentiating activity of culture supernatants from Epstein-Barr virus (EBV) transformed B cells. *Immunology* 53:207, 1984.

148. Scherr, E., et al. Binding the low affinity FcεR on B cells suppresses ongoing human IgE synthesis. *J. Immunol.* 142:481, 1989.

149. Schuler, G., and Steinman, R. M. Murine epidermal Langerhans' cells mature into potent immunostimulatory dendritic cells *in vitro. J. Exp. Med.* 161:526, 1985.

150. Sehgal, P. B., et al. Human β2 interferon and B-cell differentiation factor BSF-2 are identical. *Science* 235:731, 1987.

151. Shimizu, A., Takahashi, N., and Honjo, T. Organization of the constant region gene family of the mouse. *Cell* 28:499, 1982.

152. Slattery, J., Holowka, D., and Baird, B. Segmental flexibility of receptor-bound immunoglobulin E. *Biochemistry* 24:7810, 1985.

153. Snapper, C. M., and Paul, W. E. Interferon-γ and B cell stimulatory factor-1 reciprocally regulate Ig isotype production. *Science* 236:944, 1987.

154. Snapper, C. M., Peschel, C., and Paul, W. E. IFN-γ stimulates IgG2a secretion by murine cells stimulated with bacterial lipopolysaccharide. *J. Immunol.* 140:2121, 1988.

155. Snapper, C. M., Finkelman, F. D., and Paul, W. E. Differential regulation of IgG1 and IgE synthesis by interleukin 4. *J. Exp. Med.* 167:183, 1988.

156. Springer, T. A. Adhesion receptors of the immune system. *Nature* 346:425, 1990.

157. Stevens, T. L., et al. Regulation of antibody isotype secretion by subsets of antigen-specific helper T cells. *Nature* 334:255, 1988.

158. Stout, R. D., and Bottomly, K. Antigen-specific activation of effector macrophages by IFN-γ producing (Th1) T cell clones. Failure of IL-4-producing (Th2) T cell clones to activate effector function in macrophages. *J. Immunol.* 142:760, 1989.

159. Street, N. E., and Mosmann, T. R. Functional diversity of T lymphocytes due to secretion of different cytokine patterns. *FASEB J.* 5:171, 1991.

160. Swain, L. S., et al. The role of IL4 and IL5: Characterization of a distinct helper T cell subset that makes IL4 and IL5 (Th2) and requires priming before induction of lymphokine secretion. *Immunol. Rev.* 102:77, 1988.

161. Takahashi, N., et al. Structure of human immunoglobulin gamma genes: Implications for evolution of a gene family. *Cell* 24:671, 1982.

162. Tamir, R., Castracane, J. M., and Rocklin, R. E. Generation of suppressor cells in atopic patients during immunotherapy that modulate IgE synthesis. *J. Allergy Clin. Immunol.* 79:591, 1987.

163. Taudorf, E., et al. Specific IgE, IgG, and IgA antibody response to oral immunotherapy in birch pollinosis. *J. Allergy Clin. Immunol.* 83:589, 1989.

164. Tepper, R. I., et al. IL-4 induces allergic-like inflammatory disease and alters T cell development in transgenic mice. *Cell* 62:457, 1990.

165. TeVelde, A. A., et al. IFN-α and IFN-γ have different regulatory effects on IL-4-induced membrane expression of FcεRIIb and release of soluble FcεRIIb by human monocytes. *J. Immunol.* 144:3052, 1990.

166. Thyphronitis, G., et al. IgE secretion by Epstein-Barr virus infected purified human B lymphocytes is stimulated by interleukin-4 and suppressed by interferon-γ. *Proc. Natl. Acad. Sci. USA* 86:5580, 1989.

167. Tite, J. P., Powell, M. B., and Ruddle, N. H. Protein-antigen specific Ia-restricted cytolytic T cells: Analysis of frequency, target cell susceptibility, and mechanism of cytolysis. *J. Immunol.* 135:25, 1985.

168. Tonnel, A. B., et al. Participation of FcεRII Positive Cells in Asthma. In W. J. Pichler, et al. (eds.), *Progress in Allergy and Clinical Immunology.* Toronto: H. Huber, 1989. Pp. 325–342.

169. Tsicopoulos, A., Lassalle, P., and Joseph, M. Effect of disodium cromoglycate on inflammatory cells bearing the Fc epsilon receptor type II (FcεRII). *Int. J. Immunopharmacol.* 10:227, 1988.

170. Uchibayashi, N., et al. Recombinant soluble Fcε receptor II (FcεRII/CD23) has IgE binding activity but no B cell growth promoting activity. *J. Immunol.* 142:3901, 1989.

171. Umetsu, D. T., et al. Functional heterogeneity among human inducer T cell clones. *J. Immunol.* 140:4211, 1988.

172. Vercelli, D., et al. The B-cell binding site on human immunoglobulin E. *Nature* 338:649, 1989.

173. Vercelli, D., et al. Human recombinant interleukin-4 induces FcεR2/CD23 on normal human monocytes. *J. Exp. Med.* 167:1406, 1988.

174. Verwaerde, C., et al. Properties of serine proteases of *Schistosoma mansoni* schistosomula involved in the regulation of IgE synthesis. *Scand. J. Immunol.* 27:17, 1988.

175. Waldmann, T. A., Polmar, S. H., and Terry, W. D. IgE Levels and Metabolism in Immune Deficiency Diseases. In D. H. Dayton (ed.), *The Biological Role of the Immunoglobulin E System.* National Institute of Child Health and Human Development. Washington, D.C.: US Government Printing Office, 1976. Pp. 74–88.

175a. Wong, H. L., et al. Administration of recombinant IL-4 to humans regulates gene expression, phenotype, and function in circulating monocytes. *J. Immunol.* 148:2118, 1992.

176. Yamamura, K., et al. Functional expression of a microinjected Eα^d gene in C 57 BL/6 transgenic mice. *Nature* 316:67, 1985.

177. Yodoi, J., and Ishizaka, K. Lymphocytes bearing Fc receptors for IgE. I. Presence of human and rat T lymphocytes with Fcε receptors. *J. Immunol.* 122:2577, 1979.

178. Yokota, A., et al. Two species of human Fcε receptor II (FCεRII/CD23): Tissue-specific and IL-4-specific regulation of gene expression. *Cell* 55:611, 1988.

179. Yoshida, K., et al. Immunoglobulin switch circular DNA in the mouse infected with *Nippostrongylus brasiliensis*: Evidence for successive class switching from μ to ε via γ1. *Proc. Natl. Acad. Sci. USA* 87:7829, 1990.

180. Yukawa, K., et al. A B cell-specific differentiation antigen CD23, is a receptor for IgE (FcεR) on lymphocytes. *J. Immunol.* 138:2576, 1987.

181. Yunginger, J. W., Jones, R. T., and Leiferman, K. M. Immunological studies in beekeepers and their family members. *J. Allergy Clin. Immunol.* 61:93, 1978.

182. Zurawski, G., et al. Activation of mouse T-helper cells induces abundant preproenkephalin mRNA synthesis. *Science* 232:772, 1986.

IgE Immediate Hypersensitivity

Samuel C. Bukantz
Richard F. Lockey

8

The "classic" allergic diseases result from the interaction of a unique immunoglobulin (IgE) with a specific antigen at receptor sites on the surface of specialized cells. This cell-surface interaction releases a number of chemical mediators, both preformed and synthesized de novo. The discovery of that knowledge is one of the many extraordinary stories during the development of the field of allergy and immunology. It begins in 1921 with Prausnitz and Küstner's (PK) [48] demonstration of a serum factor (then called *reagin*) capable of transferring allergic sensitivity to the skin of nonallergic individuals. The methods of gravimetric quantitation of the immune response, which followed the electrophoretic and ultracentrifugal identification of antibodies as classes of gamma globulins, were incapable of identifying reagin. Quantitative efforts, for example, in 1940 by Loveless and Kabat, failed to measure the uptake of reagin (skin-sensitizing antibody, later identified as IgE) from sera of ragweed-sensitive patients, using a suspension of formalinized pollen [34]. Later work by the Ishizakas and Hornbrook [26] and Johansson and colleagues [32] revealed that IgE is so much more active per unit of weight than is rabbit IgG that the gravimetric method was unsuitable for the isolation of IgE. The Ishizakas and Hornbrook had also isolated reagin from the sera of ragweed-allergic patients and established that the reaginic activity (transferability) did not correspond to IgG, IgM, IgA, or IgD immunoglobulins. A rabbit antiserum against a reagin-rich fraction of allergic sera retained its antireaginic activity after complete absorption with the known immunoglobulin classes. The absorbed serum also precipitated an antigenically unique immunoglobulin found in the gamma 1 region on electrophoresis, an immunoglobulin that also bound ragweed antigen E (AgE) and the presence of which correlated with the ability to transfer a PK response [24, 25].

IgE AS A UNIQUE IMMUNOGLOBULIN CLASS

Subsequently, a human IgE myeloma protein (ND), discovered by Johansson and Bennich [31], was studied in collaboration with the Ishizakas. The IgE purified from allergic sera shared major antigenic structures with the IgE from the myeloma serum and the IgE myeloma protein blocked the PK reaction [1] (see Chap. 7).

Prior to isolation and identification of IgE as the antibody of immediate hypersensitivity, detection of this "reaginic" activity in vitro was based on passive sensitization of leukocytes or tissues [44]. The development of the radioallergosorbent test (RAST), a much simpler and specific in vitro test utilizing radioactive reagents [65], led to many investigations into the nature of the immediate hypersensitivity reaction (see Chap. 38).

HIGH- AND LOW-AFFINITY RECEPTORS FOR IgE

High-affinity receptors for IgE (FcεRI) are present on basophilic leukocytes and mast cells [30] and there is a strong correlation

between serum IgE levels and the number of basophil IgE molecules, with many more molecules per basophilic cell being found in atopic subjects with high levels of serum IgE [9]. Other inflammatory cells, including eosinophils, monocytes, alveolar macrophages, and platelets, also have receptors for IgE [5, 6, 33, 36, 38]. These receptors (FcεRII) have lower binding affinity for IgE, are enhanced in relation to cell activation, and may be upregulated by chemotactic factors. FcεRII on eosinophils may have some homology with the CD23 IgE receptor on a subpopulation of B-lymphocytes that may be associated with production of IgE [16].

IgE-DEPENDENT RELEASE MECHANISMS

IgE-dependent release mechanisms are initiated by the interaction of a specific allergen with two or more divalent IgE molecules bound firmly to specific receptors on mast cells and basophils, resulting in a cascade of cellular events leading to exocytosis and mediator secretion [21].

A number of studies have demonstrated parallel triggering mechanisms induced by anti-IgE and by specific allergen in the atopic individual [41]. Heterologous, divalent anti-IgE, first produced by the Ishizakas, triggers cellular anaphylactic responses of basophils and mast cells, leading to cell degranulation like that of cells from atopic individuals challenged with specific allergen [22, 23]. The high-affinity Fc receptor of these two cell types binds IgE molecules that can be cross-linked by anti-IgE or its F(ab)₂ fragments. Bridging two or more IgE molecules results in the elaboration of many pharmacologic mediators including histamine, leukotrienes, prostaglandins, and, except for human basophils, platelet-activating factor (PAF). Studies of these mechanisms have helped to clarify how the mediators, together with other cells of the inflammatory process, amplify the pathophysiologic changes associated with allergic reactions [41].

IMMUNOPATHOLOGIC MECHANISMS IN ASTHMA

The low-affinity IgE receptors of the macrophage, eosinophil, lymphocyte, and platelet probably bind very few single monomeric IgE molecules, and their major triggering mechanism may involve IgE immune complexes [50]. This binding of multiple IgE Fc sites to low-affinity receptors forms an avid association of antigen with the cell and serves to "bridge" two or more IgE receptors, which is the first step in activating many inflammatory cells. Low-affinity receptors for IgE on macrophages were first revealed by finding that IgE bound to the trematode schistosomes permitted rat macrophages to kill the parasites more effectively [4]. FcεRII receptors have also been directly demonstrated on macrophages and lymphocytes [37]. IgE dimers may induce the macrophage to discharge its content of lysosomal enzymes, produce superoxide, and secrete interleukin-1 and products of arachidonic acid metabolism such as prostaglandins and the potent bronchospastic leukotrienes. It is then possible that the atopic asthmatic subject could experience bronchospasm, during bronchoprovocation or after inhalation of naturally occurring airborne antigens, as the result of an antigen-IgE interaction that activates mast cells, basophils, platelets, and macrophages, causing the release and synthesis of mediators of bronchospasm and inflammation.

Platts-Mills [47a] reviewed the evidence relating IgE to the mechanisms of bronchial reactivity. These IgE antibodies are seen as a marker for a complex immune response producing cellular responses and delayed hypersensitivity (cutaneous basophil hypersensitivity) as well as mediator release from the mast cells. The suggestion is made that if T-cells are involved in lung inflammation, it is selectively those T-cells associated with IgE responses. It is those T-cells that produce interleukin-4 and probably interleukin-5. There has been a reinforcement of the correlation between asthma and IgE in a large population survey.

Of additional interest is the observation by several investigators that beta-adrenergic agonists have a greater inhibitory effect on antigen-induced peptidoleukotriene release than on histamine release from the lung [18, 45, 61]. Not only was the maximum response to isoproterenol greater but also the intrinsic efficacy of isoproterenol for inhibiting the release of arachidonic acid metabolites was three times greater compared to that of histamine [62].

IgE AND INFLAMMATORY CELLS

Much of current understanding of the immediate hypersensitivity reaction stems from the description of IgE antibody [13]. The sequence of the human epsilon heavy chain is now known, the Fcϵ gene has been cloned, a model of the Fc portion of IgE has been established, and the region of Fcϵ that interacts with the receptor has been identified. The four-chain structure of the high-affinity receptor on mast cells and basophils has been determined [39] and the receptor has been cloned and expressed [2]. The structure and synthesis pathways of many of the once-called factors of anaphylaxis, their target receptors, their pharmacology, and that of their antagonists have been established and the heterogeneity of mast cells and the T-cell control of the mucosal, bone marrow–derived mast cells have been explored.

BIOCHEMICAL EVENTS FOLLOWING THE BRIDGING OF CELL SURFACE–BOUND IgE OR IgE RECEPTORS (FcϵRI) ON HISTAMINE-CONTAINING CELLS

The initial trigger of the biochemical events resulting in the release of mediators from mast cells and basophils is the bridging of two or more IgE molecules bound to cell-surface IgE Fc receptors (FcϵRI) [29]. Identical biochemical events followed by mediator secretion will occur if anti-IgE Fc receptor antibody is used as the secretion stimulus [28] (Fig. 8-1).

Many biochemical events and the release of mediators follow the bridging event (Fig. 8-2). A very-well-established event is the influx of Ca^{++}, which is required for mediator release. The IgE cross-bridging elevates cyclic adenosine monophosphate (AMP) to methylation of membrane phospholipids, and finally to Ca^{++} influx and histamine secretion. Phosphatidylcholine, resulting from the triple methylation of phosphatidylethanolamine, moves across the cell membrane to the cell surface. Phosphatidylcho-

line is a phospholipid in which a glycerol molecule is substituted at the 2-position with arachidonic acid; see Chapter 10 for further details.

Immediate elevation of cyclic AMP follows cross-bridging before the release of granular stores of histamine. An augmentation of the catalytic site activity of adenylate cyclase (an endoenzyme) cleaves ATP to form cyclic AMP, two molecules of which bind to a separate tetramolecular complex. This releases two molecules of catalytic protein which, together with ATP (as a phosphate donor), activates the enzymes responsible for the actual secretory event (see Fig. 8-2). The rise of cyclic AMP and the methylation of phospholipids are both biochemical pathways necessary for the release of the catalytic protein, essential if phospholipid methylation is to lead to a requisite Ca^{++} influx. An increase in Ca^{++} concentration within the cytoplasm is a critical cofactor for the function of the protein kinases produced by the elevation of cyclic AMP.

The production of newly formed lipid mediators of anaphylaxis results from the biochemical events surrounding histamine secretion. Membrane-bound phospholipase A$_2$ cleaves the phosphatidylcholine produced during phospholipid methylation, which then liberates arachidonic acid both extracellularly and intracellularly. Metabolism of arachidonic acid produces the potent bronchoconstrictors including prostaglandins and leukotrienes. Acetylglycerylphosphoryl choline (AGEPC) (also referred to as platelet-activating factor) is another mediator produced by the burst of lipid synthesis following cross-bridging. Figure 8-3 represents the arachidonic acid cascade and Tables 8-1 and 8-2 list the products of the two pathways of arachidonic acid metabolism identified by the initial enzymes involved, and give the tissue source of each metabolite and its functional contribution to the hypersensitivity and/or inflammatory action. The mast cell–derived mediators may also be grouped as preformed, newly generated, or granule associated (Table 8-3). The pathologic changes possibly induced by individual mediators are tabulated in Table 8-4.

THE IgE RECEPTOR: TARGET FOR ALLERGY THERAPY

Studies over the years have characterized the immunoglobulin-binding receptor at the protein level as composed of one alpha, one beta, and two gamma subunits arranged together in the complex protein (Fig. 8-4) [2, 19, 35].

The genes that encode the three different subunits have been isolated in several species, including humans. The three genes have subsequently been introduced into cells that did not express the receptor and these cells then expressed millions of surface receptors. It is very difficult to purify basophils to work with their IgE surface receptors. The new ability to express millions of human receptors by gene transfer, however, now allows very easy characterization of the binding of human IgE to the human receptor. Practically, this means that reagents can be tested for their ability to inhibit the binding of human IgE to the human receptor. Inhibition of such binding could prevent the allergic reaction that is triggered through the IgE receptor and this inhibition could work for any type of allergen. Solid-phase assays have already been set up to be conducted by a huge robot that can test an average of 1,000 reagents per week [35]. The hope is that one or more of the many thousands of drugs to be tested may inhibit the IgE-receptor binding sufficiently well to justify additional work on the compound to make it safe and more active for human therapeutic use.

REGULATION OF IgE SYNTHESIS

T-Cell Factors

What remains of great interest is the regulation of IgE synthesis, a subject that occupied a great deal of the Ishizakas' attention

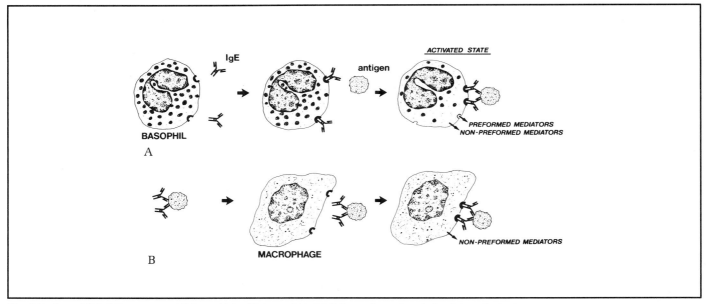

Fig. 8-1. *Basophil IgE Fc receptors (A) have high affinity and bind IgE for prolonged periods of time. Activation of the release and production of mediators occurs primarily through the binding of cell-bound IgE to antigen. Macrophage IgE Fc receptors (B) in contrast have low affinity, and cellular activation occurs primarily through multiple IgE molecules bound to antigen. Prostaglandin and leukotriene compounds are nonpreformed mediators produced by both activated basophils (mast cells) and macrophages. Basophils release preformed mediators (e.g., histamine) from cytoplasmic granules.*

Table 8-1. Cyclooxygenase products with a role in asthma and allergy

Compound	Tissue source	Action
PGD$_2$	Mast cells	Inhibits platelet aggregation, possibly prevents release of PAF Constricts pulmonary artery and airways
PGE$_2$	Many cells, macrophages	Relaxes smooth muscle of airways and microvasculature Potentiates vascular actions of LTB$_4$ and LTD$_4$ Immunosuppressant
PGF$_{2\alpha}$	Many cells	Contracts smooth muscle of airways and microvasculature
PGI$_2$ (prosta-cyclin)	Vascular endothelium, brain, lung parenchyma, kidney	Relaxes arterioles, dilates pulmonary vessels Reverses platelet aggregation Minimal effects on airways
Thromboxane	Platelets, lung parenchyma	Aggregates platelets Constricts arterioles, pulmonary vessels, and airways

PG = prostaglandin; PAF = platelet-activating factor; LT = leukotriene.

Table 8-2. Lipoxygenase products with a role in allergy and inflammation

Compound	Tissue source	Action
5-HETE	Granulocytes	Chemotaxis[a] granulocytes Chemokinesis[b] granulocytes, T-lymphocytes Augments histamine release
12-HETE	Platelets	Chemotaxis,[a] chemokinesis[b]
15-HETE	T-lymphocytes Lung	Inhibits 5-lipoxygenase WBC, 12-lipoxygenase platelets Major AA product in lung
5,12-diHETE	Granulocytes	Chemotaxis,[a] chemokinesis[b]
LTB$_4$	Granulocytes Macrophages Eosinophils	Potent chemotactant for neutrophils, eosinophils Causes adhesion of leukocytes to endothelium and migration of WBC into extravascular space Constricts airways
LTC$_4$ LTD$_4$ SRS LTE$_4$	Mast cells Macrophages Eosinophils Basophils	Constricts peripheral and central airways Constricts coronary arteries, pulmonary vessels Increases vascular permeability → edema Increases bronchial mucus, slows transport

WBC = white blood cells; AA = arachidonic acid; LT = leukotriene; HETE = hydroxyeicosatetraenoic acid; SRS = slow-reacting substance.
[a] Chemotactic potency: LTB$_4$ ≫ 5-HETE > 5,12-diHETE > 12-HETE.
[b] Chemokinesis refers to random migration leukocytes.

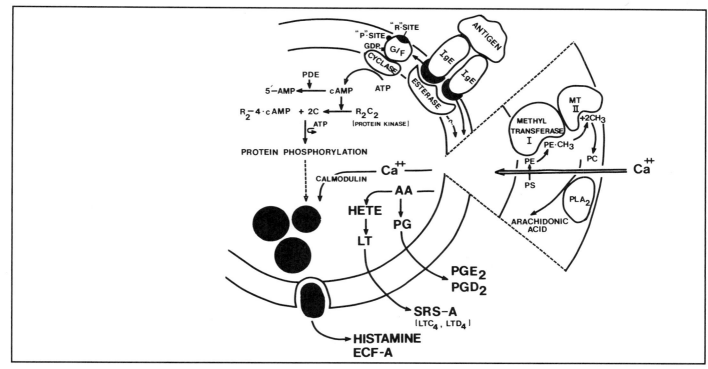

Fig. 8-2. *Mast cell schematic of the biochemical events of mediator release. PDE = phosphodiesterase; G/F = GTP binding, fluoride-activated regulatory protein; "R"-site = adenosine-binding site activated by analogs containing an unaltered ribose moiety; "P"-site = adenosine-binding site activated by adenosine analogs containing an intact purine ring; R_2C_2 = inactive protein kinase tetramere containing two catalytic (C) and two regulatory (R) proteins; AA = arachidonic acid; HETE = hydroxyeicosatetraenoic acid; PG = phosphatidylserine; PE = phosphatidylethanolamine; PE·CH_3 = monomethylphosphatidylethanolamine; +2CH_3 = addition of two methyl groups forming phosphatidylcholine (PC); PLA_2 = phospholipase A_2.*

Table 8-3. Mast cell-derived mediators

Preformed, rapidly released under physiologic conditions:
  Histamine
  Eosinophil chemotactic factors of anaphylaxis
  Neutrophil chemotactic factors
  Kininogenase
  Arylsulfatase A
Secondary or newly generated mediators:
  Superoxide and other reactive oxygen species
  Leukotrienes C_4, D_4, E_4
  Prostaglandins
  Monohydroxyeicosatetraenoic acids
  Hydroperoxyeicosatetraenoic acids
  Hydoxyheptadecatetraenoic acid
  Thromboxanes
  Prostaglandin-generating factor of anaphylaxis
  Adenosine
  Bradykinin
  Platelet-activating factor
Granule-associated mediators:
  Heparin or other proteoglycans
  Tryptase
  Chymotryptic proteinase
  Arylsulfatase B
  Inflammatory factors of anaphylaxis
  Peroxidase
  Superoxide dismutase

Source: G. L. Piacentini and M. Kaliner. The potential roles of leukotrienes in bronchial asthma. *Am. Rev. Respir. Dis.* 143:S96, 1991. Reprinted with permission.

Table 8-4. Pathologic changes in asthma and the mediators possibly responsible

Pathologic changes	Mast cell mediator responsible
Bronchial smooth muscle contraction	Histamine (H_1 response)
	Leukotrienes C_4, D_4, E_4
	Prostaglandins and thromboxane A_2
	Bradykinin
	Platelet-activating factor
	Chymotryptic proteinase
Mucosal edema	Histamine (H_1 response)
	Leukotrienes C_4, D_4, E_4
	Prostaglandin E_2
	Bradykinin
	Platelet-activating factor
Mucosal inflammation	Inflammatory factors or anaphylaxis
	Eosinophil chemotactic factors
	Neutrophil chemotactic factors
	Monohydroxyeicosatetraenoic acids
	Leukotrienes B_4
	Platelet-activating factor
Mucus secretion	Histamine (H_2 response)
	Prostaglandins and thromboxane A_2
	Chymotryptic proteinase
	Monohydroxyeicosatetraenoic acids
	Leukotrienes C_4, D_4, E_4
	Platelet-activating factor

Source: G. L. Piacentini and M. Kaliner. The potential roles of leukotrienes in bronchial asthma. *Am. Rev. Respir. Dis.* 143:S96, 1991. Reprinted with permission.

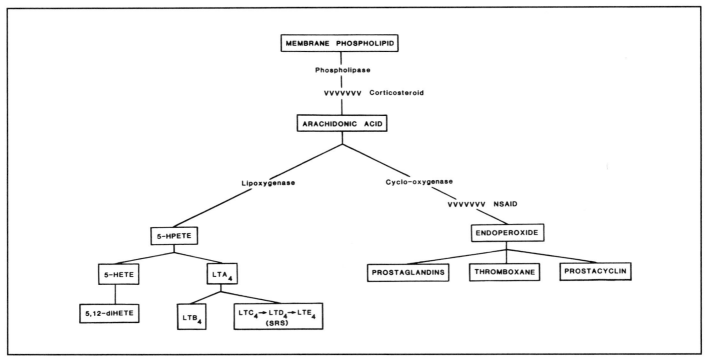

Fig. 8-3. *The arachidonic acid cascade. LT = leukotriene; NSAID = nonsteroidal antiinflammatory drugs.*

Fig. 8-4. *Model for the tetrameric high-affinity receptor for IgE. The receptor is oriented such that the large extracellular portion of the subunit is shown at the top, and the remainder of the chain on the left. To the right of the alpha subunit is the beta subunit with its four transmembrane segments, and to the right of the beta subunit is the dimer of gamma chains. The putative transmembrane segments have all been shown to consist of 21 residues and would presumably be in the alpha-helical conformation [19]. (Adapted by permission from Nature 337:187, 1989. Copyright © 1989 Macmillan Magazines Ltd.)*

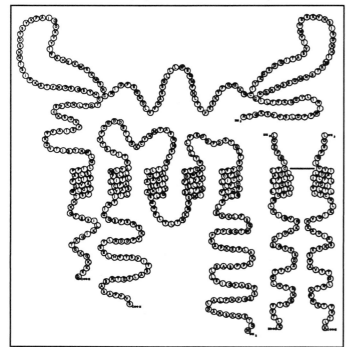

(and that of many others) following the identification of IgE as the active antibody responsible for hay fever, allergic asthma, and other allergic diseases [20]. The review by Ishizaka and colleagues of a number of attempts to suppress IgE antibody formation made through antigen-specific mechanisms led to these conclusions [27]: (1) Selective enhancement and suppression of IgE responses by various immunologic maneuvers probably share common mechanisms, that is, selective formation of either IgE-potentiating factor or IgE-suppressive factor. (2) The two IgE-binding factors are comparable in molecular weight, have affinity for IgE, and share a common determinant with FcεRI. (3) The main differences between them are their carbohydrate moieties, which play an essential role in their biologic activities. (4) The same T-cells appeared to form both IgE-potentiating and IgE-suppressive factor and the nature and biologic activities of IgE-binding factors appear to be decided by posttranslational glycosylation processes of the precursor molecules.

Regulatory Effects of Interleukin-4 and Interferon

There are apparently two regulatory influences involved in IgE synthesis, namely IgE-enhancing and IgE-suppressing factors. However, since the cloning of interleukin-4 (IL-4), it has become the major factor known to induce human IgE synthesis reproducibly [15].

Heusser and colleagues reviewed the gradually, more clearly defined steps required for the induction of an IgE response [17]. First, B-cells are stimulated to differentiate into IgE production (Fig. 8-5). In response to an antigen, B-cells are activated by a signal induced by physical interaction with T-cells [43]. Lymphokines, secreted by T-cells, then act on B-cells, inducing their differentiation [63], both processes following major histocompatibility complex (MHC) restriction [64]. It has been established that IL-4 instructs B-cells to switch to IgE production in both murine [8, 40, 45] and human [46] systems. Thus, human IgE responses are dependent on the physical contact of B-cells with activated helper T-cells as well as the presence of IL-4. In fact,

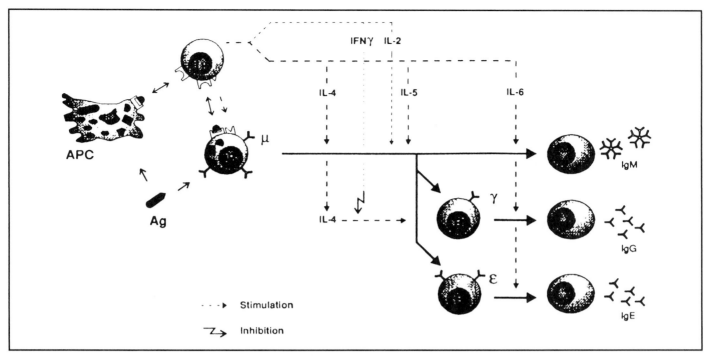

Fig. 8-5. *Mechanisms that regulate an immune response leading to specific IgE antibody formation. Ag = antigen; APC = antigen-presenting cell; IFN = interferon; IL = interleukin. (© 1989 by Hogrefe & Huber Publishers, 12 Bruce Park Avenue, Toronto, Ontario, Canada M4P 2S3. This figure has been reproduced with the permission of Hogrefe & Huber Publishers from C. H. Heusser, et al. Establishment of a memory in vivo murine IgE response to benzylpenicillin and its resistance to suppression by anti-IL-4 antibody. Int. Arch. Allergy Appl. Immunol. 90:45, 1989.)*

if IL-4 is provided by T-cells previously stimulated in an MHC restricted antigen cognate interaction, the noncognate signal can drive B-cells in a polyclonal fashion toward IgE secretion [51, 52].

Interferon gamma antagonizes the IL-4 switch induction in B-cells in both murine [7, 14, 49] and human [3, 31, 47, 60] systems. Interferon alpha blocks the IL-4–dependent IgE formation by human peripheral blood mononuclear cells (PBMCs) [10, 31]. Interferon alpha, like interferon gamma, functionally antagonizes the switch of B-cells to IgE. Interferon alpha has also been shown to reduce serum IgE levels, isotype specifically, in patients with atopic dermatitis, and leads to a transient clinical improvement [56]. An important implication of interferon alpha is that cells other than T-cells (e.g., macrophages) may also regulate B-cell activity with regard to IgE production.

Heusser's group also demonstrated that IL-4 provided by activated mast cells and basophil-like cells was able to induce the switch of B-cells to make IgE. The group concluded that it was possible that such a mast cell–dependent pathway of IgE formation is relevant in the allergen-mediated maintenance of a local allergic reaction. Thus, T-cell–activated B-cells could differentiate to IgE secretion in a mast cell–stimulated environment [17] (Fig. 8-6).

HUMAN IgE RESPONSES

In humans, PBMCs from normal nonatopic donors only produce IgE if the cells are cultured in the presence of exogenously added IL-4 [12]. However, PBMCs from atopic donors produce IgE spontaneously in vitro without the addition of IL-4 [11, 53]. PBMCs from such donors may contain activated T-cells that provide sufficient amounts of IL-4, and further investigations ascertained that the ongoing IgE response observed in vitro is dependent on

Table 8-5. Influences on IgE biosynthesis

Age
  Low level at birth
  Peaks at age 10 years
  Variably stable at ages 15–50 years
  Decreases with older age
Sex
  Possibly greater in males
Race
  Greater in Orientals, blacks, American Indians
Genetics
  Monozygotic twins have higher concordance
Infant feeding pattern
  Lower with breast-feeding

Source: Modified from P. V. Manuel and S. L. Bahna. Clinical aspects of serum total IgE level. *Immunol. Allergy Pract.* 5:212, 1983.

endogenously produced IL-4. Spontaneous IgE synthesis was not affected by the addition of a neutralizing anti–IL-4 antibody to the culture, whereas the IgE response induced by exogenously added IL-4 was completely suppressed [11]. The most likely explanation is that in an atopic situation, there are IgE-switched B-cells that have become IL-4 independent and may persist for longer periods [17].

Serum IgE concentrations are frequently elevated in patients with atopic disease, and the levels of IgE are influenced by the intensity of allergen exposure, age, sex, race, genetics, and, in infants, feeding patterns (Table 8-5). High IgE concentrations may also be found in patients with helminth infestations (*Ascaris, Necator,* and *Schistosoma*). Smaller increases in IgE concentra-

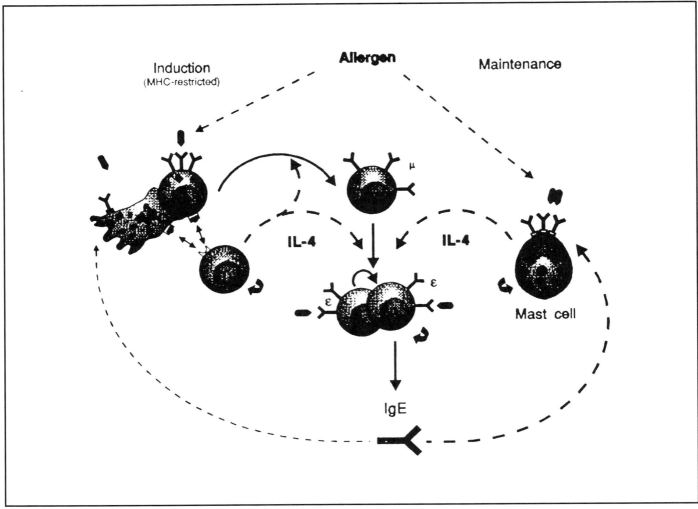

Fig. 8-6. *The pathways of T-cell–mediated induction and mast cell–mediated maintenance of a B-cell response leading to specific IgE antibody formation. IL = interleukin. (© 1989 by Hogrefe & Huber Publishers, 12 Bruce Park Avenue, Toronto, Ontario, Canada M4P 2S3. This figure has been reproduced with the permission of Hogrefe & Huber Publishers from C. H. Heusser, et al. Establishment of a memory in vitro murine IgE response to benzylpenicillin and its resistance to suppression by anti-IL-4 antibody.* Int. Arch. Allergy Appl. Immunol. *90: 45, 1989.)*

tion occur in patients with bacterial and viral infections (including acquired immunodeficiency syndrome [AIDS]), which may stimulate immunologic systems regulating IgE synthesis rather than specific antibody production [66] (Table 8-6). In an evaluation in children, a strong relationship between serum IgE levels and airway hyperresponsiveness was observed (Table 8-7). No asthma was seen in children with IgE levels lower than 32 IU/ml while 36 percent of children with IgE levels at 1,000 IU/ml or higher were reported to have asthma [54].

REGULATION OF IgE SYNTHESIS BY ANTI-IgE AUTOANTIBODIES

Another concept for human IgE regulation was proposed by Stadler's group in Bern, Switzerland [57, 59]. This concept moves away from the exclusive role of T-cells and emphasizes the role of anti-IgE autoantibodies [57, 59].

Antiidiotypic as well as antiisotypic anti-IgE autoantibodies have been described by many authors and there is substantial evidence that the naturally occurring antiisotypic anti-IgE antibodies may be composed of different functional types of autoantibodies [58, 59]. There are autoantibodies that lead to histamine release if incubated together with human basophils, and these may be regarded as anaphylactogenic antibodies (Fig. 8-7). Some, on the other hand, seem to be capable of binding to FcεRII-bound IgE without triggering histamine release. These antibodies may be of importance for the indirect regulation of IgE synthesis, for example, by inducing cytokine production from basophils and mast cells. This concept would again favor the possibility that cytokines such as IL-4 produced by mast cells are in effect the regulatory moiety. In the Swiss view, this type of IgE regulation is regarded as a feedback mechanism by the effector cells of the allergic reaction.

IgE bound to the low-affinity IgE receptor (CD23) may also be a target for autoantibodies. Using murine monoclonal anti-IgE antibodies, two distinct types of antibodies were characterized, one removing IgE from the surface and the other inhibiting the binding of IgE to CD23, depending on their epitope specificity

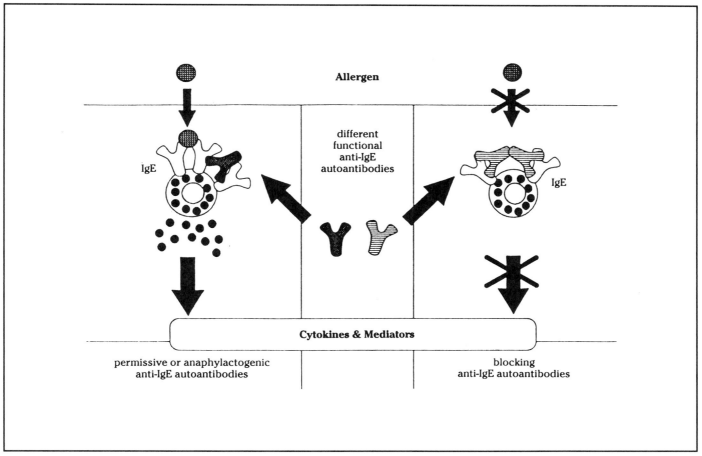

Fig. 8-7. *Anti-IgE autoantibodies and the effector phase of allergy. Anti-IgE autoantibodies that exist in serum are capable of triggering mediator release. Similarly, there may be anti-IgE autoantibodies that induce cytokine formation in basophils and mast cells, aggravating the inflammatory process. This may also represent a feedback mechanism for regulating IgE synthesis. Immune complexes consisting of anti-IgE autoantibodies and IgE are also found on the surface of basophils. Such autoantibodies may be permissive or not for allergen triggering. The ones that hinder allergen stimulation may represent the actual "blocking" antibodies in allergic reactions. (© 1991 by Hogrefe & Huber Publishers, 12 Bruce Park Avenue, Toronto, Ontario, Canada M4P 2S3. This figure has been reproduced with the permission of Hogrefe & Huber Publishers from B. M. Stadler. A new concept for human IgE regulation. Allergy Clin. Immunol. News 3:53, 1991.)*

[42]. Human anti-IgE autoantibodies isolated from natural immune complexes were demonstrated to effectively bind more IgE to CD23+ cells. Such autoantibodies may induce a signal via Fc or CD23 to the receptor-positive cells (Fig. 8-8).

The concept of the regulatory role of anti-IgE antibodies proposed by the Swiss group is depicted in Figure 8-9. It is proposed that the production of IgE and other isotypes will boost the production of antiisotype antibodies and initiate an autoimmune response. The nonatopic individual responds to allergen contact by developing "beneficial" anti-IgE autoantibodies to help clear the newly produced B_ϵ-cells or the IgE immunoglobulin itself. Secondary contact with allergen by the atopic individual results in sensitization of mast cells and basophils with IgE and anti-IgE antibodies that are nonblocking. This boosts IgE formation and a stronger autoimmune reaction against IgE with measurable accumulation in serum of "nonbeneficial" and "nonblocking" anti-IgE autoantibodies. The resultant generation of cytokines and enhancement of CD23 expression causes greater deposition of IgE and immune complexes of anti-IgE and IgE on CD23+ cells, which may represent an additional feedback or an amplifying arm for IgE regulation.

This emphasis on the role of anti-IgE autoantibodies has stimulated the Swiss investigators to generate recombinant anti-IgE autoantibodies, some of which may have therapeutic use by interfering with endogenous autoimmune responses, for example, by eliminating B-cells. They suggest that the success of hyposensitization indicates that our immune system learns to adjust to allergen, perhaps by changing the composition of the spectrum of anti-IgE autoantibodies. This, in turn, may result in a downregulation of IgE synthesis in vivo.

Additional strategies for modulating IgE synthesis have been proposed by O'Hehir and Lamb [43a]. These investigators have observed that following repeated exposure of activated house dust mite (HDM)–reactive cloned T-cells to subimmunogenic but escalating concentrations of whole HDM extract, the T-cells were partially nonresponsive to an immunogenic challenge. Similarly, pretreatment of cloned T-cells with single pulses of peptides of the Group I allergen of *D. pteronyssinus* at supraimmunogenic concentrations induced antigen-specific anergy resulting in inhibition of IL-4, but not IFN gamma, secretion on restimulation. IgE production is promoted by IL-4, whereas IFN gamma has the antagonistic effect of inhibiting IgE synthesis. Therefore, produc-

Table 8-6. Serum IgE levels in atopic and other diseases

	Mean IgE in percentage of normal	Percent patients with high IgE	U/ml*
Asthma			
Extrinsic	400–700	40–60	
Intrinsic	100		
Hay fever	200–400	20–40	
Eczema			
Atopic	300–1,100	Up to 80	
Contact	100		
Urticaria	100		
Parasites (e.g., *Ascaris*)	1,000–3,000		
Aspergillosis	Up to 1,000		
Virus infections	100		
Bacterial infections	100		
Autoimmune diseases	100		
Cancer	100		
Hyperimmuno-globulinemia E syndrome			2,150–40,000
Nezolof's syndrome			5–7,000
Wiskott-Aldrich syndrome			135–720

* Source: Data from R. H. Buckley and S. A. Fiscus. Serum IgD and IgE concentrations in immunodeficiency diseases. *J. Clin. Invest.* 55(Jan.):157, 1975.

Table 8-7. Percent of study children with airway responsiveness, according to symptoms and serum IgE levels[a]

		Any response[c]		
Serum IgE level (IU/ml)	Hyperresponsive[b]	All	No diagnosed asthma	No diagnosed asthma or wheezing
		percent (no. of children at risk)		
<32	1 (114)	2 (114)	2 (112)	0 (74)
32–99	5 (147)	10 (147)	7 (133)	8 (98)
100–315	14 (115)	23 (115)	17 (96)	13 (62)
316–999	17 (95)	26 (95)	17 (71)	18 (44)
>1000	28 (53)	38 (53)	28 (29)	21 (19)
P for trend	<0.0001	<0.0001	<0.0001	<0.0001

PC_{20} = provocation concentration of methacholine that produces a 20 percent fall in the forced expiratory volume in 1 second.
[a] Numbers in parentheses represent the children at risk. (Eighteen children given only albuterol and 20 children who declined to undergo methacholine challenge are not included.)
[b] Hyperresponsive was defined as a PC_{20} of ≤8 mg per milliliter.
[c] Any response was defined as a PC_{20} of ≤25 mg per milliliter. Numbers include children with hyperresponsiveness.
Source: M. R. Sears, et al. Relation between airway responsiveness and serum IgE in children with asthma and in apparently normal children. *N. Engl. J. Med.* 325: 1067, 1991. Reprinted by permission of the *New England Journal of Medicine*.

Fig. 8-8. *Anti-IgE autoantibodies and IgE association with CD23. There are convincing data that anti-IgE autoantibodies are capable of removing IgE from or inhibiting binding to the surface of CD23⁺ cells. Using anti-IgE autoantibodies, killing of IgE-sensitized CD23⁺ cells can be induced either by complement or killer cells. The question remains whether some anti-IgE autoantibodies may deliver a positive stimulatory signal to IgE-coated cells or, on the other hand, induce apoptosis. Thus, anti-IgE autoantibodies may be involved in clonal deletion of Bₑ-cells. ADCC = antibody-dependent cell-mediated cytotoxicity. (© 1991 by Hogrefe & Huber Publishers, 12 Bruce Park Avenue, Toronto, Ontario, Canada M4P 2S3. This figure has been reproduced with the permission of Hogrefe & Huber Publishers from B. M. Stadler. A new concept for human IgE regulation. Allergy Clin. Immunol. News 3:53, 1991.)*

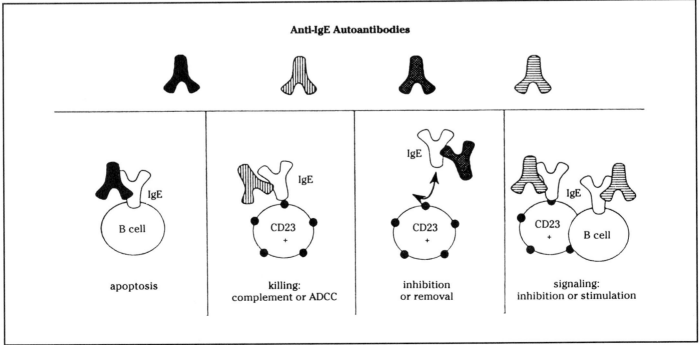

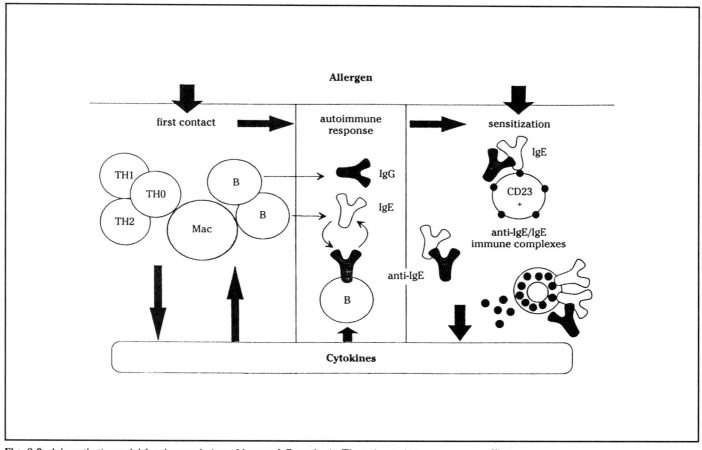

Fig. 8-9. *A hypothetic model for the regulation of human IgE synthesis. The primary immune response (first contact) to an allergen is controlled by the T-cell repertoire, and may not be significantly different in an atopic or nonatopic individual. During an autoimmune response, which depends on the B-cell repertoire, the nonatopic individual will eliminate IgE-producing cells or neutralize de novo formed IgE by anti-IgE autoantibodies. The atopic individual, in contrast, would not be capable of completely neutralizing the formed IgE, and allows IgE-producing cells to escape this internal control mechanism. A secondary contact (sensitization) with allergen leads to an accumulation of IgE and nonblocking immune complexes of IgE and anti-IgE on the effector cells of allergy, which in turn may generate more cytokines that amplify the inflammatory reaction, as well as the autoimmune response. (© 1991 by Hogrefe & Huber Publishers, 12 Bruce Park Avenue, Toronto, Ontario, Canada M4P 2S3. This figure has been reproduced with the permission of Hogrefe & Huber Publishers from B. M. Stadler. A new concept for human IgE regulation.* Allergy Clin. Immunol. News *3:53, 1991.)*

tion of IgE is dependent on the balance between the synthesis of these two lymphokines. The ability to selectively modulate lymphokine secretion by HDM-reactive T-cells, such that IL-4 production is inhibited and IFN gamma is enhanced, would be an advantage in the downregulation of allergic immune responsiveness. Experimental use of fragments of allergens for hyposensitization has already been adopted in clinical trials.

A second strategy involves modulation of specific responsiveness by antigen competition. A number of studies have confirmed that it is possible to develop nonstimulatory peptides with limited allele specificity that are able to inhibit T-cell recognition of HDM allergens. Further substitutions and modifications of structure, these investigators believe, may enhance the specificity of binding.

In summary, great advances in understanding the pathogenesis of immediate hypersensitivity reactions have followed the identification of IgE as the antibody mediator and the development of highly sensitive and specific methods for its assay. The further

characterization of the human epsilon chain, the cloning of the Fcε gene, the definition of the four-chain structure of the high-affinity receptor, and its cloning have created tremendous opportunities to define the molecular characteristics of the immediate hypersensitivity reactions. New concepts and brilliant new technologies are on the verge of providing both immunologic and pharmacologic measures to prevent and/or to obliterate the immediate hypersensitivity reaction—and without prejudice to the host's endogenous immunologic defense system.

REFERENCES

1. Bennich, H., et al. A comparative antigenic study of γE-globulin and myeloma-IgND. *J. Immunol.* 102:826, 1969.
2. Blank, U., et al. Complete structure and expression in transfected cells of high affinity IgE receptor. *Nature* 337:187, 1989.
3. Brinkmann, V., Kilchherr, E., and Heusser, C. H. Suppression of human IgE

secretion by interferon gamma and an interleukin-4 induced endogenous mechanism. Presented at the 7th International Congress of Immunology, Berlin, 1989. Abstract W-63-29.

4. Capron, A., et al. Specific IgE antibodies in immune adherence of normal macrophages to *Schistosoma mansoni* schistosomules. *Nature* 253:474, 1975.

5. Capron, M., et al. Evidence for IgE-dependent cytotoxicity by rat eosinophils. *J. Immunol.* 126:1764, 1981.

6. Capron, M., et al. Role of IgE receptors in effector function of human eosinophils. *J. Immunol.* 132:462, 1984.

7. Coffman, R. L., and Carty, J. A T cell activity that enhances polyclonal IgE production and its inhibition by interferon gamma. *J. Immunol.* 136:949, 1986.

8. Coffman, R. L., et al. B cell stimulator factor-1 enhances the IgE response of lipopolysaccharide activated B cells. *J. Immunol.* 136:4538, 1986.

9. Conroy, M. C., Adkinson, N. F., and Lichtenstein, L. M. Measurement of IgE on human basophils: Relation to serum IgE and anti-IgE induced histamine release. *J. Immunol.* 118:1317, 1977.

10. Delespessee, G., Sarfati, M., and Peleman, R. Influence of recombinant IL-4, IFN-alpha and IFN-gamma on the production of IgE-binding factor (soluble CD23). *J. Immunol.* 142:134, 1989.

11. Delespessee, G., et al. The ongoing IgE synthesis of lymphocytes from atopic individuals is IL-4 independent. Presented at the 7th International Congress of Immunology, Berlin, 1989. Abstract W-75-7.

12. Del Prete, G. F., et al. IL-4 is an essential factor for the IgE synthesis induced *in vitro* by human T cell clones and their supernatants. *J. Immunol.* 140:4193, 1988.

13. Dessaint, J. P., and Capron, A. IgE and inflammatory cells: The cellular networks in allergy. *Int. Arch. Allergy Appl. Immunol.* 90:28, 1989.

14. Finkelman, F. D., and Holmes, J. Lymphokine control of *in vivo* immunoglobulin isotype selection. *Annu. Rev. Immunol.* 8:303, 1990.

15. Finkelman, F. D., et al. IL-4 is required to generate and sustain *in vivo* IgE responses. *J. Immunol.* 141:2335, 1988.

16. Gordon, J., and Guy, G. R. The molecules controlling B lymphocytes. *Immunol. Today* 8:339, 1987.

17. Heusser, C. H., et al. Establishment of a memory *in vitro* murine IgE response to benzylpenicillin and its resistance to suppression by anti-IL-4 antibody. *Int. Arch. Allergy Appl. Immunol.* 90:45, 1989.

18. Hughes, J. M., Seale, J. P., and Temple, D. M. Effect of fenoterol on immunologic release of leukotrienes and histamine from human lung *in vitro*: Selective antagonism by B-adrenoreceptor antagonists. *Eur. J. Pharmacol.* 95:239, 1983.

19. Ishizaka, K. Basic mechanisms of IgE-mediated hypersensitivity. *Curr. Opin. Immunol.* 1:625, 1989.

20. Ishizaka, K. Regulation of IgE synthesis. *Annu. Rev. Immunol.* 2:159, 1984.

21. Ishizaka, K., and Ishizaka, T. Induction of erythema-wheal reactions by soluble antigen-γE antibody complexes in humans. *J. Immunol.* 101:68, 1968.

22. Ishizaka, K., and Ishizaka, T. Reversed type allergic skin reactions by anti-E globulin antibodies in humans and monkeys. *J. Immunol.* 100:544, 1968.

23. Ishizaka, K., and Ishizaka, T. Immune mechanisms of reversed type reaginic hypersensitivity. *J. Immunol.* 103:588, 1969.

24. Ishizaka, K., Ishizaka, T., and Hornbrook, M. M. Physiochemical properties of human reaginic antibody. IV. Presence of a unique immunoglobulin as a carrier of reaginic activity. *J. Immunol.* 97:75, 1966.

25. Ishizaka, K., Ishizaka, T., and Hornbrook, M. M. Physiochemical properties of human reaginic antibody. V. Correlation of reaginic activity with γE-globulin antibody. *J. Immunol.* 97:840, 1966.

26. Ishizaka, K., Ishizaka, T., and Hornbrook, M. M. Allergen-binding activity of γE, γG, and γA antibodies in sera from atopic patients. *In vitro* measurements of reaginic antibody. *J. Immunol.* 98:490, 1967.

27. Ishizaka, K., et al. T cell factors involved in the regulation of IgE synthesis. *Int. Arch. Allergy Appl. Immunol.* 105:383, 1987.

28. Ishizaka, T., and Ishizaka, K. Triggering of histamine release from rat mast cells by divalent antibodies against IgE receptors. *J. Immunol.* 120:800, 1978.

29. Ishizaka, T., Ishizaka, K., and Tomioka, H. Release of histamine and slow reacting substance of anaphylaxis (SRS-A) by IgE-anti-IgE reaction on monkey mast cells. *J. Immunol.* 108:513, 1972.

30. Ishizaka, T., Soto, C. S., and Ishizaka, K. Mechanisms of passive sensitiza-

tion. III. Number of IgE molecules and their receptor sites on human basophil granulocytes. *J. Immunol.* 111:500, 1973.

31. Johansson, S. G. O., and Bennich, H. Immunologic studies of an atypical (myeloma) immunoglobulin. *Immunology* 13:381, 1967.

32. Johansson, S. G. O., Bennich, H., and Wide, L. A new class of immunoglobulin in human serum. *Immunology* 14:265, 1968.

33. Joseph, M., et al. The receptor for IgE on blood platelets. *Eur. J. Immunol.* 16:306, 1986.

34. Kabat, E. A. Getting started 50 years ago—Experiences, perspectives, and problems of the first 21 years. *Annu. Rev. Immunol.* 1:14, 1983.

35. Kinet, J. P. The IgE receptor: Target for allergy therapy. *NIH Observer* 2 (Nov/Dec):3, 1990.

36. Melewicz, F. M., et al. Characterization of Fc receptors for IgE on human alveolar macrophages. *Clin. Exp. Immunol.* 49:364, 1982.

37. Melewicz, F. M., Plummer, J. M., and Spiegelberg, H. L. Comparison of the Fc receptors for IgE on human lymphocytes and monocytes. *J. Immunol.* 129:563, 1982.

38. Melewicz, F. M., and Spiegelberg, H. L. Fc receptors of IgE on a subpopulation of human peripheral blood monocytes. *J. Immunol.* 125:1026, 1980.

39. Metzger, H. Molecular aspects of receptors and binding factors for IgE. *Adv. Immunol.* 80:227, 1988.

40. Moon, H. B., et al. Regulation of IgG1 and IgE synthesis by interleukin-4 in mouse B cells. *Scand. J. Immunol.* 30:355, 1989.

41. Moqbel, R. Leucocyte Mediator Release by Anti-IgE. In F. Shakib (ed.), *Autoantibodies to Immunoglobulins. Monographs in Allergy,* Vol. 26. Basel: Karger, 1989. Pp. 103–113.

42. Nakajima, K., de Weck, A. L., and Stadler, B. M. Effect of anti-IgE antibodies on IgE binding to CD23. *Allergy* 44:187, 1989.

43. Noelle, R. J., et al. Cognate interactions between helper T cells and B cells. III. Contact-dependent, lymphokine-independent induction of B cell cycle entry by activated helper T cells. *J. Immunol.* 143:1807, 1989.

43a. O'Hehir, R. E., and Lamb, J. R. Strategies for modulating immunoglobulin E synthesis. *Clin. Exp. Allergy* 22:7, 1992.

44. Osler, A. G., Lichtenstein, L. M., and Levy, D. In vitro studies of human reaginic allergy. *Adv. Immunol.* 8:183, 1968.

45. Peachell, P. T., et al. Regulation of human basophils and lung mast cell function by cAMP. *J. Immunol.* 140:571, 1988.

46. Pène, J., et al. IgE production by normal human lymphocytes is induced by interleukin-4 and suppressed by interferons gamma and alpha and prostaglandin E2. *Proc. Natl. Acad. Sci. USA* 85:6880, 1988.

47. Pène, J., et al. IgE production by normal human B cells induced by alloreactive T cell clones is mediated by IL-4 and suppressed by IFN-gamma. *J. Immunol.* 141:1218, 1988.

47a. Platts-Mills, T. A. E. Mechanisms of bronchial reactivity: The role of immunoglobulin E. *Am. Rev. Respir. Dis.* 145:S44, 1992.

48. Prausnitz, C., and Küstner, H. Studien uber die Ueberemfindlichkeit. *Zentralbl. Bkt. Orig.* 86:160, 1921.

49. Rabin, E. M., et al. Interferon gamma inhibits the action of B cell stimulatory factor (BSF)-1 on resting B cells. *J. Immunol.* 137:1573, 1986.

50. Rocklin, R. E., and Findlay, S. R. Immunologic Mechanism and Recent Advances in Asthma. In E. B. Weiss (ed.), *Bronchial Asthma: Mechanisms and Therapeutics* (2nd ed.). Boston: Little, Brown, 1985. Pp. 41–51.

51. Romagnani, S. Regulation and deregulation of human IgE synthesis. *Immunol. Today* 11:316, 1990.

52. Romagnani, S., and Ricci, S. Present views on the regulation of human IgE synthesis. *Allergy Clin. Immunol. News* 2:192, 1990.

53. Sarfati, M., et al. The spontaneous secretion of IgE by B lymphocytes from allergic individuals: A model to investigate the regulation of human IgE synthesis. *Immunology* 53:187, 1984.

54. Sears, M. R., et al. Relation between airway responsiveness and serum IgE in children with asthma and in apparently normal children. *N. Engl. J. Med.* 325:1067, 1991.

55. Snapper, C. M., Finkelman, F. D., and Paul, W. E. Differential regulation of IgG1 and IgE synthesis by interleukin-4. *J. Exp. Med.* 167:183, 1988.

56. Souillet, G., Rousset, F., and De Vries, J. E. Alpha-interferon treatment of a patient with hyper IgE syndrome. *Lancet* 1:1384, 1989.

57. Stadler, B. M. A new concept for human IgE regulation. *Allergy Clin. Immunol. News* 3:53, 1991.

58. Stadler, B. M., et al. IgG anti-IgE autoantibodies in immunoregulation. *Int. Arch. Allergy Appl. Immunol.* 94:83, 1991.

59. Stadler, B. M., et al. Anti-isotype Regulation: Cytokines and Anti-IgE auto-

antibodies. In C. Sorg (ed.), *Cytokines*, Vol. 2. *Cytokines Regulating the Allergic Response.* Basel: Karger, 1989. Pp. 37–50.

60. Thyphronitis, G., et al. IgE secretion by Epstein-Barr virus-infected purified human B lymphocytes is stimulated by IL-4 and suppressed by IFN-gamma. *Proc. Natl. Acad. Sci. USA* 86:5580, 1989.

61. Undem, B. J., and Buckner, C. K. Effects of forskolin alone and in combination with isoproterenol on antigen-induced histamine release from guinea pig minced lung. *Arch. Int. Pharmacodyn. Ther.* 281:110, 1986.

62. Undem, B. J., Peachell, P. T., and Lichtenstein, L. M. Isoproterenol-induced inhibition of immunoglobulin E-mediated release of histamine and arachi-donic acid metabolites from the human lung mast cell. *J. Pharmacol. Exp. Ther.* 247:209, 1988.

63. Vercelli, D., and Geha, R. Regulation of IgE synthesis in humans. *J. Clin. Immunol.* 9:75, 1989.

64. Vitetta, E. S., et al. Cellular interactions in the immune response. *Adv. Immunol.* 45:1, 1989.

65. Wide, L., Bennich, H., and Johansson, S. G. O. Diagnosis of allergy by an in vitro test for allergen antibodies. *Lancet* 2:1105, 1967.

66. Wright, D. N., et al. Serum IgE and human immunodeficiency virus (HIV) infection. *J. Allergy Clin. Immunol.* 85:445, 1990.

Inflammation

9

Peter J. Barnes

In recent years, views about asthma have changed rather strikingly. In the past, asthma was viewed simply as allergen-induced mast cell degranulation, resulting in the release of mediators such as histamine and slow-reacting substance of anaphylaxis (sulfidopeptide leukotrienes) that contracted airway smooth muscle (Fig. 9-1). It has now become clear that asthma is a chronic inflammatory disease involving many interacting cells which release a whole variety of inflammatory mediators that activate several target cells in the airway, resulting in bronchoconstriction, microvascular leakage and edema, mucus hypersecretion, and stimulation of neural reflexes [13] (Fig. 9-2, Table 9-1). This chapter reviews the components of this inflammatory process.

ASTHMA AS AN INFLAMMATORY DISEASE

Inflammatory responses are concerned with defense against invasion by outside organisms and with tissue repair, and are thus beneficial. However in asthma the inflammatory response appears to have been mounted inappropriately, leading to adverse effects. Inflammation is a general process, but the type of inflammatory response may vary considerably from tissue to tissue and with different initiating stimuli. The cardinal signs of inflammation are *calor* and *rubor* (heat and redness form vasodilatation), *tumor* (swelling from plasma exudation and edema), and *dolor* (pain from sensitization of sensory nerves). More recent research has highlighted the importance of migration of inflammatory cells from the circulation into the airway tissues. Recent research has emphasized the fact that the inflammatory process in asthmatic airways appears to have common features from patient to patient, irrespective of whether asthma is allergic in origin ("extrinsic") or apparently nonallergic ("intrinsic") [68]. Thus, although there may be several ways of initiating this inflammatory response, the inflammation that is characteristic of asthma is typified by infiltration with eosinophils and lymphocytes and by shedding of airway epithelial cells. These inflammatory changes may be seen even in patients with the mildest of asthma.

Fatal Asthma

It has long been recognized that patients who die from asthma attacks have grossly abnormal lungs. Post mortem the lungs fail to deflate due to widespread occlusion of airways by tenacious mucus plugs, which resulted in fatal hypoxia. Histologic studies have demonstrated several common features, including occlusion of the airway lumen by plugs comprised of exuded plasma proteins and mucus glycoproteins, which have trapped cellular debris consisting of shed epithelial cells and inflammatory cells. The airway epithelium shows widespread shedding and there is thickening of the subepithelial layer [70] (see Chap. 28). The airway smooth muscle layer is invariably thickened, due to hypertrophy of airway smooth muscle cells [71, 180]. There is also mucous gland and goblet cell hyperplasia. The whole airway wall is thickened and edematous, and is infiltrated with various inflammatory cells, but most notably eosinophils and lymphocytes. This inflammatory response is seen throughout the length of the airways, from the trachea down to the terminal bronchioles, although the intensity of inflammation may vary from area to area. The inflammation never appears to extend into the lung parenchyma, but occasionally there is inflammation in pulmonary vessels adjacent to peripheral airways [180]. The pathologic appearance of fatal asthma is characteristic, particularly in the presence of activated eosinophils and extensive epithelial shedding.

Bronchoalveolar Lavage

Bronchoalveolar lavage (BAL), which has demonstrated many characteristic differences between normal and diseased lungs, has provided evidence that there is an active inflammatory process in asthmatic airways (see Chap. 24). Several studies have demonstrated an increase in the percentage of mast cells and eosinophils [81, 95, 124, 135, 204], whereas others have revealed increases in lymphocytes [95, 121] and epithelial cells [26, 204]. The major problem in interpreting lavage results is the variable dilution which may change the composition of the fluid collected, and there appears to be no satisfactory method for correcting this dilutional factor [202]. BAL fluid does provide a useful source of inflammatory cells for further investigation, however. Furthermore, the cellular composition of BAL material may not accurately reflect the inflammatory state in the underlying mucosa, as has become evident with interstitial lung disease. There are likely to be even greater discrepancies in asthmatic airways, since many of the lavaged cells originate in the alveolar spaces and "dilute" the inflammatory cells derived from airways. This may be overcome by selected lavage of airways using double-lumen catheters with balloons to isolate a segment of a proximal airway. This provides a more accurate assessment of the inflammatory status of a proximal airway, but does not provide sufficient cells for detailed study. Premedication and the persistence of previous antiasthma therapies may affect cell function and give misleading information about cell activation and regulation in asthma. These issues will have to be increasingly addressed as research into the cell biology of asthma progresses.

Bronchial Biopsy

Although the inflammatory nature of fatal asthma has long been recognized, it is now apparent that inflammation may be present even in patients with mild asthma. Bronchial biopsies have confirmed that similar, though less severe changes are present in the mucosa of patients with mild asthma [26, 33, 63, 94, 112, 131,

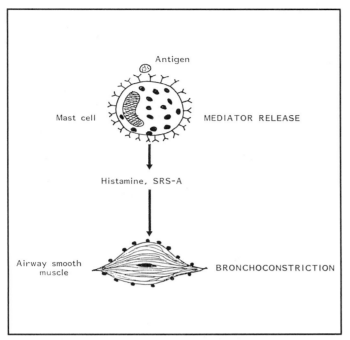

Fig. 9-1. *The traditional view of asthma emphasized mast cells and airway smooth muscle contraction. SRS-A = slow-reacting substance of anaphylaxis.*

Table 9-1. *Major events in an inflammatory response*

Pathophysiologic events	Associated structural changes
Tissue injury	Disrupted epithelium and
Mediator release	damaged subepithelial
From damaged cells	structure
Lipid peroxidation of arachidonic acid	
From activated plasma	
Complement system	
Kinin system	
Fibrinolytic system	
Coagulation system	
From tissue	
Mast cells	
Nerve endings	
Vascular response	
Increased blood flow	Congested vascular bed
Fluid exudation from microvessels	Edema
Cellular response	
Migration of inflammatory cells into the exudate	Presence of inflammatory cells in fluid exudate
Release of additional mediators	
Repair	
Stimulation of epithelium	Goblet cell metaplasia, squamous cell metaplasia, basement membrane formation
Stimulation of subepithelial connective tissue	Connective tissue deposition, increased muscle

Source: J. C. Hogg, A. L. James, and P. D. Paré. Evidence of inflammation in asthma. *Am. Rev. Respir. Dis.* 143:S39, 1991. Reprinted with permission.

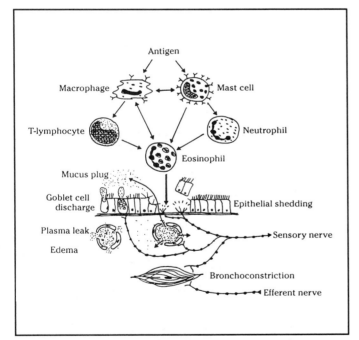

Fig. 9-2. *The current view of asthma includes several inflammatory cells which interact in a complex manner and release multiple inflammatory mediators that act on various target cells of the airways to produce the characteristic pathophysiology of asthma.*

143, 170, 175]. These studies revealed eosinophil infiltration, and a variable degree of epithelial disruption and subepithelial fibrosis. These inflammatory changes may be present in even the mildest forms of asthma and confirm the view that asthma is an inflammatory condition. However, biopsy studies have limitations. The airways from which biopsy specimens may be taken

are proximal and therefore no information is provided about inflammatory changes in the more peripheral airways known to be involved in asthma [70, 180]. The inflammatory changes have long been recognized to be patchy, and it is therefore difficult to make useful correlations with asthma severity. The biopsy procedure itself, particularly with fiberoptic bronchoscopy, may lead to artifacts and pressure distortion, making a detailed analysis of structure difficult. Finally, histologic studies do not give information about cell activity, although an increasing number of cell-surface markers are now available and may give insights into the state of activation, particularly in immune cells. The use of complementary DNA (cDNA) probes and the polymerase chain reaction may provide useful information about the synthesis of various proteins (e.g., cytokines, enzymes, receptors) by cells in the asthmatic airway.

Inflammation and Symptoms

There is compelling evidence that inflammation underlies the phenomenon of airway hyperresponsiveness (AHR), which is the hallmark of asthma [48, 159] (Fig. 9-3). The precise relationship between airway inflammation, AHR, and symptoms is still not certain and the commonly used tests of AHR, such as histamine or methacholine challenge, may not relate as closely to clinical symptoms in individual patients as had been suspected [36, 116]. This may be because inflammation may directly lead to symptoms, perhaps by activating sensitized sensory nerve endings in the inflamed airway, and resulting in symptoms such as cough and chest tightness, which may be the equivalent of inflammatory pain in other organs. Antiinflammatory treatments, such as the inhalation of steroids, are often rapidly successful in the control of asthma symptoms, yet have a relatively small effect in reducing AHR [16]! This is presumably because the control of inflammation directly reduces some symptoms and there is some reduction in AHR due to active inflammation, but residual AHR may be due to

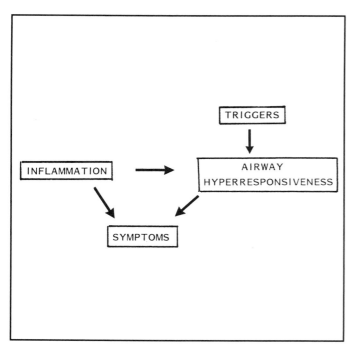

Fig. 9-3. *Interrelationship between airway inflammation, airway hyperresponsiveness, and symptoms in asthma.*

structural changes in the airway that are not reversible by any known treatment.

Animal Models

There are no satisfactory animal models of asthma, as detailed in Chapter 31, and previous "models" have proved to be very misleading, since the information provided was not applicable to either normal or asthmatic humans. Animals may be useful in modeling certain aspects of the asthmatic process, however [136, 188]. Most models of asthma have been used to investigate acute effects on airway function, yet asthma is a chronic inflammatory disease that may result in biochemical and structural changes quite distinct from those seen during short-term studies. There has been considerable debate about the choice of species for asthma research, but different species may be useful for the investigation of different aspects of asthmatic inflammation, providing it is remembered that inflammatory mediators, receptors, and innervation show marked species differences.

Human Models

Because of marked differences between species, there has recently been increasing emphasis on studies in humans. Thus, human inflammatory cells may be obtained from peripheral blood and BAL material, and human airways obtained at lung surgery. However, normal cells and airways may not behave in the same way as asthmatic tissues, which may have been modified by chronic inflammation.

In vivo studies of asthmatic patients have proved to be very valuable in elucidating the inflammatory mechanisms in asthma. Measurement of AHR is precise and can be performed repeatedly and after treatments or pharmacologic interventions. Allergen challenge has proved particularly useful. The early response after allergen inhalation is completely inhibited and reversed by beta agonists and is likely to be due to airway smooth muscle contraction. A late-phase response often follows 4 to 6 hours after allergen challenge; the airway narrowing is slower in onset and asso-

ciated with greater symptoms, which may include systemic symptoms [159, 168]. This response is more difficult to reverse with beta agonists and may be due to infiltration of inflammatory cells and submucosal edema [55, 64, 159] (see Chap. 12). The late response may be followed by a prolonged period of increased AHR, during which the patient experiences increased symptoms, such as exercise- and irritant-induced wheeze [54] and recurrent nocturnal asthma [157]. This period of increased AHR may last for 1 to 4 weeks, and is currently presumed to be due to increased inflammation in the airway resulting from allergen exposure. Although acute allergen exposure is a useful model of allergic asthma, it is somewhat artificial since asthmatic patients are rarely exposed over such a short time to such large doses of allergen. Usually the asthmatic subject is exposed to very small concentrations of allergen that may give rise to a "grumbling" chronic inflammation, which may differ in its nature and pharmacology from the acute and subacute inflammation provoked by the conventional allergen challenge.

A related question is how the inflammatory state of the airway should be assessed in asthmatic patients, particularly in the evaluation of new therapies. It is clearly impractical to consider repeated biopsy and BAL, although this may be indicated in exceptional circumstances for research purposes. Measurement of AHR by histamine or methacholine challenge may give some indication of the inflammatory state of the airways, although as noted above there may be discrepancies between exacerbations of asthma and increases in AHR. Furthermore, the effects of bronchodilator medications may interfere with these measurements. A more practical method of assessing inflammation may be the measurement of airway function during the day. Monitoring peak expiratory flow (PEF) in the morning and evening allows the measurement of diurnal variability of airway obstruction, which may be a reasonable assessment of airway inflammation. The need for beta-agonist rescue medication may also give a similar indication. Further studies are needed on the relationship between symptoms, PEF variability, AHR, and inflammation.

INFLAMMATORY CELLS

It is now clear that many different inflammatory cells are involved in asthma, although the precise role of each cell type is not yet certain.

Mast Cells

Mast cells, discussed in detail in Chapter 21, have long been associated with asthma, since they release a variety of preformed and newly synthesized mediators that could account for several features of asthma. Mast cells are activated by allergen via cross-linking of high-affinity IgE Fc receptors (FcεRI). Mast cells are superficially localized in the airway epithelium and are ideally located to respond to inhaled allergen. There is an apparent increase in mast cells in the BAL material of asthmatic patients [81, 198]. The mast cells in the bronchial mucosa and lumen belong to the MC_T type, whose secretory granules contain the neutral protease tryptase, in distinction to the connective tissue–type mast cells which contain both tryptase and chymase (MC_{TC}) [185]. There is histologic evidence for continuing mast cell activation in asthma, since mast cells in asthma biopsy specimens have an appearance of degranulation [26]. This is supported by the increased concentrations of histamine and tryptase, both derived from mast cell granules, in BAL fluid of asthma patients [43, 207]. Circumstantial evidence strongly links the mast cell with the early response to allergen, and there is good reason to think that it may also be involved in other "indirect" challenges, such as exercise and fog. Mast cells release a variety of mediators, including histamine, prostaglandin (PG) D_2, and leukotriene (LT)

C_4, which may contribute to immediate bronchoconstrictor responses. Mast cells also release enzymes such as tryptase, which may degrade bronchodilator peptides such as vasoactive intestinal peptide [44] and heparin, an important component of the granule that binds histamine. Heparin may be an important antiinflammatory mechanism and may inactivate the basic proteins released from eosinophils [164].

The role of the mast cell in the late response, AHR, and thus chronic asthma has recently been questioned, however. Cromolyn sodium was shown to stabilize rat peritoneal mast cells [59] and this seemed a reasonable explanation for its ability to prevent early and late bronchoconstrictor responses to allergen. More potent mast cell stabilizers that were later developed (more than 30 such compounds have now gone into clinical trial) failed to show any useful effect in clinical asthma and, although some of these drugs protected against early responses to allergen, they failed to prevent late responses and did not reduce subsequent AHR [191]. In addition, beta$_2$ agonists such as albuterol and terbutaline, which are potent stabilizers of human mast cells [53], fail to inhibit late responses or to reduce AHR [56, 122, 126]. Indeed, there are indications that regular therapy with beta agonists may even increase AHR in patients with chronic asthma [186, 200]. Furthermore, corticosteroids, which when given in a single dose have no effect on the early response and are highly effective in preventing the late response and in preventing the subsequent increase in AHR, have no apparent direct action on human lung mast cells [184]. Thus, although mast cells are involved in immediate responses to allergens (and probably other acute challenges, such as exercise and fog), they are less likely to play a critical role in AHR and chronic asthma.

Macrophages

There has been increasing interest in the possible role of macrophages in asthma, particularly following the observation that they may be activated by allergen via a low-affinity IgE receptor (FcϵRII) [90, 115]. Macrophages make up the majority of cells in BAL fluid and are derived from blood monocytes. Although usually referred to as alveolar macrophages, macrophages also traffic through the airways and are present in the mucosa and submucosa. There is a marked increase in the numbers of macrophages in BAL fluid after allergen challenge in asthmatic patients [150] and increased numbers of macrophages in biopsies from asthmatic patients [222]. BAL macrophages from asthmatic subjects release increased amounts of oxygen-derived free radicals [121], indicating that they have been activated by some endogenous mechanism.

Macrophages release a whole variety of mediators, and over 100 different secretory products have been identified [156]. Macrophages may release a different spectrum of mediators, depending on the type and intensity of stimulation, and in this way they may play a very important role in determining the characteristics of the inflammatory response. Thus, after allergen exposure alveolar macrophages release a variety of inflammatory mediators, including LTB$_4$, PGF$_{2\alpha}$, thromboxane (TX) B$_2$, and platelet-activating factor (PAF) [4, 146]. Macrophages also release a large variety of cytokines, peptide mediators that are now recognized to play a very important role in chronic inflammation and the communication between different inflammatory cells [120]. These cytokines include interleukin (IL) -1, IL-8, IL-10, granulocyte-macrophage colony-stimulating factor (GM-CSF), histamine-releasing factors, and tumor necrosis factor-alpha (TNF-α) (see also Chap. 13).

Macrophages may both increase and decrease inflammation, depending on the stimulus. Alveolar macrophages normally have a suppressive effect on lymphocyte function, but this may be impaired in asthma after allergen exposure [5, 189]. Macrophages may therefore play an important antiinflammatory role, preventing the development of allergic inflammation. Macrophages may also act as antigen-presenting cells that process allergen for presentation to T-lymphocytes, although alveolar macrophages are far less effective in this respect than macrophages from other sites, such as the peritoneum [101]. By contrast, dendritic cells, which are specialized macrophages in the airway epithelium, are very effective antigen-presenting cells [102] and may therefore play a very important role in the initiation of allergen-induced responses.

The pharmacology of macrophages is quite different from that of mast cells. In contrast to mast cells, release of mediators from alveolar macrophages is inhibited by corticosteroids [89], but not by beta agonists [91]. This would be consistent with a role for macrophages in the initiation of the late response and AHR.

Eosinophils

Eosinophil infiltration is a characteristic feature of asthmatic airways and differentiates asthma from other inflammatory conditions of the airway. Indeed, asthma might more accurately be termed *chronic eosinophilic bronchitis*. Allergen inhalation results in a marked increase in eosinophils in BAL fluid at the time of the late reaction [64, 151], and there is a close relationship between eosinophil counts in peripheral blood or bronchial lavage and AHR [195, 204].

Eosinophils (see Chap. 20) were originally viewed as beneficial cells in asthma, as they have the capacity to inactivate histamine and leukotrienes, but it now seems more likely that they play a damaging role, and may be linked to the development of AHR [93]. Eosinophils may be activated in a number of different ways, including allergen via FcϵRII [41, 42], PAF [127, 128], and cytokines such as GM-CSF and IL-5 [209, 214].

Eosinophils release a variety of mediators, including LTC$_4$, PAF, 15-hydroxyeicosatetraenoic acid (15-HETE), and oxygen-derived free radicals. Eosinophils from asthmatic patients produce more PAF than those from normal donors [137], which may be a reflection of this activation. Eosinophils also release basic proteins that are toxic to airway epithelium, such as major basic protein (MBP), eosinophil cationic protein (ECP), eosinophil-derived neurotoxin, and eosinophil peroxidase [93, 154]. Eosinophils cause marked epithelial shedding when they are stimulated to degranulate [212]. Activated eosinophils in the airway lumen may thus lead to the epithelial shedding that is so characteristic of asthma [26, 131]. In vitro MBP causes an increase in airway responsiveness, which appears to be due to inhibition of the release of a putative epithelium-derived relaxant factor (EpDRF) [80] (see Chap. 23). There is evidence for increased release of MBP and ECP in the BAL fluid of asthmatic subjects [64, 204], and a correlation with AHR has been reported [204].

An important area of research is now concerned with the mechanisms involved in recruitment of eosinophils into asthmatic airways. Eosinophils are derived from bone marrow precursors. After allergen challenge, eosinophils appear in BAL fluid during the late response [64], and this is associated with a decrease in peripheral eosinophil counts and with the appearance of eosinophil progenitors in the circulation [92]. The signal for increased eosinophil production is presumably derived from the inflamed airway. Eosinophil recruitment initially involves adhesion of eosinophils to vascular endothelial cells in the airway circulation, their migration into the submucosa, and their subsequent activation (Fig. 9-4). The role of individual cytokines and mediators in orchestrating these responses has yet to be clarified.

Adhesion of eosinophils involves the expression of specific glycoprotein molecules on the surface of eosinophils (integrins) and their expression of such molecules as intercellular adhesion molecule-1 (ICAM-1) on vascular endothelial cells. A recent study demonstrated that in sensitized monkeys, an antibody directed at

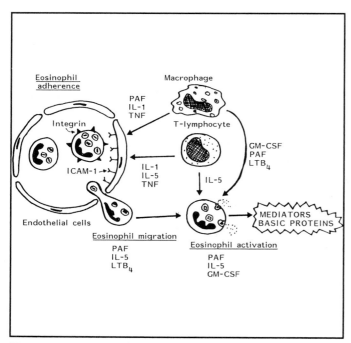

Fig. 9-4. *Mechanisms of eosinophilic inflammation. Eosinophils firstly adhere to endothelial cells in the bronchial circulation and then migrate into the tissue where they survive and are activated to release mediators and granule products. Each step is directed by specific agents that may be released from macrophages and T-lymphocytes. ICAM-1 = intercellular adhesion molecule-1; PAF = platelet-activating factor; IL = interleukin; TNF = tumor necrosis factor; GM-CSF = granulocyte-macrophage colony-stimulating factor; LTB_4 = leukotriene B_4.*

ICAM-1 markedly inhibits eosinophil accumulation in the airways after allergen exposure and also blocks the accompanying hyperresponsiveness [206]. Eosinophil migration may be due to the effects of PAF, which is selectively chemoattractant to eosinophils [205] and to the effects of cytokines such as GM-CSF, IL-3, and IL-5 [120]. These cytokines may be very important for the survival of eosinophils in the airways [163, 209] and may "prime" eosinophils to exhibit enhanced responsiveness. Eosinophils from asthmatic patients show greatly exaggerated responses to PAF and phorbol esters, compared to eosinophils from atopic nonasthmatic individuals [46], suggesting that these cells may have been primed by exposure to cytokines in the circulation. Asthmatic patients characteristically have a high proportion of hypodense eosinophils in the circulation [85]. Hypodense eosinophils may arise from activation of these cells, and it is interesting that PAF and IL-5 are able to induce hypodense eosinophils in vitro [177, 211]. Several mechanisms may lead to activation of eosinophils in the tissues. PAF is very effective at degranulating eosinophils [127, 128], but several other activating mechanisms are possible.

Eosinophils are moderately sensitive to corticosteroids in vitro [75], but steroids are remarkably effective in reducing the number of eosinophils from the blood and from airway tissues, presumably by inhibiting the release of cytokines from the airway. Inhaled steroids cause a marked reduction in the proportion of hypodense eosinophils in asthmatic patients [161], presumably by inhibiting the local release of cytokines. By contrast, eosinophils are not very effectively inhibited by beta agonists or theophylline [25, 210, 213].

Neutrophils

While neutrophil infiltration is found in some animal models of asthma [159], the role of neutrophils in human asthma is less

certain. In some experimental studies, neutrophil infiltration apparently *follows* the development of increased responsiveness, and neutrophil depletion with cyclophosphamide does not affect its development [155]. Neutrophils appear to be involved in ozone-induced AHR in dogs [160].

The role of neutrophils in human asthma is now in doubt. Neutrophils are found in the airways of patients with chronic bronchitis and patients with bronchiectasis who do not have the degree of AHR found in asthma. The neutrophil may, however, be involved in certain types of asthma (such as certain types of occupational asthma) [77] (see Chap. 46). Neutrophils may be found in BAL fluid of asthmatic subjects and may increase after allergen challenge. It is possible that neutrophils appear in the airways in association with eosinophils, since they appear to adhere to endothelial cells in response to the same stimuli, but there is no convincing evidence that they play an important role in asthmatic inflammation. Indeed after challenge with inhaled PAF, there appears to be a negative association between the increase in airway responsiveness and the number of eosinophils in the BAL fluid [203].

T-lymphocytes

Although the role of B-lymphocytes in the synthesis of IgE is well established, it is only recently that a role for T-lymphocytes in asthma has been recognized. CD4$^+$ (helper) lymphocytes are prominent in asthmatic biopsy specimens [6, 112, 170]. There is evidence that these lymphocytes are in a state of activation since they express IL-2 receptors. It seems likely that these lymphocytes may be involved in orchestrating the chronic inflammatory response in asthma through the secretion of a specific pattern of lymphokines, such as IL-3, IL-4, IL-5, and GM-CSF, which may be important in the recruitment, maintenance, differentiation of eosinophils and in the maintenance of mast cells in airway tissues. Presumably T-lymphocytes are coded to express a distinctive pattern of cytokines, possibly similar to that described in the murine Th2 type of T-lymphocyte [153, 208], which characteristically expresses IL-3, IL-4, and IL-5. This coding of T-lymphocytes is presumably due to antigen-presenting cells such as dendritic cells, which may migrate from the epithelium to regional lymph nodes (Fig. 9-5). This topic is discussed in Chapter 13.

Platelets

Various abnormalities of platelet function in asthma have been described and animal studies suggest that platelets may be implicated in certain types of AHR [60]. Platelets may release a variety of mediators such as serotonin, thromboxane, and lipoxygenase products and may also be activated by IgE-dependent mechanisms [114], although their role in asthma has not yet been determined. Platelets have been detected in BAL fluid of asthmatic subjects [151] and in bronchial biopsy specimens [112] (see Chap. 22).

INFLAMMATORY MEDIATORS

Many different mediators have been implicated in asthma and they may have a variety of effects on the airways, which could account for the pathologic features of asthma [22]. Mediators such as histamine, prostaglandins, and leukotrienes contract airway smooth muscle, increase microvascular leakage, increase airway mucus secretion, and attract other inflammatory cells (Table 9-2, Fig. 9-6). It is therefore possible that interactions between inflammatory mediators might account for AHR. Because each mediator has many effects, the role of individual mediators in the pathophysiology of asthma is not yet clear. Indeed the multiplicity of mediators makes it unlikely that antagonizing

Table 9-2. Effects of inflammatory mediators implicated in asthma

Mediator	Bronchoconstriction	Airway secretion	Microvascular leakage	Chemotaxis	Bronchial hyperresponsiveness
Histamine	+	+	+	+	−
Prostaglandins D_2, $F_{2\alpha}$	+ +	+	?	?	+
Prostaglandin E_2	−	+	−	+	−
Thromboxane	+ +	?	−	±	+
Leukotriene B_4	−	−	±	+ +	±
Leukotrienes C_4, D_4, E_4	+ +	+ +	+ +	?	±
Platelet-activating factor	+ +	+	+ +	+ +	+ +
Bradykinin	+	+	+ +	−	−
Adenosine	+	?	?	?	−
Substance P	+	+ +	+ +	±	−
Neurokinin A	+ +	?	+	−	−
Complement fragments	+	+	+	+ +	−
Serotonin	±	?	+	−	−
Oxygen radicals	+	?	+	?	−

+ + = pronounced effect; + = moderate effect; ± = uncertain effect; ? = information not available.

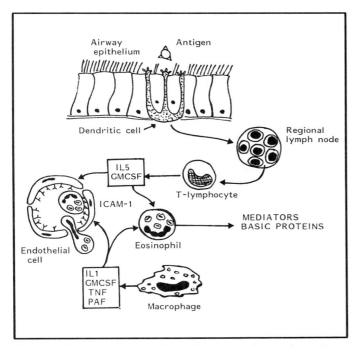

Fig. 9-5. *T-lymphocytes may play an important role in orchestrating chronic inflammation in asthma. They may be programmed in regional lymph nodes by antigen-presenting cells, such as dendritic cells in the airway epithelium, which then migrate to regional lymph nodes. See Figure 9-4 for abbreviation key.*

a single mediator will have a major impact in clinical asthma. A more detailed account of these mediators will be found in subsequent chapters of this text.

Histamine

Histamine was the first mediator implicated in the pathophysiology of asthma. It has multiple effects on the airways that are mediated by three types of histamine receptors [11]. H_1 *receptors* mediate bronchoconstriction, activation of sensory reflexes, vasoconstriction and vasodilatation of bronchial vessels [141], and airway microvascular leakage; H_2 *receptors* mediate mucus secretion and vasodilatation (some species); and H_3 *receptors*

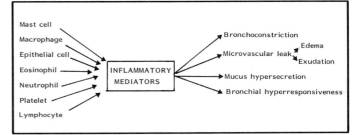

Fig. 9-6. *Mediators may be released from a variety of inflammatory cells in asthma and make up a "soup" of variable composition, which then leads to the characteristic pathology of asthma.*

mediate modulation of cholinergic and sensory nerves [104, 105, 108], but may also act as feedback inhibitory receptors to histamine secretion to mast cells [106]. Despite all these effects, antihistamines have been disappointing in the treatment of asthma [100] (see Chap. 65). Antihistamines cause a resting bronchodilatation in asthmatic patients, however, indicating a certain degree of histamine "tone," presumably due to the basal release of histamine from activated mast cells [58].

Prostaglandins

PGD_2 (via activation of thromboxane TP receptors) potentiates the bronchoconstrictor response to both histamine and methacholine in asthmatic subjects [88]. This sensitizing effect is transient and therefore unlikely to account for the sustained AHR of asthma. There is considerable interest in the role of thromboxane receptors in asthma, since prostaglandins cause contraction of airway smooth muscle by activating TP receptors. A thromboxane synthase inhibitor has been found to reduce AHR in asthmatic patients [84], although a thromboxane antagonist was without effect [27]. The role of prostaglandins and thromboxane in asthma is unlikely to be of major importance, since cyclooxygenase inhibitors do not appear to have a beneficial effect in clinical asthma [158]. Indeed in a small group of asthmatic subjects they cause a deterioration.

Leukotrienes

The sulfidopeptides LTC_4, LTD_4, and LTE_4 are potent constrictors of human airways and both LTD_4 and LTE_4 have been reported to increase AHR [3, 119] and may play an important role in asthma [139]. The recent development of potent specific leukotriene antagonists (see Chap. 66) has made it possible to evaluate the role of these mediators in asthma. Potent LTD$_4$ antagonists are remarkably effective against exercise-induced [147] and allergen-induced responses [194], suggesting that leukotrienes contribute to bronchoconstrictor responses. The role of leukotrienes in chronic asthma remains to be defined and several clinical trials with potent antagonists are currently underway.

LTB$_4$ is chemotactic for neutrophils but since neutrophil infiltration is less characteristic than eosinophil infiltration in asthmatic airways, it is not a primary causative candidate, although it may be synergistic, with other mediators. Inhalation of LTB$_4$ does not appear to have any effect on airway responsiveness in normal subjects [29].

Platelet-activating Factor

A mediator that has attracted considerable attention recently is PAF, since it mimics many of the features of asthma [21] (see Chap. 22). PAF, like prostaglandins and leukotrienes, is formed by the action of phospholipase A$_2$ on membrane phospholipids and may be produced by several of the inflammatory cells implicated in asthma, such as macrophages, eosinophils, and neutrophils. Inhaled PAF causes not only bronchoconstriction, but also a small increase in bronchial responsiveness in normal subjects, whereas lyso-PAF is without effect [62, 119]. The maximal effect is observed 3 days after inhalation and may persist for up to 4 weeks. Other studies have not observed this increased responsiveness [130], but this may be because the increase in responsiveness is small and may only be observed with careful measurements in trained volunteers. Similar changes have also been observed in asthmatic subjects, although these changes do not achieve statistical significance because of the greater variability in airway reactivity [49]. That PAF is rapidly inactivated in vivo suggests that it must trigger a chain of inflammatory events which lead to the very prolonged increase in bronchial responsiveness. Perhaps this is related to its interaction with eosinophils. PAF, like antigen, stimulates selective accumulation of eosinophils in the lungs [65, 181] and in the skin of atopic subjects [98]. PAF increases the adhesion of eosinophils to endothelial surfaces [123], which may be the initial step in eosinophil recruitment into tissues. Since eosinophils themselves are a rich source of PAF [137], they can attract further eosinophils and there is the potential for a continued inflammatory reaction. PAF is very effective in stimulating human eosinophils to release basic proteins [127, 128], which may result in epithelial damage. PAF also causes an increased expression of IgE receptors on eosinophils [152] and increased expression of low-affinity IgE receptors on monocytes [166].

PAF has other properties that may be relevant in asthma. In animals, PAF is a potent inducer of airway microvascular leakage, being the most potent mediator so far described [76], and increases airway secretions and epithelial permeability [176].

Several specific antagonists of PAF are available and their use in models of disease should now make it possible to evaluate the role of endogenous PAF. One such antagonist, ginkgolide B, is derived from Ginkgo biloba leaves, an ancient Chinese herb used as a remedy for chest disease. Ginkgolides, given orally, inhibit PAF-induced platelet aggregation and wheal and flare responses in the skin [50] and may therefore be useful in determining the role of PAF in allergic disease. These PAF antagonists also inhibit the late response to allergen in human skin, which is characterized by eosinophil infiltration [174]. Whether PAF antagonists have a role in human asthma is not yet known, but the development of several potent drugs in this class should soon answer this question. Clinical trials of the most potent antagonist, WEB 2086, which is effective in inhibiting ex vivo platelet aggregation

in response to PAF after oral administration [1], are currently underway, but preliminary reports suggest that WEB 2086 has no effect on allergen challenge [215, 216]. It is possible that this PAF antagonist, when given orally, is not potent enough to block the effects of PAF endogenously released into the airways.

Bradykinin

Bradykinin is formed from high-molecular-weight kininogens in the plasma by the action of kininogenases, which include kallikrein and tryptase from mast cells [171] (see Chap. 10). Bradykinin is a potent constrictor of asthmatic airways in vivo, but is a weak constrictor of human airways in vitro [86, 87]. Inhalation of bradykinin induces a sensation of dyspnea very similar to that experienced during an asthma attack, supporting the idea that bradykinin acts on sensory nerves in the airways [217]. The bronchoconstrictor effect of bradykinin is reduced by an anticholinergic agent and also by cromolyn sodium and nedocromil sodium, which may act on sensory nerves [67, 87]. In guinea pigs bradykinin-induced bronchoconstriction is markedly reduced by atropine and by capsaicin depletion of sensory nerves [107]. In human asthma bradykinin may be an activator of sensory nerves, producing symptoms such as cough and chest tightness. Potent antagonists have recently been developed [99], so that it may soon be possible to evaluate the role of this neglected mediator in asthma.

Oxygen-derived Free Radicals

Many inflammatory cells produce oxygen-derived free radicals such as superoxide anions. These may play an important role in asthmatic inflammation and may contribute to the epithelial damage in asthma [18]. Hydrogen peroxide causes contraction of airway smooth muscle [173] and has been implicated in AHR in animal models [118]. Oxygen radicals may lead to changes in receptor function, which could influence airway reactivity [74]. This topic is discussed in Chapter 71.

Cytokines

Cytokines are peptide mediators released from inflammatory cells that are important in signaling between cells and may determine the type and duration of an inflammatory response. It now seems increasingly likely that cytokines play a major role in the inflammation of asthma. While inflammatory mediators like histamine, leukotrienes, and PAF may be important in the acute and subacute inflammatory responses and in exacerbations of asthma, it is likely that cytokines play a dominant role in chronic inflammation. Multiple cytokines are now found in lungs [120] and almost every cell is capable of producing cytokines under certain conditions. Research in this area is hampered by the fact that there are no specific antagonists, although important observations have been made using specific neutralizing antibodies. It is beyond the scope of this chapter to review this rapidly advancing field in detail, but some of the cytokines that may be particularly important in asthma will be highlighted (Fig. 9-7); further discussion is presented in Chapter 13.

IL-3 may be important in persistence of mast cells and eosinophils in airway tissues. IL-4 may be important in programming B-lymphocytes to produce IgE. A monoclonal antibody to IL-4 inhibits IgE production without affecting the production of IgG [79]. IL-5 and GM-CSF may be involved in eosinophil recruitment, survival in tissues, and priming [163, 178, 209]. Many cells may synthesize cytokines, and although T-lymphocytes and macrophages may be the major source of cytokines in asthmatic airways, mast cells may also synthesize cytokines (GM-CSF, IL-3, and IL-5) under certain conditions [39]. Even structural cells such as epithelial cells may release cytokines [162].

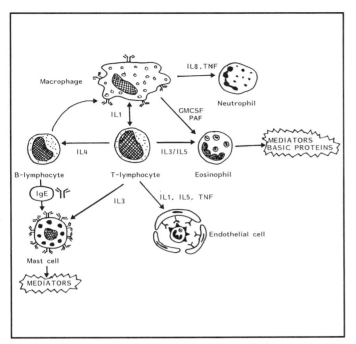

Fig. 9-7. *The role of cytokines in asthma is increasingly recognized. IL = interleukin; TNF = tumor necrosis factor; GM-CSF = granulocyte-macrophage colony-stimulating factor; PAF = platelet-activating factor.*

Although there are no effective blockers of cytokine receptors, studies with monoclonal antibodies directed at specific cytokines are beginning to reveal the roles of individual cytokines in inflammation. Thus, an antibody agonist, IL-5, inhibits eosinophilia in mice infested with worms [57].

Multiple Mediators

It is clear that no single mediator can be responsible for all the features of asthma, and it is likely that multiple mediators constitute an "inflammatory soup" which may vary from patient to patient, depending on the relative state of activation of the different inflammatory cells (see Fig. 9-6). There may be important interactions between the different mediators and the concept of "priming" may be very important, since a combination of mediators may have a much greater effect than each mediator alone. This may be particularly important in the actions of cytokines, which may have no effect in isolation but may have a very pronounced effect after a cell has been exposed to another cytokine.

EFFECTS OF INFLAMMATION ON TARGET CELLS

The chronic inflammatory response has several effects on the target cells of the airways, resulting in the characteristic pathophysiologic changes associated with asthma (see Fig. 9-2). Important advances have recently been made in understanding these changes, although their role in asthma symptoms is often not clear.

Airway Epithelium

Airway epithelial damage may be a critical feature of AHR [26, 131] (see Chap. 23), and may explain how several different mechanisms, such as ozone exposure, certain virus infections, chemical sensitizers, and allergen exposure, can lead to its develop-

ment, since all these stimuli may lead to epithelial disruption. Epithelium may be shed as a consequence of inflammatory mediators, such as eosinophil basic proteins and oxygen-derived free radicals, together with various proteases released from inflammatory cells. Epithelial cells are commonly found in clumps in the BAL fluid or sputum (Creola bodies) of asthmatic subjects, suggesting that there has been a loss of attachment to the basal layer or basement membrane. Epithelium is not always shed in asthma [143], but it is still possible that there may be abnormal functioning of airway epithelium. Epithelial damage may contribute to AHR in a number of ways.

Loss of Barrier
Epithelial shedding may remove a protective barrier, thus allowing allergens and inhaled chemicals to reach cells in the submucosa that would normally be unprotected. There is little evidence for an increase in mucosal permeability to inhaled radioactive markers in asthmatic patients [109], but this may reflect the difficulty in making measurements of *airway* as opposed to *alveolar* permeability using inhaled tracers. Increased permeability would allow inhaled allergens to reach mast cells and other inflammatory cells in the submucosa that would normally be inaccessible.

Loss of Epithelium-derived Relaxant Factor
Mechanical removal of epithelial cells in vitro results in increased responsiveness of airway smooth muscle to several spasmogens [61, 199], and suggests that epithelial cells may release a relaxant factor analogous to the EpDRF in blood vessels. Damage of epithelium would thus remove the protective effect of this relaxant factor, leading to exaggerated bronchoconstrictor responses. The nature of this putative relaxant factor (EpDRF) is not certain, although it is not an eicosanoid or nitric oxide. Its existence has been demonstrated in superfusion experiments [78], but the effects of epithelial removal on contractile responses to spasmogens are small, and the relevance of this phenomenon is not certain, particularly in vivo when the labile factor would have to diffuse across the submucosa and its blood supply to reach airway smooth muscle. Perhaps this factor may have a more important role as a vasodilator regulating airway blood flow.

Enzymatic Degradation of Mediators
Epithelial cells strongly express neutral endopeptidase [113], which is an important enzyme in degrading various bronchoconstrictor peptides, such as tachykinins, bradykinin, cholecystokinin octapeptide (CCK), and endothelin. Mechanical removal of airway epithelium greatly potentiates the bronchoconstrictor effect of tachykinins [82], bradykinin [34, 83], and CCK [192], an effect that is mimicked by the neutral endopeptidase inhibitor phosphoramidon. Several factors that lead to exacerbations of asthma appear to downregulate the function of epithelial neural endopeptidase, including virus infections [110], oxidants [72], and toluene diisocyanate [187].

Sensory Nerve Exposure
Epithelial damage will also expose sensory nerve endings, which may be activated by inflammatory mediators, leading to inflammation via an axon reflex mechanism [10] (see Chaps. 17 and 18).

Mediator Release
Epithelial cells themselves may release inflammatory mediators such as 15-lipoxygenase products, which are chemotactic for inflammatory cells [103]; PGE_2, which may protect against bronchoconstriction or may sensitize sensory nerve endings [138]; and endothelin, which is a potent bronchoconstrictor peptide [30]. Indeed, recent studies have shown that endothelin-line im-

munoreactivity is increased in the epithelium of asthmatic patients [190].

Subepithelial Fibrosis

An apparent increase in the basement membrane has been observed in fatal asthma, although similar changes have been seen in the airways in other conditions [70]. Electron microscopy of bronchial biopsy specimens from asthmatic patients demonstrates that this thickening is due to subepithelial fibrosis [175]. Type III and V collagens appear to be laid down, and may be produced by myofibroblasts situated under the epithelium [35]. The mechanism of fibrosis is not yet clear but several cytokines, including transforming growth factor-beta, may be produced by epithelial cells or macrophages in the inflamed airway [120]. The subepithelial fibrosis may be one of the factors contributing to the irreversible airway obstruction and the persisting AHR after steroid treatment, and is still present even after prolonged treatment with inhaled steroids [145].

Airway Smooth Muscle

There is still debate about the role of abnormalities in airway smooth muscle in asthmatic subjects. In vitro airway smooth muscle from asthmatic patients usually shows no increased responsiveness to spasmogens [196], although exceptions reported are increased maximal contractile effects or increased sensitivity to certain spasmogens [182]. Reduced responsiveness to beta agonists has also been demonstrated in postmortem or surgically removed bronchi from asthmatic subjects [7, 45, 96]. These abnormalities of airway smooth muscle may be a reflection of the chronic inflammatory process. For example, the reduced beta-adrenergic responses in airway smooth muscle could be due to phosphorylation of the stimulatory G-protein coupling beta receptors to adenyl cyclase, resulting from the activation of protein kinase C by the stimulation of airway smooth muscle cells by inflammatory mediators.

In asthmatic airways there is also a characteristic hypertrophy of airway smooth muscle [71, 73, 97], which is presumably the result of stimulation of airway smooth muscle cells by various growth factors, such as platelet-derived growth factor, or endothelin [125] released from inflammatory cells. Even mediators such as histamine are able to stimulate growth in airway smooth muscle cells as measured by the increase in c-*fos* expression [165] (see Chap. 25).

Vascular Responses

Vasodilatation occurs in inflammation, yet little is known about the role of the airway circulation in asthma, partly because of the difficulties involved in measuring blood flow in airway vessels. The bronchial circulation may play an important role in regulating airway caliber, since an increase in the vascular volume may contribute to airway narrowing. Passive venous congestion from left ventricular failure results in increased airway reactivity to methacholine challenge [40]. Increased venous congestion may also contribute to the increased AHR that occurs at night in association with the supine posture. Increased airway blood flow may be important in removing inflammatory mediators from the airway, and may play a role in the development of exercise-induced asthma [149].

Plasma Extravasation and Mucosal Edema

Microvascular leakage is an essential component of the inflammatory response and many of the inflammatory mediators implicated in asthma produce this leakage [22] (see Chap. 23). There is good evidence for microvascular leakage in asthma [52, 169],

since there are increased plasma proteins in BAL fluid [134, 135] and in sputum [37, 179]. Microvascular leakage occurs only at postcapillary venules and appears to be due to retraction of endothelial cells, so that plasma proteins can leave the vessel. Increased gaps between endothelial cells in bronchial venules have been directly observed by electron microscopy of bronchial biopsy specimens [132]. There are several consequences of plasma extravasation.

Effects on Airway Secretions

Exuded plasma appears to pass preferentially into the lumen of the airway by passing between epithelial cells. Plasma has an inhibitory effect on mucociliary clearance, possibly because of an increased viscosity of luminal secretions, but possibly also because of an inhibitory plasma factor [69]. In addition, plasma proteins such as albumin interact with mucus glycoproteins to form a viscous secretion [140], and together with DNA from cell debris and coagulation proteins result in the characteristic mucus plug that occludes the airways and is prominent in fatal asthma.

Generation of Plasma-derived Mediators

Plasma exuded into the airway mucosa and lumen may provide a source of new mediators. Kinins are generated from high-molecular-weight kininogens, which have been detected in asthmatic airways [47]. Anaphylatoxin complement peptides C3a and C5a may also be formed, and may act as spasmogens and potent chemoattractants of other inflammatory cells [172]. There are probably numerous other plasma-derived mediators that may amplify the inflammatory response in the airways.

Mucosal Edema

Submucosal edema is present in asthmatic airways, although it is difficult to quantify [70]. This may contribute to airway narrowing in asthma, although recent studies in animals indicate that mediators causing mucosal edema have a relatively small effect on airway resistance [142]. Of greater relevance is the effect on AHR, for geometric reasons; since the edematous mucosa is noncompressible and as airway smooth muscle contracts, the cross-sectional area of the airway lumen may markedly diminish, resulting in a large amplification of the increased airway resistance [111]. In addition, edema of the peribronchial region may loosen the parenchymal attachments that tend to keep airways open during deflation. Edema thus uncouples airways from the parenchyma, resulting in premature closure of peripheral airways, and this may result in the loss of the plateau of bronchoconstriction that occurs in asthma [66]. Mucosal edema may also be very important in the exacerbations of asthma that occur frequently at night. Nocturnal asthma may be related to circadian changes in various neurohumoral factors [23]. The falls in plasma cortisol and epinephrine levels at night may result in increased microvascular leak, since both hormones appear to regulate airway microvascular leakage [20, 31, 32, 169], in addition to mediator release from inflammatory cells. This leads to increased mucosal edema at night, which then amplifies the increase in airway resistance produced by the normal nocturnal increase in vagal cholinergic tone [12]. Support for this hypothesis is provided by the demonstration that airway inflammation increases at night in asthmatic patients with nocturnal symptoms [148] (see Chap. 76).

Adhesion Molecules

The movement of inflammatory cells from the circulation into the tissues depends on adhesion to endothelial cells. This adhesion is mediated by an interaction between specific adhesion glycoproteins expressed on the endothelial cell surface and on inflammatory cells. Several families of adhesion molecules have now been characterized [2]. The integrins are a large supergene family of adhesion molecules which include leukocyte adhesion molecules (LEUCAM) on lymphocytes, granulocytes, and macrophages and intercellular adhesion molecules on endothelial (and epithelial) cells, such as ICAM-1. A monoclonal antibody to ICAM-1 inhibits eosinophil infiltration into primate airways after allergen challenge, emphasizing the importance of cell adhesion [206]. After allergen exposure there is increased expression of ICAM-1 in bronchial endothelial and epithelial cells [206]. In other tissues, various cytokines such as IL-1 and TNF-α have been shown to increase the expression of ICAM-1 [178], and this may be regulated in part by protein kinase C activation. ICAM-1 is also involved in the recruitment and activation of T-lymphocytes, and may play a critical role in cell immunity. Another integrin, vascular cell adhesion molecule-1 (VCAM-1), may also be involved in leukocyte adhesion in inflammatory diseases and is induced by cytokines [218]. The selectins are another large family of adhesion molecules involved in the adhesion between leukocytes and endothelial cells, and include E-selectin (ELAM-1). It is clear that further investigation of adhesion molecules and their regulation in asthma may lead to novel therapeutic approaches in the future.

Mucus Hypersecretion

Mucus hypersecretion is a common inflammatory response in secretory tissues. Increased mucus secretion contributes to the viscid mucus plugs that occlude asthmatic airways, particularly in fatal asthma. There is evidence for hyperplasia of submucosal glands confined to large airways and of increased numbers of epithelial goblet cells. This increased secretory response may be due to inflammatory mediators acting on submucosal glands and due to stimulation of neural elements [144]. Little is understood about the control of goblet cells, which are the main source of mucus in peripheral airways, although recent studies investigating the control of goblet cells in guinea pig airways suggest that cholinergic, adrenergic, and sensory neuropeptides are important in stimulating secretion [129, 197] (see Chaps. 29 and 52).

Neural Effects

There has recently been a renewal of interest in neural mechanisms in asthma. In the last century, asthma was explained by neural mechanisms. Autonomic nervous control of the airways is complex, for in addition to classic cholinergic and adrenergic mechanisms, nonadrenergic noncholinergic (NANC) nerves and several neuropeptides have been identified in the respiratory tract [8, 9]. Several studies have investigated the possibility that defects in autonomic control may contribute to AHR and asthma, and abnormalities of autonomic function, such as enhanced cholinergic and alpha-adrenergic responses or reduced beta-adrenergic responses, have been proposed [117]. Current thinking suggests that these abnormalities are likely to be secondary to the disease, rather than primary defects [8, 17]. It is possible that airway inflammation may interact with autonomic control by several mechanisms [9] (see Chaps. 17 and 18).

Inflammatory Effects on Nerves

Inflammatory mediators may act on various prejunctional receptors on airway nerves to modulate the release of neurotransmitters [19]. Thus, thromboxane and PGD2 facilitate the release of acetylcholine from cholinergic nerves in canine airways [51, 193], whereas histamine inhibits cholinergic neurotransmission at both parasympathetic ganglia and postganglionic nerves via H3 receptors [108]. Inflammatory mediators may also activate sensory nerves, resulting in reflex cholinergic bronchoconstriction or release of inflammatory neuropeptides. Inflammatory prod-

ucts may also sensitize sensory nerve endings in the airway epithelium, so that the nerves become hyperalgesic. Hyperalgesia and pain (dolor) are cardinal signs of inflammation, and in the asthmatic airway may mediate cough and dyspnea, which are characteristic symptoms of asthma. The precise mechanisms of hyperalgesia are not yet certain, but mediators such as prostaglandins and certain cytokines (such as IL-1β) may be important.

Neurogenic Inflammation

Airway nerves may release not only neurotransmitters that are antiinflammatory (such as vasoactive intestinal peptide and nitric oxide), but also neurotransmitters that have inflammatory effects. Thus, neuropeptides such as substance P, neurokinin A, and calcitonin gene–related peptide may be released from sensitized inflammatory nerves in the airways, which increase and extend the ongoing inflammatory response (see Chap. 18).

IMPLICATIONS FOR THERAPY

Because airway obstruction in asthma involves more than spasm of airway smooth muscle, it follows that treatment must involve more than bronchodilators [14]. Beta2-agonist bronchodilators not only fail to reduce AHR, but may even exacerbate it [122, 126, 186, 201]. By giving acute relief of symptoms, these drugs may mask the underlying inflammatory process and overreliance on beta agonists may be a contributory factor to the recent increase in asthma morbidity and mortality. It is important that some sort of prophylactic or antiinflammatory therapy that reduces the chronic inflammation and AHR is also used in the chronic treatment of asthma [14].

Corticosteroids, which inhibit virtually every step in the inflammatory process [183], are effective in reducing AHR in asthma [16], and reduce the inflammation in the airways [133, 219, 220]. Other drugs such as cromolyn sodium and nedocromil sodium may also be useful [28] (see Chap. 63). Antiinflammatory therapies should probably be started at an earlier stage of treatment and there is a case to be made for introducing inhaled steroids, cromolyn sodium, or nedocromil sodium as the *initial* therapy, together with an inhaled beta agonist for symptom relief. Yet even high-dose steroid therapy is frequently unable to reduce the AHR and airway narrowing of asthma back to normal, suggesting that there is an irreversible component. This is most likely due to structural changes, such as hypertrophy of airway smooth muscle and subepithelial fibrosis [145, 175], which could result from the release of various growth factors (such as macrophage- and platelet-derived growth factors) from inflammatory cells. Although these changes cannot be reversed by therapy, it seems likely that they may be prevented by effective and continued suppression of the airway inflammation. Prolonged therapy with prophylactic drugs may thus prevent the later development of irreversible airflow obstruction, which may be seen in chronic asthma [38, 167] (Fig. 9-8).

New Approaches

It seems probable that there are several different types of asthma involving different mechanisms that may respond to different forms of therapy, but far more research is needed, particularly in human subjects, since animal models have proved to be so misleading in the past. Although inhaled corticosteroids are highly effective in controlling asthmatic inflammation, their side effects after continued use are increasingly recognized. There is therefore a need for alternative antiasthma therapies that lack these adverse effects, and in particular therapies that are more specific for asthmatic inflammation. Cromolyn sodium and nedocromil sodium have this increased specificity, but are only effec-

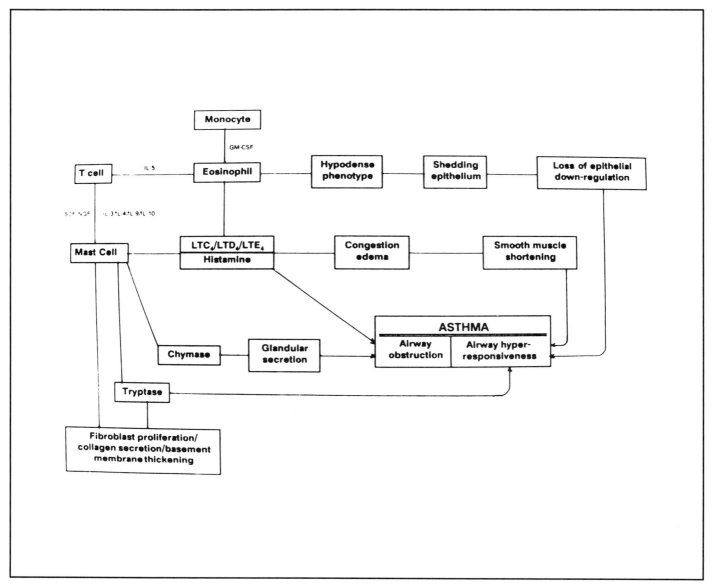

Fig. 9-8. *The relationship between airway inflammatory changes in asthma and the clinical components of the disease, for example, airway obstruction, airway hyperresponsiveness. (Reprinted with permission from T. H. Lee. Conclusions and summary.* Am. Rev. Respir. Dis. *145:S58, 1992.)*

tive in mild asthma. Several promising new drugs, such as leukotriene and PAF antagonists and selective phosphodiesterase inhibitors, may prove valuable in treating asthma in the future [15], but an improved understanding of currently effective drugs such as steroids, cromolyn, and nedocromil is also needed.

Drugs that modulate the abnormal immune response in asthma are also needed. While cyclosporine, which inhibits certain functions of T-lymphocytes, may be useful for several asthmatic patients, less toxic and more specific therapy that may block specific cytokines such as IL-4 and IL-5 may be the way forward in the future [24]. It is hopeful that a major research effort will lead to further understanding and reduced morbidity and mortality of asthma.

REFERENCES

1. Adamus, W. S., et al. Inhibitory effect of oral WEB 2086, a novel selective PAF-acether antagonist, on *ex vivo* platelet aggregation. *Eur. J. Clin. Pharmacol.* 35:237, 1988.

2. Albelda, S. M. Endothelial and epithelial cell adhesion molecules. *Am. J. Respir. Cell. Mol. Biol.* 4:195, 1991.

3. Arm, J. P., Spur, B. W., and Lee, T. H. The effects of inhaled leukotriene E4 on the airway responsiveness to histamine in subjects with asthma and normal subjects. *J. Allergy Clin. Immunol.* 82:654, 1988.

4. Arnoux, B., et al. Antigenic release of Paf-acether and beta-glucuronidase from alveolar macrophages of asthmatics. *Bull. Eur. Physiopathol. Respir.* 23:119, 1987.

5. Aubus, P., et al. Decreased suppressor cell activity of alveolar macrophages in bronchial asthma. *Am. Rev. Respir. Dis.* 130:875, 1984.

6. Azzawi, M., et al. Identification of activated T lymphocytes and eosinophils in bronchial biopsies in stable atopic asthma. *Am. Rev. Respir. Dis.* 142:1407, 1990.

7. Bai, T. R. Abnormalities in airway smooth muscle in fatal asthma: A comparison between trachea and bronchus. *Am. Rev. Respir. Dis.* 143:441, 1991.

8. Barnes, P. J. Neural control of human airways in health and disease. *Am. Rev. Respir. Dis.* 134:1289, 1986.

9. Barnes, P. J. Airway inflammation and autonomic control. *Eur. J. Respir. Dis.* 69(Suppl. 147):80, 1986.

10. Barnes, P. J. Asthma as an axon reflex. *Lancet* 1:242, 1986.

11. Barnes, P. J. Histamine receptors in airways. *Agents Actions Suppl.* 33: 103, 1991.

12. Barnes, P. J. Inflammatory mechanisms and nocturnal asthma. *Am. J. Med.* 85 (Suppl. 1B):64, 1988.

13. Barnes, P. J. New concepts in the pathogenesis of bronchial hyperresponsiveness and asthma. *J. Allergy Clin. Immunol.* 83:1013, 1989.

14. Barnes, P. J. A new approach to asthma therapy. *N. Engl. J. Med.* 321: 1517, 1989.

15. Barnes, P. J. *New Drugs for Asthma* (2nd ed.). London: IBC Technical Services, 1992.

16. Barnes, P. J. Effect of corticosteroids on airway hyperresponsiveness. *Am. Rev. Respir. Dis.* 141:S162, 1990.

17. Barnes, P. J. Neural control of airway function: New perspectives. *Mol. Aspects Med.* 11:351, 1990.

18. Barnes, P. J. Reactive oxygen species and airway inflammation. *Free Radic. Biol. Med.* 9:235, 1990.

19. Barnes, P. J. Neuromodulation in the airways. *Physiol. Rev.* In press.

20. Barnes, P. J., et al. Effects of treatment on airway microvascular leak. *Eur. J. Respir. Dis.* 3(Suppl. 12):663, 1990.

21. Barnes, P. J., Chung, K. F., and Page, C. P. Platelet-activating factor as a mediator of allergic disease. *J. Allergy Clin. Immunol.* 81:919, 1988.

22. Barnes, P. J., Chung, K. F., and Page, C. P. Inflammatory mediators and asthma. *Pharmacol. Rev.* 40:49, 1988.

23. Barnes, P., et al. Nocturnal asthma and changes in circulating epinephrine, histamine and cortisol. *N. Engl. J. Med.* 303:263, 1980.

24. Barnes, P. J. New therapeutic approaches in asthma. *Br. Med. Bull.* 48: 231, 1992.

25. Barnes, P. J., et al. Pharmacology of Eosinophils. In A. B. Kay (ed.), *Eosinophils in Allergic Disease.* Oxford: Blackwell, 1990. Pp. 144–157.

26. Beasley, R., et al. Cellular events in the bronchi in mild asthma after bronchial provocation. *Am. Rev. Respir. Dis.* 139:806, 1989.

27. Beasley, R. C. W., et al. Effects of a thromboxane receptor antagonist on PGD_2 and allergen induced bronchoconstriction. *J. Appl. Physiol.* 66: 1685, 1989.

28. Bel, E. H., et al. The longer term effects of nedocromil sodium and beclomethasone dipropionate on bronchial responsiveness to methacholine in non-atopic asthmatic subjects. *Am. Rev. Respir. Dis.* 141:21, 1990.

29. Black, P. N., et al. Effect of inhaled leukotriene B_4 alone and in combination with prostaglandin D_2 on bronchial responsiveness to histamine in normal subjects. *Thorax* 44:491, 1989.

30. Black, P. N., et al. Formation of endothelin by cultured airway epithelial cells. *FEBS Lett* 255:129, 1989.

31. Boschetto, P., et al. The effect of antiasthma drugs on microvascular leak in guinea pig airways. *Am. Rev. Respir. Dis.* 139:416, 1989.

32. Boschetto, P., et al. Corticosteroid inhibition of airway microvascular leakage. *Am. Rev. Respir. Dis.* 143:605, 1991.

33. Bousquet, J., Chanez, P., and Lacoste, J. Y. Eosinophilic inflammation in asthma. *N. Engl. J. Med.* 323:1033, 1990.

34. Bramley, A. M., Samhoun, M. N., and Piper, P. J. The role of epithelium in modulating the responses of guinea-pig trachea induced by bradykinin *in vitro. Br. J. Pharmacol.* 99:762, 1990.

35. Brewster, C. E. P., et al. Myofibroblasts and subepithelial fibrosis in bronchial asthma. *Am. J. Respir. Cell Mol. Biol.* 3:507, 1990.

36. Britton, J. R., et al. The relation between changes in airway reactivity and change in respiratory symptoms and medication in a community survey. *Am. Rev. Respir. Dis.* 138:530, 1988.

37. Brogan, T. D., et al. Soluble proteins of bronchopulmonary secretions from patients with cystic fibrosis, asthma and bronchitis. *Thorax* 30:72, 1975.

38. Brown, J. P., Greville, W. H., and Finucane, K. E. Asthma and irreversible airflow obstruction. *Thorax* 39:131, 1984.

39. Burd, P. R., et al. Interleukin 3-dependent and -independent mast cells stimulated with IgE and antigen express multiple cytokines. *J. Exp. Med.* 170:245, 1989.

40. Cabanes, L. R., et al. Bronchial hyperresponsiveness to methacholine in patients with impaired left ventricular function. *N. Engl. J. Med.* 320:1317, 1989.

41. Capron, M., et al. Role of IgE receptors in effector function of human eosinophils. *J. Immunol.* 132:462, 1984.

42. Capron, M., et al. Selectivity of mediators released by eosinophils. *Int. Arch. Allergy Clin. Immunol.* 88:54, 1989.

43. Casale, T. B., et al. Elevated bronchoalveolar lavage fluid histamine levels in allergic asthmatics are associated with methacholine bronchial hyperresponsiveness. *J. Clin. Invest.* 79:1197, 1987.

44. Caughey, G. H. Roles of mast cell tryptase and chymase in airway function. *Am. J. Physiol.* 257:L39, 1989.

45. Cerrina, J., et al. Comparison of human bronchial muscle response to histamine *in vivo* with histamine and isoproterenol agonists *in vitro. Am. Rev. Respir. Dis.* 134:57, 1986.

46. Chanez, P., et al. Generation of oxygen free radicals from blood eosinophils from asthma patients after stimulation with PAF or phorbol ester. *Eur. Respir. J.* 3:1002, 1990.

47. Christiansen, S. C., Proud, D., and Cochrane, C. G. Detection of tissue kallikrein in the bronchoalveolar lavage fluid of asthmatic patients. *J. Clin. Invest.* 79:188, 1987.

48. Chung, K. F. Role of inflammation in the hyperreactivity of the airways in asthma. *Thorax* 41:657, 1986.

49. Chung, K. F., and Barnes, P. J. Effects of platelet activating factor on airway calibre, airway responsiveness and circulating cells in asthmatic subjects. *Thorax* 44:108, 1989.

50. Chung, K. F., et al. Effect of a ginkgolide mixture (BN 52063) in antagonising skin and platelet responses to platelet activating factor in man. *Lancet* 1:251, 1987.

51. Chung, K. F., et al. Modulation of cholinergic neurotransmission in canine airways of thromboxane mimetic U46619. *Eur. J. Pharmacol.* 117:373, 1985.

52. Chung, K. F., et al. The role of increased airway microvascular permeability and plasma exudation in asthma. *Eur. Respir. J.* 3:329, 1990.

53. Church, M. K., and Hiroi, J. Inhibition of IgE-dependent histamine release from human dispersed lung mast cells by anti-allergic drugs and salbutamol. *Br. J. Pharmacol.* 90:421, 1987.

54. Cockcroft, D. W. Mechanism of perennial allergic asthma. *Lancet* 2:253, 1983.

55. Cockcroft, D. W. Airway hyperresponsiveness: Therapeutic implications. *Ann. Allergy* 59:405, 1987.

56. Cockcroft, D. W., and Murdoch, K. Y. Comparative effects of inhaled salbutamol, sodium cromoglycate and BDP on allergen-induced early asthmatic responses, late asthmatic responses and increased bronchial responsiveness to histamine. *J. Allergy Clin. Immunol.* 79:734, 1987.

57. Coffman, R. L., et al. Antibody to interleukin-5 inhibits helminth-induced eosinophilia in mice. *Science* 245:308, 1989.

58. Cookson, W. O. C. M. Bronchodilator action of the antihistamine terfenadine. *Br. J. Clin. Pharmacol.* 24:120, 1987.

59. Cox, J. S. G. Disodium cromoglycate (FPL 670) ("Intal"): A specific inhibitor of reaginic antibody-antigen mechanisms. *Nature* 216:1328, 1967.

60. Coyle, A. J., Spina, D., and Page, C. P. PAF-induced bronchial hyperresponsiveness in the rabbit: Contribution of platelets and airway smooth muscle. *Br. J. Pharmacol.* 101:31, 1990.

61. Cuss, F. M., and Barnes, P. J. Epithelial mediators. *Am. Rev. Respir. Dis.* 136:S32, 1987.

62. Cuss, F. M., Dixon, C. M. S., and Barnes, P. J. Effects of inhaled platelet activating factor on pulmonary function and bronchial responsiveness in man. *Lancet* 2:189, 1986.

63. Cutz, E., Levison, H., and Cooper, D. M. Ultrastructure of airways in children with asthma. *Histopathology* 2:407, 1978.

64. De Monchy, J. G. R., et al. Bronchoalveolar eosinophilia during allergen-induced late asthmatic reactions. *Am. Rev. Respir. Dis.* 131:373, 1985.

65. Denjean, A., Arnoux, B., and Benveniste, J. Long-lasting effect of intratracheal administration of PAF-acether in baboons. *Am. Rev. Respir. Dis.* 137:283, 1988.

66. Ding, D. J., Martin, J. G., and Macklem, P. T. Effects of lung volume on maximal methacholine-induced bronchoconstriction in normal humans. *J. Appl. Physiol.* 62:1324, 1987.

67. Dixon, C. M. S., and Barnes, P. J. Bradykinin induced bronchoconstriction: Inhibition by nedocromil sodium and sodium cromoglycate. *Br. J. Clin. Pharmacol.* 270:8310, 1989.

68. Djukanovic, R., et al. Mucosal inflammation in asthma. *Am. Rev. Respir. Dis.* 142:434, 1990.

69. Dulfano, M. J., and Luk, C. K. Sputum and ciliary inhibition in asthma. *Thorax* 37:646, 1982.

70. Dunnill, M. S. The pathology of asthma, with special reference to the changes in the bronchial mucosa. *J. Clin. Pathol.* 13:27, 1960.

71. Dunnill, M. S., Massarella, G. R., and Anderson, J. A. A comparison of the quantitative anatomy of the bronchi in normal subjects, in status asthmaticus, in chronic bronchitis and emphysema. *Thorax* 24:176, 1969.

72. Dusser, D. J., et al. Cigarette smoke induces bronchoconstrictor hyperresponsiveness to substance P and inactivates airway neutral endopeptidase in the guinea pig lung. Possible role of free radicals. *J. Clin. Invest.* 84:900, 1989.

73. Ebina, M., et al. Hyperreactive site in the airway tree of asthmatic patients recorded by thickening of bronchial muscles: A morphometric study. *Am. Rev. Respir. Dis.* 141:1327, 1990.

74. Engels, F., Oosting, R. S., and Nijkamp, F. P. Pulmonary macrophages induce deterioration of guinea-pig tracheal β-adrenergic function through release of oxygen radicals. *Eur. J. Pharmacol.* 111:143, 1985.

75. Evans, P. M., Barnes, P. J., and Chung, K. F. Effect of corticosteroids on human eosinophils *in vitro*. *Eur. J. Pharmacol.* 3:160S, 1990.

76. Evans, T. W., et al. Effect of platelet activating factor on airway vascular permeability: Possible mechanisms. *J. Appl. Physiol.* 63:479, 1987.

77. Fabbri, L. M., Boschetto, P., and Zocca, E. Bronchoalveolar neutrophilia during late asthmatic reactions induced by toluene diisocyanate. *Am. Rev. Respir. Dis.* 136:36, 1987.

78. Fernandes, L. B., Paterson, J. W., and Goldie, R. G. Coaxial bioassay of a smooth muscle relaxant factor released from guinea pig tracheal epithelium. *Br. J. Pharmacol.* 96:117, 1989.

79. Finkelman, F. D., et al. Suppression of *in vivo* polyclonal IgE responses by monoclonal antibody to the lymphokine B-cell stimulating factor 1. *Proc. Natl. Acad. Sci. USA* 83:9675, 1986.

80. Flavahan, N. A., et al. Human major basic protein causes hyperreactivity of respiratory smooth muscle. *Am. Rev. Respir. Dis.* 138:685, 1988.

81. Flint, K. C., et al. Bronchoalveolar mast cells in extrinsic asthma: A mechanism for the initiation of antigen specific bronchoconstriction. *Br. Med. J.* 291:923, 1985.

82. Frossard, N., Rhoden, K. J., and Barnes, P. J. Influence of epithelium on guinea pig airway responses to tachykinins: Role of endopeptidase and cyclooxygenase. *J. Pharmacol. Exp. Ther.* 248:292, 1989.

83. Frossard, N., Stretton, C. D., and Barnes, P. J. Modulation of bradykinin responses in airway smooth muscle by epithelial enzymes. *Agents Actions* 31:204, 1990.

84. Fujimura, M., et al. Effects of a thromboxane synthetase inhibitor (OXY-046) and a lipoxygenase inhibitor (AA-861) on bronchial responsiveness to acetylcholine in asthmatic subjects. *Thorax* 41:955, 1986.

85. Fukuda, T., et al. Increased numbers of hypodense eosinophils in the blood of patients with bronchial asthma. *Am. Rev. Respir. Dis.* 132:981, 1985.

86. Fuller, R. W., and Barnes, P. J. Kinins. In P. J. Barnes, I. M. Rodger, and N. C. Thomson (eds.), *Asthma: Basic Mechanisms and Clinical Management.* London: Academic, 1988. Pp. 259–272.

87. Fuller, R. W., et al. Bradykinin-induced bronchoconstriction in man: Mode of action. *Am. Rev. Respir. Dis.* 135:176, 1987.

88. Fuller, R. W., et al. Prostaglandin D_2 potentiates airway responses to histamine and methacholine. *Am. Rev. Respir. Dis.* 133:252, 1986.

89. Fuller, R. W., et al. Dexamethasone inhibits the production of thromboxane B_2 and leukotriene B_4 by human alveolar and peritoneal macrophages in culture. *Clin. Sci.* 67:693, 1984.

90. Fuller, R. W., et al. Immunoglobulin E-dependent stimulation of human alveolar macrophages: Significance of type 1 hypersensitivity. *Clin. Exp. Immunol.* 65:416, 1986.

91. Fuller, R. W., et al. Human alveolar macrophage activation: Inhibition by forskolin but not β-adrenoceptor stimulation or phosphodiesterase inhibition. *Pulmon. Pharmacol.* 1:101, 1988.

92. Gibson, P. G., et al. Allergen-induced asthmatic responses: Relationship between increases in airway responsiveness and increases in circulating eosinophils, basophils and their progenitors. *Am. Rev. Respir. Dis.* 143:331, 1991.

93. Gleich, G. J., et al. The eosinophil as a mediator of damage to respiratory epithelium: A model for bronchial hyperreactivity. *J. Allergy Clin. Immunol.* 81:776, 1988.

94. Glynn, A. A., and Michaels, L. Bronchial biopsy in chronic bronchitis and asthma. *Thorax* 15:142, 1960.

95. Godard, P., et al. Functional assessment of alveolar macrophages: Comparison of cells from asthmatics and normal subjects. *J. Allergy Clin. Immunol.* 70:88, 1982.

96. Goldie, R. G., et al. *In vitro* responsiveness of human asthmatic bronchus to carbachol, histamine, β-adrenoceptor agonists and theophylline. *Br. J. Clin. Pharmacol.* 22:669, 1986.

97. Heard, B. E., and Hossain, S. Hyperplasia of bronchial muscle in asthma. *J. Pathol.* 110:319, 1973.

98. Henocq, E., and Vargaftig, B. B. Skin eosinophils in atopic patients. *J. Allergy Clin. Immunol.* 81:691, 1988.

99. Hock, F. J., et al. HOE 140, a new potent and long acting bradykinin-antagonist: *In vitro* studies. *Br. J. Pharmacol.* 102:769, 1991.

100. Holgate, S. T., and Finnerty, J. P. Antihistamines in asthma. *J. Allergy Clin. Immunol.* 83:537, 1989.

101. Holt, P. G. Down-regulation of immune responses in the lower respiratory tract: The role of alveolar macrophages. *Clin. Exp. Immunol.* 63:261, 1986.

102. Holt, P. G., Schon-Hegrad, M. A., and Phillips, M. J. Ia positive dendritic cells form a tightly meshed network within the human airway epithelium. *Clin. Exp. Allergy* 19:597, 1989.

103. Hunter, J. A., et al. Predominant generation of 15-lipoxygenase metabolites of arachidonic acid by epithelial cells from human trachea. *Proc. Natl. Acad. Sci. USA* 82:4633, 1985.

104. Ichinose, M., and Barnes, P. J. Inhibitory histamine H_3-receptors on cholinergic nerves in human airways. *Eur. J. Pharmacol.* 163:383, 1989.

105. Ichinose, M., and Barnes, P. J. Histamine H_3-receptors modulate non-adrenergic non-cholinergic bronchoconstriction in guinea pig *in vivo*. *Eur. J. Pharmacol.* 174:49, 1989.

106. Ichinose, M., and Barnes, P. J. Histamine H_3-receptors modulate antigen-induced bronchoconstriction in guinea pigs. *J. Allergy Clin. Immunol.* 86:491, 1990.

107. Ichinose, M., Belvisi, M. G., and Barnes, P. J. Bradykinin-induced bronchoconstriction in guinea-pig *in vivo*: Role of neural mechanisms. *J. Pharmacol. Exp. Ther.* 253:1207, 1990.

108. Ichinose, M., et al. Histamine H_3-receptors inhibit cholinergic neurotransmission in guinea-pig airways. *Br. J. Pharmacol.* 97:13, 1989.

109. Ilowite, J. S., et al. Permeability of the bronchial mucosa to ^{99m}Tc-DPTA in asthma. *Am. Rev. Respir. Dis.* 139:1139, 1989.

110. Jacoby, D. B., et al. Influenza infection increases airway smooth muscle responsiveness to substance P in ferrets by decreasing enkephalinase. *J. Appl. Physiol.* 64:2653, 1988.

111. James, A. L., Paré, P. D., and Hogg, J. C. The mechanisms of airway narrowing in asthma. *Am. Rev. Respir. Dis.* 139:242, 1989.

112. Jeffery, P. K., et al. Bronchial biopsies in asthma: An ultrastructural, quantitative study and correlation with hyperreactivity. *Am. Rev. Respir. Dis.* 140:1745, 1989.

113. Johnson, A. R., et al. Neutral metalloendopeptidases in human lung tissue and cultured cells. *Am. Rev. Respir. Dis.* 132:564, 1985.

114. Joseph, M., et al. A new function for platelets: IgE-dependent killing of schistosomes. *Nature* 303:310, 1983.

115. Joseph, M., et al. Involvement of immunoglobulin E in the secretory process of alveolar macrophages from asthmatic patients. *J. Clin. Invest.* 71:221, 1983.

116. Josephs, L. K., et al. Non-specific bronchial reactivity and its relationship to the clinical expression of asthma. *Am. Rev. Respir. Dis.* 140:350, 1989.

117. Kaliner, M., et al. Autonomic nervous system abnormalities and allergy. *Ann. Intern. Med.* 96:349, 1982.

118. Katsumata, U., et al. Oxygen radicals produce airway constriction and hyperresponsiveness in anesthetized cats. *Am. Rev. Respir. Dis.* 141:1158, 1990.

119. Kaye, M. G., and Smith, L. J. Effects of inhaled leukotriene D4 and platelet activating factor on airway reactivity in normal subjects. *Am. Rev. Respir. Dis.* 141:993, 1990.

120. Kelley, J. Cytokines of the lung. *Am. Rev. Respir. Dis.* 141:765, 1990.

121. Kelly, C. A., et al. Numbers and activity of cells obtained at bronchoalveolar lavage in asthma, and their relationship to airway responsiveness. *Thorax* 43:684, 1988.

122. Kerrebijn, K. F., Van Essen-Zandvliet, E. E. M., and Neijens, H. J. Effect of long-term treatment with inhaled corticosteroids and beta-agonists on bronchial responsiveness in asthmatic children. *J. Allergy Clin. Immunol.* 79:653, 1987.

123. Kimani, G., Tonnesen, M. G., and Henson, P. G. Stimulation of eosinophil adherence to human vascular endothelial cells *in vitro* by platelet activating factor. *J. Immunol.* 140:3161, 1988.

124. Kirby, J. G., et al. Bronchoalveolar lavage profiles of asthmatic and non asthmatic subjects. *Am. Rev. Respir. Dis.* 136:379, 1987.

125. Komuro, I., et al. Endothelin stimulates c-fos and c-myc expression and proliferation of vascular smooth muscle cells. *FEBS Lett.* 238:249, 1988.

126. Kraan, J., et al. Changes in bronchial hyperreactivity induced by 4 weeks of treatment with antiasthmatic drugs in patients with allergic asthma: A comparison between budesonide and terbutaline. *J. Allergy Clin. Immunol.* 76:628, 1985.

127. Kroegel, C., et al. Platelet activating factor induces eosinophil peroxidase release from human eosinophils. *Immunology* 64:559, 1988.

128. Kroegel, C., et al. Stimulation of degranulation from human eosinophils by platelet activating factor. *J. Immunol.* 142:3518, 1989.

129. Kuo, H.-P., et al. Capsaicin and sensory neuropeptide stimulation of goblet cell secretion in guinea pig trachea. *J. Physiol.* 431:629, 1990.

130. Lai, C. K. W., et al. Inhaled PAF fails to induce airway hyperresponsiveness in normal human subjects. *J. Appl. Physiol.* 68:919, 1990.

131. Laitinen, L. A., et al. Damage of the airway epithelium and bronchial respiratory tract in patients with asthma. *Am. Rev. Respir. Dis.* 131:599, 1985.

132. Laitinen, L. A., and Laitinen, A. Mucosal inflammation and bronchial hyperreactivity. *Eur. Respir. J.* 1:488, 1988.

133. Laitinen, L. A., et al. Eosinophilic airway inflammation during exacerbation of asthma and its treatment with inhaled corticosteroid. *Am. Rev. Respir. Dis.* 143:423, 1991.

134. Lam, S., et al. Effect of bronchial lavage volume on cellular and protein recovery. *Chest* 88:856, 1985.

135. Lam, S., et al. Cellular and protein changes in bronchial lavage fluid after late asthmatic reaction in patients with red cedar asthma. *J. Allergy Clin. Immunol.* 80:44, 1987.

136. Larsen, G. L. Experimental Models of Reversible Airway Obstruction. In R. G. Crystal, et al. (eds.), *The Lung: Scientific Foundations.* New York: Raven, 1991. Pp. 953–966.

137. Lee, T.-C., et al. Increased biosynthesis of platelet activating factor in activated human eosinophils. *J. Biol. Chem.* 259:5526, 1984.

138. Leikhauf, G. D., Driscoll, K. E., and Wey, H. E. Ozone-induced augmentation of eicosanoid metabolism in epithelial cells from bovine trachea. *Am. Rev. Respir. Dis.* 137:435, 1988.

139. Lewis, R. A., Austen, K. F., and Soberman, R. J. Leukotrienes and other products of the 5-lipoxygenase pathway. *N. Engl. J. Med.* 323:645, 1990.

140. List, S. J., et al. Enhancement of the viscosity of mucin by serum albumin. *Biochem. J.* 175:565, 1978.

141. Liu, S. F., Yacoub, M., and Barnes, P. J. Effect of histamine on human bronchial arteries *in vitro. Naunyn Schmiedebergs Arch. Pharmacol.* 342:90, 1990.

142. Lötvall, J. O., et al. Airflow obstruction after substance P aerosol: Contribution of airway and pulmonary edema. *J. Appl. Physiol.* 69:1473, 1990.

143. Lozewicz, S., et al. Morphological integrity of the bronchial epithelium in mild asthma. *Thorax* 45:12, 1990.

144. Lundgren, J. D., and Shelhamer, J. H. Pathogenesis of airway mucus hypersecretion. *J. Allergy Clin. Immunol.* 85:399, 1990.

145. Lungren, R., et al. Morphological studies on bronchial mucosal biopsies from asthmatics before and after ten years treatment with inhaled steroids. *Eur. Respir. J.* 1:883, 1988.

146. MacDermot, J., and Fuller, R. W. Macrophages. In P. J. Barnes, I. W. Rodger, and N. C. Thomson (eds.), *Asthma: Basic Mechanisms and Clinical Management.* London: Academic, 1988. Pp. 97–114.

147. Manning, P. J., et al. Inhibition of exercise-induced bronchoconstriction by MK-571, a potent leukotriene D₄-receptor antagonist. *N. Engl. J. Med.* 323:1736, 1990.

148. Martin, R. J., et al. Airways inflammation and nocturnal asthma. *Am. Rev. Respir. Dis.* 143:351, 1991.

149. McFadden, E. R. Hypothesis: Exercise-induced asthma as a vascular phenomenon. *Lancet* 335:880, 1990.

150. Metzger, W. J., Hunninghake, G. W., and Richerson, H. B. Late asthmatic responses: Inquiry into mechanisms and significance. *Clin. Rev. Allergy* 3:145, 1985.

151. Metzger, W. J., et al. Local allergen challenge and bronchoalveolar lavage of allergic asthmatic lungs. *Am. Rev. Respir. Dis.* 135:433, 1987.

152. Moqbel, R., et al. The effect of platelet-activating factor on IgE binding to, and IgE-dependent biological properties of human eosinophils. *Immunology* 70:251, 1990.

153. Mossman, T. R., and Coffman, R. L. TH1 and TH2 cells: Different patterns of lymphokine secretion lead to different functional properties. *Annu. Rev. Immunol.* 7:145, 1989.

154. Motojima, S., et al. Toxicity of eosinophil cationic proteins for guinea pig tracheal epithelium *in vitro. Am. Rev. Respir. Dis.* 139:801, 1989.

155. Murlas, C. G., and Roum, J. H. Sequence of pathologic changes in the airway mucosa of guinea pigs during ozone-induced bronchial hyperreactivity. *Am. Rev. Respir. Dis.* 131:314, 1985.

156. Nathan, C. F. Secretory products of macrophages. *J. Clin. Invest.* 79:319, 1987.

157. Newman Taylor, A. J., et al. Recurrent nocturnal asthmatic reaction to bronchial-provocation tests. *Clin. Allergy* 9:213, 1979.

158. O'Byrne, P. M., and Fuller, R. W. The role of thromboxane A₂ in the pathogenesis of airway hyperresponsiveness. *Eur. Respir. J.* 2:782, 1989.

159. O'Byrne, P. M., Hargreave, F. E., and Kirby, J. G. Airway inflammation and hyperresponsiveness. *Am. Rev. Respir. Dis.* 136:S35, 1987.

160. O'Byrne, P. M., et al. Neutrophil depletion inhibits airway hyperresponsiveness induced by ozone exposure in dogs. *Am. Rev. Respir. Dis.* 130:214, 1985.

161. O'Connor, B. J., et al. Effect of an inhaled steroid (budesonide) on indirect airway responsiveness and eosinophils in asthma. *Am. Rev. Respir. Dis.* In press.

162. Ohtoshi, T., et al. Monocyte-macrophage differentiation induced by upper airway epithelial cells. *Am. J. Respir. Cell. Mol. Biol.* 4:255, 1991.

163. Owen, W. F., et al. Regulation of human eosinophil viability, density and function by granulocyte/macrophage colony stimulating factor in the presence of 3T3 fibroblasts. *J. Exp. Med.* 166:129, 1987.

164. Page, C. P. One explanation for the asthma paradox: Inhibition of rational anti-inflammatory mechanism by β-agonists. *Lancet* 337:717, 1991.

165. Panettieri, R. A., et al. Histamine induces proliferation and c-fos transcription in cultured airway smooth muscle. *Am. J. Physiol.* 259:L365, 1990.

166. Paul-Eugène, N., et al. Influence of interleukin-4 and platelet activating factor on the fcε RII/CD 23 expression on human monocytes. *J. Lipid Mediat.* 2:95, 1990.

167. Peat, J. K., Woolcock, A. J., and Cullen, K. Rate of decline of lung function in subjects with asthma. *Eur. J. Respir. Dis.* 70:171, 1987.

168. Pelikan, Z., and Pelikan-Filipek, M. The late asthmatic response to allergen challenge—Part 1. *Ann. Allergy* 56:414, 1986.

169. Persson, C. G. A. Plasma exudation and asthma. *Lung* 166:1, 1988.

170. Poulter, L., Power, C., and Burke, C. The relationship between bronchial immunopathology and hyperresponsiveness in asthma. *Eur. J. Respir. Dis.* 3:729, 1990.

171. Proud, D., and Kaplan, A. P. Kinin formation: Mechanisms and role in inflammatory disorders. *Annu. Rev. Immunol.* 6:49, 1988.

172. Regal, J. F. The role of C5a in hypersensitivity reactions in the lung. *Pulmon. Pharmacol.* 2:3, 1989.

173. Rhoden, K. J., and Barnes, P. J. Effect of oxygen-derived free radicals on responses of guinea-pig tracheal smooth muscle *in vitro. Br. J. Pharmacol.* 98:325, 1989.

174. Roberts, N. M., et al. The effect of a specific PAF antagonist, BN 52063, on antigen-induced cutaneous responses in man. *J. Allergy Clin. Immunol.* 93:672, 1988.

175. Roche, W. R., et al. Subepithelial fibrosis in the bronchi of asthmatics. *Lancet* 1:520, 1989.

176. Rogers, D. F., et al. Effect of platelet activating factor on formation and composition of airway fluid in the guinea pig trachea. *J. Physiol.* 431:643, 1991.

177. Rothenburg, M. E., et al. IL-5 dependent conversion of normodense human eosinophils to the hypodense phenotype uses 3T3 fibroblasts for enhanced viability, accelerated hypodensity and sustained antibody-dependent cytotoxicity. *J. Immunol.* 143:2311, 1989.

178. Rothlein, R., et al. Induction of ICAM-1 on primary and continuous cell lines by proinflammatory cytokines. *J. Immunol.* 141:1665, 1988.

179. Ryley, H. C., and Brogan, T. D. Variation in the composition of sputum in chronic chest diseases. *Br. J. Exp. Pathol.* 49:25, 1968.

180. Saetta, M., et al. Quantitative structural analysis of peripheral airways and arteries in sudden fatal asthma. *Am. Rev. Respir. Dis.* 143:138, 1991.

181. Sanjar, S., et al. Pretreatment with rh-GMCSF, but not rh-IL3, enhances PAF-induced eosinophil accumulation in guinea-pig airways. *Br. J. Pharmacol.* 100:399, 1990.

182. Schellenberg, R. R., and Foster, A. *In vitro* responses of human asthmatic airway and pulmonary vascular smooth muscle. *Int. Arch. Allergy Appl. Immunol.* 75:237, 1984.

183. Schleimer, R. P. Effects of glucocorticoids on inflammatory cells relevant to their therapeutic application in asthma. *Am. Rev. Respir. Dis.* 141:S59, 1990.

184. Schleimer, R. P., et al. Characterization of inflammatory mediator release from purified human lung mast cells. *Am. Rev. Respir. Dis.* 133:614, 1986.

185. Schwartz, L. B., and Huff, T. F. Mast Cells. In R. G. Crystal, et al. (eds.), *The Lung: Scientific Foundations.* New York: Raven, 1991. Pp. 601–616.

186. Sears, M. R., et al. Regular inhaled beta-agonist treatment in bronchial asthma. *Lancet* 336:1391, 1990.

187. Sheppard, D., et al. Toluene diisocyanate increases airway responsiveness to substance P and decreases airway and neutral endopeptidase. *J. Clin. Invest.* 81:1111, 1988.

188. Smith, H. Animal models of asthma. *Pulmon. Pharmacol.* 2:59, 1989.

189. Spiteri, M. A., et al. Alveolar macrophage-induced suppression of T-cell hyperresponsiveness in asthma is reversed following allergen exposure *in vitro. Am. Rev. Respir. Dis.* 143:A821, 1992.

190. Springall, D. R., et al. Endothelin immunoreactivity of airway epithelium in asthmatic patients. *Lancet* 337:697, 1991.

191. Stokes, T. C., and Morley, J. Prospects for an oral intal. *Br. J. Dis. Chest.* 75:1, 1981.
192. Stretton, C. D., and Barnes, P. J. Cholecystokinin octapeptide constricts guinea-pig and human airways. *Br. J. Pharmacol.* 97:675, 1989.
193. Tamaoki, J., et al. Cholinergic neuromodulation by prostaglandin D_2 in canine airway smooth muscle. *J. Appl. Physiol.* 63:1396, 1987.
194. Taylor, I. K., et al. Effect of cysteinyl-leukotriene receptor antagonist ICI 204,219 on allergen-induced bronchoconstriction and airway hyperreactivity in atopic subjects. *Lancet* 337:690, 1991.
195. Taylor, K. J., and Luksza, A. R. Peripheral blood eosinophil counts and bronchial responsiveness. *Thorax* 42:452, 1987.
196. Thomson, N. C. *In vivo* versus *in vitro* human airway responsiveness to different pharmacologic stimuli. *Am. Rev. Respir. Dis.* 136:S58, 1987.
197. Tokuyama, K., et al. Neural control of goblet cell secretion in guinea pig airways. *Am. J. Physiol.* 259:L108, 1990.
198. Tomioka, M., et al. Mast cells in bronchoalveolar lumen of patients with bronchial asthma. *Am. Rev. Respir. Dis.* 129:1000, 1984.
199. Vanhoutte, P. M. Epithelium derived relaxing factor: Myth or reality. *Thorax* 43:665, 1988.
200. Van Schayck, C. P., et al. Increased bronchial hyperresponsiveness after inhaling salbutamol during 1 year is not caused by subsensitization to salbuterol. *J. Allergy Clin. Immunol.* 86:736, 1990.
201. Vathenen, A. S., et al. Rebound increase in bronchial responsiveness after treatment with inhaled terbutaline. *Lancet* 1:554, 1988.
202. Walters, E. H., Duddridge, M., and Gardiner, P. V. Bronchoalveolar lavage: Its place in diagnosis and research. *Respir. Med.* 83:457, 1989.
203. Wardlaw, A. J., et al. Effects of inhaled PAF in man in circulating and bronchoalveolar lavage neutrophils: Relationship to bronchoconstriction and changes in airway responsiveness. *Am. Rev. Respir. Dis.* 141:386, 1990.
204. Wardlaw, A. J., et al. Eosinophils and mast cells in bronchoalveolar lavage in subjects with mild asthma. *Am. Rev. Respir. Dis.* 137:62, 1988.
205. Wardlaw, A. J., et al. Platelet activating factor. A potent chemotactic and chemokinetic factor from human eosinophils. *J. Clin. Invest.* 78:1701, 1986.
206. Wegner, C. D., et al. Intracellular adhesion molecule-1 (1 CAM-1) in the pathogenesis of asthma. *Science* 247:456, 1990.
207. Wenzel, S. E., Fowler, A. A., and Schwartz, L. B. Activation of pulmonary mast cells by bronchoalveolar allergen challenge. *In vivo* release of histamine and tryptase in atopic subjects with and without asthma. *Am. Rev. Respir. Dis.* 137:1002, 1988.
208. Wierenga, E. A., et al. Evidence for compartmentalization of functional subjects of CD4+ T lymphocytes in atopic patients. *J. Immunol.* 144:4651, 1990.
209. Yamaguchi, Y., et al. High purified murine interleukin 5 (IL-5) stimulates eosinophil function and prolongs *in vitro* saliva. *J. Exp. Med.* 167:1737, 1988.
210. Yukawa, T., et al. Effect of theophylline and adenosine on eosinophil function. *Am. Rev. Respir. Dis.* 140:327, 1989.
211. Yukawa, T., et al. Density heterogeneity of eosinophil leukocytes: Induction of hypodense eosinophils by platelet activating factor. *Immunology* 68:140, 1989.
212. Yukawa, T., et al. The effects of activated eosinophils and neutrophils on guinea pig airway epithelium *in vitro*. *Am. J. Respir. Cell Mol. Biol.* 2:341, 1990.
213. Yukawa, T., et al. Beta-adrenergic receptors on eosinophils: Binding and functional studies. *Am. Rev. Respir. Dis.* 141:1446, 1990.
214. Weller, P. F. The immunobiology of eosinophils. *N. Engl. J. Med.* 324:1110, 1991.
215. Freitag, A., et al. The effect of treatment with an oral platelet-activating factor antagonist (WEB 2086) on allergen-induced asthmatic responses in human subjects. *Am. Rev. Respir. Dis.* 143:A157, 1991.
216. Wilkens, H., et al. Effects of an inhaled PAF antagonist (WEB 2086 BS) on allergen-induced early and late asthmatic responses and increased bronchial responsiveness to methacholine. *Am. Rev. Respir. Dis.* 143:A812, 1991.
217. Barnes, P. J. Bradykinin as a mediator of asthma. *Thorax.* In press.
218. Weller, P. F., et al. Human eosinophil adherence to vascular endothelium mediated by binding to vascular cell adhesion molecule 1 and endothelial leukocyte adhesion molecule 1. *Proc. Natl. Acad. Sci. USA* 88:7430, 1991.
219. Djukanovic, R., et al. Effect of an inhaled corticosteroid on airway inflammation and symptoms of asthma. *Am. Rev. Respir. Dis.* 145:669, 1992.
220. Laitinen, L. A., Laitinen, A., and Haahtela, T. A comparative study of the effects of an inhaled corticosteroid, budesonide, and of a beta$_2$-agonist, terbutaline, on airway inflammation in newly diagnosed asthma. *J. Allergy Clin. Immunol.* 90:32, 1992.
221. Barnes, P. J. New aspects of asthma. *J. Int. Med.* 231:453, 1992.
222. Lee, T. H., and Lane, S. J. The role of macrophages in the mechanisms of airway inflammation in asthma. *Am. Rev. Respir. Dis.* 145:S27, 1992.

Biochemical Mediators: Histamine, 5-Hydroxytryptamine, Kinins, Peptide Chemotactic Factors, and Complement

10

Wayne H. Anderson

The biochemical mediators discussed in this chapter, as well as in other chapters, including platelet-activating factor (PAF), the leukotrienes, prostaglandins, tachykinins, and interleukins, form a group of interactive substances, many of which alone can mimic the symptomatology of asthma and immediate hypersensitivity responses. It is in fact difficult, if not impossible, with the current array of pharmacologic tools, to determine the role of a single mediator in allergic diseases. It is the interactive, often synergistic nature of these biochemical components that should be realized in discussing the correlation between their pharmacologic profile and physiologic role. It should also be stressed that the profile of each mediator should be viewed in the context of the species variability of the responses.

Great advances continue to be made in the understanding of these relationships and in the development of pharmacologic tools, some of which may serve as the basis of therapeutic agents, and others in providing insight into the pathophysiology of the diseases.

HISTAMINE

It has long been observed that histamine can mimic many of the symptoms of anaphylaxis [3, 14, 267], a fact that has prompted prolific investigations of this amine in allergic diseases. Many extensive reviews have been written to encompass the diverse physiologic influences of this amine [248, 249, 297]. Following extensive pharmacologic reviews by Dale and Laidlaw [63, 64], it was soon observed that antigen-antibody interactions could liberate histamine [23, 24]. The majority of histamine is stored in mast cells, with a good correlation between tissue histamine content and the number of mast cells [246]. In addition to lung tissue, histamine is present in epidermis and the central nervous system. In the gastrointestinal mucosa, histamine is not associated with mast cells but rather exists free, in a rapid turnover pool. The histamine content of fetal tissues is generally higher than that of adult tissues.

Histamine is formed from L-histidine by enzymatic decarboxylation catalyzed by a pyridoxyl 5′-phosphate–dependent enzyme [295, 306], L-histidine decarboxylase (Fig. 10-1). This enzyme is specific for histidine and can be distinguished from the nonspecific aromatic amino acid decarboxylase (dopa decarboxylase) by its susceptibility to inhibition by alpha-methyldopa, as well as by its K_m for histidine [95, 312]. Antibodies generated against histidine decarboxylase from fetal tissues demonstrated good cross-reactivity with adult enzyme from stomach tissue but cross-reacted incompletely with enzyme from brain, suggesting the presence of isozymes [295]. There was no cross-reactivity with bacterial derived enzyme. Two different isozymes have been isolated from brain and fetal tissues by isoelectric focusing and diethylaminoethylcellulose (DEAE-cellulose) chromatography

[307]. Stomach tissue contains both isozymes, explaining the partial cross-reactivity with antifetal enzyme antibodies. Each isozyme has a similar K_m for histidine and may represent mast cell and non–mast cell–derived enzymes [307].

Histidine decarboxylase is an inducible enzyme subject to environmental and mitogen-dependent regulation [72, 215, 259, 260]. In mouse lung a variety of stimuli, including epinephrine [107, 228, 262, 263], Freund's complete adjuvant [263], exercise [107], and the tumor promoter tetradecanoylphorbol-acetate [308], have been demonstrated to induce histidine decarboxylase activity. Enzyme induction did not reflect an increase in mast cells, as was demonstrated in mouse lung following repeated injection of the histamine-releasing agent compound 48/80 [253].

Histidine decarboxylase activity was also demonstrated to be increased in rat basophilic (2H3) cells and in human bone marrow following stimulation with an IgE oligomer and interleukin-3 (IL-3), respectively [195, 305]. Antigenic challenge of *Nippostrongylus brasiliensis*–infected mice resulted in a rapid increase in histidine decarboxylase activity, which could be duplicated with intravenous injections of IL-3 [170]. Protein kinase c activation appears to be associated with the increase in histidine decarboxylase activity [258, 305].

The uptake of L-histidine into the mast cell occurs via energy-independent, sodium-independent transport [166], possibly coupled to histidine decarboxylase activity [25], and is unaffected by extracellular histamine. The K_m for histidine uptake is roughly equal to plasma levels, and thus dietary histidine may influence uptake and regranulation [25]. Some cellular reincorporation of ³H-histamine can be demonstrated in culture [310]; however, the high K_m for uptake for histamine with respect to histidine favors regranulation by synthesis rather than uptake.

Granular uptake of intracellularly synthesized histamine in mast cells is ATP dependent and favored by a pH gradient across the granule membrane, resulting in ion trapping [166]. The mast cell granule, composed of approximately 60 percent protein, 30 percent heparin, 10 percent histamine, 1 to 2 percent phospholipid, and less than 0.2 percent ATP [310], functions as a cationic exchanger, with histamine binding to carboxylic acid groups [298]. Analysis by dye binding indicates that histamine may also bind to the N-sulfate or uronic carboxylic group of heparin [165]. Following release, replenishing tissue stores of histamine in tissues containing large numbers of mast cells may require weeks.

Histamine release from mast cells and basophils can be induced by a variety of compounds [180, 248]. In addition to the classic antigen bridging of IgE bound to high-affinity Fcε receptors on the cell surface, compound 48/80 (a low-molecular-weight polymer of *p*-methoxy-*N*-methylphenylethylamine), opioids, endorphins, and phospholipase A found in polymorphonuclear leukocyte granules, various venoms and toxins, neuropeptides (substance P, neurotensin, calcitonin gene–related peptide), C3a and C5a (components of the complement system),

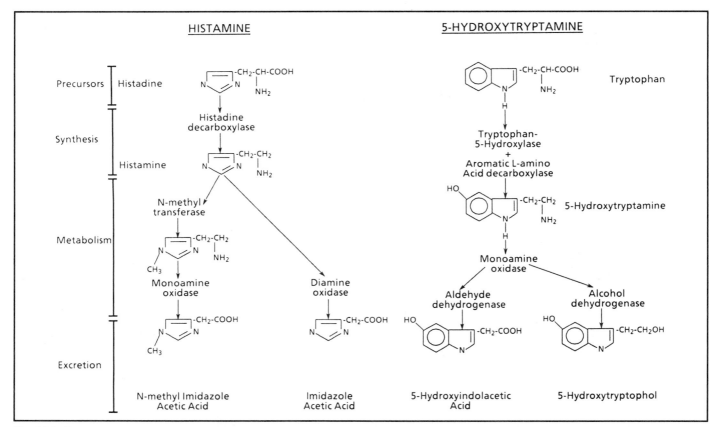

Fig. 10-1. *Biosynthesis and metabolism of histamine and 5-hydroxytryptamine.*

dextrans, and certain other plasma substitutes have all been demonstrated to induce mediator release. A great deal of information elucidating the sequence of events from stimulus to release has accumulated (see Mechanisms of Histamine Release) (see also Chap. 8).

In humans, histamine is rapidly metabolized via two major pathways (see Fig. 10-1) to pharmacologically inactive compounds that are excreted into the urine [261]. While some unmetabolized ^{14}C-histamine (2–3%) can be detected, most of the histamine (42–47%) is oxidized by monoamine oxidase and excreted as *N*-methylimidazole acetic acid. The second major pathway of catabolism involves a nonspecific diamine oxidase (histaminase), which oxidizes histamine to imidazole acetic acid, which is either excreted directly (9–11%) or conjugated with ribose and excreted (16–23%). Plasma histaminase activity increases during anaphylactic shock in a variety of species [178, 251], including humans [44]. Release of histaminase apparently occurs during the process of histamine release but does not parallel plasma histamine levels [53]. Histaminase can be liberated by heparin [186].

Pharmacologic effects of histamine are mediated by three receptor subtypes, H_1, H_2 and H_3 [8a, 10, 35]. Histamine H_1 receptors are preferentially stimulated with 2-methylhistamine and blocked by the classic antihistamines such as pyrilamine maleate and diphenhydramine. Responses elicited through H_2 receptors are preferentially stimulated with 4-methylhistamine and inhibited by burimamide and cimetidine. H_1 receptor antagonists (H_1 antagonists) are generally very lipophilic, while H_2 antagonists are polar hydrophilic compounds. Maintaining the imidazole ring of the parent histamine molecule is believed to be important for H_2 receptor recognition (Table 10-1) (see Chap. 65). A large number of histamine H_3 receptor subtypes have been found in the central nervous system [268a] and recently on eosinophils

Table 10-1. Histamine receptors and histamine action in humans

H_1 receptor
  Contraction of smooth muscle
  ↑ cGMP
  Prostaglandin generation
  ↑ Vascular permeability
  ↓ Atrioventricular node conduction time
  Activation of vagal afferents
H_2 receptor
  ↑ Lower airway mucus secretion
  Gastric acid secretion
  ↑ cAMP
  Basophil histamine release
  Neutrophil chemotaxis
  Stimulation of suppressor T-cell
H_1 + H_2 receptors
  Flushing
  Hypotension
  Headache

Source: Modified from M. V. White. The role of histamine in allergic diseases. *J. Allergy Clin. Immunol.* 86:599, 1990.

[242a]. H_3 receptor activation on eosinophils results in cellular activation, characterized by an increase in intracellular calcium.

Histamine has a variety of potent effects on the cardiovascular system, which vary remarkably between species [2, 220]. On isolated heart preparations, histamine generally has a positive ionotropic (H_1 and H_2) and chronotropic (H_2) effect. Similar effects can be observed in vivo but are complicated by varying effects of the anesthesia [2] and reflex responses elicited by histamine's stimulatory effects on sympathetic nerves. In humans, a positive chronotropic effect can be readily demonstrated [311].

The most characteristic effects of histamine are on the microvasculature. Histamine causes marked hypotension by a combined action on H_1 and H_2 receptors, causing relaxation of arterioles and precapillary sphincters. The endothelial cells of the postcapillary venules constrict to histamine, resulting in cellular separation and an increase in permeability across the exposed basement membrane [184, 213]. These actions of histamine combine to produce a phenomenon referred to as the triple response [175]. Intradermal injection of histamine causes the immediate formation of a red spot, resulting from microvessel vasodilation localized to the site of injection. This area is surrounded by a brighter red flare of irregular outline, resulting indirectly from a histamine-induced reflex vasodilation. In 1 to 2 minutes the original red spot blanches and fills with edema due to the increased vascular permeability. The pain and itch associated with the formation of the wheal and flare may in part result from histamine's ability to stimulate afferent nerve endings [156].

Histamine also has potent effects on bronchial smooth muscle. Generally, histamine causes constriction of isolated airway tissue through H_1 receptors. In sheep bronchi, however, only H_2 receptors are evident; when stimulated they produce bronchodilation [78]. In cat trachea activation of both H_1 and H_2 receptors causes relaxation [78, 183]. Even in guinea pig tracheal tissue, which is exquisitely sensitive to the contractile effects of histamine, evidence of functionally opposed histamine H_1 and H_2 receptors has been presented [216]. However, it is believed that H_2 receptors have no in vivo or in vitro physiologic significance in guinea pig airways [40].

Michoud and coworkers [104] observed that in normal human subjects, great differences existed in the sensitivity to histamine and in the effects of H_2 receptor blockade on histamine responses. In very sensitive subjects, cimetidine (H_2 receptor antagonist) decreased responsiveness to histamine, while in only modestly sensitive subjects cimetidine enhanced airway reactivity. Thus, the nature of the sample population with respect to its sensitivity to histamine may relate to the role of H_2 receptors in individual responsiveness. In asthmatic subjects who are generally very sensitive to histamine, cimetidine had little effect on baseline pulmonary function and was without effect on bronchial reactivity to aerosol histamine challenge [212]. H_2 receptor activation in basophils is inhibitory, reducing mediator release [176]. Conversely, as demonstrated in passively sensitized monkey lung [48], inhibiting H_2 receptors prior to antigen challenge increases mediator release.

Histamine is a potent inducer of prostaglandin synthesis [4, 317], which in guinea pigs and dogs results in depressed tracheal reactivity [5, 158]. In canine tracheal smooth muscle this negative feedback can actually render the tissue tachyphylactic to further histamine responsiveness [4, 6].

The in vivo pulmonary effect of histamine is both direct and indirect, the indirect effects mediated by the vagus. In unanesthetized, spontaneously breathing guinea pigs, cholinergic blockage with atropine will block resistance and compliance changes to low doses of histamine. At higher doses histamine's effects are resistant to cholinergic blockage, indicating a direct effect on airway smooth muscle [73]. Vagotomy also attenuates histamine-induced increases in resistance and decreases in compliance in spontaneously breathing anesthetized guinea pigs, but is less effective in paralyzed, artificially ventilated animals [194].

Basal plasma histamine levels have been shown to be elevated in asthmatic subjects [20, 33] and markedly increase following specific allergen aerosol challenge, but not following challenge with skin test–negative allergens or methacholine [33]. During naturally occurring asthmatic episodes, plasma histamine levels seem to correlate with decreased pulmonary function [20, 42, 272], yet antihistamines are generally considered ineffective during asthmatic episodes [152]. Many earlier studies employing antihistamines did not use a double-blind protocol, and many relied on subjective evaluation rather than objective data on pulmonary function. Antihistamine therapy with diphenhydramine hydrochloride (Benadryl) [172], neohetramine [58], Theophorin [59], and others [152] has failed to demonstrate significant improvements in pulmonary function. Intramuscular administration of thiazinamium (Multergan), however, was effective in preventing antigen-induced bronchoconstriction [36], but this result may be related to the drug's significant anticholinergic and bronchodilatory properties.

Two new oral antihistamines, terfenadine (180 mg) and astemizole (10 mg/day × 2 weeks), have been shown to produce a 35-fold and 17-fold shift in histamine responsiveness, respectively [131, 242]. Methacholine responsiveness was not affected, demonstrating the specificity of these agents. Fifty percent of the immediate response to antigen in asthmatic subjects has been demonstrated to be inhibited by a single dose of 180 mg of terfenadine [126].

In two asthma clinical trials, terfenadine (120 and 180 mg) produced significant improvement in symptom scores, peak expiratory flow rates, and with the higher dose, a 40 percent reduction in bronchodilator use [126, 290]. Clinically significant improvement was most evident in patients with pollen-sensitive asthma.

Two conclusions can be drawn: (1) Histamine is not a singularly important mediator in asthma, and (2) in light of alternative approaches, antihistamines are relatively poor therapeutic agents in managing asthma. Since antihistamines have a variety of pharmacologic activities including the ability to release histamine [9, 94] and to contract airway tissue [115, 116], especially following aerosol treatment, it is with caution that histamine's role in the pathogenesis of asthmatic symptomatology is dismissed on the sole basis of the therapeutic ineffectiveness of antihistamines.

5-HYDROXYTRYPTAMINE (SEROTONIN)

In mammals, 5-hydroxytryptamine (5-HT) is most abundant in the enterochromaffin cells of the gastrointestinal tract, with small amounts located in platelets and the central nervous system [77]. 5-HT can also be found in the pulmonary neuroendocrine cells of the airway epithelium [106, 145]. Pulmonary neuroendocrine cell hyperplasia can occur in chronic respiratory lung disease, and an increase in serotonin excretion in the urine is correlated with cough in bronchitis [275a].

Even though significant quantities of 5-HT are available from the diet, 5-HT is synthesized from tryptophan by successive hydroxylation (tryptophan-5-hydroxylase) and decarboxylation (aromatic-1-amino acid decarboxylase) (see Fig. 10-1). Once formed, it is taken up into storage granules and complexed with ATP. The storage process is very similar to catecholamine uptake and sensitive to the same blockers. A high-affinity uptake mechanism into tryptaminergic nerve endings and platelets allows the accumulation of 5-HT against a concentration gradient [37, 67].

Metabolism of 5-HT occurs by the action of monoamine oxidase forming 5-hydroxyindoleacetaldehyde. This is further metabolized, primarily by aldehyde dehydrogenase, to 5-hydroxyindoleacetic acid (5-HIAA), or by alcohol dehydrogenase to 5-hydroxytryptophol (5-HTOL). Both 5-HIAA and 5-HTOL are excreted in urine as the glucuronide or sulfate conjugate [37, 96].

The effects of 5-HT are mediated via receptors designated 5-HT_1, 5-HT_2, and 5-HT_3. The 5-HT_1 receptors have been further subdivided into four additional subtypes labeled 5-HT_{1A} to 5-HT_{1D}. Subtypes A and C have been cloned and sequenced [79, 181]. 5-HT_{1A} receptor stimulation activates adenylate cyclase via a guanosine triphosphate (GTP) –binding protein, while 5-HT_{1B} and 5-HT_{1D} receptors inhibit the enzyme [232]. The 5-HT_2 receptor has also been cloned and has been demonstrated to increase intracellular calcium via activation of phospholipase C [66, 235].

The 5-HT$_3$ receptors appear to be part of the family of ligand-gated ion channels [68], and independent of G-protein or second-messenger involvement.

The cardiovascular effects of 5-HT, as with histamine, are species variable. 5-HT has a direct positive ionotropic and chronotropic effect on isolated heart preparations, mediated by 5-HT$_1$ receptors [39]. Some cardiac effects may also occur indirectly via catecholamine release from adrenergic nerve terminals [75]. 5-HT$_3$ receptor activation on coronary vessels can result in a Benzold-Jarish reflex inhibition of sympathetic activity, resulting in vagal mediated bradycardia in vivo [96].

Intravenous administration of 5-HT causes a multiphasic blood pressure response. An early and transient depressor phase results from stimulation of the coronary chemoreceptor reflex. A short pressor response ensues due to direct effects on peripheral resistance via direct 5-HT$_2$ receptors, resulting in contraction of arteries, veins, and venules [130]. This is generally followed by a prolonged period of hypotension, resulting from vasodilation in the skeletal muscle beds [221, 222], mediated by 5-HT$_1$–induced release of endothelial-derived relaxation factor (EDRF) [207, 225].

Capillary permeability is increased in rats following an intradermal injection of 5-HT, whereas in humans there is little effect. 5-HT can induce the erythema and flare components of the triple response without any evidence of wheal formation.

The effects of 5-HT on respiration are also quite variable. Apnea often follows intravenous administration in some species [161, 317a], probably by activation of the 5-HT$_3$ receptor subtype, especially evident in the cat. In the dog and in humans an increase in minute volume is generally observed, accompanied by tachypnea. Evidence exists that monoaminergic neurons are involved in modulation of the respiratory drive, both centrally [167, 182] and peripherally [211, 219]. 5-HT has been immunohistologically localized to neuroendocrine cells and neuroendocrine bodies believed to respond to airway hypoxia and hypercapnia [106, 145]. Their presence has been demonstrated to increase in various chronic obstructive pulmonary diseases [145, 146].

Infusion of 5-HT into isolated dog lungs causes constriction predominantly of bronchial and bronchiolar smooth muscle, but also results in compression of alveoli and capillaries [250]. Short-term aerosol exposure to 5-HT in the dog increases airway reactivity to vagal stimulation and histamine [69, 113], an effect not observed after acetylcholine exposure. Bronchoconstriction results from intravenous administration of 5-HT in guinea pigs [119] and cats [54]. The bronchoconstriction in guinea pigs is blocked by the 5-HT$_2$ receptor antagonist ketanserin [43]. Repeated challenge of animals with 5-HT results in a rapidly developing tachyphylaxis, with cross-tachyphylaxis to antigen challenge in albumin-sensitized guinea pigs [120]. However, since the desensitization is a generalized decrease in mediator responsiveness, a bronchoconstrictor role for 5-HT in guinea pig anaphylaxis cannot be supported.

In vitro, human bronchioles respond to 5-HT with relaxation [41], but in vivo, humans are relatively resistant [192]. Asthmatic subjects, however, respond to aerosolized 5-HT with a prompt decrease in expiratory flow and vital capacity. In a double-blind, crossover study in patients with chronic obstructive disease, ketanserin, presumably by antagonizing 5-HT$_2$ receptors, has been shown to increase 1-second forced expiratory volume (FEV$_1$) and forced expiratory flow after 50 percent of vital capacity has been expelled (FEF$_{50\%}$) [47].

KININS

The biologically active kinins bradykinin (Arg-Pro-Gly-Phe-Ser-Pro-Phe-Arg), a nonapeptide, and kallidin, also referred to as lysylbradykinin (Lys-Arg-Pro-Gly-Phe-Ser-Pro-Phe-Arg), a decapeptide, are cleaved from two precursors called kininogens (Fig.

10-2). The kininogens exist as high-molecular-weight (MW 110,000) and low-molecular-weight (MW 50,000) alpha globulins [288], both products of the same gene [159].

Both the high- and low-molecular-weight kininogens are composed of three components: identical heavy chains, a Leu-Met-Lys-bradykinin-Ser- sequence, and a unique light chain that distinguishes the two kininogens apart, both in size as well as in activation processes. The low-molecular-weight kininogen has a light chain with a molecular weight of 4,000 while the light chain of the high-molecular-weight kininogen has a molecular weight of approximately 70,000. The light chain of the high-molecular-weight kininogen has binding sites for prekallikrein (see below) as well as a surface-binding site that confers on the high-molecular-weight kininogen the ability to be activated by surface contact, resulting in the release of bradykinin. Within the heavy chain of both kininogens has been found cysteine proteinase inhibitory activity, now demonstrated to be identical with the cysteine proteinase inhibitors found in human plasma [206, 257].

Kininogens are present in plasma at an approximate concentration of 270 μg/ml, the majority of which is the low-molecular-weight kininogen [237]. Extravascular concentrations of kininogens are probably low but have the potential to increase dramatically under conditions leading to plasma exudation. It is unlikely that kininogens are locally synthesized in the lung [239].

Several proteinases, such as tryptase from human lung mast cells [238], neutrophil-derived proteinases [202], and platelet-derived calpains (a cysteine proteinase) [121], have been demonstrated to cleave kininogens to active kinins. Other proteolytic enzymes such as trypsin, those found in snake venoms, and plasmin will form kinins from kininogens. The activity of these enzymes is generally insignificant compared with that of plasma and tissue kallikreins. The kallikreins are substrate specific for kininogens with little activity on other proteins [320].

Plasma kallikrein is a single-chain alpha globulin synthesized in the liver. It circulates in the plasma as the inactive proenzyme prekallikrein bound to the light chain of the high-molecular-weight kininogen [185]. Thus enzyme and substrate circulate as a bound complex. Prekallikrein is converted to active kallikrein by Hageman factor (Factor XII), a protease also active in the intrinsic pathway of coagulation. Hageman factor circulates in an inactive state and is activated by "solid-phase" substances such as collagen [243], monosodiumurate crystals [157], certain immune complexes [201], and in vitro by glass [243]. Negatively charged surfaces such as heparin and mucus glycoproteins also have the potential to activate Factor XII [236].

Binding of high-molecular-weight kininogen to a surface via the surface-binding site together with Factor XII in close proximity results in an accelerated activation of Factor XII. In addition, kallikrein can activate Factor XII, resulting in a positive "feedback" loop [111, 214]. Thus, contact activation results in the formation of a "nucleus" consisting of substrate, enzyme, and activation factors, resulting in the release of the proinflammatory peptide bradykinin and consequently the activation of the intrinsic pathway of coagulation via activation of Factor XII. This close association of enzyme and substrates also makes high-molecular-weight kininogen the preferred, if not the only substrate for plasma kallikrein in vivo [233], and results only in the production of bradykinin. Kallikrein is inactivated by alpha-macroglobulin and by the complement component C1 inhibitor. The C1 inhibitor also limits the activity of the high-molecular-weight kininogen/kallikrein system by inhibiting activated Factor XII [189, 265].

Tissue or glandular kallikreins are distinct proteins, smaller than the plasma kallikreins, and present in most tissues as proenzymes. Exocrine glands such as the pancreas are rich sources of these enzymes [236]; in fact, the name *kallikrein* is derived from the Greek word for pancreas [97]. Unlike plasma kallikrein, tissue kallikrein has no specificity toward low- or high-molecular-weight kininogens and results in the formation of kallidin [309].

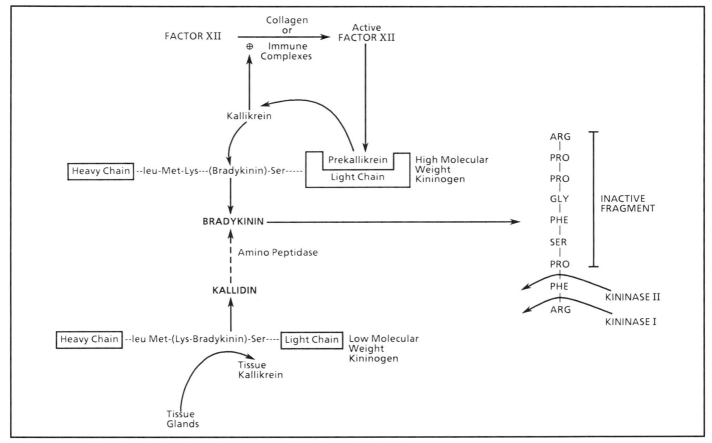

Fig. 10-2. *Activation of the kinin pathway and generation of bradykinin and kallidin. The pathway can be activated by either the activation of Factor XII or by the release of tissue kallikrein, resulting in the formation of bradykinin or kallidin, respectively. Inactivation occurs rapidly by removal of the terminal phenylalanine or phenylalanine-arginine amino acids, resulting in an inactive peptide.*

Kallidin can be converted to bradykinin by aminopeptidases found on cell membranes and in plasma [112, 223]. The rate of inactivation of both bradykinin and kallidin is however significantly more rapid than the aminopeptidase conversion of kallidin to bradykinin, and thus this pathway of bradykinin formation does not result in significant net-bradykinin formation [97]. Tissue kallikrein is poorly regulated by proteinase inhibitors, the most active being alpha$_1$-antiprotease. Therefore, kinin formation by tissue kallikreins appears to be regulated by the rate of activation and/or secretion of tissue prokallikrein as well as substrate availability [236].

The half-life of bradykinin in blood is very short (< 30 seconds), with both tissue and plasma-metabolizing enzymes (kininases) participating in the hydrolysis. Approximately 80 percent of plasma bradykinin is removed by the lungs on a single pass [86]. Metabolism occurs in or near the endothelium of the pulmonary vessels [255]. There are two primary kininases that rapidly inactivate the kinins. Kininase I (carboxypeptidase N), a plasma enzyme, removes the C-terminal amino acid arginine. Kininase II, which is synonymous with angiotensin-converting enzyme (ACE), removes the C-terminal dipeptide phenylalanine-arginine. Bradykinin is the preferred substrate for this enzyme, with a markedly lower K_m when compared to angiotensin [70]. Captopril, an ACE inhibitor, can only inhibit a maximum of 50 percent of the metabolism of bradykinin in perfused rat lung, indicating the presence of other metabolizing enzymes [19], possibly endopeptidase 24.15 [64a] (Table 10-2).

The kinins spectrum of pharmacologic activity includes vaso-

Table 10-2. Actions of bradykinin

1. Smooth muscle spasmogenesis
2. Vasodilation, microvascular leakage
3. Stimulation of inflammatory mediator release: PAF, peptidoleukotrienes, LTB$_4$, hydroxytetraenoic acids
4. Stimulation of sensory nerve endings with release of tachykinins, as substance P
5. Contribution to inflammatory response in allergy
6. Potent bronchoconstriction

dilation, bronchoconstriction, increased capillary permeability, and pain. Bradykinin receptors have been classified as B$_1$, B$_2$, and B$_3$ based on sensitivity to peptide analogs and antagonists [321–323].

In humans and many other mammals bradykinin causes dilation of arterioles, a decrease in vascular resistance, and hypotension [324–326]. The kinins induce permeability changes in the skin of many species, being 100-fold more potent than histamine in the guinea pig [327, 328]. Although differences in potency between kallidin and bradykinin can be established on certain smooth muscle preparations [329], generally kallidin and bradykinin are similar.

The hemodynamic effects of the kinins are, however, complicated by their interaction with other potent endogenous agents such as catecholamines [330], release of histamine [331], and production of endothelium-derived relaxant factor (EDRF) [332,

333], which also influence blood pressure and vascular permeability.

Bradykinin causes contraction of isolated guinea pig tracheal smooth muscle, but not rabbit, dog, or human bronchus [334]. Bradykinin is both less potent and less effective than histamine in inducing contraction of guinea pig trachea, and is not blocked by B_1 or B_2 receptor antagonists [323]. In isolated perfused guinea pig lung preparations, however, bradykinin is generally more potent than histamine, suggesting that bradykinin is more specific for peripheral airways [335]. This is supported by bronchograms demonstrating in vivo an apparent selectivity of bradykinin for narrowing bronchioles [336].

Bronchoconstriction induced by bradykinin in the guinea pig in vivo is selectively antagonized by aspirin-like drugs, suggesting that the in vivo effects may be mediated by bradykinin-stimulated prostaglandin or thromboxane synthesis [337].

A bradykinin antagonist has been demonstrated to block antigen-induced increases in airway hyperreactivity and neutrophil influx in the sheep [338], and bradykinin is a potent dilator of the tracheal circulation [339]. Asthmatic patients are hyperresponsive to bradykinin [340], and bradykinin has been detected in antigen-induced skin wheals of sensitive patients [341].

COMPLEMENT

The complement system is a cascade of activation sequences that comprises an important component of host defense. The process consists of two activation pathways (classical and alternative), an amplification reaction, and a common effector response (Fig. 10-3). Activation of the classical pathway involves nine proteins: C1 through C9. Following activation, many of the proteins become enzymatically active. Two exceptions include C1q (a subunit of C1), which serves as a recognition protein of bound immunoglobulins, and C4, which recognizes membrane-binding sites for complement and itself serves as a binding site for additional complement proteins.

The fifth protein, C5, has a high affinity for cellular membranes and initiates the assembly of the "attack" complex, comprised of proteins C5 through C9. While individual components of the attack complex may not be enzymatically active, the complex ultimately causes cell lysis. This sequential activation and assembly of plasma proteins can be achieved by both immunologic (the classical pathway) and nonimmunologic (the alternative pathway) stimuli. The end result is the conversion of inactive serum zymogens to active serine esterases and their attachment to membrane receptors, which causes damage to cellular membranes, alteration of particle surfaces for increased clearance, and the production of potent mediators of inflammation.

The classical pathway of complement activation is initiated by IgM or adjacent IgG molecules bound to a surface or membrane. IgG4, IgA, and IgE do not activate complement [203, 231]. The initial complement protein, C1, is a complex containing three separate subunits, C1q, C1r, and C1s. The C1 subunits are synthesized in epithelial cells, mononuclear phagocytes, and fibroblasts and circulate in the plasma predominantly as the C1 complex C1qr2s2 [319]. Assembly of one molecule of C1q with two molecules each of C1r and C1s forms C1. C1q is a unique molecule with six globular IgG- and IgM-binding sites joined to a common collagen-like stalk by connecting strands [179, 270]. Binding of C1q to immunoglobulins results in a conformation change, which allows binding of C1r. C1r is composed of two identical polypeptide subunits that autoactivate on binding to C1q, resulting in the expression of serine esterase activity [268, 318]. Activated C1r cleaves the single polypeptide chain of C1s into two polypeptide chains, which again results in an active serine esterase whose natural substrates are the fourth and second complement proteins C4 and C2 [204].

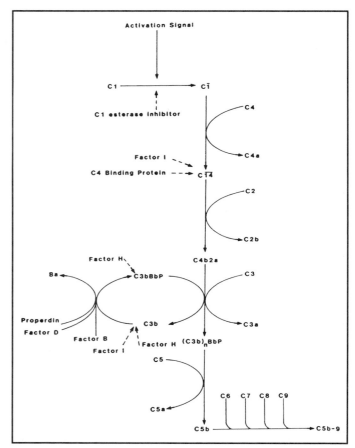

Fig. 10-3. *Overview of the complement cascade, demonstrating the alternative and classical pathways of activation. (Reprinted with permission from N. Berend. Complement. In: P. J. Barnes, I. W. Rodger, and N. C. Thompson (eds.),* Asthma: Basic Mechanisms and Clinical Management. *New York: Academic, 1988. P. 326.)*

The C1s and C1r serine esterases are inhibited by a plasma protein C1 inhibitor. C1 inhibitor appears to be synthesized in many of the same cells that produce the C1 subunits: hepatocytes, mononuclear phagocytes, and fibroblasts [264]. C1 inhibitor can also bind to kallikrein, plasmin, and clotting Factors XI and XII [65].

The enzymatic activity of C1s cleaves from C4 a small fragment, C4a, resulting in the expression of a labile site on the remaining C4b fragment for binding to cellular membranes. C4 is produced in hepatocytes, monocytes, and alveolar macrophages and synthesis can be increased by interferon gamma (IFN-γ) [163]. The small C4a fragment can increase binding of C2 to enzymatically active C1s, with subsequent hydrolysis of C2 into C2a and C2b [98, 99]. Binding of C2a to the membrane-bound C4b constitutes an enzymatic complex (C4bC2a), referred to as C3 convertase, which cleaves C3 into a small C3a and larger C3b fragment. The latter C3b fragment binds to the C4bC2a complex (C4bC2aC3b), which can then recognize and bind the fifth complement protein, C5 [104]. C3a is pharmacologically active (see below). Bacterial lipopolysaccharide, IL-1, IL-6, and IFN-γ can all increase C3 production [230, 283].

C5 is cleaved to C5a and C5b by the C5 convertase (C4bC2aC3b) complex [164, 171]. The C3 and C5 convertase complexes are covalently linked to cellular membranes via a thiolester group [169]. Free C5b binds both C6 and C7 complement proteins [164, 234] and then inserts into a cellular membrane surface, serving as a binding site for C8. C8 is composed of three polypeptide chains alpha, beta, and gamma [277]. Binding of C8 to the C5b67 complex results in the insertion of the alpha and gamma chains into the membrane, causing a 10- to 30-nm lesion [76, 188]. Binding of C9 to the complex and its insertion allows for the polymerization of additional C9 molecules. This results in a membrane lesion of approximately 100 nm [234], leading to disruption of cellular integrity. The C5-C9 complex is often referred to as the attack complex.

C3 can also be activated by the alternative or otherwise known as the properdin pathway. The alternative pathway is activated by polysaccharides, lipopolysaccharides, viruses, bacteria, DNA, C-reactive protein, and mitochondrial membranes [22, 151, 231, 281]. In addition to the proteins C3 and C5 (which are common to both pathways) and the components of the attack complex, this pathway uses five additional proteins: Factor B, Factor D, Factor H, Factor I, and properdin. Once C3b is bound to a cell surface, Factor B, a beta$_2$ globulin, binds to C3b, forming C3bB, the inactive C3 and C5 convertase of the alternative pathway. In the presence of magnesium, the C3bB complex is susceptible to enzymatic attack by Factor D, a serine esterase [80], which cleaves a small fragment Ba from B. Factor D is produced in adipocytes and mononuclear phagocytes [21, 252]. Removal of Ba unmasks an enzymatic site on the remaining Bb such that the activated C3bBb complex can bind and cleave C3 into C3a and more C3b. Additional C3b, following attachment to membrane receptor sites, can then bind more Factor B, thus repeating the positive feedback process [299]. Factor B can be produced by mononuclear phagocytes, fibroblasts, and endothelial cells and can be regulated by a variety of growth factors and cytokines [229, 230]. This amplification system can result in the generation and binding of a large number of C3b fragments. In addition, the unstable C3bBb complex can be "stabilized" by properdin, further enhancing the alternative pathway [81, 274].

Alternatively, the C3bBb complex can also bind an additional C3b fragment, which then recognizes, binds, and hydrolyzes C5. Thus, activation of C5 to C5b initiates activation of the attack complex by the alternative as well as the classical pathway [61, 300].

Two proteins, Factor H and Factor I, are responsible for controlling the alternative pathway amplification system. The system is inherently self-limiting, as discussed above, in that the binding site of activated C3b on the cellular membrane is labile. Factor H, a heat-sensitive beta globulin, is devoid of enzymatic activity. It inhibits C3b by binding to the C3b molecule, prevents access of Factor B [155], causes dissociation of existing bound Bb [205], and increases binding of Factor I [224]. Factor I is the second inhibitory protein with endopeptidase activity, which cleaves C3b to inactive fragments when Factor H is bound [224]. Factor I requires a cofactor, recently identified as membrane cofactor protein (MCP). MCP may protect cells, which express the protein from complement mediated analysis [64b, 213a], and can be released by phospholipase [41a].

In addition to the enhanced recognition and cell lysis that result from the activation of the complement pathways, two low-molecular-weight fragments, C3a (MW 9,000) and C5a (MW 17,000), cause an additional array of immunopharmacologic effects. These effects, as reported in 1929, were thought to result from toxic products (termed *anaphylatoxins*) generated by incubating guinea pig serum with antigen-antibody complexes [93]. Although differences exist in molecular weight, there are structural similarities within each anaphylatoxin molecule; that is, 40 to 45 percent of the molecule has an alpha-helix configuration stabilized by intrachain disulfide bonds. Each molecule also has six half-cysteine residues in the linear sequence, and the C-terminal end of both C3a and C5a plays a prominent role in function [84].

Binding of the anaphylatoxin C3a to cell membranes has been demonstrated [292]; this binding results in histamine release

from skin mast cells (but not lung mast cells) and basophils, and activates neutrophils [108, 109, 144, 266]. Human C3a and C5a also contract isolated guinea pig parenchymal strips and trachea, independent of histamine release since antihistamines will not attenuate the complement-induced contraction [244, 280]. In addition to histamine release, C5a has been reported to stimulate leukotriene release from guinea pig lung, suggesting that leukotrienes may mediate the guinea pig tracheal response to C5a [245, 278].

Serum carboxypeptidase removes the carboxy-terminal arginine (des Arg) from the anaphylatoxins C3a and C5a, which for human anaphylatoxins renders them ineffective in evoking histamine release or smooth muscle contraction [71, 80]. The des Arg form of porcine C5a, however, is nearly as active as C5a in stimulating smooth muscle contraction and leukotriene release [279].

C5a is chemotactic for neutrophils, eosinophils, and monocytes [302]. Plasmin, trypsin, elastase, and kallikrein can generate chemotactic fragments from both C3 and C5, resembling the activity of C5a [301]. C3a itself does not appear to be chemotactic [134, 275]. The des Arg form of human C5a does retain significant chemotactic activity [85]. Instillation of C5a, C5a des Arg, and C3a can result in lung injury characterized by edema, vascular congestion, and cellular influx [118, 168, 269]. The biology and biochemistry of the anaphylatoxins have been reviewed [133].

Three complement receptors—Type 1, Type 2, and Type 3 (CR1, CR2, and CR3)—have been identified on a variety of cells. CR1 is found on erythrocytes, lymphocytes, monocytes, and granulocytes and has a high affinity for C3b and C4b. These receptors can be upregulated in the presence of C5a, tumor necrosis factor (TNF), and some viral agents [74, 83, 162]. The primary function of CR1 appears to be regulation of the complement cascade by binding and therefore decreasing the availability of C3b and C4b. CR1 may also aid in removal of complement-fixing immune complexes via the reticuloendothelial system [291].

CR2 has a high affinity for proteolytic fragments of C3b as well as a protein found on the viral envelope of Epstein-Barr virus. Binding of the viral protein to CR2, which has some sequence homology with C3b, results in B-cell proliferation [191]. The CR2 receptor is found predominantly on lymphocytes. The C3 receptor, which binds C3bi, a proteolytic fragment of C3b, is one of the alpha chains of the leukocyte adhesion glycoprotein Mac-1 [55]. Hemodialysis has been shown to increase the expression of CR3 receptors on granulocytes and has been implicated in the sequestration of cells in the pulmonary circulation, resulting in a decrease in pulmonary function [8].

Many of the cells in the lung including alveolar macrophages, alveolar Type II cells, epithelial cells, and fibroblasts can synthesize complement proteins C1 to C5, as well as factors of the alternative pathway. Thus, the lung has the potential to locally activate the complement cascade, and such activation has been implicated as a contributing factor in adult respiratory distress syndrome (ARDS) [114, 247].

EOSINOPHIL CHEMOTACTIC FACTOR OF ANAPHYLAXIS

Eosinophil chemotactic factors are released from guinea pig and human lung over a similar time course as histamine release [153, 154]. Eosinophil chemotactic factor of anaphylaxis (ECF-A) is preformed and associated with mast cell granules [303]. Early characterization demonstrated the factor(s) to be of low molecular weight (MW 300–1,000) and inactivated by proteolytic enzymes [304]. Purification of human lung–derived ECF-A by combined chromatographic steps demonstrated two distinct acidic tetrapeptides having the amino acid sequences Val-Gly-Ser-Glu and Ala-Gly-Ser-Glu [101]. The biologic activity was confirmed using synthetic ECF-A and was demonstrated to be specific for eosinophils [103]. Chemotaxis is maximal when the ECF-A concentration is in the 10^{-7} M range, whereas deactivation, a process rendering the cells unresponsive to further chemotactic stimuli, occurs with doses as low as 10^{-10} M [102]. Binding and subsequent activation or deactivation of the eosinophil are unaffected by rearrangement of the two internal peptides glycine and serine. Removal of one of these two peptides, however, decreases the activity tenfold, indicating that spacing between the terminal NH$_2$ and COOH group is important to binding and activity [100]. In addition to attracting and holding eosinophils at a site (activation and deactivation), ECF-A was observed to increase the number of C3b receptors on eosinophils, thus enhancing the effectiveness of the complement system [7].

These tetrapeptides are not to be confused with LTB$_4$, which can be released by similar stimuli and is also chemotactic for eosinophils. However, an eosinophil chemotactic factor released from cultured, murine bone marrow–derived mast cells had a physiochemical profile of an arachidonic acid metabolite, and no preexisting activity was found in a freeze-thawed extract of nonactivated cells [1]. It has been suggested that low-molecular-weight ECF-A and LTB$_4$ are the same molecule [60].

Also released from human lung [100] and rat mast cells [18] is an intermediate-molecular-weight (MW 1,500–3,000) group of eosinophil chemotactic factors differing in charge and hydrophobicity [45]. These intermediate-molecular-weight ECF-As are also released, presumably from the granule, and have the same chemotactic and deactivation profile as the low-molecular-weight ECF-A tetrapeptides [38].

The ECF-A tetrapeptides and intermediate-molecular-weight ECF-As are relatively selective for eosinophils, whereas a high-molecular-weight chemotactic factor (MW > 750,000 daltons) is preferentially chemotactic to neutrophils. A high-molecular-weight neutrophil chemotactic factor has been isolated from human leukemic basophils [173], human lung [100], and rat peritoneal mast cells [258]. The kinetics of its release is similar to that of the release of histamine and ECF-A and can be blocked with disodium cromoglycate, suggesting that it is preformed [13]. The biologic profile of high-molecular-weight chemotactic factor for neutrophils, including chemotaxis and deactivation, is similar to that of ECF-A for eosinophils.

MECHANISMS OF HISTAMINE RELEASE

The biochemical mechanisms of activation and mediator release from mast cells have been the subject of intense research efforts for many years, often yielding conflicting results. Some of these results can be attributed to species differences or the secretagogue employed. Several review articles [30, 139, 227] highlighted the efforts made to elucidate mechanisms of activation. It seems clear that phospholipid metabolism in the membrane by phospholipases A$_2$ and C and interaction of the second messengers cyclic AMP, inositol phosphates, and calcium are involved in initiation of mast cell activation (Figs. 10-4 and 10-5).

The first step in the biochemical cascade of events leading to mast cell and basophil mediator release may be activation of a peptidase or possibly a serine esterase [16, 17, 28]. Enzymatic activity, which can be distinguished from complement C1 esterase activity, is inhibited by irreversible phosphorylating phosphonates such as diisopropylfluorophosphate (DFP) [138, 240]. Inhibition, however, requires cell activation and calcium. Washing the cells previously incubated with DFP prior to activation results in no inhibition, suggesting that the enzyme may be protected or in a proesterase form [147, 240].

Guanosine Triphosphate–Binding Proteins, Phospholipase C, and Inositol Phosphate Pathway

It is well known that many ligand-receptor interactions are coupled to an effector protein by a trimeric GTP-binding protein (G-protein); several different proteins have been identified [34, 105]. The activated receptor facilitates the binding of GTP to the Gα subunit of the G-protein, resulting in the dissociation of this subunit from the Gβγ complex. The Gα-GTP subunit binds to the effector protein and initiates the response. The reaction is terminated by the hydrolysis of GTP to guanosine diphosphate (GDP), resulting in a conformational change and reassembly of the G-protein subunits.

It is proposed that two GTP-binding proteins are involved in mast cell activation and subsequent mediator release [52]. A Gp protein activates phospholipase C, resulting in the formation of (1,4,5)inositol trisphosphate ((1,4,5)IP$_3$) and diacylglycerol (see below). A second G-protein GE, acts at a later stage of stimulus-secretion coupling possibly via calcium and activation of a calcium-binding protein [52]. GTPγ-S, a nonhydrolyzable analog of GTP, when introduced into permeabilized rat mast cells, causes histamine release in the presence of added calcium [105, 256]. The effects of GTPγ-S on histamine release are time and dose dependent [52].

The activation of phospholipase C has been demonstrated to occur following activation of a diverse number of receptors in a variety of cell types [241]. Phospholipase C catalyzes the hydrolysis of the membrane phospholipid, phosphatidylinositol 4,5-bisphosphate (PIP$_2$). PIP$_2$ is formed by sequential phosphorylation of phosphatidylinositol. The inositol phosphate metabolic pathway is quite complex and is the subject of several recent reviews [31, 132, 196].

Hydrolysis of PIP$_2$ results in the formation of (1,4,5)IP$_3$, and diacylglycerol, a lipid-soluble membrane-bound messenger. (1,4,5)IP$_3$ is water soluble and can diffuse from the membrane into the cytoplasm of the cell, triggering the rapid release of Ca^{++} from intracellular stores [32, 282]. (1,4,5)IP$_3$ can be sequentially dephosphorylated by a series of phosphatases to inositol or it can be phosphorylated to (1,3,4,5)inositol tetraphosphate ((1,3,4,5)IP$_4$) by the transfer of phosphate from ATP [135]. (1,3,4,5)IP$_4$ may affect Ca^{++} entry [137, 200] but does not appear to be an obligatory step in mast cell activation [129]. (1,3,4,5)IP$_4$ is dephosphorylated by phosphatases to inositol.

In addition to the phospholipase C–catalyzed formation of (1,4,5)IP$_3$, inositol cyclic 1:2,4,5-trisphosphate can also be formed from PIP$_2$ [313], and like (1,4,5)IP$_3$, also causes the release of intracellular calcium [136, 314]. Intracellular levels of cyclic (1:2,4,5)IP$_3$ rise slower than those of (1,4,5)IP$_3$ and it is metabolized more slowly, suggesting that it may be involved in intracellular Ca^{++} mobilization during instances of prolonged receptor stimulation.

The ubiquitous nature of (1,4,5)IP$_3$ and its relationship to receptor action has established this second messenger as an integral part of the stimulus-secretion pathway. The regulation of the synthesis and metabolism of (1,4,5)IP$_3$ and the mechanisms of its receptor-stimulated effects on intracellular calcium should result in a new understanding of the regulation of mast cell activation.

Phospholipid Methylation and Turnover

Following IgE receptor aggregation, a rapid monophasic increase in membrane phospholipid methylation has been observed [122]. Two plasma membrane enzymes, phospholipid methyltransferases I and II, sequentially methylate phosphatidylethanolamine to phosphatidylcholine [122], which can be further metabolized to lysophosphatidylcholine [125]. The localization of methyltransferases I and II to the cytoplasmic and extracellular sides of

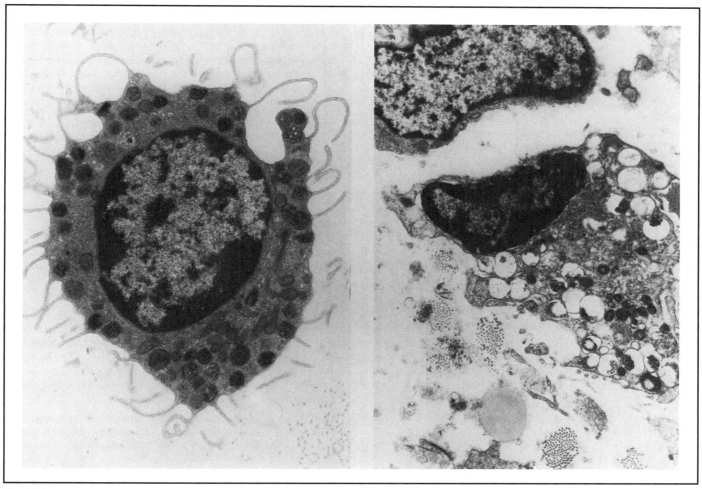

Fig. 10-4. *Mast cells from human airway. Left panel. Subepithelial mast cell from a normal volunteer. Note the crystalline ultrastructure to the granule matrix (× 13,950; Inset × 73,000). Right panel. Mast cell showing extensive degranulation in a biopsy specimen from a patient with atopic asthma (× 13,700). (Reprinted with permission from S. Holgate. New insights into airway inflammation by endobronchial biopsy. Am. Rev. Respir. Dis. 145:S2, 1992.)*

the plasma membrane, respectively, could, following activation, result in an asymmetric distribution or translocation of phospholipids in the lipid bilayer, resulting in a decrease in the microviscosity of the membrane [123, 124].

In the absence of calcium, concanavalin A induces a sustained increase in methylated products without histamine release. Readdition of calcium results in a degradation of methylated products and subsequent mediator release [125], suggesting that the turnover of phosphatidylcholine or products of this process resulted in the initiation of mediator release. Inhibitors of methylation [190, 273] and variants of the RBL cell line deficient in the membrane methyltransferase enzymes [49, 198, 199] demonstrate inhibited calcium influx and histamine release.

Rat mast cells [140] and rat leukemic basophils [56, 57] stimulated with anti-IgE receptor antibodies or anti-rat IgE both demonstrate a rapid monophasic increase in phospholipid methylation, which is followed by an increase in calcium uptake and histamine release. Other degranulating agents such as compound 48/80, the calcium ionophore A 23187, N-formyl-methionyl-leucyl-phenylalanine (FMLP), or the C5a complement component do not increase phospholipid methylation [125, 198]. Activation of human lung mast cells with IgE also failed to demonstrate any change in methylation of phospholipids [29], suggesting that

phospholipid methylation may not be obligatory for all mast cells or all stimuli.

Cyclic AMP and Mediator Release

Early studies on the pharmacologic control of mediator release demonstrated that agents capable of increasing cyclic AMP through beta-adrenergic receptor stimulation inhibited the release of histamine, with an inverse relationship between tissue cyclic AMP levels and mediator release [11, 12, 15, 141, 217, 218] (see Chap. 15). Alpha-adrenergic stimulation enhanced mediator release and concurrently decreased cyclic AMP [15, 149]. Cholinergic agents also potentiated mediator release without affecting cyclic AMP [149]. The cholinergic increase in mediator release could be mimicked with 8-bromocyclic GMP, whereas dibutyryl cyclic AMP caused dose-dependent inhibition. Similar changes in cyclic nucleotides modulating mediator release have been demonstrated in human nasal polyps [148] and human leukocytes [177].

These early studies are consistent in that each used heterogeneous lung tissue challenged with a specific antigen, the assumption being that measurable changes in cyclic nucleotide levels in such multicellular tissue reflect parallel changes in mast cells, a

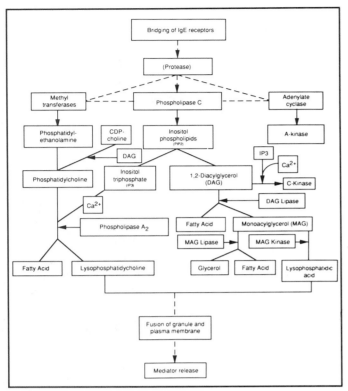

Fig. 10-5. *Biochemical cascade of IgE-dependent mediator release from mast cells and basophils. (Reprinted with permission from F. L. Pearce. Mast cells: function, differentiation and activation. Curr. Opin. Immunol. 1:630, 1989.)*

relatively small percentage of the tissue. In isolated basophils and mast cells, increasing cyclic AMP has been reported to either inhibit mediator release [226, 284, 285, 315], increase mediator release [92], or have little effect [92, 315]. Conversely, inhibition of mediator release can occur [287] unassociated with changes in cyclic AMP. Exogenous addition of dibutyryl cyclic AMP to immunologically stimulated cells has a dual effect, increasing the initial rate of mediator release, while decreasing the maximum amount released [91].

Kinetic studies on nucleotide turnover following immunologic activation demonstrate two monophasic increases in cyclic AMP and cyclic GMP [174, 208, 286]. The second phase of the cyclic AMP rise, occurring maximally at 3 minutes, as well as both cyclic GMP phases were inhibited with indomethacin [174], suggesting that they are secondary to the release of cyclooxygenase-derived products. The indomethacin-resistant initial rise in cyclic AMP peaks at 15 seconds and follows a time course identical to that of methyltransferase activation [57, 138, 140].

In purified human basophils and human lung mast cells challenged with either concanavalin A or anti-IgE, no biphasic cyclic AMP response was observed, while a functioning adenylate cyclase system was clearly evident from isoproterenol-induced increases in cyclic AMP [12].

One known mechanism for translating changes in cyclic AMP to physiologic processes is through activation of cyclic AMP–dependent protein kinases. Protein kinase isozymes, Types I and II, are tetramers containing an inhibitory regulator dimer and two catalytic subunits. The regulatory unit contains four binding sites for cyclic AMP. Increasing saturation of these sites causes dissociation of the regulator from the catalytic subunits, resulting in activation of the enzyme. Protein kinases, utilizing ATP, phosphorylate specific serine and threonine residues, including

autophosphorylation of the regulatory subunit, which attenuates the rate of reassociation of the regulatory subunit [154, 160, 210].

Approximately 94 percent of rat mast cell protein kinase is cyclic AMP activated [127], with equal amounts of Types I and II isozymes. Immunologic activation of mast cells by anti-IgE receptor antibodies increases protein kinase activity and mediator release [127, 316]. Theophylline, however, which has been demonstrated to inhibit histamine release via increases in cyclic AMP, also activates both Type I and II isozymes [128]. PGD_2 increases cyclic AMP without activating either protein kinase isozyme [315]. Thus, the observed disparities in the effects of cyclic AMP on mediator release are still apparent at the protein kinase step. Additional studies are necessary to determine whether one of the isozymes is associated with activation and one with inhibition, as suggested for lymphocyte mitogenesis [46], or whether separate pools of protein kinase can be activated [117].

Alternatively, selective substrate phosphorylation, perhaps via localized kinase activation, may provide diverse regulation of cellular function [110]. Changes in cellular events may correlate more closely with specific protein phosphorylation than with changes in intracellular messengers. In mast cells increased ^{32}P-phosphate labeling into a number of proteins of different molecular weights is observed following stimulation with compound 48/80 or A23187 [271, 294].

Thus the postulation of localized cyclic AMP pools, independently regulated protein kinases, and activation or inhibition through selective phosphorylation seems to encompass the diverse observations directed at unraveling the role of cyclic AMP in mediator release.

Calcium

Many studies have demonstrated a good correlation between calcium uptake and mediator release for a variety of stimuli [62, 89, 142, 276]. The requirement of extracellular calcium (Ca^{++}) for mediator release is apparently dependent on the stimulus [26]. Receptor-mediated release from isolated mast cells, basophils, and guinea pig chopped lung is highly dependent on extracellular calcium [197]. Barium (Ba^{++}) and strontium (Sr^{++}) can substitute for Ca^{++}, Sr^{++} having greater efficacy for maximum mediator release than either Ba^{++} or Ca^{++}.

Potentiation of immunologically stimulated mediator release with phosphatidylserine is associated with a parallel increase in $^{45}Ca^{++}$ uptake [89, 142], while inhibitors of mediator release, dibutyryl cyclic AMP [89], theophylline [89], antimycin A (an inhibitor of cytochrome electron transfer) [142], and disodium cromoglycate [276], all decrease $^{45}Ca^{++}$ uptake.

The increase in membrane permeability to Ca^{++} appears to be a transient event. Antigen stimulation of mast cells in calcium-free buffer leads to a progressive state of desensitization when the time interval between stimulus and readdition of calcium is increased [50, 88]. Desensitization to antigen becomes complete, while a portion of the compound 48/80–induced release is resistant. Complete restoration of release can be obtained by addition of a calcium ionophore, suggesting that desensitization occurs at the membrane calcium gates. Phosphatidylserine delays the onset of desensitization to antigen [88]; increasing extracellular calcium accelerates it [51]. The latter observation poses the question of whether Ca^{++} can regulate its own permeability through a membrane pool of regular Ca^{++}. Care must be exercised in the interpretation of studies where extracellular Ca^{++} is removed to determine Ca^{++} dependency of mediator release, since this can lead to marked elevation of cyclic AMP [284].

The well-documented smooth muscle calcium antagonists verapamil, D 600, and nifedipine were ineffective in inhibiting antigen-induced mediator release from human basophils [87]. These compounds are generally believed to be more effective inhibitors of voltage-sensitive calcium channels [87, 193], suggesting a difference in the mechanisms of calcium translocation in smooth muscle and mast cells. Lanthanum (La^{+++}), a trivalent cation that displaces calcium from extracellular binding sites, does however inhibit antigen-induced histamine release from mast cells [90].

Direct microinjection of Ca^{++} but not magnesium (Mg^{++}) or potassium (K^+) has been reported to cause degranulation of impaled mast cells [150], although this method has not been uniformly successful [289]. Intracellular infusion of Ca^{++} with subsequent histamine release was demonstrated by fusing Ca^{++}-containing phospholipid vesicles (liposomes) with mast cell membranes [293]. These studies suggest that increasing intracellular calcium is sufficient for mediator release.

Several recent studies have challenged the concept that increases in intracellular calcium alone are responsible for mediator release. It has been demonstrated that for equivalent increases in intracellular calcium the calcium ionophore A 23187 is less efficient for inducing histamine release from RBL-2H3 cells than is antigen [27]. Patch clamp studies with rat peritoneal mast cells demonstrated that GTPγ-S could evoke release even when the intracellular calcium concentration was zero. Increasing calcium accelerated the GTP response, but was not sufficient by itself to induce release [209]. Interestingly in these studies, (1,4,5)IP$_3$ increased intracellular calcium, but was not able to induce release in the absence of GTP, while in permeabilized rat peritoneal mast cells (1,4,5)IP$_3$ caused a dose-dependent release of histamine in the absence of free calcium [143]. Both studies agreed that GTPγ-S in the absence of calcium could induce histamine release, possible by inducing the formation of inositol phosphates.

Whole-cell, patch-clamped rat peritoneal mast cells identified two means of calcium influx [187]. Intracellular application of (1,4,5)IP$_3$ increased intracellular calcium release as well as influx. The latter was not associated with channel activity, or the channels were so small and calcium specific that detection was difficult. Agonists such as compound 48/80, substance P, or GTPγ-S activated large-conductance cation channels.

The data are still consistent with the concept that the biochemical mechanisms associated with mast cell activation and mediator release are very much agonist and cell type (and species) specific. It is also becoming apparent that these biochemical pathways function interdependently with calcium during cell activation.

REFERENCES

1. Abe, T., and Nawa, Y. Eosinophil chemotactic factor released from murine bone marrow derived cultured mast cells. *Arerugi* 39:69, 1990.
2. Altura, B. M., and Halery, S. Cardiovascular Actions of Histamine. In M. Rocha and E. Silva (eds.), *Handbook of Experimental Pharmacology.* New York: Springer, 1978.
3. Anderson, J. F., and Schultz, W. H. The cause of serum anaphylactic shock and some methods of alleviating it. *Proc. Soc. Exp. Biol.* 7:32, 1909–1910.
4. Anderson, W. H., et al. Increased synthesis of prostaglandin-like material during histamine tachyphylaxis in canine tracheal smooth muscle. *Biochem. Pharmacol.* 28:2223, 1979.
5. Anderson, W. H., et al. Characteristics of histamine tachyphylaxis in canine tracheal smooth muscle: A possible prostaglandin mediated phenomenon. *Naunyn Schmiedebergs Arch. Pharmacol.* 308:117, 1979.
6. Anderson, W. H., et al. Prostaglandins as mediators of tachyphylaxis to histamine in canine tracheal smooth muscle. *Adv. Prostaglandin Thromboxane Leukot. Res.* 7:995, 1980.
7. Anwar, A. R. E., and Kay, A. B. The ECF-A tetrapeptides and histamine selectively enhance human eosinophil complement receptors. *Nature* 269:522, 1977.
8. Arnaout, M. A., et al. In expression of an adhesion-promoting surface glycoprotein in the granulocytopenia of hemodialysis. *N. Engl. J. Med.* 312:457, 1985.
8a. Arrang, J. M., et al. Highly potent and selective ligands for histamine H$_3$-receptors. *Nature* 327:117, 1987.
9. Arunlakshana, O. Histamine release by antihistamines. *J. Physiol.* 119,47P, 1953.
10. Ash, A. S. F., and Schild, H. O. Receptors mediating some actions of histamine. *Br. J. Pharmacol.* 27:427, 1966.
11. Assem, E. S. K., and Schild, H. O. Inhibition by sympathomimetic amines of histamine release induced by antigen in passively sensitized human lung. *Nature* 224:1028, 1969.
12. Assem, E. S. K., and Schild, H. O. Antagonism by β-adrenoceptor blocking agents of the antianaphylactic effect of isoprenaline. *Br. J. Pharmacol.* 42:620, 1971.
13. Atkins, P. C., et al. Release of neutrophil chemotactic activity during immediate hypersensitivity reactions in humans. *Ann. Intern. Med.* 86: 415, 1977.
14. Auer, J., and Lewis, P. A. The physiology of the immediate reaction of anaphylaxis in the guinea pig. *J. Exp. Med.* 12:151, 1910.
15. Austen, K. F. A Review of Immunological, Biochemical and Pharmacological Factors in the Release of Chemical Mediators from Human Lung in Asthma. In K. F. Austen and L. M. Lichtenstein (eds.), *Asthma: Physiology, Immunopharmacology, and Treatment.* New York: Academic, 1977.
16. Austen, K. F. Biologic implications of the structural and functional characteristics of the chemical mediators of immediate-type hypersensitivity. *Harvey Lect.* 73:1, 1979.
17. Austen, K. F., and Brocklehurst, W. E. Anaphylaxis in chopped guinea pig lung: I. Effect of peptidase substrates and inhibitors. *J. Exp. Med.* 113: 521, 1961.
18. Austen, K. F., Wasserman, S. I., and Goetzl, E. J. Mast Cell-Derived Mediators: Structural and Functional Diversity and Regulation of Expression. In S. G. O. Johansson, V. Strandberg, and B. Uvnas (eds.), *Molecular and Biological Aspects of the Acute Allergic Reaction.* New York: Plenum, 1976.
19. Baker, C. R., et al. Kinin metabolism in the perfused ventilated rat lung. I: Bradykinin metabolism in a system modeling the normal, uninjured lung. *Circ. Shock* 33:37, 1991.
20. Baldwa, V. S., et al. Cytomorphological variations and blood histamine in bronchial asthma. *Ann. Allergy* 36:117, 1976.
21. Barnum, S. R., and Volanakis, J. E. *In vitro* biosynthesis of complement protein D by U937 cells. *J. Immunol.* 134:1799, 1985.
22. Bartholomew, R. M., and Esser, A. F. Mechanisms on antibody-independent activation of the first component of complement (C1) on retrovirus membranes. *Biochemistry* 19:2847, 1980.
23. Bartosch, R., Feldberg, W., and Nagel, E. Das Freiwerden eines histaminahnlichen Stoffes bei der Anaphylaxie des Meerschweinchens. *Pflugers Arch.* 230:129, 1932.
24. Bartosch, R., Feldberg, W., and Nagel, E. Versuche uber das Freiwerden eines histaminah nlichen Stoffes aus der durchstromten Lunge sensibiliserter Meerschweinchen. *Pflugers Arch.* 231:616, 1933.
25. Bauza, M. T., and Lagunoff, D. Histidine transport by isolated rat peritoneal mast cells. *Biochem. Pharmacol.* 30:1271, 1981.
26. Baxter, J. H., and Adamik, R. Differences in requirements and actions of various histamine-releasing agents. *Biochem. Pharmacol.* 27:497, 1978.
27. Beaven, M. A., et al. Synergistic signals in the mechanism of antigen-induced exocytosis in 2H3 cells: Evidence for an unidentified signal required for histamine release. *J. Cell Biol.* 105:1129, 1987.
28. Becker, E. L., and Austen, K. F. Mechanisms of immunologic injury of rat peritoneal mast cells. I. The effect of phosphonate inhibitors in the homocytotrophic antibody-mediated histamine release and the first component of rat complement. *J. Exp. Med.* 124:379, 1966.
29. Benyon, R. C., Church, M. K., and Holgate, S. T. IgE-dependent activation of human lung mast cells is not associated with increased phospholipid methylation. *J. Immunol.* 141:954, 1988.
30. Bernstein, J. A., and Lawrence, I. D. The mast cell: A comprehensive, updated review. *Allergy Proc.* 11:209, 1990.
31. Berridge, M. J. Inositol triphosphate and diacylglycerol: Two interacting second messengers. *Annu. Rev. Biochem.* 56:159, 1987.
32. Berridge, M. J. Inositol and calcium signaling. *Proc. R. Soc. Lond.* 234: 359, 1988.
33. Bhat, K. H., et al. Plasma histamine changes during provoked bronchospasm in asthmatic patients. *J. Allergy Clin. Immunol.* 58:647, 1976.
34. Birnbaumer, L., and Brown, A. M. G proteins and the mechanism of action of hormones, neurotransmitters, and autocrine and paracrine regulatory factors. *Am. Rev. Respir. Dis.* 141:S106, 1990.
35. Black, J. W., et al. Definition and antagonism of histamine H$_2$-receptors. *Nature* 236:385, 1972.

36. Booij-Noord, H., et al. Protection tests on bronchial allergen challenge with disodium chromoglycate and thiazinamien. *J. Allergy* 46:1, 1970.

37. Bosin, T. R. Serotonin Metabolism. In W. B. Essman (ed.), *Availability, Localization and Disposition,* Vol. 1. *Serotonin in Health and Disease.* New York: Spectrum, 1978.

38. Boswell, R. N., Austen, K. F., and Goetzl, E. J. Intermediate molecular weight eosinophil chemotactic factors in rat peritoneal mast cells: Immunologic release, granule association and demonstration of structural heterogeneity. *J. Immunol.* 120:15, 1978.

39. Bradley, P. B., et al. Proposals for the classification and nomenclature of functional receptors for 5-hydroxytryptamine. *Neuropharmacology* 25: 563, 1986.

40. Brink, C., Douglas, J. S., and Duncan, P. G. Changes in the response of guinea pig airways *in vivo* and *in vitro* to cimetidine and propranolol during development. *Br. J. Pharmacol.* 75:531, 1982.

41. Brocklehurst, W. The Action of 5-Hydroxytryptamine on Smooth Muscle. In G. P. Lewis (ed.), *5-Hydroxytryptamine.* New York: Pergamon, 1958.

41a. Brooimans, R. A. CD59 expressed by human endothelial cells functions as a protective molecule against complement mediated lysis. *Eur. J. Immunol.* 22:791, 1992.

42. Brown, M. J., et al. A sensitive and specific radiometric method for the measurement of plasma histamine in normal individuals. *Anal. Biochem.* 109:142, 1980.

43. Buckner, C. K., et al. A pharmacologic examination of receptors mediating serotonin-induced bronchoconstriction in the anesthetized guinea pig. *J. Pharmacol. Exp. Ther.* 257:26, 1991.

44. Buffoni, F. Histaminase and related amine oxidase. *Pharmacol. Rev.* 18: 1163, 1966.

45. Bunting, S., et al. Arterial walls generate from prostaglandin endoperoxides a substance (prostaglandin X) which relaxes strips of mesenteric and coeliac arteries and inhibits platelet aggregation. *Prostaglandins* 12: 897, 1976.

46. Byus, C. V., et al. Type I and type II cyclic-AMP-dependent protein kinase as opposite effectors of lymphocyte mitogenesis. *Nature* 268:63, 1977.

47. Cazzola, M., et al. Ketanserin, a new blocking agent of serotonin S2-receptors. Respiratory functional effects in chronic obstruction of the airways. *Chest* 92:863, 1987.

48. Chakrin, L. W., et al. Effect of histamine H_2-receptor antagonist on immunologically induced mediator release *in vitro. Agents Actions* 4:297, 1974.

49. Chiang, P. K., Richards, H. H., and Cantoni, G. L. S-adenosyl-L-homocysteine hydrolase: Analogs of S-adenosyl-L-homocysteine as potential inhibitors. *Mol. Pharmacol.* 13:939, 1977.

50. Cochrane, D. E., and Distel, D. L. Association of ^{45}calcium with rat mast cells stimulated by 48/80: Effects of inactivation, calcium and metabolic inhibitors. *J. Physiol. (Lond.)* 330:413, 1982.

51. Cochrane, D. E., et al. Stimulus-secretion coupling in rat mast cells: Inactivation of extracellular calcium dependent secretion. *J. Physiol. (Lond.)* 323:423, 1982.

52. Cockcroft, S., Howell, T. W., and Gomperts, B. D. Two G-proteins act in series to control stimulus-secretion coupling in mast cells: Use of neomycin to distinguish between G-proteins controlling polyphosphoinositide phosphodiesterase and exocytosis. *J. Cell Biol.* 105:2745, 1987.

53. Cody, D. T., Code, C. F., and Kennedy, J. C. Studies on the mechanism of anaphylaxis in the rat. *J. Allergy* 34:26, 1963.

54. Comroe, J. H., et al. Reflex and direct cardiopulmonary effects of 5-HT (serotonin). *Am. J. Physiol.* 173:379, 1953.

55. Corbi, A. L., et al. The human leukocyte adhesion protein Mac-1 (complement receptor type 3, CD11b) α subunit: Cloning, primary structure, and relation to the integrins, von Willebrand factor and factor B. *J. Biol. Chem.* 263:12404, 1988.

56. Crews, F. T., et al. Phospholipid methylation affects immunoglobulin E-mediated histamine and arachidonic acid release in rat leukemic basophils. *Biochem. Biophys. Res. Commun.* 93:42, 1980.

57. Crews, F. T., et al. IgE-mediated histamine release in rat basophilic leukemia cells: Receptor activation, phospholipid methylation Ca^{2+} flux, and release of arachidonic acid. *Arch. Biochem. Biophys.* 212:561, 1981.

58. Criep, L. H., and Aaron, T. H. Neohetramine: An experimental and clinical evaluation in allergic states. *J. Allergy* 19:215, 1948.

59. Criep, L. H., and Aaron, T. H. Theophorin: An experimental and clinical evaluation in allergic states. *J. Allergy* 19:304, 1948.

60. Czarnetzki, B. M., and Rosenbach, T. From eosinophil chemotactic factor of anaphylaxis to leukotriene B_4. Chemistry, biology and functional significance of eosinophil chemotactic leukotrienes in dermatology. *Dermatologica* 179(Suppl. 1):54, 1989.

61. Daha, M. B., Fearon, D. T., and Austen, K. F. C3 requirements for formation of alternative pathway C5 convertase. *J. Immunol.* 117:630, 1976.

62. Dahlquist, R. Relationship of uptake of sodium and ^{45}calcium to ATP-induced histamine release from rat mast cells. *Acta Pharmacol. Toxicol.* 35:11, 1974.

63. Dale, H. H., and Laidlaw, P. P. The physiological action of β-imidazolylethylamine. *J. Physiol.* 41:318, 1910.

64. Dale, H. H., and Laidlaw, P. P. Further observations on the action of β-imidazolylethylamine. *J. Physiol.* 43:182, 1911.

64a. Da Silva, A., et al. Endopeptidase 24.15 modulates bradykinin-induced contraction in guinea pig trachea. *Eur. J. Pharmacol.* 212:97, 1992.

64b. Davies, K. A. Complement. *Baillieres Clin. Haematol.* 4:927, 1991.

65. Davis, A. E. C1 inhibitor and hereditary angioneurotic edema. *Annu. Rev. Immunol.* 6:595, 1988.

66. de Chaffoy de Courcelles, D., et al. Evidence that phospholipid turnover is the signal transducing system coupled to serotonin-S_2 receptor sites. *J. Biol. Chem.* 260:7603, 1985.

67. De Clerck, F. F., and Vanhoutte, M. (eds.), *5-Hydroxytryptamine in Peripheral Reactions.* New York: Raven, 1982.

68. Derkach, V., Surprenant, A., and North, R. A. 5-HT$_3$ receptors are membrane ion channels. *Nature* 339:706, 1989.

69. Dixon, M., Jackson, D. M., and Richards, I. M. The effects of 5-hydroxytryptamine, histamine, and acetylcholine on the reactivity of the lung of the anesthetized dog. *J. Physiol.* 307:85, 1980.

70. Dorer, F. E., et al. Hydrolysis of bradykinin by angiotensin-converting enzyme. *Circ. Res.* 34:824, 1974.

71. Douglas, G. N. *Complement System.* La Jolla, CA: Calbiochem-Behring (a division of American Hoechst Corp.), 1977. Publication No. 8162-383.

72. Douglas, W. W. Histamine and 5-Hydroxytryptamine (Serotonin) and Their Antagonists. In A. G. Gilman, L. S. Goodman, and A. Gilman (eds.), *The Pharmacological Basis of Therapeutics.* New York: Macmillan, 1980.

73. Drazen, J. M., and Austen, K. F. Atropine modification of the pulmonary effects of chemical mediators in the guinea pig. *J. Appl. Physiol.* 38:834, 1975.

74. Dyckman, T. R., Holers, V. M., and Atkinson, J. P. The Function and Structure of the C3b/C4b Complement Receptor (CR1). In L. Levie (ed.), *Microbiology.* Washington, D.C.: ASM Publishing, 1985.

75. Erspamer, V. Peripheral Physiological and Pharmacological Actions of Indolalkylamines. In O. Eichler and A. Farah (eds.), *Handbook of Pharmacology.* New York: Springer, 1966.

76. Esser, A. F., et al. Molecular recognition of lipid bilayers by complement: A possible mechanism of membranolysis. *Proc. Natl. Acad. Sci. USA* 76: 1410, 1979.

77. Essman, W. B. Serotonin Distribution in Tissues and Fluids. In W. B. Essman (ed.), *Availability, Localization, and Disposition,* Vol. 1. *Serotonin in Health and Disease.* New York: Spectrum, 1978.

78. Eyre, P. Histamine H_2-receptors in the sheep bronchus and cat trachea. The actions of burimamide. *Br. J. Pharmacol.* 48:321, 1973.

79. Fargin, A., et al. The genomic clone G-21, which resembles a β-adrenergic receptor sequence encodes the 5-HT$_{1A}$ receptor. *Nature* 335:358, 1988.

80. Fearon, D. T. Identification of the membrane glycoprotein that is the C3b receptor of the human erythrocyte B lymphocyte and monocyte. *J. Exp. Med.* 152:20, 1980.

81. Fearon, D. T., and Austen, K. F. Properdin: Binding to C3b and stabilization of the C3b-dependent C3 convertase. *J. Exp. Med.* 142:856, 1975.

82. Fearon, D. T., Austen, K. F., and Ruddy, S. Properdin factor D: Characterization of its active site and isolation of the precursor form. *J. Exp. Med.* 139:355, 1974.

83. Fearon, D. T., and Collins, L. A. Increased expression of C3b receptors on polymorphonuclear leukocytes induced by chemotactic factors and purification procedures. *J. Immunol.* 130:370, 1983.

84. Fernandez, H. N., and Hugli, T. E. Chemical evidence of common genetic ancestry of complement components C3 and C5. *J. Biol. Chem.* 252:1826, 1977.

85. Fernandez, H. N., et al. Chemotactic response to human C3a and C5a anaphylatoxins: I. valuation of C3a and C5a leukotaxis *in vivo* and *in vitro. J. Immunol.* 120:109, 1978.

86. Ferreira, S. H., and Vane, J. R. Half-lives of peptides and amines in the circulation. *Nature* 215:1237, 1967.

87. Fleckenstein, A. Specific pharmacology of calcium in myocardium, cardiac pacemakers, and vascular smooth muscle. *Annu. Rev. Pharmacol. Toxicol.* 17:149, 1977.

88. Foreman, J. C., and Garland, L. G. Desensitization in the process of histamine secretion induced by antigen and dextran. *J. Physiol. (Lond.)* 239: 381, 1974.

89. Foreman, J. C., Hallett, M. B., and Mongar, J. L. The relationship between histamine secretion and $^{45}C^{++}$ uptake by mast cells. *J. Physiol. (Lond.)* 271:193, 1977.

90. Foreman, J. C., and Mongar, J. L. The action of lanthanum and manganese on anaphylactic histamine secretion. *Br. J. Pharmacol.* 48:527, 1973.

91. Foreman, J. C., Sobotka, A. K., and Lichtenstein, L. M. Modulation of the rate of histamine release from basophils by cyclic AMP. *Eur. J. Pharmacol.* 63:341, 1980.

92. Fredholm, B. B., et al. Cyclic AMP independent inhibition by papaverine of histamine release induced by compound 48/80. *Biochem. Pharmacol.* 25:1583, 1976.

93. Friedberger, E. Kritik de theorien uber die anaphylaxie. *Z. Immunitaetsforsch. Immunobiol.* 2:298, 1929.

94. Frisk-Holmberg, M. Drug induced changes in the release and uptake of biogenic amines: A study on mast cells. *Acta Physiol. Scand. Suppl.* 376: 1, 1972.

95. Fukui, H., Watanabe, T., and Wada, H. Immunochemical cross reactivity of the antibody elicited against L-histidine decarboxylase purified in the whole bodies of fetal rats with the enzyme from rat brain. *Biochem. Biophys. Res. Commun.* 93:333, 1980.

96. Garrison, J. C. Histamine, Bradykinin, 5-Hydroxytryptamine, and Their Antagonists. In A. G. Gilman, et al. (eds.), *The Pharmacological Basis of Therapeutics.* New York: Pergamon, 1990.

97. Garrison, J. C., and Rall, T. W. Histamine, Bradykinin, 5-Hydroxytryptamine, and Their Antagonists. In A. G. Gilman, et al. (eds.), *Goodman and Gilman's. The Pharmacological Basis of Therapeutics.* New York: Pergamon, 1990.

98. Gigli, I., and Austen, K. F. Fluid phase destruction of C2^{hu} by C1^{hu}: I. Its enhancement and inhibition by homologous and heterologous C4. *J. Exp. Med.* 129:679, 1969.

99. Gigli, I., and Austen, K. F. Fluid phase destruction of C2^{hu} by C1^{hu}: II. Unmasking by C4i^{hu} of C1^{hu} specificity for C2^{hu}. *J. Exp. Med.* 130:833, 1969.

100. Goetzl, E. J., and Austen, K. F. Specificity and Modulation of the Eosinophil Polymorphonuclear Leukocyte Response to the Eosinophil Chemotactic Factor of Anaphylaxis (ECF-A). In S. G. O. Johansson, K. Strandberg, and B. Uvnas (eds.), *Molecular and Biological Aspects of the Acute Allergic Reaction.* New York: Plenum, 1976.

101. Goetzl, E. J., and Austen, K. F. Purification and synthesis of eosinophilotactic tetrapeptides of human lung tissue: Identification as eosinophil chemotactic factor of anaphylaxis. *Proc. Natl. Acad. Sci. USA* 72:4123, 1975.

102. Goetzl, E. J., and Austen, K. F. Structural determinants of the eosinophil chemotactic activity of the acidic tetrapeptides of eosinophil chemotactic factor of anaphylaxis. *J. Exp. Med.* 144:1424, 1976.

103. Goetzl, E. J., et al. Production of a low molecular weight eosinophil polymorphonuclear leukocyte chemotactic factor by anaplastic squamous cell carcinomas of human lung. *J. Clin. Invest.* 61:770, 1978.

104. Michoud, M. C., Lelorier, J., and Amyot, B. Factors modulating the interindividual variability of airway responsiveness to histamine. The influence of H$_1$ and H$_2$ receptors. *Clin. Respir. Physiol.* 17:807, 1981.

105. Gomperts, B. D. Involvement of guanine nucleotide-binding protein in the gating of Ca^{++} by receptors. *Nature* 306:64, 1983.

106. Gould, V. E., and Warren, W. H. Immunohistochemical evaluation of neuroendocrine cells and neoplasms of the lung. *Pathol. Res. Pract.* 183:200, 1988.

107. Graham, P., Kahlson, G., and Rosengren, E. Histamine formation in physical exercise, anoxia, and under the influence of adrenaline and related substances. *J. Physiol.* 172:174, 1964.

108. Grant, J. A., et al. Complement-mediated release of histamine from human leukocytes. *J. Immunol.* 114:1101, 1975.

109. Grant, J. A., et al. Complement-mediated release of histamine from human basophils. II. Biochemical characterization of the reaction. *J. Immunol.* 117:450, 1976.

110. Greengard, P. Phosphorylated proteins as physiological effectors. *Science* 199:146, 1978.

111. Griffin, J. H., and Cochrane, C. G. Mechanisms for the involvement of high molecular weight kininogen in surface-dependent reactions of Hageman factor. *Proc. Natl. Acad. Sci. USA* 73:2554, 1976.

112. Guimaraes, J. A., et al. Kinin-converting aminopeptidases from human serum. *Biochem. Pharmacol.* 22:3157, 1973.

113. Hahn, H. L., et al. Interaction between serotonin and efferent vagus nerves in dog lungs. *J. Appl. Physiol.* 44:144, 1978.

114. Hammerschmidt, D. E., et al. Association of complement activation and elevated plasma-C5a with adult respiratory distress syndrome. Patho-

115. Hawkins, D. F. Bronchoconstrictor and bronchodilator actions of antihistamine drugs. *Br. J. Pharmacol.* 10:230, 1955.

116. Hawkins, D. F., and Schild, H. O. The action of drugs on isolated human bronchial chains. *Br. J. Pharmacol.* 6:682, 1951.

117. Hayes, J., Brunton, L. L., and Mayer, S. E. Selective activation of particulate cAMP-dependent protein kinase by isoproterenol and prostaglandin E. *J. Biol. Chem.* 255:5113, 1980.

118. Henson, P. M., et al. Complement fragments, alveolar macrophages and alveolitis. *Am. J. Pathol.* 97:93, 1979.

119. Herxheimer, H. The 5-hydroxytryptamine shock in the guinea pig. *J. Physiol.* 128:435, 1955.

120. Herxheimer, H. The 5-Hydroxytryptamine Shock in the Guinea Pig. In G. P. Lewis (ed.), *5-Hydroxytryptamine.* New York: Pergamon, 1958.

121. Higashiyama, S., et al. Kinin release from kininogens by calpains. *Life Sci.* 39:1639, 1986.

122. Hirata, F., and Axelrod, J. Enzymatic synthesis and rapid translocation of phosphatidylcholine by two methyltransferases in erythrocyte membranes. *Proc. Natl. Acad. Sci. USA* 75:2348, 1978.

123. Hirata, F., and Axelrod, J. Enzymatic methylation of phosphatidylethanolamine increases erythrocyte membrane fluidity. *Nature* 275:219, 1978.

124. Hirata, F., and Axelrod, J. Phospholipid methylation and biological signal transmissions. *Science* 209:1082, 1980.

125. Hirata, F., Axelrod, J., and Crews, F. T. Concanavalin A stimulates phospholipid methylation and phosphatidylserine decarboxylation in rat mast cells. *Proc. Natl. Acad. Sci. USA* 76:4813, 1979.

126. Holgate, S. T., and Finnerty, J. P. Antihistamines in asthma. *J. Allergy Clin. Immunol.* 83:537, 1989.

127. Holgate, S. T., Lewis, R. A., and Austen, K. F. 3',5'-Cyclic adenosine monophosphate-dependent protein kinase of the rat serosal mast cell and its immunologic activation. *J. Immunol.* 124:2093, 1980.

128. Holgate, S. T., et al. Effects of prostaglandin D$_2$ and theophylline on rat serosal mast cells: Discordance between increased cellular levels of cAMP and activation of cyclic AMP-dependent protein kinase. *J. Immunol.* 127:1530, 1981.

129. Horstman, D. A., Takemura, H., and Putney, J. W., Jr. Formation and metabolism of [^{3}H]inositol phosphates in AR42J pancreatoma cells: Substance P induced Ca++ mobilization in the apparent absence of inositol 1,4,5-triphosphate 3-kinase activity. *J. Biol. Chem.* 263:15297, 1988.

130. Houston, D. S., and Vanhoutte, P. M. Serotonin and the vascular system: Role in health and disease, and implications for therapy. *Drugs* 31:149, 1986.

131. Howarth, P. H., and Holgate, S. T. Astemizole, an H$_1$ antagonist in allergic asthma. *J. Allergy Clin. Immunol.* 75:166, 1985.

132. Hughes, A. R., et al. Inositol phosphate metabolism and signal transduction. *Am. Rev. Respir. Dis.* 141:S115, 1990.

133. Hugli, T. E. Biochemistry and biology of anaphylatoxins. *Complement* 3: 111, 1986.

134. Hugli, T. E., and Muller-Eberhard, H. J. Anaphylatoxins: C3a and C5a. *Adv. Immunol.* 26:1, 1978.

135. Irvine, R. F., et al. The inositol tris/tetrakisphosphate pathway - demonstration of Ins(1,4,5)P$_3$ 3-kinase activity in animal tissues. *Nature* 320: 631, 1986.

136. Irvine, R. F., et al. Specificity of inositol phosphate-stimulated Ca++ mobilization from swiss-mouse 3T3 cells. *Biochem. J.* 240:301, 1986.

137. Irvine, R. F., and Moor, R. M. Micro-injection of inositol 1,3,4,5-tetrakisphosphate activates sea urchin eggs by a mechanism dependent on external Ca++. *Biochem. J.* 240:917, 1986.

138. Ishizaka, T. Analysis of triggering events in mast cells for immunoglobulin E-mediated histamine release. *J. Allergy Clin. Immunol.* 67:90, 1981.

139. Ishizaka, T., White, J. R., and Saito, H. Activation of basophils and mast cells for mediator release. *Int. Arch. Allergy Appl. Immunol.* 82:327, 1987.

140. Ishizaka, T., et al. Stimulation of phospholipid methylation, Ca^{++} influx, and histamine release by bridging of IgE receptors on rat mast cells. *Proc. Natl. Acad. Sci. USA* 77:1903, 1980.

141. Ishizaka, T., et al. Pharmacologic inhibition of the antigen-induced release of histamine and slow reacting substance of anaphylaxis (SRS A) from monkey lung tissues mediated by human IgE. *J. Immunol.* 106:1267, 1971.

142. Ishizaka, T., et al. Induction of calcium flux across the rat mast cell membrane by bridging IgE receptors. *Proc. Natl. Acad. Sci. USA* 76:5858, 1979.

143. Izushi, K., and Tasaka, K. Histamine release from beta-escin-permeabilized rat peritoneal mast cells and its inhibition by intracellular Ca2+

blockers, calmodulin inhibitors and cAMP. *Immunopharmacology* 18: 177, 1989.

144. Johnson, A. R., Hugli, T. E., and Muller-Eberhard, H. J. Release of histamine from rat mast cells by the complement peptides C3a and C5a. *Immunology* 28:1069, 1975.

145. Johnson, D. E., and Georgieff, M. K. Pulmonary neuroendocrine cells. Their secretory products and their potential roles in health and chronic lung disease in infancy. *Am. Rev. Respir. Dis.* 140:1807, 1989.

146. Johnson, D. E., Wobken, J. D., and Landrum, B. G. Changes in bombesin, calcitonin, and serotonin immunoreactive pulmonary neuroendocrine cells in cystic fibrosis and after prolonged mechanical ventilation. *Am. Rev. Respir. Dis.* 137:123, 1988.

147. Kaliner, M., and Austen, K. F. A sequence of biochemical events in the antigen-induced release of chemical mediators from sensitized human lung tissue. *J. Exp. Med.* 138:1077, 1973.

148. Kaliner, M., Wasserman, S. I., and Austen, K. F. Immunologic release of chemical mediators from human nasal polyps. *N. Engl. J. Med.* 289:277, 1973.

149. Kaliner, M. A., Orange, R. P., and Austen, K. F. Immunologic release of histamine and slow reacting substance of anaphylaxis from human lung: IV. Enhancement by cholinergic and alpha adrenergic stimulation. *J. Exp. Med.* 136:556, 1972.

150. Kanno, T., Cochrane, D. E., and Douglas, W. W. Exocytosis (secretory granule extrusion) induced by injection of calcium into mast cells. *Can. J. Physiol. Pharmacol.* 51:1001, 1973.

151. Kaplan, M. H., and Volanakis, J. E. Interaction of C-reactive protein complexes with the complement system. Consumption of human complement associated with the reaction of C-reactive protein with pneumococcal C-polysaccharide and with choline phosphatides, lecithin and sphingomyelin. *J. Immunol.* 112:2135, 1974.

152. Karlin, J. M. The use of antihistamines in asthma. *Ann. Allergy* 30:342, 1972.

153. Kay, A. B., and Austen, K. F. The IgE-mediated release of an eosinophil leukocyte chemotactic factor from human lung. *J. Immunol.* 107:899, 1971.

154. Kay, A. B., Stechschulte, D. J., and Austen, K. F. An eosinophil leukocyte chemotactic factor of anaphylaxis. *J. Exp. Med.* 133:602, 1971.

155. Kazatchkine, M. D., Fearon, D. T., and Austen, K. F. Human alternative complement pathway: Membrane associated sialic acid regulates the competition between B and B1H for cell bound C3b. *J. Immunol.* 122:75, 1979.

156. Keele, C. A., and Armstrong, D. *Substances Producing Pain and Itch.* Baltimore: Williams & Wilkins, 1964.

157. Kellermeyer, R. W., and Breckenridge, R. T. Inflammatory process in acute gouty arthritis: I. Activation of Hageman factor by sodium urate crystals. *J. Lab. Clin. Med.* 657:307, 1965.

158. Kennerly, D. A., Sullivan, T. J., and Parker, C. W. Activation of phospholipid metabolism during mediator release from stimulated rat mast cells. *J. Immunol.* 122:152, 1979.

159. Kitamura, N., et al. Structural organization of the human kininogen gene and a model for its evolution. *J. Biol. Chem.* 260:8610, 1985.

160. Krebs, E. G., and Beavo, J. A. Phosphorylation-dephosphorylation of enzymes. *Annu. Rev. Biochem.* 48:923, 1979.

161. Kroeger, D. C., and Lucco, L. J. Serotonin-induced apnea. *J. Am. Pharmacol. Assoc.* 49:170, 1960.

162. Kubota, Y., et al. Characterization of the C3 receptor induced by herpes simplex virus type 1 infection of human epidermal, endothelial cell and A431 cells. *J. Immunol.* 138:1137, 1987.

163. Kulics, J., Colten, H. R., and Perlmutter, D. H. Counterregulatory effects of interferon-γ and LPS on expression of the human C4 genes. *J. Clin. Invest.* 85:943, 1990.

164. Lachman, P. J., and Thompson, R. A. Reactive lysis: The complement-mediated lysis of unsensitized cells: II. The characterization of activated reactor as C5-6 and the participation of C8 and C9. *J. Exp. Med.* 131:643, 1970.

165. Lagunoff, D. Analysis of dye binding sites in mast cell granules. *Biochemistry* 13:3982, 1974.

166. Lagunoff, D., and Bauza, M. The Formation and Storage of Histamine in the Mast Cell. In B. Uvnas and K. Tasaka (eds.), *Advances in the Biosciences,* Vol. 23. *Advances in Histamine Research.* New York: Pergamon, 1982.

167. Lambert, G. H., et al. Involvement of 5-hydroxytryptamine in the central control of respiration, blood pressure and heart rate in the anesthetized rat. *Neuropharmacology* 17:807, 1978.

168. Larsen, G. L., et al. A differential effect of C5a and C5a des Arg in the induction of pulmonary inflammation. *Am. J. Pathol.* 100:179, 1980.

169. Law, S. K., et al. Interaction between the labile binding sites of the fourth (C4) and fifth (C5) human complement proteins and erythrocyte cell membranes. *J. Immunol.* 125:634, 1980.

170. Lebel, B., et al. Antigenic challenge of immunized mice induces endogenous production of IL-3 that increases histamine synthesis in hematopoietic organs. *J. Immunol.* 145:1222, 1990.

171. Lee, C. W., et al. Oxidative inactivation of leukotriene C4 by stimulated human polymorphonuclear leukocytes. *Proc. Natl. Acad. Sci. USA* 79: 4166, 1982.

172. Levy, L., and Seabury, J. H. Spirometric evaluation of Benadryl in asthma. *J. Allergy* 18:244, 1947.

173. Lewis, R. A., et al. The release of four mediators of immediate hypersensitivity from human leukemic basophils. *J. Immunol.* 114:87, 1975.

174. Lewis, R. A., et al. Effects of indomethacin on cyclic nucleotide levels and histamine release from rat serosal mast cells. *J. Immunol.* 123:1663, 1979.

175. Lewis, T. *The Blood Vessels of the Human Skin and Their Responses.* London: Shaw, 1927.

176. Lichtenstein, L. M., and Gillespie, E. The effects of the H1 and H2 antihistamines on "allergic" histamine release and its inhibition by histamine. *J. Pharmacol. Exp. Ther.* 192:441, 1975.

177. Lichtenstein, L. M., and Margolis, S. Histamine release *in vitro:* Inhibition by catecholamines and methylxanthines. *Science* 161:902, 1968.

178. Logan, G. B. Release of a histamine-destroying factor during anaphylactic shock in guinea-pigs. *Proc. Soc. Exp. Biol. Med.* 107:466, 1961.

179. Loos, M., Martin, H., and Petry, F. The biosynthesis of C1q, the collagen-like and Fc-recognizing molecule of the complement system. *Behring Inst. Mitt.* 84:32, 1989.

180. Lorenz, W., and Doenicke, A. Histamine release in clinical conditions. *Mt. Sinai J. Med.* 45:357, 1978.

181. Lubbert, H., et al. cDNA cloning of serotonin 5-HT1C receptor by electrophysiological assays of mRNA-injected Xenopus oocytes. *Proc. Natl. Acad. Sci. USA* 84:4332, 1987.

182. Lundberg, D. B. A., Mueller, R. A., and Breese, G. R. An evaluation of the mechanism by which serotonergic activation depresses respiration. *J. Pharmacol. Exp. Ther.* 212:397, 1980.

183. Maengwyn-Davies, G. D. The dual mode of action of histamine in the cat isolated tracheal chain. *J. Pharm. Pharmacol.* 20:572, 1968.

184. Majno, G., Shea, S. M., and Leventhal, M. Endothelial contraction induced by histamine-type mediators. *J. Cell Biol.* 42:647, 1969.

185. Mandle, R., Jr., Colman, R. W., and Kaplan, A. P. Identification of prekallikrein and HMW-kininogen as a circulating complex in human plasma. *Proc. Natl. Acad. Sci. USA* 73:4179, 1976.

186. Maslinski, C. Histamine and its metabolism in mammals. II. Catabolism of histamine and histamine liberation. *Agents Actions* 5:183, 1975.

187. Matthews, G., Neher, E., and Penner, R. Second messenger-activated calcium influx in rat peritoneal mast cells. *J. Physiol. (Lond.)* 418:105, 1989.

188. Mayer, M. M. Membrane Attack by Complement (with Comments on Cell-mediated Cytotoxicity). In W. R. Clark and P. Goldstein (eds.), *Mechanisms of Cell-mediated Cytotoxicity.* New York: Plenum, 1982.

189. McConnell, D. J. Inhibitors of kallikrein in human plasma. *J. Clin. Invest.* 51:1611, 1972.

190. McGivney, A., et al. Rat basophilic leukemia cell lines defective in phospholipid methyl-transferase enzymes, Ca²⁺ influx, and histamine release: Reconstitution by hybridization. *Proc. Natl. Acad. Sci. USA* 78:6176, 1981.

191. Melchers, F., et al. Growth control of activated, synchronized murine B cells by the C3d fragment of complement. *Nature* 317:267, 1985.

192. Michelson, A. L., Hollander, W., and Lowell, F. C. The effect of 5-hydroxytryptamine (serotonin) on the respiration of nonasthmatic and asthmatic subjects. *J. Lab. Clin. Med.* 51:57, 1958.

193. Middleton, E., Drzewiecki, G., and Triggle, D. Effects of smooth muscle calcium antagonists on human basophil histamine release. *Biochem. Pharmacol.* 30:2867, 1981.

194. Mills, J. E., and Widdicombe, J. G. Role of the vagus nerves in anaphylaxis and histamine-induced bronchoconstrictions in guinea-pigs. *Br. J. Pharmacol.* 39:724, 1970.

195. Minkowski, M., et al. Interleukin 3 induces histamine synthesis in the human hemopoietic system. *Exp. Hematol.* 18:1158, 1990.

196. Mitchel, R. H., Drummond, A. H., and Downes, C. P. (eds.), *Inositol Lipids in Cell Signalling.* London: Academic, 1989.

197. Mongar, J. L., and Schild, H. O. The effect of calcium and pH on the anaphylactic reaction. *J. Physiol. (Lond.)* 140:272, 1958.

198. Morita, Y., Chiang, P. K., and Siraganian, R. P. Effect of inhibitors of

transmethylation on histamine release from human basophils. *Biochem. Pharmacol.* 30:785, 1981.

199. Morita, Y., and Siraganian, R. P. Inhibition of IgE mediated histamine release from rat basophilic leukemia cells and rat mast cells by inhibitors of transmethylation. *J. Immunol.* 127:1339, 1981.

200. Morris, A. P., et al. Synergism of inositol triphosphate and tetrakisphosphate in activating Ca++-dependent K+ channels. *Nature* 330:653, 1987.

201. Movat, H. Z., and DiLorenzo, N. L. Activation of the plasma kinin system by antigen-antibody aggregates: I. Generation of permeability factor in guinea pig serum. *Lab. Invest.* 19:187, 1968.

202. Movat, H. Z., et al. Demonstration of a kinin-generating enzyme in the lysosomes of human polymorphonuclear leukocytes. *Lab. Invest.* 29:669, 1973.

203. Muller-Eberhard, H. J. Complement. *Annu. Rev. Biochem.* 38:389, 1969.

204. Muller-Eberhard, H. J., and Lepow, I. H. C1 esterase effect on activity and physicochemical properties of the fourth component of complement. *J. Exp. Med.* 121:819, 1965.

205. Muller-Eberhard, H. J., and Schreiber, R. D. Molecular biology and chemistry of the alternative pathway of complement. *Adv. Immunol.* 29:1, 1980.

206. Muller-Esterl, W., et al. Human plasma kininogens are identical with a_2-thiol proteinase inhibitors. Evidence from immunological, enzymological and sequence data. *FEBS Lett.* 182:310, 1985.

207. Mylecharane, E. J. Mechanisms involved in serotonin-induced vasodilation. *Blood Vessels* 27:116, 1990.

208. Namm, D. H., Tadepalli, A. S., and High, J. A. Species specificity of the platelet responses to 1-0-alkyl-2-acetyl-sn-glycero-3-phosphocholine. *Thromb. Res.* 25:341, 1982.

209. Neher, E. The influence of intracellular calcium concentration on degranulation of dialysed mast cells from rat peritoneum. *J. Physiol. (Lond.)* 395:193, 1988.

210. Nimmo, H. G., and Cohen, P. L. Hormonal control of protein phosphorylation. *Adv. Cyclic Nucleotide Res.* 8:145, 1977.

211. Nishi, K. The action of 5-hydroxytryptamine on chemoreceptor discharges of the cat's carotid body. *Br. J. Pharmacol.* 55:27, 1975.

212. Nogrady, S. G., and Bevan, C. H2 receptor blockade and bronchial hyperreactivity to histamine in asthma. *Thorax* 36:268, 1981.

213. Northover, A. M. Action of histamine on endothelial cells of guinea-pig isolated hepatic portal vein and its modification by indomethacin or removal of calcium. *Br. J. Exp. Pathol.* 56:52, 1975.

213a. Oglesby, P. C., et al. Membrane cofactor protein (CD46) protects cells from complement-mediated attack by an intrinsic mechanism. *J. Exp. Med.* 175:1547, 1992.

214. Ogston, D., et al. Studies on a complex mechanism for the activation of plasminogen by kaolin or chloroform: The participation of Hageman factor and additional cofactors. *J. Clin. Invest.* 48:1786, 1969.

215. Oh, C., et al. Histamine synthesis by non-mast cells through mitogen-dependent induction of histidine decarboxylase. *Immunology* 65:143, 1988.

216. Okpako, D. T., Chand, N., and Eyre, P. The presence of inhibitory histamine H2-receptors in guinea pig tracheobronchial muscle. *J. Pharm. Pharmacol.* 30:181, 1978.

217. Orange, R. P., Austen, W. G., and Austen, K. F. Immunological release of histamine and slow-reacting substance of anaphylaxis from human lung. I. Modulation by agents influencing cellular levels of cyclic 3′,5′-adenosine monophosphate. *J. Exp. Med.* 134:136s, 1971.

218. Orange, R. P., et al. Immunological release of histamine and slow reacting substance of anaphylaxis from human lung: II. Influence of cellular levels of cyclic AMP. *Fed. Proc.* 30:1725, 1971.

219. Osborne, M. P., and Butler, P. J. New theory for receptor mechanism of carotid body chemoreceptors. *Nature* 254:701, 1975.

220. Owen, D. A. A. Histamine receptors in the cardiovascular system. *Gen. Pharmacol.* 8:141, 1977.

221. Page, I. H., and McCubbin, J. W. The variable arterial pressure response to serotonin in laboratory animals and man. *Circ. Res.* 1:354, 1953.

222. Page, I. H., and McCubbin, J. M. Modification of vascular response to serotonin. *Am. J. Physiol.* 174:436, 1953.

223. Palmieri, F. E., Petrelli, J. J., and Ward, P. E. Vascular plasma membrane aminopeptidase M. Metabolism of vasoactive peptides. *Biochem. Pharmacol.* 34:2309, 1985.

224. Pangburn, M. K., Schreiber, R. D., and Muller-Eberhard, H. J. Human complement C3b inactivator: Isolation, characterization, and demonstration of an absolute requirement for the serum protein B1H for cleavage of C3b and C4b in solution. *J. Exp. Med.* 146:257, 1977.

225. Peach, M. J., et al. Endothelium-derived vascular relaxing factor. *Hypertension* 7 (Suppl. I):I94, 1985.

226. Peachell, P. T., et al. Regulation of human basophil and lung mast cell function by cyclic adenosine monophosphate. *J. Immunol.* 140:571, 1988.

227. Pearce, F. L. Mast cells: Function, differentiation and activation. *Curr. Opin. Immunol.* 1:630, 1989.

228. Pearlman, D. S., and Waton, N. G. Observations on the histamine forming capacity of mouse tissues and of its potentiation after adrenaline. *J. Physiol.* 183:257, 1966.

229. Perlmutter, D. H. Distinct Mediators and Mechanisms Regulate Human Acute Phase Gene Expression. In M. L. Perdue, J. R. Feramisco, and S. Lundquist (eds.), *Stress-induced Proteins.* New York: Alan R. Liss, 1989.

230. Perlmutter, D. H., and Colton, H. R. Structure and expression of the complement genes. *Pharmacol. Ther.* 34:247, 1987.

231. Perlmutter, D. H., Strunk, R. C., and Colten, H. R. Complement. In R. G. Crystal, et al. (eds.), *The Lung: Scientific Foundations.* New York: Raven, 1991.

232. Peroutka, S. J. 5-Hydroxytryptamine receptor subtypes. *Annu. Rev. Neurosci.* 11:45, 1988.

233. Pierce, J. V., and Guimaraes, J. A. Further Characterization of Highly Purified Human Plasma Kininogens. In J. J. Pisano and K. F. Austen (eds.), *Chemistry and Biology of the Kallikrein-Kinin System in Health and Disease.* Washington, D.C.: 1976. DHEW Publication No. 76-791.

234. Podack, E. R., et al. The C5b-6 complex: Reaction with C7, C8, C9. *J. Immunol.* 121:484, 1978.

235. Pritchett, D. B., et al. Structure and functional expression of cloned rat serotonin 5HT-2 receptor. *EMBO J.* 7:4135, 1988.

236. Proud, D., and Kaplan, A. P. Kinin formation: Mechanisms and role in inflammatory disorders. *Annu. Rev. Immunol.* 6:49, 1988.

237. Proud, D., Pierce, J. V., and Pisano, J. J. Radioimmunoassay of human high molecular weight kininogen in normal and deficient plasmas. *J. Lab. Clin. Med.* 95:563, 1980.

238. Proud, D., Siekierski, E. S., and Bailey, G. S. Identification of human lung mast cell kininogenase as tryptase and relevance of tryptase kininogenase activity. *Biochem. Pharmacol.* 37:1473, 1988.

239. Proud, J. Production and Metabolism of Kinins. In R. G. Crystal, et al. (eds.), *The Lung: Scientific Foundations.* New York: Raven, 1991.

240. Pruzansky, J. J., and Patterson, R. The diisopropylfluorophosphate inhibitable step in antigen-induced histamine release from human leukocytes. *J. Immunol.* 114:939, 1975.

241. Putney, J. W. Calcium mobilizing receptors. *Trends Pharmacol. Sci.* 8:481, 1987.

242. Rafferty, P., and Holgate, S. T. Terfenadine (Seldane) is a potent and selective histamine H1-receptor antagonist in asthmatic airways. *Am. Rev. Respir. Dis.* 135:181, 1987.

242a. Raible, D. G., et al. Mast cell mediators prostaglandin-D2 and histamine activate human eosinophils. *J. Immunol.* 148:3536, 1992.

243. Ratnoff, O. D. Biology and pathology of the initial stages of blood coagulation. *Prog. Hematol.* 5:204, 1966.

244. Regal, J. F., Eastman, A. Y., and Pickering, R. J. C5a induced tracheal contraction: A histamine independent mechanism. *J. Immunol.* 124:2876, 1980.

245. Regal, J. F., and Pickering, R. J. C5a-induced tracheal contractions: Effect of an SRS-A antagonist and inhibitors of arachidonate metabolism. *J. Immunol.* 126:313, 1981.

246. Riley, J. F., and West, G. B. The Occurrence of Histamine in Mast Cells. In O. Eichler and A. Farah (eds.), *Handbook of Experimental Pharmacology.* Berlin: Springer, 1966.

247. Robbins, R. A., et al. Activation of the complement system in the adult respiratory distress syndrome. *Am. Rev. Respir. Dis.* 135:651, 1987.

248. Rocha, E., and Silva, M. Release of Histamine in Anaphylaxis. In O. Eichler and A. Farah (eds.), *Handbook of Experimental Pharmacology.* New York: Springer, 1966.

249. Rocha, E., and Silva, M. Histamine II and Anti-histamine. In M. Rocha and E. Silva (eds.), *Handbook of Experimental Pharmacology.* New York: Springer, 1978.

250. Rodbard, S., and Kira, S. Lobar, airway and pulmonary vascular effects of serotonin. *Angiology* 23:188, 1972.

251. Rose, B., and Leger, J. Serum histamine during rabbit anaphylaxis. *Proc. Soc. Exp. Biol. Med.* 79:379, 1952.

252. Rosen, B. S., et al. Adipsin and complement factor D activity: An immune-related defect in obesity. *Science* 244:1483, 1989.

253. Rossoni, G., et al. Bronchoconstriction by histamine and bradykinin in guinea pigs: Relationship to thromboxane A2 generation and the effect of aspirin. *Prostaglandins* 20:547, 1980.

254. Rubin, C. S., and Rosen, O. M. Protein phosphorylation. *Annu. Rev. Biochem.* 44:831, 1975.

255. Ryan, J. W., Roblero, J., and Stewart, J. M. Inactivation of bradykinin in the pulmonary circulation. *Biochem. J.* 110:795, 1968.

256. Saito, H., Ishizaka, K., and Ishizaka, T. Effect of nonhydrolyzable guanosine phosphate on IgE-mediated activation of phospholipase C and histamine release from rodent mast cells. *J. Immunol.* 143:250, 1989.

257. Salvesen, G., et al. Human low molecular weight kininogen contains three copies of a cystatin sequence that are divergent in structure and in inhibitory activity for cystein proteinases. *Biochem. J.* 234:429, 1986.

258. Saxena, S. P., et al. Synthesis of intracellular histamine in platelets is associated with activation of protein kinase C, but not with mobilization of Ca2+. *Biochem. J.* 272:405, 1991.

259. Schayer, R. W. Enzymatic Formation of Histamine from Histidine. In O. Eichler and A. Farah (eds.), *Handbook of Experimental Pharmacology.* New York: Springer, 1966.

260. Schayer, R. W. Histidine decarboxylase in mast cells. *Ann. NY Acad. Sci.* 103:164, 1968.

261. Schayer, R. W., and Cooper, J. A. D. Metabolism of C^{14} histamine in man. *J. Appl. Physiol.* 9:481, 1956.

262. Schayer, R., and Reilly, M. A. Suppression of inflammation and histidine decarboxylase by protein synthesis inhibitors. *Am. J. Physiol.* 215:472, 1968.

263. Schayer, R. W., and Reilly, M. A. Studies on the mechanism of activation and deactivation of histidine decarboxylase. *Eur. J. Pharmacol.* 20:271, 1972.

264. Schmaier, A. H., Smith, P. M., and Colman, R. W. Platelet C1 inhibitor. A secreted alpha-granule protein. *J. Clin. Invest.* 75:242, 1985.

265. Schreiber, A. D., Kaplan, A. P., and Austen, K. F. Inhibition by C1-INH of Hageman factor fragment activation of coagulation, fibrinolysis and kinin generation. *J. Clin. Invest.* 52:1402, 1973.

266. Schulman, E. S., et al. Differential effects of the complement peptides, C5a and C5a des Arg on human basophil and lung mast cell histamine release. *J. Clin. Invest.* 81:918, 1988.

267. Schultz, W. H., and Jordan, H. E. Physiological studies in anaphylaxis: III. A microscopic study of the anaphylactic lung of the guinea-pig and mouse. *J. Pharmacol. Exp. Ther.* 2:275, 1911.

268. Schumaker, V. N., Zavodszky, P., and Poon, P. H. Activation of the first component of complement. *Annu. Rev. Immunol.* 5:21, 1987.

268a. Schwartz, J. C. Histamine receptors in brain. In *ISI Atlas of Science: Pharmacology*, Vol 1. Institute for Scientific Information, Philadelphia, 1988, Pp. 185–189.

269. Shaw, J. O. Leukocytes in chemotactic-fragment-induced lung inflammation. *Am. J. Pathol.* 101:283, 1980.

270. Shelton, E., Yonemasu, K., and Stroud, R. M. Ultrastructure of the human complement component C1q. *Proc. Natl. Acad. Sci. USA* 69:65, 1972.

271. Sieghart, W., et al. Calcium-dependent protein phosphorylation during secretion by exocytosis in the mast cell. *Nature* 275:329, 1978.

272. Simon, R. A., et al. The relationship of plasma histamine to the activity of bronchial asthma. *J. Allergy Clin. Immunol.* 60:312, 1977.

273. Siraganian, R. P., et al. Variants of the rat basophilic leukemia cell line for the study of histamine release. *Fed. Proc.* 41:30, 1982.

274. Smith, C. A., et al. Molecular architecture of human properdin, a positive regulator of the alternative pathway of complement. *J. Biol. Chem.* 259:4582, 1984.

275. Snyderman, R., Gewurz, H., and Mergenhagen, S. E. Interactions of the complement system with endotoxic lipopolysaccharide. Generation of a factor chemotactic for polymorphonuclear leukocytes. *J. Exp. Med.* 128:259, 1968.

275a. Sparrow, D., et al. Relationship of urinary serotonin excretion to cigarette smoking and respiratory symptoms. The normative aging study. *Chest* 101:976, 1992.

276. Spataro, A. C., and Bosmann, H. B. Mechanism of action of disodium cromoglycate mast cell calcium ion influx after a histamine-releasing stimulus. *Biochem. Pharmacol.* 25:505, 1976.

277. Steckel, E. W., et al. The eighth component of human complement: Purification and physiochemical characterization of its unusual subunit structure. *J. Biol. Chem.* 255:11997, 1980.

278. Stimler, N. P., et al. Complement anaphylatoxin C5a stimulates release of SRS-A-like activity from guinea pig lung fragments. *J. Pharm. Pharmacol.* 32:804, 1980.

279. Stimler, N. P., et al. Release of leukotrienes from guinea pig lung stimulated by C5a$_{des\ arg}$ anaphylatoxin. *J. Immunol.* 123:2247, 1982.

280. Stimler, N. P., et al. Anaphylatoxin-mediated contraction of guinea pig lung strips: A nonhistamine tissue response. *J. Immunol.* 126:2258, 1981.

281. Storrs, S. B., et al. Characterization of the binding of purified human C1q to heart mitochondrial membranes. *J. Biol. Chem.* 256:10924, 1981.

282. Streb, H., et al. Release of Ca++ from a nonmitochondrial store in pancreatic cells by inositol-1,4,5-triphosphate. *Nature* 306:67, 1983.

283. Strunk, R. C., Whitehead, A. S., and Cole, F. S. Pretranslational regulation of the third component of complement in human mononuclear phagocytes by the lipid A portion of lipopolysaccharide. *J. Clin. Invest.* 76:985, 1985.

284. Sullivan, T. J., et al. Modulation of cyclic AMP in purified rat mat cells: I. Responses to pharmacologic, metabolic and physical stimuli. *J. Immunol.* 114:1473, 1975.

285. Sullivan, T. J., et al. Modulation of c-AMP in purified rat mast cells: II. Studies on the relationship between intracellular cyclic AMP concentrations and histamine release. *J. Immunol.* 114:1480, 1975.

286. Sullivan, T. J., et al. Modulation of cyclic-AMP in purified rat mast cells: III. Studies on the effects on concanavalin A and anti-IgE or cyclic AMP concentrations during histamine release. *J. Immunol.* 117:713, 1976.

287. Sydbom, A., and Freditolm, B. B. On the mechanism by which theophylline inhibits histamine release from rat mast cells. *Acta Physiol. Scand.* 114:243, 1982.

288. Takagaki, Y., Kitamura, N., and Nakanishi, S. Cloning and sequence analysis of cDNAs for human high molecular weight and low molecular weight prekininogens. Primary structures of two human prekininogens. *J. Biol. Chem.* 260:8601, 1985.

289. Tasaka, K., et al. Degranulation of isolated rat mast cells induced by ATP in presence of calcium ions. *Proc. Jpn. Acad.* 46:317, 1970.

290. Taytard, A., et al. Treatment of bronchial asthma with terfenadine: A randomized controlled trial. *Br. J. Clin. Pharmacol.* 24:743, 1987.

291. Tedder, T. F., Clement, L. T., and Cooper, M. D. Expression of C3d receptors during human B cell differentiation: Immunofluorescence analysis with the HB-5 monoclonal antibody. *J. Immunol.* 133:678, 1984.

292. TerLaan, B., et al. Interaction of human anaphylatoxin C3a with rat mast cells demonstrated by immunofluorescence. *Eur. J. Immunol.* 4:393, 1974.

293. Theoharides, T. C., and Douglas, W. W. Secretion in mast cells inhibited by calcium entrapped within phospholipid vesicles. *Science* 201:1143, 1978.

294. Theoharides, T. C., et al. Antiallergic drug cromolyn may inhibit histamine secretion by regulating phosphorylation of a mast cell protein. *Science* 207:80, 1980.

295. Tran, V. T., and Snyder, S. H. Histidine decarboxylase. Purification from fetal rat liver, immunologic properties, and histochemical localization in brain and stomach. *J. Biol. Chem.* 256:680, 1981.

296. Uvnas, B. Histamine storage and release. *Fed. Proc.* 33:2172, 1974.

297. Uvnas, B. (ed.), *Advances in Histamine Research.* New York: Pergamon, 1982.

298. Uvnas, B., Aborg, C., and Bergendorff, A. Storage of histamine in mast cells. Evidence for an ionic binding of histamine to protein carboxyls in the granule heparin-protein complex. *Acta. Physiol. Scand. Suppl.* 336:3, 1970.

299. Vogt, W., et al. Complement activation by the properdin system: Formation of a stoichiometric C3 cleaving complex of properdin factor B with C3b. *Immunochemistry* 14:201, 1977.

300. Vogt, W., et al. A new function of the activated third component of complement: Binding to C5, an essential step for C5 activation. *Immunology* 34:29, 1978.

301. Ward, P. A. Complement Derived Chemotactic Factors and Their Interactions with Neutrophilic Granulocytes. In D. G. Igram (ed.), *Biologic Activities of Complement.* Basel: S. Karger, 1972.

302. Ward, P. A., and Newman, L. J. A neutrophil chemotactic factor from human C5. *J. Immunol.* 102:93, 1969.

303. Wasserman, S. I., et al. Modulation of the immunological release of the eosinophil chemotactic factor of anaphylaxis from human lung. *Immunology* 26:677, 1974.

304. Wasserman, S. I., et al. Tumor-associated eosinophilotactic factor. *N. Engl. J. Med.* 290:420, 1974.

305. Watanabe, R. T., Maeyama, K., and Taguchi, Y. Release and synthesis of histamine in rat basophilic leukemia (2H3) cells. *Dermatologica* 179(Suppl. 1):45, 1989.

306. Watanabe, T., et al. Partial purification and characterization of L-histidine decarboxylase from fetal rats. *Biochem. Pharmacol.* 28:1149, 1979.

307. Watanabe, T., et al. Purification and Properties of Histidine Decarboxylase Isozymes and Their Pharmacological Significance. In B. Uvnas and K. Tasaka (eds.), *Advances in the Biosciences.* New York: Pergamon, 1982.

308. Watanabe, T., et al. Increase in histidine decarboxylase activity in mouse

skin after application of the tumor promoter tetradecanoylphorbol acetate. *Biochem. Biophys. Res. Commun.* 100:427, 1981.

309. Webster, M. E., and Pierce, J. V. The nature of the kallidins released from human plasma by kallikreins and other enzymes. *Ann. NY Acad. Sci.* 104: 91, 1963.

310. Weill, B. J., and Renoux, M. L. Study of granule reappearance and histamine synthesis in rat mast cells maintained in short term cultures. *Cell. Immunol.* 68:220, 1982.

311. Weiss, S., Robb, G. P., and Ellis, L. B. The systemic effects of histamine in man. *Arch. Intern. Med.* 49:360, 1932.

312. Weissbach, H., Lovenberg, W., and Udenfriend, S. Characteristics of mammalian histidine decarboxylating enzymes. *Biochim. Biophys. Acta.* 50:177, 1961.

313. Wilson, D. B., et al. Inositol cyclic phosphates are produced by cleavage of phosphatidylphosphoinositols (polyphosphoinositides) with purified sheep vesicle phospholipase C enzymes. *Proc. Natl. Acad. Sci. USA* 82: 4013, 1985.

314. Wilson, D. B., et al. Isolation and characterization of the inositol cyclic phosphate products of polyphosphoinositide cleavage by phospholipase C. Physiological effects in permeabilized platelets and limulus photoreceptor cells. *J. Biol. Chem.* 260:13496, 1985.

315. Winslow, C. M., and Austen, K. F. Enzymatic regulation of mast cell activation and secretion by adenylate cyclase and cyclic AMP-dependent protein kinases. *Fed. Proc.* 41:22, 1982.

316. Winslow, C. M., Lewis, R. A., and Austen, K. F. Mast cell mediator release as a function of cyclic AMP-dependent protein kinase activation. *J. Exp. Med.* 154:1125, 1981.

317. Yen, S. S., Mathe, A. A., and Dugan, J. J. Release of prostaglandins from healthy and sensitized guinea-pig lung and trachea by histamine. *Prostaglandins* 11:227, 1976.

317a. Yoshioka, M., et al. Pharmacological characterization of 5-hydroxytryptamine-induced apnea in the rat. *J. Pharmacol Exptl. Therap.* 260:917, 1992.

318. Ziccardi, R., and Cooper, N. R. Activation of C1r by proteolytic cleavage. *J. Immunol.* 116:504, 1976.

319. Ziccardi, R. J., and Cooper, N. R. Direct demonstration and quantitation of the first component of complement in human serum. *Science* 199:1080, 1978.

320. Zuber, M., and Sache, E. Isolation and characterization of porcine pancreatic kallikrein. *Biochemistry* 13:3098, 1974.

321. Regoli, D. Kinins. *Br. Med. Bull.* 43:270, 1987.

322. Steranka, L. R., Farmer, S. G., and Burch, R. M. Antagonists of B$_2$ bradykinin receptors. *FASEB J.* 3:2019, 1989.

323. Farmer, S. G., et al. Evidence for a pulmonary B$_3$ bradykinin receptor. *Mol. Pharmacol.* 36:1, 1989.

324. Page, I. H., and Olmsted, F. Hemodynamic effects of angiotensin, norepinephrine, and bradykinin continuously measured in unanesthetized dogs. *Am. J. Physiol.* 201:92, 1961.

325. Mason, D. T., and Melmon, K. L. Effects of bradykinin on forearm venous tone and vascular resistance in man. *Circ. Res.* 17:106, 1965.

326. Graham, R. C., et al. Pathogenesis of inflammation: II. In vivo observations of the inflammatory effects of activated Hageman factor and bradykinin. *J. Exptl. Med.* 121:807, 1965.

327. Carr, J., and Wilhelm, D. L. The evaluation of increased vascular permeability in the skin of guinea pigs. *Aust. J. Exp. Biol. Med. Sci.* 42:511, 1964.

328. Carr, J., and Wilhelm, D. L. Interspecies differences in response to polypeptides as permeability factors. *Nature* 208:653, 1964.

329. Sturmer, E., and Berde, B. A pharmacological comparison between synthetic bradykinin and synthetic kallidin. *J. Pharmacol. Exp. Therap.* 139: 38, 1963.

330. Feldberg, W., and Lewis, G. P. Action of peptides on adrenal medulla: Release of adrenaline by bradykinin and angiotensin. *J. Physiol.* 171:98, 1964.

331. Melmon, K. L., and Kline, M. J. Kinins. *Am. J. Med.* 43:153, 1967.

332. Furchgott, R. F., and Vanhoutte, P. M. Endothelium-derived relaxing and contracting factors. *FASEB J.* 3:2007, 1989.

333. Peach, M. J. Endothelium-derived vascular relaxing factor. *Hypertension* 7(Suppl.):I94, 1985.

334. Bhoda, V. D., et al. Actions of some peptides in bronchial muscle. *Br. J. Pharmacol.* 19:190, 1962.

335. Aarsen, P. M. The influence of analgesic antipyretic drugs on the responses of guinea-pig lungs to bradykinin. *Br. J. Pharmacol.* 27:196, 1966.

336. Jankala, E. O., and Virtama, P. Bronchographic demonstration of the bronchoconstrictor effect of bradykinin in the guinea pig. *Annales Medicinae Experimentalis et Biologiae Fenniae* 41:436, 1963.

337. Collier, H. O. J., et al. The bronchoconstrictor action of bradykinin in the guinea pig. *Br. J. Pharmacol.* 15:290, 1960.

338. Soler, M., Sielczak, M., and Abraham, W. M. A bradykinin-antagonist blocks antigen-induced airway hyperresponsiveness and inflammation in sheep. *Pulmon. Pharmacol.* 3:9, 1990.

339. Corfield, D. R., et al. The actions of bradykinin and lys-bradykinin on tracheal blood flow and smooth muscle in anaesthetized sheep. *Pulmon. Pharmacol.* 4:85, 1991.

340. Herxheimer, H., and Stressemann, E. The effect of bradykinin aerosol in guinea pigs and in man. *J. Physiol.* 158:38P, 1961.

341. Michel, B., et al. Release of kinins during wheal and flare allergic reactions. *J. Clin. Invest.* 47:68a, 1968.

Chemical Mediators: Leukotrienes and Eicosanoids

11

Jonathan P. Arm
Tak H. Lee

Leukotrienes and the prostanoids (prostaglandins and thromboxane) are lipid mediators formed from the oxidative metabolism of arachidonic acid by the lipoxygenase and cyclooxygenase enzyme cascades, respectively [209, 250]. In contrast to mediators such as histamine, which are preformed and stored in granules, the lipid mediators are newly synthesized on cell activation. Following their discovery and characterization, considerable interest has centered on the potential role of these mediators in inflammation. They have potent proinflammatory and spasmogenic properties and are present in asthmatic airways at rest and during an acute attack of asthma. With the development of potent and selective receptor antagonists and enzyme inhibitors, there is now compelling evidence that eicosanoid mediators play an important role in the pathophysiology of bronchial asthma.

LEUKOTRIENES

Synthesis, Metabolism, and Sources

Synthesis
Arachidonic acid is a 20-carbon polyunsaturated fatty acid released from membrane phospholipids by the action of phospholipase A_2. Metabolism by the lipoxygenase and cyclooxygenase pathways leads to the generation of leukotrienes and prostanoids, respectively (Fig. 11-1). The 5-lipoxygenase (5-LO) generates the unstable intermediate 5S-hydroperoxy-6-*trans*-8,11,14-*cis*-eicosatetraenoic acid (5-HPETE) [30] which is reduced to 5S-hydroxy-6-*trans*-8,11,14-*cis*-eicosatetraenoic acid (5-HETE) or is converted to an epoxide, 5,6-oxido-7,9-*trans*-11,14-*cis*-eicosatetraenoic acid (leukotriene A_4 [LTA_4]) [31, 102, 201]. LTA_4 is processed by an epoxide hydrolase to 5S,12R-dihydroxy-6,14-*cis*-8,10-*trans*-eicosatetraenoic acid (leukotriene B_4 [LTB_4]) [32] or by a glutathione-*S*-transferase to 5S-hydroxy-6R-*S*-glutathionyl-7,9-*trans*-11,14-*cis*-eicosatetraenoic acid (leukotriene C_4 [LTC_4]) [12, 13, 172]. LTC_4 is cleaved by gammaglutamyl-transpeptidase to 5S-hydroxy-6R-*S*-cysteinylglycyl-7,9-*trans*-11,14-*cis*-eicosatetraenoic acid (leukotriene D_4 [LTD_4]), which is cleaved by a dipeptidase to 5S-hydroxy-6R-*S*-cysteinyl-7,9-*trans*-11,14-*cis*-eicosatetraenoic acid (leukotriene E_4 [LTE_4]) [12, 147, 148, 171, 172, 184]. LTA_4 also undergoes nonenzymatic hydrolysis to 5S,12R- and 5S,12S-dihydroxy-6,8,10-*trans*-14-*cis*-eicosatetraenoic acid diastereoisomers (5S,12R- and 5S,12S-dihydroxy-6-*trans*-LTB_4, respectively) and to minor products, 5,6-dihydroxy-eicosatetraenoic acid diastereoisomers [33].

With the molecular cloning of 5-LO it became apparent that cellular 5-LO activity was dependent on an additional factor. Osteosarcoma cells were transfected with the complementary DNA (cDNA) for 5-LO. While cell lysates expressed active enzyme, intact cells were unable to generate leukotrienes on stimulation with the calcium ionophore A 23187 [207]. Furthermore a class of compounds that inhibit the generation of cellular leukotrienes but have no inhibitory effect on soluble 5-LO, of which MK-886 is an example, has been described [96]. The nature of this additional activity was recently characterized at the biochemical and molecular level [67, 169]. The target of the leukotriene inhibitor MK-886 was identified in neutrophil extracts by photoaffinity labeling, and by its retention on agarose gels to which analogs of MK-886 had been bound [169]. A membrane protein of relative molecular mass (M_r) 18,000 that bound to MK-886 and its analogs but not to other inhibitors of leukotriene synthesis was isolated. This protein was named *5-LO–activating protein* (FLAP) [169]. N-terminal and internal amino acid sequences were obtained and used to design oligonucleotide probes, with which cDNA clones were isolated from both rat RBL-1 cell and human HL-60 cell cDNA libraries [67]. The cDNA hybridizes to a 1-kb species of messenger RNA (mRNA) on Northern analysis, and encodes a protein of 161 amino acids with three transmembrane domains. Osteosarcoma cells transfected with 5-LO or FLAP alone did not generate leukotrienes on activation with A 23187. By contrast, activation of cells transfected with both 5-LO and FLAP resulted in significant generation of LTB_4 and other hydrolysis products of LTA_4. Expression of both 5-LO and FLAP is therefore necessary for cellular leukotriene synthesis. The mechanism of action of FLAP is unknown, but translocation of 5-LO to the cell membrane is blocked by MK-886 [67, 206]. It has therefore been proposed that a stable complex is required at the cell membrane between 5-LO, FLAP, and possibly other components of the lipoxygenase pathway (Fig. 11-2). The formation of this complex could regulate the interaction of 5-LO with arachidonic acid, thereby regulating the generation of leukotrienes.

Cellular Sources
The distribution and action of 5-LO are limited, and different cells demonstrate specificity in their metabolism of arachidonic acid. Peripheral blood neutrophils and monocytes preferentially generate LTB_4, whereas eosinophils preferentially generate LTC_4 [29, 213, 262]. Monocytes and macrophages have the capacity to generate both LTB_4 and LTC_4 [77, 162, 266]. Thus peripheral blood neutrophils generate about 50 ng of $LTB_4/10^6$ cells and only one-tenth as much LTC_4 in response to activation with the calcium ionophore A 23187 [135, 262], the quantities and ratio being reversed for eosinophils [262]. Both peripheral blood monocytes in monolayers and adherent or suspended alveolar macrophages respond to the ionophore with a substantial generation of LTB_4 and, for the former, of LTC_4. Peripheral blood monocytes produce about 70 ng of LTB_4 and 30 ng of $LTC_4/10^6$ cells [266], whereas adherent alveolar macrophages generate 100 to 400 ng of $LTB_4/10^6$ cells, in an average 20-fold excess relative to LTC_4 [77, 162]. The quantities of leukotriene generated by each of these cells in response to physiologic stimuli are generally less than those obtained with ionophore activation. For example,

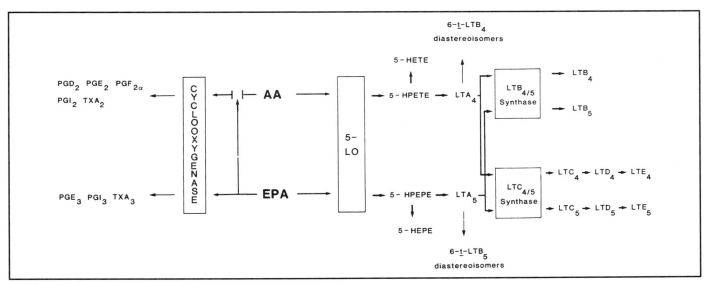

Fig. 11-1. *Metabolism of arachidonic (AA) acid and eicosapentaenoic acid (EPA) by the 5-lipoxygenase (5-LO) and cyclooxygenase pathways. PG = prostaglandin; LT = leukotriene; 5-HETE = 5-hydroxyeicosatetraenoic acid; 5-HPETE = 5-hydroperoxyeicosatetraenoic acid; 5-HEPE = 5-hydroxyeicosapentaenoic acid; 5-HPEPE = 5-hydroperoxyeicosapentaenoic acid; TXA₂ = thromboxane A₂.*

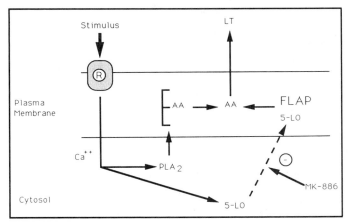

Fig. 11-2. *Proposed mechanism of action of 5-lipoxygenase–activating protein (FLAP). Following an appropriate stimulus, phospholipase A₂ (PLA₂) is activated to cleave arachidonic acid (AA) from cell membrane phospholipids. In addition, 5-lipoxygenase (5-LO) translocates from the cytoplasm to the cell membrane where it is activated by FLAP, leading to the generation of leukotrienes (LT).*

activation by unopsonized [155, 266, 267] or opsonized zymosan [47, 187, 253], and IgG-coated sepharose beads [214], acting via the IgG Fc receptor, generates approximately one-sixth to one-third of the quantity of products produced in response to ionophore. Comparable phagocytosis of particles via monocyte IgG Fc receptors causes minimal LTB_4 and LTC_4 generation, as compared with stimulation by zymosan acting at its specific receptor [266]; thus, transmembrane physiologic stimuli also differ in the magnitude of associated leukotriene generation.

Human mast cells isolated from both skin and lung generate LTC_4 in response to IgE-mediated stimulation, both in vivo [238] and in vitro [25, 152, 190, 192]. The maximal release of LTC_4 from purified human skin and lung mast cells is of the order of 4 ng and 16 ng/10^6 cells, respectively. By comparison, prostaglandin D_2 (PGD_2) is the major eicosanoid released from human mast cells, in an approximate 10-fold molar excess compared to LTC_4 [145].

The LTA_4 hydrolase enzyme that converts LTA_4 to LTB_4 is widely distributed. Thus LTA_4 may be metabolized within its cell of origin, or may be released for metabolism by other cells. Such transcellular metabolism may lead to the generation of LTB_4 by erythrocytes [167] or of LTC_4 by platelets [71, 154], endothelial cells [76], and mast cells [61].

In addition to their generation by inflammatory cells, the leukotrienes may be synthesized and metabolized by lung tissue. Thus, with the use of radiolabeled leukotrienes, the conversion of LTA_4 to LTB_4, LTC_4, LTD_4, and LTE_4 has been demonstrated in guinea pig lung [217], and of LTC_4 to LTD_4 and LTE_4 in human lung parenchyma [3, 55].

Metabolism of Leukotrienes

LTB_4 is converted intracellularly by an LTB_4-20 hydroxylase to 20-hydroxy LTB_4 (20-OH LTB_4), and by further oxidation to a biologically inactive molecule 5S,12R-dihydroxy,20-aldehyde 6,14-cis-8,10-trans-eicosatetraenoic acid (20-CHO LTB_4) [212, 225, 226]. LTB_4-20 hydroxylase is a member of the P_{450} family and is located in neutrophils. 20-CHO LTB_4 is converted irreversibly to 5S,12R-dihydroxy,20-carboxy-6,14-cis-8,10-trans-eicosatraenoic acid (20-COOH LTB_4) [232]. An aldehyde reductase in microsomes converts 20-CHO LTB_4 back to 20-OH LTB_4.

In addition to the bioconversion of LTC_4 to LTD_4 and to LTE_4, there is another mechanism for modifying the structures and functional activities of the sulfidopeptide leukotrienes, which depends on the triggering of the respiratory burst [135]. Neutrophils metabolize LTC_4, LTD_4, and LTE_4 and eosinophils metabolize LTC_4 through an extracellular hydrogen peroxide-peroxidase-chloride–dependent reaction. The six products elute as three doublets on reverse-phase high-performance liquid chromatography. More than 70 percent of the metabolites are composed of the 6-trans-LTB₄-diastereoisomers and the subclass specific diastereoisomeric leukotriene sulfoxides. The 6-trans-LTB₄-diastereoisomers are inactive as spasmogenic agents and are not immunoreactive in a sulfidopeptide leukotriene radioimmunoassay. The sulfoxides possess less than 5 percent spasmogenic activity but are fully immunoreactive.

Cellular Distribution and Leukotriene Transport

Cellular and extracellular distribution of LTB_4 generated by human neutrophils stimulated with unopsonized zymosan was compared with that generated in neutrophils activated by the calcium ionophore [267]. With zymosan stimulation, 5-HETE and the 6-*trans*-LTB_4-diastereoisomers were not released, LTB_4 was partially released, and the omega-oxidation products for LTB_4 were preferentially extracellular in distribution. In contrast, with ionophore stimulation, only 5-HETE had any duration of intracellular residence, being equally distributed intracellularly and extracellularly; 6-*trans*-LTB_4, LTB_4, and the omega-oxidation products of LTB_4 were retained at less than 19 percent.

When human eosinophils are stimulated under optimal conditions with unopsonized zymosan particles, 30 to 60 percent of the generated LTC_4 remains cell associated [155]. The amount of immunoreactive LTC_4 that remains cell associated after calcium ionophore stimulation of the eosinophils was largely cell associated in the first 5 minutes following stimulation (71%), but this figure declined to 9 percent after 15 minutes, by which time there had been a redistribution of LTC_4 to the supernatant. The finding that stimulation of neutrophils and eosinophils with unopsonized zymosan resulted in the cellular retention of 5-LO products suggests that release of these metabolites may be an event that is regulated separately from its generation.

Lam and colleagues examined the requirements for the export of LTC_4 by cultured human eosinophils [133]. Using criteria of saturability, time dependence of LTC_4 release at 37°C, competition of LTC_4 with LTC_5 for release, and the inhibition of LTC_4 at 0°C, they established that the export of LTC_4 from cells was a specific biochemical step. This was distinct from both LTA_4 uptake and the conjugation of LTA_4 with reduced glutathione by LTC_4 synthase to form LTC_4. The same investigators then proceeded to study the mechanism of LTB_4 export from human neutrophils and were able to demonstrate that the release of LTB_4 from these cells was a carrier-mediated process that was distinct from its biosynthesis [132].

Biologic Activity

Leukotriene B₄

LTB_4 is a potent proinflammatory mediator. Its in vitro activities are apparent at concentrations as low as 10^{-9} M and include chemokinesis and chemotaxis of human neutrophils and eosinophils [86, 174]; chemokinesis of monocytes [188]; aggregation of neutrophils [86]; enhanced expression of complement receptors, CR1 and CR3, on granulocytes [142]; release of lysosomal enzymes from neutrophils [216]; and augmentation of neutrophil adherence to endothelial cell monolayers [114]. In vivo, intradermal injection of LTB_4 promotes a prolonged neutrophil infiltration into human skin, the lesion being characterized by induration and tenderness which are most prominent 4 to 6 hours after injection [227]. LTB_4 is also spasmogenic for smooth muscle, acting indirectly through the stimulated biosynthesis of secondary cyclooxygenase products [218].

Sulfidopeptide Leukotrienes

Sulfidopeptide leukotrienes are potent spasmogenic agents on nonvascular smooth muscle. They also enhance mucus secretion, constrict arterioles, and enhance venopermeability. Bronchial mucosal explants respond in tissue culture by enhanced mucus secretion to as little as 10^{-9} M LTC_4 [54, 161]. Augmented postcapillary venular permeability was first shown for dermal vascular beds of the guinea pig responding to locally injected LTC_4, LTD_4, and LTE_4 in concentrations as low as 10^{-7} M [69, 148] and

was later confirmed by the leakage of intravascular dye into the tissue of the hamster cheek pouch after topical application of each leukotriene [62]. The intradermal administration of LTC_4, LTD_4, and LTE_4 in normal human subjects produces a local wheal and flare response, in which the wheal representing enhanced venopermeability is sustained for 2 to 4 hours [38, 227]. The capacity of LTC_4 and, to a lesser extent, LTD_4 to constrict arterioles was initially demonstrated in guinea pig skin at the site of intradermal administration of the leukotriene, requiring less than 10^{-7} M of either compound [69, 148], and was confirmed by the response to topical administration to the hamster cheek pouch [62] and by blanching at the injection site in normal human skin [38, 227]. The sulfidopeptide leukotrienes are potent contractile agonists for bronchial smooth muscle both in vitro and in vivo.

Receptors

Radioligand-binding studies suggest the existence of a heterogeneous population of LTB_4-binding sites on human polymorphonuclear cells on the basis of a biphasic [³H]LTB_4 dissociation curve. The K_d of the high-affinity receptor was approximately 0.5 nmol and the K_d of the low-affinity receptor was approximately 300 nmol [98]. The high-affinity receptor is believed to mediate chemotaxis, and the low-affinity receptor, lysosomal enzyme release [150].

The activity and binding of the sulfidopeptide leukotrienes in various tissues and cells have been characterized. With regard to the lung, there are limited data on human tissues and most attention has focused on guinea pig lung, in which stereospecific, reversible, and saturable binding of LTC_4, LTD_4, and LTE_4 has been demonstrated. The existence of receptor heterogeneity for these agonists is suggested by differences in the contractile properties and kinetics of action of the separate leukotrienes, the effects of leukotriene receptor antagonists, and radioligand-binding studies.

In the guinea pig, LTC_4, LTD_4, and LTE_4 are potent contractile agonists for tracheal spirals and parenchymal strips, eliciting equivalent contractions in a molar ratio of $1:1:0.1$ and $1:0.05:3$, respectively [70, 136, 148]. This reversal of potency ratios for LTD_4 and LTE_4 with airway smooth muscle from the same species suggests there are separate receptors for each. The contraction of guinea pig ileal smooth muscle strips produced by LTC_4 requires a 60-second latent period after exposure to LTC_4, whereas the contraction of guinea pig ileum produced by LTD_4 is immediate [131]. Furthermore, inhibition of the conversion of LTC_4 to LTD_4 by serine-borate complex did not inhibit the contractile response or increase the latency period required for the contractile response of LTC_4 [131], supporting the view that there are different contractile mechanisms for LTC_4 and LTD_4. Furthermore, whereas LTC_4 and LTE_4 elicit monophasic contraction in guinea pig peripheral airway strips, LTD_4 evokes a biphasic response [69]. Lee and others [136] demonstrated that exposure of guinea pig tracheal smooth muscle but not lung parenchymal strips to LTE_4 produces a hyperresponsiveness to subsequent stimulation with histamine, an effect that was not produced by LTC_4 or LTD_4.

Evidence for separate receptors for the sulfidopeptide leukotrienes also comes from radioligand-binding studies in guinea pig lung. The activity and binding of LTC_4 are insensitive to the actions of FPL 55712, which is a selective LTD_4/LTE_4 antagonist [224, 258]. The binding of LTD_4 and LTE_4 to guinea pig lung membranes is antagonized by Na^+ ions and guanosine triphosphate (GTP) analogs, and enhanced by divalent cations [199]. In contrast, the binding of LTC_4 to guinea pig lung membranes is independent of these compounds. Thus there is evidence in the guinea pig for separate LTC_4 and LTD_4 receptors.

The binding affinities of LTD_4 and LTE_4 for guinea pig lung membranes are comparable [40, 170]. Further, the inhibition of binding of radiolabeled LTD_4 and LTE_4 by unlabeled LTC_4, LTD_4, LTE_4, and FPL 55712 is also similar [40]. Studies by Cheng and Townley demonstrated biphasic dissociation kinetics for LTD_4 and Scatchard analysis suggested the existence of both low- and high-affinity receptors for LTD_4 [41]. Studies of the antagonism of $[^3H]LTD_4$ and $[^3H]LTE_4$ action on guinea pig trachea by FPL 55712 demonstrated a bimodal distribution of dissociation constants for LTD_4 [130]. Further analysis suggested that there were two distinct receptors for LTD_4 and that LTE_4 bound to the high-affinity LTD_4 receptor. The ability of LTD_4 to elicit further contraction of guinea pig trachea following a maximally effective concentration of LTE_4, but not vice versa [108], and the observation that in the presence of salbutamol, LTE_4 shifted the dose-response curve for LTD_4 to the right [108], suggest that LTE_4 may be a partial agonist at the LTD_4 receptor. Binding studies by Aharony and associates showed that the binding of $[^3H]LTE_4$ was completely reversed by an excess of LTD_4 but that the reverse was not seen [2]. The density and affinity of binding sites for LTE_4 were lower than for LTD_4. The binding of LTE_4 was also more sensitive to Na^+, divalent cations, and GTP analogs, thereby providing further evidence that LTE_4 binds to a subset of LTD_4 receptors [2].

The differences in the rank order of relative contractile potencies for the sulfidopeptide leukotrienes in various tissues, the differences in the time courses of spasmogenic responses to the three compounds in the same tissues, the distinct effect of LTE_4 in producing hyperresponsiveness, and the results of binding studies cannot be explained by interaction of these agonists for a single population of receptors, even if different affinities for each leukotriene are postulated. The data cannot be solely accounted for by differential rates of leukotriene metabolism. Thus, physiologic studies of the sulfidopeptide leukotriene subclasses in guinea pig tissues indicate that there may be different recognition mechanisms and, in view of the stereochemical requirement for agonist action, suggest the involvement of two or more distinct receptors.

In human lung, binding of $[^3H]LTD_4$ is also sensitive to guanine nucleotides and the concentration of Na^+ and divalent cations [146]. In contrast to the results in guinea pig tissues, a study conducted in the presence of bioconversion inhibitors on intralobar airways isolated from human subjects undergoing surgery for carcinoma of the bronchus did not reveal evidence for multiple leukotriene receptors [37]. FPL 55712 was an effective competitive inhibitor of contractions mediated by all three sulfidopeptide leukotrienes, with similar values for the negative log of the molar equilibrium constant (pA_2) calculated for each agonist. SK&F 104353 is also a selective LTD_4/LTE_4 antagonist in guinea pig lung, but antagonizes the actions of LTC_4, LTD_4, and LTE_4 in isolated human bronchi [107]. However, it should be emphasized that the data from human tissue are very limited. Furthermore, the effects of underlying disease on the expression of the different leukotriene receptors have not been studied and data are not available for asthmatic lung.

Leukotrienes in Bronchial Asthma

Potency

LTC_4 and LTD_4 are potent constrictors of human airways both in vitro and in vivo. Dahlen and colleagues [63] demonstrated that LTC_4 and LTD_4 were approximately 1,000-fold more potent than histamine on a molar basis in contracting isolated human bronchi in vitro. Ten micromolar histamine was required to elicit 100 percent contraction of isolated human airways whereas the same response was elicited by only 6.3 nM LTC_4. Other investigators confirmed the potent contractile properties of LTC_4 and LTD_4 both in vitro [136, 204] and in vivo [113, 259, 261] (Fig. 11-3). In normal subjects the concentrations of LTC_4 and histamine required to produce a 30 percent fall in expiratory flow at 30

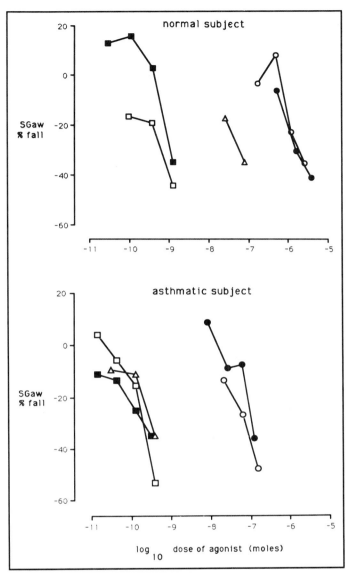

Fig. 11-3. *Dose-response curves to histamine (open circles), methacholine (closed circles), leukotriene (LT) C_4 (open squares), LTD_4 (closed squares), and LTE_4 (open triangles) in a normal individual (top panel) and an asthmatic individual (bottom panel). The dose of histamine, methacholine, LTC_4, LTD_4, and LTE_4 causing a 35 percent fall in specific airway conductance (SGaw) in the normal subject were 2.6 µmol, 3.0 µmol, 1.0 nmol, 1.4 nmol, and 90 nmol, respectively; and in the asthmatic subject, 0.09 µmol, 0.12 µmol, 0.24 nmol, 0.31 nmol, and 0.35 nmol, respectively.*

percent of baseline vital capacity ($\dot{V}_{30}$) were 2 to 20 µg/ml, and 2 to 10 mg/ml, respectively [259]. Thus, LTC_4 was 600- to 9,500-fold more potent than histamine, and LTD_4 was 6,000-fold more potent than histamine on a molar basis [261]. While LTC_4 and LTD_4 have similar potencies in human airways in vivo, they have a different time course of contraction. Maximal bronchoconstriction occurs 10 to 15 minutes after inhalation of LTC_4 and 2 minutes after inhalation of LTD_4 [261].

In asthmatic subjects the sulfidopeptide leukotrienes are also potent bronchoconstrictors. Griffin and coworkers reported that LTD_4 was 140-fold more potent than histamine in eliciting a 30 percent fall in $\dot{V}_{30}$ derived from partial expiratory flow volume curves ($\dot{V}_{30}$-P) in asthmatic subjects [100]. This contrasts with the data in normal subjects in whom LTD_4 was 6,000-fold more potent than histamine [261]. A comparison between these two groups of subjects revealed that the asthmatic subjects were only one-third more responsive to LTD_4 than the normal subjects, despite an approximate 100-fold hyperresponsiveness to inhaled histamine. Barnes and associates demonstrated a correlation between airway responses to histamine and LTD_4, and confirmed the relative lack of hyperresponsiveness to LTC_4 and LTD_4 in asthmatic subjects [14]. Adelroth and colleagues similarly showed a correlation between the airway responsiveness to methacholine and the airway responsiveness to LTC_4 and LTD_4 [1]. A correlation was also observed between airway responsiveness to methacholine and the relative responsiveness to LTC_4 and LTD_4. Thus the subjects with the most responsive airways demonstrated the lowest relative responsiveness to LTC_4 and LTD_4 as compared to methacholine [1]. The findings by Smith and others contrasts with these results, reporting that a group of asthmatic subjects who were 35-fold more responsive to methacholine than normal controls were 100-fold more responsive to LTD_4 [220].

There are only limited data on the bronchoconstrictor properties of LTE_4 in vivo. Using $\dot{V}_{30}$ as an index of airway bronchoconstriction, Davidson and coworkers demonstrated that LTE_4 is 39-fold more potent than histamine in normal subjects and 14-fold more potent than histamine in asthmatic subjects [65]. However, using specific airway conductance (SGaw) as an index of bronchoconstriction, the relative potency of LTE_4 compared with histamine and methacholine was two to three times greater in asthmatic than in normal subjects [181]. The discrepancies between these studies may be due to patient selection or due to the parameter of airway caliber used to monitor the bronchoconstrictor response. It is notable that in Davidson's study a 30 percent fall in $\dot{V}_{30}$-P induced by LTE_4 was accompanied by a 2.6 percent fall in 1-second forced expiratory volume (FEV_1) in normal subjects, but a 15 percent fall in FEV_1 in asthmatic subjects. In contrast, a 30 percent fall in $\dot{V}_{30}$-P induced by histamine was accompanied by comparable falls in FEV_1 in both groups of subjects [65]. Therefore, the relative hyperresponsiveness to LTE_4 observed by O'Hickey and colleagues [181] may be selective for the central airways.

Because of the inherent difficulties in comparing studies performed in different subjects using different methodologies, the potencies of LTC_4, LTD_4, and LTE_4 were compared to one another and to both histamine and methacholine in the same normal and asthmatic subjects [8]. The airways of asthmatic subjects were 14-fold, 15-fold, 6-fold, 9-fold, and 219-fold more responsive than the airways of normal subjects to histamine, methacholine, LTC_4, LTD_4, and LTE_4, respectively (Table 11-1). Furthermore, while LTC_4 and LTD_4 were 100- to 150-fold more potent than LTE_4 in constricting the airways of normal subjects, they were only four- to fivefold more potent than LTE_4 in asthmatic subjects. The cumulative data therefore suggest that the airways of asthmatic subjects are relatively unresponsive to LTC_4 and LTD_4, but have a marked hyperresponsiveness to LTE_4 (see Fig. 11-3).

Table 11-1. The geometric mean doses required to cause a 35 percent fall in specific airway conductance (PD_{35}), and the relative potencies between eight asthmatic and six normal subjects

	PD_{35}		Relative potency
	Asthmatic	Normal	
Histamine (μmol/L)	0.31	4.21	14
Methacholine (μmol/L)	0.12	1.85	15
Leukotriene C_4 (nmol/L)	0.14	0.87	6
Leukotriene D_4 (nmol/L)	0.16	1.45	9
Leukotriene E_4 (nmol/L)	0.64	140	219

Site of Airway Response to Inhaled Leukotrienes

Differences between asthmatic and normal individuals in the predominant site of response to leukotrienes within the tracheobronchial tree have been described. Initial studies found that the inhalation of LTC_4 and LTD_4 had an effect on $\dot{V}_{30}$ with little effect on FEV_1, suggesting a predominant peripheral site of action in normal subjects [113]. Weiss established that in normal subjects a 50-fold greater concentration of LTC_4 was required to achieve a 20 percent fall in FEV_1 compared to the concentration needed to achieve a 30 percent fall in $\dot{V}_{30}$ [260]. However, in other studies inhalation of leukotriene was noted to have a similar effect on both SGaw and $\dot{V}_{30}$ [15, 123, 220]. Studies in asthmatic subjects suggest that leukotrienes may elicit a response that is more marked in the central than the peripheral airways. Bisgaard and coworkers reported that the airways of asthmatic subjects were more responsive to LTD_4 than were those of nonasthmatic subjects [28]. The relative difference in potency between asthmatic and normal subjects was 100- to 1,000-fold when measured in terms of FEV_1 but only 15-fold in terms of $\dot{V}_{30}$. Smith and coworkers found that a 30 percent fall in $\dot{V}_{30}$ in response to LTD_4 was accompanied by a 60 percent fall in SGaw in asthmatic subjects, but only a 30 percent fall in SGaw in normal controls [220]. The study by Davidson and associates also suggested a predominantly central effect of LTE_4 in asthmatic subjects compared to normal controls [65]. Pichurko and coworkers used both density dependence of maximal expiratory flow ($\dot{V}_{max}$) and the effects of a deep breath on expiratory flow rates as indices of the predominant site of response to LTC_4 or histamine aerosols [196]. They found that there was a predominant central airway response to inhaled LTC_4 in asthmatic subjects that was not seen with histamine inhalation.

Mechanism of Leukotriene-induced Bronchoconstriction

The mechanism whereby leukotrienes produce a contractile response is unknown. The fact that prior administration of aspirin [261] or indomethacin [222] does not change leukotriene responsiveness suggests that secondary generation of cyclooxygenase products is not important. The calcium channel blocker verapamil has been shown to inhibit LTD_4-induced bronchoconstriction in normal humans, suggesting that extracellular calcium entry is required for LTD_4-induced bronchoconstriction [202]. In contrast verapamil did not inhibit the response of asthmatic subjects to inhaled LTD_4, suggesting that there may be a different mechanism of action of LTD_4 in asthmatic subjects compared to normal subjects [203].

Leukotrienes and Airway Hyperresponsiveness

The in vitro observation that slow-reacting substance of anaphylaxis (SRS-A) enhanced the contractile response of guinea pig ileum to histamine [36] suggested that the sulfidopeptide leukotrienes might contribute to the pathogenesis of airway hyperresponsiveness in asthma. This is supported by in vitro studies with guinea pig pulmonary tissue. Pretreatment of guinea pig tracheal spirals with 10 to 23 nM LTE_4, but not LTC_4 or LTD_4, enhanced the subsequent contractile response to histamine [136]. Although LTE_4 elicited a similar contractile response in parenchymal strips, there was no enhancement in the response to histamine. Pretreatment of tracheal spirals with indomethacin had no effect on the contractile response to LTE_4, but abolished the LTE_4-induced histamine hyperresponsiveness.

Studies with leukotriene analogs suggested that the capacity of LTE_4 to enhance the response of tracheal spirals to histamine was dependent on the carboxyl group at C-1, the cysteine carboxyl group, and the free NH_2-terminal amino group of the cysteine in the structure of LTE_4. The dissociation of the contractile response from the enhancement of histamine responsiveness, and the initial requirements for structure suggested that the hyperresponsiveness was mediated via a receptor distinct from that which mediated contraction. In a separate study, LTD4 enhanced the contractile response of guinea pig tracheal spirals to histamine only in the presence of low concentrations of extracellular calcium ions [57].

Further studies have shown that LTE4-induced hyperresponsiveness of guinea pig tracheal spirals is selective for histamine and is not seen for carbachol or substance P [119]. LTE4-induced hyperresponsiveness is blocked not only by indomethacin, but also by a thromboxane2/prostaglandin H2 (TP) receptor antagonist (GR 32191), atropine, and tetrodotoxin [119]. Preincubation of tracheal spirals with LTE4 also potentiated the contractile response to electrical field stimulation. These results suggest that LTE4 augments the contractile response of guinea pig tracheal spirals to histamine by facilitating cholinergic neurotransmission, and is mediated via the secondary generation of cyclooxygenase products acting at the TP receptor (Fig. 11-4). Treatment

Fig. 11-4. *Proposed mechanism of leukotriene (LT) E_4–induced hyperresponsiveness. (1) LTE_4 acts on bronchial smooth muscle to elicit contraction and (2) to release thromboxane (TX) A_2. TXA_2 acts at TXA_2/prostaglandin H_2 (TP) receptors on cholinergic nerve terminals (3) to prime them for increased release of acetylcholine (ACh) on subsequent stimulation by histamine. ACh and methacholine act directly on M_3 receptors (4) to elicit contraction of bronchial smooth muscle.*

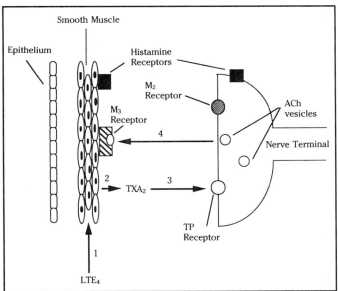

of human bronchus with 4.8 nM LTE4 produced a fourfold leftward displacement of the histamine dose-response curve [119]. This effect was blocked by 1 μM atropine and 10 μM GR 32191, suggesting a similar mechanism to that defined for guinea pig trachea.

In vivo studies support a role for the sulfidopeptide leukotrienes in enhancing airway hyperresponsiveness in asthma (Table 11-2). Inhalation of a bronchoconstricting dose of LTD4 in normal subjects produced an approximate twofold increase in airway methacholine responsiveness [123]. In a further study inhalation of a dose of LTD4 that gave a mean 57 percent fall in SGaw led to a significant increase in the airway response to methacholine in six of eight normal subjects [122]. In these six subjects the maximal effect on methacholine responsiveness was observed at Day 7, and persisted for 2 to 3 weeks in five individuals. The degree and duration of changes in the airway responsiveness to methacholine were comparable to those observed following inhalation of platelet-activating factor (PAF) in the same individuals [122]. In normal subjects inhalation of a bronchoconstricting dose of LTD4 did not significantly enhance the airway response to exercise [27]. Inhalation of a subthreshold dose of LTD4 had no effect on the airway response to histamine, although it increased the sensitivity of the airways to inhaled PGF2α by approximately sevenfold [14].

Studies in asthmatic subjects have been more limited. The inhalation of bronchoconstricting doses of LTC4 did not enhance the airway response to inhalation of distilled water in nine asthmatic individuals [26]. Because LTC4 and LTD4 may be metabolized within the airways to LTE4 [3, 55, 217], and because LTE4 may persist at the site of contraction the longest [131], Arm and coworkers focused on the effects of this mediator. Preinhalation of a bronchoconstricting dose of LTE4 in asthmatic subjects increased histamine responsiveness by approximately threefold [10] (Fig. 11-5). Changes in airway histamine responsiveness were maximal at 4 to 7 hours after inhalation of LTE4 and had returned to baseline values by 1 week. Methacholine inhalation which led to a similar decrease in SGaw as did LTE4 did not elicit any change in histamine hyperresponsiveness. Subsequent work has shown that bronchoconstricting doses of LTC4 and LTD4 elicit a comparable increase in airway responsiveness to histamine in asthmatic individuals [7]. Prior administration of indomethacin prevented the increase in airway responsiveness elicited by LTE4 [42], suggesting that the capacity of the sulfidopeptide leukotrienes to increase airway histamine responsiveness in vivo depends on the secondary generation of cyclooxygenase products. Neither LTC4, LTD4, nor LTE4 elicited any change in airway responses to histamine in normal subjects, although each mediator was administered in a dose that elicited a mean 35 percent fall in SGaw [7, 10]. The lack of effect in normal

Table 11-2. *The effect of inhaled leukotrienes on the airway responses to other bronchoconstrictor stimuli*

Leukotriene	Dose	Stimulus	Index	Effect
Normal subjects				
D4	Subthreshold	Histamine	SGaw : $\dot{V}_{max_{30}}$	None [14]
D4	Subthreshold	Prostaglandin F2α	Not stated	Increased responsiveness: 7-fold [14]
D4	Bronchoconstricting	Methacholine	$\dot{V}_{30}$-P : SGaw	Increased responsiveness: 2-fold, for 7–21 days [122, 123]
D4	Bronchoconstricting	Exercise	$\dot{V}_{max_{30}}$	None [27]
D4	Bronchoconstricting	Methacholine	FEV1; $\dot{V}_{40}$	No shift in dose-response curve; increased maximal airway narrowing [20]
				Effect abolished by steroids [19]
C4, D4, E4	Bronchoconstricting	Histamine	SGaw	None [7, 10]
Asthmatic subjects				
C4	Threshold	H2O	SGaw	None [26]
C4, D4, E4	Bronchoconstricting	Histamine	SGaw	Increased responsiveness: 3-fold for up to 7 days [7, 10]
E4	Subthreshold	Histamine	SGaw	1.5-fold increase in responsiveness [10]
C4	PD12.5*	Histamine, prostaglandin D2	FEV1; $\dot{V}_{30}$-P	Synergy [193]

* Dose required for a 12.5 percent fall in FEV1.

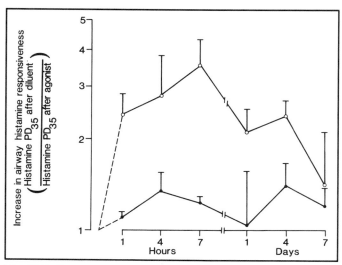

Fig. 11-5. *Time course of changes in airway histamine responsiveness after inhalation of bronchoconstricting doses of methacholine (closed circles) and leukotriene E_4 (LTE$_4$) (open circles). Results are the geometric mean ± standard error for four subjects with asthma and were calculated as the ratio of histamine provocation dose producing a 35 percent fall in SGaw (PD$_{35}$) after inhalation of diluent, to histamine PD$_{35}$ after inhalation of methacholine or LTE$_4$. (Reprinted with permission from J. P. Arm, B. W. Spur, and T. H. Lee. The effects of inhaled leukotriene E_4 on the airway responsiveness to histamine in subjects with asthma and normal subjects. J. Allergy Clin. Immunol. 82: 654, 1988.)*

individuals is in contrast to the findings of Kaye and Smith [122] and Kern and colleagues [123] (above), and may be due to a selective effect of LTD$_4$ on airway responses to methacholine (as opposed to histamine), to the timing of measurements of airway responsiveness, or to individual variability.

In addition to the capacity of inhaled leukotrienes to enhance subsequent airway responses to histamine in subjects with asthma, there is evidence that LTC$_4$ interacts synergistically with histamine and PGD$_2$ in the acute bronchoconstrictor response [193]. The doses of histamine, PGD$_2$, and LTC$_4$ required to elicit a 12.5 percent fall in FEV$_1$ (PD$_{12.5}$) and then to increase this fall in FEV$_1$ to 25 percent (PD$_{25-12.5}$) were determined. Subsequently, subjects inhaled the PD$_{12.5}$ of LTC$_4$ followed by the PD$_{25-12.5}$ of either histamine or PGD$_2$. During the first 9 minutes after LTC$_4$-histamine and LTC$_4$-PGD$_2$ inhalation there was a greater than predicted bronchoconstrictor response. Although the effect was small, these findings suggested that these pairs of mediators were synergistic in their action and not merely additive. This is in contrast to the additive effects of PGD$_2$ with histamine in asthmatic subjects [103].

Normal and asthmatic airway responses in vivo differ by their sensitivity to a wide range of pharmacologic and nonpharmacologic agents [111] and by the presence of maximal airway narrowing to histamine and methacholine in nonasthmatic subjects [229, 269]. While asthmatic subjects show a leftward shift of the dose-response curve and progressive airway narrowing with increasing doses of an agonist, the airway response in normal subjects reaches a plateau at mild degrees of airway narrowing [229, 269]. Bel and colleagues investigated the effect of LTD$_4$ on both the position of the dose-response curve to methacholine and the degree of maximal airway narrowing in normal subjects [20]. Methacholine challenges were performed 1 day before and at 1 and 3 days after inhalation of LTD$_4$ to achieve maximal airway narrowing. The degree of maximal airway narrowing was consistently greater in response to LTD$_4$ than to methacholine. After administration of LTD$_4$ there was no change in the position of

the dose-response curve to methacholine; however, the maximal airway response to methacholine increased. There was a further 4 to 6 percent fall in FEV$_1$ and a further 9 percent fall in $\dot{V}_{40}$-P in response to methacholine 1 to 3 days after inhalation of LTD$_4$. The authors suggested that the greater maximal airway narrowing caused by LTD$_4$ was due to changes in vascular permeability leading to edema of the mucosa, and possibly increased mucus production. Persistence of the mucosal changes may account for the subsequent increase in maximal airway narrowing to methacholine. This view is supported by the observation that corticosteroids prevented the LTD$_4$-induced augmentation of maximal airway narrowing. Pretreatment with inhaled budesonide for 1 week diminished the maximal response to LTD$_4$ and also abolished the LTD$_4$-induced increase in maximal airway narrowing to methacholine [19].

Release of Leukotrienes in Asthma

Physical, chemical, and immunologic methods have been employed to detect leukotrienes in bronchoalveolar lavage (BAL) fluid of asthmatic subjects, both at rest and following bronchial challenge (see Chap. 24). Lam and colleagues used fast atom bombardment mass spectroscopy to analyze the BAL fluid of asthmatic and normal subjects for LTC$_4$, LTD$_4$, LTE$_4$, and the oxidation products of LTB$_4$ [134]. LTE$_4$ was the predominant leukotriene recovered, being detected in the BAL fluid from 15 of 17 asthmatic subjects. LTD$_4$ was detected in 2 subjects, and 20-hydroxy LTB$_4$ in 12 subjects with asthma. Leukotrienes were not detected in the BAL fluid of healthy subjects. In a further study C18 SepPak extraction followed by radioimmunoassay (RIA) was used to analyze LTC$_4$, LTD$_4$, and LTB$_4$ in BAL fluid of 16 atopic asthmatic individuals, 17 subjects with various forms of interstitial lung disease, and healthy controls [257]. Significant quantities of LTC$_4$ and LTB$_4$ were detected in BAL fluid of symptomatic asthmatic subjects compared to normal controls. Increased quantities of LTB$_4$ were also detected in lavage fluid of patients with cryptogenic fibrosing alveolitis and correlated with the recovery of polymorphonuclear cells in BAL fluid. Crea and colleagues reported significantly greater quantities of LTB$_4$, but not of the sulfidopeptide leukotrienes, in BAL fluid of asthmatic subjects compared to normal controls [56a]. These results differ from those above and may relate to the selection of subjects with very mild asthma. Leukotrienes have been detected in BAL fluid following local endobronchial challenge with allergen [263] and following isocapnic hyperventilation [198]. As assessed by high-pressure liquid chromatography, the predominant sulfidopeptide leukotriene in lavage fluid of atopic asthmatic patients prior to allergen challenge was LTC$_4$, with lower amounts of LTD$_4$ and LTE$_4$. Following allergen challenge, mean LTC$_4$ levels rose from 64 pg/ml of lavage fluid to 616 pg/ml [263]. LTC$_4$ was detected in lavage fluid in one of seven atopic nonasthmatic subjects prior to challenge, and at a mean level of 88 pg/ml after challenge. Leukotrienes were undetectable in nonatopic controls before and after allergen challenge. Following asthma provoked by isocapnic hyperventilation, BAL fluid concentrations of LTB$_4$ and immunoreactive sulfidopeptide leukotrienes rose from baseline levels of 10 pg/ml and 46 pg/ml to 121 pg/ml and 251 pg/ml, respectively [198].

Automated reversed-phase high-pressure liquid chromatography with RIA has been used to analyze leukotrienes in complex biologic fluids [237]. In humans, LTC$_4$ is converted enzymatically in blood to LTD$_4$ and LTE$_4$, which is excreted in the urine [185]. Maltby and colleagues showed that following infusion of radiolabeled LTC$_4$, 12 to 20 percent appeared in the urine, of which a substantial proportion (4–6% of the total dose) was LTE$_4$, most of which appeared in the first 4 hours [157]. LTE$_4$ may be detected in the urine of both normal and asthmatic subjects. The levels of LTE$_4$ in the urine of asthmatic subjects at rest are not significantly

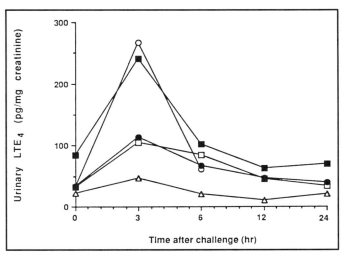

Fig. 11-6. *Urinary leukotriene E_4 (LTE_4) concentration following allergen challenge in five asthmatic subjects. Data for each individual are shown separately.*

higher than those in the urine of nonasthmatic subjects, and they do not correlate with resting FEV_1 or with airway responsiveness to histamine and methacholine [219a, 265a]. Measurement of urinary LTE_4 concentration may therefore act as a marker of systemic release of sulfidopeptide leukotrienes. Taylor and associates demonstrated that urinary LTE_4 levels increase during acute severe asthma and at 3 hours following antigen challenge of asthmatic subjects [239]. These findings were extended in a study of 72 subjects presenting with acute airway obstruction [70a]. Urinary excretion of LTE_4 was raised in 16 subjects whose peak flow increased more than twofold following treatment with inhaled albuterol, compared to 12 subjects whose peak flow failed to increase by more than 25 percent and 13 normal subjects. These findings support a role for leukotrienes in acute reversible bronchospasm. Manning and coworkers also demonstrated a rise in urinary LTE_4 in the first 3 hours following the early asthmatic response to antigen, which correlated with the severity of the bronchoconstriction. No increases in urinary LTE_4 were observed during the development of the late asthmatic response, 3 to 7 hours after challenge [159]. In the presence of the leukotriene D_4 antagonist, ICI 204,219, allowing the administration of two- to fourfold more allergen, the rise in urinary LTE_4 was augmented [131a]. Smith and coworkers also demonstrated release of urinary leukotrienes following allergen challenge (Fig. 11-6) but failed to detect a rise in urinary LTE_4 concentrations following exercise-induced asthma despite a similar fall in FEV_1 [219b]. In contrast, Kikawa and colleagues demonstrated increased excretion of urinary LTE_4 following exercise-induced asthma in 8 of 13 children [124]. The release of leukotrienes following aspirin challenge is discussed below.

Therapeutic Intervention

The action of leukotrienes may be modulated by receptor antagonists or by inhibitors of their generation. The latter may be accomplished by direct inhibition of 5-LO or by inhibiting the activation of the enzyme by FLAP. If leukotrienes play a significant role in the pathogenesis of asthma, then attempts to inhibit their generation or to antagonize their action at specific receptors should be of some benefit in asthma. Studies of the effects of 5-LO inhibitors and sulfidopeptide leukotriene antagonists on asthma induced by exercise and inhalation of antigen and of cold, dry air have now been reported. In addition, preliminary data on

the effects of these drugs on the clinical severity of day-to-day asthma have been presented.

Leukotriene Antagonists
One of the earliest leukotriene antagonists was FPL 55712. This compound is an antagonist of LTD_4 and LTE_4 in guinea pig trachea [224, 258] and of all three sulfidopeptide leukotrienes in isolated human bronchi (see above) [37]. It is a weak antagonist with a short half-life, is not bioavailable via the oral route, and has therefore been given by inhalation [143]. A pilot study of its effect in asthma proved disappointing [143].

LY 171883 is very similar in structure to FPL 55712, has a similar low potency, and can be given orally [84]. LY 171883 is only a weak antagonist of inhaled LTD_4 in nonasthmatic subjects, shifting the dose-response curve to LTD_4 to the right by approximately fivefold [194]. The administration of 400 μg of LY 171883 orally to six asthmatic subjects led to no significant change in baseline pulmonary function and inhibited the response to inhaled LTD_4 in four individuals [90]. In the same subjects there was a significant attenuation of the early response to inhaled antigen, but not of the late phase response. In a study of 19 asthmatic subjects it attenuated the response to isocapnic hyperventilation [118]. The mean respiratory heat exchange required to produce a 20 percent fall in FEV_1 rose by 20 percent from 1.00 kcal/min following placebo to 1.24 kcal/min following 2 weeks' treatment with LY 171883 (600 mg twice daily). Although small, this change was statistically significant and was accompanied by a decrease in symptoms of chest tightness. This drug has now been withdrawn due to toxicity.

Recently, highly potent and selective leukotriene antagonists have become available, allowing a more critical evaluation of the role of leukotrienes in asthma. These have included MK-571 [85], ICI 198,615 [129, 223], ICI 204,219 [128], and SK&F 104353 [247] (see also Chap. 66).

MK-571 is a racemate and both enantiomers are potent, selective, and orally active [85]. It has high affinity for the LTD_4 receptor(s) with 50 percent inhibitory concentrations (IC_{50}) of 1 nM and 8 nM in guinea pig and human lung parenchymal membranes, respectively. It is a potent antagonist of the spasmogenic activity of LTD_4 in vitro. While MK-571 is an orally active compound, early trials have been carried out with intravenous infusions, in an attempt to correlate clinical effects with blood levels. It appears to be well tolerated in normal human volunteers up to blood levels of 300 μg/ml [85]. Administration of the drug in asthmatic subjects, but not normal subjects, produces bronchodilatation, suggesting that LTD_4 may contribute to resting airway tone in asthma [92, 125]. This effect was additive to that of inhaled albuterol [92]. Complete antagonism of the bronchoconstrictor response to LTD_4 was achieved in normal subjects with blood levels as low as 1 μg/ml [125]. In asthmatic subjects more than 40-fold and more than 80-fold shifts in the dose-response curve to inhaled LTD_4 were achieved with intravenous infusions of 28 mg and 277 mg, respectively [125]. The effects of MK-571 on exercise-induced asthma were evaluated in 12 asthmatic subjects. One hundred sixty milligrams of drug or placebo was administered intravenously 20 minutes prior to exercise challenge in a double-blind, randomized, crossover design [160]. The mean fall in FEV_1 following exercise was 9.2 percent in subjects given MK-571, compared to 25.2 percent in subjects given placebo. The extent of the protection afforded by MK-571 varied from 29 to 100 percent. Preliminary data suggest that MK-571 attenuates both the early and the late asthmatic responses to inhaled allergen [168].

Inhalation of 800 μg of SK&F 104353 by normal human subjects 15 minutes prior to LTD_4 inhalation challenge [74] led to an approximate 75 percent inhibition of the fall in $V_{max_{30}}$ and SGaw. When 800 μg and 400 μg of SK&F was administered 4 hours before challenge, there was still 67 and 34 percent inhibition of the bronchoconstrictor response to LTD_4, respectively. The drug had no effect on the bronchoconstriction induced by histamine [74]. The effect in asthmatic subjects was evaluated in 12 subjects in a double-blind, placebo-controlled crossover study [121]. Following inhalation of 800 μg of SK&F 104353 there was a modest but significant 23 percent increase in baseline SGaw and 5 percent increase in baseline FEV_1. In 6 subjects who inhaled the drug 30 minutes prior to LTD_4 challenge, there was a mean shift in the dose-response curve to LTD_4 of approximately 12-fold (provocation concentration producing 20 percent fall in FEV_1 [PC_{20} FEV_1]) and 8-fold (PC_{35} SGaw). In a separate study LTC_4- and LTE_4-induced bronchoconstriction in asthmatic subjects was blocked by prior inhalation of 900 μg of aerosolized SK&F 104353 30 minutes prior to challenge [43]. The dose of either LTC_4 or LTE_4 required to induce bronchoconstriction increased at least 10-fold after prior inhalation of SK&F 104353, without changing baseline airway caliber. Interestingly, a significant inhibition of PAF-induced bronchoconstriction was noted [247], consistent with the suggestion that PAF may stimulate leukotriene generation [241, 252]. Preliminary data also indicate that this compound inhibits the bronchoconstriction induced by allergen [73] and exercise [247] in asthmatic subjects.

ICI 204,219 is a structural analog of ICI 198,615, which has an improved profile of bioavailability when given orally [128]. In normal subjects a single oral dose of 40 mg given 2 hours, 12 hours, and 24 hours prior to LTD_4 inhalation challenge increased the concentration of LTD_4 required to elicit a 35 percent fall in SGaw by 117-fold, 9-fold, and 5-fold, respectively [221]. The effect of this potent leukotriene antagonist on allergen-induced asthma was evaluated in 10 subjects in a double-blind protocol [240]. Administration of 40 mg of the antagonist 2 hours prior to challenge led to a significant attenuation of both early and late asthmatic responses, and inhibited the increase in airway responses to histamine 6 hours after allergen challenge. The mean maximal falls in FEV_1 during early reaction and late reaction were 32.4 and 27.9 percent, respectively, following placebo, and were 6.3 and 12.7 percent, respectively, following treatment with ICI 204,219. The increase in histamine responsiveness accompanying the late reaction was attenuated by about twofold. In a separate study, 40 mg of ICI 204,219 increased the dose of antigen required to elicit a 20 percent fall in FEV_1 by a mean of 10-fold [78a]. A significant attenuation of exercise-induced asthma has also been demonstrated [81a], the mean maximum percentage fall in FEV_1 following exercise being 21.6 percent following ICI 204,219, compared to 36 percent following placebo. The maximum effect of the leukotriene antagonist was seen from 5 to 30 minutes following exercise, consistent with the prolonged bronchoconstriction induced by the sulfidopeptide leukotrienes.

The effects of leukotriene antagonists in chronic asthma have now been reported. The effect of LY 171883 was evaluated in a multicenter trial of 138 subjects [48]. Subjects received 600 mg of active drug or placebo twice daily for 6 weeks in double-blind fashion. Following active treatment, mean FEV_1 rose from 78.8 percent of predicted to 83.3 percent, and was significantly different from the change in placebo-treated subjects. This was associated with a decrease in severity of both daytime and nighttime wheezing and breathlessness, though no changes in cough or chest tightness were noted. In those patients who took more than 23 mg/week of metaproterenol prior to entry into the study there was a significant decrease in its use of -22.2 mg/week compared to $+6.0$ mg/week in placebo-treated subjects. There was no change in use of inhaled $beta_2$ agonists in subjects who used less than 23 mg/week of metaproterenol prior to entry.

MK-571 has also been evaluated in chronic asthma [93]. Subjects received either placebo or 75 mg of MK-571 three times a day for 2 weeks followed by 150 mg three times a day for 4 weeks. Compared to placebo treatment, treatment with MK-571 led to a mean 8 to 14 percent improvement in FEV_1, a 30 percent decrease in morning and evening symptom scores, and an approximate 30 percent decrease in usage of albuterol.

5-Lipoxygenase Inhibitors

Compared with the data on leukotriene receptor antagonists there are relatively few data on the effects of 5-LO inhibitors in asthma. A 64077 is one such inhibitor that has been evaluated in asthma induced by cold dry air [117] and by allergen [116]. Eight hundred milligrams of inhibitor or placebo was administered 3 hours prior to challenge with cold dry air. The inhibition of 5-LO was assessed by measuring the ex vivo ionophore-induced leukotriene generation in whole blood. The ionophore-induced production of LTB_4 was inhibited by 74 percent following treatment with A 64077, with no inhibition of the generation of thromboxane B_2 (TXB_2). This was associated with an increase in the respiratory heat exchange required to produce a 10 percent fall in FEV_1. There was no significant difference in baseline lung function between placebo and active treatment. In a separate study, 800 mg of oral A 64077, administered 3 hours prior to allergen challenge, led to a mean 93 percent inhibition in the ex vivo generation of LTB_4 in response to ionophore, 4 hours after dose administration [116]. In these same individuals there was a 48 percent reduction in the urinary excretion of LTE_4 produced following allergen challenge. This was associated with a small attenuation of the early asthmatic response to allergen, which did not reach statistical significance. Nevertheless there was a correlation between the inhibition of urinary leukotriene excretion and the attenuation in the early asthmatic response, suggesting that the lack of clinical effect may have been related to an insufficient inhibition of 5-LO. Preliminary data have been reported of the effects of A 64077 in chronic asthma [117a]. Six hundred milligrams of the active drug 4 times a day for 28 days led to a significant improvement of airway function and a reduction in symptoms.

MK-886 is a potent inhibitor of the synthesis of leukotrienes by a number of cell types in vitro, and inhibits leukotriene generation in animals in vivo [85]. It is of particular interest in that it is not a direct inhibitor of 5-LO, but rather it binds to FLAP, preventing activation of 5-LO on cell activation [169, 206]. The results of clinical trials of this interesting compound are awaited.

The overall impression from the studies described above is that leukotrienes contribute to the resting airway tone in asthma, and the asthmatic response to a range of stimuli including exercise, allergen, and cold dry air. They may also contribute to the airway hyperresponsiveness induced by allergen challenge of sensitized subjects. It is notable that inhibiting effects on leukotriene actions are particularly apparent when the newer generation of potent and selective antagonists is used. Studies of the effects of these drugs in day-to-day asthma suggest a role for leukotrienes in the pathophysiology of asthma. However, further studies are needed to evaluate the possible place of leukotriene antagonists and inhibitors in the management of asthma.

PROSTAGLANDINS AND THROMBOXANE

Biosynthesis and Metabolism

Arachidonic acid may be metabolized by cyclooxygenase to the cyclic endoperoxides, PGG_2 and PGH_2, which are then converted by specific synthases to thromboxane (TX) A_2 or to the various prostaglandins PGD_2, $PGF_{2\alpha}$, PGE_2, and PGI_2 [210, 249] (see Fig. 11-1). TXA_2 is generated predominantly by platelets. It is unstable and is rapidly hydrolyzed to its inactive metabolite, TXB_2. PGI_2, prostacyclin, is generated by vascular endothelial cells and by both vascular and nonvascular smooth muscle. PGI_2 spontaneously hydrolyzes to its inactive metabolite, 6-keto-$PGF_{1\alpha}$. PGE_2 is the predominant cyclooxygenase product of a number of different types of cells, including epithelial cells and macrophages. PGD_2 is the major cyclooxygenase product of the mast cell [112, 149] and it is released after both IgE-dependent challenge and ionophore challenge of human lung fragments [112, 149, 211]. PGD_2 is metabolized by an NADPH-dependent 11-keto reductase to an active metabolite, $9\alpha,11\beta$-PGF_2, which contracts airway smooth muscle both in vitro and in vivo [16]. In addition to the specific metabolites described above, the prostaglandins may be metabolized by reduction of the 11-keto group, 15-hydroxyl dehydrogenation, beta oxidation, and omega oxidation.

Biologic Activity

The cyclic endoperoxides PGG_2 and PGH_2, and TXA_2 are labile molecules with short half-lives and appear to act at a common receptor [49]. They constrict vascular and bronchial smooth muscle and aggregate platelets [50, 156]. PGI_2 is active in many tissues, producing vasodilatation, inhibiting platelet aggregation, and relaxing bronchial smooth muscle [95, 235]. Its importance in platelet-endothelial interactions is well recognized. PGE_2 has diverse properties depending on the site of action. Its actions are mediated by at least two types of receptor [51]. It inhibits platelet aggregation, and may contract or relax vascular and nonvascular smooth muscle [52, 68]. In human airways it acts as a bronchodilator [219]. $PGF_{2\alpha}$, PGD_2, and its stable metabolite $9\alpha,11\beta$-PGF_2 are potent bronchoconstrictors [16]. The luteolytic activities of $PGF_{2\alpha}$ are also well recognized [115]. PGD_2 contracts pulmonary smooth muscle [16, 17, 106], stimulates neutrophil chemokinesis [97], causes vasodilatation, and increases postcapillary venular permeability [227]. It acts synergistically with LTB_4 in promoting neutrophil infiltration of human skin [227].

Receptors

Initial attempts to classify the prostaglandin receptors were based on comparisons of the rank order of potency of the prostanoids and the stable TXA_2-mimetic, U-44619 [51]. This led to the suggestion that there were at least five different receptors with preferential sensitivity to PGE_2, $PGF_{2\alpha}$, PGD_2, PGI_2, and TXA_2, which were designated EP, FP, DP, IP, and TP receptors, respectively. This initial classification has been strengthened and extended by the development of selective agonists and antagonists, and by radioligand-binding studies. The current classification of prostanoid receptors has recently been reviewed [94, 101]. PGE_2 may have both contractile/stimulatory and relaxant/inhibitory activities [52, 68]. The receptors for these distinct actions are designated EP-1 and EP-2, respectively. A third receptor for PGE_2, EP-3, has been proposed and appears to have stimulatory activity in some tissues and inhibitory activity in others. There is also evidence for the existence of at least two subtypes of TXA_2/PGH_2 (TP) receptor. A large number of TP receptor agonists have been synthesized and while selective for this receptor, they have different profiles of activity.

There is evidence that prostanoid receptors act via second-messenger systems. They modulate cyclic AMP levels through guanine nucleotide regulatory proteins and activate phospholipase C with subsequent hydrolysis of phosphatidyl inositol and increase of intracellular free calcium [101]. There are preliminary reports on the biochemical isolation and characterization of these important receptors, and subsequent isolation of cDNAs.

Prostaglandins and Asthma

Potency

Initial studies of the bronchoconstrictor effects of prostaglandins were directed to the properties of $PGF_{2\alpha}$. $PGF_{2\alpha}$ was shown to contract human airways in vivo, and asthmatic subjects were

shown to be more sensitive to $PGF_{2\alpha}$ than were normal controls. Smith and coworkers [219] studied 10 asthmatic subjects and 5 healthy controls and found that whereas asthmatic individuals were approximately 8 times more responsive to histamine than normal subjects, they were 160 times more responsive to $PGF_{2\alpha}$. Mathé and Hedqvist [163] compared airway responses to histamine and $PGF_{2\alpha}$ in 10 asthmatic and 10 normal individuals. Whereas asthmatic subjects were 10 times more sensitive to histamine than the control subjects, they were 8,000 times more sensitive to $PGF_{2\alpha}$. In this study $PGF_{2\alpha}$ was 2,400 times more potent than histamine on a molar basis in asthmatic subjects, and 2.6 times more potent than histamine in normal healthy controls. Thomson and colleagues [244] demonstrated that airway responsiveness to $PGF_{2\alpha}$ correlated with that to methacholine, but that the range of responsiveness to $PGF_{2\alpha}$ was greater than that to methacholine. Challenges with $PGF_{2\alpha}$ were found to be as reproducible as those with methacholine, and a cumulative dose effect was noted. However, subsequent studies suggested that the airway response to $PGF_{2\alpha}$ in vivo might not be as simple as originally described. Both Fish [83] and Beasley [17] and their respective colleagues reported complex biphasic or triphasic responses to inhaled $PGF_{2\alpha}$, possibly due to the action of $PGF_{2\alpha}$ on separate receptors mediating bronchodilatation and bronchoconstriction. Studies of the effects of cholinergic blockade on airway responses to $PGF_{2\alpha}$ have yielded conflicting results [17, 83, 163, 176, 183, 189], but the cumulative data suggest that the contribution of cholinergic pathways to $PGF_{2\alpha}$-induced bronchoconstriction is small. Neither alpha-adrenergic blockade [189] nor pretreatment with cromolyn [176, 189] inhibited airway responses to $PGF_{2\alpha}$.

In normal and asthmatic subjects, PGD_2 is a potent contractile agent when inhaled [16, 17, 106]. Hardy and associates [106] demonstrated that the potency of PGD_2 in asthmatic subjects was approximately 3.5 and 10 times greater than that of $PGF_{2\alpha}$ and histamine, respectively. In addition, there was a significant correlation between airway responsiveness to PGD_2 and histamine. Normal subjects were substantially less sensitive to PGD_2: 500 µg/ml of PGD_2 produced a mean 20 percent fall in SGaw; by comparison the same dose of $PGF_{2\alpha}$ had no discernible effect in normal subjects.

The major metabolite of PGD_2 is $9\alpha,11\beta$-PGF_2. Recent studies showed that $9\alpha,11\beta$-PGF_2 is a potent contractile agonist for human airways both in vitro and in vivo [16]. $9\alpha,11\beta$-PGF_2 was found to be approximately four times more potent than PGD_2 in contracting human bronchial smooth muscle in vitro, but these two agonists were equipotent in eliciting bronchoconstriction in vivo, suggesting that some of the contractile activity of PGD_2 may be mediated through its metabolite. A significant correlation exists between airway responses to $9\alpha,11\beta$-PGF_2 and those to both PGD_2 and histamine. Pretreatment with 1 mg of inhaled ipratropium bromide attenuated the airway response to methacholine by 70- to 200-fold, and the response to PGD_2 and $9\alpha,11$ β-PGF_2 by 12- to 23-fold [17], suggesting that some of the action of these prostaglandins was mediated through cholinergic pathways.

There are both in vitro and in vivo data to suggest that the bronchoconstrictor actions of prostaglandins within human airways are mediated through the TP receptor. The rank order of contractile agonist potency of prostanoid agonists on isolated human bronchus was U-46619 markedly greater than $9\alpha,11\beta$-PGF_2, equal to $PGF_{2\alpha}$, greater than PGD_2, greater than PGE_2, and greater than PGI_2 [53]. U-46619 was at least 300-fold more potent than other prostanoids with a mean concentration eliciting 50 percent of the maximum response (EC_{50}) of 12 nM. The rank order of potency of these agonists is similar to that reported for other tissues with TP receptors. Furthermore, the TP receptor antagonist, AH 23848, antagonized the contractile response to the prostanoids, but had no effect on carbachol-induced contractions. Because of its very short half-life, it is not possible to study the bronchoconstrictor properties of thromboxane. Therefore, the bronchoconstrictor effect of the thromboxane mimetic, U-46619, has been studied in vivo in normal subjects and in subjects with mild asthma [119a]. U-46619 was on average 178-fold more potent than methacholine, and there was a correlation between the airway responsiveness to methacholine and U-46619. No tachyphylaxis to U-46619 was observed. The effects of various competitive antagonists on prostanoid-induced contractions of isolated human bronchus are also consistent with a bronchoconstrictor response mediated predominantly through a TP receptor. GR 32191 is a specific and potent TP receptor–blocking drug. A single oral dose of 80 mg of GR 32191 did not change resting airway caliber in nine asthmatic subjects, increased the mean dose of PGD_2 required to cause a 20 percent fall in FEV_1 by more than 10-fold, and decreased the slope of the dose-response curve to PGD_2 [18]. GR 32191 had no effect on the position or slope of the dose-response curve to methacholine.

Prostaglandins of the E series are bronchodilators. The inhalation of 55 μg of PGE_1 and PGE_2 in normal human subjects led to a mean increase in SGaw of 10 and 18 percent, respectively [219]. In asthmatic subjects the same doses of these agonists led to a mean increase of 41 and 39 percent, respectively. These increases in airway caliber were comparable to those induced by 550 μg of inhaled isoprenaline. PGE_2 was also noted to speed the recovery from $PGF_{2\alpha}$-induced bronchoconstriction. However, both PGE_1 and PGE_2 were highly irritant when inhaled, making them unsuitable for therapeutic use.

PGI_2 has complex effects on the airways in humans. Precontracted human bronchus relaxes in response to PGI_2 in vitro [95]. However, the response in vivo is more complicated. Inhaled PGI_2 had no consistent effect on airway caliber as measured by changes in SGaw in normal and asthmatic subjects [105]. This was further evaluated in subjects with mild allergic asthma who inhaled PGI_2 in increasing concentrations up to 500 μg/ml [104]. The effect on SGaw was variable, with changes varying from a 50 percent fall in the subject with the most responsive airways, to a 40 percent increase in SGaw in another individual. In contrast, concentration-related falls in both FEV_1 and $\dot{V}_{max_{30}}$ were observed in all subjects, with mean maximal falls of 19 and 42 percent, respectively, at 500 μg/ml. Although PGI_2 caused a concentration-dependent bronchoconstriction, it also protected the airways against the bronchoconstrictor effects of PGD_2 and methacholine. When PGI_2 was inhaled with PGD_2, it was not possible to determine a PC_{35} SGaw to PGD_2, and there was a 10-fold and 5-fold increase in the PC_{35} $\dot{V}_{max_{30}}$, and PC_{20} FEV_1, respectively. It was proposed that the paradoxic effects of PGI_2 on the airways of asthmatic subjects might be explained by its effect on the vasculature within the airways. PGI_2 is a potent systemic vasodilator. Increased mucosal blood flow might lead to engorgement of the mucosa, leading to significant reduction in caliber of the small airways, reflected by changes in FEV_1 and $\dot{V}_{max_{30}}$, but without significantly altering large-airway caliber, as reflected by changes in SGaw. Increased mucosal blood flow might also lead to a more rapid clearance of inhaled bronchoconstrictor agonists from the airways, providing a degree of functional antagonism. A direct bronchodilator effect on smooth muscle cannot be excluded.

Prostanoids and Airway Hyperresponsiveness

The effects of several prostanoid mediators on the response of isolated human bronchi to methacholine were evaluated in human lung tissue obtained at thoracotomy from patients undergoing lung resection for treatment of pulmonary malignancy [120]. Dose-response curves to methacholine were constructed before, during, and after incubation with either subthreshold or threshold concentrations of histamine, U-46619,

PGD_2, or $PGF_{2\alpha}$. Small but significant decreases in the dose of methacholine required to elicit a 50 percent contraction of the airway preparation was noted following treatment with each mediator. The amplitude of the decrease varied from 0.03 to 0.16 log units. While the effects of histamine, $PGF_{2\alpha}$, and U-46619 were readily reversed by washing the preparation, those of PGD_2 were sustained and were only reversed by extensive washing. No effect of pretreatment with either methacholine or LTC_4 was noted.

Several studies have suggested that prostanoids may enhance airway responsiveness in both normal and asthmatic subjects in vivo. Inhalation of a subthreshold dose of $PGF_{2\alpha}$ immediately before histamine provocation enhanced the airway response to a subsequent histamine challenge in nine nonatopic normal subjects [256]. These observations were extended in a separate study of similar design in which inhalation of a subthreshold dose of $PGF_{2\alpha}$ 10 minutes before challenge enhanced airway responsiveness to histamine by approximately fourfold but had no effect on the airway response to methacholine [110].

The effects of PGD_2 on airway responses to histamine and methacholine were investigated by Fuller and coworkers [91]. Six atopic asthmatic subjects inhaled a single breath of either saline, histamine, bradykinin, or PGD_2 in doses that produced no measurable bronchoconstriction immediately before each dose of histamine or methacholine. They found that PGD_2, but not saline, bradykinin, or histamine, enhanced airway responses to subsequent histamine and methacholine challenge by approximately twofold. Hardy and others [103] confirmed the potentiating effect of PGD_2 on airway histamine responsiveness in three asthmatic subjects but suggested that the results may represent a physiologic rather than a pharmacologic effect of PGD_2. They investigated the effect of equipotent doses of two mediators given sequentially on the bronchoconstrictor response [103]. Histamine or PGD_2 was inhaled by asthmatic subjects to produce a 25 percent fall in SGaw, followed immediately by inhalation of an equipotent dose of histamine or PGD_2. The airway response to histamine given as the second agonist was the same irrespective of whether PGD_2 or histamine was given as the first agonist. Histamine and PGD_2 were therefore additive and not synergistic in their bronchoconstrictor effects on the airways of asthmatic subjects.

In view of the evidence implicating TXA_2 in the induction of airway hyperresponsiveness, the effect of the thromboxane mimetic, U-46619, on methacholine responsiveness was studied [119a]. One minute after inhalation of a subthreshold dose of saline, histamine, or U-46619, the mean fall in FEV_1 in response to a dose of methacholine previously established to cause a 10 to 15 percent fall in FEV_1 was 13.2, 12.4, and 25.7 percent, respectively. The enhanced response to methacholine was no longer apparent 1 hour after inhalation of U-46619, suggesting a transient effect. The effect on histamine responsiveness was not studied.

Measurements of Prostanoids in Biologic Fluids

In view of the proposed role of prostanoids in asthma, there have been various attempts to measure these mediators in the lungs, blood, and urine of asthmatic subjects in both stable asthma and asthma provoked by a number of stimuli.

Liu and colleagues used gas chromatography–mass spectrometry to measure the presence of a spectrum of prostanoid mediators in the BAL fluid of healthy normal subjects, subjects with allergic rhinitis, and subjects with atopic asthma [151]. Levels of PGD_2, $9\alpha,11\beta$-PGF_2, and $PGF_{2\alpha}$, were 3.8, 0.5, and 1.4 nM, respectively, in BAL fluid of asthmatic individuals, and were elevated 10- to 20-fold compared to levels in the control groups. There was an inverse correlation between levels of these mediators and the dose of methacholine required to produce a 20 percent fall in FEV_1 when all subjects were considered, but not when the asthmatic group was considered alone.

PGD_2 is the major cyclooxygenase product released by activated mast cells [145, 149], and has therefore been measured in the BAL fluid of asthmatic subjects after allergen challenge. Murray and associates performed lavage before and after local allergen challenge in five subjects with atopic asthma [173]. PGD_2 levels were measured by gas chromatography–mass spectrometry after normal-phase high-pressure liquid chromatography, and rose from basal levels of less than 8 pg/ml before challenge to 322 pg/ml after challenge, the levels increasing by between 20- and 400-fold in the five subjects studied. Wenzel and colleagues measured the spectrum of prostanoids in BAL fluid of atopic and nonatopic subjects with and without asthma [265]. No significant differences in the levels of these mediators were found before challenge between groups. Significant increases in PGD_2 and TXB_2 were detected after local allergen challenge in the atopic asthmatic subjects but not in the other groups. Levels of 6-keto-$PGF_{1\alpha}$ and PGE_2 did not change with allergen challenge. These findings were extended in a study of the relationship between mediator release and the late-phase allergic response in atopic subjects with and without asthma [264]. Subjects with asthma were challenged with inhaled allergen and divided into those with isolated early responses and those with late-phase responses, defined as a fall in FEV_1 of more than 15 percent 3 to 8 hours after challenge. On a separate study day these individuals underwent bronchoscopy and local allergen challenge, BAL fluid being sampled before and 5 minutes after instillation of allergen. PGD_2 and TXB_2 were measured by enzyme immunoassays. There were significant increases in the levels of both PGD_2 and TXB_2 following allergen instillation, and these changes were greater for subjects with isolated early responses than for subjects with late responses. Levels of mediators were unrelated to airway responsiveness to methacholine, the amount of allergen administered, the extent of the early response induced by inhaled allergen, or skin reactivity. Mediators were not measured during the late-phase response. The results suggested that the late response may be determined by factors other than mediators released during the early response.

The principal urinary metabolites of TXA_2 are 2,3-dinor-TXB_2 and 11-dehydro-TXB_2, with a small quantity of TXB_2 excreted unchanged in the urine. These metabolites together with 6-oxo-$PGF_{1\alpha}$ and its 2,3-dinor metabolite were measured in the urine during acute severe asthma and following allergen challenge by affinity chromatography followed by gas chromatography–mass spectroscopy [242]. There was a considerable range in the excretion of the prostanoid metabolites in the urine in acute severe asthma, but all were significantly elevated by 2.7- to 9.4-fold. In this study no significant increases were noted following antigen challenge. However, following inhalation of 20 μg of TXB_2, less than 2 percent was recovered in the urine, suggesting that the assay technique may not have been sensitive enough to detect small changes in the release of TXA_2. In a further study 11-dehydro-TXB_2 was assayed in urine by radioimmunoassay before and after allergen-induced asthma in five atopic subjects [131a]. Following allergen challenge, there was a modest increase in urinary excretion of 11-dehydro-TXB_2 from basal levels of 164 ± 29 ng/mmol creatinine (mean ± standard error) to a peak of 238 ± 25 ng/mmol creatinine.

Pharmacologic Modulation of Prostanoid Action

Our understanding of the role of prostanoids in asthma has been severely hampered by a lack of specific and potent receptor antagonists and specific inhibitors of the individual synthetases. Initial attempts to investigate the role of prostaglandins in asthma therefore centered on the effects of cyclooxygenase inhibitors.

Airway Tone and Acute Asthmatic Responses

Although cyclooxygenase inhibitors relax the resting tone of isolated guinea pig trachea [35, 95], a similar effect on isolated human airways has not been observed [35, 60, 66, 109]. Furthermore, incubation of human bronchial tissue with 0.17 μM indomethacin did not alter the contractile response to acetylcholine or histamine. In normal human subjects and asthmatic individuals the administration of cyclooxygenase inhibitors, thromboxane synthetase inhibitors, or TP receptor antagonists had no significant effect on resting airway caliber [59, 80, 81, 88, 89, 255]. The cumulative in vitro and in vivo evidence therefore suggests that prostanoid mediators do not contribute significantly to the regulation of airway tone in either normal or asthmatic individuals (Table 11-3).

Fish and coworkers examined the effect of indomethacin on the airway responses to allergen in atopic individuals [82]. Subjects were challenged with inhaled allergen after 4 days of pretreatment with either placebo or 50 mg of indomethacin every 6 hours. In asthmatic subjects pretreatment with indomethacin had no effect on the PD_{20} FEV_1, but resulted in a small but significant 1.5-fold increase in the PD_{35} SGaw. In a separate study 50 mg of indomethacin twice daily for 2 days had no significant effect on the acute airway response to allergen [126]. Administration of the more potent cyclooxygenase inhibitor flurbiprofen in a dose of 150 mg daily for 3 days prior to allergen challenge reduced the fall in FEV_1 in response to a single dose of allergen from 38 to 30 percent, a decrease of 21 percent [59]. In the same subjects the fall in FEV_1 after a single oral dose of the H_1 antagonist terfenadine was 21 percent, a decrease of 45 percent. In atopic nonasthmatic subjects, pretreatment with indomethacin led to a significant increase in the airway response to allergen, with a shift in the PD_{35} SGaw, and PD_{20} FEV_1 of 0.36 log units (2.3-fold) and 0.41 log units (2.6-fold), respectively [82].

The increase in airway responsiveness to allergen in atopic nonasthmatic individuals following pretreatment with indomethacin is of interest and of practical importance. The capacity of inhibitors of cyclooxygenase to cause bronchoconstriction in a proportion of asthmatic individuals is well described, and is discussed later in this chapter. In addition, the capacity of cyclooxygenase inhibitors to exacerbate the allergic response both in vitro [249] and in vivo [139] is well recognized, possibly due to a shunting of arachidonate metabolism to the lipoxygenase pathway. Pretreatment of passively sensitized human airways with indomethacin in vitro resulted in an increased release of LTC_4 in response to both antigen and anti-IgE stimulation [249]. In a guinea pig model of antigen-induced anaphylaxis, pretreatment of animals with indomethacin resulted in an augmentation of the pulmonary mechanical response to intravenous antigen, and this was accompanied by an increased generation of LTB_4 [139].

The data therefore suggest that cyclooxygenase inhibitors have minimal inhibitory action on the acute response to allergen in asthmatic subjects, and may exacerbate the response in certain individuals. This provides further grounds for caution in prescribing these agents in asthmatic subjects.

There are conflicting data on the effect of cyclooxygenase inhibitors on the late asthmatic response. An early report in a small number of individuals with late-phase responses to allergen reported that pretreatment with indomethacin 25 mg daily for 4 days consistently attenuated the late-phase response [215]. Fairfax and coauthors also reported attenuation of the late response to house dust mite in four individuals [75]. However, other workers failed to confirm these findings [126], although indomethacin inhibited the allergen-induced increases in airway hyperresponsiveness that followed the late response.

There are limited data on the effects of prostaglandin receptor antagonists in asthma, due to their toxicity or relative lack of potency. The effects of GR 32191, a specific and potent TP receptor antagonist, on the airway response to allergen has been reported. Seven asthmatic subjects inhaled a dose of allergen calculated to produce a 30 percent fall in FEV_1 after pretreatment with placebo or a single oral dose of 80 mg of GR 32191 [18]. The mean maximal fall in FEV_1 was 29 percent after GR 32191 pretreatment and 38 percent after placebo pretreatment. The overall attenuation of the acute asthmatic response, as assessed by the area under the FEV_1 time-course curve, was 25 percent.

The effects of flurbiprofen on the asthmatic response to isocapnic hyperventilation, hypertonic saline solution, and exercise have also been studied. Flurbiprofen, 100 mg administered 2 hours prior to challenge, increased the dose of hypertonic saline solution required to give a 25 percent fall in FEV_1 by approximately twofold [81]. However, flurbiprofen had no effect on the airway response to a single dose of hypertonic saline solution. By contrast, pretreatment of the same individuals with the H_1 antagonist terfenadine attenuated the dose-response curve to hypertonic saline solution by more than sevenfold, and attenuated the response to a single dose of hypertonic saline solution by 70 percent.

Administration of 50 mg of indomethacin twice daily for 3 days had no effect on exercise-induced asthma [178]. In a separate study 150 mg of flurbiprofen was administered 2 hours prior to exercise challenge [79]. The mean maximal fall in FEV_1 after exercise was attenuated from 39 percent on the control day to 27 percent after flurbiprofen treatment. This was comparable to the effect of 180 mg of terfenadine, and the effect of the two drugs was not additive. As assessed by changes in the area under the FEV_1 time-course curve, flurbiprofen attenuated the asthmatic response to exercise by 42 percent. By contrast, 120 mg of GR 32191 administered 1 hour before exercise had no significant effect on the airway response to exercise [80]. The maximal percent fall in FEV_1 was 30 percent after placebo and 32 percent after GR 32191 administration. The lack of effect of a TP receptor antagonist on exercise-induced asthma contrasts with both the small but significant effect of flurbiprofen on exercise-induced asthma and the effect of GR 32191 on allergen-induced asthma. It has been suggested that a part of the mechanism of exercise-induced asthma may be vascular in nature. Any contribution of PGI_2 to this would be modified by flurbiprofen, but not by antagonism at the TP receptor.

Refractory Period

A proportion of subjects with exercise-induced asthma demonstrate a refractory period following an initial exercise task, during which an identical exercise task will evoke significantly less bronchoconstriction [72]. A similar phenomenon is described after asthma provoked by hypertonic saline solution [23] and ultrasonically nebulized distilled water [165]. The mechanism of the refractory period is unknown, but is not related to mediator depletion or to release of protective catecholamines [21, 22]. The observation that the refractory period to exercise [178], hypertonic saline solution [182], and distilled water [164] is abolished by pretreatment with indomethacin suggests that protective prostanoids may be an important contributory factor in the mechanism of refractoriness.

Airway Hyperresponsiveness

As described above, there is evidence that prostaglandins may contribute to the airway hyperresponsiveness that is characteristic of asthma. This suggestion is supported by the observation that airway hyperresponsiveness in asthma may be affected by both inhibition of cyclooxygenase and inhibition of thromboxane synthetase. Walters investigated the effect of indomethacin on the airway responses to histamine, analyzing the response in terms of both the position (sensitivity) and the slope (reactivity) of the dose-response curve [255]. Following the administration

of indomethacin, 50 mg four times daily for 3 days, there was a significant decrease in the sensitivity of the airways of asthmatic subjects to histamine, although the slope of the dose-response curve was increased. The concentration of histamine required to elicit a 20 percent fall in FEV_1 increased from 0.4 mg/ml following placebo to 1.8 mg/ml following indomethacin treatment. These findings were confirmed in a study in which 50 mg of flurbiprofen given three times daily for 3 days led to a mean 3.3-fold decrease in the airway response to histamine [59]. Interestingly, in the same individuals there was no effect on the airway response to methacholine. These results are consistent with the observation that inhaled $PGF_{2\alpha}$ enhanced the airway response to histamine but not to methacholine in asthmatic subjects [110]. In contrast, Manning and coworkers [158] failed to find any effect of indomethacin on airway histamine responsiveness, although it did abolish histamine tachyphylaxis.

A possible role for thromboxane in airway hyperresponsiveness was suggested by studies of canine airways. In these studies the thromboxane synthesis inhibitor OKY-046 significantly attenuated the airway hyperresponsiveness induced by inhalation of ozone [4], PAF [46], LTB_4 [179], and allergen [45] in the dog, with no accompanying change in the associated influx into the airways of inflammatory cells.

Administration of the thromboxane synthetase inhibitor OKY-046, in a dose of 3 mg for 3 days, to a group of nonatopic asthmatic individuals led to a fourfold decrease in the airway response to acetylcholine [89]. A single inhaled dose of OKY-046 administered 10 minutes before challenge had no effect on the airway response to acetylcholine. In contrast, the TP receptor antagonist AA-2414, given as 40 mg daily for 4 days, led to a change in the dose of methacholine causing a 20 percent fall in FEV_1 from 0.43 mg/ml to 0.93 mg/ml [88]. A lower dose of 20 mg daily had no significant effect on airway responses to methacholine. While oral administration of OKY-046 for 4 days attenuated the airway responsiveness to methacholine in asthma, no effect was observed in normal subjects or in subjects with bronchitis and bronchiectasis [87].

As detailed in Chapter 4, the mechanism of airway hyperresponsiveness is likely to be multifactorial. Furthermore, the concept of nonspecific airway hyperresponsiveness may be misleading, since there are differences in the degree of hyperresponsiveness to various mediators, and the airway response to one agonist can be modulated without effecting changes in the response to others [59, 110, 180]. Thus, the heterogeneous mechanisms, differences in study design, and patient selection may explain some of the apparent discrepancies between different studies. However, in spite of these differences, the cumulative data support the hypothesis that prostanoids contribute to the airway hyperresponsiveness in asthma.

Cyclooxygenase inhibition has no effect on the sensitivity of the airways to histamine in nonasthmatic subjects [255], except when there is an increased airway sensitivity to histamine after viral upper respiratory tract infection [254].

In summary, it may be seen from Table 11-3 that pharmacologic studies have given somewhat conflicting results concerning the contribution of prostanoids in asthma. Nevertheless, the data suggest that prostanoids make little contribution to the acute bronchoconstrictor response to allergen, exercise, or osmotic stimuli. Prostanoids appear to play an important role in the mechanisms of refractoriness to hypertonic saline solution, exercise-induced asthma, and ultrasonically nebulized distilled water, and also of histamine tachyphylaxis. In addition, thromboxane may play a role in the induction or maintenance of airway hyperresponsiveness in asthma.

ASPIRIN-INDUCED ASTHMA

A proportion of subjects with asthma are intolerant of aspirin. In these subjects ingestion of aspirin is followed within 1 to 2 hours

Table 11-3. The effect of cyclooxygenase inhibitors, thromboxane synthetase inhibition, and TP receptor antagonists on the resting airway tone and airway responsiveness in normal and asthmatic individuals

Nonasthmatic subjects		
Resting airway tone	SGaw ↑ 10%	Indomethacin, 50 mg qds, 4 days [255]
	No effect	Indomethacin, 50 mg qds, 4 days [82]
Histamine challenge	PD_{20} FEV_1, no change; slope increased	Indomethacin, 50 mg qds, 4 days [255]
Allergen challenge in atopic nonasthmatic subjects	Increased sensitivity; PD_{20} FEV_1, ↓ 2.6-fold; PD_{35} SGaw, ↓ 2.3-fold	Indomethacin, 50 mg qds, 4 days [82]
Asthmatic subjects		
Resting airway tone	No effect	Indomethacin, 50 mg qds, 4 days [255]
		GR 32191, 120 mg, single dose [80]
		OKY-046, 3 mg, 4 days [89]
		Flurbiprofen, 150 mg, 3 days [59]
Histamine challenge	PC_{20} FEV_1, ↑ 4.5-fold	Indomethacin, 50 mg qds, 4 days [255]
	PC_{20} FEV_1, ↑ 3.3-fold	Flurbiprofen, 50 mg tds, 3 days [59]
	No effect	Indomethacin, 50 mg bd, 2 days [158]
Methacholine challenge	No effect	Flurbiprofen, 50 mg tds, 3 days [59]
		OKY-046 [87]
	PD_{20} FEV_1, ↑ 2.2-fold	AA-2414, 40 mg daily, 4 days [88]
Acetylcholine	PC_{20} FEV_1, ↑ 4-fold	OKY-046, 3 mg, 3 days [89]
	No effect	OKY-046, 30 mg, single inhaled dose [89]
Allergen challenge	PD_{20} FEV_1, no effect; PD_{35} SGaw, ↑ 1.5-fold	Indomethacin, 50 mg qds, 4 days [82]
	25% inhibition of EAR	GR 32191, 80 mg, single dose [18]
	Attenuation of LAR	Indomethacin, 25 mg qds, 4 days [215]
	Attenuation of LAR	Indomethacin, 25 mg, single dose [75]
	No effect on LAR; less hyperresponsiveness following LAR	Indomethacin, 50 mg bd, 2 days [126]
HS challenge	PD_{25} FEV_1, ↑ 2-fold, no effect on single dose of HS	Flurbiprofen, 100 mg, single dose [81]
EIA	31% inhibition	Flurbiprofen, 150 mg, single dose [79]
	No effect	Indomethacin, 50 mg bd, 3 days [178]
Refractoriness to EIA, HS, UNDW	Abolished	Indomethacin [164, 178, 182]

HS = hypertonic saline; EIA = exercise-induced asthma; UNDW = ultrasonically nebulized distilled water; EAR = early asthmatic response; LAR = late asthmatic response.

by the onset of bronchospasm that may be accompanied by rhinitis and/or urticaria [39, 166, 208] (see also Chap. 48). The majority of subjects with aspirin-induced asthma (AIA) may be desensitized to aspirin by the administration of incremental doses of aspirin orally [197, 231]. This may lead to an improvement in the severity of asthma [231] and rhinitis [230]. The mechanism of AIA may relate to inhibition of the cyclooxygenase. This has led to several hypotheses proposing a loss of protective prostaglandins or a shunting of arachidonate metabolism, leading to increased generation of leukotrienes in susceptible individuals. It is therefore appropriate to consider the role of eicosanoids in this type of asthma.

The role of cyclooxygenase inhibition in AIA is suggested by the observation that aspirin-sensitive subjects also react to other inhibitors of this enzyme [233, 234] and by the observation of cross-desensitization between these drugs [197]. Szczeklik and coauthors reported cross-reactivity between aspirin and other nonsteroidal antiinflammatory drugs (NSAIDs), which are known inhibitors of cyclooxygenase [233]. The potency of these drugs in causing asthma was related to their potencies as inhibitors of the cyclooxygenase enzyme. These observations were extended in a study of 123 patients with a history of allergic-type reactions to analgesics [234]. Eighty of these individuals had AIA, with threshold doses of aspirin between 20 and 300 mg. Of 38 subjects challenged with indomethacin, all developed asthma in response to doses from 2 to 30 mg. By comparison, only 3 of 49 patients responded adversely to acetaminophen (a weak inhibitor of cyclooxygenase) at doses between 150 and 600 mg. A correlation was observed between threshold doses of aspirin and of noramidopyrine, another cyclooxygenase inhibitor. No adverse reactions were observed in response to salicylamide, dextropropoxyphene, benzydamine, or chloroquine, analgesics that do not inhibit cyclooxygenase. Studies by workers at the Scripps Clinic, in addition to confirming the cross-reactivity between NSAIDs in subjects with AIA, demonstrated cross-desensitization [197]. They described three subjects with AIA who failed to respond to indomethacin after oral desensitization to aspirin. When these

patients stopped ingesting aspirin, asthma could be provoked by indomethacin. Following indomethacin challenge they were again refractory to aspirin. Cross-refractoriness to ibuprofen and naproxen was also demonstrated.

Thus, inhibition of cyclooxygenase appears to be central to the mechanism of AIA. The mechanism by which inhibition of cyclooxygenase leads to the occurrence of asthma, rhinitis, and/or urticaria is unclear. It has been suggested that individuals with AIA are overdependent on bronchodilator prostanoids [246, 251], though there are limited data to support this. Although prostacyclin protected against PGD_2-induced bronchoconstriction in asthmatic subjects [104], the intravenous infusion of PGI_2 failed to inhibit the development of AIA [177]. Airway responses to $PGF_{2\alpha}$, PGE_2, and histamine were compared in 27 subjects with AIA and 28 asthmatic subjects tolerant of aspirin [236]. There was a mean increase in peak expiratory flow rate (PEFR) of 13 percent immediately after inhalation of 60 μg of PGE_2 in subjects with AIA, compared with 5.5 percent in subjects without AIA. At 10 minutes after inhalation of PGE_2 the PEFR was on average 8 percent higher than at baseline in subjects with AIA, but the PEFR had returned to normal in control asthmatic subjects. Although these differences were statistically significant, the range of responses to PGE_2 was wide. There was considerable overlap in responses between subjects with and those without AIA, and the overall differences between groups were small. The same authors noted a diminished airway responsiveness to $PGF_{2\alpha}$ relative to histamine in aspirin-sensitive subjects [236]. A similar lack of responsiveness to $PGF_{2\alpha}$ relative to methacholine was noted by Thomson and colleagues in three subjects with AIA [244]. Orehek and associates, however, found no consistent difference in the bronchoconstrictor response to $PGF_{2\alpha}$ between asthmatic subjects with and those without AIA, although a comparison with airway responsiveness to histamine or methacholine was not made [183].

An alternative hypothesis for the pathogenesis of AIA is that inhibition of cyclooxygenase leads to a shunting of arachidonate metabolism with the increased generation of bronchoconstrictor leukotrienes. Ferreri and colleagues measured mediator release in the nasal lavage fluids of aspirin-sensitive asthmatic subjects after aspirin challenge [78]. Release of LTC_4 into nasal secretions was noted in four subjects in whom AIA was associated with nasoocular symptoms. In two subjects in whom the asthmatic response occurred without nasoocular symptoms there was no increase in LTC_4. Histamine release was also noted in three of four aspirin-sensitive subjects, but no increase in immunoreactive LTB_4 was detected. It is of note that PGE_2 levels in nasal washings remained unchanged during and following adverse reactions to aspirin. There were no changes in LTC_4 levels in nasal washings of subjects with AIA who had been desensitized, in aspirin-tolerant asthmatic subjects, and in normal controls following ingestion of 650 mg of aspirin. Nevertheless, in these same individuals, ingestion of 650 mg of aspirin led to a mean 75 percent decrease in PGE_2 levels. Thus, nasoocular reactions to aspirin in subjects with AIA were associated with increased generation of LTC_4 locally, and were unrelated to changes in levels of PGE_2. Ortolani and coworkers measured histamine, immunoreactive LTC_4, and SRS-A activity (by bioassay using guinea pig ileum) in nasal washings following intranasal challenge of aspirin-sensitive subjects with lysine aspirin [186]. Aspirin challenge was followed by significant increases in histamine, immunoreactive LTC_4, and bioactive SRS-A 60 minutes after challenge. No significant increases in histamine, LTC_4, or SRS-A were found in aspirin-tolerant subjects. The release of leukotrienes into the nasal airway following aspirin challenge in aspirin-sensitive subjects has subsequently been confirmed in a further study [195a].

Urinary LTE_4 was measured before and after aspirin challenge in six subjects with AIA [44] (Fig. 11-7). Following oral aspirin challenge there was a mean fourfold increase in urinary LTE_4, which was not observed following placebo challenge in the same subjects. There was no increase in urinary LTE_4 following methacholine challenge in aspirin-sensitive subjects or following either aspirin or placebo challenge in aspirin-tolerant asthmatic subjects. Raised urinary excretion of LTE_4 following aspirin-induced asthma has been confirmed in at least two subsequent reports

[127a, 131a]. An interesting observation was the increased urinary LTE_4 concentrations in subjects with AIA compared to aspirin-tolerant asthmatic subjects prior to challenge [44], a finding that has been confirmed by others [131a, 219a]. This is consistent with an upregulation of arachidonate metabolism in aspirin-sensitive subjects. Also supporting this suggestion is the finding that circulating levels of $PGF_{2\alpha}$ are raised in subjects with AIA [268] and in subjects with aspirin-induced urticaria [11]. Further work is needed to characterize the abnormalities of arachidonate release and metabolism in AIA.

An additional mechanism of AIA might be an increased sensitivity of the airways to leukotrienes released following aspirin challenge. Airway responses to LTE_4 and histamine were therefore compared between asthmatic subjects with and those without AIA [9]. Airway responses to histamine were comparable between the two groups of subjects. In contrast, the mean dose of LTE_4 causing a 35 percent fall in SGaw was 0.17 nmol in subjects with AIA, compared to 2.8 nmol in asthmatic subjects without AIA. Thus, LTE_4 was on average 145 times more potent than histamine in eliciting bronchoconstriction in aspirin-tolerant asthmatic subjects and 1,870-fold more potent than histamine in constricting the airways of aspirin-sensitive subjects. Following oral desensitization to aspirin there was a mean 20-fold decrease in the sensitivity of the airways to LTE_4 but not to histamine.

The possible role of leukotriene release in the pathogenesis of AIA was tested by the use of the $LTC_4/D_4/E_4$ receptor antagonist SK&F 104353 [43]. The prior inhalation of SK&F 104353 inhibited aspirin-induced bronchoconstriction in five of six aspirin-sensitive subjects.

In conclusion, inhibition of cyclooxygenase appears to be central to the mechanism of AIA. There is evidence that this is accompanied by release of leukotrienes. An increased sensitivity of the airways to leukotrienes, released at the time of adverse reactions to aspirin, may contribute to the mechanism of AIA. In addition, desensitization may result from a decrease in airway responsiveness to leukotrienes, combined with an attenuation of leukotriene release in response to aspirin. The role of leukotriene antagonists in the management of AIA requires further evaluation.

Fig. 11-7. *The relationship between the increase in urinary leukotriene E_4 (LTE_4) excretion and change in FEV_1 following aspirin-induced asthma.*

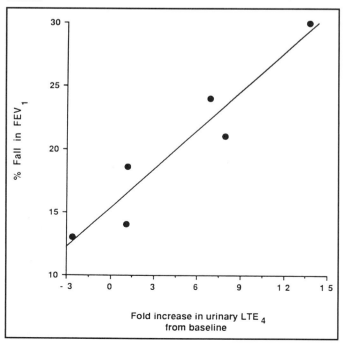

DIETARY FISH OIL IN BRONCHIAL ASTHMA

One approach to modulating the inflammatory response has been through the provision in the diet of fatty acid substrates alternative to arachidonic acid for metabolism to leukotrienes and prostanoids (see Fig. 11-1). Fatty acid nomenclature is confusing, using trivial names, chemical names, and shorthand notation of chemical structure, often interchangeably. Thus arachidonic acid is also termed *eicosatetraenoic acid* or $20:4$. $20:4$ gives the chain length (20 carbon atoms) and the number of C=C double bonds. Unsaturated fatty acids are further divided into three main classes according to the position of the first C=C double bond counting from the *methyl* end (or omega carbon) of the molecule. This describes the fatty acids as being omega or 'n' followed by the number of the carbon atom at which the first double bond occurs. The three classes of unsaturated fatty acids are the omega-9 (n-9) or oleic acid class, the omega-6 (n-6) or linoleic acid class, and the omega-3 (n-3) or alpha-linolenic acid class. Plants readily introduce double bonds between the methyl end of the fatty acid and carbon number 9, during desaturation and elongation of fatty acids. In animals, however, insertion of a double bond between the methyl end and carbon atom 9 does not occur, although further double bonds can be inserted beyond that carbon atom. Elongation and desaturation of linoleic acid ($18:2$, n-6) result in the formation of arachidonic acid ($20:4$, n-6) whereas alpha-linolenic acid ($18:3$, n-3) is converted to eicosapentaenoic acid ($20:5$, n-3; EPA) and docosahexaenoic acid ($22:6$, n-3;

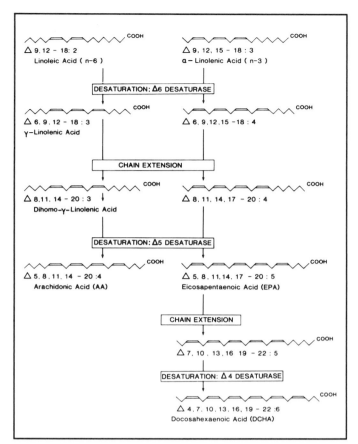

Fig. 11-8. *Desaturation and chain elongation of n-6 and n-3 fatty acids to form arachidonic acid, eicosapentaenoic acid, and docosahexaenoic acid. (Reprinted with permission from T. H. Lee and J. P. Arm. Prospects for modifying the allergic response by fish oil diets.* Clin. Allergy *16:89, 1986.)*

DCHA) (Fig. 11-8). Because animals are unable to desaturate C—C bonds between carbon atom 9 and the methyl end of fatty acids, n-3 fatty acids enter the food chain through marine phytoplankton, which are eaten by fish which readily convert alpha-linolenic to EPA and DCHA. Further, in most human tissues alpha-linolenic acid is a poor substrate, compared to linoleic acid, for chain extension and desaturation [245]. Therefore, the most efficient method of incorporating EPA and DCHA into human cell membrane phospholipids is through their provision in the diet.

In Vitro Actions and 5-Lipoxygenase Pathway Products of Fish Oil–Derived Fatty Acids

The two major types of polyunsaturated fatty acids prominent in marine fish oils, EPA (20:5, n-3) and DCHA (22:6, n-3), are incorporated into tissue phospholipids of mammals that consume a predominantly fish oil–enriched diet. EPA and DCHA competitively inhibit the conversion of arachidonic acid by the cyclooxygenase pathway to prostanoid metabolites [56, 175]. To the extent they are formed, the endoperoxides and TXA_3 derived from EPA are substantially less active than the arachidonic acid–derived counterparts in eliciting aggregation of human platelets [175]. DCHA is not metabolized to any cyclooxygenase product. With respect to the metabolism of EPA and DCHA by 5-LO, EPA is converted sequentially to LTB_5, LTC_5, LTD_5, and LTE_5. DCHA is metabolized only to the 7- and 4-hydroperoxy DCHA and their reduction products, 7- and 4-hydroxy DCHA, respectively. LTB_5 is substantially less active than LTB_4 in a number of proin-

flammatory functions [99, 140, 142, 243], but LTC_5 and LTC_4 are equiactive in constricting nonvascular smooth muscle [64, 144]. Thus EPA is capable of inhibiting the elaboration of inflammatory mediators by the cyclooxygenase pathway and is metabolized to LTB_5 with attenuated biologic activity.

The capacity of nonesterified EPA and DCHA to modulate the oxidative metabolism of membrane phospholipid-derived arachidonic acid by the 5-LO pathway in human neutrophils has been compared [141]. In these in vitro experiments, LTB_4 production was diminished throughout the EPA dose response, reaching 50 percent suppression at 10 μg/ml and 84 percent suppression at 40 μg/ml. DCHA did not alter the metabolism of membrane-derived arachidonic acid, did not inhibit LTB_4 generation, and was not a substrate for leukotriene formation. Thus, in contrast to DCHA, EPA attenuated the generation of LTB_4 [141, 200] and was converted to LTB_5.

Human leukocytes generate PAF-acether, a lipid mediator of inflammation, from membrane alkyl phospholipids through the release of arachidonic acid or other fatty acids from the 2-position and subsequent acetylation [24] (see Chap. 22). Whereas treatment of monocyte monolayers with an optimally effective concentration of arachidonic acid of 1 μg/ml resulted in a 64 percent increase of calcium ionophore–induced PAF-acether generation, treatment of monolayers with EPA at the optimal concentration of 1 μg/ml decreased PAF-acether generation by 28 percent [228]. Treatment of monocyte monolayers with DCHA did not appreciably affect PAF-acether generation.

In Vivo Incorporation of Fish Oil–derived Fatty Acids and Effects on the Generation of 5-Lipoxygenase Pathway Products and Leukocyte Function

The effects of dietary fish oil fatty acids on the 5-LO pathway activity of peripheral blood polymorphonuclear leukocytes and monocytes were studied in normal human subjects who supplemented their usual diets for 6 weeks with 3.2 gm of EPA and 2.2 gm of DCHA daily [138]. The diet increased the EPA content in polymorphonuclear neutrophils and monocytes more than sevenfold without changing the quantities of arachidonic acid and DCHA. When the neutrophils were activated in vitro with the ionophore A 23187, the release of arachidonic acid and its metabolites was reduced by a mean of 37 percent and the maximum generation of the major 5-LO metabolites, including LTB_4, was reduced by a mean of 48 percent. When monocyte monolayers were activated with the ionophore A 23187, the release of arachidonic acid and its metabolites was reduced by a mean of 39 percent and the generation of LTB_4 was suppressed by 58 percent. In addition, the generation of PAF-acether was inhibited by approximately 50 percent [228]. The adherence of neutrophils to endothelial cell monolayers that had been pretreated with LTB_4 was inhibited completely and their average chemotactic response to LTB_4 was inhibited by 70 percent, as compared with values determined before the diet was started. The leukocyte biochemical and functional suppression had recovered by 6 weeks after the diet was discontinued. Margination of leukocytes to endothelial surfaces is the initial step in the recruitment of cells by a chemotactic stimulus to an inflammatory focus. Thus, the impairment of leukocyte function caused by the dietary incorporation of fish oil fatty acids into membrane phospholipids would be expected to be antiinflammatory. This effect would be amplified by the substantial suppression of the biosynthesis of arachidonic acid–derived metabolites.

In Vivo Incorporation of Fish Oil–derived Fatty Acids and In Vivo Generation of 5-Lipoxygenase Pathway Products

In order to investigate the effects of a fish oil–enriched diet in acute anaphylaxis, pulmonary mechanical responses to intravenous allergen challenge were evaluated in two groups of mechanically ventilated and anesthetized guinea pigs [137]. The animals were pretreated with mepyramine to uncover the leukotriene and prostaglandin contributions. One group of animals was fed a fish oil diet (FFD) whereas the control group was fed a beef tallow diet (BFD). The FFD animals demonstrated incorporation of EPA and DCHA into the phospholipids of pulmonary tissue, with a ratio of EPA and DCHA to arachidonic acid of 2.5 as compared to that of BFD animals of 0.04. Intravenous allergen challenge in both groups of animals elicited a decrease in dynamic compliance (Cdyn) and pulmonary conductance (G_L). The decrease in Cdyn in the animals fed the FFD was significantly greater than that of the control animals at 1.5 to 5.0 minutes after allergen challenge. Since EPA and DCHA inhibit the cyclooxygenase pathway, these results are consistent with the view that the tissue levels of these fatty acids either partially inhibited the generation of bronchodilator prostaglandins released after allergen challenge and/or diverted EPA and arachidonic acid metabolism from the cyclooxygenase to the lipoxygenase pathway, resulting in the generation of greater quantities of bronchoconstrictor leukotrienes.

Support for the enhancement in 5-LO pathway activity in the presence of EPA comes from further studies in guinea pigs. The changes in arterial plasma concentrations of immunoreactive LTB were compared after allergen challenge of two groups of sensitized, mepyramine-treated, and mechanically ventilated guinea pigs, one group fed a diet enriched with fish oil and the other a control diet enriched with beef tallow [139]. The lung tissue of animals fed an FFD for 9 to 10 weeks incorporated EPA and DCHA to constitute 8 to 9 percent of total fatty acid content, whereas these alternative fatty acids constituted less than 1 percent of the total fatty acid content of the lung tissue of animals on a BFD. The combination of indomethacin and mepyramine markedly augmented the antigen-induced increase in arterial plasma immunoreactive LTB_4 concentrations in BFD animals, but had no effect on immunoreactive LTB levels in FFD animals. Limited in vivo measurements showed a smaller increase of plasma immunoreactive TXB_2 in the FFD compared to the BFD animals during anaphylaxis. Furthermore, ex vivo measurements showed a decreased LTB_4-stimulated (cyclooxygenase product–dependent) contractile response of pulmonary parenchymal strips from the FFD relative to the BFD animals, providing evidence for blockade of the cyclooxygenase pathway in the FFD animals. These findings in guinea pigs subjected to anaphylaxis provide further in vivo evidence of the augmented presence of 5-LO pathway products in the presence of cyclooxygenase pathway blockade.

Studies in Bronchial Asthma

In view of the likely role of airway inflammation in the pathogenesis of asthma, several investigators have evaluated the effects of fish oil–supplemented diets in bronchial asthma. In a study on the effects of dietary EPA in subjects with severe persistent asthma, two groups of six subjects received either 0.1 or 4.0 gm of purified EPA a day in a double-blind fashion for 8 weeks [127, 191]. Both doses of EPA led to a small but significant generation of LTB_5 by polymorphonuclear and mixed mononuclear leukocytes in response to the calcium ionophore A 23187. Only high-dose EPA suppressed ionophore-induced LTB_4 generation by leukocytes. High-dose EPA also suppressed neutrophil, but not mononuclear leukocyte chemotaxis to C5a, FMLP (N-formyl-L-methionyl-L-leucyl-L-phenylalanine), and LTB_4. Neither dose of EPA attenuated ionophore-induced PAF generation by mixed mononuclear cells. In addition, both low-dose and high-dose EPA led to an enhanced T-lymphocyte proliferative response to mitogen. Changes in leukocyte function were not accompanied by

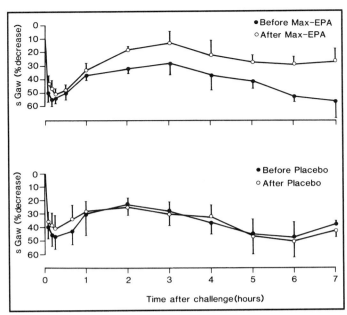

Fig. 11-9. *The time-dependent changes in specific airway conductance (s Gaw) expressed as percent fall from baseline values after allergen challenge in six subjects with late asthmatic responses before (closed circles) and after (open circles) treatment with Max-EPA (top panel) and in six subjects with late asthmatic responses before (closed circles) and after (open circles) treatment with placebo (bottom panel). See text. (Reprinted with permission from J. P. Arm, et al. The effects of dietary supplementation with fish oil lipids on the airways response to inhaled allergen in bronchial asthma. Am. Rev. Respir. Dis. 139:1395, 1989.)*

changes in severity of asthma, as assessed by history, clinical examination, or a panel of pulmonary function tests.

The effect of a fish oil–enriched diet in subjects with mild asthma has also been tested [5, 6]. Subjects received either 18 capsules a day of Max-EPA (3.2 gm of EPA and 2.2 gm of DCHA) or identical placebo capsules containing olive oil, in a double-blind fashion. EPA was incorporated into polymorphonuclear leukocyte phospholipids following dietary supplementation with fish oil. Polymorphonuclear leukocytes from these subjects demonstrated a 50 percent reduction in the generation of LTB (LTB_4 and LTB_5) in response to calcium ionophore, and a substantial attenuation of their chemotactic responses to FMLP and LTB_4. In subjects who had received placebo, the phospholipid content of EPA, LTB_4 generation, and chemotactic responses of polymorphonuclear leukocytes were unchanged. Following 10 weeks' dietary supplementation with fish oil there was a significant, approximately 35 percent attenuation of the late asthmatic response to inhaled antigen (Fig. 11-9). There were no changes in immediate cutaneous responses to antigen, total serum IgE, or airway responses to histamine in the same subjects, factors known to influence the development of the late asthmatic response [34, 58, 153, 205, 248]. There were also no changes in the immediate asthmatic response to antigen or exercise. Insofar as airway inflammation is believed to be central to the pathophysiology of the allergen-induced late asthmatic response, the attenuation of the late-phase reaction by fish oil is consistent with an antiinflammatory effect. Nevertheless, there were no changes in the severity of asthma in these individuals, as judged by diurnal peak flow measurements, symptoms, scores, and use of beta2 agonists.

The lack of any clinical benefit in subjects with either mild disease [5, 6] or severe persistent asthma [127, 191] from a fish oil–enriched diet may have been due to insufficient time for regeneration of airway epithelium and resolution of the chronic inflammatory changes in the airways to effect a change in clinical variables. Alternatively, leukocyte function and the late response may not have been altered sufficiently for a clinically significant effect to become apparent. It is also possible that the mechanisms of the late response may be irrelevant to the pathogenesis of clinical asthma.

Although there was no benefit derived from a fish oil–enriched diet on the natural history of bronchial asthma, EPA may modulate asthma in a minority of patients. Picado and associates [195] investigated the effects of a fish oil–enriched diet in subjects with AIA. Ten individuals with AIA received a control diet for 6 weeks followed by a diet containing approximately 3 gm of EPA daily for 6 weeks. There was no change in symptom scores, but there was a significant 15 to 18 percent reduction in PEFRs and an approximate 70 percent increase in bronchodilator use during the last 2 weeks of treatment with fish oil. These changes in clinical variables were accompanied by a significant 50 percent reduction in serum levels of immunoreactive TXB_2. The adverse effects of fish oil in subjects with AIA were attributed to inhibition of the cyclooxygenase.

In conclusion, a fish oil–enriched diet has potential in modulating the humoral and inflammatory components of the allergic response by inhibiting the generation of proinflammatory mediators derived from arachidonic acid and by reducing the production of PAF. In addition, EPA suppresses the responses of target cells and tissues. However, the modulating influence of alternative fatty acid substrates on arachidonic acid metabolism may not always be beneficial, as demonstrated in the animal model of antigen-induced acute anaphylaxis and the effects of fish oil in AIA. The reason for these discrepant clinical results may be related to the complex interactions between the metabolites of the cyclooxygenase and lipoxygenase pathways. Attenuation of a portion of one or both pathways would alter the relative quantities of end products and may have quite different effects depending on the type of pathobiologic mechanisms involved in the disease process.

Studies in bronchial asthma confirm the antiinflammatory potential of a fish oil–enriched diet. Dietary supplementation with EPA in subjects with asthma led to changes in leukocyte mediator generation and chemotactic responses, and a significant attenuation of the late asthmatic response to inhaled antigen. Thus the potential of a fish oil–enriched diet to modulate the inflammatory component of the allergic response is realized. However, no benefit of fish oil diets in day-to-day asthma has been demonstrated and such treatments cannot be recommended for bronchial asthma. Furthermore, fish oil supplements are contraindicated in subjects with AIA.

REFERENCES

1. Adelroth, E., et al. Airway responsiveness to leukotrienes C_4 and D_4 and to methacholine in patients with asthma and normal controls. *N. Engl. J. Med.* 315:480, 1986.
2. Aharony, D., Catanese, C. A., and Falcone, R. C. Kinetic and pharmacological analysis of [³H] leukotriene E_4 binding to receptors on guinea pig lung membranes: Evidence of selective binding to a subset of leukotriene D_4 receptors. *J. Pharmacol. Exp. Ther.* 248:581, 1989.
3. Aharony, D., Dobson, P. T., and Krell, R. D. *In vitro* metabolism of [³H]-peptide leukotrienes in human and ferret lung: A comparison with the guinea pig. *Biochem. Biophys. Res. Commun.* 131:892, 1985.
4. Aizawa, H., et al. Significance of thromboxane generation in ozone-induced airway hyperresponsiveness in dogs. *J. Appl. Physiol.* 59:1918, 1985.
5. Arm, J. P., et al. Effect of dietary supplementation with fish oil lipids on mild asthma. *Thorax* 43:84, 1988.
6. Arm, J. P., et al. The effecs of dietary supplementation with fish oil lipids on the airways response to inhaled allergen in bronchial asthma. *Am. Rev. Respir. Dis.* 139:1395, 1989.
7. O'Hickey, S. P., et al. Leukotrienes C_4, D_4, and E_4, enhance histamine responsiveness in asthmatic airways. *Am. Rev. Respir. Dis.* 144:1053, 1991.
8. Arm, J. P., et al. Asthmatic airways have a disproportionate hyperresponsiveness to LTE_4, as compared with normal airways, but not to LTC_4, LTD_4, methacholine, and histamine. *Am. Rev. Respir. Dis.* 142:1112, 1990.
9. Arm, J. P., et al. Airway responsiveness to histamine and leukotriene E_4 in subjects with aspirin-induced asthma. *Am. Rev. Respir. Dis.* 140:148, 1989.
10. Arm, J. P., Spur, B. W., and Lee, T. H. The effects of inhaled leukotriene E_4 on the airway responsiveness to histamine in subjects with asthma and normal subjects. *J. Allergy Clin. Immunol.* 82:654, 1988.
11. Asad, S. I., et al. Effect of aspirin in "aspirin sensitive" patients. *Br. Med. J.* 288:745, 1984.
12. Bach, M. K., et al. Identification of leukotriene C-1 as a major component of slow-reacting substance from rat mononuclear cells. *J. Immunol.* 125:115, 1980.
13. Bach, M. K., Brashler, J. R., and Morton, D. R. Solubilization and characterization of the leukotriene C_4 synthetase of rat basophilic leukaemia cells: A novel particulate glutathione-S-transferase. *Arch. Biochem. Biophys.* 230:455, 1984.
14. Barnes, N. C., Piper, P. J., and Costello, J. F. Actions of inhaled leukotrienes and their interactions with other allergic mediators. *Prostaglandins* 28:629, 1984.
15. Barnes, N. C., et al. Action of inhaled leukotriene C and D on large and small airways. Effect of pre-inhalation of leukotriene D on histamine dose-response curve. *Am. Rev. Respir. Dis.* 129:A1, 1984.
16. Beasley, C. R. W., et al. $9\alpha,11\beta$-Prostaglandin F_2: A novel metabolite of prostaglandin D_2 is a potent contractile agonist of human and guinea-pig airways. *J. Clin. Invest.* 79:978, 1987.
17. Beasley, R., et al. Cholinergic-mediated bronchoconstriction induced by prostaglandin D_2 and its initial metabolite $9\alpha,11\beta$-PGF_2 and $PGF_{2\alpha}$ in asthma. *Am. Rev. Respir. Dis.* 136:1140, 1987.
18. Beasley, R. C. W., et al. Effect of a thromboxane receptor antagonist on PGD_2- and allergen-induced bronchoconstriction. *J. Appl. Physiol.* 66:1685, 1989.
19. Bel, E. H., et al. The effect of inhaled budesonide on the maximal degree of airway narrowing to leukotriene D4 and methacholine in normal subjects in vivo. *Am. Rev. Respir. Dis.* 139:427, 1989.
20. Bel, E. H., et al. Maximal airway narrowing to inhaled leukotriene D4 in normal subjects. Comparison and interaction with methacholine. *Am. Rev. Respir. Dis.* 136:979, 1987.
21. Belcher, N. G., et al. Circulating concentrations of histamine, neutrophil chemotactic activity, and catecholamines during the refractory period in exercise-induced asthma. *J. Allergy Clin. Immunol.* 81:100, 1988.
22. Belcher, N. G., et al. A comparison of mediator and catecholamine release between exercise- and hypertonic saline-induced asthma. *Am. Rev. Respir. Dis.* 137:1026, 1988.
23. Belcher, N. G., et al. A comparison of the refractory periods induced by hypertonic airway challenge and exercise in bronchial asthma. *Am. Rev. Respir. Dis.* 135:822, 1987.
24. Benveniste, J., et al. Semi-synthese et strucure proposee du facteur activant les plaquettes (PAF): PAF-aceter, un alkyl ether analogue de la lysophosphatidylcholine. *CR Acad. Sci. Paris* 289D:1037, 1979.
25. Benyon, R. C., Lowman, M. A., and Church, M. K. Human skin mast cells: Their dispersion, purification, and secretory characterization. *J. Immunol.* 138:861, 1987.
26. Bianco, S., et al. Effects of Leukotriene C_4 on the Bronchial Response to an Ultrasonic Mist of Water. In H. Herzog and A. P. Perruchoud (eds.), *Progress in Respiratory Research*, Vol. 19: *Asthma and Bronchial Hyperreactivity*. Basel: Karger, 1985. Pp. 82–86.
27. Bisgaard, H., and Groth, S. Bronchial effects of leukotriene D_4 inhalation in normal human lung. *Clin. Sci.* 72:585, 1987.
28. Bisgaard, H., Groth, S., and Madsen, F. Bronchial hyperreactivity to leukotriene D_4 and histamine in exogenous asthma. *Br. Med. J.* 290:1468, 1985.
29. Borgeat, P., et al. Eosinophil-rich human polymorphonuclear leukocyte preparations characteristically release leukotriene C_4 on ionophore A23187 challenge. *J. Allergy Clin. Immunol.* 74:310, 1984.
30. Borgeat, P., and Samuelsson, B. Metabolism of arachidonic acid by polymorphonuclear leukocytes: Structural analysis of novel hydroxylated compounds. *J. Biol. Chem.* 254:7865, 1979.
31. Borgeat, P., and Samuelsson, B. Arachidonic acid metabolism in polymorphonuclear leukocytes: Unstable intermediate in the formation of dihydroxy acids. *Proc. Natl. Acad. Sci. USA* 76:3213, 1979.

32. Borgeat, P., and Samuelsson, B. Arachidonic acid metabolism in polymorphonuclear leukocytes: Effects of ionophore A23187. *Proc. Natl. Acad. Sci. USA* 76:2148, 1979.

33. Borgeat, P., and Samuelsson, B. Transformation of arachidonic acid by rabbit polymorphonuclear leukocytes. Formation of a novel dihydroxyeicosatetraenoic acid. *J. Biol. Chem.* 254:2643, 1979.

34. Boulet, L.-P., et al. Prediction of late asthmatic responses to inhaled allergen. *Clin. Allergy* 14:379, 1984.

35. Brink, C., et al. The interaction between indomethacin and contractile agents on human isolated airway muscle. *Br. J. Pharmacol.* 69:383, 1980.

36. Brocklehurst, W. E. Slow reacting substance and related compounds. *Prog. Allergy* 6:539, 1962.

37. Buckner, C. K., et al. Pharmacological evidence that human intralobar airways do not contain different receptors that mediate contractions to leukotriene C_4 and leukotriene D_4. *J. Pharmacol. Exp. Ther.* 237:558, 1986.

38. Camp, R. D. R., et al. Response of human skin to intradermal injection of leukotrienes C_4, D_4 and B_4. *Br. J. Pharmacol.* 80:497, 1983.

39. Chafee, F. H., and Settipane, G. A. Aspirin intolerance: 1. Frequency in an allergic population. *J. Allergy Clin. Immunol.* 53:193, 1974.

40. Cheng, J. B., and Townley, R. G. Evidence for a similar receptor site for binding of [^{3}H] leukotriene E_4 and [^{3}H] leukotriene D_4 to the guinea-pig crude lung membrane. *Biochem. Biophys. Res. Commun.* 122:949, 1984.

41. Cheng, J. B., and Townley, R. G. Identification of leukotriene D_4 receptor binding sites in guinea pig lung homogenates using [^{3}H] leukotriene D_4. *Biochem. Biophys. Res. Commun.* 118:20, 1984.

42. Christie, P. E., et al. The effect of indomethacin on LTE_4-induced histamine hyperresponsiveness in asthmatic patients. *Am. Rev. Respir. Dis.* In press.

43. Christie, P. E., Smith, C. M., and Lee, T. H. The potent and selective sulfidopeptide leukotriene antagonist, SK&F 104353, inhibits aspirin-induced asthma. *Am. Rev. Respir. Dis.* 144:957, 1991.

44. Christie, P. E., et al. Urinary leukotriene E_4 concentrations increase after aspirin challenge in aspirin-sensitive asthmatic subjects. *Am. Rev. Respir. Dis.* 143:1025, 1991.

45. Chung, K. F., et al. Inhibition of antigen-induced airway hyperresponsiveness by a thromboxane synthetase inhibitor (OKY-046) in allergic dogs. *Am. Rev. Respir. Dis.* 134:258, 1986.

46. Chung, K. F., et al. Airway hyperresponsiveness induced by platelet-activating factor: Role of thromboxane generation. *J. Pharmacol. Exp. Ther.* 236:580, 1986.

47. Claesson, H.-E., Lundberg, V., and Malmsten, C. Serum-coated zymosan stimulates the synthesis of leukotriene B_4 in human polymorphonuclear leukocytes. Inhibition by cyclic AMP. *Biochem. Biophys. Res. Commun.* 99:1230, 1981.

48. Cloud, M. L., et al. A specific LTD_4/LTE_4-receptor antagonist improves pulmonary function in patients with mild, chronic asthma. *Am. Rev. Respir. Dis.* 140:1336, 1989.

49. Coleman, R. A., et al. Further evidence that AH19437 is a specific thromboxane receptor blocking drug. *Br. J. Pharmacol.* 73:258, 1981.

50. Coleman, R. A., et al. Comparison of the actions of U-44619, a prostaglandin H_2-analogue, with those of prostaglandin H_2 and thromboxane A_2 on some isolated smooth muscle preparations. *Br. J. Pharmacol.* 73:773, 1981.

51. Coleman, R. A., et al. Prostanoid receptors—The development of a working classification. *Trends Pharmacol. Sci.* 5:303, 1984.

52. Coleman, R. A., Kennedy, I., and Sheldrick, R. L. G. New evidence with selective agonists and antagonists for the subclassification of PGE_2-sensitive (EP) receptors. *Adv. Prostaglandin Thromboxane Leukot. Res.* 17:467, 1987.

53. Coleman, R. A., and Sheldrick, R. L. G. Prostanoid-induced contraction of human bronchial smooth muscle is mediated by TP-receptors. *Br. J. Pharmacol.* 96:688, 1989.

54. Coles, S. J., et al. Effects of leukotrienes C_4 and D_4 on glycoprotein and lysozyme secretion by human bronchial mucosa. *Prostaglandins* 25:155, 1983.

55. Conroy, D. M., et al. Metabolism and generation of cysteinyl containing leukotrienes by human airways in vitro. *Br. J. Pharmacol.* 96:72P, 1989.

56. Corey, E. J., Shih, C., and Cashman, J. R. Docosahexaenoic acid is a strong inhibitor of prostaglandin but not leukotriene biosynthesis. *Proc. Natl. Acad. Sci. USA* 80:3581, 1983.

56a. Crea, A. E. G., Nakhosteen, J. A., and Lee, T. H. Mediator concentrations in bronchoalveolar lavage fluid of patients with mild asymptomatic bronchial asthma. *Eur. Respir. J.* 5:190, 1992.

57. Creese, R. R., and Bach, M. K. Hyperreactivity of airways smooth muscle

58. Crimi, E., et al. Predictive accuracy of late asthmatic reaction to *Dermatophagoides pteronyssinus*. *J. Allergy Clin. Immunol.* 78:908, 1986.

59. Curzen, N., Rafferty, P., and Holgate, S. T. Effects of a cyclooxygenase inhibitor, flurbiprofen, and an H_1 histamine receptor antagonist, terfenadine, alone and in combination on allergen induced immediate bronchoconstriction in man. *Thorax* 42:946, 1987.

60. Cuthbert, N. J., and Gardiner, P. J. Endogenous generation of cyclooxygenase products by human isolated lung tissue. *Br. J. Pharmacol.* 80:496P, 1983.

61. Dahinden, C. A., et al. Leukotriene C_4 production by murine mastocytoma cells: Evidence for a role for extracellular leukotriene A_4. *Proc. Natl. Acad. Sci. USA* 82:6632, 1985.

62. Dahlen, S.-E., et al. Leukotrienes promote plasma leakage and leukocyte adhesion in postcapillary venules: In vivo effects with relevance to the acute inflammatory response. *Proc. Natl. Acad. Sci. USA* 78:3887, 1981.

63. Dahlen, S.-E., et al. Leukotrienes are potent constrictors of human bronchi. *Nature* 288:484, 1980.

64. Dahlen, S.-E., Hedqvist, P., and Hammarström, S. Contractile activities of several cysteine-containing leukotrienes in the guinea pig lung strip. *Eur. J. Pharmacol.* 86:207, 1982.

65. Davidson, A. B., et al. Bronchoconstrictor effects of leukotriene E_4 in normal and asthmatic subjects. *Am. Rev. Respir. Dis.* 135:333, 1987.

66. Davis, C., et al. Control of human airway smooth muscle: In vitro studies. *J. Appl. Physiol.* 53:1080, 1982.

67. Dixon, R. A. F., et al. Requirement of a 5-lipoxygenase-activating protein for leukotriene synthesis. *Nature* 343:282, 1990.

68. Dong, Y. J., Jones, R. L., and Wilson, N. H. Prostaglandin E receptor subtypes in smooth muscle: Agonist activities of stable prostacyclin analogues. *Br. J. Pharmacol.* 87:97, 1986.

69. Drazen, J. M., et al. Comparative airway and vascular activities of leukotrienes C-1 and D in vivo and in vitro. *Proc. Natl. Acad. Sci. USA* 77:4354, 1980.

70. Drazen, J. M., et al. Pulmonary Pharmacology of the SRS-A Leukotrienes. In F. Berti, G. Folco, and G. P. Velo (eds.), *Leukotrienes and Prostacyclin*. New York: Plenum, 1983. Pp. 125–134.

70a. Drazen, J. M., et al. Recovery of leukotriene E_4 from the urine of patients with airway obstruction. *Am. Rev. Respir. Dis.* 146:104, 1992.

71. Edenius, C., Heidvall, K., and Lindgren, J. A. Novel transcellular interaction: Conversion of granulocyte-derived leukotriene A_4 to cysteinyl-containing leukotrienes by human platelets. *Eur. J. Biochem.* 178:81, 1988.

72. Edmunds, A. T., Tooley, M., and Godfrey, S. The refractory period after exercise-induced asthma: Its duration and relation to severity of exercise. *Am. Rev. Respir. Dis.* 117:247, 1978.

73. Eiser, N. M., Hayhurst, M., and Denman, W. The contribution of histamine and leukotriene release to the production of early and late asthmatic responses to antigen. *Am. Rev. Respir. Dis.* 139:A462, 1989.

74. Evans, J. M., et al. Effects of inhaled leukotriene antagonist, SK&F 104353-Z_2, on LTD_4 and histamine induced bronchoconstriction in normal man. *Br. J. Clin. Pharmacol.* 26:667P, 1988.

75. Fairfax, A. J., Hanson, J. M., and Morley, J. The late reaction following bronchial provocation with house dust mite allergen. Dependence on arachidonic acid metabolism. *Clin. Exp. Immunol.* 52:393, 1983.

76. Feinmark, S. J., and Cannon, P. J. Endothelial cell leukotriene C_4 synthesis results from intercellular transfer of leukotriene A_4 synthesized by polymorphonuclear leukocytes. *J. Biol. Chem.* 261:16466, 1986.

77. Fels, A. O., et al. Human alveolar macrophages produce leukotriene B_4. *Proc. Natl. Acad. Sci. USA* 79:7866, 1982.

78. Ferreri, N. R., et al. Release of leukotrienes, prostaglandins, and histamine into nasal secretions of aspirin-sensitive asthmatics during reaction to aspirin. *Am. Rev. Respir. Dis.* 137:847, 1988.

78a. Findlay, S. R., et al. Effect of the oral leukotriene antagonist, ICI 204,219, on antigen-induced bronchoconstriction in subjects with asthma. *J. Allergy Clin. Immunol.* 89:1040, 1992.

79. Finnerty, J. P., and Holgate, S. T. Evidence for the roles of histamine and prostaglandins as mediators in exercise-induced asthma: The inhibitory effect of terfenadine and flurbiprofen alone and in combination. *Eur. Respir. J.* 3:540, 1990.

80. Finnerty, J. P., et al. Effect of GR32191, a potent thromboxane receptor antagonist, on exercise induced bronchoconstriction in asthma. *Thorax* 46:190, 1991.

81. Finnerty, J. P., Wilmot, C., and Holgate, S. T. Inhibition of hypertonic saline-induced bronchoconstriction by terfenadine and flurbiprofen. *Am. Rev. Respir. Dis.* 140:593, 1989.

produced in vitro by leukotrienes. *Prostaglandins Leukot. Med.* 11:161, 1983.

81a. Finnerty, J. P., et al. Role of leukotrienes in exercise-induced asthma: Inhibitory effect of ICI 204219, a potent leukotriene D_4 receptor antagonist. *Am. Rev. Respir. Dis.* 145:746, 1992.

82. Fish, J. E., et al. Indomethacin modification of immediate-type immunologic airway responses in allergic asthmatic and non-asthmatic subjects. *Am. Rev. Respir. Dis.* 123:609, 1981.

83. Fish, J. E., et al. Novel effects of $PGF_{2\alpha}$ on airway function in asthmatic subjects. *J. Appl. Physiol.* 54:105, 1983.

84. Fleisch, J. H., et al. LY171883, 1-[2-hydroxy-3-propyl-4[4-(1H-tetrazol-5-yl) butoxy]phenyl]ethanone, an orally active leukotriene D_4 antagonist. *J. Pharmacol. Exp. Ther.* 233:148, 1985.

85. Ford-Hutchinson, A. W. Regulation of the production and action of leukotrienes by MK-571 and MK-886. *Adv. Prostaglandin Thromboxane Leukot. Res.* 21:9, 1990.

86. Ford-Hutchinson, A. W., et al. Leukotriene B, a potent chemokinetic and aggregating substance released from polymorphonuclear leukocytes. *Nature* 286:264, 1980.

87. Fujimura, M., Sakamoto, S., and Matsuda, T. Attenuating effect of a thromboxane synthetase inhibitor (OKY-046) on bronchial responsiveness to methacholine is specific to bronchial asthma. *Chest* 98:656, 1990.

88. Fujimura, M., et al. Effect of a thromboxane A_2 receptor antagonist on bronchial hyperresponsiveness to methacholine in subjects with asthma. *J. Allergy Clin. Immunol.* 87:23, 1991.

89. Fujimura, M., et al. Effects of a thromboxane synthetase inhibitor (OKY-046) and a lipoxygenase inhibitor (AA-861) on bronchial responsiveness to acetylcholine in asthmatic subjects. *Thorax* 41:955, 1986.

90. Fuller, R. W., Black, P. N., and Dollery, C. T. Effect of the oral leukotriene D_4 antagonist LY171883 on inhaled and intradermal challenge with allergen and leukotriene D_4 in atopic subjects. *J. Allergy Clin. Immunol.* 83:939, 1989.

91. Fuller, R. W., et al. Prostaglandin D_2 potentiates airway responsiveness to histamine and methacholine. *Am. Rev. Respir. Dis.* 133:252, 1986.

92. Gaddy, J., et al. The effects of a leukotriene D_4 (LTD_4) antagonist (MK-571) in mild to moderate asthma (abstract). *J. Allergy Clin. Immunol.* 85:197, 1990.

93. Gaddy, J., et al. A potent leukotriene D_4 antagonist (MK-571) significantly reduces airway obstruction in mild to moderate asthma (abstract). *J. Allergy Clin. Immunol.* 87:306, 1991.

94. Gardiner, P. J. Classification of prostanoid receptors. *Adv. Prostaglandin Thromboxane Leukot. Res.* 20:110, 1990.

95. Gardiner, P. J., and Collier, H. O. J. Specific receptors for prostaglandins in airways. *Prostaglandins* 19:819, 1980.

96. Gillard, J. et al. L-663,536 (MK-886) (3-[1-(4-chlorobenzyl)-3-t-butyl-thio-5-isopropylindol-2-yl]-2,2-dimethylpropanoic acid), a novel, orally active leukotriene biosynthesis inhibitor. *Can. J. Physiol. Pharmacol.* 67:456, 1989.

97. Goetzl, E. J., Weller, P. F., and Valone, F. H. Biochemical and Functional Bases of the Regulatory and Protective Roles of the Human Eosinophil. In G. Weissman, B. Samuelsson, and R. Paoletti (eds.), *Advances in Inflammation Research,* Vol. 1. New York: Raven, 1979. Pp. 157–167.

98. Goldman, D. W., and Goetzl, E. J. Specific binding of leukotriene B_4 to receptors on human polymorphonuclear leukocytes. *J. Immunol.* 129:1600, 1982.

99. Goldman, D. W., Pickett, W. C., and Goetzl, E. J. Human neutrophil chemotactic and degranulating activities of leukotriene B_5 (LTB_5) derived from eicosapentaenoic acid. *Biochem. Biophys. Res. Commun.* 117:282, 1983.

100. Griffin, M., et al. Effects of leukotriene D on the airways in asthma. *N. Engl. J. Med.* 308:436, 1983.

101. Halushka, P. V., et al. Thromboxane, prostaglandin and leukotriene receptors. *Annu. Rev. Pharmacol. Toxicol.* 10:213, 1989.

102. Hammarström, S., and Samuelsson, B. Detection of leukotriene A_4 as an intermediate in the biosynthesis of leukotrienes C_4 and D_4. *FEBS Lett.* 122:83, 1980.

103. Hardy, C. C., et al. The combined effects of two pairs of mediators, adenosine with methacholine and prostaglandin D_2 with histamine, on airway calibre in asthma. *Clin. Sci.* 71:385, 1986.

104. Hardy, C. C., et al. Bronchoconstrictor and antibronchoconstrictor properties of inhaled prostacyclin in asthma. *J. Appl. Physiol.* 64:1567, 1988.

105. Hardy, C. C., et al. Airway and cardiovascular responses to inhaled prostacyclin in normal and asthmatic subjects. *Am. Rev. Respir. Dis.* 131:18, 1985.

106. Hardy, C. C., et al. The bronchoconstrictor effect of inhaled prostaglandin D_2 in normal and asthmatic men. *N. Engl. J. Med.* 311:209, 1984.

107. Hay, D. W. P., et al. Pharmacological profile of SK&F 104353: A novel, potent and selective peptidoleukotriene receptor antagonist in guinea-pig and human airways. *J. Pharmacol. Exp. Ther.* 243:474, 1987.

108. Hay, D. W. P., et al. Functional antagonism by salbutamol suggests differences in the relative efficacies and dissociation constants of the peptidoleukotrienes in guinea pig trachea. *J. Pharmacol. Exp. Ther.* 244:71, 1988.

109. Haye-Legrand, I., et al. Histamine contraction of isolated human airway muscle preparations: Role of prostaglandins. *J. Pharmacol. Exp. Ther.* 239:536, 1986.

110. Heaton, R. W., et al. The influence of pretreatment with prostaglandin $F_{2\alpha}$ on bronchial sensitivity to inhaled histamine and methacholine in normal subjects. *Br. J. Dis. Chest* 78:168, 1984.

111. Holgate, S. T., Beasley, C. R. W., and Twentyman, O. P. The pathogenesis and significance of bronchial hyperresponsiveness in airways disease. *Clin. Sci.* 73:561, 1987.

112. Holgate, S. T., et al. Anaphylactic- and calcium-dependent generation of prostaglandin D_2 (PGD_2), thromboxane B_2 and other cyclooxygenase products of arachidonic acid by dispersed human lung mast cells and relationship to histamine release. *J. Immunol.* 133:2138, 1984.

113. Holroyde, M. C., et al. Bronchoconstriction produced in man by leukotrienes C and D. *Lancet* 2:17, 1981.

114. Hoover, R. L., et al. Leukotriene B_4 action of endothelium mediates augmented neutrophil/endothelial adhesion. *Proc. Natl. Acad. Sci. USA* 81:2191, 1984.

115. Horton, E. W., and Poyser, N. L. Uterine leuteolytic hormone: A physiological role for prostaglandin $F_{2\alpha}$. *Physiol. Rev.* 56:595, 1976.

116. Hui, K. P., et al. Effect of a 5-lipoxygenase inhibitor on leukotriene generation and airway responses after allergen challenge in asthmatic patients. *Thorax* 46:184, 1991.

117. Israel, E., et al. The effects of a 5-lipoxygenase inhibitor on asthma induced by cold, dry air. *N. Engl. J. Med.* 323:1740, 1990.

117a. Israel, E., et al. A double-blind multicenter study of Zileuton, a potent 5-lipoxygenase (5-LO) inhibitor versus placebo in the treatment of spontaneous asthma in adults (abstract). *J. Allergy Clin. Immunol.* 89:236, 1992.

118. Israel, E., et al. Effect of a leukotriene antagonist, LY171883, on cold air-induced bronchoconstriction in asthmatics. *Am. Rev. Respir. Dis.* 140:1348, 1989.

119. Jacques, C. A. J., et al. The mechanism of LTE_4-induced histamine hyperresponsiveness in guinea pig tracheal and human bronchial smooth muscle, in vitro. *Br. J. Pharmacol.* 104:859, 1991.

119a. Jones, G. L., et al. Effect of an inhaled thromboxane mimetic (U46619) on airway function in human subjects. *Am. Rev. Respir. Dis.* 145:1270, 1992.

120. Jongejan, R., et al. Effects of inflammatory mediators on the responsiveness of isolated human airways to methacholine. *Am. Rev. Respir. Dis.* 142:1129, 1990.

121. Joos, G. F., et al. The effect of aerosolized SK&F 104353-Z_2 on the bronchoconstrictor effect of leukotriene D_4 in asthmatics. *Pulmonary Pharmacol.* 4:37, 1991.

122. Kaye, M. G., and Smith, L. J. Effects of inhaled leukotriene D_4 and platelet-activating factor on airway reactivity in normal subjects. *Am. Rev. Respir. Dis.* 141:993, 1990.

123. Kern, R., et al. Characterization of the airway response to inhaled leukotriene D_4 in normal subjects. *Am. Rev. Respir. Dis.* 133:1127, 1986.

124. Kikawa, Y., et al. Urinary leukotriene E_4 after exercise challenge in children with asthma. *J. Allergy Clin. Immunol.* 89:1111, 1992.

125. Kips, J. C., et al. MK-571, a potent antagonist of leukotriene D_4-induced bronchoconstriction in the human. *Am. Rev. Respir. Dis.* 144:617, 1991.

126. Kirby, J. G., et al. Effect of indomethacin on allergen-induced asthmatic responses. *J. Appl. Physiol.* 66:578, 1989.

127. Kirsch, C. M., et al. Effect of eicosapentaenoic acid in asthma. *Clin. Allergy* 18:177, 1988.

127a. Knapp, H. R., Sladek, K., and Fitzgerald, G. A. Increased excretion of leukotriene E_4 during aspirin-induced asthma. *J. Lab. Clin. Med.* 119:48, 1992.

128. Krell, R. D., et al. The preclinical pharmacology of ICI 204,219. *Am. Rev. Respir. Dis.* 141:978, 1990.

129. Krell, R. D. et al. In vivo pharmacology of ICI 198,615: A novel, potent and selective peptide leukotriene antagonist. *J. Pharmacol. Exp. Ther.* 243:557, 1987.

130. Krell, R. D., et al. Heterogeneity of leukotriene receptors in guinea pig trachea. *Prostaglandins* 25:171, 1983.

131. Krilis, S., et al. Bioconversion of C-6 sulfidopeptide leukotrienes by the responding guinea pig ileum determines the time course of its contraction. *J. Clin. Invest.* 71:909, 1983.

131a. Kumlin, M., et al. Urinary excretion of leukotriene E₄ and 11-dehydro-thromboxane B₂ in response to bronchial provocations with allergen, aspirin, leukotriene D₄ and histamine in asthmatics. *Am. Rev. Respir. Dis.* 146:96, 1992.

132. Lam, B. K., et al. The mechanism of leukotriene B₄ export from human polymorphonuclear leukocytes. *J. Biol. Chem.* 265:13438, 1990.

133. Lam, B. K., et al. The identification of a distinct export step following the biosynthesis of leukotriene C₄ by human eosinophils. *J. Biol. Chem.* 264:12885, 1989.

134. Lam, S., et al. Release of leukotrienes in patients with bronchial asthma. *J. Allergy Clin. Immunol.* 81:711, 1988.

135. Lee, C. W., et al. The myeloperoxidase-dependent metabolism of leukotrienes C₄, D₄ and E₄ to 6-*trans*-leukotriene B₄ diastereoisomers and the subclass specific S-diastereoisomeric sulfoxides. *J. Biol. Chem.* 258:15004, 1983.

136. Lee, T. H., et al. Leukotriene E₄-induced airway hyperresponsiveness of guinea pig tracheal smooth muscle to histamine and evidence for three separate sulfidopeptide leukotriene receptors. *Proc. Natl. Acad. Sci. USA* 81:4922, 1984.

137. Lee, T. H., et al. The effects of a fish-oil enriched diet on pulmonary mechanics during anaphylaxis. *Am. Rev. Respir. Dis.* 132:1204, 1985.

138. Lee, T. H., et al. Effect of dietary enrichment with eicosapentaenoic and docosahexaenoic acid on in vitro neutrophil and monocyte leukotriene generation and neutrophil function. *N. Engl. J. Med.* 312:1217, 1985.

139. Lee, T. H., et al. Enhancement of plasma levels of biologically active leukotriene B compounds during anaphylaxis in guinea pigs pretreated by indomethacin or by a fish oil-enriched diet. *J. Immunol.* 136:2575, 1986.

140. Lee, T. H., et al. Characterization and biological properties of 5,12-dihydroxy derivatives of eicosapentaenoic acid including leukotriene B₅ and the double lipoxygenase product. *J. Biol. Chem.* 259:2383, 1984.

141. Lee, T. H., et al. Effects of exogenous arachidonic, eicosapentaenoic, and docosahexaenoic acids on the generation of 5-lipoxygenase pathway products by ionophore-activated human neutrophils. *J. Clin. Invest.* 74:1922, 1984.

142. Lee, T. H., et al. Characterization of leukotriene B₃: Comparison of its biological activities with leukotriene B₄ and leukotriene B₅ in complement receptor enhancement, lysozyme release and chemotaxis of human neutrophils. *Clin. Sci.* 74:467, 1988.

143. Lee, T. H., et al. Slow reacting substance of anaphylaxis antagonist FPL 55712 in chronic asthma. *Lancet* 2:304, 1981.

144. Leitch, A. G., et al. Immunologically induced generation of tetraene and pentaene leukotrienes in the peritoneal cavities of menhaden-fed rats. *J. Immunol.* 132:2559, 1984.

145. Leung, K. B. P., et al. Mast cells and basophils. Some further properties of human pulmonary mast cells recovered by bronchoalveolar lavage and enzymic dispersion of lung tissue. *Agents Actions* 20:213, 1987.

146. Lewis, M. A., et al. Identification and characterization of leukotriene D₄ receptors in adult and fetal human lung. *Biochem. Pharmacol.* 34:4311, 1985.

147. Lewis, R. A., et al. Slow reacting substance of anaphylaxis: Identification of leukotriene C-1 and D from human and rat sources. *Proc. Natl. Acad. Sci. USA* 77:3710, 1980.

148. Lewis, R. A., et al. Identification of the C(6)-S-conjugate of leukotriene A with cysteine as a naturally occurring slow reacting substance of anaphylaxis (SRS-A). Importance of the 11-cis-geometry for biological activity. *Biochem. Biophys. Res. Commun.* 96:271, 1980.

149. Lewis, R. A., et al. Prostaglandin D₂ generation after activation of rat and human mast cells with anti-IgE. *J. Immunol.* 129:1627, 1982.

150. Lin, A. H., Ruppel, P. L., and Gorman, R. R. Leukotriene B₄ binding to human neutrophils. *Prostaglandins* 28:837, 1984.

151. Liu, M. C., et al. Evidence for elevated levels of histamine, prostaglandin D₂, and other bronchoconstricting prostaglandins in the airways of subjects with mild asthma. *Am. Rev. Respir. Dis.* 142:126, 1990.

152. MacGlashan, D. W., et al. Generation of leukotrienes by purified human lung mast cells. *J. Clin. Invest.* 70:747, 1982.

153. MacIntyre, D., and Boyd, G. Factors influencing the occurrence of a late reaction to allergen in atopic asthmatics. *Clin. Allergy* 14:311, 1984.

154. Maclouf, J. A., and Murphy, R. C. Transcellular metabolism of neutrophil-derived leukotriene A₄ by human platelets. *J. Biol. Chem.* 263:174, 1988.

155. Mahauthaman, R., et al. The generation and cellular distribution of leukotriene C₄ in human eosinophils stimulated by unopsonized zymosan and glucan particles. *J. Allergy Clin. Immunol.* 81:696, 1988.

156. Malmsten, C. Some biological effects of prostaglandin endoperoxide analogues. *Life Sci.* 18:169, 1976.

157. Maltby, N. H., et al. Leukotriene C₄ elimination and metabolism in man. *J. Allergy Clin. Immunol.* 85:3, 1990.

158. Manning, P. J., Jones, G. L., and O'Byrne, P. M. Tachyphylaxis to inhaled histamine in asthmatic subjects. *J. Appl. Physiol.* 63:1572, 1987.

159. Manning, P. J., et al. Urinary leukotriene E₄ levels during early and late asthmatic responses. *J. Allergy Clin. Immunol.* 86:211, 1990.

160. Manning, P. J., et al. Inhibition of exercise-induced bronchoconstriction by MK-571, a potent leukotriene D₄ antagonist. *N. Engl. J. Med.* 323:1736, 1990.

161. Marom, Z., et al. Slow-reacting substances, leukotrienes C₄ and D₄, increase the release of mucus from human airways in vitro. *Am. Rev. Respir. Dis.* 126:449, 1982.

162. Martin, T. R., et al. Leukotriene B₄ production by the human alveolar macrophage: A potential mechanism for amplifying inflammation in the lung. *Am. Rev. Respir. Dis.* 129:106, 1984.

163. Mathé, A. A., and Hedqvist, P. Effects of prostaglandins F₂α and E₂ on airway conductance in healthy subjects and asthmatic patients. *Am. Rev. Respir. Dis.* 111:313, 1975.

164. Mattoli, S., et al. The effect of indomethacin on the refractory period occurring after the inhalation of ultrasonically nebulized distilled water. *J. Allergy Clin. Immunol.* 79:678, 1987.

165. Mattoli, S., et al. Refractory period to ultrasonic mist of distilled water: Relationship to methacholine responsiveness, atopic status, and clinical characteristics. *Ann. Allergy* 58:134, 1987.

166. McDonald, J. R., Mathison, D. A., and Stevenson, D. D. Aspirin intolerance in asthma: Detection by oral challenge. *J. Allergy Clin. Immunol.* 50:198, 1972.

167. McGee, J. E., and Fitzpatrick, F. A. Erythrocyte-neutrophil interactions: Formation of leukotriene B₄ by transcellular biosynthesis. *Proc. Natl. Acad. Sci. USA* 83:1349, 1986.

168. Mendeles, L., et al. Leukotriene D₄ is an important mediator of antigen-induced bronchoconstriction: Attenuation of dual response with MK-571, a specific LTD₄ receptor antagonist (abstract). *J. Allergy Clin. Immunol.* 85:197, 1990.

169. Miller, D. K., et al. Identification and isolation of a membrane protein necessary for leukotriene production. *Nature* 343:278, 1990.

170. Mong, S., et al. Leukotriene E₄ binds specifically to LTD₄ receptors in guinea pig lung membranes. *Eur. J. Pharmacol.* 109:183, 1985.

171. Morris, H. R., et al. Structure of slow reacting substance of anaphylaxis from guinea-pig lung. *Nature* 285:104, 1980.

172. Murphy, R. C., Hammarström, S., and Samuelsson, B. Leukotriene C: A slow reacting substance from murine mastocytoma cells. *Proc. Natl. Acad. Sci. USA* 76:4275, 1979.

173. Murray, J. J., et al. Release of prostaglandin D₂ into human airways during acute antigen challenge. *N. Engl. J. Med.* 315:800, 1986.

174. Nagy, L., et al. Complement receptor enhancement and chemotaxis of human neutrophils and eosinophils by leukotrienes and other lipoxygenase products. *Clin. Exp. Immunol.* 47:541, 1982.

175. Needleman, P., et al. Triene prostaglandins: Prostacyclin and thromboxane biosynthesis and unique biological properties. *Proc. Natl. Acad. Sci. USA* 76:944, 1979.

176. Newball, H. H., and Lenfant, C. The influence of atropine and cromolyn on human bronchial hyperreactivity to aerosolized prostaglandin F₂α. *Respir. Physiol.* 30:125, 1977.

177. Nizankowska, E., Czerniawska-Mysik, G., and Szczeklik, A. Lack of effect of i.v. prostacyclin on aspirin-induced asthma. *Eur. J. Respir. Dis.* 69:363, 1986.

178. O'Byrne, P. M., and Jones, G. L. The effect of indomethacin on exercise-induced bronchoconstriction and refractoriness after exercise. *Am. Rev. Respir. Dis.* 134:69, 1986.

179. O'Byrne, P. M., et al. Leukotriene B₄ induces airway hyperresponsiveness in dogs. *J. Appl. Physiol.* 59:1941, 1985.

180. O'Hickey, S. P., et al. Airway responsiveness to methacholine after inhalation of nebulized hypertonic saline in bronchial asthma. *J. Allergy Clin. Immunol.* 83:472, 1989.

181. O'Hickey, S. P., et al. The relative responsiveness to inhaled leukotriene E₄, methacholine and histamine in normal and asthmatic subjects. *Eur. Respir. J.* 1:913, 1988.

182. Hawksworth, R. J., et al. The effects of indomethacin on the refractory period to hypertonic saline-induced bronchoconstriction. *Eur. Respir. J.* 5:963, 1992.

183. Orehek, J., et al. Bronchial response to inhaled prostaglandin F₂α in patients with common or aspirin-sensitive asthma. *J. Allergy Clin. Immunol.* 59:414, 1977.

184. Örning, L., Hammarström, S., and Samuelsson, B. Leukotriene D: A slow

reacting substance from rat basophilic leukaemia cells. *Proc. Natl. Acad. Sci. USA* 77:2014, 1980.

185. Örning, L., Kaijser, L., and Hammarström, S. In vivo metabolism of leukotriene C$_4$ in man. *Biochem. Biophys. Res. Commun.* 130:214, 1985.
186. Ortolani, C., et al. Study of mediators of anaphylaxis in nasal fluids after aspirin and sodium metabisulfite nasal provocation in intolerant rhinitic patients. *Ann. Allergy* 59:106, 1987.
187. Palmer, R. M. J., and Salmon, J. A. Release of leukotriene B$_4$ from human neutrophils and its relationship to degranulation induced by N-formyl-methionyl-leucyl-phenylalanine, serum-treated zymosan, and the ionophore A23187. *Immunology* 50:65, 1983.
188. Palmer, R. M. J., et al. Chemokinetic activity of arachidonic acid lipoxygenase products on leukocytes of different species. *Prostaglandins* 20:411, 1980.
189. Patel, K. R. Atropine, sodium cromoglycate and thymoxamine in PGF$_{2\alpha}$-induced bronchoconstriction in extrinsic asthma. *Br. Med. J.* 2:360, 1975.
190. Paterson, N. A. M., et al. Release of chemical mediators from partially purified human lung mast cells. *J. Immunol.* 117:1356, 1976.
191. Payan, D. G., et al. Alterations in human leukocyte function induced by ingestion of eicosapentaenoic acid. *J. Clin. Immunol.* 6:402, 1986.
192. Peters, S. P., et al. Arachidonic acid metabolism in purified human lung mast cells. *J. Immunol.* 132:1972, 1984.
193. Phillips, G. D., and Holgate, S. T. Interaction of inhaled LTC$_4$ with histamine and PGD$_2$ in airway caliber in asthma. *J. Appl. Physiol.* 66:304, 1989.
194. Phillips, G. D., et al. Dose-related antagonism of leukotriene D$_4$-induced bronchoconstriction by p.o. administration of LY-171883 in nonasthmatic subjects. *J. Pharmacol. Exp. Ther.* 246:732, 1988.
195. Picado, C., et al. Effects of a fish oil enriched diet on aspirin intolerant asthmatic patients: A pilot study. *Thorax* 43:93, 1988.
195a. Picado, C., et al. Release of peptide leukotriene into nasal secretions after local instillation of aspirin in aspirin-sensitive asthmatic patients. *Am. Rev. Respir. Dis.* 145:65, 1992.
196. Pichurko, B. M., et al. Localization of the site of the bronchoconstrictor effects of leukotriene C$_4$ compared with that of histamine in asthmatic subjects. *Am. Rev. Respir. Dis.* 140:334, 1989.
197. Pleskow, W. W., et al. Aspirin desensitization in aspirin-sensitive asthmatic patients: Clinical manifestations and characterization of the refractory period. *J. Allergy Clin. Immunol.* 69:11, 1982.
198. Pliss, L. B., et al. Assessment of bronchoalveolar cell and mediator response to isocapneic hyperpnea in asthma. *Am. Rev. Respir. Dis.* 142:73, 1990.
199. Pong, S.-S., and DeHaven, R. N. Characterization of a leukotriene D$_4$ receptor in guinea pig lung. *Proc. Natl. Acad. Sci. USA* 80:7415, 1983.
200. Prescott, S. M. The effect of eicosapentaenoic acid on leukotriene B production by human neutrophils. *J. Biol. Chem.* 259:7615, 1984.
201. Radmark, O., et al. Leukotriene A: Isolation from human polymorphonuclear leukocytes. *J. Biol. Chem.* 255:11828, 1980.
202. Roberts, J. A., et al. In vitro and in vivo effect of verapamil on human airway responsiveness to leukotriene D$_4$. *Thorax* 41:12, 1986.
203. Roberts, J. A., Rodger, I. W., and Thomson, N. C. Effect of verapamil and sodium cromoglycate on leukotriene D$_4$ induced bronchoconstriction in patients with asthma. *Thorax* 41:753, 1986.
204. Roberts, J. A., Rodger, I. W., and Thomson, N. C. In vivo and in vitro human airway responsiveness to leukotriene D$_4$ in patients without asthma. *J. Allergy Clin. Immunol.* 80:688, 1987.
205. Robertson, D. G., et al. Late asthmatic responses induced by ragweed pollen allergen. *J. Allergy Clin. Immunol.* 54:244, 1974.
206. Rouzer, C. A., et al. MK886, a potent and specific leukotriene biosynthesis inhibitor blocks and reverses the membrane association of 5-lipoxygenase in ionophore-challenged leukocytes. *J. Biol. Chem.* 265:1436, 1990.
207. Rouzer, C. A., et al. Characterization of cloned human leukocyte 5-lipoxygenase expressed in mammalian cells. *J. Biol. Chem.* 263:10135, 1988.
208. Samter, M., and Beers, R. F. Intolerance to aspirin: Clinical studies and consideration of its pathogenesis. *Ann. Intern. Med.* 68:975, 1968.
209. Samuelsson, B. Leukotrienes: Mediators of hypersensitivity reactions and inflammation. *Science* 220:568, 1983.
210. Samuelsson, B., et al. Prostaglandins and thromboxanes. *Annu. Rev. Biochem.* 47:997, 1978.
211. Schulman, E. S., et al. Anaphylactic release of thromboxane A$_2$, prostaglandin D$_2$, and prostacyclin from human lung parenchyma. *Am. Rev. Respir. Dis.* 124:402, 1981.
212. Shak, S., and Goldstein, I. M. Omega-oxidation is the major pathway for the catabolism of leukotriene B$_4$ in human polymorphonuclear leukocytes. *J. Biol. Chem.* 259:10181, 1984.

213. Shaw, R. J., Cromwell, O., and Kay, A. B. Preferential generation of leukotriene C$_4$ by human eosinophils. *Clin. Exp. Immunol.* 56:716, 1984.
214. Shaw, R. J., et al. Activated human eosinophils generate SRS-A leukotrienes following IgG-dependent stimulation. *Nature* 316:150, 1985.
215. Shephard, E. G., et al. Lung function and plasma levels of thromboxane B$_2$, 6-ketoprostaglandin F$_1$, and thromboglobulin in antigen-induced asthma before and after indomethacin pretreatment. *Br. J. Clin. Pharmacol.* 19:459, 1985.
216. Showell, H. J., et al. Characterization of the secretory activity of leukotriene B$_4$ toward rabbit neutrophils. *J. Immunol.* 128:811, 1982.
217. Sirois, P., et al. Correlation between the myotropic activity of leukotriene A$_4$ on guinea-pig lung, trachea and ileum and its biotransformation in situ. *Prostaglandins* 30:21, 1985.
218. Sirois, P., Roy, S., and Borgeat, P. The lung parenchymal strip as a sensitive assay for leukotriene B$_4$. *Prostaglandins* 6:153, 1981.
219. Smith, A. P., Cuthbert, M. F., and Dunlop, L. S. Effects of inhaled prostaglandins E$_1$, E$_2$ and F$_{2\alpha}$ on the airway resistance of healthy and asthmatic man. *Clin. Sci.* 48:421, 1975.
219a. Smith, C. M., et al. Urinary leukotriene E$_4$ in bronchial asthma. *Eur. Respir. J.* 5:693, 1992.
219b. Smith, C. M., et al. Urinary leukotriene E$_4$ levels after allergen and exercise challenge in bronchial asthma. *Am. Rev. Respir. Dis.* 144:1411, 1991.
220. Smith, L. J., et al. The effect of inhaled leukotriene D$_4$ in humans. *Am. Rev. Respir. Dis.* 131:368, 1985.
221. Smith, L. J., et al. Inhibition of leukotriene D$_4$-induced bronchoconstriction in normal subjects by the oral LTD$_4$ receptor antagonist ICI 204,219. *Am. Rev. Respir. Dis.* 141:988, 1990.
222. Smith, L. J., et al. Mechanism of leukotriene D$_4$-induced bronchoconstriction in normal subjects. *J. Allergy Clin. Immunol.* 80:338, 1987.
223. Snyder, D. W., et al. In vitro pharmacology of ICI 198,615: A novel, potent selective peptide leukotriene antagonist. *J. Pharmacol. Exp. Ther.* 243:548, 1987.
224. Snyder, D. W., and Krell, R. D. Pharmacological evidence for a distinct leukotriene C$_4$ receptor in guinea-pig trachea. *J. Pharmacol. Exp. Ther.* 231:616, 1984.
225. Soberman, R. J., et al. Identification and functional characterization of leukotriene B$_4$ 20-hydroxylase of human polymorphonuclear leukocytes. *Proc. Natl. Acad. Sci. USA* 82:2292, 1985.
226. Soberman, R. J., et al. The identification and formation of 20-aldehyde leukotriene B$_4$. *J. Biol. Chem.* 263:7996, 1988.
227. Soter, N. A., et al. Local effects of synthetic leukotrienes (LTC$_4$, LTD$_4$, LTE$_4$ and LTB$_4$) in human skin. *J. Invest. Dermatol.* 80:115, 1983.
228. Sperling, R. I., et al. The effects of N-3 polyunsaturated fatty acids on the generation of PAF-acether by human monocytes. *J. Immunol.* 139:4186, 1987.
229. Sterk, P. J., Timmers, M. C., and Dijkman, J. H. Maximal airway narrowing in humans in vivo: Histamine compared with methacholine. *Am. Rev. Respir. Dis.* 134:714, 1986.
230. Stevenson, D. D., et al. Aspirin-sensitive rhinosinusitis asthma: A double-blind crossover study of treatment with aspirin. *J. Allergy Clin. Immunol.* 73:500, 1984.
231. Stevenson, D. D., Simon, R. A., and Mathison, D. A. Aspirin-sensitive asthma: Tolerance to aspirin after positive oral challenge. *J. Allergy Clin. Immunol.* 66:82, 1980.
232. Sutyak, J., Austen, K. F., and Soberman, R. J. Identification of an aldehyde dehydrogenase in the microsomes of human polymorphonuclear leukocytes that metabolizes 20-aldehyde leukotriene B$_4$. *J. Biol. Chem.* 264:14818, 1989.
233. Szczeklik, A., Gryglewski, R. J., and Czerniawska-Mysik, G. Relationship of inhibition of prostaglandin biosynthesis by analgesics to asthma attacks in aspirin-sensitive patients. *Br. Med. J.* 1:67, 1975.
234. Szczeklik, A., Gryglewski, R. J., and Czerniawska-Mysik, G. Clinical patterns of hypersensitivity to nonsteroidal anti-inflammatory drugs and their pathogenesis. *J. Allergy Clin. Immunol.* 60:276, 1977.
235. Szczeklik, A., et al. Circulatory and anti-platelet effects of intravenous prostacyclin in healthy man. *Pharmacol. Res. Commun.* 10:545, 1978.
236. Szczeklik, A., Nizankowska, E., and Nizankowska, R. Bronchial reactivity to prostaglandins F$_{2\alpha}$, E$_2$, and histamine in different types of asthma. *Respiration* 34:323, 1977.
237. Tagari, P., et al. Measurement of urinary leukotrienes by reversed-phase liquid chromatography and radioimmunoassay. *Clin. Chem.* 35:388, 1989.
238. Talbot, S. F., et al. Accumulation of leukotriene C$_4$ and histamine in human allergic skin reactions. *J. Clin. Invest.* 76:650, 1985.
239. Taylor, G. W., et al. Urinary leukotriene E$_4$ after antigen challenge and in acute asthma and allergic rhinitis. *Lancet* 1:584, 1989.

240. Taylor, I. K., et al. Effect of cysteinyl-leukotriene receptor antagonist ICI 204.219 on allergen-induced bronchoconstriction and airway hyperreactivity in atopic subjects. *Lancet* 337:690, 1991.

241. Taylor, I. K., et al. Inhaled PAF stimulates leukotriene and thromboxane A_2 production in humans. *J. Appl. Physiol.* 71:1396, 1991.

242. Taylor, I. K., et al. Thromboxane A_2 biosynthesis in acute asthma and after antigen challenge. *Am. Rev. Respir. Dis.* 143:119, 1991.

243. Terano, T., Salmon, J. A., and Moncada, S. Biosynthesis and biological activity of leukotriene B_5. *Prostaglandins* 27:217, 1984.

244. Thomson, N. C., et al. Comparison of bronchial responses to prostaglandin $F_{2\alpha}$ and methacholine. *J. Allergy Clin. Immunol.* 68:392, 1981.

245. Ticono, J. Dietary requirements and functions of alpha-linolenic acid in animals. *Prog. Lipid Res.* 21:1, 1982.

246. Toogood, J. H. Aspirin intolerance, asthma, prostaglandins, and cromolyn sodium. *Chest* 72:135, 1977.

247. Torphy, T. J., et al. The clinical and preclinical pharmacology of SK&F 104353, a potent and selective peptidoleukotriene receptor antagonist. *Ann. NY Acad. Sci.* 629:157, 1991.

248. Umemoto, L., et al. Factors which influence late cutaneous allergic responses. *J. Allergy Clin. Immunol.* 58:60, 1976.

249. Undem, B. J., et al. The effect of indomethacin on the immunologic release of histamine and sulfidopeptide leukotrienes from human bronchus and lung parenchyma. *Am. Rev. Respir. Dis.* 136:1183, 1987.

250. Uotila, P., and Vapaatalo, H. Synthesis, pathways and biological implications of eicosanoids. *Ann. Clin. Res.* 16:226, 1984.

251. VanArsdel, P. P., Jr. Aspirin idiosyncracy and intolerance. *J. Allergy Clin. Immunol.* 73:431, 1984.

252. Voelkel, N. F., et al. Nonimmunological production of leukotrienes induced by platelet-activating factor. *Science* 218:286, 1982.

253. Walsh, C. E., et al. Release and metabolism of arachidonic acid in human neutrophils. *J. Biol. Chem.* 256:7228, 1981.

254. Walters, E. H. Effect of inhibition of prostaglandin synthesis on induced bronchial hyperresponsiveness. *Thorax* 38:195, 1983.

255. Walters, E. H. Prostaglandins and the control of airways responses to histamine in normal and asthmatic subjects. *Thorax* 38:188, 1983.

256. Walters, E. H., et al. Induction of bronchial hypersensitivity: Evidence for a role for prostaglandins. *Thorax* 36:571, 1981.

257. Wardlaw, A. J., et al. Leukotrienes, LTC_4 and LTB_4, in bronchoalveolar lavage in bronchial asthma and other respiratory diseases. *J. Allergy Clin. Immunol.* 84:19, 1989.

258. Weichman, B. M., and Tucker, S. S. Differentiation of the mechanisms by which leukotrienes C_4 and D_4 elicit contraction of the guinea pig trachea. *Prostaglandins* 29:547, 1985.

259. Weiss, J. W., et al. Bronchoconstrictor effects of leukotriene C in humans. *Science* 216:196, 1982.

260. Weiss, J. W., et al. Comparative bronchoconstrictor effects of histamine, leukotriene C, and leukotriene D in normal human volunteers. *Trans. Assoc. Am. Physicians* 95:30, 1982.

261. Weiss, J. W., et al. Airway constriction in normal humans produced by inhalation of leukotriene D. Potency, time course, and effect of aspirin therapy. *JAMA* 249:2814, 1983.

262. Weller, P. F., et al. Generation and metabolism of 5-lipoxygenase pathway leukotrienes by human eosinophils: Predominant production of leukotriene C_4. *Proc. Natl. Acad. Sci. USA* 80:7626, 1983.

263. Wenzel, S. E., et al. Elevated levels of leukotriene C_4 in bronchoalveolar lavage fluid from atopic asthmatics after endobronchial allergen challenge. *Am. Rev. Respir. Dis.* 142:112, 1990.

264. Wenzel, S. E., Westcott, J. Y., and Larsen, G. L. Bronchoalveolar lavage fluid mediator levels 5 minutes after allergen challenge in atopic subjects with asthma: Relationship to the development of late asthmatic responses. *J. Allergy Clin. Immunol.* 87:540, 1991.

265. Wenzel, S. E., et al. Spectrum of prostanoid release after bronchoalveolar allergen challenge in atopic asthmatics and control groups: An alteration in the ratio of bronchoconstrictive to bronchoprotective mediators. *Am. Rev. Respir. Dis.* 139:450, 1989.

265a. Westcott, J. Y., et al. Urinary leukotriene E_4 in patients with asthma: Effect of airways reactivity and sodium cromoglycate. *Am. Rev. Respir. Dis.* 143:1322, 1991.

266. Williams, J. D., Czop, J. K., and Austen, K. F. Release of leukotrienes by human monocytes on stimulation of their phagocytic receptor for particulate activators. *J. Immunol.* 132:3034, 1984.

267. Williams, J. D., et al. Intracellular retention of the 5-lipoxygenase pathway product, leukotriene B_4, by human neutrophils activated with unopsonised zymosan. *J. Immunol.* 134:2624, 1985.

268. Williams, W. R., Pawlowicz, A., and Davies, B. H. In vitro tests for the diagnosis of aspirin-sensitive asthma. *J. Allergy Clin. Immunol.* 86:445, 1990.

269. Woolcock, A. J., Salome, C. M., and Yan, K. The shape of the dose-response curve to histamine in asthmatic and normal subjects. *Am. Rev. Respir. Dis.* 130:71, 1984.

Late Asthmatic Reactions

Jean-Luc Malo
André Cartier

12

After they have been exposed to a stimulus, most often a common allergen or occupational sensitizer, subjects can develop not only an immediate reaction that is maximal 10 to 30 minutes after exposure, but also a reaction several hours later. In recent years significant interest has been focused on these so-called late asthmatic reactions. The prevailing belief was that immediate asthmatic reactions were more harmful as they were clinically more noticeable and functionally more pronounced, but it is now well documented that late asthmatic reactions occur at the site of the ongoing inflammatory process that takes place in asthma. This has been widely investigated in recent years and has been the subject of many symposiums [133]. The physiopathology of the late-phase allergic reaction in the many mucosa (nose, eye, bronchi) has been extensively studied and reviewed [52] but there are numerous questions still being debated. Late asthmatic reactions have been the specific subject of several review articles in recent years [32, 51, 53, 54, 100, 105, 131, 132, 134].

HISTORICAL BACKGROUND

Pepys wrote an interesting review of the history of late allergic reactions [142]. He reported that Charles Blackley was apparently the first to describe long-lasting respiratory tract reactions to pollens in experimental challenges on himself [161]. Charles Blackley reported in 1873 [17]:

In preparing the pollen of one of the *Amentaceae* for the microscope a considerable quantity was accidentally inhaled before I was aware that it had been thrown off from the catkins so abundantly. A violent attack of sneezing came on in a few minutes. . . . Later on there was a moderately copious discharge of thin serum which kept up for some hours. After the sneezing and coryza had continued for a couple of hours the breathing became very difficult as if from constriction of the trachea or bronchial tubes. . . . A very restless night was passed. . . . Occasionally there was slight cough with expectoration of thin frothy sputum, and for twenty-four hours I felt as if passing through an unusually severe attack of influenza.

This clearly points to the fact that the reaction occurred after an inhaled challenge, and that it occurred a few hours after exposure and lasted for 24 hours. Prausnitz and Kustner as well as Cooke [39] also described late reactions. Stevens mentioned that symptoms of asthma could last several days after allergen inhalation challenges [158].

Herxheimer, however, was the first author to make a distinct comparison of late asthmatic reactions with immediate reactions. He originally described four subjects who developed late reactions on exposure to house dust [77]. One year later, he reported on a series of 62 patients who were challenged for the purpose of hyposensitization to house dust, pollen, and cat fur; he noted the occurrence of late asthmatic reactions in 21 in-

stances. He also made the point that the reactions were not reproducible in terms of their isolated immediate, late, or dual components [78]. More extensive physiologic and immunologic characterization of late reactions was later made by Pepys and coworkers who used various antigens, including common inhalants, *Aspergillus*, and various occupational sensitizers [118, 141, 143, 157]. Investigation of the physiopathology of these reactions was later carried out. It was found that these temporal reactions are the main cause of bronchial inflammation and of "eosinophilic bronchitis" [7].

DESCRIPTION, FREQUENCY, CLINICAL RELEVANCE, AND RESPONSIBLE AGENTS

Table 12-1, based on Pepys and Hutchcroft's original publication [143], summarizes the features of immediate and late reactions to occupational sensitizers. The same features apply for common allergens. Although the typical patterns of so-called immediate and late reactions were originally identified (Fig. 12-1), they are not constant, especially after exposure to occupational agents. Atypical reactions have indeed been identified [146] as shown in Figure 12-2. The physiopathology of these atypical, nonimmediate-type reactions is unknown.

As reviewed by Cockcroft [31], Bierman [14], and O'Byrne and coworkers [134], the occurrence of late reactions as assessed in the laboratory among selected groups of asthmatic subjects may reach 50 percent. As for late reactions caused by stimuli other than allergens, late reactions may occur more frequently in children. Indeed, Warner elicited late reactions in 73 percent (36/49) of children who had undergone challenges with house dust mite [169]. Late asthmatic reactions are most often preceded by immediate reactions. However, Hill gave an account of five children who developed isolated late reactions after challenges with house mites [79]. As the assessment was done using peak expiratory flow rates, which are less sensitive than 1-second forced expiratory volume (FEV_1) (see below), it is possible that the immediate component was missed. Although the reproducibility of immediate asthmatic reactions to common allergens has been assessed [95], it has not been assessed for late asthmatic reactions in a sufficiently large group of subjects [24].

For common allergens, late reactions are generally preceded by immediate reactions. By contrast, late reactions often occur without evidence of immediate reactions after exposure to occupational agents, especially the low-molecular-weight agents such as isocyanates or plicatic acid, the causal agent of Western red cedar asthma [29, 137] (see also Chap. 46).

Allergens and occupational sensitizers have been described as the primary cause of late reactions. However, there have been reports of late reactions after exposure to nonspecific agents. Although Dahl and Henriksen were unable to detect late asth-

135

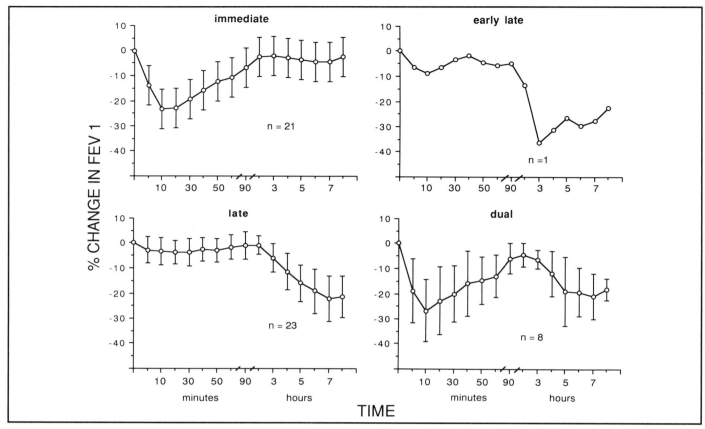

Fig. 12-1. *Mean ± standard deviation or individual values of the percent change in FEV₁ (on the ordinate) as a function of time since exposure (on the abscissa) for the four typical patterns of reactions. The numbers of individuals for each pattern are shown. (Reprinted with permission from B. Perrin, et al. Reassessment of the temporal patterns of bronchial obstruction after exposure to occupational sensitizing agents. J. Allergy Clin. Immunol. 87:630, 1991.)*

Table 12-1. Features of immediate and nonimmediate asthmatic reactions

	Immediate	Nonimmediate
Clinical and functional findings	Acute, sharp, rapid decrease in FEV₁, clinically readily evident	Slowly developing, progressively more severe, often not obvious clinically except on exertion, until fully developed, when dyspnea and wheezing appear
Onset of reaction	10–20 min	1–8 hr
Maximal decrease in FEV₁	10–20 min	3–8 hr
Duration	1–2 hr	3–96 hr
Systemic reactions	None	Malaise, myalgia, fever (rare)
White blood cell counts	Little or no change	Leukocytosis (rare)
Eosinophilia	No or slight increase	Present

Source: Modified from J. Pepys and B. J. Hutchcroft. Bronchial provocation tests in etiologic diagnosis and analysis of asthma. *Am. Rev. Respir. Dis.* 112:829, 1975.

matic reactions after exercise as compared to antigen exposure [45], several descriptions of late asthmatic responses to exercise were later made. Bierman was the first to publish (in abstract form) several cases of late reactions due to exercise as reviewed elsewhere [15]. Lee and coworkers described 15 subjects, including 13 children, who had both immediate and late reactions after exercise with a concomitant increase in neutrophil chemotactic activity during both immediate and late reactions [103]. In a subsequent publication, Bierman compared the features of late asthmatic reactions to antigens and to exercise [15]. Bierman and coauthors later described nine young adult subjects with dual (immediate and late) responses to exercise [16]. The immediate reaction was interpreted as involving the large airways, whereas the late reaction was more peripheral as assessed by the response to breathing a helium-oxygen mixture. Exposure of the peripheral airways to dry air causes bronchoconstriction as well as infiltration of eosinophils and neutrophils [64]. Horn and coworkers also saw late asthmatic reactions to exercise in eight young adults [80]. Iikura and coworkers found that the magnitude of the late reactions was related to the severity of the early component [88]. The prevalence of late asthmatic reactions was later investigated. In a sample of 24 subjects, Boulet and coworkers identified 7 (30%) with definite late responses but were unable to detect any increase in neutrophil chemotactic activity [21]. There was no change in nonspecific bronchial responsiveness to histamine as assessed 24 hours after exercise. Foresi and coworkers were also unable to detect significant changes in responsiveness to methacholine in four subjects who had late reactions

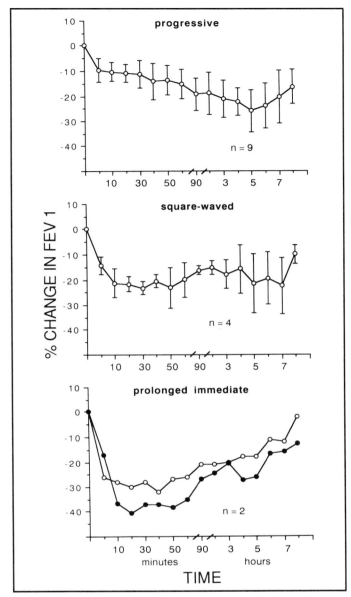

Fig. 12-2. *Mean ± standard deviation or individual values of the percent change in FEV₁ (on the ordinate) as a function of time since exposure (on the abscissa) for the three atypical patterns of reactions. The numbers of individuals for each pattern are shown. (Reprinted with permission from B. Perrin, et al. Reassessment of the temporal patterns of bronchial obstruction after exposure to occupational sensitizing agents. J. Allergy Clin. Immunol. 87:630, 1991.)*

[63]. A 15 percent (8/53) prevalence was found by another group of investigators [149]. Speelberg and coauthors described a 38 percent prevalence of dual asthmatic reactions after exercise as assessed by falls in peak expiratory flow rates greater than 10 percent as compared with rates on a control day [155]. Seven of the 33 subjects had isolated late asthmatic reactions. The fact that the reproducibility of late responses to exercise was weak suggested to some that they represented a nonspecific mechanism different from what is observed for late reactions to antigens. Moreover, it was suggested that the two reactions might be independent [171]. It was thought that the inappropriateness of a satisfactory control day might affect the likelihood of such reactions [104]. The appearance of late reactions might have been due to the study design: Medication had to be stopped a few

hours before exercise, making the asthmatic subjects more vulnerable to unstable airway caliber.

Late asthmatic responses have also been described after other stimuli. Foresi and coworkers described late reactions in five of nine subjects who had previously showed immediate bronchoconstriction after inhaling ultrasonically nebulized distilled water [63]. This was confirmed in another study by the same group of investigators. They were unable to detect significant changes in bronchial responsiveness to methacholine after the late reaction, whereas changes occurred after the immediate reaction [117].

FUNCTIONAL ASPECTS AND PHYSIOLOGIC CONSEQUENCES

It has been recognized that late reactions affect primarily the peripheral airways. This was documented by analyzing the pattern of response to a helium-oxygen mixture [109, 121]. By examining lung resistance and dynamic lung compliance in 61 asthmatic children who underwent specific challenges with house dust, Gaultier and coworkers found that the immediate reactions are more frequently located in the central airways whereas late reactions are both central and peripheral [69]. Although the patterns of response after early and late reactions are qualitatively similar, subjects with late reactions generally show more pronounced changes in FEV₁ and residual volume at the time of the immediate reaction [109]. However, MacIntyre and Boyd were unable to distinguish the site of airway obstruction, as the response to flows after breathing helium-oxygen was similar with both immediate and late reactions [110]. Similarly, Chan-Yeung and coworkers showed that subjects who were either responders or nonresponders to the helium-oxygen mixture in terms of flow rates had similar patterns of response during both immediate and late reactions [28]. There are possible explanations for these discrepancies: the timing of the assessment, the variety of allergens tested, and the intrinsic variability of the helium response test [98].

Late asthmatic reactions can be followed by recurrent and long-lasting variability in airway caliber manifested by nocturnal asthmatic episodes [46, 152, 159]. It is thought that the cause of these recurrent episodes is related to the changes in nonspecific bronchial responsiveness [33]. Increasing the dose of allergen can modify the pattern of reactions. On the one hand, by increasing the dose, an isolated immediate reaction may be followed by a late reaction. This was shown by Lai and coworkers, who blocked the immediate component of the reaction to common inhalants by giving terfenadine [96] or rimiterol [97], a short-acting beta₂-adrenergic agent. This made it possible to use increasing doses of allergens. Although increasing the dose of allergen can cause a late asthmatic reaction, this does not produce further changes in nonspecific bronchial hyperresponsiveness [97]. On the other hand, giving a low dose of allergen can cause an isolated late reaction, which will be transformed into a dual (immediate and late) reaction when the dose is increased [86]. The possibility of an isolated late reaction without a previous immediate response was confirmed in inbred rats who underwent specific challenges to ovalbumin [59]. Three of the five rats that had had no immediate reaction experienced a late reaction. Exposure to pollens during the season can result in more constant and more severe late asthmatic reactions than if the test is performed out of season [44]. Infections and pollution can also affect late asthmatic reactions. Rhinovirus upper respiratory tract infection can increase not only airway hyperreactivity but also the likelihood of developing late asthmatic reactions. Before infection, only 1 of 10 subjects developed a late asthmatic reaction after an antigen challenge, whereas 8 of the 10 had late reactions when they had the viral infection [106]. However, it was also found that in dogs, previous exposure to ozone blocks the late asthmatic response induced by *Ascaris suum* antigen [165]. The upper airways play a role in the development of late asthmatic reactions. Guinea pigs challenged through a tracheostomy failed to develop late reactions [92]. When the animals were challenged through the upper airways, and the measurement of specific airway conductance included both the upper and the lower airways, late reactions were found in 5 (28%) of 18 animals. When the measurement included only the lower airways, evidence of isolated late airway reactions could be demonstrated in only 2 (10%) of 20 animals. This study using guinea pig therefore clearly shows that a significant part of the increase in specific airway conductance during late reactions originates in the upper airways and that the occurrence of pure airway reactions is conditioned by sensitization of the upper airways.

Late asthmatic reactions also have a circadian pattern. The frequency, magnitude, and associated changes in bronchial hyperresponsiveness to methacholine are greater when the challenge is carried out in the evening as compared to the morning. Moreover, the time to onset of the reaction is shorter after an evening challenge [124]. Deep inspiration, the so-called volume history, has a greater bronchodilator effect on immediate as compared to late reactions, as was shown in 18 patients who underwent challenges to house dust mite [140].

The magnitude of an immediate asthmatic reaction to an allergen can be predicted based on the ground of the degree of immunologic sensitization and bronchial hyperresponsiveness, as was originally suspected by Tiffeneau [162] and confirmed by two studies from the same group of investigators [36, 38]. It was shown that the magnitude of immediate and late asthmatic reactions can be predicted with similar accuracy using a model that incorporates baseline FEV_1, degree of bronchial hyperresponsiveness, and immediate immunologic reactivity as assessed by

specific IgE levels [43]. The magnitude of the early reaction is also a significant determinant of the late reaction [75]. Correspondence was sought in the cutaneous and bronchial responses to an allergen. Robertson and coworkers detected serum IgE antibodies to ragweed only in subjects with late asthmatic reactions; the same subjects also had larger late cutaneous reactions to the antigen [146]. It was later found that a dual bronchial response was more likely to occur when there were higher levels of specific IgE, a small immediate cutaneous reaction followed by a late reaction, and a low antigen concentration eliciting a late cutaneous reaction [22]. Although it was originally suggested that levels of specific IgE were related to immediate reactions whereas subjects who produced IgG4 antibodies were more likely to develop late reactions [73], these findings could not be duplicated [58, 90]. Ito and coworkers failed to show a correlation between the levels of specific IgE antibodies to house dust mite and the development of late asthmatic responses in seven subjects, as compared with five subjects who experienced isolated immediate reactions [90]. However, they found that the level of IgG1 antibodies was higher in those with late reactions.

It is known that seasonal exposure to allergens can increase bronchial responsiveness [19, 107, 154]. Boulet and coworkers showed that subjects with the greatest change in bronchial responsiveness to methacholine during the pollen season where those who exhibited late asthmatic reactions after laboratory bronchoprovocation [20]. Unlike isolated immediate reactions, late reactions to common inhalant allergens change bronchial responsiveness to nonspecific agents [37], the magnitude and duration of the change being related to the severity of airway obstruction during the reaction [27]. Similar findings apply to occupational sensitizers (Fig. 12-3), especially toluene diisocya-

Fig. 12-3. *Combined monitoring of peak expiratory flow rate (PEFR) and of bronchial responsiveness assessed by the provocation concentration producing a 20 percent fall in FEV_1 (PC_{20}) in the same subjects before and after return to work. Squares represent the time spent at work, whereas lozenges illustrate the use of inhaled salbutamol (albuterol). Baseline FEV_1 values before each histamine inhalation test are given. They vary by no more than 6 percent from one test to another. (Reprinted with permission from A. Cartier, et al. Occupational asthma in snow crab-processing workers.* J. Allergy Clin. Immunol. *74:261, 1984.)*

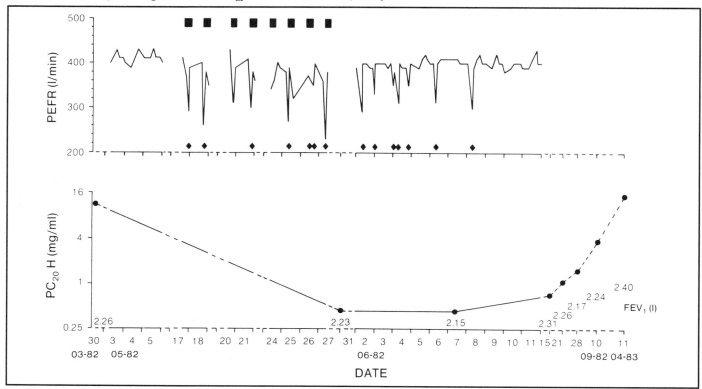

Table 12-2. Changes in bronchial responsiveness according to type of reaction

	Changes in PC_{20} in subjects with late reactions (n = 101)	Changes in PC_{20} in subjects with immediate reactions (n = 63)
Changes in PC_{20} (fold-difference)		
0–2	44	39
2–3.2	16	13
>3.2	41	11

Overall chi square = 9.63, p = 0.008.
Comparing subjects with PC_{20} changes less than twofold and more than or equal to twofold difference, chi square = 5.2, p = .02.
Odds for the presence of significant changes in PC_{20} in subjects with late reactions = 56% (95% confidence intervals = 46%–66%).
Odds for the absence of significant changes in PC_{20} in subjects with immediate reactions = 62% (95% confidence intervals = 49%–74%).

PC_{20} = provocation concentration producing a 20 percent fall in FEV_1.
Source: From J.-L. Malo et al. Late asthmatic reactions to occupational sensitizing agents: Frequency of changes in nonspecific bronchial responsiveness and of response to inhaled beta-2-adrenergic agent. *J. Allergy Clin. Immunol.* 85:834, 1990. Reprinted with permission.

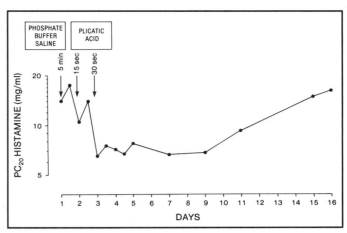

Fig. 12-4. *Changes in bronchial responsiveness as assessed by the histamine provocation concentration producing a 20 percent fall in FEV_1 (PC_{20}) as a function of time on consecutive days, before and after inhalation of phosphate buffer saline (Day 1, control day) and of plicatic acid, the active product in Western red cedar for 15 seconds and 30 seconds, on two consecutive days (Days 2 and 3). The duration of inhalation of phosphate buffer saline solution and plicatic acid is illustrated. (Reprinted with permission from A. Cartier, J. L'Archevêque, and J.-L. Malo. Exposure to a sensitizing occupational agent can cause a long-lasting increase in bronchial responsiveness to histamine in the absence of significant changes in airway caliber. J. Allergy Clin. Immunol. 78:1185, 1986.)*

nate [114]. The changes in bronchial responsiveness can last for 1 to 4 weeks after a single challenge causing a late reaction, as was shown by the same group of investigators using toluene diisocyanate [115]. The changes in bronchial responsiveness are not unique to late reactions and can occur after immediate reactions, as was demonstrated prospectively in individual patients and retrospectively in a vast number of subjects exposed to occupational sensitizers (Table 12-2) [111, 112] as well as to common inhalants [108]. It has generally been assumed that late reactions respond less well to inhaled beta$_2$-adrenergic agents than do immediate reactions, this being explained by the presence of airway inflammation [143]. However, it was recently shown that inhaled beta$_2$-adrenergic agents can restore airway caliber, although the duration of this effect is unknown [111].

Changes in bronchial responsiveness are more sensitive in detecting late asthmatic reactions than changes in airway caliber are and they can be long-lasting even in the absence of changes in airway caliber [26]. Changes in bronchial responsiveness have indeed been shown to occur before the changes in airway caliber during late reactions (Fig. 12-4). Although the changes do not seem to be present 2 hours after the immediate reaction [34], significant changes in bronchial responsiveness to histamine were documented 3 hours after the challenge [56]. Changes in bronchial caliber related to late reactions are proportional to the changes in bronchial responsiveness as assessed 3 hours after the challenge [72].

PHYSIOPATHOLOGY

The availability of fiberoptic bronchoscopy and bronchoalveolar lavage has improved our understanding of the mechanisms of immediate and late asthmatic reactions a great deal [121]. The lavage technique has made it possible for investigators to study both the cellular and the liquid content of the lavage material for immediate and late reactions. Fiberoptic bronchoscopy has made it possible to perform direct challenges of the airways [123]. Pathologic evidence has also been obtained from biopsy specimens. Several animal models of late reactions have been developed, specifically in rabbits [119], sheep [1, 149], and guinea pigs [85]. The proposed physiopathologic scheme of late- and early-phase asthmatic reactions is shown in Figure 12-5.

Pathologic Changes

An animal model of a late reaction was developed in rabbits sensitized to *Alternaria*. The immediate response was characterized by interstitial edema and vessel dilatation. The late reaction was characterized by residual edema and infiltrate of granulocytes, a mixture of neutrophils and eosinophils at 6 hours and of predominantly eosinophils at 48 hours. It was also found that the histopathologic changes were paralleled by similar changes in the histopathology of skin biopsy specimens that had also been challenged [8, 9, 101]. The presence of eosinophils within the airway walls 7 hours after the challenge was confirmed by Iijima and coworkers in guinea pigs exposed to an *A. suum* extract [87]. Although neutrophils and mononuclear cells were also found, the quantity of eosinophils was more marked in animals with late reactions than in those with isolated immediate reactions.

Late-phase allergic reactions to plicatic acid are also associated with an increase in sloughing of bronchial epithelial cells and degenerated cells, mainly epithelial cells and alveolar macrophages [99].

Cells Obtained by Bronchoalveolar Lavage

The Role of Eosinophils

The role of eosinophils and T-lymphocytes in late-phase allergic reactions was recently reviewed [66]. It has been shown that there is a fall in peripheral eosinophilia during a late reaction [41], with an increase 24 hours after the challenge [40, 57, 99]. This increase in eosinophils is not seen after isolated immediate reactions and correlates with the baseline level of bronchial hyperresponsiveness [57]. Baseline levels of eosinophils and the eosinophil cationic protein are also higher in subjects who develop late asthmatic reactions. There is a significant reduction in eosinophils after a 4-week course of inhaled steroids [167].

DeMonchy and coworkers found an increase in bronchoalveolar eosinophilia and the eosinophil cationic protein–albumin ratio in the bronchoalveolar lavage fluid at the time of late reactions in six subjects who developed dual reactions after being

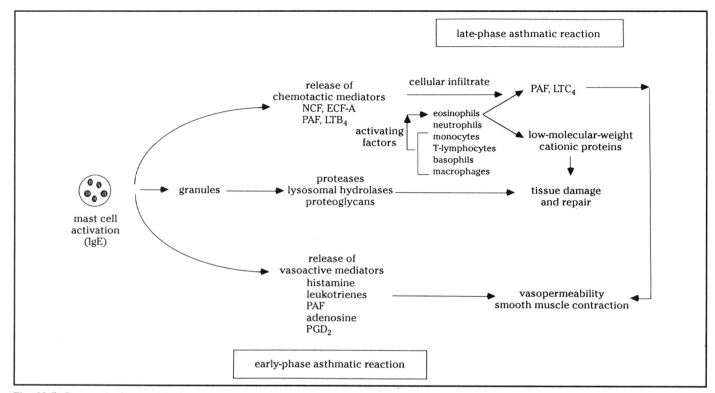

Fig. 12-5. *Proposed scheme of the late- and early-phase asthmatic reactions. NCF = neutrophil chemotactic factor; ECF-A = eosinophilic chemotactic factors of anaphylaxis; PAF = platelet-activating factor; LT = leukotriene; PG = prostaglandin. (Modified from S. I. Wasserman. The Physiopathology of Mediators in Asthma. In M. E. Gershwin (ed.), Bronchial Asthma. New York: Grune & Stratton, 1986; and H. F. Kauffman et al. Corticosteroids. In W. Dorsch (ed.), Late Phase Allergic Reaction. Boca Raton: CRC Press, 1990.)*

challenged with house dust mites [49]. The increase in eosinophils in the bronchoalveolar lavage fluid was also found in subjects with late reactions who underwent challenges with plicatic acid, the active component of Western red cedar [99]. Eosinophilia in the bronchoalveolar lavage fluid was found in the animal models (guinea pigs and sheep) of late reactions [4, 67, 82]. Pretreatment with cromolyn and nedocromil sodium blocks the dual reactions as well as the increase in bronchoalveolar eosinophilia in the late reaction [5]. Frick and coworkers showed more recently that the eosinophils, levels of which increased 24 hours after challenging subjects with common inhalants, were of the hypodense type [68]. Moreover, in a study of 38 asthmatic subjects, the same authors found that there was a correlation between the percentage of circulating hypodense eosinophils and the severity of the asthma.

Role of Neutrophils
Findings of increases in the number of neutrophils in the bronchoalveolar lavage fluid have been inconstant. Hutson and coworkers found a significant increase in neutrophil counts in the lavage 6 and 17 hours after the challenge among guinea pigs with late reactions to ovalbumin [82]. Coyle and coworkers also found increased numbers of neutrophils in rabbits challenged with ragweed [41]. In seven subjects with late asthmatic responses, Diaz and coworkers demonstrated a significant increase in the number of neutrophils, although the increase was not as marked as was the increase in eosinophil count [50]. Lam and coworkers found an increase in neutrophil counts 48 hours after challenging human subjects with plicatic acid [99]. However, Abraham and coworkers failed to detect any increase in the number of neutrophils in the lavage approximately 8 hours after challenging sheep with *A. suum* [5]. In asthma caused by toluene diisocyanate, Fab-

bri and coworkers found increased numbers of neutrophils in the lavage fluid 2 and 8 hours after the challenge in subjects who experienced late asthmatic reactions [60]. In the same subjects, eosinophil counts increased only 8 hours after the challenge. Even if there is neutrophilia in the lavage, as was confirmed in a more recent report [84], depletion of circulating neutrophils by a specific antiserum did not result in changes to the magnitude of the early and late reactions to ovalbumin. This suggests that neutrophils do not play a significant functional role in the induction of a late asthmatic reaction. However, there might be differences in the response between species. Indeed, Murphy and coworkers, who induced neutropenia in a rabbit model of asthma, showed that neutrophils were a required element of a late asthmatic reaction [125].

Role of Lymphocytes
The number of lymphocytes increases during late reactions, as was shown in seven subjects challenged with grass or house dust mites [50]. T-lymphocytes may also be involved in late asthmatic reactions, as was reviewed recently [67]. However, the proportion of helper and suppressor T-cells seems to be altered during immediate reactions but not during late reactions [71]. Challenging guinea pigs with ovalbumin resulted in an accumulation of T-lymphocytes [67]. The sensitization phase resulted in an accumulation of CD8 T-cells, but the postchallenge infiltrate in the submucosa and adventitia was predominantly of the CD3 type. Bronchoalveolar lavage fluid and peripheral lymphocyte counts were not significantly altered. The increase in T-cells was correlated with the increase in eosinophilia 17 and 72 hours after the challenge. An increase in CD3-type lymphocytes was also detected in the late-phase skin reactions of human atopic subjects by the same group of investigators [65]. Lymphokines with

specific effects on neutrophils were identified by the same workers.

Platelets

The depletion of platelets in rabbits sensitized to ragweed resulted in a marked reduction in the late asthmatic reaction and the associated changes in nonspecific bronchial responsiveness to histamine [41]. These changes were associated with a fall in the number of eosinophils, but not neutrophils, in the bronchoalveolar lavage fluid.

Others

The number of mast cells in the bronchoalveolar lavage fluid 6 hours after the challenge decreased significantly [50].

Soluble Agents and Mediators

Pituitary and Adrenal Function

Low plasma cortisol concentrations have been found during late reactions in 13 asthmatic subjects [130]. These results were later confirmed by the same group of investigators who also found no significant changes in corticotropin levels [128].

Complement

Although it was initially suspected that components of the complement activation could specifically be involved in the late asthmatic reaction [6], this was later disclosed in several publications [58, 81, 145, 156].

Histamine

Although plasma histamine concentrations are elevated during immediate reactions, this does not seem to be the case in late reactions [93]. Urinary N-tau-methylhistamine levels increased during immediate reactions, but no such change was elicited by late reactions in 16 subjects who underwent specific challenges. This suggests that a renewed degranulation of mast cells during late bronchial reactions is unlikely [94]. It should be mentioned, however, that histamine levels in the bronchoalveolar lavage fluid were increased in five of seven subjects with late reactions [50].

Neutrophil and Eosinophilic Chemotactic Activity

The increased levels of neutrophil chemotactic activity in the blood were initially detected during immediate and late-phase reactions to allergens [126] and in exercise-induced asthma [102]. Leukocytes are activated during immediate and late reactions to antigens, as was demonstrated by the number of monocyte complement rosettes [55]. The increase in neutrophil chemotactic activity during late reactions corresponded to the heat labile fraction [168]. Eosinophilic chemotactic activity can also be detected during immediate and late asthmatic reactions to inhaled allergens [122]. The quantity of neutrophil and eosinophilic chemotactic activity generated seems to be proportional to the degree of bronchoconstriction [122, 168].

Arachidonic Acid Products

Products of the Lipoxygenase Pathway: Leukotrienes. Leukotrienes (LT), including LTC_4, LTD_4, and LTE_4, are the active components of the formerly named slow-reacting substance of anaphylaxis (SRS-A). They are released by various cells including mast cells, eosinophils, and macrophages and are potent bronchoconstrictors. There has been a vast amount of research investigating the role of leukotrienes in late asthmatic reactions. This role has been reviewed extensively in recent years [1–3]. Administration of a specific antagonist prevented the development of late asthmatic reactions caused by inhaling LTD_4 among allergic sheep sensitized to *A. suum* antigen [48]. LTD_4 has also been

implicated in the development of immediate and late reactions to ovalbumin in rats; two specific antagonists have been shown to block the late reaction and, to a lesser extent, the immediate reaction [150]. Other evidence of the role of leukotrienes in the onset of late asthmatic reactions has been documented by Fairfax and colleagues, who were able to block the late reaction by administering indomethacin (an inhibitor of the cyclooxygenase pathway) or benoxaprofen (an inhibitor of both cyclooxygenase and lipoxygenase pathways) prior to challenges with house dust mites in small groups (four or less) of asthmatic subjects [62]. Finally, sheep who had been sensitized to *A. suum* and presented dual asthmatic reactions after the challenge also presented dual asthmatic reactions after a challenge with LTD_4. This dual reaction was blocked by a specific antagonist [1]. Sheep having an isolated immediate reaction to the antigen also had an isolated immediate reaction to LTD_4. The possibility that LTC_4 and LTD_4 could play a role in immediate and late-phase asthmatic reactions was challenged by Bel and coworkers; they were unable to block the reactions with a specific antagonist in 10 subjects who had been challenged with house dust mites [10].

LTD_4 and LTC_4 are potent bronchoconstrictors and are excreted in the urine as LTC_4, as has been reviewed elsewhere [23]. Studies of urinary LTC_4 concentrations have been performed during early and late reactions to allergens in humans. Taylor and coworkers found a significant immediate (within 3 hours) increase in urinary LTC_4 among eight atopic asthmatic subjects who had undergone specific inhalation challenges [160]. Similar findings were reported by Manning and coworkers [113]. They did not find significant changes in LTE_4 during late reactions (Fig. 12-6), which suggests either that LTD_4 is not implicated in late asthmatic reactions or that other metabolites of leukotrienes that were not measured may be involved. LTC_4 concentrations do not increase in the lavage, as shown by Smith and coworkers [153]. The degree of immediate bronchoconstriction was proportional to urinary LTE_4 levels for Manning and coworkers [113] but not for Taylor and coauthors [160]. LTB_4 can be implicated in late asthmatic reactions to toluene diisocyanate, an occupational sensitizer, because increased levels were detected using bronchoalveolar lavage of asthmatic subjects who had been challenged with it [172]. Subjects pretreated with oral cortisone did not have late reactions or increased LTB_4 in the lavage fluid.

Products of the Cyclooxygenase Pathways: Prostaglandins and Thromboxanes. Plasma thromboxane A_2 levels increased after immediate reactions but more so after late reactions in 12 asthmatic subjects challenged with house dust [91]. Moreover, a specific thromboxane A_2 synthetase inhibitor has been shown to inhibit both immediate and late asthmatic reactions. The fact that indomethacin inhibits late asthmatic reactions may indicate the participation of cyclooxygenase products in the reaction, although other researchers have documented the opposite effect, namely an increase in in vitro antigen-induced bronchoconstriction [89]. Thromboxane B_2 levels increase in the bronchoalveolar lavage fluid 5 minutes after allergen challenge in atopic subjects, but more so in subjects who develop dual asthmatic reactions as opposed to those subjects with isolated immediate reactions [170]. Similar findings apply for other mediators such as histamine, prostaglandin (PG) D_2 and LTC_4 [170].

Platelet-activating Factor

Although the role of the platelet-activating factor in human asthma has been the subject of numerous studies in recent years, its role in the development of late asthmatic reactions is still debatable. Using a sheep model of asthma, Abraham and coworkers were able to elicit immediate bronchospastic reactions in all seven of the animals that were challenged; however, late reactions were obtained in only three of them [5]. Concentrations of lysoform of the platelet-activating factor were significantly increased in the plasma in nine subjects 6 hours after antigen chal-

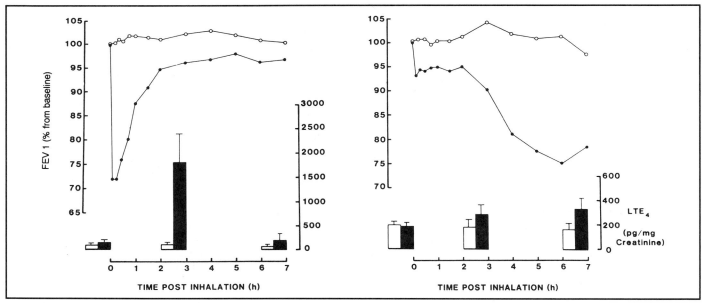

Fig. 12-6. *Changes in FEV$_1$ (%) in five subjects, each of whom developed an isolated early (left) or late (right) asthmatic reaction (closed circles) by comparison with control values (open circles). The levels of urinary leukotriene E$_4$ (LTE$_4$) (mean and standard error) measured before inhalation of the diluent (open bars) or the sensitizing agent (solid bars) and between 2 to 3 hours and between 6 to 7 hours after inhalation are also illustrated. A significant increase in urinary LTE$_4$ (p = 0.04) occurred after the isolated immediate reaction but not after the late reaction. (Reprinted with permission from P. J. Manning, et al. Urinary leukotriene LTE$_4$ levels during early and late asthmatic reactions.* J. Allergy Clin. Immunol. 86:211, 1990.)

lenges. By contrast, no significant change was seen after immediate reactions in four subjects [127].

MODULATIONS: THE ROLE OF MEDICATION AND IMMUNOTHERAPY

Antihistamines

Although it was originally thought that antihistamine preparations had no significant effect on immediate or late asthmatic reactions to allergens [143], Hamid and coworkers showed that terfenadine, a long-acting anti-H$_1$ preparation, had a blocking effect, as did flurbiprofen, which inhibits the arachidonic cyclooxygenase pathway, on the immediate and late reactions when 10 asthmatic subjects were challenged with common allergens [74]. Nakazawa and coworkers presented an interesting case report of a subject whose late reaction was not blocked by an H$_1$ or H$_2$ antagonist but in whom the blocking effect was demonstrated after using both drugs [129].

Beta$_2$-adrenergic Agents

Inhaled fenoterol can significantly reverse late asthmatic reactions, although this effect does not completely restore airway caliber [11, 111]. Beta$_2$-adrenergic agents can significantly reduce the magnitude of late asthmatic responses, but they seem to have no significant effect on the inflammatory process related to the reaction, as has been shown in animal models [83]. Administering a short-acting beta$_2$-adrenergic agent by inhalation before antigenic challenges in humans has no significant effect on the late bronchial reaction [35] although some protection has been demonstrated [76]. A new long-acting beta$_2$ agonist offers slightly more protection than short-acting beta$_2$ agonists [136].

Cromolyn and Nedocromil

It is well documented that cromolyn sodium can block immediate and late asthmatic reactions to inhaled common antigens or occupational sensitizers, as has been reviewed elsewhere [143]. Cromolyn can also block the changes in bronchial responsiveness in the pollen season [107]. These findings were later confirmed [35, 139] (Fig. 12-7). Although Mattoli and coworkers were unable to significantly reduce the magnitude of late reactions, they showed that cromolyn reduces the allergen-induced increase in nonspecific bronchial responsiveness in a dose-dependent manner [116]. Nedocromil sodium can also block early and late asthmatic responses in animals [30] and humans [42].

Corticosteroids

It is known that cortisol depletion augments the occurrence of late responses to *Ascaris* antigen in dogs [151]. The overwhelming evidence is that oral and inhaled corticosteroids block late asthmatic reactions, as has been reviewed [143] and confirmed [139] elsewhere. This effect is more pronounced than what is noticed for immediate reactions [25]. Oral corticosteroids can also block the associated increase in nonspecific bronchial hyperresponsiveness [61] and airway inflammation [18], as was shown in subjects who were challenged with toluene diisocyanate. Inhaled corticosteroids (dexamethasone isonicotinate) also block dual and late asthmatic reactions induced by toluene diisocyanate but ketotifen does not [163, 164].

Miscellaneous Agents

Theophylline and enprofylline may attenuate immediate and late asthmatic reactions, as was shown in nine subjects with asthma caused by common inhalants [138]. Atropine does not have any effect on the severity of late reactions to toluene diisocyanate [138]. The calcium antagonist gallopamil partially inhibits both

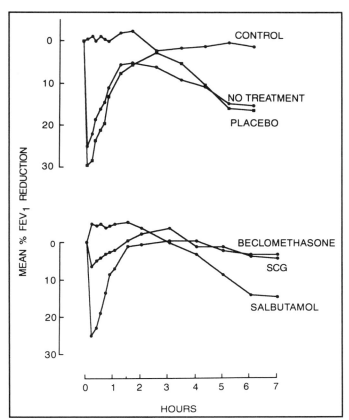

Fig. 12-7. *Mean bronchial response on the control and five allergen challenge days. FEV$_1$ (% fall) is on the vertical axis and time (hours) is on the horizontal axis. Time 0 is before challenge, and other times are after completion of challenge. The top panel includes responses to Day 1 control inhalation (control) and to allergen on Day 2 (placebo) and Day 6 (no treatment). The bottom panel demonstrates allergen response on Days 3 to 5 with pretreatments of beclomethasone dipropionate, 200 μg; salbutamol, 200 μg; and sodium cromoglycate (SCG) 10 mg. (Reprinted with permission from D. W. Cockcroft and K. Y. Murdock. Comparative effects of inhaled salbutamol, sodium cromoglycate, and beclomethasone dipropionate on allergen-induced early asthmatic responses, late asthmatic responses, and increased bronchial responsiveness to histamine. J. Allergy Clin. Immunol. 79: 734, 1987.)*

immediate and late-phase reactions to *A. suum* antigen in allergic sheep [47]. It was also recently found that inhaled furosemide blocked immediate and late asthmatic reactions in 11 subjects who had undergone challenges with common allergens [13].

Immunotherapy

Desensitizing children over the course of 1 year to house dust mites resulted in an attenuation of immediate and, more so, of late asthmatic reactions after challenges with this allergen [166]. A recurrence of the magnitude of the late response was observed 1 year after the end of immunotherapy, and a plateau effect was noticed in subjects who continued immunotherapy for a total of 2 years [12]. The effect of immunotherapy on immediate and late responses among subjects who were sensitized to and challenged with dog and cat extracts remains controversial [146].

In conclusion, late asthmatic reactions were documented more than a century ago and have been well documented since 1950. However, it is only in recent years that their relevance to the physiopathology of asthma, which involves a complex inflammatory process, has been recognized. In this regard, late asthmatic

reactions are probably more significant in contributing to the general inflammation of asthma, which has been labeled as a type of "eosinophilic bronchitis" by some [6], an entity on its own described by others [70], than immediate reactions are. The role of cells and mediators and their relationship in generating the inflammatory process remain to be elicited. The mechanism by which existing and future drugs affect this process will also have to be studied.

REFERENCES

1. Abraham, W. The role of leukotrienes in allergen-induced late responses in allergic sheep. *Ann. NY Acad. Sci.* 524:260, 1988.
2. Abraham, W. The role of eicosanoids in allergen-induced early and late bronchial responses in allergic sheep. *Adv. Prostaglandin Thromboxane Leukot. Res.* 20:201, 1990.
3. Abraham, W., and Perruchoud, A. Role of arachidonic acid metabolites in allergen-induced late response. *Respiration* 56:48, 1989.
4. Abraham, W., et al. Cellular markers of inflammation in the airways of allergic sheep with and without allergen-induced late responses. *Am. Rev. Respir. Dis.* 138:1565, 1988.
5. Abraham, W., Stevenson, J., and Garrido, R. A possible role for PAF in allergen-induced late responses: Modification by a selective antagonist. *J. Appl. Physiol.* 66:2351, 1989.
6. Arroyave, C., et al. Plasma complement changes during bronchospasm provoked in asthmatic patients. *Clin. Allergy* 7:173, 1977.
7. Barnes, P. J. General Discussion. In H. J. Sluiter and R. van der Lende, assisted by J. Gerritsen and D. S. Postman (eds.), *Bronchitis IV.* Assen The Netherlands: Van Gorcum, 1989. P. 111.
8. Behrens, B., et al. Comparison of the histopathology of immediate and late asthmatic and cutaneous responses in a rabbit model. *Chest* 87:153, 1985.
9. Behrens, B., et al. Comparison of the evolving histopathology of early and late cutaneous and asthmatic responses in rabbits after a single antigen challenge. *Lab. Invest.* 56:101, 1987.
10. Bel, E., et al. The effect of an inhaled leukotriene antagonist, L-648,051, on early and late asthmatic reactions and subsequent increase in airway responsiveness in man. *J. Allergy Clin. Immunol.* 85:1067, 1990.
11. Bever, H. V., Desager, K., and Stevens, W. The effect of inhaled fenoterol, administered during the late asthmatic reaction to house dust mite (*Dermatophagoides pteronyssinus*). *J. Allergy Clin. Immunol.* 85:700, 1990.
12. Bever, H. V., and Stevens, W. Evolution of the late asthmatic reaction during immunotherapy and after stopping immunotherapy. *J. Allergy Clin. Immunol.* 86:141, 1990.
13. Bianco, S., et al. Protective effect of inhaled furosemide on allergen-induced early and late asthmatic reactions. *N. Engl. J. Med.* 321:1069, 1989.
14. Bierman, C. A comparison of late reactions to antigen and exercise. *J. Allergy Clin. Immunol.* 73:654, 1984.
15. Bierman, C. W. Exercise-induced Asthma and Late Asthmatic Reactions. In W. Dorsch (ed.), *Late Phase Allergic Reactions.* Boca Raton: CRC Press, 1990. Pp. 169–184.
16. Bierman, C., Spiro, S., and Petheram, I. Characterization of the late response in exercise-induced asthma. *J. Allergy Clin. Immunol.* 74:701, 1984.
17. Blackley, C. *Experimental Researches on the Causes and Nature of Catarrhus Aestivus.* London: Dawson's of Pall Mall, 1959 (first published in 1873).
18. Boschetto, P., et al. Prednisone inhibits late asthmatic reactions and airway inflammation induced by toluene diisocyanate in sensitized subjects. *J. Allergy Clin. Immunol.* 80:261, 1987.
19. Boulet, L., et al. Asthma and increases in nonallergic bronchial responsiveness from seasonal pollen exposure. *J. Allergy Clin. Immunol.* 71:399, 1983.
20. Boulet, L.-P., et al. Asthma and increases in nonallergic bronchial responsiveness from seasonal pollen exposure. *J. Allergy Clin. Immunol.* 71:399, 1983.
21. Boulet, L.-P., et al. Prevalence and characteristics of late asthmatic responses to exercise. *J. Allergy Clin. Immunol.* 80:655, 1987.
22. Boulet, L.-P., et al. Prediction of late asthmatic responses to inhaled allergen. *Clin. Allergy* 14:379, 1984.
23. Bruynzeel, P., and Verhagen, J. The possible role of particular leuko-

trienes in the allergen-induced late-phase asthmatic reaction. *Clin. Allergy* 19(Suppl.):25, 1989.

24. Bundgaard, A., and Boudet, L. Reproducibility of the late asthmatic response. *Eur. J. Respir. Dis.* 68(Suppl. 143):41, 1986.

25. Burge, P., et al. Double-blind trials of inhaled beclomethasone dipropionate and fluocortin butyl ester in allergen-induced immediate and late asthmatic reactions. *Clin. Allergy* 12:523, 1982.

26. Cartier, A., L'Archevêque, J., and Malo, J. Exposure to a sensitizing occupational agent can cause a long-lasting increase in bronchial responsiveness to histamine in the absence of significant changes in airway caliber. *J. Allergy Clin. Immunol.* 78:1185, 1986.

27. Cartier, A., et al. Allergen-induced increase in bronchial responsiveness to histamine: Relationship to the late asthmatic response and change in airway caliber. *J. Allergy Clin. Immunol.* 70:170, 1982.

28. Chan-Yeung, M., et al. Effect of helium on maximal expiratory flow in patients with asthma before and during induced bronchoconstriction. *Am. Rev. Respir. Dis.* 113:433, 1976.

29. Chan-Yeung, M., and Lam, S. Occupational asthma. *Am. Rev. Respir. Dis.* 133:686, 1986.

30. Church, M., Hutson, P., and Holgate, S. Effect of nedocromil sodium on early and late phase responses to allergen challenge in the guinea-pig. *Drugs* 37(Suppl. 1):101, 1989.

31. Cockcroft, D. Allergen-induced late asthmatic responses and associated increases in nonallergic bronchial responsiveness: Clinical importance. *Immunol. Allergy Pract.* 6:92, 1984.

32. Cockcroft, D. Airway hyperresponsiveness and late asthmatic responses. *Chest* 94:178, 1988.

33. Cockcroft, D., Hoeppner, V., and Werner, G. Recurrent nocturnal asthma after bronchoprovocation with Western Red Cedar sawdust: Association with acute increase in nonallergic bronchial responsiveness. *Clin. Allergy* 14:61, 1984.

34. Cockcroft, D., and Murdock, K. Changes in bronchial responsiveness to histamine at intervals after allergen challenge. *Thorax* 42:302, 1987.

35. Cockcroft, D., and Murdock, K. Comparative effects of inhaled salbutamol, sodium cromoglycate, and beclomethasone dipropionate on allergen-induced early asthmatic responses, late asthmatic responses, and increased bronchial responsiveness to histamine. *J. Allergy Clin. Immunol.* 79:734, 1987.

36. Cockcroft, D., et al. Prediction of airway responsiveness to allergen from skin sensitivity to allergen and airway responsiveness to histamine. *Am. Rev. Respir. Dis.* 135:264, 1987.

37. Cockcroft, D., et al. Allergen-induced increase in non-allergic bronchial reactivity. *Clin. Allergy* 7:503, 1977.

38. Cockcroft, D., et al. Determinants of allergen-induced asthma: Dose of allergen, circulating IgE antibody concentration, and bronchial responsiveness to inhaled histamine. *Am. Rev. Respir. Dis.* 120:1053, 1979.

39. Cooke, R. Studies in specific hypersensitiveness. IX. On the phenomenon of hyposensitization (the clinically lessened sensitiveness of allergy). *J. Immunol.* 7:219, 1922.

40. Cookson, W., et al. Falls in peripheral eosinophil counts parallel the late asthmatic response. *Am. Rev. Respir. Dis.* 139:458, 1989.

41. Coyle, A., et al. The requirement for platelets in allergen-induced late asthmatic airway obstruction. *Am. Rev. Respir. Dis.* 142:587, 1990.

42. Crimi, E., Brusasco, V., and Crimi, P. Effect of nedocromil sodium on the late asthmatic reaction to bronchial antigen challenge. *J. Allergy Clin. Immunol.* 83:985, 1989.

43. Crimi, E., et al. Predictive accuracy of late asthmatic reaction to *Dermatophagoides pteronyssinus. J. Allergy Clin. Immunol.* 78:908, 1986.

44. Crimi, E., et al. Late asthmatic reaction to perennial and seasonal allergens. *J. Allergy Clin. Immunol.* 85:885, 1990.

45. Dahl, R., and Henriksen, J. Development of late asthmatic reactions after allergen or exercise challenge tests. *Eur. J. Respir. Dis.* 61:320, 1980.

46. Davies, R., Green, M., and Schoefield, N. Recurrent nocturnal asthma after exposure to grain dust. *Am. Rev. Respir. Dis.* 114:1011, 1976.

47. D'Brot, J., Abraham, W., and Ahmed, T. Effect of calcium antagonist gallopamil on antigen-induced early and late bronchoconstrictor responses in allergic sheep. *Am. Rev. Respir. Dis.* 139:915, 1989.

48. Delehunt, J., et al. The role of slow-reacting substance of anaphylaxis in the late bronchial response after antigen challenge in allergic sheep. *Am. Rev. Respir. Dis.* 130:748, 1984.

49. DeMonchy, J., et al. Bronchoalveolar eosinophilia during allergen-induced late asthmatic reactions. *Am. Rev. Respir. Dis.* 131:373, 1985.

50. Diaz, P., et al. Leukocytes and mediators in bronchoalveolar lavage during allergen-induced late-phase asthmatic reactions. *Am. Rev. Respir. Dis.* 139:1383, 1989.

51. Dolovich, J., et al. Late-phase airway reaction and inflammation *J. Allergy Clin. Immunol.* 83:521, 1989.

52. Dorsch, W. *Late Phase Allergic Reactions.* Boca Raton: CRC Press, 1990.

53. Durham, S. Late asthmatic responses. *Respir. Med.* 84:263, 1990.

54. Durham, S. The significance of late responses in asthma. *Clin. Exp. Allergy* 21:3, 1991.

55. Durham, S., et al. Leukocyte activation in allergen-induced late-phase asthmatic reactions. *N. Engl. J. Med.* 311:1398, 1984.

56. Durham, S., et al. Increases in airway responsiveness to histamine precede allergen-induced late asthmatic responses. *J. Allergy Clin. Immunol.* 82:764, 1988.

57. Durham, S., and Kay, A. Eosinophils, bronchial hyperreactivity and late-phase asthmatic reactions. *Clin. Allergy* 15:411, 1985.

58. Durham, S., et al. Immunologic studies in allergen-induced late-phase asthmatic reactions. *J. Allergy Clin. Immunol.* 74:49, 1984.

59. Eidelman, D., Bellofiore, S., and Martin, J. Late airway responses to antigen challenge in sensitized inbred rats. *Am. Rev. Respir. Dis.* 137:1033, 1988.

60. Fabbri, L., et al. Bronchoalveolar neutrophilia during late asthmatic reactions induced by toluene diisocyanate. *Am. Rev. Respir. Dis.* 136:36, 1987.

61. Fabbri, L., et al. Prednisone inhibits late asthmatic reactions and the associated increase in airway responsiveness induced by toluene-diisocyanate in sensitized subjects. *Am. Rev. Respir. Dis.* 132:1010, 1985.

62. Fairfax, A., Hanson, J., and Morley, J. The late reaction following bronchial provocation with house dust mite allergen. Dependence on arachidonic acid metabolism. *Clin. Exp. Immunol.* 52:393, 1983.

63. Foresi, A., et al. Late bronchial response and increase in methacholine hyperresponsiveness after exercise and distilled water challenge in atopic subjects with asthma with dual asthmatic response to allergen inhalation. *J. Allergy Clin. Immunol.* 78:1130, 1986.

64. Freed, A., and Jr, N. A. Dry air-induced late phase responses in the canine lung periphery. *Eur. Respir. J.* 3:434, 1990.

65. Frew, A., et al. T lymphocytes in allergen-induced late-phase reactions and asthma. *Int. Arch. Allergy Appl. Immunol.* 88:63, 1989.

66. Frew, A., and Kay, A. Eosinophils and T-lymphocytes in late-phase allergic reactions. *J. Allergy Clin. Immunol.* 85:533, 1990.

67. Frew, A., et al. T lymphocytes and eosinophils in allergen-induced late-phase asthmatic reactions in the guinea pig. *Am. Rev. Respir. Dis.* 141:407, 1990.

68. Frick, W., Sedgwick, J., and Busse, W. The appearance of hypodense eosinophils in antigen-dependent late phase asthma. *Am. Rev. Respir. Dis.* 139:1401, 1989.

69. Gaultier, C., et al. Immediate and late bronchial reactions to house dust in children. *Bull Eur. Physiopathol. Respir.* 15:1091, 1979.

70. Gibson, P., et al. Chronic cough: Eosinophilic bronchitis without asthma. *Lancet* 334:1346, 1989.

71. Gonzalez, M., et al. Allergen-induced recruitment of bronchoalveolar helper (OKT4) and suppressor (OKT8) T-cells in asthma. *Am. Rev. Respir. Dis.* 136:600, 1987.

72. Graneek, B., Durham, S., and Newman-Taylor, A. Late asthmatic reactions and changes in histamine responsiveness provoked by occupational agents. *Bull. Eur. Physiopathol. Respir.* 23:577, 1988.

73. Gwynn, C., et al. Bronchial provocation tests in atopic patients with allergen-specific IgG4 antibodies. *Lancet* 1:254, 1982.

74. Hamid, M., Rafferty, P., and Holgate, S. The inhibitory effect of terfenadine and flurbiprofen on early and late-phase bronchoconstriction following allergen challenge in atopic asthma. *Clin. Exp. Allergy* 20:261, 1990.

75. Hargreave, F., et al. The late asthmatic responses. *Can. Med. Assoc. J.* 110:415, 1974.

76. Hegardt, B., Pauwels, R., and Straeten, M. V. D. Inhibitory effect of KWD 2131, terbutaline and DSCG on the immediate and late allergen-induced bronchoconstriction. *Allergy* 36:115, 1981.

77. Herxheimer, H. Bronchial hypersensitization and hyposensitization in man. *Int. Arch. Allergy Appl. Immunol.* 2:40, 1951.

78. Herxheimer, H. The late bronchial reaction in induced asthma. *Int. Arch. Allergy Appl. Immunol.* 3:323, 1952.

79. Hill, D. Inter-relation of immediate and late asthmatic reactions in childhood. *Allergy* 36:549, 1981.

80. Horn, C., et al. Late response in exercise-induced asthma. *Clin. Allergy* 14:307, 1984.

81. Hutchcroft, B., and Guz, A. Levels of complement components during allergen-induced asthma. *Clin. Allergy* 8:59, 1978.

82. Hutson, P., et al. Early and late-phase bronchoconstriction after allergen challenge of nonanesthetized guinea pigs. I. The association of disor-

dered airway physiology to leukocyte infiltration. *Am. Rev. Respir. Dis.* 137:548, 1988.

83. Hutson, P., Holgate, S., and Church, M. The effect of cromolyn sodium and albuterol on early and late phase bronchoconstriction and airway leukocyte infiltration after allergen challenge of nonanesthetized guinea pigs. *Am. Rev. Respir. Dis.* 138:1157, 1988.

84. Hutson, P., et al. Evidence that neutrophils do not participate in the late-phase airway response provoked by ovalbumin inhalation in conscious, sensitized guinea pigs. *Am. Rev. Respir. Dis.* 141:535, 1990.

85. Hutson, P. A., Holgate, S. T. and Church, M. K. Late Bronchial Responses in the Guinea Pig. In W. Dorsch (ed.), *Late Phase Allergic Reactions.* Boca Raton: CRC Press, 1990. Pp. 373–384.

86. Ihre, E., Axelsson, I., and Zetterström, O. Late asthmatic reactions and bronchial variability after challenge with low doses of allergen. *Clin. Allergy* 18:557, 1988.

87. Iijima, H., et al. Bronchoalveolar lavage and histologic characterization of late asthmatic response in guinea pigs. *Am. Rev. Respir. Dis.* 136:922, 1987.

88. Iikura, Y., et al. Factors predisposing to exercise-induced late asthmatic responses. *J. Allergy Clin. Immunol.* 75:285, 1985.

89. Ill, G. A., and Lichtenstein, L. Indomethacin enhances response of human bronchus to antigen. *Am. Rev. Respir. Dis.* 131:8, 1985.

90. Ito, K., et al. IgG1 antibodies to house dust mite (*Dermatophagoides farinae*) and late asthmatic response. *Int. Arch. Allergy Appl. Immunol.* 81:69, 1986.

91. Iwamoto, I., et al. Thromboxane A2 production in allergen-induced immediate and late asthmatic responses. *J. Asthma* 25:117, 1988.

92. Johns, K., et al. Contribution of upper airways to antigen-induced late airway obstructive responses. *Am. Rev. Respir. Dis.* 142:138, 1990.

93. Kauffman, H., et al. Plasma histamine concentrations and complement activation during house dust mite-provoked bronchial obstructive reactions. *Clin. Allergy* 13:219, 1983.

94. Keyzer, J., et al. Urinary N "tau"-methylhistamine during early and late allergen-induced bronchial-obstructive reactions. *J. Allergy Clin. Immunol.* 74:240, 1984.

95. Kopferschmitt-Kubler, M., Bigot, H., and Pauli, G. Allergen bronchial challenge tests: Variability and reproducibility of the early response. *J. Allergy Clin. Immunol.* 80:730, 1987.

96. Lai, C., Beasley, R., and Holgate, S. The effect of an increase in inhaled allergen dose after terfenadine on the occurrence and magnitude of the late asthmatic response. *Clin. Allergy* 19:209, 1989.

97. Lai, C., Twentyman, O., and Holgate, S. The effect of an increase in inhaled allergen dose after rimiterol hydrobromide on the occurrence and magnitude of the late asthmatic response and the associated change in nonspecific bronchial responsiveness. *Am. Rev. Respir. Dis.* 140:917, 1989.

98. Lai, C. K. W., and Holgate, S. T. Lung Function Parameters in Late Bronchial Reaction and Chronic Bronchial Asthma. In W. Dorsch (ed.), *Late Phase Allergic Reactions.* Boca Raton: CRC Press, 1990. Pp. 391–400.

99. Lam, S., et al. Cellular and protein changes in bronchial lavage fluid after late asthmatic reaction in patients with red cedar asthma. *J. Allergy Clin. Immunol.* 80:44, 1987.

100. Larsen, G. The late asthmatic response. *Chest* 93:1287, 1988.

101. Larsen, G., et al. The inflammatory reaction in the airways in an animal model of the late asthmatic response. *Fed. Proc.* 46:105, 1987.

102. Lee, T., et al. Exercise-induced release of histamine and neutrophil chemotactic factor in atopic asthmatics. *J. Allergy Clin. Immunol.* 70:73, 1982.

103. Lee, T., et al. Exercise-induced late asthmatic reactions with neutrophil chemotactic activity. *N. Engl. J. Med.* 308:1502, 1983.

104. Lee, T., and O'Hickey, S. Exercise-induced asthma and late phase reactions. *Eur. Respir. J.* 2:195, 1989.

105. Lemanske, R. Late-phase pulmonary reactions. *J. Asthma* 27:69, 1990.

106. Lemanske, R., et al. Rhinovirus upper respiratory infection increases airway hyperreactivity and late asthmatic reactions. *J. Clin. Invest.* 83:1, 1989.

107. Lowhagen, O., and Rak, S. Modification of bronchial hyperreactivity after treatment with sodium cromoglycate during pollen season. *J. Allergy Clin. Immunol.* 75:460, 1985.

108. Machado, L. Increased bronchial hypersensitivity after early and late bronchial reactions provoked by allergen inhalation. *Allergy* 40:580, 1985.

109. Machado, L., Stalenheim, G., and Malmberg, P. Early and late allergic bronchial reactions: Physiological characteristics. *Clin. Allergy* 16:111, 1986.

110. MacIntyre, D., and Boyd, G. Site of airflow obstruction in immediate and late reactions to bronchial challenge with *Dermatophagoides pteronyssinus. Clin. Allergy* 13:213, 1983.

111. Malo, J.-L., et al. Late asthmatic reactions to occupational sensitizing agents: Frequency of changes in nonspecific bronchial responsiveness and of response to inhaled beta-2 adrenergic agent. *J. Allergy Clin. Immunol.* 85:834, 1990.

112. Malo, J.-L., L'Archevêque, J., and Cartier, A. Significant changes in nonspecific bronchial responsiveness after isolated immediate bronchospecific reactions caused by isocyanates but not after a late reaction caused by plicatic acid. *J. Allergy Clin. Immunol.* 83:159, 1989.

113. Manning, P., et al. Urinary leukotriene E4 levels during early and late asthmatic responses. *J. Allergy Clin. Immunol.* 86:211, 1990.

114. Mapp, C., et al. Late, but not early, asthmatic reactions induced by toluene-diisocyanate are associated with increased airway responsiveness to methacholine. *Eur. J. Respir. Dis.* 69:276, 1986.

115. Mapp, C., et al. Time course of the increase in airway responsiveness associated with late asthmatic reactions to toluene diisocyanate in sensitized subjects. *J. Allergy Clin. Immunol.* 75:568, 1985.

116. Mattoli, S., et al. Effects of two doses of cromolyn on allergen-induced late asthmatic response and increased responsiveness. *J. Allergy Clin. Immunol.* 79:747, 1987.

117. Mattoli, S., et al. Increase in bronchial responsiveness to methacholine and late asthmatic response after the inhalation of ultrasonically nebulized distilled water. *Chest* 90:726, 1986.

118. McCarthy, D., and Pepys, J. Allergic broncho-pulmonary aspergillosis. Clinical immunology: (2) Skin, nasal and bronchial tests. *Clin. Allergy* 1:415, 1971.

119. Metzger, W. J. Late Phase Asthma in an Allergic Rabbit Model. In W. Dorsch, (ed.), *Late Phase Allergic Reactions.* Boca Raton: CRC Press, 1990. Pp. 347–362.

120. Metzger, W. J. The Use of Bronchoalveolar Lavage (BAL) to Study Late Phase Allergic Asthma. In W. Dorsch, (ed.), *Late Phase Allergic Reactions.* Boca Raton: CRC Press, 1990. Pp. 196–210.

121. Metzger, W., Nugent, K., and Richerson, H. Site of airflow obstruction during early and late phase asthmatic responses to allergen bronchoprovocation. *Chest* 88:369, 1985.

122. Metzger, W., Richerson, H., and Wasserman, S. Generation and partial characterization of eosinophil chemotactic activity and neutrophil chemotactic activity during early and late-phase asthmatic response. *J. Allergy Clin. Immunol.* 78:282, 1986.

123. Metzger, W., et al. Local allergen challenge and bronchoalveolar lavage of allergic asthmatic lungs. Description of the model and local airway inflammation. *Am. Rev. Respir. Dis.* 135:433, 1987.

124. Mohiuddin, A., and Martin, R. Circadian basis of the late asthmatic response. *Am. Rev. Respir. Dis.* 142:1153, 1990.

125. Murphy, K., et al. The requirement for polymorphonuclear leukocytes in the late asthmatic response and heightened airways reactivity in an animal model. *Am. Rev. Respir. Dis.* 134:62, 1986.

126. Nagy, L., Lee, T., and Kay, A. Neutrophil chemotactic activity in antigen-induced late asthmatic reactions. *N. Engl. J. Med.* 306:497, 1982.

127. Nakamura, T., et al. Platelet-activating factor in late asthmatic response. *Int. Arch. Allergy Appl. Immunol.* 82:57, 1987.

128. Nakazawa, T., et al. Pituitary and adrenal functions during late asthmatic responses. *Ann. Allergy* 60:355, 1988.

129. Nakazawa, T., et al. Effect of combined H1 and H2 histamine receptor antagonists on late asthmatic response in an asthmatic patient. *J. Asthma* 24:323, 1987.

130. Nakazawa, T., et al. Low plasma cortisol concentrations during late asthmatic responses. *Br. Med. J.* 291:867, 1985.

131. Nsouli, T., Nsouli, S., and Bellanti, J. Neuroimmunoallergic inflammation: New pathogenetic concepts and future perspectives of immediate and late allergic reactions. Part I (First of two parts). *Ann. Allergy* 60:379, 1988.

132. Nsouli, T., Nsouli, S., and Bellanti, J. Neuroimmunoallergic inflammation: New pathogenetic concepts and future perspectives of immediate and late allergic reactions. Part II. *Ann. Allergy* 60:483, 1988.

133. O'Byrne, P. *Asthma as an Inflammatory Disease.* New York: Marcel Dekker, 1990.

134. O'Byrne, P., Dolovich, J., and Hargreave, F. Late asthmatic responses. *Am. Rev. Respir. Dis.* 136:740, 1987.

135. Paggiaro, P., et al. Atropine does not inhibit late asthmatic responses induced by toluene-diisocyanate in sensitized subjects. *Am. Rev. Respir. Dis.* 136:1237, 1987.

136. Palmqvist, M., et al. Late asthmatic reaction decreased after pretreatment

with salbutamol and formoterol, a new long-acting beta₂ agonist. *J. Allergy Clin. Immunol.* 89:844, 1992.

137. Pauli, G., Bessot, J., and Dietemann-Molard, A. Occupational asthma: Investigations and aetiological factors. *Bull. Eur. Physiopathol. Respir.* 22:399, 1986.

138. Pauwels, R., et al. The effect of theophylline and enprofylline on allergen-induced bronchoconstriction. *J. Allergy Clin. Immunol.* 76:583, 1985.

139. Pelikan, Z., Pelikan-Filipek, M., and Remeijer, L. Effects of disodium cromoglycate and beclomethasone dipropionate on the asthmatic response to allergen challenge II. Late response (LAR). *Ann. Allergy* 60:217, 1988.

140. Pellegrino, R., et al. Effects of deep inhalation during early and late asthmatic reactions to allergen. *Am. Rev. Respir. Dis.* 142:822, 1990.

141. Pepys, J. Inhalation challenge tests in asthma. *N. Engl. J. Med.* 293:758, 1975.

142. Pepys, J. History and Introduction: Late Phase Allergic Reactions. In W. Dorsch (ed.), *Late Phase Allergic Reactions.* Boca Raton: CRC Press, 1990. Pp. 1–8.

143. Pepys, J., and Hutchcroft, B. Bronchial provocation tests in etiologic diagnosis and analysis of asthma. *Am. Rev. Respir. Dis.* 112:829, 1975.

144. Perrin, B., et al. Reassessment of the temporal patterns of bronchial obstruction after exposure to occupational sensitizing agents. *J. Allergy Clin. Immunol.* 87:630, 1991.

145. Pryjma, J., et al. Decrease of complement hemolytic activity after an allergen-house dust-bronchial provocation test. *J. Allergy Clin. Immunol.* 70:306, 1982.

146. Robertson, D. G., et al. Late asthmatic responses induced by ragweed pollen allergen. *J. Allergy Clin. Immunol.* 54:244, 1974.

147. Rohatgi, N., Dunn, K., and Chai, H. Cat- or dog-induced immediate and late asthmatic responses before and after immunotherapy. *J. Allergy Clin. Immunol.* 82:389, 1988.

148. Rubinstein, I., et al. Immediate and delayed bronchoconstriction after exercise in patients with asthma. *N. Engl. J. Med.* 317:482, 1987.

149. Russi, E. W. Late Phase Bronchial Reaction in Sheep. In W. Dorsch (ed.), *Late Phase Allergic Reactions.* Boca Raton: CRC Press, 1990. Pp. 363–372.

150. Sapienza, S., et al. Role of leukotriene D4 in the early and late pulmonary responses of rats to allergen challenge. *Am. Rev. Respir. Dis.* 142:353, 1990.

151. Sasaki, H., et al. Late asthmatic response to ascaris antigen challenge in dogs treated with metyrapone. *Am. Rev. Respir. Dis.* 136:1459, 1987.

152. Siracusa, A., Curradi, F., and Abbritti, G. Recurrent nocturnal asthma due to toluene diisocyanate: A case report. *Clin. Allergy* 8:195, 1978.

153. Smith, H. R., et al. Inflammatory cells and eicosanoid mediators in subjects with late asthmatic responses and increases in airway responsiveness. *J. Allergy Clin. Immunol.* 89:1076, 1992.

154. Sotomayor, H., et al. Seasonal increase of carbachol airway responsiveness in patients allergic to grass pollen. *Am. Rev. Respir. Dis.* 130:56, 1984.

155. Speelberg, B., et al. Immediate and late asthmatic responses induced by exercise in patients with reversible airflow limitation. *Eur. Respir. J.* 2: 402, 1989.

156. Stalenheim, G., and Machado, L. Late allergic bronchial reactions and the effect of allergen provocation on the complement system. *J. Allergy Clin. Immunol.* 75:508, 1985.

157. Stenius, B., et al. Clinical significance of specific IgE to common allergens. *Clin. Allergy* 1:37, 1971.

158. Stevens, F. A comparison of pulmonary and dermal sensitivity to inhaled substances. *J. Allergy* 5:285, 1933–4.

159. Taylor, A. N., et al. Recurrent nocturnal asthmatic reactions to bronchial provocation tests. *Clin. Allergy* 9:213, 1979.

160. Taylor, G., et al. Urinary leukotriene E4 after antigen challenge and in acute asthma and allergic rhinitis. *Lancet* 1:584, 1989.

161. Taylor, G., and Walker, J. Charles Harrison Blackley, 1820–1900. *Clin. Allergy* 3:103, 1973.

162. Tiffeneau, R. Hypersensibilité cholinergo-histaminique pulmonaire de l'asthmatique. Relation avec l'hypersensibilité allergénique pulmonaire. *Acta Allergol. Suppl.* 5:187, 1958.

163. Tossin, L., et al. Ketotifen does not inhibit asthmatic reactions induced by toluene di-isocyanate in sensitized subjects. *Clin. Allergy* 19:177, 1989.

164. Tossin, L., et al. Dexamethasone isonicotinate inhibits dual and late asthmatic reactions but not the increase of airway responsiveness induced by toluene diisocyanate in sensitized subjects. *Ann. Allergy* 63:292, 1989.

165. Turner, C., Kleeberger, S., and Spannhake, E. Preexposure to ozone blocks the antigen-induced late asthmatic response of the canine peripheral airways. *J. Toxicol. Environ. Health* 28:363, 1989.

166. Van Bever, H., and Stevens, W. Suppression of the late asthmatic reaction by hyposensitization in asthmatic children allergic to house dust mite (*Dermatophagoides pteronyssinus*). *Clin. Allergy* 19:399, 1989.

167. Venge, P., and Dahl, R. Are blood eosinophil number and activity important for the development of the late asthmatic reaction after allergen challenge? *Eur. Respir. J.* 2 (Suppl.):430, 1989.

168. Venge, P., Dahl, R., and Hakansson, L. Heat-labile neutrophil chemotactic activity in subjects with asthma after allergen inhalation: Relation to the late asthmatic reaction and effects of asthma medication. *J. Allergy Clin. Immunol.* 80:679, 1987.

169. Warner, J. Significance of late reactions after bronchial challenge with house dust mite. *Arch. Dis. Child.* 51:905, 1976.

170. Wenzel, S. E., Wescott, J. Y., and Larsen, G. L. Bronchoalveolar lavage fluid mediator levels 5 minutes after allergen challenge in atopic subjects with asthma: Relationship to the development of late asthmatic responses. *J. Allergy Clin. Immunol.* 87:540, 1991.

171. Zawadski, D., Lenner, K., and Jr, E. M. Re-examination of the late asthmatic response to exercise. *Am. Rev. Respir. Dis.* 137:837, 1988.

172. Zocca, E., et al. Leukotriene B4 and late asthmatic reactions induced by toluene diisocyanate. *J. Appl. Physiol.* 68:1576, 1990.

Immunoregulation: Role of Macrophages and T-Cells

13

Dennis J. Beer
Ross E. Rocklin

The asthmatic diathesis is characterized by a combination of reversible airway obstruction, increased airway smooth muscle responsiveness to exogenous and endogenous stimuli, and airway inflammation. Pathologic findings in the lungs of subjects with asthma include smooth muscle hypertrophy, subepithelial membranous thickening, disruption of airway epithelium, and airway inflammation associated with mucus plugging. Histologic examination of the airways demonstrates diffuse tissue infiltration with neutrophils, eosinophils, lymphocytes, and mononuclear phagocytes. Because they have undergone degranulation in vivo, mast cells and basophils may be less conspicuous (Fig. 13-1) [57]. The precise mechanisms by which all these cells and their secretory products combine to induce and maintain the underlying airway inflammation and its associated increase in airway responsiveness to myoconstrictor stimuli remain to be determined.

In this chapter, the immunoregulation in asthma is reviewed by analyzing the experimental evidence suggesting the active participation of both lung macrophages and T-lymphocytes in the pathogenesis of airway inflammatory and bronchoconstrictor responses in asthma. The emphasis on these cell types is not meant to deemphasize the important pathogenic contributions other cells such as neutrophils, eosinophils, and metachromatic cells have in the asthma process (see Chaps. 20, 21, and 22). Rather, the biology and clinical consequences of the interactions between the mononuclear cells and the multitude of other cell types participating in the asthmatic diathesis are emphasized.

The chapter is divided into three major parts. The first part is a discussion of the background cellular physiology of macrophages and lymphocytes and their secretory products. The second part reviews the mechanisms of mononuclear cell participation in three major processes contributing to the clinical expression of asthma, namely, the regulation of immunoglobulin E (IgE) synthesis, the regulation of eosinophil production and function, and the generation of the late-phase airway response. The discussion concludes with a scheme integrating mononuclear cell physiology with the multiple other elements involved in the pathogenesis of airway inflammation associated with asthma.

MACROPHAGES

The cells in the mononuclear phagocyte system include promonocytes and their precursors in the bone marrow, monocytes in the circulation, and macrophages in tissue. In the absence of localized inflammation, migration of monocytes into different tissues appears to be a random process. Once in the tissues, monocytes probably do not reenter the systemic circulation; rather, they undergo transformation into tissue macrophages

with morphologic and functional properties that are characteristic for the tissue in which they reside. This cellular transformation is presumably modulated by tissue-specific stimuli [102].

The presence of macrophages at the air-surface interface of human airways has been documented with the technique of bronchoalveolar lavage (BAL) [162] (see Chap. 24). In this procedure, physiologic fluid is instilled and aspirated through a bronchoscope wedged in a peripheral airway. When airway lavage is performed in this manner, the cells retrieved are predominantly macrophages, which are believed to arise predominantly from the alveoli. Modification of the standard BAL technique which permits in vivo isolation and lavage of a proximal airway segment has demonstrated that viable (as defined by the ability to exclude trypan blue) macrophages, identified by Wright-Giemsa staining, nonspecific esterase staining, and transmission electron microscopy, are the predominant white blood cell recovered from both normal and asthmatic subjects [63]. It is considerably more difficult to isolate and lavage airways smaller than a main stem bronchus, but it is a reasonable assumption that macrophages are present in these smaller airways as well. In addition, when bronchial biopsy specimens obtained from asthmatic and normal subjects were examined by immunohistochemical staining with monoclonal antibodies, there was a significantly greater number of macrophages expressing HLA-DR in those specimens obtained from asthmatic subjects compared to the samples obtained from normal individuals. In the bronchial specimens from asthmatic subjects, many of the macrophages had the phenotypic characteristics of blood monocytes, suggesting the recent recruitment of mononuclear phagocytes to the airways of asthmatic subjects [133].

The most important step in the maturation of macrophages from the standpoint of function is the conversion of the normal resting or resident cell to the activated macrophage. The concept of the activated macrophage was developed in the 1960s on the basis of the work of Mackaness and associates, who noted that macrophages from animals that had acquired resistance to facultative intracellular parasite infection had increased microbicidal activity against a variety of organisms [133, 149]. These activated cells had morphologic, functional, and metabolic differences from the resting cells [1, 148]. In the context of asthma, macrophage activation can be accomplished through several pathways. Cytokines including interferon gamma (IFN-γ) [148, 218] and granulocyte-macrophage colony-stimulating factor (GM-CSF) [67, 218], and the interaction of cell surface–bound IgE with relevant antigen [26, 27, 189] are all capable of activating macrophages. Activated macrophages may participate in airway inflammation and airway smooth muscle contraction in patients with asthma through the secretion of respiratory burst products, arachidonate metabolites (prostaglandins and leukotrienes), platelet-activating factor (PAF), preformed mediators (lysosomal enzymes), and newly synthesized peptides termed *monokines*.

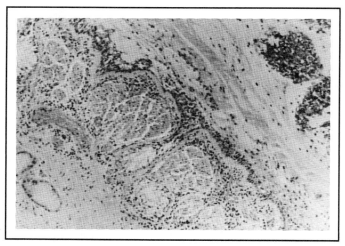

Fig. 13-1. *Bronchial wall from an asthmatic subject showing excessive mucus and cellular debris in the lumen, epithelial cell sloughing, dilated bronchial gland ducts, and a dense inflammatory cell infiltrate. (Autopsy specimen, hematoxylin-eosin, × 145.) (Reprinted with permission from R. Djukanovic, et al. Mucosal inflammation in asthma. Am. Rev. Respir. Dis. 142:434, 1990.)*

Table 13-1. *Physicochemical and biologic characteristics of the FcεRII*

Relatively low binding affinity for IgE (Ka 10^7/M)
Dimeric structure: 45–50-kd alpha chain, 25–33-kd beta chain
Structurally and antigenically distinct from FcεRI on mast cells
Present on platelets, eosinophils, lymphocytes, and macrophages
Identical to Blast-2, a B-lymphocyte–specific activation antigen (CD23)
Expression increased in atopic subjects
Inducible by interleukin-4
Provides a mechanism for IgE-dependent cell activation

MACROPHAGE RECEPTORS FOR THE Fc PORTION OF IgE

In addition to the high-affinity receptor for the Fc portion of IgE (FcεRI) present on mast cells and basophils, investigators in several laboratories [189] have demonstrated that other distinct subpopulations of inflammatory cells also possess specific cell surface membrane receptors for IgE (Table 13-1) (see also Chap. 7). The presence of these specific receptors for IgE on macrophages, eosinophils, and platelets has been documented by rosette formation with IgE-coated erythrocytes, binding of radiolabeled IgE, and use of both polyclonal and monoclonal anti-Fc IgE receptor antibodies [28, 29, 105, 189]. The most striking characteristic of this recently identified inflammatory cell receptor for IgE is its relatively low binding affinity (Ka 10^7/M) for monomeric IgE [4] compared to that of the classic IgE receptor on basophils and mast cells (Ka 10^9/M) [189], from which monomeric IgE dissociates slowly. The IgE receptor on inflammatory cells is a trypsin-sensitive dimer consisting of a 45- to 50-kd alpha chain and a 25- to 33-kd beta chain [28, 105]. This contrasts with the classic metachromatic cell IgE receptor which is a tetramer composed of an alpha, beta, and two gamma chains [189]. The inflammatory cell IgE receptor also is antigenically distinct from that on basophils and mast cells. Antibodies to inflammatory cell IgE receptors and mast cell receptors do not cross-react, whereas polyclonal and monoclonal antibodies to the inflammatory cell IgE receptor bind similarly to macrophages, eosinophils, and platelets and inhibit the interaction of IgE molecules with these cells [28, 30, 189]. Notwithstanding possible structural similarities,

these binding, structural, and antigenic distinctions justify the defining of a second class of receptors for IgE (FcεRII) which are expressed on inflammatory cells. Recently, the B-lympho-cyte–specific activation antigen (Blast-2) was shown to be identical to FcεRII and this category of cell-surface receptor/antigen is designated *CD23* [86].

Although it may be argued that the lower affinity of the FcεRII/CD23 receptor on inflammatory cells could lessen its biologic significance in IgE-dependent reactions, the affinity observed for monomeric IgE is comparable with or even higher than the affinity of the cellular receptor for the Fc portion of IgG [31]. Moreover, the increased affinity for IgE dimers or complexes (Ka 10^8/M) [31] gives this class of receptors particular significance in allergic disorders such as asthma. In addition, the number of FcεRII/CD23-bearing cells increases when IgE levels are increased pathologically or experimentally [25, 189].

The frequency of human peripheral blood monocytes bearing FcεRII/CD23 is increased in atopic subjects, particularly in the presence of high serum IgE levels, while it is negligible on monocytes from normal subjects [140, 189]. Likewise, the percentage of human alveolar macrophages expressing the FcεRII was found to be 18 to 20 percent in patients with allergic asthma, compared with 6 to 8 percent in controls [104]. The expression of FcεRII/CD23 by normal human monocytes can be induced by recombinant interleukin-4 (IL-4)/B-cell stimulatory factor-1 (BSF-1), but not by recombinant IL-1, IL-2, IL-3, IL-5, BSF-2, GM-CSF, IFN-γ, or phorbol esters [211]. Whereas IFN-γ is able to inhibit IL-4 induction of FcεRII/CD23 on B-cells [50], IFN-γ is not able to inhibit IL-4–induced expression of this receptor on monocytes [211].

The observation that IL-4 can induce the expression of FcεRII/CD23 on monocytes is of particular interest in view of the role that this lymphokine may have in the regulation of the IgE system (see below, Regulation of IgE Synthesis). The supernatant of a human alloreactive helper T-cell clone secreting IL-4, but not IFN-γ and IL-2, not only can induce IgE synthesis by normal human B-cells, but also is capable of inducing the expression of FcεRII/CD23 on monocytes and B-lymphocytes [50, 211]. Antibody to IL-4 blocks both of these activities contained within the helper cell supernatants. It is therefore likely that IL-4 plays an important role in the modulation of the IgE system by enhancing not only the synthesis of IgE, but also the expression of its receptors. An increased secretion of IL-4 in asthma may be at least partially responsible for the high percentage of circulating monocytes bearing FcεRII/CD23 observed in this disorder. The simultaneous presence of a large population of FcεRII/CD23 monocytes and high concentrations of serum and in situ IgE may augment receptor-ligand interactions on the monocyte membrane and promote the release of monocyte-derived mediators contributing to the inflammatory component of asthma.

Purified alveolar macrophages obtained by BAL from normal humans can be activated in vitro either by successive incubation with IgE and anti-IgE or by passive sensitization with the IgE-conditioned serum of allergic asthmatic subjects followed by the addition of sensitizing antigen. When anti-IgE or sensitizing antigen is added to alveolar macrophages from atopic asthmatic subjects, there is release of beta glucuronidase, generation of superoxide anion, and secretion of leukotrienes and leukocyte chemotactic factors [5, 68, 80, 104, 160, 201]. When stimulated by lipopolysaccharide, alveolar macrophages and blood monocytes from controls released IL-1 in the same amounts as alveolar macrophages and blood monocytes from allergic asthmatic subjects. After stimulation by anti-IgE or specific allergen, blood monocytes from atopic asthmatic patients released IL-1; however, under the same stimulating conditions, alveolar macrophages from these asthmatic patients did not release IL-1. In fact, the supernatants harvested from anti-IgE– or allergen-stimulated alveolar macrophages contained a 40- to 50-kd IL-1 inhibitory

Table 13-2. Macrophage-derived lipid mediators

Mediator	Other cell sources	Pathophysiologic profile
Eicosanoids		
Cyclooxygenase products		
Prostaglandins (PG)	Mast cells	Smooth muscle contraction
		Mucus secretion
		Mucosal edema (PGE_2)
Thromboxane A_2	Platelets	Smooth muscle contraction
	Mast cells	Mucus secretion
		Pulmonary vasoconstriction
		Platelet aggregation
5-Lipoxygenase products		
Leukotriene B_4	Neutrophils	Leukocyte chemotaxis
		Leukocyte activation
		Leukocyte adherence
		Mucosal inflammation
Leukotrienes C_4, D_4, E_4	Mast cells	Smooth muscle contraction
	Eosinophils	Mucus secretion
	Basophils	Mucosal edema
Platelet-activating factor	Mast cells	Smooth muscle contraction
	Neutrophils	
	Eosinophils	Eosinophil chemotaxis
	Basophils	Eosinophil activation
	Platelets	Mucosal inflammation
	Endothelial cells	Mucosal edema
		Mucus secretion
		Airway hyperresponsiveness

factor [31, 84]. These findings demonstrate a heterogeneity of response based on activating ligand and site of origin of mononuclear phagocytic cells. In addition, these findings provide a mechanism for alveolar macrophage limitation of immune and inflammatory responses to inhaled antigens.

MACROPHAGE-DERIVED LIPID MEDIATORS

The oxygenated derivatives of cell membrane arachidonic acid including prostaglandins, thromboxanes, and leukotrienes (collectively termed eicosanoids) and PAF are lipid mediators produced by multiple cells involved in inflammatory reactions. Alveolar macrophages and their precursor cell, the blood monocyte, produce both eicosanoids and PAF. These compounds have potent biologic activities relevant to the pathogenesis of asthma (Table 13-2).

Eicosanoids

Since the identification and isolation of the first prostaglandins in the 1960s, the cyclooxygenase products of arachidonic acid metabolism have been implicated in the pathogenesis of asthma. In addition to multiple other cell types involved in the asthmatic diathesis, alveolar macrophages possess the enzymatic machinery required for the generation of various prostaglandins (PGD_2, PGE_2, and $PGF_{2\alpha}$) and thromboxanes [131, 159] (see Chap. 11). In humans, whether tested in vitro or in vivo, most of the prostanoids except for those of the E series contract human airway smooth muscle [88, 89]. In human airway tissue explants, PGD_2 and $PGF_{2\alpha}$ significantly increase mucus glycoprotein release [136, 159]. Along these same lines, in normal subjects, inhalation of

$PGF_{2\alpha}$ causes increased airway secretions with the production of mucus glycoproteins [128]. The above-mentioned studies notwithstanding, there is now considerable doubt as to the magnitude of the contribution of prostaglandins to the manifestations of asthma.

In both alveolar macrophages and blood monocytes, lipoxygenation of arachidonic acid yields products with potent inflammatory and bronchoconstrictor effects that are relevant to the pathophysiology of asthma [89, 159, 161]. In particular, the leukotrienes LTC_4, LTD_4, and LTE_4, a group of closely related sulfur-containing conjugated trienes identified in the late 1970s [177], were recognized as being biologically important several decades earlier [111] when they were isolated in lung perfusates and named slow-reacting substance of anaphylaxis (SRS-A). The putative role of leukotrienes as mediators of asthma has been suggested by studies showing the presence of these lipid molecules in the sputum [205], BAL fluid [118], and plasma [150] of asthmatic individuals. Furthermore, fragments of lung [7, 48, 89] and peripheral blood leukocytes from allergic asthmatic subjects [7, 89] have been shown to be able to release leukotrienes after specific antigen challenge in vitro.

These closely related conjugated trienes derived from arachidonic acid are capable of participating in three related processes occurring in asthma. The in vitro and in vivo contractile effects of LTC_4, LTD_4, and LTE_4 on human airway smooth muscle have been adequately documented [7, 48, 49, 103]. Both in vitro and in vivo, these sulfidopeptide leukotrienes are more potent and longer-acting spasmogens than histamine and, in addition, constrict both large and small airways [7, 49, 188]. Both LTC_4 and LTD_4 are potent inducers of mucus release as measured by the output of mucus glycoprotein secretion from in vitro human airway cultures [135]. Lastly, this group of leukotrienes increases microvascular permeability in airway walls [224] and thereby produces airway wall edema and extravasation of plasma proteins into the airway lumen.

Activated macrophages also elaborate the potent chemotactic leukotriene LTB_4 [7, 131, 138] and thereby provides a mechanism for the recruitment of inflammatory leukocytes into the airways. In addition to its function as a chemotaxin, LTB_4 stimulates the release of lysosomal enzymes [66], augments the release of oxygen radicals from human neutrophils [184], and enhances the expression of surface complement (C3b) receptors on human neutrophils and eosinophils [146]. Unlike the sulfidopeptide leukotrienes, LTB_4 has no direct effect on bronchial responsiveness in humans [14]. The generation of LTB_4 by alveolar macrophages can be augmented by T-cell–derived IFN-γ [67, 90, 138]. This observation serves as another example of the interaction between mononuclear cell types in the inflammatory cascade associated with asthma.

Platelet-activating Factor

PAF was the term applied by Benveniste and colleagues to describe the platelet-aggregating activity released from anti-IgE–stimulated rabbit basophils [13]. Subsequently, several groups of investigators physicochemically defined this activity as 1-alkyl-2-acetyl-glycero-3-phosphocholine (AAGPC) [53]. PAF is synthesized de novo as a two-step process involving the generation of lyso-PAF by phospholipase A_2 cleavage of cell membrane phospholipids followed by acetylation of lyso-PAF by acetyltransferase. This process occurs in several inflammatory cells, including neutrophils, eosinophils, platelets, and macrophages. An alternative synthetic pathway involves the generation of PAF directly from the activity of a highly specific phosphocholinetransferase on ether-linked membrane phospholipids. Once generated, PAF is rapidly metabolized and inactivated by an acetylhydrolase located in the cytosol of many tissue cells as well as plasma [7].

Although unequivocal direct evidence that PAF is an important mediator of asthma and airway hyperreactivity does not exist, many observations relating to its generation and presence, as well as to its potential biologic effects, suggest that this lipid molecule contributes to the pathogenesis of asthma. Increased release of PAF and lyso-PAF has been demonstrated after in vitro allergen challenge of alveolar macrophages obtained from patients with asthma. In addition, PAF has been detected in the BAL fluid from some asthmatic individuals [45] and its major metabolite, lyso-PAF, appears in the plasma of patients experiencing a late-phase asthmatic response following allergen challenge [147]. The biologic properties of PAF include chemoattraction of eosinophils [19, 216], induction of an airway inflammatory response [214], augmentation of airway vascular permeability [64], mucus secretion [85], elicitation of airway smooth muscle contraction [47, 174], and a sustained increase in airway responsiveness [47, 174].

LYMPHOCYTES

T-lymphocytes, like B-lymphocytes, are derived from stem cells located within the hematopoietic tissues. T-cell precursors migrate to the thymus where they undergo an ordered differentiation process that can be followed both by analysis of expression of the CD4 and CD8 cell surface glycoproteins and by the determination of expression and rearrangement of the genes that encode the T-cell receptor variable and constant regions. At this stage in thymocyte development, contact with major histocompatibility complex (MHC) antigens expressed on thymic epithelial cells leads to both the selection of T-cells that can corecognize foreign antigens together with self-MHC molecules and the deletion of autoreactive T-cells [123, 193, 203].

In association with this intrathymic selection process, double positive thymocytes expressing both CD4 and CD8 develop into T-cells that express either CD4 or CD8 on their surface and increase their expression of the T-cell receptor complex polypeptides. These mature T-cells then exit the thymus and distribute to the peripheral or secondary lymphoid tissues, namely, the spleen, lymph nodes, tonsils, and unencapsulated lymphoid aggregates throughout the body. In general, CD4$^+$ T-cells function as helper or regulatory cells while CD8$^+$ T-cells function as cytotoxic or suppressor cells in immune responses [123, 193].

More recently, based on differences in their pattern of cytokine production, the CD4$^+$ T-lymphocyte population has been subdivided into helper T-cell subsets designated Th1 and Th2 [192]. This was established first in the mouse where murine T-cell clones of the Th1 subset elaborate IL-2 and IFN-γ, but not IL-4 and IL-5, and T-cell clones of the Th2 subset produce IL-4 and IL-5, but not IL-2 and IFN-γ [36, 145]. Since most alloreactive or phytohemagglutinin (PHA)-induced human CD4$^+$ T-cell clones derived from the peripheral blood of healthy donors do not fit clearly into the Th1 or Th2 subsets, this classification was thought initially not to be appropriate for the human CD4$^+$ T-lymphocyte subset. Most recently, however, several groups of investigators [134, 170] found that CD4$^+$ T-cell clones that exhibit Th1- or Th2-like profiles can accumulate in tissues or peripheral blood of patients with different disease states. For example, most CD4$^+$ T-cells infiltrating the thyroid gland in patients with autoimmune thyroiditis, when stimulated by PHA in vitro, develop into T-cell clones that produce IFN-γ, but not IL-4; most T-lymphocytes infiltrating the conjunctiva of patients with allergic vernal conjunctivitis develop into T-cell clones producing large amounts of IL-4 but no or limited amounts of IFN-γ [134, 170]. More germaine to the asthmatic diathesis, the great majority of allergen-specific T-cell clones derived from atopic donors produce IL-4 and IL-5 but no or limited quantities of IFN-γ. In contrast, virtually all T-cell clones specific for bacterial components established from the same atopic donors produced large amounts of IL-2 and IFN-γ, whereas only a portion of those clones secreted IL-4 or IL-5 [221].

Whereas the role of B-lymphocytes committed to the synthesis of antigen-specific IgE in the humoral response in allergic asthma is well established, the precise role of T-cells in the inflammatory response of asthma is in a state of evolution. Several lines of evidence support the view that T-cells are involved in the pathogenesis of asthma. Postmortem examination of the airways of patients with asthma reveals, among multiple inflammatory changes, large numbers of lymphocytes [57, 59, 60]. Study of the light and electron microscopic structure of lobar bronchial specimens taken at fiberoptic bronchoscopy from symptomatic atopic asthmatic patients reveals loss of surface epithelium, thickening of the reticular lamina of the epithelial basement membrane, and increased numbers of irregularly shaped intraepithelial lymphocytes [100, 165]. Further support for the recruitment and activation of lymphocytes in the airways of asthmatic subjects comes from the investigation of Azzawi and coworkers [6] demonstrating an increase in the number of IL-2 receptor (IL-2R, CD25)–positive T-cells in the central bronchial walls of atopic asthmatic patients, but not in the airway walls of atopic nonasthmatic and normal control subjects (Fig. 13-2).

Along these same lines, immunohistochemical staining defining lymphocyte subsets in bronchial biopsy specimens obtained from symptomatic asthmatic patients was compared to that performed on biopsy specimens obtained from asymptomatic asthmatic patients and normal controls. There was no significant difference either in any lymphocyte subset or in CD25$^+$ T-cells between the nonasthmatic control subjects and the asymptomatic asthmatic patients. By contrast, in the symptomatic asthmatic patients, the presence of CD3$^+$ T-cells, CD4$^+$ T-cells, CD25$^+$ T-cells, and natural killer (NK) cells in bronchial biopsy specimens was significantly increased compared with both the normal controls and asymptomatic asthmatic subjects [78]. This histologic picture extends to biopsy specimens obtained from both nonatopic, intrinsic asthmatic patients and atopic, extrinsic asthmatic patients [12].

Further evidence of T-cell activation in asthma comes from the studies of Corrigan and colleagues [43, 44]. Utilizing flow cytometric techniques to measure the expression of T-lymphocyte cell surface activation markers (HLA-DR, IL-2R, and very late activation-1 [VLA-1]), these investigators identified T-cells expressing these surface markers in the peripheral blood of patients with acute severe asthma. The percentage of activated blood T-cells decreased after therapy and clinical improvement. Peripheral blood T-lymphocytes from subjects with mild asthma or chronic obstructive pulmonary disease or normal subjects showed no such evidence of activation. In addition, serum concentrations of IFN-γ and soluble IL-2R, two proteins derived from activated T-cells, were elevated in patients with acute severe asthma but not in the control groups. Concentrations of these activated T-cell secretory products decreased as the patients improved clinically. Lastly, in those patients studied for 7 days, a peak expiratory flow rate of less than 50 percent of predicted was associated with higher numbers of activated CD4$^+$ lymphocytes and serum concentrations of IL-2R and IFN-γ. Taken together, these observations suggest that CD4$^+$ lymphocyte activation may contribute to the pathogenesis of ongoing, as well as acute severe asthma.

Bronchial allergen challenge studies also have provided evidence for the involvement of T-lymphocytes in the pathogenesis of asthma. After inhalation challenge of asymptomatic atopic asthmatic patients with relevant allergen, Gerblich and associates [81] observed a decrease in peripheral blood CD4$^+$ lymphocytes that persisted for at least 72 hours and after 48 hours was associated with an increase in the number of HLA-DR-positive (activated) T-cells. Further study with this model demonstrated

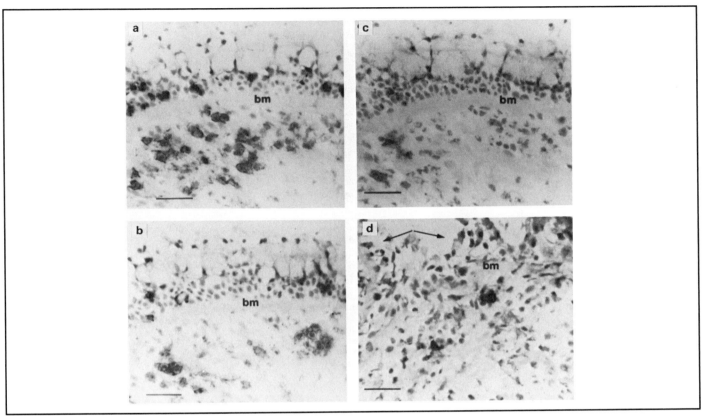

Fig. 13-2. *Bronchial mucosa from an asthmatic subject showing monoclonal antibody staining. a. CD3$^+$ T-cells above and below the epithelial basement membrane (bm). b. CD4$^+$ T-cells. c. CD8$^+$ T-cells in low frequency. d. CD25$^+$ (anti–interleukin-2 receptor)-activated T-cells beneath sloughing surface epithelium (arrows). ($\times$ 400.) Scale bar = approximately 50 μm. (Reprinted with permission from M. Azzawi, et al. Identification of activated T-lymphocytes and eosinophils in bronchial biopsies in stable atopic asthma.* Am. Rev. Respir. Dis. *142:1407, 1990.)*

that the allergen challenge–induced decrease in blood CD4$^+$ lymphocytes was associated with an increased percentage of CD4$^+$ cells recovered from the airways by BAL [83]. These data suggest a process of recruitment of peripheral CD4$^+$ lymphocytes into the respiratory tract of atopic asthmatic subjects undergoing allergen bronchoprovocation. In addition, there is a difference in the profile of regulatory T-cell subsets present in BAL fluid in subjects who respond to allergen bronchoprovocation with an early bronchoconstrictor response alone, as compared to those manifesting a dual asthmatic response. In the latter group, there is a relative inability to recruit CD8$^+$ cells into the lung [83].

MONONUCLEAR CELL–DERIVED CYTOKINES

Cytokines are a group of low-molecular-weight proteins produced by T-lymphocytes and monocytes/macrophages. These mediators have an important function in many physiologic responses and, in addition, contribute to the pathophysiology of many disease processes including asthma. Their properties include regulation of the amplitude and duration of immune and inflammatory responses, paracrine or autocrine activity at very low (picomolar) concentrations, and interaction with high-affinity receptors on cell surfaces (Fig. 13-3). Individual cytokines have multiple overlapping cell regulatory actions and work in a

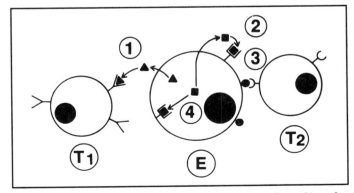

Fig. 13-3. *Modes of intercellular communication through cytokines. In the schematic, (1) a cytokine-producing effector cell (E) releases a cytokine molecule (solid triangle), which interacts with a nearby target cell (T$_1$) in a paracrine fashion; (2) by the autocrine pathway as effector cell secretes cytokine (solid squares), which interacts with its receptor on the surface of the same cell; (3) there is direct cell-cell communication via a cytokine integral to the membrane of the effector cell (solid circles), which interacts with the appropriate receptor on a contiguous target cell (T$_2$); and (4) in the modified autocrine pathway the intracellular cytokine (squares) interacts with its receptor on the inside of the cell. (Reprinted with permission from J. Kelley. Cytokines of the lung.* Am. Rev. Respir. Dis. *141:765, 1990.)*

Table 13-3. Mononuclear cell–derived cytokines

Mediator	Cell sources	Physicochemical structure	Biological profile
Platelet-derived growth factor	Macrophages Epithelial cells Platelets Endothelial cells	30-kd cationic glycoprotein Homodimer or heterodimer	Competence growth factor Inflammatory cell chemoattractant
Granulocyte-macrophage colony-stimulating factor	T-cells Endothelial cells	22-kd glycoprotein Encoded on chromosome 5	Species-specific leukocyte growth and activating factor
Interleukin-1α and β	Macrophages Endothelial cells Glial cells T- and B-cells Epithelial cells	31-kd precursors; 17.5-kd biologically active form	T- and B-cell growth and activation Macrophage and fibroblast activation Inducer of intercellular adhesion molecule-1
Interleukin-3	T-cells	15–17-kd protein Encoded on chromosome 5	Species-specific leukocyte growth factor Eosinophil activator
Interleukin-4 (IL-4)	T-cells Mast cells Fibroblasts Myeloid cell lines	20-kd glycoprotein Encoded on chromosome 5	B-cell isotype switching to IgE and IgG1 Inducer of B-cell MHC Class II and CD23 surface antigens
Interleukin-5	T-cells Mast cells Fibroblasts	18-kd glycoprotein Encoded on chromosome 5	Selective eosinophil growth and activating factor B-cell growth factor
Interleukin-6	Macrophages T-cells Fibroblasts	21–28-kd glycoprotein	Promoter of antibody secretion by B-cells Stem cell hematopoietin T-cell growth factor
Interferon gamma	T-cells	Homodimeric glycoprotein consisting of 21–24-kd subunits	Macrophage activator Inducer of MHC Class II surface antigens Inducer of intercellular adhesion molecule-1 Inhibitor of IL-4–induced IgE synthesis Inhibitor of viral replication Inhibitor of B- and T-cell growth and activation
Transforming growth factor-beta	Macrophages T-cells	25-kd protein Homodimer or heterodimer	Stimulates collagen production
Tumor necrosis factor-alpha	Macrophages Mast cells	17-kd multimer	Endothelial cell, granulocyte, and macrophage activator Stimulator of antibody secretion Cytotoxic for multiple cell types Stimulates angiogenesis
Histamine-releasing factors	Mononuclear cells Platelets	15–30-kd family of cytokines	Stimulate release of histamine and leukotrienes from mast cells and basophils

network by inducing each other; by altering cell surface receptor expression; and by synergistic, additive, or inhibitory interactions on cell function (Table 13-3). The growing awareness of these complex cytokine interactions has led to the concept that tissue homeostatic mechanisms are controlled by cytokine cascades and networks rather than by individual cytokines.

Recent studies [56, 164, 164a] investigated the cytokine messenger RNA (mRNA) profile in BAL-retrieved lymphocytes from atopic asthmatic subjects. In one study using in situ hybridization and flow cytometry, the BAL cells harvested from asthmatic subjects demonstrated increased expression of mRNA for cytokines in the IL-4 family (IL-3, IL-4, IL-5, and GM-CSF) but not IFN-γ. These observations suggested the predominant activation of the Th2-like T-cell population. Furthermore, there was a strong correlation between IL-5 mRNA-positive cells and the presence of activated (CD25⁺) CD4⁺ T-lymphocytes, which correlated with the number of eosinophils seen in the lavage fluid [164]. In another study, the percent of IL-4 mRNA-positive T-cells retrieved from allergen-challenged bronchial segments of atopic asthmatic subjects was significantly higher than those obtained from unchallenged bronchial segments [56].

In addition to detection of cytokine mRNA-positive lymphocytes harvested by BAL from asthmatic subjects, a more recent study [17a] has demonstrated the presence of tumor necrosis factor (TNF), GM-CSF, IL-2, and IL-6 in the BAL fluid harvested from symptomatic asthmatic subjects. Furthermore, macrophage-derived IL-1 has been detected in the bronchial lavage fluid obtained in the early morning hours from patients with nocturnal asthma. The amount of detectable IL-1 correlated with

disease activity and pretreatment of these individuals with corticosteroids resulted in the diminished presence of IL-1 in lavage fluid and improvement in nocturnal asthma symptoms [137].

Platelet-derived Growth Factor

Platelet-derived growth factor (PDGF) is a highly cationic glycoprotein with a molecular mass of 30 kd that is synthesized by a variety of cells including megakaryocytes, platelets, endothelial cells, epithelial cells, mesenchymal cells, and activated monocytes/macrophages [112, 144, 171]. PDGF is composed of two separate polypeptide chains (A chain and B chain) linked by multiple disulfide bonds. The biologic properties of PDGF are dependent on the composition of the intact dimer molecule (A-B heterodimers or A-A or B-B homodimers). In addition to being chemotactic for infiltrating inflammatory cells, PDGF also stimulates proinflammatory properties of these and resident lung cells [54, 112, 144, 171].

Granulocyte-Macrophage Colony-stimulating Factor

With the development of in vitro tissue culture techniques that support the clonal growth of every class of bone marrow hematopoietic cell, it has become clear that hematopoiesis is under the control of a large family of glycoprotein cytokines collectively named *hematopoietic colony-stimulating factors* [38, 185]. These cytokines work both individually and synergistically at many different ontogenetic levels of hematopoiesis and regulate not only the proliferation and differentiation of progenitor cells but also the rate at which mature blood cells exit the marrow and the functional capacity and tissue survival of these cells.

GM-CSF is a 22-kd glycoprotein produced by T-cells and endothelial cells that drives the formation of mixed colonies of granulocytes and macrophages from normal bone marrow [223]. Unlike other cytokines where cross-species activities are observed down the phylogenetic tree, the hematopoietic effects of GM-CSF are species specific. In addition to its effects on hematopoiesis, GM-CSF participates in the activation of neutrophils, eosinophils, and macrophages [41, 127].

Interleukin-1

Originally recognized for its ability to induce proliferation of murine thymocytes, IL-1 is now known to be an important mediator of inflammatory processes [112, 152]. Two forms of IL-1 (IL-1α and IL-1β) that have been identified have slightly different physicochemical properties but bind to the same target cell receptor and have similar spectra of activity [175, 186]. These interleukins are the products of two different genes and share 26 percent homology in final amino acid sequences. Both IL-1 molecules are synthesized as 31-kd precursors, and the biologically active forms are 17.5 kd. The macrophage is a major source of IL-1 and its production can be augmented by certain T-cell products such as IFN-γ [55]. IL-1 modulates hematopoietic and lymphoid cells by inducing the synthesis of colony-forming factors and contributing to the activation and clonal expansion of T- and B-cells. In addition, IL-1 indirectly contributes to inflammation by activation of macrophages, fibroblasts, and endothelial cells [112, 152].

Interleukin-3

IL-3, initially defined for its ability to induce the expression of the enzyme 20α steroid dehydrogenase in cultures of nude mouse spleen cells and to promote clonal expansion of basophil and mast cell precursors, is viewed presently as a colony-stimulating factor for most hematopoietic cell lines [92, 93]. IL-3 has a molecular mass of 15 to 17 kd, is produced by activated T-cells, and like GM-CSF has a high degree of species specificity [92, 226].

Interleukin-4

IL-4 is a multifunctional glycoprotein cytokine (molecular mass 20 kd) produced by T-cells [153], mast cells [21, 222], and some myeloid cell lines [153]. It was initially described as a B-lymphocyte stimulatory factor based on its capacity to enhance the proliferation of resting B-cells treated with low concentrations of anti-IgM antibody [116]. IL-4 also causes an increase in B-cell volume and viability [153] and induces or augments B-cell surface expression of Class II MHC molecules [172, 187], CD23 [50, 211], and its own receptor. Many of the effects of IL-4 are downregulated by IFN-γ [50, 155].

Interleukin-5

In the course of experiments designed to determine the accessory molecules necessary for B-cell replication, a factor distinct from IL-4 was isolated and called *T-cell–replacing factor* or *B-cell growth factor-2* [116, 227]. Latter designated IL-5, this cytokine has the precise molecular structure of eosinophil differentiation factor [114] and thereby is implicated in the eosinophilic tissue response that typifies asthma.

Interleukin-6

IL-6, also termed *interferon beta₂, B-cell differentiation factor,* and *hepatocyte stimulatory factor,* is a 21- to 28-kd glycoprotein cleaved from a larger precursor molecule produced by T-cells,

fibroblasts, tumor cells, and macrophages [112, 202]. This pleiotropic hormone acts in concert with other interleukins to promote B-cell secretion of immunoglobulin including IgE [210] and proliferation of the earliest of hematopoietic bone marrow stem cells [94].

Interferon Gamma

As a member of the interferon family of cytokines, IFN-γ was first described and purified on the basis of its ability to interfere with viral replication in fibroblasts [220]. This T-cell product activates macrophages and enhances cell expression of Class II MHC surface antigens, thereby promoting the interaction of various cells involved in an immune response [113, 212]. In addition, IFN-γ induces the expression of intercellular adhesion molecule-1 (ICAM-1) on airway epithelial cells, thereby promoting the adhesion of leukocytes and the subsequent development of an inflammatory cell infiltrate [217]. Lastly, IFN-γ strongly inhibits IL-4–induced IgE synthesis [155].

Transforming Growth Factor-beta

The transforming growth factors were originally defined by their ability to induce the transformed phenotype in nonneoplastic cells, whereby these cells were capable of growing in an anchorage-independent noncontact-inhibited manner [51]. Transforming growth factor-beta (TGF-β) is a 25-kd protein consisting of two identical subunit chains joined covalently by disulfide bonds. A heterodimer consisting of one chain of TGF-β₁ and -β₂ also exists. Many cells including activated T-cells and macrophages produce this molecule. TGF-β has antiproliferative effects on a wide variety of neoplastic and normal cells including T- and B-lymphocytes [110, 112, 191]. In this way, it serves an important negative feedback role. On the other hand, it potentiates an inflammatory process by its capacity to attract and activate monocytes [213].

Tumor Necrosis Factor-alpha

Tumor necrosis factor was discovered based on its ability to induce hemorrhagic necrosis in certain tumors and produce wasting (cachectin) during parasitic disease [32]. A multimer of 17 kd that is initially produced as an inactive propeptide, tumor necrosis factor-alpha (TNF-α) is a proinflammatory cytokine that is strikingly toxic and unlike most cytokines, acts both locally and systemically. In addition to cytotoxicity, TNF-α induces myriad biologic effects including endothelial cell, granulocyte, and macrophage activation [18, 24]; differentiation of myeloid cells [204]; angiogenesis [121]; and growth and antibody secretion of B-cells [101].

Histamine-releasing Factors

Histamine-releasing factors (HRFs) are an incompletely characterized group of molecules of molecular mass between 15 and 30 kd, produced by macrophages, lymphocytes, and platelets. These mediators release histamine and leukotrienes from basophils and mast cells [65, 106, 199].

REGULATION OF IgE SYNTHESIS

The IgE antibody system is a sophisticated immune defense mechanism whose specific functions are only partially understood; it is discussed in detail in Chapters 7 and 8. In a broad sense, this humoral immune system protects against offending agents coming from the respiratory and gastrointestinal tracts. IgE molecules, induced by environmental antigens (allergens),

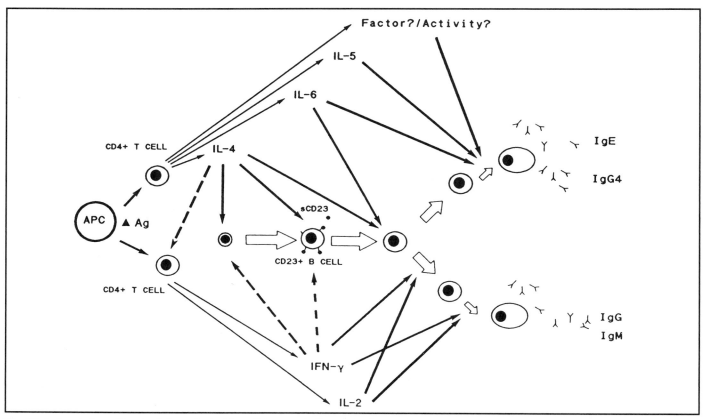

Fig. 13-4. *Regulation of human IgE synthesis. The solid arrows indicate stimulatory effects and stippled arrows, inhibitory effect. For details, see text. Ag = antigen; IFN = interferon; IL = interleukin. (Reprinted with permission from J. Pene. Regulatory role of cytokines and CD23 in the human IgE antibody synthesis. Int. Arch. Allergy Appl. Immunol. 90:32, 1989.)*

bind specifically to high-affinity receptors (FcεRI) localized on the surface of tissue mast cells and circulating basophils [96] and to low-affinity receptors (FcεRII) on B- and T-cells, eosinophils, platelets, and macrophages [25]. The reintroduction of antigen, which cross-links FcεR-bound IgE, induces the release of a variety of mediators that participate in the pathogenesis of asthma.

The induction of IgE antibody synthesis in response to allergens requires the collaboration of B-lymphocytes with macrophages and T-lymphocytes (Fig. 13-4). Class II MHC–bearing dendritic cells, similar to the Langerhans' cells of the skin, are positioned in human airway epithelium and function as an intraepithelial trap for inhaled aeroallergens [91]. Along these lines, it has been demonstrated that the number of dendritic cells in nasal epithelium of patients with grass pollen sensitivity is significantly higher during the grass pollen season [73]. Although not proven, one could postulate that a similar increase could occur in the lower respiratory tract. After antigen entrapment, the dendritic cells process allergen molecules and transport them from the airway surface to regional lymph nodes where the allergenic peptides are presented, in the context of Class II MHC, to naive T-lymphocytes [115]. The continuous, stable, and preferential presentation of certain allergenic peptides on extended surfaces of dendritic cells can considerably increase the probability of recognition by T-cells bearing a receptor specific for those peptides, with subsequent proliferation, expansion, and colonization in local lymphoid structures.

Early evidence for the requirement of T-cells in the regulation of IgE synthesis was provided by the observations that neonatally thymectomized rats [151] and athymic nude mice [97] were unable to generate IgE antibody. This defect could be corrected

by the infusion of normal thymocytes. Furthermore, subsequent animal studies in which rodents received either sublethal wholebody irradiation or low-dose cyclophosphamide demonstrated that IgE production was regulated by two functionally distinct T-cell subpopulations, namely helper/inducer and suppressor T-cells [194, 196]. Under the above-mentioned experimental circumstances, the abrogation of suppressor T-cell converted rats from their usual pattern of low-level IgE production to patterns of sustained IgE synthesis. This enhanced IgE response could be abolished by passive transfer of syngeneic T-cells. These observations provided evidence that the low level of IgE response in unmanipulated rats reflects the dominance of a suppressor T-cell regulatory control mechanism that normally limits IgE production. Of note, these experimental measures did not affect IgG production, indicating that the two antibody isotypes are subject to qualitatively or quantitatively different regulatory mechanisms.

Independent observations in humans suggest that similar to the circumstances in animals, IgE production also is under T-cell regulatory influences. First, patients with primary immunodeficiency disorders such as ataxia telangiectasia and Wiskott-Aldrich, Nezelof's, and DiGeorge's syndromes [20] have increased serum IgE levels. Second, several diseases, including the hyperIgE syndrome, severe atopic dermatitis, and acute graft-versushost disease, are associated with decreased suppressor T-cell number and function and extremely high serum IgE levels.

Our current understanding of the regulation of IgE synthesis derives from experimental animal models and in vitro human lymphocyte culture systems. Bone marrow stem cells undergo a series of maturational steps culminating in the development of B-cells committed to the production of a specific immunoglobulin isotype. This developmental process of B-cell commitment to IgE synthesis results from a complex interaction between monocytes, T-cells, and B-cells, under the control of T-cell– and monocyte-derived cytokines.

As demonstrated in experiments on cultured human blood peripheral mononuclear cells from normal donors, unlike other isotypes, IgE synthesis could not be induced by classic polyclonal activators such as pokeweed mitogen and *Staphylococcus aureus* Cowan I [71, 180, 182, 190]. This suggested either of two possibilities. First, IgE precursor B-cells are absent from the circulation of normal donors or, second, the activation of IgE-producing B-cells requires T-cell–derived signals not generated by normal T-cells under other isotype-inducing conditions. In regard to the latter possibility, supernatants from unstimulated T-cells of patients with hyper-IgE states contain a soluble helper factor that induces IgE but not IgG synthesis by normal B-cells. In contrast, supernatants from T-cells of normal individuals had no effect on IgE synthesis [180, 181].

In addition to T-cell–derived soluble factors, direct T–B-lymphocyte interactions also are involved in the induction of IgE antibody production. Normal B-cells bearing the appropriate alloantigen can be induced to synthesize immunoglobulin of all isotypic classes on cognate interaction with selected human alloreactive or autoreactive T-cell clones [119, 122, 206]. These and the above-mentioned experiments provide clear evidence for the presence, in normal individuals, of circulating B-lymphocytes with the potential to differentiate into IgE-secreting cells.

In the murine system, the T-cell–derived lymphokine IL-4 induces in vitro IgE production by lipopolysaccharide-stimulated B-cell blasts and, in addition, administration of anti–IL-4 antibody inhibits an in vivo IgE response [39, 40, 69]. These animal studies have been extended to humans. IL-4 secreted from T-cell clones or in recombinant form induces IgE synthesis by normal blood mononuclear cells but not by purified B-cells [52, 99, 155]. In this system of human T- and B-cell populations, optimal IL-4 induction of IgE synthesis requires the presence of monocytes [208]. Thus, additional soluble signals, derived from both T-cells and monocytes, are required for IL-4–induced IgE production.

Several T-cell– and monocyte-derived cytokines have been shown to influence IL-4–dependent IgE synthesis. Both IL-5 and IL-6 upregulate the IgE response induced by IL-4 and the presence of anti–IL-6 antibody in mononuclear cell culture inhibits IgE synthesis [210]. In contrast, IL-1 and TNF-α have no amplifying effect on IgE production [208, 210]. In contrast, under certain circumstances, IFN-γ inhibits IL-4–dependent IgE synthesis [155]. Although the exact molecular biology of this cytokine cascade is not defined completely, one can hypothesize a model in which the maturation of human B-cells is sequentially regulated. In this model, IL-4 activates resting B-cells and promotes isotype switching, IL-5 promotes their growth and differentiation, and IL-6 amplifies and enhances their terminal differentiation into IgE-secreting plasma cells [117].

In addition to the requirement of mononuclear cell–derived cytokines for IgE synthesis, physical contact between T- and B-cells might also be required for IL-4–dependent IgE production. If IL-4–pulsed mixtures of autologous T- and B-cells are separated in culture by a permeable membrane, IgE synthesis is abrogated [208, 209]. Likewise, IL-4–dependent IgE synthesis is inhibited by monoclonal antibodies specific for cell adhesion molecules such as CD2, CD4, and lymphocyte function–associated antigen-1 (LFA-1) [208, 209]. As evidenced by the blockade of IgE synthesis by monoclonal antibodies directed at the T-cell receptor complex, this requirement of T–B-lymphocyte contact consists of cognate interaction between the T-cell receptor/CD3 complex on T-cells and Class II MHC antigens on B-cells [209].

More recent investigation revealed a T-cell– and monocyte-independent system for induction of IgE synthesis [98]. Engagement of the B-lymphocyte antigen CD40 (a 50-kd surface glycoprotein) by F(ab')₂ fragments of a monoclonal antibody in the presence of IL-4 induces intense IgE but not IgG production by highly purified human surface IgE-negative B-cells. As seen under other culture conditions, the addition of neutralizing anti–IL-6 to this in vitro system of highly purified B-cells cultured in the presence of IL-4 and Fab fragments of antibody directed against CD40 strongly but not completely inhibited the production of IgE response.

Immunoglobulin-binding factors (Ig-BFs) modulate immunoglobulin synthesis by B-cells. IgE-BFs are produced by B- and T-lymphocytes. The role of IgE-BF from T-cells has been documented extensively in animal models [95, 107]. In humans, most of the studies in this area have focused on the IgE-BF/CD23 of B-cell origin. As mentioned previously, CD23 is the same molecule as FcεRII. Epstein-Barr virus (EBV)–transformed lymphoblastoid B-cell lines constitutively release a soluble factor that binds to IgE and reacts with monoclonal antibody directed against CD23, indicating that this factor is an IgE-BF [15, 154]. IL-4 induces from normal human B-cells the release of soluble CD23, which immunoprecipitates with anti-CD23 monoclonal antibody and is biochemically and antigenically equivalent to the soluble CD23 spontaneously released by CD23⁺ B-cell lines [15, 154]. Soluble CD23 released in the supernatants of CD23⁺ lymphoblastoid cell lines enhances the ongoing IL-4–induced IgE production by B-cells derived from atopic donors. This soluble CD23 enhancement of ongoing IgE production is indirect and requires the presence of T-cells [154, 178, 179].

Dysregulation of IgE Synthesis

As alluded to above, antibody responses of the IgE isotype are regulated by a finely tuned network of complex cellular and molecular interactions. In this network, the T-lymphocyte plays the most sophisticated regulatory role. There are helper and suppressor T-cells capable of mutually interacting with one another as well as with IgE antibody–secreting cells.

A functionally distinct subset of CD8⁺ human T-cells with suppressor capabilities has been defined by the presence of functional histamine Type 2 (H₂) receptors [10]. Several investigators [11, 139] have demonstrated decreased histamine-induced suppressor cell–activity which was paralleled by a decreased number of circulating T-cells bearing H₂ receptors [11] in patients with allergic asthma and/or rhinoconjunctivitis.

Although the relation between histamine-induced suppressor-cell dysfunction and the regulation of in vivo biosynthesis of IgE is not clear, it is possible that atopic subjects have a global in vivo deficiency in antigen-nonspecific and/or antigen-specific suppressor-cell activity, either or both of which may be necessary for the dampening of IgE antibody production. Indirect evidence for this hypothesis comes from a study [168] demonstrating that ragweed antigen–specific suppressor T-lymphocytes could be detected in ragweed-allergic individuals after 6 and 12 months of immunotherapy, but not prior to therapy. The induction of these ragweed-specific suppressor T-cells correlated with diminution of serum IgE levels. When lymphocytes were taken from treated patients and passed over columns containing insolubilized histamine, antigen-specific suppressor T-cells that could be activated by ragweed antigen were deleted. These results indicated that antigen-specific suppressor T-cells belonging to the subpopulation of lymphocytes bearing histamine receptors were generated during immunotherapy, and failure to detect these cells in untreated patients may be a reflection of a basic defect contributing to the atopic diathesis.

Rocklin and coworkers [167] analyzed the effect of fanetizole mesylate, a new immunostimulating drug similar in activity to levamisole, on histamine-induced suppressor activity and IgE synthesis in vitro. When this compound was added with histamine to mononuclear cells from atopic subjects during the generation of histamine-induced suppressor cells, their ability to suppress a subsequent mitogen-induced lymphocyte proliferation response was equivalent to that of suppressor cells from normal donors. In addition, in vitro IgE synthesis by mononuclear cells from atopic subjects was reduced significantly in the presence of fanetizole mesylate. This compound was found not to be cytotoxic for B-cells, and in fact the drug did not significantly alter pokeweed mitogen–induced IgG synthesis by atopic or normal mononuclear cells. These results suggested that fanetizole mesylate could partially correct an in vitro immunoregulatory defect in atopic individuals and could reduce IgE production. Whether this represented cause and effect has not been determined and clinical trials of this drug in the treatment of allergic subjects have not been published.

Another alteration in atopic individuals could be related to the progressive development of a greater proportion of Th2-like T-cell clones that favor IgE production by their preferential production of high amounts of cytokines like IL-4 and no or reduced amounts of IFN-γ. Supportive evidence for this hypothesis comes from an analysis of the lymphokine secretion profile of a house dust mite–specific $CD4^+$ T-cell clone generated from a patient with allergic asthma. This clone produced IL-4 but not IFN-γ and supported in vitro IgE production, which could be abrogated by supernatant derived from a house dust mite–specific T-cell clone from a nonatopic individual [163, 221].

In vitro, activated blood mononuclear cells from atopic asthmatic patients with elevated levels of IgE produce higher levels of IL-4 and lower levels of IFN-γ than mononuclear cells from healthy donors [163, 173]. In addition, the coexistent finding that atopic asthmatic subjects had enhanced concentrations of circulating soluble CD23, an IgE-BF selectively released from B-cells and monocytes on stimulation by IL-4 [173], supports the notion that IL-4 appears to be operational in vivo and that enhanced IL-4 synthesis in vivo by Th2 cells contributes to the elevated serum IgE levels observed in these patients.

This imbalance in the T-cell subsets responsible for IL-4 and IFN-γ secretion was demonstrated recently in tissue-allergic inflammatory infiltrates. The majority of T-cells isolated from conjunctival infiltrates of patients with vernal conjunctivitis consist of Th2-type lymphocytes able to secrete IL-4 and to induce IgE synthesis [134].

Having established the presence and the importance of the Th2 lymphocyte in the human IgE-mediated inflammatory response, future questions to be answered center around what conditions favor the expansion and biologic expression of this T-cell subset. Besides a particular immunogenetic constitution, such environmental factors as mode of antigen entry and dose of antigen may influence expansion of the Th2 cell subset. In addition to genetic and environmental factors, recent investigation points toward the mediator cytokine secretion inhibitory factor (CSIF, IL-10) produced by Th2 cells that inhibits Th1 function and thereby indirectly promotes Th2 growth and function [70, 192].

Dysregulation of IgE synthesis may also be related, at least in part, to the expiratory airflow obstruction noted in 10 to 25 percent of long-term survivors of bone marrow transplantation [34, 37]. The spectrum of airway obstruction ranges from asymptomatic disease of the small airways to fatal bronchiolitis obliterans. Part of the spectrum of this airway dysfunction includes clinical asthma. Recently, Agosti and associates [2] demonstrated that positive skin test reactivity to specific allergens can be transmitted from donors to recipients of allogeneic bone marrow transplants as can asthma itself. The effect extended beyond 1 year, suggesting that proliferating cells from the donor bone marrow were responsible for specific IgE hyperresponsiveness and asthma in the recipient. This may be viewed as a variant manifestation of chronic graft-versus-host disease in which a bone marrow cell, probably of lymphoid origin, provides a necessary pathogenetic link in the development of asthma.

REGULATION OF EOSINOPHIL PRODUCTION AND FUNCTION

Soon after Paul Ehrlich's initial description of the histochemical characteristics of the eosinophil [62], it became apparent that this cell was intimately associated with asthma. The earliest histopathologic descriptions of bronchial tissue from patients who had died from asthma contain vivid accounts of the heavy eosinophilic infiltration of the airway walls [57, 60, 132]. More recently, eosinophils have been noted in the bronchial walls in biopsy specimens obtained from asymptomatic individuals with mild asthma [9, 57]. For many years clinicians have recognized the presence of free eosinophils in the sputum of patients with asthma, particularly during acute exacerbations [57, 61]. The characteristic Charcot-Leyden crystals frequently observed in eosinophil-enriched sputum represent a crystallized form of the enzyme lysolecithinase derived from degenerated eosinophils [219]. The presence of blood eosinophilia in atopic and nonatopic patients with asthma [79] provides further evidence implicating these cells in the pathogenesis of the disease. Finally, several reports describe a relationship between the magnitude of airway and/or peripheral eosinophil counts and clinical disease activity [17, 197, 215] (see Chap. 20).

Along with other polymorphonuclear leukocytes, eosinophils originate from bone marrow precursor cells under the influence of growth- or colony-stimulating factors. Because the eosinophilia that normally accompanies helminthic infections is suppressed in athymic mice [156] and in normal rats or mice that have been depleted of their T-cells [8, 42], it has been concluded that eosinophilopoiesis is modulated by T-cell factors. In fact, several of these T-cell–derived cytokines have been identified and include GM-CSF, IL-3, and IL-5 [126, 141, 176, 198].

Both GM-CSF and IL-3 are multilineage hematopoietic regulators in that in addition to stimulating eosinophil growth, they also promote the differentiation of neutrophil, macrophage, and mixed neutrophil/macrophage colonies. The selectivity of eosinophil production in asthma and other allergic conditions as well as in parasitic helminthic infections suggested the possibility that a linear-specific growth factor may control the development of eosinophilia. The murine T-cell cytokine, eosinophil differentiation factor (EDF, IL-5), cross-reacts with human cells selectively stimulating the proliferation, differentiation, survival, and function of eosinophils [126], predicting the existence of a human equivalent to this molecule. Using cross-species hybridization with a murine IL-5 complementary DNA (cDNA) probe, Campbell and colleagues [23] cloned and characterized the human gene for IL-5. The human and murine proteins are highly homologous (70% identity) and the predicted size of both proteins is 115 amino acids. Recombinant human IL-5 is lineage specific for eosinophils in both liquid bone marrow cultures and the bone marrow colony assay.

Not only is recombinant human IL-5 a selective hematopoietin for eosinophil growth, it also is a potent and selective stimulator of human eosinophil function. In a dose-dependent fashion, recombinant human IL-5 induces shape changes, membrane ruffling, and granule polarization in eosinophils. These morphologic changes are accompanied by enhanced cellular cytotoxicity, phagocytosis, and superoxide generation. In contrast to eosinophils, neutrophils are not activated by this cytokine [77, 125, 225].

Another lymphokine, lymphocyte chemoattractant factor (LCF), a cationic glycoprotein consisting of four biologically active, 14-kd homomeric chains induced by histamine or specific antigen [33], recently was demonstrated to affect eosinophil function [158]. LCF binds to CD4 and previously was found to be chemoattractant for CD4$^+$ lymphocytes and monocytes [46]. Like these cell types, eosinophils express surface CD4 [129]. As demonstrated in a modified Boyden chamber assay, recombinant human LCF at low concentrations (median effective dose [ED$_{50}$] 10^{-12}–10^{-11} M) enhances both the random (chemokinetic) and directed (chemotactic) migration of eosinophils. These concentrations of LCF are 100- to 1,000-fold lower than the ED$_{50}$'s for the recognized eosinophil chemoattractants C5a and PAF [158]. Despite inducing eosinophil migration, LCF did not influence other functional responses of eosinophils such as degranulation, superoxide generation, LTC$_4$ production, in vitro survival, or cell surface expression of the adherence receptor CR3 (CD11b), HLA-DR, or IL-2R p55 (CD25) [158].

THE LATE-PHASE AIRWAY RESPONSE

The introduction of specific allergen into the skin of atopic subjects provokes an immediate local reaction consisting of pruritus, erythema, and edema. This is accompanied histologically by mast cell degranulation and increased microvascular permeability [58, 183, 195, 200]. Analogous immediate allergic reactions occur in both the upper and lower airways, producing symptoms of rhinoconjunctivitis and asthma. Several hours after the immediate response, some but not all allergen-challenged atopic subjects experience a localized delayed reaction characterized microscopically by edema and a mixed inflammatory cell infiltrate composed of both polymorphonuclear and mononuclear leukocytes [35, 72]. These allergic, IgE-dependent, late-phase responses have been recognized clinically in the skin as erythema and edema, in the nose as congestion and pruritus, in the conjunctiva as edema and pruritus, and in the lung as airway obstruction. In the lung, the clinical disorder of chronic asthma more closely parallels the pathogenesis, pathophysiology, and pharmacologic responsiveness of the late-phase reaction than of the immediate allergic response (Fig. 13-5) (see Chap. 12).

Much of our understanding of the immunopathogenesis of the allergen-induced human late-phase response comes from dermatologic studies. A small number of resident CD3$^+$/CD4$^+$ T-lymphocytes are found in the skin [16, 74]. A study of cell traffic and activation in allergen-induced human late-phase reactions in the skin revealed a lymphocytic infiltration that was almost exclusively CD4$^+$ [74]. As determined by positive staining for IL-2R, some of these T-cells were activated. Additional evidence for T-lymphocyte activation was provided by the observation that endothelial cells in the allergen-challenged biopsy specimens demonstrated increased HLA-DR expression, a presumed result of T-cell–secreted IFN-γ. The presence of activated T-cells at these sites was accompanied by the presence of activated eosinophils [74].

Fig. 13-5. *A simplified scheme to explain the relationship between early-, late-phase, and ongoing chronic asthma. The early phase is dependent on products derived from Fcε receptor–bearing mediator-releasing cells (mast cells [MC], basophils, platelets, and macrophages [Mø]). The release of chemotactic factors from these cells, as well as products derived from activated CD4$^+$ helper T-cells (T$_H$), provides the link from the early-phase bronchospastic response to the late-phase inflammatory response. Chronically activated helper T-cells and inflammatory cells amplify and perpetuate the process, thereby leading to ongoing clinical asthma. N = neutrophil; E = eosinophil; M = monocyte; Ts = suppressor T-cell; PG = prostaglandin; NCA = neutrophil chemotactic activity; INF = interferon; IL = interleukin; APC = antigen-presenting cells; LT = leukotriene; MBP = major basic protein; PAF = platelet-activating factor; ECP = eosinophil cationic protein; GM-CSF = granulocyte-macrophage colony-stimulating factor. (Reprinted with permission from A. B. Kay. Asthma and inflammation. J. Allergy Clin. Immunol. 87:893, 1991.)*

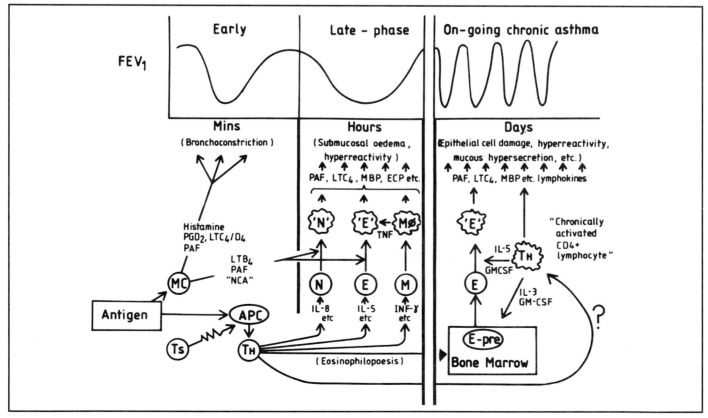

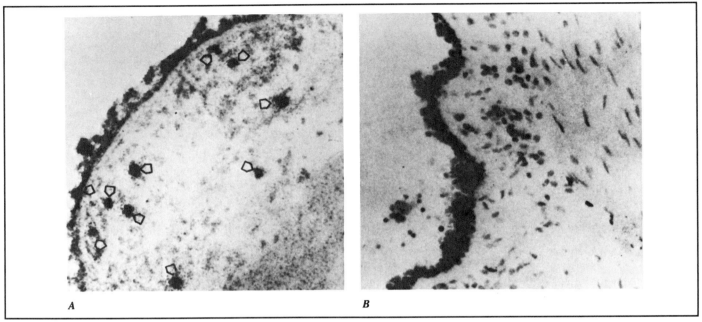

Fig. 13-6. *A. Autoradiograph of bronchial mucosa from a patient with symptomatic asthma. In situ hybridization was performed under high stringency with a ^{32}P-labeled cRNA probe encoding for interleukin-5 (IL-5) mRNA. Arrows indicate the mRNA-positive cells. ($\times$ 300.) B. Autoradiograph of bronchial mucosa from normal subject. The section was hybridized with the IL-5 cRNA probe. No hybridization signal was detected. ($\times$ 300.) (Reprinted with permission from Q. Hamid, et al. Expression of mRNA for interleukin-5 in mucosal bronchial biopsies from asthma.* J. Clin. Invest. *87:1541, 1991.)*

Using the technique of in situ hybridization, Kay and colleagues [109] determined the cytokine profile of the infiltrating CD4$^+$ T-cells seen in the late-phase skin response to allergen challenge. At the allergen-injected sites, most biopsy specimens had positive hybridization signals for IL-3, IL-4, IL-5, and GM-CSF, a group of cytokines whose genes are clustered in the region of the long arm of human chromosome 5 [207]. When the allergen-challenged site was compared with the diluent-injected site, there were significant increases in the numbers of infiltrating cells located in the upper part of the dermis expressing mRNA for the above-mentioned cytokines. In addition, at the allergen-injected sites, there were significant correlations between IL-5 mRNA-positive cells and IL-3, IL-4, and GM-CSF mRNA-positive cells. This suggests a process of linked transcription of the IL-3, IL-4, IL-5, and GM-CSF gene cluster. Because in this study [109] only the presence of cytokine mRNA was assessed, it remains to be determined whether in vivo translation and secretion of the corresponding proteins occur.

Using monoclonal antibodies combined with cytofluorimetry and immunohistochemistry, the kinetics and phenotype of T-lymphocytes infiltrating the airways of guinea pigs undergoing allergen-induced late-phase bronchoconstriction have been analyzed [76]. Challenge of sensitized animals with aerosolized albumin was followed by early (2-hour) and late (17-hour) bronchoconstriction. The numbers of total T-cells observed in the bronchial mucosa peaked at 17 and 48 hours, whereas the number of T-cells noted in the bronchial adventitia peaked at 2, 17, and 48 hours. The postchallenge infiltrating T-cells were of the CD3$^+$, CD8$^-$ phenotype. In contrast to the striking changes observed in the bronchial wall tissue, analysis of BAL and blood T-cell subsets demonstrated no significant change in this model, suggesting under certain conditions that evaluation of distant compartments (blood and bronchoalveolar fluid) may not fully reflect evolving tissue infiltration.

In humans, late-phase airway bronchoconstriction is defined as a 20 percent fall in 1-second forced expiratory volume (FEV$_1$)

or 50 percent fall in airway conductance 3 to 12 hours after a standardized allergen inhalation challenge [75, 108]. In one study of segmental bronchial allergen challenge performed via fiberoptic bronchoscopy, a selective increase in the number of CD4$^+$ T-cells in BAL fluid was observed 48 hours after challenge in subjects who had previously experienced both early and late postchallenge asthmatic responses [142]. These findings are consistent with the decrease in number of CD4$^+$ T-cells in the peripheral blood noted after allergen inhalation [81] and suggest a process of selective recruitment and retention of CD4$^+$ lymphocytes into the airways during a late-phase response.

By applying the techniques previously used in the study of the cutaneous late-phase inflammatory response, Hamid and coworkers [87] investigated the functional capabilities of the CD4$^+$ cells infiltrating the airways of asthmatic subjects (Fig. 13-6). Bronchial biopsy specimens were obtained from 10 individuals with asthma and 9 nonatopic, normal control subjects. Specific hybridization signals for IL-5 mRNA were demonstrated within the bronchial mucosa in 6 of the 10 subjects with asthma. Cells exhibiting hybridization signals were located beneath the epithelial basement membrane. In contrast, there was no detectable hybridization in the control group. In the 6 IL-5 mRNA-positive subjects, there was an accompanying increase in the infiltration of both activated T-lymphocytes and eosinophils. There was a correlation between IL-5 mRNA expression and the number of activated lymphocytes and eosinophils (Table 13-4). Taken together, these results provide evidence for airway wall localization of activated, IL-5–secreting T-cells in subjects with asthma and support the concept of cytokine participation in the local regulation of eosinophil accumulation and function.

MONONUCLEAR CELL INVOLVEMENT IN THE CASCADE OF AIRWAY INFLAMMATION

An integrated view of the pathogenetic sequences responsible for airway inflammation and its pathophysiologic effects in asthma comes from studies on the cytology and mediator content of relevant biopsy specimens and secretions, as well as from studies of inflammatory cell and mediator physiology. Data obtained from a wide variety of studies suggest that this airway inflammation results from induction, amplification, and maintenance mechanisms that originate from complex cellular and molecular interactions.

In those asthmatic subjects who are atopic and have their asthma triggered by IgE-dependent mechanisms, induction of airway inflammation starts with the local production of IgE antibody. This immune response is dependent on two main signals provided by T-lymphocytes to B-cells [169, 208]. The first signal consists of physical interaction between T- and B-cells and the second is provided by T-cell–derived IL-4. Although other cytokines or factors may enhance IgE antibody production, IL-4 is the signal required for the switch to the IgE isotype [120, 130]. The activation of the IgE-inducing cytokine network leads not only to increased synthesis of IgE, but also to augmentation of the cell types that bind IgE and to enhanced expression of FcεRI (high-affinity receptor) on mast cells and FcεRII (low-affinity receptor) on lymphocytes, eosinophils, platelets, and macrophages [25, 169, 189, 208]. This in turn results in increased binding of IgE molecules to the various effector cells. The reintroduction of antigen, which cross-links receptor-bound IgE, induces cell activation and the initiation of combined airway bronchoconstriction and inflammation (Fig. 13-7).

As part of the early-phase or immediate airway reaction that is clinically typified by bronchoconstriction induced by spasmogens (histamine, eicosanoids, PAF) released predominantly from IgE receptor–bearing cells (mast cells, macrophages, platelets, and eosinophils), potent inflammatory cell chemotactic factors such as LTB$_4$, hydroxyeicosatetraenoic acids (HETES), eosinophil chemotactic factor of anaphylaxis (ECF-A), and PAF are secreted by multiple resident cells including mast cells, macrophages, and airway epithelial cells. The stimulus for secretion of both spasmogens and chemotaxins may be either immunologic (IgE dependent) or nonimmunologic (IgE independent). The corelease of both spasmogens and inflammatory cell chemotactic factors represents an induction mechanism for airway inflammation and is the pathophysiologic link between early-phase and late-phase reactions. In addition, it is probable that activated mast cells also release proinflammatory cytokines such as IL-3, IL-4, IL-5, IL-6, and GM-CSF that contribute to the amplification and maintenance of airway inflammation [21, 157, 222].

Amplification and maintenance mechanisms of airway inflammation include further recruitment and activation of eosinophils and neutrophils; the in situ hematopoietic activities released by various resident and infiltrating cells; the induction of histamine release from metachromatic cells; secretion of proinflammatory

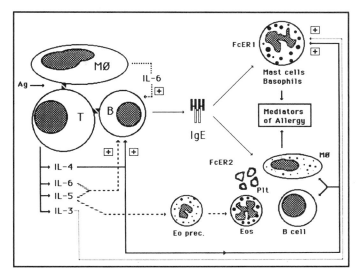

Fig. 13-7. *The IgE system as a model of allergic inflammation. Ag = antigen; IL = interleukin; Plt = platelet; B = B-cell; T = T-cell; Mø = macrophage; Eo prec. = eosinophil precursor; Eos = eosinophil. (Reprinted with permission from D. Vercelli and R. S. Geha. Regulation of IgE synthesis in humans.* J. Clin. Immunol. *9:75, 1989.)*

molecules from airway epithelium; and the activation of macrophages, endothelial cells, and fibroblasts (see Fig. 13-5).

Following their recruitment by chemotactic factors, eosinophils, neutrophils, and monocytes encounter cytokines from helper T-cells that profoundly affect their state of viability, differentiation, and activation. These include the various interleukins, GM-CSF, and IFN-γ. Continuous exposure to these cytokines drives these inflammatory cells toward terminal differentiation and maturation and ultimately leads to a state of activation and secretion of their specific granules. Proteins derived from eosinophil granules (major basic protein [MBP], eosinophil cationic protein [ECP], and neurotoxin) and neutral proteases and elastases from neutrophils and macrophages produce submucosal edema and desquamation of the bronchial epithelium [82]. These are cardinal features of the late-phase reaction, which leads to repeated and sustained airway inflammation and bronchoconstriction. Bronchial hyperreactivity to nonspecific bronchoconstrictor stimuli such as histamine or methacholine is thought to be related to this late-phase inflammatory response, but its precise relationship is still to be determined.

A group of cytokines collectively known as HRFs are produced by multiple cell types including T-cells and macrophages. These mediators release histamine and leukotrienes from basophils and mast cells. This chronic non–IgE-dependent mechanism for vasoactive and bronchoactive mediator release contributes to the perpetuation of airway inflammation. In fact, a recent study identified a strong positive correlation between the magnitude of the spontaneous production of HRFs by lymphocytes in vitro with the state of bronchial hyperreactivity in patients with asthma [3].

The bronchial epithelium has the potential for both ameliorating and exacerbating asthma. On the one hand, an intact airway epithelium limits antigen access to sensitized IgE-bearing airway wall cells and, in addition, produces smooth muscle relaxants, thereby counteracting bronchoconstrictor stimuli [22]. On the other hand, by elaborating products of the 5- and 15-lipoxygenase pathways, facilitating the release of neuropeptides, and producing growth and differentiating factors, airway epithelial cells are capable of playing an active role in the maintenance of airway inflammation [163]. In certain circumstances, epithelial cell products directly or indirectly modulate the elaboration of cytokines by macrophages or lymphocytes. In addition, the monokine IL-1

Table 13-4. Comparison of activated lymphocyte and eosinophil infiltration of the airway wall between interleukin-5 (IL-5) mRNA-positive and -negative biopsy specimens

	Total cell counts[a]		
	IL-5 mRNA-positive	IL-5 mRNA-negative	p Values[b]
Activated lymphocytes (CD25$^+$)[c]	6.8 (1–24)	0.3 (0–1)	.01–.05
Activated eosinophils (EG$^+$)[d]	10.5 (4–23)	1.3 (0–3)	.01

[a] Per millimeter length of basement membrane expressed as mean and range.
[b] Comparison of cell counts in IL-5-positive versus IL-5-negative specimens.
[c] Antibody directed against the IL-2 receptor.
[d] Antibody directed against the cleaved form of eosinophil cationic protein.
Source: Adapted from Q. Hamid, et al. Expression of mRNA for interleukin-5 in mucosal bronchial biopsies from asthma. *J. Clin. Invest.* 87:1541, 1991.

binds to specific receptors on bronchial epithelial cells and promotes the synthesis and release of GM-CSF [143] (see Chap. 23).

The release of certain cytokines by activated macrophages and lymphocytes contributes to the activation of endothelial cells and fibroblasts. In particular, TGF-β, and TNF-α activate endothelial cells, inducing a greater expression of adhesion molecules and secretion of chemotactic factors, both of which enhance inflammatory cell recruitment. The adhesion of eosinophils to endothelial cells is favored by the expression of ICAM-1. Endothelial cell-surface expression of this adhesion molecule is promoted by T-cell–derived IFN-γ. Anti–ICAM-1 antibodies inhibit eosinophilia of the bronchial mucosa and nonspecific bronchial hyperreactivity in vitro and in vivo [217]. Activation of the fibroblasts of the respiratory mucosa by mononuclear cell cytokines induces the production of interstitial proteins including collagen Types III and V and fibronectin. These proteins are responsible for the well-described thickening and fibrosis of subepithelial basement membrane seen in both allergic and nonallergic bronchial asthma [57, 166]. It has been postulated that this fibrotic process results in the transition of asthma from a completely reversible form of obstructive airway disease to one of partial fixed obstruction.

In conclusion, the causes of airway narrowing in bronchial asthma are complex and multifactorial. The histologic features are characterized by acute and chronic inflammatory changes in which many different cell types participate. One is left with the impression that no one cell or inflammatory mediator is the sole perpetrator in asthma; rather, there is a series of interactions involving many cells and many messengers. There is now considerable evidence from both in vitro and in vivo studies implicating T-cells and macrophages, as well as their cytokine networks, in the induction, amplification, and maintenance of many of the components of the asthmatic diathesis.

This recent appreciation of mononuclear cell involvement in the pathogenesis of asthma provides a background for the development of new therapeutic strategies in our treatment of the disease. Pharmacologic and other interventions aimed at manipulating these inflammatory cells and their cytokine networks in favor of the host hold out promise for disrupting the positive feedback cycle that results in chronic airway inflammation and consequent perpetuation asthma.

REFERENCES

1. Adams, D. O., and Hamilton, T. A. The cell biology of macrophage activation. *Annu. Rev. Immunol.* 2:283, 1984.
2. Agosti, J. M., et al. Transfer of allergen-specific IgE-mediated hypersensitivity with allogeneic bone marrow transplants. *N. Engl. J. Med.* 319:1623, 1988.
3. Alam, R., et al. The magnitude of the spontaneous production of histamine-releasing factor (HRF) by lymphocytes in vitro correlates with the state of bronchial hyperreactivity in patients with asthma. *J. Allergy Clin. Immunol.* 79:103, 1987.
4. Anderson, C. L., and Spiegelberg, H. L. Macrophage receptors for IgE: Binding of IgE to specific IgE receptors on a human macrophage cell line, U937. *J. Immunol.* 127:2470, 1981.
5. Arnoux, B., et al. Alveolar macrophages from asthmatics release PAF-acether and lyso-PAF-acether when stimulated with specific antigen. *Am. Rev. Respir. Dis.* 125:70A, 1982.
6. Azzawi, M., et al. Identification of activated T-lymphocytes and eosinophils in bronchial biopsies in stable atopic asthma. *Am. Rev. Respir. Dis.* 142:1407, 1990.
7. Barnes, P. J., Chung, K. F., and Page, C. P. Inflammatory mediators and asthma. *Pharmacol. Rev.* 40:49, 1988.
8. Basten, A., and Beeson, P. B. Mechanism of eosinophilia. II. Role of the lymphocyte. *J. Exp. Med.* 131:1288, 1970.
9. Beasley, R., et al. Cellular events in the bronchi in mild asthma and after bronchial provocation. *Am. Rev. Respir. Dis.* 139:806, 1989.
10. Beer, D. J., Matloff, S. M., and Rocklin, R. E. The influence of histamine on immune and inflammatory response. *Adv. Immunol.* 35:209, 1984.
11. Beer, D. J., et al. Abnormal histamine-induced suppressor-cell function in atopic subjects. *N. Engl. J. Med.* 306:454, 1982.
12. Bentley, A. M., et al. Immunohistology of the bronchial mucosa in occupational, intrinsic and extrinsic asthma. *J. Allergy Clin. Immunol.* 87:246, 1991.
13. Benveniste, J., Henson, P. M., and Cochrane, C. G. Leukocyte dependent histamine release from rabbit platelets: The role of IgE, basophils, and a platelet activating factor. *J. Exp. Med.* 136:1356, 1972.
14. Black, P. N., et al. Bronchial reactivity is not increased after inhalation of leukotriene B₄ and prostaglandin D₂. *Br. J. Clin. Pharmacol.* 25:667P, 1988.
15. Bonnefoy, J. Y., et al. Human recombinant interleukin-4 induces normal B cells to produce soluble CD23/IgE-binding analogous to that spontaneously released by lymphoblastoid B cell lines. *Eur. J. Immunol.* 18:117, 1988.
16. Bos, J. D., et al. The skin immune system: Distribution and immunophenotype of lymphocyte subpopulations in normal human skin. *J. Invest. Dermatol.* 88:569, 1987.
17. Bousquet, J., et al. Eosinophilic inflammation in asthma. *N. Engl. J. Med.* 323:1033, 1990.
17a. Broide, D. H., et al. Cytokines in symptomatic asthma airways. *J. Allergy Clin. Immunol.* 89:958, 1992.
18. Broudy, V. C., et al. Tumor necrosis factor type α stimulates human endothelial cells to produce granulocyte/macrophage colony-stimulating factor. *Proc. Natl. Acad. Sci. USA* 83:7467, 1986.
19. Bruijnzeel, P. L. B., et al. Platelet activating factor (PAF-acether) induced leukotriene C₄ formation and luminol dependent chemiluminescence of human eosinophils. *Pharmacol. Res. Commun.* 18:61, 1986.
20. Buckley, R. H., and Fiscus, S. A. Serum IgD and IgE concentration in immunodeficiency diseases. *J. Clin. Invest.* 55:157, 1971.
21. Burd, P. R., et al. Interleukin-3-dependent and independent mast cells stimulated with IgE and antigen express multiple cytokines. *J. Exp. Med.* 170:245, 1989.
22. Busk, M. F., and Vanhoutte, P. M. Epithelium-dependent Responses in Airways. In M. A. Kaliner, P. J. Barnes, and C. G. A. Persson (eds.), *Asthma: Its Pathology and Treatment.* New York: Marcel Dekker, 1991. Pp. 135–188.
23. Campbell, H. D., et al. Molecular cloning and expression of the gene encoding human eosinophil differentiation factor (interleukin-5). *Proc. Natl. Acad. Sci. USA* 84:6629, 1987.
24. Camussi, G., et al. Tumor necrosis factor/cachectin stimulates peritoneal macrophages, polymorphonuclear neutrophils, and vascular endothelial cells to synthesize and release platelet-activating factor. *J. Exp. Med.* 166:1390, 1987.
25. Capron, A., et al. From parasites to allergy: A second receptor for IgE. *Immunol. Today* 7:15, 1986.
26. Capron, A., et al. Specific IgE antibodies in immune adherence of normal macrophages to *Schistosoma mansoni* schistosomules. *Nature* 253:474, 1975.
27. Capron, A., et al. Interaction between IgE immune complexes and macrophages in the rat: A new mechanism of macrophage activation. *Eur. J. Immunol.* 7:315, 1977.
28. Capron, M., et al. Functional study of a monoclonal antibody to IgE Fc receptor (FcεR2) of eosinophils, platelets and macrophages. *J. Exp. Med.* 164:72, 1986.
29. Capron, M., et al. Cytophilic IgE on human blood and tissue eosinophils: Detection by flow microfluorometry. *J. Immunol.* 134:3013, 1985.
30. Capron, M., et al. Role of IgE receptors in effector function of eosinophils. *J. Immunol.* 232:462, 1984.
31. Capron, M., and Tonnel, A.-B. Participation of Fc Epsilon RII-positive Macrophages and Eosinophils in Asthma. In M. A. Kaliner, P. J. Barnes, and C. G. A. Persson (eds.), *Asthma, Its Pathology and Treatment.* New York: Marcel Dekker, 1991. Pp. 457–476.
32. Carswell, E. A., et al. An endotoxin-induced serum factor that causes necrosis of tumors. *Proc. Natl. Acad. Sci. USA* 72:3666, 1975.
33. Center, D. M., et al. Functional characteristics of histamine receptor-bearing mononuclear cells. I. Selective production of lymphocyte chemoattractant lymphokines with histamine used as a ligand. *J. Immunol.* 131:1854, 1983.
34. Chan, C. K., et al. Small-airways disease in recipients of allogeneic bone marrow transplants: An analysis of 11 cases and a review of the literature. *Medicine* 66:327, 1987.
35. Charlesworth, E. N., et al. Cutaneous late phase response to allergen.

Mediator release and inflammatory cellular infiltration. *J. Clin. Invest.* 83: 1519, 1989.

36. Cherwinski, H. M., et al. Two types of mouse helper T cell clone. III. Further differences in lymphokine synthesis between Th1 and Th2 clones revealed by RNA hybridization, functionally monospecific bioassays, and monoclonal antibodies. *J. Exp. Med.* 166:1229, 1987.

37. Clark, J. G., et al. Risk factors for airflow obstruction in recipients of bone marrow transplants. *Ann. Intern. Med.* 107:648, 1987.

38. Clark, S. C., and Kamen, R. The human hematopoietic colony-stimulating factors. *Science* 236:1229, 1987.

39. Coffman, R. L., and Carty, J. A T cell activity that enhances polyclonal IgE production and its inhibition by interferon-γ. *J. Immunol.* 136:949, 1986.

40. Coffman, R. L., et al. B cell stimulatory factor-1 enhances IgE response of lipopolysaccharide-activated B cells. *J. Immunol.* 136:4538, 1986.

41. Coleman, D. L., et al. Granulocyte-macrophage colony-stimulating factor enhances selective effector functions of tissue-derived macrophages. *Blood* 72:573, 1988.

42. Colley, D. G. Lymphokine-related eosinophil responses. *Lymphokine Cytokine Res.* 1:133, 1980.

43. Corrigan, C. J., Hartnell, A., and Kay, A. B. T-lymphocyte activation in acute severe asthma. *Lancet* 1:1129, 1988.

44. Corrigan, C. J., and Kay, A. B. CD4 T-lymphocyte activation in acute severe asthma: Relationship to disease severity and atopic status. *Am. Rev. Respir. Dis.* 141:970, 1990.

45. Court, E. N., et al. Platelet-activating factor in bronchoalveolar lavage fluid from asthmatic patients. *Br. J. Clin. Pharmacol.* 24:258, 1987.

46. Cruikshank, W. W., et al. Lymphokine activation of T4$^+$ T lymphocytes and monocytes. *J. Immunol.* 138:3817, 1987.

47. Cuss, F. M., Dixon, C. M. S., and Barnes, P. J. Effects of inhaled platelet activating factor on pulmonary function and bronchial responsiveness in man. *Lancet* 2:189, 1986.

48. Dahlen, S. E., et al. Allergen challenge of lung tissue from asthmatics elicits bronchial contraction that correlates with the release of leukotrienes C_4, D_4, and E_4. *Proc. Natl. Acad. Sci. USA* 80:1712, 1983.

49. Dahlen, S. E., et al. Leukotrienes are potent constrictors of human bronchi. *Nature* 288:484, 1980.

50. Defrance, T., et al. Human recombinant interleukin 4 induces Fcε receptors (CD23) on normal B lymphocytes. *J. Exp. Med.* 165:1459, 1987.

51. DeLarco, J., and Todaro, G. Growth factors from sarcoma virus-transformed cells. *Proc. Natl. Acad. Sci. USA* 75:4001, 1978.

52. Del Prete, G. F., et al. IL-4 is an essential factor for the IgE synthesis induced in vitro by human T cell clones and their supernatants. *J. Immunol.* 140:4193, 1988.

53. Demopolous, C. A., Pinckard, R. N., and Hanahan, D. J. Platelet-activating factor. Evidence for 1-0-alkyl-2-acetyl-sn-glyceryl-3-phosphorylcholine as the active component (a new class of lipid chemical mediators). *J. Biol. Chem.* 254:9355, 1979.

54. Deuel, T. F., et al. Chemotaxis of monocytes and neutrophils to platelet-derived growth factor. *J. Clin. Invest.* 69:1046, 1982.

55. Dinarello, C. A., et al. Tumor necrosis factor (cachectin) is an endogenous pyrogen and induces production of interleukin 1. *J. Exp. Med.* 163: 1433, 1986.

56. Dishuk, J., et al. Identification of interleukin 2 and 4 messenger RNA in bronchial alveolar lavage cells and allergen specific cell lines from atopic individuals. *J. Allergy Clin. Immunol.* 87:267A, 1991.

57. Djukanovic, R., et al. Mucosal inflammation in asthma. *Am. Rev. Respir. Dis.* 142:434, 1990.

58. Dorsch, W., et al. Mediator studies in skin blister fluid from patients with dual skin reactions after intradermal allergen injection. *J. Allergy Clin. Immunol.* 70:236, 1982.

59. Dunnill, M. S. The pathology of asthma with special reference to changes in the bronchial mucosa. *J. Clin. Pathol.* 13:27, 1960.

60. Dunnill, M. S., Massarella, G. R., and Anderson, J. A. A comparison of the quantitative anatomy of the bronchi in normal subjects, in status asthmaticus, in chronic bronchitis, and in emphysema. *Thorax* 24:176, 1969.

61. Durham, S. R., and Kay, A. B. Eosinophils, bronchial hyperreactivity and late phase asthmatic reactions. *Clin. Allergy* 15:411, 1985.

62. Ehrlich, P. Beitrage zur kenntnir granulirten bindegwebszellen und der eosinophilen leukocythen. *Arch. Anat. Physiol.* 166, 1897.

63. Eschenbacher, W. L., and Gravelyn, T. R. A technique for isolated airway segment lavage. *Chest* 92:105, 1987.

64. Evans, T. W., et al. Effect of platelet-activating factor on airway vascular permeability: Possible mechanisms. *J. Appl. Physiol.* 63:479, 1987.

65. Ezeamuzie, J. C., and Assem, E. S. K. A study of histamine release from basophils and lung mast cells by products of lymphocytes stimulation. *Agents Actions* 13:222, 1983.

66. Feinmark, S. J., et al. Stimulation of human leukocyte degranulation by leukotriene B_4. *FEBS Lett.* 61:136, 1981.

67. Fels, A. O. S., and Cohn, Z. A. The alveolar macrophage. *J. Appl. Physiol.* 60:353, 1986.

68. Ferreri, N. R., Howland, W. C., and Spiegelberg, H. Release of leukotrienes C_4 and B_4 and prostaglandin E_2 from human monocytes stimulated with aggregated IgG, IgA, and IgE. *J. Immunol.* 136:4188, 1986.

69. Finkleman, F. D., et al. Suppression of in vivo polyclonal IgE responses by monoclonal antibody to the lymphokine B-cell stimulatory factor 1. *Proc. Natl. Acad. Sci. USA* 83:9675, 1986.

70. Fiorentino, D. F., Bond, M. W., and Mosmann, T. R. Two types of mouse T helper cell: IV. TH2 clones secrete a factor that inhibits cytokine production by TH1 clones. *J. Exp. Med.* 170:2081, 1989.

71. Fiser, P. M., and Buckley, R. H. Human IgE biosynthesis in vitro: Studies with atopic and normal blood mononuclear cells and subpopulations. *J. Immunol.* 123:1788, 1979.

72. Fleekop, P. D., et al. Cellular inflammatory responses in human allergic skin reactions. *J. Allergy Clin. Immunol.* 80:140, 1987.

73. Fokkens, W. J., et al. Fluctuation of the number of CD-1 cells in the nasal mucosa of patients with an isolated grass-pollen allergy before, during, and after the grass-pollen season. *J. Allergy Clin. Immunol.* 84:39, 1989.

74. Frew, A. J., and Kay, A. B. The relationship between infiltrating CD4 + lymphocytes, activated eosinophils, and the magnitude of the allergen-induced late-phase cutaneous reaction in man. *J. Immunol.* 141:4158, 1988.

75. Frew, A. J., and Kay, A. B. Eosinophils and T-lymphocytes in late-phase allergic reactions. *J. Allergy Clin. Immunol.* 85:533, 1990.

76. Frew, A. J., et al. T-lymphocytes and eosinophils in allergen-induced late phase asthmatic reactions in the guinea pig. *Am. Rev. Respir. Dis.* 141: 407, 1990.

77. Fujisawa, T., et al. Regulatory effect of cytokines on eosinophil degranulation. *J. Immunol.* 144:642, 1990.

78. Fukuda, T., et al. Lymphocyte subsets in bronchial mucosa of symptomatic and asymptomatic asthmatics. *J. Allergy Clin. Immunol.* 87:302A, 1991.

79. Fukuda, T., et al. Increased numbers of hypodense eosinophils in the blood of patients with bronchial asthma. *Am. Rev. Respir. Dis.* 132:981, 1985.

80. Fuller, R. W., et al. Immunoglobulin E-dependent stimulation of human alveolar macrophages: Significance in type 1 hypersensitivity. *Clin. Exp. Immunol.* 65:416, 1986.

81. Gerblich, A. A., Campbell, A. E., and Schuyley, M. R. Changes in T-lymphocyte subpopulations after antigenic bronchial provocation in asthmatics. *N. Engl. J. Med.* 310:1349, 1984.

82. Gleich, G. The eosinophil and bronchial asthma. Current understanding. *J. Allergy Clin. Immunol.* 85:422, 1990.

83. Gonzalez, M. C., et al. Allergen-induced recruitment of bronchoalveolar (OKT4) and suppressor (OKT8) cells in asthma: Relative increases in OKT8 cells in single early responders compared with those in late-phase responders. *Am. Rev. Respir. Dis.* 136:600, 1987.

84. Gosset, P., et al. Production of an interleukin 1 inhibitory factor by human alveolar macrophages from normal and allergic patients. *Am. Rev. Respir. Dis.* 138:40, 1988.

85. Goswami, S. K., et al. Platelet activating factor enhances mucous glycoprotein release from human airways in vitro. *Am. Rev. Respir. Dis.* 135: A159, 1987.

86. Grangette, C., et al. IgE receptor on human eosinophils (FcεRII): Comparison with B cell CD23 and association with an adhesion molecule. *J. Immunol.* 143:3580, 1989.

87. Hamid, Q., et al. Expression of mRNA for interleukin-5 in mucosal bronchial biopsies from asthma. *J. Clin. Invest.* 87:1541, 1991.

88. Hardy, C. C., et al. The bronchoconstrictor effect of inhaled PGD_2 in normal and asthmatic men. *N. Engl. J. Med.* 311:209, 1984.

89. Henderson, W. R., Jr. Eicosanoids and lung inflammation. *Am. Rev. Respir. Dis.* 135:1176, 1987.

90. Henderson, W. R., Jr. Eicosanoids and platelet-activating factor in allergic respiratory disease. *Am. Rev. Respir. Dis.* 143:S86, 1991.

91. Holt, P. G., et al. Ia-positive dendritic cells form a tightly meshed network within the human airway epithelium. *Clin. Exp. Allergy* 19:587, 1989.

92. Ihle, J. N., et al. Phenotypic characteristics of cell lines requiring interleukin 3 for growth. *J. Immunol.* 129:1377, 1982.

93. Ihle, J. N., et al. Procedures for the purification of interleukin 3 to homogeneity. *J. Immunol.* 129:2431, 1982.

94. Ikebuchi, K., et al. Synergistic factors for stem cell proliferation: Further studies of the target stem cells and the mechanism of stimulation by interleukin-1, interleukin-6, and granulocyte colony-stimulating factor. *Blood* 72:2007, 1988.

95. Ishizaka, K. IgE-binding factors and regulation of the IgE antibody response. *Annu. Rev. Immunol.* 6:513, 1988.

96. Ishizaka, T., and Ishizaka, K. Biology of immunoglobulin E. *Prog. Allergy* 19:60, 1975.

97. Ito, K., et al. IgE levels in nude mice. *Int. Arch. Allergy Appl. Immunol.* 58:474, 1979.

98. Jabara, H. H., et al. CD40 and IgE: Synergism between anti-CD40 monoclonal antibody and interleukin 4 in the induction of IgE synthesis by highly purified human B cells. *J. Exp. Med.* 172:1861, 1990.

99. Jabara, H. H., Geha, R. S., and Vercelli, D. Induction of IgE synthesis by human recombinant IL-4. *FASEB J.* 2:6652, 1988.

100. Jeffery, P. K., et al. Quantitative analysis of bronchial biopsies in asthma. *Am. Rev. Respir. Dis.* 135:A316, 1987.

101. Jelinek, D. F., and Lipsky, P. E. Enhancement of human B cell proliferation and differentiation by tumor necrosis factor-α and interleukin 1. *J. Immunol.* 139:2970, 1987.

102. Johnston, R. B., Jr. Monocytes and macrophages. *N. Engl. J. Med.* 318:747, 1988.

103. Jones, T. R., Davies, C., and Daniel, E. E. Pharmacological study of the contractile activity of leukotriene C_4 and D_4 on isolated human airway smooth muscle. *Can. J. Physiol. Pharmacol.* 60:638, 1982.

104. Joseph, M., et al. Involvement of immunoglobulin E in the secretory process of alveolar macrophages from asthmatic subjects. *J. Clin. Invest.* 71:221, 1983.

105. Jouault, T., et al. Quantitative and qualitative analysis of the Fc receptor for IgE (FcεRII) on human eosinophils. *Eur. J. Immunol.* 18:237, 1988.

106. Kaplan, A. P., et al. A histamine-releasing factor from activated human mononuclear cells. *J. Immunol.* 135:2027, 1985.

107. Katz, D. H. The IgE antibody system is coordinately regulated by FcR epsilon-positive lymphoid cells and IgE-selective soluble factors. *Int. Arch. Allergy Appl. Immunol.* 77:21, 1985.

108. Kay, A. B. Asthma and inflammation. *J. Allergy Clin. Immunol.* 87:893, 1991.

109. Kay, A. B., et al. Messenger RNA expression of the cytokine gene cluster, interleukin 3 (IL-3), IL-4, IL-5, and granulocyte/macrophage colony-stimulating factor, in allergen-induced late-phase cutaneous reactions in atopic subjects. *J. Exp. Med.* 173:775, 1991.

110. Kehrl, J., et al. Production of TGFβ by human T lymphocytes and its potential role in the regulation of T cell growth. *J. Exp. Med.* 163:1037, 1986.

111. Kellaway, C. H., and Trethewie, E. R. The liberation of a slow-reacting smooth muscle-stimulating substance in anaphylaxis. *Q. J. Exp. Physiol.* 30:121, 1940.

112. Kelley, J. Cytokines of the lung. *Am. Rev. Respir. Dis.* 141:765, 1990.

113. Kelley, V. E., Fiers, W., and Strom, T. B. Cloned human interferon-γ, but not interferon-β or α, induces expression of HLA-DR determinants by fetal monocytes and myeloid leukemic cell lines. *J. Immunol.* 132:240, 1984.

114. Kinashi, T., et al. Cloning of complementary DNA encoding T-cell replacing factor and identity with B-cell growth factor II. *Nature* 324:70, 1986.

115. King, P. D., and Katz, D. R. Mechanisms of dendritic cell function. *Immunol. Today* 11:206, 1990.

116. Kishimoto, T. Factors affecting B-cell growth and differentiation. *Annu. Rev. Immunol.* 3:133, 1985.

117. Kishimoto, T., and Hirano, T. Molecular regulation of B lymphocyte response. *Annu. Rev. Immunol.* 6:485, 1988.

118. Lam, S., et al. Release of leukotrienes in patients with bronchial asthma. *J. Allergy Clin. Immunol.* 81:711, 1988.

119. Lanzavecchia, A., and Parodi, B. In vitro stimulation of IgE production at a single precursor level by human alloreactive T-helper cell clones. *Clin. Exp. Immunol.* 55:197, 1984.

120. Lebman, D. A., and Coffman, R. L. Interleukin 4 causes isotype switching to IgE in T cell-stimulated clonal B cell cultures. *J. Exp. Med.* 168:853, 1988.

121. Leibovich, S. J., et al. Macrophage-induced angiogenesis is mediated by tumour-necrosis factor. *Nature* 329:630, 1987.

122. Leung, D. Y. M., Young, M. C., and Geha, R. S. Induction of IgG and IgE synthesis in normal B cells by autoreactive T cell clones. *J. Immunol.* 136:2851, 1986.

123. Littman, D. R. The structure of the CD4 and CD8 genes. *Annu. Rev. Immunol.* 5:561, 1987.

124. Lopez, A. F., et al. Murine eosinophil differentiation factor. An eosinophil-specific colony-stimulating factor with activity for human cells. *J. Exp. Med.* 163:1085, 1986.

125. Lopez, A. F., et al. Recombinant human interleukin 5 is a selective activator of human eosinophil function. *J. Exp. Med.* 167:219, 1988.

126. Lopez, A. F., et al. Stimulation of proliferation, differentiation, and function of human cells by primate interleukin 3. *Proc. Natl. Acad. Sci. USA* 84:2761, 1987.

127. Lopez, A. F., et al. Recombinant human granulocyte-macrophage colony-stimulating factor stimulates in vitro mature human neutrophil and eosinophil function, surface receptor expression, and survival. *J. Clin. Invest.* 78:1220, 1986.

128. Lopez-Vidreiro, M. I., et al. Bronchial secretion from normal human airways after inhalation of $PGF_{2\alpha}$, acetylcholine, histamine, and citric acid. *Thorax* 32:734, 1977.

129. Lucey, D. R., et al. Human eosinophils express CD4 protein and bind human immunodeficiency virus 1 gp 120. *J. Exp. Med.* 169:327, 1989.

130. Lutzker, S., et al. Mitogen- and IL-4-regulated expression of germ-line Igγ2b transcripts: Evidence for directed heavy chain class switching. *Cell* 53:177, 1988.

131. MacDermot, J., et al. Synthesis of leukotriene B_4 and prostanoids by human alveolar macrophages: Analysis by gas chromatography/mass spectrometry. *Prostaglandins* 27:163, 1984.

132. MacDonald, I. G. The local and constitutional pathology of bronchial asthma. *Ann. Intern. Med.* 6:253, 1933.

133. Mackaness, G. B. The monocyte and cellular immunity. *Semin. Hematol.* 7:172, 1970.

134. Maggi, E., et al. Accumulation of Th-2 like helper T cells in the conjunctiva of patients with vernal conjunctivitis. *J. Immunol.* 146:1169, 1991.

135. Marom, Z., et al. Slow reacting substances LTC_4 and LTD_4 increase the release of mucus from human airways in vitro. *Am. Rev. Respir. Dis.* 126:449, 1982.

136. Marom, Z., Shelhamer, J. H., and Kaliner, M. The effect of arachidonic acid, monohydroxyeicosatetraenoic acid, and prostaglandins on the release of mucous glycoproteins from human airways *in vitro*. *J. Clin. Invest.* 67:1695, 1981.

137. Martin, R., et al. Interleukin 1β production by alveolar macrophages derived from nocturnal asthmatics. *J. Allergy Clin. Immunol.* 87:303A, 1991.

138. Martin, T. R., et al. Relative contribution of leukotriene B_4 to the neutrophil chemotactic activity produced by the resident human alveolar macrophage. *J. Clin. Invest.* 80:1114, 1987.

139. Martinez, J. D., et al. Nonspecific suppressor cell function in atopic subjects. *J. Allergy Clin. Immunol.* 64:485, 1979.

140. Melewicz, F. M., et al. Increased peripheral blood monocytes with Fc receptors for IgE in patients with severe allergic disorders. *J. Immunol.* 126:1592, 1981.

141. Metcalf, D., et al. Biologic properties *in vitro* of a recombinant human granulocyte-macrophage colony-stimulating factor. *Blood* 67:37, 1986.

142. Metzger, W. J., et al. Local allergen challenge and bronchoalveolar lavage of allergic asthmatic lungs: Description of the model and local airway inflammation. *Am. Rev. Respir. Dis.* 135:433, 1987.

143. Mezzetti, M., et al. IL1 binds to specific receptors on human bronchial epithelial cells and promotes GM-CSF synthesis and release. *J. Allergy Clin. Immunol.* 87:301A, 1991.

144. Mornex, J.-F., et al. Spontaneous expression of the c-sis gene and release of a platelet-derived growth factor-like molecule by human alveolar macrophages. *J. Clin. Invest.* 78:61, 1986.

145. Mosmann, T. R., et al. Two types of murine helper T cell clone. I. Definition according to profiles of lymphokine activities and secreted proteins. *J. Immunol.* 136:2348, 1986.

146. Nagy, L., et al. Complement receptor enhancement and chemotaxis of human neutrophils and eosinophils by leukotrienes and other lipoxygenase products. *Clin. Exp. Immunol.* 47:541, 1982.

147. Nakamura, T., et al. Platelet activating factor in late asthmatic responses. *Int. Arch. Allergy Appl. Immunol.* 82:57, 1981.

148. Nathan, C. F., et al. Activation of human macrophages: Comparison of other cytokines with interferon-γ. *J. Exp. Med.* 160:600, 1984.

149. North, R. J. The concept of the activated macrophage. *J. Immunol.* 121:806, 1978.

150. Okubo, T., et al. Plasma levels of leukotrienes C4 and D4 during wheezing attack in asthmatic patients. *Int. Arch. Allergy Appl. Immunol.* 84:149, 1987.

151. Okumura, K., and Tada, T. Regulation of homocytotropic antibody formation in the rat: III. Effect of thymectomy and splenectomy. *J. Immunol.* 106:1019, 1971.

152. Oppenheim, J. J., et al. There is more than one interleukin 1. *Immunol. Today* 7:45, 1986.

153. Paul, W. E., and Ohara, J. B-cell stimulatory factor-1/Interleukin 4. *Annu. Rev. Immunol.* 5:429, 1987.

154. Pene, J. Regulatory role of cytokines and CD23 in the human IgE antibody synthesis. *Int. Arch. Allergy Appl. Immunol.* 90:32, 1989.

155. Pene, J., et al. IgE production by normal lymphocytes is induced by interleukin 4 and suppressed by interferons γ and α and prostaglandin E_2. *Proc. Natl. Acad. Sci. USA* 85:6880, 1988.

156. Phillips, S. M., et al. Schistosomiasis in the congenitally athymic (nude) mouse: Thymic dependency of eosinophilia, granuloma formation, and host morbidity. *J. Immunol.* 18:594, 1977.

157. Plaut, M., et al. Mast cell lines produce lymphokines in response to cross-linkage of FcεR-I or to calcium ionophores. *Nature* 339:64, 1989.

158. Rand, T. H., et al. CD4-mediated stimulation of human eosinophils: Lymphocyte chemoattractant factor and other CD4-binding ligands elicit eosinophil migration. *J. Exp. Med.* 173:1521, 1991.

159. Rankin, J. A. The contribution of alveolar macrophages to hyperreactive airway disease. *J. Allergy Clin. Immunol.* 83:722, 1989.

160. Rankin, J. A., et al. IgE-dependent release of leukotriene C_4 from alveolar macrophages. *Nature* 297:329, 1982.

161. Rankin, J. A., et al. IgE immune complexes induce immediate and prolonged release of leukotriene C_4 (LTC₄) from rat alveolar macrophages. *J. Immunol.* 132:1993, 1984.

162. Reynolds, H. Y. Bronchoalveolar lavage. *Am. Rev. Respir. Dis.* 135:250, 1987.

163. Ricci, M., and Rossi, O. Dysregulation of IgE responses and airway allergic inflammation in atopic individuals. *Clin. Exp. Allergy* 20:601, 1990.

164. Robinson, D. S., et al. Cytokine mRNA profile and T-cell activation in bronchoalveolar lavage (BAL) cells from atopic asthmatics and controls. *J. Allergy Clin. Immunol.* 87:275A, 1991.

164a. Robinson, D. S., et al. Predominant T$_{H2}$-like bronchoalveolar T-lymphocyte populations in atopic asthma. *N. Engl. J. Med.* 326:298, 1992.

165. Roche, W. R., et al. Subepithelial fibrosis in the bronchi of asthmatics. *Lancet* 2:520, 1989.

166. Roche, W. R., et al. Subepithelial fibrosis in the bronchi of asthmatics. *Lancet* 1:520, 1989.

167. Rocklin, R. E., et al. Correction of *in vitro* immunoregulatory defect in atopic subjects by the immunostimulating drug fanetizole mesylate (CP-48,810). *Int. J. Immunopharmacol.* 6:1, 1984.

168. Rocklin, R. E., et al. Generation of antigen-specific suppressor cells during allergy desensitization. *N. Engl. J. Med.* 302:1213, 1980.

169. Romagnani, S. Regulation and deregulation of human IgE synthesis. *Immunol. Today* 11:316, 1990.

170. Romanagnani, S. Human T$_H$1 and T$_H$2 subsets: Doubt no more. *Immunol. Today* 12:256, 1991.

171. Ross, R., Raines, E. W., and Bowen-Pope, D. F. The biology of platelet-derived growth factor. *Cell* 46:155, 1986.

172. Rousset, F., et al. Regulation of Fc receptor for IgE (CD23) and class II MHC antigen expression on Burkitt's lymphoma cell lines by human Il-4 and IFN-gamma. *J. Immunol.* 140:2625, 1988.

173. Rousset, F., et al. Shifts in interleukin-4 and interferon-γ production by T cells of patients with elevated serum IgE levels and the modulatory effects of these lymphokines on spontaneous IgE synthesis. *J. Allergy Clin. Immunol.* 87:58, 1991.

174. Rubin, A.-H. E., Smith, L. J., and Patterson, R. The bronchoconstrictor properties of platelet-activating factor in humans. *Am. Rev. Respir. Dis.* 136:1145, 1987.

175. Rupp, E. A., et al. The specific bioactivities of monocyte derived interleukin-1 alpha and interleukin-1 beta are similar to each other on cultured murine thymocytes and cultured human connective tissue cells. *J. Clin. Invest.* 78:836, 1986.

176. Saito, H., et al. Selective differentiation and proliferation of hematopoietic cells induced by recombinant interleukins. *Proc. Natl. Acad. Sci. USA* 85:2288, 1988.

177. Samuelsson, B., et al. Leukotrienes and lipoxins: Structures, biosynthesis, and biological effects. *Science* 237:1171, 1987.

178. Sarfati, M., et al. In vitro synthesis of IgE by human lymphocytes. III. IgE potentiation activity of culture supernatants from Epstein-Barr virus (EBV) transformed B cells. *Immunology* 53:207, 1984.

179. Sarfati, M., et al. In vitro synthesis of IgE by human lymphocytes. II. Enhancement of the spontaneous IgE synthesis by IgE-binding factors secreted by RPMI 8866 lymphoblastoid B cells. *Immunology* 53:197, 1984.

180. Saryan, J. A., Leung, D. Y. M., and Geha, R. S. Induction of human IgE synthesis by a factor derived from T cells of patients with hyper-IgE states. *J. Immunol.* 130:242, 1983.

181. Saryan, J. A., et al. Regulation of human immunoglobulin E synthesis in acute graft versus host disease. *J. Clin. Invest.* 71:556, 1983.

182. Saxon, A., Morrow, C., and Stevens, R. H. Subpopulations of circulating B cells and regulatory T cells involved in in vitro immunoglobulin E production in atopic patients with elevated serum immunoglobulin E. *J. Clin. Invest.* 65:1457, 1980.

183. Schwartz, L. B., et al. Release of tryptase together with histamine during the immediate cutaneous response to allergen. *J. Allergy Clin. Immunol.* 80:850, 1987.

184. Sherhan, C. N., et al. Leukotriene B_4 is a complete secretagogue in human neutrophils: A kinetic analysis. *Biochem. Biophys. Res. Commun.* 107: 1006, 1982.

185. Sieff, C. A. Hematopoietic growth factors. *J. Clin. Invest.* 79:1549, 1987.

186. Sims, J. E., et al. cDNA expression cloning of the IL-1 receptor, a member of the immunoglobulin superfamily. *Science* 241:585, 1988.

187. Smith, C. A., and Rennick, D. M. Characterization of a murine lymphokine distinct from interleukin 2 and interleukin 3 (IL-3) possessing a T-cell growth factor activity and a mast-cell growth factor activity that synergizes with IL-3. *Proc. Natl. Acad. Sci. USA* 83:1857, 1988.

188. Smith, L. J., et al. The effect of inhaled leukotriene D_4 in humans. *Am. Rev. Respir. Dis.* 131:368, 1985.

189. Spiegelberg, H. L. Structure and function of Fc receptors for IgE on lymphocytes, monocytes, and macrophages. *Adv. Immunol.* 35:61, 1984.

190. Spiegelberg, H. L., et al. Lack of pokeweed mitogen-induced IgE formation in vitro by human peripheral blood mononuclear cells: Detection of cross-reacting idiotypic determinants on polyclonal Ig by antibodies to a single IgE myeloma protein. *J. Immunol.* 131:3001, 1983.

191. Sporn, M. B., et al. Transforming growth factor-beta: Biological function and chemical structure. *Science* 233:532, 1986.

192. Street, N. E., and Mosmann, T. R. Functional diversity of T lymphocytes due to secretion of different cytokine patterns. *FASEB J.* 5:171, 1991.

193. Swain, S. L. T cell subsets and the recognition of MHC class. *Immunol. Rev.* 74:129, 1983.

194. Tada, T., Tanaguchi, M., and Okumura, K. Regulation of homocytotropic antibody formation in the rat. II. Effect of X irradiation. *J. Immunol.* 106: 1012, 1971.

195. Talbot, S. F., et al. Accumulation of leukotriene C4 and histamine in human allergic skin reactions. *J. Clin. Invest.* 76:650, 1985.

196. Taniguchi, M., and Tada, T. Regulation of homocytotropic antibody formation in the rat. IV. Effects of various immunosuppressive drugs. *J. Immunol.* 107:579, 1971.

197. Taylor, K. J., and Luksza, A. R. Peripheral blood eosinophil counts and bronchial responsiveness. *Thorax* 42:452, 1987.

198. Thorne, K. J. I., et al. A comparison of eosinophil-activating factor (EAF) with other monokines and lymphokines. *Eur. J. Immunol.* 16:1143, 1986.

199. Thueson, D. O., et al. Histamine-releasing activity (HRA). I. Production by mitogen- and antigen-stimulated human mononuclear cells. *J. Immunol.* 123:626, 1979.

200. Ting, S., et al. Patterns of mast cell alterations and in vivo mediator release in human allergic skin reactions. *J. Allergy Clin. Immunol.* 66: 417, 1980.

201. Tonnel, M., et al. Enzyme release and superoxide anion production by human alveolar macrophages stimulated with immunoglobulin E. *Clin. Exp. Immunol.* 40:416, 1980.

202. Tosato, G., et al. Monocyte-derived human B-cell growth factor identified as interferon-β$_2$ (BSF-2, Il-6). *Science* 239:502, 1988.

203. Toyonaga, B., and Mak, T. W. Genes of the T-cell antigen receptor in normal and malignant T cells. *Annu. Rev. Immunol.* 5:585, 1987.

204. Trinchieri, G., et al. Tumor necrosis factor and lymphotoxin induce differentiation of human myeloid cell lines in synergy with immune interferon. *J. Exp. Med.* 164:1206, 1986.

205. Turnbull, L. W., et al. Mediators of immediate-type hypersensitivity in sputum from patients with chronic bronchitis and asthma. *Lancet* 2:526, 1977.

206. Umetsu, D. T., et al. Differential requirements of B cells from normal and allergic subjects for the induction of IgE synthesis by an alloreactive T cell clone. *J. Exp. Med.* 162:202, 1985.

207. van Leuwen, B. H., et al. Molecular organization of the cytokine gene cluster, involving the human IL-3, IL-4, IL-5, and GM-CSF genes, on human chromosome 5. *Blood* 73:1142, 1989.

208. Vercelli, D., and Geha, R. S. Regulation of IgE synthesis in humans. *J. Clin. Immunol.* 9:75, 1989.

209. Vercelli, D., et al. Induction of human IgE synthesis requires interleukin 4 and T/B cell interactions involving the T cell complex and MHC class II antigens. *J. Exp. Med.* 169:1295, 1989.

210. Vercelli, D., et al. Endogenous IL-6 plays an obligatory role in interleukin-4-dependent human IgE synthesis. *Eur. J. Immunol.* 8:1419, 1989.

211. Vercelli, D., et al. Human recombinant interleukin 4 induces FcεR2/CD23 on normal human monocytes. *J. Exp. Med.* 167:1406, 1988.

212. Vogel, S. N., and Friedman, R. M. Interferon and Macrophages: Activation and Cell Surface Changes. In J. Vilcek and E. DeMaeyer (eds.), *Interferons:* Vol. 2. *Interferon and the Immune System.* Amsterdam: Elsevier, 1984. Pp. 35–59.

213. Wahl, S. M., et al. Transforming growth factor type-β induces monocyte chemotaxis and growth factor production. *Proc. Natl. Acad. Sci. USA* 84: 5788, 1987.

214. Wardlaw, A. J., et al. Cellular changes in blood and bronchoalveolar lavage (BAL) and bronchial responsiveness after inhaled PAF in man. *Am. Rev. Respir. Dis.* 137:283, 1988.

215. Wardlaw, A. J., et al. Eosinophils and mast cells in bronchoalveolar lavage in mild asthma: Relationship to bronchial hyperreactivity. *Am. Rev. Respir. Dis.* 137:62, 1988.

216. Wardlaw, A. J., et al. Platelet-activating factor. A potent chemotactic and chemokinetic factor for human eosinophils. *J. Clin. Invest.* 78:1701, 1986.

217. Wegner, C. D., et al. Intercellular adhesion molecule-1 (ICAM-1) in the pathogenesis of asthma. *Science* 247:456, 1990.

218. Weiser, W. Y., et al. Recombinant human granulocyte/macrophage colony-stimulating factor activates intracellular killing of *Leishmania dono-vani* by human monocyte-derived macrophages. *J. Exp. Med.* 166:1436, 1987.

219. Weller, P. F., Bach, D. S., and Austen, K. F. Biochemical characterization of human eosinophil Charcot-Leyden crystal protein (lysophospholipase). *J. Biol. Chem.* 259:15100, 1984.

220. Wheelock, E. F. Interferon-like virus-inhibitor induced in human leukocytes by phytohemagglutinin. *Science* 149:310, 1965.

221. Wierenga, E. A., et al. Evidence for compartmentalization of functional subsets of CD4⁺ T lymphocytes in atopic patients. *J. Immunol.* 144:4651, 1990.

222. Wodnar-Filipowicz, A., Heusser, C. H., and Moroni, C. Production of the haemopoietic growth factors GM-CSF and interleukin-3 by mast cells in response to IgE receptor-mediated activation. *Nature* 339:150, 1989.

223. Wong, G. G., et al. Human GM-CSF: Molecular cloning of the complementary DNA and purification of the natural and recombinant proteins. *Science* 228:810, 1985.

224. Woodward, D. F., et al. The effect of synthetic leukotrienes on tracheal microvascular permeability. *Prostaglandins* 25:131, 1983.

225. Yamaguchi, Y., et al. Highly purified murine interleukin 5 (IL-5) stimulates eosinophil function and prolongs in vitro survival: IL-5 as an eosinophil chemotactic factor. *J. Exp. Med.* 167:1737, 1988.

226. Yang, Y.-C., et al. Human IL-3 (multi-CSF): Identification by expression cloning of a novel hematopoietic growth factor related to murine IL-3. *Cell* 47:3, 1986.

227. Yokota, T., et al. Isolation and characterization of lymphokine cDNA clones encoding mouse and human IgA-enhancing factor and eosinophil colony-stimulating factor activities: Relationship to interleukin-5. *Proc. Natl. Acad. Sci. USA* 84:7388, 1987.

Adrenergic Regulation

Andor Szentivanyi

14

This chapter describes the cellular and molecular foundations of the functioning of the mammalian adrenergic nervous system at various levels of adrenergic regulation. The discussion primarily focuses on peripheral adrenergic regulatory levels for two reasons: (1) In molecular terms, the patterns of adrenergic activities are essentially the same at central and peripheral levels of organization, and (2) a discussion of the central adrenergic influences is also included in the chapter on the immune-neuroendocrine circuitry (see Chap. 33).

THE AUTONOMIC NERVOUS SYSTEM

Interposed in the efferent pathway from the central nervous system to the visceral structures are aggregations of neurons known as the autonomic ganglia. Cells of these ganglia are in synaptic relation with fibers from the spinal cord or brain and send out axons that terminate in the three visceral effectors: smooth muscle, myocardium, and glandular epithelium. Thus unlike striated muscle, which is directly innervated by axons of centrally placed neurons, impulse transmission from the central nervous system to the viscera always involves two systems of neurons. This first neuron (preganglionic) conducts the impulse from the central nervous system to some autonomic ganglion, and although it may pass several ganglia, it forms only a single synapse. The second neuron (postganglionic) then transmits the impulse from the ganglion to the effector cells.

The autonomic ganglia may be placed in three groups: vertebral, or lateral; prevertebral, or collateral; and terminal, or peripheral. Vertebral ganglia are arranged in a segmental fashion along the ventrolateral surface of the vertebral column and are connected with each other by longitudinal fibers to form the two sympathetic trunks or ganglionated cords. Collateral ganglia are found in the mesenteric neural plexuses, whereas terminal ganglia are located within or close to the structures they innervate.

All these neurons and ganglia, as portions of the central and peripheral nervous systems, are primarily concerned with the regulation of visceral activities and are called collectively *the autonomic nervous system* (also known as the involuntary, visceral, or vegetative nervous system). Most functions so regulated are involuntary without implying that all involuntary functions are autonomic [20, 397].

Sympathetic and Parasympathetic Divisions

Three outflows of preganglionic neurons connect the central nervous system with the autonomic ganglia. The cranial outflow contains efferent visceral fibers from the oculomotor, facial, glos-

sopharyngeal, and vagus nerves, these fibers going only to the terminal autonomic ganglia. The thoracolumbar outflow is composed of neurons from the lateral sympathetic nucleus (intermediolateral column) of the spinal cord, which pass out by way of the ventral roots of the eighth cervical, all the thoracic, and the upper two or three lumbar nerves. These neurons leave the ventral roots as the white rami communicantes, enter the sympathetic trunk, and end in the vertebral ganglia of the trunk or the collateral mesenteric ganglia. The sacral outflow contains efferent visceral neurons from the inferior lateral and medial parasympathetic nuclei of the spinal cord, which pass through the ventral roots of the second, third, and fourth sacral nerves and go to the terminal ganglia associated with the pelvic organs [20, 397].

Most of the viscera receive a dual autonomic innervation, the effects of the two innervations being antagonistic as a rule. One is through the thoracolumbar outflow, which supplies all the visceral structures of the body and employs norepinephrine as its neurotransmitter agent. The other innervation is by the cranial or sacral outflow. The cranial outflow supplies the visceral structures of the head and the thoracic as well as abdominal viscera, with the exception of the pelvic organs, which are supplied by the sacral outflow.

The cranial and sacral outflows have several important features in common. Both are functionally antagonistic to the thoracolumbar outflow, react in a similar manner to drugs, and employ acetylcholine as their neurotransmitter agent. They have no white rami communicantes that enter the sympathetic trunk but their preganglionic neurons run directly to the terminal ganglia. On this basis, two main divisions comprise the autonomic nervous system: the thoracolumbar, or sympathetic, and the craniosacral, or parasympathetic, divisions [20, 397].

Complementary Sympathetic Systems

Additional sympathetic or chromaffin* tissues that functionally complement the sympathetic division of the peripheral autonomic nervous system include the adrenal medullae, paraganglia, and various other extraadrenal chromaffin cells.

The precursors of these chromaffin cells are derived from the neural crest of the embryo as primordial sympathetic ganglion cells; only after migrating outside the nervous system do some of the ganglion cells become further differentiated as adrenal medullary cells and to a lesser extent as paraganglia (including the organs of Zuckerkandl) or as the chromaffin elements of the carotid body, as well as those of homologous structures related

The work described in this chapter was supported in part by a grant from The Eleanor Naylor Dana Charitable Trust.

---

* The term *chromaffin* refers to the brown darkening effect of potassium bichromate and chromic acid on these cells, causing the formation of a pigmented granularity in their cytoplasm. Chromic acid and bichromate induce this coloration by oxidizing their catecholamine content; the oxidized products then condense to form insoluble colored polymers that resemble melanin [72].

to the great vessels of the thorax. But extraadrenal chromaffin cells may occur in any part of the more central sympathetic nervous system, including all parts of the paravertebral chain and prevertebral sympathetic plexuses. Any sympathetic ganglion may contain chromaffin elements, and isolated cells or discrete bodies may accompany any of the thoracic or intraabdominal sympathetic neurons [72].

Processing of Information in the Sympathetic and Parasympathetic Divisions

Communication between mammalian nerve cells involves a long chain of events related to initiation, conduction, and transmission of nerve impulses. The following discussion as well as later sections present only brief conceptualizations of the major processes. For their more comprehensive analysis, current reviews or texts should be consulted.

Impulse Initiation and Axonal Conduction

At rest, an electric potential exists across the cell membrane of the neuron and is referred to as the *resting potential*. This potential is present because the resting cell membrane is slightly permeable to sodium ions and highly permeable to potassium ions. The concentration of sodium ions is high on the outside surface (positive charge) and low on the inside surface (negative charge). These ionic gradients are maintained by an energy-dependent pump mechanism involving an adenosine triphosphatase (ATPase) activated by sodium at the inner surface and by potassium at the outer surface of the membrane [6, 370].

Effective stimulation makes a local region of the neuronal membrane temporarily permeable to sodium ions, which then flow freely into the axoplasm, causing decreased electronegativity on the inside. The influx of ions sets up an electrotonic current that depolarizes adjacent parts of the axolemma, giving rise to what is known as a *generator potential*, which in turn elicits an *action potential*. The action potential is self-propagating, advancing as a wave of depolarization along the axon. The nerve impulse and its conduction are therefore the migration of the change in potential from the resting to the active state in consecutive regions of the axolemma [58, 145, 146, 170, 296, 297].

In myelinated axons, the electrotonic current flow is greatly speeded up by the presence of the nodes of Ranvier. It is believed that the current remains confined to and flows forward in the axon because of the insulating myelin sheath of the internodal segment. A regeneration of the action potential cannot occur until the next node is reached, where the myelin is interrupted. Thus, the current "leaps" from one node to the next, a phenomenon called *saltatory conduction*. The electrotonic current flow is slower in nonmyelinated axons, which has been attributed to the absence of the nodes of Ranvier [170].

Junctional Transmission

Ordinarily the nerve impulse generated within the neuron travels away from the perikaryon along the axon and its branches until it reaches an anatomic end formation, the *terminal button*. This button is in contact with a centrifugally conducting perikaryon or centripetally conducting dendrites of a second neuron. This contact is an unusual one involving spatial contiguity without continuity. It is unique as a method of joining cellular elements and is found only within or in conjunction with the nervous system. This unique approximation of two cellular entities is commonly referred to as a *junction*. In general, there are two types of junctions: (1) A *synapse* is a junction involving the aforementioned two nervous elements, one a stimulating terminal of the first neuron and the other a stimulated perikaryon or dendrite of a succeeding neuron; and (2) a *neuroeffector junction* is one

between a nerve ending and a nonnervous effector cell (i.e., muscle, exocrine gland, and others).

A junctional contact therefore consists of a presynaptic membrane of the axon, the postsynaptic membrane of the dendrite or perikaryon, and an intermembranous synaptic cleft, averaging 200 to 300 Å. Because of lack of anatomic continuity, the nerve impulse is transmitted from the first to the second unit by specific chemical substances, the *neurotransmitters*. Transmission of the nerve impulse refers, therefore, to the process whereby the nerve terminal activates the second unit or transfers a stimulus to it, be the second unit a neuron or a nonnervous effector cell [28, 78, 85, 170, 171].

Similar relationships are found in the adrenal medullae. In keeping with the ganglionic ancestry, adrenal medullary cells receive their innervating fibers by way of the lesser splanchnic nerve and through direct branches from the lumbar sympathetic trunk without the interposition of postganglionic neurons [331]. Acetylcholine-containing synaptic vesicles are confined to the presynaptic terminals of the splanchnic fibers, whereas catecholamine-storing chromaffin granules are localized postsynaptically in medullary cells [176]. This arrangement is consistent with the interpretation that the nerve fibers represent the preganglionic cholinergic innervation of chromaffin cells; the limiting membranes of the chromaffin cells stand for the postganglionic membranes, whereas the cells substitute for the terminals or regular postganglionic adrenergic neurons. Shared characteristics in electrophysiologic properties [40, 223] and in sensitivities to various ganglion-blocking agents [40, 223, 283] further argue for the specific relationship between their cell membranes and authentic postganglionic membranes. This is best illustrated by the excellent agreement between the sensitivities of both membranes to methonium compounds of various chain lengths; in both cases, decamethonium (C_{10}) is ineffective and hexamethonium (C_6) is the most potent [40, 223, 283].

Thus, patterned after the two-unit architectural principle of the autonomic nervous system, the term *cholinergic* implies transmission from the first to the second unit through acetylcholine, whereas the term *adrenergic* implies transmission through adrenaline-like substances (primarily norepinephrine). By using these terms, the most widely accepted view is that all preganglionic neurons of the autonomic nervous system including the innervating fibers of the adrenal medullae, all postganglionic neurons of the craniosacral division, and some postganglionic fibers [331] of the thoracolumbar division, and all somatic motor nerves are cholinergic. On the other hand, with a few exceptions [331] the postganglionic sympathetic neurons are adrenergic [28, 85, 170].

Adrenergic Transmission

Chemically the adrenergic neurotransmitters are catecholamines. The term *catecholamine* refers generically to all compounds containing a catechol nucleus (benzene with two adjacent hydroxy groups, i.e., dihydroxybenzene, also known as catechol) and an amine group. However, use of this term is usually reserved for dihydroxyphenylethylamine (dopamine) and its metabolic products, norepinephrine and epinephrine.

Of these compounds, norepinephrine has been established as the neurotransmitter of most sympathetic postganglionic neurons and probably of certain tracts in the central nervous system. Dopamine is emerging as an important transmitter in the extrapyramidal and possibly mesolimbic systems, and epinephrine is the acknowledged major hormone of the adrenal medullae.

With the exception of the adrenal medullae, in all peripheral tissues the predominant catecholamine is norepinephrine. Its concentration in a given tissue reflects the density of adrenergic innervation and thus varies considerably. Most of the norepinephrine in peripheral tissues is localized in adrenergic nerve terminals, but small amounts are also found along the entire length of such neurons and in their perikarya in the sympathetic ganglia.

In the adrenal medullae, norepinephrine and epinephrine are stored in separate cells [94]. There are considerable species differences in medullary distribution of the two cell types and consequently in the relative proportions of the two amines. Of the total catechol contents of human medullary tissues, norepinephrine accounts for about 20 percent and epinephrine for almost 80 percent, with dopamine being present only in trace amounts [130, 283]. Medullary levels of the principal catechols, epinephrine and norepinephrine, are relatively high, with concentrations of 5 to 10 mg/gm of tissue [130, 283].

Little information is available on the catechol composition of various other extramedullary chromaffin cells. Among these, the paraganglia certainly contain catecholamines and in some cases (organs of Zuckerkandl) both norepinephrine and epinephrine [129], whereas chromaffin cells associated with the terminals of postganglionic nonadrenergic neurons probably contain only epinephrine [283].

Dopa or dopamine in most tissues can be detected only in trace amounts, since these compounds exist only as transient intermediates in catecholamine synthesis. However, in peripheral tissues of some ruminant animals, dopamine has been demonstrated to account for as much as 80 percent of the total catechol content. This dopamine is stored not in adrenergic neurons but in a specialized type of mast cell, which is chromaffin positive and occurs in abundance in dopamine-rich tissues [72, 96].

The central nervous system of mammals contains significant amounts of both norepinephrine and dopamine, which are distributed in well-defined and distinct regional patterns. The two amines are stored in different neurons, and it is likely that a new class of adrenergic neurons, in which dopamine rather than norepinephrine is the transmitter, exists in certain regions of the central nervous system. Highest levels of norepinephrine are found in the hypothalamus and other areas of central sympathetic representation, whereas dopamine is concentrated in the neostriatum, nucleus accumbens, and tuberculum olfactorium [31, 153, 256, 311]. Dopamine is also present in the superior cervical ganglion, which appears to have at least three distinct populations of neurons: cholinergic neurons, noradrenergic neurons, and small intensely fluorescent cells. The small intensely fluorescent cells are believed to be small interneurons that contain dopamine. Release of the amine from these interneurons is postulated to be responsible for hyperpolarization of the ganglion [121].

Epinephrine concentration in the central nervous system is relatively low, approximately 5 to 17 percent of the norepinephrine content. Several investigators have suggested that these estimates are erroneous and have therefore discounted the importance of the occurrence of epinephrine in the brain. Recently, however, it was demonstrated that the olfactory bulb and tubercle contain substantial amounts of phenylethanolamine-*N*-methyltransferase, indicating that these structures are capable of forming epinephrine in vivo.

Biosynthesis of Catecholamines

As with other neurotransmitters, norepinephrine is synthesized locally in the neurons that use this compound as a transmitter. In addition, norepinephrine and epinephrine are synthesized in the adrenal medullary and other chromaffin cells. In all these cells the pathway of biosynthesis is the same, and the enzymes involved appear to be identical.

Catecholamine biosynthesis is conventionally considered to begin with tyrosine, with represents a branch point for many important biosynthetic processes in mammalian tissues. Tyrosine is normally present in the circulation in a concentration of

about 5 to 8×10^{-5} M. It is taken up from the bloodstream and concentrated within the nerve or chromaffin cells by an active transport mechanism [52]. Once inside the neuron or chromaffin cell, tyrosine undergoes a series of intracellular migrations, from the cytoplasm to the mitochondria, back to the cytoplasm, and finally to a specialized subcellular organelle, the granulated vesicle or chromaffin granule. At each locus a specific enzymatic transformation occurs, resulting after three steps in the production of norepinephrine. In chromaffin cells that contain the enzyme needed to synthesize epinephrine, there is an additional intracellular migration of norepinephrine from the chromaffin granule to the cytoplasm for *N*-methylation and then back again to the chromaffin granule for storage. In dopamine-containing central neurons the last two steps of the pathway are lacking.

In the first step of the synthetic process, cytoplasmic L-tyrosine is converted to L-dihydroxyphenylalanine (dopa) by tyrosine hydroxylase in the mitochondria [242]. This enzyme is a mixed function oxidase; that is, it catalyzes a reaction of the following type:

$$RH + O_2 + XH_2 \rightarrow ROH + H_2O + X$$

In this equation RH stands for the substrate to be hydroxylated, ROH for the hydroxylated product, and XH_2 for an electron donor. Tetrahydrofolic acid together with a ferrous salt or synthetic tetrahydropteridine can act as cofactors (XH_2) for the purified enzyme. The naturally occurring cofactor is thought to be a derivative of dihydrobiopterin. Tyrosine hydroxylase shows a fairly high degree of substrate specificity; it oxidizes only the naturally occurring amino acid L-tyrosine. The Michaelis constant (K_m) for the conversion of tyrosine to dopa by purified adrenal tyrosine hydroxylase is about 2×10^{-5} M and in a preparation of brain synaptosomes, about 0.4×10^{-5} M. Tyrosine hydroxylation is the rate-limiting step in the synthesis of norepinephrine and dopamine in the central nervous system as well [233, 391].

In the second synthetic step, L-dopa is decarboxylated to dopamine (L-dihydroxyphenylethylamine) by L-dopa decarboxylase in the cytoplasm. Unlike tyrosine hydroxylase, which is a highly specific enzyme found only in catecholamine-synthesizing cells, dopa decarboxylase occurs in a wide variety of tissues. A study of purified enzyme preparations and specific inhibitors demonstrated that this dopa decarboxylase acts on all naturally occurring aromatic L-amino acids, including histidine, tyrosine, tryptophan, 5-hydroxytryptophan, and phenylalanine [218]. Therefore this enzyme is more appropriately referred to as *aromatic L-amino acid decarboxylase*. Relative to other enzymes in the catecholamine synthetic sequence, aromatic L-amino acid decarboxylase is active (V_{max} is about 1,000 times that of tyrosine hydroxylase) and requires pyridoxal phosphate as a cofactor. The enzyme has a pH optimum of 7.2 and molecular weight of 109,000. The K_m for either dopa or tyrosine is about 5×10^{-4} M [233].

The third synthetic step involves hydroxylation of the beta carbon of dopamine (the atoms separated by one carbon from the amine nitrogen), resulting in the formation of norepinephrine in the storage vesicles or chromaffin granules. This reaction is catalyzed by a mixed function oxidase, dopamine-beta-hydroxylase. The enzyme requires molecular oxygen and ascorbate and has a K_m of about 5×10^{-3} M. Dicarboxylic acids such as fumaric acid are not absolute requirements, but they stimulate the reaction. Dopamine-beta-hydroxylase is a Cu^{++}-containing protein, with about 2 mol of cupric ion per mole of enzyme, and has a molecular weight of 290,000 [105, 208, 376].

In adrenal and extramedullary chromaffin cells as well as in certain areas of the brain, norepinephrine may be further converted to epinephrine by phenylethanolamine-*N*-methyltransferase, an enzyme with a molecular weight of 30,000. Demonstration of activity requires the presence of the methyl donor *S*-adenosylmethionine. The enzyme *N*-methylates a variety of phenyletha-

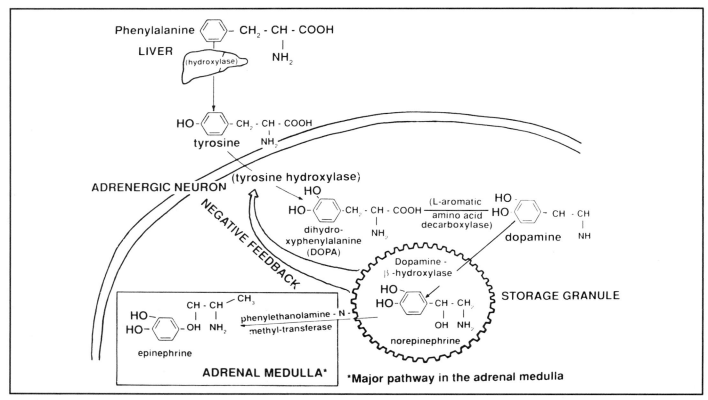

Fig. 14-1. *The major biosynthetic pathway in the formation of catecholamines. Intracellular migration and localization of specific portions of the process are depicted.*

nolamines but not phenylethylamines, a characteristic that explains its current name [233]. See Figure 14-1.

Storage of Catecholamines

After synthesis, the largest fraction of catecholamines in adrenergic neurons and adrenal medullary or other chromaffin cells is stored in cytoplasmic microvesicles (synaptic vesicles), colloquially referred to as *granules*. These specially devised subcellular organelles represent a common structural principle of neurotransmitter storage. Thus, sequestration of catecholamines in specific storage granules serves to inactivate the amines temporarily and to protect them from enzymatic destruction until they are released by an appropriate stimulus.

Of the substances that have been implicated in the granular binding of catecholamines, the adenine nucleotides are high on the list. The evidence for such a relationship rests mainly on the unusual chemical composition of the storage granules. Twenty-one percent of their dry weight is made up of catecholamines; 15 percent, of adenine nucleotides; 35 percent, of protein; and 22 percent, of lipids.* Although the principal nucleotide is adenosine triphosphate (ATP), adenosine diphosphate (ADP) and adenylic acid (AMP) are also present; their relative amounts vary from species to species. In those species in which the ATP content is not so high, the concentrations of ADP and AMP are proportionately increased, so that the total number of intragranular phosphate groups that are provided by the adenine nucleotides is approximately the same in all species examined so far. The molar ratio of catecholamines to ATP is about 4 in granules of the bovine adrenal medulla and adrenergic neurons, which means that the equivalence ratio is 1, since ATP has four negative

charges at the granular pH and the catecholamines are monocations. Nucleotides and catechols appear to be, therefore, stoichiometrically associated in the storage granules, the total number of negative charges on the adenine nucleotides being balanced by the total number of positive charges on the catecholamines [84, 304, 331].

Chromaffin and neuronal granules also contain at least eight species of a characteristic soluble protein named *chromogranin,* which is believed to participate in the storage process [36, 304]. The principal chromogranin, making up about 40 percent of the soluble protein fraction, is called *chromogranin A.* It is an acidic protein with antigenic properties [139, 140, 286, 292, 305], a molecular weight of about 77,000, and an elevated content of glutamic acid [307]. The possibility has been raised that chromogranin A is an oligomer [140], an idea that has received support by the similar amino acid composition of one of the minor species [307]. In any case, it seems likely that the anionic phosphate groups of ATP form a salt link with catecholamines, which then is reinforced by chromogranins.

Based mainly on pharmacologic evidence, current views hold that the tetracatecholamine-ATP-chromogranin complex constitutes the major storage depot of catecholamines, generally referred to as the *intragranular reserve pool.* This pool is in active equilibrium with two smaller pools, an intragranular mobile pool and a cytoplasmic mobile pool. In adrenergic nerve terminals, to effect the recapture (see the following discussion) of the previously released norepinephrine as well as to preserve the concentration gradients of de novo synthesized norepinephrine within the three pools, at least two active transport systems are believed to be operative, one from the extracellular space across the axolemma to the cytoplasmic mobile pool and the other from the cytoplasmic mobile pool through the granular membrane to the intragranular mobile pool [318, 388]. See Figure 14-2.

---

*Of the inorganic material, Ca^{++} contributes 1.6 percent and Mg^{++}, 0.36 percent [304].

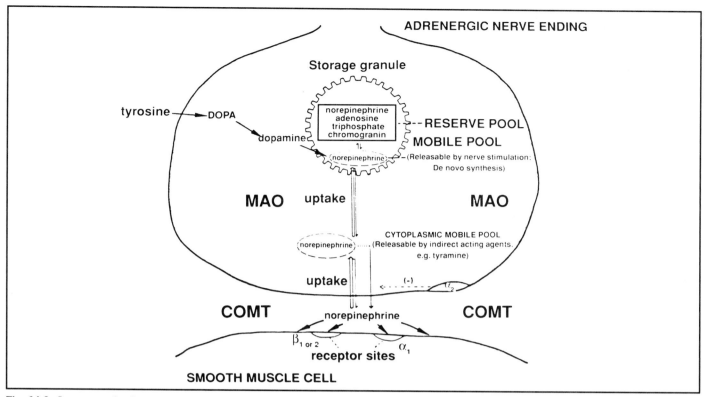

Fig. 14-2. *Storage pools of norepinephrine and their relationships in adrenergic nerve ending. Major localization of the enzymes monoamine oxidase (MAO) (mitochondrial) and catechol-O-methyltransferase (COMT) is presented.*

Release of Catecholamines

Stimulus-secretion coupling is the term coined to describe the processes involved in coupling the arrival of the action potential to the release of catecholamine from the adrenergic neuron or medullary cell [81]. The current knowledge about the stimulus-secretion coupling sequence derives primarily from study on medullary tissue and more recently on adrenergic neurons.

In the adrenal medullae, this coupling sequence is thought to consist of the following events. With activity in preganglionic (splanchnic) fibers, the preganglionic neurotransmitter acetylcholine is released and depolarizes the plasma membrane of the chromaffin cells. Depolarization produces change in membrane protein conformation, altering the permeability of this membrane to Ca^{++}. The inward movement of calcium ions is believed to promote fusion of the granular and limiting cell membranes, with the resultant discharge of granular catecholamines to the cell exterior. Release of catecholamines is then terminated on the disappearance of acetylcholine by diffusion or hydrolysis and by binding or extrusion of the calcium that has penetrated the cell [40, 58, 81, 129, 223, 283].

Calcium likewise appears to play a critical role in coupling the arrival of the nerve impulse with the release of norepinephrine at adrenergic nerve terminals [41]. Acetylcholine* release is also postulated to be an essential or facilitatory step in the neuronal liberation sequence of norepinephrine, although this is still a debated point [42, 97, 177, 214].

---

*Many postganglionic adrenergic neurons have long been known to contain cholinergic fibers and investigation has now shown that all do. Although it is not clear whether these cholinergic fibers are the same fibers in the adrenergic neuron that synthesize and store epinephrine, chances are that they are identical. If so, the adrenergic neuron is also capable of synthesizing and storing acetylcholine in addition to catecholamines [28, 29, 41, 42, 78, 85, 97, 170, 171, 177, 182, 214, 225, 331].

As to the nature of the catecholamine extrusion process, current theories suggest that granular contents are discharged directly into the junctional cleft or extracellular fluid by a process of reverse micropinocytosis or exocytosis. This is supported by findings that catecholamine discharge is accompanied by release of all soluble components of the storage granules. Thus, both catecholamines and ATP appear in the venous effluent and in approximately the same molar proportions in which they occur in the intact storage granules [82]. Moreover, under appropriate experimental conditions, ATP can escape unhydrolyzed, even though the cell and its organelles are rich in ATPases, which suggests that the nucleotide is extruded directly to the cell exterior [81, 233]. Granular proteins such as the eight species of chromogranins [36, 286, 292] and dopamine-beta-hydroxylase [253] accompany the amine release and in the same proportions as they are found in the soluble fraction of lysed granules [387]. Not only are all the soluble granular components released, but this release occurs as an all-or-none phenomenon with respect to any single granule [387]. Conversely, cytoplasmic (extragranular) proteins such as lactate dehydrogenase or phenylethanolamine-*N*-methyltransferase do not appear in the extracellular fluid in response to stimulation. Since neither ATP nor the granular proteins can readily pass through intact lipid membranes, the finding that these compounds are released on stimulation strongly favors the exocytosis model.

On the other hand, there is no evidence that the granular membrane itself is discharged during release. Electron micrographs show the membrane of the chromaffin granule fused with that of the cell [79], and stimulation produces no significant increase in the efflux of phospholipid or cholesterol, the principal lipids of the granular membrane [265, 373].

Another aspect of the problem involves the mechanism by

which the granular membrane fuses with the cytoplasmic membrane. It seems unlikely that calcium merely neutralizes net negative charges on the two membranes, allowing them to coalesce. That a metabolic process of some kind is involved is more likely. Thus, a phospholipase may be activated or ATP may be removed from the cytoplasmic membrane, permitting increased crosslinkage. Removal of cytoplasmic membranous ATP could conceivably be brought about through hydrolysis by an ATPase of the granular membrane [331].

Of further interest is whether the storage granule simply undergoes a rapid fusion with the cytoplasmic membrane or the exocytotic model of release requires insertion of the granular membrane into the cytoplasmic membrane, reappearing later by the reverse process, endocytosis. Information on the lipid and protein components of the two types of membranes suggests that there are too many differences to allow for long-term fusion-endocytosis cycles. Rapid fusion or possible contact exocytosis, therefore, seems a more plausible prospect [304, 318, 331, 388].

Metabolic Degradation of Catecholamines
Monoamine oxidase (MAO) and catechol-*O*-methyltransferase (COMT) are the two enzymes primarily involved in the metabolic degradation of catecholamines. Both act on a wide variety of amines, and each is fully active on the product of the other. Thus, an entire spectrum of metabolites of catecholamines can be identified in urine, some acted on by MAO, some by COMT, and some by both.

MAO is an enzyme that deaminates catecholamines to their corresponding aldehydes. This aldehyde intermediate is rapidly catabolized, usually by oxidation by aldehyde dehydrogenase to the corresponding acid (3,4-dihydroxymandelic acid). In some circumstances the aldehyde is reduced to the alcohol or glycol by aldehyde reductase. In the case of central norepinephrine, reduction of the aldehyde metabolite appears to be the favored route of metabolism.

MAO is widely distributed in tissues of many vertebrate species [35], where it is present primarily in the outer membrane of mitochondria [291], although a partial microsomal localization cannot be excluded [75, 273]. It has a molecular weight of about 290,000 and contains a flavoprotein and copper [106, 245]. The valence of copper does not change during the oxidative deamination of amines; thus, it appears unlikely that copper plays an active role in the reaction. Multiple forms of MAO exist (MAO-A, MAO-B), and various species of the enzyme differ in substrate specificity, heat stability, and effect of different inhibitors [59, 119, 312, 402].

The enzyme participates in the intraneuronal regulation of free neurotransmitter levels. Any norepinephrine that leaks into the axoplasm from the storage granules is catabolized to physiologically inactive products [180]. Conversely, inhibition of MAO results in an elevation of intraneuronal levels of norepinephrine and dopamine [331].

The second major enzyme in catecholamine metabolism is COMT, which converts norepinephrine and epinephrine to the corresponding 3-*O*-methylamines, normetanephrine and metanephrine. The enzyme catalyzes the transfer of the labile methyl groups from *S*-adenosylmethionine to the metahydroxyl group of catecholamines and requires a divalent cation such as Mg^{++} for activity [16]. When purified, the enzyme is labile, requires dithiothreitol for stability, and has a molecular weight of about 24,000. The K_m for any catechol substrate varies with the concentration of the second substrate, *S*-adenosylmethionine. K_m values for the latter similarly vary according to the catechol concentration, being in the range of 40 to 80 μM [8, 12].

COMT is found in many mammalian species [16], with the highest activity occurring in the liver and kidney. Distribution of COMT in the brain is asymmetric, activity being highest in the area posttrema and lowest in the cerebellar cortex [15]. Precise cellular localization of COMT has not been determined, but it is believed that the enzyme is present mainly outside the adrenergic neuron [14] in contrast to MAO, which is usually considered an intraneuronal enzyme [307].

Physiologically, COMT is involved in the metabolic degradation of catecholamines released into the circulation [14, 180] and in the inactivation of norepinephrine in tissues lacking an abundant adrenergic innervation [209]. COMT may also be associated with an extraneuronal uptake (Uptake 2) mechanism [88].

Neuronal Uptake and Inactivation of Catecholamines
COMT and MAO act on catecholamines to produce physiologically inactive metabolic products, but neither enzyme plays an important role in terminating the physiologic actions of the neurotransmitter norepinephrine or of the hormone epinephrine. The rapid inactivation of catecholamines is due to the ability of adrenergic nerve terminals to actively reaccumulate the transmitter they release.

Thus, when postganglionic adrenergic neurons are stimulated at frequencies low enough (< 10 Hz*) to be comparable to those encountered physiologically, there is little norepinephrine overflow into the circulation, indicating that local inactivation is highly efficient. This rapid local inactivation is not significantly inhibited when COMT, MAO, or both are blocked, and it involves the reuptake of the transmitter across the neuronal membrane and its subsequent retention in the storage granules described earlier [318, 388]. Although both stereoisomers of norepinephrine and epinephrine are taken up by nerve terminals, the naturally occurring levo- forms are removed more rapidly [157]. The process also shows molecular selectivity: The efficiency of uptake of norepinephrine is twice that of epinephrine, whereas little if any isoproterenol is taken up by this mechanism [318, 388].

Drugs that block this uptake across the neuronal membrane also prevent the inactivation of norepinephrine and thus prolong its physiologic actions [71]. Similarly, when postganglionic adrenergic neurons are destroyed surgically [68, 143], immunologically [369], or chemically [159, 208], the denervated tissues no longer can take up and retain norepinephrine. At the same time, the tissue response to the amine is markedly enhanced [91, 372].

Uptake through the neuronal membrane, also called *Uptake 1*, obeys saturation kinetics of the Michaelis-Menten type and involves active transport [77, 81]. Energy derived from either glycolysis or oxidation is required for the transport of norepinephrine across the neuronal membrane [389] and sodium ions must be present in the external medium [37, 160]. Norepinephrine uptake is a temperature-dependent process with a rate change to a 10°C increase (Q_{10}) of about 2 [157]. From these observations it appears that an active ion-carrier mechanism is involved in the transport of norepinephrine across the neuronal membrane.

An extraneuronal uptake process for norepinephrine called *Uptake 2* has also been demonstrated [87, 88, 112, 113, 158] and is blocked by normetanephrine and by adrenergic blocking agents [88, 117]. Uptake 2 operates at all concentrations of catecholamines to transport the amines into nonneuronal tissues where they are subsequently metabolized [212]. Compounds such as epinephrine and isoproterenol, which have a relatively low affinity for Uptake 1 and a high affinity for Uptake 2, may be inactivated primarily by Uptake 2. The termination of adrenergic amine action has been shown to be influenced by receptors (alpha$_2$) located at presynaptic sites. Activation of these alpha$_2$ sites leads to inhibition of the release of norepinephrine [93, 131, 314]. See Figure 14-2.

---

*Hz = impulse/sec.

THE ADRENOCEPTOR AS THE PHARMACOLOGICALLY SPECIFIC EFFECTOR-CELL COMPONENT OF ADRENERGIC ACTION

Adrenergic agonists elicit their characteristic effect through the activation of certain cells that are their specific effectors. These cells, called *effector cells,* are further defined as cells that are endowed with receptive membrane substances (membrane receptors) possessing sites with a steric configuration complementary to the agonist in question. The released or administered agonist combines with the complementary receptor site, thereby initiating a chain of biochemical reactions that culminates in the observable adrenergic response. From the standpoint of specificity of action, the strategically important component of the effector cell is, therefore, the membrane receptor.

The Adrenoceptors

The receptor concept implies two distinct functions: recognition of specific pharmacologically active molecules such as adrenergic agonists and activation of biologic processes through, for example, the cyclic nucleotide system and changes in ion permeability.

Pharmacologic Classification of Adrenoceptors

In 1948 Ahlquist [4] categorized the adrenoceptors as alpha and beta based on the effects and relative potencies of the adrenergic agonists norepinephrine, epinephrine, and isoproterenol on effector cells. Subsequently, the receptors were further divided into $alpha_1$, $alpha_2$, $beta_1$, and $beta_2$ subtypes [234]. The receptors classified as $alpha_1$ are located predominantly on postjunctional membranes and produce excitatory effects when stimulated by catecholamines. These receptors display a high affinity for the adrenergic antagonist prazosin. Receptors of the $alpha_2$ type are located on presynaptic nerve terminals, where they inhibit the release of neurotransmitters, and postsynaptically, where they mediate a variety of effects. These receptors have a high affinity for yohimbine. In addition, at least part of the effects produced by stimulation of $alpha_2$ receptors appears to be mediated by an inhibition of the adenylate cyclase system [7, 249]. Lands and associates [198] divided the beta receptors into $beta_1$ and $beta_2$ types based on the relative selectivity of adrenergic agonists and antagonists for these sites. The $beta_1$ receptors were believed to be the subtype distributed on cardiac muscle, whereas the $beta_2$ subtype was associated with bronchial and vascular smooth muscle. With the development of newer methods utilizing radiolabeled ligands to study the binding of a variety of agents to receptor surfaces, both $beta_1$- and $beta_2$-receptor subtypes have been reported to be widely distributed on a variety of different tissues in the body [243]. For a more complete listing of the tissue distribution and functional associations of the $alpha_1$, $alpha_2$, $beta_1$, and $beta_2$ adrenoceptors, see Table 21-1 in the chapter by Szentivanyi and coauthors in a previous publication [340]. However, there remains some doubt as to whether the selectivity of the various ligands used in such studies depends on the bioavailability of the ligands rather than on the type of receptors under investigation [202].

With the availability of more sophisticated and selective synthetic agonists and antagonists, additional improvements were made in the pharmacologic classification of adrenoceptors. Today we recognize two alpha$_1$ adrenoceptors. Of these, $alpha_{1A}$ and $alpha_{1B}$ (previous names $alpha_{1a}$ and $alpha_{1b}$) show the same potency order for the endogenous adrenergic ligands epinephrine and norepinephrine as well as the synthetic agents phenylephrine, methoxamine, and cirazoline; essentially the same applies to their selective antagonists prazosin and corynanthine. It may be added that in functional studies on smooth muscle, alpha$_1$

adrenoceptors with a high ($alpha_{1H}$) and low ($alpha_{1L}$) affinity for prazosin have been described.

Four subtypes of the $alpha_2$ adrenoceptors can be identified based on their ability to recognize various antagonist and agonist ligands. These subtypes include: (1) $alpha_{2A}$, which is the human platelet receptor exhibiting high affinity for oxymetazoline and low affinity for prazosin; (2) initially identified in neonatal rat lung, a receptor subtype $alpha_{2B}$, which exhibits low affinity for oxymetazoline and high affinity for prazosin (structural studies indicate that this receptor lacks N-linked oligosaccharide moieties); (3) $alpha_{2C}$, the OKY opossum kidney cell line $alpha_2$ receptor, which exhibits higher affinity for rauwolscine than either the $alpha_{2A}$ or $alpha_{2B}$ subtypes, intermediate affinity for oxymetazoline, and high affinity for prazosin; and (4) $alpha_{2D}$, the least well characterized of the receptor subtypes, which is expressed in rat salivary glands and exhibits 4- to 20-fold lower affinity for rauwolscine relative to the $alpha_{2A}$, $alpha_{2B}$, or $alpha_{2C}$ subtypes [200].

In the beta-adrenoceptor category, we recognize today at least three subtypes. At the beta$_1$ adrenoceptor, of the endogenous catecholamines, norepinephrine is more potent than epinephrine. In fact, norepinephrine can serve as a selective agonist together with the synthetic xamoterol; atenolol and CGP 20712A (2-hydroxy-5-(2-(hydroxy-3-(4-((1-methyl-4-trifluoromethyl)-1H-imidazol-2-yl)phenoxy)propyl)aminoethoxy)benzamide) are selective antagonists for the same receptor (beta$_1$). On the beta$_2$ adrenoceptor, epinephrine is more potent than norepinephrine and the synthetic procaterol is a selective agonist. There are two selective antagonists to the beta$_2$ adrenoceptor: alpha-methylpropranolol and ICI 118551 (erythro-DL-1-(7-methylindan-4-yloxy)-3-isopropylaminobutane-2-ol). Relaxant responses to catecholamines that are resistant to blockade by alpha- and beta-adrenoceptor antagonists have also been observed in a number of gastrointestinal smooth muscle preparations in a variety of species. In addition, this beta adrenoceptor that mediates propranolol-resistant responses is characterized by the relatively high potency of a novel class of beta-adrenoceptor agonists, that is, BRL 37344 (4-(2-((2-(3-chlorophenyl)-2-hydroxyethyl)amino)propyl)phenoxy)acetic acid). Similar beta adrenoceptors also exist in nongastrointestinal tissue, for example, in skeletal muscle and in heart, and the resistance of catecholamine responses to classic beta-adrenoceptor antagonists as well as the high potency of BRL 37344 are also features of the atypical beta adrenoceptors mediating lipolysis in rat adipocytes. In the current view, all these atypical beta receptors represent a separate subclass of beta receptors, termed the *beta$_3$ adrenoceptor* [224].

Identification of Adrenoceptors by the Radioligand Technology

Until about 20 years ago the binding of a drug or an endogenous, natural, pharmacologically active substance to its receptor had been inferred from analyses of the dose-response characteristics of specific whole-tissue responses. With the emergence of receptor-specific ligands,* radiolabeled to high specific activity, it became feasible to study directly the binding of pharmacologic agents to their receptors.

Development of the Radioligand-Binding Technology

Early radioligand-binding studies (1967–1974), using radiolabeled adrenergic agonists such as tritiated isoproterenol, epinephrine, and norepinephrine, met with methodologic problems,

---

*The term *ligand* is defined as "an atom, group of atoms or a molecule that binds to a macromolecule" (J. Stenesh. *Dictionary of Biochemistry,* New York: Wiley, 1975).

including lack of stereospecificity and poor correlation between binding data and biologic effects. In other words, the use of labeled adrenergic agonists resulted in binding to sites that did not exhibit binding characteristics of physiologically relevant beta or alpha adrenoceptors. This explains the failure of Sokol and Beall [310] to demonstrate what is described below as a substantial difference in the number of beta adrenoceptors between normal lymphocytes and those obtained from asthmatic individuals or patients with atopic dermatitis. These early experiences directed attention to the major advantages of using antagonists rather than agonists for radioligand-binding studies of adrenoceptors.

By the end of the middle 1970s, it became apparent that the first and most critical step in planning such studies is to acquire a radioligand antagonist of sufficient radiochemical specific activity, purity, stability, and biologic activity. Most receptors have equilibrium dissociation constants for ligands in the nanomolar range and below, which necessitates the use of a radioisotope with a specific activity adequate to allow measurements at these low concentrations. The most commonly used is tritium, which is incorporated into molecules either by direct synthesis or by catalytically induced tritium exchange with hydrogen atoms in the molecular structure. For molecules with an aromatic hydroxyl group, usually tyrosine residues in a peptide [^{125}I] can be incorporated to a very high specific activity without significant loss of biologic activity. With such a radioligand a theoretic specific activity of 22,500 Ci/mmol of [^{125}I] is achievable.

Based on these considerations, by 1974 three groups independently developed radioligand techniques that permitted identification and study of beta receptors with properties expected from physiologic studies, including saturability, strict stereospecificity, and parallelism between inhibition of ligand binding and activation or inhibition of adenylate cyclase. Levitsky et al. [210] used [^{3}H]propranolol; Lefkowitz et al. [205] introduced (-)[^{3}H]dihydroalprenolol; and Auerbach et al. [13] employed [^{125}I]hydroxybenzylpindolol, which is the trivial name for 1-(1-p-hydroxyphenyl-2-methyl-2-propylamino)-3-(4-indolyloxy)-2-propanol. The latter is an analog of pindolol, a clinically useful beta blocker related to propranolol (differing only by the substitution of naphthalene for the indol moiety). All these radioligands bind equally to both beta-receptor subtypes. In such situations, that is, in cases where subtype-specific radioligand is unavailable, analysis of receptor heterogeneity can only be achieved by labeling all the receptors with a nonsubtype specific ligand and analyzing inhibition curves of highly selective cold drugs, using computer-assisted iterative curve-fitting procedures [231].

Of the radioligands that became available by the late 1970s for the direct study and measurement of alpha adrenoceptors, tritiated dihydroergocryptine has been the most extensively used. This agent belongs to the group of ergot alkaloids that includes the oldest known alpha antagonists. Among them, dihydroergocryptine is particularly useful for alpha-receptor studies, since it has the highest potency as an alpha-adrenergic antagonist of all the ergot alkaloids tested. Also, it has no detectable agonist activity at concentrations as high as 10^{-7} M [147]. [^{3}H]Dihydroergocryptine ([^{3}H]DHE) is prepared by catalytic reduction of the double bond at position 9,10 of ergocryptine by the procedures of Stolls and Hofman [319] in the presence of tritium gas. This permits insertion of greater than 1 mol of tritium per mole of compound, thus assuming high specific radioactivity of the ultimate product (23.0 Ci/mmol). [^{3}H]DHE together with [^{3}H]phentolamine is a nonselective radioligand for alpha receptors, whereas [^{3}H]prazosin and [^{3}H]phenoxybenzamine are subtype-selective radioligands for alpha$_1$ receptors, and [^{3}H]yohimbine as well as [^{3}H]rauwolscine for alpha$_2$ receptors [147]. [^{3}H]Prazosin is equiselective for alpha$_{1A}$ and alpha$_{1B}$. [^{3}H]Rauwolscine, [^{3}H]yohimbine, [^{3}H]UK-14304 (5-bromo-6-(imidazolin-2-ylamino)quinoxaline) are equiselective for alpha$_{2A}$ and alpha$_{2B}$.

Kinetic Studies, Binding Isotherms, and Competitive Binding Experiments

The radioligands that have proved useful for studies of adrenoceptors in human tissues have been utilized primarily for kinetic studies, binding isotherms, and competitive binding experiments. Kinetic experiments provide information on how rapidly the ligand binds to a receptor and dissociates from it, yielding the rate constants that characterize the ligand-receptor interaction. Binding isotherms quantify the concentration of receptors and their affinity for the ligand. In such studies the ligands typically bind to receptors in a saturable manner, that is, the specific binding reaches a maximum (B$_{max}$) that reflects the total number of receptors present. The concentration of ligand that binds to half this number of receptors is the dissociation constant (K_d) and is a measure of the affinity of the receptors for the ligand. A rearrangement of the specific binding data by plotting the ratio of bound to free radioactivity against the amount bound can generate the so-called Scatchard plot. In this linear plot the intercept yields the maximum number of binding sites (B$_{max}$), and the slope is the negative reciprocal of the dissociation constant (K_d). Finally, competitive binding studies measure the ability of various compounds to compete with the ligand for binding to receptors (expressed as the dissociation constant K_d) from the binding curve. This approach is useful for studying receptor regulation and to determine whether ligand binding in a particular case involves physiologically relevant receptors. See Figure 14-3.

The G-Protein–Linked Beta Adrenoceptors

The basic approaches to the physiopharmacologic classification of adrenoceptors still utilize one of the three foregoing types of methodology: comparisons of agonist potency, comparisons of antagonist affinity, and the radioligand-binding methodology. The intensive investigation of the past decade, however, was directed toward the isolation and examination of adrenoceptors to elucidate molecular structures and composition. The types of techniques employed include the use of monoclonal antibodies, immunoaffinity chromatography, radiation inactivation/target analysis, covalent affinity labeling, and limited proteolysis. Based on the purification of these receptors, information about protein sequence from several proteolytic fragments was obtained, and the information was used to construct oligonucleotide probes that were then utilized in successful molecular cloning experiments. Consequently, the genes for the adrenoceptors have been cloned.

The human beta$_1$, beta$_2$, and beta$_3$ adrenoceptors are the products of different genes but the receptor proteins show a certain degree of homology. Whereas the complementary DNA (cDNA) for the human beta$_1$ receptor encodes a protein of 477–amino acid residues; the human beta$_2$ adrenoceptor, 413 amino acids; and the human beta$_3$ adrenoceptor is a 402–amino acid glycoprotein. There is a 54 percent homology between the human beta$_1$ and beta$_2$ adrenoceptors. The receptor traverses or spans the cell membrane seven times. The membrane-spanning regions of the adrenoceptor consist of clusters of 24 hydrophobic amino acids. There is some evidence that the cytoplasmic loops I-II and III-IV determine the ligand-binding properties. In other words, the hydrophobic amino acids within the membrane accommodate the beta agonist or antagonist. The amino acid sequences 222-229 and 258-270 have been implicated in the coupling of the receptor to the guanine nucleotide–binding regulatory proteins. Site-directed mutagenesis of the hamster beta$_2$ adrenoceptor has implicated the conserved Asp^{113} residue in the third hydrophobic domain of the receptor in the interaction with cationic amine agonists and antagonists. Substitution of Asp^{113} with a glutamic acid residue results in the partial activation of the mutant receptor by ligands that act as antagonists at the wild-type beta adre-

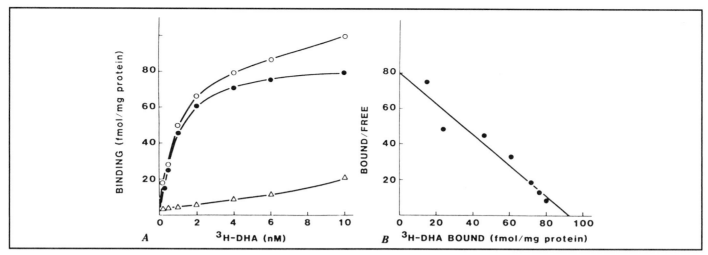

Fig. 14-3. *A. Binding isotherms of [³H]dihydroalprenolol (³H-DHA) to human lymphocyte membranes. Open circles indicate total binding; open triangles, nonspecific binding determined in the presence of 1 μM alprenolol; closed circles, specific binding. B. Scatchard plot of specific binding data shown in A. K_d = 1.1 nM; B_{max} = 91 fmol mg of protein⁻¹.*

noceptor. In other words, a single amino acid substitution in the receptor promotes partial agonist activity from antagonists [321].

Beta-adrenergic receptors are members of a large class of cell-surface receptors that alter the activity of adenylate cyclase, phospholipase C, cyclic guanosine monophosphate (cGMP) phosphodiesterase, and various ion channels indirectly via the guanosine triphosphate (GTP)–binding regulatory or "G-proteins." Agonist binding to receptors of this class promotes activation of one or more members of the G-protein family, which in turn leads to activation of specific effector units. The supergene family of G-protein–linked receptors by now contains more than 70. Of the more than 40 G-protein–linked receptors that have been described by molecular cloning, beta₂ adrenoceptors have been widely adopted as prototypes for the regulation of receptor expression [100].

In mammals, a total of eight G-proteins have been purified essentially free from each other (Gt, Gs, Gi1, Gi2, Gi3, G01, G02, and Gz/x) and the cDNAs derived from a total of nine genes encoding G-alpha subunits have been cloned and designated alpha_s, alpha_{i1}, alpha_{i2}, alpha_{i3}, alpha_o, alpha_{tr}, alpha_{tc}, alpha_{o1f}, and alpha_{z/x}, giving rise to 12 messenger RNAs (mRNAs) because of the fourfold variation in the splicing of the alpha_s precursor mRNA. In addition, there is evidence for the existence of at least seven additional G-alpha genes. Homology cloning has also revealed that there are at least four G-beta genes and three G-gamma genes [128].

The G-proteins are heterotrimeric membrane proteins (alpha, beta, gamma; 1:1:1), distinguished by unique alpha subunits, but sharing common beta subunits. Stated in a different way, G-proteins may be viewed to be composed of a unique, but homologous alpha subunit in reversible association with a complex comprised of a beta and a gamma subunit commonly shared by several different G-protein alpha subunits. Thus, the alpha subunit of Gs (the G-protein that stimulates adenylate cyclase) may share beta-gamma complex in common with the alpha subunits of the family of G-proteins that mediate inhibition of adenylate cyclase (Gi), or other G-proteins like G0, Gz, and Gt [33]. The alpha subunits bind and hydrolyze GTP, and are often the substrates for NAD⁺-dependent ADP ribosylation by bacterial toxins (i.e., pertussis, cholera). Activated beta adrenoceptors catalyze the exchange of GTP for bound guanosine diphosphate (GDP) by the alpha subunit of the holoprotein, promoting the dissociation of the GTP-bound alpha subunit from the beta-

gamma complex. It is the "free" GTP ligand alpha subunit of a G-protein that regulates the activity of the membrane-bound effector units such as adenylate cyclase [200].

The primary sequences of several G-protein–linked effectors, including adenylate cyclase [183] and phospholipase C [276], have been determined and molecular cloning of phospholipase A_2 and Ca^{++} and K^+ channels are in an advanced stage in several laboratories. As mentioned earlier G-alpha_s mediates the stimulation of adenylate cyclase and has been shown to regulate Ca^{++} channel activity. The G-proteins that mediate the inhibition of adenylate cyclase, termed *Gi*, constitute a family with at least three members, G-alpha_{i1}, G-alpha_{i2}, and G-alpha_{i3}, each the product of a separate gene. Of these, it is G-alpha_{i2} that mediates the inhibition of adenylate cyclase [200, 378].

Biochemical Consequences of Adrenergic Stimulation

The agonist–beta receptor complex promotes the high-affinity binding of GTP by Gs, which activates the nucleotide regulatory protein. A single agonist-liganded receptor could activate 6 to 10 Gs units, and the alpha_s subunit of each activated Gs is capable of producing a complex with the catalytic unit of adenylate cyclase to activate the enzyme.

The adrenergically activated adenylate cyclase, in the presence of magnesium ions, catalyzes the formation of a cyclic nucleotide and pyrophosphate from ATP (see Chap. 15). This cyclic nucleotide, adenosine-3′,5′-monophosphate (cyclic AMP), then functions as a second messenger of catecholamine or hormonal action by modifying enzyme activities and permeability barriers. This is accomplished through the activation of a class of enzymes known as protein kinases.

Two types of cyclic AMP–dependent protein kinases (Types I and II) have been identified, and both are thought to exist as tetrameres made up of two regulatory subunits and two catalytic subunits [216]. When the catalytic and regulatory subunits are associated, the kinases are inactive. Activation occurs when cyclic AMP binds to the regulatory subunits, causing dissociation and allowing the catalytic subunits to perform their function, which is the phosphorylation of endogenous substrate proteins. These phosphorylations set in motion a cascade of biochemical reactions that produce the intracellular alterations of metabolic, genetic, electrochemical, and mechanical activities that are regu-

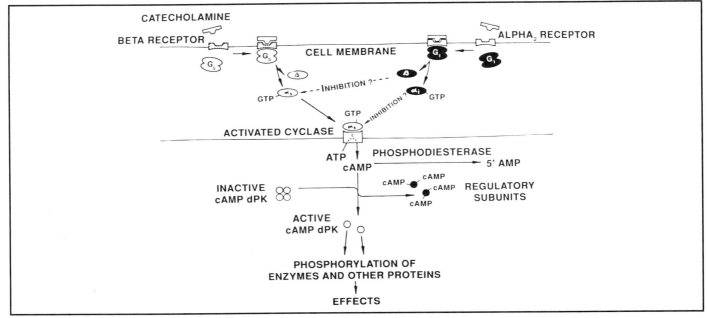

Fig. 14-4. *Conceptualization of the adenylate cyclase–cyclic AMP (cAMP) system. Certain hormones or catecholamines (first messengers) interact with specific receptor sites on the exterior surface of a cell, causing activation of adenylate cyclase on the interior surface. This increases cyclic AMP synthesis and accumulation within the cell, which leads to modification of any of several cellular activities, depending on the type of cell involved. It is believed that many, if not all, effects of cyclic AMP in different cells may be the result of activation of cyclic AMP–dependent protein kinases (cAMP dPK), which are enzymes that transfer terminal phosphate groups from ATP to amino acid (serine) residues of certain proteins. It is thought that phosphorylation of proteins at strategic locations in cells could produce alterations of metabolic, genetic, electrochemical, and mechanical activities that may be regulated by cyclic AMP. G_s and G_i = nucleotide-binding regulatory proteins. Components are not drawn to scale.*

lated by cyclic AMP. For example, in the case of smooth muscle relaxation, the above-mentioned biochemical events may lead to increased calcium sequestration within the cell or increased ATP-dependent calcium efflux from the cell [236]. Conversely, protein kinase is inactivated when the enzyme's regulatory subunits recombine with its catalytic subunits. This occurs when the concentration of cyclic AMP falls [117].

Regulation of the intracellular concentration of cyclic AMP is a function shared with adenylate cyclase by one or more specific cyclic AMP phosphodiesterases. This enzyme hydrolyzes the 3'-phosphate ester bond of cyclic AMP to yield 5'-AMP. It requires a divalent cation for catalytic activity (usually Mg^{++}), seems to be ubiquitous, and may exist in the cell in a soluble or particulate form, or both. The enzyme has been purified by a number of investigators and its characteristics reported in detail [333]. It is becoming apparent that phosphodiesterase activity in cells can be modulated by a number of regulators including calcium, calmodulin, and insulin [11, 320].

Evidence indicates that catecholamines in combination with alpha₂ receptors act by reducing endogenous levels of cyclic AMP. This can occur by interaction of the agonist-receptor complex with another component of the membrane, Gi. Gi is activated by binding GTP, and this activation can be promoted by several agonist-stimulated inhibitory receptors including the alpha₂ receptor. It is not yet clear whether Gi, once it is activated, directly inhibits adenylate cyclase or inhibits the function of Gs to activate the enzyme [144, 232, 303].

The alpha₁ receptor has been isolated from rat liver and appears to be a dimer made up of two 85,000-dalton units. Study of the affinity-labeled receptor using limited proteolysis revealed extracellular, ligand-binding, membrane, and intracellular domains quite similar to the muscarinic receptors from a variety of animal tissues. By contrast, these molecular characteristics are very different for beta₁, beta₂, beta₃, and dopaminergic (D₂) receptors [385].

When stimulated, alpha₁ receptors increase the cytosolic concentration of Ca^{++}, and this increase is thought to mediate most, if not all, of the effects of alpha₁-receptor activation in a variety of target tissues including liver, smooth muscle, salivary and lacrimal glands, heart, and cerebral cortex [95]. For example, Ca^{++} activates the calmodulin-dependent myosin light-chain kinase in smooth muscle, and phosphorylation of myosin by this kinase is in turn associated with the development of contractile tension [166]. Emerging evidence suggests that early effects on membrane phosphoinositide metabolism may be the mechanism by which alpha₁-receptor stimulation releases bound Ca^{++} from endoplasmic reticulum into the cytosol [148]. See Figure 14-4.

ADRENOCEPTORS, THEIR RESPONSIVENESS AND MECHANISMS OF THEIR REGULATION

Study of the adrenoceptors has been greatly facilitated by the development of radiolabeled ligands that bind directly to receptor surfaces as well as by our increased understanding of the molecular biology of these receptors, and consequently the mechanisms involved in their regulation. Data obtained by use of these radioligands have shown clearly that the receptors are not static entities, but are dynamic, changing with time, and regulated by a variety of biologic influences.

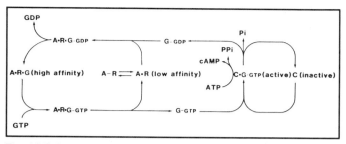

Fig. 14-5. *Interaction of components of the agonist-stimulatable adenylate cyclase system. The agonist (A) interacts with the receptor (R) on the outer surface of the effector cell. The catalytic moiety of the enzyme (C) is situated on the inner surface of the plasma membrane where it catalyzes the formation of cyclic AMP (cAMP) from ATP. See text for details. G = a nucleotide-binding regulatory protein that is an important intermediate in the activation of C; GDP = guanosine diphosphate; GTP = guanosine triphosphate.*

The Ternary Complex Model of the Agonist-Specific Binding Properties of the Adenylate Cyclase–Coupled Beta Adrenoceptor

A useful model for the adrenoceptor–adenylate cyclase interactions has been presented by DeLean and coworkers [76] based to a large extent on radioligand-binding experiments. This model envisions three principal components of the system in the cell membrane: the receptor (R), the nucleotide-binding regulatory G-protein (G), and adenylate cyclase. The binding of an agonist (A) to the receptor brings about a change that either promotes or stabilizes the formation of a ternary complex ARG (Fig. 14-5). The formation of the complex promotes the dislodging of a tightly bound GDP molecule from the G-protein and its replacement with GTP, which enables G-protein to activate adenylate cyclase, thus stimulating the formation of cyclic AMP. The GTP is subsequently hydrolyzed to GDP by guanosine triphosphatase associated with G-protein, and this leads to the inactivation of the cyclase. All three components of the system are then capable of being reactivated by renewed interactions of receptors with agonist molecules. The formation of the ternary complex ARG is of crucial importance to the functional coupling of the adrenoceptor to the cyclase in this hypothetic model. Antagonists occupy the receptor but do not promote or stabilize the formation of the ternary complex and thus do not activate the catalytic moiety of adenylate cyclase. Biochemical studies indicate that the free form of the receptor has a low affinity for agonists, while the complex of the receptor plus the nucleotide protein (RG) has a high affinity for agonists. Changes in receptor-binding properties showing a lack of high affinity of receptors for agonists are thus believed to indicate that the crucial ARG complex is not formed. Not surprisingly, there is no activation of the cyclase under these circumstances. This phenomenon resulting in the inability of agonist-stimulated beta adrenoceptors to activate adenylate cyclase is referred to as *uncoupling*, which is one of the mechanisms by which agonist-induced desensitization of beta adrenoceptors takes place [74]. See Figure 14-5.

Transcriptional and Posttranscriptional Controls of Adrenoceptor Regulation by Agonists

In connection with neuronal uptake and inactivation of catecholamines, we earlier described the mechanisms involved in the neuronal release and reuptake of norepinephrine. When considered in that framework, it is clear that neuronal reuptake of norepinephrine is one of the mechanisms by which signal transduction and consequently the responsiveness of the adrenergic receptor can be attenuated. There are additional short-term and long-term mechanisms that influence adrenoceptor responsiveness to the homologous, specific agonist. Adaptation or "desensitization" (i.e., a waning over time of an effector cell to a constant level of stimulus) typifies the short-term component.

For beta-adrenergic agonists, desensitization is characterized by the reduced ability of the beta adrenoceptor to stimulate adenylate cyclase and intracellular cyclic AMP accumulation. The major mechanism responsible for short-term desensitization is phosphorylation of the beta adrenoceptor by protein kinase A and beta adrenoceptor–specific kinase. These two enzymes alter receptor function by increasing the effective agonist concentration needed to produce 50 percent of the total response (EC_{50}) and by decreasing the V_{max} for agonist-stimulated adenylate cyclase, respectively. The molecular mechanisms underlying rapid, short-term desensitization do not require internalization of the receptors (as originally believed), but rather an alteration in the functioning of the beta adrenoceptors themselves that uncouples the receptors from Gs, the stimulatory G-protein. As stated, this uncoupling involves phosphorylation by the two kinases. Indeed, it has been shown that beta adrenoceptors are substrates for phosphorylation, and canonical sequences for recognition by protein kinase A and protein kinase C have been identified in beta adrenoceptors. Furthermore, an additional protein kinase, the earlier mentioned beta adrenoceptor–specific kinase, has also been identified and its molecular cloning shows structural similarities with the protein kinases A and C. How receptor phosphorylation alters its coupling with Gs is not known. One speculation is that phosphorylation is involved in controlling macromolecular organization of the receptor within the transmembrane-signaling assembly composed of receptors, G-proteins, and effectors [137]. As stated before, the beta$_2$ adrenoceptor spans the cell membrane seven times, and the cytoplasmic carboxyl-terminal domain has been proposed to contain molecular determinants for both the short-term desensitization as well as long-term (downregulation) agonist-specific regulatory processes. By replacement of four serine and threonine residues located within a 10–amino acid segment of this domain of beta$_2$ adrenoceptor, the agonist-promoted phosphorylation and rapid (short-term) desensitization of the adenylate cyclase response could be prevented. Thus, this small hitherto unappreciated region of the receptor molecule may selectively subserve its rapid regulation [136].

Effector cells exposed to the homologous, specific adrenergic agonist for longer periods of time display another form of beta$_2$-adrenergic subsensitivity, termed *downregulation*, which is characterized by a loss of the cellular complement of the receptor itself. This agonist-promoted downregulation of G-protein–linked adrenoceptors appears to have a major posttranscriptional element. Long-term (>4 hours) homologous agonist exposure of cells promotes a sustained downregulation (50–80%) of steady-state beta$_2$-adrenoceptor mRNA levels. The rate of transcription and the stability of the receptor mRNA may be modulated by receptor activation or intracellular cyclic AMP levels, or both. At the time of this writing, it appears that the mechanism responsible for the long-term, agonist-promoted reduction in beta-adrenoceptor mRNA levels is the destabilization of the mRNA. Thus, the loss of beta$_2$ adrenoceptors on the cell membrane is a consequence of and preceded by the loss of receptor mRNA. In contrast, the loss of radioligand-binding capacity is an early event preceding the loss of cell-surface beta$_2$ adrenoceptors.

In these examples, we have been dealing with short-term (desensitization) or long-term (downregulation) exposure of cells to adrenergic or nonadrenergic agonists that reduce the ability of the adrenoceptors to produce their characteristic biologic effects to subsequent administration of the same agonists [74, 107, 374]. Conversely, depletion of tissue catecholamines by chemical or surgical denervation [116, 262, 399] results in greater than normal responsiveness of effector cells to adrenergic agonists. This is a phenomenon of homologous upregulation. Nonadrenergic agonists can also influence responsiveness of effector cells to beta-adrenergic stimulation. For example, glucocorticoids have been found to produce complex changes (discussed later) in beta adrenoceptors, their predominant effects leading to an increase in beta-adrenoceptor gene transcription and cell-surface beta-adrenoceptor concentration [390]. This form of beta-adrenoceptor regulation is called *heterologous upregulation*. Thyroid hormones cause an increased binding of catecholamines by beta adrenoceptors and decreased binding by alpha adrenoceptors in certain tissues [54, 114, 290, 392, 396]. This is a situation where the mechanism of interconversion of adrenoceptor responsiveness is involved, which is discussed extensively later. Also, estrogens, progesterone, aging, spontaneous hypertension (rats), and a variety of other factors have been shown to influence the regulation of beta adrenoceptor–mediated responsiveness of cells to adrenergic stimulation [138, 204, 238].

In the foregoing discussions, we have been referring to examples of specific, homologous (i.e., adrenergic agonist–induced) desensitization. Another form of beta-adrenergic subsensitivity, induced by nonadrenergic agonists, has been termed *heterologous desensitization*. Paradoxically, its existence was discovered under circumstances of turkey erythrocytes' exposure to isoproterenol, that is, a bona fide beta-adrenergic agonist. Nevertheless, the isoproterenol-induced desensitization of turkey erythrocytes appeared to fall into the category of heterologous desensitization because loss of sensitivity to fluoride ion and 5′-guanylimidodiphosphate* (Gpp(NH)p), a less hydrolyzable analog that can substitute for GTP, is also produced in this situation. No decrease in beta-adrenoceptor number is detectable, but rather an uncoupling of the receptor from adenylate cyclase takes place due to impairment of the ability of occupied receptors to form a stable high-affinity ARG complex [313]. Similar refractoriness can be produced by exposure of the cells to 8-bromo-adenosine-3′,5′-cyclic monophosphate, a cyclic AMP analog, suggesting that the desensitization to isoproterenol is caused by the agonist-stimulated levels of cyclic AMP within the cells. As we shall see in the discussions below, there is considerably more experience with this phenomenon since the discovery that the allergic tissue injury itself can produce desensitization, as a consequence of the release of a variety of pharmacologic mediators in the allergic episode. Thus, heterologous desensitization of beta adrenoceptors involves uncoupling due to impairment of the ability of the receptors to form the high-affinity ARG complex and consequently to activate adenylate cyclase; this impairment is produced by the agonist-stimulated accumulation of cyclic AMP within cells.

ADRENERGIC REGULATION IN DISEASES OF ATOPIC ALLERGY

The concept of a beta-adrenergic abnormality as the constitutional basis of atopy was formulated in the 1960s [324]. In the subsequent years at least six levels of defective beta-adrenergic responses were shown to be manifestations of the beta-adrenergic subsensitivity in question, at least as the latter applies to disorders of respiratory (asthma) or cutaneous (atopic dermatitis) atopy.

These defective beta-adrenergic responses were determined to be as follows [46, 118, 174, 184, 185, 313, 324–327, 332–334, 338, 339, 341, 344, 347, 348, 354–358, 363]:

1. There is a reduction in the normal beta-adrenergic inhibition of lysosomal enzyme release, chemotaxis, phagocytosis, anti-

body-dependent cellular cytotoxicity, increased expression of Fc IgE receptors, and prostaglandin E synthesis to stimulation with histamine-induced suppressor factor, that is, effector mechanisms that are known to play an important role in immunologic inflammation.
2. There is a reduction in lymphocytic beta-adrenergic sensitivity resulting in abnormally decreased (lymphocyte transformation, E-rosette–forming cells, T-cells, suppressor cell function) and abnormally increased (IgE-producing B-cells, Fc receptor–bearing lymphocytes) lymphocyte reactivities.
3. Mast cell mediator release to immunologic or nonimmunologic stimuli, ordinarily suppressed by beta-adrenergic stimulation, is subsensitive to the same, while both cholinergic and alpha-adrenergic enhancement of mediator release is exaggerated.
4. Beta-adrenergically mediated bronchial smooth muscle dilation is reduced, while cholinergically and alpha-adrenergically mediated constriction is augmented.
5. Mucus secretion in response to alpha-adrenergic and cholinergic stimulation is increased, while sodium and water fluxes into tracheobronchial secretions in response to beta-adrenergic stimulation are reduced.
6. The beta-adrenergically mediated eosinopenia is reduced and replaced by eosinophilia.

This discussion reviews more recent findings in relation to the nature and developmental mechanisms of these reduced beta-adrenergic functions.

In the framework of the original beta-adrenergic theory of asthma [324] this reduced beta-adrenergic reactivity in response to endogenous or therapeutically applied beta-adrenergic agonists was proposed to reflect alterations at any of a number of sites in the beta-adrenergic sequence of biochemical reactions, resulting in a defective beta-adrenergic response. These include (1) abnormalities in the mobilization of endogenous catecholamines; (2) blockade of beta receptors due to microbial components, specific autoantibodies, and other possible substances interacting with the receptor; (3) changes in the affinity of beta-adrenergic agonists and their receptor sites; (4) decreases in the numbers or reactivities of beta receptors; (5) a shifting in the balance of adrenergic receptor subtypes or in their responses from the beta to alpha category; (6) alterations in the coupling of activated receptors to the catalytic units of adenylate cyclase, involving some defective participation of the so-called G-proteins or other molecular mechanisms; and (7) abnormalities in the functioning of the phosphatidylinositol messenger system. Alternatively, the lesion may occur at a point beyond the cyclic AMP generation step such as the increased catabolic activity of the phosphodiesterase system or the possible involvement of protein kinase C in allergen- or otherwise-induced nonspecific refractoriness of adenylate cyclase; in a cyclic AMP–related interacting or modulating pathway, such as that provided by acetylcholine, histamine, the prostaglandins, the thromboxanes, the leukotrienes, the interleukins, neuroactive immunoregulatory peptides, platelet-activating factor, kinins, thymic peptides, and a large group of lymphokines, monokines, and cytokines; or in any other possible intracellular system with regulatory potential. Furthermore, any of these abnormalities may be genetically determined or acquired [342, 348].

These possible abnormalities are listed herein as though they would be separate and distinct entities. In reality, they are closely interrelated with inherently overlapping features, all contributory directly or indirectly to the final pathopharmacology of airway obstruction. With this qualification and only for the convenience of the reader, the various possible biochemical sites of the beta-adrenergic dysfunction are discussed individually. However, only those for which potentially important recent advances have been made are included.

---

* 5′-guanylimidodiphosphate is an analog of GTP that contains an imidodiphosphate rather than a pyrophosphate linkage and therefore it is less hydrolyzable.

Changes in the Pattern of Mobilization of Catecholamines

Barnes and coworkers, in comparing the catecholamine response to exercise in asthmatic and nonatopic subjects, showed that the asthmatic pathology may also include abnormalities in the mobilization of catecholamines in two ways: (1) An equivalent workload in asthmatic individuals produces a smaller rise in norepinephrine than in normal subjects [18]. (2) When plasma norepinephrine levels are measured in patients with acute, severe airway obstruction, the concentrations are two to three times baseline values in the asthmatic subjects without a simultaneous increase in plasma epinephrine [154]. These findings contrast sharply with catecholamine responses seen in other acutely ill patients. Whether these observations in the first case represent a failure of sympathoadrenal activation, and in the second case a selectively impaired adrenal secretion (i.e., epinephrine versus norepinephrine), remains to be determined. A further difficulty in interpreting the significance of these findings rests with the long-established fact that if anything, it is never the exposure to decreased amounts, but the exposure to excessive amounts of the mediator (i.e., the catecholamines in this particular situation) that leads to manifestations of adrenergic subsensitivity [325, 340].

Blockade of Beta Receptors by Autoantibodies and Microbial Components

As pointed out elsewhere [17, 330, 343, 358] the concept that an autoantibody interacting with a cell membrane receptor of a hormone or neurotransmitter could cause functional derangements and subsequent disease is now becoming widely accepted, and the number of diseases that may be mediated by antireceptor antibodies is rapidly growing.

The leading examples of such diseases include myasthenia gravis involving autoantibodies directed at nicotinic acetylcholine receptors at the neuromuscular end-plates [2, 83, 213], Graves' disease involving autoantibodies to the thyrotropin receptor [222, 306], and the severe insulin resistance in Type B insulin-resistant diabetes that has been ascribed to autoantibodies to the insulin receptor [99].

Thus, the foregoing diseases may be viewed as receptor diseases, and it is possible that some subsets of asthma and other diseases of atopic allergy may ultimately be recognized as legitimate members of this group. Indeed, it has been reported that autoantibodies to beta$_2$ adrenoceptors can be identified in the plasma of some subjects with atopic allergy [103, 164, 259, 384]. Although these antibodies appear to be heterogeneous, they share the ability to affect binding of [I^{125}]protein A to calf lung membranes, to inhibit stereospecific beta-adrenergic radioligand binding to calf lung beta$_2$ adrenoceptors, and to precipitate solubilized calf lung beta-adrenergic receptors in an indirect immunoprecipitation assay. Furthermore, the presence of autoantibodies to beta$_2$ adrenoceptors in these subjects correlates well with a reduced beta$_2$- and an increased alpha-adrenergic responsiveness. It may be added that from the currently available material of these studies, even the 3 of the 19 apparently normal subjects with circulating antibodies were significantly less responsive to beta-adrenergic stimulation than the remainder of these normal controls [132]. In a study by Belcher and colleagues [22], presence of beta$_2$-adrenergic autoantibodies in pediatric asthma was also confirmed but the authors again emphasized that the existence of the autoantibodies is limited to a small number of patients. In any case, the precise frequency and distribution of these autoantibodies in various subsets of patients with asthma and other atopic diseases are currently under investigation in several American and European laboratories, as is the molecular mechanism by which they produce beta-adrenergic subsensitivity.

A discussion of blockade of beta-adrenergic receptors by microbial agents would logically follow the blockade of beta receptors by autoantibodies since autoimmunity can be the consequence of both viral as well as bacterial infections. For a discussion of this relationship, see the previously published chapter by Szentivanyi and Szentivanyi [359]. The issue that microbial components and products thereof can alter adrenergic mechanisms at a number of biochemical sites is a complex and important one that has been extensively reviewed [46, 104, 335, 336, 345, 361]. In this section, we only discuss a series of studies analyzing the structural similarities between the mammalian beta-adrenergic and reovirus Type 3 receptors [56]. This work has evolved from experiments that originally focused on the utilization of antiidiotypic antibodies in the studies of reovirus Type 3 cell receptors [56, 98]. Syngeneic monoclonal and xenogeneic polyclonal antiidiotypic antibodies with specificity for the reovirus receptor have been constructed [247, 251], and the reovirus and the antiidiotypic antibody were observed to have similar effects in limiting concanavalin A–induced stimulation of lymphocytes [248] together with inhibition of DNA synthesis as well as inhibition of reovirus binding to target cells by antireceptor antibodies in a serotype-specific manner [172]. With immunoblotting techniques it was possible to show that the virus and the antireceptor antibody bind to a 67-kd cell-surface structure obtained from lymphoid and neuronal cell membranes followed by isolation of the receptor molecule through immunoprecipitation by polyclonal antireceptor antibodies. It was further found that tissues that bind mammalian reovirus Type 3 express beta-adrenergic receptors. These tissues include brain, heart, muscle, and lymphocytes [55]. Since the reported molecular mass and isoelectric points of the beta-adrenergic receptor were comparable to those of the isolated reovirus-binding protein, the subsequent studies were targeted to examine further the structural similarities between the two receptors. Indeed, far-reaching structural similarities were found as based on the following observations. The purified beta receptor was immunoprecipitable by anti–reovirus receptor antibodies, and the purified reovirus receptor from thymoma cells and the beta-adrenergic receptors obtained from lung exhibited identical molecular masses and isoelectric points. Furthermore, digests of purified reovirus and beta-adrenergic receptors were found to display indistinguishable fragment patterns and the purified reovirus receptor was capable of binding the beta antagonist [I^{125}]iodohydroxybenzylpindolol, that is, a binding reaction that was shown to be blocked by the beta agonist isoproterenol [57].

Changes in the Affinity of Beta-Adrenergic Agonists and Their Receptor Sites

Changes in lymphocytic beta-receptor binding can also be shown in asthmatic subjects when the effects of guanine nucleotides on beta$_2$-agonist binding are studied. The normal effect of GTP and its synthetic analog Gpp(NH)p is a reduction in the apparent affinity of agonists in competing for beta-adrenergic binding sites. This was originally shown in studies on the binding of the beta agonist [^{3}H]hydroxybenzylisoproterenol ([^{3}H]HBI) to frog erythrocyte membranes [393]. In these experiments, after a steady-state level of [^{3}H]HBI binding to frog erythrocyte membranes was attained, Gpp(NH)p was added to the incubation medium, resulting in a very rapid dissociation of a large portion of the bound [^{3}H]HBI. Other nucleotides have a similar effect on agonist binding in the following order of potency: GTP > guanosine-5'-diphosphate > ATP = guanosine-5'-monophosphate. When this experimental design is used for the study of [^{3}H]HBI binding to lymphocytic membranes in the presence and absence of the guanine nucleotide, it was found that Gpp(NH)p caused a substantial decrease in [³H]HBI binding in patients without airway disease and in those with nonreversibly obstructed airway disease but an increase in patients with reversibly obstructed airway disease (asthma). At present, the nature of such a reversal in the normal effect of GPP(NH)p is unclear, but it raises the possibility of some biochemical membrane disorder possibly involving multiple receptor abnormalities [329, 358].

Another aspect of the effects of guanine nucleotides on agonist binding is that this effect is in marked contrast with the binding of a radioligand antagonist, such as [³H]DHA, which is not affected by the addition of these nucleotides to the incubation mixture. While this statement may accurately reflect the behavior of normal tissues, most recently Polson and associates [267] showed that long-term therapy (1–2 years) with ketotifen, a benzocycloheptathiophene, significantly increased the apparent equilibrium dissociation constant (K_d) for [³H]DHA binding to membrane beta receptors of lymphocytes from patients with asthma. Taken together with what has been said above on the mechanism of the reversal in the normal effect of Gpp(NH)p, the findings of Polson and colleagues [267] may further indicate the presence of some biochemical abnormality in the receptors themselves or in their membrane environment.

Finally, a decreased affinity of binding for radiolabeled beta-adrenoceptor agonists by intact circulating lymphocytes was demonstrated by Pochet, Delepesse, and DeMaubeuge [264] in atopic dermatitis.

Decreases in the Numbers or Reactivities of Beta Receptors

The first study of physiologically relevant, beta adrenoceptors with [³H]DHA in human lymphocytes was reported in 1976 by Williams and colleagues [394], followed by abstracts by Kariman and Lefkowitz in 1977 [169] and Kariman in 1980 [168] describing for the first time a reduction in the number of beta receptors in lymphocytes of asthmatic patients. In a more definitive study, this decreased specific [³H]DHA binding to lymphocytic membranes of asthmatic subjects was confirmed by Brooks and coworkers [39].

In the studies of Brooks and coworkers [39], the degree of reduction in lymphocytic beta-receptor numbers correlated well with disease severity and airway obstruction among patients. Those asthmatic patients with more severe disease and greater airway obstruction showed lower numbers of lymphocytic beta receptors. Nevertheless, it remained unclear whether this correlation could have been entirely accounted for by differences in drug treatment. Theophylline preparations were predominantly used, and administration of beta-adrenergic agonists was limited. Likewise in the studies of Kariman and Lefkowitz [169] and Kariman [168] the decrease in the numbers of beta receptors was as equally apparent in asthmatic patients receiving no adrenergic bronchodilators as was apparent in those receiving such drugs. In any case, these studies again raised the question as to whether manifestations of beta-adrenergic subsensitivities in asthma are due to the disease itself or to adrenergic medication taken by the patients [120, 165, 235, 246].

While drug-induced beta-adrenergic desensitization may clearly cause decreased beta-adrenergic reactivity or contribute in many situations to the overall beta-adrenergic subsensitivity, beta-adrenergic subsensitivity appears to be a fundamental characteristic of atopy, for the following reasons:

1. Decreased beta-adrenergic responses to catecholamines by no means represent a consistent feature of adrenergic therapy [32, 181, 201, 238, 263, 293, 301, 309, 322, 371, 395, 398].
2. There are findings to indicate that adrenoceptor susceptibility to agonist desensitization varies with the receptor subtype as

well as with the tissue involved and that some adrenoceptors may not be subject to downregulation [135, 238, 289].
3. Beta-adrenergic subsensitivity in asthma can be shown to occur also during periods without symptoms or medication or under circumstances when prior or concurrent medication can be only one contributing factor to defective beta-adrenergic function [10, 43, 44, 162, 173, 184, 199, 221, 237, 266].
4. In fact, there is evidence to suggest that atopic asthmatic and nonasthmatic atopic subjects may not develop beta-adrenergic subsensitivity as readily as do normal individuals [134, 151, 152, 161, 367]. There is no currently available explanation for this apparent paradox, but it is important to include these observations in the context of this discussion.
5. Beta-adrenergic subsensitivity is also demonstrable in atopic conditions (atopic dermatitis) in which adrenergic medication has never been involved [45, 64, 65, 111, 115, 122, 149, 150, 226, 260, 261, 264, 285, 316, 341].
6. Because of recent methodologic developments, different patterns of drug- versus host-induced beta-adrenergic subsensitivities may now be recognized in lung tissue, lymphocytes, and adipocytes in atopic asthma [287, 326–328, 334, 338, 339, 346, 363, 368]. These observations are backed up by identical findings in a number of animal experiments that are discussed below. In one of these studies, in which normal rats were chronically infused with high concentrations of catecholamines through a minipump, there was a rapid reduction in beta-adrenergic cardiac inotropy followed by loss of beta receptor–binding sites, without any change in the physiologic reactivity or number of cardiac alpha receptors [49]. Thus, agonist desensitization does not mimic and cannot account for the inverse changes in alpha and beta receptors caused by hormonal and other manipulations or disease states.
7. In harmony with the conclusions of and considerations described in Item 6 above, there are important observations indicating an alpha-receptor hyperreactivity with or without increased alpha-receptor concentration in human atopy and its animal models. Thus, pulmonary homogenates of sensitized guinea pigs that had been exposed chronically to antigen aerosol show a significant increase in alpha adrenoceptors and a decrease in beta adrenoceptors [19]. This alpha dominance is also reflected by the demonstration that alpha-adrenergic agonists produce bronchoconstriction in asthmatic patients, but not in normal subjects [9, 308]. Also, alpha-adrenergic hyperreactivity as based on vascular and pupillary responses has been demonstrated in asthma [141, 164, 206]. Moreover, enhanced phenylephrine-dependent mydriasis in medication-free asthmatic subjects has been detected. These observations suggest that alpha-adrenergic hyperreactivity cannot be attributed to medication or to the severity of airway obstruction, but might represent an intrinsic property of asthma.

In the aggregate, these findings indicate that depending on the selectivity of the agonist used, drug-induced beta-adrenergic subsensitivity may result in a reduction in the number of the relatively affected beta receptors, whereas in beta-adrenergic subsensitivity induced by the atopic state and in many other situations, some other mechanism that results in a concurrent rise in the numbers of alpha adrenoceptors or in their reactivities is involved. A most fitting and recent illustration of this conclusion can be shown by the findings of Yoshie and coworkers [400] in the experimental asthma of guinea pigs. By using midaglizole, an antagonist that selectively blocks alpha-adrenergic functions of the alpha₂ subtype, this group showed an inhibition of antigen-induced bronchoconstriction in vivo and histamine-induced isolated tracheal constriction in vitro, and that desensitization of tracheal beta₂ receptors produced by a high concentration of isoproterenol was eliminated by the administration of midaglizole. In other words, selective blockade of tracheal alpha₂ receptors restored the desensitized tracheal beta$_2$ receptors to normal reactivity. Furthermore, this alpha$_2$-receptor blocker was claimed to provide the same symptomatic relief in severe, intractable human asthma [401].

Shifting in the Balance of Adrenoceptor Subtypes or in Their Responses

Many physiologic and pathologic conditions, as shown by the discussion that follows, are associated with inverse changes in alpha- and beta-adrenoceptor responses in various tissues, which in the late 1960s and early 1970s raised the question of whether adrenoceptor subtypes are real in a physiologic and chemical anatomic sense or whether they become apparent only when certain chemicals are applied to them [5].

In the same time period, in response to this question, three different arguments were developed:

1. There is only one kind of adrenoceptor. It responds best to epinephrine. This adrenoceptor also responds to the two other natural catecholamines (dopamine and norepinephrine) and any apparent differences are due to the association of the receptor with different cells, such as smooth muscle, exocrine gland, or other effector cells.
2. There are two or more adrenoceptor subtypes because norepinephrine and epinephrine (metabolic hormone) have different functions.
3. Every adrenoceptor and their subtypes are different depending on the cell membrane on which they are located.

Today there is conclusive evidence that the various adrenoceptor subtypes that have been originally identified by classic pharmacology do in fact have physicochemically distinct molecular identities. Nevertheless, it is necessary to guide the reader through the historical progression in our thinking about the nature of these inverse, reciprocal changes in numbers and reactivities of adrenoceptor subtypes [185, 187, 191, 193, 348].

The "Interconversion" Controversy

In the pattern of receptor behavior, the mutually reciprocal changes between functionally antagonistic adrenoceptors in atopic disease and in some of its animal models are consistent enough to be reminiscent of the phenomenon of receptor "interconversion."

The Evidence Supporting the Concept of Receptor Interconversion

The existence of such a phenomenon was originally suggested by finding that the beta receptors of the frog heart could be converted to alpha receptors by cold [195]. This and subsequent observations were interpreted to indicate that alpha and beta receptors may represent different conformations of a metabolically controlled, single receptor rather than separate and independent molecular entities [326, 327].

The original observation on the effect of temperature shifting the balance of the adrenoceptors of the frog heart has been extended to include similar shifts under a number of conditions associated with low metabolic activity, including hibernation in frogs [133], low ambient temperatures, low rates of contraction, hypoxia, muscarinic cholinergic stimulation, some metabolic inhibitors, myocardial ischemia, adrenalectomy, hypothyroidism, malignant transformation [51], liver regeneration [3, 110], cholestasis [3], fasting, and nutritional status in general [90]. Furthermore, such changes are often, but not always associated with corresponding changes in the densities of alpha and beta receptor–binding sites [133, 193].

Conversely, beta-directed shifts in adrenoceptor balance appear to be operative in insulin-deficient or deprived conditions such as human and alloxan diabetes. In human diabetes, some of the noradrenergic reactions of blood vessels normally sensitive only to alpha-adrenergic antagonists can be inhibited by beta-blocking agents [365]. This beta-sensitive noradrenergic constriction, found previously in alloxan-diabetic rabbits [73], now appears to be an inherent characteristic of various diabetic vascular reactions, whether the diabetes was induced by alloxan or developed spontaneously [366, 386].

Likewise, in experiments measuring alpha- and beta-receptor concentrations with [3H]DHE and [3H]dihydroalprenolol ([3H]DHA) in myocardial homogenates of hypothyroid rats, an increase in the number of [3H]DHA-binding sites and a matching decrease in the number of [3H]DHE-binding sites, without changes in binding affinity, were found after a 6-day treatment with 0.5 mg kg^{-1} of triiodothyronine [298]. In another laboratory, similar changes were found as early as 2 days after treatment of hypophysectomized rats with 0.2 mg kg^{-1} levothyroxine. The latter treatment schedule does not lead to cardiac hypertrophy but is sufficient to reverse completely the shift from beta- to alpha-type force and rate responses of atria, which develop over several weeks after hypophysectomy. In myocardial homogenates from these rats, the density of beta receptors, identified as high-affinity [3H]DHA binding, increased from 27.5 ± 2.7 (H$_x$) to 45.5 ± 5.7 fmol mg^{-1} of protein (H$_x$ + levothyroxine), whereas the density of alpha receptors, identified as prazosin-suppressible binding of [3H]WB-4101, decreased from 38.7 ± 3.1 (H$_x$) to 18.7 ± 2.5 (H$_x$ + levothyroxine). These observations demonstrate that reciprocal changes in alpha- and beta-receptor reactivities in the rat heart are associated with similar reciprocal changes in receptor numbers [187]. It is pertinent to add that although thyroid hormones are known to induce the synthesis of a number of cell components, their effect on alpha and beta receptors may be a rapid and direct one that does not necessarily involve altered turnover of receptor protein. For instance, hypothyroidism in dogs changes the erythropoietic action of catecholamines from a beta$_2$- to an alpha-type response, and incubation of cultured bone marrow cells from hypothyroid dogs with 100 mM levothyroxine for as little as 30 minutes reverses the response pattern from alpha-type response to beta-type response [268].

There are many more examples of reciprocal changes in alpha- and beta-receptor responses in various other tissues and of factors other than thyroid state or temperature that can produce similar alterations that are discussed below [48, 70, 254, 270, 271].

Evidence Against the Concept of Receptor Interconversion

The information that has been interpreted by various workers as having provided evidence against the concept of receptor interconversion can be classed into categories.

The first involves data obtained primarily through traditional physiopharmacologic analysis or radioligand-binding studies in the years of 1975 through 1979 [23–27, 123, 255, 280, 380]. The data and their interpretation developed in these publications are limited to suggesting that in one of the many conditions associated with reciprocal changes in alpha- and beta-receptor numbers and/or reactivities, such changes may not be detected under certain experimental conditions or may be attributed to nonspecific drug effects. None of these studies was undertaken in patients with atopic disease or in their animal models.

A significantly more important category of information that has been developed involves the earlier mentioned structural analysis of beta and alpha adrenoceptors provided by a number of technical approaches including target-size analysis radiation inactivation [101, 383], receptor affinity probes [192], and immunologic studies with monoclonal and antireceptor autoantibodies [102, 103, 382, 384]. Thus, the mammalian beta$_2$ receptor is a 64-kd glycoprotein containing a 46-kd polypeptide of recently resolved sequence [80] while the molecular mass of the alpha$_1$ receptor subunit is 80 kd [192]. Taken together, these structural studies indicate that alpha and beta receptors have distinct molecular identities that are functionally linked at levels of their coupling rather than being interconvertible proteins as originally suggested [195]. Nevertheless, the reciprocal nature of the functional shifts between alpha- and beta-receptor responses in a variety of conditions suggests a common regulatory factor or a common component in the biochemistry of intercellular and intracellular communication and associated transducing systems. Several of the possibilities are examined below.

Two Questions About the Inverse, Reciprocal Adrenoceptor Reactivities

The critical questions that may be raised by the foregoing observations are as follows:

1. Are there, in fact, valid examples of reciprocal changes in alpha- and beta-receptor activities and/or in their respective concentrations?
2. If there are, what is their mechanism?

The Validity of the Early and Current Examples of Reciprocal Adrenoceptor Changes

As we discussed earlier, substantial early evidence has accumulated to suggest that indeed there are valid examples of reciprocal changes in alpha- and beta-receptor reactivities as well as in their respective concentrations. Nevertheless, additional work was required to determine the ultimate validity of these observations and their physiologic and pathologic significance, especially in studies that were carried out by radioligand-binding techniques [328].

Thus, the cells used to study adrenoceptors, primarily blood cells, often represent a mixture of several distinct populations, resulting in conflicting observations. For instance, the number of beta receptors on polymorphonuclear leukocytes seems to be normal in subjects with asthma unless they receive adrenergic agonists [108, 109, 288]. In sharp contrast, lymphocytes of asthmatic patients show a significant decrease in radioligand binding to beta receptors, independent of agonist therapy [39, 168, 169, 287–289, 326, 339, 341, 368]. The same disparity in beta-receptor behavior between polymorphonuclear leukocytes and lymphocytes can be shown to exist in patients with atopic dermatitis [109, 260, 284, 341]. Finally in a study in which polymorphonuclear lymphocytes and lymphocytes were studied simultaneously in asthmatic patients, reported for the first time in the literature [289], it was found that the patients not receiving drugs showed a significant reduction in beta-receptor concentration in lymphocytic membranes but not in polymorphonuclear membranes.

Although studies to date have not indicated any difference in beta-receptor numbers or affinities for agonists or antagonists between B- and T-cells [34, 341], there is some indication that different mononuclear cell types (T-cells and B-cells, null cells, and monocytes) do not accumulate the same amount of cyclic AMP when stimulated with isoproterenol, and the results vary with the method used to separate the cells [227, 250, 299]. It is possible that future studies emphasizing less perturbing methods to separate these various cell populations (i.e., centrifugal elutriation) will eliminate these variations in cyclic AMP concentrations [238].

Another concern that has been raised in connection with lymphocytic alpha receptors had to do with the possibility that

the [^{3}H]DHE binding in such studies represented alpha receptors on platelets that may have contaminated the cell preparations [285]. Although such a possibility cannot be entirely ruled out at the present time, it seems highly unlikely in view of the findings on adipocytes obtained from asthmatic patients and showing the same alpha$_2$-directed reciprocal shift that has been found on lymphocytes, indicating the same adrenoceptor subtype behavior in a cell preparation in which no contamination with platelets is possible [355]. The validity of these early examples of inverse reciprocal regulatory shifts in adrenoceptor reactivities has further significant support, presented in the discussions that follow. Among these, the most important examples include the receptor shifts in glycogenolytic effect of catecholamines in the liver [191, 379], in spontaneously developed as well as experimentally induced asthma and atopic dermatitis [178, 179, 228–230, 338, 339, 354, 357, 358], in the responses of pinealocytes to light [381], and in hypothalamically induced changes in adrenoceptor concentrations of cell membranes [337, 349, 350, 360, 362].

These examples are chosen to illustrate some conceptual points in our current understanding of the molecular mechanism that may be involved in the receptor shifts in question. Taken together, all these observations do provide conclusive evidence of the validity of reciprocal changes in alpha- and beta-receptor responses and in their respective concentrations. Furthermore, from such findings two consistently characteristic features of these receptor shifts have emerged: (1) Different stimuli can trigger the same change in the adrenoceptor phenotype in a given tissue, and (2) the same stimulus can elicit directionally opposite changes in alpha- and beta-adrenergic responses in different tissues of the same animal. Thus, in the rat heart, hypothyroidism reduced beta- and increased alpha-receptor responses, whereas in the rat liver it had the opposite effects. A similar increase in beta- and decrease in alpha-receptor responses in the rat liver are triggered by a number of different conditions, commonly characterized by lower levels of cellular differentiation (cellular dedifferentiation) including that produced by glucocorticoid deficiency [188, 194, 271, 302].

The Mechanism of the Reciprocal Adrenoceptor Changes

In the original conceptual framework of the interconversion hypothesis, two major mechanisms were suggested [187, 195]. One speculation was that alpha and beta receptors may represent allosteric configurations of the same structure. Furthermore, since allosteric enzymes can be influenced by compounds unrelated to the specific substrate, allosteric adrenergic receptors could be appropriately influenced by the postulated modulator substance that has been reported to alter the balance of alpha- and beta-adrenergic vascular responses in skeletal muscle [364] or by hormones. The other early conceptual approach focused on the physical state of membrane lipids, which is known to be temperature dependent and can profoundly influence many membrane-associated processes. Indeed, there is evidence that membrane lipids have an essential role in the coupling between beta-adrenergic binding sites and adenylate cyclase, and discontinuities in the Arrhenius plots of catechol-activated adenylate cyclases were found at temperatures similar to the critical temperature for changes in adrenergic receptor properties. Binding of GTP to a regulatory site, which has been implicated above in the catecholamine-induced activation of adenylate cyclase, was proposed to be the temperature-sensitive event since GTP analogs abolished the break in the Arrhenius plot [186].

Based on current studies, it appears that the potential biochemical mechanisms involved in the various experimental models of inverse regulation of alpha and beta adrenoceptors point to four possible areas of promising inquiry: (1) increased membrane phospholipase A$_2$ activity, with the resulting release of an arachidonate metabolite generated through the cyclooxygenase pathway; (2) the possible role of protein kinase C; (3) the guanyl nucleotide regulatory proteins as they relate to adrenoceptor coupling functions; and (4) existence of a protein factor regulating adrenoceptor conversion.

Increased Membrane Phospholipase A_2 Activity. Increased membrane phospholipase A_2 activity with the release of an arachidonate metabolite was suggested as a possible mechanism of an adrenoceptor shift by the finding that one of the conditions associated with the conversion of the adrenergically induced glycogenolytic response in the liver from alpha$_1$ to beta type is a glucocorticoid deficiency that is reversible by glucocorticoid treatment [48]. Glucocorticoids are known to induce the synthesis and release of a protein, called *lipomodulin* or *lipocortin*, that inhibits phospholipase A_2 with the resultant decrease in arachidonic acid (release) and its eicosanoid metabolites, a mechanism that is believed to underlie most of the pharmacologic effects of glucocorticoids (for review see [184]; see also Chap. 60). That the hypothesis on the role of phospholipase A_2 in the inverse regulation of adrenoceptors may be a promising one is supported by the following additional observations:

1. Partially purified lipomodulin acutely reverses the time-dependent conversion from alpha$_1$- to beta-adrenergic glycogenolysis in isolated liver cells, whereas melittin, an activator of phospholipase A_2, has the opposite effect [189, 379].
2. Addition of arachidonic acid to freshly isolated hepatocytes suppresses the alpha$_1$ and enhances the beta receptor–mediated activation of phosphorylase.
3. This effect of arachidonic acid may be blocked by ibuprofen, a cyclooxygenase inhibitor, but not by nordihydroguaiaretic acid, a lipoxygenase inhibitor [155].
4. Although the direction of the change in the pineal gland is opposite to that in the liver, exposure of rats to constant light increases beta- and decreases alpha$_1$-adrenoceptor responses of isolated pinealocytes, that is, changes that can be mimicked by exposure of pinealocytes from control rats to mepacrine, a phospholipase A_2 inhibitor [381].

These findings bring into focus the possible relevance of altered membrane phospholipid metabolism in the pathogenesis of asthma and in the associated glucocorticoid-sensitive adrenoceptor changes, features that may explain the unusual coexistence of a reduced beta$_2$-adrenergic sensitivity and an unusually increased glucocorticoid sensitivity in asthma and atopic dermatitis.

The Role of Protein Kinase C. Another aspect of the nature of the atopic abnormality in allergic disease has to do with the question of the relationship between the above-mentioned phospholipase–arachidonic acid mechanism and protein kinase C in the conversion of the adrenoceptor response. There are three major reasons why a discussion of this question is required. First, experimental evidence that activation of protein kinase C is involved in the culture-induced changes in adrenoceptor responses in rat hepatocytes is available [67, 69, 203, 219]. Second, it has been demonstrated that activation of protein kinase C may lead to increased release and metabolism of arachidonic acid [239] and conversely, increased release of arachidonic acid may activate protein kinase C [241]. Similarly, Kunos and Ishac [191] found cytosol to membrane translocation of protein kinase C by exposure of hepatocytes to arachidonic acid. It is also possible that arachidonic acid and protein kinase C participate in parallel, synergistic regulatory mechanisms, as it has been shown in some other biologic systems [50]. Finally, in recent experiments protein kinase C was demonstrated to have a role in allergen-induced refractoriness of adenylate cyclase in lymphocytes of patients with asthma [228].

It has been established that allergen challenge of allergic patients with asthma causes various changes in the beta$_2$-receptor adenylate cyclase system of lymphocyte membranes from these patients including uncoupling and downregulation of beta$_2$ receptors and refractoriness of adenylate cyclase as demonstrated by reduced responses to isoproterenol (beta$_2$), histamine (H_2), Gpp(NH)p, and sodium fluoride [280, 380]. Since these changes could be due to desensitization by increased plasma concentrations of catecholamines and histamine as a consequence of the allergic reaction, in subsequent experiments Meurs and associates [228] studied the effects of these agonists on the beta$_2$-receptor adenylate cyclase system in vitro with normal lymphocytes. In addition, these workers also determined the effect of phorbol 12-myristate 13-acetate (PMA) on this in vitro system, since PMA has been demonstrated to regulate several receptor systems via the activation of protein kinase C [240, 252, 300]. These studies show that both uncoupling and downregulation contribute to isoproterenol-induced beta$_2$ subsensitivity, whereas beta$_2$-receptor uncoupling, but not beta$_2$-receptor downregulation is involved in PMA-induced refractoriness. Collectively, the data suggest that the agonist-induced changes in the lymphocyte adenylate cyclase system of patients with asthma are specifically located at the beta$_2$ adrenoceptors, whereas PMA-induced adenylate cyclase refractoriness must be due to alterations distal to the receptors, probably at the stimulatory guanine nucleotide regulatory protein [123].

The Guanyl Nucleotide Regulatory Proteins. Itoh, Okajima, and Ui [156] showed that the inhibitory guanyl nucleotide–binding protein (G1) is involved in the culture-induced conversion from alpha$_1$- to beta$_2$-adrenergic glycogenolysis in rat liver cells. Primary culturing of the cells resulted in a gradual loss of the cellular substrate for pertussis toxin–induced ADP ribosylation, whereas substances that inhibit endogenous ADP ribosyltransferases delay both this loss and associated conversion of the adrenoceptor response. Based on these observations, Itoh and coworkers [156] proposed that G1 through its coupling to beta$_2$ receptors inhibits adenylate cyclase activation, and suppression of this function of G1 by the increased activity of an endogenous ADP ribosyltransferase during primary culturing leads to increased beta$_2$-receptor activity. It is also postulated by these workers that the decrease in alpha$_1$-receptor activity is secondary to the increase in beta$_2$-receptor function and therefore is also linked to G1. As Kunos and Ishac [191] correctly point out, however, this last point of the argument is not supported by some other recent observations indicating that complete inactivation of hepatic G1 by large doses of pertussis toxin had no effect on alpha$_1$-adrenergic activation of phosphorylase [220] or polyphosphoinositide breakdown, and cholera toxin was shown to be similarly ineffective [377]. These observations may suggest that guanyl nucleotide effects on hepatic alpha$_1$ receptors reflect the involvement of a novel guanyl nucleotide–binding protein, which has been tentatively named Gx [191]. There are additional reasons to believe that one or several protein factors may be involved in the regulation of adrenoceptor conversions as further discussed below.

Irrespective of the issue of whether the above-mentioned decrease in alpha$_1$-receptor activity is secondary to the increase in beta$_2$-receptor function in the adrenergic glycogenolysis of liver cells, it is established that a number of bacteria and viruses are capable of interfering with signal transduction by altering G-protein function. Thus, pertussis and cholera toxins alter G-protein function by ADP ribosylation [379], and some viral protein products, such as H-*ras* p21, are themselves G-proteins and when injected into mammalian cells, can activate second messenger–generating enzyme systems [197].

Elevation of Cyclic AMP Phosphodiesterase Activity. For the first time in 1982, it has been reported that the activity of lymphocytic cyclic AMP phosphodiesterase (i.e., the enzyme that destroys cyclic AMP) is increased in atopic dermatitis as well as in allergic respiratory disease of adults [122], and that this increased activity correlates closely with histamine release from basophils [47] (see Chap. 15). When the same enzymatic activity together with histamine release was investigated in the newborn using umbilical cord blood, the significant elevation of phosphodiesterase activity was reconfirmed in newborns with a positive atopic history in first-degree relatives, compared to newborns with a negative history. In contrast to adults, however, there was no correlation between phosphodiesterase activity and histamine release [226]. Elevation of cyclic AMP phosphodiesterase activity in cord blood leukocytes before the development of clinical manifestations of atopy would appear to suggest that increased cyclic AMP phosphodiesterase may have an important role in the pathogenesis of atopic disease. The lack of correlation between phosphodiesterase activity and histamine release in neonates may further suggest that elevated cyclic AMP phosphodiesterase activity is a genetically linked defect rather than secondary to in vivo desensitization by inflammatory mediators such as histamine and prostaglandin E_1 [285].

In addition to the foregoing, an extensive effort has been made by Hanifin and his group to determine the monocyte and lymphocyte localization of altered adrenergic receptors, cyclic AMP responses, and cyclic AMP phosphodiesterase elevated activity in atopic dermatitis [63, 65, 66, 115, 149, 150]. In these experiments, the numbers and affinities of beta-adrenergic cell-surface receptors on mononuclear leukocyte subpopulations were measured by the binding of propranolol displaceable [^{3}H]DHA to cell surfaces. Unfractionated atopic mononuclear leukocytes showed reduced numbers of beta-adrenergic receptors per cell together with the absence of a normal, lower-affinity subpopulation of high-affinity beta receptors, resulting in a linear Scatchard plot of beta-adrenergic binding to mononuclear leukocytes from atopic patients, instead of the biphasic plot seen in normal control cells. These alterations of surface receptors for cyclic AMP–elevating ligands were localized to T-cells and monocytes of patients with atopic dermatitis, whereas atopic B-cell receptor numbers and affinities were identical to those of normal B-cells [63, 64]. Of the various subpopulations of T-cells, a lymphocyte subset that is activatable by self Ia-bearing antigen-presenting monocytic cells has been identified as radiosensitive (functionally dependent on a proliferative step) OKT4$^+$, T29$^+$ helper/inducer T-cells [207, 278, 375]. A primary abnormality in the numbers and/or in the intracellular regulation of the cyclic AMP system of the radiosensitive T29$^+$ helper/inducer T-cells generated by the interaction with autologous Ia-positive antigen-presenting macrophages may explain many of the characteristic features of immune dysfunction in atopic dermatitis [65].

For instance, soluble mitogen-stimulated proliferation is critically dependent on successful macrophage–T-cell interaction, and can be reduced in patients with atopic dermatitis [89, 215]. Development of the pool of blood pokeweed mitogen–recruitable B-cells for in vitro antibody production requires induction by a radiosensitive T-cell inducer [277, 278, 317] and indeed, B-cells from patients with atopic dermatitis demonstrate decreased mitogen-stimulated antibody secretion, even when corrected for number or when normal T-cells are used to provide helper function [207]. T-cells associated with suppressor and cytotoxic functions, such as T-cells with Fc IgG receptors, OKT8 cells, and histamine H_2 receptor–bearing T-cells, often show significantly reduced values in patients with atopic dermatitis [21, 66, 167, 207, 294], which is in accord with findings indicating that the development of mature suppressor and cytotoxic effector T-cells requires induction by the aforementioned radiosensitive helper T-cells [38, 142, 279]. It may be added that development of cytotoxic T-lymphocytes is known to be dependent on Ia-positive monocyte stimulation of helper T-cell factors such as interleukin-2 [142] and a decrease in the production of interleukin-2 as well as interferon by these abnormal helper/inducer T-cells, or their

altered ability to respond to these signals may explain the reduced natural killer activity in atopic dermatitis [163, 196]. Thus, the aforementioned multiple abnormalities of the cyclic AMP system in the helper/inducer T-cells in question may account for the immune dysfunction in atopic dermatitis. Alternatively, each of the immune abnormalities listed could be due to altered immune signal processing by distal effector cells with their own malfunctioning intracellular cyclic AMP systems, as is further pointed out below.

The Role of Calcium Ions and the Inositol-Lipid Signal Pathway. Two major signal pathways are now known. One employs the widely familiar cyclic AMP second messenger, whereas the other (the inositol-lipid signal pathway) uses a combination of second messengers that includes calcium ions and two substances, inositol triphosphate (IP_3) and diacylglycerol. Both pathways have much in common: (1) The initial component is the cell-surface receptor molecule that transmits information through the membrane into the cell by the G-proteins, the activation of which requires binding of GTP; (2) in both pathways the G-proteins activate an "amplifier" enzyme on the inner surface of the membrane, an enzyme that converts precursor molecules into second messengers; and (3) the precursors are highly phosphorylated. Thus, in the case of the first pathway, the amplifier adenylate cyclase converts ATP to cyclic AMP, whereas the amplifier phospholipase C cleaves the membrane lipid phosphatidylinositol-4,5-diphosphate (PIP_2) into diacylglycerol and IP_3 [30]. This section concentrates on how the currently available information on calcium ions and the inositol-lipid signal pathway relate to each other, with special regard to the issue of beta-adrenergic subsensitivity (see also Chap. 16).

Participation of calcium in cellular processes begins with either a movement of Ca^{++} into the cell or its release from intracellular stores. Two primary pathways for Ca^{++} entry into the cell have been identified so far: (1) the potential-dependent (or voltage-dependent) channel and (2) the receptor-operated channel. Activation of the potential-dependent channel by K^+ depolarization opens the membrane channel and free Ca^{++} moves down the concentration gradient into the cell. Receptor-operated channels open when specific receptors (i.e., histaminergic, cholinergic) are activated by their corresponding agonists [148] (see Chap. 71). Regulation of intracellular Ca^{++} also involves interaction between receptors and second messengers generated by the inositol-lipid pathway. There are three myoinositol-containing phosphatides operative in this process: (1) phosphatidylinositol, (2) phosphatidylinositol-4-phosphate or diphosphoinositide (PIP), and (3) phosphatidylinositol-4,5-biphosphate or triphosphoinositide (PIP_2). It can be shown that introduction of IP_3 into the cell causes a rapid release into the cytosol of "trigger Ca^{++}" from the endoplasmic reticulum. The other phosphodiesteratic cleavage product of all the phosphoinositides, diacylglycerol, activates protein kinase C (distinct from cyclic AMP– or cyclic GMP–activated protein kinase). In addition to a requirement for diacylglycerol, protein kinase C needs phospholipids and calcium for maximal activity. The IP_3 and the diacylglycerol components of the signal cascade act synergistically to phosphorylate proteins and produce the cellular response. IP_3 achieves this by elevating cytosolic Ca^{++} to activate calmodulin-dependent protein phosphorylation, whereas diacylglycerol activates protein kinase C. A third active metabolite of the phosphoinositides is arachidonate [257, 258, 272]. The significance of protein kinase C and arachidonic acid in the reciprocal expression of alpha and beta receptors is described in the preceding section and does not require further elaboration here.

Nevertheless, these considerations complete the full circle of the core argument of this chapter and guide us back to the issue of the nature of the constitutional basis of respiratory and cutaneous atopic disease, that is, the issue of the diminished beta-adrenergic responsiveness in allergic tissues. Some of the principal features of asthma such as smooth muscle contraction, mast cell mediator release, and tissue inflammation are calcium-related phenomena, and therefore it is appropriate to consider abnormalities in Ca^{++} deposition following cell activation as a contributing factor in the development of the beta-adrenergic abnormality. Smooth muscle contraction is a case in point. As is established, the contractile activity of smooth muscle is controlled by the concentration of free intracellular Ca^{++} that increases with smooth muscle excitation. Increased cytosolic Ca^{++} activates the calcium-binding protein, calmodulin and thus myosin light-chain kinase (MLCK). Phosphorylation of myosin light chains by MLCK allows the activation by actin of myosin ATPase, and hence smooth muscle contraction. Dephosphorylation of myosin by a Ca^{++}-independent phosphatase relaxes smooth muscle. In addition, cyclic AMP–dependent protein kinase can phosphorylate MLCK; in the phosphorylated state, MLCK has reduced affinity for calmodulin and smooth muscle relaxation follows [1]. Consequently, abnormalities in Ca^{++}-dependent processes may also contribute to impaired beta-adrenergic responsiveness in asthma.

ADRENERGICALLY ACTIVE LYMPHOCYTIC PROTEINS AND THE CONSTITUTIONAL BASIS OF ATOPIC DISEASE

Inhibition of protein or mRNA synthesis by cycloheximide or actinomycin D, respectively, prevents the conversion of $alpha_1$- to beta-adrenergic glycogenolysis [244, 275, 295] as well as the inverse, reciprocal changes in $alpha_1$- and $beta_2$-receptor concentrations [295]. There is evidence that the protein involved is not the receptor protein itself [155, 190]. Furthermore, more recently Stern and Kunos [315] reported the existence of a lymphocyte-derived protein in the regulation of pulmonary beta adrenoceptors. It was shown that this lymphocytic protein upregulates $beta_2$ adrenoceptors in cultured A549 human lung cells. Depending on the experimental circumstances, this upregulation would increase the concentration of $beta_2$ adrenoceptors up to three- to fourfold, if the cells were exposed to the lymphocytic protein alone, and up to 15- to 20-fold if corticosteroids were added to the lymphocytic protein, establishing a synergistic relationship between the two. Following the preliminary confirmation of these findings by our group in 1989, we decided to establish a major effort to pursue this line of inquiry into the nature of the beta-adrenergic subsensitivity in respiratory and cutaneous atopy.

It was thought that these observations may open up a new insight into the nature of the constitutional basis of atopy. These findings were all the more attractive since after three decades of maximum effort we were unable to determine the nature of the still-elusive connecting link between the immunologic and beta-adrenergic dysregulation in atopic disease. In the beginning, following our confirmation of the basic finding of Stern and Kunos [315], we redesigned some of the features of their technology and some other aspects of their studies to serve our objectives.

Originally we retained the two cell lines used by Stern and Kunos: the A549 lung cells and the IM9 lymphocytes. The A549 cell line was initiated through explant culture of human lung carcinomatous tissue, and preparation and characterization of the cells were carried out at the American Type Culture Collection. It was found that (1) they can synthesize lecithin with a high percentage of desaturated fatty acids utilizing the cytidine-diphosphocholine pathway; (2) specific activities of choline kinase and cholinephosphate cytidyltransferase are higher in these cells than in WI-38 controls; (3) multilamellar inclusion bodies may be shown by transmission electron microscopy; and (4) the morphology is epithelial like and confirmed as human by immu-

nofluorescence and isoenzymology (glucose-6-phosphate dehydrogenase Type B and typical lactate dehydrogenase banding). Taken together, although likely, the cells cannot be definitely characterized as of Type II origin or function. The IM9 cell line was initiated from a bone marrow sample from a patient with chronic myelogenous leukemia. The cells exhibit surface markers and receptor sites characteristic of B-lymphoblasts and are capable of synthesizing immunoglobulins. It has been demonstrated that IM9 cells possess receptor sites for about 20 different hormones, neurotransmitters (including catecholamines), and immunoregulatory molecules.

By coculturing A549 cells with IM9 cells for 24 hours, we started to characterize the IM9 cells' protein components that upregulate the beta adrenoceptors of the A549 cells. For resolution of the beta-adrenoceptor upregulating activity, the lymphocyte-conditioned medium derived from IM9 cells was subjected to diethylaminoethanol (DEAE) ion-exchange high-pressure liquid chromatography [281, 282] which yielded four distinct macromolecular fractions (activity peaks). Of these, Peaks II and III possessed significant beta-adrenoceptor upregulating activity, Peak I showed significant downregulating activity, whereas Peak IV yielded no adrenergic activity [351–353]. In studying the protein components of the activity peaks of lymphocyte-conditioned medium of IM9 cells responsible for their regulatory effects on beta adrenoceptors of A549 human lung cells, three general approaches were used: (1) standard physicochemical characterization, (2) immunoneutralization using monoclonal and polyclonal antibodies to cytokines produced constitutively by lymphocytes, and (3) measurements of A549 beta-adrenoceptor concentrations to recombinant cytokines for determining whether they have the capacity to upregulate or downregulate beta adrenoceptors [282, 353].

In the activity Peak I, we identified two inhibitory factors, one of which is a secretory analog of beta-arrestin and the other one is an inhibitor of interleukin-1α (IL-1α). The existence of beta-arrestin was recently discovered when it was found that a cofactor is required for beta-adrenergic receptor kinase to inhibit beta-adrenoceptor function. The cDNA for such a cofactor was cloned and found to encode a 418–amino acid protein homologous to the retinal protein arrestin. The protein was termed *beta-arrestin* and shown to inhibit the phosphorylation of beta adrenoceptors by beta-adrenergic receptor kinase by more than 75 percent, but not that of rhodopsin. Beta-arrestin mRNA was found in all tissues examined so far, with the highest levels in brain, heart, and lung [217]. This is the first time that beta-arrestin was found to be produced by lymphocytes.

The second inhibitory factor in activity Peak I was identified as one of the IL-1 antagonists. Its characterization has not been completed, but so far it has shown essentially identical physicochemical and biologic features that were found by Eisenberg and coworkers [86]. The IL-1 receptor antagonist (IL-1RA) is a protein that blocks the binding of both IL-1α and IL-1β. It occupies the interleukin receptor but exerts no known physiologic actions on receptor function [211]; our lymphocytic IL-1RA shows the same pattern of activity and it is pertinent to add that it does not bind to A549 beta adrenoceptors or exert any modulatory activity on them. The upregulating activity Peak II was shown to be a mixture of IL-1α and IL-1β. Although both of these proteins are able to upregulate the A549 $beta_2$ adrenoceptors, Il-1α was found to be more potent. Physicochemical, immunologic, and pharmacologic analysis of the active components of the upregulating activity Peak III is currently underway.

When the lymphocyte-conditioned medium of IM9 cells was replaced by that derived from normal human peripheral blood lymphocytes and peripheral blood lymphocytes of patients with symptomatic or asymptomatic asthma, of patients with atopic dermatitis, and of patients with nonatopic skin diseases, it was found that the A549 $beta_2$-adrenoceptor upregulating capacity of the peripheral blood lymphocytes of patients with symptomatic or asymptomatic asthma and those of atopic dermatitis was significantly reduced, whereas the upregulating activity of peripheral blood lymphocytes from patients with nonatopic skin diseases was retained. The same pattern of results was obtained when lymphocyte-conditioned medium of human peripheral blood lymphocytes was replaced with that of purified T-lymphocytes derived from the same group of patients. Thus, lymphocytes of patients with atopic diseases have an impaired capacity to upregulate beta adrenoceptors in human lung cells as reflected by the behavior of the A549 cell line. On the other hand, the two downregulating proteins showed normal activity both in asthma and in atopic dermatitis [86].

The synergistic regulation of pulmonary beta adrenoceptors by glucocorticoids and IL-1α was described by Stern and Kunos [315] and Szentendrei and colleagues [323] and was also found by our group, which has had a long-time interest in the pharmacology and biochemistry of the corticosteroid potentiation of adrenergic activities (for a detailed review see previously published chapter by Szentivanyi et al. [348]). Only the most recent information is presented here. Glucocorticoids increase in vivo and in vitro the steady-state levels of pulmonary beta adrenoceptors. Conversely, glucocorticoid-deficient animals lose their ability to maintain the sensitivity of the beta-adrenoceptor adenylate cyclase system, a condition that is reversible with glucocorticoids. In response to glucocorticoids the beta-adrenoceptor mRNA levels are increased and this upregulation of receptor mRNA is due to the increased rates of gene transcription [60–62, 124–127, 390], and consensus sequences for glucocorticoid-response elements have been identified in the gene of the beta$_2$ adrenoceptor [53, 92, 175]. The following question arises then: In the synergistic regulation of beta$_2$ adrenoceptors by the upregulating lymphocytic proteins and glucocorticoids, are these substances acting on the same site or not? At the present time, depending on the experimental conditions, there is evidence that both IL-1α and corticosteroids increase the number of A549 beta adrenoceptors and the increase in receptor concentrations is preceded by an increase in beta$_2$-adrenoceptor mRNA. When, however, the DDT$_1$MF$_2$-2 cell is used, there is a dissociation between the effects of IL-1α and corticosteroids [323]. As the continuing studies on the nature of the molecular mechanisms involved in the action of these adrenergically active lymphocytic proteins unfold, we will gain a far better understanding of the nature and mechanisms of action of these adrenergically active lymphocytic proteins and consequently about the nature of the constitutional basis of atopy.

REFERENCES

1. Abdel-Latif, A. Calcium-mobilizing receptors, polyphosphoinositides, and the generation of second messengers. *Pharmacol. Rev.* 38:227, 1986.
2. Abramsky, O. Cellular immune response to acetylcholine receptor-rich fraction in patients with myasthenia gravis. *Clin. Exp. Immunol.* 19:11, 1975.
3. Aggerbeck, M., et al. Adrenergic regulation of glycogenolysis in rat liver after cholestasis. *J. Clin. Invest.* 71:476, 1983.
4. Ahlquist, R. P. A study of the adrenotropic receptors. *Am. J. Physiol.* 153:586, 1948.
5. Ahlquist, R. P. Adrenoceptor sensitivity in disease as assessed through response to temperature alteration. *Fed. Proc.* 36:2572, 1977.
6. Albers, R. W. Biochemical aspects of active transport. *Annu. Rev. Biochem.* 36:727, 1969.
7. Alexander, R. W., Cooper, B., and Handin, R. I. Characterization of the human platelet alpha-adrenergic receptor. *J. Clin. Invest.* 61:1136, 1978.
8. Anderson, P. J., and D'Iorio, A. Purification and properties of catechols-O-methyltransferase. *Biochem. Pharmacol.* 17:1943, 1968.
9. Anthracite, R. F., Vachon, L., and Knapp, P. H. Alpha-adrenergic receptors in the human lung. *Psychosom. Med.* 33:481, 1977.
10. Apold, J., and Aksnes, L. Correlation between increased bronchial responsiveness to histamine and diminished plasma cyclic adenosine monophosphate response after epinephrine in asthmatic children: Diminished plasma cyclic adenosine monophosphate response after epinephrine in moderate childhood asthma. *J. Allergy Clin. Immunol.* 59:343, 1977.
11. Appleman, M. M., and Allan, E. J., and Ariano, M. A. Insulin Control of Cyclic AMP Phosphodiesterase. In S. J. Strada and W. J. Thompson (eds.), *Advances in Cyclic Nucleotide and Protein Phosphorylation Research,* Vol. 16. New York: Raven, 1984.
12. Assicot, M., and Bohuon, C. Purification and studies of catechol-O-methyltransferase of rat liver. *Eur. J. Biochem.* 12:490, 1970.
13. Auerbach, G. D., et al. The beta-adrenergic receptor: Stereospecific interaction of iodinated beta-blocking agent with a high affinity site. *Science* 186:1223, 1974.
14. Axelrod, J. Methylation reactions in the formation and metabolism of catecholamines and other biogenic amines. *Pharmacol. Rev.* 18:95, 1966.
15. Axelrod, J., Albers, W., and Clemente, C. D. Distribution of catechol-O-methyltransferase in the nervous system and other tissues. *J. Neurochem.* 5:68, 1959.
16. Axelrod, J., and Tomchick, R. Enzymatic O-methylation of epinephrine and other catechols. *J. Biol. Chem.* 233:702, 1958.
17. Bach, J.-F. Immunologic Disturbances of Receptors in Disease. In J. W. Hadden, et al. (eds.), *Advances in Immunopharmacology 2.* Oxford: Pergamon, 1983. Pp. 293–297.
18. Barnes, P. J., et al. Circulating catecholamines in exercise and hyperventilation induced asthma. *Thorax* 36:435, 1981.
19. Barnes, P. J., Dollery, C. T., and MacDermot, A. Increased pulmonary alpha-adrenergic and beta-adrenergic receptors in experimental asthma. *Nature* 258:569, 1980.
20. Barr, M. L., and Kiernan, J.A. *The Human Nervous System: An Anatomical Viewpoint* (4th ed.). New York: Lippincott, 1983.
21. Beer, D. J., et al. Abnormal histamine induced suppressor cell function in atopic individuals. *N. Engl. J. Med.* 306:454, 1982.
22. Belcher, M., et al. Beta-blocking autoantibodies in pediatric bronchial asthma. *J. Allergy Clin. Immunol.* 74:246, 1984.
23. Benfey, B. G. Temperature dependence of phenoxybenzamine effects and the adrenoceptor transformation hypothesis. *Nature* 256:745, 1975.
24. Benfey, B. G. Temperature, phenoxybenzamine and adrenoceptor transformation. *Nature* 259:252, 1976.
25. Benfey, B. G. Cardiac adrenoceptors at low temperatures: What is the experimental evidence for the adrenoceptor interconversion hypothesis? *Fed. Proc.* 36:2575, 1977.
26. Benfey, B. G. Discussion of evidence regarding adrenoceptor interconversion. *Fed. Proc.* 37:686, 1978.
27. Benfey, B. G. The interconversion of adrenoceptors. *Trends Auton. Pharmacol.* 1:289, 1979.
28. Bennett, M. R. *Autonomic Neuromuscular Transmission.* London: Cambridge University Press, 1972.
29. Bennett, M. V. L. Electrical versus chemical neurotransmission. *Proc. Assoc. Res. Nerv. Ment. Dis.* 50:58, 1972.
30. Berridge, M. J. Inositol Phosphates as Second Messengers. In J. W. Putney (ed.), *Phosphoinositides and Receptor Mechanisms.* New York: Alan R. Liss, 1986. Pp. 24–45.
31. Bertler, A., and Rosengren, E. Occurrence and distribution of dopamine in brain and other tissues. *Experientia* 15:10, 1959.
32. Bhatia, S. P., and Davies, H. J. Evaluation of tolerance after continuous and prolonged oral administration of salbutamol to asthmatic patients. *Br. J. Clin. Pharmacol.* 2:463, 1975.
33. Birnbaumer, L., and Brown, A. M. G proteins and the mechanism of action of hormones, neurotransmitters, autocrine and paracrine regulatory factors. *Am. Rev. Respir. Dis.* 141:S106, 1990.
34. Bishopric, N. H., Cohen, H. J., and Lefkowitz, R. J. Beta-adrenergic receptors in lymphocyte subpopulations. *J. Allergy Clin. Immunol.* 65:29, 1980.
35. Blaschko, H. Amine oxidase and amine metabolism. *Pharmacol. Rev.* 4;415, 1952.
36. Blaschko, H., et al. Secretion of a chromaffin granule protein, chromogranin, from the adrenal gland after splanchnic stimulation. *Nature* 215:58, 1967.
37. Bogdanski, D. F., and Brodie, B. B. Role of sodium and potassium ions in storage of norepinephrine by sympathetic nerve endings. *Life Sci.* 5:1563, 1966.
38. Broder, S., et al. Activation of leukemic presuppressor cells to become suppressor effector cells. *N. Engl. J. Med.* 304:1382, 1981.
39. Brooks, S. M., et al. Relationship between numbers of beta-adrenergic

receptors in lymphocytes and disease severity in asthma. *J. Allergy Clin. Immunol.* 63:401, 1979.

40. Brown, G. L. Release of Sympathetic Transmitter by Nerve Stimulation. In J. R. Vane, G. E. W. Wolstenholme, and M. O'Connor (eds.), *Ciba Foundation Symposium on Adrenergic Mechanisms.* Boston: Little, Brown, 1960.

41. Burn, J. H., and Gibbons, W. R. The release of noradrenaline from sympathetic fibers in relation to calcium concentrations. *J. Physiol. (Lond.)* 181:214, 1965.

42. Burn, J. H., and Rand, M. J. Acetylcholine in adrenergic transmission. *Annu. Rev. Pharmacol.* 5:163, 1965.

43. Busse, W. W. Decreased granulocyte response to isoproterenol in asthma during upper respiratory infections. *Am. Rev. Respir. Dis.* 115:783, 1977.

44. Busse, W. W., et al. Impairment of isoproterenol, H_2 histamine, and prostaglandin D_1 response of human granulocytes after incubation in vitro with live influenza vaccines. *Am. Rev. Respir. Dis.* 119:561, 1979.

45. Busse, W. W., and Lee, T.-P. Decreased adrenergic responses in lymphocytes and granulocytes in atopic eczema. *J. Allergy Clin. Immunol.* 58:586, 1976.

46. Busse, W. W., and Reed, C. E. Asthma: Definition and Pathogenesis. In E. Middleton, C. E. Reed and E. F. Ellis (eds.), *Allergy—Principles and Practice* (3rd ed.). St. Louis: Mosby, 1988. Pp. 969–998.

47. Butler, J. M., et al. Increased leukocyte histamine release with elevated cyclic AMP-phosphodiesterase activity in atopic dermatitis. *J. Allergy Clin. Immunol.* 71:490, 1983.

48. Chan, T. M., et al. Effects of adrenalectomy on hormone action on hepatic glucose metabolism. *J. Biol. Chem.* 254:2428, 1979.

49. Chang, H. Y., Kline, R. M., and Kunos, G. Selective desensitization of cardiac beta-adrenoceptors by prolonged in vivo infusion of catecholamines in rats. *J. Pharmacol. Exp. Ther.* 221:784, 1982.

50. Chang, J. P., Graeter, J., and Catt, K. J. Coordinate actions of arachidonic acid and protein kinase C in gonadotropin-releasing hormone-stimulated secretion of luteinizing hormone. *Biochem. Biophys. Res. Commun.* 134:134, 1986.

51. Christoffersen, T., and Berg, T. Altered hormone control of cAMP formation—Isolated parenchymal liver cells from rats treated with 2-acetylaminofluorene. *Biochim. Biophys. Acta* 381:72, 1975.

52. Chrivos, M. A., Greengard, P., and Udenfriend, S. Uptake of tyrosine by rat brain in vivo. *J. Biol. Chem.* 235:2075, 1960.

53. Chung, F.-Z., et al. Cloning and sequence analysis of the human brain beta-adrenergic receptor. *FEBS Lett.* 211:200, 1987.

54. Ciaraldi, T., and Marinetti, G. V. Thyroxine and propylthiouracil effects in vivo and alpha- and beta-adrenergic receptors in rat heart. *Biochem. Biophys. Res. Commun.* 74:984, 1977.

55. Co, M. S., et al. Isolation and biochemical characterization of the mammalian reovirus type 3 cell surface receptor. *Proc. Natl. Acad. Sci. USA* 82:1494, 1985.

56. Co, M. S., et al. Structural similarities between the mammalian beta-adrenergic reovirus type 3 receptors. *Proc. Natl. Acad. Sci. USA* 82:5315, 1985.

57. Co, M. S., et al. *Hybridoma Technology in the Biosciences and Medicine.* New York: Plenum, 1985.

58. Cole, K.S. *Membranes, Ions and Impulses: A Chapter of Classical Biophysics.* Berkeley: University of California Press, 1968.

59. Collins, G. G. S., et al. Multiple forms of human brain mitochondrial monoamine oxidase. *Nature* 225:817, 1970.

60. Collins, S., et al. Genetic regulation of beta-adrenergic receptors. *Am. Rev. Physiol.* 51:203, 1989.

61. Collins, S., et al. cAMP stimulates transcription of the β_2-adrenergic receptor gene in response to short-term agonist exposure. *Proc. Natl. Acad. Sci. USA* 86:4853, 1989.

62. Collins, S., Caron, M. G., and Lefkowitz, R. J. β_2-Adrenergic receptors in hamster smooth muscle cells are transcriptionally regulated by glucocorticoids. *J. Biol. Chem.* 263:9067, 1988.

63. Cooper, K. D., Chan, S. C., and Hanifin, J. M. Differential T and B cell beta-adrenergic responsiveness implies alternative regulatory mechanisms in atopy. *Clin. Res.* 29:281A, 1981.

64. Cooper, K. D., Chan, S. C., and Hanifin, J. M. Absence of low affinity beta-adrenergic receptors in atopic dermatitis and histamine-desensitized normal leukocytes. *Clin. Res.* 30:27, 1982.

65. Cooper, K. D., Chan, S. C., and Hanifin, J. M. Lymphocyte and monocyte localization of altered adrenergic receptors, cAMP responses, and cAMP phosphodiesterase in atopic dermatitis. A possible mechanism for abnormal radiosensitive helper T cells in atopic dermatitis. *Acta Derm. Venereol. Suppl. (Stockh.)* 114:41, 1985.

66. Cooper, K. D., et al. Immunoregulation in atopic dermatitis: Functional analysis of T-B cell interactions and the enumeration of Fc receptor bearing T cells. *J. Invest. Dermatol.* 80:139, 1983.

67. Cooper, R. H., Coll, K. E., and Williamson, J. R. Differential effects of phorbol ester on phenylephrine and vasopressin-induced Ca^{2+} mobilization in isolated hepatocytes. *J. Biol. Chem.* 260:3281, 1985.

68. Cooper, T. Surgical sympathectomy and adrenergic function. *Pharmacol. Rev.* 18:611, 1966.

69. Corvera, S., et al. Phorbol esters inhibit α_1-adrenergic effects and decrease the affinity of liver cell α_1-adrenergic receptors for epinephrine. *J. Biol. Chem.* 261:520, 1986.

70. Corwin, E. J., Cho, K. W., and Malvin, E. L. Temperature-induced conversion of the renal adrenoceptor: Modulating renin release. *Am. J. Physiol.* 243:23, 1982.

71. Costa, E., et al. Interactions of drugs with adrenergic neurons. *Pharmacol. Rev.* 18:577, 1966.

72. Coupland, R. E. The Chromaffin System. In H. Blaschko and E. Muscholl (eds.), *Catecholamines.* Berlin: Springer, 1972.

73. Cseuz, R., et al. Changes of adrenergic reaction pattern in experimental diabetes mellitus. *Endocrinology* 93:752, 1973.

74. Davies, A. O., and Lefkowitz, R. J. In vitro desensitization of beta-adrenergic receptors in human neutrophils: Attenuation by corticosteroids. *J. Clin. Invest.* 71:565, 1983.

75. De Champlain, J., Mueller, R. A., and Axelrod, J. Subcellular localization of monoamine oxidase in rat tissue. *J. Pharmacol. Exp. Ther.* 166:339, 1969.

76. DeLean, A., Stadel, J. M., and Lefkowitz, R. J. A ternary complex model explains the agonist-specific binding properties of the adenylate cyclase-coupled beta-adrenergic receptor. *J. Biol. Chem.* 255:7108, 1980.

77. Dengler, H. J., et al. The uptake of labeled catecholamines by isolated brain and other tissues of the cat. *Int. J. Neuropharmacol.* 1:23, 1962.

78. DeRobertis, E. *Histophysiology of Synapses and Neurosecretion.* Oxford: Pergamon, 1964.

79. Diner, O. Cited in C. Coers. Structure and organization of the myoneural junction. *Int. Rev. Cytol.* 22:239, 1967.

80. Dixon, R. A. F., et al. Cloning of the gene and cDNA for mammalian beta-adrenergic receptor and homology with rhodopsin. *Nature* 321:75, 1986.

81. Douglas, W. W. Stimulus-secretion coupling: The concept and clues from chromaffin and other cells. *Br. J. Pharmacol.* 34:451, 1968.

82. Douglas, W. W., and Poisner, A. M. Evidence that the secreting adrenal chromaffin cell releases catecholamines directly from ATP-rich granules. *J. Physiol. (Lond.)* 183:236, 1966.

83. Drachman, D. B. Myasthenic antibodies crosslink acetylcholine receptors to accelerate degradation. *N. Engl. J. Med.* 298:1116, 1978.

84. Eccles, J. C. *The Understanding of the Brain.* New York: McGraw-Hill, 1973.

85. Eccles, J. C. *The Physiology of Synapses.* New York: Academic, 1981.

86. Eisenberg, S. P., et al. Interleukin-1 receptor antagonist is a member of the interleukin-1 gene family: Evolution of a cytokine control mechanism. *Proc. Natl. Acad. Sci. USA* 88:5232, 1991.

87. Eisenfeld, A. J., Axelrod, J., and Krakoc, L. R. Inhibition of the extraneuronal accumulation and metabolism of catecholamines by adrenergic blocking agents. *J. Pharmacol. Exp. Ther.* 156:107, 1967.

88. Eisenfeld, A. J., Landsberg, L., and Axelrod, J. Effect of drugs on the accumulation and metabolism of extraneuronal norepinephrine in the rat heart. *J. Pharmacol. Exp. Ther.* 158:378, 1967.

89. Elliott, S. T., and Hanifin, J. Lymphocyte response to phytohemagglutinin in atopic dermatitis. *Arch. Dermatol.* 115:1424, 1979.

90. El-Rafi, M. F., and Chan, T. M. Effects of fasting on hepatic catecholamine receptors. *Fed. Eur. Biochem. Soc. Lett.* 146:397, 1982.

91. Emmelin, N. Supersensitivity following "pharmacologica! denervation." *Pharmacol. Rev.* 13:17, 1961.

92. Emorine, L. J., et al. Structure of the gene for human B_2-adrenergic receptor: Expression and promoter characterization. *Proc. Natl. Acad. Sci. USA* 84:6995, 1987.

93. Enero, M. A., et al. Role of alpha adrenergic receptor in regulating noradrenaline overflow by nerve stimulation. *Br. J. Pharmacol.* 44:672, 1972.

94. Eranko, O. Cell Types of the Adrenal Medulla. In J. R. Vane, G. E. W. Wolstenholme, and M. O'Connor (eds.), *Ciba Foundation Symposium on Adrenergic Mechanisms.* Boston: LIttle, Brown, 1960.

95. Exton, J. H. Mechanism Involved in Alpha-Adrenergic Effects of Catecholamines. In G. Kunos (ed.), *Adrenoceptors and Catecholamine Action.* New York: John Wiley, 1981.

96. Falck, B., Hillarp, N. A., and Torp, A. Some observations on the histology

and histochemistry of chromaffin cells probably storing dopamine. *J. Histochem. Cytochem.* 7:323, 1959.

97. Ferry, C. B. Cholinergic link hypothesis in adrenergic neuroeffector transmission. *Physiol. Rev.* 46:420, 1966.

98. Fields, B. N., and Greene, M. I. Genetic and molecular mechanisms of viral pathogenesis—implications for prevention and treatment. *Nature* 300:19, 1982.

99. Flier, J. S. Antibodies that impair insulin receptor binding in an unusual diabetic syndrome with severe insulin resistance. *Science* 190:63, 1975.

100. Fraser, C. M. Molecular biology of adrenergic receptors: Model systems for the study of G protein-mediated signal transduction. *Blood Vessels* 28:93, 1991.

101. Fraser, C. M., et al. Autoantibodies and monoclonal antibodies in the purification and molecular characterization of neurotransmitter receptors. *J. Cell. Biochem.* 21:219, 1983.

102. Fraser, C. M., and Venter, J. C. Monoclonal antibodies to beta-adrenergic receptors: Use in purification and molecular characterization of beta receptors. *Proc. Natl. Acad. Sci. USA* 77:7034, 1980.

103. Fraser, C. M., Venter, J. C., and Kaliner, M. Autonomic abnormalities and autoantibodies to beta-adrenergic receptors. *N. Engl. J. Med.* 305:1165, 1981.

104. Friedman, H., Klein, T. W., and Szentivanyi, A. (eds.), *Immunomodulation by Bacteria and Their Products.* New York: Plenum, 1981.

105. Friedman, S., and Kaufman, S. 3,4-Dihydroxyphenylethylamine beta-hydroxylase, a copper protein. *J. Biol. Chem.* 240:PC552, 1965.

106. Gabay, S., and Valcourt, A. J. Studies of monoamine oxidases. I. Purification and properties of the rabbit liver mitochondrial enzyme. *Biochim. Biophys. Acta* 159:440, 1968.

107. Galant, S. P. Decreased beta-adrenergic receptors on polymorphonuclear leukocytes after adrenergic therapy. *N. Engl. J. Med.* 299:933, 1978.

108. Galant, S. P., et al. Beta-adrenergic receptors of polymorphonuclear particulates in bronchial asthma. *J. Clin. Invest.* 65:577, 1980.

109. Galant, S. P., et al. Beta-adrenergic receptor binding on polymorphonuclear leukocytes in atopic dermatitis. *J. Invest. Dermatol.* 72:330, 1979.

110. Garcia-Sainz, J. A., and Najera-Alvaredo, A. Hormonal responsiveness of liver cells during the liver regeneration process induced by carbon tetrachloride administration. *Biochim. Biophys. Acta.* 885:102, 1986.

111. Giannetti, A. Beta-adrenergic Blockade in Atopic Dermatitis. Evidence for an Abnormality of T-lymphocyte Beta Receptors. In *Proceedings of the International Symposium on Atopic Dermatitis.* Oslo, Norway, 1979.

112. Gillespie, J. S., and Hamilton, D. N. H. Binding of noradrenaline to smooth muscle cells in the spleen. *Nature* 212:524, 1966.

113. Gillespie, J. S., Hamilton, D. N. H., and Horie, R. J. A. The extraneuronal uptake and localization of noradrenaline in the cat spleen and the effect on this of some drugs, of cold and denervation. *J. Physiol. (Lond.)* 206:563, 1970.

114. Ginsburg, A. M. Triiodothyronine-induced thyrotoxicosis increases mononuclear leukocyte beta-adrenergic receptor density in man. *J. Clin. Invest.* 67:1785, 1981.

115. Giustina, T. A., et al. Increased leukocyte sensitivity to PDE inhibitors in atopic dermatitis: Tachyphylaxis after theophylline therapy. *J. Allergy Clin. Immunol.* 74:252, 1984.

116. Glaubiger, G. Chronic guanethidine treatment increases cardiac beta-adrenergic receptors. *Nature* 273:240, 1978.

117. Goldberg, N. D. Cyclic nucleotides and cell function. *Hosp. Pract.* 9:127, 1974.

118. Goldman, A. L., et al. Lung cyclic nucleotides in bronchospastic and nonreversible obstructive lung disease. *Am. Rev. Respir. Dis.* 115:330, 1977.

119. Gorkin, V. Z. Monoamine oxidases. *Pharmacol. Rev.* 18:115, 1966.

120. Greenacre, J. K., Schofield, P., and Connolly, M. E. Desensitization of the beta-adrenoceptor of lymphocytes from normal subjects and asthmatic patients in vitro. *Br. J. Clin. Pharmacol.* 5:199, 1978.

121. Greengard, P., and Kebabian, J. W. Role of cyclic AMP in synaptic transmission in the mammalian peripheral nervous system. *Fed. Proc.* 33:1059, 1974.

122. Grewe, S., Chan, S. C., and Hanifin, J. M. Elevated leukocyte cyclic AMP phosphodiesterase in atopic disease: A possible mechanism for cAMP agonist hyporesponsiveness. *J. Allergy Clin. Immunol.* 70:452, 1982.

123. Guellaen, G., et al. Characterization with [^{3}H]dihydroergocryptine of the alpha-adrenergic receptor of the hepatic plasma membrane. *J. Biol. Chem.* 253:1114, 1978.

124. Hadcock, J. R., and Malbon, C. C. Down-regulation of beta-adrenergic receptors: Agonist-induced reduction in receptor mRNA levels. *Proc. Natl. Acad. Sci. USA* 85:5021, 1988.

125. Hadcock, J. R., and Malbon, C. C. Regulation of beta-adrenergic receptors by "permissive" hormones: Glucocorticoids increase steady-state levels of receptor mRNA. *Proc. Natl. Acad. Sci. USA* 85:8415, 1988.

126. Hadcock, J. R., Ros, M., and Malbon, C. C. Agonist regulation of beta-adrenergic receptor mRNA: Analysis in S49 mouse lymphoma mutants. *J. Biol. Chem.* 264:13956, 1989.

127. Hadcock, J. R., Wang, H.-Y., and Malbon, C. C. Agonist-induced destabilization of beta-adrenergic receptor mRNA: Attenuation of glucocorticoid-induced upregulation of beta-adrenergic receptors. *J. Biol. Chem.* 264:19928, 1989.

128. Haeusler, G. Pharmacology of beta-blockers: Classical aspects and recent developments. *J. Cardiovasc. Pharmacol.* 16(Suppl. 5):s1, 1990.

129. Hagen, P. The storage and release of catecholamines. *Pharmacol. Rev.* 11:361, 1959.

130. Hagen, P., and Barnett, R. J. The Storage of Amines in the Chromaffin Cell. In J. R. Vane, G. E. W. Wolstenholme, and M. O'Connor (eds.), *Ciba Foundation Symposium on Adrenergic Mechanisms.* Boston: Little, Brown, 1960.

131. Haggendahl, J. Some Further Aspects on the Release of the Adrenergic Transmitter. In H. J. Schumann and G. Kroneberg (eds.), *Bayer Symposium II: New Aspects of Storage and Release Mechanisms of Catecholamines.* Berlin: Springer, 1970.

132. Halonen, M., and Kaliner, M. Determinants of Autonomic Abnormalities in Atopy. In J. W. Kerr and M. A. Ganderton (eds.), *Proceedings of Invited Symposia XI International Congress on Allergy and Immunology.* New York: Macmillan, 1983. Pp. 193–195.

133. Harker, C. T., et al. Changes in response patterns in hibernating versus active ground squirrels. *Physiologist* 27:243, 1984.

134. Harvey, J. E., and Tattersfield, A. E. Airway response to salbutamol. Effect of regular salbutamol inhalations in normal, atopic and asthmatic subjects. *Thorax* 37:280, 1982.

135. Hasegawa, M., and Townley, R. G. Differences between lung and spleen susceptibility of beta-adrenergic receptors to desensitization by terbutaline. *J. Allergy Clin. Immunol.* 71:230, 1983.

136. Hausdorff, W. P., et al. A small region of the beta-adrenergic receptor is selectively involved in its rapid regulation. *Proc. Natl. Acad. Sci. USA* 88:2979, 1991.

137. Hausdorff, W. P., Caron, M. G., and Lefkowitz, R. J. Turning off the signal: Desensitization of beta-adrenergic receptor function. *FASEB J.* 4:2881, 1990.

138. Heinsimer, J. A., and Lefkowitz, R. J. Adrenergic receptors: Biochemistry, regulation, molecular mechanism and clinical implications. *J. Lab. Clin. Med.* 100:641, 1982.

139. Helle, K. Antibody formation against soluble protein from bovine adrenal chromaffin granules. *Biochim. Biophys. Acta* 117:107, 1966.

140. Helle, K. Some chemical and physical properties of the soluble protein of bovine adrenal chromaffin granules. *Mol. Pharmacol.* 2:298, 1966.

141. Henderson, W. R., et al. Alpha-adrenergic hyperreactivity in asthma. Analysis of vascular and pupillary responses. *N. Engl. J. Med.* 300:642, 1970.

142. Henney, C. S., and Gillis, S. Cell-mediated Cytotoxicity. In W. Paul (ed.), *Fundamental Immunology.* New York: Raven, 1984.

143. Hertting, G., et al. Lack of uptake of catecholamines after chronic denervation of sympathetic nerves. *Nature* 189:66, 1961.

144. Hildebrant, J. D., Codina, J., and Rosenthal, W. Properties of Human Erythrocyte N_s and N_i, the Regulatory Components of Adenylate Cyclase, as Purified Without Regulatory Ligands. In D. M. F. Cooper and K. B. Seamon (eds.), *Advances in Cyclic Nucleotide and Protein Phosphorylation Research*, Vol. 19. New York: Raven, 1985.

145. Hodgkin, A. L., and Huxley, A. F. Currents carried by sodium and potassium ions through the membrane of the giant axon of Loligo. *J. Physiol. (Lond.)* 116:449, 1952.

146. Hodgkin, A. L., and Huxley, A. F. A quantitative description of membrane current and its application to conduction and excitation in nerve. *J. Physiol. (Lond.)* 117:500, 1952.

147. Hoffmann, B. B., and Lefkowitz, R. J. Radioligand binding studies of adrenergic receptors: New insights into molecular and physiological regulation. *Annu. Rev. Pharmacol. Toxicol.* 20:581, 1980.

148. Hokin, L. E. Receptors and phosphoinositide-generated second messengers. *Annu. Rev. Biochem.* 54:205, 1985.

149. Holden, C. A., et al. Defective cyclic nucleotide metabolism in atopic monocytes. *Clin. Res.* 32:591A, 1984.

150. Holden, C. A., Chan, S. C., and Hanifin, J. M. Adenylate cyclase activity in mononuclear leukocytes from patients with atopic dermatitis. *Acta Derm. Venereol. Suppl. (Stockh.)* 114:149, 1985.

151. Holgate, S. T., Baldwin, C. J., and Tattersfield, A. E. Beta-adrenergic resistance in normal human airways. *Lancet* 2:375, 1977.
152. Holgate, S. T., et al. Airway and metabolic resistance to intravenous salbutamol. A study in normal man. *Clin. Sci.* 59:155, 1980.
153. Hornykiewicz, O. Dopamine (beta-hydroxytyramine) and brain function. *Pharmacol. Rev.* 18:925, 1966.
154. Ind, P. W., et al. Circulating catecholamines in acute asthma. *Br. Med. J.* 290:267, 1985.
155. Ishac, E. J. N., and Kunos, G. An arachidonate metabolite is involved in the conversion from α_1- to beta-adrenergic glycogenolysis in isolated rat liver cells. *Proc. Natl. Acad. Sci. USA* 83:53, 1986.
156. Itoh, H., Okajima, F., and Ui, M. Conversion of adrenergic mechanism from alpha- to beta-type during primary culture of rat hepatocytes. Accompanying decreases in the function of the inhibitory guanine nucleotide regulatory component of adenylate cyclase identified as the substrate of islet-activating protein. *J. Biol. Chem.* 259:15464, 1984.
157. Iversen, L. L. The uptake of noradrenaline by the isolated perfused rat heart. *Br. J. Pharmacol.* 21:523, 1963.
158. Iversen, L. L. The uptake of catecholamines at high perfusion concentrations in the rat isolated heart: A novel catecholamine uptake process. *Br. J. Pharmacol.* 25:18, 1965.
159. Iversen, L. L., Glowinski, J., and Axelrod, J. Reduced uptake of tritiated noradrenaline in tissues of immunosympathectomized animals. *Nature* 206:1222, 1965.
160. Iversen, L. L., and Kravitz, E. A. Sodium dependence of transmitter uptake at adrenergic nerve terminals. *Mol. Pharmacol.* 2:360, 1966.
161. Jenne, J. W. Whither beta-adrenergic tachyphylaxis. *J. Allergy Clin. Immunol.* 70:413, 1982.
162. Jenne, J. W., et al. A comparison of beta-adrenergic function in asthma and chronic bronchitis. *J. Allergy Clin. Immunol.* 60:356, 1978.
163. Jensen, J. R., et al. Modulation of natural killer cell activity in patients with atopic dermatitis. *J. Invest. Dermatol.* 82:30, 1984.
164. Kaliner, M., et al. Autonomic nervous system abnormalities and allergy. *Ann. Intern. Med.* 96:349, 1982.
165. Kalisker, A., Nelson, H. E., and Middleton, E., Jr. Drug-induced changes of adenylate cyclase activity in cells from asthmatic and nonasthmatic subjects. *J. Allergy Clin. Immunol.* 60:259, 1977.
166. Kamm, K. E., and Stull, J. T. Function of myosin and myosin light chain kinase in smooth muscle. *Annu. Rev. Pharmacol. Toxicol.* 25:593, 1985.
167. Kang, K., et al. Immunoregulation in atopic dermatitis: T lymphocyte subsets defined by monoclonal antibodies. *Semin. Dermatol.* 2:59, 1983.
168. Kariman, K. Beta-adrenergic receptor binding in lymphocytes from patients with asthma. *Lung* 158:41, 1980.
169. Kariman, K., and Lefkowitz, R. J. Decreased beta-adrenergic receptor binding in lymphocytes from patients with bronchial asthma. *Clin. Res.* 25:503, 1977.
170. Katz, B. *Nerve, Muscle and Synapse.* New York: McGraw-Hill, 1966.
171. Katz, B. *The Release of Neural Transmitter Substances.* Springfield, Ill.: Charles C Thomas, 1969.
172. Kauffman, R. S., et al. Cell receptors for the mammalian reovirus. II. Monoclonal anti-idiotypic antibody blocks viral binding to cells. *J. Immunol.* 131:2539, 1983.
173. Keighley, J. F. Iatrogenic asthma associated with adrenergic aerosols. *Ann. Intern. Med.* 65:985, 1966.
174. Kirkman, L., et al. Enhanced in vitro sensitivity to propranolol induced beta adrenergic blockade in COPD patients. *Am. Rev. Respir. Dis.* 123:79, 1981.
175. Kobilka, B. K., et al. Delineation of the intronless nature of the genes for the human and hamster B_2-adrenergic receptor and their putative promoter regions. *J. Biol. Chem.* 262:7321, 1987.
176. Koelle, G. B. A new general concept of the neurohumoral functions and acetylcholine and acetylcholinesterase. *J. Pharm. Pharmacol.* 14:65, 1962.
177. Koelle, G. B. Current concepts of synaptic structure and function. *Ann. NY Acad. Sci.* 183:5, 1971.
178. Koeter, G. H., et al. Changes in the beta-adrenergic system in bronchial asthma induced by terbutaline. *Agents Actions* 13:259, 1983.
179. Koeter, G. H., et al. The role of the adrenergic system in allergy and bronchial hyperreactivity. *Eur. J. Respir. Dis.* 63:72, 1982.
180. Kopin, I. J. Storage and metabolism of catecholamines: The role of monoamine oxidase. *Pharmacol. Rev.* 16:179, 1964.
181. Krall, J. F., Connelly, M., and Tuck, M. L. Acute regulation of beta-adrenergic catecholamine sensitivity in human lymphocytes. *J. Pharmacol. Exp. Ther.* 214:554, 1980.
182. Krnjevic, K. Chemical nature of synaptic transmission in vertebrates. *Physiol. Rev.* 54:418, 1974.
183. Krupinski, J., et al. Adenylyl cyclase amino acid sequence: Possible channel- or transporter-like structure. *Science* 244:1558, 1989.
184. Krzanowski, J. J., et al. Reduced adenosine 3',5'-cyclic monophosphate levels in patients with reversible obstructive airways disease. *Clin. Exp. Pharmacol. Physiol.* 6:111, 1979.
185. Krzanowski, J. J., and Szentivanyi, A. Invited editorial: Reflections on some aspects of current research in asthma. *J. Allergy Clin. Immunol.* 72:433, 1983.
186. Kunos, G. Adrenoceptors. *Annu. Rev. Pharmacol.* 18:291, 1978.
187. Kunos, G. Reciprocal changes in alpha and beta adrenoceptor reactivity—Myth or reality. *Trends Pharmacol. Sci.* 1:282, 1980.
188. Kunos, G. The hepatic α_1-adrenoceptor. *Trends Pharmacol. Sci.* 5:380, 1984.
189. Kunos, G., et al. Time-dependent conversion of α_1- to beta-adrenoceptor mediated glycogenolysis in isolated rat liver cells: Role of membrane phospholipase A_2. *Proc. Natl. Acad. Sci. USA* 81:6178, 1984.
190. Kunos, G., and Ishac, E. J. N. Inverse reciprocal regulation of alpha- and beta-adrenoceptors in the rat liver: Possible mechanism. *J. Cardiovasc. Pharmacol.* 7(Suppl. 6):87, 1984.
191. Kunos, G., and Ishac, E. J. N. Mechanism of inverse regulation of α_1- and beta-adrenergic receptors. *Biochem. Pharmacol.* 36:1185, 1987.
192. Kunos, G., et al. Selective affinity labeling and molecular weight determination of hepatic α_1-adrenergic receptors with [³H] phenoxybenzamine. *J. Biol. Chem.* 258:326, 1983.
193. Kunos, G., et al. Adrenergic receptors—Possible mechanisms of inverse regulation of alpha receptors and beta reeptors. *J. Allergy Clin. Immunol.* 76:346, 1985.
194. Kunos, G., Mucci, L., and O'Regan, S. The influence of hormonal and neuronal factors on rat heart adrenoceptors. *Br. J. Pharmacol.* 71:371, 1980.
195. Kunos, G., and Szentivanyi, M. Evidence favoring the existence of a single adrenergic receptor. *Nature* 217:1077, 1968.
196. Kuscimi, N. T., and Trentin, J. J. Natural cell-mediated cytotoxic activity in the peripheral blood of patients with atopic dermatitis. *Arch. Dermatol.* 118:568, 1982.
197. Lacal, J. C., et al. Rapid stimulation of diacylglycerol production in Xenopus oocytes by microinjection of *H-ras* p21. *Science* 238:533, 1987.
198. Lands, A. M. Differentiation of receptor systems activated by sympathomimetic amines. *Nature* 214:597, 1967.
199. Lang, P., Goel, Z., and Cricco, M. H. Subsensitivity of T lymphocytes to sympathomimetic and cholinergic stimulation in bronchial asthma. *J. Allergy Clin. Immunol.* 61:248, 1978.
200. Lanier, S. M., et al. Isolation of rat genomic clones encoding subtypes of the α_2-adrenergic receptor. *J. Biol. Chem.* 266:10470, 1991.
201. Larsson, S. A., Svedmyer, N. L. V., and Thiringer, G. K. Lack of bronchial beta-adrenoceptor resistance in asthmatics during long-term treatment with terbutaline. *J. Allergy Clin. Immunol.* 59:93, 1977.
202. Leclerc, B., et al. Beta-adrenergic Receptor Subtypes. In J. W. Lamble (ed.), *Current Reviews in Biomedicine*, Vol. 1. *Towards Understanding Receptors.* Amsterdam: Elsevier, 1981. Pp. 78–83.
203. Leeb-Lundberg, L. M. F., et al. Phorbol esters promote alpha-adrenergic receptor phosphorylation and receptor uncoupling from inositol phospholipid metabolism. *Proc. Natl. Acad. Sci. USA* 82:5651, 1985.
204. Lefkowitz, R. J. Clinical physiology of adrenergic receptor regulation. *Am. J. Physiol.* 243:E43, 1981.
205. Lefkowitz, R. J., et al. Stereospecific [³H](-)alprenolol binding sites, beta-adrenergic receptors and adenyl cyclase. *Biochem. Biophys. Res. Commun.* 60:703, 1974.
206. Lemanske, R. F., and Kaliner, M. A. The Assessment of Autonomic Nervous System Function. In S. L. Spector (ed.), *Provocative Challenge Procedures: Bronchial, Oral, Nasal, and Exercise*, Vol. 2. Boca Raton, Fla.: CRC Press, 1983. Pp. 119–135.
207. Leung, D. Y. M., Rhodes, A. R., and Geha, R. S. Enumeration of T cell subsets in atopic dermatitis using monoclonal antibodies. *J. Allergy Clin. Immunol.* 67:450, 1981.
208. Levin, E. Y., Levenberg, B., and Kaufman, S. The enzymatic conversion of 3,4-dihydroxyphenylethylamine to epinephrine. *J. Biol. Chem.* 235:2080, 1960.
209. Levin, J. A., and Furchgott, R. F. Interactions between potentiating agents of adrenergic amines in rabbit aortic strips. *J. Pharmacol. Exp. Ther.* 172:320, 1970.
210. Levitsky, A., Atlas, D., and Steer, M. L. The binding characteristics and

number of beta-adrenergic receptors on the turkey erythrocyte. *Proc. Natl. Acad. Sci. USA* 71:2772, 1974.

211. Licinio, J., Wong, M.-L., and Gold, P. W. Localization of interleukin-1 receptor antagonist mRNA in rat brain. *Endocrinology* 129:562, 1991.

212. Lightman, S. L., and Iversen, L. L. The role of uptake$_2$ in the extraneuronal metabolism of catecholamines in the isolated rat heart. *Br. J. Pharmacol.* 37:638, 1969.

213. Lindstrom, J. A. Antibody to acetylcholine receptor in myasthenia gravis: Prevalence, clinical correlates and diagnostic value. *Neurology* 26:317, 1976.

214. Lloyd, D. P. C. Cholinergy and Adrenergy in the Neural Control of Sweat Glands. In D. R. Curtis and A. K. McIntyre (eds.), *Studies in Physiology.* New York: Springer, 1965.

215. Lobitz, W. C., Honeyman, J. F., and Winkler, M. W. Suppressed cell mediated immunity in two adults with atopic dermatitis. *Br. J. Dermatol.* 86:317, 1972.

216. Lohmann, S. M., and Walter, U. Regulation of the Cellular and Subcellular Concentrations and Distribution of Cyclic Nucleotide-dependent Protein Kinases. In P. Greengard and G. A. Robison (eds.), *Advances in Cyclic Nucleotide and Protein Phosphorylation Research*, Vol. 18. New York: Raven, 1984.

217. Lohse, M. J., et al. Beta-arrestin: A protein that regulates beta-adrenergic receptor function. *Science* 248:1547, 1990.

218. Lovenberg, W., Weissbach, H., and Udenfriend, S. Aromatic L-amino acid decarboxylase. *J. Biol. Chem.* 237:89, 1962.

219. Lynch, C. J., et al. Effect of islet-activating pertussis toxin on the binding characteristics of Ca^{2+}-mobilizing hormones and on agonist activity of phosphorylase in hepatocytes. *J. Biol. Chem.* 260:2844, 1985.

220. Lynch, C. J., et al. Inhibition of hepatic α_1-adrenergic effects and binding by phorbol myristate acetate. *Mol. Pharmacol.* 29:196, 1986.

221. Makino, S., et al. Comparison of cyclic adenosine monophosphate response of lymphocytes in normal and asthmatic subjects to norepinephrine and salbutamol. *J. Allergy Clin. Immunol.* 59:348, 1977.

222. Manley, S. W., Bourke, G. R., and Hawker, R. W. The thyrotropin receptor in guinea pig thyroid homogenate: Interactions with the long-acting thyroid stimulator. *J. Endocrinol.* 61:437, 1974.

223. Marley, E., and Paton, W. D. M. The output of sympathetic amines from the cat's adrenal gland in response to splanchnic nerve activity. *J. Physiol. (Lond.)* 155:1, 1961.

224. McLaughlin, D. P., and MacDonald, A. Characterization of catecholamine-mediated relaxations in rat isolated gastric fundus: Evidence for an atypical beta-adrenoceptor. *Br. J. Pharmacol.* 103:1351, 1991.

225. McLennan, H. *Synaptic Transmission* (2nd ed.). Philadelphia: Saunders, 1970.

226. McMillan, J. C., Heskel, N. S., and Hanifin, J. M. Cyclic AMP-phosphodiesterase activity and histamine release in cord blood leukocyte preparations. *Acta Derm. Venereol. Suppl. (Stockh.)* 114:24, 1985.

227. Mendelsohn, J., and Nordberg, J. Adenylate cyclase in thymus-derived and bone marrow-derived lymphocytes from normal donors and patients with chronic lymphocytic leukemia. *J. Clin. Invest.* 63:1124, 1979.

228. Meurs, H., et al. Regulation of the beta receptor adenylate cyclase system in lymphocytes of allergic patients with asthma: Possible role for protein kinase C in allergen-induced nonspecific refractoriness of adenylate cyclase. *J. Allergy Clin. Immunol.* 80:326, 1987.

229. Meurs, H., et al. The beta-adrenergic system and allergic bronchial asthma: Changes in lymphocyte beta-adrenergic receptor number and adenylate cyclase activity after an allergen-induced asthmatic attack. *J. Allergy Clin. Immunol.* 70:272, 1982.

230. Meurs, H., et al. Reduced adenylate cyclase responsiveness to histamine in lymphocyte membranes of allergic asthmatic patients after allergen challenge. *Int. Arch. Allergy Appl. Immunol.* 76:256, 1985.

231. Minneman, K. P., Pittman, R. M., and Molinoff, P. B. Beta-adrenergic receptor subtypes: Properties, distribution and regulation. *Annu. Rev. Neurosci.* 4:419, 1981.

232. Mitrius, J. C., and U'Pritchard, D. C. Regulation of α_2-Adrenoceptors by Nucleotides, Ions, and Agonists: Comparison in Cells of Neural and Nonneural Origin. In D. M. F. Cooper and K. B. Seamon (eds.), *Advances in Cyclic Nucleotide and Protein Phosphorylation*, Vol. 19. New York: Raven, 1985.

233. Molinoff, P. B., and Axelrod, J. Biochemistry of catecholamines. *Annu. Rev. Biochem.* 40:465, 1971.

234. Moran, N. C. Adrenergic Receptors. In H. Blaschko, G. Sayers, and A. D. Smith (eds.), *Adrenal Gland, Endocrinology, Handbook of Physiology*, Vol. 6, Sect. 7. Washington, D.C.: American Physiological Society, 1975. Pp. 447–472.

235. Morris, H. G., Rusnak, S. A., and Barzens, K. Leukocyte cyclic adenosine monophosphate in asthmatic children: Effects of adrenergic therapy. *Clin. Pharmacol. Ther.* 22:352, 1977.

236. Morton, I. K. M., and Halliday, J. Adrenoceptors in Smooth Muscle. In G. Kunos (ed.), *Adrenoceptors and Catecholamine Action.* New York: John Wiley, 1981.

237. Motojima, S., Fukada, T., and Makino, S. Measurement of beta-adrenergic receptors on lymphocytes in normal subjects and asthmatics in relation to beta-adrenergic hyperglycemic response and bronchial responsiveness. *Allergy* 38:331, 1983.

238. Motulsky, H. J., and Insel, P. A. Adrenergic receptors in man. *N. Engl. J. Med.* 307:18, 1982.

239. Mufson, R. A., et al. Melittin shares certain cellular effects with phorbol ester tumor promoters. *Nature* 280:72, 1979.

240. Mukhopadyay, A. K., and Schuhmacher, M. Inhibition of hCG-stimulated adenylate cyclase in purified mouse Leydig cells by the phorbol ester PMA. *FEBS Lett.* 187:56, 1985.

241. Murakami, K., and Routenberg, A. Direct activation of purified protein kinase C by unsaturated fatty acids (oleate and arachidonate) in the absence of phospholipids and Ca^{2+}. *Fed. Eur. Biochem. Soc.* 192:189, 1985.

242. Nagatsu, T., Levitt, M., and Udenfriend, S. Tyrosine hydroxylase: The initial step in norepinephrine biosynthesis. *J. Biol. Chem.* 239:2910, 1964.

243. Nahorski, S. R. Identification and Significance of Beta-adrenoceptor Subtypes. In J. W. Lamble (ed.), *Current Reviews in Biomedicine*, Vol. 1. *Towards Understanding Receptors.* Amsterdam: Elsevier, 1981. Pp. 71–77.

244. Nakamura, T., et al. Reciprocal expressions of α_1-adrenergic and beta-adrenergic receptors but constant expression of glucagon receptor by rat hepatocytes during development and primary culture. *J. Biol. Chem.* 258:9283, 1983.

245. Nara, S., Gomes, B., and Yasunobu, K. T. Amine oxidase. VII. Beef liver mitochondrial monoamine oxidase, a copper-containing protein. *J. Biol. Chem.* 241:2774, 1966.

246. Nelson, H. S., Black, J. W., and Branch, L. R. Subsensitivity to epinephrine following the administration of epinephrine and ephedrine to normal individuals. *J. Allergy Clin. Immunol.* 55:299, 1975.

247. Nepom, J. T., et al. Virus-binding receptor similarities to immune receptors as determined by anti-idiotypic antibodies. *Surv. Immunol. Res.* 1: 255, 1982.

248. Nepom, J. T., et al. Identification of a hemagglutinin specific idiotype associated with reovirus recognition shared by lymphoid and neural cells. *J. Exp. Med.* 155:155, 1982.

249. Newman, K. D., et al. Identification of alpha-adrenergic receptors in human platelets by [³H]dihydroergocryptine binding. *J. Clin. Invest.* 61: 395, 1978.

250. Niaudet, P., Beaurain, G., and Bach, M.-A. Differences in effect of isoproterenol stimulation on levels of cyclic AMP in human B and T lymphocytes. *Eur. J. Immunol.* 6:834, 1976.

251. Noseworthy, J. H., et al. Cell receptors for the mammalian reovirus. I. Syngeneic monoclonal anti-idiotypic antibody identifies a cell-surface receptor for reovirus. *J. Immunol.* 131:2533, 1983.

252. Novogrodsky, A., et al. Inhibition of beta-adrenergic stimulation of lymphocyte adenylate cyclase by phorbol myristate acetate is mediated by activated macrophages. *Biochem. Biophys. Res. Commun.* 104:389, 1982.

253. Oka, M., et al. Distribution of dopamine-beta-hydroxylase in subcellular fractions of adrenal medulla. *Life Sci.* 6:461, 1967.

254. Okajima, F., and Ui, M. Conversion of adrenergic regulation of glycogen phosphorylase and synthase from alpha to beta type during primary culture of rat hepatocytes. *Arch. Biochem. Biophys.* 213:658, 1982.

255. Page, E. D., and Neufeld, A. H. Characterization of alpha- and beta-adrenergic receptors in membranes prepared from the rabbit iris before and after development of supersensitivity. *Biochem. Pharmacol.* 27:953, 1978.

256. Papeschi, R. Dopamine extrapyramidal system, and psychomotor function. *Psychiatr. Neurol. Neurochir.* 75:13, 1972.

257. Park, S., and Rasmussen, H. Activation of tracheal smooth muscle contraction: Synergism between Ca^{2+} and activators of protein kinase C. *Proc. Natl. Acad. Sci. USA* 82:8835, 1985.

258. Park, S., and Rasmussen, H. Carbachol-induced protein phosphorylation changes in bovine tracheal smooth muscle. *J. Biol. Chem.* 261:15734, 1986.

259. Parker, C. W. Autoantibodies and beta-adrenergic receptors. *N. Engl. J. Med.* 305:1212, 1981.

260. Parker, C. W., and Eisen, A. Z. Altered cyclic AMP metabolism in atopic eczema. *Clin. Res.* 20:418, 1972.

261. Parker, C. W., Kennedy, S., and Eisen, A. Z. Leukocyte and lymphocyte cyclic AMP response in atopic eczema. *J. Invest. Dermatol.* 68:302, 1977.

262. Pik, K., and Wollemann, M. Catecholamine hypersensitivity of adenylate cyclase after chemical denervation in rat hearts. *Biochem. Pharmacol.* 26:1448, 1977.

263. Plummer, A. L. The development of drug tolerance to β_2-adrenergic agents. *Chest* 73(Suppl.):949, 1978.

264. Pochet, R., Delepesse, G., and DeMaubeuge, J. Characterization of beta-adrenoceptors on intact circulating lymphocytes from patients with atopic dermatitis. *Acta Derm. Venereol. (Stockh.)* 92:26, 1980.

265. Poisner, A. M., Trifaro, J. M., and Douglas, W. W. The fate of the chromaffin granule during catecholamine release from the adrenal medulla. II. Loss of protein and retention of lipid in subcellular fractions. *Biochem. Pharmacol.* 16:2101, 1967.

266. Polson, J. B., et al. Cyclic nucleotide phosphodiesterase activity in patients with obstructive airways disease. *Allergol. Immunopathol.* 10:101, 1982.

267. Polson, J. B., et al. Responsiveness of lymphocyte beta adrenergic receptors in patients treated with ketotifen. *Clin. Pharmacol. Ther.* 43:137, 1988.

268. Popovic, W. J., Brown, J. E., and Adamson, J. W. Modulation of in vitro erythropoiesis. Studies with euthyroid and hypothyroid dogs. *J. Clin. Invest.* 64:56, 1979.

269. Potter, L. T., and Axelrod, J. Properties of norepinephrine storage particles of the rat heart. *J. Pharmacol. Exp. Ther.* 142:299, 1963.

270. Preiksaitis, H. K., Kan, W. H., and Kunos, G. Decreased α_1-adrenoceptor responsiveness and density in liver cells of thyroidectomized rats. *J. Biol. Chem.* 257:4321, 1982.

271. Preiksaitis, H. K., and Kunos, G. Adrenoceptor-mediated activation of liver glycogen phosphorylase: Effects of thyroid state. *Life Sci.* 24:35, 1979.

272. Rasmussen, H., Takuwa, Y., and Park, S. Protein kinase C in the regulation of smooth muscle contraction. *FASEB J.* 1:177, 1987.

273. Rath, R. H., and Stjarne, L. Monoamine oxidase activity in the bovine splenic nerve granule preparation. *Acta Physiol. Scand.* 68:342, 1966.

274. Reed, C. E., Busse, W. W., and Lee, T.-P. Adrenergic mechanisms and the adenyl cyclase system in atopic dermatitis. *J. Invest. Dermatol.* 67:333, 1976.

275. Refsnes, M., et al. Mechanisms for the emergence of catecholamine-sensitive adenylate cyclase and beta-adrenergic receptors cultured hepatocytes—Dependence on protein and RNA synthesis and suppression by isoproterenol. *Fed. Eur. Biochem. Soc. Lett.* 164:291, 1983.

276. Rhee, S. G., et al. Studies of inositol phospholipid-specific phospholipase C. *Science* 244:546, 1989.

277. Rheinherz, E. L., et al. Further characterization of helper/inducer T cell subsets defined by monoclonal antibody. *J. Immunol.* 123:2984, 1979.

278. Rheinherz, E. L., et al. Subpopulations of the T4 positive inducer cell subset in man. *J. Immunol.* 126:67, 1981.

279. Rheinherz, E. L., and Schlossman, S. Regulation of the immune response-inducer and suppressor T lymphocyte subsets in humans. *N. Engl. J. Med.* 303:370, 1980.

280. Roberts, J. M., et al. Alpha-adrenoceptors but not beta-adrenoceptors increase in rabbit uterus with oestrogen. *Nature* 270:624, 1977.

281. Robicsek, S., et al. Multiple cyclic nucleotide phosphodieterase activities and the selective modulation of function in human T lymphocytes. *J. Leukoc. Biol.* Suppl. 1:232, 1990.

282. Robicsek, S. A., et al. Multiple high affinity cAMP phosphodiesterases regulate proliferation in human thymic lymphocytes. *Biochem. Pharmacol.* 42:869, 1991.

283. Robson, J. M., and Stacey, R. S. *Recent Advances in Pharmacology (3rd ed.).* Boston: Little, Brown, 1962.

284. Ruoho, A. E., DeClerque, J. L., and Busse, W. W. Characterization of granulocyte beta-adrenergic receptors in atopic eczema. *J. Allergy Clin. Immunol.* 66:218, 1981.

285. Safko, M. J., et al. Heterologous desensitization of leukocytes: A possible mechanism of beta-adrenergic blockade in atopic dermatitis. *J. Allergy Clin. Immunol.* 68:218, 1981.

286. Sage, H. J., Smith, W. J., and Kirshner, N. Mechanism of secretion from the adrenal medulla. I. A microquantitative immunologic assay for bovine adrenal storage vesicle protein and its application to studies of the secretory process. *Mol. Pharmacol.* 3:81, 1967.

287. Sano, Y., et al. Comparison of alpha and beta-adrenergic receptors in asthmatics and controls: Identification and characterization of alpha-adrenergic receptors in human lymphocytes. *Clin. Res.* 29:172, 1981.

288. Sano, Y., et al. Leukocyte beta-adrenergic receptor assay in normals and asthmatics. *Clin. Res.* 27:403, 1979.

289. Sano, Y., Watt, G., and Townley, R. G. Decreased mononuclear cell beta-adrenergic receptors in bronchial asthma: Parallel studies of lymphocytes and granulocyte desensitization. *J. Allergy Clin. Immunol.* 72:495, 1983.

290. Scarpace, P. J., and Abrass, I. B. Thyroid hormone regulation of rat heart, lymphocyte, and lung beta-adrenergic receptors. *Endocrinology* 108:1007, 1981.

291. Schnaitman, C., Erwin, V. G., and Greenawalt, J. W. The submitochondrial localization of monoamine oxidase. *J. Cell Biol.* 32:719, 1967.

292. Schneider, F. H., Smith, A. D., and Winkler, H. Secretion from the adrenal medulla: Biochemical evidence for exocytosis. *Br. J. Pharmacol. Chemother.* 31:94, 1967.

293. Schulz, V., Schnabel, K. H., and Lollgen, H. Airways resistance and haemodynamic parameters in long term therapy with the orciprenaline derivative TR 1165a (fenoterol). *Int. J. Clin. Pharmacol. Biopharm.* 4(Suppl.):167, 1972.

294. Schuster, D. L., et al. Selective deficiency of a T cell subpopulation in active atopic dermatitis. *J. Immunol.* 124:1662, 1980.

295. Schwartz, K. R., et al. Rapid reciprocal changes in adrenergic receptors in intact isolated hepatocytes during primary cell culture. *Mol. Pharmacol.* 27:200, 1985.

296. Shanes, A. M. Electrochemical aspects of physiological and pharmacological action in excitable cells. I. The resting cell and its alteration by extrinsic factors. *Pharmacol. Rev.* 10:59, 1958.

297. Shanes, A. M. Electrochemical aspects of physiological and pharmacological action in excitable cells. II. The action potential and excitation. *Pharmacol. Rev.* 10:165, 1958.

298. Sharma, V. K., and Banerjee, S. P. Alpha-adrenergic receptors in rat heart. Effects of thyroidectomy. *J. Biol. Chem.* 253:5277, 1978.

299. Sheppard, J. R., Gormus, R., and Moldow, C. F. Catecholamine hormone receptors are reduced on chronic lymphocytic leukemic lymphocytes. *Nature* 269:693, 1977.

300. Sibley, D. R., et al. Phorbol diesters promote beta-adrenergic receptor phosphorylation and adenylate cyclase desensitization in duck erythrocytes. *Biochem. Biophys. Res. Commun.* 121:973, 1984.

301. Simi, W. W., and Miller, W. C. Clinical investigation of fenoterol, a new bronchodilator, in asthma. *J. Allergy Clin. Immunol.* 59:178, 1977.

302. Simpson, W. W., Rodgers, R. L., and McNeill, J. H. Cardiac responsiveness to alpha and beta-adrenergic amines—Effects of carbachol and hypothyroidism. *J. Pharmacol. Exp. Ther.* 219:231, 1981.

303. Smigel, M. D., Ferguson, K. M., and Gilman, A. G. Control of Adenylate Cyclase Activity by G Proteins. In D. M. F. Cooper and K. D. Seamon (eds.), *Advances in Cyclic Nucleotide and Protein Phosphorylation Research*, Vol. 19. New York: Raven, 1985.

304. Smith, A. D. Biochemistry of Adrenal Chromaffin Granules. In *Biological Council Symposium on Drug Action, The Interaction of Drugs and Subcellular Components in Animal Cells.* London: Churchill, 1968.

305. Smith, A. D., and Winkler, H. Purification and properties of an acidic protein from chromaffin granules of bovine adrenal medulla. *Biochem. J.* 103:483, 1967.

306. Smith, B. R., and Hall, R. Thyroid-stimulating immunoglobulins in Grave's disease. *Lancet* 2:427, 1974.

307. Smith, W. J., and Kirshner, N. A specific soluble protein from the catecholamine storage vesicles of bovine adrenal medulla. I. Purification and chemical characterization. *Mol. Pharmacol.* 3:52, 1967.

308. Snashall, P. D., Boother, F. A., and Sterling, G. M. The effect of alpha-adrenergic stimulation on the airways of normal and asthmatic man. *Clin. Sci. Mol. Med.* 54:283, 1978.

309. Snavely, M. D., et al. Adrenergic receptors in human and experimental pheochromocytoma. *Clin. Exp. Hypertens. [A]* A4:829, 1982.

310. Sokol, W. N., and Beall, G. N. Leukocytic epinephrine receptors of normal and asthmatic individuals. *J. Allergy Clin. Immunol.* 55:310, 1975.

311. Sourkes, T. L. Central actions of dopa and dopamine. *Rev. Can. Biol.* 31:153, 1972.

312. Squires, R. F. Additional evidence for the existence of several forms of mitochondrial monoamine oxidase in the mouse. *Biochem. Pharmacol.* 17:1401, 1968.

313. Stadel, J. M. Desensitization of the beta-adrenergic receptor of frog erythrocytes: Recovery and characterization of the down-regulated receptors in sequestered vesicles. *J. Biol. Chem.* 258:3032, 1983.

314. Starke, K. Influence of alpha receptor stimulants on noradrenaline release. *Naturwissenschaften* 58:420, 1971.

315. Stern, L., and Kunos, G. Synergistic regulation of pulmonary beta-adren-

ergic receptors by glucocorticoids and interleukin-1. *J. Biol. Chem.* 263: 15876, 1988.

316. Sternberg, T. H., and Zimmerman, M. C. Stress studies in the eczema-asthma-hay fever diathesis. *Arch. Dermatol.* 65:392, 1952.

317. Stevens, R., et al. Characterization of a circulating subpopulation of spontaneous antitetanus toxoid antibody production. *J. Immunol.* 122:2498, 1980.

318. Stjarne, L. The Synthesis, Uptake and Storage of Catecholamines in the Adrenal Medulla: The Effects of Drugs. In H. Blaschko and E. Muscholl (eds.), *Catecholamines.* Berlin: Springer, 1972.

319. Stolls, A., and Hofman, A. Ergot alkaloids. IX. Dihydroderivative of naturally occurring 1-rotatory ergot alkaloids. *Helv. Chir. Acta* 26:2070, 1943.

320. Strada, S. J., Martin, M. W., and Thompson, W. J. General Properties of Multiple Molecular Forms of Cyclic Nucleotide Phosphodiesterase in the Nervous System. In S. J. Strada and W. J. Thompson (eds.), *Advances in Cyclic Nucleotide and Protein Phosphorylation Research,* Vol. 16. New York: Raven, 1984.

321. Strader, C. D., Sigal, I. S., and Dixon, R. A. F. Structural basis of beta-adrenergic receptor function. *FASEB J.* 3:1825, 1989.

322. Svedmyr, N. L. V., Larsson, S. A., and Thiringer, G. K. Development of resistance in beta-adrenergic receptors of asthmatic patients. *Chest* 69: 479, 1976.

323. Szentendrei, T., et al. Regulation of beta-adrenergic receptor gene expression by interleukin-1. *Pharmacologist* 33:225, 1991.

324. Szentivanyi, A. The beta adrenergic theory of the atopic abnormality in bronchial asthma. *J. Allergy* 42:203, 1968.

325. Szentivanyi, A. Effect of Bacterial Products and Adrenergic Blocking Agents on Allergic Reactions. In M. Samter, et al. (eds.), *Textbook of Immunological Diseases.* Boston: Little, Brown, 1971. Pp. 356–374.

326. Szentivanyi, A. The conformational flexibility of adrenoceptors and the constitutional basis of atopy. *Triangle* 18:108, 1979.

327. Szentivanyi, A. La flexibilité de conformation des adrénorécepteurs et la base constitutionelle du terrain allergique. *Rev. Fr. Allergol.* 19:205, 1979.

328. Szentivanyi, A. The radioligand binding approach in the study of lymphocytic adrenoceptors and the constitutional basis of atopy. *J. Allergy Clin. Immunol.* 65:5, 1980.

329. Szentivanyi, A. *Adrenergic and Cholinergic Receptor Studies in Human Lung and Lymphocytic Membranes and Their Relation to Bronchial Hyperreactivity in Asthma.* Darien, Conn.: Patient Care Publications, 1982.

330. Szentivanyi, A. Catecholamines, Adrenoceptors, and Anti-Receptor Antibodies. In *Proceedings of Smith, Kline and French International Symposium on the Biochemical Pharmacology of Inflammation.* Lima, Peru, 1985. Pp. 126–142.

331. Szentivanyi, A., and Fishel, C. W. Die Amin-Mediatorstoffe der allergischen Reaktion und die Reaktionsfahiegkeit ihrer Erfolgszellen. In G. Filipp (ed.), *Pathogenese und Therapie allergischer Reaktionen.* Stuttgart: Ferdinand Enke Verlag, 1966. Pp. 588–683.

332. Szentivanyi, A., and Fishel, C. W. Neurohumoral concepts of bronchial asthma. *Acta Allergol.* 29(Suppl. 11):26, 1974.

333. Szentivanyi, A., and Fishel, C. W. The Beta Adrenergic Theory and Cyclic AMP Mediated Control Mechanisms in Human Asthma. In E. B. Weiss and M. S. Segal (eds.), *Bronchial Asthma: Mechanisms and Therapeutics.* Boston: Little, Brown, 1976. Pp. 137–153.

334. Szentivanyi, A., and Fitzpatrick, D. F. The Altered Reactivity of the Effector Cells to Antigenic and Pharmacological Influences and Its Relation to Cyclic Nucleotides. II. Effector Reactivities in the Efferent Loop of the Immune Response. In G. Filipp (ed.), *Pathomechanismus und pathogenese allergischer Reaktionen.* Munich: Werk-Verlag Dr. Edmund Banachewski, 1980. Pp. 511–580.

335. Szentivanyi, A., and Friedman, H. The Biology and Physiopharmacology of Bacterial Lipopolysaccharide Endotoxins and Their Role in Immunoregulation—An Introductory Preview. In A. Szentivanyi, H. Friedman, and A. Nowotny (eds.), *The Immunobiology and Immunopharmacology of Bacterial Endotoxins. Basic and Clinical Aspects.* New York: Plenum, 1986. Pp. 3–12.

336. Szentivanyi, A., Friedman, H., and Nowotny, A. (eds.), *The Immunopharmacology of Bacterial Endotoxins. Basic and Clinical Aspects.* New York: Plenum, 1986.

337. Szentivanyi, A., et al. Hypothalamic and Other Central Influences on Antibiosis and Host Immunity. In *Proceedings of the Fourth International Conference on Immunopharmacology.* Oxford: Pergamon, 1988. P. S101.

338. Szentivanyi, A., Heim, O., and Schultze, P. Changes in adrenoceptor densities in membranes of lung tissue and lymphocytes from patients with atopic disease. *Ann. NY Acad. Sci.* 332:295, 1979.

339. Szentivanyi, A., et al. Adrenoceptor binding studies with [^{3}H] dihydroalprenolol and [^{3}H] dihydroergocryptine on membranes of lymphocytes from patients with atopic disease. *Acta. Derm. Venereol. (Stockh.)* 92:19, 1980.

340. Szentivanyi, A., Krzanowski, J. J., and Polson, J. B. The Autonomic Nervous System and Altered Effector Responses. In E. Middleton, C. E. Reed, and E. F. Ellis (eds.), *Allergy—Principles and Practice* (3rd ed.). St. Louis: Mosby, 1988. Pp. 461–483.

341. Szentivanyi, A., et al. Evolution of Research Strategy in the Experimental Analysis of the Beta Adrenergic Approach to the Constitutional Basis of Atopy. In A. Oehling, et al. (eds.), *Advances in Allergology and Clinical Immunology.* Oxford: Pergamon, 1980. Pp. 301–308.

342. Szentivanyi, A., et al. The pharmacology of microbial modulation in the induction and expression of immune reactivities. I. The pharmacologically active effector molecules of immunologic inflammation, immunity, and hypersensitivity. *Immunopharmacol. Rev.* 1:159, 1990.

343. Szentivanyi, A., Maurer, P., and Janicki, B. W. (eds.), *Antibodies: Structure, Synthesis, Function, and Immunologic Intervention in Disease.* New York: Plenum, 1987.

344. Szentivanyi, A., and Middleton, E. Asthma pharmacotherapy and why. *J. Respir. Ther.* 1:10, 1980.

345. Szentivanyi, A., et al. Effect of Microbial Agents on the Immune Network and Associated Pharmacologic Reactivities. In E. Middleton, C. E. Reed, and E. F. Ellis (eds.), *Allergy—Principles and Practice.* St. Louis: Mosby, 1983. Pp. 211–236.

346. Szentivanyi, A., Polson, J. B., and Krzanowski, J. J. Altered Reactivity of the Effector Cells to Antigenic and Pharmacological Influences and Its Relation to Cyclic Nucleotides. I. Effector Reactivities in the Afferent Loop of the Immune Response. In G. Filipp (ed.), *Pathomechanismus und pathogenese allergischer Reaktionen.* Munich: Werk-Verlag, 1980. Pp. 460–510.

347. Szentivanyi, A., Polson, J. B., and Szentivanyi, J. Issues of adrenoceptor behavior in respiratory and cutaneous disorders of atopic allergy. *Trends Pharmacol. Sci* 5:280, 1984.

348. Szentivanyi, A., Polson, J. B., and Szentivanyi, J. Adrenergic Regulation. In E. B. Weiss, M. S. Segal, and M. Stein (eds.), *Bronchial Asthma: Mechanisms and Therapeutics* (2nd ed.). Boston: Little, Brown, 1985. Pp. 126–150.

349. Szentivanyi, A., et al. Some Biochemical and Cellular Features of Adrenergic Mechanisms Induced by Bacterial Lipopolysaccharide Endotoxin in Rats with or without Chemical Sympathetic Ablation (Axotomy) Achieved by 6-Hydroxydopamine Hydrobromide (6-OHDA). In *Proceedings of International Symposium on Endotoxin.* Tochigi, Japan: Jichi Medical School Publisher, 1988. P. SV-8.

350. Szentivanyi, A., et al. The Effect of 6-Hydroxydopamine Hydrobromide (6-OHDA) on Endotoxin Induced Adrenergic Mechanisms. In *Proceedings of Second International Meeting on Respiratory Allergy.* Naples, Italy: Ospedale Regionale A. Cardarelli, 1988. P. 34.

351. Szentivanyi, A., et al. Restoration of normal beta-adrenoceptor concentrations in A549 lung adenocarcinoma cells by leukocyte protein factors and recombinant interleukin-1α. *Cytokine* 1:118, 1989.

352. Szentivanyi, J., et al. Impaired capacity of lymphocyte proteins to upregulate beta-adrenoceptors in A549 human lung adenocarcinoma cells in respiratory and cutaneous atopic disease. *Int. J. Immunopharmacol.* 13: 743, 1991.

353. Szentivanyi, A., et al. Resolution of the beta-adrenoceptor regulating activity in A549 lung cells of lymphocyte conditioned medium derived from cultured IM9 cells with DEAE ion exchange HPLC. *J. Allergy Clin. Immunol.* 87:158, 1991.

354. Szentivanyi, A., and Szentivanyi, J. Role of the sympathetic nervous system in asthma. *Respiration* 42:3, 1981.

355. Szentivanyi, A., and Szentivanyi, J. New Aspects of Receptor Behavior in Atopy. In *Proceedings of the Kongress der arztlichen Arbeitsgemeinschaft fur angewandte Allergologie.* West Berlin: Acron Verlag Manfred Bolschakoff, 1982. Pp. 4–7.

356. Szentivanyi, A., and Szentivanyi, J. Biochemical Mechanisms of Beta Adrenergic Subsensitivity in Asthma and Atopic Dermatitis. In M. Velasco (ed.), *Clinical Pharmacology and Therapeutics.* New York: Elsevier, 1983. Pp. 291–296.

357. Szentivanyi, A., and Szentivanyi, J. Neuester Stand der rezeptoren-theorie bei Atopie. *Allergologie* 6:55, 1983.

358. Szentivanyi, A., and Szentivanyi, J. Some selected aspects of the immunopharmacology of adrenoceptors. *Adv. Immunopharmacol.* 2:269, 1983.

359. Szentivanyi, A., and Szentivanyi, J. The Pathophysiology of Immunologic and Related Diseases. In W. A. Sodeman and T. M. Sodeman (eds.), *Sode-*

man's Pathologic Physiology—Mechanisms of Disease. Philadelphia: Saunders, 1985. Pp. 151–197.

360. Szentivanyi, A., et al. Nonantibiotic properties of antibiotics in relationship to immune-neuroendocrine influences. *Clin. Pharmacol. Ther.* 43: 166, 1988.

361. Szentivanyi, A., et al. Virus-associated Immune and Pharmacologic Mechanisms in Disorders of Respiratory and Cutaneous Atopy. In A. Szentivanyi and H. Friedman (eds.), *Viruses, Immunity, and Immunodeficiency.* New York: Plenum, 1986. Pp. 211–244.

362. Szentivanyi, A., et al. Changes in the Immune Parameters of Antibiotic-bacterial Interactions Induced by Hypothalamic and Other Electrolytic Brain Lesions Produced Through Stereotaxically Implanted Depth Electrodes. In G. Gillissen. et al. (eds.), *The Influence of Antibiotics on the Host-parasite Relationship*, Vol. 3. Heidelberg: Springer, 1989. Pp. 237–244.

363. Szentivanyi, A., and Williams, J. F. The Constitutional Basis of Atopic Disease. In C. W. Bierman and D. S. Pearlman (eds.), *Allergic Diseases of Infancy, Childhood, and Adolescence.* Philadelphia: Saunders, 1980. Pp. 173–210.

364. Szentivanyi, M., Kunos, G., and Juhasz-Nagy, A. Modulator theory of adrenergic receptor mechanism: Vessels of the dog hind limb. *Am. J. Physiol.* 218:869, 1970.

365. Szentivanyi, M., and Pek, L. Characteristic changes of vascular adrenergic reactions in diabetes mellitus. *Nature New Biol.* 243:276, 1973.

366. Szentivanyi, M., Takacs, K., and Botos, K. A New Aspect in Treatment of Diabetic Vascular Disease. In *Proceedings of the Seventh International Congress of Pharmacology.* Oxford: Pergamon, 1978. P. 271.

367. Tashkin, D. P., et al. Subsensitization of beta-adrenoceptors in airways and lymphocytes of healthy and asthmatic subjects. *Am. Rev. Respir. Dis.* 125:185, 1982.

368. Terpstra, G. K., Raaijmakers, J. A. M., and Van Rozen, A. G. The Involvement of First Receptor Coupling in the Pathogenesis of Asthma. In *Proceedings of the 5th International Conference on Cyclic Nucleotide and Protein Phosphorylation.* Milan, Italy: Pythagora, 1983. P. 117.

369. Thoenen, H., and Tranzer, J. P. Chemical sympathectomy by selective destruction of adrenergic nerve endings with 6-hydroxy-dopamine. *Naunyn Schmiedebergs Arch. Pharmacol. Exp. Pathol.* 261:271, 1968.

370. Thomas, R. C. Electrogenic sodium pump in nerve and muscle cells. *Physiol. Rev.* 52:563, 1972.

371. Tohmeh, J. F., and Cryer, P. E. Biphasic adrenergic modulation of beta-adrenergic receptors in man: Agonist-induced early increments and late decrements in beta-adrenergic receptor number. *J. Clin. Invest.* 65:836, 1980.

372. Trendelenburg, U. Mechanisms of supersensitivity and subsensitivity to sympathomimetic amines. *Pharmacol. Rev.* 18:629, 1966.

373. Trifaro, J. M., Poisner, A. M., and Douglas, W. W. The fate of the chromaffin granule during catecholamine release from the adrenal medulla. I. Unchanged efflux of phospholipid and cholesterol. *Biochem. Pharmacol.* 16:2095, 1967.

374. Tse, J. Isoproterenol-induced cardiac hypertrophy: Modifications in characteristics of beta-adrenergic receptor adenylate cyclase and ventricular contraction. *Endocrinology* 105:246, 1979.

375. Uchiyama, T., et al. A monoclonal antibody (anti-T) reactive with activated and functionally mature human T cells. II. Expression of Tac antigen on activated cytotoxic killer T cells. *J. Immunol.* 126:1398, 1981.

376. Udenfriend, S., and Creveling, C. R. Location of dopamine beta-oxidase in brain. *J. Neurochem.* 4:350, 1959.

377. Uhing, R. J., et al. Hormone stimulated polyphosphoinositide breakdown in rat liver plasma membranes. Roles of guanine nucleotides and calcium. *J. Biol. Chem.* 261:2140, 1986.

378. Uhl, R., Wagner, R., and Ryba, N. Watching G proteins at work. *Trends Neurosci.* 13:64, 1990.

379. Ui, M., et al. A Role of the Inhibitory Guanine Nucleotide-binding Regulatory Protein in Signal Transduction via Ca^{2+}-Mobilizing Receptors. In R. J. Lefkowitz and E. Lindenlaub (eds.), *Adrenergic Receptors: Molecular Properties and Therapeutic Implications.* Stuttgart: Schattauer, 1985.

380. U'Prichard, D. C., and Snyder, S. H. Binding of ^{3}H-catecholamines to alpha-noradrenergic receptor sites in calf brain. *J. Biol. Chem.* 252:6450, 1977.

381. Vanecek, D., et al. See-saw signal processing in pinealocytes involves reciprocal changes in the α_1-adrenergic component of the cGMP response and beta-adrenergic component of cAMP response. *J. Neurochem.* 47:678, 1986.

382. Venter, J. C., and Fraser, C. M. The Development of Monoclonal Antibodies to Beta-adrenergic Receptors and Their Use in Receptor Purification and Characterization. In R. E. Fellows and G. S. Eisenbarth (eds.), *Monoclonal Antibodies in Endocrine Research.* New York: Raven, 1981. Pp. 119–134.

383. Venter, J. C., and Fraser, C. M. The structure of alpha and beta-adrenergic receptors. *Trends Pharmacol. Sci.* 4:256, 1983.

384. Venter, J. C., Fraser, C. M., and Harrison, L. C. Autoantibodies to β_2-adrenergic receptors: A possible cause of adrenergic hyporesponsiveness in allergic rhinitis and asthma. *Science* 207:1361, 1980.

385. Venter, J. C., Fraser, C. M., and Lilly, L. Structure of Neurotransmitter Receptors (Adrenergic, Dopaminergic and Muscarinic Cholinergic). In E. Usdin, et al. (eds.), *Catecholamines: Basic and Peripheral Mechanisms.* New York: Alan R. Liss, 1984.

386. Vertesi, C., Szentivanyi, M., and Szigeti, K. Histological Evaluation of the Therapy in Diabetic Angiopathy. In *Proceedings of the Seventh International Congress of Pharmacology.* Oxford: Pergamon, 1978. P. 271.

387. Viveros, O. H., Arqueros, L., and Kirshner, N. Quantal secretion from adrenal medulla: All-or-none release of storage vesicle content. *Science* 165:911, 1969.

388. von Euler, V. W. Synthesis, Uptake and Storage of Catecholamines in Adrenergic Nerves: The Effects of Drugs. In H. Blaschko and E. Muscholl (eds.), *Catecholamines.* Berlin: Springer, 1972.

389. Wakede, A. R., and Furchgott, R. F. Metabolic requirements for the uptake and storage of norepinephrine by the isolated left atrium of the guinea pig. *J. Pharmacol. Exp. Ther.* 163:123, 1968.

390. Wang, H.-Y., et al. The biology of beta-adrenergic receptors: Analysis in human epidermoid carcinoma A431 cells. *Int. J. Biochem.* 23:7, 1991.

391. Weiner, N. Regulation of norepinephrine biosynthesis. *Annu. Rev. Pharmacol.* 10:273, 1973.

392. Williams, L. T. Thyroid hormone regulation of beta-adrenergic receptor number. *J. Biol. Chem.* 252:2787, 1977.

393. Williams, L. T., and Lefkowitz, R. J. *Receptor Binding Studies in Adrenergic Pharmacology.* New York: Raven, 1978.

394. Williams, L. T., Snyderman, R., and Lefkowitz, R. J. Identification of beta adrenergic receptors in human leukocytes with (-)[^{3}H]dihydroalprenolol. *J. Clin. Invest.* 57:149, 1976.

395. Williams, R. S., et al. Autonomic mechanisms of training bradycardia: Beta-adrenergic receptors in humans. *J. Appl. Physiol.* 51:1232, 1981.

396. Williams, R. S., and Lefkowitz, R. J. Thyroid hormone regulation of alpha-adrenergic receptors: Studies in rat myocardium. *J. Cardiovasc. Pharmacol.* 1:181, 1979.

397. Willis, W. D., and Grossman, R. G. *Medical Neurobiology: Neuroanatomical and Neurophysiological Principles Basic to Clinical Neuroscience* (3rd ed.). St. Louis: Mosby, 1981.

398. Wilson, A. F., et al. Cardiopulmonary effects of long-term bronchodilator administration. *J. Allergy Clin. Immunol.* 58:204, 1976.

399. Yamada, S., Yamamura, H. I., and Roeski, W. R. Alterations in cardiac autonomic receptors following 6-hydroxydopamine treatment in rats. *Mol. Pharmacol.* 18:185, 1980.

400. Yoshie, Y., et al. Inhibitory effect of α_2-adrenoceptor antagonist (midaglizole) on bronchial asthma. Basic studies on experimental guinea pig bronchoconstriction. *Jpn. J. Allergol.* 37:1077, 1988.

401. Yoshie, Y., Iizuka, K., and Nakazawa, T. Inhibitory effect of selective α_2 adrenoceptor antagonist on moderate and severe type asthma. *J. Allergy Clin. Immunol.* 84:747, 1989.

402. Youdim, M. B. H., Collins, G. G. S., and Sandler, M. Multiple forms of rat brain monoamine oxidase. *Nature* 223:626, 1969.

Cyclic Nucleotides

15

Ralph P. Miech

The relationship of neurotransmitters and chemical mediators to asthma can no longer be restricted to the classic concepts of an imbalance of the autonomic nervous system and the release of mediators from mast cells [14, 50]. In addition to synaptic neurotransmitters and mast cell mediators, a wide variety of autocrine and paracrine mediators released from platelets, granulocytes, monocytes, lymphocytes, macrophages, and epithelial cells trigger mechanisms that control the contractile state of bronchial smooth muscle [44, 74]. Airway patency is determined by bronchial smooth muscle tone, airway hyperreactivity, the degree and character of mucus secretion, fluctuating hormonal levels, mucociliary clearance, mucosal thickness, the local release of autocrine and paracrine mediators, and the degree of activity of the parasympathetic (cholinergic), sympathetic (adrenergic), and nonadrenergic noncholinergic (purinergic) nervous systems [25, 29, 49] (see Chaps. 17 and 18).

The nemesis of asthma is that all of the contractile signals (1) vary from individual to individual, (2) vacillate in time, (3) contribute in varying degrees to the net patency of the airways during the various stages of the disease, and (4) respond differently to pharmacologic interventions. Thus, the mechanisms controlling the initiation, maintenance, and cessation of contraction of bronchial smooth muscle in both the central and peripheral airways are multifaceted and in a state of perpetual oscillation. Yet the different cellular controls for each of these mechanisms have two common features, the involvement of cyclic nucleotides and the regulation of intracellular calcium [7, 83].

Since the discovery of cyclic nucleotides, the following axiom has evolved: The biologic actions of cyclic nucleotides vary and are highly contingent on the species, tissue, and cell type [71, 82]. The cyclic nucleotides, cyclic adenosine monophosphate (AMP) and cyclic guanosine monophosphate (GMP), are involved in hormone action, neuronal function, muscular contraction, secretory mechanisms, immune mechanisms, and release of the so-called classic chemical mediators, paracrine mediators, autocrine mediators, cytokines, and growth factors that influence cellular growth, differentiation, gene expression, and expansion of clones. This chapter presents insight into the expanding perception of the roles that cyclic nucleotides play in the regulation of the patency of airways.

CYCLIC AMP

Cyclic AMP is a ubiquitous, multifunctional regulatory molecule and the first biologic compound to be designated as an intracellular second messenger. An understanding of the multiple actions of this regulatory cyclic nucleotide is essential to the understanding of both the pathophysiology of asthma and the pharmacodynamic mechanisms of bronchodilators [49, 60].

Cyclic AMP functions in the transduction and integration of information transmitted to bronchial smooth muscle by a variety of extracellular signals (i.e., hormones, neurotransmitters, and mediators). This is a time-honored concept but is too restrictive. The role of cyclic AMP in asthma requires a panoramic view not limited to bronchial smooth muscle (Fig. 15-1). In addition to relaxation of bronchial smooth muscles, cyclic AMP is involved in numerous and diverse cellular functions, for example, inflammatory events, smooth muscle hyperplasia, IgE-dependent allergic reactions, secretion of respiratory tract fluid, production of mucus, release of neurotransmitters, vascular control of blood flow, receptor desensitization, control of ion channels, generation of cytokines, cell chemotaxis, and stabilization of the barrier function of airway epithelium and vasoactive tone of airway microvessels. A better understanding of asthma in terms of its pathophysiology and effective pharmacologic intervention will be achieved in the future with the exploration of the possible roles of cyclic nucleotides in the release of multiple types of paracrine mediators, the control of cell-surface receptors, and the differential activation of eukaryotic gene transcription in mast cells, granulocytes, lymphocytes, monocytes, platelets, and epithelial cells [27].

Synthesis of Cyclic AMP

The Beta2-Adrenergic Receptors

Depending on the tissue, different cell-surface receptors, such as beta2-adrenergic, H_2 histamine, dopamine, and vasoactive intestinal peptide (VIP) receptors, mediate the intracellular synthesis of cyclic AMP [4, 80]. Beta2-adrenergic agonists are effective bronchodilators and the most common therapeutic modality used to reverse asthmatic and nonasthmatic bronchospasm [5]. A beneficial attribute of beta2-adrenoceptor agonists is their bronchodilatory activity against a wide range of bronchoconstrictors. Unlike specific receptor antagonists that block specific receptors involved in bronchoconstriction, the sympathomimetic beta2 adrenoceptors reverse bronchoconstriction regardless of the constrictor mediator involved [55]. Beta2 agonists also stimulate adenylate cyclase activity in mast cell membranes [67]. In mast cell membranes there is an interrelationship between beta2 receptors, IgE receptors, adenylate cyclase, methyltransferases, calcium channels, and the generation of mediators from arachidonic acid [67, 85]. Even though recent studies have well characterized alpha1 and alpha2 adrenoceptors, their role in asthma is not clear [28]. The effect of alpha adrenoceptors on airways is dependent on the blockade of beta-adrenergic receptors [51].

Activation of beta2-adrenergic receptors by adrenergic agonists is invariably linked to guanine nucleotide–binding proteins known as G-proteins [24]. G-proteins in turn are linked directly to the activation of adenylate cyclase. The pharmacodynamic

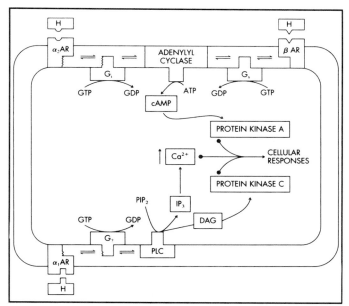

Fig. 15-1. *Activation of beta-adrenergic receptors (βAR) by a neurotransmitter or hormone (H) initiates the synthesis of cyclic AMP (cAMP) by adenylyl cyclase at the cytoplasmic surface of the cell membrane. The receptor activation of adenylyl cyclase requires that the liganded receptor interact with a stimulatory guanine nucleotide–binding regulatory protein (Gs) which in turn is activated by the nucleotide GTP. A related regulatory protein (Gi) also binds GTP but results in inhibition of adenylyl cyclase. Alpha₂-adrenergic (α₂AR) and M₂ muscarinic receptors via Gi regulatory proteins are associated with inhibition of adenylyl cyclase and also the modulation of K⁺ channels and voltage-gated Ca⁺⁺ channels. Cyclic AMP activated protein kinase A and this kinase phosphorylates a variety of cellular proteins and thereby regulates their activities. Phospholipase C (PLC) hydrolyzes a membrane phospholipid, phosphatidylinositol-4,5-bisphosphate (PIP₂) to yield two intracellular second messengers, inositol-1,4,5-trisphosphate (IP₃) and diacylglycerol (DAG). IP₃ causes release of Ca⁺⁺ from intracellular stores and diacylglycerol stimulates the activity of Ca⁺⁺-sensitive protein kinase C, which in turn regulates the activity of a variety of cellular proteins. (Reprinted with permission from Alfred G. Gilman, et al.,* Goodman & Gilman's the Pharmacological Basis of Therapeutics. *Elmsford, New York: Pergamon, 1990.)*

action of adrenergic agonists is dependent on the activation of adenylate cyclase. Adenylate cyclase enzymatically synthesizes cyclic AMP from cytosolic adenosine triphosphate (ATP). The enzyme is located within the inner lipid layer of the bilipid cell membranes of bronchial smooth muscle cells, mast cells, and synaptic junctions of central, sympathetic, and parasympathetic neurons. Activation of adenylate cyclase results in a transient increase in the intracellular concentration of cyclic AMP.

Beta₂-receptor molecules are transmembrane proteins that are embedded within the cell membrane and have three domains: a domain that is exposed to the exterior of the cell membrane, a domain that spans the bilipid cell membrane, and a domain that is exposed to the interior of the cell (Fig. 15-2) [21]. Each of these domains has a specific function. The exterior domain is responsible for the specificity of binding of both beta₂ agonists and antagonists. The order of potency of beta-adrenergic agents and the specificity of beta-receptor antagonists form the basis for differentiating beta receptors into beta₁ (heart) and beta₂ (bronchial and other tissues) subclasses. The domain of the beta₂ receptor that spans the width of the bilipid cell membrane undergoes a conformational change when the receptor is occupied by an agonist. This intramembrane domain is responsible for the activation of another membrane-bound class of proteins, the G-

protein that directly controls the activity of adenylate cyclase. The domain that is exposed to the interior of the cell is involved in the desensitization of beta₂ receptors.

Guanine Nucleotide–binding Proteins

G-proteins are linked to adenylate cyclase and belong to one of two classifications, Gs and Gi [12]. Gs-proteins stimulate adenylate cyclase and Gi-proteins inhibit adenylate cyclase (Fig. 15-3) [26, 43, 54, 63]. The inactive form of both of these G-proteins is a trimer composed of alpha, beta, and gamma subunits with guanosine diphosphate (GDP) bound to the alpha subunit [33, 40]. Gs or Gi regulation of adenylate cyclase activity requires the replacement of GDP by guanosine triphosphate (GTP) on the alpha subunit or the enzymatic phosphorylation by a nucleotide kinase of GDP to GTP while GDP remains bound to the alpha subunit of the G-protein [45]. The binding of an adrenergic agonist to the beta₂ receptor initiates a transient stabilization of a conformation of the guanine nucleotide regulatory Gs-protein. This conformational change facilitates conversion of G-alpha-GDP to G-alpha-GTP by either the release of GDP and the binding of GTP to the alpha subunit [34, 47] or direct ATP phosphorylation of the GDP bound to the alpha subunit to GTP. The GTP-alpha subunit then dissociates from the Gs complex, migrates to and binds to the regulatory site on adenylate cyclase, and activates the enzyme [57]. Activation of adenylate cyclase is terminated when the GTP-alpha subunit hydrolyzes the bound GTP to GDP [32]. This results in the dissociation of the GDP-alpha subunit from the regulatory site on adenylate cyclase and its reassociation with the beta and gamma subunits to form inactive G-protein. In the absence of the GTP-alpha subunit of the G-protein complex bound to adenylate cyclase, the enzyme is inactive. In vitro, persistent activation of adenylate cyclase by the alpha subunit can be achieved by substituting hydrolysis-resistant analogs of GTP, e.g. GMP-p(NH)p or GTP-gamma-S. Inhibition of adenylate cyclase via alpha₂-adrenergic and other types of receptors involves the Gi-protein acting by a similar but not fully elucidated mechanism [8, 61, 87].

Fig. 15-2. *The membrane topology of the beta₂-adrenergic receptor is postulated to have three domains: the free amino group terminus of the peptide as the extracellular domain, seven segments of the amino acid chain rich in lipid-soluble amino acids that undulate the cell membrane, and the free carboxy terminus of the alpha helix peptide chain projecting into the intracellular cytosol. The free carboxyl group terminus of the peptide chain is postulated to be the site of beta₂-adrenergic receptor desensitization by phosphorylation by protein kinase A (PKA) or beta-adrenergic receptor kinase (BARK).*

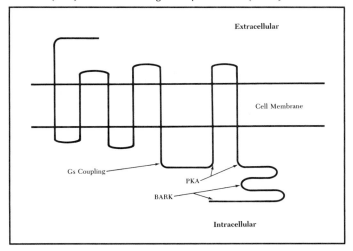

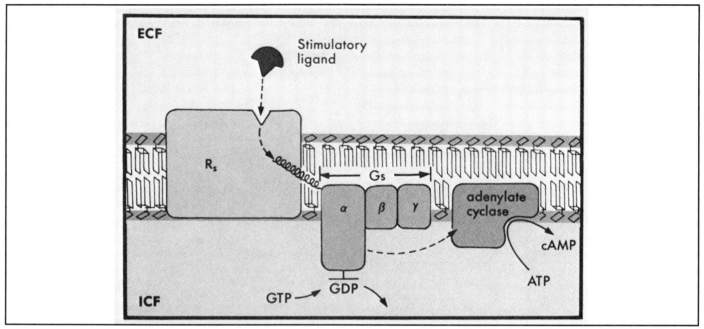

Fig. 15-3. *Binding of a stimulatory neurotransmitter or hormone ligand to the receptor protein causes a conformational change which favors an interaction with the carboxy terminus of the alpha helix domain, the subunit of the guanine nucleotide regulatory protein Gs. This interaction activates Gs by displacing bound GDP with GTP to cause Gs to dissociate so that the activated subunit of Gs can move to the location of adenylyl cyclase and activate the formation of cyclic AMP (cAMP). R_s = stimulatory receptor; ECF = extracellular fluid; ICF = intracellular fluid. (Reprinted with permission from Lemuel B. Wingard Jr., et al.,* Human Pharmacology: Molecular to Clinical. *St. Louis: Mosby-Year Book, 1991.)*

Adenylate Cyclase

A multitude of mobile receptors diffuse laterally within the cell membrane [3, 46, 53]. The beta$_2$ receptor and certain other ligand-activated receptors compete for the pool of G-proteins [54, 73]. Diversification and modulation of external cell receptors account for the ability of different hormones, neurotransmitters, and autocoids to regulate adenylate cyclase activity in smooth muscle membranes, mast cell membranes, and synaptic membranes of neurons [10]. A wide variety of naturally occurring regulatory molecules function as receptor ligands that alter the production, destruction, or biochemical action of cyclic AMP, that is, biogenic amines, polypeptides, proteins, various prostaglandins, endorphins, adenosine, and acetylcholine. Since adenylate cyclase is a ubiquitous enzyme, the characteristic response of a particular tissue to any of the above-mentioned ligands depends on the presence of the specific receptor in that tissue and the type of cellular response linked to the intracellular action of cyclic AMP.

Regulation of Beta$_2$-Adrenergic Receptors

Downregulation of beta$_2$-adrenergic receptors for the control of excessive adenylate cyclase activity is related to receptor turnover [47, 76] (see Chap. 14). Beta$_2$-adrenergic receptors are continuously being removed and reinserted, conferring a dynamic aspect of receptor turnover to the "floating receptor" model [18]. Excessive stimulation of beta$_2$ receptors is associated with "downregulation," while excessive inhibition of beta$_2$ receptors is associated with "upregulation" [59]. The turnover of receptors occurs during the life of a cell. This property of cell-surface receptors to be removed and replaced is invoked to explain a variety of hypotheses and observations in asthma, for example, Szentivanyi's hypothesis of inherent beta-receptor defects in asthmatic patients, diminution of the pharmacologic response after patient

abuse of adrenergic bronchodilator aerosols, and rebound bronchoconstriction after prolonged infusion of isoproterenol and the upregulation of beta$_2$ receptors that is associated with the delayed action of glucocorticoids [17]. In addition to affecting the number of beta receptors, exposure to glucocorticoids and the presence or absence of thyroid hormone may also affect ligand-receptor coupling to G-proteins.

Autodesensitization (tachyphylaxis) of beta$_2$-adrenergic receptors is related to agonist binding to the receptor and is reversible [62, 80]. It has been hypothesized that the tachyphylaxis is due to an autodesensitization of the beta$_2$ receptor's affinity for the agonist or the uncoupling of the ability of beta$_2$ receptors to activate Gs-proteins. Phosphorylation of the intracellular domain of the beta$_2$ receptor induces a conformational change that diminishes the affinity of the extracellular domain for adrenergic agonists (Fig. 15-4) [52]. This type of phosphorylation is catalyzed by two protein kinases, protein kinase A and beta-adrenoceptor kinase. At relatively low levels of fractional receptor occupancy, protein kinase A, the cyclic AMP–dependent protein kinase, is primarily responsible for beta-receptor desensitization. At relatively high levels of fraction receptor occupancy, the enzyme beta-adrenoceptor kinase is primarily involved in beta-receptor desensitization. Beta-adrenoceptor kinase is a cyclic AMP–independent protein kinase. Phosphorylation of the beta receptor does not appear to be a trigger for sequestration of the beta receptor.

The in vitro study of autodesensitization of beta$_2$-adrenergic receptors in guinea pig trachea showed that the autodesensitization induced by isoproterenol is concentration dependent. The concentration dependence of autodesensitization is more pronounced with salbutamol and fenoterol than with isoproterenol and epinephrine. Another study with guinea pig trachea showed that the relaxant responsiveness to the beta-adrenoceptor agonists fenoterol and norepinephrine was reduced, while theophyl-

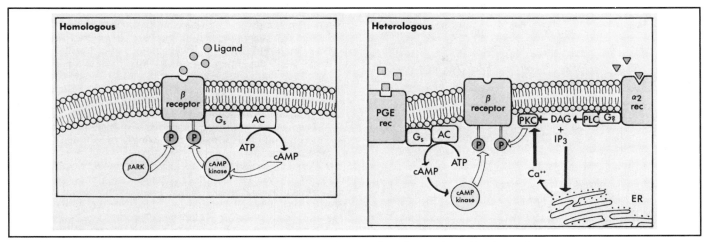

Fig. 15-4. *Beta$_2$-adrenergic receptors can be desensitized by two mechanisms, homologous desensitization and heterologous desensitization. Beta-adrenergic receptor kinase (BARK) and cyclic AMP–dependent protein kinase are involved in homologous desensitization because of the involvement of the beta$_2$-adrenergic receptor in the activation of these enzymes. Protein kinase C (PKC) and cyclic AMP–dependent protein kinase are involved in heterologous desensitization because of the involvement of another cell-surface receptor (i.e., prostaglandin receptor, PGE rec). AC = adenylyl cyclase; P = phosphorylation site; DAG = diacylglycerol; PLC = phospholipase C. (Reprinted with permission from Lemuel B. Wingard Jr., et al.,* Human Pharmacology: Molecular to Clinical. *St. Louis: Mosby-Year Book, 1991.)*

line and nitroprusside relaxant effects were unaffected. Indomethacin, a cyclooxygenase inhibitor, and mepacrine, an inhibitor of phospholipid turnover, had no significant effect on the extent of isoproterenol-induced autodesensitization. Conversely, cortisol significantly reduced desensitization and enhanced the rate of spontaneous recovery of responsiveness to isoproterenol. Autodesensitization was not accompanied by a reduction in the density of beta$_2$ adrenoceptors in the trachea, as assessed by binding and light microscopic autoradiography using [125I]iodocyanopindolol. Thus, autodesensitization is probably caused primarily by uncoupling of the beta-adrenergic/Gs-protein/adenylate cyclase complex. A change in the affinity of beta$_2$-adrenergic receptors for Gs molecules could be the cause of tachyphylaxis observed with the excessive use of beta$_2$ agonists. Downregulation, upregulation, and autodesensitization are responsible for autoregulation of the physiologic functioning of the beta$_2$-adrenergic receptors. Desensitization is the decrease or loss of ability of the ligand to activate adenylate cyclase. Thus, the control of airway caliber is achieved by (1) the adjustment of the number, type, and efficacy of surface receptors; (2) the alteration of receptor affinities for its ligand; (3) the existence of receptors that can modulate the coupling of a ligand-receptor complex to Gs; and (4) the rate of hydrolysis of GTP by the alpha subunit of the G-protein.

Cholera toxin causes an enhancement of both basal and agonist-stimulated adenylate cyclase activity [39]. Cholera toxin uses NAD$^+$ to ADP ribosylate Gs. This covalent modification of Gs by ADP ribosylation results in a loss of GTPase activity, which renders Gs capable of persistent stimulation of adenylate cyclase (Fig. 15-5). ADP-ribosylated Gs with GTP bound to the altered protein confers stability to the active form of adenylate cyclase. Thus, the reversion of the active form of the cyclase to the inactive form does not occur. This is due to the inability of the alpha subunit of the ribosylated Gs-protein to hydrolyze GTP to GDP. Hydrolysis of the bound GTP to GDP is necessary for the alpha subunit to disengage from its binding to adenylate cyclase. Certain GTP analogs, guanosine-5′-[γ-thio]triphosphate and guanosine-5′-[β,γ-imido]triphosphate (p(NH)ppG), can replace GTP in the activation of Gs [31]. Because of their structure, these GTP analogs are not substrates for the GTPase activity of Gs. Thus,

these two components when bound to Gs cause a continuous stimulation of adenylate cyclase. The beta subunit of the G-protein is believed to be the site that is activated by GTP, p(NH)ppG, fluoride ion (AlF4$^-$), and cholera toxin.

Another bacterial toxin, pertussis toxin, also causes an increase in the intracellular level of cyclic AMP via increased adenylate cyclase activity [80]. Pertussis toxin inactivates the inhibitory guanine nucleotide–binding protein Gi (see Fig. 15-5). The difference between pertussis and cholera toxins is that cholera toxin enhances the action of GTP on Gs and pertussis toxin prevents the effect of GTP on Gi. In the absence of Gi-GTP, Gs-GTP action on adenylate cyclase is unopposed. Pertussis toxin achieves this effect on Gi through ADP ribosylation of one of the subunits of Gi [72]. In contrast to these effects of cholera toxin and pertussis toxin, the diterpene forskolin has a direct stimulatory effect on the catalytic component of adenylate cyclase and does not involve guanine nucleotide–binding protein in increasing the activity of adenylate cyclase.

In some biologic systems, activation of adenylate cyclase by Gs is modulated by a cyclic AMP–dependent phosphorylation of Gs that renders Gs less active. Guanine nucleotide–dependent coupling of receptors to an effector enzyme located in the interior aspect of the cell membrane is not unique to the adenylate cyclase system. Similar systems involving G-proteins occur for other receptors and enzymes (e.g., phospholipase C [20, 23, 42]) that generate other intracellular second messengers. G-proteins couple receptors to ion channels as well as to several phospholipases that generate various second messengers.

Each component of the beta$_2$ receptor–guanine nucleotide protein–adenylate cyclase control system provides a potential for developing new classes of bronchodilator drugs. Thus, if molecules could be synthesized to reversibly mimic the action of cholera toxin, pertussis toxin, or forskolin, new classes of bronchodilator drugs would be available for the prevention and treatment of asthma.

CYCLIC AMP–DEPENDENT PROTEIN KINASES

Cyclic AMP is an intracellular second messenger that achieves regulation of a wide spectrum of cellular functions. The most

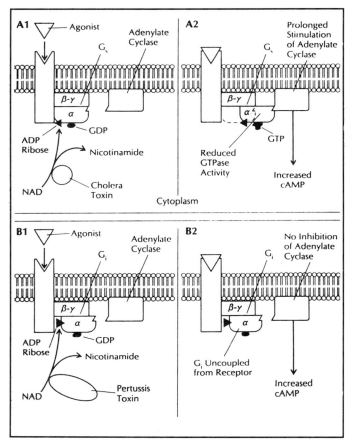

Fig. 15-5. *Cholera toxin utilizes nicotinamide adenine dinucleotide (NAD) to "ADP ribosylate" the alpha subunit of Gs. ADP ribosylation of Gs reduces GTPase activity of Gs, which in turn prevents the reversible transition of activated Gs to inactive Gs. Thus, the activated Gs continually stimulates the activation of adenylyl cyclase and its production of cyclic AMP (cAMP). Pertussis toxin also utilizes NAD for an ADP ribosylation reaction but in this case Gi is ADP ribosylated. ADP-ribosylated Gi is prevented from binding GTP, which is necessary to induce the conformational change in Gi so that Gi-GTP can inhibit adenylyl cyclase. In the absence of an active form of Gi, Gs-GTP action on adenylyl cyclase is unopposed, with a resultant increase in cyclic AMP formation. (Reprinted with permission. Spiegel, Allen M. G-Proteins in clinical medicine. Hospital Practice 23(6):106, 1988. Illustration(s) by Seward Hung.)*

typical control system for cyclic AMP regulation of intracellular functions of a multitude of proteins exploits a common biochemical mechanism, phosphorylation of tissue-specific proteins by cyclic AMP–dependent protein kinases [81]. Differential activation of eukaryotic gene transcription is regulated by a different mechanism involving cyclic AMP–binding proteins, for example, cyclic AMP receptor protein or cyclic AMP responsive element [41, 58].

Hyperpolarization and relaxation of airway smooth muscle can be induced by diverse agents that elevate cyclic AMP levels, for example, isoproterenol, forskolin, theophylline, and a variety of cyclic AMP analogs. This is consistent with the unifying hypothesis that cyclic AMP–dependent phosphorylation is involved in producing the electrical and biochemical events that implement bronchodilation [19]. When bronchial smooth muscle cells are stimulated to relax, cyclic AMP activates a cascade of protein-phosphorylating enzymes. This cascade of interdependent enzymes acts in concert to reverse the intracellular conditions necessary for the cross-bridge interaction of the contractile proteins

myosin and actin to produce bronchoconstriction. Currently two mechanisms, a decrease in myosin light-chain kinase and a decrease in cytoplasmic calcium ions, are associated with cyclic AMP–related relaxation of airway smooth muscle [11].

Cyclic AMP–dependent protein kinase (protein kinase A) and myosin light-chain kinase are integral to this cascade of enzymes that participate in the control of the functional activity of the contractile proteins (Fig. 15-6) [16]. The utilization of a cascade of enzymes as a mechanism to control contractile proteins has several advantages: amplification, fast response time, reversibility, and the potential for the cell to override or modulate external contractile signals.

Within a given cell type there are different cyclic AMP–dependent protein kinases [77]. These enzymes function as the intracellular receptors and mediators of cyclic AMP actions via phosphorylation of specific tissue proteins. Calcium-dependent K^+ channels, phosphorylase-b-kinase, glycogen synthetase, pyruvate kinase, and histones are examples of tissue proteins, other than myosin light-chain kinase, that serve as substrates for the different cyclic AMP–dependent protein kinases. In most of these phosphorylated proteins, a serine residue is the phosphorylation site. The sequence of amino acids in the vicinity of the phosphorylation site participates in determining which cyclic AMP–dependent kinase can phosphorylate the serine residue in that protein.

Cyclic AMP–dependent protein kinases are quaternary oligomers consisting of regulatory (R) subunits and catalytic (C) subunits [81]. The holoenzyme is the inactive form of cyclic AMP–dependent protein kinase and is composed of two regulatory subunits and two catalytic units. Together these subunits form a tetrameric complex, R2C2. Multiple forms of the regulatory subunits exist and the typical subunit isoform is a highly asymmetric dimer. The regulatory subunits bound to the catalytic subunits prevent the enzymatic activity of the catalytic subunit. The binding of cyclic AMP to the regulatory subunits initiates a conformation change that results in the dissociation of the regulatory subunits from the tetramer to yield two molecules of the active enzyme:

$$R2C2 + 4 \text{ cyclic AMP} \rightleftarrows 4 \text{ cyclic AMP} : 2R + 2C$$

The use of cyclic AMP to release the inhibitory effects of the regulatory subunit is unique to this type of protein kinase. Cyclic AMP–dependent protein kinases vary in (1) the affinity of the cyclic AMP–binding sites on the regulatory subunits, (2) substrate specificity of the catalytic subunits, and (3) the affinity of the holoenzyme for MgATP, and (4) the susceptibility to autophosphorylation [81]. Limited proteolysis and affinity labeling have shown that each regulatory subunit has two high-affinity binding sites for cyclic AMP. The binding of cyclic AMP to cyclic AMP–dependent protein kinase exhibits positive cooperativity; that is, the binding of the first molecule of cyclic AMP facilitates the binding of subsequent molecules of cyclic AMP. Thus activation of cyclic AMP–dependent protein kinase by cyclic AMP has the characteristics of an allosteric mechanism. One cyclic AMP–binding site has a preference for N6-substituted cyclic AMP analogs and the other binding site has a preference for C8-substituted analogs.

Several isoforms of regulatory subunits are found in most cells and their relative proportions vary from one cell type to another. Cyclic AMP analogs were used to show the existence of two classes of binding sites (A and B) of Type I (rabbit skeletal muscle) and Type II (bovine heart) cyclic AMP–dependent protein kinase. Cyclic AMP analogs discriminated between the two classes of binding sites by their binding affinities: 2-Chloro-8-methylamino-cyclic AMP had a higher affinity for BI than for AI, and 2-n-butyl-8-thiobenzyl-cyclic AMP had a higher affinity for BII than for AII [81]. The biologic significance of the different

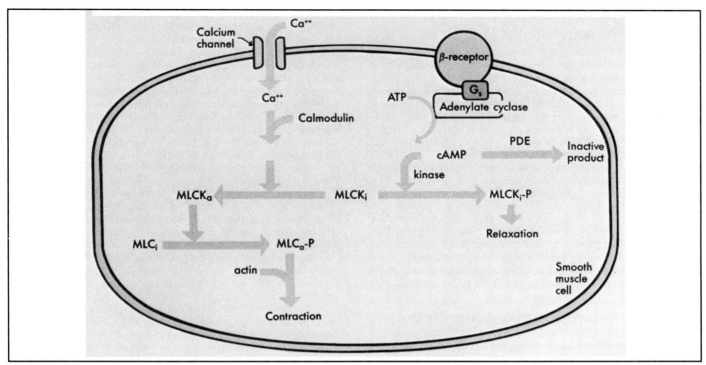

Fig. 15-6. *The proposed mechanism for cyclic AMP (cAMP)–induced relation of smooth muscle. Relaxation of smooth muscle by stimulation of beta-adrenergic receptors is initiated by the intracellular rise in cyclic AMP. This second messenger in turn activates cyclic AMP kinase which phosphorylates myosin light-chain kinase (MLCK). Relaxation is the result of the phosphorylated myosin light-chain kinase's (MLCL$_i$-P) decreased ability to bind the Ca^{++}-calmodulin complex. The Ca^{++}-calmodulin–myosin light-chain kinase complex is required for the enzymatic phosphorylation of myosin light chain so that it can interact with actin to produce the contracted smooth muscle state. MLC$_i$ = inactive myosin light chain; MLCK$_a$ = active myosin light-chain kinase; PDE = phosphodiesterase; MLC$_a$-P = active, phosphorylated myosin light chain. (Reprinted with permission from Lemuel B. Wingard Jr., et al.,* Human Pharmacology: Molecular to Clinical. *St. Louis: Mosby-Year Book, 1991.)*

holoenzymes, isoforms, and the different cyclic AMP–binding sites remains to be determined.

The C subunit designates the active enzymatic form of cyclic AMP–dependent kinase. In the case of airway smooth muscle, active cyclic AMP–dependent kinase catalyzes the phosphorylation of a specific protein, which itself is a protein kinase, known as myosin light-chain kinase. Thus, smooth muscle myosin light-chain kinase is the substrate to be phosphorylated by cyclic AMP–dependent protein kinase. The phosphorylated form of myosin light-chain kinase has reduced enzymatic activity, since it has a lower affinity for a calcium-calmodulin complex. The binding of the calcium-calmodulin complex leads to a conformational change [65] and generates active myosin light-chain kinase that is able to phosphorylate the 20-kd myosin light chain. Phosphorylation of myosin light chain is indispensable for the initiation of and/or prolongation of smooth muscle contraction [79]. Enzymatic phosphorylation of the light chain of myosin by myosin light-chain kinase is the final common step of a variety of pathways for agonists that induce smooth muscle contraction. In the absence of activated myosin light-chain kinase, phosphorylated myosin is enzymatically dephosphorylated by a phosphatase and smooth muscle fiber relaxation ensues. Thus, the phosphorylation mechanism for the inactivation of myosin light-chain kinase by cyclic AMP–dependent kinase permits smooth muscle cells to override external signals that favor contraction.

Concurrent with a decrease in the activity of myosin light-chain kinase, a reduction in cytosolic free calcium ions also occurs and a different cyclic AMP–dependent kinase is involved. This cyclic AMP–dependent kinase enzyme phosphorylates cell membrane proteins, resulting in an enhancement of sodium-cal-cium exchange across the cell membrane. Thus, multiple cyclic AMP–dependent protein kinases mediate smooth muscle relaxation by altering the affinity of myosin light-chain kinase for the calcium-calmodulin complex and by lowering the free intracellular calcium ion concentration. Even if the intracellular concentration of free calcium should rise, the decrease in the affinity of phosphorylated myosin light-chain kinase for calcium-calmodulin complex promotes relaxation of bronchial smooth muscle [2, 78]. The hydrolysis of phosphatidylinositol-4,5-bisphosphate to inositol-1,4,5-trisphosphate and 1,2-diacylglycerol is intimately involved in the regulation of the mobilization of intracellular calcium [22].

CYCLIC NUCLEOTIDES AND PHOSPHOPROTEIN PHOSPHATASES

Biologic control systems generally exploit a recycling protein phosphorylation-hydrolysis system for reversible regulation of essential electrical and biochemical functions. Enzymes, ion channels, and receptors are but a few examples of functional proteins whose cellular activities are regulated by the synchronized ATP-dependent phosphorylation (protein kinases) and hydrolysis of a phosphate ester group on serine, threonine, or tyrosine amino acid sites within the protein structure. The conformation of the protein, and hence its activation state, are determined by the presence or absence of one or more such phosphorylated amino acids. Depending on the biologic function, protein kinases and phosphoprotein phosphatases are the biochemical "on" or "off" switches or together function as a biochemical rheostat.

Smooth muscle contains at least three phosphoprotein phosphatases [19]. Phosphoprotein phosphatase 1 activity is regulated by yet another regulatory protein, known as Inhibitor 1. The inhibitory activity of Inhibitor 1 in turn is dependent on its own conformational state. A cyclic AMP–dependent protein kinase phosphorylates Inhibitor 1 and the phosphorylated Inhibitor 1 is then able to exert its maximal inhibition of phosphoprotein phosphatase 1. The enzymatic activity of the second type of phosphoprotein phosphatase is regulated by calcineurin. Calcineurin is a multisubunit protein containing a calcium-binding subunit similar to calmodulin and a catalytic unit that contains the actual phosphoprotein phosphatase activity. The active form of this enzyme consists of calcium bound to the calcium-binding subunit, which then activates the phosphoprotein phosphatase activity of the catalytic unit. Calcineurin represents the first phosphoprotein phosphatase known to be regulated by calcium. Okadaic acid, a potent protein phosphatase inhibitor, enhances and prolongs the open-state, Ca^{++}-dependent K^+ channels of tracheal myocytes initiated by the extracellular application of isoprenaline or intracellular application of protein kinase A.

CYCLIC NUCLEOTIDE PHOSPHODIESTERASES

Activation of adenylate cyclase and the inhibition of cyclic nucleotide phosphodiesterase are two pharmacologic methods for preventing or reversing bronchoconstriction. Both of these approaches are directed toward increasing or preserving an elevated intracellular level of cyclic AMP. Pharmacologic intervention is primarily directed toward smooth muscle cells and those cells which form and/or release mediators that stimulate contraction of bronchial smooth muscle. In addition to pharmacologic stimulation of adenylate cyclase via activation of the beta2 receptor, cyclic AMP levels can be increased by the second route of pharmacologic intervention, that is, the use of inhibitors of the enzymatic degradation of cyclic AMP by cyclic nucleotide phosphodiesterases [69].

Degradation of both intracellular cyclic nucleotides, cyclic AMP and cyclic GMP, is accomplished by a family of five isozymes known as cyclic nucleotide phosphodiesterases: (1) calcium-calmodulin dependent, (2) cyclic GMP stimulated, (3) cyclic GMP inhibited, (4) cyclic AMP specific, and (5) cyclic GMP specific [70]. These enzymes hydrolyze cyclic AMP and cyclic GMP to their corresponding nucleoside 5'-monophosphate derivatives. The phosphodiesterase isozymes differ in tissue distribution, intracellular location, substrate specificity, kinetic behavior, molecular weight, their susceptibility to physiologic regulation, and their susceptibility to inhibition by diverse compounds (e.g., derivatives of theophylline, phenothiazines, milrinone, rolipram, and dipyridamole). Theophylline and papaverine are classified as common nonselective inhibitors.

Substrate Specificity, Kinetic Parameters, and Cellular Regulation of Enzymatic Activity

Tracheal smooth muscle along with other tissues has several phosphodiesterase isozymes. One isozyme has a low apparent Michaelis constant (K_m) (0.29–0.49 μM) for guanosine-3':5'-cyclic monophosphate (cyclic GMP). Another isozyme from tracheal smooth muscle has both a low K_m for cyclic AMP (0.35–0.58 μM) and a high K_m for cyclic AMP (32 μM). A third phosphodiesterase isozyme is referred to as the *high K_m* form. It is responsible for the enzymatic hydrolysis of a substantial fraction of the total cyclic AMP and cyclic GMP hydrolyzed by cell extracts.

Some forms of phosphodiesterase are activated by calcium via calmodulin, which indicates that the intracellular activities of

cyclic nucleotide phosphodiesterases are under cellular control depending on the internal milieu of each cell. This is in contrast to in vitro experiments where the hydrolysis of cyclic nucleotides is usually carried out at substrate concentrations that are several orders of magnitude above physiologic concentrations, under a variety of nonphysiologic conditions, and the enzymatic hydrolysis of the cyclic nucleotide represents the combined enzymatic activity of the various isozymes. Another form of phosphodiesterase, the low K_m form, has a low K_m for cyclic AMP and very low enzymatic activity for hydrolyzing cyclic GMP. This form of phosphodiesterase is not sensitive to calmodulin, and undergoes a rapid increase in activity in some cells when they are exposed to hormones or neurotransmitters. In theory, some forms of phosphodiesterase may be interconvertible depending on the state of aggregation of the different forms of the isoenzymes.

There appears a wide variation among different tissues in the utilization of the regulation of phosphodiesterase activity to achieve biologic events. For example, light activation of rhodopsin leads to a stimulation of phosphodiesterase activity. This activation is mediated via transducin, a GTP-binding protein [56, 84]. In the retina, increased hydrolysis of cyclic GMP results in the closure of cyclic GMP–gated cation channels, which leads to a reduction in the intracellular free calcium [55]. Cyclic GMP phosphodiesterase activity is decreased in monocytes isolated from patients with atopic asthma. Polymorphonuclear and lymphocytic cells from the same group of patients with atopic asthma showed no difference in the level of cyclic GMP phosphodiesterase activity.

Structural Activity Relationships of Inhibitors

The selectivity of inhibition of the different isozymes varies with a wide range of both potency and structural characteristics of inhibitors, for example, theophylline, papaverine, M&B 22948, isobutylmethylxanthine, denfubylline, amrinone, milrinone, imazodan, CI-930, MY-5445, piroximone, and rolipram [30]. While cardiac and vascular smooth muscle phosphodiesterase isozymes are pharmacologically similar, there is pharmacologic and substrate heterogeneity with one form of phosphodiesterase isolated from aortic and from trachea smooth muscle from the same species. Isoenzyme-selective phosphodiesterase inhibitors may have a potential therapeutic role both in the prophylaxis of bronchial constriction in asthma and in the suppression of proinflammatory cell infiltration in airway tissues [86].

The xanthine derivatives 1,3-dimethylxanthine (theophylline), 1-methyl-3-propylxanthine, and 1-methyl-3-butylxanthine were evaluated for their relaxant effects on tracheal smooth muscle isolated from guinea pigs and for their pharmacokinetic characteristics in rats. The alkyl chain length correlated with the phosphodiesterase inhibition constant (K_i) value of these derivatives. The N3-alkyl chain length is significant for increasing the relaxant effect and influences the pharmacokinetic and physicochemical properties of these drugs. There were no significant differences in the volume of distribution, although the half-life showed significant differences.

Theophylline

Theophylline inhibition of phosphodiesterase activity in crude tissue extracts suggested initially the theory that this inhibition was the mechanism of action for theophylline-induced bronchodilatation [38]. This theory was supported by the observation that in isolated organ systems, theophylline in combination with a beta2-adrenergic agent potentiated the rise in cyclic AMP levels due to the beta2 agonist. Yet the definitive mechanism of action of theophylline remained obscure since the therapeutic blood levels of theophylline are well below the concentration necessary to produce significant inhibition of phosphodiesterase [66]. The interaction of theophylline with adenosine receptors had been proposed as an alternative mechanism of action for this methylated xanthine. Theophylline was shown to be an antagonist of adenosine that binds to adenosine receptors at concentrations that are within the clinical effective range [68]. Therefore, the therapeutic effectiveness of theophylline had been attributed to its ability to function as an adenosine A_1 antagonist rather than a phosphodiesterase inhibitor [9, 70] (see Chaps. 19 and 58). However, additional studies showed that there are at least two different types of cell-surface receptors for adenosine that are different from purinoceptors [36, 64]. Bronchoconstriction and a fall in intracellular cyclic AMP are associated with A_1 receptors. Bronchodilatation and a rise in cyclic AMP are associated with A_2 receptors (Fig. 15-7, Table 15-1). Bronchoconstriction can be induced in asthmatic subjects by the inhalation of adenosine. This is complicated by the fact that adenosine inhibits mediator release in human basophils but stimulates mediator release in mast cells [15]. When applied to guinea pig airways, adenosine relaxes the airways by activation of A_2 receptors. To further complicate matters, theophylline is an antagonist of both A_1 and A_2 receptors. However, it is dubious that adenosine receptor antagonism by theophylline is the major mechanism of action of theophylline since enprofylline, an analog of theophylline that produces bronchodilation, is a more potent bronchodilator than theophylline and does not have any significant adenosine antagonism.

Recent studies revealed a strong positive correlation between low K_m cyclic AMP phosphodiesterase inhibition and the tracheal smooth muscle relaxation evoked by the xanthine derivatives.

Fig. 15-7. *Purinergic receptors are subdivided into two classes, those that have an affinity for adenosine as a ligand and those that have an affinity for ATP as a ligand. In many instances the methylxanthines readily bind to the adenosine-purinergic receptors but not to the ATP-purinergic receptors. The adenosine receptors are subclassified as A_1 adenosine receptors and A_2 adenosine receptors on the basis of their ability to inhibit or stimulate adenylate cyclase. The A_2 adenosine receptors can exist in two conformational states that determine the binding affinity for adenosine; that is, A_{2a} has high affinity for adenosine and A_{1b} has low affinity for adenosine.*

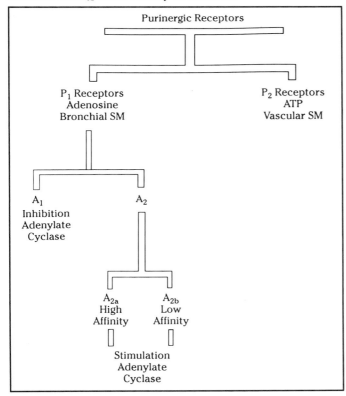

Table 15-1. Adenosine receptors

Functional classification
  P_1 Receptors
    Activated by adenosine $\gg$ ATP
    Blocked by theophylline
    Usually presynaptic receptors
  P_2 Receptors
    Activated by ATP $\gg$ adenosine
    Not blocked by theophylline
    Usually postjunctional receptors
Biochemical classification
  P-Site receptors
    Requires an unchanged purine moiety
    Intracellular site
    Inhibits adenylate cyclase
    Not blocked by theophylline
  R-Site receptors
    Requires an unchanged ribose moiety
    Mediates either activation or inhibition of adenylate cyclase
    Both subtypes R_1 and R_2 blocked by theophylline
    Subtypes
      A_1 or R_1: inhibit adenylate cyclase
      A_2 or R_2: activate adenylate cyclase

Methylation of the 1-position of several 3-alkylxanthines increased the potency of the derivative for inhibition of the low K_m cyclic AMP phosphodiesterase and relaxation of the tracheal muscle. Since a strong positive correlation was observed between the relaxant median effective concentration (EC_{50}) and the K_i value of each xanthine derivative, it suggests that low K_m cyclic AMP phosphodiesterase inhibition by xanthines may be the major effect and the explanation of the mechanism of action of theophylline as a bronchodilator. This concept would of necessity invoke a specific intracellular compartmentalization for a cyclic AMP pool that is exclusively used to initiate or maintain smooth muscle relaxation.

Since theophylline binds to the cyclic AMP–binding site on phosphodiesterase, theophylline may also bind to the cyclic AMP–binding site on the regulatory subunit of cyclic AMP–dependent protein kinase. Theoretically this could cause bronchodilation by activating or preventing the inactivation of this protein kinase without the necessity of causing a rise in the intracellular concentration of cyclic AMP. Theophylline binding to the R2C2 tetramer could cause dissociation to take place and yield the active catalytic subunit. The alternative might exist. Theophylline could bind to the free regulatory subunits and prevent the reassociation of the regulatory subunits and the catalytic subunits to form the inactive tetramer of protein kinase. This proposed mechanism of action of theophylline would also be consistent with the known synergistic effect between beta2 agonists and theophylline.

CYCLIC GMP

Cyclic GMP is also an important second messenger in virtually all cell types. Guanylate cyclase activity is found in the cell-surface plasma membrane, the cytoskeleton membrane, and the soluble fraction of cells [48]. Cell-surface receptors regulate guanylate cyclase in the plasma membrane (e.g., atrial natriuretic factor) [13]. Nitrovasodilators (e.g., nitroglycerin and nitroprusside) and the free radical (e.g., nitric oxide) also stimulate guanylate cyclase activity in the soluble fraction [75]. Nitric oxide is presumed to be an endogenous regulator (endothelium-derived relaxing factor [EDRF]) of the soluble form of guanylate cyclase and the mediator of the action of vasodilators in inducing vascular smooth muscle relaxation. The regulation of the catalytic activity of this soluble isozyme of guanylate cyclase involves calcium and calmodulin. The third type of guanylate cyclase is found

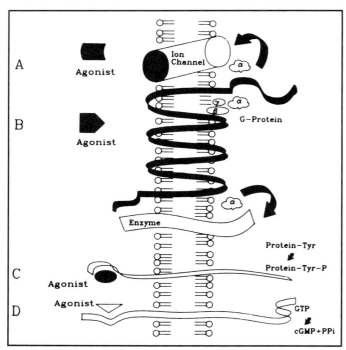

Fig. 15-8. *A depicts an agonist regulating an ion channel by interacting directly with the ion channel. B depicts an agonist binding to a beta-adrenergic receptor to release the alpha subunit of the guanine nucleotide regulatory protein (G-protein), which in turn interacts with another enzyme such as adenylate cyclase. C depicts an agonist interacting with a cell-surface receptor to stimulate the protein-tyrosine kinase activity which is the intracellular domain of the same protein that has the extracellular receptor domain. D depicts an agonist interacting with a cell-surface receptor to stimulate guanylate cyclase activity which is the intracellular domain of the same protein that has the extracellular receptor domain for the agonist depicted in D. (Reprinted with permission from Stephanie Schulz, Michael Chinkers, and David L. Garbers. The guanylate cyclase/receptor family of proteins. FASEB J. 3(9):2032, 1989.)*

in the intestinal brush border membrane and activated by *Escherichia coli* enterotoxin. The molecular targets for cyclic GMP involve cyclic GMP–dependent protein kinase. The number, type, and function of cellular proteins that are phosphorylated by cyclic GMP–dependent kinase remain to be elucidated.

There is some speculation that the combined activity of guanylate cyclase and a cyclic GMP–specific phosphodiesterase may function as a biologic unit. At first glance this combination of enzymatic activities would appear to constitute a futile cycle. However, on close scrutiny this cycle generates three protons. One proton is generated by guanylate cyclase with the conversion of GTP to cyclic GMP and inorganic pyrophosphate. A second proton is generated with the enzymatic hydrolysis of inorganic pyrophosphate. A third proton is generated with the hydrolysis of cyclic GMP to GMP. Thus, a cell could use this biochemical system as an intracellular proton generator to drive or regulate other cellular events.

Figure 15-8 illustrates the different types of cell-surface receptors and their interaction with adenylate cyclase, guanylate cyclase, protein-tyrosine kinase, and ion channels. The receptor ligand domain on the cell surface is linked to the intracellular domain via transmembrane domains of hydrophobic amino acids. Note that there is only one transmembrane domain for the receptor-activated guanylate cyclase. The transmembrane domain is structurally linked to the intracellular guanylate cyclase [75]. The single transmembrane domain of cell plasma membrane guanylate cyclase is markedly different from the seven

transmembrane domains associated with the beta₂-adrenergic receptor protein. Note that activation of adenylate cyclase involves G-proteins, whereas activation of guanylate cycle may not involve G-proteins. Thus, ligand binding results in the direct activation of guanylate cyclase without the participation of a Gs-protein. The guanylate cyclase molecule has an exterior domain that is the putative (peptide) agonist-binding portion. The complete mechanism of ligand activation of the membrane receptor form of guanylate cyclase is not understood fully but positive cooperativity has been shown for guanylate cyclase. Desensitization of the membrane receptor to regulated guanylate cyclase activity involves phosphorylation of the intracellular guanylate cyclase domain and results in the alteration of the interactions between substrate-binding sites.

The understanding of the biologic role of cyclic GMP in smooth muscle comes from the study of vascular smooth muscle. There is a paracrine relationship between vascular endothelial cells and vascular smooth muscle. Vascular endothelial cells synthesize and liberate EDRF, which initiates the following sequence of biochemical and physiologic events: interaction with a receptor on smooth muscle, activation of guanylate cyclase, a rise in the intracellular concentration of cyclic GMP, activation of a cyclic GMP–dependent protein kinase, phosphorylation of a cellular protein, a decrease in intracellular free calcium, and decreased vascular smooth muscle contraction [1]. A similar paracrine relationship between airway epithelial cells and bronchial smooth muscle is emerging. Airway epithelium exerts a profound influence on the reactivity of bronchial smooth muscle to both contractile and relaxation signals [37] (see Chap. 23). It is not surprising that there is a considerable heterogeneity in the effects of the epithelial factors at several different levels: between orders of bronchi, between species, and between pharmacologic agents. Whether or not nitric oxide has a physiologic role in regulating bronchial smooth muscle tension remains to be determined. In the presence of a high degree of cholinergic tone in airways, epithelial factors appear to exert their maximal effect for the relaxation of bronchial smooth muscle. The emerging revelations concerning the role of paracrine and autocrine mechanisms in the relationship between inflammatory processes and airway hyperresponsiveness may lead to more effective intervention in the prevention of bronchoconstriction in asthmatic patients [35].

REFERENCES

1. Adams, D. J., et al. Ion channels and regulation of intracellular calcium in vascular endothelial cells. *FASEB J.* 3:2389, 1989.
2. Adelstein, R. S., et al. Regulation of smooth muscle contractile proteins by calmodulin and cyclic AMP. *Fed. Proc.* 41:2873, 1982.
3. Barnes, P. J. Airway Receptors. In J. W. Jenne and S. Murphy (eds.), *Drug Therapy for Asthma.* New York: Marcel Dekker, 1987. Pp. 67–95.
4. Barnes, P. J. Cell-surface Receptors in Airway Smooth Muscle. In R. F. Coburn (ed.), *Airway Smooth Muscle in Health and Disease.* New York: Plenum, 1989. Pp. 77–98.
5. Barnes, P. J., Ind, P. W., and Dollery, C. T. Beta-adrenoceptors in Asthma and Their Response to Agonists. In A. B. Kay, K. F. Austen, and L. M. Lichtenstein (eds.), *Asthma, Physiology, Immunopharmacology and Treatment.* San Diego: Academic, 1984. Pp. 339–358.
6. Beavo, J. A., and Reisnyder, D. H. Primary sequence of cyclic nucleotide phosphodiesterase isozymes and the design of selective inhibitors. *Trends Pharmacol. Sci.* 11:150, 1990.
7. Berridge, M. J. Minireview—Calcium oscillations. *J. Biol. Chem.* 265:9583, 1990.
8. Bokoch, G. M., et al. Purification and properties of the inhibitory guanine nucleotide-binding regulatory component of adenylate cyclase. *J. Biol. Chem.* 259:3560, 1984.
9. Buckingham, J. C. Xanthines for asthma—Present status. *Trends Pharmacol. Sci.* 3:312, 1982.
10. Casperson, G. F., and Bourne, H. R. Biochemical and molecular genetic analysis of hormone-sensitive adenylyl cyclase. *Annu. Rev. Pharmacol. Toxicol.* 27:371, 1987.

11. Cauvin, C., et al. Beta-adrenergic Relaxation of Smooth Muscle and Second Messengers—Calcium in Smooth Muscle. In J. Morley (ed.), *Beta-adrenoceptors in Asthma.* San Diego: Academic, 1984. Pp. 25–47.

12. Cerione, R. A., et al. Functional differences in the beta gamma complexes of transducin and the inhibitory guanine nucleotide regulatory protein. *Biochemistry* 26:1485, 1987.

13. Chinkers, M., and Garbers, D. L. Signal transduction by guanylyl cyclases. *Annu. Rev. Biochem.* 60:553, 1991.

14. Chung, K. F., and Barnes, P. J. Bronchial hyperresponsiveness and inflammation in asthma. *Asthma Rev.* 1:25, 1987.

15. Church, M. K. Biochemical Basis of Pulmonary and Antiallergic Drugs. In J. P. Devlin (ed.), *Pulmonary and Antiallergic Drugs.* New York: Wiley, 1985. Pp. 43–121.

16. Coburn, R. F., and Baba, K. Coupling Mechanisms in Airway Smooth Muscle. In R. F. Coburn (ed.), *Airway Smooth Muscle in Health and Disease.* New York: Plenum, 1989. Pp. 183–197.

17. Conolly, M. E. Cyclic nucleotides, beta receptors, and bronchial asthma. *Adv. Cyclic Nucleotide Res.* 12:151, 1980.

18. Cooke, B. A. Beta-adrenoceptor-Adenylate Cyclase: Basic Mechanisms of Activation. In J. Morley (ed.), *Beta-adrenoceptors in Asthma.* San Diego: Academic, 1984. Pp. 1–24.

19. de Lanerolle, P. Cellular Control Mechanisms in Airway Smooth Muscle. In R. F. Coburn (ed.), *Airway Smooth Muscle in Health and Disease.* New York: Plenum, 1989. Pp. 99–125.

20. Dennis, E. A., et al. Role of phospholipases in generating lipid second messengers in signal transduction. *FASEB J.* 5:2068, 1991.

21. Dohlman, H. G., et al. Model systems for the study of seven-transmembrane-segment receptors. *Annu. Rev. Biochem.* 60:653, 1991.

22. Exton, J. H. Minireview—Signaling through phosphatidylcholine breakdown. *J. Biol. Chem.* 265:1, 1990.

23. Fain, J. N., Wallace, M. A., and Wojcikiewicz, R. J. H. Evidence for involvement of guanine nucleotide–binding regulatory proteins in the activation of phospholipases by hormones. *FASEB J.* 2:2569, 1988.

24. Freissmuth, M., Casey, P. J., and Gilman, A. G. G protein controls diverse pathways of transmembrane signaling. *FASEB J.* 3:2125, 1989.

25. Gabella, G. Structure of Airway Smooth Muscle and Its Innervation. In R. F. Coburn (ed.), *Airway Smooth Muscle in Health and Disease.* New York: Plenum, 1989. Pp. 1–16.

26. Gilman, A. G. G proteins: Transducers of receptor-generated signals. *Annu. Rev. Biochem.* 56:615, 1987.

27. Gomperts, B. D., Barrowman, M. M., and Cockcroft, S. Dual role for guanine nucleotides in stimulus-secretion coupling. *Fed. Proc.* 45:2156, 1986.

28. Harrison, J. K., Pearson, W. R., and Lynch, K. R. Molecular characterization of alpha-1 and alpha-2 adrenoceptors. *Trends Pharmacol. Sci.* 12:62, 1991.

29. Hay, D. W. P. Postulated Mechanisms Underlying Airway Hyperreactivity. In R. F. Coburn (ed.), *Airway Smooth Muscle in Health and Disease.* New York: Plenum, 1989. Pp. 199–235.

30. Hidaka, H., Tanaka, T., and Itoh, H. Selective inhibitors of three forms of cyclic nucleotide phosphodiesterases—Basic and potential clinical applications. *Adv. Cyclic Nucleotide Protein Phosphorylation Res.* 16:245, 1984.

31. Higashijima, T., et al. The effect of activating ligands on the intrinsic fluorescence of guanine nucleotide-binding regulatory proteins. *J. Biol. Chem.* 262:752, 1987.

32. Higashijima, T., et al. The effect of GTP and Mg^{++} on the GTPase activity and the fluorescent properties of Go. *J. Biol. Chem.* 262:757, 1987.

33. Hildebrandt, J. D., et al. Identification of a gamma-subunit associated with the adenylyl cyclase regulatory proteins Gs and Gi. *J. Biol. Chem.* 259:2039, 1984.

34. Hoffman, P. L., and Tabakoff, B. Ethanol and guanine nucleotide binding proteins: A selective interaction. *FASEB J.* 4:2612, 1990.

35. Holgate, S. T., et al. Pharmacology/Treatment. In S. T. Holgate (ed.), *The Role of Inflammatory Processes in Airway Hyperresponsiveness.* Oxford: Blackwell Scientific, 1989. Pp. 179–221.

36. Jacobson, K. A., et al. Novel therapeutics acting via purine receptors. *Biochem. Pharmacol.* 41:1399, 1991.

37. Jacoby, D. B., and Nadel, J. A. Airway Epithelial Metabolism and Airway Smooth Muscle Hyperresponsiveness. In R. F. Coburn (ed.), *Airway Smooth Muscle in Health and Disease.* New York: Plenum, 1989. Pp. 237–266.

38. Jenne, J. W. Physiology and Pharmacodynamics of the Xanthines. In J. W. Jenne and S. Murphy (eds.), *Drug Therapy for Asthma.* New York: Marcel Dekker, 1987. Pp. 297–334.

39. Johnson, G. L., Kaslow, R., and Bourne, H. R. Genetic evidence that cholera toxin substrates are regulatory components of adenylate cyclase. *J. Biol. Chem.* 253:7120, 1978.

40. Jones, D. T., et al. Biochemical characterization of three stimulatory GTP-binding proteins. *J. Biol. Chem.* 265:2671, 1990.

41. Kane-Ishii, C., and Ishii, S. Dual enhancer activities of the cyclic-AMP responsive element with cell type and promoter specificity. *Nucleic Acids Res.* 17:1521, 1989.

42. Kanoh, H., Yamada, K., and Sakane, F. Diacylglycerol kinase: A key modulator of signal transduction. *Trends Biochem. Sci.* 15:47, 1990.

43. Katada, R., et al. The inibitory guanine nucleotide-binding regulatory component of adenylate cyclase. *J. Biol. Chem.* 259:3578, 1984.

44. Kay, A. B. Cellular Mechanisms. In S. T. Holgate (ed.), *The Role of Inflammatory Processes in Airway Hyperresponsiveness.* Oxford: Blackwell Scientific, 1989. Pp. 151–179.

45. Kaziro, Y., et al. Structure and function of signal-transducing GTP-binding proteins. *Annu. Rev. Biochem.* 60:349, 1991.

46. King, C., and Cautrecasas, P. Peptide hormone-induced receptor mobility, aggregation, and internalization. *N. Engl. J. Med.* 305:77, 1981.

47. Klein, W. L., et al. Plasticity of neuronal receptors. *FASEB J.* 3:2132, 1989.

48. Krall, J. F. Receptor-mediated Regulation of Tension in Smooth Muscle Cells. In J. W. Jenne and S. Murphy (eds.), *Drug Therapy for Asthma.* New York: Marcel Dekker, 1987. Pp. 97–128.

49. Laitinen, L. A., and Laitinen, A. Pathology of Human Asthma. In M. A. Kaliner, P. J. Barnes, and C. G. A. Persson (eds.), *Asthma, Its Pathology and Treatment.* New York: Marcel Dekker, 1991. Pp. 103–134.

50. Leff, A. R. Role of the Adrenergic Nervous System in Asthma. In M. A. Kaliner, P. J. Barnes, and C. G. A. Persson (eds.), *Asthma, Its Pathology and Treatment.* New York: Marcel Dekker, 1991. Pp. 357–384.

51. Leff, A. R., et al. Physiological antagonism caused by adrenergic stimulation of canine tracheal muscle. *J. Appl. Physiol.* 60:216, 1986.

52. Lefkowitz, R. J., Hausdorff, W. P., and Caron, M. G. Role of phosphorylation in desensitization of the beta-adrenoceptor. *Trends Pharmacol. Sci.* 11:190, 1990.

53. Levitzki, A. Transmembrane signalling to adenylate cyclase in mammalian cells and in Saccharomyces cerevisiae. *Trends Biochem. Sci.* 13:298, 1988.

54. Lochrie, M. A., and Simon, M. I. G protein multiplicity in eukaryotic signal transduction systems. *Biochemistry* 27:4957, 1988.

55. Maelicke, A. The cGMP channel of the rod photoreceptor—A new type of channel structure? *Trends Biochem. Sci.* 15:39, 1990.

56. Manning, D. R., and Gilman, A. G. The regulatory components of adenylate cyclase and transducin. *J. Biol. Chem.* 258:7059, 1983.

57. Masters, S. B., et al. Carboxyl terminal domain of Gs-alpha specifies coupling of receptors to stimulation of adenylate cyclase. *Science* 241:448, 1988.

58. Merino, A., et al. Phosphorylation of cellular proteins regulates their binding to the cAMP response element. *J. Biol. Chem.* 264:21266, 1989.

59. Milligan, G., and Green, A. Agonist control of G-protein levels. *Trends Pharmacol. Sci.* 12:207, 1991.

60. Morley, J. (ed.), *Beta-adrenoceptors in Asthma.* San Diego: Academic, 1984.

61. Murphy, P. M., et al. Detection of multiple forms of Gi-alpha in HL60 cells. *FEBS Lett.* 221:81, 1987.

62. Nadel, J. A. Autonomic Regulation of Airway Smooth Muscle. In J. A. Nadel (ed.), *Physiology and Pharmacology of the Airways,* Vol. 15. New York: Marcel Dekker, 1980. P. 217.

63. Neer, E. J., and Clapham, D. E. Roles of G protein subunits in transmembrane signalling. *Nature* 333:129, 1988.

64. O'Connor, St. E., Dainty, I. A., and Leff, P. Further subclassification of ATP receptors based on agonist studies. *Trends Pharmacol. Sci.* 12:137, 1991.

65. O'Neil, K. T., and DeGrado, W. F. How calmodulin binds its targets: Sequence independent recognition of amphophilic alpha-helices. *Trends Biochem. Sci.* 15:59, 1990.

66. Pauwels, R., and Persson, C. G. A. Xanthines. In Kaliner, M. A., Barnes, P. J., and Persson, C. G. A. (eds.), *Asthma, Its Pathology and Treatment.* New York: Marcel Dekker, 1991. Pp. 503–521.

67. Pearce, F. L. Biochemical events involved in the release of anaphylactic mediators from mast cells. *Asthma Rev.* 1:95, 1987.

68. Persson, C. G. A. The pharmacology of anti-asthmatic xanthines and the role of adenosine. *Asthma Rev.* 1:61, 1987.

69. Persson, C. G. A., and Karlsson, J. In Vitro Responses to Bronchodilator Drugs. In J. W. Jenne and S. Murphy (eds.), *Drug Therapy for Asthma.* New York: Marcel Dekker, 1987. Pp. 129–176.

70. Rall, T. W. Evolution of the mechanism of action of methylxanthines: From calcium mobilizers to antagonists of adenosine receptors. *Pharmacologist* 24:277, 1982.

71. Rasmussen, R. *Calcium and cAMP as Synarchic Messengers.* New York: John Wiley, 1981.

72. Rothenberg, P. L., and Kahn, C. R. Insulin inhibits pertussis toxin-catalyzed ADP-ribosylation of G-proteins. *J. Biol. Chem.* 263:15546, 1988.

73. Sagi-Eisenberg, R. GTP-binding proteins as possible targets for protein kinase C action. *Trends Biochem. Sci.* 14:355, 1989.

74. Sanjar, S., et al. Platelet activation and airway hyperreactivity in asthma. *Asthma Rev.* 1:141, 1987.

75. Schulz, S., Yuen, P. S., and Garbers, G. L. The expanding family of guanylyl cyclases. *Trends Pharmacol. Sci.* 12:116, 1991.

76. Sibley, D. R., et al. Phosphorylation/dephosphorylation of the beta-adrenergic receptor regulates its functional coupling to adenylate cyclase and subcellular distribution. *Proc. Natl. Acad. Sci. USA* 85:9408, 1986.

77. Soderling, T. R. Minireview—Protein kinases. *J. Biol. Chem.* 265:1823, 1990.

78. Takuwa, R., Takuwa, N., and Rasmussen, H. The effects of isoproterenol on intracellular calcium concentration. *J. Biol. Chem.* 263:762, 1988.

79. Taylor, D. A., Bowman, B. F., and Stull, J. T. Cytoplasmic Ca^{++} is a primary determinant for myosin phosphorylation in smooth muscle cells. *J. Biol. Chem.* 265:6207, 1989.

80. Taylor, P., and Insel, P. A. Molecular Basis of Drug Action. In W. B. Pratt and P. Taylor (eds.), *Principles of Drug Action* (3rd ed.). New York: Churchill Livingstone, 1990. Pp. 103–200.

81. Taylor, S. S., Buechler, J. A., and Yonemoto, W. cAMP-dependent protein kinase: Framework for a diverse family of regulatory enzymes. *Annu. Rev. Biochem.* 59:971, 1990.

82. Vapaatalo, H., and Metsa-Ketela, T. Cyclic nucleotides and calcium as mediators of cellular functions. *Prog. Pharmacol.* 4: 1980.

83. Vapaatalo, H., and Tampere, T. Cyclic nucleotides and calcium mediators of cellular function. *Prog. Pharmacol.* 4:1, 1980.

84. Wessling-Resnick, M., et al. Ezymatic model for receptor activation of GTP-binding regulatory proteins. *Trends Biochem. Sci.* 12:471, 1987.

85. White, M. V., and Kaliner, M. A. Mast Cells and Asthma. In M. A. Kaliner, P. J. Barnes, and C. G. A. Persson (eds.), *Asthma, Its Pathology and Treatment.* New York: Marcel Dekker, 1991. Pp. 409–440.

86. Giembycz, M. A. Could isoenzyme-selective phosphodiesterase inhibitors render bronchodilator therapy redundant in the treatment of bronchial asthma? *Biochem. Pharmacol.* 43:2041, 1992.

87. Manji, H. K. G Proteins: Implications for Psychiatry. *Am. J. Psychiatry* 149:746, 1992.

Advances in Receptor Biochemistry

16

M. Maureen Dale
Stuart J. Hirst

This chapter deals with the receptors and signal transduction events in smooth muscle. The processes of contraction and relaxation are described, as are the various signal transduction mechanisms proposed as linking receptor activation to responses of cells in general and smooth muscle in particular. The range of receptors that initiate either contraction or relaxation in airway muscle is also considered, analyzing for each receptor and the response it elicits the extent to which the detailed signal transduction events have been determined.

CONTRACTION

Contraction of all types of muscle involves the cyclic interaction of myosin and actin whereby myosin filaments and actin filaments slide past each other without shortening. The heads of the myosin molecules link to actin filaments, forming *cross-bridges*. A conformational change in an individual head constitutes the *power stroke,* with hydrolysis of adenosine triphosphate (ATP) providing the energy. The head then disconnects and reconnects further along the actin filament and the process starts again—this is referred to as *cross-bridge cycling.* In smooth muscle, myosin activation requires phosphorylation of the 20,000-d light chains in the myosin head (Fig. 16-1). According to most studies, contraction of smooth muscle has two phases. In the first there is a rise in intracellular calcium concentration ($[Ca^{++}]_i$), which is the trigger for contraction (i.e., shortening of the muscle fiber) [195]. Ca^{++} binds to calmodulin and the main action of this complex is activation of myosin light-chain kinase (MLCK); this phosphorylates myosin, stimulating the actin-activated ATPase in the myosin head and promoting cross-bridge cycling (Figs. 16-1 and 16-2). In the second phase, maximal shortening velocity diminishes but tension is maintained although $[Ca^{++}]_i$ declines to near basal levels and myosin light-chain phosphorylation decreases (see Fig. 16-2). The data on which this model is based have been reviewed by Sommerville and Hartshorne [216]. It should be noted that some data, particularly those obtained from canine airway muscle (see below), conflict with this model [48]. The basis for the second phase of tension maintenance is still a matter of debate. A significant proposal put forward to explain the second phase was that tension is maintained by non-cycling or slowly cycling cross-bridges, termed *latch-bridges* [50]. Since a lower $[Ca^{++}]_i$ is required for tension maintenance, a second Ca^{++}-dependent regulatory mechanism with greater sensitivity to Ca^{++} than MLCK must operate. It has been suggested that this could involve roles for actin-bound caldesmon or protein kinase C (PKC), or both [102, 109, 137] (discussed below). On the other hand, some workers consider that it is not necessary to invoke a second Ca^{++}-dependent mechanism; they propose that Ca^{++}-dependent myosin phosphorylation alone is sufficient to explain latch, the suggestion being that there are two populations of cross-bridges, one that is nonphosphorylated and noncycling or slowly cycling and one that is phosphorylated and rapidly cycling, and that the balance between the two determines the tension [87, 151]. Some evidence, however, is inconsistent with this latter proposal [115].

Much of the work on the mechanism of contraction has been done on arterial and other types of smooth muscle, but similar results have been obtained in airway muscle [70, 107, 173, 194, 207, 227]. However, it should be noted that in canine airway muscle there is little alteration of myosin light-chain phosphorylation during tension maintenance [47, 114, 141] (see also Chap. 25).

Signal Transduction Mechanisms for Contraction

An increase in $[Ca^{++}]_i$ is the main biochemical event in contraction, but activation of the PKC pathway may also be implicated. The roles of these pathways in regulating airway smooth muscle contractility have been reviewed extensively in two recent articles [40, 203a].

Calcium
The main action of calcium in initiating contraction is by binding to calmodulin and activating MLCK, as explained above (see Fig. 16-1). But it may have other actions—enhancing contractility by binding directly to myosin, modulating contractility by removing the inhibitory effect of caldesmon, and activating other kinases such as PKC [2, 109].

During receptor activation the $[Ca^{++}]_i$ can rise from the resting level of 1×10^{-7} M to approximately 5×10^{-6} M [147]. $[Ca^{++}]_i$ has been measured by Ca^{++}-sensitive dyes such as aequorin [147, 225] or Fura-2-acetoxymethylester (Fura-2) [166]. Different patterns of response are reported with the two reagents. For example, in rabbit aorta, an alpha$_1$ agonist that causes maintained contraction gives a transient Ca^{++} signal with aequorin, but with Fura-2 it gives a relatively sustained increase in Ca^{++} concentration, which decreases slowly [111]. The difference may be due both to the different characteristics of the two reagents and to compartmentalization of myoplasmic Ca^{++}. Thus aequorin is thought to overrepresent the high Ca^{++} regions while Fura-2 gives the average $[Ca^{++}]_i$ [111]. Further information on this may come from using Fura-2 in digital imaging microscopy [75]. Nevertheless, data available at present indicate that in airway muscle strips, there is a reasonable correlation between the concentration of some agonists (e.g., carbachol) on the one hand and the change in Fura-2 fluorescence and contraction on the other [166]. In vascular smooth muscle cells, Morgan and colleagues correlated Ca^{++} profiles with the temporal profiles of isometric tension, myosin light-chain phosphorylation, and maximum unloaded shortening velocity [148, 149].

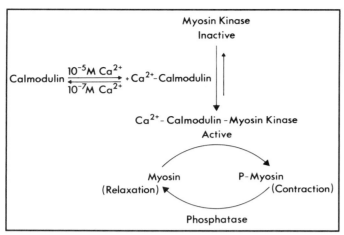

Fig. 16-1. *The regulation of smooth muscle contraction by cytosolic calcium. Elevated Ca^{++} (10^{-5} M) interacts with calmodulin. The resulting Ca^{++}-calmodulin complex binds the inactive form of myosin light-chain kinase (shown as myosin kinase). This activates the kinase, allowing it to phosphorylate myosin. Phosphorylated myosin (P-Myosin) interacts with actin (cross-bridge formation) and initiates the development of muscle tension. Lowering of the cytosolic Ca^{++} concentration to 10^{-7} M leads to dissociation of calmodulin from activated myosin light-chain kinase, returning the enzyme to its inactive form. Under these conditions phosphorylated myosin can be dephosphorylated by a phosphatase causing relaxation of the muscle. (Redrawn and adapted from R. S. Adelstein and E. Eisenberg. Regulation and kinetics of the actin-myosin-ATP interaction. Annu. Rev. Biochem. 49:921, 1980; and P. de Lanerolle. Cellular Control Mechanisms in Airway Smooth Muscle. In R. F. Coburn (ed.), Airway Smooth Muscle in Health and Disease. New York: Plenum, 1989. Pp. 99–125.)*

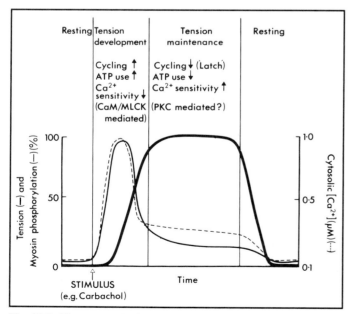

Fig. 16-2. *The proposed scheme for the contraction-relaxation cycle in smooth muscle, showing the two phases of smooth muscle contraction together with changes in cytosolic Ca^{++} and myosin phosphorylation under conditions of rest and during tension development and maintenance. (Redrawn from L. E. Sommerville and D. J. Hartshorne. Intracellular calcium and smooth muscle contraction. Cell Calcium 7: 353, 1986.)*

It should be noted that in vascular muscle, various alpha[1] agonists cause greater contraction and greater phosphorylation than does K^+ for a given $[Ca^{++}]_i$, which suggests that receptor-mediated contraction may depend not only on increased $[Ca^{++}]_i$ per se, but also on an increased sensitivity of the contractile elements to Ca^{++} [27, 111, 148, 190].

As in other cell types, the increase in $[Ca^{++}]_i$ in airway smooth muscle may be brought about by an influx of extracellular Ca^{++} (the concentration of which is 10,000-fold higher than that within the cell) and/or by a release of Ca^{++} from internal stores by enzymic mechanisms [40, 73, 194], and the contribution of these two sources varies not only with different muscles but also with different agonists in the same muscle.

Contraction due to an influx of Ca^{++} through voltage-gated Ca^{++} channels has been referred to as *electromechanical coupling*. Voltage-independent mechanisms for increasing Ca^{++} and causing contraction have been termed *pharmacomechanical coupling* [40, 194, 215]. This latter type of coupling could be considered as including both the release of Ca^{++} from internal stores and also voltage-independent, receptor-mediated influx.

It should be stressed that the Ca^{++} signal is not constant but oscillates [6, 20, 174, 230].

The homeostatic mechanisms controlling and reversing the rise in $[Ca^{++}]_i$ include Na^+-Ca^{++} exchange, Ca^{++} efflux by the Ca^{++}-Mg^{++}-ATPase, and uptake of Ca^{++} into the sarcoplasmic reticulum. Na^+-Ca^{++} exchange is driven by the movement of Na^+ down its electrochemical gradient into the cell and is linked to the Na^+-K^+-ATPase. That Na^+-Ca^{++} exchange occurs in vascular muscle is clear [26] and there is some evidence that it has a role in tracheal muscle [29]. A membrane Ca^{++}-Mg^{++}-ATPase, an electroneutral exchanger that exports Ca^{++} out of the cell in exchange for $2H^+$, occurs in the membrane of many smooth muscles including those of the airways [83]. The Ca^{++}-calmodulin complex stimulates this Ca^{++} pump, which suggests that the stimulus initiating the rise in $[Ca^{++}]_i$ also operates to modulate it [183]. In some tissues the cyclic adenosine monophosphate–dependent kinase [154, 183, 184] and PKC [124] have been shown to stimulate the pump, though incontrovertible evidence in airway smooth muscle is lacking. Ca^{++} uptake into the sarcoplasmic reticulum occurs through a specific ATPase [31]. Calsequestrin, the high-capacity, low-affinity binding protein, increases the Ca^{++} storage capacity in the sarcoplasmic reticulum [247].

The mechanisms for increasing $[Ca^{++}]_i$ are now considered.

Electromechanical Coupling. Electromechanical mechanisms are dependent on changes in the membrane potential. In smooth muscle in general, these changes can occur as a result of either receptor-mediated influx of Na^+ ions through ligand-gated ion channels or the direct effects of depolarizing agents such as K^+ (see Rang and Dale [180] for simple summary). Depolarization results in an inward Ca^{++} current through voltage-operated calcium channels and also an outward K^+ current, as reviewed by Coburn and Baron [40]. There are four types of voltage-dependent Ca^{++} channels—L, N, T, and P [189]; those found on smooth muscle are the L-type, which can be blocked by pharmacologic agents such as verapamil, nifedipine, and diltiazem—the so-called voltage-sensitive Ca^{++} channel blockers (see also Chap. 71).

Airway smooth muscle is strongly rectified (i.e., resistant to spontaneous depolarization) and action potentials are rarely evoked [41, 64]. Voltage-operated Ca^{++} channels certainly exist in airway smooth muscle and are responsible for the Ca^{++} influx induced by depolarizing agents [40]; however, there is considerable debate as to whether these Ca^{++} channels are involved in the contractile response to physiologic agonists (discussed below). There is a suggestion that though two distinct types of Ca^{++} channels (voltage operated and receptor operated) exist in some types of smooth muscle, calcium influx in airway smooth muscle may involve a single dihydropyridine-sensitive inward current not dissimilar to the slow L-type Ca^{++} current recorded in cardiac muscle cells [17].

Pharmacomechanical Coupling. Various studies have undermined the original concept that membrane depolarization resulting in the opening of voltage-dependent calcium channels was a necessary and sufficient prerequisite for increasing [Ca^{++}]$_i$ in smooth muscle. Early work by Evans and coworkers [58] demonstrated that agonists can contract ileal smooth muscle that had already been depolarized by K$^+$-containing media; a similar response is seen in airway muscle [117]. Furthermore, airway muscle can contract in Ca^{++}-free media [61], and acetylcholine-induced contractions of many types of airway muscle are resistant to the dihydropyridine calcium antagonists that block voltage-dependent calcium channels and totally inhibit K$^+$-induced contractions [73].

It has thus become clear that there are mechanisms for increasing [Ca^{++}]$_i$ that are not gated by membrane potential. As specified above, the possibilities are (1) the mobilization of intracellular calcium and (2) voltage-independent, receptor-mediated Ca^{++} influx.

It is now well established that in cells in which there is mobilization of intracellular Ca^{++}, an early event following ligand-receptor interaction is the activation of a phospholipase C (PLC), which results in the hydrolysis of phosphatidylinositol bisphosphate (PIP$_2$)—a minor phospholipid component of the cell membrane—to give diacylglycerol and inositol-1,4,5-trisphosphate (IP$_3$). Diacylglycerol activates PKC (see below) and IP$_3$ mobilizes intracellular calcium [21, 153, 158, 179] (Fig. 16-3).

There are multiple PLC enzymes in mammalian cells. As many as 13 isoforms have now been recognized, categorized into four groups designated alpha, beta, gamma, and delta [59, 123]. All isoforms can use all the phosphatidylinositols as substrates, though in general they hydrolyze phosphatidylinositol more efficiently in high Ca^{++} concentrations and PIP$_2$ at low, physiologic Ca^{++} concentrations [133]. There is evidence that this transduction mechanism can operate in smooth muscle since purified PIP$_2$ is hydrolyzed by smooth muscle membrane-bound PLC, generating IP$_3$ [67]. Furthermore, in neurally stimulated bovine tracheal muscle, the temporal relationship between inositol lipid hydrolysis and contraction supports a role for PIP$_2$ breakdown in signal transduction [145] and there is substantial evidence that receptor stimulation in intact smooth muscle preparations results in PIP$_2$ breakdown.

Many receptor types are coupled to their effector systems (enzymes or ion channels) by G-proteins. G-protein–coupled receptors have seven transmembrane spanning segments, one of the intracellular loops being able to interact with a G-protein (discussed below). G-proteins, which are freely diffusible in the plane of the membrane, consist of three subunits, alpha, beta, and gamma, the alpha subunit having guanosine triphosphatase (GTPase) activity. On binding to an agonist-occupied receptor, the alpha subunit dissociates from the other subunits and is then able to activate an effector, for example, an enzyme such as PLC (or adenylate cyclase; see later). Activation of the effector is terminated when bound GTP is hydrolyzed, which permits the alpha subunit to recombine with the beta and gamma subunits. The subject of G-proteins in transmembrane signaling is reviewed by Gilman [74], Taylor [226], and Birnbaumer et al. [23]. There is considerable indirect information that G-proteins are involved in the regulation of PLC in many cell types including smooth muscle [23, 59].

The evidence that IP$_3$ mobilizes calcium from the endoplasmic reticulum or specialized calciosomes in many cell types is now very strong [21, 53]. IP$_3$ apparently opens a calcium channel in the relevant Ca^{++}-storage organelle by binding to a specific receptor [53, 153] (see Fig. 16-3); K$^+$ uptake occurs concomitantly, ensuring electrical neutrality. Studies on rat cerebellar Purkinje

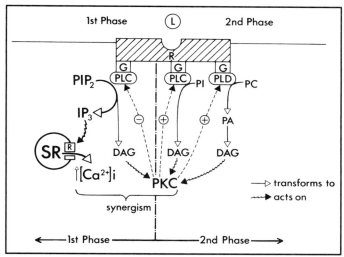

Fig. 16-3. *Proposed scheme of the signal transduction mechanisms involved in smooth muscle contraction. The initial event following interaction of a ligand (L) with a receptor (R, shown hatched) is G-protein–mediated activation of a phospholipase C (PLC) that hydrolyzes phosphatidylinositol bisphosphate (PIP$_2$) to give inositol trisphosphate (IP$_3$), which mobilizes Ca^{++}—the main internal messenger for contraction—by acting on a receptor (R) on the sarcoplasmic reticulum (SR). (The effect of the elevated intracellular calcium concentration ([Ca^{++}]$_i$) is depicted in Figs. 16-1 and 16-2.) Diacylglycerol (DAG) is generated concomitantly with IP$_3$, and activates protein kinase C (PKC), which has a negative feedback effect on the PIP$_2$-specific PLC, terminating the first phase of transduction. A second phase, operating at near basal [Ca^{++}]$_i$, is believed to occur, involving PKC. Sustained activation of PKC is produced by sustained generation of diacylglycerol, either directly from phosphatidylcholine (PC) by a PC-specific PLC (not shown) or from phosphatidylinositol (PI) by a PI-specific PLC, or indirectly from the phosphatidic acid (PA) derived from PC by the action of phospholipase D (PLD). These phospholipases can be stimulated by the PKC activated in the first phase and/or by their association, via G-proteins, with the original ligand-stimulated receptor.*

cells indicate that the receptor is a membrane glycoprotein of approximately 250 kd, occurring as a tetramer in vivo [53]. The purified protein possesses both Ca^{++} channel activity and a binding site for IP$_3$ [63]. Each of the four subunits of the receptor has an independent ligand-binding site on the N-terminal end, and the transmembrane sections form the calcium channel [143]. Binding of IP$_3$ to the N-terminal site causes a large conformational change, constituting a mechanism for channel opening [143].

Much of the work on IP$_3$ quoted above has been done on cerebellar tissue but there is clear evidence that it is relevant for smooth muscle; the mouse smooth muscle IP$_3$ receptor has been shown to be structurally and functionally similar to the mouse brain IP$_3$ receptor [135]. IP$_3$ has been shown to release calcium from skinned and/or cultured vascular and tracheal smooth muscle cells [39, 211, 221, 234, 248] and to cause both calcium release and tension development in permeabilized strips of arterial muscle [213]. Recent work has demonstrated that it opens voltage-independent Ca^{++} channels in aortic muscle sarcoplasmic reticulum incorporated into plasma lipid bilayers [57], the activity being enhanced by ATP but inhibited by heparin. Differences from the calcium-activated calcium channel in the sarcoplasmic reticulum of skeletal muscle are that it is not activated by caffeine and it has a 10-fold lower conductance (10 picosiemens) (although it should be noted that smooth muscle seems to have a separate caffeine-activated Ca^{++} channel in the sarcoplasmic reticulum) [99, 114, 248]. Single-channel analyses on isolated aortic muscle sarcoplasmic reticulum have provided clear evidence that IP$_3$ could activate the calcium channels at physiologically relevant concentrations of IP$_3$. The IP$_3$ receptor from bovine aortic muscle has been isolated and shown to be a tetramer of 224 kd [33]. Stereo-specific binding sites for IP$_3$ have been characterized in bovine tracheal muscle [37], and in dog trachea, IP$_3$ has been shown to produce both concentration-dependent Ca^{++} release [89] and contraction [114] in suitably permeabilized preparations. In such permeabilized cells, IP$_3$ stimulation of Ca^{++} release can be markedly enhanced by GTP [39, 71]. There appear to be two types of Ca^{++}-releasing vesicles, both sensitive to GTP, but only one sensitive to IP$_3$ [72, 214]. It is suggested that GTP may function to transfer Ca^{++} between intracellular compartments, possibly via some type of junctional complex and that this might regulate the size of the Ca^{++} pool on which IP$_3$ acts [53].

Although most evidence favors IP$_3$ as the main intracellular messenger responsible for mobilizing Ca^{++}, it should be stated that some studies have presented evidence for Ca^{++}-induced Ca^{++} release in ileal smooth muscle [160] and feline airway smooth muscles [103].

In the absence of changes in the membrane potential, intracellular Ca^{++} can also be elevated as a result of voltage-independent, receptor-mediated calcium influx. Several agonists stimulate Ca^{++} influx into smooth muscle cells [238], though there is some controversy on this point (discussed below). On theoretic grounds, voltage-independent Ca^{++} entry could occur through different sorts of Ca^{++} channels [193]:

1. Those that are part of a receptor-channel complex, as in the ligand-gated nicotinic receptor (e.g., at the neuromuscular junction)
2. Those coupled directly to receptors via G-proteins, as occurs with the muscarinic receptor–operated K$^+$ channel in cardiac muscle [23]
3. Those opened in the plasma membrane by a direct action of diffusible intracellular second messengers, as for the Ca^{++}-operated channel in the neutrophil [240] or the putative channel operated by an IP$_3$ metabolite [53]
4. Those linked to the Ca^{++} concentration of internal Ca^{++} pools (e.g., the putative calciosome) by second messengers such as IP$_3$ [176]

In excitable cells in general much less is known about this type of Ca^{++} influx than about voltage-gated influx. There are no potent specific ligands for most of the putative voltage-independent channels themselves, and in most tissues it has proved difficult to detect and measure the changes in individual cells or at single-channel level. However, in arterial smooth muscle cells, direct ligand gating of Ca^{++} channels by ATP without involvement of diffusible second messengers has been reported [19] and there is also other evidence for voltage-independent, receptor-mediated entry [197]. The information on voltage-independent, receptor-mediated Ca^{++} entry in airway smooth muscle is discussed in the sections on the relevant receptors.

Diacylglycerol–Protein Kinase C

PKC has a crucial role in signal transduction in many cell types [60, 158]. The enzyme requires diacylglycerol, Ca^{++}, and phospholipid (preferably phosphatidylserine) for its activation. Diacylglycerol activates PKC (see Fig. 16-3) by greatly increasing its affinity for Ca^{++} and phospholipid, and translocation of PKC to the membrane may be required for this to happen [98]. There are multiple subspecies of PKC with subtly different properties, some of which are capable of being activated by diacylglycerol in the absence of any increase of the Ca^{++} concentration (i.e., at rest-

ing Ca^{++} concentrations) [170]. Most cell types express several PKC subspecies in different ratios [60], and at least two types, with different functions, have been identified in cultured arterial smooth muscle cells [112].

Many studies have now shown that activation of PKC results in a slowly developing sustained contraction of smooth muscle. Various techniques have been used for studying the effect of PKC activation. The phorbol esters such as phorbol myristate acetate (PMA) and 4β-phorbol dibutyrate (4β-PDBu), are powerful PKC activators, 4β-PDBu being more potent in smooth muscle than PMA [45]. More physiologically relevant activators of PKC include the diacylglycerol analogs such as 1-oleoyl,2-acetylglycerol (OAG) and dioctonylglycerol (DiC$_8$). It should be emphasized that when a whole tissue is studied (e.g., smooth muscle strips), the PKC activators will stimulate not only the smooth muscle cells themselves but also numerous other cell types, and that this will complicate the interpretation of results unless suitable controls are included [162].

The role of PKC in tissue responses can also be assessed by using PKC inhibitors. A commonly used inhibitor is H7 ([1-(5-isoquinolinesulfonyl)-2 methylpiperazine]) [93] but interpretation of results with this agent is fraught with difficulty since it is equally potent against the cyclic AMP–dependent kinase. More potent and specific inhibitors are now available [233].

There have been numerous studies of the phorbol ester–induced contraction of arterial muscle, as reviewed by Obianime and Dale [161]. Different results have been obtained with different species and different vessels in terms of the necessity for external Ca^{++}, the effect on internal Ca^{++}, and the effect on voltage-operated Ca^{++} channels, but there is clear evidence that phorbol esters can cause contraction without increasing [Ca^{++}]$_i$ and that in skinned arterial muscle, contractions can be evoked at a Ca^{++} concentration that does not itself result in contraction [109]. The first study showing concentration-dependent contraction of airway smooth muscle was by Dale and Obianime [44]. Subsequent studies demonstrated that there was synergism between PKC activators and agents which raised [Ca^{++}]$_i$ [45, 168], that a response to phorbol ester still occurred in the absence of external Ca^{++} [45], and that both the phorbol ester response and the synergistic response were due to direct effects on smooth muscle and not due to activation of other cell types [162]. In some airway tissues (e.g., guinea pig trachea) phorbol esters produce biphasic responses, contraction at low and relaxation at high concentrations. Various explanations have been put forward [95, 140, 178, 203]. It is possible that PKC activation causes relaxation by releasing the potent nonadrenergic, noncholinergic inhibitory transmitter [95], now believed to be nitric oxide in some species [127, 231].

Other actions of phorbol esters in airway muscle are activation of the Na$^+$-H$^+$ antiport [217] and activation of the Na$^+$-K$^+$-ATPase [203, 217].

Studies of the phosphorylation by PKC of components of the contractile machinery of smooth muscle cells have been numerous and mostly carried out on arterial muscle preparations, as reviewed by Kamm and Stull [109]. Myosin heavy chain is phosphorylated by PKC in both arterial muscle [237] and airway muscle [109]. Myosin light chain, in addition to the crucial phosphorylation by MLCK at serine 19, is also phosphorylated by PKC at other sites, the effect being reported variously to decrease myosin ATPase activity, to inhibit the conformation change induced by MLCK [110], and to have no effect on MLCK action [209, 222]. MLCK itself is phosphorylated by PKC, which results in a reduced affinity for calmodulin [101, 109]. Myosin heavy chain is phosphorylated by PKC in both arterial muscle [237] and in airway muscle [106], as is caldesmon [236]. The significance of these diverse effects in PKC-mediated contraction is a matter of debate and has still to be resolved.

One needs to address the question as to the possible physiologic role of PKC in smooth muscle. One possibility arises from the data outlined above, that two calcium-dependent processes are implicated in contraction: an initial phosphorylation of myosin which triggers rapid cycling of cross-bridges and tension development, succeeded by a second process of tension maintenance with a lower calcium requirement. Rasmussen and colleagues [185] proposed that this second regulatory mechanism involved PKC, stressing that both agonist-induced and phorbol ester–induced maintained tensions in tracheal smooth muscle are associated with similar patterns of protein phosphorylation [169]. Furthermore, there is indirect evidence that PKC activation increases the sensitivity of the contractile apparatus for calcium in both arterial muscle [27, 105, 157] and airway muscle [37, 162, 166], although some evidence implies that it acts by increasing $[Ca^{++}]_i$ [191].

One of the proposed roles for PKC in the second phase of tension maintenance is that the downregulation by PKC of the actin-activated ATPase activity of myosin might translate into a slowing of cross-bridge turnover but not a cessation of contractile activity [2]. A more complex hypothesis was put forward by Rasmussen and colleagues [187]; it modifies the original latch-bridge hypothesis and stresses that during the sustained phase, whether due to an agonist or a PKC activator, there is phosphorylation of caldesmon, several intermediate filament proteins (including desmin and synemin), and several low-molecular-weight cytosolic proteins. It has been suggested that this actin–intermediate filament system (which is unique to smooth muscle) could be implicated in tonic contraction [210], and a role for caldesmon in latch-bridge formation has been proposed [241]. Rasmussen and colleagues further developed this suggestion by proposing that tension maintenance involves a type of latch state due to PKC-induced phosphorylation causing structural rearrangements of this system [186, 187]. If PKC *is* implicated in the sustained phase of contraction, there would need to be a sustained presence of an endogenous PKC activator. This could not be the diacylglycerol derived from PIP_2 as there is good evidence that the activation of PKC has a negative feedback effect in that it switches off agonist-stimulated PIP_2 hydrolysis and thus generation of diacylglycerol and IP_3 from PIP_2 [55] in arterial smooth muscle [205] and airway muscle [152]. This negative feedback effect is possibly the main basis for the transience of the initial calcium signal described above (see Fig. 16-2). Nevertheless, data from receptor-stimulated vascular muscle indicate that diacylglycerol production is biphasic and sustained [80]. The mechanism for the second phase could well be that PKC also initiates phosphatidylcholine degradation by a PLC pathway to give diacylglycerol directly, and by a phospholipase D (PLD) pathway to give phosphatidic acid which is cleaved to diacylglycerol by a phosphohydrolase [30, 172, 206]. Diacylglycerol generation from phosphatidylinositol by a phosphatidylinositol-specific PLC pathway can also occur. These routes to diacylglycerol formation have all been shown to occur in smooth muscle [82, 97] (see Fig. 16-3). But note that there is some initial evidence that phosphatidic acid may also function as an internal messenger in several cell types [22] including smooth muscle [164]. The role of phosphatidylcholine hydrolysis in signal transduction was recently reviewed [22, 172, 227a].

A general scheme may therefore be proposed for signal transduction for contraction of smooth muscle, as shown in Fig. 16-3.

We have shown that in guinea pig airway smooth muscle, PKC activators cause a sustained contraction that is virtually insensitive to the subsequent action of beta$_2$ agonists (which can totally reverse the histamine-induced contraction) but that is considerably more sensitive to subsequent enprofylline [163]. We have suggested on the basis of this and other circumstantial evidence, that inappropriate activation of PKC may contribute to the pathogenesis of the late phase of asthma [163]. However, it should be emphasized that although PKC is generally considered to have a

pivotal function in stimulus-response coupling [96], its precise role in ligand-stimulated transduction in smooth muscle has not yet been fully established. For one thing, the use of the powerful, unphysiologic PKC activators (such as phorbol esters) usually used to study the role of PKC may give results which themselves are unphysiologic.

The receptors mediating contraction of airway smooth muscle will now be considered.

Receptors Mediating Contraction

The physiologic and pathologic responses of airway smooth muscle depend on the interaction of transmitters or inflammatory mediators with surface receptors. The muscarinic receptor is taken as a model for this type of reaction since most of the fundamental work on transduction mechanisms in smooth muscle has been done on this receptor. Histamine H$_1$ receptors are then discussed, followed by brief consideration of leukotriene, prostanoid, tachykinin, endothelin, and adrenergic alpha$_1$ receptors.

Muscarinic Receptors

At least five distinct species of muscarinic receptors have been revealed by gene cloning [125], but three main types, M$_1$, M$_2$, and M$_3$, have been characterized by pharmacologic techniques using selective antagonists [92, 189] (see Chap. 17). Experimental evidence indicates that most muscarinic receptors are coupled to their effector systems via G-proteins, and have a structure similar to that of others in the family of G-protein–coupled receptors; this is discussed in more detail for the beta receptor, below. The M$_3$ subtype, as studied in many tissues, transduces signals through phosphoinositide hydrolysis, and the M$_2$ receptors are linked via inhibitory G-proteins to adenylate cyclase [92]. Although studies have shown that both M$_2$ and M$_3$ receptors occur in bovine airway muscle [25, 130], the evidence in human airways is that the receptors are exclusively of the M$_3$ subtype [134].

M$_3$ Receptors. The density of M$_3$ receptors is high in the smooth muscle of the large airways and decreases in the smaller airways, being virtually lacking in the smallest bronchioles [12]. Stimulation of M$_3$ receptors causes a brisk contraction of airway muscle, composed of an initial rapid increase in tension followed by a more slowly developing sustained contraction [18]. There is little evidence for the contraction being due to electromechanical coupling; it is mainly, if not entirely, due to pharmacomechanical coupling. After M$_3$ receptor stimulation a transient increase in phosphorylation of myosin light chain correlates with the transient increase in shortening velocity in rabbit and bovine tracheal preparations [70, 107] but not canine preparations [114, 141]. The main phosphorylation site in bovine trachea is the serine site known to be the site phosphorylated by MLCK [106], but other cell components, caldesmon, synemin, and desmin, are also phosphorylated [169]. A latent period of 500 msec precedes the increase in isometric tension and the phosphorylation of myosin light chain [145] in neurally stimulated bovine tracheal preparations (in which the released acetylcholine will be acting on the M$_3$ receptor). Myosin light-chain phosphorylation reaches maximum by 6 to 15 seconds and can be correlated with the rise in internal Ca^{++} concentration from 150 to 492 nM in 15 seconds, both changes being transient [227]. The increase in calcium also correlates with the percentage increase in contraction [114, 166].

The mechanisms for the release of Ca^{++} from internal stores by M$_3$ receptor activation are now well established. M$_3$ receptors are coupled to G-proteins in airway muscle [130] and there is now excellent evidence that this results in phosphoinositide hydrolysis in airway smooth muscle [196]. Muscarinic agonists evoke rapid breakdown of PIP_2 with an increase in diacylglycerol, the action being independent of external Ca^{++} [224]. The PIP_2

turnover and IP_3 accumulation correlate well with the extent of contraction and receptor occupancy [77, 142] and the generation of IP_3 occurs during the latent period for increase in tension [56, 145] and myosin phosphorylation [145]. The IP_3 concentration rises rapidly and then returns to baseline [36] as the concentrations of the IP_3 metabolites, IP_4 and IP_2, increase [35], these responses being abrogated by atropine [34]. The carbachol-induced increase in IP_3 is concentration dependent, reaches its peak in 30 seconds, and lasts about 3 minutes [114].

However, the situation regarding the role of external Ca^{++} as a source of elevated calcium is still confused. Some early studies indicated that external Ca^{++} is necessary [18, 61, 103]; others suggested that Ca^{++} influx either does not occur or does not involve voltage-dependent Ca^{++} channels—seven such studies are quoted by Giembycz and Rodger [73]. More recent experiments in canine tracheal strips suggested that external calcium is necessary for the tonic but not the phasic aspect of the M_3 receptor–mediated response [114], that the contraction is inhibited by blockers of the voltage-sensitive Ca^{++} channels [166], and that in Fura-2–loaded bovine tracheal muscle, carbachol causes Ca^{++} influx which was decreased by Ca^{++} channel blockers in a concentration-dependent manner [62]. The consensus would appear to be that Ca^{++} influx may be essential for the tonic muscarinic M_3 receptor–induced contraction but that the mechanism involved has yet to be resolved, and may differ between species. There is also some interesting evidence which implies that in porcine airways, when PIP_2 breakdown is prevented by phorbol ester–induced PKC activation by negative feedback on PLC (illustrated in Fig. 16-3), carbachol produces contractions dependent on external Ca^{++} that enters the cell through voltage-dependent channels [9]; this suggests that PKC may have a role in controlling membrane ion channels, at least in the airway muscle of some species.

M_2 Receptors. Surprisingly, most of the muscarinic receptors on bovine airway smooth muscle are of the M_2 type, coupled to adenylate cyclase by inhibitory G-proteins [130] and it has been demonstrated that muscarinic agonists reduce both basal and beta$_2$ receptor–stimulated cyclic AMP accumulation in canine tracheal preparations [114, 199] and also diminish the action of cyclic AMP–dependent kinase [229]. However, the cyclic guanosine monophosphate (GMP) system may possibly be involved in modulating M_3-induced responses in airway since in canine trachea at least, muscarinic receptor stimulation, while decreasing cyclic AMP, actually increased cyclic GMP [114].

Histamine Receptors

Three types of histamine receptors, H_1, H_2, and H_3, have been recognized on the basis of selective pharmacologic analysis using selective antagonists [68, 189, 204] and the gene for the H_2 receptor has been cloned. H_1 and H_2 receptors are coupled via G-proteins to their effector systems, which in most tissues are the Ca^{++} system and the cyclic AMP system, respectively. At present, little is known about H_3 receptors; they are reported to be found mainly in neural tissue at presynaptic sites [204]. As regards airway smooth muscle, the main histamine receptor affecting its function is the H_1 receptor, which has been identified by [^{3}H]pyrilamine binding [79]. The main action of histamine on airway smooth muscle is a sustained H_1-mediated contraction, although reviews of early work [7] included reports of H_2-mediated relaxation in some species. There may indeed be species differences in responses but there is also the possibility that H_2-mediated relaxation of *vascular* muscle in the preparations used could have been responsible for the results seen.

Histamine stimulation of canine tracheal cells and strips results in a phosphorylation of myosin light chain, which decreases only very gradually over the succeeding 30 minutes (as is the case with M_3 receptor stimulation in this species) [114]. Phos-

phorylation of myosin light chain is transient in bovine trachea [227] and correlates well with the rise in $[Ca^{++}]_i$. A main source of calcium is the internal store. Histamine releases Ca^{++} from Fura-2–loaded, cultured canine tracheal cells by an H_1 but not an H_2 receptor mechanism, the release occurring within seconds and returning to baseline within 1 minute [121]. Histamine causes a turnover of polyphosphoinositides in airway muscle [34, 88] with concentration-dependent accumulation of IP_3 [114], which reaches peak values in 30 seconds and lasts about 3 minutes, though histamine is less effective in this regard than muscarinic agonists [114, 131]. In contrast to these results, it has been reported that in saponin-permeabilized canine tracheal preparations, histamine does not cause PIP_2 hydrolysis [89].

With H_1 receptor–mediated contraction of airway muscle, as for M_3 receptor–mediated contraction, there is conflicting evidence as to the extent of calcium influx necessary for the response and the channels through which this occurs. Giembyez and Rodger [73] reviewed studies done prior to 1987, and quoted five studies supporting entry by voltage-operated channels and eight studies providing evidence against such an entry. A study using Fura-2–loaded cultured canine tracheal myocytes demonstrated that the H_1 receptor–mediated calcium transients (which peak at 16 seconds and return to baseline in 90 seconds) occur both in the presence of EGTA (ethyleneglycol-bis-(β-aminoethyl ether) N, N, N′, N′-tetraacetic acid) and in the presence of blockers of voltage-operated channels, implying that no Ca^{++} influx occurred [121]. Other recent work on tracheal strips indicated that Ca^{++} influx is required for the tonic but not the phasic aspect of the histamine response in both guinea pig [66], canine [114], and human airways [152a]. Results obtained in guinea pig tracheal strips imply that the Ca^{++} influx reported to be required for tonic contraction does not occur through voltage-dependent channels [66, 152a]. Technical factors, differences between preparations, and species differences may be the bases of these conflicting data.

There is no really substantive evidence for H_2 receptors on airway smooth muscle, and histamine stimulation in canine airways results in a decrease rather than an increase in cyclic AMP [114]. However, histamine causes a fairly marked increase in cyclic GMP, which is marginally reduced by an H_2 receptor antagonist [114], and there is evidence that pretreatment with 8-bromocyclic GMP decreases the histamine-mediated $[Ca^{++}]_i$ increase and myosin light-chain phosphorylation in cultured airway cells [227]. PKC activators in cultured canine tracheal myocytes block histamine-induced calcium transients [121]. These data imply that the histamine-induced contraction system might have two inbuilt modulatory mechanisms—the diacylglycerol-PKC pathway activated by PIP_2 hydrolysis (acting by negative feedback on PLC, see Fig. 16-3) and activation of guanylate cyclase. These factors may possibly provide part of the explanation why, dose for dose, muscarinic agonists are more effective than histamine in causing contraction of tracheal preparations [52, 114] and in stimulating inositol phosphate accumulation [131].

Agents such as the beta$_2$-adrenoceptor stimulants that are well known as being able to abrogate the histamine contraction have been shown to produce a concentration-related inhibition of histamine-induced phosphoinositide hydrolysis [88].

Leukotriene Receptors

The cysteinyl-containing leukotrienes (LT), LTC_4, LTD_4, and LTE_4, are all potent spasmogens on airway muscle [175]. There are specific antagonists for LTD_4 but not LTC_4 [189, 212], and binding sites for both LTC_4 and LTD_4 in guinea pig lung have been demonstrated, the former site being primarily the enzyme that converts LTC_4 to LTD_4 [14]. In human lung, only one specific binding site has been shown [28]. There is as yet only limited information on the structure of the receptors [54]; the genes have not been cloned, but the solubilized receptor has been characterized in the active form [242]. The signal transduction mechanism for the contraction of airway smooth muscle by both LTC$_4$ and LTD$_4$ involves PIP$_2$ hydrolysis [76, 146], LTC$_4$ being more potent than LTD$_4$.

Clinical studies with antagonists are providing evidence that the leukotrienes are implicated in the pathogenesis of asthma. Leukotrienes are dealt with in more detail in Chapters 11 and 66.

Prostanoid Receptors

There is now a rational classification of the prostanoid receptors, based on selective agonists and antagonists, and this has brought order out of the previous chaos [42]. There are five main receptors, one for each of the natural prostanoids—prostaglandin (PG) D$_2$, PGF$_{2\alpha}$, PGI$_2$, thromboxane (TX) A$_2$, and PGE$_2$—termed *DP*, *FP*, *IP*, *TP*, and *EP*, respectively—and there are three subgroups of receptors for PGE$_2$—termed *EP$_1$*, *EP$_2$*, and *EP$_3$*. Bronchoconstriction can be produced by activation of FP, TP, and EP$_1$ receptors. The ambiguous effects of PGE$_2$ in guinea pig trachea are now known to be due to the dual action of PGE$_2$ on EP$_1$ receptors (contraction) and EP$_2$ receptors (relaxation). Prostanoid-mediated contraction of human airway smooth muscle is due to activation of TP receptors [43]. Very little work has been done on the signal transduction mechanisms of prostanoid-mediated airway muscle responses. Activation of EP$_1$, FP and TP receptors is believed to involve PIP$_2$ hydrolysis [42]; however, in dog tracheal smooth muscle, PGF$_{2\alpha}$ does not affect either the PIP$_2$ or phosphatidic acid concentrations. Prostanoid actions are dealt with in more detail in Chapter 11.

Tachykinin Receptors

Tachykinins are peptides that contract airway smooth muscle; they are believed to be of significance in asthma. There are three tachykinin receptors, NK$_1$, NK$_2$, and NK$_3$, the ligands being substance P, neurokinin A (also termed *substance K*), and neurokinin B, respectively. There are selective antagonists for NK$_1$ and NK$_2$ receptors and selective agonists for all three [189]. Three distinct complementary DNA (cDNA) sequences for the three receptors have been cloned. In most tissues all three receptors are coupled by G-proteins to the PIP$_2$ hydrolysis transduction pathway [23, 84]; and there is evidence that this is the case in airway smooth muscle as well [78]. The decreasing order of potency of the tachykinins in human airway muscle is neurokinin A, substance P, and neurokinin B, and studies with selective antagonists indicate that NK$_2$ receptors are present [51]. Tachykinins are discussed further in Chapter 18.

Endothelin Receptors

Endothelin, a novel 21–amino acid peptide, was first isolated by Yanagisawa and coworkers [249]. It is the most powerful vasopressor substance known and there is now evidence that it has potent bronchoconstrictor activity. There are three subtypes of the peptide, ET-1, ET-2, and ET-3 [239] and two receptors, ET-R$_1$ and ET-R$_2$, the genes for which have been cloned [244]. The receptors have seven membrane-spanning domains, and exhibit sequence homology with other G-protein–coupled receptors such as the beta$_2$-adrenergic receptor (Fig. 16-4). They have glycosylation sites on the N-terminal region and phosphorylation sites on the cytoplasmic C3 loop and the carboxy-terminal stretch [244] (see Fig. 16-4). Specific binding sites for endothelin have been demonstrated in rat trachea [232] and on human bronchial smooth muscle cells [138] but pharmacologic studies of the receptor involved await the development of selective antagonists.

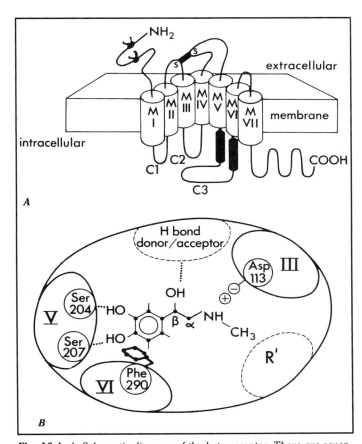

Fig. 16-4. *A. Schematic diagram of the beta receptor. There are seven membrane-spanning alpha helices (MI–MVII) forming a ligand-binding pocket (shown here opened out) with three intracellular loops (C1–C3). The thickened portions of the cytoplasmic loops indicate the areas thought to be involved in G-protein coupling. Sulfhydryl bonds may have a role in stabilizing the ligand-binding area. There are two extracellular glycosylation sites (shown as spiked beads). s = disulfide bridge. (Adapted and redrawn from R. W. Michell. Transmembrane signalling centerfold. Trends Pharmacol. Sci. 9:1988.) B. Simplified model of the interaction between a beta$_2$ adrenoceptor and epinephrine. Epinephrine is shown in the ligand-binding pocket as seen from outside the cell. Hydrogen bonds are shown between the catechol hydroxyl groups and the serine residues 204 and 207 in the membrane-spanning helix (MV). The beta-hydroxyl, critical for interaction with adrenergic receptors, is also shown interacting with a hydrogen bond donor/acceptor. A putative determinant capable of distinguishing a methyl group (as in epinephrine) from a hydrogen atom (as in norepine phrine) is designated as R'. (Modified from C. D. Strader and R. A. F. Dixon. Genetic Analysis of β-Adrenergic Receptor Structure and Function. In C. G. Cochrane and M. A. Gimbrone (eds.), Cellular and Molecular Mechanisms of Inflammation, Vol. 1. San Diego: Academic, 1990. Pp. 35–53; and J. R. Raymond, et al. Adrenergic receptors: Models for regulation of signal transduction processes. Hypertension 15:119, 1990.)*

Endothelin produces a slowly developing, long-lasting, concentration-dependent contraction of guinea pig tracheal and bronchial smooth muscle [91, 132, 235], of rat tracheal muscle [232], and ferret [126] and human [3] bronchial muscle. In the guinea pig, its spasmogenic action, which is markedly enhanced by removal of the airway epithelium [91], is not caused indirectly by a release of histamine, acetylcholine, leukotrienes, or thromboxanes [91].

There is good evidence that in many tissues, including vascular smooth muscle, the transduction mechanism involves PIP$_2$ hydrolysis [136, 192] with IP$_3$ generation and Ca^{++} influx [94], activation of PKC [46, 81], and stimulation of Na$^+$-H$^+$ exchange [120], as reviewed by Simonson and Dunn [208]. Very little work has been done on signal transduction in airway muscle, but it appears that for endothelin, PKC activity is less important in this tissue [91]. This is not supported by recent findings of Grunstein and colleagues [83a], who observed in mature rabbit airway smooth muscle a sustained (up to 10 minutes) elevation of IP$_3$ in response to endothelin. This was specific to endothelin and in contrast to the relatively transient elevation of IP$_3$ in response to other agonists such as histamine and carbachol (see earlier). The mechanism for this sustained accumulation of IP$_3$ may involve an endothelin-specific enhancement of plasma membrane PIP$_2$ content since endothelin is a potent stimulator of PKC activation in airway smooth muscle [83a].

It was originally proposed that endothelin produced contraction of vascular and airway smooth muscle by activating voltage-dependent calcium channels [235, 249] but there is now conflicting evidence on this point [91]; data obtained in the guinea pig indicate that contraction requires an influx of external Ca^{++} [132], which does not occur through voltage-dependent channels [91]. However, in studies on human bronchus it has been shown that Ca^{++} influx through voltage-dependent channels is involved in endothelin action at low concentrations (10^{-12} M–10^{-9} M) but not at higher concentrations (10^{-8} M–10^{-7} M) [3], ET-1 being the most potent of all the peptide subtypes in this tissue.

Further work in this exciting and fast-moving area of research should indicate whether or not the bronchoconstrictor action of endothelin is significant in bronchial hyperresponsiveness and whether selective antagonists could abrogate the delayed phase of asthma.

Alpha Adrenoceptors

Alpha adrenoceptors have been demonstrated in the airways of several species including humans [118], with an unexpectedly high density in the smaller airways [15]. It has been suggested that alpha receptors may be implicated in bronchial hyperresponsiveness; see the article by Barnes [14].

RELAXATION

Relaxation may be passive (i.e., due to the removal or inhibition of a contractile agonist) or active (i.e., due to the effect of a relaxant). Different relaxants may produce effects by different mechanisms.

One or more of the following processes can be considered to occur during relaxation of smooth muscle:

1. Dephosphorylation of myosin light chain.
2. Inhibition of the processes leading to myosin light-chain phosphorylation.
3. Alteration of [Ca^{++}]$_i$ through a decrease of the elevated [Ca^{++}]$_i$ to resting levels by the membrane Ca^{++}-ATPase, by Na$^+$-Ca^{++} exchange, or by Ca^{++} uptake into intracellular organelles.
4. Alteration of [Ca^{++}]$_i$ through inhibition of the processes mediating an increase in [Ca^{++}]$_i$ such as Ca^{++} influx or release from internal stores by IP$_3$. Influx could be inhibited by membrane hyperpolarization or by direct effects on Ca^{++} entry channels.
5. Alteration in the sensitivity of the contractile machinery.

It should be noted that some decrease in [Ca^{++}]$_i$ (see Figs. 16-2 and 16-3) and myosin light-chain phosphorylation (see Fig. 16-2) occurs anyway during the sustained phase of contraction in most airway muscle [69]. Phosphatases that dephosphorylate

myosin light chain have been characterized [171] (these are not calcium activated) and a reverse reaction by MLCK has also been described [100]. Myosin dephosphorylation by a phosphatase results in relaxation in chemically skinned uterine muscle [86]. In canine trachea (in which there is no marked decrease in myosin light-chain phosphorylation during tension maintenance) myosin dephosphorylation is crucial for airway muscle relaxation, and occurs during atropine antagonism of a methacholine-induced contraction (i.e., passive relaxation) as well as forskolin-induced reduction of methacholine-induced contraction (i.e., active relaxation). The latter is associated with an increase in cyclic AMP; the former is not [47]. Reduction in [Ca^{++}]$_i$ associated with agonist-induced relaxation has also been described [108, 128].

Signal Transduction Mechanisms for Relaxation

The main internal messengers implicated in active relaxation are cyclic AMP and cyclic GMP but it is possible that other mechanisms can operate in passive relaxation. Thus there is evidence for a reduction in IP$_3$ occurring before a reduction in tension when atropine antagonizes carbachol-contracted airway muscle [16].

Cyclic AMP

Cyclic AMP is derived from ATP by adenylate cyclase, which is controlled by two G-proteins, one being stimulatory (Gs) and one inhibitory (Gi) [227]. See Chapter 15 for further details. Cyclic AMP is metabolized by a phosphodiesterase to 5'-AMP. The role of cyclic AMP is assessed by measuring its tissue levels and the mechanical effects occurring during stimulation by receptor agonists, forskolin, or cyclic AMP analogs (such as dibutyryl cyclic AMP) and also during exposure to inhibitors of the phosphodiesterase. Interpretation of results with phosphodiesterase inhibitors is complicated by the fact that there are at least five distinct isoenzymes in airway smooth muscle and that these isoenzymes differ in sensitivity to activators and inhibitors [228].

It is quite clear that increases in cyclic AMP levels are associated with relaxation of airway muscle [107, 108, 113]. In general it is considered that cyclic AMP produces its effects by activating a specific kinase; the introduction of the catalytic subunit of cyclic AMP–dependent kinase, also known as protein kinase A (PKA), into skinned or permeabilized smooth muscle certainly inhibits tension development and relaxes contracted fibers [218]. In the discussion below it is taken that cyclic AMP is acting via activation of PKA. However, there is debate about the basis of the relaxant action of the cyclic AMP–PKA system [107, 108]. Possible mechanisms are discussed in the following sections.

Phosphorylation and Subsequent Decreased Action of Myosin Light-Chain Kinase by an Increase in the Ca^{++} Dependency of the Enzyme. This mechanism was proposed by Adelstein [1]. Evidence for and against was considered by Kamm and Stull [107, 108, 110] and by Rasmussen and colleagues [186]. This mechanism has been shown to operate with purified MLCK [144] and in skinned smooth muscle fibers [116, 139], but not in intact tracheal muscle strips [144]. Analysis of the data on cyclic AMP and phosphorylation of MLCK according to the rigorous criteria put forward by Krebs and Beavo for establishing phosphorylation/dephosphorylation of enzymes [122] indicates that the mechanism, as put forward by Adelstein [1], may not be critical for relaxation [108], and recent work by Stull and colleagues [219] indicates that the cyclic AMP kinase does not result in the relevant phosphorylation of MLCK.

A Decrease in Intracellular Calcium Concentration. An increase in airway muscle cyclic AMP can be shown to be associated with decreased cytosolic Ca^{++} [85]. Cyclic AMP is reported to influence several of the mechanisms outlined above that result in decreased [Ca^{++}]$_i$, including decreased entry, increased ef-

flux, and increased uptake into organelles, as reviewed by Kamm and Stull [108] and by Rasmussen and colleagues [186].

There is evidence from vascular muscle that cyclic AMP increases Ca^{++} uptake into the sarcoplasmic reticulum [243] and that in both vascular and airway smooth muscle it is implicated in hyperpolarization of the membrane through increasing the sensitivity of Ca^{++}-activated K^+ channels (mainly by increasing the probability of channel openings) [198]. In tracheal muscle, cyclic AMP is associated with an inhibition of phosphoinositide hydrolysis in response to some agonists (e.g., histamine) but not others (e.g., acetylcholine) [131]. In cerebellar tissue the IP_3 receptor is a major substrate for cyclic AMP–dependent kinase, and phosphorylation of the receptor blocks both IP_3 binding and Ca^{++} release [53]. There is also evidence for cyclic AMP effects on $[Ca^{++}]_i$ through actions on the Na^+-K^+-ATPase, with concomitant increased Ca^{++} efflux through Na^+-Ca^{++} exchange [200–202]. Although increased cyclic AMP is usually associated with decreased $[Ca^{++}]_i$, there is also paradoxic evidence in airway muscle: in the absence of spasmogen action, agents that *increase* cyclic AMP also *increase* $[Ca^{++}]_i$ but do not increase tension [225] or inhibit a subsequent carbachol-mediated rise in $[Ca^{++}]_i$ [62], although if given after carbachol, these agents cause a reduction in both the tension and the raised $[Ca^{++}]_i$ subsequently produced by this muscarinic agonist. Differential distribution of the calcium indicator and/or of Ca^{++} itself may explain these rather unusual findings.

Alteration in Sensitivity of the Contractile Machinery. Studies on permeabilized arterial smooth muscle support the proposal that cyclic AMP, probably through kinase activation, could decrease the Ca^{++} sensitivity of the contractile elements [157].

Cyclic GMP

In most tissues the increase in cyclic GMP is due to receptor activation of guanylate cyclase either directly or via a G-protein; but in some cases, guanylate cyclase itself can be the receptor [38]. The role of cyclic GMP is usually studied either by measuring cyclic GMP concentrations or by administering analogs such as 8-bromocyclic GMP, or inhibitors of cyclic GMP–dependent phosphodiesterase.

Many smooth muscle relaxants, particularly vasodilators, cause an increase of cyclic GMP. Furthermore, 8-bromocyclic GMP causes concentration-dependent relaxation of tracheal tissue [223]. However, the mechanisms whereby increased cyclic GMP is related to smooth muscle relaxation are not well understood, although cyclic GMP kinase is believed to be activated. Dephosphorylation of myosin light chain in the presence of elevated cyclic GMP has been reported [150], as has inhibition of phosphatidylinositol hydrolysis [182], a decrease in myosin light-chain phosphorylation [227], a decrease in $[Ca^{++}]_i$ [62], and increased Ca^{++} efflux [119]. The major substrate of cyclic GMP kinase in vascular smooth muscle is reported to be a membrane protein that may be coupled to or may itself be the Ca^{++} pump [11].

Perhaps the most significant finding, however, is that cyclic GMP (possibly through a specific kinase) decreases the Ca^{++} sensitivity of the contractile processes [157].

The receptors mediating relaxation of airway smooth muscle will now be discussed.

Receptors Mediating Relaxation

The beta$_2$ adrenoceptor is taken as the main model for a receptor mediating relaxation but attention is also paid to K^+ channel openers since these are likely to have clinical importance in the future. Relaxant peptides (vasoactive intestinal peptide [VIP], peptide histidine isoleucine [PHI], peptide histidine valine-42 [PHV-42]) and the putative nonadrenergic, noncholinergic inhibitory (i-NANC) transmitter are discussed briefly.

Beta$_2$ Adrenoceptors

Three types of beta receptors are recognized [189] on the basis of gene cloning, but selective antagonists are available for only the beta$_1$ and beta$_2$ subtypes.

The distribution of beta receptors was well reviewed by Barnes [13, 14]; only the beta$_2$ type has been found in human airway smooth muscle, their density increasing with decreasing size from large bronchi to terminal bronchioles. More than 90 percent of all beta receptors in the lung are found in the alveolar duct smooth muscle; the significance of this is unknown [12].

Beta-adrenergic receptors are coupled via G-proteins to adenylate cyclase and are probably the most thoroughly characterized of the family of G-protein–coupled receptors. Each receptor consists of a single polypeptide chain that includes seven stretches of hydrophobic amino acids, 20 to 25 residues in length, which form membrane-spanning alpha helices. These alternate with hydrophilic stretches that extend both extracellularly and intracellularly [220]. The transmembrane sections form a ligand-binding pocket. See Figure 16-4 for a possible model. Several residues on the intracellular portions of the receptors—on loop C3 and on the carboxy-terminal stretch—are potential sites of phosphorylation by the cyclic AMP–dependent kinase and the specific beta-adrenergic receptor kinase [90, 188]; this uncouples the receptor from its effector enzyme and results in desensitization.

Beta$_2$-receptor activation certainly attenuates the contractile properties of airway muscle and inhibits the rate and extent of both tension development and myosin light-chain phosphorylation [159, 207]. In other cell types beta$_2$ receptors interact via stimulatory G-proteins (Gs) with adenylate cyclase, as described in Chapter 15, increasing intracellular cyclic AMP; and there is good evidence that this also occurs in airway smooth muscle [108, 114, 186]. The signal transduction mechanisms therefore will be primarily those associated with increased cyclic AMP, as discussed above. However, as specified for other agents raising cyclic AMP in airway smooth muscle, beta$_2$-receptor stimulation may paradoxically, under some circumstances, be associated with a *rise* in $[Ca^{++}]_i$ [62, 225].

K$^+$ Channels

Some pharmacologic agents (e.g., cromakalim and pinacidil) produce relaxation in smooth muscle cells by increasing the permeability of the plasma membrane to K^+, that is, by opening K^+ channels. There are several types of K^+ channels in cell membranes including, among others, voltage-sensitive, Ca^{++}-activated, and receptor-operated ones [189]; but accumulating pharmacologic data suggest that the relaxant effect of the above-mentioned agents in smooth muscle is probably due to the opening of ATP-sensitive K^+ channels (K_{ATP}), which link the metabolic state of the cell to its membrane potential and excitability. This is reviewed by Quast and Cook [177] and by de Weille and coauthors [49]. The activity of these K_{ATP} channels has been well worked out in pancreatic beta cells. A rise in ATP concentration, as produced by glucose metabolism, blocks the channel, resulting in Ca^{++} influx, triggering insulin release; G-protein–linked PIP_2 hydrolysis and PKC activation also play a part. The sulfonyl ureas (e.g., glibenclamide) promote insulin release by blocking these channels.

K_{ATP} channels exist in vascular smooth muscle [19] and are believed to be the site of action of cromakalim and pinacidil, which are being tested as antihypertensives [245]. There is good evidence that these K^+ channel openers are also effective on airway smooth muscle. Most of the work has been carried out in guinea pig airway muscle, in which the compounds not only reduce spontaneous tone but also relax preparations precontracted by inflammatory mediators such as histamine, $PGF_{2\alpha}$, and LTC_4, producing about 80 percent reversal with median inhibitory concentrations (IC_{50}) of about 1 μM [4, 5, 8, 156]; they are rather less active against carbachol-induced spasm. The sulfonyl urea drug glibenclamide prevents the relaxant effect of K^+ channel openers in vitro and can effect a concentration-dependent reversal of the relaxation [155].

In in vivo studies, K^+ channel openers inhibit 5-hydroxytryptamine–induced bronchospasm and histamine-induced asphyxic collapse in the guinea pig [8]. Early studies in humans have shown that cromakalim inhibits histamine-induced bronchoconstriction [10] and can protect against nocturnal bronchoconstriction in asthmatic patients [165, 246].

These K^+ channel openers cause relaxation by a primary action considered to be the antagonism of the action of intracellular ATP, which would normally keep them closed; the channels then open and K^+ efflux and membrane hyperpolarization follow (see Rang and Dale [181] for simple summary). This would interfere with the activity of membrane Ca^{++} channels (voltage operated and receptor operated) and favor the extrusion of Ca^{++} by Na^+-Ca^{++} exchange, reducing $[Ca^{++}]_i$. An additional action may be the inhibition of the refilling of intracellular Ca^{++} stores, possibly due to the plasma membrane hyperpolarization or to a direct intracellular action on the Ca^{++}-K^+ exchange consequent on IP_3-mediated Ca^{++} release, described above.

The K^+ channel openers constitute a novel class of smooth muscle relaxants that may well have future application in the therapy of asthma and bronchial hyperresponsiveness [24]. New compounds are in development [167] and future developments in this area are awaited with interest.

Vasoactive Intestinal Peptide Receptors

VIP is a potent relaxant of isolated airway preparations taken from many species including humans (Chap. 18). VIP interacts with specific binding sites on airway smooth muscle, stimulating adenylate cyclase [65]. Autoradiographic mapping shows that VIP receptors are present on several cell types including the smooth muscle of large but not small airways [32]. In addition to VIP, related peptides such as PHI and its human counterpart, peptide histidine methionine (PHM), both derived from the same precursor molecule, prepro-VIP, and encoded by the same gene [104], are also thought to relax airway smooth muscle via VIP receptors.

VIP is also the favored candidate for the neurotransmitter of i-NANC nerves in the airways of many species including humans [12–14]. However, conclusive proof awaits the development of potent and selective antagonists of airway smooth muscle VIP receptors. Recent evidence suggests that in the airways of some species, the endothelium-derived relaxant factor, nitric oxide, may play a role in mediating the response of i-NANC nerves [127, 231]. This is discussed more fully in Chapter 18.

Whether different subtypes of VIP receptor exist in tissues such as airway smooth muscle is unknown, but no doubt will become apparent with the cloning of the receptor and the development of selective pharmacologic tools.

Adenosine Receptors

Pharmacologic analysis suggests that at least two cell-surface receptors for adenosine (also known as P_1 purinoceptors) exist on airway smooth muscle [129]. A_1 receptors are usually excitatory and inhibit adenylate cyclase activity, while A_2 receptors are inhibitory, stimulating adenylate cyclase. This class of receptor is discussed in more detail in Chapter 19.

In conclusion, airway smooth muscle expresses a wide range of pharmacologically distinct cell-surface receptors, but the diversity of the intracellular signaling mechanisms appears much more restricted. Smooth muscle is one of the few tissues in which we can follow many of the complex biochemical events from the binding of a ligand with its receptor to the final response of either contraction or relaxation. Continuing study of the signal transduction events in airway smooth muscle should enlarge our understanding of the pathogenesis of asthma and could well point the way forward to novel therapeutic approaches.

REFERENCES

1. Adelstein, R. S., and Eisenberg, E. Regulation and kinetics of the actin-myosin-ATP interaction. *Annu. Rev. Biochem.* 49:921, 1980.
2. Adelstein, R. S., and Sellers, J. R. Effects of calcium on vascular smooth muscle contraction. *Am. J. Cardiol.* 59:4B, 1987.
3. Advenier, C., et al. Contractile activity of three endothelins (ET-1, ET-2 and ET-3) on the human isolated bronchus. *Br. J. Pharmacol.* 100:168, 1990.
4. Allen, S. L., et al. Electrical and mechanical effects of BRL 34915 in guinea pig isolated trachealis. *Br. J. Pharmacol.* 89:395, 1986.
5. Allen, S. L., et al. The relaxant action of nicorandil in guinea pig isolated trachealis. *Br. J. Pharmacol.* 87:117, 1986.
6. Ambler, S. K., et al. Agonist-stimulated oscillations and cycling of intracellular free calcium in individual cultured muscle cells. *J. Biol. Chem.* 263:1952, 1988.
7. Anderson, W. H. Biochemical Mediators: Release, Chemistry, and Function. In E. B. Weiss, M. S. Segal and M. Stein (eds.), *Bronchial Asthma: Mechanisms and Therapeutics* (2nd ed.). Boston: Little, Brown, 1985. Pp. 57–87.
8. Arch, J. R. S., et al. Evaluation of the potassium channel activator cromakalim (BRL 34915) as a bronchodilator in the guinea-pig: Comparison with nifedipine. *Br. J. Pharmacol.* 95:763, 1988.
9. Baba, K., Baron, C. B., and Coburn, R. F. Phorbol ester effects on coupling mechanisms during cholinergic contraction of swine tracheal smooth muscle. *J. Physiol. (Lond.)* 412:23, 1989.
10. Baird, A., et al. Cromakalim, a potassium channel activator, inhibits histamine-induced bronchoconstriction in healthy volunteers. *Br. J. Clin. Pharmacol.* 25:114, 1988.
11. Baltensperger, K., Chiesi, M., and Carafoli, E. Substrates of cGMP kinase in vascular smooth muscle and their role in the relaxation process. *Biochemistry* 29:9753, 1990.
12. Barnes, P. J. Neural control of human airways in health and disease. *Am. Rev. Respir. Dis.* 134:1289, 1986.
13. Barnes, P. J. Cell-surface Receptors in Airway Smooth Muscle. In R. F. Coburn (ed.), *Airway Smooth Muscle in Health and Disease.* New York: Plenum, 1989. Pp. 77–97.
14. Barnes, P. J. Airway smooth muscle receptors. *Recenti Prog. Med.* 81:184, 1990.
15. Barnes, P. J., et al. Activation of α-adrenergic response in tracheal smooth muscle: A postreceptor mechanism. *J. Appl. Physiol.* 54:1469, 1983.
16. Baron, C. B., Pompeo, J., and Coburn, R. F. Decrease in Ins(1,4,5)P's pool precedes decrease in force evoked by atropine in carbachol-contracted porcine trachealis smooth muscle. *FASEB J.* 4:A1116, 1990.
17. Bean, B. P. Classes of calcium channels in vertebrate cells. *Annu. Rev. Physiol.* 51:367, 1989.
18. Bengtsson, B., Khan, A. R., and Weiber, R. Role of different calcium pools in the contraction of respiratory smooth muscle. *Acta Physiol. Scand.* 124:93, 1985.
19. Benham, C. D., and Tsien, R. W. A novel receptor-operated Ca^{2+} permeable channel activated by ATP in smooth muscle. *Nature* 328:275, 1987.
20. Berridge, M. J. Calcium oscillations. *J. Biol. Chem.* 265:9583, 1990.
21. Berridge, M. J., and Irvine, R. F. Inositol phosphates & cell signalling. *Nature* 341:197, 1989.
22. Billah, M. M., and Anthes, J. C. The regulation and cellular functions of phosphatidylcholine hydrolysis. *Biochem. J.* 269:281, 1990.
23. Birnbaumer, L., Abramowitz, J., and Brown, A. Receptor-effector coupling by G proteins. *Biochim. Biophys. Acta* 1030:163, 1990.
24. Black, J. L., and Barnes, P. J. Potassium channels and airway function: New therapeutic prospects. *Thorax* 45:213, 1990.
25. Bloom, J. W., Halonen, M., and Yamamura, H. I. Characterization of muscarinic cholinergic receptor subtypes in human peripheral lung. *J. Pharmacol. Exp. Ther.* 244:625, 1988.
26. Brading, A. F., and Aickin, C. C. Ions, Transporters, Exchangers and Pumps in Smooth Muscle Membranes. In N. Sperelakis and J. D. Wood (eds.), *Frontiers in Smooth Muscle Research.* New York: Alan R. Liss, 1990. Pp. 323–343.
27. Bruschi, G., et al. Myoplasmic Ca^{2+} force relationship studied with fura-2 during stimulation of rat aortic smooth muscle. *Am. J. Physiol.* 254: H840, 1988.
28. Buckner, C. K., et al. Pharmacological evidence that human intralobular airways do not contain different receptors that mediate contractions to leukotrienes C_4 and D_4. *J. Pharmacol. Exp. Ther.* 237:558, 1986.
29. Bullock, C. G., Fettes, J. J. F., and Kirkpatrick, C. T. Tracheal smooth

muscle—Second thoughts on sodium calcium exchange. *J. Physiol. (Lond.)* 318:46P, 1981.

30. Cabot, M. C., Huang, C., and Alton Jones, W. Hormone induced hydrolysis of cellular polyphosphoinositides by phospholipase C and phosphatidylcholine by phospholipase D: A time sequence study of the generation of second messengers. *J. Cell. Biochem. Suppl.* 14B:304, 1990.

31. Carafoli, E. Intracellular calcium homeostasis. *Annu. Rev. Biochem.* 56:395, 1987.

32. Carstairs, J. R., and Barnes, P. J. Visualisation of vasoactive intestinal peptide receptors in human and guinea pig lung. *J. Pharmacol. Exp. Ther.* 239:249, 1986.

33. Chadwick, C. C., Saito, A., and Fleischer, S. Isolation and characterization of the inositol trisphosphate receptor from smooth muscle. *Proc. Natl. Acad. Sci. USA* 87:2132, 1990.

34. Chilvers, E. R., Barnes, P. J., and Nahorski, S. R. Characterization of agonist-stimulated incorporation of myo-[^{3}H]inositol into inositol phospholipids and [^{3}H]inositol phosphate formation in tracheal smooth muscle. *Biochem. J.* 262:739, 1989.

35. Chilvers, E. R., et al. Formation of inositol polyphosphates in airway smooth muscle after muscarinic receptor stimulation. *J. Pharmacol. Exp. Ther.* 252:786, 1990.

36. Chilvers, E. R., et al. Mass changes of inositol 1,4,5-trisphosphate in trachealis muscle following agonist stimulation. *Eur. J. Pharmacol.* 164:587, 1989.

37. Chilvers, E. R., et al. Characterisation of stereospecific binding sites for inositol 1,4,5-trisphosphate in airway smooth muscle. *Br. J. Pharmacol.* 99:297, 1990.

38. Chinkers, M., et al. A membrane form of guanylate cyclase is atrial natriuretic peptide receptor. *Nature* 338:78, 1989.

39. Chopra, L. C., et al. Effects of heparin on inositol 1,4,5-trisphosphate and guanosine 5′-O-(3-thio triphosphate) induced calcium release in cultured smooth muscle cells from rabbit trachea. *Biochem. Biophys. Res. Commun.* 163:262, 1989.

40. Coburn, R. F., and Baron, C. B. Coupling mechanisms in airway smooth muscle. *Am. J. Physiol.* 258:L119, 1990.

41. Coburn, R. F., and Yamaguchi, T. Membrane potential-dependent and -independent tension in canine tracheal muscle. *J. Pharmacol. Exp. Ther.* 20:276, 1977.

42. Coleman, R. A., et al. Prostanoids and Their Receptors. In J. C. Emmett (ed.), *Comprehensive Medicinal Chemistry*, Vol. 3. *Membranes and Receptors*. Oxford: Pergamon, 1990. Pp. 643–714.

43. Coleman, R. A., and Sheldrick, R. L. G. Prostanoid-induced contraction of human bronchial smooth muscle is mediated by TP-receptors. *Br. J. Pharmacol.* 96:688, 1989.

44. Dale, M. M., and Obianime, A. W. Phorbol myristate acetate causes in guinea-pig lung parenchymal strip a maintained spasm which is relatively resistant to isoprenaline. *FEBS Lett.* 190:6, 1985.

45. Dale, M. M., and Obianime, A. W. 4β-PDBu contracts parenchymal strip and synergizes with raised cytosolic calcium. *Eur. J. Pharmacol.* 141:23, 1987.

46. Danthuluri, N. R., and Brock, T. A. Endothelin receptor-coupling mechanisms in vascular smooth muscle: A role for protein kinase C. *J. Pharmacol. Exp. Ther.* 254:393, 1990.

47. de Lanerolle, P. Cyclic AMP, myosin dephosphorylation and isometric relaxations of airway smooth muscle. *J. Appl. Physiol.* 964:705, 1988.

48. de Lanerolle, P. Cellular Control Mechanisms in Airway Smooth Muscle. In R. F. Coburn (ed.), *Airway Smooth Muscle in Health and Disease*. New York: Plenum, 1989. Pp. 99–125.

49. de Weille, J. R., et al. Pharmacology and regulation of ATP-sensitive K$^+$ channels. *Pflugers Arch.* 414(Suppl. 1):S80, 1989.

50. Dillon, P. F., et al. Myosin phosphorylation and the cross-bridge cycle in arterial smooth muscle. *Science* 211:495, 1981.

51. Dion, S., et al. Receptors for neurokinins in human bronchus and urinary bladder are of the NK-2 type. *Eur. J. Pharmacol.* 178:215, 1990.

52. Doucet, M. Y., Jones, T. R., and Ford-Hutchinson, A. W. Responses of equine trachealis and lung parenchyma to methacholine, histamine, serotonin, prostanoids and leukotrienes *in vitro*. *Can. J. Physiol. Pharmacol.* 68:379, 1990.

53. Downes, C. P., and Macphee, C. H. Myo-inositol metabolites as cellular signals. *Eur. J. Biochem.* 193:1, 1990.

54. Drazen, J. M., et al. Arachnoids and Asthma: The Role of Receptors for Leukotrienes. In M. A. Kaliner, P. J. Barnes, and C. G. A. Persson (eds.), *Asthma, Its Pathology and Treatment*. New York: Marcel Dekker, 1991. Pp. 301–325.

55. Drummond, A. H., and MacIntyre, D. E. Protein kinase C as a bidirectional regulator of cell function. *Trends Pharmacol. Sci.* 6:233, 1985.

56. Duncan, R. A., et al. Polyphosphoinositide metabolism in canine tracheal smooth muscle (CTSM) in response to a cholinergic stimulus. *Biochem. Pharmacol.* 36:307, 1987.

57. Ehrlich, B. E., and Watras, J. Inositol 1,4,5-trisphosphate activates a channel from smooth muscle sarcoplasmic reticulum. *Nature* 336:583, 1988.

58. Evans, D. H. L., Schild, H. O., and Thesleff, S. Effects of drugs on depolarized plain muscle. *J. Physiol. (Lond.)* 143:474, 1958.

59. Fain, J. N. Regulation of phosphoinositide-specific phospholipase C. *Biochim. Biophys. Acta* 1053:81, 1990.

60. Farago, A., and Nishizuka, Y. Protein kinase C in transmembrane signalling. *FEBS Lett.* 268:350, 1990.

61. Farley, J. M., and Miles, P. R. The sources of calcium of acetylcholine-induced contractions of dog tracheal smooth muscle. *J. Pharmacol. Exp. Ther.* 206:340, 1978.

62. Felbel, J., et al. Regulation of cytosolic calcium by cAMP and cGMP in freshly isolated smooth muscle cells from bovine trachea. *J. Biol. Chem.* 263:16764, 1988.

63. Ferris, C. D., et al. Purified inositol 1,4,5-trisphosphate receptor mediates calcium flux in reconstituted lipid vesicles. *Nature* 342:87, 1989.

64. Foster, R. W., Okpalugo, B. I., and Small, R. C. Antagonism of Ca^{2+} and other actions of verapamil in guinea pig isolated trachealis. *Br. J. Pharmacol.* 81:499, 1984.

65. Fransden, E. K., Krishna, G. A., and Said, S. I. Vasoactive intestinal polypeptide promotes cyclic 3′,5′-monophosphate accumulation in guinea pig trachea. *Br. J. Pharmacol.* 62:367, 1978.

66. Fukui, H., et al. Dependency of histamine induced phasic and tonic contractions on intracellular and extracellular calcium in guinea pig tracheal smooth muscle. *Jpn. J. Pharmacol.* 50:125, 1989.

67. Fulle, H. J., et al. In vitro synthesis of ^{32}P-labelled phosphatidylinositol 4,5-bisphosphate and its hydrolysis by smooth muscle membrane-bound phospholipase C. *Biochem. Biophys. Res. Commun.* 145:673, 1987.

68. Ganellin, C. R., and Parsons, M. E. (eds.), *Pharmacology of Histamine Receptors*. Bristol: Wright, 1982. P. 481.

69. Gerthoffer, W. T., and Murphy, R. A. Ca^{2+}, myosin phosphorylation and relaxation of arterial smooth muscle. *Am. J. Physiol.* 245:C271, 1983.

70. Gerthoffer, W. T., and Murphy, R. A. Myosin phosphorylation and regulation of the cross-bridge cycle in tracheal smooth muscle. *Am. J. Physiol.* 244:C182, 1983.

71. Ghosh, T. K., et al. Competitive reversible and potent antagonism of inositol 1,4,5-trisphosphate-activated calcium release by heparin. *J. Biol. Chem.* 263:11075, 1988.

72. Ghosh, T. K., et al. GTP-activated communication between distinct inositol 1,4,5-trisphosphate-sensitive and -insensitive calcium pools. *Nature* 340:236, 1989.

73. Giembycz, M. A., and Rodger, I. W. Electrophysiological and other aspects of excitation-contraction coupling and uncoupling in mammalian airway smooth muscle. *Life Sci.* 41:111, 1987.

74. Gilman, A. G. G proteins: Transducers of receptor-operated signals. *Annu. Rev. Biochem.* 56:615, 1987.

75. Goldman, W. F., Bova, S., and Blaustein, M. P. Measurement of intracellular Ca^{2+} in cultured arterial smooth muscle cells using Fura-2 and digital imaging microscopy. *Cell Calcium* 11:221, 1990.

76. Grandordy, B. M., et al. Leukotriene C$_4$ and D$_4$ induce contraction and formation of inositol phosphates in airways and lung parenchyma. *Am. Rev. Respir. Dis.* 133:A239, 1986.

77. Grandordy, B. M., et al. Phosphatidylinositol response to cholinergic agonists in airway smooth muscle: Relationship to contraction and muscarinic receptor occupancy. *J. Pharmacol. Exp. Ther.* 238:273, 1986.

78. Grandordy, B. M., et al. Tachykinin-induced phosphoinositide breakdown in airway smooth muscle and epithelium: Relationship to contraction. *Mol. Pharmacol.* 33:515, 1988.

79. Grandordy, B. M., Rhoden, K., and Barnes, P. J. Histamine H$_1$ receptors in human lung: Correlation of receptor binding and function. *Am. Rev. Respir. Dis.* 135:A274, 1987.

80. Griendling, K. K., et al. Sustained diacylglycerol formation from inositol phospholipids in angiotensin II-stimulated vascular smooth muscle cells. *J. Biol. Chem.* 261:5901, 1986.

81. Griendling, K. K., Tsuda, T., and Alexander, R. W. Endothelin stimulates diacylglycerol accumulation and activates protein kinase C in cultured vascular smooth muscle cells. *J. Biol. Chem.* 264:8237, 1989.

82. Grillone, L. R., et al. Vasopressin induces V$_1$-receptors to activate phosphatidylinositol- and phosphatidylcholine-specific phospholipase C and

stimulates the release of arachidonic acid by at least two pathways in the smooth muscle cell. *J. Biol. Chem.* 263:2658, 1988.

83. Grover, A. K. Ca-pumps in smooth muscle: One in plasma membrane and another in endoplasmic reticulum. *Cell Calcium* 6:227, 1985.

83a. Grunstein, M. M., et al. Mechanisms of action of endothelin-1 in maturing rabbit airway smooth muscle. *Am. J. Physiol.* 260:L75, 1991.

84. Guard, S., and Watson, S. P. Tachykinin receptor types: Classification and membrane signalling mechanisms. *Neurochem. Int.* 18:149, 1991.

85. Gunst, S. J., and Bandyopadhyay, S. Contractile force and intracellular Ca^{2+} during relaxation of canine tracheal smooth muscle. *Am. J. Physiol.* 257:C355, 1989.

86. Haeberle, J. R., Hathaway, F. R., and DePaoli-Roach, A. A. Dephosphorylation of myosin by the catalytic subunit of type-2 phosphatase produces relaxation of chemically skinned uterine smooth muscle. *J. Biol. Chem.* 260:9965, 1985.

87. Hai, C. M., and Murphy, R. A. Ca^{2+} crossbridge phosphorylation and contraction. *Annu. Rev. Physiol.* 51:285, 1989.

88. Hall, I. P., and Hill, S. J. β-Adrenoceptor stimulation inhibits histamine-stimulated inositol phospholipid hydrolysis in bovine tracheal smooth muscle. *Br. J. Pharmacol.* 95:1204, 1988.

89. Hashimoto, T., Hirata, M., and Ito, Y. A role for inositol 1,4,5-trisphosphate in the initiation of agonist-induced contractions of dog tracheal smooth muscle. *Br. J. Pharmacol.* 86:191, 1985.

90. Hausdorff, W. P., Caron, M. G., and Lefkowitz, R. J. Turning off the signal: Desensitization of β-adrenergic receptor function. *FASEB J.* 4:2881, 1990.

91. Hay, D. W. P. Mechanism of endothelin-induced contraction in guinea-pig trachea: Comparison with rat aorta. *Br. J. Pharmacol.* 100:383, 1990.

92. Heller Brown, J. (ed.), *The Muscarinic Receptors.* Clifton, N.J.: Humana, 1989. P. 496.

93. Hidaka, H., et al. Isoquinolinesulfonamides, novel and potent inhibitors of cyclic nucleotide dependent protein kinase and protein kinase C. *Biochemistry* 23:5036, 1984.

94. Hiley, C. R. Functional studies on endothelin catch up with molecular biology. *Trends Pharmacol. Sci.* 10:47, 1989.

95. Hirst, S. J., et al. What is the mechanism for phorbol ester-induced relaxation of guinea pig trachea? *Br. J. Pharmacol.* 97:449P, 1989.

96. Houslay, M. D. 'Crosstalk': A pivotal role for protein kinase C in modulating relationships between signal transduction pathways. *Eur. J. Biochem.* 195:9, 1991.

97. Huang, C., and Cabot, M. C. Phorbol diesters stimulate the accumulation of phosphatidate, phosphatidylethanol, and diacylglycerol in three cell types. *J. Biol. Chem.* 265:14858, 1990.

98. Huang, K.-P. The mechanism of protein kinase C activation. *Trends Neurosci.* 12:425, 1989.

99. Iino, M. Calcium release mechanisms in smooth muscle. *Jpn. J. Pharmacol.* 54:345, 1990.

100. Ikebe, M., and Hartshorne, D. J. Reverse reaction of smooth muscle myosin light chain kinase. *J. Biol. Chem.* 261:8249, 1986.

101. Ikebe, M., et al. Phosphorylation of smooth muscle myosin light chain kinase by Ca^{2+}-activated, phospholipid-dependent protein kinase. *J. Biol. Chem.* 260:4547, 1985.

102. Ito, M., and Hartshorne, D. J. Phosphorylation of Myosin as a Regulatory Mechanism in Smooth Muscle. In N. Sperelakis and J. D. Wood (eds.), *Frontiers in Smooth Muscle Research.* New York: Alan R. Liss, 1990. Pp. 57–72.

103. Ito, Y., and Itoh, T. The roles of stored Ca^{2+} in contractions of cat tracheal smooth muscle produced by electrical stimulation, acetylcholine and high K^+. *Br. J. Pharmacol.* 83:667, 1984.

104. Itoh, N., et al. Human prepro-vasoactive intestinal polypeptide contains a novel PHI-27-like peptide, PHM-27. *Nature* 304:547, 1983.

105. Itoh, T., Kubota, Y., and Kuriyama, H. Effects of a phorbol ester on acetylcholine-induced Ca^{2+} mobilization and contraction in the porcine coronary artery. *J. Physiol. (Lond.)* 397:401, 1988.

106. Kamm, K. E., et al. Phosphorylation of smooth muscle myosin heavy and light chains: Effects of phorbol dibutyrate and agonists. *J. Biol. Chem.* 264:21223, 1989.

107. Kamm, K. E., and Stull, J. T. Myosin phosphorylation, force, and maximal shortening velocity in neurally stimulated tracheal smooth muscle. *Am. J. Physiol.* 249:C238, 1985.

108. Kamm, K. E., and Stull, J. T. The function of myosin and myosin light chain kinase phosphorylation in smooth muscle. *Annu. Rev. Pharmacol. Toxicol.* 25:593, 1985.

109. Kamm, K. E., and Stull, J. T. Regulation of smooth muscle contractile elements by second messengers. *Annu. Rev. Physiol.* 51:299, 1989.

110. Kamm, K. E., and Stull, J. T. Second Messenger Effects on the Myosin Phosphorylation System in Smooth Muscle. In R. J. Paul, G. Elzinga, and K. Yamada (eds.), *Muscle Energetics.* New York: Alan R. Liss, 1989. Pp. 265–278.

111. Karaki, A. Ca^{2+} localisation and sensitivity in vascular smooth muscle. *Trends Pharmacol. Sci.* 10:320, 1989.

112. Kariya, K., et al. Two types of protein kinase C with different functions in cultured rabbit aortic smooth muscle cells. *Biochem. Biophys. Res. Commun.* 161:1020, 1989.

113. Katsuki, S., and Murad, F. Regulation of adenosine cyclic 3′5′-monophosphate and guanosine cyclic 3′5′-monophosphate levels and contractility in bovine tracheal smooth muscle. *Mol. Pharmacol.* 13:330, 1977.

114. Katsuyama, H., Suzuki, S., and Nishiye, E. Actions of second messengers synthesized by various spasmogenic agents and their relation to mechanical responses in dog tracheal smooth muscle. *Br. J. Pharmacol.* 100:41, 1990.

115. Kenney, R. E., Hoar, P. E., and Kerrick, G. L. The relationship between ATPase activity, isometric force, and myosin light-chain phosphorylation and thiophosphorylation in skinned smooth muscle fibre bundles from chicken gizzard. *J. Biol. Chem.* 265:8642, 1990.

116. Kerrick, W. G. L., and Hoar, P. E. Inhibition of smooth muscle tension by cAMP-dependent protein kinase. *Nature* 292:253, 1981.

117. Kirkpatrick, C. T. Excitation and contraction in bovine tracheal smooth muscle. *J. Physiol. (Lond.)* 244:263, 1975.

118. Kneussl, M. P., and Richardson, J. B. Alpha-adrenergic receptors in human and canine tracheal and bronchial smooth muscle. *J. Appl. Physiol.* 45:307, 1978.

119. Kobayashi, S., Kanaide, H., and Nakamura, N. Cytosolic free calcium transients in cultured vascular smooth muscle cells: Microfluorometric measurements. *Science* 229:553, 1985.

120. Koh, E., et al. Endothelin stimulates Na^+/H^+ exchange in vascular smooth muscle cells. *Biochem. Int.* 20:375, 1990.

121. Kotlikoff, M. I., Murray, P. K., and Reynolds, E. E. Histamine-induced calcium release and phorbol antagonism in cultured airway smooth muscle cells. *Am. J. Physiol.* 253:C561, 1987.

122. Krebs, E. G., and Beavo, J. A. Phosphorylation-dephosphorylation of enzymes. *Annu. Rev. Biochem.* 48:923, 1979.

123. Kriz, R., et al. Phospholipase C enzymes: Structural and functional similarities. *Ciba Found. Symp.* 150:112, 1990.

124. Lagast, H., et al. Phorbol myristate acetate stimulates ATP-dependent calcium transport by the plasma membrane of neutrophils. *J. Clin. Invest.* 73:878, 1984.

125. Lechleiter, J., et al. Distinct sequence elements control the specificity of G protein activation by muscarinic acetylcholine receptor subtypes. *EMBO J.* 9:4381, 1990.

126. Lee, H.-K., Leikauf, G. D., and Sperelakis, N. Electromechanical effects of endothelin on ferret bronchial and tracheal smooth muscle. *J. Appl. Physiol.* 68:417, 1990.

127. Li, C. G., and Rand, M. J. Evidence that part of the NANC relaxant response of guinea pig trachea to electrical field stimulation is mediated by nitric oxide. *Br. J. Pharmacol.* 102:91, 1991.

128. Lincoln, T. M., Cornwell, T. L., and Taylor, A. E. cGMP-dependent protein kinase mediates the reduction of Ca^{2+} by cAMP in vascular smooth muscle cells. *Am. J. Physiol.* 258:C399, 1990.

129. Londos, C., Copper, D. M. F., and Wolff, J. Subclasses of external adenosine receptors. *Proc. Natl. Acad. Sci. USA* 77:2551, 1980.

130. Lucchesi, P. A., et al. Ligand binding and G protein coupling of muscarinic receptors in airway smooth muscle. *Am. J. Physiol.* 258:C730, 1990.

131. Madison, J. M., and Brown, J. K. Differential inhibitory effects of forskolin, isoproterenol, and dibutyryl cyclic adenosine monophosphate on phosphoinositide hydrolysis in canine tracheal smooth muscle. *J. Clin. Invest.* 82:1462, 1988.

132. Maggi, C. A., et al. Potent contractile effect of endothelin in isolated guinea-pig airways. *Eur. J. Pharmacol.* 160:179, 1989.

133. Majerus, P. W., et al. Recent insights in phosphatidylinositol signalling. *Cell* 63:459, 1990.

134. Mak, J. C. W., and Barnes, P. J. Autoradiographic visualisation of muscarinic receptor subtypes in human and guinea pig lung. *Am. Rev. Respir. Dis.* 141:1559, 1990.

135. Marks, A. R., et al. Smooth muscle and brain inositol 1,4,5-trisphosphate receptors are structurally and functionally similar. *J. Biol. Chem.* 265:20719, 1990.

136. Marsden, P. A., et al. Endothelin action on vascular smooth muscle involves inositol trisphosphate and calcium mobilization. *Biochem. Biophys. Res. Commun.* 158:86, 1989.

137. Marston, S. B. What is latch? New ideas about tonic contraction in smooth muscle. *J. Muscle Res. Cell Motil.* 10:97, 1989.

138. Mattoli, S., et al. Specific binding of endothelin on human bronchial smooth muscle cells in culture and secretion of endothelin-like material from bronchial epithelial cells. *Am. J. Respir. Cell Mol. Biol.* 3:145, 1990.

139. Meisheri, K. D., Zlugner, C., and Ruegg, B. Ca^{2+}-cyclic AMP interactions in chemically skinned smooth muscle. *Eur. J. Pharmacol.* 129:405, 1986.

140. Menkes, H., Baraban, J. M., and Snyder, S. H. Protein kinase C regulates smooth muscle tension in guinea-pig trachea and ileum. *Eur. J. Pharmacol.* 122:19, 1986.

141. Merkel, L., Gerthoffer, W. T., and Torphy, T. J. Dissociation between myosin phosphorylation and shortening velocity in canine trachea. *Am. J. Physiol.* 258:C524, 1990.

142. Meurs, H., et al. Evidence for a direct relationship between phosphoinositide metabolism and airway smooth muscle contraction induced by muscarinic agonists. *Eur. J. Pharmacol.* 156:271, 1988.

143. Mignery, G. A., and Sudhof, T. C. The ligand binding site and transduction mechanism in the inositol 1,4,5-trisphosphate receptor. *EMBO J.* 9:3893, 1990.

144. Miller, J. R., Silver, P. J., and Stull, J. T. The role of myosin light chain kinase phosphorylation in β-adrenergic relaxation of tracheal muscle. *Mol. Pharmacol.* 24:235, 1983.

145. Miller-Hance, W. C., et al. Biochemical events associated with activation of smooth muscle contraction. *J. Biol. Chem.* 263:13979, 1988.

146. Mong, S., et al. Leukotriene-induced hydrolysis of inositol lipids in guinea-pig lung: Mechanism of signal transduction for leukotriene-D_4 receptors. *Mol. Pharmacol.* 31:35, 1987.

147. Morgan, J. P., and Morgan, K. G. Vascular smooth muscle: The first recorded Ca^{2+} transients. *Pflugers Arch.* 395:75, 1982.

148. Morgan, K. G. Calcium and vascular smooth muscle tone. *Am. J. Med.* 82(Suppl. 3B):9, 1987.

149. Morgan, K. G., Brozovich, F. V., and Jiang, M. J. Measurements of intracellular calcium concentration in mammalian vascular smooth muscle cells during agonist-induced contractions. *Biochem. Trans.* 16:493, 1988.

150. Murad, F. Cyclic guanosine monophosphate as a mediator of vasodilation. *J. Clin. Invest.* 78:1, 1986.

151. Murphy, R. A. Special topic: Contraction in smooth muscle cells. *Annu. Rev. Physiol.* 51:275, 1989.

152. Murray, R. K., et al. Mechanism of phorbol ester inhibition of histamine-induced IP_3 formation in cultured airway smooth muscle. *Am. J. Physiol.* 257:L209, 1989.

152a. Murray, R. K., and Kotlikoff, M. I. Receptor-activated calcium influx in human airway smooth muscle cells. *J. Physiol. (Lond.)* 435:123, 1991.

153. Nahorski, S. R. Receptors, inositol polyphosphates and intracellular Ca^{2+}. *Br. J. Clin. Pharmacol.* 30:23S, 1990.

154. Neyses, L., Reinlib, L., and Carafoli, E. Phosphorylation of the Ca^{2+}-pumping ATPase of heart sarcolemma and erythrocyte plasma membrane by the cAMP-dependent protein kinase. *J. Biol. Chem.* 260:10283, 1985.

155. Nielsen-Kudsk, J. E., Bang, L., and Bronsgaard, A. M. Glibenclamide blocks the relaxant action of pinacidil and cromakalim in airway smooth muscle. *Eur. J. Pharmacol.* 180:291, 1990.

156. Nielsen-Kudsk, J. E., et al. Effects of pinacidil on guinea-pig airway smooth muscle contracted by asthma mediators. *Eur. J. Pharmacol.* 157:221, 1988.

157. Nishimura, J., and Van Breemen, C. Direct regulation of smooth muscle contractile elements by second messengers. *Biochem. Biophys. Res. Commun.* 163:929, 1989.

158. Nishizuka, Y. Studies and perspectives of protein kinase C. *Science* 233:305, 1986.

159. Obara, K., and de Lanerolle, P. Isoproterenol attenuates myosin phosphorylation and contraction of tracheal muscle. *J. Appl. Physiol.* 66:2017, 1989.

160. Obara, K., Ito, Y., and Yabu, H. Ca^{2+}-induced Ca^{2+} release in skinned single smooth muscle cells isolated from guinea-pig taenia caeci. *Comp. Biochem. Physiol.* 86A:703, 1987.

161. Obianime, A. W., and Dale, M. M. The effect of relaxants working through different transduction mechanisms on the tonic contraction produced in rat aorta by 4β-PDBu. *Br. J. Pharmacol.* 97:647, 1989.

162. Obianime, A. W., Hirst, S. J., and Dale, M. M. Interactions between phorbol esters and agents which increase cytosolic calcium in the guinea pig parenchymal strip: Direct and indirect effects on the contractile response. *J. Pharmacol. Exp. Ther.* 247:262, 1988.

163. Obianime, A. W., Hirst, S. J., and Dale, M. M. The effect of smooth muscle relaxants working through different transduction mechanisms on the phorbol dibutyrate-induced contraction of the guinea-pig lung parenchymal strip: Possible relevance for asthma. *Pulm. Pharmacol.* 2:191, 1989.

164. Ohanian, J., et al. Agonist-induced production of 1,2-diacylglycerol and phosphatidic acid in intact resistance arteries. *J. Biol. Chem.* 265:8921, 1990.

165. Owen, S., et al. A randomised double blind placebo controlled crossover study of a potassium channel activator in morning dipping. *Thorax* 44:825P, 1989.

166. Ozaki, H., et al. Changes in cytosolic calcium and contraction induced by various stimulants and relaxants in canine tracheal smooth muscle. *Pflugers Arch.* 416:351, 1990.

167. Paciorek, P. M., et al. Evaluation of the bronchodilator properties of RO 31-6930, a novel potassium channel opener, in the guinea-pig. *Br. J. Pharmacol.* 100:289, 1990.

168. Park, S., and Rasmussen, H. Activation of tracheal smooth muscle contraction: Synergism between Ca^{2+} and activators of protein kinase C. *Proc. Natl. Acad. Sci. USA* 82:8835, 1985.

169. Park, S., and Rasmussen, H. Carbachol-induced protein phosphorylation changes in bovine tracheal smooth muscle. *J. Biol. Chem.* 261:15734, 1986.

170. Parker, P. F., et al. Protein kinase C—A family affair. *Mol. Cell. Endocrinol.* 65:1, 1989.

171. Pato, M. D., and Adelstein, R. S. Dephosphorylation of the 20,000-dalton light chain of myosin by two different phosphatases from smooth muscle. *J. Biol. Chem.* 255:6535, 1980.

172. Pelech, S. L., and Vance, D. E. Signal transduction via phosphatidylcholine cycles. *Trends Biochem. Sci.* 14:28, 1989.

173. Persechini, A., Kamm, K. E., and Stull, J. T. Different phosphorylated forms of myosin in contracting tracheal smooth muscle. *J. Biol. Chem.* 261:6293, 1986.

174. Petersen, O. H., and Wakui, M. Oscillating intracellular Ca^{2+} signals evoked by activation of receptors linked to inositol lipid hydrolysis: Mechanism of generation. *J. Membrane Biol.* 118:93, 1990.

175. Piper, P. J., Samhoun, M. N., and Conroy, D. M. Leukotrienes and Airway Smooth Muscle Tone. In C. L. Armour and J. L. Black (eds.), *Mechanisms in Asthma: Pharmacology, Physiology, and Management.* New York: Alan R. Liss, 1988. Pp. 47–54.

176. Putney, J. W. A model for receptor-regulated calcium entry. *Cell Calcium* 7:1, 1986.

177. Quast, U., and Cook, N. S. Moving together: K^+ channel openers and ATP-sensitive K^+ channels. *Trends Pharmacol. Sci.* 10:431, 1989.

178. Raeburn, D. Do phorbol esters produce relaxation of tracheal muscle by generation of arachidonic acid from airway epithelium? *Br. J. Pharmacol.* 98:785P, 1989.

179. Rana, R. S., and Hokin, L. E. Role of phosphoinositides in transmembrane signalling. *Physiol. Rev.* 70:115, 1990.

180. Rang, H. P., and Dale, M. M. *Pharmacology* (2nd ed.). London: Churchill-Livingstone, 1991. P. 347.

181. Rang, H. P., and Dale, M. M. *Pharmacology* (2nd ed.). London: Churchill-Livingstone, 1991, P. 355.

182. Rapoport, R. M. Cyclic guanosine monophosphate inhibition of contraction may be mediated through inhibition of phosphatidylinositol hydrolysis in rat aorta. *Circ. Res.* 58:407, 1986.

183. Rasmussen, H. The calcium messenger system. (First of two parts.) *N. Engl. J. Med.* 314:1094, 1986.

184. Rasmussen, H. The calcium messenger system. (Second of two parts.) *N. Engl. J. Med.* 314:1164, 1986.

185. Rasmussen, H., et al. TPA-induced contraction of isolated rabbit vascular smooth muscle. *Biochem. Biophys. Res. Commun.* 120:481, 1984.

186. Rasmussen, H., Kelley, G., and Douglas, J. S. Interactions between Ca^{2+} and cAMP messenger system in regulation of airway smooth muscle contraction. *Am. J. Physiol.* 258:L279, 1990.

187. Rasmussen, H., Takuwa, Y., and Park, S. Protein kinase C in the regulation of smooth muscle contraction. *FASEB J.* 1:177, 1987.

188. Raymond, J. R., et al. Adrenergic receptors: Models for regulation of signal transduction processes. *Hypertension* 15:119, 1990.

189. Receptor nomenclature supplement. *Trends Pharmacol. Sci.* 12:1, 1991.

190. Rembold, C. M. Modulation of the Ca^{2+} sensitivity of myosin phosphorylation in intact swine arterial smooth muscle. *J. Physiol. (Lond.)* 429:77, 1990.

191. Rembold, C. M., and Murphy, R. A. $[Ca^{2+}]$-dependent myosin phosphorylation in phorbol diester stimulated smooth muscle contraction. *Am. J. Physiol.* 255:C719, 1988.

192. Resink, T. J., Scott-Burden, T., and Buhler, F. R. Endothelin stimulates phospholipase C in cultured vascular smooth muscle cells. *Biochem. Biophys. Res. Commun.* 157:1360, 1988.

193. Rink, T. J. Receptor-mediated calcium entry. *FEBS Lett.* 268:381, 1990.

194. Rodger, I. W. Excitation-contraction coupling and uncoupling in airway smooth muscle. *Br. J. Clin. Pharmacol.* 20:255S, 1985.
195. Rodger, I. W. Calcium Ions and Contraction of Airways Smooth Muscle. In A. B. Kay (ed.), *Asthma: Clinical Pharmacology and Therapeutic Progress.* Oxford: Blackwell, 1986. Pp. 114–127.
196. Roffel, A. F., et al. Characterization of the muscarinic receptor subtype involved in phosphoinositide metabolism in bovine tracheal smooth muscle. *Br. J. Pharmacol.* 99:293, 1990.
197. Ruegg, U. T., et al. Receptor-operated calcium-permeable channels in vascular smooth muscle. *J. Cardiovasc. Pharmacol.* 14:S49, 1989.
198. Sadoshima, J., et al. Cyclic AMP modulates Ca-activated K channel in cultured smooth muscle cells of rat aortas. *Am. J. Physiol.* 255:H754, 1988.
199. Sankary, R. M., et al. Muscarinic cholinergic inhibition of cyclic AMP accumulation in airway smooth muscle: Role of a pertussis toxin-sensitive protein. *Am. Rev. Respir. Dis.* 138:145, 1988.
200. Scheid, C. R., and Fay, F. S. β-Adrenergic effects on transmembrane $^{45}Ca^{2+}$ fluxes in isolated smooth muscle. *Am. J. Physiol.* 246:C431, 1984.
201. Scheid, C. R., and Fay, F. S. β-Adrenergic stimulation of ^{42}K influx in isolated smooth muscle cells. *Am. J. Physiol.* 246:C415, 1984.
202. Scheid, C. R., Honeyman, T. W., and Fay, F. S. Mechanism of β-adrenergic relaxation of smooth muscle. *Nature* 277:32, 1979.
203. Schramm, C. M., and Grunstein, M. M. Mechanisms of protein kinase C regulation of airway contractility. *J. Appl. Physiol.* 66:1935, 1989.
203a. Schramm, C. M., and Grunstein, M. M. Assessment & signal transduction mechanisms regulating airway smooth muscle contractility. *Am. J. Physiol.* 262:L119, 1992.
204. Schwartz, J.-C., Arrang, J.-M., and Gabarg, M. Three classes of histamine receptors in brain. *Trends Pharmacol. Sci.* 7:24, 1986.
205. Sharma, R. V., and Bhalla, R. C. Regulation of cytosolic free Ca^{2+} concentration in vascular smooth muscle cells by A- and C-kinases. *Hypertension* 13:845, 1989.
206. Shukla, S. D., and Halenda, S. P. Phospholipase D in cell signalling and its relationship to phospholipase C. *Life Sci.* 48:851, 1991.
207. Silver, P. J., and Stull, J. T. Regulation of myosin light chain and phosphorylase phosphorylation in tracheal smooth muscle. *J. Biol. Chem.* 257:6145, 1982.
208. Simonson, M. S., and Dunn, M. J. Endothelin: Pathways of transmembrane signalling. *Hypertension* 15(Suppl. 1):I5, 1990.
209. Singer, H. A. Protein kinase C activation and myosin light chain phosphorylation in ^{32}P-labeled arterial smooth muscle. *Am. J. Physiol.* 259:C631, 1990.
210. Small, J. V., Furst, D. O., and De Mey, J. Localization of filamin in smooth muscle. *J. Cell. Biol.* 102:210, 1986.
211. Smith, J. B., Smith, L., and Higgins, B. L. Temperature and nucleotide dependence of calcium release by myo-inositol 1,4,5-trisphosphate in cultured vascular smooth muscle cells. *J. Biol. Chem.* 260:14413, 1985.
212. Smith, L. J., et al. Inhibition of leukotriene D₄-induced bronchoconstriction in normal subjects by the oral LTD₄ receptor antagonist ICI 204, 219. *Am. Rev. Respir. Dis.* 141:988, 1990.
213. Somlyo, A. V., et al. Inositol trisphosphate-induced calcium release and contraction in vascular smooth muscle. *Proc. Natl. Acad. Sci. USA* 82:5231, 1985.
214. Somlyo, A. V., et al. Heparin-sensitive Inositol Trisphosphate Signalling and the Role of G-proteins in Ca^{2+}-release and Contractile Regulation in Smooth Muscle. In N. Sperelakis and J. D. Woods (eds.), *Frontiers in Smooth Muscle Research.* New York: Alan R. Liss, 1990. Pp. 167–182.
215. Somlyo, A. V., and Somlyo, A. P. Electromechanical and pharmacomechanical coupling in vascular smooth muscle. *J. Pharmacol. Exp. Ther.* 159:129, 1968.
216. Sommerville, L. E., and Hartshorne, D. J. Intracellular calcium and smooth muscle contraction. *Cell Calcium* 7:353, 1986.
217. Souhrada, M., and Souhrada, J. F. Sodium and calcium influx induced by phorbol esters in airway smooth muscle cells. *Am. Rev. Respir. Dis.* 139:927, 1989.
218. Sparrow, M. P., et al. Effect of calmodulin, Ca^{2+} and cAMP protein kinase on skinned tracheal smooth muscle. *Am. J. Physiol.* 246:C308, 1984.
219. Stull, J. T., et al. Myosin light chain kinase phosphorylation in tracheal smooth muscle. *J. Biol. Chem.* 265:16683, 1990.
220. Strader, C. D., and Dixon, R. A. F. Genetic Analysis of β-Adrenergic Receptor Structure and Function. In C. G. Cochrane and M. A. Gimbrone (eds.), *Cellular and Molecular Mechanisms of Inflammation,* Vol. 1. San Diego: Academic, 1990. Pp. 35–53.
221. Suematsu, E., et al. Inositol 1,4,5-trisphosphate releases Ca^{2+} from intracellular store sites in skinned single cells of porcine coronary artery. *Biochem. Biophys. Res. Commun.* 120:481, 1984.
222. Sutton, T. A., and Haeberle, J. R. Phosphorylation by protein kinase C of the 20,000-dalton light chain of myosin in intact and chemically skinned vascular smooth muscle. *J. Biol. Chem.* 265:2749, 1990.
223. Suzuki, K., et al. The relationship between tissue levels of cyclic GMP and tracheal smooth muscle relaxation in the guinea-pig. *Clin. Exp. Pharmacol. Physiol.* 13:39, 1986.
224. Takuwa, Y., Takuwa, N., and Rasmussen, H. Carbachol induces a rapid and sustained hydrolysis of polyphosphoinositide in bovine tracheal smooth muscle measurements of the mass of polyphosphoinositides, 1,2-diacylglycerol, and phosphatidic acid. *J. Biol. Chem.* 261:14670, 1986.
225. Takuwa, Y., Takuwa, N., and Rasmussen, H. The effects of isoproterenol on intracellular Ca^{2+} concentration. *J. Biol. Chem.* 263:762, 1988.
226. Taylor, C. W. The role of G proteins in transmembrane signalling. *Biochem. J.* 272:1, 1990.
227. Taylor, D. A., Bowman, B. F., and Stull, J. T. Cytoplasmic Ca^{2+} is a primary determinant for myosin phosphorylation in smooth muscle cells. *J. Biol. Chem.* 264:6207, 1989.
227a. Thompson, N. T., Bonser, R. W., and Garland, L. G. Receptor-coupled phospholipase D and its inhibition. *Trends Pharmacol. Sci.* 12:404, 1992.
228. Torphy, T. J., and Cieslinski, L. B. Characterization and selective inhibition of cyclic nucleotide phosphodiesterase isozymes in canine tracheal smooth muscle. *Mol. Pharmacol.* 37:206, 1990.
229. Torphy, T. J., et al. The inhibitory effect of methacholine on drug-induced relaxation, cyclic AMP accumulation and cyclic AMP-dependent protein kinase activation in canine tracheal muscle. *J. Pharmacol. Exp. Ther.* 233:409, 1985.
230. Tsien, R. Y. Calcium channels, stores, and oscillations. *Annu. Rev. Cell Biol.* 6:715, 1990.
231. Tucker, J. F., et al. L-N^G-nitroarginine inhibits non-adrenergic, non-cholinergic relaxations of guinea pig isolated tracheal smooth muscle. *Br. J. Pharmacol.* 100:663, 1990.
232. Turner, N. C., et al. Endothelin-induced contractions of tracheal smooth muscle and identification of specific endothelin binding sites in the trachea of the rat. *Br. J. Pharmacol.* 98:361, 1989.
233. Twomey, B., et al. The effect of new potent and selective inhibitors of protein kinase C in the neutrophil respiratory burst. *Biochem. Biophys. Res. Commun.* 171:1087, 1990.
234. Twort, C. H. C., and Van Breemen, C. Human airway smooth muscle in cell culture: Control of the intracellular calcium store. *Pulm. Pharmacol.* 2:45, 1989.
235. Uchida, Y., et al. Endothelin, a novel vasoconstrictor peptide, as potent bronchoconstrictor. *Eur. J. Pharmacol.* 154:227, 1988.
236. Umekawa, H., and Hidaka, H. Phosphorylation of caldesmon by protein kinase C. *Biochem. Biophys. Res. Commun.* 132:56, 1985.
237. Umekawa, H., et al. Conformational studies of myosin phosphorylated by protein kinase C. *J. Biol. Chem.* 260:9833, 1985.
238. Van Breemen, C., and Saida, K. Cellular mechanisms regulating $[Ca^{2+}]_i$ smooth muscle. *Annu. Rev. Physiol.* 51:315, 1989.
239. Vane, J. Endothelins come home to roost. *Nature* 348:673, 1990.
240. Von Tscharner, V., Prod'Hom, B., and Baggiolini, M. Ion channels in human neutrophils activated by a rise in free cytosolic calcium concentration. *Nature* 324:369, 1986.
241. Walsh, M. P., and Sutherland, C. A model for caldesmon in latch-bridge formation in smooth muscle. *Adv. Exp. Med. Biol.* 255:337, 1988.
242. Watanabe, T., et al. Characterization of the guinea pig lung membrane leukotriene D₄ receptor solubilized in an active form. *J. Biol. Chem.* 265:21237, 1990.
243. Watras, J. Regulation of calcium uptake in bovine aortic sarcoplasmic reticulum by cyclic AMP-dependent protein kinase. *J. Mol. Cell. Cardiol.* 20:711, 1988.
244. Webb, D. J. Endothelin receptors cloned, endothelin converting enzyme characterized and pathophysiological roles for endothelin proposed. *Trends Pharmacol. Sci.* 12:43, 1991.
245. Weston, A. H. Smooth muscle K⁺ channel openers: Their pharmacology and clinical potential. *Pflugers Arch.* 414(Suppl. 1):S99, 1989.
246. Williams, A. J., et al. Attenuation of nocturnal asthma by cromakalim. *Lancet* 336:334, 1990.
247. Wuytack, F., et al. Smooth muscle endoplasmic reticulum contains a cardiac-like form of calsequestrin. *Biochim. Biophys. Acta* 899:151, 1987.
248. Yamamoto, H., and Van Breemen, C. Inositol-1,4,5-trisphosphate releases calcium from skinned cultured smooth muscle cells. *Biochem. Biophys. Res. Commun.* 130:270, 1985.
249. Yanagisawa, M., et al. A novel potent vasoconstrictor peptide produced by vascular endothelial cells. *Nature* 332:411, 1988.

Neural Control of the Airways and Cholinergic Mechanisms

17

Ronald L. Sorkness
William J. Calhoun
William W. Busse

The autonomic nervous system is composed of the sympathetic (adrenergic) and parasympathetic (cholinergic) systems (Fig. 17-1). Although the actions of the autonomic nervous system are important in the control of airway activity, the precise contributions to the control of lung function are not fully established. Furthermore, the traditional view that the autonomic nervous system exists as a balance with opposing actions on various target organs (Fig. 17-2) has been modified by evidence that the final tissue response represents a complex interaction of adrenergic, cholinergic, and nonadrenergic, noncholinergic activity. Consequently, autonomic nervous system activity is an important factor in the regulation of airway function.

This chapter focuses on the cholinergic control of the airways. It is important to realize that the cholinergic system influences bronchial smooth muscle, submucosal glands, and vascular beds as well as inflammatory cell function. Because the cholinergic nervous system is the dominant neural pathway for bronchoconstriction in human airways, there has been considerable interest that enhanced cholinergic mechanisms (see Fig. 17-2) contribute to the pathogenesis of asthma. It is our goal to review the principles of the cholinergic nervous system as they relate to airway physiology, to review how its activity is regulated, and to indicate some aspects of cholinergic system function that may contribute to the pathogenesis of asthma.

ANATOMIC BASIS OF PARASYMPATHETIC CONTROL OF AIRWAYS

Origins, Organization, Pathways, and Actions

Cholinergic outflow to the respiratory tract originates in motor nuclei located in the brain stem. Although there may be species variability, the dorsal motor nucleus of the vagus, the nucleus ambiguous, the nucleus retroambiguous, and the nucleus dorsomedialis contribute fibers supplying the respiratory tract [90, 91]. Recent functional studies in dogs indicate that neurons originating in the caudal and rostral areas of the ventrolateral medulla affect parasympathetic output to the airways [72a, 137a]. These preganglionic fibers course via the left and right vagus nerves, and innervate both left and right sides of the airway via crossovers in the posterior pulmonary plexus [31, 103]. Preganglionic fibers synapse in parasympathetic ganglia located in the adventitia of the posterior aspect of the trachea and bronchi [73]. Ganglionic neurons then give rise to short postganglionic fibers which innervate smooth muscle, epithelium, and submucosal glands.

Central-Peripheral Heterogeneity of Cholinergic Innervation

The distribution of cholinergic innervation of the respiratory tract is heterogeneous. The trachea and large airways appear to have a greater density of cholinergic fibers than do the more peripheral airways [16, 48, 140]. Similarly, autoradiographic mapping of muscarinic receptors demonstrates reduced binding in terminal bronchioles [11]. Functional studies also suggest that vagal stimulation has more prominent central than peripheral effects. Parasympathetically induced bronchoconstriction, assessed by tantalum bronchography in dogs, has been shown to affect preferentially the large airways but to produce minimal effects in small airways [132]. Likewise, human studies, using helium-oxygen mixtures, suggest that cholinergic blockade dilates central airways preferentially [117]. However, Ludwig and associates [109] demonstrated that vagal stimulation in dogs results in increases in peripheral lung resistance and viscance, the magnitudes of which were comparable to the increased resistance seen in the central compartment. These data suggest that the distribution of cholinergic influence is more extensive than previously believed.

Parasympathetic Ganglia

Intraganglionic transmission is mediated by release of the neurotransmitter acetylcholine from preganglionic nerve terminals, and can be blocked by classic nicotinic antagonists such as hexamethonium. Acetylcholine stimulates nicotinic receptors on the surface of postganglionic neurons and is rapidly degraded by acetylcholinesterase. Likewise, activated postganglionic fibers release acetylcholine in proximity to smooth muscle cells and secretory glands. In contrast to ganglionic neurotransmission, however, the end-organ receptors are muscarinic in nature, and exist as distinct biochemical and pharmacologic subtypes.

Ganglionic neurons are also heterogeneous in both histochemistry and electrophysiology [6, 31, 34]; this morphologic and physiologic heterogeneity raises the possibility of differential regulation of neurotransmission in these cells, although direct correlations among histology, electrophysiology, and neurotransmission have not been made.

Modulation of Neurotransmission

A more complete discussion of this topic follows. The goal of this brief discussion is to emphasize the anatomic connections and receptors. Factors that modulate cholinergic neurotransmission are schematized in Figure 17-9.

Adrenergic Modulation of Cholinergic Neurotransmission

Parasympathetic ganglionic neurotransmission can be modulated by adrenergic stimuli. Adrenergic nerve terminals have

This work was supported in part by grants AI-10404, AI-26609, and K08-01828 from the National Institutes of Health.

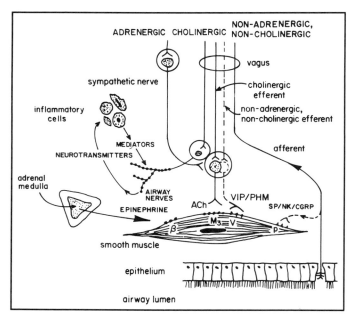

Fig. 17-1. *Simplified anatomic relationships of selected aspects of the autonomic nervous system. Cholinergic fibers synapse in ganglia close to the airway smooth muscle and mucous glands. Postganglionic fibers release acetylcholine (ACh) to stimulate muscarinic receptors (type M_3) on airway smooth muscle. VIP = vasoactive intestinal peptide; PHM = peptide histidine methionine; SP = substance P; NK = neurokinin(s); CGRP = calcitonin gene–related peptide. Airway smooth muscle expresses receptors for beta agonists (β), acetylcholine (M_3), VIP/PHM (V), and substance P (p).*

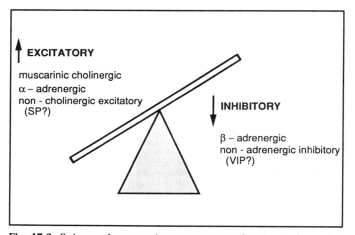

Fig. 17-2. *Balance of autonomic nervous system function in the control of airway caliber. SP = substance P; VIP = vasoactive intestinal peptide.*

been demonstrated in parasympathetic ganglia [84, 100], and there is evidence that alpha$_1$-, alpha$_2$-, and beta$_2$-adrenoreceptor agonists reduce ganglionic transmission [7, 65, 167] and inhibit the release of acetylcholine from postganglionic nerve terminals [44]. Thus, locally released and circulating catecholamines may modulate bronchial smooth muscle tone by means of inhibiting cholinergic neurotransmission; additionally, circulating catecholamines may directly result in smooth muscle relaxation via beta adrenoreceptors on the myocyte surface [150]. Further evidence for predominantly indirect actions of the sympathetic nervous system on smooth muscle function is the near absence of direct sympathetic innervation to the airway in humans [146].

Thus, adrenergic neural control of airway structures in humans (as distinguished from the direct effects of circulating catecholamines on airway smooth muscle tone) probably occurs largely by adrenergic modulation of parasympathetic transmission. In addition to adrenergic mechanisms, the sympathetic nerve fibers may modulate parasympathetic transmission by releasing neuropeptide Y in the airways [173].

Cholinergic Modulation of Cholinergic Neurotransmission
Modulation of ganglionic transmission by cholinergic mechanisms has also been proposed [82, 122]. Muscarinic receptors of the M_1 subtype facilitate neurotransmission, as selective M_1 antagonism with pirenzepine attenuates reflex bronchoconstriction to inhaled sulfur dioxide (SO_2) but not the direct smooth muscle contraction evoked by methacholine [102]. These data suggest that M_1 receptors might mediate or potentiate reflex bronchoconstriction. In contrast, selective blockade of prejunctional M_2 muscarinic receptors augments parasympathetic nervous system–activated bronchoconstriction in animals and humans [21, 121], and pilocarpine, an M_2 agonist, attenuates SO_2-induced bronchoconstriction in subjects without asthma [123]. Collectively, these data suggest that postganglionic prejunctional M_2 receptors limit the degree of bronchoconstriction induced by parasympathetic mechanisms.

Other Factors Modulating Cholinergic Neurotransmission
Cholinergic transmission may also be modulated by mediators of inflammation (see Chaps. 10 and 11). The spatial association of mast cells and ganglia [8] suggests that mediators derived from mast cells could also modulate parasympathetic ganglionic neurotransmission in a manner similar to events in sympathetic ganglia [189], although direct confirmation is lacking. For example, histamine facilitates acetylcholine release from postganglionic neurons [79] but also inhibits ganglionic transmission via H$_3$-receptor activation [75]. Serotonin [67] prostaglandin F$_{2\alpha}$ [80], prostaglandin D$_2$, and thromboxane A$_2$ [85a, 160, 177] may potentiate cholinergic effects, whereas prostaglandin E$_2$ can reduce them [43, 83, 187]. Further, the demonstration of neuropeptides in ganglia suggests that these compounds may also subserve a possible regulatory role in neurotransmission, although this postulated link has not yet been demonstrated in human tissue [29, 45]. Animal studies have demonstrated both facilitating and inhibitory effects on acetylcholine release of vasoactive intestinal peptide (VIP), depending on the dose used [158]. Moreover, the sensory neuropeptide substance P promotes acetylcholine release in animal models [18, 159, 179] (see Chap. 18). Thus, this complex network of anatomic and physiologic connections may permit fine control of cholinergic tone; however, the precise interactions among these factors require additional study. A more detailed discussion of these events follows.

Cotransmission of neuropeptides from postganglionic fibers may further modulate physiologic responses to cholinergic activation by direct actions on airway smooth muscle or mucous glands. (The roles of neuropeptides in asthma are discussed in greater detail in Chap. 18.) VIP relaxes tracheobronchial smooth muscle and consequently has been postulated as a modulator of endogenous bronchial tone in vivo [138, 152]. VIP has been demonstrated in airway cholinergic nerves, and receptors for VIP are preferentially distributed centrally rather than peripherally, a distribution reminiscent of that of cholinergic nerves [17, 101]. Consequently, Barnes postulated that cotransmission of VIP from cholinergic nerves limits the bronchoconstriction produced by activation of cholinergic nerves [15]. Confirmation of this hypothesis requires further study.

Table 17-1. Muscarinic receptor subtypes in the lung

Feature	M_1	M_2	M_3
Selective agonist(s)	—	Pilocarpine	—
Selective antagonist(s)	Pirenzepine	Gallamine AF-DX 116 Methoctramine	4-DAMP Hexahydrosiladifenidol
Pulmonary distribution (human)	Ganglia Alveolar epithelium Mucous glands	Ganglia	ASM Mucous glands
Putative function(s)	Enhance ganglionic transmission ?Induce mucus secretion	Inhibit ganglionic transmission (autoreceptor)	Induce ASM contraction Induce mucus secretion
G-protein receptor coupling	Gp	Gk, Gi	Gp

ASM = airway smooth muscle; 4-DAMP = 4-diphenylacetoxy-N-methylpiperidine methobromide.

Receptor Types in Cholinergic Neurotransmission

Nicotinic Receptors

Preganglionic (vagal) fibers on stimulation release acetylcholine, which crosses the synaptic cleft and stimulates nicotinic receptors on the postganglionic neuron. These receptors can be blocked by ganglionic blockers such as hexamethonium, but are stimulated by nicotinic agonists [13].

Muscarinic Receptors

It is now well established that muscarinic receptors are heterogeneous in structure, specificity, postreceptor coupling mechanism, and distribution (Table 17-1). At least three pharmacologic types (M_1–M_3) and five biochemical types (m_1–m_5) have been identified [50, 61, 121]. M_1 receptors are characterized by a high binding affinity for pirenzepine. M_2 receptors are selectively inhibited by gallamine and methoctramine, and M_3 muscarinic receptors are blocked by 4-diphenylacetoxy-N-methylpiperidine methobromide (4-DAMP) and hexahydrosiladifenidol [126].

Muscarinic M_1 Receptors. Muscarinic receptors with a high affinity for pirenzepine are distributed in the autonomic ganglia and specifically in the cholinergic pathways [70, 102]. Pirenzepine attenuates vagally induced bronchoconstriction in animals [19, 22] and SO_2-induced bronchoconstriction in humans [102]. However, the precise neurophysiologic role of M_1 receptors in modulating cholinergic tone remains unclear.

In human tissues, muscarinic M_1 receptors have been detected on submucosal glands by autoradiography, but have not been found on smooth muscle. Further, binding of ^{3}H-pirenzepine was observed in alveolar walls of human tissue, suggesting that M_1 receptors were also expressed peripherally [113]. The physiologic role of these peripheral (alveolar wall) M_1 receptors is not known.

Muscarinic M_2 Receptors. Muscarinic receptors of the M_2 subtype are classically expressed in the cardiac atria, and produce bradycardia when they are stimulated. They are selectively antagonized by gallamine, AF-DX 116, and methoctramine, and selectively activated by pilocarpine [14, 120]. With autoradiography, muscarinic receptors (type unspecified) can also be found in human airway nerves and ganglia [113]. Other investigators have shown that these muscarinic receptors are of the M_2 pharmacologic type, and are expressed in several species including humans. They are located prejunctionally on postganglionic nerves, and subserve an inhibitory function for acetylcholine release [53, 121]. The details of this modulation are discussed below.

Muscarinic M_3 Receptors. Autoradiographic studies have demonstrated that muscarinic M_3 receptors are expressed on human airway smooth muscle [113]. Binding of radiolabeled quinuclidinyl benzilate (QNB), a muscarinic receptor ligand, to human smooth muscle muscarinic receptors was completely inhibited by the M_3 antagonist 4-DAMP, suggesting that human smooth muscle muscarinic receptors are principally of the M_3 subtype;

species variation may exist however. Binding of radiolabeled QNB to guinea pig smooth muscle was only partially inhibited by 4-DAMP. Thus, smooth muscle in this animal may express muscarinic receptors of more than one type. Functional evidence also suggests that M_3 muscarinic receptors mediate smooth muscle contraction [148].

M_3 receptors are also found on submucosal glands [113]. Autoradiographic studies suggest that these structures express both M_1 and M_3 receptors; however, the differential functional consequences of M_1 versus M_3 receptor stimulation have not been established.

Mechanisms of Receptor-Response Coupling

Muscarinic receptors regulate intracellular events via G-proteins (Fig. 17-3). Receptors of types M_1 and M_3 couple with Gp, and M_2 receptors link primarily with Gi and Gk [61, 71, 141]. Stimulation of neuronal M_1 muscarinic receptors leads to decreased potassium-ion conductance and subsequent excitation [35]. In contrast, inhibitory M_2 receptor stimulation leads to increased potassium currents due to Gk-linked potassium channel opening and subsequent neuronal hyperpolarization [61].

M_3 receptor occupation in smooth muscle or glandular epithelium is associated with an increased turnover of phosphatidylinositol, which may be mediated by Gp. Turnover of phosphatidylinositol leads to the formation of inositol triphosphate, mobilization of intracellular calcium, calcium influx, and ultimately smooth muscle contraction or secretion [61, 62, 128] (see Chap. 71).

CHOLINERGIC CONTROL OF AIRWAY SMOOTH MUSCLE TONE

Central Origin of Efferent Neural Activity

The activity of the preganglionic efferent parasympathetic fibers to the airway smooth muscle ("bronchomotor" neurons) presumably reflects the net of excitatory and inhibitory inputs from both central and peripheral neural origins (Table 17-2). Whether there is an independent group of pattern generator neurons responsible for maintaining an intrinsic level of activity in the absence of modulating neural inputs, versus activity dependent entirely on afferent information or on pattern generators shared by other systems, is not known.

One source of central excitatory input to the bronchomotor neurons may be the inspiratory pattern generator neurons. Recordings from putative bronchomotor neurons reveal increased firing during inspiration, and this pattern becomes more prominent when peripheral chemoreceptors are stimulated [116, 192]. Changes in bronchomotor activity also are qualitatively similar to changes in breathing when pulmonary reflexes are evoked [192]. Based on these observations, Mitchell and coworkers [125]

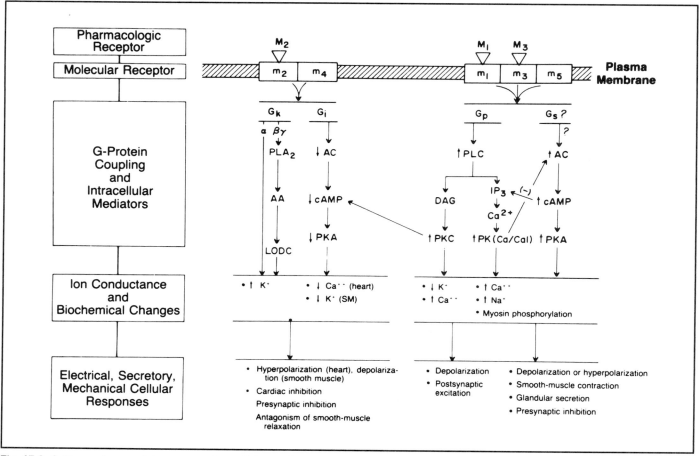

Fig. 17-3. *Subtypes of muscarinic receptors, intracellular mediators, and cellular responses. Pharmacologic receptor types M_1 and M_3 are associated with molecular types m_1 and m_3, and are linked to Gp. M_2 receptors are associated with molecular type m_2 and m_4, and couple with Gi and Gk. AA = arachidonic acid; AC = adenylate cyclase; cAMP = cyclic AMP; DAG = diacylglycerol; IP_3 = inositol triphosphate; LODC = lipoxygenase-derived compounds; PLA_2 = phospholipase A_2; PLC = phospholipase C; PKA = protein kinase A; PKC = protein kinase C. (Reprinted with permission from R. K. Goyal. Muscarinic receptor subtypes. Physiology and clinical implications. N. Engl. J. Med. 321:1022, 1989.)*

studied the relationship between tracheal smooth muscle tension and phrenic nerve activity in cats, and found the two variables to be tightly coupled throughout various maneuvers performed to enhance or inhibit inspiratory neural activity (Fig. 17-4). Although these studies were conducted under nonphysiologic conditions (anesthetized, paralyzed, hyperoxic, hypercapnic), the data are convincing that at least part of the central excitatory input to the bronchomotor neurons has an origin in common with inspiratory motoneurons. Psychologic influences may also increase cholinergic bronchomotor tone.

Peripheral Inputs to Efferent Neural Activity

In addition to the bronchomotor inputs that arise from within the central nervous system, there are peripheral sensory fibers, both pulmonary and extrapulmonary, that can evoke reflex changes in bronchomotor neural activity (see Table 17-2). The contribution of these sensory fibers to the neural control of airway smooth muscle tone is potentially great, due not only to their ability to exert powerful influence on bronchomotor efferent activity but also to the release of locally active neuropeptides from some sensory fibers. (The neuropeptide mechanisms of neural control of airways are discussed in Chap. 18.) The reflex effects of peripheral sensory neurons on bronchomotor activity have

been studied extensively, but mostly in anesthetized animals [40, 95].

Sensory fibers of nasal, epipharyngeal, and laryngeal origin are present in the trigeminal, glossopharyngeal, and superior laryngeal nerves. Except for bronchoinhibitory responses arising during gentle mechanical stimulus of the anterior nares or epipharyngeal region, stimulation of receptors in the upper airways of anesthetized animals generally produces a bronchoconstrictor reflex [40, 95]. Many of these upper airway stimuli elicit a sneeze or cough in awake animals, and the bronchomotor reflex may be a component of a reflex response involving a complex, coordinated effort of several muscle groups.

In lower airways, four categories of sensory receptors that can evoke bronchomotor reflexes have been described. The first is the slowly adapting pulmonary stretch receptor, which is a mechanoreceptor that is activated by distention of the airway wall, has a myelinated axon in the vagus nerve, and evokes inhibitory influences on both inspiratory and bronchomotor neural activity [25, 40]. The reflex inhibition evoked by the stretch receptors is apparent not only during sustained lung inflation (i.e., the Hering-Breuer reflex), but also during phasic breathing, as a function of the alveolar ventilation rate (Fig. 17-5) [169]. Awake, adult humans do not exhibit the profound inspiratory inhibition observed in some other species during lung inflation, but it is not certain to

Table 17-2. Sources of influence for bronchomotor neural activity

Source	Bronchomotor response
Central nervous system	
Inspiratory pattern generator neurons	Excitation
Psychogenic (emotional, behavioral, sensory)	Excitation/inhibition
Central chemoreceptor (CO_2)	Excitation
Airways and lungs	
Nasal afferents (irritation)	Excitation
Nasal or epipharyngeal afferents (gentle mechanical stimulus)	Inhibition
Laryngeal afferents (mechanical, osmolar, chemical, particulate, cold)	Excitation
Slowly adapting pulmonary stretch receptors (lung inflation)	Inhibition
Rapidly adapting pulmonary receptors (chemical, mechanical)	Excitation
Bronchial and pulmonary C-fiber receptors (chemical, mechanical)	Excitation
Heart	
Mechanical distention	Excitation
Coronary artery (chemical)	Excitation
Epicardial (chemical)	Inhibition
Arterial chemoreceptors (hypoxia, hypercapnia)	Excitation
Arterial baroreceptors (pressure change)	Excitation/inhibition
Skeletal muscle Group III and IV afferents (mechanical, chemical)	Inhibition
Esophagus (acid)	Excitation

what degree stretch receptors influence bronchomotor activity in humans. Although antimuscarinic drugs abolish a postinflation decrease in flow resistance in humans [186], suggesting that inflation causes a withdrawal of bronchomotor tone, this might also be explained by a preinflation decrease in airway hysteresis due to the antimuscarinic drug, and a mechanical rather than neural mechanism for the postinflation changes in resistance [28, 139].

The second category of receptors in the lower airways also has myelinated axons in the vagus nerve, and characteristically fires short bursts during mechanical stimulation (i.e., rapidly adapting), and also responds to particulate and chemical stimuli; thus, the designations *rapidly adapting receptor* and *irritant receptor* are both used to describe this category. Stimulation of rapidly adapting pulmonary receptors elicits a bronchoconstrictor reflex that may be accompanied by cough, hyperpnea, or augmented breaths [40, 95].

The remaining lower airway receptors are those with unmyelinated axons (C fibers). These receptors respond to pulmonary congestion and a variety of chemical stimuli, and are classified as bronchial C-fiber receptors if they respond to substances via the bronchial circulation, and as pulmonary C-fiber receptors (or J receptors) if they respond to substances via the pulmonary circulation [40]. C fibers also release neuropeptides, and thus serve simultaneous afferent and efferent functions (see Chap. 18). Stimulation of C-fiber receptors elicits a bronchoconstrictor reflex that typically is accompanied by a brief apnea followed by tachypnea, and sometimes by cough [40, 95].

One extrapulmonary source of influence on bronchomotor neural activity is the arterial chemoreceptors. As discussed above, the inspiratory pattern generator neurons appear to be a source of excitatory input to the bronchomotor neurons; as a

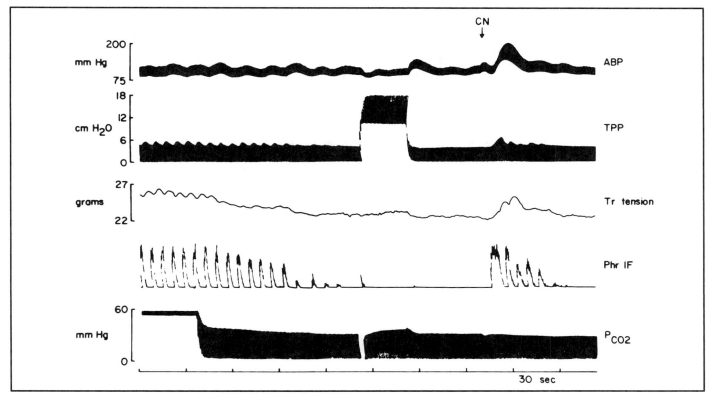

Fig. 17-4. *Relationship of tracheal tension (Tr tension) with phrenic nerve inspiratory activity (Phr IF) during reduction of PCO_2, during increased transpulmonary pressure (TPP), and after injection of cyanide (CN) in an anesthetized, ventilated cat. ABP = arterial blood pressure. (Reprinted with permission from R. A. Mitchell, D. A. Herbert, and D. G. Baker. Inspiratory rhythm in airway smooth muscle tone. J. Appl. Physiol. 58:911, 1985.)*

result, it would be expected that changes in the activity of either peripheral or central sensors to oxygen or carbon dioxide could in turn influence the activity of bronchomotor neurons [40, 124]. Whether oxygen or carbon dioxide influences bronchomotor activity independently of the effects on inspiratory pattern generator neurons cannot be resolved from data currently available. Patients with chronic lung disease exhibit atropine-sensitive airway obstruction, which is decreased with improvement of their hypoxia [3, 64, 107, 181]. No role has been defined for chemoreceptor reflexes in the airway obstruction of asthma. Although bilateral or unilateral carotid body resection has appeared as a treatment for asthma intermittently over the past 50 years, evidence for a therapeutic effect is lacking, and the blunting of ventilatory responses to hypoxia that results from glomectomy makes this surgical procedure unacceptable for asthma management [2].

In addition to chemoreceptor-evoked bronchomotor reflexes, chemoreceptor activity may modulate the response to other bronchomotor reflexes. In anesthetized dogs, reflex tracheal constriction evoked by aerosolized histamine is profoundly affected by the level of oxygenation at the time of challenge [185]. Such changes in the reflex bronchomotor response could not be attributed to histamine-induced changes in carotid body activity [184]. Hyperoxia also was found to attenuate exercise-induced airway obstruction in asthma patients with intact carotid bodies, but to have no effect in subjects who underwent carotid body resection [154].

Other bronchomotor reflexes have been identified that can be initiated by extrapulmonary sensory receptors, including mechanical distention of the heart, chemical stimulation of the coronary arteries or the epicardium, pressure changes in the carotid sinus, mechanical or chemical stimulation of the skeletal muscle Group III or IV afferent fibers in limb or diaphragm, and acid irritation of the esophagus (see Table 17-2) [40].

Preganglionic bronchomotor neuron activity appears to reflect a summation of excitatory and inhibitory inputs of both central and peripheral origin. The various inputs tend to act in a reciprocal fashion with one another, preventing large changes in bronchomotor activity under conditions where large changes in the individual inputs do occur. For example, in awake dogs bronchoconstrictor input associated with hypoxia is completely countered by bronchodilator reflexes evoked by the ventilatory

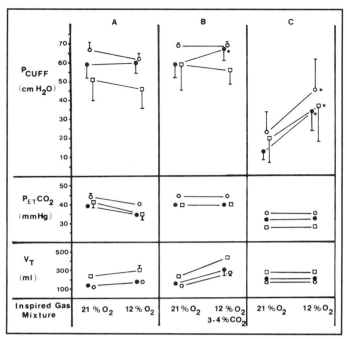

Fig. 17-6. *The effect of hypoxia on tracheal smooth muscle tone (P_{CUFF}) in three awake dogs breathing spontaneously (A), breathing spontaneously under isocapnic conditions (B), and ventilated mechanically with constant frequency and tidal volume (C). Hypoxia caused an increase in tracheal tone when ventilation was controlled, but not when the dogs were allowed to increase their alveolar ventilation. $P_{ET}CO_2$ = end-tidal PCO_2; V_T = tidal volume. (Reprinted with permission from R. L. Sorkness and E. H. Vidruk. Ventilatory responses to hypoxia nullify hypoxic tracheal constriction in awake dogs. Respir. Physiol. 66:41, 1986.)*

response to hypoxia, resulting in a negligible change in bronchomotor activity in hypoxia compared with normoxia (Fig. 17-6) [170]. However, if dogs are ventilated mechanically to maintain constant ventilation, hypoxia consistently increases bronchomotor activity [170], and if ventilation is increased without changing blood gases, bronchomotor activity consistently decreases due to pulmonary stretch receptor inputs [169]. Similarly, during lung inflation, bronchoconstrictor inputs from rapidly adapting receptors are countered by bronchodilator inputs from pulmonary stretch receptors [147], and bronchodilator inputs from limb muscle afferents may contribute to a net decrease in bronchomotor tone during exercise [108].

Modulation of Ganglionic and Junctional Transmission of Bronchomotor Activity

In addition to central and peripheral influences on bronchomotor activity in preganglionic parasympathetic neurons, a number of substances have been identified that modulate the transmission of signals from preganglionic neurons to postganglionic neurons, and can modulate the release of transmitter from the postganglionic neuron to the effector organ. In this manner, mediators, neurotransmitters, and exogenous substances may increase or decrease the amount of acetylcholine released to the effector organ by the postganglionic neuron for a given amount of preganglionic neural activity.

In recent years it has become apparent that acetylcholine, in addition to being an excitatory neurotransmitter at both the parasympathetic ganglion and the effector organ, may serve as a modulator at both sites. At the ganglion, the principal excitatory po-

Fig. 17-5. *The effect of isocapnic changes in ventilation on tracheal smooth muscle tone (Pc) in awake dogs, using changes in frequency (circles) or changes in tidal volume (squares). Tracheal tone changed as a function of alveolar ventilation (right panel). $\dot{V}_E/(\dot{V}_E)_0$ = proportional change in total ventilation rate; $\dot{V}_A/(\dot{V}_A)_0$ = proportional change in alveolar ventilation rate. (Reprinted with permission from R. Sorkness and E. Vidruk. Reflex effects of isocapnic changes in ventilation on tracheal tone in awake dogs. Respir. Physiol. 69:161, 1987.)*

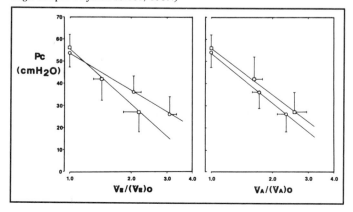

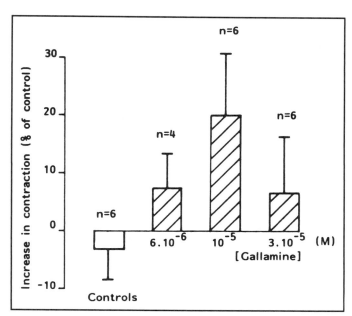

Fig. 17-7. *Percent increase in contraction of isolated human bronchial strips to electrical field stimulation with increasing concentrations of gallamine. Gallamine enhanced the contractions at concentrations that selectively inhibit M_2 muscarinic receptors. (Reprinted with permission from P. A. Minette and P. J. Barnes. Prejunctional inhibitory muscarinic receptors on cholinergic nerves in human and guinea pig airways. J. Appl. Physiol. 64:181, 1988.)*

tential occurs via interaction of acetylcholine with a nicotinic cholinergic receptor. However, in sympathetic ganglia, muscarinic cholinergic receptors of two subtypes (M_1 and M_2) also exist on the postsynaptic neuron and produce a slow excitatory potential (M_1) and a slow inhibitory potential (M_2) when activated by a cholinergic agonist [61, 134]. The M_1-selective muscarinic antagonist pirenzepine decreases the smooth muscle response to preganglionic nerve stimulation in isolated rabbit airway [22, 23] and the reflex bronchoconstriction to SO_2 in humans [102]; these observations suggest that M_1 receptor–mediated enhancement of transmission also may modulate parasympathetic ganglia of the airways.

Acetylcholine also may interact with presynaptic muscarinic cholinergic receptors and inhibit further release of acetylcholine from presynaptic terminals of either preganglionic or postganglionic fibers [61, 82, 189a]. It is not known whether presynaptic muscarinic receptors exist in airway parasympathetic ganglia; however, at the postganglionic neuron–smooth muscle junction there are prejunctional muscarinic receptors that serve as autoreceptors to suppress further release of acetylcholine. These prejunctional inhibitory receptors appear to be of the M_2 muscarinic subtype in humans, cats, guinea pigs, and rats [1, 21, 58, 121] and of the M_1 subtype in dogs [85] (Fig. 17-7). Subjects without asthma have decreased reflex bronchoconstriction to SO_2 after inhalation of the M_2-selective agonist pilocarpine at a dose that is subthreshold for smooth muscle muscarinic receptors (M_3 subtype) but that may stimulate the more sensitive prejunctional inhibitory M_2 receptors [123].

Cholinergic neurotransmission in the airways also may be inhibited by sympathetic neurotransmitters that act at presynaptic terminals in parasympathetic ganglia and/or at prejunctional terminals of postganglionic neurons. Modulation of synaptic transmission in ferret tracheal parasympathetic ganglia was demonstrated by Baker and associates [7], who found that norepinephrine could inhibit markedly the transmission of preganglionic stimuli to the postganglionic neurons. Because norep-

inephrine had no measurable effect on the postsynaptic membrane and because the modulatory effects of norepinephrine were reversed by alpha- but not beta-adrenergic antagonists, Baker and associates concluded that presynaptic alpha-receptor activation is the most likely mechanism [7].

Evidence for adrenergic inhibition of acetylcholine release from postganglionic neurons has been obtained from studies of isolated airways from guinea pigs, dogs, and humans, but there appear to be considerable differences among these three species. In canine bronchi, endogenous release of norepinephrine from sympathetic fibers suppresses acetylcholine release via activation of prejunctional beta$_1$-adrenergic receptors [44, 183]. In other studies, prejunctional inhibition was attributed to alpha$_2$-receptor activation in guinea pigs and with beta$_2$-receptor stimulation in human bronchi; however, no inhibitory effect of sympathetic fibers was demonstrable in these two species [145, 182]. Although Rhoden and coworkers speculated that circulating epinephrine, rather than sympathetic neurons, might be the mechanism by which humans achieve adrenergic modulation of airway neurotransmission, the issue is confused by the fact that the concentration of circulating epinephrine in humans is at least an order of magnitude lower than is necessary to elicit prejunctional inhibition in isolated human airways [10, 42, 145].

Other endogenous substances that inhibit cholinergic neurotransmission include prostaglandin E$_2$ [43, 45a, 81, 165, 187], nitric oxide [20a], and the neuropeptide VIP [68, 114]. Prejunctional inhibition of acetylcholine release in airways also is inhibited by agonists for the mu-type opioid receptor [20, 20b, 87]. Endogenous substances that may enhance cholinergic neurotransmission (or release acetylcholine from the nerve terminal) include serotonin [67, 163], tachykinins such as neurokinin A and substance P (via NK$_2$ receptors, Fig. 17-8) [69, 89, 128a, 173a, 178, 179], corticotropin-releasing factor [176], prostaglandin D$_2$ [177], and the thromboxane mimetic U-46619 [36, 85a]. Leukotriene E$_4$ also enhances parasympathetic neurotransmission by a mechanism involving thromboxane A$_2$ [84a]. A predominant effect of histamine appears to be the enhanced release of acetylcholine

Fig. 17-8. *Enhancement of the contractile response of isolated guinea pig trachea to vagal nerve stimulation by the addition of substance P (SP) to the bath. Ordinate = intraluminal tracheal pressure. (Reprinted with permission from A. K. Hall, et al. Facilitation by tachykinins of neurotransmission in guinea-pig pulmonary parasympathetic nerves. Br. J. Pharmacol. 97:274, 1989.)*

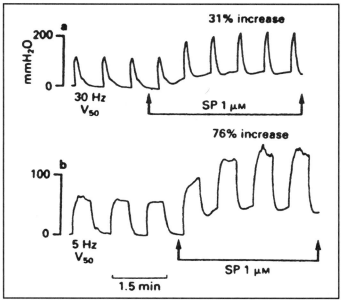

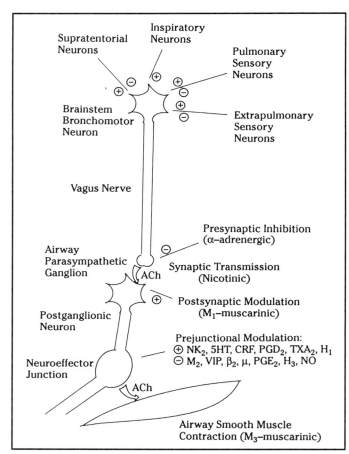

Fig. 17-9. *Central and peripheral factors that affect the amount of acetylcholine (ACh) released by the bronchomotor neuron at the effector organ in the airway. NK = neurokinin; 5HT = serotonin; CRF = corticotropin-releasing factor; PG = prostaglandin; TX = thromboxane; H = histamine; M = muscarinic; VIP = vasoactive intestinal polypeptide; β = beta adrenergic; μ = mu opioid; NO = nitric oxide.*

from postganglionic neurons via H_1 histamine receptors; if H_1 receptors are blocked, histamine may instead cause prejunctional inhibition via H_3 receptors [75, 166]. A synthetic analog of bacterial chemotactic peptide, formyl-methionine-leucine-phenylalanine (FMLP), is another substance that can facilitate cholinergic neurotransmission in airways; while FMLP is not an endogenous substance in healthy airways, these observations may be relevant to conditions involving bacterial colonization or infection [94]. Figure 17-9 is a summary of mechanisms that control parasympathetic output to airway smooth muscle.

In addition to substances that may modulate neurotransmission, there exist substances that, when inhaled, can activate postganglionic parasympathetic neurons independently of preganglionic input. Examples of this mechanism are nicotine, which directly stimulates postsynaptic nicotinic receptors [72], and red tide (*Ptychodiscus brevis*) toxin, which activates sodium ion channels in the neuron [164].

Cholinergic Modulation of Epithelium-Derived Relaxant Factor

Isolated airway smooth muscle often is more responsive to contractile agonists if the adjacent epithelium is disrupted, and it has been proposed that epithelium secretes mediators capable of attenuating airway smooth muscle contraction (see Chap. 23).

Guinea pig tracheas with intact epithelium produce a substance that can relax precontracted vascular smooth muscle. The relaxant factor is produced in the presence of cholinergic agonists, but no relaxation occurs if the tracheas are denuded of epithelium or pretreated with atropine [54, 76]. Lev and coauthors [106] reported that rabbit airways with intact epithelium were less sensitive to acetylcholine-induced contraction in the presence of the selective M_1 muscarinic receptor antagonist pirenzepine and, conversely, more sensitive to acetylcholine in the presence of the selective M_2 receptor antagonist gallamine. The airway contractile response to acetylcholine was not affected by either antagonist after the removal of airway epithelium [106]. This observation implies that a dominant M_2 effect would enhance the production of epithelium-derived relaxant factor, while a dominant M_1 effect would inhibit such a response. Because the effect of intact epithelium in these studies was to attenuate the airway smooth muscle response to acetylcholine, one might speculate that the M_2 receptor effects predominate over the M_1 receptor actions in intact epithelium exposed to acetylcholine.

WHY IS AIRWAY SMOOTH MUSCLE TONE REGULATED?

The fact that cholinergic parasympathetic innervation of airway smooth muscle exists in all mammals, along with complex systems that can influence central parasympathetic activity and modulate peripheral neural transmission, implies that precise regulation of airway smooth muscle tone is of great importance to the survival of the species. However, despite our vast knowledge of maneuvers and substances that influence cholinergic regulation of airway smooth muscle, we have yet to identify a means by which the cholinergic neurons unequivocally and independently determine a state of either lung health or lung disease. Nonetheless, here we summarize first the potential benefits of cholinergic stimulation of airway smooth muscle, and second the possible mechanisms by which the cholinergic system might precipitate or aggravate obstructive airway disease.

One beneficial role of cholinergic airway smooth muscle contraction may be to stabilize the airways and to enhance the expulsion of intraluminal material during a cough. Transient reflex airway smooth muscle contraction accompanies coughing in awake dogs [174] and probably in humans [95] (see Chap. 50). Although increased smooth muscle tone would narrow the lumen of the airways, it would also make the airways less compliant and thus less compressible from high intrathoracic pressures generated during coughing [37, 135–137] such that patency might be better maintained during coughing. The higher linear velocities and turbulence that would occur in constricted large airways might favor dislodging fluid or particulate matter from within the lumen [95, 112].

However, it seems unlikely that such a complex control system would evolve only to make coughing more efficient; there must be additional reasons for adjusting bronchomotor tone during normal breathing. Widdicombe and Nadel [193] proposed that bronchomotor tone might serve to achieve an optimal balance between anatomic dead space and airway resistance, so as to minimize the total work of breathing. For example, during quiet breathing, resistive work is low due to low flow rates, whereas elastic work is relatively high due to the dead space being a larger proportion of the small tidal volume. A modest bronchoconstriction during quiet breathing would reduce dead space with a minimal effect on resistive pressures, thus decreasing total work of breathing. Conversely, during exercise, with large tidal volumes and high flow rates, bronchodilation would reduce resistive work considerably, while increasing elastic work minimally. Although subsequent studies in humans have confirmed that bronchodilation decreases work of breathing during hyperpnea, they could detect no increase in work due to bronchodilation and increased dead space during quiet breathing [86, 156]. Consequently, any benefit realized in terms of work of breathing from stimulation of airway smooth muscle remains unproved.

Another beneficial role proposed for bronchomotor tone is that some degree of airway smooth muscle contraction creates a more uniform distribution of a tidal volume within the lungs, and an optimal interdependence between airways and lung parenchyma [52, 66]. Engel and coworkers studied the effect of changes in airway smooth muscle tone on the distribution of xenon inhaled from residual lung volume and found that the gas was distributed preferentially to the upper lung regions after bronchodilation, compared with more uniform upper and lower lung distribution after bronchoconstriction [52]. They proposed that airway smooth muscle tone widens the distribution of opening pressures throughout the lungs, so that there is more interregional overlap and less dependency on gravitational influences. It should, however, be noted that there is minimal airway closure in healthy lungs during normal tidal breathing from functional reserve volume (as opposed to residual volume); how bronchomotor tone might benefit the distribution of a normal tidal volume is unclear. Hahn and associates [66] studied the relationship between airway diameter and lung volume in anesthetized dogs and found that vagal stimulation decreased the diameter-pressure compliance of the airways and increased the diameter-pressure hysteresis of the airways. Vagal stimulation resulted in marked changes in the interdependence between airways and lung parenchyma, such that at intermediate levels of vagal tone, airway diameter and lung volume hysteresis became more similar, and relative changes in airway diameter with lung volume became homogeneous among airways of 3- to 15-mm diameter [66]. Conversely, when vagal tone was absent or high, hysteresis of airways and lung parenchyma was mismatched, and large and small airways were less homogeneous with respect to relative changes of diameter with lung volume [66]. Recently there has been renewed interest in the potential role of relative airway and parenchymal hysteresis in postinflation changes in airway conductance [28, 78]; it is possible that the cholinergic control of airway smooth muscle tone might serve to adjust airway smooth muscle for some optimal interdependence of airways with lung parenchyma in normal lungs.

POSSIBLE MECHANISMS OF CHOLINERGIC CONTRIBUTION TO ASTHMA

Clinical Background

There is considerable evidence that the cholinergic nervous system might have a major influence in asthma. Airways exhibit a resting tone that can be reduced with atropine [46]. Further, in asthma, there is hyperresponsiveness to cholinergic agonists, and airway obstruction can be relieved by anticholinergic agents [24].

Other factors besides cholinergic tone or excessive neural release of acetylcholine must be considered important in the development of airway obstruction. These factors are reviewed in detail elsewhere in this book. However, smooth muscle responses can be characterized by increased sensitivity to stimulus, by increased maximal response, or by a combination of the two (Fig. 17-10). There is now evidence that isolated tracheal (but not bronchial) smooth muscle from asthma patients is hyperresponsive to contractile stimuli [4, 5]. Likewise, the development of airway obstruction (in distinction to smooth muscle response) to cholinergic stimuli in asthma subjects may show increased maximal response, heightened sensitivity to agonists, or a combination of the two [127]. In addition, it is important to recognize

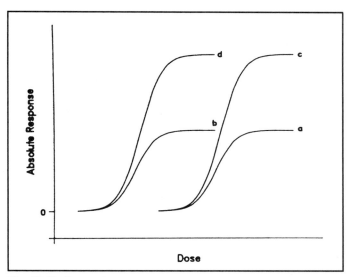

Fig. 17-10. *Types of agonist responses. a = normal response; b = deviation supersensitivity, resulting from increased activity of agonist at receptor site; c = nondeviation supersensitivity, characterized by increased maximal response; d = mixed pattern. (Reprinted with permission from R. H. Moreno, J. C. Hogg, and P. D. Paré. Mechanics of airway narrowing. Am. Rev. Respir. Dis.* 133:1171, 1986.)

that other factors, which may or may not be influenced by cholinergic tone, can be important determinants of airflow limitation in the intact airway. These factors include the thickness of the airway wall (particularly that component on the luminal side of the airway smooth muscle), the presence of increased luminal secretions, and reduced baseline airway caliber [85c, 127, 194]. Thus, dissecting the precise contribution of cholinergic stimuli to the development of airway hyperresponsiveness and obstruction in the intact human airway remains extremely difficult.

If abnormalities in parasympathetic control of the airway were universally seen in asthma, increased cholinergic airway tone should exist. However, there is little direct evidence of increased cholinergic-dependent airway tone in asthma. The observation that asthma patients are also hyperresponsive to cholinesterase inhibitors is consistent with increased cholinergic outflow or with airway smooth muscle hyperresponsiveness to acetylcholine (reviewed in [24]). Recent data indicate that tracheal airway smooth muscle from patients with fatal asthma contracts more vigorously to acetylcholine than that from control subjects [4, 5]. However, previous investigations have not shown differences in response to contractile agonists, so additional study will be required to clarify this point [60, 190]. Although asthmatic subjects have bronchial hyperresponsiveness to cholinergic stimuli, they do to irritants as well. Thus, whether or not increased cholinergic outflow regularly contributes to excess airway smooth muscle contraction in asthma remains unclear.

Possible Parasympathetic Abnormalities in Asthma

Increased Central Output

Sleep-related or circadian increases in cholinergic bronchomotor activity have been hypothesized, based on the frequency of nocturnal exacerbations of asthma. However, unequivocal data demonstrating a parasympathetic origin of nighttime airway obstruction are lacking due to both technical factors and the complexity of the parasympathetic system.

Direct assessment of vagal tone in humans is not possible with current techniques. Nonetheless, indirect indices of vagal tone (heart rate variability, sweating, and pupillary response to cholinergic agonists) are increased in asthma [92, 93]. Using heart rate as a physiologic index of "vagal" activity, a correlation between increased nocturnal vagal activity and decreased peak expiratory flows in asthma has been demonstrated [12, 142]. However, efferent fibers in the cardiac branches of the vagus nerve have strikingly different firing patterns than do efferent fibers from the pulmonary branches of the vagus, and cardiac and airway vagal efferents have different origins in the brain stem [116]; consequently, heart rate may not be an entirely reliable index of parasympathetic bronchomotor activity. Until direct measurements of airway cholinergic tone in humans are made, this question will remain open.

Heightened circadian variability in airway caliber, discussed in Chapter 76, is also a characteristic of asthma. Some patients with asthma exhibit less dramatic nocturnal changes in peak flows after inhaling an antimuscarinic drug compared with placebo [38], consistent with cholinergic contribution to nocturnal obstruction. However, it is not certain that this effect is due to a greater central bronchomotor tone in asthma. Circadian variation in lower airway resistance, which varies in parallel with indirect measures of vagal tone, is not appreciably altered by the stage of sleep. Further, sleep (versus wakefulness) is associated with increased lower airway resistance, but numerous alternative explanations besides increased cholinergic tone are possible [9, 115]. Moreover, studies in unmedicated dogs revealed that although tracheal smooth muscle tone changed erratically during rapid eye movement (REM) sleep, the maximal tone during REM sleep was similar to that observed during quiet awake periods, and the tracheal tone during deeper stages of sleep generally was lower than that during quiet wakefulness [174]. Thus, increased vagal tone at night exists as a possible contributing factor in nocturnal bronchial obstruction, but direct confirmation is lacking.

Besides heightened cholinergic activity, other explanations for increased nocturnal airway obstruction have been proposed. Subjects with asthma exhibit nocturnal decreases in circulating epinephrine that correlate with changes in peak flow rates [10]. Varying catecholamine concentrations could result in an increase in airway smooth muscle tone by removal of the physiologic antagonism of bronchomotor tone by epinephrine at the smooth muscle [10] and possibly by removal of epinephrine-induced inhibition of acetylcholine release (see above discussion of neuromodulation). Other mediators produced by airway tissues and inflammatory cells are also capable of altering parasympathetic neurotransmission, airway smooth muscle responsiveness, and lung mechanics. Thus, changes in the local mediator milieu or in circulating levels of epinephrine could explain nocturnal changes of airways and heart rate, without having to implicate nighttime changes in central cholinergic activity.

Another putative source of central excitatory input to bronchomotor neurons is psychogenic factors. In a series of studies in patients with asthma, an atropine-sensitive bronchoconstriction response was evoked reproducibly in half the subjects after they were given a placebo aerosol which they believed to be a bronchoprovocative substance. The placebo-induced bronchoconstriction was then reversed with a second dose of placebo aerosol, which the subjects believed to be a bronchodilator (Fig. 17-11)[111, 118, 171]. A subsequent study, more stringently controlled and including physiologic indices of emotional responses, confirmed the ability of suggestion to elicit an airway response in some subjects, and furthermore showed correlations between the changes in airway resistance and emotional responses [74]. In another interesting report, pulmonary resistance in two hypnotized asthmatic subjects was increased during suggestions of anger, fear, or asthma attack, and was decreased during suggestions of relaxation [168]. More recently, emotional events have been cited as precipitating or exacerbating factors in a subgroup of severe, rapid-onset, short-duration asthma attacks [188]. Thus,

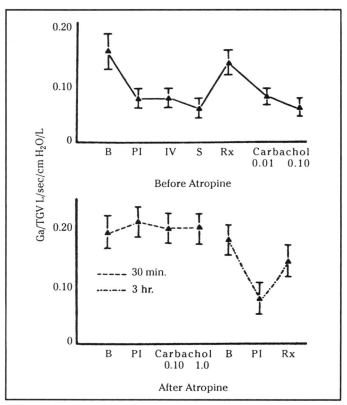

Fig. 17-11. *Changes in specific airway conductance (Ga/TGV) in response to suggestion in patients with asthma, before and after treatment with atropine. Conductance decreased from baseline (B) after the administration of bogus antigen (PI and S) and an intravenous placebo injection which they believed to be a substance that would enhance an allergic response (IV). Conductance returned toward baseline after administration of a placebo that the patients believed to be a bronchodilator (Rx), and decreased again after administration of carbachol. Thirty minutes after administration of atropine (lower), which patients believed to be a substance that would enhance an allergic response, no change in conductance occurred in response to either bogus antigen or carbachol administration, but 3 hours after atropine administration the conductance again changed in response to suggestion. (Reprinted with permission from E. R. McFadden, Jr., et al. The mechanism of action of suggestion in the induction of acute asthma attacks. Psychosom. Med. 31:134, 1969. © by American Psychosomatic Society.)*

it appears that in some persons with preexisting hyperresponsive airways, psychogenic inputs to bronchomotor neurons may evoke significant changes in airway resistance, presumably via increased cholinergic tone.

Altered Output from Peripheral Receptors

As discussed, vagal afferent fibers arise from at least three receptor types: slowly adapting (stretch) receptors, rapidly adapting (irritant) receptors, and C-fiber endings. However, the distinction between rapidly adapting receptor and C-fiber endings is somewhat blurred. Activation of the slowly adapting receptors may promote bronchodilation, and initiates the Hering-Breuer reflex [13, 133]. Inhibition of stretch receptor activity might therefore be postulated to lead to bronchoconstriction, but direct data addressing this point in humans are lacking.

Rapidly adapting receptors appear to mediate coughing and bronchoconstriction. Receptors located in the larynx and trachea show increased sensitivity to particulate stimuli, and their stimulation produces coughing. Irritant receptors located more peripherally may mediate bronchoconstrictor responses [129, 191]. Increased output from or sensitivity of the irritant receptors might therefore be associated with bronchoconstriction. Although direct evidence that increased rapidly adapting receptor output is a universal concomitant of asthma is lacking, some data do suggest that these receptors contribute to bronchoconstriction in certain situations. For example, viral respiratory tract infections, known exacerbants of asthma, are associated with heightened irritant receptor responses [51] (see Chap. 44). Histamine, serotonin, and prostaglandin $F_{2\alpha}$ all stimulate irritant receptors [153]. Further, low doses of histamine produce vagally mediated reflex bronchoconstriction [47]. Thus, inflammatory mediators may cause airway obstruction in part via reflex cholinergic mechanisms in asthma. However, vagal blockade does not entirely abrogate bronchial obstruction following antigen challenge in humans or animals, suggesting that mechanisms other than cholinergic reflex bronchoconstriction also participate [27, 149]. Damage to or disruption of epithelium has also been postulated to increase irritant receptor output, by exposing them to luminal irritants [13].

C-fiber endings are nonmyelinated, and have been demonstrated in the epithelium of human airways [13, 99]. They are sensitive to bradykinin and capsaicin [39, 97] and to compounds that also stimulate irritant receptors [41]. Stimulation of C fibers is thought to have physiologic consequences similar to those produced by irritant receptors [105]. Furthermore, C fibers contain neuropeptides including substance P [110], which Barnes suggests are released via an axon reflex [13]. Because substance P can increase acetylcholine release from postganglionic nerves [69], its liberation may cause cholinergic-mediated bronchial obstruction. Factors that enhance release or activity of this sensory neuropeptide, including airway epithelial injury or disruption, might increase parasympathetically mediated bronchial constriction. Further, the degradation enzyme neutral endopeptidase rapidly cleaves and inactivates neurokinins, including substance P, and is localized to the airway epithelium [88, 157]. Reduced activity of neutral endopeptidase could thereby heighten airway responses to substance P [130]. Thus, because removal of airway epithelium, viral respiratory tract infections, and exposure to toluene diisocyanate increase airway responsiveness, it is possible that this heightened activity is due to reduced neutral endopeptidase activity [130, 131].

Altered Ganglionic or Postganglionic Transmission
Several other mechanisms might also contribute to increased cholinergic effect in asthma in the absence of increased central outflow. Ganglionic and postganglionic neurotransmissions are reduced by beta agonists via specific receptors [167, 183]. Studies have suggested that beta-adrenoreceptor function is reduced in asthma [26, 30, 162] (see Chap. 14) and made more abnormal by allergen challenge [119]. Other investigators, however, have not clearly identified abnormal beta-receptor function in asthma [59, 180]. If beta-receptor function is subnormal in asthma, cholinergic neurotransmission would increase via a loss of inhibitory adrenergic control. The observation that beta-adrenoceptor antagonists provoke severe or fatal asthma suggests that this mechanism may be important in some patients. Recent data demonstrating the effectiveness of oxitropium bromide in propranolol-induced bronchoconstriction in asthmatic subjects are further evidence of the potential clinical import of this control mechanism [77]. However, other investigators have been unable to demonstrate significant protection against propranolol-induced asthma by ipratropium [104]. Whether this discrepancy relates to the agent used, the population studied, or the variability of asthma is unclear.

Administration of beta-receptor antagonists in several forms can precipitate severe asthma [33, 55]. Some authors have suggested that asthma exacerbations related to the administration of beta-receptor blockers are mediated by a loss of beta-receptor agonist inhibition of cholinergic transmission, coupled with a muscarinic M_2 receptor defect [14, 77]. Although this hypothesis is attractive, other investigators have been unable to demonstrate clear protection from beta blocker–induced asthma by anticholinergic agents [104]. Thus, the role of cholinergic tone in asthma exacerbations induced by beta-receptor blockade remains controversial.

Altered cholinergic neurotransmission might also be produced by abnormalities in muscarinic receptor function. Enhanced expression or avidity of the potentiating M_1 ganglionic receptors, or reduced expression or activity of the inhibitory M_2 receptor, would potentiate cholinergic bronchoconstriction. The lack of a protective effect of the M_2 agonist pilocarpine on SO_2- or histamine-induced bronchospasm in asthmatic but not in normal subjects has been suggested as evidence for a defect in M_2 receptor activity in asthma [14, 123]. Additional data are required to clarify this point. However, recent observations have shown a reduced affinity of M_2 muscarinic receptors following in vitro incubation of lung tissue with Type 1 parainfluenza virus, suggesting a possible link between viral infections and abnormality in the regulation of cholinergic airway tone [56]. Moreover, in vivo parainfluenza Type 3 infection in guinea pigs reduces M_2 autoreceptor function [57]. In addition, M_2 autoreceptors in guinea pig airways appear to be damaged by the inflammatory response to repeated allergen challenge [58a].

Other interactions have been postulated. VIP, possibly cotransmitted with acetylcholine, is a potent bronchial smooth muscle relaxant [138, 151, 152]. Proteolytic enzymes, including mast cell–derived tryptase and chymase, may degrade VIP and thus enhance the effect of released acetylcholine by removing a relaxing factor [32].

Inflammatory mediators released during immediate or late-phase asthmatic responses could promote cholinergic neurotransmission, and hence worsen bronchial obstruction. Histamine, prostaglandin $F_{2\alpha}$, prostaglandin D_2, and thromboxane A_2 can all facilitate postganglionic acetylcholine release. Enlarged airway parasympathetic transmission due to ozone exposure or allergen-activated alveolar macrophages in dogs has been associated with thromboxane A_2 [85b, 175]. Moreover, because high-dose VIP inhibits, whereas low-dose VIP promotes acetylcholine release [158], partial degradation of cotransmitted VIP might also potentiate cholinergic bronchial obstruction by enhancing acetylcholine release.

Anticholinergic Therapy in Asthma: Clues to Cholinergic Function

Insight for a potential role of the cholinergic system in asthma can be gained by examining anticholinergic therapy in obstructive lung disease. The preceding discussion outlined the rationale for anticholinergic therapy in obstructive lung disease, and indicated that the contribution of cholinergic tone and reflex activity to overall bronchoconstriction in clinical situations remains unknown [63].

In subjects with emphysema, Gross and Skorodin [64] found that an inhaled anticholinergic agent, atropine methonitrate, gave significantly greater bronchodilation than a beta agonist, salbutamol. Further, the anticholinergic agent produced additional bronchodilation following maximal effects with salbutamol. From these observations, it was concluded "that parasympathetic activity is the dominant reversible component of airway obstruction in" emphysema. Because clinically used anticholinergic agents produce blockade of all muscarinic receptor subtypes, the site and mechanism of bronchodilation or its extension to other forms of lung disease cannot be made.

Evaluation of anticholinergic therapy in asthma, rather than other forms of obstructive lung disease, has added to the confusion of cholinergic regulation of airway function (see Chap. 64). Initially, Storms and coworkers [172] found equivalent bronchodilation with an isopropyl derivative of atropine, Sch 1000, and isoproterenol in inhalation form. Bronchodilation with the anticholinergic agent had different kinetics than that of the beta agonist: slower onset but longer duration. Similar responses in asthma were found with another anticholinergic aerosol, glycopyrrolate, in studies by Schroeckenstein and coworkers [155]. Taken at face value, these data support the concept that resting cholinergic tone is inherent in symptomatic asthma and contributes to underlying bronchial obstruction. In contrast, anticholinergic therapy in acute asthma produces little reversal of airway obstruction except when given with a beta agonist [49, 96, 143, 144]. Thus, by examining therapeutic responses to anticholinergics, it is difficult to assess precisely the contribution of cholinergic airway function in asthma.

In summary, the cholinergic innervation and regulation of airway function are complex and unresolved. However, the influence of cholinergic function on airway activity cannot be determined simply by examining postganglionic innervation of bronchial smooth muscle; this is only one component of its activity. As illustrated in Figure 17-9, the cholinergic system is regulated at many levels—central, ganglia, and neuroeffector junction—to control airway smooth muscle. It may also influence other tissues important to normal airway function, for example, inflammatory cells, epithelium, and secretory glands. Until these many interactions can be identified and isolated for study, and more specific antagonists for muscarinic receptor subtypes made available, the full impact of the cholinergic system in obstructive lung diseases, including asthma, will remain unappreciated. Nevertheless, this most important control system for bronchomotor tone is likely critical in normal and pathologic function in human airways.

REFERENCES

1. Aas, P., and Maclagan, J. Evidence for prejunctional M2 muscarinic receptors in pulmonary cholinergic nerves in the rat. *Br. J. Pharmacol.* 101: 73, 1990.
2. American Academy of Allergy and Immunology position statement. Carotid body resection. *J. Allergy Clin. Immunol.* 78:273, 1986.
3. Astin, T. W., and Penman, R. W. B. Airway obstruction due to hypoxemia in patients with chronic lung disease. *Am. Rev. Respir. Dis.* 95:567, 1967.
4. Bai, T. R. Abnormalities in airway smooth muscle in fatal asthma. *Am. Rev. Respir. Dis.* 141:552, 1990.
5. Bai, T. R. Abnormalities in airway smooth muscle in fatal asthma: A comparison between trachea and bronchus. *Am. Rev. Respir. Dis.* 143: 441, 1991.
6. Baker, D. G. Parasympathetic motor pathways to the trachea: Recent morphologic and electrophysiologic studies. *Clin. Chest Med.* 7:223, 1986.
7. Baker, D. G., et al. Transmission in airway ganglia in ferrets: Inhibition by norepinephrine. *Neurosci. Lett.* 41:139, 1983.
8. Baker, D. G., et al. The architecture of nerves and ganglia of the ferret trachea as revealed by acetylcholinesterase histochemistry. *J. Comp. Neurol.* 246:513, 1986.
9. Ballard, R. D., et al. Effect of sleep on nocturnal bronchoconstriction and ventilatory patterns in asthmatics. *J. Appl. Physiol.* 67:243, 1989.
10. Barnes, P., et al. Nocturnal asthma and changes in circulating epinephrine, histamine, and cortisol. *N. Engl. J. Med.* 303:263, 1980.
11. Barnes, P. J., et al. Muscarinic receptors in lung and trachea: Autoradiographic localization using ^{3}H-quinuclidinyl benzilate. *Eur. J. Pharmacol.* 86:103, 1983.
12. Barnes, P. J. Circadian variation in airway function. *Am. J. Med.* 79(Suppl. 6A):5, 1985.
13. Barnes, P. J. Neural control of human airways in health and disease. *Am. Rev. Respir. Dis.* 134:1289, 1986.
14. Barnes, P. J. Muscarinic receptors in airways: Recent developments. *J. Appl. Physiol.* 68:1777, 1990.
15. Barnes, P. J. Neuropeptides and asthma. *Am. Rev. Respir. Dis.* 143:S28, 1991.
16. Barnes, P. J., Basbaum, C. B., and Nadel, J. A. Autoradiographic localization of autonomic receptors in airway smooth muscle: Marked differences between large and small airways. *Am. Rev. Respir. Dis.* 127:758, 1983.
17. Barnes, P. J., and Dixon, C. M. S. The effect of inhaled vasoactive intestinal peptide on bronchial hyperreactivity in man. *Am. Rev. Respir. Dis.* 130: 162, 1984.
18. Barnes, P. J., MacLagan, J., and Meldrum, L. A. Effects of tachykinins on cholinergic neural responses in guinea-pig trachea. *Br. J. Pharmacol.* 90: 138P, 1987.
19. Beck, K. C., et al. Muscarinic M_1 receptors mediate the increase in pulmonary resistance during vagus nerve stimulation in dogs. *Am. Rev. Respir. Dis.* 136:1135, 1987.
20. Belvisi, M. G., Stretton, C. D., and Barnes, P. J. Modulation of cholinergic neurotransmission in guinea-pig airways by opioids. *Br. J. Pharmacol.* 100:131, 1990.
20a. Belvisi, M. G., Stretton, C. D., and Barnes, P. J. Nitric oxide as an endogenous modulator of cholinergic neurotransmission in guinea-pig airways. *Eur. J. Pharmacol.* 198:219, 1991.
20b. Belvisi, M. G., et al. Inhibition of cholinergic neurotransmission in human airways by opioids. *J. Appl. Physiol.* 72:1096, 1992.
21. Blaber, L. C., Fryer, A. D., and Maclagan, J. Neuronal muscarinic receptors attenuate vagally-induced contraction of feline bronchial smooth muscle. *Br. J. Pharmacol.* 86:724, 1985.
22. Bloom, J. W., et al. A muscarinic receptor subtype modulates vagally stimulated bronchial contraction. *J. Appl. Physiol.* 65:2144, 1988.
23. Bloom, J. W., et al. A muscarinic receptor with high affinity for pirenzepine mediates vagally induced bronchoconstriction. *Eur. J. Pharmacol.* 133:21, 1987.
24. Boushey, H. A., et al. Bronchial hyperreactivity. *Am. Rev. Respir. Dis.* 121: 389, 1980.
25. Bowes, G., et al. An efferent pathway mediating reflex tracheal dilation in awake dogs. *J. Appl. Physiol.* 57:413, 1984.
26. Brooks, S. M., et al. Relationship between numbers of beta adrenergic receptors in lymphocytes and disease severity in asthma. *J. Allergy Clin. Immunol.* 63:401, 1979.
27. Brown, K. J., et al. Physiological and pharmacological properties of canine trachealis muscle in vivo. *J. Appl. Physiol.* 49:84, 1980.
28. Burns, C. B., Taylor, W. R., and Ingram, R. H., Jr. Effects of deep inhalation in asthma: Relative airway and parenchymal hysteresis. *J. Appl. Physiol.* 59:1590, 1985.
29. Burnstock, G., Allen, T. G. J., and Hassall, C. J. S. The electrophysiologic and neurochemical properties of paratracheal neurones in situ and in dissociated cell culture. *Am. Rev. Respir. Dis.* 136:S23, 1987.
30. Busse, W. W. Decreased granulocyte response to isoproterenol in asthma during upper respiratory infections. *Am. Rev. Respir. Dis.* 115:783, 1977.
31. Cameron, A. R., and Coburn, R. F. Electrical and anatomic characteristics of cells of ferret paratracheal ganglion. *Am. J. Physiol.* 246:C450, 1984.
32. Caughey, G. H., et al. Substance P and vasoactive intestinal peptide degradation by mast cell tryptase and chymase. *J. Pharmacol. Exp. Ther.* 224: 133, 1988.
33. Chester, E. H., Schwartz, H. J., and Fleming, G. M. Adverse effect of propranolol on airway function in non-asthmatic chronic obstructive lung disease. *Chest* 79:540, 1981.
34. Chiang, C.-H., and Gabella, G. Quantitative study of the ganglion neurones of the mouse trachea. *Cell Tissue Res.* 246:243, 1986.
35. Christie, M. J., and North, R. A. Control of ion conductances by muscarinic receptors. *Trends Pharmacol. Sci.* 9(Suppl.):30, 1988.
36. Chung, K. F., et al. Modulation of cholinergic neurotransmission in canine airways by thromboxane mimetic U46619. *Eur. J. Pharmacol.* 117:373, 1985.
37. Coburn, R. F., Thornton, D., and Arts, R. Effect of trachealis muscle contraction on tracheal resistance to airflow. *J. Appl. Physiol.* 32:397, 1972.
38. Coe, C. I., and Barnes, P. J. Reduction of nocturnal asthma by an inhaled anticholinergic drug. *Chest* 90:485, 1986.
39. Coleridge, H. M., Coleridge, J. C. G., and Luck, J. C. Pulmonary afferent fibers of small diameter stimulated by capsaicin and by hyperinflation of the lungs. *J. Physiol. (Lond.)* 179:248, 1965.
40. Coleridge, H. M., Coleridge, J. C. G., and Schultz, H. D. Afferent pathways involved in reflex regulation of airway smooth muscle. *Pharmacol. Ther.* 42:1, 1989.
41. Coleridge, J. C. G., and Coleridge, H. M. Afferent vagal C fibre innervation

of the lung and airways and its functional significance. *Rev. Physiol. Biochem. Pharmacol.* 99:1, 1984.

42. Cryer, P. E. Physiology and pathophysiology of the human sympatho-adrenal neuroendocrine system. *N. Engl. J. Med.* 303:436, 1980.

43. Daniel, E. E., and Davis, C. Effects of endogenous and exogenous prostaglandin in neurotransmission in canine trachea. *Can. J. Physiol. Pharmacol.* 65:1433, 1987.

44. Danser, A. H. J., et al. Prejunctional beta-adrenoreceptors inhibit cholinergic neurotransmission in canine bronchi. *J. Appl. Physiol.* 62:785, 1987.

45. Day, R. D., Shannon, W. R., and Said, S. I. Localization of VIP-immunoreactive nerves in airways and pulmonary vessels of dogs, cats, and human subjects. *Cell Tissue Res.* 229:231, 1981.

45a. DeLisle, S., et al. Effects of prostaglandin E_2 on ganglionic transmission in the guinea pig trachea. *Resp. Physiol.* 87:131, 1992.

46. deTroyer, A., Yernault, J.-C., and Rodenstein, D. Effects of vagal blockade on lung mechanics in normal man. *J. Appl. Physiol.* 46:217, 1979.

47. Dixon, M., Jackson, D. M., and Richards, I. M. The effects of H_1 and H_2 receptor antagonists on total lung resistance, dynamic lung compliance, and irritant receptor discharge in the anaesthetized dog. *Br. J. Pharmacol.* 66:203, 1979.

48. Doidge, J. M., and Satchell, D. G. Adrenergic and non-adrenergic inhibitory nerves in mammalian airways. *J. Auton. Nerv. Syst.* 5:83, 1982.

49. Easton, P. A., et al. A comparison of the bronchodilating effects of a beta-2 adrenergic agent (albuterol) and an anticholinergic agent (ipratropium bromide), given by aerosol alone or in sequence. *N. Engl. J. Med.* 315:735, 1986.

50. Eglen, R. M., and Whiting, R. L. Muscarinic receptor subtypes: A critique of the current classification and a proposal for a working nomenclature. *J. Auton. Pharmacol.* 5:323, 1986.

51. Empey, D. W., et al. Mechanisms of bronchial hyperreactivity in normal subjects after upper respiratory tract infection. *Am. Rev. Respir. Dis.* 113:131, 1974.

52. Engel, L. A., et al. Influence of bronchomotor tone on regional ventilation distribution at residual volume. *J. Appl. Physiol.* 40:411, 1976.

53. Faulkner, D., Fryer, A. D., and MacLagan, J. Post-ganglionic muscarinic inhibitory receptors in pulmonary parasympathetic nerves in guinea pig. *Br. J. Pharmacol.* 88:181, 1986.

54. Fernandes, L. B., Paterson, J. W., and Goldie, R. G. Co-axial bioassay of a smooth muscle relaxant factor released from guinea-pig tracheal epithelium. *Br. J. Pharmacol.* 96:117, 1989.

55. Fraunfeder, F. T., and Barker, A. F. Respiratory effects of timolol. *N. Engl. J. Med.* 311:1411, 1984.

56. Fryer, A. D., El-Fakahany, E. E., and Jacoby, D. B. Parainfluenza virus type 1 reduces the affinity of agonists for muscarinic receptors in guinea-pig lung and heart. *Eur. J. Pharmacol.* 181:51, 1990.

57. Fryer, A. D., and Jacoby, D. B. Parainfluenza virus infection damages inhibitory M_2 muscarinic receptors on pulmonary parasympathetic nerves in the guinea pig. *Br. J. Pharmacol.* 102:267, 1991.

58. Fryer, A. D., and MacLagan, J. Muscarinic inhibitory receptors in pulmonary parasympathetic nerves in the guinea-pig. *Br. J. Pharmacol.* 83:973, 1984.

58a. Fryer, A. D., and Wills-Karp, M. Dysfunction of M_2-muscarinic receptors in pulmonary parasympathetic nerves after antigen challenge. *J. Appl. Physiol.* 71:2255, 1991.

59. Galant, S. P., et al. Decreased beta-adrenergic receptors on polymorphonuclear leukocytes after adrenergic therapy. *N. Engl. J. Med.* 299:933, 1978.

60. Goldie, R. G., et al. *In vitro* responsiveness of human asthmatic bronchus to carbachol, histamine, β-adrenoceptor agonists and theophylline. *Br. J. Clin. Pharmacol.* 22:669, 1986.

61. Goyal, R. K. Muscarinic receptor subtypes. Physiology and clinical implications. *N. Engl. J. Med.* 321:1022, 1989.

62. Grandordy, B. M., and Barnes, P. J. Phosphoinositide turnover in airway smooth muscle. *Am. Rev. Respir. Dis.* 136:17, 1987.

63. Gross, N. J. Ipratropium bromide. *N. Engl. J. Med.* 319:486, 1988.

64. Gross, N. J., and Skorodin, M. S. Role of the parasympathetic systemic airway obstruction due to emphysema. *N. Engl. J. Med.* 311:421, 1984.

65. Gundstrom, N., and Andersson, R. G. G. Inhibition of the cholinergic neurotransmission in human airways via prejunctional α_2-adrenoceptors. *Acta Physiol. Scand.* 125:513, 1985.

66. Hahn, H. L., Graf, P. D., and Nadel, J. A. Effect of vagal tone on airway diameters and on lung volume in anesthetized dogs. *J. Appl. Physiol.* 41:581, 1976.

67. Hahn, H. L., et al. Interaction between serotonin and efferent vagus nerves in dog lung. *J. Appl. Physiol.* 44:144, 1978.

68. Hakoda, H., and Ito, Y. Modulation of cholinergic neurotransmission by the peptide VIP, VIP antiserum and VIP antagonists in dog and cat trachea. *J. Physiol. (Lond.)* 428:133, 1990.

69. Hall, A. K., et al. Facilitation by tachykinins of neurotransmission in guinea-pig pulmonary parasympathetic nerves. *Br. J. Pharmacol.* 97:274, 1989.

70. Hammer, R., and Giachetti, A. Muscarinic receptor subtypes: M_1 and M_2 biochemical and functional characterization. *Life Sci.* 31:2991, 1982.

71. Harden, T. K., Tanner, L. I., and Martin, M. W. Characteristics of two biochemical responses to stimulation of muscarinic cholinergic receptors. *Trends Pharmacol. Sci.* 7(Suppl.):14, 1986.

72. Hartiala, J. J., et al. Nicotine-induced respiratory effects of cigarette smoke in dogs. *J. Appl. Physiol.* 59:64, 1985.

72a. Haselton, J. R., Padrid, P. A., and Kaufman, M. P. Activation of neurons in the rostral ventrolateral medulla increases bronchomotor tone in dogs. *J. Appl. Physiol.* 71:210, 1991.

73. Honjin, R. On the ganglia and nerves of the lower respiratory tract of the mouse. *J. Morphol.* 95:263, 1954.

74. Horton, D. J., et al. Bronchoconstrictive suggestion in asthma: A role for airways hyperreactivity and emotions. *Am. Rev. Respir. Dis.* 117:1029, 1978.

75. Ichinose, M., et al. Histamine H_3 receptors inhibit cholinergic transmission in guinea pig airways. *Br. J. Pharmacol.* 97:13, 1989.

76. Ilhan, M., and Sahin, I. Tracheal epithelium releases a vascular smooth muscle relaxant factor: Demonstration by bioassay. *Eur. J. Pharmacol.* 131:293, 1986.

77. Ind, P. W., et al. Anticholinergic blockade of beta-blocker induced bronchoconstriction. *Am. Rev. Respir. Dis.* 139:1390, 1989.

78. Ingram, R. H., Jr. Physiological assessment of inflammation in the peripheral lung of asthmatic patients. *Lung* 168:237, 1990.

79. Inoue, T., and Ito, Y. Characteristics of neuroeffector transmission in the smooth muscle layer of dog bronchiole and modifications by autocoids. *J. Physiol. (Lond.)* 370:551, 1986.

80. Itahn, R. A., and Patil, P. N. Salivation induced by $PGF_{2\alpha}$ and modification of the response by atropine and physostigmine. *Br. J. Pharmacol.* 44:527, 1972.

81. Ito, I., et al. Pre-junctional inhibitory action of prostaglandin E2 on excitatory neuro-effector transmission in the human bronchus. *Prostaglandins* 39:639, 1990.

82. Ito, Y., and Yoshitomi, T. Autoregulation of acetylcholine release from vagus nerve terminals through activation of muscarinic receptors in the dog trachea. *Br. J. Pharmacol.* 93:636, 1988.

83. Ito, Y. Prejunctional control of excitatory neuroeffector transmission by prostaglandins in the airway smooth muscle tissue. *Am. Rev. Respir. Dis.* 143:S6, 1991.

84. Jacobowitz, D., et al. Histofluorescent study of catecholamine containing elements in cholinergic ganglion from the calf and dog lung. *Proc. Soc. Exp. Biol. Med.* 144:464, 1973.

84a. Jacques, C. A. J., et al. The mechanism of LTE_4-induced histamine hyper-responsiveness in guinea-pig tracheal and human bronchial smooth muscle. *Br. J. Pharmacol.* 104:859, 1991.

85. Janssen, L. J., and Daniel, E. E. Pre- and postjunctional muscarinic receptors in canine bronchi. *Am. J. Physiol.* 259:L304, 1990.

85a. Janssen, L. J., and Daniel, E. E. Pre- and postjunctional effects of a thromboxane mimetic in canine bronchi. *Am. J. Physiol.* 261:L271, 1991.

85b. Janssen, L. J., O'Bryne, P. M., and Daniel, E. E. Mechanism underlying ozone-induced in vitro hyperresponsiveness in canine bronchi. *Am. J. Physiol.* 261:L55, 1991.

85c. Jeffery, P. K. Morphology of the airway wall in asthma and in chronic obstructive pulmonary disease. *Am. Rev. Respir. Dis.* 143:1152, 1991.

86. Jennings, S. J., Warren, J. B., and Pride, N. B. Airway caliber and the work of breathing in humans. *J. Appl. Physiol.* 63:20, 1987.

87. Johansson, I. G. M., Grundstrom, N., and Andersson, R. G. G. Both the cholinergic and non-cholinergic components of airway excitation are inhibited by morphine in the guinea-pig. *Acta Physiol. Scand.* 135:411, 1989.

88. Johnson, A. R., et al. Neutral metalloendopeptidase in human lung tissue and cultured cells. *Am. Rev. Respir. Dis.* 132:664, 1985.

89. Joos, G. F., Pauwels, R. A., and Van der Straeten, M. E. The mechanism of tachykinin-induced bronchoconstriction in the rat. *Am. Rev. Respir. Dis.* 137:1038, 1988.

90. Kalia, M., and Mesulam, M. M. Brain stem projections of sensory and motor components of the vagus complex in the cat: II. Laryngeal, tracheobronchial, cardiac, and gastrointestinal branches. *J. Comp. Neurol.* 193:467, 1980.

91. Kalia, M. P. Organization of central control of airways. *Annu. Rev. Physiol.* 49:595, 1987.

92. Kaliner, M., et al. Autonomic nervous system abnormalities and allergy. *Ann. Intern. Med.* 96:349, 1982.

93. Kallenbach, J. M., et al. Reflex heart rate control in asthma. *Chest* 87:644, 1985.

94. Kanemura, T., et al. The effect of N-formyl-methionyl-leucyl-phenylalanine on cholinergic neurotransmission and its modulation by enkephalinase in rabbit airway smooth muscle. *Regul. Pept.* 26:107, 1989.

95. Karlsson, J.-A., Sant'Ambrogio, G., and Widdicombe, J. Afferent neural pathways in cough and reflex bronchoconstriction. *J. Appl. Physiol.* 65:1007, 1988.

96. Karpel, J. P., et al. A comparison of atropine sulfate and metaproterenol sulfate in the emergency treatment of asthma. *Am. Rev. Respir. Dis.* 133:727, 1986.

97. Kaufman, M. P., et al. Bradykinin stimulates afferent vagal C-fibers in intrapulmonary airways of dogs. *J. Appl. Physiol.* 48:511, 1980.

98. Knowles, M., et al. Bioelectric properties and ion flow across excised human bronchi. *J. Appl. Physiol.* 56:868, 1984.

99. Laitinen, A. Ultrastructural organisation of intraepithelial nerves in the human airway tract. *Thorax* 40:488, 1985.

100. Laitinen, A., et al. Electron microscopic study on the innervation of the human lower respiratory tract: Evidence of adrenergic nerves. *Eur. J. Respir. Dis.* 67:209, 1985.

101. Laitinen, A., et al. VIP-like immunoreactive nerves in human respiratory tract. Light and electron microscopic study. *Histochemistry* 82:313, 1985.

102. Lammers, W. J., et al. The role of pirenzipine-sensitive (M_1) muscarinic receptors in vagally mediated bronchoconstriction in humans. *Am. Rev. Respir. Dis.* 139:446, 1989.

103. Larsell, O., and Mason, M. L. Experimental degeneration of the vagus nerve and its relation to the terminations in the lung of the rabbit. *J. Comp. Neurol.* 33:509, 1921.

104. Latimer, K. M., and Ruffin, R. E. The effect of inhaled fenoterol and ipratropium bromide on propranolol induced bronchoconstriction in the asthmatic airways. *Clin. Exp. Pharmacol. Physiol.* 17:627, 1990.

105. Leff, A. R. Endogenous regulation of bronchomotor tone. *Am. Rev. Respir. Dis.* 137:1198, 1988.

106. Lev, A., et al. Epithelial effects on tracheal smooth muscle tone: Influence of muscarinic antagonists. *Am. J. Physiol.* 258:L52, 1990.

107. Libby, D. M., Briscoe, W. A., and King, T. K. C. Relief of hypoxia-related bronchoconstriction by breathing 30 per cent oxygen. *Am. Rev. Respir. Dis.* 123:171, 1981.

108. Longhurst, J. C. Static contraction of hindlimb muscles in cats reflexly relaxes tracheal smooth muscle. *J. Appl. Physiol.* 57:380, 1984.

109. Ludwig, M. S., et al. Partitioning of pulmonary resistance during constriction in the dog: Effects of volume history. *J. Appl. Physiol.* 62:807, 1987.

110. Lundberg, J. M., et al. Substance-P immunoreactive sensory nerves in the lower respiratory tract of various mammals including man. *Cell Tissue Res.* 235:252, 1984.

111. Luparello, T., et al. Influences of suggestion on airway reactivity in asthmatic subjects. *Psychosom. Med.* 30:819, 1968.

112. Macklem, P. T., and Mead, J. Factors determining maximum expiratory flow in dogs. *J. Appl. Physiol.* 25:159, 1968.

113. Mak, J. C., and Barnes, P. J. Autoradiographic visualization of muscarinic receptor subtypes in human and guinea pig lung. *Am. Rev. Respir. Dis.* 141:1559, 1990.

114. Martin, J. G., et al. The effects of vasoactive intestinal polypeptide on cholinergic neurotransmission in an isolated innervated guinea pig tracheal preparation. *Respir. Physiol.* 79:111, 1990.

115. Martin, R. J. The sleep-related worsening of lower airways obstruction: Understanding and intervention. *Med. Clin. North Am.* 74:701, 1990.

116. McAllen, R. M., and Spyer, K. M. Two types of vagal preganglionic motoneurones projecting to the heart and lungs. *J. Physiol. (Lond.)* 282:353, 1978.

117. McFadden, E. R., Jr., et al. Predominant site of flow limitation and mechanisms of postexertional asthma. *J. Appl. Physiol.* 42:746, 1977.

118. McFadden, E. R., Jr., et al. The mechanism of action of suggestion in the induction of acute asthma attacks. *Psychosom. Med.* 31:134, 1969.

119. Meurs, H., et al. The beta-adrenergic system and bronchial asthma: Changes in lymphocyte beta-adrenergic receptor number and adenylate cyclase activity after an allergen-induced attack. *J. Allergy Clin. Immunol.* 70:272, 1982.

120. Michel, A. D., and Whiting, R. L. Methocramine, a polymethylene terramine, differentiates three subtypes of muscarinic receptor in direct binding studies. *Eur. J. Pharmacol.* 145:61, 1988.

121. Minette, P. A., and Barnes, P. J. Prejunctional inhibitory muscarinic receptors on cholinergic nerves in human and guinea pig airways. *J. Appl. Physiol.* 64:181, 1988.

122. Minette, P. A., and Barnes, P. J. Muscarinic receptor subtypes in lung: Clinical implications. *Am. Rev. Respir. Dis.* 141:S162, 1990.

123. Minette, P. A. H., et al. A muscarinic agonist inhibits reflex bronchoconstriction in normal but not in asthmatic subjects. *J. Appl. Physiol.* 67:2461, 1989.

124. Mitchell, G. S., and Vidruk, E. H. Neural and humoral factors in control of tracheal caliber. *J. Appl. Physiol.* 59:198, 1985.

125. Mitchell, R. A., Herbert, D. A., and Baker, D. G. Inspiratory rhythm in airway smooth muscle tone. *J. Appl. Physiol.* 58:911, 1985.

126. Mitchelson, F. Muscarinic receptor differentiation. *Pharmacol. Ther.* 37:357, 1988.

127. Moreno, R. H., Hogg, J. C., and Paré, P. D. Mechanics of airway narrowing. *Am. Rev. Respir. Dis.* 133:1171, 1986.

128. Moummi, C., et al. Muscarinic receptors in smooth muscle cells from gastric antrum. *Biochem. Pharmacol.* 37:1363, 1988.

128a. Myers, A. C., and Undem, B. J. Functional interactions between capsaicin-sensitive and cholinergic nerves in the guinea-pig bronchus. *J. Pharmacol. Exp. Ther.* 259:104, 1991.

129. Nadel, J. A. Parasympathetic nervous control of airway smooth muscle. *Ann. NY Acad. Sci.* 221:99, 1974.

130. Nadel, J. A. Regulation of neurogenic inflammation by neutral endopeptidase. *Am. Rev. Respir. Dis.* 145:S48, 1992.

131. Nadel, J. A., and Borson, D. B. Modulation of neurogenic inflammation by neutral endopeptidase. *Am. Rev. Respir. Dis.* 143:S33, 1991.

132. Nadel, J. A., Cabezas, G. A., and Austin, J. H. M. In vivo roentgenographic examination of parasympathetic innervation of small airways: Use of powdered tantalum and a fine focal spot x-ray tube. *Invest. Radiol.* 6:9, 1971.

133. Nadel, J. A., and Tierney, D. F. Effect of a previous deep inspiration on airway resistance in man. *J. Appl. Physiol.* 16:717, 1961.

134. Newberry, N. R., and Priestly, T. Pharmacological differences between two muscarinic responses of the rat superior cervical ganglion in vitro. *Br. J. Pharmacol.* 92:817, 1987.

135. Olsen, C. R., DeKock, M. A., and Colebatch, H. J. H. Stability of airways during reflex bronchoconstriction. *J. Appl. Physiol.* 23:23, 1967.

136. Olsen, C. R., Stevens, A. E., and McIlroy, M. B. Rigidity of tracheae and bronchi during muscular constriction. *J. Appl. Physiol.* 23:27, 1967.

137. Olsen, C. R., et al. Structural basis for decreased compressibility of constricted tracheae and bronchi. *J. Appl. Physiol.* 23:35, 1967.

137a. Padrid, P. A., Haselton, J. R., and Kaufman, M. P. Role of caudal ventrolateral medulla in reflex and central control of airway caliber. *J. Appl. Physiol.* 71:2274, 1991.

138. Palmer, J. B., Cuss, F. M. C., and Barnes, P. J. VIP and PHM and their role in non-adrenergic inhibitory responses in isolated human airways. *J. Appl. Physiol.* 61:1322, 1986.

139. Parham, W. M., et al. Analysis of time course and magnitude of lung inflation effects on airway tone: Relation to airway reactivity. *Am. Rev. Respir. Dis.* 128:240, 1983.

140. Partanen, M., et al. Catecholamine and acetylcholinesterase containing nerves in human lower respiratory tract. *Histochemistry* 76:175, 1982.

141. Peralta, E. G., et al. Differential regulation of PI hydrolysis and adenyl cyclase by muscarinic receptor subtypes. *Nature* 334:434, 1988.

142. Postma, D. S., et al. Influence of the parasympathetic and sympathetic nervous system on nocturnal bronchial obstruction. *Clin. Sci.* 69:251, 1985.

143. Rebuck, A. S., et al. Nebulized anticholinergic and sympathetic treatment of asthma and chronic obstructive airways disease in the emergency room. *Am. J. Med.* 82:59, 1987.

144. Rebuck, A. S., Gent, M., and Chapman, K. R. Anticholinergic and sympathomimetic combination therapy of asthma. *J. Allergy Clin. Immunol.* 71:317, 1983.

145. Rhoden, K. J., Meldrum, L. A., and Barnes, P. J. Inhibition of cholinergic neurotransmission in human airways by β2-adrenoceptors. *J. Appl. Physiol.* 65:700, 1988.

146. Richardson, J. B. Nerve supply to the lung. *Am. Rev. Respir. Dis.* 119:758, 1979.

147. Roberts, A. M., Coleridge, H. M., and Coleridge, J. C. G. Reciprocal action of pulmonary vagal afferents on tracheal smooth muscle tension in dogs. *Respir. Physiol.* 72:35, 1988.

148. Roffel, A. F., Elzinga, C. R. S., and Zaagsma, J. Muscarinic M3 receptors mediate contraction of human central and peripheral airway smooth muscle. *Pulm. Pharmacol.* 3:47, 1990.

149. Rosenthal, R. R., et al. Role of the parasympathetic system in antigen induced bronchospasm. *J. Appl. Physiol.* 42:600, 1977.
150. Russel, J. A. Tracheal smooth muscle. *Clin. Chest Med.* 7:189, 1986.
151. Said, S. I. Vasoactive intestinal peptide in the lung. *Ann. NY Acad. Sci.* 527:450, 1988.
152. Said, S. I. Neuropeptides (VIP and tachykinins). VIP as a modulator of lung inflammation and airway constriction. *Am. Rev. Respir. Dis.* 143:S22, 1991.
153. Sampson, S. R., and Vidruk, E. T. I. Properties of 'irritant' receptors in canine lung. *Respir. Physiol.* 25:9, 1975.
154. Schiffman, P. L., et al. Hyperoxic attenuation of exercise-induced bronchospasm in asthmatics. *J. Clin. Invest.* 63:30, 1979.
155. Schroeckenstein, D. C. et al. Twelve-hour bronchodilation in asthma with a single dose of the anticholinergic compound glycopyrrolate. *J. Allergy Clin. Immunol.* 82:115, 1988.
156. Sekizawa, K., et al. Effect of bronchomotor tone on work rate of breathing. *J. Appl. Physiol.* 57:7, 1984.
157. Sekizawa, K., et al. Enkephalinase inhibitor potentiates mammalian tachykinin-induced contraction in ferret trachea. *J. Pharmacol. Exp. Ther.* 243:1211, 1987.
158. Sekizawa, K., et al. Modulation of cholinergic neurotransmission by vasoactive intestinal peptide in ferret trachea. *J. Appl. Physiol.* 64:2433, 1988.
159. Sekizawa, K., et al. Enkephalinase inhibitor potentiates substance P and electrically induced contraction in ferret trachea. *J. Appl. Physiol.* 63:1401, 1987.
160. Serio, R., and Daniel, E. E. Thromboxane effects on canine trachealis neuromuscular function. *J. Appl. Physiol.* 64:1979, 1988.
161. Shelhamer, J., Marom, Z., and Kaliner, M. Immunologic and neuropharmacologic stimulation of mucous glycoprotein release from human airways in vitro. *J. Clin. Invest.* 66:1400, 1980.
162. Shelhamer, J. H., et al. Abnormal beta-adrenergic responsiveness in allergic subjects: Analysis of isoproterenol-induced cardiovascular and plasma cyclic adenosine monophosphate responses. *J. Allergy Clin. Immunol.* 66:52, 1980.
163. Sheller, J. R., et al. Interaction of serotonin with vagal and ACh-induced bronchoconstriction in canine lungs. *J. Appl. Physiol.* 52:964, 1982.
164. Shimoda, T., et al. In vitro red tide toxin effects on human bronchial smooth muscle. *J. Allergy Clin. Immunol.* 81:1187, 1988.
165. Shore, S., Collier, B., and Martin, J. G. Effect of endogenous prostaglandins on acetylcholine release from dog trachealis muscle. *J. Appl. Physiol.* 62:1837, 1987.
166. Shore, S., et al. Mechanisms of histamine-induced contraction of canine airway smooth muscle. *J. Appl. Physiol.* 55:22, 1983.
167. Skoogh, B.-E., and Svedmyr, N. Beta$_2$-adrenoceptor stimulation inhibits ganglionic transmission in ferret trachea. *Pulm. Pharmacol.* 1:167, 1989.
168. Smith, M. M., Colebatch, H. J. H., and Clarke, P. S. Increase and decrease in pulmonary resistance with hypnotic suggestion in asthma. *Am. Rev. Respir. Dis.* 102:236, 1970.
169. Sorkness, R., and Vidruk, E. Reflex effects of isocapnic changes in ventilation on tracheal tone in awake dogs. *Respir. Physiol.* 69:161, 1987.
170. Sorkness, R. L., and Vidruk, E. H. Ventilatory responses to hypoxia nullify hypoxic tracheal constriction in awake dogs. *Respir. Physiol.* 66:41, 1986.
171. Spector, S., et al. Responses of asthmatics to methacholine and suggestion. *Am. Rev. Respir. Dis.* 113:43, 1976.
172. Storms, W. W., DoPico, G. A., and Reed, C. E. Aerosol SCH 1000: An anticholinergic bronchodilator. *Am. Rev. Respir. Dis.* 111:419, 1975.
173. Stretton, D., and Barnes, P. J. Modulation of cholinergic neurotransmission in guinea pig trachea by neuropeptide Y. *Br. J. Pharmacol.* 93:672, 1988.
173a. Stretton, D., Belvisi, M. G., and Barnes, P. J. The effect of sensory nerve depletion on cholinergic neurotransmission in guinea pig airways. *J. Pharmacol. Exp. Ther.* 260:1073, 1992.
174. Sullivan, C. E., et al. Regulation of airway smooth muscle tone in sleeping dogs. *Am. Rev. Respir. Dis.* 119:87, 1979.
175. Tamaoki, J., et al. IgE-dependent activation of alveolar macrophages augments neurally mediated contraction of small airways. *Br. J. Pharmacol.* 103:1458, 1991.
176. Tamaoki, J., et al. Corticotropin-releasing factor potentiates the contractile response of rabbit airway smooth muscle to electrical field stimulation but not to acetylcholine. *Am. Rev. Respir. Dis.* 140:1331, 1989.
177. Tamaoki, J., et al. Cholinergic neuromodulation by PGD$_2$ in canine smooth muscle. *J. Appl. Physiol.* 63:1396, 1987.
178. Tanaka, D. T., and Grunstein, M. M. Mechanisms of substance P-induced contraction of rabbit airway smooth muscle. *J. Appl. Physiol.* 57:1551, 1984.
179. Tanaka, D. T., and Grunstein, M. M. Effects of substance P on neurally mediated contraction of rabbit airway smooth muscle. *J. Appl. Physiol.* 60:458, 1986.
180. Tashkin, D. P., et al. Subsensitization of beta-adrenoceptors in airways and lymphocytes of healthy and asthmatic subjects. *Am. Rev. Respir. Dis.* 125:185, 1982.
181. Teague, W. J., et al. An acute reduction in the fraction of inspired oxygen increases airway constriction in infants with chronic lung disease. *Am. Rev. Respir. Dis.* 137:861, 1988.
182. Thompson, D. C., Diamond, L., and Altiere, R. J. Presynaptic alpha adrenoceptor modulation of neurally mediated cholinergic excitatory and nonadrenergic noncholinergic inhibitory responses in guinea pig trachea. *J. Pharmacol. Exp. Ther.* 254:306, 1990.
183. Vermiere, P. A., and Vanhoutte, P. M. Inhibitory effects of catecholamines in isolated canine bronchial smooth muscle. *J. Appl. Physiol.* 46:787, 1979.
184. Vidruk, E., and Sorkness, R. Questionable involvement of carotid body chemoreceptors in hypoxic potentiation of histamine-induced bronchoconstriction. *Am. Rev. Respir. Dis.* 129:A262, 1984.
185. Vidruk, E. H., and Sorkness, R. L. Histamine-induced reflex tracheal constriction is attenuated by hyperoxia and exaggerated by hypoxia. *Am. Rev. Respir. Dis.* 132:287, 1985.
186. Vincent, N. J., et al. Factors influencing pulmonary resistance. *J. Appl. Physiol.* 29:236, 1970.
187. Walters, E. H., et al. Control of neurotransmission by prostaglandins in canine trachealis smooth muscle. *J. Appl. Physiol.* 57:129, 1984.
188. Wasserfallen, J.-B., et al. Sudden asphyxic asthma: A distinct entity? *Am. Rev. Respir. Dis.* 142:108, 1990.
188a. Watson, N., Barnes, P. J., and MacLagan, J. Actions of methoctramine, a muscarinic M$_2$ receptor antagonist, on muscarinic and nicotinic cholinoceptors in guinea-pig airways in vivo and in vitro. *Br. J. Pharmacol.* 105:107, 1992.
189. Weinrich, D., and Undem, B. J. Immunologic regulation of synaptic transmission in isolated guinea pig autonomic ganglia. *J. Clin. Invest.* 79:1529, 1987.
189a. Wessler, I., et al. Release of [^{3}H]acetylcholine from the isolated rat or guinea-pig trachea evoked by preganglionic nerve stimulation: A comparison with transmural stimulation. *Naunyn Schmiedebergs Arch. Pharmacol.* 344:403, 1991.
190. Whicker, S., Armour, C., and Black, J. Responsiveness of bronchial smooth muscle from asthmatic subjects to contractile and relaxant agonists. *Pulm. Pharmacol.* 1:25, 1988.
191. Widdicombe, J. G. Receptors in the trachea and bronchi of the cat. *J. Physiol. (Lond.)* 123:71, 1954.
192. Widdicombe, J. G. Action potentials in parasympathetic and sympathetic efferent fibres to the trachea and lungs of dogs and cats. *J. Physiol. (Lond.)* 186:56, 1966.
193. Widdicombe, J. G., and Nadel, J. A. Airway volume, airway resistance, and work and force of breathing: Theory. *J. Appl. Physiol.* 18:863, 1963.
194. Wiggs, B. R., et al. A model of airway narrowing in asthma and in chronic obstructive pulmonary disease. *Am. Rev. Respir. Dis.* 145:1251, 1992.

Nonadrenergic, Noncholinergic Nerves and Neuropeptides

Peter J. Barnes

Neural control of the airways is complex. In addition to the classic cholinergic, adrenergic, and afferent nerves are neural effects not blocked by adrenergic or cholinergic antagonists and therefore termed *nonadrenergic, noncholinergic* (NANC). While the neurotransmitters of NANC neural effects are not yet certain, there is increasing evidence that neuropeptides are at least contributory.

A diverse collection of neuropeptides are localized to sensory, parasympathetic, and sympathetic neurons in the respiratory tract (Table 18-1). These peptides have potent effects on bronchomotor tone, airway secretions, the bronchial circulation, and inflammatory and immune cells (Table 18-2). The precise physiologic role of each peptide is still not known, but some clues are provided by the localization and functional effects of the peptides. The purpose of this chapter is to discuss what is known of these peptides, particularly in the human respiratory tract, and to speculate on their possible pathophysiologic role in asthma.

Many neuropeptides have been isolated from the gut, where they are involved in the regulation of gut motility, sphincters, and secretion. There is convincing evidence that these neuropeptides are neurotransmitters or neuromodulators, and appear to be involved in the complex integrative regulation of the gastrointestinal tract. Since the airways are derived embryologically from the foregut, it is not surprising that similar peptides are also found in the respiratory tract [14, 15, 23, 227, 269, 295].

NONADRENERGIC, NONCHOLINERGIC NERVES

NANC nerves were first demonstrated in the gut and therefore their existence in the respiratory tract is to be expected. NANC nerves were initially conceived as a "third" nervous system in the lungs [11, 237], but it rapidly became apparent that several distinct neural mechanisms are included. NANC mechanisms result in both bronchodilatation and bronchoconstriction, vasodilation and vasoconstriction, and mucus secretion, indicating that several types of neurotransmitters are involved.

Inhibitory Nonadrenergic, Noncholinergic Nerves

Inhibitory NANC (i-NANC) nerves relax airway smooth muscle. They have been demonstrated in vitro by electrical field stimulation after adrenergic and cholinergic blockade in several species, including humans [12, 13, 149a, 238]. In human airway smooth muscle the NANC inhibitory system is the only neural bronchodilator pathway, since there is no functional sympathetic innervation to airway smooth muscle. Because NANC innervation is the sole inhibitory pathway from the trachea to the smallest bronchi, there has been considerable research into the identity of the neurotransmitter.

Inhibitory NANC nerves have also been demonstrated in vivo in some species by electrical stimulation of the vagus after adrenergic and cholinergic blockade [71, 126]. Stimulation of this pathway produces pronounced and long-lasting bronchodilatation, which may be inhibited by ganglion blockers. This pathway may be activated reflexly by mechanical or chemical stimulation of the larynx [282]. In human subjects in vivo mechanical stimulation of the larynx and chemical stimulation with capsaicin in the presence of adrenergic and cholinergic blockers have also demonstrated reflex reversal of induced tone [124, 150, 201] (Fig. 18-1).

Purines

At first it was believed that purines may be the neurotransmitters in i-NANC nerves in airways, but the evidence does not support this view. Although exogenous adenosine triphosphate (ATP) may relax airway smooth muscle, the antagonist quinidine fails to block NANC relaxation in vitro and in vivo and the purine uptake inhibitor dipyridamole does not enhance i-NANC responses [127, 137]. Similarly, adenosine fails to mimic NANC relaxation and antagonists such as theophylline have no blocking effect [128, 137]. In human airways there is a prominent i-NANC response in vitro, particularly in proximal airways. However, ATP analogs do not mimic this relaxant response, and reactive blue 2, an antagonist of the inhibitory P_{2y} receptor, has no effect on i-NANC responses [34].

Nitric Oxide

Recent evidence has demonstrated that nitric oxide may be a neurotransmitter of some NANC responses [47, 229a]. The enzyme nitric oxide synthase, which produces nitric oxide from the precursor L-arginine, is localized to several peripheral nerves [44]. Inhibition of nitric oxide synthase by L-N^Gnitroarginine markedly reduces i-NANC responses in guinea pig trachea in vitro [156, 291]. In human trachea this nitric oxide synthase inhibitor largely abolishes i-NANC responses, indicating that nitric oxide is the major transmitter of i-NANC responses in human airways [34, 356].

Vasoactive Intestinal Peptide

Evidence also favors a neuropeptide as a neurotransmitter of i-NANC nerves. Of the several neuropeptides identified in airways, only vasoactive intestinal peptide (VIP) and the related family of peptides (see below) relax airway smooth muscle and are therefore the only identified peptide candidates. In guinea pig trachea there is compelling evidence that VIP contributes to the i-NANC response, since this is partially reduced by alpha-chymotrypsin, which degrades VIP [79], and by preincubation with a specific antiserum to VIP [80, 156]. It now seems likely that both nitric oxide and VIP contribute to the i-NANC response in airways and it is possible that they are differentially released from airway

Table 18-1. *Neuropeptides in the respiratory tract*

Peptide	Localization
Vasoactive intestinal peptide Peptide histidine isoleucine/methionine Peptide histidine valine-42 Helodermin Pituitary adenylate cyclase–activating peptide-27 Galanin	Parasympathetic (afferent)
Substance P Neurokinin A Neuropeptide K Calcitonin gene–related peptide Gastrin-releasing peptide	Afferent
Neuropeptide Y	Sympathetic
Somatostatin Enkephalin Cholecystokinin octapeptide	Afferent/uncertain

nerves under different conditions of nerve stimulation. Thus, VIP may only be released at high frequencies of stimulation, whereas nitric oxide may be released at all frequencies.

Excitatory Nonadrenergic, Noncholinergic Nerves

Electrical stimulation of guinea pig bronchi, and occasionally trachea in vitro, and vagus nerve in vivo produces a component of bronchoconstriction that is not inhibited by atropine [7, 173]. This bronchoconstrictor response has been termed the *excitatory NANC* (*e-NANC*) *response* [22a]. There is now convincing evidence that tachykinins released retrogradely from a certain population of sensory nerves mediate e-NANC responses. A similar e-NANC response has occasionally been observed in human airways in vitro, but this is not consistent [10, 173].

Other Nonadrenergic, Noncholinergic Responses

Other NANC responses in airways, in addition to effects on airway smooth muscle, have been described. NANC-mediated secretion of mucus has been demonstrated in cats in vivo using vagal nerve stimulation [224] and in ferret airways in vitro using electrical field stimulation [39]. NANC regulation of airway blood flow has been demonstrated in several species [188, 313], with both vasodilator and vasoconstrictor effects. NANC neurally mediated plasma extravasation has also been shown in some species. These NANC secretory and vascular effects are likely to be mediated by a variety of neuropeptides, and in some instances by purines and nitric oxide.

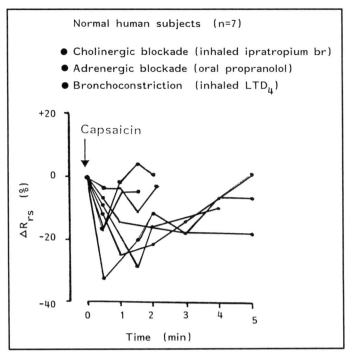

Fig. 18-1. *Inhibitor nonadrenergic, noncholinergic bronchodilator reflex in normal human subjects.* ΔR_{rs} = *change in total respiratory resistance (%)*; LTD_4 = *leukotriene D_4.*

Cotransmission

Although NANC nerves were originally envisaged as an anatomically separate nervous system, it is now more likely that NANC neural effects are mediated by the release of neurotransmitters from classic autonomic nerves. Thus, the i-NANC responses in airway smooth muscle are likely to be mediated by the release of cotransmitters such as nitric oxide and VIP from cholinergic nerves. NANC vasoconstrictor responses are mediated by the release of neuropeptide Y (NPY) from adrenergic nerves. Excitatory NANC bronchoconstrictor responses are mediated by the release of tachykinins from unmyelinated sensory nerves. The physiologic relevance of cotransmission is likely to be related to the "fine-tuning" of classic autonomic nerves, but the role of the cotransmitters may become more apparent in disease [18].

Coexistence of several peptides within the same nerve is commonly seen in the peripheral nervous system, and multiple combinations are possible, giving rise to the concept of "chemical

Table 18-2. *Effects of neuropeptides on airway functions*

Peptide	ASM	Mucus secretion	Vessels	Nerves	Other cells
VIP*	Relax	Increase/decrease	Dilate	↓ Chol/e-NANC	↓ Mast cells/T-lymphocytes
SP	(Contract)	Increase	Dilate ↑ Leak	(↑ Chol)	↑ Macrophage/monocytes
NKA	Contract	(Increase)	(Dilate)	↑ Chol	↑ Macrophage
CGRP	(Contract)	(Increase)	Dilate	?	↓ Macrophage
NPY	(Contract)	Increase	Constrict	↓ Chol/e-NANC	?
GRP	Contract	Increase	Constrict	?	↑ Epithelial growth
CCK₈	Contract	?	?	No effect	?
Galanin	No effect	?	No effect	↓ e-NANC	?

Definition of abbreviations: ASM = airway smooth muscle; VIP = vasoactive intestinal peptide; SP = substance P; NKA = neurokinin A; CGRP = calcitonin gene–related peptide; NPY = neuropeptide Y; GRP = gastrin-releasing peptide; CCK₈ = cholecystokinin; e-NANC = excitatory nonadrenergic noncholinergic. Parentheses indicate small or uncertain effects.
* VIP-related peptides PHI/M, PACAP-27, and helodermin have similar effects.
Source: P. Barnes, et al. Neuropeptides in respiratory tract. *Am. Rev. Respir. Dis.* 144:1187, 1991. Reprinted with permission.

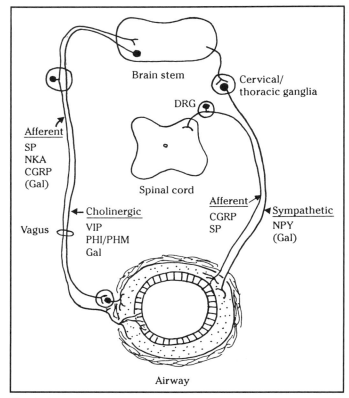

Fig. 18-2. *Innervation of the lower respiratory tract, showing neuropeptide colocalization in autonomic nerves.* DRG = *dorsal root ganglion;* SP = *substance P;* NKA = *neurokinin A;* CGRP = *calcitonin gene–related peptide;* Gal = *galanin;* VIP = *vasoactive intestinal peptide;* PHI/PHM = *peptide histidine isoleucine/methionine;* NPY = *neuropeptide Y.*

coding" of nerve fibers. VIP and peptide histidine isoleucine (PHI) usually coexist since they are derived from the same precursor peptide coded by a single gene. Galanin is often present with VIP in cholinergic neurons [56, 68]. In sensory nerves substance P, neurokinin A (NKA), and calcitonin gene–related peptide (CGRP) often coexist, but some sensory nerves may also contain galanin and VIP [176]. Similarly adrenergic nerves that contain NPY may also contain somatostatin, galanin, VIP, and enkephalin [157]. Thus, there is a complex distribution of neuropeptides in the innervation of the airways, with the same peptides occurring in different types of nerves (Fig. 18-2). The physiologic significance of this complexity is not yet clear, but it seems likely that there may be functional interactions between the multiple neuropeptides released and the classic transmitters that allow complex integration and regulation of the functions in the airway.

Neuropeptides are often released by high-frequency firing and therefore may only be coreleased with classic neurotransmitters with certain patterns of neural activation. Little is known about the optimal conditions for neuropeptide release, but it seems likely that release may be favored by certain physiologic and pathophysiologic conditions. Furthermore, little is known about the effect of repeated neural activation on the synthesis and release of neuropeptides, but it is possible that in certain diseases, when chronic nerve irritation may occur, there may be increased neuropeptide gene expression, synthesis, and release.

Peptidergic Neurotransmission

Peptides are stored in nerves as large electron-dense granules ("p-type" granules) [146]. The peptides are synthesized in the neuronal cell body and processed during transport peripherally for storage and release. The recent cloning of several genes that code for neuropeptides has made it possible to identify the sites of peptide gene transcription and to study the various factors that may regulate synthesis. For example, tachykinins in the airway sensory nerves are predominantly synthesized in the neuronal cell bodies in the nodose ganglia. Using in situ hybridization it has been possible to localize tachykinin messenger RNA (mRNA) in a population of these neurons [114].

Neuropeptide Receptors

Neuropeptide receptors have proved to be more difficult to study than the receptors for classic transmitters because of a relative lack of specific antagonists. More potent antagonists, including nonpeptide antagonists, are now being developed and this greatly assists the investigation of the role of neuropeptides. Thus, a potent nonpeptide selective tachykinin antagonist was recently developed and may be very useful in elucidating the roles of tachykinins in human disease in the future [268]. The recent cloning of certain neuropeptide receptors, such as three different tachykinin receptors [187, 262, 321], should now lead to more rapid advances in understanding the regulation of these receptors in health and disease.

Neuropeptide Effects

Neuropeptides produce many different effects mediated by surface receptors, and the functional responses in the respiratory tract depend on the localization of receptors and the second messengers linked to receptor activation in the target cells. In addition to acute effects, such as contraction and relaxation of airway smooth muscle, there may be chronic effects of neuropeptides, such as effects on growth and development [316]. It is now apparent that there are complex interactions between neuropeptides and the immune system, and these interactions are likely to be relevant in asthma [64a]. Several neuropeptides, most notably gastrin-releasing peptide and bombesin, have already been implicated in airway epithelial growth, and it is likely that the trophic effects of neuropeptides will be increasingly recognized.

VASOACTIVE INTESTINAL PEPTIDE

VIP is a 28–amino acid peptide that was originally extracted from porcine duodenum as a vasodilator peptide [249]. VIP is localized to several types of nerve in the respiratory tract of several species, including humans. It has potent effects on airway and pulmonary vascular tone and on airway secretion, which suggests that it may have an important regulatory role [16, 246].

Localization

VIP has been isolated from lung extracts of several species, including humans, and is one of the most abundant of the neuropeptides found in the lungs [104]. VIP-like immunoreactivity is localized to nerves and ganglia in airways and pulmonary vessels [70, 168, 227, 295]. VIP immunoreactivity is present in ganglion cells in the posterior trachea and around intrapulmonary bronchi, diminishing in frequency as the airways become smaller. Usually VIP-immunoreactive neurons occur in parasympathetic ganglia, but isolated ganglion cells are also seen. These cells give rise to intrinsic VIP-ergic motor nerves that are largely cholinergic.

VIP-immunoreactive nerves are widely distributed throughout the respiratory tract. There is a rich VIP-ergic innervation in the proximal airways, but the density of innervation diminishes peripherally so that few VIP-ergic fibers are found in the bronchioles

[168, 227, 295]. The pattern of distribution largely follows that of cholinergic nerves in airways, consistent with the colocalization of VIP and acetylcholine in human airways [147]. VIP-ergic nerves are found within airway smooth muscle and around bronchial vessels and surrounding submucosal glands. VIP-ergic fibers are also found in the adventitia of pulmonary vessels, particularly medium-size arteries. VIP may be localized to some sensory nerves, including subepithelial nerves in the airways, which may arise in the jugular and nodose ganglia [168, 269]. VIP, at least in some species, may also be localized to sympathetic nerves [176]. VIP-immunoreactive nerves are markedly depleted in older animals [102], which may have important clinical implications in terms of airway disease in the elderly.

Vasoactive Intestinal Peptide Receptors

VIP receptors have been identified in the lung of several species by receptor-binding techniques using [^{125}I]VIP [239]. Binding of VIP to its receptor activates adenylyl cyclase, and VIP stimulates cyclic adenosine monophosphate (AMP) formation in lung fragments [92]. The actions of VIP are, therefore, similar to those of beta-adrenoceptor agonists and any differences in response of different tissues to VIP or beta agonists depend on the relative densities or coupling of their respective receptors. The distribution of VIP receptors in the lungs has been investigated using an autoradiographic method to map out specific VIP-binding sites [52]. VIP receptors are found in high density in pulmonary vascular smooth muscle and in the smooth muscle of large, but not small airways. VIP receptors are also found in high density in airway epithelium and submucosal glands. The distribution of receptors is consistent with the known functions of VIP.

The distribution of VIP receptors has also been studied by a functional immunocytochemical method using an antibody to cyclic AMP. After stimulation by VIP, cyclic AMP increases in those cells with specific receptors. This technique confirms the autoradiographic findings by demonstrating VIP receptors in airway smooth muscle, epithelium, and submucosal glands of several species [152].

Effects on Airway Smooth Muscle

VIP is a potent relaxant of airway smooth muscle in vitro and this relaxation is independent of adrenergic receptors [246]. VIP is more potent than isoproterenol in relaxing human bronchi, making it one of the most potent endogenous bronchodilators [218]. The rich VIP-ergic innervation of human bronchi suggests that VIP may be an important regulator of bronchial tone and may be involved in counteracting the bronchoconstriction of asthma. The response to VIP may depend on the size of the airway. In human airways, bronchi are potently relaxed by VIP, while bronchioles are unaffected. In contrast, both relax to an equal degree with isoproterenol [218]. This response of human airways is consistent with the distribution of VIP receptors, since receptors are seen in bronchial smooth muscle but not in bronchiolar smooth muscle [52]. This peripheral diminution of VIP receptors is also consistent with the distribution of VIP-immunoreactive nerves, which diminish markedly as the airways become smaller [168]. These studies suggest that VIP, while regulating the caliber of large airways, is unlikely to influence small airways.

VIP causes bronchodilatation in vivo. Given intravenously, it causes potent bronchodilatation in cat airways [71, 72]. Inhaled VIP protects against the bronchoconstrictor effects of histamine and prostaglandin (PG) $F_{2\alpha}$ in dogs [248]. In asthmatic patients, however, inhaled VIP has no bronchodilator effect, although a beta-adrenergic agonist in the same subjects is markedly effective [27]. Inhaled VIP has only a small protective effect against the bronchoconstrictor effect of histamine [220] and has no effect against exercise-induced bronchoconstriction [48]. This lack of potency of inhaled VIP may be explained by the epithelium, which possesses proteolytic enzymes and may present a barrier to diffusion. Infused VIP has no bronchodilator effect in normal subjects who readily bronchodilate with isoproterenol [220]. However, infusion of VIP produces flushing, marked hypotension, and reflex tachycardia. These effects limit the dose that can be given by infusion and because VIP has a more potent relaxant effect on vessels than on airway smooth muscle, a sufficient bronchodilating dose cannot be administered. Infused VIP causes bronchodilation in asthmatic subjects, but the effect is trivial [205] and might be explained by the reflex sympathoadrenal activation secondary to the profound cardiovascular effects. Thus, although VIP has potent bronchodilator effects in vitro, it has no significant action in vivo, and therefore has little therapeutic potential. More stable analogs or novel compounds that activate VIP receptors may have little advantage over existing beta$_2$ agonists.

Effects on Airway Secretion

VIP-immunoreactive nerves are closely associated with airway submucosal glands and form a dense network around the gland acini. VIP potently stimulates mucus secretion, as measured by ^{35}S-labeled glycoprotein secretion, in ferret airway in vitro, being significantly more potent than isoproterenol [223]. VIP increases cyclic AMP formation in submucosal gland cells, and there is some suggestion that as with beta-adrenergic agonists, there may be preferential effects on mucous rather than serous cells of these glands [152], indicating that VIP may stimulate the secretion of mucus rich in glycoprotein in some species. VIP receptors have been localized to human submucosal glands, suggesting that VIP-ergic nerves may regulate mucus secretion in human airways [52]. VIP has an inhibitory effect on glycoprotein secretion from human tracheal explants [62], which is surprising since agonists that stimulate cyclic AMP formation would be expected to stimulate secretion. More recently the effects of VIP on mucus secretion have been found to be more complex and may depend on the drive to gland secretion. Mucus secretion stimulated by cholinergic agonists is inhibited in ferret trachea but stimulated in cat trachea, whereas secretion stimulated with the alpha-adrenergic agonist phenylephrine is augmented [264, 309] (see Chap. 29).

VIP is a potent stimulant of chloride ion transport and therefore of water secretion in dog tracheal epithelium [209], suggesting that VIP may be a regulator of airway water secretion and therefore mucociliary clearance. The high density of VIP receptors on epithelial cells of human airways suggests that VIP may regulate ion transport and other epithelial functions in human airways [52].

Vascular Effects

VIP is a potent dilator of pulmonary vessels [110]. The relaxation is independent of endothelial cells, indicating that VIP acts directly on vascular smooth muscle cells rather than by releasing a relaxant factor from endothelial cells [26, 110]. This is confirmed by autoradiographic studies showing the high density of receptors in smooth muscle with no labeling of endothelial cells [26, 52].

VIP increases airway blood flow in dogs and pigs, and is more potent on tracheal than on bronchial vessels [188, 313]. There is convincing evidence that VIP is a mediator of NANC vasodilatation in the trachea, whereas in more peripheral airways other neuropeptides are involved [189]. Since VIP is likely to have a greater effect on bronchial vessels than on airway smooth muscle, it may provide a mechanism for increasing blood flow to contracted smooth muscle. Thus, if VIP is released from cholinergic nerves, it may improve muscular perfusion during cholinergic

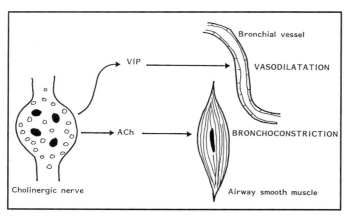

Fig. 18-3. *Vasoactive intestinal peptide (VIP) is released from cholinergic nerves in the airways. Since VIP is a potent vasodilator, it may increase the blood flow to airways that are contracted with acetylcholine (ACh).*

contraction (Fig. 18-3). Perhaps the apparent protective effect of inhaled VIP against histamine-induced bronchoconstriction in human subjects [27], despite a lack of effect on bronchomotor tone, can be explained by an increase in bronchial blood flow, which would more rapidly remove inhaled histamine from the sites of deposition in the airways.

Neuromodulatory Effects

VIP is localized to nerves that surround airway ganglia, suggesting a possible neuromodulatory effect on cholinergic neurotransmission. VIP appears to modulate cholinergic neurotransmission in guinea pig parasympathetic ganglia [181] and postganglionic nerves [81, 254, 278], as it has a greater inhibitory effect on neurally induced bronchoconstriction than on an equivalent contractile response induced by exogenous acetylcholine. VIP also modulates the release of peptides from sensory nerves in guinea pig bronchi in vitro [278].

Antiinflammatory Actions

VIP inhibits the release of mediators from pulmonary mast cells [299] and may have several other antiinflammatory actions in airways. VIP may interact with T-lymphocytes and has the potential to act as a local immunomodulator in airways [214]. VIP may protect the lung against hydrochloric acid–induced pulmonary edema [89, 247] and may act as a free radical scavenger.

Vasoactive Intestinal Peptide as an Inhibitory Nonadrenergic, Noncholinergic Transmitter

Several lines of evidence implicate VIP as a neurotransmitter of i-NANC nerves in airways. VIP produces prolonged relaxation of airway smooth muscle, which is unaffected by adrenergic or neural blockade and has a time course similar to that of i-NANC responses both in vitro and in vivo in several species. VIP mimics the electrophysiologic changes in airway smooth muscle produced by NANC nerve stimulation [51, 128]. Electrical field stimulation of tracheobronchial preparations releases VIP into the bathing medium and this release is blocked by tetrodotoxin, proving that it is derived from nerve stimulation [51, 193]. Furthermore, the amount of VIP released is related to the magnitude of nerve stimulation. Several antagonists of VIP receptors have been developed, but whereas these may weakly inhibit some actions of VIP, they do not inhibit the effects of VIP on airway smooth muscle [80]. In the absence of potent specific blockers

of VIP receptors, other strategies have been adopted. Incubation of cat and guinea pig trachea with high concentrations of VIP induces tachyphylaxis and also reduces the magnitude of NANC nerve relaxation, while responses to sympathetic nerve stimulation and isoproterenol are unaffected [128, 193, 303]. VIP relaxes airway smooth muscle by increasing intracellular cyclic AMP and its effects are therefore potentiated by a selective inhibitor of cyclic AMP phosphodiesterase, which normally degrades intracellular cyclic AMP [235]. Under the same experimental conditions, this phosphodiesterase also potentiates i-NANC responses in guinea pig trachea, whereas an inhibitor of cyclic guanosine monophosphate (GMP) phosphodiesterase does not, supporting the idea that the i-NANC transmitter activates adenylyl cyclase. Perhaps the most convincing evidence that VIP is a transmitter of i-NANC nerves in airways comes from studies with enzymes that degrade this peptide. VIP is rapidly broken down into inactive fragments by trypsin and alpha-chymotrypsin and also by mast cell tryptase [54, 55, 284]. Incubation of guinea pig trachea with alpha-chymotrypsin, under conditions that completely block responses to exogenous VIP, results in a significant reduction in i-NANC responses [79]. However, this inhibition is incomplete, indicating that some other transmitter may be involved. A similar experimental design in feline airways showed no effect of alpha-chymotrypsin on i-NANC responses [4], suggesting that there may be differences in the i-NANC transmitter between species. In human airways the i-NANC response is unaffected by alpha-chymotrypsin, but it is possible that the enzyme does not have good access to the sites where VIP is released [34]. The close association between responses to VIP and NANC relaxation in human airways of different sizes [218] provides supportive evidence for VIP as a neurotransmitter.

Some evidence argues against VIP as a neurotransmitter of i-NANC in airways. After pretreatment of guinea pig trachea with maximally effective concentrations of VIP, there is no diminution of i-NANC relaxation, which would be expected if all VIP receptors were occupied [137]. However, exogenous VIP may not have ready access to the VIP receptors related to VIP-ergic nerves. Removal of the epithelium potentiates the bronchodilator action of VIP in vitro, but has no enhancing effect on i-NANC responses [85, 234]. This might be because VIP is released from cholinergic nerves distant from the airway epithelium. In addition, there is convincing evidence from guinea pig and human airways that nitric oxide contributes to bronchodilator i-NANC responses [34, 35b, 156, 291]. The precise role of VIP as an i-NANC transmitter can only be resolved when potent and specific VIP antagonists become available.

Cotransmission with Acetylcholine

VIP coexists with acetylcholine in some cholinergic nerves supplying exocrine glands, and potentiates the salivary secretory response to acetylcholine [164]. VIP may be released from cholinergic nerves only with high-frequency firing and may serve to increase the blood flow to exocrine glands under conditions of excessive stimulation. VIP appears to coexist with acetylcholine in airways [147], and it seems likely that there is a functional relationship between VIP and cholinergic neural control.

It is possible that excessive stimulation of cholinergic nerves and certain patterns of firing result in VIP release. In bovine tracheal smooth muscle, VIP has an inhibitory effect on cholinergic nerve–induced contraction only with high-frequency firing, and also reduces the contractile effect of exogenous acetylcholine [217]. This does not involve any change in muscarinic receptor density or affinity, and may be due to functional antagonism. VIP also has an inhibitory effect on the release of acetylcholine from airway cholinergic nerves [81, 181, 254, 278]. Conversely, alpha-chymotrypsin, which degrades VIP, potentiates cholinergic nerve–induced contractions in guinea pig airways [31]. VIP and

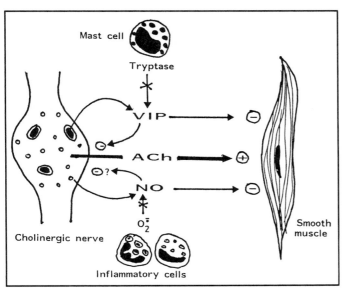

Fig. 18-4. *Vasoactive intestinal peptide (VIP) and nitric oxide (NO) may be coreleased from cholinergic nerves and act as functional antagonists of cholinergic bronchoconstriction. In addition, they may act prejunctionally to inhibit acetylcholine (ACh) release. In asthma, enzymes such as tryptase released from airway mast cells may rapidly degrade VIP, and oxygen free radials such as superoxide anions (O_2^-) from inflammatory cells may inactivate nitric oxide, thus leading to exaggerated cholinergic neural bronchoconstriction.*

nitric oxide seem to counteract the bronchoconstrictor effect of cholinergic bronchoconstriction and thus may function as the "braking" mechanism for airway cholinergic nerves [17, 31, 35a] (Fig. 18-4). If this mechanism were to be deficient with either reduced release or increased breakdown of VIP, then an exaggerated bronchoconstrictor response may result.

Possible Abnormalities in Asthma

Whether dysfunction of VIP-ergic innervation contributes to human airway disease is uncertain. VIP-immunoreactive nerves are strikingly absent in lung tissue largely obtained postmortem from patients with asthma [215]. The loss of VIP immunoreactivity from all tissues including pulmonary vessels is so complete that it seems unlikely to represent a fundamental absence of VIP-immunoreactive nerves in asthma. More likely is the possibility that enzymes, such as mast cell tryptase, are released from inflammatory cells in asthma and that these rapidly degrade VIP when sections are cut [19]. In biopsy specimens taken from patients with mild asthma, VIP-immunoreactive nerves appear normal [119]. VIP antibodies, which would neutralize the effects of VIP, have also been detected in the plasma of asthmatic patients [221]. They are found with the same prevalence in nonasthmatic patients, so their significance is doubtful. While it seems unlikely that there would be any primary abnormality in VIP innervation in the airways of patients with asthma, it is possible that a secondary abnormality may arise as a result of the inflammatory process in the airway.

Mast cell tryptase is particularly active in degrading VIP [54, 284] and is known to be present in elevated concentrations in asthmatic airways [312]. Inhibition of tryptase potentiates the bronchodilator response to VIP in human airways in vitro [285]. Mast cell tryptase reverses the relaxation of airways induced by VIP [91] and markedly increases the in vitro responsiveness of canine airways [253]. Tryptase released from mast cells in the asthmatic airway may then more rapidly degrade VIP and related peptides released from airway cholinergic nerves. This would

remove a "brake" from cholinergic nerves and lead to exaggerated cholinergic reflex bronchoconstriction (see Fig. 18-4). This may also have the effect of increasing inflammatory responses in the airway, since VIP has antiinflammatory actions. In addition, nitric oxide may also be more rapidly degraded by oxidants such as superoxide anion released from activated inflammatory cells, further adding to the increase in cholinergic tone and inflammatory effects.

Whether i-NANC responses are impaired in asthma is not yet certain. There is evidence for dysfunction of i-NANC responses after allergen inhalation in sensitized cats [203a]. In patients with mild asthma, no evidence for an impaired NANC bronchodilator reflex has been observed [150, 201]. However, this does not preclude a defect in patients with more severe asthma in whom the degree of airway inflammation may be greater. In sensitized guinea pigs exposed to allergen, a reduction in i-NANC responses has been found [203]. This is presumably due to the release of enzymes or oxygen free radicals from inflammatory cells in the airways. However, as discussed above, the contribution of VIP to i-NANC responses in human airways is not yet established, and increased degradation of this peptide in asthma may have a relatively minor effect on airway tone.

VASOACTIVE INTESTINAL PEPTIDE–RELATED PEPTIDES

Several other peptides that are similar in structure and effect to VIP have now been identified in the mammalian nervous system.

Peptide Histidine Isoleucine

PHI and its human equivalent peptide histidine methionine (PHM) have a marked structural similarity to VIP, with 50 percent amino acid sequence homology. PHI and PHM are encoded by the same gene as VIP and both peptides are synthesized in the same prohormone [287]. It is therefore not surprising to find that compared to VIP, PHI has a similar immunocytochemical distribution in the lungs and that PHI-immunoreactive nerves supply airway smooth muscle (especially larger airways), bronchial and pulmonary vessels, submucosal glands, and airway ganglia [60, 157, 164a]. The amount of PHI immunoreactivity is very similar to that obtained for VIP immunoreactivity in the respiratory tract [60]. Like VIP, PHI stimulates adenylyl cyclase and appears to activate the same receptor as VIP [239].

There are some differences between VIP and PHI. PHI is less potent as an airway vasodilator [149, 313] and more potent as a stimulant of secretion than VIP [307]. Like VIP, PHI potentiates cholinergic and inhibits alpha-adrenergic stimulation of mucus secretion in vitro [307]. In human bronchi in vitro PHM is a potent relaxant and is equipotent to VIP [218]. It is likely that PHI/PHM is released with VIP from airway nerves and may also be a contributory neurotransmitter in i-NANC nerves.

Peptide Histidine Valine

Peptide histidine valine (PHV-42) is an N-terminally extended precursor of VIP. PHV is a potent bronchodilator of guinea pig airways in vitro [320], but when infused in asthmatic patients, it has no demonstrable bronchodilator effect [57]. It is not yet clear whether this peptide is released from airway nerves.

Helodermin

Helodermin is a 35–amino acid peptide of similar structure to VIP. It has been isolated from the salivary gland venom of the Gila monster lizard. Helodermin-like immunoreactivity has been localized to airway nerves and has effects similar to those of

VIP, but has a longer duration of action. Helodermin is a potent relaxant of airway smooth muscle in vitro, and helodermin-like immunoreactivity has been found in the trachea [88]. Helodermin appears to activate a high-affinity form of the VIP receptor [239].

Pituitary Adenylate Cyclase–Activating Peptide

Pituitary adenylate cyclase–activating peptide (PACAP), a 38–amino acid peptide isolated from sheep hypothalamus, and PACAP-27, a truncated fragment, have marked sequence homology with VIP and have been demonstrated in the peripheral nervous system [204]. PACAP-like immunoreactivity has a similar distribution to VIP in airways of several species, and may be localized to cholinergic and also to capsaicin-sensitive afferent nerves [177]. The effects of PACAP-27 are likely to be similar to those of VIP. There appears to be a particularly high density of receptors for PACAP in lung tissue [108].

TACHYKININS

While substance P was isolated over 50 years ago, structurally related peptides (tachykinins) called *neurokinin A* (NKA) and *neurokinin B* (NKB) have now been identified in the mammalian nervous system [117, 207]. Tachykinins are a family of peptides with the common C-terminal sequence Phe-X-Gly-Leu-Met-NH$_2$. NKA and substance P are coded by the same preprotachykinin (PPT) gene. This gene produces three mRNAs: alpha-PPT produces substance P alone; beta-PPT codes for substance P, NKA, and its N-terminally extended form neuropeptide K (NPK); and gamma-PPT produces substance P, NKA, and a novel N-terminally extended form of NKA termed *NP-gamma* [283]. A fourth splicing variant of the PPT gene termed *delta-PPT* has also been identified in rat tissues; it predicts the existence of a novel tachykinin NP-delta [115]. NKB is coded by a different gene.

Localization

Substance P is localized to sensory nerves in the airways of several species, including humans [161, 283, 295], although there has been debate about whether substance P can be demonstrated in human airways [146]. Rapid enzymatic degradation of substance P in airways, and the fact that its concentrations may decrease with age and possibly after cigarette smoking, could explain the difficulty in demonstrating this peptide in some studies. Substance P–immunoreactive nerves in the airway are found beneath and within the airway epithelium, around blood vessels, and to a lesser extent, within airway smooth muscle. Substance

P–immunoreactive nerve fibers innervate parasympathetic ganglia, suggesting a sensory input that may modulate ganglionic transmission and so result in ganglionic reflexes.

Substance P appears to be localized predominantly to capsaicin-sensitive unmyelinated nerves in the airways. It is predominantly synthesized in the nodose ganglion of the vagus nerve and then transported down the vagus to peripheral branches in the lungs. Some substance P–immunoreactive nerves also arise in the dorsal root ganglia [166], but whether this population of nerves has a similar distribution and function as those arising from the nodose ganglion is not certain. Treatment of animals with capsaicin, bradykinin, histamine, the nicotinic agonist dimethylphenylpiperazinium, and electric nerve stimulation causes acute substance P, NKA, and CGRP release from sensory nerves in the lungs and heart [103, 173, 251]. Chronic administration of capsaicin only partially depletes the lungs of tachykinins and CGRP, indicating the presence of a population of capsaicin-resistant substance P–immunoreactive nerves, as in the gastrointestinal tract [173]. Similar capsaicin denervation studies are not possible in human airways, but after extrinsic denervation by heart-lung transplantation there appears to be a loss of substance P–immunoreactive nerves in the submucosa [270]. NKA-like immunoreactivity has been demonstrated in human airways, and appears to be colocalized with substance P [186]. NPK is also present in the airways. NKB does not appear to be present in airways [186], and it is not certain whether NP-gamma or NP-delta are present.

Tachykinin Receptors

Tachykinin effects on target cells are mediated by specific receptors and each tachykinin appears to selectively activate a distinct subtype of receptor: NK$_1$ receptors are activated preferentially by substance P; NK$_2$ receptors, by NKA; and NK$_3$ receptors, by NKB [231] (Fig. 18-5). Three distinct tachykinin receptors have now been cloned [187, 262, 321]. A fourth subtype of receptor has been suggested based on the potency of a series of synthetic tachykinin analogs in guinea pig trachea [200]. With the development of selective agonists and antagonists, it has been possible to differentiate subtypes of the NK$_2$ receptor; thus, the NK$_2$ receptor in tracheal smooth muscle appears to differ from that in urinary bladder and pulmonary artery [46, 178].

Autoradiographic studies have mapped the widespread distribution of substance P receptors in guinea pig and human lungs [53]. Substance P receptors are found in high density in airway smooth muscle from the trachea down to the small bronchioles and vascular endothelium, whereas pulmonary vascular smooth

Fig. 18-5. *Tachykinins and their receptors. At least three types of tachykinin receptors are now recognized, based on the relative potencies of naturally occurring tachykinins. Originally called SP-P, SP-E, and SP-N receptors, they are now known as NK$_1$, NK$_2$, and NK$_3$ receptors, respectively.*

```
● NK-1 (SP-P):   SP > NKB > E > NKA

● NK-2 (SP-E):   NKA > E > NKB > SP

● NK-3 (SP-N):   NKB > NKA > SP
```

Substance P	SP	Arg-Pro-Lys-Pro-Gln-Gln-Phe-Phe-Gly-Leu-Met-NH$_2$
Physalaemin	PHY	Glp-Ala-Asp-Pro-Asn-Lys-Phe-Tyr-Gly-Leu-Met-NH$_2$
Eledoisin	E	Glp-Pro-Ser-Lys-Asp-Ala-Phe-Ile-Gly-Leu-Met-NH$_2$
Kassinin	KAS	Asp-Val-Pro-Lys-Ser-Asp-Gln-Phe-Val-Gly-Leu-Met-NH$_2$
Neurokinin A	NKA	His-Lys-Thr-Asp-Ser-Phe-Val-Gly-Leu-Met-NH$_2$
Neurokinin B	NKB	Asp-Met-His-Asp-Phe-Phe-Val-Gly-Leu-Met-NH$_2$

muscle and epithelial cells are less densely labeled. Submucosal glands in human airways are also labeled.

Metabolism

Tachykinins are subject to degradation by at least two enzymes, angiotensin-converting enzyme (ACE; EC 3.4.15.1, kininase I) and neutral endopeptidase (NEP; EC 3.4.24.11, enkephalinase) [267]. ACE is predominantly localized to vascular endothelial cells and therefore breaks down intravascular peptides. ACE inhibitors, such as captopril, enhance bronchoconstriction due to intravenously administered substance P [182, 266], but not inhaled substance P [161]. NKA is not a good substrate for ACE, however. NEP appears to be the most important enzyme for the breakdown of tachykinins in tissues. Inhibition of NEP by phosphoramidon or thiorphan markedly potentiates bronchoconstriction in vitro [38, 255, 273] and after inhalation in vivo in rodents [78, 161]. Thiorphan also potentiates the bronchoconstrictor response to inhaled NKA in humans in vivo [56a]. NEP inhibition also potentiates mucus secretion in response to tachykinins [40, 175, 240]. NEP inhibition enhances e-NANC and capsaicin-induced bronchoconstriction, due to the release of tachykinins from airway sensory nerves [76, 95].

The activity of NEP in the airways appears to be an important factor in determining the effects of tachykinins; any factors that inhibit the enzyme or its expression may be associated with enhanced tachykinin effects. Reductions in NEP activity occur after respiratory tract infections [130, 198, 225] and exposures to cigarette smoke [77], ozone [319], and high doses of toluene diisocyanate [260].

Another endopeptidase (EC 3.4.24.15) that effectively degrades tachykinins has also been demonstrated in rat airway epithelium and nerves [58]. This enzyme is not inhibited by drugs that inhibit NEP and its role in regulating tachykinin effects in the airway is not yet clear.

Effects on Airway Smooth Muscle

While substance P contracts the airway smooth muscle of several species, including humans [87, 170], NKA is considerably more potent [1, 38, 186, 217], indicating that an NK_2 receptor is likely to be involved. This is confirmed by the use of selective synthetic agonists that are resistant to enzymatic degradation. The NK_2-selective agonist $[Nle^{10}]$-NKA(4-10) is a potent constrictor of human bronchi in vitro, whereas NK_1- and NK_3-selective agonists are ineffective [178, 208, 236]. Furthermore, an NK_2-selective antagonist L659,877 also has a high potency [236]. The NK_2-selective competitive antagonist R-396 appears to be 100 times more potent in hamster tracheal smooth muscle than MEN 10207, whereas the reverse is true in rabbit pulmonary artery, demonstrating that different subtypes of the NK_2 receptor must exist [178]. In guinea pig trachea bronchoconstriction is mediated by NK_1 as well as NK_2 receptors [236] and there is also evidence for an atypical "NK_4" receptor [200]. The contractile response to NKA is significantly greater in smaller human bronchi than in more proximal airways, indicating that tachykinins may have a more important constrictor effect on more peripheral airways [94], whereas cholinergic constriction tends to be more pronounced in proximal airways. In vivo substance P does not cause bronchoconstriction either by intravenous infusion [83, 98] or by inhalation [98, 133], whereas NKA causes bronchoconstriction after intravenous administration [83] and after inhalation in asthmatic subjects [133]. Surprisingly the bronchoconstrictor effect of nebulized NKA in asthmatic patients is inhibited by prior treatment with cromolyn sodium, indicating that it is mediated indirectly rather than by a direct effect on airway smooth muscle [135]. Like most other spasmogens, tachykinins cause contraction of airway smooth muscle by stimulating phosphoinositide

hydrolysis and increasing the formation of inositol-1,4,5-trisphosphate, which releases calcium ions from intracellular stores in airway smooth muscle [109]. As expected, NKA is more potent than substance P in this respect.

Interactions with Epithelium

Airway epithelium modulates the bronchoconstrictor effect of many spasmogens, possibly by releasing a relaxant substance termed *epithelium-derived relaxant factor* (EpDRF), which may be similar but not identical to endothelium-derived relaxant factor (see Chap. 23). This may be of functional relevance in asthma since airway epithelium is often shed, even in patients with relatively mild asthma [148]. Mechanical removal of epithelium markedly potentiates the bronchoconstrictor effect of tachykinins [67, 86, 95, 109, 290]. For NKA, the effect of epithelium removal can be mimicked by inhibiting NEP with phosphoramidon. Since NEP is localized to airway epithelium, mechanical denudation may remove the major site of tachykinin metabolism [95]. The situation for substance P is more complex, since in addition substance P may interact with NK_1 receptors on epithelial cells to release the putative EpDRF and other bronchodilators such as PGE_2. Epithelium removal also potentiates the effects of capsaicin, indicating that endogenous tachykinin effects are also enhanced [76, 95]. If epithelium is shed in asthmatic airways, any effects of tachykinins may be more pronounced, not only effects on airway smooth muscle, but also inflammatory effects in the mucosa and submucosa (Fig. 18-6).

Airway Secretion

Substance P stimulates mucus secretion from submucosal glands in animal and human airways in vitro [40, 240]. In canine trachea, substance P is one of the most potent stimulants of mucus secretion described, and at low concentrations appears to stimulate secretion without morphologic effects on secretory cells. This suggests that substance P may cause the myoepithelial cells that surround submucosal glands to contract and expel mucus from the glands and ducts, rather like toothpaste is squeezed from a tube [61]. Direct measurement of gland duct secretion in cats confirms this suggestion [265]. Morphologic studies in ferret suggest that substance P at higher concentrations stimulates serous cells [100]. This is confirmed by functional studies that demonstrated an increased output of lysozyme, a serous cell marker [308]. Substance P is much more potent than NKA in stimulating airway mucus secretion, indicating that NK_1 receptors are involved [240, 308], and these have been localized by autoradiography to submucosal glands in human bronchi [53].

Stimulation of the vagus nerve causes a discharge from goblet cells in guinea pig trachea, as measured by a morphometric technique [289]. This response is almost completely abolished by capsaicin pretreatment, indicating that the release of sensory neuropeptides is involved. Of the sensory neuropeptides, substance P is by far the most potent in stimulating goblet cell secretion [143], indicating that an NK_1 receptor is involved. Since goblet cells are the only source of mucus in peripheral airways, it is possible that substance P plays an important role in mucus secretion in peripheral airways in patients with asthma and in cigarette smokers. Indeed cigarette smoking in guinea pigs results in marked goblet cell discharge, which is partly mediated by the vapor phase which activates capsaicin-sensitive nerves [142].

Tachykinins also stimulate ion transport in airway epithelium, with substance P being more potent than NKA [230], indicating that NK_1 receptors are involved. Substance P also releases PGE_2 and possibly EpDRF from airway epithelial cells [66, 95]. Tachykinins also increase mucociliary clearance in airways [317, 318]

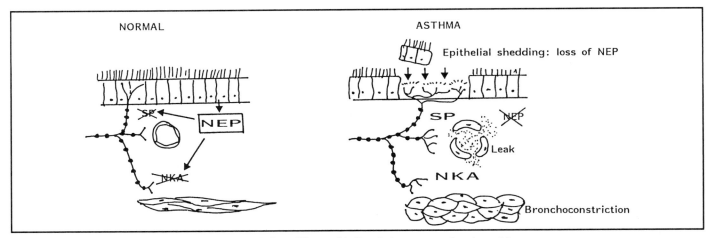

Fig. 18-6. *Interaction of tachykinins with airway epithelium. When epithelium is intact, neutral endopeptidase (NEP) degrades substance P (SP) and neurokinin A (NKA) released from sensory nerves (left panel). In asthmatic airways when epithelium is shed or NEP downregulated, any tachykinins released will have an exaggerated effect (right panel).*

and this response may be secondary to an increase in airway secretions.

Vascular Effects

Stimulation of the vagus nerve in rodents causes microvascular leakage, which is prevented by prior treatment with capsaicin or by a tachykinin antagonist, indicating that the release of tachykinins from sensory nerves mediates this effect [153a, 171]. Among the tachykinins, substance P is the most potent at causing leakage in guinea pig airways [242] and NK_1 receptors have been localized to postcapillary venules in the airway submucosa [257]. This has recently been confirmed by the inhibitory effect of the selective NK_1-receptor antagonist CP-96,345 on neurogenic plasma exudation in guinea pig airways [153a]. The distributions of leakage after vagus nerve stimulation and after intravenous administration of substance P are similar, with maximal effect in the lower trachea and main bronchi, indicating some differential distribution of NK_1 receptors in postcapillary venules in different airways [84]. Inhaled substance P also causes microvascular leakage in guinea pigs and its effect on the microvasculature is more marked than its effect on airway smooth muscle [160]; inhaled substance P causes an increase in airway resistance in anesthetized guinea pigs, but unlike the increased resistance seen after administration of a cholinergic agonist, this is not reversed by a full inflation. Whether tachykinins cause microvascular leakage in human airways is not yet certain, since no direct measurements have been made. Nevertheless, substance P injected intradermally causes a wheal in human skin, which indicates the capacity to cause microvascular leak in human postcapillary venules; NKA is less potent, indicating that an NK_1 receptor mediates this effect [96].

Tachykinins have potent effects on airway blood flow. Indeed the effect of tachykinins on airway blood flow may be their most important physiologic and pathophysiologic role in airways. In canine and porcine trachea both substance P and NKA cause a marked increase in blood flow [149, 189, 250]. Tachykinins also dilate canine bronchial vessels in vitro, probably via an endothelium-dependent mechanism [196]. Tachykinins also regulate bronchial blood flow in pig; stimulation of the vagus nerve causes a vasodilatation mediated by the release of sensory neuropeptides, and it is likely that CGRP as well as tachykinins are involved [189]. CGRP and VIP act as arterial dilators and have synergistic effects on substance P–induced vascular permeability in skin [42, 99, 139].

Effects on Inflammatory Cells

Tachykinins may also interact with inflammatory and immune cells [199], although whether this is of pathophysiologic significance remains to be determined. Substance P degranulates certain types of mast cells, such as those in human skin [90, 112]. Substance P injected into human skin causes a wheal and flare response; the latter is likely to be due to histamine release from dermal mast cells since the response is abolished by antihistamines. This is confirmed by the release of histamine into veins draining the area of skin injected [25]. This response is not mediated by a classic tachykinin receptor, since it is dependent on the N-terminal sequence of the peptide [162], whereas receptor binding is determined by the C-terminal sequence. The N-terminal region of substance P is highly basically charged and may interact with cell membrane phosphate moieties while the hydrophobic tail inserts itself into hydrophobic sites [232]. Furthermore, NKA injected in equimolar doses fails to induce any flare in human skin [96]. It is unlikely that substance P release causes mast cell degranulation under physiologic circumstances, however, since the injection of capsaicin intradermally to stimulate the release of substance P from sensory nerves in the skin fails to induce the same rise in venous histamine [25]. However, human lung mast cells do not degranulate in response to substance P [3]. In rats the bronchoconstrictor response to tachykinins is reduced by blocking the effect of 5-hydroxytryptamine released from mast cells (rather than histamine) and also by cromolyn sodium and ketotifen, which may act by stabilizing mast cells [134]. Furthermore, tachykinins increase the concentration of histamine in the bronchoalveolar fluid of guinea pigs, indicating that tachykinins may directly activate airway mast cells [222]. Surprisingly, NKA is more potent than substance P in this respect, indicating that an NK_2 receptor is involved. While similar measurements have not been made in human airways, indirect evidence that a similar phenomenon applies may be the demonstration that the bronchoconstrictor response to nebulized NKA in asthmatic patients is reduced by pretreatment with cromolyn sodium [134].

This raises questions about the functional innervation of mast cells in airways. Histologic studies have demonstrated a close proximity between mast cells and sensory nerves in airways [36]. There is also evidence that antidromic stimulation of the vagus nerve leads to mast cell mediator release in canine airways [153]. Furthermore, allergen exposure has effects on ion transport in guinea pig airways that are dependent on capsaicin-sensitive nerves [258].

Substance P has a degranulating effect on eosinophils [141]; again, the degranulation is related to high concentrations of peptide and is dependent on the N-terminal sequence. Tachykinins have effects on macrophage function in vitro and an NK$_2$ receptor appears to be involved [45]. Tachykinins may activate monocytes to release inflammatory cytokines, such as interleukin-6 (IL-6) [163], and cause transient vascular adhesion of neutrophils in the airway circulation [298]. In the skin, substance P induces an infiltration with neutrophils, which appears to be dependent on the degranulation of dermal mast cells [191], but this may not be relevant in the airways for the reasons discussed above.

Effects on Nerves

In rabbit and ferret, the bronchoconstrictor effect of tachykinins is partly mediated by the release of acetylcholine from postganglionic cholinergic nerves, since atropine reduces this response [256, 286]. In guinea pig trachea, tachykinins also potentiate cholinergic neurotransmission at postganglionic nerve terminals, and an NK$_2$ receptor appears to be involved [113]. The potentiation is more marked at subthreshold voltages, suggesting that tachykinins may facilitate the *spread* of cholinergic transmission through postganglionic terminals. Endogenous tachykinins may also facilitate cholinergic neurotransmission, as capsaicin pretreatment results in a significant reduction in cholinergic neural responses both in vitro and in vivo [183, 275]. Interestingly, capsaicin pretreatment also enhances i-NANC responses in airways, indicating that endogenous tachykinins may inhibit i-NANC mediated bronchodilatation [276]. Substance P–immunoreactive nerves appear to innervate parasympathetic ganglia in the airways, suggesting that endogenous tachykinins may also have a facilitatory effect on cholinergic neurotransmission at a ganglionic level. Indeed, substance P and capsaicin appear to enhance ganglionic neurotransmission [300]. The interaction between tachykinins and human airway nerves is less certain. Although tachykinins do not facilitate cholinergic nerve–induced contraction of human bronchi under resting conditions, NKA has a facilitatory effect in the presence of potassium channel blockers [37].

CALCITONIN GENE–RELATED PEPTIDE

CGRP is a 37–amino acid peptide formed by the alternative splicing of the precursor mRNA coded by the calcitonin gene. There are two forms of CGRP, which differ by three amino acids [272, 314]. Both alpha-CGRP and beta-CGRP are expressed in sensory neurons [212] and both are potent vasodilators.

Localization

CGRP-immunoreactive nerves are abundant in the respiratory tract of several species. CGRP is costored and colocalized with substance P in afferent nerves [165, 184]. CGRP has been extracted from and is localized to human airways [219]. CGRP-immunoreactive nerve fibers appear to be more abundant than substance P–immunoreactive fibers, possibly because CGRP has greater stability and is also present in some nerves that do not contain substance P. CGRP is found in trigeminal, nodose-jugular, and dorsal root ganglia [292]. Unlike substance P, it has also been detected in neuroendocrine cells of the lower airways [50].

Calcitonin Gene–Related Peptide Receptors

CGRP binds to specific surface receptors that are linked via Gs to adenyl cyclase, thus increasing intracellular cyclic AMP concentrations. CGRP receptors have been detected in the lungs by direct binding studies [206] and have been localized by autoradiographic mapping [180]. At least two subtypes of receptors

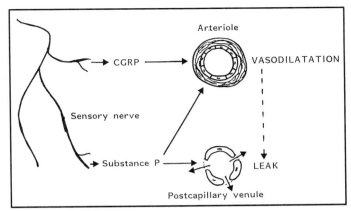

Fig. 18-7. *Effect of sensory neuropeptides in airway vessels. Substance P causes vasodilatation and plasma exudation, whereas calcitonin gene–related peptide (CGRP) causes vasodilatation of the arterioles, which may theoretically increase plasma extravasation by increasing blood delivery to leaky postcapillary venules.*

have been suggested on the basis of structure activity studies with CGRP analogs [65].

Vascular Effects

CGRP is a potent vasodilator that has long-lasting effects [314]. After intradermal injection in human skin, CGPR induces a long-lasting flare response [43]. CGRP is an effective dilator of human pulmonary vessels in vitro and acts directly on receptors on vascular smooth muscle [195]. It also potently dilates canine bronchial vessels in vitro [195] and produces a marked and long-lasting increase in airway blood flow in anesthetized dogs [250] and conscious sheep [211]. Receptor-mapping studies have demonstrated that CGRP receptors are localized predominantly to bronchial vessels rather than to smooth muscle or epithelium in human airways [180]. It is possible that CGRP may be the predominant mediator of arterial vasodilatation and increased blood flow in response to sensory nerve stimulation in the bronchi [189]. CGRP may be an important mediator of airway hyperemia in asthma.

By contrast, CGRP has no direct effect of airway microvascular leak [242]. In the skin, CGRP potentiates the leakage produced by substance P, presumably by increasing the blood delivery to the sites of plasma extravasation in the postcapillary venules [99, 139]. This does not occur in the airway when CGRP plus substance P is administered intravenously, possibly because blood flow in the airways is higher [242]. It is possible that potentiation of leakage may occur when the two peptides are released together from sensory nerves (Fig. 18-7).

Effect on Airway Smooth Muscle

CGRP causes constriction of human bronchi in vitro [219]. This is surprising since CGRP normally activates adenylate cyclase, an event that is usually associated with bronchodilatation. Receptor-mapping studies suggest few, if any, CGRP receptors over airway smooth muscle in humans or guinea pigs and this suggests that the paradoxic bronchoconstrictor response reported in human airways may be mediated indirectly. In guinea pig airways, CGRP has no consistent effect on tone [185].

Other Airway Effects

CGRP has a weak inhibitory effect on cholinergically stimulated mucus secretion in ferret trachea [310] and on goblet cell discharge in guinea pig airways [143]. This is probably related to the low density of CGRP receptors on mucus secretory cells, but does not preclude the possibility that CGRP might increase mucus secretion in vivo by increasing blood flow to the submucosal glands.

CGRP injection into human skin causes a persistent flare, but biopsy studies have revealed an infiltration of eosinophils [226]. CGRP itself does not appear to be chemotactic for eosinophils, but proteolytic fragments of the peptide are active [116], suggesting that CGRP released into the tissues may lead to eosinophilic infiltration.

CGRP inhibits the proliferative response of T-lymphocytes to mitogens and specific receptors have been demonstrated on these cells [296]. CGRP also inhibits macrophage secretion and the capacity of macrophages to activate T-lymphocytes [213]. This suggests that CGRP has potential antiinflammatory actions in the airways.

NEUROGENIC INFLAMMATION

Pain, heat, redness, and swelling are the cardinal signs of inflammation. Sensory nerves may be involved in the generation of each of these signs. There is now considerable evidence that sensory nerves participate in inflammatory responses. This "neurogenic inflammation" is due to the antidromic release of neuropeptides from nociceptive nerves or C fibers via an axon reflex. The phenomenon is well documented in several organs, including the skin, eyes, gastrointestinal tract, and bladder [118, 179]. There is also increasing evidence that neurogenic inflammation occurs in the respiratory tract [21] and that it may contribute to the inflammatory response in asthma [12].

Neurogenic Inflammation in Asthma

There are several lines of evidence that neurogenic inflammation may be important in asthma.

Sensory Neuropeptide Effects

Sensory neuropeptides mimic many of the pathophysiologic features of asthma. NKA is a very potent constrictor of human airways and enhances cholinergic neurotransmission; substance P is a vasodilator, causes microvascular leakage, and stimulates mucus secretion from submucosal glands and epithelial goblet cells; CGRP is a potent and long-lasting vasodilator (Fig. 18-8). In addition, these peptides may have effects on the regulation of local mucosal immunity.

Sensory Nerve Activation

Sensory nerves may be activated in airway disease. In asthmatic airways the epithelium is often shed, thereby exposing sensory nerve endings. Sensory nerves in asthmatic airways may be "hyperalgesic" as a result of exposure to inflammatory mediators such as prostaglandins and certain cytokines. Hyperalgesic nerves may then be activated more readily by other mediators, such as kinins.

Bradykinin is a potent bronchoconstrictor in asthmatic patients and also induces coughing and a sensation of chest tightness, which closely mimics a naturally occurring asthma attack [97, 229]. Yet bradykinin is a weak constrictor of human airways in vitro, suggesting that its potent constrictor effect is mediated indirectly. Bradykinin is a potent activator of bronchial C fibers in dogs [138] and releases sensory neuropeptides from perfused rodent lungs [251]. In guinea pigs bradykinin instilled into the airways causes bronchoconstriction, which is reduced significantly by a cholinergic antagonist (as in asthmatic patients [97]) and also by capsaicin pretreatment [122]. This indicates that bradykinin activates sensory nerves in the airways and that part of the bronchoconstrictor response is mediated by the release of constrictor peptides from capsaicin-sensitive nerves. Whether the bronchoconstrictor response to bradykinin seen in asthmatic patients is also due to sensory peptide release is not certain, since specific tachykinin antagonists have not yet been studied

Fig. 18-8. *Possible neurogenic inflammation in asthmatic airways via retrograde release of peptides from sensory nerves by an axon reflex. Substance P (SP) causes vasodilatation, plasma exudation, and mucus secretion, whereas neurokinin A (NKA) causes bronchoconstriction and enhanced cholinergic reflexes and calcitonin gene–related peptide (CGRP) causes vasodilatation. v/d = vasodilatation.*

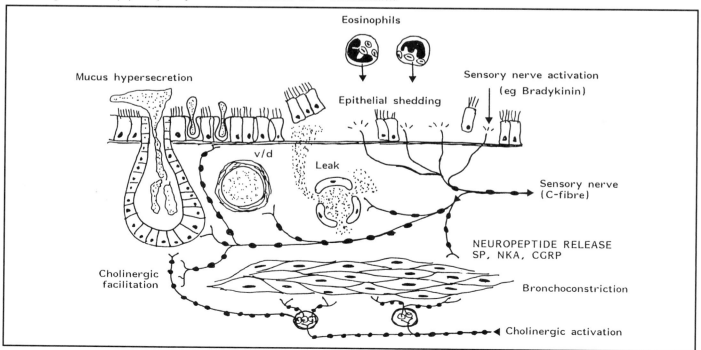

in this situation. The inhibitory effects of cromolyn sodium and nedocromil sodium on bradykinin-induced bronchoconstriction provide supportive evidence [73, 97].

Pattern of Innervation
Chronic inflammation may lead to changes in the pattern of innervation, through the release of neurotrophic factors from inflammatory cells. Thus in chronic arthritis and inflammatory bowel disease there is an increase in the density of substance P–immunoreactive nerves [118, 155]. A striking increase in nerves with substance P–like immunoreactivity has been demonstrated in the airway of patients with fatal asthma [216]. This increased density of nerves is particularly noticeable in the submucosa. Whether this increase is due to proliferation of sensory nerves or is due to increased synthesis of tachykinins has not yet been established. Cultured sensory neurons are stimulated by nerve growth factor (NGF), which markedly increases the gene transcription of beta-PPT, the major precursor peptide for tachykinins [158]. Since NGF may be released from several types of inflammatory cells, it is possible that this could lead to increased tachykinin synthesis and increased nerve growth. Several other neurotrophic factors have also recently been identified. However, studies of bronchial biopsy specimens from patients with mild asthma have not revealed any evidence of increased substance P–immunoreactive nerves. This may indicate that the increased innervation [216] is a feature of either prolonged or severe asthma.

Neuropeptide Metabolism
The metabolism of sensory neuropeptides may be impaired in asthmatic airways or airways affected by chronic obstructive pulmonary disease (COPD). The activity of NEP may be an important determinant of the extent of neurogenic inflammation in airways. Certain virus infections enhance e-NANC responses in guinea pigs [245] and *Mycoplasma* infection enhances neurogenic microvascular leakage in rats [197], an effect that is mediated by the inhibition of NEP activity. Influenza virus infection of ferret trachea in vitro and of guinea pigs in vivo inhibits the activity of epithelial NEP and markedly enhances the bronchoconstrictor responses to tachykinins [130]. Similarly, Sendai virus infection potentiates neurogenic inflammation in rat trachea [225]. This may explain why respiratory tract virus infections are so deleterious to patients with asthma. Hypertonic saline solution also impairs epithelial NEP function, leading to exaggerated tachykinin responses [297], and cigarette smoke exposure has a similar effect, which can be explained by an oxidizing effect on the enzyme [77]. Toluene diisocyanate, albeit at rather unrealistic doses, also reduces NEP activity, and this may be a mechanism contributing to the airway hyperresponsiveness that may follow exposure to this chemical [260]. Thus, many of the agents that lead to exacerbations of asthma appear to reduce the activity of NEP at the airway surface, resulting in exaggerated responses to tachykinins (and other peptides) and to increased airway inflammation. The role of NEP in human airway disease remains to be investigated.

Sensory Nerve Depletion
In several animal models of asthma, the role of neurogenic inflammation has been explored by selectively depleting sensory neuropeptides with capsaicin. In rat trachea, capsaicin pretreatment inhibits the microvascular leakage induced by irritant gases, such as cigarette smoke [172], and inhibits goblet cell discharge and microvascular leakage induced by cigarette smoke in guinea pigs [144]. Capsaicin pretreatment also reduces the vasodilator response to allergen in pig bronchi [5] and to toluene diisocyanate in rat airways [288]. Capsaicin-sensitive nerves may also contribute to the bronchoconstrictor response to hypocap-

nia in rodents [233], but not to the acute bronchoconstrictor response to allergen [159]. However, more prolonged exposure of sensitized guinea pigs to aerosolized antigen results in a pronounced increase in airway responsiveness, which is completely abolished by capsaicin pretreatment [192]. This suggests that capsaicin-sensitive nerves may play an important role in chronic inflammatory responses to allergen. It is probably not possible to apply capsaicin in high concentrations to human lower airways in order to study the role of capsaicin-sensitive nerves in asthma, but preliminary studies in which capsaicin was topically applied to the nasal mucosa under local anesthesia indicated that this treatment may be effective in controlling vasomotor rhinitis [1, 271, 315].

Modulation of Neurogenic Inflammation

There are several ways in which neurogenic inflammation may be modulated [24] (Fig. 18-9), and these may provide novel approaches to antiinflammatory therapy in the future.

Inhibition of Sensory Neuropeptide Effects
Antagonists of tachykinin or CGRP receptors should be effective. However, it has proved difficult to develop antagonists that are potent and selective. An NK$_2$-receptor antagonist that has reasonable potency in human bronchi in vitro has been developed [236], but this antagonist is a peptide and would therefore present problems with airway delivery. More potent tachykinin antagonists are now under development and an NK$_1$ antagonist would be particularly useful, since the NK$_1$ receptor mediates most of the mucosal inflammatory effects of tachykinins. A potent nonpeptide NK$_1$ antagonist was recently developed and may prove very useful in the future [268]. No CGRP antagonists have yet been reported. Since multiple peptides are released from sensory nerves (and there is no evidence for selective release), it is likely that antagonism of a single peptide may not be entirely effective. A more attractive approach may be to inhibit the release of all peptides.

Inhibition of Sensory Neuropeptide Release
Several different agonists act on prejunctional receptors on sensory nerves in airways to inhibit the release of sensory neuropeptides, thus inhibiting neurogenic inflammation. Opioids are the most effective agonists in this respect, and perhaps this is not surprising as they inhibit the release of substance P from nociceptive fibers in the central nervous system (CNS) [132]. Opioids inhibit e-NANC bronchoconstriction in guinea pig bronchi in vitro [33, 93] and in vivo [29, 32] while having no effect on equivalent tachykinin-induced bronchoconstriction, thereby indicating an effect on the release of tachykinins. The effects of opioids are mediated by opioid receptors, since they are inhibited by naloxone. A mu-opioid receptor is involved since mu-selective agonists are effective, whereas delta and kappa agonists are not [29, 32, 33, 93]. A mu-opioid agonist also modulates cholinergic neurotransmission in guinea pig airways, but this is largely via an inhibitory effect on the facilitatory action of e-NANC nerves [33]. Opioids also inhibit neurogenic microvascular leakage in guinea pig airways [29, 32], mucus secretion from human bronchi in vitro [241], cholinergic neurotransmission in human airways in vitro [29], and cigarette smoke–induced goblet cell discharge from guinea pig airways in vivo [144].

Several other agonists are also effective. These include the inhibitory central neurotransmitter gamma-aminobutyric acid (GABA) which acts by a GABA$_B$ receptor [30], NPY [190, 277], alpha$_2$ agonists [111, 190], galanin [107], corticotropin-releasing factor [311], beta$_2$ agonists [136, 304], adenosine acting by A$_2$ receptors [136, 305], and histamine acting by an H$_3$ receptor [120, 123]. The fact that so many different receptors have an inhibitory

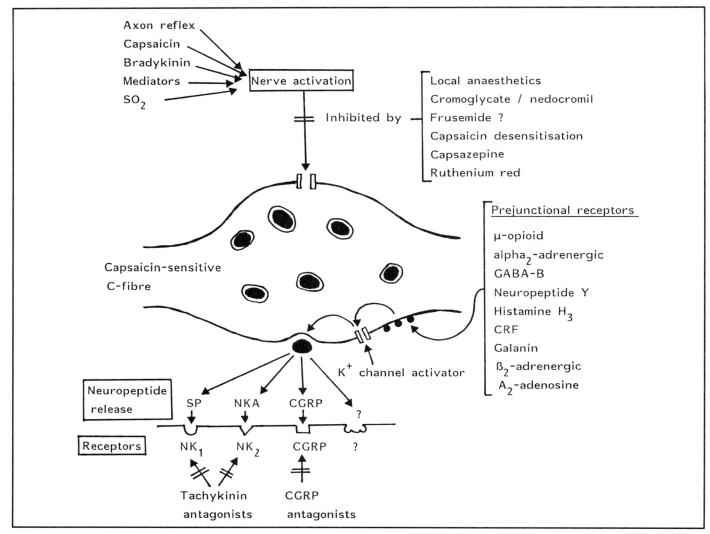

Fig. 18-9. *Modulation of neurogenic inflammation (see text). Neurogenic inflammation may be reduced by blocking neuropeptide receptors or by inhibiting the release of neuropeptide from sensory nerves by agonists such as mu opioids. In addition, activation of sensory nerves may be possible using drugs such as cromolyn sodium. CRF = corticotropin-releasing factor; SP = substance P; NKA = neurokinin A; CGRP = calcitonin gene–related peptide.*

effect raises the question of whether there is a common inhibitory mechanism. In the CNS, several of the agonists that are inhibitory to neuropeptide release have been found to open a common K^+ channel [59]. The K^+ channel activator cromakalim and its active stereoisomer lemakalim are effective in inhibiting e-NANC bronchoconstriction in guinea pigs in vivo and in vitro. Their effects are inhibited by blockers of ATP-sensitive channels [121, 280]. However, a potent ATP-sensitive channel blocker completely inhibits the effect of lemakalim but has no effect against the inhibitory actions of an opioid or alpha$_2$ agonist. By contrast, charybdotoxin, an inhibitor of large conductance Ca^{++}-activated K^+ channels, is extremely effective in inhibiting these inhibitory actions, indicating that a common Ca^{++}-activated K^+ channel that hyperpolarizes the sensory nerve and inhibits neuropeptide release may be involved.

Another agent that inhibits neuropeptide release from sensory nerves in airways is the dye ruthenium red. Ruthenium red is a selective inhibitor of capsaicin-induced contraction of guinea pig airways in vitro [6, 46], but has no effect against e-NANC bronchoconstriction induced by electrical field stimulation or bradykinin.

Inhibition of Sensory Nerve Activation

Activation of sensory nerves may be inhibited by local anesthetics, but it has proved to be very difficult to achieve adequate local anesthesia of the respiratory tract. Inhalation of local anesthetics, such as lidocaine, has not been found to have consistent inhibitory effects on various airway challenges, and indeed may even promote bronchoconstriction in some patients with asthma [194]. This paradoxic bronchoconstriction may be due to the greater anesthesia of laryngeal afferents linked to a tonic nonadrenergic bronchodilator reflex [150, 151]. Other drugs may inhibit the activation of airway sensory nerves. Cromolyn sodium and nedocromil sodium may have direct effects on airway C fibers [75, 129] and this might contribute to their antiasthma effect. Nedocromil sodium is highly effective against bradykinin-induced and sulfur dioxide–induced bronchoconstriction in asthmatic patients [74, 75], which is believed to be mediated by the activation of sensory nerves in the airways. In addition, nedocromil sodium and, to a much lesser extent, cromolyn sodium inhibit e-NANC bronchoconstriction in guinea pig bronchi in vitro, indicating an effect on the release of sensory neuropeptides as well as on the activation [306]. The loop diuretic furosemide given by nebulization behaves in a fashion similar to that of nedocromil sodium and inhibits metabisulfite-induced bronchoconstriction in asthmatic patients [210] and also e-NANC and cholinergic bronchoconstriction in guinea pig airways in vitro [82]. In addition, nebulized furosemide also inhibits certain types of cough [302], providing further evidence for an effect on sensory nerves.

Replacement of Neutral Endopeptidase

Since a defective function of NEP may be critical in amplifying neurogenic inflammation, another strategy would be to replace the enzyme. Indeed, recombinant human NEP has been shown to inhibit cough induced by tachykinins in guinea pig [140]. It may also be possible to increase the activity of NEP in the airways. Thus, corticosteroids appear to increase the activity of NEP in airways, and this may be at the level of gene expression in epithelial cells [41]. Perhaps one of the potential beneficial actions of inhaled corticosteroids in asthma is increased expression of NEP activity.

Sensory Denervation

Exposure of adult animals to high concentrations of capsaicin depletes sensory neuropeptides, which are only slowly repleted. Topical application of capsaicin might therefore be a useful approach to controlling neurogenic inflammation in the respiratory tract. While this may be difficult to achieve in the lower airways, it appears to be feasible in the nose. Nasal application of capsaicin is reported to be effective in controlling nonallergic vasomotor rhinitis for periods of over a year [101, 271, 315].

NEUROPEPTIDE Y

NPY is a 36–amino acid peptide that is a cotransmitter with norepinephrine in adrenergic nerves and usually amplifies its effects [228].

Localization

The distribution of NPY follows the distribution of adrenergic nerves and is predominantly to nasal vessels and bronchial vessels and glands, with less marked innervation of airway smooth muscle [8, 261, 294, 295]. After extrinsic denervation in heart-lung transplant recipients, there is an apparent increase in NPY-like–immunoreactive nerves, suggesting that there may normally be some descending inhibitory influence to the expression of this peptide [270]. In rodents, depletion of sensory neuropeptides with capsaicin is associated with an increase in adrenergic nerves, indicating that there may be a reciprocal interaction between sensory and adrenergic innervation in the lungs [301]. NPY may also be found within parasympathetic ganglia, where it coexists with VIP, since sympathectomy does not completely deplete NPY. This suggests that there is a small population of NPY-immunoreactive fibers in the respiratory tract that are not sympathetic in origin.

Effects on Airway Tone

NPY has no direct effect on the airway smooth muscle of guinea pig [279], but may cause bronchoconstriction via release of prostaglandins [49]. NPY has a modulatory effect on the cholinergic transmission of postganglionic cholinergic nerves [279]. This appears to be a direct effect on prejunctional NPY receptors, rather than secondary to any effect on alpha adrenoceptors. NPY also has a modulatory effect on e-NANC bronchoconstriction both in

vitro and in vivo, and this effect is surprisingly long-lasting [192, 279].

Vascular Effects

NPY is a potent vasoconstrictor in some vascular beds, acting predominantly on the resistance arterioles. It causes a long-lasting reduction in tracheal blood flow in anesthetized dogs [250], but has no direct effect on canine bronchial vessels in vitro [196], suggesting a preferential effect on resistance vessels in the airway. NPY also causes long-lasting vasoconstriction in the nose, and is released with sympathetic nerve stimulation, particularly at higher frequencies [145]. NPY may constrict resistance vessels reducing mucosal blood flow, and reducing microvascular leakage through the reduction in the perfusion of permeable postcapillary venules.

Effects on Secretion

NPY has no direct effect on secretion from ferret airways, although it has complex effects on stimulated secretion. NPY enhances both cholinergic and adrenergic stimulation of mucus secretion, but inhibits stimulated serous cell secretion [307].

GASTRIN-RELEASING PEPTIDE

Gastrin-releasing peptide (GRP) is a 27–amino acid peptide, and is the mammalian form of the amphibian peptide bombesin [63, 281]. Other shorter peptides that share the common C-terminal sequence have been described [63] and these peptides interact with specific receptors.

Localization

GRP/bombesin-like immunoreactivity is localized to neuroendocrine cells in human and animal lower airways [64, 202]. Bombesin-like immunoreactive peptides have been recovered from the bronchoalveolar lavage fluid from smokers [2]. GRP-containing nerve fibers have been demonstrated around blood vessels and submucosal glands in the airways of several species [293]. GRP/bombesin-binding sites are present on bronchial epithelial cells and submucosal glands [9, 174].

Airway Effects

GRP and bombesin-like peptides may play important roles in lung maturation. GRP mRNA production in the lungs is increased on the day prior to birth and then declines [64]. Bombesin-like immunoreactivity decreases with maturation [64, 105]. Bombesin has a trophic effect on several cell types and may be important in epithelial growth [63, 316].

Bombesin is a potent bronchoconstrictor in guinea pigs in vivo [35, 125]. However, in vitro it has no effect on either proximal airways or on lung strips, indicating that it produces bronchoconstriction indirectly. The bronchoconstrictor response is not blocked by an antihistamine, cyclooxygenase inhibitor, lipoxygenase inhibitor, platelet-activating factor antagonist, or serotonin antagonist, indicating that mediator release is unlikely, nor is it inhibited by capsaicin pretreatment or by cholinergic antagonists, suggesting that neural reflex mechanisms are not involved. The bronchoconstrictor response is inhibited by a bombesin receptor antagonist, BIM 26159, indicating that bombesin/GRP receptors are involved [35]. Bombesin reduces tracheal blood flow in dogs, indicating a vasoconstrictor action [250].

GRP and bombesin are potent stimulants of mucus secretion in human and cat airways in vitro [9, 174].

OTHER PEPTIDES

Cholecystokinin

Cholecystokinin octapeptide (CCK$_8$) has been identified in low concentration in the lungs and airways of several species [104]. It may be localized to sensory nerves [118].

CCK$_8$ is a potent constrictor of guinea pig and human airways in vitro [274]. The bronchoconstrictor response is potentiated by epithelial removal and by phosphoramidon, suggesting that it is degraded by epithelial NEP. The bronchoconstrictor effect of CCK$_8$ is also potentiated in guinea pigs sensitized and exposed to inhaled allergen, possibly because allergen exposure reduces epithelial NEP function. CCK$_8$ acts directly on airway smooth muscle and is potently inhibited by the specific CCK antagonist L363,851, indicating that CCK$_A$ receptors (peripheral type) are involved. CCK$_8$ has no apparent effect on cholinergic neurotransmission either at the level of parasympathetic ganglia or at postganglionic nerve terminals. While few CCK-immunoreactive nerves are present in the airways, CCK$_8$ may still have a significant effect on airway tone if these particular neural fibers are activated selectively.

Somatostatin

Somatostatin has been localized to some afferent nerves [131], but the concentration detectable in the lungs is low [104, 295]. Somatostatin has no direct action on airway smooth muscle in vitro, but appears to potentiate cholinergic neurotransmission in ferret airways [252]. While somatostatin has a modulatory effect on neurogenic inflammation in the rat foot pad [154], no modulation of e-NANC nerves in airways is apparent (C. D. Stretton and P. J. Barnes, unpublished observations).

Galanin

Galanin is a 29–amino acid peptide named after its N-terminal glycine and C-terminal *alanine* [243]. Galanin is widely distributed in the respiratory tract innervation of several species. It is colocalized with VIP in cholinergic nerves of airways and is present in parasympathetic ganglia [56, 69]. It is also colocalized with substance P and CGRP in sensory nerves and dorsal root, nodose, and trigeminal ganglia [295]. Galanin has no direct effect on airway tone in guinea pigs, but modulates e-NANC neurotransmission [107]. It has no effect on airway blood flow in dogs [250], and its physiologic role in airways remains a mystery.

Enkephalins

Leucine-enkephalin has been localized to neuroendocrine cells in airways [64], and [met]enkephalin-Arg[6]-Gly[7]-Leu[8]–immunoreactive nerves have been demonstrated in guinea pig and rat lungs [106, 131], with a distribution similar to that for VIP [263]. The anatomic origins and functional roles of the endogenous opioids are not clear since the opioid antagonist naloxone has no effect on neurally mediated airway effects [29, 32]. However, it is possible that these opioid pathways may be selectively activated from brain stem centers under certain conditions. Exogenous opioids potently modulate the neuropeptide release from sensory nerves in airways [29, 32, 93] via mu-opioid receptors, and may also modulate cholinergic neurotransmission via mu- or delta-opioid receptors [244].

ROLE OF NEUROPEPTIDES IN ASTHMA

The presence of so many neuropeptides in the respiratory tract raises questions about their physiologic role. It is now appreci-ated that many of these peptides are cotransmitters in classic autonomic nerves and may be regarded as modulators of autonomic effects, perhaps acting to fine-tune airway functions [20] and to modulate the release of other neurotransmitters [22]. Although much of the research on neuropeptides in the airways previously concentrated on their effects on airway smooth muscle [18], it is now clear that the most potent effects of many of the relevant peptides are on airway vasculature and secretions, and that neuropeptides may have an important role in regulating the mucosal surface of the airways. The lack of understanding of the physiologic role of individual peptides is largely due to the lack of specific antagonists that can be given safely to humans, but rapid advances in peptide chemistry are making the discovery of such antagonists possible, and recently nonpeptide antagonists have been developed [268, 306a].

Whether neuropeptides contribute to the pathophysiology of asthma has not yet been elucidated, although there are indications that increased effects of some peptides or defective function of other peptides may affect the inflammatory process and symptoms [17, 28].

VIP appears to act as an antiinflammatory peptide in general, as it acts as an antioxidant [247], inhibits mucus glycoprotein secretion from human airways [62], and inhibits mediator release from mast cells [299]. VIP is also a potent bronchodilator of proximal airways and may mediate part of the i-NANC response. Thus, if VIP is more rapidly degraded in asthma by the action of enzymes such as tryptase released from mast cells, then inflammatory effects and bronchoconstriction may be exaggerated. Indeed, a complete absence of VIP-immunoreactive nerves in the lungs of patients with severe asthma supports this possibility [215], although it is likely that this reflects the breakdown of VIP seen in histologic sections by the action of mast cell tryptase [19]. The distribution and density of VIP receptors appear to be normal in asthmatic airways [259]. Although VIP is an effective bronchodilator in vitro, it has little or no effect on airway caliber in humans, probably because of degradation by the action of NEP and in asthmatic patients by tryptase in the airways. It is therefore unlikely that VIP or even more stable analogs would have any therapeutic value in asthma.

There has been considerable interest in the possibility that sensory neuropeptides may contribute to the inflammatory response in asthmatic airways, but to date there is little direct evidence for this. Tachykinin-immunoreactive nerves are rather sparse in human airways, although it is possible that these nerves may be proliferated or sensitized or may show increased neuropeptide expression in patients with severe asthma. It is also possible that the degradation of tachykinins may be impaired in asthma due to functional defects in NEP or other degradative enzymes. An understanding of the role of sensory neuropeptides in asthma may depend on the development of specific receptor antagonists or strategies to inhibit peptide release from these nerves [24]. It is possible that neurogenic inflammation may only be relevant in certain types of asthma or in asthma of a certain degree of severity. This does point toward a need for more research on the distribution and effects of endogenous neuropeptides in the asthmatic patient, rather than reliance on animal models in which the importance of these neural mechanisms may be overemphasized.

In conclusion, many neuropeptides have been localized to the respiratory tract, and almost certainly more will be discovered. These peptides often have potent actions on airway and vascular tone and on lung secretions, but the presence of so many peptides raises questions about their physiologic role. Unique combinations of peptides are colocalized and coreleased from the various subpopulations of sensory, parasympathetic, and sympathetic nerve fibers. The neuropeptides may produce synergistic and/or antagonist events at both presynaptic and postsynaptic neurons, and on any surrounding target cells that possess the appropriate spectrum of peptide receptors. In this way, neuropeptides may act as subtle regulators of tissue activities under physiologic conditions. However, in inflammatory diseases such as asthma, they may have important pathogenetic roles. Alterations of degrading enzymes such as NEP may result in unopposed actions of proinflammatory neuropeptides. Until specific antagonists have been developed, it will be difficult to evaluate the precise roles of each of the neuropeptides in disease. It is certainly possible that pharmacologic agents which interact with neuropeptides by affecting their release, metabolism, or receptors may be developed in the future, with therapeutic potential.

REFERENCES

1. Advenier, C., et al. Relative potencies of neurokinins in guinea pig and human bronchus. *Eur. J. Pharmacol.* 139:133, 1987.
2. Aguayro, S. M., et al. Increased levels of bombesin-like peptides in the lower respiratory tract of asymptomatic smokers. *J. Clin. Invest.* 84:1105, 1989.
3. Ali, H., et al. Comparison of histamine releasing activity of substance P on mast cells and basophils from different species and tissues. *Int. Arch. Allergy Appl. Immunol.* 79:121, 1986.
4. Altiere, R. J., Szarek, J. L., and Diamond, L. Neurally mediated nonadrenergic relaxation in cat airways occurs independent of cholinergic mechanisms. *J. Pharmacol. Exp. Ther.* 234:590, 1985.
5. Alving, K., et al. Allergen challenge induces vasodilation in pig bronchial circulation via a capsaicin sensitive mechanism. *Acta Physiol. Scand.* 134:571, 1988.
6. Amman, R., and Lembeck, F. Ruthenium red selectively prevents capsaicin induced nociceptor stimulation. *Eur. J. Pharmacol.* 161:227, 1989.
7. Andersson, R. G., and Grundstrom, N. The excitatory noncholinergic, nonadrenergic nervous system of the guinea-pig airways. *Eur. J. Respir. Dis.* 131(Suppl.):141, 1983.
8. Baraniuk, J. N., et al. Neuropeptide Y (NPY) in human nasal mucosa. *Am. J. Respir. Cell. Mol. Biol.* 3:165, 1990.
9. Baraniuk, J. N., et al. Gastrin releasing peptide (GRP) in human nasal mucosa. *J. Clin. Invest.* 85:998, 1990.
10. Barlinski, J., Riquet, M., and Frossard, N. Electrically-induced non-adrenergic non-cholinergic contraction in human bronchial strips in vitro. *Am. Rev. Respir. Dis.* 141:A664, 1990.
11. Barnes, P. J. The third nervous system in the lung: Physiology and clinical perspectives. *Thorax* 39:561, 1984.
12. Barnes, P. J. Asthma as an axon reflex. *Lancet* 1:242, 1986.
13. Barnes, P. J. Nonadrenergic, noncholinergic neural control of human airways. *Arch. Int. Pharmacodyn. Ther.* 280:208, 1986.
14. Barnes, P. J. Neuropeptides in human airways: Function and clinical implications. *Am. Rev. Respir. Dis.* 136:S77, 1987.
15. Barnes, P. J. Neuropeptides in the lung: Localization, function and pathophysiological implications. *J. Allergy Clin. Immunol.* 79:285, 1987.
16. Barnes, P. J. Vasoactive Intestinal Peptide and Pulmonary Function. In M. A. Hollinger (ed.), *Current Topics in Pulmonary Pharmacology and Toxicology.* New York: Elsevier, 1987. Pp. 156–173.
17. Barnes, P. J. Neuropeptides and asthma. *Am. Rev. Respir. Dis.* 143:S28, 1991.
18. Barnes, P. J. Neuropeptide and airway smooth muscle. *Pharmacol. Ther.* 36:119, 1988.
19. Barnes, P. J. Vasoactive intestinal peptide and asthma. *N. Engl. J. Med.* 321:1128, 1989.
20. Barnes, P. J. Airway neuropeptides: Roles in fine tuning and in disease. *News Physiol. Sci.* 4:116, 1989.
21. Barnes, P. J. Neurogenic inflammation in airways and its modulation. *Arch. Int. Pharmacodyn. Ther.* 303:67, 1990.
22. Barnes, P. J. Neuromodulation in the airways. *Physiol. Rev.* 72:699, 1992.
22a. Barnes, P. J. Sensory nerves, neuropeptides and asthma. *Ann. N. Y. Acad. Sci.* 629:193, 1991.
23. Barnes, P. J., Baraniuk, J., and Belvisi, M. G. Neuropeptides in the respiratory tract. *Am. Rev. Respir. Dis.* 144:1187 (Part I) and 1391 (Part II), 1991.
24. Barnes, P. J., Belvisi, M. G., and Rogers, D. F. Modulation of neurogenic inflammation: Novel approaches to inflammatory diseases. *Trends Pharmacol. Sci.* 11:185, 1990.
25. Barnes, P. J., et al. Histamine is released from skin by substance P but does not act as the final vasodilator in axon reflex. *Br. J. Pharmacol.* 88:741, 1986.
26. Barnes, P. J., et al. Vasoactive intestinal peptide in bovine pulmonary

artery: Localisation, function and receptor autoradiography. *Br. J. Pharmacol.* 89:157, 1986.
27. Barnes, P. J., and Dixon, C. M. S. The effect of inhaled vasoactive intestinal peptide on bronchial reactivity to histamine in man. *Am. Rev. Respir. Dis.* 130:162, 1984.
28. Barnes, P. J., and Lundberg, J. M. Airway Neuropeptides and Asthma. In M. Kaliner, P. J. Barnes, and C. G. A. Persson (eds.), *Asthma: Its Pathology and Treatment.* New York: Marcel Dekker, 1991. Pp. 385–408.
29. Belvisi, M. G., et al. Opioid modulation of non-cholinergic neural bronchoconstriction in guinea-pig in *in vivo. Br. J. Pharmacol.* 95:413, 1988.
30. Belvisi, M. G., Ichinose, M., and Barnes, P. J. Modulation of non-adrenergic non-cholinergic neural bronchoconstriction in guinea-pig airways via GABA-β receptors. *Br. J. Pharmacol.* 97:1125, 1989.
31. Belvisi, M. G., et al. Endogenous vasoactive intestinal peptide and nitric oxide modulate cholinergic neurotransmission in guinea pig trachea. *Eur. J. Pharmacol.* In press.
32. Belvisi, M. G., Rogers, D. F., and Barnes, P. J. Neurogenic plasma extravasation: Inhibition by morphine in guinea pig airways in *vivo. J. Appl. Physiol.* 66:268, 1989.
33. Belvisi, M. G., Stretton, C. D., and Barnes, P. J. Modulation of cholinergic neurotransmission in guinea-pig airways by opioids. *Br. J. Pharmacol.* 100:131, 1990.
34. Belvisi, M. G., Stretton, C. D., and Barnes, P. J. Nitric oxide is the endogenous neurotransmitter of bronchodilator nerves in human airways. *Eur. J. Pharmacol.* 210:221, 1992.
35. Belvisi, M. G., Stretton, C. D., and Barnes, P. J. Bombesin-induced bronchoconstriction in the guinea pig: Mode of action. *J. Pharmacol. Exp. Ther.* 258:36, 1991.
35a. Belvisi, M. G., Stretton, C. D., and Barnes, P. J. Nitric oxide is an endogenous modulator of cholinergic neurotransmission in guinea pig airways. *Eur. J. Pharmacol.* 198:219, 1991.
35b. Belvisi, M. G., et al. Inhibitory NANC nerves in human tracheal smooth muscle: A quest for the neurotransmitter. *J. Appl. Physiol.* In press.
36. Bienenstock, J., et al. Inflammatory cells and epithelium: Mast cell/nerve interactions in lung in vitro and in vivo. *Am. Rev. Respir. Dis.* 138:S31, 1988.
37. Black, J. L., et al. Neurokinin A with K^+ channel blockade potentiates contraction to electrical stimulation in human bronchus. *Eur. J. Pharmacol.* 180:311, 1990.
38. Black, J. L., Johnson, P. R. A., and Armour, C. L. Potentiation of the contractile effects of neuropeptides in human bronchus by an enkephalinase inhibitor. *Pulm. Pharmacol.* 1:21, 1988.
39. Borson, D. B., et al. Neural regulation of $^{35}SO_4$-macromolecule secretion from glands of ferrets. *J. Appl. Physiol.* 57:457, 1984.
40. Borson, D. B., et al. Enkephalinase inhibitors potentiate substance P-induced secretion of 35S-macromolecules from ferret trachea. *Exp. Lung Res.* 12:21, 1987.
41. Borson, D. B., Jew, S., and Gruenert, D. C. Glucocorticoids induce neutral endopeptidase in transformed human trachea epithelial cells. *Am. J. Physiol.* 260:L83, 1991.
42. Brain, S. D., and Williams, T. J. Inflammatory oedema induced by synergism between calcitonin gene-related peptide (CGRP) and mediators of increased vascular permeability. *Br. J. Pharmacol.* 86:855, 1985.
43. Brain, S. D., et al. Calcitonin gene related peptide is a potent vasodilator. *Nature* 313:54, 1985.
44. Bredt, D. S., Hwang, P. M., and Snyder, S. H. Localization of nitric oxide synthase indicating a neural role for nitric oxide. *Nature* 347:768, 1990.
45. Brunelleschi, S., et al. Tachykinins activate guinea pig alveolar macrophages: Involvement of NK_2 and NK_1 receptors. *Br. J. Pharmacol.* 100:417, 1990.
46. Buckley, T. L., Brain, S. L., and Williams, T. J. Ruthenium red selectively inhibits oedema formation and increased blood flow induced by capsaicin in rabbit skin. *Br. J. Pharmacol.* 99:7, 1990.
47. Bult, H., et al. Nitric oxide as an inhibitory non-adrenergic non-cholinergic neurotransmitter. *Nature* 345:346, 1990.
48. Bungaard, A., Enehjelm, S. D., and Aggestrop, S. Pretreatment of exercise-induced asthma with inhaled vasoactive intestinal peptide. *Eur. J. Respir. Dis.* 64:427, 1983.
49. Cadieux, A., et al. Bronchoconstrictive action of neuropeptide Y (NPY) on isolated guinea pig airways. *Neuropeptides* 13:215, 1989.
50. Cadieux, A., et al. Occurrence, distribution and ontogeny of CGRP-immunoreactivity in the rat lower respiratory tract: Effect of capsaicin treatment on surgical denervation. *Neuroscience* 19:605, 1986.
51. Cameron, A. R., et al. Search for the inhibitory neurotransmitter in bovine tracheal smooth muscle. *Q. J. Exp. Physiol.* 68:413, 1983.

52. Carstairs, J. R., and Barnes, P. J. Visualization of vasoactive intestinal peptide receptors in human and guinea pig lung. *J. Pharmacol. Exp. Ther.* 239:249, 1986.

53. Carstairs, J. R., and Barnes, P. J. Autoradiographic mapping of substance P receptors in lung. *Eur. J. Pharmacol.* 127:295, 1986.

54. Caughey, G. H. Roles of mast cell tryptase and chymase in airway function. *Am. J. Physiol.* 257:L39, 1989.

55. Caughey, G. H., et al. Substance P and vasoactive intestinal peptide degradation by mast cell tryptase and chymase. *J. Pharmacol. Exp. Ther.* 244: 133, 1988.

56. Cheung, A., et al. The distribution of galanin immunoreactivity in the respiratory tract of pig, guinea pig, rat, and dog. *Thorax* 40:889, 1985.

56a. Cheung, D., et al. An effect of an inhaled neutral endopeptidase inhibitor, thiorphan, on airway responses to neurokinin A in normal humans in vivo. *Am. Rev. Respir. Dis.* 145:1275, 1992.

57. Chilvers, E. R., et al. Effect of peptide histidine valine on cardiovascular and respiratory function in normal subjects. *Thorax* 43:750, 1988.

58. Choi, H.-S. H., et al. Immunohistochemical localization of endopeptidase 24.15 in rat trachea, lung tissue and alveolar macrophages. *Am. J. Respir. Cell Mol. Biol.* 3:619, 1990.

59. Christie, M. J., and North, R. A. Agonists at μ-opioid, M_2-muscarinic, and $GABA_B$-receptors increase the ionic potassium conductance in rat lateral paratracheal nerves. *Br. J. Pharmacol.* 95:896, 1988.

60. Christofides, N. O., et al. Distribution of peptide histidine isoleucine in the mammalian respiratory tract and some aspects of its pharmacology. Endocrinology 115:1958, 1984.

61. Coles, S. J., Neill, K. H., and Reid, L. M. Potent stimulation of glycoprotein secretion in canine trachea by substance P. *J. Appl. Physiol.* 57:1323, 1984.

62. Coles, S. J., Said, S. I., and Reid, L. M. Inhibition by vasoactive intestinal peptide of glycoconjugate and lysozyme secretion by human airways in vitro. *Am. Rev. Respir. Dis.* 124:531, 1981.

63. Cuittitta, F., et al. Gastrin releasing peptide gene associated peptides are expressed in normal human fetal lung and small cell lung cancer: A novel peptide family in man. *J. Clin. Endocrinol. Metab.* 67:576, 1988.

64. Cutz, E. Neuroendocrine cells of the lung—An overview of morphological characteristics and development. *Exp. Lung Res.* 3:185, 1982.

64a. Daniels, R. P., et al. Neuroimmune interactions in the lung. *Am. Rev. Respir. Dis.* 145:1230, 1992.

65. Dennis, T., et al. Structure activity profile of calcitonin gene-related peptide in peripheral and brain tissues. Evidence for receptor multiplicity. *J. Pharmacol. Exp. Ther.* 251:718, 1989.

66. Devillier, P., et al. Respiratory epithelium releases relaxant prostaglandin E2 through activation of substance P (NK1) receptors. *Am. Rev. Respir. Dis.* 139:A351, 1991.

67. Devillier, P., et al. Comparison of the effects of epithelium removal and of an enkephalinase inhibitor on the neurokinin-induced contractions of guinea pig isolated trachea. *Br. J. Pharmacol.* 94:675, 1988.

68. Dey, R. D., Hoffpauir, J., and Said, S. I. Colocalization of vasoactive intestinal peptide in substance P containing nerves in cat bronchi. *Neuroscience* 24:275, 1988.

69. Dey, R. D., Mitchell, H. W., and Coburn, R. F. Organization and development of peptide-containing neurons in the airways. *Am. J. Respir. Cell Mol. Biol.* 3:187, 1990.

70. Dey, R. D., Shannon, W. A., and Said, S. I. Localization of VIP-immunoreactive nerves in airways and pulmonary vessels of dogs, cats and human subjects. *Cell Tissue Res.* 220:231, 1981.

71. Diamond, L., and O'Donnell, M. A nonadrenergic vagal inhibitory pathway to feline airways. *Science* 208:185, 1980.

72. Diamond, L., et al. *In vivo* bronchodilatory activity of vasoactive intestinal peptide in the cat. *Am. Rev. Respir. Dis.* 128:827, 1991.

73. Dixon, C. M. S., and Barnes, P. J. Bradykinin induced bronchoconstriction: Inhibition by nedocromil sodium and sodium cromoglycate. *Br. J. Clin. Pharmacol.* 27:831, 1989.

74. Dixon, C. M. S., Fuller, R. W., and Barnes, P. J. The effect of nedocromil sodium on sulphur dioxide induced bronchoconstriction. *Thorax* 42:462, 1987.

75. Dixon, N., Jackson, D. M., and Richards, I. M. The effect of sodium cromoglycate on lung irritant receptors and left ventricular receptors in anesthetized dogs. *Br. J. Pharmacol.* 67:569, 1979.

76. Djokic, T. D., et al. Inhibitors of neutral endopeptidase potentiate electrically and capsaicin-induced non-cholinergic contraction in guinea pig bronchi. *J. Pharmacol. Exp. Ther.* 248:7, 1989.

77. Dusser, D. J., et al. Cigarette smoke induces bronchoconstrictor hyperresponsiveness to substance P and inactivates airway neutral endopeptidase in the guinea pig lung. Possible role of free radicals. *J. Clin. Invest.* 84:900, 1989.

78. Dusser, D. J., et al. Airway neutral endopeptidase-like enzyme modulates tachykinin-induced bronchoconstriction in vivo. *J. Appl. Physiol.* 65: 2585, 1988.

79. Ellis, J. L., and Farmer, S. G. Effects of peptidases on nonadrenergic, noncholinergic inhibitory responses of tracheal smooth muscle: A comparison with effects on VIP- and PHI-induced relaxation. *Br. J. Pharmacol.* 96:521, 1989.

80. Ellis, J. L., and Farmer, S. G. The effects of vasoactive intestinal peptide (VIP) antagonists, and VIP and peptide histidine isoleucine antisera on nonadrenergic, noncholinergic relaxations of tracheal smooth muscle. *Br. J. Pharmacol.* 96:513, 1989.

81. Ellis, J. L., and Farmer, S. G. Modulation of cholinergic neurotransmission by vasoactive intestinal peptide and peptide histidine isoleucine in guinea pig tracheal smooth muscle. *Pulm. Pharmacol.* 2:107, 1989.

82. Elwood, W., et al. Loop diuretics inhibit cholinergic and non-cholinergic nerves in guinea pig airways. *Am. Rev. Respir. Dis.* 143:1340, 1991.

83. Evans, T. W., et al. Comparison of neurokinin A and substance P on cardiovascular and airway function in man. *Br. J. Pharmacol.* 25:273, 1988.

84. Evans, T. W., et al. Regional and time-dependent effects of inflammatory mediators on airway microvascular permeability in guinea pigs. *Clin. Sci.* 76:479, 1989.

85. Farmer, S. G., and Togo, J. Effects of epithelium removal on relaxation of airway smooth muscle induced by vasoactive intestinal peptide and electrical field stimulation. *Br. J. Pharmacol.* 100:73, 1990.

86. Fine, J. M., Gordon, T., and Sheppard, D. Epithelium removal alters responsiveness of guinea pig trachea to substance P. *J. Appl. Physiol.* 66: 232, 1989.

87. Finney, M. J. B., Karlson, J. A., and Persson, C. G. A. Effects of bronchoconstriction and bronchodilation on a novel human small airway preparation. *Br. J. Pharmacol.* 85:29, 1985.

88. Foda, H. D., Higuchi, J., and Said, S. I. Helodermin, a VIP-like peptide, is a potent long-acting pulmonary vasodilator. *Am. Rev. Respir. Dis.* 141: A486, 1990.

89. Foda, H. D., et al. Vasoactive intestinal peptide protects against HCl-induced pulmonary edema in rats. *Ann. NY Acad. Sci.* 527:633, 1988.

90. Foreman, J. C., et al. Structure-activity relationships for some substance P-related peptides that cause wheal and flare reactions in human skin. *J. Physiol. (Lond.)* 335:449, 1983.

91. Franconi, G., et al. Mast cell tryptase and chymase reverse airway smooth muscle relaxation induced by vasoactive intestinal peptide in ferret. *J. Pharmacol. Exp. Ther.* 248:947, 1989.

92. Frandsen, E. K., Krishina, G. A., and Said, S. I. Vasoactive intestinal polypeptide promotes cyclic adenosine 3',5' monophosphate accumulation in guinea pig trachea. *Br. J. Pharmacol.* 62:367, 1978.

93. Frossard, N., and Barnes, P. J. μ-Opioid receptors modulate non-cholinergic constrictor nerves in guinea-pig airways. *Eur. J. Pharmacol.* 141: 519, 1987.

94. Frossard, N., and Barnes, P. J. Effects of tachykinins on small human airways and the influence of thiorphan. *Am. Rev. Respir. Dis.* 137:195A, 1988.

95. Frossard, N., Rhoden, K. J., and Barnes, P. J. Influence of epithelium on guinea pig airway responses to tachykinins: Role of endopeptidase and cyclooxygenase. *J. Pharmacol. Exp. Ther.* 248:292, 1989.

96. Fuller, R. W., et al. Sensory neuropeptide effects in human skin. *Br. J. Pharmacol.* 92:781, 1987.

97. Fuller, R. W., et al. Bradykinin-induced bronchoconstriction in man: Mode of action. *Am. Rev. Respir. Dis.* 135:176, 1987.

98. Fuller, R. W., et al. The effects of substance P on cardiovascular and respiratory function in human subjects. *J. Appl. Physiol.* 62:1473, 1987.

99. Gamse, R., and Saria, A. Potentiation of tachykinin-induced plasma protein extravasation by calcitonin gene-related peptide. *Eur. J. Pharmacol.* 114:61, 1985.

100. Gashi, A. A., et al. Neuropeptides degranulate serous cells of ferret tracheal glands. *Am. J. Physiol.* 251:C223, 1986.

101. Geppetti, P., et al. Secretion, pain, and sneezing with and without allergic rhinitis. *Br. J. Pharmacol.* 93:509, 1988.

102. Geppetti, P., et al. Age related changes in vasoactive intestinal peptide levels and distribution in rat lung. *J. Neural Transm.* 74:1, 1988.

103. Geppetti, P., Maggi, C. A., and Perretti, F. Simultaneous release by bradykinin of substance P and calcitonin gene related peptide immunoreactivities from capsaicin-sensitive guinea pig heart. *Br. J. Pharmacol.* 94:288, 1988.

104. Ghatei, M. A., et al. Regulatory peptides in the mammalian respiratory tract. *Endocrinology* 111:1248, 1982.

105. Ghatei, M. A., et al. Bombesin and vasoactive intestinal peptide in the developing lung: Marked changes in acute respiratory distress syndrome. *J. Clin. Endocrinol. Metab.* 57:1226, 1983.

106. Gibbins, I. L., Furness, J. B., and Costa, M. Pathway specific patterns of coexistence of substance P, calcitonin gene related peptide, cholecystokinin, and dynorphin in neurons of the dorsal root ganglion of the guinea pig. *Cell Tissue Res.* 248:417, 1987.

107. Guiliani, S., et al. Modulatory action of galanin on responses due to antidromic activation of peripheral terminals of capsaicin-sensitive sensory nerves. *Eur. J. Pharmacol.* 163:91, 1989.

108. Gottschall, P. E., et al. Characterization and distribution of binding sites for the hypothalamic peptide pituitary adenylate cyclase activating polypeptide. *Endocrinology* 127:272, 1990.

109. Grandordy, B. M., et al. Tachykinin-induced phosphoinositide breakdown in airway smooth muscle and epithelium: Relationship to contraction. *Mol. Pharmacol.* 33:515, 1988.

110. Greenberg, B., Rhoden, K., and Barnes, P. J. Relaxant effects of vasoactive intestinal peptide and peptide histidine isoleucine in human and bovine pulmonary arteries. *Blood Vessels* 24:45, 1987.

111. Grundstrom, N., and Andersson, R. G. G. In vivo demonstration of α_2-adrenoceptor mediated inhibition of the excitatory non-cholinergic neurotransmission in guinea pig airways. *Naunyn Schmiedebergs Arch. Pharmacol.* 328:236, 1985.

112. Haggermark, O., Hokfelt, T., and Pernow, B. Flare and itch induced by substance P in human skin. *J. Invest. Dermatol.* 71:233, 1978.

113. Hall, A. K., et al. Facilitation of tachykinins of neurotransmission in guinea-pig pulmonary parasympathetic nerves. *Br. J. Pharmacol.* 97:274, 1989.

114. Hamid, Q., et al. Localization of β-pre-protachykinin mRNA in nodose ganglion of the rat. *Neuropeptides* 20:145, 1991.

115. Harmar, A. J., Hyde, V., and Chapman, K. Identification and cDNA sequence of δ-preprotachykinin, a fourth splicing variant of the rat substance P precursor. *FEBS Lett.* 275:22, 1990.

116. Haynes, L. W., and Manley, C. Chemotactic response of guinea pig polymorphonucleocytes in vivo to rat calcitonin gene related peptide and proteolytic fragments. *J. Physiol. (Lond.)* 43:79P, 1988.

117. Helke, C. J., et al. Diversity in mammalian tachykinin peptidergic neurons: Multiple peptides, receptors, and regulatory mechanisms. *FASEB J.* 4:1606, 1990.

118. Holzer, P. Local effector functions of capsaicin-sensitive sensory nerve endings: Involvement of tachykinins, calcitonin gene related peptide, and other neuropeptides. *Neuroscience* 24:739, 1988.

119. Howarth, P. H., et al. Neuropeptide containing nerves in human airways in vivo: A comparative study of atopic asthma, atopic non-asthma and non-atopic non-asthma (abstract). *Thorax* 45:786, 1990.

120. Ichinose, M., and Barnes, P. J. Histamine H_3-receptors modulate nonadrenergic non-cholinergic bronchoconstriction in guinea pig *in vivo*. *Eur. J. Pharmacol.* 174:49, 1989.

121. Ichinose, M., and Barnes, P. J. A potassium channel activator modulates both noncholinergic and cholinergic neurotransmission in guinea pig airways. *J. Pharmacol. Exp. Ther.* 252:1207, 1990.

122. Ichinose, M., Belvisi, M. G., and Barnes, P. J. Bradykinin-induced bronchoconstriction in guinea-pig *in vivo*: Role of neural mechanisms. *J. Pharmacol. Exp. Ther.* 253:1207, 1990.

123. Ichinose, M., Belvisi, M. G., and Barnes, P. J. Histamine H_3-receptors inhibit neurogenic microvascular leakage in airways. *J. Appl. Physiol.* 68:21, 1990.

124. Ichinose, M., et al. Possible sensory receptor of non-adrenergic inhibitory nervous system. *J. Appl. Physiol.* 63:923, 1987.

125. Impicciatore, M., and Bertaccini, G. The bronchoconstrictor action of the tetradecapeptide bombesin in the guinea pig. *J. Pharm. Pharmacol.* 25:812, 1973.

126. Irvin, C. G., et al. Bronchodilatation: Noncholinergic, nonadrenergic mediation demonstrated in vivo in the cat. *Science* 207:791, 1980.

127. Irvin, C. G., Martin, R. R., and Macklem, P. T. Nonpurinergic nature and efficacy of nonadrenergic bronchodilatation. *J. Appl. Physiol.* 52:562, 1982.

128. Ito, Y., and Takeda, K. Nonadrenergic inhibitory nerves and putative transmitters in the smooth muscle of cat trachea. *J. Physiol. (Lond.)* 330:497, 1982.

129. Jackson, D. M., Norris, A. A., and Eady, R. P. Nedocromil sodium and sensory nerves in the dog lung. *Pulm. Pharmacol.* 2:179, 1989.

130. Jacoby, D. B., et al. Influenza infection increases airway smooth muscle

131. Jancso, G., et al. Immunohistochemical studies on the effect of capsaicin on spinal and medullary peptide and monoamine neurons using antisera to substance P, gastrin/CCK, somatostatin, VIP, enkephalin, neurotensin, and 5-hydroxytryptamine. *J. Neurocytol.* 10:963, 1981.

132. Jessel, T. M., and Iversen, L. L. Opiate analgesics inhibit substance P release from rat trigeminal nucleus. *Nature* 268:549, 1977.

133. Joos, G., Pauwels, R., and van der Straeten, M. E. Effect of inhaled substance P and neurokinin A in the airways of normal and asthmatic subjects. *Thorax* 42:779, 1987.

134. Joos, G. F., Pauwels, R. A., and van der Straeten, M. E. Mechanisms of tachykinin-induced bronchoconstriction. *Am. Rev. Respir. Dis.* 137:1038, 1988.

135. Joos, G. F., Pauwels, R. A., and van der Straeten, M. E. The effect of nedocromil sodium on the bronchoconstrictor effect of neurokinin A in subjects with asthma. *J. Allergy Clin. Immunol.* 83:663, 1989.

136. Kamikawa, Y., and Shimo, Y. Adenosine selectively inhibits noncholinergic transmission in guinea pig bronchi. *J. Appl. Physiol.* 66:2084, 1991.

137. Karlsson, J. A., and Persson, C. G. A. Neither vasoactive intestinal peptide (VIP) nor purine derivatives may mediate nonadrenergic tracheal inhibition. *Acta Physiol. Scand.* 122:589, 1984.

138. Kaufman, M. P., et al. Bradykinin stimulates afferent vagal C-fibres in intrapulmonary airways of dogs. *J. Appl. Physiol.* 48:511, 1980.

139. Khalil, Z., Andrews, P. V., and Helme, R. D. VIP modulates substance P induced plasma extravasation in vivo. *Eur. J. Pharmacol.* 151:281, 1988.

140. Kohrogi, H., et al. Recombinant human enkephalinase (neutral endopeptidase) prevents cough induced by tachykinins in awake guinea pigs. *J. Clin. Invest.* 84:781, 1989.

141. Kroegel, C., Giembycz, M. A., and Barnes, P. J. Characterization of eosinophil activation by peptides. Differential effects of substance P, mellitin, and f-met-leu-phe. *J. Immunol.* 145:2581, 1990.

142. Kuo, H.-P., et al. Cigarette smoke induced goblet cell secretion: Neural involvement in guinea pig trachea. *Eur. Respir. J.* 3:1895, 1990.

143. Kuo, H.-P., et al. Capsaicin and sensory neuropeptide stimulation of goblet cell secretion in guinea pig trachea. *J. Physiol. (Lond.)* 431:629, 1990.

144. Kuo, H.-P., et al. Morphine inhibition of cigarette smoke induced goblet cell secretion in guinea pig trachea in vivo. *Respir. Med.* 84:425, 1990.

145. Lacroix, J. S. Adrenergic and non-adrenergic mechanisms in sympathetic vascular control of the nasal mucosa. *Acta Physiol. Scand.* Suppl. 581:1, 1989.

146. Laitinen, A., et al. Electron microscopic study on the innervation of human lower respiratory tract. *Eur. J. Respir. Dis.* 67:209, 1985.

147. Laitinen, A., et al. VIP-like immunoreactive nerves in human respiratory tract. Light and electron microscopic study. *Histochemistry* 82:313, 1985.

148. Laitinen, L. A., et al. Damage of the airway epithelium and bronchial respiratory tract in patients with asthma. *Am. Rev. Respir. Dis.* 131:599, 1985.

149. Laitinen, L. A., et al. Vascular actions of airway neuropeptides. *Am. Rev. Respir. Dis.* 136:559, 1987.

149a. Lammers, J.-W. J., Barnes, P. J., and Churg, K. E. Nonadrenergic noncholinergic airway inhibitory nerves. *Eur. Respir. J.* 5:239, 1992.

150. Lammers, J.-W. J., et al. Capsaicin-induced bronchodilatation in mild asthmatic subjects: Possible role of nonadrenergic inhibitory system. *J. Appl. Physiol.* 67:856, 1989.

151. Lammers, J.-W. J., et al. Nonadrenergic bronchodilator mechanisms in normal human subjects in vivo. *J. Appl. Physiol.* 64:1817, 1988.

152. Lazarus, S. C., et al. Mapping of VIP receptors by use of an immunocytochemical probe for the intracellular mediator cyclic AMP. *Am. J. Physiol.* 251:C115, 1986.

153. Leff, A. R., et al. Augmentation of respiratory mast cell secretion of histamine caused by vagal nerve stimulation during antigen challenge. *J. Immunol.* 136:1066, 1982.

153a. Lei, Y.-H., Barnes, P. J., and Rogers, D. F. Inhibition of neurogenic plasma exudation in guinea pig airways by CP-96,345, a new nonpeptide NK_1-receptor antagonist. *Br. J. Pharmacol.* 105:261, 1992.

154. Lembeck, F., Donnerer, J., and Bartho, L. Inhibition of neurogenic vasodilation and plasma extravasation by substance P antagonists, somatostatin and [D-Met^2, Pro^5]-enkephalinamide. *Eur. J. Pharmacol.* 85:171, 1982.

155. Levine, J. D., et al. Contribution of sensory afferents and sympathetic efferents to joint injury in experimental arthritis. *J. Neurosci.* 6:3423, 1986.

156. Li, C. G., and Rand, M. J. Evidence that part of the NANC relaxant response

of guinea-pig trachea to electrical field stimulation is mediated by nitric oxide. *Br. J. Pharmacol.* 102:91, 1991.

157. Lindh, B., Lundberg, J. M., and Hokfelt, T. NPY-, galanin-, VIP/PHI-, CGRP- and substance P-immunoreactive neuronal populations in cat autonomic and sensory ganglia and their projections. *Cell Tissue Res.* 256:259, 1989.

158. Lindsay, R. M., and Harmar, A. J. Nerve growth factor regulates expression of neuropeptide genes in sensory neurons. *Nature* 337:362, 1989.

159. Lötvall, J. O., et al. Capsaicin pretreatment does not inhibit allergen-induced airway microvascular leakage in guinea pig. *Allergy* 46:105, 1991.

160. Lötvall, J. O., et al. Airflow obstruction after substance P aerosol: Contribution of airway and pulmonary edema. *J. Appl. Physiol.* 69:1473, 1990.

161. Lötvall, J. O., et al. Effects of aerosolized substance P on lung resistance in guinea pigs: A comparison between inhibition of neutral endopeptidase and angiotensin-converting enzyme. *Br. J. Pharmacol.* 100:69, 1990.

162. Lowman, M. A., Benyon, R. C., and Church, M. K. Characterization of neuropeptide-induced histamine release from human dispersed skin mast cells. *Br. J. Pharmacol.* 95:121, 1988.

163. Lotz, M., Vaughn, J. H., and Carson, D. M. Effect of neuropeptides on production of inflammatory cytokines by human monocytes. *Science* 241:1218, 1988.

164. Lundberg, J. M. Evidence for coexistence of vasoactive intestinal peptide (VIP) and acetylcholine in nerves of cat exocrine glands: Morphological, biochemical and functional studies. *Acta Physiol. Scand. Suppl.* 496:1, 1981.

164a. Lundberg, J. M., Fahrenberg, J., and Hokfelt, T. Coexistence of peptide HI (PHI) and VIP in nerves regulating blood flow and bronchial smooth muscle in various animals, including man. *Peptides* 5:593, 1984.

165. Lundberg, J. M., et al. Coexistence of substance P and calcitonin gene-related peptide-like immunoreactivities in sensory nerves in relation to cardiovascular and bronchoconstrictor effects of capsaicin. *Eur. J. Pharmacol.* 108:315, 1985.

166. Lundberg, J. M., Brodin, E., and Saria, A. Effects and distribution of vagal capsaicin-sensitive substance P neurons with special reference to the trachea and lungs. *Acta Physiol. Scand.* 119:243, 1983.

168. Lundberg, J. M., et al. Coexistence of peptide histidine isoleucine (PHI) and VIP in nerves regulating blood flow and bronchial smooth muscle tone in various mammals including man. *Peptides* 5:593, 1984.

169. Lundberg, J. M., et al. Substance P-immunoreactive sensory nerves in the lower respiratory tract of various mammals including man. *Cell Tissue Res.* 235:251, 1984.

170. Lundberg, J. M., Martling, C. R., and Saria, A. Substance P and capsaicin induced contraction of human bronchi. *Acta Physiol. Scand.* 119:49, 1983.

171. Lundberg, J. M., et al. A substance P antagonist inhibits vagally induced increase in vascular permeability and bronchial smooth muscle contraction in the guinea-pig. *Proc. Natl. Acad. Sci. USA* 80:1120, 1983.

172. Lundberg, J. M., and Saria, A. Capsaicin-induced desensitization of the airway mucosa to cigarette smoke, mechanical and chemical irritants. *Nature* 302:251, 1983.

173. Lundberg, J. M., et al. *Bioactive Peptides in Capsaicin-sensitive C-fiber Afferents of the Airways: Functional and Pathophysiological Implications.* New York: Marcel Dekker, 1987. P. 417.

174. Lundgren, J. D., et al. Gastrin releasing peptide stimulates glycoconjugate release from feline tracheal explants. *Am. J. Physiol.* 258:L68, 1990.

175. Lundgren, J. D., et al. Substance P receptor mediated secretion of respiratory glycoconjugate from feline airways in vitro. *Exp. Lung Res.* 15:17, 1989.

176. Luts, A., and Sundler, F. Peptide containing nerve fibres in the respiratory tract of the ferret. *Cell Tissue Res.* 258:259, 1989.

177. Luts, A., et al. PACAP, a new VIP-like peptide in the respiratory tract. *Cell Tissue Res.* In press.

178. Maggi, C. A., et al. Competitive antagonists discriminate between NK2 tachykinin receptor subtypes. *Br. J. Pharmacol.* 100:588, 1990.

179. Maggi, C. A., and Meli, A. The sensory efferent function of capsaicin sensitive sensory nerves. *Gen. Pharmacol.* 1:43, 1988.

180. Mak, J. C. M., and Barnes, P. J. Autoradiographic localization of calcitonin gene-related peptide binding sites in human and guinea pig lung. *Peptides* 9:957, 1988.

181. Martin, J. G., et al. The effects of vasoactive intestinal polypeptide on cholinergic neurotransmission in isolated innervated guinea pig tracheal preparations. *Respir. Physiol.* 79:111, 1990.

182. Martins, M. A., et al. Peptidase modulation of the pulmonary effects of tachykinins in tracheal superfused guinea pig lungs. *J. Clin. Invest.* 85:170, 1990.

183. Martling, C., et al. Capsaicin pretreatment inhibits vagal cholinergic and

184. Martling, C. R. Sensory nerves containing tachykinins and CGRP in the lower airways: Functional implications for bronchoconstriction, vasodilation, and protein extravasation. *Acta Physiol. Scand. Suppl.* 563:1, 1987.

185. Martling, C. R., et al. Calcitonin gene related peptide and the lung: Neuronal coexistence and vasodilatory effect. *Regul. Pept.* 20:125, 1988.

186. Martling, C. R., Theodorsson-Norheim, E., and Lundberg, J. M. Occurrence and effects of multiple tachykinins: Substance P, neurokinin A, and neuropeptide K in human lower airways. *Life Sci.* 40:1633, 1987.

187. Masu, Y., et al. cDNA cloning of bovine substance K receptor through oocyte expression system. *Nature* 329:836, 1987.

188. Matran, R., et al. Vagally mediated vasodilatation by motor and sensory nerves in the tracheal and bronchial circulation of the pig. *Acta Physiol. Scand.* 135:29, 1989.

189. Matran, R., et al. Effects of neuropeptides and capsaicin on tracheobronchial blood flow in the pig. *Acta Physiol. Scand.* 135:335, 1989.

190. Matran, R., Martling, C.-R., and Lundberg, J. M. Inhibition of cholinergic and nonadrenergic, noncholinergic bronchoconstriction in the guinea-pig mediated by neuropeptide Y and alpha$_2$-adrenoceptors and opiate receptors. *Eur. J. Pharmacol.* 163:15, 1989.

191. Matsuda, H., et al. Substance P induces granulocyte infiltration through degranulation of mast cells. *J. Immunol.* 142:927, 1989.

192. Matsuse, T., et al. Capsaicin inhibits airway hyperresponsiveness, but not airway lipoxygenase activity nor eosinophilia following repeated aerosolized antigen in guinea pigs. *Am. Rev. Respir. Dis.* 144:368, 1991.

193. Matsuzaki, Y., Hamasaki, Y., and Said, S. I. Vasoactive intestinal peptide: A possible transmitter of nonadrenergic relaxation of guinea pig airways. *Science* 210:1252, 1980.

194. McAlpine, L. G., and Thomson, N. C. Lidocaine-induced bronchoconstriction in asthmatic patients. Relation to histamine airway responsiveness and effect of preservative. *Chest* 96:1012, 1989.

195. McCormack, D. G., et al. Calcitonin gene-related peptide vasodilation of human pulmonary vessels: Receptor mapping and functional studies. *J. Appl. Physiol.* 67:1265, 1989.

196. McCormack, D. G., Salonen, R. O., and Barnes, P. J. Effect of sensory neuropeptides on canine bronchial and pulmonary vessels *in vitro. Life Sci.* 45:2405, 1989.

197. McDonald, D. M. Neurogenic inflammation in the respiratory tract: Actions of sensory nerve mediators on blood vessels and epithelium of the airway mucosa. *Am. Rev. Respir. Dis.* 136:S65, 1987.

198. McDonald, D. M. Respiratory tract infections increase susceptibility to neurogenic inflammation in the rat trachea. *Am. Rev. Respir. Dis.* 137:1432, 1988.

199. McGillis, J. P., Organist, M. L., and Payan, D. G. Substance P and immunoregulation. *Fed. Proc.* 14:120, 1987.

200. McKnight, A. T., et al. Characterization of receptors for tachykinins using selectivity of agonists and antagonists: Evidence for a NK-4 receptor in guinea pig isolated trachea. *J. Physiol. (Lond.)* 409:30p, 1989.

201. Michoud, M.-C., et al. Reflex decrease of histamine-induced bronchoconstriction after laryngeal stimulation in asthmatic patients. *Am. Rev. Respir. Dis.* 138:1548, 1988.

202. Miller, Y. E. Bombesin-like peptides: From frog skin to human lung. *Am. J. Respir. Cell Mol. Biol.* 3:189, 1990.

203. Miura, M., et al. Effect of nonadrenergic, noncholinergic inhibitory nerve stimulation on the allergic reaction in cat airways. *Am. Rev. Respir. Dis.* 141:29, 1990.

203a. Miura, M., et al. Dysfunction of nonadrenergic noncholinergic inhibitory system after antigen inhalation in actively sensitized cat airways. *Am. Rev. Respir. Dis.* 145:70, 1992.

204. Miyata, A., et al. Isolation of a neuropeptide corresponding to the N-terminal 27 residues of the pituitary adenylate cyclase activating polypeptide with 38 residues (PACAP38). *Biochem. Biophys. Res. Commun.* 170:643, 1990.

205. Morice, A., Unwin, R. J., and Sever, P. S. Vasoactive intestinal peptide causes bronchodilation and protects against histamine-induced bronchoconstriction in asthmatic subjects. *Lancet* 2:1225, 1983.

206. Nakamuta, H., Fukuda, Y., and Koida, M. Binding sites of calcitonin gene-related peptide (CGRP): Abundant occurrence in visceral organs. *Jpn. J. Pharmacol.* 42:175, 1986.

207. Nakanishi, S. Substance P precursor and kininogen: Their structures, gene organizations, and regulation. *Physiol. Rev.* 67:1117, 1987.

208. Naline, E., et al. Characterization of neurokinin effects on receptor selectivity in human isolated bronchi. *Am. Rev. Respir. Dis.* 140:679, 1989.

209. Nathanson, I., Widdicombe, J. H., and Barnes, P. J. Effect of vasoactive

noncholinergic control of pulmonary mechanisms in guinea pig. *Naunyn Schmiedebergs Arch. Pharmacol.* 325:343, 1984.

intestinal peptide on ion transport across dog tracheal epithelium. *J. Appl. Physiol.* 55:1844, 1983.

210. Nichol, G. M., et al. Effect of inhaled furosemide on metabisulfite- and methacholine induced bronchoconstriction and nasal potential difference in asthmatic subjects. *Am. Rev. Respir. Dis.* 142:576, 1990.

211. Nichol, G. M., et al. Effect of neuropeptides on bronchial blood flow and pulmonary resistance in conscious sheep. *Thorax* 44:884p, 1989.

212. Noguchi, K., et al. Coexistence of alpha-CGRP and beta-CGRP mRNAs in rat dorsal root ganglion cells. *Neurosci. Lett.* 108:1, 1990.

213. Nong, Y. H., et al. Peptides encoded by the calcitonin gene inhibit macrophage function. *J. Immunol.* 143:45, 1989.

214. O'Dorisio, M. S., et al. Identification of high affinity receptors for vasoactive intestinal peptide on human lymphocytes of B cell lineage. *J. Immunol.* 142:3533, 1989.

215. Ollerenshaw, S., et al. Absence of immunoreactive vasoactive intestinal polypeptide in tissue from the lungs of patients with asthma. *N. Engl. J. Med.* 320:1244, 1989.

216. Ollerenshaw, S. L., et al. Substance P immunoreactive nerve fibres in airways from patients with and without asthma. *Am. Rev. Respir. Dis.* 139:A237, 1989.

217. Palmer, J. B. D., and Barnes, P. J. Neuropeptides and airway smooth muscle function. *Am. Rev. Respir. Dis.* 136:S50, 1987.

218. Palmer, J. B. D., Cuss, F. M. C., and Barnes, P. J. VIP and PHM and their role in nonadrenergic inhibitory responses in isolated human airways. *J. Appl. Physiol.* 61:1322, 1986.

219. Palmer, J. B. D., et al. Calcitonin gene-related peptide is localized to human airway nerves and potently constricts human airway smooth muscle. *Br. J. Pharmacol.* 91:95, 1987.

220. Palmer, J. B. D., et al. The effect of infused vasoactive intestinal peptide on airway function in normal subjects. *Thorax* 41:663, 1986.

221. Paul, S., et al. Characterization of autoantibodies to vasoactive intestinal peptide in asthma. *J. Neuroimmunol.* 23:133, 1989.

222. Pauwels, R. A., Joos, G. F., and van der Straeten, M. E. The effect of different tachykinins on airway calibre and histamine release. *J. Allergy Clin. Immunol.* 83:A299, 1989.

223. Peatfield, A. C., et al. Vasoactive intestinal peptide stimulates tracheal submucosal gland secretion in ferret. *Am. Rev. Respir. Dis.* 128:89, 1983.

224. Peatfield, A. C., and Richardson, P. S. Evidence for noncholinergic, nonadrenergic nervous control of mucus secretion into the cat trachea. *J. Physiol. (Lond.)* 342:335, 1983.

225. Piedimonte, G., et al. Sendai virus infection potentiates neurogenic inflammation in the rat trachea. *J. Appl. Physiol.* 68:754, 1990.

226. Pietrowski, W., and Foreman, J. C. Some effects of calcitonin gene related peptide in human skin and on histamine release. *Br. J. Dermatol.* 114:37, 1986.

227. Polak, J. M., and Bloom, S. R. Regulatory peptides of the gastrointestinal and respiratory tracts. *Arch. Int. Pharmacodyn. Ther.* 280:16, 1986.

228. Potter, E. K. Neuropeptide Y as an autonomic neurotransmitter. *Pharmacol. Ther.* 37:251, 1988.

229. Proud, D., and Kaplan, A. P. Kinin formation: Mechanisms and role in inflammatory disorders. *Annu. Rev. Immunol.* 6:49, 1988.

229a. Rand, M. Nitrergic transmission: Nitric oxide as a mediator of nonadrenergic, noncholinergic neuro-effector transmission. *Clin. Exp. Pharmacol. Physiol.* 19:147, 1992.

230. Rangachari, P. K., and McWade, D. Effects of tachykinins on the electrical activity of isolated canine tracheal epithelium: An exploratory study. *Regul. Pept.* 12:9, 1985.

231. Regoli, D. Pharmacological receptors for substance P and neurokinins. *Life Sci.* 403:66, 1987.

232. Reptke, H., and Beinert, M. Structural requirements for mast cell triggering by substance P-like peptides. *Agents Actions* 23:207, 1988.

233. Reynolds, A. M., and McEvoy, R. D. Tachykinins mediate hypocapnia-induced bronchoconstriction in guinea pigs. *J. Appl. Physiol.* 67:2454, 1989.

234. Rhoden, K., and Barnes, P. J. Epithelial modulation of NANC and VIP-induced responses: Role of neutral endopeptidase. *Eur. J. Pharmacol.* 171:247, 1989.

235. Rhoden, K. J., and Barnes, P. J. Potentiation of non-adrenergic non-cholinergic relaxation in guinea pig airways by a cAMP phosphodiesterase inhibitor. *J. Pharmacol. Exp. Ther.* 282:396, 1990.

236. Rhoden, K. J., and Barnes, P. J. Classification of tachykinin receptors on guinea pig and human airway smooth muscle. *Am. Rev. Respir. Dis.* 141: A726, 1990.

237. Richardson, J. B. Nerve supply to the lung. *Am. Rev. Respir. Dis.* 119:785, 1979.

238. Richardson, J. B. Nonadrenergic inhibitory innervation of the lung. *Lung* 159:315, 1981.

239. Robberecht, P., et al. Pharmacological characterization of VIP receptors in human lung membranes. *Peptides* 9:339, 1988.

240. Rogers, D. F., Aursudkij, B., and Barnes, P. J. Effects of tachykinins on mucus secretion on human bronchi *in vitro. Eur. J. Pharmacol.* 174:283, 1989.

241. Rogers, D. F., and Barnes, P. J. Opioid inhibition of neurally mediated mucus secretion in human bronchi: Implications for chronic bronchitis therapy. *Lancet* 1:930, 1989.

242. Rogers, D. F., et al. Effects and interactions of sensory neuropeptides on airway microvascular leakage in guinea pigs. *Br. J. Pharmacol.* 95:1109, 1988.

243. Rokaeus, A. Galanin: A newly isolated biologically active peptide. *Trends Neurosci.* 10:158, 1987.

244. Russell, J. A., and Simons, E. J. Modulation of cholinergic neurotransmission in airways by enkephalin. *J. Appl. Physiol.* 58:853, 1985.

245. Saban, R., et al. Enhancement of parainfluenza 3 infection of contractile responses to substance P and capsaicin in airway smooth muscle from guinea pig. *Am. Rev. Respir. Dis.* 136:586, 1987.

246. Said, S. I. Vasoactive peptides in the lung, with special reference to vasoactive intestinal peptide. *Exp. Lung Res.* 3:343, 1982.

247. Said, S. I. Neuropeptides as modulators of injury and inflammation. *Life Sci.* 47:PL19, 1990.

248. Said, S. I., Geumi, A., and Hara, N. Bronchodilator Effect of VIP In Vivo: Protection Against Bronchoconstriction Induced by Histamine and Prostaglandin $F_{2\alpha}$. In S. I. Said (ed.), *Vasoactive Intestinal Peptide.* New York: Raven, 1982. Pp. 185–191.

249. Said, S. I., and Mutt, V. Long acting vasodilator peptide from lung tissue. *Nature* 224:699, 1969.

250. Salonen, R. O., Webber, S. E., and Widdicombe, J. G. Effects of neuropeptides and capsaicin on the canine tracheal vasculature in vivo. *Br. J. Pharmacol.* 95:1262, 1988.

251. Saria, A., et al. Release of multiple tachykinins from capsaicin-sensitive nerves in the lung by bradykinin, histamine, dimethylphenylpiperazinium, and vagal nerve stimulation. *Am. Rev. Respir. Dis.* 137:1330, 1988.

252. Sekizawa, K., Graf, P. D., and Nadel, J. A. Somatostatin potentiates cholinergic neurotransmission in ferret trachea. *J. Appl. Physiol.* 67:2397, 1989.

253. Sekizawa, K., et al. Mast cell tryptase causes airway smooth muscle hyperresponsiveness in dogs. *J. Clin. Invest.* 83:175, 1989.

254. Sekizawa, K., et al. Modulation of cholinergic transmission by vasoactive intestinal peptide in ferret trachea. *J. Appl. Physiol.* 69:2433, 1988.

255. Sekizawa, K., et al. Enkephalinase inhibitors potentiate mammalian tachykinin-induced contraction in ferret trachea. *J. Pharmacol. Exp. Ther.* 243:1211, 1987.

256. Sekizawa, K., et al. Enkephalinase inhibitor potentiates substance P and electrically induced contraction in ferret trachea. *J. Appl. Physiol.* 63: 1401, 1987.

257. Sertl, K., et al. Substance P: The relationship between receptor distribution in rat lung and the capacity of substance P to stimulate vascular permeability. *Am. Rev. Respir. Dis.* 138:151, 1988.

258. Sestini, P., et al. Ion transport in rat tracheal ganglion in vitro. Role of capsaicin-sensitive nerves in allergic reactions. *Am. Rev. Respir. Dis.* 141: 393, 1990.

259. Sharma, R. K., and Jeffery, P. K. Airway VIP receptor number is reduced in cystic fibrosis but not asthma. *Am. Rev. Respir. Dis.* 140:A726, 1990.

260. Sheppard, D., et al. Toluene diisocyanate increases airway responsiveness to substance P and decreases airway and neutral endopeptidase. *J. Clin. Invest.* 81:1111, 1988.

261. Sheppard, M. N., et al. Neuropeptide tyrosine (NPY), a newly discovered peptide, is present in the mammalian respiratory tract. *Thorax* 39:326, 1984.

262. Shigemoto, R., et al. Cloning and expression of a rat neuromedin K receptor cDNA. *J. Biol. Chem.* 265:623, 1990.

263. Shimosegawa, T., Foda, H. D., and Said, S. I. [Met]enkephalin-Arg[6]-Gly[7]-Leu[8]-immunoreactive nerves in guinea pig and rat lungs: Distribution, origin, and coexistence with vasoactive intestinal polypeptide immunoreactivity. *Neuroscience* 36:737, 1990.

264. Shimura, S., et al. VIP augments cholinergic-induced glycoconjugate secretion in tracheal submucosal glands. *J. Appl. Physiol.* 65:2537, 1988.

265. Shimura, S., et al. Effect of substance P on mucus secretion of isolated submucosal glands from feline trachea. *J. Appl. Physiol.* 63:646, 1987.

266. Shore, S. A., et al. Substance P induced bronchoconstriction in guinea pig. Enhancement by inhibitors of neutral metalloendopeptidase and angiotensin converting enzyme. *Am. Rev. Respir. Dis.* 137:331, 1988.

267. Skidgel, R. A., et al. Hydrolysis of substance P and neurotensin by converting enzyme and neutral endopeptidase. *Peptides* 5:767, 1989.

268. Snider, R. M., et al. A potent nonpeptide antagonist of the substance P (NK₁) receptor. *Science* 251:435, 1991.

269. Springall, D. R., Bloom, S. R., and Polak, J. M. Neural, Endocrine and Endothelial Regulatory Peptides. In *The Lung: Scientific Foundations*. New York: Raven, 1991. P. 69.

270. Springall, D. R., et al. Persistence of intrinsic neurones and possible phenotypic changes after extrinsic denervation of human respiratory tract by heart-lung transplantation. *Am. Rev. Respir. Dis.* 141:1538, 1990.

271. Stammberger, H., and Wolfe, G. Headaches and sinus disease: The endoscopic approach. *Ann. Otol. Rhinol. Laryngol. Suppl.* 134:3, 1989.

272. Steenbergh, P. H., et al. Structure and expression of the human calcitonin/CGRP genes. *FEBS Lett.* 209:97, 1986.

273. Stimler-Gerard, N. P. Neutral endopeptidase-like enzyme controls the contractile activity of substance P in guinea pig lung. *J. Clin. Invest.* 79:1819, 1987.

274. Stretton, C. D., and Barnes, P. J. Cholecystokinin octapeptide constricts guinea-pig and human airways. *Br. J. Pharmacol.* 97:675, 1989.

275. Stretton, C. D., Belvisi, M. G., and Barnes, P. J. The effect of sensory nerve depletion on cholinergic neurotransmission in guinea pig airways. *Br. J. Pharmacol.* 98:782P, 1989.

276. Stretton, C. D., Belvisi, M. G., and Barnes, P. J. Sensory nerve depletion potentiates inhibitory NANC nerves in guinea pig airways. *Eur. J. Pharmacol.* 184:333, 1990.

277. Stretton, C. D., Belvisi, M. G., and Barnes, P. J. Neuropeptide Y modulates non-adrenergic non-cholinergic neural bronchoconstriction *in vivo* and *in vitro*. *Neuropeptides* 17:163, 1990.

278. Stretton, C. D., Belvisi, M. G., and Barnes, P. J. Modulation of neural bronchoconstrictor responses in the guinea pig respiratory tract by vasoactive intestinal peptide. *Neuropeptides* 18:149, 1991.

279. Stretton, D., and Barnes, P. J. Modulation of cholinergic neurotransmission in guinea pig trachea by neuropeptide Y. *Br. J. Pharmacol.* 93:672, 1988.

280. Stretton, D., et al. Calcium activated potassium channels mediate prejunctional inhibition of peripheral sensory nerves. *Proc. Natl. Acad. Sci. USA* 89:1325, 1992.

281. Sunday, M. E., et al. Gastrin releasing peptide (mammalian bombesin) gene expression in health and disease. *Lab. Invest.* 59:5, 1988.

282. Szarek, J. L., et al. Reflex activation of the non-adrenergic non-cholinergic inhibitory nervous system in feline airways. *Am. Rev. Respir. Dis.* 133:1159, 1986.

283. Takeda, Y., et al. Regional distribution of neuropeptide gamma and other tachykinin peptides derived from the substance P gene in the rat. *Regul. Pept.* 28:323, 1990.

284. Tam, E. K., and Caughey, G. H. Degradation of airway neuropeptides by human lung tryptase. *Am. J. Respir. Cell Mol. Biol.* 3:27, 1990.

285. Tam, E. K., et al. Protease inhibitors potentiate smooth muscle relaxation induced by vasoactive intestinal peptide in isolated human bronchi. *Am. J. Respir. Cell Mol. Biol.* 2:449, 1990.

286. Tanaka, D. T., and Grunstein, N. M. Effect of substance P on neurally mediated contraction of rabbit airway smooth muscle. *J. Appl. Physiol.* 60:458, 1986.

287. Tatemoto, K. PHI—a new brain-gut peptide. *Peptides* 5:151, 1984.

288. Thompson, J. E., et al. Tachykinins mediate the acute increase in airway responsiveness by toluene diisocyanate in guinea-pigs. *Am. Rev. Respir. Dis.* 136:43, 1987.

289. Tokuyama, K., et al. Neural control of goblet cell secretion in guinea pig airways. *Am. J. Physiol.* 259:L108, 1990.

290. Tschirhart, E., and Landry, Y. Epithelium releases a relaxant factor: Demonstration with substance P. *Eur. J. Pharmacol.* 132:103, 1986.

291. Tucker, J. F., et al. L-Nᴳ-nitro arginine inhibits nonadrenergic, noncholinergic relaxations of guinea-pig isolated tracheal smooth muscle. *Br. J. Pharmacol.* 100:663, 1990.

292. Uddman, R., Luts, A., and Sundler, F. Occurrence and distribution of calcitonin gene related peptide in the mammalian respiratory tract and middle ear. *Cell Tissue Res.* 214:551, 1985.

293. Uddman, R., Moghimzadeh, E., and Sundler, F. Occurrence and distribution of GRP-immunoreactive nerve fibres in the respiratory tract. *Arch. Otorhinolaryngol.* 239:145, 1984.

294. Uddman, R., and Sundler, F. Innervation of the upper airways. *Clin. Chest Med.* 7:201, 1986.

295. Uddman, R., and Sundler, F. Neuropeptides in the airways: A review. *Am. Rev. Respir. Dis.* 136:S3, 1987.

296. Umeda, Y., and Arisawa, H. Characterization of the calcitonin gene related peptide receptor in mouse T lymphocytes. *Neuropeptides* 14:237, 1989.

297. Umeno, E., McDonald, D. M., and Nadel, J. A. Hypertonic saline increases vascular permeability in the rat trachea by producing neurogenic inflammation. *J. Clin. Invest.* 85:1905, 1990.

298. Umeno, E., et al. Inhibition of neutral endopeptidase potentiates neurogenic inflammation in the rat trachea. *J. Appl. Physiol.* 66:2647, 1989.

299. Undem, B. J., Dick, E. C., and Buckner, C. K. Inhibition by vasoactive intestinal peptide of antigen-induced histamine release from guinea pig minced lung. *Eur. J. Pharmacol.* 88:247, 1983.

300. Undem, B. J., et al. Vagal innervation of guinea pig bronchial smooth muscle. *J. Appl. Physiol.* 69:1336, 1991.

301. van Ranst, L., and Lauweryns, J. M. Effects of long-term sensory vs. sympathetic denervation on the distribution of calcitonin gene-related peptide and tyrosine hydroxylase immunoreactivity in the rat lung. *J. Neuroimmunol.* 29:131, 1990.

302. Ventresca, G. P., et al. Inhaled furosemide inhibits cough induced by low chloride content solutions but not by capsaicin. *Am. Rev. Respir. Dis.* 142:143, 1990.

303. Venugopalan, C. S., and O'Malley, N. A. Cross desensitization of VIP- and NANC-mediated inhibition of guinea pig tracheal pouch. *J. Auton. Pharmacol.* 8:53, 1988.

304. Verleden, G. M., et al. Inhibition of nonadrenergic noncholinergic neural bronchoconstriction in guinea pig airways in vitro by β₂-adrenoceptors (abstract). *Am. Rev. Respir. Dis.* In press.

305. Verleden, G. M., et al. Modulation of neurotransmission in guinea pig airways by purinoceptors (abstract). *Am. Rev. Respir. Dis.* In press.

306. Verleden, G. M., et al. Nedocromil sodium modulates non-adrenergic non-cholinergic bronchoconstrictor nerves in guinea-pig airways *in vitro. Am. Rev. Respir. Dis.* 143:114, 1991.

306a. Watling, K. Nonpeptide antagonists herald a new era in tachykinins. *Trends Pharmacol. Sci.* 13:266, 1992.

307. Webber, S. E. The effects of peptide histidine isoleucine and neuropeptide Y on mucous volume output from ferret trachea. *Br. J. Pharmacol.* 55:40, 1988.

308. Webber, S. E. Receptors mediating the effect of substance P and neurokinin A on mucous secretion and smooth muscle tone of the ferret trachea: Potentiation by enkephalinase inhibition. *Br. J. Pharmacol.* 98:1197, 1989.

309. Webber, S. E., and Widdicombe, J. G. The effect of vasoactive intestinal peptide on smooth muscle tone and mucous volume output from ferret trachea. *Br. J. Pharmacol.* 91:139, 1987.

310. Webber, S. G., Lim, J. C. S., and Widdicombe, J. G. The effects of calcitonin gene related peptide on submucosal gland secretion and epithelial albumin transport on ferret trachea in vitro. *Br. J. Pharmacol.* 102:79, 1991.

311. Wei, E. T., and Kiang, J. C. Inhibition of protein exudation from the trachea by corticotropin releasing factor. *Eur. J. Pharmacol.* 140:63, 1987.

312. Wenzel, S. E., Fowler, A. A., and Schwartz, L. B. Activation of pulmonary mast cells by bronchoalveolar allergen challenge. In vivo release of histamine and tryptase in atopic subjects with and without asthma. *Am. Rev. Respir. Dis.* 137:1002, 1988.

313. Widdicombe, J. G. The NANC system and airway vasculature. *Arch. Int. Pharmacodyn. Ther.* 303:83, 1990.

314. Williams, G., Cardosa, H., and Ball, J. A. Potent and comparable vasodilator actions of A- and B-calcitonin gene related peptides on the superficial subcutaneous vasculature of man. *Clin. Sci.* 75:309, 1988.

315. Wolfe, G. Neue aspekte zur pathogenese und therapie der hyperflektorischen rhinopathie. *Laryngol. Rhinol. Otol.* 67:438, 1988.

316. Woll, P. J., and Rozengurt, E. Neuropeptides as growth regulators. *Br. Med. Bull.* 45:492, 1989.

317. Wong, L. B., Miller, I. F., and Yeates, D. B. Is substance P a mediator of irritant stimulation of ciliary beat frequency? *Am. Rev. Respir. Dis.* 139:A466, 1989.

318. Wong, L. B., Miller, I. F., and Yeates, D. B. Stimulation of tracheal ciliary beat frequency by capsaicin. *J. Appl. Physiol.* 68:2574, 1990.

319. Yeadon, M., Wilkinson, D., and Payne, A. N. Ozone induces bronchial hyperreactivity to inhaled substance P by functional inhibition of enkephalinase. *Br. J. Pharmacol.* 99:191p, 1990.

320. Yiangou, Y., et al. Isolation, characterization, and pharmacological actions of peptide histidine valine 42, a novel prepro-vasoactive intestinal peptide derived peptide. *J. Biol. Chem.* 262:14010, 1987.

321. Yokota, Y., et al. Molecular characterization of a functional cDNA for rat substance P receptor. *J. Biol. Chem.* 264:17649, 1989.

Role of Adenosine and Adenosine Receptors

19

Stephen T. Holgate
Riccardo Polosa
Gerrard D. Phillips

A large number of different chemical entities have been described as candidate mediators of asthma. Some of these such as histamine are preformed, while others are generated de novo on appropriate cell stimulation. Some are produced as primary products of the inflammatory tissue response, whereas others are secondary (see Chap. 9). Adenosine is a purine nucleoside that serves an autocoid function in a large number of physiologic systems including the airways, and falls into the secondary class of mediator. Extracellular adenosine is largely derived from the cleavage of adenosine 5'-monophosphate (AMP) by the membrane-located enzyme 5'-nucleotidase. Other important metabolic pathways for generating adenosine include the demethylation of S-adenosylmethionine and de novo synthesis. Once generated, extracellular adenosine is rapidly scavenged by cells involving a mechanism of facilitated uptake, which may be blocked by such drugs as dipyridamole and hexobendine. Adenosine produces most of its cell-surface effects by stimulating specific cell-surface receptors, leading to either an increase or a decrease in cellular levels of cyclic 3'5'-adenosine monophosphate (cyclic AMP) by stimulating (A_2) or inhibiting (A_1) adenylate cyclase activity respectively [57]. The inhibitory actions of adenosine on adenylate cyclase involve at least three G-proteins, whereas excitation through the A_2 receptor involves only a single G-protein. Two further functions of adenosine have recently been described: the opening of K^+-Na^+ channels [57] and the opening of Ca^{++} channels [53]. The receptor exhibiting the latter function is a newly described receptor termed A_3. Available evidence indicates that individual cells possess only a single class of adenosine receptor that serves the autocoid functions of this mediator, although at high concentrations adenosine has profound effects on intracellular metabolic pathways relating to methylation and phosphorylation.

AIRWAY EFFECTS OF ADENOSINE

Adenosine and related analogs exert a number of different effects on the airways. On guinea pig tracheal preparations they exhibit a preferential activity at A_2 purinoceptors to produce a transient contraction followed by relaxation [25]. Since the small contractile effect is inhibited by atropine, it is probably mediated by cholinergic nerves. Subsequent relaxation of an established contraction occurs through an increase in cellular levels of cyclic AMP. On the basis of these animal studies, it seemed reasonable to propose a bronchodilator action for this purine. However, events proved to the contrary. When inhaled by asthmatic but not normal subjects, adenosine produced dose-related bronchoconstriction measured as a fall in specific airway conductance [14]. This response was observed in subjects with both allergic (extrinsic) and nonallergic (intrinsic) asthma, but not when the related nucleosides inosine and guanosine were inhaled. This indicated some selectivity for the constrictor response and was compatible with an interaction of the nucleoside with purinoceptors.

Since adenosine has a low solubility in isotonic sodium chloride, the parent nucleotides AMP and adenosine diphosphate (ADP) proved to be more suitable for airway challenge [34]. Both agents caused dose-related bronchoconstriction in asthmatic subjects over a similar concentration range. Since AMP is rapidly hydrolyzed in vivo to adenosine, the airway effects of AMP and ADP are likely to be mediated by the nucleoside (adenosine) after dephosphorylation. A single inhalation of adenosine or AMP produces bronchoconstriction, achieving a maximum 3 to 5 minutes after the challenge, which in contrast to the early response with allergen was not accompanied by a late phase of bronchoconstriction or an increase in "nonspecific" bronchial responsiveness [44]. Responsiveness of the airways to inhaled adenosine and AMP correlates only weakly with more direct indices of airway responsiveness measured with such agonists as histamine [34] and methacholine [32]. Taken together, these findings indicate that bronchoconstriction produced by adenosine is not a mere reflection of nonspecific bronchial hyperresponsiveness but involves a selective interaction with cells in asthmatic but not normal airways.

MECHANISMS OF ADENOSINE-INDUCED BRONCHOCONSTRICTION

Bronchoconstriction provoked by a wide range of agonists occurs through a combination of receptor-mediated contraction of airway smooth muscle, stimulation of sensory nerves with excitation of cholinergic and peptidergic reflex pathways, and vascular engorgement and leakage. To investigate the contribution of cholinergic mechanisms to bronchoconstriction triggered by adenosine, the influence of prior treatment with the inhaled muscarinic antagonist ipratropium bromide has been studied [32]. At an inhaled dose of 1 mg, ipratropium bromide produced an approximate 200-fold protection of asthmatic airways against the dose-related fall in 1-second forced expiratory volume (FEV_1) produced by inhaled methacholine, but failed to protect against inhaled adenosine. In a repeat of this experiment using AMP rather than adenosine as the provocative stimulus, ipratropium bromide produced a small but significant additive protection beyond that achieved with the H_1 antagonist terfenadine [50]. These data indicate that activation of muscarinic vagal reflexes by adenosine plays only a minor role in its ability to provoke bronchoconstriction and therefore differs from observations made in certain rat strains.

Since adenosine and AMP produce many of their pharmacologic effects through the activation of cell-surface purinoceptors, the effect of antagonism of this receptor class on AMP-induced

253

bronchoconstriction has been studied. Theophylline (2,3-dimethylxanthine) is a weak competitive antagonist of purinoceptors in addition to being an inhibitor of cyclic nucleotide phosphodiesterase. On the other hand, enprofylline has no reported effects at adenosine receptors, but is a potent inhibitor of phosphodiesterase and a relaxant of airway smooth muscle [31]. In a placebo-controlled study [7], infusions of theophylline and enprofylline at concentrations that produced equivalent bronchodilatation resulted in a similar degree of protection against the fall in FEV_1 with inhaled histamine. However, theophylline was more active than enprofylline in protecting the airways against the constrictor effect of AMP. Enprofylline's protective action against histamine and AMP could be accounted for by functional antagonism, while for theophylline, the additional protection afforded against AMP indicated an additional action as a purinoceptor antagonist. We obtained a similar selective protective effect of theophylline against the airway effects of adenosine when the drug was administered by inhalation [15] or orally [33]. The importance of theophylline interactions with adenosine receptors was recently highlighted by demonstrating rebound hyperresponsiveness to inhaled adenosine on withdrawal of chronic theophylline therapy. One explanation of this is an upregulation of adenosine receptors [58].

For adenosine to mediate its bronchoconstrictor action by interacting with cell-surface purinoceptors, any drug that inhibits cellular uptake would be expected to augment the bronchoconstrictor response. One such drug is dipyridamole. When administered to asthmatic patients by intravenous infusion [13] or by inhalation [8], dipyridamole enhances the bronchoconstrictor response to inhaled adenosine. Thus, by increasing extracellular concentrations, the enhancing effect of these maneuvers provides additional evidence that this nucleoside mediates its effect through a cell-surface interaction.

While these data implicate purinoceptors in the airway response to adenosine, they do not indicate the receptor subclass involved or the effector cells of the response. Some insight into this has been obtained using sodium cromoglycate, which, when inhaled prior to adenosine challenge, effectively inhibits the ensuing bronchoconstrictor response [12]. The inhibitory effect is dose dependent [55]. In a series of studies, inhaled nedocromil sodium was also shown to be a powerful inhibitor of the airway response to AMP in both allergic [54] and nonallergic [47] asthmatic subjects. In molar terms, nedocromil sodium is about two to five times more active than sodium cromoglycate as an inhibitor of the AMP response. Nedocromil sodium also has a preferential inhibitory action when administered by inhalation rather than orally or intravenously, indicating an action on the surface of the airways [59]. Since both sodium cromoglycate and nedocromil sodium have inhibitory effects against airway mast cells, an attempt has been made to determine the contribution of mast cell mediators to the constrictor response of AMP.

In a series of studies, we showed that potent and selective histamine H_1-receptor antagonists attenuate bronchoconstriction produced by a variety of stimuli involving activation of airway mast cells (see Chap. 65). When administered as a single dose of 180 mg 3 hours before challenge, terfenadine produced a mean 35-fold displacement of the concentration-FEV_1-response curve with inhaled histamine [52] and partially protected the airways against the early response to inhaled allergen [11], exercise [21], hypertonic saline solution [23], and isocapnic hyperventilation [20]. The same dose of terfenadine almost totally inhibited the fall in FEV_1 produced by a concentration of AMP, which in the presence of placebo, reduced this index of airway caliber by more than 20 percent of baseline [51] (Fig. 19-1). Similar results were obtained with the longer-acting antihistamine astemizole [27]. With both of these antihistamines, maximum inhibition of the AMP response was observed during the first 5 minutes of the challenge, with a diminishing effect thereafter.

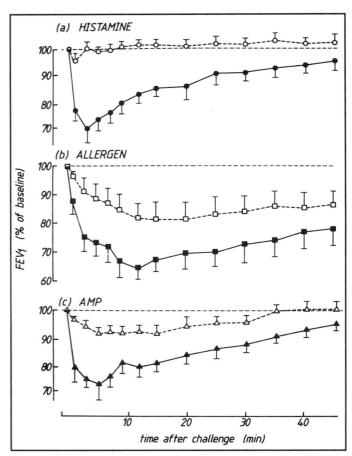

Fig. 19-1. *Inhibitory effect of terfenadine (open symbols), 120 mg orally, and placebo (closed symbols) on bronchoconstriction provoked by inhaled histamine, allergen, and AMP.*

Thus, it is likely that histamine released from airway mast cells is a major mediator of the AMP response and that in primed mast cells, AMP is serving as an "incomplete" agonist. Accordingly, we undertook a study in which venous plasma concentrations of histamine in patients with mild asthma were measured before and after challenge with methacholine, allergen, and AMP. Allergen and methacholine both produced a 25 to 30 percent maximum fall in FEV_1, but only with allergen was a threefold to fivefold increase in plasma histamine concentrations observed [46]. However, provocation of the airways with AMP to produce a similar decrease in FEV_1 resulted in a significant increase in plasma histamine, but this was considerably less than that observed with allergen. One interpretation of these findings is that histamine released by adenosine requires the participation of other mediators to produce its maximum effect on the airways; possibilities include prostanoids [48]. As already discussed, part of this additional response may also be reflex mediated as suggested by experimental evidence in rodents [41].

When applied to isolated human lung, histamine can initiate prostanoid synthesis via stimulation of both H_1 and H_2 receptors [46]. To investigate the role of prostanoids in AMP-provoked bronchoconstriction, the effect of flurbiprofen, an inhibitor of cyclooxygenase that is approximately 5,000 times more potent than aspirin, alone and in combination with terfenadine, was observed [45]. When compared to placebo, flurbiprofen inhibited the AMP response by approximately 50 percent. However, when combined with terfenadine, only a small further inhibition of the response was observed, particularly over the first few minutes following challenge. Indomethacin administered prior to adenosine challenge also inhibits bronchoconstriction provoked by adenosine [9]. These data support the view that the release of prostanoids comprises an important component of the AMP-mediated bronchial response, but this only applies to histamine when it is released endogenously, because flurbiprofen has no effect on the airway response to exogenously administered histamine [45].

EFFECT OF ADENOSINE AND ITS ANALOGS ON MAST CELL RESPONSES

When incubated with rat serosal mast cells, adenosine and 2-chloroadenosine augment histamine release when triggered by the calcium ionophore A 23187 [37]. Subsequent studies on rodent mast cells showed that adenosine and related analogs could also enhance IgE-triggered mediator release in parallel with stimulation of adenylate cyclase [26]. A direct relationship between adenosine's capacity to enhance mediator secretion and stimulation of adenylate cyclase in rat mast cells was recently questioned when 8-phenyltheophylline, a purinoceptor antagonist free of cyclic nucleotide phosphodiesterase activity, was shown to inhibit the cyclic AMP response but not the enhancement of concanavalin A–induced histamine secretion [28]. Thus, on rodent mast cells, adenosine may operate through a separate receptor that is not linked to adenylate cyclase, possibly the A_3 receptor linked to Ca^{++} flux. Crimi and coworkers failed to show that pretreatment of asthmatic subjects with the potent calcium antagonist nifedipine had any effect on the constrictor response to inhaled adenosine [10]. Thus, the Ca^{++} channel involved in enhancing activation-secretion coupling in mast cells is likely to be receptor rather than voltage operated.

The intracellular mechanism for purinoceptor-mediated enhancement of mast cell histamine release is not known, although in interleukin-3 (IL-3)–dependent, mouse bone marrow–derived mast cells, Marquardt and Walker [38] found evidence for stimulation of a protein kinase C involved in cell signaling. Adenosine and synthetic analogs preferentially augmented the release of granule-derived mediators such as beta-hexosaminidase rather than the newly formed oxidation products of arachidonic acid, indicating that the biochemical pathway on which adenosine has an influence is downstream from that activated by cross-linkage. Such a mechanism explains why atopic subjects, when compared to nonatopic subjects, are relatively more responsive to adenosine and AMP than they are to methacholine (Fig. 19-2).

Human basophils and lung mast cells also respond to adenosine and synthetic analogs with augmented IgE-triggered histamine release, but only if the autocoid is present when or after the immunologic stimulus has been applied [5, 29]. Different from rodent mast cells, the purinoceptor-mediated augmentation of mediator release from human lung mast cells extends to the newly formed mediators prostaglandin (PG) D_2 and leukotriene (LT) C_4 [42], suggesting some interspecies differences. That the human mast cell response to adenosine is accompanied by a transient stimulation of adenylate cyclase and may be antagonized by 8-phenyltheophylline also indicates an A_2 receptor–mediated function and further highlights a difference from the rodent system [6, 42]. The capacity of adenosine to augment mediator release from mast cells in the presence of a low-level second stimulus, which may be immunologic or nonimmunologic, raises the possibility that the nucleoside produces mediator release in asthmatic human airways by interacting with cytokine-"primed" mast cells on the surface of inflamed airways. There is strong evidence that mast cells recovered from asthmatic airways by bronchoalveolar lavage (BAL) are increased in number [24, 30] and that these cells have an increased capacity to release their mediators both spontaneously and in the pres-

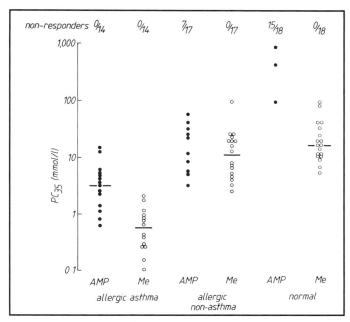

Fig. 19-2. *Provocative concentrations of AMP (closed circles) and methacholine (open circles) that produce a 35 percent fall in specific airway conductance in three groups of subjects: allergic asthmatic subjects, allergic nonasthmatic subjects, and nonallergic normal volunteers. Note the increased AMP responsiveness relative to methacholine in the allergic nonasthmatic subjects.*

ence of a secretory stimulus [24]. That this occurs in vivo is shown by the increased concentration of histamine measured in the BAL fluid phase of asthma [3] and by the bronchodilator action of selective histamine H_1 antagonists [60].

A recent study by Bjorek and coworkers [2a] has shown that airway specimens obtained from asthmatic lung tissue at surgery are hyperresponsive to adenosine in vitro, the contractile response being effectively inhibited by both adenosine A_1 and dual A_1 and A_2 antagonists. In addition, they have shown that the combination of leukotriene antagonism using the receptor blocker ICI 198615, or the biosynthesis inhibitor MK886, and histamine antagonism using the antihistamines mepyramine and metiamide block the contractile effects of adenosine, suggesting that this nucleotide acts indirectly by liberation of leukotrienes and histamine from mast cells. These findings therefore add to both the isolated cell and in vivo evidence that adenosine-induced bronchoconstriction is a mast cell–dependent event.

CLINICAL IMPLICATIONS OF ADENOSINE-INDUCED BRONCHOCONSTRICTION

An interesting observation that has been made with AMP is the ease with which the airways are rendered refractory to the bronchoconstrictor response on repeated challenge [17]. The ability to induce this refractoriness to AMP is inversely related to the basal level of nonspecific bronchial responsiveness, providing evidence that the dose of AMP reaching the airways rather than their sensitivity to it is important in determining the loss of responsiveness [43]. Refractoriness to AMP shows no cross-reaction with inhaled histamine, making it unlikely that the re-fractoriness results from fatigue of airway smooth muscle or downregulation of histamine H_1 receptors. In a group of subjects in whom AMP refractoriness could be shown, repeated histamine provocation with increasing doses of the agonist on three consecutive occasions failed to produce a consistent downregulation of the response, which differed from the experience of Manning and colleagues [36]. Following two to three dose-response challenges with AMP, loss of airway response to the nucleoside persists for 4 to 6 hours [17]. The mechanism responsible for AMP refractoriness in asthmatic airways is not known, but possibilities include depletion of preformed mediators from airway mast cells, A_2-purinoceptor downregulation, and elaboration of an inhibitory substance. In support of receptor downregulation, Marquardt and coworkers [39] showed that only a single exposure of mast cells to the A_2-agonist N^5-ethylcarboxamide adenosine (NECA) is sufficient to render them completely refractory to subsequent stimulation with adenosine. This in vitro tachyphylaxis could be reversed by washing and returning the cells to culture for 4 hours, a time to regain sensitivity similar to that observed in our human experiments [17].

Two observations regarding adenosine refractoriness have proved difficult to explain. The first is the demonstration of cross-refractoriness between AMP and exercise since these two stimuli are considered to be quite different [22]. The second is cross-tachyphylaxis between inhaled bradykinin and AMP. Repeated inhalation of bradykinin results in a progressive loss of airway response to this agonist, with cross-tachyphylaxis being observed with lysyl-bradykinin (kallidin) [49]. When airways have been rendered nonresponsive to bradykinin, they are also nonresponsive to AMP. One possible explanation for these findings is that during the induction of exercise or bradykinin refractoriness, a "protective substance" that extends the protection to AMP is released. However, this inhibitory substance would have to exhibit some selectivity since cross-refractoriness does not extend to histamine. For exercise, this substance is suggested to be either PGE_2 or PGI_2 [40]. Another explanation for refractoriness following repeated exercise challenge of asthmatic airways is depletion of constrictor mediators from mast cells. However, for loss of the AMP response this is unlikely because airways rendered refractory to AMP respond to allergen provocation, with enhanced rather than reduced bronchoconstriction [43]. This is likely to be a reflection of adenosine's capacity to augment mediator release, but does not support the mediator depletion hypothesis.

Although we have provided some evidence that adenosine is released into venous plasma following allergen provocation of asthma airways [34], the known rapid uptake of this nucleoside by vascular endothelium and erythrocytes might indicate that the plasma adenosine measured originated from blood cells possibly ex vivo. In isolated human peripheral blood leukocytes, the calcium ionophore A 23187, or the more specific chemoattractant peptide stimulus formyl-methionine-leucine-phenylalanine (FMLP), releases adenosine in parallel with that of histamine from basophils [52]. Thus, the presence of elevated plasma concentrations of adenosine following airway challenge in asthma might be a reflection of peripheral blood leukocyte activation rather than release from the lung.

Adenosine released into the airways is likely to be of pathophysiologic relevance only in moderate to severe asthma, which places the airway tissue under hypoxic and metabolic stress. In this regard the recently reported cases of severe asthma provoked by intravenously administered dipyridamole in the thallium-dipyridamole stress test for coronary insufficiency are of concern and relevant to adenosine's possible mediator role in asthma [19].

From a mechanistic point of view, adenosine may prove to be of some interest as a marker for mast cell priming in asthma. The demonstration of bronchoconstriction occurring with AMP in normal subjects, but only if they are atopic, adds further evidence for an interaction between this nucleoside and the mast cell IgE system [4]. Endobronchial biopsy studies recently showed that the airways of atopic nonasthmatic subjects without bronchial hyperresponsiveness may exhibit some of the features of inflammation seen in asthma, for example, mast cell degranulation, eosinophil infiltration, and sub–basement membrane collagen deposition [27]. Thus, bronchoconstriction provoked in atopic asthmatic and normal subjects may well affect the state of airway mast cell priming and, indeed, may be an in vivo test for this. Cytokine-primed mast cells may also account for their participation in bronchoconstriction by such stimuli as exercise, isocapnic hyperventilation, and hypertonic saline solution, and may help explain the cross-refractoriness between these stimuli, although in atopics the skin wheal response to AMP is not enhanced [18]. The capacity of adenosine to act as an incomplete stimulus for primed mast cells also explains the inhibitory action of inhaled furosemide on AMP-induced bronchoconstriction, since this inhibitor of the Na^+-Cl^- antiport also has a preferential suppressive effect on other mast cell–dependent airway events including the allergen-induced early- and late-phase response [1], fog-induced bronchoconstriction [56], and exercise-induced asthma [2].

In conclusion, provocation of the airways with adenosine and its parent nucleotide AMP has provided a unique insight into the potential role of mast cells as effector cells in provoked asthma. Recent work suggests that the airway response to these agents may be an index of mast cell priming and therefore may provide a useful tool to further explore the inflammatory and immunologic processes in this and related diseases. In providing this additional information, adenosine and AMP provocation is gaining increasing acceptance as an additional measure of disease activity in asthma [16].

REFERENCES

1. Bianco, S., et al. Protective effect of inhaled frusemide on allergen-induced early and late asthmatic reactions. *N. Engl. J. Med.* 321:1069, 1989.
2. Bianco, S., et al. Prevention of exercise-induced bronchoconstriction by inhaled frusemide. *Lancet* 2:252, 1988.
2a. Bjorck, T., Gustafsson, L., and Dahlen, S.-V. Isolated bronchi from asthmatics are hyperresponsive to adenosine, which apparently acts indirectly by liberation of leukotrienes and histamine. *Am. Rev. Respir. Dis.* 145:1087, 1992.
3. Casale, T. B., et al. Elevated bronchoalveolar lavage fluid histamine levels in allergic asthmatics are associated with methacholine responsiveness. *J. Clin. Invest.* 79:1197, 1987.
4. Church, M. K., and Holgate, S. T. Adenosine and asthma. *Trends Pharmacol. Sci.* 7:49, 1986.
5. Church, M. K., Holgate, S. T., and Hughes, P. J. Inosine inhibits and potentiates IgE-dependent histamine release from human basophils by an A_2-receptor mediated mechanism. *Br. J. Pharmacol.* 80:719, 1983.
6. Church, M. K., Hughes, P. J., and Varley, C. J. Studies on the receptor mediating cyclic AMP-independent enhancement by adenosine of IgE-dependent mediator release from rat mast cells. *Br. J. Pharmacol.* 87:233, 1986.
7. Clarke, H., et al. The protective effects of intravenous theophylline and enprofylline against histamine- and adenosine 5'-monophosphate-provoked bronchoconstriction: Implications for the mechanisms of action of xanthine derivatives in asthma. *J. Pulm. Pharmacol.* 2:147, 1989.
8. Crimi, N., et al. Enhancing effect of dipyridamole inhalation on adenosine-induced bronchospasm in asthmatic patients. *Allergy* 43:179, 1988.
9. Crimi, N., Palermo, F., and Polosa, R. Effect of indomethacin on adenosine-induced bronchoconstriction. *J. Allergy Clin. Immunol.* 83:921, 1989.
10. Crimi, N., Palermo, F., and Vancheri, C. Effect of sodium cromoglycate and nifedipine on adenosine-induced bronchoconstriction. *Respiration* 53:74, 1988.
11. Curzen, N., Rafferty, P., and Holgate, S. T. Effects of a cyclooxygenase inhibitor, flurbiprofen, and an H_1-histamine receptor antagonist, terfenadine, alone and in combination on allergen-induced immediate bronchoconstriction. *Thorax* 42:946, 1987.
12. Cushley, M. J., and Holgate, S. T. Adenosine-induced bronchoconstriction in asthma: Role of mast cell mediator release. *J. Allergy* 75:272, 1985.
13. Cushley, M. J., Tallant, N., and Holgate, S. T. The effect of single dose intravenous dipyridamole on histamine and adenosine-induced broncho-

constriction in normal and asthmatic subjects. *Eur. J. Respir. Dis.* 86:185, 1986.

14. Cushley, M. J., Tattersfield, A. E., and Holgate, S. T. Inhaled adenosine and guanosine on airway resistance in normal and asthmatic subjects. *Br. J. Clin. Pharmacol.* 15:161, 1983.

15. Cushley, M. J., Tattersfield, A. E., and Holgate, S. T. Adenosine-induced bronchoconstriction in asthma: Antagonism by inhaled theophylline. *Am. Rev. Respir. Dis.* 129:380, 1984.

16. Daillarguelo, C., Quinores, E., and Menardo, J.-L. Adenosine, exercise and fog bronchial challenges in asthmatic children. *J. Allergy Clin. Immunol.* 87:338, 1991.

17. Daxun, Z., et al. Airway refractoriness to adenosine 5'-monophosphate after repeated inhalation by atopic non-asthmatic subjects. *J. Allergy* 83:152, 1989.

18. Djukanovic, R., Finnerty, J. P., and Holgate, S. T. Wheal-and-flare responses to intradermally injected adenosine 5'-monophosphate, hypertonic saline, and histamine: Comparison of atopic and nonatopic subjects. *J. Allergy Clin. Immunol.* 84:373, 1989.

19. Eagle, K. A., and Boucher, C. A. Intravenous dipyridamole infusion causes severe bronchospasm in asthmatic patients. *Chest* 95:258, 1989.

20. Finnerty, J. P., Harvey, A., and Holgate, S. T. The contribution of histamine and prostanoids to bronchoconstriction provoked by isocapnic hyperventilation in asthma. *Eur. Respir. J.* Submitted.

21. Finnerty, J. P., and Holgate, S. T. Role of histamine and prostaglandins in EIA. *J. Allergy* 81:240, 1988.

22. Finnerty, J. P., and Holgate, S. T. The effect of repeat bronchial challenge with adenosine monophosphate (AMP) on exercise-induced bronchoconstriction in asthma. *Thorax* 44:865P, 1989.

23. Finnerty, J. P., Wilmot, C., and Holgate, S. T. Inhibition of hypertonic saline-induced bronchoconstriction by terfenadine and flurbiprofen: Evidence for the predominant role of histamine. *Am. Rev. Respir. Dis.* 140:593, 1989.

24. Flint, K. C., et al. Bronchoalveolar mast cells in extrinsic asthma: A mechanism for the initiation of antigen specific bronchoconstriction. *Br. Med. J.* 291:923, 1985.

25. Fredholm, B. B., Brodin, K., and Strandberg, K. On the mechanism of relaxation of tracheal muscle by theophylline and other cyclic nucleotide phosphodiesterase inhibitors. *Acta Pharmacol.* 45:336, 1979.

26. Holgate, S. T., Lewis, R. A., and Austen, K. F. Role of adenylate cyclase in immunologic release of mediators from rat mast cells: Agonist and antagonist effects of purine- and ribose-modified analogs. *Proc. Natl. Acad. Sci. USA* 70:6800, 1980.

27. Howarth, P. H., et al. The influence of atopy on the endobronchial appearance in atopic asthma: A comparison between atopic asthma, atopic non-asthma and non-atopic non-asthma. *Am. Rev. Respir. Dis.* 141(Suppl.):501, 1990.

28. Hughes, P. J., and Church, M. K. Separate purinoceptors mediate enhancement by adenosine of concanavalin A-induced mediator release and the cyclic AMP response in rat mast cells. *Agents Actions* 18:81, 1986.

29. Hughes, P. J., Holgate, S. T., and Church, M. K. Adenosine inhibits and potentiates IgE-dependent histamine release from human lung mast cells by an A_2-purinoceptor mediated mechanism. *Biochem. Pharmacol.* 33:3847, 1984.

30. Kirby, J. G., et al. Bronchoalveolar cell profiles of asthmatic and non-asthmatic subjects. *Am. Rev. Respir. Dis.* 136:379, 1987.

31. Lunell, E., et al. A novel bronchodilator xanthine apparently without adenosine antagonism or tremorgenic effect. *Eur. J. Respir. Dis.* 64:333, 1983.

32. Mann, J. S., Cushley, M. J., and Holgate, S. T. Adenosine-induced bronchoconstriction in asthma: Role of parasympathetic stimulation and adrenergic inhibition. *Am. Rev. Respir. Dis.* 132:1, 1985.

33. Mann, J. S., and Holgate, S. T. Specific antagonism of adenosine induced bronchoconstriction in asthma by oral theophylline. *Br. J. Clin. Pharmacol.* 19:685, 1985.

34. Mann, J. S., et al. Airway effects of purine nucleosides and nucleotides and release with bronchial provocation in asthma. *J. Appl. Physiol.* 61:1667, 1986.

35. Mann, J. S., Renwick, A. G., and Holgate, S. T. Release of adenosine and its metabolites from activated human leucocytes. *Clin. Sci.* 70:461, 1986.

36. Manning, P. J., Jones, G. L., and O'Byrne, P. M. Tachyphylaxis to inhaled histamine in asthmatic subjects. *J. Appl. Physiol.* 63:1572, 1987.

37. Marquardt, D. L., Parker, C. W., and Sullivan, T. J. Potentiation of mast cell mediator release by adenosine. *J. Immunol.* 120:871, 1978.

38. Marquardt, D. L., and Walker, L. L. Pretreatment with phorbol esters abrogates mast cell adenosine responsiveness. *J. Immunol.* 142:1268, 1989.

39. Marquardt, D. L., Walker, L. L., and Wasseman, S. I. Adenosine receptors on mouse bone marrow derived mast cells. Functional significance and regulation by aminophylline. *J. Immunol.* 133:932, 1984.

40. O'Byrne, P. M., and Jones, G. L. The effect of indomethacin on exercise-induced bronchoconstriction and refractoriness after exercise. *Am. Rev. Respir. Dis.* 134:69, 1986.

41. Pauwels, R. A., and van der Straeten, M. E. An animal model for adenosine-induced bronchoconstriction. *Am. Rev. Respir. Dis.* 136:374, 1987.

42. Peachell, P. T., et al. Inosine potentiates mediator release from human lung mast cells. *Am. Rev. Respir. Dis.* 138:1143, 1988.

43. Phillips, G. D., et al. The influence of refractoriness to adenosine 5'-monophosphate on allergen-provoked bronchoconstriction in asthma. *Am. Rev. Respir. Dis.* 140:321, 1989.

44. Phillips, G. D., and Holgate, S. T. Absence of a late response or increase in histamine responsiveness following bronchial provocation with adenosine 5'-monophosphate in atopic and non-atopic asthma. *Clin. Sci.* 75:429, 1988.

45. Phillips, G. D., and Holgate, S. T. The effect of oral terfenadine alone and in combination with flurbiprofen on the bronchoconstrictor response to inhaled adenosine 5'-monophosphate in non-atopic asthma. *Am. Rev. Respir. Dis.* 129:463, 1989.

46. Phillips, G. D., et al. The response of plasma histamine to bronchoprovocation with methacholine, adenosine 5'-monophosphate, and allergen in atopic non-asthmatic subjects. *Am. Rev. Respir. Dis.* 141:9, 1990.

47. Phillips, G. D., et al. Effect of nedocromil sodium and sodium cromoglycate against bronchoconstriction induced by inhaled adenosine 5'-monophosphate. *Eur. Respir. J.* 2:210, 1989.

48. Platshon, L. F., and Kaliner, M. The effect of the immunologic release of histamine on human lung cyclic nucleotide levels and prostaglandin generation. *J. Clin. Invest.* 62:1113, 1978.

49. Polosa, R., and Holgate, S. T. Cross tachyphylaxis to inhaled kinins in asthma and its implications for a receptor-mediated mechanism. *Eur. Respir. J.* 3(Suppl. 10):2795, 1990.

50. Polosa, R., et al. The effect of inhaled ipratropium bromide alone and in combination with oral terfenadine on bronchoconstriction provoked by adenosine-5'-monophosphate and histamine in asthma. *J. Allergy Clin. Immunol.* In press.

51. Rafferty, P., Beasley, C. R., and Holgate, S. T. The contribution of histamine to bronchoconstriction produced by inhaled allergen and adenosine 5'-monophosphate in asthma. *Am. Rev. Respir. Dis.* 136:369, 1987.

52. Rafferty, P., and Holgate, S. T. Terfenadine (Seldane) is a potent and selective H_1-histamine receptor antagonist in asthmatic airways. *Am. Rev. Respir. Dis.* 135:181, 1987.

53. Riberio, J. A., and Sebastico, A. M. Adenosine receptors and calcium: Basis for proposing a third (A_3) adenosine receptor. *Prog. Neurobiol.* 26:179, 1986.

54. Richards, R., Phillips, G. D., and Holgate, S. T. Nedocromil sodium is more potent than sodium cromoglycate against AMP-induced bronchoconstriction in atopic asthmatic subjects. *Clin. Exp. Allergy* 19:285, 1989.

55. Richards, R., et al. Inhalation rate of sodium cromoglycate determines plasma pharmacokinetics and protection against AMP-induced bronchoconstriction in asthma. *Eur. Respir. J.* 1:896, 1988.

56. Robuschi, M., et al. Inhaled frusemide is highly effective in preventing ultrasonically nebulised water bronchoconstriction. *Pulm. Pharmacol.* 1:187, 1989.

57. Scharabe, V. Subclassification of Adenosine Receptors (Pi-purinoceptors): Structure-activity Relationships, Transduction Mechanisms. In G. Burnstock (ed.), *Adenosine and ATP Receptors.* In press.

58. Srikiatkhachorn, A., White, D., and Strunk, R. C. Bronchial hyperreactivity to adenosine increases when theophylline is discontinued. *J. Allergy Clin. Immunol.* 87:312, 1991.

59. Summers, Q. A., et al. The protective efficacy of inhaled oral and intravenous nedocromil sodium against adenosine 5'-monophosphate induced bronchoconstriction in asthmatic volunteers. *J. Pulm. Pharmacol.* 3:190, 1990.

60. Wood-Baker, R., and Holgate, S. T. A comparative efficacy and adverse effect profile of single doses of H_1-receptor antagonists in the airways and skin of asthmatic subjects. *J. Clin. Exp. Ther.* In press.

Eosinophil

Andrew J. Wardlaw
A. Barry Kay

20

The association of eosinophils with asthma has been recognized since the beginning of this century [37], and necropsy studies done in patients dying of asthma have demonstrated a clear inflammatory component to the disease [35]. At one stage, eosinophils were thought to have an antiallergic effect because of their potential ability to degrade metabolites such as histamine [156]. In the last 10 years, in vitro studies have highlighted the capacity of the eosinophil to elaborate large amounts of potent inflammatory mediators with a potential for inducing the pathologic changes characteristic of asthma. In parallel with this, reports of clinical studies, particularly those using the fiberoptic bronchoscope to obtain samples of the airways from patients with mild asthma, have emphasized the presence of airway inflammation even in asymptomatic asthmatic patients. The characteristic changes in the airways in asthma, as detailed in Chapter 28, consist of collagen deposition beneath the basement membrane, epithelial desquamation, and increased numbers of activated eosinophils and T-lymphocytes. Although the patient populations in most studies have consisted of young atopic asthmatics, preliminary studies in patients with occupational and intrinsic asthma have yielded similar findings. A unifying hypothesis has therefore emerged, suggesting that the changes in the mucosa in asthma are largely the result of eosinophil products and that the eosinophil is recruited and activated by cytokines secreted by activated T-lymphocytes, and possibly other cells. Some general properties of eosinophils are reviewed in this chapter, as well as findings yielded by clinical studies which indicate that eosinophils play a role in the pathogenesis of asthma.

EOSINOPHIL MORPHOLOGY

Eosinophils are nondividing, granule-containing cells that arise principally in the bone marrow. They are 8 μm in diameter, and their granules avidly take up acidic dyes such as eosin, from which they got their name. The eosinophil granule is characteristic. Human eosinophils contain about twenty refractile granules that are often spherical or ovoid and are about 0.5 to 1.0 μm in diameter [89]. Ultrastructural studies have shown that the granules are bounded by a double-layered membrane, containing a rectangular or square, crystalline-like core that is surrounded by a less electron-dense matrix [12, 95]. The core is composed of major basic protein (MBP), and the matrix contains a number of other biologic agents, including the other three eosinophilic basic proteins. Mature eosinophils also contain a smaller granule that stains intensely for acid phosphatase and arylsulfatase [104]. The eosinophil nucleus is bilobed. Eosinophils have mitochondria, Golgi apparatus, ribosomes, and an endoplasmic reticulum which is better developed than that found in the neutrophil [62].

EOSINOPHIL DIFFERENTIATION

Eosinophils, like other leukocytes, differentiate myeloid from precursor cells in the bone marrow under the control of cytokine growth factors, of which interleukin-3 (IL-3), granulocyte/macrophage–colony stimulating factor (GM-CSF), and IL-5 are the ones active in promoting eosinophil differentiation [26, 116]. IL-5 is produced principally, if not solely, by T-lymphocytes [117]. In mice, a subset of cloned CD4$^+$ T-lymphocytes, termed *Th2 lymphocytes*, is characterized by the ability to secrete IL-4 and IL-5. This is in contrast to Th1 cells that secrete IL-2 and interferon gamma (IFN-γ) [99]. The genes encoding IL-3, GM-CSF, IL-4, and IL-5 are all located on the long arm of chromosome 5 [140]. There is some evidence, discussed later, that a similar pattern exists in humans, with the Th2 type predominating in allergic reactions and Th1-type responses seen in classic delayed-type hypersensitivity. Eosinophilia may therefore result from the activation of Th2 lymphocytes that are responding to parasite- or allergy-associated antigens. IL-3 and GM-CSF act on a number of leukocyte lineages, whereas human IL-5 appears to effect only eosinophil differentiation. Eosinophils appear to be related to basophils. In colony-forming assays, eosinophil and basophil colonies can appear together, suggesting a common precursor cell [87]. Furthermore, basophils also contain MBP and Charcot-Leyden crystals (CLCs) and are activated by IL-5 [13]. Neutrophil and monocyte differentiation appears to be quite distinct from eosinophilopoiesis.

It has long been recognized that the eosinophilia associated with parasitic helminth infections is T-cell dependent. Eosinophil proliferation in parasitized mice was found to be abolished by thymectomy, thoracic duct drainage, and antilymphocyte serum [10], and this effect was mediated by soluble factors released from sensitized lymphocytes [27]. It seems almost certain that this effect was due to one or more of the mediators already mentioned. The findings from in vitro studies suggested that IL-5 was only active on the committed eosinophil precursor that was acting as an eosinophil-differentiating factor, and that the proliferation of less committed precursors toward eosinophil differentiation was under the influence of other growth factors such as IL-3 and GM-CSF [26, 117, 164]. This idea has now been challenged by the observation that transgenic mice expressing the gene for IL-5 become markedly eosinophilic and exhibit increased numbers of eosinophil precursors in their bone marrow [32, 134]. Increased synthesis of IL-3 and GM-CSF was not observed in these animals, suggesting that IL-5 alone is sufficient to generate an eosinophilia from stem-cell precursors. Interestingly, the IL-5 transgenic mice appeared to be perfectly healthy. In addition, an antibody directed against IL-5 was able to abolish parasite-induced eosinophilia in mice [123]. If IL-5 alone were sufficient to mediate the eosinophilia observed in parasite infection, allergy, and other diseases, it would explain why eosino-

258

philia is often seen in isolation, without the expansion of other cell lineages.

Eosinophils can be cultured from human umbilical cord blood [116]. After 28 days in culture with IL-5 and IL-3, mononuclear cells in cord blood differentiate into eosinophils that are up to 95 percent pure. Cord blood eosinophils are morphologically and functionally similar to peripheral blood eosinophils [143]. Eosinophils can also be induced to differentiate from adult peripheral blood. The number of eosinophil precursors appears to be increased in the blood of atopic subjects after allergen challenge [53, 54]. The morphologic features of eosinophils as they differentiate have been well described, focusing in particular on the development of eosinophil granules [130]. Uncommitted stem cells express CD34, a cell-surface receptor of unknown function. As they differentiate, these cells become CD34$^-$, at which stage they are still mononuclear. They then develop nongranular, pink-staining cytoplasm with immature indented nuclei, as shown by May-Grünwald/Giemsa staining, and so become more mature, bilobed, granulated cells that stain with eosinophilic dyes [40, 115]. At present, little is known about the changes that occur in gene transcription and membrane receptor expression as the eosinophil differentiates.

There is also little information on eosinophil turnover in vivo. The results of labeling of blood eosinophils in normal individuals have suggested that their half-life in the circulation is 13 to 18 hours, similar to neutrophils, and it is prolonged in the presence of eosinophilia [130]. It is believed that eosinophils reside principally in the tissues, with approximately 500 eosinophils in the connective tissue for every circulating eosinophil. The effect of glucocorticoids (GCs), which cause a rapid eosinopenia, on eosinophil kinetics has not been studied.

EOSINOPHIL HETEROGENEITY

Peripheral blood eosinophils from normal individuals consist of dense cells that separate out from other leukocytes in the lower bands of Percoll or metrizamide, discontinuous-density gradients. These differences in density form the basis for one method of purifying eosinophils [138]. A proportion of eosinophils from individuals with a raised eosinophil count exhibit a lower density than do eosinophils from normal subjects [9]. Although the mechanism for this heterogeneity is not clear, it has been suggested that low-density eosinophils are degranulated. Low-density eosinophils appear to be vacuolated and contain smaller-sized granules, although their numbers are the same as those of normal-density eosinophils. Membrane ruffling, leading to changes in cell volume, may also lead to a decrease in density. The presence of low-density (or hypodense) eosinophils appears to be a nonspecific phenomenon that occurs in any eosinophilic condition, including asthma [50]. It is generally thought that low-density eosinophils are more activated. They exhibit increased oxygen consumption [162] and increased cytotoxicity toward helminthic targets [106]; they also release more leukotriene C$_4$ (LTC$_4$) after physiologic stimulation [122]. In vitro activation of eosinophils with inflammatory mediators such as platelet-activating factor (PAF), as well as long-term culture with cytokines, was also associated with a decrease in eosinophil density [49, 103, 112]. Eosinophils obtained by bronchoalveolar lavage (BAL) from patients with pulmonary eosinophilia showed a low density [107]. In contrast, there was no difference in receptor expression between normal- and low-density eosinophils [66]. The function of normal-density eosinophils from patients with eosinophilia is enhanced compared with the function of eosinophils from normal individuals. It is possible that the association between the low density and activation is coincidental, with the lower-density cells representing more immature cells. One of the problems in directly comparing normal- and low-density eosinophils is the difficulty in obtaining purified populations of low-density eosinophils, as the layers in which they are found are heavily contaminated with neutrophils and mononuclear cells.

EOSINOPHIL RECEPTORS

Like all leukocytes, eosinophils express a large number of membrane receptors through which they communicate with the extracellular environment (Fig. 20-1). This includes the recognition of soluble mediators, immunoglobulin complexes, and insoluble structures such as other leukocytes, vascular endothelium, and parasite targets. The expression of eosinophil receptors may be modulated by increased expression, a conformational change in the receptor moving from an unresponsive to a responsive state, or de novo expression. These changes in eosinophil phenotype may come about through the recruitment of receptors from intracellular stores, the synthesis of new receptors, or changes in the activation state of the receptor triggered by processes such as phosphorylation under the influence of inflammatory mediators.

Adhesion Receptors

A key aspect of leukocyte function is its ability to migrate from the vascular space into extracellular tissue. The initial step in this process is adherence to postvenular endothelium. This occurs as the result of an interaction between receptors on the surface of leukocytes and their ligands on the endothelial cell surface. An increasingly complex array of receptors is involved in this process (Table 20-1). They are grouped into several gene superfamilies, and include the integrin superfamily, members of the immunoglobulin superfamily, and another gene family termed the *selectins*. This last family is characterized by a lectin-binding domain, which is a domain homologous to the epithelial growth factor receptor, and repetitive motifs related to those found in complement regulatory proteins, such as decay-accelerating factor and C4-binding protein [128, 145]. Expression of the endothelial adhesion receptors, including intercellular adhesion molecule 1 (ICAM-1, CD54), endothelial-leukocyte adhesion molecule 1 (ELAM-1), and vascular-cell adhesion molecule 1 (VCAM-1), is markedly increased when the endothelial cell is stimulated for several hours with inflammatory mediators such as IL-1 or tumor necrosis factor-alpha (TNF-α).

The integrin superfamily consists of three members, defined by distinct though related beta chains: β1(CD29), β2(CD18), and β3 (GpIIIa, CD61). Each beta chain associates at the cell surface with a variable number of alpha chains. The β1 family has six members (α1 to α6 [CD49a–f]), the β2 integrin family, termed the *leukocyte integrins*, has three members (LFA-1, Mac-1, and p150,95 [CD11a–c]), and the β3 integrins have two members (GpIIB [CD41] and CD51). This convenient classification has become more complex with the characterization of alternate beta chains (β4 to β6). Mac-1 also functions as the complement receptor CR3, which binds one of the complement fragments, C3bi. In vitro assays of leukocyte adhesion to cultured human umbilical vein endothelial cells (HUVEC) have clarified the role of the individual receptors and their ligands in adhesion. Eosinophil adhesion to unstimulated HUVEC is upregulated by inflammatory mediators, including PAF [79]. This increase in adhesion appears to be mediated primarily through Mac-1, as it is almost totally abolished by anti–Mac-1 monoclonal antibodies (mAbs) [86]. IL-5 and IL-3 also upregulate eosinophil, but not neutrophil, adhesion to unstimulated endothelium, offering a selective pathway of eosinophil adhesion [142]. The adherence of both stimulated and unstimulated eosinophils to IL-1–stimulated HUVEC is increased compared with resting HUVEC. This adhesion is inhibited by mAbs directed against ICAM-1 and ELAM-1 on the endothelium and by mAb directed against LFA-1 and Mac-1 on the eosinophil

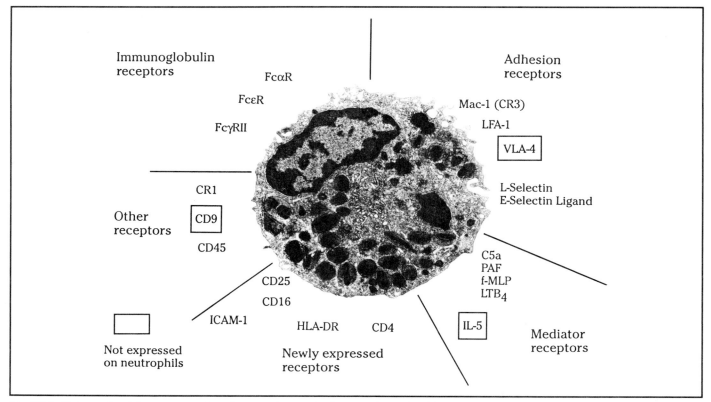

Fig. 20-1. *Major eosinophil receptors and an electron micrograph of a normal peripheral blood eosinophil. The characteristic granules can be clearly identified.* LFA-1 = *lymphocytic function–associated antigen 1;* ICAM-1 = *intercellular adhesion molecule 1;* PAF = *platelet-activating factor;* f-MLP = *formyl-methionyl-leucyl-phenylalanine;* LTB$_4$ = *leukotriene B$_4$;* IL-5 = *interleukin-5. (Kindly prepared by Ann Dewar, National Heart & Lung Institute, × 10,500.)*

Table 20-1. Adhesion receptors

Endothelial receptor	Gene family	Counter receptor	Gene family	Leukocyte
ICAM-1	Ig	LFA-1 + Mac-1	Integrin	All leukocytes
ICAM-2	Ig	LFA-1	Integrin	All leukocytes
VCAM-1	Ig	VLA-4	Integrin	EO + LO + MO
PECAM	Ig	PECAM + integrin	?	?
E-Selectin	Selectin	Sialated Lewis X	Carbohydrate	? all leukocytes
P-Selectin	Selectin	Sialated and nonsialated Lewis X	Carbohydrate	? all leukocytes
Sialated Lewis X	Carbohydrate	L-Selectin	Selectin	? all leukocytes

ICAM-1, ICAM-2 = intercellular adhesion molecule 1 and 2, respectively; VCAM-1 = vascular-cell adhesion molecule 1; LFA-1 = lymphocytic function–associated antigen 1; EO = eosinophil; LO = lymphocyte; MO = monocyte.

[84]. To this extent, the mechanism of eosinophil adhesion is very similar to that described for neutrophils. However, eosinophils, but not neutrophils, express α4β1 (VLA-4), which binds VCAM-1 on the surface of IL-1–stimulated endothelium. Eosinophil, but not neutrophil, adhesion to both IL-1–stimulated HUVEC and COS cells transfected with the VCAM-1 complementary DNA (cDNA) was observed to be inhibited by mAbs raised against α4β1 [144]. That this pathway may be functionally important has been suggested by observations made in patients with leukocyte adhesion deficiency (LAD), a rare autosomal recessive immuno-deficiency disease, which is due to mutations in the β2 chain as a result of which none of the leukocyte integrins (Mac-1, LFA-1, p150,95) are expressed on the leukocyte cell surface [4]. These patients are subject to life-threatening infections because their neutrophils cannot migrate out of the vascular space. At least one patient with LAD had eosinophils in their tissues, suggesting

that eosinophils were able to adhere to the endothelium. Expression of α4β1 by eosinophils but not neutrophils offers a second selective adhesion pathway for eosinophils that could explain in part why eosinophils, but not neutrophils, accumulate preferentially in tissues in the presence of diseases such as asthma and helminth infections (Fig. 20-2).

Eosinophils, like neutrophils, may also be able to adhere to extracellular matrix proteins such as fibronectin, collagen, and hyaluronate by means of specific receptors. These include α4β1, which also functions as a receptor for fibronectin, and CD44, which binds hyaluronate and is expressed on eosinophils. Interaction with matrix proteins may be important when the eosinophil has traversed the endothelium into the extracellular space.

The expression of Mac-1 on neutrophils, as detected by staining with a specific mAb and flow cytometry, can be rapidly and markedly increased by stimulation with inflammatory mediators

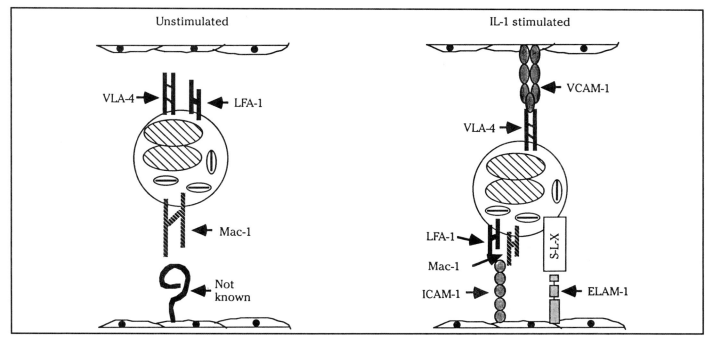

Fig. 20-2. *The adhesion receptors potentially involved in eosinophil migration from peripheral blood into tissue. Eosinophils can potentially use all three selectins for the initial adhesion and rolling step. The second step of flattening and transmigration could involve Mac-1 binding to an unidentified ligand on unstimulated endothelium and Mac-1, LFA-1, and VLA-4 binding to their respective ligands, ICAM-1, ICAM-2, and VCAM-1, on stimulated endothelium. Having migrated into the extracellular matrix, eosinophils could interact with fibronectin through VLA-4 and with other matrix proteins through as yet unidentified ligands. IL-1 = interleukin-1; LFA-1 = lymphocytic function–associated antigen 1; VCAM-1 = vascular-cell adhesion molecule 1; ICAM-1 = intercellular adhesion molecule 1; ELAM-1 = endothelial-leukocyte adhesion molecule 1.*

such as PAF [11]. This is because the Mac-1 is recruited from intracellular stores on the membrane of intracytoplasmic granules [7]. Increased membrane expression also occurs in eosinophils, but to a much lesser extent, and eosinophils have been shown to contain very little in the way of intracellular Mac-1 [20]. The Mac-1 on eosinophils is much more convincingly upregulated by incubation with IL-3, IL-5, and GM-CSF over a 24-hour period. This appears to be due to protein synthesis and is inhibited by dexamethasone at physiologic concentrations.

Immunoglobulin Receptors

The eosinophil expresses receptors for IgG, IgA, and IgD. The eosinophil also binds IgE in a specific manner [20], and eosinophils can undertake a number of IgE-dependent functions, including killing of schistosomes opsonized with specific IgE [21]. It was thought that the eosinophil IgE receptor was related to the low-affinity IgE receptor found on B-lymphocytes, platelets, and macrophages—FcεRII (CD23) [22]. However, peripheral blood eosinophils do not express messenger RNA (mRNA) for CD23 and do not stain with a panel of mAbs directed against this receptor [A. Hartnell, Personal communication, 1991]. The nature of eosinophil IgE binding therefore remains to be clarified.

There are three receptors for IgG: the high-affinity receptor FcγRI (CD64) and two low-affinity receptors FcγRII (CDw32) and FcγRIII (CD16) [137]. CD16 is expressed as two forms that are transcribed from two distinct, though closely related, genes. One form, found on neutrophils, is anchored to the cell membrane by a phosphatidylinositol linkage and the other form, found on natural killer cells, has a transmembrane anchor [21]. The functional significance of these two forms of CD16 is not clear. Only CD32 is constitutively expressed by eosinophils to any significant degree [103]. A number of eosinophil functions are mediated via this receptor, including schistosome killing, phagocytosis, the secretion of granule proteins, and the generation of newly formed, membrane-derived lipid mediators such as PAF and LTC₄. The different expressions of Fc receptors by freshly isolated eosinophils and neutrophils can be effectively utilized as an alternative to density-gradient centrifugation for purifying eosinophils from neutrophils by panning with a mAb directed against CD16. After stimulation for 2 days with IFN-γ, eosinophils express CD16 and CD64 as well as CD32, an example of the eosinophil-changing phenotype brought about by cytokine stimulation of protein synthesis.

The eosinophil also expresses IgA receptors that, when engaged by IgA-coated Sepharose beads, can trigger a substantial release of eosinophil granule proteins [1]. As eosinophils are often found at mucosal surfaces, this may be of physiologic importance.

Complement and Other Receptors

Eosinophils express low levels of CR1, a polymorphic single-chain glycoprotein of about 250 kd that binds the complement fragment C3b [42]. As noted already, CR3 (Mac-1), which binds C3bi, is strongly expressed on eosinophils.

The eosinophil receptor phenotype has still not been as exhaustively analyzed as the phenotypes of other leukocytes, and eosinophils likely express many receptors other than those already described. Few, if any, of these receptors are likely to be specific to eosinophils. An interesting feature of the eosinophil is its ability to express new receptors after prolonged (>48 hr) culture in a number of cytokines. For example, after culture in GM-CSF, eosinophils express HLA-DR antigens and increased amounts of ICAM-1 [91, 120; A. Hartnell, Personal communication, 1991]. This implies that the eosinophil has the potential to present antigen, and the findings from in vitro studies have suggested that eosinophils expressing HLA class II antigens do indeed have this function. In addition, eosinophils express CD4 after cytokine culture and can be infected with human immuno-deficiency virus [92].

Eosinophils express a number of antigens, such as CD9, of uncertain function that are also expressed by platelets. Some caution needs to be exercised in interpreting the expression of receptors found on platelets, as this expression could be due to platelet contamination. In addition, eosinophils respond to soluble mediators such as f-MLP (formyl-methionyl-leucyl-phenylalanine), C5a, C3a, and cytokines, as well as to lipid mediators such as PAF and IL-5, by means of specific receptors [25, 59, 82]. Receptors for the anaphylatoxins f-MLP and PAF belong to the rhodopsin family of guanosine 5'-triphosphate (GTP)–binding proteins [51, 70].

EOSINOPHIL MIGRATION

After differentiation in the bone marrow, eosinophils are released into the circulation and then migrate into tissue. The inhibition of eosinophil accumulation at sites of allergic inflammation is an obvious target for therapeutic manipulation, and the mechanism of eosinophil locomotion has been the subject of considerable study. Eosinophil locomotion is thought to be under the influence of chemotactic agents released at the inflammatory focus. Chemotaxis is an in vitro phenomenon usually demonstrated in a Boyden chamber, in which cells are placed in the top of the chamber and separated by a filter from the potential chemoattractant in the lower half of the chamber. Cells migrate through the filter along a concentration gradient under the influence of the chemoattractant. A large number of eosinophil chemotactic agents have been described. However, there are few that are very effective and none of these is specific (Table 20-2) [147]. The two most effective and fully characterized eosinophil chemotactic mediators are PAF and C5a [147]. Leukotriene B_4 (LTB_4), 5,15-dihydroxy-eicotetraenoic acid (5,15-DIHETE), and 8,15-DIHETE are chemotactic for eosinophils, although their activity is relatively weak. LTB_4 is more active against neutrophils. In the guinea pig, LTB_4 is very active against eosinophils but not neutrophils, and the reverse is the case for PAF [119]. In the early 1970s came the first reports of an eosinophilotactic activity in the supernatants of chopped lung from sensitized guinea pigs challenged with antigen [95]. This eosinophilic chemotactic factor of anaphylaxis (ECF-A) has been identified recently as a combination of 8,15-DIHETE and LTB_4 [119].

Table 20-2. Eosinophil chemotactic factors

Factor	Activity	Selective
Lipids		
PAF	High	No
LTB_4	Moderate	No
5,15-DIHete	Moderate	No
8,15-DIHete	Moderate	No
Peptides		
C5a	High	No
f-MLP	Weak	No
ECF-A tetrapeptides	Negligible	—
Cytokines		
IL-5[a,b]	Weak	Yes
IL-3[a,b]	Weak	Yes
GM-CSF[a]	Weak	No
IL-8	Weak	No

[a] Active only on eosinophils from normal individuals.
[b] IL-5 and IL-3 selectively and effectively prime eosinophils for increased response to other chemoattractants.
PAF = platelet-activating factor; LTB_4 = leukotriene B_4; 5,15- and 8,15-DIHETE = 5,15- and 8,15-dihydroxy-eicotetraenoic acid, respectively; GM-CSF = granulocyte/macrophage–colony stimulating factor; ECF-A = eosinophilic chemotactic factor of anaphylaxis; IL = interleukin; f-MLP = formyl-methionyl-leucyl-phenylalanine.

A similar, though weaker, activity was observed in human chopped lung tissue. Purification of this activity resulted in the isolation of two ECF-A tetrapeptides: Val-Gly-Ser-Glu and Ala-Gly-Ser-Glu [61]. However, these peptides proved ineffective in vivo and, when compared with PAF in the Boyden chamber assay, showed negligible activity [151]. The nature of human ECF-A is therefore uncertain. In addition, histamine and f-MLP exhibit very little chemotactic activity against unstimulated eosinophils.

A number of papers have reported eosinophilic chemotactic activity in mononuclear cell supernatants, which suggested that peptide cytokines may be active in promoting eosinophil locomotion [141]. Recombinant IL-5, GM-CSF, and IL-3 have been reported to have eosinophilic chemotactic activity in vitro against eosinophils purified from normal donors without an eosinophilia. However, the activity of IL-5 was only comparable to that of f-MLP [96, 152]. IL-2 and a 56-kd lymphocyte-derived chemotactic factor, which binds CD4 and is released after stimulation of lymphocytes with histamine, have been reported as being selectively chemotactic for eosinophils [155]. We have compared the activity of PAF with the activity of a number of purified cytokines, including IL-1, IL-2, IL-3, IL-5, IL-8, and GM-CSF, on eosinophils purified from subjects with a mild to moderate eosinophilia, and could only demonstrate negligible activity. IL-5, IL-3, and GM-CSF were weakly chemotactic for eosinophils from individuals with a normal eosinophil count, and IL-5 effectively primed the chemotaxis of these eosinophils toward PAF, LTB_4, and f-MLP. This difference in response to IL-5 between eosinophils from subjects with a mild eosinophilia and subjects with a normal blood eosinophil count may be due to in vivo desensitization.

There are relatively few studies investigating the in vivo effect of potential chemotactic agents in humans. PAF injected into the skin caused the accumulation of eosinophils in atopic individuals, but neutrophils were prominent in nonatopic subjects [69]. Increased numbers of neutrophils, but not eosinophils, appeared in BAL fluid 4 to 6 hours after the inhalation of PAF in a group of eight normal subjects, three of whom were atopic. Two of the atopic individuals did show a modest increase in eosinophil counts compared with controls who inhaled lyso-PAF [150]. It is possible that a highly effective but nonspecific mediator such as PAF combines with a selective but weakly chemotactic agent such as IL-5 to promote the specific accumulation of eosinophils in allergic disease.

PROLONGED TISSUE SURVIVAL

An alternative mechanism for a specific accumulation of eosinophils in tissue would be prolonged survival at the site of inflammation. The tissue survival time of eosinophils in vivo is not known. However, eosinophils, unlike neutrophils, can be maintained in culture for several days in the presence of IL-3, IL-5, and GM-CSF [103, 113, 114].

The fate of eosinophils in inflammatory reactions is not well understood. One possibility is that, on reaching their target, they degranulate and die. Alternatively, following degranulation they may recover, resynthesize their mediators, and undergo further degranulation. A third possibility is that they undergo apoptosis and phagocytosis by macrophages.

EOSINOPHIL MEDIATORS

Eosinophils have the capacity to secrete a number of potent mediators (Fig. 20-3). These include the basic proteins stored in eosinophil granules, lipid mediators that are newly formed after eosinophil stimulation, various eosinophil proteases, and components of the oxygen burst, including superoxide and hydrogen peroxide.

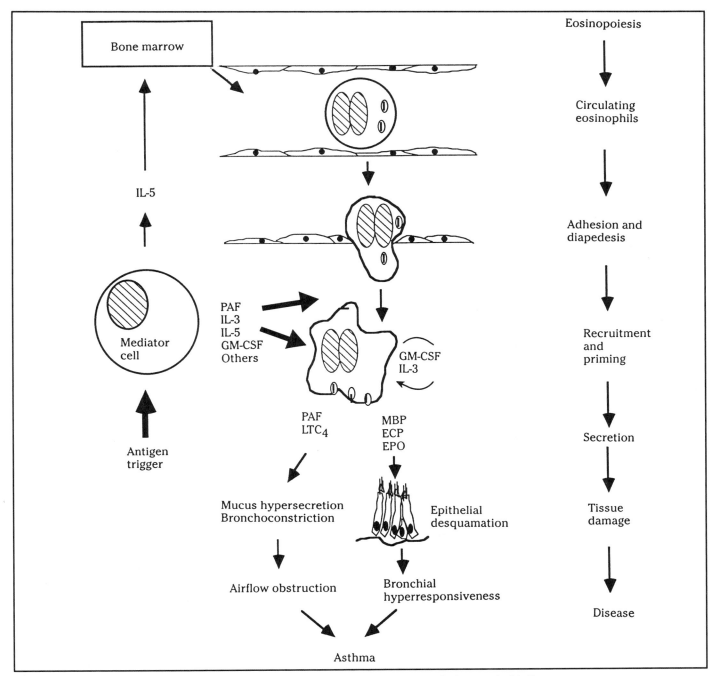

Fig. 20-3. *The possible mechanism of action of eosinophils in the pathogenesis of asthma. IL-5 = interleukin-5; PAF = platelet-activating factor; GM-CSF = granulocyte/macrophage colony–stimulating factor; LTC₄ = leukotriene C₄; MBP = major basic protein; ECP = eosinophil cationic protein; EPO = eosinophil peroxidase.*

Lipid Mediators

Eosinophils release relatively large amounts of the sulfidopeptide leukotriene LTC_4 (5S-hydroxy-6R,S-glutathionyl-7,9-*trans*-11,14-*cis*-eicosatetraenoic acid) [121, 158]. After stimulation with the calcium ionophore A23187, normal-density eosinophils generated up to 40 ng/10^6 cells of LTC_4 and light-density eosinophils generated up to 70 ng/10^6 cells, whereas neutrophils, monocytes, alveolar macrophages, and mast cells generated 7, 30, 10, and 25 ng/10^6 cells, respectively. In contrast, eosinophils produce only 6 ng/10^6 cells of LTB_4 (5S,12R-dihydroxy-6,14-*cis*-8,10-*trans*-eicosatetraenoic acid) compared with up to 200 ng/10^6 cells from

neutrophils. Eosinophils can also generate substantial quantities of 15-HETE via the 15-lipoxygenase pathway. LTC_4 generation by human eosinophils was also observed after stimulation with both opsonized zymosan and via an FcγII-dependent mechanism using Sepharose beads coated with IgG [122]. Release was maximal at 45 minutes, greater in hypodense eosinophils than in normal-density eosinophils, and enhanced by f-MLP.

PAF (1-O-alkyl-2-acetyl-*sn*-glycerol-3-phosphatidylcholine) is a potent phospholipid mediator that causes leukocyte activation and a prolonged increase in bronchial hyperresponsiveness in humans (Chap. 22). Eosinophils generate large amounts of PAF after both stimulation with calcium ionophore, zymosan, and

IgG-coated Sepharose beads [29, 51, 68, 88]. After IgG stimulation, eosinophils released up to 2 ng/10⁶ cells of PAF. Neutrophils released about 0.5 ng/10⁶ cells. About 25 ng/10⁶ cells were released after stimulation with calcium ionophore. Much of the PAF remained cell associated and was either intracellular, possibly acting as an intracellular messenger, or was bound to PAF receptors on eosinophils and acted as an autocrine agent. Interestingly, stimulation of eosinophils with f-MLP did not augment PAF release, and hypodense eosinophils from patients with a marked eosinophilia released less PAF than did normal eosinophils. [³H]PAF was added to normal- and low-density eosinophils, together with calcium ionophore, and the products analyzed by DIOL-HPLC. The [³H]PAF added to the hypodense cells was much more rapidly incorporated into the phospholipid pool than was the [³H]PAF from the normal-density cells. This suggests that the hypodense cells were metabolizing the exogenous PAF at a greater rate than were the normal-density cells, and may explain why stimulation with f-MLP did not result in an increased generation of PAF. As with leukotriene synthesis, release of PAF was maximal at 45 minutes.

Eosinophils also generate mediators of the cycloxygenase pathway, including prostaglandins E_1 and E_2 and thromboxane B_2. This pathway has not been so well studied as the lipoxygenase pathway. In addition, Morita and colleagues [98] reported that eosinophils release a lipid mediator similar but distinct from 5,15-DIHETE upon incubation with arachidonic acid. This mediator had potent eosinophilic chemotactic activity.

Eosinophil Granule Proteins

A characteristic feature of eosinophils are the four basic proteins stored in the crystalloid granules found in the eosinophil cytoplasm. MBP is found in the electron-dense granule core, and eosinophil-derived neurotoxin (EDN), eosinophil cationic protein (ECP), and eosinophil peroxidase (EPO) are located in the surrounding matrix [56].

The cDNA for MBP has been obtained and the full amino acid sequence deduced [8]. MBP has a molecular weight of 13.801 and a pI of 10.9. It contains 17 arginine residues, which accounts for its basicity. MBP is initially synthesized as a proprotein. The proprotein is acidic and may neutralize MBP's toxicity while it is stored in the eosinophil granule. The function of MBP and the other basic proteins has recently been reviewed by Gleich [55]. Purified MBP was shown to be cytotoxic for the schistosomes of *Schistosoma mansoni*, and adherence of eosinophils to IgG-coated schistosomes resulted in the secretion of MBP onto the integument of the larvae, which were killed shortly afterward [18]. MBP at a concentration as low as 10 μg/ml has also been shown to be toxic for both guinea pig and human respiratory epithelial cells, as well as for rat and human pneumocytes [5, 47, 57, 67, 100]. MBP caused exfoliation and bleb formation of epithelial cells in guinea pig tracheal organ cultures as soon as 6 hours after incubation with 50 μg/ml of both native and alkylated MBP (MBP contains at least four reactive sulfhydryl groups that are stabilized by alkylation). Partial ciliostasis was observed by 12 hours. The mechanism of action of MBP on epithelial cells appears to be mediated through the inhibition of ATPase activity. When MBP was applied to the mucosal surface of dog tracheal membranes, it caused an increase in chloride secretion that was not due to a cytotoxic effect, as lactate dehydrogenase was not detected [72]. The inhalation of MBP, albeit at high concentrations (1 mg/ml), caused bronchial hyperresponsiveness in a nonhuman primate model of asthma [64]. The effect of MBP as well as the other basic proteins does not appear to be simply a function of their negative charge, as other cationic proteins such as polylysine and polyarginine do not have the same effect. MBP and EPO have recently been shown to be strong agonists for platelet activation [109]. Basophils also contain MBP, but only about 140 ng/10⁶ cells compared with up to 5,000 ng/10⁶ cells for normal-density eosinophils.

EPO is a heme-containing protein composed of a 14,000 (light)– and a 58,000 (heavy)–dalton subunit derived from the same mRNA and subsequently cleaved. The cDNA also demonstrates the presence of a prosequence. EPO shares a 68 percent amino acid identity with human neutrophil myeloperoxidase as well as other peroxidase enzymes. EPO is toxic for parasites, respiratory epithelium, and pneumocytes, both in its own right and even more potently when combined with H_2O_2 and halide, the preferred ion in vivo being bromide [55].

ECP is an arginine-rich protein with a pI of 10.8. The cDNA encodes for a 27 amino acid leader sequence and a 133 amino acid, mature polypeptide with a molecular mass of 15.6 kd. ECP shows 66 percent amino acid homology with EDN and 31 percent homology with human pancreatic ribonuclease [110]. Like EDN, it has ribonuclease activity but is 100-fold less active [126]. It appears to be expressed only in eosinophils or eosinophilic cell lines. ECP is toxic for helminthic parasites, isolated myocardial cells, and guinea pig tracheal epithelium, although the effect in the guinea pig preparation was not marked and was only seen at high concentrations [55]. ECP also inhibits lymphocyte proliferation in vitro [105]. Both ECP and EDN produce neurotoxicity (the Gordon phenomenon) when injected into the cerebrospinal fluid of experimental animals. ECP may damage cells by a colloid osmotic process, as it can introduce non-ion-selective pores in both cellular and synthetic membranes [166]. The secreted form of ECP differs structurally and antigenically from the stored form. This difference has been used to differentiate between resting eosinophils and activated eosinophils in which active secretion is occurring, with mAb EG1 recognizing the stored form and mAb EG2 the activated state [131].

EDN, also called EPX, is a 16-kd glycosylated protein possessing marked ribonuclease activity. The cDNA predicts a 134 amino acid, mature polypeptide which is identical to that reported for human urinary ribonuclease. Like ECP, it is a member of a ribonuclease multigene family [111]. EDN expression is not restricted to eosinophils, as it is found in mononuclear cells and possibly neutrophils. It is also probably secreted by the liver. It does not appear to be toxic to parasites or mammalian cells and its only known function, other than its ribonuclease activity, is the neurotoxicity exhibited in the Gordon phenomenon [45].

A major constituent of eosinophils is CLC protein whose characteristic crystals have been recognized since the nineteenth century as being pathognomonic of a tissue eosinophilia. CLC has been shown to be lysophospholipase. It constitutes up to 10 percent of eosinophil protein and is also found in large quantities in basophils, thus highlighting the similarities between these two cell types. Its function is not clear [157].

Other Eosinophil-derived Mediators

In addition to the basic proteins and CLC, eosinophils may be able to synthesize a number of other peptides with mediator function. One study demonstrated mRNA expression for vasoactive intestinal peptide in granulomas from mice infected with schistosomes and, using in situ hybridization, localized expression to eosinophils in the granuloma [154]. Another study, also using in situ hybridization, detected mRNA expression of IL-1 in murine peritoneal–derived eosinophils [30]. Activated eosinophils have also been shown to secrete significant amounts of transforming growth factor-alpha [163]. We, and others, have demonstrated that, after stimulation with calcium ionophore and IFN-γ, eosinophils express mRNA for GM-CSF and IL-3, which is translated into protein and then secreted [87, 97]. The full secretory potential of eosinophils is likely to be considerable.

The eosinophil contains a number of granule-stored enzymes whose role in eosinophil function is not clear. These have been reviewed by Spry [129]. They include acid phosphatase (large amounts of which have been isolated from eosinophils), collagenase, arylsulfatase B, histaminase, phospholipase D, catalase, nonspecific esterases, vitamin B_{12}–binding proteins, and glycosaminoglycans. Eosinophils, unlike neutrophils, do not appear to contain elastase or other nonspecific neutral proteases. Eosinophils can undergo a respiratory burst with release of superoxide ion and H_2O_2 in response to stimulation with both particulate stimuli, such as opsonized zymosan, and soluble mediators, such as LTB_4 and phorbol myristate acetate. Eosinophils can generate twice as much chemoluminescence as neutrophils, and the capacity of the eosinophil to generate chemoluminescence and reactive oxygen species is increased in the presence of allergic rhinitis and hookworm infections [124, 159]. This process is assumed to play an important part in eosinophil cytotoxicity.

EOSINOPHIL CYTOTOXICITY

It has generally been considered that the teleologic role of eosinophils is to combat parasitic helminth infections [16]. The ability of eosinophils to kill parasites such as the schistosomes of *S. mansoni* [17] and the observation that larvae in tissue are surrounded by eosinophils have supported this concept, although it has been undermined recently by findings from studies in which the parasite-induced eosinophilia in mice was abolished by anti–IL-5 antibodies without any clear effect on the response to parasite infection [123].

Eosinophils can kill schistosomes after they have been opsonized with IgG, IgE, or complement. Eosinophils activated by a wide range of inflammatory mediators are more effective at killing schistosomes, and indeed schistosome killing has been a very useful assay for the identification of eosinophil-active mediators. Schistosome killing appears to involve an adherence stage, which is quite rapid, followed by close attachment of the eosinophil to the tegument of the schistosome. Over about a 3-hour period, the eosinophil secretes its proteins onto the surface of the larvae, the tegument is breached, and eosinophils appear to crawl under it and strip the tegument away [93]. Eosinophils are relatively ineffective at killing bacteria, possibly because they phagocytose small particles poorly. Neutrophils can also kill schistosomes, but less effectively than eosinophils, at least after opsonization with IgG. In contrast, monocytes and neutrophils are much more effective than eosinophils in killing both hybridoma cells, which secrete antibody against the individual Fcγ receptors, and chicken erythrocytes, which are opsonized with heterotypic antibodies directed against the individual Fcγ receptors and the cell surface of the erythrocyte [39]. The reasons for the discrepancy between schistosome killing and cytotoxicity against other targets is not clear. A further illustration of the target specificity of granulocyte killing was illustrated by another study in which eosinophils were more effective at killing Daudi lymphoma cells coated with specific IgG than were neutrophils via a FcγRII–dependent pathway [139].

EOSINOPHIL SECRETION AND ACTIVATION

One of the most striking features of eosinophil-rich inflammatory reactions is the marked deposition of large amounts of granule proteins, demonstrated by immunofluorescence with specific mAbs, often in the presence of relatively small numbers of intact eosinophils. Secretion appears to be more pronounced if the eosinophil is confronted by a large target such as a parasite or Sepharose bead rather than by phagocytizable stimuli such as zymosan. In vitro, secretion can be triggered physiologically by means of the engagement of the IgG and IgA Fc receptors [1]. IgE-dependent secretion has also been described [19]. The role of other receptors in triggering eosinophil secretion, particularly the CR3 and CR1 receptors, is less certain. The killing of schistosomes opsonized with serum is thought to be mediated via the CR3 and CR1 receptors, and incubation of eosinophils with serum-coated Sepharose beads resulted in the release of 15 percent of the ECP [161]. Again, secretion was presumed to be mediated through the C3 complement receptors. This low amount of secretion is characteristic of the release of eosinophil granule proteins, suggesting that other pathways may be involved, although recovery of granule proteins may be artificially low due to their inherent stickiness. Similarly, opsonized zymosan interacts with eosinophils, causing the generation of hydrogen peroxide and the phagocytosis of zymosan [165]. Soluble mediators such as PAF and LTB_4 elicit both the direct secretion of granules and the new formation of mediators [48], although this is a relatively ineffective stimulus. They also enhance secretion mediated through Fc receptor triggering [80]. Interestingly, differential secretion of granule proteins depending on the stimulus has been reported. IgG complexes induced the secretion of ECP but not EPO, whereas IgE complexes induced the secretion of EPO but not ECP [23, 78]. Secretion was low in both instances, however. If differential secretion does occur in vivo, it may explain the different pathologic conditions associated with eosinophil infiltration. It is not clear what leads to eosinophil secretion in vivo, particularly in those circumstances in which immune complexes do not obviously play a part, as in asthma.

The intracellular events leading to secretion were studied by Nusse and coworkers [102] who measured secretion of the lysosomal enzyme hexosaminidase from guinea pig eosinophils permeabilized with streptolysin-O and by whole-cell patch-clamp capacitance measurements. Eosinophils release their granule components by exocytosis, with individual granules fusing with the plasma membrane. This process involves a GTP-binding protein and is modulated by the intracellular calcium concentration. The mechanism of release is therefore very similar to that observed for neutrophils and mast cells.

Several cytokines have a marked effect on eosinophil function. IL-5, besides being a growth factor for eosinophils, also selectively stimulates a number of mature human eosinophil functions, including prolonged survival, cytotoxicity toward helminth targets, and increased adhesion to vascular endothelium [90, 114, 144]. IL-3 and GM-CSF have similar though less specific activities [103, 113]. The effects of IFN-γ appear to be more restricted to functions associated with Fcγ receptors. TNF-α stimulated eosinophil cytotoxicity toward schistosomes, oxidant production, and toxicity toward endothelium [125, 127]. IL-3, IL-5, and GM-CSF have both short-term effects on eosinophils, which are maximal within an hour and do not depend on protein synthesis, and more long-term effects, which are seen with in vitro culture of eosinophils including increased receptor expression and depend on protein synthesis. The biochemical basis for these differences is not known.

EOSINOPHILS AND ASTHMA

The association between eosinophils, asthma, and allergic disease has been known for many years. It is well established that large numbers of eosinophils together with mononuclear cells are frequently found in and around the bronchi in patients who have died of asthma. The immunostaining of bronchial tissue from such patients has revealed the existence of large amounts of MBP deposited in the airways [41]. The presence of increased numbers of peripheral blood eosinophils in both atopic and nonatopic chronic asthma is well known, although this elevation is not as great as that seen in other eosinophil-associated diseases and the eosinophil count is often normal in asthmatic individuals. Horn and colleagues [71], in a longitudinal study of 14 oral corticosteroid–dependent asthmatics being treated at a chest clinic, on 44 separate occasions found that eosinophil counts correlated with several measurements of airflow obstruction. Durham and Kay [36] found that the degree of bronchial hyperreactivity inversely correlated with the peripheral blood eosinophil count in patients developing a late-phase response after antigen challenge, and these observations were supported by findings from a cross-sectional study of asthmatics seen at a routine chest clinic where a similar correlation was observed [132].

Full appreciation of the extent of eosinophil involvement in asthma has come with the use of fiberoptic bronchoscopy which can obtain tissue specimens from the airways in patients with mild to moderate asthma. Over the last 10 years, a number of studies have been performed on both steady-state asthmatics and in patients after allergen challenge, performing both BAL and endobronchial biopsy of the large airways. This has proved to be a safe approach in experienced hands when appropriate selection procedures are used and adequate precautions taken [101, 146]. However, this technique is potentially hazardous, particularly in asthmatics with marked bronchial hyperresponsiveness. The ability to select subjects for study has made possible controlled trials of nonsmoking individuals, with asthma of carefully documented severity.

Antigen Challenge Studies

When challenged with inhaled antigen, sensitized asthmatics exhibit an early response of short duration. About 40 percent of subjects then exhibit a further fall in their 1-second forced expiratory volume (FEV_1), which is delayed by about 6 hours and lasts for 6 to 12 hours. This is termed the *late-phase response*. The early response is thought to be due to the release of bronchoconstrictor mediators from mast cells, whereas the late response is thought to result from a secondary influx of inflammatory cells, thereby more closely mimicking the pathologic characteristics of day-to-day asthma (see Chap. 12 for details).

An early study of BAL in patients with asthma revealed that the late response to allergen challenge was associated with the migration of large numbers of eosinophils into the airways and an increased ECP–albumin ratio in the lavage fluid [31]. Eosinophilia was not seen in subjects who had only a single early reaction or those lavaged before the development of the late response. This suggested that eosinophils were important for the development of the late-phase response. Diaz and associates [33] lavaged 14 asthmatics 6 hours after allergen challenge, seven of whom had a late-phase response. They found increased numbers of eosinophils and, to a lesser extent, neutrophils only in those subjects who had a dual response. This observation was confirmed by Metzger and coworkers [94] using a technique of local allergen challenge administered through the bronchoscope. They found increased numbers of both eosinophils and neutrophils, as did Casale and colleagues [24], who used the same technique, as well as two groups of researchers working with patients who had occupational asthma. Lam and associates [85] found an increased number of eosinophils and epithelial cells, and, after 48 hours, neutrophils in patients with red cedar asthma. Fabbri and colleagues [38] found that the numbers of neutrophils and eosinophils were increased in lavage fluid obtained from patients with asthma induced by toluene diisocyanate; in these patients, eosinophil influx occurred a few hours after the appearance of neutrophils. The pathologic changes that take place in the airways after allergen challenge therefore seem similar to those in the skin and nose, in that there is a brief initial reaction, probably due to the bronchospasm secondary to the release of mast cell–derived mediators, and then a more delayed response characterized by the influx of inflammatory cells, including activated lymphocytes, eosinophils, and neutrophils [46].

The pathologic changes that occur in patients with day-to-day asthma have also been intensively studied. Godard and associates [60] found that patients with asthma and idiosyncratic reactions to aspirin had large numbers of eosinophils in lavage fluid. Tomioka [135] and Flint [43] and their coworkers, though primar-

ily interested in the role of mast cells in asthma, both found increased numbers of eosinophils as well as mast cells in the lavage fluid from mild atopic asthmatics. We performed a cross-sectional study in 17 patients with mild atopic asthma [149]. Nine were symptomatic at the time of lavage, requiring only daily inhaled β2 agonists, and eight were asymptomatic. There was a significant increase in the number of eosinophils in the symptomatic asthmatics compared with the findings in subjects with allergic rhinitis but no asthma and nonatopic nonasthmatic subjects. There were no differences in the eosinophil counts in the asymptomatic group compared with that in controls. However, those subjects who were asymptomatic but showed airway hyperresponsiveness (methacholine PC_{20} < 4 mg/ml [provocation concentration producing a 20 percent fall in FEV_1]) did have increased eosinophil counts. The concentration of MBP in the BAL fluid was increased and levels correlated with the eosinophil counts in BAL fluid. A number of other studies have confirmed that eosinophils are consistently increased in BAL fluid from asthmatic subjects [44, 77, 80]. This BAL eosinophilia in the absence of interstitial lung disease appears to be a relatively specific feature of asthma [3]. The numbers of eosinophils in BAL fluid are generally only modestly raised in patients with asthma, ranging from 1 to 5 percent (normals, <1%), although occasionally eosinophil counts can be in the range of 30 to 50 percent.

Endobronchial biopsy specimens from asthmatics have told a similar story, with increased numbers of activated eosinophils in the submucosa as shown by positive staining with the mAb EG2, which stains the secreted form of ECP [6, 34]. Most studies have been performed on atopic asthmatics. However, it is likely that the cellular profiles in the airways of patients with occupational asthma and intrinsic asthma are similar. Our group compared the airway immunohistologic characteristics of seven atopic asthmatics with those of 10 patients with intrinsic asthma, 9 with occupational asthma, and 12 control subjects. The control subjects had no eosinophils in the submucosa as determined by staining with EG2, whereas the three groups of asthma patients had activated eosinophils in the submucosa; however, the occupational asthmatics had slightly less than the extrinsic and intrinsic asthmatics [A. M. Bentley, Personal communication, 1991].

It is therefore clear that eosinophils are closely associated with the development of asthma and bronchial hyperresponsiveness. The evidence that this is a cause-and-effect relationship is still largely circumstantial, although inhibition of the migration of eosinophils into the airways of allergen-challenged nonhuman primates, using an mAb directed against the adhesion molecule ICAM-1, also inhibited the development of airway hyperresponsiveness [153]. We found that the eosinophil counts were increased only in asthmatics who had airway hyperresponsiveness. Similarly, Bousquet and colleagues [14], in a study of 45 asthmatics and 10 controls, found that there was an increased number of eosinophils in the peripheral blood, BAL fluid, and bronchial biopsy specimens in asthmatics and that there was a significant increase in the level of eosinophilia, with increasing clinical severity as measured by a nonlinear scoring system described by Aas. However, there does not appear to be a direct linear correlation between the degree of bronchial hyperresponsiveness and the degree of eosinophilic inflammation in asthmatics. For example, in our study, the most hyperresponsive subject had one of the lowest BAL eosinophil counts. This suggests that another factor, independent of airway inflammation, controls the degree of airway hyperresponsiveness.

If eosinophils are required for the development of airflow obstruction and hyperresponsiveness, are these abnormalities an inevitable consequence of eosinophilic inflammation of the airways? Eosinophils are present in the airways of some atopic individuals with rhinitis who do not have airflow obstruction and have a PC_{20} in the normal range. One study investigated a group of patients with chronic productive cough responsive to corticosteroids who had eosinophils in the sputum but no evidence of asthma [52]. For eosinophils to cause tissue damage in the airways, they need to be actively secreting their mediators. Measurements of eosinophilic basic proteins may therefore be a better gauge of eosinophilic inflammation than numbers of eosinophils. We found that, although the number of eosinophils in BAL fluid from some asymptomatic asthmatics and atopic non-asthmatics was in the symptomatic asthmatic range, none of the patients had increased amounts of MBP. In addition, Adelroth and coworkers [2] found that, whereas inhaled corticosteroids had no effect on the number of eosinophils in BAL fluid from asthmatics, they markedly reduced the amounts of ECP in lavage fluid.

Glucocorticoids are highly effective drugs for the treatment and prevention of asthma. They are also able to inhibit the migration of eosinophils into sites of allergic inflammation and cause a marked eosinopenia, thus providing a further link between eosinophils and asthma [118]. In addition, inhaled GCs ameliorate bronchial hyperresponsiveness [73]. The mechanism of action of GCs in asthma is not clear. Most reports of the effects of GC on eosinophils in vitro have noted that only high concentrations of GC inhibit eosinophil function, although eosinophils do possess GC receptors and we have found that GCs inhibit the cytokine upregulation of eosinophil receptor expression at physiologic doses. A possible source of action is through inhibition of the release of eosinophil-active cytokines from activated T-cells, as it is well recognized that GCs are potent inhibitors of T-cell function.

For many years it was believed that mast cell–derived mediators were responsible for the accumulation of eosinophils in the airways in patients with asthma. However, this now appears to be less likely. Although the numbers of mast cells are increased in BAL fluid from asthmatics, the proportions remain small (0.2% in asthmatics versus 0.02% in normal controls). This is also a nonspecific finding, as similar numbers were found in a range of lung diseases [148]. Effective inhibitors of mast cell degranulation in vitro, such as sodium cromoglycate and nedocromil sodium, are relatively ineffective in treating patients with asthma when compared to corticosteroids, which do not inhibit IgE-mediated degranulation of lung mast cells in vitro and fail to prevent the early response to inhaled allergens in sensitized individuals, which is thought to be mediated by mast cells. In addition, although mast cell–derived supernatants do have eosinophilotactic activity, this is not specific for eosinophils, and the ECF-A tetrapeptides, which were once thought to play a major part in eosinophil recruitment, are ineffective in promoting eosinophil migration. In contrast, there is increasing evidence for T-cell activation in asthma (Chap. 13) [74]. Activated T-cells, as defined by the expression of the IL-2 receptor CD25, are found in increased numbers in the peripheral blood from patients with acute severe asthma [28] and in the BAL fluid and endobronchial biopsy specimens from mild asthmatics [6, 108]. We have found that sites of allergic inflammation, including BAL-derived leukocytes from atopic asthmatics, are characterized by expression of mRNA for IL-5, IL-4, IL-3, and GM-CSF, as detected by in situ hybridization; there were low levels of expression of mRNA for IL-2 and IFN-γ [65, 76, 108]. This pattern of cytokines is particularly intriguing, as it corresponds to the pattern seen in Th2-cell subsets described in mice. Tuberculin reactions in the skin, as a model of delayed-type hypersensitivity reactions, showed a different pattern of expression that was consistent with a Th1 pattern of T-cell activation; in this setting, there was a high expression of IL-2 and IFN-γ and negligible expression of IL-3, IL-4, IL-5, and GM-CSF [136]. In addition, T-cell clones from atopic individuals, raised against house-dust-mite antigen, secreted IL-2 and IL-4, whereas T-cell clones from nonatopic individuals, raised against the same antigen, secreted IL-2 and IFN-γ [160]. Thus, exposure to allergens in atopic individuals may be associated with activation of a subset of T-cells that preferentially expresses eosinophil-active cytokines. If this is the case, then intrinsic asthma may be due to a response to an antigen, not recognized as an allergen, which stimulates a Th2-type response in some individuals. However, it should be noted that mast cells have been shown to secrete a large number of cytokines, including those active on eosinophils after IgE-mediated stimulation [63]. The evidence implicating the eosinophil and CD4+ helper T-lymphocytes in allergic asthma has been recently reviewed by Kay [167].

In conclusion, the eosinophil is able to release large amounts of potent mediators, the effects of which could produce the pathologic changes characteristic of asthma. In particular, the basic proteins have been shown to cause epithelial desquamation, and PAF and LTC$_4$, to cause mucus hypersecretion and bronchoconstriction. Activated eosinophils appear to be almost invariably present in increased numbers in the airways of asthmatics, although there are anecdotal reports of patients dying of asthma who exhibit no evidence of eosinophils in their airways [58]. While it must not be forgotten that eosinophils may be innocent bystanders in the airways, or even play a reparative role, a convincing hypothesis has emerged which proposes that asthma is due to eosinophilic inflammation of the airways, possibly brought about by the release of eosinophil-active cytokines from a Th2 subset of activated T-lymphocytes (see Fig. 20-3). This offers several targets for therapeutic action, including inhibition of T-cell–derived mediator release; inhibition of eosinophil migration, possibly by blocking eosinophil-specific adhesion to vascular endothelium; inhibition of eosinophil activation; or antagonism of eosinophil-derived mediators. The development of drugs that have these properties will help to determine if this hypothesis is correct.

REFERENCES

1. Abu-Ghazaleh, R. I., et al. IgA-induced eosinophil degranulation. *J. Immunol.* 142:2393, 1989.
2. Adelroth, E., et al. Inflammatory cells and eosinophilic activity in asthma investigated by bronchoalveolar lavage. The effects of anti-asthmatic treatment with budesonide or terbutaline. *Am. Rev. Respir. Dis.* 142:91, 1990.
3. Allen, J. N., Davis, W. B., and Pacht, E. R. Diagnostic significance of increased bronchoalveolar lavage fluid eosinophils. *Am. Rev. Respir. Dis.* 142:642, 1990.
4. Anderson, D. C., and Springer, T. A. Leukocyte adhesion deficiency: an inherited defect in the Mac-1, LFA-1 and p150,95 glycoproteins. *Annu. Rev. Med.* 38:175, 1987.
5. Ayars, G. H., et al. Eosinophil and eosinophil granule–mediated pneumocyte injury. *J. Allergy Clin. Immunol.* 76:595, 1985.
6. Azzawi, M., et al. Identification of activated T lymphocytes and eosinophils in bronchial biopsies in stable atopic asthma. *Am. Rev. Respir. Dis.* 142:1407, 1990.
7. Bainton, D. F., et al. Leukocyte adhesion receptors are stored in peroxidase-negative granules of human neutrophils. *J. Exp. Med.* 166:1641, 1987.
8. Barker, R. L., Gleich, G. J., and Pease, L. R. Acidic precursor revealed in human eosinophil granule major basic protein cDNA. *J. Exp. Med.* 168:1493, 1988.
9. Bass, D. A., et al. Comparison of human eosinophils from normals and patients with eosinophilia. *J. Clin. Invest.* 66:1265, 1980.
10. Basten, A., and Beeson, P. B. Mechanism of eosinophilia. II. Role of the lymphocyte. *J. Exp. Med.* 131:1288, 1970.
11. Berger, M., et al. Human neutrophils increase expression of C3bi as well as C3b receptors upon activation. *J. Clin. Invest.* 74:1566, 1984.
12. Bessis, M., and Thiery, H. Electron microscopy of human white blood cells and their stem cells. *Int. Rev. Cytol.* 12:199, 1961.
13. Bischoff, S. C., et al. Interleukin 5 modifies histamine release and leukotriene generation by human basophils in response to diverse agonists. *J. Exp. Med.* 172:1577, 1990.
14. Bousquet, J., et al. Eosinophilic inflammation in asthma. *N. Engl. J. Med.* 323:1033, 1990.

15. Burke, L. A., et al. Comparison of the generation of platelet-activating factor and leukotriene C_4 in human eosinophils stimulated by unopsonized zymosan and by the calcium ionophore A23187: the effects of nedocromil sodium. *J. Allergy Clin. Immunol.* 85:26, 1990.

16. Butterworth, A. E. Cell-mediated damage to helminths. *Adv. Parasitol.* 23:143, 1984.

17. Butterworth, A. E., et al. Eosinophils as mediators of antibody-dependent damage to schistosomula. *Nature* 256:727, 1975.

18. Butterworth, A. E., et al. Damage to schistosomula of *S. mansoni* induced directly by eosinophil major basic protein. *J. Immunol.* 122:221, 1979.

19. Capron, M., and Capron, A. The IgE Receptor of Human Eosinophils. In A. B. Kay (ed.), *Allergy and Inflammation.* London: Academic Press, 1987, P. 151.

20. Capron, M., et al. Fc receptors for IgE on human and rat eosinophils. *J. Immunol.* 126:2087, 1981.

21. Capron, M., et al. Role of IgE receptors in effector function of human eosinophils. *J. Immunol.* 132:462, 1984.

22. Capron, M., et al. Functional study of a monoclonal antibody to IgE Fc receptor (Fc R2) of eosinophils, platelets and macrophages. *J. Exp. Med.* 164:72, 1986.

23. Capron, M., et al. Immunoglobulin-mediated Activation of Eosinophils. In J. Morley and I. Colditz (eds.), *Eosinophils in Asthma.* London: Academic Press, 1989. P. 49.

24. Casale, T. B., et al. Direct evidence for a role of mast cells in the pathogenesis of antigen-induced bronchoconstriction. *J. Clin. Invest.* 80:1507, 1987.

25. Chihara, J., et al. Characterization of a receptor for interleukin 5 on human eosinophils: variable expression and induction by granulocyte-macrophage colony–stimulating factor. *J. Exp. Med.* 172:1347, 1990.

26. Clutterbuck, E. J., Hirst, E. M. A., and Sanderson, C. J. Human interleukin 5 (IL-5) regulates the production of eosinophils in human bone marrow cultures: comparison and interaction with IL-1, IL-3, IL-6 and GM-CSF. *Blood* 73:1504, 1988.

27. Colley, D. Lymphokine-related eosinophil responses. Lymphokine Cytokine Res 1:133, 1980.

28. Corrigan, C. J., Hartnell, A., and Kay, A. B. T-lymphocyte activation in acute severe asthma. *Lancet* 1:1129, 1988.

29. Cromwell, O., et al. IgG-dependent generation of platelet activating factor by normal and low density eosinophils. *J. Immunol.* 145:3862, 1990.

30. Del Pozo, V., et al. Murine eosinophils and IL-1: αIL-1 mRNA detection by in situ hybridization. Production and release of IL-1 from peritoneal eosinophils. *J. Immunol.* 144:3117, 1990.

31. De Monchy, J. G. R., et al. Bronchoalveolar eosinophilia during allergen-induced late asthmatic reactions. *Am. Rev. Respir. Dis.* 131:373, 1985.

32. Dent, L. A., et al. Eosinophilia in transgenic mice expressing interleukin 5. *J. Exp. Med.* 172:1425, 1990.

33. Diaz, P., et al. Leukocytes and lipid mediators in bronchoalveolar lavage during allergen-induced late-phase asthmatic reactions. *Am. Rev. Respir. Dis.* 139:1383, 1989.

34. Djukanovic, R., et al. Quantitation of mast cells and eosinophils in the bronchial mucosa of symptomatic atopic asthmatics and healthy subjects using immunohistochemistry. *Am. Rev. Respir. Dis.* 142:863, 1990.

35. Dunnill, M. S. The pathology of asthma with special reference to changes in the bronchial mucosa. *J. Clin. Pathol.* 13:27, 1960.

36. Durham, S. R., and Kay, A. B. Eosinophils, bronchial hyperreactivity and late-phase asthmatic reactions. *Clin. Allergy* 15:411, 1985.

37. Ellis, A. G. The pathological anatomy of bronchial asthma. *Am. J. Med. Sci.* 136:407, 1908.

38. Fabbri, L. M., et al. Bronchoalveolar neutrophilia during late asthmatic reactions induced by toluene diisocyanate. *Am. Rev. Respir. Dis.* 136:36, 1987.

39. Fanger, M. W., et al. Cytotoxicity mediated by human Fc receptors for IgG. *Immunol. Today* 10:92, 1989.

40. Favre, C., et al. Human eosinophil ontogeny: isolation and characterization of committed precursors (submitted for publication).

41. Filley, W. V., et al. Identification by immunofluorescence of eosinophil granule major basic protein in lung tissue of patients with bronchial asthma. *Lancet* 2:11, 1982.

42. Fischer, E., et al. Human eosinophils express CR1 and CR3 complement receptors for cleavage fragments of C3. *Cell Immunol.* 97:297, 1986.

43. Flint, K. C., et al. Bronchoalveolar mast cells in extrinsic asthma: a mechanism for the initiation of antigen specific bronchoconstriction. *Br. Med. J.* 291:923, 1985.

44. Foresi, A., et al. Inflammatory markers in bronchoalveolar lavage and in bronchial biopsy in asthma during remission. *Chest* 98:528, 1990.

45. Fredens, K., Dahl, R., and Venge, P. The Gordon phenomenon induced by eosinophil cationic protein and eosinophil protein X. *J. Allergy Clin. Immunol.* 70:361, 1982.

46. Frew, A. J., and Kay, A. B. The relationship between infiltrating CD4 + lymphocytes, activated eosinophils, and the magnitude of the allergen induced late-phase response in man. *J. Immunol.* 141:4158, 1988.

47. Frigas, E., et al. Elevated levels of eosinophil granule major basic protein in the sputum of patients with asthma. *Mayo Clin. Proc.* 56:345, 1981.

48. Fujisawa, T., et al. Regulatory effect of cytokines on eosinophil degranulation. *J. Immunol.* 144:642, 1990.

49. Fukuda, T., and Makino, S. Eosinophil Heterogeneity. In J. Morley and I. Colditz (eds.), *Eosinophils in Asthma.* London: Academic Press, 1989. P. 125.

50. Fukuda, T., et al. Increased numbers of hypodense eosinophils in the blood of patients with bronchial asthma. *Am. Rev. Respir. Dis.* 132:981, 1985.

51. Gerard, N. P., and Gerard, C. The chemotactic receptor for human C5a anaphylotoxin. *Nature* 349:614, 1991.

52. Gibson, P. G., et al. Chronic cough: eosinophilic bronchitis without asthma. *Lancet* 1:1346, 1989.

53. Gibson, P. G., et al. The inflammatory response in asthma exacerbation: changes in circulating eosinophil, basophils and their progenitors. *Clin. Exp. Allergy* 20:661, 1990.

54. Gibson, P. G., et al. Allergen-induced asthmatic responses. Relationship between increases in airway responsiveness and increasing eosinophils, basophils and their progenitors. *Am. Rev. Respir. Dis.* 143:331, 1991.

55. Gleich, G. J. The eosinophil and bronchial asthma: current understanding. *J. Allergy Clin. Immunol.* 85:422, 1990.

56. Gleich, G. J., and Adolphson, C. R. The eosinophil leucocyte. *Annu. Rev. Immunol.* 39:177, 1986.

57. Gleich, G. J., et al. Cytotoxic properties of eosinophil major protein. *J. Immunol.* 123:2925, 1979.

58. Gleich, G. J., et al. The eosinophilic leukocyte and the pathology of fatal bronchial asthma: evidence for pathologic heterogeneity. *J. Allergy Clin. Immunol.* 80:412, 1987.

59. Glovsky, M. M., et al. Anaphylotoxin-induced histamine release with human leukocytes: studies of C3a leukocyte binding and histamine release. *J. Clin. Invest.* 64:804, 1979.

60. Godard, P., et al. Functional assessment of alveolar macrophages: comparison of cells from asthmatics and normal subjects. *J. Allergy Clin. Immunol.* 70:88, 1982.

61. Goetzl, E. J., and Austen, K. F. Purification and synthesis of eosinophilotactic tetrapeptides of human lung: identification as human eosinophil chemotactic factor of anaphylaxis. *Proc. Natl. Acad. Sci. USA* 72:4123, 1975.

62. Goodman, J. R., Reilly, E. B., and Moore, R. E. Electron microscopy of formed elements of normal human blood. *Blood* 12:428, 1957.

63. Gordon, J. R., Burd, P. R., and Galli, S. J. Mast cells as a source of multifunctional cytokines. *Immunol. Today* 11:458, 1990.

64. Gundel, R. H., Letts, L. G., and Gleich, G. J. Human eosinophil major basic protein induces airway constriction and airway hyperresponsiveness in primates. *J. Clin. Invest.* 87:1470, 1991.

65. Hamid, Q., et al. Expression of mRNA for interleukin-5 in mucosal bronchial biopsies from asthma. *J. Clin. Invest.* 87:1541, 1991.

66. Hartnell, A., et al. Fc gamma and CD11/CD18 receptor expression on normal density and low density human eosinophils. *Immunology* 69:264, 1990.

67. Hastie, A. T., et al. The effect of purified human eosinophil major basic protein on mammalian ciliary activity. *Am. Rev. Respir. Dis.* 135:848, 1987.

68. Henderson, W. R., Harley, J. B., and Fauci, A. S. Arachidonic acid metabolism in normal and hypereosinophilic syndrome human eosinophils: generation of leukotrienes B_4, C_4, D_4 and 15-lipoxygenase products. *J. Immunol.* 124:1383, 1984.

69. Henocq, E., and Vaargaftig, B. B. Accumulation of eosinophils in response to intracutaneous PAF-acether and allergens in man. *Lancet* 1:1378, 1986.

70. Honda, Z., et al. Cloning by functional expression of platelet activating receptor from guinea-pig lung. *Nature* 349:342, 1991.

71. Horn, B. R., et al. Total eosinophil counts in the management of bronchial asthma. *N. Engl. J. Med.* 292:1152, 1975.

72. Jacoby, D. B., et al. Effect of human eosinophil major basic protein on

ion transport in dog tracheal epithelium. *Am. Rev. Respir. Dis.* 137:13, 1988.

73. Juniper, E. F., et al. Effect of long-term treatment with an inhaled corticosteroid (budesonide) on airway hyperresponsiveness and clinical asthma in non-steroid-dependent asthmatics. *Am. Rev. Respir. Dis.* 142: 832, 1990.

74. Kay, A. B. Asthma and inflammation. *J. Allergy Clin. Immunol.* 87:893, 1991.

75. Kay, A. B., Stechschulte, D. J., and Austen, K. F. An eosinophil leukocyte chemotactic factor of anaphylaxis. *J. Exp. Med.* 133:602, 1971.

76. Kay, A. B., et al. Messenger RNA expression of the cytokine gene cluster, IL-3, IL-4, IL-5 and GM-CSF in allergen-induced late-phase cutaneous reactions in atopic subjects. *J. Exp. Med.* 173:775, 1991.

77. Kelly, C., et al. Number and activity of inflammatory cells in bronchoalveolar lavage fluid in asthma and their relation to airway responsiveness. *Thorax* 43:684, 1988.

78. Khaliffe, J., et al. Role of specific IgE antibodies in peroxidase (EPO) release from human eosinophils. *J. Immunol.* 137:1659, 1986.

79. Kimani, G., Tonnesen, M. G., and Henson, P. M. Stimulation of eosinophil adherence to human vascular endothelial cells *in vitro* by platelet activating factor. *J. Immunol.* 140:3161, 1988.

80. Kirby, J. G., et al. Bronchoalveolar cell profiles of asthmatic and non-asthmatic subjects. *Am. Rev. Respir. Dis.* 136:379, 1987.

81. Kroegel, C., et al. Stimulation of degranulation from human eosinophils by platelet-activating factor. *J. Immunol.* 142:3518, 1989.

82. Kurihara, K., et al. Inhibition of platelet-activating factor (PAF)–induced chemotaxis and PAF binding to human eosinophils and neutrophils by the specific ginkgolide-derived PAF antagonist, BN 52021. *J. Allergy Clin. Immunol.* 83:83, 1989.

83. Kita, H., et al. GM-CSF and interleukin 3 release from human peripheral blood eosinophils and neutrophils. *J. Exp. Med.* 174:745, 1991.

84. Kyan-Aung, U., et al. Endothelial leukocyte adhesion molecule-1 and intercellular adhesion molecule-1 mediate adhesion of eosinophils to endothelial cells *in vitro* and are expressed by endothelium in allergic cutaneous inflammation *in vivo J. Immunol.* 146:521, 1991.

85. Lam, S., et al. Cellular and protein changes in bronchial lavage fluid after late asthmatic reaction in patients with red cedar wood asthma. *J. Allergy Clin. Immunol.* 80:44, 1987.

86. Lamas, A. M., Mulroney, C. M., and Schleimer, R. Studies of the adhesive interaction between purified human eosinophils and cultured vascular endothelial cells. *J. Immunol.* 140:1500, 1988.

87. Leary, A. G., and Ogawa, M. Identification of pure and mixed basophil colonies in culture of human peripheral blood and marrow cells. *Blood* 64:78, 1984.

88. Lee, T., et al. Increased biosynthesis of platelet activating factor in activated human eosinophils. *J. Biol. Chem.* 259:5526, 1984.

89. Lazlo, J., and Rundles, R. W. Morphology of Granulocytes and Their Precursors. In W. J. Williams, et al. (eds.), *Hematology.* New York: McGraw-Hill, 1972. P. 563.

90. Lopez, A. F., et al. Recombinant human interleukin 5 is a selective activator of human eosinophil function. *J. Exp. Med.* 167:219, 1988.

91. Lucey, D. R., Nicholson-Weller, A., and Weller, P. F. Mature human eosinophils have the capacity to express HLA-DR. *Proc. Natl. Acad. Sci. USA* 86:1348, 1989.

92. Lucey, D. R., et al. Human eosinophils express CD4 protein and bind human immunodeficiency virus 1 gp120. *J. Exp. Med.* 169:327, 1989.

93. McLaren, D. J., Mackenzie, C. D., and Ramalho-Pinto, F. J. Ultrastructural observations on the *in vitro* interaction between rat eosinophils and some parasitic helminths (*Schistosoma mansoni, Trichinella spiralis* and *Nippostrongylus brasiliensis*). *Clin. Exp. Immunol.* 30:105, 1977.

94. Metzger, W. J., et al. Local allergen challenge and bronchoalveolar lavage of allergic asthmatic lungs: description of the model and local airway inflammation. *Am. Rev. Respir. Dis.* 135:433, 1987.

95. Miller, F., de Harven, E., and Palde, G. E. The structure of eosinophil leukocyte granules in rodents and man. *J. Cell. Biol.* 31:349, 1966.

96. Ming Wang, J., et al. Recombinant human interleukin 5 is a selective eosinophil chemoattractant. *Eur. J. Immunol.* 19:701, 1989.

97. Moqbel, R., et al. Expression of mRNA and immunoreactivity for the granulocyte/macrophage–colony stimulating factor (GM-CSF) in activated human eosinophils. *J. Exp. Med.* 174:749, 1991.

98. Morita, E., Schroder, J.-M., and Christophers, E. Identification of a novel and highly potent eosinophil chemotactic lipid in human eosinophils treated with arachidonic acid. *J. Immunol.* 144:1893, 1990.

99. Mosmann, R., and Coffman, R. L. Th1 and Th2 cells: different patterns of lymphokine secretion lead to different functional properties. *Annu. Rev. Immunol.* 7:145, 1989.

100. Motojima, S., et al. Toxicity of the eosinophil cationic proteins for guinea pig tracheal epithelium *in vitro. Am. Rev. Respir. Dis.* 139:801, 1989.

101. NHLBI Workshop Summaries: summary and recommendations of a workshop on the investigative use of fiberoptic bronchoscopy and bronchoalveolar lavage in asthmatics. *Am. Rev. Respir. Dis.* 132:180, 1985.

102. Nusse, O., et al. Intracellular application of guanosine-5'-O-(3-thiotriphosphate) induces exocytic granule fusion in guinea-pig eosinophils. *J. Exp. Med.* 171:775, 1990.

103. Owen, W. F., et al. Regulation of human eosinophil viability, density and function by granulocyte/macrophage colony–stimulating factor in the presence of 3T3 fibroblasts. *J. Exp. Med.* 166:129, 1987.

104. Parmley, R. T., and Spicer, S. S. Cytochemical ultrastructural identification of a small type granule in human late eosinophils. *Lab. Invest.* 30: 557, 1974.

105. Peterson, C. G. B., Scoog, V., and Venge, P. Human eosinophil cationic proteins (ECP and EP-X) and their suppressive effects on lymphocyte proliferation. *Immunobiology* 171:1, 1986.

106. Prin, L., et al. Heterogeneity of human peripheral blood eosinophils: variability in cell density and cytotoxic ability in relation to the level and origin of hypereosinophilia. *Int. Arch. Allergy Appl. Immunol.* 72: 336, 1983.

107. Prin, L., et al. Eosinophilic lung disease. Immunological studies of blood and alveolar eosinophils. *Clin. Exp. Immunol.* 63:249, 1986.

108. Robinson, D. S., et al. Cytokine gene expression in bronchoalveolar lavage cells from atopic asthmatics and normal controls (submitted for publication).

109. Rohrbach, M. S., et al. Activation of platelets by eosinophil granule proteins. *J. Exp. Med.* 172:1271, 1990.

110. Rosenberg, H. F., Ackerman, S. J., and Tenen, D. G. Human eosinophil cationic protein. Molecular cloning of a cytotoxin and helminthotoxin with ribonuclease activity. *J. Exp. Med.* 170:163, 1989.

111. Rosenberg, H. F., Tenen, D. G., and Ackerman, S. J. Molecular cloning of the human eosinophil–derived neurotoxin: a member of the ribonuclease gene family. *Proc. Natl. Acad. Sci. USA* 86:4460, 1989.

112. Rothenburg, M. E., et al. Eosinophils co-cultured with endothelial cells have increased survival and functional properties. *Science* 237:645, 1987.

113. Rothenburg, M. E., et al. Human eosinophils have prolonged survival, enhanced functional properties and become hypodense when exposed to human interleukin 3. *J. Clin. Invest.* 81:1986, 1988.

114. Rothenburg, M. E., et al. IL-5 dependent conversion of normodense human eosinophils to the hypodense phenotype uses 3T3 fibroblasts for enhanced viability, accelerated hypodensity and sustained antibody-dependent cytotoxicity. *J. Immunol.* 143:2311, 1989.

115. Saeland, S., et al. Combined and sequential effects of human IL-3 and GM-CSF on the proliferation of CD34 + ve hematopoietic cells from cord blood. *Blood* 73:1195, 1989.

116. Saito, H., et al. Selective differentiation and proliferation of haematopoietic cells induced by recombinant human interleukins. *Proc. Natl. Acad. Sci. USA* 85:2288, 1988.

117. Sanderson, C. J., Warren, D. J., and Strath, M. Identification of a lymphokine that stimulates eosinophil differentiation *in vitro*: its relationship to interleukin 3 and functional properties of eosinophils produced in cultures. *J. Exp. Med.* 162:60, 1985.

118. Schleimer, R. P. Effects of glucocorticoids on inflammatory cells relevant to their therapeutic applications in asthma. *Am. Rev. Respir. Dis.* 141:S59, 1990.

119. Sehmi, R., et al. The identification of guinea-pig eosinophil chemotactic factor of anaphylaxis (ECF-A) as leukotriene B₄ and 8(S)15(S)-diHete. *J. Immunol.* 147:2276, 1991.

120. Selveraj, P., et al. The major Fc receptor in blood has a phosphatidylinisotol anchor and is deficient in paroxysmal nocturnal haemaglobinuria. *Nature* 333:565, 1988.

121. Shaw, R. J., Cromwell, O., and Kay, A. B. Preferential generation of leukotriene C₄ by human eosinophils. *Clin. Exp. Immunol.* 56:716, 1984.

122. Shaw, R. J., et al. Activated human eosinophils generate SRS-A leukotrienes following physiological (IgG-dependent) stimulation. *Nature* 316:150, 1985.

123. Sher, A., et al. Interleukin 5 is required for the blood and tissue eosinophilia but not granuloma formation induced by infection with *Schistosoma mansoni. Proc. Natl. Acad. Sci. USA* 87:61, 1990.

124. Shult, P. A., Graziano, F. M., and Busse, W. W. Enhanced eosinophil lu-

minol–dependent chemoluminescence in allergic rhinitis. *J. Allergy Clin. Immunol.* 77:702, 1985.

125. Silberstein, D. S., and David, J. R. Tumor necrosis factor enhances eosinophil toxicity to *Schistosoma mansoni* larvae. *Proc. Natl. Acad. Sci. USA* 83:1055, 1986.

126. Slifman, N. R., et al. Ribonuclease activity associated with human eosinophil–derived neurotoxin and eosinophil cationic protein. *J. Immunol.* 137:2913, 1986.

127. Slungard, A., et al. Tumor necrosis factor α/cachectin stimulates eosinophil oxidant production and toxicity towards human endothelium. *J. Exp. Med.* 171:2025, 1990.

128. Springer, T. A. Adhesion receptors of the immune system. *Nature* 346: 425, 1990.

129. Spry, C. *Eosinophils.* Oxford and London: Oxford University Press, 1988. P. 29.

130. Spry, C. Eosinopoiesis. In *Eosinophils. A Comprehensive Review and Guide to the Scientific and Medical Literature.* New York and London: Oxford University Press, 1988. P. 10.

131. Tai, P. C., et al. Monoclonal antibodies distinguish between storage and secreted forms of eosinophil cationic protein. *Nature* 309:182, 1984.

132. Taylor, K. J., and Luksza, A. R. Peripheral blood eosinophil counts and bronchial responsiveness. *Thorax* 42:452, 1987.

133. Ten, R. M., et al. Molecular cloning of the human eosinophil peroxidase. *J. Exp. Med.* 169:1757, 1989.

134. Tominaga, A., et al. Transgenic mice expressing a B cell growth and differentiation factor gene (interleukin 5) develop eosinophilia and auto-antibody production. *J. Exp. Med.* 173:429, 1991.

135. Tomioka, M., et al. Mast cells in bronchoalveolar lumen of patients with bronchial asthma. *Am. Rev. Respir. Dis.* 129:1000, 1984.

136. Tsicopoulos, A., et al. Evidence for Th1-type cells (mRNA IFN-gamma +, IL-2 +, IL-4 −, IL-5 −), in classical delayed-type (tuberculin) hypersensitivity reactions in human skin (submitted for publication).

137. Unkeless, J. C., Scigliano, E., and Freedman, V. H. Structure and function of human and murine receptors for IgG. *Annu. Rev. Immunol.* 6:251, 1988.

138. Vadas, M. A., et al. A new method for the purification of human eosinophils and neutrophils and a comparison of the ability of these cells to damage schistosomula of *Schistosoma mansoni. J. Immunol.* 122:1228, 1979.

139. Valerius, T., et al. Effects of interferon on human eosinophils in comparison with other cytokines. *J. Immunol.* 145:2950, 1990.

140. Van Leuwen, B. H., et al. Molecular organization of the cytokine gene cluster, involving the human IL-3, IL-4, IL-5 and GM-CSF genes on chromosome 5. *Blood* 73:1142, 1989.

141. Wadee, A. E., and Sher, R. The effect of a soluble factor released by sensitized mononuclear cells incubated with *S. haematobium* ova on eosinophil migration. *Immunology* 41:989, 1980.

142. Walsh, G. M., et al. IL-5 enhances the *in vitro* adhesion of human eosinophils, but not neutrophils, in a leucocyte integrin (CD11/18)–dependent manner. *Immunology* 71:258, 1990.

143. Walsh, G. M., et al. Receptor expression and functional status of cultured human eosinophils derived from umbilical cord blood mononuclear cells. *Blood* 76:105, 1990.

144. Walsh, G. M., et al. Human eosinophil, but not neutrophil, adherence to IL-1 stimulated HUVEC is α4β1 (VLA-4) dependent. *J. Immunol.* 146:3419, 1991.

145. Wardlaw, A. J. Leucocyte adhesion to endothelium. *Clin. Exp. Allergy* 20: 619, 1990.

146. Wardlaw, A. J., Collins, J. V., and Kay, A. B. Mechanisms in asthma using the technique of bronchoalveolar lavage. *Int. Arch. Allergy Appl. Immunol.* 82:518, 1987.

147. Wardlaw, A. J., and Kay, A. B. Neutrophil and Eosinophil Chemotaxis and Cutaneous Inflammatory Reactions. In M. W. Greaves and S. Shuster (eds.), *Pharmacology of the Skin* I. Berlin: Springer-Verlag, 1989. P. 395.

148. Wardlaw, A. J., et al. Morphological and secretory properties of bronchoalveolar lavage mast cells in respiratory diseases. *Clin. Allergy* 16: 163, 1986.

149. Wardlaw, A. J., et al. Eosinophils and mast cells in bronchoalveolar lavage fluid and mild asthma: relationship to bronchial hyperreactivity. *Am. Rev. Respir. Dis.* 137:62, 1988.

150. Wardlaw, A. J., et al. Effects of inhaled PAF in humans on circulating and bronchoalveolar lavage fluid neutrophils. *Am. Rev. Respir. Dis.* 141:386, 1990.

151. Wardlaw, A. J., et al. Platelet activating factor. A potent chemotactic and chemokinetic factor for human eosinophils. *J. Clin. Invest.* 78:1701, 1986.

152. Warringa, R. J., et al. Modulation and induction of eosinophil chemotaxis by granulocyte–macrophage colony stimulating factor and interleukin 3. *Blood* 77:2694, 1991.

153. Wegner, C. D., et al. Intercellular adhesion molecule-1 (ICAM-1) in the pathogenesis of asthma. *Science* 247:456, 1990.

154. Weinstock, J. V., and Blum, A. M. Detection of vasoactive intestinal peptide and localization of its mRNA within granulomas of murine schistosomiasis. *Cell Immunol.* 125:291, 1990.

155. Weller, P. F. Immunobiology of eosinophils. *N. Engl. J. Med.* 324:1110, 1991.

156. Weller, P. F., and Goetzl, E. J. The regulatory and effector roles of eosinophils. *Adv. Immunol.* 27:339, 1979.

157. Weller, P. F., Goetzl, E. J., and Austen, K. F. Identification of human eosinophil lysophospholipase as the constituent of Charcot-Leyden crystals. *Proc. Natl. Acad. Sci. USA* 77:7440, 1980.

158. Weller, P. F., et al. Generation and metabolism of 5-lipoxygenase pathway leukotrienes by human eosinophils: predominant production of leukotriene C4. *Proc. Natl. Acad. Sci. USA* 80:7625, 1983.

159. White, C. J., Maxwell, C. J., and Gallin, J. I. Changes in the structural and functional properties of human eosinophils during experimental hookworm infection. *J. Infect. Dis.* 154:778, 1986.

160. Wierenga, E. A., et al. Evidence for compartmentalization of functional subsets of CD4 + T lymphocytes in atopic patients. *J. Immunol.* 144:4651, 1990.

161. Winquist, I., Olofsson, T., and Olsson, I. Mechanisms for eosinophil degranulation. Release of the eosinophil granule protein. *Immunology* 51: 1, 1984.

162. Winquist, I., et al. Altered density, metabolism and surface receptors of eosinophils in eosinophilia. *Immunology* 47:531, 1982.

163. Wong, D. T., et al. Human eosinophils express transforming growth factor α. *J. Exp. Med.* 172:673, 1990.

164. Yamaguchi, Y., et al. Purified interleukin 5 supports the terminal differentiation and proliferation of murine eosinophilic precursors. *J. Exp. Med.* 167:43, 1988.

165. Yazdanbakhsh, M., Eckmann, C. M., and Roos, D. Characterization of the interaction of human eosinophils and neutrophils with opsonized particles. *J. Immunol.* 135:1378, 1985.

166. Young, J. D. E., et al. Mechanism of membrane damage mediated by human eosinophil cationic protein. *Nature* 321:613, 1986.

167. Kay, A. B. Helper (CD4 +) T cells and eosinophils in allergy and asthma. *Am. Rev. Respir. Dis.* 145:S22, 1992.

Mast Cell and Basophil

David Lagunoff

The mast cell, by virtue of its store of inflammatory mediators, its capacity to generate additional mediators, its abundance of high-affinity immunoglobulin E (IgE) receptors, and its proximity to blood vessels, smooth muscle, and mucosal surfaces, is recognized as the central effector cell of allergic reactions (Fig. 21-1). The basophil, which is the least prevalent of the circulating granulocyte types in humans, resembles the tissue mast cell in a number of respects: its metachromatic secretory granules, its histamine, and its high-affinity IgE receptors. Unlike mast cells, which are propitiously situated in connective tissue to perform their inflammatory functions, basophils must be recruited from the circulation across the endothelial layer to the interstitium. The small number of circulating basophils and the time required to infiltrate the connective tissue suggest that the component of acute allergic inflammation attributable to basophils may be delayed.

In humans, as in most mammals, mast cells are widely distributed in the connective tissue, and related cells have also been found in animals of the other vertebrate classes. Comparative histochemical evidence suggests that the mast cell has undergone extensive evolutionary modifications in its specialized constituents [36]. For instance, histamine, seemingly so crucial to mast cell function in humans, is found in the mast cells of mammals, birds, and reptiles, but not in fish or amphibian mast cells. Other amines, serotonin [15] and dopamine [131], are present in the mast cells of a few rodent species and cows, respectively.

The structure of the mature mast cell, as shown by both light and electron microscopy, is dominated by its secretory granules. An unusual staining property of these granules was responsible for the primary identification of the mast cell as a distinct cell type: "Man kann von diesen Standpunkt aus die granulirten Zellen gewissermaasen als Producte der Mastung der Bindegewebeszellen ansehen und sie dem entsprechend als Mastzellen bezeichnen." [64a] (From this perspective, the granular cells may be considered the result of the engorgement of connective tissue cells, and accordingly they can be called mast cells.) Ehrlich [64] observed that certain cells in the connective tissue stained in an anomalous manner with a number of aniline dyes. He coined the term *Metachromasie* for the modification in color that occurs when these dyes bind to mast cell granules. The metachromatic shift in the absorbance spectrum depends on the stacking of multiple planar cationic dye molecules on an anionic polymer possessing a sufficiently high linear-charge density.

Mast cells are preeminently secretory, and a wide variety of stimuli cause the extrusion of mast cell granules, with the accompanying release of histamine and the formation of prostaglandin D_2, leukotriene B_4, and leukotriene C_4. Histamine is released from the granule matrix when the granules are discharged by exocytosis. Prostaglandin D_2 and the leukotrienes are not stored in a preformed state but are synthesized from arachidonic acid in response to a secretory stimulus (see Chaps. 10 and 11).

Mast cell histamine is strongly implicated in hay fever and hives. Mast cell–derived leukotriene and platelet-activating factor (PAF), another phospholipid-derived mediator produced by stimulated mast cells, have been proposed to be more important than histamine in the asthmatic reactions of bronchial constriction. Some observations appear to implicate the basophil in the late-phase allergic reactions [8, 204, 220, 244], when their appearance together with eosinophils and neutrophils is likely to depend on mediators released by indigenous mast cells.

ULTRASTRUCTURE OF THE GRANULE

A mature human-lung mast cell contains approximately 1,000 granules [101]; rat peritoneal mast cells contain a similar number of granules [102, 108]. The secretory granules in their intracellular habitat are coherent structures, each surrounded by a membrane and in aggregate occupy about 50 percent of the total rat cell volume [102]. Upon stimulation, the granules are extruded from the cell and unravel in the extracellular milieu [23, 35, 156, 157, 234]. The ultrastructure of human mast cell granules is complex, with several distinctive patterns discernible. The most prevalent of these is a curved beaded sheet. Short lengths of these sheets are arranged in concentric clusters, often at the outer margins of granules, and may appear as either arcs or straight lines, depending on the plane of section. Larger lengths of the sheets are wrapped in scrolls that are evident in electron micrographs as spirals or groups of parallel lines. The spacing between the sheets or lamellae (approximately 150 nm) is usually greater than the distance (approximately 75 nm) between the beads [35], but, in some images, a secondary lamella exists between the primary sheets. Well-formed spiral arrays have been referred to as *complete scrolls* and the curved parallel arrays and other imperfect scrolls, which often meld into other granule constituents, as *incomplete* or *nondiscrete scrolls* (Fig. 21-2). A second pattern is crystalline and presents as either gratings, consisting of a set of parallel electron-dense lines, or lattices, appearing as two or more intersecting arrays of such lines. The spacing between these lines closely approximates that seen between the elements of the scrolls. A third pattern is less orderly, ranging from an amorphous collection of irregular densities to a reticular distribution of more-or-less discrete particles, which has been variously termed as *reticular, beaded,* or *ropey*. These several patterns do not segregate completely, either in different cells or even in granules in the same cell [35, 156, 181, 290]. Any hope of understanding this diversity of structure must rely on the identification of the underlying molecular determinants of the structures.

The electron microscopy immunochemical studies of Schwartz and collaborators [50, 51, 123, 251] indicate that the complete scrolls contain tryptase alone and the gratings and lattices con-

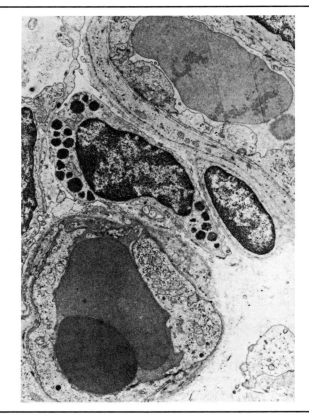

Fig. 21-1. *Electron micrograph of a portion of the submucosa from a normal human rectal biopsy. A mast cell is situated between two small blood vessels. Close association of mast cells with the microcirculation is common. (× 6,500.)*

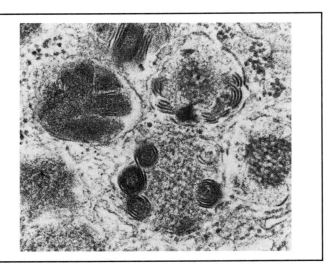

Fig. 21-2. *Electron micrograph of a human rectal submucosal mast cell granule. Several cross sections of complete scrolls are evident, together with amorphous material in one granule. Typical incomplete scrolls are evident in another granule, and longitudinal sections of complete scrolls are seen in two granules. (× 23,400.)*

sistently contain chymase plus tryptase. Most mast cells have a predominant granule structure, consistent with the immuno-chemical identification of the proteases present. Granules containing complete scrolls occur almost exclusively in the mast cells containing only tryptase (MC_T), whereas lattices and gratings have only been found in those mast cells containing chymase and carboxypeptidase in addition to tryptase (MC_TC). Both MC_T and MC_TC contain incomplete scrolls and reticular granules, and the granules are either tryptase positive or doubly positive according to the cell type—MC_T or MC_TC, respectively. As yet there is no report on the immunohistochemical characterization at the electron microscopy level of the granules in those infrequent cells that contain lattices or gratings, or both, along with well-formed scrolls. Craig and colleagues [50] have reported that immature MC_T contain reticular granules and scrolls, whereas the granules in immature MC_TC are amorphous and have electron-dense cores. The limited conclusions that can be drawn at this point are that lattices and gratings require the presence of both tryptase and chymase, and perhaps also carboxypeptidase, and most if not all discrete scrolls occur when only tryptase is present. The observation that imperfect scrolls, which so closely resemble discrete scrolls, can contain either tryptase alone or both proteases is puzzling if the main determinant of granule substructure is the protein component. It is conceivable that the glycosaminoglycan constituents contribute significantly to the varying appearance of the granules in electron micrographs.

Mature rat mast cell granules in situ appear as dense, homogeneous spheres that resolve into a network of filaments when the granules are extruded from their protective membrane by active secretion or when isolated granules are placed into a solution of

sufficiently high salt concentration [156]. Mast cell granules, like other secretory granules, originate in the Golgi apparatus. In the rat, some 1,000 Golgi-derived progranules coalesce to form a single-unit secretory granule [102]. These unit granules fuse slowly to form an array of granule sizes. A multimodal distribution of granule sizes occurs in human and rat mast cells [6, 101–104] and appears to be a common feature of all secretory cells. A sequence for the formation of granules in connective-tissue mast cells of the rat and mouse has been described by Combs and colleagues [47, 48].

GRANULE CONSTITUENTS

Heparin

The identification of the metachromatic substance of the granules as a highly sulfated mucopolysaccharide was initially proposed by Lison [183]. This was later confirmed by the observation of a positive correlation between heparin content and mast cell number in different tissues [118]; the best evidence has come from the extraction of heparin from mast cell tumors [192], normal mast cells [138], and isolated mast cell granules [165]. Heparin, unlike the interstitial connective tissue glycosaminoglycans, is essentially an intracellular component that has only a transitory extracellular existence after it has been released from the granule. Extruded granule matrices have been found in macrophages [75, 78, 80] and fibroblasts [76, 105].

The heparin polymer is constructed largely of repeating disaccharide units of N-substituted glucosamine and uronic acid [147]. The saccharide units are joined by $1{\rightarrow}4$ glycosidic bonds. Although the uronic acid in heparin has long been considered to be glucuronic, there is now clear evidence for a preponderance of iduronic acid moieties [180, 217, 218]. Preparations of heparin vary in their overall sulfate content, ranging from 2 to 2.5 sulfate groups per disaccharide repeat unit. A 2-N-sulfate and a 6-O-sulfate on glucosamine are constant; a variable sulfate occurs at position 2 of iduronic acid. An oligosaccharide end-piece, Gal-Gal-Xyl. is interposed between the covalently associated protein core and the reducing end of the glycosaminoglycan, with xylosylserine bonds joining multiple heparin chains to a short polypeptide core [147]. Commercial heparin extracted by standard methods from hog intestinal mucosa or bovine pleura occurs as individual glycosaminoglycan chains unattached to any protein, with molecular weights ranging between 10,000 and 20,000, whereas the intact human heparin–proteoglycan complex has a molecular weight of between 60,000 and 100,000 [270], and the molecular weight of rat heparin proteoglycan ranges from 750,000 to 1,000,000 [119, 193].

Heparin, with its high-charge density, binds divalent cations such as Ca^{++} and histamine (at pHs below the pKa of the imidazole nitrogen) as well as multivalent basic proteins. Most biologic activities of heparin can be traced to this property, although a specific heparin-binding site for antithrombin III has been identified [181]. In spite of heparin's considerable potential for biologic activity, little convincing evidence has been adduced for an extracellular, physiologic function of the endogenous form. In the dog, massive degranulation of hepatic mast cells is associated with incoagulability of the blood, presumably because of the release of heparin into the circulation. Heparin at concentrations lower than those required to inhibit coagulation elicits lipoprotein lipase activity [151], but again evidence that endogenous mast cell heparin exerts this action is meager [161]. Heparin acts on endothelial cells to stimulate motility [9] and avidly binds basic growth factors [73] that induce endothelial cell replication. In most instances of mast cell secretion, because of the stable complexes formed between granule proteins and heparin, it is unlikely that very much soluble heparin ever gains access to the circulation despite the proximity of mast cells to the microcirculation. The intrinsic functional properties of heparin are likely to be markedly modified by the bound protein. In turn, the behavior of the bound proteins are likely modified by their attachment to heparin; for instance, human mast cell tryptase is stabilized by heparin [250].

Heparin serves as a major structural component of the mast cell granule through its protein-binding properties. It also binds much of the granule histamine. The capacity of heparin to bind to and inhibit polypeptide and protein toxins led Higginbotham and coworkers [43, 112, 113] to propose mast cell heparin as a general antagonist of noxious cationic agents that gain access to the connective tissue. Another property of secreted heparin emphasized by Selye and colleagues [258] is manifested in the complex reactions of mastocalciphylaxis and mastocalcergy. In these reactions, calcification of tissues follows the induction of mast cell secretion. The local release of histamine increases vascular permeability, and the secreted heparin may serve as a nidus for the precipitation of calcium and other salts.

In recent years, glycosaminoglycans other than heparin have been identified in mast cells (Table 21-1) [270]. Chondroitin-4-sulfate and chondroitin sulfate E have been isolated from human-lung mast cells [271, 277] and colonic mucosal mast cells [65]. These two chondroitin sulfates occur in cultured mouse mast cells [90, 260] and have also been described as minor granule

constituents of rat peritoneal mast cells [138]. Chondroitin-6-sulfate [54] and dermatan sulfate [138, 257] have also been found in mast cells under various conditions. The chondroitin sulfates have *N*-acetylgalactosamine in place of heparin's *N*-SO_4-glucosamine, and the glycosidic bond linking the uronic acid to the galactosamine is $1 \rightarrow 3$ instead of the $1 \rightarrow 4$ bond found in heparin [77]. Dermatan sulfate, like heparin, has an iduronic acid group in place of the glucuronic acid found in the chondroitin sulfates [77]. A common feature of the non–heparin glycosaminoglycans present in mast cells is a disaccharide with two sulfate groups instead of the one typical of extracellular glycosaminoglycans. In the mast cell dermatan sulfate derivative, the second sulfate is found at the 2 position of iduronic acid [257]; in chondroitin E sulfate, both the 4 and 6 positions of *N*-acetylgalactosamine are sulfated [226]. Chondroitin sulfate D is chondroitin-6-sulfate, with the extra sulfate at the 2 position of glucuronic acid. It must be noted that the estimated proportions of the various glycosaminoglycan species reported for mast cells are derived from experiments that depend on the incorporation of $^{35}SO_4$, so the values obtained reflect the relative rates of sulfate incorporation and are not necessarily an accurate estimate of the relative mass of preformed glycosaminoglycan present in the granules.

Histamine

The mast cell was largely a cytologic curiosity until Riley and West [54] demonstrated the association of mast cells and tissue histamine, thus establishing the cell as the major source of tissue histamine and thereby implicating it in the allergic inflammatory reactions dependent on this mediator. However compelling the logic, evidence is still lacking that mast cell histamine acts on blood vessels and smooth muscle in a manner more subtle than is evident in the setting of allergic inflammation. The availability of a potent, nontoxic, specific inhibitor of mast cell histidine decarboxylase, α-fluoromethylhistidine [12], provides a means of maintaining reduced levels of mast cell histamine for a long time [167, 289] and allows for experiments designed to identify the potential function of histamine. Rats, under laboratory conditions, seem to tolerate prolonged suppression of histamine synthesis with no evident untoward effects. The findings from experiments in which animals with chronically depressed histidine decarboxylase levels are subjected to specific challenges designed to test for a specific homeostatic function of mast cell histamine have yet to be reported. Reliable evidence has also not been derived from studies of mice genetically deficient in mast cells that sheds light on an essential physiologic role of mast cell histamine.

Mast cell histamine is synthesized from histidine by cytoplasmic histidine decarboxylase [12, 159, 240]. In the rat mast cell, there does not seem to be a special transport system for taking up histidine [11, 159]. Instead, several amino acid trans-

Table 21-1. Mast cell glycosaminoglycans

Glycosaminoglycans	Uronic acid	Hexosamine	Uronic–hexosamine bond	N-substituent	O-SO_4	Mast cell type
Heparin	Idu	*N*-Glu	α 1-4	SO_4	*N*-Glu-2, *N*-Glu-6, Idu-2	MC_{TC}, rat peritoneal, RBL
Chondroitin-4-sulfate	Glu	*N*-Gal	β 1-3	Ac	*N*-Gal-4	MC_T, mouse BM, RBL
Chondroitin sulfate E	Glu	*N*-Gal	β 1-3	Ac	*N*-Gal-4, *N*-Gal-6	MC_T, mouse BM
Chondroitin sulfate D	Glu	*N*-Gal-*N*	β 1-3	Ac	*N*-Gal-6, Glu-2	Rat LN
Dermatan sulfate (chondroitin sulfate di-B)	Idu	*N*-Gal	α 1-3	Ac	*N*-Gal-4, Idu-2	Rat BM, RBL

Idu = iduronic acid; Glu = glucuronic acid; *N*-Glu = glucosamine; *N*-Gal = galactosamine; Ac = acetate; BM = bone marrow–derived culture; LN = lymph node–derived culture; RBL = rat basophilic leukemia cell line; MC_{TC} = mast cells containing chymase, carboxypeptidase, and tryptase; MC_T = tryptase-containing mast cells.

porters are utilized, and their effectiveness is markedly enhanced by the rapid removal of intracellular histidine through conversion to the amine and sequestration of the amine within the granules [11, 184].

The bulk of histamine normally present in the mast cell is in the granules. Much of this granule histamine is bound to the granule proteoglycan by ionic bonds involving the two positive charges of histamine (pKa's of 9.47 and 5.84 at 35°C), at the pH of 5.0 to 5.5 estimated for the granule matrix [135, 168]. Based on the findings from nuclear magnetic resonance studies, a small fraction of the histamine seems to be free in the granule water [222]. A gradient of free amine across the granule membrane is maintained by the steep pH gradient. Nigericin, which collapses the gradients intracellularly, leads to the release of histamine into the cytoplasm. Because of its relatively weak binding to heparin, histamine is readily displaced from the granule by competing cations when the granules are extruded from the mast cell [153]. Serotonin, with its single positive charge, binds comparatively poorly to heparin, and much of it may be free in the granule, sequestered largely by the proton gradient (see also Chap. 10).

Lipid Mediators

Products of the lipoxygenase and cyclooxygenase pathways of arachidonic acid metabolism are not stored in mast cells but are synthesized and released following stimulation of the mast cells. This group of mediators includes leukotriene C_4 [40, 176, 178, 219, 243], a vascular permeability factor; leukotriene B_4, chemotactic for neutrophils [219, 243]; and prostaglandin D_2, a vasodilator identified as a major product of arachidonic acid in human mast cells (Table 21-2) [40, 177, 233]. In the past, it was assumed that much of the arachidonic acid utilized for lipid mediator synthesis was provided by the combined action of phospholipase C followed by diacylglycerol (DAG) lipase [139, 140] or of phospholipase A_2 alone [187, 297]. Recent evidence raises the possibility of a significant contribution by phospholipase D [59, 179], in concert with phosphatidic acid phosphatase, to the formation of arachidonic acid as well as DAG. PAF, a potent mediator capable of augmenting vascular permeability and inducing neutrophils to adhere to endothelial cells, among other functions, is made by human lung mast cells but is not apparently released from the cell [243]. Nitric oxide, a recently discovered nonlipid mediator first described as an endothelial cell product and a potent vasodilator, has been reported to be generated by stimulated mast cells (see Chap. 11) [238].

Chemotactic Factors

Several chemotactic peptides appear to be associated with the granule matrix. Eosinophilic chemotactic factor of anaphylaxis is a tetrapeptide (Val/Ala-Gly-Ser-Glu) that selectively attracts eosinophils [86, 87, 288]. Because of the limited amounts of the tetrapeptide and its weak chemotactic activity, doubt has been cast on the significance of this peptide [255]. At least one interme-

diate-molecular-weight polypeptide chemotactic for eosinophils [25] and several larger proteins chemotactic for neutrophils have been obtained from mast cells [87]. Histamine itself has some effect as a chemotaxin for eosinophils [44].

Cytokines

The class of cytokines includes an ever-enlarging group of factors; they are all proteins of modest size that are active as mediators of inflammation, plus serve as modulators of the immune response and as growth factors for hematopoietic cells. The cytokines act by binding to specific receptors on their target cell surfaces. The recognition of anti–tumor cell cytotoxicity of mast cells led to the identification of tumor necrosis factor alpha (TNF-α) in mouse mast cells [269]. The mast cell's preformed TNF-α is apparently stored in the secretory granules and released by standard secretagogues [94]. However, tenfold greater amounts of TNF-α than are stored in the cells are synthesized and released in response to stimulation by an IgE-dependent mechanism [95]. Experiments using a specific antibody have shown that TNF-α is responsible for at least part of the IgE-dependent accumulation of leukocytes in the late-phase allergic response [292]. Indirect evidence for the release of TNF-α by human skin mast cells has also been reported [148]. The possibility that mast cells are capable of providing other cytokines is suggested by the identification of several other cytokine messenger RNAs in mouse mast cells in culture (Chap. 13) [97, 158].

Proteases

The first evidence that mast cells contained an unusual hydrolytic enzyme was provided by Gomori [91]. Using histochemical methodology, he demonstrated that the chloracetyl ester of naphthol AS was hydrolyzed more rapidly by mast cells than by any other cell type. Studies of extracts of rat mast cells and granules [14], as well as detailed histochemical analysis [212], established that the enzyme responsible for mast cell staining was a serine esteroprotease with many similarities to α-chymotrypsin. Fibrinolytic activity extractable from dog mast cell tumors was consistent with the presence of a second protease, a trypsin-like enzyme [66]. The third distinct type of protease identified in mast cells was carboxypeptidase [98, 284]. The capacity of these enzymes for selectively cleaving peptide bonds endows them with the potential for a variety of potent biologic actions, including the formation [221] and inactivation [155] of kinins, conversion of angiotensin I to angiotensin II [227], activation of collagenases [21], participation in the hemostatic process [190, 252], degradation of low-density lipoprotein [149, 150], inactivation of complement components [83], and proteolysis of connective tissue matrix proteins [20, 87, 286]. The presence of several proteases in a single granule makes possible the concerted actions of these enzymes [149]. Which, if any, of the potential functions are actually performed by the mast cell proteases is not established. Unlike the lysosomal hydrolytic enzymes, the proteases of mast cell granules have alkaline pH optima.

The identification of a second chymotrypsin-like protease [228] in a subset of mast cells present in rat bowel and airway mucosa presaged the existence of multiple, related enzymes in human and mouse mast cells. There is cathepsin G in human mast cells [242], and as many as four homologous chymases have been identified in the mouse [198, 199, 208]. The selective expression of the closely related genes for these chymase variants, together with those responsible for the other proteases, has been used to define the phenotypic heterogeneity among mast cells. How much of this heterogeneity represents fixed differentiation and how much is attributable to maturational or extrinsic modulation, or both, are as yet undetermined [81].

The term *mast cell chymase* was originally proposed to avoid

Table 21-2. Mediator content of human mast cells

Site	Histamine (pg/cell)	PGD_2 (fg/cell)	LTC_4 (fg/cell)	LTB_4 (fg/cell)	PAF (fg/cell)
Skin	3.5	144	15	?	?
Lung	3.6	55	50	4	?
Intestine	2.8	21	4	?	?
Uterus	2.1	89	45	?	?
Basophil	0.5	<1	21	6	0.4

PGD_2 = prostaglandin D_2; LTC_4 = leukotriene C_4; LTB_4 = leukotriene B_4; PAF = platelet-activating factor.

referring to the enzyme as "a chymotrypsin-like esterase of mast cells," and to imply that the enzyme might belong to a distinct family of proteases [211]. The parallel term *tryptase* for the trypsin-like esterase was proposed at the same time.

Rat mast cell chymase I contains 227 amino acids with considerable homology in its three-dimensional structure with pancreatic chymotrypsin and related enzymes [173]. The human form of chymase has been isolated and characterized [239, 241]. The sequence homology of the mast cell chymases with lymphocyte proteases and neutrophil cathepsin G is greater than that with pancreatic chymotrypsin. Both the sequence of the proenzyme form of rat mast cell chymase II, adduced from its complementary DNA sequence, and the distribution of its three disulfide bonds further indicate the existence of an inflammatory cell serine protease family [16]. Unlike pancreatic chymotrypsinogen, the chymase in the mature secretory granule requires no proteolytic activation. The active site is available in situ for reaction with such inhibitors as phenylmethylsulfonyl fluoride or diisopropyl fluorophosphate [168]. The low pH of the granule matrix restricts the enzyme activity, and enzyme activity may also be limited through immobilization by matrix heparin. Le Trong and colleagues [172] have proposed that the activity of chymase following secretion is limited by a granule matrix barrier that excludes proteins with molecular weights of 15,000 or less. Observations from experiments suggest that expansion of the granule matrix in the normal extracellular ionic milieu effectively eliminates any limitation of access to the granule-bound chymase of most soluble extracellular proteins, including the inhibitor α_1-antiprotease (D. Lagunoff and A. Rickard. Unpublished observations, 1991).

Mast cell tryptase is distinct from chymase in several ways, besides its substrate specificity. Its active form in the three species in which it has been studied is a tetramer with a molecular weight of 135,000 to 156,000. Based on the sequence of tryptase determined from a dog tumor, there are 245 amino acids in the active enzyme [285]. The human enzyme and a variant form have also been cloned [200, 201]. The dog and human enzymes are stabilized by heparin [34, 122], and, once tryptase separates from the glycosaminoglycan, it dissociates to its inactive monomers. The small amount of tryptase in the rat mast cell is weakly bound to the granule matrix, and enzyme activity is rapidly lost following secretion [169]. In human mast cells, tryptase is the predominant protease in both the MC_T and MC_{TC} types [251, 253].

Mast cell carboxypeptidase, which was first found in the rat [46, 98], has since been identified in human [90, 229] and mouse mast cells [229, 230]. MC_T lacks identifiable carboxypeptidase, but, as in the rat peritoneal mast cell, it is a major granule protein in the human MC_{TC} [125]. Although the enzyme has greater sequence homology with pancreatic carboxypeptidase B, its substrate specificity more closely resembles that of pancreatic carboxypeptidase A, with its predilection for C-terminal phenylalanine and leucine residues [229]. The substrate specificity of mast cell carboxypeptidase suggests a capacity to work together with chymase, cleaving C-terminal residues exposed by the prior action of chymase [149]. The molecular weight of mast cell carboxypeptidase is 35,000. An aminopeptidase first observed histochemically in rat mast cells [28] has been rediscovered in mouse mast cells [259]. Rat mast cells also contain a trypsin inhibitor, trasylol [79, 141, 142], that is complexed to tryptase; the tryptase nevertheless largely retains its activity, particularly at pH 7.5 [141, 169].

Lysosomal Enzymes

The absence of ultrastructural evidence for the existence of lysosomes in mast cells prompted investigation for the presence and distribution in the rat mast cell of the acid hydrolases found in these organelles. N-acetyl-β-hexosaminidase appears to be exclusively a secretory granule enzyme [166]. Most, but not all, mast cell β-glucuronidase also exists in the granules. Of the three enzymes initially studied, only acid phosphatase is apparently not present in the specific secretory granules of the mast cells, and thus can serve as a marker for the cell's lysosomes [166]. The localization of N-acetyl-β-hexosaminidase and β-glucuronidase to the secretory granule has been confirmed in the rat and human by the demonstration of its corelease with histamine upon stimulation of cell secretion [248, 249, 254]; both enzymes are largely diffusible during granule exocytosis. Arylsulfatase, another hydrolase with an acid pH optimum, also exists in mast cell granules [185].

Other Granule Constituents

Peroxidase [111] and superoxide dismutase [58, 111] have both been reported to be present in rat mast cell granules. Studies in my laboratory have yielded data indicating that the peroxidase activity is attributable to contamination of the cell and granule preparations with eosinophils and eosinophil granules rich in this enzyme (D. Lagunoff and A. Rickard. Unpublished observations, 1991). Mast cell granules avidly bind eosinophil peroxidase [110].

GRANULE STRUCTURE

Because human mast cell granules have not yet been isolated, the information available on aspects of the granule structure has been derived from studies of rat mast cell granules. The striking differences in the morphology between the rat and human granule ultrastructure suggest a high likelihood of important differences in the molecular details of the granule structure in the two species as well.

Rat mast cell granules are readily isolated with their surrounding membranes intact [152, 223]. Removal of the perigranule membrane in hypotonic solution, with or without use of the detergent triton X-100, leaves the granule matrix intact, as observed by electron microscopy. Removal of the membrane in a low-ionic-strength medium releases some histamine as well as most of the tryptase and N-acetyl-β-hexosaminidase. Treatment of the granule with sodium chloride solutions of increasing ionic strength to 3.0 M progressively solubilizes the components of the granule: residual histamine, glucuronidase, chymase, and carboxypeptidase, in that order. At a salt concentration of 0.15 M, equivalent to that in the extracellular milieu, little chymase and essentially no carboxypeptidase are released from the granule matrix (D. Lagunoff and A. Rickard. Unpublished observations, 1991). In the process of secretion, the swelling of the granule, evident on electron micrographs, has been elegantly documented in video images using image enhancement [202]. The reversible salt-dependent swelling is associated with increased access of the protein substrates and inhibitors to the matrix-bound proteases (D. Lagunoff and A. Rickard. Unpublished observations, 1991). Simultaneous patch-clamp measurements and video monitoring indicate that granule swelling consistently occurs after secretion and not before [5, 29, 72, 298]. The swelling is not associated with proteoglycan cleavage [225].

In studies of granules isolated without membranes, neither my colleagues and I [165] nor Berqvist's group [19] identified more than just traces of phospholipid in the granules. In contrast, Chock and Schmauder-Chock [38] claimed that rat granules isolated with intact membranes contain three times the quantity of phospholipid required to envelop the granules with a lipid bilayer. They proposed that the excess phospholipids are located in the granule matrix in a non-bilayer form and that this phospholipid is the source of much of the arachidonic acid that is converted to lipid mediators by stimulated cells [37, 245]. It may be that these workers have captured lipid bodies [63, 101] in their granule preparations.

MECHANISM OF GRANULE SECRETION

A wide range of stimuli can induce granule secretion and histamine release, including firm stroking of the skin and cold in sensitive individuals [164]. The activity of many of the medically significant stimuli is determined by the presence of specific IgE antibodies on the mast cell surface [128, 129]. Substances that act independently of IgE can be classified as cytotoxic agents, enzymes, polysaccharides, lectins, anaphylatoxins, polybasic compounds, or paucibasic compounds [164]. However, even such an extended classification does not completely suffice, because adenosine triphosphate (ATP) [18], fluoride [213, 257], formylmethionine peptides [83], calcium ionophores [17, 45], and histamine-releasing factors [10, 137] are also active (Table 21-3).

Early observations made by light microscopy of mast cell granule discharge misled some investigators to believe that the cell was disrupted in the process (Fig. 21-3). Detailed biochemical studies [133, 134], carefully performed light microscopy evaluations [120, 234], and use of the electron microscope [23, 263] corrected this error in thinking and established that histamine release in most instances depends on an active organized process of granule extrusion by a viable cell. After an extensive loss of granules, the mast cell can reinitiate granule synthesis and reconstitute its supply of mediators [104, 203].

Cell secretion considered in topological terms poses the problem of transferring secretory material from the inside to the outside of the cell without interrupting the continuity of the cell membrane. In the case of the mast cell granule, as with other secretory granules, a second boundary, the perigranule membrane, is interposed between the cytoplasm and the granule. This perigranule membrane simplifies the secretory process, as the granule inside its membrane is already topologically outside the cell. Secretion thus requires only that continuity be established between the membrane-limited extracellular compartment in which the granule is lodged and the extended extracellular compartment outside the cell. Detailed studies of the process with the electron microscope have indicated that the two compartments initially join through the focal fusion of the cell membrane and perigranule membrane [156]. A subsequent rearrangement creates a cell membrane extended by the insertion of the perigranule membrane. Further fusions of adjacent perigranule membranes place the granules in channels of extracellular medium, deep within the domain of the cell (Fig. 21-4) [156, 234]. Nothing as yet is known of the molecular events that occur at the site of membrane fusion, although a substantial amount of research has been devoted to identifying factors that initiate, facilitate, or inhibit histamine secretion.

When mast cells are deprived of their usual content of ATP [56, 57, 132] or are depleted of calcium [82, 216], secretion does not

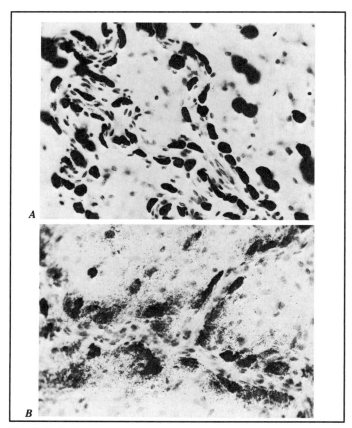

Fig. 21-3. *Light micrographs of perivascular mast cells in the subcutaneous connective tissue of rat foot skin. The connective tissue spreads were stained with toluidine blue. A. Tissue incubated in balanced salt solution. The mast cells are densely stained and have distinct margins; only a few extracellular granules are evident. B. A spread from skin incubated in the presence of 2.5 mg/ml of ovomucoid, a mast cell–degranulating protein present in egg white. The mast cells have extensively discharged their granules. (× 260.)*

proceed. The role of adenosine 3':5'-cyclic phosphate (cAMP) in mast cell secretion has also been examined intensively. The first wave of investigations led to the proposal that increases in the cAMP content were associated with a decreased capacity of mast cells for secretion. This hypothesis was beset with discrepant results and inconsistencies [272] and was replaced by the concept that a transient elevation in the cAMP concentration occurs in association with secretion, but inconsistencies remain [114–117] and the controversy continues [215].

At least four mast cell proteins are phosphorylated after the induction of secretion [261, 262]. One of these has been proposed as an inhibitory factor responsible for limiting the secretory response [262, 275]. The presence of a kinase that is under the influence of cAMP has not been demonstrated.

Since Michell and colleagues [171, 195, 196] first called attention to the increased turnover of phosphatidylinositol in a variety of cells in association with secretion, there has been intense interest in the role of membrane inositol phospholipid metabolism in secretion. In the mast cell, Kennerly and colleagues [139, 140] authenticated the increased turnover of phospholipid and proposed that an accumulation of DAG may be essential in mast cell secretion. The inhibitory effects on secretion of eicosatetraenoic acid [206], an inhibitor of both the cyclooxygenase and lipoxygenase pathways of arachidonic acid metabolism, implicated one or the other of these pathways in secretion, but several instances of dissociation of arachidonic acid metabolism and

Table 21-3. *Secretory stimuli for human mast cells*

Tissue source	Secretory stimulus				
	IgE	FMLP	C5a	Substance P	Morphine
Skin	+	+	+	+	+
Lung	+	−	−	−	−
Intestine	+	−	−	−	−
Uterus	+	−	−	−	?
Basophil	+	+	+	−	−

IgE = immunoglobulin E; FMLP = formyl-methionyl-leucyl-phenylalanine; + = positive; − = negative.

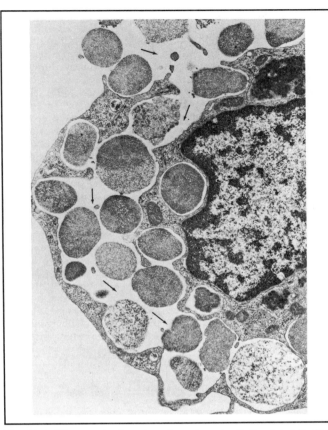

Fig. 21-4. *Micrograph of a rat peritoneal mast cell stimulated in vitro with polymyxin B sulfate. A deep channel is seen that contains granules in different stages of dissolution (arrows). The cytoplasm forming the outer boundary of the channel, although extremely attenuated, is obviously intact. (× 13,000.)*

secretion are inconsistent with a requirement for either pathway products in secretion [39, 41, 194]. An attractive feature of the inositol phosphate pathway as a possible critical part of the secretory mechanism is the generation of two complementary agents, DAG, an activator of protein kinase C, and inositol trisphosphate, a Ca^{++}-releasing agent. In the case of the mast cell, relatively little of the DAG produced during a secretory response derives from phosphatidylinositol; most of it comes from phosphatidylcholine via the actions of phospholipase D and phosphatidic acid phosphatase [59, 179]. Also damaging to the proposal for involvement of the inositol phosphate pathway with activation of protein kinase C in mast cell secretion is the evidence that ATP, and thus phosphorylation, is not essential for the terminal events of mast cell secretion, at least in the permeabilized cell [186].

A great number of experimental results support a critical intermediary role for an increased cytoplasmic Ca^{++} concentration in mast cell secretion. For many secretagogues, adequate levels of extracellular Ca^{++} or a substitute are essential for secretion; for others, depletion of intracellular Ca^{++} in the absence of extracellular Ca^{++} prevents secretion. The strong secretory activity shown by Ca^{++} ionophores [17, 45, 74] and by Ca^{++} when introduced by microinjection [136] or liposome fusion [276] further supports the hypothesis that elevated intracellular levels of Ca^{++} can trigger the secretory process.

Of a substantial number of exogenous enzymes examined, only phospholipase A_2 [15, 282] and chymotrypsin [163, 235, 282] were found to stimulate mast cell secretion at concentrations below 1 mg/ml. Neither enzyme is cytotoxic at effective concentrations.

An interesting feature of the histamine release caused by chymotrypsin is that it can be inhibited by prior treatment of the mast cells with trypsin [163]; however, the trypsin neither releases histamine nor inhibits the release caused by polymyxin B sulfate. An endogenous esterase with characteristics similar to those of chymase has been implicated in mast cell secretion using specific inhibitors [126]. The putative enzyme apparently cannot be inhibited before the secretory mechanism is activated, and it is presumed that conversion from a precursor to an active form occurs during secretion. Failure to demonstrate the enzyme directly has dampened the enthusiasm for this concept.

The identification of microtubules and microfilaments in mast cells and the availability of drugs that derange the structure of these elements have generated much interest in the role of these cytoskeletal elements in secretion. Colchicine, vinblastine sulfate, and griseofulvin, which cause the dissociation of microtubules, have been reported to inhibit mast cell secretion. However, unusually high concentrations of the drugs are required, only moderate inhibition is achieved, and there is no association between disruption of the microtubules and interference with secretion [162], so that microtubules do not appear to be essential for granule secretion.

Cytochalasins B and D have been used to dissociate microfilaments and to implicate actin participation in cytokinesis, morphogenetic events, and other cell activities. Actin filaments are found in mast cells, but the results of studies that examine the effect of cytochalasins on mast cell secretion have been contradictory; inhibition of secretion has been reported [212], but, in my laboratory, we found that cytochalasin B had no effect on rat peritoneal mast cell secretion when stimulated by polymyxin B sulfate at concentrations of cytochalasin B that caused a major loss of microfilaments. In addition, a decrease in the filamentous actin concentration has been shown to occur in parallel with secretion in permeabilized mast cells [94]. Botulinum toxin C_2, which causes the breakdown of actin filaments by blocking adenosine diphosphate–ribosylation of actin, partially inhibits histamine release induced by some secretagogues, but does not affect that induced by A23187 [26].

Two recent methods that allow access to the cytoplasmic domain of the cell have substantially helped in adding to the information on the mechanism of mast cell secretion: the whole-cell patch-clamp electrode [3, 5, 71] and membrane permeabilization [93]. In the whole-cell patch-clamp method, an electrode in the form of a micropipette is first sealed to the cell membrane and the patch of membrane within the pipette tip is then ruptured, leaving the pipette sealed in the membrane. This arrangement allows exchange of cytoplasmic material with the solution in the micropipette and the simultaneous measurement of secretion as an increase in capacitance caused by insertion of granule membrane into the plasma membrane. The second technique, membrane permeabilization, entails disrupting the plasma membrane as a barrier to the free exchange of small charged molecules and macromolecules, while preserving the secretory capability of the cell. Bacterial lysins, most commonly streptolysin O or agents such as digitonin or saponin, which perturb membrane structure by virtue of their aggregation of cholesterol, have been used [121, 158, 267]. The most important finding derived from the application of these methods is the central importance of guanosine triphosphate (GTP) in mast cell secretion [92]. The addition of GTP or its analogs, including those that are nonhydrolyzable by cell enzymes, can, in the presence of permissive levels of free Ca^{++}, induce mast cell exocytosis [121, 158]. In the permeabilized cell, only levels of Ca^{++} greater than 100 μM induce secretion in the absence of GTP [158]. The general inability of pertussis toxin to inhibit secretion of the permeabilized cell induced by GTP rules out participation of the specific G-protein target of this toxin [182]. Under some conditions, ATP can be demonstrated to regulate permeabilized mast cell secretion [42], but its reduction to very low levels of approximately 10 nM does not prevent secretion [158]. It has been possible to restore the capacity for secretion to permeabilized cells that have lost this ability by replenishing the ATP [42]. Such cells require Ca^{++}, but surprisingly not GTP, for the induction of secretion. Because treatment with okadaic acid, a specific protein phosphatase inhibitor, maintains the requirement for GTP in the absence of ATP, Churcher and associates [42] have proposed that protein dephosphorylation is a permissive step in secretion and that the role of GTP is to activate a putative protein phosphatase. Based on studies with permeabilized rat basophilic leukemia (RBL) cells, the elevated cytoplasmic pH has been proposed as another critical signal for secretion [4]. It is obvious that no coherent picture of the biochemical events involved in the terminal stages of mast cell secretion can yet be drawn, but an inventory of the molecular participants is painstakingly being drawn up.

MAST CELL HETEROGENEITY

From the time of their first description by Heidenhain [107], the granular cells of the digestive tract have created confusion. Weill [291] made an early attempt to distinguish among the several different cell types that fell into the group. Following Maximow's proposal, he considered one of these cell types to be atypical mast cells. The term *atypical mast cell* has now largely been replaced by *mucosal mast cells* [70]. My attention was first drawn to these cells by their unexpected appearance when rat stomach and intestine tissue was stained with histochemical chymase substrates [160]. Present both within the epithelium and the lamina propria, these cells were the only strongly chymase-positive cells other than connective tissue mast cells; the cells stained only faintly with acidic toluidine blue and contained fewer granules than do connective tissue mast cells. Enerbäck [67] definitively demonstrated the atypical mast cells in rat gut tissue by fixation in Carnoy's solution or a diluted acid formaldehyde solution and staining with alcian blue. An improved staining method was more recently introduced by Wingren and Enerbäck [293] and uses conventional formaldehyde fixation with staining in 0.5% toluidine blue at pH 0.5 for a week. They have proposed that the difference between the staining of cells which contain heparin and those which contain non-heparin proteoglycan after formalin fixation is a function of differential blocking of staining that depends on the penetration of the granule by the dye rather than on a loss of the proteoglycan in the fixative.

Enerbäck [67, 69] observed that not only did the mucosal mast cells fail to stain after standard formalin fixation, but their granules are consistently positive for alcian blue using the alcian blue–safranin method, and the cells are unresponsive to compound 48/80 [68]. In contrast, typical connective tissue mast cells are safranin positive and degranulate on exposure to compound 48/80. Combs and colleagues [48] proposed that safranin staining of mast cells depends on the presence of *N*-sulfated heparin, as the selective removal of *N*-sulfated glycosaminoglycan with nitrous acid converted safranin-positive mast cells to alcian blue–positive cells. Tas and Berndsen [273] provided evidence that the removal of *N*-sulfated heparin allowed the macromolecular alcian blue aggregates to penetrate the granule matrix, there bind to residual glycosaminoglycan, and thereby block safranin staining. The chemical basis for the anomalous staining of mucosal mast cells was explained by the identification of an over-sulfated dermatan sulfate in rat mucosal mast cells [70]. The same glycosaminoglycan is found in RBL cells [257].

Woodbury and coworkers [296] discovered that mucosal mast cells and connective tissue mast cells in the rat harbor distinct chymases [296]. Irani and coworkers [123] showed that two types of human mast cells could be distinguished by the presence of chymase in one (MC$_{TC}$) but not in the other (MC$_T$). The presence of carboxypeptidase in MC$_{TC}$ but not in MC$_T$ further distinguishes the two types of mast cells [124]. The two cell types in humans contain heparin plus chondroitin sulfate E [271], but in different proportions; MC$_{TC}$ in skin contain more heparin than chondroitin sulfate, whereas MC$_T$ in lung contain predominantly chondroitin sulfate. A complete absence of heparin has been reported in gut mast cells, with only chondroitin sulfate E present [65]. The difference in responsiveness to the polyamine class of secretagogues between connective tissue and mucosal mast cells [68, 70] is also reflected by the two types of human mast cells [81]. Ratios of prostaglandin D$_2$ to leukotriene C$_4$ generated on stimulation differ among mast cells from different tissues; skin cells have a higher ratio than do lung and intestine. As far as the origin of the differences in mast cells, Michels [197] observed in his monograph of 1938 that "variations in the morphology of the tissue mast cell may be due to various factors, intrinsic or extrinsic. Among the former may be listed a) genetic origin, b) ameboid movement, c) physiologic condition of the cell; among the latter a) environmental or media conditions, b) fixation, embedding and staining." The current formulation of the problem of mast cell heterogeneity is couched in terms of phenotypic variation, differentiation, and transdifferentiation, and the indicators of variability are the glycosaminoglycans, the proteases, and the appearance of the granules on electron micrographs [81]. Results of studies of the generation of mast cells in mice strongly indicate that the two mast cell phenotypes are, to a great extent, interconvertible [144].

DISTRIBUTION OF MAST CELLS

Mast cells in human tissues can be found wherever there is loose connective tissue; mast cells are excluded from cartilage and bone matrix. In most tissues, because the preponderance of histamine is stored in mast cells, the quantity of histamine in a tissue can be used as a rough indicator of mast cell frequency. Histamine levels above 5 μg/gm occur in the skin, lungs, and gastrointestinal tract of humans. Intermediate levels of 1 to 5 μg/gm are found in most other organs. The central nervous system contains less than 1 μg/gm, and not all of the histamine originates from the mast cell [89].

Soter [268] counted 12.1 $\pm$ 5.1 $\times 10^6$ mast cells per cubic millimeter in human dermis. Mast cells in the dermis, as elsewhere, have a predilection for associating with small blood vessels and nerves. Although frequently situated close to the blood vessel wall, mast cells do not reside within the endothelial basal lamina. In nerves, mast cells are frequently found inside the endoneurium. The results of a number of studies have indicated interactions between the nervous system and mast cells, particularly nerve terminals that secrete substance P [22, 209, 264].

In the gastrointestinal tract, MC$_{TC}$ predominate in the submucosa [266], where they may be found in association with blood vessels and nerves, as in the skin. In the mucosa, most of the mast cells are of the MC$_T$ type. In the lung, mast cells which are largely of the MC$_{TC}$ type are prevalent in the submucosa of the bronchi and bronchioles, as well as in association with the large blood vessels. Mucosal mast cells in both tissues are capable of penetrating the basal lamina and taking up residence in the epithelium.

The numbers of mast cells are plentiful in the pleura, limited in normal alveolar septa, and notably increased in the context of interstitial pulmonary fibrosis. The findings from quantitative studies of mast cell frequency in the larynx, trachea, and mainstem bronchi of human embryos have been reported [127]. The most thorough study of mast cell distribution in the adult primate lung is that of Guerzon and associates [96], who examined the monkey *Macaca fascicularis*. Eighty-three percent of the total lung mast cells were found in the conducting airways. The mast cell frequency was essentially the same from the trachea to the small bronchi and ranged from 250 to 500 cells/mm^3, but the frequency increased to 1,000 cells/mm^3 in the bronchioles. Gold and his collaborators [88] found that, in the dog airway, there is a progressive increase in the number of cells per cubic millimeter as the airway diameter decreases. The only quantitative study of human lung mast cells is that of Connell [49], who observed no notable difference between the number of mast cells post mortem in proximal airways of different sizes; there was no mention of the number of mast cells in the bronchioles.

Less attention has been directed to the distribution of mast cells through the thickness of the walls of airways. Connell [49] found mast cells at the ends of cartilage segments, between cartilage and muscle, and outside the basement membrane of mucous glands. Guerzon and coworkers [96] noted the distribution in monkey airways for three levels, epithelium, basement membrane to cartilage, and outside the cartilage, to be 0 to 15 percent, 40 to 60 percent, and 40 to 50 percent, respectively.

While the wall of the airways is not as clearly segregated into mucosa and submucosa by its smooth muscle as the wall of the gastrointestinal tract is divided by the muscularis mucosa, a lamina propria in the human airways can be distinguished from the submucosal connective tissue. When the airways are fixed with the smooth muscle in a contracted state, the lamina propria is particularly obvious as the substance of the ridges that protrude into the airway lumen. I have examined the distribution of lung mast cells in tissues in three persons who died suddenly of trauma without known antecedent disease. Mast cells are far more prevalent in the submucosa between the smooth muscle and the cartilage than in the lamina propria. Some, but by no means most, of the mast cells are close to the walls of small veins. A few mast cells are intimately associated with mucous glands. No predilection for nerves is evident. Occasionally mast cells are present within fascicles of smooth muscle cells.

In the trachea and main-stem bronchi of the rat, the lamina propria in the uninflamed state is quite narrow, containing capillaries, a few venules, and little else; few mast cells are present in this site. As in human airways, submucosal mast cells are found close to small veins, within smooth muscle bundles, or simply scattered in the loose connective tissue. Outside the cartilage, the mast cells are found in fat, occasionally within nerves, and scattered throughout the loose connective tissue. Within the actual epithelial layer of both the trachea and bronchus, there are cells with metachromatic granules and the ultrastructural appearance of mast cells. Cells with these characteristics have been observed by Brinkman [30] and Cutz and colleagues [53] in the epithelium in human biopsy material.

Patterson and coworkers have obtained mast cells by bronchial lavage from rhesus monkeys [279] and humans [214]. These cells secrete histamine in response to several stimuli. It is plausible that the source of luminal mast cells is the intraepithelial mast cell population. Patterson and coworkers have proposed that the mast cells in the alveoli are responsible for the ability of inhaled high-molecular-weight, poorly permeant allergens to elicit histamine release.

GENESIS OF MAST CELLS

The development sequence of mast cells in the mammalian embryo has been most thoroughly studied in the rat [48]. Cells with metachromatic granules first appear at 15 days after conception in the cephalad mesenchyme of the rat and become most numerous in the limb buds. Subsequently, mast cells increase in number, both by differentiation from precursors and by mitosis of incompletely differentiated forms. These two mechanisms for cell increase are retained in adult connective tissue. The earliest cells in the developmental sequence, identifiable as mast cells

by the presence of a few granules positive for chymase, stain blue with the alcian blue–safranin method. As the cells accumulate granules, there is a shift to increasing proportions of safranin-positive granules. The specific identification of the glycosaminoglycans present during this process has not been undertaken. The observation that the least mature mast cells identifiable in the mast cell lineage in the peritoneal fluid of rat pups are well endowed with high-affinity IgE-binding sites suggests that these cell-surface receptors may be useful for the identification and isolation of the earliest stages in the sequence of mast cell development [170].

Kitamura and associates [145, 146] have carried out a series of experiments to identify the source of precursors of mast cells in the mouse. A critical part of their approach has been the use of two mouse strains, W/W^v and SL/SL^d, that possess complementary genetic defects in the production of mast cells. They found the largest number of precursors in adult bone marrow and spleen as well as fetal liver. Lymphoid tissues, including the thymus, contain only a small fraction, less than 0.1 percent, of the number of precursors present in the hematopoietic tissues on a per gram basis. Evidence against a lymphoid precursor to the connective tissue mast cell includes a normal number of connective tissue mast cells in T-cell–deficient nude mice [189, 294] and the failure of anti–Thy 1,2 antibodies in the presence of complement to deplete the bone marrow of mast cell precursors. However, the importance of an intact lymphoid system for mucosal mast cell differentiation is attested to by the following facts: the increase in mast cell numbers in the bowel wall in response to nematode infection does not occur in nude mice [189]; mucosal mast cells are depleted in patients with DiGeorge syndrome [189], who congenitally lack a thymus; and T-cell deficiency in humans is associated with the selective absence of MC$_T$ [122]. Using spleen colonies formed in irradiated mice, Kitamura and coworkers [146] showed that colony-forming unit–spleen stem cells are capable of differentiating to mast cells as well as erythrocytes, granulocytes, megakaryocytes, and B-lymphocytes. Unlike other derivatives of the multipotential hematopoietic stem cells, mast cell precursors normally leave the hematopoietic tissues and complete their differentiation in connective tissues.

A major advance in understanding the control of mast cell differentiation were the independent discoveries that supernatants from WEHI cells [210, 274], mouse spleen cells exposed to concanavalin A [203, 224], and rat lymphocytes from *Nippostrongylus brasiliensis*–infected rats stimulated with specific antigen [99] are able to induce the differentiation of mast cells from immature hematopoietic cells in vitro. The cells that develop under these circumstances have been variously proposed to be immature, incompletely developed, or mucosal mast cells. Such cells have low levels of histamine, predominantly contain chondroitin sulfate E rather than heparin [226] and possess plasma membrane receptors for IgE [224, 274]. In the case of bone marrow–derived mast cells in the rat, chymase II is present in the cells [99], a characteristic of the mucosal type of mast cell. The factor responsible for the appearance of these mast cells in culture has been identified as interleukin-3 (IL-3). Repeated IL-3 injections are able to induce mast cell proliferation in the nude mouse intestine [1]. Transforming growth factor-beta prevents the proliferation but not the differentiation induced in mast cell precursors by IL-3 [31].

Subsequent studies have adduced evidence for additional factors active in stimulating the expression of the mast cell phenotype. IL-4 [100, 265] in the presence of IL-3 enhances the proliferation of mouse mast cells and contributes to the differentiation of the cells but seems to add little to the effect of IL-3 on human mast cells and basophil precursors. The cell responsive to IL-3 in human bone marrow has been identified as CD34 positive [143]. Antibodies to IL-3 and IL-4 administered to mice prevent the considerable increase in intestine mucosal mast cells induced by parasitic infection [186]. IL-3 also stimulates mast cell motility [188], and IL-4 increases mast cell attachment to the endothelial intercellular adhesion molecule protein [283].

The coculture of mast cell precursors with embryonic fibroblasts was a component of the first successful strategy for culturing mast cells in vitro [85]. The 3T3 line of presumptive fibroblasts was subsequently shown to produce a factor, or factors, that support differentiation of connective tissue mast cells [130, 175]. Most recently, exploitation of the genetic defect in the mast cell–deficient SL/SL^d mouse led to the characterization of a factor, the stem cell factor (SCF), also called *mast cell growth factor* or *kit ligand*, which is produced variously by fibroblasts, fetal liver, and bone marrow, that induces both proliferation of an early mast cell precursor and mast cell differentiation [280, 281]. The W/W^v mouse, which also expresses a severe mast cell deficiency, lacks the transmembrane protein kinase receptor to which SCF binds [81].

MAST CELL NEOPLASMS

Human mast cell neoplasms, although rare, present in a perplexing array of proliferations, varying from circumscribed, solitary, and nodular benign tumors of the skin to diffuse, multifocal, infiltrative malignancies (Table 21-4) [191, 236, 278]. A modification of the classification of Travis and associates has been proposed to encompass this variety of disorders [182]. Uncomplicated papular urticaria pigmentosa is the most common lesion. Systemic symptoms of widespread flushing, tachycardia, nausea, vomiting, headache, and, less frequently, shock, fever, colic, duodenal ulcers, diarrhea, and malabsorption may occur as complications of urticaria pigmentosa and of other variants of mastocytosis or mast cell malignancies. Some of these symptoms are attributable to the effects of histamine or prostaglandin D$_2$, or both substances, released by the mast cells [232, 233]. Antihistamines, cromolyn sodium, and corticosteroids have been used effectively for treatment [192]. Skin mast cell neoplasms (mast cell sarcomas) are common in dogs [143], with a particularly high frequency in the Boston bull and the boxer. Mastocytomas occur in cats and have been reported in cattle.

BASOPHILS

The similarity in the metachromatic staining characteristics between the circulating blood basophil and the mast cell was apparent to Ehrlich [64], and the homology is now known to extend to several granule constituents. Histamine was found to exist in basophils at the same time as in tissue mast cells, but at a lower concentration [61], and an esterase with the substrate specificity of trypsin has been identified in rat basophils [154]. The level of tryptase in human basophils has been estimated at $\frac{1}{300}$ of that in MC$_{TC}$ [33]. Protease activity attributable to neither chymase nor

Table 21-4. Mast cell proliferative lesions

Cutaneous mastocytosis
  Mastocytoma
  Urticaria pigmentosa
  Diffuse cutaneous mastocytosis
  Telangiectasia macularis eruptiva perstans
Systemic mastocytosis
  Indolent mastocytosis: cutaneous infiltrate, gastrointestinal disease, bone marrow involvement, skeletal disease, hepatosplenomegaly, lymphadenopathy
  Hematologic mastocytosis: myeloproliferation, myelodysplasia
  Aggressive mastocytosis
  Leukemic mastocytosis

tryptase has been noted in human basophils [154, 207]. Basophils, like mast cells, have high-affinity receptors for IgE and can be induced to secrete granules when the appropriate antigen combines with IgE on the cell surface [13, 61, 62, 105, 109].

There are important morphologic differences between mature basophils and mast cells [81]. Mast cells possess a single-lobed nucleus, whereas the smaller basophils typically display a polymorphic nucleus. The fine structure of the granules differs between the two cells in humans. Basophil granules are universally particulate [61, 106]. The constituents also differ, in that the glycosaminoglycan of human basophil granules is chondroitin-4-sulfate and the basophil produces no prostaglandin D$_2$ and little leukotriene B$_4$ [287], although it does manufacture leukotriene C$_4$ and PAF. Basophils, unlike mast cells, contain two proteins originally described in eosinophils: lysophospholipase (Charcot-Leyden crystal material) and eosinophil major basic protein [2, 174]. Basophil differentiation like that of the mast cell is induced by IL-3 [284], but, in contrast to the process in the mast cell, completion of the differentiation program appears to depend on granulocyte/macrophage colony–stimulating factor (GM-CSF) [246] rather than on IL-4 or SCF. It is notable that GM-CSF inhibits the proliferation of mast cell precursors [31]. Evidence has recently been adduced that IL-5 may contribute to basophil differentiation [55].

Basophils are the least common cell normally circulating in humans. Decreased basophil counts have been reported to be associated with acute urticaria [295]. True basophil leukemias are very rare, but basophilia is common early in the chronic form of myelogenous leukemia [84]. Increases in the number of circulating basophils stemming from other causes are uncommon. Intense local infiltrations of basophils occur in the Jones-Mote hypersensitivity reaction to protein antigens observed in guinea pigs [61, 231]. Similar infiltrates in humans in hypersensitivity states have been demonstrated in Rebuck skin windows [295] and in lesions of contact hypersensitivity [61]. Substantial numbers of basophils are also seen in late-phase IgE-mediated inflammatory reactions, and mediators released by basophils have been proposed to be responsible for the late-phase reaction in the nasal mucosa [204, 244] and skin [220]. Like neutrophils, basophils carry the integrin antigens CD11 and CD18 on their surface. Several inflammatory mediators can act on basophils to increase adhesion to the endothelial cells; the effect can be inhibited by anti-CD18 antibody [24], as in the case of the neutrophil.

ROLE OF THE MAST CELL IN ASTHMA

Since the discovery of the IgE-dependent activation of mast cells by antigen, the possibility that mast cells play a role in asthma has been pursued. The arguments for a central role of mast cells, that mast cells were plentiful in the bronchial wall and that antigens capable of eliciting histamine release from skin and nasal mast cells in atopic individuals could also precipitate asthmatic attacks, were initially undermined by the ineffectiveness of antihistamines in antagonizing asthmatic bronchiolar constriction. Subsequent evidence that mast cells could produce significant amounts of leukotriene C$_4$, PAF, TNF, and interleukins has reactivated interest in the contribution of mast cells to the asthmatic reaction.

Pioneering studies of Salvato [237] and Connell [49] that used bronchial biopsy and autopsy material, respectively, provided evidence for mast cell degranulation in asthmatics. Salvato [237] reported a higher frequency of cells that exhibited degranulation after the provocation of asthmatics with compound 48/80 or allergens. Connell [49] demonstrated a marked decrease in bronchial mast cell numbers in patients dying in status asthmaticus, compared with patients dying of other causes. In their dog model of asthma, Gold and his collaborators [88] observed a decrease in mast cell numbers upon aerosol introduction of antigen into the lungs of *Ascaris*-sensitive dogs. These workers were also able to measure concomitant decreases in the lung histamine level and increases in the plasma histamine level. Increases in the blood histamine concentration have also been found in patients during spontaneous asthmatic attacks and following deliberate provocation of bronchial constriction [7].

With the introduction of bronchoalveolar lavage and fiberoptic bronchoscopic biopsy as tools in the study of asthma, there has been a substantial increase in the evidence for mast cell secretion as an integral part of the bronchial inflammatory reaction in asthma. Broide and colleagues [32] compared the cells and mediators present in the bronchoalveolar lavage fluid from symptomatic asthmatics with those from asymptomatic asthmatics and controls. They found greatly increased histamine levels and moderately increased (though not statistically significant) tryptase activity. Values for asymptomatic patients did not differ from those of control subjects. The numbers of airway mast cells were no different among the three groups, but the mast cells in the asymptomatic group released considerably more histamine during incubation after recovery than was observed for the other two groups. Neither Bradley and associates [27] nor Djukanovic and coworkers [60] were able to demonstrate differences between the mast cell numbers in bronchial biopsy specimens obtained from asthmatics and those of nonasthmatic subjects, but Djukanovic's group described changes and provided electron micrographs of findings they considered indicative of ongoing mast cell secretions. Crimi and colleagues [52] studied the changes in asthmatic patients observed following allergen inhalation challenge. Four hours after challenge, the total number of mast cells in bronchial biopsy specimens was unchanged, but the number of degranulated cells increased. In biopsy specimens obtained at 24 hours after challenge, those patients who exhibited a late-phase response had increased numbers of mast cells compared with the count in asthmatics who failed to show a late-phase response.

The obvious importance of eosinophils in asthma, the presence of lymphocytes and macrophages in asthmatic bronchial wall, and the well-known neurogenic effects, argue for considerable complexity of the asthmatic response. The time is ripe for a rigorous and critical sorting out of the mediators involved in the asthmatic reaction, their cell sources, and the interaction between the cells. Whatever the outcome of future studies, any new data are unlikely to controvert the abundant evidence that the mast cell, though not acting alone, must be a central character in the asthmatic scenario.

Mast cells of varying phenotypes share with basophils the common attributes of high-affinity receptors for IgE and secretion. Secretion by this family of cells characteristically takes place in response to antigens that cross-link receptor-bound IgE on the cell surface and thus bring together the receptors and bring about the consequential influx of Ca^{++}. The multiplicity of mediators contained within the mast cell's secretory granules assures a wide range of actions attendant on activation of the secretory mechanism. The catalog of mediators has expanded substantially in the past 10 years, and no doubt a few surprises are still left. We do not have very reliable concepts of how the currently identified components released by the cells act either in physiologic or pathologic contexts. Our ignorance of the actual functions of the abundant supply of active proteases harbored in the granules of these cells is particularly galling. As our knowledge of mast cells and basophils has enlarged, so too has our understanding of the functional range of potential cell targets for their mediators, endothelial cells, epithelial cells, smooth muscle cells, and the circulating leukocytes.

The diversity of phenotypes, although long intimated, has been thoroughly documented in recent years. Even if much of the observed variation turns out to stem from the plasticity of a single cell type that is affected by diverse conditions and stimuli, more like a fibroblast's ability to assume different functional forms than the distinct lineages of lymphocytes, the variability still permits a wide range of activities in different sites under different circumstances. While each new mediator discovered sooner or later prompts the development of a new set of antagonists, hope remains that a thorough dissection of the secretory mechanism will provide the basis for a global interruption of mast cell mediator release without having to resort to counteracting each agonist with a separate, specific drug.

REFERENCES

1. Abe, T., et al. Induction of intestinal mastocytosis in nude mice by repeated injection of interleukin-3. *Int. Arch. Allergy Appl. Immunol.* 86:356, 1988.
2. Ackerman, S. J., et al. Localization of eosinophil major basic protein in human basophils. *J. Exp. Med.* 158:946, 1983.
3. Ahnert-Hilger, G., and Gratzl, M. Controlled manipulation of the cell interior by pore-forming proteins. *Trends Pharmacol. Sci.* 9:195, 1988.
4. Ali, H., Collado-Escobar, D. M., and Beaven, M. A. The rise in concentration of free Ca and of pH provides sequential synergistic signals for secretion in antigen-stimulated rat basophilic leukemia (RBL-2H3) cells. *J. Immunol.* 143:2626, 1989.
5. Almers, W. Exocytosis. *Annu. Rev. Physiol.* 52:607, 1990.
6. Alvarez de Toledo, G., and Fernandez, J. M. Patch-clamp measurements reveal multimodal distribution of granule sizes in rat mast cells. *J. Cell Biol.* 110:1033, 1990.
7. Atkins, P. C., et al. Comparison of plasma histamine and cyclic nucleotides after antigen and metacholine inhalation in man. *J. Allergy Clin. Immunol.* 66:478, 1980.
8. Atkins, P. C., et al. In vivo antigen induced cutaneous mediator release; simultaneous comparisons of histamine, tryptase and prostaglandin D_2 release and the efficacy of oral corticosteroid administration. *J. Allergy Clin. Immunol.* 80:371, 1990.
9. Azizkhan, R. G., et al. Mast cell heparin stimulates migration of capillary endothelial cells in vitro. *J. Exp. Med.* 152:931, 1980.
10. Baeza, M. L., et al. Relationship of one form of human histamine–releasing factor to connective tissue activating peptide-III. *J. Clin. Invest.* 85:1516, 1990.
11. Bauza, M. T., and Lagunoff, D. Histidine transport by isolated rat peritoneal mast cells. *Biochem. Pharmacol.* 30:1271, 1981.
12. Bauza, M. T., and Lagunoff, D. Histidine uptake by isolated rat peritoneal mast cells: effect of inhibition of histidine decarboxylase by α-fluoromethylhistidine. *Biochem. Pharmacol.* 32:59, 1982.
13. Becker, K. E. et al. Surface IgE on human basophils during histamine release. *J. Exp. Med.* 138:394, 1973.
14. Benditt, E. P., and Arase, M. An enzyme in mast cells with properties like chymotrypsin. *J. Exp. Med.* 110:451, 1959.
15. Benditt, E. P., et al. 5-Hydroxytryptamine in mast cells. *Proc. Soc. Exp. Biol. Med.* 90:303, 1955.
16. Benfey, P. N., Yin, F. H., and Leder, P. Cloning of the mast cell protease, RMCP II. Evidence for cell-specific expression and a multi-gene family. *J. Biol. Chem.* 262:5377, 1987.
17. Bennett, J. P., Crockcroft, S., and Gomperts, B. D. Ionomycin stimulates mast cell histamine secretion by forming a lipid-soluble calcium complex. *Nature* 282:851, 1979.
18. Bennett, J. P., Crockcroft, S., and Gomperts, B. D. Rat mast cells permeabilized with ATP secrete histamine in response to calcium ions buffered in the micromolar range. *J. Physiol.* 317:335, 1981.
19. Berqvist, U., Samuelson, G., and Uvnas, B. Chemical composition of basophil granules from isolated mast cells. *Acta Physiol. Scand.* 83:362, 1971.
20. Bienenstock, J., et al. Mast cell/nerve interactions in vitro and in vivo. *Am. Rev. Respir. Dis.* 143:S55, 1991.
21. Birkedal-Hansen, H., et al. Activation of fibroblast procollagenase by mast cell proteases. *Biochim. Biophys. Acta* 438:273, 1976.
22. Blennerhasset, M. G., Tomioka, M., and Bienenstock, J. Formation of contacts between mast cells and sympathetic neurons in vitro. *Cell Tissue Res.* 265:121, 1991.
23. Bloom, G. D., and Haegermark, O. A study on morphological changes and histamine release induced by 48/80 in rat peritoneal mast cells. *Exp. Cell Res.* 40:637, 1965.

24. Bochner, B. S., et al. Adherence of human basophils to cultured umbilical vein endothelial cells. *J. Clin. Invest.* 81:1355, 1988.
25. Boswell, R. N., Austen, N. F., and Goetzl, E. J. Intermediate molecular weight eosinophil chemotactic factors in rat peritoneal mast cells: Immunologic release, granule association, and demonstration of structural heterogeneity. *J. Immunol.* 120:15, 1978.
26. Bottinger, H., Reuner, K.-H., and Aktories, K. Inhibition of histamine release from rat mast cells by botulinum C2 toxin. *Int. Arch. Allergy Appl. Immunol.* 84:380, 1987.
27. Bradley, B. L., et al. Eosinophils, T-lymphocytes, mast cells, neutrophils, and macrophages in bronchial biopsy specimens from atopic subjects with asthma: comparison with biopsy specimens from atopic subjects without asthma and normal control subjects and relationship to bronchial hyperresponsiveness. *J. Allergy Clin. Immunol.* 88:661, 1991.
28. Braun-Falco, O., and Salfeld, K. Leucine aminopeptidase activity in mast cells. *Nature* 183:51, 1959.
29. Breckenridge, L. J., and Almers, W. Final steps in exocytosis observed in a cell with giant secretory granules. *Proc. Natl. Acad. Sci.* 84:1945, 1987.
30. Brinkman, G. L. The mast cell in normal human bronchus and lung. *J. Ultrastruct. Res.* 23:115, 1968.
31. Broide, D. H., et al. Transforming growth factor-β1 selectively inhibits Il-3–dependent mast cell proliferation without affecting mast cell function or differentiation. *J. Immunol.* 143:1591, 1989.
32. Broide, D. H., et al. Evidence of ongoing mast cell and eosinophil degranulation in symptomatic asthma airway. *J. Allergy Clin. Immunol.* 88:637, 1991.
33. Castells, M. C., Irani, A., and Schwartz, L. B. Evaluation of human peripheral blood leukocytes for mast cell tryptase. *J. Immunol.* 138:2184, 1987.
34. Caughey, G. H., et al. Dog mastocytoma tryptase: affinity purification, characterization, and amino-terminal sequence. *Arch. Biochem. Biophys.* 258:555, 1987.
35. Caulfield, J. P., et al. Secretion of dissociated human pulmonary mast cells: evidence for solubilization of granule's contents before discharge. *J. Cell Biol.* 85:229, 1980.
36. Chiu, H., and Lagunoff, D. Histochemical comparison of vertebrate mast cells. *Histochemistry* 4:135, 1972.
37. Chock, S. P., and Schmauder-Chock, E. A. Synthesis of prostaglandins and eicosanoids by the mast cell secretory granule. *Biochem. Biophys. Res. Comm.* 156:1308, 1988.
38. Chock, S. P., and Schmauder-Chock, E. A. Phospholipid storage in the secretory granule of the mast cell. *J. Biol. Chem.* 264:2862, 1989.
39. Church, M. K., et al. Allergy or inflammation? From neuropeptide stimulation of human skin mast cells to studies on the mechanism of the late asthmatic response. *Agents Actions* 26:22, 1989.
40. Church, M. K., et al. Plenary lecture: mast cells, neuropeptides and inflammation. *Agents Actions* 27:8, 1989.
41. Churcher, Y., Allan, D., and Gomperts, B. D. Relationship between arachidonate generation and exocytosis in permeabilized mast cells. *Biochemistry* 266:157, 1990.
42. Churcher, Y., Kramer, I. M., and Gomperts, B. D. Evidence for protein dephosphorylation as a permissive step in GTP-γ-S-induced exocytosis from permeabilized mast cells. *Cell Regul.* 1:523, 1990.
43. Clark, J. M., and Higginbotham, R. D. Cottonmouth moccasin venom: Fractionation of toxic and allergenic components and interaction with tissue mast cells. *Tex. Rep. Biol. Med.* 29:181, 1971.
44. Clark, R. A., Gallin, J. I., and Kaplan, A. P. The selective eosinophil chemotactic activity of histamine. *J. Exp. Med.* 142:1462, 1975.
45. Cochrane, D. E., and Douglas, W. W. Calcium-induced extrusion of secretory granules (exocytosis) in mast cells exposed to 48/80 or the ionophores A-23187 and X-537A. *Proc. Natl. Acad. Sci.* 71:408, 1974.
46. Cole, K. R., et al. Rat mast cell carboxypeptidase: amino acid sequence and evidence of enzyme activity within mast cell granules. *Biochemistry* 30:648, 1991.
47. Combs, J. W. Maturation of rat mast cells: an electron microscopy study. *J. Cell Biol.* 31:563, 1966.
48. Combs, J. W., Lagunoff, D., and Benditt, E. P. Differentiation and proliferation of embryonic mast cells of the rat. *J. Cell Biol.* 25:577, 1965.
49. Connell, J. T. Asthmatic deaths: role of the mast cell. *JAMA* 215:769, 1971.
50. Craig, S. S., Schechter, N. M., and Schwartz, L. B. Ultrastructural analysis of maturing human T and TC mast cells in situ. *Lab. Invest.* 60:147, 1989.
51. Craig, S. S., and Schwartz, L. B. Tryptase and chymase, markers of distinct types of human mast cells. *Immunol. Res.* 8:130, 1989.
52. Crimi, E., et al. Increased numbers of mast cells in bronchial mucosa after the late-phase asthmatic response to allergen. *Am. Rev. Respir. Dis.* 144:1282, 1991.
53. Cutz, E., Levison, H., and Cooper, D. M. Ultrastructure of airways in children with asthma. *Histopathology* 2:407, 1978.
54. Davidson, S., et al. Synthesis of chondroitin sulfate D and heparin proteoglycans in murine lymph node derived mast cells. The dependency on fibroblasts. *J. Biol. Chem.* 265:12324, 1990.
55. Denburg, J. A., Silver, J. E., and Abrams, J. S. Interleukin-5 is a human basophilopoietin: induction of histamine content and basophilic differentiation of HL-60 cells and of peripheral blood basophil–eosinophil progenitors. *Blood* 77:1462, 1991.
56. Diamant, B. Energy production in rat mast cells and its role for histamine release. *Int. Arch. Allergy Appl. Immunol.* 49:155, 1975.
57. Diamant, B., and Uvnas, B. Evidence for energy-requiring processes in histamine release and mast cell degranulation in the rat tissues induced by compound 48/80. *Acta. Physiol. Scand.* 53:315, 1961.
58. Dileepan, K. N., Simpson, K. M., and Stechschulte, D. J. Modulation of macrophage superoxide–induced cytochrome c reduction by mast cells. *J. Lab. Clin. Med.* 113:577, 1989.
59. Dinh, T. T., and Kennerly, D. A. Assessment of receptor-dependent activation of phosphatidylcholine hydrolysis by both phospholipase D and phospholipase C. *Cell Regul.* 2:299, 1991.
60. Djukanovic, R., Wilson, J. W., Britten, K. M., et al. Quantitation of mast cells and eosinophils in the bronchial mucosa of symptomatic atopic asthmatics and healthy control subjects using immunohistochemistry. *Am. Rev. Respir. Dis.* 142:863, 1990.
61. Dvorak, A. M. Biology and Morphology of Basophilic Leukocytes. In M. K. Bach (ed.), *Immediate Hypersensitivity: Modern Concepts and Developments.* New York: Marcel Dekker, 1978.
62. Dvorak, A. M. Anaphylactic degranulation of guinea pig basophilic leukocytes. *Lab. Invest.* 44:174, 1981.
63. Dvorak, A. M., et al. Lipid bodies: cytoplasmic organelles important to arachidonate metabolism in macrophages and basophils. *J. Immunol.* 131:2965, 1983.
64. Ehrlich, P. Beitrage zur Kenntniss der Anilinfarbungen und ihrer Verwendung in der mikroskopischen Technik. *Arch. Mikrosk. Anat.* 13:263, 1877.
64a. Ehrlich, P. Beitrage zur Kenntniss der granulirten Bindegewebeszellen und der eosinophilen leukocythen. *Arch. Anat. Physiol.* 3:166, 1879.
65. Eliakim, R., et al. Histamine and chondroitin sulfate E proteoglycan released by cultured human colonic mucosa: indication for possible presence of E mast cells. *Proc. Natl. Acad. Sci. USA* 83:461, 1986.
66. Ende, N., and Auditore, J. Fibrinolytic activity of human tissues and dog mast cell tumors. *Am. J. Clin. Pathol.* 36:16, 1991.
67. Enerbäck, L. Mast cells in rat gastrointestinal mucosa: I. Effects of fixation. *Acta Pathol. Microbiol. Scand.* 66:289, 1966.
68. Enerbäck, L. Mast cells in rat gastrointestinal mucosa: III. Reactivity towards compound 48/80. *Acta Pathol. Microbiol. Scand.* 66:313, 1966.
69. Enerbäck, L. Mast cells in rat gastrointestinal mucosa: II. Dye-binding and metachromatic properties. *Acta Pathol. Microbiol. Scand.* 66:303, 1966.
70. Enerbäck, L. The gut mucosal mast cell. *Monogr. Allergy* 17:222, 1981.
71. Fernandez, J. M., Neher, E., and Gomperts, B. D. Capacitance measurements reveal stepwise fusion events in degranulating mast cells. *Nature* 312:453, 1984.
72. Finkelstein, A., Zimmerberg, J., and Cohen, F. S. Osmotic swelling of vesicles: its role in the fusion of vesicles with planar phospholipid bilayer membranes and its possible role in exocytosis. *Annu. Rev. Physiol.* 48:163, 1986.
73. Folkman, J. How is blood vessel growth regulated in normal and neoplastic tissue. *Cancer Res.* 46:467, 1986.
74. Foreman, J. C., Hallett, M. B., and Mongar, J. D. The relationship between histamine secretion and calcium uptake by mast cells. *J. Physiol.* 271:193, 1977.
75. Foreman, J. C., and Mongar, J. L. Effect of calcium on dextran-induced histamine release from isolated mast cells. *Br. J. Pharmacol.* 46:767, 1972.
76. Foreman, J. C., Mongar, J. L., and Gomperts, B. D. Calcium ionophores and movement of calcium ions following the physiological stimulus to a secretory process. *Nature* 245:249, 1973.
77. Fransson, L. A. Structure and function of cell-associated proteoglycans. *Trends Biochem. Sci.* 12:406, 1987.
78. Fredholm, B. B. Cyclic AMP independent inhibition by papaverine of histamine release induced by compound 48/80. *Biochem. Pharmacol.* 25:1583, 1975.
79. Fritz, H., et al. Immunofluorescence studies indicate that the basic trypsin-kallikrein inhibitor of bovine organs (trasylol) originates from mast cells. *Z. Physiol. Chem.* 360:437, 1979.

80. Fruhman, G. J. In vitro ingestion of zymosan particles by mast cells. *J. Reticuloendothel. Soc.* 13:424, 1973.

81. Galli, S. J. New insights into "the riddle of the mast cells": microenvironmental regulation of mast cell development and phenotypic heterogeneity. *Lab. Invest.* 62:5, 1990.

82. Garland, L. G., and Payne, A. N. The role of cell-fixed calcium in histamine release by compound 48/80. *Br. J. Pharmacol.* 65:609, 1979.

83. Gervasoni, J. E., Jr., et al. Degradation of human anaphylatoxin C3a by rat peritoneal mast cells: a role for the secretory granule enzyme chymase and heparin proteoglycan. *J. Immunol.* 136:285, 1986.

84. Gilead, L., et al. Cultured human bone marrow-derived mast cells, their similarities to cultured murine E-mast cells. *J. Immunol.* 63:669, 1988.

85. Ginsburg, H., and Lagunoff, D. The in vitro differentiation of mast cells. *J. Cell Biol.* 35:685, 1967.

86. Goetzl, E. J., and Austen, K. F. Purification and synthesis of eosinophilotactic tetrapeptides of human lung tissue: identification as eosinophil chemotactic factor of anaphylaxis. *Proc. Natl. Acad. Sci. USA* 72:4123, 1975.

87. Goetzl, E. J., and Austen, K. F. Structural determinants of the eosinophil chemotactic activity of the acidic tetrapeptides of eosinophil chemotactic factor of anaphylaxis. *J. Exp. Med.* 144:1424, 1976.

88. Gold, W. M., et al. Changes in airway mast cells and histamine caused by antigen aerosol in allergic dogs. *J. Appl. Physiol.* 43:271, 1977.

89. Goldschmidt, R. C., Hough, L. B., and Glick, S. D. Rat brain mast cells: contribution to brain histamine. *J. Neurochem.* 44:1943, 1985.

90. Goldstein, S. M., et al. Human mast cell carboxypeptidase purification and characterization. *J. Clin. Invest.* 83:1630, 1989.

91. Gomori, G. Chloracyl esters as histochemical substrates. *J. Histochem. Cytochem.* 1:469, 1953.

92. Gomperts, B. D. GE: a GTP-binding protein mediating exocytosis. *Annu. Rev. Physiol.* 52:591, 1990.

93. Gomperts, B. D. Exocytosis: the role of Ca2+, GTP and ATP as regulators and modulators in the rat mast cell model (current status review). *J. Exp. Pathol.* 71:423, 1990.

94. Gordon, J. R., and Galli, S. J. Mast cells as a source of both preformed and immunologically inducible TNF-α/cachectin. *Nature* 346:274, 1990.

95. Gordon, J. R., and Galli, S. J. Release of both preformed and newly synthesized tumor necrosis factor α (TNF-α)/cachectin by mouse mast cells stimulated via the FCεRI. A mechanism for the sustained action of mast cell–derived TNF-α during IgE-dependent biological responses. *J. Exp. Med.* 174:103, 1991.

96. Guerzon, G. M. The number and distribution of mast cells in monkey lungs. *Am. Rev. Respir. Dis.* 119:59, 1979.

97. Gurish, M. F., et al. Cytokine and mRNA are preferentially increased relative to secretory granule protein mRNA in mouse bone marrow–derived mast cells that have undergone IgE-mediated activation and degranulation. *J. Immunol.* 146:1527, 1991.

98. Haas, R., Heinrich, P. C., and Sasse, D. Proteolytic enzymes of rat liver mitochondria: evidence for a mast cell origin. *FEBS Lett.* 103:168, 1979.

99. Haig, D. M. Generation of mucosal mast cells is stimulated in vitro by factors derived from T cells of helminth-infected rats. *Nature* 300:188, 1982.

100. Hamaguchi, Y., et al. Interleukin 4 as an essential factor for in vitro clonal growth of murine connective tissue–type mast cells. *J. Exp. Med.* 165:268, 1987.

101. Hammel, I., et al. Differences in the volume distributions of human lung mast cell granules and lipid bodies: evidence that the size of these organelles is regulated by distinct mechanisms. *J. Cell Biol.* 100:1488, 1985.

102. Hammel, I., et al. Periodic, multimodal distribution of mast cell granule volumes. *Cell Tissue Res.* 228:51, 1983.

103. Hammel, I., Lagunoff, D., and Kruger, P. G. Studies on the growth of mast cells in rats: changes in granule size between 1 and 6 months. *Lab. Invest.* 59:549, 1988.

104. Hammel, I., Lagunoff, D., and Kruger, P. G. Recovery of rat mast cells after secretion: a morphometric study. *Exp. Cell Res.* 184:518, 1989.

105. Hastie, R. The antigen-induced degranulation of basophil leucocytes from atopic subjects, studied by phase-contrast microscopy. *Clin. Exp. Immunol.* 8:45, 1971.

106. Hastie, R. A study of the ultrastructure of human basophil leukocytes. *Lab. Invest.* 31:223, 1974.

107. Heidenhain, R. Beitrage zur Histologie und Physiologie der Dunndarmschleimhaut. *Arch. f.d. ges. Physiol.* Suppl. 1, 43: 1888.

108. Helander, H. F., and Bloom, G. D. Quantitative analysis of mast cell structure. *J. Microsc.* 100:315, 1974.

109. Hempstead, B. L., Parker, C. W., and Kulczycki, A. Characterization of the IgE receptor isolated from human basophils. *J. Immunol.* 123:2283, 1979.

110. Henderson, W. R., Jong, E. C., and Klebanoff, S. J. Binding of eosinophil peroxidase to mast cell granules with retention of peroxidase activity. *J. Immunol.* 124:1383, 1980.

111. Henderson, W. R., and Kaliner, M. Mast cell granule peroxidase: location, secretion, and SRS-S inactivation. *J. Immunol.* 122:1322, 1979.

112. Higginbotham, R. D. Mast cells and local resistance to Russell's viper venom. *J. Immunol.* 95:867, 1965.

113. Higginbotham, R. D., and Karnella, S. The significance of the mast cell response to bee venom. *J. Immunol.* 106:233, 1971.

114. Holgate, S. T., Lewis, R. A., and Austen, K. F. Role of adenylate cyclase in immunologic release of mediators from rat mast cells: agonist and antagonist effects of purine- and ribose-modified adenosine analogs. *Proc. Natl. Acad. Sci. USA* 77:6800, 1980.

115. Holgate, S. T., Lewis, R. A., and Austen, K. F. 3′,5′-Cyclic adenosine monophosphate–dependent protein kinase of the rat serosal mast cell and its immunologic activation. *J. Immunol.* 124:2093, 1980.

116. Holgate, S. T., et al. Effects of prostaglandin D2 on rat serosal mast cells: discordance between immunologic mediator release and cyclic AMP levels. *J. Immunol.* 125:1367, 1980.

117. Holgate, S. T., et al. Effects of prostaglandin D2 and theophylline on rat serosal mast cells: discordance between increased cellular levels of cyclic AMP and activation of cyclic AMP–dependent protein kinase. *J. Immunol.* 127:1520, 1981.

118. Holmgren, H., and Wilander, O. Beitrag zur kenntnis der Chemie und Funktion der Ehrlichschen Mastzellen. *Z. Mikrosk. Anat. Forsch.* 42:242, 1937.

119. Horner, A. A. Macromolecular heparin from rat skin: isolation, characterization and depolymerization with ascorbate. *J. Biol. Chem.* 246:231, 1971.

120. Horsfield, G. I. The effect of compound 48/80 on the rat mast cell. *J. Pharmacol. Bacteriol.* 90:599, 1966.

121. Howell, T. W., Cockcroft, S., and Gomperts, B. D. Essential synergy between Ca2+ and guanine nucleotides in exocytotic secretion from permeabilized rat mast cells. *J. Cell Biol.* 105:191, 1987.

122. Irani, A.-M., et al. Deficiency of the tryptase-positive, chymase-negative mast cell type in gastrointestinal mucosa of patients with defective T lymphocyte function. *J. Immunol.* 138:4381, 1987.

123. Irani, A. A., et al. Detection of MC and MC types of human mast cells by immunohistochemistry using new monoclonal anti-tryptase and anti-chymase antibodies. *J. Histochem. Cytochem.* 37:1509, 1989.

124. Irani, A. A., et al. Human mast cell carboxypeptidase selective localization to MCTC cells. *J. Immunol.* 147:247, 1991.

125. Irani, A. A., et al. Human mast cell carboxypeptidase. *J. Immunol.* 147: 247, 1991.

126. Ishizaka, T. Biochemical analysis of triggering signals induced by bridging of IgE receptors. *Fed. Proc.* 41:17, 1982.

127. Ishizaka, T., et al. Morphologic and immunologic characterization of human basophils developed in cultures of cord blood mononuclear cells. *J. Immunol.* 134:532, 1985.

128. Ishizaka, T., and Ishizaka, K. Triggering of histamine release from rat mast cells by divalent antibodies against IgE-receptors. *J. Immunol.* 120: 800, 1978.

129. Ishizaka, T., Ishizaka, K., and Tomioka, H. Release of histamine and slow-reacting substance of anaphylaxis (SRS-A) by IgE–anti-IgE reactions on monkey mast cells. *J. Immunol.* 108:513, 1972.

130. Jarboe, D. L., et al. Mast cell–committed progenitor 1. Description of a cell capable of IL-3 independent proliferation and differentiation without contact with fibroblasts. *J. Immunol.* 142:2405, 1989.

131. Jenkinson, D. M. Histochemical studies on mast cells in cattle skin. *Histochem. J.* 2:419, 1970.

132. Johansen, T. Energy metabolism in rat mast cells in relation to histamine secretion. *Pharmacol. Toxicol.* 61:1, 1987.

133. Johnson, A. R., and Moran, N. C. Release of histamine from rat mast cells. A comparison of the effects of 48/80 and two antigen-antibody systems. *Fed. Proc.* 28:1716, 1969.

134. Johnson, A. R., and Moran, N. C. Selective release of histamine from rat mast cells by compound 48/80 and antigen. *Am. J. Physiol.* 216:453, 1969.

135. Johnson, R. G., et al. The internal pH of mast cell granules. *FEBS Lett.* 120:75, 1980.

136. Kanno, T., Cochrane, D. E., and Douglas, W. W. Exocytosis (secretory granule extrusion) induced by injection of calcium into mast cells. *Can. J. Physiol. Pharmacol.* 51:1001, 1973.

137. Kaplan, A. P., et al. A histamine releasing factor from activated human mononuclear cells. *J. Immunol.* 135:2027, 1985.

138. Katz, H. R., et al. Secretory granules of heparin-containing rat serosal mast cells also possess highly sulfated chondroitin sulfate proteoglycans. *J. Biol. Chem.* 261:13393, 1986.

139. Kennerly, D. A. Diacyl glycerol metabolism in mast cells: a potential role in membrane fusion and arachidonic acid release. *J. Exp. Med.* 150:1039, 1979.

140. Kennerly, D. A., Sullivan, T. J., and Parker, C. W. Activation of phospholipid metabolism during mediator release from stimulated rat mast cells. *J. Immunol.* 122:152, 1979.

141. Kido, H., Fukusen, N., and Katunuma, N. Chymotrypsin- and trypsin-type serine proteases in rat mast cells: properties and functions. *Arch. Biochem. Biophys.* 239:436, 1985.

142. Kido, H., Yokogoshi, Y., and Katunuma, N. Kunitz-type protease inhibitor found in rat mast cells. *J. Biol. Chem.* 263:18104, 1988.

143. Kirshenbaum, A. S., et al. Demonstration of the origin of human mast cells from CD34+ bone marrow progenitor cells. *J. Immunol.* 140:1410, 1991.

144. Kitamura, Y., et al. Mutual phenotypic changes between connective tissue type and mucosal mast cells. *Int. Arch. Allergy Appl. Immunol.* 82:244, 1987.

145. Kitamura, Y., et al. Distribution of mast cell precursors in hematopoietic and lymphopoietic tissues of mice. *J. Exp. Med.* 150:482, 1979.

146. Kitamura, Y., et al. Spleen colony–forming cell as common precursor for tissue mast cells and granulocytes. *Nature* 291:159, 1981.

147. Kjellen, L., and Lindahl, U. Proteoglycans: structures and interactions. *Ann. Rev. Biochem.* 60:443, 1991.

148. Klein, L. M., et al. Degranulation of human mast cells induces an endothelial antigen central to leukocyte adhesion. *Proc. Natl. Acad. Sci.* 86:8972, 1989.

149. Koffer, A., Tatham, P. E. R., and Gomperts, B. D. Changes in the state of actin during the exocytotic reaction of permeabilized rat mast cells. *J. Cell. Biol.* 111:919, 1990.

150. Kokkonen, J. O., and Kovanen, P. T. Low density lipoprotein degradation by rat mast cells—demonstration of extracellular proteolysis caused by mast cell granules. *J. Biol. Chem.* 260:14756, 1985.

151. Korn, E. D. Clearing factor, a heparin-activated lipoprotein lipase. I. Isolation and characterization of the enzyme from normal rat heart. *J. Biol. Chem.* 215:1, 1955.

152. Kruger, P. G., Lagunoff, D., and Wan, H. Isolation of rat mast cell granules with intact membranes. *Exp. Cell Res.* 129:83, 1980.

153. Lagunoff, D. Structural Aspects of Histamine Binding: The Mast Cell Granule. In U. S. von Euler, S. Rosell, and B. Uvnas (eds.), *Mechanisms of Release of Biogenic Amines.* New York: Pergamon, 1966, p. 79.

154. Lagunoff, D. Histochemistry of proteolytic enzymes. In E. Bajusz and G. Jasmin (eds.), *Methods and Achievements in Experimental Pathology.* Basel, New York: Karger, 1967, P. 55.

155. Lagunoff, D. The properties of mast cell proteases. *Biochem. Pharmacol.* Suppl. 221: 221, 1968.

156. Lagunoff, D. Contributions of electron microscopy to the study of mast cells. *J. Invest. Dermatol.* 58:296, 1972.

157. Lagunoff, D. Membrane fusion during mast cell secretion. *J. Cell Biol.* 57:252, 1973.

158. Lagunoff, D. Control of mast cell secretion. *Adv. Cell Biol.* 3:177, 1990.

159. Lagunoff, D., and Bauza, M. The formation and storage of histamine in the mast cell. *Adv. Biosciences* 33:29, 1982.

160. Lagunoff, D., and Benditt, E. P. Histochemical examinations of chymotrypsin-like esterases. *Nature* 192:1198, 1961.

161. Lagunoff, D., Benditt, E. P., and Arase, M. Effect of mast cell granules on heparin-activated tissue lipase. *Proc. Soc. Exp. Biol. Med.* 121:864, 1966.

162. Lagunoff, D., and Chi, E. Effect of colchicine on rat mast cells. *J. Cell Biol.* 71:182, 1976.

163. Lagunoff, D., Chi, E. Y., and Wan, H. Effects of chymotrypsin and trypsin on rat peritoneal mast cells. *Biochem. Pharmacol.* 24:1573, 1975.

164. Lagunoff, D., Martin, T. W., and Read, G. W. Agents that release histamine from mast cells. *Ann. Rev. Pharmacol. Toxicol.* 23:331, 1983.

165. Lagunoff, D., et al. Isolation and preliminary characterization of rat mast cell granules. *Lab. Invest.* 13:1331, 1964.

166. Lagunoff, D., Pritzl, P., and Mueller, L. N-Acetyl-β-glucosaminidase in rat mast cell granules. *Exp. Cell Res.* 61:129, 1970.

167. Lagunoff, D., Ray, A., and Rickard, A. Effect on mast cell histamine of inhibiting histamine formation in vivo with α-fluoromethylhistidine. *Biochem. Pharmacol.* 34:1205, 1985.

168. Lagunoff, D., and Rickard, A. Evidence for control of mast cell protease in situ by low pH. *Exp. Cell Res.* 144:353, 1984.

169. Lagunoff, D., Rickard, A., and Marquardt, C. Rat mast cell tryptase. *Arch. Biochem. Biophys.* 291:52, 1991.

170. Lagunoff, D., et al. Flow Cytofluorometric Studies of IgE Binding Sites on Rat Peritoneal Mast Cells. In A. D. Befus, J. Bienenstock, and J. A. Denburg (eds.), *Mast Cell Differentiation and Heterogeneity.* New York: Raven Press, 1986, Pp. 289–299.

171. Lapetina, E. G., and Michell, R. H. Phosphatidylinositol metabolism in cells receiving extracellular stimulation. *FEBS Lett.* 31:1, 1973.

172. Le Trong, H., Neurath, H., and Woodbury, R. G. Substrate specificity of the chymotrypsin-like protease in secretory granules isolated from rat mast cells. *Proc. Natl. Acad. Sci. USA* 84:364, 1987.

173. Le Trong, H., et al. Amino acid sequence of rat mast cell protease I (chymase). *Biochemistry* 26:6988, 1987.

174. Leiferman, K. M., et al. Differences between basophils and mast cells: failure to detect Charcot-Leyden crystal protein (lysophospholipase) and eosinophil granule major basic protein in human mast cells. *J. Immunol.* 136:852, 1986.

175. Levi-Schaffer, F., et al. Co-culture of human lung–derived mast cells with mouse 3T3 fibroblasts: morphology and IgE-mediated release of histamine, prostaglandin D2, and leukotrienes. *J. Immunol.* 139:494, 1987.

176. Lewis, R. A. Slow-reacting substances of anaphylaxis identification of leukotrienes C-1 and D from human and rat sources. *Proc. Natl. Acad. Sci. USA* 77:3710, 1980.

177. Lewis, R. A. Preferential generation of prostaglandin D_2 by rat and human mast cells. In: E. L. Becker, A. S. Simon, and K. F. Austen (eds.), *Biochemistry of Acute Allergic Reactions: Fourth International Symposium* (Kroc Foundation Series). New York: Alan R. Liss, 1981.

178. Lewis, R. A., and Austen, K. F. Mediation of local homeostasis and inflammation by leukotrienes and other mast cell–dependent compounds. *Nature* 293:103, 1981.

179. Lin, P., Wiggan, A., and Gilfillan, A. M. Activation of phospholipase D in a rat mast (RBL 2H3) cell line: a possible unifying mechanism for IgE-dependent degranulation and arachidonic acid metabolite release. *J. Immunol.* 146:1609, 1991.

180. Lindahl, U., and Axelsson, O. Identification of iduronic acid as the major sulfated uronic acid of heparin. *J. Biol. Chem.* 246:74, 1971.

181. Lindahl, U., et al. *J. Biol. Chem.* 259:12368, 1984.

182. Lindau, M., and Nube, O. Pertussis toxin does not affect the time course of exocytosis in mast cells stimulated by intracellular application of GTP-γ-S. *FEBS Lett.* 222:317, 1987.

183. Lison, L. Etudes sur la metachromasie: colorants metachromatiques et substances chromotropes. *Arch. Biol.* 46:599, 1935.

184. Ludowyke, R., and Lagunoff, D. Amine uptake into intact mast cell granules in vitro. *Biochemistry* 25:6287, 1986.

185. Lynch, S. M., Austen, K. F., and Wasserman, S. I. Release of arylsulfatase A but not B from rat mast cells by noncytolytic secretory stimuli. *J. Immunol.* 121:1394, 1978.

186. Madden, K. B., et al. Antibodies to IL-3 and IL-4 suppress helminth-induced intestinal mastocytosis. *J. Immunol.* 147:1387, 1991.

187. Martin, T. W., and Lagunoff, D. Rat mast cell phospholipase A2: activity towards exogenous phosphatidylserine and inhibition by N-(4-nitro-benzo-2-oxa-1,3 diazole) phosphatidylserine. *Biochemistry* 21:1254, 1982.

188. Matsuura, N., and Zetter, B. R. Stimulation of mast cell chemotaxis by interleukin 3. *J. Exp. Med.* 170:1421, 1989.

189. Mayrhofer, G., and Bazin, H. Nature of the thymus dependency of mucosal mast cells: III. Mucosal mast cells in nude mice, nude rats, in B rats and in a child with the DiGeorge syndrome. *Int. Arch. Allergy. Appl. Immunol.* 64:320, 1981.

190. Meier, H. L., et al. Release of elastase from purified human lung mast cells and basophils. *Inflammation* 13:295, 1989.

191. Metcalfe, D. D. Classification and diagnosis of mastocytosis: current status. *J. Invest. Dermatol.* 96:1s, 1991.

192. Metcalfe, D. D. The treatment of mastocytosis; an overview. *J. Invest. Dermatol.* 96:55S, 1991.

193. Metcalfe, D. D., Smith, J. A., and Austen, K. F. Polydispersity of rat mast cell heparin. *J. Biol. Chem.* 255:11753, 1980.

194. Metzger, H. The high affinity receptor for IgE on mast cells. *Clin. Exp. Allergy* 21:269, 1991.

195. Michell, R. H. Inositol phospholipids and cell surface receptor function. *Biochim. Biophys. Acta* 415:81, 1975.

196. Michell, R. H. Inositol phospholipids in membrane function. *Trends Biochem. Sci.* 4:128, 1979.

197. Michels, N. A. The mast cells. In H. Downey (ed.), *Handbook of Hematology Section IV.* New York: Hoeber, 1938, Pp. 231–372.

198. Miller, H. R. P., et al. Mouse and rat: granule chymases and the characteri-

zation of mast cell phenotype and function in rat and mouse. *Monogr. Allergy* 27:1, 1990.

199. Miller, H. R. P., et al. Granule proteinases define mast cell heterogeneity in the serosa and the gastrointestinal mucosa of the mouse. *Immunol.* 65:559, 1988.

200. Miller, J. S., Moxley, G., and Schwartz, L. B. Cloning and characterization of a second complementary DNA for human tryptase. *J. Clin. Invest.* 86:864, 1990.

201. Miller, J. S., Westin, E. H., and Schwartz, L. B. Cloning and characterization of complementary DNA for human tryptase. *J. Clin. Invest.* 84:1188, 1989.

202. Monck, J. R., et al. Is swelling of the secretory granule matrix the force that dilates the exocytotic fusion pore? *Biophys. J.* 59:39, 1991.

203. Nabel, G., et al. Inducer T lymphocytes synthesize a factor that stimulates proliferation of cloned mast cells. *Nature* 291:332, 1981.

204. Naderio, R. M., et al. Inflammatory mediators in late antigen-induced rhinitis. *N. Engl. J. Med.* 313:65, 1985.

205. Nadel, J. Biologic effects of mast cell enzymes. *Am. Rev. Respir. Dis.* 145:S37, 1992.

206. Nemeth, E. F., and Douglas, W. W. Differential inhibitory effects of the arachidonic acid analog ETYA on rat mast cell exocytosis evoked by secretagogues utilizing cellular or extracellular calcium. *Eur. J. Pharmacol.* 67:439, 1980.

207. Newball, H. H., et al. Anaphylactic release of a basophil kallikrein-like activity: I. Purification and characterization. *J. Clin. Invest.* 64:457, 1979.

208. Newlands, G. F. J., et al. Heterogeneity of murine bone marrow-derived mast cells: analysis of their proteinase content. *Immunology* 72:434, 1991.

209. Newsom, B., et al. Suggestive evidence for a direct enervation of mucosal mast cells. *Neuroscience* 10:565, 1983.

210. Nogao, K., Yokoro, K., and Aaronson, S. A. Continuous lines of basophil mast cells derived from normal mouse bone marrow. *Science* 212:333, 1981.

211. Orr, T. S. C. The effect of disodium cromoglycate on the release of histamine and degranulation of rat mast cells induced by compound 48/80. *Life Sci.* 10:805, 1971.

212. Orr, T. S. C., Hall, D. E., and Allison, R. C. Role of contractile microfilaments in the release of histamine from mast cells. *Nature* 236:350, 1972.

213. Patkar, S. A., Kazimierczak, W., and Diamant, B. Sodium fluoride: a stimulus for a calcium-triggered secretory process. *Int. Arch. Allergy Appl. Immunol.* 55:193, 1977.

214. Patterson, R., et al. Living histamine-containing cells from the bronchial lumens of humans. *J. Clin. Invest.* 59:217, 1977.

215. Peachell, P. T., et al. Regulation of human basophil and lung mast cell function by cyclic adenosine monophosphate. *J. Immunol.* 140:571, 1988.

216. Pearce, F. L. Role of intra- and extracellular calcium in histamine release from rat peritoneal mast cells. *Agents Actions* 11:51, 1981.

217. Perlin, A. S. The 13C fourier transform spectrum of heparin: evidence for a biose repeating sequence of residues. *Can. J. Chem.* 50:2437, 1972.

218. Perlin, A. S., Mackie, D. M., and Dietrich, C. P. Evidence for a (aT4)-linked 4-O-(α-L-idopyranosyluronic acid 2-sulfate)-(2-deoxy-2-sulfoamino-D-glucopyranosyl 6-sulfate) sequence in heparin. *Carbohydr. Res.* 18:185, 1971.

219. Peters, S. P., et al. Arachidonic acid metabolism in purified human lung mast cells. *J. Immunol.* 132:1972, 1984.

220. Pienkowski, M. M., et al. Prostaglandin D2 and histamine during the immediate and late phase components of allergic cutaneous response. *J. Allergy Clin. Immunol.* 82:95, 1985.

221. Proud, D., et al. Immunoglobulin E–mediated release of a kininogenase from purified human lung mast cells. *Am. Rev. Respir. Dis.* 132:405, 1985.

222. Rabenstein, D. L., Ludowyke, R., and Lagunoff, D. Proton nuclear magnetic resonance studies of mast cell histamine. *Biochemistry* 26:6923, 1987.

223. Raphael, G. D., Henderson, W. R., and Kaliner, M. Isolation of membrane-bound rat mast cell granules. *Exp. Cell Res.* 115:428, 1978.

224. Razin, E., Cordon-Cardo, C., and Good, R. A. Growth of a pure population of mouse mast cells in vitro with conditioned medium derived from concanavalin A–stimulated splenocytes. *Proc. Natl. Acad. Sci. USA* 79:4665, 1982.

225. Razin, E., et al. Interleukin-3: a differentiation and growth factor for the mouse E-mast cell. *J. Immunol.* 132:1479, 1984.

226. Razin, E., et al. Culture from mouse bone marrow of a subclass of mast cells possessing a distinct chondroitin sulfate proteoglycan with glycosaminoglycans rich in *N*-acetylgalactosamine-4,6-disulfate. *J. Biol. Chem.* 257:7229, 1982.

227. Reilly, C. F., et al. Rapid conversion of angiotensin I to angiotensin II by neutrophil and mast cell proteinases. *J. Biol. Chem.* 257:8619, 1982.

228. Remington, S. J., et al. The structure of rat mast cell protease II at 1.9-A resolution. *Biochemistry* 27:8097, 1988.

229. Reynolds, D. S., et al. Cloning of cDNAs that encode human mast cell carboxypeptidase A, and comparison of the protein with mouse mast cell carboxypeptidase A and rat pancreatic carboxypeptidases. *Proc. Natl. Acad. Sci. USA* 86:9480, 1989.

230. Reynolds, D. S., et al. Isolation and molecular cloning of mast cell carboxypeptidase A: a novel member of the carboxypeptidase gene family. *J. Biol. Chem.* 264:20094, 1989.

231. Richerson, H. B., Dvorak, H. F., and Leskowitz, S. Cutaneous basophil hypersensitivity: I. A new look at the Jones-Mote reaction, general characterics. *J. Exp. Med.* 132:546, 1970.

232. Roberts, L. J. Carcinoid syndrome and disorders of systemic mast-cell activation including systemic mastocytosis. *Endocrin. Metabol. Clinics North Am.* 17:415, 1988.

233. Roberts, L. J., et al. Increased production of prostaglandin D2 in patients with systemic mastocytosis. *N. Engl. J. Med.* 303:1400, 1980.

234. Rohlich, P., Anderson, P., and Uvnas, B. Electron microscope observations on compound 48/80–induced degranulation in rat mast cells. *J. Cell Biol.* 51:465, 1962.

235. Saeki, K. Effects of compound 48/80, chymotrypsin and antiserum on isolated mast cells under aerobic and anaerobic conditions. *Jpn. J. Pharmacol.* 45:375, 1964.

236. Sagher, F., and Even-Paz, Z. Mastocytosis (Urticaria Pigmentosa). In S. M. Bluefarb (ed.), *Cutaneous Manifestations of the Reticuloendothelial Granulomas* (Am. Lect. Series No. 263). Springfield, Ill.: Thomas, 1960.

237. Salvato, G. Mast cells in bronchial connective tissue of man: their modifications in asthma and after treatment with histamine liberator 48/80. *Int. Arch. Allergy Appl. Immunol.* 18:348, 1961.

238. Salvemini, D., et al. Synthesis of a nitric oxide–like factor from L-arginine by rat serosal mast cells: stimulation of guanylate cyclase and inhibition of platelet aggregation. *Biochem. Biophys. Res. Comm.* 169:596, 1990.

239. Sayama, S., et al. Human skin chymotrypsin-like proteinase chymase subcellular localization to mast cell granules and interaction with heparin and other glycosaminoglycans. *J. Biol. Chem.* 262:6808, 1987.

240. Schayer, R. W. Formation and binding of histamine by free mast cells of rat peritoneal fluid. *Am. J. Physiol.* 186:199, 1956.

241. Schechter, N. M., et al. Identification of a chymotrypsin-like proteinase in human mast cells. *J. Immunol.* 137:962, 1986.

242. Schechter, N. M., et al. Identification of a cathepsin G–like proteinase in the MCTC type of human mast cell. *J. Immunol.* 145:2652, 1990.

243. Schleimer, R. P., et al. Characterization of inflammatory mediator release from purified human lung mast cells. *Am. Rev. Respir. Dis.* 133:614, 1986.

244. Schleimer, R. P., et al. Inflammatory mediators and mechanisms of release from purified human basophils and mast cells. *J. Allergy Clin. Immunol.* 74:473, 1984.

245. Schmauder-Chock, E. A., and Chock, S. P. Localization of cyclooxygenase and prostaglandin E2 in the secretory granule of the mast cell. *J. Histochem. Cytochem.* 37:1319, 1989.

246. Schneider, et al. Histamine producing cell stimulatory activity. Interleukin 3 and granulocyte macrophage colony stimulating factor induce de novo synthesis of histidine decarboxylase in hemopoietic progenitor cells. *J. Immunol.* 139:3710, 1987.

247. Schwartz, L. B. Cellular inflammation in asthma: neutral proteases of mast cells. *Am. Rev. Respir. Dis.* 145:518, 1992.

248. Schwartz, L. B., and Austen, K. F. Acid Hydrolases and Other Enzymes of Rat and Human Mast Cell Secretory Granules. In E. L. Becker, A. S. Simon, and K. F. Austen (eds.), *Biochemistry of the Acute Allergic Reaction: Fourth International Symposium* (Kroc Foundation Series, Vol. 14). New York: Alan R. Liss, 1981, Pp. 103–121.

249. Schwartz, L. B., Austen, K. F., and Wasserman, S. I. Immunologic release of β-hexosaminidase and β-glucuronidase from purified rat serosal mast cells. *J. Immunol.* 123:1445, 1979.

250. Schwartz, L. B., and Bradford, T. R. Regulation of tryptase from human lung mast cells by heparin. *J. Biol. Chem.* 261:7372, 1986.

251. Schwartz, L. B., et al. The major enzymes of human mast cell secretory granules. *Am. Rev. Respir. Dis.* 135:1186, 1987.

252. Schwartz, L. B., et al. The fibrinogenolytic activity of purified tryptase from human lung mast cells. *J. Immunol.* 135:2762, 1985.

253. Schwartz, L. B., et al. Quantitation of histamine, tryptase, and chymase in dispersed human T and TC mast cells. *J. Immunol.* 138:2611, 1987.

254. Schwartz, L. B., et al. Acid hydrolases and tryptase from secretory granules of dispersed human lung mast cells. *J. Immunol.* 126:1290, 1981.

255. Sehmi, R., et al. Identification of guinea pig eosinophil chemotactic factor of anaphylaxis as leukotriene B4 and 8(S),15(S)-dihydroxy-5,9,11,13(Z,E,Z,E)-eicosatetraenoic acid. *J. Immunol.* 147:2276, 1991.

256. Sekizawa, K., et al. Mast cell tryptase causes airway smooth muscle hyperresponsiveness in dogs. *J. Clin. Invest.* 83:175, 1989.

257. Seldin, D. C., Austen, K. F., and Stevens, R. L. Purification and characterization of protease-resistant secretory granule proteoglycans containing chondroitin sulfate Di-B and heparin-like glycosaminoglycans from rat basophilic leukemia cells. *J. Biol. Chem.* 260:11131, 1985.

258. Selye, H. Mastocalciphylaxis. *Ann. Allergy* 22:645, 1964.

259. Serafin, W. E., et al. Identification of aminopeptidase activity in the secretory granules of mouse mast cells. *Proc. Natl. Acad. Sci. USA* 88:5984, 1991.

260. Serafin, W. E., et al. Complexes of heparin proteoglycans, chondroitin sulfate E proteoglycans, and [3H] diisopropyl fluorophosphate–binding proteins are exocytosed from activated mouse bone marrow–derived mast cells. *J. Biol. Chem.* 261:15017, 1986.

261. Sieghart, W. Calcium-dependent protein phosphorylation during secretion by exocytosis in the mast cell. *Nature* 275:329, 1978.

262. Sieghart, W. Phosphorylation of a single mast cell protein in response to drugs that inhibit secretion. *Biochem. Pharmacol.* 30:2737, 1981.

263. Singleton, E. M., and Clark, S. L., Jr. The response of mast cells to compound 48/80 studied with the electron microscope. *Lab. Invest.* 14:1744, 1965.

264. Skofitsch, G., Savitt, J. M., and Jacobwitz, D. M. Suggestive evidence for a functional unit between mast cells and substance P fibers in the rat diaphragm and mesentery. *Histochemistry* 82:5, 1985.

265. Smith, C. A., and Rennick, D. M. Characterization of a murine lymphokine distinct from interleukin 2 and interleukin 3 (IL-3) possessing a T-cell growth factor activity and a mast cell growth factor activity that synergizes with IL-3. *Proc. Natl. Acad. Sci. USA* 83:1857, 1986.

266. Sorenson, L. S., et al. Propagation and characterization of human blood basophils. *Int. Arch. Allergy Appl. Immunol.* 86:267, 1988.

267. Sorimachi, M., Nishimura, S., and Sadano, H. Role of guanine nucleotide regulatory protein in histamine secretion from digitonin-permeabilized rat mast cells. *Biomed. Res.* 8:205, 1987.

268. Soter, N. A. Cutaneous necrotizing vasculitis; a segmental analysis of the morphological alterations occurring after mast cell degranulation in a patient with a unique syndrome. *Clin. Exp. Immunol.* 32:46, 1978.

269. Steffen, M., et al. Presence of tumour necrosis factor or a related factor in human basophil/mast cells. *Immunology* 66:445, 1989.

270. Stevens, R. L., and Austen, K. F. Proteoglycans of the Mast Cell. In E. L. Becker, A. S. Simon, and K. F. Austen (eds.), *Biochemistry of the Acute Allergic Reaction: Fourth International Symposium* (Kroc Foundation Series, Vol. 14). New York: Alan R. Liss, 1988. Pp. 69–88.

271. Stevens, R. L., et al. Identification of chondroitin sulfate E proteoglycans and heparin proteoglycans in the secretory granules of human lung mast cells. *Proc. Natl. Acad. Sci. USA* 85:2284, 1988.

272. Sydbom, A., Fredholm, B., and Uvnas, B. Evidence against a role of cyclic nucleotides in the regulation of anaphylactic histamine release in isolated rat mast cells. *Acta Physiol. Scand.* 112:47, 1981.

273. Tas, J., and Berndsen, R. G. Does heparin occur in mucosal mast cells of the rat small intestine? *J. Histochem. Cytochem.* 25:1058, 1977.

274. Teritan, G. Long-term in vitro culture of murine mast cells: I. Description of a growth factor–dependent culture technique. *J. Immunol.* 127:788, 1981.

275. Theoharides, T. C. Antiallergic drug cromolyn may inhibit histamine secretion by regulating phosphorylation of a mast cell protein. *Science* 207:80, 1980.

276. Theoharides, T. C., and Douglas, W. W. Secretion in mast cells induced by calcium entrapped within phospholipid vesicles. *Science* 201:1143, 1978.

277. Thompson, H. L., Schulman, E. S., and Metcalfe, D. D. Identification of chondroitin sulfate E in human lung mast cells. *J. Immunol.* 140:2708, 1988.

278. Travis, W. D., et al. Systemic mast cell disease analysis of 58 cases and literature review. *Medicine* 67:345, 1988.

279. Ts'ao, C., et al. Histamine-containing cells in bronchial lavage fluid: I. Ultrastructural characterization and comparison with mast cells in three types of tissues of rhesus monkeys. *Int. Arch. Allergy Appl. Immunol.* 52:315, 1976.

280. Tsai, M., et al. The rat c-kit ligand, stem cell factor, induces the development of connective tissue-type and mucosal mast cells in vivo. Analysis by anatomical distribution, histochemistry and protease phenotype. *J. Exp. Med.* 174:125, 1991.

281. Tsai, M., et al. Induction of mast cell proliferation, maturation and heparin synthesis by the rat c-kit ligand, stem cell factor. *Proc. Natl. Acad. Sci. USA* 88:6382, 1991.

282. Uvnas, B., and Antonsson, J. Triggering action of phospholipase A and chymotrypsins on degranulation of rat mesentery mast cells. *Biochem. Pharmacol.* 12:867, 1963.

283. Valent, P., et al. Interleukin 4 promotes expression of mast cell ICAM-1 antigen. *Proc. Natl. Acad. Sci. USA* 88:3339, 1991.

284. Valent, P., et al. Interleukin-3 is a differentiation factor for human basophils. *Blood* 73:1763, 1989.

285. Vanderslice, P., et al. Molecular cloning of dog mast cell tryptase and a related protease: structural evidence of a unique mode of serine protease activation. *Biochemistry* 28:4148, 1989.

286. Vartio, T., Seppa, H., and Vaheri, A. Susceptibility of soluble and matrix fibronectins to degradation by tissue proteinases, mast cell chymase and cathepsin G. *J. Biol. Chem.* 256:471, 1981.

287. Warner, J. A., et al. Purified human basophils do not generate LTB4. *Biochem. Pharmacol.* 36:3195, 1987.

288. Wasserman, S. I., Goetzl, E. J., and Austen, K. F. Preformed eosinophil chemotactic factor of anaphylaxis (ECF-A). *J. Immunol.* 112:351, 1974.

289. Watanabe, T., et al. Pharmacology of α-fluoromethylhistidine, a specific inhibitor of histidine decarboxylase. *Trends Pharmacol. Sci.* 11:363, 1990.

290. Weidner, N., and Austen, K. F. Evidence for morphologic diversity of human mast cells. *Lab. Invest.* 63:63, 1990.

291. Weill, P. Uber die leukocytaren Elemente der Darmschleimhaut der Saugetiere. Ein Beitrage zur Beurteilung der Granulationen in Leukocyten. *Arch. f. mikr. Anat.* 93:1, 1919.

292. Wershil, B. K., et al. Recruitment of neutrophils during IgE-dependent cutaneous late phase reactions in the mouse is mast cell–dependent: partial inhibition of the reaction with antiserum against tumor necrosis factor-alpha. *J. Clin. Invest.* 87:446, 1991.

293. Wingren, U., and Enerbäck, L. Mucosal mast cells of the rat intestine: a re-evaluation of fixation and staining properties, with special reference to protein blocking and solubility of the granular glycosaminoglycan. *Histochem. J.* 15:571, 1983.

294. Wlodarski, D. Mast cells in the pinna of the Balb/c 'nude' (nu/nu) and heterozygotes (nu/+) mice. *Experientia* 32:1591, 1976.

295. Wolf-Jurgenson, P. The basophilic leukocyte. *Series Haematologica* 1:45, 1968.

296. Woodbury, R. G., Gruzenski, G. M., and Lagunoff, D. Immunofluorescent localization of a serine protease in rat small intestine. *Proc. Natl. Acad. Sci. USA* 75:2785, 1978.

297. Yamada, K., et al. A major role for phospholipase A2 in antigen-induced arachidonic acid release in rat mast cells. *Biochemistry* 247:95, 1987.

298. Zimmerberg, J., et al. Simultaneous electrical and optical measurements show that membrane fusion precedes secretory granule swelling during exocytosis of beige mouse mast cells. *Proc. Natl. Acad. Sci. USA* 84:1585, 1987.

Platelet-Activating Factor, Platelets, and Asthma

Clive P. Page
John Morley

22

PLATELET ACTIVATION IN ASTHMA

Platelets in Allergic Reactions

Platelets have not received much emphasis as constituents of the inflammatory reaction to allergen in the lung and elsewhere in the body. In part, this may reflect the small size of platelets, whose presence, other than as constituents of a thrombus, may be easily overlooked. Furthermore, there has been no body of evidence furnished by studies of antiplatelet drugs that implicates platelets in allergic reactions. For instance, iloprost, a prostacyclin analog, strongly inhibits the activation of platelets but has not been reported to diminish the clinical manifestations of acute allergic reactions. In consequence, it might be presumed that platelets play no major role in allergic reactions other than as an incidental element of inflammatory cell activation.

Both theoretical considerations and experimental observations refute such conclusions. For example, it is now evident that endothelial cells can express adhesion molecules which interact with integrins expressed on the surface of activated platelets as well as neutrophils [128]. Such adhesion molecules enter endothelial cell membranes at their luminal surface following fusion of Wielbel-Palade bodies. In consequence, endothelial cell activation by allergic reactions might reasonably be anticipated to result in an adherence of platelets to endothelial cells. Whether such events would be primary elements of an allergic reaction or ancillary sequelae cannot be predicted; however, there is evidence that sensitized platelets are activated following contact with antigen. Thus, binding studies and the measurement of platelet-mediated cytotoxicity have implicated immunoglobulin E (IgE) as a recognition molecule that binds directly to the platelet plasmalemma [118]. On this basis, IgE might reasonably be anticipated to participate in acute allergic reactions, and there are several observations that accord with such expectations. Direct observation of platelets from sensitized animals has revealed that allergen or anti-IgE cause activation, as indicated by an oxidative burst or manifestation of cytotoxicity [118]. An in vivo counterpart of these findings was provided by the evidence that serum from convalescent animals would only protect naive animals from infection with *Schistosoma* if intact platelets were present in the circulation [55]. The protection afforded by platelets is not necessarily dependent on platelet aggregation, even though platelet aggregation can be demonstrated in vitro and in vivo in association with interactions between antigen and IgG [54]. Intravenous injection of antigen induces platelet accumulation in the thorax of sensitized guinea pigs, but such effects have not been shown to depend on IgE [91]. A morphologic counterpart of these findings is the influx of platelets into the extrapulmonary compartment of the airways, presumably as a prelude to emigration into the airway lumen (see later discussion). Again, however, such events have not yet been shown to depend on IgE.

In Vitro Evidence for Platelet Activation in Asthma and Allergic Disease

Platelets isolated from patients with allergic asthma show an in vitro response to specific allergens and to stimulation with anti-IgE antibodies by releasing cytotoxic mediators such as oxygen free radicals [54]. Interestingly, asthmatic patients who exhibit bronchospasm following the ingestion of nonsteroidal antiinflammatory drugs (NSAIDs) have platelets that respond to NSAID by releasing free radicals; this occurs both in vitro [54] and ex vivo [56]. These changes are not observed with platelets from patients who are asthmatic but do not have NSAID sensitivity, and furthermore are not observed for other blood elements from aspirin-sensitive asthmatics. This abnormal responsiveness of platelets to NSAID in this subset of asthmatic patients has been suggested to be secondary to abnormal prostaglandin endoperoxide behavior [1] or to altered hydrogen peroxide metabolism within the platelet membrane [95].

Over the past 15 years, there have been a number of studies that ascertained the responsiveness of asthmatic platelets to a wide range of stimuli, using the technique of platelet aggregometry (Table 22-1). Some of these in vitro studies have reported abnormalities in platelet function [9, 37, 76, 93, 105, 113, 121, 125], while others have not been able to distinguish between the behavior of platelets from asthmatic and nonasthmatic patients [40–43, 79]. Platelet aggregometry, although widely used to investigate platelet function in vitro, is a technique with inherent variability and low sensitivity, so that a variation in results might be anticipated given the wide range of methodologies used by different investigators. Differences reported in the literature have been attributed to discrepancies in methodology. However, those overall abnormalities that have been detected might be accounted for by platelet exhaustion, presumably due to overstimulation of platelets in vivo [41].

Apart from the abnormalities detected using platelet aggregometry, a range of other variables has been investigated in vitro, and these studies have revealed abnormal function in platelets obtained from asthmatics (Table 22-2) [7, 14, 24, 30, 33, 69, 70, 74, 133]. These include reports that platelets from asthmatics have abnormal arachidonic acid metabolism, reduced uptake of serotonin, and abnormal resting levels of second messenger molecules, such as Ca^{++} and inositol trisphosphate.

In Vivo Evidence from Platelet Activation Asthmatics

The predictability of in vitro results in platelet research is increasingly being questioned, and so it is usually necessary to seek in vivo evidence for the definitive implication of platelet involvement in any particular condition. It is therefore of considerable interest that platelet activation has been detected in vivo

Table 22-1. In vitro platelet aggregation in human asthma

Patients (no.)	Aggregating agent	Results	References
n.s.	ADP	Abnormal (2nd phase)	Fishel et al., 1970 [37]
26	Epinephrine	Abnormal (2nd phase)	Solinger et al., 1973 [113]
10	Epinephrine ADP Streptococcal M protein	Normal	Harwell et al., 1973 [42]
15	Collagen	Sensitivity to aspirin	Schwartz et al., 1973 [105]
41	Epinephrine	Normal	McDonald et al., 1974 [76]
33	Epinephrine ADP Thrombin Collagen	Abnormal Abnormal Abnormal (±) Abnormal (±)	Maccia et al., 1977 [70]
12	PAF Collagen	Abnormal Normal	Thompson et al., 1984 [125]
6	ADP	Normal	Greer et al., 1984 [40]
31	Collagen ADP PAF	Abnormal Abnormal Normal	Szczeklik et al., 1986 [121]
10	PAF + Collagen	Normal	Menz et al., 1987 [79]
n.s.	PAF + Collagen	Abnormal	von Felton and Beer, 1983 [136]
73	ADP Epinephrine Collagen AA	Abnormal (±) Abnormal (±) Abnormal (±) Abnormal (±)	Palma-Carlos et al., 1989 [93]
10	Epinephrine AA PAF	Normal Normal Normal	Hemmendinger et al., 1989 [43]

n.s. = not specified; ADP = adenosine diphosphate; PAF = platelet-activating factor; AA = amino acid.
Source: Modified from P. Gresele. The Platelet in Asthma. In C. P. Page (ed.), *The Platelet in Health and Disease.* Oxford: Blackwell, 1991, Pp. 132–157.

in asthmatics under a variety of circumstances using a range of techniques (Table 22-3). Storck and his colleagues [119] first showed the existence of platelet activation in 1955 when they demonstrated that thrombocytopenia may accompany allergen challenge of allergic subjects. This finding has recently been confirmed by another laboratory [71], although still other investigators have reported an increased incidence of circulating platelet aggregates in asthmatic subjects. There have been numerous attempts to measure concentrations of platelet-derived mediators in biologic fluids obtained from asthmatic subjects [41, 71,

119]. Some of these investigators have reported increased plasma concentrations of platelet-specific proteins, such as platelet factor 4 [52, 59] and β-thromboglobulin [41, 80]; they have also demonstrated the release of thromboxane B_2 which might be presumed to originate from activated platelets [68, 85, 107]. When platelet activation does occur, it is not secondary to the bronchoconstriction observed in asthma. Although such changes have been observed in patients following both challenge with allergen and exercise or in cases of nocturnal asthma [49, 52, 132], they are not seen in asthma patients after exposure to substances that contract smooth muscle directly [52]. Recently, platelet-derived markers have also been demonstrated in bronchoalveolar lavage fluid after local antigen challenge in allergic asthmatics [134].

Platelet activation in the circulation leads to trapping of platelets within the microvasculature of the lung [75]. Although this has not been detected using ^{111}indium-labeled platelets in a small number of patients [43, 50], platelets have been observed in lung biopsy specimens collected from asthmatics during allergen-induced late-onset airway obstruction [8]. Features of diseases that involve platelet activation can include abnormal platelet survival times and hemostatic defects [41], and abnormal platelet survival times have been reported for allergic subjects in studies using both isotopic [123] and nonisotopic [41] methods. Such changes in the platelet survival time can be influenced by therapy with antiasthma drugs such as glucocorticoids and ketotifen [122]. Asthmatic subjects have also been observed to have increased platelet size, counts, and mass, as well as moderately prolonged bleeding times [121]. Whether this is due to platelet abnormalities or to elevated levels of circulating heparin-like material [63, 64] (possibly originating from increased mast cell degranulation [90]) remains to be resolved. Nonetheless, a number of investigators have speculated that the reduced incidence of cardiovascular abnormalities in patients with asthma may be related to such hemostatic defects [63, 99].

Several groups have used lung biopsy to study the histopathologic features of mild asthma. These studies have provided direct evidence of the existence of activated platelets in these airways [8], and platelets have been identified that are undergoing diapedesis through gap junctions in the bronchial microvasculature of asthmatic subjects [61]. The inference that platelets can migrate like leukocytes has been confirmed by the finding that platelets dwell on the epithelial surface of symptomatic, but not asymptomatic, asthmatics [51], and hence are present in bronchoalveolar lavage fluid recovered from asthmatic subjects [20, 80]. Whether extravascular platelets participate in the repair of epithelial damage that characterizes asthma, or whether they participate in the recruitment of eosinophils into the airway lumen, is

Table 22-2. Various variables of in vitro platelet function in human asthma

Patients (no.)	Variable studied	Results	References
33	Release of 5-HT, PF_4 (by collagen, epinephrine, and ADP)	Dec.	Maccia et al., 1977 [70]
2	Intraplatelet nucleotides	Dec.	D'Souza and Glueck, 1977 [33]
18	Uptake of 5-HT	Dec.	Malmgren et al., 1982 [74]
n.s.	Platelet β-adrenergic response	Dec.	Fishel and Zwemer, 1970 [37]
40	Platelet β-adrenergic response	Dec.	Coffey and Middleton, 1975 [24]
10	Platelet α_2-adrenergic response	N	Davis and Lieberman, 1982 [30]
9	Resting cytoplasmic Ca^{++} and IP_3	Inc.	Block et al., 1988 [14]
n.s.	Oxygen generation by platelets challenged with antigen	Inc.	Capron et al., 1986 [18]
19	Platelet lipo/cyclooxygenase	Inc.	Yen and Morris, 1981 [133]
11	Platelet lipo/cyclooxygenase	Inc.	Audera et al., 1988 [7]
10	PAF production	N	Lurie et al., 1987 [69]
n.s.	Altered hydrogen peroxide	Dec.	Pearson and Suarez-Mendez, 1990 [95]
31	Altered platelet mass	Inc.	Szczeklik et al., 1986 [121]

n.s. = not specified; 5-HT = serotonin; PF_4 = platelet factor 4; IP_3 = inositol trisphosphate; N = normal; Inc. = increased; Dec. = decreased.
Source: Modified from P. Gresele. The Platelet in Asthma. In C. P. Page (ed.), *The Platelet in Health and Disease.* Oxford: Blackwell, 1991, Pp. 132–157.

Table 22-3. In vivo platelet functions in human asthma

Patients (no.)	Clinical condition	Variable studied	Results	References
13	Antigen challenge	PF4	Inc.	Knauer et al., 1981 [59]
15	Antigen challenge	β-TG	Inc.	Gresele et al., 1982 [41]
			Inc.	Gresele et al., 1985 [41]
20	Antigen challenge	β-TG	Inc.	Metzger et al., 1985
		PF4	N	
9	Exercise challenge	β-TG	Inc.	Johnson et al., 1986 [52]
		PF4	Inc. ($\pm$)	
6	Antigen challenge	β-TG	N	Greer et al., 1985 [40]
13	Antigen challenge	β-TG	N	Durham et al., 1985 [41]
		PF4	N	
8	Antigen challenge	β-TG	N	Shephard et al., 1985 [107]
10	Antigen challenge	β-TG	N	Hemmendinger et al., 1989 [43]
		PF4	N	
15	Antigen challenge	Circulating platelet aggregate	Inc.	Gresele et al., 1982 [41]
				Gresele et al., 1985 [41]
8	Spontaneous attack	Circulating activated platelets	Inc.	Traietti et al., 1984 [127]
19	Exercise challenge	TXB_2	Inc.	Morris et al., 1980 [85]
8	Antigen challenge	TXB_2	Inc.	Ind et al., 1985 [50]
3	Antigen challenge	Platelet survival (^{111}In)	N	Taytard and Vuillemain
10	Antigen challenge	Platelet survival (^{111}In)	Dec.	Gresele et al., 1987
7	Spontaneous attack	Platelet regeneration time (MDA)	Dec.	Taytard et al., 1986 [123]
5	Antigen challenge	Platelet survival (^{111}In)	N	Hemmendinger et al., 1989 [43]
33	Asymptomatic	Bleeding time	N	Maccia et al., 1977 [70]
n.s.	Asymptomatic	TXB_2	Inc.	Lupinetti et al., 1989 [68]
n.s.	Asymptomatic	PF4	Inc.	Wilkins et al., 1990 [132]
		β-TG	Inc.	
31	Asymptomatic	Bleeding time	Inc.	Szczeklik et al., 1986 [121]
12	Antigen challenge	Platelets in BAL fluid	Inc.	Metzger et al., 1987 [80]
3	Status asthmaticus	Megakaryocytes in lung	Inc.	Slater et al., 1985 [135]
n.s.	Antigen challenge	Platelets in BAL fluid	Inc.	Choi et al., 1990 [20]

n.s. = not specified; PF_4 = platelet factor 4; β-TG = β-thromboglobulin; TXB_2 = thromboxane B_2; MDA = malionaldehyde; BAL = bronchoalveolar lavage; Inc. = increased; N = normal; Dec. = decreased.
Source: Modified from P. Gresele. The Platelet in Asthma. In C. P. Page (ed.), *The Platelet in Health and Disease*. Oxford: Blackwell, 1991, Pp. 132–157.

unresolved. Some [25, 67], but not all [104], investigators have reported that the selective depletion of circulating platelets reduces the extent of both eosinophil infiltration and bronchial hyperresponsiveness in both normal animals treated with platelet-activating factor (PAF) and allergic animals treated with allergen [28, 67]. The nature of the mechanism whereby platelets or platelet products interact with eosinophils primed with interleukin (IL-5) or other cytokines requires investigation. Similarly, the observation that the extent of neonatal thrombocytopenia correlates with umbilical cord IgE levels and can identify those infants who will later develop atopy [72] indicates that the interaction between platelet products and lymphocytes responding to IL-4 and interferon merits investigation. Even if platelet changes mirror rather than determine changes in eosinophilia or IgE, these cell types could provide convenient diagnostic aids.

PAF IN ASTHMA

PAF as a Mediator of Allergy

Dale and Laidlaw introduced the concept that the allergic response might be attributed to the release of an endogenous autocoid, and recognized that histamine would mimic many of the clinical manifestations of an allergic reaction. The realization that a single simple chemical could evoke several of the more prominent characteristics of an allergic response prompted a search for substances that might efficiently and selectively inhibit the action of histamine. However, although reactions to applied histamine are very efficiently inhibited by such drugs, the manifestations of allergy are only partially suppressed. As a consequence, attention was directed toward alternative, or supplementary, mediators, reemploying those same test systems that had

been used to characterize histamine. Such tests focused on the contraction of smooth muscle (gut, vascular, and lung) and on edema, and this research led to recognition of the contribution of other amines (serotonin), peptides (kallikrein and lysyl-brady-kinin), and eicosanoids (prostacyclin, thromboxane, and peptidoleukotrienes) to the genesis of allergic reactions. Processes such as leukocyte accumulation were not measured, and this neglect led to leukocytes being relegated to an incidental role. Hence, the absence of an effect on inflammatory cells did not debar consideration of a role for a mediator in allergy and, instead, pharmaceutical research proposals focused on antagonists of smooth muscle spasmogens. The attraction to PAF as a mediator of asthma and allergy arose because this substance appeared unique in overcoming the deficiency of lung allergic mediators, in that it contracted smooth muscle, induced airway resistance, and attracted and activated inflammatory cells.

PAF had originally been identified and proposed as a mediator of platelet activation during acute allergic reactions in the rabbit [10]. Anaphylaxis in the rabbit is dominated by cardiovascular collapse and, to a lesser extent, by airway obstruction. These effects of intravenously administered allergen were minimicked faithfully by intravenously administered PAF [45]. In this respect, PAF might be categorized as an allergic mediator of the same type as peptidoleukotrienes, which were identified on the basis of slow contraction of smooth muscle. However, studies of the effects of intracutaneously injected PAF in guinea pig skin revealed that increased vascular permeability [82] and platelet [94] and neutrophil accumulation were succeeded by mononuclear cell accumulation along with macrophage activation [32], properties hitherto attributed to large-molecular-weight cytokines. This finding allowed PAF to be proposed as a mediator of allergic and other forms of inflammation in the airways. It was also realized that the singular effects of PAF could contribute to, or account for, the occurrence of acute bronchospasm as well as subsequent cellular infiltration and associated airway hyperreactivity (i.e., the constellation of symptoms that can be observed when allergic asthmatics react to inhaled allergen) [84].

Chemistry and Nomenclature

PAF was identified in 1979 by three independent groups of researchers as the ether-linked phospholipid 1-O-alkyl-2-acetyl-sn-glycero-3-phosphorylcholine (Fig. 22-1) [11, 13, 31].

Cell damage or disruption does not yield substantial amounts of PAF, suggesting that this material is neither pre-formed nor stored [124]. In several cell types, there is coincidental formation of PAF and a nonacylated compound termed *lyso-PAF* [12, 78]. Lyso-PAF has similar physiochemical properties to PAF, but is essentially devoid of biologic activity. Lyso-PAF has been shown to be released in vitro by macrophages [78], neutrophils [57], and platelets [12] in response to activation by a variety of agents, and the formation of lyso-PAF can be abolished by inhibitors of phospholipase A_2, indicating the involvement of this enzyme in the synthesis of PAF [129].

A number of observations have lent support to the concept that lyso-PAF is a precursor of PAF; it can be shown that the addition of synthetic lyso-PAF and acetylcoenzyme A to rat macrophages yields PAF [86]. This observation is consistent with the proposition that PAF is formed as a consequence of acylation of lyso-PAF, and is further substantiated by the observation that platelets incorporate radiolabeled acetate into PAF [19]. It is now recognized that acetylation of lyso-PAF can be achieved by an acetyltransferase enzyme that has been described for a number of cell types [66, 77, 96]; this enzyme acts as a rate-limiting enzyme for PAF synthesis [111]. This pathway is sometimes referred to as the "remodeling pathway."

More recently, a second pathway, sometimes called the "de novo pathway," has been described for PAF synthesis and involves the transfer of phosphorylcholine from ether-linked phospholipids (plasmalogens) [98, 112]. This is a single-step reaction

catalyzed by the enzyme phosphocholinetransferase [98, 111]. The extent to which these enzymes participate in the production of PAF in vivo is not fully understood, but it appears that, in inflammatory cells, the two-step synthetic pathway involving the rate-limiting acetyltransferase enzyme predominates [112], whereas in cell types such as renal cells, in which PAF may be produced continuously to serve as a physiologic hormone, the phosphocholine transferase appears active [112]. However, it is now known that certain cell types such as neurons may be able to synthesize PAF via both pathways, although the precise role for each pathway in nerves remains to be established [39].

The lability of PAF in vivo is due to the widespread distribution of a cytosolic acetylhydrolase enzyme [36] (phosphatide-2-acetylhydrolase), which is able to cleave the acetate moiety at the sn-2 position to leave lyso-PAF. Recent evidence has suggested that a group of Japanese asthmatic children have a genetic deficiency for this enzyme, and that the degree of the deficiency correlates with the severity of their asthma [81]. In experimental animals, acetylhydrolase rapidly degrades [³H]PAF to lyso-PAF, such that, 1 minute following a bolus intravenous injection of PAF, 70 percent is present as lyso-PAF [62]. An acetylhydrolase enzyme has also been identified on the surface of platelets [120]. Furthermore, when [³H]PAF is instilled into the airways, it is very rapidly metabolized to [³H]lyso-PAF, suggesting the existence of a related enzyme residing in pulmonary tissue, although the present cellular location of this enzyme in the lung has not been investigated. Lyso-PAF is further metabolized by removal of the O-alkyl group by an enzyme that is similar, or identical, to the well-characterized tetrahydropteridine-dependent alkylmonooxygenase enzyme isolated from rat liver [65]. This process generates a fatty aldehyde and the hydrosoluble glyceryl-3-phosphorylcholine.

The total synthesis of PAF has led to the synthesis of a wide range of analogs of PAF, permitting the formulation of structure–activity relationships to determine the optimum requirements for the biologic activity of PAF. This has been extensively reviewed elsewhere [16], but, in particular, it is known that the presence of the ether linkage and the length of the alkyl side chain at position 2 of the molecule is less critical. PAF derived from biologic origin, including human skin, is mainly a mixture of C_{16} and C_{18} types [73], and the biologic activities of C_{16}PAF and C_{18}PAF do not appear to be qualitatively or quantitatively different [3]. Structure–activity studies have also allowed a putative structure of the binding site for PAF to be put forward [15].

Properties of PAF Relevant to Asthma

Increased Vascular Permeability
In a number of species, the intracutaneous injection of PAF proved to be a potent stimulus of plasma protein extravasation [4, 97]; in the guinea pig, PAF was about 100 times more potent than bradykinin, which formerly had been considered the most potent agent causing increased vascular permeability [82, 94]. In addition to defining the potency of PAF, this study also established that the response of skin vessels to PAF was accompanied by, but independent of, platelet accumulation [94, 97]. It has therefore been proposed that PAF exerts a direct action on vascular endothelium, presumably to cause endothelial discontinuity [48]. Certainly the findings from the analysis of interactions between vasodilator agents and PAF in the skin of a number of species accord with such an interpretation [5, 82]. PAF has also been reported to induce the leakage of plasma proteins into the airways, presumably by means of an effect on the bronchial vasculature [34, 88].

Airway Obstruction
PAF induces airflow obstruction in a number of species, including humans, whether administered by inhalation [29] or intravenous

Fig. 22-1. *A. Structure of platelet-activating factor (PAF). B. Biosynthesis of PAF. AA = arachidonic acid; PLA_2 = phospholipase A_2; PKC = protein kinase C; GPC = glycerylphosphorylcholine. (Reprinted with permission from L. Smith. The role of platelet-activating factor in asthma. Am. Rev. Respir. Dis. 143[Suppl.]:100, 1991.)*

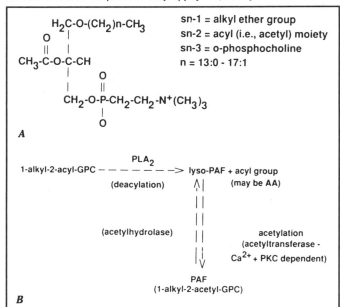

injection ([2] and reviewed in [89]). Airway obstruction in response to the intravenous injection of PAF is associated with, and slightly antecedes, intrathoracic platelet accumulation [2]. In these circumstances, airway obstruction may be due to platelet activation and the concomitant release of airway spasmogens, as airway obstruction is abolished when animals have been pretreated with lytic antiplatelet antiserum [130]. In this phase of the response, neither neutrophils nor increased vascular permeability contributes substantially to the occurrence of airway obstruction. Hence, prior treatment with lytic antineutrophil antiserum has little effect on the airway obstruction evoked by PAF, and, although there is a marked decrease in compliance, this is a transient change that abates within minutes. More protracted responses to PAF can be observed, in which the infiltration and activation of inflammatory cells are prominent features, and, in these circumstances, edema, mucous secretion, and the inflammatory consequences of tissue damage may contribute to the cause of airway obstruction. Marked changes in compliance support the presumption that progressive edema may be of substantial importance (J. Morley, personal communication, 1992). In humans, PAF-induced bronchospasm is independent of histamine release [23, 109] or the cyclooxygenase metabolites of arachidonic acid metabolism [109], but it is partially reduced by antagonists of peptidoleukotrienes [58, 114].

Airway Hyperreactivity

When PAF was proposed as a potential mediator of asthma, there was no clear evidence of any defined allergic mediator that had the capacity to induce airway hyperreactivity; rather, there has been a consensus that narrowing of the airways could account for airway hyperreactivity. In that context, all allergic mediators that cause increased vascular permeability might be expected to evoke airway hyperreactivity. In practice, the development of airway hyperreactivity in the guinea pig is not related to changes of basal compliance, and, moreover, airway hyperreactivity is selective for particular airway spasmogens.

The intravenous infusion of PAF induces airway obstruction in the guinea pig that is accompanied by intrathoracic platelet accumulation. However, whereas the magnitude of platelet accumulation decreases progressively with successive injections, the associated airway obstruction increases progressively. By way of contrast, both platelet accumulation and airway obstruction in response to the intravenous injection of adenosine diphosphate (ADP) show parallel diminution [108]. It can be inferred from these findings that airway obstruction due to PAF increases because of enhanced airway reactivity, and this conclusion is reinforced by the evidence that airway obstruction brought about by the intravenous injection of histamine is also increased. This effect of PAF is dependent on the presence of intact circulating platelets, which are absent in animals depleted of platelets by the intravenous injection of lytic antiserum, which does not prevent the induction of airway hyperreactivity by other substances (e.g., (±)isoproterenol) [83]. This finding poses a paradox, since other agents of platelet activation, including collagen and thrombin as well as ADP and the thromboxane mimetic U46619, cause platelet accumulation without attendant airway hyperreactivity [102]. It follows, therefore, that *both* platelets and PAF are implicated in the processes that determine altered airway hyperreactivity. As PAF only induces airway hyperreactivity in animals with intact platelets, it was possible to ascertain whether the interaction between PAF and platelets might yield an intermediary substance that was capable of precipitating airway hyperreactivity directly, without the intervention of platelets. To test this possibility, platelets were incubated briefly with PAF and the supernatants tested in animals that had been depleted of platelets. This maneuver allowed for the demonstration of such an intermediary, termed *platelet-derived hyperreactivity factor* (PDHF) [103].

This material has not been characterized but is not released by mechanical disruption of platelets nor following incubation with thrombin.

The capacity of PDHF to produce airway hyperreactivity without any changes in basal airway mechanics further argues against edema being significantly involved in the genesis of airway hyperreactivity following the intravenous injection of PAF. This conclusion is supported by other observations. Firstly, the increased airway hyperreactivity evoked by PAF is considerably greater than that which results when intravenous infusion of dextran (i.e., obstruction of the airways by engorged vessels) or histamine (to induce airway edema) is used to evoke a comparable change of basal pulmonary mechanics. Secondly, airway hyperreactivity due to PAF is demonstrably enhanced when histamine is used as a spasmogen but is diminished if acetylcholine is the test spasmogen. Furthermore, airway hyperreactivity caused by PAF can be reversed immediately following injection of potassium channel openers, whereas the reduction of edema is a slower process, taking hours rather than seconds. It is likely that the cellular basis of altered airway reactivity is some manifestation of changed neural function; this conclusion is reinforced by the observation that PAF-induced airway hyperreactivity is inhibited by capsaicin, a substance thought to specifically interfere with the action of sensory C-fiber nerves [116]. PAF has also been reported by some groups to elicit bronchial hyperresponsiveness in normal human subjects [29], although this has not been universally observed [60, 115, 117]. However, the effects of PAF in asthmatic subjects have not been widely studied [21].

Airway Eosinophilia

Several substances have been purported to induce eosinophilia in allergic reactions and, by inference, may be involved in the pathogenesis of asthma. However, possibly the most noteworthy characteristic of these materials was an absence of or, at best, limited efficacy in vivo. When initially studied as an inflammatory mediator, PAF gave no indication of having any capacity to evoke selective eosinophil accumulation. However, study of PAF in skin window preparations in allergic subjects did reveal a selective eosinophilia that was comparable to that evoked by allergen [35, 44], a finding not observed in the skin of normals.

PAF had previously been observed to elicit an eosinophil accumulation in the lungs of baboons [6], and, more recently, inhalation of PAF was shown to cause a selective eosinophilia in the airway lumen, which was maximal at 2 days and persisted for 1 week [26, 104, 106]. However, although highly significant when compared with vehicle-treated animals, these responses were modest when compared with the airway eosinophilia seen in sensitized animals that responded to allergen in doses otherwise insufficient to elicit clinical symptoms. The inference that cells might be primed by allergen to become more reactive to PAF or other substances has been confirmed, so that PAF might reasonably be considered a putative mediator of airway eosinophilia in allergy.

It is interesting to consider the potential mechanism whereby this is achieved. Directed chemotaxis seems implausible, as subcutaneous or intraperitoneal injections are similarly effective. Rather, it must be concluded that PAF influences (i.e., activates) the behavior of eosinophils sufficiently to cause their retention in the pulmonary circulation, with their selective emigration to the airway lumen governed by undefined endogenous processes. In this context, the emigration of platelets might be considered a device for ensuring selective eosinophilia. The inability of PAF to match responses to allergen suggests it has a role as an enhancer of primed cells rather than as a priming agent per se, and, in this context, leukotriene B_4 and PAF were similarly effective (though less effective than allergen) in causing eosinophil emigration into the cornea. There is evidence that several cytokines can cause eosinophilia of the airways, but it can be presumed that these substances act via the induction of IL-5 synthesis, as has been shown for IL-3. PAF antagonists have been reported by some [106], but not all [104], investigators to inhibit allergen-induced airway eosinophilia, suggesting that PAF does not serve as an obligatory intermediary. The possibility that PAF provides a priming signal that might substitute for IL-5 does not accord with our findings; we have found PAF shows little or no response under these conditions in certain batches of animals. When antisera to guinea pig IL-5 becomes available, this problem may be resolved.

Of particular interest, however, is the ability of a range of chemically unrelated prophylactic antiasthma drugs (cromoglycate, theophylline, ketotifen, and glucocorticoids), but not β_2 agonists, to inhibit PAF-induced eosinophil infiltration [56], suggesting a common mechanism of action for these agents.

PAF Antagonists

There is now a wide range of selective synthetic and naturally occurring PAF antagonists available as experimental tools to help unravel the physiologic and pathophysiologic roles of PAF (reviewed in [46]) (see also Chap. 66).

All of the PAF antagonists described are capable to varying extents of inhibiting the wide array of PAF-induced pathologic effects, both in vitro and in vivo (reviewed in [46]). This includes the ability of some to inhibit PAF-induced bronchial hyperresponsiveness [26, 106] and eosinophil infiltration in experimental animals [26, 106]. Several of the PAF antagonists have also been observed to counteract allergen-induced bronchoconstriction in experimental animals (reviewed in [92]). Furthermore, a number of PAF antagonists have been reported to reverse allergen-induced, late-onset responses in various animal models, including the rabbit [27, 110] and sheep [118]. In addition, there have now been many investigations into the ability of PAF antagonists to inhibit allergen-induced cell infiltration and bronchial hyperresponsiveness in a range of animal models (reviewed in [92]). Such studies have revealed that PAF antagonists can, in certain circumstances, suppress the recruitment of inflammatory cells such as eosinophils and neutrophils into airway tissues and the bronchial hyperresponsiveness associated with this airway infiltration. However, not all investigators have noted such inhibitory effects, and the basis of these discrepancies is likely in part to reflect the wide array of sensitization methods utilized and the different routes used for the administration of the drugs or antigen.

Ginkgolides have been demonstrated to possess PAF antagonistic activity, and the oral pretreatment of healthy volunteers with a ginkgolide mixture (BN 52063) was found to inhibit PAF-induced wheal and flare responses in the skin as well as PAF-induced aggregation of platelets removed from these individuals [22]. However, there was no significant effect on histamine-induced wheal and flare responses or ADP-induced platelet aggregation. Orally administered BN 52063 was shown to have only modest effects on PAF-induced bronchoconstriction or neutropenia in normal volunteers, suggesting that it is not potent enough for use in the treatment of asthma [100]. Orally administered BN 52063 has also been observed to reduce allergen-induced late responses in the skin of allergic volunteers [101], indicating that PAF may be involved in the late response in the skin in which there is a similar pathology to the late response in the airways. Clinical studies in the airways using more potent PAF antagonists such as WEB 2086 and MK-571 have failed to inhibit allergen-induced early or late responses in the airways of allergic asthmatics [38, 131]. Nonetheless, other potent orally active antagonists are under development; these include WEB 2170 [47] and UK 74,505, which evoke a prolonged inhibition against the

bronchoconstrictor and neutropenic responses induced by inhaled PAF [87]. Even the most potent PAF antagonists may not be effective in asthma, however, as it may be difficult to achieve a high enough local concentration of antagonist at sites of PAF release in the airways, and the inhaled route may be preferable for the delivery of the PAF antagonists. Theoretically, it may be better to develop inhibitors of PAF synthesis, particularly if it is shown that intracellular PAF has effects on cell function operating through mechanisms other than activation of the cell-surface receptor for PAF, which all of the existing PAFs have been screened against. Ultimately, however, only double-blind studies in patients with chronic asthma can decide the precise role of PAF in the pathogenesis of chronic asthma.

The Place of PAF in Asthma

When PAF was proposed as a potential mediator of asthma in 1984, the concept proved attractive, presumably because a singular mechanism accounted for such diverse pathologic processes as airway smooth muscle spasm, airway hyperreactivity, smooth muscle hyperplasia, abnormal platelet function, and airway eosinophilia. Not surprisingly, such far-reaching claims prompted investigations to test the validity of this proposition, and these investigations have been considerably aided by the availability of selective PAF-receptor antagonists. What has emerged from these studies is confirmation of the capacity of PAF to mimic several aspects of asthma pathogenesis, coupled with a clear recognition that other allergic mediators can share certain of these properties. Thus, even though PAF remains impressive because of its capacity to evoke a plethora of effects related to asthma, PAF is now not unique in this regard. One consequence has been to quell hope that PAF receptor antagonists will serve as a panacea for asthma, which, with hindsight, was an unjustified expectation. Another, more interesting, issue is the need to define the significance of PAF in the pathologic processes of asthma.

That PAF might account for the more protracted airway hyperreactivity that persists in asthma irrespective of treatment is an interesting possibility, especially as it might be linked to events close to birth when the airways are subjected to high concentrations of the substance [53]. Furthermore, PAF has been shown to induce fibrosis [17] and smooth muscle thickening in the airways of animals [126], both of which are recognized structural changes present in the airways of asthmatic individuals. Regarding eosinophilia, it has also become apparent that intracellular adhesion molecules may be central to the process of margination, but, again, the unusual capacity of PAF to influence platelet emigration may provide a second signal system to ensure selective emigration.

Over the past 25 years, there has been a progressive accumulation of observations that implicate the involvement of platelets in allergic responses and, more recently, the pathogenesis of asthma. As is commonplace in science, unusual and unexpected findings are contested and disputed and such has been the case in the study of platelets, in that there is still no general acceptance that platelets contribute to the cause of asthma. Nonetheless, it must be recognized that the body of evidence implicating platelets in the genesis of asthma is continuing to grow, so it is now unreasonable to portray an asthma pathology that excludes this blood element.

REFERENCES

1. Ameisen, J. C. Aspirin sensitive asthma: a model for a role of platelets in hypersensitivity reactions. *Ann. Inst. Pasteur Immunol.* 137D:141, 1986.
2. Ameisen, J. C., et al. Aspirin sensitive asthma: abnormal platelet response to drugs inducing asthmatic attacks. Diagnostic and physiopathological implications. *Int. Arch. Allergy Appl. Immunol.* 78:438, 1985.

3. Archer, C. B., Cunningham, F. M., and Greaves, M. W. Comparison of the inflammatory action of C18 isomers and C16 isomers of platelet activating factor. *Br. J. Dermatol.* 113:779, 1986.

4. Archer, C. B., et al. Inflammatory characteristics of platelet activating factor (Paf-acether) in human skin. *Br. J. Dermatol.* 110:45, 1984.

5. Archer, C. B., et al. Synergistic interactions between prostaglandins and Paf-acether in experimental animals and man. *Prostaglandins* 27:495, 1984.

6. Arnoux, B., et al. Pulmonary effects of Paf-acether in baboons, inhibition by ketotifen. *Am. Rev. Respir. Dis.* 137:855, 1988.

7. Audera, C., et al. Altered arachidonic acid metabolism and platelet size in atopic subjects. *Clin. Immunol. Immunopathol.* 46:352, 1988.

8. Beasley, R., et al. Cellular events in the bronchi in mild asthma following bronchial provocation. *Am. Rev. Respir. Dis.* 140:806, 1989.

9. Beer, J., and von Felten, A. Synergismus zwischen dem "platelet activating factor" (PAF) und Adrenalin, Kollagen und ADP bei der Aktivierung humaner Thrombozyten: Die Freisetzungsreaktionen, nicht aber die Aggregation, sind Thromboxan-abhangig (abstract). *Schweiz. Med. Wochenschr.* 113:1483, 1983.

10. Benveniste, J., Henson, P. M., and Cochrane, C. G. Leukocyte dependent histamine release from rabbit platelets: the role of IgE, basophils and platelet activating factor. *J. Exp. Med.* 136:1356, 1972.

11. Benveniste, J., et al. Semie-synthese et structure propose des facteur activat les plaquettes (PAF): Paf-acether, un alkyl ether analogue de la phosphotidylcholine. *C. R. Acad. Sci.* (Paris) 289:1037, 1979.

12. Benveniste, J., et al. Biosynthesis of platelet activating factor (PAF-acether). II. Involvement of phospholipase A2 in the formation of PAF-acether and lyso-PAF-acether from rabbit platelets. *Thromb. Res.* 25:375, 1982.

13. Blank, M. L., et al. Anti-hypertensive activity of and alkyl ether analogue of phosphatidylcholine. *Biochem. Biophys. Res. Commun.* 90:1194, 1979.

14. Block, L. H., Imhof, E., and Perruchoud, A. P. Platelets of asthmatics show increased phosphatidyl-inositol turnover in response to PAF (abstract). *Am. Rev. Respir. Dis.* 137:235, 1988.

15. Braquet, P., and Godfroid, J. J. Platelet activating factor (PAF-acether) specific binding sites: 2. design of specific antagonists. *Trends Pharmacol. Sci.* 7:397, 1986.

16. Braquet, P., et al. Perspectives in platelet activating factor research. *Pharmacol. Rev.* 39:97, 1987.

17. Camussi, G., et al. Acute lung inflammation induced in the rabbit by local instillation of native platelet activating factor. *Am. J. Pathol.* 112:78, 1983.

18. Capron, M., et al. Functional study of a monoclonal antibody to IgE Fc receptor (FceRII) of eosinophils, platelets and macrophages. *J. Exp. Med.* 164:72, 1986.

19. Chap, H., et al. Biosynthetic labelling of platelet activating factor (Paf-acether) from radioactive acetate by stimulated platelets. *Nature* 289: 312, 1981.

20. Choi, B. W., et al. Platelets in bronchoalveolar lavage of allergic asthmatics (abstract). *Am. Rev. Respir. Dis.* 141:A657, 1990.

21. Chung, K. F., and Barnes, P. J. Effects of platelet activating factor on airway calibre, airway responsiveness, and circulating cells in asthmatic subjects. *Thorax* 44:108, 1989.

22. Chung, K. F., et al. Effects of a specific antagonist of platelet activating factor (BN 52063) in man. *Lancet* 1:248, 1987.

23. Chung, K. F., et al. Ketotifen inhibits the cutaneous but not the airway responses to platelet activating factor in man. *J. Allergy Clin. Immunol.* 81:1192, 1988.

24. Coffey, R. G., and Middleton, E. Increased adenosine triphosphatase activity in platelets of asthmatic children. *Int. Arch. Allergy Appl. Immunol.* 48:171, 1975.

25. Coyle, A. J., Spina, D., and Page, C. P. The contribution of platelets and airway smooth muscle to PAF-induced bronchial hyperresponsiveness in the rabbit. *Br. J. Pharmacol.* 101:31, 1990.

26. Coyle, A. J., et al. The effect of the selective PAF antagonist BN 52021 on antigen-induced eosinophil infiltration and bronchial hyperreactivity. *Eur. J. Pharmacol.* 148:51, 1988.

27. Coyle, A. J., et al. Modification of the late asthmatic response and bronchial hyperreactivity by BN 52021, a platelet activating factor antagonist. *J. Allergy Clin. Immunol.* 84:960, 1988.

28. Coyle, A. J., et al. The role of platelets in antigen-induced late phase asthma, eosinophil accumulation and heightened airway responsiveness in an allergic rabbit model. *Am. Rev. Respir. Dis.* 142:587, 1990.

29. Cuss, F. M., Dixon, C. M., and Barnes, P. J. Inhaled platelet activating factor in man: effects on pulmonary function and bronchial responsiveness. *Lancet* 2:189, 1986.

30. Davis, P. B., and Lieberman, P. Normal alpha$_2$-adrenergic responses in platelets from patients with asthma. *J. Allergy Clin. Immunol.* 69:35, 1982.

31. Demopolous, C. A., Pinckard, R. N., and Hanahan, D. J. Platelet activating factor: evidence for 1-o-alkyl-2-acetyl-sn-glyceryl-3-phosphorylcholine as the active component of platelet activating factor (a new class of lipid chemical mediators). *J. Biol. Chem.* 254:9355, 1979.

32. Dewar, A., et al. Cutaneous and pulmonary histopathological responses to platelet activating factor (Paf-acether) in the guinea pig. *J. Pathol.* 144: 25, 1984.

33. D'Souza, L., and Glueck, H. I. Measurement of nucleotide pools in platelets using high pressure liquid chromatography. *Thromb. Haemost.* 38: 990, 1977.

34. Evans, T. W., et al. Effects of a PAF antagonist, WEB 2086, on airway microvascular leakage in guinea pigs and vascular permeability in man. *Br. J. Pharmacol.* 94:164, 1988.

35. Fadel, R., et al. In vivo effects of citirizine on cutaneous reactions and eosinophil migration induced by platelet activating factor (Paf-acether) in man. *J. Allergy Clin. Immunol.* 86:314, 1990.

36. Farr, R. S., et al. Preliminary studies of an acid-labile factor (ALF) in human sera that inactivates platelet activating factor (PAF). *Clin. Immunol. Pathol.* 15:318, 1980.

37. Fishel, C. W., and Zwemer, R. J. Aggregation of platelets from B. pertussis–infected mice and atopically sensitive human individuals. *Fed. Proc.* 29:640, 1970.

38. Freitag, A., et al. The effect of treatment with an oral platelet activating factor antagonist (WEB 2086) in allergen-induced asthmatic responses in human subjects. *Am. Rev. Respir. Dis.* 143:A157, 1981.

39. Goracci, G., and Francescangeli, E. Properties of PAF-synthesising phospholine transferase and evidence for lyso-PAF acetyltransferase activity in rat brain. *Lipids* 26:986, 1991.

40. Greer, I. A., et al. Platelets in asthma. *Lancet* 2:1479, 1984.

41. Gresele, P. The Platelet in Asthma. In C. P. Page (ed.), *The Platelet in Health and Disease.* Oxford: Blackwell, 1991, Pp. 132–157.

42. Harwell, W. B., et al. Platelet aggregation in normal and atopic subjects. *J. Allergy Clin. Immunol.* 51:274, 1973.

43. Hemmendinger, S., et al. Platelet function: aggregation by PAF or sequestration in lung is not modified during immediate or late allergen-induced bronchospasm in man. *J. Allergy Clin. Immunol.* 83:990, 1989.

44. Henocq, E., and Vargaftig, B. B. Skin eosinophilia in atopic patients. *J. Allergy Clin. Immunol.* 81:691, 1988.

45. Henson, P. M., and Pinckard, R. N. Basophil-derived platelet activating factor (PAF) as an in vivo mediator of acute allergic reactions: demonstration of specific desensitization of platelets to PAF during IgE-induced anaphylaxis in the rabbit. *J. Immunol.* 119:2179, 1977.

46. Hosford, D., et al. PAF Receptor Antagonists. In P. J. Barnes, C. P. Page, and P. M. Henson (eds.), *Platelet Activating Factor and Human Disease.* Oxford: Blackwell, 1989, Pp. 82–116.

47. Heuer, H., et al. Pharmacologic effects of Bepafant (WEB 2170), a new selective hetrazepinic antagonist of platelet activating factor. *J. Pharmacol. Exp. Ther.* 255:962, 1990.

48. Humphrey, D. M., et al. Morphological basis of increased vascular permeability induced by acetyl glyceryl ether phosphorylcholine. *Lab. Invest.* 50:16, 1984.

49. Inacci, L., et al. Platelet desensitization to PAF in nocturnal asthma. *Am. Rev. Respir. Dis.* 141:A477, 1990.

50. Ind, W., et al. Pulmonary platelet kinetics in asthma. *Thorax* 40:412, 1985.

51. Jeffery, P. K., et al. Bronchial biopsies in asthma. An ultrastructural, quantitative study and correlation with hyperreactivity. *Am. Rev. Respir. Dis.* 140:1745, 1989.

52. Johnson, C. E., et al. Platelet activation during exercise induced asthma: effect of prophylaxis with cromoglycate and salbutamol. *Thorax* 41:290, 1986.

53. Johnston, J. M., and Maki, N. PAF and Foetal Development. In P. J. Barnes, C. P. Page, and P. M. Henson (eds.), *PAF and Human Disease.* Oxford: Blackwell, 1989, Pp. 297–324.

54. Joseph, M. The Involvement of Platelets in Allergic Responses. In C. P. Page (ed.), *The Platelet in Health and Disease.* Oxford: Blackwell, 1991, Pp. 120–131.

55. Joseph, M., et al. A new function for platelets: IgE-dependent killing of schistosomes. *Nature* 303:810, 1983.

56. Joseph, M., et al. Inhalation of nedocromil sodium, but not sodium cromoglycate, inhibits the abnormal in vitro response to aspirin of platelets from aspirin-sensitive asthmatics (abstract). *Am. Rev. Respir. Dis.* 137:29A, 1988.

57. Jouvin-Marche, E., et al. Effect of the calcium antagonist on the release

of platelet activating factor (Paf-acether), and slow reacting substance SRS and beta-glucuronidase from human neutrophils. *Eur. J. Pharmacol.* 89:19, 1983.

58. Kidney, J. C., et al. Inhibition of PAF-induced bronchoconstriction by the oral leukotriene antagonist ICI 204,219 in normal subjects. *Am. Rev. Respir. Dis.*, 143:A811, 1991.

59. Knauer, K. A., et al. Platelet activation during antigen-induced airway reactions in asthmatic subjects. *N. Engl. J. Med.* 304:1404, 1981.

60. Lai, L. K. W., et al. Inhaled PAF fails to induce airway hyperresponsiveness in normal human subjects. *J. Appl. Physiol.* 68:919, 1990.

61. Laitinen, L. The pathology of asthma. In C. P. Page and P. J. Barnes (eds.), *The Pharmacology of Asthma* (Handbook of Experimental Pharmacology, Vol. 99). Heidelberg: Springer-Verlag, 1991. Pp. 1–20.

62. Lartigue-Mattei, C., et al. Pharmacokinetic study of 3H-labelled PAF-acether II. Comparison with 3H-labelled lyso-PAF acether after intravenous administration in the rabbit and protein binding. *Agents Actions* 15: 643, 1984.

63. Lasser, E. C., Berry, C., and Kortman, K. Diminished atherosclerotic calcifications in asthma. *Allergy* 42:549, 1987.

64. Lasser, E. D., et al. Heparin-like anticoagulants in asthma. *Allergy* 42:619, 1987.

65. Lee, T. C., et al. Substrate specificity in the biocleavage of the 1-alkyl-2-acetyl-sn-glyceryl-3-phosphorylcholine (a hypotensive and platelet activating lipid) and its metabolites. *Arch. Biochem. Biophys.* 208:353, 1981.

66. Lee, T.-C., et al. Increased biosynthesis of platelet activating factor in activated human eosinophils. *J. Biol. Chem.* 259:5526, 1984.

67. Lellouch-Tubiana, A., et al. Eosinophil recruitment into guinea pig lungs after Paf-acether and allergen administration. Modulation by prostacyclin, platelet depletion and selective antagonists. *Am. Rev. Respir. Dis.* 137:948, 1988.

68. Lupinetti, M. D., et al. Thromboxane biosynthesis in allergen-induced bronchospasm. Evidence for platelet activation. *Am. Rev. Respir. Dis.* 140:9932, 1989.

69. Lurie, A., et al. Exercise- and allergen-induced asthma do not change the production of PAF-acether by neutrophils and platelets. *Bull. Eur. Physiopathol. Respir.* 23:347, 1987.

70. Maccia, C. A., et al. Platelet thrombopathy in asthmatic patients with elevated immunoglobulin E. *J. Allergy Clin. Immunol.* 59:101, 1977.

71. Maestrelli, P., et al. Venous blood platelets decrease during allergen-induced asthmatic reactions. *Clin. Exp. Allergy* 20:367, 1990.

72. Magnusson, C. G. M., and de Weck, A. L. Is thrombocytopenia in cord blood indicative of intra-uterine sensitization? *Allergy* 44:143, 1989.

73. Mallet, A. J., Cunningham, F. M., and Daniel, F. Rapid isocratic high performance liquid chromatographic purification of platelet activating factor (PAF) and lyso-PAF from human skin. *J. Chromatogr.* 309:160, 1985.

74. Malmgren, R., et al. Defective serotonin (5-HT) transport mechanism in platelets from patients with endogenous and allergy asthma. *Allergy* 37: 29, 1982.

75. May, G. R., et al. The role of nitric oxide as an endogenous regulator of platelet and neutrophil activation within the pulmonary circulation of the rabbit. *Br. J. Pharmacol.* 102:759, 1991.

76. McDonald, J. R., et al. Platelet aggregation in asthmatic and normal subjects. *J. Allergy Clin. Immunol.* 54:200, 1974.

77. Mencia-Huerta, J. M., and Benveniste, J. Platelet activating factor (PAF-acether) and macrophages. II. Phagocytosis-associated release of PAF-acether from rat peritoneal macrophages. *Cell Immunol.* 57:281, 1981.

78. Mencia-Huerta, J. M., et al. Is platelet activating factor (PAF-acether) synthesis by murine peritoneal cells (Pc) a two step process? *Agents Actions* 11:556, 1981.

79. Menz, G., et al. Lack of PAF release in extrinsic asthma. *Agents Actions* 21(suppl.):139, 1987.

80. Metzger, W. J., et al. Platelets in bronchoalveolar lavage from asthmatic patients and allergic rabbits with allergen induced late phase responses. *Agents Actions* 21:151, 1987.

81. Miwa, M., et al. Characterization of serum platelet activating factor (PAF) acetylhydrolase: correlation between deficiency of serum PAF acetylhydrolase and respiratory symptoms in asthmatic children. *J. Clin. Invest.* 82:1983, 1988.

82. Morley, J., Page, C. P., and Paul, W. Inflammatory actions of platelet activating factor (Paf-acether) in guinea pig skin. *Br. J. Pharmacol.* 80: 503, 1983.

83. Morley, J., and Sanjar, S. Isoprenaline induces increased airway reactivity in the guinea pig (abstract). *J. Physiol.* 390:180, 1987.

84. Morley, J., Sanjar, S., and Page, C. P. The platelet in asthma. *Lancet* 2: 1142, 1984.

85. Morris, H. G., et al. Radioimmunoassay of thromboxane B2 in plasma of normal and asthmatic subjects. *Adv. Prostaglandin Thromboxane Res.* 8:1759, 1980.

86. Ninio, E. W., et al. Biosynthesis of platelet activating factor: evidence for acetyl-transferase activity in murine macrophages. *Biochim. Biophys. Acta.* 710:23, 1982.

87. O'Connor, B. J., et al. Complete inhibition of airway and neutrophil responses to inhaled platelet activation by an oral PAF antagonist UK74,505. *Am. Rev. Respir. Dis.* 143:A156, 1991.

88. O'Donnell, S. R., Erjefalt, I., and Persson, C. G. A. Early and late tracheo-bronchial plasma exudation by platelet activating factor administered to the airway mucosal surface in guinea pigs: effects of WEB 2086 and enprophylline. *J. Pharmacol. Exp. Ther.* 254:65, 1990.

89. Page, C. P. The role of platelet activating factor in asthma. *J. Allergy Clin. Immunol.* 81:144, 1988.

90. Page, C. P. One explanation of the asthma paradox: inhibition of natural anti-inflammatory mechanism by β_2 agonists. *Lancet* 337:717, 1991.

91. Page, C. P., Paul, W., and Morley, J. Platelets and bronchospasm. *Int. Arch. Allergy Clin. Immunol.* 74:347, 1984.

92. Page, C. P., Spina, D., and Coyle, A. J. The involvement of PAF in allergic inflammation. *Pulm. Pharmacol.* 2:13, 1989.

93. Palma-Carlos, M., Coneicao-Santos, M., Palmo-Carlos, A. G. Aggregation plaquettaire dans l'asthme. *Allergic Immunol.* 21:177, 1989.

94. Paul, W., et al. The plasma protein extravasation response to Paf-acether is independent of platelet accumulation. *Agents Actions* 15:80, 1984.

95. Pearson, D. J., and Suarez-Mendez, V. J. Abnormal hydrogen peroxide metabolism in aspirin hypersensitivity. *Clin. Exp. Allergy* 20:157, 1990.

96. Pirotzky, E., et al. Biosynthesis of platelet activating factor. VI. Precursor of platelet activating factor and acetyl-transferase activity in isolated rat kidney cells. *Lab. Invest.* 51:567, 1984.

97. Pirotzky, E., et al. Paf-acether induced plasma exudation is independent of platelets and neutrophils in rat skin. *Microcirc. Endothelium Lymphatics* 1:107, 1984.

98. Renooij, W., and Snyder, F. F. Biosynthesis of 1-alkyl-2-acetyl-sn-glycero-3-phosphorylcholine (platelet activating factor and a hypotensive lipid) by choline phosphotransferase in various rat tissues. *Biochim. Biophys. Acta* 663:545, 1981.

99. Rhatigan, R. M., and Torre, A. Myocardial necrosis and bronchial asthma. *Ann. Allergy* 28:434, 1970.

100. Roberts, N. M., et al. Effect of a PAF antagonist, BN 52063, on PAF-induced bronchoconstriction in human subjects. *Br. J. Clin. Pharmacol.* 26:65, 1988.

101. Roberts, N. M., et al. Effects of BN 52063 on antigen-induced early and late cutaneous responses in volunteers. *J. Allergy Clin. Immunol.* 81:236, 1988.

102. Robertson, D. N., and Page, C. P. Effect of platelet agonists on intrinsic platelet accumulation and airway reactivity. *Br. J. Pharmacol.* 92:105, 1987.

103. Sanjar, S., Smith, D., and Kristersson, A. Incubation of platelets with PAF produces a factor which causes airway hyperreactivity in guinea pigs. *Br. J. Pharmacol.* 96:75P, 1989.

104. Sanjar, S., et al. Eosinophil accumulation in pulmonary airways of guinea pigs induced by exposure to an aerosol of platelet activating factor: effect of anti-asthma drugs. *Br. J. Pharmacol.* 99:267, 1990.

105. Schwartz, H. J., and Bennett, B. The differential effect of acetylsalicylic acid on in vitro aggregation of platelets from normal, asthmatic and aspirin-sensitive subjects. *Int. Arch. Allergy* 45:899, 1973.

106. Seeds, E. A. M., Coyle, A. J., and Page, C. P. The effect of the selective PAF antagonist WEB 2170 on PAF and antigen induced airway hyperresponsiveness and eosinophil infiltration. *J. Lipid Med.* 4:111, 1991.

107. Shephard, E. G., et al. Lung function and plasma levels of thromboxane B2, 6-ketoprostaglandin F1α and β-thromboglobulin in antigen-induced asthma before and after indomethacin pretreatment. *Br. J. Clin. Pharmacol.* 19:459, 1985.

108. Smith, D., Sanjar, S., and Morley, J. Platelet activation and PAF-induced airway hyperreactivity in the anaesthetised guinea pig. *Br. J. Pharmacol.* 96:74P, 1989.

109. Smith, I. J., Rubin, A. E., and Patterson, R. Mechanism of platelet activating factor–induced bronchoconstriction in humans. *Am. Rev. Respir. Dis.* 137:1015, 1988.

110. Smith, H. R., et al. Effect of the PAF antagonist L-659,989 on the late asthmatic response and increased airway reactivity in the rabbit. *Am. Rev. Respir. Dis.* 137:A283, 1988.

111. Snyder, F. Chemical and biochemical aspects of platelet activating factor:

a novel class of acetylated ether-linked choline phospholipids. *Med. Res.* 5:107, 1985.

112. Snyder, F. The significance of dual pathways for the biosynthesis of platelet activating factor: 1-alkyl-2-lyso-sn-glycero-3-phosphate as a branch point. In C. M. Winslow, and M. L. Lee (eds.), *New Horizons in Platelet Activating Research.* New York: Wiley, 1987, Pp. 13–26.

113. Solinger, A., Bernstein, I. L., and Glueck, H. I. The effect of epinephrine on platelet aggregation in normal and atopic subjects. *J. Allergy Clin. Immunol.* 51:29, 1973.

114. Spencer, D. A., et al. Bronchospasm induced by platelet activating factor is reduced by a selective cysteinyl-leukotriene antagonist in normal man. *Am. Rev. Respir. Dis.* 141:A218, 1990.

115. Spencer, D. A., et al. Platelet activating factor does not cause a reproducible increase in bronchial responses in normal man. *Clin. Exp. Allergy* 20:525, 1990.

116. Spina, D., et al. Effect of capsaicin on PAF-induced bronchial hyperresponsiveness and pulmonary cell accumulation in the rabbit. *Br. J. Pharmacol.* 103:1268, 1991.

117. Stenton, S. C., et al. The actions of GR 32191B, a thromboxane receptor antagonist, on the effects of inhaled PAF on human airways. *Clin. Exp. Allergy* 20:311, 1990.

118. Stevenson, J. S., et al. The effect of the PAF antagonist WEB 2086 on the early and late response in allergic sheep. *Fed. Proc.* 46:6683, 1987.

119. Storck, H., Hoigne, R., and Koller, F. Thrombocytes in allergic reactions. *Int. Arch. Allergy* 6:372, 1955.

120. Suzuki, Y., et al. Acetylhydrolase released from platelets of aggregation with PAF. *Eur. J. Biochem.* 172:1117, 1988.

121. Szczeklik, A., et al. Prolonged bleeding time, reduced platelet aggregation altered PAF sensitivity and increased platelet mass are a trait of asthma and hay fever. *Thromb. Haemost.* 56:183, 1986.

122. Taytard, A., et al. Platelet kinetics in stable asthmatics: effect of corticosteroid therapy (abstract). *Am. Rev. Respir. Dis.* 131:A285, 1985.

123. Taytard, A., et al. Platelet kinetics in stable asthmatic subjects. *Am. Rev. Respir. Dis.* 134:983, 1986.

124. Tence, M., et al. Release, purification, and characterisation of platelet activating factor (PAF). *Biochimie* 62:251, 1980.

125. Thompson, P. J., et al. Platelets, platelet activating factor and asthma (abstract). *Am. Rev. Respir. Dis.* 129:3A, 1984.

126. Touvey, C., et al. Effect of long term infusion of platelet activating factor on pulmonary responses and morphology in the guinea pig. *Pulm. Pharmacol.* 4:43, 1991.

127. Traietti, S., et al. Circulating platelet aggregates in respiratory disease: differences between arterial and venous blood in COLD and asthmatic patients. *Respiration* 46(suppl. 1):62, 1984.

128. Tuffin, D. P. The Platelet Surface Membrane: Ultrastructure, Receptor Binding and Future. In C. P. Page (ed.), *The Platelet in Health and Disease.* Oxford: Blackwell, 1991. Pp. 10–60.

129. Vargaftig, B. B., Chignard, M., and Benveniste, J. Present concepts on the mechanisms of platelet aggregation. *Biochem. Pharmacol.* 30:263, 1981.

130. Vargaftig, B. B., et al. Platelet activating factor induces a platelet dependent bronchoconstriction unrelated to the formation of prostaglandin elements. *Eur. J. Pharmacol.* 65:185, 1980.

131. Wilkens, H., et al. Effects of an inhaled PAF antagonist (WEB 2086) on allergen-induced early and late response and increased bronchial responses to methacholine. *Am. Rev. Respir. Dis.* 143:A812, 1991.

132. Wilkins, J. H., et al. Effect of a PAF antagonist (BN 52063) on bronchoconstriction and platelet activation during exercise-induced asthma. *Br. J. Clin. Pharmacol.* 29:85, 1990.

133. Yen, S. S., and Morris, H. G. An imbalance of arachidonic acid metabolism in asthma. *Biochem. Res. Commun.* 103:774, 1981.

134. Averill, F. J., et al. Platelet activation in the lung after antigen challenge in a model of allergic asthma. *Am. Rev. Respir. Dis.* 145:571, 1992.

135. Slater, D. N., Trowbridge, E. A., and Martin, J. F. The platelet in asthma. *Lancet* 1:110, 1985.

136. von Felton, A., and Beer, J. Reduced threshold synergism between PAF-acether and collagen: Sensitive test system to detect desensitization of human platelets to PAF-acether in vitro and in vivo. In F. Russo-Marie, J. M. Mencia Huerta, and M. Chignard (eds.), Advances in Inflammation Research. New York: Raven, 1983. Pp. 323–325.

Role of Epithelium

23

Lauri A. Laitinen
Annika Laitinen
Carl G. A. Persson

Epithelia serve to protect the body against damaging factors such as microorganisms, abrasion, and excessive loss of heat and moisture. The airway epithelium especially serves as a primary target organ for exogenous inhaled luminal irritants, and its structure and cellular profile may undergo certain changes resulting from a pathologic process in the airways. The recognition of changes in the airway epithelium, even of living asthmatic patients whose disorder is fairly mild [39], has led to studies of airway structure in asthma through the use of endoscopical bronchial biopsing techniques [73]. The possible relationship between increased bronchial reactivity and epithelial airway damage is schematized in Figure 23-1.

Recent work has given new insights into the barrier functions of the respiratory epithelial lining and into the ability of epithelial cells to release biologically active compounds [52a]. The main emphasis of this chapter is on the structure of airway epithelium in asthma. We will also discuss other aspects of airway epithelium, including the exudation of plasma proteins across the epithelial lining and how this process may relate to the absorption ability of the airway mucosa.

THE STRUCTURE OF NORMAL AIRWAY EPITHELIUM

Epithelium in Different Levels of the Airways

The airways are divided into bronchi and bronchioli, depending on the distribution of cartilage. The bronchi are defined as those airways that are proximal to the last plate of cartilage located along the airway wall. The bronchioli, whose diameter is less than 1 mm, are distal to the last plate of cartilage and proximal to the alveolar region. The terminal bronchiolus is located immediately before a respiratory bronchiolus, and it represents the most distal part of the airway with a complete lining of airway epithelium.

In the large airways, the lining of the human tracheobronchial tree consists of pseudostratified, ciliated columnar epithelium; the lining changes into the simple columnar ciliated type, with goblet cells in the smaller bronchi. In the bronchioles, the epithelium changes to a simple cuboidal, ciliated and nonciliated type, without goblet cells in the terminal bronchioles [2].

The cell types composing the bronchial epithelium differ somewhat for different species. In the normal human, most often seen are four main cell types of bronchial epithelium, all of which rest on a basement membrane [23, 65]; these are: ciliated cells, basal cells, secretory (mucous or goblet) cells, and Kulchitsky (neuroendocrine) cells. The Clara cells, which are secretory cells, are seen in the bronchioles. Serous cells can be observed in pathogen-free rat airways as well as in the airways of human fetuses and newborn infants. In adults, the serous cells have been

transformed to mucous cells [2]. In general, mucous and serous cells are considered to represent different phenotype expressions of a common cell type [30, 50]. Ciliated and secretory cells reach the lumen, as do some of the neuroendocrine cells. There are roughly three to five ciliated cells for every mucous cell [50]. In the airways of healthy nonsmokers, even such a high ratio of ciliated cells to goblet cells as 10:1 has been reported [71]. The ciliated cells diminish in number toward the periphery, but they still occur as far as the respiratory bronchiole.

Nonciliated, columnar epithelial cells that contain no obvious secretory granules, or "intermediate cells," may be presecretory or preciliated cells. In addition, there are cells that cannot be classified; these "indeterminate cells" are described in the literature, and may be undifferentiated cells [50].

Nerves in the Epithelium

In the larger airways, the human airway epithelium contains nerves near the lumen and basement membrane. In the smaller airways, intraepithelial nerves are located deeper, close to the basement membrane [32]. The neuroendocrine cells usually are triangular and rest on the basement membrane. Their basal part is filled with dense-cored vesicles (Fig. 23-2). The basal part of the cells is innervated by nerves making synapse-like contacts with the cells. Even in large human airways, the individual neuroendocrine cells have been found to reach the lumen [33].

The Vasculature and the Epithelium

The epithelium is an avascular tissue. A basement membrane gives support to the epithelium and connects it to the underlying tissue. Just beneath the epithelial lining within the airways is a rich network of microvessels [38], with the blood supply providing nutrition for the mucosa. In addition, this vasculature, which is so close to the epithelium (Fig. 23-3), may possess other functions, such as playing a part in the respiratory defense mechanism, either by means of plasma exudation or, possibly, by absorbing epithelium-derived substances or inhaled drugs and distributing them along the airways or deeper into the mucosa.

Inflammatory Cells in the Epithelium

Biopsy studies of normal human airways have suggested that the absence or presence of a negligible number of inflammatory cells could be a reliable criterion for differentiating between healthy and diseased airways [71] (Chap. 24). When asthmatics, long-time smokers, and healthy control subjects were compared, the normal airway epithelium differed from that of asthmatics and smokers in that the numbers of mast cells, eosinophils (Fig. 23-4), and neutrophils (Fig. 23-5) were lower [34].

STRUCTURAL CHANGES IN THE AIRWAY EPITHELIUM AND BRONCHIAL HYPERRESPONSIVENESS

Asthma

In bronchial specimens obtained from patients dying in status asthmaticus, it is difficult to find normal areas of bronchial epithelium. A prominent feature in such cases is shedding of airway columnar epithelial cells. In many areas, only a layer of basal or reserve cells is left [11]. More recently, bronchial biopsy specimens from living asthmatics have been investigated using light and electron microscopy, and epithelial changes have been revealed [5, 18, 39, 46]. Histologic specimens (Fig. 23-6), which show the columnar epithelial cells still attached to each other at

Fig. 23-1. *Scheme showing possible relationships between epithelial damage and increased bronchial responsiveness. (Reprinted with permission from F. M. Cuss and P. J. Barnes. Epithelial mediators. Am. Rev. Respir. Dis. 136:S34, 1987.)*

Fig. 23-2. *Transmission electron micrograph from the upper lobe bronchus of a patient with mild asthma. A neuroendocrine-like cell (NE) is seen near the basement membrane in the epithelium. The cell contains numerous dense-cored vesicles (arrows). (× 13,000, bar = 1 μm.)*

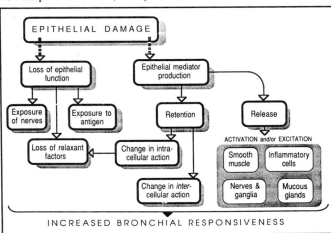

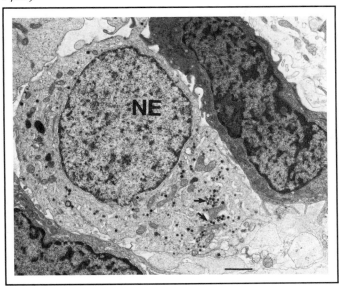

Fig. 23-3. *An electron micrograph from a patient with newly detected asthma shows the thickened basement membrane (B) forming a relatively cell-free area between the epithelium (E) and lamina propria (LP). Inflammatory cells are only occasionally seen in this area. The microvessels (V) come close to the epithelium but remain separated from it by the basement membrane. (×7,800, bar = 2 μm.)*

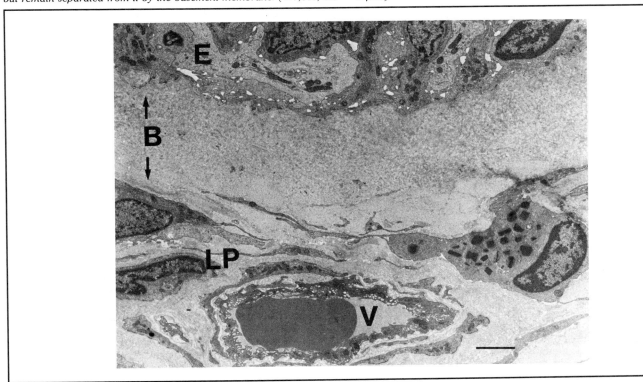

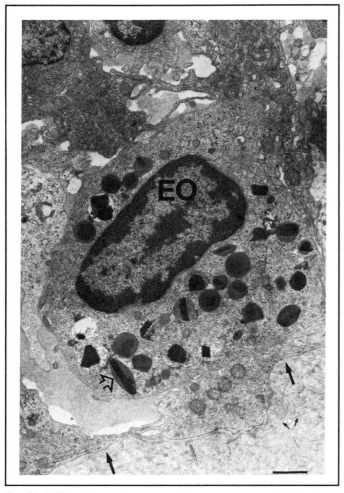

Fig. 23-4. *This electron micrograph shows an eosinophil (EO) with typical crystalloid core granules (open arrow) at the base of the airway epithelium in an asthmatic airway. Black large arrows point to the basal lamina immediately beneath the epithelium. The small arrows show collagenous fibers in the basement membrane. (×13,000, bar = 1 μm.)*

the luminal side, but separated in the middle of the epithelium by homogeneous fluidlike material, may relate to an ongoing shedding process affected by edema fluid [39]. The possibility that plasma exudation occurs in these airways is supported by findings of vascular endothelial gaps [35]. However, it remains speculative whether it is plasma exudation per se that is causing the disruption or shedding of the epithelium. Eosinophil-released toxic proteins may damage epithelial cells [5, 17], but it is not known whether they can serve as a mechanism by which whole epithelial cells are shed (see Chap. 20).

An important question is to what extent is there a loss of columnar epithelial cells in patients with asthma. The presence of shed epithelial cells in the sputum of asthmatic subjects is well described (Chap. 52); these take the form of Creola bodies and Curschmann's spirals [10, 55]. This finding has been considered a characteristic of asthma. Asthmatic subjects have shown greater numbers of shed epithelial cells in bronchoalveolar lavage (BAL) fluid than have nonasthmatic control subjects [4]. Based on histologic evaluations, several authors have reported epithelial shedding in the airways of patients with mild to severe asthma [24, 39, 44]. However, the mechanical denudation of the epithelium caused by the biopsy procedure itself, as described in control

subjects [71], may be difficult to distinguish from the real epithelial shedding caused by the disease. Unsolved problems with fiberoptic biopsing techniques that lead to the artifactual loss of epithelium have precluded quantitative assessment of the extent of epithelial shedding [4, 44, 71]. It has also been difficult to secure evidence of structural epithelial changes other than epithelial shedding.

In a recent study, bronchial biopsy specimens from newly diagnosed asthmatics were taken by means of rigid-tube bronchoscopy [36]. This method allows the study of larger uniform areas of epithelium with less artifactual loss of the epithelial cells than is seen with the fiberoptic technique. When the epithelium was analyzed with respect to ciliated, goblet, and other epithelial cells reaching the airway lumen, clear changes in its structure were noticed. These included an increased number of inflammatory cells, goblet cell hyperplasia, with or without ciliated cells, and squamous metaplasia (Figs. 23-7 and 23-8). Both the epithelial structure and the number and location of blood-borne or resident cells in the mucosa in asthmatic airways were different from those of the control subjects [36], and the findings in asthmatics were consistent with those typical of chronic inflammation. Perhaps more important than the actual epithelial shedding is a more continuous replacement of the ciliated epithelium by another type of epithelium in asthmatic airways in the early stage of the disease.

Morphologic studies on bronchial biopsy specimens have led to our present understanding of asthma as an inflammatory airway disease, as discussed in Chapter 9. Even mild asthmatics with a relatively short duration of the disease can have infiltration of different kinds of inflammatory cells to the epithelium and lamina propria [4, 5, 24, 39, 44]. Assessment of the condition of the epithelium may be of primary importance when evaluating the treatment effects on the disease. The disappearance of inflammatory cells from the mucosa may be insufficient when it comes to treating asthma. If the appearance of such cells is secondary to epithelial alterations, restoration of normal epithelium may be a primary therapeutic goal.

Viral Infections in the Lower Respiratory Tract

Asthma often begins or becomes worse during respiratory tract infections [42, 53] (see also Chap. 44). It has been speculated that viral infections are associated with bronchial hyperresponsiveness and represent the pathogenetic mechanism behind asthma [12, 40]. Animal studies have shown that an influenza virus preferentially attaches itself to, and subsequently infects, ciliated cells—but not secretory cells—in the epithelium of mature airways; this process has been observed even during early stages of ciliation [63]. The initial step in influenza infection before penetration is attachment of the virus to the host cell surfaces. This attachment is mediated by the specific binding of hemagglutinin, a viral envelope glycoprotein, to sialic acid–containing receptors in the apical membrane of airway cells [78]. In dogs infected by influenza C virus, histologic studies have revealed diffuse epithelial damage in the central airways; however, counts of infiltrated cells within the airway tissue were not significantly different between infected animals and noninfected control dogs. The luminal mast cell number was established from examination of BAL fluid, and the epithelial damage score correlated with the increase in airway responsiveness in the group of infected dogs [54]. However, the numbers of other inflammatory cells, such as neutrophils and eosinophils, were not increased 2 weeks after viral inoculation, when the animals had become most hyperreactive to inhaled acetylcholine. Viral respiratory tract infections provide mechanisms by which the structure of the epithelium may be injured initially, an event accompanied by an increase in absorption permeability and bronchial hyperresponsiveness to inhaled agents. This acute hyperresponsiveness may be different

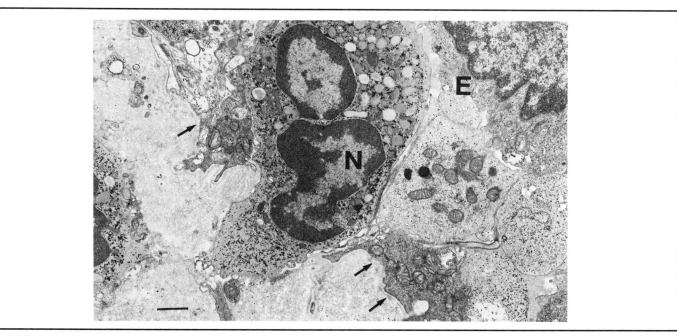

Fig. 23-5. *A specimen from a patient with clinically severe asthma of several years' duration. A neutrophil (N) is seen penetrating through the basal lamina (arrows) into the epithelium (E). (×13,000, bar = 1 μm.)*

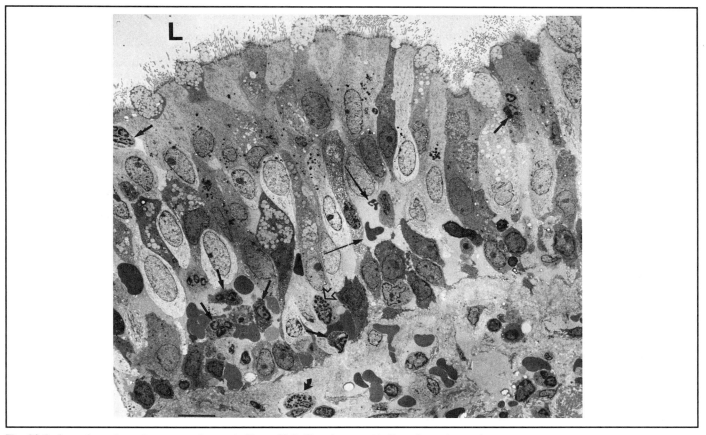

Fig. 23-6. *A specimen from the same patient as in Figure 23-5. The airway epithelium shows destructive changes, consisting of widening of intercellular spaces and shedding of the epithelium focally. Some of the ciliated and goblet cells are separated from the base by homogeneously staining material (long thin arrows). The epithelium is infiltrated by inflammatory cells, especially neutrophils (short black arrows). A capillary containing an eosinophil (curved arrow) is seen in the lamina propria close to the basement membrane. L = lumen; open arrow = eosinophil. (×1,300, bar = 10 μm.)*

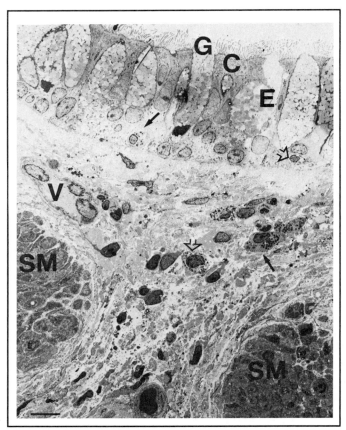

Fig. 23-7. *Specimen from a patient with clinically mild, extrinsic, newly detected asthma. The epithelium (E) shows goblet cell hyperplasia. Inflammatory cells, consisting mainly of eosinophils (black arrows) and lymphocytes as well as partly degranulated mast cells (open arrows), are detected both in the epithelium and lamina propria. Microvessels (V) are seen between the epithelium and airway smooth muscle (SM). C = ciliated cell; G = goblet cell. (×1,300, bar = 10 μm.)*

from that associated with an allergic or a chronic inflammatory reaction.

Bronchial reactivity during an influenza infection has been found to rise initially, but to return to normal within 7 weeks [12].

Patients suffering from influenza virus infections have been reported to exhibit a reddened bronchial mucosa and epithelial shedding [24]. In contrast to the findings of Hers [24], Söderberg and colleagues [70] did not find any major disturbances with regard to airway epithelium in bronchial biopsy specimens taken from patients with viral respiratory tract infections 1 to 6 weeks after the onset of the disease. The only differences between the influenza-infected patients and control subjects when the biopsies were done 3 to 6 weeks after the onset of the disease were that the epithelium was thicker and there was a slight lymphocytosis in the subepithelial tissue. However, the only patient in their study from whom biopsy tissue was taken 1 week after the onset of the disease showed areas of thin epithelium and an absence of cilia, which were assumed to represent a phase of regeneration after injury. In infected mice, regeneration of epithelium was recognized as soon as 5 days after the onset of infection; after 10 days, the epithelium was thin but contained both ciliated and nonciliated cells [64]. Hence, morphologic studies done in both humans and animals suggest that influenza viruses can indeed cause epithelial changes, but that these changes appear to be of short duration.

AIRWAY EPITHELIAL REGENERATION

Spontaneous Regeneration

Epithelial Turnover
Under normal conditions, the tracheobronchial lining is well differentiated and only a few cells undergo mitosis at the same time. However, a marked increase in proliferation and phenotypic modulation can occur in connection with an inflammatory process.

It is believed that, in the context of epithelial injury and damage, either basal cells [28] or secretory cells [31], or both, are the progenitor cells for epithelial regeneration. Of the three major epithelial cell types, only the basal and secretory cells have the capacity to divide and differentiate. The ciliated cells are considered to represent end-stage cells and are incapable of cell division [51]. The secretory cells are capable of proliferating into ciliated and secretory (goblet, serous, and Clara) cells. During differentiation, the postmitotic secretory cells may exhibit features of ciliogenesis (pre-ciliated cell) (Fig. 23-9) or a few mucous droplets (pre-secretory cell) before final differentiation into either cell [50]. In denuded rat tracheal grafts, it has been found that the secretory cells are capable of reestablishing a new epithelium composed of basal, secretory, and ciliated cells, whereas the basal cells are capable only of basal and ciliated cell differentiation [30]. In the rat bronchi, a renewal of the epithelium occurs in the absence of basal cells [15].

During inflammation and repair, adhesion glycoproteins and matrix macromolecules such as fibronectin and fibrinogen are thought to play an important role in cell recruitment, attachment, growth, and differentiation [68].

Epithelial Integrity and Cellular Adhesion
The function and integrity of the epithelium are dependent on specific cell-surface adhesion molecules. In addition, several adhesion molecules participate in airway processes such as inflammation and wound healing. Operationally, epithelial adhesion-mediating proteins can be considered as (1) those on the abluminal, basement membrane side of the cell functioning as cell substratum adhesion receptors, (2) those at the cell borders of adjacent epithelial cells maintaining cell-to-cell adhesion, and (3) those on the luminal side of the cell during inflammation functioning as cell-to-cell adhesion molecules in white blood cells.

The best characterized of the cell adhesion molecules are the glycoproteins which are members of the integrin family of receptors. Various types of integrin receptors with different alpha and beta subunits have been found in human airway epithelial cells; these include $alpha_2$, $alpha_3$, $alpha_6$, and $beta_1$ collagen-laminin receptors and $alpha_v$ fibronectin-fibrinogen receptors [1]. Differences have been noted in the pattern of integrins expressed by cultured cells compared with those expressed by some cells in tissue. In addition, other proteins, such as the 67- to 69-kd laminin/elastin/collagen receptors and the CD44 receptor binding to hyaluronic acid may be involved in the epithelial cell-to-substratum adhesion.

Extracellular Matrix
The extracellular matrix (ECM) is composed of a mixture of macromolecules, including (1) polysaccharide glycosaminoglycans (which are usually found covalently linked to protein in the form of proteoglycans) and (2) fibrous proteins of two functional types, one of which is mainly structural (e.g., collagen and elastin) and the other, mainly adhesive (e.g., fibronectin and laminin). The glycosaminoglycan and proteoglycan molecules form a highly hydrated, gellike "ground substance" in which the fibrous proteins are embedded. The major collagen composing the ECM

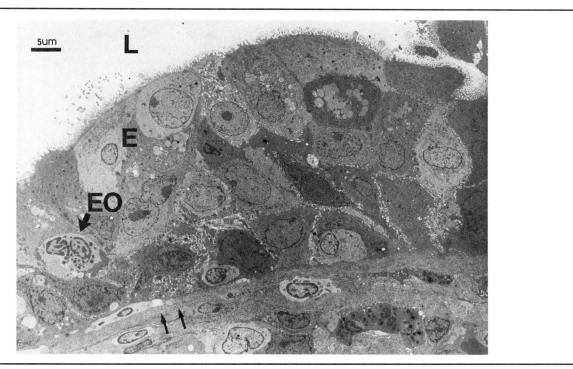

Fig. 23-8. *Electron micrograph showing structural changes in the airway epithelium (E) during spontaneous exacerbation of asthma in an intrinsic asthmatic patient. The epithelium consists mainly of undifferentiated cells possessing microvilli. The ciliated cells are lost and only a few cells contain mucous granules. Both the epithelium and lamina propria are highly invaded by eosinophils (EO). L = lumen; arrows = basement membrane. (×2,600.)*

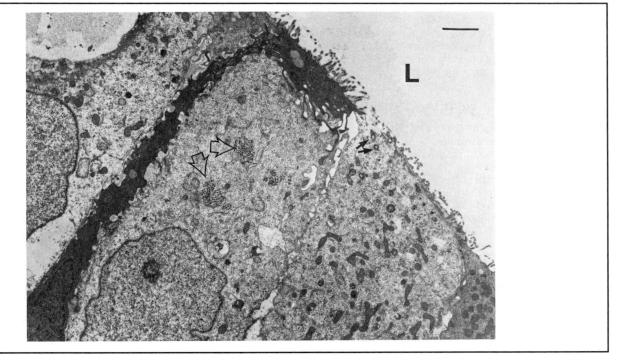

Fig. 23-9. *Electron micrograph showing signs of ciliogenesis in the epithelium in an asthmatic patient during beta₂-agonist therapy. One pre-ciliated cell shows fibrogranular areas (open arrows) and the other shows basal bodies (small black arrows) close to its luminal surface. L = lumen. (×7,800, bar = 2 μm.)*

is Type IV. The macromolecules of the ECM are mainly secreted locally by cells in the matrix. In most connective tissues, these macromolecules are secreted largely by fibroblasts. Bronchial epithelial cells have been shown to produce Type IV collagen, fibronectin, and laminin [72]. Some ECM proteins can function as intermediaries by binding both to the cell through a receptor and to other matrix proteins, such as collagen. Laminin and fibronectin can interact with collagenous structures. During epithelial repair, it is thought that a provisional matrix is formed by fibronectin and vitronectin in the wounded area [7, 22].

Many of the proteins that can interact directly with specific cell-surface receptors contain a tripeptide, arginine-glycine-aspartic acid (RGD), at the cell-recognition site. Cell-binding proteins include fibronectin, laminin, vitronectin, and the collagens. The RGD segment found in each of these adhesive proteins is recognized by at least one of the members of a family of integrin receptors. However, recent investigations have shown that epithelial cells attach to proteins of the ECM by means of more than one mechanism, including an RGD-mediated and a non-RGD–mediated process [66]. Although the RGD tripeptide is a major cell-recognition site for the integrin receptors, some integrin receptors can use other sites for attachment. In addition, cells may have non–integrin receptors for matrix proteins.

Basement Membrane

Not very much is known about the ECM and basement membrane in the airway mucosa of asthmatic subjects. Some studies have, through ultrastructural analysis and direct measurements from electron micrographs, suggested that the epithelial basement membrane in asthmatics is thickened by up to 7.95 (± 1.78 S.E.) μm compared to that in controls, or 4.17 (± 0.59 S.E.) μm [67]. Several other investigators have also described a thickened basement membrane to be characteristic of asthma [11]. It is, however, difficult in morphologic terms to define the exact limits of the epithelial basement membrane. In a biopsy study of 37 normal control subjects, the thickness of the basement membrane was reported to range between 3 to 17.5 μm, with a median value of 8.5 μm [71], which is greater than that in the asthmatic subjects in the above-mentioned study [67]. This question has become important because it has been suggested to be relevant to the treatment of asthma. It has been proposed that the thickening of the epithelial basement membrane in asthma could be one cause for the disease becoming more persistent.

Effect of Treatment on Airway Epithelial Structure

There have not been many controlled studies reporting changes in the airway epithelial structure of asthmatic airways either in different clinical stages of the disease or during pharmacologic intervention [23, 41].

The results of animal studies suggest that the type of epithelium which appears during regeneration may be different, depending on which cells (basal or secretory, or both) serve as the stem cells for the regeneration process [30]. This may be relevant to the changes noticed in the epithelium of asthmatics, and explain the diversity of epithelial changes observed during injury, spontaneous regeneration, and treatment. Abrupt epithelial shedding, in which both ciliated and goblet cells are lost, may be followed by a regeneration process that differs from a long-standing irritation process in the epithelium. Low-grade irritation in the epithelium could lead to goblet cell hyperplasia with loss of the vulnerable ciliated cells, representing a simultaneous degeneration–regeneration process. In support of this view, a low-dose exposure to toluene-diisocyanate produced no visible injury but induced goblet cell hyperplasia (periodic–acid-shift–positive cells) in guinea pig tracheobronchial airways several weeks after exposure [62].

In a recent study of newly diagnosed asthmatics who had not been treated with previous continuous medication, the major difference in epithelial structure, compared to that of nonsmoking nonallergic control subjects, was the clear decrease in the number of ciliated cells and increase in the number of goblet cells [37]. These asthma patients were further randomized into two parallel study groups in a double-blind manner; one group received an inhaled steroid (600 μg b.i.d.) and the other received an inhaled beta$_2$ agonist (375 μg b.i.d.) for 3 months. Bronchial biopsy specimens were taken both before and after treatment. They showed an increased number of ciliated cells in the epithelium of patients who had undergone inhaled steroid treatment (Fig. 23-10), the ciliated goblet cell ratio being similar to that of the healthy control group. In a comparison made after inhalation of the beta$_2$ agonist, no statistically significant change was found in the relative numbers of ciliated and goblet cells, although some inflammatory cell parameters changed. These findings support the idea that there is a slow "destructive" process of the epithelium along with some kind of a regeneration process going on in asthmatic patients. Ciliated cells are probably the first to disappear upon injury, and they may not be replaced with their own kind until the injurious stimulation is over [50]. It is possible that the regeneration process in asthmatic airways does not reach a mature state of ciliated epithelium, but remains in an earlier phase of regeneration until the inflammatory driving forces of the disease have ceased or been well suppressed by the treatment.

FUNCTIONS OF THE AIRWAY EPITHELIUM

Epithelium-Derived Agents

The airway epithelium may produce a wide range of biologically active compounds. These range from smooth muscle–active factors to mediators of acute and chronic inflammation. By analogy with the interaction between vascular endothelium and vascular smooth muscle, it has been suggested that tracheobronchial epithelial cells release factors that may control airway tone (Fig. 23-11). Epithelium-derived relaxing factors, which would be lost if the epithelium were shedded, have been suggested as being important components of the pathophysiology of asthma [6] (Fig. 23-12). Some of the findings appear to be inconsistent [45], and in vivo support for this particular hypothesis is lacking. Table 23-1 summarizes some of the effects of epithelial removal on airway tissues.

The interest in what epithelial cells may produce and release has led to the demonstration of epithelium-derived prostaglandins and leukotrienes [27]. These mediators may affect nearby structures, including the sensory innervation and the superficial airway microcirculation. However, the role of the epithelium in providing mediators of acute inflammation, as compared with other sources, remains to be established.

It has recently been demonstrated in vitro cultures that the epithelium in the human airway has a significant capacity to produce and release cytokines. The structural cells of the airway lining, through their great number and strategic position, may orchestrate immune and inflammatory responses of the airways. Cox and associates [9] have demonstrated that cultured human bronchial epithelial cells, through generation of the granulocyte/macrophage colony–stimulating factor (GM-CSF), increase eosinophil survival. The majority of the cells exhibited reduced granularity and increased vacuolation, consistent with an activated phenotype of eosinophils. Interleukin-1 (IL-1), which may be produced by bronchial epithelial cells [48], increases the epithelial production of GM-CSF [9]. The baseline and the IL-1–induced production of GM-CSF, as well as the subsequent increased eosinophil survival [9], can be inhibited by a synthetic glucocorti-

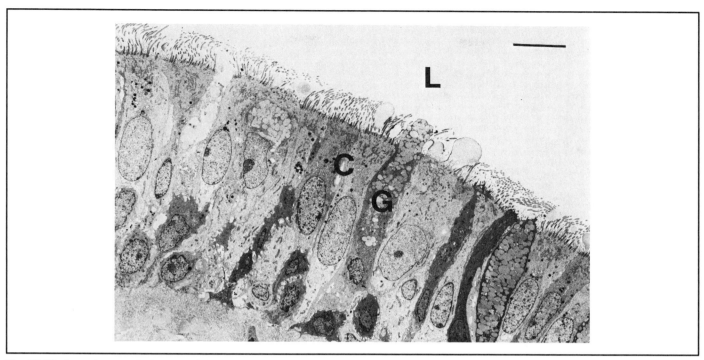

Fig. 23-10. *A nearly normal airway epithelium with ciliated (C) and goblet cells (G) in an asthmatic patient after 3 months of inhaled corticosteroid therapy. Before treatment, the epithelium was highly destroyed and was invaded with eosinophils, lymphocytes, and mast cells. L = lumen. (×2,000, bar = 10 μm.)*

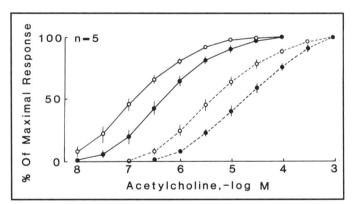

Fig. 23-11. *Effect of removal of the epithelium on concentration-response curves to acetylcholine in canine bronchi. (Closed circles = rings with epithelium; open circles = rings without epithelium; dashed lines = responses under control conditions; solid lines = responses after inhibition of acetylcholinesterase, the major enzyme responsible for the breakdown of the cholinergic transmitter.) Note in both cases a marked shift to the left of the concentration-response curve after removal of the epithelium. (Reprinted with permission from N. A. Flavahan, et al. The respiratory epithelium inhibits bronchial smooth muscle. J. Appl. Physiol. 58:834, 1985.)*

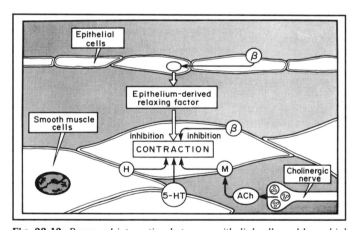

Fig. 23-12. *Proposed interaction between epithelial cells and bronchial smooth muscle. Under basal conditions, the epithelium secretes epithelium-derived relaxing factor, which acts as a functional antagonist on the bronchial smooth muscle, causing a comparable depression of the response to a variety of bronchoconstrictor agonists. The release of the factor can be activated by stimulation of β-adrenoceptors on the endothelial cells. (ACh = acetylcholine; β = β-adrenoceptors; H = histaminergic receptor; 5-HT = serotonergic receptor; M = muscarinic receptor.) (Reprinted with permission from P. M. Vanhoutte. Epithelium-derived relaxing factors. Am. Rev. Respir. Dis. 138:S24, 1988.)*

coid budesonide. Simultaneous work by Marini and coworkers [48] demonstrated that IL-1, by binding to specific surface receptors on human bronchial epithelial cells, upregulates the synthesis and release of GM-CSF. They further showed that 1 μM hydrocortisone abolished the baseline and IL-1–induced epithelial release of GM-CSF. Working with human upper airway epithelial cells, Ohtoshi and associates [57] have demonstrated that these cells have a capacity to induce monocytic differentiation of human hematopoietic progenitors, and that this capacity is increased in epithelial cells obtained from inflamed airways. They

could not identify the responsible factor or cytokine but demonstrated GM-CSF, granulocyte-CSF, and IL-6 in the epithelial cells.

Thus, there is increasing evidence that epithelial cells can release various kinds of biologically active compounds [3, 27, 69]. However, there has not been much information as to which type of epithelial cell releases these compounds. In a recent study, Takizawa and colleagues [75], investigating cultured bovine epithelial cells, observed a marked difference between ciliated and

Table 23-1. Effects of epithelial removal on airway tissue*

CONTRACTION

Tissue	Histamine	Cholinergic	5-HT	K+
Dog	↑	↑	↑	—
Cow	↑ (↑ max)	↑ (↑ max)	↑ (↑ max)	0
GP	↑	0	—	0
GP	↑	↑	↑	↑
GP	↑	↑	↑	0
GP	—	↑ (↑ max)	↑	—
GP	↑ (↑ max)	↑ (MCh)	—	↑ (↓ max)
Rat	—	0 (CCh)	↑	—
Rabbit	↑	↑ (MCh)	—	0
Rabbit	—	↑ (BCh)	—	—
Human	—	↑ (MCh)	—	0

RELAXATION

Tissue	Contractile agent/relaxant
Dog	ACh/ISO (↓ max)
Cow	ACh/ISO (0) 5-HT/ISO (↓) HIST/ISO (0)
GP	CCh/ISO (↓ max) CCh/forskolin (↓ max)
	CCh/Theo (↓ max) CCh/nitroglycerin (0)
GP	Resting tone/ISO (↑) adenosine (0)
GP	Adenosine (↑) nitroprusside (↑) papaverine (0) salbutamol (0)
	Salbutamol (0) resting tone/ISO (↑) (blocked by corticosterone)
Rat	Antigen/SP (↓)
Rabbit	Hist/verapamil (↓ max) MCh/verapamil (↓ max)
Rabbit	Arachidonic acid (↓ max)
Human	MCh/verapamil (↓ max)

BLOCKADE

Tissue	Contractile agent		
Dog	ACh	INDO (↑ max Ep+)	Bay G6575 (0)
Cow	ACh ↑	INDO (0)	Mepacrine (0)
GP	Hist	INDO (↑ max Ep+ > Ep−)	DTT (↑ Ep+) phenindione (↑)
GP	ACh/Hist/EFS	INDO (↑ Ep− > Ep+)	
GP	ACh/5-HT		SKF 525 (↑ max Ep+)
GP	ACh/Hist	INDO (↑ + ↑ max/ ↑ max Ep+)	
Rabbit	BCh	INDO (↑ Ep+)	

GP = guinea pig; 5-HT = serotonin; ISO = isoproterenol; Hist = histamine; CCh = carbamoylcholine; MCh = methacholine; BCh = bethanechol; ACh = acetylcholine; EFS = electrical field stimulation; Theo = theophylline; SP = substance P; INDO = indomethacin; (0) = no effect; (↑ max) = increased or (↓ max) = decreased efficacy after epithelial removal; (↑) = increased or (↓) = decreased potency after epithelial removal. (Ep+) = intact tissue; (Ep−) = deepithelialized tissue.
* The effects of epithelial removal on airway tissues and summary of results; specific references are cited in F. M. Cuss and P. J. Barnes. Epithelial mediators. *Am. Rev. Respir. Dis.* 136:S32, 1987. Reproduced with permission.

nonciliated cells with regard to the quantitative release of fibronectin. The ciliated cells released much less fibronectin than did the nonciliated, mainly basal, cells. This suggests that the ciliated and nonciliated cells may have different roles in the repair process following tissue injury.

Many cell types expressing the class II major histocompatibility complex may be present in or just beneath the epithelium in inflammatory diseases. These cells, including dendritic cells, Langerhan's cells, monocytes/macrophages, B-cells, and sometimes epithelial cells, are thus possible antigen-presenting cells [26]. The importance of this property of the epithelial cells, together with their cytokine-producing ability, remains largely unexplored. A well-developed capacity for antigen presentation may represent a more important change in airway disease than the reputed general increase in perviousness of the epithelial lining.

Absorption Permeability Across the Airway Mucosa

In 1910, Meltzer [52] described "bronchial asthma as a phenomenon of anaphylaxis." This view led to an explicit interest in the absorptive function of the airway mucosa. A particular concern was the mucosal penetration of allergic material. Experimental studies showed that allergens can be absorbed across the airway mucosa, and this property appeared to be well developed in healthy subjects. Cohen and associates [8] examined the Prausnitz-Küstner reactions in passively sensitized skin sites after the administration of ragweed pollen into the nostrils of normal and allergic subjects. Their data suggested that atopic patients with rhinitis and asthma absorb less allergenic material than do control subjects. However, during the 1960s through the 1980s, an idea prevailed which suggested that the allergic or inflamed airway mucosa is characterized by "absorption hyperpermeability" [25]. Later, many attempts to relate asthma and bronchial hyperresponsiveness to an increased absorption of inhaled tracer molecules failed [56].

Recently, methods have been developed that allow for specific studies of inflammatory processes and mucosal absorption in guinea pig tracheobronchial airways and in human nasal airways [14, 19]. In the studies conducted in humans, a compressible nasal-pool device is used to create an "organ bath" in one of the nasal cavities. Using this method, allergen and histamine-type mediators have been noted to produce immediate inflammatory or exudative effects in the nasal and tracheobronchial mucosa, but, even at high doses, this acute response is not associated with any change in the rate of absorption of small or large tracer molecules [20]. More sustained inflammatory responses may not increase the mucosal absorptive ability. Indeed, late in the pollen season, patients with active allergic rhinitis absorb tracer molecules less readily than they do before the season [21]. The airway mucosa may be asymmetrical in its barrier function [61], and it may allow the luminal entry of different-sized plasma macromolecules without increasing its absorptive ability.

Increased bronchial absorption rates may not characterize asthma. Especially early in the disease, the predominating structural changes occurring in the epithelial lining may not be a widespread shedding of cells but only a gradual replacement of ciliated epithelium with goblet cells, which would be compatible with a maintained absorption barrier of the bronchial mucosa.

Exudation Permeability Across the Airway Mucosa

Topically administered challenges of the airway mucosa with allergens, occupational agents, and inflammatory mediators produce extravasation of plasma from the subepithelial microcirculation [59]. Inflammatory stimulus–induced extravasation is suggested to be a specific defense or inflammatory response. In human airways, extravasation of plasma may not be produced by irritants that evoke neurally mediated effects [60].

The mechanism of inflammatory extravasation may be an active separation of venular endothelial cells that produces holes in the microvascular wall [35]. Hydrostatic pressure then moves unfiltered plasma through these holes, which open only for a short while unless the challenge is continued or escalated. The extravasated plasma in the airways appears to be regulated by a flux across the epithelial lining (Fig. 23-13).

It has been believed that a significant entry of large plasma proteins into the airway lumen occurs only after the epithelium has been severely disrupted. Dunnill [11] has suggested that the mucosal crossing of plasma is an epithelium-damaging process. It is also a widespread notion that the extravasated plasma will produce marked airway edema before its luminal entry. However, recent observations show that such mediators as platelet-activating factor, histamine, leukotriene D4, and bradykinin, when applied to the tracheobronchial mucosa of guinea pigs, produce

exudation of plasma into both the tissue and lumen [13] (Fig. 23-14). The luminal entry of plasma is graded and dose-dependent, and occurs without the formation of edema. Sustained inflammatory responses such as those occurring after topical challenge with allergen or toluene-diisocyanate are reflected by the continuous luminal entry of plasma macromolecules [60].

In subjects with allergic asthma, endobronchial allergen challenge has produced the exudation of large plasma proteins such as fibrinogen, with increased levels in BAL samples. The levels of plasma proteins have also been increased in BAL liquids obtained from asthmatic subjects during the late sequelae of challenges with allergen [43] and occupational agents such as toluene-diisocyanate [16]. Van de Graaf and associates [76] have reported that the prolonged treatment of asthmatic subjects with an inhaled glucocorticoid (budesonide) reduced the levels of large plasma proteins in BAL liquids. Similarly, Svensson and colleagues [74] have demonstrated glucocorticoid-induced inhibition (budesonide) of mucosal exudation of fibrinogen in patients with seasonal allergic rhinitis.

The composition of mucous plugs and sputum supports the view that plasma proteins may be abundant in the bronchial lumen, particularly in severe asthma (see Chap. 29). Plasma exudation is a specific sign of ongoing inflammation, compared with many other tissue responses such as hypersecretion, hyperemia, mucociliary activity, and cough, which may simply reflect irritant

Fig. 23-14. *Suggested sequence of events initiated by the release or arrival of inflammatory mediators in the vicinity of tracheobronchial microvessels. (Reprinted with permission from C. G. A. Persson. Leakage macromolecules from microcirculation. Am. Rev. Respir. Dis. 135:S71, 1987.)*

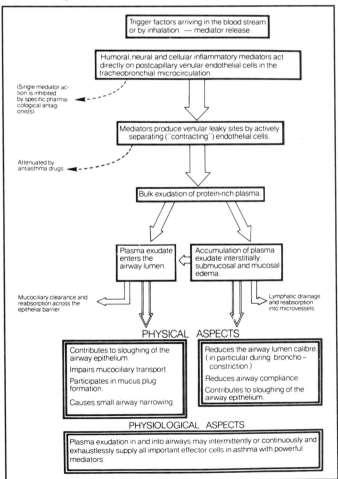

Fig. 23-13. *Illustration of a leaky microvessel and a leaky epithelial barrier with free movement of large solutes from the vascular compartment into the luminal airway compartment. (Reprinted with permission from C. G. A. Persson. Leakage macromolecules from microcirculation. Am. Rev. Respir. Dis. 135:S71, 1987.)*

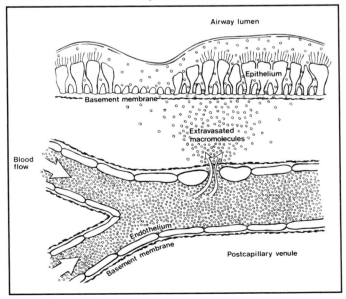

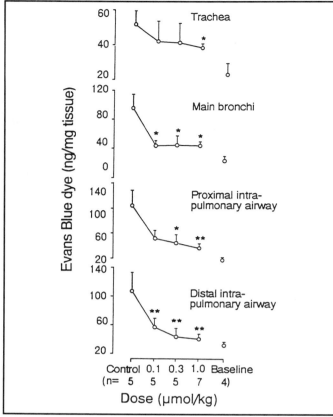

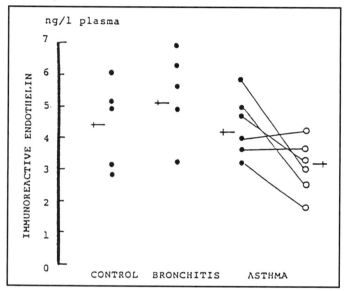

Fig. 23-17. *Evaluation of immunoreactive endothelins in peripheral blood of patients with asthma or chronic bronchitis and in normal volunteers (control subjects); amounts of circulating endothelin-like material recovered in normal subjects, in patients with chronic bronchitis, and in patients with symptomatic asthma before treatment (●); concentrations of immunoreactive endothelins in plasma from patients with asthma after treatment with corticosteroids and bronchodilators (○). (Bars indicate mean values for each group.) (Reprinted with permission from S. Mattoli, et al. Levels of endothelin in the bronchoalveolar lavage fluid of patients with symptomatic asthma and reversible airflow obstruction. J. Allergy Clin. Immunol. 88: 376, 1991.)*

Fig. 23-15. *Effect of a 5-lipoxygenase inhibitor, A-63162, on Evans blue extravasation induced by ovalbumin allergen challenge at different airway levels. The baseline group consisted of unsensitized guinea pigs treated with vehicle alone, and the control group consisted of sensitized animals treated with vehicle (DMSO). Values are mean ± SEM of n animals. *$P < 0.05$ and **$P < 0.01$, comparing each A-63162–treated group with the control group. (Reprinted with permission from K. P. Hui, et al. Attenuation of inhaled allergen-induced airway microvascular leakage and airflow obstruction in guinea pigs by a 5-lipoxygenase inhibitor. Am. Rev. Respir. Dis. 143: 1015, 1991.)*

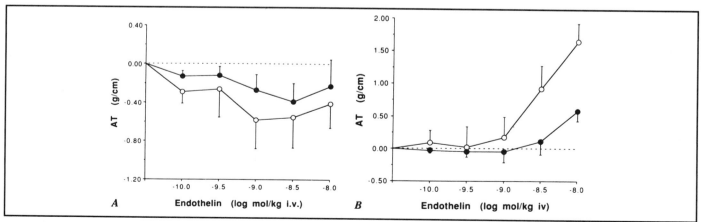

Fig. 23-16. *Effect of epithelium removal on tracheal smooth muscle response elicited by intravenously administered endothelin-1. A. Relaxation phase of the response. Tracheal smooth muscle relaxation was not altered significantly by removal of the epithelium of the isolated tracheal segment (closed circles) compared with animals with an intact epithelium (open circle; AT = active tension). B. Contractile phase of the response. Tracheal smooth muscle contraction was attenuated substantially after removal of the epithelium of the isolated tracheal segment (N = 6) (closed circles) compared with animals with an intact epithelium (N = 6) (open circles). (Reprinted with permission from S. R. White, et al. Epithelial modulation of airway smooth muscle response to endothelin-1. Am. Rev. Respir. Dis. 144:373, 1991.)*

neural responses [62a]. Furthermore, plasma exudation may have an important role in the pathogenesis of asthma [58]. The potential physical effects of an exudate located beneath and above the airway epithelium, and the exudate's abundant content of inflammatory plasma–derived factors and mediators, may contribute to the asthmatic diathesis, even if edema and epithelial disruption are not induced (Fig. 23-15).

Endothelin

Endothelin is a 21–amino acid peptide with potent vasoconstrictor properties. Isopeptide endothelin-1, which is isolated from supernatants of cultured vascular endothelial cells, also exhibits potent effects on airway smooth muscle. In situ airway smooth muscle responses in the guinea pig following intravenous administration of endothelin-1 exhibit a biphasic response during active tracheal tension. This consists of a brief initial relaxation, not mediated by eicosanoids, that is followed by a prolonged contractile response, which appears to be eicosanoid mediated. Removal of the contiguous epithelium results in responses that are blunted compared to airway segments with intact epithelium, suggesting the epithelium adjacent to the airway smooth muscle modulates contraction induced by endothelin-1 [77] (Fig. 23-16).

Human bronchial smooth muscle cells exhibit a single class of binding sites for endothelin-1 with a molecular weight of 1.13×10^{-10} mol/liter and a maximal binding capacity of 22.1 fmol/10^6 cells [47]. In a recent clinical evaluation, the release of endothelin from the airway mucosa, as shown by radioimmunoassay in BAL fluid, revealed increased amounts of immunoreactive endothelin in asthmatics compared with findings in normal subjects and patients with chronic bronchitis [49]. Antiasthma therapy with oral corticosteroids and inhaled beta agonists maintained for 15 days resulted in both clinical improvement and a greater than threefold reduction of the endothelin content in the BAL samples [49] (Fig. 23-17).

In conclusion, it is widely thought that dramatic epithelial changes, such as shedding, represent a major mechanism in the pathogenesis of asthma and bronchial hyperresponsiveness. However, due to difficulties in obtaining proper biopsy samples, it has not yet been established to what extent epithelial shedding really occurs in preterminal stages of asthma. Indeed, results from studies of airway barrier function using inhaled tracer molecules suggest that the tightness of the epithelial lining is not compromised in asthma. This barrier may be little affected by the plasma exudation process that characterizes ongoing airway inflammation. In line with this, recent animal data have suggested that plasma exudates do not produce edema, but may readily enter the airway lumen, also across a normal epithelial lining.

The attachment of the epithelial cells to each other and to ECM macromolecules is probably regulated by adhesion glucoproteins. We need to learn more about the function of these adhesion molecules in asthma, both to improve our understanding of the exudation and absorption asymmetry of the airway mucosa and to better assess the role of structural epithelial changes in this disease.

Bronchial biopsy specimens from living asthmatics with mild cases of the disease have revealed that normal ciliated epithelium is altered, such that goblet or other nonmatured epithelial cells predominate. These structural intraepithelial changes may reflect a stereotyped response to a long-standing irritation in the epithelium. The epithelium in asthmatic subjects is further characterized by the presence of abnormally high numbers of inflammatory cells, particularly eosinophils and lymphocytes. It cannot be excluded that the appearance of these cells is secondary to initial events in the epithelial lining itself, which, besides structural changes, may consist of a changed capacity of the epithelial cells to release biologically active agents, including leukotrienes and cytokines. The epithelium may also participate in antigen presentation. If the epithelium orchestrates significant components of inflammation in asthma, it may not be sufficient to direct the antiinflammatory therapy only against lymphocytes, inflammatory cells, and the microcirculation. We may also have to find ways of normalizing the structure and biologic activity of the epithelial lining in order to achieve an optimal treatment of bronchial asthma.

REFERENCES

1. Albelda, S. M. Endothelial and epithelial cell adhesion molecules. *Am. J. Respir. Cell Mol. Biol.* 4:195, 1991.
2. Ayers, M., and Jeffery, P. K. Proliferation and differentiation in mammalian airway epithelium. *Eur. Respir. J.* 1:58, 1988.
3. Barnett, K., et al. The effects of epithelial cell supernatant on contractions of isolated canine tracheal smooth muscle. *Am. Rev. Respir. Dis.* 138:780, 1988.
4. Beasley, R., et al. Cellular events in the bronchi in mild asthma and after bronchial provocation. *Am. Rev. Respir. Dis.* 139:806, 1989.
5. Bousquet, J., et al. Eosinophilic inflammation in asthma. *N. Engl. J. Med.* 323:1033, 1990.
6. Busk, M. F., and Vanhoutte, P. M. Epithelium-dependent Responses in Airways. In M. A. Kaliner, P. J. Barnes, and C. G. A. Persson (eds.), *Asthma: Its Pathology and Treatment* (Lung Biology in Health and Disease). New York: Dekker, 1991, Pp. 135–188.
7. Clark, R. A., et al. Fibronectin and fibrin provide a provisional matrix for epidermal cell migration during wound reepithelialization. *J. Invest. Dermatol.* 79:264, 1982.
8. Cohen, M. B., et al. The rate of absorption of ragweed pollen material from the nose. *J. Immunol.* 18:419, 1930.
9. Cox, G., et al. Promotion of eosinophil survival by human bronchial epithelial cells and its modulation by steroid. *Am. J. Respir. Cell Mol. Biol.* 4:525, 1991.
10. Curschmann, H. Einige Bemerkungen über die im Bronchialsekret vorkommenden Spiralen. *Dtsch. Arch. Klin. Med.* 36:578, 1885.
11. Dunnill, M. S. The pathology of asthma with special reference to changes in the bronchial mucosa. *J. Clin. Pathol.* 13:27, 1960.
12. Empey, D. W., et al. Mechanisms of bronchial hyperreactivity in normal subjects after upper respiratory tract infection. *Am. Rev. Respir. Dis.* 113:131, 1976.
13. Erjefält, I., and Persson, C. G. A. Inflammatory passage of plasma macromolecules into airway tissue and lumen. *Pulm. Pharmacol.* 2:93, 1989.
14. Erjefält, I., and Persson, C. G. A. Pharmacological control of plasma exudation in guinea-pig lower airways. *Am. Rev. Respir. Dis.* 143:1008, 1991.
15. Evans, M. J., et al. Renewal of the terminal bronchiolar epithelium in the rat following exposure to NO_2 or O_3. *Lab. Invest.* 35:246, 1976.
16. Fabbri, L. M., et al. Bronchoalveolar neutrophilia during late asthmatic reactions induced by toluene diisocyanate. *Am. Rev. Respir. Dis.* 136:36, 1987.
16a. Farmer, S. G., and Hay, D. W. P. *The Airway Epithelium: Physiology, Pathophysiology, and Pharmacology.* New York: Dekker, 1991.
17. Gleich, G. J., et al. Comparative properties of Charcot-Leyden crystal protein and the major basic protein from human eosinophils. *J. Clin. Invest.* 57:633, 1976.
18. Glynn, A. A., and Michaels, L. Bronchial biopsy in chronic bronchitis and asthma. *Thorax* 15:142, 1960.
19. Greiff, L., et al. The nasal pool device applies controlled concentrations of solutes on human nasal airway mucosa and samples its surface exudations/secretions. *Clin. Exp. Allergy* 20:253, 1990.
20. Greiff, L., et al. Different patterns of inflammatory effects on airway barriers: plasma exudation with and without increased absorption of small or large luminal solutes. *Thorax* 46:700, 1991.
21. Greiff, L., et al. Reduced mucosal absorption permeability in allergic rhinitis. *Clin. Exp. Allergy* (in press).
22. Hayman, E. G., et al. Serum spreading factor (vitronectin) is present at the cell surface and in tissue. *Proc. Natl. Acad. Sci. U.S.A.* 80:4003, 1983.
23. Heino, M. Morphological changes related to ciliogenesis in the bronchial epithelium in experimental conditions and clinical course of disease. *Eur. J. Respir. Dis.* 151(suppl):1, 1987.
24. Hers, J. F. P. H. Disturbances of the ciliated epithelium due to influenza virus. *Am. Rev. Respir. Dis.* 93:162, 1966.
25. Hogg, J. C. Bronchial mucosal permeability and its relationship to airways hyperreactivity. *J. Allergy Clin. Immunol.* 67:421, 1981.

26. Holt, P. G., Schon-Hegrad, M. A., and McMenamin, P. G. Dendritic cells in the respiratory tract. *Int. Rev. Immunol.* 6:139, 1990.
27. Holtzman, M. J. Arachidonic acid metabolism. Implications of biological chemistry for lung function and disease. *Am. Rev. Respir. Dis.* 143:188, 1991.
28. Inayama, Y., et al. The differentiations potential of tracheal basal cells. *Lab. Invest.* 58:706, 1988.
29. Jeffery, P. K., et al. Bronchial biopsies in asthma: an ultrastructural quantification study and correlation with hyperreactivity. *Am. Rev. Respir. Dis.* 140:1745, 1989.
30. Johnson, N. F., and Hubbs, A. F. Epithelial progenitor cells in rat trachea. *Am. J. Respir. Cell Mol. Biol.* 3:579, 1990.
31. Keenan, K. P., Combs, J. W., and McDowell, E. M. Regeneration of hamster tracheal epithelium after mechanical injury. Focal lesions: quantitative morphologic study of cell proliferation. *Virchows Arch. B Cell Pathol.* 41:193, 1982.
32. Laitinen, A. Ultrastructural organization of intraepithelial nerves in the human airway tract. *Thorax* 40:488, 1985.
33. Laitinen, L. A. Detailed Analysis of Neural Elements in Human Airways. In M. Kaliner and P. Barnes (eds.), *Neural Regulation of the Airways in Health and Disease.* New York: Dekker, 1988, Pp. 35–36.
34. Laitinen, L. A. Epithelial Damage. In J. L. Malo, F. Hargreave, and J. Hogg (eds.), *Glucocorticoids and Mechanisms of Asthma.* Amsterdam: Excerpta Medica, 1989, Pp. 215–229.
35. Laitinen, L. A., and Laitinen, A. Pathology of Human Asthma. In M. Kaliner, P. Barnes, and C. Persson (eds.), *Asthma. Its Pathology and Treatment* (Lung Biology and Health and Disease). New York: Dekker, 1991, Pp. 103–134.
36. Laitinen, L. A., Laitinen, A., and Haahtela, T. Inflammatory cell population in the airways of newly diagnosed asthmatic patients; a quantitative ultrastructural study. *Eur. Respir. J.* 3(suppl 10):156A, 1990.
37. Laitinen, L. A., Laitinen, A., and Haahtela, T. Treatment of eosinophilic airway inflammation with inhaled corticosteroid in newly diagnosed asthmatic patients. *J. Allergy Clin. Immunol.* 90:32, 1991.
38. Laitinen, L. A., Laitinen, A., and Widdicombe, J. G. Effects of inflammatory and other mediators on airway vascular beds. *Am. Rev. Respir. Dis.* 135:567, 1987.
39. Laitinen, L. A., et al. Damage of the airway epithelium and bronchial reactivity in patients with asthma. *Am. Rev. Respir. Dis.* 131:599, 1985.
40. Laitinen, L. A., et al. Bronchial hyperresponsiveness in normal subjects during attenuated influenza virus infection. *Am. Rev. Respir. Dis.* 143:358, 1991.
41. Laitinen, L. A., et al. Eosinophilic airway inflammation during exacerbation of asthma and its treatment with inhaled corticosteroid. *Am. Rev. Respir. Dis.* 143:423, 1991.
42. Little, J. W., et al. Airway hyperreactivity and peripheral airway dysfunction in influenza A infection. *Am. Rev. Respir. Dis.* 118:295, 1978.
43. Liu, M. C., et al. Immediate and late inflammatory responses to ragweed antigen challenge of the peripheral airways in allergic asthmatics. *Am. Rev. Respir. Dis.* 144:51, 1991.
44. Lozewicz, S., et al. Morphological integrity of the bronchial epithelium in mild asthma. *Thorax* 45:12, 1990.
45. Lundblad, K. A. L., and Persson, C. G. A. The epithelium and the pharmacology of guinea-pig tracheal tone in vitro. *Br. J. Pharmacol.* 93:909, 1988.
46. Lundgren, R., et al. Morphological studies of bronchial mucosal biopsies from asthmatics before and after ten years of treatment with inhaled steroids. *Eur. Respir. J.* 1:883, 1988.
47. Marini, M., et al. Specific binding of endothelin on human bronchial smooth muscle cells in culture and secretion of endothelin-like material from bronchial epithelial cells. *Am. J. Respir. Cell Mol. Biol.* 3:145, 1990.
48. Marini, M., et al. Interleukin-1 binds to specific receptors on human bronchial epithelial cells and upregulates granulocytes/macrophage colony-stimulating factor synthesis and release. *Am. J. Respir. Cell Mol. Biol.* 4:519, 1991.
49. Mattoli, S., et al. Levels of endothelin in the bronchoalveolar lavage fluid of patients with symptomatic asthma and reversible airflow obstruction. *J. Allergy Clin. Immunol.* 88:376, 1991.
50. McDowell, E. M., and Beals, T. F. *Biopsy Pathology of the Bronchi.* Philadelphia: Saunders, 1987.
51. McDowell, E. M., and Trump, B. F. Conceptual review: histogenesis of preneoplastic and neoplastic lesions in tracheobronchial epithelium. *Surv. Synth. Pathol. Res.* 2:235, 1984.
52. Meltzer, S. J. Bronchial asthma as a phenomenon of anaphylaxis. *JAMA* 50:1021, 1910.
52a. Miller, Y. E. Epithelial cell biology and airway disease. *Chest* 101:3S, 1992.
53. Minor, T. E., et al. Rhinovirus and influenza type A infections as precipitants of asthma. *Am. Rev. Respir. Dis.* 113:149, 1976.
54. Miura, M., et al. Increase in luminal mast cell and epithelial damage may account for increased airway responsiveness after viral infection in dogs. *Am. Rev. Respir. Dis.* 140:1738, 1989.
55. Naylor, B. The shedding of the mucosa of the bronchial tree in asthma. *Thorax* 17:69, 1962.
56. O'Byrne, P. M., et al. Lung epithelial permeability. Relation to non-specific airway responsiveness. *J. Appl. Physiol.* 57:77, 1984.
57. Ohtoshi, T., et al. Monocyte-macrophage differentiation induced by human upper airway epithelial cells. *Am. J. Respir. Cell Mol. Biol.* 4:255, 1991.
58. Persson, C. G. A. Role of plasma exudation in asthmatic airways. *Lancet* 2:1126, 1986.
59. Persson, C. G. A. Plasma exudation and asthma. Plus commentary. *Lung* 169:S133, 1991.
60. Persson, C. G. A. Plasma Exudation from Tracheobronchial Microvessels in Health and Disease. In J. Butler (ed.), *The Bronchial Circulation.* New York: Dekker, (in press).
61. Persson, C. G. A., et al. Review: plasma exudation as a first line respiratory mucosal defence. *Clin. Exp. Allergy* 21:17, 1991.
62. Persson, C. G. A., et al. Toluene diisocyanate produces an increase in airway tone that outlasts the inflammatory exudation phase. *Clin. Exp. Allergy* 21:715, 1991.
62a. Persson, C. G. A., et al. Editorial: the use of the nose to study the inflammatory response of the respiratory tract. *Thorax* (in press).
63. Piazza, F. M., et al. Attachment of influenza A virus to ferret tracheal epithelium at different maturational stages. *Am. J. Respir. Cell Mol. Biol.* 4:82, 1991.
64. Ramphal, R., et al. Murine influenzal tracheitis: a model for the study of influenza and tracheal epithelial repair. *Am. Rev. Respir. Dis.* 120:1313, 1979.
65. Reid, L., and Jones, R. Bronchial mucosal cells. *Fed. Proc.* 38:191, 1979.
66. Rickard, K. A., et al. Attachment characteristics of bovine bronchial epithelial cells to extracellular matrix components. *Am. J. Respir. Cell Mol. Biol.* 4:440, 1991.
67. Roche, W. R., et al. Subepithelial fibrosis in the bronchi of asthmatics. *Lancet* 1:520, 1989.
68. Ruoslahti, E., Engwall, E., and Hayman, E. H. Fibronectin: current concepts of the structures and functions. *Coll. Relat. Res.* 1:95, 1981.
69. Shoji, S., et al. Bronchial epithelial cells produce lung fibroblast chemotactic factor: fibronectin. *Am. J. Respir. Cell Mol. Biol.* 1:13, 1989.
70. Söderberg, M., et al. Bronchial epithelium in humans recently recovering from respiratory infections caused by influenza or mycoplasma. *Eur. Respir. J.* 3:1023, 1990.
71. Söderberg, M., et al. Structural characterization of bronchial mucosal biopsies from healthy volunteers: a light and electron microscopical study. *Eur. Respir. J.* 3:261, 1990.
71a. Sokolovsky, M. Endothelins and sarafotoxins: physiologic regulation, receptor, subtypes, and transmembrane signaling. *Pharmacol. Ther.* 54:129, 1992.
72. Stoner, G. D., et al. Cultured human bronchial epithelial cells: blood group antigens, keratin, collagens and fibronectin. *In Vitro* 17:577, 1981.
73. Summary and recommendations of a workshop on the investigative use of bronchoscopy and bronchoalveolar lavage in asthmatics. *J. Allergy Clin. Immunol.* (in press).
74. Svensson, C., et al. A topical glucocorticoid reduces the levels of fibrinogen and bradykinins on the allergic mucosa during natural pollen exposure. *J. Allergy Clin. Immunol.* 87:147, 1991.
75. Takizawa, H., et al. Separation of bovine bronchial epithelial cell subpopulations by density centrifugation: a method to isolate ciliated and nonciliated cell fractions. *Am. J. Respir. Cell Mol. Biol.* 3:553, 1990.
76. Van de Graaf, E. A., et al. Respiratory membrane permeability and bronchial hyperreactivity in patients with stable asthma. *Am. Rev. Respir. Dis.* 143:362, 1991.
77. White, S. R., et al. Epithelial modulation of airway smooth muscle response to endothelin-1. *Am. Rev. Respir. Dis.* 144:373, 1991.
78. Wiley, D. C., and Skehel, J. J. The structure and function of the hemagglutinin membrane glycoprotein of influenza virus. *Annu. Rev. Biochem.* 56:365, 1987.

Bronchoalveolar Lavage

Gianni Marone
Vincenzo Casolaro
Giuseppe Spadaro
Arturo Genovese

24

Bronchial asthma is an atopic disorder characterized by three hallmarks: (1) dysregulation of immunoglobulin E (IgE) synthesis; (2) increased "releasability" of primary effector cells of allergic reactions (peripheral blood basophils and tissue mast cells); and (3) nonspecific bronchial hyperresponsiveness to various immunologic and nonimmunologic stimuli [28].

A feature of asthma is chronic inflammation in the bronchial airways. The cellular profile of bronchial inflammation was originally yielded by several autopsy studies performed in patients dying of asthma [12, 16, 29]. Techniques are now available to study several aspects of airway inflammation in vivo. Flexible fiberoptic bronchoscopy is an improved and convenient technique for making an endobronchial diagnosis and for washing the lungs with a physiologic saline solution. The concept of endobronchial lavage was not new to the field of clinical allergy, as it was first used for therapeutic purposes in patients with severe bronchial asthma. The rationale was that it was a "last resort" measure for patients with refractory disease who were thought to have extensive impaction of viscid mucus in the terminal airways [1a, 6, 22].

Flexible fiberoptic bronchoscopy offers a new way of doing bronchoalveolar lavage (BAL) in patients with pulmonary diseases. Experience with this technique has led to significant improvements in the study of the immunologic pathogenesis of various lung disorders such as pulmonary fibrosis, allergic alveolitis, sarcoidosis, and the pneumonitis seen in patients with AIDS. The clinical and research experience gained from the study of these disorders has contributed to the rapid accumulation of information on inflammatory cells and the release of proinflammatory mediators in BAL fluid from patients with asthma. The BAL technique has given us a better understanding of the alterations of inflammatory cells and of mediator release in patients with different types (extrinsic and intrinsic) or degrees (mostly mild and asymptomatic) of bronchial asthma, both in baseline conditions and after bronchial challenge with specific allergens.

Because the BAL techniques used by different groups of investigators have varied somewhat, just sufficiently to explain some of the differences between reports, guidelines were published following a workshop at the National Institutes of Health on the investigative use of fiberoptic bronchoscopy and BAL in individuals with asthma [33]. These recommendations should be followed carefully by investigators in this field to better standardize their techniques and to make the results obtained from different studies comparable (see also Chap. 84).

Currently, fiberoptic bronchoscopy and BAL are safe and useful tools for research purposes in most patients with asymptomatic and mild asthma [42a]. Although appealing data are rapidly accumulating, it appears at this time that BAL and fiberoptic bronchial biopsy in patients with asthma have no practical application for diagnostic purposes.

INFLAMMATORY CELLS IN BAL FLUID OF ASTHMATICS

Initial studies have been performed over the last two decades to recover respiratory cells and other components of the airway-lining fluid from stable asthmatics who had been, in general, free of bronchospasm for at least one week [10, 21, 23, 40, 42]. A variety of lavage techniques were used and no severe complications were reported. These studies focused on the identification and counting of immune cells from BAL fluid in normal donors and asthmatics. Many studies converged on the identification of metachromatic cells in BAL fluid, based on the common belief that these cells are primary effector cells of atopic disorders [27, 28, 42]. More recently, however, attention has been paid to eosinophils, which are considered important inflammatory cells in the pathogenesis of bronchial asthma, starting with the association between eosinophilia and asthma that was observed soon after eosinophils were first described [17]. Metachromatic cells (basophils and mast cells) were first identified in BAL fluid by bright-field and dark-field microscopy (Fig. 24-1) [37].

Patterson and coworkers [37] also found that histamine-containing cells in BAL fluid release histamine after immunologic stimulation and amount to less than 1 percent of the total cells. In a subsequent study in normal donors and asthmatic patients, mast cells were observed only in asthmatic patients who also exhibited a higher percentage of eosinophils [23]. A significant increase in the percentages of mast cells and eosinophils in patients with stable bronchial asthma was found, whereas the percentages of alveolar macrophages, lymphocytes, and neutrophils were the same as those in controls [42]. Similar findings were reported by Flint and colleagues [18], who also evaluated the in vitro IgE-mediated response of BAL mast cells in patients with asthma and normal donors. They first reported that BAL mast cells from asthmatic patients were exquisitely sensitive to IgE cross-linking by anti-IgE, a finding confirmed by our group [8].

Eosinophils circulate in the blood and can migrate into inflamed tissues, where they play a role through the release of proinflammatory mediators such as major basic protein (MBP). There is compelling evidence that the percentage of eosinophils in the BAL fluid of asthmatics is higher than the percentage in normal donors [23, 24, 43]. Kirby and associates [24] found a significant correlation only between the number of metachromatic cells and the airway responsiveness to methacholine, but no correlation between methacholine PC_{20} (i.e., the concentration inducing a 20% decrease in peak expiratory flow rate) and lavage MBP levels. Another study found a significant increase in

Supported in part by grants from the CNR (Project FATMA: Subproject Prevention and Control of Disease Factors; Project No. 91.00081.PF41), the MURST, and "Ministero Sanità-Istituto Superiore di Sanità" AIDS Project 1990 (Rome, Italy).

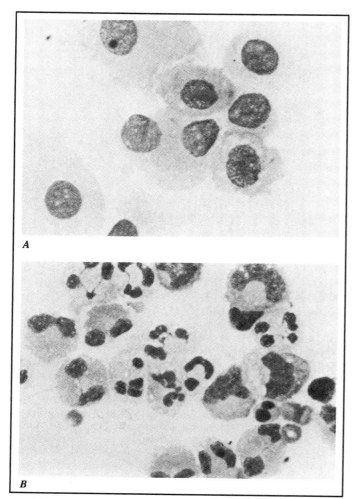

Fig. 24-1. *A. Light micrograph showing baseline (pre-local challenge) cellular content of bronchoalveolar lavage specimen from allergic asthmatic patient. Most of the cells are alveolar macrophages. Few neutrophils or eosinophils are present. B. Cells obtained from challenged subsegment of the same patient 48 hours after local instillation of antigen. In addition to alveolar macrophages, a large percentage of the cells are neutrophils and eosinophils. (Reprinted with permission from W. J. Metzger, et al. Methods for bronchoalveolar lavage in asthmatic patients following bronchoprovocation and local antigen challenge. Chest 87(Suppl.):165, 1985.)*

the percentage of mast cells in both symptomatic and asymptomatic asthmatics with mild disease [43]; in addition, there was a significant elevation in the eosinophil count and in the concentration of MBP in the BAL fluid of the symptomatic asthmatic patients. An inverse correlation between the methacholine PC_{20} and the percentages of mast cells, eosinophils, epithelial cells, and the amount of MBP in BAL fluid was also seen. These results suggest that bronchial hyperresponsiveness could be secondary to epithelial damage induced by eosinophil- and mast cell–derived granule products.

In a more recent study, the percentages of peripheral blood eosinophils and levels of eosinophil cationic protein (ECP) were correlated with the clinical severity of asthma and pulmonary function in patients with chronic asthma of different degrees of severity [4]. There was a significant increase in the number of peripheral blood eosinophils in asthmatic patients, which correlated with both the clinical severity and the alterations of pulmonary function. Eosinophils and ECP levels were increased in the BAL specimens from asthmatics and also correlated with the

severity of the disease. In the same study, intraepithelial eosinophils were found only in patients with asthma. Taken together, these data support the notion that eosinophilia and eosinophil activation are present in peripheral blood, BAL fluid, and bronchial biopsy specimens in patients with asthma, and are related to the severity of asthma.

Fiberoptic bronchoscopy biopsy specimens taken in asthmatics during remission showed that markers of inflammation are present in stable asthmatic patients [2] and even during clinical remission [19]. Using immunochemistry and monoclonal antibodies, the phenotypic composition and activation status of the cellular infiltrate in such biopsy specimens from asthmatic patients were examined. Mucosal biopsy material from central and subsegmental bronchi showed a significantly higher number of interleukin-2 receptor (CD25)–positive cells (a marker of lymphocyte activation) in the asthmatic group compared with the findings in controls [2]. These findings correlated with the increase in the percentage of tissue eosinophils. In addition, eosinophil infiltration in the submucosa can be found in patients with mild asthma even during remission [3, 19]. In these studies, the number of mast cells in the epithelium was also increased, whereas the number of mast cells in the submucosa was similar in both groups [19], as previously reported [3, 25]. These data confirm that bronchial inflammation is present and detectable both by BAL and bronchial biopsy in asthma even during prolonged clinical remission.

INFLAMMATORY MEDIATORS IN BAL FLUID OF ASTHMATICS

Another series of studies evaluated the presence of proinflammatory mediators in the BAL fluid of asthmatics in resting conditions or at different intervals after allergen challenge or both. Several studies looked at the release of proinflammatory mediators after endobronchial antigen challenge in patients with respiratory allergies, whereas only a few have documented the resting levels of mediators in the BAL fluid of asthmatics. Although a preliminary study reported that subjects with asthma had normal numbers of BAL mast cells and histamine levels [39], we and others have clearly demonstrated that the histamine levels in BAL specimens from asthmatics are higher than those in controls [8, 26, 43, 47]. The resting levels of histamine in the BAL fluid of controls ranged from 52 to 271 pg/ml versus 337 pg/ml in one study, and 2,400 pg/ml in another [8, 26, 43, 47]. In general, histamine levels in BAL fluid were four to 12 times higher in asthmatics than in normal subjects.

Prostaglandin D_2 (PGD_2) is the main arachidonic acid metabolite synthesized through the cyclooxygenase pathway by human mast cells [36] but not by basophils. BAL specimens from patients with mild asthma yielded significantly higher concentrations of PGD_2 than did those from controls [26, 47]. Levels of PGD_2 were approximately twelve times higher in asthmatics.

Thus, even in patients with mild asthma there is evidence of airway inflammation caused by some degree of activation of metachromatic cells, presumably mast cells, in BAL fluid. It also appears that the degree of activation in asthmatic patients is greater than that in normal subjects. To test this, we compared the releasability of peripheral blood basophils and BAL mast cells from normal and mild asthmatic donors. An altered releasability of human basophils and mast cells is an important parameter and, as mentioned, is one of the three hallmarks of atopic disorders [27, 28]. The histamine content of BAL mast cells (2.5 ± 0.3 pg/cell) was higher than that in peripheral blood basophils (1.3 ± 0.1 pg/cell), and the "spontaneous" releasability of BAL mast cells was higher than that of basophils in both asthmatic and normal donors.

We then studied histamine release from basophils and BAL mast cells challenged with various concentrations of anti-IgE, the formyl-containing tripeptide f-Met-Leu-Phe (FMLP), and the Ca^{++} ionophore A23187 to obtain complete dose-response curves for each donor. BAL mast cells from asthmatics were highly sensitive to anti-IgE, which, however, caused little release of histamine from the BAL mast cells of control subjects. The IgE-mediated releasability of BAL mast cells of asthmatics was increased at all concentrations of anti-IgE (Fig. 24-2). BAL mast cells were essentially unresponsive to FMLP, which caused histamine release from the peripheral blood basophils of normal donors and asthmatics. Interestingly, the releasability of basophils from mild asthmatic patients was very similar to that of control donors, presumably due to the mild activity of the disease. These results led us to conclude that BAL mast cell releasability may be increased in mild asthmatic patients even in the absence of increased basophil releasability, the latter occurring only in patients with more severe disease [7]. It thus appears that metachromatic cells in the BAL fluid of asthmatics possess some degree of activation that is probably responsible for the higher concentrations of histamine and PGD_2 found in the BAL specimens from asthmatic subjects.

Other investigators have focused their attention on the presence of proinflammatory mediators released by eosinophils in asthmatic BAL fluid. Activated eosinophils can release granule-derived proteins, the most cytotoxic of which are ECP [34] and MBP [20]. Significantly elevated MBP levels have been found in the BAL fluid of symptomatic asthmatic patients [43]. The ECP level was higher in BAL specimens from patients with asthma than that in controls, and the levels correlated with the severity of asthma [4]. These findings support the theory that eosinophils, through the release of cytotoxic mediators, play a role in the airway inflammation observed in asthma.

Different groups of investigators have set out to demonstrate the presence of other mediators in asthmatic BAL fluid; these include the peptide leukotrienes C_4 (LTC_4), D_4, and E_4 or platelet-activating factor (PAF). However, the results indicated that peptide leukotrienes and PAF were undetectable, under resting conditions, in BAL fluid from asthmatics using the analytical techniques so far available.

Fig. 24-2. *Histamine release included by anti–immunoglobulin E (0.1-3 μg/ml) in bronchoalveolar lavage mast cells from 17 normal donors (open circles) and 19 patients with asthma (closed circles). Values are mean ± standard error in the mean. (Redrawn from V. Casolaro, et al. Human basophil/mast cell releasability. V. Functional comparisons of cells obtained from peripheral blood, lung parenchyma, and bronchoalveolar lavage in asthmatics. Am. Rev. Respir. Dis. 139:1375, 1989.)*

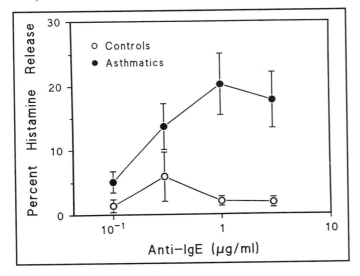

INFLAMMATORY CELLS AND MEDIATORS IN BAL SPECIMENS OF ASTHMATICS AFTER ANTIGEN CHALLENGE

Techniques are now available to evaluate various parameters in BAL fluid after antigen challenge in asthmatic patients. BAL can be performed in asthmatic patients after aerosol challenge with allergen, to which the patients have known skin test reactivity [13, 30]. Coughing is a common reaction, but no major complications have been reported. BAL was performed before and 10 minutes after inhalation challenge with plicatic acid in five patients with red cedar asthma [9]. The release of histamine and leukotriene B_4 into BAL fluid was significant in all patients after challenge.

The majority of investigators in this field used a different technique for collecting BAL specimens after *local airway challenge* with antigen. In this model, airway responsiveness to allergen in asthmatics is evaluated after local instillation of the specific allergen on subsegmental airways. The bronchoscopic instillation of allergen into the respiratory epithelium permits the direct assessment of the airway response to antigen and the collection of airway cells and fluid from non-allergen-exposed and allergen-exposed airways. In one study, BAL was performed in five patients with chronic stable asthma before and 9 minutes after local airway challenge with *Dermatophagoides pteronyssinus*. The lavage fluid was analyzed for products of arachidonic acid metabolism and exhibited a 150-fold increase in the PGD_2 levels after local instillation of the antigen [32].

This model of local airway challenge with antigen has been used to evaluate, in sequence, the alterations of inflammatory cells and the release of proinflammatory mediators. In asthmatics, the eosinophil and neutrophil BAL levels rose significantly 48 hours after local allergen challenge, as did helper T-lymphocytes [31]. At 96 hours, the neutrophil count returned to normal, but the numbers of eosinophils and helper T-cells remained elevated. Electron microscopy revealed degranulation of mast cells and eosinophils, both immediately and later (48 and 96 hours) after local antigen challenge. These results suggest that, when allergen is introduced into allergic asthmatic airways, there is an immediate local response and significant locally induced cellular inflammation, which can persist for at least 4 days [21a].

The sequence of inflammatory events after allergen inhalation challenge in asthmatic patients was recently described in detail. BAL specimen examined 6 hours after challenge showed a significant increase in the numbers of lymphocytes, neutrophils, and eosinophils, and a significant reduction in the percentage of mast cells [14]. The histamine concentrations in BAL fluid increased in the majority of patients. In the model of local airway challenge with antigen, there was a significant increase above baseline in the concentrations of histamine, PGD_2, and tryptase 5 minutes after challenge [44–46]. In one of these studies, the LTC_4 level was also increased in BAL fluid examined after allergen challenge [45].

To determine whether a link exists between the recruitment of inflammatory cells in the airways and the development of the late-phase asthmatic reaction to allergen (LAR), Rossi and co-workers [41] studied BAL fluid from asthmatic patients, either at baseline or 4, 24, and 72 hours after inhalation challenge. Both the number and percentage of BAL eosinophils were increased in patients with LAR 4 hours after allergen challenge and in patients without LAR 24 hours after allergen inhalation. The same group of investigators reported that allergen inhalation in mild asthmatics increases the number of mast cells in the bronchial mucosa, provided the allergic stimulus is sufficiently strong to trigger the LAR [11].

Several important questions arise from the recent observation

Table 24-1. Cellular and biochemical composition of bronchoalveolar lavage and bronchial wash fluid obtained by fiberoptic bronchoscopy in atopic asthmatics: comparison with nonasthmatic control subjects[a,b]

Type of lavage	Total cells (N)	Cell populations					Epithelial cells	Other findings in BAL fluid	Reference
		Macrophages	Mast cells	Eosinophils	Neutrophils	Lymphocytes			
BAL, five 20-ml aliquots	—	—	↑	↑	—	—	—	No difference in supernatant MBP	Kirby et al., 1987 [24]
BW, 20 ml	—	—	↑	↑	—	—	—		
BAL, three to five 50-ml aliquots	NA	NA	—	NA	NA	NA	NA	No difference in supernatant histamine and mast cell histamine content	Agius et al., 1985 [1]
BAL, 180 ml	—	NA	NA	NA	NA	↑ Total lympho- cytes ↑ T_8 lympho- cytes	NA	T_8 lymphocytes correlated with PC_{20}	Kelly et al., 1989 [23a]
BAL, three 60-ml aliquots	—	—	↑	↑	—	—	NA	↑ Histamine/mast cell ↑ Spontaneous histamine release	Flint et al., 1985 [18]
BW, 50 ml	—	—	NA	—	—	—	↑	Epithelial cell number correlated with PC_{20} histamine	Beasley et al., 1989 [3]
BAL, 180 to 240 ml	—	—	↑	↑	—	—	↑	↑ Histamine release in symptomatic and hyperreactive asthmatics	Wardlaw et al., 1988 [43]
BW, 20 ml	—	—	↑	↑	—	—	↑	No difference in histamine/mast cell ↑ Supernatant MBP	
BW, 20 ml	—	—	NA	↑	—	—	↑	↑ Supernatant LTE_4	Lam et al., 1987 [25a]
BAL, five 20-ml aliquots	—	—	↑	↑	—	—	NA	↑ Supernatant histamine	Casale et al., 1987 [6a]
BAL, two to eight 50-ml aliquots	—	↓	NA	↑	↑	↑	—		Godard et al., 1982 [21]

BAL = bronchoalveolar lavage; BW = bronchial wash; MBP = major basic protein; LTE_4 = leukotriene E_4; NA = not analyzed; ↑ = increased in asthmatics by comparison to normal subjects; ↓ = decreased in asthmatics by comparison to normal subjects.
[a] Includes patients with lung cancer and atopic nonasthmatics.
[b] Dashes indicate no significant difference.
Source: R. Djukanovic et al. Mucosal inflammation in asthma. *Am. Rev. Respir. Dis.* 142:434, 1990. Reprinted with permission.

that inflammatory changes (i.e., cellular infiltration and release of mediators) occur not only immediately but even several days after antigen challenge [37] and that markers of inflammation persist in BAL fluid and bronchial biopsy specimens from asthmatics even during clinical remission [19]. Furthermore, in some asthmatic patients sensitive to toluene-diisocyanate (TDI), BAL and biopsy of bronchial mucosa 3 to 39 months after they had stopped work showed increased numbers of eosinophils, epithelial damage, and thickening of the basement membrane [35]. These findings suggest that, even long after cessation of exposure, evidence of inflammatory reactions can persist in asthmatic subjects sensitized to TDI.

BAL has also been employed to study inflammatory cells and mediators in patients with exercise-induced asthma (EIA), or to assess the response to isocapnic hyperpnea (ISH) in asthma. Pre- and postexercise BAL fluid in atopic subjects with EIA showed no differences in histamine, tryptase, and PGD_2 levels [5]. ISH in asthmatics caused a significant increase in BAL concentrations of peptide leukotrienes, but not of histamine, and an increase in the number of eosinophils and epithelial cells [38]. Table 24-1 illustrates some cellular and biochemical constituents in BAL specimens of asthmatics.

During the last decades, fiberoptic bronchoscopy, BAL, and bronchial biopsy have entered the domain of research for the study of many aspects of bronchial asthma. BAL and bronchial biopsy in patients with stable asthma can be safely accomplished, but should be done under control conditions by experienced persons, including before and after allergen bronchoprovocation [15]. Significant information has been gained about the qualitative and quantitative evaluation of inflammatory cells and about the identification of inflammatory mediators in BAL fluid under resting conditions and at different intervals after antigen challenge. Some information has already been obtained, and certainly more will be yielded in the near future, on the ultrastructural and immunologic characteristics of inflammatory cells in different parts of the bronchial tree.

BAL, local allergen challenge, and bronchial biopsy offer enormous potential as investigative tools in the study of asthma, although they have no role as yet in the diagnosis and staging of the disease. These techniques are now being used to characterize the inflammatory changes during the immediate and late-phase responses of asthma. It is already evident that some of the discrepancies between the findings of different studies are related to the selection of asthmatic patients (e.g., atopic versus nonatopic, in remission, mild cases, and so on), and future studies should take this important aspect into account. These techniques have already greatly extended our understanding of the basic inflammatory aspects of asthma and will provide important insights into its pathogenetic mechanisms.

REFERENCES

1. Agius, R. M., Godfrey, R. C., and Holgate, S. T. Mast cell and histamine content of human bronchoalveolar lavage. *Thorax* 40:760, 1985.
1a. Ambiavagar, M., and Jones, E. S. Resuscitation of the moribund asthmatic. Use of intermittent positive pressure ventilation, bronchial lavage, and intravenous infusions. *Anaesthesia* 22:375, 1967.
2. Azzawi, M., et al. Identification of activated T lymphocytes and eosinophils in bronchial biopsies in stable atopic asthma. *Am. Rev. Respir. Dis.* 142:1407, 1990.
3. Beasley, R., et al. Cellular events in the bronchi in mild asthma and after bronchial provocation. *Am. Rev. Respir. Dis.* 139:806, 1989.
4. Bousquet, J., et al. Eosinophilic inflammation in asthma. *N. Engl. J. Med.* 323:1033, 1990.
5. Broide, D., et al. Airway levels of mast cell–derived mediators in exercise-induced asthma. *Am. Rev. Respir. Dis.* 141:563, 1990.
6. Broom, B., and Lond, M. B. Intermittent positive-pressure respiration and therapeutic bronchial lavage in intractable status asthmaticus. *Lancet* 1:899, 1960.
6a. Casale, T. B., et al. Elevated bronchoalveolar lavage fluid histamine levels in allergic asthmatics are associated with methacholine bronchial responsiveness. *J. Clin. Invest.* 79:1197, 1987.
7. Casolaro, V., Spadaro, G., and Marone, G. Human basophil releasability. VI. Changes in basophil releasability in patients with allergic rhinitis or bronchial asthma. *Am. Rev. Respir. Dis.* 142:1108, 1990.
8. Casolaro, V., et al. Human basophil/mast cell releasability. V. Functional comparisons of cells obtained from peripheral blood, lung parenchyma, and bronchoalveolar lavage in asthmatics. *Am. Rev. Respir. Dis.* 139:1375, 1989.
9. Chan-Yeung, M., et al. Histamine and leukotriene release in bronchoalveolar fluid during plicatic acid–induced bronchoconstriction. *J. Allergy Clin. Immunol.* 84:762, 1989.
10. Crimi, E., et al. Total and specific IgE in serum, bronchial lavage, and bronchoalveolar lavage of asthmatic patients. *Allergy* 38:553, 1983.
11. Crimi, E., et al. Increased numbers of mast cells in bronchial mucosa after the late-phase asthmatic response to allergen. *Am. Rev. Respir. Dis.* 144:1282, 1991.
12. Cutz, E., Levison, H., and Cooper, D. M. Ultrastructure of airways in children with asthma. *Histopathology* 2:407, 1978.
13. DeMonchy, J. G. R., et al. Bronchoalveolar eosinophilia following allergen-induced delayed asthmatic reactions. *Am. Rev. Respir. Dis.* 131:373, 1985.
14. Diaz, P., et al. Leukocytes and mediators in bronchoalveolar lavage during allergen-induced late-phase reactions. *Am. Rev. Respir. Dis.* 139:1383, 1989.
15. Djukanović, R., et al. The safety aspects of fiberoptic bronchoscopy, bronchoalveolar lavage, and endobronchial biopsy in asthma. *Am. Rev. Respir. Dis.* 143:772, 1991.
16. Dunnill, M. S. The pathology of asthma, with special references to changes in the bronchial mucosa. *J. Clin. Pathol.* 13:27, 1960.
17. Ellis, A. G. The pathological anatomy of bronchial asthma. *Am. J. Med. Sci.* 136:407, 1908.
18. Flint, K. C., et al. Bronchoalveolar mast cells in extrinsic asthma: a mechanism for the initiation of antigen specific bronchoconstriction. *Br. Med. J.* 291:923, 1985.
19. Foresi, A., et al. Inflammatory markers in bronchoalveolar lavage and in bronchial biopsy in asthma during remission. *Chest* 98:528, 1990.
20. Gleich, G. J., et al. Comparative properties of the Charcot-Leyden crystal protein and the major basic protein from human eosinophils. *J. Clin. Invest.* 57:633, 1976.
21. Godard, P., et al. Functional assessment of alveolar macrophages: comparison of cells from asthmatic and normal subjects. *J. Allergy Clin. Immunol.* 70:88, 1982.
21a. Gratziou, C. A., et al. Early changes in T lymphocytes recovered by bronchoalveolar lavage after local allergen challenge of asthmatic airways. *Am. Rev. Respir. Dis.* 145:1259, 1992.
22. Helm, W. H., Barran, K. M., and Mukerjee, S. C. Bronchial lavage in asthma and bronchitis. *Ann. Allergy* 30:518, 1972.
23. Joseph, M., et al. Involvement of IgE in the secretory processes of alveolar macrophages from asthmatic patients. *J. Clin. Invest.* 71:221, 1983.
23a. Kelly, C. A., et al. Lymphocyte subsets in bronchoalveolar lavage fluid obtained from stable asthmatics and their correlations with bronchial responsiveness. *Clin. Exp. Allergy* 19:169, 1989.
24. Kirby, J. G., et al. Bronchoalveolar cell profiles of asthmatic and nonasthmatic subjects. *Am. Rev. Respir. Dis.* 136:379, 1987.
25. Laitinen, L. A., and Laitinen, A. Mucosal inflammation and bronchial hyperreactivity. *Eur. Respir. J.* 10:488, 1988.
25a. Lam, S., LeRiche, J., Phillips, D., and Chan-Yeung, M. Cellular and protein changes in bronchial lavage fluid after late asthmatic reaction in patients with red cedar asthma. *J. Allergy Clin. Immunol.* 80:44, 1987.
26. Liu, M. C., et al. Evidence of elevated levels of histamine, prostaglandin D_2, and other bronchoconstricting prostaglandins in the airways of subjects with mild asthma. *Am. Rev. Respir. Dis.* 142:126, 1990.
27. Marone, G., et al. Pathophysiology of human basophils and mast cells in allergic disorders. *Clin. Immunol. Immunopathol.* 50:S24, 1989.
28. Marone, G., et al. Releasability in Allergic Disorders. In G. Melillo, P. S. Norman, and G. Marone (eds.), *Respiratory Allergy. Clinical Immunology*, Vol. 2. Toronto: Decker, 1990, P. 67.
29. Messer, J. W., Peters, G. A., and Bennet, W. A. Causes of death and pathologic findings in 304 cases of bronchial asthma. *Dis. Chest* 38:616, 1960.
30. Metzger, W. J., et al. Methods for bronchoalveolar lavage in asthmatic patients following bronchoprovocation and local antigen challenge. *Chest* 87(Suppl.):165, 1985.
31. Metzger, W. J., et al. Local allergen challenge and bronchoalveolar lavage of allergic asthmatic lungs. *Am. Rev. Respir. Dis.* 135:433, 1987.
32. Murray, J. J., et al. Release of prostaglandin D_2 into human airways during acute antigen challenge. *N. Engl. J. Med.* 315:800, 1986.
33. National Institutes of Health Workshop Summary. Summary and recommendations of a workshop on the investigative use of fiberoptic bronchoscopy and bronchoalveolar lavage in individuals with asthma. *J. Allergy Clin. Immunol.* 76:145, 1986.
34. Ollson, I., et al. Arginine-rich cationic proteins of human eosinophil granules: comparison of the constituents of eosinophilic and neutrophilic leukocytes. *Lab. Invest.* 36:493, 1977.
35. Paggiaro, P., et al. Bronchoalveolar lavage and morphology of the airways after cessation of exposure in asthmatic subjects sensitized to toluene diisocyanate. *Chest* 98:536, 1990.
36. Patella, V., et al. Protein L: a bacterial Ig-binding protein that activates human basophils and mast cells. *J. Immunol.* 145:3054, 1990.
37. Patterson, R., et al. Living histamine-containing cells from the bronchial lumens of humans. *J. Clin. Invest.* 59:217, 1977.
38. Pliss, L. B., et al. Assessment of bronchoalveolar cell and mediator response to isocapnic hyperpnea in asthma. *Am. Rev. Respir. Dis.* 142:73, 1990.
39. Rankin, J. A., Kaliner, M., and Reynolds, H. Y. Histamine levels in bronchoalveolar lavage from patients with asthma, sarcoidosis, and idiopathic pulmonary fibrosis. *J. Allergy Clin. Immunol.* 79:371, 1987.
40. Rankin, J., et al. Bronchoalveolar lavage. Its safety in subjects with mild asthma. *Chest* 85:723, 1984.
41. Rossi, G. A., et al. Late-phase asthmatic reaction to inhaled allergen is associated with early recruitment of eosinophils in the airways. *Am. Rev. Respir. Dis.* 144:379, 1991.
42. Tomioka, M., et al. Mast cells in bronchoalveolar lumen of patients with bronchial asthma. *Am. Rev. Respir. Dis.* 129:1000, 1984.
42a. Vyve, T., et al. Safety of bronchoalveolar lavage and bronchial biopsies in patients with asthma of variable severity. *Am. Rev. Respir. Dis.* 146:116, 1992.
43. Wardlaw, A. J., et al. Eosinophils and mast cells in bronchoalveolar lavage in subjects with mild asthma. *Am. Rev. Respir. Dis.* 137:62, 1988.
44. Wenzel, S. E., Fowler, A. A., and Schwartz, L. B. Activation of pulmonary mast cells by bronchoalveolar allergen challenge. *Am. Rev. Respir. Dis.* 137:1002, 1988.
45. Wenzel, S. E., Westcott, J. Y., and Larsen, G. L. Bronchoalveolar lavage fluid mediator levels 5 minutes after allergen challenge in atopic subjects with asthma: relationship to the development of late asthmatic responses. *J. Allergy Clin. Immunol.* 87:540, 1991.
46. Wenzel, S. E., et al. Spectrum of prostanoid release after bronchoalveolar allergen challenge in atopic asthmatics and in control groups. *Am. Rev. Respir. Dis.* 139:450, 1989.
47. Zehr, B. B., et al. Use of segmental airway lavage to obtain relevant mediators from the lungs of asthmatics and control subjects. *Chest* 95:1059, 1989.

Airway Smooth Muscle: Physiology, Bronchomotor Tone, Pharmacology, and Relation to Asthma

25

Newman L. Stephens
Chun Y. Seow

Undoubtedly the greatest impetus to research in elucidating the fundamental biophysics and biochemistry of airway smooth muscle (ASM) has been provided by the need to understand how these are altered in asthma. Many of the biophysical and biochemical properties of this muscle have been reviewed before [72, 92, 93, 95, 96, 98]. They resemble those of striated muscle. However, while mechanical properties are very similar, there are differences in biochemistry. For example, in smooth muscle, calcium-sensitive regulation of contraction is not mediated by the familiar troponin-tropomyosin system but by a calmodulin/myosin-light-chain kinase/phosphatase system [2, 23, 36, 71]. Thus the molecular mechanisms to be investigated in understanding disorders of smooth muscle relaxation, which occur in allergic bronchospasm [91] for example, may be quite different from those in striated muscle.

Much of the following material is based on studies of canine tracheal smooth muscle (TSM), since there is evidence [52] that it serves as a model—at least with respect to contractility—for ASM down to the sixth generation of airways. Studies of isolated smooth muscle from smaller airways [84] are few and are based mainly on studies of lung strips [68]. We have recently developed a bronchial smooth muscle preparation (fifth generation) that allows the precise study of those airways that are involved in allergic bronchospasm [114].

Considerable work has been carried out on ASM from a variety of animal models of asthma (see Chap. 31). Incidentally, it should be pointed out that none of these reproduces the human disease exactly, which should really be identified as an example of nonspecific hyperreactivity. Be that as it may, the nonspecificity found in human patients in vivo and in animals [40, 79] suggests that the primary cause of asthma may reside at the muscle cell level. Whether it is the cell membrane, the excitation-contraction coupling apparatus, or the contractile machinery that is primarily involved is not known.

The general approach for what follows will be to discuss fundamentals first and then the pathophysiology of asthma. The electric properties of ASM will not be exhaustively dealt with; however, they will be mentioned in discussing the conversion of multiunit properties of ASM to single-unit properties, a process felt to be important in the pathogenesis of allergic bronchoconstriction [49].

MECHANICAL PROPERTIES OF AIRWAY SMOOTH MUSCLE

Length-Tension Relationships: Reduced Activation at Shorter Muscle Lengths

Length-Tension Curves

Isometric studies of force (or tension) and length provide information about the ability of the muscle to stiffen and support loads and about muscle elasticity. Length-tension curves obtained by supramaximal electrical stimulation of isolated isometric canine tracheal smooth muscle strips are shown in Figure 25-1. The resting tension curve shows the shape expected of complex biologic tissues; it results from the presence of collagen and elastin [82]. Since smooth muscles generally possess a variable degree of resting tone, passive length-tension curves are obtained after treatment with appropriate pharmacologic relaxants or metabolic inhibitors of energy production. Canine TSM demonstrates stress-relaxation; its magnitude is a direct function of length change and the period of time the muscle is held isometric at high tensions. Length change in excess of 25 percent of the initial length results in stress-relaxation. Because of stress-relaxation, length-tension curves show hysteresis; repeated cycling of tissue length narrows the loop.

Figure 25-1 also shows total and active tension curves. Active tension is the important one to consider, since it provides insight into the working of the contractile element of the muscle. The curve shows a maximum at a unique length which is defined as optimal length (l_o). In skeletal muscle l_o has the additional quality of representing the muscle's in vivo length. It has recently been determined that this is so for the TSM [70]. The maximum active tension (P_o) elicited is 1.10 kg/cm^2 (1.10 $\times$ 10^5 N/M^2) + 0.059 (S.E.). This value of P_o is obtained when the bathing medium is at 37°C and has a 2 mM calcium concentration; when the latter is raised to 4.75 mM, P_o increases to 1.980 kg/cm$_2$ + 0.123 (S.E.), which represents an 80 percent increment [101]. When the concentration is raised to beyond 4.75 mM, P_o decreases presumably because of the stabilization of the muscle cell membrane. Both smooth [93] and heart [54] muscle differ from skeletal muscle in which there is no increase of P_o (at l_o) with Ca^{++} concentration above 2 mM. The TSM data confirm Murphy's observation [2] that smooth muscle cross-bridges develop the same force as those of skeletal. Since the former muscle possesses only one-fifth the myosin of the latter, this performance is remarkable.

Another noteworthy feature is the ability of the TSM to "supercontract," i.e., to shorten much more than skeletal muscle, which can only shorten to 65 percent of l_o; the TSM shortens to 10 percent of l_o. The mechanism enabling this is unknown; nor is it easy to see what is its in vivo significance. Macklem (personal communication, 1991) has speculated that the capacity for supercontraction raises the question as to why severe asthmalike bronchoconstriction does not occur normally. He suggests that shortening is abbreviated by the activation of a nonadrenergic, noncholinergic inhibitory nervous system. We believe that it is the phenomenon of reduced activation of the muscle at short lengths ($l<l_o$), discussed below, that is responsible. Another concept put forward by Macklem (personal communication, 1991) is that alteration in the elastic recoil forces that the lung parenchyma exerts on the airways is responsible for allergic bronchospasm.

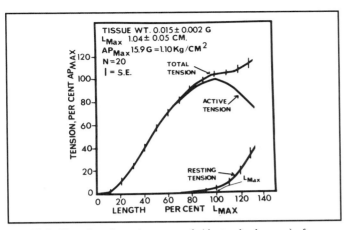

Fig. 25-1. *Mean length-tension curves (with standard errors) of tracheal smooth muscle. Note: full curve not shown. (Reprinted with permission from N. L. Stephens, et al., Force-velocity characteristics of respiratory airway smooth muscle. J. Appl. Physiol. 26:685, 1969.)*

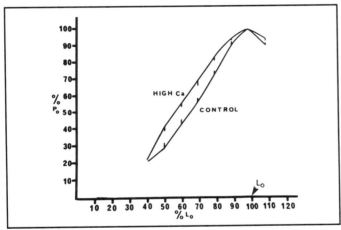

Fig. 25-2. *Mean length-tension curves for tracheal smooth muscle. Length and tension are expressed as percentages of L_o and P_o, respectively. Standard errors are shown. Calcium concentration for the upper curve is 4.75 mM and for the lower control is 2.0 mM. (Reprinted with permission from N. L. Stephens, et al., Nature of Contractile Unit: Shortening Inactivation, Maximum Force Potential, Relaxation, Contractility. In N. L. Stephens (ed.), Smooth Muscle Contraction. New York: Marcel Dekker, 1984. Courtesy of Marcel Dekker, Inc.)*

In length-tension curves, the maximum isometric tetanic tension developed at any length is influenced by the history of the contraction. We have reported [102] that isometric active tension curves differ from those derived from freeloaded or afterloaded contractions. At any given length, the tension developed by muscles that contracted is always less than that of muscles in which no shortening occurred.

Reduced Activation at Short Lengths

Taylor [83, 108] has observed that at $l < l_o$ there is reduced mechanical activation in single skeletal muscle fibers. Jewell [54] has reported that the same phenomenon exists in cat heart whole papillary muscle. Siegman (personal communication, 1986) has obtained similar findings for smooth muscle. Figure 25-2 shows two active tension (P) versus length (*l*) curves. Length and tension are expressed as percentages of l_o and P_o, respectively. The curve to the right was obtained from muscles incubating in a

bathing medium containing 2 mM Ca^{++} at 37°C. The curve to the left was elicited from a muscle incubating in medium containing 4.75 mM Ca^{++}. The shift to the left indicates that at lengths between 40 percent l_o and 85 percent l_o the muscle was not maximally activated. The mechanism underlying this phenomenon in smooth muscle is not known but it suggests that the muscle could be mechanically unstable at these lengths. Another speculation is that as the smooth muscle shortens—for example, during expiration—the airway undergoes critical closure. The associated reduction in activation would minimize this.

Force-Velocity Relationships at Loads Less than P_o

Length-tension curves are of limited value since they only deal with static conditions. They do not enable one to assess the power production of the muscle. For this, force-velocity curves are needed. A mean force-velocity curve, derived from records of isotonic afterloaded shortening in TSM, is shown in Figure 25-3 [27]. It is fitted by Hill's equation [43]:

$$(P + a)(v + b) = (P_o + a)b$$

where v is the maximum velocity for a given load; a is a constant with units of force and is an index of numbers of force-generating sites in the muscle's cross-section; and b has units of velocity and is an index of the rate of energy liberation or of actomyosin ATPase activity. These constants can be calculated from the slope ($1/b$) and intercept (a/b) of a plot of $(P_o - P)/V$ versus P (*dashed line* in Figure 25-3), which is a linearizing transform of Hill's equation. There is doubt as to the usefulness of this equation because the a constant appears to be load dependent. However, Woledge [113] has shown that for smooth muscle a is a true constant. The final constant obtained from the data is V_{max}, which is the velocity of shortening at a hypothetical zero load. V_{max} is obtained from the equation $P_o b/a$. The curve shows that P_o is not too dissimilar from that of skeletal muscle; however, V_{max} is almost a hundred times slower.

Changes in V_{max} in a given muscle suggest changes in actomyosin ATPase activity. Antonissen and associates [6] have shown that V_{max} is increased in TSM from a canine model of allergic

Fig. 25-3. *Mean force-velocity curve of tracheal smooth muscle. Standard error bars shown. All experiments conducted at l_o. (Reprinted with permission from N. L. Stephens, et al., Force-velocity characteristics of respiratory airway smooth muscle. J. Appl. Physiol. 26:685, 1969.)*

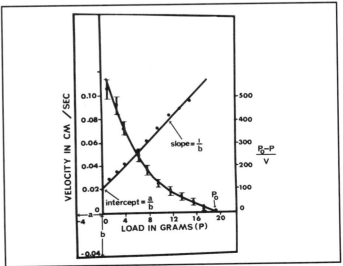

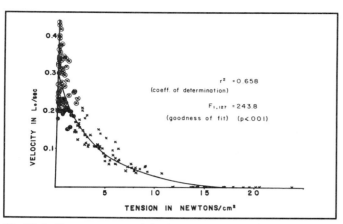

Fig. 25-4. *The mean curve of the force-velocity relationships with all the raw data points. Both afterloaded (loads greater than the preload, denoted by x's) and load-clamped (to loads less than preload and including zero-load clamps, denoted by open circles) data points are plotted. Both afterloaded and load-clamped sets of data fall on the same curve.*

Table 25-1. Constants from Hill's force-velocity relationship

	Afterloaded	Pooled, afterloaded, and load-clamped
a (N/cm^2)	3.563 ± .390	3.971 ± .295
b (l_o/sec)	.073 ± .010	.075 ± .009
a/P$_o$	.225 ± .031	.241 ± .023
V$_{max}$ (l_o/sec)	.328 ± .021	.313 ± .020
V$_o$ (l_o/sec) (zero load-clamp)	—	.301 ± .022
	P$_o$ = 16.869 ± .849 N/cm^2	
	n = 15	

Note: These constants were determined by afterloading force-velocity points and by using afterloaded data points as well as the load-clamped (to loads less than preload) data pooled together for each TSM. No significant differences could be determined by paired, two-tailed *t*-tests between any of the constants.

bronchospasm. This is important because it suggests that the underlying alteration is in the ATPase and points the way to biochemical research.

It must be pointed out that estimation of V$_{max}$ involves mathematic or graphic extrapolation. Brutsaert and colleagues [17] have suggested such extrapolations could be inaccurate and have devised a method for directly measuring velocity at zero load by applying an abrupt zero load clamp. In this way, velocity points have been obtained between zero load and the preload that was needed to set the muscle at its l_o. Using a muscle lever built by Brutsaert for us, we have obtained velocity data points for this range of loads as shown in Figure 25-4. Analysis of the data shown in Table 25-1 demonstrates the V$_{max}$ obtained by analysis of the conventional afterloaded data or of the entire set of afterloaded and load-clamped data, or by direct measurement (zero load), is the same. From these results, two useful conclusions follow—that the conventional analysis of afterloaded isotonic shortening curves is valid for TSM, and that V$_{max}$ can be accurately obtained by a single (zero load clamp) measurement.

The conventional analysis of force-velocity curves yields erroneous results for high load values because the bridges responsible for force development seem different from those responsible for the velocity of shortening. While the values of velocity at low loads are accurate, those at high loads are not. This problem is resolved by measuring force-velocity curves for the two types of

bridges separately. This is facilitated by using so-called abrupt load-clamping techniques.

Normally Cycling and Latch (or Slowly Cycling) Bridges

Recent discoveries by Murphy's group [23] have shown that the skeletal muscle approach cannot be applied when analyzing the mechanical properties of smooth muscle, because of the differences in cross-bridges for the two types of muscles. Two types of bridges are recruited sequentially in smooth muscle. Those activated first manifest maximum cycling activity and are called *normally cycling cross-bridges*. They are activated by phosphorylation of the 20,000-dalton myosin light chain. This phosphorylation enables actin activation of myosin ATPase activity. Calcium-calmodulin activation of myosin-light-chain kinase is responsible for the phosphorylation. The normally cycling cross-bridges are soon replaced by very slowly cycling bridges that consume about one-quarter the energy of the former. They have been termed *latch bridges* and reduce the muscle's velocity by retarding the normally cycling cross-bridges. However, this notion is disputed and some believe what is really happening is that the normally cycling cross-bridges slow progressively with time and latch bridges do not develop. According to this view, these bridges should be termed *slowly cycling cross-bridges* [20]. Results of studies of the energetics of smooth muscle contraction by our group support the notion.

We have shown that normally cycling cross-bridges and latch bridges also exist in canine [97] and murine [115] TSM and in the canine coronary artery [110] and saphenous vein [111].

These cross-bridges are recognized by their unloaded shortening velocities. Figure 25-5 shows the results from the application of so-called zero-load clamps to a tracheal muscle shortening isotonically under a load just sufficient to stretch it to its l_o. The loads were applied at 0.5-second intervals using a special electronic muscle lever system devised by Brutsaert and colleagues [17]. The response shown in the figure consists of a rapid transient resulting from elastic recoil of the series elastic component followed by a slow transient due to shortening of the contractile element. The maximum slope of this component is represented by V$_o$. Scrutiny of the slow transients demonstrates a progressive decline in V$_o$.

Fig. 25-5. *Plot of isotonic shortening versus time in an electrically stimulated canine tracheal smooth muscle. The muscle shortens from 1.0 to approximately 0.65 l/l$_o$, as depicted by the heavy sigmoidal curve. During similar subsequent isotonic contractions, zero loads were always abruptly applied at 0.5-sec intervals. The rapid transients for these releases represent the recoil of the series elastic component. The maximum slopes of the succeeding slow transients represent the maximum velocity of shortening (V$_o$).*

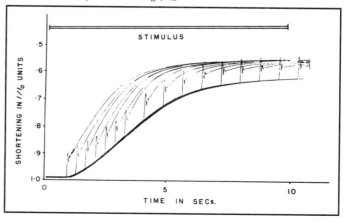

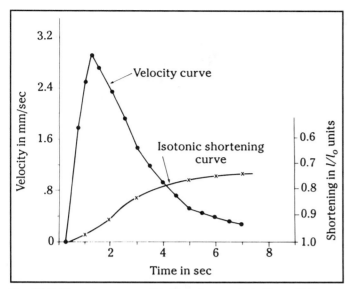

Fig. 25-6. *The instantaneous V_o's from the records in Figure 25-5 are plotted as a function of time. The isotonic shortening curve is also reproduced.*

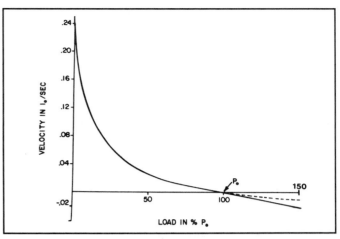

Fig. 25-7. *Mean force-velocity curves elicited during shortening and elongation of activated tracheal smooth muscle. The broken curve is an estimated one. (Reprinted with permission from B. S. R. Hanks and N. L. Stephens, Mechanics and energetics of lengthening of active airway smooth muscle. Am. J. Physiol. 241:C42, 1981.)*

Figure 25-6 shows a plot of the V_o's versus time. The isotonic shortening curve is also displayed. V_o rises to a maximum at 1.75 seconds. The ascending part of the curve results from the progressive increase in the muscle's active state and the peak denotes normally cycling cross-bridge activity. Thereafter the V_o's drop to a very low level at 7 seconds. The low V_o is due to latch-bridge activity.

These data confirm that normally cycling and latch bridges are also present in ASM. Analysis has also shown that, in the normally preloaded muscle, 75 percent of the isotonic shortening is due to normally cycling cross-bridge activity and that most of the maximum isometric force developed is due to latch-bridge activity. Speculatively, it almost appears that smooth muscle has developed discrete, dedicated cross-bridges—at least in a functional sense—to its two major activities of shortening and stiffening. The implications are fairly important because they indicate that, in asthma for example, in order to elucidate the mechanism of bronchoconstriction it is the normally cycling cross-bridges that must be studied, i.e., studies must be conducted within the first 2 to 3 seconds of isotonic contraction.

Force-Velocity Relationships at Loads Greater than P_o

While considerable effort has gone into the study of shortening muscle, very little has gone into the study of muscle that is being forcibly elongated while activated. Yet antagonist skeletal muscles are precisely in this situation every time an agonist shortens. Since it is possible a similar situation could be obtained for ASM, we investigated the relation between force and velocity in a muscle forcibly elongated by applying a series of loads greater than P_o. Conventional quick-release methods using loads below and above P_o were employed. The force-velocity curve obtained is shown in Figure 25-7. Loads greater than 150 percent P_o could not be elicited since the length changes were too great to permit measurement of maximum velocity of shortening at a constant starting length (l_o).

The *broken line* represents the predicted curve for elongation; it was obtained by using the constants obtained from the $P<P_o$ part of the curve. The *solid line* depicts the experimentally measured curve. These curves are significantly different ($p<.05$). The

curve for $P > P_o$ resembles that reported by Johansson and associates (personal communication, 1983) for urinary bladder.

Analysis of the curve shows interestingly that at a lengthening velocity of 0.03 l_o/sec (this is shown as a negative velocity) the smooth muscle can support a load of 150 percent P_o. However, at a similar velocity during shortening, it can only support a load of 50 percent P_o. This testifies to the surprisingly considerable strength of the elongating muscle. Our biochemical studies have also demonstrated that the elongating muscle consumes considerably less energy than the shortening muscle at equivalent velocities [39].

The physiologic significance of this finding can only be speculated upon. It is possible that tonically contracted ASM in vivo may be forcibly elongated during an inspiration. This does not produce the mechanical instabilities expected because of the operation of the process mentioned in the preceding paragraph. The phenomenon may also be recruited if relaxation is not synchronous among the contractile units in series, those cells that are less strongly activated being forcibly lengthened by those that are more strongly activated.

The Series Elastic Component

Mechanical records of smooth muscle contraction indicate that its series elastic component (SEC) is longer (or more compliant) than that of striated muscle. We have published the properties of the SEC of TSM [100]. The studies showed that when the isometric muscle developed a force equal to P_o, the internal elongation of the SEC was 7.5 percent l_o. Similar values have been reported for vascular smooth muscle [55], but on the whole larger values are seen in the majority of smooth muscles. Alterations in these properties in hypoxia [62, 94] were correlated with changes in P_o, suggesting that the SEC resides in active components, most likely the cross-bridges.

The Parallel Elastic Component

The Internal Resistance to Shortening

This will be dealt with later when studies are described to determine the mechanism for the increased shortening of sensitized ASM.

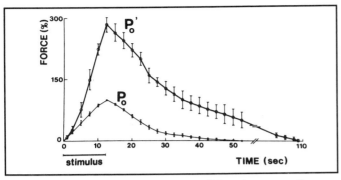

Fig. 25-8. *Maximum force potential curve (P'_o) and corresponding isometric myogram (P_o) for canine tracheal smooth muscle. Means and standard errors are shown. Muscle length for all experiments was set at l_o. N = 18. Note 100 percent on the time axis is 13 sec. (Reprinted with permission from N. L. Stephens and D. L. Brutsaert, Maximum force potential of tetanized mammalian smooth muscle. Am. J. Physiol. 242:C283, 1982.)*

Maximum Force Potential (Active State)

Brutsaert and Housmans [18] have coined the term *maximum force potential* to describe the maximum load-bearing capacity of a muscle contracting isometrically. In essence it is similar to the active state curve of striated muscle described by Jewell and Wilkie [53]. The load-clamp method of eliciting the maximum force potential curve is superior to the quick-stretch or quick-release methods generally employed, since in these the length of the SEC is constantly changing, thus obscuring the mechanical behavior of the contractile element. The advantage of the abrupt load-clamp technique is that the length of the SEC is held constant during contractile element activity.

Maximum force potential curves are shown in Figure 25-8. The curve designated P_o is the mean isometric tetanic, active tension curve. The P'_o curve is the maximum force potential curve obtained with the abrupt load clamp. It has a slow onset and a time course similar to that of the tetanus itself. The P'_o/P_o ratio is 2:86, which is much higher than that of skeletal [42] and of cardiac [54] muscle and suggests very strong cross-bridges. Another interesting fact is that while the P_o curve returns to zero at about 52 seconds, the P'_o curve does so at about 104 seconds. Work done by Siegman and associates [87] and by Dillon and coworkers [23] indicates that cross-bridges maintaining tension in the latter half of all isometric tetani are of a noncycling, nonenergy (or low-energy)–requiring type. These have been termed *latch bridges* by analogy to the catch bridges of molluscan muscle. It is very likely that similar latch bridges are present in tracheal smooth muscle also. Our data suggest that these latch bridges are made at a speed at least twice as slow as regular cycling smooth-muscle bridges; and that even though the muscle appears to be at rest at least as judged by the tetanic curve, its cross-bridges are not in a normal resting state.

Contractility

Contractility has been most rigorously defined by Brutsaert and colleagues [17] for heart muscle as the instantaneous relationship between force, velocity, length, and time. The last-mentioned variable is particularly important because of the fact that normally heart muscle only undergoes twitch contractions and hence the intensity of the ability to develop force or to shorten wanes rapidly. Alternatively, this is expressed by saying that the intensity of the active state wanes. The mechanism responsible is that with cessation of muscle activation by the electric stimulus, energy-liberating biochemical reactions rapidly decrease. This

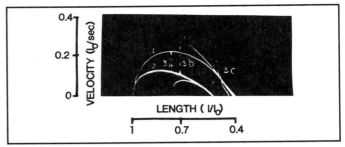

Fig. 25-9. *Length-velocity phase planes for three contractions elicited from canine tracheal smooth muscle.*

of course influences the relation between force and velocity in the shortening muscle. In skeletal and smooth muscle, tetanization ensures that these reactions are held at a steady maximum. Hence at constant muscle length the relation between force and velocity adequately serves as an index of contractility. However, since the manner and timing of load application to a shortening muscle may reduce the active state's intensity, it becomes necessary to demonstrate the force-velocity-length-time relationship in these muscles also. Brutsaert and coworkers [17] have studied these relationships using the abrupt load-clamp technique. They showed that the force-velocity-length relationship was unchanged for most of the duration of muscle shortening and for about 15 percent of the extent of shortening of the muscle.

Figure 25-9 depicts length-velocity phase planes for electrically stimulated TSM. In curves 1 and 2 the muscle is shortening with loads of 8 mN and 28 mN, respectively. In curve 3a the load was abruptly (within 3 msec) changed from 8 to 28 mN midway through shortening. After the initial artifact it is clear that the muscle follows the 28 mN phase plane exactly. Toward the end of shortening the load was changed back to 8 mN. The shortening now follows the 8 mN curve. In 3b the load was clamped from 8 to 28 mN very early in the shortening (not visible in figure). At about 0.5 l_o, load was changed back to 8 mN. Coincidence of the curves, after the overshoot, is clearly seen. In 3c where load is changed from 8 to 28 mN again very early in shortening, coincidence of trajectories is seen. At 0.7 l_o load was changed back to 8 mN, but this time the appropriate phase plane was not regained and an undershoot is in evidence.

The upper section of Figure 25-10 shows phase planes for a TSM contracting from different initial lengths. Schematics of these tracings are shown below. The different lengths are set by applying varying preloads. The records show that the maximum velocity of shortening at the different loads is different also. However, comparisons are not valid since not only the initial length but also the initial loads are different. When zero load-clamp velocities are applied at each length (set by preloads ranging from 1 to 16 mN), it is evident that the trajectories coincide. It is only at 1.3 l_o (set by a preload of 3 mN) that maximum velocities decrease. These data show that the length-velocity phase planes are the same for muscle lengths ranging from 0.75 to 1.0 l_o.

These experiments confirm that a steady state of contractility does exist for tracheal smooth muscle also. This extends for most of the duration of shortening and for about 30 percent of the extent of shortening from l_o.

Relaxation

Relaxation in smooth muscle has not received the attention it deserves. For example, Shibata has found (personal communication) in caudal artery strips from spontaneously hypertensive rats that, while P_o is unaffected, relaxation time is considerably prolonged. This is of obvious importance in the pathogenesis of hypertension.

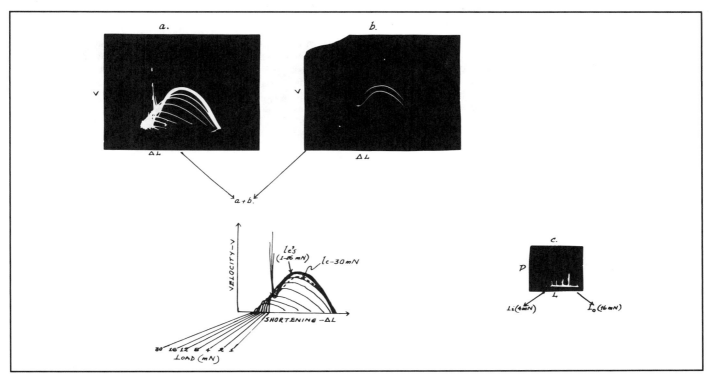

Fig. 25-10. *The upper section shows oscilloscopic records of length-velocity phase planes for a tracheal smooth muscle contracting from different initial lengths. Schematics of these tracings are shown below.*

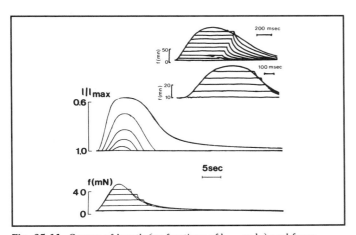

Fig. 25-11. *Curves of length (as fractions of l_{max} or l_o) and force versus time during conventional afterloaded isotonic contractions taken from a single experiment on canine tracheal smooth muscle. The inset shows similar force versus time curves for cat heart papillary muscle (above) and for ventricular muscle (below). (Reprinted with permission from N. L. Stephens, et al., Nature of Contractile Unit: Shortening Inactivation, Maximum Force Potential, Relaxation, Contractility. In N. L. Stephens (ed.), Smooth Muscle Contraction. New York: Marcel Dekker, 1984. Courtesy of Marcel Dekker, Inc.)*

Shortening and force data obtained from afterloaded isotonic force-velocity experiments enable us to analyze the relaxation process. Figure 25-11 shows that initially isotonic relaxation occurs; when the muscle has returned to its starting length, isometric relaxation follows. The latter phase seems to consist of two components—an initial fast one and a following slow one. The upper panel in the inset to Figure 25-11 shows curves for twitching cat heart papillary muscle. Relaxation pathways for the different loads differ from each other and from that of the isometric

contraction (the uppermost). Brutsaert feels that this type of relaxation is seen in muscles with a well-developed and efficient calcium-resequestrating apparatus, by which the muscle's active state is terminated rapidly and the time course of relaxation is then dictated by the load. He has termed this *load-dependent relaxation*. The lower panel represents similar curves but for frog ventricular muscle whose relaxation pathways are all almost identical. This has been ascribed to a poor calcium-resequestrating apparatus. Relaxation is load independent and depends on termination of the active state. This has been termed *inactivation-dependent relaxation*.

The rest of the figure shows curves from TSM. It is evident that relaxation is of the inactivation-dependent type, which is not unexpected because of the paucity of sarcoplasmic reticulum in this muscle. We have shown [101] that the relaxation is not affected either by the time at which the isotonic load is applied or by the manner (abruptly increased or decreased to the value chosen for study) in which it is applied.

Studies of the type described need to be carried out in ASM from animal models of allergic bronchospasm and in blood vessels from spontaneously hypertensive rats.

Length-Tension Curves and Hysteresis

As airway diameters change during respiration, it becomes necessary to determine the behavior of the smooth muscle under external length forcing, especially at frequencies and amplitudes that are likely to be imposed during breathing maneuvers. Such experiments show considerable force-length hysteresis. Sasaki and Hoppin [86] have conducted careful studies of this problem and conclude that ASM, cycled as it may be during respiration, shows great stiffness for small cycles and considerable hysteresis for larger cycles, consistent with the idea that muscle-shortening velocity is very slow relative to the imposed length cycling and that it reversibly slips or yields at a variable threshold force.

Mechanical Heterogeneity of Airway Smooth Muscle

Differences in Smooth Muscle Mechanics at Different Levels of Airway

Though Russell [84] showed that muscle strips from canine trachea and from 5 mm and 1.5 mm diameter airways produced qualitatively similar length-tension curves and that sensitivities to acetylcholine were also similar, the ratio of maximal tension produced by supramaximal electric stimulation and maximal doses of acetylcholine decreased from the trachea to the 1.5 mm diameter bronchus. This may result from a poorer vagal innervation of the smaller airways or alternatively from increasing inhibitory innervation (beta-adrenergic or nonadrenergic inhibitory).

Pharmacologic heterogeneity also exists. Central airways are constricted due to cholinergic (predominantly) and alpha-adrenergic activity. Peripheral airways demonstrate very weak alpha-adrenoceptor activity but strong histamine activity.

Species-Engendered Differences

Because of the well-known species differences in ASM function, one must be careful about extrapolating from data obtained from dogs, cats, monkeys, rats, and guinea pigs to humans. An example of such heterogeneity is that histamine produces marked constriction in guinea pig trachea, results in relaxation of cat trachea, and has no effect on rat and rabbit tracheas [30].

Heterogeneity is also produced by differences in the nonadrenergic inhibitory system. Thus it is known that, while such a system exists in human lungs [81], it is absent from canine.

Other sources of heterogeneity are agents liberated in feedback loops. Examples of these are leukotrienes and prostaglandins, and the release of transmitters from the presynapse. With respect to the last, histamine appears to interact with presynaptic H_1 receptors in TSM [5]. This releases acetylcholine, which contributes about 15 percent to the overall contractile response to histamine (see Chaps. 10 and 11).

Effect of Age, Temperature, and Hormones

Fleisch and colleagues [31] have reported that alpha-adrenergic responses of TSM are greater in 9-month-old rats than in 6-week-old rats. Additionally, Kunos and Szentivanyi [64] found that epinephrine and norepinephrine in rats are blocked by an alpha-receptor antagonist at low temperatures and by a beta-receptor antagonist at higher temperatures. Miller and Marshall [69] showed that adrenoceptors in estrogen-treated myometrium are predominantly of the alpha type but in progesterone-treated myometrium predominantly of the beta type.

Mechanics of Cat Lung Strips; Interstitial Cells

Lulich and associates [68] have developed the cat lung strip as an in vitro model of peripheral airways and have studied its mechanical and pharmacologic properties. The obvious shortcoming of the model is that it contains smooth muscle from airways, blood vessels, and the so-called interstitial cells described by Kapanci and coworkers [56]. Nevertheless, by using suitable pharmacologic blockers, it is possible to study the responses of the airways. Perhaps the best critique of the lung strip has been provided by Evans (personal communication), who concludes that it is not a very good model.

At any rate, the studies of Lulich and colleagues show that cat lung strip possessed tone that could be reduced by catecholamines, aminophylline, and flufenamate. It was contracted by histamine, prostaglandin $F_{2\alpha}$, and electric stimulation. TSM from the same animal was unreactive to histamine and prostaglandin $F_{2\alpha}$. Isoprenaline and epinephrine exerted a stronger effect on the lung strip than on the tracheal muscle. Experiments indicated

predominance of beta$_2$ adrenoceptors in the lung strip and beta$_1$ adrenoceptors in the trachea.

Both tissues could be sensitized, and a Schultz-Dale reaction could be elicited from them. The initial component of the isometric tension response from the lung strip was due to histamine. It was absent in tracheal muscle. The slow response which appeared leukotriene-mediated was seen in both preparations.

In passing, a comment should be made about the interstitial cells described by Kapanci and colleagues [56]. These are located in alveolar septa in relation to pre- and postcapillary vessels. They possess thin and thick filaments as judged by histochemical techniques employing antibodies to actin and myosin. They are claimed to act as a fine control mechanism with respect to optimizing ventilation-perfusion relationships. However, whether enough contractile material is present to exert significant control is moot.

In recent times, the lung strip seems to have fallen out of favor. This is because attempts are being made to study the small airway smooth muscle directly. Furthermore, because of the heterogeneity of the musculature in the lung strip, analysis of the data has proved difficult.

Physiologic Role of Airway Smooth Muscle

In spite of much speculation there is no concrete idea as to what the role of ASM is. The most reasonable notion is that it controls regional ventilation and thus optimizes ventilation-perfusion ratios in the lung [74].

AIRWAY SMOOTH MUSCLE IN ASTHMA

Having delineated the normal mechanical properties of ASM, we now pass to a consideration of the changes that occur in these as a result of sensitization with a specific antigen. The model (ovalbumin-dinitrophenol–sensitized pups) was developed by Kepron and coworkers [59] and is a very satisfactory one, only the Basenji greyhound being better because of the presence of a congenital component in the hyperreactivity. The former demonstrates high antibody titers, which are well sustained. The sensitized animals react to aerosol challenge of specific antigen with significant reduction in specific airway conductance (see Chap. 31).

Before describing the changes we find in sensitized ASM, some remarks regarding asthmatic bronchoconstriction are in order. After many years of research, it is now recognized that the increased responsiveness of sensitized ASM to histamine is really a very nonspecific one [40]. From this has developed the idea that the primary pathophysiologic abnormality in asthma may be at the muscle cell level. In this connection, Wardlaw [112] has suggested that the hyperreactivity of asthma may arise from smooth muscle changes induced by an autosomal dominant at a single gene locus. Levitt and Mitzner [65] have arrived at a similar conclusion with respect to an inbred rat model of acetylcholine hyperresponsiveness. Holme and Piechuta [46], working with Sprague-Dawley rats, have also developed a model of inbred hyperreactivity, but have concluded the changes are induced by polygenic influences.

With respect to alterations in mechanical properties, Souhrada and Dickey [91] have found in ovalbumin-sensitized guinea pig TSM no change in isometric tension (P_o) but an increased relaxation time. Using the model referred to above, we also found no change in P_o, but an increase in the ability of the muscle to shorten and in its maximum velocity of shortening (V_{max}). We have not studied relaxation time.

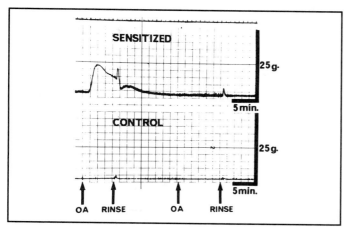

Fig. 25-12. *Isometric tension versus time records for sensitized and control tracheal smooth muscle strips. The former shows a Schultz-Dale response (a phasic contraction) to ovalbumin (OA). (The second spike is a washout artifact.) The control strip shows no response to a similar OA challenge. (Reprinted with permission from L. A. Antonissen, et al., Mechanical alterations of airway smooth muscle in a canine asthmatic model.* J. Appl. Physiol. *46:681, 1979.)*

Schultz-Dale Reaction in Sensitized Canine Tracheal Smooth Muscle

Seen in Fig. 25-12, sensitized TSM contracted vigorously on challenge with specific antigen. The TSM obtained from a littermate control showed no response The contraction seen in the sensitized TSM is completely blocked by pretreatment with pyrilamine maleate ($10^{-8} M$), an H_1 antagonist, indicating that histamine is the major mediator. Leukotrienes do not appear to be involved in the response. We found no evidence of a delayed response such as is seen in human asthma. When the antihistamine is applied at the peak of the mechanical response, the latter is reduced to the baseline level much more rapidly than in the spontaneous relaxation.

Tachyphylaxis develops very rapidly, and in fact the Schultz-Dale response can be elicited only once. This could be due to depletion of histamine stores in the isolated muscle. However, we also noted tachyphylaxis to exogenously applied histamine in both sensitized and control muscles. Szentivanyi [96] has indicated that tachyphylaxis is due to the liberation of relaxant prostaglandins. We have confirmed his observations that indomethacin completely eliminates the tachyphylaxis.

Pathophysiology of Sensitized Airway Smooth Muscle

Isometric Studies

Electric stimulus–response and carbachol dose–response curves showed no difference between control and sensitized TSMs. These results were surprising because we had expected to obtain evidence of nonspecific hyperresponsiveness of the type seen in vivo. Incidentally, hyperresponsiveness as used in this chapter includes hypersensitivity (a leftward shift of the dose-response curve) and hyperreactivity (an upward shift).

In spite of these negative results, the sensitized TSM showed some unique changes in its isometric myogram. In Figure 25-13, the prolonged plateau of the myogram from sensitized TSM is evident. To elucidate the cause of the prolonged plateau, the response to $5 \times 10^{-4} M$ histamine was studied, since it consisted of an initial rapid phase (phasic) and a final slow phase (tonic) (Fig. 25-14). On incubation in zero-calcium-containing solution only the phasic response was seen. On restoring 2 mM calcium

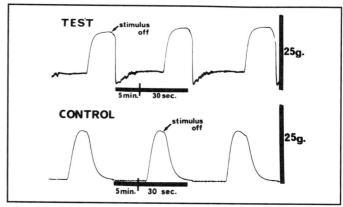

Fig. 25-13. *Isometric tension myograms from sensitized test and control tracheal smooth muscle specimens. Supramaximal electrical stimulation was used. (Reprinted with permission from L. A. Antonissen, et al., Mechanical alterations of airway smooth muscle in a canine asthmatic model.* J. Appl. Physiol. *46:681, 1979.)*

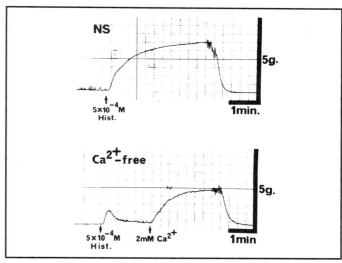

Fig. 25-14. *Isometric tension versus time records from a single experiment. The top trace was obtained from a control tracheal smooth muscle bathed in normal (NS) Krebs-Henseliet solution. The bottom panel shows the mechanical responses when the muscle was in Ca^{++}-free solution initially and then when Ca^{++} was added. (Reprinted with permission from N. L. Stephens, Histamine pharmacology in airway smooth muscle from a canine model of asthma.* J. Pharmacol. Exp. Ther. *213:150, 1980.)*

only the tonic response was obtained. Adding these two responses we obtain the same response as seen in the upper panel. We surmise that the prolonged plateau of the sensitized TSM may be due to extracellular calcium.

Another characteristic of sensitized TSM is the development of spontaneous phasic activity. Additionally, a myogenic response can be elicited. This is not seen in the control muscle.

Isotonic Studies

Isotonic studies are of greater importance than the isometric since the development of asthma can only stem from narrowing of the airways. Force-velocity curves from control and sensitized TSMs are shown in Figure 25-15. They show that, though P_o is not different between the two, V_{max} is increased in the sensitized muscle. The caveat mentioned before about the validity of velocity points at heavy loads must be kept in mind. Table 25-2 com-

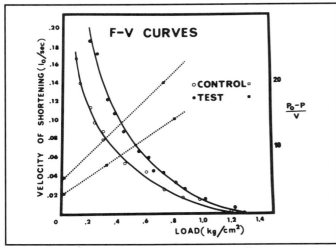

Fig. 25-15. *Load (or force)-velocity (F-V) data for sensitized and control tracheal smooth muscle, both set at their predetermined optimal lengths. The straight lines are linearized transforms of the hyperbolas. The righthand ordinate and the abscissa are the coordinates for the linear transforms. (Reprinted with permission from L. A. Antonissen, et al., Mechanical alterations of airway smooth muscle in a canine asthmatic model. J. Appl. Physiol. 46:681, 1979.)*

Table 25-2. Force-velocity constants for sensitized test and control TSMs

Force-velocity parameters	Test (n = 11)	Control (n = 9)
V_{max} (l_o/sec)	.346 ± .043*	.234 ± .022*
b (l_o/sec)	.062 ± .004*	.047 ± .003*
a (kg/cm^2)	.238 ± .030	.263 ± .032
P_o (kg/cm^2)	1.161 ± .056	1.211 ± .071
a/P_o	.212 ± .032	.230 ± .040

* $p < .05$.
Source: L. A. Antonissen, et al. Mechanical alterations of airway smooth muscle in a canine asthmatic model. *J. Appl. Physiol.* 46:681, 1979. Reprinted with permission.

pares muscle constants for the two muscles obtained from the force-velocity hyperbolas. No significant changes were found in the *a* constant which, as pointed out before, is an index of the number of force-generating sites in the muscles' cross-sections. These negative findings are important because they indicate that at the time of the experiment there was no hypertrophy or hyperplasia. This proves that the changes in velocity constants (V_{max} and *b*) are not secondary to structural muscle changes. The faster V_{max} of the sensitized TSM indicates a faster rate of energy utilization, which in turn leads to the tentative hypothesis that in asthma the properties of the actomyosin ATPase are altered. However, particularly in smooth muscle the role of calcium must also be kept in mind, since it has been shown that smooth muscle actomyosin ATPase is stimulated by Ca^{++}.

Analysis of the muscle-shortening data from which velocities were computed reveals that sensitized TSM shortens more than control (Fig. 25-16). This finding is of considerable significance since it is the counterpart to in vivo bronchoconstriction. Thus one can conclude that changes develop in sensitized TSM that precede ultrastructural change. This in turn makes it more likely that the primary pathophysiologic alteration in asthma is at the smooth muscle level.

The changes in function of the sensitized TSM described above suggest that the first component of the attack may be a rapid and increased shortening of ASM, resulting in a greater than normal

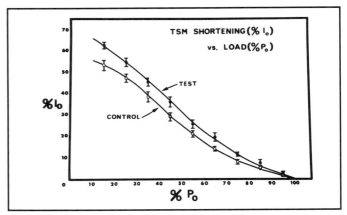

Fig. 25-16. *Mean (with standard errors) tracheal smooth muscle (TSM) shortenings versus tension plots (N = 11). Tension and length changes are shown in percentage units. (Reprinted with permission from L. A. Antonissen, et al., Mechanical alterations of airway smooth muscle in a canine asthmatic model. J. Appl. Physiol. 46:681, 1979.)*

Table 25-3. Canine tracheal smooth muscle

Variables	Sensitized	Control
P_o (kg/cm^2)	1.482	1.50
Δl_{max} (l_o)	0.643	0.531
t_T (sec)	8.33	5.50
V_o–3 sec (l_o/sec)	0.401	0.296
V_o–8 sec (l_o/sec)	0.121	0.128

P_o = maximum active tension; Δl_{max} = change in optimal length; l_o = optimal length; t_T = time to peak tension; V_o = zero-load shortening velocity.

fall in specific airway conductance or 1-second forced expiratory volume. Spontaneous phasic activity and the development of a myogenic response could further increase the bronchoconstriction.

Table 25-3 shows data from studies of the mechanical properties of tracheal muscle obtained from ragweed pollen–sensitized dogs and their littermate controls. Several features are worthy of note. First, it is the increased shortening capacity (Δl_{max}) that is the most important finding, as it accounts for the severe bronchospasms of allergy. Also noteworthy is the fact that only the normally cycling cross-bridges show increased cycling activity. Though not shown in the table, the data also demonstrated that most of the increased shortening (Δl_{max}) of the sensitized muscle is complete in the first 2 seconds of contraction. This demonstrates that the in vitro studies of asthma or allergic bronchoconstriction must be conducted in the isotonic or auxotonic mode, and it is only the mechanical change occurring in the first 2 to 3 seconds that is important. The importance of such changes strongly indicates that, for elucidating mechanisms, myosin-light-chain phosphorylation must be studied.

In conditions in which latch bridges are affected, the process to study is myosin-light-chain dephosphorylation, which is affected by the activity of a specific phosphatase. A caveat must be entered to the effect that the relationship of dephosphorylation to the development of latch bridges has not yet been clearly established.

In Table 25-3, Δl_{max} and V_o at 2 seconds are shown to be significantly different on the basis of a two-tailed paired *t*-test (<.05). V_o and P_o measured at 8 seconds showed no differences between control and sensitized muscles. The absence of a difference in P_o is interesting, as it shows that isometric parameters are insensitive indicators of pathophysiology. In early disease—and the whole purpose of our work has been to work with models of early disease as they would more likely provide information regarding primary causes—the isotonic parameters are all-important.

Given the existence of changes in mechanical properties, the next step is to elucidate the underlying cellular and molecular mechanisms.

Biochemistry of Sensitized Tracheal Smooth Muscle

The two major changes in the mechanical properties of sensitized ASM that we have detected, increased Δl_{max} and V_o, require two different biochemical methods of analysis.

Increased Δl_{max}

The major consideration in detecting increased Δl_{max} is the resistance to shortening that does not permit a muscle cell to contract maximally. This resistance could reside within muscle cells or be located between the cells or cell bundles. Such a resistance has been demonstrated in cardiac muscle. Its presence can be demonstrated simply by taking a strip of smooth muscle and stimulating it to shorten isotonically at peak shortening; if the stimulus is abruptly withdrawn, the muscle does not remain shortened but reelongates to exactly its initial length.

The possible sources of the internal resistor are the collagen, elastin, or basement membrane tissues between the cells or cytoskeletal proteins, such as desmin, vimentin, α-actinin, and filamin, to name a few. Studies are being initiated to evaluate the importance of these factors.

Berner and coworkers [11] have shown that, in a model of smooth muscle hypertrophy, the first change to occur is an increase in the concentration of cytoskeletal proteins.

An increase in the compliance properties of the cytoskeleton could account for the increased bronchoconstriction of asthma.

Increased V_o

Normally one would not think that an increase in V_o should affect Δl_{max}, provided adequate time is available for completion of shortening. A striking exception is that of cardiac muscle, which, since it cannot be tetanized, must complete its shortening in less than a second. In this case, a reduced V_o would not permit shortening to be completed. In smooth muscle, which can be tetanized, and in which contraction time is at least 10 seconds, such a limitation should not exist. However, the finding that 75 percent of isotonic shortening is complete within 2 seconds indicates that velocity must play a fairly important part. Because of this consideration, our finding that V_o is greater in sensitized TSM than in the control is significant.

We carried out the following experiments in an attempt to elucidate the pathogenesis of the measured V_o.

The first assessed myofibrillar ATPase activity. The biochemical counterpart to V_o is myofibrillar ATPase activity. Figure 25-17 shows that specific ATPase activity is increased in the sensitized muscle (*STSM*) compared to control (*CTSM*).

Myosin-heavy-chain isoenzyme distribution was also analyzed. In striated muscle, the presence of myosin-heavy-chain isoenzymes has been demonstrated. Increases in V_o have been shown to be associated with changes in isoenzyme distribution. In rat cardiac muscle, for example, two isoenzymes have been demonstrated [104]: V_1 and V_3; V_1 has a higher molecular weight and higher ATPase activity. When ventricular hypertrophy develops, V_o diminishes and the isoenzyme distribution changes from being predominantly V_1 (with respect to V_3) to V_3.

We have studied TSM extracts using SDS-polyacrylamide gel electrophoresis and shown that myosin-heavy-chain isoenzymes are present in this muscle. Studies with molecular-weight markers indicated the molecular weights of the two bands are 204 kd and 200 kd, respectively. Densitometry of nine gel patterns showed no differences between the two muscle extracts. On the

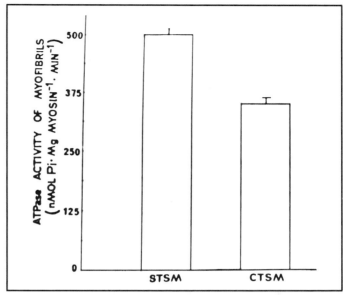

Fig. 25-17. *Histograms (standard error bars shown) of myofibrillar ATPase activity of tracheal smooth muscle from sensitized (STSM) and control (CTSM) animals.*

basis of these experiments, we concluded that the cause of the increased myofibrillar ATPase activity was not due to a change in myosin-heavy-chain isoenzyme distribution. The remaining possibility was that phosphorylation of the sensitized muscle's myosin light chain (20,000 daltons) was increased, thus accounting for the increased ATPase activity.

Figure 25-18 shows Coomassie Blue–stained 10 percent polyacrylamide gel electrophoretograms of crude muscle extracts. The 20,000-dalton light chains are seen in gels from sensitized (A) and control (B) TSM. The muscles had been equilibrated with ^{32}P-labeled ATP. The two lower gels represent autoradiograms of the gels shown in the top panel. Increased phosphorylation (*lane A*) of myosin light chain from the sensitized muscles is clearly seen.

Figure 25-19 shows the two-dimensional gel electrophoresis patterns of proteins from control and sensitized TSM. The figure reveals that the first dimension is isoelectric with a pH range from 5.7 to 5.3. The second dimension is for separation by molecular weight and uses SDS-polyacrylamide gels. In the upper lefthand panel, *arrows* indicate the unphosphorylated (*UP-LC*) and phosphorylated (*P-LC*) light chains stained with Coomassie-Blue from control canine TSM. The lower lefthand panel shows similar light chains, but these were from muscles incubated with ^{32}P-labeled ATP. The extent of phosphorylation of the light chain is visible. Both the *B* panels on the righthand side are similar to the *A* panels, but are from muscles obtained from ragweed pollen–sensitized dogs. The upper *B* panel suggests greater phosphorylation of the light chain than that shown in panel *A*. The lower *B* panel clearly demonstrates the increased phosphorylation of the light chain compared to that in panel *A*. We conclude that, in ragweed pollen–sensitized canine ASM, myosin-light-chain (20,000-dalton) phosphorylation is increased. This could account for the increased myofibrillar ATPase activity and the increased V_o.

Currently we are conducting studies to determine whether myosin-light-chain kinase (the enzyme responsible for phosphorylation) activity is increased as a result of sensitization. Preliminary experiments using appropriate antibodies and the Western blotting technique indicate that this activity is increased. Furthermore, we have found from a pilot experiment that messenger RNA for the kinase is also increased.

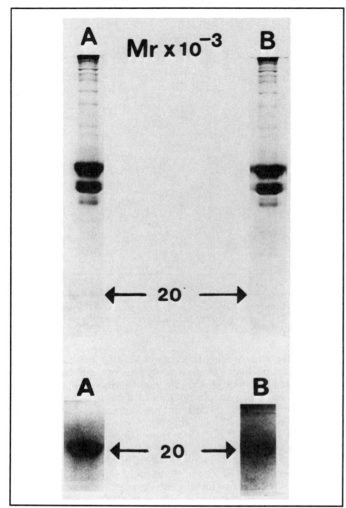

Fig. 25-18. *Upper panel shows Coomassie blue–stained 10 percent SDS-polyacrylamide gels. Arrows indicate the position of 20,000-dalton myosin light chains. Lower panel shows autoradiograms of the upper gels. A = sensitized canine tracheal smooth muscle; B = control canine tracheal smooth muscle.*

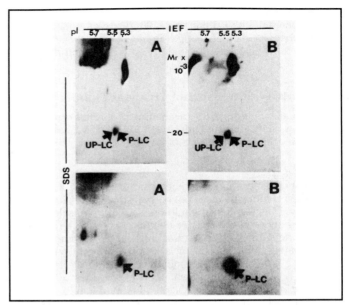

Fig. 25-19. *Upper panel shows increase in myosin light chain (MLC) phosphorylation in sensitized tracheal smooth muscle. Lower panel shows autoradiograms of the 20,000-dalton MLC separated by two-dimensional electrophoresis. See text for discussion.*

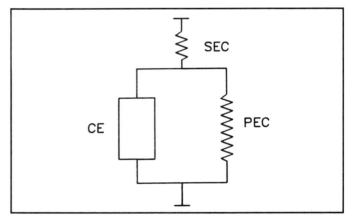

Fig. 25-20. *Schematic representation of Voigt model of muscle. (SEC = series elastic component; PEC = parallel elastic component; CE = contractile element.)*

Determining the Mechanism for Increased Shortening of Sensitized Airway Smooth Muscle

Although many studies have been carried out in a variety of striated and smooth muscles to determine the cause for changes in maximum velocity of shortening, very few have been designed to elucidate the mechanism responsible for increased shortening. This is even more true for smooth muscle.

One factor that could influence the magnitude of shortening is an internal resistance to shortening. The evidence that such a phenomenon exists is straightforward. If one stretches a muscle to beyond l_{max} and then releases it, it returns to l_{max}. Furthermore, if one allows a stimulated muscle to shorten maximally and then removes the stimulus, the muscle reelongates to its original length. It is as if there was an elastic resistance to shortening and stretching. In the shortening mode, this resistor undergoes compression and stores potential energy. When the stimulus is stopped, the resistor reexpands and restores the muscle to its original length.

The hypothesis we tested is whether increased compliance of the internal resistor would facilitate increased shortening of the muscle. To test this, a method was developed to delineate the length-tension curve of the internal resistor, using the Voigt model for contraction (Fig. 25-20). When a load is applied to an activated muscle, it is transferred to the muscle's contractile element via the springlike series elastic component (SEC). The maximal velocity attained by the contractile element would then be an inverse function of the magnitude of the load. If, however, the external load were suddenly changed to zero by application of a so-called zero-load clamp, the muscle would shorten at maximum velocity. It is evident, however, that as shortening develops the spring denoting the parallel elastic component would relax from its slightly stretched state at l_{max}. With further shortening of the contractile element, the parallel component would be compressed further, thus imposing an internal load on the contractile element whose velocity would be diminished proportionately.

The critical assumption we make at this point is that the force-velocity curve for the muscle's contractile element is the same whether loaded internally via the compressed parallel elastic component or externally via the SEC.

It is possible to measure maximum velocities of shortening at

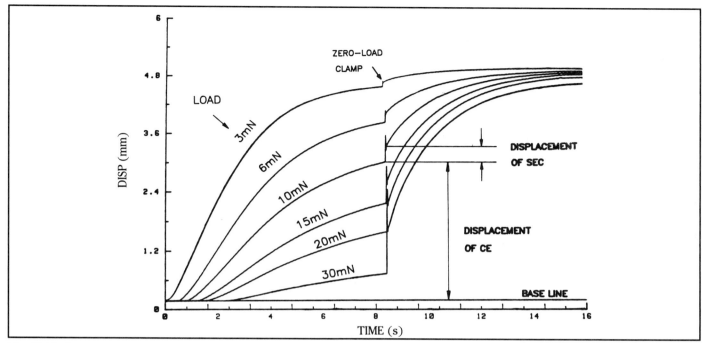

Fig. 25-21. *Experimental records of shortening versus time of a strip of canine tracheal smooth muscle set at optimal length (l_o) initially. The contractile element (CE) length was obtained by subtracting the displacement of the CE and the series elastic component (SEC) from the l_o. The maximum velocity (V_o) for each length was obtained by measuring the slope of the shortening curve 100 msec after the onset of the zero load clamp. The time chosen was arbitrary.*

different contractile element lengths when the external load has been clamped to zero. Figure 25-21 shows a series of shortening records in which the maximally stimulated muscle was allowed to shorten isotonically. At any point in time, the length of the contractile element was a function of the magnitude of the load. At the instant shown in the records, zero-load clamps were applied. A rapid transient due to the shortening of the unclamped SEC is seen in each trace, followed by a slower transient that represents shortening of the contractile element. The maximum velocity attained during this phase is plotted against the calculated contractile element length. Once a suitable range of contractile element lengths had been explored, velocity–contractile element length curves with a curvilinear relationship were obvious (Fig. 25-22). A quadratic function best fitted the data. In terms of physiologic significance, it is evident that, for the first 25 percent of shortening, velocity is almost independent of length.

Conventional force-velocity curves were obtained. These were elicited by applying a range of loads after quick-release at the same time at which the studies of the internal resistor had been conducted.

Figure 25-23 shows such force-velocity curves (elicited from control tracheal smooth muscle) superimposed on Figure 25-22. At isovelocity points, corresponding length and load values must depict tension-compression points for the parallel elastic component (PEC) as shown in Figure 25-24. This segment of the PEC is the same as the internal resistance to shortening. Figure 25-25 shows the curve of Figure 25-24 along with a curve elicited from sensitized tracheal smooth muscle. The increased compliance of the PEC is evident, which could account for the greater ability to shorten that we have found in the past for the sensitized muscle.

Pharmacology of Sensitized Tracheal Smooth Muscle

We have reported [5, 6] that carbachol dose-response curves were unchanged in sensitized TSM. This was surprising since

methacholine dose-response studies in humans have shown increased responsiveness [25, 40, 61]. We have no explanation for these differences; they result from differences either in species (dogs versus humans) or preparations (in vitro versus in vivo). Another possibility is that carbachol maximally stimulates all cholinergic receptors in control and sensitized muscles and obscures any differences due to the esterase inactivation of acetylcholine (see Chap. 17).

Histamine

Dose-Response Curves. Figure 25-26 shows that the histamine dose-response curve for sensitized TSM was shifted leftward and upward with respect to control. Normalizing the data (see Fig. 10-26B) reveals the statistically significant persistence of the leftward shift. Shifts of this type to histamine have been reported in ASM from several other animal models of asthma.

With respect to histamine, H_1 (constrictor) and H_2 (dilator) receptors have been reported in horse and rat by Eyre [29]. In the canine TSM, however, only H_1 receptors are present. The contractile response to a maximal dose of histamine was abolished by pyrilamine maleate ($10^{-8}\ M$).

An interesting finding was that sensitized TSM did not respond to ovalbumin (specific antigen) challenge when the muscle had been previously challenged with histamine. This may represent feedback inhibition of histamine release by histamine itself. Lichtenstein and Gillespie [67] suggest that this may be an H_2 receptor–mediated effect. Since we have not detected any H_2 receptors (nor have Bradley and Russell [14]), this could not explain the inhibition.

Cholinergic Component of Histamine Response. The idea that asthma was predominantly due to acetylcholine released via an irritant receptor reflex was an historically important one in the field. But, while several studies have shown that increased bronchomotor responses to histamine can be blocked by atropine [5, 47, 88], others have disputed this [21, 50].

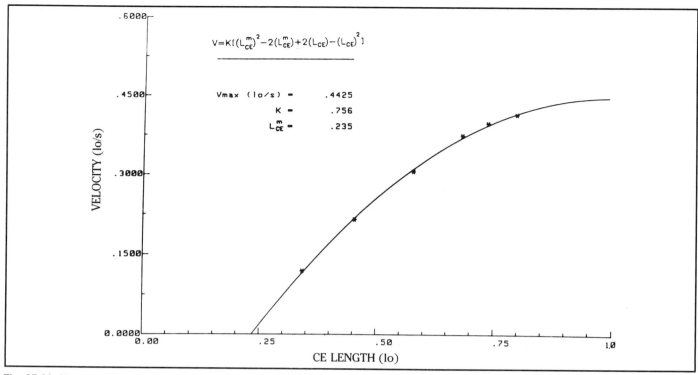

Fig. 25-22. *Velocity versus contractile element (CE) length curve obtained from data in Fig. 25-21.*

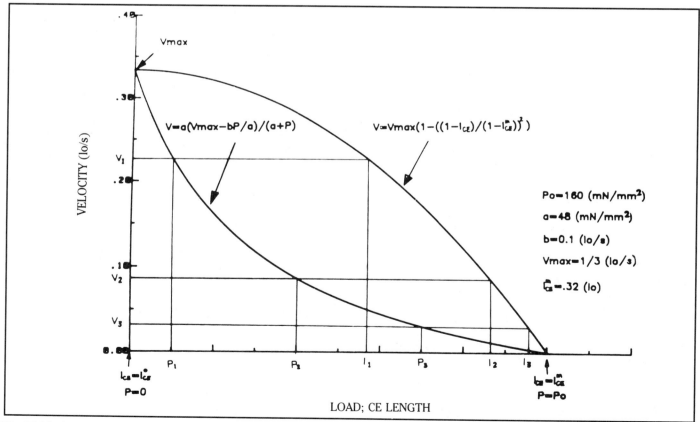

Fig. 25-23. *Curves of Fig. 25-22 superimposed on a force-velocity curve for the same muscle. Note that the abscissa represents load for the force-velocity curve and contractile element (CE) length for the length-velocity phase plane.*

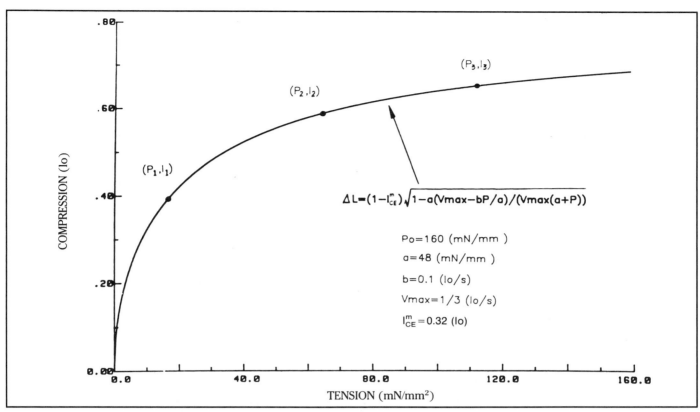

Fig. 25-24. *Tension-compression curve for the parallel elastic component obtained from Fig. 25-23.*

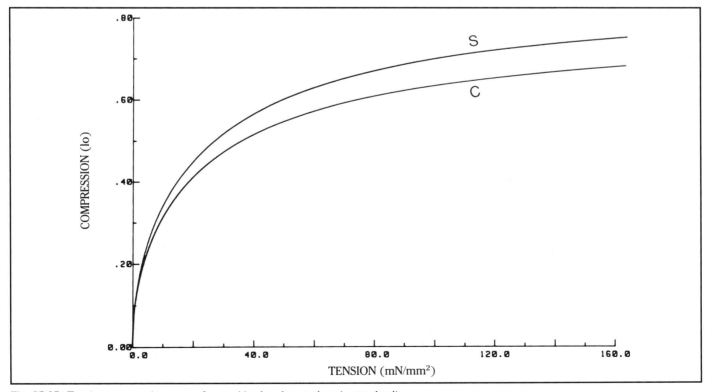

Fig. 25-25. *Tension-compression curves for sensitized and control canine trachealis.*

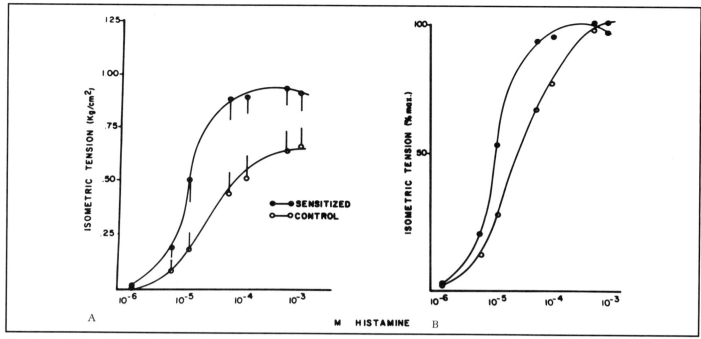

Fig. 25-26. *A. Mean histamine log dose–response curves for control and sensitized tracheal smooth muscles. Standard error bars are shown. B. Same data, normalized. See text. (Reprinted with permission from N. L. Stephens, Histamine pharmacology in airway smooth muscle from a canine model of asthma.* J. Pharmacol. Exp. Ther. *213:150, 1980.)*

Work with isolated sensitized canine TSM has provided some fresh insights. Antonissen and coworkers [5] reported that about 20 to 30 percent of the histamine response is atropine sensitive. This in turn suggests that presynaptic histamine response is atropine sensitive. This in turn suggests that presynaptic histamine receptors exist on cholinergic fibers innervating the muscle. Therefore histamine could induce TSM contraction by direct stimulation of the sarcolemmal receptors and by releasing acetylcholine from the presynapse.

Histamine Tachyphylaxis. Tachyphylaxis to histamine develops rapidly in vitro. The mechanism responsible seems related to the action of prostaglandins, as Anderson and colleagues [3, 4] have shown that it is eliminated by pretreatment with indomethacin. Orehek [77, 78] and Grodzinska [37] and their associates have obtained similar evidence to ours. The role of leukotrienes in the elimination of tachyphylaxis has not been conclusively determined. We find (unpublished data) that a small part of the increased tension after indomethacin treatment can be blocked by FLP55712, an SRS-A antagonist. SRA-A is the slow-reacting substance of anaphylaxis and recent evidence suggests it consists of leukotrienes C_4 and D_4 (see Chaps. 11 and 66).

Role of Histamine in Allergic Bronchoconstrictions. For a long time it was felt that histamine was the major mediator of the allergic reaction that resulted in asthma. The failure of antihistamines to relieve asthma was explained by postulating that the tissue concentration of these drugs in tolerable oral therapeutic doses was inadequate. Reports from Samuelsson's [22] and Austen's [113] laboratories have indicated that the response to aerosolized leukotrienes in human asthmatics resembles clinical asthma while that to histamine aerosol does not. Evidence of this kind has served to strengthen the concept that clinical asthma results in great part from leukotriene production and not histamine.

The Role of Airway Smooth Muscle Adrenoceptors
While the status of the role of adrenoceptors in the pathogenesis of asthma is still far from clear, as is the question of their neuro-

genic control, there is no doubt about the potent effect of catecholamines in the relief of asthma.

The presence of alpha and beta adrenoceptors in human ASM has been reported by Kneussel and Richardson [60], Russell [85], and Simonsson and associates [89]. The variability of their distribution between different species and between different parts of the airway has been alluded to by Brocklehurst [15, 16] and Golla and Symes [35].

Alpha Adrenoceptors. Evidence seems to indicate that alpha adrenoceptors are sparse [31, 32]. There are, however, several reports that alpha-adrenoceptor activity may be contributing to part of the allergic bronchospasm. For example, Simonsson and coworkers [88] found in asthmatic patients that alpha-adrenoceptor stimulation with phenylepinephrine during beta-adrenoceptor blockade resulted in bronchoconstriction. Barnes and colleagues [9] using prazosin, an alpha-adrenoceptor blocker, obtained evidence for the activity of such receptors in the development of exercise-induced asthma. Several other alpha adrenoceptors have been found in ASM from humans, guinea pigs, rabbits, cats and old rats [7, 30, 31]. All these studies have led to the possibility that an increased number or activity of alpha adrenoceptors may be unmasked in asthmatics (see Chap. 14).

Beta Adrenoceptors. $Beta_2$ adrenoceptors that specifically control airways and blood vessels have been found in the respiratory tree. $Beta_1$ adrenoceptors whose main effects are to stimulate lipolysis and cardiac function are also present. However, the ratio of $beta_2$ to $beta_1$ receptors appears to vary between animal species and between different locations in the airways (see Chap. 14).

The powerful bronchodilator action of $beta_2$ agonists has been known for a long time; such drugs are a major component of the therapy of acute allergic bronchospasm.

Beta-receptor stimulation is modulated by the release of other transmitters. In experiments where postganglionic nerve fibers were blocked with guanethidine, the effect of histamine was potentiated [13].

Beta-Adrenoceptor Desensitization. Szentivanyi [106] has put forward the theory that beta-adrenoceptor desensitization may be responsible for the bronchospasm of asthma (see Chap. 14). Keighley [57], Patterson and associates [79], and Tashkin and colleagues [107] have noted the development of refractoriness to adrenergic bronchodilator aerosols in asthma. Jenne [52] has also reported a reduced beta-adrenoceptor response in patients on prolonged terbutaline therapy. Similar block of salbutamol effect has been reported by Holgate et al. [45]. However, controversy exists in the field since Furchgott [33] and Svedmyr and coworkers [103] have shown that, while tachyphylaxis to oral terbutaline exists with respect to muscle tremor in patients, none exists to bronchodilator response. Holgate and colleagues [45] state that tachyphylaxis to beta-adrenergic agonists has been produced in dog, guinea pig, and human ASM but not in rat. Tachyphylaxis to inhaled beta-adrenergic agonists has been produced in vivo in dogs [52] and normal humans [34, 103]. However, mild asthmatics showed no such tachyphylaxis [41]. Holgate and associates [45] conclude, "These results suggest that airway smooth muscle beta-receptor function is if anything protected in asthmatic subjects, which is quite contrary to the predictions of Szentivanyi." The reasons for the discrepancy are not clear but may be due to differences in bronchodilator dosage, variability in patient hyperresponsiveness, or concomitant administration of other drugs. The status of beta-adrenoceptor blockade therapy remains open at this time.

Tone and Adrenergic Responses of Airway Smooth Muscle. An important consideration in asthma research is that the response of ASM depends qualitatively and quantitatively on the basal conditions of the muscle. Since these differ between in vitro and in vivo situations, it is easy to see how research controversies develop.

Bergen and Kroeger [10], for example, found that the isolated resting TSM did not contract in response to norepinephrine even in the presence of beta-adrenoceptor blockade. However, they found that, if the tissue was pretreated with 22.8 mM K$^+$ such that a small contraction developed, then contraction to norepinephrine in the presence of atropine and propranolol was readily elicited. This contraction was seen at norepinephrine concentrations ranging between $10^{-9} M$ and $10^{-6} M$. At higher concentrations a propranolol-sensitive relaxation was seen. They concluded that canine TSM possesses both alpha and beta adrenoceptors postjunctionally and that the alpha adrenoceptors are primed by raising intracellular levels of free calcium. Douglas and associates [24] have reported similar data for sensitized guinea pig ASM; they found that phentolamine prevented bronchoconstriction in sensitized animals but had little effect in control animals. These findings again suggest that alpha adrenoceptors may be important in the development of asthma.

The Nonadrenergic Inhibitory System

The reader is referred to Chapter 18 for discussion of the nonadrenergic inhibitory system. It is said to be the major relaxant system for human ASM, and its impairment could result in asthma. Its putative transmitter is said to be vasoactive intestinal peptide. For purposes of this chapter suffice it to say that the dog does not appear to possess such a system. In humans this system is present, but its role may be minor.

The Nonadrenergic, Noncholinergic Excitatory System

This system has been identified recently. Uchida and coworkers [105] have identified the transmitter involved and named it *endothelin*; it is a potent bronchoconstrictor. Whether it has a role to play in the pathogenesis of asthma has yet to be determined.

The Role of Conversion of Multiunit Airway Smooth Muscle to Single-unit Muscle

TSM in the dog is of the multiunit type [19], and is characterized by tonic activity, an absent myogenic response, absent action potentials, and a paucity of low-impedance gap injections. It should be richly innervated but is not and for this reason is really an intermediate type of smooth muscle. Single-unit smooth muscle is phasically active from a mechanical point of view; it possesses action potentials and a myogenic response. There are a large number of gap junctions and a paucity of nerves.

The idea has been put forward that the pathogenesis of asthma is based on conversion of ASM from multiunit to single unit [49], it being implied that under these circumstances the muscle becomes hyperresponsive to a number of stimuli. The basis for this idea is a report by Akasaka and colleagues [1]. Using a specially designed intraluminal electrode they recorded action potentials from human bronchial muscle during an asthmatic attack. This was supported by data published by Kroeger and Stephens [63] that canine TSM in vitro is of a multiunit or intermediate type with no action potentials. However, on treatment with tetraethylammonium bromide it developed single-unit properties with decrementally conducted complex action potentials. They also found that the action potentials were carried by Ca^{++}.

While the concept of conversion to single-unit muscle is attractive and suggests that inhibitors of Ca^{++} uptake may be of value in asthma, sufficient grounds do not exist to accept the idea. Inspection of Akasaka's records show that while asthmatics certainly show phasic electric activity, the controls also showed occasional spikes. Secondly, Kroeger and Stephens' [63] data must be evaluated bearing in mind that they were obtained from in vitro experiments. It is possible that the process of removing TSM from in vivo to in vitro also causes it to change from multiunit to single-unit. Bergen and Kroeger [10] have shown that when TSM is bathed in plasma it displays powerful single-unit activity. Hence it is not unlikely that in vivo TSM is of the single-unit type. A third piece of evidence which suggests that TSM in vivo is of the single-unit type comes from the work of Hakansson and Toremalm [32]. They showed that normal rabbit TSM was of the single-unit type. While no action potentials were found, the membrane potential showed well-defined oscillations. The peaks of the oscillations were associated with mechanical responses.

All this (in vitro, animal) evidence does not support the idea that asthma is produced by conversion of ASM from multiunit to single-unit but rather indicates that normally present single-unit characteristics become amplified with development of the asthmatic attack.

The Role of Changes in the Operation of the Contractile Machinery

The large variety of stimuli (cold, exercise, emotion, histamine, methacholine, leukotrienes) that induce increased bronchoconstriction in patients with asthma also support the idea that the hyperresponsiveness of sensitized ASM is nonspecific and related to changes occurring within the cell. Furthermore, there appears to be no clear correlation between IgE levels and bronchospasm, which indicates that changes in ASM are not specific to sensitization. Hence excitation-contraction coupling or the contractile machinery itself could be the source of the primary disorder in asthma. Our mechanical studies showed an increase in V$_{max}$ in sensitized canine TSM. The simplest explanation for this would be an increase in the actomyosin isoenzyme patterns in which isoenzymes with faster ATPase activity become dominant. It could also be due to a change in the degree of phosphorylation of the myosin light chain.

The Role of the Pulmonary Circulation

Interest is developing in the idea that asthma may be primarily a disease of the pulmonary blood vessels. The idea that dilatation of the smaller vessels encroaches on the airways resulting in narrowing and altered compliance has been put forward by Hogg et al. and coworkers [44]. The concept mentioned in the first sentence is based on the fact that while the changes in the early part of the asthmatic attack are those of reduced airway conductance (stemming from constriction of central airways), those after the initial 5 to 10 minutes are associated with changes in lung compliance because of narrowing of smaller bronchioles in the periphery with alveolar collapse. This delayed response is probably triggered by leukotrienes. It could, goes the argument, be secondary to pulmonary venoconstriction with dilatation upstream. It is notable that drugs used in the relief of bronchospasm could also relieve the vasoconstriction.

In some support of the above speculation is a publication of Kong and colleagues [61] in which a well-defined Schultz-Dale response was reported in the intralobar pulmonary veins of ovalbumin-sensitized dogs. Histamine dose-response curves from such tissues show increased sensitivity and reactivity. These authors also found that while the pulmonary artery showed no Schultz-Dale response, it demonstrated increased sensitivity and reactivity to histamine. Furthermore, force-velocity curves displayed an increased maximum velocity of shortening when compared to controls. Eyre [29] has also noted pharmacologic changes in blood vessels from sensitized sheep. Since current evidence suggests that leukotrienes are the major transmitters in allergic response, it is of some significance that Smedegard et al. [90] report that leukotriene C$_4$ (LTC$_4$) causes transient pulmonary and systemic hypertension initially.

Leukotrienes and Allergic Bronchospasm

The existence of a second slow contractile response of sensitized ASM after the initial rapid response to an antigen has subsided has been well known for many years [16, 30, 51, 59]. The agent responsible for this was termed *slow-reacting substance of anaphylaxis* (SRS-A). Because of the small amounts available, all that was known chemically about SRS-A was that it was an acidic, highly polar lipid [22] of molecular weight under 700 and containing a sulfur atom in its structure [66].

Important studies of this substance were carried out by several investigators [8, 26, 75, 76], culminating in the studies of Borgeat and Samuelsson [12], which demonstrated the presence of a metabolite of arachidonic acid, 5,12-di-hydroxyeicosatetraenoic acid. They recognized the relevance of its three conjugated double bands to the absorption spectrum of SRS-A. Murphy, Hammerstrom, and Samuelsson [73] defined the parent SRS generated by ionophore activation of mouse mastocytoma cells as 5-hydroxy,6S-glutathionyl-7,9,11,14-eicosatetraenoic acid—LTC$_4$. Three groups of workers [89–91] have described an even more active spasmogen—the 6-sulfido-cysteinyl-glycine metabolite (LTD$_4$). Rat SRS-A has been found to contain three leukotrienes—LTC$_4$, LTD$_4$, and LTE$_4$. These possess vasoactive and spasmogenic activities that are more potent than those of histamine [66], at least with respect to small airway smooth muscle. A preferential action of partially purified SRS-A in guinea pig parenchymal strips as compared to tracheal preparations [26] was confirmed with purified and synthetic constituents of SRS-A [26, 66]. Furthermore, with respect to the site of action, it was found that intravenous administration of partially purified SRS-A [26] and of synthetic leukotrienes resulted in a marked fall in the dynamic compliance of peripheral airways in intact, unanesthetized guinea pigs, whereas only minor increments in resistance occurred in the more central airways. Though histamine seems as potent at LTC$_4$ and LTE$_4$ but not LTD$_4$, its effect on compliance

lacks the duration of the leukotriene effects and is accompanied by an even more marked effect on central airways. Some idea of the potency of the leukotrienes and hence of their importance may be gained from the observation that in human bronchi LTC$_4$ and LTD$_4$ are 1,000 times as potent as histamine and 500 times more potent than prostaglandin F$_2$ on a molar basis [22].

Samuelsson [22] and Austen [113] and their associates have recently reported important studies carried out with leukotrienes. They found that the clinical picture of the response of ASM to aerosolized histamine in human asthmatics is characterized by central airway constriction and considerable irritation of the upper respiratory passages. This is unlike an asthmatic attack, where upper airway irritation is minimal and, after the central bronchospasm subsides, respiratory distress is mainly associated with alterations in dynamic lung compliance, suggesting that small airways or blood vessels are constricted or that interstitial edema is developing. Furthermore, both aerosolized antigen and leukotriene C produce pictures strongly resembling the clinical one. All this provides evidence to support the idea that leukotrienes may be one of the most important group of agonists involved in human asthma (see Chap. 11).

The possibility that ASM may play a greater role in the primary causation of asthma has not received sufficient attention in the past since the field was dominated by immunologic and neurologic considerations. As matters stand, these are still the major contenders in the field. The roles of alpha-adrenoceptor overactivity and beta-adrenergic blockade await clarification. However, the findings that the maximum velocity and magnitude of shortening of sensitized ASM are increased [6] and that relaxation time is prolonged [91] suggest that asthma could be originating at the muscle cell level.

The possibility that the change in smooth muscle mechanics underlying asthma is a conversion from multiunit properties to single-unit ones is interesting but needs more research to evaluate its role.

REFERENCES

1. Akasaka, K., Konno, K., and Ono, Y. Electromyograph of study of bronchial smooth muscle in bronchial asthma. *Tohoku J. Exp. Med.* 117:55, 1975.
2. Aksoy, M. O., Murphy, R. A., and Kamm, K. E. Role of Ca^{++} and myosin light chain phosphorylation in regulation of smooth muscle. *Am. J. Physiol.* 242:109, 1982.
3. Anderson, W., et al. Differences in histamine responsiveness of canine trachea and small airways (abstract). *Fed. Pro.* 39:1094, 1980.
4. Anderson, W. H., et al. Decreased synthesis of prostaglandin-like material during histamine tachyphylaxis in canine tracheal smooth muscle. *Biochem. Pharmacol.* 28:2223, 1979.
5. Antonissen, L. A., et al. Histamine pharmacology in airway smooth muscle from a canine model of asthma. *J. Pharmacol. Exp. Ther.* 213:150, 1980.
6. Antonissen, L. A., et al. Mechanical alterations of airway smooth muscle in a canine asthmatic model. *J. Appl. Physiol.* 46:681, 1979.
7. Anthracite, R. F., Vachon, L., and Knapp, P. H. Alpha adrenergic receptors in the human lung. *Psychomat. Med.* 33:481, 1971.
8. Bach, M. K., Braschlen, J. R., and Gorman, R. R. On the structure of slow-reacting substance of anaphylaxis: Evidence of biosynthesis from arachidonic acid. *Prostaglandins* 14:21, 1977.
9. Barnes, P. J., Wilson, N. M., and Vickers, H. Prazosin, an α_1-adrenoceptor antagonist, partially inhibits exercise-induced asthma. *J. Allergy Clin. Immunol.* 68:411, 1981.
10. Bergen, J. M., and Kroeger, E. A. Isometric tension responses to norepinephrine in canine tracheal smooth muscle (TSM). *Fed. Proc.* 39:1175A, 1980.
11. Berner, P. F., Somlyo, A. V., and Somlyo, A. P. Hypertrophy induced increase of intermediate filaments in vascular smooth muscle. *J. Cell Biol.* 88:96, 1981.
12. Borgeat, P., and Samuelsson, B. Metabolism of arachidonic acid in poly-

morphonuclear leukocytes: Structural analysis of novel hydroxylated compounds. *J. Biol. Chem.* 254:7865, 1979.

13. Boushey, H. A. Acquired hyper-reactivity. In F. E. Hargreave (ed.), Mississauga, Ontario: Astra, 1980. Pp. 145–150.

14. Bradley, S. L., and Russell, J. A. Distribution of histamine H1 and H2 receptors in dog airway smooth muscle (abstract). *Physiologist* 20:11, 1977.

15. Brocklehurst, W. The Action of 5-Hydroxytryptamine on Smooth Muscle. In C. P. Lewis (ed.), *5-Hydroxytryptamine.* London: Pergamon, 1958. Pp. 172–176.

16. Brocklehurst, W. E. J. The release of histamine and formation of a slow-reacting substance (SRS-A) during anaphylactic shock. *J. Physiol. (Lond.)* 151:416, 1960.

17. Brutsaert, D. L., Claes, V. A., and Sonnenblick, E. H. Effects of abrupt load alterations on force-velocity-length and time relations during isotonic contractions of heart muscle: Load clamping. *J. Physiol. (Lond.)* 216:319, 1971.

18. Brutsaert, D. L., and Housmans, P. R. Load-clamp analysis of maximal force potential of mammalian cardiac muscle. *J. Physiol. (Lond.)* 271:587, 1977.

19. Burnstock, G. Purinergic nerves. *Pharmacol. Rev.* 24:509, 1972.

20. Butler, T. M., Siegman, M. J., and Mooers, S. U. Chemical energy usage during shortening and work production in mammalian smooth muscle. *Am. J. Physiol.* 244:C234, 1983.

21. Casterline, C. L., Evans, R., III, and Ward, G. W., Jr. The effect of atropine and albuterol aerosols on the human bronchial response to histamine. *J. Allergy Clin. Immunol.* 58:607, 1976.

22. Dahlen, S. E., et al. Leukotrienes are potent constrictors of human bronchi. *Nature* 288:484, 1980.

23. Dillon, P. F., et al. Myosin phosphorylation and the cross-bridge cycle in arterial smooth muscle. *Science* 211:495, 1981.

24. Douglas, J. S., et al. Airway constriction in guinea pigs: Interaction of histamine and autonomic drugs. *J. Pharmacol. Exp. Ther.* 184:169, 1973.

25. Drazen, J. M. Airway Responses to a Combined Local and Reflex Stimulus. In F. E. Hargreave, (ed.), *Airway Reactivity.* Mississauga, Ontario: Astra, 1980. Pp. 136–142.

26. Drazen, J. M., and Austen, K. F. Effects of intravenous administration of slow-reacting substance of anaphylaxis, histamine, bradykinin and PGF_2 on pulmonary mechanics in the guinea pig. *J. Clin. Invest.* 53:1679, 1974.

27. Drazen, J. M., et al. Comparative airway and vascular activities of leukotrienes C-1 and D in vivo and in vitro. *Proc. Natl. Acad. Sci. USA.* 77:4354, 1980.

28. Everitt, B. J., and Carincross, K. D. Adrenergic receptors in the guinea pig trachea. *J. Pharm. Pharmacol.* 21:97, 1969.

29. Eyre, P. Pulmonary Histamine in H1 and H2 Receptor Studies. In L. M. Lichtenstein and K. F. Austen (eds.), *Asthma: Physiology, Immunopharmacology and Treatment.* New York: Academic, 1977. Vol. 2, p. 169.

30. Feldberg, W., Holden, H. F., and Kellaway, C. H. Formation of lysolecithin and of muscle stimulating substance by snake venoms. *J. Physiol. (Lond.)* 94:232, 1938.

31. Fleisch, J. H., Maling, A. M., and Brodie, B. B. Evidence for existence of alpha-adrenergic receptors in the mammalian trachea. *Am. J. Physiol.* 218:596, 1970.

32. Fleisch, J. H., Kent, K. M., and Cooper, T. Drug Receptors in Smooth Muscle. In L. M. Lichtenstein and K. F. Austen (eds.), *Asthma: Physiology, Immunopharmacology and Treatment.* New York: Academic, 1973. Pp. 139–167.

33. Furchgott, R. F. The pharmacological differentiation of adrenergic receptors. *Ann. N.Y. Acad. Sci.* 139:553, 1967.

34. Gibson, G. J., Tattersfield, A. E., and Pride, N. B. The effects of oral salbutamol on response to inhaled isoprenaline in asthmatic subjects. *Bull. Physiopath. Res.* 8:5657, 1972.

35. Golla, F. L., and Symes, W. L. The reversible action of adrenaline and some kindred drugs on the bronchioles. *J. Pharmacol. Exp. Ther.* 5:87, 1913.

36. Gorecka, A., Aksoy, M. O., and Hartshorne, D. J. The effect of phosphorylation of gizzard myosin on actin activation. *Biochem. Biophys. Res. Commun.* 71:325, 1974.

37. Grodzinska, L., Banczenko, B., and Gruglewski, R. J. Generation of prostaglandin E–like material by the guinea pig trachea contracted by histamine. *J. Pharm. Pharmacol.* 27:88, 1975.

38. Hakansson, C. H., and Toremalm, N. G. Studies on the physiology of the trachea: V. Histology and mechanical activity of the smooth muscles. *Ann. Otol. Rhinol. Laryngol.* 77:255, 1968.

39. Hanks, B. S. R., and Stephens, N. L. Mechanics and energetics of lengthening of active airway smooth muscle. *Am. J. Physiol.* 241:C42, 1981.

40. Hargreave, F. E., et al. Allergen-induced Airway Responses and Relationships with Nonspecific Airway Reactivity. In F. E. Hargreave (ed.), *Airway Reactivity.* Mississauga, Ontario: Astra, 1980. Pp. 145–150.

41. Harvey, J. E., et al. Airway and metabolic responses to intravenous salbutamol in asthma: Effect of regular inhaled salbutamol. *Clin. Sci.* 60:579, 1981.

42. Hill, A. V. *First and Last Experiments in Muscle Mechanics.* Cambridge: Cambridge University Press, 1970.

43. Hill, A. V. The heat of shortening and the dynamic constants of muscle. *Proc. R. Soc. Lond. [Biol.]* 126:136, 1938–1939.

44. Hogg, J. C., et al. Distribution of airway resistance with developing pulmonary edema in dogs. *J. Appl. Physiol.* 32:20, 1972.

45. Holgate, S. H., Baldwin, C. J., Tattersfield, A. T. Beta-adrenergic agonist resistance in normal human airways. *Lancet* 2:375, 1977.

46. Holme, G., and Piechuta, H. The derivation of an inbred line of rats which develop asthmalike symptoms following challenge with aerosolized antigen. *Immunology* 42:19, 1981.

47. Holtzman, M., et al. Effect of ganglionic blockade on bronchial reactivity in atopic subjects. *Am. Rev. Respir. Dis.* 122:17, 1980.

48. Horwits, R., et al. A physiological role for titin and nebulin in skeletal muscle. *Nature* 323:160, 1986.

49. Irvin, C. G., et al. Bronchodilatation: Non-cholinergic, nonadrenergic mediation demonstrated in vivo in the cat. *Science* 107:791, 1980.

50. Itkin, I. H., and Anand, S. C. The role of atropine as a mediator blocker of induced bronchial obstruction. *J. Allergy* 45:178, 1970.

51. Jakschik, B. A., Falkenstein, S., and Parker, C. W. Precursor role of arachidonic acid in release of slow reacting substance from rat basophilic leukaemia cells. *Proc. Natl. Acad. Sci. USA* 74:4577, 1977.

52. Jenne, J., et al. Induction of β-receptor tolerance by terbutaline. *J. Allergy Clin. Immunol.* 55:96, 1975.

53. Jewell, B. R., and Wilkie, D. R. The mechanical properties of relaxating muscle. *J. Physiol. (Lond.)* 152:30, 1960.

54. Jewell, B. R. Discussion of S. R. Taylor, Decreased Activation in Skeletal Muscle Fibers at Short Lengths. In R. Porter and D. W. Fitzsimons (eds.), *The Physiological Basis of Startlings' Law of the Heart.* Ciba Symposium 24 (new series). London: Elsevier/Excerpta, Medica/North Holland, 1974. Pp. 93–116.

55. Johansson, R., Hellstrand, P., and Uvelius, B. Responses of smooth muscle to quick load change studied at high time resolution. *Blood Vessels* 15:65, 1978.

56. Kapanci, Y., Costabello, P. M., and Gabbiani, G. Location and Function of Contractile Interstitial Cells of the Lungs. In A. Bouhuys (ed.), *Lung Cells in Disease.* New York: Elsevier/North Holland, 1976. Pp. 69–84.

57. Keighley, J. F. Iatrogenic asthma associated with adrenergic aerosols. *Ann. Intern. Med.* 65:985, 1966.

58. Kellaway, C. H., and Trethewie, E. R. Liberation of slow-reacting smooth muscle-stimulating substance in anaphylaxis. *Q. J. Exp. Physiol.* 30:121, 1940.

59. Kepron, W., et al. A canine model for reaginic hypersensitivity and allergic bronchoconstriction. *J. Allergy Clin. Immunol.* 59:64, 1977.

60. Kneussel, M. P., and Richardson, J. B. Alpha-adrenergic receptors in human and canine tracheal and bronchial smooth muscle. *J. Appl. Physiol.* 45:307, 1978.

61. Kong, S. K., and Stephens, N. L. Pharmacological studies of sensitized canine pulmonary blood vessels. *J. Pharmacol. Exp. Ther.* 219:551, 1981.

62. Kroeger, E. A., and Stephens, N. L. Effect of hypoxia on energy and calcium metabolism in airway smooth muscle. *Am. J. Physiol.* 220:1199, 1971.

63. Kroeger, E. A., and Stephens, N. L. Effect of tetraethylammonium on tonic airway smooth muscle: Initiation of phasic electrical activity. *Am. J. Physiol.* 228:633, 1975.

64. Kunos, G., and Szentivanyi, M. Evidence favouring the existence of a single adrenergic receptor. *Nature* 217:1077, 1968.

65. Levitt, R. C., and Mitzner, W. Expression of airway hyperreactivity to acetylcholine as a simple autosomal recessive trait in mice. *FASEB J.* 2:2605, 1988.

66. Lewis, R. A., et al. Identification of the C(6)-S-conjugate of leukotriene A with cysteine as a naturally occurring slow-reacting substance of anaphylaxis (SRS-A). Importance of the 11-cis-geometry for biological activity. *Biochem. Biophys. Res. Commun.* 96:271, 1980.

67. Lichtenstein, L. M., and Gillespie, E. Histamine receptors—inhibition of histamine release is controlled by an H2 receptor. *Nature* 244:287, 1973.

68. Lulich, K. M., Mitchell, H. W., and Sparrow, M. P. The cat lung strip as an in vitro preparation of peripheral airways: A comparison of alpha-adrenoceptor agonists, autocoids and anaphylactic challenge on the lung strip and trachea. *Br. J. Pharmacol.* 58:71, 1976.

69. Miller, M. D., and Marshall, J. M. Uterine response to nerve stimulation: Relation to hormonal status and catecholamines. *Am. J. Physiol.* 209:859, 1976.

70. Moreno, R. H., Hogg, J. C., and Pare, P. D. Mechanics of airway narrowing. *Am. Rev. Respir. Dis.* 133:1171, 1980.

71. Mrwa, U., and Ruegg, J. C. Myosin-linked calcium regulation in vascular smooth muscle. *FEBS Lett.* 60:81, 1975.

72. Mulvany, M. J. The undamped and damped series elastic components of a vascular smooth muscle. *Biophys. J.* 26:401, 1979.

73. Murphy, R. C., Hammerstrom, S., and Samuelsson, B. Leukotriene C: A slow-reacting substance from murine mastocytoma cells. *Proc. Natl. Acad. Sci. USA* 76:4275, 1979.

74. Olson, C. R., et al. Structural basis for decreased compressibility of constricted trachea and bronchi during muscular contraction. *J. Appl. Physiol.* 23:35–39, 1967.

75. Orange, R. P., et al. The physiochemical characteristics and purification of slow-reacting substance of anaphylaxis. *J. Immunol.* 110:760, 1973.

76. Orange, R. P., Valentine, M. D., and Austen, K. F. Antigen induced release of slow-reacting substance of anaphylaxis (SRS-A rat) in rats prepared with homologous antibody. *J. Exp. Med.* 127:767, 1968.

77. Orehek, J., Douglas, J. S., and Bouhuys, A. Contractile responses of the guinea pig trachea in vitro: Modification by prostaglandin synthesis inhibiting drugs. *J. Pharmacol. Exp. Ther.* 194:554, 1975.

78. Orehek, J., et al. Prostaglandin regulation in airway smooth muscle tone. *Nature [New Biol.]* 245:84, 1973.

79. Paterson, J. W., Evans, R. J. C., and Prime, F. J. Selectivity of bronchodilator action of salbutamol in asthmatic patients. *Br. J. Dis. Chest* 65:22, 1971.

80. Rasmussen, H., Tukuwd, Y., and Park, S. Protein kinase C in the regulation of smooth muscle contraction. *FASEB J.* 1(3):177, 1987.

81. Richardson, J. B. The Neural Control of Human Tracheobronchial Smooth Muscle. In L. M. Lichtenstein and K. F. Austen (eds.), *Asthma: Physiology, Immunopharmacology and Treatment.* New York: Academic, 1977. Pp. 237–247.

82. Roach, M. R., and Burton, A. C. The reason for the shape of the distensibility curves of arteries. *Can. J. Biochem. Physiol.* 35:681, 1957.

83. Rudel, R., and Taylor, S. R. Striated muscle fibers: Facilitation of contraction at short lengths by caffeine. *Science* 172:387, 1971.

84. Russell, J. A. Responses of isolated canine airways to electric stimulation and acetylcholine. *J. Appl. Physiol.* 45:690, 1978.

85. Russell, J. A. Innervation of beta-adrenergic receptors in airway smooth muscle of dog. *Fed. Proc.* 37:81A, 1978.

86. Sasaki, H., and Hoppin, F. G., Jr. Hysteresis of contracted airway smooth muscle. *J. Appl. Physiol.* 47:1251, 1979.

87. Siegman, N. J., Butler, T. M., Mooers, S. U., and Davies, R. E. Mechanical and Energetic Correlates of Isometric Relaxation. In R. Casteels, T. Godfraind, and J. C. Ruegg (eds.). *Excitation-Contraction Coupling in Smooth Muscle.* New York: Elsevier/North-Holland, 1977. Pp. 449–453.

88. Simonsson, B. G., Jacobs, F. M., and Nadel, J. A. Role of autonomic nervous system and the cough reflex in the increased responsiveness of airways in patients with obstructive airway disease. *J. Clin. Invest.* 46:1812, 1967.

89. Simonsson, B. G., et al. In vivo and in vitro studies on alpha-receptors in human airway: Potentiation with bacterial endotoxin. *Scand. J. Respir. Dis.* 53:227, 1972.

90. Smedegard, G., et al. Leukotriene C4 affects pulmonary and cardiovascular dynamics in monkey. *Nature* 295:327, 1982.

91. Souhrada, J. F., and Dickey, D. C. Effect of antigen challenge on sensitized guinea pig trachea. *Respir. Physiol.* 27:241, 1976.

92. Souhrada, J. F., and Loader, J. Changes of Airway Smooth Muscle in Experimental Asthma. In M. A. deKock, J. A. Nadel, and C. M. Lewis (eds.), *Mechanisms of Airways Obstruction in Human Respiratory Disease.* Capetown: A. A. Balkema, 1979. Pp. 195–207.

93. Stephens, N. L. The Mechanics of Isolated Airway Smooth Muscle. In A. Bouhuys (ed.), *Airway Dynamics.* Springfield, Ill.: Thomas, 1970. Pp. 191–208.

94. Stephens, N. L. Mechanism of Action of Hypoxia in Tracheal Smooth Muscle (TSM) with a Note on the Role of the Series Elastic Component. In E. Betz (ed.), *Vascular Smooth Muscle.* Berlin: Springer, 1972. Pp. 153–156.

95. Stephens, N. L. Physical properties of contractile systems. In E. E. Daniel and D. M. Paton (eds.), *Methods in Pharmacology.* Vol. 3 *Smooth Muscle.* New York: Plenum, 1975. Pp. 165–196.

96. Stephens, N. L. Airway Smooth Muscle: Biophysics, Biochemistry and Pharmacology. In L. M. Lichtenstein and K. F. Austen (eds.) *Asthma: Physiology, Immunopharmacology and Treatment.* New York: Academic, 1977. Pp. 147–167.

97. Stephens, N. L., Kagan, M. L., and Packer, C. S. Time dependence of shortening velocity in tracheal smooth muscle. *Am. J. Physiol.* 251:C435, 1980.

98. Stephens, N. L., and Kroeger, E. A. Ultrastructure, biophysics and biochemistry of airway smooth muscle. In J. A. Nadel (ed.), *Physiology and Pharmacology of the Airways.* New York: Marcel Dekker, 1980. Pp. 31–121.

99. Stephens, N. L., Kroeger, E. A., and Mehta, J. A. Force-velocity characteristics of respiratory airway smooth muscle. *J. Appl. Physiol.* 26:685, 1969.

100. Stephens, N. L., and Kromer, U. Series elastic component of tracheal smooth muscle. *Am. J. Physiol.* 220:1890, 1971.

101. Stephens, N. L., Mitchell, R., and Brutsaert, D. L. Nature of Contractile Unit: Shortening Inactivation, Maximum Force Potential, Relaxation, Contractility. In N. L. Stephens (ed.), *Smooth Muscle Contraction.* New York: Marcel Dekker, in press.

102. Stephens, N. L., and Van Niekerk, W. Isometric and isotonic contractions in airway smooth muscle. *Can. J. Physiol. Pharmacol.* 55:933, 1977.

103. Svedmyr, N., Larsson, A. L., and Thiringer, G. K. Development of "resistance" in beta adrenergic receptors of asthmatic patients. *Chest* 69:479, 1976.

104. Swynghedauw, B. Development and functional adaptation of contractile proteins in cardiac and skeletal muscle. *Physiol. Rev.* 66:710, 1986.

105. Uchida, Y., et al. Endothelin: a novel vasoconstrictor peptide as potent bronchoconstrictor. *Eur. J. Pharmacol.* 154:227, 1988.

106. Szentivanyi, A. The β-adrenergic theory of the atopic abnormality in bronchial asthma. *J. Allergy* 42:203, 1968.

107. Tashkin, D. P., et al. Subsensitization of β-adrenoceptors in airways and lymphocytes of healthy and asthmatic subjects. *Am. Rev. Respir. Dis.* 125:185, 1982.

108. Taylor, S. R. Decreased Activation in Skeletal Muscle Fibers at Short Lengths. In R. Porter and D. W. Fitzsimons (eds.), *The Physiological Basis of Startling's Law of the Heart.* Ciba Symposium 24 (new series). London: Elsevier/Excerpta, Medica North Holland, 1974. Pp. 93–116.

109. Wang, H., and Ramirez-Mitchell, C. A network of transverse and longitudinal intermediate filaments is associated with sarcomeres of adult vertebrate skeletal muscle. *J. Cell Biol.* 96:562, 1983.

110. Wang, Z., Seow, C. Y., and Stephens, N. L. Mechanical properties of isolated canine coronary artery. *FASEB J.* 2(4):A333, 1988.

111. Wang, Z., and Stephens, N. L. Normally cycling and latchbridges in venous smooth muscle. *Blood Vessels.* 26:272, 1989.

112. Wardlaw, A. C. Inheritance of responsiveness to pertussis HSF in mice. *Int. Allergy* 38:573, 1970.

113. Weiss, J. W., et al. Bronchoconstrictor effects of leukotriene C in humans. *Science* 216:196, 1982.

114. Woledge, R. C. The energetics of tortoise muscle. *J. Physiol. (Lond.)* 155:685, 1968.

115. Xu, J., et al. Mechanical properties of inbred hyperactive rat trachealis. *FASEB J.* 4(3):A269, 1990.

Physiology and Gas Exchange

Adrian J. Williams

26

Asthma, although a disease of airways, causes derangements in virtually all aspects of lung function [9, 18, 49, 59, 75a, 113, 114, 121, 126], spanning the breadth of severity. Therapy of a severe episode will lead through multiple phases, varying from widespread obstruction, through small airways dysfunction, to complete normality [18, 113]. Typical changes may be summarized as follows: Attendant on airways obstruction, there is an increase in total lung capacity (TLC) along with a much greater increase in residual volume (RV); the maximum expiratory flow volume shows severe obstruction; specific conductance is reduced along with conductance at all lung volumes despite hyperinflation; and ventilation-perfusion ($\dot{V}/\dot{Q}$) relationships are deranged with consequential alterations in gas exchange. These events are the subject of this chapter, and are summarized in Figure 26-1.

PHYSIOLOGIC CONSIDERATIONS

Lung Compliance or Distensibility

The lungs are elastic structures. Since they are encased in a closed and relatively rigid thorax, they tend to retract from the chest wall, creating a negative pressure in the pleural space [1]. This is really a potential space, because under normal conditions the visceral pleura that covers the lung and the parietal pleura that lines the thoracic wall are separated by a very thin film of lubricating fluid [2].

The strength of retraction of the lung, i.e., the elastic recoil, is related to the degree of stretching of the lungs. That is, the greater the lung volume, the greater the elastic recoil; therefore, the more negative is the intrapleural pressure.

The slope of the line relating the change in lung volume to the change in the distending or transpulmonary pressure ($\Delta V/\Delta P$) is termed *lung compliance* or *distensibility*, and it is measured in liters per cmH₂O. The relationship between lung volume and pressure is not constant. At lower lung volumes, a large volume change is associated with a small pressure change—the compliance is high; that is, the lung is distensible. At high lung volumes, a small volume change is associated with a huge pressure change—the compliance is low; that is, the lung is stiff [137]. Pressure-volume relationships in normal subjects are depicted in Figure 26-2; note that, in some asthmatics with prolonged bronchospasm, a reversible leftward and upward shift in the pressure-volume relationship has been observed.

Airflow Resistance

When pressure is measured during breathing, there is a greater pressure change than is required to overcome the elasticity of the lung alone. The additional pressure is needed to overcome the friction between molecules of the gas and between the gas molecules and the airway wall—i.e., the resistance to airflow offered by the airways [107], which is influenced by the flow rate, caliber of the airways, the nature of the gas breathed, and the type of flow (turbulent or laminar). Thus, to move air, the pressure created is dissipated in overcoming elasticity and resistance (inertia is negligible). Both elasticity and resistance can be directly measured during submaximal respiratory maneuvers (elasticity as compliance, and airways resistance by relating alveolar pressure to airflow using a body plethysmograph). They can also be derived indirectly from maximal respiratory efforts, i.e., spirometry (Fig. 26-3) and its derivative, the maximum expiratory flow-volume curve (MEFVC).

Spirometry is technically simple to perform and consequently is widely applied, but, despite this experience, the findings yielded are difficult to interpret completely because the method is influenced by a variety of factors; these include airway caliber, the elastic recoil of the lung, the volume of air in communication, the muscle power generated, and the level of patient cooperation. The determinants of maximum flow are most simply considered, however, as an interplay of airways resistance and static recoil. Isovolume pressure-flow curves have been useful in examining the relationships between intrathoracic pressure, lung volume, and airflow [51] (Fig. 26-4). The maximum flow for each lung volume (at lung volumes of less than 78% vital capacity [VC]) shows that flow is independent of the effort applied. At critical intrathoracic pressures, further increases in the pressure driving airflow (alveolar pressure) are counterbalanced by increasing airways resistance (created by increases in the pleural pressure surrounding the intrathoracic airways). This was eloquently expounded by Mead and associates [91] as the Equal Pressure Point Theory, along with Pride and colleagues [112], and was more "scientifically" defined by the Choke Point Theory proposed by Dawson and Elliott [36].

The very simplicity of spirometry makes it the most commonly used measurement, but it is important to stress quality control issues. The device used must meet published standards [35, 52, 152], including a starting point for the spirogram that is back-extrapolated from the steep portion of the curve to correct for inertia, along with the performance of three adequate maneuvers and selection of the "curve" with the highest sum of forced vital capacity (FVC) and forced expiratory volume (FEV) [52, 101, 129]. The ratio of FEV to FVC, when reduced, is a specific index for airways obstruction [97]. Other measurements from the spirogram are useful but subject to wider normal ranges, such as midflow rates, or to effort dependence, such as the peak flow rate [97], which is consequently not recommended by the American Thoracic Society [45] for diagnostic use.

Factors other than equipment or technique also influence the results of spirometry. The time of day can affect flow rates [6, 30,

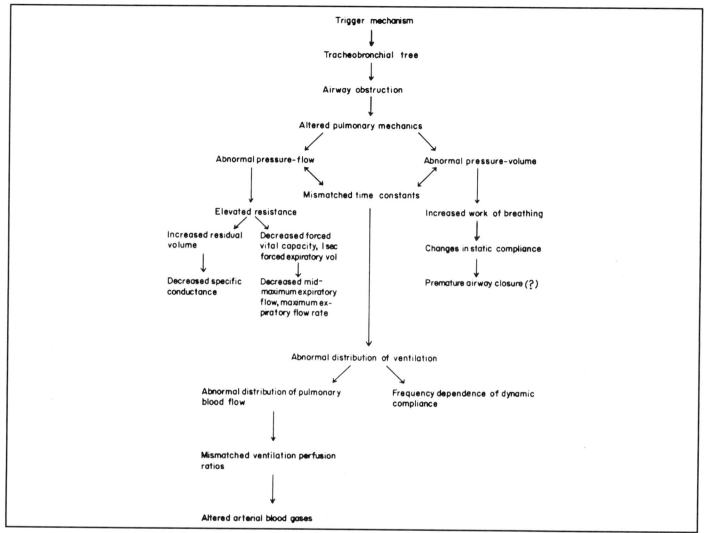

Fig. 26-1. *Diagram of the functional defects that are seen during an acute exacerbation of asthma and their interrelations. A complete explanation is given in the text.*

34]. Such a circadian rhythm was shown by Hetzel and Clark [63], who demonstrated that the peak flow varies by 8 percent about the mean in normal individuals and also that this circadian effect was exaggerated in asthmatics whose peak flow rates varied by 50 percent about the mean. They further proposed that such excess variability could be used as a diagnostic standard for asthma, suggesting as abnormal a variability of greater than 20 percent about the mean [62].

The effect of the deep inspiration prior to forced expiration on airway caliber has also been studied. In normal subjects with induced bronchoconstriction, transient bronchodilatation (of 1–2 minutes' duration) is seen [100, 106], and this effect may occur mainly in peripheral airways [13]. However, although some asthmatics may respond in this way, it is more usual that little change occurs, or indeed that bronchoconstriction results [105, 153]. Froeb and Mead [50] wondered if the airways and parenchyma had different hysteresis patterns, such that when airway exceeds lung bronchodilation results, while when lung exceeds airway bronchoconstriction results. Whether this may also be due to vagal reflexes [150] is unclear. Most recently, a calcium channel blocker has been shown to attenuate the bronchoconstriction induced by deep inspiration.

Distribution of Ventilation

The facility with which a lung unit ventilates depends on the resistance to airflow into that unit (R) and on the compliance or distensibility of the unit (C). The product of resistance and compliance ($R \times C$) has the dimension of time, and is called the *time constant*. The greater the time constant of a lung unit, the lower its ventilation. The lung can be considered as being made up of millions of lung units, each with its own time constant. When the lungs are normal, all the units have similar short time constants. When disease is present, not all units are affected to the same degree, such that some units will have relatively normal time constants and others will have abnormal time constants. Thus, in the presence of disease, because not all units have the same time constants, ventilation will be unevenly distributed (Fig. 26-5). Distributional inhomogeneity seen in acute asthma is well depicted in classic simple nitrogen washout curve analysis (Fig. 26-6).

Collateral Ventilation

Access of gas to air spaces beyond collapsed or closed airways in chronic airflow obstruction may be possible through collateral channels such as the pores of Kohn [38, 93]. This mechanism presumably accounts for the rarity of atelectasis in chronic airflow obstruction. However, ventilation via the collateral channels is inefficient because of the increased distance required for molecular diffusion. This results in impaired gas mixing. In addition, the air going into the collaterally ventilated unit has also traversed the normal unit, and so has already taken part in gas exchange. Thus, the air going into the collaterally ventilated unit will have a higher partial pressure of carbon dioxide (PCO_2) and a low partial pressure of oxygen (PO_2). This unit thus appears to be hypoventilating relative to the normal unit.

PHYSIOLOGIC CONSEQUENCES

Reduced Flow Rates

The hallmark of asthma is short-term variability of airway narrowing, especially in the early hours of the morning [63]. Studies of the acute reaction to antigen challenge have helped expand the understanding of the physiologic events and consequences of bronchoconstriction alone (with the recognition that, in more prolonged attacks, plugging of the airways with mucus is an important factor). From these studies, it has been appreciated that asymptomatic subjects have residual physiologic abnormalities [12], and that in symptomatic subjects there is increased airways resistance (up by 50%) [60] with consequential reduced expiratory flow. Along with this, there is some airway closure [85, 89] and hyperinflation [70, 81, 92, 148, 151], as evidenced by an increase in the RV along with functional residual capacity (FRC), and a reduction in VC. TLC changes less, if at all (the demonstrated increase may be due to measurement errors; see later discussion). Recent work has also suggested "that moderate amounts of airway wall thickening, which have little effect on baseline resistance, can profoundly affect the airway narrowing caused by smooth muscle shortening" and that such "airway wall thickening (and a loss of lung recoil) can partially explain the airway hyperresponsiveness observed in patients with asthma" [145a].

Fig. 26-2. *Static pressure-volume curves showing the shift in slope that can occur with asthma. By moving to a new relationship, air can be moved with less work.*

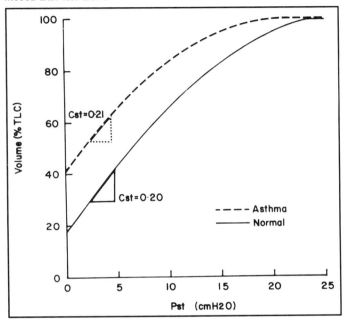

Fig. 26-3. *Spirometry. A. A maximum expiration showing the forced vital capacity (FVC) and 1-second forced expiratory volume (FEV₁). The former is the absolute amount of air that can be expelled irrespective of time, whereas the latter is the volume expired in 1 second. B. Maximum midexpiratory flow rate (MMF), defined as the slope of a line connecting the first and last quarter of a forced vital capacity, and as such it represents the flow rate in the mid-vital capacity range. C. Maximum expiratory flow rate (MEFR), defined as a slope of a line tangent to the steepest part of a forced vital capacity. It represents the maximum flow that can be achieved. The first 200 cc of expiration is ignored because it represents the acceleration of gas in the instrument tubing, etc. (Adapted from R. C. Kory, et al., Clinical spirometry. Dis. Chest 43:1963.)*

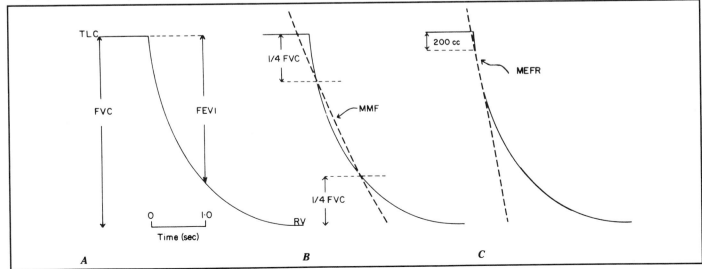

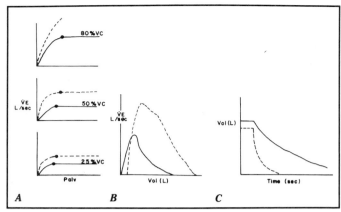

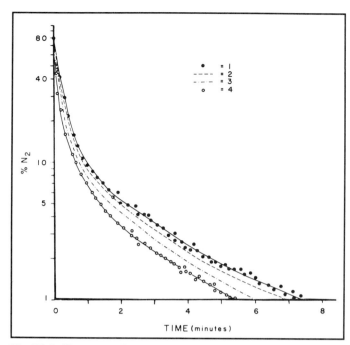

Fig. 26-4. *A. Isovolume pressure-flow curves at 80, 50, and 25 percent of the vital capacity (VC) in the normal state (broken line) and during an asthma attack (solid line). The black circles represent P_{alv}'. B. Maximum expiratory flow volume curves. By expressing the ordinate in absolute terms, one can appreciate that during an episode of asthma (solid curve), even though the patient starts from a higher volume, lung emptying is severely impaired. The point at which flow stops indicates the new residual volume. C. Spirogram. The same phenomenon occurs as outlined in B, but here it is expressed as a function of time.*

Fig. 26-6. *Nitrogen washout curves in a patient with asthma. The numbers 1 through 4 represent data that were collected serially from the time of acute illness until the patient had recovered (4 = recovery.)*

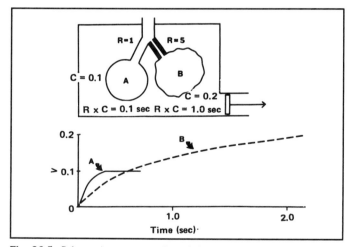

Fig. 26-5. *Schematic representation of time constant discrepancies in parallel lung units and the effects of time-dependent behavior. (R = resistance; C = compliance.) Unit B has a time constant 10 times that of unit A. If a square wave of negative pressure is created in the box by pulling the plunger, unit B fills more slowly because of its increased resistance. If the pressure is maintained over time, unit B fills more than A because of its increased compliance. Thus, rapid maneuvers magnify resistive abnormalities, and slow or maintained maneuvers amplify compliance abnormalities. (Reprinted with permission from E. R. McFadden and R. H. Ingram. Clinical Application and Interpretation of Airway Physiology. In J. Nadel (ed.), Physiology and Pharmacology of the Airways. New York: Dekker, 1980.)*

In addition, since it is known that some airways are closed at TLC [43, 44], it is therefore likely that more will be closed during expiration, which may explain the increased convexity of the MEFVC just after the peak flow (the "contraction" of the flow-volume curve). Other mechanisms seem less likely. Widespread airway narrowing without airway closure would lead to a reduction in the slope of the MEFVC with little change in the VC. If there

were complete closure of some airways while others remained normal, a parallel shift in the MEFVC would result [103]. Progressive closure of many airways would also explain the increase in RV.

The airway narrowing of asthma leads to the generation of an increase in negative pressure and, as a consequence, to an increase in the airway size (by radial tension on intrapulmonary airways), which increases the work of breathing [90, 144] (Fig. 26-7). Static pressure-volume curves illustrate this. The thorax is held in an inspiratory position to maintain equivalent flows, which is achieved by use of the accessory muscles of respiration. The reader can easily appreciate how tiring this can be by the simple experiment of breathing spontaneously at a higher-than-normal FRC.

Localization of Airflow Obstruction
Many attempts have been made to define the site of airway narrowing, whether predominantly in the large or small airways. In 1972, Despas and associates [37], using a helium-oxygen mixture (Fig. 26-8), found that maximum flow does not increase in some asthmatics, a feature particularly true of smokers [3] and indicative of airflow limitation in the peripheral airways [72]. An increased loss of density dependence has been shown with increasing disease severity [15, 28, 46]. However, a complete understanding of the usual change in asthmatics is difficult to reach because the disease itself is so variable.

Upper airway changes are also postulated. Collett and coworkers [33] have reported that, in 12 asymptomatic asthmatics given histamine or water by inhalation, expiratory flow was reduced to 36 percent along with a reduction in glottic cross-sectional area up to 45 percent. Continuous positive airway pressure of 10 cm H_2O abolished the glottic constriction. Others have also noted changes in the glottic area in asthmatics [67, 120] and in normal subjects given histamine [66].

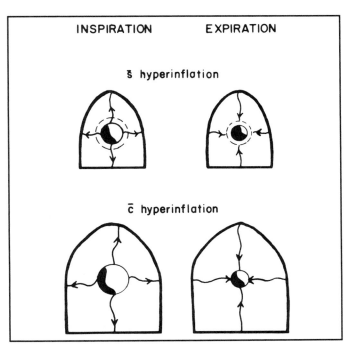

Fig. 26-7. *The effect of an episode of asthma on airway caliber, and the compensations brought about by hyperinflation. The broken circles represent the normal resting airway dimensions during inspiration and expiration. The arrows indicate the direction of the dilating or compressive forces. When asthma strikes, bronchoconstriction and intraluminal obstruction combine to decrease the lumen of the airways. Hyperinflation of the lung compensates for this by increasing the lateral traction on the walls of the bronchi, thereby enlarging their intrinsic caliber.*

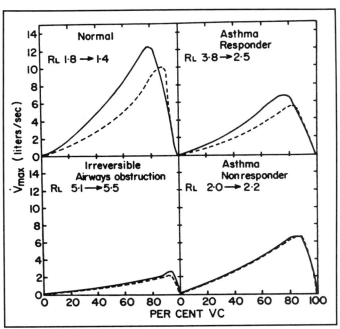

Fig. 26-8. *Representative maximum expiratory flow-volume curves while breathing air (broken lines) and He-O_2 mixture (solid lines) for normal subject, patient with COPD (irreversible airway obstruction), and asthmatic subjects with (responder) and without (nonresponder) density dependence of maximum flow ($\dot{V}_{max}$). Pulmonary resistance (R_L) in cmH$_2$O·liter^{-1}·s indicated (air $\rightarrow$ He-O$_2$) for each subject. Volume measured with subject in body plethysmograph and expressed as percent of vital capacity (VC) remaining to be expired. (Adapted from P. J. Despas, M. Leroux, and P. T. Macklem, Site of airway obstruction in asthma as determined by measuring maximum expiratory flow breathing air and a helium-oxygen mixture. J. Clin. Invest. 51:3235, 1972.)*

Reversibility of Airflow Obstruction

The diagnosis of asthma rests heavily on the reversibility of airflow obstruction, and therefore a consideration of the physiologic definition is appropriate. Aside from historical evidence of reversible airways obstruction (of, for example, intermittent severe wheezing on exposure to aeroallergens), such diagnostic information may consist of exaggerated peak flow variability [6], response to inhaled bronchodilator [69, 77, 108], or response to a trial of corticosteroids. The most studied is the response to inhaled bronchodilators. The question of what constitutes a significant increase in flow rates over any that might occur spontaneously within a testing period was answered by Pennock [108], who established that, on repeat testing, a mean change in FVC or FEV of 5 percent was seen, with a maximum ($+2$ S.D.) of 9.5 percent. This implies that a change in the FVC or FEV of greater than 10 percent is statistically significant. However, experience gathered over time has led to a consensus that changes equal to or greater than 15 percent are more indicative of true asthma. Such a change may occur in the measured lung volume or the flow rates, or both. Ramsdell and Tisi [115] found that one-third of the significant changes were in volume alone, with the potential therefore for worsening of the FVC/FEV ratio [55, 80, 147]. Recommended criteria for bronchodilator responses are summarized in Table 26-1.

Other tests of reversibility are more sensitive. The plethysmographic determination of airway resistance [17, 80] avoids the problems of dynamic airway compression and, in a recent study, was shown to identify on additional 15 percent of patients with reversible airway obstruction—patients who reported subjective

Table 26-1. *Recommended criteria for response to a bronchodilator in adults*

Organization	FVC (%)	FEV$_1$ (%)	FEF$_{25-75\%}$ (%)	Comments
American College of Chest Physicians	15–25	15–25	15–25	% of baseline in at least two of three tests
Intermountain Thoracic Society	15	12	45	% of baseline
American Thoracic Society	12	12	—	% of baseline and an absolute change of 200 ml

FVC = forced vital capacity; FEV$_1$ = 1-second forced expiratory volume; FEF$_{25-75\%}$ = mean forced expiratory flow during middle half of FVC.
Source: Medical Section of the American Lung Association. Lung function testing. *Am. Rev. Respir. Dis.* 144:1202, 1991. Reprinted with permission.

benefit after bronchodilator treatment despite no objective spirometric improvement [126a]. The isovolume midflow rate (i.e., the slope of the MEFVC at the same volume below TLC) is another [32, 104], but is subject to a wider range of normal values. However, changes in the FEV and FVC remain the most useful indicators [79].

Lung Volumes

Many studies have demonstrated abnormal lung volumes in asthma [12, 61, 79, 148]. Typically, the VC is reduced while others (RV, TLC) are increased, along with an increase in the RV/TLC ratio. As noted before, hyperinflation reduces airway resistance, but at the expense of increased "elastic" work. Some controversy about this exists, however. Measurements yielded by body plethysmography are greater than those from helium dilution [151] because the body "box" may overestimate volumes [20, 32, 61, 79, 87, 104, 125, 192]. In this method, pressure changes at the mouth (which equal the alveolar pressure) are plotted against box pressure changes (calibrated as volume changes) during panting. The slope of the relationship gives a measure of FRC [42]. With airways obstruction, mouth pressure does not equal alveolar pressure, and an overestimate results [20–22, 125]. This can be corrected for by substituting the esophageal pressure for mouth pressure.

Additionally, abdominal gas contributes to the total (and thus thoracic) gas volume [23, 58], but Dubois [14, 41] has concluded that the original studies of lung volume are valid. Changes in abdominal pressure are small [23, 58], and the important problem is poor transmission of alveolar pressure to the mouth in the presence of airways obstruction [14, 20].

The increases in RV and FRC are quite characteristic [87, 148]. The elevation in FRC may be related to progressive airway closure [111] because, during the acute event, the RV often exceeds the patient's normal FRC. Tachypnea accompanying the episode may be an added adverse factor, but the precise mechanisms leading to hyperinflation are poorly understood. One major cause is an increase in the tonic activity of the inspiratory muscles [84]. This activity results in a higher lung volume with a greater tissue radial traction force on the airway favoring its patency. Nevertheless, a mechanical disadvantage may ensue when breathing occurs at such markedly elevated lung volumes. Concurrently, this phenomenon may also be responsible for the development of the severe dyspnea that patients with advanced asthma experience. For example, Permutt [109] has pointed out that an increase in the FRC of 2.5 liters leads to an 11-fold rise in the inspiratory work of breathing, thereby contributing to the sensation of clinical dyspnea. The increased inspiratory muscle force needed to overcome the larger elastic recoil of the lungs and thorax at these high volumes also explains the sternocleidomastoid muscle retraction observed in severe asthma. That the diaphragm may also be actively involved in maintaining an increased lung volume has been reported by Muller and associates [98] during experimental histamine-induced hyperinflation.

Another factor in allowing the increase in lung volumes is the loss of some elastic recoil, as reported by Gold and coworkers [56] and others [48, 54, 86, 149]. This results in a shift in the volume-pressure curve up and to the left (see Fig. 26-2). Compliance (the slope near FRC) is, however, the same or even decreased [5, 47, 109], and the change reverses with treatment [48, 89]. This could be explained by stress relaxation due to prolonged air trapping or reducing surface forces [54]. Closure of peripheral airways may, by the closing of lung units, limit their contribution to the elastic recoil [82].

The patterns of abnormal lung volumes in acute asthma (Fig. 26-9) are therefore those of large elevations in RV and FRC (of the order of 378 ± 21% and 222 ± 113%, respectively) with more modest rises in TLC (124 ± 38%). With recovery, RV (141 ± 83%) and FRC (140 ± 47%) are still abnormal, whereas the TLC is normal. This, of course, implies persistent obstruction with a potential for maldistribution of air and hypoxemia [78]. These figures will go some way to underline the variability of these findings.

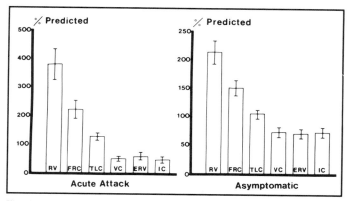

Fig. 26-9. *Pattern of abnormalities seen in lung volumes during an acute episode of asthma and after recovery. (RV = residual volume; FRC = functional residual capacity; TLC = total lung capacity; VC = vital capacity; ERV = expiratory reserve volume; IC = inspiratory capacity.) The height of the bars indicates mean values and the brackets, the standard error.*

Large changes in intrathoracic pressure with the increased work of breathing and alterations in cardiac preload and afterload may occur [146]. The inspiratory reduction in intrathoracic pressure is transmitted to the heart, resulting in a proportional inspiratory reduction in intracardiac pressures. When this occurs, the left ventricle may not develop enough increased force on the subsequent beat to maintain arterial pressure, and blood pressure may drop transiently with each inspiration, returning to its previous level at expiration. This phenomenon is known as *pulsus paradoxus;* its magnitude has been shown to be roughly proportional to the severity of obstruction [124]. Measurement of TLC during acute asthma may also be obtained by planimetric radiography [16].

Gas Exchange

The advanced airway obstruction leads to gross maldistribution of inspired air, with adverse effects on $\dot{V}/\dot{Q}$ relationships, and hence on arterial blood gases and pH. Airway obstruction in asthma is not uniform throughout the lungs; there is preferential distribution of ventilation to areas with the least involvement, leaving obstructed regions relatively hypoventilated. Local hypoxic vasoconstriction results in redistribution of blood flow to some extent, but this compensation is imperfect and V/Q inequality can result, with subsequent hypoxemia.

The abnormal gas exchange in asthma has been reviewed recently by Wagner and Rodriguez-Roisin [139]. In asymptomatic asthma, the following were noted: (1) A well-preserved arterial $PO_2(PaO_2)$; (2) considerable V/Q mismatch, often apparent as a clear population of low V/Q units; (3) absence of shunt; (4) lack of improvement in response to potent bronchodilators that simultaneously normalize airflow rates; and (5) dissociation between airflow rate and gas exchange abnormalities. The altered distribution of ventilation and perfusion has been shown by Wagner and coworkers [140] using the multiple inert gas infusion technique. In experimental animal models, mild asthma resulted in a broader than normal unimodal pattern of V/Q distribution, but, in more severe bronchospasm, a bimodal pattern is seen whereby collateral ventilation to areas occluded by mucous plugs leads to very low V/Q values (Fig. 26-10). In patients with acute severe asthma [8, 53, 134] or chronic symptomatic asthma

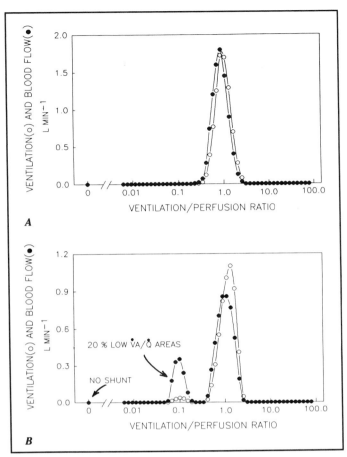

Fig. 26-10. *A. Distribution of ventilation-perfusion ratios in an upright, young, normal subject. There is little inequality evident and, in particular, no areas of very low or very high ventilation-perfusion ratio. Shunt is absent. B. An example of the distribution of ventilation-perfusion ratios in an asthmatic subject. Note the separate population of areas of low ventilation-perfusion ratio distinct from the main mode. The size of the low ratio of alveolar ventilation to perfusion ($\dot{V}_A/\dot{Q}$) varies considerably among individuals, but it commonly comprises about 20 percent of the cardiac output, as indicated. Shunt is notably absent in most patients with asthma. (Reprinted with permission from P. D. Wagner, Clinical advances in pulmonary gas exchange. Am. Rev. Respir. Dis. 143:883, 1991.)*

Table 26-2. Changes in blood gas tensions and pH with varying degrees of severity of asthma as defined by the degree of airways obstruction

	Airways obstruction		
	Mild	*Moderate*	*Severe*
FEV_1 (% predicted)	>60%	30–60%	<30%
PaO_2	Normal/mild hypoxemia	Mild/moderate hypoxemia	Severe hypoxemia
$PaCO_2$	Normal/mild hypocapnia	Normal/moderate hypocapnia	Hypercapnia in some, hypocapnia in others
pH	Normal	Normal/respiratory alkalosis	Respiratory acidosis/mixed respiratory and metabolic alkalosis

FEV_1 = 1-second forced expiratory volume; PaO_2, $PaCO_2$ = arterial O_2 and CO_2 tension, respectively.

Arterial Blood Gases

Dangerous levels of hypoxemia, occasionally developing with alarming speed, may ensue. This hypoxemia may initially be unassociated with carbon dioxide retention. The degree of arterial hypoxemia roughly correlates with the severity of airways obstruction (Table 26-2), and significant hypoxemia ($PaO_2 < 60$ mmHg) is generally seen when the FEV_1 is less than 1.0 liter. For example, in 101 patients, McFadden and Lyons [88] found a mean FEV_1 that was 59, 39, and 18 percent of predicted and a mean PaO_2 of 83, 71, and 63 mmHg, respectively. In another series, a PaO_2 of less than 60 mmHg was common with an FEV_1 of less than 0.5 liter, or 30 percent of predicted.

Hypocapnia (i.e., a low arterial PCO_2) is usual during bronchospasm. The reason for this is unclear, but it may be the result of reflexes originating in the airways (perhaps histamine induced), lung parenchyma, or chest wall. It does not appear to be secondary to hypoxic peripheral chemoreceptor stimulation, since it is present in patients who do not have hypoxemia. With very severe bronchospasm, the patient may fatigue and hypercarbia supervene, reflecting alveolar hypoventilation. The transition from hypocarbia to normocarbia during an asthma attack should be regarded as a danger signal, since respiratory failure with a high $PaCO_2$ may rapidly follow [143].

The relationship between $PaCO_2$ and FEV_1 is not linear. When the FEV_1 exceeds 0.75 liter or 30 percent of predicted, hypercapnia is rarely seen. As the FEV_1 falls below these levels, hypercapnia is observed with increasing frequency. These observations stress the limited value of ventilatory function tests in differentiating various levels of gas exchange in persons with severe asthma. While the absolute incidence of such hypercapnia may be as low as 10 percent or as high as 50 percent, depending on the reported patient series, prompt identification of this hypoventilatory stage is required because of its potentially high mortality rate.

No one single pattern of PaO_2, $PaCO_2$, or pH is characteristic of severe asthma (Fig. 26-11). Several experimental [122] and clinical studies [8, 76, 87, 118, 141] have demonstrated dissociation between maximal expiratory airflow rates and pulmonary gas exchange in both acute and chronic forms of bronchial asthma. Accordingly, it has been suggested that airflow rates are

[138], the PO_2 is accurately predicted by the degree of V/Q imbalance, implying that the source of hypoxemia is imbalance, whereas airflow rates and V/Q are not correlated even in a single patient [8]. The corollary of this, of course, is that V/Q is not correlated with clinical severity [83, 112, 140, 142] and week-by-week variability is unrelated to symptoms, airflow [138], or aerobic fitness as measured by maximal oxygen uptake [52a].

A variable effect of hypoxic vasoconstriction can be demonstrated by rebreathing 100% oxygen, and a variable response of V/Q balance to bronchodilators such as salbutamol and fenoterol has been shown, although in general administering oxygen and bronchodilators leads to worsening V/Q and improved spirometry [8, 53, 134]. However, there is a broad relationship between the physiologic and clinical severity, as evidenced by lower PO_2's and lower FEVs at 1 second (FEV_1) in those patients admitted to the hospital. To fully evaluate patients with asthma, clinical and spirometric indices may not be sufficient and evaluation of gas exchange is important.

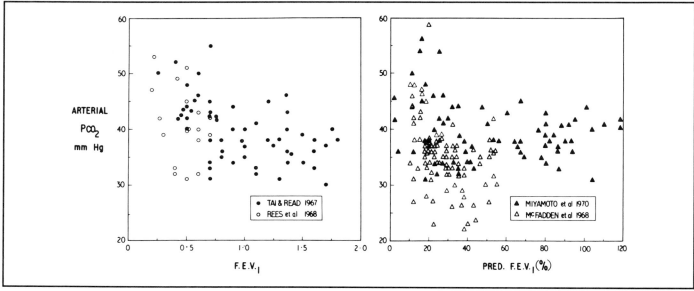

Fig. 26-11. *Relationships between the arterial PCO₂ and FEV₁ (lefthand side) or FEV₁ as percentage of the predicted normal value (righthand side) in asthmatic patients.*

determined mostly by properties of the larger airways, whereas gas exchange is more related to peripheral airway obstruction [118].

Such blood gas profiles serve as the most reliable basis for assessing asthma severity. Hypoxemia with mild hypocapnia and respiratory alkalemia (due to hyperventilation from hypoxia, anxiety, and metabolic stress) characterizes the least severe gas exchange disturbance, or Stage I. Here, V/Q abnormalities are insufficient to precipitate ventilatory failure, and respiratory work remains effective in eliminating carbon dioxide. Oxygen supplementation and a sound therapeutic program generally support such patients. In Stage II, which reflects more severe airway obstruction, advanced hypoxemia with augmented hyperventilation is observed; these patients are typically tachypneic and dyspneic and exhibit frank respiratory distress. Many of these patients respond to proper bronchodilator therapy and other supportive measures. Regrettably, other patients may remain refractory to such therapy and progress to graver stages of gas exchange impairment in association with pharmacologic resistance.

Stage III is a critical point in the evolution of airway obstruction. It may serve as a clinically reliable index of progressive respiratory failure heralding frank ventilatory instability and respiratory acidosis [143]. The salient feature is the finding of normal PaCO₂ and pH values despite the patient's obvious continued clinical deterioration. This normalization of PaCO₂–pH relationships reflects progressive failure of effective alveolar ventilation, and is, in fact, a state of relative hypoventilation. This is the crossover phase. It is stressed to alert physicians to the evolution of hypoventilation (Stage IV) from hyperventilation Stages I and II. Because Stage IV, consisting of overt alveolar hypoventilation and respiratory acidosis, is most critical in terms of morbidity or even survival, and can develop with alarming rapidity, the crossover phase is a major clinical signal and cause for concern. At this point, serial arterial blood gas observations are mandatory in addition to intensification of therapeutic modalities. Stage IV patients with advanced hypoxemia complicated by hypercapnia and respiratory acidosis may exhibit limited responses to bron-

chodilator drugs and other conservative measures. While some patients presenting in Stage IV of the disease may be successfully managed with conservative measures, as dictated by the individual clinical conditions, other patients require intubation and mechanical ventilator support if they are exhausted, obtunded, or have critical PaO₂, PaCO₂, or pH values.

Metabolic acidosis due to lactic acid accumulation may occur in some patients with acute severe asthma. The lactic acidosis is believed to be due to a continued overproduction of lactic acid by the respiratory muscles and diminished hepatic removal of lactate [4]. Alterations in cardiac function may also lead to diminished peripheral perfusion with resulting anaerobic metabolism. Lactic acidosis results in a low pH and increased anion gap, and is indicative of a severe state of asthma likely to produce severe ventilatory difficulties. However, it is not generally appreciated that a non–anion gap metabolic acidosis may have been seen more commonly in asthmatic patients in the days prior to hospital admission, with the acidosis stemming from renal bicarbonate loss in compensation for the hypocapnia induced by hyperventilation [102]. Acid-base changes in acute severe asthma are detailed in Chapter 73, which deals with status asthmaticus, and are summarized in Figure 26-12.

Diffusing Capacity

The diffusing capacity tests for carbon monoxide are not as greatly affected by the abnormal V/Q distribution as are the arterial blood gases. While steady-state measurements of carbon monoxide diffusing capacity (DLCO-SS) are sometimes reduced if bronchospasm is present, the single-breath measurement (DLCO-SB) [24] is usually normal even in the presence of significant airflow obstruction. The DLCO-SB is therefore useful in distinguishing asthma from emphysema. Some studies of an increase in DLCO-SB in acute asthma suggest that regional shifts in perfusion to the lung apices enhance diffusion-perfusion ratios, and possibly explain a higher DLCO-SB (Fig. 26-13).

Table 26-3 provides some physiologic changes, as discussed

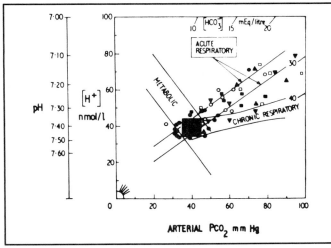

Fig. 26-12. *Acid-base relationships in severe asthma. Closed symbols are from adults, open symbols from children in various series of severe asthma. Ninety-five percent confidence limits of these relationships in pure metabolic acid-base disturbances and in acute and chronic respiratory disturbances are shown. (Reprinted with permission from D. C. Flenley, Blood gas tensions in severe asthma. Proc. R. Soc. Med. 64:1149, 1971.)*

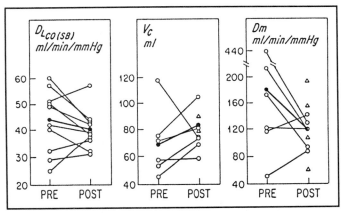

Fig. 26-13. *Changes in asthma in single-breath diffusing capacity (DLCO), capillary blood volume (VC), and membrane-diffusing capacity (D$_M$) after 10 days of intensive steroid therapy. Open circles are individual subjects; closed circles are mean values. (Data from J. L. Ohman, et al., The diffusing capacity in asthma: effect of airflow obstruction. Am. Rev. Respir. Dis. 107:932, 1973.)*

Table 26-3. Physiologic changes in acute asthma

Parameter	Units	Control	Acute attack	Percent control
VC	cc	5,560	1,460	26
FEV$_1$	cc	2,630	718	27
FEV$_1$/FVC	%	47	49	104
PaO$_2$	mmHg	81	54	67
PaCO$_2$	mmHg	32	36	113
Q̇s/Q̇t	%	4	25	625
V̇O$_2$	cc/m^2	111	179	161
Q̇	liters/min/m^2	2.5	4	160
A–V	O$_2$ vol%	4.5	4.5	100
V$_D$/V$_T$	%	34	48	141

VC = vital capacity; FEV$_1$ = 1-second forced expiratory volume; FEV$_1$/FVC = forced expiratory volume in 1 second divided by forced vital capacity × 100; Q̇s/Q̇t = percent of shunted pulmonary blood flow to total pulmonary blood flow; V̇O$_2$ = oxygen consumption (ml/min); Q̇ = cardiac index; A–V = arterial – venous oxygen content difference; V$_D$/V$_T$ = percent of dead space ventilation to total minute ventilation.
Source: W. A. Sumner, In E. B. Weiss (ed.), *Status Asthmaticus.* Baltimore, MD: University Park Press, 1978.

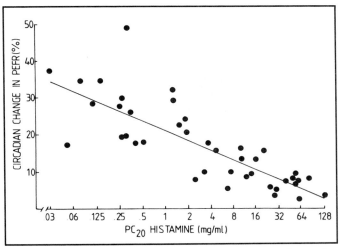

Fig. 26-14. *Relationship between circadian change in peak flow and histamine responsiveness in asthmatics. (Data from N. J. Douglas and D. C. Flenley, Breathing during sleep in patients with obstructive lung disease. Am. Rev. Respir. Dis. 141:1055, 1990.)*

previously, and these are profiled for one patient with acute asthma.

Nocturnal Asthma and Hypoxemia

The FEV and peak flow rates fall overnight in patients with asthma [30, 116, 131], the fall being as much as 50 percent in some—the so-called morning-dippers [135]. The correlation of nocturnal asthma with bronchial reactivity to histamine is shown in Figure 26-14. Evidence exists that nocturnal worsening of asthma can be serious [31, 64] and was shown by Turner-Warwick [136] to be common. In this survey of 7,729 asthmatic patients, 94 percent responded that they awoke at least one night a month with symptoms of asthma, 74 percent at least one night a week, and 39

percent every night. Serious consequences of such attacks may be explained by a blunted arousal mechanism, as shown in two subjects [68], and possibly induced by the sleep deprivation accompanying nocturnal asthma [7] (see also Chap. 76).

The reason for such nocturnal worsening is unclear. Factors that have been suggested, but seem unlikely, include the sleeping posture [30], interruption of bronchodilator treatment [135], and allergens in the bedding [30]. The last factor is unlikely, since increased wheeze is not abolished by avoiding such allergens [116, 123]. However, it must be recognized that antigen exposure may modify the severity of nocturnal asthma [110, 116, 123]. The effect of sleep itself can be discounted, since the nocturnal worsening persists if wakefulness is imposed on subjects [26]. Neither is the sleep stage important. In a large study [75], it was shown that asthmatic attacks were distributed throughout the stages of sleep in proportion to the amount of time spent in each sleep stage. Expiratory time, which would lengthen during bronchospasm, although initially thought to be increased in rapid-eye-movement sleep [75] (Fig. 26-15), has subsequently been

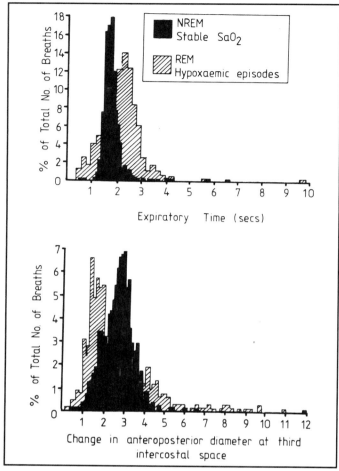

Fig. 26-15. *(Upper panel) expiratory times of all breaths during non-REM (NREM) sleep with stable ear oxygen saturation (SaO_2; dark areas) and during REM sleep with hypoxemic episodes (diagonally lined areas). (Lower panel) chest wall movement (anteroposterior diameter at the level of the third intercostal space anteriorly, in arbitrary units) in a chronic stable asthmatic. (Reprinted with permission from J. R. Catterall, et al., Irregular breathing and hypoxaemia during sleep in chronic stable asthma.* Lancet *1:301, 1982.)*

shown to be unchanged overall [95]. Changes in mean ventilation between wakefulness and the different stages of sleep are similar to those in normal individuals [40]. Other disturbances of ventilation, such as apneas, have been variably reported as being more prevalent [25] or normal [94, 133] in asthmatics, but most recently intriguing evidence has been presented that obstructive apneas may precipitate lower airway obstruction, which is relieved by nasally administered continuous positive airway pressure [27] (see Fig. 26-16).

Circadian variations in hormone levels seem to be much more relevant. Peak flow rates parallel changes in the levels of circulating steroids [128], though the relationship is not causal since infused hydrocortisone does not prevent the change. Synchronous troughs also exist for peak flow rates and catecholamine levels, along with rises in the plasma histamine levels [10]. These two may act in unison to cause the change. Some controversy exists, however, since questions about the histamine assay used have been raised [74] and sodium chromoglycate has been found to have little or no effect on nocturnal asthma [65, 74], suggesting that mast cell mediator release may not be central to nocturnal bronchoconstriction.

Other mechanisms may also contribute. Parasympathetic tone tends to increase at night [11], with changes in heart rate paralleling peak flow in some asthmatics [130] and cyclic GMP levels falling in children [117]. It has also been reported that breathing warm, humid air (37°C, 100% saturated) abolished nocturnal bronchoconstriction in six of seven asthmatics [29]. Finally, there seems to be a high incidence of gastroesophageal reflux in persons with asthma [15], especially those with nocturnal wheeze. A small but significant change in nocturnal symptoms has been produced by the H_2-receptor blocker in 18 patients [57].

The consequences of nocturnal bronchoconstriction include disturbed sleep, hypoxemia, and probably death. There is sleep disruption [25, 43, 44, 94] which may interfere with daytime performance, and sleep deprivation has been known to reduce ventilatory drive [145]. The undoubted hypoxemia [25, 94, 127] is rarely severe, with saturations ranging from 85 to 95 percent in stable asthma (Fig. 26-17). The extent of this is best predicted by the daytime PO_2 [25] (Fig. 26-18). Unstable asthma may be different, as illustrated in one report in which prolonged desaturation, lasting 5 minutes, occurred [94].

Death rates in asthmatics are rising, and, although two studies showed no increase in deaths at night [3, 73], combining the four largest series [19, 31] reveals an excess of such deaths, such that a 28 percent increase in death rate is seen compared with 5 percent in the general population [39].

Fig. 26-16. *Diagram of causes of nocturnal asthma. (Reprinted with permission from N. J. Douglas and D. C. Flenley, Breathing during sleep in patients with obstructive lung disease.* Am. Rev. Respir. Dis. *141:1055, 1990.)*

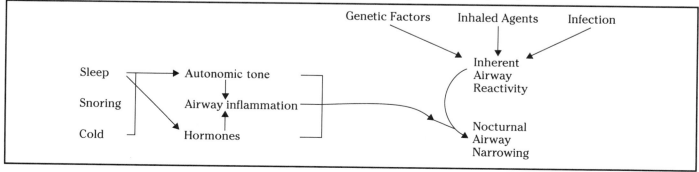

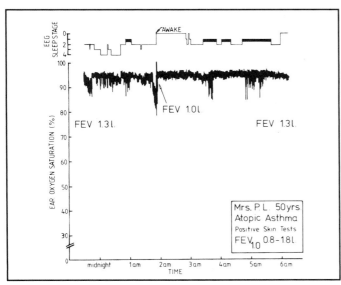

Fig. 26-17. *Recordings of EEG sleep stage (Stages 0 to 4 representing progressive stages of sleep from awake to deep sleep, solid bars indicating periods of REM sleep) and ear oxygen saturation (SaO₂%) during sleep in a chronic stable asthmatic, showing falls in SaO₂ during REM sleep. Airways obstruction increased during the night, as shown by a fall in the 1-second forced expiratory volume* (FEV₁.₀) *recorded at approximately 2 A.M. when the patient awoke spontaneously.*

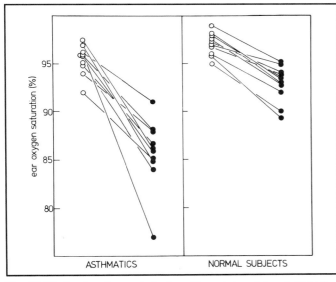

Fig. 26-18. *Presleep* (open circles) *and lowest sleep* (closed circles) *ear oxygen saturation* (%) *in asthmatics and age-matched healthy subjects. (Reprinted with permission from J. R. Catterall, et al., Irregular breathing and hypoxaemia during sleep in chronic stable asthma.* Lancet *1:301, 1982.)*

REFERENCES

1. Agostini, E. Mechanics of the pleural space. In P. T. Macklem and J. Mead (eds.), *Handbook of Physiology,* Sect. 3, Vol. 3, Pt. 2. Bethesda: American Physiological Society, 1986.
2. Agostini, E., Miserocchi, G., and Bonanni, M. V. Thickness and pressure of the pleural liquid in some mammals. *Respir. Physiol.* 6:245, 1969.
3. Antic, R., and Macklem, P. T. The influence of clinical factors on site of airway obstruction in asthma. *Am. Rev. Respir. Dis.* 114:851, 1976.
4. Appel, D., et al. Lactic acidosis in severe asthma. *Am. J. Med.* 75:580, 1983.
5. Backlund, L., and Irnell, L. Compliance in bronchial asthma. *Acta Med. Scand.* 183:281, 1968.
6. Bagg, L. R., and Hughes, D. T. D. Diurnal variation in peak expiratory flow in asthmatics. *Eur. J. Respir. Dis.* 61:298, 1980.
7. Ballard, R. D., Kelly, P. L., and Tan, W. C. Effects of sleep, before and after sleep deprivation, on ventilatory and arousal responses to induced bronchoconstriction. *Am. Rev. Respir. Dis.* 134(4):A54, 1988.
8. Ballester, E., et al. Ventilation-perfusion mismatching in acute severe asthma: effects of salbutamol and 100% oxygen. *Thorax* 44:258, 1989.
9. Barnes, P. J. New concepts in the pathogenesis of bronchial hyperresponsiveness and asthma. *J. Allergy Clin. Immunol.* 8:1013, 1989.
10. Barnes, P., et al. Nocturnal asthma and changes in circulating epinephrine, histamine and cortisol. *N. Engl. J. Med.* 303:263, 1980.
11. Baust, W., and Bohnert, B. The regulation of heart rate during sleep. *Exp. Brain Res.* 7:169, 1969.
12. Beale, H. D., Fowler, W. S., and Comroe, J. H. Jr. Pulmonary function studies in 20 asthmatic patients in the symptom-free interval. *J. Allergy* 23:1, 1952.
13. Beaupre, A., and Orehek, J. Factors influencing the bronchodilator effect of a deep inspiration in asthmatic patients with provoked bronchoconstriction. *Thorax* 37:124, 1982.
14. Bedell, G. N., et al. Measurement of the volume of gas in the gastrointestinal tract. Values in normal subjects and ambulatory patients. *J. Clin. Invest.* 35:336, 1956.
15. Benater, S. R., Clark, T. J. H., and Cochrane, G. M. Clinical relevance of the flow response to low density gas breathing in asthmatics. *Am. Rev. Respir. Dis.* 111:126, 1975.
16. Blackie, S. P., et al. Changes in total lung capacity during acute spontaneous asthma. *Am. Rev. Respir. Dis.* 142:79, 1990.
17. Boushy, S. F. The use of expiratory forced flows for determining response to bronchodilator therapy. *Chest* 62:534, 1972.
18. Briscoe, W. A. A method for dealing with data concerning uneven ventilation of the lung and its effect on gas transfer. *J. Appl. Physiol.* 14:291, 1959.
19. British Thoracic Association. Death from asthma in two regions of England. *Br. Med. J.* 285:1251, 1982.
20. Brown, R., Ingram, R. H. Jr., and McFadden, E. R. Jr. Problems in the plethysmographic assessment of changes in total lung capacity in asthma. *Am. Rev. Respir. Dis.* 118:685, 1978.
21. Brown, R., Scharf, S. M., and Ingram, R. Jr. Nonhomogeneous alveolar pressure swings: effect of different respiratory muscles. *J. Appl. Physiol.* 52:638, 1982.
22. Brown, R., Scharf, S., and Ingram, R. H. Jr. Nonhomogeneous alveolar pressure swings in the presence of airway closure. *J. Appl. Physiol.* 49:398, 1980.
23. Brown, R., et al. Influence of abdominal gas on the Boyle's law determination of thoracic gas volume. *J. Appl. Physiol.* 44:469, 1978.
24. Burrows, B., Kasik, J. E., and Niden, A. H. Clinical usefulness of the single-breath pulmonary diffusing capacity test. *Am. Rev. Respir. Dis.* 84:789, 1961.
25. Catterall, J. R., et al. Irregular breathing and hypoxaemia during sleep in chronic stable asthma. *Lancet* 1:301, 1982.
26. Catterall, J. R., et al. Effect of sleep deprivation on overnight bronchoconstriction in nocturnal asthma. *Thorax* 41:676, 1986.
27. Chan, C. S., Woolcock, A. J., and Sullivan, C. E. Nocturnal asthma: role of snoring and obstructive sleep apnea. *Thorax* 42:733, 1987.
28. Chan-Yeung, M., et al. Effect of helium on maximal expiratory flow in patients with asthma before and during induced bronchoconstriction. *Am. Rev. Respir. Dis.* 113:433, 1976.
29. Chen, W. Y., and Chai, H. Airway cooling and nocturnal asthma. *Chest* 81:675, 1982.
30. Clark, T. J. H., and Hetzel, M. R. Diurnal variation of asthma. *Br. J. Dis. Chest* 71:87, 1977.
31. Cochrane, G. M., and Clark, T. J. H. A survey of asthma mortality in patients between ages 35 and 65 in the greater London hospitals in 1971. *Thorax* 30:300, 1975.
32. Cockcroft, D. W., and Berscheid, B. A. Volume adjustment of maximal midexpiratory flow: importance of changes in total lung capacity. *Chest* 78:595, 1980.
33. Collett, P. W., Brancatisano, T., and Engel, L. A. Changes in the glottic aperture during bronchial asthma. *Am. Rev. Respir. Dis.* 128:719, 1983.
34. Connolly, C. K. Diurnal rhythms in airway obstruction. *Br. J. Dis. Chest* 73:357, 1979.

35. Crapo, R. O., Morris, A. H., and Gardner, R. M. Reference spirometric values using techniques and equipment that meets ATS recommendations. *Am. Rev. Respir. Dis.* 123:659, 1981.
36. Dawson, S. V., and Elliott, E. A. The wave speed limitation of expiratory flow—a unifying concept. *J. Appl. Physiol.* 43:498, 1977.
37. Despas, P. J., Leroux, M., and Macklem, P. T. Site of airway obstruction in asthma as determined by measuring maximal expiratory flow breathing air and a helium-oxygen mixture. *J. Clin. Invest.* 51:3235, 1972.
38. Desplechain, C., et al. Les pores de Kohn des alveoles pulmonares. *Bull. Eur. Physiopathol. Respir.* 19:59, 1983.
39. Douglas, N. J. Asthma. In M. H. Kryger, T. Roth, W. C. Dement (eds.), *Principles and Practice of Sleep Medicine.* P. 597.
40. Douglas, N. J., et al. Respiration during sleep in normal man. *Thorax* 37:840, 1982.
41. DuBois, A. B., Botelho, S. Y., and Comroe, J. H. Jr. A new method for measuring airway resistance in man using a body plethysmograph: values in normal subjects and in patients with respiratory disease. *J. Clin. Invest.* 35:327, 1956.
42. DuBois, A. B., et al. A rapid plethysmographic method for measuring thoracic gas volume: a comparison with a nitrogen washout method for measuring functional residual capacity in normal subjects. *J. Clin. Invest.* 35:322, 1956.
43. Dunnill, M. S. The Pathology of Asthma. In R. Porter and J. Birch (eds.), *Identification of Asthma.* London: Churchill Livingstone, 1971, Pp. 35–40.
44. Dunnill, M. S. *Pulmonary Pathology.* Edinburgh: Churchill Livingstone, 1982, Pp. 50–62.
45. Eichenhorn, M. S., et al. An assessment of three portable peak flow meters. *Chest* 82:306, 1982.
46. Fairshter, R. D., and Wilson, A. F. Relationship between the site of airflow limitation and localization of the bronchodilator response in asthma. *Am. Rev. Respir. Dis.* 122:27, 1980.
47. Finucane, K. E., and Colebatch, H. J. H. Elastic behavior of the lung in patients with airway obstruction. *J. Appl. Physiol.* 26:330, 1969.
48. Freedman, S., Tattersfield, A. E., and Pride, N. B. Changes in lung mechanics during asthma induced by exercise. *J. Appl. Physiol.* 38:974, 1975.
49. Frigas, E., and Gleich, G. J. The eosinophil and the pathophysiology of asthma. *J. Allergy Clin. Immunol.* 77:527, 1986.
50. Froeb, H. F., and Mead, J. Relative hysteresis of the dead space and lung in vivo. *J. Appl. Physiol.* 25:244, 1968.
51. Fry, D. L., and Hyatt, R. E. Pulmonary mechanics: a unified analysis of the relationship between pressure, volume and gasflow in the lungs of normal and diseased human subjects. *Am. J. Med.* 29:672, 1960.
52. Gardner, R. M., et al. ATS statement—Snowbird Workshop on Standardization of Spirometry. *Am. Rev. Respir. Dis.* 119:831, 1979.
52a. Garfinkel, S. K., et al. Physiologic and nonphysiologic determinants of aerobic fitness in mild to moderate asthma. *Am. Rev. Respir. Dis.* 145:741, 1992.
53. Gazioglu, K., Condemi, J. J., and Hyde, R. W. Effect of isoproterenol on gas exchange during air and oxygen breathing in patients with asthma. *Am. J. Med.* 50:185, 1971.
54. Gibson, G. J., and Pride, N. B. Lung distensibility: the static pressure-volume curve of the lungs and its use in clinical assessment. *Br. J. Dis. Chest* 70:143, 1976.
55. Girard, W. M., and Light, R. W. Should the FVC be considered in evaluating response to bronchodilator? *Chest* 84:87, 1983.
56. Gold, W. M., Kaufman, H. S., and Nadel, J. A. Elastic recoil of the lungs in chronic asthmatic patients before and after therapy. *J. Appl. Physiol.* 23:433, 1967.
57. Goodall, R. J. R., et al. Relationship between asthma and gastro-oesophageal reflux. *Thorax* 36:116, 1981.
58. Habib, M. P., and Engel, L. A. Influence of the panting technique on the plethysmographic measurement of thoracic gas volume. *Am. Rev. Respir. Dis.* 117:265, 1978.
59. Hargreave, F. E., Ryan, G., and Thomson, N. C. Bronchial responsiveness to histamine or methacholine in asthma: measurement and clinical significance. *J. Allergy Clin. Immunol.* 68:347, 1981.
60. Hedstrand, U. Ventilation, gas exchange, mechanics of breathing and respiratory work in acute bronchial asthma. *Acta. Soc. Med. Ups.* 76:248, 1971.
61. Herschfus, J. A., Bresnick, E., and Segal, M. S. Pulmonary function studies in bronchial asthma. I. In the control state. *Am. J. Med.* 14:23, 1953.
62. Hetzel, M. R. The pulmonary clock. *Thorax* 36:481, 1981.
63. Hetzel, M. R., and Clark, T. J. H. Comparison of normal and asthmatic circadian rhythms in peak expiratory flow rate. *Thorax* 35:732, 1980.
64. Hetzel, M. R., Clark, T. J. H., and Branthweite, M. A. Asthma: analysis of sudden deaths and ventilatory arrests in hospital. *Br. Med. J.* 1:808, 1977.
65. Hetzel, M. R., Clark, T. J. H., and Gillam, S. J. Is sodium cromoglycate effective in nocturnal asthma. *Thorax* 40:793, 1984.
66. Higenbottam, T. Narrowing of glottis opening in humans associated with experimentally induced bronchoconstriction. *J. Appl. Physiol.* 49:403, 1980.
67. Higenbottam, T., and Payne, J. Glottis narrowing in lung disease. *Am. Rev. Respir. Dis.* 125:746, 1982.
68. Hudgel, D. W., Kellum, R., and Martin, R. F. Depressed arousal response to airflow obstruction: a possible factor in near-fatal nocturnal asthma. *Am. Rev. Respir. Dis.* 125(S):202, 1982.
69. Hume, K. M., and Gandevia, B. Forced expiratory volume before and after isoprenaline. *Thorax* 12:276, 1957.
70. Hurtado, A., and Kaltreider, N. L. Studies of total pulmonary capacity and its subdivisions: VII. Observations during the acute respiratory distress of bronchial asthma and following the administration of epinephrine. *J. Clin. Invest.* 13:1053, 1934.
71. Hyatt, R. E., Schilder, D. P., and Fry, D. L. Relationship between maximum expiratory flow and degree of lung inflation. *J. Appl. Physiol.* 13:331, 1958.
72. Ingram, R. H. Jr., and McFadden, E. R. Jr. Localization and mechanisms of airway responses. *N. Engl. J. Med.* 297:596, 1977.
73. Ingram, R. H., Jr., and McFadden, E. R. Jr. Localization and mechanisms of airway responses. *N. Engl. J. Med.* 297:596, 1977.
74. Ino, P. W., Barnes, P. J., and Causon, R. Plasma levels of histamine in asthma. *Br. J. Clin. Pharmacol.* 15:145, 1983.
75. Kales, A., et al. Sleep studies in asthmatic adults: relationship of attacks to sleep stage and time of night. *J. Allergy* 41:164, 1968.
75a. Kamp, D. W. Physiologic evaluation of asthma. *Chest* 101:396S, 1992.
76. Kelsen, S. G., Kelsen, D. P., and Fleegler, F. B. Emergency room assessment and treatment of patients with acute asthma: adequacy of the conventional approach. *Am. J. Med.* 64:622, 1978.
77. Kennedy, M. C. S., and Thursby-Pelham, D. C. Cortisone in treatment of children with chronic asthma. *Br. Med. J.* 1:1511, 1956.
78. Levin, G., Housey, E., and Macklem, P. Gas exchange abnormalities in mild asthma. *N. Engl. J. Med.* 282:1277, 1970.
79. Light, R. W., Conrad, S. A., and George, R. B. The one best test for evaluating the effects of bronchodilator therapy. *Chest* 72:512, 1977.
80. Lonky, S. A., and Tisi, G. M. Determining changes in airway caliber in asthma: the role of submaximal expiratory flow rates. *Chest* 77:741, 1980.
81. Mayfield, J. D., Paez, P. N., and Nicholson, D. P. Static and dynamic lung volumes and ventilation perfusion abnormalities in adult asthma. *Thorax* 26:591, 1971.
82. Mansell, A., Dubrawsky, C., and Levison, H. Lung mechanics in antigen induced asthma. *J. Appl. Physiol.* 37:297, 1974.
83. Marthan, R., et al. Gas exchange alterations in patients with chronic obstructive lung disease. *Chest* 87:470, 1985.
84. Martin, J. The role of respiratory muscles in the hyperinflation of bronchial asthma. *Am. Rev. Respir. Dis.* 121:441, 1980.
85. McCarthy, D., and Millic-Emili, J. Closing volume in asymptomatic asthma. *Am. Rev. Respir. Dis.* 107:559, 1973.
86. McCarthy, D. S., and Sigurdson, M. Lung elastic recoil and reduced airflow in clinically stable asthma. *Thorax* 35:298, 1980.
87. McFadden, E. R. Jr., Kiser, R., and DeGroot, W. J. Acute bronchial asthma: relations between clinical and physiologic manifestations. *N. Engl. J. Med.* 288:221, 1973.
88. McFadden, E. R. Jr., and Lyons, H. A. Arterial blood-gas tension in asthma. *N. Engl. J. Med.* 278:1027, 1968.
89. McFadden, E. R. Jr., and Lyons, H. A. Serial studies of factors influencing airway dynamics during recovery from acute asthma attacks. *J. Appl. Physiol.* 27:452, 1969.
90. McIlroy, M. B., and Marshall, R. The mechanical properties of the lungs in asthma. *Clin. Sci.* 15:345, 1956.
91. Mead, J., et al. Significance of the relationship between lung recoil and maximum expiratory flow. *J. Appl. Physiol.* 22:95, 1967.
92. Meisner, P., and Hugh-Jones, P. Pulmonary function in bronchial asthma. *Br. Med. J.* 1:470, 1968.
93. Menkes, H. A., et al. Influence of surface forces on collateral ventilation. *J. Appl. Physiol.* 31:544, 1971.
94. Montplaisir, J., Walsh, J., and Malo, J. L. Nocturnal asthma features of attacks, sleep and breathing patterns. *Am. Rev. Respir. Dis.* 125:18, 1982.
95. Morgan, A. D., Rhind, G. B., and Connaughton, J. J. Breathing and oxygenation during sleep in nocturnal asthma. *Thorax* 42:600, 1987.
96. Morgan, A. D., et al. Sodium cromoglycate in nocturnal asthma. *Thorax* 41:39, 1986.

97. Morris, J. F., Temple, W. P., and Koski, A. Normal values for the ratio of one-second force expiratory volume to forced vital capacity. *Am. Rev. Respir. Dis.* 108:1000, 1973.

98. Muller, N., Bryan, A. C., and Zamel, N. Tonic inspiratory muscle activity as a cause of hyperinflation in histamine-induced asthma. *J. Appl. Physiol.* 49:869, 1980.

99. Mushkin, G. J. Time factor in the measurement of response to bronchodilators. *Thorax* 22:538, 1967.

100. Nadel, J. A., and Tierney, D. F. Effect of a previous deep inspiration on airway resistance in man. *J. Appl. Physiol.* 16:717, 1961.

101. Nathan, S. P., Lebowitz, M. D., and Knudson, R. J. Spirometric testing: number of tests required and selection of data. *Chest* 76:384, 1979.

102. Okrent, G. D., et al. Metabolic acidosis not due to lactic acidosis in patients with severe acute asthma. *Crit. Care Med.* 15:1098, 1984.

103. Olive, J. T. Jr., and Hyatt, R. E. Maximal expiratory flow and total respiratory resistance during induced bronchoconstriction in asthmatic subjects. *Am. Rev. Respir. Dis.* 106:366, 1972.

104. Olsen, C. R., and Hale, F. C. A method for interpreting acute response to bronchodilators from the spirogram. *Am. Rev. Respir. Dis.* 98:301, 1968.

105. Orehek, J., et al. Influence of the previous deep inspiration on the spirometric measurement of provoked bronchoconstriction in asthma. *Am. Rev. Respir. Dis.* 123:269, 1981.

106. Parham, W. M., et al. Analysis of time course and magnitude of lung inflation effects on airway tone: relation to airway reactivity. *Am. Rev. Respir. Dis.* 128:240, 1983.

107. Pendley, T. J., and Drazen, J. M. Aerodynamic Theory. In A. P. Fishman, et al. (eds.), *Handbook of Physiology, The Respiratory System.* Sect. 3, Vol. 3, Part 1. Bethesda: American Physiological Society, 1986.

108. Pennock, B. E., Rogers, R. M., and McCaffree, D. R. Changes in measured spirometric indices. What is significant? *Chest* 80:97, 1981.

109. Permutt, S. Physiologic changes in the acute asthmatic attack. In K. F. Austen and L. M. Lichtenstein (eds.), *Asthma, Physiology, Immunopharmacology and Treatment.* New York; Academic, 1973, P. 15.

110. Platts-Mills, T. A. E., et al. Reduction of bronchial hyper-reactivity during prolonged allergen avoidance. *Lancet* 2:675, 1982.

111. Pride, N. B., and Macklem, P. T. Lung mechanics in disease. In A. P. Fishman, et al. (eds.), *Handbook of Physiology, The Respiratory System.* Sect. 3, Vol. 3, Part 2. Bethesda: American Physiological Society, 1986, Pp. 659–692.

112. Pride, N. B., Permutt, S., and Bromberger-Barnea, B. Determinants of maximum expiratory flow from the lungs. *J. Appl. Physiol.* 23:646, 1967.

113. Rahn, H., and Fenn, W. O. *A Graphical Analysis of the Respiratory Gas Exchange.* Washington, DC: American Physiological Society, 1955.

114. Raine, J. M., and Bishop, J. M. A-a difference in O_2 tension and physiological dead space in normal man. *J. Appl. Physiol.* 18:284, 1963.

115. Ramsdell, J. W., and Tisi, G. M. Determination of bronchodilation in the clinical pulmonary function laboratory: role of changes in static lung volumes. *Chest* 76:622, 1979.

116. Reinberg, A., and Gervais, P. Circadian rhythms in respiratory functions, with special reference to human chronophysiology and chronopharmacology. *Bull. Physiopathol. Respir.* 8:663, 1972.

117. Reinhardt, D., et al. Comparison of the effects of theophylline, prednisolone and sleep withdrawal on airway obstruction and urinary cyclic AMP/cyclic GMP excretion of asthmatic children with and without nocturnal asthma. *Int. J. Clin. Pharmacol. Ther. Toxicol.* 18:399, 1980.

118. Roca, J., et al. Serial relationships between Va/Q inequality and spirometry in acute severe asthma requiring hospitalization. *Am. Rev. Respir. Dis.* 137:605, 1988.

119. Roca, J., et al. Serial relationships between ventilation-perfusion inequality and spirometry in acute severe asthma requiring hospitalization. *Am. Rev. Respir. Dis.* 137:1055, 1988.

120. Rodenstein, D. O., Francis, C., and Stanescu, D. C. Emotional laryngeal wheezing, a new syndrome. *Am. Rev. Respir. Dis.* 127:354, 1983.

121. Rodman, D. M., and Voelkel, N. F. Regulation of vascular tone. In R. A. Crystal and J. B. West (eds.), *The Lung: Scientific Foundations.* New York: Raven, 1990.

122. Rodriguez-Roisin, R., et al. Gas exchange responses to bronchodilators following methacholine challenge in dogs. *Am. Rev. Respir. Dis.* 130:617, 1984.

123. Scherr, M. S., and Peck, L. W. The effects of high efficiency air filtration system on night time asthma attacks. *W. Va. Med. J.* 73:144, 1977.

124. Shim, C., and Williams, M. H. Jr. Pulsus paradoxus asthma. *Lancet* 1:530, 1978.

125. Shore, S., Milic-Emili, J., and Martin, J. G. Reassessment of body plethysmography technique for the measurement of thoracic gas volume in asthmatics. *Am. Rev. Respir. Dis.* 118:685, 1978.

126. Sly, R. M. Mortality from asthma 1979–1984. *J. Allergy Clin. Immunol.* 82:705, 1988.

126a. Smith, H. R., Irvin, C. G., and Cherniack, R. M. The utility of spirometry in the diagnosis of reversible airways obstruction. *Chest* 101:1577, 1992.

127. Smith, T. H., and Hudgel, D. W. Arterial oxygen desaturation during sleep in children with asthma and its relation to airway obstruction and ventilatory drive. *Pediatrics* 66:746, 1980.

128. Smolensky, M., Halberg, F., and Sargent, F. Chronobiology of the life sequence. In S. Itoh, K. Ogata, and H. Yoshimura (eds.), *Advances in Climatic Physiology.* Berlin, Springer-Verlag, 1972, Pp. 281–318.

129. Sorensen, J. B., et al. Selection of the best spirometric values for interpretation. *Am. Rev. Respir. Dis.* 122:802, 1980.

130. Soutar, C. A., Carruthers, M., and Pickering, C. A. C. Nocturnal asthma and urinary adrenaline and noradrenaline excretion. *Thorax* 32:677, 1977.

131. Soutar, C. A., Costello, J., and Ijaduola, O. Nocturnal and morning asthma. *Thorax* 30:436, 1975.

132. Stanescu, D. C., et al. Failure of body plethysmography in bronchial asthma. *J. Appl. Physiol.* 52:939, 1982.

133. Tabachnik, E., et al. Chest wall mechanics and patterns of breathing during sleep in asthmatic adolescents. *Am. Rev. Respir. Dis.* 124:269, 1981.

134. Tai, E., and Read, J. Response of blood gas tensions to aminophylline and isoprenaline in patients with asthma. *Thorax* 22:543, 1967.

135. Turner-Warwick, M. On observing patterns of airflow obstruction in chronic asthma. *Br. J. Dis. Chest* 71:73, 1977.

136. Turner-Warwick, M. Epidemiology of nocturnal asthma. *Am. J. Med.* 85:1B:6–8, 1988.

137. Vawter, D. L., Matthew, S. L., and West, J. B. Effect of shape or size of the lung and chest wall on stresses in the lung. *J. Appl. Physiol.* 39:9, 1975.

138. Wagner, P. D., Hedenstierna, G., and Bylin, G. Ventilation-perfusion inequality in chronic asthma. *Am. Rev. Respir. Dis.* 136:605, 1987.

139. Wagner, P. D., and Rodriguez-Roisin, R. Clinical advances in pulmonary gas exchange. *Am. Rev. Respir. Dis.* 143:883, 1991.

140. Wagner, P. D., Saltzman, H. H., and West, J. B. Measurement of continuous distributions of ventilation-perfusion ratios: theory. *J. Appl. Physiol.* 36:588, 1974.

141. Wagner, P. D., et al. Ventilation-perfusion inequality in asymptomatic asthma. *Rev. Respir. Dis.* 118:304, 1978.

142. Wagner, P. D., et al. Ventilation-perfusion inequality in asymptomatic asthma. *Am. Rev. Respir. Dis.* 118:511, 1978.

143. Weiss, E. B., and Faling, L. J. Clinical significance of $PaCO_2$ during status asthma: the cross-over point. *Ann. Allergy* 26:545, 1968.

144. Wells, R. R. Jr. Mechanics of respiration in bronchial asthma. *Am. J. Med.* 26:384, 1959.

145. White, D. P., et al. Sleep deprivation and the control of ventilation. *Am. Rev. Respir. Dis.* 128:984, 1983.

145a. Wiggs, R., et al. A model of airway narrowing in asthma and in chronic obstructive pulmonary disease. *Am. Rev. Respir. Dis.* 145:1251, 1992.

146. Williams, M. H. Jr., and Schim, C. S. Clinical Evaluation of Asthmatic. In E. B. Weiss, M. S. Segal, and M. Stein (eds.), *Bronchial Asthma: Mechanics and Therapeutics,* 2nd ed. Boston: Little, Brown, 1985, Pp. 310–317.

147. Woolcock, A. J. Improvement in bronchial asthma not reflected in forced expiratory volume. *Lancet* 2:1323, 1965.

148. Woolcock, A. J., and Read, J. Lung volumes in exacerbations of asthma. *Am. J. Med.* 41:259, 1966.

149. Woolcock, A. J., and Read, J. The static elastic properties of the lungs in asthma. *Am. Rev. Respir. Dis.* 98:788, 1968.

150. Woolcock, A. J., et al. Influences of the autonomic nervous system on airway resistance. *J. Appl. Physiol.* 26:814, 1969.

151. Woolcock, A. J., et al. Lung volume changes in asthma measured concurrently by two methods. *Am. Rev. Respir. Dis.* 104:703, 1971.

152. Zamel, N., Altose, M. D., and Speir, W. A. Jr. Statement on spirometry. A report of the Section on Respiratory Pathophysiology. *Chest* 83:547, 1983.

153. Zamel, N., et al. Partial and complete maximum expiratory flow-volume curves in asthmatic patients with spontaneous bronchospasm. *Chest* 83:35, 1983.

Control of Breathing

David W. Hudgel

27

Clinical presentations of some patients with chronic bronchial asthma may suggest abnormalities in control of breathing. For instance, a patient who is cyanotic but not dyspneic; a patient who does not recognize his own wheezing; and one who does not awaken at night during a severe bronchoconstrictive attack may all have an abnormality in the mechanisms that control breathing. The clinician is challenged with a difficult but important diagnostic task, for if the etiology of these characteristics is not identified and the situation corrected, the patient may develop severe complications of hypoxemia or even die as a result of these circumstances.

During acute asthma, bronchoconstriction and mucous plugging of airways lead to disruption of the normal ventilation-perfusion match within the lung. Thus, ventilation becomes inefficient. Work of breathing and alveolar ventilation must increase in order to preserve oxygenation and carbon dioxide elimination. Ventilatory drive mechanisms are responsible for (1) the detection of both altered arterial blood gas tensions and the resistive load to breathing placed on the respiratory system by asthma; and (2) the stimulation of the ventilatory neuromuscular system to produce the appropriate level of enhanced ventilation. Without this response, severe hypoxemia and respiratory failure could occur.

There are three components of the ventilatory control system that are important for asthmatic patients: (1) chemical control of breathing, (2) mechanical control of breathing, and (3) conscious awareness of altered blood gas tensions and/or of loaded breathing. In the following discussion the normal and abnormal physiology of these mechanisms will be reviewed.

GENERAL PRINCIPLES OF THE VENTILATORY CONTROL SYSTEM

For the three components of the ventilatory control system that was just mentioned, there must be (1) afferent receptors, which are responsible for detection of gas tensions or work of breathing, (2) a central controller, which is made up of several nuclei located in the medullopontine area of the brain, (3) an efferent effector system made up of the muscles of ventilation, the chest wall, and the lungs, which together provide the ventilation needed, and (4) all neural connections between these three components. The afferent sensors for the chemical control of breathing are the carotid body and a chemoreceptor located in juxtaposition to the fourth ventricle in the brainstem. Loaded breathing is detected by mechanoreceptors located in the respiratory muscles and by yet undefined receptors in the respiratory tract. In addition to these receptors, cerebral cortical function is responsible for the conscious awareness of worsening asthma. The medullopontine respiratory center is made up of nuclei composed of stimulatory and inhibitory neurons. Simply speaking, this center integrates unconscious and conscious afferent input and generates an increased or decreased neural output to ventilatory muscles and thus directs a given change in the level of alveolar ventilation (Fig. 27-1). The efferent limb is common to all three levels of drive discussed here. An abnormality of any of the components of the efferent limb such as muscle weakness due to physical inactivity or excessive corticosteroid administration, chest cage structural abnormalities such as kyphoscoliosis or obesity, and airflow limitation may interfere with the ability of a particular patient to generate the appropriate level of ventilation called for by a given ventilatory drive neural stimulus.

The ventilatory control system also is modulated by extrinsic factors—for instance, those that affect metabolic rate [10] and thyroid status [37]—such that stimulants of metabolism enhance responsiveness to ventilatory stimuli and metabolic suppressants diminish responsiveness. Chronic high-altitude residence [31] and long-term physical conditioning [32] also decrease responses. We have demonstrated that familial, presumably genetic, factors also influence the activity of the ventilatory control system [17]. This finding has been substantiated by several subsequent investigations [1, 7, 20, 26]. Impaired consciousness, natural or drug induced, and brainstem diseases also affect the ventilatory control system.

Thus, a defect in the afferent sensors, the respiratory center, the respiratory muscles, the chest wall, lungs, the neurologic connections between these components, or systemic illness that affects drive mechanisms could result in an abnormally decreased response to ventilatory stimuli.

MEASUREMENT OF VENTILATORY DRIVES

A detailed discussion of the technical aspects of ventilatory drive measurements is beyond the scope of this text but general comments will be provided. In the laboratory the patient who cannot recognize a ventilatory stimulus can be distinguished from the patient who recognizes but cannot respond to such a stimulus because of a mechanical impediment to breathing. By measuring the neuromuscular output, recognition can be analyzed; by evaluating the ventilation produced in relation to the neuromuscular output, a mechanical problem can be detected.

To measure the responses to hypoxemia and hypercapnia, either an open or closed system can be used. We prefer the latter (Fig. 27-2). During the hypoxic exposure, for patient safety it is best to have two instruments to measure oxygenation such as an oxygen meter and ear or finger oximeter. Electrocardiogram also should be monitored. During a hypoxic challenge the end-tidal oxygen tension is lowered to about 40 mmHg; isocapnia is maintained since hypercapnia will augment and hypocapnia suppress the response. During a hypercapnic challenge, the end-tidal carbon dioxide tension is increased from 15 to 20 mmHg; oxygenation is kept above a level that might enhance ventilation.

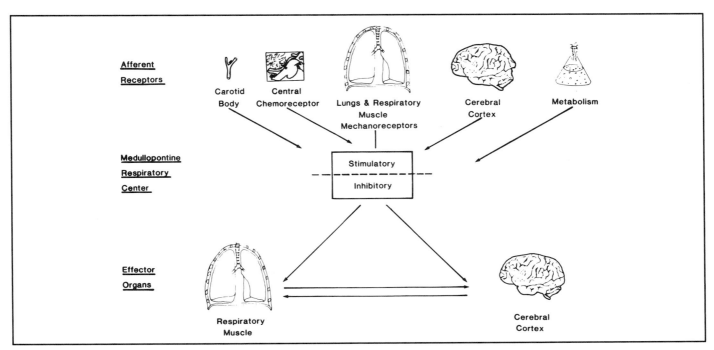

Fig. 27-1. *Concepts of control of breathing. Several afferent inputs stimulate or inhibit the respiratory center. Accordingly, neural output drives the respiratory pump and leads to conscious recognition of mechanical load or altered arterial blood gas status.*

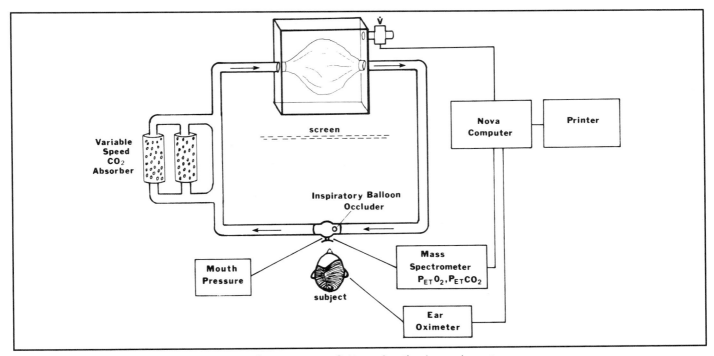

Fig. 27-2. *Closed system used for ventilatory control measurements. Subject rebreathes isocapnic gas to produce hypoxemia or normoxic gas without carbon dioxide absorption to produce hypercapnia.*

By measuring the mouth pressure at 100 msec of inspiration (P_{100}) against an occluded airway [21, 34], the total inspiratory neuromuscular effort is assessed. The measurement is made before conscious recognition of the occlusion occurs. Since there is no airflow present during the occlusion, P_{100} is not affected by abnormal lung mechanics. Ventilatory output is measured as minute ventilation and may be corrected for body size.

Generation of the normal amount of inspiratory pressure by the inspiratory muscles in response to a ventilatory drive stimulus requires normal-functioning respiratory muscles. Thus, if the ventilatory pump muscles are weak, the inspiratory muscles may receive a strong efferent neural stimulus but not be able to respond fully, resulting in decreased inspiratory transpulmonary driving pressure and, consequently, ventilatory output. If unrecognized, this situation could be falsely interpreted as indicating depressed ventilatory control, when the problem is really centered around the respiratory muscles. Problems with respiratory muscle function can be analyzed by (1) tests of respiratory muscle strength (maximal inspiratory and expiratory pressure generation) and (2) by measuring the chest wall electromyogram in response to mechanical or chemical stimuli to breathing. In a human, the ventilatory system response to a stimulus can be analyzed one step closer to the respiratory center by the electromyogram, thereby bypassing the pressure-generation response. It must be remembered that muscle electrical activity depends on normal efferent neural pathways; phrenic nerve paralysis would surely alter this measurement.

To measure the ventilatory response to added resistive loads to breathing, a series of external resistors can be applied to the inspiratory, expiratory, or both the inspiratory and expiratory lines which are connected to a three-way mouth valve. Loading can also be produced with methylcholine or histamine inhalation. Mouth occlusion pressure and ventilation responses can be measured to detect the extent of the drive and ventilation compensation for a given load. The ability to (1) detect loaded breathing, or (2) rate the degree of discomfort produced can be assessed by adding small increments of increased resistance to breathing and asking the subject to (1) signal when he or she recognizes the increased load, or (2) rate the sensation of dyspnea, respectively. A wide range of normality exists for these responses; each laboratory should develop its own set of normal predicted values for these tests.

CHEMICAL STIMULI TO BREATHING IN ASTHMA

In essence, the carotid body is the only organ that monitors oxygenation in humans. The carotid body senses changes in tissue oxygen tension, not oxygen saturation. Normally the relationship between ventilation (or mouth occlusion pressure or venti-

Fig. 27-3. *Normal hypoxic drive. Minute ventilation ($\dot{V}E$) is plotted against end-tidal (alveolar) oxygen tension ($P_{A}O_2$). (Reprinted with permission from J. V. Weil, et al., Hypoxic ventilatory drive in normal man. J. Clin. Invest. 49:1061, 1970.)*

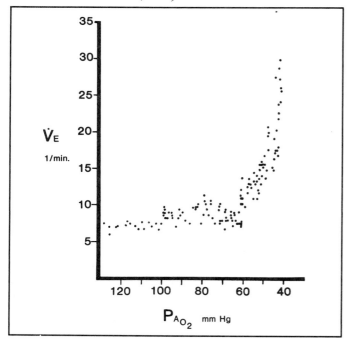

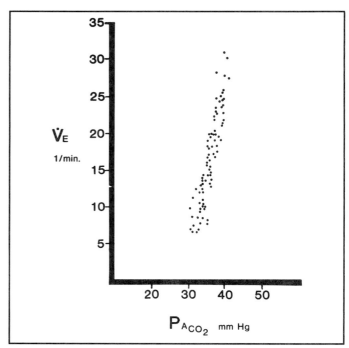

Fig. 27-4. *Normal hypercapnic drive. Minute ventilation ($\dot{V}E$) is plotted against end-tidal (alveolar) carbon dioxide tension ($P_{A}CO_2$).*

latory muscle electrical activity) and oxygen tension is hyperbolic (Fig. 27-3). Little stimulation of ventilation occurs until the arterial oxygen tension decreases to a level below approximately 60 mmHg. As oxygen tension decreases below 60 mmHg, large increases in ventilation occur for small changes in oxygen tension. The carotid body is also partially responsible for the recognition of hypercapnia, detected as changes in tissue hydrogen ion concentration. The central chemoreceptor also recognizes changes in the hydrogen ion concentration. Unlike the hypoxic response, the relationship between ventilation (and mouth occlusion pressure and ventilatory muscle electrical activity) and carbon dioxide tension is linear (Fig. 27-4).

Carotid body function can be adversely affected by certain circumstances. Severe acute hypoxemia that might occur during an asthma attack can decrease ventilation by suppressing carotid body function and/or depressing central nervous system function. In addition, glomectomy, at one time advocated as a treatment for chronic asthma, entirely removes one's awareness of, and ability to respond to, hypoxemia [5, 25]. The procedure also impairs exercise hyperpnea [12, 25]. Glomectomy has never been objectively demonstrated to help asthma; therefore, it is not recommended as a therapeutic consideration [8, 30].

Respiratory muscle weakness and obesity secondary to long-term systemic corticosteroid therapy and physical inactivity impair the ability of the ventilatory pump to respond to neural stimuli from the respiratory center. Likewise, bronchoconstriction or mucus accumulation in the airways reduces the ability of the respiratory pump to respond to such neural input. We have found evidence that asthmatic patients may have some difficulty recognizing or responding to hypoxemia. When hypoxemia is produced in these patients in the presence of low-grade airflow obstruction, there is a failure to heighten the neuromuscular drive, resulting in a depressed ventilatory response [13]. Thus, two acute ventilatory stimuli, hypoxemia and chronically present loaded breathing, appear not to be handled concurrently. A depressed P_{100} response to chemical stimuli can be enhanced with a respiratory stimulant such as medroxyprogesterone or acetazolamide. If the P_{100} response is normal or high but the ventilatory response is low, the effector organ (i.e., lungs and/or rib cage) needs to be unloaded. If bronchoconstriction is present, an appropriate bronchodilator and/or corticosteroid program is needed. If respiratory muscles are weak, strength training of these muscles needs to be undertaken. If the patient is obese, weight loss may be helpful.

The relationship between oxygen therapy and the ventilatory control system needs to be discussed in relation to asthma. Too little oxygen is often administered in acute asthma because of the fear of depressing ventilation with high-flow oxygen. Asthmatic patients who do not have chronic carbon dioxide retention do not hypoventilate with oxygen administration unless concentrations near 100 percent are administered. Since the increased work of breathing required to combat acute asthma increases the metabolic oxygen demand substantially, one should not restrict oxygen therapy for the severely ill asthmatic patient, even in the face of acute hypercapnia. One should use enough oxygen to ensure adequate tissue oxygenation and prevent metabolic acidosis.

MECHANICAL STIMULI TO BREATHING IN ASTHMA (RESPONSIVENESS TO RESISTIVE LOADING)

Most investigations examining the response to loading breathing involve the application of external loads, usually during inspiration. With the addition of a resistive load to breathing, the normal response is characterized by an increase in inspiratory neuromuscular activity [2, 18, 24]. However, in most subjects, ventilation is decreased by external load application. Based on studies in paraplegic patients, both chest wall and diaphragm receptors are important in load detection [9].

How do asthmatic patients compensate for the resistive load of asthma? During chronic stable airflow limitation, asthmatic patients have a heightened neuromuscular drive [13, 22], and alveolar ventilation is higher than normal [13]. At this time oxygenation is satisfactory, so it is assumed that the hyperventilation is due to a stimulus of chronic airflow limitation. However, during acute bronchoconstriction when there is an increased resistive load and likely hypoxemia, the respiratory center must coordinate the response to both chemical and mechanical stimuli to breathing by heightening the neural output to respiratory muscles. Kelsen and associates [22] found a greater increase in ventilation during acute bronchoconstriction than during the application of external resistive loads. We showed that asthmatic patients had a high enough increase in neuromuscular activity during both normoxia and hypoxemia to maintain ventilation during acute bronchoconstriction (Fig. 27-5). During spontaneous acute asthma, Zackon [36] found a slight decrease in ventilation although neuromuscular activity was increased. These three studies imply that there are afferent receptors that detect mechanical loads which act in conjunction with those that detect altered blood gas tension in acute asthma. The major drawback to these studies is that the load to breathing was not severe. With a greater degree of acute airflow limitation, there may or may not be adequate compensation. It is apparent that some asthmatic patients do not possess this compensatory hyperventilation.

Although not specifically studied in asthmatics, studies performed in emphysema patients with chronic alveolar hypoventilation suggest that endogenous endorphins play a role in this load-induced hypoventilation [28]. It is possible that endorphins suppress ventilation in some asthmatics, even during an acute exacerbation. During severe hypoxia with a PO_2 of 28 to 35 mmHg, ventilation in adult awake dogs was increased after the administration of naloxone, an opiate antagonist [29]. In humans, naloxone does not change the ventilatory response to acute hypoxia [19], but the level of hypoxemia in these studies was not as severe as that reached in the dogs, nor was it the level that

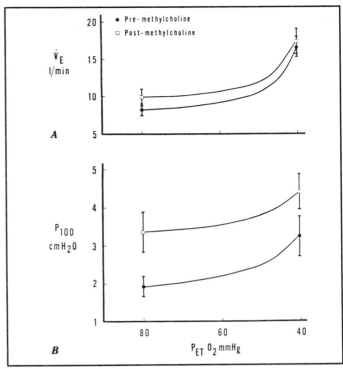

Fig. 27-5. *Effect of methylcholine loading on hypoxic drive in asthma. Minute ventilation ($\dot{V}E$) (A) and inspiratory neuromuscular output (P_{100}) (B) are plotted against end-tidal oxygen tension ($P_{ET}O_2$) before and after bronchoconstriction. P_{100} increases in order to preserve ventilation with methylcholine loading.*

might occur in a severe asthma attack. It is known that, when hypoxemia becomes prolonged in humans, ventilation decreases in both the awake state [19] and during sleep [6]. This effect could be mediated by endogenous respiratory depressants. In some studies, the hypercapnic ventilatory drive in hyperoxia was enhanced in both normal humans and patients with lung disease by naloxone administration [27]. However, the latter findings have not been consistently confirmed. In these studies, if a change in ventilatory response was seen after naloxone administration, it was concluded that endogenous endorphins were involved in depressing the ventilatory response to the stimulus. However, this conclusion may not be totally valid because naloxone may antagonize other ventilatory depressing mediators. In addition, naloxone per se may have some ventilatory stimulatory activity. Thus, endogenous respiratory depressants may affect the asthmatic patient's response to added resistive loads and to hypoxemia. Clinically these patients are difficult to identify because those with impaired load response may not be alarmed and may appear relatively comfortable to both family members and their physicians in the face of severe load and subsequent hypoxemia.

It has been shown that the activity of endogenous opiates was increased under conditions of severe methacholine-induced bronchoconstriction; concurrently, the sensation of dyspnea and the ventilatory output were observed to be decreased [2a].

These potential defects in the hypoxic ventilatory response and the ability to respond to loaded breathing dictate that clinicians must be aware of the oxygenation status of their asthmatic patients, even those appearing to be in only mild distress. A good rule of thumb is to administer supplemental oxygen during an acute exacerbation of asthma, even when symptoms appear rather mild. At the present time no good therapy for enhancing the response to loaded breathing exists, other than assisting the overloaded lung and rib cage, as mentioned above.

IMPORTANCE OF CONSCIOUS RECOGNITION OF WORSENING ASTHMA, ALTERED BLOOD GAS TENSION, OR LOADED BREATHING

A discussion of the complicated mechanisms of dyspnea is beyond the scope of this text, except to state that the sensation of dyspnea surely plays a role in the conscious recognition of altered blood gas tensions or loaded breathing. Recognition of worsening asthma is important so that patients can assess the severity of their asthma and initiate the appropriate therapy or seek medical attention.

The determination of threshold detection can be used to evaluate patients' ability to detect loaded breathing. The level of baseline airways resistance [35], inspiratory muscle activity [23], genetic factors [20], time of testing, and behavioral style [14] affect recognition of added loads. Thus, although this measurement is affected by several factors and consequently is somewhat variable, we [14] and others [4] have shown that, as a group, the ability of asthmatic patients to detect loads to breathing does not differ from that of normal subjects. These findings suggest that asthmatic patients who are obviously wheezing or laboring to breathe and are otherwise asymptomatic may, indeed, have impaired load responsiveness; more likely, they really do recognize the load but, for some as yet undetermined reason, they fail to cope with worsening asthma in a healthy fashion. These findings from a group of asthmatics do not rule out the possibility that the impaired ventilatory responsiveness of some asthmatic patients may have an organic basis, in that, regardless of their ability to recognize loaded breathing, they may truly not be able to respond to mechanical or chemical stimuli to breathing. These patients need to be taught to pay attention to physical clues that indicate the status of the asthma. Use of a peak-flow meter can routinely help this type of patient be more objective in his or her self-awareness.

In contrast, clinicians are aware of the anxious patient who complains of worsening asthma, but upon evaluation find no objective signs of deterioration. In this situation, the patient is not supersensitive to physical signs but is probably erroneously interpreting psychological or other nonpulmonary physical stress as asthma. Training to properly identify asthma symptoms and relaxation training will help this type of patient. The physician must thoroughly evaluate such a patient when he or she complains of worsening asthma, because if the asthma is not really objectively worse, therapy will not help. When symptoms worsen in spite of increased therapy, the underlying psychological problem needs to be identified and treated.

Since many asthmatic patients experience nocturnal worsening of their disease, we need to be concerned about the ventilatory compensation and the arousal response to the loaded breathing of asthma (see Chapter 76). Compared to wakefulness, the ventilatory response to hypoxemia is markedly depressed during all stages of sleep [3, 11]. However, we now know that part of this depression is due to the increase in upper airway resistance that occurs normally during sleep [15]. Nevertheless, there may be a real depression of ventilatory drives, as assessed by the mouth occlusion technique in rapid-eye-movement sleep [33]. Since metabolic rate is decreased during sleep, we might anticipate some diminution in drives, but not to the level we have observed. In addition, hypoxemia appears to be a poor arousal stimulus in humans, since one study showed that decrease in arterial oxygen saturation to 70 percent did not awaken about one-half of one group studied [3]. Resistive loading during sleep produces less neuromuscular effort output than during wakefulness [19]. The arousal response to loaded breathing has not been specifically studied, but predictably large resistances would be required for arousal. If the arousal responses to hypoxemia and

Table 27-1. Arousal time from airway occlusion[a]

	R.K.[b]		D.K.[b]		Control (N = 8)
Stage 2 sleep					
# Occlusions	5		5		22
Mean time (sec)	9.8		7.7		8.6
S.D.	3.8		1.8		4.9
P		NS		NS	
REM sleep					
# Occlusions	11		8		7
Mean time (sec)	26.5		8.6		5.4
S.D.	20		4.1		2.8
P		0.5[c]		NS	

P = p value; NS = nonsignificant; REM = rapid eye movement.
[a] Arousal time is the time from the first inspiration after the occlusion until alpha waves appeared in the EEG tracing.
[b] Asthmatic identical twins. R.K. had history of respiratory arrests at night; D.K. did not.
[c] In REM sleep R.K. had significantly longer arousal time than D.K. and nonasthmatic controls.

loaded breathing are normally blunted in order to preserve sleep, then asthmatic patients may be at some risk during sleep if their disease worsens during this time. They may have a lower ventilatory response to bronchoconstriction than during wakefulness, leading to hypoxemia which, in turn, may not awaken and thus alert them that a problem exists. Thus, it is not surprising that most asthmatic deaths occur at night. In a few patients who have a history of awakening with a severe asthma attack resulting in a respiratory arrest that we have studied, a delayed arousal response to total airway occlusion in some sleep stages has been found. An example is shown in Table 27-1. Identical twin male adolescents both had asthma, but only one had severe nocturnal attacks. The twin with these attacks had experienced cardiopulmonary arrests during some of these episodes, and often his brother would have to awaken him during the wheezing episodes. In the laboratory, the twin with the nocturnal attacks showed a delayed arousal response to loaded breathing during rapid-eye-movement sleep. We concluded that he had an impaired arousal response to respiratory distress. Thus, some asthmatic patients may not sense worsening airflow obstruction until a severe life-threatening situation is reached. We have attempted to treat some of these patients by awakening them at night for an inhaled bronchodilator treatment or by administering a ventilatory stimulant such as medroxyprogesterone. At this time we do not have enough clinical experience with this problem to make definitive therapeutic recommendations.

REFERENCES

1. Arkinstall, W. W., et al. Genetic differences in the ventilatory response to inhaled CO_2. *J. Appl. Physiol.* 36:6, 1974.
2. Barnett, T. B., and Rasmussen, B. Ventilatory and occlusion pressure response to CO_2 and hypoxia with resistive loads. *Acta Physiol. Scand.* 105: 23, 1979.
2a. Bellofiore, S. B. et al. Endogenous opiates modulate the increase in ventilatory output and dyspnea during severe acute bronchoconstriction. *Am. Rev. Respir. Dis.* 142:812, 1990.
3. Berthon-Jones, M., and Sullivan, C. E. Ventilatory and arousal responses to hypoxia in sleeping humans. *Am. Rev. Respir. Dis.* 125:632, 1982.
4. Burki, N. K., Chaudhary, B. A., and Zeckman, F. W. The ability of asthmatics to detect added resistive loads. *Am. Rev. Respir. Dis.* 117:71, 1978.
5. Chang, K. C., Morrill, C. G., and Chai, H. Impaired responses to hypoxia after bilateral carotid body resection for treatment of bronchial asthma. *Chest* 73:667, 1978.
6. Chin, K., et al. Breathing during sleep with mild hypoxia. *Appl. Physiol.* 67:1198, 1989.

7. Collins, D. D., et al. Hereditary aspects of decreased hypoxic responses. *J. Clin. Invest.* 62:105, 1978.

8. Curran, W. S., and Graham, W. G. B. Long term effects of glomectomy. *Am. Rev. Respir. Dis.* 103:566, 1971.

9. Davis, J. N. Contribution of somatic receptors in the chest wall to detection of added inspiratory airway resistance. *Clin. Sci.* 33:249, 1967.

10. Doekel, R. C., et al. Clinical semi-starvation. *N. Engl. J. Med.* 295:358, 1976.

11. Douglas, N. J., et al. Hypoxic ventilatory response decreases during sleep in normal man. *Am. Rev. Respir. Dis.* 125:286, 1982.

12. Honda, Y., et al. Decreased exercise hyperpnea in patients with bilateral carotid chemoreceptor resection. *J. Appl. Physiol.* 46:908, 1979.

13. Hudgel, D. W., Capehart, M., and Hirsch, J. E. Ventilation response and drive during hypoxia in adult patients with asthma. *Chest* 76:294, 1979.

14. Hudgel, D. W., Cooperson, D. M., and Kinsman, R. A. Recognition of added resistive loads in asthma. *Am. Rev. Respir. Dis.* 126:121, 1982.

15. Hudgel, D. W., et al. Mechanics of the respiratory system and breathing pattern during sleep in normal humans. *J. Appl. Physiol.* 56:133, 1984.

16. Hudgel, D. W., et al. Neuromuscular and mechanical responses to inspiratory resistive loading during sleep. *J. Appl. Physiol.* 63:603, 1987.

17. Hudgel, D. W., and Weil, J. V. Asthma associated decreased hypoxic ventilatory drive: a family study. *Ann. Intern. Med.* 80:622, 1974.

18. Iber, C., et al. Ventilatory adaptations to resistive loading during wakefulness and non-REM sleep. *J. Appl. Physiol.* 52:607, 1982.

19. Kagawa, S., et al. No effect of naloxone on hypoxia-induced ventilatory depression in adults. *J. Appl. Physiol.* 52:1030, 1982.

20. Kawakami, Y., et al. Control of breathing in young twins. *J. Appl. Physiol.* 52:537, 1982.

21. Kelsen, S. G., et al. Effect of hypoxia on the pressure developed by inspiratory muscles during airway occlusion. *J. Appl. Physiol.* 40:372, 1976.

22. Kelsen, S. G., et al. Comparison of the respiratory responses to external resistive loading and bronchoconstriction. *J. Clin. Invest.* 67:1761, 1981.

23. Killman, K. J., Bucens, D. D., and Campbell, E. J. M. Effect of breathing patterns on the perceived magnitude of added loads to breathing. *J. Appl. Physiol.* 52:578, 1982.

24. Kryger, M. H., Yacoub, O., and Anthonisen, N. R. Effect of inspiratory resistance on occlusion pressure in hypoxia and hypercapnia. *Respir. Physiol.* 24:241, 1975.

25. Lugliani, R., et al. Effect of bilateral carotid-body resection on ventilatory control at rest and during exercise in man. *N. Engl. J. Med.* 285:1105, 1971.

26. Moore, G. C., et al. Respiratory failure associated with familial depression of ventilatory response to hypoxia and hypercapnia. *N. Engl. J. Med.* 295:861, 1976.

27. Mvztabona, Ambrosino, N., and Barnes, P. J. Endogenous opiates and the control of breathing in normal subjects and patients with chronic airflow obstruction. *Thorax* 38:834, 1982.

28. Santiago, T. V., et al. Endorphins and the control of breathing: ability of naloxone to restore flow-resistive load compensation in chronic obstructive pulmonary disease. *N. Engl. J. Med.* 304:1190, 1981.

29. Schaeffer, J. I., and Haddad, G. G. Ventilatory response to moderate and severe hypoxia in adult dogs: role of endorphins. *J. Appl. Physiol.* 65:1383, 1988.

30. Wasserman, K. The carotid bodies—pathologic or physiologic? *Chest* 73:564, 1978.

31. Weil, J. V., et al. Acquired attenuation of chemoreceptor function in chronically hypoxic man at high altitude. *J. Clin. Invest.* 50:186, 1971.

32. Weil, J. V., et al. Ventilatory control in normal man: effects of acute exercise, chronic physical conditioning and chronic hypoxia. *Chest* 61:45s, 1972.

33. White, D. P. Occlusion pressure and ventilation during sleep in normal humans. *J. Appl. Physiol.* 61:1279, 1986.

34. Whitelaw, W. A., Derenne, J. P., and Milic-Emili, J. Occlusion pressure as a measure of respiratory center output in conscious man. *Respir. Physiol.* 23:181, 1975.

35. Wiley, R. L., and Zeckman, F. W. Perception of added airflow resistance in humans. *Respir. Physiol.* 2:73, 1966.

36. Zackon, H., Despas, P. J., and Anthonisen, N. R. Occlusion pressure responses in asthma and chronic obstructive pulmonary disease. *Am. Rev. Respir. Dis.* 114:917, 1976.

37. Zwillich, C. W., et al. Ventilatory control in myxedema and hypothyroidism. *N. Engl. J. Med.* 292:662, 1975.

Pathology

James C. Hogg

28

The concept that asthma is an inflammatory disease of the conducting airways is now widely held and has been the subject of at least two books [12, 22]. This chapter will briefly review the anatomy of the normal airways and the structural changes that occur in them in the presence of a chronic inflammatory process. A comparison of the inflammatory features of asthma and chronic obstructive pulmonary disease is presented in Table 28-1. The mechanism by which these structural changes lead to the reduction in airways function associated with asthma will then be summarized.

FUNCTIONAL ANATOMY OF THE CONDUCTING AIRWAYS

Quantitative examination of the human airways [3, 28] has shown that there is considerable variation in the length of the pathway from the trachea to the terminal airways (Fig. 28-1A and B). It has also been shown that small bronchi and bronchioles 2 mm in diameter are spread out from the fourth to the fourteenth generations of airway branching, and that the total cross-sectional area at each airway generation increases rapidly beyond the airways that are 2 mm in diameter (see Fig. 28-1C and D). This means that the central conducting airways are relatively narrow in order to optimize mass flow, whereas the peripheral airways have a wide cross-sectional area in order to optimize rapid diffusion of gas to the exchanging surface [28]. Both direct measurements [11] are predictive analysis of the distribution of resistance [23] of the human tracheobronchial tree have confirmed this arrangement by showing that the central airway accounts for most of the airways resistance and that the resistance offered by airways 2 mm or less in internal diameter is small.

Examination of the histologic characteristics of the conducting airways (Plate 2) shows that they are lined by a pseudostratified epithelium which covers the lumen and extends into the bronchial glands. This epithelium overlies the submucosal connective tissue, smooth muscle, and cartilage and is supplied by the bronchial vasculature. Quantitative studies [7, 27], which are summarized in Figure 28-2, show that the main-stem airways are made up of about 30 percent cartilage, 15 percent mucous glands, and 5 percent smooth muscle, with the remainder consisting of other connective tissue elements and the bronchial vascular system. With progression along the intrapulmonary airways, the amount of cartilage and glands decreases but the percentage of smooth muscle increases to account for 20 percent of the total wall thickness in the bronchioles. The degree to which the smooth muscle surrounds the airway lumen also increases from the central to the peripheral airway. In the trachea and main-stem bronchi, the muscle is found only in the posterior membranous sheath, whereas the lumen of the bronchioles is completely encircled by smooth muscle [20]. This means that the same degree of muscle

shortening will have much less effect on the airway caliber of the trachea and main-stem airways than it will on the more distal bronchi and bronchioles. As we shall see, this anatomic fact is an important consideration in determining the site of airways obstruction in disease.

The bronchial circulation supplies the tissue in the conducting airways (Plate 3). These vessels originate from the ventral side of the upper part of the thoracic aorta on the left. The right bronchial artery is the most variable in its origin and may arise from the first to third intercostal, the right internal mammary, or even the right subclavian artery. Miller's classic anatomic studies [20] show that two to three branches of the bronchial artery accompany each of the larger bronchi and divide with each subdivision of the bronchial tree, and that anastomoses between the main branches form an arterial plexus which runs at right angles to the muscular layer. Small branches of this plexus penetrate the muscular layer to form a capillary network possessing the same long axis as the bronchial tree. These capillaries empty into venous radicals that form a venous plexus on the inner side of the muscle layer. Short branches extend from this venous plexus through the muscular layer to form a second plexus of larger vessels along the outer surface of the smooth muscle. Recent studies from Widdicombe's laboratory [10] have shown that this outer plexus contains large venous sinuses which are submucosal in the major bronchi, where the muscle is entirely located in the posterior membranous sheath and the vessels are found next to the cartilage. The venous blood draining from the first two or three subdivisions of the bronchial tree empties into the azygos and hemiazygos venous system and then to the right heart. However, most of the intrapulmonary bronchial venous flow drains into the pulmonary circulation. Airways disease markedly increases the anastomotic flow between bronchial vascular and pulmonary systems. For example, when contrast material is injected into the bronchial arterial system in patients with bronchiectasis, it is possible to fill the pulmonary arterial tree all the way to the pulmonic valve [4].

STRUCTURAL CHANGES IN ASTHMA

The structural changes that occur in the airways in asthma are a result of chronic inflammation, where inflammation is defined as the reaction of living vascularized tissue to injury [3] (see Chap. 9). Local injury results in vascular congestion, exudation of plasma from the vascular to the interstitial space, migration of inflammatory cells from the microvessels into the interstitial tissue, and proliferation of epithelial, vascular, and connective tissue wherever this process occurs [3]. In structures such as the bronchial tree, where the lumen is covered with a mucus-secreting membrane, two additional features of inflammation are present [8]. These include an increased secretion of mucus and

Table 28-1. Comparison of the principal pathologic features of asthma and COPD

Feature	Asthma	COPD
Site of inflammation	Entire bronchial tree but not alveoli; relative importance of various sites uncertain	Small airways and alveoli
Infiltrating inflammatory cells	Predominance of eosinophils, monocytes, and T-lymphocytes; mast cells and neutrophils also implicated	Predominance of neutrophils and monocytes
Trigger factors	Immunologically specific: allergens, occupational agents, aspirin. Nonspecific: dust, fog, cold air	Immunologically nonspecific: cigarette smoke, (?) dust, and air pollution
Proinflammatory substances implicated in disease pathogenesis	Leukotrienes, PAF-acether, prostaglandins, histamine, eosinophil basic proteins, neutrophil and monocyte granule proteases, lymphokines	Leukotrienes, superoxide ions, neutrophil and monocyte granule proteases
Evidence for involvement of specific immunologic mechanisms	Considerable	None

COPD = chronic obstructive pulmonary disease; PAF = platelet-activating factor.
Source: C. J. Corrigan and A. B. Kay. The roles of inflammatory cells in the pathogenesis of asthma and of chronic obstructive lung disease. *Am. Rev. Respir. Dis.* 143:1165, 1991. Reprinted with permission.

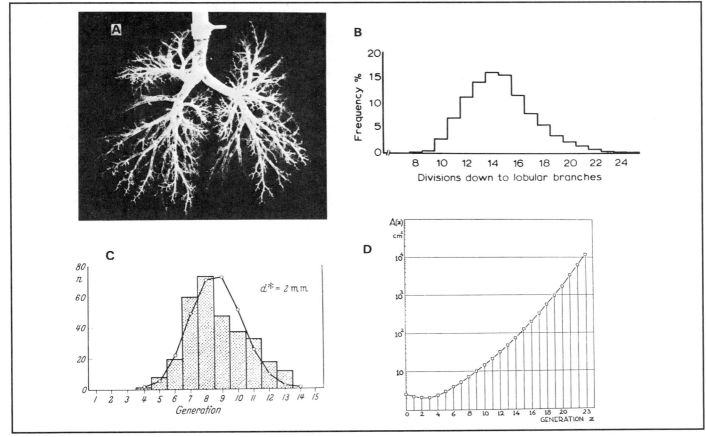

Fig. 28-1. A. A normal human postmortem bronchogram. The trachea is considered generation zero and the branches of the bronchial tree are numbered sequentially as various pathways are followed to the gas-exchanging surface. B. Data from [13], showing that the terminal or lobular branches of the airways can be reached in as few as eight generations, if a short pathway is followed (i.e., to the apical segment of the lower lobe), or as many as 23 generations, if a longer pathway is taken (i.e., to the basal segments of a lower lobe). C. Data from [28], showing that airways 2 mm in internal diameter are spread out from the fourth to the fourteenth generation of branching. This occurs because the airways in the tracheobronchial tree (see A) narrow in such a way that makes the distance from the trachea to a 2-mm airway depend on the pathway followed. D. Data from [28], showing that the cross-sectional area of the trachea is about 2.5 cm² and that this decreases slightly in the main-stem airways and then increases rapidly. Note that airways which exceed 2 mm in diameter (i.e., beyond generation 14) show a rapid increase in the total cross-sectional area at each generation.

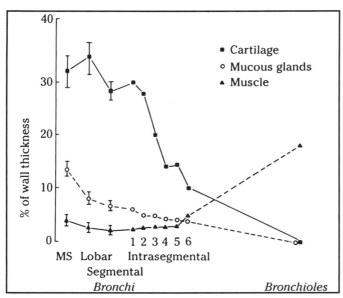

Fig. 28-2. *Data modified from [8, 27], showing that the wall thickness of central airways contains large amounts of cartilage and mucous glands, and that these elements disappear in the peripheral airways where a greater proportion of wall area is taken up by smooth muscle.*

sloughing of epithelial cells from the surface into the lumen. As this response becomes chronic, the vascular bed expands, and there is remodeling of the airways structure as the amount of connective tissue increases in the injured area as part of the repair process [3].

In patients who die of asthma, the bronchial vasculature is markedly dilated and the inflammatory exudate often completely occludes the airways lumen (Plates 4 and 5A). This luminal material is frequently referred to as a *mucous plug*, but it actually consists of fluid, proteins, migrating inflammatory cells, and sloughed epithelium, all of which are components of the exudate. Although mucus is present, it accounts for only a small amount of the plug. In severe cases of asthma, the exudate forms casts of the airways, which can be coughed up in the sputum. These have been called *Curschmann spirals* [5] because they tend to coil up when they lose their attachments to the airways. Sputum specimens from asthmatics also contain compact clusters of sloughed epithelial cells, which are referred to as *Creola bodies* [21] after a patient named Creola Jones in whom they were first described. The exudate also contains numerous eosinophils (see Plate 5B and C), many of which are necrotic and release granules with elongated eosinophilic bodies called *Charcot-Leyden crystals* (see Chap. 52).

The inflammatory process also changes the airway wall. The normal pseudostratified columnar epithelium which is sloughed away during the inflammatory process is frequently replaced by goblet cells (goblet cell metaplasia) or squamous cells (squamous cell metaplasia). The increase in the number of goblet cells in the epithelium contributes to the excess mucus secretion into the lumen, but a substantial portion of the mucus also comes from the enlarged glands [7]. The appearance of squamous cells is part of the repair process required to cover over areas of epithelium that have been sloughed away. The nature of the mechanism of the epithelial sloughing is controversial. Gleich and associates [9] believe that the major basic protein present in the eosinophils damages the epithelium directly. Others (J. Widdicombe, personal communication) have suggested that very high pressures might develop in the swollen submucosa brought about by contracting airway smooth muscle, and that these pressures might separate the epithelium from the airway surface. The

basement membrane upon which the epithelium sits is markedly increased in thickness (see Plate 5) due to an excess production of Type IV collagen.

The comparison of asthmatic to nonasthmatic airways requires a method of categorizing airways by size. James and associates [16] have shown that the internal perimeter of the airways can be used as a yardstick of airways size because they found that this remains constant with the contraction and relaxation of airway smooth muscle. Comparison of normal and asthmatic lungs using this method shows (Fig. 28-3) that the wall thickness is increased in most of the conducting airways of asthmatic patients compared to that in controls. These studies confirm that a chronic inflammatory process in the conducting airways of asthmatics fills the airway lumen with exudate and increases the volume of the tissue in the airway wall.

Quantitative studies of the airway wall have also shown that dilatation of the bronchial vessels accounts for a proportion of the increase in wall thickness [18]. The exudate of fluid and cells from the bronchial vasculature expands the tissue volume, as does the increase in connective tissue, particularly smooth muscle, which can be increased by two to three times its normal amount [7, 14, 16, 27]. These changes in the wall are also associated with a generalized increase in the number of epithelial cells, suggesting that the epithelial, connective, and vascular tissues all contribute to the increase in the volume of tissue in the walls of asthmatic airways (see Fig. 28-3).

There has been considerable controversy as to whether the lesions seen in patients that die of asthma are present in living patients with mild to moderate disease. This question has been partially answered by bronchographic studies performed by Leo Rigler in the 1930s [24], which confirmed that many patients with chronic asthma had extensive plugging of their airways. Other studies have addressed this question by examining the lungs of asthmatic patients who died of causes not related to their asthma [6, 17, 25]. More recently biopsy of the airways of living subjects has been done in the study of this issue [2, 19]. The studies of Laitinen and associates [19] were based on biopsy of three sites in the right major bronchi, and showed that the epithelium was destroyed and the epithelial nerves were exposed. More recent studies by Beasley and coworkers [2] have shown that patients with mild asthma have an excess deposition of connective tissue in the submucosa of the biopsied airways. These studies confirm that the epithelial damage and submucosal deposition of connective tissue so clearly demonstrated in autopsy studies are also

Fig. 28-3. *Data from James and colleagues [16], showing where the square root of wall area is plotted against the internal perimeter of the airway. The internal perimeter is a measure of airway size and the data show that the airways of asthmatic subjects (open circles) have thicker walls than the airways of control subjects (crosses) for every sized airway.*

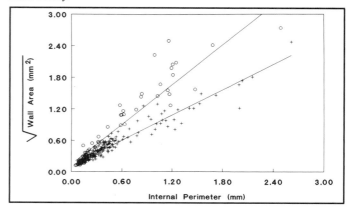

present in patients with mild stable asthma who have volunteered to undergo bronchial biopsy.

FUNCTIONAL CONSEQUENCES OF THE DISORDERED ANATOMY IN ASTHMA

Bates and colleagues [1] have summarized the abnormalities in lung function seen in patients with asthma. They found that some patients who are in clinical remission have mild but measurable defects in their lung function. Other patients have completely normal lung function, but show an increase in airways responsiveness compared with nonasthmatic subjects when challenged with a nonspecific stimulus. When symptoms and signs of asthma are present, patients usually have more severe abnormalities in lung function that include changes in the subdivisions of lung volume, a reduced forced expiratory volume at 1 second, and evidence of abnormal gas distribution. As the asthmatic state becomes more severe, lung function continues to deteriorate until it is reduced to a level that is life-threatening (Chaps. 26 and 73).

It is curious that patients who die a sudden violent death when their asthma is in remission can exhibit pathologic changes in the airways that are as severe as those in patients who die of an unremitting asthmatic attack. A recent analysis of a model of the human bronchial tree [29] may partially explain this discrepancy. This model has shown [30] that even the marked increase in airway wall thickness seen in asthma need not reduce the airways caliber when the airway smooth muscle is at its resting length because this thickening does not encroach on the airway lumen. However, even minimal increases in wall thickness reduce the airway lumen excessively when the muscle shortens. Smooth muscle is capable of shortening up to 70 percent of its resting length [26], and James and coworkers' [15] studies of human lungs have shown that the smooth muscle in asthmatic airways needs to shorten by only about 40 percent of its resting length to completely occlude the airway lumen. This means that the substantial increase in airway wall thickness in asthmatic lungs leads to narrowing and closure of the airway lumen when the smooth muscle shortening is well within its normal range. It also means that the smaller bronchi and bronchioles are particularly vulnerable to closure because they are encircled by smooth muscle.

Reevaluation of the clinical pathologic correlation in the light of data obtained by anatomic study [15] and the computer model [26, 30] provides insight into observations that are otherwise difficult to explain. For example, the severe airways disease found in patients who die a violent death while their asthma is in remission could be explained by a full relaxation of the airway smooth muscle where the thickened wall may not encroach on the airway lumen. At the other end of the spectrum, patients with normal airway function but a minimal increase in wall thickness might show an excess narrowing of the airway lumen when the airway smooth muscle is stimulated to shorten. The important outcome from the analysis of this model has been a shift in emphasis from abnormal smooth muscle function to the inflammatory changes in the airway wall and lumen to explain the abnormal physiology. It also suggests that, in treating asthma, therapy designed to reduce the structural defects produced in the airway wall and lumen by the inflammatory process may be as important as drugs that relax smooth muscle.

REFERENCES

1. Bates, D. V., Macklem, P. T., and Christie, R. V. *Respiratory Function in Disease*, 2nd ed. Philadelphia: Saunders, 1971. P. 111.
2. Beasley, R., et al. Cellular events in the bronchi in mild asthma and after bronchial provocation. *Am. Rev. Respir. Dis.* 139:806, 1989.
3. Cotran, R. S., Kumar, V., and Robbins, S. L. Inflammation and repair. In *Pathologic Basis of Disease*, Philadelphia: Saunders, 1989, Pp. 39–86.
4. Cudkowicz, L. *The Human Bronchial Circulation in Health and Disease.* Baltimore: Williams & Wilkins, 1968.
5. Curschmann, H. Ueber Bronchiolitis exsudativa und ihr Verhaltnis zum Asthma nervosum. *Dtsch. Arch. Klin. Med.* 32:1, 1883.
6. Dunnill, M. S. Pathology of Asthma. In *Transactions of the World Asthma Conference*, London: Chest and Heart Assoc., 1965.
7. Dunnill, M. S., Massarella, G. R., and Anderson, J. A. A comparison of the quantitative anatomy of the bronchi in normal subjects, in status asthmatics, in chronic bronchitis, and in emphysema. *Thorax* 24:176, 1969.
8. Florey, H. The Secretion of Mucus and Inflammation in Mucus Membranes. In H. Florey (ed.), *General Pathology*, 3rd ed. London: Lloyd-Luke, 1962, Pp. 167–196.
9. Gleich, G. J., et al. Cytotoxic properties of eosinophil major basic protein. *J. Immunol.* 123:2925, 1979.
10. Hill, P., et al. Blood sinuses in the submucosa of the large airways of the sheep. *J. Anat.* 162:235, 1989.
11. Hogg, J. C., Macklem, P. T., and Thurlbeck, W. M. The site and nature of airways obstruction in chronic obstructive lung disease. *N. Engl. J. Med.* 278:1355, 1968.
12. Holgate, S. T. (ed.), *The Role of the Inflammatory Process in Airways Hyperresponsiveness.* Boston: Blackwell, 1989.
13. Horsfield, K., and Cumming, G. Morphology of the bronchial tree in man. *J. Appl. Physiol.* 24:373, 1968.
14. Huber, H. L., and Koessler, K. K. The pathology of bronchial asthma. *Arch. Intern. Med.* 30:689, 1922.
15. James, A. L., Pare, P. D., and Hogg, J. C. The mechanics of airway narrowing in asthma. *Am. Rev. Respir. Dis.* 139:242, 1989.
16. James, A. L. et al. The use of internal perimeter to compare airway size and to calculate smooth muscle shortening. *Am. Rev. Respir. Dis.* 138:136, 1988.
17. Kleinerman, J., and Abelson, L. A study of asthma deaths in a coroner's population. *J. Allergy Clin. Immunol.* 80:406, 1987.
18. Kuwano, K., et al. Morphometric dimensions of small airways in asthma and chronic obstructive pulmonary disease (COPD). *Am. Rev. Respir. Dis.* 143:A428, 1991.
19. Laitinen, L. A., et al. Damage to the airway epithelium and bronchial reactivity in patients with asthma. *Am. Rev. Respir. Dis.* 131:599, 1985.
20. Miller, W. F. *The Lung*, 3rd ed. Springfield, Ill. and Baltimore: Thomas, 1943.
21. Naylor, B. The shedding of the mucosa of the bronchial tree in asthma. *Thorax* 17:69, 1962.
22. O'Byrne, P. (ed.), *Asthma as an Inflammatory Disease.* New York: Marcel Dekker, 1990.
23. Pedley, T. J., Schroter, R. C., and Sudlow, M. F. The prediction of pressure drop and variation of resistance within the human bronchial airways. *Respir. Physiol.* 9:387, 1970.
24. Rigler, L. G., and Koucky, R. Roentgen studies of pathological physiology of bronchial asthma. *Am. J. Roentgenol.* 39:353, 1938.
25. Sobonya, R. E. Concise clinical study: quantitative structural alterations in long-standing allergic asthma. *Am. Rev. Respir. Dis.* 130:289, 1984.
26. Stephens, N. L., and Van Nickerk, W. Isometric and isotonic contractors in airway smooth muscle. *Can. J. Physiol. Pharmacol.* 55:833, 1977.
27. Takizawa, T., and Thurlbeck, W. M. Muscle and mucous gland size in the major bronchi of patients with chronic bronchitis, asthma and asthmatic bronchitis. *Am. Rev. Respir. Dis.* 104:331, 1971.
28. Weibel, E. R. Morphometry of the Human Lung. New York: Academic, 1963.
29. Wiggs, B. R., et al. A model of the mechanics of airway narrowing. *J. Appl. Physiol.* 69:849, 1990.
30. Wiggs, B. R., et al. A Model of the Mechanics of Airway Narrowing in Asthma. In M. A. Kaliner, P. J. Barnes, and K. G. A. Persson (eds.), *Asthma: Its Pathology and Treatment* (Lung Biology in Health and Disease Series). New York: Marcel Dekker, 1991. Pp. 73–101.

Bronchial Mucus

Maria Teresa Lopez-Vidriero
K. Ramakrishnan Bhaskar
Lynne M. Reid

29

IMPORTANCE OF BRONCHIAL MUCUS TO CLINICAL PROBLEMS OF ASTHMA

Asthma is characterized by widespread narrowing of the airways, which can change rapidly either spontaneously or under treatment. Pathophysiologic and clinical studies have shown that while airway narrowing results mainly from smooth muscle contraction, airway lumen obstruction by mucosal edema and secretions often also contributes [44, 47, 54, 66, 74, 75]. In a given patient their relative contribution to narrowing of airway lumen varies, not only between attacks but at different stages of an attack and, at a given stage, at different levels of the tracheobronchial tree [106]. The relative importance of these factors varies between the various types of asthma, since these represent a wide range of pathologic processes. The role of genetic regulation is not yet understood but, with the recent developments in molecular biology, is currently being explored.

The term bronchial mucus signifies total bronchial liquid or secretion. Its contents are important for the understanding of the pathophysiologic features of the patient with asthma both during and between attacks. In the normal airway, bronchial mucus can be considered to have a protective role, in that the presence of bronchial mucus is necessary for bronchial toilet by mucociliary clearance; antigenic and chemical irritants are both cleared in this way (see Chap. 30). Mucus contains antibodies and enzymes such as lysozyme that destroy infective agents. It also contains the mediators of inflammation, whether cell or serum derived, and these contribute to the overreactivity of airway muscle and the secretion of mucus [3]. These changes are the expression of the patient's hypersensitivity to the environment and cause the disability of the asthma attack. Typically, in asthmatic subjects between attacks tracheobronchial clearance is slower than that in normal subjects or those with mucoid chronic bronchitis. This points to an underlying abnormality of mucociliary clearance, suggesting that in some way bronchial mucus is abnormal [9].

Casts of the airways may form quickly from bronchial mucus and be a sudden life-threatening event. In fatal cases of status asthmaticus, the plugging of airways by highly viscous casts is a major cause of suffocation and failure of bronchodilators to penetrate the airways (see Chap. 73). That mechanical plugging of small airways can be important even in quiescent stages of asthma is suggested by the demonstration of mucous plugging of peripheral airways in children during remission [48] and by the impairment of lung function that persists for some days after an attack has clinically resolved.

This report refers to studies supported by National Institutes of Health Research Grants 5R01 HL 22444 and NIH HL 19170.

BRONCHIAL MUCUS IN SITU

Mucus Lining the Airways

Bronchial mucus as it lines the airway is conveniently considered in three layers, of which only the first two are always present: a periciliary layer of low viscosity that bathes the cilia, a surface mucus film, and rafts or gobs of secretion that on occasion float on the surface of the mucus film [124] (Fig. 29-1). The contribution of the periciliary layer to expectorated secretions or bronchial lavage fluid is not clear. The cilia probably move to and fro in the periciliary layer and do not move this layer when they shift the surface mucus film.

The mucus film varies at different levels of the airways. In normal conditions it forms a thin layer, but if the airways are stimulated acutely by inhalation of an irritant, the film becomes thicker and the common term mucus blanket is justifiably applied. Whether the normal surface film represents secretion from the serous and mucous cells of the gland is still a matter of speculation. The glycoconjugate in normal mucus seems to be a proteoglycan.

After freeze fracture the surface film is demonstrated as a three-dimensional network of fibers [138]. The fibers could be the gel secretion, while the open spaces of the network represent the sol. In peripheral airways the fibers are thinner and the mesh more expanded, possibly due to the presence of alveolar surfactant acting as a fiber conditioner [64]. Phospholipids may well contribute to the formation of the film by facilitating spreading of the secretion.

The rafts and gobs of mucus that are visible at bronchoscopy sit upon this mucus film. In normal airways responding acutely to irritation, they may represent discharge from the mucous cells of the surface epithelium. In disease they probably come from the hypertrophied submucosal glands as well as from mucous cells of the surface epithelium. In the normal airway the total volume of the submucosal glands is about 4.0 ml, about 40 times that of the surface mucous cells.

Volume of Secretion and Diurnal Variation

Airway mucus is propelled by the cilia toward the larynx and is then swallowed. The amount of airway liquid produced by a normal unstimulated tracheobronchial tree is still debated. A much-quoted figure is 10 ml/day (0.1–0.3 ml/kg body weight), an estimate derived from laryngectomized patients [144]. Although often used as controls, the airways of laryngectomized patients are not actually normal, and the mucus collected probably represents stimulated rather than baseline secretion, since stimulation of the larynx promotes reflex mucus secretion from the trachea. Extrapolation from animal studies gives even higher figures [37,

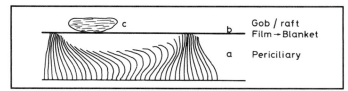

Fig. 29-1. *Liquid lining of bronchial tree: periciliary layer (a) and the surface film (b), which in normal persons is thin, virtually a liquid–gas interface. With hypersecretion, the surface film becomes thicker and justifies the term* blanket. c = *discrete gobs of secretion.*

115]. From the theoretical calculations based on the thickness of the mucus layer, the surface area of the tracheobronchial tree, and the rate of ciliary transport, an estimate as high as 355 ml for the daily volume of airway liquid has been suggested by Van As [147].

Although a diurnal variation in sputum production has been described in chronic bronchitis, information on bronchial mucus production in healthy subjects is lacking [90]. The diurnal variation shows a gradual decrease in the rate of sputum production and in the macromolecular concentration as the day progresses. A circadian variation has also been described in mucociliary clearance. In normal individuals, clearance of secretions is markedly reduced during sleep [9, 110]. Reduced mucus production and reduced ciliary activity could each be contributory. In some way this circadian effect is mediated by sleep, since the slower clearance does not occur if the patient stays awake.

Physical Properties

A solid responds to stress by deformation that recovers when the stress is removed; this represents elasticity, the ability to store energy. While stress is applied, a fluid is continuously deformed (i.e., it flows), but when the stress is removed, there is no recovery; this represents viscosity, the ability to dissipate energy. Mucus behaves both as a solid and as a fluid—that is, it is viscoelastic. Initial elastic deformation (Go), total elastic deformation (Ge), total recoverable strain (SR), and compliance (Jo) are measures of elasticity. The various instruments used for testing measure different aspects of its physical properties [87, 103]. Several mechanical models have been used to analyze the viscoelastic properties of mucus, such as the Maxwell model of the spring (elastic component) and dashpot (viscous component) [103].

Airway mucus performs many functions [120], but perhaps its main role is to form a mechanical coupling with cilia, converting ciliary movement into effective transport [1, 76, 132]. Mucus from different sources such as the gut, airway, or cervix shares with synthetic polymers the physical properties that make them coupling agents. Any material capable of cross-linking and forming a gel that is viscoelastic can be transported by cilia.

An observation probably relevant to the complex mechanical role of bronchial mucus is that its elasticity increases with shear rate, the degree of change being more marked at high rates ($0.1–0.791_s{}^{-1}$ [139]). Concerning its viscosity, airway mucus is a nonnewtonian pseudoplastic material—that is, its viscosity decreases with increasing shear rate, the inverse of the pattern for elasticity. The shear rate exerted by cilia has been estimated to be on the order of $1_s{}^{-1}$ [87].

When mucus is discharged from gland cells into the gland duct and from the duct into the airway lumen, the elastic component should be relatively low in order for the mucus to flow easily; when acting as a coupling agent to the cilia, it needs a high elasticity and should behave more like a solid. Elasticity has been shown to be much more important than viscosity for mucus transport [36, 76, 132]. Other physical properties of airway mucus relevant to its protective functions of trapping and transporting particles are its adhesiveness and spinnability [120].

Bronchial constriction in asthma doubtless applies shear forces to bronchial mucus. When sputum is sheared at low rates ($0.01–1_s{}^{-1}$), its viscosity decreases, but if the mucus is left in the instrument for 30 minutes and then retested at ascending shear rates, the viscosity increases between eight- and eightyfold [139]. Dehydration of mucus is not the cause since, when a sample is dried to about half its weight, the viscosity only increases two- to threefold. Retention of mucus within airways and shearing as the result of bronchial smooth muscle contraction could contribute to the high viscosity of casts, which is not directly related to macromolecular concentration.

CHEMICAL CONSTITUENTS OF BRONCHIAL MUCUS AND THEIR SECRETION

The chemical composition of bronchial mucus (total bronchial liquid) is very different in the normal from that in disease and varies widely between diseases. Thus, our recent studies of bronchial aspirate from normal subjects indicate that mucous glycoprotein of typical buoyant density is probably not a constituent of normal airway mucus but evidence of bronchial stimulation, be it neural or irritant.

We first describe separately the various chemical constituents found in bronchial mucus (see Chap. 52). In considering total bronchial mucus, we refer when possible to human studies and to secretions from asthmatic subjects. As baseline we will consider mucus obtained from normal airways and from other diseases, in particular from chronic bronchitis (a disease marked by mucus hypersecretion), in either its mucoid or purulent phase. Chemical studies of bronchial mucus obtained either as aspirate or as sputum and analysis of the secretory product of human airway in organ culture as well as experimental animal studies will also be discussed.

The epithelial glycoprotein in bronchial mucus typifies the viscoelastic sticky secretion that is termed sputum. We are learning more of the structure of the native or undegraded mucous glycoprotein macromolecule and of the units from which it is assembled. It is emerging that the linkage of this glycoprotein to lipid and other macromolecules is important in determining the physical properties of bronchial mucus. Certain linkages seem characteristic of asthma, and partition of the macromolecules and lipids between sol and gel is different in the various diseases, indicating significant biologic differences.

Bronchial or airway mucus consists of water and dialyzable and nondialyzable constituents [89, 90]. Epithelial mucous glycoprotein, plasma-type glycoproteins, proteins, and lipids are the major nondialyzable constituents. Recent studies of airway mucus, both normal human and canine, in vivo and in vitro, have shown that components of proteoglycans are also present ([15, 41], Bhaskar, K. R., et al. Constituents of normal bronchial mucus aspirate from a) healthy volunteers and b) tracheostomized patients, manuscript in preparation). Deoxyribonucleic acid (DNA) is not usually found in secretions from normal airways but is present in infected secretions [114]. Although water is the major constituent of airway mucus (90–95% by weight), little information is available about its physicochemical features. It is present in free and bound forms, and there is rapid exchange between these compartments. Water molecules can bind to macromolecules, particularly to the sugar residues of the mucous glycoprotein, and the number of bound water molecules influences viscosity [88].

Inorganic Ions and pH

Electrolytes in the form of sodium, potassium, calcium, and chloride are present in airway mucus and are bound to both the soluble and insoluble macromolecular components.

The viscoelastic properties of mucus and ciliary activity are influenced by pH; acidic pH increases viscosity and reduces ciliary beat frequency [53, 87]. The pH of airway mucus has been measured in healthy subjects in vivo during bronchoscopy [26, 62, 137] and in vitro in expectorated secretion [96]; the pH measured in situ was 6.58, while that of expectorated secretion was 8.28. The discrepancy between the in situ and in vitro measurements could be due to loss of carbon dioxide in the expectorated sputum. On the other hand, the measurements taken in situ are likely to represent epithelial-surface pH, since in normal airways the amount of secretion is too small to be measured with the probe.

Proteins

Proteins represent 10 to 25 percent of the nondialyzable material of bronchial mucus studied as sputum and are its best characterized macromolecular constituents [10, 31, 79, 105, 123, 149, 155]. Albumin and lysozyme are proteins, but the term protein is often also taken to include plasma-type glycoproteins such as the immunoglobulins that have a protein content that is relatively higher than that of mucous glycoprotein.

The major proteins identified in normal bronchial mucus are albumin, lysozyme, and bronchotransferrin. The plasma-type glycoproteins include immunoglobulins A, G, M, and D, secretory IgA (SIgA), free secretory piece, 2-macroglobulin, complement (C3, C4), haptoglobulin, amylase, and the antiproteases 1-antitrypsin and antichymotrypsin. Albumin and the immunoglobulins (particularly SIgA, IgA, and IgG) are probably the most important because they are present in the highest concentration, contribute to the viscoelastic properties of the mucus, and have a role in the defense of the airways.

Lipids

Lipids contribute 20 to 30 percent of the nondialyzable contents, but in spite of this considerable contribution, little is known of their nature. Information derives mostly from studies carried out in abnormal airway mucus [13, 59, 85, 86, 133, 134, 148]. The lipids identified in sputum or bronchoalveolar lavage fluid from patients contain neutral lipids (free fatty acids, triglycerides, diglycerides, cholesterol, and cholesterol esters), phospholipids (mainly phosphatidylcholine and phosphatidylethanolamine), and glycolipids.

Recent studies of secretion produced by human bronchial explants [41] show that here also lipids contribute significantly to the nondialyzable component, indicating that they derive from airway mucosa, not just from the alveolar serum. Among nonpolar lipids glycerides, free fatty acids, cholesterol, and palmitate are identified; phospholipids, lysolecithin, phosphatidylcholine and phosphatidylethanolamine, and several glycolipids are also present.

Glycoconjugates

The term glycoconjugate describes polymeric substances consisting of carbohydrate covalently linked to lipid or protein. Glycoproteins and proteoglycans are glycoconjugates, but they differ in the size and shape of the carbohydrate component as well as the type of sugars present. A proteoglycan contains long, straight polysaccharide chains with 30 to 50 repeating units of disaccharide that are known as *glycosaminoglycans* and are linked to protein through the sugar xylose. With the exception of keratan sulfate, all proteoglycans contain hexuronic acid. By contrast, a glycoprotein contains less carbohydrate and the sugar chains are smaller, with reported lengths ranging from 3 to 30 monosaccharide units. The oligosaccharide side chains are usu-

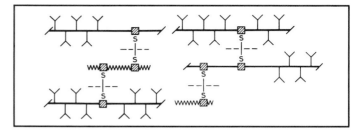

Fig. 29-2. *The naked peptide regions of bronchial epithelial glycoprotein. Disulfide bonds (S-S) and a small peptide (vvvvv) seem responsible for the aggregation of the glycoprotein monomers to polymer.*

ally branched, have few or no repeating units, and do not contain hexuronic acid [121].

Glycoproteins are divided into two types: mucous glycoprotein and plasma-type glycoprotein. They differ in the types of amino acid present in the protein core, the carbohydrate content, the type of linkage, and the presence of specific sugars. Plasma glycoproteins contain less carbohydrate than the mucous glycoprotein (about 25% compared with more than 50%), the linkage is mostly N-glycosidic, and they are rich in mannose, while fucose and N-acetylgalactosamine are absent or present in very small amounts. Of more than 60 so-called proteins that have been isolated from human plasma, only serum albumin and prealbumin are not in fact glycoproteins of plasma type.

Epithelial Mucous Glycoprotein

Epithelial or mucous glycoproteins are glycoconjugates in which carbohydrate side chains are linked to a polypeptide backbone by an O-glycosidic bond between N-acetylgalactosamine and serine or threonine. They are rich in carbohydrate (more than 50% by weight); the sugars most commonly identified are fucose, galactose, N-acetylglucosamine, sialic acid (N-acetylneuraminic acid), and N-acetylgalactosamine. Serine, threonine, and proline represent 40 percent of the amino acid content.

The bronchial mucous glycoproteins isolated without degradation as by DGU (see subsequent discussion) are large macromolecules with molecular weights of the order of 3 to 7×10^6. They have high sedimentation coefficients, and sedimentation-velocity experiments indicate considerable polydispersity. The polypeptide core contains regions devoid of oligosaccharide side chains known as naked peptide regions [125] that have an important role in the formation of insoluble aggregates (Fig. 29-2).

When the undegraded epithelial glycoprotein is treated with dithiothreitol (DTT) to reduce the disulfide bonds, the reduced molecule is smaller ($0.5–1.3 \times 10^6$), the sedimentation coefficient is almost halved, and the viscosity is considerably reduced [46]. The increase observed in buoyant density of the reduced material indicates that a small but significant amount of peptide has been lost, and amino acid analysis suggests that the relevant peptide is rich in acidic amino acids (aspartic and glutamic acids). The epithelial glycoprotein molecules are disulfide-linked aggregates, and it seems that a small cross-linking protein is involved in the aggregation (see Fig. 29-2).

It has been suggested that the cross-linking peptides released during thiol reduction represent a fragment of the naked peptide regions that have been cleaved by proteolytic enzymes released by the thiol reagents [23, 67, 84]. Our recent studies comparing the effect of thiol reduction and proteolytic digestion indicate that a similar fraction is removed by both treatments, suggesting that intermolecular disulfide cross-linkages (covalent bonds) are mainly responsible for the gel structure of mucus [12].

Proteins can interact with epithelial glycoproteins through hydrogen bonds, other ionic bonds, and Van der Waals forces. Entanglement of glycoprotein subunits has also been postulated as being important for gel formation. Lipid-epithelial glycoprotein complexes have been identified in airway mucus [13, 14], suggesting that the hydrophilic groups of the phospholipids and the epithelial glycoprotein are bound through hydrogen bonds.

Proteoglycans

Until recently, proteoglycans were considered questionable constituents of bronchial mucus, but recent studies have established them as secretory products of the airway epithelium. In secretions from unstimulated human bronchial and canine tracheal explants, 80 percent of radiolabeled [¹⁴C]glucosamine was associated with chondroitin sulfate and hyaluronic acid [18]. Proteoglycans have also been identified in secretions from the primary culture of hamster tracheal epithelial cells [75] and were found to be the major secretory product of bovine tracheal serous cells in culture [109]. The identification of proteoglycans in human [16, 17] and canine [19] bronchial aspirates suggests that the above findings are not due to artifacts of the in vitro system. The role of proteoglycans in normal mucociliary function and in the pathobiology of mucus hypersecretions needs to be studied in more detail.

DENSITY GRADIENT ULTRACENTRIFUGATION

Because bronchial mucus is intractable to handle, isolation and characterization of the bronchial epithelial glycoprotein is difficult. Several methods have been used to solubilize the secretion, including proteolytic digestion [82], sonication, and thiol reduction [23, 130], but since these actions represent degradation of macromolecules, these methods are not ideal to characterize mucous glycoprotein [90]. Even the use of a fairly mild chaotropic agent such as urea, the mildest yet applied when Roberts [126] used it, has some drawbacks, since it facilitates thiol-disulfide exchange. The introduction of density gradient ultracentrifugation (DGU) in cesium salts to isolate epithelial glycoproteins from an ovarian cyst [45] opened a new era for the study of the epithelial glycoproteins, and has been especially important for the study of those from bronchial sources [46].

DGU separates the various constituents of mucus according to relative buoyant density (Fig. 29-3). The low-density components (lipids, proteins, plasma-type glycoprotein) separate in the upper third of the tube (density 1.3 g/ml). The typical mucous glycoprotein, which is rich in sugars (60–80%), bands in the middle (1.5 gm/ml). The high-density components, such as proteoglycans and DNA, separate in the lower third of the tube (1.5 gm/ml). The method gives complete recovery of the various nondialyzable molecules in as near an undegraded state as possible at present.

MARKERS OF MACROMOLECULAR COMPONENTS INCLUDING ASTHMA

The material most commonly used to study the chemical composition and rheologic properties of airway mucus in asthma is sputum. Bronchial lavage fluid is less readily available and is only suitable for chemical analysis [90]. Sputum represents airway mucus that has reached the trachea and is expectorated mixed with saliva. Saliva contributes little to the chemical composition of airway mucus, and although care should be taken during collection of sputum to minimize salivary contamination, sputum is a suitable material for chemical and rheologic studies. The main problem in characterizing bronchial mucus in asthma is that most asthma patients produce sputum only during an acute attack. Even during an attack, particularly if it is severe, the patient usually produces sputum only after 24 to 48 hours.

Asthma patients tend to produce less sputum than patients with chronic bronchitis. In one study we attempted to collect sputum every 4 hours from six asthmatics and eight bronchitics over a period of 12 hours (6 A.M. to 6 P.M.). The asthmatics produced fewer samples, and the volume of sputum was less in asthma (6 ± 2 ml) than in chronic bronchitis (14 ± 1.5 ml) [94].

Certain simple chemical molecules can be taken as markers of the macromolecular constituents of airway mucus—fucose and sulfate for epithelial glycoprotein, and albumin and mannose for tissue fluid, whether transudate or exudate. Since neuraminic acid (NANA) is present in both epithelial and plasma-type glycoproteins, the fucose/NANA ratio gives an indication of the relative proportion of these two components [90, 92]. When comparing the chemical constituents of sputum between various diseases or between different types or stages of a given disease, it is important to compare the same macroscopic type of sputum—mucoid,

Fig. 29-3. *The density gradient method of separation as applied to sputum. Sputum dispersed in cesium bromide (CsBr) before (left) and after (right) ultracentrifugation at 40,000 rpm for 48 to 72 hours. CsBr, initially present at a uniform density (left), has formed a gradient (right) under the centrifugal field, and the different macromolecular species in sputum (left) have separated according to their buoyant densities (right). (Adapted from W. Szybalski, Equilibrium Sedimentation of Viruses, Nucleic Acids and Other Macromolecules. In Fractions. Palo Alto, Calif.: Beckman, 1968, P. 1.)*

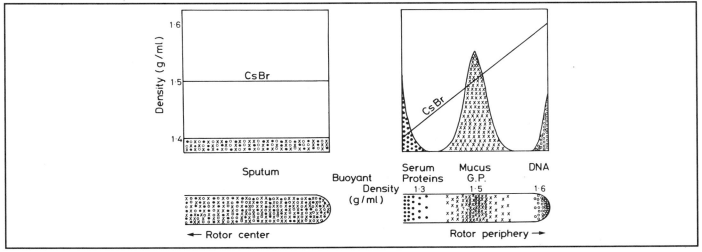

mucopurulent, or purulent. Differences in chemical markers between these macroscopic types of sputum are more marked than between diseases for a given macroscopic type. The absolute levels of dry weight of nondialyzable material and of the markers of epithelial glycoprotein and tissue fluid in mucoid sputum from unclassified asthmatics are similar to those found in mucoid chronic bronchitic sputum, but the asthmatic group shows a greater variance (Table 29-1).

When the asthma group is divided into extrinsic and intrinsic asthma, and then into patients with or without chronic mucus hypersecretion, the chemical composition of sputum from extrinsic asthma without hypersecretion shows less variance; there is greater uniformity in this than in the other three groups (Tables 29-2 and 29-3). In extrinsic and intrinsic asthma, each without chronic mucus hypersecretion, the proportion of epithelial glycoprotein is similar, but the tissue fluid component is higher in extrinsic than in intrinsic asthma. When chronic mucus hypersecretion (chronic bronchitis) is present, whether the asthma is extrinsic or intrinsic, the epithelial glycoprotein component is similar and higher than when the disease is not associated with chronic bronchitis, presumably reflecting submucosal gland hypertrophy.

Histochemical and immunofluorescence studies have demonstrated the presence of considerable amounts of proteins in intraluminal mucus from postmortem specimens. Most of the proteinaceous material is albumin; immunoglobulins, particularly IgG and IgE, are also present [54].

The protein content of mucoid asthmatic sputum is higher than that of chronic bronchitis and falls within the range found in

Table 29-1. *Dry weight and chemical constituents of mucoid sputum from patients with chronic bronchitis, asthma, and cystic fibrosis*

	Chronic bronchitis	Asthma	Cystic fibrosis
Dry weight (mg/ml)			
Mean	15.04	17.96	13.40
SE	0.84	1.84	1.40
Range	26.10–5.00	45.5–2.70	25.7–3.60
Fucose (μmole/ml)			
Mean	5.11	5.08	3.00
SE	0.39	0.39	0.40
Range	10.70–1.20	10.60–0.80	7.90–0.90
Sulfate (μmole/ml)			
Mean	1.80	1.30	0.90
SE	0.40	0.30	0.10
Range	4.50–0.30	4.20–0.30	1.50–0.20
Mannose (μmole/ml)			
Mean	0.90	0.70	0.50
SE	0.20	0.10	0.06
Range	1.60–0.40	1.40–0.21	1.10–0.20
NANA (μmole/ml)			
Mean	2.17	2.49	1.90
SE	0.21	0.22	0.20
Range	3.60–0.40	5.50–0.30	3.40–0.40
NANA/fucose ratio			
Mean	0.42	0.51	0.60
SE	0.03	0.04	0.10
Range	0.80–0.08	1.20–0.20	0.90–0.40

Comparisons using "Student's" t test	Chronic bronchitis/ cystic fibrosis	Asthma/cystic fibrosis
Fucose	9.140 ($p < 0.001$)	9.130 ($p < 0.001$)
NANA	NS	2.069 ($p < 0.05$)

NANA = N-acetylneuraminic acid; NS = difference not significant.
Source: M. T. Lopez-Vidriero and L. Reid, Chemical markers of bronchial and serum glycoproteins in mucoid and purulent sputum from various hypersecretory diseases. *Am. Rev. Respir. Dis.* 117:465, 1978. Reprinted with permission.

Table 29-2. *Dry weight and chemical markers of mucoid sputum from patients with asthma*

	EA	IA	EA + CB	IA + CB
Dry weight (mg/ml)				
Mean	14.38	20.10	15.00	20.50
SE	1.70	5.20	1.80	3.20
Range	28.80–5.00	45.50–2.70	17.40–11.40	42.20–4.80
Fucose (μmole/ml)				
Mean	5.00	4.30	7.30	5.20
SE	0.60	0.80	1.70	0.60
Range	7.90–2.10	7.60–0.80	10.60–4.80	9.10–1.40
Sulfate (μmole/ml)				
Mean	1.66	0.60		
SE	0.45	0.14		
Range	4.20–0.62	0.94–0.31		
Mannose (μmole/ml)				
Mean	0.97	0.49		
SE	0.15	0.28		
Range	1.40–0.72	0.77–0.21		
NANA (μmole/ml)				
Mean	2.50	2.50	2.50	2.40
SE	0.20	0.70	0.70	0.40
Range	5.50–1.00	5.50–0.30	3.90–1.70	4.80–0.80
NANA/fucose ratio				
Mean	0.60	0.50	0.30	0.40
SE	0.10	0.10	0.04	0.03
Range	1.20–0.30	0.95–0.20	0.40–0.20	0.70–0.20

EA = extrinsic asthma without chronic bronchitis; IA = intrinsic asthma without chronic bronchitis; EA + CB = extrinsic asthma with chronic bronchitis; IA + CB = intrinsic asthma with chronic bronchitis; NANA = N-acetylneuraminic acid.
Source: M. T. Lopez-Vidriero and L. Reid, Chemical markers of bronchial and serum glycoproteins in mucoid and purulent sputum from various hypersecretory diseases. *Am. Rev. Respir. Dis.* 117:465, 1978. Reprinted with permission.

Table 29-3. *Dry weight and chemical constituents of mucopurulent sputum from patients with asthma*

	IA (n = 8)	EA + CB (n = 4)	IA + CB (n = 14)
Dry weight (mg/ml)			
Mean	32.20	46.40	31.30
SE	6.90	6.10	3.60
Range	57.40–16.00	62.80–42.50	47.70–9.20
Fucose (μmole/ml)			
Mean	10.30	9.80	6.80
SE	2.28	1.40	0.90
Range	20.10–4.70	14.00–7.30	11.10–1.70
Sulfate (μmole/ml)			
Mean	3.29	3.02	3.71
SE	0.79	0.98	0.28
Range	4.18–1.70	4.00–2.04	4.10–3.16
Mannose (μmole/ml)			
Mean	2.96		3.00
SE	1.04		0.28
Range	4.00–0.88		3.80–2.50
NANA (μmole/ml)			
Mean	5.40	8.40	4.80
SE	0.80	1.30	0.80
Range	8.60–2.40	12.20–5.80	8.40–0.20
NANA/fucose ratio			
Mean	0.60	0.90	0.70
SE	0.10	0.10	0.10
Range	0.80–0.40	1.00–0.60	1.50–0.10

IA = intrinsic asthma without chronic bronchitis; EA + CB = extrinsic asthma with chronic bronchitis; IA + CB = intrinsic asthma with chronic bronchitis; NANA = N-acetylneuraminic acid.
Source: M. T. Lopez-Vidriero and L. Reid, Chemical markers of bronchial and serum glycoproteins in mucoid and purulent sputum from various hypersecretory diseases. *Am. Rev. Respir. Dis.* 117:465, 1978. Reprinted with permission.

grossly infected cystic fibrosis sputum [31]. The albumin content is six times higher than that found in sputum from chronic bronchitis and is even higher than that in infected cystic fibrosis. Other proteins derived from plasma (IgG, transferrin, 1-antitrypsin, antichymotrypsin, and haptoglobin) are also considerably higher in asthma than in chronic bronchitis, indicating an inflammatory exudate. In contrast, the content of proteins produced by the mucus-secreting cells of the airways (lysozyme and bronchotransferrin) is similar to that of chronic bronchitic sputum.

Protein content has not been analyzed separately for extrinsic and intrinsic asthma or for asthma with or without chronic mucus hypersecretion. It has been suggested that in extrinsic asthma the airway mucus contains more IgE than in intrinsic asthma, but these findings are based on a small number of patients [50, 68].

Bronchorrhea

Bronchorrhea is a condition characterized by the production of a large volume of sputum (more than 100 ml/day in the convention we follow for diagnosis) that is transparent, resembles egg white, and is usually topped by a layer of froth. The concentration of nondialyzable material is low, in most cases being less than 1 percent of the total weight; water represents as much as 98 to 99 percent of the airway mucus expectorated by these patients. The daily production of epithelial glycoprotein is within the range found in chronic bronchitis, but the water tissue fluid transudate is well above chronic bronchitic levels. This is important for the management of these patients, since they respond better to corticosteroids than to atropine [73].

In some bronchorrhea specimens, the secretion separates spontaneously into two layers, a thicker opaque gel floating on a thin clear watery fluid [95]. Unlike other diseases, in bronchorrhea some sputum samples become more viscous with time, suggesting that intermolecular cross-linkage is taking place when the mucus is outside the airways.

Bronchial Casts

Bronchial casts are sometimes found in sputum from asthma patients and are often seen in their bronchial lavage fluid. Two types of bronchial casts have been identified [73]. One is characterized by an extremely high content of nondialyzable material (211–336 mg/ml) and high NANA content (6.29–16.6 mg/ml). In the other, the casts chemically resemble chronic bronchitic sputum in dry weight yield (15.4 mg/ml) and NANA content (0.56 mg/ml). The first type of bronchial cast is probably formed by retention of secretion and slow dehydration, while in the second other factors must be involved that change the physical state of the secretion.

Constituents of Sol and Gel Phases

Airway mucus has the appearance of a fibrillar network, including open spaces filled with liquid [138]. By means of high-speed ultracentrifugation, the liquid or soluble component of the mucus (the sol phase) can be squeezed out of the mesh made by the nondispersed component or gel phase.

The pattern of separation of sputum into sol and gel phases by high-speed ultracentrifugation has been studied in various diseases including asthma [91, 93]. Complete separation into sol and gel is achieved in all diseases at 160,000 g, but the centrifugal speed at which separation starts varies between diseases. In bronchorrhea, separation starts at 5,000 g, while in chronic bronchitis it is only at the higher speed of 60,000 g. In bronchorrhea states, much of the sputum volume (the water) is in the sol phase. When the sol phase represents 85 percent or more of the mucus, we describe the pattern of separation as the bronchorrhea or sol type; when the gel phase accounts for 40 to 60 percent of the total secretion, as it does in chronic bronchitis, we consider it the chronic bronchitic or gel type. Noninfected chronic bronchitic sputum typically separates as the gel type, while asthmatic sputum sometimes separates as the gel and sometimes as the sol type. Whether this variation reflects different degrees of gland hypertrophy, inflammatory reaction, or the effect of drugs is not known. In general, proteins, epithelial glycoprotein, and DNA have been identified in both phases, while lipids are present only in the gel.

In patients with bronchorrhea, the chemical markers of tissue fluid transudate, albumin, transferrin, and IgG show a different pattern of distribution in extrinsic versus intrinsic asthma. In extrinsic asthma, albumin and IgG are considerably higher in the sol phase than in the gel. In intrinsic asthma, they are present in similar amounts in both phases. In extrinsic asthma, immunoglobulin A, measured as total IgA (7S + 11S) follows the pattern of separation of albumin—that is, being higher in the sol compared to the gel phase. In intrinsic asthma the reverse exists; the gel contains more IgA than the sol phase, indicating that in intrinsic asthma the epithelium is predominantly secreting IgA that is strongly bound to the epithelial glycoprotein. In extrinsic asthma perhaps the IgA derives from plasma transudate (7S) and separates with the other plasma proteins. Fucose, a marker of epithelial glycoprotein, is present in both phases, although the gel contains 10 to 40 times more than the sol. The sol phase of extrinsic asthma contains less fucose than that of intrinsic asthma, suggesting that in extrinsic asthma most of the epithelial glycoprotein is forming insoluble aggregates.

It is of interest to note that in patients with asthma and without bronchorrhea epithelial glycoprotein has not been identified in the sol phase [13]. From chronic bronchitics, however, a soluble mucous glycoprotein in always recovered from the sol phase [14]. Since it is tempting to assume that the sol phase constitutes the periciliary layer, this finding points to a major difference in this liquid layer between the two diseases. In bronchorrhea the rate of secretion is increased, and it is possible that the synthesis of the epithelial glycoprotein molecule is not complete.

The mucous glycoprotein in the asthma gel is insoluble and seems to resemble that recovered from chronic bronchitics. In extrinsic asthma its concentration is less than that in intrinsic asthma. In intrinsic asthma its concentration is reminiscent of chronic bronchitis secretions. The chemical composition is similar in both types of asthma.

PHYSICOCHEMICAL STUDIES OF BRONCHIAL MUCUS

Normal Bronchial Mucus

The application of the DGU technique to analysis of bronchial mucus aspirated from normal volunteers [11] has revealed some unexpected results concerning the nature of bronchial mucus in situ in normal airways. In a study of unpooled, individual bronchial aspirates obtained by fiberoptic bronchoscopy ([17] and additional subjects examined since then), epithelial glycoprotein of typical buoyant density was not detected in nine of ten such aspirates from healthy nonsmoking volunteers. Supporting this notion that normal bronchial mucus contains little if any typical epithelial glycoprotein is a similar finding in aspirates from normal canine trachea [19]. Twenty-seven pre-SO_2 aspirates from 17 different dogs did not contain epithelial glycoprotein of typical buoyant density. The glycoconjugate present, besides having a higher buoyant density, seemed a "hybrid," in that it had features of both glycoprotein and proteoglycan. A similar high-density component was present in the mucus from acute quadriplegic patients, in addition to a component of buoyant density typical of epithelial glycoprotein. The amino acid composition (glycine

⟩ serine ⟩ threonine) of the high-density component was different from that of typical glycoprotein (threonine ⟩ serine ⟩ glycine). The high-density component reacted positively to a monoclonal antibody raised to keratan sulfate but the glycoprotein did not.

The proteoglycan structure includes O-linked oligosaccharides, as is typical of epithelial glycoproteins, in the region where keratan sulfate chains are present: the hybrid glycoconjugate of normal bronchial mucus could very well be this part of the proteoglycan polymer. In support of this is a recent report that "rabbit tracheal surface epithelium secretes glycosaminoglycans and a novel high molecular weight glycoprotein resembling keratan sulfate" [25]. In heavy smokers, as in post-SO_2 aspirates from dogs, glycoprotein of typical buoyant density and composition was recovered even before yields of nondialyzable material had reached the high levels characteristic of hypersecretory conditions such as chronic bronchitis. Further support for the postulate that typical epithelial glycoprotein is not a component of normal mucus but appears only upon irritation came from studies using a monoclonal antibody raised to typical bronchial epithelial glycoprotein: it was found that there were relatively low mean titers to this antibody in the canine pre-exposure aspirates, but significantly increased titers after prolonged SO_2 exposure [78]. Immunohistochemical analysis of airway tissue from control dogs whose aspirates did not react with the antibody showed little or no staining, whereas SO_2-exposed dogs whose bronchial aspirates reacted positively with the antibody showed patchy staining of the mucous glands and airway secretory cells as well as dense staining of the supraciliary mucus layer in the airway lumen (Plate 6).

Recently this has been confirmed in another species. Davies and colleagues [49] in the cat found typical mucus in pilocarpine-stimulated secretion but not in basal secretion; in the latter, they identified a glycoconjugate of higher buoyant density that was not DNA but contained keratanase-sensitive material.

The lipid profile of normal mucus is also markedly different from that seen in hypersecretory mucus. In both human and canine normal mucus, neutral lipids are predominant, with lesser amounts of phospholipids; glycolipids have not been detected. In hypersecretory mucus from several human diseases, glycolipids are usually the predominant species [20, 21, 65]. The presence of glycolipids in the mucus of the normal smoker as well as their early appearance in canine mucus after exposure to SO_2 indicate that glycolipids are an early marker of hypersecretion. Tracheostomy findings suggest that either the surgical procedure or repeated aspiration is sufficient to induce mucus hypersecretion. The bronchial mucus aspirated from the normal smoker probably includes a surface mucus film plus periciliary layer, while that from the heavier smoker comes from a thicker surface film, one thick enough perhaps to be considered a blanket.

Other attempts to obtain normal secretions can be compared with the above findings. From normal volunteers, secretion of bronchial mucus was stimulated by inhalation of PGF_2 [96]. The material expectorated contained tissue fluid transudate. Fucose also was found and taken to be a marker of mucous glycoprotein, but since IgA contains fucose (as does α_2-macroglobulin and haptoglobin, not to mention fucoglycolipids), and since in our recent study typical glycoprotein was not found in the normal, there must be some doubt about this interpretation. Aspirates obtained after exposure to SO_2, 200 ppm and 50 ppm, contain epithelial glycoprotein, indicating that some degree of epithelial stimulation is necessary to recover typical mucous glycoprotein.

Some investigators claim to have found epithelial glycoprotein in secretions from normal subjects, but the nature of the samples or the techniques used in these studies is not adequate to disprove the above results. Williams and coworkers [156] reported the presence of high-molecular-weight glycoprotein in the bronchial aspirates from healthy nonsmoking volunteers. The criteria they used, namely, absorption at 280 nm, void volume elution,

Table 29-4. Percentage composition of the gel phases (obtained by centrifugation) of AsEXT and AsINT sputa

	AsEXT	AsINT
Protein	42 (1.0)*	30 (0.7)
Insoluble gel	23 (0.6)	13 (0.3)
Mucous glycoprotein	35 (0.9)	57 (1.4)

* Numbers in parentheses indicate percent yields of wet weight of gel.
AsEXT = extrinsic asthma; AsINT = intrinsic asthma.
Source: K. R. Bhaskar and L. Reid, Application of density gradient methods for the study of mucus glycoprotein and other macromolecular components of the sol and gel phases of asthmatic sputa. *J. Biol. Chem.* 256:7583, 1982. Reprinted with permission.

Table 29-5. Physical properties of native and reduced mucous glycoprotein isolated from AsEXT and AsINT gels

	AsEXT		AsINT	
	Native	Reduced	Native	Reduced
Buoyant density, ρ_0 (gm/ml)	1.505	1.522	1.518	1.530
Sedimentation coefficient, s_{20}*	11.3	7.5	19.7	10.1
η_{red} (ml/gm)	258	82	317	63

* s_{20} and η_{red} determined on solutions of 1 mg/ml concentration.
AsEXT = extrinsic asthma; AsINT = intrinsic asthma.
Source: K. R. Bhaskar and L. Reid, Application of density gradient methods for the study of mucus glycoprotein and other macromolecular components of the sol and gel phases of asthmatic sputa. *J. Biol. Chem.* 256:7583, 1982. Reprinted with permission.

and alcian blue staining, are also characteristic of glycosaminoglycans. The study of Sachdev and associates [131] identified epithelial glycoprotein in aspirate from nonsmoking volunteers, but this finding was made in pooled aspirates. More recently, Thornton and coworkers [142] reported that the size and macromolecular architecture of tracheal mucins isolated from mucous airway samples of patients undergoing dental surgery under general anesthesia was similar to that of mucin from chronic bronchitic sputum, but no amino acid compositions were reported.

Asthma, Extrinsic and Intrinsic

Studies on asthmatic mucus have been limited because of the small volumes produced by patients, but in recent years information on this subject has been increasing [13, 55, 129]. Gels from asthmatic sputa are recalcitrant to dispersion in cesium bromide (CsBr), much more so than the even more viscous gels from cystic fibrosis sputa [13] (Tables 29-4 and 29-5). This difference seems to be related to the presence of infection rather than to the disease. In one patient with chronic bronchitis, for example, we examined a sputum sample during infection and after recovery [14]. The gel from the mucoid (not infected) sample was refractory to dispersion as in asthma, and the lipids were bound to their glycoprotein. In contrast, the gel from the infected sputum, although more viscous than the gel from the mucoid sputum, dispersed quickly, and the glycoprotein separated easily. Repeated DGU, however, eventually separates from insoluble lipids the soluble epithelial mucous glycoproteins that have been characterized in detail (Fig. 29-4).

Glycoproteins isolated from asthmatic sputa, both extrinsic and intrinsic, have features similar to those of epithelial glycoproteins from airway mucus from other diseases such as cystic fibrosis and chronic bronchitis (Fig. 29-5). Fucose, galactose, N-acetylglucosamine, and N-acetylgalactosamine are the predominant sugars and make up 80 percent of the total (Table 29-6).

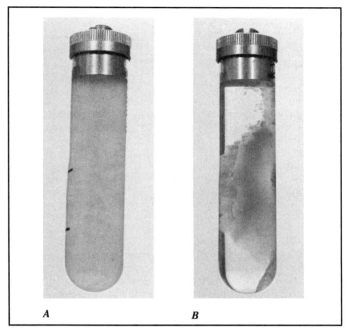

Fig. 29-4. *Density gradient ultracentrifugation (DGU) of gel from extrinsic asthma sputum. Centrifuge tube contains gel dispersed in CsBr (initial density, 1.41 gm/ml) before (A) and after (B) DGU (40,000 rpm for 48 hours at 15°C). Clear liquid at top contained most of the serum proteins. Insoluble gel together with clear liquid at bottom contained all mucous glycoprotein, lipids, and some protein (this was subjected to DGU II).*

Amino acids constitute the rest of the molecule, and of these serine, threonine, and proline make up 45 percent. Buoyant densities in CsBr ($\sim$1.5 gm/ml) are typical of epithelial mucous glycoproteins [7]. Sedimentation coefficients are high, especially for intrinsic asthma, implying large molecular weights of the order of 3 to 7 $\times$ 10^6. The glycoproteins give rise to very viscous solutions, much more so than glycoproteins isolated from cystic fibrosis sputum at similar concentrations. Treatment with the disulfide bond-breaking reagent DTT produces marked changes in the glycoprotein: Solution viscosities and sedimentation coefficients are lower, suggesting reduction in molecular weights; buoyant densities are higher, indicating loss of peptide, while molar ratios of sugars remain practically unchanged [13]. These results indicate that the native glycoprotein is an aggregate formed by disulfide bonds, possibly through a cross-linking peptide.

The marked reduction in solution viscosity brought about by thiol treatment gives a molecular basis for the use of thiol reagents as mucolytics. The intractable nature of the lipid glycoprotein complex, however, suggests that such interactions through electrostatic and/or hydrophobic forces between the glycoprotein and lipids are equally important in the stabilization of the gel structure, perhaps even more than disulfide-bond aggregation.

Even after the third DGU of the gel from intrinsic asthma, some lipids remained bound to the mucous glycoprotein. However, when the gel resulting from the second DGU was reduced with DTT before a third DGU was run, no such lipid-bound glycoprotein was recovered. It seems that the region of the disulfide bonds is also the region where lipids attach. Since this region appears to have a cross-linking peptide relatively enriched in the acidic amino acids, it would favor charge interactions (Table 29-7). Rose and colleagues [129] also found that the gel from an asth-

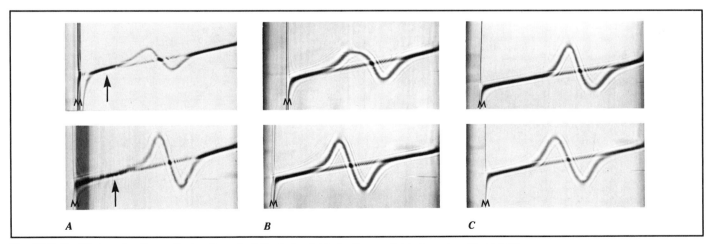

Fig. 29-5. *Equilibrium density gradient patterns in CsBr. A. Insoluble fraction containing mucous glycoprotein (after density gradient ultracentrifugation [DGU] II). B. Native mucous glycoprotein isolated from it by DGU III. C. Reduced mucous glycoprotein isolated from it by DGU III'. (Upper row) extrinsic asthma; (lower row) intrinsic asthma. Initial density: B and C, lower row, 1.535 gm/ml; all others, 1.5 gm/ml; 40,000 rpm at 20°C. In both rows, A shows a dark band at the meniscus (M) region; this arises partly from the insoluble layer of lipids and partly from protein that accumulates in this region. The pronounced curvature near the meniscus seen in A of the upper row is also protein. Mucous glycoprotein in both cases forms a distinct zone in the middle (two-lobed pattern). The initial density for DGU III and III' to separate mucous glycoprotein from the rest was chosen to correspond to the region of separation seen here (arrows). B and C of isolated mucous glycoprotein, both native and reduced, show negligible material at the meniscus. Reduced mucous glycoprotein bands are farther to the right than are those of native mucous glycoprotein because of their high buoyant densities.*

Table 29-6. Chemical composition of native and reduced mucous glycoprotein isolated from AsEXT and AsINT gels[a]

	AsEXT		AsINT	
	Native	Reduced	Native	Reduced
Fucose	7 (0.9)[b]	8 (0.9)	13 (2.3)	15 (2.4)
Galactose	23 (2.6)	26 (2.6)	29 (4.9)	33 (4.8)
N-Acetylglucosamine	21 (1.9)	23 (1.8)	22 (3.0)	26 (3.1)
N-Acetylgalactosamine	11 (1.0)	12 (1.0)	7 (1.0)	8 (1.0)
N-Acetylneuraminic acid	16 (1.1)	17 (1.0)	10 (1.0)	14 (1.2)
Sulfate	1	1	1	1
Amino acids	24	18	17	12

[a] Compositions are expressed as grams of component/100 gm of glycoprotein.
[b] Numbers in parentheses indicate molar ratios of sugars with respect to N-acetylgalactosamine.
AsEXT = extrinsic asthma; AsINT = intrinsic asthma.
Source: K. R. Bhaskar and L. Reid, Application of density gradient methods for the study of mucus glycoprotein and other macromolecular components of the sol and gel phases of asthmatic sputa. *J. Biol. Chem.* 256:7583, 1982. Reprinted with permission.

Table 29-7. Amino acid composition of native and reduced mucous glycoprotein isolated from AsEXT and AsINT gels[a]

	AsEXT		AsINT	
	Native	Reduced	Native	Reduced
Aspartic acid	7.1	5.5	5.8	3.7
Threonine	17.9	22.5	20.4	25.6
Serine	12.1	13.7	12.1	14.1
Glutamic acid	9.7	7.8	8.7	6.1
Proline	12.7	13.7	12.5	14.2
Glycine	8.1	7.6	8.9	7.8
Alanine	7.1	7.5	8.4	9.0
Half-cystine	1.1	1.5[b]	1.3	1.5[b]
Others	24.2	20.2	21.9	18.0
Aspartic acid + glutamic acid	16.8	13.3	14.5	9.8
Serine + threonine + proline	42.7	49.9	45.0	53.9

[a] Values are expressed as micromoles of amino acid/100 μmol of total amino acids.
[b] As S-carboxymethylcysteine.
AsEXT = extrinsic asthma; AsINT = intrinsic asthma.
Source: K. R. Bhaskar and L. Reid, Application of density gradient methods for the study of mucus glycoprotein and other macromolecular components of the sol and gel phases of asthmatic sputa. *J. Biol. Chem.* 256:7583, 1982. Reprinted with permission.

matic sputum that was not solubilized by thiol reagent could be solubilized by dissociating salts such as guanidine chloride, urea, and sodium dodecyl-sulfate. It would therefore appear that gel formation is a two-step process, involving both disulfide-bond formation between glycoprotein molecules and charge forces between glycoprotein and other molecules.

Status Asthmaticus

Bronchial mucus taken from the airways of a fatal case of status asthmaticus has recently been analyzed (K. R. Bhaskar, et al. Characterization of airway mucus from a fatal case of status asthmaticus, manuscript in preparation). Analysis of the freeze-dried mucus by DGU showed no material in the buoyant density region (1.5 gm/ml) typical of mucous glycoprotein. Over 90 percent of the nondialyzable material was recovered in the region to which lipids and proteins migrate. Most of this material was present as an insoluble sticky layer at the very top of the tube (lowest density) and contained appreciable amounts of lipids. Thin-layer chromatography of the $CHCl_3:MeOH$ extract of this insoluble fraction indicated that the main lipids were phosphatidylcholine,

sphingomyelin, phosphatidylethanolamine, lysophosphatidylethanolamine, cholesterol, and cholesterol esters, and in addition, in lesser amounts, dihexosyl ceramide and tetrahexosyl ceramide, ganglioside (GM_3), phosphatidic acid, phosphatidylserine, and phosphatidylinositol (Plate 7). The presence of glycolipids and ganglioside is interesting and suggests possible parasympathetic nerve breakdown; the acidic phospholipids also suggest membrane instability or premature degranulation.

Surprisingly, the residue left after the extraction of lipids from this insoluble fraction contained all the sugars typical of mucous glycoproteins. In addition, oligosaccharides, 3 to 12 sugars long, were cleaved by treatment with alkaline borohydride, implying that these were O-glycosidically linked as in typical glycoproteins. It has been shown recently that mucous glycoproteins can be strongly associated with lipids [13, 157], such associations often being resistant to cesium salt gradients and effectively pulling the mucous glycoprotein into regions of buoyant density lower than is typical of the free glycoprotein. This is especially true of asthmatic mucus. This strong linkage between the lipid and glycoprotein could occur within or without the cell, the latter being more likely. Besides the usual sugars, the residue also contained glucose and methylmannuronate, which are not associated with mucous glycoprotein. The glucose may be degraded glucosamine.

A small proportion of the nondialyzable content of the mucus (7%) was found in the high-density region (1.58 gm/ml). This component also contained all the sugars typical of epithelial glycoprotein but in addition contained xylose and glucose. It remains to be established whether these disparate components occur in the same molecule due to an aberration of the synthetic process or are parts of different molecules tightly bound together.

Physical Properties of Bronchial Mucus in Asthma

In asthma the physical properties of expectorated bronchial mucus range from a copious watery secretion to an extremely viscid mucus that is difficult or impossible to expectorate. This range is reflected in higher viscosity levels than those seen in chronic bronchitis, cystic fibrosis, or bronchiectasis [34, 92]. Sputum from patients with intrinsic asthma and chronic mucus hypersecretion shows the widest variation and tends to be more viscous than that produced by patients with extrinsic asthma without or with chronic mucus hypersecretion or intrinsic asthma without chronic sputum production [92]. When infection is present, asthmatic sputum is significantly more viscous than that from patients with chronic bronchitis, cystic fibrosis, or bronchiectasis. Once again, intrinsic asthma sputum shows the highest variance, but extrinsic asthma sputum tends to be more viscous. The elasticity of asthmatic sputum, measured at low frequencies (less than 1 cycle/sec), falls within the levels found in other diseases [107]. It is of interest to note that asthmatic sputum is more resistant to shear than that from chronic bronchitis or cystic fibrosis, indicating that molecular cross-linking is stronger than that in other diseases.

CELLS OF ORIGIN OF AIRWAY MUCUS

The surface epithelial lining of the airways includes eight cell types, although not all are found at all levels. The submucosal glands, found only in the trachea and bronchi (that is, in about the proximal two-thirds of the axial intrasegmental airways), include an additional five cell types as well as the surface epithelial cell types in the first few millimeters of the gland opening. Mucous and serous cells are found in surface epithelium and in the gland but should be considered distinct cell types, since the regulation of their secretion is different. Serous cells from bovine

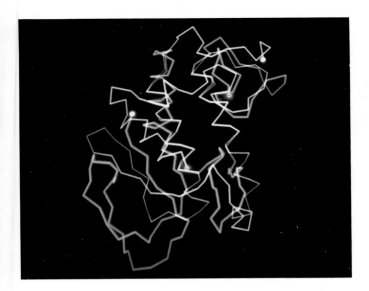

Plate 1. *Backbone Cα traces of bee venom (blue) and bovine pancreatic (orange) phospholipase A₂. The blue and white dots represent, respectively, the N- and C-termini of these proteins. The different shades of blue or orange represent relative depth from the plane of the photo. The pink tracings represent regions of similarity of the two proteins. (Reprinted with permission from D. L. Scott, et al. Crystal structure of bee venom phospholipase A2 in a complex with a transition-state analogue. Science 250:1563, 1990. Copyright 1990 by the AAAS.)*

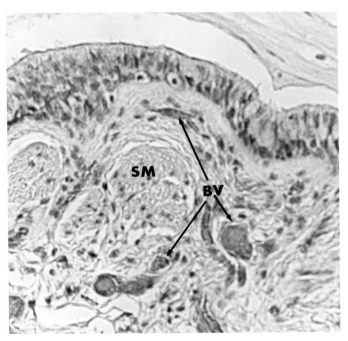

Plate 3. *A histologic section of an airway from an asthmatic lung. Note the smaller dilated vessels in the submucosa joined by interconnecting vessels that pass between the muscle bundles and join the larger bronchial venous plexus outside the muscle. (SM = smooth muscle; BV = bronchial vessels; hematoxylin-eosin, ×900.)*

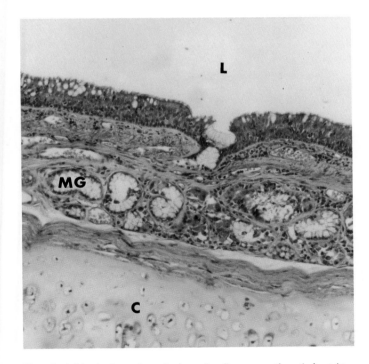

Plate 2. *A histologic section of a bronchus from an asthmatic lung in which the pseudostratified epithelium is present on the surface; the opening to a bronchial gland duct is also shown. The gland itself is in the submucosa and occupies a large proportion of the space between the bronchial cartilage and the basement membrane. (L = lumen; MG = mucous gland; C = cartilage; Masson, ×620.)*

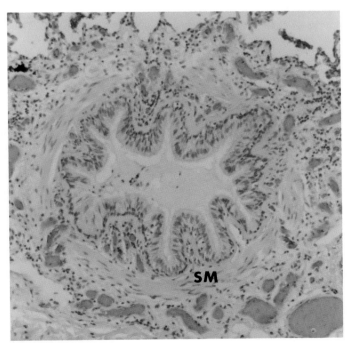

Plate 4. *A histologic section showing a bronchiole, in which the lumen is filled with an inflammatory exudate, and a markedly dilated bronchial vasculature. Note that the vessels inside the muscle layer are smaller than those outside. (SM = smooth muscle; hematoxylin-eosin, ×760.)*

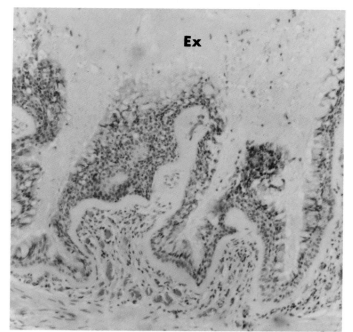

A

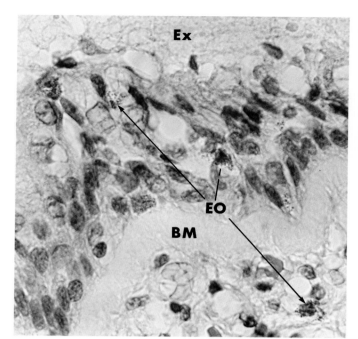

B

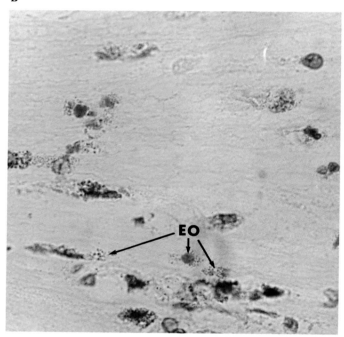

C

Plate 5. *Histologic sections from an asthmatic airway. A. A disrupted epithelium due to shedding and regeneration of the epithelial surface. Note the very markedly thickened basement membrane, the inflammatory exudate in the lumen, and the dilatation of the bronchial vessels. (Ex = exudate in the bronchial lumen; hematoxylin-eosin, ×760.) B. A close-up showing the markedly thickened basement membrane with eosinophils present both below the basement membrane and in the epithelium. (Ex = exudate in the bronchial lumen; BM = basement membrane; EO = eosinophils; hematoxylin-eosin, ×960.) C. A close-up of the exudate in the airway lumen where there are large numbers of cells, many of which are eosinophils in various states of degranulation. (EO = eosinophils; hematoxylin-eosin, ×1200.)*

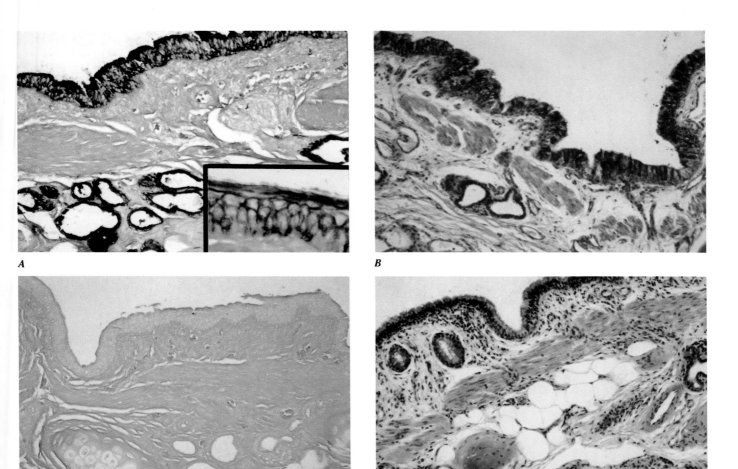

Plate 6. *Immunoperoxidase (A) and periodic acid–Schiff (PAS) staining of SO$_2$-exposed (B) and control (D) dog lungs. In the experimental dog, there is dense reaction in the surface epithelium and glandular cells, as well as in the airway lumen. Inset in A shows the detail of the immunohistochemical reaction pattern in airway epithelial cells. There is little or no reaction in the immunostained control dog section (C). PAS-stained sections show numerous positive cells in the airway epithelium of the SO$_2$-exposed dog. Generally, there was mucous gland hypertrophy and hyperplasia in experimental dog lungs. (×200; inset: ×500). (Reprinted with permission from T. Koshino, et al., Recovery of an epitope recognized by a novel monoclonal antibody from airway lavage during experimental induction of chronic bronchitis.* Am. J. Respir. Cell Mol. Biol. *2:453, 1990.)*

Orcinol spray: yellow to brown = phospholipid
purple = glycolipid

Cholesterol and cholesterol esters

Glycolipid-1 (GL-1) (double spot)

Phosphatidylethanolamine (PE)

Glycolipid-2 (GL-2) (double spot)

Sulfatide

Glycolipid-3 (GL-3)

Phosphatidylcholine (PC)

Phosphatidylserine (PS)

Sphingomyelin

Lysophosphatidylcholine (LPC)
Phosphatidylinositol (PI)

Gangliosides (four spots) e.g., GM-3

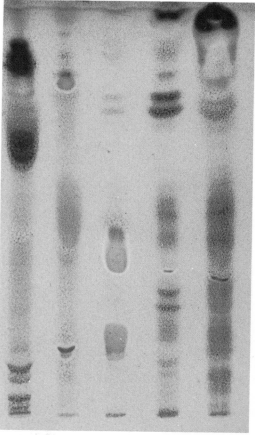

Brain glyco-lipid std	PE PC PI	GL-2 PC PS LPC	Trache-ostomy	Stat asth

Plate 7. *Thin-layer chromatography of lipids from mucous plugs from a fatal case of status asthmaticus* (Stat asth) *(right) and from a tracheostomy aspirate from a patient with neurologic disease (second from right). Appropriate standards are also shown, and their abbreviations are given in the lefthand column.*

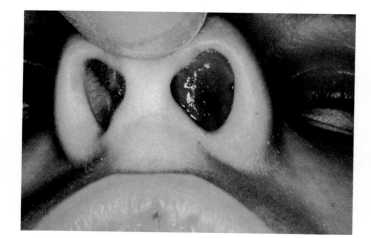

Plate 8. *Nasal polyp.*

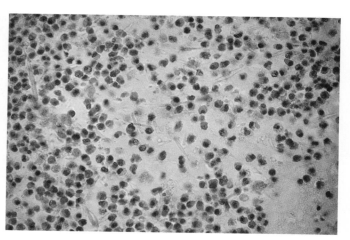

Plate 9. *Photomicrograph of sputum from a patient with allergic bronchopulmonary aspergillosis. Eosinophils and Charcot-Leyden crystals are present. Fungal hyphae are not seen.*

tracheal glands have been shown to produce proteoglycans [109]. They have also been shown to secrete an albumin-like protein [69]. Most agents that are secretagogues for the glands have no effect on the surface cells. The Clara cell found in small airways also secretes glycoprotein [112]. Under conditions of prolonged stimulation or irritation, Clara and serous cells of the surface epithelium can each rapidly develop into a mucous cell [71].

Proteins present in airway mucus derive from tissue fluid transudate and are also locally produced by the mucous and serous cells of the submucosal glands (lysozyme, bronchotransferrin, secretory piece) or by plasma cells (immunoglobulins) [27, 28, 30]. Although lipids in airway liquid are partly derived from alveolar surfactant and tissue fluid transudate, they are also produced by the airway mucosal cells in human and canine tracheobronchial explants [41]. Proteoglycans probably derive from connective tissue and cell membranes, but further studies of their origin and the regulation of their secretion are needed. Isolated hamster tracheal epithelial cells in culture also produce a wide range of lipids [75].

The intracellular types of epithelial glycoproteins have been extensively studied in the mucous and serous cells of the submucosal glands and the surface epithelium [72, 80, 81]. By means of various histochemical techniques, either singly or in combination, several types of glycoprotein have been identified. These include two main types, neutral and acidic. The acidic glycoproteins are sialylated and/or sulfated, and within the sialylated type they can be sensitive or resistant to the action of neuraminidase. Each of these glycoproteins is identified in the secretory cells of the human airways, both in health and disease, but they exist only in certain combinations [72, 80, 81]. The Clara cell found in the bronchioli is also a secretory cell. Although the nature of its secretion is not fully established, it contains proteins and neutral sugars.

CONTROL OF PRODUCTION OF BRONCHIAL MUCUS

Understanding of the control of bronchial mucus production in man and animals has come mainly from in vitro analysis [8, 22, 33, 40, 113, 141], although a limited number of in vivo studies have also been performed [60, 146] (Table 29-8). Most studies focused on the effect of exogenous secretagogues on the secretion of the macromolecular constituents of bronchial mucus, particularly glycoproteins, usually after radiolabeling in vitro with radioactive carbohydrates or sulfate. An estimate of the labeled macromolecules released into the culture medium can be combined with biochemical analysis.

The surface epithelium and submucosal glands can be studied separately, as can the variety of secretory cell types at each site, and the normal can be compared with the hypertrophied bronchitic gland. By labeling the glycoprotein, morphometric techniques, and precursor autoradiographic analysis of secretory cells, precursor uptake, glycoprotein synthesis, and granule transport and discharge can be analyzed [39]. Such methods have not been used extensively. A large number of agents, including cholinergic and adrenergic agonists, neuropeptides, and inflammatory mediators, are now known to induce bronchial mucus secretion, but the specific cell types in the airway mucosa upon which most of these act are not known. It cannot be assumed that an agent that increases airway mucus secretion does so by stimulating macromolecular discharge from secretory cells in either the submucosal gland or epithelium. Preliminary studies carried out in this laboratory show that two of the newly identified potent agonists for airway mucus secretion, leukotrienes and substance P, have little or no effect on secretory cell discharge. At least one of these, substance P, appears to act by constricting

Table 29-8. *In vitro studies of control of airway secretion in humans*

	Mucus constituent	Effect	Reference
Neurotransmitters			
Cholinergic	Gp	↑	Sturgess & Reid, 1972 [141]
	Gp	↑	Coles & Reid, 1978 [39]
	Gp	↑	Shelhamer et al., 1980 [136]
	Ions	↑	Knowles et al., 1982 [77]
Beta-adrenergic	Gp	−	Sturgess & Reid, 1972 [141]
	Gp	−	Boat & Kleinerman, 1975 [22]
	Gp	↑	Phipps et al., 1982 [113]
	Ions	−	Knowles et al., 1982 [77]
Alpha-adrenergic	Gp	↑	Phipps et al., 1982 [113]
	Gp	↑	Shelhamer et al., 1980 [136]
	Ions	−	Knowles et al., 1982 [77]
Opioid agonists			
Morphine	Gp	↑	Rogers & Barnes, 1989 [127]
Regulatory peptides			
VIP	Gp	↓	Coles et al., 1981 [40]
Substance P	Gp	↑	Coles et al., 1984 [38]
Calcitonin gene–related peptide	Gp	↑	Mak & Barnes, 1988 [100]
Neurokinin A	Gp	↑	Lundberg et al., 1985 [98]
Chemical mediators			
Histamine	Gp	−	Sturgess & Reid, 1972 [141]
	Gp	↑	Shelhamer et al., 1980 [136]
Arachidonic acid	Gp	↑	Marom et al., 1982 [102]
Prostaglandins			
$PGF_{2\alpha}$, PGA_2, PGD_2	Gp	↑	Marom et al., 1982 [102]
PGE_2	Gp	↓	Marom et al., 1982 [102]
Monohydroxyeicosatetraenoic acid	Gp	↑	Marom et al., 1981 [101]
Leukotrienes C_4, D_4	Gp	↑	Shelhamer et al., 1982 [135]
	Gp	↑	Coles et al., 1983 [42]
Bradykinin	Gp	↑	Proud & Kaplan, 1988 [116]
Platelet-activating factor	Gp	↑	Barnes et al., 1988 [6]

VIP = vasoactive intestinal peptide; Gp = glycoprotein; ↑ = increase; ↓ = inhibitory; − = no effect.

the collecting duct and/or secretory tubules of the submucosal gland, resulting in clearance of their intraluminal mucus into the airway; this effect may be due to contraction of the myoepithelial cell sheath of the secretory tubules and gland ducts.

The rate of clearance of mucus from the submucosal glands seems also to be influenced by the concentration of calcium (Ca^{++}) or possibly of other divalent cations bound to the mucous glycoprotein. A reduction in Ca^{++} concentration increases mucus clearance from the glands, while an increase in Ca^{++} reduces it [37]. The Ca^{++} changes the physical properties of airway mucus, in particular its solubility, viscoelasticity, and degree of hydration [24, 56, 57, 104].

The contribution of macromolecules derived from a transudate of serum to the total volume of mucus secreted may also be of considerable significance in vivo. Many agents known to increase airway mucus secretion in vitro, including substance P, neurokinin A, histamine, prostaglandins, leukotrienes, bradykinins, and platelet-activating factor (PAF), also increase airway vascular permeability in vivo, potentially increasing transudation of serum macromolecules into the airway lumen. These not only increase the macromolecular content of respiratory mucus but also modify its physicochemical properties.

A recent study of bronchial mucus hypersecretion in victims of acute quadriplegia indicated that neuronal regulation of bronchial mucus secretion may be of considerable importance [16]. Many quadriplegic patients develop excessive bronchial mucus secretions soon after injury. The onset of hypersecretion is, however, too sudden to result from gland hypertrophy, and yet analysis showed that, in both macromolecular yields and chemical composition, the mucus resembled that from established hypersecretory diseases such as chronic bronchitis. Further, there is spontaneous recovery from hypersecretion after several months in many such patients. This points to a disturbance of regulation as the critical cause.

Neural Control

Administration of cholinergic agonists in vivo [60, 146] and in vitro [8, 39, 140] and stimulation of vagal efferent nerves in vivo [62] induce secretion of mucous glycoproteins and lysozyme by the airway mucosa of man and animals. Cholinergic agonists in vitro cause discharge of radiolabeled macromolecules and degranulation of both mucous and serous cells of the submucosal glands [8, 36] but do not cause secretion from epithelial goblet cells. Methacholine induces goblet cell secretion in human airways in vitro [7]. The role of adrenergic innervation is less well understood [46, 119, 122]. Earlier, in vitro studies of human airways and those of other species showed adrenergic agonists had little effect on glycoprotein secretion [8, 33] or on discharge of radiolabeled material from mucous cells of the submucosal gland [140]. Recent in vivo studies of the cat airway [60] and in vitro studies of human bronchial mucosa [113] demonstrate that both alpha- and beta-adrenergic agonists stimulate secretion of radiolabeled macromolecules. Morphometric studies of the ferret tracheal glands show that alpha- but not beta-adrenergic agonists cause degranulation of serous cells, a finding paralleled by their stimulation of lysozyme release [8, 143]. Such studies also illustrate the high degree of species variability.

Neuropeptides

Regulatory peptides, first identified in brain and intestine, are now known to be present also in the airway mucosa of man and other mammals, either in nerve endings or in cells of the diffuse endocrine system (see Chap. 18). Nerves containing immunoreactive vasoactive intestinal peptide (VIP) [52, 145] or substance P [51, 97, 153] are present in proximity to the airway submucosal glands and within the airway surface epithelium, while bombesin– [152], leu-enkephalin– [47], and calcitonin– [47] immunoreactive neuroendocrine cells are present in the surface epithelium. This leads to the suggestion that these peptides contribute to the regulation of airway mucus secretion.

In normal human airway in vitro, VIP at concentrations as small as 10 ng/ml reduces baseline and methacholine-stimulated release of radiolabeled glycoprotein and lysozyme by an effect that seems partly, but not entirely, due to inhibition of macromolecule discharge from mucous and serous cells of the submucosal glands [40]. In contrast, in bronchial explants of patients with chronic bronchitis, VIP did not inhibit radiolabeled glycoprotein secretion and produced less inhibition of lysozyme secretion than in explants of normal airways. These findings suggest that, not only does VIP have an inhibitory role in the regulation of mucus secretion by the normal airway, but also that this inhibitory mechanism is less effective in the bronchitic airway, a factor that may contribute to mucus hypersecretion.

The effects of VIP on airway secretion in other mammals have not yet been widely studied, although it has been reported to stimulate in vitro secretion of ^{35}S-labeled macromolecule by ferret trachea [111]. Preliminary studies in our laboratory suggest that in canine trachea VIP increases radiolabeled glycoprotein release. The VIP response varies with species.

Substance P has been reported to increase the in vitro secretion of radiolabeled mucous gel by canine trachea, an effect accompanied by an increase in mucosal galactosyl transferase activity [4]. It could not be established whether increased mucus secretion represented an increased rate of synthesis or of secretion. Recent studies carried out in our laboratory indicate that substance P, when incubated with canine tracheal explants for only a few minutes at concentrations as low as $10^{-10} M$, stimulates the release of radiolabeled glycoproteins [38]. This effect is not inhibited by cholinergic, adrenergic, or histaminergic antagonists and is augmented by preincubation with the cholinergic agonist methacholine. Studies of secretory kinetics and morphometric analyses indicate that substance P has no effect on macromolecular discharge from mucous or serous cells in the submucosal glands and goblet cells in the airway surface epithelium. They do suggest that it induces mucus secretion by constricting the collecting ducts and/or secretory tubules of the submucosal glands, thus increasing the rate of clearance of mucus from the gland duct into the airway. Such a mechanism represents the most rapid way to release mucus from the submucosal glands into the airways in response to airway irritation or immune events like anaphylaxis.

Calcitonin gene–related peptide (CGRP), a 37–amino acid peptide that has been recently identified in bronchial smooth muscle, submucosal glands, and airway epithelium [100], is a weak secretagogue [151]. In ferret trachea, CGRP stimulates basal serous cell secretion as well as epithelial albumin transport. Neurokinin A has been localized to sensory nerves in human airways, including smooth muscle, blood vessels, and epithelium, as well as around submucosal glands [98]. In vitro studies conducted in ferret trachea have shown that neurokinin A stimulates submucosal gland secretion and increases albumin transport across the epithelium [150]. The effect of neurokinin A on mucous gland secretion is approximately 20 times less potent than that of substance P. The effect of neurokinin A on airway muscle is probably mediated through NK-1 receptors. Opioid receptors have been demonstrated on unmyelinated capsaicin sensory nerve fibers [2], and opioid agonists (morphine) can inhibit mucus secretion induced by stimulation of sensory nerves [127].

Inflammatory Mediators

Mediators released in the airway structures in response to inflammation or immunologic challenge have been shown to stimulate airway mucus secretion. At micromolar concentrations, histamine [136] and prostaglandins A_2, D_2, and F_2 [101] cause release of radiolabeled glycoprotein from human bronchial explants, while PGE_2 is inhibitory. By far the most potent stimulants, however, are the lipoxygenase products of arachidonic acid, including 5-, 8-, 11-, and 12-HETEs [101, 135] and the sulfidopeptide leukotrienes C_4, D_4, and E_4 [42, 102]. These leukotrienes at nanomolar concentrations cause release of glycoprotein into airways and are about 100-fold more potent than methacholine, though in contrast to methacholine they do not increase lysozyme secretion. Surprisingly, it seems that the sulfidopeptide leukotrienes do not interact with a stereospecific secretory receptor, since we have shown that the minimal structural requirements necessary to elicit a maximal secretory response are eight eicosanoid carbon atoms and an ionized C-1 carboxylate group [42]. The hydrophobic omega domain is of minimal importance to the secretory effect.

Bradykinin and kallidin, which are inflammatory mediators formed by the proteolytic action of kallikreins and other kininkinases on tissue and plasma kininogens [116], have been identified in nasal secretions following allergen challenge [117] and during the late-phase reaction [108]. In asthmatic patients, inhalation of bradykinin induces bronchoconstriction [58]. In human nasal mucosa, bradykinin has a weak effect on mucus secretion, which seems to occur via an indirect stimulation of the arachidonic acid pathway since its effect is blocked by nonsteroidal antiinflammatory agents [5]. PAF has been implicated as a key inflammatory mediator in the pathogenesis of asthma [6]. It induces mucus secretion in vivo in the ferret [83] and in human bronchi in vitro [128].

The mechanism(s) by which inflammatory mediators induce airway mucus secretion are unknown. Histamine has no significant effect on radiolabeled macromolecule discharge from mucous cells in the human submucosal glands [140], and our preliminary studies indicate that the sulfidopeptide leukotrienes have no effect on discharge from secretory cells in the submucosal glands or epithelium of the human airway. Possibly, inflammatory mediators, as described above for substance P, act by constriction of gland tubules as a rapid way to mobilize gland mucus into the airway.

The relative importance of these mediators in the mucus hypersecretion accompanying an asthma attack is not known. One study has shown that supernatant fluids from human lung exhibiting anaphylaxis increase mucus secretion in vitro, while antigen and anti-IgE antibody increase mucus secretion in IgE-sensitized airways [136]. Inflammatory mediators could induce mucus secretion indirectly, since many stimulate airway irritant receptors [154]; additionally, mucus secretion is increased by exposure of the airway mucosa to gaseous, particulate, or chemical irritants [124]. The mechanism of irritant-induced mucus secretion is not well understood, although it could be mediated in part by vagovagal reflexes or by local mucosal axonal reflexes involving the release of substance P [97].

Prostaglandins

Preliminary results of the effects of prostaglandins F_2 and E_2 show that both drugs have a stimulatory effect but apparently only in some explants, not in all (personal communication); this is not due to patient sensitivity. These agents affect mucous and serous cells, not goblet cells. When a prostaglandin stimulates, only some cells and acini are affected. While the effect of any stimulatory drug is focal, what is peculiar to the prostaglandins is the size of the territory that, at a given time, is sensitive or insensitive. A much larger group of cells or acini seems to be in the same phase of sensitivity to prostaglandins than is the case for other drugs.

The secretion of the gland is the end product of activity by a variety of cells: The collecting duct cell is likely to control water and electrolytes; the secretory cells control the macromolecules of glycoprotein and protein. A variety of stages of cell activity need also to be considered, since these are to some extent dissociated and represent phases that are separately controlled: precursor uptake, molecular synthesis, secretory granule formation, intracellular migration, cell discharge, mixing molecules, and duct emptying.

It seems justified to extrapolate from the above in vitro studies to the likely in vivo events. Increased release of mucus from the gland does not necessarily mean increased synthesis. Change(s) in the physical state of the mucus or agents that act on myoepithelial cells may lead to its release.

Basal gland secretion does not necessarily include macromolecules from all cell types. The fastest and largest response to acute challenge is achieved by duct emptying. Duct emptying is not necessarily associated with an increase in cell mucus synthesis or discharge. Agents that have proved highly effective in emptying the ducts are eicosanoid mediators of inflammation and substance P, a regulatory neuropeptide; these are likely to be important in the pathophysiologic disturbances seen during an asthmatic attack. The vagal component, also important in asthma, contributes to increased secretory cell activity of the submucosal glands. None of these regulatory drugs has any effect on goblet cells of surface epithelium. This leads to a longer-term increase in glycoprotein synthesis and discharge.

Genes Encoding the Mucin Polypeptides

Gum and coworkers [63] have screened a human small intestine complementary DNA (cDNA) library with antisera prepared against the deglycosylated protein backbone of human-colon-cancer xenograft mucin. Three cDNAs were characterized from this screening, SMUC 40 to 42. These clones all contained tandem repeats of 69 nucleotides and encode a threonine- and proline-rich protein consensus sequence. RNA from colon, small intestine, and colon cancer cells all hybridized with SMUC 41. Their results indicate the presence of restriction-fragment-length polymorphisms in the intestinal mucin gene.

The genetic control of the structure of bronchial mucus, particularly the genes encoding for the polypeptide core, is currently being explored. Gerard and colleagues [61] have constructed a cDNA library from a cystic fibrosis trachea. They probed this with a synthetic oligonucleotide containing a consensus sequence recently identified in human intestinal mucin [62]. One of the isolated lung clones that they have characterized extensively (AMN 22) was similar but not identical to that of the gut. In the cystic fibrosis trachea, the messenger RNA hybridizing to this AMN 22 is extremely polydisperse. A similar pattern with less abundant message was found in the bronchiectatic parenchyma of the cystic fibrosis lung. The lung cDNA hybridized with RNA of colon but not of stomach or lymphoma. Restriction digests of genomic DNA indicated a single polymorphic locus for the mucin gene expressed in lung and intestine. The further studies of Gum's group suggest a chromosomal localization for this mucin gene to human chromosome 11, within the 11p13–11pTer region. It appears that a polymorphic gene encodes a mucin core polypeptide expressed in both lung and intestine.

Gum and colleagues presented the results of Northern blot analysis, which indicated a lack of cross-hybridization between colon and stomach RNA [69]. This group later showed that one of the original SMUC isolates hybridized to polydisperse transcripts of bronchus, cervix, gallbladder, and mammary gland [69]. Recently, they carried out a similar study of deglycosylated normal mucus from human small intestine and identified a new gene on chromosome 7 that includes a 51-nucleotide tandem repeat encoding a 17–amino acid repetitive peptide with a constant sequence of HSTPSFTSSITTTETTS. At present, it is unclear whether this second mucin gene is expressed in lung tissues.

REFERENCES

1. Adler, K. et al. Physical properties of sputum. *Am. Rev. Respir. Dis.* 106: 85, 1972.
2. Atweh, S. F., Murrin, L. C., and Kuhar, M. J. Presynaptic localization of opiate receptors in the vagal and accessory optic systems: an autoradiographic study. *Neuropharmacology* 17:101, 1981.
3. Austen, K. F., et al. Generation and Release of Chemical Mediators of Immediate Hypersensitivity in Human Cells. In M. Stein (ed.), *New Directions in Asthma.* Park Ridge, Ill: American College of Physicians, 1975.
4. Baker, A. P., et al. Effect of kallidin, substance P and other basic polypeptides on the production of respiratory macromolecules. *Am. Rev. Respir. Dis.* 115:811, 1977.
5. Baraniuk, J. N., et al. Bradykinin and respiratory mucous membranes. *Am. Rev. Respir. Dis.* 141:706, 1990.
6. Barnes, P. J., Chung, K. F., and Page, C. P. Inflammatory mediators and asthma. *Pharmacol. Rev.* 40:49, 1988.
7. Barnes, P. J., et al. Effect of vagus nerve stimulation on goblet-cell secretion in guinea-pig trachea in vivo. *J. Physiol.* 442:99P, 1990.
8. Basbaum, C. B., et al. Tracheal submucosal gland serous cells stimulated in vitro with adrenergic and cholinergic agonists. *Cell Tissue Res.* 220: 481, 1981.
9. Bateman, J. R. M., Pavia, D., and Clarke, S. W. The retention of lung secretions during the night in normal subjects. *Clin. Sci.* 55:523, 1978.
10. Bell, D. Y., et al. Plasma proteins of the broncho-alveolar surface of the lungs of smokers and nonsmokers. *Am. Rev. Respir. Dis.* 124:72, 1981.
11. Bhaskar, K. R., and Creeth, J. M. The macromolecular properties of blood-group specific glycoproteins. Characterization of a series of fractions obtained by density-gradient ultracentrifugation. *Biochem. J.* 143:669, 1974.
12. Bhaskar, K. R., O'Sullivan, D. D., and Reid, L. The effect of thiol reduction and proteolysis on bronchial mucus glycoprotein isolated by density gradient methods (abstract). Presented at Symposium on Glycoconjugates. Lund-Ronneby, Sweden, July, 1983.
13. Bhaskar, K. R., and Reid, L. Application of density gradient methods for the study of mucus glycoprotein and other macromolecular components of the sol and gel phases of asthmatica sputa. *J. Biol. Chem.* 256:6583, 1982.
14. Bhaskar, K. R., et al. Characterization of Sol and Gel Phases of Infected and Mucoid Samples from a Chronic Bronchitic Patient. In E. N. Chantler, J. B. Elder, and M. Elstein (eds.), *Mucus in Health and Disease.* New York and London: Plenum Press, 1982, Vol. 2, Pp. 361–364.
15. Bhaskar, K. R., et al. Characterization of canine bronchial mucus before and after exposure to SO_2. *Chest* 81:39S, 1982.
16. Bhaskar, K. R., et al. Bronchial mucus hypersecretion in acute quadriplegia: macromolecular yields and glycoconjugate composition. *Am. Rev. Respir. Dis.* 143:640, 1991.
17. Bhaskar, K. R., et al. Density gradient study of bronchial mucus aspirates from healthy volunteers (smokers and nonsmokers) and from patients with tracheostomy. *Exp. Lung Res.* 9:289, 1985.
18. Bhaskar, K. R., et al. Density gradient analysis of secretions produced in vitro by human and canine airway mucosa: identification of lipids and proteoglycans in such secretions. *Exp. Lung Res.* 10:401, 1986.
19. Bhaskar, K. R., et al. Transition from normal to hypersecretory bronchial mucus in a canine model of bronchitis: changes in yield and composition. *Exp. Lung Res.* 14:101, 1988.
20. Bhaskar, K. R., et al. Lipids in airway secretions. *Eur. J. Respir. Dis.* 71(suppl. 153):215, 1987.
21. Bhaskar, K. R., et al. Characterization of airway mucus from a fatal case of status asthmaticus. *Pediatr. Pulmonol.* 5:176, 1988.
22. Boat, T. F., and Kleinerman, J. I. Human respiratory tract secretions: II. Effect of cholinergic and adrenergic agents on in vitro release of protein and mucous glycoprotein. *Chest* 67(suppl.):32, 1975.
23. Boat, T. F., et al. Human respiratory tract secretions: mucous glycoproteins of non-purulent tracheobronchial secretions and sputum of patients with bronchitis and cystic fibrosis. *Arch. Biochem. Biophys.* 177:95, 1976.
24. Boat, T. F., et al. Hydration of tracheal mucus: the role of calcium. *Am. Rev. Respir. Dis.* 121:284, 1980.
25. Boat, T. F., et al. Identification of glycoconjugates (G) secreted by rabbit tracheal surface epithelium (RTSE). *Am. Rev. Respir. Dis.* 137(4):8, 1988.
26. Bodem, C. R., et al. Endobronchial pH: relevance to aminoglycoside activity in gram-negative bacillary pneumonia. *Am. Rev. Respir. Dis.* 127:39, 1983.
27. Bowes, D., Clark, A. E., and Corrin, B. Ultrastructural localization of lac-toferrin and glycoprotein in human bronchial glands. *Thorax* 36:108, 1977.
28. Bowes, D., and Corrin, B. Ultrastructural immunocytochemical localization of lysozyme in human bronchial glands. *Thorax* 32:163, 1977.
29. Boyd, E. M., and Ronan, A. Excretion of respiratory tract fluid. *Am. J. Physiol.* 135:383, 1943.
30. Brandtzaeg, P. Review and Discussion of IgA Transport across Mucosal Membranes. In W. Strober, L. A. Hanson, and K. W. Sell (eds.), *Recent Advances in Mucosal Immunity.* New York: Raven, 1982, Pp. 267.
31. Brogan, T. D., et al. Soluble proteins of bronchopulmonary secretions from patients with cystic fibrosis, asthma and bronchitis. *Thorax* 30:72, 1975.
32. Carlsted, I., et al. Isolation and Purification of the Mucin Component of Human Cervical Mucus. In E. N. Chantler, J. B. Elder, and M. Elstein (eds.), *Mucus in Health and Disease.* New York: Plenum, 1982, Vol. 2.
33. Chakrin, L. W., et al. Effect of cholinergic stimulation on the release of macromolecules by canine trachea in vitro. *Am. Rev. Respir. Dis.* 108:69, 1973.
34. Charman, J., and Reid, L. Sputum viscosity in chronic bronchitis, bronchiectasis, asthma and cystic fibrosis. *Biorheology* 9:185, 1972.
35. Chen, T. M., and Dulfano, M. J. Mucus viscoelasticity and mucociliary transport rate. *J. Lab. Clin. Med.* 91:423, 1978.
36. Coles, S. Regulation and Secretory Cycles of Mucous and Serous Cells in the Human Bronchial Gland. In M. Elstein and D. V. Parke (eds.), *Mucus in Health and Disease* (Advances of Experimental Medicine and Biology). New York: Plenum, 1977.
37. Coles, S. J., Judge, J., and Reid, L. Differential effects of calcium ions on glycoconjugate secretion by canine tracheal explants. *Chest* 81(suppl.): 34S, 1982.
38. Coles, S. J., Neill, K. H., and Reid, L. M. Potent stimulation of glycoprotein secretion in canine trachea by substance P. *J. Appl. Physiol.* 57:1323, 1984.
39. Coles, S. J., and Reid, L. Glycoprotein secretion in vitro by human airway: normal and chronic bronchitis. *Exp. Mol. Pathol.* 29:326, 1978.
40. Coles, S. J., Said, S. I., and Reid, L. M. Inhibition by vasoactive intestinal peptide of glycoconjugate and lysozyme secretion by human airways in vitro. *Am. Rev. Respir. Dis.* 124:531, 1981.
41. Coles, S. J., et al. Macromolecular Composition of Secretion Produced by Human Bronchial Explants. In E. N. Chantler, J. B. Elder, and M. Elstein (eds.), *Mucus in Health and Disease.* New York: Plenum, 1982.
42. Coles, S. J., et al. Effects of leukotrienes C_4 and D_4 on glycoprotein and lysozyme secretion by human bronchial mucosa. *Prostaglandins* 25:155, 1983.
43. Conner, M. W., and Reid, L. M. Mapping of beta-adrenergic receptors in rat lung: effect of isoproterenol. *Exp. Lung Res.* 6:91, 1984.
44. Cosio, M., et al. The relations between structural changes in small airways and pulmonary-function tests. *N. Engl. J. Med.* 298:1277, 1978.
45. Creeth, J. M., and Denborough, M. A. The use of equilibrium-density-gradient methods for the preparation and characterisation of blood group specific glycoprotein. *Biochemistry* 117:879, 1970.
46. Creeth, J. M., et al. The separation and characterisation of bronchial glycoprotein by density gradient methods. *Biochem. J.* 167:557, 1977.
47. Cutz, E., Chan, W., and Trach, N. S. Bombesin, calcitonin and leu-enkephalin immunoreactivity in endocrine cells of human lung. *Experientia* 37: 765, 1981.
48. Cutz, E., Levison, H., and Cooper, D. M. Ultrastructure of airways in children with asthma. *Histopathology* 2:407, 1978.
49. Davies, J. R., et al. Mucins in cat airway secretions. *Biochem. J.* 275:663, 1991.
50. Deuschl, H., and Johansson, S. G. O. Immunoglobulins in tracheobronchial secretion with special reference to IgE. *Clin. Exp. Immunol.* 16:401, 1974.
51. Dey, R. D., and Said, S. I. Localization of substance P–like immunofluorescence in nerves within dog airways and pulmonary vessels. *Fed. Proc.* 40:595, 1981.
52. Dey, R. D., Shannon, W. A., and Said, S. I. Localization of VIP immunoreactive nerves in airways and pulmonary vessels of dogs, cats, and human subjects. *Cell Tissue Res.* 220:231, 1981.
53. Dulfano, M. J., and Luk, C. K. Sputum and ciliary inhibition in asthma. *Thorax* 37:646, 1982.
54. Dunnill, M. S. The Morphology of the Airways in Asthma. In M. Stein (ed.), *New Directions in Asthma.* Park Ridge, Ill: American College of Chest Physicians, 1975.
55. Feldhoff, P. A., Bhavanandan, V. P., and Davidson, E. A. Purification prop-

erties, and analysis of human asthmatic bronchial mucin. *Biochemistry* 18:2430, 1979.

56. Forstner, J. F., et al. Interaction of mucins with calcium, H+ ion and albumin. *Mod. Probl. Paediatr.* 19:54, 1977.

57. Forstner, J. F., and Forstner, G. G. Effects of calcium on intestinal mucins: implications for cystic fibrosis. *Pediatr. Res.* 10:609, 1976.

58. Fuller, R. W., et al. Bradykinin-induced bronchoconstriction in human. Mode of action. *Am. Rev. Respir. Dis.* 135:176, 1987.

59. Galabert, C., Filliat, M., and Lamblin, G. Lipid analysis of sputum from patients with chronic bronchial diseases. *Bull. Eur. Physiopathol. Respir.* 17:197, 1981.

60. Gallagher, J. T., et al. The composition of tracheal mucus and the nervous control of its secretion in the cat. *Proc. R. Soc. Lond.* [Biol.] 192:49, 1975.

61. Gerard, C., Eddy, R. L., and Shows, T. B. The core polypeptide of cystic fibrosis tracheal mucin contains a tandem repeat structure: evidence for a common mucin in airway and gastrointestinal tissue. *J. Clin. Invest.* 86:1921, 1990.

62. Guerrin, F., et al. Resultats de la pH metrie bronchique in situ. Hypersecretion Bronchique Colloque International de Pathologie Thoracique, Lille, 1968, P. 249.

63. Gum, J. R. et al. Molecular cloning of human intestinal mucin cDNAs: sequence analysis and evidence for genetic polymorphism. *J. Biol. Chem.* 264(11):6480, 1989.

64. Hills, B. A. What is the role of the surfactant in the lung? *Thorax* 36:1, 1981.

65. Hincman, H. O., et al. Lipids in airway mucus of acute quadriplegic patients. *Exp. Lung Res.* 16:369, 1990.

66. Hogg, J. C., Macklem, P. T., and Thurlbeck, W. M. Size and nature of airway obstruction in chronic obstructive lung disease. *N. Engl. J. Med.* 278:1355, 1968.

67. Houdret, N., et al. Comparative action of reducing agents on fibrillar human bronchial mucus under dissociating and nondissociating conditions. *Biochem. Biophys. Acta* 668:413, 1981.

68. Ishizaka, K., and Newcomb, P. W. Presence of IgE in nasal washings and sputum from asthmatic patients. *J. Allergy* 46:197, 1970.

69. Jacquot, J., et al. Modulation of albumin-like protein and lysozyme production by bovine tracheal gland serous cells: dependence on culture conditions. *Fed. Eur. Biochem. Soc.* 269(1):65, 1990.

70. Jany, B. H. et al. Human bronchus and intestine express the same mucin gene. *J. Clin. Invest.* 87:77, 1991.

71. Jeffery, P. K., and Reid, L. The effect of tobacco smoke, with or without phenylmethyloxadiazole (PMO) on rat bronchial epithelium: a light and electron microscopy study. *J. Pathol.* 133:341, 1981.

72. Jones, R., and Reid, L. M. Experimental chronic bronchitis. *Int. Rev. Exp. Pathol.* 24:335, 1983.

73. Keal, E. E. Biochemistry and rheology of sputum in asthma. *Postgrad. Med. J.* 47:171, 1971.

74. Keal, E. E., and Reid, L. Pathological Alterations in Mucus in Asthma Within and Without the Cell. In M. Stein (ed.), *New Directions in Asthma.* Park Ridge, Ill: American College of Chest Physicians, 1975, Pp. 223–239.

75. Kim, K. C., Opackkar-Hincman, H., and Bhaskar, K. R. Secretions from primary hamster tracheal epithelial cells in culture: mucins, proteoglycans and lipids. *Exp. Lung Res.* 15:299, 1989.

76. King, M., et al. On the transport of mucus and its rheologic stimulants in ciliated systems. *Am. Rev. Respir. Dis.* 110:740, 1974.

77. Knowles, M. R., et al. Ion transport in excised human bronchi and its neuro-humoral control. *Chest* 81:11S, 1982.

78. Koshino, et al. Recovery of an epitope recognized by a novel monoclonal antibody from airway lavage during experimental induction of chronic bronchitis. *Am. J. Resp. Cell. Mol. Biol.* 2:453, 1990.

79. Laine, A., and Hayem, A. Identification et caracterisation des constituents proteiques de la secretion bronchique humaine. *Clin. Chim. Acta* 67:159, 1969.

80. Lamb, D., and Reid, L. Histochemical types of acidic glycoprotein produced by mucous cells of the tracheobronchial glands in man. *J. Pathol.* 98:213, 1969.

81. Lamb, D., and Reid, L. Quantitative distribution of various types of acid glycoprotein in mucous cells of human bronchi. *Histochem. J.* 4:91, 1972.

82. Lamblin, G., et al. Mucins from cystic fibrosis sputum. *Mod. Probl. Paediatr.* 19:153, 1977.

83. Lang, M., Hansen, D., and Hahn, H. L. Effects of the PAF-antagonist CV-3988 on PAF-induced changes in mucus secretion and in respiratory and circulatory variables in ferrets. *Agents Actions* 21(suppl.):245, 1987.

84. LeTreut, A., et al. Reevaluation of the action of reducing agents on soluble

85. Lewis, R. W. Lipid composition of human bronchial mucus. *Lipids* 6:859, 1971.

86. Lhermitte, M., et al. Affinity of bronchial secretion glycoproteins and cells of human bronchial mucosa for *Ricinus communis* lectins. *Biochimie* 59:611, 1977.

87. Litt, M. L. Physicochemical determinants of mucociliary flow. *Chest* 80:846, 1981.

88. Lofdahl, C. G., and Odeblad, E. Biophysical variables relating to viscoelastic properties of mucus secretions, with special reference to NMR-methods for viscosity measurement. *Eur. J. Respir. Dis.* 61(suppl. 110):113, 1980.

89. Lopez-Vidriero, M. T. Bronchial mucus in obstructive lung disease. *Scand. J. Respir. Dis.* Suppl. 103:33, 1979.

90. Lopez-Vidriero, M. T., Das, I., and Reid, L. Airway Secretions. Source, Biochemical and Rheological Properties. In J. D. Brain, D. F. Proctor, and L. M. Reid (eds.), *Respiratory Defense Mechanisms,* New York: Dekker, 1977, Part I. P. 289.

91. Lopez-Vidriero, M. T., Das, I., and Reid, L. Bronchorrhoea—separation of mucus and serum components in sol phases. *Thorax* 34:512, 1979.

92. Lopez-Vidriero, M. T., and Reid, L. Chemical markers of bronchial and serum glycoproteins in mucoid and purulent sputum from various hypersecretory diseases. *Am. Rev. Respir. Dis.* 117:465, 1978.

93. Lopez-Vidriero, M. T., and Reid, L. Respiratory tract fluid—chemical and physical properties of airway mucus. *Eur. J. Respir. Dis.* Suppl. 61:21, 1980.

94. Lopez-Vidriero, M. T., and Reid, L. Pathological Changes in Asthma. In T. J. H. Clark and S. Godfrey (eds.), *Asthma.* Philadelphia: Saunders, 1983.

95. Lopez-Vidriero, M. T., et al. Bronchorrhoea. *Thorax* 30:624, 1975.

96. Lopez-Vidriero, M. T., et al. Bronchial secretion from normal human airways after inhalation of prostaglandin F_2 alpha, acetylcholine, histamine and citric acid. *Thorax* 32:734, 1977.

97. Lundberg, J. M., and Saria, A. Capsaicin-induced desensitization of airway mucosa to cigarette smoke, mechanical and chemical irritants. *Nature* 152:183, 1983.

98. Lundberg, J. M., et al. Co-existence of substance P and calcitonin gene–related peptide-like immunoreactivities in sensory nerves in relation to cardiovascular and bronchoconstrictor effects of capsaicin. *Eur. J. Pharmacol.* 108:315, 1985.

99. Lundberg, J. M., et al. Substance P immunoreactive sensory nerves in the lower respiratory tract of various mammals including man. *Cell Tis. Res.* 235:251, 1984.

100. Mak, J. C., and Barnes, P. J. Autoradiographic localization of calcitonin gene–related peptide (CGRP) binding sites in human and guinea-pig lung. *Peptides* 9:957, 1988.

101. Marom, Z., Shelhamer, J. H., and Kaliner, M. Effects of arachidonic acid, monohydroxy-eicosatetraenoic acid and prostaglandins on the release of mucous glycoprotein from human airways in vitro. *J. Clin. Invest.* 67:1695, 1981.

102. Marom, Z., et al. Slow-reacting substances, leukotrienes C_4 and D_4, increase the release of mucus from human airways in vitro. *Am. Rev. Respir. Dis.* 126:449, 1982.

103. Marriott, C. The viscoelastic nature of mucus secretion. *Chest* Suppl. 80:804, 1981.

104. Marriott, C., Shih, C. K., and Litt, M. Changes in the gel properties of tracheal mucus induced by divalent cations. *Biorheology* 16:331, 1979.

105. Masson, P. L., and Heremans, J. F. Sputum Proteins. In M. J. Dulfano (ed.), *Sputum Fundamentals and Clinical Pathology.* Springfield, Ill: Thomas, 1973, Pp. 412.

106. McFadden, E. R., Jr. Some Observations on the Pathophysiology of Acute Bronchial Asthma. In M. Stein (ed.), *New Directions in Asthma.* Park Ridge, Ill: American College of Chest Physicians, 1975.

107. Mitchell-Heggs, P., Palfrey, A. J., and Reid, L. The elasticity of sputum at low shear rates. *Biorheology* 11:417, 1974.

108. Naclerio, R. M., et al. Inflammatory mediators in late antigen-induced rhinitis. *N. Engl. J. Med.* 313:65, 1985.

109. Paul, A. et al. Glycoconjugates secreted by bovine tracheal serous cells in culture. *Arch. Biochem. Biophys.* 260:75, 1988.

110. Pavia, D., et al. Lung Mucociliary Transport in Man. In G. Cumming and G. Bonsignore (eds.), *Cellular Biology of the Lung.* New York: Plenum, 1982.

111. Peatfield, A. C., et al. Vasoactive intestinal peptide stimulates tracheal submucosal gland secretion in ferrets. *Am. Rev. Respir. Dis.* 128:89, 1983.

112. Petrik, P., and Collet, A. J. Quantitative electron microscopic autoradiography of in vivo incorporation of ^{3}H-leucine, ^{3}H-acetate and ^{3}H-galactose in non-ciliated bronchiolar (Clara) cells of mice. *Am. J. Anat.* 139:519, 1974.

113. Phipps, R. J., et al. Adrenergic stimulation of mucus secretion in human bronchi. *Chest* 81(suppl.):19S, 1982.

114. Picot, R., Das, I., and Reid, L. Pus, deoxyribonucleic acid and sputum viscosity. *Thorax* 33:235, 1978.

115. Policard, A., and Galy, P. *Les Bronches.* Paris: Masson, 1945.

116. Proud, D., and Kaplan, A. P. Kinin formation: mechanisms and role in inflammatory disorders. *Annu. Rev. Immunol.* 6:49, 1988.

117. Proud, D., et al. Kinins are generated in vivo following nasal airway challenge of allergic individuals with allergen. *J. Clin. Invest.* 72:1678, 1983.

118. Puchelle, E., Zahm, J. M., and Aug, F. Viscoelasticity, protein content and ciliary transport rate of sputum in patients with recurrent and chronic bronchitis. *Biorheology* 18:659, 1981.

119. Reid, L. M. The lung and its receptors. *J. Lab. Clin. Med.* 103:161, 1984.

120. Reid, L., Bhaskar, K. R., and Coles, S. J. Clinical aspects of respiratory mucus. In E. N. Chantler, J. B. Elder, and M. Elstein (eds.), *Mucus in Health and Disease,* 2nd ed. New York: Plenum, 1982.

121. Reid, L., and Clamp, J. R. The biochemical and histochemical nomenclature of mucus. *Br. Med. Bull.* 34:1, 1978.

122. Reid, L. M., and Coles, S. J. The Bronchial Epithelium of Humans: Cytology, Innervation and Function. In K. L. Becker and A. F. Gadzar (eds.) *The Endocrine Lung.* London: Saunders, 1983, Chap. 3.

123. Reynolds, H. Y., and Newball, H. H. Analysis of proteins and respiratory cells obtained from human lungs by bronchial lavage. *J. Lab. Clin. Med.* 84:559, 1974.

124. Richardson, P. S., et al. The Role of Mediators, Irritants and Allergens in Causing Mucin Secretion from the Trachea. In R. Porter, J. Rivers, and M. O'Connor (eds.), *Respiratory Tract Mucus* (Ciba Foundation Symposium 54, new series). Amsterdam: Elsevier, 1978, P. 111.

125. Roberts, G. P. The role of disulfide bonds in maintaining the gel structure of bronchial mucus. *Arch. Biochem. Biophys.* 173:528, 1976.

126. Roberts, G. P. Isolation and characterisation of glycoproteins from sputum. *Eur. J. Biochem.* 50:265, 1974.

127. Rogers, D. F., and Barnes, P. J. Opioid inhibition of neurally mediated mucus secretion in human bronchi. *Lancet* 1:930, 1989.

128. Rogers, D. F., et al. Effect of platelet activating factor on formation and composition of airway fluid in the guinea-pig trachea. *J. Physiol.* 431:643, 1990.

129. Rose, M. C., Lynn, W. S., and Kaufman, B. Resolution of the major components of human lung mucosal gel and their capabilities for reaggregation and gel formation. *Biochemistry* 18:4030, 1979.

130. Roussel, P., et al. Heterogeneity of the carbohydrate chains of sulfated glycoproteins isolated from a patient suffering from cystic fibrosis. *J. Biol. Chem.* 260:2114, 1975.

131. Sachdev, G. P., et al. Isolation, chemical composition and properties of the major mucin component of normal human tracheobronchial secretions. *Biochem. Med.* 24:82, 1980.

132. Sade, J., et al. The role of mucus in transport by cilia. *Am. Rev. Respir. Dis.* 102:48, 1970.

133. Sahu, S., and Lynn, W. S. Lipid composition of airway secretions from patients with asthma and patients with cystic fibrosis. *Am. Rev. Respir. Dis.* 115:233, 1977.

134. Schlimmer, P., Augsten, M., and Ferber, E. Classification and possible function of phospholipids obtained from central airways. *Eur. J. Respir. Dis.* 64(suppl. 128):318, 1983.

135. Shelhamer, J. H., et al. The effects of arachinoids and leukotrienes on the release of mucus from human airways. *Chest* 81:36S, 1982.

136. Shelhamer, J. H., Marom, Z., and Kaliner, M. Immunologic and neuropharmacologic stimulation of mucous glycoprotein release from human airways in vitro. *J. Clin. Invest.* 66:1400, 1980.

137. Steinman, E. La secretion bronchique et le pH. *Les Bronches* 6:126, 1956.

138. Sturgess, J. Bronchial mucus secretion in cystic fibrosis. *Mod. Probl. Paediatr.* 19:129, 1977.

139. Sturgess, J., Palfrey, A. J., and Reid, L. Rheological properties of sputum. *Rheologica Acta* 10:36, 1971.

140. Sturgess, J., and Reid, L. An organ culture study of the effect of drugs on the secretory activity of the bronchial submucosal gland. *Clin. Sci.* 43:533, 1972.

141. Sturgess, J., and Reid, L. Secretory activity of the human bronchial mucous glands in vitro. *Exp. Mol. Pathol.* 16:362, 1972.

142. Thornton, D. J., et al. Mucus glycoproteins from "normal" human tracheobronchial secretion. *Biochem. J.* 265:179, 1990.

143. Tom-Moy, M., Basbaum, C., and Nadel, J. Localization of lysozyme and release of lysozyme by cholinergic and adrenergic agonists in the ferret trachea. *Chest* 81:22S, 1982.

144. Toremalm, N. G. The daily amount of tracheo-bronchial secretions in man. *Acta Otolaryngol.* Suppl. 158:43, 1960.

145. Uddman, R., et al. Occurrence and distribution of VIP nerves in the nasal mucosa and tracheobronchial wall. *Acta Otolaryngol.* 367:1, 1978.

146. Ueki, I., German, V. F., and Nadel, J. A. Micropipette measurement of airway submucosal gland secretion. Autonomic effects. *Am. Rev. Respir. Dis.* 121:351, 1980.

147. Van As, A. Pulmonary clearance mechanisms: a reappraisal. *Am. Rev. Respir. Dis.* 115:721, 1977.

148. Warembourg, H., et al. Les lipides de l'expectoration: Isolement et caractérisation du surfactant pulmonaire dans l'expectoration. Hypersecretion Bronchique Colloque International de Pathologie Thoracique, Lille, 1968, P. 181.

149. Warr, G. A., et al. Normal human bronchial immunoglobulins and proteins. *Am. Rev. Respir. Dis.* 116:25, 1977.

150. Webber, S. E. Receptors mediating the effect of substance P and neurokinin A on mucus secretion and smooth muscle tone of the ferret trachea: potentiation by an enkephalinase inhibitor. *Br. J. Pharmacol.* 98:1197, 1989.

151. Webber, S. E., Lim, J. C. S., and Widdicombe, J. G. The effects of calcitonin gene–related peptide on submucosal gland secretion and epithelial albumin transport in the ferret trachea *in vitro. Br. J. Pharmacol.* 102:79, 1991.

152. Wharton, J., et al. Bombesin-line immunoreactivity in the lung. *Nature* 273:769, 1978.

153. Wharton, J., et al. Substance P–like immunoreactive nerves in mammalian lung. *Invest. Cell Pathol.* 2:3, 1979.

154. Widdicombe, J. G. Receptors in the trachea and bronchi of the cat. *J. Physiol.* (Lond.) 123:71, 1954.

155. Wiggins, J., Hill, S. L., and Stockley, R. A. Lung secretion sol-phase proteins: comparison of sputum with secretions obtained by direct sampling. *Thorax* 28:102, 1983.

156. Williams, I. P., et al. Analyses of human tracheobronchial mucus from healthy subjects. *Eur. J. Resp. Dis.* 63:510, 1982.

157. Woodward, H., et al. Isolation, purification and properties of respiratory mucus glycoproteins. *Biochemistry* 21:694, 1982.

Mucociliary Function

Alejandro D. Chediak
Adam Wanner

30

It has long been recognized that excessive airway secretions play an important role in the pathophysiology of various types of obstructive airway disease and contribute to the clinical manifestations of these disorders [60]. Bronchial asthma clearly belongs to this group of diseases. Cough productive of mucoid sputum is common in patients with bronchial asthma, and mucous plugs in the airways can be observed either directly by endoscopy or indirectly by chest radiography revealing atelectasis. These clinical features are in keeping with the histologic lesions of asthma, which involve primarily the epithelium and mucus-producing structures of the conducting airways. Indeed, the extent of mucous plugging found at autopsy in patients who died from status asthmaticus is so impressive that pathologists consider it to be the cause of death. Thus, the clinical and pathologic findings in bronchial asthma suggest abnormal production and elimination of airway secretions. The purpose of the following discussion is to review the pathogenesis and physiologic consequences of mucociliary dysfunction associated with bronchial asthma.

NORMAL FUNCTION OF THE MUCOCILIARY APPARATUS

The airway mucociliary system contributes to pulmonary defenses by physical removal of inhaled foreign material from the conducting airways and by biochemical and immunologic processes that protect against invasion of the mucosa by infectious agents. The respiratory tract is lined by a ciliated epithelium extending from the proximal trachea to the terminal bronchioles [60]. Most of the surface of the larynx is covered by mucus-secreting squamous epithelium; cilia are present only in the posterior commissure. There is no convincing evidence of direct nervous or hormonal control of ciliary beat frequency. Respiratory mucus in the tracheobronchial tree is produced by both submucosal glands and goblet cells interspersed with ciliated columnar cells. The ratio of ciliated columnar cells to goblet cells is approximately five to one. The absolute numbers of both decrease from the trachea to the peripheral airways (Figs. 30-1 and 30-2). Submucosal glands are only found in cartilaginous airways. In the most peripheral bronchi, goblet cells are also absent, and the small number of ciliated cells are characterized by fewer and shorter cilia than in the larger bronchi.

In the larger airways, the major part of the epithelium is ciliated but with focal areas as large as 1 mm in diameter devoid of cilia. These areas are covered with nonciliated, microvillous, columnar cells or submucosal gland duct openings. The surface of each ciliated columnar cell contains approximately 200 cilia with an average length of 6 μ and an average diameter of 0.2 μ. Each cilium contains longitudinal microtubules; these contractile elements are responsible for ciliary bending. The cilia beat in one plane with a fast effective stroke (power stroke) and a recovery

stroke that is two to three times slower. The motion of adjacent cilia on an individual cell and the motion among cilia of adjacent cells are coordinated.

Respiratory secretions consist of mucus (gel) produced by submucosal glands and goblet cells and periciliary fluid that is probably supplied by transepithelial ion and water transport (see Fig. 30-1 and Chap. 29). Goblet cells seem to secrete on direct irritation. The daily volume of respiratory secretions has been reported to be between 10 and 100 ml. Human respiratory secretions are approximately 95 percent water, with the rest consisting of micromolecules (electrolytes and amino acids) and macromolecules (lipids, carbohydrates, nucleic acids, mucins, immunoglobulins, enzymes, and albumin). Mucociliary interaction depends on the rheologic properties and depth of the mucous layer and the depth of the periciliary fluid layer. The viscoelastic properties of mucus are determined by biochemical characteristics (disulfide cross-linking and hydrogen bonding between glycoprotein molecules and water). In the central airways, the "normal" mucous layer is approximately 5 μ deep and the cilia beat at approximately 1,000 beats/min. This results in a surface transport velocity in the trachea of approximately 10 mm/min, with a gradual decline toward the lung periphery (see Fig. 30-2). Mucus is absent in the peripheral airways. The velocity of liquid transport in peripheral airways is unknown but must be much lower than in central airways [50]. In the normal tracheobronchial tree, the clearance of mucus from the airways is not influenced by gravity. Exercise has been reported to stimulate mucociliary clearance slightly [68]; hyperoxia appears stimulatory [74].

Normal respiratory secretions contain secretory IgA and several enzymes (e.g., lysozyme) that also appear to serve as a defense system in the conducting airways. Phagocytes (macrophages, neutrophils) can also be found in the airway lumen. Their role in tracheobronchial defense remains unclear, but they are likely to contribute to the clearance of colonizing bacteria.

Neural mechanisms play a role in the regulation of respiratory secretions. There is evidence that submucosal glands are innervated by the parasympathetic, sympathetic, and nonadrenergic, noncholinergic nervous systems [19, 55, 65]. However, there is no known neural innervation of goblet cells. In humans, stimulation of cholinergic and alpha- and beta-adrenergic neurons results in an increased secretion of mucins from submucosal glands. Nonadrenergic, noncholinergic neural pathways have also been implicated in the regulation of airway mucus, and their action is possibly mediated by vasoactive intestinal peptide, which inhibits the secretion of mucus from normal human bronchus in vitro [13] (see Chap. 18). Therefore, depletion of this neurotransmitter in the airways and thus removal of an inhibitory factor of mucus secretion may play a role in the pathogenesis of airway diseases characterized by mucus hypersecretion. The tachykinins, notably substance P, stimulate the contraction of glandular ducts and cause a degranulation of serous cells in fer-

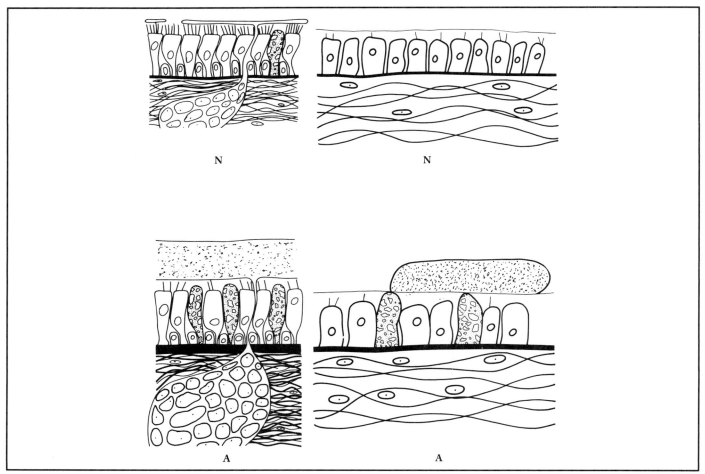

Fig. 30-1. *Normal mucosa* (N) *and the typical abnormalities of the mucosa in bronchial asthma* (A)*. Note differences between central* (left) *and peripheral* (right) *airways: In central airways, asthma is characterized by an increase in the quantity of mucus-producing elements (submucosal glands and goblet cells) and luminal mucus. In the peripheral airways, goblet cells and luminal mucus are present only in asthma. (Adapted with permission from A. Wanner. The role of mucociliary dysfunction in bronchial asthma. Am. J. Med. 67:477, 1979.)*

rets [12, 22]. The secretory response to substance P can be markedly enhanced by inhibiting neutral endopeptidase, an observation that has led some investigators to suggest that infections may augment mucus release by reducing the levels of neutral endopeptidase, thus prolonging the effect of tachykinins [5, 34]. The effect of other peptides (gastrin-releasing peptides, endorphins) on the release of mucus in human airways has not been fully assessed.

MUCOCILIARY DYSFUNCTION

The structure-function relationships of the mucociliary apparatus are incompletely understood. On the one hand, abnormal clearance of airway mucus has been clearly demonstrated in individuals with primary ciliary dyskinesia in whom structural defects of the cilia lead to abnormal ciliary function and hence defective mucociliary transport. In this instance, it is easy to understand how the primary structural abnormality is responsible for the impaired function. On the other hand, Battista and colleagues [4] have demonstrated that during the early regeneration period after mechanical denudation of the tracheal epithelium, 30 to 50 percent of mucus transport activity is present at a time when only 10 percent of the regenerating epithelium is cil-

iated, and that ciliary function is completely intact by 14 days after denudation, when complete regeneration has not yet occurred. These findings show that structure is not always intimately related to function in the mucociliary system and that mechanisms other than ciliary beating may move airway secretions. For example, airway secretions, if present in excessive quantities, could be transported by air liquid pumping at air velocities attained during quiet breathing (not only coughing).

Structure of the Mucociliary Apparatus

The pathologic lesions in the airways of patients with bronchial asthma strongly suggest the presence of mucociliary dysfunction. In status asthmaticus, the mucosa is characterized by edema and disruption of epithelial cells, a decrease in the number of ciliated cells, and an increase in the number of goblet cells, along with goblet cell metaplasia in peripheral airways (see Fig. 30-1). Detachment of superficial epithelial cells can be seen in some areas. The basement membrane is thickened. Submucosal tissues show edema, dilated capillaries, and cellular infiltration with eosinophils, neutrophils, and mononuclear cells [18]. There is a decrease in the number of mast cells, with partial degranulation of those remaining. IgE deposits can be demonstrated in lymphocytes and eosinophils within the bronchial wall [8]. There

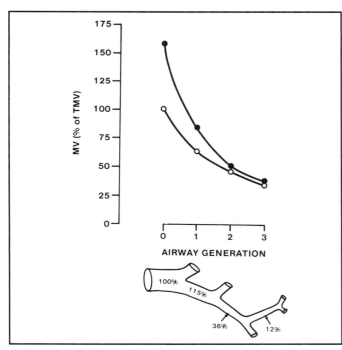

Fig. 30-2. *Relationship between mucus velocity (MV) and airway generation (0 = trachea) in normal dogs. Corresponding ciliary density of surface epithelium is also shown. Data are expressed as percent of tracheal mucus velocity (TMV) and percent of tracheal ciliary density. Open circles show mucus velocities before and closed circles, after intravenous administration of aminophylline (4 mg/kg). Note the diminished responsiveness to pharmacologic mucociliary stimulation in higher airway generations.*

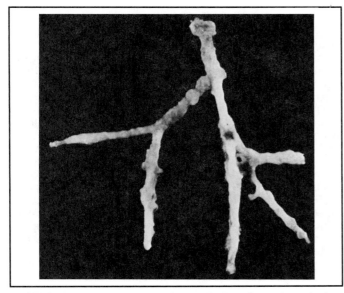

Fig. 30-3. *Bronchial mucus cast obtained by bronchoscopic aspiration from an asthmatic patient with bronchopulmonary aspergillosis. The proximal end of cast was located in the distal portion of the left main bronchus. (Courtesy T. Ahmed, M.D.)*

is hyperplasia and hypertrophy of the submucosal glands [18]. Widespread mucous plugging of the bronchi is usually seen (Fig. 30-3). It should be pointed out that none of these lesions is pathognomonic for bronchial asthma; they can also be seen in chronic bronchitis.

The pathologic features of stable bronchial asthma and of asthma in remission differ only quantitatively from those of status asthmaticus (Fig. 30-4). The destructive changes of the epithelium are not as evident and the amount of luminal mucus is less in the former. However, spotty obstruction of smaller airways with mucous plugs has been clearly demonstrated, mainly in bronchi greater than 1 mm in diameter, but also in smaller peripheral airways [14] (Fig. 30-5). Thus, with respect to mucociliary function, the relevant pathologic findings in bronchial asthma are excessive mucus in large airways, the presence of mucus in small airways that in the normal lung do not contain mucus, and disruption of the ciliated epithelium.

Mucociliary Transport

Normal clearance of mucus from the airways depends primarily on how well cilia interact with mucus. The slowing or cessation of mucociliary transport in bronchial asthma could theoretically result from an abnormality in ciliary performance or in the physical characteristics of airway secretions (mucus and periciliary fluid). Based on the currently available information, the latter appears to be more important than the former.

Cilia

Because of the incomplete destruction of the ciliated surface epithelium and the impressive functional reserve of the ciliary apparatus [4], it is unlikely that an insufficient number of cilia is principally responsible for mucociliary dysfunction in bronchial asthma.

A primary disturbance of ciliary motility is difficult to assess by in vivo techniques that measure ciliary beat frequency or by in vitro techniques using airway segments because of the presence of mucus, which has an effect on ciliary beat frequency. It cannot be determined to what extent a stimulus applied to the system affects ciliary motility directly or indirectly by altering the physical properties of mucus. To determine if a primary abnormality of ciliary function contributes to allergic mucociliary dysfunction, Maurer and associates [33] used an in vitro technique. In conscious sheep with *Ascaris suum* hypersensitivity, ciliated cells were obtained with a cytology brush, and the recovered cells (also containing mast cells) were suspended in a perfusion chamber. Ciliary activity was viewed microscopically and recorded on videotape for subsequent slow-motion analysis of ciliary beat frequency. Ciliary beat frequency increased on in vitro exposure to various concentrations of *A. suum* antigen. This effect was completely blocked by cromolyn sodium and specific antagonists of slow-reacting substance of anaphylaxis (SRS-A) [33] (Fig. 30-6). The H_1 and H_2 histamine receptor–blocking agents mepiramine and cimetidine failed to modify antigen-induced ciliostimulation. These observations suggested that antigen-induced release of chemical mediators, including leukotrienes but not histamine, causes a transient increase in ciliary beat frequency. This was subsequently confirmed by assessing the effects of selected chemical mediators of anaphylaxis in the same preparation [53]. Leukotriene C_4 and D_4, and the prostaglandins E_1 and E_2 caused dose-dependent increases in ciliary beat frequency between concentrations of 10^{-5} and 10^{-3} M, while histamine caused ciliostimulation only at the relatively high concentrations of 10^{-3} and 10^{-5} M. Prostaglandin $F_{2\alpha}$ was without effect. Leukotriene C_4 was the most potent of all the mediators tested. These ciliostimulatory effects of several prostaglandins and the relative insensitivity of cilia to histamine have been reported by other investigators [25, 58, 59].

Physiologic and inflammatory stimuli may have different effects on the various components of mucociliary function. Seybold and coworkers demonstrated dose-dependent increases in ciliary beat frequency after stimulation with acetylcholine and epi-

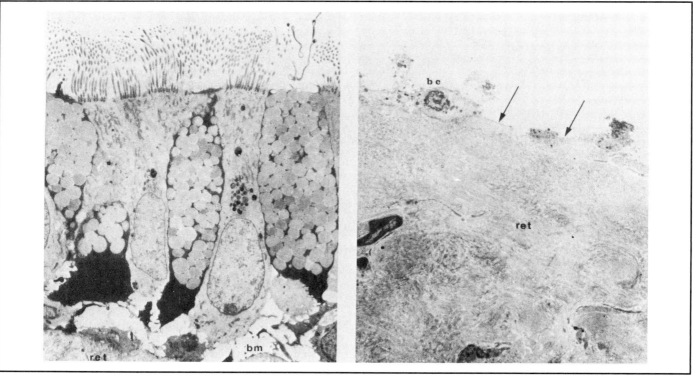

Fig. 30-4. *Airway mucosal biopsy specimens obtained at fiberoptic bronchoscopy showing electron microscopic appearances of* (left) *normal control epithelium with mucous and ciliated cells and basal* (bm) *and reticular* (ret) *laminae (× 2,170), and* (right) *patient with symptomatic asthma whose mucosal biopsy specimen shows complete sloughing of the surface epithelium but for occasional basal cells* (bc), *which remain attached to an intact basal lamina* (arrows). *There is marked thickening of the reticular lamina* (ret) *(× 2,170). All tissues for electrom microscopy fixed in glutaraldehyde and osmium tetroxide. (Reprinted with permission from P. K. Jeffery. Morphology of the airway wall in asthma and in chronic obstructive pulmonary disease. Am. Rev. Respir. Dis. 143:1152, 1991.)*

nephrine [51]. Acetylcholine increased surface liquid velocity while platelet-activating factor produced the opposite effect and decreased ciliary beat frequency. Antigen challenge increased ciliary beat frequency but reduced surface liquid velocity. None of these stimuli produced a significant change in the viscoelastic properties of mucus. These data suggest that an alteration of one component of mucociliary transport may not be translated into a complementary change of another parameter (Fig. 30-7).

The effectiveness of ciliary action in transporting mucus depends on several characteristics of ciliary beating, of which the beat frequency is but one. The coordination of the beating patterns, for instance, is also an important determinant of ciliary performance. It may thus be possible that a given stimulus causes at the same time an increase in ciliary beat frequency and ciliary discoordination, thereby producing ineffective ciliary activity. Ciliary discoordination has not been reported in in vitro preparations either after antigen challenge or under the influence of chemical mediators of anaphylaxis [32, 33, 53]. In allergic asthma, changes in ciliary beat frequency may therefore be translated into changes in mucociliary transport, provided the physical properties of respiratory secretions remain unaltered.

One can conclude from these studies that several chemical mediators of anaphylaxis stimulate ciliary beat frequency, with leukotrienes being the most potent, and that none of the chemical mediators tested to date depress ciliary activity. Primary ciliary dysfunction therefore does not appear to play a major role in the abnormality of mucociliary clearance in allergic bronchial asthma. Some studies have suggested that ciliodepression may occur secondarily through the release of several proteins from eosinophils [17, 21].

Airway Secretions

Theoretically, the transportability of airway mucus depends on the rheologic properties and quantity of mucus and periciliary fluid. Ross and Corssin [45] developed a mathematical model to describe the effects of physical factors on mucociliary transport. Their theoretic considerations (assuming the classic two-layer concept of mucus and periciliary fluid) suggested that within a moderate range of deviation from "normal" values, and with ciliary beat frequency and wave velocity held constant, the mucus transport velocity is directly related to mucus elasticity and the depth of periciliary fluid and inversely related to mucus viscosity and the depth of the mucous layer. Viscosity appears to play a less important role than elasticity. Ross and Corsin also predicted that the effect of gravity is negligible under normal conditions. Some of these factors have been tested experimentally. Stewart [54] investigated the weight-carrying capacity of ciliated epithelium. He found that up to a weight of 20 mg/mm² there was no decrease in test particle transport, and that no acceleration of particle transport occurred with lighter weights. Above this value, impairment of transport was observed. The relationship between the viscoelasticity and transportability of mucus has also been demonstrated by determining the viscosity and the elastic modulus of sputum from patients with chronic bronchitis and measuring the transport rate of the same sputum on the frog palate [16]. It was shown that sputum with a viscosity between 1,000 and 3,000 poise and an elastic modulus between 10 and 25 dynes/cm² was transported at the fastest rate [11]. The role of physical characteristics of periciliary fluid in determining mucus transport remains theoretic because experimental verification is technically difficult and has thus far not been accomplished.

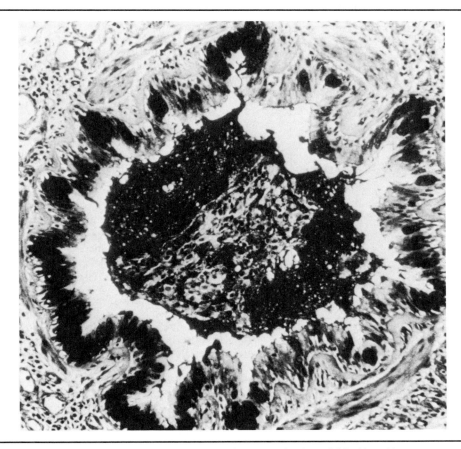

Fig. 30-5. *Small airway (inner diameter = 0.15 mm) with an intraluminal mucous plug in a child with stable asthma. Note the numerous macrophages encased in the mucous plug. (Lung biopsy, × 240, reprinted with permission from E. Cutz, H. Levison, and D. M. Cooper. Ultrastructure of airways in children with asthma.* Histopathology *2:407, 1978.)*

Periciliary fluid being a sol, changes in its rheologic properties appear to be less important than changes in its depth. Although theoretic predictions postulate an increase in mucus transport rates as the depth of the periciliary fluid layer increases, this relationship can only exist until the depth of the periciliary fluid layer exceeds the length of the ciliary shafts. Once this occurs, a diminution of mucus transport would be expected.

Several of the physical changes of airway secretions that theoretically impair mucus transport have been demonstrated in patients with bronchial asthma and in animal models of allergic bronchoconstriction.

Mucus. Qualitative changes of airway mucus in bronchial asthma have been reported [61] (see Chap. 29). Glycoproteins seem to determine the rheologic properties of mucus to a great extent. Increased concentrations of unusual polysaccharides and cross-binding between transudated serum protein and secretory IgA have been found in the sputum of patients with bronchial asthma [23, 47, 49]. Changes in electrolyte concentrations including increases in calcium have also been reported, and serum proteins appear to accumulate in the sol phase of asthmatic sputum [24, 47]. These distinguishing biochemical characteristics of respiratory secretions in asthma could have an effect on their rheologic properties. Unfortunately, this has not been adequately studied. The best known observation was made on expectorated sputum that may not be representative of lower airway secretions [10]. In that study, sputum from asthmatic patients tended to be more viscous than that from patients with other types of obstructive airway disease; a marked increase in viscosity at a low shear

rate was particularly characteristic for sputum obtained from asthmatic patients. If mucus in the lower airways indeed possesses abnormal rheologic properties, this abnormality may well alter transport rates. One study demonstrated that sputum obtained from patients with asthma can also impair ciliary activity through biochemical rather than rheologic factors [17]. Ciliary beat frequency measured photoelectrically in a bronchial explant was reduced when expectorated sputum from allergic and nonallergic asthmatic patients was placed on the preparation. The cilioinhibitory effect of sputum was more pronounced during clinical exacerbations of asthma.

In addition, mucociliary interaction also depends on the depth (weight) of the mucus. Mucus hypersecretion is not only indirectly suggested by the presence of excessive mucus in the airway lumina but has also been experimentally demonstrated in in vivo and in vitro models of bronchial asthma. Yamatake and coworkers [71] demonstrated hypersecretion of respiratory tract fluids after inhalation challenge with specific antigen in allergic dogs. By using IgE-sensitized human airway fragments, Shelhamer and colleagues [52] found a 35 percent increase in radiolabeled glycoprotein secretion after the addition of antigen to the preparation. In subsequent experiments, the same group of investigators showed that the anaphylactic release of glycoproteins is mediated primarily by lipoxygenase products of arachidonic acid [30, 31]. Monohydroxyeicosatetraenoic acid, leukotriene C_4, and leukotriene D_4 were all found to stimulate glycoprotein secretion in this model. Similar observations were made by Phipps and associates [43]. They studied the effects of purified *A. suum*

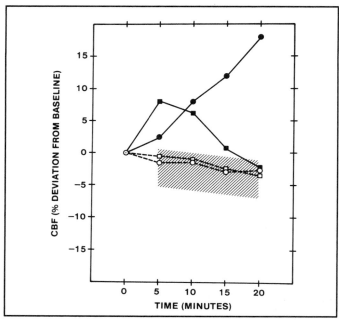

Fig. 30-6. *Effect of in vitro challenge with specific antigen (10^{-2} dilution) on ciliary beat frequency (CBF) of tracheal cells in the absence of pharmacologic agents (■), and in the presence of cromolyn sodium (□) and the slow-reacting substance of anaphylaxis (SRS-A) antagonist FPL 55712 (○). The effect of leukotriene C_4 (10^{-8} M) is also shown (●). Shaded area reflects normal range of CBF over time. (Adapted with permission from D. R. Maurer, et al. The role of ciliary motility in acute allergic mucociliary dysfunction. J. Appl. Physiol. 52: 1018, 1982.)*

antigen on tracheal glycoprotein secretion in vitro by using pieces of trachea obtained from allergic sheep who had responded previously with bronchoconstriction to inhalation of *A. suum* antigen. Glycoprotein secretion was assessed by adding ^{35}S-sulfate and ^3H-threonine to the submucosal side of the tissue and monitoring the output of macromolecular bound ^{35}S and ^3H on the luminal side. *A. suum* antigen increased the secretion of bound ^{35}S by 57 percent and of bound ^3H by 78 percent. FPL 57231, an antagonist of SRS-A, blocked these effects. Prostaglandin-generating factor of anaphylaxis and possibly platelet-activating factor are products generated during airway anaphylaxis that may exert their effects on mucus secretion by amplification of eicosanoid production [27, 29]. The role of other chemical mediators of anaphylaxis in mediating mucus hypersecretion is not well established. For example, several investigators have reported inconsistent effects of histamine on mucus secretion [9, 26, 40, 52, 55]. In one of these studies [52], a marked stimulation of mucous glycoprotein release from human airways in vitro was found in response to histamine, and this effect was mediated primarily through H_2 histamine receptors.

These in vitro and in vivo experiments strongly suggest that bronchial asthma is characterized by excessive secretion of mucus with abnormal rheologic and biochemical properties and that, at least in allergic asthma, the mucus hypersecretion is caused by chemical mediators of anaphylaxis, notably SRS-A.

Periciliary Fluid. If one assumes that periciliary fluid is produced by the airway epithelium, quantitative information about the production of this fluid could be obtained by analyzing active epithelial ion and water transport. Phipps and Denas [41, 43] determined the effects of antigen challenge on epithelial fluxes of water, chloride, and sodium in vitro using pieces of sheep trachea obtained from allergic sheep. Immediately after antigen challenge, there was a net absorption of water from the luminal

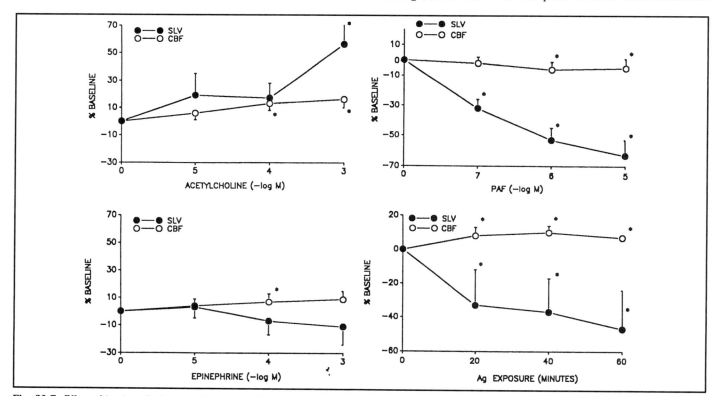

Fig. 30-7. *Effect of in vitro challenge with acetylcholine, epinephrine, platelet-activating factor (PAF), and antigen (Ag) on surface liquid velocity (SLV) and ciliary beat frequency (CBF) in the trachea of allergic sheep. (Adapted with permission from Z. Seybold, et al. Mucociliary interaction in vitro: Effects of physiologic and inflammatory stimuli. J. Appl. Physiol. 68:1421, 1990.)*

side followed by a transient increase of water flux toward the lumen. Changes in sodium fluxes paralleled those of water fluxes, while there was an initial absorption of chloride from the luminal side with a subsequent transient increase in chloride secretion toward the lumen. This study indicates that antigen challenge is associated with transient changes in water fluxes across the airway epithelium. These changes may alter the thickness of the periciliary fluid such that mucociliary interaction is impaired. Histamine appears to be an important mediator of active water transport toward the lumen [28, 39]. However, other mediators may also be involved.

Mucociliary Interaction

From the disturbances in mucus secretions, one might expect impaired mucociliary interaction, and hence abnormal mucus transport in bronchial asthma (Tables 30-1 and 30-2). This has indeed been described by different investigators who studied groups of asthmatic patients in different stages of their disease (Table 30-3). Mezey and coworkers [37, 72] measured tracheal mucus velocity by using discrete surface markers of mucus transport in six asymptomatic patients with ragweed asthma. In these patients, mean tracheal mucus velocity was lower than in normal age-matched nonsmokers. In patients with mild (symptomatic) bronchial asthma, Bateman and colleagues [3] also observed impaired clearance of an inhaled radioaerosol. In their study, patients who were in remission had clearance values that were not different from those in normal controls. In stable asthma, Foster and associates [20] also reported impaired tracheal and bronchial clearance of inhaled insoluble radioactive particles. Finally, three elderly patients with late-onset asthma were studied in another investigation [48]. Their tracheal mucus transport rates were markedly reduced as compared with normal age-matched controls and indistinguishable from values seen in patients with chronic bronchitis.

The pathogenesis of asthma-associated mucociliary dysfunction has been extensively studied in animal models of allergic bronchoconstriction and in allergic subjects, and it appears that mucociliary dysfunction is intimately related to chemical mediators of anaphylaxis. In the study of Mezey and colleagues [37]

Table 30-1. Effect of antigen and inflammatory mediators on mucociliary function in allergic airways

Function	Agonist	Species	Effect
Tracheal mucus velocity	Antigen	Man	Depression
	Antigen	Dog	Depression
	Antigen	Sheep	Depression
	Leukotriene D_4	Sheep	Depression
	Histamine	Dog	Stimulation
Ciliary beat frequency	Antigen	Sheep	Stimulation
	Leukotriene C_4 and D_4	Sheep	Stimulation
	Histamine	Sheep	Stimulation
	Prostaglandin E_1 and E_2	Sheep	Stimulation
	Prostaglandin $F_{2\alpha}$	Sheep	None
	Platelet-activating factor	Sheep	Depression
Mucus secretion*	Antigen	Sheep	Stimulation
	Leukotriene D_4	Sheep	Stimulation
	Substance P	Man	Stimulation
	Substance P	Ferret	Stimulation
Epithelial water transport	Antigen	Sheep	Absorption, then secretion
	Leukotriene D_4	Sheep	Absorption
	Histamine	Sheep	Secretion

* Mucus secretory responses in man are summarized in Table 30-2.

Table 30-2. Human respiratory mucus secretory responses

Agent	Airway mucus
Methacholine	↑
Atropine	NE*
Methacholine + atropine	NE
Alpha-adrenergic agonists	↑
Beta-adrenergic agonists	NE
Cyclic guanosine monophosphate	↑
Cyclic adenosine monophosphate	NE
Arachidonic acid	↑
Prostaglandins E_1, $F_{2\alpha}$, D_2, I_2, A_2	↑
Prostaglandin E_2	↓
Aspirin	↑
Indomethacin	↑
Eicosatetraenoic acid	↓
5-,8-,9-,11-, or 15-hydroxyeicosatetraenoic acid	↑
5- and 9-hydroperoxyeicosatetraenoic acid	↑
Leukotriene C_4 or D_4	↑
Anaphylaxis	↑
Histamine	↑
Prostaglandin-generating factor	↑
Macrophage or monocyte mucus secretagogue	↑
C3a	↑
Vasoactive intestinal peptide	↓

* No net effect on mucus secretion.
Source: M. Kaliner. Human respiratory mucus. *Am. Rev. Respir. Dis.* 134:612, 1986. Reprinted with permission.

Table 30-3. Mucociliary clearance in asthma

Severity of asthma	Mucociliary clearance (%)*	Reference
In remission	54	37
Stable		
Mild	69	3
Moderate	15	48

* Group mean expressed as percent of age-matched controls (nonsmokers).

involving asymptomatic patients with a history of ragweed asthma, bronchial challenge with ragweed extract reduced the mean tracheal mucociliary transport rate to 72 percent of baseline immediately after completion of bronchial challenge when mean specific airway conductance was reduced by 35 percent. One hour later, mean specific airway conductance had returned to its baseline values; however, the mean tracheal mucociliary transport rate was further reduced to 47 percent of baseline at this time. These changes in mucus transport were prevented by pretreatment with 20 mg of cromolyn sodium by inhalation (Fig. 30-8). Thus, in patients with allergic asthma and antigen-induced bronchospasm, the decrease in tracheal mucus transport appears to be independent of bronchospasm and to be related to airway anaphylaxis and the release of chemical mediators. Similar observations have been made in animal models of allergic bronchoconstriction. In dogs with *A. suum* hypersensitivity, the inhalation of aerosolized *A. suum* extract has been shown to have differential effects on airway function and mucociliary transport [63]. Although only 50 percent of the dogs responded with bronchospasm to inhalation of *A. suum* antigen, tracheal mucociliary transport rates decreased in all animals by a mean of 70 percent within 30 to 45 minutes of antigen challenge regardless of whether bronchospasm occurred; tracheal mucociliary transport rates were still decreased at the end of 2 hours. No changes in airway function or mucociliary transport occurred in control animals that inhaled ragweed, an antigen to which they were not sensitive. This observation again underscores the lack of interdependence between changes in airway mechanics and mucociliary transport during allergic bronchoconstriction. Sheep

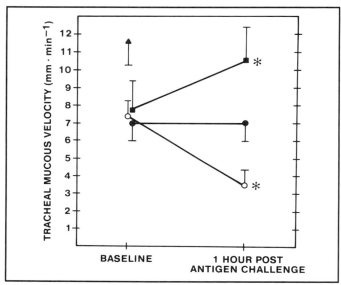

Fig. 30-8. *Effect of inhalation challenge with ragweed extract on mean tracheal mucus velocity in asymptomatic patients with ragweed asthma. Brackets indicate the standard error of the mean. Asterisks denote significant change from baseline. Ragweed challenge was performed without premedication (○), after inhalation of cromolyn sodium (●), and after inhalation of the SRS-A antagonist FPL 55712 (■). Mean tracheal mucus velocity of normal controls is also shown for comparison (▲).*

with *A. suum* hypersensitivity exhibit airway responses to the inhalation of aerosolized *A. suum* antigen that are similar to those in allergic dogs [62]. Mucociliary transport has also been shown to be reduced to 55 percent of baseline 1 hour and to 51 percent of baseline 2 hours after antigen challenge in these animals [66]. This decrease in mucociliary transport has not been observed in the same animals when challenged with a control antigen (ragweed) and was completely prevented by prior inhalation of cromolyn sodium or the beta-adrenergic agonist terbutaline sulfate, both of which presumably protect against the development of allergic mucociliary dysfunction by inhibition of mast cell degranulation.

Several chemical mediators released from mast cells during anaphylaxis may be responsible for mucociliary dysfunction. Identification of the putative mediator has been attempted both in animal models and in patients with bronchial asthma. In the allergic dog model, the questions of whether histamine and leukotrienes, two major chemical mediators, play a role in mucociliary dysfunction, and whether the effect of these mediators on the mucociliary apparatus is direct or involves a cholinergic reflex, were addressed [63]. Inhalation of histamine or acetylcholine aerosols in concentrations that produced a degree of bronchospasm comparable to that observed after antigen challenge resulted in a transient increase in tracheal mucociliary transport rates, thereby excluding these substances as mediators of the observed mucociliary impairment after antigen challenge. On the other hand, inhalation of *A. suum* antigen together with compound FPL 55712, an antagonist of SRS-A, produced a transient, nearly threefold increase in tracheal mucus velocity regardless of whether bronchospasm was elicited. FPL 55712, when given alone or with a control antigen, had no effect on tracheal mucociliary transport rates, thereby excluding a nonspecific stimulatory action. These results suggest that mucociliary dysfunction is related to the release of SRS-A and does not involve a vagal reflex. One might speculate that the stimulation of tracheal mucus transport rates by the combined administration of specific antigen and FPL 55712 was related to an inhibition of the depres-

sant effect of leukotrienes, thereby unmasking the stimulatory effects of other mediators such as histamine.

The results of this animal study were later confirmed in patients with ragweed asthma [1]. By administering FPL 55712 in conjunction with antigen challenge, it was found that the expected decrease in tracheal mucus velocity after ragweed challenge was not only prevented but also reversed to an increase above baseline (see Fig. 30-8). This effect was observed with both 0.5% and 1% solutions of FPL 55712, and there was no difference between the two doses.

Aerosol challenge with leukotriene D_4 decreased tracheal mucus velocity in conscious sheep with (allergic) and without (nonallergic) *A. suum* hypersensitivity [46]. In contrast, only the allergic animals exhibited bronchial smooth muscle responses following challenge with leukotriene D_4. The maximal decline in mucus clearance and the duration of the effect were similar to that observed after antigen challenge in allergic sheep. Pretreatment with the leukotriene antagonist FPL 55712 failed to inhibit the leukotriene D_4–induced decrease in tracheal mucus velocity but blocked the airway response in allergic sheep. These observations suggest that the allergic state is characterized by airway smooth muscle hyperresponsiveness to leukotriene D_4. Considering that leukotriene D_4 stimulates the output of radiolabeled mucin and ciliary activity in the trachea of sheep (in vitro) [42], it is suspected that leukotriene D_4–induced impairment of mucus transport is related to its potent effects as a mucus secretagogue.

Studies in cultured cells with Fura-2 revealed increases in ciliary beat frequency associated with elevated $[Ca^{++}]_i$; the effects of therapeutic agents may be evaluated by this approach [73].

CLINICAL CONSEQUENCES OF MUCOCILIARY DYSFUNCTION

The sequence of events outlined above leads to the accumulation of mucus in the airways because of increased secretion combined with reduced clearance. The accumulation of mucus has several pathophysiologic consequences that are potentially of clinical significance. Of these, cough, airflow obstruction, and increased susceptibility to respiratory infections are particularly important as they have a direct bearing on the symptoms of the patient with bronchial asthma.

Cough

If airway mucociliary transport fails, cough assumes an important role as a backup defense system that removes retained respiratory secretions and hence inhaled foreign materials that have been deposited in the airways. It is unclear to what extent excessive airway mucus contributes to the cough of the patient with bronchial asthma, as the cough reflex may also be triggered by inflammatory changes of the epithelium. The relation between the quantity and rheologic properties of airway mucus on the one hand and cough frequency and efficiency on the other has thus far not been examined experimentally (see Chap. 50).

Airflow Obstruction

While structure-function correlations have not been directly established with respect to the effects of excessive airway mucus on airflow obstruction in bronchial asthma, there is circumstantial evidence for such a relationship. The postmortem findings of widespread mucous plugging in the airways of patients who die in status asthmaticus have long been considered the major cause of death [2, 18, 44]; in these cases the contribution of the mucous plugs to the increased airflow resistance hardly requires experimental proof. To what extent excessive airway secretions contribute to airflow obstruction in patients with stable bronchial asthma is not known, but such obstruction appears to be a possibility if one considers the histologic demonstration of mucous plugs in intermediate and small airways [14]. McFadden and

Lyons [36] suggested that the residual airway dysfunction found in patients with asthma in remission is partially related to the presence of excessive mucus in peripheral airways. Frequency dependence of dynamic lung compliance and altered density dependence of the maximum expiratory flow volume curve are frequently observed in asymptomatic asthmatic patients with normal or near-normal spirometry values and airway resistance [15, 70]. It has been shown that these and similar functional abnormalities suggestive of peripheral airway obstruction are not reversed or only partially reversed by the administration of bronchodilators [7, 35], which implicates excessive airway mucus, mucosal edema, or both, rather than increased bronchomotor tone, as the causes of airflow obstruction. In this regard, the observations of Foster and coworkers [20], which suggested abnormal mucus clearance in peripheral airways of such patients, assume major importance. This defect presumably results from a mismatch between excessive amounts of mucus and the poorly developed ciliary apparatus in peripheral airways where ordinarily little or no mucus is secreted.

Increased Susceptibility to Respiratory Infection

Based on epidemiologic studies, Trendelenburg [56] and others suggested a relation between asthma and respiratory infections. However, this has not been tested experimentally. The mucociliary dysfunction in bronchial asthma may predispose patients to respiratory infections by prolonged residence of infectious agents on the respiratory mucosa because of impaired mucus transport, the creation of a favorable milieu for the multiplication of infectious agents in pools of airway secretions, epithelial damage favoring bacterial attachment to epithelial cells, changes in the biochemical composition of respiratory secretions that reduce their bactericidal properties, or an inhibitory effect of airway mucus on cellular defense mechanisms. The last was recently suggested by Woodside and associates [69]. Macrophages are found in the airways and may exist either in the periciliary fluid layer or embedded in mucus [6]. Mucous plugs in bronchial asthma contain large numbers of macrophages [14]; however, the viability of these cells has until recently been reported. In an attempt to evaluate the effects of mucus on macrophage function, Woodside and colleagues [69] obtained alveolar macrophages from sheep by lung lavage and incubated them in vitro with and without airway mucus obtained from the same animal by tracheal aspiration after systemic administration of the secretagogue pilocarpine. The phagocytic activity of macrophages treated with mucus (10% by volume) was compared with their phagocytic activities in the absence of any additions and after the addition of small amounts of pilocarpine to mimic the presence of pilocarpine in mucus aspirated from the sheep after systemic administration of pilocarpine. The rates of phagocytosis were measured with 1.09-μ polystyrene latex particles at nonsaturating and saturating levels [57]. Mucus inhibited phagocytosis at nonsaturating levels of particles by 75 percent and at saturating levels by 47 percent (Fig. 30-9). Pilocarpine had no effect on phagocytosis. These findings suggest impairment of an important macrophage function in the tracheobronchial tree, particularly in airway diseases associated with mucus hypersecretion, including bronchial asthma. It remains to be demonstrated if and how this impairment may alter the susceptibility to respiratory infections.

Another possible mechanism of increased susceptibility to respiratory infections in bronchial asthma is the impaired mechanical removal of inhaled infectious agents that are deposited in the tracheobronchial tree. Most animal studies that have addressed this question have used a protocol of previous injury to the mucociliary apparatus by various inhalants followed by a bacterial load by inhalation to determine bacterial clearance. Unfortunately, this approach is not capable of determining the contribution of mucociliary transport per se because of the effect of the inhalant on other pulmonary defense systems. However, the im-

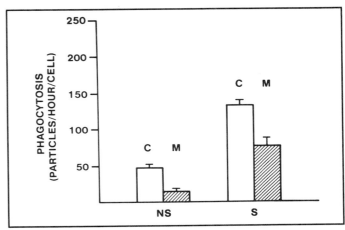

Fig. 30-9. *Effect of airway mucus* (M) *(10% by volume) on the phagocytic activity of lung macrophages in vitro. Phagocytosis was measured with polystyrene latex particles at nonsaturating* (NS) *and saturating* (S) *levels. Brackets reflect standard error of the mean. The difference between control* (C) *and M is significant at both levels. (Adapted with permission from K. Woodside, et al. Inhibition of pulmonary macrophage function by airway mucus. J. Appl. Physiol. 54: 94, 1983.)*

Table 30-4. *Effect of atropine sulfate on persistence of inhaled bacteria in the trachea*[a]

	Average tracheal mucus transport rate (mm/min)[b]	Time required for complete sterility (hr)[b]
Control	10.5 ($\pm$0.5)	3 ($\pm$1)
Atropine sulfate treated (0.2 mg/kg qh)	6.0 ($\pm$0.3)	14 ($\pm$4)

[a] After controlled inhalation challenge with aerosolized solution of *Pasteurella haemolytica*.
[b] Mean ($\pm$ S.E.) for five sheep.

portance of mucociliary transport in this regard is exemplified in patients with primary ciliary dyskinesia [38]. These persons have akinetic or dyskinetic cilia in their airways and markedly depressed or absent mucociliary clearance. The ciliary dyskinesia is caused by a genetically determined structural abnormality of cilia. Since patients with primary ciliary dyskinesia are born with this abnormality, it is reasonable to assume that the characteristic clinical manifestations of recurrent respiratory infections, chronic bronchitis, and bronchiectasis are sequelae of the primary ciliary dysfunction. Thus a primary disturbance of mucociliary transport seems to facilitate the development of respiratory infection and chronic airway disease.

Whiteside and associates [67] used a sheep model to test this relationship experimentally. The sheep inhaled a standard bacterial aerosol with or without the administration of atropine sulfate, which reduces tracheal mucociliary transport rates by approximately 40 percent. The subsequent persistence of the bacteria (*Pasteurella haemolytica*) in the trachea was assessed by semiquantitative sampling with a sterile catheter-protected brush. The impairment of mucociliary transport after atropine sulfate administration was associated with a prolonged persistence of bacteria (Table 30-4). Atropine sulfate may have interfered with the normal function of the mucosa in more ways than by impairment of mucus transport. However, this experiment further supports the importance of mucociliary function in bacterial clearance from the conducting airways and indicates that a breakdown of mucociliary clearance such as in bronchial asthma may render the lungs more susceptible to infection.

REFERENCES

1. Ahmed, T., et al. Abnormal mucociliary transport in allergic patients with antigen-induced bronchospasm: Role of slow reacting substance of anaphylaxis. *Am. Rev. Respir. Dis.* 124:110, 1981.
2. Alexander, H. L. A historical account of death asthma. *J. Allergy* 34:305, 1980.
3. Bateman, J. R. M., et al. Tracheobronchial clearance in asthma. *Thorax* 38:463, 1983.
4. Battista, S. P., Denine, E. P., and Kensler, C. J. Restoration of tracheal mucosa and ciliary particle transport activity after mechanical denudation in the chicken. *Toxicol. Appl. Pharmacol.* 22:56, 1972.
5. Borson, D. B., Corrales, R., and Varsano, S. Enkephalinase inhibitors potentiate substance P-induced secretion of $^{35}SO_4^-$ macromolecules from ferret trachea. *Exp. Lung Res.* 12:21, 1987.
6. Brain, J. D., Sorokin, S. P., and Godleski, J. J. Quantification, Origin, and Fate of Pulmonary Macrophages. In J. D. Brain (ed.), *Respiratory Defense Mechanisms.* New York: Marcel Dekker, 1977. P. 849.
7. Bullow, K., et al. Changes in volume of trapped gas in the lungs during provoked asthma followed by beta-2 receptor stimulation. *Respiration* 36: 19, 1978.
8. Callerama, J. L., et al. Immunoglobulins in bronchial tissues from patients with asthma, with special reference to immunoglobulin. *Eur. J. Allergy* 47: 187, 1971.
9. Chakrin, L. W., et al. Effect of cholinergic stimulation on the release of macromolecules by canine trachea in vitro. *Am. Rev. Respir. Dis.* 108:69, 1973.
10. Charman, J., and Reid, L. Sputum viscosity in chronic bronchitis, bronchiectasis, asthma, and cystic fibrosis. *Biorheology* 9:185, 1972.
11. Chen, T. M., and Dulfano, M. J. Mucus viscoelasticity and mucociliary transport rate. *J. Lab. Clin. Med.* 91:423, 1978.
12. Coles, S. J., Neil, K. H., and Reid, L. M. Potent stimulation of glycoprotein secretion in canine trachea by substance P. *J. Appl. Physiol.* 57:1323, 1984.
13. Coles, S. J., Said, S. I., and Reid, L. M. Inhibition by vasoactive intestinal peptide of glycoconjugate and lysozyme secretion by human airways in vitro. *Am. Rev. Respir. Dis.* 124:531, 1981.
14. Cutz, E., Levison, H., and Cooper, D. M. Ultrastructure of airways in children with asthma. *Histopathology* 2:407, 1978.
15. Despas, P. J., Leroux, M., and Macklem, P. T. Site of airway obstruction in asthma as determined by measuring maximal expiratory flow breathing air and a helium oxygen mixture. *J. Clin. Invest.* 51:3235, 1972.
16. Dulfano, M. J., and Adler, K. B. Physical properties of sputum: VII. Rheologic properties and mucociliary transport. *Am. Rev. Respir. Dis.* 112:341, 1975.
17. Dulfano, M. J., and Luk, C. K. Sputum and ciliary inhibition in asthma. *Thorax* 37:646, 1982.
18. Dunnil, M. S., Massarella, G. R., and Anderson, J. A. A comparison of the quantitative anatomy of the bronchi in normal subjects, in status asthmaticus, in chronic bronchitis, and in emphysema. *Thorax* 24:176, 1969.
19. Florey, H., Carleton, H. M., and Wells, A. Q. Mucus secretion in the trachea. *Br. J. Exp. Pathol.* 13:269, 1932.
20. Foster, W. M., et al. Quantitation of mucus clearance in peripheral lung and comparison with tracheal and bronchial mucus transport velocities in man: Adrenergics return depressed clearance and transport velocities in asthmatics to normal. *Am. Rev. Respir. Dis.* 117:337, 1978.
21. Frigas, E., et al. Elevated levels of the eosinophil granule major basic protein in the sputum of patients with bronchial asthma. *Mayo Clin. Proc.* 56:345, 1981.
22. Gashi, A. A., et al. Neuropeptides degranulate serous cells of ferret tracheal glands. *Am. J. Physiol.* 251:C223, 1986.
23. Gurgis, H. A., and Townley, R. G. Biochemical study on sputum in asthma and emphysema. *J. Allergy Clin. Immunol.* 51:86, 1973.
24. Hoffnianvou, H., and Ebelt, H. Der Elektrolytgehalt des Sputums und des Serums bein Patientem mit Asthma und chronischer Bronchitis. *Allerg. Asthmaforsch.* 14:227, 1968.
25. Iravani, J., and Melville, G. N. Mucociliary activity in the respiratory tract as influenced by prostaglandin E_1. *Respiration* 32:305, 1975.
26. Lopez-Vidriero, M. T., et al. Bronchial secretion from normal human airways after inhalation of prostaglandin F_2, acetylcholine, histamine, and citric acid. *Thorax* 32:734, 1977.
27. Lundgren, J. D., et al. Platelet-activating factor releases lipoxygenase metabolites and glucoconjugates from human airway tissue in vitro. *FASEB J.* 3:A609, 1989.
28. Marin, M. G., Davis, B., and Nadel, J. A. Effect of histamine on electrical and ion transport properties of tracheal epithelium. *Am. J. Physiol.* 42:735, 1977.
29. Marom, Z., et al. Prostaglandin-generating factor of anaphylaxis induces mucus glycoprotein release and the formation of lipoxygenase products of arachidonate from human airways. *Prostaglandins* 28:79, 1984.
30. Marom, Z., et al. Slow-reacting substances, leukotrienes C_4 and D_4, increase the release of mucus from human airways in vitro. *Am. Rev. Respir. Dis.* 126:449, 1982.
31. Marom, Z., Shelhamer, J. H., and Kaliner, M. Effects of arachidonic acid, monohydroxyeicosatetraenoic acid and prostaglandins on the release of mucous glycoproteins from human airways in vitro. *J. Clin. Invest.* 67: 1695, 1981.
32. Maurer, D. R., et al. Ciliary motility in airway anaphylaxis. *Cell Motil.* 1(Suppl.):67, 1982.
33. Maurer, D. R., et al. Role of ciliary motility in acute allergic mucociliary dysfunction. *J. Appl. Physiol.* 52:1018, 1982.
34. McDonald, D. M. Respiratory tract infections increase susceptibility to neurogenic inflammation in the rat trachea. *Am. Rev. Respir. Dis.* 137: 1432, 1988.
35. McFadden, E. R., Jr. Exertional dyspnea and cough as preludes to acute attacks of bronchial asthma. *N. Engl. J. Med.* 29:555, 1975.
36. McFadden, E. R., Jr., and Lyons, H. A. Airway resistance and uneven ventilation in bronchial asthma. *J. Appl. Physiol.* 25:365, 1968.
37. Mezey, R. J., et al. Mucociliary transport in allergic patients with antigen-induced bronchospasm. *Am. Rev. Respir. Dis.* 118:677, 1978.
38. Mossberg, B., et al. On the pathogenesis of obstructive lung disease: A study on the immotile-cilia syndrome. *Scand. J. Respir. Dis.* 59:55, 1978.
39. Olver, R. E., et al. Active transport of Na^+ and Cl^- across the canine tracheal epithelium in vitro. *Am. Rev. Respir. Dis.* 112:811, 1975.
40. Parke, D. V. Pharmacology of mucus. *Br. Med. Bull.* 34:89, 1978.
41. Phipps, R. J., and Denas, S. M. Epithelial water fluxes in sheep trachea. *Physiologist* 25:224, 1982.
42. Phipps, R., Denas, S., and Wanner, A. Leukotriene D_4 stimulates secretion of glycoproteins, ions and water in sheep trachea. *FASEB J.* 42:461, 1983.
43. Phipps, R., Denas, S., and Wanner, A. Antigen stimulates tracheal glycoprotein secretion and ion fluxes in allergic sheep. *J. Appl. Physiol.* 55:1593, 1983.
44. Rezek, P. R., and Millard, M. *Autopsy Pathology.* Springfield, Ill.: Thomas, 1963. P. 364.
45. Ross, S. M., and Corrsin, S. Results of an analytical model of mucociliary pumping. *J. Appl. Physiol.* 37:333, 1974.
46. Russi, E. W., et al. Effects of leukotriene D_4 on mucociliary and respiratory function in allergic and non-allergic sheep. *J. Appl. Physiol.* 59:1416, 1985.
47. Ryley, H. C., and Brongan, T. D. Variation in the composition of sputum in chronic chest disease. *Br. J. Exp. Pathol.* 49:625, 1968.
48. Santa Cruz, R., et al. Tracheal mucous velocity in normal man and patients with obstructive lung disease: Effects of terbutaline. *Am. Rev. Respir. Dis.* 109:458, 1974.
49. Savato, G. Some histological changes in chronic bronchitis and asthma. *Thorax* 23:168, 1968.
50. Serafini, S. M., Wanner, A., and Michaelson, E. D. Mucociliary transport in central and intermediate size airways: Effect of aminophylline. *Bull. Physiopathol. Respir.* 12:415, 1976.
51. Seybold, Z. V., et al. Mucociliary interaction in vitro: Effects of physiologic and inflammatory stimuli. *J. Appl. Physiol.* 68:1421, 1990.
52. Shelhamer, J. H., Marom, Z., and Kaliner, M. Immunologic and neuropharmacologic stimulation of mucous glycoprotein release from human airways in vitro. *J. Clin. Invest.* 66:1400, 1980.
53. Sielczak, M., et al. Effect of chemical mediators of anaphylaxis on ciliary function. *J. Allergy Clin. Immunol.* 72:663, 1983.
54. Stewart, W. C. Weight-carrying capacity and excitability of excised ciliary epithelium. *Am. J. Physiol.* 152:1, 1948.
55. Sturgess, J., and Reid, L. An organ culture study of the effect of drugs on the secretory activity of the human bronchial submucosal gland. *Clin. Sci.* 43:533, 1972.
56. Trendelenburg, F. Bacteriology of chronic lung disease. *Respiration* 27(Suppl.):199, 1970.
57. Vassalli, J. D., Hamilton, J., and Reich, E. Macrophage plasminogen activator: Modulation of enzyme production by anti-inflammatory steroids, mitotic inhibitors and cyclic nucleotides. *Cell* 8:271, 1978.
58. Verdugo, P. Ca^{2+}-dependent hormonal stimulation of ciliary activity. *Nature* 283:764, 1980.

59. Verdugo, P., Rumery, R. E., and Tam, P. Y. Hormonal control of oviductal ciliary activity: Effect of prostaglandins. *Fertil. Steril.* 33:193, 1980.

60. Wanner, A. State of the art: Clinical aspects of mucociliary transport. *Am. Rev. Respir. Dis.* 116:73, 1977.

61. Wanner, A. The role of mucociliary dysfunction in bronchial asthma. *Am. J. Med.* 67:477, 1979.

62. Wanner, A., et al. Antigen-induced bronchospasm in conscious sheep. *J. Appl. Physiol.* 47:917, 1979.

63. Wanner, A., et al. Tracheal mucous transport in experimental canine asthma. *J. Appl. Physiol.* 39:950, 1975.

64. Wanner, A., et al. Ciliary responsiveness in allergic and non-allergic airways. *J. Appl. Physiol.* 60:1967, 1986.

65. Webber, S. E., and Widdicombe, J. G. The actions of methacholine, phenylephrine, salbutamol, and histamine on mucus secretion from the ferret in vitro trachea. *Agents Actions* 22:82, 1987.

66. Wessberger, D., et al. Impaired tracheal mucous transport in allergic bronchoconstriction: Effect of terbutaline pre-treatment. *J. Allergy Clin. Immunol.* 67:357, 1981.

67. Whiteside, M., et al. Effect of atropine on tracheal mucociliary clearance and bacterial counts. *Bull. Eur. Physiopathol. Respir.* 20:347, 1984.

68. Wolff, R. K., et al. Effects of exercise and eucapnic hyperventilation on bronchial clearance in man. *J. Appl. Physiol.* 43:46, 1977.

69. Woodside, K. H., et al. Inhibition of pulmonary macrophage function by airway mucus. *J. Appl. Physiol.* 54:94, 1983.

70. Woolcock, A. J., Vincent, N. J., and Macklem, P. T. Frequency dependence of compliance as a test for obstruction in the small airways. *J. Clin. Invest.* 48:1097, 1969.

71. Yamatake, Y., et al. Allergy induced asthma with *Ascaris suum* administration to dogs. *Jpn. J. Pharmacol.* 27:285, 1977.

72. O'Riordan, T. G., Zwang, J., and Smaldone, G. C. Mucociliary clearance in adult asthma. *Am. Rev. Respir. Dis.* 149:598, 1992.

73. Sanderson, M. J., Lansly, A. B., and Dirkson, E. R. Regulation of ciliary beat frequency in respiratory tract cells. *Chest* 101:69S, 1992.

74. Harrison, R. A., Wong, L. B., and Yeates, D. B. Short-term interaction of airway and tissue oxygen tensions on ciliary beat frequency in dogs. *Am. Rev. Respir. Dis.* 146:141, 1992.

Experimental Asthma in Animals

Carol A. Hirshman
Hall Downes

31

To better understand asthma, we need to identify the causal agents or conditions and to unravel the underlying pathogenic mechanisms. Animal models are needed to accomplish this goal and to develop new therapeutic approaches. Theoretically, potential animal models are of two types: those that develop spontaneous episodes of bronchoconstriction, and those in which bronchoconstriction is produced by experimental conditions, such as challenge with antigen, pharmacologic agents, or inhaled irritants. Since, with rare exceptions, populations of laboratory animals with spontaneous asthma have not been identified, almost all animal models of asthma are based on experimentally induced bronchoconstriction. One exception would be the "heaves" in ponies, which is a naturally occurring asthma-like disorder [261] that is precipitated by environmental exposure to hay [273]. Bronchospasm induced by acute antigen challenge in the laboratory has been the basis of most animal models of asthma. Some, but not all, of such models may show a delayed as well as an initial obstructive phase and/or nonspecific airway hyperreactivity. In addition, models with spontaneously occurring and persistent nonspecific airway hyperreactivity have been developed on the basis of selective breeding. These various models emphasize different aspects thought to contribute to human asthma, for example, allergy, airway inflammation, nonspecific hyperreactivity, and genetic predisposition. Which species—the mouse, the rat, the guinea pig, the dog, the sheep, the monkey, or the pony—is the "best" model of human asthma at present? Each species has advantages and disadvantages. The species chosen for use in a particular study depends on the question to be answered. This chapter focuses on the advantages and disadvantages of these species as experimental models of human asthma.

ANTIGEN CHALLENGE

Experimentally induced airway constriction in previously sensitized animals by challenge with specific antigen has been clearly demonstrated in the guinea pig [24, 27, 87, 169, 329], the rat [56, 75, 138, 389, 390], the dog [152, 227, 229, 241, 318, 323, 345, 412, 434, 442], the monkey [303, 317], and the sheep [415]. The most common antigens employed are ovalbumin in the guinea pig [24, 27, 87, 169, 329] and *Ascaris suum* in the dog [152, 227, 229, 241, 318, 323, 438], sheep [412, 415], and monkey [303, 317]. Dogs, monkeys, and sheep are often natively allergic to *A. suum* as a result of a prior parasitic infection with round worms, which cross-react with *A. suum*.

The traditional immunologic model of antigen-induced airway constriction has been the guinea pig [27], which is easily sensitized to foreign proteins and in which the lung is the primary target organ in the anaphylactic reaction. Although a variety of mediators are involved in the pulmonary response to anaphylaxis in the guinea pig [87, 133, 301, 327], histamine plays a particularly important role and antihistamines afford a much higher degree of protection [41] than in many other species.

Rats are difficult to sensitize to foreign proteins [258, 355], and furthermore the primary target organ during anaphylaxis is the intestine rather than the lung [355]. Nevertheless, systemic anaphylaxis can be produced by appropriate challenge in animals sensitized to foreign proteins using adjuvants such as *Bordetella pertussis* [264, 286] or in animals infested with the nematode *Nippostrongylus brasiliensis* [76, 297]. Antigen-induced bronchoconstriction in the rat has been the subject of numerous studies [57, 58, 138, 192, 194, 324, 389, 390], and an inbred strain that has been developed shows a more homogeneous asthma-like response during antigen challenge than is found in the usual laboratory strains [192, 194]. The pulmonary response to antigen in the rat differs from that in humans and in most of the animal models of asthma in that it is mediated primarily by serotonin and is most effectively treated with a serotonin antagonist such as methysergide [76, 138, 324, 390]. Although other mediators may also be involved, histamine plays little or no role in the pulmonary response in this model.

The dog is unusual in that a well-defined atopic disease related to aeroallergens possibly occurs spontaneously [305] in some dogs. Three decades ago Patterson and coworkers [313] described spontaneous allergy to ragweed pollen in dogs, with the major clinical signs of conjunctivitis, rhinitis, and dermatitis rather than respiratory problems. The association of dermatitis and aeroallergens has been so striking that this condition is commonly referred to as *canine allergic inhalant dermatitis* [20]. Butler and coworkers [54] demonstrated these skin lesions in every dog in a population of dogs with airway hyperreactivity that had been sensitized to *Ascaris* antigen by the aerosol route.

In contrast to dogs, rhesus monkeys demonstrating airway reactivity to *Ascaris* antigen are rare, constituting only about 5 percent of the population [312]. Although intuitively one finds it easier to relate studies from monkeys rather than nonprimate species to humans, there seems little in our literature to suggest any great advantage to the monkey over more readily available laboratory animals. Sheep can be massively and chronically instrumented and do not require anesthesia for aerosol challenge studies. However, the immunology of *Ascaris*-induced airway responses in sheep has not been defined.

Immunology

An IgE-mediated reaction that causes the release of bronchoactive substances is thought to play a major role in the pathogenesis of atopic human asthma [219], whereas the importance of IgG-mediated reactions in asthma is not yet clear. In the guinea pig, some sensitizing procedures used to produce anaphylactic bronchoconstriction produce IgG-type rather than IgE-type antibodies [23], whereas in the rat, antigen-induced bronchoconstriction is mediated primarily by IgE-type antibodies [324, 389].

Ascaris-induced airway constriction in the dog also is mediated by an IgE-like antibody [228, 318, 323]. The anti-*Ascaris* antibodies are heat labile and nonprecipitating. Passive transfer of serum from highly allergic dogs to hyporeactive dogs causes skin reactions [39] and respiratory reactions [228] in the recipient animal. Schwartzman and coworkers observed a high incidence of spontaneous atopic hypersensitivity in the progeny of these atopic dogs [360]. Further studies by Patterson and colleagues [315] showed that the canine respiratory tract responds with local antibody synthesis to inhaled *Ascaris* antigen aerosol. Both IgA and presumably IgE *Ascaris*-specific antibodies have been measured in the respiratory secretions of the dog [315].

Although there are populations of atopic dogs, dermatitis rather than respiratory symptoms constitutes the major allergic manifestation in the mongrel dog [312]. Moreover, to obtain a colony of such dogs, it has been necessary to screen large numbers of animals, and attempts to induce reaginic hypersensitivity in adult mongrel dogs have met with varying degrees of success. For example, Schwartzman and coworkers [360] were able to sensitize only half of their atopic dogs and none of the nonatopic dogs to dinitrophenylated (DNP) pollen antigens. Kepron and coworkers [227] were more successful at sensitizing newborn mongrel puppies to a conjugate of 2,4-dinitrobenzine ovalbumin and an adjuvant. They demonstrated the presence of specific serum IgE antibodies, a relationship between the bronchial response to inhalation challenge and the level of serum IgE antibodies for as long as 7 months, and suppression of the response by the administration of tolerogenic conjugates of DNP and a carrier [403]. More recently, this same group [32, 266] established a colony of mongrel dogs that had been neonatally sensitized to ragweed antigen.

Studies in rhesus monkeys have demonstrated immunologic responses similar to those in the dog. Some monkeys have positive results of skin tests with *Ascaris* antigen and presumably have become sensitized by prior infestation with nematodes [219, 315]. Some of these monkeys undergo airway constriction when challenged with aerosols of *Ascaris* antigen. The antibody mediating the reactions is like IgE. Skin reactivity and airway reactivity to *Ascaris* aerosols can be passively transferred to nonreactive monkeys by the administration of serum [219] or bronchial lumen cells [316] from highly reactive monkeys. Moreover, rhesus monkeys can be passively sensitized with human IgE antibodies and exhibit cutaneous and even airway responses when appropriately challenged. However, these animals require sensitization for every challenge, which greatly limits the usefulness of this procedure [219]. Sensitized ponies, when housed in barns and exposed to hay containing mold spores, develop bronchoconstriction and airway hyperresponsiveness [26, 103], but the antigen involved has not yet been identified.

Pulmonary Mechanics

Changes in Airway Caliber

In the guinea pig, the simplest measure for estimating the intensity of antigen-induced bronchoconstriction is the time needed to produce asphyxial convulsions, that is, the "preconvulsion time" [172]. The overflow ventilation technique of Konzett and Rossler is another older method that has been extensively employed for pharmacologic studies in guinea pigs. In this procedure, as described in the English literature [90, 191, 235], an anesthetized, tracheotomized animal is ventilated at a constant-volume. A side arm from the tracheal cannula permits some of the ventilator output to escape from a water valve offering a fixed resistance, and the escaping air operates a piston recorder. When compliance of the lungs is reduced, more air escapes (overflows) through the side arm. Changes in tidal volume have also been

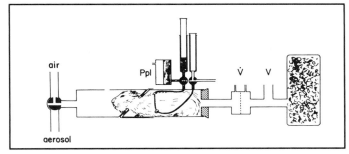

Fig. 31-1. *The body plethysmograph for the measurement of tidal volume, flow, and intrapleural pressure in an unanesthetized, spontaneously breathing guinea pig. Ppl = intrapleural pressure; V = tidal volume; V̇ = flow. (Reprinted with permission from J. S. Douglas, et al. Airway dilation and constriction in spontaneously breathing guinea pigs.* J. Pharmacol. Exp. Ther. *180:98, 1972.)*

employed as a measure of the pulmonary response to antigen challenge in the guinea pig [329], and the decrease in tidal volume (rapid, shallow breathing) roughly correlates with the decrease in dynamic compliance. This method is noninvasive and allows repeated studies in unanesthetized animals.

Pulmonary resistance (R_L) and dynamic compliance (C_{dyn}) can be measured in all species, either awake or anesthetized, using recordings of pleural pressure, tidal volume, and airflow. In dogs, monkeys, and sheep an esophageal balloon is used to record pleural pressure. In small animals (Fig. 31-1), a catheter can be introduced into the pleural space [19, 110], through a small incision in the chest wall; however, a variety of noninvasive, plethysmographic techniques have been developed for use in small animals to measure pulmonary resistance and compliance without the need for a direct measure of intrapleural pressure [11, 218, 322]. Apparatus for application of these techniques is commercially available and has been extensively employed to measure pulmonary mechanics in uninstrumented animals breathing through the nose.

In addition, Holroyde and coworkers [193] described a technique in which anesthetized guinea pigs are forced to undergo an inspiratory-expiratory maneuver in response to externally applied pressure, which allowed measurement of peak expiratory flow rates, forced vital capacity, forced expiratory volume in the first 0.1 second ($FEV_{0.1}$), and maximal midexpiratory flow rates. All values were decreased after exposure to antigen, but the reduction was especially notable in forced vital capacity and $FEV_{0.1}$. Guinea pigs and sheep are generally studied in the conscious state, while dogs and monkeys are usually studied anesthetized. However, changes in airway caliber after antigen challenge are similar in conscious [96, 255] and anesthetized dogs [152, 227, 229, 241, 318, 323, 346, 412, 434, 442] and monkeys [303, 425].

Antigen challenge provokes a diffuse constriction involving large, medium, and small airways and a corresponding increase in pulmonary resistance and decrease in dynamic compliance. In the dog, Kessler and coworkers [229], using tantalum bronchograms, found that the constriction in the dog was most marked in airways 1 to 8 mm in diameter. Antigen-induced bronchoconstriction is associated with decreases in oxygen tension [152, 303, 346, 412, 415] and the initial (immediate response) increase in resistance can be prevented or reversed by beta-adrenergic agonists [152, 173, 390, 442].

The time course for antigen-induced bronchoconstriction depends on the species and the methods employed for immunization and subsequent challenge, and can involve both an immediate and a delayed response. In the guinea pig, maximal changes in dynamic compliance occur 2 minutes after challenge and dynamic compliance returns to normal after 30 to 60 minutes [87, 194, 329]. In dogs, monkeys, and sheep [152, 187, 303, 415], airflow resistance increases within 5 minutes of challenge, peaks in 10 to 15 minutes, and gradually returns to baseline levels within 45 minutes to a few hours. Decreases in dynamic compliance follow a similar time course. As discussed in a subsequent section, bronchoconstriction may recur as one or even two delayed responses a number of hours after resolution of the immediate response.

Among the mechanisms involved in the pulmonary response to inhaled allergen in both humans and experimental animals, much interest has focused on the relative roles of direct and reflex bronchoconstriction. Direct bronchoconstriction results from the effects of mediators that are released from sensitized cells and that act directly on the airways [116]. In reflex bronchoconstriction these mediators stimulate subepithelial irritant receptors [150], with resulting bronchoconstriction. The antigen-antibody complex itself, as well as distortion of smooth muscle during contraction, is thought to stimulate irritant receptors to produce reflex bronchoconstriction [150]. In addition to the irritant receptors and centrally mediated reflex bronchoconstriction, another population of sensory receptors in the airway (C fibers) appears to be able to influence smooth muscle tone by a purely peripheral mechanism, involving the release of substance P from the sensory nerve ending itself [30, 265, 270]. This tachykinin-type peptide can act directly on smooth muscle or by facilitating cholinergic neurotransmission (see Chap. 18).

In the dog, the guinea pig, and the monkey, the role of vagal reflexes in antigen-induced bronchoconstriction has been controversial, as have been the implications for human asthma. Studies employing vagal blockade (by atropine or physical methods) have demonstrated variable effects on the pulmonary response to inhaled allergen. In the guinea pig, Drazen and Austen [118] found that atropine prevented the decrease in conductance and, to a much lesser extent, the decrease in dynamic compliance produced by ovalbumin challenge; similarly, Advenier and coworkers [10], using smaller doses of atropine, found that atropine reduced the increase in pulmonary resistance by 30 percent, with no protective effect on compliance changes. Gold and coworkers [151] and Kessler and coworkers [229] found that in dogs, vagal section, efferent block with atropine, and afferent block by vagal cooling all markedly reduced or actually prevented increases in pulmonary resistance elicited by *Ascaris* antigen aerosols. Yamatake and coworkers [435] also found that atropine reduced the response to *Ascaris* antigen in mongrel dogs, and Zimmermann and Ulmer [437, 439] had similar results with vagal cooling in boxer dogs. In contrast, we [181] and Krell and coworkers [241] using dogs and Patterson and Harris [307] and Miller and coworkers [281] using rhesus monkeys found that large intravenous doses of atropine did not usually result in a marked reduction in the response to *Ascaris* antigen. In ponies, a large component of the spontaneous bronchoconstriction appears to be mediated by cholinergic pathways since atropine largely reduces the airway obstruction [44]. The conflicting results of vagal block on antigen-induced pulmonary resistance may reflect differences in the purity of antigen preparations, in the reactivity of individual animals, or in the experimental conditions in different studies. For example, in dogs extensive parasympathetic control of the airway has been demonstrated, but considerable differences exist between individual animals [431].

Deep anesthesia can suppress airway reflexes [214] and may mask the importance of reflex bronchoconstriction. In contrast, light anesthesia with ultra-short-acting intravenous barbiturates produces little depression of airway reflexes in humans [388] or dogs [33]. Although the effects of vagal blockade on antigen-induced changes in pulmonary resistance have been controversial, none of the investigators have been able to prevent the antigen-induced fall in dynamic compliance by vagal blockade [118, 151, 181, 241, 434, 435, 439]. This implies that a substantial

component of pulmonary response to antigen challenge is not mediated by vagal reflexes.

The possible role of substance P or other tachykinins released from afferent nerve endings within the lung is just beginning to be appreciated. Capsaicin, the active ingredient in hot peppers, has provided a powerful tool with which to study such effects, since capsaicin releases and depletes substance P from sensory nerve endings [48]. Capsaicin pretreatment in guinea pigs (to deplete substance P) both attenuates antigen-induced bronchoconstriction [265] and prevents the atropine-insensitive bronchoconstriction elicited by antidromic stimulation of vagal afferents [270], emphasizing the potential importance of C fibers and tachykinin release in experimentally induced bronchoconstriction (see Chap. 18).

Changes in Lung Volume

In humans, acute attacks of asthma are usually accompanied by increases [385] in the volume of gas trapped in the lung. This has not been reproduced by allergic bronchoconstriction in the mongrel dog [152, 229, 255] or in the monkey [303]. In contrast, sensitized guinea pigs challenged with antigen aerosols show increases in functional residual capacity, decreases in total lung capacity, and increases in residual volume [120, 304] in the immediate postchallenge period. However, chronic exposure does not lead to long-term changes in lung volumes [304]. The sheep is another species that usually shows an increase in functional residual capacity after antigen aerosol challenge [415].

The variable effects on lung volumes have been attributed to species differences in the extent of collateral ventilation [274]. It is also possible that the absence of an increase in the volume of gas trapped in the lung in experimental asthma in the mongrel dog, for example, reflects the mild degree of bronchoconstriction provoked by the challenge [152, 229, 346], since the more intense bronchoconstriction elicited in basenji-greyhound dogs by *Ascaris* antigen aerosols is associated with increases in residual volume [185]. Other explanations include interspecies differences in chest wall mechanics, effects of general anesthetics and muscle relaxants, and the methods used to measure lung volume. The latter may be of particular importance in view of the work by Stănescu and coworkers [386] demonstrating that changes in lung volume in the presence of acute airway obstruction are grossly overestimated when measured by body plethysmographic compared with gas dilution techniques.

Ventilation-Perfusion Abnormalities

Hypoxemia with normocapnia is frequently seen in acute severe asthma in humans [347]. Antigen-induced airway constriction in the sheep [415], the monkey [236, 307], and the dog [152, 346] also is accompanied by decreases in arterial oxygen tension with normocapnia. Arterial hypoxemia is probably due to regional ventilation-perfusion abnormalities, since arterial carbon dioxide tension is normal and arterial oxygen tension increases appropriately when animals are ventilated with oxygen.

In studies of pulmonary circulation and gas exchange in the mongrel dog, the changes in pulmonary mechanics induced by antigen challenge have been very mild [82, 229, 346, 347], and their relationship to ventilation-perfusion abnormalities in status asthmaticus in humans is tenuous. Nevertheless, evidence is accumulating that chemical mediators of asthma may have direct effects on the pulmonary vasculature as well as on the airways [82, 347, 379]. This may result in a compensatory constriction of the pulmonary vasculature in areas of alveolar hypoxia. On the other hand, mediators could prevent hypoxic pulmonary vasoconstriction and worsen ventilation-perfusion abnormalities. Evidence for the protective effect of mediators in limiting ventilation-perfusion abnormalities was recently supplied by Boynton

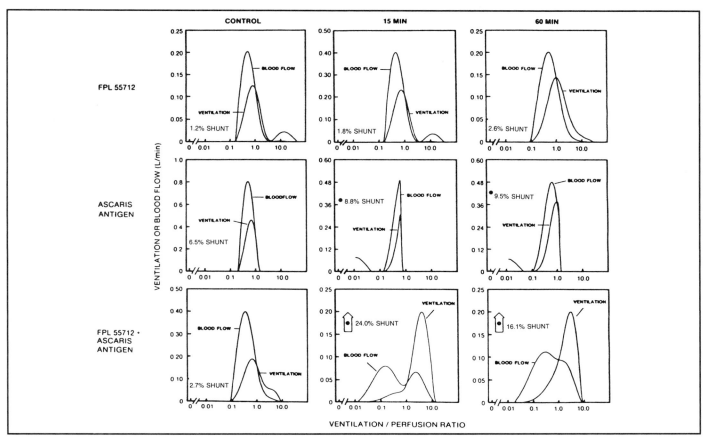

Fig. 31-2. *Representative distribution of the ratio of ventilation to perfusion recovered from a single basenji-greyhound dog before (10 minutes) and after (15 minutes and 60 minutes) aerosol administration of FPL 55712, Ascaris suum antigen, and FPL 55712 plus A. suum antigen. (Reprinted with permission from B. R. Boynton, et al. The deleterious effect of FPL 55712 on gas exchange in the basenji-greyhound dog model of asthma.* J. Crit. Care *2:27, 1987.)*

and coworkers [42], who studied the interaction of FPL 55712 and antigen on ventilation-perfusion relationships in *Ascaris*-sensitive basenji-greyhound dogs. Pretreatment with a leukotriene receptor antagonist, FPL 55712, prior to antigen challenge resulted in marked impairment of gas exchange (Fig. 31-2). These findings are consistent with the idea that mediators released by antigen challenge constrict blood vessels as well as airways, resulting in the preservation of ventilation-perfusion ratios.

Mediators

Using passively sensitized guinea pig tracheal chains, Adams and Lichtenstein [9] elegantly demonstrated that both histamine and leukotrienes were involved in the airway response to antigen (Fig. 31-3): The early phase of contraction was antagonized by diphenhydramine, an H_1 antagonist; the later phase, by FPL 55712, a leukotriene receptor antagonist [133]. Inhibition of antigen-induced contraction by this combination was marked but not complete, so that mediators other than histamine and leukotrienes probably also contributed to the response. In addition, diphenhydramine and FPL 55712 are only moderately selective as antagonists of histamine and leukotrienes, respectively, and other actions may have contributed to the inhibition of antigen-induced contraction [50].

The kinetics of histamine appearance in blood after antigen aerosol challenge is similar in dogs [71, 153, 188, 440] and humans [35]. Histamine increases immediately after the start of antigen challenge, peaks early, and then rapidly decreases to control levels (Fig. 31-4). The persistence of bronchoconstriction in the face of decreasing plasma levels of histamine [71, 188] and the poor correlation between plasma histamine concentration and degree of bronchoconstriction [188, 440] indicate the importance of other mediators in the canine pulmonary response to inhaled allergens. The inability of antihistamines to inhibit antigen-induced airway constriction in dogs [237] and monkeys [314] further supports this view. Sheep [8] and guinea pigs [41, 87, 173], however, differ in this regard, since pretreatment with histamine (H_1) antagonists protects against antigen-induced airway constriction. In guinea pigs, H_1 antagonists protect against antigen challenge in animals immunized to produce either IgG alone or both IgG and IgE [24].

A mixture of leukotrienes (LTC_4, LTD_4, and LTE_4) is released from the lungs after antigen challenge in vitro in many species, and leukotriene receptor antagonists reduce the intensity of antigen-induced bronchoconstriction in rats [138] and guinea pigs [24], but not in sheep [8], dogs [188], or monkeys [311]. These differences, however, may reflect the short half-life of FPL 55712, the antagonist most commonly used, and the consequent difficulty in obtaining adequate concentrations in vivo rather than true species differences in the importance of leukotrienes in anaphylactic bronchoconstriction.

Prostaglandins and other cyclooxygenase products also are released from the lungs after antigen challenge in vitro, but pretreatment with indomethacin or other inhibitors of the cyclooxygenase pathway often has not afforded protection against antigen-induced bronchoconstriction in vivo. Although Collier and

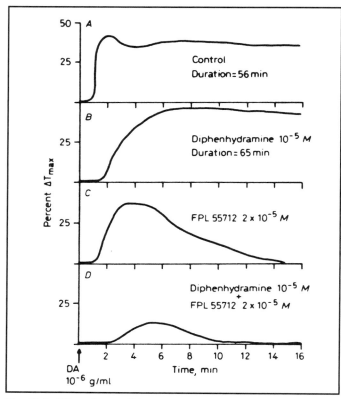

Fig. 31-3. *Effect of an antihistamine and a slow reactive substance of anaphylaxis (SRS-A) antagonist, alone and in combination, on response of guinea pig tracheal chains to antigen. Four chains were prepared from a single sensitized trachea. Dog albumin (DA) was administered at t = 0 minutes. ΔT_{max} represents tension change resulting from treatment with 10^{-3} M methacholine. Record A is the control tracing. The tissue depicted in record B was treated with 10^{-5} M diphenhydramine; in record C, 2×10^{-5} M FPL 55712; in record D, both diphenhydramine and FPL 55712. The antagonists were added to the baths 5 minutes before antigen administration. Selective antagonism of the early and protracted phases of the contraction resulted from treatment with diphenhydramine and FPL 55712, respectively. The combination of antihistamine and SRS-A antagonist reduced the amplitude of both phases and decreased the duration of the response. (Reprinted with permission from G. K. Adams and L. Lichtenstein. In vitro studies of antigen-induced bronchospasm: Effect of antihistamine and SRS-A antagonist on response of sensitized guinea pig and human airways to antigen. J. Immunol. 122:555, 1979.)*

James [87] found that meclofenamate sodium suppressed part of the bronchoconstrictor response to antigen challenge in guinea pigs, other studies employing indomethacin showed no protection against antigen challenge in the guinea pig [278] or an actual enhancement of the bronchoconstrictor response [24]. Indomethacin also has been ineffective in attenuating antigen-induced bronchoconstriction in the rat [138, 390], sheep [8], monkey [309], and pony [157]. However, in the lung periphery of the mongrel dog, both cyclooxygenase inhibition [230] and thromboxane synthetase inhibition [231] significantly decreased airway responses to *Ascaris* antigen inhalation.

Serotonin [138, 390], bradykinin [87], and platelet-activating factor (PAF) [407] all have been shown to participate in anaphylactic bronchoconstriction, at least in some species. Thus, multiple mediators are released from the lungs after immunologic challenge, and these probably interact to regulate further release of mediators. The development of more specific antagonists will, we hope, increase our knowledge in this area.

Mucociliary Dysfunction

Studies in both animal models [410, 414, 426] and asthmatic patients [277] have demonstrated an impairment of mucociliary transport. This impairment is not related to changes in airway mechanics as the hypoxemia associated with antigen aerosol challenge and may persist for days [411]. Cromolyn sodium and terbutaline sulfate [426] prevent this impairment in sheep, which suggests the involvement of mediators in this response, and studies in allergic dogs [414] implicate leukotrienes in this response since FPL 55712 prevents the fall in mucus velocity provoked by antigen challenge.

Late-Phase Reactions

It has been recognized for over a hundred years that inhaled antigen could produce a delayed as well as an immediate worsening of clinical asthma [294]. The late response, as described in 1974 by Robertson and coauthors [341], in asthmatic patients inhaling ragweed pollen allergen began after 4 to 6 hours, peaked at 8 to 12 hours, and either resolved within 24 hours or persisted for several days. A late asthmatic response is observed in about half of asthmatic patients receiving antigen aerosols and is believed to represent a response to an inflammatory infiltrate (see Chap. 12).

Despite the early recognition of the importance and frequency of the late-phase response in humans, similar delayed responses in animals were not reported until relatively recently—first in rabbits [365] in 1982 and then in sheep [4] in 1983. However, in the succeeding years, late-phase responses were demonstrated in most of the species that have been used as animal models of asthma—although special procedures may be needed to "unmask" the late phase or permit its expression.

In previously sensitized guinea pigs, late-phase responses have been produced by three basically different experimental protocols: (1) intratracheal instillation of ovalbumin coupled to Sepharose (approximately 100 μM) beads in anesthetized animals [270, 422]; (2) inhalation of *Ascaris* aerosols administered by face mask in unanesthetized and unpremedicated animals [205]; and (3) inhalation of ovalbumin aerosols, also administered by face mask in unanesthetized animals, but after premedication with an antihistamine [77, 202]. The reason for use of the antihistamine is that it mutes the immediate response to antigen challenge, which is frequently lethal in the guinea pig, and thereby permits administration of a sufficiently large dose of antigen to produce consistent late-phase responses [77, 202]. Virtually all of the animals challenged by the third protocol [77, 202] show late-phase responses, whereas only about 40 percent of the animals studied under the second protocol [205], which employs a different and possibly less-intense antigen challenge, go on to show a late response. The advantage of studying airway responses in unanesthetized guinea pigs (in the second and third protocols) is in part offset by the very prominent contribution of the upper airway to antigen-induced increases in respiratory resistance [220]. Indeed, when awake antihistamine-premedicated guinea pigs inhaled ovalbumin antigen aerosols through the nose and were then subsequently anesthetized and intubated for the recording of pulmonary mechanics, only 10 percent of the animals showed a late response, in contrast to a late-phase response in 78 percent of animals when the airway response to the same challenge was evaluated in unanesthetized animals breathing through the nose [131].

The late-phase responses elicited by antigen challenge in these various guinea pig models are quantitatively different and intriguingly out of phase, suggesting that there may be significant differences in their pathogenesis. In the animals pretreated with antihistamine and challenged with ovalbumin aerosols, there were two late responses, one peaking at 17 hours and the other at 72

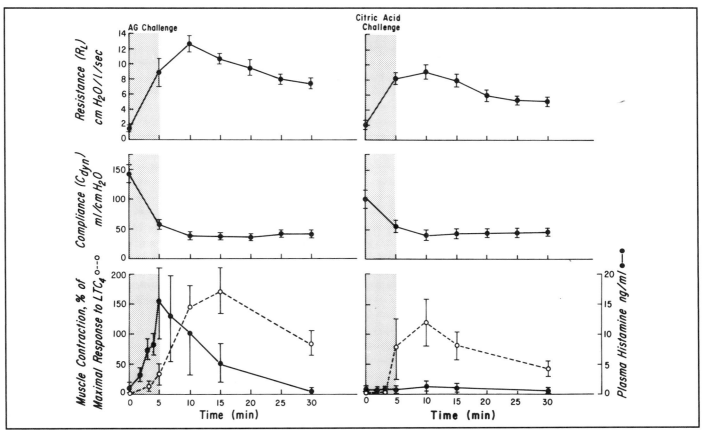

Fig. 31-4. *Pulmonary resistance, dynamic compliance, plasma histamine concentrations (●), and plasma SRS-A activity (○) before and after the* Ascaris *antigen (AG) (left) and citric acid (right) 5-minute challenge in basenji-greyhound dogs. Each point represents mean ± standard error for five dogs. Abscissa is the elapsed time from start of the aerosol challenge. SRS-A activity is expressed as percent of contraction produced by leukotriene C_4 (LTC$_4$) (3 × 10⁻⁸ M).*

hours after challenge [203]. However, in the guinea pigs that were challenged with *Ascaris* antigen aerosols without antihistamine pretreatment [205], the single late-phase response (that was observed) peaked in the obstruction-free interval (6–9 hours after challenge) of the preceding model. The explanation of these phase differences remains to be determined and could reflect the different antigens employed, the relative contributions of upper versus lower airway obstruction, and the presence or absence of medications (antihistamines); clearly, however, the delayed response in the guinea pig has a variable expression, and the predominant sites of airway obstruction (upper or lower airway) are uncertain. Clear identification of the site of obstruction is particularly important, since attempts at correlating the late-phase response with an inflammatory infiltrate have been based on cellular changes in the lower airway, as assessed by bronchoalveolar lavage (BAL) or histologic section.

All of the guinea pig models in which a late-phase airway obstruction is elicited by antigen challenge show an inflammatory infiltrate in the lower airway at the time of the delayed response. This infiltrate contains both polymorphonuclear leukocytes (PMNs) and eosinophils [77, 202, 203, 205, 270, 422]. The PMN infiltrate, however, does not appear to be essential to the late-phase obstruction. Thus, in the *Ascaris*-challenged animals (no antihistamine), there was no significant difference in neutrophil infiltration of the airway walls between animals that showed a late response (40%) and those that did not; that is, infiltration also occurred in animals not showing a late response [205]. Similarly, in the ovalbumin-challenged animals (pretreated with anti-

histamine), inhalation of albuterol before the antigen challenge inhibited the PMN influx but had no significant effect on either of the late-phase airway obstructions [203], and cromolyn administered after the initial bronchoconstrictor response partially inhibited both late-phase obstructions but not the PMN influx [203].

The possible role of eosinophils in the late-phase obstructions is difficult to assess, in part because the guinea pig is a relatively "eosinophilic animal" [203] with a high background level of eosinophils in BAL fluid. Since there was no consistent relationship between the inhibition by cromolyn of (1) the first late-phase response and (2) the inhibition of eosinophil accumulation in BAL fluid, it seems likely that "eosinophil accumulation per se is not responsible for the reduction of airways function at 17 hours" [203]. In contrast, cromolyn did inhibit both airway obstruction and eosinophil accumulation at the late, late phase (72 hours), without reducing PMN accumulation [203]. However, in evaluating these temporal associations and dissociations between drug effects on airway function and BAL fluid, it should be remembered that there might be a substantial time lag between infiltration into the airway wall and accumulation of a cell type in the BAL fluid, and that the obstruction is not necessarily in the lower airway.

In sensitized, inbred rats—intubated and anesthetized—inhalation of ovalbumin aerosols produced an immediate lower airway obstruction in most animals (67%) followed by a gradual recovery during the next hour [131]. However, the postchallenge pulmonary resistance was higher than in control animals throughout the observation period of up to 12 hours, and in some animals, it fluctuated up and down through a series of minor peaks. The investigators defined a late response as an increase in "R_L exceeding the mean plus 2 standard deviations of all the R_L measurements taken from 1 hour after challenge to the end of the experiment." By this criterion, most animals (67%) showed a delayed response, with onset varying between 120 to 600 minutes after challenge. There was no correlation between the intensities of the immediate and late responses, and 20 percent of the animals showed a late response without a detectable immediate response. Cellular infiltrates after antigen challenge were not evaluated in this study, but have been described for antigen challenge in the rat by other investigators [37], who observed parenchymal and airway inflammation with a time course similar to the onset of the late-phase obstruction and persisting for up to 24 hours.

In the rabbit [365], the tendency to maintain some increase in pulmonary resistance throughout most of the postchallenge study period appears to be even more pronounced than in the rat. Thus, in previously sensitized rabbits, aerosol challenge with *Alternaria tenius* (a saprophytic mold) extracts leads to an immediate obstructive response followed by a delayed obstructive response, with onset as early as 105 minutes after challenge. The latter develops progressively for the remainder of the experimental period [365]. The peak intensity of this late-phase response is substantially greater than that of the immediate response, and averaged data do not show a pronounced recovery phase intervening between the immediate-phase response and the steadily progressing late-phase response. The late-phase obstruction is associated with an increase in granulocytes in the airways, both PMNs and eosinophils, which declines by 48 hours and resolves by 7 days after challenge [246]. This granulocyte infiltrate shows a progressive increase in the number of eosinophils throughout the first 48 hours, ranging from 20 to 40 percent at 6 hours to more than 80 percent at 48 hours [246]. In antigen-sensitized rabbits made neutropenic by the administration of nitrogen mustard, subsequent antigen challenge elicits an immediate but not a late-phase obstructive airway response [246, 289]; replacement with a neutrophil-rich infusion prior to antigen challenge restored the late-phase response, suggesting that granulocytes and especially neutrophils are important in its pathogenesis.

In dogs, antigen aerosols frequently have been used to elicit a rapid-onset bronchoconstriction, but without any evidence of a more delayed response. Even in dogs with a marked immediate airway response, pulmonary resistance at 6 hours after antigen challenge was not significantly different than in the control period [74]. However, recent studies showed that a late-phase response can be elicited in the canine airway under special conditions, such as pretreatment with metyrapone [356], a cortisol synthesis inhibitor, or topical administration of a large challenge dose of antigen to a limited portion of the airway using a wedged bronchoscope technique [404]. The rationale for the use of metyrapone [356] is that endogenous steroid production might play a major role in determining the extent of the late-phase response, since pretreatment with exogenous steroid curtails late-phase responses in both humans and animal models. After pretreatment with the cortisol synthesis inhibitor, most dogs did show a late-phase response, comparable in intensity to the immediate response, and with an onset within 4 to 6 hours after challenge. At the time of the late-phase response, BAL fluid showed a significant increase in neutrophils but not of other cell types, and there was a significant correlation between intensity of the late-phase airway response and the neutrophil accumulation. Histologic studies also showed a prominent neutrophil accumulation in the bronchiolar walls. In contrast to many other studies of inflammatory infiltrates following antigen challenge, eosinophils were not increased either in BAL fluid or histologic sections at the time of the delayed increase in pulmonary resistance. The late-phase response, as seen with the wedged bronchoscope technique, was

also accompanied by a large influx of PMNs into the airway wall [404], but the relative contribution of neutrophils and eosinophils was not determined.

In awake sheep, without medication other than topical anesthesia for placement of an endotracheal tube and an esophageal balloon catheter, the inhalation of antigen aerosols elicits a well-defined dual response [2, 3, 7, 129] in some but not all animals. The initial bronchoconstriction begins shortly after challenge and lasts about 4 hours [2, 4], which is a relatively long duration in comparison to the initial response in humans and most other animals. The late response begins at about 6.5 hours, peaks at 6.5 to 7.5 hours, starts to remit by 8 hours, and resolves by 24 hours after challenge. The late phase represents an increase in pulmonary resistance without significant changes in thoracic gas volume and is substantially less intense than the immediate response to antigen inhalation [4]. BAL fluid obtained during the late-phase airway response [5] showed a significant increase in neutrophils and eosinophils, compared to unchallenged controls; moreover, when compared to BAL fluid obtained at the same time (after challenge) from sheep that had shown only an immediate response, the increase in eosinophils was three to five times greater in the dual responders, whereas the increase in neutrophils was not significantly different, suggesting that eosinophils might be particularly important in the pathogenesis of the late-phase response in this species.

The late-phase responses to allergen challenge in these animal models of asthma have a number of common characteristics, although all have not been thoroughly evaluated in all models. They are IgE dependent [205, 246, 365]; they are associated with granulocytic influx into the BAL fluid and bronchiolar wall [202, 203, 246, 356, 404]; and they are inhibited by glucocorticoids [2, 4, 404] and cromolyn sodium [4, 203]. On the other hand, there are marked differences between models (even within the same species) with respect to time course, possible sites of airway obstruction, the occurrence of an obstruction-free interval between the immediate and late responses, and the presence of a significant influx of eosinophils. These differences suggest that while the late-phase response is an "inflammatory response," its cellular mechanisms are not necessarily the same in all models.

PHARMACOLOGIC CHALLENGE

A variety of endogenously produced substances can be administered as drugs to elicit experimental bronchoconstriction in vivo or to contract isolated preparations of trachea, bronchus, or lung. The potency, efficacy, and even the mechanism of action of these substances can vary enormously among species, among the different sites in the airway of the same species, and among different routes of administration. Such differences clearly affect the relevance of agonist-induced bronchoconstriction in a particular animal model to the pathophysiology or treatment of clinical asthma. The major agonists used to elicit experimental bronchoconstriction have been histamine, cholinergic drugs (acetylcholine, carbachol, or methacholine), serotonin, prostaglandin (PG) $F_{2\alpha}$, LTC_4 and LTD_4, and PAF.

Histamine

Histamine acting at H_1 receptors can trigger bronchoconstriction by stimulation of vagal pathways [408], as well as by a direct action on bronchial smooth muscle. These actions may be partially antagonized by histamine-stimulated release of catecholamines from the adrenal medulla [387] or intrapulmonary nerve endings [13, 263]. In addition, histamine acting at H_2 receptors has been shown to increase cyclic adenosine monophosphate (AMP) levels and impair mediator release [256], and to relax airway smooth muscle, at least in some species. These latter effects have suggested that histamine may modulate as well as initiate pathophysiologic events in the lungs during allergic bronchoconstriction [64, 124].

In healthy human subjects, administration of an adequate dose of histamine, by either aerosol inhalation or parenteral injection, elicits a marked pulmonary response [161, 171, 209, 222], which has been variously measured as decreases in vital capacity, expiratory flow rates, specific airway conductance, or dynamic or static pulmonary compliance, or as increases in pulmonary resistance. The dose of histamine needed to produce a pulmonary response of a given intensity is usually less in asthmatic patients than in normal volunteers [93, 94, 171, 209, 383, 402]; however, there is a wide range of airway sensitivity to histamine in nonasthmatic subjects [161]. In animal studies a wide range of histamine sensitivity is also apparent in normal populations without overt pulmonary disease. Sensitivity to histamine aerosol challenge in large populations of mongrel dogs (n = 102) (Fig. 31-5) [373] and female albino guinea pigs (n = 131) [111] was found to be log normally distributed, with a 40-fold range in dogs and a nearly 100-fold range in guinea pigs in the concentrations that elicited comparable pulmonary responses in the most and the least sensitive individuals. A wide variation in histamine sensitivity was also demonstrated in smaller populations of sheep [178, 200] and rhesus monkeys [279]. Ponies with a history of heaves show increased sensitivity to histamine [103, 104] following environmental exposure to hay, but do not show increased histamine sensitivity during clinical remission.

Studies in isolated preparations of airway smooth muscle obtained from humans, guinea pigs, and dogs (Fig. 31-6) show that in these species, histamine produces a contractile response in all parts of the airway, but that relative to the maximal response elicited by cholinergic agonists, histamine produces its greatest effect in the lung parenchymal strip, a preparation thought to reflect drug effects on small airways [122, 154, 232]. A prominent effect on peripheral airways is also indicated by the marked decreases in compliance elicited by histamine challenge in most species [84, 85, 110, 200, 240, 259, 279], including humans [161, 243].

Part of the pulmonary response to histamine is vagally mediated. Pretreatment with anticholinergic drugs has diminished the pulmonary response to histamine challenge in some clinical studies [80, 321], although in others anticholinergic drugs afforded little or no protection [60, 210, 429]. Conflicting results also have been obtained in dog studies. Vagal block, vagotomy,

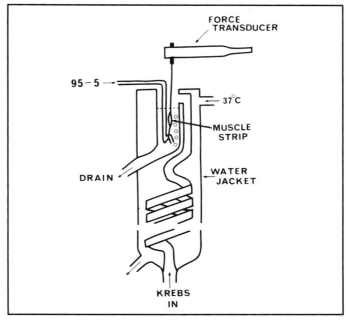

Fig. 31-6. *Apparatus for isometric experiments that allows recording of tension development under various stimuli. The muscle strip is suspended in Krebs physiologic saline solution, aerated with 95 percent oxygen and 5 percent carbon dioxide. (Reprinted with permission from L. A. Antonissen et al., Mechanical alterations of airway smooth muscle in a canine asthmatic model. J. Appl. Physiol. 46:681, 1979.)*

or anticholinergic drugs have virtually abolished the pulmonary response to histamine in some studies [96, 151], suggesting that the major effect of histamine in these studies was vagally mediated. Other investigators, however, found that vagal block or vagotomy had no consistent effect on the pulmonary response to histamine in the dog [259, 374] or in the pony [44], or that massive doses of atropine (1 mg/kg intravenously) produced only a slight shift to the right (dose ratio, 3.6) of the dose-response curve for histamine-induced increases in pulmonary resistance [241]. In the dog, which is usually studied while anesthetized, deep barbiturate anesthesia depresses the vagally mediated component of the pulmonary response to histamine [214]. This component involves the increase in pulmonary resistance elicited by histamine aerosol rather than the fall in dynamic compliance. Although depth and type of anesthesia may explain some of the differences among experiments, histamine challenges delivered to fully conscious dogs have shown a dominant vagal component in some studies [96] and little or no vagally mediated effect in others [259]. These discrepancies perhaps are explained best on the basis of individual variation, since in dogs, large differences have been demonstrated in both the extent and the character of histamine-vagal interactions [260, 436].

Nearly all studies in the guinea pig, beginning with the initial observations of histamine-induced bronchoconstriction by Dale and Laidlaw [97], have shown that atropine or vagotomy reduces, but does not abolish the bronchoconstriction elicited by histamine [110, 119, 191, 282]. After intravenous administration of histamine, which both increases resistance and decreases dynamic compliance, atropine attenuates both responses but has the greatest effect on resistance [119]. Changes in resistance and compliance elicited by low doses are totally blocked by atropine, which suggests a primarily reflex action; at high doses histamine elicits marked changes in resistance and compliance despite atropine pretreatment, which indicates a direct action on central and peripheral airways. In spontaneously breathing guinea pigs, intravenous administration of histamine elicits rapid shallow

Fig. 31-5. *Histogram and estimated distributions of histamine responses in 102 dogs studied in terms of log $ED_{65} C_{dyn}$. $ED_{65} C_{dyn}$ is the concentration of histamine producing a decrease in dynamic compliance (C_{dyn}) to 65 percent of the control value. (Reprinted with permission from J. R. Snapper, et al. Distribution of pulmonary responsiveness to aerosol histamine in dogs. J. Appl. Physiol. 44:738, 1978.)*

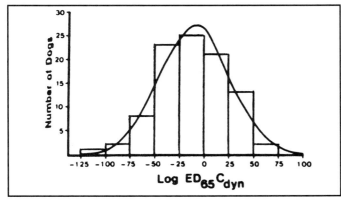

breathing; this effect is abolished or markedly reduced by atropine [282]. Although anesthetics have been variously observed to depress [110] or enhance [10] the response to histamine challenge in guinea pigs, strong responses involving both resistance and compliance can be elicited in both anesthetized and unanesthetized animals.

The rat differs dramatically from most other laboratory animals in that histamine, even in massive doses, does not contract airway smooth muscle either in intact animals [75] or in isolated preparations of trachea, bronchi, or lung parenchyma [51, 262]. In the rat, histamine is released from the lungs and other sites during anaphylaxis [138] and contributes to the systemic response but has little or no stimulatory effect on the airway response to other bronchoactive mediators. The mouse is similar to the rat in its responses to histamine in vivo [269] and in vitro [421].

In the rhesus monkey, sheep, and rabbit, histamine challenge in intact animals produces bronchoconstriction, but the effect on isolated portions of the airway demonstrates a marked heterogeneity of smooth muscle response [69, 135, 140]. Thus, in the sheep [135], histamine contracts the trachea and major bronchi while relaxing lesser bronchi and bronchioles. Such heterogeneous responses, which depend on differences in the distribution of pharmacologic receptors within the airway, are found in many other species [64]. However, histamine has elicited contraction of the lung parenchymal strip in all species reported on so far, with the sole exception of the rat, which is unresponsive. Contractile responses are mediated by H_1 receptors and blocked by H_1 antagonists. The relaxant responses to histamine (or more specific H_2 agonists) are in some instances clearly mediated by H_2 receptors and competitively blocked by H_2 antagonists [233], but in other instances are not, which suggests either a nonspecific relaxant effect of high drug doses or an atypical H_2 receptor [136].

Even in species such as the guinea pig in which histamine produces contractile responses throughout the airway, H_2 receptors are widely distributed and H_2 agonists such as dimaprit can relax tracheal or lung parenchymal tissue contracted by carbachol [123]. Pretreatment with H_2-receptor antagonists has been reported to potentiate histamine-induced bronchoconstriction in humans [291], dogs [375], sheep [12], monkeys [159], and guinea pigs [127], but negative results have also been obtained in several human studies [132].

Isolated preparations of airway tissue obtained from dogs showing marked in vivo airway hyperreactivity to histamine and from control dogs without in vivo hyperreactivity showed similar in vitro sensitivity to histamine [112, 113]. This suggests that an abnormality in the contractile mechanism of the airway smooth muscle to histamine is not the cause of in vivo histamine hyperreactivity.

Cholinergic Agonists

Cholinergic agonists (methacholine, carbachol, and acetylcholine), on the other hand, are believed to have little or no irritant effect but to act directly on cholinergic receptors on smooth muscle. Binding studies show both M_2 and M_3 muscarinic receptor subtypes in airway smooth muscle. However, contraction of airway smooth muscle is probably mediated by the M_3 (sensitive to 4-diphenyl-acetoxy-N-methyl-piperidine and hexahydrosiladifenidol) receptors [343]. Functional studies demonstrate M_2 receptors on the parasympathetic nerves in the lung where they function to inhibit the release of acetylcholine [146].

Isolated preparations of airway smooth muscle obtained from humans [154], guinea pigs [122, 167], pigs [154], dogs [348], rhesus monkeys [69], sheep [135], rats [409], baboons [280], and mice [421] show a contractile response to cholinergic agonists in all parts of the airway. However, in contrast to histamine,

cholinergic agonists in most instances produce their greatest effects on the larger airways (trachea and bronchus), rather than the fine peripheral airways (bronchiole and parenchymal strip); dogs [348] and baboons [280] may be exceptions.

In humans [383, 402, 429], monkeys [236, 279, 281, 319], guinea pigs [329, 330], sheep [413], dogs [187, 374], and ponies [26], aerosol administration of cholinergic agonists elicits airway constriction that is totally inhibited by cholinergic antagonists. Intravenous infusion of methacholine in dogs [333] also produces marked airway constriction. The effect abates within 5 to 15 minutes of terminating the infusion or aerosol.

Despite pharmacologic dissimilarities between histamine and cholinergic agonists and their predilections for different sites of action in the airway, pulmonary reactivity to cholinergic agonists and histamine is closely correlated, both in experimental animals [374] and humans [383], which indicates that airway hyperreactivity is not restricted to responses initiated by a specific receptor.

Most dog models of asthma fail to demonstrate the airway hyperreactivity characteristic of human asthma [116, 239], and animals are often selected for use on the basis of allergic sensitivity to *Ascaris* antigen rather than airway hyperreactivity. By selecting animals at the high end of the distribution of airway hyperreactivity, we can perhaps come closer to reproducing human asthma and to identifying the mechanisms underlying airway hyperreactivity. Indeed, we [187] demonstrated marked nonspecific airway hyperreactivity in a highly inbred population of basenji-greyhound dogs selected on the basis of response to inhalational challenges. Takino and coworkers [397] selectively bred two lines of guinea pigs on the basis of airway sensitivity to chemical mediators, and Holme and Piechuta [192] did the same in rats with respect to the intensity of the pulmonary response to antigen aerosol challenge.

Airway hyperreactivity does not appear to result from increased smooth muscle sensitivity to cholinergic agonists. Downes and coworkers [112] studied in vitro contractile responses in tracheal muscle from basenji-greyhound dogs that were allergic and showed in vivo airway hyperreactivity to methacholine, and from greyhounds and basenjis that served as nonallergic and allergic control populations. Trachealis muscle from basenji-greyhounds and from allergic control dogs was significantly less sensitive, not more sensitive, to methacholine than was trachealis muscle from the nonallergic control dogs (Fig. 31-7). Broadstone and colleagues [43] had similar findings in horses.

Fig. 31-7. *Cumulative dose-response curves for methacholine-induced contraction in thoracic trachealis muscle from five basenji-greyhounds (BG), greyhounds (G), and basenjis (B). Methacholine was less potent in trachealis preparations from the basenji-greyhound and basenji dogs than in those from the greyhound dogs (p < .05).*

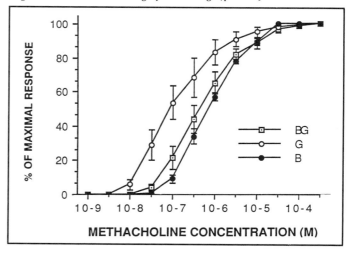

In vitro, airway smooth muscle from horses with in vivo cholinergic airway hyperreactivity showed decreased, not increased, sensitivity to acetylcholine. Weinmann and associates [421] found that tracheal tissue from mice with in vivo cholinergic airway hyperreactivity [252] did not show increased in vitro sensitivity. It is interesting to note that several studies have examined the relationship of in vivo airway hyperreactivity and pharmacologic responsiveness of human asthmatic airway tissue in vitro and failed to find a positive correlation [29, 61, 155, 399, 427]. In fact, Whicker and coworkers [427] and Goldie and associates [155] showed decreased in vitro sensitivity to cholinergic agonists in bronchial preparations obtained from asthmatic subjects. These studies, however, unlike the studies in animal models, are difficult to interpret because of the confounding factors of prior drug therapy and end-stage disease.

Serotonin

Humans show exceptionally little airway reactivity to serotonin (5-hydroxytryptamine [5HT]), and inhalation of serotonin aerosols does not usually produce bronchoconstriction in normal subjects [174, 267, 302], although responses are frequently elicited in patients with asthma [38, 149, 163, 174]. In contrast, serotonin produces bronchoconstriction in most laboratory animals. Its effects, like those of histamine, are produced in part by interaction with vagal pathways and in part by direct effects on airway smooth muscle. In addition, although serotonin contracts isolated preparations of airway smooth muscle from most laboratory animals, relaxant effects have been demonstrated in human bronchus [154, 262, 271], guinea pig airway [31], goat trachea [67], and amphibian lung [115, 271, 358]. Since both the contractile [51, 65, 69, 75, 87, 135] and the relaxant responses [31, 67, 115, 271] are antagonized by $5HT_2$-receptor antagonists, they appear to be mediated by the same type of serotonin receptor.

In autonomic ganglia, serotonin has a presynaptic effect on the release of acetylcholine [128, 179] and can either facilitate or depress ganglionic transmission. In lungs, serotonin potentiates the bronchomotor effect of electrical stimulation of vagal efferent nerves [106, 162, 367], and could be important as a modulator of synaptic transmission in bronchomotor pathways, even in species in which its other airway effects are inconsequential. Further, it has been proposed [367] that amplification of efferent cholinergic traffic by serotonin "could contribute to the nonspecific hyperreactivity characteristic of asthma." Serotonin, however, does not release neuropeptides in the guinea pig airway, as pretreatment with capsaicin (at concentrations that deplete tissues of neuropeptides) does not modify serotonin-induced contraction of guinea pig trachea [31].

Aside from its possible role as a neuromodulator, serotonin elicits pronounced bronchoconstriction in the dog [162, 208, 239, 332, 367], sheep [16], cat [85, 91, 235], guinea pig [87, 191, 235, 352], rat [75, 352], and mouse [253, 269]; in some species, the rat, for example, serotonin is of major importance as a bronchoactive mediator in anaphylaxis. Both in vivo and in vitro [51, 65, 66, 68, 167, 232, 238, 433] airway responses to serotonin are often not as intense as those to histamine or to cholinergic agonists, may show tachyphylaxis, and may be partially or completely inhibited by pretreatment with atropine. Nevertheless, serotonin (if administered in a high enough dose) has a direct effect on airway smooth muscle since isolated preparations are contracted by serotonin in the presence of concentrations of atropine that are adequate to block the effects mediated by stimulation of intramural cholinergic efferent pathways [31, 36, 51, 65, 213, 366].

The relative importance of vagal pathways in the in vivo response to serotonin varies considerably among species but is especially pronounced in the dog. Although canine bronchi respond to low concentrations of serotonin in vitro [271], aerosol challenges that elicit marked bronchoconstriction in vivo act largely or entirely through vagal interactions. Vagal cooling reduces the in vivo response by two thirds [162], and atropine pretreatment abolishes it [208, 241].

Serotonin, like histamine, increases lung irritant receptor discharge, but the level of this discharge does not correlate well with the intensity of neurally mediated bronchoconstriction [106]. On the other hand, serotonin markedly potentiates the increase in pulmonary resistance elicited by electrical stimulation of vagal efferents [107, 162]. This suggests an action at one or more sites in efferent vagal pathways. Since serotonin potentiates the response to vagal stimulation without altering the response to methacholine aerosols [367], the interaction appears to involve efferent nerves rather than muscarinic receptors on smooth muscle. Histamine has been found to have similar potentiating effects in some studies [107] but not in others [162]. Atropine and vagotomy also have been shown to decrease the pulmonary response to serotonin in cats [235], guinea pigs [175, 191], mice [253], and rats [75], but in these species the protection is less complete, and direct effects presumably contribute to low-dose bronchoconstrictor responses.

Prostaglandins

Cyclooxygenase products such as prostaglandins and thromboxanes contribute to the intrinsic tone of airway smooth muscle [299, 300, 426], modulate transmission in intrapulmonary vagal efferents [211, 212], mediate or modulate some of the effects of other bronchoactive autacoids [326, 344], and are released as part of the anaphylactic response [100, 165, 301, 327, 328, 359, 391]. Pulmonary effects of prostaglandins are the subject of several recent reviews [204, 362, 378, 379, 418] (see Chap. 11). This section considers only a few topics that are of particular importance to the interpretation of results in the commonly used animal models of asthma.

Most experimental studies of prostaglandin-induced bronchoconstriction have employed $PGF_{2\alpha}$ because of its relative stability in solution. Challenge with $PGF_{2\alpha}$ by the aerosol [15, 199, 272, 371, 372] or intravenous [47] route elicits bronchoconstriction in normal and asthmatic human subjects. $PGF_{2\alpha}$ contracts isolated preparations of human bronchi [170, 199, 262, 271, 394], which shows a direct action on smooth muscle; however, in asthmatic patients, pretreatment with anticholinergic drugs attenuates the response [15, 272, 298], which demonstrates a vagally mediated component.

As with histamine and serotonin, the pulmonary response to $PGF_{2\alpha}$ varies considerably among the different species employed as animal models of asthma. The rat, for example, appears insensitive to the pulmonary effects of $PGF_{2\alpha}$ as well as to histamine. Intravenous administration of $PGF_{2\alpha}$ produces only minimal bronchoconstriction in the intact rat [75], and isolated preparations of rat trachea and lung are unresponsive to concentrations of $PGF_{2\alpha}$ that produce marked contraction in similar preparations of human tissue [262]. In the guinea pig, $PGF_{2\alpha}$ elicits a more pronounced bronchoconstriction [34, 164, 170, 393] and contracts both tracheal chains [396] and lung parenchymal strips [66, 357]; these effects, however, require relatively high concentrations and are of lesser intensity than responses to histamine or cholinergic agonists. In contrast, in the dog, $PGF_{2\alpha}$ is a potent bronchoconstrictor [239, 331, 374, 380, 381, 416, 418]. In most dog studies, atropine or vagal block has attenuated, but not prevented $PGF_{2\alpha}$-induced bronchoconstriction [239, 374, 381, 417, 418]. Canine lung parenchymal strips are strongly contracted by $PGF_{2\alpha}$ [68] but canine bronchial preparations, unlike human bronchi, are unresponsive [238] or relaxed [432].

Although relatively little is known about its synthesis in vivo [379], PGD_2 contracts bronchial preparations [99], and it is a more potent bronchoconstrictor in vivo than is $PGF_{2\alpha}$ in the dog [310, 380, 419], the guinea pig [164], and the monkey [310]. Rabbit aorta contracting substance (a mixture of thromboxane A_2 and prostaglandin endoperoxides) and the endoperoxides per se, although rapidly inactivated, are potent constrictors of airway smooth muscle from humans [170, 328] and guinea pigs [164, 165, 393], and endoperoxide analogs that are less rapidly inactivated have been shown to be potent bronchoconstrictors in vivo in the dog [382, 418]. As assayed on the guinea pig tracheal chain, thromboxane A_2 was five times more potent than the endoperoxide PGH_2 [393], which in turn was nine times more potent than $PGF_{2\alpha}$ [164]. In the guinea pig, thromboxane A_2 plays a particularly important role in experimentally induced bronchoconstriction, since it is released from lung tissue not only during antigen challenge [100, 301] but also after administration of other bronchoactive autacoids [134, 301, 326, 344, 405]. Thromboxane A_2 appears to be one of the major cyclooxygenase products of arachidonic acid in the guinea pig lung, but not in the human or rat lung [18, 284, 326] and not in the guinea pig trachea [284]. In guinea pig lung, the major effect of exogenously administered bradykinin and slow-reacting substance of anaphylaxis (SRS-A), or its component leukotrienes, appears to be due to stimulation of thromboxane A_2 synthesis [326, 344] and is greatly reduced by pretreatment with cyclooxygenase inhibitors or specific inhibitors of thromboxane synthetase [88, 89, 158, 326, 344, 405]. Although thromboxane A_2 can be produced by human lung tissue [359], there is no evidence that it plays as important a role in humans as in guinea pigs.

Leukotrienes

LTC_4, LTD_4, and LTE_4 contract airway smooth muscle preparations [9, 45]; impair pulmonary mechanics in intact guinea pigs [125, 126, 420], monkeys [59, 370], some dogs [190], sheep [298], and humans [195, 423]; stimulate arachidonic acid metabolism in isolated lung preparations [134, 363]; and alter vascular permeability [95]. The critical question of how important leukotrienes are in causing the symptoms of asthma remains to be answered.

Guinea pig parenchymal strips are exquisitely sensitive to leukotrienes [325]. However, leukotriene-induced contractions of guinea pig parenchymal strips are blocked or greatly reduced by indomethacin or thromboxane synthetase inhibitors, which indicates that a large part of this response is due to a leukotriene-induced release of thromboxane A_2 from the parenchyma [325, 420]. Leukotrienes do not stimulate the release of thromboxane A_2 from guinea pig trachea, which may account for the lower sensitivity of this tissue to leukotrienes. Parenchymal strips from human and rat lungs contract in response to LTC_4 and LTD_4, but much higher concentrations are required than for guinea pig, and the contractions, unlike those in guinea pig lung strips, are not reduced by thromboxane synthetase inhibitors [325].

Studies in intact animals are also consistent with the above-cited results from in vitro experiments. In guinea pigs, LTC_4 and LTD_4 produce marked bronchoconstriction that is largely blocked by pretreatment with nonsteroidal antiinflammatory agents [406]. These findings suggest that leukotrienes stimulate the formation of prostaglandins, which are at least partly responsible for the bronchoconstrictor effect. In contrast to the guinea pig, leukotrienes produce rather modest changes in pulmonary mechanics in humans [195, 423], primates [59, 370], and dogs [190]. Thus, both in vivo and in vitro evidence suggests that cyclooxygenase products play an important role in the marked bronchoconstriction produced by leukotrienes in the guinea pig and perhaps the sheep [81] but not in most other species.

Platelet-Activating Factor

PAF (acetyl glyceryl ether phosphorylcholine) induces the contraction of airway smooth muscle [55], provokes acute reversible bronchoconstriction, and increases airway reactivity in primates [102, 306, 308], dogs [73], sheep [72], and guinea pigs [21] when it is given either intravenously or intratracheally (see Chap. 22). The mechanisms involved are poorly understood but release of prostaglandins and leukotrienes is thought to be involved. In the guinea pig, PAF-induced histamine hyperreactivity was reduced by pretreatment with a leukotriene synthesis inhibitor or a leukotriene receptor antagonist [21], but not by a cyclooxygenase blocker [22]. In the dog, the acute airway constriction and the increased reactivity to acetylcholine induced by PAF were reduced by OKY-046, a thromboxane synthetase inhibitor [73], whereas in the monkey, PAF-induced airway constriction was unaffected by cyclooxygenase blockers and airway reactivity was not evaluated [102].

Although PAF has been shown to increase airway reactivity in animals, the time course for this increase is unclear and at the present time there is considerable disagreement over whether or not a similar effect can be seen in humans.

PHYSICAL AND CHEMICAL CHALLENGES

Inhalation of irritant gases and chemically inert dusts constricts airways in humans [290] and animals [350] by stimulating sensory receptors in the epithelium of the trachea and bronchi. Physiologic studies have distinguished three separate types of sensory receptors [428], but aerosol challenge studies often do not identify the specific sensory structures involved. One of these receptors, a structure with large mitochondria and many neurotubules that lies just underneath the tight junctions of the epithelial cells, is often referred to as the *irritant receptor* [353, 428]. The afferent connections of these receptors run in the vagus nerve [108, 428, 441, 443]. Single-fiber recordings show that the action potential discharge is stimulated by the inhalation of irritant gases, inert dusts, and cigarette smoke. The irritant receptors are mainly localized to the intrapulmonary airways [285]; their concentration increases markedly from the upper trachea to the lobar bronchi and then decreases peripherally [285]. The other two classes of airway sensory receptors are stretch receptors and free nerve endings (C fibers) [428].

Unusually small doses of various inhaled irritants [17, 369] provoke airway constriction in asthmatic humans, whereas much higher concentrations are needed in normal humans. The mongrel dog is similar to the normal human in this respect. Mongrel dogs are relatively unreactive to irritant substances such as ammonia vapor, ether, and cigarette smoke [353]. Basenji-greyhound dogs, which demonstrate airway hyperreactivity to a variety of substances including hypotonic aerosols [189], show marked pulmonary reactivity to citric acid aerosols, whereas mongrel dogs show no response to this challenge [187] when it is administered to the whole lung. Ponies with airway hyperreactivity to methacholine [26] and rats with airway hyperreactivity to antigen [166] also show airway hyperreactivity to citric acid aerosols.

In the basenji-greyhound dog, the mechanism of citric acid–induced bronchoconstriction involves calcium chelation. We [114] found that Na_2 ethylenediaminetetraacetic acid (EDTA), which is also a calcium chelator, induced bronchoconstriction, while $CaNa_2$ EDTA did not. Acidity alone did not provoke the bronchoconstriction, since acetic acid had no effect on lung resistance, yet a mixture of citric acid and sodium citrate buffered to the same pH produced a response. Atropine inhibited the bronchoconstrictor response to a 2-minute challenge of citric acid [181], yet had no effect on the response to a 5-minute challenge [189]. A low dose (2-minute challenge) may act primarily through irritant receptors that activate vagal pathways, while a high dose (5-minute challenge) acts through some mechanism independent of vagal input. That mechanism seems to involve the release of mediators, since cromolyn sodium, a drug that is thought to stabilize membranes and inhibit mediator release, attenuated the response to the 5-minute challenge [189].

Hyperventilation with cold dry air provokes airway constriction in patients with asthma [101]. Administration of dry air to the lung periphery of dogs results in airway constriction with a time course similar to that found in exercising humans [137]. Hyperventilation with cold dry air has also been shown to elicit bronchoconstriction in cats [216], rabbits [217], and guinea pigs [70, 335]. The mechanisms underlying the airway constriction in these four models differ. In the mongrel dog, the mechanism is not known but epithelial cell injury may be involved, as the degree of airway cooling correlated with the magnitude of the airway response [143] and increases in epithelial cells and PGD_2 were found in the lavage fluid following the challenge [142]. In the cat and the rabbit, the responses were entirely abolished by sectioning the vagus nerve [216, 217], whereas in the guinea pig neither vagotomy nor atropine altered the response [335]. In the guinea pig, capsaicin pretreatment attenuated and phosphoramindon (a neutral endopeptidase inhibitor) pretreatment potentiated the response [334], implicating tachykinin release as an important mechanism in the guinea pig. The relevance of any of these models in exercise-induced asthma in humans remains to be established.

ADRENERGIC AND NONADRENERGIC RESPONSES

Two types of adrenergic receptors in airway smooth muscle have been described: alpha and $beta_2$ receptors. Stimulation of alpha receptors constricts airway smooth muscle, while stimulation of $beta_2$ receptors relaxes it. Studies support the existence of alpha receptors in the airway smooth muscle of experimental animals [233, 248] and humans [233, 271], although the response generated by stimulation of these receptors is small (10–20% of the maximal response elicited by acetylcholine). Thus, alpha-receptor stimulation probably results in only mild bronchoconstriction. Although ganglionic stimulants can elicit sympathetically mediated airway relaxation in adrenalectomized animals [249], and exogenous norepinephrine causes relaxation of airway smooth muscle in vitro, the adrenergic innervation of the lung is sparse and norepinephrine, the predominant neurotransmitter released from adrenergic nerve terminals, is much less potent than epinephrine as a $beta_2$ agonist [62]. Therefore, it seems likely that the major sympathetic control of bronchomotor tone is mediated by circulating epinephrine. This view is supported by the similar effects of adrenalectomy and beta-adrenergic blockade on the pulmonary response to airway challenge in animals [83, 105, 117, 183, 247, 250, 411].

Propranolol increases airway tone and reactivity in asthmatic humans, but not in nonasthmatic humans. Allergic sheep [411] and sensitized ponies exposed to hay containing mold [361] develop baseline airway constriction after beta-adrenergic blockade. Similarly, basenji-greyhound dogs develop increases in baseline tone [183] and increases in airway reactivity [400, 401]. In contrast, enhanced airway tone and reactivity after beta-adrenergic blockade are not seen in mongrel dogs [292, 376, 401] or in monkeys [312].

In the guinea pig, however, high doses of propranolol increase pulmonary resistance and decrease dynamic compliance in most animals [110, 330], and propranolol potentiates the response to histamine challenge, particularly in those animals that are initially less sensitive to histamine [110]. These findings suggest that differences in beta-adrenergic tone in this species may be critically important in determining its wide range of histamine sensitivity. The pharmacologic responses of guinea pig airways in vitro and in vivo are consistent with this explanation: There is a much greater variability in the histamine response in the intact animal than in the isolated tracheal preparations, and histamine sensitivity in vivo is inversely correlated with isoproterenol sensitivity in vitro and unrelated to histamine sensitivity in vitro [109].

The intracellular events involved in the relaxation of airway smooth muscle are not completely understood, but increased accumulation of cyclic AMP is thought to play a pivotal role. Beta-adrenergic agonists increase cyclic AMP levels in airway muscle [28, 340, 354, 430] via activation of the catecholamine-sensitive adenylyl cyclase complex [221, 339]. Since Szentivanyi [395] proposed in 1968 that asthma might be due to an inherited or acquired deficit in beta-adrenergic function, much research has focused on the beta-adrenergic receptor and the beta-adrenergic cascade (see Chap. 14). However, over 20 years later the question is still unsettled because research has largely focused on the leukocyte, and a great deal of evidence indicating that the leukocyte is a poor model of human asthma has accumulated. Although several studies have demonstrated that leukocytes from asthmatics [46, 92, 257] or allergic dogs with chronic airway hyperreactivity [63] show reduced cyclic AMP responses to beta agonists, similar responses are seen in leukocytes from normal individuals following treatment with beta agonists [148, 398], in atopic individuals who do not have asthma [160, 336], and in atopic dogs [186] that do not have airway hyperreactivity. In addition, leukocytes from some asthmatic patients show this beta deficit only after allergen exposure [234, 275]. Moreover, beta-adrenergic receptors on lung tissue and on leukocytes show markedly different susceptibilities to desensitization by beta agonists [168].

However, compelling evidence in favor of decreased beta-adrenergic sensitivity in asthma comes from studies of bronchial muscle tissue obtained from animal models of asthma [113, 224, 225, 283, 342, 345, 377] and from studies of human tissues (obtained either at surgery or at autopsy) from asthmatic subjects which showed a deficit in beta-adrenergic function. These results have largely been buried in studies showing a poor correlation between in vivo and in vitro responses to contractile agonists [61, 155, 384, 399] in asthma and have led to the present bias that an intrinsic defect does not reside in the smooth muscle of the airway. However, close examination of these data reveals significant differences in relaxation between tissue from asthmatic and nonasthmatic subjects. Cerrina and associates [61] related airway reactivity to aerosolized histamine in vivo to the effects produced by isoproterenol in histamine-preconstricted airways in vitro. Four of the 19 subjects were asthmatic. Asthmatic airways showed in vitro insensitivity to isoproterenol with an inverse relationship to in vivo responses, suggesting that beta-adrenergic function decreased as the level of in vivo airway hyperreactivity increased. Goldie and coworkers [155], using human bronchial preparation obtained at autopsy from 32 nonasthmatic and from 7 asthmatic subjects, preconstricted with carbachol, found that asthmatic tissue was 3- to 20-fold less sensitive to isoproterenol than control tissue, whereas sensitivity to theophylline was similar.

Similarly, trachealis muscle obtained from the basenji-greyhound dog model of chronic airway hyperreactivity showed decreased sensitivity to isoproterenol compared to control trachealis when the muscle was precontracted with methacholine [112, 113] (Fig. 31-8). This decreased sensitivity to isoproterenol could not be related to prior drug therapy since no animal had ever received beta-adrenergic or steroid therapy. Moreover, this beta-adrenergic deficit in airway smooth muscle was not seen in a control population of allergic dogs lacking airway hyperreactivity, suggesting that the decreased sensitivity to beta-adrenergic agonists was related in some way to the airway hyperreactivity.

Aside from the classic adrenergic pathways, nonadrenergic inhibitory nerves have also been demonstrated in many species

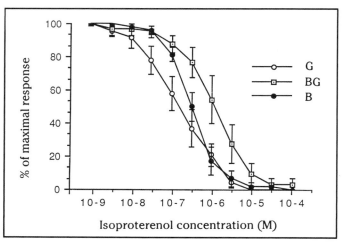

Fig. 31-8. *Cumulative dose-response curves for isoproterenol-induced relaxation in thoracic trachealis muscle from five basenji-greyhounds (BG), greyhounds (G), and basenjis (B). Preparations were precontracted with methacholine (EC$_{50}$). Isoproterenol was less potent in trachealis preparations from the basenji-greyhounds than in those from the basenjis and greyhounds (p < .05).*

[52, 53]. Stimulation of these nerves promotes airway relaxation, which is blocked by tetrodotoxin but not propranolol. This type of inhibitory innervation to the lungs is prominent in amphibians and many reptiles [52, 53] and was first demonstrated in mammals in the guinea pig [79, 86, 338], in which it is especially well developed. Nonadrenergic inhibitory nerves also are present in humans [337], baboons [280], cats [207], and ponies [342], but not in dogs [212, 251, 349, 392]. The relative importance of this system (or the absence of it) in the pathophysiology of reactive airway disease remains to be defined.

AIRWAY HYPERREACTIVITY

Inflammation

The mechanisms underlying airway hyperreactivity are still unknown, but a role for airway inflammation in both its development and perpetuation has been suggested. The hypothesis arose from observations that humans dying in status asthmaticus—and even those with mild asthma—show pathologic evidence of epithelial damage and airway inflammation [129, 242] and that exogenous factors increasing airway reactivity also can cause airway inflammation (see Chap. 9). This relationship has been pursued in many animal models by attempting to correlate the degree of inflammation, as measured either histologically or by analysis of BAL fluid, with accompanying changes in airway reactivity. However, while hyperreactivity is often accompanied by airway inflammation, a pronounced increase in airway reactivity can occur in the absence of any evidence of inflammation or, conversely, a pronounced inflammatory response may occur without hyperreactivity. Moreover, inbred strains of a number of species, including mice [252], rats [192], guinea pigs [397], and dogs [188], can show marked airway hyperreactivity with respect to other strains, without receiving any sort of treatment that might lead to airway inflammation.

Guinea Pig

In the guinea pig, airway hyperreactivity has been induced by antigen challenge [25, 139, 223] and by inhalation of toluene diisocyanate (TDI) [78, 156], ozone [287, 288], or cigarette smoke [198, 293]. Allergen-induced increases in airway reactivity to

pharmacologic stimuli have been observed both after resolution of the late-phase obstruction [139, 223] and in animals that did not develop a delayed obstructive response [25]. Inhalation of relatively high concentrations of TDI (2 ppm) produced airway hyperreactivity to acetylcholine at 2 and 6 hours but not at 24 hours after exposure [156]. The total number of PMNs in bronchial epithelium was increased only at 2 hours, but eosinophil counts were increased at 6 and 24 hours. TDI also produced epithelial disruption, observable at all time points. Guinea pigs exposed to only 1 ppm show increased numbers of PMNs at 2 hours, but did not develop airway hyperreactivity. Further studies in this model by another group using 3 ppm of TDI showed that depletion of PMNs by pretreatment with cyclophosphamide had no effect on either the incidence or the degree of airway hyperreactivity to acetylcholine, suggesting that TDI-induced hyperreactivity in this species is independent of circulating or airway PMNs [78]. Studies with ozone or cigarette smoke exposure in guinea pigs also suggested that factors other than an influx of PMNs are involved in the resulting airway hyperreactivity. Ozone increases airway reactivity to intravenous administration of acetylcholine between 2 hours and 3 days. Although epithelial damage is seen at 2 hours (at the start of hyperreactivity), the PMN influx occurs 4 hours after the development of airway hyperreactivity and persists long after the hyperreactivity has resolved [287]. Moreover, PMN depletion by cyclophosphamide fails to inhibit the ozone-provoked hyperreactivity [288]. Similarly, when airway hyperreactivity is produced in guinea pigs by exposure to cigarette smoke, the hyperreactivity precedes the migration of PMNs into the bronchial epithelium [198]. Furthermore, other investigators, exploring the dose-response relationships between cigarette smoke, hyperreactivity, and inflammatory infiltrates [293], found that a 20-puff dose in guinea pigs increased airway reactivity to methacholine, both immediately and at 5 hours after smoke exposure, without evidence of inflammation, eosinophilia, or increased vascular permeability in the airway epithelium. These studies with ozone- and cigarette smoke–induced hyperreactivity suggest that the appearance of PMNs in the postchallenge period (if it occurs) is a response to tissue damage, but not the cause of increased airway responsiveness. Studies with endotoxin-induced injury of guinea pig lung provided a complementary set of data, in which there is a marked PMN influx, but no increase in airway reactivity to histamine [141].

Rat

In sensitized rats, repeated challenge with antigen aerosols has been shown to increase airway reactivity to methacholine [131]. However, hyperreactivity to methacholine was not observed at 1 week after a single antigen challenge, even though late-phase obstructive responses occurred in most animals and roughly half of the animals in the series died [131]. Thus, despite the intensity of the airway response to antigen challenge, hyperreactivity either did not develop or did not persist until the time of testing. In other studies, inhalation of endotoxin [320] was found to produce an impressive influx of PMN at 1.5 hours after the exposure. However, of three rat strains tested, although all showed the inflammatory response, only one showed airway hyperreactivity to intravenously administered serotonin.

Rabbit

In the rabbit, airway hyperreactivity has been induced by inhalation of C5A [206] or by antigen in sensitized animals [268]. In both instances, the hyperreactivity appears to be associated with an influx of PMNs; however, airway reactivity induced by other (nonallergic) pathways has received little study in this species. In antigen-challenged rabbits, airway hyperreactivity (6.5-fold shift) to histamine can be demonstrated at 3 days after antigen challenge, when the pronounced late-phase changes in pulmonary mechanics have returned to normal [268]. At this time, the inflammatory infiltrate has partially resolved, but the numbers of PMNs and monocytes are still increased in BAL fluid. By 7 days after antigen challenge, both airway reactivity and BAL fluid have returned to normal or near normal. When such rabbits were made granulocytopenic at the time of antigen challenge, neither a late-phase obstruction nor an increase in airway reactivity occurred, but when granulocytes were restored at the time of antigen challenge by an infusion of neutrophil-rich white cells, both a late-phase obstruction and airway hyperreactivity could be observed [289].

Dog

Hyperreactivity in dog models can occur on a genetic basis [184] or be induced by antigen challenge [190] or ozone inhalation [222, 226]. Highly inbred basenji-greyhound dogs have persistent airway hyperreactivity to aerosol challenges, including methacholine and citric acid [187], which is transmitted to their offspring [184]. In addition, these dogs show increased percentages of luminal mast cells, lymphocytes [180], and eosinophils [98] in the BAL fluid. Daily treatment with methylprednisolone, 2 mg/kg, for 6 weeks decreased airway reactivity to methacholine and abolished reactivity to citric acid aerosols. This was associated with marked decreases in circulating and BAL fluid eosinophils [98]. Although the mechanisms by which glucocorticoids exert their protective effects in this model are not known, it is likely that part of their action is through their antiinflammatory effects.

Antigen challenge in sensitized dogs can produce a substantial increase in airway reactivity, whether or not a late-phase airway obstruction is seen. In inbred ragweed-sensitized dogs challenged with aerosols of ragweed extract, mean pulmonary resistance increased 11-fold at 5 minutes after challenge and had returned to baseline by 1.5 hours [74]. These animals showed no evidence of a late-phase obstruction, and the pulmonary resistance at 6 hours after challenge was similar to that in the control period. When tested with acetylcholine aerosols at 2 hours after the antigen challenge (after resolution of the immediate response), there was no evidence of hyperreactivity; however, at 6 hours after antigen challenge, all of the dogs that had shown an immediate response to the antigen now showed hyperreactivity to acetylcholine (6.6-fold shift). Hyperreactivity persisted for from less than 4 days to as long as 16 weeks. BAL fluid showed a significant increase in neutrophils (approximately 6-fold) at both 2 and 6 hours after antigen challenge, and in the latter period there was a significant correlation between the change in responsiveness and the influx of neutrophils. However, in contrast to the progressive influx of eosinophils in the guinea pig and rabbit models, the eosinophil counts in the canine BAL fluid were significantly less at 6 hours after antigen challenge (time of airway hyperreactivity) than at 2 hours after antigen challenge (before onset of hyperreactivity).

Other investigators pretreated dogs with metyrapone to facilitate expression of a late-phase obstruction [356]. They observed a late-phase obstruction in 8 of 10 dogs so pretreated, and were able to show an increased sensitivity to acetylcholine even in the 2 dogs that had not undergone a late-phase increase in pulmonary resistance. There was a significant increase in neutrophil but not eosinophil counts in the BAL fluid of the metyrapone-treated animals. A control group that was challenged with antigen without pretreatment with metyrapone did not show late responses or an influx of neutrophils into the BAL fluid, and in contrast to the preceding study, no increase in airway reactivity was observed in these dogs. These studies [74, 356] agree, however, in that increased reactivity occurred against a background of neutrophilic but no eosinophilic influx into the BAL fluid.

Dogs exposed to ozone, 1.0 to 2.2 ppm for up to 2 hours, developed increases in airway reactivity to acetylcholine aerosols 1 hour, and in some animals 24 hours, but not 1 week following exposure [196, 197]. Dogs that showed increased airway reactivity also developed a marked and reversible increase in the number of PMNs in the airway epithelium [196] and increased numbers of PMNs and epithelial cells in the BAL fluid [137]. Hydroxyurea pretreatment, which depletes PMNs (and perhaps other cells), prevented the increase in airway hyperreactivity following ozone exposure [296], suggesting PMN involvement. Moreover, in indomethacin-pretreated dogs, ozone exposure was associated with an influx of PMNs into the airways but increases in airway reactivity failed to develop [295]. Similarly, pretreatment with a thromboxane synthetase inhibitor prevented the ozone-induced airway hyperreactivity, again without altering the PMN influx [14]. These three studies taken together suggest that cyclooxygenase-derived products of inflammatory cells (largely thromboxane) are necessary for the development of airway hyperreactivity in dogs following ozone exposure. Again, this is in contrast to the guinea pig studies in which PMN depletion did not inhibit the development of hyperreactivity [288].

Despite the apparently close association in dogs between a PMN influx and antigen- or ozone-induced hyperreactivity, chronic exposure to sulfur dioxide produces a persistent infiltration of PMNs and mononuclear cells [364] but decreases rather than increases airway reactivity to histamine aerosols [121]. More recent studies failed to show a relationship between the onset of inflammation (as measured by increases in PMNs in BAL fluid) and the decrease in reactivity to methacholine aerosols [368]. Since the airway reactivity to intravenously administered methacholine was unchanged, the decreased reactivity to the aerosols presumably reflects an enhanced mucoepithelial barrier. A similar decrease in airway reactivity, coupled with airway inflammation, also has been observed in dogs repeatedly exposed to nitric acid aerosols [147].

Sheep

In sheep, challenge with antigen aerosols produces an increase in airway reactivity to carbachol (approximately twofold shift) at 2 hours after antigen challenge in most animals, whether or not they subsequently develop a late-phase obstruction [3]. However, when tested at 24 hours after antigen challenge, only the animals that developed a late-phase obstruction (dual responders) were hyperreactive to carbachol (approximately twofold shift) [245]. Both dual responders and sheep with only an immediate response (acute responders) had similar increases in PMNs in the BAL fluid at 7 to 8 hours after antigen challenge, but eosinophil counts were significantly increased only in the dual responders [1]. At 24 hours after antigen challenge, the PMN counts in the BAL fluid remained elevated in both acute and dual responders; eosinophil numbers in these groups [245] were not significantly different at that time. A number of drugs influencing the cyclooxygenase or lipoxygenase pathways have been shown to inhibit the development of hyperreactivity to carbachol in dual responders at the 24-hour test period; these include both indomethacin [245] and several leukotriene antagonists [1, 245]. Since inhalation of LTD$_4$ itself induces both acute and delayed bronchoconstriction in dual, but not acute responders [6], it has been proposed that lipoxygenase products released during the acute exposure to antigen play a role in the subsequent development of the late response and, by inference, the increased airway reactivity [1]. "Antiallergic" agents such as cromolyn [1] and nedrocromil also effectively inhibit the antigen-induced development of airway hyperreactivity in this model; but most curiously, budesonide (an inhaled glucocorticosteroid) did not prevent antigen-induced airway hyperreactivity, even though it blocked the late-phase obstruction [244]. This would suggest that the hyperreactivity is not that tightly linked to the inflammatory events of the late-phase response, and is consistent with the early development of hyperreactivity at the 2-hour test period (before the beginning of the late-phase response) [245].

The extent of airway hyperreactivity provoked by antigen challenge in sheep is relatively slight (approximately twofold shift). Infusion of endotoxin in sheep produces a substantially greater increase in airway reactivity when tested 5 hours later with histamine aerosols (37-fold shift) [201], and the hyperreactivity occurs at a time when there is a marked pulmonary influx of granulocytes and lymphocytes [276]. Endotoxin also produces an increase in pulmonary resistance and a decrease in dynamic compliance, which peak shortly after termination of the infusion [81, 201]; by 5 hours after infusion, pulmonary resistance has returned toward normal, although dynamic compliance remains reduced. Endotoxin infusion produces high concentrations of cyclooxygenase and lipoxygenase products of arachidonic acid metabolism in both blood and lung lymph, and it has been proposed that the lipoxygenase products act as a stimulus for the cyclooxygenase pathway [81]. L-651,392 (an inhibitor of the lipoxygenase pathway) attenuates the endotoxin-induced changes in pulmonary resistance and dynamic compliance, as well as the increase in lung lymph of cyclooxygenase and lipoxygenase products [81]. Thus, as with antigen challenge in this species, lipoxygenase products, presumably generated by the inflammatory infiltrate, appear to play a critical role in endotoxin-induced changes in pulmonary function. The importance of granulocytes in the pulmonary response to endotoxin was tested by depleting the granulocytes with hydroxyurea before infusing the endotoxin. This attenuated the alteration in pulmonary mechanics [177] induced by endotoxin, but the effect on airway reactivity during endotoxemia was not assessed. In normal sheep, however, granulocyte depletion reduced the reactivity to histamine aerosols [176]. These studies show that the granulocyte is essential for the genesis of endotoxin-induced changes in pulmonary mechanics and for maintenance of the normal reactivity of the airway to histamine; but they do not establish that a granulocytic influx underlies the endotoxin-induced airway hyperreactivity.

Viruses

A number of investigators recently focused attention on the possible role of peptidergic sensory nerve endings in the pathogenesis of some types of airway hyperreactivity, in particular that induced by viral respiratory infections [144]. Viral infections potentiate the spasmogenic effect of substance P [130, 215, 351], apparently by decreasing the activity of an enzyme (neutral endopeptidase) responsible for the catabolism of substance P (Fig. 31-9). Viral infections have been shown to reduce neutral endopeptidase (also called enkephalinase) in a number of species,

including rats [40], ferrets [215], and guinea pigs [130], with an accompanying accentuation of airway reactivity and neurogenic inflammation. Reduction of endopeptidase activity, however, does not appear to be the only effect of viral infection on the neural control of airway smooth muscle. Bronchoconstriction invoked by electrical stimulation of the efferent vagus nerves is potentiated by viral infection but the response of the airway smooth muscle is unchanged [49]. Release of acetylcholine from vagal nerve endings is subject to feedback inhibition mediated by M_2 muscarinic receptors [146], and selective blockade of M_2 receptors with gallamine can markedly increase vagally mediated bronchoconstriction (see Fig. 31-9). However, following viral infection in guinea pigs, the M_2 receptor loses its ability to inhibit acetylcholine release [145]. Thus, viral infections can increase airway reactivity by effects on both sensory and motor nerve endings.

Genetic Factors

Biologic variability in responses to aerosol challenges must be determined in part by genetic factors. The familial aggregation of human asthma is well known [254]. We [187] demonstrated marked nonspecific airway hyperreactivity in a highly inbred population of basenji-greyhound dogs selected on the basis of response to inhalational challenges. Takino and coworkers [397] selectively bred two lines of guinea pigs on the basis of airway sensitivity to chemical mediators, and Holme and Piechuta [192] did the same in rats with respect to the intensity of the pulmonary response to antigen aerosol challenge.

If airway hyperreactivity is an inherited trait, it should be possible to identify genes that determine airway responses. Inbred strains of mice that are hyperreactive to acetylcholine [252] and to serotonin [253] have been identified. However, the pattern of airway hyperreactivity to serotonin and acetylcholine differed in the nine inbred strains screened. These studies suggest that in mice, nonspecific airway hyperreactivity to agonists is determined by multiple genes, that these traits are inherited independently, and that the genes controlling the serotonin and acetylcholine loci are not closely linked.

In summary, pulmonary responsiveness to markedly dissimilar aerosol challenges closely correlates in both experimental animals [182, 239, 374] and humans [383], which indicates that airway hyperreactivity is not restricted to responses elicited by a specific receptor. Unusually small concentrations of inhaled irritants [17, 369], histamine, and methacholine [369] provoke airway constriction in asthmatic humans; much higher concentrations are needed in nonasthmatic humans. Unselected populations of mongrel dogs [373], guinea pigs [111], and rats [192] are relatively unresponsive to nonspecific aerosol challenges. However, the unimodal distribution of airway responsiveness in experimental animals [111, 373], as well as humans [424], allows selection of groups of animals at the spectrum's reactive end.

It is currently believed that inflammation plays a crucial role in airway hyperreactivity and much research has focused on the role of injury and inflammation in the pathogenesis of airway hyperreactivity. Airway injury and inflammation can certainly modulate airway reactivity in animal models and humans. However, there are inbred strains of mice [252], rats [192], guinea pigs [397], and dogs [184] that show marked airway hyperreactivity in the absence of any obvious inflammation. The airway consists of many different structures and cells that can contribute to airway hyperreactivity. A damaged epithelium, an increased release of acetylcholine from parasympathetic nerves, or a decreased sensitivity of the airway smooth muscle to relaxing agonists may all play a role.

Animal models have been useful and will continue to be useful to test hypotheses concerning mechanisms of airway hyperreac-

Fig. 31-9. *Mechanisms of virus-induced hyperreactivity of the airways. See text.*

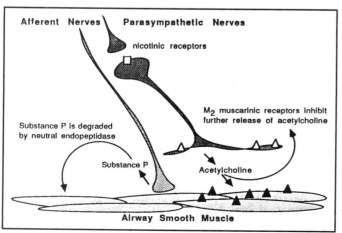

tivity that are untestable in humans. In animal models, invasive studies are feasible, airway tissue is easily obtained, and environmental and genetic factors can be reasonably controlled. Studies in animal models are needed to provide insights into the pathogenesis and treatment of airway hyperreactivity in humans.

REFERENCES

1. Abraham, W. M. The importance of lipoxygenase products of arachidonic acid in allergen-induced late responses. *Am. Rev. Respir. Dis.* 135:S49, 1987.
2. Abraham, W. M. The role of leukotrienes in allergen-induced late responses in allergic sheep. *Ann. NY Acad. Sci.* 524:260, 1988.
3. Abraham, W. M., et al. Antigen-induced airway hyperresponsiveness does not contribute to airway late responses. *Am. Rev. Respir. Dis.* 135:A97, 1987.
4. Abraham, W. M., et al. Characterization of a late phase pulmonary response after challenge in allergic sheep. *Am. Rev. Respir. Dis.* 128:839, 1983.
5. Abraham, W. M., et al. Bronchoalveolar lavage fluid from allergic sheep with allergen-induced late responses contains increased inflammatory cells and slow reacting substance of anaphylaxis (SRS-A). *Am. Rev. Respir. Dis.* 133:A240, 1986.
6. Abraham, W. M., et al. Production of early and late pulmonary responses with inhaled leukotriene D$_4$ in allergic sheep. *Prostaglandins* 29:715, 1985.
7. Abraham, W. M., Stevenson, J. S., and Garrido, R. A leukotriene and thromboxane inhibitor (Sch 37224) blocks antigen-induced immediate and late responses and airway hyperresponsiveness in allergic sheep. *J. Pharmacol. Exp. Ther.* 247:1004, 1988.
8. Abraham, W. M., et al. Effect of pharmacologic agents on antigen-induced decreases in specific lung conductance in sheep. *Am. Rev. Respir. Dis.* 124:554, 1981.
9. Adams, G. K., and Lichtenstein, L. *In vitro* studies of antigen-induced bronchospasm: Effect of antihistamine and SRS-A antagonist on response of sensitized guinea pig and human airways to antigen. *J. Immunol.* 122:555, 1979.
10. Advenier, C., et al. The effects of pentobarbitone and urethane on pulmonary airway resistance in guinea-pigs and their interactions with drugs. *Br. J. Pharmacol.* 64:519, 1978.
11. Agrawal, K. P. Specific conductance in guinea pigs: Normal values and histamine-induced fall. *Respir. Physiol.* 43:23, 1981.
12. Ahmed, T., et al. Role of H$_1$- and H$_2$-receptors in airway reactions to histamine in conscious sheep. *J. Appl. Physiol.* 49:826, 1980.
13. Ainsworth, G. A., Garland, L. G., and Payne, A. N. Modulation of bronchoconstrictor responses to histamine in pithed guinea pigs by sympathetic nerve stimulation. *Br. J. Pharmacol.* 77:249, 1982.
14. Aizawa, H., et al. Significance of thromboxane generation in ozone-induced airway hyperresponsiveness in dogs. *J. Appl. Physiol.* 59:1918, 1985.
15. Alanko, K., and Poppius, H. Anticholinergic blocking of prostaglandin-induced bronchoconstriction. *Br. Med. J.* 1:294, 1973.
16. Alexander, F., et al. Effects of histamine and 5-hydroxytryptamine on sheep. *J. Comp. Pathol.* 77:1, 1967.
17. Allegra, L., and Bianco, S. Non-specific bronchoreactivity obtained with an ultrasonic aerosol of distilled water. *Eur. J. Respir. Dis.* 61(Suppl. 106):41, 1980.
18. Al-Ubaidi, F., and Bakhle, Y. S. Differences in biological activation of arachidonic acid in perfused lungs from guinea pig, rat, and man. *Eur. J. Pharmacol.* 62:89, 1980.
19. Amdur, M. O., and Mead, J. Mechanics of respiration in unanesthetized guinea pigs. *Am. J. Physiol.* 192:364, 1958.
20. Anderson, W. Atopic dermatitis in the dog. *Cutis* 15:955, 1975.
21. Andersson, G. P., White, H. L., and Fennessy, M. R. Increased airway responsiveness to histamine induced by platelet activating factor in the guinea pig: Possible role of lipoxygenase metabolites. *Agents Actions* 24:1, 1988.
22. Andersson, G. P., White, H. L., and Fennessy, M. R. Lipoxygenase metabolites mediate increased airway responsiveness to histamine after platelet activating factor exposure in the guinea pig. *Agents Actions* 24:8, 1988.
23. Andersson, P. Antigen-induced bronchial anaphylaxis in actively sensitized guinea-pigs: Pattern of response in relation to immunization regimen. *Allergy* 35:65, 1980.
24. Andersson, P. Effects of inhibitors of anaphylactic mediators in two

25. Andersson, P., and Bergstrand, H. Antigen-induced bronchial anaphylaxis in actively sensitized guinea pigs: Effect of long-term treatment with sodium cromoglycate and aminophylline. *Br. J. Pharmacol.* 74:601, 1981.
26. Armstrong, P. J., et al. Airway responses to aerosolized methacholine and citric acid in ponies with recurrent airway obstruction (heaves). *Am. Rev. Respir. Dis.* 133:357, 1986.
27. Auer, J., and Lewis, P. A. The physiology of the immediate reaction of anaphylaxis in the guinea pig. *J. Exp. Med.* 12:151, 1910.
28. Austin, D. R., et al. Cyclic nucleotide function in trachealis muscle of dogs with and without airway hyperresponsiveness. *J. Appl. Physiol.* 63:2309, 1987.
29. Bai, T. R. Abnormalities in airway smooth muscle in fatal asthma. *Am. Rev. Respir. Dis.* 141:552, 1990.
30. Barnes, P. J. Asthma as an axon reflex. *Lancet* 1:242, 1986.
31. Baumgartner, R. A., et al. Serotonin induces constriction and relaxation of the guinea pig airway. *J. Pharmacol. Exp. Ther.* 255:165, 1990.
32. Becker, A. B., et al. Development of chronic airway hyperresponsiveness in ragweed-sensitized dogs. *J. Appl. Physiol.* 66:2691, 1989.
33. Bernstine, M. L., Berker, E., and Cullen, M. The bronchomotor effects of certain intravenous barbiturates on vagal stimulation in dogs. *Anesthesiology* 18:866, 1957.
34. Berry, P. A., and Collier, H. O. J. Bronchoconstrictor action and antagonism of a slow-reacting substance from anaphylaxis of guinea pig isolated lung. *Br. J. Pharmacol.* 23:201, 1964.
35. Bhat, K. N., et al. Plasma histamine changes during provoked bronchospasm in asthmatic patients. *J. Allergy Clin. Immunol.* 58:647, 1976.
36. Bhattacharya, B. K. A pharmacological study on the effect of 5-hydroxytryptamine and its antagonists on the bronchial musculature. *Arch. Int. Pharmacodyn. Ther.* 103:357, 1955.
37. Blythe, S., et al. IgE antibody mediated inflammation of rat lung: Histologic and bronchoalveolar lavage assessment. *Am. Rev. Respir. Dis.* 134:1246, 1986.
38. Booij-Noord, H., Orie, N. G. M., and deVries, K. Serotonin (5-hydroxytryptamine) inhalation in patients with chronic nonspecific lung disease. *Scand. J. Respir. Dis.* 50:301, 1969.
39. Booth, B. H., Patterson, R., and Talbot, C. H. Immediate-type hypersensitivity in dogs: Cutaneous, anaphylactic, and respiratory responses to *Ascaris*. *J. Lab. Clin. Med.* 76:181, 1970.
40. Borson, D. B., et al. Neutral endopeptidase and neurogenic inflammation in rats with respiratory infection. *J. Appl. Physiol.* 66:2653, 1989.
41. Bovet, D. Introduction to antihistamine agents and Antergan derivatives. *Ann. NY Acad. Sci.* 50:1089, 1950.
42. Boynton, B. R., et al. The deleterious effect of FPL 55712 on gas exchange in the basenji-greyhound dog model of asthma. *J. Crit. Care* 2:27, 1987.
43. Broadstone, R. V., et al. *In vitro* responses to acetylcholine and electrical stimulation of airways from horses with recurrent obstructive pulmonary disease. *Physiologist* 32:180, 1989.
44. Broadstone, R. V., et al. Effects of atropine in ponies with recurrent airway obstruction. *J. Appl. Physiol.* 65:2720, 1988.
45. Brocklehurst, W. E. The release of histamine and formation of a slow reacting substance (SRS-A) during anaphylactic shock. *J. Physiol. (Lond.)* 151:416, 1960.
46. Brooks, S. M., et al. Relationship between numbers of beta-adrenergic receptors in lymphocytes and disease severity in asthma. *J. Allergy Clin. Immunol.* 63:401, 1979.
47. Brown, R., Ingram, R. H., and McFadden, E. R. Effects of prostaglandin F$_{2\alpha}$ on lung mechanics in nonasthmatic and asthmatic subjects. *J. Appl. Physiol.* 44:150, 1978.
48. Buck, S. H., and Burks, T. F. The neuropharmacology of capsaicin: Review of some recent observations. *Pharmacol. Rev.* 38:179, 1986.
49. Buckner, C. K., et al. *In vivo* and *in vitro* studies on the use of the guinea pig as a model for virus provoked airway hyperreactivity. *Am. Rev. Respir. Dis.* 132:305, 1985.
50. Burka, J. F., and Paterson, N. A. M. The effects of SRS-A and histamine antagonists on antigen-induced contraction of guinea pig trachea. *Eur. J. Pharmacol.* 70:489, 1981.
51. Burns, J. W., and Doe, J. E. A comparison of drug-induced responses on rat tracheal, bronchial and lung strip *in vitro* preparations. *Br. J. Pharmacol.* 64:71, 1978.
52. Burnstock, G. Evolution of the autonomic innervation of visceral and cardiovascular systems in vertebrates. *Pharmacol. Rev.* 21:247, 1969.
53. Burnstock, G. Comparative studies of purinergic nerves. *J. Exp. Zool.* 194:103, 1975.

54. Butler, J. M., et al. Pruritic dermatitis in asthmatic basenji-greyhound dogs: A model for human atopic dermatitis. *J. Am. Acad. Dermatol.* 8:33, 1983.

55. Camussi, G., et al. Platelet activating factor mediated contraction of rabbit lung strips: Pharmacologic modulation. *Immunopharmacology* 6:87, 1983.

56. Carswell, F., and Oliver, J. The respiratory response in sensitized rats to aerosol challenge. *Immunology* 34:465, 1978.

57. Carswell, F., and Oliver, J. Site of respiratory reaction in allergic rats challenged via the airways. *Int. Arch. Allergy Appl. Immunol.* 57:358, 1978.

58. Casey, F. B., and Abboa-Offei, B. E. Pulmonary function changes in normal rats induced by antibody against rat IgE. *Clin. Exp. Immunol.* 36:473, 1979.

59. Casey, L., et al. Cardiovascular, Respiratory, and Hematologic Effects of Leukotriene D$_4$ in Primates. In B. Samuelsson and R. Paoletti (eds.), *Leukotrienes and Other Lipoxygenase Products.* New York: Raven, 1982. Pp. 201–211.

60. Casterline, C. L., Evans, R., and Ward, G. W. The effect of atropine and albuterol aerosols on the human bronchial response to histamine. *J. Allergy Clin. Immunol.* 58:607, 1976.

61. Cerrina, J., et al. Comparison of human bronchial muscle responses to histamine *in vivo* with histamine and isoproterenol agonists *in vitro.* Am. Rev. Respir. Dis. 134:57, 1986.

62. Chahl, L. A., and O'Donnell, S. R. The interaction of cocaine and propranolol with catecholamines on guinea pig trachea. *Eur. J. Pharmacol.* 2:77, 1967.

63. Chan, S. C., et al. Elevated leukocyte phosphodiesterase as a basis for depressed cyclic adenosine monophosphate responses in the basenji-greyhound dog model of asthma. *J. Allergy Clin. Immunol.* 76:148, 1985.

64. Chand, N. Distribution and classification of airway histamine receptors: The physiological significance of histamine H$_2$-receptors. *Adv. Pharmacol. Chemother.* 17:103, 1980.

65. Chand, N. Reactivity of isolated trachea, bronchus and lung strip of cats to carbachol, 5-hydroxytryptamine and histamine: Evidence for the existence of methysergide-sensitive receptors. *Br. J. Pharmacol.* 73:853, 1981.

66. Chand, N., and De Roth, L. Response of guinea-pig lung parenchymal strips to prostaglandins and some selected autacoids. *J. Pharm. Pharmacol.* 31:712, 1979.

67. Chand, N., De Roth, L., and Eyre, P. Relaxant response of goat trachea to 5-hydroxytryptamine mediated by D-tryptamine receptors. *Br. J. Pharmacol.* 66:331, 1979.

68. Chand, N., De Roth, L., and Eyre, P. Pharmacology of Schultz-Dale reaction in canine lung strip *in vitro*: Possible model for allergic asthma. *Br. J. Pharmacol.* 66:511, 1979.

69. Chand, N., et al. Reactivity of trachea, bronchi, and lung strips to histamine and carbachol in rhesus monkeys. *J. Appl. Physiol.* 49:729, 1980.

70. Chapman, R. W., and Danko, G. Hyperventilation-induced bronchoconstriction in guinea pigs. *Int. Arch. Allergy Appl. Immunol.* 78:190, 1985.

71. Chiesa, A., et al. Histamine release during antigen inhalation in experimental asthma in dogs. *Am. Rev. Respir. Dis.* 111:148, 1975.

72. Christman, B. W., Lefferts, P. L., and Snapper, J. R. Effect of platelet activating factor on aerosol histamine responsiveness in awake sheep. *Am. Rev. Respir. Dis.* 135:1267, 1987.

73. Chung, K. F., et al. Airway hyperresponsiveness induced by platelet activating factor: Role of thromboxane generation. *J. Pharmacol. Exp. Ther.* 236:580, 1986.

74. Chung, K. F., et al. Antigen-induced airway hyperresponsiveness and pulmonary inflammation in the allergic dog. *J. Appl. Physiol.* 58:1347, 1985.

75. Church, M. K. Response of rat lung to humoral mediators of anaphylaxis and its modification by drugs and sensitization. *Br. J. Pharmacol.* 55:423, 1975.

76. Church, M. K., Collier, H. O. J., and James, G. W. L. The inhibition by dexamethasone and disodium cromoglycate of anaphylactic bronchoconstriction in the rat. *Br. J. Pharmacol.* 46:56, 1972.

77. Church, M. K., Hutson, P. A., and Holgate, S. T. Effect of nedocromil sodium on early and late phase responses to allergen challenge in the guinea pig. *Drug* 37:101, 1989.

78. Cibulas, W., et al. Toluene diisocyanate-induced airway hyperreactivity in guinea pigs depleted of granulocytes. *J. Appl. Physiol.* 64:1773, 1988.

79. Coburn, R. F., and Tomita, T. Evidence for nonadrenergic inhibitory nerves in the guinea pig trachealis muscle. *Am. J. Physiol.* 224:1072, 1973.

80. Cockcroft, D. W., et al. Protective effect of drugs on histamine-induced asthma. *Thorax* 32:429, 1977.

81. Coggeshall, J. W., et al. Effect of inhibition of 5-lipoxygenase metabolism of arachidonic acid on response to endotoxemia in sheep. *J. Appl. Physiol.* 65:1351, 1988.

82. Cohn, M. A., Baier, H., and Wanner, A. Failure of hypoxic pulmonary vasoconstriction in the canine asthma model. *J. Clin. Invest.* 61:1463, 1978.

83. Colebatch, H. J. H., and Engel, L. A. Constriction of the lung by histamine before and after adrenalectomy in cats. *J. Appl. Physiol.* 37:798, 1974.

84. Colebatch, H. J. H., and Mitchell, C. A. Constriction of isolated living liquid-filled dog and cat lungs with histamine. *J. Appl. Physiol.* 30:691, 1971.

85. Colebatch, H. J. H., Olsen, C. R., and Nadel, J. A. Effect of histamine, serotonin and acetylcholine on the peripheral airways. *J. Appl. Physiol.* 21:217, 1966.

86. Coleman, R. A., and Levy, G. P. A nonadrenergic inhibitory nervous pathway in guinea pig trachea. *Br. J. Pharmacol.* 52:167, 1974.

87. Collier, H. O. J., and James, G. W. L. Humoral factors affecting pulmonary inflation during acute anaphylaxis in the guinea-pig *in vivo.* Br. J. Pharmacol. 30:283, 1967.

88. Collier, H. O. J., James, G. W. L., and Piper, P. J. Antagonism by fenamates and like-acting drugs of bronchoconstriction induced by bradykinin or antigen in the guinea-pig. *Br. J. Pharmacol.* 34:76, 1968.

89. Collier, H. O. J., and Shorley, P. G. Analgesic antipyretic drugs as antagonists of bradykinin. *Br. J. Pharmacol.* 15:601, 1960.

90. Collier, H. O. J., et al. The bronchoconstrictor action of bradykinin the guinea pig. *Br. J. Pharmacol.* 15:290, 1960.

91. Comroe, J. H., et al. Reflex and direct cardiopulmonary effects of 5-OH-tryptamine (serotonin). *Am. J. Physiol.* 173:379, 1953.

92. Conolly, M. E., and Greenacre, J. K. The lymphocyte β-adrenoceptors in normal subjects and patients with bronchial asthma. *J. Clin. Invest.* 58:1307, 1976.

93. Curry, J. J. The action of histamine on the respiratory tract in normal and asthmatic subjects. *J. Clin. Invest.* 25:785, 1946.

94. Curry, J. J., and Lowell, F. C. Measurement of vital capacity in asthmatic subjects receiving histamine and acetyl-beta-methylcholine. *J. Allergy* 19:9, 1948.

95. Dahlen, S.-E., et al. Leukotrienes promote plasma leakage and leukocyte adhesion in postcapillary venules: *In vivo* effects with relevance to the acute inflammatory response. *Proc. Natl. Acad. Sci. USA* 78:3887, 1981.

96. Dain, D., and Gold, W. M. Mechanical properties of the lungs and experimental asthma in conscious allergic dogs. *J. Appl. Physiol.* 38:96, 1975.

97. Dale, H. H., and Laidlaw, P. P. The physiological action of β-iminazolyethylamine. *J. Physiol. (Lond.)* 41:318, 1910.

98. Darowski, M. J., Hannon, V. M., and Hirshman, C. A. Corticosteroids decrease airway hyperresponsiveness in the basenji-greyhound dog model of asthma. *Am. Rev. Respir. Dis.* 66:1120, 1989.

99. Dawson, W., et al. Potent bronchoconstrictor activity of 15-keto prostaglandin F$_{2\alpha}$. *Nature* 250:331, 1974.

100. Dawson, W., et al. Release of novel prostaglandins and thromboxanes after immunological challenge of guinea pig lung. *Nature* 262:699, 1976.

101. Deal, E. C., et al. Airway responsiveness to cold air and hyperpnea in normal subjects and in those with hay fever and asthma. *Am. Rev. Respir. Dis.* 121:621, 1980.

102. Denjean, A., et al. Acute effects of intratracheal administration of platelet activating factor in baboons. *J. Appl. Physiol.* 55:799, 1983.

103. Derkson, F. J., et al. Airway reactivity in ponies with recurrent airway obstruction (heaves). *J. Appl. Physiol.* 58:598, 1985.

104. Derkson, F. J., et al. Intravenous histamine administration in ponies with recurrent airway obstruction (heaves). *Am. J. Vet. Res.* 46:774, 1985.

105. Diamond, L. Potentiation of bronchomotor responses by beta-adrenergic agonists. *J. Pharmacol. Exp. Ther.* 181:434, 1972.

106. Dixon, M., Jackson, D. M., and Richards, I. M. The effects of histamine, acetylcholine and 5-hydroxytryptamine on lung mechanics and irritant receptors in the dog. *J. Physiol. (Lond.)* 287:393, 1979.

107. Dixon, M., Jackson, D. M., and Richards, I. M. The effects of 5-hydroxytryptamine, histamine and acetylcholine on the reactivity of the lung of the anaesthetized dog. *J. Physiol. (Lond.)* 307:85, 1980.

108. Dixon, M., Jackson, D. M., and Richards, I. M. A study of the afferent and efferent nerve distribution to the lungs of dogs. *Respiration* 39:144, 1980.

109. Douglas, J. S., Ridgway, P., and Brink, C. Airway responses of the guinea pig *in vivo* and *in vitro.* J. Pharmacol. Exp. Ther. 202:116, 1977.

110. Douglas, J. S., et al. Airway dilatation and constriction in spontaneously breathing guinea pigs. *J. Pharmacol. Exp. Ther.* 180:98, 1972.

111. Douglas, J. S., et al. Airway constriction in guinea pigs: Interaction of histamine and autonomic drugs. *J. Pharmacol. Exp. Ther.* 184:169, 1973.

112. Downes, H., et al. Comparison of drug responses *in vivo* and *in vitro* in airways of dogs with and without airway hyperresponsiveness. *J. Pharmacol. Exp. Ther.* 237:214, 1986.

113. Downes, H., et al. Comparison of *in vitro* drug responses in airways of atopic dogs with and without *in vivo* hyperresponsiveness. *Pulm. Pharmacol.* 2:209, 1989.

114. Downes, H., and Hirshman, C. A. Importance of calcium in citric acid-induced airway constriction. *J. Appl. Physiol.* 55:1496, 1983.

115. Downes, H., and Taylor, S. M. Distinctive pharmacological profile of a nonadrenergic inhibitory system in bullfrog lung. *Br. J. Pharmacol.* 78:339, 1983.

116. Drazen, J. M. Pulmonary Physiologic Abnormalities in Animal Models of Acute Asthma. In L. M. Lichtenstein and K. F. Austen (eds.), *Asthma: Physiology, Immunopharmacology and Treatment.* New York: Academic, 1977. Pp. 249–264.

117. Drazen, J. M. Adrenergic influences on histamine-mediated bronchoconstriction in the guinea pig. *J. Appl. Physiol.* 44:340, 1978.

118. Drazen, J. M., and Austen, K. F. Pulmonary response to antigen infusion in the sensitized guinea pig: Modification by atropine. *J. Appl. Physiol.* 39:916, 1975.

119. Drazen, J. M., and Austen, K. F. Atropine modification of the pulmonary effects of chemical mediators in the guinea pig. *J. Appl. Physiol.* 38:834, 1975.

120. Drazen, J. M., Loring, S. H., and Venugopalan, C. Lung volumes after antigen infusion in the guinea pig *in vitro*: Effects of vagal section. *J. Appl. Physiol.* 45:957, 1978.

121. Drazen, J. M., O'Cain, C. F., and Ingram, R. H. Experimental induction of chronic bronchitis in dogs: Effects on airway obstruction and responsiveness. *Am. Rev. Respir. Dis.* 126:75, 1982.

122. Drazen, J. M., and Schneider, M. W. Comparative responses of tracheal spirals and parenchymal strips to histamine and carbachol *in vitro. J. Clin. Invest.* 61:1441, 1978.

123. Drazen, J. M., Schneider, M. W., and Venugopalan, C. S. Bronchodilator activity of dimaprit in the guinea-pig *in vitro* and *in vivo. Eur. J. Pharmacol.* 55:233, 1979.

124. Drazen, J. M., Venugopalan, C. S., and Soter, N. A. H₂-receptor mediated inhibition of immediate type hypersensitivity reactions *in vivo. Am. Rev. Respir. Dis.* 117:479, 1978.

125. Drazen, J. M., et al. Comparative airway and vascular activities of leukotrienes C-1 and D *in vivo* and *in vitro. Proc. Natl. Acad. Sci. USA* 77:4354, 1980.

126. Drazen, J. M., et al. Effects of leukotriene E on pulmonary mechanics in the guinea pig. *Am. Rev. Respir. Dis.* 125:290, 1982.

127. Dulabh, R., and Vickers, M. R. The effects of H₂-receptor antagonists on anaphylaxis in the guinea-pig. *Agents Actions* 8:559, 1978.

128. Dun, N. J., and Karczmar, A. G. Evidence for a presynaptic inhibitory action of 5-hydroxytryptamine in a mammalian sympathetic ganglion. *J. Pharmacol. Exp. Ther.* 217:714, 1981.

129. Dunnell, M. S., Massarella, G. R., and Anderson, J. A. A comparison of quantitative anatomy of the bronchi in normal subjects, in status asthmaticus, in chronic bronchitis and in emphysema. *Thorax* 24:176, 1969.

130. Dusser, D. J., et al. Virus induces airway hyperresponsiveness to tachykinins: Role of neutral endopeptidase. *J. Appl. Physiol.* 67:1504, 1989.

131. Eidelman, D. H., Bellofiore, S., and Martin, J. G. Late airway responses to antigen challenge in sensitized inbred rats. *Am. Rev. Respir. Dis.* 137:1033, 1988.

132. Eiser, N. M. Histamine antagonists and asthma. *Pharmacol Ther.* 17:239, 1982.

133. Engineer, D. M., et al. Release of mediators of anaphylaxis: Inhibition of prostaglandin synthesis and the modification of release of slow-reacting substance of anaphylaxis and histamine. *Br. J. Pharmacol.* 62:61, 1978.

134. Engineer, D. M., et al. The release of prostaglandins and thromboxanes from guinea-pig lung by slow-reacting substance of anaphylaxis, and its inhibition. *Br. J. Pharmacol.* 64:211, 1978.

135. Eyre, P. The pharmacology of sheep tracheobronchial muscle: A relaxant effect of histamine on the isolated bronchi. *Br. J. Pharmacol.* 36:409, 1969.

136. Eyre, P., and Besner, R. N. Cimetidine fails to block functional antagonism or carbachol by histamine in rat trachea. *Res. Commun. Chem. Pathol. Pharmacol.* 24:457, 1979.

137. Fabbri, L. M., et al. Airway hyperresponsiveness and changes in cell counts in bronchoalveolar lavage after ozone exposure in dogs. *Am. Rev. Respir. Dis.* 129:288, 1984.

138. Farmer, J. B., et al. Mediators of passive lung anaphylaxis in the rat. *Br. J. Pharmacol.* 55:57, 1975.

139. Featherstone, R. L., et al. Active sensitization of guinea pig airways *in vivo* enhances *in vitro* responsiveness. *Eur. Respir. J.* 1:839, 1988.

140. Fleisch, J. H., and Calkins, P. J. Comparison of drug-induced responses of rabbit trachea and bronchus. *J. Appl. Physiol.* 41:62, 1976.

141. Folkerts, G., Henricks, P. A. J., and Nijkamp, F. P. Inflammatory reactions in the respiratory airways of the guinea pig do not necessarily induce bronchial hyperreactivity. *Agents Actions* 23:94, 1988.

142. Freed, A. N., Peters, S. P., and Menkes, H. A. Airflow-induced bronchoconstriction: Role of epithelium and eicosanoid mediators. *J. Appl. Physiol.* 62:574, 1987.

143. Freed, A. N., Wang, D., and Menkes, H. A. Dry air-induced constriction: Effects of pharmacologic intervention and temperature. *J. Appl. Physiol.* 62:1794, 1987.

144. Fryer, A. D., and Jacoby, D. B. Abnormalities in neural control of smooth muscle in virus-infected airways. *Trends Pharmacol. Sci.* 11:393, 1990.

145. Fryer, A. D., and Jacoby, D. B. Parainfluenza virus infection damages inhibitory M₂ muscarinic receptors on pulmonary parasympathetic nerves in the guinea pig. *Br. J. Pharmacol.* 102:267, 1991.

146. Fryer, A. D., and Maclagan, J. Muscarinic inhibitory receptors in pulmonary parasympathetic nerves in the guinea pig. *Br. J. Pharmacol.* 83:973, 1984.

147. Fujita, M., Schroeder, M. A., and Hyatt, R. E. Canine model of chronic bronchial injury: Lung mechanics and pathologic changes. *Am. Rev. Respir. Dis.* 137:429, 1988.

148. Galant, S. P., et al. Decreased beta-adrenergic receptors on polymorphonuclear leukocytes after adrenergic therapy. *N. Engl. J. Med.* 299:933, 1978.

149. Girard, J. P., and Moret, P. Action de la serotonine et de la bradykinine en aerosols chez les asthmatiques. *Helv. Med. Acta* 30:520, 1963.

150. Gold, W. M. Experimental Models of Asthma. In M. Stein (ed.), *New Directions in Asthma.* Park Ridge, Ill.: American College of Chest Physicians, 1975. P. 241.

151. Gold, W. M., Kessler, G.-F., and Yu, D. Y. C. Role of vagus nerves in experimental asthma in allergic dogs. *J. Appl. Physiol.* 33:719, 1972.

152. Gold, W. M., et al. Pulmonary physiologic abnormalities in experimental asthma in dogs. *J. Appl. Physiol.* 33:496, 1972.

153. Gold, W. M., et al. Changes in airway mast cells and histamine caused by antigen aerosols in allergic dogs. *J. Appl. Physiol.* 43:271, 1977.

154. Goldie, R. G., Paterson, J. W., and Wale, J. L. Pharmacological responses of human and porcine lung parenchyma, bronchus and pulmonary artery. *Br. J. Pharmacol.* 76:515, 1982.

155. Goldie, R. G., et al. *In vitro* responsiveness of human asthmatic bronchus to carbachol, histamine, β-adrenoceptor agonists and aminophylline. *Br. J. Clin. Pharmacol.* 22:669, 1986.

156. Gordon, T., et al. Airway hyperresponsiveness and inflammation induced by toluene diisocyanate in guinea pigs. *Am. Rev. Respir. Dis.* 132:1106, 1985.

157. Gray, P. R., et al. The role of cyclooxygenase products in the acute airway obstruction and airway hyperreactivity of ponies with heaves. *Am. Rev. Respir. Dis.* 140:154, 1989.

158. Greenberg, R., Antonaccio, M. J., and Steinbacher, T. Thromboxane A₂ mediated bronchoconstriction in the anesthetized guinea pig. *Eur. J. Pharmacol.* 80:19, 1982.

159. Greenberger, P., Harris, K., and Patterson, R. The effect of histamine-1 and histamine-2 antagonists on airway responses to histamine in the rhesus monkey. *J. Allergy Clin. Immunol.* 64:189, 1979.

160. Greive, S. R., Chan, S. C., and Hanifin, J. M. Elevated leukocyte cAMP-phosphodiesterase in atopic disease: A possible mechanism for cAMP agonist hyporesponsiveness. *J. Allergy Clin. Immunol.* 70:452, 1982.

161. Habib, M. P., Pare, P. D., and Engel, L. A. Variability of airway responses to inhaled histamine in normal subjects. *J. Appl. Physiol.* 47:51, 1979.

162. Hahn, H. L., et al. Interaction between serotonin and efferent vagus nerves in dog lungs. *J. Appl. Physiol.* 44:144, 1978.

163. Hajos, M. K. Clinical studies on the role of serotonin in bronchial asthma. *Acta Allergol.* 17:358, 1962.

164. Hamberg, M., et al. Prostaglandin endoperoxides: IV. Effects on smooth muscle. *Life Sci.* 16:451, 1975.

165. Hamberg, M., et al. Involvement of endoperoxides and thromboxanes in anaphylactic reactions. *Adv. Prostaglandin Thromboxane Res.* 1:495, 1976.

166. Hamel, R., and Ford-Hutchinson, A. W. Pulmonary and cardiovascular changes in hyperreactive rats from citric acid aerosols. *J. Appl. Physiol.* 59:354, 1985.

167. Hanna, C. J., and Roth, S. H. The guinea pig tracheobronchial spiral strip: Responses to selected agonists. *Can. J. Physiol. Pharmacol.* 56:823, 1978.

168. Hasegawa, M., and Townley, R. G. Difference between lung and spleen susceptibility of beta-adrenergic receptors to desensitization by terbutaline. *J. Allergy Clin. Immunol.* 71:230, 1983.

169. Hedman, S. E., and Andersson, R. G. G. The cyclic AMP system in sensitized and desensitized guinea-pig tracheal smooth muscle. *Eur. J. Pharmacol.* 83:107, 1982.

170. Hedqvist, P., Strandberg, K., and Hamberg, M. Bronchial and cardiovascular actions of prostaglandin endoperoxides and an endoperoxide analogue. *Acta Physiol. Scand.* 103:299, 1978.

171. Herxheimer, H. Bronchial obstruction induced by allergens, histamine and acetyl-beta-methylcholinechloride. *Int. Arch. Allergy Appl. Immunol.* 2:27, 1951.

172. Herxheimer, H. Repeatable 'microshocks' of constant strength in guinea pig anaphylaxis. *J. Physiol. (Lond.)* 117:251, 1952.

173. Herxheimer, H. The protective action of antihistaminic and sympathomimetic aerosols in anaphylactic microshock of the guinea pig. *Br. J. Pharmacol.* 8:461, 1953.

174. Herxheimer, H. Further observations on the influence of 5-hydroxytryptamine on bronchial function. *J. Physiol. (Lond.)* 122:49, 1953.

175. Herxheimer, H. The 5-hydroxytryptamine shock in the guinea pig. *J. Physiol. (Lond.)* 128:435, 1955.

176. Hinson, J. M., et al. Effects of granulocyte depletion on pulmonary responsiveness to aerosol histamine. *J. Appl. Physiol.* 56:411, 1984.

177. Hinson, J. M., et al. Effect of granulocyte depletion on altered lung mechanics after endotoxemia in sheep. *J. Appl. Physiol.* 55:92, 1983.

178. Hinson, J. M., et al. Role of circulating granulocytes in pulmonary responsiveness to aerosol histamine in the awake sheep. *Physiologist* 25:331, 1982.

179. Hirai, K., and Koketsu, K. Presynaptic regulation of the release of acetylcholine by 5-hydroxytryptamine. *Br. J. Pharmacol.* 70:499, 1980.

180. Hirshman, C. A., et al. Increased metachromatic cells and lymphocytes in bronchoalveolar lavage fluid of dogs with airway hyperreactivity. *Am. Rev. Respir. Dis.* 133:482, 1986.

181. Hirshman, C. A., and Downes, H. The basenji-greyhound dog model of asthma: Influence of atropine on antigen-induced bronchoconstriction. *J. Appl. Physiol.* 50:761, 1981.

182. Hirshman, C. A., and Downes, H. Airway responses to methacholine and histamine in basenji-greyhound and other purebred dogs. *Respir. Physiol.* 63:339, 1986.

183. Hirshman, C. A., et al. The basenji-greyhound dog model of asthma: Pulmonary responses after β-adrenergic blockade. *J. Appl. Physiol.* 51:1423, 1981.

184. Hirshman, C. A., Downes, H., and Veith, L. Airway responses in offspring of dogs with and without airway hyperreactivity. *J. Appl. Physiol.* 56:1272, 1984.

185. Hirshman, C. A., Leon, D. A., and Bergman, N. A. The basenji-greyhound dog: Antigen-induced changes in lung volume. *Respir. Physiol.* 43:377, 1981.

186. Hirshman, C. A., et al. Elevated mononuclear leukocyte phosphodiesterase in allergic dogs with and without airway hyperresponsiveness. *J. Allergy Clin. Immunol.* 79:46, 1987.

187. Hirshman, C. A., Malley, A., and Downes, H. The basenji-greyhound dog model of asthma: Reactivity to *Ascaris suum*, citric acid and methacholine. *J. Appl. Physiol.* 49:953, 1980.

188. Hirshman, C. A., et al. Role of mediators in allergic and nonallergic asthma in dogs with hyperreactive airways. *J. Appl. Physiol.* 54:1108, 1983.

189. Hirshman, C. A., et al. Citric acid airway constriction in dogs with hyperreactive airways. *J. Appl. Physiol.* 54:1101, 1983.

190. Hirshman, C. A., et al. Airway constrictor effects of leukotriene D_4 in dogs with hyperreactive airways. *Prostaglandins* 25:481, 1983.

191. Holgate, J. A., and Warner, B. T. Evaluation of antagonists of histamine, 5-hydroxytryptamine and acetylcholine in the guinea-pig. *Br. J. Pharmacol.* 15:561, 1960.

192. Holme, G., and Piechuta, H. The derivation of an inbred line of rats which develop asthma-like symptoms following challenge with aerosolized antigen. *Immunology* 42:19, 1981.

193. Holroyde, M. C., Smith, S. Y., and Holme, G. Evaluation of pulmonary mechanics in guinea pigs during respiratory anaphylaxis. *J. Pharmacol. Exp. Ther.* 212:162, 1980.

194. Holroyde, M. C., Smith, S. Y., and Holme, G. Analysis of antigen-induced changes in pulmonary mechanics in sensitized inbred rats. *Can. J. Physiol. Pharmacol.* 60:644, 1982.

195. Holroyde, M. C., et al. Bronchoconstriction produced in man by leukotrienes C and D. *Lancet* 2:17, 1981.

196. Holtzman, M. J., et al. Importance of airway inflammation for hyperresponsiveness induced by ozone. *Am. Rev. Respir. Dis.* 127:686, 1983.

197. Holtzman, M. J., et al. Time course of airway hyperresponsiveness induced by ozone in dogs. *J. Appl. Physiol.* 55:1232, 1983.

198. Hulbert, W. M., McLean, T., and Hogg, J. C. The effect of acute airway inflammation on bronchial reactivity in guinea pigs. *Am. Rev. Respir. Dis.* 132:7, 1985.

199. Hutas, I., et al. Relaxation of human isolated bronchial smooth muscle. *Lung* 159:153, 1981.

200. Hutchison, A. A., Brigham, K. L., and Snapper, J. R. Effect of histamine on lung mechanics in sheep: Comparison of aerosol and parenteral administration. *Am. Rev. Respir. Dis.* 126:1025, 1982.

201. Hutchison, A. A., et al. Effect of endotoxin on airway responsiveness to aerosol histamine in sheep. *J. Appl. Physiol.* 54:1463, 1983.

202. Hutson, P. A., et al. Early and late-phase bronchoconstriction after allergen challenge of nonanesthetized guinea pigs. *Am. Rev. Respir. Dis.* 137:548, 1988.

203. Hutson, P. A., Holgate, S. T., and Church, M. K. The effect of cromolyn sodium and albuterol on early and late phase bronchoconstriction and airway leukocyte infiltration after allergen challenge of nonanesthetized guinea pigs. *Am. Rev. Respir. Dis.* 138:1157, 1988.

204. Hyman, A. L., et al. Prostaglandins and the lung. *Med. Clin. North Am.* 65:789, 1981.

205. Iijima, H., et al. Bronchoalveolar lavage and histologic characterization of late asthmatic response in guinea pigs. *Am. Rev. Respir. Dis.* 136:922, 1987.

206. Irvin, C. G., Berend, N., and Henson, P. M. Airway hyperreactivity and inflammation produced by aerosolization of human C5A desarg. *Am. Rev. Respir. Dis.* 134:777, 1986.

207. Irvin, C. G., et al. Bronchodilation: Noncholinergic nonadrenergic mediation demonstrated *in vivo* in the cat. *Science* 207:791, 1980.

208. Islam, M. S., Melville, G. N., and Ulmer, W. T. Role of atropine in antagonizing the effect of 5-hydroxytryptamine (5-HT) on bronchial and pulmonary vascular systems. *Respiration* 31:47, 1974.

209. Itkin, I. H. Bronchial hypersensitivity to mecholyl and histamine in asthma subjects. *J. Allergy* 40:245, 1967.

210. Itkin, I. H., and Anand, S. C. The role of atropine as a mediator blocker of induced bronchial obstruction. *J. Allergy* 45:178, 1970.

211. Ito, Y., and Tajima, K. Spontaneous activity in the trachea of dogs treated with indomethacin: An experimental model for aspirin-related asthma. *Br. J. Pharmacol.* 73:563, 1981.

212. Ito, Y., and Tajima, K. Actions of indomethacin and prostaglandins on neuro-effector transmissions in the dog trachea. *J. Physiol. (Lond.)* 319:379, 1981.

213. Ito, Y., and Tajima, K. Dual effects of catecholamines on pre- and postjunctional membranes in the dog trachea. *Br. J. Pharmacol.* 75:433, 1982.

214. Jackson, D. M., and Richards, I. M. The effects of pentobarbitone and chloralose anaesthesia on the vagal component of bronchoconstriction produced by histamine aerosol in the anaesthetized dog. *Br. J. Pharmacol.* 61:251, 1977.

215. Jacoby, D. B., et al. Influenza infection causes airway hyperresponsiveness by decreasing enkephalinase. *J. Appl. Physiol.* 64:2653, 1988.

216. Jammes, Y. P., Barthelemy, P., and Delpierre, S. Respiratory effects of cold air breathing in anesthetized cats. *Respir. Physiol.* 54:41, 1983.

217. Jammes, Y. P., et al. Cold air-induced bronchospasm in normal and sensitized rabbits. *Respir. Physiol.* 63:347, 1986.

218. Johanson, W. G., and Pierce, A. K. A noninvasive technique for measurement of airway conductance in small animals. *J. Appl. Physiol.* 30:146, 1971.

219. Johansson, S. G. O., and Foucard, T. IgE in Immunity and Disease. In E. Middleton, C. E. Reed, and E. T. Ellis (eds.), *Allergy: Principles and Practice*, Vol. 2. St. Louis: Mosby, 1978. P. 551.

220. Johns, K., et al. Contribution of upper airways to antigen-induced late airway obstructive responses in guinea pigs. *Am. Rev. Respir. Dis.* 142:138, 1990.

221. Jones, C. A., et al. Muscarinic cholinergic inhibition of adenylate cyclase in airway smooth muscle. *Am. J. Physiol.* 253:C97, 1987.

222. Kamburoff, P. L., Griffin, J. P., and Bianco, S. The use of histamine induced bronchoconstriction as a method for investigating bronchodilator drugs. *Br. J. Dis. Chest* 66:21, 1972.

223. Karlsson, J.-A., Zackrisson, C., and Erjefält, J. Effects of histamine and citric acid in guinea pigs with immediate and late bronchoconstrictor responses to *Ascaris* serum. *Am. Rev. Respir. Dis.* 139:A463, 1989.

224. Kaukel, E., et al. Mechanical and biochemical alterations in guinea pig tracheae caused by sensitization. *Respiration* 45:255, 1984.

225. Kaukel, E., and Rieckenberg, B. Partial beta-adrenergic receptor blockade in experimental bronchial asthma. *Biochem. Biophys. Res. Commun.* 96: 1626, 1980.

226. Kenakin, T. P., and Beek, D. A quantitative analysis of histamine H_2-receptor-mediated relaxation of rabbit trachea. *J. Pharmacol. Exp. Ther.* 220:353, 1982.

227. Kepron, W., et al. A canine model for reaginic hypersensitivity and allergic bronchoconstriction. *J. Allergy Clin. Immunol.* 59:64, 1977.

228. Kessler, G. F., Frick, O. L., and Gold, W. M. Immunologic and physiologic characterization of the role of reaginic antibodies in experimental asthma in dogs. *Int. Arch. Allergy Appl. Immunol.* 47:313, 1974.

229. Kessler, G. F., et al. Airway constriction in experimental asthma in dogs: Tantalum bronchographic studies. *J. Appl. Physiol.* 35:703, 1973.

230. Kleeberger, S. R., et al. Central role of cyclooxygenase in the response of canine lung peripheral airways to antigen. *J. Appl. Physiol.* 61:1309, 1986.

231. Kleeberger, S. R., et al. Thromboxane contributes to the immediate antigenic response of canine peripheral airways. *J. Appl. Physiol.* 62:1589, 1987.

232. Kleinstiver, P. W., and Eyre, P. The lung parenchyma strip preparation of the cat and dog: Responses to anaphylactic mediators and sympathetic bronchodilators. *Res. Commun. Chem. Pathol. Pharmacol.* 27:451, 1980.

233. Kneussl, M. P., and Richardson, J. B. Alpha-adrenergic receptors in human and canine tracheal and bronchial smooth muscle. *J. Appl. Physiol.* 45:307, 1978.

234. Koeter, G. H., et al. The role of the adrenergic system in allergy and bronchial hyperreactivity. *Eur. J. Respir. Dis.* 63(Suppl.):72, 1982.

235. Konzett, H. The effects of 5-hydroxytryptamine and its antagonists on tidal air. *Br. J. Pharmacol.* 11:289, 1956.

236. Krell, R. D. Airway hyperreactivity to pharmacologic agents in rhesus monkeys cutaneously hypersensitive to *Ascaris* antigen. *Life Sci.* 19:1777, 1976.

237. Krell, R. D. Investigation of the role of histamine in antigen-induced bronchoconstriction in *Ascaris*-hypersensitive dogs. *Br. J. Pharmacol.* 62:519, 1978.

238. Krell, R. D. Pharmacologic characterization of isolated canine bronchial smooth muscle. *Eur. J. Pharmacol.* 49:151, 1978.

239. Krell, R. D., and Chakrin, L. W. Canine airway responses to acetylcholine, prostaglandin $F_{2\alpha}$, histamine, and serotonin after chronic antigen exposure. *J. Allergy Clin. Immunol.* 58:664, 1976.

240. Krell, R. D., and Chakrin, L. W. The effect of metiamide in *in vitro* and *in vivo* canine models of Type 1 hypersensitivity reactions. *Eur. J. Pharmacol.* 44:35, 1977.

241. Krell, R. D., Charkrin, L. W., and Wardell, J. R. The effect of cholinergic agents on a canine model of allergic asthma. *J. Allergy Clin. Immunol.* 58:19, 1976.

242. Laitinen, L. A., et al. Damage of the airway epithelium and bronchial reactivity in patients with asthma. *Am. Rev. Respir. Dis.* 131:599, 1985.

243. Laitinen, L. A., et al. Effects of intravenous histamine on static lung compliance and airway resistance in normal man. *Am. Rev. Respir. Dis.* 114: 291, 1976.

244. Lanes, S., et al. Effects of Budesonide on Late Bronchial Response and the Associated Airway Hyperresponsiveness in Allergic Sheep. In J. C. Hogg, R. Ellul-Micallef, and R. Brattsand (eds.), *Glucocorticosteroids, Inflammation and Bronchial Hyperreactivity.* New York: Excerpta Medica, 1985. Pp. 38–50.

245. Lanes, S., et al. Indomethacin and FPL-57231 inhibit antigen-induced airway hyperresponsiveness in sheep. *J. Appl. Physiol.* 61:864, 1986.

246. Larsen, G. L., et al. The inflammatory reaction in the airways in an animal model of the late asthmatic response. *Fed. Proc.* 46:105, 1987.

247. Leff, A. R. Pathogenesis of asthma: Neurophysiology and pharmacology of bronchospasm. *Chest* 81:224, 1982.

248. Leff, A. R., and Munoz, N. M. Evidence for two subtypes of alpha-adrenergic receptors in canine airway smooth muscle. *J. Pharmacol. Exp. Ther.* 217:530, 1981.

249. Leff, A. R., and Munoz, N. M. Selective autonomic stimulation of canine trachealis with dimethylphenyl piperazinium. *J. Appl. Physiol.* 51:428, 1981.

250. Leff, A. R., and Munoz, N. M. Interrelationship between alpha and beta-adrenergic agonists and histamine in canine airways. *J. Allergy Clin. Immunol.* 68:300, 1981.

251. Leff, A. R., Munoz, N. M., and Hendrix, S. G. Sympathetic inhibition of histamine-induced contraction of canine trachealis *in vivo. J. Appl. Physiol.* 53:21, 1982.

252. Levitt, R. C., and Mitzner, W. Expression of airway hyperreactivity to acetylcholine as a simple autosomal recessive trait in mice. *FASEB J.* 2: 2605, 1988.

253. Levitt, R. C., and Mitzner, W. Autosomal recessive inheritance of airway hyperreactivity to 5-hydroxytryptamine. *J. Appl. Physiol.* 67:1125, 1989.

254. Levitt, R. C., Mitzner, W., and Kleeberger, S. R. A genetic approach to the study of lung physiology: Understanding biological variability in airway responsiveness. *Am. J. Physiol.* 258:L157, 1990.

255. Lewis, A. J., et al. *Ascaris*-induced allergic asthma in the conscious dog: A model for the pharmacologic modulation of immediate type hypersensitivity. *J. Pharmacol. Methods* 7:35, 1982.

256. Lichtenstein, L. M., and Gillespie, E. Inhibition of histamine release by histamine controlled by H_2-receptor. *Nature* 224:287, 1973.

257. Logsdon, P. J., Middleton, E., and Coffrey, R. G. Stimulation of lymphocyte adenylyl cyclase by hydrocortisone and isoproterenol in asthmatic and nonasthmatic subjects. *J. Allergy Clin. Immunol.* 50:45, 1972.

258. Longcope, W. T. Insusceptibility to sensitization and anaphylactic shock. *J. Exp. Med.* 36:627, 1922.

259. Loring, S. H., Drazen, J. M., and Ingram, R. H. Canine pulmonary response to aerosol histamine: Direct versus vagal effects. *J. Appl. Physiol.* 42:946, 1977.

260. Loring, S. H., et al. Vagal and aerosol histamine interactions on airway responses in dogs. *J. Appl. Physiol.* 45:40, 1978.

261. Lowell, F. C. Observations on heaves: An asthma-like syndrome in the horse. *J. Allergy* 35:322, 1964.

262. Lulich, K. M., and Paterson, J. W. An *in vitro* study of various drugs on central and peripheral airways of the rat: A comparison with human airways. *Br. J. Pharmacol.* 68:633, 1980.

263. Maengwyn-Davies, G. D. The dual mode of action of histamine in the cat isolated tracheal chain. *J. Pharm. Pharmacol.* 20:572, 1968.

264. Malkiel, S., and Hargis, B. J. Histamine sensitivity and anaphylaxis in the pertussis-vaccinated rat. *Proc. Soc. Exp. Biol. Med.* 81:689, 1952.

265. Manzini, S., et al. Capsaicin desensitization protects from antigen-induced bronchospasm in conscious guinea-pigs. *Eur. J. Pharmacol.* 138: 307, 1987.

266. Mapp, C., et al. Airway responsiveness to inhaled antigen, histamine, and methacholine in inbred, ragweed-sensitized dogs. *Am. Rev. Respir. Dis.* 132:292, 1985.

267. Marcelle, R., et al. Evaluation de l'activite bronchomotrice de la 5-hydroxytryptamine (5HT) chez les sujets normaux et asthmatiques. *Acta Allergol.* 23:1, 1968.

268. Marsh, W. R., et al. Increases in airway reactivity to histamine and inflammatory cells in bronchoalveolar lavage after the late asthmatic response in an animal model. *Am. Rev. Respir. Dis.* 131:875, 1985.

269. Martin, T. R., et al. Pulmonary responses to bronchoconstrictor agonists in the mouse. *J. Appl. Physiol.* 64:2318, 1988.

270. Martling, C.-R., et al. Capsaicin pretreatment inhibits vagal cholinergic and non-cholinergic control of pulmonary mechanics in the guinea pig. *Naunyn Schmiedebergs Arch. Pharmacol.* 325:343, 1984.

271. Mathé, A. A., Astrom, A., and Persson, N. A. Some bronchoconstricting and bronchodilating responses of human isolated bronchi: Evidence for the existence of α-adrenoceptors. *J. Pharm. Pharmacol.* 23:905, 1971.

272. Mathé, A. A., and Hedqvist, P. Effect of prostaglandin $F_{2\alpha}$ on airway conductance in healthy subjects and asthmatic patients. *Am. Rev. Respir. Dis.* 111:313, 1975.

273. McPherson, E. A., et al. Chronic obstructive pulmonary disease (COPD) in horses: Aetiological studies; responses to intradermal and inhalation antigenic challenge. *Equine Vet. J.* 11:159, 1979.

274. Menkes, H. A., and Traystman, R. J. Collateral ventilation. *Am. Rev. Respir. Dis.* 116:287, 1977.

275. Meurs, H., et al. The beta-adrenergic system and allergic bronchial asthma: Changes in lymphocyte beta-adrenergic number and adenylate cyclase activity after an allergen asthmatic attack. *J. Allergy Clin. Immunol.* 70:272, 1982.

276. Meyrick, B., and Brigham, K. L. Acute effects of E. coli endotoxin on the pulmonary microcirculation of anesthetized sheep: Structure-function relationships. *Lab. Invest.* 48:458, 1983.

277. Mezey, R. J., et al. Mucociliary transport in allergic patients with antigen-induced bronchospasm. *Am. Rev. Respir. Dis.* 118:677, 1978.

278. Michoud, M.-C., et al. Effect of indomethacin and atropine in experimental asthma in conscious guinea pigs. *J. Appl. Physiol.* 40:889, 1976.

279. Michoud, M.-C., et al. Airway responses to histamine and methacholine in *Ascaris suum*-allergic rhesus monkeys. *J. Appl. Physiol.* 45:846, 1978.

280. Middendorf, W. F., and Russell, J. A. Innervation of airway smooth muscle in the baboon: Evidence for a nonadrenergic inhibitory system. *J. Appl. Physiol.* 48:947, 1980.

281. Miller, M. M., Patterson, R., and Harris, K. E. A comparison of immunologic asthma to two types of cholinergic respiratory responses in the rhesus monkey. *J. Lab. Clin. Med.* 88:995, 1976.

282. Mills, J. E., and Widdicombe, J. G. Role of the vagus nerves in anaphylaxis and histamine-induced bronchoconstriction in guinea-pigs. *Br. J. Pharmacol.* 39:724, 1970.

283. Mirbahar, K. B., and Eyre, P. Autacoid and autonomic reactivity of bovine and ovine bronchus: Modifications by antigenic sensitization. *Arch. Int. Pharmacodyn. Ther.* 258:60, 1982.

284. Mitchell, H. W., and Denborough, M. A. The metabolism of arachidonic acid in the isolated tracheal and lung strip preparations of guinea-pigs. *Lung* 158:121, 1980.

285. Mortola, J., Santambrogio, G., and Clement, M. G. Localization of irritant receptors in the airways of the dog. *Respir. Physiol.* 24:107, 1975.

286. Mota, I. The mechanism of anaphylaxis: I. Production and biological properties of 'mast cell sensitizing' antibody. *Immunology* 7:681, 1964.

287. Murlas, C. G., and Roum, J. H. Sequence of pathologic changes in the airway mucosa of guinea pigs during ozone-induced bronchial hyperreactivity. *Am. Rev. Respir. Dis.* 131:314, 1985.

288. Murlas, C. G., and Roum, J. H. Bronchial hyperreactivity occurs in steroid-treated guinea pigs depleted of leukocytes by cyclophosphamide. *J. Appl. Physiol.* 58:1630, 1985.

289. Murphy, K. R., et al. The requirement for polymorphonuclear leukocytes in the late asthmatic response and heightened airway reactivity in an animal model. *Am. Rev. Respir. Dis.* 134:62, 1986.

290. Nadel, J. A., et al. Mechanism of bronchoconstriction during inhalation of sulfur dioxide. *J. Appl. Physiol.* 20:164, 1965.

291. Nathan, R. A., et al. The effects of H_1 and H_2 antihistamines on histamine inhalation challenges in asthmatic patients. *Am. Rev. Respir. Dis.* 120; 1251, 1979.

292. Nisam, M. R., et al. Distribution and pharmacological release of histamine in canine lung *in vivo*. *J. Appl. Physiol.* 44:455, 1978.

293. Nishikawa, M., et al. Acute exposure to cigarette smoke induces airway hyperresponsiveness without airway inflammation in guinea pigs. *Am. Rev. Respir. Dis.* 142:177, 1990.

294. O'Byrne, P. M., Dolovich, J., and Hargreave, F. E. Late asthmatic responses. *Am. Rev. Respir. Dis.* 136:740, 1987.

295. O'Byrne, P. M., et al. Indomethacin inhibits the airway hyperresponsiveness but not the neutrophil influx by ozone in dogs. *Am. Rev. Respir. Dis.* 130:220, 1984.

296. O'Byrne, P. M., et al. Neutrophil depletion inhibits airway hyperresponsiveness induced by ozone exposure. *Am. Rev. Respir. Dis.* 130:214, 1984.

297. Ogilvie, B. M. Reagin-like antibodies in rats infected with the nematode parasite *Nippostrongylus brasiliensis*. *Immunology* 12:113, 1967.

298. Ogletree, M. L., Snapper, J. R., and Brigham, K. L. Immediate pulmonary vascular and airway responses after intravenous leukotriene (LT) D$_4$ injections in awake sheep. *Physiologist* 25:275, 1982.

299. Orehek, J., Douglas, J. S., and Bouhuys, A. Contractile responses of the guinea-pig trachea *in vitro*: Modification by prostaglandin synthesis-inhibiting drugs. *J. Pharmacol. Exp. Ther.* 194:554, 1975.

300. Orehek, J., et al. Prostaglandin regulation of airway smooth muscle tone. *Nature New Biol.* 245:84, 1973.

301. Palmer, M. A., Piper, P. J., and Vane, J. R. Release of rabbit aorta contracting substance (RCS) and prostaglandins induced by chemical or mechanical stimulation of guinea pig lungs. *Br. J. Pharmacol.* 49:226, 1973.

302. Panzani, R. 5-Hydroxytryptamine (serotonin) in human bronchial asthma. *Ann. Allergy* 20:271, 1962.

303. Pare, P. D., Michoud, M. C., and Hogg, J. C. Lung mechanics following antigen challenge of *Ascaris suum*-sensitive rhesus monkeys. *J. Appl. Physiol.* 41:668, 1976.

304. Pare, P. D., et al. Pulmonary effects of acute and chronic antigen exposure of immunized guinea pigs. *J. Appl. Physiol.* 46:346, 1979.

305. Patterson, R. Investigation of spontaneous hypersensitivity of the dog. *J. Allergy* 31:351, 1960.

306. Patterson, R., et al. Airway responses to sequential challenges with platelet activating factor and leukotriene D$_4$ in rhesus monkeys. *J. Lab. Clin. Med.* 104:340, 1984.

307. Patterson, R., and Harris, K. E. The effect of cholinergic and anticholinergic agents on the primate model of allergic asthma. *J. Lab. Clin. Med.* 87:65, 1976.

308. Patterson, R., and Harris, K. E. The activity of aerosolized and intracutaneous synthetic platelet activating factor (AGEPC) in rhesus monkeys with IgE mediated airway responses and normal monkeys. *J. Lab. Clin. Med.* 102:933, 1983.

309. Patterson, R., Harris, K. E., and Greenberger, P. A. The effect of arachidonic acid on airway responses of rhesus monkeys. *Life Sci.* 22:389, 1978.

310. Patterson, R., Harris, K. E., and Greenberger, P. A. Effect of prostaglandin D$_2$ and I$_2$ on the airways of rhesus monkeys. *J. Allergy Clin. Immunol.* 65: 269, 1980.

311. Patterson, R., Harris, K. E., and Krell, R. D. Effect of a leukotriene D$_4$ (LTD$_4$) antagonist on LTD$_4$ and *Ascaris* antigen-induced airway response in rhesus monkeys. *Int. Arch. Allergy Appl. Immunol.* 86:440, 1988.

312. Patterson, R., and Kelly, J. F. Animal models of the asthmatic state. *Annu. Rev. Med.* 25:53, 1974.

313. Patterson, R., Pruzansky, J. J., and Chang, W. W. Y. Spontaneous canine hypersensitivity to ragweed: Characterization of the serum factor transferring skin, bronchial and anaphylactic sensitivity. *J. Immunol.* 90:35, 1963.

314. Patterson, R., Pruzansky, J. J., and Harris, K. E. An agent that releases basophil and mast cell histamine but blocks cyclooxygenase and lipoxygenase metabolism of arachidonic acid inhibits immunoglobulin E-mediated asthma in rhesus monkeys. *J. Allergy Clin. Immunol.* 67:444, 1981.

315. Patterson, R., Roberts, M., and Pruzansky, J. J. Comparisons of reaginic antibodies from three species. *J. Immunol.* 102:466, 1969.

316. Patterson, R., Suszko, I. M., and Harris, K. E. The *in vivo* transfer of antigen-induced airway reactions by bronchial lumen cells. *J. Clin. Invest.* 62:519, 1978.

317. Patterson, R., and Talbot, C. H. Respiratory responses in sub-human primates with immediate type hypersensitivity. *J. Lab. Clin. Med.* 73:924, 1969.

318. Patterson, R., et al. Airway responses of dogs with ragweed and *Ascaris* hypersensitivity. *Chest* 65:488, 1974.

319. Patterson, R., et al. Reagin-mediated asthma in rhesus monkeys and relation to bronchial cell histamine release and airway reactivity to carbacholine. *J. Clin. Invest.* 57:586, 1976.

320. Pauwels, R., Pelman, R., and Van Der Straeten, M. Airway inflammation and non-allergic bronchial responsiveness. *Eur. J. Respir. Dis.* 68(Suppl.144):137, 1986.

321. Pegelow, K.-O. Bronchial reactivity to inhaled histamine in asthmatic patients before and after administration of atropine, phentolamine or disodium cromoglycate. *Acta Allergol.* 29:365, 1974.

322. Pennock, B. E., et al. A noninvasive technique for measurement of changes in specific airway resistance. *J. Appl. Physiol.* 46:399, 1979.

323. Peters, J. E., Hirshman, C. A., and Malley, A. The basenji-greyhound dog model of asthma: Leukocyte histamine release, serum IgE, and airway response to inhaled antigen. *J. Immunol.* 129:1245, 1982.

324. Piechuta, H., et al. The respiratory response of sensitized rats to challenge with antigen aerosols. *Immunology* 38:385, 1979.

325. Piper, P. J. Pharmacology and biochemistry of the leukotrienes. *Eur. J. Respir. Dis.* 63(Suppl. 122):54, 1982.

326. Piper, P. J., and Samhoun, M. N. The mechanism of action of leukotrienes C$_4$ and D$_4$ in guinea-pig isolated perfused lung and parenchymal strips of guinea pig, rabbit, and rat. *Prostaglandins* 21:793, 1981.

327. Piper, P. J., and Vane, J. R. Release of additional factors in anaphylaxis and its antagonism by anti-inflammatory drugs. *Nature* 223:29, 1969.

328. Piper, P. J., and Walker, J. L. The release of spasmogenic substances from human chopped lung tissue and its inhibition. *Br. J. Pharmacol.* 47:291, 1973.

329. Popa, V., Douglas, J. S., and Bouhuys, A. Airway responses to histamine, acetylcholine, and antigen in sensitized guinea pigs. *J. Lab. Clin. Med.* 84:225, 1974.

330. Popa, V., Douglas, J. S., and Bouhuys, A. Airway response to histamine, acetylcholine, and propranolol in anaphylactic hypersensitivity in guinea pigs. *J. Allergy Clin. Immunol.* 51:344, 1973.

331. Quan, S. F., Moon, M. A., and Lemen, R. J. Effects of arachidonic acid, PGF$_{2\alpha}$ and a PGH$_2$ analogue on airway diameters in dogs. *J. Appl. Physiol.* 53:1005, 1982.

332. Rahamimoff, R., and Bruderman, I. Changes in pulmonary mechanics induced by melatonin. *Life Sci.* 4:1383, 1965.

333. Ramsdell, J. W., and Georghiou, P. F. Prolonged methacholine-induced bronchoconstriction in dogs. *J. Appl. Physiol.* 47:418, 1979.

334. Ray, D. W., et al. Tachykinins mediate bronchoconstriction elicited by isocapnic hyperpnea in guinea pigs. *J. Appl. Physiol.* 66:1108, 1989.

335. Ray, D. W., et al. Bronchoconstriction elicited by isocapnic hyperpnea in guinea pigs. *J. Appl. Physiol.* 65:934, 1988.

336. Reed, C. E., Busse, W. W., and Lee, T. P. Adrenergic mechanisms and the adenyl cyclase system in atopic dermatitis. *J. Invest. Dermatol.* 67:333, 1976.

337. Richardson, J., and Beland, J. Nonadrenergic inhibitory nervous system in human airways. *J. Appl. Physiol.* 41:764, 1976.

338. Richardson, J. B., and Bouchard, T. Demonstration of a nonadrenergic inhibitory nervous system in the trachea of the guinea pig. *J. Allergy Clin. Immunol.* 56:473, 1975.

339. Rinard, G. A., and Jenson, A. Preparation of hormone-sensitive airway smooth muscle adenylate cyclase from dissociated canine trachealis cells. *Biochim. Biophys. Acta* 678:207, 1981.

340. Rinard, G. A., et al. Depressed cyclic AMP levels in airway smooth muscle from asthmatic dogs. *Proc. Natl. Acad. Sci. USA* 76:1472, 1979.

341. Robertson, D. G., et al. Late asthmatic responses induced by ragweed pollen allergen. *J. Allergy Clin. Immunol.* 54:244, 1974.

342. Robinson, E. H., et al. Isoproterenol and electrically stimulated relaxation of airways from horses with recurrent obstructive pulmonary disease. *Physiologist* 32:179, 1989.

343. Roffel, A. D., et al. Muscarinic M_2 receptors in bovine tracheal smooth muscle: Discrepancies between binding and function. *Eur. J. Pharmacol.* 153:73, 1988.

344. Rossoni, G., et al. Bronchoconstriction by histamine and bradykinin in guinea pigs: Relationship to thromboxane A_2 generation and the effect of aspirin. *Prostaglandins* 20:547, 1980.

345. Rubinfeld, A. R., Rinard, G. A., and Mayer, S. E. Responsiveness of isolated tracheal smooth muscle in a canine model of asthma. *Lung* 160:99, 1982.

346. Rubinfeld, A. R., Wagner, P. D., and West, J. B. Gas exchange during acute experimental canine asthma. *Am. Rev. Respir. Dis.* 118:525, 1978.

347. Rudolf, M., et al. Arterial blood gas tensions in acute severe asthma. *Eur. J. Clin. Invest.* 10:55, 1980.

348. Russell, J. A. Responses of isolated canine airways to electric stimulation and acetylcholine. *J. Appl. Physiol.* 45:690, 1978.

349. Russell, J. A. Nonadrenergic inhibitory innervation of canine airways. *J. Appl. Physiol.* 48:16, 1980.

350. Russell, J. A., and Lai-Fook, S. J. Reflex bronchoconstriction induced by capsaicin in the dog. *J. Appl. Physiol.* 47:961, 1979.

351. Saban, R., et al. Enhancement by parainfluenza 3 infection of contractile responses to substance P and capsaicin in airway smooth muscle from the guinea pig. *Am. Rev. Respir. Dis.* 136:586, 1987.

352. Sadavongvivad, C. Pharmacological significance of biogenic amines in the lung: 5-Hydroxytryptamine. *Br. J. Pharmacol.* 38:353, 1970.

353. Sampson, S. R., and Vidruk, E. H. Properties of 'irritant' receptors in canine lung. *Respir. Physiol.* 25:9, 1975.

354. Sankary, R. M., et al. Muscarinic cholinergic inhibition of cyclic AMP accumulation in airway smooth muscle: Role of a pertussis-sensitive protein. *Am. Rev. Respir. Dis.* 138:145, 1988.

355. Sanyal, R. K., and West, G. B. Anaphylactic shock in the albino rat. *J. Physiol. (Lond.)* 142:571, 1958.

356. Sasaki, H., et al. Late asthmatic response to *Ascaris* antigen challenge in dogs treated with metyrapone. *Am. Rev. Respir. Dis.* 136:1459, 1987.

357. Schneider, M. W., and Drazen, J. M. Comparative *in vitro* effects of arachidonic acid metabolites on tracheal spirals and parenchymal strips. *Am. Rev. Respir. Dis.* 121:835, 1980.

358. Schnizer, W., Hoang, N. D., and Brecht, K. Transmitter in der Froschlunge. *Pflugers Arch.* 304:271, 1968.

359. Schulman, E. S., et al. Anaphylactic release of prostaglandins, thromboxane A_2 and prostacyclin from human lung. *Fed. Proc.* 39:444, 1980.

360. Schwartzman, R. M., Rockey, J. H., and Halliwell, R. E. Canine reaginic antibody characterization of spontaneous anti-ragweed and induced anti-dinitrophenyl reaginic antibodies of the atopic dog. *Clin. Exp. Immunol.* 9:549, 1971.

361. Scott, J. S., et al. β-Adrenergic blockade in ponies with recurrent obstructive pulmonary disease. *J. Appl. Physiol.* 64:2324, 1988.

362. Seale, J. P. Prostaglandins, slow-reacting substances (leukotrienes) and the lung. *Aust. NZ J. Med.* 11:550, 1981.

363. Seale, J. P., and Piper, P. J. Stimulation of arachidonic acid metabolism by human slow-reacting substances. *Eur. J. Pharmacol.* 52:125, 1978.

364. Seltzer, J., et al. Morphologic correlations of physiologic changes caused by SO_2-induced bronchitis in dogs: The role of inflammation. *Am. Rev. Respir. Dis.* 129:790, 1984.

365. Shampain, M. P., et al. An animal model of late pulmonary responses to *Alternaria* challenge. *Am. Rev. Respir. Dis.* 126:493, 1982.

366. Sheller, J. R., and Brigham, K. L. Bronchomotor responses of isolated sheep airways to electrical field stimulation. *J. Appl. Physiol.* 53:1088, 1982.

367. Sheller, J. R., et al. Interaction of serotonin with vagal- and ACh-induced bronchoconstriction in canine lungs. *J. Appl. Physiol.* 52:964, 1982.

368. Shore, S. A., et al. Sulfur dioxide-induced bronchitis in dogs: Effects on airway responsiveness to inhaled and intravenously administered methacholine. *Am. Rev. Respir. Dis.* 135:840, 1987.

369. Simonsson, B. G., Jacobs, F. M., and Nadel, J. A. Role of autonomic nervous system and the cough reflex in the increased responsiveness of the airways in patients with obstructive airway diseases. *J. Clin. Invest.* 46: 1812, 1967.

370. Smedegard, G., et al. Leukotriene C_4 affects pulmonary and cardiovascular dynamics in the monkey. *Nature* 295:327, 1982.

371. Smith, A. P., and Cuthbert, M. F. Antagonistic action of aerosols of prostaglandins $F_{2\alpha}$ and E_2 on bronchial muscle tone in man. *Br. Med. J.* 3:212, 1972.

372. Smith, A. P., Cuthbert, M. F., and Dunlop, L. S. Effects of inhaled prostaglandins, E_1, E_2, and $F_{2\alpha}$ on the airway resistance of healthy and asthmatic man. *Clin. Sci. Mol. Med.* 48:421, 1975.

373. Snapper, J. R., et al. Distribution of pulmonary responsiveness to aerosol histamine in dogs. *J. Appl. Physiol.* 44:738, 1978.

374. Snapper, J. R., et al. Vagal effects on histamine, carbachol, and prostaglandin $F_{2\alpha}$ responsiveness in the dog. *J. Appl. Physiol.* 47:13, 1979.

375. Snapper, J. R., et al. *In vivo* effect of cimetidine on canine pulmonary responsiveness to aerosol histamine. *J. Allergy Clin. Immunol.* 66:70, 1980.

376. Snapper, J. R., et al. Effects of beta-adrenergic blockade on muscarinic and prostaglandin responsiveness in the dog. *J. Allergy Clin. Immunol.* 67:199, 1981.

377. Souhrada, J. F. Changes of airway smooth muscle in experimental asthma. *Respir. Physiol.* 32:79, 1978.

378. Spannhake, E. W., Hyman, A. L., and Kadowitz, P. J. Dependence of the airway and pulmonary vascular effects of arachidonic acid upon route and rate of administration. *J. Pharmacol. Exp. Ther.* 212:584, 1980.

379. Spannhake, E. W., Hyman, A. L., and Kadowitz, P. J. Bronchoactive metabolites of arachidonic acid and their role in airway function. *Prostaglandins* 22:1013, 1981.

380. Spannhake, E. W., et al. Effects of arachidonic acid and prostaglandins on lung function in the intact dog. *J. Appl. Physiol.* 44:397, 1978.

381. Spannhake, E. W., et al. 15(S)-15-methyl prostaglandin $F_{2\alpha}$ elicits marked peripheral airway constriction in the intact dog. *J. Pharmacol. Exp. Ther.* 207:83, 1978.

382. Spannhake, E. W., et al. Analysis of airway effects of a PGH_2 analogue in the anesthetized dog. *J. Appl. Physiol.* 44:406, 1978.

383. Spector, S. L., and Farr, R. S. A comparison of methacholine and histamine inhalations in asthmatics. *J. Allergy Clin. Immunol.* 56:308, 1975.

384. Spina, D., et al. Autoradiographic localization of beta-adrenoceptors in asthmatic human lung. *Am. Rev. Respir. Dis.* 140:1410, 1989.

385. Stânescu, D. C., and Teculescu, D. B. Pulmonary function in status asthmaticus: Effect of therapy. *Thorax* 25:581, 1970.

386. Stânescu, D. C., et al. Failure of body plethysmography in bronchial asthma. *J. Appl. Physiol.* 52:939, 1982.

387. Staszewska-Barczak, J., and Vane, J. R. The release of catecholamine from the adrenal medulla by histamine. *Br. J. Pharmacol.* 25:728, 1965.

388. Steinhaus, J. E., and Gaskin, L. A study of intravenous lidocaine as a suppressant of cough reflex. *Anesthesiology* 24:285, 1963.

389. Stotland, L. M., and Share, N. N. Active bronchial anaphylaxis in the rat. *Can. J. Physiol. Pharmacol.* 52:1114, 1974.

390. Stotland, L. M., and Share, N. N. Pharmacological studies on active bronchial anaphylaxis in the rat. *Can. J. Physiol. Pharmacol.* 52:1119, 1974.

391. Sullivan, T. J., et al. Modulation of cyclic AMP in purified rat mast cells: II. Studies on the relationship between intracellular cyclic AMP concentrations and histamine release. *J. Immunol.* 114:1480, 1975.

392. Suzuki, H., Morita, K., and Kuriyama, H. Innervation and properties of the smooth muscle of the dog trachea. *Jpn. J. Physiol.* 26:303, 1976.

393. Svensson, J., et al. Thromboxane A_2: Effects on airway and vascular smooth muscle. *Prostaglandins* 14:425, 1977.

394. Sweatman, W. J. F., and Collier, H. O. J. Effects of prostaglandins on human bronchial muscle. *Nature* 217:69, 1968.

395. Szentivanyi, A. The beta-adrenergic theory of the atopic abnormality in bronchial asthma. *J. Allergy* 42:203, 1968.

396. Takano, S., et al. A comparison of responses of guinea-pig isolated trachea to six prostaglandins. *Prostaglandins* 15:485, 1978.

397. Takino, Y., Sugahara, K., and Horino, I. Two lines of guinea pigs sensitive and nonsensitive to chemical mediators and anaphylaxis. *J. Allergy* 47: 247, 1971.

398. Tashkin, D. P., et al. Subsensitization of beta-adrenoceptors in airways and lymphocytes of healthy and asthmatic subjects. *Am. Rev. Respir. Dis.* 125:185, 1982.

399. Thomson, N. C. Airway disease and bronchodilators: *In vivo* versus *in*

vitro human airway responsiveness to different pharmacologic stimuli. *Am. Rev. Respir. Dis.* 136:S58, 1987.

400. Tobias, J. D., Sauder, R. A., and Hirshman, C. A. Pulmonary reactivity to methacholine during β-adrenergic blockade: Propranolol vs. esmolol. *Anesthesiology* 73:132, 1990.

401. Tobias, J. D., Sauder, R. A., and Hirshman, C. A. Methylprednisolone prevents propranolol-induced airway hyperreactivity in the basenji-greyhound dog. *Anesthesiology.* In press.

402. Townley, R. G., Dennis, M., and Itkin, I. H. Comparative action of acetylbeta-methylcholine, histamine, and pollen antigens in subjects with hay fever and patients with bronchial asthma. *J. Allergy* 36:121, 1965.

403. Tse, K. S., Kepron, W., and Sehon, A. H. A canine model of the study of allergic asthma and suppression of hapten-specific IgE antibody response. *Monogr. Allergy* 14:38, 1979.

404. Turner, C. R., and Spannhake, E. W. Acute topical steroid administration blocks mast cell increase and the late asthmatic response of the canine peripheral airways. *Am. Rev. Respir. Dis.* 141:421, 1990.

405. Ueno, A., Tanaka, K., and Katori, M. Possible involvement of thromboxane in bronchoconstrictive and hypertensive effects of LTC_4 and LTD_4 in guinea pigs. *Prostaglandins* 23:865, 1982.

406. Vargaftig, B. B., Lefort, J., and Murphy, R. C. Leukotriene C and D induce aspirin-sensitive bronchoconstriction in the guinea pig. *Agents Actions* 11:574, 1981.

407. Vargaftig, B. B., et al. Platelet-activating factor induces a platelet-dependent bronchoconstriction unrelated to the formation of prostaglandin derivatives. *Eur. J. Pharmacol.* 65:185, 1980.

408. Vidruk, E. H., et al. Mechanism by which histamine stimulates rapidly adapting receptors in dog lungs. *J. Appl. Physiol.* 43:397, 1977.

409. Vornanen, M., and Tirri, R. Cholinergic responses in different sections of rat airways. *Acta Physiol. Scand.* 113:177, 1981.

410. Wanner, A. The role of mucociliary dysfunction in bronchial asthma. *Am. J. Med.* 67:477, 1979.

411. Wanner, A., and Abraham, W. M. Experimental models of asthma. *Lung* 160:231, 1982.

412. Wanner, A., Friedman, M., and Baier, H. Study of the pulmonary circulation in a canine model of asthma. *Am. Rev. Respir. Dis.* 115:241, 1977.

413. Wanner, A., and Reinhart, M. E. Respiratory mechanics in conscious sheep: Response to methacholine. *J. Appl. Physiol.* 44:479, 1978.

414. Wanner, A., et al. Tracheal mucus transport in experimental canine asthma. *J. Appl. Physiol.* 39:950, 1975.

415. Wanner, A., et al. Antigen-induced bronchospasm in conscious sheep. *J. Appl. Physiol.* 47:917, 1979.

416. Wasserman, M. A. Bronchopulmonary effects of prostaglandin $F_{2\alpha}$ and three of its metabolites in the dog. *Prostaglandins* 9:959, 1975.

417. Wasserman, M. A. Bronchopulmonary responses to prostaglandin $F_{2\alpha}$, histamine and acetylcholine in the dog. *Eur. J. Pharmacol.* 32:146, 1975.

418. Wasserman, M. A. Bronchopulmonary pharmacology of some prostaglandin endoperoxide analogs in the dog. *Eur. J. Pharmacol.* 36:103, 1976.

419. Wasserman, M. A., Griffin, R. L., and Marsalisi, F. B. Potent bronchoconstrictor effects of aerosolized prostaglandin D_2 in dogs. *Prostaglandins* 20:703, 1980.

420. Weichman, B. M., et al. *In vivo* and *in vitro* mechanisms of leukotriene-mediated bronchoconstriction in the guinea pig. *J. Pharmacol. Exp. Ther.* 222:202, 1982.

421. Weinmann, C. G., et al. *In vitro* tracheal responses from mice chosen for *in vivo* lung cholinergic sensitivity. *J. Appl. Physiol.* 69:274, 1990.

422. Weislander, E., et al. Importance of particulate antigen for induction of dual bronchial reaction in guinea pigs. *Agents Actions* 16:37, 1985.

423. Weiss, J. W., et al. Bronchoconstrictor effects of leukotriene C in humans. *Science* 216:196, 1982.

424. Weiss, S. T., et al. The distribution of airway responsiveness in a population sample of adults and children. *Am. Rev. Respir. Dis.* 123(Suppl.):130, 1981.

425. Weissberg, R. M. Conscious primate model for evaluating antiallergic drugs. *Monogr. Allergy* 14:324, 1979.

426. Weissberger, D., et al. Impaired tracheal mucus transport in allergic bronchoconstriction: Effect of terbutaline pretreatment. *J. Allergy Clin. Immunol.* 67:357, 1981.

427. Whicker, S. D., Armour, C. L., and Black, J. L. Responsiveness of bronchial smooth muscle from asthmatic patients to relaxant and contractile agonists. *Pulm. Pharmacol.* 2:25, 1989.

428. Widdicombe, J. G. Some experimental models of acute asthma. *J. R. Coll. Physicians Lond.* 11:141, 1977.

429. Woenne, R., et al. Bronchial hyperreactivity to histamine and methacholine in asthmatic children after inhalation of SCH 1000 and chlorpheniramine maleate. *J. Allergy Clin. Immunol.* 62:119, 1978.

430. Wong, S. K., and Buckner, C. K. Studies on β-adrenoceptors mediating changes in mechanical events and adenosine 3',5'-monophosphate levels: Guinea pig trachea. *Eur. J. Pharmacol.* 47:273, 1978.

431. Woolcock, A. J., et al. Effect of vagal stimulation on central and peripheral airways in dogs. *J. Appl. Physiol.* 26:806, 1969.

432. Yamaguchi, T., Hitzig, B., and Coburn, R. F. Endogenous prostaglandins and mechanical tension in canine trachealis muscle. *Am. J. Physiol.* 230:1737, 1976.

433. Yamatake, Y., Sasagawa, S., and Yanauura, S. Drug responses of canine trachea, bronchus and bronchiole. *Chem. Pharm. Bull.* (Tokyo) 26:318, 1978.

434. Yamatake, Y., et al. Allergy-induced asthma with *Ascaris suum* administration to dogs. *Jpn. J. Pharmacol.* 27:285, 1977.

435. Yamatake, Y., et al. Involvement of histamine H_1- and H_2-receptors in induced asthma in dogs. *Jpn. J. Pharmacol.* 27:791, 1977.

436. Yanta, M. A., et al. Direct and reflex bronchoconstriction induced by histamine aerosol inhalation in dogs. *J. Appl. Physiol.* 50:869, 1981.

437. Zimmermann, I., and Ulmer, W. T. Effect of unilateral vagus blockade on allergen-induced airway obstruction. *Respiration* 34:69, 1977.

438. Zimmermann, I., and Ulmer, W. T. Influence of low concentrations of allergens on bronchial system. *Respiration* 35:87, 1978.

439. Zimmermann, I., and Ulmer, W. T. Therapeutic influence of vagus blockade on antigen-induced airway obstruction. *Respiration* 37:1, 1979.

440. Zimmermann, I., and Ulmer, W. T. Effect of intravenous histamine, allergen (*Ascaris suum* extract) and compound 48/80 and inhaled allergen-aerosol on bronchoconstriction and histamine release. *Respiration* 42:30, 1981.

441. Zimmermann, I., Ulmer, W. T., and Weller, W. The role of upper airways and of sensoric receptors on reflex bronchoconstriction. *Res. Exp. Med.* (Berl.) 174:253, 1979.

442. Zimmermann, I., Walkenhorst, W., and Ulmer, W. T. The site of action of bronchodilating drugs (β2-stimulators) on antigen-induced bronchoconstriction. *Respiration* 38:65, 1979.

443. Zimmermann, I., Walkenhorst, W., and Ulmer, W. T. The location of sensoric bronchoconstricting receptors in the upper airways. *Respiration* 38:1, 1979.

Aerosols

Joseph D. Brain
James D. Blanchard

32

Aerosols are important to the asthmatic patient both as irritants and as therapeutic substances. On the one hand, inhaled antigens can trigger bronchoconstriction. On the other hand, bronchodilators, steroids, and mediator antagonists given as aerosols can be an essential aspect of the treatment of asthma. Aerosols may also be used for provocation testing and to help diagnose airway disease. For each of these applications, it is important to describe aerosol retention accurately. Quantification of dose is also essential for the comparison of results among different laboratories. The effectiveness of therapies utilizing inhaled aerosols cannot be compared unless the dose and preferably the distribution of dose can be described.

The availability of pharmacologic aerosols in respiratory therapy illustrates some of the key issues. Pharmaceutical companies manufacture and promote aerosols that are intended to relieve bronchospasm, congestion, edema, allergy, and inflammation, as well as reduce the viscosity of mucus, treat sinus infection, activate macrophages, inhibit proteases, and so on. Other aerosolized agents can elicit bronchoconstriction.

A major concern with most inhaled aerosols is whether they reach the desired location in the respiratory tract. Deposition site is highly dependent on the particle size of the aerosol and the breathing pattern used. These are not always adequately controlled. Particles may be too large or individuals may inhale too quickly to allow particles to pass the oropharynx and larynx into the lungs. Thus, in many cases it is difficult to estimate or calculate the dose of a drug given to a patient by aerosol.

Aerosols for drug therapy may be produced by nebulizers, pressurized metered-dose inhalers (MDIs), or dry-powder inhalers. Although a variety of aerosol generators are made, in many cases there are insufficient data regarding the size distribution of the particles produced and the efficiency of generation. Furthermore, nebulizers of the same design and model may not perform alike [200, 214]. Accurate characterization of many freshly generated therapeutic aerosols is quite complex because the size of the particles may change rapidly due to evaporation, hygroscopic growth, or agglomeration. A large fraction of the fresh aerosol may be too large to penetrate into the lungs. Unfortunately, much data on particle size distribution are collected by methods that do not account for these dynamic changes.

Dose estimation is further complicated by other factors. Many devices require intelligent use by the patient and they are frequently misused [45, 206]. There is often little known about the distribution and metabolism of the drugs given. Comprehensive studies describing the accumulation of drugs in blood or urine, or the site of action within the respiratory tract, are seldom available. Also lacking is adequate knowledge of the anatomic distribution of receptor sites throughout the respiratory tract. So even when a drug is delivered to the lungs, it is not always known if it reached the desired region. For example, stiffened parts of the lungs or regions served by obstructed airways receive little or no drug.

During aerosol therapy or challenge, considerable effort is given to measuring the appropriate responses, frequently changes on pulmonary function tests. Responses can also be measured at the level of a cell (degranulation of mast cells), at the level of an enzyme (increased phosphodiesterase), or a receptor (the leukotriene [LT] D_4 receptor on the plasma membrane). Descriptions of responses are of little value, however, without accurate measurements of the dose, preferably at the site of action. Aerosol exposures present a special problem since the actual dose retained is often difficult to determine. Many investigators fail to try. They report the dose to an animal or person as the concentration in the nebulizer fluid, the amount of aerosol generated, or the amount in the exposure chamber. Since exposure dose does not equal retained dose, it is important to adequately describe the variables that determine exposure-dose relationships.

In this review we summarize particle deposition and clearance mechanisms and how they influence retention. We also discuss strategies that can be used to deliver aerosols and to describe the amount and distribution of dose, as well as factors that are known to influence the amount and distribution of retained particles. Although gases accompanying inhaled drugs and gas-particle interactions are sometimes important, the effects and uptake of inhaled gases are not covered.

MECHANISMS OF PARTICLE DEPOSITION

Deposition is the process that determines the fraction of the inspired particles that is caught in the respiratory tract and thus fails to exit with expired air. Deposited dose is equal to the amount of material inhaled times the fraction of material that deposits. All particles that touch a surface are assumed to deposit at the site of initial contact. Distinct physical mechanisms operate on inspired particles to move them across streamlines of air and toward the surface of the respiratory tract; these are gravitational sedimentation, inertia, brownian diffusion, and electrostatic forces. Which mechanisms contribute to the deposition of a specific particle depend on the particle's physicochemical characteristics, the subject's breathing pattern, the geometry of the respiratory tract, and the flow and mixing pattern of the aerosol. For most aerosols, the first three mechanisms are the most important. More detailed treatments on particle deposition are available [1, 25, 78, 93, 97, 99, 140, 145, 161, 192, 223, 227]. Comprehensive treatises on aerosol behavior are also available [49, 71, 111, 195].

The transport and deposition of a particle larger than 1.0 μm in the respiratory system are largely determined by aerodynamic characteristics: particle size, density, and shape plus gas velocity [93]. A 2-μm-diameter sphere with a density of 4.0 gm/cm³ behaves aerodynamically the same as a 4-μm sphere with a density

405

of 1 gm/cm³. Such particles may be compared by their aerodynamic equivalent diameter (d$_{ae}$). Aerodynamic diameter is the diameter of the unit-density (1 gm/cm³) sphere that has the same gravitational settling velocity in air as the particle in question. Aerodynamic diameter is proportional to dρ$^{1/2}$, where d is the geometric diameter and ρ is the particle density. Thus, in the above example, both particles have a d$_{ae}$ of 4 μm. The d$_{ae}$ can be used to describe the size of particles larger than 0.4 μm, the particle size that deposits least in the respiratory tract [95]. For particles of unknown density or shape, d$_{ae}$ must be determined experimentally.

Gravity accelerates falling bodies downward, and the terminal settling velocity of a particle is reached when viscous resistive forces of the air are equal and opposite in direction to gravitational forces. Respirable particles reach this constant terminal sedimentation velocity in less than 1.0 msec. Particles are removed when their settling causes them to strike airway walls or alveolar surfaces. The probability that a particle will deposit by gravitational settling increases with increasing d$_{ae}^2$t, where t is the residence time in the respiratory tract [93]. Thus, breath holding enhances deposition by sedimentation. Sedimentation is important for particles larger than about 0.1 μm and within the peripheral airways and alveoli where airflow rates are slow and residence times are long [97].

Inertia is the tendency of a moving particle to resist changes in direction and speed and is related to momentum: the product of the particle's mass and velocity. High air velocities and abrupt changes in the direction of airflow occur in the nose and oropharynx and at central airway bifurcations. Inertia causes a particle entering bends at these sites to continue in its original direction instead of following the curvature of the airflow. If the particle has sufficient mass and velocity, it will cross airflow streamlines and impact on the airway wall. The probability that a particle will deposit by inertial impaction increases with increasing product of d$_{ae}^2$Q, where Q is the respired flow rate [93, 141]. Impaction probability also increases with increasing angle of airstream deflection. Inertial impaction is an important deposition mechanism for particles with a d$_{ae}$ larger than 2 μm [97] and may occur both during inspiration and during expiration in the extrathoracic airways (oropharynx, nasopharynx, and larynx) and central airways. In obstructed airways the enhanced linear velocities at narrowed sites may cause smaller particles to deposit by impaction.

Aerosol particles also undergo brownian diffusion—a random motion in three dimensions caused by their collisions with gas molecules; this motion can lead to contact and deposition on respiratory surfaces. Diffusion is significant for particles with diameters less than 1 μm so that their size is similar to the mean free path of gas molecules. Unlike inertial or gravitational displacement, diffusion is independent of airflow rate or particle density; however, it is affected by particle shape and size [103]. For diffusing particles that are 0.4 μm and smaller, size can be expressed in terms of the thermodynamic equivalent diameter, d$_{te}$, the diameter of a sphere that has the same average diffusional velocity in the air as the actual particle [95]. The probability that a particle will be deposited by diffusion increases with decreasing particle size or increasing values of (t/d$_{te}$)$^{1/2}$ [93]; deposition is dependent on the square root of residence time. Diffusion, like sedimentation, is usually most important in the peripheral airways and alveoli [97], but can also occur in the nose and mouth [84].

As particle size decreases, inertia and sedimentation become less important, but diffusion increases in importance. For example, a 2-μm unit-density spherical particle will be displaced by diffusion (brownian displacement) only about 5 μm in 1 second; it will settle by gravity about 120 μm in the same period. However, as particle size drops to 0.2 μm, the diffusional displacement increases to 22 μm, whereas gravitational displacement

Table 32-1. Root mean square brownian displacement in 1 second compared to distance fallen in air in 1 second for unit-density particles of different diameters[a]

	Diameter (μm)	Brownian displacement in 1 sec (μm)	Distance fallen in 1 sec (μm)
Settling greater in 1 sec	50	0.978	71,700
	20	1.55	11,500
	10	2.20	2,910
	5	3.14	740
	2	5.10	124
	1	7.50	33.7
Diffusion greater in 1 sec	0.5	11.4	9.71
	0.2	21.6	2.23
	0.1	38.1	0.871
	0.05	71.4	0.382
	0.02	172	0.141
	0.01	339	0.0689
	0.00037[b]	9060	0.00249

[a] Values are for air at 37°C and 100 percent relative humidity; air viscosity = 1.906 × 10^{-5} Pa s; air density = 1.112 kg/m³; Cunningham slip correction calculated according to Jennings [119a].
[b] Diameter of a typical "air molecule" [111].

decreases to only about 2 μm. A comparison of settling and diffusion displacements for a range of particle sizes is shown in Table 32-1. It can also be seen that although a 0.01-μm particle diffuses about 340 μm in 1 second, this distance is still only about 4 percent of the distance a typical gas molecule travels in the same amount of time. Generally, gravity and inertia dominate the transport and deposition of particles larger than 1.0 μm in diameter, and diffusion dominates the transport and deposition of particles smaller than 0.1 μm. For particles between 0.1 and 1.0 μm, sedimentation and diffusion are both important [95].

Electrical forces may cause charged particles to deposit in the respiratory tract. The surfaces of the respiratory tract are uncharged but electrically conducting. When an electrically charged particle approaches the lung surface, the particle induces an image charge of the opposite polarity in that surface which attracts the particle. This attraction may cause the particle to deposit, and thus the deposition of charged particles is increased relative to that of neutral particles. Experimental [153] and theoretic [256] studies show that electrostatic attraction may be an important deposition mechanism in the lung periphery for particles (especially fibers) that are both charged above a certain threshold and have a diameter, d (d$_{ae}$ or d$_{th}$), of 0.1 to 1.0 μm [245]. Melandri and colleagues [153] established that the probability of electrostatic deposition is proportional to (q^2/d)$^{1/3}$, where q is the electrical charge on the particle. For 1-μm charged particles, deposition is increased over that of uncharged particles once there are about 40 charges on the particle; for 0.3-μm particles only 10 charges are needed. Other forces acting to affect deposition, such as acoustic forces, magnetic forces, or thermal forces, are normally not significant in the respiratory tract.

Deposition can also occur in the lungs when particles have dimensions that are significant relative to those of the air spaces. As particles move into smaller and smaller air spaces, some may reach a point where the distance to a surface from the center of a particle is less than the particle size. The resulting contact is called *interception*. Interception is particularly important for the deposition of fibers [91, 237].

CLEARANCE AND RETENTION OF PARTICLES

The lungs' response to aerosols depends not only on the amount of particles deposited there but also on the amount retained over time. Retention is the amount of material present in the lungs at any time and equals deposition minus clearance. An equilibrium concentration or retention is reached during continuous exposure to aerosols when the rate of deposition equals the rate of clearance. It is both the amount of particles retained within a specific lung region over time and those properties of the retained particles that determine the magnitude of the pharmacologic response.

As discussed elsewhere, such factors as particle size, hygroscopicity, and breathing pattern affect the site of deposition within the respiratory tract. In turn, where particles deposit in the lungs determines which mechanisms are used to clear them and how fast they are cleared. This influences the amount retained over time. Examples of the implications of particle characteristics on integrated retention were given by Brain and Valberg [24] using a model developed by the Task Group on Lung Dynamics [235]. They showed that the total amount as well as the distribution of retained dose among the nose and pharynx, trachea and bronchi, and pulmonary and lymphatic compartments were dramatically altered by particle size and solubility.

Particles that deposit on the ciliated airways are cleared primarily by the mucociliary escalator. Those particles that penetrate to and deposit in the peripheral, nonciliated areas of the lung can be cleared by many mechanisms, including phagocytosis by alveolar macrophages, particle dissolution, and movement of free particles or particle-containing cells directly into the interstitium or the lymphatics. Excellent reviews discuss these clearance processes in detail [29, 138, 145, 176, 180, 208].

Mucociliary Transport

Less-soluble particles that deposit on the mucus blanket covering pulmonary airways and the nasal passages are moved toward the pharynx by the cilia. Also present in this moving carpet of mucus are cells and particles that have been transported from the nonciliated alveoli to the ciliated airways. Mucus, cells, and debris coming from the nasal cavities and the lungs meet at the pharynx, mix with salivary secretions, and enter the gastrointestinal tract after being swallowed. In humans the ciliated epithelium extends from the trachea down to the terminal bronchioles. The particles are removed with half-times of minutes to hours; the rate depends on the speed of the mucus blanket. The speed is faster in the trachea than in the small airways [212]. There is little time for solubilization of slowly dissolving materials. In contrast, particles deposited in the nonciliated compartments have much longer residence times; there, small differences in in vivo solubility can have great significance. A number of factors can have great significance. The speed of mucus flow can be affected either by factors influencing the cilia or by the amount and quality of mucus.

Ciliary action may be affected by the number of strokes per minute, the amplitude of each stroke, the time course and form of each stroke, the length of the cilia, the ratio of ciliated to nonciliated area, and the susceptibility of the cilia to intrinsic and extrinsic agents that modify their rate and quality of motion. The characteristics of the mucous layer are also critically important. The thickness of the mucous layer and its rheologic properties may vary widely. In asthmatic subjects, tracheobronchial clearance can be retarded, possibly because of a combination of ciliary dysfunction and altered mucus rheologic properties [156a]. Wanner [250] and Camner and Mossberg [30] reviewed many of these factors that influence clearance and discussed their clinical implications.

Mucociliary transport has been studied by a variety of techniques such as monitoring the movement of inert or radiolabeled particles deposited on the tracheal mucus via a bronchoscope or as an inhaled bolus. Tracheal mucus velocity (TMV) can then be estimated from the distance the particles moved over time as observed either with movies filmed through the bronchoscope or by a gamma camera [203, 255]. Bronchoscopic techniques yield higher numbers for TMV (15–21 mm/min) than do the noninvasive bolus techniques (4.4 mm/min). These values are only characteristic for the trachea and large central airways. Transport in the small peripheral airways is slower probably due to the discontinuous mucous layer [242].

Many investigators have estimated mucociliary transport from whole-lung clearance curves. These curves are generated by monitoring the amount of radioactivity in the lungs over time (hours to days) following the inhalation of a radiolabeled aerosol. Albert and Arnett [4] first used this method and noted that the clearance curve can be divided into two phases: a rapid and a slow phase. The fast phase was complete within 24 to 48 hours and has generally been attributed to tracheobronchial clearance; the slow phase has been attributed to alveolar clearance [16, 141, 163]. This approach has been used to study clearance in normal and abnormal individuals [31, 147, 187, 204, 220]. However, evidence indicates that clearance from the airways might not be complete in the first 24 hours; this may be even more pronounced in patients with lung disease. Gore and Patrick [83] noted that particles instilled into the trachea can be sequestered in epithelial cells. Geiser and associates [77] found latex particles trapped in the periciliary fluid below the mucus blanket. The particles may have been displaced there by surface tension forces in the airways [76, 209a]. Stahlhofen and coworkers [222] noted both fast and slow phases of clearance even in humans given a bolus of particles delivered only 45 cm^3 beyond the larynx. Wolff and associates [252a] deposited radiolabeled particles with a bronchoscope to airway generations 6 through 10 in dogs and found that about 20 percent of the particles were cleared slowly.

Another approach is to examine the deposition and clearance of particles in central versus peripheral lung regions [217]. The uses of this type of analysis in the interpretation of clearance curves have been noted in an editorial by Foster [67].

More studies are needed to elucidate the best methodology used to model mucociliary clearance and to understand its role and importance in patients with pulmonary disease. Clearly, it is also essential to understand the initial deposition pattern of inhaled particles in order to determine the importance of mucociliary clearance on the disappearance of the particles from the lungs. See Chapter 30 for further information on mucociliary transport.

Nonciliated Regions

Particles deposited in the nonciliated portion of the lungs either are moved toward the ciliated region, primarily within alveolar macrophages, or enter the lung connective tissue as free particles or within macrophages [122]. Macrophages are credited with keeping the alveolar surfaces clean and sterile. These cells rest on the continuous epithelial layer of the lung. It is their phagocytic and lytic potentials that provide most of the bactericidal properties of the lungs. Rapid endocytosis of insoluble particles prevents particle penetration through the alveolar epithelia and facilitates alveolar-bronchiolar transport. Particles in connective tissue may slowly dissolve or may be transported to new sites through lymphatic pathways. Particles remaining on alveolar surfaces are cleared with biologic half-times estimated to be days to weeks in humans, while particles that have penetrated into fixed tissues are cleared with half-times ranging from a few days to thousands of days, depending on their solubility. The biology of lung macrophages has been reviewed [20, 212a, 240] and an editorial [21] emphasized that many kinds of lung macrophages exist. These include alveolar, airway, connective tissue, pleural, and intravascular macrophages.

CHARACTERIZING AND DELIVERING THERAPEUTIC AEROSOLS

Important considerations in exposing human subjects or experimental animals to pharmacologic aerosols include techniques of aerosol generation; characterization of the aerosol mass, size distribution, and dynamic properties; delivery of the aerosol; and delineation of the factors that influence the amount of material deposited in the lungs including breathing pattern and characteristics of the subject. Different subjects breathing the same aerosol frequently retain quite different amounts, and variations in breathing pattern are often responsible; thus, an important challenge for physicians is to train patients in the proper aerosol inhalation technique [152a].

Many chemical and physical processes can be used to generate liquid and solid pharmacologic aerosols. Several texts describe both theoretic and practical aspects of aerosol generation and measurement [44, 49, 51, 111, 137, 154, 246, 251, 251a]. Surveys of typical devices and possible future devices have been published [3a, 25, 27, 28, 55, 73, 81, 160, 168, 185]. Aerosol methods for inhalation challenges have also been described [40a, 40b]. The technique used to generate pharmacologic aerosols depends on the physical properties of the drug. If the drug is water soluble, a nebulizer that is driven either by compressed air or by ultrasonic energy is commonly used. If the material is water insoluble, an MDI or a dry-powder inhaler is often used to aerosolize it. The choice of generation device also depends on practicality. Nebulizers are simple to prepare and use, especially in hospitals, whereas MDIs are cheaper, convenient, and inconspicuous; hold multiple doses; require less time for dosing; and are safe from contamination by pathogens [166]. However, some subjects have difficulty using an MDI [45, 206]. Ultrasonic nebulizers have high drug output per unit of time but can also degrade some labile drugs. Dry-powder inhalers have many of the same advantages as MDIs, though dry-powder inhalers may be easier to use since they are breath actuated and some devices, such as the Turbuhaler, deliver pure drug.

Characterization of the aerosol in terms of the particle size distribution as well as the mass concentration is needed to estimate total and regional dose. Particle size helps determine the fraction of inhaled particles that deposits in each lung region; it also influences the fraction of the particles that are small enough to penetrate past the oropharynx into the lungs. The mass concentration is proportional to the amount of particles that deposits in each region. Size distributions can be described in terms of particle number, surface area, or mass; most dose estimates use mass. Particle mass distributions are often characterized by two values, the mass median aerodynamic diameter $(d_{ae,mm})$ and the geometric standard deviation (σ_g) [95]. The $d_{ae,mm}$ denotes the particle size (d_{ae}) at which half of the total aerosol mass is contained in larger particles and half in smaller particles. Since the $d_{ae,mm}$ is expressed as an aerodynamic diameter, it describes how the aerosol behaves in the respired air and can be used to estimate where and by what processes the particles deposit in the respiratory tract.

The σ_g denotes the spread of particle size. Most aerosols have particles of sizes that are distributed lognormally: On a frequency distribution versus log particle diameter plot, the distribution looks gaussian. An aerosol that is composed of identical particles would have a σ_g of 1.0. An aerosol with a σ_g of 1.22 or lower is considered monodisperse [72]; to a first approximation, all the particles behave aerodynamically alike. An aerosol with a σ_g above 1.22 is polydisperse; there are significant differences in aerodynamic behavior among the particles. Most therapeutic aerosols are polydisperse. An aerosol with a $d_{ae,mm}$ of 2 μm and a σ_g of 2 would have 1 geometric standard deviation or 68 percent of its mass contained in particles with a d_{ae} between 1 and 4 μm.

An important implication of a lognormal distribution is that much of the aerosol mass can be contained in the large particles since mass is proportional to the cube of the diameter. Where these large particles deposit in the respiratory tract will govern where much of the dose is deposited.

The mass output of a device per unit of time or per actuation can be measured by pulling the generated aerosol through an absolute filter at a known volumetric flow rate [218]. Mass output is often measured gravimetrically; however, if the drug is combined with other ingredients, measurements of bioactivity, chemical structure, or a tightly bound fluorescent or radioactive tag can be more meaningful. The outputs of nebulizers are often based on the weight or volume change of the solution, but this output may be erroneous if evaporative losses of the solute are neglected [155]. In addition, optical methods using light scattering can give continuous estimates of particle concentration.

The mass output of a nebulizer or an MDI is used to calculate its delivery efficiency. Delivery efficiency helps determine how much drug to use and may also be a criterion for selecting among different types of devices, especially when expensive drugs are aerosolized [214]. For a nebulizer the delivery efficiency is the fraction of drug initially within the nebulizer that is delivered to the mouthpiece over the treatment period. For an MDI the delivery efficiency is the fraction of the total mass aerosolized during each actuation that is delivered to the actuator outlet or the spacer mouthpiece. Delivery efficiencies vary markedly among nebulizers: For one ultrasonic and two jet nebulizers, the efficiencies ranged from 5 to 22 percent, with much of the losses occurring within the tubing and nebulizer surfaces [218].

Freshly generated aerosols are dynamic, which is an important consideration when it comes to measurements of size distribution and mass concentration. Evaporation, agglomeration, and losses in tubing or spacers cause rapid changes in $d_{ae,mm}$ and σ_g. From the moment droplets become airborne, evaporation causes immediate shrinkage of water droplets from a nebulizer or Freon propellant droplets from an MDI. The $d_{ae,mm}$ for one MDI changed from 43 μm at the outlet to 10 μm only 25 cm downstream [159]. Particle agglomeration is an important consideration for dry-powder inhalers. Furthermore, once hydrophilic particles such as drug salts mix with the warm, humid air in the lungs, they may start to gain water and grow, a process known as *hygroscopic growth*. Thus, there are two particle size distributions of interest when calculating inhaled dose of drugs: the distribution at the mouthpiece and the distribution in the lungs after the particles have equilibrated within the lungs. The size distribution at the mouthpiece determines the fraction of particles that are sufficiently small to be inhaled past the oropharynx. Less than half the particles larger than 8 μm penetrate past the mouth during tidal breathing [97].

The particle size distribution within the lungs determines the fraction of particles that deposit in the airways versus the parenchyma. For hydrophobic particles from an MDI, this size distribution depends on how rapidly the propellant evaporates, which may be on the order of seconds. For hydrophilic particles, estimation of the size distribution in the lungs is complex since it must account for hygroscopic growth. The relative humidity in the lungs beyond the upper bronchi is about 99.5 percent [62], which causes dry sodium chloride (NaCl) particles with a d_{ae} from 0.1 to 10.0 μm to increase in diameter by factors of 2.5 to 4.4, respectively [63]. Hygroscopic growth is discussed in more detail later.

The particle size distributions from devices are based on measurements either of the freshly generated particles, such as the spray droplets from a nebulizer or an MDI or the particles from a dry-powder inhaler, or of the particles remaining after spray evaporation. Techniques to analyze droplet sizes within sprays were addressed in detail by Lefebvre [137]. Optical methods for characterizing sprays include high-speed photography [52, 87], holography, and laser diffraction [39]. These optical methods offer the advantage of direct and continuous measurements of high-concentration sprays without interfering with the aerosol. Droplets can also be collected on slides and analyzed by light or electron microscopy combined with image analysis systems [88]. Since all these optical measurements are based on the particles' surface area, the particle density must also be known to compute the $d_{ae,mm}$. Droplets from MDIs and dry-powder inhalers have been measured with multistage liquid impingers in ways that mimic inhalation [12, 89]. One consideration with any measurement of fresh aerosol is that if tubing or spacers are used, it is more meaningful to make the measurements at the mouthpiece since these will account for droplet evaporation and losses within the system [127].

Alternatively, characterization of the dry-particle size distribution after evaporation of water or Freon offers the advantages that (1) the size distribution is stable, and thus fast-responding devices are not needed; (2) one can calculate the size distribution of the initial spray droplets based on the composition of the original solution [61, 65, 156]; (3) for hygroscopic particles, one can calculate the equilibrium droplet size in the lungs based on the molar composition of the solution and physicochemical properties of the particle [64]; and (4) for hydrophobic particles, the dry-particle size distribution is the size distribution in the lungs, to the extent that evaporation and agglomeration occur quickly.

In addition to the measurement techniques listed above, the $d_{ae,mm}$ and σ_g of dry particles can be measured with cascade impactors [129, 218], cascade impactors with piezoelectric crystals, centrifugal aerosol spectrometers [236], inertial spectrometers [191], and electrical mobility analyzers [224]. All of these analyzers can analyze undiluted aerosols, but some may require additional makeup air since they sample at higher airflows than many devices produce. The size distributions of lower-concentration dry particles can be measured with light-scattering devices, time-of-flight analyzers [17], and single-particle aerodynamic relaxation time (SPART) [108] analyzers. Light-scattering devices report particle size distributions based on particle surface area; time-of-flight and SPART analyzers measure $d_{ae,mm}$. Fresh spray droplets can also be analyzed by these devices; however, any added makeup or dilution air must be either at the same humidity as the aerosol, in order to prevent changing particle size, or at a known humidity from which the final size can be calculated. To the extent that the measurement and adjustment of high-humidity atmospheres is difficult, these analyzers are more easily and reliably used with dry aerosols. Experimental systems for studying hygroscopic droplet growth in a surrogate lung were recently described [138a, 152]. Also any device that must withdraw the aerosol from the air is subject to isokinetic sampling effects and the loss of large particles to the walls of the sampling inlet [225, 246].

Aerosol size distribution measurements for MDIs have been made by a number of investigators [17, 108, 109, 129, 202]. Kim and associates [129] measured the outputs of 10 drugs from MDIs with a cascade impactor both after evaporation and in a relative humidity of 90 percent. They found $d_{ae,mm}$'s of 2.4 to 5.5 µm and σ_g's of 1.7 to 2.5. At 90 percent relative humidity, the $d_{ae,mm}$ generally increased 1 to 10 percent, whereas σ_g remained unchanged. Drugs for MDIs are usually milled and then suspended in a mixture of Freon propellants, so the final particle size reflects the size of the primary milled particles, their agglomerates, plus any nonvolatile additives or lubricants. The size distribution of initial droplets is influenced by the metering volume, the actuator design, the types and amounts of propellants, and cosolvents [28, 87].

Spacers of various designs are added to MDIs to make it easier for patients to coordinate MDI actuation with inspiration, to allow more time for droplet evaporation, and to decrease the linear velocity of the droplets. Linear velocities drop from a peak of 15 to about 5 m/sec at 10 cm from the actuator [52]. Spacers can reduce the dose deposited in the oropharynx, but usually fail to dramatically increase the dose delivered to the lungs, which is only about 10 percent [56, 171, 244]. However, reduction of oropharyngeal dose is important for inhaled corticosteroids, which can cause oral candidiasis (thrush), hoarseness, and bronchospasm [165, 243]. The effects of spacers on inhaled aerosol size and mass have been an active area of study and are covered in more detail in Chapter 56.

For aerosols produced from isotonic saline solution by jet nebulizers, the effect of evaporation on inhaled droplet size is minimized since the relative humidity at the nebulizer outlet is about 99 percent; the consequent droplet shrinkage from the point of formation is usually about 20 percent or less [61]. Size distribution data for nebulizers come from a number of studies [39, 65, 110, 155, 200, 218, 224]. Sterk and colleagues [224] analyzed the aerosols generated from isotonic saline solution by 11 jet nebulizers and found $d_{ae,mm}$'s from 1.6 to 4.9 µm and σ_g's from 1.8 to 2.3.

For aerosols produced by ultrasonic nebulizers, the water mass output per unit of air volume is about three times that of jet nebulizers [224]. The relative humidity at the outlet is high enough to prevent droplet evaporation so these aerosols tend to maintain the same size after formation. Sterk and colleagues [224] analyzed the outputs from nine ultrasonic nebulizers and found $d_{ae,mm}$'s from 2.9 to 7.1 µm and σ_g's from 1.8 to 2.2.

Dry-powder inhalers use the inhaled air through the device to aerosolize the drug powder, with particle size decreasing with increasing inhaled flow rate [119, 129]. An increase from 0.8 to 1.3 L/min caused the $d_{ae,mm}$ of a powder from a Spinhaler to decrease from 5.6 to 3.3 µm, while the σ_g decreased from 2.8 to 2.3 [129].

Once an adequately characterized pharmacologic aerosol has been produced, the aerosol particles may be deposited in the lungs by a variety of strategies. In animal models, a nose-only or head-only exposure minimizes the amount of aerosol needed and the extent of contamination. Alternatively, the aerosol can be delivered to a human subject or animal directly through the nose, the mouth, or an endotracheal tube [185, 192a].

In addition to delivery by aerosol, a solution or suspension of the drug can be placed directly into the lumen of an airway by intratracheal or transtracheal instillation [22]. The fluid and particles, propelled by gravity and sometimes airflow, run down into the dependent areas of the lungs. The carrier liquid is rapidly absorbed into the pulmonary circulation, leaving the particles on the internal surfaces of the lungs. This approach is being used with some success to deliver surfactants to animals [120] and human babies [79] with respiratory distress syndrome. When drugs are instilled with a surfactant carrier, they are more evenly distributed in the lungs because of the lower surface tension forces of the surfactant [129a].

FACTORS INFLUENCING PARTICLE DEPOSITION

The physical mechanisms responsible for deposition have already been discussed. The effectiveness of these mechanisms depends on various factors, some of which can be controlled by the clinician or scientist, such as particle size and breathing pattern. Others such as airway geometry and disease are uncontrollable. Many aspects of particle deposition in mammalian lungs have captured the energy and imagination of investigators; these studies are reviewed in many papers and books [3, 6, 23, 25, 36, 92, 93, 97, 99, 140, 144, 145, 160, 192, 223, 227]. Other excellent sources of information on deposition are published works from the International Symposia on Inhaled Particles [47,

48, 54, 247–249]. Particle deposition from a more clinical perspective was featured at the recent Symposia on Respiratory Drug Delivery [29a–29c] and at the International Congresses on Aerosols in Medicine [190, 190a]. Some major influences on the fraction of the inspired particles that deposit within the respiratory tract and the anatomic distribution of retained particles are now discussed.

Anatomy of the Respiratory Tract

The configuration of the lungs and airways is important since the efficiency of deposition depends, in part, on the diameters of the airways, their angles of branching, and the average distances of particles to lung surfaces in the alveoli. Along with the volumetric flow rate, airway anatomy specifies the local linear velocity of the airstream and thus determines whether the flow is laminar or turbulent. For example, an air jet is formed at the laryngeal aperture, which creates turbulent and unstable airflows that enhance particle impaction in the trachea [32, 143]. There are interspecies and intraspecies differences in lung morphometry [175, 185, 209, 219]; even within the same individual, the dimensions of the respiratory tract change with lung volume, age, and pathologic processes. Among normal individuals breathing in the same manner, total deposition has a coefficient of variation as large as 27 percent. This is largely due to intersubject differences in airway geometry [14, 98, 100, 258]. Gender differences in laryngeal and airway geometries may cause women to have greater upper airway deposition by impaction compared to men [189]. Within a person, decreasing lung volume not only increases deposition, but also causes the major site of particle deposition within the airways to shift from the lung periphery to more central airways [1]. At low lung volumes, airways have smaller cross-sectional areas, higher linear velocities, and thus enhanced deposition by impaction in central airways for a given flow rate. As a person ages, anatomic changes of the respiratory tract also appear to affect deposition. Children less than 8 years old have higher total, head, and tracheobronchial deposition and lower alveolar deposition of particles at rest than adults [10, 112, 254, 261].

Choice of Pathway

Most people breathe nasally at rest. However, as ventilation rate rises above 35 to 40 L/min, the high-resistance nasal pathway starts to be combined with the low-resistance oral pathway [31a, 173, 203a]. As ventilation rate continues to increase, the oral path tends to take on a greater percentage of the total ventilation, but this percentage varies considerably among subjects, ranging from only 10 percent to as much as 80 percent [31a, 174, 250a].

A highly significant change in the effective anatomy of the respiratory tract occurs when air is inhaled through the mouth instead of the nose, or when the nose is bypassed because of a tracheostomy or an endotracheal tube. The nose has a major role as an upstream filter that prevents inhaled particles from penetrating into the lungs. The combination of high velocities, sharp curves, nasal hairs, and secondary flows all combine to collect inhaled particles in the nose. Excellent reviews of particle deposition in the nose are available [114, 140, 205, 223, 259]. The deposition and clearance of particles in the head during nasal breathing have been extensively studied by several investigators [25a, 101, 113, 118, 132, 133, 139, 150, 179, 194, 211, 232a, 233, 259]. Collectively, these reports indicate that the anterior portion of the nose collects particles larger than 1 μm by impaction, with the probability of impaction increasing with increasing d_{ae}^2Q, though there is some evidence that impaction probability is better described by $d_{ae}^2p^{2/3}$, where p is the pressure drop across the nose [113, 223]. Particles may also be intercepted by nasal hairs. Finally, the nose collects significant fractions of particles smaller than 0.005 μm by diffusion [34, 84, 207, 211, 232a]. This size range is relevant to radon progeny, an indoor air pollution problem (see Chap. 45).

Among individuals there are large variations in particle deposition in the nose, which are bigger than those found for deposition in the lungs [194]. These variations may be due to intersubject differences in nasal distensibility and geometry including the number and shape of nasal hairs. Most studies show that particles larger than 10 μm are completely trapped in the nose. Besides being an upstream filter, the nose also humidifies the inspired air. It does so more effectively than the mouth because the inhaled air passes by the large surface area of the turbinates. The nose also contains the smallest cross section of the respiratory tract. Hygroscopic particles ($d_{ae} > 1$ μm) grow more rapidly when inhaled by the nose than the mouth and thus have enhanced deposition [63].

The shift from high filtering efficiency during nasal breathing to decreased filtering efficiency during oronasal breathing may potentiate asthma attacks during exercise. Large volumes of air are inhaled by mouth during exercise, so that more and more antigenic particles, such as pollen, penetrate to and deposit in the lungs. This increased exposure of airways increases the risk of allergic responses. With exercise the amount of particles depositing in the lungs may increase in excess of that predicted by the increased ventilation. Although airway cooling and drying are central features of exercise-induced asthma [33, 50], if allergens are present in the inspired air, increased penetration and deposition of allergens because of mouth breathing may also be involved. The nose is an efficient filter for large particles, but the mouth, due to its simpler geometry, is not. The tracheal and airway doses of 10-μm pollen particles can be increased by an order of magnitude as patients shift from nose to mouth breathing [97].

When breathing orally through a tube, substantial particle deposition can occur by impaction at the larynx; the configuration of the vocal cords influences the extent of deposition. Rudolf and colleagues [196] found that the probability of particles depositing at the larynx is related to $d_{ae}^2Q^{2/3}V^{-1/4}$, where V is the tidal volume. When breathing oronasally without a tube, oral deposition of particles is higher, but is sensitive to changes in oral configuration with ventilation level [19]. Diffusional deposition in the mouth may be significant for particles less than 0.05 μm [34a, 84]. Reviews of particle deposition in the oropharynx are available [223, 259].

When breathing through an endotracheal tube, so that the larynx is bypassed, both airway and pulmonary depositions of particles are increased relative to nasal breathing [130]. An increasingly common practice with intubated patients is to deliver drugs from MDIs directly through the endotracheal tube. In these instances, the drug is delivered with peak delivery efficiencies ranging from 11 to 32 percent for adult-size tracheal tubes [44a, 58a] and from about 1 percent up to 97 percent for pediatric-size tubes [84a, 175a, 235b].

Particle Size and Size Distribution

A major factor governing the effectiveness of deposition mechanisms is the size of the inspired particles. The aerodynamic equivalent diameter (d_{ae}) is a function of the size, density, and shape of the particles and affects the magnitude of forces acting on them. For example, while inertial and gravitational effects increase with increasing particle size, the displacements produced by diffusion decrease. The importance of particle size is clearly seen in Table 32-2, which lists the total and regional deposition of particles in three healthy subjects. Depending on particle size, total deposition varies from 98 to 11 percent; regional deposition is similarly sensitive. As is discussed later, selection of particle size is one way to target particles to desired lung regions. The importance of particle size on total and regional

Table 32-2. Total and regional deposition of stable unit-density spheres in the human respiratory tract during oral breathing from FRC at two tidal volumes (V) and flow rates (Q)

Particle diameter (μm)	Percent deposition							
	Q = 250 cm³/sec, V = 500 cm³				Q = 750 cm³/sec, V = 1,500 cm³			
	Total	Larynx	Airways*	Alveolar*	Total	Larynx	Airways	Alveolar
0.005	67				87			
0.010	62				84			
0.050	33	0	0	33	45	0	0	45
0.100	21	0	0	21	25	0	0	25
0.200	13	0	0	13	14	0	0	14
0.400	11	0	0	11	11	0	0	11
0.700	12	0	0	12	12	0	0	12
1	15	0	0	15	15	0	0	15
2	28	2	1	25	39	1	1	37
3	44	8	4	32	63	8	5	50
4	56	16	7	33	77	21	11	45
5	65	24	11	30	86	40	17	29
6	72	34	15	23	90	52	20	18
7	78	43	18	17	93	61	22	10
8	82	52	20	10	95	69	21	5
9	84	59	19	6	96	77	17	2
10	86	65	17	4	97	82	14	1
12	87	74	12	1	98	89	9	0
15	89	81	8	0				

* The airway and alveolar region designations are based on fast- and slow-clearing compartments, respectively.
Source: Modified from J. Heyder, et al. Deposition of particles in the human respiratory tract in the size range 0.005–15 μm. *J. Aerosol. Sci.* 17:811, 1986.

dose is featured prominently in discussions of particle deposition in the respiratory tract [23, 25, 92, 97, 99, 140, 145, 192, 223, 227].

Our ability to predict the impact of varying particle size is confounded by the fact that most therapeutic aerosols are polydisperse. One can estimate total and regional deposition on the basis of the aerosol's $d_{ae,mm}$ regardless of the geometric standard deviation (σ_g), but theoretic studies show that for many $d_{ae,mm}$'s, this approach significantly overestimates or underestimates total and regional deposition of particles [53, 80, 183, 197]. Diu and Yu [53] found that increasing polydispersity increased the deposition of particles from aerosols with $d_{ae,mm}$'s between 0.04 and 2.00 μm, and decreased the deposition of particles from aerosols with $d_{ae,mm}$'s outside this range. Thus, the overall effect of increasing polydispersity is to decrease the dependency of deposition on particle size; that is, it flattens out the saddle in the deposition curves [80].

Hygroscopicity and Evaporation

In many situations there are dynamic changes in particle size as an aerosol moves through the delivery system and the respiratory tract. Volatile droplets composed of Freon propellant or water shrink through evaporation while hygroscopic droplets such as NaCl particles may grow dramatically, especially as the relative humidity nears 100 percent [35, 60, 63]. Since the relative humidity is 99.5 percent in the lungs beyond the upper airways during normal breathing [62], hygroscopicity has an important effect on particle size and deposition in the lungs. Salt particles grow by factors of 2.0 to 4.4 in the lungs [63]. Many inhaled drugs are hygroscopic [85, 107, 129]; for example, dry 1-μm particles of atropine sulfate and histamine grow in the lungs by factors of 2.2 and 3.5, respectively [64].

The effect of hygroscopicity on particle deposition in humans has been studied both experimentally [9, 15, 105, 239] and theoretically [60, 63, 151, 183, 253, 261], and has been recently reviewed [106, 162, 188]. The overall theme suggested by these studies is that with increasing particle hygroscopicity and relative humidity, the curve describing the relation between deposi-

tion fraction and particle size is shifted to smaller particle sizes. That is, whereas the deposition minimum for nonhygroscopic particles is about 0.4 μm (see Table 32-2), the minimum for dry NaCl particles is about 0.1 μm [253]. Consequently, the total deposition of dry hygroscopic particles with diameters greater than 0.1 μm exceeds the deposition of nonhygroscopic particles of the same size (Table 32-3). In addition, hygroscopicity affects regional deposition (see Table 32-3); it more than doubles the bronchial and pulmonary deposition of drug particles with initial dry sizes of about 0.5 to 2.0 μm [64].

The rate of hygroscopic particle growth is dependent on particle size. Dry particles less than 1 μm reach their full size in about 2 seconds, whereas particles 3 μm and larger take more than 10 seconds [65]. The time lag for the growth of large particles offers an attractive means to enhance deposition in the airways and pulmonary region while minimizing deposition in the oropharynx. Fifty percent of 5-μm (initially dry) NaCl particles deposit in the airways during tidal oral breathing, whereas only 23 percent of nonhygroscopic 5-μm particles deposit there, even though both particles have the same deposition in the oropharynx [65].

The osmolality of the nebulized solution governs hygroscopic growth when the hygroscopic material is inhaled. Inhaled hygroscopic droplets reach equilibrium size when the water vapor pressures at the droplet surface and in the lungs are equal. The water vapor pressure in the lungs is controlled by the osmolality of the liquid lining the lung surface, which is approximately isosmotic with serum [16a]. Thus, inhaled droplets absorb or desorb water until the droplet solution is isosmotic with the surface liquid: Solid hygroscopic particles or hyperosmotic droplets gain water and grow, hyposmotic droplets lose water and shrink (pure water droplets completely evaporate), and isosmotic droplets change little in size. The measurement and adjustment of the osmolality of the nebulized solution comprise a valuable, yet underutilized strategy to predict and optimize drug delivery [85, 184]. However, one must also remember that marked hyperosmotic or hyposmotic concentrations may cause cough and bronchoconstriction in asthmatic subjects [59].

Table 32-3. Total and regional deposition of stable unit-density spheres and NaCl particles in the human respiratory tract during oral and nasal breathing from FRC[a]

Initial particle diameter (μm)	Type	Percent deposition							
		Oral breathing				Nasal breathing			
		Total	Larynx	Airways[b]	Alveolar[b]	Total	Larynx	Airways	Alveolar
0.1	Stable	43	0	8	35	43	0	8	35
	NaCl	22	0	4	18	22	0	4	18
0.4	Stable	17	0	3	15	19	2	2	14
	NaCl	37	0	4	34	40	3	4	33
1.0	Stable	25	0	3	22	28	4	3	21
	NaCl	76	0	11	65	79	15	10	54
2.0	Stable	52	0	6	46	62	23	5	35
	NaCl	84	0	24	61	89	31	17	40
5.0	Stable	84	11	23	50	91	53	12	26
	NaCl	90	11	50	28	94	55	26	12
10.0	Stable	91	30	47	15	96	77	19	5
	NaCl	93	30	60	3	96	77	19	0

[a] Tidal volume = 1,000 cm³; flow rate = 250 cm³/sec.
[b] The airway and alveolar region designations are based on fast- and slow-clearing compartments, respectively.
Source: Modified from G. A. Ferron, W. G. Kreyling, and B. Haider. Inhalation of salt aerosol particles. II. Growth and deposition in the human respiratory tract. *J. Aerosol. Sci.* 19:611, 1988.

Breathing Pattern

When a subject changes the breathing pattern, particle deposition may be affected profoundly. Minute volume defines the total number of particles that enter the lungs. Flow rate affects the probability of particle impaction, whereas flow rate, tidal volume, and lung volume affect the particle residence time in each lung region and hence the probability of deposition by gravitational and diffusional forces [93]. Tidal volume and flow rate also influence the motion of the larynx and affect particle deposition there [196]. Flow rate determines the degree and extent of turbulent flow in the upper airways that enhances particle deposition. Changing lung volume also alters the dimensions of the airways and parenchyma. High levels of ventilation compared to breath holding represent extremes of breathing patterns; they give rise to markedly different deposition patterns.

Many of these breathing pattern interactions are represented in Table 32-2, which shows total and regional deposition data for two breathing patterns that differ in flow rate and tidal volume by a factor of 3. The larger tidal volume increases the proportion of the breath that goes to the alveoli, and the higher flow rate causes the particles to spend less time in the airways and more time in the alveoli. Both of these factors enhance deposition by diffusion and sedimentation for particles less than 5 μm in diameter in the alveoli. The higher flow rate also enhances deposition by impaction for particles 4 μm and larger at the larynx. Yet, despite the large change in breathing pattern, the deposition in the airways hardly changes. Thus, when airflow velocities increase, such as in physical exertion or labored respiration consequent to an asthma attack, inertial deposition increases. During slow, relaxed breathing, particle sedimentation and diffusion are the primary deposition processes, and aerosol collection in the alveoli and distal lung units increases due to the proximity of lung surfaces there.

The optimal breathing pattern for drug delivery may depend on the type of device used. For MDIs used with bronchodilators, it is recommended that the inspiratory flow rate be less than 500 cm³/sec, the inspired volume be large but not to total lung capacity, and there be a 10-second breath hold at end-inspiration [170]. With this maneuver about 10 to 20 percent of the aerosolized drug deposits in the lungs; a large amount of the drug deposits by impaction in the oropharynx due to the high velocity of the aerosol as it leaves the MDI [168]. For jet nebulizers used with continuous flow, it is recommended that the inspiratory flow rate also be slow (<550 cm³/sec) as higher flow rates enhance drug deposition in the oropharynx [135]. Tidal breaths should be large (1–2 liters) to enhance the dose of drug delivered to the pulmonary region [181, 184]. Minute ventilations should be 12 to 14 L/min for optimum deposition of particles ($d_{ae,mm}$ = 1.1 μm) in obstructed patients [115], though deposition in restricted patients is less dependent on ventilation [214]. If nebulization is continuous, breath holding is not suggested since it wastes drug and is not as effective as continually breathing the drug over the same length of time [184]. Like MDIs, jet nebulizers deposit about 10 percent of the nebulized drug in the lungs, but with nebulizers most of the drug is lost in the apparatus and tubing rather than the oropharynx [168].

In contrast to MDIs and nebulizers, dry-powder inhalers require rapid inspirations. Peak inspiratory flow rates of 500 cm³/sec and greater aid in dispersing the drug powder into smaller particles which enter the lungs and improve the effectiveness of drug delivered; however, breath holding or inspirations from residual volume have no added benefit [90, 119, 182]. Deposition of drug in the lungs with dry-powder inhalers averages about 15 percent, which is comparable to the levels for MDIs and nebulizers [168a, 169, 244].

Disease

Respiratory diseases are often heterogeneously distributed and influence the distribution of inspired particles. Bronchoconstriction or obstruction of airways due to mucus or inflammation diverts more airflow to nonobstructed airways. With advancing disease the remaining healthy alveoli and airways are increasingly exposed to inspired particles. Particle deposition in these healthy regions also increases due to (1) higher flow rates, which increase particle impaction in airways; and (2) longer residence times in the lung periphery, which favor sedimentation and diffusion [125, 126, 238]. Furthermore, deposition at obstructed sites is also enhanced despite the reduced airflow through these regions. However, the regions downstream of the obstructions have less deposition [116, 117, 126, 148, 193, 234, 238]. Similar heterogeneous deposition patterns are found in asthmatic subjects [2, 136, 227a], patients with cystic fibrosis [134], and smokers [58].

At sites of mild to severe obstruction, high linear velocities and flow turbulence enhance particle deposition by impaction and turbulent diffusion, which combine to create focal deposition "hot spots" immediately downstream [116, 125, 126, 148]. Sites of obstruction may also be dynamic: The passing airflow can create mucus waves that increase particle losses due to turbulent diffusion [124]; similarly, flow limitation and dynamic compression of airways during exhalation enhance particle deposition in patients with bronchitis or emphysema [216]. Decreased particle deposition in the lung regions downstream of obstructions can be explained by the filtering of the constricted sites plus the lower airflow entering the region [126]. Overall, deposition in obstructed patients is greater than in healthy persons and increases with the severity of disease as indicated by pulmonary function or clinical diagnosis [5, 7, 128, 142, 149]. The net result for the asthma patient, particularly during an acute episode, is increased heterogeneity of lung retention, with a predominance of central deposition. In restrictive disease, there is an irregular peripheral deposition pattern in patients with diffuse interstitial fibrosis [117]; however, patients with sarcoidosis have the same deposition of submicrometric particles as healthy subjects [8].

SELECTING DEPOSITION PATTERNS

Some of the factors just discussed that are known to influence particle deposition may be exploited to target drugs to diseased lung regions with greater control of dose while simultaneously decreasing systemic side effects [167]. Probably the most powerful is the combination of a preselected breathing pattern with a particular particle size. Stahlhofen and coworkers [221], based on their studies in healthy subjects, recommend that to target the nose or oropharynx or larynx, rapid breaths (Q > 750 cm^3/sec) of particles with a 9-μm $d_{ae,mm}$ or larger be used. This strategy will deposit more than 80 percent of the mass in these regions due to enhanced particle impaction. To target the alveoli, slow, deep breaths (1,000-cm^3 breaths, 8/min) of 2-μm particles could be used. This enhances particle settling and deposits about 50 percent of the mass in the lung periphery, with most of the remaining mass being exhaled.

Targeting the tracheobronchial region by selecting breathing pattern and particle size, without appreciable deposition in other regions, is not possible. Particles with a $d_{ae,mm}$ of 6 to 8 μm are useful since about 20 percent of the mass deposits in the airways. However, when these particles are inhaled with rapid, shallow breathing, there is also enhanced head deposition, whereas when inhaled with slow, deep breathing, alveolar deposition is also enhanced. One proven way to target the airways is to inhale smaller particles (2–3 μm) and use forced exhalations or coughing to enhance deposition at flow-limiting segments during exhalation [13, 68, 86, 215, 232]. In diseased patients with narrowed or obstructed airways, enhanced deposition of particles at sites of obstruction helps target these areas [126], while particles may need to be smaller than 1 μm to successfully pass through obstructed sites to reach downstream lung regions.

Several investigators have tailored the particle size, breathing pattern, or both in attempts to enhance drug or particle deposition in the airways or lung periphery [37, 38, 57, 74, 86, 121, 135, 158, 167, 181, 201, 213, 226]. Many studies appeared successful; those that were not may have failed because the range of particle sizes, breathing patterns, or lung penetrations were insufficient to favor deposition in one region over another. Furthermore, as mentioned above, the airways cannot be targeted exclusively [221].

There are other strategies to target particles [12a, 81]. Breath holding increases both airway and alveolar deposition of particles. Increased aerosol monodispersity allows better prediction and control of deposition sites [53, 80, 183, 197], or particle sizes, such as 2 μm, that have deposition patterns independent of polydispersity could be used [53, 197]. Hygroscopic particles can be produced that are initially small enough to escape deposition in the mouth or nose, but they grow in the airways and thus enhance deposition of particles in the airways [184]. Conversely, hygroscopic growth can be decreased when particles are mixed with hydrophobic materials [104, 177, 252]. To minimize deposition in conducting airways, the aerosolized drug can be delivered at the beginning of inspiration or as an aerosol bolus that is followed by clean air [172, 198, 199, 201]. Boluses introduced at the end of the breath enhance deposition of particles in the airways. Boluses offer the advantages of reducing the total dose of drug delivered to the lungs as well as decreasing the likelihood of side effects and cost. Bolus delivery may also help those patients who are unable to do the respiratory gymnastics required for targeted delivery.

How direct instillation of particles can be used to achieve selected location concentrations has already been discussed [22]. Using catheters, one can place drugs directly onto the tracheal surface, into the left or right bronchi, or in other localized sites. Injection of particles containing drugs into the circulation could be used. The caliber of the blood vessel in which the drug particle lodges can be controlled by selecting the appropriate diameter of the injected microspheres. Depending on the surgical skills available, one could selectively expose specific regions of the respiratory tract by picking a specific branch of the pulmonary or bronchial circulation. Other drugs may also be removed from the circulating blood by endothelial cells or by resident phagocytic cells in lung capillaries.

There is the possibility, mostly theoretic at this point, that one could enhance deposition mechanisms locally and thus influence local collection efficiency and regional deposition. Magnetic and acoustic forces such as shock waves are possibilities.

When choosing a targeting method, one should also consider how to calculate delivered drug dose and the local distribution of dose. Delivered drug dose may be calculated on the basis of inhaled mass per unit of time and the fraction that deposits in the targeted region, which is based on the $d_{ae,mm}$ and breathing pattern. Yet this compartmental approach neglects the substantial disparity in the surface area of the airways and parenchyma. For example, Sweeney and associates [228] analyzed the deposition of drug from an MDI on the basis of anatomic compartments and surface area. About half of the drug was deposited in the lungs; of that, 82 percent deposited in the parenchyma and only 18 percent in the intrapulmonary airways. However, when surface area was accounted for, the airway dose per unit of surface area was about 280 times greater than the parenchymal dose. Often the deposition of particles is enhanced in certain airway generations, in which case the disparity between airway and parenchymal surface dose would be even greater [78].

The anatomic distribution of particle deposition on the lung surface is influenced by the deposition mechanism, disease, and lung geometry. Particle impaction creates enhanced areas of deposition at bifurcations and immediately downstream of lung obstructions [126, 143]. Sedimentation deposits particles on only the bottom half of lung surfaces, while diffusion deposits particles on all surfaces. In humans and dogs theoretic studies suggest there is a uniform pattern of deposition at alveolar ducts [257], but in rodents experimental studies show there is nonuniform deposition at duct bifurcations [26] and between ducts and alveoli [262].

Animal models of chronic pulmonary disease have been used to study the effect of the developing disease on the site of deposition within the lungs. Sweeney and colleagues [229–231] studied the progressive influence of emphysema, chronic bronchitis, and fibrosis on the distribution of deposition of submicrometric particles throughout rodent lungs. One common result in all three diseases is that the presence of detectable pulmonary disease always results in less uniform patterns of particle deposition throughout the lungs.

MEASURING PARTICLE RETENTION

Once aerosols have been introduced into the respiratory tract, the challenge of quantifying the amount and distribution of dose must be faced. Not only are the technologic solutions frequently complex, but also the nature of the problem to be solved is frequently obscure. How should the dose to the respiratory tract be calculated? Should it be averaged over the whole lung, or should the local airway or alveolar epithelial dose be estimated?

At the outset it is essential to remember that the initial deposition pattern is continuously modified by clearance processes. Loss and redistribution of deposited particles is the rule, not the exception, unless the aerosol exposure period is brief and the interval between exposure and analysis is short.

An extensive menu of measurement techniques is available. The approaches vary in expense, resolution, and the extent to which the subject must be disturbed. There are advantages in using nondestructive, noninvasive methods of detection. They allow repeated measurements on the same animal or person, and thus permit replications and serial measurements. For human experimentation such detection methods are essential. However, measurements of retention in whole animals may not provide adequate details about the distribution of dose to structures of interest. The greatest precision is achieved by killing and dissecting animals. By freezing or drying, the lungs can be made rigid and then sliced or dissected. It is then possible to physically divide the respiratory tract into individual pieces or specific lung compartments and analyze the particle content of each piece. Depending on one's patience and the sensitivity of the detection method, the distribution of particle retention can be described with increasing detail. These approaches permit an identification of anatomic location of retained particles. Recent articles and a review from our laboratory [227b, 229, 262] detailed these methods.

Actual detection of particles can rely on any distinctive property of the aerosol. Particles may be radioactive, fluorescent, radiopaque, magnetic, or pharmacologically active. They may have a characteristic visual appearance that can be identified with light and electron microscopy. Their elemental or molecular nature may be identified by a repertoire of techniques including colorimetry, atomic absorption, neutron activation, nuclear magnetic resonance, electron energy loss spectrometry (EELS), and other procedures. The type of question being asked suggests which properties of the particle can be exploited for ease and specificity of detection.

Various approaches that can be used were reviewed in greater detail by Brain and Valberg [25] and in the accompanying references. The first approach is to estimate the dose based on measurements of inspired particle size and concentration. The minimum characterization of any aerosol exposure should include its concentration, size, and composition. Although it is essential to describe the aerosol inhaled, it is important to realize that many factors such as species, age, level of activity, and disease will influence the fraction of the inspired particles deposited in each subject and its distribution.

Modeling

If ventilation is measured well, one can estimate deposition based on theoretic predictions and models. Early attempts at models that could be used to predict deposition were made by Findeisen [66], Landahl [131], Altshuler [5a], and Beeckmans [11]. More recent deposition models include those of Taulbee, Yu, and Diu [235a, 258]; Egan and Nixon [58b]; and Koblinger and Hofmann [111a, 130a]. The deposition of hygroscopic particles was modeled by Ferron and coworkers [63]. The general concepts of several deposition models, including some just mentioned, were explained in a review by Heyder and Rudolf [102]. The International Commission on Radiological Protection (ICRP) Task Group [235] model includes both theoretic predictions and experimental data and represents the Committee's best estimates of deposition at the time. The model has been converted to convenient equations, nomograms, and computer programs by Brain and Valberg [24] so that total integrated exposure to particles can be calculated when particle solubility, size, and concentration are known. Recently the ICRP model has been revised to include new experimental deposition data and to model deposition in adults and children at different activity levels [9a]. Many of the considerations that enter dosimetric modeling of inhaled particles were recently discussed [44, 46a, 176a].

Prediction of total and regional deposited dose in healthy persons has become much easier with recently developed semiempirical deposition formulas that are based on data like those shown in Table 32-2 [196, 223]. These formulas are designed for individuals breathing well-characterized aerosols in a known manner and are customized for each individual based on his or her functional residual capacity. Other equations have been developed to predict the regional deposition of particles in persons of different ages [261a] and in adults at a variety of activity levels and for oronasal breathing [157].

Photometry

Another approach is to measure experimentally the difference in the aerosol content of inspired and expired air using light-scattering methods [75] or filters [115]. By adding a measurement of ventilation, one can determine the total amount of material that is deposited in the respiratory tract. No information regarding the sites of deposition, however, is obtained. Information regarding airway size and convective transport in the respiratory tract can be obtained [94, 96].

Bronchoalveolar Lavage

Bronchoalveolar lavage is a technique accessible to most clinicians that can provide some information about retention of drugs that are not rapidly absorbed across the lung epithelium. For example, Smaldone and coworkers [214] found that deposition of pentamidine was correlated with the drug concentration lavaged from the middle lobe airways 24 hours after exposure.

Radioactivity

Radioactivity has been used frequently for studies of particle deposition because of its potential for noninvasive measurement and its sensitivity and resolution. Hundreds of radioisotopes are produced, and labeled drugs can be synthesized with a wide spectrum of energies, type of radiation (alpha, beta, gamma, positrons), and half-lives. Gamma emitters penetrate through tissue and are therefore suitable for making measurements externally. Alpha or beta emitters are better suited for producing autoradiographs; their short path-length, which makes them unsuitable for external detection, produces high resolution on film in contact with particle-laden tissue.

Descriptions of the technologies involved are widely available. Several books summarize the applications of radioactivity to imaging [70, 82]. Frequently it is useful to restrict the field of view of the detector to a region of interest. This can be achieved with a collimator constructed of lead, which blocks most radiation coming to the detector except that from a selected region of the body. A variety of shielded counters that utilize large sodium iodide crystals and appropriate lead shielding have been constructed [46, 164].

Gamma Cameras

Gamma cameras are similar but utilize a stationary detector, which simultaneously collects information from a large area. As first described by Anger (see [178]), this device uses a single, large scintillation crystal, which is masked with a honeycomb, parallel-hole lead collimator with as many as 15,000 holes. Each part of the crystal looks at a small area of the patient or animal and scintillations are produced in different parts of the crystal. An array of phototubes senses the light pulses produced in the crystal by incoming gamma rays and the relative pulse sizes from different photomultiplier tubes give the position of the scintillation. From this the two-dimensional position of the labeled particle in the respiratory tract can be estimated and displayed on a cathode-ray tube screen or stored in a computer. Images are often divided into central and peripheral lung regions; a penetration index that represents the relative deposition in these two areas can then be calculated [58]. Methodologic considerations for the use of gamma cameras to measure lung dose were recently discussed [45a, 235c].

Tomography

Tomography is used to map and follow the distribution of retained particles in three dimensions. In the two-dimensional view of the lung provided by a gamma camera, the central lung region, which is taken to represent the central airways, also contains overlapping small airways and alveoli. Thus, one cannot discriminate among particle deposition in these regions, and deposition in central airways may be overestimated [186]. In contrast, central airways and peripheral lung regions can be resolved when tomography is used. There are two types of tomography for measuring regional particle retention: single-photon emission computed tomography (SPECT) and positron emission tomography (PET). With SPECT the subject inhales gamma-emitting particles and lies over a gamma camera, and a scan is made [146]. Then the camera is rotated a few degrees and another scan is made; the process is repeated until the lung has been scanned from 64 angles [186]. Since each radiolabeled particle releases multiple photons, which the camera detects from other positions, there are several emission lines with the particle at their intersection. After the scan, a computer program reconstructs the series of two-dimensional scans into a three-dimensional image, and particle retention in desired lung slices can be compared [43].

To date PET has not been used for particle retention studies, but it is readily adaptable [210]. The subject would inhale a positron-emitting radionuclide, such as carbon 11–containing particles or gallium oxide ($^{68}Ga_2O_3$) aggregates, and lie in the PET. A positron travels 2 to 5 mm before it combines with an electron; the ensuing annihilation process produces two gamma photons at 180 degrees relative to each other. A series of paired scintillation detectors surrounding the subject record the site of interaction of these photons; then the line along which decay events originate can be reconstructed. Since the particle creates multiple photon pairs, which other detector pairs detect, there are several emission lines, with the particle at their intersection. After the scan is complete, these multiple emission lines are analyzed by tomographic computer analysis to generate the three-dimensional particle deposition pattern. Since PET determines the origin of photon emission based on the coincident detection by detector pairs, as opposed to the collimation required by SPECT, PET ignores less of the emitted radiation and is more efficient than SPECT [210]. Another advantage is that the positron-emitting isotopes have short half-lives, so it is easier to make repeated studies in the same subject.

Magnetopneumography

Some aerosols are magnetizable, and sensitive magnetopneumography can be used to measure their concentration and distribution in the lungs [241]. The technique consists of applying a magnetic field to the whole thorax or to localized areas and detecting the resulting alignment of ferromagnetic domains in retained lung particles. Accumulations of magnetic particles have been measured in foundry workers, arc welders, coal miners, and asbestos miners [42, 69, 123]. The greatest advantage of this technique is that the duration of measurement is not limited by radioactive decay. Measurements can be made as long as sufficient dust remains in the lungs. Thus, one can noninvasively describe clearance kinetics over years [41]. Two magnetic dusts suitable for studying retention of dust in the lung are Fe_3O_4 (magnetite) and gamma-Fe_2O_3 (a magnetic form of hematite). Both are inert and relatively insoluble at physiologic pH, and can be produced as aerosols. The magnitude of the remnant field can be used to quantify the amount of dust remaining in the lungs.

DEPOSITION PATTERNS AND CLINICAL EFFECTS

Even if specific deposition patterns of drug aerosols can be selected, we are left with the key question: "Does it make a difference?" If deposition is mainly in large airways, will the distribution of response differ importantly from that seen when the same drug or allergen is placed in small airways or alveoli? The answer may well depend on the mechanisms and pathways involved.

For example, if the distribution of responses was relatively uniform, in spite of changing particle deposition patterns, that would suggest that there may be a uniform reflex bronchoconstriction. It could also suggest that there may be drug absorption and transport via the bronchial circulation. It should be remembered that the anatomic distribution of response depends not exclusively on the distribution of particle deposition, but also on the distribution of mast cells as well as other inflammatory cells in the airways and the distribution of receptors throughout the airway epithelia. The regional distribution of many receptor classes is still too ill-defined to evaluate the effectiveness of targeting strategies. Furthermore, the properties of the mucus and bronchial epithelium are important, since many drugs or antigens must breach these barriers in order to come into contact with more reactive cells, nerves, or smooth muscle. It remains to be shown conclusively whether widely varying retention patterns importantly influence the extent and distribution of the airway responsiveness.

Determining the distribution of pharmacologic aerosols within the respiratory tract is one segment of the more general problem of correlating drug concentrations at their site of action with a measured response. It is possible that much of the variability in drug responses among different pharmaceutic preparations, different individuals, and various animal species may result from differences in concentration of the drug at the site of action rather than to variation in responsiveness of specific active tissues [214]. Different drug preparations may be deposited at different sites and absorbed at different rates from airway and alveolar surfaces. The chemical stability of the drug at different sites within the respiratory tract is important, as are enzymes throughout the respiratory tract that may be involved in drug metabolism. Looking for the drug and its metabolites in blood, urine, and feces may provide important clues to its fate. Such studies of drug disposition and metabolism within the respiratory tract will continue to be central to the use of therapeutic drugs and provocation challenges. They will be an essential step in determining the proper form of the drug and the appropriate dosages. Such considerations will also be central to the search for mechanisms that underlie drug effects, interactions between drugs, and adverse drug reactions. Investment in a thorough description of the location of aerosols in the respiratory tract will be rewarded since improved understanding of the effects of aerosols stems from the recognition of factors important to their uptake and fate.

REFERENCES

1. Agnew, J. E. Physical Properties and Mechanisms of Deposition of Aerosols. In S. W. Clarke and D. Pavia (eds.), *Aerosols and the Lung: Clinical and Experimental Aspects*. Boston: Butterworths, 1984. Pp. 49–70.
2. Agnew, J. E., et al. Radionuclide demonstration of ventilatory abnormalities in mild asthma. *Clin. Sci.* 66:525, 1984.
3. Aharonson, E. F., Ben-David, A., and Klingberg, M. A. (eds.), *Air Pollution and the Lung*. New York: Halsted Press-Wiley, 1976.
3a. Aiache, J.-M. The ideal drug delivery system: A look into the future. *J. Aerosol Med.* 4:323, 1991.
4. Albert, R. E., and Arnett, L. C. Clearance of radioactive dust from the lung. *Arch. Environ. Health* 12:99, 1955.
5. Albert, R. E., et al. Bronchial deposition and clearance of aerosols. *Arch. Intern. Med.* 131:115, 1973.
5a. Altschuler, B. Calculation of regional deposition of aerosol in the respiratory tract. *Bull. Math. Biophys.* 21:257, 1959.
6. Altshuler, B., et al. Aerosol deposition in the human respiratory tract. I. Experimental procedures and total deposition. *AMA Arch. Ind. Health* 15:293, 1957.
7. Anderson, P. J., et al. Aerosol bolus dispersion and deposition in cystic fibrosis patients and healthy nonsmokers. *Am. Rev. Respir. Dis.* 140:1317, 1989.
8. Anderson, P. J., Wilson, J. D., and Hiller, F. C. Respiratory tract deposition of ultrafine particles in subjects with obstructive or restrictive lung disease. *Chest* 97:1115, 1990.
9. Anselm, A., et al. Human Inhalation Studies of Growth of Hygroscopic Particles in the Respiratory Tract. In W. Schikarski, H. Fissan, and S. Friedlander (eds.), *Aerosols—Formation and Reactivity*. Elmsford, N.Y.: Pergamon, 1986. Pp. 252–255.
9a. Bair, W. J. The revised International Commission on Radiological Protection (ICRP) dosimetric model for the human respiratory tract—An overview. Presented at the 7th International Symposium on Inhaled Particles, September 1991, Edinburgh. Abstracted in *J. Aerosol Med.* 5:51, 1992.
10. Becquemin, M. H., et al. Deposition of Inhaled Particles in Healthy Children. In W. Hofmann (ed.), *Deposition and Clearance of Aerosols in the Human Respiratory Tract*. Vienna: Facultas, 1987. Pp. 22–27.
11. Beeckmans, J. M. The deposition of aerosols in the respiratory tract. I. Mathematical analysis and comparison with experimental data. *Can. J. Physiol. Pharmacol.* 43:157, 1965.
12. Bell, J. H., Hartley, P. S., and Cox, J. S. G. Dry powder inhalers. 1. A new powder inhalation device. *J. Pharm. Sci.* 10:1559, 1971.
12a. Bennett, W. D. Targeting respiratory drug delivery with aerosol boluses. *J. Aerosol Med.* 4:69, 1991.
13. Bennett, W. D., and Ilowite, J. S. Dual pathway clearance of Tc99m-DPTA from the bronchial mucosa. *Am. Rev. Respir. Dis.* 139:1132, 1989.
14. Blanchard, J. D., et al. Aerosol-derived lung morphometry: Comparisons with a lung model and lung function indexes. *J. Appl. Physiol.* 71:1216, 1991.
15. Blanchard, J. D., and Willeke, K. Total deposition of ultrafine sodium chloride particles in human lungs. *J. Appl. Physiol.* 57:1850, 1984.
16. Booker, D. V., et al. Elimination of 5 micron particles from the human lung. *Nature* 215:30, 1967.
16a. Boucher, R. C., et al. Regional differences in airway liquid composition. *J. Appl. Physiol.* 50:613, 1981.
17. Bouchikhi, A., et al. Particle size study of nine metered dose inhalers, and their deposition probabilities in the airways. *Eur. Respir. J.* 1:547, 1988.
18. Bowes, S. M., III, Frank, R., and Swift, D. L. The head dome: A simplified method for human exposures to inhaled air pollutants. *Am. Ind. Hyg. Assoc. J.* 51:257, 1990.
19. Bowes, S. M., III, and Swift, D. L. Deposition of inhaled particles in the oral airway during oronasal breathing. *Aerosol Sci. Technol.* 11:157, 1989.
20. Brain, J. D. Macrophages in the Respiratory Tract. In A. P. Fishman and A. B. Fisher (eds.), *Handbook of Physiology*, Vol. 1. *Circulation and Nonrespiratory Functions*. Bethesda, Md.: American Physiological Society, 1985. Pp. 447–471.
21. Brain, J. D. Lung macrophages—How many kinds are there? What do they do? *Am. Rev. Respir. Dis.* 137:507, 1988.
22. Brain, J. D., et al. Pulmonary distribution of particles given by intratracheal instillation or by aerosol inhalation. *Environ. Res.* 11:13, 1976.
23. Brain, J. D., Proctor, D. F., and Reid, L. M. (eds.), *Lung Biology in Health and Disease*, Vol. 5. *Respiratory Defense Mechanisms*. New York: Marcel Dekker, 1977.
24. Brain, J. D., and Valberg, P. A. Models of lung retention based on the ICRP Task Group. *Arch. Environ. Health* 28:1, 1974.
25. Brain, J. D., and Valberg, P. A. Deposition of aerosol in the respiratory tract. *Am. Rev. Respir. Dis.* 120:1325, 1979.
25a. Breysse, P. N., and Swift, D. L. Inhalability of large particles into the human nasal passage: In vivo studies in still air. *Aerosol Sci. Technol.* 13:459, 1990.
26. Brody, A. R., and Roe, M. W. Deposition pattern of inorganic particles at the alveolar level in the lungs of mice and rats. *Am. Rev. Respir. Dis.* 128:724, 1983.
27. Byron, P. R. Aerosol Formulation, Generation, and Delivery Using Nonmetered Systems. In P. R. Byron (ed.), *Respiratory Drug Delivery*. Boca Raton, Fla.: CRC Press, 1990. Pp. 143–165.
28. Byron, P. R. Aerosol Formulation, Generation, and Delivery Using Metered Systems. In P. R. Byron (ed.), *Respiratory Drug Delivery*. Boca Raton, Fla.: CRC Press, 1990. Pp. 167–205.
29. Byron, P. R., and Phillips, E. M. Absorption, Clearance, and Dissolution in the Lung. In P. R. Byron (ed.), *Respiratory Drug Delivery*. Boca Raton, Fla.: CRC Press, 1990. Pp. 107–141.
29a. Byron, P. R. (ed.), *Respiratory Drug Delivery*. Boca Raton, Fla.: CRC Press, 1990.
29b. Byron, P. R. (ed.), *Proceedings of Respiratory Drug Delivery II*. Lexington: University of Kentucky College of Pharmacy, 1991.
29c. Byron, P. R. (ed.), Proceedings of Respiratory Drug Delivery III. *J. Biopharm. Sci.* 3(1–2), 1992.
30. Camner, P., and Mossberg, B. Mucociliary disorders: A review. *J. Aerosol Med.* 1:21, 1988.
31. Camner, P., and Philipson, M. S. Human alveolar deposition of 4 micron Teflon particles. *Arch. Environ. Health* 33:181, 1978.
31a. Chadha, T. S., Birch, S., and Sackner, M. A. Oronasal distribution of ventilation during exercise in normal subjects and patients with asthma and rhinitis. *Chest* 92:1037, 1987.
32. Chan, T. L., Shreck, R. M., and Lippmann, M. Effect of the laryngeal jet on particle deposition in the human trachea and upper bronchial airways. *J. Aerosol Sci.* 11:447, 1980.
33. Chen, W. Y., and Horton, D. J. Heat and water loss from the airways and exercise-induced asthma. *Respiration* 34:305, 1977.
34. Cheng, Y.-S., et al. Diffusional deposition of ultrafine aerosols in a human nasal cast. *J. Aerosol Sci.* 19:741, 1988.
34a. Cheng, Y.-S., et al. Deposition of ultrafine particles in a human oral cast. *Aerosol Sci. Technol.* 3:1075, 1990.
35. Cinkotai, F. F. The behavior of sodium chloride particles in moist air. *J. Aerosol Sci.* 2:325, 1971.
36. Clarke, S. W., and Pavia, D. (eds.), *Aerosols and the Lung*. Boston: Butterworths, 1984.
37. Clay, M. M., and Clarke, S. W. Effect of nebulized aerosol size on lung deposition in patients with mild asthma. *Thorax* 42:190, 1987.
38. Clay, M. M., Pavia, D., and Clarke, S. W. Effect of aerosol particle size on bronchodilation with nebulized terbutaline in asthmatic patients. *Thorax* 41:364, 1986.
39. Clay, M. M., et al. Factors influencing the size distribution of aerosols from jet nebulizers. *Thorax* 38:755, 1983.
40. Clay, M. M., et al. Assessment of jet nebulizers for lung aerosol therapy. *Lancet* 2:592, 1983.
40a. Cloutier, Y., et al. New methodology for specific inhalation challenges with occupational agents in powder form. *Eur. Respir. J.* 2:769, 1989.
40b. Cloutier, Y., and Malo, J.-L. Update on an exposure system for particles in the diagnosis of occupational asthma. *Eur. Respir. J.* 5:887, 1992.
41. Cohen, D., Arai, S., and Brain, J. D. Smoking impairs longterm dust clearance from the lungs. *Science* 204:514, 1979.
42. Cohen, D., et al. Magnetic lung measurements in relation to occupational exposure in asbestos miners and millers of Quebec. *Environ. Res.* 26:535, 1981.
43. Coleman, R. E., et al. Regional Dosimetry of Inhaled Particles Using SPECT. In J. D. Crapo, et al. (eds.), *Extrapolation of Dosimetric Relationships to Inhaled Particles and Gases*. San Diego: Academic, 1989. Pp. 201–210.
44. Crapo, J. D., et al. (eds.), *Extrapolation of Dosimetric Relationships to Inhaled Particles and Gases*. San Diego: Academic, 1989.
44a. Crogan, S. J., and Bishop, M. J. Delivery efficiency of metered dose aerosols given via endotracheal tubes. *Anesthesiology* 70:1008, 1989.
45. Crompton, G. K. Problems patients have using pressurised aerosol inhalers. *Eur. J. Respir. Dis.* 63(Suppl. 119):101, 1982.
45a. Cross, C. E., et al. Aerosol deposition: Practical considerations of method-

ology for the direct measurement of aerosol delivery to the lung bronchiolar-alveolar surfaces. *J. Aerosol Med.* 5:39, 1992.

46. Cuddihy, R. G., and Boecker, B. B. Controlled administration of respiratory tract burdens of inhaled radioactive aerosols in beagle dogs. *Toxicol. Appl. Pharmacol.* 25:597, 1973.

46a. Dahl, A. R., et al. Comparative dosimetry of inhaled materials: Differences among animal species and extrapolation to man. Symposium overview. *Fund. Appl. Toxicol.* 16:1, 1991.

47. Davies, C. N. (ed.), *Inhaled Particles and Vapours.* Elmsford, N.Y.: Pergamon, 1961.

48. Davies, C. N. (ed.), *Inhaled Particles and Vapours II.* Elmsford, N.Y.: Pergamon, 1964.

49. Davies, C. N. (ed.), *Aerosol Science.* New York: Academic, 1966.

50. Deal, E. C., Jr., et al. Role of respiratory heat exchange in production of exercise-induced asthma. *J. Appl. Physiol.* 46:467, 1979.

51. Dennis, R. (ed.), *Handbook on Aerosols.* National Technology Information Service. Washington, D.C.: U.S. Department of Commerce, 1976.

52. Dhand, R., et al. High speed photographic analysis of aerosols produced by metered dose inhalers. *J. Pharm. Pharmacol.* 40:429, 1988.

53. Diu, C. K., and Yu, C. P. Respiratory tract deposition of polydisperse aerosols in humans. *Am. Ind. Hyg. Assoc. J.* 44:62, 1983.

54. Dodgson, J., et al. (eds.), Inhaled Particles VI. *Ann. Occup. Hyg.* 32(Suppl. 1):1, 1988.

55. Dolovich, M. Physical properties underlying aerosol therapy. *J. Aerosol Med.* 2:171, 1989.

56. Dolovich, M., et al. Optimal delivery of aerosols from metered dose inhalers. *Chest* 80(Suppl.):911, 1981.

57. Dolovich, M., Ryan, G., and Newhouse, M. T. Aerosol penetration into the lung: Influence of airway responses. *Chest* 80(Suppl.):834, 1981.

58. Dolovich, M. B., et al. Aerosol penetrance: A sensitive index of peripheral airways obstruction. *J. Appl. Physiol.* 40:468, 1976.

58a. Donna, E., et al. Delivery efficiency of 3 metered dose inhaler aerosols and 2 actuators via an endotracheal tube (abstract). *Anesthesiology* 69: A838, 1988.

58b. Egan, M. J., and Nixon, W. A model of aerosol deposition in the lung for use in inhalation dose assessments. *Radiat. Prot. Dosim.* 11:5, 1985.

59. Eschenbacher, W. L., Boushey, H. A., and Sheppard, D. Alteration in osmolarity of inhaled aerosols causes bronchoconstriction and cough, but absence of a permanent anion causes cough alone. *Am. Rev. Respir. Dis.* 129:211, 1984.

60. Ferron, G. A. The size of soluble aerosol particles as a function of the humidity of the air: Application to the human respiratory tract. *J. Aerosol Sci.* 8:251, 1977.

61. Ferron, G. A., and Gebhart, J. Estimation of the lung deposition of aerosol particles produced with medical nebulizers. *J. Aerosol Sci.* 19:1083, 1988.

62. Ferron, G. A., Haider, B., and Kreyling, W. G. Inhalation of salt aerosol particles. I. Estimation of the temperature and relative humidity of the air in the human upper airways. *J. Aerosol Sci.* 19:343, 1988.

63. Ferron, G. A., Kreyling, W. G., and Haider, B. Inhalation of salt aerosol particles. II. Growth and deposition in the human respiratory tract. *J. Aerosol Sci.* 19:611, 1988.

64. Ferron, G. A., Oberdörster, G., and Henneberg, R. Estimation of the deposition of aerosolized drugs in the human respiratory tract due to hygroscopic growth. *J. Aerosol Med.* 2:271, 1989.

65. Ferron, G. A., Weber, J., and Kerrebijn, K. F. Properties of aerosols produced with three nebulizers. *Am. Rev. Respir. Dis.* 114:899, 1976.

66. Findeisen, W. Über das Absetzen kleiner, in der Luft suspendierter Teilchen in der menschlichen Lunge bei der Atmung. *Pflugers Arch.* 236:367, 1935.

67. Foster, W. M. Editorial: Is 24 hour lung retention an index of alveolar deposition? *J. Aerosol Med.* 1:1, 1988.

68. Foster, W. M., et al. Flow limitation on expiration induces central particle deposition and disrupts effective flow of airway mucus. *Ann. Occup. Hyg.* 32(Suppl. 1):101, 1988.

69. Freedman, A. P., Robinson, S. E., and Johnston, R. J. Noninvasive magnetopneumographic estimation of lung dust loads and distribution in bituminous coal workers. *J. Occup. Med.* 26:613, 1980.

70. Freeman, L. M., and Johnson, P. M. (eds.), *Clinical Scintillation Imaging* (2nd ed.). New York: Grune & Stratton, 1975.

71. Fuchs, N. A. *The Mechanics of Aerosols.* Elmsford, N.Y.: Pergamon, 1964 (reprinted by Dover, New York, 1989).

72. Fuchs, N. A., and Sutugin, A. G. Generation and Use of Monodisperse Aerosols. In C. N. Davies (ed.), *Aerosol Science.* New York: Academic, 1966. Pp. 1–30.

73. Ganderton, D., and Jones, T. (eds.), *Drug Delivery to the Respiratory Tract.* New York: VCH, 1987.

74. Gayrard, P., et al. Different bronchoconstrictor effects of carbachol boluses inhaled near residual volume or total lung capacity. *Respiration* 51: 81, 1987.

75. Gebhart, J., et al. The use of light scattering photometry in aerosol medicine. *J. Aerosol Med.* 1:89, 1988.

76. Gehr, P., et al. The fate of particles deposited in the intrapulmonary conducting airways. *J. Aerosol Med.* 4:349, 1991.

77. Geiser, M., et al. Histological and stereological analysis of particle deposition in the conducting airways of hamster lungs. *J. Aerosol Med.* 3:131, 1990.

78. Gerrity, T. R. Pathophysiological and Disease Constraints on Aerosol Delivery. In P. R. Byron (ed.), *Respiratory Drug Delivery.* Boca Raton, Fla.: CRC Press, 1990. Pp. 1–38.

79. Gitlin, J. D., et al. Randomized controlled trial of exogenous surfactant for the treatment of hyaline membrane disease. *Pediatrics* 79:31, 1987.

80. Gonda, I. Study of the effects of polydispersity of aerosols on regional deposition in the respiratory tract. *J. Pharm. Pharmacol.* 33(Suppl.):52P, 1981.

81. Gonda, I. Aerosols for delivery of therapeutic and diagnostic agents to the respiratory tract. *Crit. Rev. Ther. Drug Carrier Systems* 6:273, 1990.

82. Goodwin, P. N., and Dandamud, V. R. *An Introduction to the Physics of Nuclear Medicine.* Springfield, Ill.: Charles C Thomas, 1977.

83. Gore, D. J., and Patrick, G. A quantitative study of the penetration of insoluble particles into the tissues of the conducting airways. *Ann. Occup. Hyg.* 26:149, 1982.

84. Gradon, L., and Yu, C. P. Diffusional particle deposition in the human nose and mouth. *Aerosol Sci. Technol.* 11:213, 1989.

84a. Grigg, J., et al. Delivery of therapeutic aerosols to intubated babies. *Arch. Dis. Child.* 67:25, 1992.

85. Groom, C. V., and Gonda, I. Equilibrium diameters of inhalation aerosol droplets. *J. Pharm. Pharmacol.* 32(Suppl.):1P, 1980.

86. Guillemi, S., Jones, A. L., and Pare, P. D. Effect of breathing pattern during inhalation challenge on the shape and position of the dose-response curve. *Lung* 167:95, 1987.

87. Hallworth, G. W. The Formulation and Evaluation of Pressurised Metered-dose Inhalers. In D. Ganderton and T. Jones (eds.), *Drug Delivery to the Respiratory Tract.* New York: VCH, 1987. Pp. 87–118.

88. Hallworth, G. W., and Hamilton, R. R. Size analysis of metered suspension pressurized aerosols with the Quantimet 720. *J. Pharm. Pharmacol.* 28: 890, 1976.

89. Hallworth, G. W., and Westmoreland, D. G. The twin impinger: A simple device for assessing the delivery of drugs from metered dose pressurized aerosol inhalers. *J. Pharm. Pharmacol.* 39:966, 1987.

90. Hansen, O. R., and Pedersen, O. R. Optimal inhalation technique with terbutaline Turbuhaler. *Eur. Respir. J.* 2:637, 1989.

91. Harris, R. L., and Fraser, D. A. A model for deposition of fibers in the human respiratory tract. *Am. Ind. Hyg. Assoc. J.* 37:73, 1976.

92. Hatch, T. F., and Gross, P. *Pulmonary Deposition and Retention of Inhaled Aerosols.* New York: Academic, 1964.

93. Heyder, J. Particle transport onto human airway surfaces. *Eur. J. Respir. Dis.* 63(Suppl. 119):29, 1982.

94. Heyder, J. Assessment of airway geometry with inert aerosols. *J. Aerosol Med.* 2:89, 1989.

95. Heyder, J. Definitions and standards related to aerosols in medicine: Aerosols. *J. Aerosol Med.* 4:217, 1991.

96. Heyder, J., et al. Convective mixing in human respiratory tract: Estimates with aerosol boli. *J. Appl. Physiol.* 64:1273, 1988.

97. Heyder, J., et al. Deposition of particles in the human respiratory tract in the size range 0.005–15 µm. *J. Aerosol Sci.* 17:811, 1986.

98. Heyder, J., Gebhart, J., and Scheuch, G. Influence of human lung morphology on particle deposition. *J. Aerosol Med.* 1:81, 1988.

99. Heyder, J., Gebhart, J., and Stahlhofen, W. Inhalation of Aerosols: Particle Deposition and Retention. In K. Willeke (ed.), *Generation of Aerosols and Facilities for Exposure Experiments.* Ann Arbor: Ann Arbor Science, 1980. Pp. 65–103.

100. Heyder, J., et al. Biological variability of particle deposition in the human respiratory tract during controlled and spontaneous mouth-breathing. *Ann. Occup. Hyg.* 26:137, 1982.

101. Heyder, J., and Rudolf, G. Deposition of Aerosol Particles in the Human Nose. In W. H. Walton (ed.), *Inhaled Particles IV.* Oxford: Pergamon, 1977. Pp. 107–125.

102. Heyder, J., and Rudolf, G. Mathematical models of particle deposition in the human respiratory tract. *J. Aerosol Sci.* 15:697, 1984.

103. Heyder, J., and Scheuch, G. Diffusional transport of nonspherical aerosol particles. *Aerosol Sci. Technol.* 2:41, 1983.

104. Hickey, A. J., et al. The effect of hydrophobic coating upon the behavior of a hygroscopic aerosol powder in an environment of controlled temperature and humidity. *J. Pharm. Sci.* 79:1009, 1990.

105. Hicks, J. F., et al. Experimental Evaluation of Aerosol Growth in the Human Respiratory Tract. In W. Schikarski, H. J. Fissan, and S. K. Friedlander (eds.), *Aerosols: Formation and Reactivity.* New York: Pergamon, 1986. Pp. 244–247.

106. Hiller, F. C. Health implications of hygroscopic particle growth in the human respiratory tract. *J. Aerosol Med.* 4:1, 1991.

107. Hiller, F. C., Mazumder, M. K., and Bone, R. C. Physical properties, hygroscopicity, and estimated pulmonary retention of various therapeutic aerosols. *Chest* 77(Suppl.):318S, 1980.

108. Hiller, F. C., et al. Aerodynamic size distribution of metered dose bronchodilator aerosols. *Am. Rev. Respir. Dis.* 118:311, 1978.

109. Hiller, F. C., et al. Effect of low and high relative humidity on metered-dose bronchodilator solution and powder aerosols. *J. Pharm. Sci.* 69:334, 1980.

110. Hiller, F. C., et al. Physical properties of therapeutic aerosols. *Chest* 80(Suppl.):901, 1981.

111. Hinds, W. C. *Aerosol Technology—Properties, Behavior, and Measurement of Airborne Particles.* New York: Wiley-Interscience, 1982.

111a. Hofmann, W., and Koblinger, L. Monte Carlo modeling of the aerosol deposition in human lungs. Part II: Deposition fractions and their sensitivity to parameter variations. *J. Aerosol Sci.* 21:675, 1990.

112. Hofmann, W., Martonen, T. B., and Graham, R. C. Predicted deposition of nonhygroscopic aerosols in the human lung as a function of subject age. *J. Aerosol Med.* 2:49, 1989.

113. Hounam, R. F., Black, A., and Walsh, M. Deposition of aerosol particles in the nasopharyngeal region of the human respiratory tract. *Nature* 221:1254, 1969.

114. Hounam, R. F., and Morgan, A. Particle Deposition. In J. D. Brain, D. F. Proctor, and L. M. Reid (eds.), *Respiratory Defense Mechanisms.* New York: Marcel Dekker, 1977. Pp. 125–156.

115. Ilowite, J. S., Gorvoy, J. D., and Smaldone, G. C. Quantitative deposition of aerosolized gentamicin in cystic fibrosis. *Am. Rev. Respir. Dis.* 136:1445, 1987.

116. Isawa, T., Wasserman, K., and Taplin, G. V. Lung scintigraphy and pulmonary function studies in obstructive airway disease. *Am. Rev. Respir. Dis.* 102:161, 1970.

117. Itoh, H., et al. Clinical observations of aerosol deposition in patients with airways obstruction. *Chest* 80(Suppl.):837, 1981.

118. Itoh, H., et al. Mechanisms of aerosol deposition in a nasal model. *J. Aerosol Sci.* 16:529, 1985.

119. Jaegfeldt, H., et al. Particle Size Distribution from Different Modifications of Turbuhaler. In S. P. Newman, F. Morén, and G. K. Crompton (eds.), *A New Concept in Inhalation Therapy.* Brussels: Medicom, 1987. Pp. 90–99.

119a. Jennings, S. G. The mean free path in air. *J. Aerosol Sci.* 19:159, 1988.

120. Jobe, A., et al. Duration and characteristics of treatment of premature lambs with natural surfactant. *J. Clin. Invest.* 67:370, 1981.

121. Johnson, M. A., et al. The optimum aerosol size and dose of salbutamol in the treatment of asthma (abstract). *Thorax* 42:730, 1987.

122. Jones, J. G. Clearance of Inhaled Particles from the Alveoli. In S. W. Clarke and D. Pavia (eds.), *Aerosols and the Lung: Clinical and Experimental Aspects.* Boston: Butterworths, 1984. Pp. 170–196.

123. Kalliomaki, K., et al. Instrumentation for measuring the magnetic lung contamination of steel workers. *Ann. Occup. Hyg.* 23:175, 1980.

124. Kim, C. S., et al. Influence of two-phase gas-liquid interaction on aerosol deposition in airways. *Am. Rev. Respir. Dis.* 131:618, 1985.

125. Kim, C. S., et al. Deposition of aerosol particles and flow resistance in mathematical and experimental airway models. *J. Appl. Physiol.* 55:154, 1983.

126. Kim, C. S., et al. Aerosol deposition in the lungs with asymmetric airways obstruction: In vivo observation. *J. Appl. Physiol.* 67:2579, 1989.

127. Kim, C. S., Eldridge, M. A., and Sackner, M. A. Oropharyngeal deposition and delivery aspects of metered-dose inhaler aerosols. *Am. Rev. Respir. Dis.* 135:157, 1987.

128. Kim, C. S., Lewars, G. A., and Sackner, M. A. Measurement of total lung aerosol deposition as an index of lung abnormality. *J. Appl. Physiol.* 64:1527, 1988.

129. Kim, C. S., Trujillo, D., and Sackner, M. A. Size aspects of metered-dose inhaler aerosols. *Am. Rev. Respir. Dis.* 132:137, 1985.

129a. Kharasch, V. S., et al. Pulmonary surfactant as a vehicle for intratracheal

130. Knight, V., et al. Ribavirin aerosol dosage according to age and other variables. *J. Infect. Dis.* 158:443, 1988.

130a. Koblinger, L., and Hofmann, W. Monte Carlo modeling of aerosol deposition in the human lungs. Part I: Simulation of particle transport in a stochastic lung structure. *J. Aerosol Sci.* 21:661, 1990.

131. Landahl, H. D. On the removal of air-borne droplets by the human respiratory tract. I. The lung. *Bull. Math. Biophys.* 12:43, 1950.

132. Landahl, H. D., and Black, S. Penetration of air-borne particulates through the human nose. I. *J. Ind. Hyg. Toxicol.* 29:269, 1947.

133. Landahl, H. D., and Tracewell, T. Penetration of air-borne particulates through the human nose. II. *J. Ind. Hyg. Toxicol.* 31:55, 1949.

134. Laube, B. L., et al. Homogeneity of bronchopulmonary distribution of ⁹⁹ᵐTc aerosol in normal subjects and cystic fibrosis patients. *Chest* 95:822, 1989.

135. Laube, B. L., Swift, D. L., and Adams, G. K., III. Single-breath deposition of jet-nebulized saline aerosol. *Aerosol Sci. Technol.* 3:97, 1984.

136. Laube, B. L., et al. The effect of bronchial obstruction on central airway deposition of a saline aerosol in patients with asthma. *Am. Rev. Respir. Dis.* 133:740, 1986.

137. Lefebvre, A. H. *Atomization and Sprays.* New York: Hemisphere, 1989.

138. Lehnert, B. E. Lung defense mechanisms against deposited dusts. *Probl. Respir. Care* 3:130, 1990.

138a. Li, W., Montassier, N., and Hopke, P. K. A system to measure the hygroscopicity of aerosol particles. *Aerosol Sci. Technol.* 17:25, 1992.

139. Lippmann, M. Deposition and clearance of inhaled particles in the human nose. *Ann. Otol. Rhinol. Laryngol.* 79:519, 1970.

140. Lippmann, M. Regional Deposition of Particles in the Human Respiratory Tract. In D. H. K. Lee, H. L. Falk, and S. D. Murphy (eds.), *Handbook of Physiology,* Sect. 9, *Reactions to Environmental Agents.* Bethesda, Md.: American Physiological Society, 1977. Pp. 213–232.

141. Lippmann, M., and Albert, R. E. The effect of particle size on the regional deposition of inhaled aerosols in the human respiratory tract. *Am. Ind. Hyg. Assoc. J.* 30:257, 1969.

142. Lippmann, M., Albert, R. E., and Peterson, H. T., Jr. The Regional Deposition of Inhaled Aerosols in Man. In W. H. Walton (ed.), *Inhaled Particles III,* Vol. I. Surrey, England: Unwin, 1971. Pp. 105–122.

143. Lippmann, M., and Altshuler, B. Regional Deposition of Aerosols. In E. F. Aharonson, A. Ben-David, and M. A. Klingberg (eds.), *Air Pollution and the Lung.* New York: Halsted Press-Wiley, 1976. Pp. 25–48.

144. Lippmann, M., and Esch, J. Effect of lung airway branching pattern and gas composition on particle deposition. I. Background and literature review. *Exp. Lung. Res.* 14:311, 1988.

145. Lippmann, M., Yeates, D. B., and Albert, R. E. Deposition, retention, and clearance of inhaled particles. *Br. J. Ind. Med.* 37:337, 1980.

146. Logus, J. W., et al. Single photon emission tomography of lungs imaged with Tc-labeled aerosol. *J. Can. Assoc. Radiol.* 35:133, 1984.

147. Lourenço, R. V., Klimek, M. F., and Borowski, C. J. Deposition and clearance of 2 micron particles in the tracheo-bronchial tree of normal subjects—Smokers and nonsmokers. *J. Clin. Invest.* 50:1411, 1971.

148. Lourenço, R. V., Loddenkemper, R., and Cargon, R. W. Patterns of distribution and clearance of aerosols in patients with bronchiectasis. *Am. Rev. Respir. Dis.* 106:857, 1972.

149. Love, R. G., and Muir, D. C. F. Aerosol deposition and airway obstruction. *Am. Rev. Respir. Dis.* 114:891, 1976.

150. Märtens, A., and Jacobi, W. Die in-vivo Bestimmung der Aerosolteilchendeposition im Atemtrakt bei Mund—bzw. Nasenatmung. In *Aerosole in Physik, Medizin und Technik.* Bad Soden, West Germany: Gesellschaft für Aerosolforschung, 1973. Pp. 117–121.

151. Martonen, T. B. Analytical model of hygroscopic particle behavior in human airways. *Bull. Math. Biol.* 44:425, 1982.

152. Martonen, T. B. Development of surrogate lung systems with controlled thermodynamic environments to study hygroscopic particles: Air pollutants and pharmacologic drugs. *Part. Sci. Technol.* 8:1, 1990.

152a. Mas, J. C., et al. Misuse of metered dose inhalers by house staff members. *Am. J. Dis. Child.* 146:783, 1992.

153. Melandri, C. V., et al. Deposition of charged particles in the human airways. *J. Aerosol Sci.* 14:657, 1983.

154. Mercer, T. T. *Aerosol Technology in Hazard Evaluation.* New York: Academic, 1973.

155. Mercer, T. T. Production of therapeutic aerosols; principles and techniques. *Chest* 80(Suppl.):813, 1981.

156. Mercer, T. T., Goddard, R. F., and Flores, R. L. Output characteristics of several commercial nebulizers. *Ann. Allergy* 23:314, 1965.

156a. Mezey, R. J., et al. Mucociliary transport in allergic patients with antigen-induced bronchospasm. *Am. Rev. Respir. Dis.* 118:677, 1978.

157. Miller, F. J., et al. Influence of breathing mode and activity level on the regional deposition of inhaled particles and implications for regulatory standards. *Ann. Occup. Hyg.* 32(Suppl. 1):3, 1988.

158. Mitchell, D. M., et al. Effect of particle size on bronchodilator aerosols on lung distribution and pulmonary function in patients with chronic asthma. *Thorax* 42:457, 1987.

159. Morén, F. Pressurized aerosols for oral inhalation. *Int. J. Pharm.* 8:1, 1981.

160. Morén, F., Newhouse, M. T., and Dolovich, M. B. (eds.), *Aerosols in Medicine—Principles, Diagnosis, and Therapy.* New York: Elsevier, 1985.

161. Morgan, W. K. C., Clague, H. W., and Vinitski, S. On paradigms, paradoxes, and particles. *Lung* 161:195, 1983.

162. Morrow, P. E. Factors determining hygroscopic aerosol deposition in airways. *Physiol. Rev.* 66:330, 1986.

163. Morrow, P. E., Gibb, F. R., and Gazioglu, K. M. A study of particulate clearance from the human lungs. *Am. Rev. Respir. Dis.* 96:1209, 1968.

164. Morsy, S. M., et al. A detector of adjustable response for the study of lung clearance. *Health Phys.* 32:243, 1977.

165. Newhouse, M. Aerosol therapy of obstructive and parenchymal pulmonary disease: Principles and clinical aspects. *J. Aerosol Med.* 2:187, 1989.

166. Newhouse, M., and Dolovich, M. Aerosol therapy: Nebulizer vs. metered dose inhaler. *Chest* 91:799, 1987.

167. Newhouse, M. T., and Ruffin, R. E. Deposition and fate of aerosolized drugs. *Chest* 73:936, 1978.

168. Newman, S. P. Therapeutic Aerosols. In S. W. Clarke and D. Pavia (eds.), *Aerosols and the Lung: Clinical and Experimental Aspects.* Boston: Butterworths, 1984. Pp. 197–224.

168a. Newman, S. P., et al. Terbutaline sulphate Turbuhaler: Effect of inhaled flow rate on drug deposition and efficacy. *Int. J. Pharm.* 74:209, 1991.

169. Newman, S. P., et al. Deposition and clinical efficacy of terbutaline sulphate from Turbuhaler, a new multi-dose powder inhaler. *Eur. J. Respir. Dis.* 2:247, 1989.

170. Newman, S. P., et al. Effects of various inhalation modes on the deposition of radioactive pressurised aerosols. *Eur. J. Respir. Dis.* 63(Suppl. 119):57, 1982.

171. Newman, S. P., et al. Deposition of pressurized aerosols in the human respiratory tract. *Thorax* 36:52, 1981.

172. Nieminen, M. M., et al. Aerosol deposition in automatic dosimeter nebulization. *Eur. J. Respir. Dis.* 71:145, 1987.

173. Niinimaa, V., et al. The switching point from nasal to oronasal breathing. *Respir. Physiol.* 42:62, 1980.

174. Niinimaa, V., et al. Oronasal distribution of respiratory airflow. *Respir. Physiol.* 43:69, 1981.

175. Nikiforov, A. T., and Schlesinger, R. B. Morphometric variability of the human upper bronchial tree. *Respir. Physiol.* 59:289, 1985.

175a. O'Callaghan, J., et al. Evaluation of techniques for delivery of steroids to lungs of neonates using a rabbit model. *Arch. Dis. Child.* 67:20, 1992.

176. Oberdörster, G. Lung clearance of inhaled insoluble and soluble particles. *J. Aerosol Med.* 1:289, 1988.

176a. Oberdörster, G. Lung dosimetry and extrapolation of results of animal inhalation studies to man. *J. Aerosol Med.* 4:335, 1991.

177. Otani, Y., and Wang, C. S. Growth and deposition of saline droplets covered with a monolayer of surfactant. *Aerosol Sci. Technol.* 3:155, 1984.

178. Park, R. P., Smith, P. H. S., and Taylor, D. M. *Basic Science of Nuclear Medicine.* New York: Churchill-Livingstone, 1978.

179. Pattle, R. E. The Retention of Gases and Particles in the Human Nose. In C. N. Davies (ed.), *Inhaled Particles and Vapors.* Elmsford, N.Y.: Pergamon, 1977. Pp. 302–311.

180. Pavia, D. Lung Mucociliary Clearance. In S. W. Clarke and D. Pavia (eds.), *Aerosols and the Lung: Clinical and Experimental Aspects.* Boston: Butterworths, 1984. Pp. 127–155.

181. Pavia, D., et al. Effect of lung function and mode of inhalation on penetration of aerosol into the human lung. *Thorax* 32:194, 1977.

182. Pedersen, S., and Steffensen, G. Fenoterol powder inhaler technique in children: Influence of inspiratory flow rate and breath-holding. *Eur. J. Respir. Dis.* 68:207, 1986.

183. Persons, D. D., et al. Airway deposition of hygroscopic heterodispersed aerosols: Results of computer calculation. *J. Appl. Physiol.* 63:1195, 1987.

184. Persons, D. D., Hess, G. D., and Scherer, P. W. Maximization of pulmonary hygroscopic aerosol deposition. *J. Appl. Physiol.* 63:1205, 1987.

185. Phalen, R. F. (ed.), *Inhalation Studies: Foundations and Techniques.* Boca Raton, Fla.: CRC Press, 1984.

186. Phipps, P. R., et al. Comparison of planar and tomographic gamma scintigraphy to measure the penetration of inhaled aerosols. *Am. Rev. Respir. Dis.* 139:1516, 1989.

187. Poe, N. D., Cohen, M. B., and Yanda, R. L. Application of delayed lung imaging following radioaerosol inhalation. *Radiology* 122:739, 1977.

188. Pritchard, J. N. Particle Growth in the Airways and the Influence of Airflow. In S. P. Newman, F. Morén, and G. K. Crompton (eds.), *A New Concept in Inhalation Therapy.* Brussels: Medicom, 1987. Pp. 3–24.

189. Pritchard, J. N., Jefferies, S. J., and Black, A. Sex differences in the regional deposition of inhaled particles in the 2.5–7.5 μm size range. *J. Aerosol Sci.* 17:385, 1986.

190. Proceedings of the Seventh International Congress on Aerosols. *J. Aerosol Med.* 2:81, 1989.

190a. Proceedings of Consensus Seminars on Issues of Aerosol Therapy: Definitions and standards related to aerosols in medicine. *J. Aerosol Med.* 4:217, 1991.

191. Prodi, V., et al. An inertial spectrometer for aerosol particles. *J. Aerosol Sci.* 10:411, 1979.

192. Raabe, O. G. Deposition and Clearance of Inhaled Aerosols. In H. Witschi and P. Nettesheim (eds.), *Mechanisms in Respiratory Toxicology,* Vol. I. Boca Raton, Fla.: CRC Press, 1982. Pp. 27–75.

192a. Raeburn, D., Underwood, S. L., and Villamil, M. E. Techniques for drug delivery to the airways, and the assessment of lung function in animal models. *J. Pharmacol. Toxicol. Methods* 27:143, 1992.

193. Ramanna, L., et al. Radioaerosol lung imaging in chronic obstructive pulmonary disease. *Chest* 68:634, 1975.

194. Rasmussen, T. R., et al. Influence of nasal passage geometry on aerosol particle deposition in the nose. *J. Aerosol Med.* 3:15, 1990.

195. Reist, P. C. *Introduction to Aerosol Science.* New York: Macmillan, 1984.

196. Rudolf, G., et al. An empirical formula describing aerosol deposition in man for any particle size. *J. Aerosol Sci.* 17:350, 1986.

197. Rudolf, G., et al. Mass deposition from inspired polydisperse aerosols. *Ann. Occup. Hyg.* 32(Suppl. 1):919, 1988.

198. Ruffin, R. E., et al. The preferential deposition of inhaled isoproterenol and propranolol in asthmatic patients. *Chest* 80(Suppl.):904s, 1981.

199. Ruffin, R. E., et al. The effects of preferential deposition of histamine in the human airway. *Am. Rev. Respir. Dis.* 117:485, 1978.

200. Ryan, G., et al. Standardization of inhalation provocation tests: Influence of nebulizer output, particle size, and method of inhalation. *J. Allergy Clin. Immunol.* 67:156, 1981.

201. Ryan, G., et al. Standardization of inhalation provocation tests: Two techniques of aerosol generation and inhalation compared. *Am. Rev. Respir. Dis.* 123:195, 1981.

202. Sackner, M. A., Brown, L. K., and Kim, C. S. Basis of an improved metered aerosol delivery system. *Chest* 80(Suppl.):915, 1981.

203. Sackner, M. A., Rosen, M. J., and Wanner, A. Estimation of tracheal mucous velocity by bronchofiberscopy. *J. Appl. Physiol.* 34:495, 1973.

203a. Saibene, F., et al. Oronasal breathing during exercise. *Pflügers Arch.* 378:65, 1978.

204. Sanchis, J., et al. Quantitation of regional aerosol clearance in the normal human lung. *J. Appl. Physiol.* 33:757, 1972.

205. Sato, Y. A review of aerosol therapy in otorhinolaryngology. *J. Aerosol Med.* 1:133, 1988.

206. Saunders, K. B. Misuse of inhaled bronchodilator agents. *Br. Med. J.* 1:1037, 1965.

207. Schiller, C. F., et al. Deposition of monodisperse insoluble aerosol particles in the 0.005 to 0.2 μm size range within the human respiratory tract. *Ann. Occup. Hyg.* 32(Suppl. 1):41, 1988.

208. Schlesinger, R. B. Clearance from the respiratory tract. *Fund. Appl. Toxicol.* 5:435, 1985.

209. Schlesinger, R. B., and McFadden, L. Comparative morphometry of the upper bronchial tree in six mammalian species. *Anat. Rec.* 199:99, 1981.

209a. Schürch, S., et al. Surfactant displaces particles toward the epithelium in airways and alveoli. *Respir. Physiol.* 80:17, 1990.

210. Schuster, D. P. Positron emission tomography: Theory and its applications to the study of lung disease. *Am. Rev. Respir. Dis.* 139:818, 1989.

211. Scott, W. R., Taulbee, D. B., and Yu, C. P. Theoretical study of nasal deposition. *Bull. Math. Biol.* 40:581, 1978.

212. Serafini, S. M., Wanner, A., and Michaelson, E. D. Mucociliary transport in central and intermediate size airways and effect of aminophyllin. *Bull. Eur. Physiopathol. Respir.* 12:415, 1976.

212a. Sibelle, Y., and Reynolds, H. Y. Macrophages and polymorphonuclear neutrophils in lung defense and injury. *Am. Rev. Respir. Dis.* 141:471, 1990.

213. Simonds, A. K., et al. Alveolar targeting of aerosol pentamidine. *Am. Rev. Respir. Dis.* 141:827, 1990.

214. Smaldone, G. C., et al. Factors determining pulmonary deposition of aerosolized pentamidine in patients with human immunodeficiency virus infection. *Am. Rev. Respir. Dis.* 143:727, 1991.

215. Smaldone, G. C., and Messina, M. S. Enhancement of particle deposition by flow-limiting segments in humans. *J. Appl. Physiol.* 59:509, 1985.

216. Smaldone, G. C., and Messina, M. S. Flow limitation, cough, and patterns of aerosol deposition in humans. *J. Appl. Physiol.* 59:515, 1985.

217. Smaldone, G. C., et al. Interpretation of "24 hour lung retention" in studies of mucociliary clearance. *J. Aerosol Med.* 1:11, 1988.

218. Smaldone, G. C., Perry, R. J., and Deutsch, D. G. Characteristics of nebulizers used in the treatment of AIDS-related *Pneumocystis carinii* pneumonia. *J. Aerosol Med.* 1:113, 1988.

219. Soong, T. T., et al. A statistical description of the human tracheobronchial tree geometry. *Respir. Physiol.* 37:161, 1979.

220. Stahlhofen, W., Gebhart, J., and Heyder, J. Experimental determination of the regional deposition of aerosol particles in the human respiratory tract. *Am. Ind. Hyg. Assoc. J.* 41:385, 1980.

221. Stahlhofen, W., et al. Deposition pattern of droplets from medical nebulizers in the human respiratory tract. *Bull. Eur. Physiopathol. Respir.* 19:459, 1983.

222. Stahlhofen, W., et al. Measurement of lung clearance with pulses of radioactively labelled aerosols. *J. Aerosol Sci.* 17:333, 1986.

223. Stahlhofen, W., Rudolf, G., and James, A. C. Intercomparison of experimental regional aerosol deposition data. *J. Aerosol Med.* 2:285, 1989.

224. Sterk, P. J., et al. Physical properties of aerosols produced by several jet and ultrasonic nebulizers. *Bull. Eur. Physiopathol. Respir.* 20:65, 1984.

225. Stöber, W. Aerosol Sampling and Characterization for Inhalation Exposure Studies with Experimental Animals. In W. Willeke (ed.), *Generation of Aerosols and Facilities for Exposure Experiments.* Ann Arbor: Ann Arbor Science, 1980. Pp. 31–63.

226. Strohl, K. P., et al. Inhalation pattern and predominant site of bronchoconstriction in healthy subjects. *J. Appl. Physiol.* 50:575, 1981.

227. Stuart, B. O. Deposition and clearance of inhaled particles. *Environ. Health Perspect.* 55:369, 1984.

227a. Svartengren, M., et al. Regional deposition of 3.6-μm particles and lung function in asthmatic subjects. *J. Appl. Physiol.* 71:2238, 1991.

227b. Sweeney, T. D., and Brain, J. D. Pulmonary deposition: Determinants and measurement techniques. *Toxicol. Pathol.* 19:384, 1991.

228. Sweeney, T. D., et al. Delivery of aerosolized drugs to the lungs with a metered-dose inhaler: Quantitative analysis of regional deposition. *J. Aerosol Sci.* 21:350, 1990.

229. Sweeney, T. D., et al. Emphysema alters the deposition pattern of inhaled particles in hamsters. *Am. J. Pathol.* 128:19, 1987.

230. Sweeney, T. D., et al. Chronic bronchitis produced by SO_2 alters the deposition pattern of inhaled aerosol in rats. *Am. Rev. Respir. Dis.* 131:A195, 1985.

231. Sweeney, T. D., et al. Retention of inhaled particles in hamsters with pulmonary fibrosis. *Am. Rev. Respir. Dis.* 128:138, 1983.

232. Swift, D. L. A New Method for Aerosol Delivery to the Bronchial Airways. In W. Hofmann (ed.), *Deposition and Clearance of Aerosols in the Human Respiratory Tract.* Vienna: Facultas, 1987. Pp. 207–211.

232a. Swift, D. L., et al. Inspiratory deposition of ultrafine particles in human nasal replicate cast. *J. Aerosol Sci.* 23:65, 1992.

233. Swift, D. L., and Proctor, D. F. Human respiratory deposition of particles during oronasal breathing. *Atmos. Environ.* 16:2279, 1982.

234. Taplin, G. V. et al. Early detection of chronic obstructive pulmonary disease using radionuclide lung-imaging procedure. *Chest* 71:567, 1977.

235. Task Group on Lung Dynamics. Deposition and retention models for internal dosimetry of the human respiratory tract. *Health Phys.* 12:173, 1966.

235a. Taulbee, D. B., and Yu, C. P. A theory of aerosol deposition in the human respiratory tract. *J. Appl. Physiol.* 38:77, 1975.

235b. Taylor, R. H., and Lerman, J. High-efficiency delivery of salbutamol with a metered-dose inhaler in narrow tracheal tubes and catheters. *Anesthesiology* 74:360, 1991.

235c. Thomas, S. H. L., et al. Variability in the measurement of nebulized aerosol deposition in man. *Clin. Sci.* 81:767, 1991.

236. Tillery, M. I. Aerosol Centrifuges. In D. A. Lundgren, et al. (eds.), *Aerosol Measurement.* Gainesville: University of Florida Press, 1979. P. 3.

237. Timbrell, V. The inhalation of fibrous dusts. *Ann. NY Acad. Sci.* 132:255, 1965.

238. Trajan, M., et al. Relationship between regional ventilation and aerosol deposition in tidal breathing. *Am. Rev. Respir. Dis.* 130:64, 1984.

239. Tu, K. W., and Knutson, E. O. Total deposition of ultrafine hydrophobic and hygroscopic aerosols in the human respiratory system. *Aerosol Sci. Technol.* 3:453, 1984.

240. Valberg, P. A., and Blanchard, J. D. Pulmonary Macrophage Physiology: Origin, Motility, and Endocytosis. In R. A. Parent (ed.), *Comprehensive Treatise on Pulmonary Toxicology: Comparative Biology of the Normal Lung.* Boca Raton, Fla.: CRC Press, 1991.

241. Valberg, P. A., and Brain, J. D. Lung particle retention and lung macrophage function evaluated using magnetic aerosols. *J. Aerosol Med.* 1:331, 1988.

242. Van As, A. Pulmonary airway clearance mechanisms: A reappraisal. *Am. Rev. Respir. Dis.* 115:721, 1977.

243. Velasquez, D. J. Toxicologic Responses to Inhaled Aerosols and Their Ingredients. In P. R. Byron (ed.), *Respiratory Drug Delivery.* Boca Raton, Fla.: CRC Press, 1990. P. 39.

244. Vidgren, M., et al. In-vitro and in-vivo deposition of drug particles inhaled from pressurised aerosol and dry powder inhalers. *Drug Dev. Ind. Pharm.* 14:2649, 1988.

245. Vincent, J. H. On the practical significance of electrostatic lung deposition of isometric and fibrous aerosols. *J. Aerosol Sci.* 16:511, 1985.

246. Vincent, J. H. *Aerosol Sampling: Science and Practice.* New York: John Wiley, 1989.

247. Walton, W. H. (ed.), *Inhaled Particles III.* Surrey, England: Unwin, 1971.

248. Walton, W. H. (ed.), *Inhaled Particles IV.* Elmsford, N.Y.: Pergamon, 1977.

249. Walton, W. H. (ed.), Inhaled Particles V. *Ann. Occup. Hyg.* 26:1, 1982.

250. Wanner, A. Clinical Aspects of Mucociliary Transport. In J. F. Murray (ed.), *Lung Disease State of the Art.* New York: American Lung Association, 1978.

250a. Wheatley, J. R., Amis, T. C., and Engel, L. A. Oronasal partitioning of ventilation during exercise in humans. *J. Appl. Physiol.* 71:546, 1991.

251. Willeke, K. (ed.), *Generation of Aerosols and Facilities for Exposure Experiments.* Ann Arbor: Ann Arbor Science, 1980.

251a. Willeke, K., and Baron, P. (eds.), *Aerosol Measurement.* New York: Van Nostrand Reinhold, 1992.

252. Wojciak, J. F., Notter, R. H., and Oberdörster, G. Size stability of phosphatidylcholine-phosphatidylglycerol aerosols and a dynamic film compression state from their interfacial tension. *J. Colloid Interface Sci.* 106:547, 1985.

252a. Wolff, R. K., et al. Deposition and clearance of radiolabeled particles from small ciliated airways in beagle dogs. *J. Aerosol Med.* 2:261, 1989.

253. Xu, G. B., and Yu, C. P. Theoretical lung deposition of hygroscopic NaCl aerosols. *Aerosol Sci. Technol.* 4:455, 1985.

254. Xu, G. B., and Yu, C. P. Effects of age on deposition of inhaled aerosols in the human lung. *Aerosol Sci. Technol.* 5:349, 1986.

255. Yeates, D. B., et al. Mucociliary transport rates in man. *J. Appl. Physiol.* 39:487, 1975.

256. Yu, C. P. Theories of electrostatic lung deposition. *Ann. Occup. Hyg.* 29:219, 1985.

257. Yu, C. P., and Cai, F. S. Calculated particle deposition at the alveolar duct. *J. Aerosol Med.* 2:69, 1989.

258. Yu, C. P., and Diu, C. K. A probabilistic model for intersubject deposition variability of inhaled particles. *Aerosol Sci. Technol.* 1:355, 1982.

259. Yu, C. P., Diu, C. K., and Soong, T. T. Statistical analysis of aerosol deposition in nose and mouth. *Am. Ind. Hyg. Assoc. J.* 42:726, 1981.

260. Yu, C. P., and Xu, G. B. Predictive models for deposition of diesel exhaust particulates in human and rat lungs. *Aerosol Sci. Technol.* 5:337, 1986.

261. Yu, C. P., and Xu, G. B. Deposition of Hygroscopic Aerosol Particles in Growing Human Lungs. In W. Hofmann (ed.), *Deposition and Clearance of Aerosols in the Human Respiratory Tract.* Vienna: Facultas, 1987. Pp. 111–117.

261a. Yu, C. P., et al. Algebraic modeling of total and regional deposition of inhaled particles in the human lung of various ages. *J. Aerosol Sci.* 23:73, 1992.

262. Zeltner, T. B., et al. Retention and clearance of 0.9-μm particles inhaled by hamsters during rest and exercise. *J. Appl. Physiol.* 70:1137, 1991.

Immune-Neuroendocrine Circuitry and Its Relation to Asthma

33

Andor Szentivanyi

Of the various evolving views on immunologic inflammation, immunity, and hypersensitivity, this chapter discusses the irrevocable shift and turnabout in our concepts of immunoregulation as connected with our growing understanding of the immune-neuroendocrine circuitry. This network, which is powerful enough both conceptually and in de facto functioning to bring about a radical change in our perceptions of the human immune, endocrine, and nervous systems, has already enlisted the minds and resources of a large number of leading laboratories in many areas of life sciences on an international scale.

THE DISCOVERY OF THE IMMUNE-NEUROENDOCRINE CIRCUITRY AND THE CONCEPTS OF PREVAILING IMMUNOLOGIC THOUGHT THAT IMPEDED THE TIMELY RECOGNITION OF ITS ROLE IN IMMUNE HOMEOSTASIS

The integrative center of this awesome edifice is the hypothalamus. The hypothalamus is a small, anatomically complex region of the diencephalon, which in a variety of ways contributes to a large number of regulatory systems. The functional and anatomic complexity of the hypothalamus results in part from its role as a nodal region for (1) convergence of input from the limbic system, which contributes to an association between visceral and behavioral functions; (2) bidirectional bundles of nerve fibers with their cell bodies (perikarya) in the telencephalon or brain stem; and (3) local neurons coordinating distant organ system activities through the effector functions of the endocrine and autonomic nervous systems.

The role of hypothalamic influences in the induction and expression of immunologic inflammation, immunity, and hypersensitivity was first discovered in my laboratory in the fall of 1951 at the University of Debrecen School of Medicine in Hungary. The rationale behind the decision for a systematic exploration of the hypothalamus was as follows. Historically, the interpretation of the symptomatology and the underlying reaction sequence of human asthma was patterned after those of the anaphylactic guinea pig. However, the range of atopic responsiveness in asthma includes a variety of stimuli that are nonimmunologic in nature. Foremost among these are a broad range of pharmacologically active mediators that today could be considered as the chemical organizers of central and peripheral autonomic regulation. Therefore, I believed (A. Szentivanyi) that anaphylaxis could not be used as a model for the investigation of the constitutional basis of atopy in asthma. It was postulated that such a model, if it was to be meaningful, must be able to imitate both the immunologic and autonomic abnormalities of the disease. Since at that early time (1951) none of the current neuroactive agents (ago-nists, antagonists, etc.) that one could conceivably use as an experimental tool to induce an autonomic imbalance were in existence, it was concluded that the best chance to develop such a condition would be through various manipulations at the neuroendocrine regulatory level of the hypothalamus. Consequently, hypothalamically imbalanced anaphylactic animals were used. Such animals were produced by the electrolytic lesion, and conversely, the electrical stimulation of various nuclear groupings in the hypothalamus through permanently implanted depth electrodes placed stereotaxically into the hypothalamus. The resulting cumulative findings obtained with such a model indicated that the hypothalamus has a modulatory influence on all cellular and humoral immune reactivities and that both neural as well as endocrine pathways are required for hypothalamic modulation of immune responses [28–33, 89, 96, 97, 99, 100, 104–106, 108–114, 117–122, 125–133, 136–139].

Concurrently with these developments, however, an unparalleled expansion of information on the basic aspects of immunology in general and on the nature of antibody diversity in particular started to occupy the center stage of immunologic interest. Most importantly, the new perceptions surrounding the nature of antibody diversity began to surface in the late 1950s, with the first conclusive genetic studies having been completed and a new set of concepts defined. These circumstances led to a total transformation of prevailing immunologic thought, ultimately leading to the replacement of instructionist theories by the selective theories as advanced by D. W. Talmage (in the Spring of 1957) and M. Burnet (in the Fall of 1957).

Three major postulates were implicit in these theories of heritable cellular commitment: (1) The antigen-receptor site and the antibody combining site whose synthesis that cell controls are identical and are derived at least partially from the same structural gene; (2) the condition guaranteeing the correspondence of the immunoglobulin (Ig) synthesized with the antigen is that they are limited to the same cell that is the cell specialized for the synthesis of a single antibody; and (3) the cell specialization stipulated in Item 2 is inherited and therefore clonal (the clonal selection theory of acquired immunity). Subsequently, it became established that virtually all antibody diversity and specificity encoded in the immune system can be accounted for in genetic terms and thus the controls for the antibody response must reside largely within the major histocompatibility complex (MHC) where different genes appear to code for immune response, suppression, and cell interaction [115]. An impediment in the timely recognition of the significance of the immune-neuroendocrine circuitry in immune homeostasis was the ability to have immune reactivities to proceed in vitro. This further supported the concept that the immune system is a totally autonomous and self-regulating unit (this view overlooked the rich neurohormonal milieu in which most in vitro immune responses occur). Sporadic refutations of these postulates have occurred and continue to surface in the literature, but the great bulk of the evidence is supportive of the clonal selection theory. The theory's sheer eloquence, however, has probably been most responsible for its dominant role in immunologic thought and its acceptance as dogma since the early 1960s. In any case, these concepts and the large body of supportive evidence have so permeated the field that it became difficult, if not impossible, to think of immunology outside of this framework [101].

In the late 1950s and throughout the 1960s the two conceptual centers of these ideas were under the leadership of Talmage at the University of Chicago and later at Colorado, and the group at Walter and Eliza Hall Institute in Australia under Burnet. Because of the close association with Talmage, extending over a period of 10 years, I was very much under the influence of these views and developed reservations against the significance of our hypothalamic findings in immunoregulation. Nevertheless, by 1966 in a chapter of a German text [109], through an extensive analysis of our findings and the dominant immunologic concepts, I came to articulate the following conclusions: (1) The significance of the immunopharmacologic mediators of immune manifestations in normal mammalian physiology is that they are the chemical organizers of central and peripheral autonomic action; (2) the preceding suggests the inseparability of the immune response system from the neuroendocrine system; (3) such inseparability indicates the de facto existence of immune-neuroendocrine circuits and the necessity for a bidirectional flow of information between the two systems; (4) one must distinguish between the concepts of autoregulation as one that primarily revolves around one effector molecule of immunity, the antibody, and satisfies the requirements of antibody diversity and specificity, in contrast to the more complex requirements of immune homeostasis; (5) in contrast to autoregulation that is always self-contained, homeostatic control is always beyond the constraints of one single cell or tissue system; and (6) thus, immune homeostasis must represent a far more sophisticated level of control than autoregulation, and is based on immune-neuroendocrine circuits. Indeed, as Schechter [88] pointed out, no bodily system is as simple, sacred, or singular as once thought. Instead, as in any good relationship, the separate components strive for sensitivity, synchrony, and synergy. Recognition and communication among the immune, endocrine, and nervous systems exemplify the formula for harmony and homeostasis.

While the manifold similarities between the immune and nervous systems are fully realized (see below), the immune system has a major additional level of complexity over that of the nervous system. Although the nervous system with its spectacular masses of much-revealing and well-defined projection patterns is well moored in the body in a static web of axons, dendrites, and synapses, the elements of the immune system are in a continuously mobile phase, incessantly scouring over and percolating through the body tissues, returning via an intricate system of lymphatic channels, and then blending again in the blood. This dynamism is relieved only by scattered concentrations called *lymphoid organs*. These circumstances would appear to indicate that the functional plasticity of the immune system is far greater than that of the nervous system, and consequently, its regulation must require a more complex and sophisticated level of control. For these reasons, in the 1966 text I raised the frivolous question of whether the immune system is more "intelligent" than the brain.

When these conclusions were reached (in the 1960s), our understandings of cellular immunology were in an early phase. The 1970s saw the discovery of the lymphokines, monokines, and a broad range of other effector molecules of immunologic inflammation, immunity, and hypersensitivity, but it was only in the 1980s that we recognized that the cells of the immune system, primarily the lymphocytes, synthesize, store, and release neurotransmitters, hypothalamohypophyseal hormones, and so on,

and by all criteria serve as neuroendocrine cells "par excellence" [46, 109, 110, 114, 117]. For additional analysis of the significance of lymphocytes in neuroendocrine regulation with special regard to human bronchial asthma, see Chapter 13 and the discussion below.

DEVELOPMENTAL INTERRELATIONSHIPS AMONG THE CELLULAR AND HUMORAL COMPONENTS

The developmental interrelationships among the cellular and humoral components of the immune-neuroendocrine circuitry may be briefly stated through a discussion of (1) the cells involved in the synthesis, storage, secretion, and/or release of the effector molecules of immunologic reactivities; (2) neural crest interactions in the development of the immune system; (3) cerebral dominance or lateralization and the immune system; (4) the ancient superfamily of immune recognition molecules and the neural cell adhesion molecule (N-CAM); (5) the immune system and the nervous system sharing the capacity to remember; and (6) the unique recognition and communication powers of the immune and nervous systems as shared characteristics.

The Cells Involved in the Synthesis, Storage, Secretion, and/or Release of the Effector Molecules of Immunologic Reactivities

The functions of the immune system are the properties of cells distributed throughout the body. They include (1) free or circulating cells of the blood, lymph, and intravascular spaces; (2) similar cells collected into units that allow for close interaction with lymph or circulating blood—lymph nodes, spleen, liver, and bone marrow; and (3) two major control organs for the system, the thymus gland and the hypothalamic-pituitary-adrenal complex.

The cells involved in the synthesis, storage, secretion, and/or release of the effector molecules of immunologic inflammation, immunity, and immunologically based hypersensitivity (allergy) represent a continuous spectrum of related cell types specialized in the production and storage of various physiopharmacologically active effector substances in variable proportions, that is, of cells that have a common developmental origin, with differentiation being determined by the specific requirements of the local neurohumoral regulation [114]. Accounting only for those effector molecules for which the cell type has been identified, this incomplete spectrum of cells and effector substances includes macrophages and lymphocytes (interleukins [IL] 1–11, interferons [IFN], tumor necrosis factors [TNF], lysosome and complement components, prostaglandins, leukotrienes, acid hydrolases, neutral proteinases, arginase, nucleotide metabolites, various neuroactive immunoregulatory peptides including corticotropin [ACTH], corticotropin-releasing factor [CRF]–like activity, bombesin, endorphins, enkephalins, thyrotropin [TSH], growth hormone, prolactin, neurotensin, chorionic gonadotropin, vasoactive intestinal peptide [VIP], tachykinin neuropeptides including substance P [SP], substance K, neuromedin K, somatostatins [SOMs], mast cell growth factor, suppressin, etc.); neutrophil leukocytes (slow-reacting substance of anaphylaxis [SRS-A], eosinophilic chemotactic factors of anaphylaxis [ECF-A], enzymes, platelet-activating factor [PAF] and other vascular permeability factors, kinin-generating substances, a complement-activating factor, histamine releasers, a neutrophil inhibitory factor, VIP, 5-hydroxyeicosatetraenoic acid [5-HETE], etc.); basophilic leukocytes (histamine, SRS-A, ECF-A, neutrophil chemotactic factor [NCF], PAF, SP, SOMs, etc.); murine basophilic leukocytes (the same as in humans plus serotonin); eosinophilic leukocytes (PAF,

8,15-diHETE, SRS-A, eosinophil peroxidase, major basic protein, etc.); serosal, connective tissue or TC mast cells (histamine, SRS-A, ECF-A, NCF, PAF, VIP, SP, SOMs, etc.); mucosal or T mast cells (histamine, SRS-A, ECF-A, NCF, PAF, VIP, SP, SOMs, etc.); "chromaffin-positive" mast cells (dopamine in ruminants; in other species possibly norepinephrine and neuropeptide Y); the so-called P-cells (histamine, serotonin); enterochromaffin cells (serotonin); chromaffin cells (epinephrine, norepinephrine, dopamine, neuropeptide Y, IL-1α, etc.); platelets (depending on species, histamine, serotonin, catecholamines, prostaglandins, 12-HETE); neurosecretory cells (histamine, serotonin, catecholamines, acetylcholine, prostaglandins, and other eicosanoids, kinins, the various hypothalamic substances that release or inhibit the release of the anterior pituitary hormones, and the group of neuroactive immunoregulatory peptides including ACTH, bombesin, neurotensin, endorphins, enkephalins, TSH, growth hormone, prolactin, luteinizing hormone [LH], LH-releasing hormone [LHRH], chorionic gonadotropin, VIP, the tachykinin neuropeptides, SOMs, neuropeptide Y, ILs 1–6, suppressin, etc.); the medullary thymic epithelial cells and the Hassall's corpuscles (thymosins and other thymic factors, oxytocin, vasopressin, etc.); the serum inhibitory factor cells (dopamine); and other nerve cells including essentially all the effector molecules listed under the neurosecretory cells. These various cells produce their effector molecules either constitutively or on induction. For more detailed information on all the foregoing cell types and effector molecules, see other publications [46, 109, 110, 114, 117].

Many of these cell types possess different morphologic, physicochemical, and general biologic characteristics. Nevertheless, in passing from one member of this cell spectrum to another, obvious transitions are seen in all these characteristics. Furthermore, when one surveys their properties and their probable physiologic function in the higher organism, significant cohesive features become apparent and set them apart from other body constituents as a distinct single class of cells that must be included in current concepts of neurosecretion.

Some workers postulated that the cellular components of the immune-neuroendocrine circuitry and their effector molecules could be viewed as two different divisions of this network. The two major divisions according to these workers may be defined as involved in neurovascular immunology and neuroendocrine immunology. Neurovascular immunology is concerned with immune response–related actions of vasoactive neurotransmitter substances that function as potent, short-lived local "hormones," first identified and studied as mediators of immunologic inflammation and hypersensitivity. They also play important roles in blood flow, vascular permeability, and pain transmission. These soluble effector molecules are simple compounds (i.e., amine mediators), short-chain peptides (i.e., kinins, SP, etc.), and short-chain lipids (i.e., prostaglandins, leukotrienes) and have a long evolutionary history in biologic defense. They use paracrine and synaptic signaling on their effector cells. The second major division, defined above as involved in neuroendocrine immunology, represents all the immune response–related hypothalamic, pituitary, and other hormones that use endocrine signaling and are primarily immunomodulatory in character. This perhaps convenient but arbitrary functional separation of these two divisions is intrinsically incorrect, as discussed by my colleagues and me [134].

Neural Crest Interactions in the Development of the Immune System

In discussing neural crest interactions in the development of the immune system, first I must briefly characterize the developmental biology of this structure. The neural crest is produced from ectodermal cells, which are released from the apical portions of the neural folds at about the time fusion occurs to form the neural tube and a separate overlying ectodermal layer. The basement membrane underlying the neural crest cells breaks down, the cellular characteristics change, and they become separated from the other components of the neural fold. There is a change in relative spatial relationship, or migration, of the neural crest cells to varied associations and destinies [44].

The portion of the neural crest pertinent to this discussion is that which is closely associated with the developing brain, specifically the hind brain. Crest cells in this cranial portion (anterior to the fifth somite) differentiate into mesenchyme, in addition to other connective tissue, muscular, and nervous components. Neural crest cells migrate ventrolaterally through the bronchial arches and contribute mesenchymal cells to a number of structures. It is this mesenchyme that forms the layers around the epithelial primordia of the thymus [57].

The full significance of the foregoing will be even more appreciated when viewed in the context of three additional considerations: (1) The thymus is formed by contributions from different sources that must interact in a precisely timed sequence for proper development; (2) ablation of small portions of the neural crest prevents or alters the development of the thymus; and (3) formation of the thymus precedes that of the more secondary, peripheral lymphoid tissues, reflecting a critical thymic role already in the early development of the immune system. Taken together, development of the immune system is inherently linked to the neural crest and any aberration in this link results in defective immune development such as that seen for instance in DiGeorge's syndrome.

Cerebral Dominance or Lateralization and Immune Disorders

The recognition of cerebral lateralization grew out of the discovery in the last century of cerebral dominance, that is, the superior capacity of each side of the brain to acquire particular skills. Over the past 120 years, it was believed that hemispheric dominance was based on functional asymmetry, on the differences in function of the two sides of the brain and of specific regions within them. In the face of the prevalent belief that cerebral dominance lacked an anatomic correlate, work over the past three decades has conclusively established that cerebral dominance is based on asymmetries of structure. An early example of this is the early detectable asymmetry in the human brain that involves the upper surface of the posterior portion of the left temporal lobe, the *planum temporale*. The larger size of the left planum temporale reflects the greater extent of a particular temporoparietal cytoarchitectonic area on the left. There are other asymmetries in the human brain and the same applies to the findings throughout the animal kingdom. In addition to genetic, several other factors in the course of development, both prenatal and postnatal, influence the direction and extent of these structural differences [41].

Associations of anomalous cerebral dominance include not only developmental disorders such as dyslexia, autism, stuttering, mental retardation, and learning disorders, as well as some extraordinary musical, mathematic, athletic, and other talents,* but also alterations in many bodily systems including the immune system. In these situations, the same influences that modify structural asymmetry in the brain also modify other systems such as the immune system. The suspected molecular mechanisms involved in the influence of structural asymmetry on the development of immune reactivities are discussed in more detail in a larger review [102]. Here I shall only mention that there is good evidence that left-handedness more frequently occurs in persons with diseases of atopic allergy (asthma, allergic

---

* It is difficult to speak of extraordinary talents as the "pathology of superiority" but that is what the evidence dictates.

rhinitis, atopic dermatitis), and that animal experiments in the past 10 years provided some insight into the nature of the association between anomalous hemispheric dominance and immune reactivities.

Thus, beginning in 1980 and continuing throughout the decade, Renoux and coworkers showed in a series of studies that immunomodulation of the T-cell lineage in rodents can be a phenomenon of hemispheric lateralization. In 1980, the initial observation presented data indicating that lesioning the left cerebral neocortex depresses T-cell–mediated responses in mice without affecting B-cell responses. These observations were extended in experiments where animals with a right cortical lesion served as controls for animals with a left cortical ablation. The findings demonstrated a balanced brain asymmetry in which the right hemisphere controls the inductive influence of T-cells of signals emitted by the left hemisphere. In addition, most recent studies found that ditiocarb sodium (Imuthiol), an immunostimulant specifically active on the T-cell lineage, can replace the signals emitted by the left neocortex, since mice without a left neocortex were stimulated to increased T-cell–dependent responses by treatment with ditiocarb sodium, whereas the agent did not modify the responses already increased in right decorticates. B-cell–dependent and some macrophage-dependent responses are not affected by either neocortical ablation or ditiocarb sodium. This lateralization of cortical influences on immune function in rodents is likely to be predictive of an even greater influence in humans with more profound and complex cortical functions [80].

The Ancient Superfamily of Immune Recognition Molecules and the Neural Cell Adhesion Molecule

The ancient superfamily of immune recognition molecules and the N-CAM represent another aspect of the interrelationships among the cellular and molecular components of the immune-neuroendocrine circuitry. Most of the glycoproteins that mediate cell-cell recognition or antigen recognition in the immune system contain related structural elements, suggesting that the genes that encode them have a common evolutionary history. Included in this Ig superfamily are antibodies; T-cell receptors; MHC glycoproteins; the CD2, CD4, and CD8 cell-cell adhesion proteins; some of the polypeptide chains of the CD3 complex associated with T-cell receptors; and the various Fc receptors on lymphocytes and other white blood cells—all of which contain one or more Ig-like domains (Ig homology units). Each Ig homology unit is usually encoded by a separate exon, and it seems likely that the entire supergene family evolved from a gene coding for a single Ig homology unit similar to that encoding Thy-1 or beta$_2$-microglobulin which may have been involved in mediating cell-cell interactions. Since a Thy-1–like molecule has been isolated from the brain of squids, it is probable that such a primordial gene arose before vertebrates diverged from their invertebrate ancestors some 400 million years ago. New family members presumably arose by exon and gene duplications, and similar duplication events probably gave rise to the multiple gene segments that encode antibodies and T-cell receptors [17].

An increasing number of cell-surface glycoproteins that mediate Ca^{++}-independent cell-cell adhesion in vertebrates are being discovered to belong to the Ig superfamily. One of these is the so-called N-CAM, which is a large, single-pass transmembrane glycoprotein (about 1,000–amino acid residues long). N-CAM is expressed on the surface of nerve cells and glial cells and causes them to stick together by a Ca^{++}-independent mechanism. When these membrane proteins are purified and inserted into synthetic phospholipid vesicles, the vesicles bind to one another, as well as to cells that have N-CAM on their surface; the binding is blocked if the cells are pretreated with monovalent anti–N-CAM antibodies. Thus, N-CAM binds cells together by a homophilic interaction that directly joins two N-CAM molecules [68].

Anti–N-CAM antibodies disrupt the orderly pattern of retinal development in tissue culture and when injected into the developing chick eye, disturb the normal growth pattern of retinal nerve cell axons. These observations suggest that N-CAM plays an important part in the development of the central nervous system by promoting cell-cell adhesion. In addition, the neural crest cells that form the peripheral nervous system have large amounts of N-CAM on their surface when they are associated with the neural tube, lose it while they are migrating, and then reexpress it when they aggregate to form a ganglion, suggesting that N-CAM plays a part in the assembly of the ganglion.

There are several forms of N-CAM, each encoded by a distinct messenger RNA (mRNA). The different mRNAs are generated by alternative splicing of an RNA transcript produced from a single large gene. The large extracellular post of the polypeptide chain (~680–amino acid residues) is identical in most forms of N-CAM and is folded into five domains characteristic of antibody molecules. Thus, N-CAM belongs to the same ancient superfamily of recognition proteins to which antibodies belong [147].

I mentioned earlier the guidance provided by the neural crest in the development of the thymus, that is, a central regulatory organ for the immune system. The converse also appears to be true: The immune system has a special role in the development of the nervous system. In this context, the most critical feature of the immune system is its tremendous polymorphism so that lymphocytes that are produced can recognize enormous numbers of different antigens. For this reason, the immune system is ideally suited to provide markers or "anchoring sites" that enable developing structures to be built up in precisely the correct form. In no organ system is this type of detailed anchorage mechanism as important as in the developing nervous system in which many millions of nerve fibers traverse great distances and establish connections with particular groups of target cells. Marking by means of histocompatibility antigens provides exactly such a system, as indeed the original function of the MHC antigens has been defined already in the 1970s as the general plasma membrane anchorage site of organogenesis-directing proteins [23].

The Immune System and the Nervous System Sharing the Capacity to Remember

The immune system and the nervous system possess short- or long-term memory, or both. The latter may be defined as the recording of experiences that can modify behavior. This general definition encompasses a broad spectrum of phenomena from the bacterial capacity of sensing chemical gradients to cognitive learning in humans.

The clonal selection theory of acquired immunity provides a useful conceptual framework for understanding the cellular basis of immunologic memory. According to this scheme, immunologic memory is generated during the primary immune response because (1) the proliferation of antigen-triggered virgin cells creates a large number of memory cells—a process known as *clonal expansion*; (2) the memory cells have a much longer life span than do virgin cells and recirculate between the blood and secondary lymphoid organs; and (3) each memory cell is able to respond more readily to antigen than does a virgin cell.

One reason, if not the most important reason, for the increased responsiveness of memory B-cells is the higher affinity (avidity) of their antibody receptors for the homologous antigen. Thus, with the passage of time after immunization, there is a progressive increase in the affinity of antibodies produced against the immunizing antigen. This phenomenon is known as *affinity maturation*, and it is due to the accumulation of somatic mutations in variable (V) region coding sequences after antigen stimulation of B-lymphocytes. The rate of somatic mutation in these sequences is estimated to be 10^{-3} per nucleotide pair per cell generation, which is about a million times greater than the spontaneous mutation rate in other genes [115]. This process is called *somatic hypermutation*. Since B-cells are stimulated to proliferate by the binding of antigen, any mutation occurring during the course of an immune response that increases the affinity of a cell-surface antibody molecule will cause the preferential proliferation of the B-cell making the antibody, especially when antigen concentration decreases with increasing time after immunization. Thus, affinity maturation is the consequence of repeated cycles of somatic hypermutation followed by antigen-driven selection in the course of an antibody response.

Research in the field of neuronal memory is still in an early phase, primarily because of methodologic difficulties and the validity of approaches currently used. The human brain is extraordinarily complex (10^{12} neurons) and intricate (an average neuron may have 10,000 dendrites interacting with other neurons), dictating the use of reductionist approaches which always require a correlation with the whole organism to verify the conclusions reached at the molecular level. Such relationship emphasizes the importance relating the biochemical events in single cells to the more complex organisms such as Aplysia, Drosophila, rodents, cats, and humans. The fact, however, that adjacent neurons are practically never identical means that the quantity of material needed for biochemical analysis necessitates a cell-line approach. Both bacteria and neural cell lines provide a homogeneous population of cells that can be studied biochemically. Bacteria detect chemical gradients using a memory obtained by the combination of a fast excitation process and a slow adaptation process. This model system, which has the advantages of extensive genetic and biochemical information, shows no features of long-term memory.

To study long-term memory, other biologic systems that exhibit two phenomena associated with learning and memory, habituation and potentiation, must be used. *Habituation* is defined as the decreased responsiveness to a stimulus when it is presented repetitively over time. *Potentiation*, on the other hand, is defined as the increased responsiveness to a stimulus when that stimulus is presented repetitively over time. In the mammalian brain, the hippocampus plays a special role in learning: When it is destroyed on both sides of the brain, the ability to form new memories is largely lost, although previous long-established memories remain. The evidence obtained on hippocampal slices indicates that the biochemical changes in the synapse represent the molecular bases for long-term memory [5, 62]. Despite the wealth of information provided by investigations in mammalian brain slices, it became increasingly clear that the study of cultured neural cells is more desirable because only in such a system could one be certain that the complete biochemical pathway, that is, the complete signal transduction pathway from stimulatory input to a behavioral output, could be analyzed. To study memory, however, some modifiable behavior needs to be observed. Because neurons communicate with each other chemically through the release of a neurotransmitter, the secretion of neurotransmitters (the output) evoked by various chemical stimuli (the input) could be used to monitor the responsiveness of the cell. This experimental system was used to study the input-output properties of a particular neuron, and both habituation and potentiation could be demonstrated in neuronal cell lines, indicating that they can serve as good model systems for the memory process except that they do not possess synaptic connections. In the early phase of these studies, the absence of synaptic connections posed a substantial problem for two major reasons: (1) As stated before, current evidence favors (in more organized neural tissue such as brain slices) the idea that the biochemical changes in the synapse are the molecular basis of long-term memory, and (2) the synapse is a unique anatomic

association of two cells that occurs only in the nervous system and therefore represents a special *sui generis* neuronal feature.

Whether memories, however, are generally recorded in presynaptic changes or in postsynaptic changes, in synaptic chemistry or in synaptic structure, or indeed in synapses at all, are still open questions. Regardless of the validity of any of these questions, it appears that the biochemical features of all memory-forming processes (i.e., habituation, potentiation, and associative learning in invertebrates, mammalian brain slices, and cultured clonal neural cell lines) are highly similar (the PC 12 cells [65, 66] and HT4 cells [70, 71]). They can be characterized as follows: A monoamine (primarily serotonin) and a glutamate receptor (known as NMDA receptor because it is selectively activated by the artificial glutamate analog *N*-methyl-D-aspartate) are involved; (2) binding of the neurotransmitter (serotonin, glutamate) by these receptors initiates a cascade of enzymatic reactions; (3) the first step in this cascade is the activation of a G-protein, which may either interact directly with ion channels or control the production of cyclic adenosine monophosphate (AMP) or Ca^{++}; (4) the two second messengers in turn regulate ion channels directly or activate kinases that phosphorylate various proteins including ion channels; (5) at many synapses both channel-linked and non-channel-linked receptors are present, responding either to the same or to different neurotransmitters; (6) responses mediated by nonchannel-linked receptors (serotonin) have a slow onset and long duration, and modulate the efficacy of subsequent synaptic transmission, providing the basis for memory formation; (7) channel-linked receptors that allow Ca^{++} to enter the cell (NMDA receptor) also mediate long-term memory effects; and (8) either too much or too little cyclic AMP can interfere with memory formation [21].

In all these processes, the interaction between serotonin and glutamate and their respective receptor systems can be illustrated by the studies carried out on the HT4 neural cell line [71]. The HT4 cells do not habituate to repetitive membrane depolarization, but after exposure of these cells to various neurotransmitters, serotonin has the capacity to potentiate cellular responsiveness. Depending on the strength of the serotonin stimulus, both short- and long-term potentiation can be induced. For instance, a 2-minute exposure to serotonin results in the transient increase in cellular responsiveness, where a 5-minute presentation gives rise to a more permanent potentiation, the difference between the two involving the activation of NMDA receptors. Thus, the stronger (5-minute) serotonin stimulus results in the endogenous release of excitatory amino acids with activation of NMDA receptors. Consistent with this mechanism, long-term secretory potentiation can also be produced with a 2-minute stimulus of serotonin only if glutamate or NMDA is given simultaneously.

As I now begin a comparison of immunologic versus neuronal memory, I have to return to an earlier statement that immunologic memory is due to clonal selection and lymphocyte maturation. Although this is correct in cellular terms, in molecular terms the problem of clonal selection and expansion reduces to the issue of affinity maturation of the antibody on the surface of the lymphocyte. In other words, the entire antigen-driven selection of antibody-producing lymphocytes is based on the strength of the antibody-antigen interaction, which depends on both the affinity and the number of binding sites. The affinity of an antibody reflects the strength of binding of an antigenic determinant to a single antigen-binding site, and it is independent of the number of sites. However, the total avidity of an antibody for a multivalent antigen, such as a polymer with repeating subunits, is defined as the total binding strength of all of its binding sites together. When a multivalent antigen combines with more than one antigen-binding site on an antibody, the binding strength is greatly increased because all the antigen-antibody bonds must be broken simultaneously before the antigen and antibody can dissociate. Thus, a typical IgG molecule will bind at least 1,000 times more strongly to a multivalent antigen if both antigen-binding sites are engaged than if only one site is involved. For the same reason, if the affinity of the antigen-binding sites in an IgG and an IgM molecule is the same, the IgM molecule (with ten binding sites) will have a much greater avidity for a multivalent antigen than an IgG molecule (which has two sites). This difference in avidity, often 10^4-fold or more, is important because antibodies produced early in an immune response usually have much lower affinities than those produced later. Because of its high total avidity, IgM—the major Ig class produced early in immune responses—can function effectively even when each of its binding sites has only a low affinity [115].

In the late 1950s, an excellent correlation was shown between the body temperature of rabbits and the affinity and avidity of the antibody produced against the radiolabeled antigen as tested in equilibrium dialysis experiments [107]. The higher the body temperature was, the greater the affinity and avidity were. In the beginning of these studies, commercially available *Escherichia coli* endotoxin was used, but later the rise in temperature was reproduced by electrical stimulation of the posterior hypothalamus or hippocampus through stereotaxically implanted, permanent depth electrodes in studies without endotoxin administration [140]. Discovery of the peptidoglycan and its derivatives as powerful immunologic adjuvants opened up a new window for the consideration of the relationship between immunologic and neuronal memory. The peptidoglycan, which is the basal layer of the bacterial cell wall, is a rigid macromolecule surrounding the cytoplasmic membrane. It is formed by the polymerization of a disaccharide tetrapeptide subunit; in the intact peptidoglycan, disaccharides form linear chains, whereas peptides are linked by interpeptide linkages [46]. The recognition of the immunomodulating properties of peptidoglycans and peptidoglycan fragments is the result of the work aimed at identifying the structure responsible for the adjuvant activity of the mycobacterial cells in Freund's adjuvant [37]. Simple active molecules were soon produced by organic synthesis followed by a vast array of analogs and derivatives that can be classified into several categories. The one that is most pertinent to this discussion is the group of "simple muramyl peptides." Of these the smallest immunoactive synthetic muramyl peptide is *N*-acetylmuramyl-L-alanyl-D-isoglutamine (MDP) [53, 116]. This substance has a pyrogenic effect that originally was attributed to its ability to induce the release of endogenous pyrogen from mononuclear phagocytes. However, a direct central nervous system action could not be excluded since MDP was found to be active by the intracerebroventricular route (MDP was shown to cross the blood-brain barrier [55]), and in rabbits made leukopenic by nitrogen mustard treatment [46]. In addition, it was subsequently shown that MDP can also induce sleep, and the somnogenic effect can be separated from its pyrogenic activity. MDP's pyrogenic activity does not affect brain temperature changes that are tightly coupled to sleep states [56]. More importantly, with respect to the direct central nervous system neuronal effects of MDP, this substance is capable of specific binding to serotonin receptors of synaptosomal membranes of brain tissue and competes with serotonin for these binding sites, and the kinetics of serotonin binding to brain homogenates is altered after sleep deprivation [34]. Additional findings on the capacity of MDP to act directly and specifically on central neurons include the following: MDP alters neuronal firing rates in different regions of the brain [20]; humoral antibody responses are enhanced by lowering serotonin levels in the brain [26]; and administration of *para*-chlorophenylalamine, which markedly decreases the level of brain serotonin, completely abolishes the MDP-induced rise in body temperature as well as the somnogenic effect [63]. Finally, it has been established that immunization decreases the concentration of serotonin in the hypothalamus and the hippocampus [145].

Although the foregoing evidence is fragmentary, it does estab-

lish a set of future reference points to begin to undertake a more informed comparison of the molecular mechanisms involved in immune and neuronal memory.

The Unique Recognition and Communication Powers of the Immune and Neuroendocrine Systems as Shared Characteristics

Earlier I cited Schechter, pointing out that a good relationship between two biologic systems must be sensitive, synchronized, and synergistic [88]. There are no two biologic systems where such characterization of an ideal relationship would be more valid than in case of the immune and neuroendocrine systems, as reflected by their unique recognition and communication powers as shared characteristics. The latter are based on four critical features shared by both: (1) They are composed of extraordinarily large numbers of phenotypically distinct cells organized into intricate networks. Moreover, the size of this extensive cellular arsenal continuously increases as new sequence information becomes available and enormous numbers of new members of the Ig supergene family surface each year. Within these cell networks, the individual cells can interact either positively or negatively, and the response of one cell reverberates through the system by affecting many other cells. (2) Cells of both systems synthesize, secrete, and/or release the same effector molecules. (3) Recognition of these effector molecules is realized by the same cellular receptors and second messenger mechanisms of both cell systems. (4) These cellular and molecular determinants make a continuous, bilateral flow of information, the sine qua non of the unique interactions within the immune-neuroendocrine circuitry, possible.

A more amplified view on the basic biochemistry and molecular biology of receptor-effector coupling by G-proteins (i.e., the fundamental mechanism used by hormones, neurotransmitters, and the immunomodulatory cytokines for signal transmission by G-proteins) is presented in Chapter 14 and by Lochrie and Simon [60] and Birnbaumer and Brown [10]. Here, I shall only mention that about 80 percent of all known neurohormones, neurotransmitters, immunomodulatory lymphokines, and other autocrine and paracrine factors that regulate cellular interactions in the immune-neuroendocrine circuitry, called *"primary"* messengers, elicit cellular responses by combining with specific receptors that are coupled to effector functions by G-proteins. Although the primary messengers are many, the number of physicochemically and biologically distinct receptors that mediate their action is even larger. So far about 80 distinct receptors that recognize 40 hormones, neurotransmitters, and so on, can be identified. It is reasonable to assume that the total number of distinct receptors coupled by G-proteins will be 100 to 150 (Table 33-1). In contrast to receptors, the number of final effector functions regulated by these receptors and the number of G-proteins that provide for receptor-effector coupling are much lower, probably not much more than 15 each.

At the time of writing, receptors for simple substances, such as the amine mediators and short-chain peptides as well as lipids, and for more than 20 different hypothalamopituitary peptides have been identified in the cells of the immune system, essentially in lymphocytes. In addition, to the hypothalamopituitary hormones, lymphocytes also express receptors for peptides secreted from neurons together with other neurotransmitters. These neuropeptides take on added significance as immunomodulators, since it is now known that lymphoid organs are directly innervated with nerves secreting these agents. From the standpoint of the integration of information in the immune-neuroendocrine circuitry, future studies will have to examine these parallel signaling pathways in isolation. In other words, it will be necessary to determine how an individual cell completely processes and integrates information from these individual pathways. This

Table 33-1. Examples of receptors acting on cells via G-proteins

Type of receptor	Membrane function/system affected	Effect	Coupling protein involved	Examples of target cell(s)/organs
A. *Neurotransmitters*				
1. Adrenergic				
Beta-1	AC	Stimulation	G_s	Heart, fat, sympathetic synapse
	Ca channel	Stimulation	G_s	Heart, skeletal muscle
Beta-2	AC	Stimulation	G_s	Liver, lung
Alpha-1	PhL C	Stimulation	G_{plc}	Smooth muscle, liver
	PhL A_2	Stimulation	G_{pla}	FRTL-5 cells
Alpha-2A, -2B	AC	Inhibition	G_i	Platelet, fat (human)
	Ca channel	Closing	G_o (G_p)?	NG-108, sympathetic presynapse
2. Dopamine				
D-1	AC	Stimulation	G_s	Caudate nucleus
D-2	AC	Inhibition	G_i	Pituitary lactotrophs
3. Acetylcholine				
Muscarinic M_1	PhL C	Stimulation	G_{plc}	Pancreatic acinar cell
	K channel (M)	Closing	?	CNS, sympathetic ganglia
Muscarinic M_2	AC	Inhibition	G_s	Heart
	K channel	Opening	G_k (G_i?)	Heart, CNS
	PhL C	Stimulation	G_p	Heart, transfected cells
4. GABAB	Ca channel	Closing	G_o (G_p?)	Neuroblastoma N1E
	K channel	Opening	G_i (G_k?)	Sympathetic ganglia
5. Purinergic P_1				
Adenosine A-1 or Ri	AC	Inhibition	G_i	Pituitary, CNS, heart
	K channel	Opening	G_k (G_i?)	Heart
Adenosine A-2 or Ra	AC	Stimulation	G_s	Fat, kidney, CNS
6. Purinergic P_{2X} and P_{2Y}	PhL C (PIP_2)	Stimulation	G_{pic}	Turkey erythrocytes
	PhL C (PC)	Stimulation	G-(?)	Liver
	AC	Inhibition	G_i	Liver
7. Serotonin (5HT)				
S-1a (5HT-1a)	AC	Inhibition	G_i	Pyramidal cells
	K channel	Opening	(G_i?)	Pyramidal cells
S-1b (5HT-1b)	AC	Inhibition	G_i	
	DNA synthesis	Stimulation	G(ptx)	
S-1c (5HT-1c)	PhL C	Stimulation	G_{pic}	Aplysia
S-2 (5HT-2)	AC	Stimulation	G_s	Skeletal muscle
8. Histamine				
H-1	PhL C	Stimulation	G_{pic}	Smooth muscle, macrophages
	PhL A_2 (?)	Stimulation	G_{pla}	
H-2	AC	Stimulation	G_s	Heart
H-3	AC	Inhibition	G_i	Presynaptic CNS, lung; mast
B. *Peptide hormones*				
1. Pituitary				
Adrenocorticotropin (ACTH)	AC	Stimulation	G_s	Fasciculata, glomerulosa
Opioid (mu, kappa, delta)	AC	Inhibition	G_i	NG-108
	Ca channel	Closing	G_o (G_p?)	NG-108
Luteinizing hormone (LH)	AC	Stimulation	G_s	Granulosa, luteal, Leydig
Follicle stimulating hormone (FSH)	AC	Stimulation	G_s	Granulosa
Thyrotropin (TSH)	AC	Stimulation	G_s	Thyroid, FRTL-5
	PhL?	Stimulation	G_p (?)	Thyroid
Melanocyte stimulating hormone (MSH)	AC	Stimulation	G_s	Melanocytes
2. Hypothalamic				
Corticotropin releasing hormone (CRH)	AC	Stimulation	G_s	Corticotroph, hypothalamus
Growth hormone releasing hormone (GRH)	AC	Stimulation	G_s	Somatotroph
Gonadotropin releasing hormone (GnRH)	PhL A_2	Stimulation	G_{pla}	Gonadotroph
	PhL C	Stimulation	G_{plc}	Gonadotroph
	Ca channel	Opening	G_i-type	GH_3
Thyrotropin releasing hormone (TRH)	PhL C	Stimulation	G_{plc}	Lactotroph, thyrotroph
	AC	Inhibition	G_i	GH_4C_1
Somatostatin (SST or SRIF)	AC	Inhibition	G_i	Pituitary cells, endocrine pancreas
	K channel	Opening	G (G_i?)	Pituitary cells, endocrine pancreas
	Ca channel	Closing	?	Pituitary cells
Vasopressin				
V-1a (vasopressor, glycogenolytic)	PhL C	Stimulation	G_{plc}	Smooth muscle, liver, CNS
	AC	Inhibition	G_i	Liver
V-1b (pituitary)	PhL C	Stimulation	G_{plc}	Pituitary
V-2 (antidiuretic)	AC	Stimulation	G_s	Distal and collecting tubule
Oxytocin	PhL C	Stimulation	G_{plc}	Uterus, CNS

Table 33-1. (continued)

Type of receptor	Membrane function/system affected	Effect	Coupling protein involved	Examples of target cell(s)/organs
B. *Peptide hormones* (cont.)				
3. Other hormones				
Glucagon	AC	Stimulation	G_s	Liver, fat, heart
	Ca pump	Inhibition	G_s (?)	Liver, heart (?)
	PhL C	Stimulation	?	Liver
Cholecystokinin (CCK)	PhL C	Stimulation	G_{plc}	Pancreatic acini
Secretin	AC	Stimulation	G_s	Pancreatic duct, fat
Vasoactive intestinal peptide (VIP)	AC	Stimulation	G_s	Pancreatic duct, CNS
	PhL C	Stimulation	G_{plc}	Sensory ganglia, CNS
Angiotensin II	PhL C	Stimulation	G_{plc}	Liver, glomerulosa cells
	AC	Inhibition	G_i	Liver, glomerulosa cells
	Ca channel	Stimulation	G_i-type	Y1 adrenal cells
Chorionic gonadotropin	AC	Stimulation	G_s	Granulosa, luteal, Leydig
C. *Other regulatory factors*				
1. Chemoattractant (fMet-Leu-Phe or fMLP)	PhL C	Stimulation	G_{plc}	Neutrophils, HL-60 cells
2. Thrombin	PhL C	Stimulation	G_{plc}	Platelets, fibroblasts
	AC	Inhibition	G_i	Platelets
3. Bombesin	PhL C	Stimulation	G_{plc}	Fibroblasts
4. IgE	PhL C	Stimulation	G_{plc}	Mast cells
5. Bradykinin	PhL C	Stimulation	G_{plc}	Lung, fibroblasts, NG-108
	PhL A_2	Stimulation	G_{pla}	Fibroblasts, endothelial cells
	K channel	Stimulation	G_k (G_i?)	NG-108
	AC	Inhibition	G_i	NG-108
6. Neurokinin/tachykinin				
NK1 (substance P)	PhL C	Stimulation	G_{plc}	CNS, salivary gland, endothelial
NK2 (neurokinin A or substance K)	PhL C	Stimulation	G_{plc}	CNS, sympathetic, smooth muscle
NK3 (neurokinin B)	PhL C (?)	Stimulation	G_{plc}	CNS, smooth muscle
7. Neuropeptide Y	K channels	Stimulation	G_k	Heart
	Ca channels	Inhibition	G_o	Sensory ganglia
8. Tumor necrosis factor (TNF)	?	?	?	Monocytes
9. Colony-stimulating factor (CSF-1)	?	?	?	Monocytes
D. *Prostanoids*				
1. Prostaglandin E_1, E_2	AC	Inhibition	G_i	Fat, kidney
2. Prostacyclin (PGI_2, PGE_1, PGE_2)	AC	Stimulation	G_s	Luteal cells, endothelial, kidney
3. Thromboxanes	PhL C	Stimulation	G_{plc}	Platelets
4. Platelet activating factor (PAF)	PhL C	Stimulation	G_{plc}	Platelets
5. Leukotriene D_4, C_4	PhL A_2	Stimulation	G_{pla}	Endothelial cells
E. *Sensory*				
1. Light (rhodopsins)	cGMP-PDE	Stimulation	Tr(G_t-r)	Retinal rod cells (night)
	cGMP-PDE	Stimulation	Tc(G_t-c)	Retinal cone cells (color)
2. Olfactory signals	AC	Stimulation	G_{olf}	Olfactory cilia
	PhL's?	Stimulation	G_p?	
3. Taste signals	AC	Stimulation	G_s	Taste epithelium
	PhL's	Stimulation	G_p?	

AC = adenylyl cyclase; PhL C = unless denoted otherwise, phospholipase C with specificity for phosphatidylinositol bisphosphate; PhL A_2 = phospholipase A_2 (substrate specificity unknown); PIP_2 = phosphatidylinositol bisphosphate; PC = phosphatidylcholine.
Source: L. Birnbaumer and A. M. Brown. G proteins. *Am. Rev. Respir. Dis.* 141:S106, 1990. Reprinted with permission.

is all the more remarkable because the cell is faced with the task of balancing the need to communicate with other cells, with the need for growth and maintenance of the differentiated state while preserving adequate flexibility to support regulation, sensitivity, and gain. One early result of such inquiries is the demonstration of cross-regulation (cross-talk) between the various G-protein–mediated signaling pathways. Thus, it was shown that in the cross-regulation between alpha$_1$- and beta$_2$-adrenergic receptor–mediated pathways, activation of beta$_2$-adrenergic receptors increased alpha$_1$-adrenergic receptor mRNA levels [72]. Conversely, activation of the G1α-mediated inhibitory pathway of adenylate cyclase cross-regulates the stimulatory (Gsα-mediated) beta-adrenergic–sensitive adenylate cyclase system by (1) upregulating beta$_2$-adrenergic receptors and enhancing the activation of the stimulatory (Gsα-mediated) adenylate cyclase pathway, and (2) downregulating elements of the inhibitory adenylate cyclase pathway, G1α2 and A$_1$ adenosine receptor binding, respectively [45]. It may be added that cross-regulation is also

observed between signaling pathways that do not share the same effectors. Although much more work remains to be done to unravel the complexities of the coordinated regulation of information processing and integration by the cell, it is already possible to state that there is cross-regulation between neurally derived substances and lymphokines.

In the foregoing sections, discussions of the reciprocal, regulatory interplay between the immune and neuroendocrine systems have mainly covered the peripheral pathways by which the neuroendocrine influences are able to affect immune functions. However, as stated earlier, the flow of information in the immune-neuroendocrine circuitry is bidirectional, and there is conclusive evidence that products of the immune system are capable of modulating neuroendocrine processes. There are two lines of evidence indicating that the products of the immune system can influence the brain or the pituitary gland, or both. The first is provided by correlational studies, which show that changes occur in the brain during the course of an immune response.

Along this line, Korneva and Klimenko [54] recorded single-unit activity in the hypothalamus, showing significant changes in the neuronal firing patterns in the posterior, ventromedial, and supramaxillary nuclei during the course of an immune response. These observations were independently confirmed by Besedovsky and coworkers [9] who found a considerable increase in the firing rate of neurons in the ventromedial hypothalamus 1 to 5 days following sensitization to trinitrophenol-hemocyanin. Srebro and associates [93] found a significant increase in the nuclear volume of neurosecretory cells in the supraoptic nucleus during skin allograft rejection. Changes in the serotonin levels occur in the hypothalamus and hippocampus following immunization with typhoid antigen [145], whereas increases in dopamine-stimulated adenylate cyclase activity in caudate homogenates are found following bacille Calmette-Guérin (BCG) antigen administration [15]. In recent years, these observations have been expanded by the findings on the effects of Newcastle disease virus on the metabolism of cerebral biogenic amines [22], and similar changes have also been observed with influenza virus.

The second line of evidence implicating the immune system in regulating physiologic processes at the level of the brain or the pituitary gland, or both, is derived from studies in which products of the cells of the immune system were administered to experimental animals or added to cultured neuronal or pituitary cells. IL-1 stimulation of ACTH secretion was first shown in a mouse pituitary cell line, AtT-20 cells [148] and subsequently confirmed on primary pituitary cells [8, 52]. In addition, IL-1 alters the release of TSH, growth hormones, and prolactin [81]; stimulates astroglial proliferation following brain injury [42]; stimulates somatostatin synthesis in the fetal brain [87]; inhibits progesterone secretion in cultures of granulosa cells [39]; and elicits the production of CRF by the hypothalamus [7, 86]. In these neuronal interactions, IL-1 acts on specific receptors in the brain [27]. IL-1 shows complex, multitargeted effects on insulin secretion: (1) It has direct glucose-dependent inhibitory and stimulatory effects on pancreatic B-cell function [150], (2) IL-1 induces hyperinsulinemia by a central action [14], and (3) it acts as a hypoglycemic agent independently from effects on insulin release [19]. Other lymphokines also have effects on the neuroendocrine system. IL-2 stimulates oligodendroglial proliferation and maturation [6] and also induces ACTH secretion in pituitary cells [91]. TNF-α and IL-6 augment ACTH secretion in vivo together with numerous other effects on the neuroendocrine system [27, 67, 74, 90, 94], and the thymic hormone, thymosin fraction 5, stimulates prolactin and growth hormone release from anterior pituitary cells [92].

THE LYMPHOCYTE AS THE UNIFYING REGULATORY CELL COMPONENT OF THE IMMUNE-NEUROENDOCRINE CIRCUITRY AND ITS RELATION TO HUMAN ASTHMA

In the past 10 years the lymphocyte in general, and in the past 3 years the T-lymphocyte in particular, emerged as both the basic regulatory unit of the immune-neuroendocrine network and as a fundamental cell in the pathogenesis of bronchial asthma. This view is connected with our growing realization of T-lymphocyte's role in the development of the bronchial obstructive process not only as an immunoregulator but also as the inflammatory cell of possibly central significance, the cell with a key involvement in bronchial hyperresponsiveness, the effector cell of the delayed-type hypersensitivity (DTH) reaction in the genesis of airway hyperreactivity, and a genetically defective neuroendocrine cell that may be specifically responsible for the immunologic, inflammatory, and beta-adrenergic dysregulation in contrast to the large number of other factors that may and do contribute secondarily to the beta-adrenergic deficit in this disorder (see Chap. 14).

The T-lymphocyte as a Critical Cell of Bronchial Inflammation

The role of IgE in immunologically based asthma has been known for a long time, as was the demonstration that its production clearly depended on multiple subsets of lymphocytes (see Chaps. 7 and 13). With the discovery of soluble immunoregulatory molecules (i.e., monokines and lymphokines), it has also been established that the T-cell–derived lymphokines, IL-4, IL-5, and IFN-γ, are intimately involved in the regulation of IgE production [59]. Until recently, however, the critical role of T-cell–derived lymphokines in the regulation and expression of the inflammation associated with allergy and asthma of both the extrinsic and intrinsic varieties has not been established. Our current understanding now clearly shows a coordinated regulation of immune and inflammatory responses by T-cell–derived lymphokines [69]. Indeed, T-cells appear to orchestrate the bronchial inflammatory response to inhaled allergens and other stimuli in asthma by the production of several lymphokines with widely varying attributes such as IL-1, IL-3, IL-5, and granulocyte-macrophage colony-stimulating factor (GM-CSF). Of these, IL-5 has selective and the most pronounced effects on eosinophils including chemokinetic, chemotactic, phagocytic, cytotoxic, superoxide, and complement receptor–inducing activities, together with prolongation of survival and activation [61, 77, 85]. The chemotactic factors released by T-cells recruit eosinophils to the sites of airway inflammation, whereas other lymphokines activate eosinophils and indirectly regulate the release of their products [50, 58]. Also, T-lymphocytes have chemotactic activity for neutrophils, basophil granulocytes, as well as monocytes, and can activate or degranulate these effector cells [16, 51]. Furthermore, production of eosinophils by bone marrow is dependent on T-cells and their lymphokines [36]. Of the latter, IL-4 may require special note, since this substance promotes the synthesis of IgE by B-lymphocytes [69] and induces the production of an IgE-binding factor (a cleavage fragment of the IgE receptor, FcRII [18]). Lymphocytes from asthmatic patients are capable of spontaneously producing the IgE-binding factor [149]. The principal cytokines and their function are summarized in Table 33-2.

T-lymphocytes also play a role in the proliferation and activation of mast cells, and in fact an intact immune system is a requirement for the development of a functional mucosal mast cell system; the latter cells require a T-cell–derived factor to divide after stimulation. T-cells also produce substances that enhance the release of histamine from mast cells. Thus, IFN-γ, IL-1, IL-3, and GM-CSF can prime mast cells to increase their release of histamine to appropriate stimulation. In addition, T-cells produce histamine-releasing factors (HRFs) as well as a histamine-release inhibitory factor, which directly or indirectly participate in the release of histamine from mast cells or in its inhibition, respectively [1–3]. The issue of these lymphocytic HRFs is further discussed below.

The Involvement of T-lymphocytes in Bronchial Hyperresponsiveness in Asthma

Nonspecific bronchial hyperresponsiveness is usually defined as an increased reactivity of the airways to physical, thermal, chemical, immunologic, microbial (both bacterial and viral), pharmacologic, and otherwise physiologic stimuli. This manifestation has been interpreted as a characteristic of asthma and associated with airway inflammation. In the past decade, the lymphocytes, most specifically the T-lymphocytes, have become conspicuous among the inflammatory cells infiltrating the bronchi in asthmatic patients [75, 139] (Table 33-3).

Two most recently published extensive studies demonstrated the relationship of T-lymphocytes to other inflammatory cells and to bronchial hyperresponsiveness. The first of these [146]

Table 33-2. The principal cytokines

Name	Target cell/organ	Function
Interleukin 1α and β	T cells	Activation; cytokine release
IL-1α and IL-1β	B cells	Proliferation and differentiation
	Bone marrow	Induction GM-CSF, G-CSF, IL-6 by stromal cells
	Fibroblasts	Proliferation; prostaglandin release
	Hepatocytes	Acute phase protein release
	Muscle	Proteolysis
	Osteoclasts	Resorption bone
	CNS	Slow wave sleep
Interleukin 2	T cells	Progression to proliferation
IL-2	B cells	Growth and Ig synthesis
	NK cells	Proliferation; augmentation of non MHC restricted killing
	Monocytes	Increased cytotoxicity
Interleukin-3	Pluripotent stem cells	Growth/differentiation
IL-3		
	Basophils/mast cells	Growth; cytokine release
	Monocytes	Enhanced cytotoxicity; phagocytosis
	Eosinophils	ADCC; phagocytosis; activation
Interleukin 4	T cells	Growth
IL-4	B cells	Induction Class II MHC, enhancement IgG and IgE synthesis; induction FcεRII (CD23)
	Mast cells	Growth
	Macrophages	Induction MHC Class I and II: activation; growth
Interleukin-5	B cells	Growth; enhancement IgA and IgM synthesis; enhancement IL-4 induced IgE production
IL-5		
	Eosinophils	Growth/differentiation progenitor cells; ADCC, degranulation
Interleukin 6	B cells	Stimulation of immunoglobulin synthesis
IL-6		
	T cells	IL-2 synthesis; growth; differentiation
	Pluripotent stem cells	Differentiation
	Hepatocytes	Acute phase protein release
Interleukin 7	Pre-B cells	
IL-7	Thymocytes	Proliferation
	T cells	
Interleukin 8	Neutrophils	
IL-8	T cells	Chemotaxis
Granulocyte colony stimulating factor	Neutrophil progenitors	Proliferation; differentiation
G-CSF	Neutrophils	Activation
Macrophage colony stimulating factor	Monocyte progenitors	Proliferation; differentiation
M-CSF	Monocyte/macrophages	Proliferation; activation
Granulocyte-macrophage colony stimulating factor, FM-CSF	Pluripotent stem cells	Growth factor for myelogenous cells
	Neutrophils	
	Monocyte/macrophage	Activation
	Eosinophils	
Interferon γ	B cells	
IFN-γ	Macrophages	Induces Class I and Class II MHC expression
	Endothelial cells	
	Epithelial cells	
Tumour necrosis factor α and β	T cells	Growth; activation
TNF α and β	B cells	Growth; Ig synthesis
	Monocytes	Activation; cytokine synthesis
	Neutrophils	Activation
	Fibroblasts	Growth; cytokine synthesis; induction Class I MHC expression
Transforming growth factor-β	Macrophages	
TGF-β	T cells	Inhibits functions
	B cells	
	Neutrophils	
	NK cells	Enhances cytotoxicity

Source: A. S. Hamblin. Cytokines in asthma. *Ann. NY Acad. Sci.* 629:250, 1991. Reprinted with permission.

studied the regulatory role of activated T-lymphocytes in eosinophilic inflammation, investigating T-cell activation and eosinophilia in blood and bronchoalveolar lavage (BAL) fluid from patients with asthma not receiving steroid treatment. Compared to that from normal individuals, BAL fluid from asthmatic patients contained markedly increased numbers of both lymphocytes and eosinophils (see Chap. 24). The lymphocytosis consisted of increased numbers of both CD4$^+$ and CD8$^+$ T-cells, and the T-cell populations expressed elevated levels of T-cell activation markers such as IL-2 receptor (IL-2R) (CD25), HLA-DR, and very

late activation antigen-1 (VLA-1). Close correlation was found between CD4$^+$ IL-2R-positive T-cells, eosinophil concentrations, and the degree of bronchial hyperresponsiveness. In the second recent publication [11], T-lymphocytes, eosinophils, mast cells, neutrophils, and macrophages were studied in bronchial biopsy specimens from subjects with or without asthma and their relationship to bronchial hyperresponsiveness determined using immunohistochemical techniques and monoclonal antibodies at two airway levels. There were no significant differences in the numbers of mucosal-type or connective tissue–type mast cells,

Table 33-3. Inflammatory cytokines

Cytokine	Activities induced
Local	
IL-1 α/β	Secretion from neutrophils; endothelial cell adhesion of neutrophils
IL-2	Cytotoxicity of monocytes; chemotaxis monocytes
IL-8	Chemotaxis neutrophils and T cells; adhesion monocytes to endothelium
G-CSF	Production of superoxide by neutrophils
M-CSF	Macrophage secretion of plasminogen activator
GM-CSF	Production cytokines, chemotaxis, superoxide production and phagocytosis by neutrophils. Production cytokines by macrophages.
IFN-γ	Synergistic with TNF for neutrophil and macrophage activation
TNF α/β	Chemotactic for neutrophils, macrophages. Superoxide production, endothelial cell adhesion, phagocytosis of neutrophils
Systemic	
IL-1	Haematopoiesis and acute phase protein synthesis Fever induction
IL-6	Haematopoiesis and acute phase protein synthesis Fever induction
TNF α/β	Fever induction Acute phase protein synthesis

Source: A. S. Hamlin. Cytokines in asthma. *Ann. NY Acad. Sci.* 629:250, 1991. Reprinted with permission.

elastase-positive neutrophils, or Leu-M3⁺ cells in the airways in asthma patients compared to controls. Conversely, at both proximal and subsegmental biopsy sites, significantly more IL-2R-positive (CD25⁺) cells and "activated" (EG2⁺) eosinophils were present in the airways of patients with asthma. There were positive correlations between numbers of T-lymphocytes, activated (CD25⁺) cells, eosinophils, CD3 and EG2, CD3 and CD25, and CD25 and EG2⁺ in the airways of asthmatic patients. Furthermore, the ratio of EG2⁺ to CD45⁺ cells correlated with the bronchial hyperresponsiveness as measured by the provocative concentration of methacholine that caused a 20 percent decrease of 1-second forced expiratory volume (FEV_1). This supports the view that activated (CD25⁺) T-lymphocytes release products that regulate recruitment of eosinophils into the airway wall and that the eosinophils may be responsible for airway mucosal damage, particularly shedding of epithelial cells, which are believed to be a factor in precipitating bronchial hyperreactivity [38, 43]. These considerations are in harmony with findings indicating that asthmatic bronchial mucosal biopsy specimens contain T-cells expressing mRNA for IL-5 and their numbers correlate with those of CD25⁺ cells and the number of eosinophils in the biopsy specimens [47]. Thus, these and other studies were interpreted to mean that the prominent eosinophilic infiltration in atopic asthma and the eosinophil-mediated damage result in bronchial hyperresponsiveness. It was further proposed that eosinophil accumulation is under the control of T-lymphocytes or mast cell products, or both, and that neutrophils and macrophages further amplify mucosal inflammation through release of their own mediators.

The T-lymphocytes as the Effector Cells of the Delayed-type Hypersensitivity (DTH) Reaction in the Genesis of Airway Hyperreactivity

In the early 1980s, a murine model of pulmonary DTH was established through immunization with picryl chloride (PCL) [24] and revealed a peribronchial and perivascular mononuclear cell infil-

trate as well as an increase in mucus-producing cells. This pulmonary DTH was shown to be antigen specific, T-cell and serotonin dependent, and associated with increased vascular permeability. Subsequent analysis of this model showed that mice with PCL-induced pulmonary DTH developed T-cell–dependent, antigen-specific airway hyperreactivity, as determined by the measurement of pulmonary resistance in vivo and of tracheal reactivity to carbachol in vitro [40]. It is not known whether the inflammation found in late-phase bronchial reactions represents a T-cell–mediated DTH response or whether some immediate hypersensitivity reactions might be triggered by non-IgE, antigen-specific factors analogous to the PCL factor (PCL-F) identified in cutaneous DTH in mice. Nor is it clear whether the phenotypic subtypes of T-cells in murine pulmonary or cutaneous DTH are the same as those involved in manifestations discussed in the preceding sections. What is clear, however, is that all the available data taken together support a central role of T-lymphocytes in the pathogenesis of asthma and in the development of bronchial hyperresponsiveness.

Bronchial Hyperresponsiveness and Lymphokines

The foregoing considerations resulted in a perception that asthma (both extrinsic and intrinsic), bronchial inflammation, bronchial hyperresponsiveness, and the bronchial influx of lymphocytes are interrelated, in fact inseparable, features in the genesis of asthma. These views, however, could not account for the following observations: (1) Profound inflammation of the airways is present without airway hyperresponsiveness [35, 78]; (2) prevention of airway inflammation does not block the development of airway hyperresponsiveness [13, 73, 141]; (3) bronchial hyperresponsiveness is not a common feature of other inflammatory conditions (i.e., sarcoidosis) that are characterized by lymphocyte infiltration of the lungs [84]; (4) the quantitatively increased and qualitatively altered end-organ sensitivity to a broad range of specific as well as nonspecific stimuli is not restricted to asthma but is also present in allergic rhinitis and atopic dermatitis [98]; (5) airways hyperresponsive to methacholine challenge represent a frequent finding in patients with atopic dermatitis without airway inflammation or symptomatic asthma [4]; (6) there is evidence that bronchial hyperresponsiveness usually precedes the development of asthma [49]; (7) bronchial hyperresponsiveness correlates with the production of T-lymphocyte products and not directly with IgE antibody synthesis [144]; and (8) there is evidence in twins that bronchial hyperresponsiveness, total serum IgE, and skin test scores are separately controlled by genetic factors [48, 79].

Although additional investigations are needed to clarify further the profile and kinetics of appearance of lymphocytes in bronchial biopsy specimens and/or in the bronchial lavage fluid of patients with asthma, some important generalizations can already be made at this time. Thus, we know that these lymphocytes are "activated," thereby supporting a functional role for lymphocytes, or more specifically for their lymphokines, in airway walls and in lung lining fluid, in the pathogenesis of airway hyperreactivity associated with asthma. The "activated state" of these lymphocytes and their lymphokines must reflect a specifically altered functional capacity that is directly related to the developmental mechanism of bronchial hyperresponsiveness. This altered functional capacity of these lymphocytes and the role of their lymphokines in nonspecific bronchial hyperresponsiveness are further supported by a series of observations, some of which have been already mentioned but require some further consideration. One of these is the lymphokine HRF that lymphocytes from patients with intrinsic and extrinsic asthma spontaneously produce and release even under in vitro conditions. HRF releases histamine from basophils and mast cells together with leukotriene C_4 and its production can be further enhanced by preincubating lymphocytes from patients with extrinsic asthma or intrinsic asthma, with skin test–positive allergens or antigenic bacterial antigens, respectively. Furthermore, the magnitude of its spontaneous production by lymphocytes in vitro correlates with bronchial hyperresponsiveness in asthma of both varieties [1–3, 12]. The roles of two other lymphokines, IL-4 and IL-5, have already been adequately reviewed in preceding sections. In many viral respiratory infections precipitating asthma there is an increased IFN-γ production by lymphocytes [25], which in turn releases PAF that is known to be involved in bronchial hyperresponsiveness. It has also been shown that IFN-γ activation of alveolar macrophages leads to the release of more thromboxane B_2, prostaglandin $F_{2\alpha}$, and leukotriene B_4, which have the capacity to induce bronchial hyperresponsiveness [76, 142]. As mentioned earlier, lymphocytes from asthmatic patients are capable of spontaneously producing an IgE-binding factor that increases IgE synthesis by B-cells and enhances antigen-induced histamine release [150]. Finally, when challenged with antigen, the lymphocytes from patients with asthma produce more IL-2 than those from the controls, and viral respiratory infections in asthmatic patients can further enhance IL-2 production after exposure to the antigen [143]. The role of the lymphokines in the developmental mechanism of bronchial hyperresponsiveness and in relation to the constitutional basis of asthma is further discussed below from the perspective of the lymphocyte as a neuroendocrine cell.

Emergence of the Lymphocyte as a Neuroendocrine Cell and Its Significance for Asthma

As pointed out in preceding sections, the entire concept of the nature and role of the lymphocyte in immunology, immunologic inflammation, and allergy has so radically changed in the past 10 years that it requires the listing again of the effector molecules that must be expected to play a regulatory influence in both health and disease (primarily asthma) of the human airways. These include interleukins; interferons; tumor necrosis factors; nucleotide metabolites; various neuroactive immunoregulatory peptides including hypothalamic CRF-like activity, ACTH, TSH, growth hormone, prolactin, chorionic gonadotropin, bombesin, endorphins, enkephalins, neurotensin, and VIP; and tachykinin neuropeptides including substance P, substance K, neuromedin K, SOMs, mast cell growth factor, suppressin, and so on. In the past 4 years an additional group of lymphocytic proteins with highly potent adrenergic regulatory activities was also discovered. This vast array of effector molecules makes the lymphocyte a veritable, mobile, neuroendocrine and/or neurosecretory cell with a range of activities that are bound to have a dominant regulatory participation in both the pathogenesis as well as the constitutional basis of asthma. Although the recently discovered adrenergically active lymphocytic proteins were briefly described in Chapter 14, it is necessary to continue to discuss some important aspects and activities of these substances.

Three macromolecular fractions with adrenergic activity can be identified in lymphocyte-conditioned medium by diethylaminoethanol (DEAE) ion-exchange high-performance liquid chromatography (HPLC), immunoneutralization, molecular mass, sequence analysis, and biologic characterizations. One of these fractions contains a secretory variant of beta-arrestin and an IL-1α antagonist, both of which downregulate beta$_2$-adrenergic receptors in A549 human lung epithelial cells. The two other fractions represent protein components that upregulate beta$_2$-adrenergic receptors. One of these contains a mixture of IL-1α and IL-1β, whereas the adrenergically active component of the remaining fraction is currently being characterized (Fig. 33-1A through E). The first question that may be asked in the context

of this chapter is whether the adrenergically highly active IL-1α obtained from the corresponding macromolecular fraction of lymphocyte-conditioned medium has a specific receptor on airway cells. Recent studies designed to explore this question used human bronchial epithelial cells isolated and cultured from the normal bronchi of patients undergoing surgery (for standard clinical reasons) essentially as described by Mattoli and coauthors [64]. Using this method, 99 percent of the final cell population contains epithelial cells. The latter were then incubated with IL-1α radiolabeled by a modified chloramine-T method. In addition to binding of specific, single-class IL-1α receptors, the latter were also identified by internalization of the receptor, affinity cross-linking, and sodium dodecyl sulfate–polyacrylamide gel electrophoresis (SDS-PAGE). Using unlabeled IL-1α and [^{3}H]dihydroalprenolol for measuring beta-adrenergic mRNA with the guanidium thiocyanate method, the IL-1α-induced accumulation of beta$_2$-adrenoceptor mRNA is demonstrable within 2 hours and an increase in beta-adrenoceptor concentration within 4 hours. In other words, concentrated Il-1α derived from human T-lymphocytes binds to a specific, single-class surface receptor on human bronchial epithelial cells and induces the production of beta$_2$-adrenoceptor mRNA via an associated or separate receptor-linked signaling pathway leading to an increase in epithelial beta$_2$-adrenoceptor concentration [83].

Subsequently, it was shown that lymphocytic IL-1α is a cell- and species-specific factor in increasing beta-adrenoceptor concentration and induction of its gene. In this study [103], we used A549 human lung epithelial cells, the A431 human epidermoid cells, the DDT$_1$MF$_2$ hamster smooth muscle cells, cultured human bronchial epithelial cells and smooth muscle cells, and cultured canine tracheal epithelial and tracheal smooth muscle cells. Concentrated human lymphocytic IL-1α was then cocultured with these various cell populations for 24 hours and beta$_2$-adrenoceptors measured radioactively. The originally shown synergistic beta-adrenoceptor upregulation between IL-1α and cortisol [95] was present in the A549 and A431 cells, as well as the human bronchial epithelial cells. Northern blot hybridization showed that levels of beta$_2$-adrenoceptors and beta$_2$-adrenoceptor mRNAs increased significantly by both IL-1α and cortisol, whereas Gsα, Gi2α, Gi3α mRNA levels remained unchanged. In all these situations, the increase in beta$_2$-adrenoceptor mRNAs always preceded the enhanced expression of the receptor. When DDT$_1$MF$_2$ cells and human and canine tracheal smooth muscle cells were used, IL-1α had no effect either on beta$_2$-adrenoceptors or beta$_2$-adrenoceptor mRNAs, whereas cortisol remained active [103]. This extraordinary degree of cell and species specificity of the beta$_2$-adrenoceptor upregulating effect of lymphocytic IL-1α makes these observations highly important both for normal airway physiology as well as for the possible nature of the beta-adrenergic dysregulation in asthma. Thus, it raises the possibility that the primary beta-adrenergic abnormality is restricted to cells that are derived from the neural crest (i.e., bronchial epithelial cells) and that *sui generis* atopic asthma occurs only in humans.

THE FUTURE

The immune-neuroendocrine circuitry represents an immensely complex, powerful, and wide-ranging charter of human physiologic and pathologic possibilities, which among others is working its way to the creation of a new kind of immunology based on a vastly enlarged vision of immunologic potential in health and disease. The emergence of this new interdisciplinary field will require a critical reexamination of some of our basic current views on the pathophysiologic and immunopharmacologic realities surrounding the problems of human asthma.

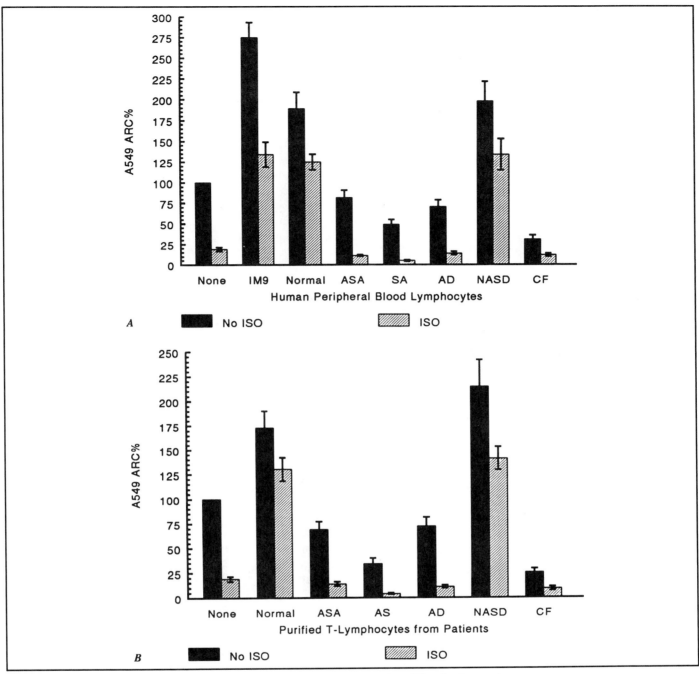

Fig. 33-1A and 33-1B. *Effect of lymphocyte-conditioned medium (LCM) derived from IM9 cells of normal human peripheral blood lymphocytes (HPBLs), HPBLs of patients with asthma (asymptomatic [ASA], symptomatic [SA]), HPBLs of patients with atopic dermatitis (AD), HPBLs of patients with nonatopic skin diseases (NASD), and HPBLs of patients with cystic fibrosis (CF) on beta-adrenoceptor concentrations (ARC) of cultured A549 cells. Notes: A549 cells were incubated with the test substance for 24 hours. 100% represents 202 ± 18 receptors/A549 cell (1.82 ± 0.22 fmol/mg of protein). Values are expressed as percent of the beta-adrenoceptor concentrations in untreated controls when cultured alone. For normal HPBLs, equieffective amounts of LCM of IM9 cells were used. There were five male subjects in each group (normal or diseased) except for the group with cystic fibrosis, where there were only four male subjects. NASDs consist of bullous pemphigoid, dermatitis herpetiformis, psoriasis, contact dermatitis, and seborrheic dermatitis. Isoproterenol (ISO) pretreatment of A549 cells was done to approximate the pathopharmacologic realities of asthma [135]. Effect of LCM derived from purified normal human T-lymphocytes (PTLs), PTLs of patients with asthma (asymptomatic [ASA], symptomatic [SA]), PTLs of patients with atopic dermatitis (AD), PTLs of patients with nonatopic skin disease (NASD), and PTLs of patients with cystic fibrosis (CF) on beta-adrenoceptor concentrations (ARC) of cultured A549 cells. See "Notes" in A. For normal PTLs, equieffective amounts of LCM of IM9 cells were used. There were five male subjects in each group (normal or diseased) except for the group with cystic fibrosis, where there were only four male subjects. NASDs consist of bullous pemphigoid, dermatitis herpetiformis, psoriasis, contact dermatitis, and seborrheic dermatitis. Isoproterenol (ISO) pretreatment of A549 cells was done to approximate the pathopharmacologic realities of asthma [135].*

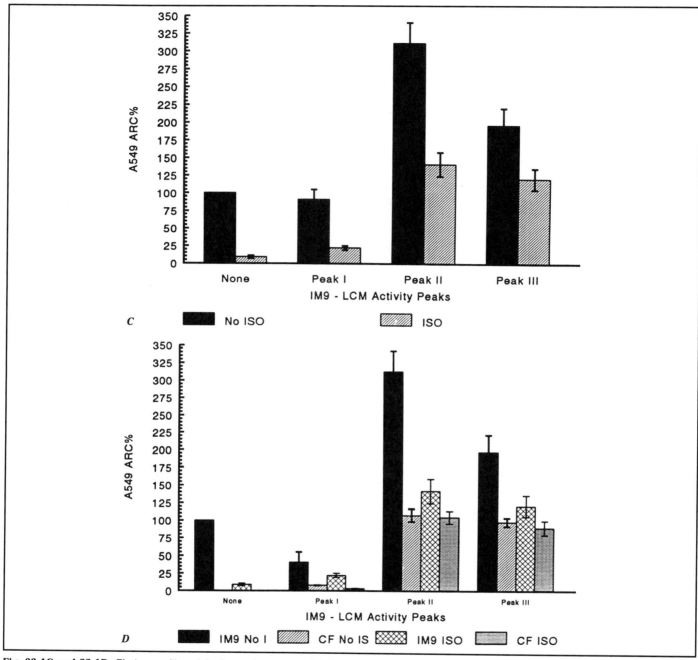

Fig. 33-1C and 33-1D. *Elution profiles of the beta-adrenoceptor* (ARC) *upregulating activity of the LCM of IM9 cells by diethylaminoethanol (DEAE) ion-exchange high-performance liquid chromatography (HPLC) using A549 cells in vitro as adrenergic effector cells. Notes: Activity peaks are distinguished by three criteria: (1) retention time on DEAE ion exchange column (time post-injection of LCM), (2) relative ability to increase beta-adrenoceptor density above that of untreated A549 cells when cultured alone, and (3) immunoneutralization of the A549 beta-adrenoceptor upregulating effect of LCM activity peaks by polyclonal or monoclonal antibodies to recombinant human cytokines. A549 cells were incubated with the test substance for 24 hours. 100% represents 283 ± 21 receptors/A549 cell (2.12 ± 0.26 fmol/mg of protein). Values are expressed as percent of the beta-adrenoceptor concentrations in the untreated controls when cultured alone. Isoproterenol (ISO) pretreatment of A549 cells was done to approximate the pathopharmacologic realities of asthma [123, 124]. No I, No IS = no isoproterenol pretreatment; CF = cystic fibrosis.*

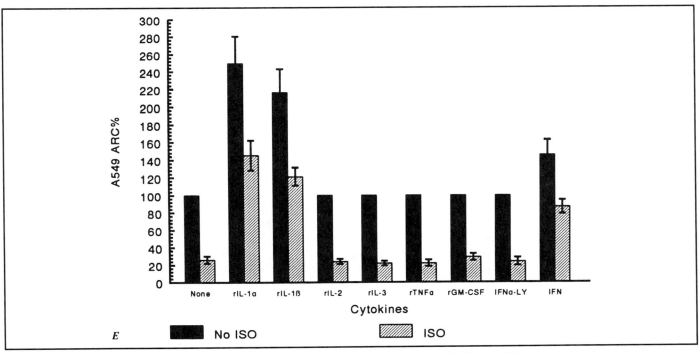

Fig. 33-1E. *Effects of cytokines on beta-adrenoceptor concentrations (ARC) of cultured A549 cells. Notes: A549 cells were incubated with the test substance for 24 hours. 100% represents 202 ± 18 receptors/A549 cell (1.82 ± 0.22 fmol/mg of protein). Values are expressed as percent of the beta-adrenoceptor concentrations in the untreated controls when cultured alone [82]. Isoproterenol (ISO) pretreatment of A549 cells was done to approximate the pathopharmacologic realities of asthma. rIL = recombinant interleukin; rTNFα = recombinant tumor necrosis factor-alpha; rGM-CSF = recombinant granulocyte-macrophage colony-stimulating factor; IFN = interferon.*

REFERENCES

1. Alam, R., Grant, J. A., and Lett-Brown, M. A. Identification of a histamine release inhibitory factor produced by human mononuclear cells in vitro. *J. Clin. Invest.* 82:2056, 1988.
2. Alam, R., and Rozniecki, J. A mononuclear cell-derived histamine-releasing factor (HRF) in asthmatic patients. II. Activity in vivo. *Allergy* 40:124, 1985.
3. Alam, R., Rozniecki, J., and Selmaj, K. A mononuclear cell-derived histamine-releasing factor (HRF) in asthmatic patients. I. Histamine release from basophils in vitro. *Ann. Allergy* 53:66, 1984.
4. Barker, A. F., et al. Airway responsiveness in atopic dermatitis. *J. Allergy Clin. Immunol.* 87:780, 1991.
5. Bekkers, J. M., and Stevens, C. F. Presynaptic mechanism for long-term potentiation in the hippocampus. *Nature* 346:724, 1990.
6. Benveniste, E. N., and Merrill, J. E. Stimulation of oligodendroglial proliferation and maturation by interleukin-2. *Nature* 321:610, 1986.
7. Berkenbosch, F., et al. Corticotropin-releasing factor producing neurons in the rat activated by interleukin-1. *Science* 238:524, 1987.
8. Bernton, E. W., et al. Release of multiple hormones by direct action of interleukin-1 on pituitary cells. *Science* 238:519, 1987.
9. Besedovsky, H. O., et al. Hypothalamic changes during the immune response. *Eur. J. Immunol.* 7:325, 1977.
10. Birnbaumer, L., and Brown, A. M. G proteins and the mechanism of action of hormones, neurotransmitters, and autocrine and paracrine regulatory factors. *Am. Rev. Respir. Dis.* 141:S106, 1990.
11. Bradley, B. L., et al. Eosinophils, T-lymphocytes, mast cells, neutrophils, and macrophages in bronchial biopsy specimens from atopic subjects with asthma: Comparison with biopsy specimens from atopic subjects without asthma and normal control subjects and relationship to bronchial hyperresponsiveness. *J. Allergy Clin. Immunol.* 88:661, 1991.
12. Chonmaitree, T., Lett-Brown, M. A., and Grant, J. A. Respiratory viruses induce production of histamine-releasing factor by mononuclear leukocytes: A possible role in the mechanism of virus-induced asthma. *J. Infect. Dis.* 164:592, 1991.
13. Cibulas, W., et al. Toluene diisocyanate-induced airway hyperreactivity in guinea pigs depleted of granulocytes. *J. Appl. Physiol.* 64:1773, 1988.
14. Cornell, R. P. Central interleukin-1 elicited hyperinsulinemia is mediated by prostaglandin but not autonomics. *Am. J. Physiol.* 257:R839, 1989.
15. Cotzias, G. C., and Tang, L. C. Adenylate cyclase of brain reflects propensity for breast cancer in mice. *Science* 197:1094, 1977.
16. Crump, J. W., Pueringer, R. J., and Hunninghake, G. W. Bronchoalveolar lavage and lymphocytes in asthma. *Eur. Respir. J.* 4(Suppl. 13):39s, 1991.
17. Cunningham, B. A., et al. Neural cell adhesion molecule: Structure, immunoglobulin-like domains, cell surface modulation, and alternative RNA splicing. *Science* 236:799, 1987.
18. Delespesse, G., Sarfati, M., and Peleman, R. Influence of recombinant IL-4, IFN-α and IFN-γ on the production of human IgE binding factor (soluble CD23). *J. Immunol.* 142:134, 1989.
19. Del Rey, A., and Besedovsky, H. Antidiabetic effects of interleukin-1. *Proc. Natl. Acad. Sci. USA* 86:5943, 1989.
20. Dougherty, P. M., and Dafny, N. Central opioid systems are differentially affected by products of the immune response. *Soc. Neurosci. Abstr.* 13:1437, 1987.
21. Dudai, Y. Neurogenetic dissection of learning and short-term memory in Drosophila. *Annu. Rev. Neurosci.* 11:537, 1988.
22. Dunn, A. J., et al. Effects of Newcastle disease virus administration to mice on the metabolism of cerebral biogenic amines, plasma corticosterone, and lymphocyte proliferation. *Brain Behav. Evol.* 1:216, 1987.
23. Edelman, G. M. *Neural Darwinism.* New York: Basic Book, 1987.
24. Enander, I., et al. Sensitizing ability of derivatives of picryl chloride after exposure of mice on the skin and in the lung. *Int. Arch. Allergy Appl. Immunol.* 72:59, 1983.
25. Ennis, F. A., et al. Interferon induction and increased natural killer cell activity—Influenza infections in man. *Lancet* 2:891, 1981.
26. Eremina, O. F., and Devoino, L. V. Production of humoral antibodies in rabbits following destruction of the nucleus of the midbrain raphe. *Bull. Exp. Biol. Med.* 74:258, 1973.
27. Farrar, W. L., et al. Visualization and characterization of interleukin-1 receptors in brain. *J. Immunol.* 139:459, 1987.

28. Filipp, G., and Szentivanyi, A. Frage der Organlokalisation der allergischen Reaktion. *Wien. Klin. Wochenschr.* 65:620, 1953.

29. Filipp, G., and Szentivanyi, A. Experimentelle Data zur regulativen Rolle des Neuroendokriniums in experimenteller Anaphylaxie. I. Relazioni e Communicazioni. *Rome II Pansiero Scientifico* 229:1, 1956.

30. Filipp, G., Szentivanyi, A., and Mess, B. Anaphylaxis and nervous system. *Acta Med. Hung.* 2:163, 1952.

31. Filipp, G., and Szentivanyi, A. Die Wirkung von Hypothalamuslasionen auf den anaphylaktischen Schock des Meerschweinchens. *Allergie Asthmaforsch. Bd.* 1:12, 1957.

32. Filipp, G., and Szentivanyi, A. Anaphylaxis and the nervous system. Part III. *Ann. Allergy* 16:306, 1958.

33. Filipp, G., and Szentivanyi, A. Anaphylaxis and the Nervous System. Part III. In S. Locke, et al. (eds.), *Foundations of Psychoneuroimmunology.* Hawthorne, NY: Aldine, 1985. Pp. 1–12.

34. Fillion, M. P., et al. Hypothetical Role of the Serotonergic System in Neuroimmunomodulation: Preliminary Molecular Studies. In J. W. Hadden, K. Masek, and G. Nistico (eds.), *Interactions Among Central Nervous System, Neuroendocrine and Immune Systems.* Rome: Pythagora, 1989. Pp. 235–250.

35. Folkerts, G., et al. Endotoxin-induced inflammation and injury of the guinea pig respiratory airways cause bronchial hyporeactivity. *Am. Rev. Respir. Dis.* 137:1441, 1988.

36. Frew, A. J., et al. T lymphocytes in allergen-induced late-phase reactions and asthma. *Int. Arch. Allergy Appl. Immunol.* 88:63, 1989.

37. Friedman, H., Klein, T. W., and Szentivanyi, A. (eds.), *Immunomodulation by Bacteria and Their Products.* New York: Plenum, 1981.

38. Frigas, S. E., Loegering, D. A., and Gleich, G. J. Cytotoxic effects of the guinea pig eosinophil major basic protein on tracheal epithelium. *Lab. Invest.* 43:35, 1980.

39. Fukuoka, M., et al. Interleukin-1 stimulates growth and inhibits progesterone secretion in cultures of porcine granulosa cells. *Endocrinology* 124:884, 1989.

40. Garssen, J., et al. T-cell mediated induction of airway hyperreactivity in mice. *Am. Rev. Respir. Dis.* 144:931, 1991.

41. Geschwind, N., and Galaburda, A. M. Cerebral lateralization: Biological mechanisms, associations, and pathology. Parts I–III. *Arch. Neurol.* 42:428, 1985.

42. Giulian, D., and Lachman, L. B. Interleukin-1 stimulation of astroglial proliferation after brain injury. *Science* 228:497, 1985.

43. Gleich, G. J., et al. Cytotoxic properties of the eosinophil major basic protein. *J. Immunol.* 123:2925, 1979.

44. Goodman, C. S., and Pearson, K. G. Neuronal development: Cellular approaches in invertebrates. *Neurosci. Res. Program Bull.* 20:777, 1982.

45. Hadcock, J. R., Port, J. D., and Malbon, C. C. Cross-regulation between G-protein mediated pathways. Activation of the inhibitory pathway of adenylyl/cyclase increases the expression of β₂-adrenergic receptors. *J. Biol. Chem.* 266:11915, 1991.

46. Hadden, J. W., and Szentivanyi, A. (eds.), *The Pharmacology of the Reticuloendothelial System.* New York: Plenum, 1985.

47. Hamid, Q. A., et al. Localization of beta₂-adrenoceptor messenger RNA in human and rat lung using in situ hybridization: Correlation with receptor autoradiography. *Eur. J. Pharmacol.* 206:133, 1991.

48. Hopp, R. J., et al. Specificity and sensitivity of methacholine inhalation challenge in normal and asthmatic children. *J. Allergy Clin. Immunol.* 74:154, 1984.

49. Hopp, R. J., et al. The presence of airway reactivity before the development of asthma. *Am. Rev. Respir. Dis.* 141:2, 1990.

50. Kay, A. B. Leucocytes in asthma. *Immunol. Invest.* 17:679, 1988.

51. Kay, A. B. T-lymphocytes and their products in atopic allergy and asthma. *Int. Arch. Allergy Appl. Immunol.* 94:189, 1991.

52. Kehrer, P., et al. Human recombinant interleukin-1β and -α, but not recombinant tumor necrosis factor-α stimulate ACTH release from rat anterior pituitary cells in vitro in a prostaglandin E₂ and cAMP independent manner. *Neuroendocrinology* 48:160, 1988.

53. Klein, T. W., et al. (eds.), *Biological Response Modifiers in Human Oncology and Immunology.* New York: Plenum, 1983.

54. Korneva, E. A., and Klimenko, V. M. Neuronale hypothalamusaktivitt und homoostat-ische rektionen. *Ergeb. Exp. Med.* 23:373, 1976.

55. Krueger, J. M., et al. Endogenous Slow-wave Sleep Substances: A Review. In C. Dugsovic and A. Wauquier (eds.), *Current Trends in Slow-wave Sleep Research.* New York: Raven, 1988.

56. Krueger, J. M., et al. Immune Response Modifiers and Sleep. In J. W. Hadden, K. Masek, and G. Nistico (eds.), *Interactions Among Central Nervous System, Neuroendocrine and Immune Systems.* Rome: Pythagora, 1989. Pp. 323–350.

57. LeDouarin, N. *The Neural Crest.* Cambridge, England: Cambridge University Press, 1982.

58. Lee, F., et al. Isolation and characterization of a mouse interleukin cDNA clone that expresses B cell stimulatory factor-1 activities and T-cell and mast cell-stimulating activities. *Proc. Natl. Acad. Sci. USA* 83:2061, 1986.

59. Leung, D. Y. M., and Geha, R. S. Regulation of the human IgE antibody response. *Int. Rev. Immunol.* 2:75, 1987.

60. Lochrie, M. A., and Simon, M. I. G protein multiplicity in eukaryotic signal transduction systems. *Biochemistry* 17:4957, 1988.

61. Lopez, A. G., et al. Recombinant human interleukin 5 is a selective activator of human eosinophil function. *J. Exp. Med.* 167:219, 1988.

62. Malinow, R., and Tsien, R. W. Presynaptic enhancement shown by whole-cell recordings of long-term potentiation in hippocampal slices. *Nature* 346:177, 1990.

63. Masek, K., et al. The Interactions Between Neuroendocrine and Immune Systems at the Receptor Level. The Possible Role of Serotonergic System. In J. W. Hadden, K. Masek, and G. Nistico (eds.), *Interactions Among Central Nervous System, Neuroendocrine and Immune Systems.* Rome: Pythagora, 1989. Pp. 225–234.

64. Mattoli, S., et al. Bronchial epithelial cells exposed to isocyanates potentiate activation and proliferation of T cells. *Am. J. Physiol.* 259:L320, 1990.

65. McFadden, P. N., and Koshland, D. E., Jr. Habituation in the single cell: Diminished secretion of norepinephrine with repetitive depolarization in PC12 cells. *Proc. Natl. Acad. Sci. USA* 87:2031, 1990.

66. McFadden, P. N., and Koshland, D. E., Jr. Parallel pathways for habituation in repetitively stimulated P12 cells. *Neuron* 4:615, 1990.

67. Mealy, K., et al. Hypothalamic-pituitary-adrenal (HPA) axis regulation by tumor necrosis factor. *Prog. Leukoc. Biol.* 10B:225, 1990.

68. Milner, R. J., et al. Expression of Immunoglobulin-like proteins in the Nervous System: Properties of the Neural Protein 1B236/MAG. In E. J. Goetzl and N. H. Spector (eds.), *Neuroimmune Networks: Physiology and Diseases.* New York: Alan R. Liss, 1989. Pp. 9–15.

69. Miyajima, A., Miyatake, S., and Schreurs, J. Coordinate regulation of immune and inflammatory responses by T-cell-derived lymphokines. *FASEB J.* 2:2462, 1988.

70. Morimoto, B. H., and Koshland, D. E., Jr. Excitatory amino acid uptake and N-methyl-D-aspartate-mediated secretion in a neural cell line. *Proc. Natl. Acad. Sci. USA* 87:3518, 1990.

71. Morimoto, B. H., and Koshland, D. E., Jr. Induction and expression of long- and short-term neurosecretory potentiation in a neural cell line. *Neuron* 5:875, 1990.

72. Morris, G. M., Hadcock, J. R., and Malbon, C. C. Cross-regulation between G-protein-coupled receptors. Activation of β₂-adrenergic receptors increases α₁-adrenergic receptor mRNA levels. *J. Biol. Chem.* 266:2233, 1991.

73. Murlas, C., and Roum, J. H. Bronchial hyperactivity occurs in steroid-treated guinea pigs depleted of leukocytes by cyclophosphamide. *J. Appl. Physiol.* 58:1630, 1985.

74. Naitoh, Y., et al. Interleukin-6 stimulates the secretion of adrenocorticotropic hormone in conscious, freely-moving rats. *Biochem. Biophys. Res. Commun.* 155:1459, 1988.

75. Nijkamp, F. P., and Henricks, P. A. J. Beta-adrenoceptors in lung inflammation. *Am. Rev. Respir. Dis.* 141:145s, 1990.

76. O'Sullivan, M. G., et al. Modulation of arachidonic acid metabolism by bovine alveolar macrophages exposed to interferons. *J. Leukoc. Biol.* 44:116, 1988.

77. Owen, W. F., Rothenberg, M. E., and Silberstein, D. S. Regulation of human eosinophil viability, density, and function by granulocyte/macrophage colony-stimulating factor in the presence of 3T3 fibroblasts. *J. Exp. Med.* 166:129, 1987.

78. Pauwels, R., Peleman, R., and Van Der Straeten, M. Airway inflammation and non-allergic bronchial responsiveness. *Eur. J. Respir. Dis.* 68:137, 1986.

79. Pauwels, R. A. Genetic factors controlling airway responsiveness. *Clin. Rev. Allergy* 7:235, 1989.

80. Renoux, G., et al. Consequences of bilateral brain neocortical ablation on imuthiol-induced immunostimulation in mice. *Ann. NY Acad. Sci.* 496:346, 1987.

81. Rettori, V., Jurcovicova, J., and McCann, S. M. Central action of interleukin-1 in altering the release of TSH, growth hormone and prolactin in the male rat. *J. Neurosci. Res.* 18:179, 1987.

82. Robicsek, S., et al. Characterization of the A549 β-adrenoceptor regulat-

ing protein components of lymphocyte conditioned medium of IM9 cells. *J. Allergy Clin. Immunol.* 87:307, 1991.

83. Robicsek, S., et al. Concentrated IL-1α derived from human T-lymphocytes binds to a specific single class surface receptor on human bronchial epithelial cells and induces the production of beta-adrenoceptor mRNA via an associated or separate receptor-linked signalling pathway. *J. Allergy Clin. Immunol.* 89:212, 1992.

84. Rochester, C. L., and Rankin, J. A. Is asthma T-cell mediated? *Am. Rev. Respir. Dis.* 144:1005, 1991.

85. Rothenberg, M. E., et al. Human eosinophils have prolonged survival, enhanced functional properties, and become hypodense when exposed to human interleukin-3. *J. Clin. Invest.* 81:1986, 1988.

86. Sapolsky, R., et al. Corticotropin-releasing factor-producing neurons in the rat activated by interleukin-1. *Science* 238:522, 1987.

87. Scarborough, D. E., et al. Interleukin-1β stimulates somatostatin biosynthesis in primary cultures of fetal rat brain. *Endocrinology* 124:549, 1989.

88. Schechter, G. A good relationship: Sensitive, synchronized and synergistic. *Prog. Neuro-endocr. Immunol.* 2:35, 1989.

89. Schwartz, M. E., et al. Further Observations on the Cellular and Molecular Mechanisms Involved in the Reciprocal Histamine-catecholamine Counterregulatory Interplay in Relation to Induction of Histidine Decarboxylase Synthesis by Interleukin-3 and Granulocyte-macrophage Colony Stimulating Factor. In *Proceedings of XIII International Congress of Allergology and Clinical Immunology.* Montreux, Switzerland, 1988. Abstract 64. St. Louis, Mo.: Mosby-Year Book.

90. Sherry, B., and Cerami, A. Cachectin/tumor necrosis factor exerts endocrine, paracrine, and autocrine control of inflammatory responses. *J. Cell Biol.* 107:1269, 1988.

91. Smith, L. R., Brown, S. L., and Blalock, J. E. Interleukin-2 induction of ACTH secretion: Presence of an interleukin-2 receptor α-chain-like molecule on pituitary cells. *J. Neuroimmunol.* 21:249, 1989.

92. Spangelo, B. L., et al. Thymosin fraction 5 stimulates prolactin and growth hormone release from anterior pituitary cells in vitro. *Endocrinology* 121:2035, 1987.

93. Srebro, Z., Spisak-Plonka, I., and Szirmai, E. Neurosecretion in mice during skin allograft rejection. *Agressologie* 15:125, 1974.

94. Sternberg, E. M. Monokines, Lymphokines and the Brain. In J. M. Cruse and J. E. Lewis (eds.), *The Year in Immunology,* Vol. 5. Basel: Karger, 1989. Pp. 205–217.

95. Szentendrei, T., et al. Regulation of beta-adrenergic receptor gene expression by interleukin-1. *The Pharmacologist* 33:225, 1991.

96. Szentivanyi, A. Allergie und Zentralnervensystem. *Acta Allergol.* 6:27, 1953.

97. Szentivanyi, A. Hypothalamic Influences on Antibody Formation and on Bronchial Responses to Histamine. In *Proceedings of the Fourth Aspen Conference on Research in Emphysema and Asthma.* Aspen, Colorado, 1961. P. 78.

98. Szentivanyi, A. The beta-adrenergic theory of the atopic abnormality in bronchial asthma. *J. Allergy* 42:203, 1968.

99. Szentivanyi, A. The Discovery of Immune-neuroendocrine Circuits and the Concepts of Prevailing Immunologic Thought That Impeded the Timely Recognition of Their Role in Immune-homeostasis. In *Proceedings of the International Symposium on Interactions Between the Neuroendocrine and Immune Systems.* Montepaone Lido, Italy, 1988. Rome: Pythagora. Pp. 23–24.

100. Szentivanyi, A. Plenary Lecture: Natural Neuropeptides in the Immunologic Inflammation of the Airways in Asthma. In *Proceedings of XIV World Congress of Natural Medicines.* Malaga, Spain. 1988. Madrid: Editorial Garsi. P. 1.

101. Szentivanyi, A. The Discovery of Immune-neuroendocrine Circuits in the Fall of 1951. In J. W. Hadden, G. Nistico, and K. Masek (eds.), *Interactions Among the Central Nervous System, Neuroendocrine and Immune Systems.* Rome, Italy: Pythagora, 1989. Pp. 1–5.

102. Szentivanyi, A. Beta-adrenergic subsensivity in asthma and atopic dermatitis: A status report. *Acta Biomed. Hung. Amer.* 1:1, 1991.

103. Szentivanyi, A., et al. Cell- and species-specific dissociation in the beta-adrenoceptor upregulating effects of IL-1α derived from lymphocyte conditioned medium and cortisol. *J. Allergy Clin. Immunol.* 89:274, 1992.

104. Szentivanyi, A., and Filipp, G. Experimentelle Data zur regulativen Rolle des Neuroendokriniums in experimenteller Anaphylaxic. II. Relazionie e Communicazioni. *Rome Il Pansiero Scientifico* 237:1, 1956.

105. Szentivanyi, A., Filipp, G., and Legeza, I. Investigations on tobacco sensitivity. *Acta Med. Hung.* 2:175, 1952.

106. Szentivanyi, A., and Filipp, G. Anaphylaxis and the nervous system. Part II. *Ann. Allergy* 16:143, 1958.

107. Szentivanyi, A., and Filipp, G. *Propriètès Immuno-Chimiques et Physico-Chimiques des Anticorps.* Paris: Editions Mèdicales Flammarion, 1962.

108. Szentivanyi, A., and Fishel, C. W. Effect of Bacterial Products on Responses to the Allergic Mediators. In M. Samter (ed.), *Immunological Diseases.* Boston: Little, Brown, 1965. Pp. 226–241.

109. Szentivanyi, A., and Fishel, C. W. Die Amin-Mediatorstoffe der allergischen Reaktion und die Reaktionsfahiegheit ihrer Erfolgeszellen. In G. Filipp and A. Szentivanyi (eds.), *Pathogenese und Therapie allergischer Reaktionen. Grundlagenforschung und Klinik.* Stuttgart, Germany: Ferdinand Enke, 1966. Pp. 588–683.

110. Szentivanyi, A., and Fitzpatrick, D. F. The Altered Reactivity of the Effector Cells to Antigenic and Pharmacological Influences and Its Relation to Cyclic Nucleotides. II. Effector Reactivities in the Efferent Loop of the Immune Response. In G. Filipp (ed.), *Pathomechanismus und Pathogenese allergischer Reaktionen.* Munich: Werk-Verlag Dr. Edmund Banachewski, 1980. Pp. 511–580.

111. Szentivanyi, A., et al. Hypothalamic and Other Central Influences on Antibiosis and Host Immunity. In *Proceedings of the Fourth International Conference on Immunopharmacology.* Osaka, Japan, 1988. Abstract 5101. Oxford: Pergamon.

112. Szentivanyi, A., Krzanowski, J. J., and Polson, J. B. The Autonomic Nervous System: Structure, Function, and Altered Effector Responses. In E. Middleton, C. E. Reed, and E. F. Ellis (eds.), *Allergy: Principles and Practice.* St. Louis: CV Mosby, 1978. Pp. 256–300.

113. Szentivanyi, A., Krzanowski, J. J., and Polson, J. B. The Autonomic Nervous System and Altered Effector Responses. In E. Middleton, C. E. Reed, and E. F. Ellis (eds.), *Allergy: Principles and Practice* (3rd ed.). St. Louis: CV Mosby, 1988. Pp. 461–493.

114. Szentivanyi, A., et al. The pharmacology of microbial modulation in the induction and expression of immune reactivities. I. The pharmacologically active effector molecules of immunologic inflammation, immunity, and hypersensitivity. *Immunopharmacol. Rev.* 1:159, 1990.

115. Szentivanyi, A., Maurer, P., and Janicki, B. W. (eds.), *Antibodies: Structure, Synthesis, Function, and Immunologic Intervention in Disease.* New York: Plenum, 1987.

116. Szentivanyi, A., et al. Effect of Microbial Agents on the Immune Network and Associated Pharmacologic Reactivities. In E. Middleton, C. E. Reed, and E. F. Ellis (eds.), *Allergy: Principles and Practice.* St. Louis: CV Mosby, 1983. Pp. 211–236.

117. Szentivanyi, A., Polson, J. B., and Krzanowski, J. J. The Altered Reactivity of the Effector Cells to Antigenic and Pharmacological Influences and Its Relation to Cyclic Nucleotides. I. Effector Reactivities in the Efferent Loop of the Immune Response. In G. Filipp (ed.), *Pathomechanismus und Pathogenese allergischer Reaktionen.* Munich: Werk-Verlag Dr. Edmund Banachewski, 1980. Pp. 460–510.

118. Szentivanyi, A., et al. The Influence of Anterior Hypothalamic Lesions on the Kinetic Parameters of ^{125}I-VIP (Vasoactive Intestinal Peptide) Binding to Murine Mononuclear Cells. In *Proceedings of Workshop 12 on Mediators in Asthma, XII World Congress of Asthmology.* Barcelona, Spain, 1987. Madrid: Editorial Garsi. P. 41.

119. Szentivanyi, A., et al. Some Biochemical and Cellular Features of Adrenergic Mechanisms Induced by Bacterial Lipopolysaccharide Endotoxin in Rats With or Without Chemical Sympathetic Ablation Achieved by 6-Hydroxydopamine Hydrobromide (6-OHDA). In *Proceedings of International Symposium on Endotoxin.* Tochigi, Japan, 1988. Abstract SV-8. Tochigi: Jichi Medical School Press.

120. Szentivanyi, A., et al. The Effect of 6-Hydroxydopamine Hydrobromide on Endotoxin-induced Adrenergic Mechanisms. In *Proceedings of Second International Meeting on Respiratory Allergy.* Sorrento, Italy, 1988. Abstract 311. Rome: Pythagora.

121. Szentivanyi, A., et al. The effect of sympathetic ablation [6-hydroxydopamine hydrobromide (6-OHDA); axotomy] on endotoxin induced adrenergic mechanisms. *The Pharmacologist* 31:118, 1989.

122. Szentivanyi, A., et al. Restoration of normal beta adrenoceptor concentrations in A549 lung adenocarcinoma cells by leukocyte protein factors and recombinant interleukin-1α. *Cytokine* 1:118, 1989.

123. Szentivanyi, A., et al. The nature of the adrenergically active constituents of lymphocyte conditioned medium (LCM) of IM9 cells. *Int. J. Immunopharmacol.* 13:70, 1991.

124. Szentivanyi, A., et al. The elution profile of the A549 beta-adrenergic (βAR) regulating activity of lymphocyte conditioned medium (LCM) of IM9 cells developed by DEAE ion exchange HPLC. *Int. J. Immunopharmacol.* 13:68, 1991.

125. Szentivanyi, A., and Szekely, J. Effect of injury to, and electrical stimula-

tion of hypothalamic areas on the anaphylactic and histamine shock of guinea pig. *Ann. Allergy* 14:259, 1956.

126. Szentivanyi, A., and Szekely, J. Uber den Effekt der Schadigung und der elektrischen Reizung der hypothalamischen Gegenden auf den anaphylaktischen und Histamin-Schock des Meerschweinchens. *Allergie Asthmaforsch. Bd.* 1:28, 1957.

127. Szentivanyi, A., and Szekely, J. Wirkung der konstanten Reizung hypothalamischer Strukturen durch Tiefenelektroden auf den histaminbedingten Schock des Meerschweinchens. *Acta Physiol. Hung.* 11(Suppl. V):41, 1957.

128. Szentivanyi, A., and Szekely, J. Anaphylaxis and the nervous system. Part IV. *Ann. Allergy* 16:389, 1958.

129. Szentivanyi, A., and Szentivanyi, J. Immunomodulatory Effects of Central and Peripheral Autonomic Mechanisms Mediated by Neuroeffector Molecules. In *Proceedings of International Symposium on Biological Response Modifiers in Clinical Oncology and Immunology.* Tampa, Fla., 1982. New York: Plenum. P. 8.

130. Szentivanyi, A., and Szentivanyi, J. The Emergence of Neuroendocrine Disorders as a New Group of Autoimmune Diseases. In *Proceedings of Symposium on Clinical Laboratory Immunology.* Clearwater, Fla., 1982. New York: Plenum. P. 3.

131. Szentivanyi, A., and Szentivanyi, J. Immune-neuroendocrine Circuits in Antibiotic-bacterial Interactions. In *Proceedings of Third International Symposium on the Influence of Antibiotics on the Host-Parasite Relationship.* Cologne, Germany, 1987. Abstract 40. Heidelberg: Springer-Verlag.

132. Szentivanyi, A., and Szentivanyi, J. Antibiotic-bacterial Interactions in Relation to Immune-neuroendocrine Circuits. In *Proceedings of XIII International Congress of Allergology and Clinical Immunology.* Montreux, Switzerland, 1988. Abstract 986. St. Louis, Mo.: Mosby-Year Book.

133. Szentivanyi, A., et al. Nonantibiotic properties of antibiotics in relationship to immune-neuroendocrine influences. *Clin. Pharmacol. Ther.* 43: 166, 1988.

134. Szentivanyi, A., et al. The pharmacology of microbial modulation in the induction and expression of immune reactivities. II. Effector mechanisms in the afferent and efferent limbs of the immune response. *Immunopharmacol. Rev.* In press.

135. Szentivanyi, J, et al. Similarities and differences in patterns of beta-adrenergic regulation by lymphocytic proteins in respiratory and cutaneous atopy versus cystic fibrosis. *J. Allergy Clin. Immunol.* 89:162, 1992.

136. Szentivanyi, J., et al. Hypothalamic and other central influences on antibiotic modulated bacterial immunogenicity. *The Pharmacologist* 31:193, 1989.

137. Szentivanyi, J., et al. The effect of hypothalamic and extrahypothalamic nuclear groupings on the antibiotic modulated bacterial immunogenicity and production of IL-1, IFN and TNF. *Cytokine* 1:364, 1989.

138. Szentivanyi, J., et al. Changes in the Immune Parameters of Antibiotic-bacterial Interactions Induced by Hypothalamic and Other Electrolytic Brain Lesions Produced Through Stereotaxically Implanted Depth Electrodes. In G. Gillissen, et al. (eds.), *The Influence of Antibiotics on the Host-parasite Relationship.* Heidelberg, Germany: Springer, 1989. Pp. 237–244.

139. Szentivanyi, J., et al. Influences of Hypothalamic and Extrahypothalamic Brain Structures on the Immunogenicity of Antibiotic-pretreated Bacteria. In *Proceedings of Annual Meeting of the International Society for Interferon Research.* Kyoto, Japan, 1988. Abstract 5-30. Kanagawa, Japan: Japanese Society for Interferon Research.

140. Szentivanyi, J., et al. Virus Associated Immune and Pharmacologic Mechanisms in Disorders of Respiratory and Cutaneous Atopy. In A. Szentivanyi and H. Friedman (eds.), *Viruses, Immunity and Immunodeficiency.* New York: Plenum, 1986. Pp. 211–244.

141. Thompson, J. E., et al. Hydroxyurea inhibits airway hyperresponsiveness in guinea pigs by a granulocyte-independent mechanism. *Am. Rev. Respir. Dis.* 134:1213, 1986.

142. Valone, F. H., and Epstein, L. B. Biphasic platelet activating factor synthesis by human monocytes stimulated with IL-1β, tumor necrosis factor or interferon-γ. *J. Immunol.* 141:3945, 1988.

143. Van Oosterhout, A. J. M., and Nijkamp, F. P. Lymphocytes and bronchial hyperresponsiveness. *Life Sci.* 46:1255, 1990.

144. Van Oosterhout, A. J. M., and Nijkamp, F. P. Effect of lymphokines on beta-adrenoceptor function of human peripheral blood mononuclear cells. *Br. J. Clin. Pharmacol.* 30:150S, 1990.

145. Vekshina, N., and Magaeva, S. V. Changes in the serotonin concentration in the limbic structures of the brain during immunization. *Bull. Exp. Biol. Med.* 77:625, 1974.

146. Walker, C., et al. Activated T cells and eosinophilia in bronchoalveolar lavages from subjects with asthma correlated with disease severity. *J. Allergy Clin. Immunol.* 88:935, 1991.

147. Williams, A. F., and Barclay, A. N. The immunoglobulin superfamily—domains for cell surface recognition. *Annu. Rev. Immunol.* 6:381, 1988.

148. Woloski, B. M. R. N. J., et al. Corticotropin-releasing activity of monokines. *Science* 230:1035, 1985.

149. Yanagihara, Y., et al. Enhancement of IgE synthesis and histamine release by T-cell factors derived from atopic patients with bronchial asthma. *J. Allergy Clin. Immunol.* 79:448, 1987.

150. Zawalich, W. S., Zawalich, K. C., and Rasmussen, H. Interleukin-1α exerts glucose-dependent stimulatory and inhibitory effects on islet cell phosphoinositide hydrolysis and insulin secretion. *Endocrinology* 124:2350, 1989.

II Diagnostics and Laboratory

Clinical Incitants

Paul P. VanArsdel, Jr.

34

Anyone concerned with understanding and managing asthma must be struck not only with the wide variation in the expression of asthma among a population of patients, but also with the frequency with which several factors are involved in the production of asthma in a single patient. It is unlikely that a single causal factor ever is responsible for abnormalities associated with asthma—although one agent may, of course, be the ultimate trigger responsible for producing the symptoms of asthma. This chapter introduces a broad perspective of the common clinical causes of asthma, which are discussed in greater detail in subsequent sections.

Many attempts have been made to develop appropriate classifications of asthma based on provoking factors, degree of bronchial reactivity (as provoked by exercise, cold air, methacholine, or histamine), pathophysiology, response to therapy, or various permutations. No single classification has become generally accepted. Perhaps the oldest, and certainly the most durable, is the one developed in the decade following the report by Meltzer that asthma was associated with anaphylactic sensitivity [31]. It soon became apparent that the clinical sensitivity of some patients with asthma was associated with positive results on skin tests with environmental antigens (allergens). The importance of specific sensitivity was further strengthened by a report in 1919 of horse dander asthma produced passively by transfusing blood from a sensitive donor [38]. These patients were classified as having *extrinsic* asthma by Rackemann in 1918; the remainder, a group whose asthma had no well-defined cause, were considered to have *intrinsic* asthma [37]. This classification was still useful in considering causal factors in asthma, although it is obviously oversimplified. The term *intrinsic asthma* is confusing to many because it applies to such a heterogeneous group of patients, but there is little or no disagreement among most authorities regarding extrinsic asthma. Even the apparently simple association of extrinsic asthma with atopic (IgE antibody–mediated) sensitivity that was established years ago has been complicated by the recognition of a subclass of extrinsic asthma, caused by occupational agents, that is not associated with an atopic diathesis and often is not associated with specific IgE antibodies (Table 34-1). Furthermore, one can argue that any asthma that is induced or aggravated by inhaled irritants or ingested drugs is, in part at least, extrinsic.

The anaphylactic concept supplanted, in part at least, an older notion that asthma was a "neurotic" disorder related perhaps to autonomic dysfunction. Nevertheless, there is continuing interest in autonomic imbalance as a possible common denominator in asthma regardless of classification. The airways of asthmatic patients are hyperreactive to a variety of stimuli. There is some evidence that this reactivity is caused by a relatively poor beta-adrenergic compensatory response to the bronchoconstricting action of parasympathetic, and perhaps alpha-adrenergic, stimuli. This concept is discussed in detail in Chapter 14. Possibly a

factor in the genesis of intrinsic asthma, it may be necessary for the expression of extrinsic asthma as well. Among a group of patients with a similar degree of sensitivity immunologically, some will react to allergen exposure with asthma, but most have only allergic rhinitis or hay fever. An asthmatic reaction to inhaled allergen can be induced, in the latter group, by pretreatment with the beta-blocking drug propranolol [35]. In the last 5 years, both clinicians and investigators have shifted their attention from autonomic regulation to inflammation and epithelial injury as major factors in the pathogenesis of asthma [26a]. The roles of eosinophils, inflammatory mediators, and the epithelium are discussed in Chapters 9, 20, and 23. Inflammation, rather than bronchospasm, plays a major role in the production of the late-phase asthmatic reaction, discussed in Chapter 12. This is usually more important than the immediate reaction in asthma produced by the inhaled allergens, to be discussed next.

ALLERGENS AND ASTHMA

By definition, atopic patients with extrinsic asthma react to substances in the environment that are innocuous to the general population and to other asthmatic subjects (excluding nonspecific irritants). Such patients tend to be young, with onset of symptoms usually in childhood. Sensitivity is of the immediate or anaphylactic (Type I) class and thus is associated with specific wheal and erythema skin reactions to the offending allergens and with circulating antibodies of the IgE immunoglobulin class. Such patients also have a strong personal and family history of atopic disease (i.e., extrinsic asthma, allergic rhinitis, infantile eczema, atopic dermatitis). The allergens to which any single individual will become sensitive are unpredictable and variable; once a sensitivity develops, it persists indefinitely, although clinical expression of the sensitivity may change and often diminishes from childhood to adult life. The important categories of allergens implicated in the production of asthma symptoms are pollens and other inhalants such as house dust, epidermal allergens, molds, and insects, as listed in Table 34-2. Characterizing the allergens contained in these substances has been a slow and tedious job. For example, to develop the first international standard for birch pollen alone required the collaborative efforts of 20 laboratories in 11 countries [3]. By a combination of biologic and immunochemical methods, the important allergens in a few common pollens, molds, house mites, and some animal danders have now been highly purified and chemically characterized. Sufficient progress has been made so that the International Union of Immunological Societies has established a new nomenclature system for these allergens. For example, ragweed antigen E is now called *Amb a* I [28]. These results provide the hope that at long last, a reliable system for standardization of allergenic

Table 34-1. Classification of extrinsic and intrinsic asthma

| | Extrinsic asthma | | Intrinsic (idiopathic) asthma |
	Atopic	Nonatopic	
Age at onset	Usually childhood	Adult	Usually after age 25
Symptoms	Variable with environment and season	Usually occupation related	Unpredictable fluctuations, often chronic
Associated conditions	Allergic rhinitis, atopic dermatitis	None	Bronchitis, sinusitis, nasal polyps
Family history of atopic disease	Strong	Minor	Asthma only (?)
Skin test results (wheal-erythema)	Several positive, related to history	Negative, or one reaction only	Usually negative
Total IgE	High	Usually normal	Normal
Eosinophilia	High during allergen exposure	Sometimes high during allergen exposure	High
Prognosis	Good, especially with allergen avoidance	Good, especially with allergen avoidance	Fair, remissions uncommon

Table 34-2. Common allergens used for diagnostic skin testing

Pollens*	Other inhalants
Trees	Epidermal allergens
Alder	Cat
Ash	Cattle
Birch	Dog
Cottonwood	Horse
Elm	Bird
Hazel	Others
Hickory	Molds
Juniper	*Alternaria*
Maple	*Aspergillus*
Mountain cedar	*Cladosporium*
Oak	*Fusarium*
Pecan	*Helminthosporium*
Poplar	*Monilia*
Sycamore	*Penicillium*
Grasses	*Rhizopus*
Bermuda	Algae
Blue	Insects
Fescue	Cockroach
Orchard	Caddis fly (limited
Rye	distribution)
Timothy	Mayfly
Vernal	Mite
Weeds	
Dock	
English plantain	
Lamb's-quarters	
Marsh elder	
Pigweed	
Ragweed	
Russian thistle	
Sagebrush	

* Major allergens in at least some regions of the United States. See Solomon and Mathews [43] and Appendix A for geographic breakdown.

extracts for clinical use is within reach [39]. See Chapters 38, 39, 40, and 42.

Pollens of most plant species may sensitize atopic individuals. Those from flowering plants, being insect borne, heavy, and sticky, are of little clinical importance. Wind-borne pollens can be disseminated hundreds of miles and are clinically important roughly in proportion to the prevalence of the species in a given region. Although scores of species have been implicated, only a few are major offenders. As a rule, trees pollinate early in the spring, grasses later in the spring, and weeds in the summer. Detailed information on the range, prevalence, and seasonal production of many pollen species has been collected from airborne pollen surveys and is available in standard texts [43].

Pollen grains range in size from 20 μ in diameter (ragweed) to about 60 μ. They contain water-soluble allergens that are low-molecular-weight proteins. Only a few have been isolated and characterized chemically. The major allergen of ragweed (antigen E) is a globular protein with a molecular weight of 37,800. The molecular weights of other major allergens fall between 20,000 and 40,000, but those of minor allergens may range from a few thousand to 70,000 [25]. Some very-low-molecular-weight ragweed allergens are rapidly released from pollen grains and may contribute greatly to symptoms [22] (see Chap. 5).

The mechanism by which pollens produce asthma is not entirely clear. The traditional explanation has been that antigen reacts with IgE antibody on bronchial mast cells, with the release of mediators such as histamine, leukotrienes, and chemotactic factors that produce bronchoconstriction and inflammation; these mediators are reviewed in detail in Chapters 10 and 11. On theoretic grounds alone, this concept is questionable: The pollen grains should be too large to reach the lower airways. Wilson and colleagues [53] observed the distribution of radiolabeled whole grass pollen grains after inhalation; no radioactivity was found in the bronchi or even in the trachea—all of the pollen was in the mouth or had been swallowed. By contrast, about 10 percent of a nebulized aqueous pollen extract reached the lung after inhalation. There is no evidence, however, that any major natural exposure to soluble aerosols occurs. It is possible that pollen fragments small enough to reach the lungs are responsible; in fact, airborne particles smaller than 5 μ in diameter containing ragweed allergen have been identified during the pollen season [2] and rye grass allergens have recently been identified in starch granules from osmotically ruptured pollen grains [45a] (see also Chap. 42).

The major allergenic molds belong to the class Fungi Imperfecti and include numerous genera; *Alternaria* and *Cladosporium* (*Hormodendrum*) are typical of those that grow on plants and decaying vegetation, and *Aspergillus* and *Penicillium* are the most common ones found indoors. Mold spores vary greatly in size. Some are less than 5 μ in diameter and probably do reach the lower airways, though no direct evidence exists on this point. *Penicillium* spores are as small as 2 μ in diameter, whereas *Helminthosporium* spores may reach 75 μ in length (Fig. 34-1). Theoretically, small spores such as those of *Aspergillus* and *Penicillium* should be more likely to produce asthma symptoms than the larger spores. There is no clinical evidence that this is so; *Alternaria*, in particular, is a major offender in many parts of the country. As with pollens, it appears that intact spores do not need to reach the lower airways to produce symptoms. There is no well-defined season; spore counts in the air are at a minimum during freezing weather and reach their highest levels during dry, windy periods after a rainy season.

As with pollens, mold spores contain numerous potential aller-

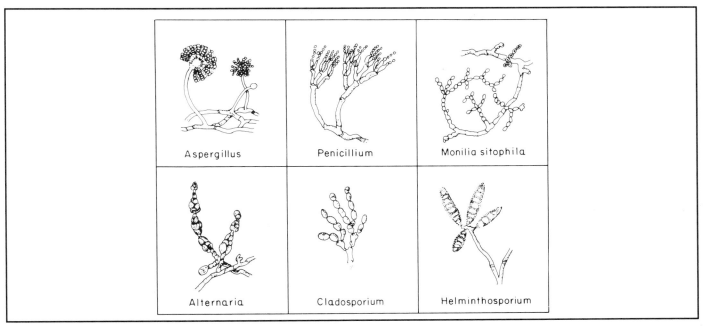

Fig. 34-1. *Typical fungi and their spores. The top three are members of the family Monilaceae. Note the small spore size. The bottom three, family Dematiaceae, have much larger spores. Spore size does not seem to be a factor in allergenicity or symptom provocation. (Reprinted with permission from J. M. Sheldon, R. G. Lovell, and K. P. Mathews [eds.], A Manual of Clinical Allergy [2nd ed.]. Philadelphia: Saunders, 1967. Chap. 16. By courtesy of William R. Solomon, M.D., and the publisher.)*

gens, and much work is now being done to characterize them. A major *Alternaria* allergen (*Alt a* I) has recently been purified [36a].

Molds, as well as pollens and other allergens, can produce dual asthmatic reactions that occur immediately and again several hours later, as discussed in Chapter 12. Most authorities now believe that both phases are consequences of the reaction of allergen with IgE antibody. In addition, some molds, particularly *Aspergillus fumigatus*, can in a few patients produce dual reactions, in which both Type I and Type III mechanisms may be involved. The condition is discussed in detail in Chapter 49.

House dust in large concentrations can act as a primary irritant, as can any dust. Its importance as an allergen may not be recognized. The unfortunate result is that the problem of asthma in sensitive patients associated with exposure to small amounts of invisible house dust in the air may go unrecognized. The size of dust particles extends over a wide range; some are small enough to reach the bronchioles and even alveoli. Asthma related to house dust allergy may be perennial; typically, symptoms are worse in the fall when homes are closed up and the forced-air furnace is turned on. The major allergens in house dust are derived from the mites of the genus *Dermatophagoides*. The prevalent species are *D. pteronyssinus* and *D. farinae*. Allergens derived from these two species cross-react, but not completely [15]. One major mite allergen is a glycoprotein with a molecular weight of 24,000 and was first identified and called antigen P_1 by Platts-Mills and his associates [49]. Antigen P_1 is now called *Der p* I. About 95 percent of the allergen is found in mite feces, which are similar in size to allergenic pollen grains.

Cockroach allergy can be a significant cause of asthma, especially among children living in high-density, inner-city dwellings and in subtropical climates. The German species, which is ubiquitous, and American species, prevalent in the southern United States, share allergens, which have molecular weights varying from less than 10,000 to over 600,000 [24, 24a].

Epidermal allergens, which include animal danders and feathers, are contained in a wide range of particle sizes, some certainly small enough to reach the lower airways. There is little immunologic cross-reaction, and clinical sensitivity is often restricted to one species. Animal hair itself is inert except as a primary irritant. Thus, wool and processed furs cannot be incriminated clinically as allergens, though extracts made from them may produce positive skin test results. Ohman and his associates [26] identified a major cat allergen several years ago that they labeled allergen 1. Although it was extracted from the cat pelt, the main source was eventually found to be saliva. A glycoprotein with a molecular weight of 37,000 [26], it is called *Fel d* I. Monoclonal antibodies have been prepared against this allergen, and is now used to measure its concentration in air samples and other environmental materials [27]. The major allergens in laboratory rats and mice are found in their urine [34], while cat urinary allergens, different from allergen 1, may be of some clinical importance [30]. Only recently has a major dog dander allergen been identified. It is common to several dog breeds and is termed *Can f* I [40a]. An allergen in horse dander is a glycoprotein with a molecular weight of about 34,000. The allergenic activity in feathers is associated with an extremely polydisperse mixture of keratinous protein components [8].

The role of food allergens in provoking asthma is a limited one, despite frequent claims to the contrary (see Chap. 43). Older children and adults who are atopic frequently show positive results on skin tests with common allergenic foods such as grains, milk, egg white, nuts, legumes, and seafood. Those who have any symptoms after ingestion of such foods are in the minority, and those who have asthma symptoms are rare indeed. Claims that foods may be responsible for chronic asthma on some other, nonatopic basis have not been supported when subjected to well-controlled studies [51]. Ingested food allergens probably do aggravate asthma in very young atopic children, who absorb more undigested allergens than do older persons. One of the few studies supporting this impression was done by Aas in Norway [1]. Aas confirmed an association between codfish allergy and asthma in children, both by provocation meals and by inhalation challenge, and found an increased tolerance with increasing age.

The problem of diagnosing food sensitivity was reviewed critically by Bock [9]. By far the clearest association between food allergy and asthma, however, is found in occupational exposure, in which the material is inhaled rather than ingested. Bakers' asthma, related usually to wheat flour inhalation, is a relatively common problem [47]. These patients do not develop symptoms after they eat wheat products. Asthma is also a common problem among sensitized workers handling coffee beans, soybeans, castor beans, cottonseed, and other foods that contain potent allergens. As with wheat flour, these products cause problems as inhaled allergens but do not produce asthma when eaten by the sensitive consumer.

OCCUPATIONAL ASTHMA

The discussion above on foods as inhaled allergens leads naturally to a more general discussion of asthma as an occupational health problem. The provoking agents fall into three categories: protein allergens, low-molecular-weight chemicals, and nonspecific primary irritants.

The development of atopic sensitivity is an important health problem, not only to food handlers, but also to anyone whose job requires exposure to the common allergens discussed above. Veterinarians and those who work with laboratory animals may become sensitized to animal danders and be forced to make major occupational changes. Any foreign protein used in industry is capable of sensitizing some persons. If conditions are such that inhalation of the protein occurs, the sensitized worker usually develops respiratory symptoms, including asthma. Such conditions did exist when the soap and detergent industry began to add proteolytic enzymes to their detergents. The enzymes are prepared from cultures of *Bacillus subtilis* and *B. licheniformis* and provided in powder form for mixing with detergent in the factory. As many as 25 percent of workers handling the enzyme powder developed asthma symptoms associated with skin test sensitivity [42]. This experience should serve as a warning that conventional industrial precautions will not be adequate for operations involving the use of foreign protein that may disperse in the ambient air. Problems continue to appear. Recently a paper from Spain reported asthma in some pharmaceutical-manufacturing employees provoked by alpha-amylase inhalation [26b].

Wood dust may act as a primary irritant, aggravating preexisting asthma, but some individuals react specifically to inhalation challenge with some extracts or dusts and others do not [44]. Asthma is particularly prevalent among cedar workers. Symptoms can be reproduced consistently by inhalation of an aqueous extract of western red cedar; the active ingredient is a low-molecular-weight chemical, plicatic acid. The sensitivity is acquired and develops in only about 5 percent of exposed workers. Specific IgE antibodies to crude extract or to a plicatic acid–human serum albumin conjugate have been found in the serum of some workers. These antibodies are more likely to be present in workers who have bronchial hyperreactivity by methacholine challenge than those who do not [52].

Among the many simple chemicals reported to induce asthma, the best known is toluene diisocyanate (TDI), which is used as a polymerizing agent in the production of polyurethane foams and other substances. In high enough concentrations it is a primary respiratory irritant. However, in some workers who have used TDI without trouble for weeks or months, asthma develops and recurs on exposure to very small concentrations. This suggests strongly that these subjects have become specifically sensitized, although specific IgE antibody has been found in only a small proportion of affected workers [7]. For other simple chemicals, the separation of sensitization reactions from primary irritant reactions also remains imprecise in the absence of reproducible objective tests for allergy. Some exceptions should be noted.

Anhydrides in particular are highly reactive chemically and readily form stable covalent bonds with carrier proteins in vivo. Positive immediate skin reactions and specific IgE antibodies have been found in workers sensitized to phthalic, trimellitic, and other anhydrides [54]. By some other mechanism, complex platinum salts can also sensitize workers, producing specific IgE-mediated skin sensitivity [14]. Asthma in workers using phenylglycine acid chloride in the synthesis of ampicillin was associated with positive immediate skin sensitivity that could be passively transferred to normal recipients [23]. Positive skin test results have also been noted in subjects with asthma reactions to nickel salts [29].

Patients with preexisting asthma, whatever the cause, are particularly susceptible to primary respiratory irritants of any sort, occupational or otherwise, including dusts, tobacco smoke, other types of smoke, strong odors, cold air, and the various general atmospheric pollutants such as sulfur dioxide [17a, 20]. Formaldehyde, in particular, has received considerable attention as a possible irritant or even allergen. There is suggestive clinical evidence that a few workers have become sensitized through prolonged occupational exposure to relatively high levels of formaldehyde [16]. However, efforts to find immunologic abnormalities that have any correlation with clinical disease have been negative [19]. There is no convincing evidence that asthma is caused or even provoked by the relatively low concentrations of formaldehyde found in dwellings that contain urea formaldehyde foam insulation or the particle board that was used extensively at one time in the manufacture of mobile homes [17, 21]. Irritants need not reach the lower airways to produce symptoms. Introducing nonspecific irritants to the upper airway alone can induce vagally mediated bronchospasm [41]. As a rule symptoms occur the first time a person is exposed to a primary irritant and will continue as long as the exposure continues.

A unique situation exists with byssinosis, in which symptoms of obstructive airway disease occur after inhalation of textile dust by workers in cotton mills. Symptoms are worst on Monday and diminish in severity thereafter, a pattern that is not characteristic of the usual irritant dusts. The explanation may be that a histamine-releasing agent in cotton dust depletes the lung mast cells of histamine, and the worker becomes tolerant [10]. It is also possible that symptoms are produced by endotoxins that can activate the alternative complement pathway, microbial enzymes, or both. Allergic factors may also play a role, at least in some workers. Occupational asthma is discussed in more detail in Chapter 46.

DRUGS AND ASTHMA

Asthma may develop in association with anaphylactic drug reactions but is rarely if ever the only manifestation of allergy after oral or parenteral administration. Drugs administered by inhalation that may sensitize the patient and induce asthma include penicillin and posterior pituitary powder. These reactions are now rare since nebulized antibacterial therapy has become restricted to unusual circumstances and since posterior pituitary powder has been supplanted by synthetic desmopressin. Other agents administered by inhalation, such as proteolytic enzymes and acetylcysteine, are likely to produce bronchospasm as primary irritants and are contraindicated in asthma treatment [50]. Drug-induced asthma, including adverse reactions to aspirin, other nonsteroidal antiinflammatory agents, and the yellow dye tartrazine, is discussed in detail in Chapter 48.

EXERCISE BRONCHOSPASM

Wheezing dyspnea develops in some young asthmatic patients after (but not during) vigorous exercise; exercise may be the only major provoking factor. Other subjects with a history of asthma or hay fever may show a major reduction in ventilatory flow rates after exercise without experiencing symptoms. This is a very common phenomenon, discussed in detail in Chapter 47, that was recently studied extensively in many clinics and laboratories. Despite the reproducibility and apparent simplicity of the exercise response, much conflicting information in the literature regarding its mechanism remains to be resolved. In contrast to hyperventilation-induced airway cooling, exercise bronchospasm is associated with the release of mediators such as those released during antigen-induced bronchospasm.

NOCTURNAL ASTHMA

Asthma is often worse at night. Not only are patients awakened at night with acute attacks, but those with daytime symptoms are likely to suffer more at night. About a third of patients in one report had their lowest airflow rates in the early hours of the day (the "morning dippers"). In this group there is probably an increased risk of nocturnal death [4]. Although continued exposure to the household mite and other allergens in the bedroom may play some role in aggravating asthma at night, most evidence indicates that the pattern of nocturnal asthma does not correlate well with the presence or absence of specific inhalant allergy. Compared with normal control subjects, asthmatic patients sleep less well and have more irregular breathing and a greater fall in oxygen saturation. Classic sleep apnea has not been observed in two independent studies. Asthma attacks are least likely to occur during deep (electroencephalogram Stages 3 and 4) sleep than at other times. An association has been observed with Stage 5 (rapid eye movement) by some observers, but not by others [12, 32]. Prevention of sleep at night does not prevent attacks or morning dips.

Nocturnal asthma may be caused by a circadian fall in plasma epinephrine. In asthmatic patients Barnes and coworkers observed that such a fall is associated with a rise in plasma histamine [6]. The observed nocturnal drop in plasma cortisol has also been proposed as contributing to the problem. Unfortunately for these concepts, neither epinephrine nor cortisol replacement is very effective in preventing nocturnal asthma. Another possibility is that a reduction in body temperature triggers asthma. In one recent study nocturnal asthma was prevented by the breathing of warm humidified air, which provides support for this idea [13]. See Chapter 76 for further discussion.

OTHER FACTORS

Respiratory infection and psychological factors are commonly thought to aggravate asthma, but the relationships are so complex and variable as to preclude a concise discussion in this chapter. These important subjects are covered in later chapters. It is a common clinical impression that asthma can be aggravated by weather conditions such as high humidity, rapid temperature or pressure changes, or the notorious dry winds of Europe (*Föhnen*) and the Middle East (*siroccos*). Efforts to prove any direct association have met with little success. Most weather-related increases in asthma complaints are better explained by the associated increase in air pollution caused by irritants [18], allergens [40], or both. See Chapters 44 and 45.

Tobacco smoke is generally recognized as a respiratory irritant. Furthermore, there is increasing evidence that passive exposure to smoke can significantly increase asthma morbidity, particularly among children with smokers in the household. In addition to the aggravating effect on preexisting asthma, exposure to smoke may increase the prevalence of allergic sensitization, as measured by IgE levels [46], and has been found to in-

crease the risk of developing asthma in children with atopic dermatitis [33]. Adults with asthma differ significantly in their airway reactivity to cigarette smoke. In one study, only 7 of 21 subjects showed a significant reduction in ventilatory function following smoke inhalation challenge. There was no evidence for IgE-mediated tobacco leaf allergy in these reactive subjects [45].

Certain associated conditions may aggravate or even induce asthma; though uncommon, they should not be overlooked. Bronchopulmonary irritation from a foreign body in the tracheobronchial tree or a pulmonary embolus may produce diffuse reflex bronchospasm. Another cause of reflex bronchospasm that is not so generally recognized is gastroesophageal reflux. Patients with this problem usually, but not always, have a hiatus hernia demonstrated radiographically. Since aspiration of gastric acid is rare in asthmatic patients, the association between gastroesophageal reflux and asthma needs to be explained on some other basis, such as reflex bronchoconstriction triggered by acid receptors in the esophagus. However, experimental evidence that reflux indeed causes asthma is inconclusive, though there is no doubt that the two conditions frequently exist in the same patient [36]. (See Chap. 75.)

Adrenal insufficiency theoretically should aggravate coexisting asthma, but the condition is extremely rare except after injudicious withdrawal of adrenal corticosteroid treatment. Occasionally, hyperthyroidism may aggravate coexisting asthma. The mechanism is not established. Possibly the accelerated metabolism of glucocorticoids by thyroxine contributes; in rats prostaglandin breakdown is inhibited. Thyrotropin-releasing hormone has produced an attack of wheezing in an asthmatic patient [5, 48].

The following list of causal and precipitating factors in asthma is illustrative only; it is not intended as a comprehensive compilation.

1. Allergens
   Pollens, fungal spores, house dust, dust mites, insect parts (scales, emanations), animal danders (cat, dog, horse), foods (including inhaled products), drugs (penicillin, pituitary snuff), vaccines, parasites, etc. These are identified usually by a specific seasonal or episodic clinical history and confirmed by skin tests.
2. Occupational
   Organic dusts, isocyanates, anhydrides, dyes, antibiotic drug manufacturing, complex metal salts.
3. Drugs (pharmacologic or unknown mechanism)
   Propranolol and other beta-adrenergic blockers, methacholine, isoproterenol metabolites, reserpine, narcotics, aspirin, other nonsteroidal antiinflammatory drugs, anesthetic agents, food additives.
4. Exercise
   Sports, sexual activity. (Exercise-related or exercise-induced asthma differs from hyperventilation.)
5. Irritants
   Odors and chemical fumes, air pollutants, tobacco smoke, cold air, paints, cosmetics, perfumes, weather (barometric pressure and humidity) changes, irritative dusts, aspiration (gastric), reflex (vagal) from foreign body.
6. Infection
   Viral, not often bacterial.
7. Psychogenic
   Fatigue, anxiety, stress, laughter.
8. Coexistent conditions
   Ear, nose, or throat disease (sinusitis, nasal polyp), hyperthyroidism, vagal reflexes, premenstrual state.
9. Heredity, familial predisposition
10. Circadian (nocturnal) rhythms

REFERENCES

1. Aas, K. Studies of hypersensitivity to fish. *Int. Arch. Allergy* 29:346, 1966.
2. Agarwal, M. K., et al. Airborne ragweed allergens: Association with various particle sizes and short ragweed plant parts. *J. Allergy Clin. Immunol.* 74: 687, 1984.
3. Arntzen, F. C., et al. The international collaborative study on the first international standard of birch (*Betula verrucosa*)-pollen extract. *J. Allergy Clin. Immunol.* 83:66, 1989.
4. Asthma at night. *Lancet* 1:220, 1983.
5. Ayres, J., and Clark, T. J. H. Asthma and the thyroid. *Lancet* 2:1110, 1981.
6. Barnes, P., et al. Nocturnal asthma and changes in circulating epinephrine, histamine, and cortisol. *N. Engl. J. Med.* 303:263, 1980.
7. Bernstein, I. L. Isocyanate-induced pulmonary diseases: A current perspective. *J. Allergy Clin. Immunol.* 70:24, 1982.
8. Berrens, L. Allergens from Epithelial Tissue. In P. Kallos, T. M. Inderbitzin, and B. H. Waksman (eds.), *The Chemistry of Atopic Allergens* (Monographs in Allergy, vol. 7). New York: Karger, 1971. P. 104.
9. Bock, S. A. Food sensitivity. *Am. J. Dis. Child.* 134:973, 1980.
10. Bouhuys, A. Byssinosis: Scheduled asthma in the textile industry. *Lung* 154:3, 1976.
11. Budd, T. W., et al. Antigens of *Alternaria*: I. Isolation and partial characterization of a basic peptide allergen. *J. Allergy Clin. Immunol.* 71:277, 1983.
12. Catterall, J. R., et al. Irregular breathing and hypoxaemia during sleep in chronic stable asthma. *Lancet* 1:301, 1982.
13. Chen, W. Y., and Chai, H. Airway cooling and nocturnal asthma. *Chest* 81: 675, 1982.
14. Cromwell, O., et al. Specific IgE antibodies to platinum salts in sensitized workers. *Clin. Allergy* 9:109, 1979.
15. Dailey, F., Stier, R., and Featherstone, L. Incomplete cross reactivity between the mites *Dermatophagoides farinae* and *D. pteronyssimus*. *J. Allergy Clin. Immunol.* 69:127, 1982.
16. Feinman, S. E. *Formaldehyde Sensitivity and Toxicity*. Boca Raton, CRC Press, 1988. Pp. 135–148.
17. Frigas, E., and Reed, C. E. Formaldehyde gas bronchial challenge does not provoke asthma. *J. Allergy Clin. Immunol.* 71:136, 1983.
17a. From, L. J., et al. The effects of open leaf burning on spirometric measurements in asthma. *Chest* 101:1236, 1992.
18. Girsh, I. S., et al. A study on the epidemiology of asthma in children in Philadelphia. *J. Allergy* 39:347, 1967.
19. Grammer, L. C., et al. Clinical and immunologic evaluation of 37 workers exposed to gaseous formaldehyde. *J. Allergy Clin. Immunol.* 86:177, 1990.
20. Harries, M. G., et al. Role of bronchial irritant receptors in asthma. *Lancet* 1:5, 1981.
21. Harving, H., et al. Pulmonary function and bronchial reactivity in asthmatics during low-level formaldehyde exposure. *Lung* 168:15, 1990.
22. Hussain, R., Norman, P. S., and Marsh, D. G. Rapidly released allergens from ragweed pollen: II. Identification and partial purification. *J. Allergy Clin. Immunol.* 67:217, 1981.
23. Kammermeyer, J. K., and Mathews, K. P. Hypersensitivity to phenylglycine acid chloride. *J. Allergy Clin. Immunol.* 52:73, 1973.
24. Kang, B. C. Cockroach allergy. *Clin. Rev. Allergy* 8:87, 1990.
24a. Kang, B. C., and Wu, C. W. Characteristics and diagnosis of cockroach-sensitive bronchial asthma. *Ann. Allergy* 68:237, 1992.
25. King, T. P. Immunochemical properties of some atopic allergens. *J. Allergy Clin. Immunol.* 64:159, 1979.
26. Leiterman, K., and Ohman, J. L. Cat allergen I: Biochemical, antigenic and allergenic properties. *J. Allergy Clin. Immunol.* 74:147, 1984.
26a. Lemanske, R. F. Mechanisms of airway inflammation. *Chest* 101:373S, 1992.
26b. Losada, E., et al. Occupational asthma caused by α-amylase inhalation: Clinical and immunological findings and bronchial response patterns. *J. Allergy Clin. Immunol.* 89:118, 1992.
27. Luczynska, C. M., et al. Airborne concentrations and particle size distribution of allergen derived from domestic cats (*Felis domesticus*). *Am. Rev. Respir. Dis.* 141:361, 1990.
28. Marsh, D. G., et al. Allergen nomenclature. *J. Allergy Clin. Immunol.* 80: 639, 1987.
29. McConnell, I. H., et al. Asthma caused by nickel sensitivity. *Ann. Intern. Med.* 78:888, 1973.
30. McElhinney, M. E., et al. Cat urinary allergens. *J. Allergy Clin. Immunol.* 69:144, 1982.
31. Meltzer, S. J. Bronchial asthma as a phenomenon of anaphylaxis. *JAMA* 55:1021, 1910.
32. Montplaisir, J., Walsh, J., and Malo, J. L. Nocturnal asthma: Features of attacks, sleep and breathing patterns. *Am. Rev. Respir. Dis.* 125:18, 1982.
33. Murray, A. B., and Morrison, B. J. It is children with atopic dermatitis who develop asthma more frequently if the mother smokes. *J. Allergy Clin. Immunol.* 86:732, 1990.
34. Newman Taylor, A., Longbottom, J. L., and Pepys, J. Respiratory allergy to urine proteins of rats and mice. *Lancet* 2:847, 1977.
35. Ouellette, J. J., and Reed, C. E. The effect of partial beta-adrenergic blockade on the bronchial response of hay fever subjects to ragweed aerosol. *J. Allergy* 39:160, 1967.
36. Pack, A. I. Acid: A nocturnal bronchoconstrictor? *Am. Rev. Respir. Dis.* 141:1391, 1990.
36a. Paris, S., et al. The 31 KD major allergen ALTαI$_{1563}$ of *Alternaria alternata*. *J. Allergy Clin. Immunol.* 88:902, 1991.
37. Rackemann, F. M. A clinical study of one hundred fifty cases of bronchial asthma. *Arch. Intern. Med.* 22:517, 1918.
38. Ramirez, M. A. Horse asthma following blood transfusion. *JAMA* 73:984, 1919.
39. Reed, C. E., and Yuninger, J. W. Quality assurance and standardization of allergy extracts in allergy practice. *J. Allergy Clin. Immunol.* 84:4, 1989.
40. Salvaggio, J., Seaburg, J., and Schoenhart, E. A. New Orleans asthma: V. Relationship between Charity Hospital admission rates, semiquantitative pollen and fungal spores count, and total particulate aerometric sampling data. *J. Allergy Clin. Immunol.* 48:96, 1971.
40a. Schou, C., et al. Assay for the major dog allergen, Can f I: Investigation of house dust samples and commercial dog extracts. *J. Allergy Clin. Immunol.* 88:847, 1991.
41. Simonsson, B. G., Jacobs, F. M., and Nadel, J. A. Mechanism of changes in airway size during inhalation of various substances in asthmatics. *Am. Rev. Respir. Dis.* 95:873, 1967.
42. Slavin, R. G., and Lewis, C. R. Sensitivity to enzyme additives in laundry detergent workers. *J. Allergy* 48:262, 1971.
43. Solomon, W. R., and Mathews, K. P. Aerobiology and Inhalant Allergens. In E. Middleton, Jr., et al. (eds.), *Allergy: Principles and Practice* (3rd ed.). St. Louis: Mosby, 1988. Pp. 312–372.
44. Sosman, A. J., et al. Hypersensitivity to wood dust. *N. Engl. J. Med.* 281: 977, 1969.
45. Stankus, R. P., et al. Cigarette smoke–sensitive asthma: Challenge studies. *J. Allergy Clin. Immunol.* 82:331, 1988.
45a. Suphioglu, C., et al. Mechanism of grass pollen-induced asthma. *Lancet* 339:569, 1992.
46. Tager, I. B. Passive smoking—Bronchial responsiveness and atopy. *Am. Rev. Respir. Dis.* 138:507, 1988.
47. Thiel, H., and Ulmer, W. T. Bakers' asthma: Development and possibility for treatment. *Chest* 78:400, 1980.
48. Thyroid disease and asthma. *Br. Med. J.* 2:1173, 1977.
49. Tovey, E. R., Chapman, M. D., and Platts-Mills, T. A. E. Mite faeces are a major source of house dust allergens. *Nature* 289:592, 1981.
50. VanArsdel, P. P., Jr. Adverse Drug Reactions. In E. Middleton, Jr., C. E. Reed, and E. F. Ellis (eds.), *Allergy: Principles and Practice* (2nd ed.). St. Louis: Mosby, 1983. Pp. 1389–1414.
51. Van Metre, T. E., Jr., et al. A controlled study of the effects on manifestations of chronic asthma of a rigid elimination diet based on Rowe's cereal-free diet 1,2,3. *J. Allergy* 41:195, 1968.
52. Vedal, S., et al. Longitudinal study of the occurrence of bronchial hyperresponsiveness in western red cedar workers. *Am. Rev. Respir. Dis.* 137:651, 1988.
53. Wilson, A. E., et al. Deposition of inhaled pollen and pollen extract in human airways. *N. Engl. J. Med.* 288:1056, 1973.
54. Zeiss, C. R., et al. Clinical and immunological evaluation of trimellitic anhydride workers in multiple industrial settings. *J. Allergy Clin. Immunol.* 70:15, 1982.

Clinical Evaluation

M. Henry Williams, Jr.
Chang Shim

35

The diagnosis of asthma is based on the presence of variable airway obstruction. Assessment of the severity of illness and hence the need for treatment requires an estimate of the degree of airway obstruction. Such an estimate is best achieved by a measurement of expiratory flow rate, as will be discussed, but can also be based on the patient's symptoms and physical findings.

In asthma, airway obstruction may be induced by a variety of naturally occurring or artificial events and, if present, can be reversed by bronchodilator drugs. Thus, there are many strategies for making an accurate diagnosis. Symptoms may be a surprisingly accurate indication of severity of obstruction and in addition may reflect disability or discomfort that requires therapy even in the absence of major limitation of airflow.

The key to the detection and clinical evaluation of asthma is a careful history. Not only can the physician usually elicit a description of symptoms that are sufficiently characteristic to make a diagnosis, but it may be possible to obtain important information about agents that are responsible for worsening symptoms so they can be avoided. Equally important, a thoughtful history gives the physician the opportunity to establish a trusting relationship with the patient, so the therapeutic program will be followed and amplified by the positive effect of the physician's optimism and reassurance.

PRESENTING SYMPTOMS

Characteristically patients with asthma have some combination of dyspnea, wheeze, chest tightness, and cough. The salient feature is not so much the actual description of the symptom, which will be discussed, but the episodic and variable nature of the complaint. There is as much variability from time to time in a given patient as between patients.

The diagnosis can often be made quickly and accurately from the patient's description of complaints, although it should be confirmed by appropriate measurement of expiratory flow rates (see later). Symptoms may follow exposure to specific agents, such as inhaled or ingested antigens or viral infections. More often symptoms develop without identifiable cause. Rarely are symptoms so severe at the onset as to require medical attention, and when the patient first comes to a physician the diagnosis has often been correctly made by others. One of the common features is development or worsening of symptoms at night (see Chap. 76). It is known that both normal people and asthmatic patients have circadian rhythms of peak expiratory flow rate (PEFR) [24, 25]; PEFR is lowest between 3 and 6 A.M. [63]. As a result, it is common for patients to wake in the early morning with symptoms of asthma.

In some patients the symptoms may be relatively sustained and chronic. Although asthma may develop at any age, from the first to the eighth decade, it is common for older patients in whom cough and dyspnea first develop to be given a mistaken diagnosis of chronic obstructive pulmonary disease (COPD). Particular attention must be paid to the establishment of the correct diagnosis in these patients since proper therapy is so important. Clues to asthma include the presence of eosinophils in blood and sputum, and substantial improvement of expiratory flow rates after inhalation of a bronchodilator. In some individuals, it may be necessary to give a short course of corticosteroids to exclude an asthmatic component in the illness.

Dyspnea

Shortness of breath is an extremely common but not invariable complaint of patients with asthma. The nature of this symptom has been studied and discussed for years but remains poorly understood. It is likely, however, that it is related in some fashion to the sense of effort required to achieve adequate ventilation and is, to a degree, a function of the severity of airway obstruction. Nevertheless, there is a poor correlation between the sense of dyspnea and measurable airway resistance, in part because the degree of hyperventilation associated with asthma varies. The greater the ventilation, the greater the respiratory effort and, perhaps, the attendant distress. Since all types of intrathoracic airway obstruction are more severe during expiration than inspiration, one might expect that patients would complain of greater difficulty expiring than inspiring. In fact in one survey 78 percent of physicians reported believing that dyspnea was predominantly expiratory [42]. In the same study, however, only 19 percent of the patients complained of expiratory dyspnea, the majority indicating that the difficulty was most notable during inspiration. This is probably due to the fact that one of the characteristic features of asthma is sustained and tonic activity of the inspiratory muscles [43]. The chest is maintained in a relatively inflated position so as to make it possible to expire from the increased elastic recoil of the distended lung. In fact there is tonic activity of the inspiratory muscles throughout expiration as well as inspiration, and this excessive, much of it wasted, inspiratory muscle activity is undoubtedly a major cause of the sense of shortness of breath.

Wheeze

The high velocity of flow through narrowed large airways produces wheeze, which is often just as audible to the patient as to the physician. Many patients note wheeze during periods of asthma, but it is by no means present all of the time, and its absence should not exclude consideration of the diagnosis.

Patients are quite accurate in their perception of wheezing. We found that of 165 occasions when patients reported that they had wheezing, a wheeze was heard by a physician 95 percent of the time [58]. When patients claimed that they were free of wheeze (132 occasions), they were correct 71 percent of the time. The PEFR was significantly lower (39% of normal) when wheeze was present than when it was absent (63% of normal). See also Chapter 51.

Tightness

One of the characteristic symptoms of asthma, probably the most common one, is the sense of chest tightness. Patients commonly volunteer that their symptoms are associated with this sensation of tightness; if they do not do so, when asked they will almost always say they have tightness. It is likely that this sensation reflects the excessive activity of the vagal irritant receptors known to be a fundamental feature of asthma. In experimental animals, rapid shallow breathing can be induced by inhalation of bronchoconstricting drugs even if bronchoconstriction is prevented by inhalation of a bronchodilator, and it is possible to record increased afferent activity from the vagus nerve from this stimulation of the irritant receptors (see Chap. 17). In patients it is quite likely that a component of this sensory stimulus relates to bronchoconstriction, but since tightness can occur without wheeze or dyspnea or, for that matter, without reduction of expiratory flow rates, tightness is probably a direct reflection of irritant receptor activity rather than of airway obstruction.

Cough

Cough is a common feature of asthma. Cough often develops as patients start to improve and the inspissated mucous plugs that have occluded airways are dislodged into the tracheobronchial tree so that they can be expectorated. In addition, however, cough may occur early and, in fact, may be the only symptom in some patients. McFadden described two interesting groups of patients with asthma who complained either of cough alone or of exertional dyspnea at a time when they were free of audible wheeze [35]. In the group with cough, there was evidence that the obstruction was primarily in the larger airways; substantial improvement after inhalation of bronchodilators suggested that the cough was largely due to contraction of bronchial smooth muscle. In contrast, the patients complaining of dyspnea had a marked increase in residual volume and reduced expiratory flow rates suggestive of peripheral airway obstruction, perhaps by mucosal edema or secretions. The important clinical point, however, is that cough, like dyspnea, may be the sole manifestation of asthma [11], and patients with unexplained cough should be given a trial of bronchodilators even if expiratory flow rates are normal [22].

Since cough, like chest tightness, need not be associated with a reduction of expiratory flow rates, it may well be a reflection of irritant receptor activity. On the other hand, one of the notable effects of inhaled atropine is a reduction of cough. Since this drug acts on the muscarinic receptors in smooth muscle and has little if any afferent activity, one must presume that bronchoconstriction is an important contributor to the symptom. See also Chapter 50.

Upper Airway Symptoms

Although asthma is primarily a disorder of the intrathoracic airways, some patients do indicate that their symptoms originate in the region of the larynx. Lisboa and associates produced evidence that there is narrowing of the extrathoracic upper airways in asthma and that this may contribute to the reduction of inspiratory and expiratory flow rates [31]. They described a patient in whom inspiratory stridor was induced by a bronchoscopy at which time the vocal cords were noted to come into close apposition, particularly during inspiration. Rarely, vocal cord dysfunc-

tion simulates asthma. Christopher and associates described five such patients in whom wheeze and dyspnea were due to adduction of the vocal cords, probably because of an emotional disturbance [8]. We recently saw such a patient who was intubated because of marked respiratory distress and the incorrect diagnosis of asthma. A useful clue to the correct diagnosis is the ability of patients with vocal cord dysfunction to hold their breath, in contrast to asthmatic patients [38]. Psychotherapy and speech therapy may offer effective treatment. See also Chapter 41.

Cor Pulmonale

Rarely, asthma presents as cor pulmonale [12]. We have seen three such patients who apparently ignored their symptoms of asthma or were not troubled by them enough to seek medical assistance so that they continued to have airflow obstruction for long enough to get chronic pulmonary hypertension and right-sided heart failure, which disappeared after treatment of the asthma. This is but one illustration of the many faces of asthma, which can range from trivial to life-threatening spasmodic disease to various types of chronic airway obstruction.

HISTORY

As discussed above, careful description of the nature and timing of symptoms is extremely important in suggesting a diagnosis of asthma. In addition, other historical information may contribute to an understanding of the patient's illness and make it possible to advise avoidance of conditions associated with worsening symptoms.

Clearly, genetic factors are involved in the development of asthma (see Chap. 3), and a large percentage of patients have a family history of asthma or allergic disease. What is not clear is the degree to which familial factors are due to inheritance rather than a common environment. There is evidence for independent inheritance of asthma and atopy [59], and there are a few studies of identical twins reporting that one twin had asthma and the other was perfectly normal, even with respect to airway reactivity. In exploring the family history, the physician has the opportunity to gain understanding of the patient's own perceptions of the condition, which are often associated with anxiety and fear based on experience with a parent or sibling.

In some patients, asthma appears by history to be related to seasons of the year, to exposure to pets (notoriously cats), and to ingestion of certain foods. This should prompt the suspicion of an allergic basis for the condition and, possibly, study of specific antigens by skin testing or bronchial provocation (see Chaps. 39 and 40). Sensitivity to mites, detailed in Chapter 42, is being increasingly recognized in asthmatics [47], and such patients may be effectively treated by desensitization [33]. In adults, however, it appears that specific antigens are rarely of major importance in causing symptoms and disability. The most common cause of an exacerbation of asthma in adults is a viral infection (see Chap. 44). In fact, there is a great deal of epidemiologic and clinical evidence that viral but not bacterial infections are a major cause of worsening of asthma [7, 52]. If worsening can be clearly related to upper respiratory tract infections, it may be wise to intensify therapy at the first sign of such an illness to prevent severe airway obstruction. The history is of great importance in making this decision. There is a long list of substances in the working environment and in the natural environment that are associated with worsening asthma [3], and a careful occupational history is obviously extremely important (see Chap. 46). A wide variety of agents, ranging from simple elements such as nickel [4] to more complex organic chemicals, can produce asthma by allergic or other means. In many patients symptoms appear to result from strong odors!

One of the most common causes of worsening asthma is exercise or breathing of cold air (see Chap. 47). These events are coupled because it has now been shown that the bronchoconstriction that almost invariably follows exercise is related to heat loss in the respiratory tract [37]. Thus, the severity of bronchoconstriction becomes a function of temperature and humidity of the inspired air as well as of the magnitude of the ventilation induced by exercise. A history of exercise-induced symptoms, particularly in cold weather, is strongly suggestive of asthma and may necessitate either avoidance or prophylactic therapy.

In the clinical evaluation, it is important to remember that other diseases may be important in inducing symptoms of asthma. Many patients have associated sinusitis; if this is successfully treated, the asthma may improve [60] (see Chap. 41). There have been a number of reports of an association between asthma and gastroesophageal reflux [10, 30]. This may be one mechanism for the nocturnal worsening discussed in the previous section (see Chap. 75). Very commonly in women asthma is worse just before the onset of the menstrual period, and this has been documented by a reduction of PEFR at that time [15, 21]. The mechanism is unknown but probably relates to arachidonic acid metabolism and may turn out to be responsive to appropriate pharmacologic therapy.

Most physicians are convinced that emotional factors are extremely important in causing worsening or improvement of asthma (see Chap. 85). This is very difficult to prove, and there is little evidence of specific psychological profiles or psychodynamic events common to patients with asthma. On the other hand, suggestion can cause a measurable change in airway resistance and, at the least, the positive attitude of the physician can reinforce and amplify the pharmacologic action of drugs. If, in taking a history, the physician can uncover specific events that are associated with asthma, he or she may be able to provide valuable advice or even, in some cases, suggest major changes in life-style so as to enhance self-esteem and satisfaction, which may be followed by improvement.

A great many drugs may be associated with asthma (see Chap. 48). Two groups of compounds are particularly important. Aspirin and to a lesser extent nonsteroidal antiinflammatory drugs and azo dyes may produce a particularly explosive form of asthma in sensitive subjects [65]. Such a reaction is common among women with sinusitis but may occur in others. The azo dyes that produce this reaction are present in a variety of preserved foods and drugs so that a detailed history may be very important [61]. The mechanism of this reaction is not clear. It is not immunologic but rather apparently relates to effects on arachidonic acid metabolism. Nonetheless, patients sensitive to aspirin may be desensitized so that they can take the drug without having symptoms develop and may even experience improvement of asthma [48]. The other important group of provocative agents are the beta-adrenergic blocking drugs. Although bronchoconstriction does not occur in normal subjects when given doses producing full beta blockade, it does in patients with asthma [68]. In fact, asthma may first develop after the ingestion of these drugs [18] or even after their application as eye drops for the treatment of glaucoma [51]. Careful questioning is important to learn whether or not the patient is under the effect of any beta-blocking agent. The fact that beta blockers have no effect on normal subjects but do have such an explosive one in asthmatics suggests that in patients with asthma, endogenous catecholamines are essential in maintaining bronchodilation in the face of the powerful cholinergic stimuli that characterize the disease. The effect is so common and so important—potentially lethal—that beta blockers should be avoided by all patients with asthma or, at the very least, given only under careful supervision.

As mentioned above, some patients appear to be allergic to certain foods, particularly shellfish, chocolates, and peanuts. In addition, metabisulfites, used to preserve the color of salad greens and to stabilize wines and beers, may precipitate explosive asthma in sensitive subjects [14]. See Chapter 43 for further details.

Finally, it is very important to learn whether a patient has ever experienced severe asthma requiring respiratory therapy or intubation. Although such life-threatening asthma is rare, probably occurring no more commonly than in 0.2 percent of patients with asthma per year, and although it generally does not occur until a patient has had asthma for many years, once it occurs it is apt to happen again [67]. In fact, about 10 percent of patients who have life-threatening asthma experience a recurrence each year. Such high-risk individuals must be identified and treated with extra care when their symptoms worsen.

PHYSICAL FINDINGS

On physical examination, the well-known hallmark of asthma is the presence of wheezing in the chest. Because of turbulent airflow through narrowed airways, wheeze is produced during both inspiration and expiration. This wheeze is typically polyphonic, of differing intensity and tone from time to time and place to place over the chest. It is apt to be more notable during expiration, when the airways are narrower, than during inspiration, and it may improve after inhalation of a bronchodilator. But, as emphasized above, a wheeze is not always present. It is particularly important to remember that patients may have such severe airway obstruction as to be unable to generate sufficiently rapid airflow to produce the characteristic sound. We have performed 320 auscultatory examinations of 93 patients with asthma to learn whether there were any features that correlated with the severity of airway obstruction [58]. We found that wheeze was not usually restricted to expiration but was twice as commonly present on both inspiration and expiration. Wheezing on both inspiration and expiration was associated with a significantly lower PEFR (36% normal) than expiratory wheezing alone (49% normal). Wheeze was rarely confined to inspiration. There was a significant correlation between the intensity (loudness) of wheeze and the reduction of PEFR, and low-pitch wheezing was associated with a significantly higher PEFR than high-pitch wheezing. Finally, holoexpiratory wheezing was associated with a lower PEFR than wheeze occurring either early or late in expiration. Although these data are interesting, the scatter was large. Accurate assessment of the severity of airway obstruction in an individual patient requires a measurement of expiratory flow rate such as PEFR. See also Chapter 51, dealing with wheezing in asthma.

Wheezing is obviously not diagnostic of asthma. Chapter 37 details the differential considerations required for proper clinical evaluation.

Other important physical findings relate to the severity of the airway obstruction. As discussed previously, excessive activity of the inspiratory muscles serves to maintain maximal inflation of the chest so as to allow elastic recoil to produce expiration but leads to hyperinflation of the chest. Although there may be some increase of total lung capacity in acute asthma, radiographic measurements have failed to confirm this finding [49] and much of the hyperinflation is chronic. Of more importance is detection of the activity of the inspiratory muscles, notably the scalenes and the sternocleidomastoid if the obstruction is severe. We believe that there is a general relationship between the severity of airway obstruction and the palpable activity of scalene muscles, notable only during inspiration in mild cases but present throughout the respiratory cycle in patients with severe asthma [43]. In fact, this activity is so great as to limit generation of expiratory flow rate [62] and may be a major factor in the ultimate development of respiratory muscle fatigue and respiratory arrest. This activity of the inspiratory muscles is reflected in the general appearance of the patient who makes rapid forceful inspiratory efforts and then more slowly expires against pursed lips. The appearance is one of active inspiratory distress rather than work during expiration.

Although these findings of inspiratory muscle activity are characteristic of asthma and obviously absent between attacks, they are not useful in evaluating the severity of asthma [56]. It has been suggested that the development of pulsus paradoxus is a useful means of identifying patients with severe asthma. It is known that the very negative pleural pressure generated during an acute attack of asthma is associated with a fall of blood pressure during inspiration, and that the amount of this fall bears a rough relationship to the severity of airway obstruction. However, this relationship is imperfect; patients with severe airway obstruction may not have pulsus paradoxus and patients with pulsus paradoxus need not have marked reduction of expiratory flow rates [55]. The magnitude of the pulsus paradoxus is, as mentioned, a function of the pleural pressure swing, which in turn depends on the respiratory effort developed by the patient. An anxious patient, working very hard to breathe against moderately obstructed airways, may generate very negative pleural pressure and pulsus paradoxus; conversely, a patient with respiratory muscle fatigue and severe obstruction may fail to have this finding. Thus, the time and effort required to obtain an accurate measurement of pulsus paradoxus are probably not warranted clinically and should not replace the simple measurement of PEFR.

LABORATORY STUDIES

Pulmonary Function Studies

The most important laboratory studies in asthma are measurements of pulmonary function, since they reflect the severity and document the reversibility of the airway obstruction. The diagnosis of asthma is generally based on a 25 percent or greater increase of expiratory flow rate after inhalation of a bronchodilator (see later). The physiologic and gas exchange abnormalities characteristic of asthma, detailed in Chapter 26, all stem from airway obstruction [36]. Obviously the degree of spirometric disturbance depends on the severity of obstruction, ranging from absent to pronounced in an individual patient as well as among different patients. The most important abnormalities are slowing of the expiratory flow rate, reflected in reduction of forced expiratory volume in 1 second (FEV_1), PEFR, and maximal midexpiratory flow rate. Any one of these measurements may provide an accurate indication of the severity of obstruction, and there is a rough correlation among them. Although the PEFR is effort dependent, it is quite reproducible, even in sick patients, and is particularly useful because it can be measured without a forced, complete expiration, which is apt to produce cough and worsening of obstruction. In addition the peak flow meter is inexpensive and portable and allows the patient to obtain measurements at home so as to gauge the severity of obstruction and regulate therapy [13, 66]. Spirometric abnormalities include reduction of vital capacity, stemming from closure of airways at larger than normal lung volumes, which generally parallels the decreased flow rates. Airway resistance, more difficult to measure, may be elevated as much during inspiration as in expiration in asthma, in contrast to other types of obstructive lung disease. To maintain expiratory flow rates, patients with asthma breathe at a larger lung volume, so that functional residual capacity is increased. In chronic cases, the total lung capacity is increased, which is reflected in hyperinflation on the roentgenogram. In general, simple spirometric measurements are all that are needed to evaluate the clinical severity of asthma, but in some patients other tests may be useful to assess the presence of emphysema. These include the diffusing capacity and lung recoil, both of which are reduced in proportion to the extent of emphysema.

Two important features of ventilatory function should be emphasized. In some patients with asthma, some airways appear to be completely occluded, with relatively little limitation of expiratory flow rate through other bronchi, so that the spirometric pattern is one of restrictive rather than obstructive lung disease [28]. The characteristic spirometric finding is relative preservation of the FEV_1/FVC.* Patients hospitalized with asthma generally have a higher FEV_1/FVC than those with other types of obstructive lung disease [9], because the totally occluded airways cause similar reductions of FEV_1 and vital capacity without detectable slowing of the rest of the expiration. Patients manifesting this phenomenon may develop total atelectasis, either of one lung or of a lobe, occasionally without wheeze or detectable airway obstruction [26]. This is interesting evidence that the formation of occluding secretions may be independent of generalized bronchoconstriction, although obviously the two are often associated.

Another important consideration is that patients with asthma who have had a tracheostomy or endotracheal intubation are later at risk of developing upper airway obstruction. This is often associated with stridor, particularly during inspiration, audible over the trachea or larynx and can best be confirmed by measuring inspiratory as well as expiratory flow rates [53]. In patients with upper airway obstruction, the inspiratory flow rate is more reduced than is the expiratory flow rate, in contrast to other types of obstructive lung disease, in which expiration is much more affected.

Arterial Blood Gases

Although measurements of arterial blood gases are not useful in diagnosing asthma, they do reflect the severity and ventilatory status. Irritant receptor activity, resulting from inhalation of agents producing asthma or from bronchoconstriction, and anxiety cause hyperventilation in patients with asthma [40]. When the airway obstruction becomes severe, the patient may not be able to maintain the required alveolar ventilation, or respiratory muscle fatigue may develop so that the arterial carbon dioxide tension ($PaCO_2$) tends to rise, a well-known feature of severe asthma that necessitates intensive observation and care. Because of this hyperventilation, most patients with asthma have a respiratory alkalosis until the $PaCO_2$ rises, at which time the pH may become acidemic. In addition, acidosis resulting from lactic acid accumulation may be present in some patients with hypocapnia [1]. Lactic acidosis apparently results from increased respiratory muscle activity and, possibly, diminished hepatic function, either from elevated venous pressure or from diminished hepatic artery blood flow. It has been shown, furthermore, that the development of lactic acidosis, characterized by a pH lower than predicted from the $PaCO_2$ and an anion gap in excess of 15 mEq/L, indicates severe asthma that is apt to lead to ventilatory failure.

The arterial oxygen tension is almost always reduced in acute asthma but uncommonly to levels less than 50 mmHg [40]. The hypoxemia is not as severe as generally encountered in patients with exacerbations of COPD and may not require therapy with oxygen. Hypoxemia results from abnormalities of ventilation-perfusion ratios in various parts of the lung, resulting from variable degrees of obstruction to the airways. It will improve with therapy. Hypoxemia may paradoxically worsen after administration of bronchodilator drugs, but this is not of sufficient consequence to withhold such medication.

X-ray

The radiographic findings in asthma that assist in the clinical appraisal are discussed in Chapter 53. The main feature is hyper-

---

* Forced vital capacity.

inflation, particularly in patients with chronic symptoms. Otherwise, roentgenographic abnormalities relate to complications such as pneumonia, barotrauma (pneumomediastinum and pneumothorax), or atelectasis from mucoid impaction of bronchi [6]. In most patients the roentgenogram is normal, and there is evidence that radiography is not always necessary in patients with acute symptoms [16]. Radiographic examination may be important in evaluating a precipitating pneumonia, but certainly every patient presenting to an emergency room with worsening symptoms does not have to undergo radiography on each visit.

It is very common for patients with acute asthma to have perfusion defects in the lung [29]. These defects probably result from hyperinflation of some of the alveolar capillaries distal to partially obstructed airways and possibly from hypoxic vasoconstriction in such units. The perfusion defects are important because they are so common and have frequently led to a misdiagnosis of pulmonary embolism. But they are of little consequence with regard to the course and treatment of asthma.

Electrocardiogram

Asthma is associated with relative pulmonary hypertension owing to the hyperinflated lungs and markedly negative pleural pressure. As a result, electrocardiographic changes are very common, P pulmonale being present in up to 50 percent of patients with asthma, depending on severity [19]. Right axis deviation is less common. These changes generally return toward normal within 2 to 5 days. Cardiac interactions in asthma are discussed further in Chapter 78.

Blood Cell Count

Leukocytosis is very common in asthma, a total white blood cell count of 20,000/mm³ being average for hospitalized patients. This may result from the stress of asthma, from repeated injections of epinephrine, or from corticosteroids. The leukocytosis may also reflect augmented leukocyte chemotactic activity, one of the products of mast cell release in asthma [44].

The eosinophil count is elevated in asthma, generally in excess of 300/mm³, regardless of whether there is an associated allergic or atopic component [27]. The count generally falls within 24 to 36 hours after administration of corticosteroids [32]. Eosinophilia is considered by some an indication that larger doses of corticosteroids are necessary for the treatment of asthma. In some patients, however, the asthma remains severe despite eosinopenia. A more rational approach to management is therefore based on expiratory flow rates rather than the eosinophil count. Thus, although eosinophilia suggests the need for more steroids, some patients may benefit from steroid therapy even though the eosinophil count is already suppressed.

Sputum

Patients with asthma characteristically expectorate mucous plugs easily visible when the sputum is suspended in water. Microscopic examination reveals Curschmann's spirals and, generally, clumps of eosinophils. Like blood eosinophilia, sputum eosinophilia does not necessarily signify allergic disease and may be present in patients with bronchitis [46]. In some patients with obstructive lung disease, clumps of eosinophils in the sputum may indicate responsiveness to corticosteroids [54] (see Chap. 52 for detailed discussion).

Blood Chemistry

There are no characteristic abnormalities of blood chemistry in patients with acute or chronic asthma except for elevation of serum creatine phosphokinase [20]. This enzyme is released from

Table 35-1. Diagnosis of asthma

Patient's condition	Criterion
Asymptomatic	Induce 25% fall in expiratory flow rate by provocation (exercise, inhalation challenge) with reversal by bronchodilator
Symptomatic	Observe 25% or greater improvement of expiratory flow rate with bronchodilator

the overactive respiratory muscles and may reach levels close to 1,000 units. It is simply another indirect marker of clinical severity.

DIAGNOSIS

The diagnosis of asthma is based on the demonstration of variable and reversible airway obstruction. As indicated, this diagnosis may be strongly suggested by a characteristic history but must be confirmed by the demonstration of variability of and reversibility of reduced expiratory flow rates. Clearly the approach to the asymptomatic patient differs from that used when the patient is symptomatic (Table 35-1).

Asymptomatic Patient

When the patient is asymptomatic at the time of examination, the history is particularly important in raising the suspicion of asthma. Then if expiratory flow rates are normal, as they often are, the diagnosis should be based on a demonstration of reduced expiratory flow rates after suitable provocation. This should be followed by a return to normal values after inhalation of an adrenergic aerosol. There are a variety of methods for demonstrating abnormal reactivity of the airways. These are outlined in Chapters 4, 36, and 39, and in the superb monograph edited by Hargreave [23]. A simple test that can be employed by the physician is based on the fact that almost all patients with asthma, even while asymptomatic, have reduced expiratory flow rates after exercise [37]. (Exercise-associated asthma is discussed in Chap. 47.) The physician may utilize this phenomenon by having the patient perform exercise, such as running up and down stairs, and then measuring PEFR. If immediately after exercise, the PEFR has fallen by 20 percent and promptly returns to normal after inhalation of a beta agonist, the diagnosis of asthma is highly likely.

An alternative approach is to have patients measure their own PEFR with a peak flow meter during daily activities at home. PEFR is known to fall in the early morning, and substantial diurnal variation is strongly suggestive of asthma. If, in addition, the patient records a low PEFR at the time of symptoms, after exercise or inhalation of cold air, or after exposure to agents that are thought to produce tightness, dyspnea, and wheeze, and if there is return to baseline after inhalation of a beta agonist, the diagnosis is well established.

Symptomatic Patient

In patients who present with the typical history and symptoms, in whom the physical examination reveals wheezing and the other findings noted above, the diagnosis of asthma is established by measuring a reduction of expiratory flow rates with at least a 25 percent improvement after inhalation of a beta agonist (see Table 35-1). The difficulties with such a diagnostic approach relate to the marked variability in the effect of such drugs from time to time in a given patient. For example, very mild airway obstruction may show little improvement since the patient is near normal, or if the obstruction is very severe, from mucous plugging and inflammatory changes that are not immediately reversible, there may be little, if any, improvement. For this reason, the measurements should be obtained several times, at each visit to the physician or in between by the patient at home with a portable peak flow meter. Since patients with COPD generally reveal some improvement with bronchodilators, it is difficult to say just how much improvement warrants a diagnosis of asthma. Asthma is likely if a single inhalation of the beta agonist produces an immediate improvement of greater than 25 percent, but patients with COPD can, during the course of the day, demonstrate as much as 70 percent improvement in expiratory flow rates in conjunction with therapy and mobilization of obstructing secretions by cough.

In testing the effects of adrenergic aerosols, one must be certain that the patient has developed a good inhalation technique. It is surprising how many patients with asthma who have used aerosols for months or years simply do not know how to use the medication properly [57]. Obviously both in the physician's office and in the home, good inhalation technique is essential if one is to draw a correct conclusion from this test.

It is often difficult to distinguish patients with asthma from those with COPD. Since, as mentioned above, asthma can develop late in life, since symptoms may be relatively chronic and persistent, and since on many occasions there may be little response to beta agonists, it is essential that multiple measurements be obtained before and after inhalation of bronchodilator aerosol to help distinguish these groups. In some patients it is helpful to obtain more detailed studies of pulmonary function since emphysema, in contrast to asthma, is characterized by a reduction of diffusing capacity and lung elastic recoil. But the overlap is great, and it is often a matter of judgment as to whether or not the patient should be diagnosed as having asthma or COPD. Often one is left with the conclusion that a patient has COPD with a reversible component, which requires the same vigorous therapy as for asthma. It is particularly important to learn whether or not there is a steroid-responsive component to the COPD; recent data indicate that a substantial number of patients with COPD respond to corticosteroids [41]. Although such patients are apt to have a better response to bronchodilators and are more likely to have sputum eosinophilia [54] than patients who do not respond to steroids, this is not always the case, and it is probably wise to give all patients with COPD a therapeutic trial of corticosteroids. Since improvement should be evident within 2 or 3 days, generally reaching a maximum within 8 days [64], a 2-week trial is more than adequate. But it must be coupled with measurements of expiratory flow rates, preferably daily by the patient at home, to evaluate the response properly.

The differential diagnosis of asthma is discussed in detail in Chapter 37. Two conditions that are said to offer the most difficulty are pulmonary embolism and pulmonary edema. Despite some reports, wheezing is very rare in pulmonary embolism, and the dyspnea is rarely associated with major airway obstruction. Cardiac asthma has long been described as a feature of pulmonary edema, but again it is unlikely that wheezing is a common feature of pulmonary edema unless the patient has underlying obstructive lung disease. Studies of ventilatory function characteristically reveal a marked reduction of vital capacity in pulmonary edema with little if any decrease of expiratory flow rates. To reiterate a note of caution, asthmatic patients with mucous plugging may have a restrictive pattern on spirometry. However, the characteristic appearance of a patient with pulmonary edema—cold, sweating, and with inspiratory crackles—contrasted with the anxious, labored breathing with wheeze of the asthmatic patient usually offers little clinical difficulty. Vascular redistribution and, in advanced cases, alveolar infiltrate on

x-ray film characterize pulmonary edema, while blood or sputum eosinophilia may be a helpful indication of asthma. If the diagnosis is still not clear, administration of a beta agonist by aerosol and low doses of theophylline (0.5 mg/kg/hr) by vein may be useful.

The need for assessing upper airway obstruction by measurement of inspiratory flow rate was discussed above.

EVALUATION OF SEVERITY

Chronic

Although not proved, it is generally believed that asthma should be treated early, when it is mild, and that if left untreated it may become more refractory to therapy. If this is so, it is extremely important to identify and treat early airway obstruction before it becomes severe. There is substantial evidence that physicians are unable, by examining the patient, to make an accurate assessment of the severity of airway obstruction [56]. The only way that this can be done accurately is to measure expiratory flow rates. For this reason spirometry values, PEFR, or both should always be measured when a patient with asthma is seen by a physician. If asthma proves refractory to therapy, the patient should measure his or her own PEFR at home and regulate therapy accordingly. Patients trained to measure their own peak flow can actually estimate this value with surprising accuracy [56]. As a result, with appropriate training the patient can learn to identify symptoms of asthma when the obstruction is mild. In addition, as mentioned above, there are some patients in whom tightness and cough warrant therapy even in the absence of airway obstruction.

Acute

Physicians vary greatly in their assessment of the severity of airway obstruction, and their assessment correlates poorly with lung function [39, 56]. While it is true that contraction of the sternocleidomastoid muscles and the presence of pulsus paradoxus generally indicate severe asthma, even these indices are imperfect. Hence it is essential that severity be evaluated by measurements of expiratory flow rate (Table 35-2).

As mentioned above, hypercapnia, or even a normal $PaCO_2$, in the presence of airway obstruction, indicates that asthma is very severe, as does metabolic acidosis. But it is impractical to measure arterial blood gases in the patient severely ill with asthma

Table 35-2. Severe asthma

Feature	Finding
Expiratory flow rate	PEFR reduced to ≤100 L/min
Wheeze	Usually high-pitched, throughout both inspiration and expiration; may be absent ("silent chest")
Pulsus paradoxus	Often >20 mmHg; may not be present when respiratory effort decreases
Contraction of accessory muscles	Palpable, sustained contraction of scalenes; visible inspiratory contraction of sternocleidomastoid
Arterial blood gases	
$PaCO_2$	Generally <40 torr with alkaline pH; increase of $PaCO_2$ (respiratory acidosis) indicates very severe asthma
PaO_2	50–80 torr; mild to moderate hypoxemia
Metabolic acidosis	Acid pH with normal or reduced $PaCO_2$ and anion gap >15 mEq/L suggests lactic acidosis caused by severe asthma

PEFR = peak expiratory flow rate; $PaCO_2$ = arterial carbon dioxide tension; PaO_2 = arterial oxygen tension.

as frequently as necessary to guide therapy, and, in fact, such measurements are generally not necessary. If at the first examination the $PaCO_2$ is reduced and the pH is normal or alkaline, measurements of blood gases need not be repeated unless there is a deterioration of PEFR [5, 34] or unless severe asthma persists for several hours with evidence that the patient is becoming fatigued or obtunded. Blood gas measurements need not be obtained for all asthma patients appearing at the emergency room but are indicated if admission is necessary or if expiratory flow rates fail to respond to the initial treatment.

In assessing acute clinical severity, Banner and his associates pointed out that patients with severe airway obstruction (reflected in a PEFR less than 16% of predicted) who had less than 16 percent improvement after injection of epinephrine almost always required hospitalization; such patients should be admitted promptly [2]. Similar guidelines have been published by others [45]. Fischl and associates developed an index based on several factors, including PEFR, that they found to be highly predictive of need for hospitalization [17]. They found that the initial evaluation was more predictive than was the response to treatment after 1 hour, but clearly there are patients in whom dramatic improvement may follow the administration of beta agonist. It has become our policy to admit patients to a hospital if the PEFR remains less than 100 L/min after an hour of therapy. Other indicators of severe asthma requiring hospitalization include hypercapnia, metabolic acidosis, and a history of severe, life-threatening asthma, since it is known that such an episode is frequently followed by a recurrence [67].

Once a patient has been hospitalized, the course of the asthma must be continuously followed by measurements of PEFR and intermittent measurements of arterial blood gases. It is sometimes very difficult to decide which patients require intubation and artificial ventilation. Since most patients with asthma maintain maximal respiratory activity until the time of respiratory arrest (probably caused by respiratory muscle fatigue and failure, which may develop with great rapidity), the goal is to anticipate impending arrest and need for artificial ventilation. There is no level of respiratory function or of arterial blood gas derangement that mandates intubation, but criteria include sustained, severe obstruction; hypercapnia; obtundation; and distress (see Chap. 73). The judgment of the physician is critical in deciding when the respiratory muscles are about to fail. Clues to respiratory muscle failure include incoordinate movement of the diaphragm and intercostals, reflected in intermittent and irregular abdominal protrusion during inspiration. However, this whole problem requires much more study so that impending respiratory muscle failure can be detected and treated with artificial ventilation [50].

REFERENCES

1. Appel, D., et al. Lactic acidosis in severe asthma. *Am. J. Med.* 75:580, 1983.
2. Banner, A. S., Shah, R. S., and Addington, W. W. Rapid prediction of need for hospitalization in acute asthma. *JAMA* 235:1337, 1976.
3. Bernstein, I. L. Occupational asthma. *Clin. Chest Med.* 2:255, 1981.
4. Block, G. T., and Yeung, M. Asthma induced by nickel. *JAMA* 247:1600, 1982.
5. Bondi, E., and Williams, M. H., Jr. Severe asthma. *NY State J. Med.* 77:350, 1977.
6. Braman, S. S., and Whitcomb, M. E. Mucoid impaction of the bronchus. *JAMA* 223:641, 1973.
7. Busse, W. W. Respiratory infections: Their role in airway responsiveness and the pathogenesis of asthma. *J. Allergy Clin. Immunol.* 85:671, 1990.
8. Christopher, K. L., et al. Vocal-cord dysfunction presenting as asthma. *N. Engl. J. Med.* 308:1566, 1983.
9. Colp, C., and Williams, M. H., Jr. Total occlusion of airways producing a restrictive pattern of ventilatory impairment. *Am. Rev. Respir. Dis.* 108:118, 1973.
10. Cooper, D. N., Bernstein, A., and Temple, J. G. Relationship between asthma and gastro-oesophageal reflux. *Thorax* 36:116, 1981.
11. Corrao, W. M., Braman, S. S., and Irwin, R. S. Chronic cough as the sole presenting manifestation of bronchial asthma. *N. Engl. J. Med.* 300:633, 1979.
12. Corris, P. A., and Gibson, C. J. Asthma presenting as cor pulmonale. *Br. Med. J.* 288:299, 1984.
13. Daman, H. R. Peak expiratory flow rate. *NY State J. Med.* 80:1125, 1980.
14. Delohery, J., et al. The relationship of inhaled sulfur dioxide reactivity to ingested metabisulfite sensitivity in patients with asthma. *Am. Rev. Respir. Dis.* 130:1027, 1984.
15. Eliasson, O., Scherzer, H. H., and Degraff, A. C., Jr. Morbidity in asthma in relation to the menstrual cycle. *J. Allergy Clin. Immunol.* 77:87, 1986.
16. Findley, L. J., and Sahn, S. A. The value of chest roentgenograms in acute asthma in adults. *Chest* 80:535, 1981.
17. Fischl, M. A., Pitchenik, A., and Gardner, L. B. An index predicting relapse and need for hospitalization in patients with acute bronchial asthma. *N. Engl. J. Med.* 305:783, 1981.
18. Fraley, D. S., et al. Propranolol related bronchospasm in patients without history of asthma. *South. Med. J.* 73:238, 1980.
19. Gelb, A. F., et al. P pulmonale in status asthmaticus. *J. Allergy Clin. Immunol.* 64:18, 1979.
20. Gualde, N., et al. Serum creatine phosphokinase activity in asthma. *Am. Rev. Respir. Dis.* 116:327, 1977.
21. Hanley, S. P. Asthma variation with menstruation. *Br. J. Dis. Chest* 75:306, 1981.
22. Hannaway, P. J., and Hopper, D. K. Cough variant asthma in children. *JAMA* 247:206, 1982.
23. Hargreave, F. E. (ed.), *Airway Reactivity.* ASTRA Pharmaceutical, 1980.
24. Hetzel, M. R., and Clark, T. J. H. Does sleep cause nocturnal asthma? *Thorax* 34:749, 1979.
25. Hetzel, M. R., and Clark, T. J. H. Comparison of normal and asthmatic circadian rhythms in peak expiratory flow rate. *Thorax* 35:732, 1980.
26. Hopkirk, J. A. C., and Stark, J. E. Unilateral pulmonary collapse in asthmatics. *Thorax* 33:207, 1978.
27. Horn, B. R., et al. Total eosinophil counts in the management of bronchial asthma. *N. Engl. J. Med.* 292:1152, 1975.
28. Hudgel, D. W., Cooper, D., and Souhrada, J. Reversible restrictive lung disease simulating asthma. *Ann. Intern. Med.* 85:328, 1976.
29. Hyde, J. S., et al. Technetium Tc 99m macroaggregated albumin lung scans. *JAMA* 235:1125, 1976.
30. Kjellen, G., et al. Oesophageal function in asthmatics. *Eur. J. Respir. Dis.* 62:87, 1981.
31. Lisboa, D., et al. Is extrathoracic airway obstruction important in asthma? *Am. Rev. Respir. Dis.* 122:115, 1980.
32. Lowell, F. C. The total eosinophil count in obstructive pulmonary disease. *N. Engl. J. Med.* 292:1182, 1975.
33. Machiels, J. J., et al. Allergic bronchial asthma due to *Dermatophagoides pteronyssimus* hypersensitivity can be efficiently treated by inoculation of allergen-antibody complexes. *J. Clin. Invest.* 85:1024, 1990.
34. Martin, T. G., Elenbaas, R. M., and Pingleton, S. H. Use of peak expiratory flow rates to eliminate unnecessary arterial blood gases in acute asthma. *Ann. Emerg. Med.* 11:70, 1982.
35. McFadden, E. R., Jr. Exertional dyspnea and cough as preludes to acute attacks of bronchial asthma. *N. Engl. J. Med.* 292:555, 1975.
36. McFadden, E. R., Jr. Asthma: Pathophysiology. *Semin. Respir. Med.* 1:297, 1980.
37. McFadden, E. R., Jr. An analysis of exercise as a stimulus for the production of airway obstruction. *Lung* 159:3, 1981.
38. McFadden, E. R., Jr. Glottic function and dysfunction. *J. Allergy Clin. Immunol.* 79:707, 1987.
39. McFadden, E. R., Jr., Kiser, R., and DeGroot, W. J. Acute bronchial asthma. *N. Engl. J. Med.* 288:221, 1973.
40. McFadden, E. R., Jr., and Lyons, H. A. Arterial-blood gas tension in asthma. *N. Engl. J. Med.* 278:1027, 1968.
41. Mendella, L. A., et al. Steroid response in stable chronic obstructive pulmonary disease. *Ann. Intern. Med.* 96:17, 1982.
42. Morris, M. J. Asthma: Expiratory dyspnea? *Br. Med. J.* 283:838, 1981.
43. Muller, N., Bryan, A. C., and Zamel, N. Tonic inspiratory muscle activity as a cause of hyperinflation in asthma. *J. Appl. Physiol.* 50:279, 1981.
44. Nagy, L., Lee, T. H., and Kay, A. B. Neutrophil chemotactic activity in antigen-induced late asthmatic reactions. *N. Engl. J. Med.* 306:497, 1982.
45. Nowak, R. M., et al. Comparison of peak expiratory flow and FEV_1 admission criteria for acute bronchial asthma. *Ann. Emerg. Med.* 11:64, 1982.
46. O'Connell, J. M., Baird, L. I., and Campbell, A. H. Sputum eosinophilia in chronic bronchitis and asthma. *Respiration* 35:65, 1978.

47. Platts-Mills, T. A. E. Dust mite allergens and asthma—A worldwide problem. *J. Allergy Clin. Immunol.* 83:416, 1989.
48. Pleskow, W. W., et al. Aspirin desensitization in aspirin-sensitive asthmatic patients: Clinical manifestations and characterization of the refractory period. *J. Allergy Clin. Immunol.* 69:11, 1982.
49. Rothstein, M. S., et al. Radiographic measurement of total lung capacity in acute asthma. *Thorax* 44:510, 1989.
50. Roussos, C. The failing ventilatory pump. *Lung* 160:59, 1982.
51. Schoene, R. B., et al. Timolol-induced bronchospasm in asthmatic bronchitis. *JAMA* 245:1458, 1981.
52. Sherter, C. B., and Polintsky, C. A. The relationship of viral infections to subsequent asthma. *Clin. Chest Med.* 2:67, 1981.
53. Shim, C., et al. Pulmonary function studies in patients with upper airway obstruction. *Am. Rev. Respir. Dis.* 106:233, 1972.
54. Shim, C., Stover, D. E., and Williams, M. H., Jr. Response to corticosteroids in chronic bronchitis. *J. Allergy Clin. Immunol.* 62:363, 1978.
55. Shim, C., and Williams, M. H., Jr. Pulsus paradoxus in asthma. *Lancet* 1:530, 1978.
56. Shim, C., and Williams, M. H., Jr. Evaluation of the severity of asthma: Patients versus physicians. *Am. J. Med.* 68:11, 1980.
57. Shim, C., and Williams, M. H., Jr. The adequacy of inhalation of aerosol from canister nebulizers. *Am. J. Med.* 69:891, 1980.
58. Shim, C. S., and Williams, M. H., Jr. Relationship of wheezing to the severity of asthma. *Arch. Intern. Med.* 143:890, 1983.
59. Sibbald, B., et al. Genetic factors in childhood asthma. *Thorax* 35:671, 1980.
60. Slavin, R. G., et al. Sinusitis and bronchial asthma. *J. Allergy Clin. Immunol.* 66:250, 1980.
61. Smith, L. J., and Slavin, R. G. Drugs containing tartrazine dye. *J. Allergy Clin. Immunol.* 58:456, 1976.
62. Stalcup, S. A., and Mellins, R. B. Mechanical forces producing pulmonary edema in acute asthma. *N. Engl. J. Med.* 297:592, 1977.
63. Todisco, T., et al. Circadian rhythms of respiratory function in asthmatics. *Respiration* 40:128, 1980.
64. Webb, J., Clark, T. J. H., and Chilvers, C. Time course of response to prednisolone in chronic airflow obstruction. *Thorax* 36:18, 1981.
65. Weber, R. W., et al. Incidence of bronchoconstriction due to aspirin, azo dyes, non-azo dyes, and preservatives in a population of perennial asthmatics. *J. Allergy Clin. Immunol.* 64:32, 1979.
66. Williams, M. H., Jr. Evaluation of asthma (editorial). *Chest* 76:3, 1979.
67. Williams, M. H., Jr. Life-threatening asthma. *Arch. Intern. Med.* 140:1604, 1980.
68. Zaid, G., and Beall, G. N. Bronchial response to beta-adrenergic blockade. *N. Engl. J. Med.* 275:580, 1966.

Methods of Assessing Bronchoreversibility: Site of Airway Obstruction and Bronchodilator Response

Archie F. Wilson

While the response of obstructed airways to therapy can often be successfully assessed by strictly clinical tools such as symptom evaluation and physical examination or, in the critical care unit, by ventilator pressures and blood gas values, the magnitude and major site(s) of airway response to bronchodilators are best evaluated by pulmonary function tests. It is now evident that predominant narrowing of the large airways characterizes mild asthma, while marked narrowing of the small airways is found in more severe asthma [11]. Since specific pulmonary function tests change with bronchodilator administration differently [17a, 18] and are affected by degree [16] and probably by site [11] of obstruction, selection of the appropriate pulmonary function tests is essential for analysis of the bronchodilator response.

SELECTION OF PULMONARY FUNCTION TESTS

Many respiratory maneuvers and tests have been utilized to measure the effects of bronchodilators on pulmonary function. Tests employed for this purpose include forced expiration and inspiration (spirometry, peak expiratory flow rate [PEFR], flow-volume relationships), body plethysmography (airway resistance [Raw] and thoracic gas volume at functional residual capacity [V_{TG}] plus the derived relationship, specific conductance [SGaw]), and helium dilution (subdivisions of total lung capacity [TLC], functional residual capacity [FRC], and residual volume [RV]). In most asthmatic patients, all of these values are abnormal and change markedly after a bronchodilator is administered [1, 4, 6, 9–12, 16–20, 26–30]. Hence, if only simple quantitation of the bronchodilator effect is wanted, a single test of forced expiration such as PEFR or 1-second forced expiratory volume (FEV_1) may be sufficient. However, in patients with chronic obstructive pulmonary disease (COPD), particularly those with airway collapse (see below), more complicated measures such as body plethysmography may be necessary to assess bronchomotor response [3]. If an analysis of the site of airway obstruction is desired, a measurement of density dependence of airflow, a comparison of maximum airflow at high and low lung volumes, and a measurement of RV are useful [13, 17]. Since maximal respiratory maneuvers themselves can produce a change in bronchomotor tone [23, 33], consideration may also be given to the performance of partial expiratory flow maneuvers.

As noted above, the concomitant presence or absence of emphysema is another important factor in choosing pulmonary function tests for evaluation of the bronchodilator response. While the anatomic lesion of emphysema does not change after bronchodilator administration, small airway bronchodilatation may be associated with major changes in pulmonary function, even though emphysema is also present [1, 15, 26]. For example, it is not uncommon for forced vital capacity (FVC) to increase more than twice the increase of FEV_1 after bronchodilator administration in patients with mixed emphysema, bronchitis, and bronchospasm (COPD) [1, 15]. This predominant volume response pattern to bronchodilators in COPD patients is in marked contrast to the predominant flow response of asthmatic patients without emphysema [11, 26]. The mechanism of this volume response phenomenon is thought to be due to greater (compared to values before bronchodilator use) collapse of large airways during forced expiration because of higher flow rates resulting from bronchodilatation of small, peripheral airways [15]. The results of pulmonary function tests that require forced expiration may also fail to improve after bronchodilator administration because of a reduction of bronchomotor tone in large, central airways [2]. Under these circumstances, forced expiration may produce increased collapse of large airways and mask improvement in the resting airway caliber. However, Raw and SGaw, tests performed during a panting maneuver and hence not associated with airway collapse, often still demonstrate considerable improvement after bronchodilator administration [3].

BRONCHODILATOR ADMINISTRATION

Bronchodilators may be given to patients with both acute and chronic symptoms by injection, by mouth, or by inhalation. Rapid onset of activity is produced by either intravenous injection or inhalation [4, 29]. While either an injected or an oral bronchodilator will eventually be transported by the bloodstream to airways and produce bronchodilatation, these modes of administration are inconvenient because of a delay in response, a greater likelihood of undesirable side effects, and the necessity of trained medical personnel to administer the drug (if given parenterally) or monitor drug side effects (when given by any route other than inhalation). Hence, virtually every laboratory employs the inhalation route to administer bronchodilators.

As discussed in detail in Chapter 56, several types of aerosol generator can be utilized to deliver the drug to test bronchoreversibility. While either a jet or an ultrasonic nebulizer reliably dispenses sufficient drug to allow assessment of the bronchodilator response, these modalities require more equipment and effort, require longer exposure times, run the potential risk of infection, and are much less standardized when compared to the metered-dose inhaler (MDI). Hence, the MDI is the most commonly used modality for dispensing a test bronchodilator. However, it is important to note that the administration technique of an MDI must be carefully monitored to ensure that it is used properly [5]. A large amount of effort has been expended to study the most appropriate means of using MDIs [7, 8, 24, 28]. An effective and relatively easy protocol for patient use is as follows:

1. Place the MDI in the mouth and close the lips around the opening.
2. Exhale normally (to FRC).
3. While breathing in slowly (for at least 5 seconds steadily), activate the MDI canister either at the onset of inhalation or shortly before inhalation begins.

4. Without stopping inhalation, breathe in completely (to TLC).
5. Hold the breath (at TLC) for 10 seconds if possible.
6. Repeat about 1 minute later.

Variations that individual laboratories follow include:

1. Place the MDI about 4 to 5 cm from the open mouth.
2. Begin inhalation at RV.
3. Have laboratory personnel activate the MDI canister to ensure proper timing.
4. Repeat two or more times.
5. Wait 10 minutes before repeating inhalation of the MDI contents.

Usually when an adrenergic agonist is used, the peak effect is normally achieved at about 10 to 30 minutes after inhalation [29]; with some agents, activity declines rapidly after 60 minutes while other inhaled bronchodilators cause significant effects for hours [29].

SIGNIFICANCE OF CHANGES AFTER BRONCHODILATOR ADMINISTRATION

Despite the obvious practical value of establishing firm criteria for determining the magnitude of pulmonary function changes that indicate significant bronchodilatation, only tentative recommendations can be made. Studies of normal populations revealed small but definite responses to bronchodilators [6]. In one large epidemiologic study, 95 percent of normal subjects had an average increase of FEV_1 of less than 9 percent expressed as percent increase over baseline divided by predicted baseline [6]. In a study of 75 normal subjects, the response to inhaled bronchodilator averaged 2.5 percent for FEV_1, 16 percent for maximal mid-volume expiratory flow rate ($FEF_{25-75\%}$), and 24 percent for SGaw [32]. However, variability of pulmonary function test results is directly related to the magnitude of the measured bronchodilator response [20]. Pulmonary function measurements also have intrinsic variability. In a group of 54 normal subjects, FEV_1 varied 190 ml over a 20-minute test and retest period [31]. In asthmatic subjects, variability of the bronchodilator response may be very large [20]; however, it has been pointed out that the variation is reduced if the change is expressed as a percentage of the predicted value rather than the usual practice of expressing change as a percentage of the baseline value [18a, 20].

When comparison between several types of measurement is made based on the signal-noise ratio (change-variability ratio), FEV_1 had the best ratio of change to variability [18]. However, in individual patients [30], lung volumes [20], FVC [1], or SGaw [29a] (see above) may demonstrate changes not readily apparent from FEV_1 measurements.

One set of recommendations offered to establish true bronchodilator improvement [27] is as follows (see also Chap. 26):

FEV_1—increases at least 15 percent of baseline and more than 200 ml
$FEF_{25-75\%}$—increases at least 20 percent of baseline
Vital capacity—increases at least 10 percent (even without major change in flow rates)

PARTIAL EXPIRATORY FLOW-VOLUME MANEUVERS

It is well established that airways exhibit hysteresis; that is, airway tone is influenced by the preceding volume history [23]. In normal persons (especially in the presence of pharmacologically induced bronchoconstriction), inspiration to TLC reduces airway tone [23]. Conversely, in most asthmatic patients, inspiration to TLC increases bronchomotor tone [33]. Since inspiration to TLC

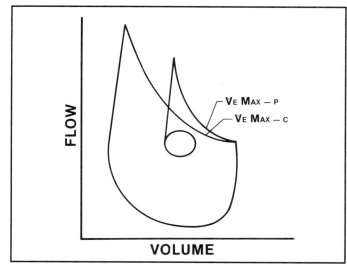

Fig. 36-1. *Partial and maximal expiratory flow-volume maneuvers in a patient with mild asthma. On the partial flow-volume maneuver, expiratory flow was initiated at the end of a tidal inspiration (about 60% of vital capacity). The subject exhaled forcibly to residual volume, immediately inhaled to total lung capacity, and again exhaled maximally to residual volume. Flow rates at 25 percent of the complete vital capacity were compared on the partial ($\dot{V}_EMax$-p) and maximal ($\dot{V}_EMax$-c) flow-volume maneuvers.*

conventionally precedes FVC and maximal expiratory flow-volume (MEFV) maneuvers, results of these tests are influenced by the effects of lung inflation on bronchomotor tone. The influence of a TLC volume history can be avoided by using tests (such as Raw or partial expiratory flow-volume [PEFV] curves) that do not require a preceding deep breath. PEFV maneuvers are initiated at about 60 percent of vital capacity (Fig. 36-1). Flow rates are then measured at a point in the PEFV curve beyond the initial flow transits [33].

Recent data in asthmatic subjects demonstrate that flow rates at 25 percent of FVC are often higher on PEFV curves ($\dot{V}_EMax_{25}$-p) compared to flow rates from complete MEFV curves ($\dot{V}_EMax_{25}$-c) (see Fig. 36-1) [33]. After inhalation of isoproterenol or atropine, $\dot{V}_EMax_{25}$-p usually increases more than $\dot{V}_EMax_{25}$-c [33]. Hence, detection of bronchoreversibility may be facilitated by utilizing PEFV maneuvers. On the other hand, since $\dot{V}_EMax_{25}$-p also increases more than $\dot{V}_EMax_{25}$-c in normal subjects after inhalation of a bronchodilator [9], it is necessary to compare changes in partial expiratory flow rates in normal subjects relative to asthmatics to determine whether prebronchodilator and postbronchodilator PEFV measurements actually enhance the detection of bronchodilator responses. In addition, since methodology and technical requirements of PEFV determinations are more exacting and coefficients of variation are generally larger, the criteria for a bronchodilator response are less well defined when flow rates are measured at low lung volume. Consequently, prebronchodilator and postbronchodilator PEFV maneuvers probably should not be used as a routine test to assess bronchoreversibility. Under special circumstances, such as spirometry-associated bronchospasm [14], assessment of bronchoreversibility using PEFV maneuvers may be helpful.

SITE OF AIRFLOW LIMITATION AND LOCALIZATION OF BRONCHODILATOR RESPONSE

Previous studies have indicated that flow rates measured at high lung volumes (PEFR, FEV_1) and Raw mainly reflect the caliber

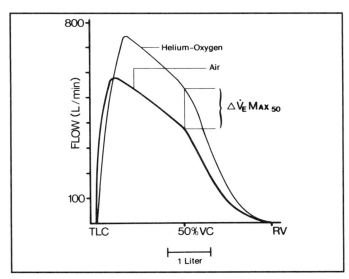

Fig. 36-2. *Example of maximal expiratory flow-volume curves produced after breathing air and a helium-oxygen mixture (He-O₂) in a normal subject. Flow rates are higher after breathing He-O₂. At 50 percent of vital capacity (VC), the difference between maximal expiratory flow ($\dot{V}_EMax_{50}$) breathing air and He-O₂ can be quantitated as:*

$$\Delta\dot{V}_EMax_{50}\ (\%) = \frac{\dot{V}_EMax_{50}(He\text{-}O_2) - \dot{V}_EMax_{50}(air)}{\dot{V}_EMax_{50}(air)} \times 100.$$

(TLC = total lung capacity; RV = residual volume.)

of large airways [13]; conversely, flow rates at middle (forced expiratory flow at mid–expiratory phase [FEF₂₅₋₇₅%]) and, to an even greater extent, low lung volumes (FEF₇₅₋₈₅%) are appreciably influenced by resistance to airflow in the smaller peripheral airways [13]. It has been suggested that reductions in flow rates at low lung volumes coupled with normal values of Raw and FEV₁ indicate peripheral airway obstruction. However, if peripheral airways are severely narrowed, resistance to airflow will be reduced at all lung volumes and Raw will be increased and FEV₁ reduced. Similarly, application of an external orifice with a very small diameter at the mouth will reduce expiratory flow rates throughout the entire exhaled volume [21]. Thus, site of airway obstruction frequently cannot be clearly delineated, particularly when Raw, FEV₁, FEF₂₅₋₇₅%, and FEF₇₅₋₈₅% are all abnormal.

Lung volume abnormalities may also reflect an alteration in airway caliber. The caliber of peripheral airways probably influences both closing volume and RV [19, 25]. Although RV has multiple determinants, elevation of RV with near-normal flow rates is a relatively early sign of peripheral airway dysfunction [25]; since TLC does not usually increase in these patients, elevation of RV is often associated with reduced vital capacity. Since peripheral airway narrowing is thought to be a determinant of RV, a reduction in RV after bronchodilator administration is compatible with peripheral airway dilatation.

Studies of the density dependence of maximal expiratory flow have been used to identify the predominant site of airflow limitation [8, 10–12, 17]. These measurements are made by comparing the maximum expiratory flow at 50 percent of vital capacity ($\dot{V}_EMax_{50}$) after breathing a low-density mixture of gas (80% helium and 20% oxygen, He-O₂) to maximum airflow while breathing room air. The difference between $\dot{V}_EMax_{50}$(He-O₂) and $\dot{V}_EMax_{50}$(air) is quantitated; this difference is termed $\Delta\dot{V}_EMax_{50}$ (Fig. 36-2) [8]. Density dependence of airflow ($\Delta\dot{V}_EMax_{50} \geq 20\%$) suggests predominantly large airway flow limitation, whereas reduced values ($\Delta\dot{V}_EMax_{50} < 20\%$) are compatible with predominantly peripheral sites of airflow limitation [8]. The rationale is as follows:

Flow-related pressure losses in the large airways are due to turbulence, convective acceleration, or both; both turbulence and convective pressure losses are reduced by breathing low-density gas mixtures such as He-O₂ [8, 22]. In contrast, pressure losses in peripheral airways are thought to be related to the viscosity rather than the density of a respired gas (He-O₂ is more viscous than air) [8]. Accordingly, breathing He-O₂ does not reduce flow-resistive losses (and in fact may increase the resistance to airflow) in the peripheral airways. Although there are questions regarding the validity of these concepts [22], evidence compatible with the theory has been found. In asthma, density dependence appears to decrease in proportion to the reduction in airflow, which suggests that flow limitation may become more peripheral as the severity of asthma increases [11]. Bronchodilator administration usually produces a major response in those airways most obstructed [11].

Ingram and associates suggested that postbronchodilator changes in density dependence may be useful in assessing the predominant site of bronchodilatation [17]. In this regard, Ingram and colleagues regarded the upstream resistance (toward the alveoli) from the site of flow limitation as containing large and small (i.e., peripheral) airways in series. The total resistance (Rt) of that segment is the sum of the resistances of the large and peripheral airways (Rt = Rl + Rp). As previously discussed, Rp is considered primarily viscosity dependent, whereas Rl is considered density dependent. Accordingly, the overall density dependence of flow should be inversely related to the ratio Rp/Rl (the larger the ratio, the lower the density dependence). If $\dot{V}_EMax$ increases after bronchodilator administration, bronchodilatation can be assumed. If density dependence ($\Delta\dot{V}_EMax_{50}$) also changes, then changes in Rp/Rl are assumed. For example, if predominantly peripheral airway bronchodilatation occurs, Rp/Rl will diminish (overall Rt would decrease but because of a relatively larger increase in the size of the peripheral airways, Rp would decrease more than Rl). The result would be an increase in $\Delta\dot{V}_EMax_{50}$. Hence, according to these concepts [17], the combination of improved flow rates and increased density dependence suggests predominantly peripheral airway bronchodilatation. In contrast, postbronchodilator improvements in airflow associated with reduced values of $\Delta\dot{V}_EMax_{50}$ are thought to be compatible with predominantly large airway bronchodilatation. The combination of improved flow rates after bronchodilator use and no change in $\Delta\dot{V}_EMax_{50}$ is thought to indicate proportionately equal bronchodilatation of large and peripheral airways [17]. Based on these concepts (summarized in Table 36-1), it has been suggested that sympathomimetic and antimuscarinic compounds are capable of dilating both large and peripheral airways [10–12]. Furthermore, since significant inverse relationships have been observed between initial (prebronchodilator) values of $\Delta\dot{V}_EMax_{50}$ and changes in that parameter after bronchodilator use, it is possible that the predominant site of bronchodilatation may be related to the major site of airflow limitation before drug administration [10–12].

Table 36-1. Interpretation of changes in density dependence after bronchodilator administration[a]

Expiratory flow[b]	Density dependence[b]	Interpretation
Increased	Increased	Predominant peripheral airway bronchodilatation
Increased	Decreased	Predominant large airway bronchodilatation
Increased	Unchanged	Proportionately equal large and peripheral airway bronchodilatation

[a] As per Ingram et al. [17].
[b] Compared with prebronchodilator values.

REFERENCES

1. Bellamy, D., and Hutchinson, D. C. S. The effects of salbutamol aerosol on lung function in patients with pulmonary emphysema. *Br. J. Dis. Chest* 75: 190, 1981.
2. Bouhuys, A., and van de Woestijne, K. P. Respiratory mechanics and dust exposure in byssinosis. *J. Clin. Invest.* 49:106, 1970.
3. Burrows, B., Saksena, F., and Diener, C. F. Carbon dioxide tension and ventilatory mechanics in chronic obstructive pulmonary disease. *Ann. Intern. Med.* 65:685, 1966.
4. Clark, T. J. H. Factors Influencing the Route of Administration of Airway Therapy. In P. Sadoul, et al. (eds.), *Small Airways in Health and Disease.* Amsterdam: Excerpta Medica, 1979.
5. Crompton, G. K. Problems patients have using pressurized aerosol inhalers. *Eur. J. Respir. Dis.* 63(Suppl. 119):109, 1982.
6. Dales, R. E., et al. Clinical interpretation of airway response to a bronchodilator. *Am. Rev. Respir. Dis.* 138:317, 1988.
7. Newman, S. P., et al. Improving the bronchial deposition of pressurized aerosols. *Chest* 80(Suppl.):909, 1981.
8. Dolovich, M., et al. Optimal delivery of aerosols from metered dose inhalers. *Chest* 80(Suppl.):911, 1981.
9. Douglas, N. J., Sudlow, M. F., and Flenley, D. C. Effect of an inhaled atropine-like agent on normal airway function. *J. Appl. Physiol.* 46:256, 1979.
10. Fairshter, R. D., Habib, M. P., and Wilson, A. F. Inhaled atropine sulfate in acute asthma. *Respiration* 42:263, 1981.
11. Fairshter, R. D., and Wilson, A. F. Relationship between the site of airflow limitation and localization of the bronchodilator response in asthma. *Am. Rev. Respir. Dis.* 122:27, 1980.
12. Fairshter, R. D., and Wilson, A. F. Relationship between the sites of airflow limitation and severity of chronic airflow obstruction. *Am. Rev. Respir. Dis.* 123:3, 1981.
13. Gelb, A. F., and Zamel, N. Simplified diagnosis of small airway obstruction. *N. Engl. J. Med.* 288:395, 1973.
14. Gimeno, F., et al. Spirometry-induced bronchial obstruction. *Am. Rev. Respir. Dis.* 105:68, 1972.
15. Healy, F., Wilson, A. F., and Fairshter, R. D. Physiologic correlates of airway collapse in chronic airflow obstruction. *Chest* 85:476, 1984.
16. Hume, K. M., and Gandevia, B. Forced expiratory volume before and after isoprenaline. *Thorax* 12:276, 1957.
17. Ingram, R., Jr., et al. Relative contributions of large and small airways to flow limitation in normal subjects before and after atropine and isoproterenol. *J. Clin. Invest.* 59:696, 1977.
17a. Laube, B. L., Norman, P. S. and Adams III, G. K. The effect of aerosol distribution on airway responsiveness to inhaled methacholine in patients with asthma. *J. Allergy Clin. Immunol.* 89:510, 1992.
18. Light, R. W., Conrad, S. A., and George, R. B. The one best test for evaluating the effects of bronchodilator therapy. *Chest* 72:512, 1977.
18a. Lurie, A., et al. Best mode of expression of acute reversibility of airway obstruction in patients with asthma: Application to a new beta-2 agonist, RU 42 173. *Meth. Find. Exp. Clin. Pharmacol.* 14:29, 1992.
19. McCarthy, D. S., et al. Measurement of "closing volume" as a simple and sensitive test for early detection of small airways disease. *Am. J. Med.* 52: 747, 1972.
20. Meslier, N., and Racineux, J. L. Tests of reversibility of airflow obstruction. *Eur. Respir. Rev.* 1:34, 1991.
21. Miller, R. D., and Hyatt, R. E. Obstructing lesions of the larynx and trachea: Clinical and physiological characteristics. *Mayo Clin. Proc.* 44:145, 1969.
22. Mink, S., Ziesmann, M., and Wood, L. D. H. Mechanisms of increased maximal expiratory flow during He-O_2 breathing in dogs. *J. Appl. Physiol.* 47:490, 1979.
23. Nadel, J. A., and Tierney, D. F. Effect of a previous deep inspiration on airway resistance in man. *J. Appl. Physiol.* 16:717, 1961.
24. Newman, S. P., Pavia, D., and Clarke, S. W. Improving the bronchial deposition of pressurized aerosols. *Chest* 80(Suppl.):909, 1981.
25. Pride, N. B., et al. Determinants of maximal expiratory flow from the lung. *J. Appl. Physiol.* 23:646, 1967.
26. Ramsdell, J. W., and Tisi, G. M. Determination of bronchodilatation in the clinical pulmonary function laboratory. *Chest* 76:622, 1979.
27. Ries, A. L. Response to Bronchodilators. In J. Clausen (ed.), *Pulmonary Function Testing: Guidelines and Controversies.* New York: Academic, 1982.
28. Riley, D. J., Weitz, B. W., and Edelman, W. H. The response of asthmatic subjects to isoproterenol inhaled at different volumes. *Am. Rev. Respir. Dis.* 114:509, 1976.
29. Roth, M., Wilson, A. F., and Novey, H. S. A comparative study of the aerosolized bronchodilators, isoproterenol, metaproterenol and terbutaline. *Ann. Allergy* 38:16, 1977.
29a. Smith, H. R., Irvin, C. G., and Cherniack, R. M. The utility of spirometry in the diagnosis of reversible airways obstruction. *Chest* 101:1577, 1992.
30. Tashkin, D. P. Measurement and Significance of the Bronchodilator Response. In J. W. Jenne and S. Murphy (eds.), *Drug Therapy for Asthma.* New York: Dekker, 1985.
31. Tweedale, P. M., et al. Short term variability in FEV_1: Relation to pretest activity, level of FEV_1, and smoking habits. *Thorax* 39:928, 1984.
32. Watanabe, S., et al. Airway responsiveness to a bronchodilator aerosol. I. Normal human subjects. *Am. Rev. Respir. Dis.* 109:530, 1974.
33. Zamel, N., et al. Partial and complete maximum expiratory flow volume curves in asthmatic patients with spontaneous bronchospasm. *Chest* 83: 35, 1983.

Differential Diagnosis

Kenneth F. MacDonnell
Henry D. Beauchamp

37

The differential diagnosis of asthma is one of the most vexing problems in clinical medicine. The diagnosis of asthma traditionally calls to mind paroxysms of wheezing and shortness of breath. However, there are patients who have reversible airway obstruction (asthma) without substantial wheezing. These patients may complain of episodes of shortness of breath, or perhaps spasms of coughing or chest tightness, and in rare instances chest pain. It is now known that cough without dyspnea or wheezing may be the only manifestation of asthma. Furthermore, some suffer asthma only after exercise, and these episodes may be subtle, with dyspnea and chest tightness as the only symptoms. Other patients complain of classic wheezing, which makes the diagnosis more apparent. When the presentation is not typical, challenge testing is indicated [316]. In general, however, in establishing the diagnosis of asthma the physician is confronted with the differential diagnosis of wheezing, dyspnea, and perhaps cough [310]. In a recent article, the prevalence of wheezing was 19.2 percent, and 8 years later in the same population group studied, it was 21.4 percent [11, 249]. The association between wheezing and asthma is even ingrained in the lay literature; witness the definition of wheezing in *Webster's New World Dictionary*, "to breathe hard with a whistling breathing sound as in asthma." However, equating a symptom with a diagnosis is not taught and should not be practiced, as illustrated by Jackson's dictum—"All that wheezes is not bronchial asthma."

Stated differently, all that wheezes is obstruction. However, it is apparent that wheezing and shortness of breath are nonspecific and merely reflect obstruction to airflow. The unique anatomy of the lung, with its large cross-sectional area in the peripheral airways, requires that the obstruction to airflow be strategically located if a wheeze is to result, and certainly the larger the airway, the larger the wheeze. The reverse is also true to the extent that those portions of the lungs in which the airways are less than 2 mm in diameter constitute silent zones. These are areas in which extensive disease may yield a minimum of findings on physical examination, and the clinician should be reminded that the absence of wheezing does not exclude the diagnosis of asthma. In fact, when there is a marked increase in airway obstruction, there is such a diminution of airflow that Reynold's number is decreased below auditory perception. Wheezing is characteristically absent in such patients. The patency of airways and the maintenance of laminar flow (and thus quiet flow) depend on a variety of related forces including the tone of the bronchial musculature, the integrity of the supporting cartilage, and the amount and character of secretions (see Chap. 51). Turbulent gas flow and wheezing may result when the integrity of the mucous membrane is altered in airways of sufficient size, as happens in chronic bronchitis with its attendant bronchial mucous gland hypertrophy and increased mucous secretions.

Edema of the mucous membrane as seen with congestive heart failure can greatly narrow the caliber of the airway. Pulmonary embolic disease may result in the release of bronchoactive amines that affect the tone of the tracheobronchial tree, occasionally resulting in diffuse polyphonic wheezing. An intraluminal abnormality, be it a tumor or a foreign body, may cause intermittent or continuous obstruction and monophonic wheezing. Thus, it is quite clear that wheezing, the hallmark of asthma, merely reflects obstruction in the airway, whatever the cause.

An understanding of the event surrounding the onset of the symptoms is critical to sorting out the various illnesses capable of producing an asthmatic picture. For example, it is important to remember that transient periods of bronchial hyperreactivity can be seen in patients with viral infections and possibly mycoplasma [326] of the respiratory tract [144]. This hyperreactivity can last up to 8 weeks. In such instances, the patient should not be labeled as suffering from asthma. Equally, an initial diagnosis of bronchial asthma is not justified in the patient who arrives in the emergency room with burns around the face, respiratory wheezing, dyspnea, and a recent exposure to toxic fumes. Rather, a diagnosis of thermal injury to the respiratory tract is indicated. Conversely, the 8-year-old with eczema and the family history of asthma who starts wheezing when the family purchases a new pet does not suggest the diagnosis of pulmonary embolic disease. Probably the most difficult problems arise in the middle-age group, often cigarette smokers, with a strong history of chronic bronchitis. They may work at hazardous occupations and live in smog-infested cities. Thus, when they are seen in the emergency room with wheezing and dyspnea, the differential diagnosis among heart failure, pulmonary embolus, and bronchial asthma may be exceedingly difficult.

Among the group of asthma masqueraders fall those groups of patients whose tendency to asthma manifests when exposed to certain medications or diseased states that unmask the asthma. Such cases of "hidden asthma" are not uncommon as a variety of commonly used medicines may be the culprit [313]. Most notable among these are the beta blockers that can be used systemically, for example, to control hypertension, and also topically as eyedrops in the treatment of glaucoma, when the instilled solution is absorbed systemically through the conjunctival sac and may worsen or precipitate asthma [307, 325]. The use of eyedrops is frequently overlooked in the history. The potential adverse effects of beta-adrenergic competitive antagonism are illustrated in a number of patient reports describing the therapeutic misadventure of these drugs. Because of their extensive therapeutic indications and their potential for increasing airway resistance, these beta-adrenergic blocking agents should be on the checklist used by physicians confronted with a wheezing patient. Similarly, the hyperthyroid state can have adverse effects in asthmatic patients. Several reports have linked the onset of hyperthyroidism with the exacerbation of existing asthma [29, 142, 245, 338]. Restoration to the euthyroid state resulted in significant improvement [50]. The nature of the underlying bio-

Table 37-1. *Features helpful in the differential diagnosis of laryngeal dysfunction, bronchial asthma, and factitious asthma*

Feature	Laryngeal dysfunction	Bronchial asthma	Factitious asthma
Wheeze	Maximal intensity over the larynx	Diffuse, scattered over lung fields	Maximal intensity over the larynx
Pulmonary function test results	May be inconsistent	Obstructive pattern	Normal
Provocation test results	Negative	Positive	Negative
Bronchoscopy findings	Expiratory and inspiratory vocal cord adduction	Normal	Intermittent vocal cord adduction
Bronchoscopy findings after anesthesia with intravenous diazepam	Abnormal expiratory and inspiratory vocal cord apposition may persist	Normal	Vocal cord apposition disappears
Response to conventional asthma therapy	Poor	Good	Poor
Response to psychotherapy and speech therapy	Good	Poor	Good (other manifestations of malingering may be associated, e.g., gastrointestinal complaints, headache)

chemical interaction remains obscure despite several suggested explanations: (1) the increased degradation of hydrocortisone, increased urinary excretion of conjugated steroid metabolites, and reduced free plasma cortisol concentrations noted in hyperthyroid patients; (2) the impaired breakdown of prostaglandin F, a potent bronchoconstricting agent, noted in vitro in lungs of hyperthyroid rats; and (3) increased airway reactivity [50]. However, it has been found that in nonasthmatic subjects, hyperthyroidism protects against nonspecific bronchial hyperreactivity [127] and hypothyroidism increases nonspecific bronchial hyperreactivity [287]. Whatever the underlying mechanism, it is prudent to ensure that a euthyroid state has been established.

Historic features often resolve many difficulties in clarifying the causes of wheezing and dyspnea. A careful and detailed physical examination, along with a selective and logical use of the clinical laboratory, often helps to establish the correct diagnosis. Unfortunately, there are a number of cases in which distinction is not only difficult but also impossible, and the clinician must then resort to a therapeutic trial (Table 37-1).

This chapter concerns the illnesses that must be considered in the differential diagnosis of wheezing and dyspnea. No attempt is made to list the differential diagnosis of cough, chest tightness, or chest pain. Rather the clinician is reminded that asthma must be considered and appropriate laboratory studies, used judiciously, will help confirm or exclude the diagnosis (Fig. 37-1).

NONASTHMATIC DISEASES

Pulmonary Embolism

The startling frequency of pulmonary embolism has been appreciated only in the past two decades. In a recent review, it was estimated that 5,000,000 patients per year have a deep venous thrombosis, 10 percent of whom develop a pulmonary embolism, 10 percent of whom die [191]. However, when clinically apparent pulmonary embolism is successfully diagnosed and appropriately treated, it is an uncommon cause of death [304]. Difficulty in establishing the diagnosis of pulmonary embolism is also well recognized. Until the advent of lung scanning and pulmonary angiography, only 11 to 12 percent of patients with a pulmonary embolism were successfully diagnosed antemortem [278]. Even now only 30 percent of patients with a major pulmonary embolism are successfully diagnosed antemortem [238]. In a study by Goldhaber, only 10 percent of the patients over the age of 70 with a major pulmonary embolism were successfully diagnosed antemortem, and no patient who had pneumonia and a major pulmonary embolism were successfully diagnosed antemortem

[101]. Compounding the problem is the fact that pulmonary embolism occurring in young patients tends to have a more subtle presentation [311], and many of the clinical and laboratory findings of pulmonary embolisms are also seen with bronchial asthma [16, 118]. Establishing whether a patient is having an episode of bronchial asthma or has a pulmonary embolism is of more than casual academic interest, for once the diagnosis is made, energetic therapy sometimes hazardous to the alternative condition must be instituted. Wheezing was formerly thought to be common in patients with a pulmonary embolism [286]; it is not [16, 118]. However, the ability of pulmonary embolisms to produce significant dyspnea allows pulmonary emboli to masquerade as bronchial asthma [82, 240, 286, 293].

The postulated pathophysiologic mechanisms of embolic wheezing include (1) the release of bronchoactive amines (e.g., serotonin, prostaglandins) from platelet aggregations in the thrombus [274], an effect that can be blocked with heparin [241]; and (2) the release of certain chemical mediators (prostaglandins) in response to microspheric emboli, as demonstrated in dog lungs [157]. Several mechanisms are known to result in hypoxia due to pulmonary embolism [191], including ventilation-perfusion (V/Q) inequalities [135], decreased cardiac output from right ventricular failure resulting in a widening of the arteriovenous oxygen difference [135, 165], and shunting either through a patent foramen ovale [115] or through an intrapulmonary shunt [60].

In establishing the diagnosis of pulmonary embolism, many valuable clues can be obtained from the clinical history, for example, predisposing factors such as congestive heart failure, occult cancer, thrombophlebitis, trauma, immobility, increased clotting tendencies, pregnancy, varicose veins, and the use of oral contraceptive pills (OCPs).* These factors should be contrasted with the usual asthmatic history, which centers around the many manifestations of allergy or related irritants.

The major symptoms of pulmonary emboli with or without infarction, in order of decreasing frequency, are dyspnea, pleural pain, apprehension, cough, diaphoresis, hemoptysis, and syncope. This constellation of symptoms is not observed in uncomplicated asthma. The cardinal findings of pulmonary embolism on physical examination may include tachypnea, tachycardia, bilateral heart failure or ipsilateral rales of infarction, pleural friction rub, increased S_2P or S_3/S_4 gallop or both, phlebitis, sweating, cyanosis, fever, and hypotension [16, 118].

The laboratory tests most frequently employed in establishing

---

* OCPs with low-dose estrogen (<100 μg) are associated with a lower incidence of venous thromboembolism [236]. Current studies are evaluating the risk of venous thromboembolism with very-low-dose-estrogen (<30 μg) OCPs [275].

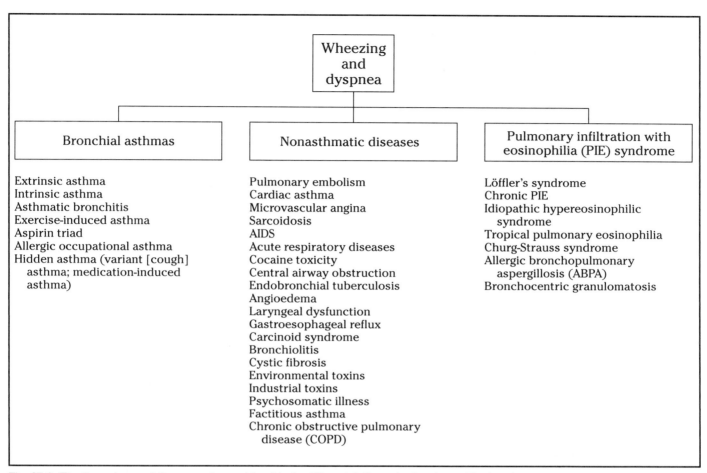

Fig. 37-1. *The three classes of diseases to be considered in the differential diagnosis of patients with wheezing and dyspnea.*

the diagnosis of pulmonary embolism vary in specificity and sensitivity, with the pulmonary arteriogram remaining the definitive procedure. A number of abnormalities have been recognized on the chest x-ray films. A common finding is an elevated diaphragm reflecting a loss of lung volume, a situation quite contrary to the hyperinflated lung seen in asthma. The other major abnormalities related to pulmonary embolism include the following:

1. Oligemia
   Local oligemia resulting from occlusion of a large vessel
   Peripheral oligemia resulting from occlusion of a large vessel
   Unilateral oligemia of the entire lung resulting from occlusion of the main pulmonary vessels or widespread small-vessel occlusions
2. Increase in the size of the proximal pulmonary artery
3. Alteration in the size and configuration of the heart, reflecting acute cor pulmonale

Unfortunately, these findings are nonspecific and can be seen in a variety of disorders including asthma and emphysema [108]. The electrocardiogram (ECG) is also nonspecific, but occasionally classic signs of acute right ventricular strain due to pulmonary embolism may be seen, such as P pulmonale $S_1Q_3T_3$ and right axis deviation [179]. The measurement of arterial blood gases may be helpful in patients suspected of having a pulmonary embolism. Arterial hypoxemia, that is, arterial oxygen tension (PaO_2) less than 80 mmHg, is usually seen. In one series, 9 per-

cent of patients with pulmonary embolism had PaO_2 values greater than 90 mmHg [241]. Of 55 patients with pulmonary embolism documented by pulmonary angiography, the PaO_2 on room air was 90 mmHg or greater in 6 percent and 80 mmHg or greater in 14 percent [16]. Dantzker reviewed arterial blood gases following pulmonary embolism and concluded that the severity and mechanism of blood gas abnormalities depend on the size and location of the embolism, the presence or absence of cardiopulmonary disease, and the time elapsed since the embolism occurred [61]. More recently, the value of an increased alveolar-arterial oxygen gradient and hypocapnia in diagnosing acute pulmonary embolism was studied. Of 78 patients with angiographically proved pulmonary embolism and arterial blood gases drawn on room air, hypoxemia was present in 59 (76%), hypoxemia or hypocapnia was present in 73 (93%), an increased alveolar-arterial oxygen gradient was present in 74 (95%), and an increased alveolar-arterial oxygen gradient or hypocapnia was present in 77 patients (98%) [57]. The sensitivity of arterial blood gas analysis in the evaluation of acute pulmonary embolism is thus increased by considering the partial pressure of carbon dioxide and the alveolar-arterial oxygen gradient. However, it is apparent that the arterial blood gas abnormalities described above are nonspecific, and seen in a variety of diseases.

Serum levels of fibrinogen degradation products (FDPs)—specifically D-dimer—have been found to be diagnostically useful by some investigators when measured in patients with suspected pulmonary embolism [22, 27]. However, others have not found this test to be sensitive or specific [102, 265].

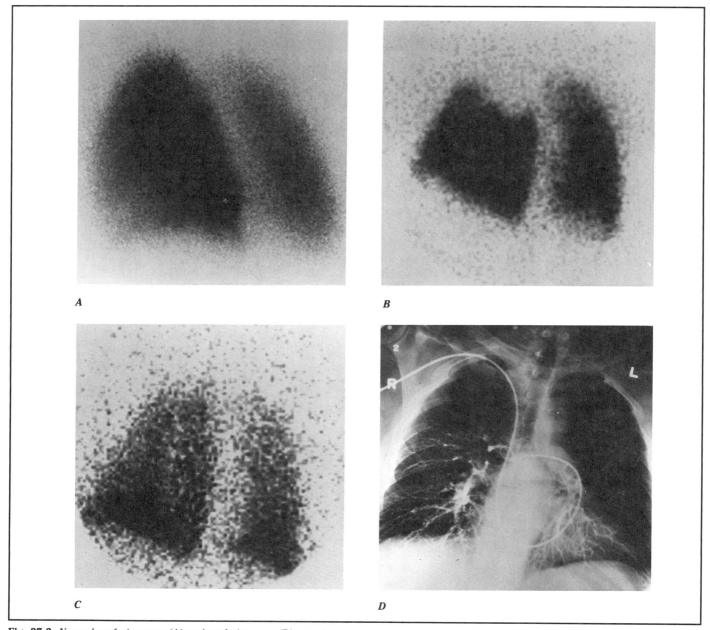

Fig. 37-2. *Normal perfusion scan (A) and perfusion scan (B), ventilation scan (C), and arteriogram (D) of a patient with pulmonary embolus. B. A perfusion defect involving the right upper lobe is seen. C. The ventilation scan is normal. D. The catheter is seen in the right pulmonary artery with injection of contrast material. This representative film shows contrast outlining the arterial system of the right lung with no perfusion in the upper branch of the right lung.*

For example, Goldhaber found elevated levels of D-dimer to be present in 56 percent of patients suspected of pulmonary embolism but who had a normal-appearing lung scan [102]. Further trials are necessary to establish the exact role of FDPs in the diagnosis of acute pulmonary embolism.

Ventilation-perfusion (V/Q) scans are one of the most valuable diagnostic tests available for the evaluation of a patient with suspected pulmonary embolism (Fig. 37-2). The results of the prospective investigation of pulmonary embolism diagnosis trial conclude that: (1) A normal or near-normal V/Q scan makes the diagnosis of pulmonary embolism very unlikely (4% have an embolism); however, of the 21 patients who had normal Q scans, none of them had a pulmonary embolism by angiography or clini-

cally at follow-up (thus confirming a larger previous study of 515 patients with completely normal Q scans, where 1 of the 515 patients studied subsequently developed a pulmonary embolism when anticoagulant therapy was withheld [123]). Thus, a normal Q scan virtually rules out pulmonary embolism. (2) Of patients with a high probability V/Q scan, 12 percent did not have angiographic evidence of a pulmonary embolism. (3) Of patients with a low probability V/Q scan, only 12 percent had angiographic evidence of an embolism [20, 239]. It should be noted that V/Q inequality is also seen in bronchial asthma [282, 330] (Fig. 37-3).

Since the primary source of pulmonary embolism is from a deep venous thrombosis of the lower extremities, studies of the venous system of the lower extremities should be done on all

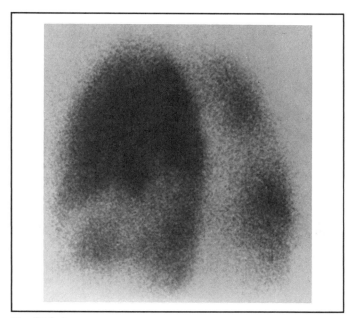

Fig. 37-3. *Perfusion scan in patient with extrinsic asthma. Note the asymmetric decrease in perfusion with an almost total loss in the left middle lung zone and right lower lung zone.*

patients suspected of pulmonary embolism to help guide management. However, 30 percent of patients with angiographic evidence of a pulmonary embolism have negative findings on a venogram [122].

Finally, in clinical situations in which clear diagnostic distinction is impossible, a pulmonary arteriogram must be performed (see Fig. 37-2). The pulmonary arteriogram has proved to be the most reliable method of diagnosing pulmonary embolisms. Technical advantages in arteriography employing selective catheterization of the pulmonary arteries and magnification techniques have further increased the diagnostic accuracy of the procedure [58, 123].

In summary, pulmonary embolisms can masquerade as bronchial asthma because the two illnesses share many of the same signs and symptoms. The diagnostic dilemma is further compounded by the lack of specificity in the generally employed laboratory tests. Various clinical clues such as the presence of predisposing factors, hemoptysis, and pleural pain may help the physician in arriving at the correct diagnosis. The most valuable differential laboratory tests are radioisotope lung scanning and definitive pulmonary arteriogram.

Cardiac Asthma

Cardiac asthma is left ventricular failure manifested in the lung by wheezing and dyspnea. Left ventricular failure and pulmonary edema are such frequent manifestations of heart disease that cardiac asthma is often confused with true bronchial asthma.

In 1835, Hope coined the term *cardiac asthma* when he wrote that "an immense proportion of asthmas—and of the most dangerous and distressing cases, result from disease of the heart. . .If the cause be overlooked, the asthmatic is harassed with a farrago of inappropriate and unavailing, not to say pernicious remedies. . ." [120]. The term was initially used in the original Greek sense ("gasping") to describe the sudden suffocating breathlessness that afflicts patients with heart failure [205]. The expression *cardiac asthma* is still used to describe the symptoms and clinical bronchial signs of pulmonary edema. The triad of dyspnea, cough, and wheezing is as characteristic of exacerbations of chronic left ventricular failure as it is of bronchial asthma [297].

Under normal circumstances, the lung interstitium can accommodate approximately 500 ml of fluid. When this capacity is surpassed, intraalveolar edema results. Furthermore, with accumulation of mucosal edema, there is a narrowing of the airways. To a major extent, the narrowing of airways is not caused by spasm of bronchial smooth muscles as in asthma, but rather by mechanical obstruction by edema fluid in the conducting airways per se. Extrinsic compression and therefore reduction in the airway lumen are caused by peribronchial edema, which is seen in the early stages of congestive heart failure (CHF). This is the hemodynamic hypothesis [76, 93, 189, 284]. However, airway obstruction can also result from the mechanical deformation of the bronchial wall [284]. Recently, Cabanes found frequent bronchial hyperreactivity to methacholine in 21 of 23 nonatopic patients in the New York Heart Association functional Class III, with a mean left ventricular ejection fraction of 26 percent [30]. These 21 patients were then retested with methacholine; 6 of 21 received pretreatment with the alpha agonist methoxamine, which resulted in a normal methacholine challenge test; another 6 received the alpha blocker phentolamine before receiving methoxamine and were then challenged with methacholine. It was found that phentolamine blocked the protective effect of methoxamine, thus resulting in a positive result on the methacholine challenge test. It was therefore proposed that methoxamine exerted its protective action via alpha receptors. The protective effect of methoxamine in these patients with left ventricular dysfunction is in contrast to the increased airway obstruction to methoxamine reported in bronchial asthmatics. Cabanes suggested that the bronchial hyperreactivity seen in patients with left ventricular dysfunction was due to the dilation of bronchial vessels, and that this could be blocked by the vasoconstrictor effects of methoxamine [30]. This vasomotor hypothesis is thought to be an extension of the hemodynamic hypothesis [76]. Pison also found bronchial hyperreactivity in patients with left ventricular dysfunction [217]. Other investigators have not found bronchial hyperreactivity in patients with left ventricular dysfunction [78, 244]. This may be due to a loss of bronchial hyperreactivity as left ventricular dysfunction progresses [225], and is supported by Plotz's observation that the response to bronchodilator drugs is lost as CHF progresses [218]. An abnormality of neural control of bronchial smooth muscle [12] has been proposed to help explain the bronchial hyperreactivity, involving a reflex mediated by nonmyelinated "J" fibers [225]. Such bronchospasm may account for the limited but observable response to bronchodilator therapy seen in some patients. It is unclear just how much each of these physiologic derangements contributes to the production of turbulent airflow and thus wheezing.

If these events occur precipitously during sleep, the familiar clinical syndrome of paroxysmal nocturnal dyspnea (PND) results. In its classic form PND is unmistakable. Typically the patient is well on retiring but awakens abruptly a few hours later acutely short of breath and experiencing severe air hunger. The patient assumes an upright posture and frequently obtains symptomatic relief. While the patient may return to bed without any further difficulty, in some instances florid pulmonary edema results. The asthmatic patient, on the other hand, may awaken at any time during the night, and his or her distress usually does not subside simply as a result of a change in posture. Nocturnal dyspnea associated with bronchial asthma may, however, improve with cough and sputum clearance, or with the use of an inhaler. A cardinal symptom of heart failure is dyspnea. Evaluation of the factors that precipitate and relieve it may provide valuable diagnostic clues. Ankle edema is a common complaint of patients with heart failure, but not of patients with uncomplicated asthma. Another important symptom is orthopnea. This condition is more common as a symptom of advanced heart failure in patients with heart disease; however, it may be seen in select patients with asthma and chronic obstructive pulmonary disease (COPD), generally in advanced cases. Sitting up and leaning forward increases the intraabdominal pressure pushing up the diaphragm. This increases the muscle fiber length and improves the tension-generating capability of the diaphragm. Prime abnormalities on physical examination of a patient with heart failure include tachycardia, elevated jugular venous pulsation, bilateral basal crackles, displaced apex beat, S_3 or S_4 gallop rhythm, tender hepatomegaly, and dependent edema—sacral or of the ankle. However, many studies have shown a poor correlation of physical findings with CHF [40, 73, 204]. Such findings, with the exception of tachycardia, are not part of the usual uncomplicated asthmatic presentation. Unfortunately, in some patients with long-standing asthma, cor pulmonale may develop, thus confusing the clinical picture.

The diagnosis of heart failure can be made without the aid of the laboratory; yet in complex cases valuable clues can be obtained by a careful and detailed analysis of the laboratory profile. Typically, the chest roentgenogram of the patient in cardiac failure shows enlargement of the heart with an increased cardiothoracic ratio. Interstitial edema may be present, as reflected by Kerley's B lines. There may also be an enlargement of upper-lobe pulmonary veins and an increase in the caliber of the pulmonary arteries. Pleural effusions and the typical butterfly pattern of pulmonary edema may be seen with florid heart failure. Hyperinflation of the pulmonary parenchyma is not a characteristic finding, as it is in bronchial asthma. Occasionally, other clues such as valve or vessel calcification may be observed.

No ECG changes are diagnostic of heart failure, but supporting evidence either for heart disease or for bronchial asthma might be uncovered. For example, the patient with an acute myocardial infarction may display typical ECG changes; however, reversible ECG abnormalities have been reported in acute asthmatic attacks [306, 336].

A diagnostic maneuver that may be successful in patients with histories of both heart disease and bronchial asthma, and in whom standard testing techniques have failed, employs the Swan-Ganz catheter. Elevations of pulmonary arterial pressure may be observed with acute asthmatic episodes, but in uncomplicated cases the pulmonary wedge pressure remains normal. Conversely, an elevated pulmonary wedge pressure establishes the diagnosis of cardiac failure, provided the plasma oncotic pressure is normal [222]. Such invasive diagnostic maneuvers should be reserved for those critically ill patients for whom diagnostic confusion is profound.

In ambulatory patients and in patients in whom the use of a Swan-Ganz catheter is not deemed fit, a noninvasive test that may be helpful is multiple-gated acquisition radioisotopes angiography (MUGA scan). The ejection fraction obtained by contrast ventriculoangiograms and two-dimensional echocardiograms correlates well with the results of the MUGA scan [119]. An ejection fraction of less than 55 percent (normal, 55–65%) is an indicator of decreased myocardial performance and points to cardiac dysfunction.

Pulmonary function testing in patients with acute CHF typically reveals a combined obstructive and restrictive defect that improves with treatment of the CHF. However, a study by Light [156] revealed that as many as half of such patients were left with a residual obstructive defect, despite symptomatic improvement with treatment of the CHF.

In emergencies when the physician is faced with an anxious, diaphoretic patient complaining of severe dyspnea and orthopnea who has diffuse expiratory and inspiratory wheezing, the distinction between cardiac asthma and bronchial asthma is difficult. Indeed, it may be impossible to establish either diagnosis with certainty, and the clinician must resort to a therapeutic trial. If such is the case, treatment with diuretics, aminophylline, beta₂-agonist nebulizers, and oxygen is appropriate. Morphine sulfate, because of its deleterious effects in bronchial asthma, must be used selectively and with caution. It should be remembered that acute CHF may respond to the bed rest, theophylline, and nebulized bronchodilators prescribed to treat acute bronchial asthma [297]. It must be stressed that a diagnosis of cardiac asthma requires a high index of suspicion in the appropriate clinical setting.

Microvascular Angina

Approximately 10 to 30 percent of patients with anginalike pain have no lesions demonstrated at cardiac catheterization. Many of these patients have increased resistance in the small microvascular coronary vessels. Some of these patients have demonstrated a generalized abnormality of smooth muscle, both vascular and nonvascular, including coronary microvasculature and bronchial wall smooth muscle. Fourteen (45%) of 31 patients described by Cannon also demonstrated a positive response to methacholine inhalation challenge testing. The author concluded that the increased incidence of airway hyperresponsiveness may account for the disproportionate degree of dyspnea that these patients exhibit [33].

If dyspnea dominates the clinical presentation, and the patient demonstrates increased airway hyperresponsiveness, confusion with bronchial asthma is possible. A careful analysis of the total picture should clarify the issue.

Sarcoidosis

Cough, wheeze, and dyspnea are seen in both bronchial asthma and sarcoidosis. This may present difficulty in a differential diagnosis. In 1941, the first case of intrabronchial sarcoidosis was described: "[T]he picture clinically was that of asthma with universal wheezing and rhonchi" [17]. Since then there have been many reports of patients presenting with wheeze, dyspnea, and cough secondary to sarcoidosis [110, 166, 185, 267, 292]. Airway obstruction due to sarcoidosis occurs more frequently than is generally accepted [154, 246, 247]. Obstructive lesions can occur anywhere in the respiratory tract, and are commonly seen in Stage I (hilar adenopathy) and Stage II (hilar adenopathy with parenchymal involvement) sarcoidosis [6, 66, 167].

The mechanisms of airway obstruction in sarcoidosis are varied [25, 154, 247] and include (1) bronchial fibrosis [185]; (2) granuloma that may compress or intrude on the lumen of large airways; (3) granulomas formed in the interstitium that may modify the supporting structure around terminal and respiratory bronchioles; and (4) as described more recently [15, 167], a hyperreactivity of the airways as shown by a positive result on the methacholine inhalation test [246].

Recent investigations propose that the bronchoactive mediators, prostaglandin E_2, leukotriene B_4, and histamine are released by cells present in the alveoli [49, 219, 223]. Whether this is the mechanism of wheezing in sarcoidosis remains speculative.

The total clinical picture and laboratory profile with features such as hilar and paratracheal adenopathy on chest x-ray films, elevated angiotensin-converting enzyme (ACE) levels, and positive findings on gallium scans are associated with active sarcoidosis and help differentiate it from bronchial asthma. In addition, one is reminded that airway obstruction due to sarcoidosis generally does not respond to bronchodilators, whereas asthma does. Airway obstruction due to asthma typically has a high single breath diffusion capacity, believed to be a hallmark of asthma [152], whereas airway obstruction due to sarcoidosis usually has a low single breath diffusion capacity, but this is not always the case [246].

It should be remembered that if granulomas are strategically located, cough, wheeze, and spirometry demonstrating obstruction may result. Therefore, any illness characterized by pulmonary granulomatosis (e.g., Wegener's granulomatosis [52, 89, 233]) may produce this pattern.

Adult Respiratory Distress Syndrome

Adult respiratory distress syndrome (ARDS) was first described in 1967 by Ashbaugh and coauthors [7]. Currently accepted definitions rely mainly on the presence of hypoxia, diffuse pulmonary infiltrates on chest x-ray films, and poorly compliant ("stiff") lungs [59]. Many physicians attempt to exclude cardiogenic pulmonary edema by documenting a normal pulmonary capillary wedge pressure. More recently, an expanded definition was proposed [174, 194, 214], supported by data from a study in England [75, 231]. The expanded definition first categorizes the parenchymal lung injury into acute or chronic, and then into mild to moderate or severe, and finally associates the injury with the event that caused it or was associated with it [194]. Thus, the expanded definition takes into account causes known and unknown, the possibility of a chronic nature to the disease, and a spectrum of disease severity, with ARDS representing the most severe form.

A number of mediators have been implicated in ARDS [171, 227, 230, 270]; however, no unifying mediator has been uncovered.

Occasionally, wheezing and airway obstruction can be seen with this syndrome. Bronchial asthma can usually be easily differentiated from ARDS based on the total clinical picture. In follow-up of ARDS survivors, some patients developed airway obstruction [80, 99, 296] and increased bronchial hyperreactivity [255]. Elliot and colleagues reported abnormal values for 1-second forced expiratory volume (FEV_1)–forced vital capacity (FVC) in 4 of 16 previously healthy nonsmokers recovering from ARDS [81]. The pulmonary function of most ARDS survivors returns to normal in 5 to 7 months after the event [213]. Of particular importance are those ARDS survivors who required especially high PEEP values, some of whom seem to be at higher risk for developing laryngotracheal stenosis, a condition that may be confused with bronchial asthma (see section on central airway obstruction). The clinical spectra of bronchial asthma and ARDS are distinct and not confusing. Nevertheless, the obstructive sequela of ARDS requires careful definition and longitudinal follow-up.

Acquired Immunodeficiency Syndrome

Airway obstruction has been found in patients with the acquired immunodeficiency syndrome (AIDS) [288]. Wheezing and chest tightness are common in some AIDS populations [202]. In one study, 4 of 61 AIDS patients presented with a cough and a normal-appearing chest x-ray film. Spirometry revealed reversible airway obstruction, and all patients had symptomatic and spirometric improvement with bronchodilators [268]. Another study noted that 44 percent of patients with AIDS had either a low forced expiratory flow rate or a significant improvement after bronchodilator treatment. There was a significant association between symptoms of wheeze, cough, and chest tightness and the presence of abnormal airway function [202].

Patients with Kaposi's sarcoma may present with wheeze, dyspnea, and nonproductive cough [180, 299] due to the presence of endobronchial lesions, or microscopic compromise of small airways due to the perivascular and peribronchial location of Kaposi's sarcoma [180]. In one study, 6 of 11 AIDS patients studied at autopsy had prior evidence of airflow obstruction by pulmonary function testing; 4 of these 6 had endobronchial lesions [180]. However, the pattern and tempo of chest x-ray findings along with the appropriate clinical setting should distinguish this disease entity. Endobronchial lesions may also be seen with cytomegalovirus [125], *Pneumocystis carinii* pneumonia [97], tuberculosis [285], and *Mycobacterium avium* complex infection [207] occurring in AIDS patients. Other proposed mechanisms for airway obstruction could be infection-induced bronchospasm, especially viral [144], or a hypersensitivity phenomenon as seen with the high incidence of reactions to trimethoprim-sulfamethoxazole in AIDS patients [103]. In a recent study of 100 HIV-infected patients, 26 were found to have evidence of airway obstruction by spirometry and visual analogue scale [317].

Cocaine Toxicity

Reports of pulmonary toxicity, temporally related to cocaine abuse, are occurring with increasing frequency as smoking of the cocaine alkaloid, commonly known as *crack*, has become more popular [86, 195, 272]. Included among these complications is the association of asthma with cocaine [224, 237]. Asthma can be provoked by cocaine, as was first suggested in 1932 [283], and Suhl reported wheezing in a third of cocaine smokers [269]. Mild airway obstruction has been demonstrated on pulmonary function tests [64, 128] and bronchospasm in nonasthmatic patients has also been described [141]. Possible mechanisms of cocaine-induced bronchospasm include cocaine-induced bronchial smooth muscle contraction and a direct irritant effect of the inhaled noxious gas on airway epithelium [272].

Central Airway Obstruction

Central airway obstruction represents a group of disorders characterized by airflow obstruction in larger airways. This important group of asthma masqueraders may require surgery. The clinical manifestations can range from wheezing spells, frequently associated with terrifying episodes of stridor and gasping respirations, to severe spasms of coughing and even syncope, or to focal wheezing with few other complaints. In addition, focal central lesions may induce, via an irritative reflex mechanism, diffuse bronchoconstriction resulting in widespread polyphonic wheezing. Symptoms with exercise usually occur when the airway diameter is reduced to about 8 mm. Stridor at rest may occur when the airway diameter is narrowed to 5 mm. The importance of distinguishing a lesion of the central airway from asthma is obvious, but the distinction is possible only if the clinician undertakes a careful systematic analysis of the clinical circumstances, physical findings, and laboratory data. For example, in the middle-aged cigarette-smoking man, suffering from the recent onset of hoarseness and a palpable wheeze or rhonchus over the larynx, a lesion at this level of the airway must clearly be suspected and requires an entirely different diagnostic and therapeutic regimen from that for bronchial asthma.

The lung, when viewed in longitudinal section, has been likened to a trumpet [32], the glottis being analogous to the mouthpiece and the lung parenchyma to the horn portion. The predominance of inspiratory or expiratory dysfunction depends on whether a lesion is extrathoracic or intrathoracic. Normally, intrathoracic airways become narrow and short with expiration, and long and wide during inspiration. Therefore, wheezing associated with intrathoracic disease is predominantly expiratory. If the obstructed airway is extrathoracic, the pressure differential on the affected region caused by a vigorous inspiratory effort results in a substantial narrowing of the airway and inspiratory stridor [186].

The pulmonary function profile of a patient with extrathoracic disease may show an abnormal inspiratory limb to the vital capacity of the flow-volume curve (Fig. 37-4). Central airway lesions classically produce a marked increase in airway resistance with normal distribution of ventilation as measured by nitrogen or xenon. Breathing a mixture of helium and oxygen increases flow in density-dependent areas, that is, large airways [51, 160, 186].

Leape [148] noted a number of clues that may point to a nonallergic or mechanical cause of wheezing: (1) sudden onset of wheezing; (2) history of aspiration; (3) nocturnal asthma; (4)

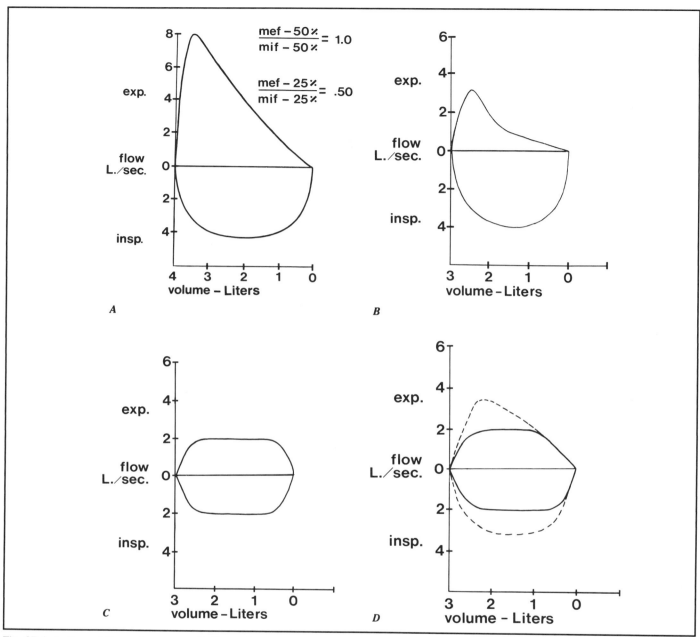

Fig. 37-4. *A. Normal flow-volume curve. B. Flow-volume curve in chronic obstructive pulmonary disease, showing a decrease in expiratory flow. C. Flow-volume curve in a patient with fixed extrathoracic obstruction. No change in flow is noted during inspiration and expiration. D. Flow-volume curve in a patient with extrathoracic obstruction breathing room air* (solid lines) *and helium* (dotted lines). *Note the improvement in flow with helium.* exp. = *expiration;* insp. = *inspiration;* mef = *maximum expiratory flow;* mif = *minimum inspiratory flow.*

absence of allergic markers, that is, history of atopy, hay fever, or eczema; (5) absence of specific triggering mechanism or cause; (6) fair to poor response to bronchodilator therapy; and (7) presence of other signs of associated disease, for example, stridor, fever, cellulitis of the neck, and hemoptysis.

The initial onset of symptoms and signs, which may be insidious or abrupt, is characterized by continuous or paroxysmal episodes of wheezing and shortness of breath. Some lesions may be pedunculated and thus provoked by positional changes. This is illustrated by the not uncommon history of unilateral or diffuse wheezing with recumbency. Some patients may even be able to identify the location of the lesion.

The physical examination may be particularly helpful in pointing to the large airways as the involved area. For example, the palpation of a mass (e.g., thyroid, tumor), signs of venous obstruction (although neck vein distention may be seen with acute asthma), or perhaps deviation of the trachea by a mass lesion may indicate the cause of wheezing.

A focal monophonic wheeze that is loudest at the level of involvement, often audible and palpable, generally spreads with decreasing intensity away from the focal point. This produces the combination of focal noisy breathing with clear lung fields and is most suggestive of central airway obstruction. Thus, it is not unusual to find normal diaphragmatic motion and remarkably silent peripheral lung fields. On the contrary, during an episode of bronchial asthma, one may be unable to detect any diaphragmatic motion, and the peripheral lung fields usually disclose widespread polyphonic wheezing [289], except during severe episodes resulting in insufficient air movement to generate a wheeze. With central airway lesions, if rales or rhonchi are present, they do not disappear with coughing. On the other hand, the patient may complain of wheezing when none is heard on auscultation, and it is only with rapid deep breathing or position change that one may evoke the characteristic monophonic wheeze.

The problem of tracheal stricture continues to be of concern because of the frequent use of endotracheal tubes and tracheostomies [150].

Broncholithiasis due to chronically inflamed adjacent lymph nodes may erode into the airways, causing a central airway obstruction. The causes of the adjacent lymphadenopathy can be infectious, such as tuberculosis or fungi, or noninfectious, such as silicosis [303].

Thoracic malignancies can also be confused with bronchial asthma. Classically endobronchial tumors, primary or metastatic, can present with wheezing, cough, and dyspnea [13, 26, 124, 248]. Lymphomas can present as wheezing due to endobronchial obstruction [87]. Hodgkin's disease is one of the more common tumors of the young, 60 percent of whom have mediastinal involvement. Tumors that are strategically located may give rise to symptoms and signs of airway obstruction. A recent article reported on 6 patients with Hodgkin's disease presenting with life-threatening airway obstruction due to endobronchial disease. All responded well to steroids, chemotherapy, or radiotherapy [132]. Lymphangitic carcinomatosis of the lung may present with wheezing, both paroxysmal and continuous; however, the pathogenesis remains unclear [14, 181].

A chest x-ray film should be obtained for every patient in whom a diagnosis of asthma is made for the first time. This may reveal abnormalities such as radiopaque foreign bodies that classically occur in children, but can also be seen in adults [31, 36]; focal atelectasis; or compression of a major airway. A flow volume loop usually reveals evidence of intra- or extrathoracic airway obstruction, and body plethysmography can help define the lesion [329].

The CT scan provides detailed structural visualization of the trachea and larynx. However, bronchoscopy is definitive. Finally, the clinician should be alert to the development of an upper airway lesion in a patient with established asthma. The causes and clinical presentation of central airway obstruction are summarized in Table 37-2.

Endobronchial Tuberculosis

Nonproductive cough, wheeze, and dyspnea are well described manifestations of endobronchial tuberculosis [279, 290]. The ability of tuberculosis to masquerade as bronchial asthma [290] should not be surprising given the extensive variety of known presentations of tuberculosis.

Endobronchial tuberculosis was first described by the English physician Richard Morton in 1689 [190], but this was not commonly appreciated until the advent of bronchoscopy in the late 1920s. Since then, it has been estimated that 10 to 20 percent of patients with pulmonary tuberculosis who have undergone bronchoscopy have endobronchial tuberculosis [178, 261, 279], and as many as 60 to 70 percent of patients with pulmonary tuberculosis are found to have evidence of endobronchial involvement at postmortem examination [9].

Early findings of endobronchial tuberculosis include mucosal granularity and ulcers, progressing to hyperplastic inflammatory polyps occurring in the region of previous ulcers, eventually progressing to fibroid stenosis [260]. This occurs as a result of (1)

Table 37-2. Diagnosis of wheezing caused by central airway obstruction

Symptoms
  Hacking "metallic" cough
  Hoarseness (or voice change)
  Diaphoresis
  Anxiety (may be marked)
  Dyspnea
Signs
  Wheezing: monophonic, polyphonic
  Respiratory rales
  Inspiratory stridor
  Cyanosis (a very late manifestation)
Causes
  Extrathoracic
    Extrinsic
      Thyroid
        Goiter
        Hashimoto's thyroiditis
        Tumor
      Lymphoma
      Edema of subcutaneous tissues of neck
      Postoperative hemorrhage (e.g., after thyroid surgery)
      Retropharyngeal compression by edema
      Mediastinal compression by edema (trauma, postoperative)
      Vascular anomalies
        Congenital
        Aortic aneurysm
      Hematoma secondary to trauma (e.g., internal jugular cannulation)
      Infections
        Ludwig's angina
        Peritonsillar abscess
        Diphtheria
    Intrinsic
      Burns
      Supraglottitis
      Tracheobronchitis
      Acute bronchitis
      Epiglottitis
      Foreign body
        Vegetative: acute inflammation, cough, septic fever
        Nonvegetative: sharp or blunt
      Tracheal fracture
      Tracheal stricture
      Tracheomalacia
      Pertussis
      Laryngeal trauma
      Laryngeal edema (anaphylaxis)
      Laryngeal spasm
      Hematoma
      Cyst
      Fungal infections of trachea (e.g., mucormycosis)
      Tracheobronchial tumor
        Benign: papilloma, fibrolipoma, angioma, adenoma
        Malignant: epithelioma, sarcoma
  Intrathoracic
    Stricture
    Tumor, especially squamous cell
    Foreign body
    Polyps
    Vascular rings
    Hematoma (e.g., subclavian vein cannulation)

direct implantation of the tubercle bacillus into the bronchus from infected sputum, blood, or lymphatics; or (2) extension from adjacent infiltrate, occurring more commonly in adults, or from adjacent mediastinal lymph nodes, occurring more commonly in children [126, 260, 290]. More recently, a hypersensitivity to endobronchial granulomas was proposed for those patients who have wheezing despite adequately treated tuberculosis [290].

On examination, auscultation may reveal the classic low-pitched localized wheeze always heard at the same site. However, as the endobronchial lesion increases in size, the airway becomes so compromised that the wheeze may decrease in intensity and even disappear. Also, bronchostenosis and the wheeze it produces may persist and indeed progress, despite adequate antituberculosis therapy [1].

In addition, there are reports of patients with appropriately treated primary pulmonary tuberculosis who clinically deteriorated 6 to 26 weeks after starting treatment, presenting with wheezing that was unresponsive to bronchodilators. The wheezing was found to be the result of sterile endobronchial granuloma. Both wheeze and granuloma responded to cortical steroids and the authors proposed a hypersensitivity component as the cause for the wheezing [290].

Sputum smears and culture should differentiate endobronchial tuberculosis from bronchial asthma and in the case of a localized wheeze, bronchoscopy with biopsy should prove diagnostic.

Angioedema

Angioedema is a local, well-circumscribed inflammation, with edema and vascular congestion involving the deep layers of the skin and submucosa. There are two major categories of angioedema, one common, the other rare. The pathogenesis of the common form is unknown. The rare form is due to a deficiency of normal-functioning C1 esterase inhibitor (C1INH), and can be hereditary—hereditary angioneurotic edema (HAE) [62, 68]—or acquired [3, 96].

The differentiation of the common form of angioedema from the rare form rests on the detection of a low serum level of normal-functioning C1INH seen in the rare form.

The common form of angioedema can affect up to 15 percent of the population [175, 259], most commonly women in their 20s and 30s [109]. It can be a result of an allergic reaction (Type I Gell and Coombs) and multiple factors, including trauma, food, drugs, infections (viral, parasitic, and bacterial), inhalants, and psychogenic factors, have been found to induce it [175]. In addition, there is a common association of angioedema with asthma, including that 40 percent of angioedema attacks are induced by aspirin [109, 234] and exercise [151, 153]. In addition to cough, angioedema can also occur as a side effect of ACE inhibitor therapy. However, the incidence of angioedema induced by ACE inhibitor is rare, occurring in 0.1 to 0.2 percent of patients receiving ACE inhibitor therapy [312, 315].

C1INH is a serum alpha$_2$ globulin and has an inhibitory action on four systems: (1) complement, (2) intrinsic pathway of coagulation, (3) fibrinolysis, and (4) kinin-generating enzyme system [96]. The precise pathophysiologic mechanisms remain controversial and the mediators of symptoms have been difficult to determine. Bradykinin is thought to be the primary mediator, but other mediators such as the peptide identified by Donaldson [67] are also thought to be involved.

Patients with angioedema frequently complain of paroxysms of shortness of breath and wheezing, presenting at first glance a picture very similar to asthma. To confuse matters further, patients with HAE are frequently young and have strong family histories of similar episodes that may be reported as family histories of asthma; such patients may also have asthma as well as angioedema [109, 151, 153, 234].

Angioedema due to C1INH deficiency (HAE) may occur in multiple sites, and is not painful except when there is gastrointestinal tract involvement. Patients with gastrointestinal tract involvement present with crampy abdominal pain, which may be useful in distinguishing this angioedema from other causes of airway obstruction. However, the laryngeal involvement is the issue. Because the larynx is so frequently involved, the clinical presentation of both the hereditary and the nonhereditary forms of

C1INH deficiency may be episodic wheezing, during which fatal asphyxiation may occur. The typical picture of central airway obstruction is seen with inspiratory stridor, crowing respirations, hoarseness, and apprehension to the point of panic. There may or may not be a history of recent local trauma, such as dental extraction or tonsillectomy, or emotional stress, factors known to incite this syndrome.

There is no biochemical test available for identifying the common form of angioedema. The diagnosis of the rare form of angioedema is most reliably determined by the detection of a low level of normal-functioning C1INH in the serum. HAE is distinguished from the acquired form of C1INH deficiency by the presence of a low C1q subunit in the acquired form and a normal level in HAE.

In patients with C1INH deficiency, a high index of suspicion is critical to the proper diagnosis. C1INH deficiency is distinguished from asthma by a low serum level of normal-functioning C1INH.

Laryngeal Dysfunction

Over the past few years, numerous reports have appeared of patients initially misdiagnosed as having bronchial asthma and subsequently found to have vocal cord dysfunction [28, 45] and, more recently, pharyngeal constriction [324] without an identifiable organic cause. Vocal cord dysfunction is an episodic upper airway obstruction where no organic lesion can be found. It is believed by some to be a manifestation of a conversion disorder [45].

Patients present with wheezing episodes that are often dramatic, and may be associated with dyspnea. Such episodes are usually unresponsive to bronchodilators. On examination, wheezing is heard maximally over the anterior part of the neck and may be transmitted to the chest. Hypoxia may be present [42], but is usually not. Pulmonary function tests reveal the classic upper airway obstructive pattern during an attack and normal findings between attacks. When performed, methacholine challenge testing shows negative results. Laryngoscopy performed between attacks shows normal anatomy and function, but during an attack reveals adduction of the vocal cords that may [28] or may not [42] be abolished by intravenous diazepam. EMG of the laryngeal muscles is helpful [322]. Occasionally tracheostomy may be necessary [42, 51]. There is a good response to speech therapy and psychotherapy [319]. In addition, the patient may have bronchial asthma as well as vocal cord dysfunction; such cases can be even more difficult to differentiate (see Table 37-1). The subject of laryngeal dysfunction masquerading as bronchial asthma has recently been extensively reviewed [203, 308] (see Chap. 79).

Gastroesophageal Reflux

The association of gastroesophageal reflux (GER) with asthma has been observed since the late nineteenth century [183, 205]. In 1946, Mendelson's classic paper described intraoperative aspiration presenting as an asthma-like syndrome with wheezing [182]. Since then a great deal of attention has been placed on the role of GER in the provocation of bronchial asthma [170, 321].

There are two major mechanisms by which GER provokes wheezing. The first involves inhalation of stomach contents into the lungs [24, 55], especially acid [206]. The second involves a reflex mechanism mediated by the vagus nerve in response to the presence of acid in the lower esophagus [168] or upper airways [24, 206, 305]. This second mechanism is supported by an increased response to methacholine challenge with intraesophageal perfusion of acid [116]. Other reflex mechanisms have been proposed involving gastric distention [170] but not much data are available (see Chap. 75).

Patients may not volunteer symptoms of GER and close questioning of such symptoms is vital. Patients may note such classic symptoms of GER as heartburn, indigestion, and chest pain, but may also note worsening of their "asthma" after a large meal, ingestion of alcoholic beverages, or when they lie down. These patients frequently have nocturnal wheezing. Symptoms that start in adulthood, obese body habitus, absence of a history of allergy, and symptoms that worsen with aminophylline therapy [19, 121, 294] are all useful diagnostic clues. The physical examination may reveal monophonic wheezing if aspiration of food contents has occurred in a focal area; if not, then GER-induced bronchospasm may be indistinguishable from the bronchospasm of true bronchial asthma. The most accurate diagnostic tool for GER is the 24-hour pH monitor, which is able to detect the presence of acid reflux into the esophagus. In addition, scintigraphy of the lungs the morning after ingestion of a radiolabeled meal may be used to detect microaspiration into the lung. In treating the pulmonary symptoms related to GER, it should be remembered that the commonly used bronchodilators, beta-adrenergic agonists, anticholinergic agents, and aminophylline, can relax the lower esophageal sphincter and promote reflux [19, 121, 294]. In treating the GER, medical therapy may provide some improvement in the patient's wheezing [79]. There are reports of cures of such wheezing after surgical treatment of the GER; these cures were predominantly of nocturnal wheezing [37, 212, 263, 335].

It should be remembered while GER can cause or worsen bronchial asthma, bronchial asthma can in turn trigger GER by increasing transdiaphragmatic pressure [24, 71, 206]. The extent of the role of GER in bronchial asthma is still a matter of debate [206, 271].

Carcinoid Syndrome

The carcinoid syndrome, originally described by Thorsen in 1954 [276], is a constellation of clinical signs and symptoms resulting from the release of various humoral agents from carcinoid tumors. The major clinical characteristics are paroxysmal episodes of flushing, watery diarrhea, wheezing, and hypotension. When wheezing and shortness of breath are prominent, confusion with bronchial asthma is possible [173, 251, 281].

Carcinoid tumors are neoplasms of low-grade malignancy originating in Kulchitzky's cells, commonly known as *argentaffin cells.* Carcinoid tumors can present clinically because of obstruction of the organ system where the primary tumor is located, or from endocrine symptoms resulting from the release of humoral substances such as serotonin or bradykinin. Whether a carcinoid tumor causes the carcinoid syndrome depends on its ability to release vasoactive hormones and its anatomic location. The carcinoid syndrome only occurs when large amounts of the biologically active substances reach the systemic circulation. Carcinoid tumors of the gastrointestinal tract most often cause the carcinoid syndrome only after metastases to the liver have occurred because most of their venous drainage is into the portal circulation. Bronchial carcinoid tumors, on the other hand, can cause the carcinoid syndrome without metastases occurring because of the release of mediators directly into the systemic circulation. However, since the incidence of metastasis is less than 2 percent when carcinoid tumors are smaller than 1 cm and 100 percent when larger than 2 cm [281] and because the carcinoid syndrome can occur only when a tumor is large enough to produce sufficient quantities of hormone, by the time a primary carcinoid tumor has produced the carcinoid syndrome, metastases have usually already occurred.

There are two mechanisms by which carcinoid tumors can present difficulty in the differential diagnosis of a wheezing patient. The first is by airway obstruction from a primary bronchial carcinoid tumor [5, 133, 301], occurring in 10 to 20 percent of patients with carcinoid tumors [173, 281, 298]. The second is by bronchospasm induced by the mediators released by the carci-

noid tumor (i.e., the carcinoid syndrome), occurring in less than 10 percent of all patients with carcinoid tumors [173, 281].

Most carcinoid tumors do not produce the carcinoid syndrome [173, 281]. However, when the syndrome is present, serotonin and bradykinin are the mediators most frequently responsible for the clinical manifestations.

The major symptoms related to the lung are cough, fever, chest pain, dyspnea, hemoptysis, and wheezing. Patients most likely to have pulmonary symptoms are those with prominent flushing episodes. A flush is initially red, followed by a violaceous hue that spreads progressively from the face to the trunk—bradykinin is the mediator responsible [200, 229]. The wheezing and dyspnea of the carcinoid syndrome may respond to steroids when the carcinoid tumor is of foregut origin, thus rendering the therapeutic separation from asthma of no diagnostic value. Furthermore, both illnesses may occur paroxysmally and may be triggered by similar events such as anxiety, anger, or exercise. However, the presence of watery or explosive diarrhea, hypotension, abdominal pain, or urinary urgency indicates the carcinoid syndrome. Dermatologic manifestations such as telangiectasia are helpful. Heart valve lesions including fibrosis of the pulmonic and tricuspid valves are late but distinct manifestations of this syndrome.

The diagnosis of the carcinoid syndrome depends on a strong clinical suspicion in patients with the symptoms mentioned above, and is established by the detection of considerably elevated levels of mediators or their breakdown products in the serum or urine. Of the implicated mediators, serotonin is the only one that can be measured routinely. When serotonin is measured in the serum or urine, or its breakdown product 5-hydroxyindoleacetic acid (5-HIAA) is measured in the urine, there is an 85 percent sensitivity for detecting patients with carcinoid tumor. Urinary 5-HIAA levels alone have 73 percent sensitivity and 100 percent specificity [281]. Normal blood contains approximately 0.05 to 0.50 μg/ml of serotonin. It is oxidatively deaminated by monoamine oxidase and appears in the urine as 5-HIAA. The normal range for 5-HIAA secretion in the urine is 2 to 8 mg/24 hr. In some cases of the carcinoid syndrome, the levels of urinary 5-HIAA may be normal, and a careful search for other conjugated by-products of 5-HIAA, such as glucuronides and ethereal sulfates, must be undertaken. If these values are found to be normal, then provocative testing may be employed. Alcohol ingestion, infusions of norepinephrine, dopamine, histamine or calcium may elevate serotonin and 5-HIAA concentrations to diagnostic levels [136]. The other diagnostic method is, of course, tissue biopsy.

Note that certain foods (bananas, tomatoes, pineapples, and walnuts) are capable of elevating urinary 5-HIAA levels, as are the malabsorptive states (sprue, Whipple's disease, and blind loop syndrome). Patients taking acetaminophen or cough syrup containing guaifenesin may have spuriously elevated 5-HIAA levels, but not of the same magnitude as usually seen with the carcinoid syndrome. No single measure detects all cases of carcinoid syndrome, but the 24-hour urine collection for 5-HIAA appears to be the best screening procedure.

Chest radiograph or CT scan usually detects primary bronchial carcinoid tumors [281]. Abdominal CT detects liver metastases, but locating the primary carcinoid tumor in the gastrointestinal tract is more difficult. Recently, scintigraphy using iodine 131 metaiodobenzylguanidine (MIBG) has been used successfully to help locate gastrointestinal carcinoid tumors [281].

In treating the carcinoid syndrome, various modalities, including a long-acting somatostatin analog, interferon, and hepatic arterial embolization, have been successfully employed [53, 143, 172].

Bronchiolitis

Bronchiolitis is an acute inflammatory obstruction of the small airways [84]. Originally described in 1901 [146], the term has been applied most often to infants with severe lower respiratory tract infection, usually due to the respiratory syncytial virus (RSV). However, bronchiolitis also occurs in adults [69, 138] and is a major cause of decreased long-term survival in heart-lung transplant recipients [273]. A number of causes have been incriminated and include viral infection, connective tissue disorders, various medications, and inhalation of noxious gases; in those patients for whom no cause is found, the term *idiopathic bronchiolitis* is applied. RSV infection, especially in the winter, accounts for most of the bronchiolitis seen in children but in adults most cases are idiopathic. See also Chapter 44.

The clinical picture in bronchiolitis may be indistinguishable from that of acute bronchial asthma. Adult patients present with an accelerated form of obstructive lung disease of rapid onset that fails to improve with bronchodilator therapy. Many children with bronchiolitis do not require hospital admission, although the classic presentation is of a critically ill infant with hyperinflation and chest wall recession, often with cyanosis and sometimes carbon dioxide retention. Wheezing is a prominent sign [43, 193]. Viral bronchiolitis is usually preceded by the signs and symptoms of an upper respiratory tract infection. Frequently other members of the family are also ill. In this setting a therapeutic trial with epinephrine, which results in a dramatic clinical remission, would be most consistent with but not diagnostic of bronchial asthma. The chest radiographs in both asthma and bronchiolitis may show hyperinflation, but with bronchiolitis areas of atelectasis and thickened bronchi are much more common. A negative history or marker for atopy or extrinsic allergy, such as blood or sputum eosinophilia, is more suggestive of bronchiolitis. The distinguishing features of bronchiolitis and bronchial asthma are summarized in Table 37-3.

Diagnostic confusion is further compounded because many infants with acute bronchiolitis develop asthma [114, 177, 187, 258]. Henry looked at 55 children who had documented RSV infection and a clinical diagnosis of bronchiolitis, found that 75 percent had subsequent episodes of wheezing in a 2-year follow-up period, and suggested that this was a result of increased bronchial hyperreactivity [114]. Subsequent studies showed a role for prophylactic nebulized topical steroids to prevent the high incidence of respiratory problems, especially wheezing, in infants and small children recovering from bronchiolitis [34]. The clinical improvement with inhaled steroids was sustained even after discontinuing the inhaled steroid, implying a different mechanism of bronchial hyperreactivity to that observed in bronchial asthma. Such a therapeutic response to inhaled steroids in patients with bronchiolitis is important, as bronchiolitis can have unfavorable responses to $beta_2$ agonists [187] and anticholinergic [113] bronchodilators. More studies are needed to confirm these findings and to establish dosing and delivery [74, 201].

Open lung biopsy may be necessary to make a definitive diagnosis of bronchiolitis, and reveals varying degrees of inflammation of the bronchioles with or without airway obliteration. However, an elevated neutrophil count of greater than 25 percent in bronchoalveolar lavage (BAL) fluid from patients with a high clinical suspicion of bronchiolitis may exempt the necessity for open lung biopsy [69, 138]. The results of open lung biopsy and the use of BAL in patients with bronchiolitis suggest a central role for the neutrophil.

Cystic Fibrosis

Cystic fibrosis is a systemic disorder transmitted in an autosomal recessive manner. Carriers occur in 5 percent of the U.S. white population and are asymptomatic. The cystic fibrosis gene was recently isolated and sequenced and the major mutation identified [137, 228, 232]. The incidence of cystic fibrosis is approximately 1 in 2,000 births. It is characterized by chronic pulmonary disease, pancreatic exocrine insufficiency, and in increase in the concentration of sweat electrolytes. The excessive absorption of sodium and defective regulation of the secretory chloride channel in patients with cystic fibrosis [21, 155] lead to the dehydration of airway secretions and probably contribute to the ineffective clearance of airway secretions, airway obstruction, and chronic bacterial infection [295]. The physicochemical proper-

Table 37-3. Differentiation of bronchiolitis and bronchial asthma

Feature	Bronchiolitis	Bronchial asthma

Associated with	Viral infection
	  Respiratory syncytial virus
	  Influenza
	  Adenoviruses 7 and 21
	  Measles
	Heart-lung transplantation
	Toxic vapors, fumes, and chemicals (e.g., nitric, sulfuric, and hydrochloric acid fumes; talcum powder; zinc stearate)
	Collagen diseases (e.g., rheumatoid arthritis after penicillamine therapy, scleroderma)
	Interstitial pneumonitis
	Miscellaneous
	  Myasthenia gravis
	  Lymphoma
	  Pulmonary alveolar proteinosis
		Respiratory syncytial virus infection in children
		Postnasal drip from chronic sinusitis
		Gastroesophageal reflux
		Hay fever, atopy

Airway obstruction	Usually irreversible	Reversible
Bacterial superinfection	Common	Uncommon
Pulmonary function testing	Obstructive pattern and/or restrictive pattern may also be seen	Mild to marked obstructive pattern
Chest x-ray	Hyperinflation Disseminated small nodular shadows in both lungs Disseminated tram lines in bilateral lower lung fields	Restrictive pattern with associated pneumothorax Hyperinflation Associated pneumothorax and/or pneumomediastinum may rarely be seen in severe cases
Response to bronchodilator therapy	Corticosteroids, if given early, may be beneficial in patients exposed to toxic fumes	Good

ties of mucus in patients with cystic fibrosis were compared with those of mucus from bronchial asthmatics, and it was found that mucus in patients with cystic fibrosis formed larger aggregates of mucin than did mucus from the bronchial asthmatics, thus further impairing the clearance of airway secretion [39].

The clinical spectrum may vary from primarily gastrointestinal complaints to cough, wheezing, and dyspnea. Pulmonary involvement may dominate the clinical picture, especially in patients who manifest the fibrosis in late adolescence or adulthood. When the initial clinical manifestations are confined to the respiratory system, cystic fibrosis can easily be mistaken for asthma or asthmatic bronchitis. Early symptoms of cystic fibrosis can be confused with asthma, whereas later the distinction is not difficult. Wheezing, dyspnea, and perhaps cough may be present continuously or episodically during the mild and moderate stages of the illness. In a 10-year study of 194 patients with cystic fibrosis, chronic cough, pneumonia, and wheezing were the most common clinical features [235]. Although wheezing was more common in patients diagnosed before the age of 1 year [235], it was also observed in adults. The adult with cystic fibrosis is also prone to allergic bronchopulmonary aspergillosis [253, 254]. The cough is productive of variable amounts of sputum that does not contain large numbers of eosinophils or Charcot-Leyden crystals, as in bronchial asthma.

Severe cases of cystic fibrosis are characterized by protracted coughing spasms productive of thick viscid sputum. These patients appear cachectic and have stooped shoulders. They have a barrel chest with a low flat diaphragm, distant breath sounds, scattered rales, rhonchi and wheezes, digital clubbing, cyanosis, and cor pulmonale in the later stage. Distinction from bronchial asthma is not very difficult when confronted with such advanced clinical disease. Hemoptysis, which may be seen in cystic fibrosis, is a symptom not seen in uncomplicated bronchial asthma. Systemic steroids have been used in cystic fibrosis in an attempt to reduce inflammation. Although short-term systemic steroid therapy is of no proven benefit in adults [208], in children alternate-day systemic steroid therapy appears to help [8], but long-term follow-up is required. In addition, 15 percent of adult patients with cystic fibrosis can develop the complication of the "meconium ileus equivalent" [111], and the bronchodilator ipratropium bromide used for bronchial asthma has been cited as a possible cause [192].

The sweat test is crucial in establishing the diagnosis of cystic fibrosis. Shwachman noted that in the presence of symptoms and a family history of cystic fibrosis, the sweat test establishes the diagnosis with a reliability of 98 percent in the age group between 3 to 4 weeks and 17 years [250]. Sodium and chloride concentrations in human sweat increase with age, yet even in adults the sweat test is an excellent diagnostic marker of cystic fibrosis [235]. The sweat test (pilocarpine iontophoresis) as described by Gibson and Cooke [100] reveals a sweat chloride concentration greater than 60 mEq/L in 98 percent of cystic fibrosis patients and between 50 and 60 mEq/L in 1 to 2 percent; only 1 in 1,000 patients with cystic fibrosis has a sweat chloride concentration less than 50 mEq/L [235]. Elevated levels of sweat chloride are seen in clinically unrelated conditions such as Addison's disease, ectodermal dysplasia, nephrogenic diabetes insipidus, and untreated hypothyroidism [63]. The implications of a positive sweat test result are so serious that a diagnosis of cystic fibrosis should only be made in the face of the overall clinical picture and at least two positive sweat test results [161, 252].

Environmental and Industrial Toxins

Inhalation of toxic gases can cause respiratory disease that can be confused with bronchial asthma. Irritant gases cause a laryngotracheobronchitis that may result in laryngeal edema, causing wheezing or stridor. Irritant gas inhalation may also cause bronchiolitis obliterans weeks after the exposure and such patients may then present with cough, wheeze, and dyspnea [84]. Diagnosis rests on the clinical manifestations in an appropriate setting and the characteristic odor of the gas. Treatment involves 100% oxygen and bronchodilator drugs if there is evidence of bronchial spasm, with careful attention to potential secondary bacterial infection.

Smoke inhalation is one of the most common irritant gas inhalation injuries seen. In a recent study it was shown that airway obstruction and bronchial hyperresponsiveness are common after smoke inhalation, although it is unclear how long these abnormalities persisted as the follow-up period was only 3 months [140]. Nitrogen dioxide is also an irritant gas and even short-term exposure to concentrations as low as 1.5 ppm increases bronchial reactivity in normal subjects [95].

Allergic asthma (Type I hypersensitivity reaction) can be caused by an industrial or environmental agent acting as a complete allergen. The affected worker usually complains of wheezing and shortness of breath in the evening after a day's exposure. This acute wheezing and dyspnea may be quite protracted and severe. If removal from the affected environment results in clinical remission, and if rechallenge causes an exacerbation of symptoms, then a presumptive diagnosis can be made. Unfortunately, the duration of time necessary to effect a remission is quite variable and may range up to several months. There may be no family or personal history of atopy. On the other hand, a moderate eosinophilia of 5 to 15 percent is frequently observed [164]. Some patients demonstrate an immediate wheal-and-flare reaction with skin testing. The pulmonary function profile is nonspecific as is the chest roentgenogram, and specific bronchoprovocation testing with the appropriate allergen may be required if a definitive diagnosis is necessary.

The diagnosis of occupational asthma is suggested by the onset of a wheezing illness in a population for which there is a clear industrial exposure [41]. However, in other cases the distinction may not be so obvious. The "do-it-yourselfer" who is working with substances such as toluene diisocyanate (TDI) may not even realize that he or she is being exposed to a provocative agent, and must be asked specifically what substances he or she handles, not just at work but also outside the workplace.

The extrinsic allergic pneumonias in general do not pose a problem in the differential diagnosis of asthma. Most of their symptoms such as fever, shortness of breath, and diffuse aches and pains are ascribed to a Type III (Gell and Coombs classification) hypersensitivity reaction (see Chap. 6). Wheezing is characteristically absent. In some cases, however, there may be a good deal of diagnostic confusion. For example, approximately 10 percent of patients with farmer's lung may have episodes of extrinsic asthma with exposure to moldy hay [198]. The laboratory findings in these instances may be the only method of separating these episodes from uncomplicated bronchial asthma, but one should keep in mind that dual reactions (Types I and III) can occur. The laboratory hallmarks of extrinsic allergic pneumonias include (1) the presence of serum-precipitating antibody to thermophilic actinomycetes, (2) a positive but delayed response (6–8 hour) to antigenic challenge by inhalation, and (3) x-ray findings of a nodular or reticular-nodular pattern.

Confusion may arise when the exposure is subtle, as exemplified by the case report of a patient developing hypersensitivity pneumonitis after exposure to air from a humidifying system contaminated with thermophilic actinomycetes [91].

Psychosomatic Illness

Patients with emotional illness frequently complain of respiratory distress. A common symptom is the inability to take a deep breath. This may be associated with repeated deep sighing and may be observed during the physician's interview. In addition, a typical hyperventilation syndrome, with paresthesia of the hands and face and a sense of light-headedness, may be present in some of these patients. Reassurance that no catastrophe is about to occur, along with an explanation of the physiologic alterations responsible for the patient's symptoms, frequently solves the problem. Reproduction of the symptoms with voluntary hyperventilation or their prevention (e.g., using a rebreathing device) on occasion can be quite useful. No evidence of airway obstruction is demonstrable either on physical examination or by pulmonary function studies. Occasionally, some difficulty may be encountered in distinguishing psychogenic breathing disorders from postexercise asthma. Patients with a psychosomatic illness are to be contrasted with the conscious malingerers (those with factitious asthma).

Factitious Asthma

Factitious asthma is a term that implies the patient is consciously malingering, and may easily be initially misdiagnosed as bronchial asthma [18, 70, 188, 211, 266]. Such patients are usually young females and have the same personality types as patients who have factitious fever and factitious gastrointestinal complaints. These patients have full control of their symptoms and signs, unlike patients with laryngeal dysfunction [45, 51]. A thorough clinical evaluation and appropriate investigatory studies in these patients reveal a wheeze of maximal intensity over the anterior part of the neck and transmitted to the chest, and no evidence of hypoxia or increased alveolar arterial oxygen gradient. A V/Q scan is normal and there is no evidence of hyperinflation on chest x-ray films. A negative result on the methacholine challenge test is seen. On bronchoscopy voluntary adduction of the vocal cords may be seen; this is abolished, along with the wheeze, with intravenous administration of diazepam. A history of previous factitious disorders or other psychiatric manifestations helps distinguish factitious asthma from true bronchial asthma (see Table 37-1). Such distinction between factitious asthma and bronchial asthma is necessary to avoid inappropriate steroid therapy and possible tracheostomy [188]. Appropriate psychiatric evaluation and therapy are indicated, but seldom accepted by the patient.

Chronic Bronchitis, Emphysema, and Small Airway Disease

As defined by the American Thoracic Society criteria, COPD incorporates three disorders: emphysema, chronic bronchitis, and peripheral airway disease [4]. When airway obstruction is prominent, there may be considerable diagnostic confusion with bronchial asthma and routine reversibility testing for airway obstruction, such as methacholine inhalation, may be of no value in distinguishing chronic bronchitis from bronchial asthma [184].

PULMONARY INFILTRATION WITH EOSINOPHILIA

Eosinophilia associated with bronchial asthma is well known but its precise role has not yet been identified [23, 72]. The pulmonary infiltration with eosinophilia (PIE) syndromes have as their common denominator pulmonary infiltration and peripheral blood eosinophilia. Patients with allergic backgrounds are especially prone to the PIE syndromes, which in many instances may be mistaken for typical bronchial asthma. Asthma-like symptoms may be very prominent features of the following members of the PIE group [83, 90, 98, 215]: (1) Löffler's syndrome, (2) chronic

eosinophilic pneumonia, (3) idiopathic hypereosinophilic syndrome, (4) tropical eosinophilia, (5) allergic bronchopulmonary mycosis (see Chap. 49), and (6) Churg-Strauss syndrome.

Löffler's Syndrome

In 1932, Löffler described a syndrome of transient pulmonary infiltrates and peripheral eosinophilia associated with *Ascaris lumbricoides,* the helminthic parasite, infection. Since then, drug sensitivity has been frequently incriminated as the cause, although extrapulmonary manifestations of hypersensitivity such as skin, joint, and kidney ailments are lacking. The suspected drugs are legion, including such common agents as penicillin; disodium chromoglycate, which is commonly used in asthma [262]; acetylsalicylic acid (ASA) and NSAIDs [309], which are also known to exacerbate bronchial asthma. In a review of 5,702 consecutive patients with asthma, Ford noted 20 with PIE [94].

Löffler's syndrome is a self-limiting disease usually lasting less than 4 weeks. Patients can present with cough, wheeze, and dyspnea [83]. The findings on physical examination may be variable, ranging from normal to the acutely ill with tachypnea and diffuse wheezing. In some instances, however, there may be a marked decrease in breath sounds over the area of the chest affected by the pulmonary infiltrate, a finding not typical of uncomplicated bronchial asthma (i.e., without secondary pneumonia or atelectasis). The chest x-ray pattern is that of a fleeting or fluffy infiltrate, frequently peripheral or segmental in location and distribution. Such lesions may last for days, or shift in 24 hours. Mild to moderate blood eosinophilia is observed.

The diagnosis of Löffler's syndrome is based on the demonstration of peripheral eosinophilia and a consistent radiographic evaluation, and on occasion is reinforced by a therapeutic steroid trial. Thus, Löffler's syndrome may be confused with typical asthma. Compounding the confusion, this syndrome also occurs frequently in patients with atopy.

Chronic Pulmonary Infiltration with Eosinophilia

A persistent pulmonary infiltration with eosinophilia that does not clear in 6 weeks is known as chronic PIE. These patients have a more severe protracted course than do patients with Löffler's syndrome, if left untreated. Chronic PIE is twice as common in females and occurs with the peak incidence in patients in their 30s [131]. The relationship between asthma and chronic PIE has been verified in a number of studies. In a recent report of 19 patients and a review of the literature, Jederlinic found that asthma preceded chronic PIE in 7 of 19 patients and that the asthma was most often extrinsic in nature associated with allergic rhinitis and nasal polyps [131]. However, wheezing was reported in one-third of patients after recovery from chronic PIE with no history of bronchial asthma [131]. In another study, follow-up of 7 patients for more than 3 years revealed a positive result on the methacholine challenge test [139].

Patients present most commonly with the insidious onset of cough, fever, and dyspnea. Wheezing occurs in one-third of patients with no history of asthma [131]. Findings on physical examination range from normal to grossly abnormal with percussion, dullness, moist crackles, and wheezing. The peripheral eosinophilia varies widely from 1 to 90 percent, with a mean of 25 percent [35, 131]. The chest radiograph is frequently characteristic enough to suggest the diagnosis. Typically, it shows dense pneumonic infiltrates arranged in a peculiar peripheral pattern (Fig. 37-5), known as the photographic negative of pulmonary edema [176]. These infiltrates may be extensive and progressive. However, this classic picture is seen on chest radiographs in less than 50 percent of patients [131]. When the chest x-ray film is not typical, chest CT is helpful [176]. Approximately one-third of patients with chronic PIE present with subacute upper respira-

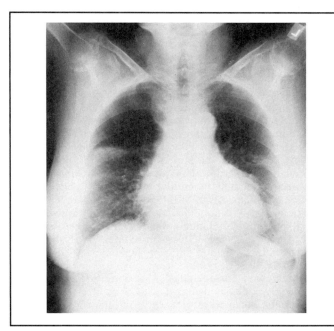

Fig. 37-5. *Chronic pulmonary infiltration with eosinophilia. Note the diffuse, essentially symmetric interstitial infiltrates throughout both lungs, with marked involvement of the peripheral basal portions.*

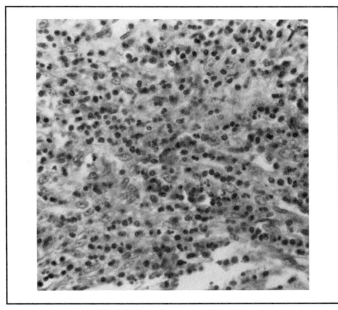

Fig. 37-6. *Lung biopsy specimen demonstrates a diffuse infiltrate composed of eosinophils and histocytes. The character of the infiltrate is dense enough to obliterate normal alveolar structure. (Hematoxylin-eosin, × 400 before 33% reduction.)*

tory tract infection and/or constitutional symptoms, a serum eosinophilia, and a chest radiograph or CT scan that reveals a peripheral infiltrate [131]. A lung biopsy specimen demonstrates alveoli filled with a mixture of large mononuclear cells and eosinophils, edematous interstitium with a similar cellular infiltration, and some plasma cells in the interstitium (Fig. 37-6). Focal areas of fibrosis are found in 50 percent of patients [131]. Spirometry reveals a combined restrictive and obstructive pattern accompanied by hypoxemia and a reduction in diffusion capacity. In dis-

tinguishing this syndrome from bronchial asthma, the critical observations are the persistence in untreated chronic PIE of an abnormal-appearing chest radiograph with its characteristic pattern, and the presence of a prominent or spectacular peripheral eosinophilia. Chronic PIE may be subtle and easily overlooked, masquerading as asthma or asthmatic bronchitis.

Thus in Löffler's syndrome and chronic PIE, two important variants, wheezing and dyspnea may be due to a disorder other than bronchial asthma, and the differentiation may depend on the clinical setting and radiographic and temporal features.

Recently, there have been a number of reports of an acute form of chronic PIE [2, 10, 77, 107, 162]. The acute form was not associated with asthma and no precipitating cause was found. Symptoms, signs, and chest x-ray findings were similar to those for chronic PIE, but the onset was less than a week, much faster than classic chronic PIE, and the condition progressed rapidly to acute respiratory failure; 3 of 6 patients required mechanical ventilation. The pneumonia resolved in 1 to 8 days, much faster than the 2 to 72 months for chronic PIE, and there were no recurrences. This acute form of chronic PIE further confuses the clinician's ability to differentiate this disease from bronchial asthma.

Idiopathic Hypereosinophilic Syndrome

Idiopathic hypereosinophilic syndrome is characterized by idiopathic persistent eosinophilia (1,500 eosinophils/mm^{-3}, or more for a period of at least 6 months) and evidence of organ dysfunction caused by cellular infiltration [48]. The diagnosis requires the exclusion of known causes of eosinophilia (parasites, allergies, etc.). Hypereosinophilic syndrome is a rare condition; most patients are men and have cardiac involvement [88]. Pulmonary manifestations include cough and dyspnea [130], and thus, this syndrome may be mistaken for asthma. Treatment is aimed at lowering the eosinophil count with prednisone and hydroxyurea, and where this fails alpha interferon is used [300]. However, consideration of the total clinical picture and evidence of organ dysfunction, which is not seen in asthma, assist in the differentiation.

Tropical Pulmonary Eosinophilia

First described in 1916 by Low [163], tropical pulmonary eosinophilia is a clinical syndrome of respiratory symptoms, peripheral eosinophilia, and pulmonary infiltrate. It is thought to be a hypersensitivity reaction to the human filarial parasites *Wuchereria bancrofti* and *Brugia malayi* [197]. Tropical pulmonary eosinophilia occurs frequently in areas where filariasis is endemic: India, Southeast Asia, Africa, and South America. With the increasing availability of air travel, there have been increasing numbers of case reports from nonendemic areas, of patients who had recently spent a few months in an endemic area [44, 65, 134, 158]. The diagnostic criteria include (1) recent residence in the tropics; (2) predominantly pulmonary symptoms, especially wheezing and dyspnea; (3) blood eosinophil count in excess of 2,000/mm^{-3}; (4) antifilarial antibodies; (5) elevated IgE; (6) predominantly restrictive pattern seen on pulmonary function tests; and (7) a clinical response to diethylcarbamazine citrate characterized by the disappearance of symptoms in 2 weeks and a fall in the eosinophil count within a month.

The association of eosinophilia and pulmonary symptoms with other helminthic infestations has been well recognized for many years (Table 37-4). This is especially true of worms that migrate through the host, such as *Ascaris*. Experimentally produced *Ascaris* infestations of the lungs produce symptoms by two separate mechanisms: (1) primary infection with *Ascaris* larvae followed by mechanical damage of pulmonary capillaries and subsequent infestation of pulmonary tissue; and (2) reinfection resulting in

Table 37-4. Eosinophilia and pulmonary diseases

Allergic (atopic) asthma
Intrinsic asthma
Granulomatous infection
   Tuberculosis
   Histoplasmosis
   Coccidioidomycosis
   Brucellosis
Bacterial infection
Allergic aspergillosis
Hypersensitivity pneumonitis
Helminth infestation
   Visceral larvae migrans
   Ascariasis
   Amebiasis
   Clonorchiasis
   Filariasis
   Paragonimiasis
   Schistosomiasis
   Strongyloidiasis
   Tropical eosinophilia
Hodgkin's disease
Sarcoidosis
Vasculitis
   Periarteritis nodosa
   Churg-Strauss syndrome
Rheumatoid arthritis
Drug sensitivity
   Nitrofurantoin
   Sulfonamides
   Para-aminosalicylate
   Methotrexate
   Chlorpropamide*
   Imipramine*
   Mephenesin carbamate*
   Penicillin*
Idiopathic pulmonary eosinophilia syndromes
   Löffler's syndrome
   Chronic eosinophilic pneumonia
   Hypereosinophilic syndrome

* Rare association may not necessarily be a cause-effect relationship.

a potent immune response as reflected in brisk eosinophilia, an increase in circulating antibody, and pulmonary infiltrates that in lung biopsy specimens show a substantial eosinophilic component along with edema. The latter type of reaction may be accompanied by considerable wheezing and may be misdiagnosed as bronchial asthma.

Patients typically present with cough, wheeze, and dyspnea, especially at night, and may have fever, sweats, and weight loss. Chest radiographs may show a variety of patterns [145], including interstitial infiltrates that may have a reticular nodular pattern, with a predominance for the middle and lower lobes. The peripheral eosinophilia is marked and is also seen in BAL fluid from patients with acute tropical pulmonary eosinophilia, that reverses with treatment [216]. Another study showed higher levels of polyclonal IgG and IgE in BAL fluid from patients with acute tropical pulmonary eosinophilia than in that from bronchial asthmatics [199]. Pulmonary function testing usually reveals a combined restrictive and obstructive pattern [196, 220, 256] often in the presence of an impaired diffusion capacity [129, 280]. Bronchial hyperreactivity has been shown in two patients with acute tropical pulmonary eosinophilia [38], adding further confusion to the difficulty of distinguishing it from acute bronchial asthma.

The overall clinical picture of worm infestation usually suggests an infectious cause and is characterized by fever and cough. The specific diagnosis, and thus the distinction from bronchial asthma, rests on the isolation and demonstration of the worms or, indirectly, serologic mechanisms.

Churg-Strauss Syndrome

Rackemann and Green [221] first described the association of vasculitis, eosinophilia, and asthma. In reviewing 245 cases of polyarteritis occurring between 1866 and 1939, they demonstrated 27 cases in which asthma played a prominent role. However, sparing of the pulmonary vasculature (pulmonary and bronchial vessels) is so consistent a finding in classic polyarteritis that a predominance of pulmonary involvement prompted a sep

Fig. 37-7. *A pulmonary vein with a perivascular granulomatous reaction characterized by epithelial cells and giant cells. There is an associated mixed inflammatory cell infiltrate composed of lymphocytes and eosinophils. (Hematoxylin-eosin, × 250 before 53% reduction.)*

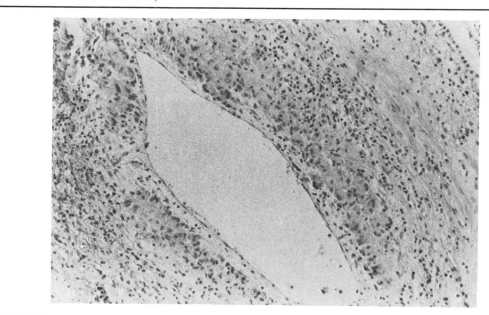

Table 37-5. Differential diagnosis of bronchial asthma

Diagnosis	History	Findings on physical examination	Laboratory tests	Differential diagnostic signs
Bronchial asthmas Extrinsic asthma	Paroxysms of wheezing and dyspnea Family history of atopy Younger age	Polyphonic wheezing, mainly expiratory Rhonchi scattered throughout	Modest blood eosinophilia Sputum eosinophils, Charcot-Leyden crystals, Curschmann's spirals Chest x-ray film shows hyperinflation Positive results on methacholine challenge test	Positive results on skin tests with various antigens Increased levels of IgE
Intrinsic asthma	Paroxysms of wheezing and dyspnea No family history of atopy Older age group, usually > 30 yr	Polyphonic wheezing, mainly expiratory Rhonchi Nasal polyps in some cases	Blood eosinophilia may or may not be present Few eosinophils in sputum Positive results on methacholine inhalation test	Generally negative skin test results Normal or low IgE levels Frequently sensitive to aspirin
Asthmatic bronchitis	Chronic productive cough Older age group, usually > 30 yr Smoking history is frequent	Polyphonic wheezing, both inspiratory and expiratory, with coarse rhonchi throughout	Chest x-ray film may show signs of chronic infection with peribronchial thickening and increased markings Sinusitis may be present Sputum polymorphonuclear leukocytes; bacteria may be present	Typical history of bronchitis with negative results on allergy workup Sputum shows few eosinophils
Exercise-induced asthma	May be only symptom of asthma Type of exercise that induces attack may be variable	May be unremarkable	Decrease in $FEV_{1.0}$ after exercise	Induction of episode with exercise and/or isocapneic hyperventilation with cold air
Aspirin sensitivity, nasal polyps, and asthma	Asthma, usually intrinsic Temporal relation More common in females than in males	Polyphonic wheezing and rhonchi Rhinitis Nasal polyps	X-ray film shows sinusitis in some cases IgE generally normal	Possible positive skin test reaction to aspirin and positive response to challenge with aspirin ingestion
Variant asthma	Paroxysmal coughing Vague or nonexistent history of allergy	May be normal	Reversible decrease in $FEV_{1.0}$ Mild to moderate blood eosinophilia Positive response to methacholine inhalation challenge	Marked response to steroids
Hidden asthma Medication-induced	Use of beta blockers	Scattered wheezes on auscultation	Decrease in flow rates on pulmonary function tests	History of beta-blocker use
Variant (cough) asthma	Cough as the sole symptom	May be negative	Normal results on pulmonary function tests, positive results on methacholine inhalation challenge test	Responds to bronchodilator
Nonasthmatic diseases Pulmonary embolism	Predisposition: pregnancy, postoperative state, stasis, oral contraceptive use Sudden dyspnea Pleuritic chest pain Hemoptysis Apprehension Cough	Polyphonic wheezing Signs of right-sided heart failure with large embolus Increased S_2P Shock Tachypnea Tachycardia Rales (focal) Cyanosis	Hypoxemia High probability ventilation-perfusion scan Positive impedance phlebography findings Pulmonary arteriogram showing compatible filling defects Abnormal electrocardiogram Chest x-ray film shows local and general oligemia; atelectasis; increased size of pulmonary artery; focal pleural effusion	Pulmonary arteriogram is definitive for most cases

Table 37-5. (continued)

Diagnosis	History	Findings on physical examination	Laboratory tests	Differential diagnostic signs
Nonasthmatic diseases (cont.)				
Cardiac asthma	Heart disease Paroxysmal nocturnal dyspnea Orthopnea Pedal edema	Polyphonic wheezing may be prominent during inspiration Fine moist inspiratory rales S_3/S_4 gallop, cardiomegaly Jugular vein distention Hepatojugular reflux (if right-sided failure is present)	Increased venous pressure Increased pulmonary wedge pressure Electrocardiographic evidence of heart disease Chest x-ray film shows increased heart size, vascular congestion, effusions MUGA scan ejection fraction < 55%	History of cardiac disease, absence of previous episodes of asthma; if both illnesses are present, differential diagnosis is most difficult Response to diuretics and cardiac support
Microvascular angina	Angina with disproportionate dyspnea	May be unremarkable	Normal spirometry results Positive results on methacholine challenge test	History of angina and dyspnea with positive results on methacholine challenge test
Sarcoidosis	Cough Dyspnea Skin rash	Scattered wheezing, or rales in advanced cases Erythema nodosum, hepatosplenomegaly and lymphadenopathy in some cases	Elevated ACE level Positive results on gallium scan of lung Chest x-ray film may show bilateral hilar and/or paratracheal adenopathy	Hilar adenopathy on chest x-ray film Elevated ACE level
Adult respiratory distress syndrome (noncardiogenic pulmonary edema)	Associated with gram-negative sepsis, shock, trauma, infections, aspiration, etc.	Rales with scattered wheezes	Hypoxemia: $PaO_2 < 60$ mmHg with FIO_2 50% Diffuse bilateral infiltrate on chest x-ray film Decreased lung compliance Normal pulmonary capillary wedge pressure	History of underlying precipitating cause No response to bronchodilator drugs
Acquired immunodeficiency syndrome	Intravenous drug abuse Homosexual activity Blood transfusions	Diffuse focal wheeze	HIV positive	History of risk factors and HIV positive
Cocaine toxicity	Temporal relationship with cocaine use	Diffuse wheeze	Toxic screen positive for cocaine metabolites	Recent cocaine use and positive results on toxic screen
Central airway obstruction	Foreign body aspiration May be unremarkable	Stridor may be present, focal absence of breath sounds Occasional click over foreign body	Flow-volume curve may be abnormal, chest x-ray, fluoroscopy, and CT scan may reveal site of obstruction and collapse of lobe or segment, bronchoscopy reveals the site of obstruction; chest x-ray film may show foreign body	Bronchoscopy, although definitive, should be done with caution as it may cause total obstruction Poor response to bronchodilator therapy
Endotracheal tuberculosis	Fever, chills, nightsweats, malaise	Positive findings for purified protein derivative and acid–fast bacillus on sputum smear	Localized wheeze Positive findings for purified protein derivative	Systemic symptoms Positive acid–fast bacillus
Angioedema	Occurs spontaneously or after trauma Gastrointestinal colic Episodic shortness of breath Family history of sudden death may be present	Inspiratory stridor, crowing respirations	In uncommon form, C1 esterase inhibitor deficiency Fluoroscopy, laminagram, or CT scan of upper airways may show decrease in lumen size	In the uncommon form, diagnosis rests on demonstration of decrease or ineffectiveness of C1 esterase inhibitor In the common form of angioedema, no specific laboratory test is available, although history of exposure to offending agent may be obtained
Laryngeal dysfunction	Emotional disorder Barking cough	Wheeze, maximal over the larynx	Abnormal flow-volume curve, may be inconsistent Negative results on methacholine inhalation test	May have persistence of vocal cord spasm despite deep intravenous diazepam anesthesia

Table 37-5. (continued)

Diagnosis	History	Findings on physical examination	Laboratory tests	Differential diagnostic signs
Nonasthmatic diseases (cont.)				
Gastroesophageal reflux	Predisposing factors: neurologic disease, e.g. cardiovascular accident or seizures; esophageal disease, e.g., hiatus hernia with reflux; alcoholism Nocturnal wheezing	Monophonic or polyphonic wheeze Reflux bronchoconstriction with diffuse wheezing	Gastroesophageal reflux documented by 24-hr pH monitor or barium swallow	Consider aspiration as cause of cough and wheeze in infants and elderly patients with recent-onset asthma
Carcinoid syndrome	Gastrointestinal symptoms, e.g., diarrhea Episodes of wheezing and hemoptysis Violaceous skin rash	Red-violaceous rash spreading from face to trunk Hypotensive spells Tricuspid and pulmonic murmurs	Increased 5-HIAA in urine; increased serotonin in blood; increased serum bradykinin X-ray gastrointestinal series may show tumor; chest x-ray film may show coin lesion	Systemic complaints Elevated 24-hr urine 5-HIAA Provocative testing: alcohol ingestion and injection; catecholamines; norepinephrine; dopamine; histamine and calcium infusion* Biopsy of tumor
Bronchiolitis	Infants < 2 yr (usually); may occur in adults 1–2 days of upper respiratory tract infection, then sudden respiratory distress	Diffuse polyphonic wheezing Fine inspiratory and expiratory rales Severe retractions Nasal flaring Cyanosis (in severe cases) Fever	Immunofluorescent identification of respiratory syncytial virus Chest x-ray film shows hyperinflation, focal atelectasis Transient hyperreactivity (6–8 wk)	Asthma generally rare in infancy Not associated with development of asthma in adults History of exposure to noxious gases
Cystic fibrosis	Meconium ileus Rectal prolapse Pancreatic infections Recurrent infections Failure to thrive Cough	Diffuse inspiratory and expiratory rhonchi and wheezing Barrel chest (in advanced cases) Cachexia (in advanced cases) Digital clubbing Cyanosis	Thick viscid sputum Positive results on sweat test Chest x-ray film variable from hyperinflation to bronchiectasis Metachromatic staining of skin fibroblasts	Diagnostic test is the sweat test, reliable in adults and children May be associated with allergic bronchopulmonary aspergillosis
Environmental, and industrial toxins (e.g., toluene diisocyanate, smoke inhalation, nitrogen dioxide)	Exposure history may be quite subtle	Diffuse polyphonic wheezing	Blood eosinophilia may be present Response to skin or inhalation challenge may be positive	Detailed geographic and work history is necessary Possible Type I or Type III hypersensitivity reaction
Psychosomatic illness	Hysterical personality Recent stress	Normal	Normal Negative results on challenge test with exercise and methacholine inhalation	Frequent deep sighing respirations Voluntary hyperventilation PaO_2 normal (or high)
Factitious asthma	Hysterical personality Other complaints present	Wheeze, maximal over larynx	Negative results on methacholine inhalation test	Disappearance of vocal cord spasm with deep intravenous diazepam anesthesia
Chronic bronchitis	Chief complaint: cough with sputum production Dyspnea mainly during exacerbations caused by superimposed infections	Coarse rales, scattered wheezing	Increased bronchial markings on chest x-ray film Total lung capacity normal or increased $PaCO_2$ may be chronically elevated Pulmonary artery pressure may be elevated at rest	History, physical examination, and laboratory profile
Emphysema	Chief complaint: slowly progressive dyspnea Minimal cough with scant sputum production Major weight loss	Breath sounds decreased End-expiratory wheeze	Overinflated, hyperlucent lungs with low flat diaphragm on chest x-ray film, unchanged between episodes Total lung capacity increased $PaCO_2$ normal until late in disease Pulmonary artery pressure may be normal or elevated at rest	History, physical examination, and laboratory profile Emphysema is a destructive disease; therefore, reversible components are not prominent

Table 37-5. (continued)

Diagnosis	History	Findings on physical examination	Laboratory tests	Differential diagnostic signs
Pulmonary infiltration with eosinophilia (PIE)				
Löffler's syndrome	Drug ingestion, e.g., penicillin Shortness of breath Prior infectious illness	Wheezing may be present Areas of decreased breath sounds	Chest x-ray film shows migratory infiltrates Mild to moderate blood eosinophilia Pulmonary function tests show combined obstructive and restrictive pattern	Fluffy infiltrates (lasting up to 6 wk) associated with peripheral eosinophilia Response to corticosteroids good
Chronic PIE	May last for weeks or years	Normal Percussion dullness, moist rales	Modest to spectacular eosinophilia Dense pneumonic infiltrates in peripheral pattern	On lung biopsy specimen, alveoli filled with large mononuclear cells and eosinophils Eosinophil count may be normal
Idiopathic hypereosinophilic syndrome	Nonspecific complaints, cough, dyspnea Eosinophilia discovered on routine examination	Wheezing S_3/S_4 gallop; hepatomegaly may be present	Eosinophilia of unknown cause of > 6-mo duration Diffuse organ dysfunction, e.g., cardiac, neurologic	Diagnosis by exclusion of secondary causes of eosinophilia and evidence of multiple-organ dysfunction
Tropical eosinophilia	Recent residence in tropics Predominantly pulmonary symptoms	Diffuse, polyphonic wheezing	Eosinophilia Positive results on filarial complement fixation test	Clinical response to diethylcarbamazine citrate within 2 wk Other worms such as *Ascaris* may be involved
Churg-Strauss syndrome	Middle-aged men most commonly Evidence of systemic vasculitis	Diffuse wheezing	Eosinophilia Hematuria	Tissue biopsy specimen shows granulomatous vascular reactions
Allergic bronchopulmonary aspergillosis	Allergy Cough	Diffuse, polyphonic wheezing	Brown sputum with eosinophils Total IgE markedly increased Identification of fungus in sputum, increased serum titers of precipitins Recurrent infiltrate on x-ray film	Positive Type I skin test results; Type III, Type IV reactions may also occur Marked increase in IgE Therapeutic response to steroids
Bronchocentric granulomatosis	Cough	Wheezing Tachypnea	Mucoid impaction with heavy eosinophilic infiltration and destruction of distal airways	Paranasal sinuses not involved Bronchiectasis and characteristic features on lung biopsy specimen not seen in asthma
Systemic mastocytosis	Fatigue, malaise, rash flushing, abdominal pain Bronchospasm is rare	Peripheral lymphadenopathy, hepatosplenomegaly, skin lesion	Elevated serum alkaline phosphate Bone marrow and/or liver biopsy specimen shows mast cell infiltration	Mast cell infiltration on tissue biopsy specimen

* May elevate serum serotonin and 5-HIAA to diagnostic levels.
$FEV_{1.0}$ = forced expiratory volume in 1 second; MUGA = multiple-gated acquisition radioisotopes angiography; PaO_2 = arterial oxygen tension; FIO_2 = inspired oxygen concentration; CT = computed tomography; 5-HIAA = 5-hydroxyindoleacetic acid; $PaCO_2$ = arterial carbon dioxide tension; ACE = angiotensin-converting enzyme.

arate classification by Churg and Strauss [47], who reported a syndrome of asthma and extensive involvement of the pulmonary vessels in granulomatous vascular and extravascular reactions that occurred predominantly in middle-aged men, although recently the case of a 68-year-old man was described [54]. In a review of the literature, Lanham and colleagues reported on 118 patients with Churg-Strauss syndrome, all with evidence of asthma [147], but there are rare case reports of the Churg-Strauss syndrome without asthma [159]. The asthma associated with these conditions tends to be progressive and resistant to treatment, but single episodes of wheezing and dyspnea may respond to routine asthma therapy.

Constitutional symptoms such as fever, weakness, malaise, and weight loss point to a widespread systemic involvement. Eosinophilia ($>5,000/mm^3$) associated with an elevated erythrocyte sedimentation rate, anemia, and elevated IgE levels is characteristic of exacerbations of systemic disease [46, 242].

Hemoptysis, pleural pain, anemia, hematuria, and other extrapulmonary manifestations suggestive of vasculitis indicate that the patient is suffering from something other than typical bronchial asthma. Distinction from late-onset bronchial asthma may be difficult, especially early in the course of the vasculitis.

There are no pathognomonic laboratory tests for Churg-Strauss syndrome. Chest radiography may be helpful but is not sufficiently specific to be diagnostic. Patchy consolidations, often with peripheral distribution or perhaps a nodular or reticular-

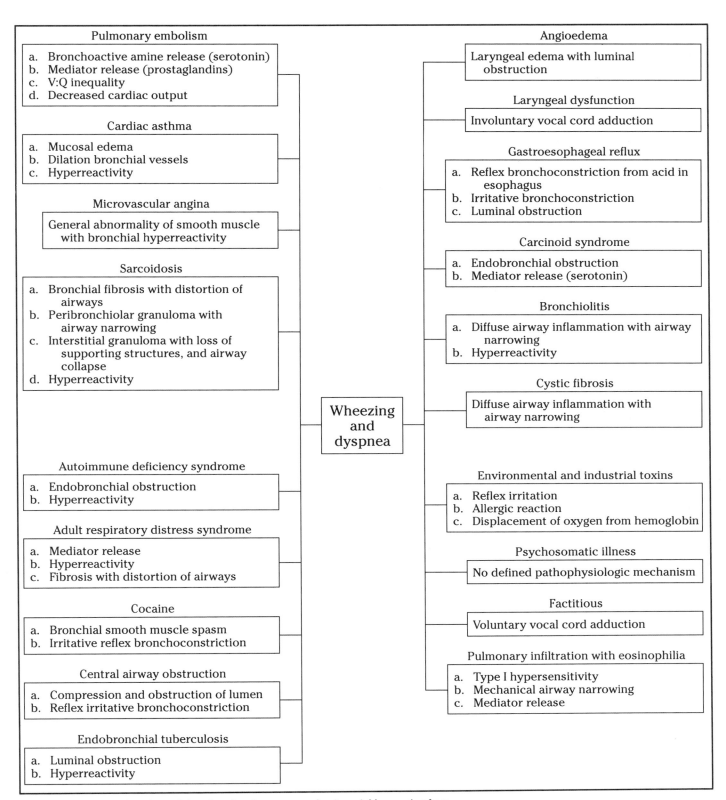

Fig. 37-8. *The pathophysiology of the wheezing-dyspnea complex is variable, ranging from bronchoconstriction, edema, and hyperventilation to mechanical compression.*

nodular pattern, may be seen. Hilar adenopathy may also be seen. Pleural effusions occur commonly and are acidic and exudative in nature, with a low glucose and high eosinophil count [85]. Tissue biopsy remains the only method of absolutely establishing the diagnosis (Fig. 37-7). Eosinophilia and bronchospasm may occur in systemic mastocytosis (Table 37-5), although they are not classified under the PIE syndrome.

Allergic Bronchopulmonary Aspergillosis

The association of *Aspergillus fumigatus* with pulmonary infiltrates, eosinophilia, and asthma was first described in 1952 by Hinson and associates [117], and is the most common cause of the PIE syndrome [243]. Allergic bronchopulmonary aspergillosis (ABPA) generally occurs with a background of allergy. In one study 22 percent of bronchial asthmatics in England were thought to have ABPA [112]. Five stages of ABPA are recognized: acute, remission, exacerbation, corticosteroid-dependent asthma, and fibrotic lung disease. Pathologically, a marked inflammatory process that is mainly bronchocentric is seen [257].

The clinical picture is of recurrent febrile episodes with severe cough and wheezing and a characteristic brown sputum. Examination of this sputum may disclose mycelial plugs from which one can easily culture the organism. Peripheral eosinophilia may be mild, modest, or spectacular. Of some interest is the marked elevation of serum IgE that may be observed at diagnosis irrespective of the stage of ABPA [105, 226, 257]. There is no individual test to establish the diagnosis of ABPA, and a combination of clinical, radiologic, and immunologic criteria is currently used for diagnosis [104, 210], and includes (1) the presence of asthma, (2) pulmonary infiltrates with eosinophilia, (3) Type I skin reaction to *Aspergillus* antigen, (4) precipitin antibodies against *Aspergillus* antigen, (5) elevated serum IgE levels, and (6) central or apical bronchiectasis.

Delay in the recognition of ABPA may lead to the development of fibrotic lung disease (Stage V) [149], believed to be preventable with the use of systemic corticosteroids [92, 106, 209]. This subject is detailed in Chapter 49.

A similar clinical picture may be seen with other fungi, and the term *allergic bronchopulmonary mycosis* has been used for such diseases.

BRONCHIAL ASTHMA

There are various forms of bronchial asthma, which may be a source of confusion. Included are the following categories: (1) extrinsic asthma; (2) intrinsic asthma; (3) asthmatic bronchitis; (4) exercise-induced asthma; (5) the triad of aspirin sensitivity, nasal polyps, and asthma; (6) variant asthma; and (7) hidden asthma. These illnesses are covered extensively in other chapters, but salient features are reviewed in Table 37-5. Figure 37-8 summarizes conditions that may masquerade as asthma.

REFERENCES

1. Albert, R. K. Endobronchial TB progressing to bronchial stenosis. *Chest* 70:537, 1976.
2. Allen, J. N. Acute eosinophilic pneumonia as a reversible cause of noninfectious respiratory failure. *N. Engl. J. Med.* 321:569, 1989.
3. Alsenz, J. Autoantibody-mediated acquired deficiency of C1 inhibitor. *N. Engl. J. Med.* 316:1360, 1987.
4. American Thoracic Society Official Statement. Standards for the diagnosis and care of patients with COPD and asthma. *Am. Rev. Respir. Dis.* 135:225, 1986.
5. Andrassy, R. J. Bronchial carcinoid tumors in children and adolescents. *J. Pediatr. Surg.* 12:513, 1977.
6. Argyropoulou, P. K. Airway function in Stage I and Stage II pulmonary sarcoidosis. *Respiration* 46:17, 1984.
7. Ashbaugh, D. G., et al. Acute respiratory distress in adults. *Lancet* 2:319, 1967.
8. Auerbach, H. S. Alternate-day prednisone reduces morbidity and improves pulmonary function in cystic fibrosis. *Lancet* 2:686, 1985.
9. Auerbach, O. Tuberculosis of the trachea and major bronchi. *Am. Rev. Tuberc.* 60:604, 1949.
10. Badesch, D. B. Acute eosinophilic pneumonia: A hypersensitivity phenomenon. *Am. Rev. Respir. Dis.* 139:249, 1989.
11. Barbee, R. A. A longitudinal study of respiratory symptoms in a community population sample. *Chest* 99:20, 1991.
12. Barnes, P. J. Neural control of human airways in health and disease. *Am. Rev. Respir. Dis.* 134:1289, 1986.
13. Baumgartner, W. A., and Mark, J. B. D. Metastatic malignancies from distant sites to the tracheobronchial tree. *J. Thorac. Cardiovasc. Surg.* 79:499, 1980.
14. Beamis, J. F. Case records of the MGH. *N. Engl. J. Med.* 321:1738, 1989.
15. Bechtel, J. J. Airway hyperreactivity in patients with sarcoidosis. *Am. Rev. Respir. Dis.* 124:759, 1981.
16. Bell, W. R. The clinical features of submassive and massive pulmonary emboli. *Am. J. Med.* 62:355, 1977.
17. Benedict, E. B. Sarcoidosis with bronchial involvement. *N. Engl. J. Med.* 224:186, 1941.
18. Bernstein, J. A. Potentially fatal asthma and syncope: a new variant of Munchausen's syndrome in sports medicine. *Chest* 99:763, 1991.
19. Berquist, W. E. Effect of theophylline on gastroesophageal reflux in normal adults. *J. Allergy Clin. Immunol.* 67:407, 1981.
20. Bone, R. C. Ventilation : perfusion scan in pulmonary embolism (editorial). *JAMA* 263:2794, 1990.
21. Boucher, R. C. Evidence for reduced Cl$^-$ and increased Na$^+$ permeability in cystic fibrosis human primary cell cultures. *J. Physiol.* 405:77, 1988.
22. Bounameaux, H. Diagnostic value of plasma D-dimer in suspected pulmonary embolism. *Lancet* 2:628, 1988.
23. Bousquet, J. Eosinophilic inflammation in asthma. *N. Engl. J. Med.* 323:1033, 1990.
24. Boyle, J. T. Mechanisms for the association of gastroesophageal reflux and bronchospasm. *Am. Rev. Respir. Dis.* 131S:S16, 1985.
25. Bradvik, I. Lung mechanics and their relationship to lung volumes in pulmonary sarcoidosis. *Eur. Respir. J.* 2:643, 1989.
26. Braman, S. S., and Whitcomb, M. E. Endobronchial metastasis. *Arch. Intern. Med.* 135:543, 1975.
27. Bridey, F. Plasma D-dimer and pulmonary embolism. *Lancet* 1:791, 1989.
28. Brown, T. M., Merritt, W. D., and Evans, D. L. Psychogenic vocal cord dysfunction masquerading as asthma. *J. Nerv. Ment. Dis.* 176:308, 1988.
29. Bush, R. K. Thyroid disease and asthma. *J. Allergy Clin. Immunol.* 59:398, 1977.
30. Cabanes, L. R. Bronchial hyperresponsiveness to methacholine in patients with impaired left ventricular function. *N. Engl. J. Med.* 320:1317, 1989.
31. Caglayan, S., et al. Bronchial foreign body vs asthma. *Chest* 96:509, 1989.
32. Cameron, J. L., and Zuidema, G. D. Aspiration pneumonia. *JAMA* 219:1194, 1972.
33. Cannon, R. O. Airway hyperresponsiveness in patients with microvascular angina. *Circulation* 82:2011, 1990.
34. Carlsen, K. H. Nebulised beclomethasone dipropionate in recurrent obstructive episodes after acute bronchiolitis. *Arch. Dis. Child.* 63:1428, 1988.
35. Carrington, C. B. Chronic eosinophilic pneumonia. *N. Engl. J. Med.* 280:789, 1969.
36. Casson, A. G., and Guy, J. R. F. Foreign-body aspiration in adults. *Can. J. Surg.* 30:193, 1987.
37. Castell, D. O. Asthma and gastroesophageal reflux (editorial). *Chest* 96:2, 1989.
38. Chabra, S. K. Airway hyperreactivity in tropical pulmonary eosinophilia. *Chest* 93:1105, 1988.
39. Chace, K. V. Comparison of physicochemical properties of purified mucus glycoproteins isolated from respiratory secretions of cystic fibrosis and asthmatic patients. *Biochemistry* 24:7334, 1985.
40. Chako, S. Clinical, radiographic and hemodynamic correlations in chronic congestive heart failure. *Am. J. Med.* 90:353, 1991.
41. Chan-Yeung, M. Occupational asthma update. *Chest* 93:407, 1988.
42. Chawla, S. S., Upadhyay, B. K., and MacDonnell, K. F. Laryngeal spasm mimicking bronchial asthma. *Ann. Allergy* 53:319, 1984.

43. Cherian, T. Evaluation of simple clinical signs for the diagnosis of acute lower respiratory tract infection. *Lancet* 333:125, 1988.
44. Chitkara, R. K. Tropical eosinophilia. *Chest* 97:253, 1990.
45. Christopher, K. L., et al. Vocal cord dysfunction presenting as asthma. *N. Engl. J. Med.* 308:1566, 1983.
46. Chumbley, L. C., et al. Allergic granulomatosis and angiitis: Churg-Strauss syndrome. *Mayo Clin. Proc.* 52:477, 1977.
47. Churg, J., and Strauss, L. Allergic granulomatosis, allergic angiitis and periarteritis nodosa. *Am. J. Pathol.* 27:277, 1951.
48. Chusid, M. J. The hypereosinophilic syndrome. *Medicine* 54:1, 1975.
49. Clancy, L. Arachidonic acid metabolites and small airways disease in non-smoking sarcoidosis patients. *Eur. J. Respir. Dis.* 69:199, 1986.
50. Cockcroft, D. W. Decrease in non-specific bronchial reactivity in an asthmatic following treatment of hyperthyroidism. *Ann. Allergy* 41:160, 1978.
51. Cohen, J. I. Upper airway obstruction in asthma. *John Hopkins Med. J.* 147:233, 1980.
52. Cordier, J. F. Pulmonary Wegener's granulomatosis. *Chest* 97:906, 1990.
53. Coupe, M. Therapy for symptoms in the carcinoid syndrome. *Q. J. Med.* 271:1021, 1989.
54. CPC. Churg-Strauss syndrome. *NY State J. Med.* April:190, 1990.
55. Crausaz, F. M. Aspiration of solid food particles into lungs of patients with gastroesophageal reflux and chronic bronchial disease. *Chest* 93:376, 1988.
56. Cregler, L., and Mark, H. Medical complications of cocaine abuse. *N. Engl. J. Med.* 315:1495, 1986.
57. Cvitanic, O. Improved use of arterial blood gas analysis in suspected pulmonary embolism. *Chest* 95:48, 1989.
58. Dalen, J. E. Pulmonary angiography in acute PE. *Am. Heart J.* 81:175, 1971.
59. Dal Nogare, A. R. Southwestern Internal Medicine Conference: Adult respiratory distress syndrome. *Am. J. Med. Sci.* 298:413, 1989.
60. D'Alonzo, G. E. The mechanisms of abnormal gas exchange in acute massive pulmonary embolism. *Am. Rev. Respir. Dis.* 128:170, 1983.
61. Dantzker, D. R. Alterations in gas exchange following pulmonary embolism. *Chest* 81:4, 1982.
62. Davis, A. E. C1 Inhibitor and hereditary angioneurotic edema. *Annu. Rev. Immunol.* 6:595, 1988.
63. Davis, P. B. Clinical notes on respiratory disease. *Cystic Fibrosis* 21:1, 1983.
64. Dean, N. C. Pulmonary function in heavy users of freebase cocaine (abstract). *Am. Rev. Respir. Dis.* 137:489, 1988.
65. DeBlic, J. Persisting "asthma" in tropical pulmonary eosinophilia. *Thorax* 39:398, 1984.
66. Dines, D. E. Obstructive disease of the airways associated with stage I sarcoidosis. *Mayo Clin. Proc.* 53:788, 1978.
67. Donaldson, V. H. Permeability-increasing activity in hereditary angioneurotic edema plasma. *J. Clin. Invest.* 48:642, 1969.
68. Donaldson, V. H. The challenge of hereditary angioneurotic edema (editorial). *N. Engl. J. Med.* 308:1094, 1983.
69. Dorinsky, P. M. Adult bronchiolitis. *Chest* 88:58, 1985.
70. Downing, E. T. et al. Factitious asthma. *JAMA* 248:2878, 1982.
71. Ducolone, A. Gastroesophageal reflux in patients with asthma and chronic bronchitis. *Am. Rev. Respir. Dis.* 135:327, 1987.
72. Durham, S. R. Blood eosinophils and eosinophil-derived proteins in allergic asthma. *J. Allergy Clin. Immunol.* 84:931, 1989.
73. Editorial. Clinical signs in heart failure. *Lancet* 2:309, 1989.
74. Editorial. Inhaled steroids and recurrent wheeze after bronchiolitis. *Lancet* 334:999, 1989.
75. Editorial. ARDS times. *Lancet* 1:140, 1989.
76. Editorial. Cardiac asthma. *Lancet* 335:693, 1990.
77. Editorial. Acute eosinophilic pneumonia. *Lancet* 335:947, 1990.
78. Eichacker, P. Q. Methacholine bronchial reactivity testing in patients with chronic congestive heart failure. *Chest* 93:336, 1988.
79. Ekstrom, T. Effects of ranitidine treatment on patients with asthma and a history of gastro-oesophageal reflux. *Thorax* 44:19, 1989.
80. Elliot, C. G. Pulmonary sequelae in survivors of the adult respiratory distress syndrome. *Clin. Chest Med.* 11:789, 1990.
81. Elliot, C. G., et al. Prediction of pulmonary function abnormalities after ARDS. *Am. Rev. Respir. Dis.* 135:634, 1987.
82. Emery, J. L. Pulmonary embolism in children. *Arch. Dis. Child.* 37:591, 1962.
83. Enright, T. Pulmonary eosinophilic syndromes. *Ann. Allergy* 62:277, 1989.
84. Epler, G. R. The spectrum of bronchiolitis obliterans (editorial). *Chest* 83:161, 1983.
85. Erzurum, S. C., et al. Pleural effusion in Churg-Strauss syndrome. *Chest* 95:1357, 1989.
86. Ettinger, N. A. A review of the respiratory effects of smoking cocaine. *Am. J. Med.* 87:664, 1989.
87. Fanburg, B. L. Case records of the MGH. *N. Engl. J. Med.* 310:1653, 1984.
88. Fauci, A. S. The idiopathic hypereosinophilic syndrome. *Ann. Intern. Med.* 97:78, 1982.
89. Fauci, A. S. Wegener's granulomatosis. *Ann. Intern. Med.* 98:76, 1983.
90. Feigin, D. S. Allergic diseases in the lungs. *CRC Crit. Rev. Diagn. Imaging* 25:159, 1985.
91. Fink, J., et al. Interstitial pneumonitis due to hypersensitivity to an organism contaminating a heating system. *Ann. Intern. Med.* 74:80, 1971.
92. Fink, J. N. ABPA. *Chest* 87:81S, 1985.
93. Fishman, A. P. Cardiac asthma—A fresh look at an old wheeze. *N. Engl. J. Med.* 320:1346, 1989.
94. Ford, R. Transient pulmonary eosinophilia and asthma. *Am. Rev. Respir. Dis.* 93:797, 1966.
95. Frampton, M. W. Effects of nitrogen dioxide exposure on pulmonary function and airway reactivity in normal humans. *Am. Rev. Respir. Dis.* 143:522, 1991.
96. Frigas, E. Angioedema with acquired deficiency of the C1 inhibitor. *Mayo Clin. Proc.* 64:1269, 1989.
97. Gagliardi, A. J., Stover, D. E., and Zaman, M. K. Endobronchial pneumocystis carinii infection in a patient with AIDS. *Chest* 91:463, 1987.
98. Geddes, D. M. Pulmonary eosinophilia. *J. R. Coll. Physicians Lond.* 20:139, 1986.
99. Ghio, A. J., et al. Impairment after adult respiratory distress syndrome. *Am. Rev. Respir. Dis.* 139:1158, 1989.
100. Gibson, L. E., and Cooke, R. E. A test for concentration of electrolytes in sweat in cystic fibrosis of the pancreas utilizing pilocarpine by electrophoresis. *Pediatrics* 23:545, 1959.
101. Goldhaber, S. Z. Factors associated with correct antemortem diagnosis of major pulmonary embolism. *Am. J. Med.* 73:822, 1982.
102. Goldhaber, S. Z. Utility of cross-linked fibrin degradation products in the diagnosis of pulmonary embolism. *Am. Heart J.* 116:505, 1988.
103. Gordin, F. M. Adverse reactions to trimethoprim-sulfa-methoxazole in patients with AIDS. *Ann. Intern. Med.* 100:495, 1984.
104. Greenberger, P. A., and Patterson, R. Diagnosis and management of ABPA. *Ann. Allergy* 56:444, 1986.
105. Greenberger, P. A., and Patterson, R. ABPA. *Chest* 91:165S, 1987.
106. Greenberger, P. A., and Patterson, R. J. ABPA and the evaluation of the patient with asthma. *J. Allergy Clin. Immunol.* 81:646, 1988.
107. Greenburg, M. Acute eosinophilic pneumonia. *N. Engl. J. Med.* 322:635, 1990.
108. Greenspan, R. H. Accuracy of the chest radiograph in diagnosis of pulmonary embolism. *Invest. Radiol.* 17:539, 1982.
109. Haddad, A. Angioedema of the head and neck. *J. Otolaryngol.* 14:14, 1985.
110. Hadfield, J. W. Localized airway narrowing in sarcoidosis. *Thorax* 37:443, 1982.
111. Hanly, J. G. Meconium ileus equivalent in older patients with cystic fibrosis. *Br. Med. J.* 286:1411, 1983.
112. Henderson, A. H., English, M. P., and Vecht, R. J. Pulmonary aspergillosis. *Thorax* 23:513, 1968.
113. Henry, R. L. Ineffectiveness of ipratropium bromide in acute bronchiolitis. *Arch. Dis. Child.* 58:925, 1983.
114. Henry, R. L. Respiratory problems 2 years after acute bronchiolitis in infancy. *Arch. Dis. Child.* 58:713, 1983.
115. Herve, P. The mechanisms of abnormal gas exchange in acute massive pulmonary embolism. *Am. Rev. Respir. Dis.* 128:1101, 1983.
116. Herve, P. Intraesophageal perfusion of acid increases the bronchomotor response to methacholine and to isocapnic hyperventilation in asthmatic subjects. *Am. Rev. Respir. Dis.* 134:986, 1986.
117. Hinson, K. F. W., Moon, A. J., and Plummer, N. S. Bronchopulmonary aspergillosis. *Thorax* 7:317, 1952.
118. Hoellerich, V. L. Diagnosing pulmonary embolism using clinical findings. *Arch. Intern. Med.* 146:1699, 1986.
119. Holland, E. D. Assessment of left ventricular ejection fraction by cineangiographic and radionuclide techniques. *Circulation* 60:760, 1979.
120. Hope, J. *A Treatise on the Diseases of the Heart and Great Vessels* (2nd ed.). London: W. Kidd, 1835. P. 345.
121. Hubert, D. Effect of theophylline on gastroesophageal reflux in patients with asthma. *J. Allergy Clin. Immunol.* 81:1168, 1988.
122. Hull, R. D. Pulmonary angiography, ventilation lung scanning, and venography for clinically suspected pulmonary embolism with abnormal perfusion lung scan. *Ann. Intern. Med.* 98:891, 1983.

123. Hull, R. D. Clinical validity of a normal perfusion lung scan in patients with suspected pulmonary embolism. *Chest* 97:23, 1990.

124. Hyde, L., and Hyde, C. I. Clinical manifestations of lung cancer. *Chest* 65: 299, 1974.

125. Imoto, E. M., et al. Central airway obstruction due to CMV induced necrotizing tracheitis in a patient with AIDS. *Am. Rev. Respir. Dis.* 142:884, 1990.

126. Ip, M. S. M. Endobronchial TB revisited. *Chest* 89:727, 1986.

127. Israel, R. M. Hyperthyroidism protects against carbachol induced bronchospasm. *Chest* 91:242, 1987.

128. Itkonen, J. Pulmonary dysfunction in 'freebase' cocaine users. *Arch. Intern. Med.* 144:2195, 1984.

129. Jain, S. K. Tropical eosinophilia (editorial). *Indian J. Chest Dis. Allied Sci.* 30:V, 1988.

130. Jameson, M. D. Idiopathic hypereosinophilic syndrome. *Postgrad. Med.* 84:93, 1988.

131. Jederlinic, P. J. Chronic eosinophilic pneumonia. *Medicine* 67:154, 1988.

132. Jeffrey, G. M. Life-threatening airways obstruction at the presentation of Hodgkin's disease. *Cancer* 67:506, 1991.

133. Johnson, R. C. A patient referred for steroid-resistant asthma. *Chest* 98: 1495, 1990.

134. Jones, D. A. Persisting "asthma" in tropical pulmonary eosinophilia. *Thorax* 38:692, 1983.

135. Kapitan, K. S. Mechanisms of hypoxemia in chronic thromboembolic pulmonary hypertension. *Am. Rev. Respir. Dis.* 139:1149, 1989.

136. Kaplan, E. A new provocative test for the diagnosis of the carcinoid syndrome. *Am. J. Surg.* 123:173, 1972.

137. Kerem, B. Identification of the cystic fibrosis gene: Genetic analysis. *Science* 245:1073, 1989.

138. Kindt, G. C. Bronchiolitis in adults. *Am. Rev. Respir. Dis.* 140:483, 1989.

139. Kino, T. Prognosis of prolonged eosinophilic pneumonia—Possibly acquired bronchial hyperreactivity. *Nippon Kyobu Shikkan Gakkai Zasshi* 26:868, 1988.

140. Kinsella, J. Increased airways reactivity after smoke inhalation. *Lancet* 337:595, 1991.

141. Kissner, D. G. Crack lung: Pulmonary disease caused by cocaine abuse. *Am. Rev. Respir. Dis.* 136:1250, 1987.

142. Korsager, S. Iodine-induced hypothyroidism and its effect on the severity of asthma. *Acta Med. Scand.* 205:115, 1979.

143. Kvols, L. K. Treatment of the malignant carcinoid syndrome. *N. Engl. J. Med.* 315:663, 1986.

144. Laitinen, L. A. Bronchial hyperresponsiveness in normal subjects during attenuated influenza virus infection. *Am. Rev. Respir. Dis.* 143:358, 1991.

145. Lal, C. Everything that wheezes is not asthma. *Chest* 96:1418, 1989.

146. Lange, W. Ueber eine eigenthumliche erkrankung der kleinen bronchien und bronchiolen (bronchitis et bronchiolitis obliterans). *Dtsche. Arch. Klin. Med.* 70:342, 1901.

147. Lanham, J. G., et al. Systemic vasculitis with asthma and eosinophilia. *Medicine* 63:65, 1984.

148. Leape, L. Surgical Causes of Asthma. In B. Berman and K. MacDonnell (eds.), *Differential Diagnosis and Treatment of Pediatric Allergy.* Boston: Little, Brown, 1981. P. 117.

149. Lee, T. M., et al. Stage V (fibrotic) ABPA. *Arch. Intern. Med.* 147:319, 1987.

150. LeFemine, A., MacDonnell, K., and Moon, R. Tracheal stenosis following cuffed tube tracheostomy: Anatomical variation and selected treatment. *Ann. Thorac. Surg.* 15:456, 1973.

151. Leung, A. K. C. Exercise-induced angioedema and asthma. *Am. J. Sports Med.* 17:442, 1989.

152. Levine, B. W. Case records of the Mass. Gen. Hosp. *N. Engl. J. Med.* 320: 108, 1989.

153. Lewis, J. Exercise-induced urticaria, angioedema, and anaphylactoid episodes. *J. Allergy Clin. Immunol.* 68:432, 1981.

154. Lewis, M. I. Airflow obstruction in sarcoidosis (editorial). *Chest* 92:582, 1987.

155. Li, M. Cyclic AMP-dependent protein kinase opens chloride channels in normal but not cystic fibrosis airway epithelium. *Nature* 331:358, 1988.

156. Light, R. W. Serial pulmonary function in patients with acute heart failure. *Arch. Intern. Med.* 143:429, 1983.

157. Lindsey, H. E. Release of prostaglandins from embolized lungs. *Br. J. Surg.* 57:783, 1970.

158. Lipton, S. V. Tropical PIE in Boston. *Pediatr. Infect. Dis. J.* 7:742, 1988.

159. Lipworth, B. J., et al. Allergic granulomatosis without asthma. *Respir. Med.* 83:249, 1989.

160. Lisboa, C., et al. Is extrathoracic airway obstruction important in asthma? *Am. Rev. Respir. Dis.* 122:115, 1980.

161. Littlewood, J. M. The sweat test. *Arch. Dis. Child.* 61:1041, 1986.

162. Llibre, J. M. Acute eosinophilic pneumonia. *N. Engl. J. Med.* 322:634, 1990.

163. Low, G. L. An interesting case of eosinophilia. *Trans. Soc. Trop. Med. Hyg.* 9:77, 1916.

164. Lowell, F. Antigenic dusts and respiratory disease. *N. Engl. J. Med.* 281: 1012, 1969.

165. Manier, G. Determinants of hypoxemia during the acute phase of pulmonary embolism in humans. *Am. Rev. Respir. Dis.* 132:332, 1985.

166. Manning, P. J. Bronchostenosis due to sarcoidosis. *Ir. Med. J.* 77:210, 1984.

167. Manresa Presas, F. Bronchial hyperreactivity in fresh Stage I sarcoidosis. *Ann. NY Acad. Sci.* 465:523, 1986.

168. Mansfield, L. E. The role of the vagus nerve in airway narrowing caused by intraesophageal hydrochloric acid provocation and esophageal distention. *Ann. Allergy* 47:431, 1981.

169. Mansfield, L. E. The effects of acute gastric distension on the pulmonary functions of asthmatic subjects. *J. Asthma* 22:191, 1985.

170. Mansfield, L. E. Gastroesophageal reflux and respiratory disorders. *Ann. Allergy* 62:158, 1989.

171. Marks, J. D., et al. Plasma tumor necrosis factor in patients with septic shock. *Am. Rev. Respir. Dis.* 141:94, 1990.

172. Marlink, R. G. Hepatic arterial embolization for metastatic hormone-secreting tumors. *Cancer* 65:2227, 1990.

173. Maton, P. N. The carcinoid syndrome. *JAMA* 260:1602, 1988.

174. Matthay, M. A. The adult respiratory distress syndrome; Definition and prognosis. *Clin. Chest Med.* 11:575, 1990.

175. Matthews, K. P. Urticaria and angioedema. *J. Allergy Clin. Immunol.* 72: 1, 1983.

176. Mayo, J. R. Chronic eosinophilic pneumonia. *AJR* 153:727, 1989.

177. McConnochie, K. M. Wheezing at 8 and 13 years. *Pediatr. Pulmonol.* 6: 138, 1989.

178. McIndoe, R. B. Routine bronchoscopy in patients with active pulmonary TB. *Am. Rev. Tuberc.* 39:617, 1939.

179. McIntyre, K. M. Relation of the electrocardiogram to hemodynamic alterations in pulmonary embolism. *Am. J. Cardiol.* 30:205, 1972.

180. Meduri, G. U. Pulmonary Kaposi's sarcoma in AIDS. *Am. J. Med.* 81:11, 1986.

181. Mendeloff, A. I. Severe asthmatic dyspnea as the sole presenting symptom of generalized endolymphatic carcinomatosis. *Ann. Intern. Med.* 22:386, 1945.

182. Mendelson, C. L. The aspiration of stomach contents into the lungs during obstetric anaesthesia. *Am. J. Obstet. Gynecol.* 52:191, 1946.

183. Mermod, E. Dilatation diffuse de l'oesophage sans retrecissement organique. *Rev. Med. Suisse Romande* 7:422, 1887.

184. Meslier, N. Diagnostic value of reversibility of chronic airway obstruction to separate asthma from chronic bronchitis: A statistical approach. *Eur. Respir. J.* 2:497, 1989.

185. Miller, A. Airway function in chronic pulmonary sarcoidosis with fibrosis. *Am. Rev. Respir. Dis.* 109:179, 1974.

186. Miller, R. D., and Hyatt, R. E. Obstructing lesions of the larynx and trachea. *Mayo Clin. Proc.* 44:145, 1969.

187. Milner, A. D. Acute bronchiolitis in infancy (editorial). *Thorax* 44:1, 1989.

188. Mitchell, D. M., Spiro, S. G., and Doyle, P. M. Munchausen's syndrome with multiple pulmonary manifestations. *R. Soc. Med.* 78:681, 1985.

189. Moreno, R. H. Mechanics of airway narrowing. *Am. Rev. Respir. Dis.* 133: 1171, 1986.

190. Morton, R. Phthisiologica Seu Exercitationes de phthisi. London: S. Smith, 1689.

191. Moser, K. M. Venous thromboembolism. *Am. Rev. Respir. Dis.* 141:235, 1990.

192. Mulherin, D. Meconium ileus equivalent in association with nebulized ipratropium bromide in cystic fibrosis. *Lancet* 335:552, 1990.

193. Mulholland, E. K. Clinical findings and severity of acute bronchiolitis. *Lancet* 335:1259, 1990.

194. Murray, J. F., et al. An expanded definition of the adult respiratory distress syndrome. *Am. Rev. Respir. Dis.* 138:720, 1988.

195. National surveillance of cocaine use and related health consequences. *MMWR* 31:265, 1982.

196. Nesarajah, M. S. Pulmonary function in tropical eosinophilia. *Thorax* 27: 185, 1972.

197. Neva, F. A. Tropical (filarial) eosinophilia. *N. Engl. J. Med.* 298:1129, 1978.

198. Nicholson, D. Extrinsic allergic pneumonias. *Am. J. Med.* 53:131, 1972.

199. Nutman, T. B. Tropical pulmonary eosinophilia. *J. Infect. Dis.* 160:1042, 1989.

200. Oates, J., et al. Release of kinin peptide in carcinoid syndrome. *Lancet* 1: 514, 1964.

201. O'Callaghan, C. Inhaled steroids and recurrent wheeze after bronchiolitis. *Lancet* 334:1458, 1989.

202. O'Donnell, C. R. Abnormal airway function in individuals with AIDS. *Chest* 94:945, 1988.

203. O'Hollaren, M. T. Masqueraders in clinical allergy: Laryngeal dysfunction causing dyspnea. *Ann. Allergy* 65:351, 1990.

204. O'Neill, T. W. Diagnostic value of the apex beat. *Lancet* 1:410, 1989.

205. Osler, W. B. *The Principles of Medicine.* New York: Appleton, 1892.

206. Pack, A. I. Acid: A nocturnal bronchoconstrictor (editorial). *Am. Rev. Respir. Dis.* 141:1391, 1990.

207. Packer, S. J., Cesario, T., and Williams, J. H. Mycobacterium avium complex infection presenting as endobronchial lesions in immunosuppressed patients. *Ann. Intern. Med.* 109:389, 1988.

208. Pantin, C. Prednisolone in the treatment of airflow obstruction in adults with cystic fibrosis. *Thorax* 41:34, 1986.

209. Patterson, R., et al. Prolonged evaluation of patients with corticosteroid dependent asthma stage of ABPA. *J. Allergy Clin. Immunol.* 80:663, 1987.

210. Patterson, R., Greenberger, P. A., and Radir, R. C. ABPA: Staging as an aid to management. *Ann. Intern. Med.* 99:18, 1983.

211. Patterson, R., Schatz, M., and Horton, M. Munchausen's stridor: Non-organic laryngeal obstruction. *Clin. Allergy* 4:307, 1974.

212. Perrin-Fayolle, M. Long-term results of surgical treatment for gastroesophageal reflux in asthmatic patients. *Chest* 96:40, 1989.

213. Peters, J. I., et al. Clinical determinants of abnormalities in pulmonary functions in survivors of the adult respiratory distress syndrome. *Am. Rev. Respir. Dis.* 139:1163, 1989.

214. Petty, T. L. ARDS. Refinement of concept and redefinition (editorial). *Am. Rev. Respir. Dis.* 138:724, 1988.

215. Pierce, C. P. C. Asthma and eosinophilia. *Am. J. Med.* 87:439, 1989.

216. Pinkston, P. Acute tropical pulmonary eosinophilia. *J. Clin. Invest.* 80: 216, 1987.

217. Pison, C. Bronchial hyperresponsiveness to inhaled methacholine in subjects with chronic left heart failure. *Chest* 96:230, 1989.

218. Plotz, M. Bronchial spasm in cardiac asthma. *Ann. Intern. Med.* 26:521, 1947.

219. Plusa, T. In vivo evaluation of BAL fluid in atopic bronchial asthma, chronic bronchitis and sarcoidosis patients. *Allerg. Immunol.* 36:11, 1990.

220. Poh, S. C. The course of lung function in treated tropical pulmonary eosinophilia. *Thorax* 29:710, 1974.

221. Rackemann, F. M., and Green, J. E. Periarteritis nodosa and asthma. *Trans. Assoc. Am. Physician* 54:112, 1939.

222. Rackow, E. C. Colloid osmotic pressure as a prognostic indicator of pulmonary edema and mortality in the critically ill. *Chest* 72:709, 1977.

223. Rankin, J. A. Histamine levels in BAL from patients with asthma, sarcoidosis, and idiopathic pulmonary fibrosis. *J. Allergy Clin. Immunol.* 79:371, 1987.

224. Rebhun, J. Association of asthma and freebase smoking. *Ann. Allergy* 60: 339, 1988.

225. Remetz, M. S. Pulmonary and pleural complications of cardiac disease. *Clin. Chest Med.* 10:545, 1989.

226. Ricketti, A. J., Greenberger, P. A., and Patterson, R. Serum IgE as an important aid in management of ABPA. *J. Allergy Clin. Immunol.* 74:68, 1984.

227. Rinaldo, J. E., and Christman, J. W. Mechanisms and mediators of the adult respiratory distress syndrome. *Clin. Chest Med.* 11:621, 1990.

228. Riordan, J. R. Identification of the cystic fibrosis gene: Cloning and characterization of complementary DNA. *Science* 245:1066, 1989.

229. Robbins, T. *Basic Pathology.* Philadelphia: Saunders, 1971. Pp. 261, 351, 437–439.

230. Roberts, D. J., et al. Tumor necrosis factor and adult respiratory distress syndrome. *Lancet* 2:1043, 1989.

231. Rocker, G. M., et al. Diagnostic criteria for adult respiratory distress syndrome: Time for reappraisal. *Lancet* 1:120, 1989.

232. Rommens, J. M. Identification of the cystic fibrosis gene: Chromosome walking and jumping. *Science* 245:1059, 1989.

233. Rosenberg, D. M. Functional correlates of lung involvement in Wegener's granulomatosis. *Am. J. Med.* 69:387, 1980.

234. Rosenblatt, J. Upper airway angioedema. *Aust. Fam. Physician* 14:775, 1985.

235. Rosenstein, B. J. Cystic fibrosis: Diagnostic considerations. *John Hopkins Med. J.* 150:113, 1982.

236. Royal College of General Practitioners Oral Contraception Study. Oral contraceptives, venous thrombosis and varicose veins. *J. R. Coll. Gen. Pract.* [*Occas. Pap.*] 28:393, 1978.

237. Rubin, R. B. Cocaine-associated asthma. *Am. J. Med.* 88:438, 1990.

238. Rubinstein, I. Fatal pulmonary emboli in hospitalized patients. *Arch. Intern. Med.* 148:1425, 1988.

239. Saltzman, H. A. Valve of the ventilation:perfusion scan in acute pulmonary embolism. *JAMA* 263:2753, 1990.

240. Sasahara, A. A. Clinical and physiologic studies in pulmonary thromboembolism. *Am. J. Cardiol.* 20:10, 1967.

241. Sasahara, A. A. The urokinase pulmonary embolism trial. *Circulation* 2(Suppl.):1, 1973.

242. Schatz, M., Wasserman, S., and Patterson, R. The eosinophil and the lung. *Arch. Intern. Med.* 142:1515, 1982.

243. Seaton, A., Seaton, D., and Leitch, A. G. Pulmonary Eosinophilia. In *Crofton and Douglas's Respiratory Diseases*, Vol. 28 (4th ed.). Oxford: Blackwell, 1989. P. 734.

244. Seibert, A. F. Normal airway responsiveness to methacholine in cardiac asthma. *Am. Rev. Respir. Dis.* 140:1805, 1989.

245. Settipane, G. A. Asthma and hyperthyroidism. *J. Allergy Clin. Immunol.* 49:348, 1972.

246. Sharma, O. P. Airway obstruction in sarcoidosis. *Chest* 94:343, 1988.

247. Sharma, O. P. The importance of airway obstruction in sarcoidosis. *Sarcoidosis* 5:119, 1988.

248. Shepherd, M. P. Endobronchial metastatic disease. *Thorax* 37:362, 1982.

249. Sherman, C. B. What causes cough and wheeze (editorial). *Chest* 99:1, 1991.

250. Shwachman, H. Cystic Fibrosis. In E. L. Kendig and V. Cherniack (eds.), *Disorders of the Respiratory Tract in Children* (4th ed.). Philadelphia: Saunders, 1972. P. 640.

251. Silkoff, P. Respiratory arrest in the carcinoid syndrome due to severe bronchospasm. *J. Asthma* 24:361, 1987.

252. Simmonds, E. Fractional measurements of sweat osmolality in patients with cystic fibrosis. *Arch. Dis. Child.* 64:1717, 1989.

253. Simmonds, E. J. Allergic bronchopulmonary aspergillosis. *Lancet* 335: 1229, 1990.

254. Simmonds, E. J. Cystic fibrosis and allergic bronchopulmonary aspergillosis. *Arch. Dis. Child.* 65:507, 1990.

255. Simpson, D. L. Long-term follow-up and bronchial reactivity testing in survivors of the adult respiratory distress syndrome. *Am. Rev. Respir. Dis.* 117:449, 1978.

256. Singh, R. P. Ventilatory functions in tropical pulmonary eosinophilia. *JAPI* 37:775, 1989.

257. Slavin, R. G., et al. A pathological study of ABPA. *J. Allergy Clin. Immunol.* 81:718, 1988.

258. Sly, P. D. Childhood asthma following hospitalization with acute viral bronchiolitis in infancy. *Pediatr. Pulmonol.* 7:153, 1989.

259. Small, P. Chronic urticaria and angioedema. *Clin. Allerg.* 28:131, 1982.

260. Smith, L. S. Endobronchial TB. *Chest* 91:644, 1987.

261. So, S. Y. Rapid diagnosis of suspected pulmonary tuberculosis by fiberoptic bronchoscopy. *Tubercle* 63:195, 1982.

262. Soda, R. A case of bronchial asthma and PIE syndrome induced by disodium cromoglycate. *Nippon Kyoba Shikkan Gakkai Zasshi* 27:89, 1989.

263. Sontag, S. Is gastroesophageal reflux a factor in some asthmatics? *Am. J. Gastroenterol.* 82:119, 1987.

264. Soria, R. Les modifications de L'electrocardiogramme dans L'etat de mal asthmatique. *Ann. Cardiol.* 3:153, 1984.

265. Speiser, W. Plasm D-Dimer and pulmonary embolism. *Lancet* 1:792, 1989.

266. Spiro, H. R. Chronic factitious illness: Munchausen's syndrome. *Arch. Gen. Psychiatry* 18:569, 1968.

267. Stjernberg, N. Pulmonary function in patients with endobronchial sarcoidosis. *Acta Med. Scand.* 215:121, 1984.

268. Stover, D. E. Spectrum of pulmonary diseases associated with AIDS. *Am. J. Med.* 78:429, 1985.

269. Suhl, J. Pulmonary function in male freebase cocaine smokers (abstract). *Am. Rev. Respir. Dis.* 137:488, 1988.

270. Swank, D. W., and Moore, S. B. Roles of the neutrophil and other mediators in adult respiratory distress syndrome. *Mayo Clin. Proc.* 64:1118, 1989.

271. Tan, W. C. Effects of spontaneous and simulated gastroesophageal reflux on sleeping asthmatics. *Am. Rev. Respir. Dis.* 141:1394, 1990.

272. Taylor, R. F., and Bernard, G. R. Airway complications from free-basing cocaine. *Chest* 95:476, 1989.

273. Theodore, J. Obliterative bronchiolitis. *Clin. Chest Med.* 11:309, 1990.

274. Thomas, D. Humoral Factors Mediated by Platelets in Experimental Pul-

monary Embolism. In A. Sasahara and M. Stein (eds.), *Pulmonary Embolic Disease.* New York: Grune & Stratton, 1965. P. 59.

275. Thorogood, M. An epidemiologic survey of cardiovascular disease in women taking oral contraceptives. *Am. J. Obstet. Gynecol.* 163(Suppl. 1, pt. 2):274, 1990.

276. Thorsen, A. Malignant carcinoid of the small intestine with metastases to the liver, valvular disease of the right side of the heart, peripheral vasomotor symptoms, bronchoconstriction and an unusual type of cyanosis. A clinical and a pathological syndrome. *Am. Heart J.* 47:795, 1954.

277. Tuchman, D. N. Comparison of airway responses following tracheal or esophageal acidification in the cat. *Gastroenterology* 87:872, 1984.

278. Uhland, H. Pulmonary embolism. A commonly missed clinical entity. *Dis. Chest* 45:533, 1964.

279. Van den Brande, P. M. Clinical spectrum of endobronchial TB in elderly patients. *Arch. Intern. Med.* 150:2105, 1990.

280. Vijayan, V. K. Diffusing capacity in acute untreated tropical eosinophilia. *Indian J. Chest Dis. Allied Sci.* 30:71, 1988.

281. Vinik, A. I. Clinical features, diagnosis, and localization of carcinoid tumors and their management. *Gastroenterol. Clin. North Am.* 18:865, 1989.

282. Wagner, P. D. Ventilation:perfusion inequality in chronic asthma. *Am. Rev. Respir. Dis.* 136:605, 1987.

283. Waldbott, G. L. Asthma due to a local anaesthetic. *JAMA* 99:1942, 1932.

284. Wanner, A. Circulation of the airway mucosa. *J. Appl. Physiol.* 67:917, 1989.

285. Wasser, L. S., Shaw, G. W., and Talavera, W. Endobronchial tuberculosis in AIDS. *Chest* 94:1240, 1988.

286. Webster, J. R. Wheezing due to pulmonary embolism. *N. Engl. J. Med.* 274:931, 1966.

287. Weishammer, S. Effects of hypothyroidism on bronchial reactivity in nonasthmatic subjects. *Thorax* 45:947, 1990.

288. White, D. A., and Matthay, R. A. Noninfectious pulmonary complications of infection with the HIV. *Am. Rev. Respir. Dis.* 140:1763, 1989.

289. Widdecombe, J. The autonomic nervous system and breathing. *Arch. Intern. Med.* 126:311, 1970.

290. Williams, D. J. Endobronchial TB presenting as asthma. *Chest* 93:836, 1988.

291. Wilson, N. V. Bronchoscopic observations in TB tracheobronchitis. *Dis. Chest* 11:36, 1945.

292. Wilson, R. Upper respiratory tract involvement in sarcoidosis and its management. *Eur. Respir. J.* 1:269, 1988.

293. Windebank, W. J. Pulmonary thromboembolism presenting as asthma. *Br. Med. J.* 1:90, 1973.

294. Wong, R. K. H. The effect of terbutaline sulfate, nitroglycerin and aminophylline on lower esophageal sphincter pressure and radionuclide esophageal emptying in patients with achalasia. *J. Clin. Gastroenterol.* 9: 386, 1987.

295. Wood, R. E. Cystic fibrosis. *Am. Rev. Respir. Dis.* 113:833, 1976.

296. Wright, P. E., and Bernard, G. R. The role of airflow resistance in patients with the adult respiratory distress syndrome. *Am. Rev. Respir. Dis.* 139: 1169, 1989.

297. Yernault, J. C. Dyspnoea, wheezing and respiratory insufficiency in pregnancy: Was it bronchial or cardiac asthma? *Eur. Respir. J.* 3:247, 1990.

298. Zeitels, J., et al. Carcinoid tumors: A 37-year experience. *Arch. Surg.* 117: 732, 1982.

299. Zibrak, J. D., et al. Bronchoscopic and radiologic features of Kaposi's sarcoma involving the respiratory system. *Chest* 90:476, 1986.

300. Zielinski, R. M. Alpha interferon for the hypereosinophilic syndrome. *Ann. Intern. Med.* 113:716, 1990.

301. Zwerdling, R. G. Case records of the Mass. Gen. Hosp. *N. Engl. J. Med.* 321:1665, 1989.

302. Austen, K. F. Systemic mastocytosis. *N. Engl. J. Med.* 326:639, 1992.

303. Cahill, B. C., et al. Tracheobronchial obstruction due to silicosis. *Am. Rev. Respir. Dis.* 145:719, 1992.

304. Carson, J. L., et al. The clinical course of pulmonary embolism. *N. Engl. J. Med.* 326:1240, 1992.

305. Cunningham, E. T. et al. Vagal reflexes referred from the upper aerodigestive tract: An infrequently recognized cause of common cardiorespiratory responses. *Ann. Intern. Med.* 116:575, 1992.

306. Efthimiou, J., et al. Reversible T-wave abnormality in severe acute asthma: An electrocardiographic sign of severity. *Respir. Med.* 85:195, 1991.

307. Fraunfelder, F. T., and Barker, A. F. Respiratory effects of timolol. *N. Engl. J. Med.* 311:1441, 1984.

308. Goldman, J., and Muers, M. Vocal cord dysfunction and wheezing (editorial). *Thorax* 46:401, 1991.

309. Goodwin, S. D., and Glenny, R. W. Nonsteroidal anti-inflammatory drug-associated pulmonary infiltrates with eosinophilia. *Arch. Intern. Med.* 152:1521, 1992.

310. Grammer, L. C., and Greenberger, P. A. Diagnosis and classification of asthma. *Chest* 101:393S, 1992.

311. Green, R. M., et al. Pulmonary embolism in younger adults. *Chest* 101: 1507, 1992.

312. Hedner, T., et al. Angioedema in relation to treatment with angiotensin converting enzyme inhibitors. *Br. Med. J.* 304:941, 1992.

313. Hunt, L. W., and Rosenow, E. C. Asthma-producing drugs. *Ann. Allergy* 68:453, 1992.

314. Iamandescu, I. B. NSAIDs-induced asthma. *Allergol. Immunopathol.* 6: 285, 1989.

315. Iraili, Z. H., and Hall, W. D. Cough and angioneurotic edema associated with angiotensin-converting enzyme inhibitor therapy. *Ann. Intern. Med.* 117:234, 1992.

316. Kang, B. C., Grizz, V., and Phillips, B. Nonwheezing bronchial asthma diagnosed by methacholine challenge. *Am. J. Med.* 88:675, 1990.

317. Katzman, M., et al. High incidence of bronchospasm with regular administration of aerosolized pentamidine. *Chest* 101:79, 1992.

318. Kaufman, J., et al. Angiotensin-converting enzyme inhibitors in patients with bronchial responsiveness and asthma. *Chest* 101:922, 1992.

319. Kivity, S., et al. Vocal cord dysfunction presenting as wheezing and exercise-induced asthma. *J. Asthma* 23:241, 1986.

320. Kluin-Nelemans, H. C., et al. Response to interferon alpha-2b in a patient with systemic mastocytosis. *N. Engl. J. Med.* 326:619, 1992.

321. Larrain, A., et al. Medical and surgical treatment of nonallergic asthma associated with gastroesophageal reflux. *Chest* 99:1330, 1991.

322. Marion, M., et al. Strider and focal laryngeal dystonia. *Lancet* 1:457, 1992.

323. Marshall, G. M., and White, L. Effective therapy for a severe case of the idiopathic hypereosinophilic syndrome. *Am. J. Pediatr. Hematol. Oncol.* 11:178, 1989.

324. Nagai, A., et al. Functional upper airway obstruction: Psychogenic pharyngeal constriction. *Chest* 101:1460, 1992.

325. Odeh, M., Oliven, A., and Bassan, H. Timolol eyedrop-induced fatal bronchospasm in an asthmatic patient. *J. Fam. Prac.* 32:97, 1991.

326. Petrovsky, T. Mycoplasma pneumonia infection and post-infection asthma. *Med. J. Aust.* 152:391, 1990.

327. Popa, V. Captopril-related (and induced?) asthma. *Am. Rev. Respir. Dis.* 136:999, 1987.

328. Rao, A. N., Polos, P. G., and Walther, F. A. Crack abuse and asthma: A fatal combination. *N.Y. State. J. Med.* 90:511, 1990.

329. Reinoso, M. A., Jett, J. R., and Beck, K. C. Body plethysmography in the evaluation of intrathoracic airway abnormalities. *Chest* 101:1674, 1992.

330. Rodriguez-Roisin, R. et al. Ventilation-perfusion mismatch after methacholine challenge in patients with mild bronchial asthma. *Am. Rev. Respir. Dis.* 144:88, 1991.

331. Schwartz, H. J., and Greenberger, A. The prevalence of allergic bronchopulmonary aspergillosis in patients with asthma, determined by serologic and radiologic criteria in patients at risk. *J. Lab. Clin. Med.* 117:138, 1991.

332. Semple, P. F., and Herd, G. W. Cough and wheeze caused by inhibitors of angiotensin-converting enzyme. *N. Engl. J. Med.* 314:61, 1986.

333. Simon, S. R., et al. Cough and ACE inhibitors. *Arch. Intern. Med.* 152:1698, 1992.

334. Small, D., et al. Exertional dyspnea and ventilation in hyperthyroidism. *Chest* 101:1268, 1992.

335. Sontag, S. J. Gut feelings about asthma: The burp and the wheeze (editorial). *Chest* 99:1321, 1991.

336. Siegler, D. Reversible electrocardiographic changes in severe acute asthma. *Thorax* 32:328, 1977.

337. Symposium. Similarities and discrepancies between asthma and chronic obstructive pulmonary disease. *Am. Rev. Respir. Dis.* 143:1149–96, 1421–72, 1991.

338. White, N. W., Raine, R. I., and Bateman, E. D. Asthma and hyperthyroidism. *S. Afr. Med. J.* 78:750, 1990.

Laboratory Methods for Diagnosing Allergic Asthma

38

Lawrence M. Du Buske
Doris S. Pennoyer
Albert L. Sheffer

Allergic asthma may be defined as reversible airway disease due to exogenous antigen-induced release of chemical mediators from IgE-sensitized mast cells and basophils. It is the most commonly encountered immunologic pulmonary disease, affecting nearly 50 percent of adults and 80 percent of children who have asthma [4].

An increase in hospital admissions for children with asthma in the last 10 years has been correlated with an increase in the prevalence of atopic dermatitis and allergic rhinitis among children [143]. High levels of serum IgE and multiple positive radioallergosorbent test (RAST) scores are associated with more severe and chronic asthma and higher medication requirements [202]. Studies of older children have demonstrated that increasing atopy is associated with an increasing tendency toward steroid dependency for control of asthma. Children with severe chronic asthma are easily sensitized to form IgE antibodies to a variety of aeroallergens, which then perpetuate their asthmatic responses [203]. The incidence of allergic rhinitis is highest in those individuals with the most severe asthma [95].

The necessity of aeroallergen avoidance to prevent the progression of asthma is well documented. In some populations the prevalence of dust mite sensitivity has been estimated to be responsible for up to 85 percent of all asthma episodes [194]. Similar studies have associated exposures to cat dander, cockroach, and grass pollen with an increased risk of asthma attacks in individuals sensitized to these allergens [143].

To diagnose allergic asthma, an IgE-related mechanism must be demonstrated, since many exogenous substances may cause otherwise clinically indistinguishable syndromes including bronchospasm by mechanisms not related to IgE sensitization of mast cells and basophils. Immunologic reactions can be classified according to the participating immunoreactants as IgE-mediated, complement- or immune complex–mediated, eicosanoid-mediated, or lymphocyte-mediated reactions (Table 38-1). A late cutaneous or bronchial reaction to antigen challenge may be IgE mediated [175] but it can also signal immune complex formation with complement activation [150] or when the reaction is delayed, possibly a cell-mediated immune response as in hypersensitivity pneumonitis [82]. The diagnosis of allergic asthma may be further complicated by the elaboration of metabolites of arachidonic acid such as is seen in patients who are intolerant to aspirin and nonsteroidal antiinflammatory agents [108, 170].

To establish the immunologic mechanisms for asthma clinically, it is necessary to demonstrate allergen-specific IgE or inflammatory mediator release following appropriate antigen challenge. However, such responses may be considered clinically relevant only if there is a history compatible with symptoms induced by exposure to the allergen. A thorough patient history is critical, not only in selecting the appropriate allergens for testing, but also in interpreting the test results. All test results must be intrepreted in the context of the test sensitivity (the ability to detect true positives, specificity (the ability to detect only true positives), efficiency (likelihood of the test detecting only true positives or true negatives), and positive or negative predictive value (likelihood that a positive or negative test result truly means a positive or negative assessment of disease presence) [230]. The absence of an antigen-specific, IgE-induced response argues against an allergic mechanism as a cause for the responses.

Appreciation that the chronic inflammation associated with asthma may be due to the perpetuation of inflammation in the lungs secondary to chronic late-phase inflammation has had a dramatic impact on asthma therapy. It is now appreciated that mast cell activation secondary to the reaction of an antigen with membrane-bound IgE not only is essential for the development of the immediate bronchospasm seen during a classic allergic response, but also is necessary for the more delayed bronchospasm that can occur 3 to 12 hours after an allergic challenge. This late phase of bronchospasm is associated with a significant increase in airway hyperresponsiveness to a variety of bronchoconstrictor mediators, including environmental allergens [132].

Careful historical documentation for the presence of allergens, which are then correlated with allergen-specific sensitivity through proper allergy testing, may allow for avoidance of those allergens that can perpetuate asthma by inducing chronic and recurrent late-phase reactions in the lungs. A recent study of dust mite–allergic asthmatic subjects demonstrated that low respiratory thresholds to acetylcholine-induced bronchospasm are associated with high levels of basophil histamine release induced by dust mite antigens and high serum IgE levels. This suggests that the perpetuation of inflammation and the subsequent development of persistent and severe asthma are related to this exquisite sensitivity to dust mite in these individuals [90]. Even among individuals having seasonal allergic rhinitis without known asthma, bronchial reactivity to methacholine increases during the pollen season, suggesting that natural exposure to aeroallergens in nonasthmatic atopic subjects may induce significant airway inflammation in the lungs [32].

For a large population of individuals with asthma, the prevalence of asthma is closely related to the serum IgE level standardized for age and sex, with no asthma being present among those individuals with the lowest IgE levels. The division of asthma into extrinsic or allergic and intrinsic or nonallergic types may not be as clear as was previously believed. It now appears that most patients with asthma probably had some allergic basis initially inducing their disease, even though the presence of this allergic factor may not be evident once the patient has had asthma for many years [42]. Thus, an assessment for allergens inducing asthma is essential for the proper diagnosis and treatment of asthma. This assessment should include clinically relevant allergens such as dust mite, cockroach, cat dander, dog dander, locally common pollens, and common molds inducing inhalant

Table 38-1. Laboratory methods for diagnosing allergic asthma

I. IgE mediated
  A. Antigen challenge
    1. In vivo
      a. Direct
        (1) Skin test
        (2) Bronchopulmonary challenge
      b. Indirect
        (1) Prausnitz-Küstner passive transfer
    2. In vitro
      a. Direct
        (1) Antigen-specific IgE
          (a) RAST
          (b) FEIA
          (c) CLIA
          (d) RAST inhibition
          (e) CRIE
          (f) Immuno-blotting
        (2) Total IgE PRIST/IRMA/ELISA
        (3) Antigen-induced basophil histamine release
        (4) Spontaneous basophil histamine releasability
        (5) Antigen-induced cellular proliferation
        (6) Antigen-induced lymphokine or mediator release
      b. Indirect
        Passive sensitization of normal nonallergic human basophils
  B. Mediator measurement
    1. With antigen challenge
      a. Histamine
      b. Tryptase
      c. Leukotrienes
      d. Prostaglandins/thromboxanes
      e. Cytokines
      f. Eosinophil factors: ECP, EDN, MBP
      g. Neutrophil factors: MPO
      h. Other: PAF, NCF-A, ECF-A
    2. Sources
      a. Urine: PGD_2, LTE_4
      b. Blood: NCF-A, ECF-A, PAF, LTC_4, Histamine, Tryptase, ECP, EDN, MPO
II. Complement mediated
  A. Immune-complex detection
  B. Measurement of complement components
  C. Pathologic examination of tissue
III. Arachidonate mediated (i.e., aspirin, tartrazine, and nonsteroidal antiinflammatory agents)
  A. In vivo: arachidonate metabolite measurements
  B. In vitro: bronchoalveolar lavage cellular metabolites in presence of ASA
IV. Lymphocyte mediated
  A. Bronchopulmonary challenge
  B. Bronchoalveolar lavage
  C. Transbronchial biopsy
V. Direct mast cell– or basophil-mediated release
  A. In vivo
    1. Skin test
    2. Bronchoalveolar lavage
    3. Nasal pharyngeal lavage
  B. In vitro
    1. Basophil histamine release
    2. Human lung fragment histamine release

RAST = radioallergosorbent test; PRIST = paper radioimmunosorbent test; PAF = platelet-activating factor; ELISA = enzyme-linked immunosorbent assay; IRMA = immunoradiometric assay; LTE_4 = leukotriene E_4; LTC_4 = leukotriene C_4; NCF-A = neutrophil chemotactic factor of anaphylaxis; ECF-A = eosinophil chemotactic factor of anaphylaxis; PGD_2 = prostaglandin D_2; ASA = acetylsalicylic acid; FEIA = fluorescence enzyme immunoassay; CLIA = chemiluminescent immunoassay; CRIE = crossed radio immuno-electrophoresis; ECP = eosinophil cationic protein; EDN = eosinophil-derived neurotoxin; MBP = major basic protein; MPO = myeloperoxidase.

allergy, with evaluation for more obscure allergens seldom yielding significant positive results in individuals who otherwise manifest no allergic reactivity [231]. Allergens chosen as clinically relevant should be historically related to the development of asthma symptoms on exposure, as a positive skin test to an inhal-

ant allergen does not guarantee that this allergen truly induces asthmatic responses [214].

SKIN TESTING

Skin testing relevant to a patient history of allergen-induced symptoms remains the diagnostic method of choice in IgE-mediated allergic disease. A clinically significant allergy is confirmed by the development of an immediate wheal-and-flare reaction following the introduction of small amounts of suspected allergen into the skin [31]. The simplicity, efficiency, and relatively low cost of the technique have made it preferable to other approaches in defining an individual's specific allergies. With proper controls and good technique, skin testing provides rapid, reliable, and reproducible results. Longitudinal stability of skin test results obtained by skin prick testing to aeroallergens is extremely high, with less than 5 percent conversion of negative to positive results noted in studies of patients tested yearly over a three-year period [221].

Procedure

Selection of Allergens

Testing with appropriately selected allergens chosen on the basis of a thorough patient history usually provides the necessary information for the diagnosis and treatment of allergic disease. Routine testing with allergens that are not clinically relevant based on the patient's exposure is considered inappropriate. The history should include a thorough inventory of allergens in the patient's environment, exposures thought to induce symptoms and changes in the environment relative to the onset of symptoms. Inquiry regarding seasonal exacerbation of symptoms can provide guidance about pollens to be tested. The regional patterns of tree, grass, and weed pollination must be considered when considering allergens. At times, perennial allergens can produce a seasonal exacerbation of symptoms that may be confused with pollen-induced symptoms. For example, perennial symptoms may increase with dust mite proliferation in the late summer and early fall concomitant with the ragweed season. Similarly, allergy due to a rise in outdoor mold counts in the springtime and the late fall can be confused with allergy to trees and weeds that also occur during these times of the year.

Skin testing should only be performed with great caution with any allergen to which a patient appears to have had an anaphylactic reaction, as cutaneous rechallenge may induce a systemic reaction [72]. Clinical examples of anaphylactic allergies that can induce significant reactions on skin testing include allergies to some food to which the patient may be highly sensitive, such as nuts, shellfish, and cottonseed. Due to the danger of systemic reactions, these food allergens should be administered by scratch rather than intradermal testing [41]. Care should also be taken to avoid simultaneous testing with allergens to which the patient appears highly sensitive by history. When skin testing is performed, a physician should be immediately available in case an anaphylactic event occurs. Treatment for such anaphylaxis would normally include the subcutaneous administration of epinephrine, which should be readily available at the time of allergy skin testing.

Patient Preparation

All medications with antihistaminic action should be omitted for an appropriate period of time before testing [142]. The effect of most antihistamines will have disappeared after 48 to 72 hours, but the effect of others such as hydroxyzine can persist up to

96 hours. The long-acting antihistamine astemizole can have a persistent antihistaminic effect for 4 to 6 weeks after discontinuation. The use of H_2 antagonists such as cimetidine, ranitidine, and famotidine can inhibit skin test reactivity. Tricyclic antidepressants can have a fairly prolonged antihistaminic effect, at times lasting for weeks after withdrawal. Phenothiazines used as psychotropic agents are also antihistamines. Topical corticosteroids suppress skin test reactivity, but systemically administered corticosteroids do not. Asthma medications should not be discontinued. Theophylline, beta-adrenergic agonists, inhaled corticosteroids, and cromolyn have not been shown to effect skin test results significantly [33, 47, 78].

In the asthmatic patient who is tolerating a beta-adrenergic blocker, the question of whether skin testing should be performed in the presence of this agent is controversial at this time. The risk of anaphylaxis appears increased in asthma if a beta-adrenergic blocking agent is present, as such a drug would antagonize epinephrine were it needed in the event of a systemic reaction consequent to the allergy skin testing [93]. The risk of refractory hypotension in a patient with cardiovascular problems in particular must be considered.

The patient with asthma should be under satisfactory control at the time of skin testing. Testing should not be done in the presence of an acute illness since symptoms or sequelae might inappropriately be attributed to the testing procedure. The skin of the testing site should be clear. Dermatographic skin can give false-positive results. Lichenified skin, such as can be seen with severe psoriasis and eczema, can give false-negative results. Mild eczema does not preclude skin testing, as there is good reproducibility of significant positive skin prick tests for inhalants in such individuals [235]. In cases of either dermatographism or severe systemic dermatosis, in vitro diagnostic testing such as RAST is an appropriate alternative for skin testing.

Technique

The two methods for application of skin tests are epicutaneous and intracutaneous, also known as intradermal testing. Epicutaneous techniques include scratch, prick, and puncture methods. The epicutaneous method is 1,000 times less sensitive than the intradermal method [27]. Commercial extracts are available for either epicutaneous or intradermal methodologies. Standardized and conventional nonstandardized extracts may give similar results, especially in instances of strong reaction positivity; however, results obtained using different extract preparations for the same allergens are not directly interchangeable [222]. When an extract prepared for epicutaneous testing is used, care must be taken that it not be introduced through the epidermis into the dermis, thus giving the patient a larger than intended dose resulting in a potentially serious reaction if the individual is highly sensitive to the antigen. Reproducibility of prick and intradermal testing is affected by the age of the patient, the area of skin tested, circadian rhythms, skin pigmentation, the presence of antihistamines, and the potency and stability of the extract. In general, infants and elderly patients are the least reactive; the greatest reactivity occurs on the upper part of the back compared to the lower back, and on the back compared to the volar aspect of the forearms. The least reactivity occurs in the early morning hours; hyperpigmentation of the skin or abnormalities in skin pigmentation can affect the reliability of readings; and the presence of antihistamines or drugs with antihistaminic properties may cause false-negative results.

Epicutaneous Test. Epicutaneous tests may be introduced by scratch, prick, or puncture techniques. Although the scratch technique was the earliest approach to cutaneous challenge, it has limited applicability now. In this method a small amount of the suspected allergen contained in an extract is dropped on a 1- to 2-mm bloodless scratch that involves only the superficial layer of the epidermis. The antigen may be wiped off once a reaction begins, thus avoiding further allergen absorption. This low level of exposure makes this technique a very useful modality for patients who, by history, appear to have extreme hypersensitivity to a given antigen.

The prick technique is faster and simpler and when used with proper care, is safe and reproducible [33, 129]. A drop of allergenic extract of appropriate concentration is placed on the skin, which has been cleansed with alcohol and allowed to dry. The tip of a needle is depressed parallel to the skin through the drop of extract to introduce it superficially into the corneum. The needle tip is then lifted upward through the superficial layer of the skin to complete the inoculation. If more than one extract is being tested, a fresh hypodermic needle must be used for each extract. Other nonhollow needles must be wiped clean with an alcohol sponge between each inoculation and then discarded or sterilized when the patient's testing is completed. The prick should be made through the diluent as a negative control and through 1% histamine solution as a positive control.

Attempts have been made to develop flanged needles that prevent the point from penetrating beyond the epidermis when introduced vertically by a puncture technique. Commercially available products include a disposable adaptation of the Morrow-Brown needle and a shortened variant of the disposable hematology lancet [38, 152]. An evaluation of nine different prick puncture test devices or methods revealed coefficient of variation between 8 percent and 21 percent, devices that were lancets, such as Phazet, producing less variable results than more needle-like pointed devices such as the Morrow-Brown needle [211]. A multipronged apparatus, the Multitest, permits preloading of a disposable plastic applicator having eight clusters of tine-type prongs so that all eight allergens can be introduced simultaneously to the skin. These devices may yield an increasing number of positive tests, however, when greater mechanical pressure is applied to them in performing skin testing [226]. A recent comparison of the precision and accuracy of commonly used epicutaneous devices reveals some false-positive reactions with the Multitest device [5]. When the Multitest device is used in children for expediency, positive results may require confirmation by one of the single-needle methods of epicutaneous testing should the degree of positivity be questionable. A difficulty noted with the Multitest device is the close proximity of the individual allergen testing sites. This proximity allows a potentiation of reactions to occur. A strongly positive reaction placed next to an allergen that would otherwise cause a negative result could cause that adjacent allergen site to present as a false-positive reading.

Intracutaneous Tests. Intracutaneous tests, also known as intradermal tests, are used when increased test reliability, sensitivity, and reproducibility are required. This procedure identifies a larger population of reactive patients, including those with negative puncture test results. The test is more sensitive than prick testing, requiring the use of extracts significantly more dilute than those used in prick testing. A 26 to 30 gauge hypodermic needle is used with 0.01 to 0.05 ml of extract introduced into the dermis, forming a small bleb intracutaneously. The maximum recommended extract concentration for intradermal tests is 1:1,000 dilution (weight/volume), roughly being 50- to 100-fold more dilute than the concentrated extract used in prick testing. With glycerinated extract solutions, care must be taken to test a glycerinated extract control, as the glycerin component may give a false-positive reaction. A positive histamine and negative buffer diluent control test should also be performed. For the more dilute extracts used in intradermal testing, stability and potency are more important factors than is the case with the concentrated solutions used for prick testing. Extracts that are more dilute tend to degrade and lose antigenicity more rapidly than do concentrated allergy extracts. The risks of anaphylaxis and systemic reactions are greater in intradermal testing due to the larger quantity of antigen injected. Associated with the enhanced sensitivity of intradermal testing, false-positive reactions are more likely to occur. These positive reactions may not in fact be false, but may indicate allergic reactivity in patients who have not as yet demonstrated clinical signs of allergy. Individuals who have positive skin test results but who do not demonstrate current signs of allergy are more likely to develop symptoms of allergy than are individuals who test negative on skin tests when followed over a 5- to 10-year period. False-positive reactions, however, may also occur due to the histamine content of some extracts, most notably Box elder, Johnson grass, ragweed, and a variety of foods and venoms that contain histamine as a naturally occurring contaminant [237].

Intradermal testing is preferred for the biologic standardization of allergenic extracts, as the intradermal method produces a steeper dose-response line than do the epicutaneous or puncture methods, allowing more accurate and precise data for the evaluation of allergen potency. Intracutaneous testing generally requires only a single allergen concentration, serial testing with increasing concentrations being used clinically for the diagnosis of venom or drug sensitivity. The utilization of threshold dilution testing, wherein an "end point" is established as the lowest concentration that produces a positive skin test result, is useful for allergen standardization and clinical research but is not necessary for the evaluation of allergic disease. In particular, end point titration methods of administration of allergen immunotherapy, such as the Rinkel method, have not been scientifically proven to be of use in multiple prospective investigations [230].

In the evaluation of the potentially allergic patient, testing should first be performed with the epicutaneous prick puncture method to identify those individuals exquisitely sensitive to a given allergen. Those individuals, negative by epicutaneous testing, can then be evaluated by intracutaneous or intradermal testing, performed only with those antigens showing no reactivity on the initial epicutaneous test. When properly performed, the intracutaneous allergy skin test has high sensitivity and specificity for the diagnosis of allergic disease [30].

Preparation of Extracts

Commercially prepared extracts of the most common inhalant allergens are available. Food extracts are also available and clinical correlation with a limited panel applied epicutaneously has been established [18, 161]. The intradermal route is generally avoided for food testing because of the potential for systemic reactions in highly sensitive individuals and the possibility of a false-positive reaction due to the irritant effects of some of the extracts. Foods can be applied directly without extraction over a scratch made in the skin or by pricking first the food and then the skin.

The potency and stability of the extracts must be assured [14]. Extracts should be refrigerated when not in use. Concentrated extracts are usually stable for the period indicated by the company that prepared them. More dilute solutions deteriorate more rapidly. Stability is increased by the addition of glycerin or albumin to the diluent. Extracts stored in 50% glycerin retain their potency better than those stored in 10% glycerin or 0.03% albumin [124]. Glycerinated extracts can be used for epicutaneous testings, but are too irritating for intradermal use if they are stored in a solution above 5% glycerin. If glycerinated extracts are used, the skin test must be compared with a similar 5% glycerinated buffer control that would act as a negative control in order to avoid a false-positive interpretation. A saline diluent containing 0.03% albumin can be used for intradermal testing. Extremely dilute extract should be prepared at the time of use. While standardized extracts are comparable from lot to lot and company to company [148], there are relatively few standardized

extracts available at this time. Results of testing using standardized and nonstandardized extracts are not directly interchangeable [222]. There is often great variation in allergenic potency from lot to lot of a given unstandardized extract, even when prepared by the same company.

Grading of Test Results

Systems for grading skin test results are based on the area of both the wheal and the erythematous flare that occur 15 to 20 minutes after injection of the antigen [30]. It is helpful to compare the skin test result with the negative control result, in the form of a diluent that is used for the extract, and a positive control, in the form of histamine. A histamine control is satisfactory if the reaction area is larger than 10 mm. A negative diluent control is satisfactory if the reaction area is smaller than 5 mm. Areas of reaction to allergenic extracts that are less than 50 percent larger than the size of the diluent negative control reaction area are of questionable significance. Similarly, reaction areas that are less than half the size of the histamine control area are of lesser significance than those that are greater than 50 percent the size of the histamine control area. Results of skin testing may be uninterpretable if the response to the controls is unsatisfactory. With dermatographism, there may be excessive reactivity to the diluent, making it impossible to distinguish between positive and negative controls.

False-positive skin reactivity may result from (1) overlapping reaction from an adjacent strongly positive result, (2) contamination of the needle or injection site with another extract, (3) the irritant effect of other constituents in the extract, (4) too great a concentration or volume of the extract itself, (5) penetration of epidermal extract into the dermis, (6) air bleeding into the injection site, (7) unrecognized dermatographism, or (8) histamine presence as a contaminant of the extract [237]. False-negative skin test results may occur from (1) outdated or improperly stored extract, (2) subcutaneous injection of intradermal extract, (3) failure to adequately inoculate the epidermis in the prick or puncture technique, (4) denaturation of extract by alcohol used in cleansing, (5) loss of extract through bleeding from the site, (6) persistent unrecognized antihistaminic effect, (7) pretreatment of the skin with topical corticosteroids, (8) lichenification or adjacent eczematous changes in the skin, or (9) lack of relevant antigen in the extract. Late-phase skin reactions have long been recognized and are now known to be IgE mediated. Production of late-phase skin reactions generally requires injection of a larger amount of allergen than needed to produce an immediate-phase reaction. The patient should be instructed to report late reactions since they may sometimes occur despite a negative immediate skin test result [33, 173, 191, 195].

Clinical Interpretation

The skin test reaction must be interpreted with care. Only results that correlate with the patient's history can be considered meaningful.

Although direct skin testing has only limited quantitative precision, this bioassay is highly cost-effective, sensitive, and safe in experienced hands [129]. Its sensitivity is greater than the alternative in vitro assay, such as the RAST [6], although lack of standardization of commercially available extracts adds to the imprecision [158]. Lack of standardized procedures makes it difficult to compare results. The need for better standardization of materials, equipment, and technique has been recognized and measures are currently being formulated to provide for greater standardization [151, 179].

THE PRAUSNITZ-KÜSTNER REACTION (PASSIVE TRANSFER REACTION)

The Prausnitz-Küstner reaction is the classic method of passive sensitization of a normal nonallergenic recipient's skin by injection of the allergic patient's serum [146]. Concern for the presence of human immunodeficiency virus (HIV) antibody or hepatitis-associated antigens make the Prausnitz-Küstner reaction test less acceptable as a viable technique today. However, passive sensitization of normal nonallergic lung fragments, basophils, or mast cells is possible in vitro. These procedures are mainly used for research purposes [94, 107, 135].

BRONCHIAL PROVOCATION TEST

Theoretically, inhalation challenge studies should increase precision in a diagnosis of allergic asthma. In the practical application of these tests, however, several potential problems limit their usefulness. Their major disadvantages include (1) the uncertainty about the comparability of the challenge with natural exposure, (2) the diminutive particle size needed to penetrate small airways, (3) the inability to test more than one allergen per day, (4) the variability in the amount of allergen needed to provoke a response dependent on the patient's nonspecific airway reactivity, and (5) the possibility of inducing a severe asthma attack either during the course of the study or after a delay of 4 to 12 hours [85].

False-negative results can occur if (1) the challenge particles are too large to penetrate the small airways, (2) the challenge doses fail to approximate levels actually encountered in the patient's environment, (3) the test antigen differs from that to which the patient is actually allergic, and (4) the patient's airway reactivity is different when tested from its reactivity in allergen season. False-positive results can occur because of (1) nonspecific irritation from the antigen solution, (2) a dose much higher than that naturally encountered by the patient, and (3) different reactivity to the antigen at various times of the year. Overlap has been reported between bronchial provocation results of ragweed-sensitive asthmatic patients and ragweed-sensitive hay fever patients [40, 141]. European investigators have long thought inhalation challenge to be the most accurate ways to identify the allergen-sensitive asthmatic patient and have used this method extensively for diagnostic purposes [2, 3]. Others also have reported positive results on bronchial antigen challenge testing despite negative skin test results [176] and negative RAST test results, though the clinical significance of such positive bronchial challenges remains questionable [233]. Differences in technique may explain conflicting results [122]. With more standardized procedures, data have begun to show skin testing, RAST, and bronchial provocation to be roughly comparable [24, 49, 118, 139]. Most allergists, therefore, favor skin testing related to the patient's history as the most economical and efficient method of the three. Bronchial provocation testing is used mainly when the results of skin testing and RAST conflict with the patient's history. Provocation testing is also proving helpful in diagnosing occupational asthma caused by workplace allergens, particularly when antigens are not available for skin testing or RAST [48, 64, 156, 157].

Bronchial challenge is also useful in establishing the presence and degree of sulfite sensitivity [172]. Assays of chemical mediators in plasma, serum, urine, and bronchoalveolar lavage fluid may further enhance the clinical application of bronchial provocation, which is primarily investigational at this point [99, 147]. A recent study of tryptase in the bronchoalveolar lavage fluid revealed markedly higher levels in the atopic asthmatic patient compared to atopic nonasthmatic patients and control subjects following endobronchial allergen challenge [199]. Other mediators, such as cytokines, not readily detected in serum may best be detected in bronchoalveolar lavage fluid [208].

ORAL CHALLENGE TESTS

Oral provocation with food or drugs can be monitored with direct patient observation, pulmonary function studies, and possibly measurement of released mediators. Double-blind or single-blind placebo-controlled oral food challenges are considered the most definitive procedures for the diagnosis of food allergies [159]. Demonstration of specific IgE to the food by prick test confirms the cause of the reaction [200]. Adverse food reactions can occur by many mechanisms [97]. A rise in plasma histamine has been demonstrated with positive results on food challenge [160]. As with skin testing, challenge with a food known to have caused anaphylaxis should only be attempted with great caution. RAST provides an acceptable and safe alternative mode for establishing a diagnosis in such individuals.

Drug challenges are usually contraindicated unless there is no acceptable alternative for a vitally needed medication [155]. Except for aspirin intolerance, drug-induced asthma usually occurs as part of an anaphylactic reaction to agents such as penicillin and radiocontrast media. Special protocols for testing and desensitization are available for such specific instances [11, 62, 138]. Challenge, coupled with examination of bronchoalveolar lavage cells, has been helpful in the diagnosis of propranolol-induced hypersensitivity pneumonitis [9].

MEASUREMENT OF TOTAL SERUM IgE

Techniques

Techniques generally used for the assessment of immunoglobulin concentration such as radial immunodiffusion cannot be used to establish IgE concentrations because total serum IgE levels are normally extremely low. Three methods currently employed to measure total serum IgE include the radioimmunosorbent test (RIST), the paper immunosorbent test (PRIST), and the enzyme-linked immunosorbent assay (ELISA). The RIST is a competitive inhibition procedure, also known as a competitive displacement radioimmunoassay (RIA), that measures the capacity of IgE to block the reaction between a defined amount of radioisotope-labeled IgE and specific antibodies to IgE, wherein the more IgE there is in the sample, the less radioisotope will be bound to the antibody. False elevations in apparent IgE levels can occur in the lower range of this assay due to an interference from serum factors, limiting the accuracy of this assay in situations of total IgE levels less than or equal to 40 IU/ml [50]. The PRIST is a double-antibody, sandwich-type assay, also known as a two-site immunoradiometric assay (IRMA). In this type of assay, IgE from test serum reacts with anti-IgE bound to a solid-phase paper disk. Complexes are formed on the disk between the anti-IgE and the serum IgE. These complexes are then exposed to radiolabeled anti-IgE. The bound radioactivity is directly proportional to concentrations of IgE in the unknown serum [80]. This assay is highly sensitive, specific, and reproducible. Modifications of this assay allow a sensitivity to as low as 0.24 μg/ml or 0.1 IU/ml of IgE [186]. A variety of other IRMAs utilize techniques wherein serum samples are incubated with two anti-IgE antibodies directed against different antigenic sites. One of these anti-IgE antibodies is radiolabeled. Inaccurate falsely low results can occur in the presence of high levels of serum IgE due to saturation of the recognition sites on both the unlabeled, or captured, and the labeled antibodies. Dilution of the specimen can correct this deficit if this technical problem is properly recognized [163].

The ELISA method of measuring total serum IgE uses a nonradioactive colorimetric end point [168]. An enzyme-derived fluorescent product may be formed in the fluorescence enzyme immunoassay (FEIA) variant of this method. Typically, a solid phase is used and a sandwich technique similar to the IRMA technique is employed. The method uses anti-IgE antibodies insolubilized on an immunosorbent surface. A sample containing IgE is reacted with the insolubilized anti-IgE. Then, following washing to remove unbound IgE, anti-IgE conjugated to an enzyme is added. After unbound enzyme is washed away, the bound enzymatic activity is related to the total IgE by a standard curve [192, 197]. The correlation between enzyme immunoassay and RIA for measuring total IgE is very high, with a correlation coefficient greater than 0.97 reported for some commercially available methods that have a sensitivity to allow determination of 0.5 IU/ml of IgE [111, 181]. Recently, a nonenzymatic chemiluminescence immunoassay (CLIA) has been devised for total IgE determination, acridinium ester hydrolysis forming a chemiluminiscent product. The natural occurrence of anti-IgE antibodies in some patients with very high total IgE levels may falsely lower total IgE results [189].

Importance of Serum IgE

The mean serum IgE level in patients with atopic disease is within the normal range, making the determination of total IgE not a sensitive diagnostic test for establishing an absolute determination of the presence or absence of atopy. Though the distribution of IgE levels is different among the skin test–positive and skin test–negative patients, the range of IgE levels is extremely wide in age-defined groups such that no single level of IgE clearly distinguishes atopic from nonatopic individuals [98]. The mean total serum IgE concentration in normal subjects is 60 μg/ml (25 IU/ml), with an upper 95 percent confidence limit at 900 μg/ml (375 IU/ml) [186]. Total IgE levels in 60 to 80 percent of atopic patients are above the normal range [89, 129, 136]. A total serum IgE level less than 50 μg/ml (21 IU/ml) helps exclude atopy, except in instances such as penicillin drug allergy, Hymenoptera sensitivity, or allergy restricted to only a few antigens. Many individuals with clinical allergy and demonstrable allergen-specific IgE have IgE levels in the normal range [29, 68]. Normal values for total IgE vary with age, with infants having the lowest and adolescents generally the highest IgE levels. Levels higher than 10 IU/ml at less than 1 year old or higher than 100 IU/ml at 13 to 16 years old carry a sensitivity of 83 percent and specificity of 91 percent for the diagnosis of atopy [111].

Population analyses of IgE levels have demonstrated higher levels in men than women among older subjects. In men, cigarette smoking is the highest, strongest correlate with IgE levels, whereas in women a personal allergy history is the strongest correlate [111]. In children of smokers, a similar analysis has noted both eosinophilia and IgE levels to be more prevalent in male children of smoking parents than male children of nonsmoking parents [53]. Associations between IgE level and subjective symptoms of chronic cough and chronic rhinitis are not conclusively present in studies of large populations when factors such as smoking status are considered [22].

In a study of a large population of self-reported asthmatic patients and patients having allergic rhinitis, the prevalence of asthma was correlated closely with serum IgE level standardized for age and sex, with no asthma present in those subjects with the very lowest serum IgE levels. The presence of allergic rhinitis in this same study was independent of IgE level, however, and associated primarily with skin test reactivity to common aeroallergens. The implication of this is that in some way the presence of IgE is indicative of a tendency to have the subsequent development of asthma, leading to the speculation that an underlying atopic state may, in fact, be present in most individuals with asthma irrespective of skin test negativity to common aeroallergens [42].

A high total serum IgE level, over 900 μg/ml (375 IU/ml), is usually associated with a sensitivity to multiple aeroallergens. Very high total serum IgE levels, often higher than 2,000 μg/ml (833 IU/ml), are seen in immunodeficiency states and some states of parasitism. Defects in the T-cell regulation of IgE synthesis or an absence of T-cells leads to very high IgE levels. Individuals with Wiskott-Aldrich syndrome or the hyper-IgE syndrome associated with staphylococcal infections often have total IgE levels higher than 60,000 μg/ml (25,000 IU/ml) [186]. Patients with malignancies such as Hodgkin's disease who have impaired cellular immunity, patients receiving cytotoxic chemotherapy for bone marrow transplants, and patients with graft-versus-host disease also have very high total IgE levels [168]. Helminthic parasites produce a specific antibody response including IgE as part of the host defense. Other nonallergic states associated with high total IgE levels include Kawasaki's disease and IgE myeloma [197]. Very high IgE levels also occur with some allergic states such as allergic bronchopulmonary aspergillosis or severe atopic dermatitis associated with asthma [186]. Total IgE level may fluctuate during the allergy season in atopic individuals, with an increase during the pollen season or with initiation of immunotherapy. Ultimately, over the course of immunotherapy, total IgE level after an initial rise gradually declines, though this decline may take several years to occur [52].

The utility of obtaining a total serum IgE level for the diagnosis of allergy has been shown to be related to the prior probability of allergy based on the clinical diagnosis, with high total IgE levels increasing the likelihood of allergy, especially if the initial clinical assessment indicates that allergy is unlikely, whereas a low total IgE decreases the likelihood of allergy if there is not a strong initial clinical suspicion of allergy [197].

In a study demonstrating good concordance between the results of intradermal skin tests and RAST for most allergens, there was no significant correlation between total IgE and RAST scores to *Dermatophagoides pteronyssinus,* ragweed, or Bermuda grass. There was a high correlation between total serum IgE and RAST scores to *D. farinae,* however, indicating that the correlation of total serum IgE to specific IgE against an individual allergen may differ depending on the allergen selected for analysis [178]. In a study of tree pollen allergy, a positive correlation was noted between the scores on skin prick testing and RAST and serum IgE levels, with patients having the highest total IgE demonstrating the highest RAST scores [61, 123]. A correlation between total serum IgE and number of allergens positive on the RAST among atopic patients has also been demonstrated.

Elevated serum IgE levels in neonatal cord blood are strongly associated with the subsequent development of allergy in more than 50 percent of infants with a family history of atopy [25, 54]. In areas of endemic parasitism, however, high baseline maternal total IgE levels may make such analysis impossible [81].

An elevated IgE level is among the diagnostic criteria for allergic bronchopulmonary aspergillosis, with falling IgE levels seen with successful glucocorticoid therapy and rising IgE levels seen with disease exacerbations [86, 154, 183, 193].

The clearest indications for determining serum IgE levels are (1) to predict the development of allergic disease in infants, (2) for the diagnosis and treatment of allergic bronchopulmonary aspergillosis, (3) for the evaluation of immunodeficiency states, and (4) to screen for infestation with tissue-invading parasites [201]. Other proposed uses of a serum total IgE level include (1) as a predictive factor for the presence or absence of atopy, (2) as an assessment of the degree of atopy present, and (3) as an index of the efficacy of allergy immunotherapy. Unfortunately, the large amount of overlap between normal individuals and atopic individuals makes the use of a total serum IgE as the sole criteria to determining atopy impossible. Any utilization of a serum IgE level must be in the clinical context of the likelihood of the presence of an allergic disease [52, 72, 197].

DIRECT MEASUREMENT OF ANTIGEN-SPECIFIC IgE

Radioallergosorbent Test

The RAST was first developed in 1967 by Wide as a method to quantify allergen-specific IgE in serum, the initial commercial development occurring shortly thereafter [227]. The test is performed by incubating a patient's serum with a solid-phase matrix that has been coupled to the allergen to be evaluated. The patient's allergen-specific IgE will bind to the antigen-matrix complex in direct proportion to the amount of allergen-specific IgE in the serum. Radiolabeled anti-IgE is added to quantify the amount of allergen-specific IgE present, resulting in a "sandwich" being formed containing the matrix-coupled antigen, the antigen-specific IgE from the patient's serum, and the radiolabeled anti-IgE antibody. The amount of allergen-specific IgE is estimated with reference to a standard curve and graded from 1 to 4 based on arbitrary divisions of a birch allergen reference curve [168]. Recent advances include the use of a World Health Organization standard for total IgE as the reference material used in formulating a standard curve, allowing for the quantification of antigen-specific IgE in more meaningful and reproducible units [217].

The modified RAST (mRAST) system uses a single point calibration curve determined by the time required for the production of 25,000 counts detected by a gamma scintillation counter upon incubation of 25 U/ml of IgE standard with ^{125}I anti-IgE [238]. In mRAST scoring, all results are quantified by extrapolation from the single standard point to zero, results being mathematically "derived," whereas in standard RAST scoring, all results are quantified by comparison to a multipoint standard curve generally containing three to five dilutions of a standard. As the mRAST allows extrapolation of results to IgE levels below conventional standard dilutions, very low thresholds for antigen specific IgE determinations have been claimed; however, this lower threshold for positive reactions induces an overdiagnosis of allergic disease in an attempt to gain greater sensitivity than standard RAST methodology allows [220, 238]. False-positive results occur at the lower end of the mRAST assay range due to technical factors such as incomplete washing away of unbound radiolabeled anti-IgE [168]. The mRAST is not appropriate for clinical or research settings where high specificity is required [238].

Due to the lack of standardization of the allergens coupled to the solid phase, low values reported in most RAST systems must be interpreted with caution. Results of RAST testing correlate better with prick skin testing results than with the more sensitive but less specific intradermal skin testing results [227]. In comparison to skin testing and in comparison to in vitro leukocyte histamine release assays, 10 to 25 percent of individuals positive for allergy on these other bioassays will be negative by RAST [168]. Results of RASTs are semi-quantitative, as scoring for a given allergen is valid only for testing within that specific assay system [168].

Instances where the RAST is clearly indicated include dermatologic diseases associated with overreactivity of the skin such as dermatographism or physical urticaria, where false-positive results could occur simply by scratching the skin even in the absence of an allergen. Additionally, widespread dermatologic diseases with significant lichenification of the skin may result in significant hyporeactivity of the skin and false-negative results. Individuals with widespread skin diseases such as generalized eczema or psoriasis or individuals with highly pigmented skin may also present significant difficulties in scoring and reading skin prick test results, and thus would be candidates for the RAST. Other instances where the RAST would be indicated include those situations where medications interfere with skin testing, such as a requirement for the chronic use of antihistamines or antidepressants which the patient is unable to discontinue for a sufficient time prior to skin testing. Additionally, instances when administered medications might make any resuscitative efforts difficult due to an anaphylactic reaction to a skin test would be a relative contraindication to skin testing; these include patients who require systemic beta-adrenergic blockers that cannot be discontinued prior to skin testing. Proposed advantages of the RAST include (1) safety of the procedure with lack of the risk of anaphylaxis associated with skin testing; (2) quantification of the relative degree of reactivity based on the total amount of allergen-specific IgE identified; (3) convenience to the patient, which is especially important in young children or very apprehensive patients; (4) the ability to follow the long-term results of immunotherapy, as the ultimate development of lower specific IgE levels tends to correlate with clinical results, especially for dust mite and ragweed immunotherapy [69, 180]; and (5) the good correlation noted between skin testing, basophil histamine release, and the severity of allergic disease and the RAST in multiple studies [90, 178, 180, 187]. Disadvantages of the RAST include (1) the lower sensitivity for the diagnosis of allergy—skin tests potentially measure minute amounts of antigen-specific IgE that may not be detected by RAST, which only detects IgE that is in significant quantities in the serum; (2) the longer wait for test results compared to the immediately available results from a skin test; (3) the interference caused by high levels of allergen-specific IgE antibodies, giving false-negative results (a problem rectified by diluting the patient's serum to be tested); (4) the lack of sufficient sensitivity to diagnose the presence of life-threatening allergic states such as Hymenoptera sensitivity or penicillin sensitivity for which skin testing is the diagnostic test of choice [144]; (5) lack of standardization of methodologies and reported results, allowing for difficulty comparing results from one method or laboratory to another; (6) lack of sufficient quality control; and (7) lack of sufficient clinical data comparing results of RAST testing to clinically significant allergic disease [227]. Further criticisms of the RAST include its use for the remote practice where the diagnosis of allergy is established based on the blood test result without a physician gathering historical information or physical evidence correlating the signs and symptoms of allergic disease with the result of the in vitro allergy evaluation [227]. Allergy immunotherapy administered solely on the basis of a RAST result is an example of the abuse potential for in vitro allergic diagnostic testing [17].

Enzyme-linked Immunoassays

Enzymatic markers with longer stability are gradually replacing radioactive markers in many assay procedures. The ELISA uses the same basic format as the RAST, with a solid-phase–coupled antigen incubated with the patient's serum and then subsequently reacted with anti-IgE coupled to an enzyme, which then reacts with a specific substrate to produce either visible light or fluorescence as the product that is quantified. A variety of commercially available systems differ in the allergosorbent used, the detection system, and the enzyme employed [30]. These include the enzyme allergosorbent test (EAST), using paper disks in test tubes or microtiter wells and a visible enzyme product; the fluorescence allergosorbent test (FAST), using antigen bound to a plastic absorbent and a fluorescent enzyme product; and the CAP system, employing a capsule containing a hydrophilic cellulose polymer covalently bonded to antigen, available in standard radiolabeled or fluorescent enzyme formats. The CLIA systems are not actually ELISA methods as no enzymatic reaction occurs. A variety of reports compared the sensitivity and specificity of each of these systems to either skin testing or the RAST.

Difficulties exist in comparing results obtained using these different allergen-specific IgE testing systems. A study comparing three commercially available systems gave concordant results only 30 percent of the time, largely due to differences in the antigens bound on the solid-phase matrix of the systems [140]. A study comparing FAST to RAST and skin testing in 36 patients yielded identical results between the FAST and RAST in only 42 percent of the patients and between the FAST and skin testing in 54 percent if identical scoring results are sought, thus giving identical quantification [166]. The significance of low-positive or equivocal results in the FAST and some other methods may be questionable, as scoring systems that enhance sensitivity of these assays to greater than 90 percent frequently decrease the specificity to under 50 percent, rendering the results of such testing clinically questionable [216]. Scoring for individual allergens reveals that the sensitivity and specificity of each of these systems vary significantly from allergen to allergen [140]. The cellulose foam matrix to which antigen is coupled in the CAP system has enhanced binding capacity for antibody compared to systems wherein antigen is bound to test tubes, microtiter wells, or paper disks, the CAP binding 40-fold greater amounts of antibody than a paper disk. Additionally, the CAP results are reported quantitatively in units that are based on a World Health Organization standard for IgE which is used to form the standard curve for this assay. Compared to RAST testing, the CAP has been reported to have enhanced sensitivity, of up to 95 percent, and specificity, of up to 98 percent, using skin prick testing as the reference standard [224]. Studies comparing the CAP [217] to mRAST have shown similar sensitivity with greater specificity of CAP results compared to skin tests [217] suggesting that the threshold for detection in mRAST is too low [239]. The correlation coefficient between the CAP system and the conventional RAST for a variety of antigens is reported to be between 0.85 and 0.98, with a specificity, sensitivity, and efficiency greater than 85 percent [34]. The CAP test results are positive in 78 percent of subjects with positive skin test results, compared to RAST being positive in 65 percent of those with positive skin test results. The concordance of CAP and RAST results is 91 percent, nearly 90 percent of the discordant results being positive CAP with negative RAST results to a given antigen, suggesting enhanced sensitivity of CAP compared to conventional paper disk-based RAST. For instance, 4.8 percent of tests in one series demonstrated positive findings for allergen-specific IgE by the CAP system but negative findings by both the RAST and direct skin testing. These positive results occurred predominantly in individuals who gave a history compatible with sensitivity to the allergen identified on the CAP tests, suggesting the possibility that the CAP test may be more sensitive in certain instances than skin prick testing. That the CAP test results have been uniformly negative when done on neonatal cord blood known not to contain antigen-specific IgE lends further credence to this possibility [106].

An immunochemiluminescent assay for antigen specific IgE, the Magic Lite SQ system, has been developed using paramagnetic particles coupled with standardized allergens as a solid phase and specific anti-IgE antibody labeled with acridinium ester, with pH change producing a chemiluminescent product. Correlation of results using this technology with results of CAP testing yields correlation coefficients from 0.7 to 0.9, depending on the antigen being tested [219]. Other CLIA tests are under development using a variety of substances for production of light emission. These assays have the potential advantage of significantly enhanced sensitivity allowing detection of up to 1000-fold less analyte than these other technologies [238].

To settle such questions regarding the sensitivity and specificity of the currently available allergen-specific IgE assays, further study utilizing techniques such as basophil histamine release and bronchial provocation may be necessary to elucidate the reasons for the discrepancy between skin test results and in vitro specific

IgE test results. Analysis of sensitivity and specificity using receiver operating characteristic (ROC) curves has improved the evaluation of new antigen-specific IgE detection technologies, demonstrating the loss of sensitivity inherent in applications where utmost specificity is required [215]. Laboratories may have to establish appropriate lower levels of detectability for antigen-specific IgE based on assay of allergen-specific negative control serum to determine the appropriate lower threshold of clinical significance [212, 239]. Furthermore, there is a definite need to standardize the reagents used for both skin testing and specific IgE in vitro testing. Both the standardization of laboratory methods and the introduction of comparisons to standardized reference serum may be required before test results obtained by ELISAs are universally accepted as valid [140].

Crossed Radioimmunoelectrophoresis, Immunoblotting, and RAST Inhibition

In crossed radioimmunoelectrophoresis (CRIE), allergen extract is first electrophoresed into an agarose gel and then electrophoresed into a gel containing a rabbit antibody directed toward the relevant allergens. This crossed immunoelectrophoresed gel is reacted with the human serum containing IgE antibody toward the allergenic extract. The human IgE antibody that binds to the allergens in the gel is identified by incubation with ^{125}I-labeled anti-IgE, which is detected through use of autoradiography. Although this technique offers high resolution, it is difficult to perform and requires a rabbit antiserum with high titers of antibody toward the relevant allergens. Additionally, significant variation can occur in the pattern of rabbit antibody binding to the electrophoresed allergens, thereby causing a significant change in CRIE patterns.

In immunoblotting techniques, polyacrylamide gel electrophoresis and thin layer isoelectric focusing are combined with Western immunoblotting in order to separate allergenic proteins. After either electrophoretically or passively blotting the allergenic proteins on nitrocellulose paper, washing with an aluminum containing buffer is performed and the nitrocellulose paper incubated with IgE antibody–containing sera and radiolabeled anti-IgE. Autoradiographic techniques allow detection of the IgE antibody. A variety of patterns of reactivity may be noted, due to differing antibodies being formed to selected components of the allergenic material [240]. Quantification of allergen-specific IgE is more difficult in immunoblotting than in CRIE, but immunoblotting has the advantage of not requiring rabbit antibodies to the allergen. Both CRIE and immunoblotting are generally reserved for research application.

In the RAST-inhibition test, serum is mixed with increasing amounts of allergen extract. The nonbound IgE is assayed by RAST, the inhibition of which is expressed in inhibition units. By comparing a reference extract to an unknown extract, a 50% inhibition concentration may be used to denote allergenicity of the extracts. RAST inhibition is used in research settings and as a method of standardizing allergen extracts [236].

ANTIGEN-SPECIFIC IgG SUBCLASS DETERMINATION

The clinical utility of measuring antigen-specific IgG subclasses is under investigation. Investigational studies have demonstrated a significant rise in allergen-specific IgG1 and IgG4 levels, along with a decrease in late-phase skin reactivity, associated with successful results of inhalant immunotherapy [1]. The presence of IgG4 antibodies in serum from patients with suspected food allergy has not been proved to be of diagnostic value [83]. The frequency of IgG4 antibodies to common foods and inhalant allergens is similar in healthy adults and those with asthma [84]. Though IgG4 may be more common in allergic than in nonallergic children, the frequency in nonallergic individuals makes the presence or absence of these antibodies not useful either to establish a diagnosis of asthma or to make prognostic implications with regard to the subsequent course of asthma in such individuals [79].

MEASUREMENTS OF MEDIATORS OF INFLAMMATION

Measurement of the mediators of inflammation include assays for those mediators that are preformed and stored in secretory granules of mast cells such as histamine and tryptase. Histamine is also released on degranulation of basophils. The concentration of tryptase in basophils is much lower than the concentration in mast cells, making tryptase primarily an indicator of mast cell degranulation [164].

Assays for histamine initially were bioassays such as the contraction of guinea pig ileum, but now a variety of newer and quantitative assays exist [26, 39, 103, 171]. These histamine assays include (1) gas chromatography–mass spectrometry; (2) high-performance liquid chromatography (HPLC); (3) enzymatic single-isotope assays; (4) enzymatic double-isotope assays; (5) fluorometric-fluoroenzymatic assays; and (6) RIAs. Significant interlaboratory variation due to quality control and reference standards may occur when comparing values quantifying histamine [133]. A new fluorometric assay for histamine depends on the binding of histamine to a glass-fiber matrix, which potentially allows for the rapid analysis of samples. In this assay the total performance time is under 3 hours and a sensitivity to as low as 3 ng/ml of histamine has been observed, with a variation of 5 ng/ml within the assay and a correlation with conventional methods of histamine assay that is greater than 90 percent [15, 174]. An RIA for histamine has been developed using succinyl glycinamide derivatization of histamine to allow for accurate measurement of both plasma and urinary histamine levels within a range of concentration from 0.1 to 5.0 ng/ml, with great reproducibility [116, 120]. Determination of urinary N-methyl histamine by RIA may allow retrospective analysis of mast cell or basophil involvement in anaphylaxis, as 10 percent of histamine release is metabolized by N-methylation and may be detected in the urine up to 6 hours after anaphylaxis [177].

Airway obstruction in allergic asthma is related to a subject's baseline responsiveness to histamine and the absolute changes in plasma histamine level after allergen challenge in investigational studies [43]. Thus, measurement of plasma histamine may serve as a valuable investigational tool in studying allergic asthma.

Tryptase levels are more than 100-fold higher in mast cells than in basophils, whereas histamine levels are twice as high in mast cells and basophils. This allows tryptase to be used as an index of mast cell activation when it is measured in peripheral blood [164]. Elevated tryptase levels have been noted in allergic and nonallergic anaphylaxis [88] and systemic mastocytosis. Analysis of tryptase in biologic fluids such as nasal lavage and cutaneous skin blisters gives evidence of the relative mast cell involvement in complex inflammatory processes [20, 167]. Tryptase levels generally rise higher over baseline and are detectable longer after allergen challenge than are corresponding histamine levels [45]. A sandwich ELISA is used to quantitate the levels of tryptase [198]. Elevated levels of tryptase have been noted in bronchoalveolar lavage fluid of atopic patients with symptomatic asthma [207]. Rapid elevations of tryptase after allergen challenge with return to baseline within 48 hours in bronchoalveolar lavage studies suggest a pivotal role for the mast cell in immediate bronchospastic events [229].

Assays for mediators of allergic inflammation may include assessment of not only mast cell– and basophil-derived mediators but also factors released by eosinophils, neutrophils, macrophages, and lymphocytes which are especially prominent during late-phase inflammation. Quantification of eosinophil-derived factors, discussed later, may correlate with ongoing allergic inflammation in asthmatics.

Other mediators of the immediate hypersensitivity response include neutrophil chemotactic factor (NCF) [19, 85]; thromboxane B_2 [71, 99]; platelet-activating factor [55]; prostaglandin D_2 [92]; the leukotrienes (LT) including LTB_4, LTC_4, LTD_4, and LTE_4 [108]; and cytokines including tumor necrosis factor (TNF), granulocyte-macrophage colony stimulating factor (GM-CSF), interleukin (IL)-1γ, IL-1β, IL-2, IL-4, and IL-6 [208]. These assays are generally performed by either HPLC, RIA, or ELISA, cytokine assays often requiring specific cytotoxic or proliferation assays with confirmation of the cell source of the individual cytokines by using RNA-polymerase chain reaction technology [208]. Studies of eosinophils from asthmatic subjects have noted an increase in LTC_4 generation compared to those from healthy donors [7]. Bronchial lavage fluids from asthmatics have higher concentrations of LTE_4 compared to lavage fluids from nonasthmatic individuals [101]. Urinary leukotriene E_4 levels, reflecting production of LTC_4 and LTD_4, may significantly rise in children with exercise-induced asthma after exercise challenge, suggesting a role for assay of this analyte in specific research evaluations [218]. During symptomatic asthma attacks, elevated levels of specific cytokines including TNF, GM-CSF, IL-1β, IL-2, and IL-6 have been noted, suggesting a role for T-cells and alveolar macrophages in asthmatic inflammation [208]. These types of studies indicate the research utility of determining specific mediator levels.

COMPLEMENT DETERMINATIONS

Complement components act as acute-phase reactants, as levels are often increased in acute inflammation. Low complement levels can occur with decreased synthesis as in congenital complement deficiencies, liver diseases, or malnutrition, or due to increased utilization as in autoimmune diseases such as systemic lupus erythematosus (SLE) or necrotizing vasculitis. Measurements of total hemolytic activity (CH_{50}) is the most useful screening test for complement deficiency, with individual component deficiencies often associated with discrete syndromes [112]. In clinical allergy, fluctuations in complement levels following challenge with allergens have not been proved to be of clinical relevance and measurements of these levels is not a valid method to categorize the reaction following antigen challenge [50].

IMMUNE COMPLEX ASSAYS

Immune complexes can occur in association with a variety of disease states including (1) rheumatologic conditions such as rheumatoid arthritis and SLE; (2) systemic vasculitis such as Henoch-Schönlein purpura; (3) infectious diseases such as hepatitis B antigenemia, Lyme arthritis, infectious endocarditis, and acquired immunodeficiency syndrome (AIDS); (4) malignant processes such as breast cancer, ovarian cancer, Hodgkin's disease, acute and myeloid leukemia; and (5) endocrine disorders such as hyperthyroidism [185]. Occasionally useful to establish a diagnosis or monitor disease activity and efficacy of therapy, in general, the presence of immune complexes is not conclusively diagnostic of any disease entity. Current assays do not detect the antigen, but rather the immunoglobulin or the complement component in the antigen-antibody complexes. These assays include complement-dependent assays such as (1) the C1q-binding assay, which detects preferentially IgG-containing immune complexes dependent on the size and concentration of the circulating immune complexes based on the ability of C1q to bind aggregated immunoglobulins [185]; (2) the Raji cell assay, which detects complement-containing immune complexes based on the high avidity of the C3b and C3d receptors on the Raji lymphoblastoid B-cell line; (3) conglutinin-binding assay, which binds complement factor C3b in immune complexes; and (4) anti-C3 assay [185]. Other immune complex assays include precipitation assays such as (1) polyethylene glycol precipitation, which uses radiolabeled antiimmunoglobulin or anticomplement antibodies to selectively determine the constituents of labeled immune complexes that have been precipitated by the polyethylene glycol [185] and (2) assays such as the cryoglobulin assay based on the decreased solubility of immune complexes [185]. Still other assays available include immunoglobulin constant region–dependent assays such as monoclonal rheumatoid factor and platelet aggregation assays [102]. Results of the immune complex assays are affected by the freezing and thawing of samples, leading to potential false-positive and -negative results. Laboratory to laboratory variance may exist, but collaborative standardization reference materials are under development. Up to 10 percent of normal subjects may have detectable immune complexes, generally in low titers [185]. The presence of immune complexes, including attempts to quantify circulating IgE-containing complexes, has not been found useful in clinical allergy to date [50, 186]. In particular, the presence or absence of IgG or IgE food-related immune complexes has not been shown to be useful in clinical practice, as there is a lack of proof that such complexes do not occur normally or are qualitatively or quantitatively different in allergic disease states [169].

LYMPHOCYTE TRANSFORMATION

Cell-mediated reactions may be studied by blast transformation of lymphocytes exposed to antigens or mitogens. The clinical utility includes transplant compatibility screening, evaluation of immunodeficiency, and evaluation of specific drug sensitivity [23, 119, 134]. Mixed lymphocyte reactions are a modification of this test to assess the compatibility of a donor and recipient prior to transplantation. Blastogenesis and lymphokine production have been used in research-oriented laboratories. Significant variation exists from laboratory to laboratory, with variations in validity and reproducibility noted [50]. Investigative use includes studies of atopic dermatitis and cellular immunity [59].

MEASUREMENT OF LYMPHOCYTE SUBSETS

Measurement of T-cell and B-cell subsets is useful for evaluating immunodeficiency such as AIDS and lymphoproliferative disease entities. These techniques may be useful in investigative work including studies of IgE synthesis, studies of the response to allergen immunotherapy, and research regarding the cellular elements of asthmatic late-phase reactions [50]. Currently, these measurements of specific T-cell and B-cell numbers are not clinically useful in the routine evaluation and management of asthma associated with environmental allergens [115].

IN VITRO ANTIGEN-INDUCED LEUKOCYTE HISTAMINE RELEASE

An in vitro test of antigen-induced leukocyte histamine release has potential advantages over specific IgE serum assays since IgE is preferentially bound to basophils and mast cells. Histamine release from basophils exposed to a specific allergen is due to

antigen interaction with surface-bound specific IgE, degranulating the basophils in a noncytolytic process. Histamine release from basophils is a functional biologic assay, as both IgE-mediated and non–IgE-mediated histamine release can occur. Although non–IgE-dependent stimuli such as opiates, highly charged antibiotics, muscle relaxants, dextrans, and radiologic contrast media also cause basophil degranulation, antigen-induced histamine release is a very specific assay of sensitivity to specific allergens [50]. Recent advances in histamine assays, combined with automated microtiter well technology for performance of whole blood leukocyte histamine release, have produced a rapid advance in the clinical study of basophil histamine release as a tool for allergy diagnosis [204].

Basophil Histamine Release

Studies comparing basophil histamine release with RASTs and skin prick tests have indicated a concordance between these tests of 85 to 95 percent, with positive predictive values of basophil histamine release of greater than 90 percent for pollen and house dust mite based on a comparison with bronchial provocation, and the sensitivity of basophil histamine release being equivalent to the sensitivity of the RAST [128]. The sensitivity of basophil histamine release in dander allergy is also greater than 90 percent but the specificity is lower than that of either RASTs or skin tests for animal dander allergy [128]. Combining basophil histamine release with more sensitive methods of performing a histamine assay improves the diagnostic capability of basophil histamine release procedures. A study of 68 asthmatic children with dust mite and animal dander allergy demonstrated an 87 percent concordance between bronchial provocation tests and basophil histamine release [137]. In children with asthma, basophil histamine release shows a 90 percent concordance with RAST results [128]. A higher correlation between basophil histamine release and bronchial provocation testing than between either specific IgE testing or allergen skin testing and bronchial provocation has been reported for dust mite allergy [76] and occupational allergens [100]. Thus, in asthmatic children or subjects at high risk, basophil histamine release may be considered as a substitute for bronchial challenge [96, 196]. For food allergy evaluation, an 87 percent concordance between RASTs and basophil histamine release and a 74 percent concordance between skin prick testing and basophil histamine release have been reported [126, 145], although the sensitivity of basophil histamine release is not as great as skin prick testing for the diagnosis of food allergy. Additionally, discordance between gut mast cell histamine release and basophil histamine release upon allergen challenge has been noted, suggesting a heterogeneity of mast cell and basophil responses to allergen [126]. Basophil histamine release is affected by medications used by the patient, some of which must be discontinued for up to 3 weeks before testing is performed [128]. Basophil histamine release is also adversely affected by sample handling time and conditions, more rapid processing of sample allowing for more reproducible and accurate results. Delays in processing can result in nonviable cells and false-negative results. As up to 10 percent of normal individuals fail to respond to anti-IgE challenge of basophils, an unacceptably high false-negative rate exists with current basophil histamine release techniques [223]. The intracellular mechanism of this nonresponsivity of basophils appears to be heterogeneous, involving signal translation events following the crosslinking of IgE on basophil membranes [220].

Passive Sensitization of Basophils

Passive sensitization of normal basophils with patient's serum IgE in vitro is an in vitro equivalent to the Prausnitz-Küstner reaction. Passive sensitization of basophils can be used to evaluate the presence of antigen-specific IgE as a research method. In a study of children with dust mite allergy documented by bronchial provocation testing and skin testing, but whose basophils did not respond in a conventional basophil histamine release, the results of passive sensitization by the patient's serum of basophils harvested from normal nonatopic donors have been shown to correlate highly with RAST and bronchial provocation results [127]. For evaluation of drug allergy, histamine release from basophils passively sensitized with patient blood has been used to investigate the presence of immediate hypersensitivity without the risk potentially entailed in doing direct patient challenges with the questioned drug [125].

Spontaneous Basophil Histamine Release

Spontaneous in vitro basophil histamine release may be affected by a variety of factors including the presence of asthma, allergic asthmatics having higher basophil histamine release in D_2O buffer-based systems than do control subjects [182]. Spontaneous histamine release from basophils is also higher in asthmatics than in normal individuals [8, 63], spontaneous release of histamine from basophils correlating with elevated serum histamine levels after allergen challenge [213]. Presence of food allergies and atopic dermatitis may also increase spontaneous basophil histamine release [228]. The complexity of analyzing the significance of spontaneous basophil histamine release has limited its use to primarily research investigational settings.

EOSINOPHIL COUNTS AND FACTORS

Eosinophils play a critical role in the development and perpetuation of chronic allergic asthma [70]. Eosinophils accumulate in airways during late asthmatic responses, promoting airway obstruction, injury, and hyperresponsivity [209]. On migration to the airway, eosinophils become activated, characterized by a decrease in the cellular density and expression of cell-surface activation markers such as EG2, and release toxic pro-inflammatory, newly generated and preformed mediators [209]. Prominent among the newly generated mediators are leukotrienes, such as LTC_4. The preformed factors include the secretory granule proteins such as major basic protein (MBP), eosinophilic cationic protein (ECP), and eosinophil-derived neurotoxin (EDN), all potentially pro-inflammatory factors. Bronchoalveolar lavage studies of patients with symptomatic versus asymptomatic asthma reveal elevated percentages of eosinophils and significantly greater amounts of eosinophil-derived factors such as MBP and EDN [207].

Elevated ECP level in bronchoalveolar lavage fluid and increased asthma disease severity have also been correlated, whereas neutrophil mediators such as myeloperoxidase (MPO) are not clearly related to asthma severity [205]. Activated eosinophils expressing the EG2 surface marker have been correlated with IL-2 receptor–positive ($CD25^+$) T-lymphocytes in biopsy specimens of patients with atopic asthma, suggesting that activated T-lymphocytes release products that regulate recruitment and activation of eosinophils in the airway walls of asthmatics [206].

Similarly, in skin blister models wherein allergen is presented for a prolonged period at a skin site, MBP and EDN accumulate between 2 and 5 hours after antigen challenge, consistent with an influx of eosinophils following the immediate allergic response [241]. Eosinophilia may occur in a large number of diseases that are not a consequence of immediate hypersensitivity. Pulmonary diseases, other than allergic asthma, with concomitant elevations in eosinophil counts in the blood and IgE levels in the serum include allergic granulomatosis with angiitis (Churg-Strauss syndrome), Löffler syndrome, allergic bronchopulmonary aspergil-

losis, hypereosinophilic syndrome, and tropical eosinophilia. At times, allergic drug reactions may also be associated with eosinophilia and pulmonary manifestations [131].

There is a correlation in asthmatic patients between lung function and the number of circulating eosinophils when eosinophilia is pronounced, whereas eosinophil factors such as serum ECP level correlate better with disease activity when eosinophilia in the blood is less pronounced [77]. ECP may be measured in the serum by RIA, the normal level in healthy individuals being 6.0 $\mu g/L$, with a 95 percent confidence range of 2.3 to 15.9 $\mu g/L$, and an elimination rate t½ in vivo of 65 minutes [225]. Levels of EDN, eosinophil peroxidase, and MBP are elevated during late asthmatic responses and may be superior markers to absolute eosinophil counts in the blood during the late phase of an allergic asthmatic response [60, 88]. Reduction in serum ECP levels has been correlated with a decrease in the number of asthma attacks and improvement in pulmonary function, especially in patients with ECP levels greater than 30 to 40 $\mu g/L$ [232]. In exercise-induced asthma, an initial rise in ECP occurs immediately after exercise, followed by a fall in ECP levels by 1 hour after exercise, similar to the pattern of ECP fluctuations seen after antigen challenges [234]. Steroid treatment, even in inhaled low doses, can decrease ECP and EDN levels [190]. Irrespective of lung function, eosinophils obtained from pollen-allergic asthmatics release more ECP and EDN during the pollen season than prior to the pollen season, suggesting a priming of eosinophils consequent to allergen exposure [210]. In population studies, the combination of eosinophilia with positive skin test results is more significantly associated with recurrent asthmatic attacks and persistent wheeze than is a positive skin test result without associated eosinophilia [117]. A general leukocytosis, including neutrophilia, has also been associated with bronchial hyperreactivity in similar investigations of asthma [16], though neutrophil-derived mediator levels are less clearly related to asthma severity than are eosinophil-derived mediators.

Increased sputum eosinophil counts have been associated with acute exacerbations of asthma. Compared with blood eosinophil counts, a higher inverse correlation with peak flow rate in asthmatics has been reported for sputum eosinophil counts [10].

Nasal eosinophilia on nasal cytologic investigation is useful to classify rhinitis into eosinophilic and noneosinophilic forms. Eosinophilic nonallergic rhinitis associated with nasal polyps and aspirin-induced asthma is more amenable to therapy than noneosinophilic vasomotor rhinitis [121]. Estimation of eosinophil counts or percentages in sputum and nasal secretions are limited by staining techniques and sampling procedures used. The value of measuring eosinophils in either blood, sputum, or nasal secretions in relationship to a specific antigen challenge is questionable, as the relative degree of response in terms of eosinophil counts observed is highly variable [50].

UNPROVEN TECHNIQUES

Cytotoxic food testing, now available commercially in many parts of the country, has been vigorously evaluated in large, well-controlled studies and found to yield neither clinically consistent nor reproducible results [28, 46, 66, 74, 105, 110, 113, 114, 188]. Similar deficiencies have been found in sublingual provocative food testing [35, 36, 73, 104, 162]. Subcutaneous provocation-neutralization testing has also been shown to be of unknown diagnostic value [37, 51, 58, 87, 91].

Determination of circulating IgG and IgE food-related immune complexes has also no proven value at this time [153]. A process of controlled trials is mandatory prior to the clinical use of any procedure that is proposed as being diagnostic of allergic disease. Any procedure that has not been proved effective by proper studies should not be employed [13, 149].

REFERENCES

1. Aalberse, R. C., Van der Gaag, and Van Leeuwen, J. Serologic aspects of IgG⁴ antibodies I prolonged immunization results in an IgG⁴-restricted response. *J. Immunol.* 130(Suppl. 2):S722, 1983.

2. Aas, K. Bronchial provocation tests in asthma. *Arch. Dis. Child.* 45:221, 1970.

3. Aas, K. Diagnosis of immediate type respiratory allergy. *Pediatr. Clin. North Am.* 22:23, 1975.

4. Aas K. Immunotherapy of Bronchial Asthma. In L. M. Lichtenstein and K. F. Austen (eds.), *Asthma: Physiology, Immunopharmacology, and Treatment* (Second International Symposium). New York: Academic, 1977. P. 365.

5. Adinoff, A. D., et al. A comparison of six epicutaneous devices in the performance of immediate hypersensitivity skin testing. *J. Allergy Clin. Immunol.* 84:168, 1989.

6. Adkinson, N. F., Jr. The radioallergosorbent test: Use and abuses. *J. Allergy Clin. Immunol.* 65:1, 1980.

7. Aizawa, T., et al. Eosinophil and neutrophil production of leukotriene C₄ and B₄: Comparison of cells from asthmatic subjects and healthy donors. *Ann. Allergy* 64:287, 1990.

8. Akagi, K., and Townley, R. G. Spontaneous histamine release and histamine content in normal subjects and subjects with asthma. *J. Allergy Clin. Immunol.* 83:742, 1989.

9. Akoun, G. W., et al. Provocation test coupled with bronchoalveolar lavage in diagnosis of propranolol-induced hypersensitivity pneumonitis. *Am. Rev. Respir. Dis.* 139:247, 1989.

10. Alfaro, C., et al. Inverse correlation of expiratory lung flows and sputum eosinophils in status asthmaticus. *Ann. Allergy* 63:251, 1989.

11. Anderson, J. A., and Adkinson, N. F. Allergic reactions to drugs and biological agents. *JAMA* 258:2891, 1987.

12. Anderson, J. A., et al. American Academy of Allergy and Immunology physician statement. The remote practice of allergy. *J. Allergy Clin. Immunol.* 77:651, 1986.

13. Anderson, J. A., et al. American Academy of Allergy and Immunology physician statement: Unproven procedures for diagnosis and treatment of allergic and immunologic diseases. *J. Allergy Clin. Immunol.* 78:275, 1986.

14. Anderson, W. C., and Baer, H. Antigenic and allergenic changes during storage of a pollen extract. *J. Allergy Clin. Immunol.* 69:310, 1982.

15. Andersson, N., et al. *Measurement of Histamine in Nasal Lavage Fluid: Comparison of a Glass Fibre Based Fluorometric Method with Two Radio Immunoassays.* Roche Biomedical Laboratories, 1990.

16. Annesi, I., et al. Leukocyte count and bronchial hyperresponsiveness. *J. Allergy Clin. Immunol.* 82:1006, 1988.

17. A position paper. American College of Physicians. Allergy testing. *Ann. Intern. Med.* 110:317, 1989.

18. Atkins, F. M., Steinberg, S. F., and Metcalfe, D. D. Evaluation of immediate adverse reactions to foods in adults: I. Correlation of demographic, laboratory, and prick skin test data with response to controlled oral food challenge. *J. Allergy Clin. Immunol.* 75:348, 1985.

19. Atkins, P. C., Norman, M. E., and Zweiman, B. Antigen-induced neutrophil chemotactic activity in man. *J. Allergy Clin. Immunol.* 62:149, 1978.

20. Atkins, P. C., et al. In vivo antigen-induced cutaneous mediator release: Simultaneous comparisons of histamine, tryptase and prostaglandin D₂ release and the effect of oral corticosteroid administration. *J. Allergy Clin. Immunol.* 86:360, 1990.

21. Austen, K. F., and Sheffer, A. L. Detection of hereditary angioneurotic edema by demonstration of a reduction in the second component of human complement. *N. Engl. J. Med.* 272:649, 1965.

22. Barbee, R. A., et al. A longitudinal study of respiratory symptoms in a community population sample (correlations with smoking, allergen skin test reactivity and serum IgE). *Chest* 99:20, 1991.

23. Battisto, J. R., and Ponxio, N. M. Autologous and syngeneic mixed lymphocyte reaction and their immunologic significance. *Prog. Allergy* 28:160, 1981.

24. Baur, X., et al. Clinical symptoms and results of skin tests, RAST, and bronchial provocation tests in 33 papain workers: Evidence of strong immunogenic potency and clinically relevant proteolytic affect of airborne papain. *Clin. Allergy* 12:9, 1982.

25. Bazaral, N., Orgel, H. A., and Hamburger, R. N. Immunoglobulin E level in normal infants and mothers and an inheritance hypothesis. *J. Immunol.* 107:791, 1971.

26. Beaven, M. A., Jacobsen, S. J., and Horakova, Z. Modification of the enzymatic isotopic assay of histamine and its application to measurement of histamine in tissues, serum and urine. *Clin. Chim. Acta* 37:91, 1972.

27. Belin, L. G. A., and Norman, P. S. Diagnostic test in the skin and serum of workers sensitized to *B. subtilis* enzymes. *Clin. Allergy* 7:55, 1977.

28. Benson, T. E., and Arkins, J. A. Cytotoxic testing for food allergy: Evaluations of reproducibility and correlations. *J. Allergy* 58:471, 1976.

29. Berg, T., and Johansson, S. G. O. Immunoglobulin levels during childhood with special regard to IgE. *Acta Paediatr. Scand.* 58:513, 1969.

30. Bernstein, I. L. Proceedings of the Task Force on Guidelines for Standardizing Old and New Technologies Used for the Diagnosis and Treatment of Allergic Disease. National Institute of Allergy and Infectious Disease. *J. Allergy Clin. Immunol.* 82(Suppl. III):487, 1987.

31. Blackley, C. H. Hay Fever: Its Causes, Treatment, and Effective Prevention. In *Experiment Researchers* (2nd ed.). London: Balliere, Tindell, and Cox, 1973.

32. Boulet, L.-P., et al. Bronchial responsiveness increases after seasonal antigen exposure in non-asthmatic subjects with pollen-induced rhinitis. *Ann. Allergy* 63:114, 1989.

33. Bousquet, J. In Vivo Methods for Study of Allergy Skin Test, Techniques, and Interpretation. In E. Middleton, Jr., et al. (eds.); *Allergy: Principles and Practice* (3rd ed.). St. Louis, Mosby, 1988. P. 419.

34. Bousquet, J., et al. Comparison between RAST and Pharmacia CAP system: A new automated specific IgE assay. *J. Allergy Clin. Immunol.* 85:1039, 1990.

35. Breneman, J. C., et al. Report of the food allergy committee on the sublingual method of provocative testing for food allergy. *Ann. Allergy* 31:382, 1973.

36. Breneman, J. C., et al. Final report of the food allergy committee of the American College of Allergists on the clinical evaluation of sublingual provocation testing methods for diagnosis of food allergy. *Ann. Allergy* 33:164, 1974.

37. Bronsky, E. A., Burkley, D. B., and Ellis, E. F. Evaluation of the provocative skin test technique. *J. Allergy* 47:104, 1971.

38. Brown, H. M., Su, S., and Thantrey, N. Prick testing for allergens standardized by using a precision needle. *J. Clin. Allergy* 11:95, 1981.

39. Brown, N. J., et al. Sensitive and specific radiometric method for the measurement of plasma histamine in normal individuals. *Anal. Biochem.* 109:42, 1980.

40. Bruce, C. A., et al. Quantitative inhalation bronchial challenge in ragweed, hay fever patients: A comparison with ragweed allergic asthmatics. *J. Allergy Clin. Immunol.* 56:338, 1975.

41. Buckley, R. H., and Metcalfe, D. Food allergy. *JAMA* 248:2527, 1982.

42. Burrows, B., et al. Association of asthma and serum IgE levels and skin test reactivity to allergens. *N. Engl. J. Med.* 320:272, 1989.

43. Busse, W. W., and Swenson, C. A. The relationship between plasma histamine concentrations and bronchial obstruction to antigen challenge in allergic rhinitis. *J. Allergy Clin. Immunol.* 84:658, 1989.

44. Caldwell, J. R., et al. Acquired I inhibitor deficiency in lymphosarcoma. *Clin. Immunol. Immunopathol.* 1:39, 1972.

45. Castells, M., and Schwartz, L. B. Tryptase levels in nasal-lavage fluid as an indicator of the immediate allergic response. *J. Allergy Clin. Immunol.* 82:348, 1988.

46. Chambers, V. V., Hudson, B. H., and Glaser, J. A study of the reaction of human polymorphonuclear leukocytes to various antigens. *J. Allergy* 29:93, 1958.

47. Chipps, B. E., et al. The effect of theophylline and terbutaline on immediate skin test and basophil histamine release. *J. Allergy Clin. Immunol.* 61:171, 1978.

48. Cockcroft, D. W. Bronchial inhalation test II: Measurement of allergic (and occupational) bronchial responsiveness. *Ann. Allergy* 59:89, 1987.

49. Cockcroft, D. W., et al. Prediction of airway responsiveness to allergen from skin sensitivity to allergen and airway responsiveness to histamine. *Am. Rev. Respir. Dis.* 135:514, 1987.

50. Council on Scientific Affairs. In vitro testing for allergy. Report II of the allergy panel. *JAMA* 258:1639, 1987.

51. Crawford, L. V., et al. A double-blind study of subcutaneous food testing sponsored by The Food Committee of the American Academy of Allergy. *J. Allergy Clin. Immunol.* 57:236, 1976.

52. Creticos, P. S., et al. Dose response of IgE and IgG antibodies during ragweed immunotherapy. *J. Allergy Clin. Immunol.* 73:94, 1984.

53. Criqui, M. H., et al. Epidemiology of immunoglobulin E levels in a defined population. *Ann. Allergy* 64:308, 1990.

54. Croner, S., et al. IgE screening in 1701 newborn infants and the development of atopic disease during infancy. *Arch. Dis. Child.* 57:364, 1982.

55. Cuss, F. M., Dixon, C. M. S., and Barnes, P. J. Effects of inhaled platelet

activating factor on pulmonary function and bronchial responsiveness in man. *Lancet* 2:189, 1986.

56. Donaldson, V. H., and Hess, E. V. A biochemical abnormality in hereditary angioneurotic edema. *Am. J. Med.* 35:37, 1963.

57. Donaldson, V. H., Hess, E. V., and McAdams, P. J. Lupus erythematosus-like disease in three unrelated women with hereditary angioneurotic edema. *Ann. Intern. Med.* 86:312, 1977.

58. Draper, L. W. Food testing and allergy: Intradermal provocative versus deliberate feeding. *Arch. Otolaryngol.* 95:169, 1972.

59. Duke-Cohan, J., et al. Use of an autologous reaction in vitro to assess contributions of TB lymphocytes to immune hyperreactivity of atopics. *Clin. Exp. Allergy* 19:163, 1989.

60. Durham, S. R., et al. Blood eosinophil and eosinophil-derived proteins in allergic asthma. *J. Allergy Clin. Immunol.* 84:931, 1989.

61. Eriksson, N. E. Total IgE influences, the relationship between skin tests and RAST. *Ann. Allergy* 63:65, 1989.

62. Farr, R. S., et al. Evaluation of aspirin and tartrazine idiosyncrasy. *J. Allergy Clin. Immunol.* 64:667, 1979.

63. Findlay, S. R., and Lichtenstein, L. N. Basophil "releasibility" in patients with asthma. *Am. Rev. Respir. Dis.* 122:53, 1980.

64. Fink, J. N. Evaluation of the patient for occupational lung disease. *J. Allergy Clin. Immunol.* 70:11, 1982.

65. Finnerty, J. P., Summerell, S., and Holgate, S. T. Relationship between skin prick test, the multiple allergosorbent tests and symptoms of allergic disease. *Clin. Exp. Allergy* 19:51, 1989.

66. Franklin, W., and Lowell, F. C. Failure of ragweed pollen extract to destroy wide cells from ragweed-sensitive patients. *J. Allergy* 20:375, 1949.

67. Geha, R. S., et al. Acquired C1-inhibitor deficiency associated with antiidiotypic antibody to monoclonal immunoglobulin. *N. Engl. J. Med.* 312:534, 1985.

68. Gerrard, J. W., et al. Serum IgE levels in parents and children. *J. Pediatr.* 85:660, 1974.

69. Gleich, G., et al. Effect of immunotherapy on immunoglobulin E and immunoglobulin G antibodies to ragweed antigens: A six-year prospective study. *J. Allergy Clin. Immunol.* 70:261, 1982.

70. Gleich, G. J., Loegering, D. A., and Adolphson, C. R. Eosinophils and bronchial inflammation. *Chest* 85(Suppl. 1):105, 1985.

71. Godard, P., et al. Functional assessment of alveolar macrophages: Comparison of cells from asthmatic and normal subjects. *J. Allergy Clin. Immunol.* 70:88, 1982.

72. Golbert, T. N. Food Allergy and Immunologic Diseases of the Gastrointestinal Tract. In R. Patterson (ed.), *Allergic Diseases, Diagnosis and Management* (2nd ed.). Philadelphia: Lippincott, 1980. P. 409.

73. Goldbert, T. M. Sublingual desensitization. *JAMA* 217:11703, 1971.

74. Goldbert, T. M. A review of controversial diagnostic and therapeutic techniques employed in allergy. *J. Allergy Clin. Immunol.* 56:170, 1975.

75. Golden, D. B. K., Muyers, D. A., and Kagey-Sobtka, A. Clinical relevance of the venom specific immunoglobulin G antibody level during immunotherapy. *J. Allergy Clin. Immunol.* 69:489, 1982.

76. Griese, M., Kusenbach, G., and Reinhardt, D. Histamine release test in comparison to standard test in diagnosis of children with allergic asthma. *Ann. Allergy* 65:46, 1990.

77. Griffin, E., et al. Blood eosinophil number and activity in relation to lung function in patients with asthma and eosinophilia. *J. Allergy Clin. Immunol.* 87:548, 1991.

78. Gronneberg, R., Hagermark, O., and Strandberg, K. Effect in man of oral terbutaline on cutaneous reactions induced by allergen and cold stimulation. *Allergy* 35:143, 1980.

79. Gwyn, C. M., et al. IgE and IgG₄ subclass in atopic families. *Clin. Allergy* 9:119, 1979.

80. Hamilton, R. G., and Adkinson, N. F., Jr. Clinical laboratory methods for the assessment and management of human allergic disease. *Clin. Lab. Med.* 6:117, 1986.

81. Haus, N., et al. The influence of ethnicity, and atopic family history, and maternal ascariasis on cord blood serum IgE concentrations. *J. Allergy Clin. Immunol.* 82:179, 1988.

82. Hensley, G. T., Fink, J. N., and Barboraak, J. J. Hypersensitivity, pneumonitis in the monkey. *Arch. Pathol.* 97:33, 1974.

83. Homburger, H. A. Diagnosis of allergy: In vitro testing. *CRC Crit. Rev. Lab. Sci.* 23:279, 1986.

84. Homburger, H. A., et al. Serum IgG₄ concentrations in allergen-specific IgG₄ antibodies compared in adults and children with asthma and nonallergic subjects. *J. Allergy Clin. Immunol.* 77:427, 1986.

85. Howarth, P. H., et al. The relationship between mast cell mediator released and bronchial reactivity in allergic asthma. *J. Allergy Clin. Immunol.* 80:703, 1987.

86. Imbeau, S. A., et al. Relationships between prednisone therapy, disease activity and a total serum IgE level in allergic bronchopulmonary aspergillosis. *J. Allergy Clin. Immunol.* 62:91, 1978.

87. Jewett, D. W., Feing, G., and Greenberg, M. H. A double-blind study of symptom provocation to determine food sensitivity. *N. Engl J. Med.* 323:429, 1990.

88. Johansson, S. G. O. The future of allergy diagnostic techniques. *Clin. Exp. Allergy* 21(Suppl. 1):123, 1991.

89. Johansson, S. G. O., Bennich, H., and Berg, T. The Clinical Significance of IgE. In: R. S. Schwartz (ed.), *Progress in Clinical Immunology,* Vol. 1. New York: Grune & Stratton, 1972. P. 157.

90. Juji, F., et al. Clinical study of asthma in adolescents and in young adults. Correlation between laboratory findings and severity of asthma. *Ann. Allergy* 63:427, 1989.

91. Kailin, E. W., and Collier, R. Relieving therapy for antigen exposure. *JAMA* 217:78, 1971.

92. Kaliner, M. Mast cell mediators in asthma. *Chest* 87(Suppl. 1):2S, 1985.

93. Kaplan, A. P., et al. American Academy of Allergy and Immunology position statement: Beta-adrenergic blockers, immunotherapy and skin testing. *J. Allergy Clin. Immunol.* 84:129, 1989.

94. Kay, A. B., and Austen, K. F. The IgE-mediated release of an eosinophil leukocyte chemotactic factor from human lung. *J. Immunol.* 107:899, 1971.

95. Kelly, W. J. W., et al. Atopy in subjects with asthma followed to the age of 28 years. *J. Allergy Clin. Immunol.* 85:548, 1990.

96. Kerrebijn, K. S., Begenhart, H. J., and Hammers, A. Relation between skin test, inhalation test, and histamine release from leukocytes and IgE in house dust mite allergy. *Arch. Dis. Child.* 51:252, 1976.

97. Kettlehut, B. V., and Metcalfe, D. D. Adverse Reactions to Foods. In E. Middleton, Jr., et al. (eds.); *Allergy: Principles and Practice* (3rd ed.). St. Louis: Mosby, 1988. P. 148.

98. Klink, M., et al. Problems in defining normal limits for serum IgE. *J. Allergy Clin. Immunol.* 85:440, 1990.

99. Knauer, K. A., et al. Platelet activation during antigen-induced airway reaction in asthmatic subjects. *N. Engl. J. Med.* 304:1404, 1981.

100. Kurosawa, M., et al. Antigen-induced histamine release from peripheral leukocytes of "Konnyaku asthmatic patients." *Ann. Allergy* 64:319, 1990.

101. Lam, S., et al. Release of leukotrienes in patients with bronchial asthma. *J. Allergy Clin. Immunol.* 81:711, 1988.

102. Ledford, D. K. Autoimmune diseases, serologic testing and immune complex assessment. *J. Allergy Clin. Immunol.* 84:1082, 1989.

103. Lee, T. H., et al. Exercise-induced release of histamine and neutrophil chemotactic factor in atopic asthmatics. *J. Allergy Clin. Immunol.* 70:73, 1982.

104. Lehman, C. W. A double-blind study of sublingual provocative food testing: A study of its efficacy. *Ann. Allergy* 45:144, 1980.

105. Lehman, C. W. Leukocytic food allergy tests: A study of its reliability and reproducibility. Effect of diet and sublingual food drops on this test. *Ann. Allergy* 45:150, 1980.

106. Leimgruber, A., et al. Clinical evaluation of a new in-vitro assay for specific IgE, the Immuno CAP system. *Clin. Exp. Allergy* 21:127, 1991.

107. Levy, D. A., and Osler, A. G. Studies on the mechanisms of hypersensitivity phenomena. XIV. Passive sensitization *in vitro* of human leukocyte to ragweed pollen antigen. *J. Immunol.* 97:203, 1976.

108. Lewis, R. A. Leukotrienes and other lipid mediators of asthma. *Chest* 87(Suppl. 1):5S, 1985.

109. Lewis, R. A., and Austen, K. F. Mediation of local homeostasis and inflammation by leukotrienes and other mast cell-dependent compounds. *Nature* 293:103, 1981.

110. Lieberman, P., et al. Controlled study of the cytotoxic food tests. *JAMA* 231:728, 1974.

111. Lindberg, R. E., and Arroyave, C. Levels of IgE in serum from normal children and allergic children as measured by an enzyme immunoassay. *J. Allergy Clin. Immunol.* 78:614, 1986.

112. Lopez, M. Laboratory tests. *J. Allergy Clin. Immunol.* 84:1040, 1989.

113. Lowell, F. C. Some untested diagnostic and therapeutic procedures in clinical allergy. *J. Allergy Clin. Immunol.* 56:168, 1975.

114. Lowell, F. C., and Heimer, D. C. Food allergy cytotoxic diagnostic technique not proven. *JAMA* 220:1624, 1972.

115. Marshall, E. Immune system theories on trial. *Science* 234:1490, 1986.

116. McBride, P., Bradley, D., and Kaliner, M. Evaluation of a radioimmunoassay for histamine measurement in biologic fluids. *J. Allergy Clin. Immunol.* 82:638, 1988.

117. Mensinga, T. T., et al. The relationship of eosinophilia and positive skin test reactivity to respiratory symptom prevalence in a community-based population study. *J. Allergy Clin. Immunol.* 86:99, 1990.

118. Metzger, W. J., et al. Local allergen challenge and bronchoalveolar lavage of allergic asthmatic lungs: Description of the model and local airway inflammation. *Am. Rev. Respir. Dis.* 135:433, 1987.

119. Moller, G., and Coutinho, A. Role of C_3 and Fc receptors in B lymphocyte activation. *J. Exp. Med.* 141:647, 1975.

120. Morel, A. N., and Delaage, M. A. Immunoanalysis of histamine through a novel chemical derivatization. *J. Allergy Clin. Immunol.* 82:646, 1988.

121. Mullarkey, M. F., Hill, J. S., and Webb, D. R. Allergic and non-allergic rhinitis: Their characterization with attention to the meaning of nasal eosinophilia. *J. Allergy Clin. Immunol.* 65:122, 1980.

122. Naclerio, R. W., Norman, P. S., and Fish, J. D. In Vivo Methods for Study of Allergy: Mucosal Tests, Techniques, and Interpretation. In E. Middleton, Jr., et al. (eds.); *Allergy: Principles and Practices* (3rd ed.). St. Louis: Mosby, 1988. P. 437.

123. Nagaya, H. Relationship between antigen-specific IgE antibody (RAST) and total serum IgE levels. *Ann. Allergy* 43:267, 1979.

124. Nelson, H. S. Effect of preservatives and condition of storage on the potency of allergy extracts. *J. Allergy Clin. Immunol.* 67:64, 1982.

125. Nolte, H., Carstensen, H., and Hertz, H. VM-26 (teniposide) induced hypersensitivity and degranulation of basophils in children. *Am. J. Pediatr. Hematol. Oncol.* 10:308, 1989.

126. Nolte, H., et al. Comparison of intestinal mast cell and basophil histamine release in children with food allergic reactions. *Allergy* 44:554, 1989.

127. Nolte, H., et al. Passive sensitization of basophil leukocytes from a non-atopic adult by plasma from allergic children. *Allergy* 43:32, 1988.

128. Nolte, H., Storm, K., and Schiotz, P. O. Diagnostic value of a glass fibre-based histamine analysis for allergy testing in children. *Allergy* 45:213, 1990.

129. Norman, P. S. In Vivo Methods for Study of Allergy. In E. Middleton, T. E. Reed and E. F. Ellis (eds.); *Allergy: Principles and Practice.* St. Louis: Mosby, 1978. P. 256.

130. Norman, P. S., Lichtenstein, L. M., and Ishizaka, K. Diagnostic tests in ragweed hay fever. *J. Allergy Clin. Immunol.* 52:210, 1973.

131. Nutman, T. B., Ottesen, E. A., and Cohen, S. G. The eosinophil, eosinophilia and eosinophil-related disorders III. Clinical assessments and eosinophil-related disorders. *Allergy Proc.* 10:33, 1989.

132. O'Byrne, P. M. Allergen-induced airway hyperresponsiveness. *J. Allergy Clin. Immunol.* 81:119, 1988.

133. Oosting, E., et al. Determination of histamine in human plasma: The European External Quality Control Study 1988. *Clin. Exp. Allergy* 20:349, 1990.

134. Oppenheim, J. J., and Schechta, S. Lymphocyte Transformation. In N. R. Rose and H. Friedmann (eds.), *Manual of Clinical Immunology.* Washington, D.C.: American Society for Microbiology, 1980. P. 233.

135. Orange, R. P., Austen, W. G., and Austen, K. F. Immunological release of histamine and slow reacting substance from anaphylaxis from human lung. I. Modulation by agents influencing cellular levels of cyclic 3',5' adenosine monophosphate. *J. Exp. Med.* 134:136S, 1971.

136. Orsel, H. A., et al. Development of IgE and allergy in infancy. *J. Allergy Clin. Immunol.* 55:66, 1975.

137. Ostergaard, P. A., et al. Basophil histamine release in the diagnosis of house dust mite and dander allergy of asthmatic children. *Allergy* 45:231, 1990.

138. Patterson, R., and Anderson, J. Allergic reactions to drugs and pharmacologic agents. *JAMA* 248:2637, 1982.

139. Pelikan, Z., and Pelikan-Filipek, M. A diagnostic study of immediate hypersensitivity in asthmatic patients: A comparison of bronchial challenge and serum RAST. *Ann. Allergy* 49:112, 1982.

140. Perelmutter, L., and Emanuiel, I. Assessment of in vitro IgE testing to diagnose allergic disease. *Ann. Allergy* 55:762, 1985.

141. Permutt, S., et al. Bronchial Challenge in Ragweed-Sensitive Patients. In L. M. Lichtenstein and K. F. Austen (eds.), *Asthma: Physiology, Immunopharmacology, and Treatment* (International Symposium). New York: Academic, 1977. P. 265.

142. Pipkorn, U. Pharmacologic influence of anti-allergic medication on in vivo testing. *Allergy* 43:81, 1988.

143. Platts-Mills, T. A. E. Allergens and asthma. *Allergy Proc.* 11:269, 1990.

144. Position statement of The American Academy of Allergy and Immunology: Skin testing and radioallergosorbent testing (RAST) for diagnosis of specific allergens for IgE-mediated disease. *J. Allergy Clin. Immunol.* 72: 515, 1983.

145. Prahl, P., et al. Basophil histamine release in children with adverse reactions to cow milk. *Allergy* 43:442, 1988.

146. Prausnitz, C., and Küstner, H. Studien Uber Uberempsindickheit. *Zentralbl. Bakteriol.* 86:160, 1921.

147. Prijma, J. R., et al. Decrease of complement hemolytic activity after an allergen-house dust bronchial provocation test. *J. Allergy Clin. Immunol.* 70:306, 1982.

148. Reed, C. E., Yuninger, J. W., and Evans, R. Quality assurance and standardization of allergy extracts in allergy practice. *J. Allergy Clin. Immunol.* 84:4, 1989.

149. Reisman, R. E. American Academy of Allergy: Physician's statement: Controversial techniques. *J. Allergy Clin. Immunol.* 67:333, 1981.

150. Richerson, H. B., Cheng, F. H., and Bauserman, S. C. Acute experimental hypersensitivity pneumonitis in rabbits. *Respir. Dis.* 104:568, 1971.

151. Rodriguez, G. E., Dyson, M. C., and Mohagheghi, H. The art and science of allergy skin testing. *Ann. Allergy* 61:428, 1988.

152. Roovers, W. H., et al. Phazet skin prick test versus conventional prick test with allergen and histamine in children. *Ann. Allergy* 64:166, 1990.

153. Rosen, F. S., Alper, C. A., and Pensky, J. Genetic heterogeneity of C1 esterase inhibitor in patients with hereditary angioneurotic edema. *J. Clin. Invest.* 50:2143, 1971.

154. Rosenberg, N., et al. Clinical and immunologic criteria for diagnosis of allergic bronchopulmonary aspergillosis. *Ann. Intern. Med.* 86:405, 1977.

155. Rosenow, E. C., III. Drug-induced Hypersensitivity Disease of the Lungs. In C. H. Kirkpatrick and H. Y. Reynolds (eds.), *Immunologic & Infectious Reactions in the Lungs. Lung Biology in Health and Disease,* Vol. 1. New York: Marcel Dekker, 1976. P. 261.

156. Rosenthal, R. R., et al. Indications for inhalation challenge. *J. Allergy Clin. Immunol.* 64:603, 1979.

157. Salvaggio, J. E. Occupational asthma: Overview of mechanism. *J. Allergy Clin. Immunol.* 64:646, 1975.

158. Sampson, H. A. Comparative study of promotional food antigen extracts for the diagnosis of food hypersensitivity. *J. Allergy Clin. Immunol.* 82: 718, 1988.

159. Sampson, H. A., Buckley, R. H., and Metcalfe, D. D. Food allergy, *JAMA* 258:2886, 1987.

160. Sampson, H. A., and Jolie, P. L. Increased plasma histamine concentration, food challenges in children with atopic dermatitis. *N. Engl. J. Med.* 31:372, 1984.

161. Sampson, H. A., and McCaskill, C. M. Food hypersensitivity and atopic dermatitis: Evaluation of 114 patients. *J. Pediatr.* 107:669, 1985.

162. Samter, M. M. Sublingual desensitization for allergy not recommended. *JAMA* 215:1210, 1972.

163. Saryan, J. A., Garrett, P. E., and Kurtz, S. R. Failure to detect extremely high levels of serum IgE with an immunoradiometric assay. *Ann. Allergy* 63:322, 1989.

164. Schwartz, L. B., et al. Time course of appearance and disappearance of human mast cell tryptase in the circulation after anaphylaxis. *J. Clin. Invest.* 83:1551, 1989.

165. Scolozzi, R., et al. Correlation of MAST chemiluminescent assay (CLA) with RAST and skin prick test for diagnosis of inhalant allergic disease. *Ann. Allergy* 62:193A, 1989.

166. Seltzer, J. M., Halperin, G. M., and Tsay, Y. G. Correlation of allergy test results obtained by IgE FAST, RAST, and prick puncture methods. *Ann. Allergy* 54:25, 1985.

167. Shalit, N., et al. Release of histamine and tryptase during continuous and interrupted cutaneous challenge with allergen in humans. *J. Allergy Clin. Immunol.* 86:117, 1990.

168. Shearer, W. T. Specific diagnostic modalities: IgE, skin tests, and RAST. *J. Allergy Clin. Immunol.* 84(Suppl. II):1112, 1989.

169. Sheffer, A. L., et al. Measurement of circulating IgG and IgE food immune complexes. *J. Allergy Clin. Immunol.* 81:758, 1988.

170. Sheffer, A. L., and Wasserman, S. I. Anaphylaxis. In A. S. Cowen (ed.), *Rheumatology and Immunology. The Science and Practice of Clinical Medicine,* Vol. 4. New York: Grune & Stratton, 1979. P. 468.

171. Sheffer, A. L., et al. Chemical mediators in exercise-induced anaphylaxis: A distinct form of physical allergy. *J. Allergy Clin. Immunol.* 71:311, 1983.

172. Simon, R. Sulfite challenge for the diagnosis of sensitivity. *Allergy Proc.* 10:537, 1989.

173. Skassa-Brociek, W., et al. Skin test reactivity to histamine from infancy to old age. *J. Allergy Clin. Immunol.* 80:711, 1987.

174. Skov, P. S., et al. A new method for detecting histamine release. *Agents Actions* 14:414, 1985.

175. Solley, G. O., et al. The late phase of the immediate wheal and flare reaction: Its dependence on IgE antibodies. *J. Clin. Invest.* 58:408, 1976.

176. Spector, S. L., and Farr, R. Bronchial inhalation challenge with antigens. *J. Allergy Clin. Immunol.* 64:580, 1979.

177. Stephan, B., et al. Determination of N-methylhistamine in urine as an indicator of histamine release in immediate allergic reactions. *J. Allergy Clin. Immunol.* 86:862, 1990.

178. Tang, R. B., and Wu, K. K. Total serum IgE, allergy skin testing and the radioallergosorbent test for the diagnosis of allergy in asthmatic children. *Ann. Allergy* 62:432, 1989.

179. Thomas, L. L., and Lichenstein, L. M. Laboratory Diagnosis of Immediate Hypersensitivity Disorders. In G. Sudhir and R. A. Good (eds.), *Cellular, Molecular, and Clinical Aspects of Allergic Disorders.* New York: Plenum, 1979. P. 569.

180. Tsai, L. C., Hung, N. W., and Tang, R. B. Changes of serum-specific IgE antibody titer during hyposensitization in mite-sensitive asthmatic children. *J. Asthma* 27:95, 1990.

181. Tsay, Y. G., and Halpern, G. M. IgE fluoroallergosorbent (IgE FAST) tests: Concept and clinical applications. *Immunol. Allergy Pract.* 6:27, 1984.

182. Tung, R., and Lichenstein, L. N. In vitro histamine release from basophils of asthmatic and atopic individuals in D_2O. *J. Allergy Clin. Immunol.* 128:2067, 1982.

183. Turner, K. J., et al. The association of lung shadowing with hypersensitivity responses in patients with allergic bronchopulmonary aspergillosis. *Clin. Allergy* 4:149, 1974.

184. Urbanek, R., et al. Venom specific IgE and IgG antibodies as a measure of the degree of protection in insect sting-sensitive patients. *Clin. Allergy* 13:229, 1983.

185. Valentijn, R. M., Daha, M. R., and Vanes, L. A. Clinical significance of laboratory investigations for immune complexes. *Clin. Immunol. Allergy* 5:649, 1985.

186. Van Arsdel, P. P., Jr., and Larson, E. B. Diagnostic tests for patients with suspected allergic disease. *Ann. Intern. Med.* 110:304, 1989.

187. van der Zee, J. S., et al. Discrepancies between the skin tests and IgE antibody assays: Study of histamine release, complement activity in vitro, and occurrence of allergen-specific IgE. *J. Allergy Clin. Immunol.* 82:270, 1988.

188. Van Metre, T. E. The advancement of the knowledge and practice of allergy. *J. Allergy Clin. Immunol.* 64:235, 1979.

189. Vasella, C. C., DeWeck, A. L., and Stadler, B. M. Natural anti-IgE autoantibodies interfere with diagnostic IgE determination. *Clin. Exp. Allergy* 20:295, 1990.

190. Venge, R., Dahl, R., and Peterson, C. G. B. Eosinophil granule proteins in serum after allergen challenge of asthmatic patients and the effects of anti-asthmatic medication. *Int. Arch. Allergy Appl. Immunol.* 87:306, 1988.

191. Vichvanond, P., and Nelson, H. S. Circadian variation of skin reactivity and allergy skin tests. *J. Allergy Clin. Immunol.* 83:1101, 1989.

192. Walker, C. L., and Lawrence, I. The detection of IgE antibody. *N. Engl. Reg. Allergy Proc.* 11:172, 1990.

193. Wang, J. L. F., et al. The management of allergic bronchopulmonary aspergillosis. *Am. Rev. Respir. Dis.* 120:87, 1979.

194. Warner, J. O., and Price, J. A. Aero-allergen avoidance in the prevention and treatment of asthma. *Clin. Exp. Allergy* 20(Suppl. 3):15, 1990.

195. Weeks, B., Wadsen, S., and Frelund, L. Reproducibility of challenge tests at different times. *Chest* 91(Suppl. 1):838, 1987.

196. Wegner, F., et al. Superiority of the histamine release test above case history, prick test, and radio-allergosorbent test in predicting bronchial reactivity to the house dust mite in asthmatic children. *Klin. Wochenschr.* 61:43, 1983.

197. Weltman, J. K. Laboratory tests for a total and allergen-specific immunoglobulin E. *N. Engl. Reg. Allergy Proc.* 9:129, 1988.

198. Wenzel, S., et al. Immunoassay of tryptase from human mast cells. *J. Immunol. Methods* 86:139, 1986.

199. Wenzel, S. E., Fowler, A. A., and Schartz, L. B. Activation of pulmonary mast cells by bronchoalveolar allergen challenge. In vivo release of histamine and tryptase in atopic subjects with and without asthma. *Am. Rev. Respir. Dis.* 137:1002, 1988.

200. Yunginger, J. W. Proper application of available laboratory tests for adverse reactions to foods and food additives. *J. Allergy Clin. Immunol.* 78:220, 1986.

201. Yunginger, J. W. Clinical Significance of IgE. In E. Middleton, Jr., et al. (eds.), *Allergy: Principles and Practice* (3rd ed.). St. Louis: Mosby, 1988. P. 849.

202. Zimmerman, B., Chambers, C., and Forsyth, S. Allergy in asthma. II. The highly atopic infant and chronic asthma. *J. Allergy Clin. Immunol.* 81:71, 1988.

203. Zimmerman, B., et al. Allergy in asthma. I. The dose relationship of allergy to severity of childhood asthma. *J. Allergy Clin. Immunol.* 81:63, 1988.

204. Andersson, M., et al. Measurement of histamine in nasal lavage fluid: Comparison of a glass-fiber based fluorometric method with two radioimmunoassays. *J. Allergy Clin. Immunol.* 86:815, 1990.

205. Bousquet, J., et al. Indirect evidence of bronchial inflammation assessed by titration of inflammatory mediators in BAL fluid of patients with asthma. *J. Allergy Clin. Immunol.* 88:649, 1991.

206. Bradley, B. L., et al. Eosinophils, T-lymphocytes, mast cells, neutrophils, and macrophages in bronchial specimens from atopic subjects with asthma and normal control subjects and relationship to bronchial hyperresponsiveness. *J. Allergy Clin. Immunol.* 88:661, 1991.

207. Broide, D. H., et al. Evidence of ongoing mast cell and eosinophil degranulation in symptomatic asthma airway. *J. Allergy Clin. Immunol.* 88:637, 1991.

208. Broide, D. H., et al. Cytokines in symptomatic asthma airways. *J. Allergy Clin. Immunol.* 89:958, 1992.

209. Busse, W. W., and Sedgwick, J. B. Eosinophils in asthma. *Ann. Allergy* 68:286, 1992.

210. Carlson, M., et al. Degranulation of eosinophils from pollen-atopic patients with asthma is increased during pollen season. *J. Allergy Clin. Immunol.* 89:131, 1992.

211. Demoly, P., et al. Precision of skin prick and puncture tests with nine methods. *J. Allergy Clin. Immunol.* 88:758, 1991.

212. Dolan. Immunoassay of specific IgE: Low level assays require measurement of allergen specific assay background. *Ann. Allergy* 69:151, 1992.

213. Djukanovic, R. et al. The effect of inhaled allergen on circulating basophils in atopic asthma. *J. Allergy Clin. Immunol.* 90:175, 1992.

214. Editorial: What characterizes allergic asthma? *Ann. Allergy* 68:371, 1992.

215. Editorial: Why mix ROC with RAST? *Ann. Allergy* 68:3, 1992.

216. Emanuel, I. A. A comparison of in-vitro allergy diagnostic assays. *Ear Nose Throat J.* 69:1990.

217. Kelso, J. M., et al. Diagnostic performance characteristics of the standard Phadebas RAST, modified RAST, and Pharmacia CAP system versus skin testing. *Ann. Allergy.* 67:511, 1991.

218. Kikawa, Y., Miyanomae, T., and Inoie, Y. Urinary leukotriene E_4 after exercise challenge in children with asthma. *J. Allergy Clin. Immunol.* 89:1111, 1992.

219. Kleine-Tebbe, J., et al. Comparison between MAGIC LITE- and CAP-system: Two automated specific IgE antibody assays. *Clin. Exp. Allergy* 22:475, 1991.

220. Knol, E. F., et al. Intracellular events in anti-IgE nonreleasing human basophils. *J. Allergy Clin. Immunol.* 90:92, 1992.

221. Kuehr, J., et al. Longitudinal variability of skin prick test results. *Clin. Exp. Allergy* 22:839, 1992.

222. Lavins, B. J., Dolen, W. K., and Nelson, H. S. Use of standardized and conventional allergen extracts in prick skin testing. *J. Allergy Clin. Immunol.* 89:658, 1992.

223. Nolte, H. Update: Clinical aspects of basophil histamine release. *Immunol. Allergy Pract.* 14:255, 1992.

224. Pastorello, E. A., et al. A multicentric study on sensitivity and specificity of a new *in vitro* test for measurement of IgE antibodies. *Ann. Allergy* 67:365, 1991.

225. Peterson, C. G. B., et al. Radioimmunoassay of human eosinophil cationic protein (ECP) by an improved method. Establishment of normal levels in serum and turnover *in vivo*. *Clin. Exp. Allergy* 21:561, 1991.

226. Phagoo, S. B., Wilson, N. M., and Silverman, M. Skin prick testing using allergen-coated lancets: A comparison between a multiple lancet device and a single lancet applied with varying pressure. *Clin. Exp. Allergy* 21:589, 1991.

227. Position statement. The use of in vitro tests for IgE antibody in the specific diagnosis of IgE-mediated disorders and in the formulation of allergen immunotherapy. *J. Allergy Clin. Immunol.* 90:263, 1992.

228. Sampson, H. A., Broadbent, K. R., and Bernhisel-Broadbent, J. Spontaneous release of histamine from basophils and histamine-releasing factor in patients with atopic dermatitis and food hypersensitivity. *N. Engl. J. Med.* 321:228, 1989.

229. Schwartz, L. B. Cellular inflammation in asthma: Neutral proteases of mast cells. *Am. Rev. Respir. Dis.* 145:S18, 1992.

230. Smith, T. F. Allergy testing in clinical practice. *Ann. Allergy* 68:293, 1992.

231. Sue, M. A., Gordon, E. H., and Freund, L. H. Utility of additional skin testing in "nonallergic" asthma. *Ann. Allergy* 68:395, 1992.

232. Sugai, T., Sakiyama, Y., and Matumoto, S. Eosinophil cationic protein in peripheral blood of pediatric patients with allergic diseases. *Clin. Exp. Allergy* 22:275, 1991.

233. Tamura, G., et al. Do diagnostic procedures other than inhalation challenge predict immediate bronchial responses to inhaled allergen? *Clin. Exp. Allergy* 21:497, 1991.

234. Venge, P., Henriksen, J., and Dahl, R. Eosinophils in exercise-induced asthma. *J. Allergy Clin. Immunol.* 88:699, 1991.

235. Wagenpfeil, S., et al. Reproducibility of skin prick test reactions to common allergens in patients with atopic eczema. *J. Allergy Clin. Immunol.* 89:143, 1992.

236. Weeke, B., and Poulsen, L. K. Diagnostic Test for Allergy. In S. T. Holgate and M. K. Church (eds.), *Allergy.* New York: Raven, 1993. P. 12.

237. Williams, P. B. The histamine content of allergen extracts. *J. Allergy Clin. Immunol.* 89:738, 1992.

238. Williams, P. B., et al. Immunoassay of specific IgE: Use of a single point calibration curve in the modified radioallergosorbent test. *Ann. Allergy* 69:48, 1992.

239. Williams, P. B., et al. Comparison of skin testing and three *in vitro* assays for specific IgE in the clinical evaluation of immediate hypersensitivity. *Ann. Allergy* 68:35, 1992.

240. Yunginger, J. W., and Adolphson, S. R. Standardization of Allergens. In N. R. Rose and E. Conway, et al. (eds.), *Manual of Clinical Laboratory Immunology* (4th ed.). Washington: American Society for Microbiology, 1991. Chapter 99.

241. Zweiman, B., et al. Release of eosinophil granule proteins during IgE-mediated allergic skin reactions. *J. Allergy Clin. Immunol.* 87:984, 1991.

Bronchial Provocation Tests

Sheldon L. Spector

39

An inhaled substance can be administered to humans for a variety of reasons. For example, it can help mobilize secretions, bronchodilate airways, or produce bronchial obstruction. Inhaled substances that produce bronchoconstriction can be used to help clarify the role of mediators and other factors that determine airway hyperreactivity. The most widely employed bronchial provocation tests measure nonspecific airway reactivity, which reflects the extent to which the airways are generally irritable or reactive to nonallergic agents. Bronchial provocation tests can also be used to measure the effects of specific allergenic substances found in the environment or in occupational settings. Even though the distinctions are not always clear, it is convenient to talk about the challenges by subcategorizing them into nonspecific and specific challenges. In general, asthmatic subjects are considerably more reactive to the so-called nonspecific stimuli than are normal nonasthmatic controls.

This chapter will review current concepts in bronchial provocation testing using the above-mentioned bronchoconstrictive substances. Discussion will focus on a variety of agents used to produce airway obstruction, the advantages and limitations of the techniques employed, and suggestions to circumvent side effects and ensure patient safety.

PREPARATION OF PATIENT FOR CHALLENGE

Smoking of cigarettes and the ingestion of cola, coffee, and chocolate should be treated in a similar way to the taking of medication, and stopped at least 6 hours before testing. In reality, caffeine in a dose equivalent to about three cups of coffee has a minimal, if any, effect on histamine challenge [35]. Exercise and exposure to irritants should also be avoided 2 hours before the bronchial challenge, so that the patient can remain in a relatively asymptomatic state. Ideally, patients should not be told they will receive a bronchodilator or bronchoconstrictor, as the suggestion itself could influence the result [107, 217]. Challenges should be performed at a consistent time of the day, if possible, since circadian rhythms can also influence the results of challenge [82]. Human susceptibility to antigens may also be greater during menstruation [205]. Ideally, all medications should be stopped prior to challenge, but, since this is not always practical, realistic suggestions for withholding medications or dealing with other possible influences have been made (Table 39-1).

SAFETY CONSIDERATIONS

Although methacholine and histamine inhalation challenges can be safely adapted to an office practice, antigen inhalation challenges require experienced personnel and are thereby rarely suitable for general office use. Inhalation challenge with concentrated antigens can cause severe or prolonged asthma attacks.

It is rare that a positive bronchial challenge will provoke a permanent decrement in lung function, especially if standardized techniques using step-wise increases in concentration are used. Patients undergoing antigen challenges require constant observation, especially in view of the possible late-phase reactions. A physician or nurse familiar with challenges should be directly at hand. Ideally, technicians who administer antigen bronchial challenges should not have an allergic background or have a personal or family history of asthma. A well-ventilated room helps to prevent excessive antigen exposure from the air. Persons with moderate to severe impairment of lung function (e.g., a 1-second forced vital capacity [FEV_1] of 1 liter or less) should only be tested if the necessary precautions are taken. A person with asthmatic symptoms should not be given a potential bronchoconstrictor, which can further compromise pulmonary function. The biggest potential decrement of lung function occurs within minutes after a histamine or methacholine challenge. There are a few individuals who experience a prolonged reaction (lasting less than 1 hour) to the methacholine challenge, for reasons that are not clear. Antigen inhalation challenges can provoke prolonged or late reactions that require more precautions. They should not be done routinely in an office setting, especially by inexperienced personnel. The guidelines for performing an antigen challenge is an initial antigen concentration that produces a 2+ reaction on intracutaneous injection. A 2+ equals a wheal greater than 5 mm in diameter, minus the diameter of the wheal produced by the diluent control. Using the puncture technique, a 5% solution of 1:20 w/v diluent of aqueous solutions of antigen is usually applied to the skin. A wheal greater than 2 mm in diameter is considered equivalent to a positive intradermal test, with the solution having a concentration of antigen of 1:10,000 ± one dilution.

When allergen skin tests are performed, a negative diluent control and a positive histamine control should accompany the skin test with antigens. For doing intradermal tests, the injected histamine solution consists of 0.02 ml of 0.1% base solution. For prick tests, a 1% solution of histamine base is recommended.

To treat a patient who shows an unusually severe or prolonged response to a bronchial challenge, follow the same guidelines as you would use to treat any patient suffering from an acute asthma attack. In general, patients receiving beta-adrenergic blocking agents should not be challenged with aerosolized antigens or pharmacologic bronchoconstrictors, due to a possible prolonged or exaggerated response to the stimulus. Additionally, such patients may show either an inadequate response to the beta-adrenergic agonist therapy or an exaggerated alpha effect.

After an antigen inhalation challenge, corticosteroids may be given to prevent a late bronchoconstrictive response (if monitoring for such a response is not part of the protocol). Safety considerations also require the presence of resuscitation equipment,

Table 39-1. *Factors influencing bronchial inhalation challenges*

Potential influence	Time of avoidance
Smoking	A few hours
Suggestion	Prior to challenge
Caffeine, cola, chocolate	At least 8 hr
Exercise and air pollution	At least 8 hr
Beta-adrenergic stimulating agents (aerosols)	At least 8 hr
Sustained-release beta agonists*	At least 24 hr
Short-acting theophylline derivatives*	At least 24 hr
Sustained-release theophylline derivatives*	At least 24 hr
Alpha-adrenergic blocking agents	At least 8 hr
Anticholinergic agents	At least 8 hr
Cromolyn sodium	At least 24 hr
Common antihistamines	At least 48 hr
Hydroxyzine or long-acting antihistamines*	At least 96 hr
Prior antigen challenge	Days
Vaccination	Weeks
Exposure to viral infection	Weeks

* Medications presumably will still be present in the bloodstream.

oxygen, and appropriate medication, including aerosolized bronchodilators.

INFLUENCE OF THE PULMONARY FUNCTION MEASUREMENT ITSELF

Different methods used to measure airway response, including maximal expiratory flow maneuvers and submaximal flow maneuvers such as airway resistance, are often included. The disadvantage of a forced expiratory maneuver, as measured by spirometry, is a reduction in normal tone that occurs after inspiration to total lung capacity [91, 238], or after induced bronchoconstriction in normals [155] and asthmatic subjects [171]. In contrast, a deep inspiration or expiration causes bronchoconstriction in asthmatic patients, which is prevented by anticholinergics such as atropine [79, 83, 170]. Body plethysmography is expensive and therefore not widely available. The panting maneuver itself may be affected by laryngeal narrowing that is induced by a particular drug administered during bronchial provocation. Measurements of airway resistance and maximum flow should be made at the same lung volume [112, 113, 215]. Although the FEV_1 maneuver can be effort-dependent, it has survived the test of time as a minimally variable test of pulmonary function.

In deciding on the proper pulmonary function tests, one must bear in mind that certain substances primarily affect small airways, while others primarily affect large airways [170, 237]. If such information is known, it might determine which pulmonary function test is ideal for a given challenge. If this information is not known, parameters that assess both small and large airways should be included in the testing. An adequate baseline pulmonary function must be obtained, and the nature and time of the last bronchodilator usage recorded. Even if a bronchodilator cannot be completely discontinued, it can be given in a similar manner in subsequent challenges. The timing of the measurement may also be important, since pulmonary function tests of both spirometry and body plethysmography may be technically difficult to perform if data must be collected quickly.

A pulmonary function test should be relatively sensitive and specific. A change in specific airway conductance (SGaw), for example, during a methacholine challenge, may be five times greater than the change in FEV_1. Any relatively large change must be considered in relation to the wide variability of the test and its standard error. Although the SGaw may appear to be more sensitive, it is also quite variable and cumbersome. Smoking only one cigarette can decrease SGaw more than 35 percent in normal

subjects, and certain asthmatic patients may have a 35 percent or greater fall with just the suggestion that they may experience bronchial obstruction. Various standardization panels have advocated a minimal acceptable change in FEV_1 of 20 percent and SGaw of 35 percent; however, these values are somewhat arbitrary. FEV_1 has less variability from day to day compared with SGaw. A significant difference from normal is usually defined as the value that would be expected in less than 5 percent of normal subjects. Changes observed should exceed 2 standard deviations (S.D.) for repeated measures before statistical significance is reached. Ideally, coefficients of variation should be done for measurements within a given day, as well as from week to week (Table 39-2).

Pennock and coworkers [180] suggested that a significant change in expiratory volumes or flow after administration of a bronchodilator is 1 S.D. outside the limits of normal intertrial variability. Thus, a significant change would be greater than 5 percent for FEV_1 and forced vital capacity (FVC), and greater than 13 percent for mean forced expiratory flow during the middle half of the FVC (FEF_{25-75}) in normal persons. In obstructed persons, it would be greater than 13 percent for FEV_1, greater than 11 percent for FVC, and greater than 23 percent for FEF_{25-75}. I suggest that the FEV_1, even with its limitations, should be included as one of the measurements of a bronchoconstrictor response after administration of occupational agents, methacholine, or histamine. Pulmonary function measurements can be added, depending on their availability and the need for other information about the bronchoconstrictive response. Factors affecting response include environmental influences as well as viruses, vaccines, and recent exposure to allergens.

Various investigators have suggested that baseline airway caliber has the potential of modifying bronchial hyperreactivity during the pollen season, although present data are not very convincing. Vedal and associates [236] also postulated that airway caliber and possibly immunologic sensitivity to plicatic acid are associated with the occurrence of bronchial hyperresponsiveness in red cedar workers. Hume and Gandevia [110] reported that, as the FEV_1 and FVC improve, so does the absolute response until it reaches a maximum. Absolute response is poor if the initial value is low. Goldberg and Cherniack [89] reported that the greatest changes after therapy take place when airway resistance is highest.

Herxheimer [103] and Tiffeneau [226] postulated that hyposensitization by the inhalation route can occur if very dilute antigens are given initially and progression with more concentrated antigen follows. In other words, less antigen would be required to produce a positive response, due to previous exposure to the antigen. A contrasting phenomenon is the priming effect characterized by a heightened reactivity to an allergen due to previous exposure, which usually occurs after exposure to a high concentration of antigen. Neither of these phenomena has been well studied, but they are not thought to be a problem during a routine antigen challenge.

Table 39-2. *Proposed minimal changes in pulmonary function after bronchial provocation challenge*

Pulmonary function test	Percent change from baseline
Vital capacity	−10
FEV_1	−20
Maximal midexpiratory flow rate ($FEV_{25-75\%}$) or $\dot{V}_{max_{50}}$	−25
Peak expiratory flow rate	−25
Specific airways resistance	+35 to +40
Specific airways conductance	−35 to −40
Functional residual capacity	+25

BRONCHIAL INHALATION CHALLENGE WITH DILUENT

It is important that the vehicle or diluent in which the broncho-constrictive substance is dissolved does not itself cause bronchial obstruction. If it does, the subject must be tested on another day. The phenomenon of diluent-induced bronchoconstriction was acknowledged by the panel from the Asthma and Allergic Disease Centers of the National Institutes of Health (NIH). We advocated excluding individuals from a standardized bronchial challenge who had a greater than 10 percent fall in FEV_1 "ten minutes following inhalation of five breaths of diluent" [40]. Mechanisms behind such a response have not been thoroughly studied. The method of delivery, pH, and osmolarity may be important. The preservatives in a diluent such as a glycerol are known to cause bronchial obstruction [94].

Studies by Klaustermeyer and associates [128] have emphasized these differences among asthmatics, in that most of their asthmatic patients tolerated saline without bronchoconstriction yet an important subgroup had a different response. In one of their studies consisting of 31 men with asthma, 50 percent responded to five inhalations of diluent with less than a 10 percent variation from baseline, yet 20 percent of the patients responded with more than a 25 percent decrease from baseline in SGaw or flow at 50 percent of vital capacity (V50VC). The diluent was 0.45% NaCl, 0.275% $NaHCO_3$, and 0.4% phenol administered through a DeVilbiss No. 42 nebulizer driven by a compressor at a 10-L/min flow. Four measurements were obtained: (1) SGaw by body plethysmography; (2) V50VC from the maximal expiratory flow-volume (MEFV) curve; (3) maximal expiratory flow ($\dot{V}_{max}$) from the peak of the MEFV curve; and (4) peak flow, measured with a Wright peak-flow meter. The authors considered the first two as the most sensitive and less variable than peak flow. If a response to diluent was present at the 5-minute reading, it was usually present at 10 and 20 minutes. Of some interest were two distinctly different response patterns [128]: patients can have a progressive fall in SGaw and V50VC with increasing numbers of inhalations of diluent, or patients can have an initial reduction in flow rates without further decline, in spite of additional diluent inhalations. The pattern of airway response to diluent has been reported to be reproducible and not dependent on the baseline airway obstruction [129]. Although this assertion was based on a study of only eight subjects, the authors' conclusions were based on three measurements of airway response done at three time intervals. It is not clear, however, why all eight patients, including the so-called nonresponders to diluent, had a greater than 26 percent fall from baseline in at least one measurement at one time interval.

STORAGE AND STANDARDIZATION OF PHARMACOLOGIC BRONCHOCONSTRICTIVE AGENTS

Data often are lacking regarding the proper storage of broncho-constrictive agents. A few comments will be made here regarding the most common agents used. These are: histamine, methacholine, carbachol, and serotonin. Histamine, methacholine, and carbachol are usually available as dry powders. Some methacholine chloride may still be on shelves in vials containing 25 mg/ml, since it used to be so marketed as Mecholyl. Thus, the original rationale for using 25 mg/ml as the maximum concentration was largely because this was how it was commercially available. The diluent used should be sterile and buffered to maintain the final pH of the solution at 7.0. An aqueous diluent containing 0.9% NaCl and 0.4% phenol is a commonly available example. Although there is a potential for an adverse reaction to phenol, this has not been convincingly described. Data regarding stability are often meager. The Merck Index [151] recommends that aqueous methacholine solutions be stored under refrigeration for no longer than 2 weeks, and reports that decay is hastened by alkalinity. MacDonald [138] studied the loss of potency of methacholine under various circumstances. At room temperature, it lost 10 percent of its potency after 48 days and 50 percent of its potency after 297 days. At 4°C, a 10 percent reduction in potency occurred after 128 days. The frozen solution probably retains its stability for years. Suppliers of methacholine and histamine powder especially designed for use in animal studies include the J. T. Baker Chemical Corp., Phillipsburg, NJ, ordered through McKesson-Robbins, Amfac, or other wholesalers such as Spectrum Chemicals (Los Angeles). Roche Labs licenses 100 mg of powdered methacholine chloride in sterile vials called *Provocholine*. The company provides easy instructions for making the dilutions suggested. Histamine powder (chemically pure) is furnished by Sigma Chemicals for animal use. Eli Lilly and Co. (Indianapolis) provides vials of histamine with the maximum concentration of 2.75 mg/ml histamine phosphate USP, which is a 1 mg/ml histamine base. Histamine solutions remain stable for months. Serotonin creatinine phosphate is not stable and degrades quickly. If frozen, it can be used in 8 to 12 hours. Serotonin hydrochloride is more soluble and more expensive. Both are provided by Sigma Chemicals.

Refrigerated aqueous solutions of carbachol are extremely stable over long periods [151]. It is generally not a good idea to perform an inhalation challenge with these bronchoconstrictors in a patient who is receiving beta-adrenergic blocking agents, since responses might be exaggerated or prolonged.

INHALATION CHALLENGES WITH BRONCHOCONSTRICTIVE AGENTS OTHER THAN ANTIGENS

Acetylcholine

Acetylcholine was one of the first agents to be used clinically. It was first popularized by Tiffeneau [223, 225] and is still occasionally used by investigators in Europe [41] and the Far East [153]. Its main disadvantages are its rapid inactivation in the body by cholinesterases and its short half-life, with the associated difficulty in obtaining serial measurements.

Carbamylcholine

Carbamylcholine (carbaminocholine chloride) is a derivative of acetylcholine that is not metabolized by acetylcholinesterase and thereby has a longer duration of action. It has the advantage of being stable in solution. Although certain European investigators still describe its use [169], it has never been popular among American investigators. Moreover, Cropp (personal communication, 1979) noted adverse reactions after its use, which further dampened enthusiasm for it in the United States.

Methacholine

Methacholine (acetyl-β-methylcholine [Mecolyl]) is also an analog of acetylcholine but lacks its nicotinic action. It is not as stable in solution as carbamylcholine but has become one of the most widely used bronchoconstrictors to assess nonspecific reactivity. Spector and Farr [40, 212] popularized the concept of keeping the number of breaths constant and increasing the concentration, a method later accepted by an NIH panel to standardize bronchial inhalation challenges. Tachyphylaxis does not appear to occur when methacholine is inhaled at the concentrations commonly used by asthmatic subjects.

Histamine Phosphate

Histamine (beta-imidazolylethylamine phosphate) is similar in popularity to methacholine and probably constricts airway smooth muscle, both directly [53] and reflexly [55]. Although the effects of methacholine and histamine have been compared and most individuals show similar reactivity [121], certain subjects have disparate responses [211], which implies a different mechanism of action between histamine and methacholine. Tachyphylaxis may occur following repeated histamine challenges when they are separated by up to 6 hours [141], moreover, prior histamine inhalation reduces airway responsiveness to other bronchoconstrictor stimuli such as acetylcholine [142] or exercise [98].

Hypertonic Saline

Hypertonic saline may cause bronchoconstriction in asthmatic subjects [5], and its action is probably mediated predominantly through the release of histamine from mast cells, with a minor contribution made by prostanoids [68].

Prostaglandins

Asthmatic subjects are hyperresponsive to prostaglandin D_2 [99]. They are nearly 8,000 times more sensitive to prostaglandin $F_{2\alpha}$ ($PGF_{2\alpha}$) than are healthy controls. This compares with an increased sensitivity to histamine of 10- to 100-fold. Although the F series of prostaglandins produce bronchoconstriction, many of the E family of prostaglandins produce bronchodilation [52, 110, 145]. On the other hand, both $PGF_{2\alpha}$ and PGE have proved irritating to many individuals and commonly cause cough in asthmatic subjects. Theories put forth to explain the idiosyncrasy associated with the use of aspirin and other nonsteroidal antiinflammatory agents in asthmatic subjects often involve prostaglandins and other products of arachidonic acid metabolism [102, 220]. One explanation suggests the enhancement of the metabolism of the lipoxygenase pathway, leading to increased leukotriene formation [87, 216]. Aspirin-sensitive asthmatics are reported to be more sensitive to histamine than to $PGF_{2\alpha}$ [146]. They also show a selective and marked increase in airway responsiveness to leukotriene E_4 (LTE_4) compared to histamine. After desensitization with aspirin, an average 33-fold reduction in LTE_4 responsiveness can be found [11]. Anticholinergic agents such as atropine and beta$_2$ stimulants can significantly inhibit the bronchoconstrictive response to $PGF_{2\alpha}$, while cromolyn sodium, thymoxamine, and ipratropium bromide have no blocking effect [80].

Leukotrienes

Inhaled LTC_4 produces a prominent central and slight peripheral airway response. By contrast, inhaled histamine results in a predominantly peripheral airway constriction [183]. LTD_4 may mediate cold-air isocapnic bronchoconstriction [114]. LTB_4 probably does not have an important role in bronchial hyperresponsiveness [19].

Serotonin

Although the exact role of serotonin in human bronchial constriction is not known, it may potentiate vagal effects on airway smooth muscle in dogs [95]. Certain salt solutions of serotonin appear to decompose rapidly. It is not found in the mast cells of humans per se, but is released from human platelets [97].

Adenosine

Adenosine and its metabolite, adenosine 5′-monophosphate (AMP), may produce bronchoconstriction partially through the release of histamine. Selective H_1-antihistamines, such as terfenadine and astemizole, inhibit AMP-induced bronchoconstriction by more than 80 percent and displace the concentration response curve to the right [182].

Other Bronchoconstrictive Substances

It would be impractical to give detailed descriptions here of all possible agents that have been employed to induce bronchoconstriction in normal or asthmatic subjects. Almost any agent given in large enough quantities or without ideal physiologic characteristics (e.g., too low or high a pH) can serve as a potential irritant to an asthmatic or even a healthy subject. Obstruction can be produced with cold air, hypotonic saline, and a variety of medications such as propranolol [81, 161, 235, 240].

Bradykinin is thought to act directly on smooth muscle. However, given as an aerosol, its primary action in humans may involve vagal reflexes [202]. Exercise can also produce nonspecific bronchial provocation. It can be performed in an office setting by having a patient run up and down the stairs or, for example, run on a sophisticated treadmill. Cold air is thought to be the initial stimulus for this bronchoconstriction. Possible drawbacks of exercise provocation is the rendered refractory period after the initial stimulus and the standardization of humidity and temperature ideally required [86].

COMPARISON OF DIFFERENT BRONCHOCONSTRICTIVE CHALLENGES

Although good correlation might exist between various tests of bronchial obstruction, the dissimilarities between certain responses are often more interesting than the similarities, since different mechanisms of bronchoconstriction are implied when the expected comparable reactivity between two agents is not seen in a given individual. For example, some asthmatic subjects have a negative response to exercise challenge yet have a significant fall in FEV_1 after a methacholine or histamine challenge [6, 64, 127, 149]. Other differences are also present often for technical reasons (Table 39-3). During an upper respiratory infection, normal individuals develop a transient hyperreactivity of their airways in response to exercise with cold air as well as to histamine [9]. Although both of these tests of hyperreactivity are well correlated and can be blocked by atropine, certain individuals exhibit a disparity in their recovery from the two stimuli. After 6 weeks, exercise with cold air no longer produced a decrease in SGaw ($p<.05$), yet, by 6 weeks, airway reactivity to histamine remained decreased in 9 of 13 subjects [9]. Certain individuals

Table 39-3. Comparison of exercise and aerosolized bronchoconstrictive challenges

Feature	Exercise	Methacholine or histamine
Sensitivity	Good	Better
Ease of administration	Good	Excellent
Cost of equipment (standard test)	High	Low
Reproducibility	Good	Excellent
Side effects	Minimal	Minimal, except at high concentrations
Influenced by site of deposition	No	Yes
Influenced by temperature	Yes	No
Influenced by humidity	Yes	No
Consistently blocked by cromolyn sodium	Yes	No

Table 39-4. Comparison of methacholine and histamine bronchial inhalation challenge

Feature	Histamine	Methacholine
Cumulative effect	None	Yes
Reproducibility	A type of tolerance develops in a few patients	Highly reproducible
Blocked by hexamethonium	Yes	No
Blocked by antihistamines	Yes	No
Blocked by atropine-like agents	No	Yes
Side effects at high doses	Many	Fewer

are more responsive to methacholine than to respiratory heat loss, and vice versa [101]. Hajos [96] studied 158 asthmatic subjects and found 18 percent reacted only to serotonin (0.2%) and not to histamine or acetylcholine. Most investigators feel that histamine and acetylcholine given by inhalation produce similar bronchial reactivity, especially if used in comparable doses [140, 186].

Although the similarities between the responsiveness to methacholine and histamine have been mentioned, Spector and Farr [211] found a small group of asthmatic subjects who could tolerate increasing doses of histamine without a corresponding fall in FEV_1 and who eventually became unresponsive to the highest test dose. Similar observations have been made by others [115, 141, 199]. Spector and Farr [211] also reported on one patient who was highly reactive to histamine inhalation; the patient had a fall in FEV_1 after a very low concentration but subsequently showed marked improvement after ingestion of an antihistamine.

Histamine and methacholine reactivity can also be distinguished by the ability of hexamethonium (a ganglionic blocking agent) to block the former but not the latter [106].

In general, anticholinergics such as ipratropium bromide prevent methacholine-induced but not histamine-induced bronchoconstriction, and antihistamines such as chlorpheniramine prevent histamine-induced but not methacholine-induced bronchoconstriction. It is thereby presumed that the receptor sites involved in bronchial provocation by these two agents are different [243]. It has also been observed that there is a significant cumulative dose effect with methacholine and not with histamine (Table 39-4).

INDICATIONS FOR PERFORMING BRONCHIAL CHALLENGE WITH BRONCHOCONSTRICTIVE SUBSTANCES (OTHER THAN ANTIGENS)

Defining the Hyperreactive State, or Atypical Asthma

Virtually all individuals with asthma, with rare exceptions, have hyperreactive airways [208]. Even though this finding is characteristic of asthma, it is not unique to this diagnosis. For example, a small number of healthy subjects and up to 50 percent of patients with hay fever have an abnormally exaggerated response [208]. It may be that humans are born with bronchial hyperresponsiveness and genetic or environmental factors influence its subsequent loss [135]. Hyperreactivity might also be acquired, since it is found with conditions such as bronchitis, sarcoidosis, tuberculosis, silicosis, and cystic fibrosis [208]. The acute respiratory distress syndrome is often associated with hyperreactive airways [203]. Interestingly, those patients who experience cough while on angiotensin-converting enzyme (ACE) inhibitors appear to be those with underlying bronchial hyperreactivity. Often the bronchial hyperreactivity persists despite cessation of the ACE

inhibitors [124]. Lindgren and coworkers [136] reported that, after 1 to 2 weeks of enalapril therapy, the provocation concentration producing a 20 percent fall in FEV_1 (PC_{20}) for histamine challenge was reduced, along with an increased dermal response to antihuman IgE.

Correlating Hyperreactivity with Other Factors

Histamine Inhalation Challenge
Various investigators have related histamine reactivity to other factors, such as the severity and duration of asthma [50, 51, 208]. Townley and colleagues [230] did not find a relationship between the level of reactivity and the duration of symptoms, but did find the reactivity was less in patients free of symptoms for more than 2 years. On the other hand, Spector and coworkers [218] noted that the greatest reactivity to histamine or methacholine was found in those admitted for intensive inpatient care at a younger age who had an earlier age of onset and had had asthma longer than was the case in patients with less airway reactivity. Townley and coworkers [228] reported that hay fever sufferers had intermediate methacholine reactivity compared with normals who could tolerate high concentrations and asthmatics who could only tolerate low concentrations.

Spector and Farr [211] reported that patients who were not very methacholine reactive statistically had the least severe asthma, as measured by their discharge doses of corticosteroids. Cockcroft and coworkers [45] also related heightened reactivity to the more severe asthmatic.

A correlation has also been noted with the degree of hyperresponsiveness and the amount of treatment needed to control symptoms [120]. Staudenmayer and coworkers [219] found that asthmatic patients who were highly reactive to histamine and who had a low panic-fear profile were those who were hospitalized at exceptionally high rates relative to others. Regardless of the findings from previous studies there is still debate regarding the relationship between the reactivity to methacholine or histamine and the severity of asthma. In fact, Josephs and coworkers [118] assessed the relationship between nonspecific reactivity and the day-to-day clinical expression of asthma by measuring methacholine reactivity every 2 to 3 weeks over a period of 12 to 18 months. They concluded that the association of nonspecific reactivity with exacerbations of bronchial asthma was not sufficiently close to be of practical use (see also Chap. 40).

Antigen Inhalation Challenge
The greater the nonspecific reactivity of an asthmatic subject, the more likely a reaction will occur to an aerosolized allergen mixture. For example, the mean bronchial threshold dose to mite antigen is significantly higher in the asymptomatic individual than in an asthmatic subject who is highly reactive to histamine. There is also a relationship between histamine responsiveness and bronchial responsiveness to other allergens. Investigators must be cautious about giving too high a concentration of antigen in order to produce a decrease in pulmonary function, i.e., a positive response. Even asymptomatic or hay fever patients can be induced to wheeze for the first time when the concentration of antigen is pushed high enough. Additionally, this can prove potentially dangerous [213]. At least two factors have been related to a positive bronchial inhalation challenge: nonspecific airway hyperreactivity and a positive skin test [159]. One must always keep in mind the clinical meaning of the challenge result as it relates to the history and nature of the patient's illness.

The pulmonary function tests employed can influence the results. For instance, a differential response has been noted between patients with allergic rhinitis (hay fever) and asthma [30]. Fish and associates [71] speculated that there might be hyperreactivity of both central and peripheral airways in asthmatic subjects, but only hyperreactivity of central airways in nonasthmatic subjects. However, there might also be a difference in the physiologic response to the test itself [7, 69, 70].

Other Tests of Bronchial Lability
Reactivity to nonspecific substances and exercise can be compared as a means of better understanding the mechanisms that have been previously discussed [208].

Response to Medications
Various investigators have tried to demonstrate a relationship between nonspecific reactivity and the response to certain medications such as prednisone. Oppenheimer and coworkers [167] were unsuccessful in doing so, but they only studied a small number of subjects. Hargreave and coworkers [101, 120] reported that the lower the peak flow values in the morning (along with high histamine hyperreactivity), the greater the response to albuterol. This Canadian group has noted the relationship between bronchial responsiveness and the level of treatment required to control symptoms, with the amount and strength of medication increasing for those who are the most reactive [101, 120].

Assessing Effectiveness of Treatment Modalities by Their Ability to Block Hyperreactive Airway Disease

It would be logical to assume that, if a new agent can block or normalize hyperreactivity to, for example, methacholine or histamine, this agent might have potential usefulness in the treatment of asthma. Those agents that seem to best block hyperreactivity over the long term are the corticosteroid aerosols [62, 120, 126, 131], even though some investigators feel that the reduction of bronchial responsiveness may be minimal or of questionable clinical relevance [195]. Cromolyn sodium can also block hyperreactivity, especially if treatment is given for longer than 12 weeks [44, 105]. Surprisingly, the antibiotic troleandomycin raises an asthmatic subject's threshold to methacholine and can sometimes dramatically diminish asthmatic symptoms [207, 214] (see Chap. 67). Prolonged treatment is associated with the best effect on hyperreactivity. It is not clear whether improvements in airway responsiveness and clinical asthma are maintained with prolonged use. Juniper and coworkers [123] reduced or discontinued budesonide in their patients after 1 year of vigorous therapy, and found that, even though improvements in airway responsiveness could be maintained for at least 3 months, deterioration in spirometry and symptoms may occur as a forerunner of increased responsiveness. Immunotherapy can also affect not only late-phase reactions but bronchial hyperresponsiveness as well [13]. In pollen-sensitive individuals given birch pollen immunotherapy, bronchial responsiveness to histamine became less in the immunotherapy-treated group but did not decrease in the control group [189].

Placing Occupational Asthma in Perspective

Contact with certain occupational agents has been associated with a subsequent increased reactivity to methacholine or histamine [197]. In fact, a continued reactivity implies continued exposure to the presumed offender [47, 133]. Unfortunately, almost any noxious stimulus such as a pollutant or virus can cause the same increased nonspecific responsiveness. Thus, any assumptions about cause-and-effect relationships must be made cautiously.

The initial exposure to an agent can cause either a temporary or more sustained change in nonspecific reactivity, depending on the strength and duration of the initial exposure. Histamine inhalations before and after exposure to dimethyl ethanolamine, red cedar sawdust, and pyrolysis products of polyvinyl chloride

have been associated with an increased reactivity [26, 27, 43, 233]. In many circumstances, several months after removal from exposure to such agents as California redwood, grain dust, and isocyanates, reactivity in affected subjects decreases, only to increase again with reexposure. In certain individuals, increased reactivity remains even when the initial exposure or continued exposure is not obvious [27].

Brooks and coworkers [29] have described an asthmalike illness called *reactive airways dysfunction syndrome* (RADS). Presumed normal individuals developed symptoms of shortness of breath, cough, wheezing, and chest tightness within 24 hours after exposure to high levels of noxious irritants such as vapors, fumes, and smoke [28]. Despite this brief exposure, symptoms and increased airway responsiveness continued for more than 1 year. Tarlo and colleagues [222] suggested an expanded definition to include exposure that was not limited to a single accident or incident at work. However, the distinction between RADS and other types of occupational exposures needs to be further clarified and better understood.

ALLERGEN INHALATION CHALLENGES

Provocation challenge with allergens is less widely employed than are challenges with other bronchoconstrictive substances. They are conducted in a similar manner to a histamine or methacholine challenge, but with increasing concentrations of antigens using dilutions of allergens predicted from the skin-prick method as a built-in safety feature. In contrast to the "nonspecific" provocations, the airway response to allergen occurs more slowly. Immediate reactions typically occur after 15 or 20 minutes, followed in many circumstances by a late-phase reaction (discussed subsequently).

Perhaps the most common use of allergen challenge currently is to improve our understanding of allergic mechanisms as they relate to early and late-phase reactions in asthma. The potential benefit of a new agent for the treatment of asthma might also be based on its ability to block these early and late-phase reactions. Standardized allergen extracts have made these challenges more reproducible, and the introduction of lyophilized extracts has solved a storage problem that had often been associated with loss of stability.

If allergen inhalation challenge (AIC) provides different information than a skin test or in vitro test, then there is rationale for its use [1, 209]. This is of particular interest in patients with occupational asthma if a new agent is suspected, since skin testing to that agent may not have been standardized. Mast cells themselves have different sensitivities in different parts of the body, in that there is mast cell heterogeneity [175] (see Chap. 21). There is also a difference in the basophil response compared to the tissue mast cell response [148]. It is still not clear if there is local production of IgE in the tracheobronchial tree, so that a skin test per se would not provide the same information as an immunoglobulin E (IgE) challenge to the organ of interest.

Huggins and Brostoff [109] concluded that there is a local production of IgE in nasal secretions. They found patients with a positive clinical history and positive nasal provocation despite negative skin tests and negative radioallergosorbent test (RAST) to dust mite. In looking at a possible causal relationship between an allergen and clinical symptoms, an important decision must be made regarding the maximum dose of antigen that should be used to clarify this relationship. This point is illustrated by studies of Townley and coworkers [228], who performed AIC in normal subjects and patients with hay fever and asthma. When they used an antigen concentration of 10,000 PNUs, 11 of 14 patients with hay fever had a positive bronchial inhalation challenge response even though they had never wheezed before. This implies that too high a concentration was used to differentiate hay fever patients from asthmatics, even though asthma was the condition sought for clarification [228].

Cavanaugh and colleagues [37] reported similar results and concluded that patients who upon inhalation challenge respond only to a high concentration of antigens behave as a separate population, in that they have a higher incidence of negative skin test reactions compared with other subjects tested. When we first performed antigen challenges, we also noticed severe reactions if the allergen extract concentration given was too high, such that a positive AIC was yielded but with no clinical meaning. In fact, it led us to recommend bronchial challenges using dilutions of antigens greater than 10^{-2} w/v or 10,000 PNU [212]. As mentioned previously, there is a relationship between responses to, for example, histamine or methacholine and the allergic response [159]. When there is increased reactivity, a more severe allergic reaction would be anticipated. If too high a concentration of antigen leads to a late asthmatic response, there is potential to perpetuate and accentuate the hyperreactivity.

SUBSTITUTES FOR SKIN TESTS IF THEY CANNOT BE PERFORMED

Skin disorders such as severe eczema might rule out skin testing. In vitro testing, which is a more expensive and less-sensitive alternative to skin testing, may have to be employed under such circumstances. It also may have to be used if a patient is on one of the long-acting antihistamines that suppress skin test reactivity for weeks or months.

COMPARISON OF SKIN TESTS, IN VITRO TESTS, AND OTHERS

Allergen provocation tests have been touted by some as an absolute standard to which other tests should be compared, since they measure the locally secreted IgE in the organ of involvement—the lung in an asthmatic subject. Occasionally an in vitro test may be negative despite a positive antigen inhalation test or skin test, or both.

Aas and coworkers [1] compared pollen and house dust reactivity using skin tests and AIC. They found that the type of antigen and the degree of skin test reactivity both influence the results of an AIC response. However, there was a greater likelihood for a positive bronchial challenge response in patients with pollen reactivity compared to those with house dust reactivity. Interestingly, patients with positive skin test results and negative bronchial challenge responses had nasal allergies to the pollens. This implies that skin tests reveal IgE reactivity but do not identify which organ is susceptible to this IgE effect. These researchers also studied the relationship between skin test reactivity and AIC. They found that the greater the skin test reactivity, the greater the chance for a subsequently positive AIC. We often find historical data are not very helpful, because many of our patients have perennial symptoms. On the other hand, if a patient has a positive skin test with an accompanying strong history of a reaction to that antigen, the AIC will give a predictably positive response in more than 90 percent of the circumstances [209, 210]. The level of skin test reactivity will often allow one to predict the result of a subsequent AIC, especially if the nonspecific reactivity is known.

CLARIFICATION OF MEDIATORS AND MECHANISMS

Antigen inhalation challenges have been associated with elevated histamine levels and a sustained or biphasic release of neutrophil chemotactic factor [18]. Investigators have also found liberation of what was formerly called *slow-reacting substance of anaphylaxis* (SRS-A) [4] and the purified equivalents, the leukotrienes, especially C_4 and D_4 [143]. Schwartz and coworkers [200] described a method to assess mast cell activation in vivo as contrasted with the activation of basophils. They found that an elevated plasma or serum tryptase level had diagnostic value for indicating mast cell–related events, such as would occur with anaphylactic reactions. The serum complement level falls during bronchospasm induced by antigen but not by methacholine. However, Arroyave and associates [12] also found a decrease in complement levels in some of their controls, making interpretation of these data difficult. Other investigators have also reported a drop in the hemolytic complement level after AIC, which cromolyn could prevent in a small number of patients [188]. Although platelets are activated after allergen challenge, the platelet-derived thromboxane A_2 does not appear to be important in the early bronchoconstrictor response [137].

Deal and coworkers [54] have contrasted the results from AIC with those from hyperventilation after cold air exposure. The former challenge produced a prolonged release of neutrophil chemotactic factor; the latter did not.

LOCATION OF RESPONSE

The pattern of change in the lung mechanics of gas exchange during AIC has been examined by various investigators. Olive and Hyatt [166] noted that the first effect of inhaled antigen was to cause a parallel shift in the MEFV curve with no change in slope. Not all patients showed the same pattern. One-third of the 15 subjects had closure of the units with no change in MEFV slope; another third initially showed the same pattern but displayed a MEFV slope change at the height of the response, which suggests that other airways increased their resistance. Finally, one-third had an immediate change of slope, with all but one showing an increase in residual volume. Thus, the site of airway obstruction may be different among some asthmatic subjects. Some investigators have suggested that an indicator of small airway response such as the flow isovolume ($\dot{V}iso/V$) would be a better indicator of airway response to AIC than a measurement of large airways such as SGaw [3].

Olgiati and coworkers [165] found a greater involvement of peripheral airways in the seven patients they studied. There was a decrease in the mean arterial oxygen saturation after ragweed challenge, but not after methacholine challenge for a comparable severity of bronchospasm as measured by SGaw.

IMMEDIATE VERSUS LATE ASTHMATIC RESPONSE: IMPLICATION FOR MECHANISM

Following exposure to allergens, an immediate or late-phase reaction, or both, may develop. Typically, the immediate component occurs within minutes, followed thereafter by a late phase, which is thought to be inflammatory in nature and is often associated with a hyperreactive state (see Chap. 12). In fact, allergen inhalation increases the maximum response plateau of the methacholine dose response curve in subjects who have a late asthmatic response [248]. The late-phase reaction has been defined as occurring from 4 to 12 hours after the immediate reaction and can occur in organs other than the lungs, such as the skin and nose. The prevalence of these late-phase responses usually ranges from 40 to 60 percent [23, 173, 187, 191]. Some of the variables that determine the differences in prevalence involve: (1) the parameter used to determine a positive response, such as FEV_1 versus another pulmonary function; (2) what percent fall is considered positive; (3) the IgE reactivity of the patient; and (4) the quantity of antigen administered. Bundgaard and Boudet [32] did not find the late asthmatic response to be very reproducible, since only one of the five subjects studied had similar positive allergen challenge when done on a second occasion. Ihre and associates [111] could change isolated late reactions following allergen challenge to dual reactions by increasing the allergen dose. Thus, late asthmatic responses are more likely in association with certain antigens compared to others, high concentrations of allergens, and high levels of circulating IgE in the early response as measured by skin tests or mediator release. There is not necessarily a correlation between the late-onset skin reaction compared to the bronchial reaction [14].

Other investigators have suggested that there is no need to perform AIC if the skin test reactivity and nonspecific reactivity are known [48]. However, such predictability would not carry over to late asthmatic responses after occupational exposure or after exposure to a new substance in the environment. This has important implications, since the late-phase reaction might help explain the perpetuation of asthma in an individual. The inhalation of allergens, either experimentally or through natural exposure, can increase the nonspecific bronchial responsiveness to substances such as histamine and methacholine [192, 224]. This increasing reactivity can be demonstrated shortly after the immediate airway response or during the interval following the late asthmatic response. The increased responsiveness may then persist for days or even weeks after the initial exposure.

Durham and colleagues [61] found that, in subjects who developed a late asthmatic response after exposure to occupational agents, there was an increase in the nonspecific bronchial responsiveness to methacholine 2 to 3 hours after the challenge. Clinically there is an increase in the nonspecific bronchial responsiveness during seasonal pollen exposure [25], and a reduction in reactivity can occur after prolonged allergen avoidance [185] or after immunotherapy [152, 238].

Although mediator release has been noted during early phase reactions, certain mediators are also released during late-phase responses. Neutrophil chemotactic factor activity has been consistently found with late-phase responses [134, 156]. Histamine has only been found sporadically [134].

Metabolites of arachidonic acid have been noted [88, 154]. LTB_4, which is a potent neutrophil chemotactic factor in humans, has been found in plasma specimens obtained during the development of both an early and a late asthmatic response following AIC [88, 134]. Using a sheep model, Abraham [2] found that dual responders produced more leukotrienes and were more sensitive to them than were early responders.

Those patients with a late asthmatic response had a significantly increased concentration of the lyso form of platelet-activating factor (PAF) compared with patients who had a single immediate response 6 hours after the antigen challenge [157]. There were no differences in the PAF level at 20 minutes, however.

Immunoglobulin levels have also been measured, and in six or seven patients with dual reactions to dust mite there was a higher IgG_1 antibody level compared to the five patients with isolated immediate reactions [117]. In addition there was a propensity to develop a late asthmatic response in the presence of high IgG_1 antibodies.

Gonzalez and coworkers [90] measured the number of helper (OKT4) and suppressor (OKT8) T-cells in blood and lavage fluid from patients with immediate or dual reactions. There was a significant increase in the percentage of OKT4 cells in the blood from the single early responders. The percentage of OKT4 cells was much lower ($p<.005$) on the antigen day in the early responders than on the antigen day in the late-phase responders. This suggests that suppressor T-cells are mobilized into the lung after antigen-induced single early reactions, and that this might

be associated with the presence of a subsequent late-phase response.

Diaz and coworkers [58] found a significant increase in the number of lymphocytes, neutrophils, and eosinophils ($p<.05$) in late-phase responders compared to the isolated early responders, also supporting the role of eosinophils and their products in late-phase injury responses. Frick and colleagues [77] reported an increase in the proportion of hypodense peripheral blood eosinophils only in those patients with both immediate and late asthmatic responses. They concluded that the percentage of hypodense eosinophils better reflects the severity of asthma than the concentration of total peripheral blood eosinophils.

Various medications can affect both the immediate and late response to allergen challenge. The pharmaceutical industry has utilized blocking properties to predict their possible effectiveness in various allergic diseases, especially asthma. Corticosteroids taken orally classically block a late response very well but do not block the immediate response in most systems. On the other hand, oral steroids given 3 hours before an AIC in sheep blocked both [56]. Martin and coworkers [144] found that prednisone blocked both the immediate antigen response to pollens when given at 40 mg daily for 7 days before and on the day of challenge.

In an Italian study, prednisone not only inhibited the late asthmatic response and the increased airway responsiveness after toluene diisocyanate exposure, but also normalized the number of leukocytes and the concentration of albumin in the bronchioalveolar lavage fluid [24]. Unlike oral steroids, steroid aerosols more consistently inhibit both the immediate and late response. Cromolyn also inhibits both according to most investigators [33, 147, 179]. Theophylline can block the late response, and only slightly alter the early one [178]. Pauwels [177] suggests that theophylline has activity on airway inflammation. Nedocromil, which has not yet been released for use in the United States, blocks both early and late-phase reactivity to antigen [20]. Classically, beta agonists only block the early response; however, many long-acting beta agonists have not been adequately studied using this model [108]. Ipratropium bromide has little if any effect on the immediate response to antigen challenge [108].

Specific PAF antagonists block early bronchoconstriction with a tendency toward blocking residual bronchial hyperreactivity for 6 hours after an AIC [92]. Guinot and associates [92] considered a specific PAF inhibitor to be a potentially useful medication in the treatment of asthma. Interestingly, indomethacin is reported by some to inhibit the late-phase response but not the early response [66, 119].

Although the late-phase response model has served as a possible explanation for the persistence of hyperreactivity, future studies and further clarifications are necessary to put immediate and late responses in proper perspective, for the following reasons. First, the concentration of antigen itself may be responsible for the production of certain late-phase reactions [100]. This has been demonstrated by various investigators who were able to convert an early allergen response to a dual response just by administering a large dose of allergen, for example, with a short-acting beta$_2$ agonist. Interestingly, when a beta agonist was used in conjunction with the allergen challenge, there was no accompanying increase in nonspecific hyperresponsiveness [132]. Second, nonasthmatic allergic subjects (e.g., hay fever patients) can show hyperreactivity after an allergen challenge, and many nonallergic asthmatics have hyperresponsiveness, so it is unclear which environmental factor perpetuates the symptoms of these two groups [204]. Third, in some studies of occupational exposure, increased airway responsiveness may occur after an early response alone and the late-phase response is not necessary [139]. Exercise and possibly distilled water have been associated with an increased late asthmatic response without increased nonspecific responsiveness. Fourth, and lastly, certain medica-

Table 39-5. Comparison of immediate and late asthmatic responses

Characteristic	Immediate reaction	Late reaction
Time sequence		
Begins	Within 10 min	After 4–6 hr
Peaks	In 20–30 min	In 8–12 hr
Clears	In 1–3 hr	Within 24–36 hr
IgE dependent	Yes	Probably
Influenced by IgE titer	Yes	Yes
Influenced by concentration of antigen	Yes	Yes
Inhibited by cromolyn sodium	Yes	Yes
Inhibited by oral corticosteroids	No* (?)	Yes
Inhibited by steroid aerosols	Yes	Yes
Theophylline	Slightly	Slightly
Beta agonists	Yes	No
Indomethacin	No	Yes

* Inhibition may occur with prolonged usage.

tions, such as indomethacin, inhibit the late responses, yet are not a useful treatment for asthma [66, 119] (Table 39-5).

In summary, the late-phase model has proved interesting and provocative. It may explain the perpetuation of hyperreactivity in certain individuals, yet there are certain questions with respect to its usefulness as a model which have not yet been answered.

EVALUATION OF NEW ALLERGENS IN PULMONARY DISEASE

The literature is swelling with papers on new allergens that may produce pulmonary disease. Although many are organic substances, some are not. Some of these agents are discussed in subsequent chapters of this text.

EVALUATION OF NEW TREATMENTS THAT BLOCK PROVOCATIVE CHALLENGES

Pharmaceutical manufacturers typically test new medications for their ability to block an early or a late (or both) antigen inhalation challenge. Such studies should take into account the peak action and duration of action of the blocking agent that is to be examined. If too high a concentration of antigen is used, erroneous conclusions might be drawn regarding the ability of a blocking agent to accomplish its goal, especially if the challenge itself has no clinical meaning for the patient.

EVALUATION OF THE THERAPEUTIC EFFICACY OF IMMUNOTHERAPY

As already discussed briefly, allergen challenges have been used to evaluate the benefit of hyposensitization, as reflected by a decrease in bronchial reactivity after treatment. In many instances, improvement is associated with loss of the late reaction. Immunotherapy to dust mite and cat dander in particular has been shown to cause a change in late-phase reactivity and clinical improvement.

Recently, Van Bever and Stevens [234] reported the complete resolution of the late asthmatic response in 5 of 15 children after 1 year of house dust immunotherapy. Furthermore, as a group, the subjects showed a less severe late response after 1 year of house dust immunotherapy. Although the PC_{20} of the immediate

response was not changed, the severity of the immediate response was also reduced after 1 year of house dust immunotherapy.

CONVINCING THE PATIENT OF CAUSE-AND-EFFECT RELATIONSHIPS

Occasionally, a physician uses a double-blind challenge to convince a patient that he or she is symptomatic after exposure to that allergen.

STANDARDIZATION OF ALLERGENIC EXTRACTS

Currently, allergenic extracts are complex biologicals containing certain nonallergenic antigens, irritants, crude materials, and allergens. Eventually standards for the potency of all allergenic extracts will be established, such as now exists for antigen E [85].

A variety of techniques involving in vivo and in vitro procedures are used to standardize allergenic extracts. Skin testing is the simplest and most sensitive procedure for determining the potency of allergenic extracts that incorporate end-point titration procedures. However, the technique itself is somewhat imprecise, and skin testing requires sensitive patients. Most authors record the wheal size. The reproducibility of the procedure can be improved by the use of a micrometer syringe and quantitation of the size of the reaction by planimetry [206].

Another in vivo technique for determining allergen potency is popular in Europe and was originally proposed by Aas and other members of the Nordic Council of Medicine [162]. This is the histamine equivalent potency (HEP) activity of an allergen extract. One HEP provokes a specific skin reaction to a prick test, with the wheal of the same median size as a positive reference consisting of 5.43 mM histamine. This requires a pool of sensitive subjects on whom the procedure is performed in anatomically corresponding sites. An equivalent designation for the concentration of the preparation is 1,000 biologic units (1 HEP = 1,000 BU/ml). Although histamine is often proposed as a control, it is probably better to use a mast cell–degranulating agent, such as codeine phosphate [49, 150] or compound 48/80 [244], to determine the standardized releasability of mediators from the mast cells.

In vitro potency measurements use the weight per volume (w/v) unit system, which assumes that 1 mg of a pollen contains 1,000 units. However, the activity of raw pollen materials may vary considerably with season, year of collection, and storage procedures. Protein nitrogen units (PNUs), which are precipitable by phosphotungstic acid, are another common way of expressing in vitro potency. However, the total protein in a mixture may represent only a small proportion of the actual allergenic substance [76]. Therefore, the PNU is a poor correlate of in vivo potency.

The method proposed as the reference in the United States is based on the study of Turkeltaub and coworkers [231, 232]. A proficiency study using two strengths of histamine was designed to assess the capability of a laboratory to perform correctly the standardization protocol. A screening test with the allergen extract to be tested should be performed by the puncture method, making it possible to select highly sensitized individuals. The standardization procedure requires five patients who receive several intradermal injections of dilutions of the allergen extract; the dilutions are given in threefold increments and the flare is recorded. Both a reference extract and the extract to be tested are injected and the results of the flare are compared by parallel-line bioassay. This technique is very sensitive but time-consuming, and results are given in allergy units (AU). The three main units (IU, international unit; AU, allergy unit; and BU, biologic unit) have not yet been fully compared, although present data show that they are not comparable [60].

The RAST has been adapted to the standardization of allergen extracts. Two different methods have been used: direct RAST titration [39] and RAST inhibition [74, 75, 84]. In general, there is excellent agreement between direct RAST inhibition and skin test potencies. Histamine release assays can also determine allergen potency. In this method, sensitized leukocytes are exposed to various concentrations of different extracts, and the quantity of extract required to release 50 percent of the total histamine is measured. The biggest limitation of this method is the need for fresh leukocytes from a previously identified sensitive population willing to donate their leukocytes. Two other techniques, radial immunodiffusion and double-antibody radioimmunoassay (RIA), delineate purified materials in crude extracts. The RIA requires a radiolabeled antigen and can measure very small quantities of antigen in an extract. Radial immunodiffusion requires only precipitating antibody and the standard antigen. However, both approaches to standardization are limited by the small number of stable, purified allergens available (see Chap. 38).

These in vitro procedures can be used to study cross-reactivity among various allergen groups. These techniques may also be used in conjunction with bronchial provocation tests in clinical trials.

STORAGE OF ANTIGENS

Most antigens are packaged as concentrated solutions in vials or as freeze-dried extracts. Freeze-drying should prolong the half-life almost indefinitely. A diluent containing 50% glycerol protects the antigen from degradation, perhaps by preventing enzyme activity. Glycerin significantly prolongs the original strength [160]. Although phenol is often used as an alternative, its deleterious effect becomes more marked at lower concentrations. The use of stabilizers such as albumin improves extract stability [163], as does the nonionic detergent polysorbate 80 (Tween 80). Allergens should be kept in concentrated form if possible, since loss can occur through absorption of dilute solutions into the walls of containers. Storage at 4°C also aids in maintaining stability.

EFFECTS OF MEDICATIONS

Theophylline Derivatives

According to Cockcroft and coworkers [46], theophylline blocks a nonspecific challenge with blood levels of greater than 10 mg/L. No blocking effect occurs at levels less than this. Both enprofylline and theophylline, given intravenously, cause a small dose-related increase in the methacholine PC_{20} threshold [130]. Theophylline reduces antigen-induced bronchospasm, as well as the rise in the plasma histamine level and the serum neutrophil chemotactic activity [144]. The protective effect is also related to the serum theophylline level [67, 178].

Beta Agonists and Antagonists

Oral or inhaled albuterol can protect against an aerosolized histamine provocation challenge, or shift histamine reactivity [36, 46]. Propranolol given systemically or by inhalation produces little if any bronchoconstriction in healthy subjects [229, 246]. Yet, certain investigators have reported a mild bronchoconstriction even in normals when given this agent [168]. There is general agreement that asthmatic subjects may develop severe bronchial obstruction after propranolol treatment [196]. Beta-adrenergic agonists such as inhaled fenoterol (800 μg) are reported to be more effective than cholinergic antagonists such as ipratropium bromide (80 μg) in preventing early allergen-induced bronchospasm [22]. Martin and associates [144] reported that terbutaline sulfate (2.5 mg every 6 hours for 36 hours) significantly blocked the early phase of an AIC.

Cromolyn Sodium

With short-term administration, cromolyn has partially or completely blocked methacholine or histamine challenge [242]. After long-term treatment, there have been reports of reduced bronchial hyperresponsiveness as measured by histamine challenge in patients with perennial asthma [42]. Although most studies indicate that cromolyn blocks the immediate bronchial challenge response to allergens, not all patients demonstrate such an inhibition [65, 78, 104]. Cromolyn usually blocks late reactions.

Corticosteroids

Oral corticosteroids do not appear to alter airway reactivity to inhaled parasympathomimetic drugs in asthmatic patients [10, 227]. Inhaled steroids have a significant blocking effect with time according to most investigators, although one group found that methacholine reactivity was unaffected by beclomethasone [63, 195]. With respect to allergens, many studies have shown that oral corticosteroids do not block bronchoconstriction produced by high concentrations of house dust and wheat flour antigens [21, 158]. Martin and coworkers [144] reported that oral prednisone (40 mg for 7 days) inhibited the immediate effects of bronchial challenge with pollen antigens in their subjects. Aerosol beclomethasone dipropionate, given 30 minutes before allergen challenge, inhibits the late, but not the immediate, allergen-induced reaction [181], but early reactions can also be blocked [33].

Anticholinergic Agents

As reviewed elsewhere [208], anticholinergic agents abolish bronchial constriction induced by aerosols of methacholine, citric acid, and carbon dust. It also completely or partially blocks inhalation of cold air, exercise, antigen challenges, and the effect of suggestion. When various doses of atropine are used, it minimally or completely blocks the effect of histamine and antagonizes the effect of propranolol. It partially blocks the bronchoconstrictor response to $PGF_{2\alpha}$ in asthmatic subjects but not in normals. Ipratropium bromide (SCH1000), an analog of atropine, can block methacholine-induced asthma better than histamine-induced asthma in aerosol doses of 40 and 80 μg. The protective effect of ipratropium against histamine seems less than the beta-agonist effect such as fenoterol, and they both have the ability to block histamine challenges.

Atropine blockade of antigen inhalation challenge (AIC) is a more controversial topic, especially since there is an implication regarding the role of reflexes in airway constriction of asthmatic subjects. Most investigators have not found significant blockade by atropine of antigen-induced bronchoconstriction, although Yu and associates [245] reported that 1.5 to 2.5 mg of atropine could block antigen reactions when given intravenously. There may also be patient variability, since some investigators have found complete blockade while others have found only partial blockade [72, 116, 193]. The dose of antigen may also influence results. The cholinergic effect may be more obvious at a lower antigen dose [59, 193]. At least two factors of nonspecific airway reactivity and skin test positivity influence an antigen challenge. These variables may also play a role as to the degree of blockade [31,

159], and may help explain why, in certain patients, aerosolized atropine blocks a histamine challenge better than in others [36].

Alpha-Adrenergic Blocking Agents

Although alpha-adrenergic receptors in human airway smooth muscle are sparse, their numbers may increase in the presence of lung disease [8, 93]. In any case, their role is presumed to be minimal in asthma. Nevertheless, alpha-receptor antagonists such as phentolamine or thymoxamine can block exercise or histamine challenge in asthmatic subjects [16, 17, 125]. Thymoxamine can inhibit AIC when given intravenously and even to a small degree when given by inhalation [174].

OTHER MEDICATIONS

Inhibitors of prostaglandin synthesis do not block immediate decrements in pulmonary function after AIC in asthmatic patients [73].

Nifedipine, a potent inhibitor of transmembrane calcium ion flux, can inhibit histamine provocative challenges and exercise-induced asthma [38, 241].

Pretreatment with aerosolized lidocaine blocks methacholine-induced bronchoconstriction [239]. The response to inhaled histamine is correlated with the 24-hour urinary excretion of sodium, in that a high rate of sodium excretion is associated with increased airway reactivity. It may even explain the increased infant mortality as it relates to table salt purchases [34].

Treatment with ascorbic acid can block methacholine-induced bronchoconstriction. This ameliorative action of ascorbic acid can be blocked by the ingestion of indomethacin, implicating prostaglandin pathways [164]. Ascorbic acid can protect histamine-induced airway constriction according to some investigators, but not others [247].

Cromakalim, a potassium channel blocker, protects against histamine-induced bronchoconstriction in nonasthmatic subjects [15] and produces some inhibition of early morning bronchoconstriction in asthmatic patients [172].

EMOTIONAL FACTORS

Emotional factors in asthma are thought to be mediated mainly through the parasympathetic nervous system. Bronchoconstriction occurs in a significant number of asthmatic subjects in response to psychologic stimuli [107, 217]. Those asthmatic patients with the most hyperreactive airways are the ones most likely to respond to bronchoconstrictive suggestion [107, 217]. Cholinergic antagonists such as atropine can block this bronchoconstriction, thus implicating the parasympathetic nervous system.

Other Factors

A premenstrual exacerbation of asthma has been noted by various investigators [152]. Pauli and coworkers [176] did not find a change in methacholine reactivity throughout the menstrual cycle to explain this deterioration in asthma.

CIRCADIAN AND OTHER BODY RHYTHMS

An increase in histamine hyperreactivity has been found in asthmatic and bronchitic subjects during nighttime hours [57] (see Chap. 76). Bronchial reactivity to histamine and acetylcholine follows a circadian pattern [190, 221].

OTHER DISEASE STATES

Congestive heart failure is also associated with bronchial hyperresponsiveness [184, 198]. Yet, Seibert and coworkers [201] found normal airway responsiveness to methacholine in patients with cardiac-related asthma.

PREGNANCY

Juniper and coworkers [122] found a twofold improvement in airway responsiveness during pregnancy in the 16 females they studied, which corresponded to an associated improvement in clinical asthma as indicated by a reduction in medication. Symptoms and spirometry remained unchanged during pregnancy. They also found no correlation of the asthma with progesterone or estrogen levels.

AEROSOL GENERATION, DELIVERY, AND PENETRANCE

Large particles tend to sedimentate in proximal airways and smaller particles tend to penetrate into the peripheral airways. Particles less than 0.3 μm and greater than 5 μm in diameter exhibit decreased deposition. Ideally, inhaled particles should range between 0.3 and 4 μm. Individual nebulizers may vary considerably in the median aerodynamic diameter of the particles produced (see Chap. 32).

Two popular aerosol delivery systems include the dosimeter method and continuous-flow method. Details regarding their use and comparison studies have been described [194, 217] (see also Chap. 56). Spacer devices or cones favor a more peripheral alveolar distribution and also have certain disadvantages. The particle size and distribution of the dose may not be as critical as was once thought; however, they are two variables that should be considered for their potential influence on patient response, especially during disease states.

INTERPRETATION AND EXPRESSION OF RESULTS

A standard way of expressing data on bronchoconstrictive substances, including allergens, is by the calculation of cumulative doses. This is based on the assumption that the dose of the substance generated is retained and cumulated, which in reality is not always correct. An antigen typically is accumulated, and, to a small degree, methacholine might also be accumulated in the body.

Histamine and other substances may have relatively short-lived effects that are completely dissipated in the body. Much of the generated dose is not only inhaled and exhaled, but lost in equipment, metabolized, or removed from the sites of distribution. Ideally, the baseline FEV_1 prior to starting a challenge should be 80 percent or greater of a previously observed highest value, and not so low as to compromise a minimal reserve in pulmonary function.

According to standardization protocols, five successive breaths of a bronchoconstrictive substance such as methacholine or antigen are administered to the patient. Table 39-6 shows an unabridged and abridged bronchoconstrictive change challenge for methacholine. A positive result for a methacholine challenge is a 3-minute sustained fall in FEV_1 of 20 percent or more from the control FEV_1 value. If the test result is negative, five breaths of the next dilution are given. If the result is borderline, then less than five breaths of the next dilution may be given.

Table 39-6. Cumulative doses for bronchial inhalation challenge by bronchoconstrictive agents at five breaths per dilution

Serial concentration (mg/ml)	No. of breaths	Cumulative units per concentration	Total cumulative units
LENGTHY PROTOCOL			
0.03	5	0.15	0.15
0.06	5	0.30	0.45
0.12	5	0.60	1.05
0.25	5	1.25	2.30
0.50	5	2.50	4.80
1.0	5	5.00	9.80
2.0	5	10.00	19.80
5.0	5	25.00	44.80
10.0	5	50.00	94.80
25.0	5	125.00	219.80
SHORTENED PROTOCOL (FOR METHACHOLINE)			
0.025	5	0.125	0.125
0.25	5	0.125	0.125
0.25	5	1.25	1.375
2.5	5	12.5	13.88
10.0	5	50.0	63.88
25.0	5	125.0	188.88

Table 39-7. Cumulative doses for bronchial inhalation challenge with antigen at five breaths per dilution

Antigen concentration* (w/v)	No. of breaths	Cumulative units per concentration	Total cumulative units
1:1,000,000	5	0.025	0.025
1:500,000	5	0.05	0.075
1:100,000	5	0.25	0.325
1:50,000	5	0.5	0.825
1:10,000	5	2.5	3.32
1:5,000	5	5.0	8.32
1:1,000	5	25.0	33.3
1:500	5	50.0	83.3
1:100	5	250.0	300.3

* At concentrations of antigens of 1:100 and above, the clinical meaning is unclear.

Table 39-7 shows the sequence for an antigen inhalation challenge. A positive result for an antigen challenge is a 10-minute fall in FEV_1 of 20 percent or more that is sustained for at least 10 minutes. Results are expressed by a dose-response curve using a semilogarithmic plot (Fig. 39-1), and the cumulated dose is plotted on the logarithmic abscissa. On the linearly expressed ordinate, the response is measured by the percentage of the diluent control aerosol. The plot shows a best-lined fit curve, and the cumulative dose at which lung function has deteriorated by at least 2 S.D. below control values is considered the provocation dose. The antigen or other provocative substance is multiplied by the number of breaths (usually five) to get the cumulative dose for each exposure. Sensitivity is determined by the provocation dose itself, while reactivity is determined by the slope. Abbreviated protocols have been suggested by some, but have the disadvantages of less safety and less standardization. Other ways of expressing data other than the dose-response plot would be the area under the curve, which has the advantage of defining the degree of sensitivity. After certain occupational exposures, such as to western red cedar, patients may continue to exhibit increased bronchial responsiveness to inhaled methacholine or histamine even years after their exposure to red cedar.

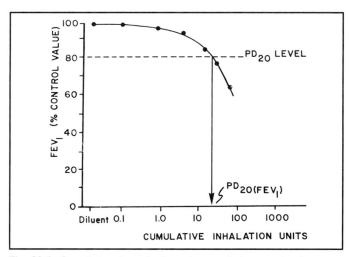

Fig. 39-1. *Cumulative dose of a bronchoconstrictive agent such as methacholine (abscissa) versus response expressed as percent of diluent control aerosol (ordinate). The PD_{20} (FEV_1) refers to the cumulative dose of bronchoconstrictor that corresponds to a 20 percent fall in FEV_1.*

REFERENCES

1. Aas, K. The bronchial provocation test. Springfield, Ill.: Thomas, 1975.
2. Abraham, W. The importance of lipoxygenase products of arachidonic acid in allergen-induced late responses. *Am. Rev. Respir. Dis.* 135:S49, 1987.
3. Ahmed, T., Fernandez, R. J., and Wanner, A. Airway responses to antigen challenge in allergic rhinitis and allergic asthma. *J. Allergy Clin. Immunol.* 67:135, 1981.
4. Ahmet, T., et al. Abnormal mucociliary transport in allergic patients with antigen-induced bronchospasm: role of slow reacting substance of anaphylaxis. *Am. Rev. Respir. Dis.* 124:110, 1981.
5. Anderson, S. D., Schoeffel, R. E., and Finney, M. Evaluation of ultrasonically nebulized solutions as a provocation in patients with asthma. *Thorax* 38:284, 1983.
6. Anderton, R. C., et al. Bronchial responsiveness to inhaled histamine and exercise. *J. Allergy Clin. Immunol.* 63:315, 1979.
7. Ankin, M. G., Peterman, V. I., and Fish, J. E. Effects of lung inflation on maximum flow responses to methacholine and antigen in hay fever and asthma subjects. *Am. Rev. Respir. Dis.* 119(Suppl.2):55, 1979.
8. Anthracite, R. F., Vachon, L., and Knapp, P. H. Alpha-adrenergic receptors in the human lung. *Psychosomat. Med.* 33:481, 1971.
9. Aquilina, A. T., et al. Airway reactivity in subjects with viral upper respiratory tract infections: the effects of exercise and cold air. *Am. Rev. Respir. Dis.* 122:3, 1980.
10. Arkins, J. A., Schleuter, D. P., and Fink, J. N. The effect of corticosteroids on methacholine inhalation in symptomatic bronchial asthma. *J. Allergy* 41:209, 1968.
11. Arm, J. P., et al. Airway responsiveness to histamine and leukotriene E_4 in subjects with aspirin-induced asthma. *Am. Rev. Respir. Dis.* 140:148, 1989.
12. Arroyave, C. C. M., et al. Plasma complement changes during bronchospasm provoked in asthmatic patients. *Clin. Allergy* 7:173, 1977.
13. Assen, E. S. K., and McAllen, M. D. Changes in challenge tests following hyposensitization with mite extract. *Clin. Allergy* 3:161, 1973.
14. Atkins, P. C., et al. Late onset reactions in humans. Correlation between skin and bronchial reactivity. *Ann. Allergy* 60:27, 1988.
15. Baird, A., et al. Cromakalim, a potassium channel activator, inhibits histamine induced bronchoconstriction in healthy volunteers. *Br. J. Clin. Pharmacol.* 25:114P, 1988.
16. Beil, M., and DeKock, A. Role of alpha-adrenergic receptors in exercise-induced bronchoconstriction. *Respiration* 35:78, 1978.
17. Bianco, S., et al. The effect of thymoxamine on histamine-induced bronchospasm in man. *Br. J. Dis. Chest* 66:27, 1972.
18. Bhat, K. N., et al. Plasma histamine changes during provoked bronchospasm in asthmatic patients. *J. Allergy Clin. Immunol.* 58:647, 1976.
19. Black, P. N., et al. Effect of inhaled leukotriene B4 alone and in combina-

tion with prostaglandin D2 on bronchial responsiveness to histamine in normal subjects. *Thorax* 44:491, 1989.

20. Bonifazi, F., et al. Double-blind crossover trial to compare the activity of nedocromil sodium and placebo in antigen challenge. *Allergol. Immunopathol.* (Madr.) 15:151, 1987.

21. Booij-Noord, H., Orle, N. G. M., and DeVries, K. Immediate and late bronchial obstructive reactions to inhalation of house dust and protective effects of disodium cromoglycate and prednisone. *J. Allergy Clin. Immunol.* 48:344, 1971.

22. Booij-Noord, H., Quanjer, P. H., and DeVries, K. Protektive Wirkung von berotec bei Provokation-stetsen mit spezfisher Allergen Inhalation und Histamin. *Int. J. Clin. Pharmacol.* 6(Suppl. 4):69, 1972.

23. Booij-Noord, H., et al. Late bronchial obstruction reaction to experimental inhalation of house dust extract. *Clin. Allergy* 2:43, 1972.

24. Boschetto, P., et al. Prednisone inhibits late asthmatic reactions and airway inflammation induced by toluene diisocyanate in sensitized subjects. *J. Allergy Clin. Immunol.* 80:261, 1987.

25. Boulet, L. P., et al. Asthma and increases in nonallergic bronchial responsiveness from seasonal pollen exposure. *J. Allergy Clin. Immunol.* 71:399, 1983.

26. Boushey, H. A., Empey, D. W., and Laitinen, L. A. Meat wrapper's asthma: effect of fumes of polyvinyl chloride on airways function. *Physiologist* 18: 148, 1975.

27. Boushey, H. A., et al. Bronchial reactivity: state of the art. *Am. Rev. Respir. Dis.* 121:389, 1980.

28. Braman, S. S., and Corrao, W. M. Bronchoprovocation testing. *Clin. Chest Med.* 10:165, 1989.

29. Brooks, S. M., Weiss, M. A., and Bernstein, I. L. Reactive airways dysfunction syndrome (RADS). *Chest* 88:376, 1985.

30. Bruce, C. A., et al. Quantitative inhalation bronchial challenge in ragweed hay fever patients: a comparison with ragweed-allergic asthmatics. *J. Allergy Clin. Immunol.* 56:331, 1975.

31. Bryant, D. H., and Burns, M. W. S. Bronchial histamine reactivity: its relationship to the reactivity of the bronchi to allergens. *Clin. Allergy* 6: 523, 1976.

32. Bundgaard, A., and Boudet, L. Reproducibility of the late asthmatic response (abstract). *Eur. J. Respir. Dis.* 137:284, 1988.

33. Burge, P. S., et al. Double blind trials of inhaled beclomethasone dipropionate and fluocortin butyl ester in allergen-induced immediate and late asthmatic reactions. *Clin. Allergy* 12:523, 1982.

34. Burney, P. G. J., et al. Effect of changing dietary sodium on airway response to histamine. *Thorax* 44:36, 1989.

35. Calacone, A., et al. Effect of caffeine on histamine bronchoprovocation in asthma. *Thorax* 45:630, 1990.

36. Casterline, C. L., Evans, R., and Ward, G. W. The effect of atropine and albuterol aerosols on the human bronchial response to histamine. *J. Allergy Clin. Immunol.* 58:607, 1976.

37. Cavanaugh, M. J., Bronsky, E. A., and Buckley, J. M. Clinical value of bronchial provocation testing in childhood asthma. *J. Allergy Clin. Immunol.* 59:41, 1977.

38. Cerrina, J., et al. Inhibition of exercise-induced asthma by a calcium antagonist, nifedipine. *Am. Rev. Respir. Dis.* 123:156, 1981.

39. Ceska, M., Ericksson, R., and Varga, J. M. Radioimmunosorbent assay of allergens. *J. Allergy* 49:1, 1972.

40. Chai, H., et al. Standardization of bronchial inhalation challenge procedures. *J. Allergy Clin. Immunol.* 56:323, 1975.

41. Chapman, T. T. Hypersensitivity to inhalation of acetylcholine related to asthma. *Ir. J. Med. Sci.* 443:507, 1962.

42. Chhabra, S. K., and Gaur, S. N. Effect of long-term treatment with sodium cromoglycate on nonspecific bronchial hyperresponsiveness in asthma. *Chest* 95:1235, 1989.

43. Cockcroft, D. W., Cotton, D. J., and Mink, J. T. Nonspecific bronchial hyperreactivity after exposure to western red cedar. *Am. Rev. Respir. Dis.* 119:505, 1979.

44. Cockcroft, D. W., and Murdock, K. Y. Comparative effects of inhaled salbutamol, sodium cromoglycate, and beclomethasone dipropionate on allergen-induced early asthmatic responses, late asthmatic responses, and increased bronchial responsiveness to histamine. *J. Allergy Clin. Immunol.* 79:734, 1987.

45. Cockcroft, D. W., et al. Bronchial reactivity to inhaled histamine: a clinical survey. *Clin. Allergy* 7:235, 1977.

46. Cockcroft, D. W., et al. Protective effect of drugs on histamine-induced asthma. *Thorax* 32:429, 1979.

47. Cockcroft, D. W., et al. Asthma caused by occupational exposure to a furan based binder system. *J. Allergy Clin. Immunol.* 66:458, 1980.

48. Cockcroft, D. W., et al. Prediction of airway responsiveness to allergen from skin sensitivity to allergen and airway responsiveness to histamine. *Am. Rev. Respir. Dis.* 135:264, 1987.

49. Conroy, M. C., and DeWeck, A. L. Codeine: a probe of basophil and mast cell reactivity. *Immunopathology* 8:249, 1980.

50. Curry, J. J. Comparative action of acetyl-beta-methylcholine and histamine on the respiratory tract in normals, patients with hay fever, and subjects with bronchial asthma. *J. Clin. Invest.* 26:430, 1947.

51. Curry, J. J., and Lowell, F. C. Measurement of vital capacity in asthmatic subjects receiving histamine and acetyl-beta-methylcholine: a clinical study. *J. Allergy* 19:9, 1948.

52. Cuthbert, M. F. Bronchodilator activity of aerosols of prostaglandin E_1 and E_2 in asthmatic subjects. *Proc. R. Soc. Med.* 64:15, 1971.

53. Dale, H. H., and Laidlaw, P. P. The physiological action of beta-iminazolylethylamine. *J. Physiol.* (Lond.) 41:318, 1910.

54. Deal, E. C. Jr., et al. Evaluation of role played by mediators of immediate hypersensitivity in exercise-induced asthma. *J. Clin. Invest.* 65:659, 1980.

55. DeKock, M. A., et al. New method for perfusing bronchial arteries: histamine bronchoconstriction and apnea. *J. Appl. Physiol.* 21:185, 1966.

56. Delehunt, J. C., et al. Inhibition of antigen-induced bronchoconstriction by methylprednisolone succinate. *J. Allergy Clin. Immunol.* 73:479, 1984.

57. DeVries, K., et al. Changes during 24 hours in the lung function and histamine hyperreactivity of the bronchial tree in asthmatic and bronchitic patients. *Int. Arch. Allergy* 20:93, 1962.

58. Diaz, P., et al. Leukocytes and mediators in broncho-alveolar lavage during allergen-induced late-phase asthmatic reactions. *Am. Rev. Respir. Dis.* 139:1383, 1989.

59. Drazen, J. M., and Austen, K. F. Atropine modification of the pulmonary effects of chemical mediators in the guinea pig. *J. Appl. Physiol.* 38:834, 1975.

60. Dreborg, S., et al. Results of biological standardization with standardized allergen preparations. *Allergy* 42:109, 1987.

61. Durham, S. R., et al. Mechanisms of early and late asthmatic reactions. In C. E. Reed (ed.), *Proceedings XII International Congress of Allergology and Clinical Immunology.* St. Louis: Mosby, 1987, Pp. 229–236.

62. Dutoid, J. I., Salome, C. M., and Woolcock, A. J. Inhaled corticosteroids reduce the severity of bronchial hyperresponsiveness in asthma, but oral theophylline does not. *Am. Rev. Respir. Dis.* 136:1174, 1987.

63. Easton, J. G. Effect of an inhaled corticosteroid on methacholine airway reactivity. *J. Allergy Clin. Immunol.* 67:388, 1981.

64. Eggleston, P. A. A comparison of asthmatic response to methacholine and exercise. *J. Allergy Clin. Immunol.* 63:104, 1979.

65. Engstrom, I., and Vejinolovna, J. The effect of disodium cromoglycate on allergen challenge in children with bronchial asthma. *Acta Allergol.* 25: 382, 1970.

66. Fairfax, A. J. Inhibition of the late asthmatic response to house dust mite by non-steroidal antiinflammatory drugs. *Prostaglandins Leukot. Med.* 8: 239, 1982.

67. Falliers, C. Assessment of oral antiasthmatic drugs by inhalation challenge. *J. Allergy Clin. Immunol.* 64:685, 1979.

68. Finnerty, J. P., Wilmot, C., and Holgate, S. T. Inhibition of hypertonic saline–induced bronchoconstriction by terfenadine and flurbiprofen. *Am. Rev. Respir. Dis.* 140:593, 1989.

69. Fish, J. E., and Kelly, J. F. Measurements of responsiveness in bronchoprovocation testing. *J. Allergy Clin. Immunol.* 64:592, 1979.

70. Fish, J. E., Peterman, V. I., and Cugell, D. W. Effect of deep inspiration on airway conductance in subjects with allergic rhinitis and allergic asthma. *J. Allergy Clin. Immunol.* 60:41, 1977.

71. Fish, J. E., et al. Airway responses to methacholine in allergic and nonallergic subjects. *Am. Rev. Respir. Dis.* 113:579, 1976.

72. Fish, J. E., et al. The effect of atropine on acute antigen-mediated airway constriction in subjects with allergic asthma. *Am. Rev. Respir. Dis.* 115: 371, 1977.

73. Fish, J. E., et al. Indomethacin modification of immediate-type immunologic airway responses in allergic asthmatic and non-asthmatic subjects. *Am. Rev. Respir. Dis.* 123:609, 1981.

74. Foucard, T., Bennich, H., and Johansson, S. G. O. Studies on the stability of diluted allergen extracts using the radio-allergosorbent test (RAST). *Clin. Allergy* 3:91, 1975.

75. Foucard, T., et al. In vitro estimation of allergens by a radioimmune antiglobulin using IgE antibodies. *Int. Arch. Allergy* 43:360, 1976.

76. Frick, O. L. Perspectives in Allergen Standardization. In E. Mathow, T. Sindo, and P. Naranjo (eds.), *Allergy and Clinical Immunology.* Amsterdam: Excerpta Medica, 1976, P. 98.

77. Frick, W. E., Sedgwick, J. B., and Busse, W. W. The appearance of hypo-

dense eosinophils in antigen-dependent late phase asthma. *Am. Rev. Respir. Dis.* 139:1401, 1989.

78. Frith, P. A., et al. Inhibition of allergen-induced asthma by three forms of sodium cromoglycate. *Clin. Allergy* 11:67, 1981.

79. Gayrard, P., et al. Bronchoconstrictor effects of a deep inspiration in patients with asthma. *Am. Rev. Respir. Dis.* 111:433, 1975.

80. Georgopoulos, D., et al. Effect of salbutamol, ipratropium bromide and cromolyn sodium on prostaglandin F_{2a}-induced bronchospasm. *Chest* 96: 809, 1989.

81. Gerritsen, J., et al. Propranolol inhalation challenge in relation to 'histamine' response in children with asthma. *Thorax* 43:451, 1988.

82. Gervais, P., et al. Twenty-four-hour rhythm in the bronchial hyperreactivity to house dust in asthmatics. *J. Allergy Clin. Immunol.* 59:207, 1977.

83. Gimeno, F., et al. Spirometry-induced bronchial obstruction. *Am. Rev. Respir. Dis.* 105:66, 1972.

84. Gleich, G. J., et al. Measurement of potency of allergenic extracts by their inhibitory capacities in the radioallergosorbent test. *J. Allergy Clin. Immunol.* 53:158, 1974.

85. Gleich, G. J., et al. Differences in the reactivity of short and giant ragweed with immunoglobulin E antibodies. *J. Allergy Clin. Immunol.* 65:110, 1980.

86. Godfrey, S. Bronchial challenge by exercise or hyperventilation. In S. L. Spector (ed.), *Provocative Challenge Procedures: Background and Methodology.* Mount Kisco, NY: Futura, 1989, Pp. 365–394.

87. Goetzl, E. J. Mediators of immediate hypersensitivity derived from arachidonic acid. *N. Engl. J. Med.* 303:822, 1980.

88. Goetzl, E. J., and Pickett, W. C. Novel structural determinants of the human neutrophil chemotactic activity of leukotriene. *Br. J. Exp. Med.* 153;482, 1981.

89. Goldberg, I., and Cherniack, R. M. The effect of nebulized bronchodilator delivered with and without IPPB on ventilatory function in chronic obstructive emphysema. *Am. Rev. Respir. Dis.* 91:13, 1965.

90. Gonzalez M. C., et al. Allergen-induced recruitment of bronchoalveolar helper (OKT4) and suppressor (OKT8) T-cells in asthma. *Am. Rev. Respir. Dis.* 136:600, 1987.

91. Green, M., and Mead, J. Time dependence of flow volume curves. *J. Appl. Physiol.* 37:793, 1974.

92. Guinot, P., et al. Effect of BN 52063, a specific PAF-acether antagonist, on bronchial provocation test to allergens in asthmatic patients: a preliminary study. *Prostaglandins* 34:723, 1987.

93. Guirgis, H. M., and McNeill, R. S. The nature of adrenergic receptors in isolated human bronchi. *Thorax* 24:613, 1969.

94. Haahtela, T., and Lahdensuo, A. Non-specific reactions caused by diluents containing glycerol in nasal and bronchial challenge tests. *Clin. Allergy* 9:225, 1979.

95. Hahn, H. L., et al. Interaction between serotonin and efferent vagus nerves in dog lungs. *J. Appl. Physiol.* 44:144, 1978.

96. Hajos, M.-K. Clinical studies on the role of serotonin in bronchial asthma. *Acta Allergol.* 17:358, 1962.

97. Halpern, B. N., Neveu, T., and Spector, S. L. On the nature of the chemical mediators involved in anaphylactic reactions in mice. *Br. J. Pharmacol.* 20:389, 1963.

98. Hamilec, C. M., Manning, P. F., and O'Byrne, P. M. Exercise refractoriness post histamine bronchoconstriction in asthmatic subjects. *Am. Rev. Respir. Dis.* 138:794, 1988.

99. Hardy, C. C., et al. The bronchoconstrictor effect of inhaled prostaglandin D2 in normal and asthmatic men. *N. Engl. J. Med.* 311:209, 1984.

100. Hargreave, F. E., et al. The late asthmatic responses. *Can. Med. Assoc. J.* 110:415, 1974.

101. Hargreave, F. E., et al. Bronchial responsiveness to histamine or methacholine in asthma: measurement and clinical significance. *J. Allergy Clin. Immunol.* 68:347, 1981.

102. Harnett, J. C., Spector, S. L., and Farr, R. S. Aspirin idiosyncrasy, asthma and urticaria. In E. Middleton Jr., C. E. Reed, and E. F. Ellis (eds.), *Allergy: Principles and Practice.* St. Louis: Mosby, 1978, Pp. 1002–1021.

103. Herxheimer, H. Bronchial hypersensitization and hyposensitization in man. *Int. Arch. Allergy* 2:40 1951.

104. Herxheimer, H. G. J., and Brewersdorff, H. Disodium cromoglycate in the prevention of induced asthma. *Br. Med. J.,* 2:220, 1969.

105. Hoag, J. E., and McFadden, E. R. Long-term effect of cromolyn sodium on nonspecific bronchial hyperresponsiveness: a review. *Ann. Allergy* 66:1, 1991.

106. Holtzman, M. J., et al. Effect of ganglionic blockade on bronchial reactivity in atopic subjects. *Fed. Proc.* 38:1110, 1979.

107. Horton, D. G., et al. Bronchoconstrictive suggestion in asthma: a role for

airways hyperreactivity and emotions. *Am. Rev. Respir. Dis.* 117:1029, 1978.

108. Howard, P. H., et al. Influence of albuterol, cromolyn sodium and ipratropium bromide on the airway and circulating mediator responses to allergen bronchial provocation in asthma. *Am. Rev. Respir. Dis.* 132:986, 1985.

109. Huggins, K. G., and Brostoff, J. Local production of specific IgE antibodies in allergic rhinitis patients with negative skin tests. *Lancet* 2:148, 1975.

110. Hume, K. M., and Gandevia, B. Forced expiratory volume before and after isoprenaline. *Thorax* 12:276, 1957.

111. Ihre, E., Axelsson, I. G. K., and Zetterstrom, O. Late asthmatic reactions and bronchial variability after challenge with low doses of allergen. *Clin. Allergy* 18:557, 1988.

112. Ingram, R. H. Jr., and McFadden, E. R. Jr. Localization and mechanisms of airway responses. *N. Engl. J. Med.* 297:596, 1977.

113. Ingram, R. H. Jr., et al. Relative contributions of large and small airways to flow limitation in normal subjects before and after atropine and isoproterenol. *J. Clin. Invest.* 49:696, 1977.

114. Israel, E., et al. Effect of leukotriene antagonist, LY171883, on cold air–induced bronchoconstriction in asthmatics. *Am. Rev. Respir. Dis.* 140:1348, 1989.

115. Itkin, I. H. Bronchial hypersensitivity to mecholyl and histamine in asthma subjects. *J. Allergy* 40:245, 1967.

116. Itkin, I. H., and Anand, S. C. The role of atropine as a mediator blocker of induced bronchial obstruction. *J. Allergy* 45:178, 1970.

117. Ito, K., et al. IgG1 antibodies to house dust mite Dermatophagoides farinae and late asthmatic response. *Int. Arch. Allergy Appl. Immunol.* 81:69, 1986.

118. Josephs, L. K., et al. Nonspecific bronchial reactivity and its relationship to the clinical expression of asthma. *Am. Rev. Respir. Dis.* 140:350, 1989.

119. Joubert, J. R., et al. Non-steroidal anti-inflammatory drugs in asthma: dangerous or useful therapy? *Allergy* 40:202, 1985.

120. Juniper, E. F., Frith, P. A., and Hargreave, F. E. Airway responsiveness to histamine and methacholine relationship to minimum treatment to control symptoms of asthma. *Thorax* 36:575, 1981.

121. Juniper, E. F., et al. Reproducibility and comparison of responses to inhaled histamine methacholine. *Thorax* 33:705, 1978.

122. Juniper, E. F., et al. Improvement in airway responsiveness and asthma severity during pregnancy. *Am. Rev. Respir. Dis.* 140:924, 1989.

123. Juniper, E. F., et al. Reduction of budesonide after a year of increased use. *J. Allergy Clin. Immunol.* 87:483, 1991.

124. Kaufman, J., et al. Bronchial hyperreactivity and cough due to angiotensin-converting enzyme inhibitors. *Chest* 95:544, 1989.

125. Kerr, J. W., Govindaraj, M., and Patel, K. R. Effect of alpha-receptor blocking drugs and disodium cromoglycate on histamine hypersensitivity in bronchial asthma. *Br. Med. J.* 2:139, 1970.

126. Kerrebijn, J. F., van Essen-Zandvliet, E. E. M., and Neijens, H. J. Effect of long-term treatment with inhaled corticosteroids and beta agonists on the bronchial responsiveness in children with asthma. *J. Allergy Clin. Immunol.* 79:653, 1989.

127. Kiviloog, J. Bronchial reactivity to exercise and methacholine in bronchial asthma. *Scand. J. Respir. Dis.* 54:347, 1973.

128. Klaustermeyer, W. B., Hale, F. C., and Prescott, E. J. Characteristics of the asthmatic airway response to inhaled diluent. *Ann. Allergy* 43:14, 1979.

129. Klaustermeyer, W. B., Hale, F. C., and Prescott, E. J. Reproducibility of the response to diluent challenge in adult asthma. *Ann. Allergy* 43:84, 1979.

130. Koeter, G. H., et al. Effect of theophylline and enprofylline on bronchial hyperresponsiveness. *Thorax* 44:1022, 1989.

131. Kraan, J., et al. Changes in bronchial hyperreactivity induced by 4 weeks of treatment with antiasthmatic drugs in patients with allergic asthma: a comparison between budesonide and terbutaline. *J. Allergy Clin. Immunol.* 76:628, 1985.

132. Lai, C. K. W., Twentyman, O. P., and Holgate, S. T. The effect of an increase in inhaled allergen dose after rimiterol hydrobromide on the occurrence and magnitude of the late asthmatic response and the associated change in nonspecific bronchial responsiveness. *Am. Rev. Respir. Dis.* 140:917, 1989.

133. Lam, S., Wong, R., and Yeung, M. Nonspecific bronchial reactivity in occupational asthma. *J. Allergy Clin. Immunol.* 63:28, 1979.

134. Lemanske, R. F. Jr., and Kaliner, M. Late-phase IgE-mediated reactions. *J. Clin. Immunol.* 8:1, 1988.

135. Lesouef, P. N., et al. Response of normal infants to inhaled histamine. *Am. Rev. Respir. Dis.* 139:62, 1989.

136. Lindgren, B. R., et al. Increased bronchial reactivity and potentiated skin responses in hypertensive subjects suffering from cough during ACE-inhibitor therapy. *Chest* 95:1225, 1989.
137. Lupinetti, M. D., et al. Thromboxane biosynthesis in allergen-induced bronchospasm. *Am. Rev. Respir. Dis.* 140:932, 1989.
138. MacDonald, N. C. Stability of methacholine chloride in normal saline solution. Creighton University Ph.D. Thesis, 1979.
139. Machado, L. Increased bronchial hypersensitivity after early and late bronchial reactions provoked by allergen inhalation. *Allergy* 40:580, 1985.
140. Makino, S. Clinical significance of bronchial sensitivity to acetylcholine and histamine in bronchial asthma. *J. Allergy* 38:127, 1966.
141. Manning, P. J., Jones, G. L., and O'Byrne, P. M. Tachyphylaxis to inhaled histamine in asthmatic subjects. *J. Appl. Physiol.* 63:1572, 1987.
142. Manning, P. F., and O'Byrne, P. M. Histamine bronchoconstriction reduces airway responsiveness in asthmatic subjects. *Am. Rev. Respir. Dis.* 137:1323, 1988.
143. Marom, Z., et al. Slow-reacting substances, leukotrienes C4 and D4 increase the release of mucus from human airways in vitro. *Am. Rev. Respir. Dis.* 126:449, 1982.
144. Martin, G. L., et al., Effects of theophylline, terbutaline, and prednisone on antigen-induced bronchospasm and mediator release. *J. Allergy Clin. Immunol.* 66:204, 1980.
145. Mathe, A. A., and Hedqvist, P. Effects of prostaglandin F_2 alpha and E_2 on airway conductance in healthy subjects and asthmatic patients. *Am. Rev. Respir. Dis.* 111:313, 1975.
146. Mathe, A. A., et al. Bronchial hyperreactivity to prostaglandin F_2 alpha and histamine in patients with asthma. *Br. Med. J.* 1:193, 1973.
147. Mattoli, S., et al. Effects of two doses of cromolyn on allergen-induced late asthmatic response and increased responsiveness. *J. Allergy Clin. Immunol.* 79:747, 1987.
148. May, C. D., and Williams, C. S. Further studies concerning the fluctuating insensitivity of peripheral leukocytes to unrelated allergens and the meaning of nonspecific "desensitization." *Clin. Allergy* 3:319, 1973.
149. Mellis, C. M., et al. Comparative study of histamine and exercise challenges in asthmatic children. *Am. Rev. Respir. Dis.* 117:911, 1978.
150. Menardo, J. L., Bousquet, J., and Michel, F. B. Standardization of skin tests. In C. Molina (ed.), *Proceedings of the Annual Meeting of the European Academy of Allergology and Clinical Immunology. Technique et Documentation.* Paris: Lavoisier, 1983, Pp. 1018–1023.
151. Merck & Co., Inc.: *The Merck Index* (9th ed.). Rahway, NJ, 1976.
152. Metzger, W. J., Donnelly, A., and Richerson, H. B. Modification of late asthmatic responses during immunotherapy for Alternaria-induced asthma. *J. Allergy Clin. Immunol.* 75:121A, 1983.
153. Muranaka, M., Nakajima, K., and Suzuki, S. Bronchial responsiveness to acetylcholine in patients with bronchial asthma after long-term treatment with gold salt. *J. Allergy Clin. Immunol.* 67:350, 1981.
154. Murray, J. J., et al. Release of prostaglandin D_2 into human airways during acute antigen challenge. *N. Engl. J. Med.* 315:800, 1986.
155. Nadel, J. A., and Tierney, D. F. Effect of a previous deep inspiration on airway resistance in man. *J. Appl. Physiol.* 16:717, 1961.
156. Nagy, L., Lee, T. H., and Kay, A. B. Neutrophil chemotactic factor activity in antigen-induced late asthmatic reactions. *N. Engl. J. Med.* 306:497, 1982.
157. Nakamura, T., et al. Platelet-activating factor in late asthmatic response. *Int. Arch. Allergy Appl. Immunol.* 82:57, 1987.
158. Nakazawa, T., et al. Inhibitory effects of various drugs on dual asthmatic responses in wheat flour–sensitive subjects. *J. Allergy Clin. Immunol.* 58:1, 1976.
159. Nathan, R. A., et al. Relationship between airways response to allergens and nonspecific bronchial reactivity. *J. Allergy Clin. Immunol.* 64:491, 1979.
160. Nelson, J. S. The effect of preservatives and dilution on the deterioration of Russian Thistle (*Salsola perifer*), a pollen extract. *J. Allergy Clin. Immunol.* 63:417, 1979.
161. Newball, H. H., and Keiser, H. R. Relative effects of bradykinin and histamine on the respiratory system of man. *J. Appl. Physiol.* 35:552, 1973.
162. Nordic Council of Medicine. *Guidelines for the Registration of Allergen Preparations.* Uppsala, Sweden, 1980.
163. Norman, P. S., and Marsh, D. G. Human serum albumin and Tween 80 as stabilizers of allergen solutions. *J. Allergy Clin. Immunol.* 62:314, 1978.
164. Ogilvy, C. S., DuBois, A. B., and Douglas, J. S. Effects of ascorbic acid and indomethacin on the airways of healthy male subjects with and without induced bronchoconstriction. *J. Allergy Clin. Immunol.* 67:363, 1981.
165. Olgiati, R., et al. Differential effects of methacholine and antigen challenge on gas exchange in allergic subjects. *J. Allergy Clin. Immunol.* 67:325, 1981.
166. Olive, J. R. Jr., and Hyatt, R. E. Maximal expiratory flow and total respiratory resistance during induced bronchoconstriction in asthmatic subjects. *Am. Rev. Respir. Dis.* 106:366, 1972.
167. Oppenheimer, E. A., Rigatto, M., and Fletcher, C. M. Airways obstruction before and after isoprenaline, histamine, and prednisolone in patients with chronic obstructive bronchitis. *Lancet* 1:552, 1968.
168. Orehek, J., et al. Effect of beta-adrenergic blockade on bronchial sensitivity to inhaled acetylcholine in normal subjects. *J. Allergy Clin. Immunol.* 55:164, 1975.
169. Orehek, J., et al. Airway response to carbachol in normal and asthmatic subjects. *Am. Rev. Respir. Dis.* 115:937, 1977.
170. Orehek, J., et al. Bronchomotor effect of bronchoconstriction-induced deep aspirations in asthmatics. *Am. Rev. Respir. Dis.* 121:297, 1980.
171. Orehek, J., et al. Influence of the previous deep inspiration on the spirometric measurement of provoked bronchoconstriction in asthma. *Am. Rev. Respir. Dis.* 123:269, 1981.
172. Owen, S., et al. A randomized double blind placebo controlled crossover study of a potassium channel activator in morning dipping (abstract). *Thorax* 44:852P, 1989.
173. Paggiaro, P. L., and Chan Yeung, M. Pattern of specific airway responses in asthma due to western red cedar (*Thuja plicata*): relationship with length of exposure and lung function measurement. *Clin. Allergy* 17:333, 1987.
174. Patel, K. R., et al. The effect of thymoxamine and cromolyn sodium on post-exercise bronchoconstriction in asthma. *J. Allergy Clin. Immunol.* 57:285, 1976.
175. Patterson, R., Suszko, I. M., and Zeiss, C. R. Jr. Reactions of primate respiratory mast cells. *J. Allergy Clin. Immunol.* 50:7, 1972.
176. Pauli, B. D., et al. Influence of the menstrual cycle on airway function in asthmatic and normal subjects. *Am. Rev. Respir. Dis.* 140:358, 1989.
177. Pauwels, R. The effects of theophylline on airway inflammation. *Chest* 92:32A, 1987.
178. Pauwels, R., et al. The effect of theophylline and enprofylline on allergen-induced bronchoconstriction. *J. Allergy Clin. Immunol.* 76:583, 1985.
179. Pelikan, Z., et al. Effects of disodium cromoglycate and beclomethasone dipropionate on the asthma response to allergen challenge. I. Immediate response (IAR). *Ann. Allergy* 60:211, 1988.
180. Pennock, B. E., Rogers, R. M., and McCaffree, D. D. R. Changes in measured spirometric indices. What is significant? *Chest* 80:97, 1980.
181. Pepys, J., et al. The effects of inhaled beclomethasone dipropionate (Becotide) and sodium cromoglycate on asthmatic reactions to provocation tests. *Clin. Allergy* 4:12, 1974.
182. Phillips, G. D., Polosa, R., and Holgate, S. T. The effect of histamine-H_1 receptor antagonism with terfenadine on concentration-related AMP-induced bronchoconstriction in asthma. *Clin. Exp. Allergy* 19:405, 1989.
183. Pichurko, B. M., et al. Localization of the site of the bronchoconstrictor effects of leukotriene C_4 compared with that of histamine in asthmatic subjects. *Am. Rev. Respir. Dis.* 140:334, 1989.
184. Pison, C., et al. Bronchial hyper-responsiveness to inhaled methacholine in subjects with chronic left heart failure at a time of exacerbation and after increasing diuretic therapy. *Chest* 96:230, 1989.
185. Platts-Mills, T. A., et al. Reduction of bronchial hyperreactivity during prolonged allergen avoidance. *Lancet* 2:675, 1982.
186. Popa, V., Douglas, J. S., and Bouhuys, A. Airway responses to histamine, acetylcholine, and antigen in sensitized guinea pigs. *J. Lab. Clin. Med.* 84:226, 1974.
187. Price, J. F., et al. Controlled trial of hyposensitization to Dermatophagoides pteronyssinus in children with asthma. *Lancet* 2:912, 1978.
188. Pyrjma, J., et al. Decrease of complement hemolytic activity after an allergen-house dust-bronchial provocation test. *J. Allergy Clin. Immunol.* 70:306, 1982.
189. Rak, S., Lowhagen, O., and Venge, P. The effect of immunotherapy on bronchial hyperresponsiveness and eosinophil cationic protein in pollen-allergic patients. *J. Allergy Clin. Immunol.* 82:470, 1988.
190. Reinberg, A., et al. Circadian Rhythms in the Threshold of Bronchial Response to Acetylcholine in Healthy and Asthmatic Subjects. In. L. Scheving, F. Halberg, and J. Pauly (eds.), Tokyo: Igaku Shoin, 1974, P. 174.
191. Robertson, D., et al. Late asthmatic responses induced by ragweed pollen. *J. Allergy Clin. Immunol.* 54:244, 1974.
192. Rosenthal, R. R., Norman, P. S., and Summer, W. R. Bronchoprovocation: effect on priming and desensitization phenomena in the lung. *J. Allergy Clin. Immunol.* 56:338, 1975.

193. Rosenthal, R. R., et al. Role of the parasympathetic system in antigen-induced bronchospasm. *J. Appl. Physiol.* 42:600, 1977.

194. Ryan, G., et al. Standardization of inhalation provocation tests: two techniques of aerosol generation and inhalation compared. *Am. Rev. Respir. Dis.* 123:195, 1981.

195. Ryan, G., et al. Effect of beclomethasone dipropionate on bronchial responsiveness to histamine in controlled nonsteroid-dependent asthma. *J. Allergy Clin. Immunol.* 75:25, 1985.

196. Ryo, U. Y., and Townley, R. G. Comparison of respiratory and cardiovascular effects of iso-proterenol, propranolol, and practolol in asthmatic and normal subjects. *J. Allergy Clin. Immunol.* 57:12, 1976.

197. Salvaggio, J. E., and Hendrick, D. J. The Use of Bronchial Inhalation Challenge in the Investigation of Occupational Asthma. In S. L. Spector (ed.), *Provocative Challenge Procedures: Background and Methodology.* Mount Kisco, NY: Futura, 1989, Pp. 417–450.

198. Sasaki, F., et al. Bronchial hyperresponsiveness in patients with chronic congestive heart failure. *Chest* 97:534, 1990.

199. Schoeffel, R. E., et al. Multiple exercise and histamine challenge in asthmatic patient. *Thorax* 35:164, 1980.

200. Schwartz, L. B., et al. Tryptase levels as an indicator of mast-cell activation in systemic anaphylaxis and mastocytosis. *N. Engl. J. Med.* 316:1622, 1987.

201. Seibert, A. E., et al. Normal airway hyperresponsiveness to methacholine in cardiac asthma. *Am. Rev. Respir. Dis.* 140:1805, 1989.

202. Simonsson, B. G., et al. In vivo and in vitro effect of bradykinin on bronchial motor tone in normal subjects. *Respiration* 30:378, 1973.

203. Simpson, D. L., et al. Long-term follow-up and bronchial reactivity testing in survivors of the adult respiratory distress syndrome. *Am. Rev. Respir. Dis.* 117:449, 1978.

204. Smith, R. M., and Richerson, H. B. A longitudinal study of airway responsiveness to methacholine in ragweed hay fever patients (abstract). *Am. Rev. Respir. Dis.* 137:284, 1988.

205. Smolensky, M., Reinberg, A., and Quent, J. T. The chronobiology and chronopharmacology of allergy. *Ann. Allergy* 47:234, 1981.

206. Spector, S. L. Effect of a selective beta-2 adrenergic agonist and theophylline on skin test reactivity and cardiovascular parameters. *J. Allergy Clin. Immunol.* 64:23, 1979.

207. Spector, S. L. Use of provocation techniques for the evaluation of drug efficacy. *J. Allergy Clin. Immunol.* 64:677, 1979.

208. Spector, S. L. Bronchial Inhalation Challenges with Aerosolized Bronchoconstrictive Substances. In S. L. Spector (ed.), *Provocative Challenge Procedures: Bronchial, Oral, Nasal and Exercise: Vol. I.* Boca Raton, FL: CRC Press, 1983, Pp. 137–176.

209. Spector, S. L. Bronchial Provocation Tests. In E. B. Weiss, M. S. Segal, and M. Stein (eds.), *Bronchial Asthma: Mechanisms and Therapeutics,* (2nd ed.). Boston, Little, Brown, 1985, Pp. 360–379.

210. Spector, S. L., and Farr, R. S. Bronchial inhalation procedures in asthmatics. *Med. Clin. North Am.* 58:71, 1974.

211. Spector, S. L., and Farr, R. S. A comparison of methacholine and histamine inhalations in asthmatics. *J. Allergy Clin. Immunol.* 56:308, 1975.

212. Spector, S. L., and Farr, R. S. Bronchial provocation tests. In E. B. Weiss and M. S. Segal (eds.), *Bronchial Asthma: Mechanisms and Therapeutics.* Boston: Little, Brown, 1976, Pp. 639–647.

213. Spector, S. L., and Farr, R. S. Bronchial inhalation challenge with antigen. *J. Allergy Clin. Immunol.* 64:580, 1979.

214. Spector, S. L., Katz, F. H., and Farr, R. S. Troleandomycin: effectiveness in steroid dependent asthma and bronchitis. *J. Allergy Clin. Immunol.* 54:367, 1974.

215. Spector, S. L., and Souhrada, J. F. Maximal midexpiratory flow as an index of acute airway changes. *Chest* 68:851, 1975.

216. Spector, S. L., Wangaard, C. H., and Farr, R. S. Aspirin and concomitant idiosyncrasies in adult asthmatic patients. *J. Allergy Clin. Immunol.* 64:500, 1979.

217. Spector, S. L., et al. Response of asthmatics to methacholine challenge and suggestion. *Am. Rev. Respir. Dis.* 113:43, 1976.

218. Spector, S. L., et al. Methacholine and histamine inhalation challenges in asthma: relationship to age of onset, length of illness, and pulmonary function. *Allergy* 34:167, 1979.

219. Staudenmayer, H., et al. Medical outcome in asthmatic patients: effects of airway hyperreactivity and symptom-focused anxiety. *Psychosom. Med.* 41:109, 1979.

220. Szczeklik, A., et al. Aspirin-induced asthma and urticaria. *J. Allergy Clin. Immunol.* 58:10, 1976.

221. Tammeling, G. J., DeVries, K., and Kruyt, E. W. The Circadian Pattern of the Bronchial Reactivity to Histamine in Healthy Subjects and in Patients with Obstructive Lung Disease. In J. P. McGovern, M. Smolensky, and A. Reinberg (eds.), *Chronobiology in Allergy and Immunology.* Springfield, Ill.: Thomas, 1976.

222. Tarlo, S. M., and Broder, I. Irritant-induced occupational asthma. *Chest* 96:297, 1989.

223. Tiffeneau, R. Hypersensibilite pulmonaire de l'asthmatique a l'acetylcholine et a l'histamine. Similitude, differentiation pharmacodynamique. *Therapie* 11:715, 1956.

224. Tiffeneau, R. Hypersensibilite cholinergo-histaminique pulmonaire de l'asthmatique. *Acta Allergol.* 13:187, 1958.

225. Tiffeneau, R. Hyperexcitabilite bronchomotrice de l'asthmatique, sequelle des agressions bronchoconstrictive allergiques. *Acta Allergol.* 14:416, 1959.

226. Tiffeneau, R. Amples variations due degre de l'allergie pulmonaire produites par administration d'allergenes par voie respiratoire. *Int. Arch. Allergy* 17:193, 1960.

227. Tiffeneau, R., and Dunoyer, P. Action de la cortisone sur l'hypersensibilite cholinergique pulmonaire de l'asthmatique. *Presse Med.* 64:719, 1956.

228. Townley, R. G., Dennis, M., and Itkin, I. H. Comparative action of acetyl-beta-methylcholine, histamine and pollen antigens in subjects with hay fever and patients with bronchial asthma. *J. Allergy* 36:121, 1965.

229. Townley, R. G., McGeady, S., and Bewtra, A. The effect of beta-adrenergic blockade on bronchial sensitivity to acetyl-beta-methacholine in normal and allergic rhinitis subjects. *J. Allergy Clin. Immunol.* 57:358, 1976.

230. Townley, R. G., et al. Bronchial sensitivity to methacholine in current and former asthmatic and allergic rhinitis patients and control subjects. *J. Allergy Clin. Immunol.* 56:429, 1975.

231. Turkeltaub, P. C. Allergic Extracts: In Vivo Standardization. In: E. Middleton Jr., et al. (eds.), *Allergy, Principles and Practice* (3rd ed.). St. Louis: Mosby, 1988, Pp. 388–401.

232. Turkeltaub, P. C. et al. A standardized, quantitative skin test assay of allergen potency: studies on the allergen dose response curve and effects of wheal, erythema and patient selection on assay results. *J. Allergy Clin. Immunol.* 70:343, 1982.

233. Valliers, M., et al. Dimethyl ethanolamine–induced asthma. *Am. Rev. Respir. Dis.* 115:867, 1977.

234. Van Bever, H. P., and Stevens, W. J. Suppression of the late asthmatic reaction by hyposensitization in asthmatic children allergic to house dust mite (Dermatophagoides pteronyssinus). *Clin. Exp. Allergy* 19:399, 1988.

235. Varonier, H. S., and Panzani, R. The effect of inhalations of bradykinin on healthy and atopic (asthmatic) children. *Int. Arch. Allergy Appl. Immunol.* 34:293, 1968.

236. Vedal, S. S., et al. A longitudinal study of the occurrence of bronchial hyperresponsiveness in western red cedar workers. *Am. Rev. Respir. Dis.* 27:651, 1988.

237. Vincent, N. J., et al. Factors influencing pulmonary resistance. *J. Appl. Physiol.* 29:236, 1970.

238. Warner, J. O., et al. Controlled trial of hyposensitisation to Dermatophagoides pteronyssinus in children with asthma. *Lancet* 2:912, 1978.

239. Weiss, E. B., and Patwardhan, A. V. The response to lidocaine in bronchial asthma. *Chest* 72:429, 1977.

240. Wells, R. E., Walker, J. E. C., and Hickler, R. B. Effects of cold air on respiratory air flow resistance in patients with respiratory tract disease. *N. Engl. J. Med.* 303:822, 1980.

241. Williams, D. O., et al. Effect of nifedipine on bronchomotor tone on histamine reactivity in asthma. *Br. Med. J.* 283:348, 1981.

242. Woenne, R., Kattan, M., and Levison, H. Sodium cromoglycate-induced changes in the dose-response curve of inhaled methacholine and histamine in asthmatic children. *Am. Rev. Respir. Dis.* 119:927, 1979.

243. Woenne, R., et al. Bronchial hyperreactivity to histamine and methacholine in asthmatic children after inhalation of SCH1000 and chlorpheniramine maleate. *J. Allergy Clin. Immunol.* 62:119, 1978.

244. Woorhorst, R., and Spieksma, T. T. M. Recent progress in the house dust mite problem. *Acta Allergol.* 24:115, 1969.

245. Yu, D. T. C., Galant, S. P., and Gold, W. M. Inhibition of antigen-induced bronchoconstriction by atropine in asthmatic patients. *J. Appl. Physiol.* 32:823, 1972.

246. Zaid, G., and Beall, G. N. Bronchial response to beta-adrenergic blockade. *N. Engl. J. Med.* 275:580, 1966.

247. Zuskin, E., Lewis, A. J., and Bouhuys, A. Inhibition of histamine-induced airway constriction by ascorbic acid. *J. Allergy Clin. Immunol.* 51:218, 1973.

248. Boonsawat, W., et al. Effect of allergen inhalation on the maximal response plateau of the dose-response curve to methacholine. *Am. Rev. Respir. Dis.* 146:565, 1992.

Correlation Between History, Skin Test, and Inhalation Test Results in Allergic Asthma

40

Valentin T. Popa

The etiologic diagnosis of allergic asthma is currently made by assessing the physiologic effect of the immunoglobulin E (IgE)–allergen interaction on different target organs or, rarely, target cells. These sites include the bronchial tree (history, bronchial challenge with allergen), the skin (prick or intradermal tests with allergen), or the peripheral basophils (allergen-induced histamine release). In selected cases, these diagnostic modalities are complemented by the measurement of specific IgE levels in serum.

The history of asthma includes two sets of data: (1) the description of symptoms suggestive of this disease (Areteus the Cappadocian, second century A.D.) and (2) the possible relationship between these symptoms and various triggering factors. These triggering factors may be physical (Maimonides, twelfth century A.D.), allergic (Ramazzini, who in the sixteenth century described flour-induced asthma in bakers), pharmacologic (e.g., β_2 agonist [106] or angiotensin converting enzyme inhibitors [131]), and so forth.

Skin testing and inhalation testing with pollen grains were studied in the context of hay fever by Blackley (1873). He proposed that the pollen held responsible for a patient's hay fever, if brought in contact with the skin or inhaled, may produce a skin or nasal reaction, respectively. The latter duplicates the complaints elicited by natural exposure [19].

It was Rackemann who clarified the role of skin testing and history in the diagnosis of asthma. His statement from 1918 still forms the basis of the etiologic diagnosis of allergic asthma: "Skin tests alone are of no value, unless reasonably compatible with the patient's history and experience" [146].

Allergen solutions, similar to those used in skin testing, were applied in inhalation tests in the 1930s (Stevens [158]). The respiratory manifestations induced by these inhalation tests were first assessed clinically (Stevens [158]) and subsequently physiologically, by recording the vital capacity (Herxheimer in late 1940s and early 1950s [70]) or the forced expiratory volume in 1 second (FEV_1) (Tiffeneau in the 1950s [166]). Since then, a multitude of pulmonary function tests have been used to assess the changes induced by allergen provocation [41, 68]. The most sensitive and specific are the tests measuring either directly or indirectly the flow resistive properties of the bronchi: pulmonary and airway resistance/conductance (e.g., SGaw) or FEV_1, respectively. The superior performance of these tests is explained by the equation describing the mechanical changes in airway caliber: resistance = pressure/flow. The method of quantitative nebulization of increasing concentrations of allergen initiated by Tiffeneau [166] was subsequently modified by several authors [35, 38, 130] (Chap. 39). The FEV_1 end point in allergen challenge tests was initially set at −10 percent or greater [166] and, more recently, at −20 percent [35, 38]. This latter change is possibly too large. Indeed, in diagnostic bronchoprovocation with histamine or cholinergic agents, the end point fulfills two functions: (1) it ascer-

tains the presence of an acute credible bronchoconstriction and (2) it discriminates between normal and asthmatic subjects [139]. In challenges with allergens or physical agents, one is solely interested in achieving the first goal. The second goal does not apply because these challenges, which are generally negative in normals, are used in known asthmatic patients to document the role of certain triggering factors. Thus, the smallest change that is physiologically convincing should suffice.

Experiments with purified and standardized allergens have shown that the aerosol particles that are the most likely to penetrate and deposit deep into the lung actually contain the major component of this allergen [53]. This legitimizes the use of allergen nebulization as a means of mimicking the natural exposure to the same allergen. The study by Findlay and colleagues [53], along with previous [130] or subsequent reports [24, 50, 175], has indicated that the usual dose of inhaled allergen during challenge test is of the nanogram order and is up to ten times larger than that reported during natural exposure. If purified allergens are appropriately standardized, the biologically equivalent dose of inhaled allergen is similar for different allergens in different subjects. So far, the bronchial responses to the purified allergens tested have had a similar lognormal distribution, with a similar median [50].

Despite major accomplishments in the standardization of allergens and allergen response, there are still basic limitations in our ability to identify the offending allergen in asthma. One of these limitations is that the etiologic diagnosis of allergic asthma is based on the correlation between IgE-mediated responses in different compartments, usually the skin and the lung; however, IgE–mast cell interaction may be heterogeneous in these compartments. A second limitation is that the amount of allergen inhaled, and hence the amount of mediator released, are ostensibly different in the naturally induced attack (as revealed by history) and the iatrogenically induced airway response to allergen (bronchial) challenge. A third limitation is that the large dose of allergen used in the iatrogenically induced response may favor the appearance of a biphasic asthmatic reaction [117] and prevent the development of another variety of late asthmatic response, apparently with clinical relevance—the isolated reaction produced by small doses of allergen [79].

A clear understanding of the relationship between history, skin tests, and bronchial tests is of paramount importance in the evaluation and treatment of asthma since in this country 58 to 87 percent of asthmatics may have an allergic component [82, 160].

THE MAIN FACTORS INVOLVED IN IgE-MEDIATED REACTIONS TO ALLERGEN IN THE SKIN AND BRONCHI

This section will examine the immunopharmacologic coordinates of the relationship between skin and bronchial sensitivity to allergen.

In the lung and skin, the reaction between allergen and IgE antibody involves two immune factors (the allergen and the specific IgE), the mast cell on which IgE is attached via a high affinity antibody [109] and which releases bronchoconstrictor mediators, and the bronchial and vascular smooth muscle [32]. In the lung, the early phase of allergen-IgE reaction is essentially spasmogenic and edematous, reflecting the action of mast cell mediators on bronchial smooth muscle and vascular permeability. The responsiveness of this muscle is a major modulator of the spasmogenic response to allergen [137, 140, 166]. In the skin, the early phase is a wheal and flare reaction, with histamine and substance P being, respectively, the major mediators involved [56]. The early phase is followed both in the skin and in the lung by a late phase [49, 70, 117, 144]. Anatomically, it is characterized by an infiltrate containing neutrophils, eosinophils, macrophages, lymphocytes and mast cells [57, 117], and also by edema [89] and muscular spasm [70]. The mediators of this late phase are not well understood. They seem to include the same mediators released during the early phase [117]. The differences between early and late phase response in time course, pharmacologic modulation and participation of bronchial nonspecific responsiveness suggest the involvement of other factors. So far, such factors remain hypothetical (e.g., the possible release of other mediators, the possible continuous rate of liberation of histamine, prostanoids and leukotrienes, or the indirect influence of various cytokines on mediator release).

The mediators and cytokines released during allergen-IgE antibody reaction act on many other cells besides the smooth muscle and inflammatory cells. For instance, the bronchial (epithelial) and vascular (endothelial) permeability as well as the secretions of bronchial glands [32] are generally increased while the bronchial arteries are dilated [182].

At the present time, it is not clear how many of the complex events observed in allergen-IgE antibody reaction influence the relationship between skin and bronchial sensitivity in asthma. For this reason, the focus of this section will be on the immunologic and cellular factors that are absolutely essential in the allergen-IgE antibody reaction in these tissues: allergen, specific IgE, mast cell, and smooth muscle. Since the same allergen is used to compare skin and bronchial sensitization, its mode of presentation rather than its nature is important for this diagnostic comparison. Consequently, three of the basic factors in allergen-IgE reaction will be reviewed in this section, while the allergen presentation will be discussed in the section comparing skin and bronchial test results.

The Mast Cell

In comparing the role of skin and lung responses to allergen one needs to consider the main properties of the mast cell: heterogeneity, releasability, and sensitivity.

Mast Cell Heterogeneity

There are many similarities but also many differences in the structural and functional aspects of mast cells, of different species and in the same species, across organs and even within the same organ [18, 79, 97, 122]. For instance, although most lung mast cells belong to the mucosal group (Mm), there are also a few of the connective tissue type (Mct) [79, 97, 122]. Moreover, mast cells of the same type may be heterogeneous in the same individual; a pertinent example is the partial functional difference between mucosal lung mast cells of normal and atopic individuals [18, 79]. The similarity in histamine content and mediators released by skin and lung mast cells during the early phase of allergen-IgE reaction—histamine, prostanoids, and leukotrienes—explains why the skin tests can provide indications regarding bronchial sensitization. In addition, in both skin and lung,

allergen challenge produces a graded response taking the form of a log dose response curve [35, 159]; these curves display a large interindividual variability and might be flatter in the skin than in the bronchi [35, 100], but in the lung and skin they have the same important modulator: the histamine responsiveness of the bronchial muscle and skin vessels [162]. However, unlike in the lung, in the skin, histamine responsiveness of the smooth muscle is not increased [179].

Some differences between skin mast cells and bronchoalveolar or parietal lung mast cells [36, 37, 91, 97, 122] may explain in part why the dose of allergen capable of stimulating the mast cells is much smaller in the lung than in the skin. For instance, following anti-IgE challenge, the lung mast cells, compared to the homologous skin cells, release a higher concentration of constrictor mediators (e.g., five times more histamine and nine times more leukotrienes) and with a higher proportion of potent LTD4/LTE4 constrictor agents [148].

Two differences in the lung mast cell populations, both potentially magnifying the response to inhaled allergen, may be clinically relevant. First, the intraluminal mast cells as compared to parietal mast cells appear to be a thousand times more sensitive to anti-IgE, although they do not release leukotrienes [63, 79, 167]. Second, the spontaneous mast cell release of histamine and arachidonic acid metabolites in the lung of asthmatic subjects [33, 55, 61, 86, 91], an excellent illustration of lung mast cell heterogeneity within the same species, may increase the responsiveness of the bronchial muscle to various constrictor mediators [33, 55]. Such an effect may be achieved in two ways: (1) a progressive increase in the lung concentration of histamine may augment airway obstruction as measured by FEV_1 [55]; and (2) these bronchoconstrictor mediators may potentiate the action of other constrictor agents, independent of the changes in the smooth muscle length [68]. The heterogeneity in IgE responsiveness between skin and lung mast cells (see above), together with the just mentioned heterogeneity of lung mast cells in terms of spontaneous release of mediators and increased sensitivity to immunologic secretagogues, tends to increase the response to inhaled allergen. One may speculate that these two aspects of mast cell heterogeneity, in conjunction with an increased histamine releasability and bronchial hyperresponsiveness to mast cell mediators, may explain in part why a positive bronchial test, requiring relatively small doses of allergen in comparison with skin testing, is usually associated with a positive skin test [2, 34, 41, 52, 141, 155]. Indeed, the nanograms of allergen needed to produce a bronchial response—apparently covering a surface of ten, if not hundreds of, square centimeters—may be only a few times higher than the dose required for a small skin response [24, 50, 53, 130, 175]. These observations may also explain why a positive bronchial test is usually associated with a positive skin test and why the opposite (a positive bronchial test associated with a negative skin test) would not be expected to be true. Considering that history represents a natural bronchial test, the above considerations should also apply to the relationship between positive history and positive or negative skin tests [141].

There are, however, many other structural and functional differences between skin (Mct) and lung mast cells (Mm) or between parietal and bronchoalveolar mast cells, but to date, these discrepancies do not seem to affect the relationship between skin and lung sensitivity to allergen. Examples of such discrepancies include the ability of skin mast cells to react to some neurotransmitters (e.g., substance P) or basic peptides of eosinophil [36, 97, 122], which are all released during attacks of asthma or the wheal and flare reaction to allergen. The selective responsiveness of lung mast cells to cromolyn glycate [37, 93] is therapeutically relevant but has no diagnostic corollary.

Mast Cell Releasability

The amount [42] and speed [148] of mediator release from mast cells or basophils (i.e., releasability) may vary from individual to individual. As a typical example, the histamine released by allergens from mast cells or basophils is not related directly to the amount of IgE antibody circulating or located on the cellular surface, but is related to an intrinsic property of these cells [42, 103]. Releasability thus connotes the characteristic capacity of the mast cells or basophils of different subjects to release variable amounts of histamine or other mediators in response to the same dose of secretagogue. I think it is essentially similar to intrinsic activity, a now classic property of drug receptors. The peripheral basophil [11] and the intraluminal mast cell [33, 53, 61, 86, 91] may have a superior releasability of histamine via IgE receptor in atopic and asthmatic subjects [103]. Thus, releasability may contribute to the enhanced responses to allergen of these subjects.

Peripheral basophils, although easy to obtain, are no substitute for bronchoalveolar or lung mast cells. Despite many similarities, the nature, dynamics, and proportion of mediators released from peripheral basophils and lung mast cells seem to be markedly different [79, 97, 122]. Thus, peripheral basophils may be used to determine whether an individual has circulating specific IgE—which is attached to its surface—but not as a substitute for intraluminal or intrabronchial mast cells. Since mediator release from basophils is not modulated by the degree of bronchial responsiveness to these agents, IgE-mediated histamine release from basophils could hardly reflect bronchial responses to allergen. Interestingly, in the nose, the IgE-mediated allergic reaction involves the participation of basophils in the late reaction [78].

Mast Cell Sensitivity

Another factor that could influence the correlation between skin and mast cell responses to allergen is mast cell sensitivity [97]. This new parameter is different from releasability, as it pertains to the mast cell response to small rather than large doses of allergen. It is conceptually challenging but of undetermined clinical relevance.

Specific IgE. In principle, the correlation between skin and bronchial sensitivity to allergen could be affected by the serum concentration of IgE and its affinity either for antigen, via the Fab fragment, or for mast cell and basophil membrane, via the Fc fragment. Considering the complex technical problems raised by the isolation of the IgE receptor, only the concentration of serum-specific IgE could be shown to influence bronchial and skin sensitivity to allergen. A high concentration of this immunoglobulin, as assessed, for instance, by passive transfer [88] or commonly by the radioallergosorbent test (RAST), is associated with an increased response of both skin and bronchi to allergen [4, 8, 13–15, 31, 40, 50, 76, 172] (Fig. 40-1). The basic implication of these findings is that, the higher the concentration of circulating IgE, the higher the number of molecules of this immunoglobulin located on the skin or lung mast cells. However, the "dose" of IgE affixed to the surface of these cells is not the only determinant of the cellular response to allergen. As noted before, releasability, a functional mast cell parameter, is an important modulator of this IgE-dependent response.

As will be discussed later, it is possible that the interface between the specific IgE and the IgE receptor of the lung mast cell could be disease specific. This is purely hypothetical, because the receptor affinity for IgE has yet to be correlated with the results of bronchial tests.

Bronchial Nonspecific Responsiveness. Compared to normal individuals, asthmatic subjects exhibit a characteristic airway hyperreactivity to chemical or physical constrictor agents [5]. The hyperresponsiveness of bronchial muscle in asthma contrasts with the usual normal responsiveness of the nasal or skin vascular muscle in hay fever or in normal and asthmatic subjects [107, 179]. As initially proposed by Tiffeneau [166], bronchial hyperresponsiveness may magnify the action of the various mediators released during the immediate allergic reaction. Tiffeneau also made the disconcerting observation that, in some subjects, bronchial allergy is comparatively much weaker than bronchial nonspecific responsiveness, whereas, in other sub-

Fig. 40-1. *Correlation between concentrations of specific IgE (in ng/ml) and bronchial sensitivity to allergen (birch pollen). Note that bronchial sensitivity increases after circulating specific IgE exceeds 500 ng/ml. w/v = weight per volume. (Reprinted with permission from T. Berg and S. G. O. Johansson, Allergy diagnosis with the radioallergosorbent test.* J. Allergy Clin. Immunol. *56:209, 1974.)*

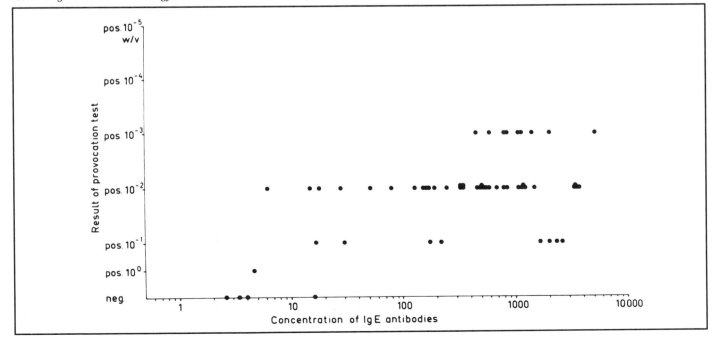

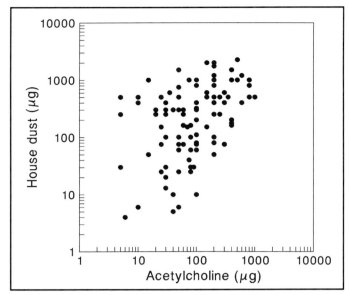

Fig. 40-2. *Correlation between bronchial sensitivity to allergen, expressed as micrograms of qualitatively delivered house dust extract, and bronchial responsiveness to acetylcholine, expressed as micrograms of quantitatively delivered dose. The numerical data of Tiffeneau [166] were plotted on the log–log axis.*

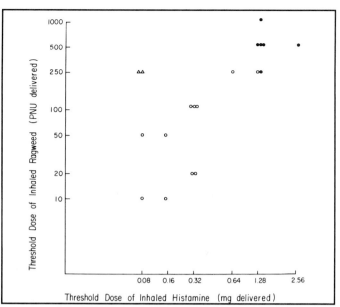

Fig. 40-3. *Correlation between threshold dose of inhaled (strictly quantitative nebulization) histamine and threshold dose (expressed as dose delivered and inhaled) of inhaled ragweed. In this study, 1000-PNU (protein nitrogen unit) ragweed extract had 2.2 mg of antigen E. Note the low-threshold dose to histamine contrasting with the high-threshold dose to allergen in two asthmatic patients who had hay fever only during ragweed season (triangles). Open circles = bronchial asthma; closed circles = hay fever only. (Reprinted with permission from V. Popa, Respiratory allergy to ragweed: correlation of bronchial responses to allergen and bronchial responses to histamine and circulating immunoglobulin E. J. Allergy Clin. Immunol. 65:389, 1980.)*

jects, the former is considerably greater than the latter. Figure 40-2, representing a plot on a log–log axis of Tiffeneau's numerical results [166], shows that the relationship between allergic sensitivity (expressed as micrograms of house dust extract inhaled) and acetylcholine responsiveness (expressed as micrograms of drug inhaled) has indeed a large interindividual variability; at times, more than two log units of allergen concentration correspond to the same degree of acetylcholine responsiveness. In the 1960s and 1970s, with rare dissenting opinions [28, 29], other authors have subsequently found that bronchial responses to allergen correlate closely with bronchial responses to histamine or cholinergic agents (Table 40-1). Taken together, the studies shown in Table 40-1 are convincing, although there is probably no single ideal study combining the use of a large population sample with optimal physiologic and immunologic methods. A major objection that may be leveled at some of these studies pertains to the use of different allergens in the subjects tested;

without immunologic and biologic standardization [3, 23, 50, 159], one cannot confidently compare the bronchial responses produced by different allergens in the same subject, let alone in different individuals.

The only study using standardized allergen and reproducible airway responses supports the positive correlation between nonspecific bronchial responsiveness and bronchial allergic sensitivity [130] (Fig. 40-3). The study suggests that an additional factor may modulate this relationship—the interface between the lung mast cell and specific IgE. As shown in Figure 40-3, two asthmatic subjects with high bronchial sensitivity to histamine who had

Table 40-1. *Studies indicating a relationship between nonspecific bronchial responsiveness and bronchial sensitivity to allergen*

			Method		Allergen			
Reference	No. of subj.	Diagnosis	Reprod.	Quant.	Diff.	Same	Mono	NSBR
Tiffeneau, 1958 [166]	100	A	No	Yes	No	Yes	No	ACh
Popa, 1967 [140]	98	A	No	No	Yes	No	No	ACh
Zuidema, 1969 [184]	80	A	No	No	No	Yes	No	H
Popa et al., 1969 [135]	28	A	No	No	No	No	Yes	ACh
Kreukniet, 1973 [87]	740	A	No	No	Yes	No	No	H
Bryant and Burns, 1975 [31]	15	A	No	No	Yes	No	No	H
Kilian et al., 1976 [85]	9	A	No	No	Yes	No	No	H
Nathan et al., 1979 [114]	54	A	No	No	Yes	No	No	H, M
Neijens et al., 1979 [115]	30	A	No	No	No	Yes	No	H
Popa, 1980 [130]	20	A + HF	Yes	Yes	No	Yes*	No	H
Cockcroft et al., 1979 [40]	25	A	No	No	Yes	No	No	H

Reprod. = reproducibility; Quant. = quantitative; Diff. = different allergens in different subjects; Same = same allergen in all subjects; Mono = the only allergen producing positive inhalation tests (monosensitization); NSBR = nonspecific bronchial responsiveness; H = histamine; ACh = acetylcholine; M = methacholine; A = asthma; HF = hay fever; * = standardized as ragweed antigen E.

severe asthma attacks when exposed to animals, but complained of hay fever during ragweed season, exhibited only a mild bronchial sensitivity to nebulized ragweed extract; their bronchial sensitivity to this allergen was comparable to that observed in subjects with ragweed hay fever but without asthma. Unlike the two asthmatics with hay fever, the hay fever subjects displayed, as expected, a low bronchial responsiveness to histamine. This discrepancy in the correlation between nonspecific responsiveness and allergic sensitivity of the bronchi should not be surprising; many patients with allergic asthma, presumably with high nonspecific bronchial responsiveness and high bronchial sensitivity to allergen, may develop skin rashes rather than wheezing when exposed to other allergens (e.g., sulfa drugs, food). Considered together, the limited experimental and clinical evidence mentioned previously raise the possibility that the interface between lung mast cells and IgE may be disease specific.

Other data suggest that the interaction between specific IgE and mast cells may be organ specific. For instance, hay fever patients may harbor specific IgE antibodies in their nasal secretions without displaying a positive skin test to the corresponding allergen [77, 108, 126]. Then, the IgE-mediated biphasic reaction may involve different organs in different subjects [145]. Finally, asymptomatic subjects with circulating anti–bee venom antibodies may not have these antibodies in their nasal secretions [84]. More recently, a genetic basis has been proposed for the localization to the nose of pollen sensitization [20].

The organ or disease-specific heterogeneity, or both, of the IgE–mast cell interaction may reflect, among many possible causes, a heterogeneity of the IgE molecules. This is suggested by the results of at least three series of experiments: (1) the increased release of histamine by anti-IgE from leukocytes of asthmatic patients [11]; (2) the intersubject variability of antibody-combining sites for the same antigen [143]; and (3) the variable effect of heating on IgE-inhibition curves across subjects [138]. Obviously, refined biochemical arguments are needed to establish the concept of IgE heterogeneity and its clinical relevance. A first step is the discovery of a new IgE isoform bound to cell membranes [124].

The relationship between bronchial nonspecific responsiveness and bronchial sensitivity to allergen represents a fundamental aspect of airway immunology, since it can be demonstrated not only in humans but also in animals. In animals, it was initially observed in the guinea pig [137] and subsequently extended to other animal species (e.g., the monkey [21]). Thus, when IgE or IgG antibodies against allergens are attached to lung mast cells, allergen-induced bronchoconstriction is modulated by bronchial nonspecific responsiveness. Intriguingly, as indicated by Figure 40-4, the ratio of bronchial sensitivity to allergen nonspecific bronchial responsiveness is several degrees of magnitude lower in animals, which cannot develop spontaneous asthma, than in humans. This further emphasizes the importance of the IgE– (or IgG–) mast cell interface.

The curve relating bronchial responsiveness to histamine or cholinergic agents and bronchial sensitivity to allergen seems to be linear on log–log plots or on arithmetic coordinates. Its steepness may vary with the degree of bronchial nonspecific responsiveness: If bronchial nonspecific responsiveness is high (i.e., in most asthmatics), the curve's angle is approximately 45 degrees [30, 40, 130]; if it is mild (some asthmatics [130] and in hay fever subjects [30]) or even normal (asymptomatic subjects with nonclinical sensitization [30]), the allergen responses seem to plateau.

The concept that in both humans and animals, the degree of bronchial responsiveness to mast cell mediators modulates the airway responsiveness to allergen needed 20 years before it was accepted (1960s and 1970s). Even more difficult to accept was the clinical relevance of bronchial nonspecific hyperresponsiveness for allergic asthma. This enhanced responsiveness to bron-

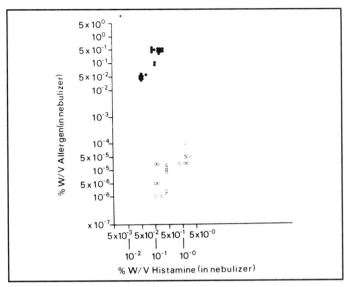

Fig. 40-4. *Correlation between threshold dose of inhaled histamine and threshold dose of inhaled allergen in anaphylactic asthma of the guinea pig (closed circles), and in human asthma and hay fever (open circles). %W/V = percent weight per volume concentration. (Reprinted with permission from V. Popa, Respiratory allergy to ragweed: correlation of bronchial responses to allergen and bronchial responses to histamine and circulating immunoglobulin E. J. Allergy Clin. Immunol. 65:389, 1980.)*

choconstrictor mediators of mast cells or other chemical or physical agents is clinically relevant for two reasons. First, the mast cell mediators released during allergen-specific IgE reaction play an important role in the genesis of bronchoconstriction. After H_1 blockers were able to blunt allergen-induced asthma [72, 131], various competitive antagonists for leukotrienes (e.g., ICI 204219 for leukotrienes LTD4/LTE4 [163]) or thromboxane antagonists acting on T1 receptors (e.g., GR32191 [16, 54]) were found to have a similar action. Animal experiments with an antagonist of platelet-activating factors seem promising. Second, the release of mast cell mediators (and other inflammatory cells?) may increase bronchial nonspecific hyperreactivity in both humans and animals following the early [137, 166] as well as the late phase [38, 117]. The pathogenesis of nonspecific bronchial hyperresponsiveness is still not elucidated. One possible mechanism may be a post-receptor enhancement of receptor signals [132, 133]. It is conceivable that the histamine and leukotrienes liberated spontaneously during intercritical periods [33, 55, 61, 86, 91] may enhance bronchial hyperresponsiveness.

Consider that the bronchodilation produced by H_1 blockers is a reliable index of the histamine concentration bathing the bronchi. As shown many years ago, chlorpheniramine-induced bronchodilation is usually seen in asthmatic subjects [129, 133] who show hyperresponsiveness to histamine. However, the former is unrelated to the latter [133]. Furthermore, patients with similar histamine hyperresponsiveness may or may not bronchodilate after chlorpheniramine [131, 133], suggesting that the concentration of histamine in the bronchi is not a determinant of histamine hyperresponsiveness. Incidentally, this may be a more general phenomenon since bronchial hyperresponsiveness to cholinergic agonist is not related to the degree of atropine-induced bronchodilation in normal or in asthmatic subjects [132]. In essence, nonspecific bronchial responsiveness may play an important role in localizing to the bronchi an IgE-mediated process by augmenting the effect of the constrictor mast cell mediators and being itself enhanced for variable periods of time by these mediators.

Nonspecific bronchial responsiveness remains the factor that best explains, though still insufficiently, the localization of asthma to the bronchi. As mentioned before, it appears that genetic factors related to mast cell-IgE interface or to mast cell heterogeneity and releasability in atopic subjects may contribute to the localization of allergy to bronchi.

In summary, this section suggests that basic science findings are consistent with many important clinical observations regarding the correlation between history, bronchial test results, and skin test results. With the caution that they are the product of extrapolation rather than direct demonstration and are pertinent to the early phase only, one may advance the following propositions:

1. A positive history or bronchial provocation test is expected to be associated with a positive skin test because (a) the various mast cell populations are more sensitive to allergen stimulation than their skin counterpart, the concentration of potent bronchoconstrictor mediators being higher in the former than in the latter; (b) the lung mast cells release histamine and possibly prostaglandins during intercritical periods, and these agents may increase the resting bronchial tone and the degree of resting bronchoconstriction, thereby augmenting allergen responsiveness; (c) bronchial hyperresponsiveness to the bronchoconstrictor mediators released by mast cells augments bronchial responses to allergen; and (d) lung mast cells may have an increased releasability to histamine.

2. A positive history and a positive skin test would be expected, for the same reasons mentioned previously, to be associated with a positive bronchial test.

3. A negative skin test is expected to be associated with a negative history and a negative bronchial test because there is no evidence that any of the previously listed factors could make the skin tests more sensitive than the bronchial response to allergen.

4. A positive skin test would not be expected to be invariably associated with a positive history or a positive bronchial test because we know only one of the localizing factors of bronchial asthma, bronchial responsiveness. For example, assuming that bronchial responsiveness is normal, its localizing effect may be overcome by increasing the concentration of inhaled allergen. This may account, at least in part, for the positive bronchial tests in hay fever or atopic dermatitis subjects (i.e., negative history of asthma but positive bronchial and skin test results). There are, however, many patients with hay fever who have mild bronchial hyperreactivity and yet do not wheeze.

Conditions Affecting the Relationship Between Skin and Bronchial Test Results. Many agents (physical, immunologic, or pharmacologic) acting on the four essential factors participating in allergen-induced skin and bronchial reactions (i.e., allergen, specific IgE, mast cell, and vascular or bronchial muscle) may alter the relationship between skin and bronchial sensitivity to allergen.

In practice, the agents that interfere most frequently with this relationship are allergen-related: allergen avoidance, seasonal exposure to allergen, immunotherapy, and the actual moment of the allergen response (early versus late). The outgrowing of asthma, with its characteristic blunting of asthma attacks, may also affect bronchial and possibly cutaneous sensitivity. It is for this reason that the relationship between history and skin and bronchial sensitivity to allergen will be examined separately for the early and late phase of allergen response, or during interventions meant to change the allergen exposure or action. The effect of the agents modulating primarily IgE, the mast cells, or the smooth muscle independent of allergen action will not be discussed since most if not all of these agents may not be diagnostically relevant.

GENERAL CHARACTERISTICS OF HISTORY, SKIN, AND PROVOCATION TESTS WITH ALLERGEN

For the diagnosis of allergic attacks of asthma, the natural exposure to allergen (history) or the reproduction of this exposure in the laboratory (provocation tests) offers important etiopathogenic information: Etiologically, history and provocation tests relate the attacks of asthma to an identifiable agent; pathophysiologically, the agent revealed by history and challenge tests is considered to be an allergen, either according to the current consensus or directly by testing the patient under consideration. As an example of how current consensus operates, if the agent is present in low concentration, both under natural and laboratory conditions, and it leads to extrapulmonary allergic symptoms in the patient evaluated, an allergic mechanism appears very likely.

In contrast to history and provocation tests, the information provided by skin tests is primarily pathogenic. If performed using an ideal technique, a positive skin test implies that the offending agent has reacted with skin-sensitizing antibodies; these antibodies, generally but not exclusively, belong to the IgE class. Thus, the correlation between history, skin and bronchial responses to allergen establishes a probable etiopathogenic diagnosis for the attacks of allergic IgE-mediated asthma. A definitive etiopathogenic diagnosis would require, in addition, the demonstration of a specific IgE antibody against the offending allergen. Such a measurement, generally performed on serum, is not only expensive but also redundant, considering the ostensible rarity of non–IgE-mediated allergic asthma.

The validity of these three diagnostic methods (history, skin tests, and bronchial provocation tests) depends on their quality control, i.e., control (test or situational), precision, reproducibility, and accuracy.

Since skin and bronchial tests using allergens can be measured objectively and quantitatively, while history represents a subjective and qualitative assessment, there are substantial similarities and differences between the quality control parameters of these diagnostic methods. For history, the control is represented by a comparable environment but without the targeted allergen; for example, the same geographic location, with and without seasonal exposure to a certain pollen, or the same home, with and without exposure to cat or seasonal multiplication of mites. Precision is the ability to reproduce the same results, or in the case of history, the demonstration that under natural conditions an agent repeatedly produces attacks of asthma. Reproducibility is the deviation from results when the method (history) is applied over a finite period of time. Accuracy reflects how close the historical observation is to the true relationship between agent and asthma.

History as well as skin and bronchial tests with allergen may be considered truly positive when the physiologic and etiopathogenic information indicates that an agent produces attacks of asthma most likely through an allergic mechanism. Any one of these three clinical parameters may become falsely positive when the response is present but for various reasons it is not produced by an allergic mechanism. These clinical parameters are considered negative when the response is absent; this absence of response may be real (truly negative) or, if due to inappropriate observation or testing, spurious (falsely negative).

The following is a brief illustration of the conditions under which the history as well as skin and bronchial tests with allergen are truly or falsely positive and truly or falsely negative.

History

Positive Results

A true positive means that natural exposure to an allergen is consistently associated with attacks of asthma. History, however, is not equally convincing (accurate) for every allergen. At times (i.e., a highly suggestive history [141]), the attacks of asthma can be convincingly related to a specific allergen because the exposure is confined in space and time and the allergen is present in high concentration. A typical example of a highly suggestive history is the exposure to most occupational allergens or pollens with a short, well-defined seasonal peak. Another example is the immediate attack of asthma on exposure to a cat. The cat allergen is present indoors in higher concentrations than the house dust or cockroach allergen [45, 128]. This may explain why cat allergy usually goes with a highly suggestive history. At other times (i.e., suggestive history [141]), the attacks of asthma occur during exposure to a mixture of allergens, making it impossible to distinguish them according to their clinical relevance. For instance, concomitant exposure to cockroaches and house dust mite [83], flour and storage mite [135], or nocturnal attacks due to house dust or unidentified nonallergic factors [141] may produce for each of these allergens a suggestive rather than very suggestive history. A standardized grading of history, on the basis of allergy workup with standardized allergens, would help the etiologic diagnosis of allergic asthma.

In a falsely positive result, intentionally or unintentionally, the patient's history points to the wrong allergen or to an irritant.

Negative Results

In a truly negative response, the patient cannot establish a clear relationship between his or her asthma attack and a well-known allergen.

In a falsely negative result, some allergists contend that many times the offending allergen, particularly if present in food, cannot be correctly identified by patients. For example, when challenged orally with the food usually consumed, such patients may develop attacks of asthma [123]. A similar argument has been offered for occult "sensitization" to such agents as aspirin, sodium benzoate, and sulfites. While the role of occult allergens cannot be dismissed, I would like to see additional provocation studies that document the reproducibility of these responses.

Skin Tests

Positive Results

A truly positive skin response is of convincing magnitude, is produced by nonirritant concentrations of allergen, *and* is clinically relevant. The third proviso is not redundant, since it may not be fulfilled even when the responses are truly allergic, for two reasons. The first is that the extract applied may contain minor rather than major allergen components or substantial amounts of contaminating protein [177]. The variable content in major allergen components is still an unsolved problem for many extracts, such as for most mold extracts [98, 99]. The use of purified extracts with a standardized content in their major allergen can avoid these clinically irrelevant tests; unfortunately, these are available only for a limited number of allergens. A second reason for dismissing the clinical relevance of a response is that the extract may contain the natural mix of minor and major allergens, but the truly allergic reaction in the skin has no clinical relevance, in that the patient has no allergic manifestation when exposed under natural conditions to this allergen (i.e., latent allergy [81]). It is important to note that latent allergy represents an IgE-mediated reaction, since it is transferable by the Prausnitz-Küstner technique [96, 149].

In a falsely positive response, the response is present but it recognizes a dermographic or irritant rather than an allergic mechanism. High concentrations of an allergen may frequently be associated with irritant responses; the use of relatively high concentrations of allergen tends to identify all subjects sensitized to an allergen but in some subjects these solutions may be irritant. Ideally, a balance between sensitivity and specificity needs to be achieved for each allergen concentration [119, 159].

Negative Results

In a truly negative result, the skin test elicits no reaction even at high concentrations.

In a falsely negative result, the absence of response reflects the application of an insufficient concentration of allergen. This may stem from a poor technique of pricking the skin, poor mediator liberation from skin mast cells, poor responsiveness of vessels to histamine, or a very low concentration of skin-sensitizing antibodies. The false negative rate of skin tests can be decreased by use of a correct technique, positive controls for histamine and codeine, and allergen solutions concentrated in a major allergen, or allergens. Compared with the prick testing method, intradermal testing allows the detection of lower concentrations of specific IgE attached to skin mast cells.

Inhalation Tests

Positive Results

In a truly positive reaction, similar to the allergic reaction in the skin, the bronchial response to an inhaled allergen needs to be physiologically convincing, produced by nonirritant concentrations, *and* clinically relevant. Indeed, the bronchoconstrictor response recorded during inhalation challenge in the laboratory may not duplicate the respiratory complaints occurring under natural conditions. Here are three examples of this. In the first, the patient suffers from rhinitis but the high concentration of allergen used in inhalation tests may lead to bronchoconstriction. In the second, the patient is a former and not current asthmatic; that is, his or her attacks have disappeared following immunotherapy, allergen avoidance, or simply because of a spontaneous, favorable evolution of the disease (see below). Yet, the high concentrations of allergen used in the laboratory may elicit an attack of asthma. In the third, a normal subject, or conceivably an asthmatic patient allergic to a different agent may have a positive bronchial test to an allergen producing only latent sensitization [30].

In a falsely positive result, the physiologic response is convincing but it reflects an irritant action (e.g., secondary to the use of an irritant preservative or a high irritant concentration of allergen).

Negative Results

In a truly negative result, using ideal technical conditions the inhalation of allergen fails to constrict the airways.

In a falsely negative result, there is a negative response in an asthmatic sensitized to an allergen indicated by history. This usually results form the inhalation of an inappropriately low concentration of allergen due to several different factors (e.g., nonstandardized allergen extract, excessively long storage, reluctance to increase the allergen concentration). The recent technologic progress in the purification and analysis of extracts, as well as the implementation of strict standardization criteria, have allowed the standardization of several allergen extracts (e.g., rye grass, birch pollen, ragweed, house dust mite, *Cladosporium*, cat, dog). For such standardized extracts, the rate of false negative results is lower than that for other nonstandardized solutions [19, 159]. It is important to remember the wide range of bronchial sensitivity, from 1 to 10,000 BU for standardized allergens [50]. Note that 10,000 BU produces a wheal of the same size with 10 mg/ml of histamine.

CORRELATION OF ALLERGEN SKIN TEST RESULTS WITH CLINICAL HISTORY AND ALLERGEN INHALATION TEST RESULTS

Early Asthmatic Responses

Most studies addressing the relationship between history, skin test results, and inhalation test results are based on early asth-

Table 40-2. History, skin test results, and inhalation test results in respiratory allergy

Reference	No. of subjects	Percent with positive inhalation test*				
		Hx + +, SKT +	Hx +, SKT +	Hx +, SKT −	Hx −, SKT +	Hx −, SKT −
Bronchial asthma						
Stevens, 1934 [158]	45	—	15 (34)	0 (11)	—	—
Juhlin-Dannfeldt, 1950 [81]	153	—	39 (99)	—	0 (66)	—
Colldahl, 1959 [41]	44	—	20 (25)	2 (5)	24 (80)	6 (5)
Gronemeyer & Fuchs, 1959 [62]	340	—	80 (97)	51 (92)	70 (99)	48 (52)
Popa et al., 1968 [141]	230 (p)	100 (33)	23 (339)	2 (52)	0 (162)	0 (11)
Aas, 1970 [2]	1035 (p)	—	55 (952)	19 (426)	—	—
Spector & Farr, 1974 [155]	100 (p)	—	92 (27)	62 (8)	39 (44)	17 (24)
Eriksson, 1977 [52]	397 (p)	—	87 (?)	31 (?)	40 (?)	9 (?)
Allergic rhinitis						
Popa & Al-George, 1969 [135]	120 (p)	100 (21)	22 (249)	0 (3)	—	0 (5)

* The numbers in parentheses are the total number of inhalation tests performed.
Hx = history; SKT = skin test result; (p) = prospective study; + + = highly suggestive; + = positive; − = negative; ? = not clearly specified.

Table 40-3. Correlation between prick test and inhalation test results[a]

Bronchial challenge tests (reference)	Dx	Size of skin R × n (mm)	Percent with positive inhalation test			Size of skin R × n (mm)	Percent with positive inhalation test		
			Pollen	Molds	H. dust		Pollen	Molds	H. dust
Holman et al., 1972 [73]	A	?	55	94	71	− prick	13	18	19
Hobday, 1972 [71]	A	4	71	—	—	?(prick?)	40	—	—
Spector & Farr, 1974 [155]	A	2	—	—	25[b]-	—	—	—	—
		5	—	—	35[b]-	—	—	—	—
		9	—	—	50[b]-	—	—	—	—
Bryant et al., 1975 [31]	A	3	13	15	17	—	—	—	—
		3	87	85	83	—	—	—	—
Cavanaugh et al., 1977 [34]	A	5	15	42	11	5	0	—	0
		5	54	92	93	5	10	42	18
		9	80	100	100	9	40	34	49

[a] This table indicates that a positive prick test result is associated in most cases with a positive inhalation test result. However, there can be positive inhalation test results even when the prick test result is negative; in such cases, when performed, the intradermal test result is positive (see last columns). For prick test responses of 3 to 5 mm in diameter, the inhalation test results are negative in 5 to 50 percent of the cases, depending on the allergen used.
[b] Various allergens including house dust.
Dx = diagnosis; + = positive; − = negative; H. dust = house dust; A = asthma; R = rhinitis; R × n = reaction; ? = not clearly specified in the paper; — = not mentioned in the paper.

matic responses. Table 40-2 summarizes reports in which more than three allergens were studied for this purpose. Following is a brief presentation of the reasons which, in our experience, account for the concordant or discordant relationship between history, skin and bronchial test results to the incriminated allergen [141]. Similar observations were made in the only prospective study that examined the role of these methods in the etiologic diagnosis of nasal allergy [135].

Very Suggestive History, Positive Skin Test Results, Positive or Negative Inhalation Test Results

If the clinical history indicates that natural exposure to an allergen consistently elicits an attack of asthma and this allergen elicits a positive skin test result, the inhalation test will invariably be positive [141]. This observation is clinically relevant, since it suggests that in these conditions the etiologic diagnosis of asthma can be firmly established by history and skin tests (a high positive predictive value for history and skin test).

Suggestive History, Positive Skin Test Results, Positive or Negative Inhalation Test Results

If the history is only suggestive, the inhalation tests are often negative despite positive skin test results (see Table 40-2). Indeed, if history cannot accurately identify the offending allergen from a mixture of allergens located in the same place at the same time, the skin tests and at times the inhalation tests may not be very helpful. Both these tests may be positive for the offending

or the coexistent allergen, reflecting either clinically relevant or clinically latent allergy, respectively. Since they may be positive in both conditions, the inhalation tests are particularly helpful when negative; in this way they rule out the irrelevant allergen.

From a practical standpoint, the combination of a suggestive history and positive skin test may lead to over- or misdiagnosis of allergy (relatively low positive predictive value). Without resorting to inhalation tests, the alternative solution is to increase the specificity of both the history and the skin test. For instance, grading the history in suggestive and very suggestive cases may improve its specificity in some subjects [141]. The specificity of the skin tests can be increased by using techniques or criteria of positivity that require high concentrations of specific IgE: selecting prick over intradermal testing (Table 40-3) because the former requires a hundred to a thousand times more allergen than the latter [34, 155]; increasing the size of response required for a positive response to a standard concentration [31, 34, 156]; or applying by the prick or intradermal testing method progressively lower concentrations of allergen [2, 39, 155, 156]. All these maneuvers are based on the observation that the asthmatic patients with high skin sensitivity to the allergen suggested by history tend to have a much higher frequency of positive inhalation tests than do those with relatively low skin sensitivity [2, 31, 34, 71, 73, 155, 156] (see Table 40-3).

In an attempt to improve the correlation between skin and inhalation test results, four additional tests have been applied. The least useful is the RAST (see also Chap. 38). This test is less sensitive than the skin test, in that approximately 15 percent of the patients with a positive intradermal test have a negative RAST. As repeatedly shown, only a high RAST score (3 or 4) has a high positive predictive value for inhalation test results with allergen [46, 52]. A RAST with such a high score is usually associated with a high skin sensitivity to allergen, making RAST not only expensive but also redundant. New developments in immunoassay methods may improve the diagnostic sensitivity of the in vitro tests but not enough to make skin testing redundant.

The determination of histamine release from leukocytes, a measurement more difficult and expensive than RAST, let alone the skin test, correlates with inhalation tests with allergen [28, 115, 157]. There is no convincing evidence that, in subjects with a positive skin or RAST test, histamine release from leukocytes increases the likelihood of the former tests being associated with positive bronchial tests. A recent study claims that, if circulating specific IgE is not detectable in serum by a RAST technique, IgE antibodies adsorbed on circulating basophils can be detected by allergen-induced histamine release [171]. Whether this finding is clinically applicable is not clear, since these authors did not conduct inhalation tests with allergen in their subjects who displayed a negative RAST but positive histamine release test from basophils.

The Prausnitz-Küstner reaction correlates with the results of the inhalation tests [88, 142]. However, this test is impractical and, because of the risk of transmitting infectious agents, outright dangerous. Additionally, the passive transfer is valuable in determining the presence of sensitizing antibodies but not their clinical relevance. Latent (nonclinical) allergy is transferable [96, 149].

Considering that bronchial sensitivity to allergen is modulated by bronchial nonspecific responsiveness [31, 40, 85, 87, 114, 115, 130, 135, 140, 166, 188], in an asthmatic patient with a suggestive history and a positive skin test, a high degree of nonspecific bronchial responsiveness supports or may even predict a positive inhalation test [39] (see later for critique).

It thus seems possible to achieve a balance between the sensitivity and specificity of the skin test [159] and its ability to predict the results of the bronchial provocation test. Plotting the true positive rate of skin tests (i.e., positive skin tests with positive bronchial response to allergen) as a function of their false positive rate (i.e., positive skin test with negative bronchial response), Ollier and colleagues [119] were able to determine the concentration of *Dermatophagoides pteronyssinus* with the highest discriminant ability between latent and manifest bronchial allergy ($0.56–1.2 \times 10^6$ U allergen ml^{-1}). This method needs to be extended to other purified allergens. It seems more promising than the attempt to predict the degree of bronchial responses to allergen based on the skin tests and bronchial response to histamine or cholinergic agents [39]. The latter predictive equation is based on the use of different nonstandardized allergens in different asthmatic subjects. This procedure will lead to a substantial variability across subjects for the same allergen and within the same subject for various allergens [3, 50]. Then, whatever the predictor, or predictors, of bronchial sensitivity to allergen, the skin test alone or the histamine/methacholine challenge in combination with the skin test, the equation does not have general applicability since it pertains only to known asthmatics, that is, patients with high nonspecific responsiveness. Such an attempt should fail in cases of latent (nonclinical) allergy: normal subjects with nonclinical allergy [30], patients with hay fever who have only mild airway responsiveness [30, 130], and as shown in Table 40-2, asthmatics with bronchial hyperresponsiveness but positive skin tests without clinical relevance.

Suggestive History, Negative Skin Test Results, Positive or Negative Inhalation Test Results

A small percentage of patients with allergic rhinitis [77, 123, 157] or asthma (see Table 40-2) may have a true positive inhalation

response despite a negative skin reaction. This may be explained by a preferential, local production of specific IgE (compartmentalization), a situation better studied in the human nose [77, 83, 108, 126] and animal lung [17] than in the human lung. For the purposes of clinical practice, instead of determining the local (pulmonary or nasal) concentration of specific IgE [77, 83, 108, 126], one may resort to techniques that increase the sensitivity of skin testing [2, 7, 159]: application of extracts that are more concentrated or contain standardized allergen, intradermal injection of the allergen extract, and, to rule out a deficient skin response, control skin tests with histamine and codeine.

For myself [141] and other authors, a negative skin test in subjects who offer a seemingly suggestive history practically rules out clinically relevant allergy (high negative predictive value).

Negative History, Positive Skin Test Results, Negative or Positive Inhalation Test Results

A positive skin test to an allergen not suggested by history connotes a latent allergy [65, 81, 96]. In this case, the use of high doses of inhaled allergen may produce positive responses that are physiologically positive but clinically irrelevant. Another example of physiologically positive but clinically irrelevant (false positive) inhalation tests is that observed in patients with only rhinitis [52, 130, 168], in "normal" (asymptomatic) subjects with positive skin tests and circulating specific IgE [30], and in subjects with atopic dermatitis but without respiratory symptoms [48].

Negative History, Negative Skin Test Results, Negative Inhalation Test Results

In my experience, the inhalation tests with allergen are invariably negative if both the history and the skin test results are negative. In essence, a negative history, regardless of the skin response to allergen, has a high negative predictive value.

Discrepancies Between Studies Correlating History, Skin Tests, and Inhalation Tests to Allergens

The only discrepancy for which a plausible explanation can be advanced concerns the high proportion of positive bronchial challenge results reported by Gronemeyer and Fuchs [62], Aas [2], Spector and Farr [155], and Eriksson [52] in subjects with both a positive history and positive skin results. A sampling effect, possibly magnified by lumping together subjects with a highly suggestive history and those with a simply suggestive history, might account for this discrepancy.

Other discrepancies are practically impossible to explain (see Table 40-2).

1. Negative history plus negative skin test and positive inhalation test results [62, 155].
2. Negative history plus positive skin test and positive inhalation test results [41, 51, 62, 155].
3. Positive history plus negative skin test and positive inhalation test results [62, 155].

In all these conditions, the authors propose that physiologically positive inhalation test results ascertain the presence of clinically relevant allergy (true positivity), even though the natural exposure or the skin test, or both, fail to suggest it. It would be disturbing if bronchoprovocation with allergen were positive in 19 to 31 percent of the cases either with a negative history or skin tests to the allergen tested, respectively; or, in 6 to 48 percent of the cases when both history and skin tests are negative [155] (see Table 40-2). If these numbers were representative for the general population with allergic asthma, the current allergy evaluation based on history and skin tests would have no place in clinical practice. Only the studies reported by Stevens [158], Juhlin-Dannfeldt [81], Colldahl [41], and my colleagues and I [141] are in agreement with the current consensus [7] or previous recommendations [146] regarding the combination of negative history–negative skin test results or negative history–positive skin test results. For practical purposes, allergy is considered absent in the former and clinically irrelevant in the latter. These discrepancies are not addressed in the current guidelines for bronchial allergy testing; these guidelines concentrate on the methodologic aspects but not the clinical relevance of the results [35].

IMMUNOTHERAPY

Few controlled studies have been devoted to the effect of immunotherapy on the clinical features of asthma (reviewed in [26] and Chap. 70). Even fewer studies mention the changes occurring in the skin and bronchial tests with allergen or constrictor drugs.

As indicated by Tables 40-4 to 40-6, immunotherapy frequently decreases the skin responses, as well as the natural or intentional bronchial responses to allergen. These changes may alter the relationship between history, allergen inhalation, and skin tests observed in the same patient prior to hyposensitization. At the same time, immunotherapy may be associated with alterations in some of the important determinants of these three parameters, for example, humoral and cellular immunity, and cytokine production and/or action.

During immunotherapy, the concentration of specific IgE may increase temporarily and then revert to the preimmunization level [95, 99, 105] or may remain essentially unchanged [120]. The correlation between the in vivo sensitivity to allergen and circulating specific IgE level noted prior to treatment may be abolished. For instance, barely positive or even negative skin or bronchial tests to allergen may be associated after immunotherapy with a substantial level of circulating specific IgE.

During immunotherapy, the concentration of specific IgG, belonging in particular [113, 151] but not exclusively [105] to IgG$_4$, usually increases. This may interfere with the reaction between allergen and specific IgE in the skin but not necessarily in the lung [67].

The decrease in histamine releasability from peripheral basophils is not a consistent event [118, 174, 180]. However, at least in the nasal model of respiratory allergy, immunotherapy decreases the immunologically induced release of mediators [43]. If this holds true for bronchial mast cells, this form of treatment may alter the relationship between bronchial sensitivity to allergen and bronchial nonspecific responsiveness.

Bronchial nonspecific responsiveness is frequently but unpredictably influenced by immunotherapy; furthermore, there is no clear relationship between clinical improvement and the change in bronchial nonspecific responsiveness (Tables 40-4 to 40-6).

The seasonal increase in the cytokine levels, favoring bronchial colonization with eosinophils and neutrophils and indirectly modulating bronchial nonspecific responsiveness, is blunted during immunotherapy [147]. Although attenuated, the respiratory symptoms persist, indicating that these changes in the cytokine levels are important but not decisive.

For the purpose of this chapter, a brief review of the changes in the history as well as the skin tests and bronchial provocation tests with allergen or constrictor drugs brought about by immunotherapy is particularly instructive. As indicated by Table 40-4, most studies have found that immunotherapy with purified or standardized allergen extract of cat and, at times, dog decreases the skin and bronchial responses to these allergens, as well as the respiratory effect of natural exposure to these animals.

Table 40-5 indicates that the effect of immunotherapy with purified extracts of *Cladosporium* and *Alternaria* on natural exposure as well as skin and bronchial challenge results is essentially similar to the effect observed after immunotherapy with purified or standardized cat (and dog) allergen.

After immunotherapy with house dust or house dust mite extract, the symptoms of asthma abated in the subjects of six of seven studies (see Table 40-5), and so did the skin and bronchial sensitivity to allergen. Some [170], but not all investigators [110], found that the late asthmatic response might be more influenced than the early response. For reasons which are not clear, the clinical effect of immunotherapy with house dust or house dust mite extract is apparently less consistent and possibly less dramatic than that produced by immunotherapy with animal extracts (see Table 40-4).

Immunotherapy with pollen generally decreases allergen responses in the skin and often in the lung as well; it also frequently blunts the corresponding seasonal peak in asthma attacks (Table 40-6).

In the controlled studies tabulated, the discrepant group changes in the history as well as skin and bronchial test results following immunotherapy do not seem to be affected by the age of subjects, duration of treatment, and, to a large extent, the nature of the allergen. The relationship between the history, skin tests, and inhalation tests is substantially influenced by the wide intersubject variability in the response to immunotherapy. To exemplify this point, consider Figure 40-5, which depicts the intersubject variability in the results of carbachol tests following immunotherapy with mite allergen [26]. Table 40-7, which is based on the raw data of Rohatgi and coworkers [152] regarding immunotherapy with dog allergen, illustrates the intersubject

Table 40-4. Effect of immunotherapy with animal hair on asthmatic symptoms, skin and bronchial allergic responses, and nonspecific bronchial responsiveness

Reference	No. of subj.	Age	Allergen	Duration of Rx	Changes after immunotherapy			
					Sympt.	ST	ABPT	NSBR
Taylor et al., 1978 [164]	5	A	Cat(S)	3–4 mo	?	↓	↓	↔
Ohman et al., 1984 [118]	9	A, C	Cat(S)	weeks	↓	↓	↓	↔
Sundin et al., 1986 [161]	41	A, C	Cat, dog(P)	12 mo	↓	↓	↓	↓
Valavirta et al., 1986 [169]	15	C	Dog(P)	12 mo	↓	↓	↓	↔
Rohatgi et al., 1988 [152]	13	A	Cat, dog	3 mo	↓	↓	↓	↕
Van Metre et al., 1988 [174]	11	A	Cat(S)	12 mo	?	↓	↓	↔
Lilja et al., 1989 [95]	35	A	Cat, dog(P)	2 yr	?	↓	↓	↓
Haugaard and Dahl, 1992 [66]	37	A	Cat, dog(P)	1 yr	↓ (cat)	?	↓	↔(5 mo), ↓ (12 mo)
					↔(dog)	?	↔	↔

Rx = treatment; A = adults; C = children; ST = skin tests; ABPT = allergen bronchial provocation test; NSBR = nonspecific bronchial responsiveness; (S) = standardized; (P) = purified and standardized; ? = not specified; ↑, ↓, ↔ = increased, decreased, unchanged, respectively.

Table 40-5. *Effect of immunotherapy with house dust, house dust mite or mold extracts on asthmatic symptoms, skin, and bronchial allergic responses and nonspecific bronchial responsiveness*

Reference	No. of subj.	Age	Allergen	Duration of Rx	Sympt.	ST	ABPT	NSBR
							Changes after immunotherapy	
Aas et al., 1971 [1]	52	C	H. dust	30 mo	↓	?	↓	?
McAllen, 1961 [104]	60	C, A	H. dust	12 wk	↓	?	↓	?
Newton et al., 1978 [116]	14	A	D. farinae	12 mo	↔	↔	↓	?
Warner et al., 1978 [181]	27	C	D. pter.	12 mo	↓	?	↓ LAR	?
Bousquet et al., 1989 [24]	20	A	D. pter.	7 wk	↓	↓	↓	?
Wahn et al., 1988 [180]	24	C	D. pter.	24 mo	↓	↓	↓ LAR	?
Van Bever & Stevens, 1989 [170]	15	C	D. pter.	12 mo	↓	↓	↓ LAR	?
Mosbach et al., 1989 [110]	46	A	D. pter.	24 mo	↓	?	Occ	↓
Murray et al., 1985 [112]	13	C	D. farinae	12 mo	↓	?	↓	↑
Dreborg et al., 1986 [51]	16	C	Cladosporium (S)	5–7 mo	↓	↓	↓	?
Malling et al., 1986, 1987 [98, 99]	11	A	Cladosporium (S)	12 mo	↓	↓	↓	?
Horst et al., 1990 [75]	13	C, A	Alternaria (S)	12 mo	↓	↓ (nasal)	↓	?

Occ = occasional; LAR = late asthmatic reaction; H. dust = house dust; *D. pter.* = *Dermatophagoides pteronyssinus*. See Table 40-4 for additional abbreviations.

Table 40-6. *Effect of immunotherapy with pollen extracts on asthmatic symptoms, skin and bronchial allergic responses, and nonspecific bronchial responsiveness**

Reference	No. of subj.	Age	Pollen allergen	Duration of Rx	Symptoms	ST	ABPT	NSBR
							Changes after immunotherapy	
McAllen, 1961 [104]	40 pollen	C, A	Mixed	12 wk	↓	↓ ↑ ↔	↓	?
Bruce et al., 1977 [29]	39	A	Ragweed	2 yr	↔	↔	↔	?
Osterballe, 1986 [121]	40	A	Grass	2 yr	↓	↓	↓ (N)	?
Ortolani et al., 1984 [120]	15	A	Grass	20 mo	↓	?	↔	?
Rak et al., 1990 [147]	40	A	Birch	1 yr	↓	↓	↓ (N)	↑
Van Bever & Stevens, 1989 [170]	9	C	Grass	1 yr	↓	↓	↓	?
Bousquet et al., 1990 [25]	57	C, A	Grass	1 yr	↓	↓	↓ (N)	?

* For abbreviations see Table 40-4; (N) = nasal test.

Table 40-7. *Intersubject variability in the effect of immunotherapy with cat allergen on skin tests and allergen and methacholine provocation tests**

Skin tests			ABPT			MBPT		
↓	↑	↔	↓	↑	↔	↓	↑	↔
4	—	—	2	1	1	1	1	2
—	0	—	0	0	0	0	0	0
—	—	4	1	2	0	3	0	1

* Data from [152]. ABPT and MBPT = allergen and methacholine bronchial provocation test, respectively; ↓, ↑, ↔ = decreased, increased, unchanged, respectively. Numbers represent numbers of patients.
Note: (1) The eventual improvement in skin sensitivity is not consistently associated with an increased tolerance to allergen or methacholine inhalation; and (2) nonspecific bronchial responsiveness may worsen after immunotherapy, despite an improvement shown by the results of skin or allergen tests (see Tables 40-4 to 40-6).

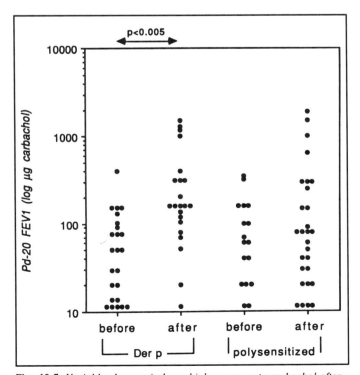

Fig. 40-5. *Variable changes in bronchial responses to carbachol after immunotherapy with Dermatophagoides pteronyssinus (Der p). (Reprinted with permission from J. Bousquet, et al., Specific immunotherapy in asthma.* J. Allergy Clin. Immunol. *86:292, 1990.)*

disparity produced by this form of treatment in skin tests, allergen provocation tests, and methacholine provocation tests. It cannot be explained why the good correlation between the clinical effect of immunotherapy and the change in bronchoprovocation with allergen that has been reported by others [1, 25] is frequently but not invariably seen. Following immunotherapy (e.g., with cat and dog hair), despite a good relationship between the degree of clinical improvement and the decrease in the size of allergen skin tests, the changes in skin tests do not correlate with the changes in bronchial provocation tests with allergen, circulating specific IgG, or specific IgE [67]. Even patients who fail to respond to immunotherapy may have a diminished skin response to allergen [67].

SEASONAL EXPOSURE TO POLLEN AND AVOIDANCE

Natural exposure to pollen allergen increases bronchial nonspecific responsiveness [6, 22, 38, 154], skin and bronchial sensitivity to allergen [44], and the level of circulating specific IgE [183]. Thus, in pollen-sensitive patients, the relationship between these four parameters may vary according to the level of antigen exposure.

The effects of allergen avoidance can be surmised from the postseasonal changes in the clinical and immunologic measurements reported in pollen allergy. It is not clear how intentional avoidance affects skin and bronchial sensitivity to other allergens; avoiding exposure to an occupational allergen may decrease the skin sensitivity [60]. Bronchial nonspecific hyperresponsiveness decreases in patients removed from an environment rich in house dust mites [127] or in an occupational allergen [178].

OUTGROWING ASTHMA

In adults who outgrow their childhood asthma, the skin and bronchial reactions to allergen as well as the bronchial nonspecific hyperresponsiveness may persist, although to a lesser degree [60, 112]. Children who exhibit a late asthmatic response when challenged with allergen usually fail to outgrow their asthma. Part of the decrease in bronchial hyperresponsiveness may be simply age related [74]. Thus, a former asthmatic who has outgrown his or her allergic asthma and currently has a negative history to the previous offending allergen may still have positive skin and bronchial test results and even some degree of bronchial nonspecific hyperresponsiveness [60]. In conclusion, the patients who outgrow their asthma, those who successfully undergo immunotherapy, and, to some extent, those who are temporarily not exposed to the offending allergen tend to resemble subjects with latent allergy, in terms of current history, skin, and bronchial response. However, the similarity in the directional changes in these conditions seems to be subtended by entirely different pathogenetic mechanisms.

LATE ASTHMATIC REACTION

Compared to the early response to allergen, the late asthmatic reaction is more severe and protracted, increases more readily the bronchial nonspecific responsiveness—which implicitly enhances bronchial susceptibility to subsequent allergen exposure—and responds well to steroids but relatively poorly to β_2 agonists (reviewed in [117] and Chap. 12).

Could suggestive history and positive skin tests predict the occurrence of late asthmatic reaction as they predict the early response? One study addressing this question found that, in 41 percent of the cases, history could not identify the offending allergen producing a late asthmatic reaction (i.e., history was negative in 41% of the cases) [123]. Even more intriguing, under natural conditions, such a late reaction could be detected in only 17 percent of the patients. The skin tests performed with a standard concentration of allergen are usually but not invariably positive. Thus, a late asthmatic reaction could be associated with positive or negative history and positive or negative skin responses. In addition, a delayed skin response to allergen predicted a late asthmatic reaction in only a minority of patients [123]. These surprising observations need to be confirmed. It is important to note that the vast majority of studies on late asthmatic reactions have been performed in patients known to have a positive history and positive skin tests. In essence, because of insufficient data, it is impossible to compare the diagnostic yield of history, skin, and bronchial tests in the context of early and late asthmatic reactions.

SKIN AND INHALATION TESTS IN ASTHMATIC PATIENTS WITH CONCOMITANT OR EXCLUSIVE BRONCHIAL SENSITIZATION CAUSED BY NON–IgE-DEPENDENT MECHANISMS

It has been postulated that short-term skin-sensitizing antibodies (see Chap. 6) belong ostensibly to the IgG_4 subclass [176], the only IgG thought to have receptors on mast cells. For some authors, these IgG_4 antibodies seem to be clinically important, since results of inhalation tests with the corresponding antigen are positive even in the absence of circulating specific IgE [64]. The skin tests need to be performed intradermally. The inhalation test responses generally require large quantities of allergen and are chronologically late [64]. Recent data indicate that IgG-IgE complexes may be attached via IgE on human circulating basophils. When challenged with any of the four IgG subclasses, particularly IgG_3, these IgG-IgE complexes liberate histamine [74]. This important observation suggests an additional mechanism for humoral hypersensitivity.

More than ten years ago, my colleagues and I reported on the intriguing features of a group of asthmatic patients exposed occupationally to simple chemicals [142]. These patients had chronologically late asthma that was triggered either by occupational exposure or by the inhalation of nonirritant concentrations of allergens. They all had negative immediate responses to prick or intradermal injection but positive patch test results. For the following reasons, the respiratory reaction of these patients to inhalation of simple chemicals was considered to represent a delayed hypersensitivity response: (1) we used nonirritant concentrations of simple chemicals; (2) the chronology of the skin-patch test reaction and respiratory responses was similar; (3) as indicated by the use of different isomers, the chemical structure of the agents producing positive patch test responses and respiratory responses was identical; (4) intradermal injection of the suspected simple chemical led to delayed skin and asthma reactions that occurred at the same time; (5) the positive patch test was eczematous and histologically consistent with delayed hypersensitivity; and (6) the nonirritant bronchial concentrations of simple chemicals were high, as they usually are when applied for patch tests, rather than low, as expected for IgE-mediated reactions. It is not clear if these late bronchial reactions reflect an exclusive delayed hypersensitivity of the bronchi to the offending simple chemicals.

Indeed, a possible concomitant participation of circulating antibodies in this delayed reaction could not be formally ruled out in these cases. With this caution, in these subjects with asthma induced by simple chemicals, a positive history may or may not be associated with positive patch test or positive bronchial test results. Some of the subjects exposed to the three agents previously listed had irritant asthma; unlike the other, sensitized subjects, the patch tests and the bronchial tests with nonirritant concentrations remained negative. In these subjects with irritant asthma, only the occupational exposure to the chemicals incriminated produced a bronchoconstrictor response.

No previous or subsequent report has tested the hypothesis that in the same asthmatic subject, the delayed asthmatic response could be associated with a delayed hypersensitivity reaction in the skin. This is intriguing, since many simple chemicals known for their ability to elicit delayed hypersensitivity responses in the skin [10] may also produce delayed bronchial reactions. In addition to the agents mentioned above [69, 142], nickel salts [101] and azodicarbonamide [102] are capable of producing such delayed bronchial reactions (see review in [12]).

It is surprising that although T-lymphocytes play an important role in allergic asthma [151], the lung parenchyma rather than the large bronchi seem to be able to mount a delayed hypersensitivity response. Indeed, in the animal experiments triggered by our report with simple chemicals, a lymphocytic infiltrate was observed in the terminal airways but not in the large bronchi [59, 111; Popa and Lehmann, unpublished observations]. In humans, delayed hypersensitivity is one, if not the main, immune mechanism in berryliosis, hypersensitivity pneumonitis, and tuberculosis, for example, and they are all diseases with a peripheral, alveolo-interstitial granulomatous infiltrate. It is difficult to understand why the terminal airways and alveoli are involved in delayed hypersensitivity due to inhaled allergen, rather than the large and medium-size bronchi where most of the inhaled agents producing these diseases are actually deposited. IgE-mediated and delayed hypersensitivity responses seem to involve different airway segments.

REFERENCES

1. Aas, K. Hyposensitization in house dust allergy asthma. *Acta Paediatr. Scand.* 60:264, 1971.
2. Aas, K. The bronchial provocation test. Springfield, Ill.: Thomas, 1975.
3. Aas, K., and Belin, K. Suggestions for biologic quantitative testing and standardization of allergens extracts. *Acta Allergol.* 29:238, 1976.
4. Aas, K., and Johansson, S. G. O. The radioallergosorbent test in the in vitro diagnosis of multiple reaginic allergy: a comparison of diagnostic approaches. *J. Allergy Clin. Immunol.* 48:134, 1981.
5. Alexander, H. L., and Paddock, R. Bronchial asthma: response to pilocarpine and epinephrine. *Arch. Intern. Med.* 27:184, 1921.
6. Altounyan, R. E. C. Changes in Histamine and Atropine Responsiveness as a Guide to Diagnosis and Evaluation of Therapy in Obstructive Airways Disease. In J. Pepys, and A. W. Frankland (eds.), *Disodium Cromoglycate in Allergic Airways Disease*. London, Butterworth, 1969.
7. American College of Physicians. Allergy testing. *Am. Intern. Med.* 110: 317, 1989.
8. Apold, J., et al. The radioallergosorbent test (RAST) in the diagnosis of reaginic allergy: a comparison between provocation tests, skin tests and RAST employing allergosorbents which were arbitrarily prepared with commercial allergen extracts. *Clin. Allergy* 6:601, 1974.
9. Arm, J., and Lee, T. H. The pathobiology of bronchial asthma. In F. J. Dixon, *Advances in Immunology* (vol. 51). San Diego: Academic, 1992.
10. Askenase, P. W. Effector and regulatory mechanisms in delayed-type hypersensitivity. In E. Middleton Jr., et al. (eds.), *Allergy: Principles and Practice* (3rd ed.). St. Louis: Mosby, 1988.
11. Assem, E. S. K., and Attalah, N. A. Increased release of histamine by anti-IgE from leucocytes of asthmatic patients and possible heterogeneity of IgE. *Clin. Allergy* 11:367, 1981.
12. Bardana, E. J., Montanaro, A., and O'Hollaren, M. T. *Occupational Asthma*. Philadelphia: Hanley & Belfus, 1992.
13. Berg, T., and Johansson, S. G. O. Allergy diagnosis with the radioallergosorbent test. *J. Allergy* 56:209, 1974.
14. Baur, X., Fruhman, R., and Von Liebe, V. Allergologishe Untersuchungsmethoden (inhalativer Provokations Test, Haut-test) in die Diagnose des Asthma bronchiale. *Klin. Wochenschr.* 56:1205, 1978.
15. Baur, X., et al. Clinical symptoms and results of skin tests, RAST, and bronchial provocation tests in 33 papain makers. *Clin. Allergy* 12:9, 1982.
16. Beasley, R. C. W., et al. The effect of a thromboxane receptor antagonist GR32191 on PGD_2 and allergen-induced bronchoconstriction. *J. Appl. Physiol.* 66:1685, 1989.
17. Bergstrand, H., et al. Antigen-induced release of histamine from rat tissues in vitro: dissociation in development of serosal mast cells, lung tissue. *Int. Arch. Allergy Appl. Immunol.* 68:342, 1982.
18. Bienenstock, J., et al. Comparative aspects of mast cell heterogeneity in different species and sites. *Int. Arch. Allergy Appl. Immunol.* 77:126, 1985.
19. Blackley, C. H. *Experimental Research on the Causes and Nature of Catarrhus Aestives (Hay Fever or Hay Asthma)* (1st ed.). London: Bailliere, Tindall & Cox, 1873.
20. Blumenthal, M., et al. HLA-DR2, (HLA-B7, SC31, DR2), and HLA-B8, SC01, DR3 haplotypes distinguish subjects with asthma from those with rhinitis only in ragweed pollen allergy. *J. Immunol.* 148:411, 1992.
21. Boucher, R. C., Pare, P. D., and Hogg, H. C. Relationship between airway hyperreactivity and hyperpermeability in *Ascaris*-sensitive monkeys. *J. Allergy Clin. Immunol.* 64:197, 1979.
22. Boulet, L. P., et al. Asthma and increases in nonallergic bronchial responsiveness from seasonal pollen exposure. *J. Allergy Clin. Immunol.* 71:399, 1983.
23. Bousquet, J., Guerin, B., and Michel, F. B. Standardization of Allergens. In S. L. Spector (ed.), *Provocative Challenge Procedures: Background and Methodology*. Mount Kisco, NY: Futura, 1989.
24. Bousquet, J., et al. Specific immunotherapy with a standardized *Dermatophagoides pteronyssinus* extract, II. Prediction of efficacy of immunotherapy. *J. Allergy Clin. Immunol.* 828:971, 1988.
25. Bousquet, J., et al. Double-blind placebo controlled immunotherapy with mixed grass pollen allergoids. IV. Comparison of the safety and efficacy of two dosages of a high-molecular-weight allergoid. *J. Allergy Clin. Immunol.* 85:490, 1990.
26. Bousquet, J., et al. Specific immunotherapy in asthma. *J. Allergy Clin. Immunol.* 86:292, 1990.
27. Bruce, R. A. Bronchial and skin sensitivity in asthma. *Int. Arch. Allergy* 22:294, 1963.
28. Bruce, C. A., et al. Diagnostic tests in ragweed allergic asthma: a comparison of direct skin tests, leucocyte histamine release and quantitative bronchial challenge. *J. Allergy Clin. Immunol.* 53:230, 1974.
29. Bruce, C. A., et al. The role of ragweed pollen in autumnal asthma. *J. Allergy Clin. Immunol.* 59:449, 1977.
30. Bryant, D. H., and Burns, M. W. The relationship between bronchial histamine reactivity and atopic status. *Clin. Allergy* 6:673, 1976.
31. Bryant, D. H., Burns, M. W., and Lazarus, L. The correlation between skin tests and the serum level of IgE specific for common allergens in patients with asthma. *Clin. Allergy* 5:145, 1975.
32. Carrol, M. P., Gratziou, C., and Holgate, S. T. Inflammation and inflammatory mediators in asthma. In T. J. H. Clark, S. Godfrey, and T. H. Lee, *Asthma* (3rd ed.). London: Chapman & Hall Medical, 1992.
33. Casale, T. B., et al. Elevated bronchoalveolar lavage fluid histamine levels in allergic asthmatics are associated with methacholine bronchial hyperresponsiveness. *J. Clin. Invest.* 79:1197, 1987.
34. Cavanaugh, M. J., Bronsky, E. A., and Buckley, J. M. Clinical value of bronchial provocation testing in childhood asthma. *J. Allergy Clin. Immunol.* 59:41, 1977.
35. Chai, H., et al. Standardization of bronchial inhalation challenge procedures. *J. Allergy Clin. Immunol.* 56:323, 1975.
36. Church, M. K., El-Lati, S., and Okayama, Y. Biological properties of human skin mast cells. *Clin. Exper. Allergy* 21(suppl. 3):1, 1991.
37. Clegg, S. A., et al. Histamine secretion from skin slices induced by anti-IgE and artificial secretagogues and the effects of sodium cromoglycate and salbutamol. *Clin. Allergy* 15:321, 1985.
38. Cockcroft, D. W., et al. Allergen-induced increase in non-allergic bronchial reactivity. *Clin. Allergy* 7:50, 1977.
39. Cockcroft, D. W., et al. Prediction of airway responsiveness to allergen from skin sensitivity to allergen and airway responsiveness to histamine. *Am. Rev. Respir. Dis.* 125:264, 1987.
40. Cockcroft, D. W., et al. Determinants of allergen-induced asthma: dose of allergen, circulating IgE antibody concentration and bronchial responsiveness to inhaled histamine. *Am. Rev. Respir. Dis.* 170:1053, 1979.
41. Colldahl, H. Provocation tests for the etiological diagnosis of asthma. *Acta Allergol.* 14:42, 1959.
42. Conroy, M. C., Adkinson, N. F. Jr., and Lichtenstein, L. M. Measurement of IgE on human basophils: relation to serum IgE and anti-IgE-induced histamine release. *J. Immunol.* 118:1317, 1977.
43. Creticos, P. S., et al. Nasal challenge with ragweed pollen in hay fever patients: effect of immunotherapy. *J. Clin. Invest.* 76:2247, 1985.
44. Crimi, E., et al. Effect of seasonal exposure to pollen on specific bronchial sensitivity in allergic patients. *J. Allergy Clin. Immunol.* 85:1014, 1990.
45. De Blay, F., et al. Airborne dust mite allergens: comparison of group II allergens with group I mite allergens and cat allergen Fel d I. *J. Allergy Clin. Immunol.* 89:1046, 1992.
46. Debelic, M. Bronchial Provocation Tests with Allergens in Clinical Practice. In G. Melillo, P. S. Norman, and G. Marone (eds.), *Respiratory Allergy* (Clinical Immunology, Vol. 2). Toronto:Decker, 1990.
47. Deve, N. K., et al. Persistence of increased nonspecific bronchial reactiv-

ity in allergic children and adolescents. *J. Allergy Clin. Immunol.* 86:147, 1990.

48. Dohi, M., et al. Bronchial responsiveness to mite allergen in atopic dermatitis without asthma. *Int. Arch. Allergy Appl. Immunol.* 92:138, 1992.
49. Dolovich, J., et al. Late cutaneous allergic responses in isolated IgE-dependent reactions. *J. Allergy Clin. Immunol.* 52:38, 1973.
50. Dreborg, S. Bronchial Provocation Tests with Biologically Standardized Allergenic Preparations. In G. Melillo, P. S. Norman, and G. Marone (eds.), *Respiratory Allergy* (Clinical Immunology, Vol. 2). Toronto: Decker, 1990.
51. Dreborg, S., et al. A double-blind, multicenter immunotherapy trial in children using a purified and standardized *Cladosporium herbarum* preparation. I. Clinical results. *Allergy* 41:131, 1986.
52. Eriksson, N. E. Diagnosis of reaginic allergy with house dust, animal dander and pollen allergens in adult patients. *Int. Arch. Allergy Appl. Immunol.* 53:341, 1977.
53. Findlay, S. R., et al. Allergens detected in association with airborne particles capable to penetrate into the peripheral lung. *Am. Rev. Respir. Dis.* 128:1008, 1983.
54. Finnerty, J. P., et al. Effect of GR32191, a potent thromboxane receptor antagonist, on exercise-induced bronchoconstriction in asthma. *Thorax* 46:190, 1991.
55. Flint, K. C., et al. Bronchoalveolar mast cells in extrinsic asthma: a mechanism for the initiation of antigen specific bronchoconstriction. *Br. Med. J.* 291:925, 1985.
56. Foreman, J. C., et al. Structure-activity relationship for same substance. *J. Physiol.* 335:449, 1983.
57. Frew, A. J., et al. Inflammatory Cell Infiltration in Late-phase Asthmatic Reactions. In G. Melillo, P. S. Norman, and G. Marone (eds.), *Respiratory Allergy* (Clinical Immunology, Vol. 2). Toronto: Decker, 1990.
58. Fuller, R. W., et al. Prostaglandin D2 potentiates airway responsiveness to histamine and methacholine. *Am. Rev. Respir. Dis.* 133:252, 1986.
59. Garssen, J., et al. Regulation of delayed-type hypersensitivity-like responses in the mouse lung, determined with histological procedures: serotonin, T-cell suppressor-induced factor and high antigen dose tolerance regulate the magnitude of T-cell dependent inflammatory reactions. *Immunology* 68:51, 1989.
60. Gerritsen, J., et al. Change in airway responsiveness to inhaled dust from childhood to adulthood. *J. Allergy Clin. Immunol.* 85:1083, 1990.
61. Godard, P., et al. Histamine release by bronchoalveolar cells of allergic asthmatic patients. *Am. Rev. Respir. Dis.* 125:A75, 1982.
62. Gronemeyer, W., and Fuchs, E. Der inhalative Antigen-Pneumometrie Test als Standard-Methode in der Diagnose allergisher Krankheiten. *Int. Arch. Allergy* 14:217, 1959.
63. Gurish, M. F., and Austen, K. F. Different Mast Cell Mediators Produced by Different Mast Cell Phenotypes. In D. Chadwick, D. Evered, and J. Wheelan (eds.), *IgE, Mast Cells and the Allergic Response.* New York, Wiley, 1989.
64. Gwynn, C. M., Ingram, J., and Almousawi, T. Bronchial provocation tests in atopic patients with allergen specific IgG₄ antibodies. *Lancet* 1:259, 1982.
65. Hagy, G. W., and Settipane, G. A. Prognosis of positive allergy skin tests in an asymptomatic population. *J. Allergy* 68:200, 1971.
66. Haugaard, L., and Dahl, R. Immunotherapy in patients allergic to cat and dog dander. I. Clinical results. *Ann. Allergy* 47:249, 1992.
67. Hedlin, G., et al. Immunotherapy with cat- and dog-dander extracts. II. In vivo and in vitro immunologic effects observed in a one-year double blind placebo study. *J. Allergy Clin. Immunol.* 77:488, 1986.
68. Hedstrand, V. Ventilation, gas exchange: mechanics of breathing and respiratory work in acute bronchial asthma. *Acta Med. Uppsala* 76:248, 1971.
69. Hendrick, D. J., and Lane, O. J. Occupational formalin asthma. *Br. J. Ind. Med.* 34:11, 1977.
70. Herxheimer, H. The late bronchial reaction in induced asthma. *Int. Arch. Allergy Appl. Immunol.* 3:189, 1952.
71. Hobday, J. D. The incidence of pollen sensitivities on skin test and bronchial challenge in asthmatic children in Perth, Western Australia. *Med. J. Aust.* 1:161, 1972.
72. Holgate, S. T., et al. Astemizole and other H₁ antihistamine drug treatment in asthma. *J. Allergy Clin. Immunol.* 76:375, 1985.
73. Holman, T. G., Molk, L., and Mickilich, D. Bronchial challenge and skin test correlation. *Ann. Allergy* 30:250, 1972.
74. Hopp, R., et al. Effect of age on methacholine response. *J. Allergy Clin. Immunol.* 73:178, 1984.

75. Horst, M., et al. Double-blind, placebo-controlled immunotherapy with a standardized *Alternaria* extract. *J. Allergy Clin. Immunol.* 85:460, 1990.
76. Houri, M., et al. Correlation of skin, nasal and inhalation tests with the IgE in the serum, nasal fluid and sputum. *Clin. Allergy* 2:285, 1972.
77. Huggins, K. J., and Brostoff, J. Local production of specific IgE antibodies in allergic-rhinitis patients with negative skin tests. *Lancet* 2:148, 1975.
78. Iliopoulos, O., et al. Histamine-containing cells obtained from the nose hours after antigen challenge have functional and phenotypic characteristics of basophils. *J. Immunol.* 148:2223, 1992.
79. Irani, A.-M., and Schwartz, L. B. Mast cell heterogeneity. *Clin. Exp. Allergy* 19:143, 1989.
80. Iure, E., et al. Late asthmatic reactions and bronchial variability after challenges with low doses of allergen. *Clin. Allergy* 18:557, 1988.
81. Juhlin-Dannfeldt, C. On the significance of exposure and provocation tests in allergic diagnosis. *Acta Med. Scand.* (suppl.) 239:320, 1950.
82. Kalliel, J. N., et al. High frequency of atopic asthma in a pulmonary clinic population. *Chest* 96:1336, 1989.
83. Kang, B. C., Wu, C. W., and Johnson, J. Characteristics and diagnoses of cockroach-sensitive bronchial asthma. *Ann. Allergy* 68:237, 1992.
84. Kemeny, D. M., et al. The immune response to bee venom: comparison of the antibody response to phospholipase A₂ with the response to inhalant allergens. *Int. Arch. Allergy Appl. Immunol.* 68:268, 1982.
85. Kilian, D., et al. Factors in allergen-induced asthma: relevance of the intensity of the airways allergic reaction for non-specific bronchial reactivity. *Clin. Allergy* 6:219, 1976.
86. Kirby, J., et al. Bronchoalveolar cell profiles of asthmatic and non-asthmatic subjects. *Am. Rev. Respir. Dis.* 136:379, 1987.
87. Kreukniet, J., and Pijper, M. M. Response to inhaled histamine and to inhaled allergens in atopic patients. *Respiration* 30:345, 1973.
88. Kurimoto, Y., and Baba, S. Specific IgE estimations by RAST in Japanese asthmatics compared with skin, passive transfer and bronchial provocation tests. *Clin. Allergy* 8:175, 1978.
89. Laitinen, A. Ultrastructural organization of intraepithelial nerves in the human airway tract. *Thorax* 40:488, 1985.
90. Lam, S., et al. Release of leukotrienes in patients with bronchial asthma. *J. Allergy Clin. Immunol.* 81:711, 1988.
91. Lefel, B., et al. Spontaneous and non-specific releasability of histamine (H) by bronchoalveolar lavage (BAL) cells in asthmatics. *J. Allergy Clin. Immunol.* 79:A165, 1987.
92. Lehrer, S. B., et al. Passive cutaneous anaphylaxis inhibition: evidence for heterogeneity in IgE–mast cell interaction. *Immunology* 44:711, 1981.
93. Leung, K. B. P., et al. A comparison of nedocromil sodium and sodium cromoglycate on human lung mast cells obtained by bronchoalveolar lavage and by dispersion of lung fragments. *Eur. J. Respir. Dis.* 69(suppl. 149):223, 1986.
94. Lichtenstein, L. M., et al. Antihuman IgG causes basophil histamine release by acting on IgG-IgE complexes bound to IgE receptors. *J. Immunol.* 148:3929, 1992.
95. Lilja, G., et al. Immunotherapy with cat- and dog-dander extracts. IV. Effects of two years of treatment. *J. Allergy Clin. Immunol.* 83:37, 1989.
96. Lindblad, J. H., and Farr, R. S. The incidence of positive intradermal reaction and the demonstration of skin-sensitizing antibody to extract of ragweed and dust in humans without history of rhinitis and asthma. *J. Allergy* 32:392, 1961.
97. MacGlashan, D. W., Jr., et al. Biomechanical Mechanisms Underlying Human Basophil and Mast Cell Responsiveness. In G. Melillo, P. S. Norman, and G. Marone (eds.), *Respiratory Allergy* (Clinical Immunology, Vol. 2). Toronto, Decker, 1990.
98. Malling, J., et al. Diagnosis and immunotherapy of mould allergy. V. Clinical efficacy and side effects of immunotherapy with *cladosporium herbarum.* *Allergy* 41:507, 1986.
99. Malling, H. J., et al. Diagnosis and immunotherapy of mould allergy. VI. IgE-mediated parameters during a one-year placebo-controlled study of immunotherapy with *Cladosporium.* *Allergy* 42:305, 1987.
100. Malling, H. J., Dreborg, S., and Weeke, B. Diagnosis and immunotherapy of mould allergy. *Allergy* 41:57, 1986.
101. Malo, J. L., et al. Isolated asthmatic reaction due to nickel sulfate without antibodies to nickel. *Clin. Allergy* 15:95, 1985.
102. Malo, J. L., Pineau, L., and Cartier, A. Occupational asthma due to azobisformamide. *Clin. Allergy* 15:261, 1985.
103. Marone, G., et al. Releasability in Allergic Disorders. In G. Melillo, P. S. Norman, and G. Marone (eds.), *Respiratory Allergy* (Clinical Immunology, Vol. 2). Toronto, Decker, 1990.

104. McAllen, K. Bronchial sensitivity testing in asthma: an assessment of the effect of hyposensitization in house dust and pollen-sensitive asthmatic subjects. *Thorax* 16:30, 1961.

105. McHugh, S. M., et al. A placebo-controlled trial of immunotherapy with two extracts of *Dermatophagoides pteronyssinus* in allergic rhinitis, comparing clinical outcome with changes in antigen-specific IgE, IgG, and IgG subclasses. *J. Allergy Clin. Immunol.* 86:521, 1990.

106. McNeil, R. S. Effect of β-adrenergic blocking agent, propranolol, on asthmatics. *Lancet* 2:1101, 1964.

107. McLean, J. A., et al. Effect of histamine and methacholine on nasal airway resistance in atopic and nonatopic subjects. *J. Allergy Clin. Immunol.* 59:165, 1977.

108. Merrett, T. G., et al. Measurement of specific IgE antibodies in nasal secretions: evidence for local production. *Clin. Allergy* 6:69, 1976.

109. Metzger, H. High affinity receptor is similar to growth factors. *Immunol. Rev.* 125:34, 1992.

110. Mosbach, H., et al. Hyposensitivity in asthmatics with mPEG modified and unmodified house dust mite extract. I. Clinical effect evaluated by diary cards and a retrospective assessment. *Allergy* 44:487, 1989.

111. Miyamoto, T., et al. Physiologic and pathologic respiratory changes in delayed-type hypersensitivity reactions in guinea pigs. *Am. Rev. Respir. Dis.* 103:509, 1971.

112. Murray, A. B., et al. Non-allergic bronchial hyperreactivity in asthmatic children decreases with age and increases with mite immunotherapy. *Ann. Allergy* 54:541, 1985.

113. Nagakawa, T., et al. IgG$_4$ antibodies in patients with house dust mite sensitive bronchial asthma: relationship with antigen-specific immunotherapy. *Int. Arch. Allergy Appl. Immunol.* 71:122, 1983.

114. Nathan, R. A., et al. Comparison of bronchial reactivity to allergens and non-specific agents. *J. Allergy Clin. Immunol.* 63:150, 1979.

115. Neijens, H. J., et al. Study on the significance of bronchial hyperreactivity in the bronchus obstruction after inhalation of cat dander allergen. *J. Allergy Clin. Immunol.* 64:504, 1979.

116. Newton, D. A. G., et al. House dust mite hyposensitization. *Br. J. Dis. Chest* 72:21, 1978.

117. O'Byrne, et al. Late asthmatic responses: state of the art. *Am. Rev. Respir. Dis.* 136:740, 1987.

118. Ohman, J. L., et al. Immunotherapy in cat-induced asthma. Double-blind trial with evaluation of in vivo and in vitro responses. *J. Allergy Clin. Immunol.* 74:230, 1984.

119. Ollier, S., et al. Skin-prick test preparations of *Dermatophagoides pteronyssinus* for prediction of a positive response to provocation testing. *Clin. Exp. Allergy* 19:457, 1989.

120. Ortolani, C., et al. Grass pollen immunotherapy: a single year double-blind, placebo-controlled study in patients with grass pollen–induced asthma and rhinitis. *J. Allergy Clin. Immunol.* 73:283, 1984.

121. Osterballe, O. Immunotherapy in hay fever with two major allergens, 19, 25, and partially purified extract of timothy grass pollen. *Allergy* 15:473, 1986.

122. Pearce, F. L. Mast Cell Heterogeneity: An Overview. In A. B. Kay (ed.), *Asthma: Clinical Pharmacology and Therapeutic Progress.* Oxford: Blackwell, 1986.

123. Pelikan, Z., and Pelikan-Filipak, M. Bronchial response to the food ingestion challenge. *Ann. Allergy* 58:164, 1987.

124. Peng, C., et al. A new isoform of human membrane-bound IgE. *J. Immunol.* 148:129, 1992.

125. Peters, S. P., et al. Arachidonic acid metabolism in purified human lung mast cells. *J. Immunol.* 131:1972, 1984.

126. Platts-Mills, T. A. E. Local production of IgG, IgA and IgE antibodies in grass pollen hay fever. *J. Immunol.* 122:2218, 1979.

127. Platts-Mills, T. A. E., et al. Reduction of bronchial hyperreactivity during prolonged allergen avoidance. *Lancet* 2:675, 1982.

128. Platts-Mills, T. A. E., et al. Dust mite allergen and asthma: report of a second international workshop. *J. Allergy Clin. Immunol.* 89:1046, 1992.

129. Popa, V. Bronchodilating activity of an H$_1$ blocker, chlorpheniramine. *J. Allergy Clin. Immunol.* 59:54, 1977.

130. Popa, V. Respiratory allergy to ragweed: correlation of bronchial responses to allergen and bronchial responses to histamine and circulating immunoglobulin E. *J. Allergy Clin. Immunol.* 65:389, 1980.

131. Popa, V. Effect of an H$_1$ blocker, chlorpheniramine, on inhalation tests with histamine and allergen in allergic asthma. *Chest* 78:442, 1980.

132. Popa, V. Bronchial cholinergic tone and sensitivity in normal and asthmatic subjects. *Clin. Pharmacol. Ther.* 40:326, 1986.

133. Popa, V. Pharmacodynamic aspects of chlorpheniramine-induced bronchodilation. *Chest* 93:952, 1988.

134. Popa, V. Captopril-related (or induced?) asthma. *Am. Rev. Respir. Dis.* 136:999, 1987.

135. Popa, V., and Al-George, S. Nasal provocation tests in allergic perennial rhinitis: a preliminary study. *Ann. Allergy* 27:45, 1969.

136. Popa, V., Al-George, S., and Gavanescu, O. Occupational and nonoccupational respiratory allergy in bakers. *Acta Allergol.* 25:159, 1970.

137. Popa, V., Douglas, J. S., and Bouhuys, A. Airway responses to histamine, acetylcholine, and propranolol in anaphylactic hypersensitivity in guinea pigs. *J. Allergy Clin. Immunol.* 51:344, 1973.

138. Popa, V., and Reardon, M. The effect of thermal treatment of IgE measured with competitive and noncompetitive assays. Is circulating IgE serologically heterogeneous? *Int. Arch. Allergy Appl. Immunol.* 77:349, 1985.

139. Popa, V., and Singleton, J. Provocation dose and discriminant analysis in histamine bronchoprovocation. *Chest* 93:952, 1988.

140. Popa, V., et al. La valeur du test bronchomoteur pour le diagnostic de l'asthme bronchique professionnel et non professionnel. *Rev. Roum. Med. Int.* 4:279, 1967.

141. Popa, V., et al. The value of inhalation tests in perennial bronchial asthma. *J. Allergy* 42:130, 1968.

142. Popa, V., et al. Bronchial asthma and asthmatic bronchitis determined by simple chemicals. *Dis. Chest* 56:395, 1969.

143. Prahl, R., and Nexo, E. Human serum IgE against two major allergens from cat hair and dander: determination of affinity and quantity of antigen specific IgE. *Allergy* 37:49, 1982.

144. Prausnitz, C., and Kustner, H. Studien uber die Uberempfindlichkeit. *Zentralbl. Bakteriol.* 86:160, 1921.

145. Price, J. F., Hey, E. N., and Soothill, J. F. Antigen provocation to the skin, nose and lung in children with asthma: immediate and dual hypersensitivity reactions. *Clin. Exp. Immunol.* 47:587, 1982.

146. Rackemann, F. H. A clinical study of one hundred and fifty cases of bronchial asthma. *Arch. Intern. Med.* 22:552, 1918.

147. Rak, S., et al. Immunotherapy abrogates the generation of eosinophil and neutrophil chemotactic activity during pollen season. *J. Allergy Clin. Immunol.* 86:706, 1990.

148. Ring, J., et al. Histamine and Allergic Diseases. In J. Ring and G. Burg (eds.), *New Trends in Allergy* II. Berlin: Springer, 1986.

149. Roane, J., et al. Intradermal tests in non-atopic children. *Ann. Allergy* 26:443, 1968.

150. Robinson, C., et al. The IgE- and calcium-dependent release of eicosanoids and histamine from human purified cutaneous mast cells. *J. Invest. Dermatol.* 93:397, 1989.

151. Rochester, G. L., and Rankin, J. A. Is asthma T-cell mediated? *Am. Rev. Respir. Dis.* 144:1005, 1991.

152. Rohatgi, N., et al. Cat- or dog-induced immediate and late asthmatic responses before and after immunotherapy. *J. Allergy Clin. Immunol.* 82:389, 1988.

153. Rowntree, S., et al. A subclass IgG$_4$ specific antigen-binding radioimmunoassay (RIA): comparison between IgG and IgG$_4$ antibodies to food and inhaled antigens in adult atopic dermatitis after desensitization treatment and during development of antibody responses in children. *J. Allergy Clin. Immunol.* 80:622, 1987.

154. Sotomayor, H., et al. Seasonal increase of carbachol airways responsiveness in patients allergic to grass pollen. *Am. Rev. Respir. Dis.* 130:56, 1984.

155. Spector, S. L., and Farr, R. S. Bronchial inhalation procedures in asthmatics. *Med. Clin. North Am.* 58:71, 1974.

156. Spector, S. L., and Farr, R. S. Bronchial inhalation challenge with antigen. *J. Allergy Clin. Immunol.* 64:580, 1979.

157. Stenius, B., and Wide, L. Reaginic antibody (IgE), skin, and provocation tests to *D. culinae* and house dust in respiratory allergy. *Lancet* 2:455, 1981.

158. Stevens, F. Comparison of pulmonary and dermal sensitivity to inhaled substances. *J. Allergy* 5:285, 1934.

159. Subcommittee on skin tests of the European Academy of Allergology and Clinical Immunology (S. Dreborg, ed.). Skin tests used in type I allergy testing (position paper). *Allergy* 47(suppl. 10):13, 1989.

160. Sue, M. A., Gordon, E. H., and Freund, L. H. Utility of additional skin testing in non "allergic" asthma. *Ann. Allergy* 68:393, 1992.

161. Sundin, B., et al. Immunotherapy with partially purified and standardized animal dander extracts. *J. Allergy Clin. Immunol.* 77:478, 1986.

162. Swain, H. H., and Becker, E. L. Quantitative studies in skin testing. V. The whealing reactions of histamine and ragweed pollen extract. *J. Allergy* 23:441, 1952.

163. Taylor, I. K., et al. Effect of cysteinyl-leukotriene receptor antagonist ICI

204219 on allergen-induced bronchoconstriction and airway hyperreactivity in atopic subjects. *Lancet* 337:690, 1991.

164. Taylor, W., et al. Immunotherapy in cat-induced asthma. *J. Allergy Clin. Immunol.* 61:283, 1978.

165. Thompson, K. A., et al. The current status of allergen immunotherapy (hypersensitization). A report of a WHO/IUIS working group. *Allergy* 44:369, 1989.

166. Tiffeneau, R. Hypersensibilite cholinergo-histaminique pulmonaire de l'asthmatique. *Acta Allergol.* 187(suppl. 5): 187, 1958.

167. Tomioka, M., et al. Mast cells in bronchoalveolar lumen of patients with bronchial asthma. *Am. Rev. Respir. Dis.* 129:1000, 1984.

168. Townley, R. G., Dennis, M., and Itkin, I. Comparative action of acetyl-beta-methylcholine, histamine, and pollen antigens in subjects with hay fever and subjects with bronchial asthma. *J. Allergy* 36:121, 1965.

169. Valavirta, M., et al. Immunotherapy in allergy to dog: immunologic and clinical findings of a double-blind study. *Ann. Allergy* 57:173, 1986.

170. Van Bever, H., and Stevens, W. J. Suppression of the late asthmatic reaction by hyposensitization in asthmatic children allergic to house dust mite (*Dermatophagoides pteronyssinus*). *Clin. Exp. Allergy* 19:399, 1989.

171. Van der Zee, J. S., et al. Discrepancies between the skin test and IgE antibody assays: study of histamine release, complement activation in vitro and occurrence of allergen-specific IgG. *J. Allergy Clin. Immunol.* 82:270, 1988.

172. Van Hage-Hamster, M., et al. Bronchial provocation studies in farmers with positive RAST to the storage mite *Lepidoglyphus destructor*. *Allergy* 43:545, 1988.

173. Van Lookeren Campagne, J. G., Knoll, K., and de Vries, K. House dust provocation in children. *Scand. J. Respir. Dis.* 50:76, 1969.

174. Van Metre, T. E., et al. Immunotherapy for cat asthma. *J. Allergy Clin. Immunol.* 82:1055, 1988.

175. Van Metre, T. E. Jr., et al. Immunotherapy decreases skin sensitivity to cat extract. *J. Allergy Clin. Immunol.* 83:888, 1989.

176. Van Toorenenbergen, A. W., and Aalbarese, A. C. IgG$_4$ and passive sensitization of basophil leucocytes. *Int. Arch. Allergy Appl. Immunol.* 65:432, 1981.

177. Vanto, T., et al. RAST in the diagnosis of dog dander allergy: a comparison between three allergen preparations using two variants of RAST. *Allergy* 37:175, 1982.

178. Venables, K. M., et al. Immunologic and functional consequences of chemical (tetrachlorophtalic anhydride)–induced asthma after four years of avoidance of exposure. *J. Allergy Clin. Immunol.* 80:212, 1987.

179. Voorhorst, R., and Van der Hooft-Van Asbeck, M. C. Atopic skin test reevaluated. VI. Skin reactions to compound 48/80 and histamine in patients with atopic and non-atopic chronic respiratory complaints and in normal volunteers. *Ann. Allergy* 42:185, 1979.

180. Wahn, U., et al. Prospective study on immunologic changes induced by two different *Dermatophagoides pteronyssinus* extracts prepared from whole mite culture and mite bodies. *J. Allergy Clin. Immunol.* 82:360, 1988.

181. Warner, J. O., et al. Controlled trial of hyposensitization to *Dermatophagoides pteronyssinus* in children with asthma. *Lancet* 2:912, 1978.

182. Webber, S. E., et al. Effects of antigen on tracheal circulation and smooth muscle in sheep of different ages. *J. Appl. Physiol.* 67:1256, 1989.

183. Yunginger, J. W., and Aleick, G. I. Seasonal changes in serum and nasal IgE concentration. *J. Allergy Clin. Immunol.* 51:174, 1973.

184. Zuidema, P. Value of inhalation tests in bronchial asthma. *Respiration* (suppl. 26):141, 1969.

Upper Respiratory Tract

Raymond G. Slavin

41

Bronchial asthma is largely thought of as a disease of the lower respiratory tract, involving mucosal edema, smooth muscle contraction, and mucosal gland hypersecretion of the bronchi and bronchioles. In this chapter, I will try to show how the upper respiratory tract relates to bronchial asthma.

The upper respiratory tract comprises the nose, paranasal sinuses, oral cavity, pharynx, and larynx. Diseases of the upper respiratory tract relate to asthma in two ways, by mimicking bronchial asthma and by causing true bronchospasm.

DISEASES OF THE UPPER RESPIRATORY TRACT THAT SIMULATE BRONCHIAL ASTHMA

The common denominator of upper respiratory tract conditions that simulate bronchial asthma is obstruction. Chapter 37, dealing with the differential diagnosis of asthma, includes many of these conditions that clinically may mimic the bronchospasm of asthma. It may be advantageous, however, to categorize by anatomic location conditions of the upper respiratory tract that produce noisy respirations which may be confused with asthma (Table 41-1). In particular, acute bouts of noisy respiration may occur in these conditions because of mucosal edema or piling up of mucus. Table 41-1 is by no means an exhaustive compendium of these conditions. It is intended only as a guide. Details of differential diagnosis can be found in Chapter 37. In general, however, noisy respirations heard best at the mouth, wheezing occurring predominantly when the patient is lying down or with varying body positions, and an overall poor response to bronchodilators should alert one to the possibility of upper airway obstruction.

DISEASES OF THE UPPER RESPIRATORY TRACT THAT EITHER CAUSE ASTHMA OR ARE ASSOCIATED WITH ASTHMA

The human airway has been traditionally divided into upper and lower segments that possess clear structural and functional distinctions. Diseases of the upper and lower airways may coexist, rhinitis and bronchial asthma being good examples. Up to 80 percent of patients with asthma have rhinitis symptoms, while 5 to 15 percent of patients with perennial rhinitis have asthma. However, until recently little attention has been paid to the possibility that the upper airway may play an important role in the pathogenesis of bronchial asthma. There are data from both experimental animal and human studies indicating that distinctions between the upper and lower airways are not as great as previously imagined. There may be important interrelationships, with

lessons to be learned about the mechanism of disease in one segment of the airway through study of the other segment.

The list that follows summarizes the possible relationships between upper and lower airway diseases. A detailed discussion of upper respiratory tract conditions will appear later in this chapter.

Allergic rhinitis
    Filter function failure: increases allergen/irritant burden on lower airway
    Heat and humidification failure: exercise-induced asthma
    Improvement in pulmonary symptoms by treatment of nasal symptoms
    Increased lower airway responsiveness: specific and nonspecific
Nasal polyps and asthma
Viral upper respiratory tract infection
Nasal sinus–bronchial reflex

Filter Function Failure of the Nose

The nose serves as an important filter of inspired air, since all inhaled particles and gases pass through the nose. Relatively large particles are captured by the hairs within the nostrils while other noxious substances are trapped in the mucus [46]. Obviously, any nasal obstruction or a failure in the filter function would increase the allergen or irritant burden to the lower airway, thus potentiating lower airway hyperresponsiveness.

Heat and Humidification Failure

The heating and humidification of inspired air is an important function of the nose. This is largely provided by the highly vascularized mucosa of the turbinates and septum. If inspired air bypasses the warming and humidification provided by the nose, then cooler, dryer air is delivered to the lung. This potentiates the phenomenon referred to as *exercise-induced asthma* (EIA) (see Chap. 47). Exercise is an important trigger for bronchial asthma, and it is the loss of water and heat from the lower airway that is thought to be responsible. Patients can reduce the severity of EIA by breathing through their nose rather than their mouth during exercise [54].

Improvement in Pulmonary Symptoms by Treatment of Nasal Symptoms

In a study comparing the efficacy of beclomethasone nasal solution, flunisolide, and cromolyn in relieving symptoms in 120 patients with ragweed allergy, it was noted that 58 patients in this group also had asthma [69]. Surprisingly, all of the intranasal treatments considerably reduced the symptoms of seasonal

Table 41-1. Upper respiratory tract conditions that may simulate asthma

Location	Condition
Nose	Mucus vibrating in nasal passages, foreign body, polyps, neoplasm
Oral cavity and pharynx	Hypertrophied adenoids and tonsils, polyps, retropharyngeal or peritonsillar abscess, choanal atresia, macroglossia, neoplasm
Larynx	Foreign body, croup, laryngotracheobronchitis, flaccid epiglottis, vocal cord abnormality, neoplasm

asthma. The authors speculated that intranasally administered drugs restore normal nasal physiologic conditions, including the warming, humidification, and filtration of airborne allergens [69]. It has been shown that a large proportion of ragweed allergen is contained in particles small enough to penetrate the bronchi. These aeroallergens are more likely to deposit in the airways during mouth breathing than during nasal breathing [1]. Another explanation for the improvement in lower airway symptoms occurring with topical nasal medications is seen in a recent study demonstrating that intranasal beclomethasone has a protective effect on bronchial responsiveness as determined by carbachol challenge [2a].

Increased Lower Airway Responsiveness in Nasal Diseases

Specific Responsiveness
Lower airway sensitivity may be increased in patients who only have clinical evidence of allergic rhinitis. In bronchial challenge studies performed with ragweed allergen, there was considerable overlap in lower airway sensitivity when patients with ragweed asthma were contrasted with patients who have allergic rhinitis. In other words, antigen challenge cannot be used to distinguish patients with hay fever only from those with asthma [40].

Nonspecific Responsiveness
Methacholine, a parasympathomimetic drug, is frequently used in the diagnosis of asthma when spirometry is normal (see Chap. 39). Asthmatics show an increased bronchoconstrictor response to inhalation of this agent. Twenty-five patients with rhinitis but no evidence of asthma were challenged with methacholine, and 10 of them showed an increased methacholine response. In five of these patients, there was also bronchoconstriction in response to hyperventilation and a further two demonstrated increased variability of peak flow rates. Thus, in 7 of 10 patients, increased bronchial responsiveness was confirmed by two different methods, although the patients were asymptomatic. The results indicate that methacholine responsiveness in the asthmatic range is seen in a significant number of patients with rhinitis alone, and that it is associated with variable air flow obstruction and subclinical asthma [44].

Nasal Polyps and Asthma
In a study by Settipane and Chaffee [52] published in 1977, 5,000 patients with asthma or allergic rhinitis were analyzed. Of the asthma group, 16.7 percent had nasal polyps and, of the 211 total patients with nasal polyps, 70 percent had asthma. It is estimated that patients with polyps have a 25 to 30 percent chance of developing bronchial asthma and vice versa [33]. Experiments conducted by Kaliner and associates [25] demonstrated that polyps from patients with allergic rhinitis will, on proper stimulation with appropriate antigen, release histamine, leukotrienes, and eosinophilic chemotactic factor of anaphylaxis. Interestingly,

when polyps from patients with chronic sinusitis are passively sensitized with immunoglobulin E (IgE) and then challenged with antigen, there is a greater release of the leukotrienes than of histamine. Several studies have offered conflicting evidence for the prevalence of bronchial hyperreactivity in patients with nasal polyps and no history of asthma. One group [15] demonstrated a low response to methacholine challenge in such subjects, while the other showed the opposite effect; that is, bronchial hyperreactivity seemed to be high in these patients, especially in nonatopics [34].

The association of nasal polyps, bronchial asthma, and aspirin sensitivity has been well described. These patients begin with vasomotor rhinitis and profuse rhinorrhea. This is associated later with intense nasal congestion and the development of nasal polyps. Following this, bronchial asthma develops and then finally, aspirin sensitivity. This subject is further detailed later in this chapter.

Increased Lower Airway Reactivity During Upper Respiratory Infections

Upper respiratory tract infections (URIs) provoke wheezing in many patients who have asthma, both children and adults. It has only recently been appreciated that respiratory viruses most commonly trigger these attacks. Respiratory syncytial virus is most common in young children with rhinovirus, and influenza virus is more prevalent in older children and adults [9]. The obstructive changes in small airway function of the lung associated with viral illness may persist for up to 5 weeks after the clinical illness has resolved. Viral URIs also cause airway hyperreactivity. The bronchial response to both a specific antigen challenge and a nonspecific challenge with methacholine or histamine is enhanced during a viral URI [16]. (See also Chapter 44 for added discussion.)

A number of mechanisms may explain how viral URIs contribute to airway reactivity, wheezing, and the pathogenesis of asthma.

1. Exfoliation of bronchial epithelium: A viral URI inflames the bronchial epithelium. This rapidly sensitizes adapting sensory vagus fibers located primarily in the epithelium of the large airways. Exposure of these sensitized fibers to an irritant such as histamine causes reflex bronchospasm.
2. Increased permeability of mucous membranes: The inflammation of the bronchial epithelium allows for increased permeability of antigen.
3. Effect on beta-adrenergic function: It is well known that there is a diminished beta-adrenergic responsiveness in asthmatics. This basic adrenergic block is enhanced in the presence of a viral URI.
4. Augmentation of mediator release: It has been demonstrated that leukocytes from asthmatic patients release increased amounts of histamine when they are incubated with respiratory viruses. This enhanced basophil-mediator release appears to be associated with the production of interferon by the viruses.
5. Stimulates synthesis of anti-viral IgE: Some respiratory viruses, in particular respiratory syncytial virus and parainfluenza virus, stimulate the production of allergic antibody IgE to virus [68]. The IgE attaches to exfoliated respiratory cells and reacts with the virus to increase the release of histamine, which causes wheezing. Enhanced histamine release causes the virus to produce interferon, which in turn enhances the release of histamine.

Nasal Sinus–Bronchial Reflex

A large number of studies have been done over the years that explored the relationship of the nose and paranasal sinuses to

Table 41-2. Evidence for nasobronchial reflex

Reference	Species	Stimulus	Intervention
Kratchmer, 1870 [30]	Cat	Ether, SO_2	—
Dixon & Brodie, 1903 [13]	Cat	Electrical	Sever vagus nerve
Ogura & Harvey, 1971 [38]	Humans	Anatomic	Surgery
Speizer & Frank, 1966 [60]	Humans	SO_2	—
Kaufman & Wright, 1969 [27]	Humans	Silica	Atropine

Table 41-3. Evidence against nasobronchial reflex

Reference	Stimulus	Lower airway
Schumacher et al., 1986 [50]	Grass or histamine	No effect
Rosenberg et al., 1983 [46a]	Ragweed	No effect
Hoehne & Reed, 1971 [23]	Ragweed	No effect

the cause of asthma (Table 41-2). Most of these studies are predicated on the fact that there are receptors in the nose, the nasopharynx, and presumably the sinuses that, on proper stimulation, result in bronchoconstriction. As long ago as 1870, Kratchmer [30], a French physiologist, demonstrated a substantial increase in lower airway resistance by stimulating the nose of cats with either ether or sulfur dioxide. In 1903, Dixon and Brodie [13] showed that electrical stimulation of the nose can also result in increased lower airway resistance in cats. They subsequently extended these observations to demonstrate that section of the vagus nerve blocked the changes in lower airway resistance.

Ogura and Harvey [38], in looking for an association between nasal resistance and bronchial asthma, conducted a series of experiments in both animals and human subjects. They were able to restore the lower airway to normal in some patients simply by correcting a nasal septal deviation [38]. Speizer and Frank [60] exposed healthy human volunteers to intranasally administered sulfur dioxide and showed an increase in lower airway reactivity.

In a well-controlled study, Kaufman and Wright [27] obtained uniform increases in lower airway resistance by blowing silica particles into the nasopharynx in 10 nonsmoking adults who had no chest complaints and normal pulmonary function tests. They repeated the experiments after the injection of atropine and demonstrated that the lower airway response was totally abolished.

Could allergy-inducing particles deposited in the nose give rise to a bronchial reflex? No such connection was found in some experimental studies (Table 41-3). When patients with grass- or ragweed-induced allergic rhinitis were subjected to intranasal challenge with specific allergens, no effect on lower airway performance could be demonstrated [23]. Schumacher and associates [50], using histamine for intranasal challenge in patients with allergic rhinitis, were similarly unable to show any effect on lower airway responsiveness.

Yan and Salome [70] performed similar studies on 12 patients with perennial rhinitis. When challenged intranasally with histamine, these patients showed a significant fall in the forced expiratory volume at 1 second (FEV_1) (six had a 20% decrease and two had a 10–17% decrease). This would suggest that a certain critical threshold of nasal disease severity may be necessary to provoke reflex changes in the lower airway as a response to nasal challenge. It was the conclusion of these authors that "the airways of some asthmatics narrow in response to nasal stimulation."

Relationship of Sinusitis and Asthma

The frequent association of paranasal sinus disease and bronchial asthma has been noted for a great many years, but there

has been a resurgence of interest in this association only during the past decade. A high incidence of radiographic evidence of sinusitis, on the order of 40 to 60 percent, has been demonstrated in asthmatic patients in several studies [5, 26]. The overriding question is, does this association represent an epiphenomenon; that is, are sinusitis and asthma manifestations of the same underlying disease process in different parts of the respiratory tract, or is there a causal relationship in that sinusitis triggers the bronchial asthma [56]?

That an association exists between sinus disease and obstructive lung disease has been established, but obviously more objective evidence that sinusitis triggers or exacerbates asthmatic systems is needed. Nevertheless, there are data which indicate that patients with difficult-to-control asthma will improve when coexistent sinusitis is eliminated by medical or surgical treatment, or both. This can be considered as strong evidence for an etiologic role of sinusitis in lower airway disease.

Evidence that sinusitis may have an important etiologic role in asthma may be obtained by examining the effects of adequate medical or surgical treatment of sinusitis on asthmatic manifestations.

Studies by Rachelefsky and associates [42] have demonstrated that children with combined sinusitis and lower airway hyperreactivity show significant improvement in their asthmatic state when they receive appropriate medical treatment for their sinusitis. Table 41-4 presents the disease characteristics observed before and after treatment for sinusitis in 48 children with hyperreactive airway disease. Only seven of these children needed sinus lavage. The rest received appropriate medical therapy. As can be seen, 79 percent of these children were able to discontinue bronchodilators once their sinusitis resolved. Pulmonary function tests showed normal results in 67 percent of those with pretreatment abnormalities. It should be emphasized that medical treatment, including appropriate antibiotics and decongestants (oral or topical), generally proves adequate in children with coexistent sinusitis and asthma, and surgical intervention is only rarely necessary in these cases. Similar results were reported for another group of children with asthma and sinusitis from the University of Pittsburgh [21].

At the St. Louis University Medical Center, we have had an opportunity to observe a large group of adult patients who had coexistent sinusitis and asthma, and who also exhibited evidence that the sinusitis played an important role in the pathogenesis of the asthma. The characteristics of this group of patients are shown in Table 41-5. The history in more than 90 percent indi-

Table 41-4. Disease characteristics before and after treatment for sinusitis in 48 children with hyperreactive airway disease

Characteristic	Before	After
Cough	100%	29%
Wheeze	100%	15%
Normal pulmonary function tests	0	67%
Bronchodilator treatment	100%	21%

Source: Data from G. S. Rachelefsky, R. M. Katz, and S. C. Siegel. Chronic sinus disease with associated reactive airway disease in children. *Pediatrics* 783:529, 1984.

Table 41-5. Characteristics of adult patients with combined sinus disease and bronchial asthma

Characteristic	Percentage
Asthma preceded by sinusitis (based on history)	>90%
Presence of atopy (based on history and skin tests)	<40%
Aspirin sensitivity (based on history)	>50%
Corticosteroid requirement	>90%

Table 41-6. Long-term follow-up of bilateral intranasal sphenoethmoidectomy effects on asthma

	Asthma symptoms	Medications	PFT	Nose
2 years post BSE	70%	65%	—	85%
5 years post BSE	63%	60%	20%	81%

PFT = pulmonary function test; BSE = bilateral intranasal sphenoethmoidectomy.

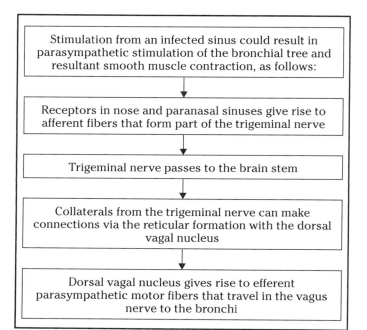

Fig. 41-1. *The postulated neural pathways involved in sinusitis-induced bronchospasm.*

cated that the sinusitis preceded the development of asthma symptoms. Based on history and a battery of allergy skin tests to common St. Louis aeroallergens, two-thirds of the patients were judged to be nonatopic and more than 50 percent had a history of aspirin sensitivity. Most importantly, more than 90 percent of these patients were receiving corticosteroids. Corticosteroid dependency furnishes an important clue to those patients who have an underlying sinus disease that may act as a trigger for the development of asthma. Our patients were uniformly resistant to medical therapy; that is, their sinusitis either recurred or never sufficiently cleared during aggressive medical management [57].

Our early results obtained with bilateral intranasal sphenoethmoidectomy revealed that 65 percent of our patients showed significant improvement in their asthmatic state following the procedure [57]. We have found that patients who showed improvement within the 2 years following surgery were likely to experience continued improvement throughout a 5-year observation period. As can be seen from Table 41-6, more than 80 percent of the patients reported that they had experienced moderately or greatly improved nasal symptomatology and 60 percent felt that their asthma symptoms had abated. Pretreatment pulmonary function test results improved an average of 20 percent [35].

Possible Mechanisms Explaining the Relationship Between Sinusitis and Asthma

Vagal Reflex
The postulated neuroanatomic pathways that could reflexly connect the paranasal sinuses to the lungs are shown in Figure 41-1. Receptors in the nose, and presumably in the paranasal si-

nuses, give rise to afferent fibers that in turn form part of the trigeminal nerve. The trigeminal nerve passes to the brain stem, where it can connect with the dorsal vagal nucleus via the reticular formation. From the vagal nucleus, parasympathetic efferent fibers travel in the vagus nerve to the bronchi. The cholinergic (parasympathetic) nervous system plays an integral part in maintaining resting bronchial muscle tone as well as in mediating acute bronchospastic responses. The vagus nerve provides the cholinergic motor supply to airway smooth muscle [11].

The Eosinophil
Evidence suggests that the eosinophil plays an important role in mediating injury to the bronchial epithelium in chronic asthma (see also Chap. 20). In a recent study, the role of the eosinophil in chronic inflammatory disease of the paranasal sinuses was investigated using tissue from patients who had undergone surgery for chronic sinusitis. As seen in Table 41-7, sinus tissue from patients with sinusitis who also had chronic asthma or allergic rhinitis, or both, was found to be extensively infiltrated with eosinophils. In contrast, sinus tissue from patients with chronic sinusitis alone had no eosinophils. Immunofluorescence studies demonstrated a striking association between the presence of extracellular deposition of major basic protein and damage to the sinus mucosa. In addition, the histopathology of the paranasal respiratory epithelium appeared similar to that described in bronchial asthma. These findings suggest that the eosinophil acts as an effector cell in chronic inflammatory disease in paranasal respiratory epithelium. This points to the fact that the sinus disease in patients with asthma may be due to the same mechanisms that cause damage to bronchial epithelium [22].

Inflammatory Mediators
Another proposed mechanism for sinusitis as an aggravator of asthma is local stimulation of irritant receptors by inflammatory mediators, with resultant reflex bronchospasm. In a recent study (Table 41-8), the levels of leukotrienes, prostaglandin D_2 (PGD_2), and histamine were measured in maxillary sinus lavage fluid obtained during surgery for chronic sinusitis. These results were compared to levels of mediators in nasal lavage fluid obtained from a group of atopic subjects. The results indicated that the levels of leukotrienes, histamine, and PGD_2 were significantly elevated over those in the control lavage fluid and were in the range associated with local inflammation and irritant receptor stimulation [61].

Table 41-7. Tissue eosinophilia in 26 patients with chronic sinusitis

Group 1	Chronic sinusitis and bronchial asthma in 5 patients, marked in all
Group 2	Chronic sinusitis, bronchial asthma, and allergic rhinitis in 8 patients, marked in all
Group 3	Chronic sinusitis and allergic rhinitis in 7 patients, marked in 6
Group 4	Chronic sinusitis marked in 0

Source: Data from S. L. Harlin, et al. A clinical and pathologic study of chronic sinusitis: the role of the eosinophil. *J. Allergy Clin. Immunol.* 81:867, 1988.

Table 41-8. Inflammatory mediators in lavage fluid

	$LTC_4/D_4/E_4$	Histamine	PGD_2
Sinus lavage in chronic sinusitis	1,110	258	84
Nasal lavage in allergic rhinitis	73	6	12

$LTC_4/D_4/E_4$ = leukotrienes C_4, D_4, and E_4, respectively; PGD_2 = prostaglandin D_2.
Source: Data from B. D. Stone, J. W. Georgitis, and B. Matthews. Inflammatory mediators in sinus lavage fluid (abstract). *J. Allergy Clin. Immunol.* 85:22, 1990.

A recent study from South Africa indicates that aspiration of fluid from the paranasal sinuses does not take place into the lower airway [3].

Allergic Rhinitis

Characteristics

Allergic rhinitis can exist in two forms, seasonal and nonseasonal. The causes of seasonal rhinitis are largely inhalants, such as tree, grass, and weed pollen and mold spores. The nonseasonal or perennial form of allergic rhinitis is due to substances such as house dust, feathers, and animal antigens, both from dander and saliva, that are encountered on a year-round basis. Foods as causes of allergic rhinitis are controversial, but probably do exist, although not nearly to the extent of inhalants. The three pathophysiologic hallmarks of allergic rhinitis are (1) dilatation of the vascular bed with edema formation, (2) engorgement of mucous glands and goblet cells, and (3) infiltration of the submucosa and mucosa with eosinophils.

Mygind [37] has elegantly described the possible pathogenetic steps in allergic rhinitis. The interaction of an allergen and IgE on the mast cells near the epithelial surface of the nose results in the release of histamine and other chemical mediators. Histamine, the most important mediator of allergic rhinitis, has several important biologic effects. It increases epithelial permeability and decreases the efficiency of the tight junction. This results in better penetration of the nasal epithelial surface by inhalant allergens. Histamine also dilates blood vessels via cell receptors and stimulates epithelial nerve endings, which initiates a parasympathetic reflex in the trigeminal nerve. Centers in the central nervous system are then activated, and this results in sneezing, which further activates the reflex arch. Impulses are then generated in parasympathetic fibers to glands and blood vessels. Acetylcholine is released from nerve terminals and subsequently activates cholinergic receptors. This results in marked mucus hypersecretion and an increase in vasodilatation. All of these changes lead to the clinical condition of allergic rhinitis.

The process by which inhalant allergens sensitize the nose is thought to occur in the following manner. Inhalant allergens are trapped in the nasal secretions and penetrate the mucosal barrier. Penetration of the nasal mucosal barrier is probably aided by relative secretory IgA deficiency [64] and a basic increase in mucosal permeability [48] thought to exist in allergic patients. In addition, the previously described effect of released histamine may play a role. After penetration of the nasal mucosal barrier, the antigen or allergen is processed by macrophages, with resultant stimulation of the lymphocytes destined to produce IgE. Helper and suppressor T-cell subpopulations regulate this process. Finally IgE is formed by the plasma cells evolving from the B-lymphocytes. IgE antibody is then distributed to blood and tissue fluids, resulting in generalized mast cell sensitization.

The clinical features of allergic rhinitis consist of sneezing, clear watery rhinorrhea, nasal pruritus, and nasal congestion [51]. Physical findings include the craniofacial abnormalities associated with chronic mouth breathing. Examination of the nose in uncomplicated allergic rhinitis will often reveal markedly swollen nasal turbinates that appear pale. This so-called typical appearance is not always seen. A patient with allergic rhinitis may have a superimposed infection, which will render the nasal mucosa red. A condition that will be discussed later, termed *nonallergic rhinitis with eosinophilia syndrome* (NARES), is nonallergic and is associated with a pale nasal mucosa.

The diagnosis of allergic rhinitis is based largely on the history and physical examination. The presence of eosinophils in the nasal secretions may be of some help, but the presence or absence of eosinophils does not confirm or rule out the diagnosis of allergic rhinitis. Infectious rhinitis as a complication of allergic rhinitis will cause the influx of many polymorphonuclear leukocytes, which will dilute out the eosinophils. On the other hand, the presence of large numbers of eosinophils may mean NARES rather than allergic rhinitis. Skin tests are helpful but must be interpreted in the proper clinical context. The clinician performing skin tests must understand the reasons for false negative results, false positive results, and results that are positive but biologically insignificant [55]. Radioimmunoassay tests are available for the determination of total circulating IgE (paper radioimmunosorbent test—PRIST) and for specific IgE directed to a particular antigen (radioallergosorbent test—RAST). These tests are not particularly cost effective and, except in unusual circumstances, should not be substituted for skin tests. (See Chap. 38.)

Nasal provocation tests do not have great usefulness in the diagnosis of allergic rhinitis. First, the measurement of nasal airway resistance is quite difficult, requiring the use of cumbersome and complicated equipment. Recently developed devices offer some hope but will have to be subjected to more study. Second, there is no evidence that nasal provocation tests offer any diagnostic advantage over the carefully taken history and properly interpreted skin tests.

Allergic rhinitis is distinctly not an innocuous medical condition. Because of the contiguous nature of the sinus mucosa and the nasal mucosa, allergic inflammation of the nose will often cause sinusitis. In addition, allergic inflammation of the nose will tend to obstruct the sinus ostium, the opening through which the sinus cavities drain into the lateral wall of the nose. With this obstruction of the opening and an increase in mucus production, the mucociliary defense mechanism of the sinuses does not function effectively, and infection of the sinuses may result.

For the same mechanical reasons, allergic inflammation of the nose may lead to obstruction of the eustachian tube with resultant chronic *serous otitis media*.

While the majority of *nasal polyps* are due to infection, there certainly is no question that polyp formation in the nose may be due to allergy.

Chronic mouth breathing caused by allergic rhinitis may result in marked *craniofacial abnormalities:* a typical thin pinched face and high arched palate.

The marked discomfort of allergic rhinitis caused by sneezing, itching, and nasal obstruction with rhinorrhea obviously interferes greatly with the patient's life. These patients do not sleep well because of nasal obstruction and eat poorly because of loss of taste and smell. It is no wonder, therefore, that patients with allergic rhinitis, children in particular, may be irritable, moody, and fatigued, with resultant *behavior problems*.

The management of allergic rhinitis generally follows one or more of three approaches. Symptomatic relief may be afforded by antihistamines, decongestants, cromolyn sodium, and nasal or systemic corticosteroids. The second approach is environmental control, which basically means avoidance of the responsible allergen or allergens. This may include air conditioning, removal of a pet from the home, or house dust avoidance. The third form of management is immunotherapy, which can be used if the above two approaches fail. Immunotherapy involves the subcutaneous injection of increasing quantities of the inhalant allergen to which the patient is sensitive. An abundance of studies attest to the efficacy of immunotherapy in the treatment of allergic rhinitis [31, 47].

Other Forms of Rhinitis

Vasomotor Rhinitis

The term *vasomotor rhinitis* is falling out of favor. Preferred terms are *perennial nonallergic rhinitis, vasoconstrictive rhinitis* [24], or *vasomotor instability* [49]. The last term is particularly graphic, for it describes the disease in terms of the basic pathogenesis, that is, a vasomotor instability caused by an abnormality of autonomic control of the vasculature and mucous gland secretion.

The parasympathetic system predominates in this instance. Secondary forms of this condition occur during pregnancy, with particular problems encountered in the second and third trimester, and in hypothyroidism.

Vasomotor rhinitis is characterized by marked nasal congestion and postnasal drainage. Frequently, the nasal blockage alternates from one side to the other. A host of triggers may precipitate symptoms illustrating vasomotor instability. These include cold weather or changes in the weather, spicy foods, sunlight, odors, fumes, dust, cigarette smoke, emotions, and on and on. The physical examination of the nose generally reveals marked edema with an erythematous nasal mucosa. The results of skin tests are either negative or clinically meaningless. The management of vasomotor rhinitis includes nasal decongestants and saline nasal lavage. Particularly important is a prescribed program of regular exercise, which results in a decrease in nasal airway resistance [45].

Nonallergic Rhinitis with Eosinophilia Syndrome
NARES is a recently described condition thought by some to comprise as much as 20 percent of the cases of chronic rhinitis [36]. It is associated with sneezing, profuse rhinorrhea, and pruritus with little in the way of nasal blockage. The symptoms are intermittent, varying from mild to severe, and sporadic, occurring from 10 to 20 times a day to 3 to 5 times a year. The results of physical examination are very similar to those in allergic rhinitis. Skin test results are either negative or clinically unimportant, and RAST results are negative, both in the blood and nasal secretions. NARES generally responds extremely well to topical steroids.

Chronic Rhinitis of Non–IgE-associated Asthma
An intriguing form of chronic rhinitis is commonly associated with so-called intrinsic or nonallergic asthma [24]. The rhinitis and the asthma are thought to represent the same basic respiratory tract abnormality. The symptoms are perennial and appear to cluster nocturnally with recurrence in the morning. The major symptoms are nasal congestion, some sneezing, rhinorrhea, and pruritus. Skin test and RAST results are either negative or clinically unimportant.

Table 41-9 summarizes seven common clinical conditions affecting the nose. In addition to the above-described forms of rhinitis, this table also includes rhinitis medicamentosum caused by the overuse of topical decongestants, structural rhinitis, and neutrophilic rhinosinusitis.

Nasal Polyps

Although nasal polyps were first described more than 3,000 years ago, a good many questions still exist with regard to incidence, causes, pathogenesis, and treatment.

Characteristics
Nasal polyps seem to be outgrowths of the nasal mucosa (Plate 8). The mass of the polyp is made up chiefly of edema fluid with sparse fibrous cells and few mucous glands. The surface epithelium generally reveals squamous metaplasia. The supporting structure is interspersed with masses of lymphocytes, plasma cells, eosinophils, and, less often, mast cells. Nasal polyp fluid contains concentrations of IgA, IgE, IgG, and IgM that are greater than one would expect from passive filtration [12]. Taylor [63] performed studies comparing nasal polyps with the adjacent normal respiratory mucosa. Using 12 stains to determine the histochemical composition of polyps, he found the same characteristics for both polyps and normal nasal epithelium. Nasal polyps, therefore, appear to be derived from and contain most of the cellular and chemical elements normally found in the respiratory

Table 41-9. Chronic rhinitis syndromes

	Allergic rhinitis	Vasomotor instability	NARES	Chronic rhinitis associated with intrinsic asthma	Rhinitis medicamentosum	Structural rhinitis	Neutrophilic rhinosinusitis
Cause or mechanisms	Allergens	Vascular hyperreactivity	Unknown	?Hyperreactivity	Medication	Septal abnormalities	Infection
Sneezing and pruritus	+ + +	–	+ + + +	+ +	–	–	–
Rhinorrhea	+ + +	±	+ + + +	+ +	–	–	Purulent
Congestion	+ +	+ + + +	±	+ + +	+ + +	+ + +	+ +
Postnasal drainage	+	+ + + +	±	+ +	–	–	+ + +
Seasonal variation	Seasonal or perennial	Perennial	Perennial	Perennial	Perennial	Perennial	Perennial
Eosinophils in nasal secretion	+	–	+	+	–	–	–
Skin test results	Positive	Negative	Negative	Negative	Negative	Negative	Negative
Total IgE	Increased	Normal	Normal	Normal	Normal	Normal	Normal
Response to methacholine challenge	Positive	Negative	Negative	Positive	Negative	Negative	Negative
Age at onset	Childhood	Adult	All ages	All ages	Adult	All ages	All ages
Associated factors	Family history Pale mucosa	Pregnancy Thyroid disorder	Pale mucosa	Pale mucosa	Use of topical decongestants, antihypertensives	Unilateral obstruction History of nasal trauma	Associated with upper respiratory infection
Treatment	Symptomatic Environmental control Immunotherapy	Decongestant Nasal saline Exercise	Topical steroids	Topical steroids	Stop medication	Surgery	Antibiotics

NARES = nonallergic rhinitis with eosinophilia syndrome; + + + + = marked; + + + = moderate; + + = mild; + = slight; ± = questionable; – = absent.
Source: R. G. Slavin, Clinical disorders of the nose and their relationship to allergy. *Ann. Allergy* 49:123, 1982.

mucosa. They do seem to be devoid of sensory vasomotor and secretomotor innervation.

It has generally been thought that there is marked uniformity in the histologic pattern of all nasal polyps, no matter what the cause or origin [67]. Recently, attempts have been made to distinguish nasal polyps histologically or histochemically. Oppenheimer and Rosenstein [39] have reported a histologic triad in the nasal polyps of cystic fibrosis patients, consisting of a barely visible basement membrane, a lack of eosinophils, and preponderance of acid mucin. In contrast, nasal polyps from atopic patients demonstrated a thickened basement membrane, numerous eosinophils, and a neutral mucin. Baumgarten and colleagues [4] have examined the cellular infiltrates in nasal polyps. While an eosinophilic and round cell infiltrate is present in all types of polyps, they maintain that a ratio of eosinophils to plasma cells of less than 5 is indicative of an allergy, and a ratio of greater than 5 corresponds more closely to infection. In other words, infection is associated with relatively more eosinophils and atopy is associated with relatively more plasma cells.

Bumsted and associates [8] have found the histamine content to be significantly greater in polyps than in normal mucosa. The norepinephrine content in the base of the polyps was greater than that in normal nasal mucosa. There were no differences in the levels of histamine, serotonin, and norepinephrine in the polyps of atopic and nonatopic patients. However, these researchers did find that the polyps of patients with nasal polyps, aspirin sensitivity, and asthma, the so-called ASA triad, had a much lower histamine concentration than did the nasal polyps of other patients. A great deal of work remains to be done on the histologic and histochemical characterization of nasal polyps.

Nasal polyps are located on the lateral wall of the nose, usually in the middle meatus or along the middle and superior turbinates. Most arise from within the ethmoid sinus, with some originating in the maxillary or sphenoid sinus. The ethmoid ostia are the smallest of the sinus ostia, measuring 1 to 2 mm. Perhaps the small diameter makes the ostium susceptible to occlusion by mucosal edema or the growth of polypoid granulation tissue.

Clinically, most patients with polyps have a long history of symptoms of perennial rhinitis. They complain chiefly of nasal airway obstruction and rhinorrhea. Total obstruction may be associated with anosmia. Symptoms are frequently exaggerated by physiologic stimuli such as temperature changes, fumes, odors, dusts, and chemicals. Polyps appear rounded or pear shaped and translucent. They are soft and gelatinous.

Incidence

The true incidence of nasal polyps is not known. Men outnumber women 2 : 1 in the occurrence of nasal polyps. The great majority of polyps occur after age 40. Nasal polyps are a rare occurrence under the age of 10, and when they do occur in a child, serious thought should be given to the possibility of cystic fibrosis. As many as 20 percent of children with cystic fibrosis have been reported to have nasal polyps [65].

Early studies of the incidence of nasal polyps in allergic disease suggested a marked correlation between polyps and allergy [29]. However, an immunologic mechanism was not demonstrated in many cases considered to be allergic, such as in patients with perennial asthma, perennial rhinitis, and vasomotor rhinitis. More recently there has been increasing evidence that there is no particular association between nasal polyps and atopy [2, 10]. The incidence of nasal polyps is quite low in uncomplicated seasonal allergic rhinitis [14]. Settipane and associates [55] analyzed 5,000 patients with asthma or allergic rhinitis. Of the 5,000, 211, or 4.2 percent, had nasal polyps. Of those with asthma, 16.7 percent had polyps; the allergic rhinitis group included 2.2 percent with polyps. Of the 211 patients with nasal polyps, 70 percent has asthma and 29.4 percent had allergic rhinitis.

To summarize, there appears to be a high incidence of nasal polyps in any type of chronic nasal disease. The increased association of nasal polyps with perennial bronchial asthma and aspirin sensitivity will be discussed later and in Chap. 48.

Pathogenesis

The pathogenesis of nasal polyps is not known. A number of mechanisms have been offered, including chronic inflammation of the nasal mucosa, an abnormal vasomotor response, increased interstitial fluid pressure and edema, and dysfunction of carbohydrate metabolism. The abnormal vasomotor response appears to be due to autonomic imbalance. This results in the previously described exaggerated response to physiologic stimuli. In many instances, there seems to be a self-perpetuating cycle. The nasal polyps interfere with sinus drainage. Subsequent sinusitis causes more venous stasis and mucosal edema, which leads to further enlargement of polyps.

Treatment

The management of nasal polyps may include medical and surgical approaches. Antihistamines, decongestants, and cromolyn sodium are generally of little benefit, and simple polypectomy alone is associated with an extremely high recurrence rate. A number of intranasal corticosteroid preparations have been shown to be effective in managing nasal polyps [62]. Significant improvement in 80 percent of patients with moderate to severe polyposis can be achieved using these preparations. In addition to decreasing polyp size and increasing nasal airway conductance, there is also a decrease in the number of eosinophils in the nasal smear, with a decrease in the albumin, IgG, and IgE levels in the secretions. The reasons for the failure of intranasal steroids in managing nasal polyps may be due to the extensive nasal mucosa and polyp swelling that prevents entrance of the drug. In this case, systemic steroids must be administered first to reduce mucosa and polyp size. Associated rhinosinusitis requires the use of antibiotics.

In a recent study from Scandinavia, surgical removal of nasal polyps was compared with the use of systemic steroids [32]. After initial treatment with either surgery or systemic steroids, both groups of patients were given topical steroids and followed for 1 year. Both groups experienced a similar increase in nasal expiratory peak flow and sense of smell, but there was a statistically significant increase in the benefit obtained from medications. The two major conclusions of the authors, who were otolaryngologists, were: (1) "the continued post-operative use of topical steroids postpones or prevents recurrence of nasal polyps," and (2) "surgical removal should be reserved for those few cases in which the presence of residual or recurrent polyps justifies the inherent risks and discomfort for the patient" [32].

Based on these and other studies, it would appear that a reasonable medical approach to the management of nasal polyps would be a 10- to 14-day course of oral prednisone followed by intranasal corticosteroids.

Sinuses

Structure and Function

The sinuses are four paired structures surrounding the nasal cavities. Each sinus has an opening or ostium on the lateral side of the nose through which drainage occurs. The maxillary sinus is located in the general area of the cheek. The floor is part of the tooth-bearing area of the maxilla and is below the floor of the nasal cavity. The base of the orbit composes the roof of the maxillary sinus. Its ostium opens into the middle meatus between the middle and inferior turbinates. The frontal sinus forms the medial portion of the roof of the orbit and is within the frontal bone. Its ostium opens into the anterior part of the middle meatus. The ethmoidal sinus lines the medial wall of the orbit close to the cranial cavity, which is separated by the cribriform plate. Bony septi divide the ethmoid sinuses into anterior, middle, and posterior sections. The anterior and middle ethmoidal cells open into the middle meatus, and the posterior ethmoidal cells drain into the superior meatus. The sphenoidal sinus empties into the sphenoethmoidal recess above the superior turbinate. Its roof is the pituitary fossa, and its lateral aspect is formed by the cavernous venous sinuses.

Developmentally, the maxillary and ethmoidal sinuses are present at birth, and the sphenoid and frontal sinuses appear by the second to third year of life.

The sinus cavities are lined by the same mucosa as the nose; the mucosa contains cilia and mucous glands.

The precise functions of the paranasal sinuses are not clear; however, some suggestions have included roles in olfaction, voice response, production of protective mucus, the dampening of sudden pressure changes in the nose during respiration, and lessening of skull weight.

Infection

The sinuses protect themselves against infection largely by the mucociliary apparatus. Microorganisms and foreign particles are trapped in the mucus and removed by constant movement of the mucus layer propelled by the underlying cilia. In this fashion, mucus is carried out to the sinus ostium. As stated earlier, the maxillary sinus base is below the floor of the nasal cavity. Its ostium is located at the highest point of the maxillary antrum (cavity). Therefore, in an upright position, in order for discharge to occur into the nose, the antrum must be completely filled or ciliary action must move secretions cephalad to the ostium. Thus ciliary action acquires tremendous importance in reducing sinus infection. Other protective factors include lysozymes and secretory IgA.

The following conditions predispose to the development of sinus disease:

Nasal allergy
Respiratory infection
Overuse of topical decongestants
Adenoids—hypertrophied
Deviated nasal septi
Polyps
Tumors
Foreign bodies
Swimming and diving
Cystic fibrosis

Viral infections and allergic inflammation resulting in rhinitis will cause an inflammatory response in the sinuses because of the contiguity of the nose and sinuses. Because of an increase in sinus mucus production and obstruction of the ostium owing to the nasal mucosal edema, the mucociliary defense mechanism will not function effectively. The severity and duration of the inflammation and consequent impairment of sinus drainage will determine whether bacterial superinfection develops.

Knowledge of the true microbiologic picture in sinusitis has emerged from studies in which sinus aspirates were aseptically obtained by direct antral puncture or by sampling directly from the involved sinus during surgery. Nasal cultures are meaningless because of contamination. Normal sinuses do not yield any bacteria. Cultures from acute sinusitis grow predominantly aerobic organisms [17], whereas positive cultures are anaerobes in 70 percent of cases of chronic sinusitis [19].

Cultures from sinus cavities in children with acute sinusitis have yielded *Streptococcus pneumoniae, Hemophilus influenzae,* and *Branhamella catarrhalis* [66]. Cultures from adults with acute disease grow *H. influenzae, S. pneumoniae, S. viridans,* and *Staphylococcus aureus* [7]. Chronic sinus disease yields largely anaerobes, including alpha streptococcus, *Bacteroides, Veillonella,* and *Corynebacterium* [19].

Diagnosis of Sinusitis

Clinical Presentation. Sinus infection may occur without fever or facial pain. Several authors have commented on the poor correlation between clinical characteristics and results of antral puncture. In adults [17], the typical asymmetric, dull facial pain aggravated by stooping may occur with a normal puncture result, and a typical purulent sinus by puncture may be entirely asymptomatic. In children [41], the common clinical presentation of sinusitis includes nasal obstruction, thick green or yellow nasal discharge and postnasal drainage, night and day coughing, sore throat, and an associated negative nasal smear for eosinophils. Headache, fever, facial pain, and earache are infrequent complaints.

Radiographic Appearance. The correlation, or lack thereof, of radiologic evidence of sinusitis and positive antral culture along with clinical evidence of sinusitis has been the subject of many publications. Earlier studies reported radiographic evidence of maxillary sinus abnormality in 26 percent of asymptomatic normal subjects [17] and in 52 percent of asthmatic patients [6]. The latter study reported only a 20 percent positive bacterial growth in antral cultures in association with positive radiographs. It has been suggested that this discrepancy, in contrast with later studies, is due to the fact that the roentgenographic diagnosis of sinusitis was made on the basis of only minor degrees of mucosal thickening, that is, 2 to 6 mm.

In a study of adults with sinusitis, Evans and colleagues [17] reported abnormal sinus aspirates in 17 of 18 patients with radiographic opacity of the sinuses, and abnormal aspirates in all subjects with mucosal thickening greater than 8 mm. Rachelefsky and associates [43] reported abnormal sinus x-ray studies in 53 percent of allergic children, with 21 percent having complete opacification of one or more sinus cavities. It appears therefore that radiographic evidence of mucosal thickening of 6 to 8 mm or greater (Fig. 41-2), air fluid levels (Fig. 41-3), or opacification (Fig. 41-4) indicates bacterial infection of the sinuses.

Transillumination. Studies [59] have indicated that transillumination of the sinuses is of limited usefulness in the diagnosis of sinusitis. While frontal sinus transillumination is a better predic-

Fig. 41-2. *Marked mucoperiosteal thickening of both maxillary sinuses.*

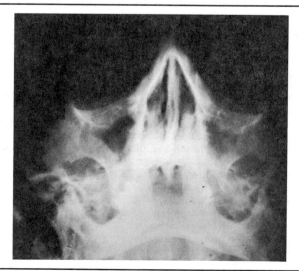

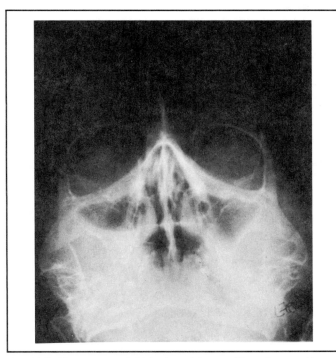

Fig. 41-3. *Mucoperiosteal thickening of the maxillary sinuses with an air fluid level on the right.*

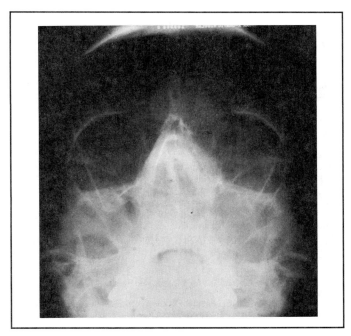

Fig. 41-4. *Opacification of both maxillary sinuses.*

tor of roentgenographically demonstrated sinus disease than is maxillary transillumination, there is still considerable error. Transillumination is not an adequate substitute for roentgenography.

Ultrasonography. Ultrasonography consists of transmitting low-power, pulsed ultrasound into the selected sinus cavity by direct contact of the transducer on the patient's face. At the frequency used, ultrasound does not propagate through air. When the sinus is healthy and filled with air, no echo appears from the back wall. If fluid is present, a strong echo will be re-

flected by the back wall of the sinus. Advantages of ultrasonography are that it is noninvasive, nonionizing, and painless. However, to date, no consensus has been reached as to the diagnostic accuracy and validity of this method. More studies and improvements in technology will be necessary before this technique can be recommended for general use.

Fig. 41-5. *Value of computed tomography in diagnosing sinus disease. A. Normal sinus film. B. CT scan in same patient revealing marked ethmoidal disease. (Films courtesy of Paul Toffel, M.D.)*

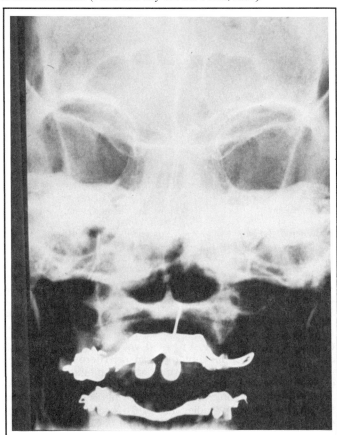

A

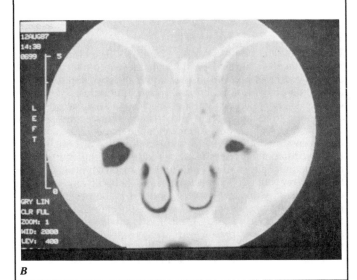

B

Table 41-10. Medical management of sinusitis: sample regimens

Therapy	Purpose	Regimen for children	Regimen for adults
Steam and saline	Prevent nasal crusting, liquify secretions, and have a mild decongestant effect	Steam inhalation several times a day. Saline administered by nasal spray (several sprays in each nostril q.i.d.) or saline lavage (¼ tsp of salt in 8 oz of warm water delivered by bulb syringe)	
Decongestants			
Oral phenylpropanolamine	Increases ostial diameter	2 to 6 years of age: 6.25 mg q4h; 6 to 12 years of age: 12.5 mg q4h, not to exceed 75 mg/day	25 mg q4h or 50 mg q8h, not to exceed 150 mg/day
Oxymetazoline	Increases ostial diameter	2 to 5 years of age: 2 to 3 drops of 0.025% solution in each nostril b.i.d.; 6 years of age and older: 2 to 3 sprays or 2 to 3 drops of 0.05% solution in each nostril b.i.d.	2 to 3 sprays or 2 to 3 drops of 0.05% solution in each nostril b.i.d.
Phenylephrine	Increases ostial diameter	2 to 6 years of age: 1 drop of 0.125% to 0.2% solution in each nostril q2–4h; 6 years of age and older: 1 to 2 sprays of 0.25% solution in each nostril q3–4h	1 to 2 sprays of 0.25% solution in each nostril q4h (0.5% and 1.0% solutions may also be used)
Topical corticosteroids			
Beclomethasone	Reduces mucosal inflammation	6 to 12 years of age: 1 spray in each nostril t.i.d.; 12 years of age and older: 1 spray in each nostril 2 to 4 times a day	1 spray in each nostril 2 to 4 times a day
Flunisolide	Reduces mucosal inflammation	6 to 14 years of age: 1 spray in each nostril t.i.d. (or 2 sprays b.i.d.)	2 sprays in each nostril b.i.d.
Mucoevacuants			
Guaifenesin	Thins and clears mucus secretions	6 to 12 years of age: 100 to 200 mg q4h, not to exceed 300 mg/day	100 to 400 mg q3–6h, not to exceed 2.4 g/day
Iodinated glycerol	Thins and clears mucus secretions	Up to one-half the adult dosage, based on weight	60 mg q.i.d.
Potassium iodide	Thins and clears mucus secretions	150 to 500 mg after meals 2 to 3 times a day	300 to 1,000 mg after meals 2 to 3 times a day (if tolerated, 1.0 to 1.5 gm t.i.d.)
Antibiotics	Manage bacterial infection	(see Table 41-11)	(see Table 41-11)

Source: R. G. Slavin. Recalcitrant asthma: could sinusitis be the culprit? *J. Respir. Dis.* 12:191, 1991. Reprinted with permission.

Computed Tomography. A major development in the diagnosis of sinusitis is the application of CT scans. There is no question that disease of the sinuses, particularly of the ethmoids, may be missed on ordinary roentgenography. CT scans can demonstrate the ostiomeatal complex and detect subtle disease not demonstrated on sinus x-ray studies (Fig. 41-5). A major problem in the past has been the rather prohibitive cost of CT scans. Through improvement in technology and the use of limited scans, the price of the technique has been lowered to a much more reasonable level and, in some centers, is quite close to that for ordinary sinus x-ray studies.

Treatment

The medical therapy of sinusitis (Table 41-10) includes promoting drainage of the sinuses through the use of decongestants such as pseudoephedrine and hot washcloths applied to the face, as well as control of infection through antibiotics. The drug of choice is ampicillin or amoxicillin. The organisms previously mentioned that cause acute and chronic sinusitis are sensitive to these drugs, and there is good evidence that adequate mucosal and even sinus fluid levels of these antibiotics are obtained. In the case of penicillin sensitivity, trimethoprim-sulfamethoxazole is an adequate alternative. One study reported a limited response to erythromycin [41]. The incidence of beta-lactam–producing organisms in acute and chronic sinusitis is increasing. In these instances, antibiotics such as amoxicillin clavulanate or cefuroxime must be used [66a]. Unlike otitis media and pharyngitis, sinusitis should be treated with an appropriate antibiotic for 3 to 4 weeks to ensure eradication of the infection. Patients with sinusitis may become asymptomatic despite persistence in the sinuses of purulent material containing high titers of bacteria.

Table 41-11. Sample antibiotic regimens for sinusitis*

Drug	Dosage for children	Dosage for adults
Amoxicillin	40 mg/kg/day	500 mg t.i.d.
Amoxicillin clavulanate	40 mg/kg/day	500 mg t.i.d.
Ampicillin	50 mg/kg/day in divided doses q6–8h	500 mg q.i.d.
Cefaclor	40 mg/kg/day	500 mg t.i.d.
Erythromycin and sulfisoxazole	50 mg/kg/day of erythromycin and 150 mg/kg/day of sulfisoxazole, in divided doses q.i.d.	
Trimethoprim sulfamethoxazole (TMP-SMX)	8 mg/kg/day of TMP and 40 mg/kg/day of SMX	160 mg of TMP and 800 mg of SMX b.i.d.

* Treat patients with acute sinusitis for 2 weeks, and treat those with chronic sinusitis for 3 weeks or more.
Source: R. G. Slavin. Recalcitrant asthma: could sinusitis be the culprit? *J. Respir. Dis.* 12:191, 1991. Reprinted with permission.

Follow-up sinus radiographs are necessary to exclude persistence of disease [17] (Table 41-11).

If there is no major clinical and radiographic improvement after 1 month, the patient should be referred to an otolaryngologist. The task of the otolaryngologist in the treatment of sinusitis is largely mechanical and consists of (1) relieving obstruction, (2) resecting diseased tissue, and (3) providing a nasal airway with drainage for all the nasal and sinus compartments [58]. When sinusitis resists medical therapy, mechanical treatment is indicated. This may be as simple as the creation of a nasoantral window in the inferior meatus to provide drainage for the maxillary antrum. A Caldwell-Luc procedure includes the creation of antral windows in the maxillary sinuses and an opportunity for the surgeon to resect diseased tissue. Anterior ethmoidectomy, which can be regarded as a mechanical extension of polypectomy, is performed when suppurative, mucopurulent disease remains in the middle meatus after polypectomy. In the hands of an experienced otolaryngologist, bilateral intranasal sphenoethmoidectomy may prove to be extremely beneficial [19].

Functional endoscopic sinus surgery is gaining increasing acceptance for the treatment of medically resistant sinus disease. The purpose is to reestablish ventilation and mucociliary clearance of the sinuses. This is accomplished by the endoscopic removal of diseased tissue from the key areas of the anterior ethmoidal sinus, middle turbinate, and middle meatus. The objective is to remove, in a limited resection, the inflammatory and anatomic defects that interfere with normal mucociliary clearance and that produce the resistant inflammation. The technique has been used successfully to treat chronic and recurrent sinusitis of the maxillary, ethmoidal, and frontal sinuses. Its advantages are minimal trauma to the normal nasal and sinus structures and conservative removal of diseased tissue. Restoration of the natural physiology as well as mucociliary clearance and function of the sinuses is thus made possible [28].

REFERENCES

1. Agarwal, M. K., et al. Airborne ragweed allergens; association with various particle sizes and short ragweed plant parts. *J. Allergy Clin. Immunol.* 74: 687, 1984.
2. Archer, G. J. Rhinitis and nasal polyps in asthma. *Clin. Allergy* 4:323, 1974.
2a. Aubier, M., et al. Different effects of nasal and bronchial glucocorticosteroid administration on bronchial hyperresponsiveness in patients with allergic rhinitis. *Am. Rev. Respir. Dis.* 146:122, 1992.
3. Bardin, P. G., Van Heerden, B. B., and Joubert, J. R. Absence of pulmonary aspiration of sinus contents in patients with asthma and sinusitis. *J. Allergy Clin. Immunol.* 85:82, 1990.
4. Baumgarten, C., et al. Histopathologic examination of nasal polyps of different etiology. *Arch. Otorhinolaryngol.* 226:187, 1980.
5. Berman, S. Maxillary sinusitis and bronchial asthma: correlation of roentgenograms, cultures and thermograms. *J. Allergy Clin. Immunol.* 53:311, 1974.
6. Berman, S. Z., et al. Maxillary sinusitis and bronchial asthma: correlation of roentgenographs, culture and thermograms. *J. Allergy Clin. Immunol.* 53:311, 1974.
7. Blackley, C. H. *Experimental Researches on the Causes and Nature of Catarrhus Aestives (Hay Fever or Hay Asthma)* (1st ed.). London: Bailliere, Tindall & Cox, 1873.
8. Bumsted, R. H., et al. Histamine, norepinephrine and serotonin content of nasal polyps. *Laryngoscope* 89:832, 1979.
9. Busse, W. E. The precipitation of asthma by upper respiratory infections. *Chest* 87(suppl.):44, 1987.
10. Caplin, I., et al. Are nasal polyps an allergy phenomenon? *Ann. Allergy* 29: 631, 1971.
11. Casale, T. Neuromechanisms of asthma. *Ann. Allergy* 59:391, 1987.
12. Chandra, R. K., and Abol, B. M. Immunopathology of nasal polypi. *J. Laryngol. Otol.* 88:1019, 1974.
13. Dixon, W. E., and Brodie, T. G. The bronchial muscles, their innervation, and the action of drugs upon them. *J. Physiol.* (London) 29:93, 1903.
14. Donovan, R. Immunoglobulins in nasal polyp fluid. *Int. Arch. Allergy Appl. Immunol.* 37:154, 1970.
15. Downing, E. Bronchial reactivity in patients with nasal polyps before and after polypectomy (abstract). *J. Allergy Clin. Immunol.* 69:102, 1983.
16. Eggleston, P. A., and Fish, J. E. Upper airway disease and bronchial hyperreactivity. *Clin. Rev. Allergy* 2:429, 1984.
17. Evans, F. O. Jr., et al. Sinusitis of the maxillary antrum. *N. Engl. J. Med.* 293:735, 1975.
18. Fascinelli, F. Maxillary sinus abnormality: radiographic evidence in an asymptomatic population. *Arch. Otolaryngol.* 90:98, 1969.
19. Frederick, J., and Braude, A. I. Anaerobic infection of the paranasal sinuses. *N. Engl. J. Med.* 290:135, 1974.
20. Friedman, W. H. Surgery for chronic hyperplastic rhinosinusitis. *Laryngoscope* 95:1999, 1975.
21. Friedman, R., Ackerman, M., and Wald, E. Asthma and bacterial sinusitis in children. *J. Allergy Clin. Immunol.* 74:185, 1984.
22. Harlin, S. L., et al. A clinical and pathologic study of chronic sinusitis: the role of the eosinophil. *J. Allergy Clin. Immunol.* 81:867, 1988.
23. Hoehne, J. H., and Reed, C. E. Where is the allergic reaction in ragweed asthma? *J. Allergy Clin. Immunol.* 48:36, 1971.
24. Jacobs, R. L. A practical classification of chronic rhinitis. *J. Respir. Dis.* 9: 20, 1981.
25. Kaliner, M., Wasserman, S. I., and Austen, K. F. Immunologic release of chemical mediators from human nasal polyps. *N. Engl. J. Med.* 289:277, 1973.
26. Katz, R. Sinusitis in children with respiratory allergy. *J. Allergy Clin. Immunol.* 61:190, 1978.
27. Kaufman, J., and Wright, G. W. The effect of nasal and nasopharyngeal irritation on airway resistance in man. *Am. Rev. Respir. Dis.* 100:626, 1969.
28. Kennedy, D. W. Functional endoscopic sinus surgery techniques. *Arch. Otolaryngol.* 3:643, 1985.
29. Kern, R. A., and Schenck, H. P. Allergy: a constant factor in the etiology of so-called mucous nasal polyps. *J. Allergy* 4:485, 1923.
30. Kratchmer, I. Cited in Kiyoski. Physiologic relationships between nasal breathing and pulmonary function. *Laryngoscopy* 76:30, 1966.
31. Lichtenstein, L. M., et al. A single year of immunotherapy for ragweed hay fever: immunologic and clinical studies. *Ann. Intern. Med.* 75:663, 1971.
32. Lildholdt, T., et al. Surgical versus medical treatment of nasal polyps. *Acta Otolaryngol.* 105:140, 1988.
33. Maloney, J., and Collins, J. Nasal polyps and bronchial asthma. *Br. J. Dis. Chest* 41:1, 1977.
34. Miles, L. R. Methacholine sensitivity in nasal polyposis and effects of polypectomy (abstract). *J. Allergy Clin. Immunol.* 69:102, 1982.
35. Mings, R., et al. Five year follow-up of the effects of bilateral intranasal sphenoethmoidectomy in patients with sinusitis and asthma. *Am. J. Rhinology* 71:123, 1988.
36. Mullarkey, M. F., et al. Allergic and non-allergic rhinitis: their characterization with attention to the meaning of nasal eosinophilia. *J. Allergy Clin. Immunol.* 65:122, 1980.
37. Mygind, N. *Nasal Allergy* (2nd ed.). Oxford: Blackwell, 1979.
38. Ogura, J. H., and Harvey, J. E. Nasopulmonary mechanisms. Experimental evidence of the influence of the upper airway upon the lower airway. *Acta Otolaryngol.* 71:123, 1971.
39. Oppenheimer, E. H., and Rosenstein, B. J. Differential pathology of nasal polyps in cystic fibrosis and atopy. *Lab. Invest.* 40:445, 1979.
40. Permutt, S. M. Bronchial Challenge in Ragweed Sensitive Patients. In K. F. Austen and L. M. Lichtenstein (eds.), *Asthma: Physiology, Immunopharmacology and Treatment.* New York: Academic, 1977, Chap. 17.
41. Rachelefsky, G. S., Katz, R. M., and Siegel, S. C. Chronic sinusitis in children with respiratory allergy: the role of antimicrobials. *J. Allergy Clin. Immunol.* 69:382, 1982.
42. Rachelefsky, G. S., Katz, R. M., and Siegel, S. C. Chronic sinus disease with associated reactive airway disease in children. *Pediatrics* 783:529, 1984.
43. Rachelefsky, G. S., et al. Sinus disease in children with respiratory allergy. *J. Allergy Clin. Immunol.* 61:310, 1978.
44. Ramsdale, E. H., et al. Asymptomatic bronchial responsiveness in rhinitis. *J. Allergy Clin. Immunol.* 75:573, 1985.
45. Richerson, H. B., and Seebohm, P. M. Nasal airway response to exercise. *J. Allergy* 41:269, 1968.
46. Ricketti, A. J. Allergic Rhinitis. In R. Patterson (ed.), *Allergic Diseases: Diagnosis and Management* (3rd ed.). Philadelphia: Lippincott, 1985, Pp. 207–231.
46a. Rosenberg, G. L., et al. Inhalation challenge with ragweed pollen in ragweed-sensitive asthmatics. *J. Allergy Clin. Immunol.* 71:302, 1983.
47. Sadan, N., et al. Immunotherapy of polyposis in children: investigation of the immunologic basis of clinical improvement. *N. Engl. J. Med.* 280:623, 1969.
48. Salvaggio, J. E., et al. A comparison of the immunologic responses of normal and atopic individuals to intranasally administered antigen. *J. Allergy* 35:62, 1964.
49. Schatz, M., and Zeiger, R. S. Chronic rhinitis: a therapeutic challenge. *Consultant* 22:61, 1980.
50. Schumacher, M. J., Cota, B. S., and Taussig, L. D. Pulmonary response to nasal challenge testing of atopic subjects with stable asthma. *J. Allergy Clin. Immunol.* 78:30, 1986.
51. Seebohm, P. M. Allergic Rhinitis and Non-allergic Rhinitis. In E. Middleton, Jr., C. E. Reed, and E. F. Ellis (eds.), *Allergy: Principles and Practice.* St. Louis: Mosby, 1978, Vol. 2, Pp. 868–876.

52. Settipane, G. A., and Chaffee, F. H. Nasal polyps in asthma and rhinitis: a review of 6,037 patients. *J. Allergy Clin. Immunol.* 59:17, 1977.

53. Settipane, G. A., Chaffee, R. H., and Klein, D. E. Aspirin intolerance: a prospective study in an atopic and normal population. *J. Allergy Clin. Immunol.* 53:200, 1974.

54. Shturman-Ellstein, R., et al. The beneficial effect of nasal breathing on exercise induced bronchoconstriction. *Am. Rev. Respir. Dis.* 118:76, 1978.

55. Slavin, R. G. Diagnostic tests in clinical allergy. *Postgrad. Med.* 67:72, 1980.

56. Slavin, R. G. Relationship of nasal disease and sinusitis to bronchial asthma. *Ann. Allergy* 49:76, 1982.

57. Slavin, R. G., Cannon, R. E., and Friedman, W. H. Sinusitis and bronchial asthma. *J. Allergy Clin. Immunol.* 66:250, 1980.

58. Slavin, R. G., et al. Sinusitis and bronchial asthma. *J. Allergy Clin. Immunol.* 66:250, 1980.

59. Spector, S. L., et al. Comparison between transillumination and the roentgenogram in the diagnosis of paranasal sinus disease. *J. Allergy Clin. Immunol.* 67:22, 1981.

60. Speizer, F. E., and Frank, N. R. A comparison of changes in pulmonary flow resistance in health volunteers actively exposed to SO_2 by mouth and nose. *Br. J. Ind. Med.* 23:75, 1966.

61. Stone, B. D., Georgitis, J. W., and Matthews, B. Inflammatory mediators in sinus lavage fluid (abstract). *J. Allergy Clin. Immunol.* 85:22, 1990.

62. Taft, A., et al. Double-blind comparison between beclomethasone diproprionate as aerosol and as powder in patients with nasal polyposis. *Clin. Allergy* 12:391, 1982.

63. Taylor, M. Histochemical studies of nasal polypi. *J. Laryngol. Otol.* 77:326, 1973.

64. Taylor, B., et al. Transient IgA deficiency and pathogenesis of infantile atopy. *Lancet* 2:111, 1973.

65. Taylor, B., et al. Upper respiratory tract in cystic fibrosis: ENT survey of children. *Arch. Dis. Child.* 49:133, 1979.

66. Wald, E. R., et al. Acute maxillary sinusitis in children. *N. Engl. J. Med.* 304:749, 1981.

66a. Wald, E. R. Sinusitis in children. *N. Engl. J. Med.* 326:319, 1992.

67. Weisskopf, A., and Burn, H. F. Histochemical studies of the pathogenesis of nasal polyps. *Ann. Otol. Rhinol. Laryngol.* 68:509, 1959.

68. Welliver, R. C. Upper respiratory infection in asthma. *J. Allergy Clin. Immunol.* 72:341, 1983.

69. Welsh, P. W., et al. The efficacy of beclomethasone nasal solution, flunisolide, and cromolyn in relieving symptoms of ragweed allergy. *Mayo Clin. Proc.* 62:125, 1987.

70. Yan, K., and Salome, C. The response of the airways to nasal stimulation in asthmatics with rhinitis. *Eur. J. Respir. Dis.* 128(suppl.):105, 1983.

Inhalant Aerobiology and Antigens

42

Robert W. Ausdenmoore
Michelle B. Lierl
Thomas J. Fischer

As discussed in Chapter 1, asthma is best defined in physiologic terms as reversible obstructive lung disease. There are many triggers for asthmatic episodes (Chap. 34), including infection, cold and dry air, psychologic stimuli, environmental changes or, in that type of asthma traditionally classified as "extrinsic," exposure to aeroallergens.

Asthma of the extrinsic type may often be suspected on the basis of clinical criteria including early onset; family history of allergy; other allergic problems such as allergic rhinitis, urticaria, or eczema; and a definitive seasonal pattern. Supporting laboratory evidence often includes nasal, sputum, and peripheral eosinophilia, a high serum level of IgE, positive skin tests, and positive radioallergosorbent (RAST) or other in vitro tests for allergens (Chap. 38).

Episodes of asthma in such individuals often occur in association with allergic rhinitis. The allergen, when identified, is one to which the patient has previously been sensitized. It is useful, then, to identify the allergens to which an asthmatic is sensitized in order to reduce his or her exposure to and/or to attempt to build up a tolerance to that specific allergen by means of immunotherapy.

That an allergen to which a person is specifically sensitized can trigger an asthma attack upon direct exposure is clear, as demonstrated by bronchial challenge (see Chap. 39). In addition, elimination of an allergen from the environment of the sensitized person often reduces the frequency and severity of that person's asthma. The precise physiologic mechanism by which the exposure to an allergen provokes asthma is not yet completely understood, however.

Evidence suggests that virtually all identified aeroallergens deposit on the nose, eyes, and oropharynx (see Fig. 42-1). It is postulated that bronchospasm and the lower airway inflammatory response result from an antigen-antibody reaction in the upper airway, resulting in a release of chemical mediators such as histamine, thromboxanes, prostaglandins, and leukotrienes into the systemic circulation [5, 91].

Alternatively, it has been suggested that antigens might be eluted from the aeroallergen, then absorbed and transported via the hematogenous route to sensitized cells surrounding the bronchi and bronchioles, at which point the chemical mediators are released.

In 1972, Busse and colleagues [16] presented evidence to suggest that pollen fragments and plant fragments of a much smaller size (<5 μm) could be important allergens, especially in asthma. Such particles or aerosols, with eluted allergens, thus might reach the bronchi where allergic reactions take place.

In 1983, Agarwal and associations [1] reported on the *immunochemical quantitation* of airborne ragweed, antigen E, *Alternaria*, and Alt-1. Special high-volume air samplers were used to eliminate the large particles and allow for the collection of the small particles (<10 μm) on small-pore filters. The allergenic activity

of eluates from these small particles correlated more closely with the mean symptom scores of patients than did the pollen and mold counts. In the case of ragweed, for instance, the peak allergen level measured by this technique is reached somewhat later than the peak of the pollen count and correlates more closely with the peak of clinically recognized ragweed asthma.

Solomon and coworkers [85] have also presented evidence that ragweed pollen antigen with particle size less than 5 μm, or even submicronic, has marked allergenic activity based on both skin tests and in vitro methods.

Understanding allergic mechanisms operative in asthma, assessing the role of allergens in each asthmatic individual, and identifying these allergens where indicated are indispensable tools for the proper prophylactic treatment of asthmatic patients.

TERMINOLOGY

The term *allergy* was coined in 1906 by Clement von Pirquet to designate *altered* reactivity in some individuals in response to the introduction of a foreign substance into their bodies. As the term is now used, it refers to a state of *heightened* reactivity occurring in humans and some lower animals upon contact with a substance that is ordinarily innocuous to most other individuals of that species. *Antigen*, a more modern term, is defined as a foreign substance that, when introduced into the body of an animal, elicits the formation of antibodies capable of reacting specifically with that substance. We customarily use the term *allergen* to describe those antigens capable of eliciting allergic reactions.

AEROALLERGENS

Animal dander, insect parts, plant fragments, pollens, mold spores, mites, dust, and algae are often referred to as *aeroallergens*, but, in reality, these substances are rather large and complex particles that are identified in air samples, when collected and carefully examined (Fig. 42-2). Only a few of the many molecular components of these particles are actually antigenic. When characterized, these antigens are usually protein in nature with some carbohydrate subunits and have a molecular weight of 10,000 to 40,000 daltons. The spatial configuration and chemical groupings of the molecules determine their antigenicity, but the prevalence in nature of the whole particle and the suitability of the particle size for impingement on the respiratory mucosa are also major factors in determining the clinical importance of an aeroallergen (see Chaps. 5, 8, and 32).

AIR SAMPLING

The aeroallergens just mentioned represent the identifiable biogenic particles in air samples. Amorphous debris is also seen and consists of dirt particles, salts, and hydrocarbons as well as specific environmental contaminants from industry or farming operations in the near vicinity. It is probable that these nonbiogenic particulate substances modify responses to acknowledged aeroallergens or, in many cases, trigger asthmatic episodes by direct irritation of the airway. Substances in the air, not visible as particulate matter (see Fig. 42-2) can also trigger asthmatic attacks or modify, usually adversely, an asthmatic response to an aeroallergen. Some gaseous substances may be suspected or identified by their characteristic color or odor (chlorine, hydrogen sulfide, formaldehyde, kerosene, gasoline, woodsmoke, tobacco smoke, or cooking odors). Others may be virtually colorless and odorless, such as nitrogen dioxide, sulfur dioxide, or carbon monoxide (industrial and photochemical smog; see Chap. 87).

Particulate matter in the air can be collected and measured in air samplers by taking advantage of their gravitational or inertial forces, or both. Gravitational samplers simply collect particles that settle on them. Impactors make use of an obstacle that is placed on a stream of air that forces particles to settle on their surfaces.

Biogenic particles such as insect parts, mite feces, disintegrating pollen and mold particles, and animal dander are not identifiable in air samples by microscopic examination but have great clinical allergic importance. Air samples collected by high-volume volumetric samplers (Fig. 42-3) onto fiberglass filters collect virtually all these particles, which can then be eluted and quantified by immunochemical assay.

A few of the commonly used samplers currently in use are shown in Figures 42-3 to 42-6. Table 42-1 lists some of the distributors and manufacturers of sampling equipment. The Durham sampler (Fig. 42-4) has long been used as a simple collecting tool. In this method, soft glycerin jelly* is placed on a slide which is then placed on a holder between two other metal plates and exposed in a horizontal position to the air. Particles deposited by gravity or turbulent airflow are identified, counted, and reported as particles per cubic centimeter. Although useful, this collector does not yield accurate quantitative results, as the deposition of particles is strongly influenced by wind velocity and

Fig. 42-1. *Deposition efficiency curves illustrating the relative likelihood of particles the size of pollens and mold spores to deposit on the nasopharyngeal mucosa. (Adapted from B. O. Stuart, Deposition of inhaled aerosols. Arch. Intern. Med. 131:60, 1973).*

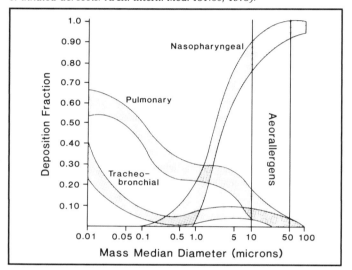

* Consisting of 2 parts gelatin, 12 parts water, 11 parts glycerine, and 2% phenol, which is warmed to mix, left to settle, and strained. To facilitate pollen identification, one may add 2 ml of Calberla's solution (5 ml of glycerine, 10 ml of 95% ethanol, 15 ml of water, and 2 gt saturated, aqueous basic fuchsin).

Fig. 42-2. *Types and sizes of commonly encountered aerosols, illustrating the relative size of pollens and mold spores compared to other substances in the air. (Adapted from D. V. Bates, et al. Deposition and retention models for internal dosimetry of human respiratory tract. Health Phys. 12:173, 1966.)*

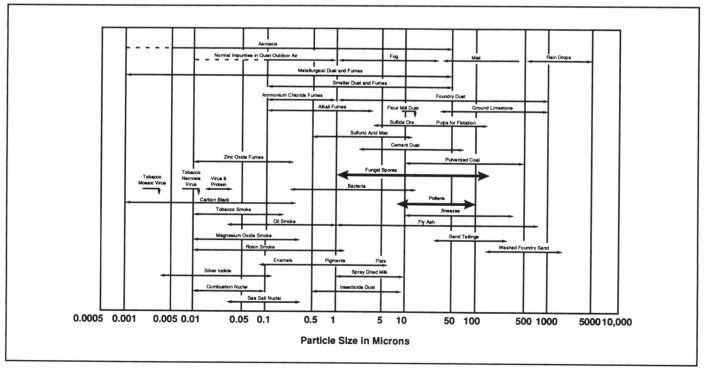

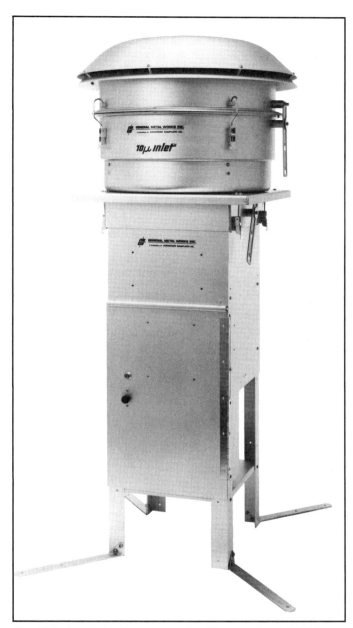

Fig. 42-3. *Accu Vol volumetric sampler. (Courtesy General Metal Works, Inc. Cleves, Ohio.)*

Table 42-1. Distributors and manufacturers of sampling equipment

Anderson Samplers 45 Wendell Drive Atlanta, Georgia tel: (800) 241-6898	General Metal Works, Inc. 45 S. Miami Drive Cleves, Ohio 45002 tel: (513) 941-2229
Biotest Diagnostics 6 Daniel Road East Fairfield, New Jersey 07006 tel: (201) 575-4560	Nucleopore Corporation 7035 Commerce Circle Pleasanton, California 94566 tel: (800) 882-7711
Burkhard Manufacturing Co., Ltd. Woodcock Hill Industrial Estate Rickmensworth, Hertfordshire England W.D. 31 P.J.	Sampling Technologies, Inc. (formerly Ted Brown & Associates) 26338 Esperanza Drive Los Altos Hills, California 94022 tel: (415) 941-1232

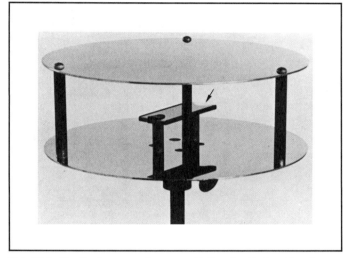

Fig. 42-4. *The Durham sampler, a gravitational collector. (Courtesy Air Pollution Training Institute, Triangle Park, North Carolina.)*

direction, by raindrops, and by condensation. Even at their best, gravitational methods favor the deposition of larger, heavier particles.

A rotating arm impactor is currently recommended by the American Academy of Allergy and Immunology as a cost-effective and reasonably accurate volumetric air sampler [2]. The Rotorod sampler, originally described by Perkins [72], is one such sampler and utilizes clear acrylic collecting rods coated with a thin layer of silicone grease. Newer modifications, illustrated in Fig. 42-5, provide automatic shields to protect the collecting surfaces between cycling periods. Collecting periods can be varied from a few seconds to several minutes, and the cycle may be repeated as often as desired (usually every 10 minutes). These features allow for convenience in counting by adjusting the collecting period in an inverse relationship to the anticipated pollen and mold concentrations. The volume of air sampled is calculated by the formula: M^3 = (collecting area [cm^2] × swing diameter [cm]

× RPM × time [min] × 3.1416)/[10^6 cm^3] [81]. In most instances, all values in this formula are constant (i.e., swing diameter, RPM, collecting surface, and the time generally remain the same). Counts are then made and expressed by the standard formula for volumetric air sampling: particles/m^3 = total particles in the sample/total volume of air sample.

Inertial suction samplers are often used when highly accurate counts are needed. In this approach, a specific volume of air is drawn through an orifice of defined pore size and particles impinge on a collecting plate within the sampler. Modifications of this collecting method permit a timed rotation of the collecting plate to provide information reflecting the variations of particle counts within the collecting periods. The Hirst spore trap (Fig. 42-6) is one such collector.

Particulate matter, whether identifiable or not microscopically, can be sized in the collection apparatus by passing the air through successively smaller filters. Directing the air through successive right-angle paths while decreasing the aperture after each bend (thus increasing the velocity of the air) results in separation of different-sized particles (the longer ones depositing at lower velocities, the smaller ones at greater velocities). This is the principle used by Cascade impactors. The particles thus separated may be counted, if identifiable, or the allergens within the particles may be eluted and measured by RAST inhibition or inhibition radioimmunoassay. These techniques have been refined and modified so that they are simple and reproducible, and virtually any allergen can be measured by them.

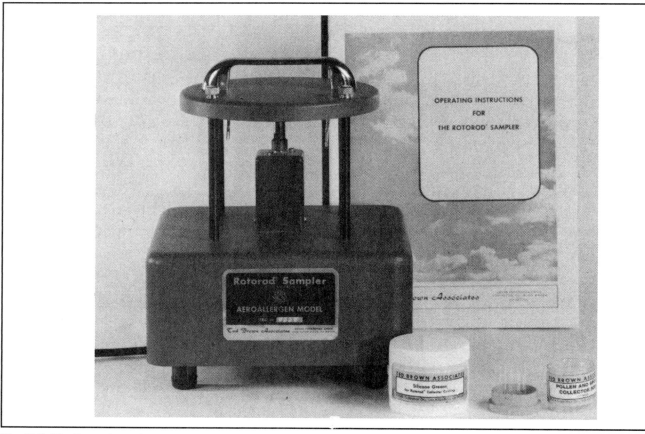

Fig. 42-5. *The Rotorod sampler, a simple impactor with intermittent rotation and shields to protect the collecting surfaces between sampling periods. (Courtesy Sampling Technologies, Inc., Los Altos Hills, California.)*

Most large particles (>2 µm in diameter) can be readily identified on slides obtained by any of the methods described above. Identification guidelines are available for comparison and increasing one's skill in counting [65, 81]. Data for many areas of North America and a few other countries are regularly compiled and reported in the statistical report of the pollen and mold committee of the American Academy of Allergy and Immunology [2]. A regional map of the United States, together with data concerning principal pollens found within geographic regions (adapted from the Hollister-Stier pollen guide), is provided in Appendix A. Caution is required when attempting to correlate pollen counts with clinical symptoms, as wide fluctuations within a small area might occur due to wind direction, cloud covers, local moisture, cutting of grass, roadwork, excavation, and the like.

GENERAL CONSIDERATIONS REGARDING POLLENS

Pollen grains are male reproductive structures of seed-bearing plants. They serve as a means by which the male gametes are transferred to the female gametes, which remain on the plant. Pollens of allergenic importance are adapted for windborne transfer (anemophily). They are typically small, light, nonadhesive, smooth, and symmetrical. Most pollen is shed in the early morning hours, but dispersal and reflotation by winds usually result in maximal pollen concentration in the afternoon and early evening. Viability of the pollen (usually 2–4 hours) does not influence its antigenicity. The light, fluffy nature of windborne pollens enables them to be refloated even by gentle air currents and to be blown for miles by the wind. Thus, even urban areas may have

pollen counts nearly equivalent to those of rural areas. Plant sources of windborne pollen typically include plants that are widespread and dull in appearance, and have small inconspicuous and nearly odorless flowers (e.g., ragweed, trees, and grass), in contrast to the colorful and fragrant flowers that will attract bees and other insects (or even other animals) which, in turn, effect the pollen transfer (entomophily). Insect-borne pollen is generally larger, more sticky, and heavier than windborne pollen.

The magnitude of pollen production by anemophilous plants is enormous: A single ragweed plant can release one billion pollen grains in a single season. One square mile of ragweed (as might be seen around road construction sites) can produce 16 tons of pollen. One million tons may be released yearly in the United States [65].

CHARACTERISTICS AND PREVALENCE OF INDIVIDUAL POLLENS

Pollen production occurs only during growing seasons, not while the plant is dormant. Remembering that pollination (transport of pollen) occurs before fertilization and seed formation, one can predict that peak pollen production occurs just before and during flowering. The time of flowering varies with the plant involved, but useful generalizations may be made.

Wild-Pollinating Trees

Wind-pollinating trees include plants from a wide variety of plant species. Each species varies with respect to the seasonal pattern, intensity, and duration of its pollination. Pollen morphology is also species specific, and very little cross-antigenicity is noted

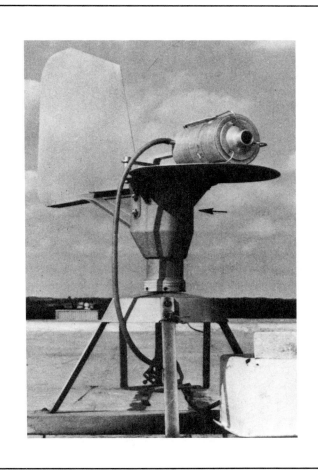

Fig. 42-6. *The Hirst Spore Trap, an inertial suction sampler utilizing a weather vane to correct for wind direction. (Courtesy Air Pollution Training Institute, Triangle Park, North Carolina.)*

between pollens of different tree species [8, 32]. Significant cross-reactivity does occur between pollens of the Betalaceae (birch) and Fagaccae (beech) families; among the Salicaceae (willows, poplars, and aspens); and among the Oleaceae (olive, ash, and privet) [15]. The important allergy-producing trees are largely deciduous, since the anemophilous conifers have pollen that has a thick outer covering (exine) that virtually precludes solubilization of the internal antigens. However, some conifers (cedars, cypresses, and junipers) are considered to be regionally important sources of allergenic pollen.

In general, deciduous trees in the northeastern coastal states and the inland, north central states have relatively brief periods of pollination in the early spring to early summer just before or during "leafing out." Individual species tend to occur in clusters or groves, so that an individual patient may be exposed (at least intensely) to relatively few species of these trees. This clustering effect, together with the brief periods of exposure to species-specific antigens, usually produces a characteristic pattern of brief, but intense, springtime symptoms in tree-sensitive persons. The season of tree pollination in the southern, southeast coastal, and western coastal states extends through the winter and spring months but, there too, relatively brief, intense, and sometimes multiple periods of difficulty are seen.

Grasses

Grasses are all species of the family, Gramineae, and are all wind-pollinating plants. Grasses are probably the leading worldwide

cause of extrinsic allergic problems because they are so widespread. The pollen is virtually indistinguishable morphologically from one species to another, so that pollination patterns for individual species are deduced from the growth patterns of the plant itself in relation to the total grass pollen concentrations observed on the slide. Bermuda grass predominates in the southern and Pacific coastal states, and pollination occurs throughout the year, with fluctuations that reflect climatic conditions. In the northern states, the pollen of blue, orchard, red top, and, especially, timothy grasses predominates, with a seasonal pattern that usually occurs in May and June. Cross-reactivity among the grasses is the rule, but Johnson, Bahia, and Bermuda grasses do not cross-react well with other grasses.

The term *weed* does not refer to a botanic classification of plants but, generally, to a horticulturist designates an unwanted plant. To an allergist, *weed* usually refers to a plant of the family Compositae and, specifically, *Ambrosia* (ragweed). These plants are most prevalent in the central plains and eastern agricultural regions of the United States and usually appear as the first plant after land cultivation and road clearing. Qualitatively and quantitatively, ragweed is one of the most important causes of allergic rhinitis and bronchial asthma in the United States, especially in the Midwest. There is a strong seasonal prevalence of ragweed pollen in late August and September. Pollen of other weedy plants, such as plantain, lambsquarter, sagebrush, marshelder, dock/sorrel, Russian thistle, cocklebur, and false and western ragweed, constitutes a significant quantity of windborne pollen throughout the summer and early fall, and is also responsible for a significant amount of allergic illness. Plantain (Plantaginiceae) is a very commonly found weed in the midcentral states and has a long pollinating schedule (May through October). Skin reactivity is frequently found, but pollen counts are consistently low in proportion to grass and ragweed species.

Figures 42-7 and 42-8 illustrate the appearance of typical allergy-inducing pollens and their parent plants.

PURIFIED ANTIGENS FROM POLLENS

Progress toward the isolation and purification of important antigens in ragweed was reported in the early 1960s by King and Norman [44]. Antigen E (MW 37,800) was described and, although this represented only 0.5 percent of the extractable solids (6% of the extractable protein), it was found to have 200 times the allergenic activity of the whole ragweed extract. Antigen K (MW 38,200; 3% of the extractable protein) was also purified and was found to be less reactive than antigen E, but was reactive in nearly all ragweed-sensitive individuals. These antigens continue to be regarded as the most important allergens within the ragweed pollen.

Timothy grass pollen has also been studied extensively and purified fractions have been isolated. Antigen B[25] has been described as the most important allergen in this pollen [34]. The major rye grass allergen, Lol pl, has been isolated and characterized [70]. Lol pl, and the similar antigens found in pollens of other members of the Festucoideae family of grasses, are referred to as the *grass group I* allergens; 85 to 95 percent of grass-sensitive patients are reactive to these allergens [12, 24]. Allergens from birch, cedar, oak, and orchard grass pollen have also been isolated and purified.

In addition to a better understanding of pollen activity, information gained from the isolation and purification of antigens will undoubtedly soon be used clinically in testing and treating patients. Technology now exists that allows isolation and purification of allergens from any source.

FUNGI AS AEROALLERGENS

Among the identifiable biogenic materials found in air samples, fungi are often the most numerous. As early as 1873, Blackley

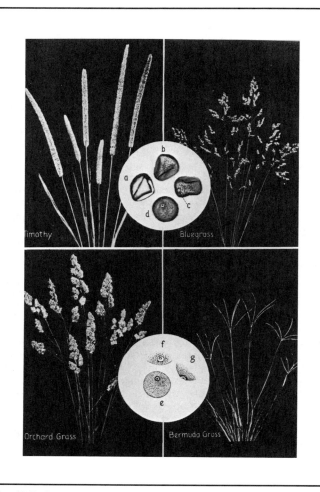

Fig. 42-7. *Grass plants and typical pollen. a, b, c = unexpanded timothy pollen; d = expanded pollen; e, f, g = detail of germinal pore; 30 to 40 μm for allergenic grass pollens. (Reprinted with permission from J. M. Sheldon,* Clinical Allergy. *Philadelphia: Saunders, 1967.)*

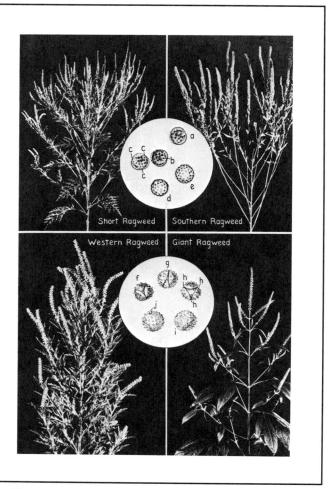

Fig. 42-8. *Ragweed plants and typical pollen. a, b, c = unexpanded pollen; d, e = expanded, stained pollen; f, g, h = typical lines caused by shrinkage from drying and the position of the tree germinal pores; i, j = expanded stained ragweed pollen; 20 to 25 μm. (Reprinted with permission from J. M. Sheldon,* Clinical Allergy. *Philadelphia: Saunders, 1967.)*

[12] performed a bronchial challenge on himself using *Penicillium* spores, and this produced "bronchial catarrh." Over the years since then, many authors have stressed the importance of fungal spores in allergic asthma, including Strom van Leuwen (1924) [90], Feinberg (1935) [25], and Van der Werff (1958) [96]. Progress in understanding the role of fungi has been relatively slow, however, in comparison to the study of pollen. There are currently great differences of opinion with regard to the importance of fungal allergy in general, as well as the relative importance of individual fungi [75].

Fungi are considered by some biologists to be distinct from the plant and animal kingdom, but the majority regard them as simple plants that are devoid of stems, leaves, roots, and chlorophyll. They are either unicellular (yeasts) or multicellular, have a rigid cell wall, and require an external source of carbohydrate for nutrition. The multicellular fungi have cells that form branching chains called *hyphae*. Most fungi produce both asexual (simple division of a cell) spores and sexual spores (fusion of two compatible cells to form a zygote followed by reduction division). The spores are adapted to airborne dispersion. The term *mold* correctly refers to the appearance of a fungal growth on a substance, but has come to be synonymous with *fungi* in the allergist's parlance. Perhaps because of their simplicity, fungi are among the most successfully adapted organisms on earth. They

are ubiquitous and can be found in completely arid or moist areas, in areas of wide temperature extremes, in soil, and in fresh or salt water. Fungi are either saprophytes (obtaining nutrients from dead organic material), parasites (feeding on viable tissue), or facultative parasites (able to infect a living host or to live outside the host).

Identification

The identification of fungi in air samples is considerably more difficult than the identification of pollen. Over 100,000 species have been identified or suspected. There are often only subtle morphologic differences between spores of different species, so that culture techniques have characteristically been used in helping identify the mold [83]. However, because of the diversity of optimal culture growth characteristics, colony counts that truly represent the proportion of the various molds in the air sample are difficult to achieve. As mentioned previously in this chapter, gravitational collectors tend to be skewed toward higher proportions of larger particles, thus minimizing the proportion of small spored species. In the past few years, however, more accurate data have been acquired using spore traps and other volumetric samplers [1, 75, 77, 82, 83, 86].

Highly purified mold spore extracts are not yet available. Standardization of mold extracts is poor and identification of the most important mold spore antigens is just now being accomplished in detail. Antigen Alt-1, from *Alternaria* (a leaf mold) [1, 85, 108] and important antigens from *Aspergillus* (an indoor mold) [54], *Calvatia cyathiformis* [38] (a basidiomycete), and *Cladosporium* (another important leaf mold) have recently been identified. In the near future, it is probable that improved standardization and identification of fungal allergens will lead to clinical studies which will more clearly establish the role of fungal allergens in asthma.

Classification

The classification of fungi is most frequently accomplished by a scheme using morphology and the method of production of their sexual spores. By this method, mycologists can group fungi into three different classes: Ascomycetes, Basidiomycetes, and Zygomycetes. Subclassification is often made on the basis of the morphologic differences of asexual spores (form classification). Such classification should not be expected to reflect the true botanic groupings or antigenic similarity. Over time, spores are regrouped as new observations about their life cycle are made. Many spores, formerly not easily classifiable, have been identified as asexual spores of molds belonging to one of the major classes. Recently spores of *Alternaria*, *Aspergillus*, and *Penicillium* have been identified as asexual spores of ascomycetes and are now regarded as belonging to a subclass called *Hyphomycetes*.

There is strong evidence that molds from the class Basidiomycetes are among the most prevalent molds. Recent studies found positive skin tests to basidiospores in 19 to 30 percent of allergic individuals [51, 52].

The majority of fungi, though widely different from one another in terms of their optimal needs for growth, do seem to require some source of elemental oxygen, moderate temperature (18–32°C), and some moisture to flourish. Requirements for survival, however, are few; some spores tolerate temperature extremes from −56° to +70°C and relative humidity from virtually 0 to 100 percent.

Dispersion of some fungi is favored by abundant moisture in the atmosphere or even by rain or dew splash, whereas others are better dispersed by high winds and low humidity. Many fungi (especially basidiomycetes and ascomycetes) have active mechanisms that operate to discharge their spores into the air stream, but most of the saprophytes (in which group many of the indoor fungi reside) require air disturbance for dispersion.

The spore content of indoor air roughly parallels that of the outside air, particularly when the doors and windows are open. Air conditioning modifies this fact but does not preclude the entrance of fungi from the outdoors [83]. Some fungi, however, arise indoors, particularly in garbage containers, food storage areas, furnace humidifiers, upholstery, wallpaper, damp basements, cool-mist vaporizers, and greenhouses [14, 56, 82, 83].

Clinically, mold sensitivity is often characterized by sporadic exacerbations that are associated with (1) fluctuations in rainfall and/or temperature, (2) intense local exposure such as during camping, harvesting, cutting grass, or raking leaves, (3) abnormally wet or musty home environments (old homes, poor insulation, wet foundations, or condensation around doors and windows), and (4) persistent symptoms during low pollen seasons.

During early, developing years of life (ages 1 to 5 years), when asthma and allergic rhinitis are often first recognized, mold sensitivity (along with other indoor inhalant sensitivity) is frequently suspected and verified by skin or in vitro testing.

Specific occupational exposures frequently occur as well. Grain workers, papermill workers, tobacco strippers, mushroom harvesters, and farmers during harvesting operations are exposed to enormous quantities of molds and can present with work-related allergic problems.

The already mentioned ubiquity of molds precludes complete avoidance in the normal pursuit of daily activities. Nonetheless, attempts to control mold exposure in the home, vehicle, and workplace are desirable and can be effective in managing patients. Such measures generally are suggested empirically, with emphasis on advice that pertains to the specific patient. Chapter 87 describes the procedures for mold control. Table 42-2 summarizes information about common molds and their relative importance.

HOUSE DUST AND HOUSE DUST MITES

Particulate matter in the indoor environment, usually referred to as *house dust*, is a composite of animal dander, indoor molds, vegetable fibers, food particles, algae, dirt, and insect parts. Mathison and colleagues [56] have provided a review of indoor inhalants as they affect asthma.

The common house dust mite (*Dermatophagoides farinae*) [95] is found in mattress stuffing, carpeting, bedding, clothing, and furniture stuffing with which humans come in contact (Fig. 42-9).

In 1928, Dekker [22] reported on mites in bedding which, he concluded, were a major cause of asthma. Human epithelial scales are the preferred substrate for mite growth, both in the laboratory and clinically. More detailed studies on mites were reported by Voorhorst and coworkers [98, 99]. Subsequent reports from Europe, North America, Africa, and Asia have tended to confirm the importance of mites as allergens [88, 95].

Dermatophagoides pteronyssinus is the most frequently found species in Europe, whereas *D. farinae* is more commonly found in the United States. Chapman and Platts-Mills [19] have characterized and purified an antigen, P1, from *D. pteronyssinus*, which accounts for most of the antigenic activity of the mite. P1 was later further characterized by them [18] to have a molecular weight of 24,000 daltons with two epitopes. *D. farinae* extracts have been shown to contain an antigen, der F1, that cross-reacts with der P1. Der P1 and der F1 are referred to as *Group I antigens*. Group II allergens have also been isolated from their respective mites. Both have molecular weights of approximately 15,000 daltons and cross-react extensively with one another. There is no cross-reactivity between Group I and Group II allergens. It is

Fig. 42-9. *An electron microphotograph of the common house dust mite (*Dermatophagoides farinae*). (Courtesy of Allergy Laboratories of Ohio.)*

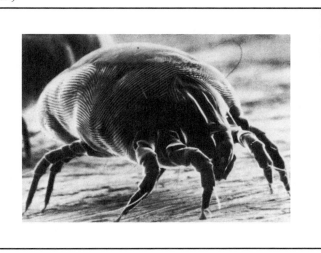

Table 42-2. Common molds and their relative clinical importance

ASCOMYCETES
>15,000 species; prevalent in wood pulp mills and on bark and deadwood; locally heavy clouds of spores are sometimes seen.
Alternaria: perhaps the most common mold identified in air samples, often exceeding pollen counts; saprophytes of leaves, plants, and other decaying organic material; high counts on hot, dry, windy days; indoor concentration reflects outdoor concentration usually by a factor of 25 percent; major problem for allergic patients, especially in the late summer months.
Aspergillus: most common indoor mold; substrate is spoiled food and other organic debris; very thermotolerant, especially where humidity is high; may colonize the respiratory tract and cause major hypersensitivity problems (allergic bronchopulmonary aspergillosis; Chap. 49).
Penicillium: indoor concentration often ≥*Aspergillus* concentrations; natural substrate includes spoiled food, cheeses, and other organic debris; allergic sensitivity to *Penicillium* not predictive of penicillin sensitivity.
Cladosporium (includes Hormodendrum): saprophyte on compost and decaying vegetables; counts often ≥ counts of *Alternaria*; hot, dry, windy days; indoor concentration usually 25 percent of outdoor concentration; major problem in late summer months.
Helminthosporium: prevalence level generally lower than that for *Alternaria* and *Cladosporium* but skin reactivity is frequent; especially common in southern states; parasite of many plants.
Aureobasidium: found in soil and on leaves but also colonizes lumber and paper; widespread in distribution but levels usually lower than those of the other prominent outdoor molds.

BASIDIOMYCETES
>12,000 species; colonize wild and cultivated plants. These are among the most prevalent molds identified by most states in the American Academy of Allergy and Immunology aeroallergen network. Positive skin prick tests to these allergens may be seen in 19 to 30 percent of individuals tested [22, 25, 38, 54]. Identification of a specific cause and effect relationship between these molds and clinical allergic situations has not yet been made.
Smuts: high concentrations in contaminated fields of grain; significant respiratory irritant allergen, especially in rural atopic people.
Rusts: lower concentrations than smuts around contaminated fields but significant exposure for rural workers, especially in dry, windy situations.
Mushrooms: prevalent in damp, forested areas, especially in wet weather; allergenic importance undetermined.

ZYGOMYCETES
Relatively few species (N = 250) are important allergically.
Rhizopus: prominent in damp interiors; contaminant of bread and sugary foods; moderate allergic importance.
Mucor: in damp interiors; contaminant of bread and sugary foods; moderate allergic importance.

OOMYCETES
>250 species identified in air samples; include "downy mildews," which infect grasses and grape or onion crops; spores become airborne in dry, breezy weather; not a proven aeroallergen.

---

likely that other antigens of clinical importance may also be present in mite extract, but this is not well established [50, 53].

Heaviest concentrations of mites are usually found in the bedroom [94], and the prevalence is usually greater where relatively high temperatures and humidity are noted; conversely, the concentration of mites tends to be lower at high altitudes [97]. A house dust mite concentration of greater than 100 mites per gram of dust in a home constitutes a major risk factor for asthma [48]. Exposure to house dust mite antigen in childhood has been shown to be associated with the subsequent development of asthma [88]. Purified mite extracts have been found to be more provocative than house dust, both by nasal and bronchial challenge. However, it is apparent that not all the antigenic activity of house dust resides in the mite fraction. Control measures for house dust are discussed in Chapter 87. A study of preventive measures in house dust allergy has been conducted by Korsgaard [48].

EPIDERMAL ALLERGENS

Sensitivity to animal dander is seen in many allergic individuals. Approximately 25 percent of allergic patients show skin sensitivity to animal protein [21]. Household pets account for the bulk of the clinical sensitivity to dander. Many of the antigens in the dander of such pets are also found in their urine and saliva [37, 63]. Close exposure increases the likelihood of sensitivity, and reactions are often denied or understated by patients because of an intense affection for the animal. Although antigens are shared by the hair and dander (epithelial fragments), the presence of hair in air samples or on surfaces within the home (i.e., shedding) is not essential for sensitization. Frequent bathing of the animal does reduce shedding of scales but it does not represent a practical method for effectively reducing sensitization or provocation. Even with removal of the animal, a considerable amount of time can be required for effective reduction of antigen expo-

sure. Careful cleaning of rugs, stuffed furniture, and, often, bedding is needed.

Immunotherapy with animal danders has been disappointing and can even be provocative. Recent placebo-controlled studies, however, have shown some efficacy of immunotherapy using cat and dog extracts, with reduction in bronchial responsiveness and skin test reactivity to the animal antigens [13, 52, 66].

Most dander exposure is a problem in the home environment, but, occasionally, occupational exposures are also serious problems (e.g., laboratory workers, veterinarians, taxidermists, and the like). Taylor and associates [93] have suggested that immunotherapy can effectively reduce the symptoms in these individuals.

Cat Dander

Cats are probably the most allergenic pet [37]. At least seven cat-derived allergens have been identified. The major allergen (Fel dI) is found in pelt, saliva, sebaceous glands, and male urine [20, 63]. Levels of Fel dI will gradually decline over a 5- to 6-month period after removal of the cat [106]. Aggressive environmental control measures, such as the removal of carpets and furniture [106] or use of tannic acid spray [59], can significantly improve the elimination of Fel dI from the environment. Airborne Fel dI allergen is present on particles that vary in size, 25 percent being less than 2.5 μm in diameter [55]. It is likely that the particle's small size and the consequental decrease in falling rate are responsible for its continuous presence as an aerosol even in undisturbed rooms. Clinically, a rapid onset of symptoms is often experienced by cat-sensitive people. By contrast, people with mite sensitivity (involving a larger particle size) most frequently require prolonged exposure or disturbance of the air before symptoms arise. Cat allergens also tend to exhibit a "stickiness," so that they often cling to walls, furniture, clothing, and so on [105]. Widespread exposure to cat (and dog) allergens occurs in the community, so that exposure is not limited to pet owners. Fel dI has been detected in schoolrooms [23], shopping malls, hospitals, and even in model homes and allergists' offices [78].

Dog Dander

Twenty-one different allergens have been identified in dog dander and hair, at least four of which appear to be major allergens [28]. Five to thirty percent of allergic individuals are found to be clinically allergic to dogs and, in some, the sensitivity is breed specific [63]. Sensitivity after the first year of life shows no correlation with dog ownership [63, 74], presumably because of the widespread exposure in the community [23].

Horse Dander

Horse dander has a great potential for sensitization, but the diminishing numbers of horses, the concomitant reduction in the use of pelts for stuffings, and the reduction in the use of horse serum for biologicals have reduced the problem. The importance of this allergen is greatest for agricultural workers, stable attendants, and riders.

Cattle Dander

Cattle dander also has a large potential for sensitization. However, the use of cattle hair for such purposes as stuffing and rug padding has been largely replaced by synthetic fibers. Most intense exposures occur among stockyard workers, farmers, and ranch hands.

Sheep Wool

Sheep wool has long been considered an important inhalant allergen. Many allergic individuals have positive skin test reactions and experience increasing symptoms upon exposure to wool, but most of this represents an irritant effect or contamination by other inhalant allergens such as mites.

Feathers

Feathers from chickens and ducks are less often used as stuffing in pillows, comforters, and quilts than formerly. When sensitivity is encountered, control measures are easily accomplished (i.e., no feather pillows). Experiments with feather-sensitive individuals have shown that the potential for sensitization increases as feathers age or are stored, suggesting that contamination by mite growth or the presence of degradation products of feathers is more important than the feathers themselves [98, 99]. Avian hypersensitivity pneumonitis (pigeon breeder's disease) is discussed in Chapters 37 and 49.

OTHER ALLERGENS

Algae

Algae have been implicated as a cause of hypersensitivity in humans. They are widely distributed and can be identified in indoor and outdoor air samples. The *Chlorella* species closely resembles pollen in size, produces positive skin tests in a significant number of atopic individuals (60% in one study) [7, 84], and results in positive bronchial challenges in some. Seasonal peaks of exposure occur from late spring to late fall. Closely related species show little cross-antigenicity, so that local exposures likely determine individual sensitivity [7, 84].

Table 42-3. Arthropods and allergic asthma

Class	Order	Example
Hexapoda	Orthoptera	Cockroach, locusts, crickets, grasshoppers
	Isoptera	Termites
	Dermaptera	Earwigs
	Hemiptera	Bedbugs, box elder bugs
	Coleoptera	Beetles, mealworms, weevils
	Lepidoptera	Moths, butterflies
	Diptera	Flies, cheronomides (midges)
	Ephemeroptera	May flies
	Hymenoptera	Ants, wasps, bees
	Siphofera	Fleas
	Tricoptera	Caddis flies
Arachnida	—	Mites, ticks
Crustacea	—	Sowbugs

Arthropods

Arthropods are well-known sources of allergic problems. Sensitivity to the venom of Hymenoptera (e.g., wasps, yellow jackets, bees, hornets, and fire ants) causing anaphylaxis in humans is an important and sometimes fatal phenomenon. Further, biting insects may cause marked local allergic reactions by virtue of absorption of their salivary secretions. Inhalation of insect parts from the caddis fly [68–69], may fly [26], moth and butterfly [4, 46, 47, 89, 107], midge [6, 31, 40, 42], and cockroach [9, 10, 45] has been documented as a cause of respiratory problems in sensitized individuals, especially in endemic areas.

Many other flying insects have been reported to cause sensitization by inhalation [3, 104], including mushroom flies [43], moths [71], and beetles [80]. Much of this information has been based on observations of allergic individuals during endemics of infestation with these insects and positive skin tests.

The role of insects as aeroallergens has historically been difficult to document because of the inability to identify insect particles through examination of air samples. With the recent advent of immunochemical assays (RAST, enzyme-linked immunosorbent assay, and the like) of air samples, there has been a renewed interest in their assessment. Indoor samples [17, 92] as well as outdoor samples [47, 107] have been examined carefully and have shown concentrations comparable to those of pollens and molds.

Nasal and bronchial challenges with cockroach [11, 41, 45], moth and butterfly [46, 47], beetle, mosquito [33], and fruit fly [87] particles have shown positive results as well. It is likely that airborne insect allergen is indeed a significant cause of allergic asthma. Table 42-3 lists the arthropods that have been implicated in respiratory allergy.

Viruses

Viruses are frequently implicated as causative agents in asthma, especially in young children and elderly patients [36, 39, 62]. The initial episode of asthma is often ushered in by a viral infection [61]. Asthmatic children have more viral infections than do their normal siblings [58, 60]. The viruses most frequently isolated in children with respiratory infections associated with wheezing are respiratory syncytial virus (RSV), parainfluenza virus, and adenovirus [36]. Welliver and colleagues have shown anti-RSV [100] and anti-parainfluenza [101] IgE antibody, respectively, in the majority of patients who had evidence of airway obstruction associated with their RSV or parainfluenza infections; patients with these infections who did not exhibit wheezing had no RSV- or parainfluenza-specific IgE. In these same studies, increased histamine secretion was demonstrated in the nasopharyngeal secretions from patients who exhibited anti-viral IgE [101, 102] and these studies also showed that virus-specific IgE was predictive

Table 42-4. The principal indoor pollutants, their sources, and typical concentrations†

Pollutant	Typical sources	Pollutant concentrations	Relevant standards	Comments
Respirable particles	Tobacco smoke, unvented kerosene heaters, wood and coal stoves, fireplaces, outside air, attached facilities, occupant activities	>500 $\mu g/m^3$ bars, meetings, waiting rooms with smoking 100 to 500 $\mu g/m^3$ typical for smoking sections of planes 10 to 100 $\mu g/m^3$ typical of homes 1,000 $\mu g/m^3$ with burning food or fireplaces	265 $\mu g/m^3$ EPA 24-hr standard ambient air 75 $\mu g/m^3$ EPA annual standard ambient air 150 $\mu g/m^3$ Japanese indoor standard	Current EPA standards are for total, and not only respirable, suspended particles
NO, NO_2	Gas ranges and pilot lights, unvented kerosene and gas space heaters, gasoline engines, some gas floor furnaces, outside air	25 to 75 ppb typical range for homes with gas stoves 100 to 500 ppb peak values for kitchens with gas stoves or kerosene gas heaters	160 ppb 1-hr maximum, WHO guideline 50 ppb annual average EPA ambient standard	No current EPA short-term standard
CO	Gas ranges and pilot lights, unvented kerosene and gas space heaters, tobacco smoke, back drafting of water heater or furnace or woodstove, gasoline engines, camping lanterns and stoves, attached garages, street level intake vents, hockey rinks	>50 ppm when oven used for heating >50 ppm attached garages, air intakes, arenas 2 to 15 ppm cooking with gas stove 2 to 10 ppm heavy smoking in homes, bars, and other locations	35 ppm EPA 1-hr standard 9 ppm EPA 8-hr standard	—
CO_2	People, unvented kerosene and gas space heaters, tobacco smoke, outside air	320 to 400 ppm outdoor air 2,000 to 5,000 ppm crowded indoor environment, inadequate ventilation	1,000 ppm Japanese indoor air standard	CO_2 concentrations below 1,000 ppm usually indicate adequate fresh air supply for buildings
Infectious, allergenic, irritating biologic materials	Dust mites and cockroaches, animal dander, bacteria, fungi, viruses, pollens	Few systematic measurements of spores, bacteria, and viruses indoors Homes with mold problem, offices with water damage: >1,000 cfu/m^3* Homes and offices without obvious problem: 500 ± 200 cfu/m^3	None	Interpretations of a level depend on the specific agent; cfu/m^3 is only an indicator
Formaldehyde	Urea formaldehyde foam insulation (UFFI), glues, fiberboard, pressed board, plywood, particle board; carpet backing and fabrics	0.1 to 0.8 ppm homes with UFFI 0.5 ppm average in mobile homes >1 ppm in a few homes and mobile homes	0.2 to 0.5 ppm adopted by several states 0.1 ppm Sweden, new homes 0.7 ppm Sweden, maximum in old buildings 3 ppm U.S. OSHA 8-hr time-weighted average	Formaldehyde concentrations in homes with UFFI decline by 50% every 2 to 3 yr
Radon and radon daughters	Ground beneath a home, domestic water, and some utility natural gas	1.5 pCi/l estimated average in U.S. homes >8 pCi/l in 3% to 5% of homes	8 pCi/l NCRP action level 4 pCi/l EPA limit for uranium processing site homes 2 pCi/l ASHRAE guidelines 5 pCi/l Sweden, maximum, existing buildings 3 pCi/l Sweden, maximum, new buildings	Radon or radon daughters can be measured. Standards are for radon. Lung cancer risk results from radon daughters.
Volatile organic compounds; benzene, styrene, tetrachloroethylene; dichlorobenzene; methylene chloride; chloroform	Outgassing from water, plasticizers, solvents, paints, cleaning compounds, mothballs, resins, glues, gasoline, oils, combustion, art materials, photocopiers, personal care products	Typical indoor concentrations of selected compounds: benzene—15 $\mu g/m^3$; 1,1,1 trichloroethylene—20 $\mu g/m^3$; chloroform—2 $\mu g/m^3$; tetrachloroethylene—5 $\mu g/m^3$; styrene—2 $\mu g/m^3$; m,p-dichlorobenzene—4 $\mu g/m^3$; m,p-xylene—15 $\mu g/m^3$	No indoor standards for nonoccupational settings	EPA Carcinogenic Assessment Group potency factors available for many of the volatile organics
Semivolatile organics: chlorinated hydrocarbons, DDT, heptachlor, chlordane	Pesticides, transformer fluids, termicides, combustion of wood, tobacco, kerosene, and charcoal; wood preservatives, fungicides	Only limited data available	No indoor standards	—
Semivolatile organics: polycyclic compounds, benzo(a)pyrene, polychlorinated biphenols	Herbicides, insecticides	—	—	—
Asbestos	Insulation on building structural components; asbestos plaster around pipes and furnaces; tiles	No systematic measurements to determine typical fiber concentrations. >1,000 ng/ m^3 when friable asbestos	2 fibers/cc OSHA 8-hr time-weighted average	EPA and state attention has been on schools and office buildings; domestic problems not evaluated

* cfu/m^3 = colony-forming units/m^3.
† Source: J. M. Samet, M. C. Marbury, and J. D. Spengler. Health effects and sources of indoor air pollution. Part I. *Am. Rev. Respir. Dis.* 136:1486, 1987. Reprinted with permission.

for recurrent wheezing episodes following these infections [103]. The strong implication is that some children with these viral infections exhibit mast cell degranulation with a specific IgE response and airway obstruction, suggesting that the virus is acting as an allergen in these individuals rather than that these clinical findings are simply the direct effect of the viral infection.

Frick and associates [30] prospectively studied infants of atopic parents in comparison to a like number of infants from nonatopic parents. They found increased clinical allergy symptoms and positive allergy tests in the atopic group within 3 months of a rise in the anti-RSV and/or anti-parainfluenza virus antibodies, whereas the nonatopic children showed no allergic symptoms or laboratory evidence of allergy following similar infections. It would appear that viral infections often trigger an atopic response, but only in individuals with a genetic predisposition to allergy. Experiments in dogs tend to support this theory [29]. Viral infections also play a role in exacerbations of asthma in many ways other than IgE-mediated mast cell degranulation, as discussed in Chapter 44.

Bacteria

Bacteria have long been thought to either precipitate or complicate bronchial asthma. Bacterial sinusitis appears to exacerbate asthma (Chap. 41). The role of bacteria as a direct cause of allergic difficulty, however, has not been established in spite of extensive research in this area. Positive immediate skin tests using bacterial antigens can be elicited in atopic individuals [35]. Bacterial vaccines have been used in an attempt to "desensitize" individuals with "bacterial allergy," but have produced inconsistent results [49, 64]. "Autogenous" vaccines (i.e., vaccines made from the patient's throat culture) have also been used, but there is no physiologic rationale for this, especially since the bacterial flora in the throat is constantly changing. Chapter 44 describes the role of infection in asthma in more detail.

Exposure to detergent enzymes made from bacteria (*Bacillus subtilis*) has been shown to cause sensitivity in occupational exposures [27], and even sensitivity resulting from casual exposure in consumers has been suspected in a few instances [79].

Plant Allergens

Plant allergens (other than pollens) also constitute a significant threat to the allergic population.

Kapok (seed hair from kapok trees) is still frequently used as stuffing for throw pillows, mattresses, and sleeping bags. It is also used for life jackets and boat cushions but, in this case, it is sealed to prevent soaking and subsequent loss of buoyancy. Sen-

Table 42-5. Control measures for pollutants

Pollutant	Control measures	
	Equipment and materials	Ventilation and design
Respirable particles	High efficiency filters	Zone and ventilate for smoking
	Tight-sealing doors and grates	Supply outside combustion air to heater and fireplace
	Properly drafting chimney	Relocate air intakes
	Electrostatic precipitators	Maintain filter system
NO, NO$_2$	Remove gasoline engine	Effective hood vent over source
	Pilotless ignition	Isolate garage from indoor space
CO	Pilotless ignition	Supply outside combustion air
	Restrict heater use to uninhabited space	Vent emission outside
	Use catalytic converter	Kitchen/hood vent
	Replace indoor gasoline engines with electric	Relocate vents
		Provide smoking zones
		Isolate garage from indoor place
CO$_2$	Check static pressure in return air ducts to make sure return is not overriding fresh air intake	Isolate garage from indoor space
Agents from biologic sources	Insulate to prevent condensation	Maintain inside relative humidities of 35–50%
	Damp-proof foundation, ducts	Exhaust bath and kitchen
	Proper drainage of drip pans under condenser coils	Vent crawl spaces
	Add bacteriocides to steam and water for humidifiers and cooling towers	
	Proper maintenance of filters and ducts	
	Routine cleaning	
	Discard water-damaged floor coverings	
	Do not use cool-mist humidifiers and vaporizers	
Formaldehyde	Substitute products such as phenolic resin plywood	Increase air exchange to house or office
	Seal sources	
	Removal of materials	
Radon and radon daughters	Vapor barrier around foundation	Vent crawl space
	Damp-proof basement and crawl space	Vent sumphole to exterior
	Seal cracks and holes in floor traps and drains	Subslab depressurization
	Install charcoal water-scrubber for well water	Vent bathroom and laundry to exterior
	Completely seal foundation	
Volatile organic compounds	Substitute products	Use only with adequate ventilation
	Isolate storage area	Ventilate laundry, shop
	Apply only according to specifications	Provide separate ventilation to storage area
	Do not locate transformers indoors	
Asbestos	Removal	Ventilation does not provide adequate protection
	Injection sealant	
	Wrap pipes with plastic and duct tape	

Source: J. M. Samet, M. C. Marbury, and J. D. Spengler. Health effects and sources of indoor air pollution. Part I. *Am. Rev. Respir. Dis.* 136:1486, 1987. Reprinted with permission.

sitivity to kapok increases in proportion to its age, just as does feather sensitivity, suggesting to many that contamination by mites is the most relevant factor in determining sensitivity.

Orrisroot (from iris rhizomes), once widely used for cosmetics, has largely been supplanted by more innocuous substances. However, allergic individuals and, especially, parents of allergic children must read cosmetic labels carefully, since some cosmetics do still contain orrisroot. These inexpensive cosmetics are often sold in children's kits or by mail order.

Pyrethrum (from the flowerheads of chrysanthemums) is included in many insecticides. Its close botanic relationship to ragweed often results in cross-sensitivity in ragweed-sensitive individuals.

Cottonseed, a potent allergen, is still used as an ingredient in dog and cattle feeds as well as in pan-greasing compounds. Less often it is found as a contaminant in inexpensive cotton-stuffed upholstery.

Other inhalant allergens cause difficulty in a few highly sensitive individuals. Some fish-sensitive patients are strongly reactive to fish odors. Occupational asthma has been seen in coffee workers, pharmacists (ipecac), woodworkers, foam manufacturing workers (toluene diisocyanate), photographers (platinum salts), printers (vegetable gum), meat wrappers (pyrolysis products of plastic), rubber workers (ethylenediamine), and pharmaceutical workers and medical assistants (penicillin and other drugs). Chapter 46 deals with these problems in greater detail.

Indoor Environmental Pollutants

Chapter 45 deals with environmental pollution and Chapter 87 with environmental control measures. There is increasing concern among environmentalists as well as allergists and other scientists that the advent of "tight" buildings and homes has resulted in higher concentrations of many indoor pollutants and allergens. Tables 42-4 and 42-5 summarize the principal indoor pollutants, their sources, and concentrations.

REFERENCES

1. Agarwal, M. K., et al. Immunochemical quantitation of airborne short ragweed, *Alternaria*, antigen E and Alt.-1 allergens: a two-year prospective study. *J. Allergy Clin. Immunol.* 72:40, 1983.
2. American Academy of Allergy and Immunology. *Pollen and Mold Counts.* 1989, Courtesy of the University of Michigan Allergy Research Laboratory.
3. Baldo, B. A., and Panzani, R. C. Detection of IgE antibodies to a wide range of insect species in subjects with suspected inhalant allergies to insects. *Int. Arch. Allergy Appl. Immunol.* 85:278, 1988.
4. Balyeat, R. M., Stemen, T. R., and Taft, C. E. Comparative pollen, mold, butterfly and moth emanation content of the air. *J. Allergy* 58(3):227, 1983.
5. Bates, D. V., et al. Deposition and retention models for internal dosimetry of human respiratory tract. *Health Phys.* 12:173, 1966.
6. Baur, X., et al. Hypersensitivity to chironomids (non-biting midges): localization of the antigenic determinants within certain polypeptide sequences of hemoglobins (erythrocruorins) or *Chironomus thummi thummi* (Diptera). *J. Allergy Clin. Immunol.* 69:66, 1982.
7. Bernstein, I. L., and Safferman, R. S. Sensitivity of skin and bronchial mucosa to green algae. *J. Allergy* 38:166, 1966.
8. Bernstein, I. L., et al. In-vitro cross-allergenicity of major aeroallergen pollens by the radioallergosorbent technique. *J. Allergy Clin. Immunol.* 57:141, 1976.
9. Bernton, H. S., and Brown, H. Insect allergy—preliminary studies of the cockroach. *J. Allergy* 35(6):506, 1964.
10. Bernton, H. S., and Brown, H. Cockroach allergy. II—The relation of infestation to sensitization. *South. Med. J.* 60:852, 1967.
11. Bernton, H. S., McMahon, T. F., and Brown, H. Cockroach asthma. *Br. J. Dis. Chest.* 66:61, 1972.
12. Blackley, C. *Experimental Researches on the Causes and Nature of Catarrhus Aestives (Hay Fever and Hay Asthma).* London: Bailliere, Tindall and Cox, 1873.
13. Bucur, J., et al. Immunotherapy with dog and cat allergen preparations in dog-sensitive and cat-sensitive asthmatics. *Ann. Allergy* 62:355, 1989.
14. Burge, H. A., Solomon, W. R., and Muilenberg, M. S. Evaluation of indoor plantings as allergen exposure sources. *J. Allergy Clin. Immunol.* 70:101, 1982.
15. Bush, R. K. Aerobiology of pollen and fungal allergens. *J. Allergy Clin. Immunol.* 84:1120, 1989.
16. Busse, W. W., Reed, C. E., and Hoehne, J. H. Where is the allergy reaction in ragweed asthma? II. Demonstration of ragweed antigen in airborne particles smaller than pollen. *J. Allergy Clin. Immunol.* 50:289, 1972.
17. Campbell, R., et al. Aeroallergens in dairy barns near Cooperstown, New York and Rochester, Minnesota. *Am. Rev. Respir. Dis.* 140:317, 1989.
18. Chapman, M. D., Sutherland, W. M., and Platts-Mills, T. A. E. Recognition of two *Dermatophagoides pteronyssinus*–specific epitopes on antigen P1 by using monoclonal antibodies: binding to each epitope can be inhibited by serum from dust mite–allergic patients. *J. Immunol.* 133:2488, 1984.
19. Chapman, M. D., and Platts-Mills, T. A. E. Purification and characterization of the major allergen from *Dermatophagoides Pteronyssinus*–antigen P1. *J. Immunol.* 125:587, 1980.
20. Dabrowski, A. J., et al. Cat skin as an important source of Fel d 1 allergen. *J. Allergy Clin. Immunol.* 86:462, 1990.
21. deGroot, H., Stapel, S. O., and Aalberse, R. C. Statistical analysis of IgE antibodies to the common inhalant allergens in 44, 496 sera. *Ann. Allergy* 65:97, 1990.
22. Dekker, H. Asthma und Milben. *Munch. Med. Wochenschr.* 75:515, 1928.
23. Dybendal, T., et al. Dust from carpeted and smooth floors. I. Comparative measurements of antigenic and allergenic proteins in dust vacuumed from carpeted and noncarpeted classrooms in Norwegian schools. *Clin. Exp. Allergy* 19:217, 1987.
24. Esch, R. E., and Klapper, D. G. Isolation and characterization of a major cross-reactive grass group I allergenic determinant. *Mol. Immunol.* 26:557, 1989.
25. Feinberg, S. Mold allergy: its importance in asthma and hay fever. *Wis. Med. J.* 34:254, 1935.
26. Figley, K. D. Asthma due to the mayfly. *Am. J. Med. Sci.* 178:338, 1929.
27. Flind, M. L. H. Pulmonary diseases due to inhalation of derivatives of *Bacillus subtilis* containing proteolytic enzymes. *Lancet* 1:1177, 1969.
28. Ford, A. W., Altermen, L., and Kemeny, D. M. The allergens of dog. I. Identification using crossed immunoelectrophoresis. *Clin. Exp. Allergy* 19:183, 1989.
29. Frick, O. L., and Brooks, D. L. Immunoglobulin E antibodies to pollens augmented in dogs by virus vaccines. *Am. J. Vet. Res.* 44:440, 1983.
30. Frick, O. L., German, D. F., and Mills, J. Development of allergy in children. Association with virus infection. *J. Allergy Clin. Immunol.* 64:228, 1979.
31. Gad El Rab, M. O., and Kay. A. B. Widespread immunoglobulin E–mediated hypersensitivity in the Sudan to the "Green Nimitti" midge *Cladotanytarsus lewisi* (Diptera: Chironomidae) I. Diagnosis by radioallergosorbent test. *J. Allergy Clin. Immunol.* 66(3):190, 1980.
32. Gregory, P. H. *Microbiology of the Atmosphere* (2nd ed.). New York: Wiley, 1973.
33. Gupta, S., et al. Role of insects as inhalant allergens in bronchial asthma with special reference to clinical characteristics of patients. *Clin. Exp. Allergy* 20:519, 1990.
34. Haas, A., Becker, W. M., and Measch, H. J. Analysis of allergen components in grass pollen extracts using immunoblotting. *Int. Arch. Allergy Appl. Immunol.* 79:434, 1986.
35. Hampton, S. F., Johnson, M. C., and Galakatos, E. Studies of bacterial hypersensitivity in asthma. *J. Allergy* 34:63, 1963.
36. Henderson, F. W., et al. Etiology and epidemiologic spectrum of bronchiolitis in pediatric practice. *J. Pediatr.* 95:83, 1979.
37. Hoffman, D. R. Dog and cat allergens, urinary or dander proteins? *Ann. Allergy* 45:205, 1980.
38. Horner, W. E., Ibanez, M. D., and Lehrer, S. B. Immunoprint analysis of *Calvatia cyathiformis* allergens. I. Reactivity with individual sera. *J. Allergy Clin. Immunol.* 83(4):784, 1989.
39. Hudjel, D. W., et al. Viral and bacterial infections in adults with chronic asthma. *Am. Rev. Respir. Dis.* 120:393, 1979.
40. Ito, K., et al. Skin test and radioallergosorbent test with extracts of larval and adult midges of *Tokunagayusurika akamus* (Diptera chironomidae)

in asthmatic patients of the metropolitan area of Tokyo. *Ann. Allergy* 57: 199, 1986.

41. Kang, B. Study on cockroach antigen as a possible causative agent in bronchial asthma. *J. Allergy Clin. Immunol.* 58:357, 1976.

42. Kay, A. B., et al. The prevalence of asthma and rhinitis in a Sudanese community seasonally exposed to a potent airborne allergen (the "green nimitti" midge), *cladotanytarsus lewisi. J. Allergy Clin. Immunol.* 71(3): 345, 1983.

43. Kern, R. A. Asthma due to sensitization to a mushroom fly *(Aphiochaeta agarici). J. Allergy* 9:604, 1938.

44. King, T. P., and Norman, P. S. Isolation studies of allergens from ragweed pollen. *Biochemistry* 1:709, 1962.

45. Kivity, S., et al. Cockroach allergen: an important cause of perennial rhinitis. *Allergy* 44:291, 1989.

46. Kino, T., and Oshima, S. Allergy to insects in Japan. I. The reaginic sensitivity to moth and butterfly in patients with bronchial asthma. *J. Allergy Clin. Immunol.* 61(1):10, 1978.

47. Kino, T., et al. Allergy to insect in Japan. III. High frequency of IgE antibody responses to insects (moth, butterfly, and chironomid) in patients with bronchial asthma and immunochemical quantitation of the insect-related airborne particles smaller than 10 μm in diameter. *J. Allergy Clin. Immunol.* 79:257, 1987.

48. Korsgaard, J. Preventive measures in house dust allergy. *Am. Rev. Respir. Dis.* 125:80, 1982.

49. Kowikko, A. Bacterial vaccine in childhood asthma. A double-blind study. *Acta Allergol.* 28:202, 1973.

50. Krilis, S., Baldo, B. A., and Basten, A. Antigens and allergens from the common house dust mite *Dermatophagoides pteronyssinus.* II. Identification of the major IgE-binding antigens by crossed radioimmunoelectrophoresis. *J. Allergy Clin. Immunol.* 74:142, 1984.

51. Lehrer, S. B., et al. Basidiomycete mycelial and spore-allergen extracts: skin test reactivity in adults with symptoms of respiratory allergy. *J. Allergy Clin. Immunol.* 78:478, 1986.

52. Lilja, G., et al. Immunotherapy with cat- and dog-dander extracts. IV. Effects of 2 years of treatment. *J. Allergy Clin. Immunol.* 83:37, 1989.

53. Lind, P. Purification and partial characterization of two major allergens from the house dust mite *Dermatophagoides pteronyssinus. J. Allergy Clin. Immunol.* 76:753, 1985.

54. Longbottom, J. L., Harvey, C., and Taylor, M. L. Characterization of immunologically important antigens and allergens of *Aspergillus fumigatus. Int. Arch. Allergy Appl. Immunol.* 88:185, 1989.

55. Luczynska, C. M., et al. Airborne concentration and particle size distribution of allergen derived from domestic cats *(Feles domesticus). Am. Rev. Respir. Dis.* 141:361, 1990.

56. Mathison, D. A., Stevenson, D. D., and Simon, R. A. Asthma and the home environment. *Ann. Intern. Med.* 97:128, 1982.

57. McCants, M. L., et al. Prevalence of basidiospore skin test reactivity in Europe. *J. Allergy Clin. Immunol.* 85:249, 1990.

58. McIntosh, K., et al. The association of viral and bacterial respiratory infections with exacerbations of wheezing in young asthmatic children. *J. Pediatr.* 82:578, 1973.

59. Miller, J. D., et al. Effect of tannic acid spray on cat allergen levels in carpets (abstract). *J. Allergy Clin. Immunol.* 85(1)S:226, 1990.

60. Minor, T. E., Baker, J. W., and Dick, E. C. Greater frequency of viral respiratory infections in asthmatic children as compared with their non-asthmatic siblings. *J. Pediatr.* 85:472, 1974.

61. Minor, T. E., et al. Viruses as precipitants of asthmatic attacks in children. *JAMA* 227:292, 1974.

62. Minor, T. E., et al. Rhinovirus and influenza A infections as preipitants of asthma. *Am. Rev. Respir. Dis.* 113:149, 1976.

63. Montanaro, A. House dust, animal proteins, pollutants and environmental controls. *J. Allergy Clin. Immunol.* 84:1125, 1989.

64. Mueller, H. L., and Lang, H. Hyposensitization with bacterial vaccine in infectious asthma. *JAMA* 208:1379, 1969.

65. Odgen, E. C., et al. *Manual for Sampling Airborne Pollen.* New York: Hafner Press, 1974.

66. Ohman, J. L., Findlay, S. R., and Leiterman, K. M. Imunotherapy in cat-induced asthma. Double-blind trial evaluation of in-vivo and in-vitro responses. *J. Allergy Clin. Immunol.* 74:230, 1984.

67. Osgood, H. Allergy to caddis fly (trichoptera). II. Clinical aspects. *J. Allergy Clin. Immunol.* 28(4):292, 1957.

68. Partlato, S. J. A case of coryza and asthma due to sand flies (caddis fly). *J. Allergy* 1:35, 1929.

69. Partlato, S. J. The sand fly (caddis fly) as an exciting cause of allergic coryza and asthma. *J. Allergy* 1(4):307, 1930.

70. Perez, M., et al. CDNA cloning and immunological characterization of the ryeglass allergen Lol pl. *J. Biol. Chem.* 265:16210, 1990.

71. Phanichyakan, P., Dockhorn, R. J., and Kirkpatrick, C. H. Asthma due to inhalation of moth flies *(Psychoda). J. Allergy* 44(1):51, 1969.

72. Perkins, W. A. *The Rotorod Sampler, 2nd Semiannual Report* (CML 186). Stanford, CA: Aerosol Laboratory, Stanford University, 1957.

73. Platts-Mills, T. A. E., et al. Dust mite allergens and asthma—a worldwide problem. *J. Allergy Clin. Immunol.* 83:416, 1989.

74. Popp, W., et al. Risk factors for sensitization to furred pets. *Allergy* 45: 75, 1990.

75. Salvaggio, J., and Aukrust, L. Mold-induced asthma. *J. Allergy Clin. Immunol.* 68:327, 1981.

76. Samet, J. M., Marbury, M. C., and Spengler, J. D. Health effects and sources of indoor air pollution. Part I. *Am. Rev. Respir. Dis.* 136:1486, 1987.

77. Sayer, W. J., Shean, D. B., and Glossieri, J. Estimation of airborne fungal flora by the Anderson sampler versus the gravity settling plate. *J. Allergy Clin. Immunol.* 44:214, 1969.

78. Shamie, S., et al. The consistent presence of cat allergens (Fel d 1) in various types of public places (abstract). *J. Allergy Clin. Immunol.* 85(1)S: 226, 1990.

79. Shapiro, R. S., and Eisenberg, B. C. Sensitivity to proteolytic enzymes in laundry detergents. *J. Allergy* 47:76, 1971.

80. Sheldon, J. M., and Johnston, J. H. Hypersensitivity to beetles (Coleoptera). Report of a case. *J. Allergy* 12:493, 1940–41.

81. Smith, E. G. *Sampling and Identifying Allergenic Pollens and Molds.* San Antonio, Texas: Bluestone Press, 1984, Vol. I; 1986, and Vol. II.

82. Solomon, W. R. Fungus aerosols arising from cold-mist vaporizers. *J. Allergy Clin. Immunol.* 54:222, 1974.

83. Solomon, W. R. Assessing fungus prevalence in domestic interiors. *J. Allergy Clin. Immunol.* 56:235, 1975.

84. Solomon, W. R., Bernstein, I. L., and Safferman, R. S. *Impact of Aeroallergens in Aerobiology. The Ecological Systems Approach* (U. S. I.B.P. Synthesis Series 10). Stroudsberg, Pennsylvania: Dowden, Hutchinson and Ross, 1979.

85. Solomon, W. R., Burge, H. A., and Muilenberg, M. L. Allergenic properties of *Alternaria* spores, mycelial and "metabolic" extracts. *J. Allergy Clin. Immunol.* 65:229, 1980.

86. Solomon, W. R., and Gilliam, J. A simplified application of the Anderson sampler to the study of airborne fungus particles. *J. Allergy Clin. Immunol.* 45:1, 1970.

87. Spieksma, F. Th. M., et al. Respiratory allergy to laboratory fruit flies *(Drosophila melanogaster). J. Allergy Clin. Immunol.* 77:108, 1986.

88. Sporek, R., et al. Exposure to house dust mite allergen (der P1) and the development of asthma in childhood, a prospective study. *N. Engl. J. Med.* 323:502, 1990.

89. Stevenson, D. D., and Mathews, K. P. Occupational asthma following inhalation of moth particles. *J. Allergy* 39(5):274, 1967.

90. Strom Van Leuwen W. Bronchial asthma in relation to climate. *Proc. R. Soc. Med.* 17:19, 1924.

91. Stuart, B. O. Deposition of inhaled aerosols. *Arch. Intern. Med.* 131:60, 1973.

92. Swanson, M. C., Agarwal, M. K., and Reed, C. E. An immunochemical approach to indoor aeroallergen quantitation with a new volumetric air sampler: studies with mite, roach, cat, mouse and guinea pig antigens. *J. Allergy Clin. Immunol.* 76:724, 1985.

93. Taylor, E. R., Longbottom, J. L., and Pepys, J. Respiratory allergy to urine proteins of rats and mice. *Lancet* 2:847, 1977.

94. Tovey, E. R., et al. The distribution of dust mite allergens in houses of patients with asthma. *Am. Rev. Respir. Dis.* 124:630, 1981.

95. van Bronswijk, J. E. M. H. Rasterlek-tronenmikroskipische Untersuchungen an *Dermatophagoides pteronyssinus. Acta Allergol.* 28:180, 1973.

96. Van der Werff, P. *Mold Fungi and Bronchial Asthma.* Springfield, Ill: Thomas, 1958.

97. Vervloet, D., et al. Altitude and house dust mites. *J. Allergy Clin. Immunol.* 69:290, 1982.

98. Voorhorst, R. To what extent are house dust mites *(Dermatophagoides)* responsible for complaints in asthma patients? *Allerg. Immunol.* 18:9, 1972.

99. Voorhorst, R., Spieksma, F. Th. M., and Varekamp, H. *House Dust Atopy and the House Dust Mite Dermatophagoides pteronyssinus (Troussart, 1877).* London: Stafleu's Scientific Publishing Company, 1969.

100. Welliver, R. C., Kaul, T. N., and Ogra, P. L. The appearance of cell-bound IgE in respiratory tract epithelium after respiratory syncytial virus infection. *N. Engl. J. Med.* 303:1198, 1980.

101. Welliver, R. C., et al. Role of parainfluenza virus–specific IgE in the pathogenesis of croup and wheezing subsequent to infection. *J. Pediatr.* 94: 370, 1979.

102. Welliver, R. C., et al. The development of respiratory syncytial virus–specific IgE and the release of histamine in nasopharyngeal secretion after infection. *N. Engl. J. Med.* 305:841, 1981.

103. Welliver, R. C., et al. Predictive value of respiratory syncytial virus–specific IgE responses for recurrent wheezing following bronchiolitis. *J. Pediatr.* 109:776, 1986.

104. Wiseman, R. D., et al. Insect allergy as a possible cause of inhalant sensitivity. *J. Allergy Clin. Immunol.* 30:191, 1959.

105. Wood, R. A., Mudd, K. E., and Eggleton, P. A. The distribution of cat allergen on verticle surfaces (abstract). *J. Allergy Clin. Immunol.* 85:225, 1990.

106. Wood, R. A., et al. The effect of cat removal on allergen content in household dust samples. *J. Allergy Clin. Immunol.* 83:730, 1989.

107. Wynn, S. R., et al. Immunochemical quantitation, size distribution and cross-reactivity of lepidoptera (moth) aeroallergens in southeastern Minnesota. *J. Allergy Clin. Immunol.* 82:47, 1988.

108. Yunginger, J. W., Jones, R. T., and Nesheim, M. E. S. Studies on *Alternaria* allergens. III. Isolation of major allergenic factor (ALT-1). *J. Allergy Clin. Immunol.* 66:138, 1980.

109. International workshop. Dust mite allergens and asthma: Report of second international workshop. *J. Allergy Clin. Immunol.* 89:1046, 1992.

110. Hamilton, R. G. House dust aeroallergen measurements in clinical practice: A guide to allergen-free home and work environments. *Immunol. Allergy Pract.* 14:96, 1992.

Food Allergens

Michael K. Farrell

43

The concept that certain foods may produce allergic reactions in susceptible persons dates back to antiquity, the aphorism "one man's meat is another man's poison" being attributed to Lucretius (c. 100 B.C.). Numerous reports and anecdotes throughout the ages have attributed virtually every imaginable malady to food allergy. The result has been fanaticism countered by skepticism. There is no doubt that there are individuals who, when exposed to specific allergens, develop classic allergic symptoms including respiratory symptoms. However, the lack of objective, reproducible, and properly controlled studies that eliminate patient and observer bias has made food allergy confusing and complex. The confusion and uncertainty increase when pulmonary symptoms are considered, since patients with reactive airway disease may react identically to a variety of environmental stimuli [2].

The terminology of reactions to food is also confusing and a potential source of bias. The terminology used in this chapter, although a bit simplistic, is an attempt to describe reactions on the basis of mechanisms [24]. Food *allergy* is used to describe IgE-mediated responses. Food *sensitivity* includes both reaginic and nonreaginic immune responses to ingested antigens. Food *intolerance* describes any nonimmunologic reaction, usually gastrointestinal in origin, such as disaccharidase deficiency.

There are also pharmacologic reactions to foods or food components. The ingestion of methylxanthines such as caffeine can result in tachycardia, sweating, gastrointestinal changes, and tachypnea mediated via catecholamine release.

Pulmonary reactions to food can also be mediated via other factors. Dohi and colleagues [9] recently reported on 11 patients with food-dependent, exercise-induced anaphylaxis. In 7, specific foods (shellfish, wheat, grape) were implicated; in 4, the act of eating followed by exercise predisposed to anaphylaxis [9].

The exact prevalence of food sensitivity is unknown and has been reported to range from 0.5 to 8.0 percent. Careful studies have placed the prevalence at approximately 0.5 to 1.0 percent of the general population [3]. Food sensitivity is more common in infants and children. Gastrointestinal reactions are the most common, followed by skin and respiratory tract involvement; there is a tendency for the type of reaction to change with increasing age [3, 4, 25]. Thus, gastrointestinal symptoms are more common in children and respiratory symptoms become more prominent in adults. Reactions can also be categorized based on the time until onset of symptoms: Immediate reactions occur within 1 hour of ingestion, intermediate reactions occur within 24 hours, and late reactions occur longer than 24 hours after exposure. Respiratory symptoms tend to be intermediate in nature.

The natural history of food sensitivity in many individuals is a gradual loss of clinical or symptomatic reactions, even though immunologic markers such as skin test reactivity remain. This phenomenon is particularly common in children. Thus, children who, as infants have an intense reaction to cow's milk, may be able to tolerate it several years later. In several studies, 75 to 80 percent of infants with documented cow's milk sensitivity tolerated milk by the age of 4 years [16, 17]. The development of this tolerance is due to a complex interaction of antigen absorption from the gastrointestinal tract, mucosal immunity, and alterations in cell antigen-antibody reactions [29].

IMMUNOLOGY AND SENSITIZATION

The body is constantly bombarded by a vast array of foreign antigens; one of the major portals is the gastrointestinal tract. Normal immunologic defense mechanisms, digestive processes, and local factors such as peristalsis, mucus, the indigenous flora, and digestive enzymes neutralize many ingested antigens and decrease the antigen load potentially available for absorption [33].

Macromolecules can be transported across the gut epithelium several ways. "M"-cells overlying Peyer's patches are specialized for antigen uptake [27]; macromolecule uptake also occurs via the enterocyte (endocytosis/exocytosis) and by passage through the intracellular gaps [40]. Macromolecule absorption occurs more frequently in infants and malnourished patients although some absorption does occur in adults [35, 37]. Most of the absorbed macromolecules are digested by intraepithelial lysozymes, but some are extravasated into the basilar interstitial space; from there, they enter the lamina propria [40]. The next line of defense is Peyer's patches. Lymphocyte sensitization and blast formation occur there; lymphocytes migrate to the lymphatic circulation and return via the systemic circulation [36]. IgE antibodies may then be produced but the majority of sensitized lymphocytes produce IgA and are the major local defense mechanism, extruding secretory IgA into the intestinal lumen [18, 27]. Specific secretory IgA induced by oral immunization with horseradish peroxidase and bovine serum albumin markedly decreases gastrointestinal uptake of these antigens. This effect is not seen following parenteral immunization [39].

Several mechanisms have been postulated to explain clinical symptoms following antigen ingestion. These include alterations in bowel permeability, decreased local IgA production, specific gastrointestinal IgE antibodies, and decreased immune tolerance [10].

Anti–milk IgG antibodies are present in virtually all children under 3 years old who drink cow's milk. Levels peak between 3 and 7 months, decline after 2 years, and are virtually undetectable in adults [23]. Neither increased cellular uptake nor decreased lysosomal proteolysis has been demonstrated in neonatal rats. In healthy human infants, the cause of the increased anti–cow's milk antibodies has not been demonstrated to be due to any particular factor. Walker and Isselbacher demonstrated increased macromolecule movement through injured mucosal cells [40]. Hence, infections and resultant mucosal injury may be an important predecessor to sensitization.

Continuous food antigen exposure can cause the normally immunologically responsive individual to develop T-cell suppression of the antibody response; this may result in an immunologically tolerant adult [26, 30]. The clinical correlate is the person with demonstrable circulating specific antibodies but no symptoms after ingestion of that food. Alterations in local IgA production and local IgE response may play a role in food sensitivity, but their role in the human remains incompletely defined [32].

DIAGNOSIS

The possibility that an individual symptom or a group of symptoms is related to a food sensitivity is usually first suggested by the clinical history. During the evaluation of suspected food sensitivity, the objective must be the rational, unbiased confirmation or refutation of the history. This is accomplished by a thorough medical history, physical examination, consideration of the differential diagnosis, and the appropriate use of specific laboratory studies. The diagnosis involves three steps: (1) proof that the adverse reaction is caused by food, (2) differentiation from other causes of adverse reactions, and (3) identification of the immunologic processes involved.

A detailed allergy history, including the family history of atopy, is vital. The incidence of food sensitivity increases by 50 percent when there is a positive family history. The precise temporal relationship between the ingestion of the suspected food and the onset of symptoms must be clarified. Specific attention must be given to any precipitating or aggravating factors. The onset of food sensitivity following acute enteritis suggests sensitization through a damaged gastrointestinal mucosa. Cross-reacting food sensitivities must also be considered (Fig. 43-1). Patients who have reacted to one member of a food family may react to other members of the same family; 10 to 20 percent of patients with documented sensitivity to cow's milk protein also react to soy

Fig. 43-1. *Evaluation of suspected food sensitivity. (Modified from S. A. Bock. Food sensitivity: A critical review and practical approach. Am. J. Dis. Child. 134:973, 1980.)*

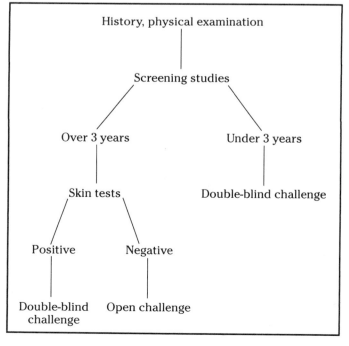

Table 43-1. *Food additives and asthmatic reactions*

Additive	Asthmatic reaction
Antimicrobials	
Sodium benzoate	Asthma
Benzoic acid	Asthma
Sorbic acid	Asthma
Antioxidants	
Sulfur dioxide	Asthma
Sulfite	Asthma
Bisulfite	Asthma, anaphylaxis
Metabisulfite	Asthma, anaphylaxis
Coloring and flavoring agents	
Tartrazine	Asthma
Azo dyes	Asthma
Monosodium glutamate	Asthma

protein [28]. Patients with aspirin-associated asthma often react to the food additive tartrazine (FD&C dye no. 5) [31]. Many drugs contain tartrazine (see Chap. 48).

The following foods often contain tartrazine:

1. Breakfast cereals
2. Refrigerated rolls, quick breads
3. Cake mixes
4. Commercial pies, gingerbread, frostings
5. Chocolate, butterscotch chips
6. Puddings
7. Certain ice creams, sherbets
8. Candy (drops, hard candies)
9. Colored marshmallows
10. Flavored carbonated beverages and drink mixes

Sulfites are commonly found in foods; many asthmatic patients have bronchospasm when challenged. Severe reactions have been reported. Patients must be instructed to read all labels carefully (Table 43-1). Sulfites, now removed from salad bars, may still be found in dried fruits, beer and wine, shrimp, and processed potatoes.

Many patients with suspected food sensitivity have gastrointestinal as well as pulmonary symptoms. Gastrointestinal symptoms tend to be more common in infants and children; in adults the initial reaction to an ingested antigen is frequently angioedema or bronchospasm [10]. A detailed history regarding vomiting, abdominal pain, infantile colic, diarrhea, and constipation should be obtained [3]. In breast-fed infants, the maternal diet must be scrutinized for potential allergens since antigens absorbed from the mother's gastrointestinal tract can pass into the breast milk and cause symptoms in the infant. This has been best documented for cow's milk [21]. The clinician must also remember that other substances such as caffeine and other drugs may pass into the breast milk and cause a variety of nonspecific symptoms.

The age at the time of onset of symptoms should be determined. Infants are more likely to have associated gastrointestinal symptoms than adults. Likewise, infants are more likely to develop tolerance to the incriminated food. The type of foods responsible for documented reactions also varies with age. In children under the age of 3 years, milk and soy are the most commonly confirmed foods, while in those over 3 years old, peanuts, other nuts, eggs, and milk are more frequently implicated [4, 6, 35]. In adults, tomato, milk, and chocolate are the most commonly incriminated foods [2] (Table 43-2).

In infants and children, growth must be monitored carefully. Food sensitivity should not result in growth failure or malnutrition; if present, another primary disease or the overzealous use of elimination diets must be excluded. Unfortunately, we have

Table 43-2. Foods more commonly associated with asthma[a]

Fish	Wheat
Shellfish	Eggs[b]
Peanuts	Milk[b]
Other nuts	Soy[b]
Tomatoes	Chocolate

[a] In general, isolated asthma as a reaction to food is uncommon. The pulmonary reaction is usually part of a generalized reaction including urticaria and gastrointestinal symptoms.
[b] More common in children.

recently seen numbers of children whose nutrition and thus subsequent growth are compromised by their parents overzealous application of restricted diets.

Heights and weights should be obtained for all children at each visit and plotted on standard growth charts. Any deviation from previously established growth patterns is a cause for concern and should prompt further investigation.

The diagnosis of food sensitivity is confirmed by carefully selected laboratory studies, skin tests, and the response to specific food challenges. Certain preliminary studies may be useful in suspected food sensitivity pulmonary disease. Soft tissue radiographs of the upper airway and a barium swallow exclude anatomic problems and vascular malformations. If growth failure and/or gastrointestinal symptoms are present, cystic fibrosis should be excluded. In patients with pulmonary disease, liver disease, or a family history of pulmonary disease, the alpha$_1$-antitrypsin phenotype should be determined. Serum alpha$_1$-antitrypsin concentrations alone are not sufficient since alpha$_1$-antitrypsin is an acute-phase reactant and may be elevated in stress states. The homozygous deficiency state, Pi ZZ phenotype, is associated with the early development of severe obstructive lung disease in adults [34]. Children may have recurrent bronchitis, wheezing, and diminished pulmonary function [8]. However, children may have little or no lung disease; the major manifestation is neonatal cholestasis. Heterozygous adults appear to be at increased risk for lung disease, especially if they smoke. Children with the heterozygous state also have pulmonary dysfunction [38]. Pi variant phenotypes are more common in children with asthma than in the general population [19].

The total eosinophil count and serum IgE concentration identify a patient as atopic; they are not specific for food sensitivity. Circulating antigen-specific IgE antibodies can be assayed by the radioallergosorbent test (RAST). However, the exact role of the RAST in the diagnosis of food sensitivity remains unclear. The RAST measures circulating IgE antibodies, not the cell-bound antibodies responsible for mediator release. Positive RAST results must be correlated with the history and confirmed by double-blind food challenges [2, 5]. The RAST is useful in patients with severe eczema and widespread dermatographism in whom skin tests are not feasible. A disadvantage to the RAST is that results are not immediately available. On balance, the RAST is more expensive, slower, and not as sensitive as skin testing (see Chap. 38).

Skin testing is performed with water-soluble food extracts. Skin tests are either epicutaneous (puncture or scratch) or intradermal. For food sensitivity testing, epicutaneous testing at concentrations of 1:10 or 1:20 weight/volume is preferred. Intradermal tests require a more dilute concentration, will have numerous false-positive results, and carry the risk of systemic reactions including anaphylaxis. Considerable controversy has been generated regarding the role of skin testing in food sensitivity [7, 42]. Much of the confusion has resulted from improper antigen preparation, standardization, and storage. The results of the skin testing are only as good as the quality of the antigen used; unfortunately, there is a wide range in specificity in commercially available antigens. Antigen solutions must be refrigerated and prepared every 2 to 3 weeks. Bock demonstrated that food extract

skin testing does not cause nonspecific irritation and does detect specific antibodies [3].

When skin testing is performed, a physician and appropriate medication and equipment must be immediately available in case of a systemic reaction. Ideally, tests are applied to the arm so that a tourniquet can be applied in the event of systemic reaction. In infants and small children, the back can be used. Controls are applied simultaneously and include testing with the diluent to determine nonspecific reactivity. A histamine control is used to assess reactivity. Results are determined 10 to 15 minutes later by measuring the wheal size. A positive reaction is a wheal 3 mm or larger after any reaction caused by the diluent is subtracted.

Interpretation is the most important aspect of the skin test. The crucial distinction is that the presence of sensitization (as detected by specific antibody responses) does not predict the presence of current clinical symptoms caused by that food. The positive skin test result indicates the presence of antigen-specific IgE on the mast cell surface but does not indicate current symptomatic food sensitivity. A food should not be removed from the diet because of a positive skin test result. All positive skin test results should be confirmed by double-blind food challenge.

Assay of circulating hemagglutinating and precipitating antibodies has not been useful. These antibodies, for example, milk precipitins, are commonly found in asymptomatic individuals. Their presence does not indicate clinical sensitivity, and they may be absent in patients with documented food sensitivity [23].

Several other areas of immunology have been investigated in food sensitivity. These include serum complement levels, circulating immune complexes, and cell-mediated immunity. However, these techniques are cumbersome, require extensive laboratory facilities, and have not been rigorously investigated. They should be considered research tools at the present time.

FOOD CHALLENGE

Suspected food sensitivity reactions must be confirmed by objective food challenges [1, 2, 6]. This is the only way that a precise diagnosis can be established and rational therapy begun. Goldman's criteria were initially proposed for the documentation of cow's milk allergy [15]. They have subsequently been modified for other foods. The criteria require (1) that symptoms subside after elimination of the suspected food; (2) that symptoms occur within 48 hours of reintroducing the food; (3) that there be three positive responses to challenge that are similar in onset, duration, and clinical features; and (4) that symptoms subside after removal of the food. With these strict criteria, milk allergy could be confirmed in only 20 percent of patients previously diagnosed as having milk allergy. While these criteria can be helpful, they are cumbersome and impractical for everyday clinical practice. False-positive and -negative challenges occur; the accuracy of the challenges can be influenced by the fact that they are open and hence subject to potential biases of both observers and patients. Other nonimmunologic causes of adverse reactions may occur under similar circumstances, for example, diarrhea due to lactose intolerance. After an initial hypersensitivity reaction, the patient's immunologic status may be altered. For example, antibody production may be reduced, which would reduce reactivity in subsequent challenges. Hence, challenges should be conducted at 2-week intervals.

For the above-mentioned reasons, food sensitivity suspected from the clinical history and skin test results should be confirmed by double-blind challenge as described by Bock [5]. Before the challenge, the patient follows an elimination diet for 2 weeks (Table 43-3). The patient should not have any intercurrent illnesses and be as symptom free as possible. Antihistamine or antiinflammatory medications should not be administered during the challenge since they may blunt the response. *Patients with a*

Table 43-3. Suggested elimination diet

Foods allowed at mealtime
  Cereal: rice, puffed rice, rice flakes, Rice Krispies
  Fruit and juices: apricots, cranberries, peaches, pears
  Meat: lamb, chicken
  Vegetables: asparagus, beets, carrots, lettuce, sweet potatoes
  Miscellaneous: tapioca, white vinegar, olive oil, honey, cane sugar, salt,
    margarine (without milk)
  Beverages: water, juices (see above), dye-free beverages
Foods to avoid
  Any food suspected of causing reactions
  Any food not on this list
  Pepper and spices
  Coffee and tea
  Chewing gum
Check with pharmacists regarding food colorings and dyes in any medica-
  tions, both prescribed and over-the-counter.

history of an anaphylactic reaction should not be challenged. Most challenges can be performed on an outpatient basis. Hospitalization is occasionally required when the history suggests a period of 1 or more days between ingestion of the suspected food and the onset of symptoms.

The challenge is performed by placing increasing amounts of the suspected food in gelatin capsules and administering them prior to a meal. It is important that neither the patient nor the observer know the content of the capsules. Any of the commonly incriminated foods such as milk, egg, and wheat can be obtained in dry form. Peanuts and other nuts can be crushed. Wet foods should be freeze-dried and powdered. The amount of food initially administered ranges from 20 to 200 mg in dry weight, depending on the age of the patient and the severity of the reported reaction. Children over the age of 6 years will usually swallow the capsules; in younger children the blind challenge is performed by having another observer place the suspected food in a tolerated food such as applesauce.

The patient is observed after the challenge; symptoms usually occur within 2 minutes to 2 hours. Pulmonary function studies may be helpful in defining bronchospasm. If no reaction occurs in 24 hours, the dose is doubled. The process is repeated until 8 gm of the food is ingested. The food is then openly introduced into the diet.

Placebo challenges are usually not necessary if the challenge is carried out in a double-blind manner, especially if more than one food is being evaluated. If only a single food is in question or there are any doubts about the reported reactions, a placebo challenge may be helpful. Vague and subjective complaints such as fatigue may be clarified by the use of identical capsules containing glucose. Great care must be taken to obscure the order of presentation.

In suspected tartrazine sensitivity, a challenge test may be useful. Tartrazine is administered orally in increasing doses (1, 5, 15, 20, 50 mg). Forced expiratory volume in 1 second (FEV_1) is measured at 0, 0.5, 1, 2, 3, and 4 hours after the challenge dose. A 20 percent decrease in FEV_1 in 4 hours is a positive reaction.

A single unequivocally positive reaction is definitive. Failure to react to 8 gm usually means that the food will be tolerated without immediate-type symptoms when usual portions are included in the diet.

Bock has used double-blind food challenges extensively to evaluate suspected food sensitivities [3, 5, 6]. In children 3 years or older, food sensitivity was confirmed in only 22 percent. Reactions occurred within 2 hours. This is remarkable, since this was a highly selected population referred to a national allergy center. The most common reactions were to peanuts, other nuts, eggs, and milk. In these children, the skin puncture test response had been positive for all foods tested. Gastrointestinal symptoms

were the most common, followed by skin reactions. Respiratory reactions were least common. Significantly, when the food sensitivity was not confirmed by the double-blind challenge, it was subsequently tolerated in the diet, despite the history of previous reactions [2]. These data support the necessity of confirming the suspected food sensitivity before eliminating it from the diet.

In infants under 3 years old, the results of 32 percent of food challenges were positive. The most common reactions were to milk, soy, and peanuts. The majority of infants experienced symptoms within 2 hours, and skin test results were positive in 85 percent. A small percentage of children had the onset of symptoms more than 4 hours after the challenge; the reactions involved the gastrointestinal tract and the skin [3]. Bernstein and coworkers applied the double-blind challenge to 22 adults [2]. Forty-six challenges were performed; 13 (28%) were positive. Respiratory symptoms such as rhinitis, asthma, and angioedema occurred within 1 hour of the challenge.

In summary, the double-blind challenge is very helpful in confirming food sensitivity and correlating it with a particular symptom. Many patients who claim to have a reaction to specific food will not have this confirmed on double-blind challenge. Figure 43-1 outlines an approach to the patient with suspected food sensitivity.

THERAPY

Therapy for documented food sensitivity is simple and yet potentially treacherous. The treatment of choice is the elimination of the offending food (see Table 43-3). Potentially cross-reacting foods should also be eliminated since potentially allergenic proteins may be hidden in seemingly innocuous foods. For example, Gern and associates [14] recently reported on six patients with a history of milk allergy who developed allergic symptoms including wheezing after eating frozen desserts labeled "dairy free." Analysis showed the presence of milk proteins [14]. Hence, patients must be instructed to carefully read food product labels. Although complete elimination of the offending food is the goal, reduced intake frequently provides symptomatic relief.

Since patients, especially infants and children, may lose their symptomatic reactions with time, the offending foodstuff can be gradually reintroduced into the diet [13]. However, patients with proven anaphylaxis, especially older children and adults, should not be rechallenged. A typical rechallenge in an infant with milk allergy would be to give 0.5 to 5.0 ml of milk and to observe the child carefully. If no reaction occurs, the volume is doubled hourly until 4 to 6 oz is being taken. This rechallenge is best done at approximately 2 years of age in a setting where close medical supervision is possible [11].

The challenge is to eliminate the offending food and at the same time, provide a nutritionally sound diet. This is vital in young children and infants who require an adequate diet for normal growth. The advice of a professional nutritionist is invaluable. Assistance is even more necessary if multiple foods must be eliminated. Iatrogenic malnutrition must be avoided. I have seen children whose nutrition and growth have been severely compromised by a "no milk, no eggs, no meat, no beef, *no calorie* diet." Lloyd-Still documented a failure to thrive secondary to the improper use of elimination diets in 15 percent of children referred for chronic nonspecific diarrhea, a benign self-limited disorder [22]. Similar problems have been reported following the institution of elimination diets for the treatment of eczema in children [12].

The food-sensitive patient with malabsorption and poor nutritional status should receive prompt nutritional repletion either prior to or concurrent with further diagnostic evaluation. Infants with severe enteritis are also in this category.

Pharmacologic therapy for food sensitivity is still under intense investigation. Antihistamines are not effective. Corticosteroids are indicated only for severe intractable disease and should be used as a last resort because of their well-known toxicity. Oral cromolyn sodium, 40 to 100 mg three times a day, taken 1 hour before meals may be helpful [20]. Immunotherapy and oral hyposensitization are of unproven effectiveness in the treatment of food sensitivity.

The interested reader is referred to a workshop detailing experimental methods for clinical studies of adverse reactions to foods and food additives [41].

REFERENCES

1. Atkins, F. M., and Metcalfe, D. D. The diagnosis and treatment of food allergy. *Annu. Rev. Nutr.* 4:233, 1984.
2. Bernstein, M., Day, J. H., and Welsh, A. Double-blind food challenge in the diagnosis of food sensitivity in the adult. *J. Allergy Clin. Immunol.* 70:205, 1982.
3. Bock, S. A. Food sensitivity: A critical review and practical approach. *Am. J. Dis. Child.* 134:973, 1980.
4. Bock, S. A. Natural history of severe reactions to foods in young children. *J. Pediatr.* 107:676, 1985.
5. Bock, S. A. A critical evaluation of clinical trials in adverse reactions to foods in children. *J. Allergy Clin. Immunol.* 78:165, 1986.
6. Bock, S. A. Prospective appraisal of complaints of adverse reactions to food in children during the first 3 years of life. *Pediatrics* 79:683, 1987.
7. Bock, S. A., et al. Appraisal of skin tests with food extracts for the diagnosis of food hypersensitivity. *Clin. Allergy* 8:559, 1978.
8. Buist, A. S., et al. Pulmonary function in young children with alpha$_1$-antitrypsin deficiency. *Am. Rev. Respir. Dis.* 122:817, 1980.
9. Dohi, M., et al. Food dependent exercise induced anaphylaxis: A study on 11 Japanese cases. *J. Clin. Allergy Immunol.* 87:34, 1991.
10. Eastham, E. J., and Walker, W. A. Adverse effects of milk formula ingestion on the gastrointestinal tract: An update. *Gastroenterology* 76:365, 1979.
11. David, T. J. Anaphylactic shock during elimination diets for severe atopic eczema. *Arch. Dis. Child.* 59:983, 1984.
12. David, T. J., et al. Nutritional hazards of elimination diets in children with atopic eczema. *Arch. Dis. Child.* 59:323, 1984.
13. Foucard, T. Developmental aspects of food sensitivity in childhood. *Nutr. Rev.* 42:96, 1984.
14. Gern, J. E., et al. Allergic reactions to milk contaminated "non-dairy" products. *N. Engl. J. Med.* 324:976, 1991.
15. Goldman, A. S., et al. Oral challenge with milk and isolated milk proteins in allergic children. *Pediatrics* 32:425, 1963.
16. Hill, D. J., et al. The spectrum of cow's milk allergy in childhood. *Acta Paediatr. Scand.* 68:847, 1979.
17. Jakobsson, I., and Lindberg, T. A prospective study of cow's milk protein intolerance in Swedish infants. *Acta Paediatr. Scand.* 68:853, 1979.
18. Jarrett, E. E. Activation of IgE regulatory mechanisms by transmucosal absorption of antigen. *Lancet* 2:223, 1977.
19. Katz, R. M., et al. Alpha$_1$-antitrypsin levels and prevalence of Pi variant phenotypes in asthmatic children. *J. Allergy Clin. Immunol.* 57:41, 1976.
20. Kocoshis, S., and Grybowski, J. D. Use of cromolyn in combined gastrointestinal allergy. *JAMA* 242:1169, 1979.
21. Lake, A. M., et al. Dietary protein induced colitis in breastfed infants. *J. Pediatr.* 101:906, 1982.
22. Lloyd-Still, J. D. Chronic diarrhea of childhood and the misuses of elimination diets. *J. Pediatr.* 95:10, 1979.
23. May, C. D., et al. A study of serum antibodies to isolated milk proteins and ovalbumin in infants and children. *Clin. Allergy* 7:583, 1977.
24. McCarty, E. P., and Frick, O. L. Food sensitivity: Keys to diagnosis. *J. Pediatr.* 102:645, 1983.
25. Metcalfe, D. D. Food hypersensitivity. *J. Allergy Clin. Immunol.* 73:749, 1984.
26. Mowat, A. M. The regulation of immune responses to dietary protein antigens. *Immunol. Today* 8:93, 1987.
27. Owens, R. L., and Jones, A. L. Epithelial cell specialization within human Peyer's patches. An ultrastructural study of intestinal lymphoid follicles. *Gastroenterology* 66:189, 1974.
28. Powell, G. K. Milk and soy-induced enterocolitis of infancy: Clinical features and standardization of challenge. *J. Pediatr.* 93:553, 1978.
29. Proujansky, R., et al. Gastrointestinal syndromes associated with food sensitivity. *Adv. Pediatr.* 35:219, 1988.
30. Richman, L. K., et al. Enterically induced immunologic tolerance: 1. Induction of suppressor T lymphocytes by intragastric administration of soluble proteins. *J. Immunol.* 121:2429, 1978.
31. Settipane, G. A. Adverse reactions to aspirin and related drugs. *Arch. Intern. Med.* 141:328, 1981.
32. Shiner, M., et al. The small intestinal mucosa in cow's milk allergy. *Lancet* 1:136, 1975.
33. Stern, M. Gastrointestinal Allergy. In W. A. Walker, et al. (eds.), *Pediatric Gastrointestinal Disease*. Philadelphia: B. C. Decker, 1991. Pp. 557–573.
34. Sveger, T. Alpha$_1$-antitrypsin deficiency in early childhood. *Pediatrics* 62: 22, 1978.
35. Teichberg, S., et al. Development of the neonatal rat small intestinal barrier to nonspecific macromolecular absorption: Effect of early weaning to artificial diets. *Pediatr. Res.* 28:31, 1990.
36. Tomasi, T. B., et al. Mucosal immunity: The origin and migration patterns of cells in the secretory system. *J. Allergy Clin. Immunol.* 65:22, 1980.
37. Udall, J., et al. Development of gastrointestinal barrier: 1. The effect of age on intestinal permeability. *Pediatr. Res.* 15:241, 1981.
38. Vance, J. C., et al. Heterozygous alpha$_1$-antitrypsin deficiency and respiratory function in children. *Pediatrics* 69:262, 1977.
39. Walker, W. A., et al. Macromolecular absorption: Mechanism of horseradish peroxidase uptake and transport in adult and neonatal rat intestine. *J. Cell Biol.* 54:195, 1972.
40. Walker, W. A., and Isselbacher, K. J. Uptake of macromolecules by the intestine: Possible role in clinical disorders. *Gastroenterology* 67:531, 1974.
41. Metcalfe, D. D., and Sampson, H. A., (eds.). Workshop on experimental methodology for clinical studies of adverse reactions to foods and food additives. *J. Allergy Clin. Immunol.* 86:421, 1990.
42. Bernhisel-Broadbent, J., Strause, D., and Sampson, H. A. Fish hypersensitivity II: Clinical relevance of altered fish allergenicity caused by various preparation methods. *J. Allergy Clin. Immunol.* 90:622, 1992.

Bacteria and Viruses in Etiology and Treatment

44

William J. Hall
Caroline Breese Hall

Ever since the great pandemic of Asian influenza infection in the late 1950s, one of the most frequently reported complications of this acute respiratory tract infection has been severe exacerbations of bronchial asthma [112]. These early clinical observations led to studies from a wide variety of scientific disciplines, which have subsequently established the key role of inflammation in the pathogenesis of asthma [34, 121]. As part of this larger body of work, studies of acute infection in asthma have confirmed a causal relationship between respiratory tract infection, especially viral infection, and exacerbations of bronchial asthma, and moreover may be providing some important clues to a more global understanding of the pathogenesis of asthma. Recent refinements in epidemiologic methods, viral isolation techniques, investigative fiberoptic bronchoscopy, and pulmonary function testing have provided the tools to characterize this relationship more precisely. In this chapter we review the evidence suggesting that viral respiratory tract infection is a major precipitating factor in acute exacerbations of asthma, and that these same infections may play a role in the actual pathogenesis of at least some chronic asthma states. Some recent data describing both the pathophysiology and immunology of infection-induced bronchospasm are reviewed. Finally, some practical diagnostic and therapeutic considerations in dealing with respiratory tract infectious syndromes in the asthmatic patient are emphasized.

INFECTION IN INFANCY AND THE PATHOGENESIS OF ASTHMA

For many years there has been considerable study of the potential importance of respiratory tract infection early in life to the subsequent development of chronic lung disease. In infancy and early childhood, respiratory viruses are the most common etiologic agents, and these infections are nearly ubiquitous [44]. Certain specific pathogens seem to have a much greater association with long-term effects than do others. For example, respiratory syncytial virus and parainfluenza virus are the most frequently documented pathogens. Bacterial infection is relatively uncommon. During the first 2 years of life, during the peak incidence of viral respiratory infections, the clinical syndrome of bronchiolitis due to respiratory syncytial virus infection is clearly the most serious and most important lower respiratory tract infection [60]. It is known that even when these viral illnesses seem clinically to be limited to the upper airway, sophisticated pulmonary function studies demonstrate significant lower airway obstruction [85]. These are "wheezy" illnesses, involving peripheral airways at critical growth and maturation periods, and are therefore prime suspects for a possible relationship to the subsequent development of obstructive airway syndromes, particularly reversible airway obstruction, hence the relevance to this chapter [18].

These potential relationships have been explored in a variety

of ways. Morbidity and mortality statistics have been examined, particularly in the United Kingdom [5, 30, 73, 109]. These investigators hypothesized that the extremely high mortality from chronic bronchitis seen in some parts of England and Wales might have definable antecedents in various common risk factors, especially the occurrence of respiratory tract illness in infancy and early childhood. The mortality from respiratory disease in cohorts of infants born from 1921 to 1925 was correlated with mortality rates from adult chronic bronchitis and emphysema in the same population during the years 1959 to 1978. A strong correlation between adult mortality and infant mortality rates from respiratory tract disease was found. In fact, infection in early childhood had a greater influence than cigarette smoking in determining the geographic distribution of obstructive airway disease.

Another approach has been to evaluate childhood respiratory tract infection as a determinant of subsequent airflow obstruction in adults. While such studies have generally described a strong association, they are complicated by the concurrence of other risk factors including family history of allergy, familial and personal smoking histories, and air pollution. It is of interest, therefore, that in addition to studies from the more industrialized areas of the world, similar associations have been observed in such diverse places as New Guinea and Micronesia [14, 86] where contemporary environmental risk factors, especially air pollutants, are not as common as in the western world.

In one of the largest such studies, Burrows and colleagues [19] evaluated the relationship of a history of childhood respiratory illness to obstructive airway disease and ventilatory impairment in 2,626 adults who were part of a population sample of adults in Tucson, Arizona. This study indicated close relationships between histories of childhood respiratory disorders and prevalences of symptoms of obstructive airway diseases, as well as ventilatory impairment. Furthermore, these subjects seemed to show that over time there was more rapid decline in lung function compared to those without childhood history, suggesting that childhood respiratory illnesses may cause the adult lung to be unusually susceptible to the adverse effects of a variety of bronchial irritants and infectious agents. Follow-up studies published a decade later [18] suggested that adults with subsequent chronic asthmatic bronchitis report a history of childhood respiratory problems more frequently than do normal adults or those with chronic obstructive lung disease related to smoking. However, studies such as these may be subject to the flaws of recall bias and cannot in and of themselves provide a direct link between childhood infection and asthma.

Other investigators, mostly from England and Wales [29, 71], have done either longitudinal or cross-sectional studies of children to relate observed ventilatory impairment to a history of childhood respiratory tract infection. Antecedent lower respiratory tract infection emerges as a major risk factor for obstructive ventilatory impairment in children.

564

In an effort to reduce the possible recall bias to which the above studies are prone because of their dependence on parental recollection, several ongoing cohort studies in the United States have used more precise means of documentation of the occurrence, frequency, and severity of antecedent childhood illness. McConnochie and coworkers [88–91] developed strict physician-based criteria for a diagnosis of bronchiolitis in a community pediatric practice in Rochester, New York. The cohort was then followed for as long as 9 years. These studies are of particular interest because these children had milder illnesses, not requiring hospitalization, and were thereby much more representative of the vast majority of infections seen in early childhood. The investigators found a highly significant increase in current wheezing in children from the bronchiolitis group, even in this cohort with relatively mild disease.

Gold and associates [47] investigated the relationship of acute lower respiratory tract illness to the absolute level and change in level of forced expiratory volumes in a cohort of 801 children followed longitudinally for a maximum of 13 years. The concurrence of a respiratory illness before the age of 2 years and two lower respiratory tract illnesses or more during a single surveillance year was associated with a 20.3 percent lower mean cross-sectional level of expiratory flow volumes and with reduced longitudinal growth in these volumes, principally in boys.

The association between lower respiratory tract infection in early childhood and impaired lung function and growth was further explored recently by Martinez and colleagues [84]. They prospectively studied 124 infants enrolled as newborns to assess the relationship between initial lung function and the subsequent incidence of lower respiratory tract illness during the first year of life. The risk of having a wheezing illness was 3.7 times higher among infants whose lung function was in the lowest third compared with infants in the upper third. The investigators concluded that a smaller initial lung size may predispose infants to wheezing in association with common viral infections, and might explain why children might have persisting abnormalities of lung function years later.

Another approach to the relationship of respiratory tract infection in early childhood and the subsequent development of asthma is represented by studies that combined precise virus isolation techniques and more sensitive methods of pulmonary function testing [51, 69, 70, 106, 117]. Respiratory syncytial virus was specifically identified as the pathogen in the development of bronchiolitis, the children were followed for a decade, and tests that assess bronchial reactivity were used [51, 69, 119]. These studies documented a high prevalence of bronchial lability, even a decade after acute infection occurred, without a strong correlation with manifestations of atopy as defined by prick test reactions to common antigens, eosinophil counts, IgE determinations, and clinical history.

Another common viral syndrome of early life, viral laryngotracheobronchitis (croup), has been studied. Several investigators independently demonstrated an increased prevalence of bronchial lability independent of allergy some 10 years after the acute viral illness occurred [80, 85, 139, 140].

In contrast to viral respiratory infection, bacterial pathogens do not appear to have a major role in the pathogenesis of asthma. In a previous era when whooping cough was common, *Bordetella pertussis* infection was considered a frequent harbinger of recurrent bronchospasm. However, common infections such as those caused by *Streptococcus pneumoniae* and *Hemophilus influenzae* have not been associated with recurrent bronchospasm.

Therefore, from the data available, several cautious generalizations seem warranted. First, viral, as opposed to bacterial, respiratory pathogens commonly herald the onset of wheezing in both atopic and nonatopic children. Infants who have documented lower respiratory tract viral infections have a much higher tendency to have wheezing later in life. This is true not only for those children inflicted with a more serious episode of bronchiolitis requiring hospitalization, but also for those with the more common lower respiratory tract illness managed in pediatric offices. Alternatively, more recent evidence suggests that infants with somewhat diminished lung function at birth may be predisposed to such infections and to wheezing. Definitive clarification will require long-term observations [115], and such studies are currently in progress [47]. Later in this chapter we outline several mechanisms that have been hypothesized to explain these relationships.

INFECTION AND ACUTE EXACERBATIONS OF ASTHMA

While the ultimate importance of respiratory infection in infancy on the subsequent development of asthma awaits more definitive epidemiologic studies, there seems little doubt that respiratory viruses commonly induce acute exacerbations of bronchospasm in patients with known asthma [147] (Table 44-1). This is in contradistinction to the observation that bacterial respiratory infections are not associated with this predilection.

In earlier prospective studies, McIntosh and associates [92, 93] reported the relationship between exacerbations of wheezing and infection in hospitalized asthmatic children. Of 139 episodes of wheezing, 58 (42%) were associated with identifiable viral respiratory infections. Respiratory syncytial virus was the most common pathogen, followed by parainfluenza virus and coronavirus. Infection with pathogenic bacteria was not statistically associated with exacerbations of wheezing.

Table 44-1. Factors responsible for altered airway reactivity after viral respiratory infection

Mechanism	References
Anatomic narrowing of airway lumen	
Inflammatory debris	13, 24
Enhanced parasympathetic neural activity	
Sensitization of airway irritant receptors	94, 98
Histamine, parasympathomimetic hyperresponse	13, 37, 54–56, 77, 78
Enhanced response to cold air, pollutants	4, 128
Neuraminidase enhancement of acetylcholine release	41
Diminished beta-adrenergic airway tone	
Inhibition of lysosomal enzyme release	17, 20–22
Attenuation of receptor activation of adenyl cyclase	28, 66, 116–117, 124
Noncholinergic, nonadrenergic system enhancement	66
Enhanced contractile response to substance P	7, 16, 66, 75, 107, 113, 116
Degradation of neutral endopeptidase activity	8, 9, 12, 36, 67, 82
Increased vascular permeability	8, 12
IgE mediator release	
Prolonged virus-specific IgE production	137, 138
Enhanced IgE-mediated histamine release	134, 135
Interferon-modulated histamine and kinin release	8, 27, 63, 76, 129
Altered T-cell regulation of IgE production	38, 132
Enhanced late-phase hyperreactivity	74

Minor and coworkers [97] prospectively studied a group of asthmatic children in an ambulatory setting during a typical fall through spring season in Wisconsin, and established several important points. Of the 61 documented episodes of acute asthma, 42 were coincident with an apparent symptomatic respiratory infection, and in 23 a specific viral cause was established by culture and serologic study. Of interest, asthma occurred with 38 of 49 clinically severe infections, while only 4 of 22 mild infections were similarly associated. No asthmatic episodes occurred during episodes of asymptomatic viral infection. Bacterial infections were not similarly associated with exacerbations. In these series, therefore, viral respiratory infections were responsible for approximately 40 percent of exacerbations of asthma in children. Moreover, the more severe (in terms of systemic manifestations) the viral infection was, the more likely that an exacerbation of asthma occurred. In terms of exact etiologic agents, in children under 2 years old, respiratory syncytial virus was the most common pathogen, followed by parainfluenza virus and influenza virus infection. In studies looking at somewhat older children, rhinovirus was the most important pathogen, followed by influenza A virus, mycoplasma, and possibly chlamydia [96, 112].

Prospective studies that concentrated on acute exacerbations of asthma in the adult population showed a smaller but still significant role for respiratory viral infection in asthma. Most of these studies are somewhat difficult to interpret because many investigators included patients with chronic bronchitis and emphysema in the study populations. However, several studies concentrating on adult asthma suggested that approximately 10 to 20 percent of acute exacerbations of asthma may be attributable to acute viral infection, especially with influenza A virus, rhinovirus, and parainfluenza virus [61, 62, 96]. Beasley and coauthors [9] reported on a controlled study of the relationship of viral respiratory tract infection and exacerbations of asthma in adult atopic patients, using more sensitive techniques for viral identification than available for earlier cited studies. They reported detailed clinical, functional, and virologic findings in 31 patients with atopic asthma aged 15 to 56 years who were followed prospectively for 11 months. Of the 30 viral identifications observed, 18 (60%) were associated with an exacerbation of asthma. Viral infection was documented in 18 (10%) of 178 exacerbations of asthma, and in 10 (36%) of the 28 severe exacerbations. The frequency of viral identification in the control subjects was no different than that observed in the asthmatic subjects. Fourteen (46%) of the 30 viral isolates were identified as respiratory syncytial virus. This pathogen was responsible for 44 percent of all asthmatic exacerbations and 33 percent of severe exacerbations.

Perhaps the most convincing study showing the lack of association between bacterial respiratory infection and asthma was done by Berman and coworkers [11]. They obtained transtracheal aspirates from 27 adult asthmatic patients with acute exacerbations as well as from a control group. There was no correlation between bacterial isolates and clinical illnesses, suggesting that overt bacterial infection of the lower respiratory tract did not contribute to the exacerbation of asthma.

The relative importance of respiratory infections in adult asthma would no doubt be considerably clarified if experimentally induced infection in human subjects could be studied. However, the ability to reproduce with experimental infection the pulmonary function changes seen in naturally acquired infection has been variable. Halpern and colleagues [57] exposed young adult volunteers to an experimental rhinovirus infection, and in those subjects developing clinical illness, documented lower respiratory involvement by obtaining rhinovirus isolates from cells harvested in the lower respiratory tract by fiberoptic bronchoscopy. However, in a later study, these investigators [58] were able to correlate airway hyperreactivity and clinical wheezing in only a minority of similar rhinovirus-infected asthmatic volunteers. These authors concluded that this very common respiratory virus was not an important factor in contributing to exacerbations of asthma. Other investigators [74], as discussed later in this chapter, documented substantial enhancement of bronchial hyperreactivity with experimental rhinovirus infection in atopic individuals. It was previously observed that experimentally induced respiratory viral infections, even influenza virus infection, do not usually cause either clinical illness or airway hyperreactivity of the same order of magnitude easily documented in the naturally acquired infection [79]. This may be related to the less virulent strains generally used for inducing experimental infection, the route of administration, or many unknown factors. In fact, the observation of attenuated illness with experimental infection is a cardinal principle behind vaccine development.

These studies also documented that when an asthmatic adult has a symptomatic viral illness, there is a 50 to 75 percent chance that the most predominant manifestation will be prolonged wheezing. Lambert and Stern [72] pointed out the importance of family clustering to this relationship. They described a threefold increase in the number of viral-induced, acute asthmatic attacks in asthmatic adults who lived in a family cluster including children compared with asthmatic adults who did not live with children. It is likely, therefore, that the most common cause of acute exacerbations of asthma in the asthmatic adult who has young children in his or her family may well be viral respiratory infection. This distinction becomes important in considering the role of preventative measures, outlined later in this chapter.

There does not seem to be any evidence to suggest that the asthmatic child or adult is uniquely susceptible to any specific respiratory pathogens. Rather, the viral agent responsible for the exacerbation of wheezing is primarily a function of the age of the patient. One controlled study suggested that there is an increased frequency of viral respiratory infections in asthmatic children compared with their nonasthmatic siblings [97]. In general, however, it is more likely that the asthmatic responds to viral infection with more obvious clinical manifestations of cough and dyspnea than does the nonasthmatic, and is therefore more likely to seek medical attention [125]. The possible exceptions to this generalization would be the individual with asthma who has a specific immunoglobulin deficiency, the asthmatic patient who becomes susceptible to allergic bronchopulmonary aspergillosis (see Chap. 49), and the patient with persistent bacterial sinusitis (see Chap. 41) [40, 108, 118].

Little is known of the relative importance of viral respiratory pathogens in the bronchospastic exacerbations observed in the geriatric population, despite the impressive data on the clinical importance of influenza virus and respiratory syncytial virus as causes of severe pneumonia in this age group [6, 32, 87]. However, it is known from recent studies that for individuals 65 years old or older, both asthmatic hospitalizations and mortality demonstrate increases during December through February, corresponding to the usual seasonal peak incidence of influenza virus and respiratory syncytial virus infections in this age group [131]. Newer techniques of viral identification will likely further define the role of viral respiratory infection in this age group [146, 147].

PATHOPHYSIOLOGY OF BRONCHOSPASM INDUCED BY VIRAL INFECTION

For many years it has been recognized that viral respiratory illnesses are often associated with seemingly inappropriately prolonged respiratory symptoms. These observations prompted a number of studies involving serial pulmonary function tests during and after viral respiratory infection [25, 31, 55, 68, 102]. Of particular interest in defining the relationship of these infections to airway reactivity have been paradoxically those studies that have by design excluded known asthmatic patients. These populations could have possibly allowed clearer relationships between viral infections and bronchospasm to be shown by eliminating the important but confusing coexistence of atopy. A wide variety of probably interrelated pathophysiologic mechanisms have been identified (see Table 44-1). Initial reports indicated prolonged abnormalities of lung function exclusively of an obstructive nature, presumably related to viral replication and inflammation. However, several observations subsequently suggested that these are inadequate explanations. First, pulmonary function abnormalities in adults with viral respiratory illness are generally more pronounced 7 to 10 days after the onset of symptoms—a time when the clinical "inflammatory" manifestations are waning [55]. Second, the abnormalities of pulmonary function may last for weeks or even months beyond the period of viral shedding.

An imbalance of the autonomic nervous system has been hypothesized not only as a mechanism of action of asthma itself, but also as a mechanism of further enhanced bronchospasm associated with viral infection, chiefly by diminished beta-adrenergic response of bronchial smooth muscle. This hypothesis began with the early work of Szentivanyi [124], which was based on experimental *B. pertussis* infection in animals. More recently, Busse and associates [17, 20–22] studied the effect of viral infection on the beta-adrenergic response. Their in vitro system evaluates enzyme release from incubated polymorphonuclear leukocytes. Isoproterenol normally inhibits lysosomal enzyme release in this cell system. This inhibition is mediated through the adenosine 3′,5′-cyclic phosphate pathway. The system may then serve as a barometer of beta-adrenergic sensitivity. Isoproterenol inhibition of lysosomal enzyme release has been found to be diminished in asthmatic patients, compared with normal subjects, and during viral infection the response is even further diminished. Busse [141] suggested that a similar change in the beta-adrenergic tone of the airways could partially explain the exaggerated bronchoconstrictor response observed during viral infection. Infection with parainfluenza virus in vivo may cause a selective blockade of the beta-adrenergic–mediated inhibition of antigen-induced contraction of airway smooth muscle. These abnormalities are not limited to those subjects with known atopy but may also be demonstrated in cell systems from normal subjects. The mechanisms of possible interaction between respiratory virus and the beta-adrenergic system are not known; however, it is of interest that cell-surface beta-adrenergic receptors can be similar to virus receptors [28]. Viral infection may also impair airway function through an attenuation of receptor and postreceptor activation of adenylate cyclase activity [116]. This area was recently reviewed [66].

The parasympathetic neurogenic hypothesis was initially proposed by Empey and colleagues [37] who studied a group of nonasthmatic subjects during and after upper respiratory tract infections. They demonstrated that these persons uniformly showed enhanced and rather dramatic airway hyperreactivity to histamine aerosol challenge after viral respiratory tract infections. These subjects were also noted to have a decreased cough threshold after challenge with aerosolized citric acid, a provocative test of airway irritability and cough threshold. The investigators postulated on the basis of these observations that respiratory viral infection caused initial epithelial damage to the tracheobronchial mucosa. This epithelial damage in turn resulted in the sensitization of rapidly adapting airway receptors, which had previously been described in studies on the neurophysiology of the mammalian lung [94]. These subepithelial receptors are primarily distributed in larger airways. Extensive work in animal models suggested that most of the stimuli known to cause bronchospasm and cough in asthmatic subjects do stimulate these receptors, resulting in a vagally mediated airway response (cough and bronchoconstriction) [98]. This hypothesis gains further credence when one recognizes that the characteris-

tic histologic marker of viral respiratory infection is epithelial destruction. Serial bronchial biopsies in patients with proven influenza A virus infection have demonstrated that cellular repair takes, on the average, about 5 weeks, which corresponds very closely to the mean duration of hyperreactivity noted in studies of viral respiratory tract infection [130].

Similarly, Carson and coworkers [24] found dysmorphic cilia on nasal brush-biopsied specimens from children with acute viral respiratory infections. Normal epithelial organization and ciliary ultrastructure appeared to be reestablished during the convalescent period, from 2 to 10 weeks after infection. In some cases these inflammatory changes may persist for even longer periods of time. Heino and associates [59] performed biopsies from the main carina in schoolchildren with chronic cough for 3 months who had a history of early lower respiratory tract infection. These children were found to have a marked increase in inflammatory cells, suggesting a close association of early lower respiratory tract infection and epithelial inflammation during chronic cough.

Other investigators studying the altered pulmonary mechanics in young adults after a variety of respiratory viral infections extended these observations in humans, and supported a vagally mediated neurogenic mechanism [13, 54]. When nonspecific bronchial hyperreactivity is evaluated, individuals with respiratory viral illnesses but no prior predilection to atopy or asthma demonstrate a transient increase in airway reactivity to aerosol challenge with cholinergic agents or histamine. In general, the duration of this reactivity is appoximately 3 to 4 weeks [77] (Fig. 44-1). Those studies, which were designed to include patients with an atopic history, did not demonstrate differences in the magnitude or duration of hyperreactivity in these patients, compared with nonatopic individuals [77, 78]. In two studies the antiviral agent amantadine hydrochloride was administered to patients with documented influenza A infection [77, 78]. This treatment brought about a more rapid resolution of clinical symptoms and improvement in results on pulmonary function tests designed to detect obstruction in smaller airways as might be associated with acute inflammation. However, amantadine hydrochloride administration had no effect on the magnitude or duration of airway reactivity.

Although major attention has focused on influenza virus infec-

Fig. 44-1. *Mean time course of airway hyperreactivity to carbacholamine aerosol challenge in 100 subjects with uncomplicated influenza virus infection tested at time of presentation and 1, 3, and 7 weeks thereafter. Airway reactivity is expressed as the numerical difference between total pulmonary resistance values before and after inhalation of carbacholamine ($\Delta R_T C$).*

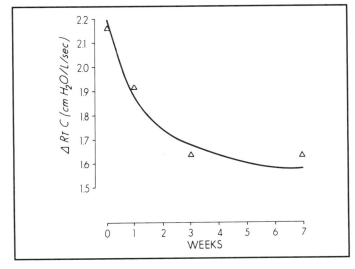

tion, it also seems likely that other viral respiratory infections of adults, as well as other nonspecific stimuli, provoked broncho-constriction in otherwise normal people during and after viral infection. In one study of pediatric house officers, widespread respiratory syncytial virus infection was associated with exaggerated airway reactivity to cholinergic challenge in a group of healthy, nonatopic individuals [56].

Other nonspecific stimuli are also associated with probable neurogenic airway hyperreactivity in the setting of viral illness. In a study of nonasthmatic subjects with probable rhinovirus infection, transient hyperreactivity to cold air inhalation and exercise was noted [4]. It is likely that airway responses to common air pollutants are exaggerated during viral respiratory illness. Utell and coworkers [128] exposed subjects to a sodium nitrate aerosol before, during, and after a naturally acquired influenza A virus infection. Although subjects showed no abnormalities in airway reactivity in response to inhalation before infection, for 3 to 4 weeks after infection the same aerosol produced exaggerated bronchoconstriction.

All of these human studies suggest that one important mechanism for virus-induced bronchoconstriction may be epithelial damage and sensitization of vagally mediated airway receptors. In the past few years these clinical findings have been confirmed by both in vivo and in vitro experiments utilizing animal models of airway reactivity. For example, it is known that the lung contains multiple muscarinic receptor subtypes. Fryer and associates [41] discovered that the enzyme neuraminidase, which is elaborated by both parainfluenza virus and influenza virus, decreases the affinity of agonists to the receptor subtype M_2, which inhibits acetylcholine release. This results in enhanced agonist activity on the M_3 muscarinic receptors, which cause muscular contraction in the presence of viral infection (see Chap. 17).

Hyperreactivity to histamine has been demonstrated in bronchiolitis in beagle puppies infected with canine parainfluenza 2 and adenovirus 2 [75, 107]. Buckner and coworkers [16] used the parainfluenza virus 3–infected guinea pig as a model for virus-provoked airway hyperreactivity. They found enhanced bronchial contractility in response to intravenously administered histamine that could be blocked by cutting the vagus nerve. However, contractile responses of isolated parenchymal strips from infected animals to the stimuli were not altered by viral infection, suggesting that no change in intrinsic muscle function could be documented with intercurrent viral infection. The exaggerated airway response to histamine could not be blocked by pretreatment with doses of atropine sufficient to cause cholinergic blockade. However, when ganglionic blockade was induced, the hyperreactivity to histamine could be blocked, which suggested that a noncholinergic neurogenic mechanism might be operative.

The observation that noncholinergic mechanisms might be playing a role in the pathogenesis of respiratory virus–induced bronchoconstriction may be especially significant. Neural pathways that do not seem to involve either the classic adrenergic or the cholinergic systems were recently demonstrated in the respiratory tract and may be especially important in asthma [7]. Stimulation of this pathway results in a cascade sometimes referred to as *neurogenic inflammation*. These responses are modulated by a novel class of polypeptide molecules, the tachykinins, one of which, substance P, has been especially well studied in asthma [144]. Substance P seems localized to the unmyelinated sensory nerves (C-fibers) in the epithelium, smooth muscle, and blood vessels of the human respiratory tract. Stimulation of the epithelial receptors can lead to an elaboration of substance P and other tachykinins, with resultant smooth muscle constriction, an increase in microvascular permeability, mast cell degradation, and enhanced chemotaxis of inflammatory cells [7].

Degradative mechanisms that modulate the effects of released tachykinins, analogous to the effect of acetylcholinesterase on acetylcholine effect, are present in the airway tissue. One enzyme, neutral endopeptidase, also known as enkephalinase, has

been characterized in airways. This enzyme is bound to the membranes of airway cells that have tachykinin receptors. The enzyme acts by cleaving substance P and other tachykinins, thereby inactivating them. Thus, the enzyme modulates the various effects of tachykinins as described above [99] (see Chap. 18).

Respiratory viral infection may have important interactions with this system. As previously described, Buckner and colleagues [16] postulated that virus-provoked airway hyperreactivity in the guinea pig infected with parainfluenza 3 might be in part regulated by the nonadrenergic noncholinergic system. In subsequent studies from the same laboratory, enhancement in airway contractile responses to substance P were documented [113]. Jacoby and associates [67] studied the effect of influenza virus using ferret tracheal strips and found a 300 percent enhancement of muscle contraction to substance P that was associated with a reduction in the enzymatic activity of neutral endopeptidase. Pretreatment with a neutral endopeptidase inhibitor abolished this enhanced muscular reactivity, further suggesting that respiratory viral infection potentiates the effect of substance P by virtue of degradation of neutral endopeptidase activity. Similar findings were seen in an in vivo guinea pig model infected with Sendai virus [36, 103]. Other manifestations of neurogenic inflammation are also affected by viral infection, including increased vascular permeability and neutrophil adhesion to the postcapillary venular endothelium [12].

Thus, neuropeptides may prove to be a particularly important pathophysiologic mechanism of virus-induced alterations in pulmonary function, and information derived from this "infection model" of asthma may have broad applications to a better understanding of the precipitating mechanisms for asthma overall. Additionally, new therapeutic measures may be forthcoming. Recombinant neutral endopeptidase (rNEP) was recently cloned, and preliminary studies do indicate that aerosolized rNEP can inhibit cough provoked by substance P in guinea pigs [82, 145].

RESPIRATORY VIRUS INFECTION AND ALTERATIONS OF IMMUNE RESPONSE

While it is recognized that not all subjects who wheeze with viral respiratory illness have evidence of atopy, the relationship between viral infection and the development of immunologic abnormalities is still quite strong. In recent years several groups of investigators combined clinical and experimental studies aimed at elucidating the possible causal links between infection and immunologic abnormalities relevant to the development of asthma. Frick and coworkers prospectively studied 13 children, all of whom had a biparental allergic history [39]. They were able to monitor a variety of external events such as infection, immunizations, introduction of new foods, and environmental factors associated temporally with the onset of allergy. Over 4 years of follow-up, immunologic evidence for allergic sensitization was found in 11 of these 13 children by means of standard tests such as radioallergosorbent tests (RASTs), IgE determination, antigen-induced leukocyte histamine release, and lymphoblastogenesis. In all of the 11 children, a viral upper respiratory tract infection occurred 1 to 2 months before the onset of allergic sensitization. The viruses identified by serologic methods were predominantly respiratory syncytial virus and parainfluenza virus. This coincidence suggested that certain viruses may contribute to allergic sensitization. Frick [38] then studied an animal model and demonstrated that dogs experimentally infected with canine parainfluenza virus vaccine had markedly enhanced IgE antibody production to subsequent pollen inhalation, compared to nonimmunized control animals. He postulated that respiratory viral infection may have caused a perturbation in the customary T-cell regulatory mechanisms for IgE production. Huftel and colleagues [143] have recently demonstrated that the enhanced basophil histamine release following influenza virus incubation is dependent on T-cells and their cytokine products.

Perhaps the most intriguing observations have been made by Welliver and colleagues [133–137] over the past decade or so. Noting that viral infections were frequently associated with clinical episodes of wheezing in infants and children, they initially studied the development of respiratory syncytial virus–specific IgE in 42 infants with the usual clinical spectrum of respiratory illness, ranging from uncomplicated upper respiratory to more severe lower respiratory tract illness (i.e., bronchiolitis and pneumonia) [137]. They found respiratory syncytial virus–specific IgE bound to nasopharyngeal epithelial cells in almost all patients, regardless of the clinical severity or anatomic localization of their infection. However, the continued presence over a subsequent 2-month follow-up period was more common in those infants with the clinical syndrome of bronchiolitis than in those with symptoms limited to upper respiratory tract infection. Moreover, persistence of IgE was also related to the incidence of prior wheezing episodes in the infants and their families. These investigators [137] postulated that IgE might cause the release of the various chemical mediators of bronchospasm, and the persistence of antibody might explain the predilection for some infants to have recurrent episodes of bronchospasm following an episode of respiratory syncytial virus bronchiolitis.

In a subsequent study [135], this hypothesis was tested. Seventy-nine infants were studied for the development of respiratory syncytial virus–specific IgE as before, only in addition the histamine content of the nasopharyngeal secretions was measured. The investigators found that peak titers of respiratory syncytial virus–specific IgE correlated significantly with concentrations of histamine and with the degree of hypoxemia experienced by these infants. Thus, there seemed to be a link between the viral infection, appearance of respiratory syncytial virus–specific IgE, chemical mediators of bronchoconstriction, and clinical severity. Similar findings were observed in croup caused by parainfluenza virus, another common "precursor" clinical illness of children. Parainfluenza virus–specific IgE was correlated with histamine levels in nasopharyngeal secretions [134].

Cohorts of these infants with bronchiolitis were subsequently followed through 48 months of life, and those children with a respiratory syncytial virus–specific IgE response during their acute illness had significantly more frequent episodes of recurrent wheezing than did infants who did not mount a respiratory syncytial virus–specific IgE response, suggesting that the IgE response at the time of bronchiolitis may be a useful prognostic indicator for the development of reactive airways [133].

To further define the mechanisms for enhanced respiratory syncytial virus–specific IgE production in infants with bronchiolitis, these same investigators studied T-cell interactions in infants with bronchiolitis. They reported a reduced number of suppressor T-cells and function in infants with bronchiolitis, which may explain the exaggerated production of IgE; that is, they speculated a "genetic" predisposition to virus-inducible IgE production [132,136].

These potential links between infection and IgE production require further confirmation and study, but do provide an intriguing potential link in this relationship. Hogg [142] has recently postulated the possibility of persistent and latent virus infections as a mechanism of prolonged bronchospasm following viral respiratory infection.

Other investigators have postulated another mechanism for enhanced IgE production following viral respiratory infection. Sakamoto and associates [114] studied allergic sensitization to aerosolized ovalbumin in mice previously infected with influenza virus. The infected mice demonstrated an enhanced IgE production relative to noninfected mice. The research group was impressed with the characteristic inflammatory response in the airways of these infected mice and postulated that the associated loss of bronchial epithelium enhanced the permeability of in-

haled antigen. Of interest, it has been established in fowl that experimentally induced viral laryngotracheitis results in a disruption of airway epithelium, which causes increased permeation of horseradish peroxidase [110]. It is therefore possible that an alternative explanation to disordered T-cell modulation of IgE production may be the enhanced presentation of aerosolized antigen in experimental animals and children following viral respiratory infection.

Respiratory virus infection may affect other cell lines involved in inflammatory and immune responses. Ida and coworkers [63] demonstrated that interferon elaborated during viral infection from leukocytes harvested from patients with ragweed allergy may induce histamine release. Other investigators [27] found that respiratory viruses are capable of enhancing IgE-mediated histamine release from human leukocytes with or without interferon. The basophil has also been identified as a target cell for mediator release during intercurrent viral infection [76]. Enhanced secretion of many other inflammatory mediators, including leukotriene C_4 [129] and kinins [8] in addition to histamine, has been described in various animal and human studies.

The relationship between airway response to respiratory viral infection and response to inhaled antigens in atopic humans has not been extensively studied. To address this issue, Lemanske and associates [74] studied 10 ragweed allergic adults and evaluated immediate airway response to histamine and ragweed antigen inhalation as well as late reactions to inhaled antigen. One month after baseline studies, patients were inoculated intranasally with live rhinovirus 16. All subjects became infected, and all had a significant increase in airway reactivity to both histamine and ragweed antigen. Of special interest, while only 1 of the 10 had a late asthmatic response to inhaled antigen at baseline, 8 did manifest this response during intercurrent viral infection. Moreover, the development of a late reaction was independent of the magnitude of immediate hypersensitivity. The authors speculated that airway responses to inhaled antigen are altered during intercurrent viral infection, probably by virtue of the cellular migration into the airways. They postulated that enhanced basophil secretion may play a key role in this phenomenon, which of course closely mirrors the common clinical complaints of atopic individuals who have the misfortune of acquiring an acute respiratory viral syndrome during times of high ragweed pollen counts. Figure 44-2 provides a schematic diagram of these various mechanisms.

CLINICAL APPROACH TO INFECTION IN THE ASTHMATIC PATIENT

A compilation of all the potential respiratory infections possibly encountered by the asthmatic patient is beyond the scope of this chapter. However, certain pathogens and clinical syndromes are of particular, and in some cases unique, concern in the patient with asthma. These situations are emphasized here. Certain general principles have particular clinical relevance. Since respiratory viruses are the leading pathogens when respiratory infection induces bronchospasm, the epidemiologic patterns of infection identifiable with these agents are highly clinically relevant. Age alone is a very important predictor of which specific virus may be the pathogen in any given respiratory tract infection (Table 44-2).

In North America the respiratory disease season is primarily from September through April. During this time, usually one of the major epidemic viruses predominates. In the fall, parainfluenza Type 1 virus is epidemic on alternate years. In the winter, respiratory syncytial virus outbreaks occur, usually followed by influenza A and/or B viruses, and in the spring, parainfluenza Type 3 virus tends to predominate. Therefore, recognition of the patterns of activity of these viruses in the community often allows prediction of which viral pathogen may be involved in a patient's illness (Table 44-3).

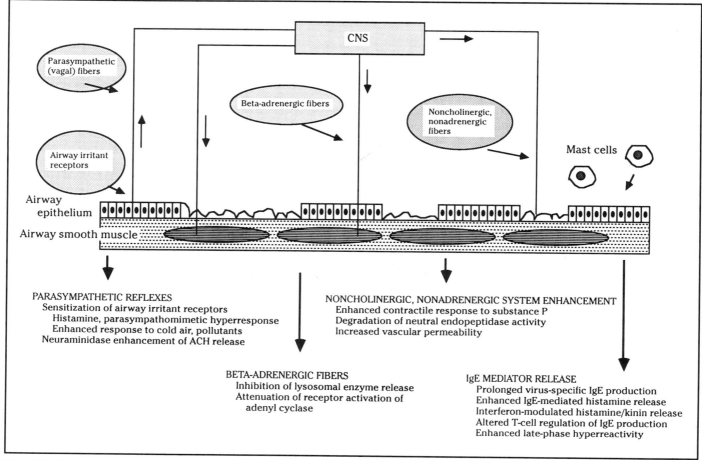

Fig. 44-2. *Factors responsible for altered airway reactivity after viral respiratory infection. The initial inflammatory response results in epithelial cell destruction, which leads to an enhanced sensitivity of airway irritant receptors. Vagally mediated bronchoconstriction is potentiated in response to external stimuli including inhaled antigens, cold air, and air pollutants. Viral infection may also be associated with a diminished beta-adrenergic response of bronchial smooth muscle. There is experimental evidence that the noncholinergic, nonadrenergic system is also transiently potentiated during intercurrent viral infection, resulting in enhanced bronchoconstriction and increased vascular permeability. Activation of IgE in response to viral infection may result in alterations in histamine release, possibly via interferon mediation, altered T-cell regulation of IgE production, and late-phase hypersensitivity.*

Table 44-2. Predominant nonbacterial agents causing exacerbations of asthma according to age of patient

Age	Agent*
Preschool (0–4 yr)	Respiratory syncytial virus
	Parainfluenza virus Types 1–3
	Influenza virus
	Rhinovirus
	Coronavirus
School age (5–16 yr)	Rhinovirus
	Influenza virus
	Mycoplasma pneumoniae
	Parainfluenza virus Types 1–3
	Respiratory syncytial virus
Adult	Influenza virus
	Rhinovirus
	Mycoplasma pneumoniae
	Chlamydia pneumoniae
	Respiratory syncytial virus

* Agents are listed for each group in descending order of incidence.

Table 44-3. Predominant seasons of infectious agents associated with exacerbations of asthma

Agent	Season
Nonbacterial	
Respiratory syncytial virus	Winter to early spring
Parainfluenza virus	Fall, spring
Influenza virus	Winter
Rhinovirus	Fall, spring to summer
Coronavirus	Winter
Adenovirus	All seasons
Mycoplasma pneumoniae	All seasons
Chlamydia pneumoniae	All seasons
Bacterial	
Hemophilus influenzae	All seasons
Streptococcus pneumoniae	Winter, spring

Infections in the Infant and Young Child

Lower respiratory tract infection in the first couple of years of life is very frequent, even in children without an atopic predisposition. During the first 3 years of life, one-fourth to one-third of children in a pediatric practice are seen for acute lower respiratory tract infections [46]. The attack rate is highest during the first year of life, mostly from viral pneumonia and bronchiolitis. These viral lower respiratory tract syndromes occurring early in life, especially those from respiratory syncytial virus, have been implicated as being "asthmatogenic," suggesting that these children are subsequently at risk for recurrent bronchospasm and lower respiratory tract illness.

Bronchiolitis and Viral Pneumonia

The peak incidence of acute lower respiratory tract disease occurs during the first year of life; this is a major cause of hospitalization in young children. Respiratory syncytial virus is the major respiratory pathogen in young children, and the rate of hospitalization for lower respiratory tract disease during the first 2 years of life correlates with the yearly outbreaks of respiratory syncytial virus in the community. The second most frequent causes of lower respiratory tract disease in this young age group are the parainfluenza viruses, especially parainfluenza Type 3 virus. Bronchiolitis tends to be the slightly more frequent manifestation of these viral infections compared to pneumonia, but both are frequent and often cannot be differentiated from each other clinically. The illness usually starts with upper respiratory tract symptoms, fever, and cough. After several days of the prodrome, lower respiratory tract signs, such as tachypnea and wheezing, develop. Although hyperinflation and wheezing are the hallmarks of bronchiolitis, both of these signs may also be present in pneumonia, as may crackles. The chest roentgenogram, especially with lower respiratory tract disease due to respiratory syncytial virus, most frequently shows air trapping and increased perihilar markings. Infiltrates are commonly present, and may be from either atelectasis or inflammation. A subsegmental area of consolidation, usually in the right upper lobe or right middle lobe, occurs in about one-fourth of patients. The x-ray picture may be relatively mild in comparison to the severity of the child's illness and the degree of hypoxemia.

The clinical findings of tachypnea, wheezing, and hyperinflation correlate with the pathologic findings of inflammation and necrosis of the bronchiolar epithelium. The sloughed material causes plugging of the lumina of the small airways and impedes the flow of air. Peripheral to these sites of partial obstruction, air trapping occurs by a ball-valve mechanism, resulting in hyperinflation. With complete obstruction of the bronchiolar lumina, the trapped air may be absorbed, leaving multiple areas of focal atelectasis. The viral infection may progress to produce a picture of pneumonia, with the characteristic findings of an interstitial infiltration of mononuclear cells. The inflammation of the lung parenchyma can produce alveolar filling and consolidation. In contrast to bacterial agents, the virus tends to spread throughout the lung of a young infant, which accounts for the hypoxemia that is almost always present in these young infants hospitalized with viral lower respiratory tract disease. Bacterial pneumonia is markedly less frequent in this age group and less likely to cause hypoxemia. However, the clinical appearance and the x-ray picture, especially if a consolidated area is present, make it difficult to differentiate from bacterial infection. In children presenting primarily with bronchospasm, asthma is the major diagnosis in the differential and often cannot be differentiated in a child with a first episode of wheezing.

Specific diagnosis of the viral agent is important, especially now that specific antiviral therapy is available. Advances in technology have engendered a number of rapid viral diagnostic assays, especially for respiratory syncytial virus. Although viral isolation in tissue culture remains the "gold standard," several of these rapid antigen tests have a high rate of specificity and sensitivity and may be performed in a variety of laboratories, including those not previously experienced in viral diagnosis.

For most children with bronchiolitis and/or pneumonia, supportive treatment is all that is necessary, and recovery usually occurs after several days to a week, except for the lingering cough. In the more severely ill children who require hospitalization, supportive therapy should include careful monitoring of the oxygen saturation and administration of supplemental oxygen as needed. The use of bronchodilators in children with bronchiolitis remains controversial. Most studies suggest that for the majority of children, the response to bronchodilators is minimal, especially in the child under 18 months old [95, 105]. Bronchodilators may also occasionally have adverse effects in the young infant. However, a subgroup of patients may respond, and hence a trial with aerosolized bronchodilators is frequently given. Systemic steroids have not been shown to be effective [122], but recently there has been interest in the possible benefits of inhaled steroids in the treatment of bronchiolitis, especially for the recurrent wheezing following bronchiolitis. While this area remains controversial, several studies have suggested symptomatic improvement in bronchospasm following the acute episode of bronchiolitis [23, 81].

For children hospitalized with respiratory syncytial virus–associated bronchiolitis and/or pneumonia the aerosolized antiviral drug ribavirin offers specific therapy. In controlled studies, this drug was associated with significant clinical benefit and improvement in the arterial oxygen saturation [53, 111]. A recent controlled study of infants with respiratory syncytial lower respiratory tract disease who required mechanical ventilation also showed significant improvement in those children treated with ribavirin. The durations of mechanical ventilation and of supplemental oxygen were significantly less for those who received ribavirin [120].

Acute Laryngotracheobronchitis (Croup)

Croup, another age-specific viral infection, presents with signs of acute inspiratory obstruction of the airway. This syndrome is characterized by inflammation in the subglottic area, resulting in dyspnea with inspiratory stridor. Croup predominantly occurs in the preschool-age child, with the peak incidence occurring in the second year of life. Parainfluenza virus Type 1 is the major cause of croup, and since it occurs in epidemic form every other year in the autumn, the number of cases of croup in outpatients and in hospitalized children fluctuates accordingly. The other important agents of croup are parainfluenza virus Type 3, respiratory syncytial virus, and the influenza viruses.

The inflammation associated with the viral infection in croup involves the epithelial surfaces at all levels of the tracheobronchial tree. Airway obstruction is the greatest at the subglottic area, as anatomically this is the least distensible part of the airway since it is encircled by cartilage. However, hypoxemia, which implies lower airway involvement, occurs in 80 percent of children hospitalized with croup [101].

In addition to the characteristic seal's bark, croup is notable for its fluctuating course. Periods of severe airway obstruction may alternate with relatively quiet breathing. Diagnosis can usually be made on clinical grounds, but if necessary neck roentgenograms will demonstrate the characteristic narrowing of the tracheal air shadow in the subglottic area.

Therapy for most children is supportive. However, even the benefit of the various modes of supportive treatment, such as mist and cold air, remain of unproven efficacy. Therapy for croup is particularly difficult to study because of the usual fluctuation in the clinical course and in the degree of airway obstruction. One of the few animal studies of croup suggested that cold dry, cold moist, and warm dry air were more effective in decreasing airway resistance in the dog model than was warm moist air which contains a high water content [138]. All the former types of air have a low moisture content, which would cool the airway, suggesting this may be the mechanism of benefit and may explain the improvement many children with croup experience when taken outside to breathe cold night or winter air. In the more seriously ill child with hypoxemia, supplemental oxygen administration is important. Nebulized racemic epinephrine administered either by intermittent positive pressure breathing or by mask has been shown to produce clinical improvement [126]. Clinical improvement is, however, transient, and the racemic epinephrine treatment does not alter the arterial oxygen saturation, but may result in fewer children requiring intubation. The use of systemic steroids in croup is controversial and studies have produced conflicting results. A critical review of most of these studies concluded that none was without flaws [127]. For the majority of children with croup, steroids are not warranted. However, in those with severe obstruction, steroids are frequently used in hope that they may be useful in avoiding the need for intubation. As previously mentioned, children with a history of croup have been shown to have a higher prevalence of increased bronchial reactivity, which occurs irrespective of allergy and baseline lung function abnormalities [50, 69, 80].

Infections in the Older Child and Adult

As previously mentioned, respiratory viruses are commonly associated with acute exacerbations of bronchospasm in all age groups. For the most part, the clinical epidemiology of these infections is no different in the asthmatic and the nonasthmatic patients. A few characteristics of specific infectious agents, however, are of particular relevance in caring for the asthmatic patient.

Mycoplasma pneumoniae Infection

Mycoplasma pneumoniae is the most common cause of community-acquired pneumonia in school-age children and young adults. Infection, however, does occur at all ages, and repetitive infections may occur over time [65, 100]. This pathogen has been frequently associated with exacerbations of asthma and is a major cause of tracheobronchitis in both children and adults [10, 26, 33, 62].

M. pneumoniae infection tends to spread through families with an incubation period of 2 to 3 weeks. Illness may start with predominantly nonrespiratory symptoms, such as headache and myalgia, or frequently with pharyngitis and low-grade fever. The classic "cold" signs of nasal congestion and sneezing are not usually part of *M. pneumoniae* infection. Most characteristic of this infection is a nonproductive cough that tends to be prolonged and often severe. If the infection progresses to pneumonia, the x-ray picture characteristically has segmental pulmonary infiltrates, which tend to progress little, and consolidation is unusual. Although occasionally minimal amounts of pleural effusion may be present, those that are easily demonstrable are unlikely to be from *M. pneumoniae*. Diagnosis is often made on the basis of the epidemiology and of the clinical features of a marked, nonproductive cough, low-grade fever, and the x-ray picture if pneumonia is present, with a normal white blood cell count.

Making the diagnosis is often difficult initially, especially since the prolonged cough is such a characteristic feature. The organism is difficult to culture, and thus diagnosis is usually made on a serologic basis. Cold agglutinins are nonspecific, but are present in over half of those with lower respiratory tract signs. Although cold agglutinins may be positive in other infections, including influenza and mononucleosis, a high titer ($>1:256$) is more suggestive of *M. pneumoniae* infection. A bedside test for

cold agglutinins can be used as a simple, screening procedure; it gives a positive result primarily when titers are higher than $1:64$. More specific serologic diagnosis can be made by the testing of acute and convalescent sera by the enzyme-linked immunosorbent assay (ELISA) and the complement fixation tests, as well as several other assays less frequently available. The caveats of serologic diagnosis are first that the protracted course brings many patients to the physician at a time when an antibody rise may already have occurred. Cold agglutinins are the first to rise (10 days–2 weeks), with antibody assayed by other tests rising 2 to 4 weeks after onset. Second, the sensitivities of these serologic tests vary. Complement fixation tests, which are most frequently available, may quite commonly give false-positive results. Furthermore, complement fixation antibodies tend to decline rather quickly.

Antibiotic therapy has been shown to be most effective if given within the first few days of illness, which often is not possible. Such treatment shortens the duration of illness, but shedding of the organism may continue for several months, despite antibiotic therapy. Erythromycin or tetracycline are equally effective, but tetracycline may not be used in young children or women who are pregnant or nursing. Treatment is usually for 2 to 3 weeks.

Influenza Virus Infection

Influenza viruses are probably the most important respiratory viral pathogens in the asthmatic patient because of their pronounced ability to exacerbate bronchospasm and because of the epidemiology of influenza. Over recent years, more than one type of influenza virus has generally caused an outbreak each year, prolonging the influenza season. Second, the ability of influenza viruses, especially influenza A virus, to drift antigenically each year results in the repeated susceptibility of all age groups. Epidemiologic studies conducted over many influenza seasons in Houston clearly demonstrated the high risk that influenza poses for the patient with asthma [42, 43, 45]. The risk of hospitalization during an outbreak of influenza is markedly increased for a patient with asthma, even for those with relatively mild disease who have not previously been hospitalized.

The onset of influenza is generally abrupt with sudden systemic symptoms, including fever, chills, myalgia, and headache. In the asthmatic patient, an irritating, dry cough and wheezing tend to develop over the ensuing 24 to 48 hours. As previously described, bronchospasm is most probably related to a sensitization of epithelial receptors secondary to respiratory epithelial destruction. Regeneration of the epithelial lining may take 3 to 6 weeks, and frequently the exacerbation of bronchospasm and tracheobronchitis may persist for a similar period, well after the systemic symptoms have subsided. Secondary bacterial infection occurs more frequently after influenza viral infection than after other common respiratory viral agents, but relative to the frequency of influenza infections, bacterial superinfection is still uncommon. If such occurs, pneumococci are the most frequent secondary invaders, followed by *H. influenzae,* and staphylococci. Treatment of an acute exacerbation of bronchospasm associated with influenza infection is no different than for any other exacerbation. However, influenza-induced exacerbations may be unusually prolonged, necessitating a continuance of aggressive therapy for weeks.

Amantadine hydrochloride may be used for the treatment of acute influenza A viral infection. Amantadine and rimantadine have been shown to reduce the severity and shorten the course of influenza A viral illness in healthy subjects. No data, however, are currently available to prove the efficacy of amantadine treatment in preventing the complications of influenza A viral infection in high-risk patients [1].

The most effective means of protecting asthmatic patients from the yearly onset of influenza is annual immunization with the inactivated influenza vaccine formulated each year [1, 35]. These inactivated influenza vaccines are 70 to 80 percent effective in reducing the occurrence of disease if the epidemic strains and those in the vaccine are closely matched. Even in years in which the vaccine is less well matched to the circulating strains, vaccine usually produces an anamnestic response in school-age children and adults who have had previous experience with similar strains, and may provide protection against the complications of influenza infection. These influenza vaccines have been shown to be safe in asthmatic patients and produce few side effects and no alterations in airway reactivity or any other measurable index of pulmonary function [2, 3, 123]. Patients with asthma should receive yearly immunization according to the guidelines published each year by the Advisory Committee on Immunization Practices of the Centers for Disease Control [1]. Amantadine may also be used for prophylaxis and appears to be most effective if it is used in conjunction with immunization.

Chlamydia pneumoniae Infection

The TWAR strain of chlamydia (*Chlamydia pneumoniae*) was recently shown to be a common cause of atypical pneumonia and may be second in frequency to *M. pneumoniae* as a cause of the "primary atypical pneumonia" syndrome. This organism appears to infect primarily adolescents and adults. Antibody to *C. pneumoniae* is infrequently seen in preschool-age children, but the frequency of specific antibody rises thereafter to close to 60 percent among adults. The organism appears to be ubiquitous and may occasionally cause outbreaks [48, 49, 83]. The clinical manifestations associated with *C. pneumoniae* appear to be similar to those caused by *M. pneumoniae*. Laryngitis and pharyngitis appear to be more frequent with *C. pneumoniae* than with *M. pneumoniae*. Tracheobronchitis, pneumonia, and sinusitis are also common manifestations. The severity of illness can be quite variable, but it is often relatively mild, and clinical manifestations may be prolonged. Some patients may have a biphasic illness of upper respiratory tract disease, usually pharyngitis and fever, followed a couple weeks later by lower respiratory tract signs of pneumonia and tacheobronchitis. As with *M. pneumoniae,* the cough tends to be nonproductive and the laboratory findings are not distinctive. The diagnosis is currently difficult to make, as commercial serologic tests generally are not yet available and cultures are not generally feasible or available. Roentgenographic findings when pneumonia is present tend to be similar to those of *M. pneumoniae* infection. The treatment of *C. pneumoniae* infection requires further study, but erythromycin or tetracycline may be beneficial if given for 10 days or more.

Of perhaps even greater interest is the recently described relationship between serologic evidence of infection with *C. pneumoniae* and wheezing, asthmatic bronchitis, and adult-onset asthma. Human respiratory infection with *C. pneumoniae,* as described above, is not a new phenomenon, but has only recently received attention with the development of accurate tests for circulating antibody. Hahn and colleagues [52] studied *C. pneumoniae* infections in patients enrolled in primary care practices in Madison, Wisconsin. They found that 47 percent of the patients with symptomatic lower respiratory tract infections due to *C. pneumoniae* had bronchospasm during these infections, an association previously pointed out for a variety of other nonbacterial agents, as described above. However, the investigators also noted that there was a strong quantitative association of *C. pneumoniae* titers with wheezing at the time of study enrollment. Thirty-four percent of subjects with antibody titers greater than or equal to 1:128 had chronic wheezing. Among those subjects with acute *C. pneumoniae* respiratory infection, there was a strong association between *C. pneumoniae* exposure and the new onset of asthmatic bronchitis in a 6-month follow-up period. These data suggest that *C. pneumoniae* infection may be a pre-

cipitating agent of acute bronchospasm, but in addition may be a risk factor for the development of chronic bronchospasm. This association, if confirmed in subsequent population-based studies, might define *C. pneumoniae* infection as an important etiologic factor in the development of bronchospasm.

COUGH AS A MANIFESTATION OF INFECTIOUS ASTHMA

One special aspect of a viral infection in asthma bears special emphasis. For a number of years, cough has been described as an asthma "variant" [64, 104]. Some investigators have postulated that patients with intractable cough even without demonstrable bronchospasm have hyperreactive airways when confronted with one of the conventional challenge tests. Many of these patients are probably showing the long-term sequela of respiratory viral illness. It has been our experience that many patients will complain of recurring cough for up to 6 months or even a year after influenza A infection. Generally, this cough responds to conventional bronchodilator administration.

USE OF CORTICOSTEROIDS IN ASTHMATIC EXACERBATIONS DUE TO VIRAL RESPIRATORY INFECTION

As detailed elsewhere in this text, the use of systemic corticosteroids in more intractable exacerbations of asthma has demonstrated therapeutic efficacy. Moreover, it is likely that the indications for both inhaled and systemic steroids in asthma will be broadened, as the significance of the inflammatory component of this disease is more appreciated. Since especially in younger children, many if not most exacerbations of asthma will be related to viral respiratory infection, the issue of efficacy and lack of deleterious side effects associated with steroid use in patients with active respiratory viral infection is an important one. At present, there does not seem to be any evidence that short-term systemic steroid use is associated with any harmful effects clinically or in terms of host defense mechanisms. In fact, in one recent study, a short course of prednisone was administered to asthmatic children as soon as the initial symptoms of an upper respiratory tract infection developed, even before symptomatic wheezing was present [15]. Over a 1-year observation period, steroid-treated children had a marked decrease in the number of wheezing days, asthma attacks, emergency room visits, and hospitalizations, compared to a control group who were treated conventionally. These observations will require further confirmation, but studies such as these suggest that the decision to use steroids should not be influenced by the possibility that the patient has an intercurrent respiratory viral infection.

REFERENCES

1. Advisory Committee on Immunization Practices (ACIP). Prevention and control of influenza. *MWWR* 39:1, 1990.
2. Albazzaz, M. K., et al. Subunit influenza vaccination in adults with asthma: Effect on clinical state, airway reactivity, and antibody response. *Br. Med. J.* 294:1196, 1987.
3. American Academy of Pediatrics. Report of the Committee on Infectious Diseases. In *Red Book* (21st ed.). Elk Grove City, Ill.: American Academy of Pediatrics, 1988. Pp. 243–251.
4. Aquilina, A. T., et al. Airway reactivity in subjects with viral upper respiratory tract infections: The effects of exercise and cold air. *Am. Rev. Respir. Dis.* 122:3, 1980.
5. Barker, D. J. P., and Osmond, C. Childhood respiratory infection and adult chronic bronchitis in England and Wales. *Br. Med. J.* 293:1271, 1986.

6. Barker, W. H. Excess pneumonia and influenza associated hospitalization during influenza epidemics in the United States, 1970–78. *Am. J. Public Health* 76:761, 1986.

7. Barnes, P. J. Neuropeptides and asthma. *Am. Rev. Respir. Dis.* 143:S28, 1991.

8. Barnett, J. K. C., Cruse, L. W., and Proud, D. Kinins are generated in nasal secretions during influenza A infections in ferrets. *Am. Rev. Respir. Dis.* 142:162, 1990.

9. Beasley, R., et al. Viral respiratory tract infection and exacerbations of asthma in adult patients. *Thorax* 43:679, 1988.

10. Berkovich, S., Millian, S. J., and Snyder, R. D. The association of viral and *Mycoplasma* infections with recurrence of wheezing in the asthmatic child. *Ann. Allergy* 28:43, 1970.

11. Berman, S. Z., et al. Transtracheal aspiration studies in asthmatic patients in relapse with "infective" asthma and in subjects without respiratory disease. *J. Allergy Clin. Immunol.* 56:206, 1975.

12. Borson, D. B., et al. Viral infection increases tracheal permeability response to substance P (SP) in rats by decreasing neutral endopeptidase (NEP). *J. Cell Biochem. Suppl.* 12B:295, 1988.

13. Boushey, H. A., et al. Bronchial hyperreactivity. *Am. Rev. Respir. Dis.* 121:389, 1980.

14. Brown, P., Sadowsky, D., and Gajdusek, D. C. Ventilatory lung function studies in Pacific Island Micronesians. *Am. J. Epidemiol.* 108:259, 1978.

15. Brunette, M. G., Lands, L., and Thibodeau, L. Childhood asthma: Prevention of attacks with short-term corticosteroid treatment of upper respiratory tract infection. *Pediatrics* 81:624, 1988.

16. Buckner, C. K., et al. In vivo and in vitro studies on the use of the guinea pig as a model for virus-provoked airway hyperreactivity. *Am. Rev. Respir. Dis.* 132:305, 1985.

17. Buckner, C. K., et al. Parainfluenza 3 infection blocks the ability of a beta adrenergic receptor agonist to inhibit antigen-induced contraction of guinea pig isolated airway smooth muscle. *J. Clin. Invest.* 67:376, 1981.

18. Burrows, B., et al. The course and prognosis of different forms of chronic airways obstruction in a sample from the general population. *N. Engl. J. Med.* 317:1309, 1987.

19. Burrows, B., Knudson, R. J., and Lebowitz, M. D. The relationship of childhood respiratory illness to adult obstructive airway disease. *Am. Rev. Respir. Dis.* 115:751, 1977.

20. Busse, W. W. Decreased granulocyte response to isoproterenol in asthma during upper respiratory infections. *Am. Rev. Respir. Dis.* 115:783, 1977.

21. Busse, W. W., et al. Effect of influenza A virus on leukocyte histamine release. *J. Allergy Clin. Immunol.* 71:382, 1983.

22. Busse, W. W., et al. Reduced granulocyte response to isoproterenol, histamine, and prostaglandin E₁ after in vitro incubation with rhinovirus 16. *Am. Rev. Respir. Dis.* 122:641, 1980.

23. Carlsen, K. H., et al. Nebulized beclomethasone dipropionate in recurrent obstructive episodes after acute bronchiolitis. *Arch. Dis. Child.* 63:1428, 1988.

24. Carson, J. L., Collier, A. M., and Hu, S. S. Acquired ciliary defects in nasal epithelium of children with acute viral upper respiratory infections. *N. Engl. J. Med.* 312:463, 1985.

25. Cate, T. R., et al. Effects of common colds on pulmonary function. *Am. Rev. Respir. Dis.* 108:858, 1973.

26. Chapman, R. S., et al. The epidemiology of tracheobronchitis in pediatric practice. *Am. J. Epidemiol.* 114:786, 1981.

27. Chonmaitree, T., et al. Role of interferon in leukocyte histamine release caused by common respiratory viruses. *J. Infect. Dis.* 157:127, 1988.

28. Co, M. S., et al. Structural similarities between the mammalian β-adrenergic and reovirus type 3 receptors. *Proc. Natl. Acad. Sci. USA* 82:5315, 1985.

29. Colley, J. R., et al. Respiratory function of infants in relation to subsequent respiratory disease: An epidemiologic study. *Bull. Eur. Physiopathol. Respir.* 12:651, 1976.

30. Colley, J. R. Respiratory disease in childhood. *Br. Med. Bull.* 27:9, 1971.

31. Collier, A. M., et al. Spirometric changes in normal children with upper respiratory infections. *Am. Rev. Respir. Dis.* 117:47, 1978.

32. Dearwater, S., et al. The incidence and impact of infections in ambulatory elderly. *Gerontologist* 28:77A, 1988.

33. Denny, F. W., and Clyde, W. A. Acute lower respiratory tract infections in nonhospitalized children. *J. Pediatr.* 108:635, 1986.

34. Djukanovic, R., et al. Mucosal inflammation in asthma. *Am. Rev. Respir. Dis.* 142:434, 1990.

35. Douglas, R. G., Jr. Prophylaxis and treatment of influenza. *N. Engl. J. Med.* 322:443, 1990.

36. Dusser, D. J., et al. Virus induces airway hyperresponsiveness to tachykinins: Role of neutral endopeptidase. *J. Appl. Physiol.* 67:1504, 1989.

37. Empey, D. W., et al. Mechanisms of bronchial hyperreactivity in normal subjects after upper respiratory tract infection. *Am. Rev. Respir. Dis.* 113:131, 1976.

38. Frick, O. L. Effect of respiratory and other virus infections on IgE immunoregulation. *J. Allergy Clin. Immunol.* 78:1013, 1980.

39. Frick, O. L., German, D. F., and Mills, J. Development of allergy in children: I. Association with virus infections. *J. Allergy Clin. Immunol.* 63:228, 1979.

40. Friedman, R., et al. Asthma and bacterial sinusitis in children. *J. Allergy Clin. Immunol.* 74:185, 1984.

41. Fryer, A. D., El-Fakahany, E. E., and Jacoby, D. B. Parainfluenza virus type 1 reduces the affinity of agonists for muscarinic receptors in guinea-pig lung and heart. *Eur. J. Pharmacol.* 181:51, 1990.

42. Glezen, W. P. Consequences to children from influenza virus infections. *Pediatr. Virol.* 4:1, 1989.

43. Glezen, W. P., Decker, M., and Perrotta, D. M. Survey of underlying conditions of persons hospitalized with acute respiratory disease during influenza epidemics in Houston, 1978–1981. *Am. Rev. Respir. Dis.* 136:550, 1987.

44. Glezen, W. P., and Denny, F. W. Epidemiology of acute lower respiratory disease in children. *N. Engl. J. Med.* 288:498, 1973.

45. Glezen, W. P., et al. Acute respiratory disease associated with influenza epidemics in Houston 1981–83. *J. Infect. Dis.* 155:1119, 1987.

46. Glezen, W. P., et al. Epidemiological patterns of acute lower respiratory disease of children in pediatric group practice. *J. Pediatr.* 78:397, 1971.

47. Gold, D. R., et al. Acute lower respiratory illness in childhood as a predictor of lung function and chronic respiratory symptoms. *Am. Rev. Respir. Dis.* 140:877, 1989.

48. Grayston, J. T. *Chlamydia pneumoniae*, strain TWAR. *Chest* 95:664, 1989.

49. Grayston, J. T., et al. A new respiratory tract infection: *Chlamydia pneumoniae* strain TWAR. *J. Infect. Dis.* 161:618, 1990.

50. Gurwitz, D., Corey, J., and Levison, H. Pulmonary function and bronchial reactivity in children after croup. *Am. Rev. Respir. Dis.* 122:95, 1980.

51. Gurwitz, D., Mindorff, C., and Levison, H. Increased incidence of bronchial reactivity in children with a history of bronchiolitis. *J. Pediatr.* 98:551, 1981.

52. Hahn, D. L., Dodge, R. W., and Goldubjatnikov, V. R. Association of *Chlamydia pneumoniae* (strain TWAR) infection with wheezing, asthmatic bronchitis, and adult onset asthma. *JAMA* 226:225, 1991.

53. Hall, C. B., et al. Aerosolized ribavirin treatment of infants with respiratory syncytial viral infection. *N. Engl. J. Med.* 308:1443, 1983.

54. Hall, W. J., and Hall, C. B. Alterations in pulmonary function following respiratory viral infection. *Chest* 76:458, 1979.

55. Hall, W. J., et al. Pulmonary mechanics after uncomplicated influenza A infection. *Am. Rev. Respir. Dis.* 113:141, 1976.

56. Hall, W. J., Hall, C. B., and Speers, D. M. Respiratory syncytial virus infection in adults: Clinical, virologic, and serial pulmonary function studies. *Ann. Intern. Med.* 88:203, 1978.

57. Halperin, S. A., et al. Pathogenesis of lower respiratory tract symptoms in experimental rhinovirus infection. *Am. Rev. Respir. Dis.* 128:806, 1983.

58. Halperin, S. A., et al. Exacerbations of asthma in adults during experimental rhinovirus infection. *Am. Rev. Respir. Dis.* 132:976, 1985.

59. Heino, M., et al. Bronchial epithelial inflammation in children with chronic cough after early lower respiratory tract illness. *Am. Rev. Respir. Dis.* 141:428, 1990.

60. Henderson, F. W., et al. The etiologic and epidemiologic spectrum of bronchiolitis in pediatric practice. *J. Pediatr.* 95:183, 1979.

61. Hudgel, D. W., et al. Viral and bacterial infections in adults with chronic asthma. *Am. Rev. Respir. Dis.* 120:393, 1979.

62. Huhti, E., et al. Association of viral and mycoplasma infections with exacerbations of asthma. *Ann. Allergy* 33:145, 1974.

63. Ida, S., et al. Enhancement of IgE-mediated histamine release from human basophils by viruses: Role of interferon. *J. Exp. Med.* 145:892, 1977.

64. Irwin, R. S., Curley, F. J., and French, C. L. The spectrum and frequency of causes, key components of the diagnostic evaluation, and outcome of specific therapy. *Am. Rev. Respir. Dis.* 141:640, 1990.

65. Iyumikawa, K., and Hara, K. Clinical features of mycoplasmal pneumonia in adults. *Yale J. Biol. Med.* 56:505, 1983.

66. Jacoby, D. B., and Fryer, A. D. Abnormalities in neural control of smooth muscle in virus-infected airways. *Trends in Pharmacol. Sci.* 11:393, 1990.

67. Jacoby, D. B., et al. Influenza infection causes airway hyperresponsiveness by decreasing enkephalinease. *J. Appl. Physiol.* 64:2653, 1988.

68. Johanson, W. G., Jr., Pierce, A. K., and Sanford, J. P. Pulmonary function in uncomplicated influenza. *Am. Rev. Respir. Dis.* 100:141, 1969.

69. Kattan, M. Long-term sequelae of respiratory illness in infancy and childhood. *Pediatr. Clin. North Am.* 26:525, 1979.

70. Kattan, M., et al. Pulmonary function abnormalities in symptom-free children after bronchiolitis. *Pediatrics* 59:683, 1977.

71. Kiernan, K. E., et al. Chronic cough in young adults in relationship to smoking habits, childhood environment, and chest illness. *Respirations* 33:236, 1976.

72. Lambert, H. P., and Stern, H. Infective factors in exacerbations of bronchitis and asthma. *Br. Med. J.* 3:323, 1972.

73. Leeder, S. R. Role of infection in the cause and course of chronic bronchitis and emphysema. *J. Infect. Dis.* 131:731, 1975.

74. Lemanske, R. F., et al. Rhinovirus upper respiratory infection increases airway hyperreactivity and late asthmatic reactions. *J. Clin. Invest.* 83:1, 1989.

75. Lemen, R. J., et al. Canine parainfluenza type 2 bronchiolitis increases histamine responsiveness in beagle puppies. *Am. Rev. Respir. Dis.* 141:199, 1990.

76. Lett-Brown, M. A., et al. Enhancement of basophil chemotaxis in vitro by virus-induced interferon. *J. Clin. Invest.* 67:547, 1981.

77. Little, J. W., et al. Airway hyperreactivity and peripheral airway dysfunction in influenza A infection. *Am. Rev. Respir. Dis.* 118:295, 1978.

78. Little, J. W., et al. Amantadine effect on peripheral airways abnormalities in influenza. *Ann. Intern. Med.* 85:177, 1976.

79. Little, J. W., et al. Attenuated influenza produced by experimental intranasal inoculation. *J. Med. Virol.* 3:177, 1979.

80. Loughlin, G. M., and Taussig, L. M. Pulmonary function in children with a history of laryngotracheobronchitis. *J. Pediatr.* 94:365, 1979.

81. Maayan, D., et al. The functional response of infants with persistent wheezing to nebulized beclomethasone dipropionate. *Pediatr. Pulmonol.* 2:9, 1986.

82. Malfroy, B., et al. Molecular cloning and amino acid sequence of rat enkephalinase. *Biochem. Biophys. Res. Commun.* 144:59, 1987.

83. Marrie, T. J., et al. Pneumonia associated with the TWAR strain of chlamydia. *Ann. Intern. Med.* 106:507, 1987.

84. Martinez, F. D., et al. Diminished lung function as a predisposing factor for wheezing respiratory illness in infants. *N. Engl. J. Med.* 319:1112, 1988.

85. Martinez, F. D., Taussig, L. M., and Morgan, W. J. Infants with upper respiratory illnesses have significant reductions in maximal expiratory flow. *Pediatr. Pulmonol.* 9:91, 1990.

86. Master, K. M. Air pollution in New Guinea. *JAMA* 228:1653, 1974.

87. Mathur, U., Bentley, D. W., and Hall, C. B. Concurrent respiratory syncytial virus and influenza A infections in the institutionalized elderly and chronically ill. *Ann. Intern. Med.* 93:49, 1980.

88. McConnochie, K. M., and Roghmann, K. J. Bronchiolitis as a possible cause of wheezing in childhood: New evidence. *Pediatrics* 74:1, 1984.

89. McConnochie, K. M., and Roghmann, K. J. Predicting clinically significant lower respiratory tract illness in childhood following mild bronchiolitis. *Am. J. Dis. Child.* 139:625, 1985.

90. McConnochie, K. M., and Roghmann, K. J. Parental smoking, presence of older siblings, and family history of asthma increase risk of bronchiolitis. *Am. J. Dis. Child.* 140:806, 1986.

91. McConnochie, K. M., et al. Normal pulmonary function: Measurements and airway reactivity in childhood after mild bronchiolitis. *J. Pediatr.* 107:54, 1985.

92. McIntosh, K. Bronchiolitis and asthma: Possible common pathogenetic pathways. *J. Allergy Clin. Immunol.* 57:595, 1976.

93. McIntosh, K., et al. The association of viral and bacterial respiratory infections with exacerbations of wheezing in young asthmatic children. *J. Pediatr.* 82:578, 1973.

94. Mills, J. E., Sellick, M., and Widdicombe, J. C. Epithelial Irritant Receptors in the Lung in Breathing. In R. Porter (ed.), *Breathing: Herring-Breuer Centenary Symposium.* London: Churchill-Livingstone, 1970.

95. Milner, A. D., and Murray, M. Acute bronchiolitis in infancy: Treatment and prognosis. *Thorax* 44:1, 1989.

96. Minor, T. E., et al. Rhinovirus and influenza type A infections as precipitants of asthma. *Am. Rev. Respir. Dis.* 113:149, 1976.

97. Minor, T. E., et al. Viruses as precipitants of asthmatic attacks in children. *JAMA* 227:292, 1974.

98. Nadel, J. A. Structure-function relationships in the airways: Bronchoconstriction mediated via vagus nerves in bronchial asthma. *Med. Thoracis* 22:231, 1963.

99. Nadel, J. A., and Borson, D. B. Modulation of neurogenic inflammation by neutral endopeptidase. *Am. Rev. Respir. Dis.* 143:S33, 1991.

100. Nagayama, Y., et al. Isolation of *Mycoplasma pneumoniae* from children with lower respiratory tract infections. *J. Infect. Dis.* 157:911, 1988.

101. Newth, C. J. L., Levison, H., and Bryan, A. C. The respiratory status of children with croup. *J. Pediatr.* 81:1068, 1972.

102. Picken, J. J., Niewoehner, D. E., and Chester, E. H. Prolonged effects of viral infections of the upper respiratory tract upon small airways. *Am. J. Med.* 52:738, 1972.

103. Piedimonte, G., et al. Sendai virus infection potentiates neurogenic inflammation in the rat trachea. *J. Appl. Physiol.* 68:754, 1990.

104. Poe, R. H., et al. Chronic cough: Bronchoscopy or pulmonary function testing. *Am. Rev. Respir. Dis.* 126:160, 1982.

105. Prendiville, A., Green S., and Silverman, M. Paradoxical response to nebulized salbutamol in wheezy infants, assessed by partial expiratory flow-volume curves. *Thorax* 42:86, 1987.

106. Pullan, C. R., and Hey, E. N. Wheezing, asthma, and pulmonary dysfunction 10 years after infection with respiratory syncytial virus in infancy. *Br. Med. J.* 284:1665, 1982.

107. Quan, S. F., et al. Acute canine adenovirus 2 infection increases histamine airway reactivity in beagle puppies. *Am. Rev. Respir. Dis.* 141:414, 1990.

108. Rachelefsky, G. S., Katz, R. M., and Siegel, S. C. Chronic sinus disease with associated reactive airway disease in children. *Pediatrics* 73:526, 1985.

109. Reid, D. D. The beginning of bronchitis. *Proc. R. Soc. Med.* 62:311, 1969.

110. Richardson, J. B., et al. Electron microscopic localization of antigen in experimental bronchoconstriction in guinea pigs. *Chest* 63:44S, 1973.

111. Rodriquez, W. J., et al. Aerosolized ribavirin in the treatment of patients with respiratory syncytial virus disease. *Pediatr. Infect. Dis. J.* 6:159, 1987.

112. Roldaan, A. C., and Masural N. Viral respiratory infections in asthmatic children staying in a mountain resort. *Eur. J. Respir. Dis.* 63:140, 1982.

113. Saban, R., et al. Enhancement by parainfluenza 3 infection of contractile responses to substance P and capsaicin in airway smooth muscle from the guinea pig. *Am. Rev. Respir. Dis.* 136:586, 1987.

114. Sakamoto, M., Ida, S., and Takishima, T. Effect of influenza virus infection on allergic sensitization to aerosolized ovalbumin in mice. *J. Immunol.* 132:2614, 1984.

115. Samet, J. M., Tager, I. B., and Speizer, F. E. The relationship between respiratory illness in childhood and chronic air-flow obstruction in adulthood. *Am. Rev. Respir. Dis.* 127:508, 1983.

116. Scarpace, P. J., and Bender, B. S. Viral pneumonia attenuates adenylate cyclase but not beta-adrenergic receptors in murine lung. *Am. Rev. Respir. Dis.* 130:1602, 1989.

117. Sims, E. G., et al. Study of 8-year-old children with a history of respiratory syncytial virus bronchiolitis in infancy. *Br. Med. J.* 1:11, 1978.

118. Slavin, R. G., et al. Sinusitis and bronchial asthma. *J. Allergy Clin. Immunol.* 66:250, 1980.

119. Sly, P. D., and Hibbert, M. E. Childhood asthma following hospitalization with acute viral bronchiolitis in infancy. *Pediatr. Pulmonol.* 7:153, 1989.

120. Smith, D. W., et al. Aerosolized ribavirin in infants requiring mechanical ventilation for severe lower respiratory tract infection caused by respiratory syncytial virus. *Clin. Res.* 39:59A, 1991.

121. Snapper, J. R. Inflammation and airway function: The asthma syndrome. *Am. Rev. Respir. Dis.* 141:531, 1990.

122. Stecenko, A. A. Treatment of viral bronchiolitis: Do steroids make sense? *Contemp. Pediatr.* 4:121, 1987.

123. Stenius-Aarniala, B., et al. Lack of clinical exacerbations in adults with chronic asthma after immunization with killed influenza virus. *Chest* 89:786, 1986.

124. Szentivanyi, A. The beta-adrenergic theory of atopic abnormality in bronchial asthma. *J. Allergy* 42:203, 1968.

125. Tarlo, S., Broder, I., and Spence, L. A prospective study of respiratory infection in adult asthmatics and their normal spouses. *Clin. Allergy* 9:293, 1979.

126. Taussig, L. M., Castro, O., and Beaudry, P. H. Treatment of laryngotracheobronchitis (croup): Use of intermittent positive pressure breathing and racemic epinephrine. *Am. J. Dis. Child.* 129:790, 1975.

127. Tunnessen, W. W., Jr., and Feinstein, A. R. The steroid-croup controversy: An analytic review of methodologic problems. *J. Pediatr.* 96:751, 1980.

128. Utell, M. J., et al. Development of airway reactivity to nitrates in subjects with influenza. *Am. Rev. Respir. Dis.* 121:233, 1980.
129. Volovitz, B., Faden, H., and Ogra, P. Release of leukotriene C_4 in respiratory tract during acute viral infection. *J. Pediatr.* 112:218, 1988.
130. Walsh, J. J., Dielein, L. F., and Low, F. N. Tracheobronchial response in human influenza. *Arch. Intern. Med.* 108:376, 1961.
131. Weiss, K. B. Seasonal trends in US asthma hospitalizations and mortality. *JAMA* 263:2323, 1990.
132. Welliver, R. C., et al. Defective regulation of immune responses in respiratory syncytial virus infection. *J. Immunol.* 133:1925, 1984.
133. Welliver, R. C., et al. Predictive value of respiratory syncytial virus-specific IgE responses for recurrent wheezing following bronchiolitis. *J. Pediatr.* 109:776, 1986.
134. Welliver, R. C., et al. Role of parainfluenza virus-specific IgE in pathogenesis of croup and wheezing subsequent to infection. *J. Pediatr.* 101:889, 1982.
135. Welliver, R. C., et al. The development of respiratory syncytial virus-specific IgE and the release of histamine in nasopharyngeal secretions after infection. *N. Engl. J. Med.* 305:841, 1981.
136. Welliver, R. C., Kaul, A., and Ogra, P. L. Cell-mediated immune response to respiratory syncytial virus infection: Relationship to the development of reactive airway disease. *J. Pediatr.* 94:370, 1979.
137. Welliver, R. C., Kaul, T. N., and Ogra, P. L. The appearance of cell-bound IgE in respiratory-tract epithelium after respiratory-syncytial-virus infection. *N. Engl. J. Med.* 303:1198, 1980.
138. Wolfsdorf, J., and Swift, D. L. An animal model simulating acute infective airway obstruction of childhood and its use in the investigation of croup therapy. *Pediatr. Res.* 12:1062, 1978.
139. Zach, M., Erben, A., and Olinsky, A. Croup, recurrent croup, allergy, and airways hyper-reactivity. *Arch. Dis. Child.* 56:336, 1981.
140. Zach, M. S., Schnall, R. P., and Landau, L. I. Upper and lower airway hyperreactivity in recurrent croup. *Am. Rev. Respir. Dis.* 121:979, 1980.
141. Busse, W. W., Lemanske, R. F. Jr., and Dick, E. C. The relationship of viral respiratory infection and asthma. *Chest* 101(Suppl. 6):385S, 1992.
142. Hogg, J. C. Persistent and latent viral infections in the pathology of asthma. *Am. Rev. Respir. Dis.* 145:S7, 1992.
143. Huftel, M. A., et al. The effect of T-cell depletion on enhanced basophil histamine release after in vitro incubation with live influenza A virus. *Am. J. Respir. Cell. Mol. Biol.* 7:434, 1992.
144. Jarreau, P., et al. Effects of neuraminidase on airway reactivity in the guinea pig. *Am. Rev. Respir. Dis.* 145:906, 1992.
145. Nadel, J. A. Regulation of neurogenic inflammation by neutral endopeptidase. *Am. Rev. Respir. Dis.* 145:S48, 1992.
146. Nagayama, Y. Infection and asthma. V. Study of childhood asthma and viral infection by cytologic analysis of nasal smears. *Arerugi* 41:485, 1992.
147. Pattemore, P. K., Johnston, S. L., and Bardin, P. G. Viruses as precipitants of asthma symptoms. I. Epidemiology. *Clin. Exp. Allergy* 22:325, 1992.

Environmental Factors: Air Pollution, Weather, and Noxious Gases

45

Jack D. Hackney
William S. Linn

Most if not all asthmatics suffer from an impairment of their airways' ability to deal with certain stresses in the external air environment. This chapter reviews the known effects of common stresses—man-made air pollutants, unfavorable temperatures, and unfavorable humidity levels. The immediately preceding and following chapters discuss the effects of naturally-occurring airborne allergens, occupational pollutant exposures, and temperature and humidity as they relate to exercise. Clinical management of asthma by control of the patient's air environment is discussed in this chapter and in Chapter 87. Various chapters in Part I discuss relevant mechanistic issues. The mechanisms of response to most air pollutants are not fully understood. Therefore, this chapter emphasizes the empirical information likely to be useful in clinical medicine: the known bronchoconstrictive and symptomatic responses to specific environmental factors, the known effects of asthma medications in mitigating those responses, and the potentially useful therapeutic measures based on protection of the patient from an unfavorable environment.

ISSUES IN SCIENTIFIC AND CLINICAL EVALUATION

The scientific literature relating air pollution to asthma is extensive. Only a brief and highly selective review is possible here. Comprehensive reviews of health research are published periodically by the U.S. Environmental Protection Agency in air quality criteria documents [21–23]. A number of more concise general reviews [3, 10, 12, 37, 68] and specialized reviews [5, 15, 25, 31, 46–48, 50, 54, 55, 63] on the health effects of air pollution are available. Most published scientific evidence is only indirectly useful to the clinicians who must identify etiologic factors and plan treatment for specific patients. Manifestations of asthma vary markedly among individuals and vary over time in the same individual, so that even the best-designed investigations can answer only small parts of the broad fundamental question "Does asthma become worse when pollution (or weather) becomes worse?"

Research can employ either a laboratory approach, an epidemiologic approach, or a combination of both. Controlled laboratory investigations of volunteers can relate specific environmental stresses to specific asthmatic responses, and determine dose-response relationships. A few laboratory studies have addressed the issue of clinical variation, but most of them deal with small homogeneous groups studied briefly in atypical environments, so their results may not be relevant to a broad range of patients. Epidemiologic studies can relate more directly to real-life experiences and encompass a broader range of patients, but must deal with larger populations under less favorable observing conditions. Thus, their measurements of exposures, health responses, and confounding factors are limited in precision and scope. Even when a strong statistical association between environment and asthma is demonstrated, the specific cause and the clinical implications may be unclear. Any laboratory or epidemiologic findings require careful evaluation to judge their validity and relevance to clinical medicine.

Ideally, susceptibility to environmental factors should be tested scientifically as part of the clinical evaluation of every asthmatic patient. In practice, this is seldom feasible. Nevertheless, clinicians and patients can employ scientific investigative principles to help identify adverse environmental influences. For example, a suspected pollution-sensitive patient may be asked to keep a detailed diary of symptoms, medication use, activities, geographic location, and stresses experienced (environmental or otherwise) for a period of days or weeks. The diary may then be compared with published pollution and weather data to address the important practical questions: Does clinical exacerbation (increased symptoms or increased medication requirement) consistently follow unfavorable changes in the air environment (higher pollution levels or bad weather)? Can other precipitating factors (e.g., emotional stress, allergens, infection) be ruled out? If the answers are "Yes," there is a sound basis for therapeutic intervention to protect the patient from the air environment.

Either outdoor air, indoor air, or both may present risk to a particular asthmatic patient [72]. The indoor environment protects against the extremes of weather and may protect against some outdoor pollutants. On the other hand, typical indoor environments contain many pollution sources and may become severely contaminated when air exchange with the outside is slow. Furthermore, most people spend far more time indoors than outdoors, increasing the relative importance of indoor respiratory hazards.

OUTDOOR AIR POLLUTION

The level of outdoor pollution in a given community depends strongly on local fuel-burning activity (in "stationary sources" and motor vehicles) and on local atmospheric conditions, which govern how rapidly the combustion products are dispersed. Even where local emission rates are low, prevailing winds may transport pollutants from sources hundreds of kilometers away. Rarely, natural sources such as volcanos emit pollution more severe than the man-made variety. Knowledge of the physical and chemical nature, concentrations, and sources of local pollutants is essential for judging their potential risks to health. In evaluating specific patients, it is important to consider the air quality in the various personal "microenvironments" they inhabit

Supported in part by the Electric Power Research Institute, Health Effects Institute, Southern California Edison Company, National Institute of Environmental Health Sciences, and American Petroleum Institute.

at home, at work, and elsewhere, as well as the overall air quality in the community. Different microenvironments may vary greatly in air quality. Airborne biologic agents—allergens and pathogenic microorganisms—must receive attention along with man-made pollutants, because in the aggregate the biologic agents probably cause far more respiratory illness [31]. Any attempt to protect an asthmatic patient by improving his or her microenvironmental air quality should address both man-made pollutants and biologic agents.

Combustion of any common fuel produces carbon monoxide (CO) and hydrocarbons from incompletely burned fuel, and nitric oxide (NO) from atmospheric nitrogen. The comparatively innocuous NO reacts with atmospheric oxygen to produce more toxic nitrogen dioxide (NO_2). The health risks from NO_2 and CO are discussed in the section on indoor air pollution. Oxides of nitrogen, hydrocarbons, and sunlight interact to produce a mixture of "photochemical oxidants," the most important of which is ozone (O_3) [65]. "Photochemical smog" is often associated with Los Angeles, which has the highest known ambient O_3 concentrations. However, many other urban and rural areas also experience levels high enough to present a health concern, especially during prolonged warm, sunny weather.

Coal and oil usually contain sulfur and noncombustible trace mineral constituents. When burned, they release a mixture of sulfur dioxide (SO_2) gas and fine mineral particles—the *sulfur oxide–particulate complex.* The SO_2 may react with atmospheric oxygen and water vapor to form sulfuric acid (H_2SO_4), which may in turn react with atmospheric ammonia to form sulfate salts. Particles formed by atmospheric reactions of gases are known as *secondary particles,* in contrast to *primary particles* directly emitted from pollution sources. Secondary-particle formation is also important in photochemical smog. Most secondary particles are small (≤ 1 μm in diameter) and thus when inhaled are deposited in the lower respiratory tract. Unlike photochemical smog, the sulfur oxide–particulate complex is often associated with cold or foggy weather. However, these two major categories of air pollution are not mutually exclusive: SO_2 may react with coexisting photochemical O_3 to form H_2SO_4, and even in the absence of sulfur compounds, strongly acidic particulate pollution may form as NO_2 is converted to nitric acid (HNO_3). "Acid summer haze," containing O_3, SO_2, and acidic particulate matter, is common in eastern North America and has shown some association with an increased incidence of respiratory illness [14].

Table 45-1 lists common outdoor air pollutants likely to affect the cardiopulmonary system, and short-term National Ambient Air Quality Standards (NAAQS) established by the U.S. Environmental Protection Agency. These standards are intended to protect the health of sensitive people and to include a margin of safety. Nevertheless, measurable physiologic and clinical effects are possible under exposure conditions that do not violate the NAAQS (see later).

Table 45-1. Common outdoor air pollutants and short-term ambient air quality standards

Pollutant	NAAQS[a]
Ozone	0.12 ppm, 1-hr average
Sulfur dioxide	0.14 ppm, 24-hr average
Nitrogen dioxide	0.25 ppm, 1-hr average[b]
Carbon monoxide	9 ppm, 8-hr average
Particulate matter[c]	150 μg/m^3, 24-hr average

[a] Primary National Ambient Air Quality Standard (NAAQS) established by the U.S. Environmental Protection Agency to protect the health of sensitive people; not to be exceeded more than 3 times in 3 years; equivalent to a Pollutant Standard Index (PSI) of 100, as reported by air-monitoring agencies.
[b] California state standard; no short-term NAAQS has been established.
[c] Particles of less than 10 μm mass median aerodynamic diameter (PM_{10}).

Respiratory Effects of Sulfur Dioxide and Particulate Matter

SO_2 and H_2SO_4 aerosol are potent respiratory irritants at concentrations above the range experienced in ambient air pollution. In past severe pollution episodes accompanied by markedly increased rates of illness and death, concentrations of SO_2 and particulate matter were shown to be very high, and H_2SO_4 concentrations probably were high also, although few specific monitoring data were available. In London in December 1952, 4 days of fog and intense pollution was associated with 3,500 to 4,000 premature deaths, occurring concurrently and during the next 2 weeks, among 8 million residents [49]. Most deaths occurred in people with preexisting chronic cardiorespiratory disease. Bronchitis was by far the most common pulmonary condition reported as a cause of death. Asthma was reported as a cause of death only infrequently and did not figure prominently in the reports of nonfatal illness related to the fog. Whether asthma played any part in the bronchitis deaths is not known. Ambient SO_2 concentrations during this episode exceeded 1 part per million by volume (ppm), and concentrations of particulate pollution reached several thousand micrograms per cubic meter of air, as 24-hour averages. Under somewhat similar atmospheric conditions in Donora, Pennsylvania in 1948, a population of 14,000 experienced 18 deaths attributed to pollution, as well as a very high rate of respiratory illness [1]. In a retrospective survey, more than 80 percent of asthmatics reported being ill, compared with about 40 percent of those without chronic respiratory problems. Present-day SO_2 and particulate levels during North American pollution episodes have decreased by 80 or 90 percent compared to those during the London and Donora incidents. The highest ambient concentrations now usually occur near metal smelters or large power plants, rather than in large cities.

Despite greatly reduced ambient SO_2 and particulate exposures, epidemiologic studies have continued to show statistical associations between ambient pollution levels and mortality or respiratory illnesses, including asthmatic attacks [3, 12, 13, 23, 25, 37, 46, 48, 51, 63] (Fig. 45-1). These associations may reflect the true effects of monitored pollutants (individually or in combination) on health, or influences of unidentified environmental factors that vary concurrently with pollution levels. In a detailed cross-sectional comparison of schoolchildren from six U.S. cities, spirometric measurements and asthma prevalence rates did not differ significantly between cities in relation to air quality [19]. However, rates of physician-diagnosed bronchitis increased significantly with the cities' pollution levels, relating most strongly to fine particulate matter or to particulate sulfate (which likely included H_2SO_4). In children with asthma or persistent wheeze, both the overall bronchitis rate and the pollution-associated increase were markedly larger than in healthy children (Fig. 45-2) [19]. Short-term longitudinal studies have suggested temporary losses in spirometric performance in generally healthy populations of schoolchildren during pollution episodes with 24-hour ambient concentrations of 0.1 to 0.2 ppm for SO_2 and 200 to 400 μg/m^3 for total particulate matter [17, 18]. The implications for asthmatic individuals are not known. A cross-sectional study of nonsmoking women in a coal-burning region showed that reports of wheezing increased with ambient SO_2 levels [57]. On the other hand, a longitudinal analysis of urban hospital admissions for asthma showed no relationship to SO_2 pollution [26].

In controlled exposures to SO_2, asthmatic individuals are consistently more reactive than healthy volunteers, in terms of bronchoconstriction and symptoms [42, 60]. Some atopic individuals without clinical asthma are especially SO_2 reactive also [42]. At SO_2 concentrations in the 0.3- to 0.5-ppm range, most asthmatic volunteers show no effect at rest but develop clinically meaningful bronchoconstriction after 3 to 5 minutes of vigorous exercise with oronasal breathing. Such concentrations are uncommon in

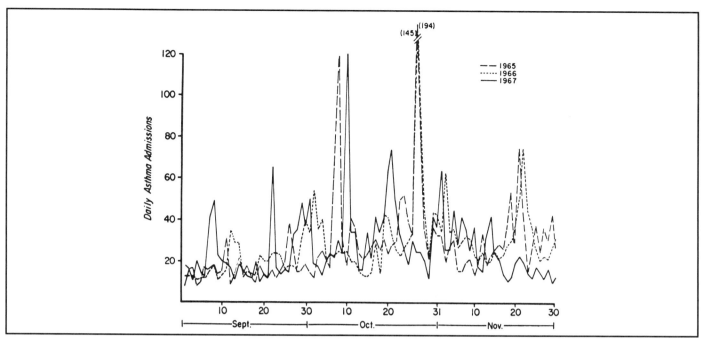

Fig. 45-1. *Daily asthma admissions to a large New Orleans hospital during three successive fall seasons. Although the sudden substantial increases in asthma morbidity strongly suggest an effect of unfavorable air quality, the complexity and variability of the air environment preclude identification of any specific causal agent (man-made or natural) in this and in most other community-based studies. (Reprinted with permission from J. Salvaggio, et al. New Orleans asthma: II. Relationship of climatologic and seasonal factors to outbreaks. J. Allergy 45:257, 1970.)*

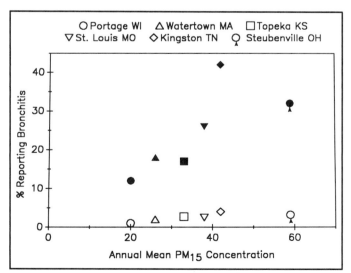

Fig. 45-2. *Percentage of 10- to 12-year-old schoolchildren who experienced at least one episode of bronchitis during a year (as reported by parents on a questionnaire), versus the annual average concentration of airborne particles less than 15 μm in diameter (PM$_{15}$), in six cities surveyed. Solid symbols indicate children with asthma or persistent wheezing (about 10% of survey population); open symbols, all other children. (Redrawn from D. W. Dockery, et al. Effects from inhalable particles on respiratory health of children. Am. Rev. Respir. Dis. 139:587, 1989.)*

ambient air, but may occur for short periods even when the 24-hour-average concentration meets the ambient air quality standard. SO_2-induced bronchoconstriction typically reverses within an hour after stopping exercise, even if exposure continues. The bronchoconstriction seems not to increase with increasing exposure time, and has not been associated with prolonged or delayed asthmatic attacks: It is exacerbated by low temperature and relative humidity [43] and is prevented or mitigated by inhaled beta-adrenergic bronchodilators (Fig. 45-3) [36, 44], by cromolyn [59], and by atropine [62] but apparently not by inhaled corticosteroids [70]. According to indirect evidence [44], minimum therapeutic doses of theophylline do not protect against SO_2 effects, except in that they improve baseline lung function. Higher doses have not been tested. In most of these respects, SO_2-induced bronchoconstriction resembles exercise-induced bronchoconstriction, discussed in Chapter 47. In ordinary circumstances, any effects from ambient SO_2 exposure probably would appear after exercise. However, the SO_2 response is a function of the inhaled dose rate (the product of ventilation rate and concentration), not of exercise per se. Concentrations experienced in polluted workplaces or in accidental outdoor SO_2 releases might induce bronchoconstriction even at rest.

Ambient particulate pollution is too complex to reproduce in the laboratory, so controlled exposure studies commonly employ aqueous H_2SO_4 aerosols to model the respiratory irritant fraction. (Less acidic aerosol substances generally have shown no respiratory irritant properties at ambient-like exposure concentrations.) Most investigations have used H_2SO_4 particles well within the respirable size range—1 μm or less in average diameter—comparable with typical ambient acid aerosols. A few studies have modeled acid-polluted fog, with average particle sizes of the order of 10 μm. In adult asthmatic volunteers exposed for 1 hour or less, H_2SO_4 concentrations of 400 μg/m³ or higher, either with small or with large particle sizes, are necessary to induce meas-

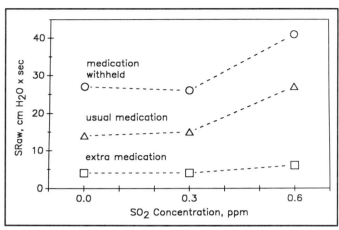

Fig. 45-3. *Mean specific airway resistance (SRaw) of 21 adult asthmatic volunteers after 10-minute exposures to SO₂ with vigorous exercise. The upper curve represents exposures with medication completely or partly withheld; the middle curve, exposures while subjects were taking their regular medication (most commonly oral theophylline) on their regular schedule; and the lower curve, exposures with subjects on regular medication supplemented with a normal adult dose of inhaled metaproterenol sulfate just prior to exposure. (Data from W. S. Linn, et al. Responses to sulfur dioxide and exercise by medication-dependent asthmatics: Effect of varying medication levels.* Arch. Environ. Health *45:24, 1990.)*

urable bronchoconstriction and irritant symptoms [8, 45, 66]. Ambient H_2SO_4 concentrations seldom exceed 40 µg/m³ when averaged over 12 to 24 hours [63]; shorter-term peak concentrations are difficult to measure. One series of studies with asthmatic adolescents showed mild bronchoconstriction after 10 minutes of exercise at exposure concentrations near the ambient range—60 to 100 µg/m³ [35]. Another presumably similar investigation showed little response [9].

In summary, laboratory dose-response information demonstrates that many asthmatics are unusually reactive to inhaled SO_2 and may experience bronchoconstriction even in very brief exposures under "worst case" ambient exposure conditions (i.e., when exercising outdoors near a pollution source). Epidemiologic evidence associates asthma and related respiratory illnesses with particulate pollution (respirable acidic aerosols in particular), and less strongly with SO_2. Laboratory studies indicate that asthmatic subjects are less likely to react to H_2SO_4 aerosol than to SO_2 at ambient concentrations. However, there is some evidence that younger asthmatics are especially susceptible to H_2SO_4, and may react to brief exposures at maximum ambient concentrations. Prolonged exposures to acid (>1 hour) have not been studied extensively in the laboratory, but are common in ambient pollution episodes.

Respiratory Effects of Photochemical Oxidants

Epidemiologic evidence is less extensive for oxidants than for SO_2 and particulates. One early study of a panel of asthmatic subjects in the Los Angeles area showed increasing reports of attacks when total oxidant (primarily O_3) levels were high (around 0.25 ppm as a 1-hour average). A small minority of the subject population accounted for all the increase [58]. A later, larger-scale panel study again showed a significant association between asthma attack rate and daily peak O_3 concentration [69]. Somewhat similar findings were obtained in Houston, where O_3 pollution is less intense than in Los Angeles but still violates ambient air quality standards frequently [32]. A panel of asthmatic subjects in Tucson, where O_3 levels usually meet air quality standards, showed significant negative associations between

daily measurements of lung function and outdoor concentrations of both O_3 and NO_2 [40]. An investigation of Los Angeles asthmatic children indicated that emergency room visits did not increase with rising O_3 concentrations, although lung function tended to decrease with increasing O_3 [52]. All these studies probably reflect exposures to O_3 without much sulfur pollution. In the Northeast, O_3 occurs at lower concentrations but may be accompanied by SO_2 and H_2SO_4. As mentioned previously, this "acid summer haze" mixture has shown some association with increased hospital admissions for respiratory illness [14]. Several studies of generally healthy children attending summer camps, both in the Northeast and in the Los Angeles area, have indicated that lung function tends to decrease slightly when ambient O_3 levels increase [30, 47]. The implications for asthmatics are not known.

Numerous controlled exposure studies have shown lung dysfunction and respiratory irritant symptoms at O_3 exposure concentrations within the ambient range [29, 47, 34a]. Unlike the SO_2 effect, the O_3 effect is primarily a restrictive ventilatory dysfunction rather than an obstructive one, is comparatively slow in onset, and becomes more intense with increasing duration of exposure. With heavy exercise, 1 to 2 hours of exposure at 0.15 to 0.20 ppm induces measurable effects in some healthy volunteers. Such exposure levels occur frequently in Los Angeles and occasionally in many other places. In longer exposures with sustained heavy exercise, measurable effects occur at or below the air quality standard concentration of 0.12 ppm [24]. Bronchoalveolar lavage studies indicate appreciable inflammatory responses in the lower respiratory tract after O_3 exposure [38]. The implications of these acute responses for the development or aggravation of chronic diseases, including asthma, are uncertain. However, many possible mechanisms of oxidative injury have been associated with O_3, NO_2, and other common pollutants [16b]; at least some of them may relate meaningfully to chronic disease. Clinical susceptibility to O_3 effects varies widely among individuals, for unknown reasons. Controlled exposures of asthmatic subjects have suggested that their responses to O_3 are similar to those of healthy volunteers and do not often include asthma attacks. However, in one study focusing on the most and least reactive individuals from a large volunteer group, asthmatic subjects and atopic subjects were significantly overrepresented in the most reactive segment [27]. Thus, asthmatics may have a moderately increased risk of respiratory disturbances from ambient O_3 exposure, and the risk is appreciable even for healthy people.

INDOOR AIR POLLUTION

Pollutants found indoors may have outdoor sources, indoor sources, or both. Chemically reactive outdoor pollutants, including SO_2 and O_3, tend to react with wall and furniture surface coatings; hence, their concentrations are often (but not always) lower indoors than outdoors. Outdoor particulate pollutants may also show decreased concentrations indoors because of deposition on indoor surfaces. Indoor levels of NO_2 and CO depend on their outdoor concentrations, the amounts produced by indoor combustion, and the rate of indoor-outdoor air exchange. Either indoor or outdoor sources may predominate. Gases and aerosols released indoors by structural elements, furnishings, or consumer products typically occur at very low concentrations outdoors, so their indoor concentrations are more or less inversely proportional to air exchange rates.

Because detailed air monitoring at numerous sites is seldom practical, most epidemiologic studies of indoor pollution have characterized exposures according to specific pollution sources in subjects' homes, for example, smokers, gas kitchen stoves, fireplaces, and unvented or incompletely vented space heaters (whether gas, oil, wood, or coal fired) [5, 15, 37, 54, 55].

"Second-hand" tobacco smoke contains a variety of gas and particulate pollutants. Most of the relevant epidemiology relates to children of smoking parents (see also Chap. 2). The majority of studies, though not all, have indicated that smoke exposure at home increases children's incidence of wheezing and other respiratory symptoms and/or decreases their rate of lung function growth [54]. Of the few controlled studies of asthmatic volunteers exposed to tobacco smoke, some have indicated lung dysfunction at exposure levels attainable in poorly ventilated rooms with multiple smokers, and others have not shown function changes [64, 71].

Among indoor-polluting home appliances, gas stoves are most common. One of the most important pollutants emitted by gas stoves is NO_2. Numerous epidemiologic investigations on the effects of gas stoves have been conducted in adults and children. The results have been mixed, but the more recent and comprehensive investigations generally have shown no significant effect, or only very small negative effects, on lung function or respiratory illness rates [54]. Short-term effects of NO_2 on asthmatics have been studied fairly extensively in controlled exposures. As in the case of H_2SO_4, most investigations of NO_2 have shown little effect at realistic exposure levels. However, some evidence indicates that a subgroup of asthmatic subjects may be susceptible to bronchoconstriction when exposed briefly to as little as 0.3 ppm of NO_2 during exercise [55]. Concentrations above 0.3 ppm may occur in poorly ventilated kitchens even when the outdoor air is clean. They also occur occasionally outdoors in Los Angeles, the city with the most severe NO_2 pollution.

Portable liquid-fueled unvented heaters may release substantial quantities of SO_2 if the fuel contains sulfur [39]. However, CO presents the most important health risk from unvented or malfunctioning heaters, causing an appreciable number of accidental deaths and acute illnesses [54]. Asthmatics are not unusually susceptible to CO, except in that carboxyhemoglobin formation will exacerbate any preexisting problems of oxygen delivery, including those related to airway obstruction. The best-documented effect of CO at moderate exposure levels is an increased susceptibility to exercise angina in persons with coronary artery disease [2].

A wide variety of potentially toxic substances can be emitted into indoor air by components of the building itself or its contents. Few of these have been investigated thoroughly; careful clinical evaluation seems the only practical way to judge a given substance's effect on an asthmatic patient. One common indoor contaminant that may be of special concern to asthmatics is formaldehyde (HCHO) [28, 54]. Particle board, plywood, foam insulation, floor coverings, and tobacco smoke are among the numerous possible sources of HCHO in indoor air. Indoor concentrations are well below 0.1 ppm in typical well-ventilated homes, but may exceed 1 ppm in poorly ventilated homes with large indoor sources. Nonspecific irritant responses to HCHO in homes may induce asthma symptoms, but specific immunologic sensitization to HCHO has been documented only in patients exposed occupationally [54].

Radon (a chemically inert radioactive gas) and radon decay products (which become attached to airborne particles) are fairly common indoor pollutants that present a long-term risk of lung cancer. Asthmatics who live in homes with elevated radon levels may be especially at risk if they spend an unusually high percentage of time indoors or keep their homes more tightly closed than usual. Mitigation of radon and of other indoor pollution problems may require increased ventilation with outdoor air, and thus may increase exposure to outdoor pollutants and biologic agents.

WEATHER

Weather-related factors may have a broad range of effects on asthmatic patients. Existing weather may induce a direct physio-logic response or a psychologically mediated response. A change in weather may induce a response by itself or by changing the concentrations of airborne pollutants or allergens. Long-term weather characteristics (i.e., climate) determine the nature of vegetation in a given area and thus the nature and quantity of airborne allergens. To determine the influence of these various factors separately is difficult, since any clinical intervention usually affects several of them at once.

Cold, damp, or windy/dusty weather conditions are often thought to exacerbate asthma, but epidemiologic evidence relating asthma attacks to short-term weather changes is equivocal [11]. A longer-term influence of climate on asthma is suggested by the observation that the age of onset seems appreciably greater in tropical southern Asia than in temperate western nations. Differences in heredity and life-styles complicate the interpretation, however [11].

Temperature and relative humidity are the weather factors most easily isolated and studied in the laboratory. Their short-term effects have been elucidated in some detail in studies of exercise-induced bronchoconstriction, discussed in Chapter 47. In many asthmatic patients, the degree of airway cooling by inspired air predicts the degree of bronchoconstriction experienced during exercise. Cooling is promoted by high ventilation rates, mouth breathing, low air temperature, and low relative humidity (which increases evaporative cooling within the airways). In some individuals the bronchoconstrictive effects of exercise in cold air can be mitigated by breathing through a mask that warms and humidifies the inspired air [56]. On the other hand, some asthmatics' airways constrict with exercise even in warm humid air [6], and humidification therapy has been reported to affect some asthmatic children favorably and others unfavorably, in terms of respiratory mechanics [53]. Thus, although temperature and humidity levels clearly have important influences on asthma, their effects in specific situations are difficult to predict. Relatively high temperature and humidity in themselves may often have a favorable effect, but they may also facilitate the production of allergens and disease organisms. In the previously mentioned six-city study of schoolchildren, chronic dampness was found in more than half the homes surveyed, and was strongly associated with lung function decrements and respiratory symptoms [16].

A change of residence, either temporary or permanent, is sometimes recommended to mitigate asthma. A long-distance move substantially changes the outdoor air environment, the indoor air environment, and the psychological and social environment, any of which may affect the patient's condition importantly. Since all factors change concurrently, the specific cause of any clinical improvement or deterioration usually cannot be documented. Little objective evidence exists concerning the long-term benefits of residence changes. One survey of asthmatic and allergic college alumni indicated that those who moved to distant areas with fewer airborne allergens experienced rapid and long-lasting clinical improvement. Those who did not move far improved to a lesser extent [61]. A group of middle-aged asthmatic and bronchitic patients from a cold, damp environment reported clinical improvement after attending a residential treatment center in a warmer, drier climate; however, objective measures of improvement were less convincing [33].

PROTECTION FROM UNFAVORABLE AIR ENVIRONMENTS

Therapeutic measures to mitigate the ill effects of an asthmatic's air environment may depend on avoidance (separating the patient from the unfavorable environmental factor) or personal protection (conditioning or purifying the air before the patient breathes it) [4]. Few of these therapeutic measures have been subjected to well-controlled clinical trials. The physician must exercise creativity and good judgment to design a treatment appropriate to the individual patient's physiologic and clinical status and compatible with the psychological, economic, and cultural characteristics of the patient and his or her family [41]. Before recommending any action, the physician should verify, to the extent possible, that the environmental exposure in question actually worsens the patient's disease, that the action contemplated will substantially reduce exposure, and that harmful side effects of the action will not outweigh its expected benefits.

Avoidance

The most straightforward course of action may be to remove the patient from the unfavorable environment or to modify the patient's behavior to reduce the level of environmental stress. Staying indoors will reduce or eliminate exposure to some outdoor pollutants and to extreme temperature or humidity. Advice to remain indoors presupposes due care to maintain good indoor air quality. Avoiding exercise will reduce the effective dose of pollutants or of cold stress, to the extent that ventilatory requirement is reduced. Change of residence is the most drastic common avoidance action. As discussed previously, there is some but not much evidence of benefit from changing residence. This should be recommended only when there is strong evidence that the patient's existing environment is deleterious and that the proposed new environment is substantially better. In some cases, avoidance is easily accomplished by keeping particular offending materials (e.g., consumer products with irritating vapors) away from the patient. The potential benefit from such simple actions should be explored thoroughly before more drastic measures are contemplated.

Personal Protection

Often the first priority in personal protection will be to maintain good air quality in the patient's home. Air quality in the workplace should be given attention also, even when there are no occupational exposures of concern. These issues are discussed further in Chapters 46 and 87. See also Tables 42-4 and 45-2. The American Thoracic Society has published a guide to the identification and correction of indoor air quality problems [5].

As suggested previously, air conditioning may benefit some asthmatics by maintaining favorable temperature and humidity levels. If they are poorly designed or poorly maintained, air conditioners also can disseminate harmful biologic agents. Most of them have little or no provision for removing man-made air pollutants, but effective air-cleaning accessories sometimes may be added to central heating and cooling systems. Typical centralized systems recirculate about 90 percent of their air; thus, if purification is applied only to the small proportion of outside "makeup" air, indoor pollution sources will remain essentially uncontrolled. Ideally the entire output of the air conditioner should be treated to remove pollutants, allergens, and pathogens (Table 45-3; see also Table 42-5).

In the absence of central air conditioning with air purification, a portable device may be used to clean a patient's immediate environment. In the typical portable air cleaner, a blower forces air through an electrostatic precipitator, filters, or both before discharging it to the user's breathing zone. Only a limited space can be cleaned effectively—at most, one room or the interior of an automobile. If the device's output of clean air is low, or if indoor pollution sources are present, or if the inside air exchanges rapidly with the polluted outside air, no benefit can be expected unless the patient breathes very near the clean air outlet. This is most practical while in bed. In a panel of young asth-

Table 45-2. Specific building-related illness

Disease	Etiologic agent	Building source of etiologic agent
Biologic agents		
Infectious diseases		
Legionellosis and related diseases	*Legionella pneumophila* (and related bacteria)	Water reservoirs
		Warm moist environment
Tuberculosis	*Mycobacterium tuberculosis*	Inadequate ventilation
Influenza, respiratory viruses	Virus	Inadequate ventilation
		Crowding
Hypersensitivity pneumonitis	Birds (pigeons, parakeets)	Pigeon droppings in air intakes
	Thermophilic actinomycetes	Contaminated water and slime in air-conditioning systems
	Contaminated cold organisms	
	Miscellaneous fungi in stagnant water	
Asthma	Arthropods (house dust mites, cockroaches)	Increased humidity, old carpet
	Animals (cats, dogs, rodents)	Water leaks
	Fungus	Poor sanitation
Chemical agents		
Carbon monoxide intoxication and poisoning	Carbon monoxide	Combustion products
		Faulty furnace
		Vehicular exhaust
		Nonvented combustion sources
		Liquid paint strippers
Asthma	TDI	Occupational or home hobby exposure to substances
	Platinum	
	Nickel	
	Cobalt salts	
	Formaldehyde	
Physical agents		
Lung cancer	Asbestos fibers	Asbestos fibers in home/building construction
	Cigarette smoke	Smoking
Radioactive agents		
Lung cancer	Radon	Radon in soil leaking into house

TDI = toluene diisocyanate.
Source: American Thoracic Society. Environmental controls and lung disease. *Am. Rev. Respir. Dis.* 142:915, 1990.

Table 45-3. *Comparision of modular ETS-cleaning devices*

	Units tested (n)	Costs of device	Replacement filter costs	Flow rate (cfm)	Particulate ECR (cfm)	Gas cleaning
Flat filter	LBL 3	$30–$40	$4–$6	10–29	0–3	Not effective
	CR 12	$15–$100	$4–$6 ($15–$41)	20–100	2–8 (14)	
With ion generator	LBL 1	$150	$12	17	7	Not effective
	CR 1	$299	$16	40–60	47	
Pleated filter	LBL 1	$395	$77	157	180	Not effective
	CR 4	$45–$140	$5–$20	10–90	6–33	
With ion generator	LBL 1	$295	$16	66	57	Not effective
	CR 2	$100	$7–$15	20–100	13–47	
Electrostatic precipitators	LBL 2	$370–$395	$15	200–215	116–122	Not effective
	CR 1	$158	$7	40–90	19	
Ion generators	LBL 2	$80–$120	—	—	1–30	Not effective
	CR 3	$44–$79	—	—	13–58	
Fan	LBL 1	$52	—	1,800	1	
No cleaning	CR				2	

Definition of abbreviations: ETS = environmental tobacco smoke; ECR = effective clearance rate; LBL = Lawrence Berkeley Laboratory [50a]; CR = Consumer Reports [16a]; cfm = cubic feet per minute.
Source: American Thoracic Society. Environmental controls and lung disease. *Am. Rev. Respir. Dis.* 142:915, 1990.

matic subjects sensitive to house dust mites, use of an air-cleaning bed attachment resulted in a decreased need for medication [67].

Negative ion generation is sometimes claimed to benefit respiratory health. Objective evidence of benefit in asthmatics is very limited and equivocal [34]. If negative ion generators do provide any benefit, it may relate either to the physiologic effects of the ions per se or to the removal of airborne particles by electrostatic precipitation.

In some circumstances, masks may be of use for personal protection. Warming and humidifying masks to mitigate exercise-induced bronchoconstriction have been mentioned previously. Masks to remove pollutants are common in industry, but clinical applications have been rare. Surgical masks or similar pollen-and-dust masks may protect well against biologic agents but not against noxious gases or small particles. "Nuisance odor masks" designed for occupational use may provide significant protection against inhaled O_3 [7]. These are similar to disposable surgical masks but incorporate activated carbon to remove pollutant gases, as well as filter media to remove particles. Problems posed by masks include ineffectiveness owing to poor fit, unattractive appearance, interference with speech, and increased work of breathing—of particular importance to people with airway obstruction.

Any protective device must be both qualitatively and quantitatively adequate for its intended application: It must have the inherent physical or chemical properties necessary to remove the existing pollutants, and it must be able to supply cleaned air at a rate sufficient to meet the existing demands. To remove particulate matter, either electrostatic precipitators or fiber-mat (usually paper) filters may be appropriate. Their effectiveness is best measured by their percentage efficiency in removing particles of the size range in question (see also Chap. 32). Airborne allergens are commonly 10 μm or larger in diameter, and so can be captured efficiently by relatively crude filters or precipitators. Smaller, combustion-related particles deposit readily in the human lower respiratory tract but are difficult to capture on filter fibers or electrostatically charged collector plates. To remove them requires high-efficiency (HEPA) filters, commonly found only in industrial clean rooms and in some small portable air cleaners.

Particulate filters and precipitators are ineffective against pollutant gases. Many gases can be removed from air by "chemical filter" media. The most common of these is activated carbon, which catalytically decomposes O_3 to molecular oxygen, and adsorbs many other pollutant gases. Another common medium, consisting of aluminum oxide impregnated with potassium permanganate, is more effective against SO_2 and NO_2. To remove CO, high-temperature catalytic oxidation is usually required. For long-term effectiveness, all the aforementioned air-cleaning devices require regular servicing or replacement.

REFERENCES

1. *Air Pollution in Donora, Pennsylvania: Epidemiology of the Unusual Smog Episode of October 1948.* Washington, D.C.: U.S. Public Health Service, 1949.
2. Allred, E. N., et al. Short-term effects of carbon monoxide exposure on the exercise performance of subjects with coronary artery disease. *N. Engl. J. Med.* 321:1426, 1989.
3. American Lung Association. *Health Effects of Ambient Air Pollution.* New York: American Lung Association, 1989.
4. American Thoracic Society. *Personal Protection Against Air Pollution: The Physician's Role.* New York: American Lung Association, 1981.
5. American Thoracic Society. Environmental controls and lung disease. *Am. Rev. Respir. Dis.* 142:915, 1990.
6. Anderson, S. D., et al. Sensitivity to heat and water loss at rest and during exercise in asthmatic patients. *Eur. J. Respir. Dis.* 63:459, 1982.
7. Avol, E. L., et al. Laboratory evaluation of a disposable half-face mask for protection against ozone. *Am. Rev. Respir. Dis.* 126:818, 1982.
8. Avol, E. L., et al. Respiratory dose-response study of normal and asthmatic volunteers exposed to sulfuric acid aerosol in the submicrometer size range. *J. Toxicol. Ind. Health* 4:173, 1988.
9. Avol, E. L., et al. Respiratory responses of young asthmatic volunteers in controlled exposures to sulfuric acid aerosol. *Am. Rev. Respir. Dis.* 142: 343, 1990.
10. Balmes, J. R. Emerging issues in ambient air quality and respiratory health. *Probl. Respir. Care* 3:163, 1990.
11. Barbee, R. A. The epidemiology of asthma. *Monogr. Allergy* 21:21, 1987.
12. Bates, D. V. *Respiratory Function in Disease* (3rd ed.). Philadelphia: Saunders, 1989. Pp. 165–171.
13. Bates, D. V., Baker-Anderson, M., and Sizto, R. Asthma attack periodicity: A study of hospital emergency visits in Vancouver. *Environ. Res.* 51:51, 1990.
14. Bates, D. V., and Sizto, R. Air pollution and hospital admissions in southern Ontario: The acid summer haze effect. *Environ. Res.* 43:317, 1987.
15. Boleij, J. S. M., and Brunekreef, B. Domestic pollution as a factor causing respiratory health effects. *Chest* 96:368S, 1989.
16. Brunekreef, B., et al. Home dampness and respiratory morbidity in children. *Am. Rev. Respir. Dis.* 140:1363, 1989.
16a. Consumer Reports. Air cleaners. *Consumer Reports* 50(1):7, 1985.
16b. Crapo, J., et al. Environmental lung diseases: Relationship between acute

inflammatory responses to air pollutants and chronic lung disease. *Am. Rev. Respir. Dis.* 145:1506, 1992.

17. Dassen, W., et al. Decline in children's pulmonary function during an air pollution episode. *J. Air Pollut. Control Assoc.* 36:1223, 1986.

18. Dockery, D. W., et al. Change in pulmonary function of children associated with air pollution episodes. *J. Air Pollut. Control Assoc.* 32:937, 1982.

19. Dockery, D. W., et al. Effects of inhalable particles on respiratory health of children. *Am. Rev. Respir. Dis.* 139:587, 1989.

20. Environmental Protection Agency. *Air Quality Criteria for Oxides of Nitrogen.* Research Triangle Park, N. C.: Environmental Protection Agency, 1982.

21. Environmental Protection Agency. *Air Quality Criteria for Carbon Monoxide.* Research Triangle Park, N.C.: Environmental Protection Agency, 1984.

22. Environmental Protection Agency. *Air Quality Criteria for Ozone and Other Photochemical Oxidants.* Research Triangle Park, N.C.: Environmental Protection Agency, 1986.

23. Environmental Protection Agency. *Second Addendum to Air Quality Criteria for Particulate Matter and Sulfur Oxides.* Research Triangle Park, N. C.: Environmental Protection Agency, 1986.

24. Folinsbee, L. J., McDonnell, W. F., and Horstman, D. H. Pulmonary function and symptom responses after 6.6-hour exposure to 0.12 ppm ozone with moderate exercise. *J. Air Pollut. Control Assoc.* 38:28, 1988.

25. Goldstein, I. F., and Hartel, D. Critical Assessment of Epidemiologic Studies of Environmental Factors and Asthma. In J. Goldsmith (ed.), *Environmental Epidemiology: Community Studies.* Boca Raton, Fla.: CRC Press, 1986. Pp. 101–114.

26. Goldstein, I. F., and Weinstein, A. L. Air pollution and asthma: Effects of exposures to short-term sulfur dioxide peaks. *Environ. Res.* 40:332, 1986.

27. Hackney, J. D., et al. Responses of Selected Reactive and Nonreactive Volunteers to Ozone Exposure in High- and Low-pollution seasons. In T. Schneider, et al. (eds.), *Atmospheric Ozone Research and Its Policy Implications.* Amsterdam: Elsevier, 1989. Pp. 745–753.

28. Hart, R. W., Terturro, A., and Neimeth, L. (eds.), Report of the consensus workshop on formaldehyde. *Environ. Health Perspect.* 58:323, 1984.

29. Hazucha, M. J. Relationship between ozone exposure and pulmonary function changes. *J. Appl. Physiol.* 62:1671, 1987.

30. Higgins, I. T. T., et al. Effect of exposures to ozone on ventilatory lung function in children. *Am. Rev. Respir. Dis.* 141:1136, 1990.

31. Hinkle, L. E., Jr., and Murray, S. H. The importance of the quality of indoor air. *Bull. NY Acad. Med.* 57:827, 1981.

32. Holguin, A. H. et al. Effects of Ozone on Asthmatics in the Houston Area. In S. D. Lee (Ed.), *Evaluation of the Scientific Basis for Ozone/Oxidants Standards.* Pittsburgh: Air Pollution Control Association, 1985. Pp. 262–280.

33. Johansson, M., Simonsson, B. G., and Skoogh, B. E. Subjective effects of a change of environment in patients with chronic airways obstruction. *Scand. J. Respir. Dis.* 53:77, 1972.

34. Jones, D. P., et al. Effect of long-term ionized air treatment on patients with bronchial asthma. *Thorax* 31:428, 1976.

34a.Kleinman, M. T. Effects of ozone on pulmonary function: The relationship of response to dose. *J. Expos. Anal. Environ Epidemiol.* 1:309, 1991.

35. Koenig, J. Q., Covert, D. S., and Pierson, W. E. Effects of inhalation of acidic compounds on pulmonary function in allergic adolescent subjects. *Environ. Health Perspect.* 79:173, 1989.

36. Koenig, J. Q., et al. Effects of albuterol on sulfur-dioxide-induced bronchoconstriction in allergic adolescents. *J. Allergy Clin. Immunol.* 79:54, 1987.

37. Koenig, J. Q., Pierson, W. E., and Bierman, C. W. The effects of atmospheric air pollution. *Immunol. Allergy Clin. North Am.* 10:463, 1990.

38. Koren, H. S., et al. Ozone-induced inflammation in the lower airways of human subjects. *Am. Rev. Respir. Dis.* 139:407, 1989.

39. Leaderer, B. P. Air pollutant emissions from kerosene space heaters. *Science* 218:1113, 1982.

40. Lebowitz M. D., et al. Respiratory symptoms and peak flow associated with indoor and outdoor air pollutants in the Southwest. *J. Air Pollut. Control Assoc.* 35:1154, 1985.

41. Leffert, F. Management of chronic asthma. *J. Pediatr.* 97:875, 1980.

42. Linn, W. S., et al. Replicated dose-response study of sulfur dioxide effects in normal, atopic, and asthmatic volunteers. *Am. Rev. Respir. Dis.* 136:1127, 1987.

43. Linn, W. S., et al. Combined effect of sulfur dioxide and cold in exercising asthmatics. *Arch. Environ. Health* 39:339, 1984.

44. Linn, W. S., et al. Responses to sulfur dioxide and exercise by medication-dependent asthmatics: Effect of varying medication levels. *Arch. Environ. Health* 45:24, 1990.

45. Linn, W. S., et al. Effect of droplet size on respiratory responses to inhaled sulfuric acid in normal and asthmatic volunteers. *Am. Rev. Respir. Dis.* 140:161, 1989.

46. Lipfert, F. W. Mortality and air pollution: Is there a meaningful connection? *Environ. Sci. Technol.* 19:764, 1985.

47. Lippmann, M. Health effects of ozone: A critical review. *J. Air Waste Mgmt. Assoc.* 39:672, 1989.

48. Lippmann, M., and Lioy, P. J. Critical issues in air pollution epidemiology. *Environ. Health Perspect.* 62:243, 1985.

49. Ministry of Health. *Morbidity and Mortality during the London Fog of December 1952.* London: Her Majesty's Stationery Office, 1954.

50. Morrow, P. E. Toxicological data on NO_2: An overview. *J. Toxicol. Environ. Health* 13:205, 1984.

50a.Offermann, F. J., et al. Control of respirable particles in indoor air with pactable air cleaners. *Atmos. Environ.* 19:1761, 1985.

51. Pope, C. A. Respiratory disease associated with community air pollution and a steel mill, Utah Valley. *Am. J. Public Health* 79:623, 1989.

52. Richards, W., et al. Los Angeles air pollution and asthma in children. *Ann. Allergy* 47:348, 1981.

53. Rodriguez, G. E., Branch, L. B., and Cotton, E. K. Use of humidity in asthmatic children. *J. Allergy Clin. Immunol.* 56:133, 1975.

54. Samet, J. M., Marbury, M. C., and Spengler, J. D. Health effects and sources of indoor air pollution. *Am. Rev. Respir. Dis.* 136:1486, 1987; 137: 221, 1988.

55. Samet, J. M., and Utell, M. J. The risk of nitrogen dioxide: What have we learned from epidemiological and clinical studies? *Toxicol. Ind. Health* 6:247, 1990.

56. Schachter, E. N., Lach, E., and Lee, M. Protective effect of a cold-weather mask on exercise-induced asthma. *Ann. Allergy* 46:12, 1981.

57. Schenker, M. B., et al. Health effects of air pollution due to coal combustion in the Chestnut Ridge region of Pennsylvania. *Arch. Environ. Health.* 38:325, 1983.

58. Schoettlin, C. E., and Landau, E. Air pollution and asthmatic attacks in the Los Angeles area. *Public Health Rep.* 76:545, 1961.

59. Sheppard, D., Nadel, J. A., and Boushey, H. A. Inhibition of sulfur-dioxide-induced bronchoconstriction by sodium cromoglycate in asthmatic subjects. *Am. Rev. Respir. Dis.* 124:257, 1981.

60. Sheppard, D., et al. Lower threshold and greater bronchomotor responsiveness of asthmatics to sulfur dioxide. *Am. Rev. Respir. Dis.* 122:873, 1980.

61. Smith, J. M. Long-term effect of moving on patients with asthma and hay fever. *J. Allergy Clin. Immunol.* 48:191, 1971.

62. Snashall, P. D., and Baldwin, C. Mechanisms of sulfur dioxide induced bronchoconstriction in normal and asthmatic man. *Thorax* 37:118, 1982.

63. Spengler, J. D., Brauer, M., and Koutrakis, P. Acid air and health. *Environ. Sci. Technol.* 24:946, 1990.

64. Stankus, R. P., et al. Cigarette-smoke-sensitive asthma: Challenge studies. *J. Allergy Clin. Immunol.* 82:331, 1988.

65. Stern, A. C. (ed.), *Air Pollution,* Vol. 1 (3rd ed.). New York: Academic Press, 1977.

66. Utell, M. J., et al. Airway responses to sulfate and sulfuric acid aerosols in asthmatics. *Am. Rev. Respir. Dis.* 128:444, 1983.

67. Verrall, B., et al. Laminar flow air cleaner bed attachment: A controlled trial. *Ann. Allergy* 61:117, 1988.

68. Waller, R. E. Atmospheric pollution. *Chest* 96:363S, 1989.

69. Whittemore, A. S., and Korn, E. L. Asthma and air pollution in the Los Angeles area. *Am. J. Public Health* 70:687, 1980.

70. Wiebicke, W., Jörres, R., and Magnussen, H. Comparison of the effects of inhaled corticosteroids on the airway response to histamine, methacholine, hyperventilation, and sulfur dioxide in subjects with asthma. *J. Allergy Clin. Immunol.* 86:915, 1990.

71. Wiedemann, H. P., et al. Acute effects of passive smoking on lung function and airway reactivity in asthmatic subjects. *Chest* 89:180, 1986.

72. Pierson, W. E., and Koenig, J. Q. Respiratory effects of air pollution on allergic disease. *J. Allergy Clin. Immunol.* 90:557, 1992.

Occupational Asthma

Stuart M. Brooks

46

Occupational asthma is a disorder in which there is induced specific and/or nonspecific airway hyperresponsiveness, which may be reversible, caused by an acute or chronic inhalation of substances or materials that a worker manufactures or uses directly or that are incidentally present at the work site. This definition encompasses a variety of disorders of airways, regardless of their cause, and includes processes that occur as a result of both immunologic and nonimmunologic mechanisms. Clinically, occupational asthma is manifested by work-related symptoms of chest tightness, wheezing, and cough but may occur as predominant nocturnal manifestations. Physiologically, there are alterations in lung mechanics that change with time. There is characteristically an increased sensitivity to many and varied nonspecific airborne physical, chemical, and pharmacologic agents. While airway obstruction is initially intermittent and reversible, continued exposure to the inciting agent may lead to irreversible airway obstructive disease, persistent nonspecific bronchial hyperresponsiveness, and chronic respiratory symptoms. The diagnosis of occupational asthma is based on clinical, physiologic, and laboratory characteristics. Occupational asthma must be differentiated from other types of obstructive pulmonary disease such as chronic bronchitis and, more important, bronchial asthma of nonoccupational origin.

DEFINITION

It seems periphrasis to undergo the endless attempts at refining a definition [17, 25, 52, 108, 147, 161, 165, 187]. The realization of the importance of a nonallergic mechanism for occupational asthma has contributed to the difficulty in arriving at a consensus opinion on definition [28, 52, 93, 165, 189]. In the context of this chapter, *allergic occupational asthma* is defined as a "condition occurring after a preceding latent period of exposure when allergic sensitization to a substance or material present in the work site occurs and is characterized physiologically by variable and work-related airflow limitation and the presence of both specific and nonspecific airway hyperresponsiveness." At present, at least 200 agents have been documented to cause allergic occupational asthma. *Nonallergic occupational asthma* is "a condition that develops without a preceding latent period, occurring after an inordinate workplace irritant exposure, and is distinguished physiologically by persistent nonspecific airway hyperresponsiveness."

The two distinguishing clinical features pertinent to these definitions are *latency* and *specific airway hyperresponsiveness* (present in allergic and absent in nonallergic occupational asthma). Both types of occupational asthma demonstrate nonspecific bronchial hyperresponsiveness and both types show pathologic changes depicting bronchial mucosal injury and inflammation [28].

OCCURRENCE

Occupational asthma is a consequential occupational respiratory ailment, in terms of total numbers of cases, morbidity, and disability [138]. Over 200 agents have been shown to provoke allergic occupational asthma and the number will no doubt continue to grow rapidly in the future. It is becoming the most commonplace occupational lung disease in western countries. In 1988, it was the major occupational respiratory disease to be awarded compensation in Canada, surpassing asbestosis and silicosis [138]. While the entity "bronchial asthma" has been estimated to affect about 10 million persons, or 5 percent of the general population in the United States, the exact prevalence of occupational asthma is not known. It has been approximated to be between 2 and 15 percent [119, 177] (see Chap. 2). More is known concerning the prevalence of specific exposures or occupations, which can vary from 1 percent to nearly 100 percent and depends on a sundry of factors [24, 57, 85, 94, 159, 186]. For example, studies have noted that approximately 4 percent of workers exposed to western red cedar developed asthma [57]. A very similar percentage of workers exposed to volatile isocyanates developed occupational asthma [159]. Clinical symptoms of asthma in workers exposed to proteolytic enzymes have been estimated to occur in 10 to 45 percent [24]. Allergic symptoms developed in approximately 70 percent of flight crews dispersing irradiated sterile male screwworm flies [94]. Almost all workers in the power plants along the Mississippi River eventually become sensitized to river flies [85].

The difficulty in obtaining accurate numbers for determining disease prevalence stems from a number of factors [186]. Cross-sectional studies usually underestimate the problem, due to the "healthy worker" effect. In such a situation, affected workers leave the industry, leaving the unaffected to be surveyed. Criteria for identifying the asthmatic state have been especially lacking. Most epidemiologic studies employ questionnaires. Unfortunately, well-validated questionnaires for asthma have not been available in the past.

PREDISPOSING AND HOST FACTORS

A number of factors are important for the development of occupational asthma (Fig. 46-1). *Exposure factors* are consequential; particularly pertinent is the chemical type and reactivity, chemical source, and chemical concentration. Heavy exposures have been implicated in the pathogenesis of toluene diisocyanate (TDI) asthma [28, 152] and the development of reactive airway dysfunction syndrome (RADS) [30, 31]. Workers with exposures to frequent TDI spills are more likely to report asthma symptoms or show changes in lung function tests [34, 114] (Fig. 46-2). A positive association between a higher level of exposure and a greater likelihood of allergic sensitization has also been recounted for western red cedar [35, 194], isocyanates [199], colophony [39, 40], baking products [155], and acid anhydrides [195] (Fig. 46-3).

Industrial factors embody operations and processes, unique working conditions, industrial hygiene practices, and engineering features of an industrial site. Hexamethylene diisocyanate (HDI) and TDI, with about the same vapor pressures, are comparatively volatile at room temperature. Diphenylmethane diisocyanate (MDI) has a lower vapor pressure and is not volatile at room temperature. Heating MDI, such as with foundry work, makes it

Fig. 46-1. *A number of influencing factors are important in the pathogenesis of occupational asthma.*

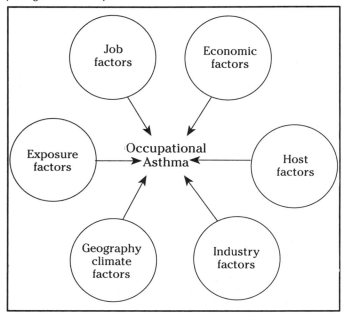

more volatile and raises its vapor pressure in the work environment; this event may lead to greater worker exposure [111, 204]. TDI asthma is more prevalent among polyurethane-processing workers compared to employees in TDI manufacturing [75, 201]. A "mill effect" or plant effect might explain noted differences in the frequency of TDI asthma among workers with similar exposures [75, 201].

Job type or activity can influence disease inauguration. Potentially dangerous job activities are pouring, grinding, blasting, sanding, sawing, and heating. Unsafe work practices can lead to spills or accidents with resultant high-level exposures. Spray painting is especially hazardous, since high levels of vapors (HDI, TDI) and particulates (MDI) become airborne [181].

Geographic and climatic factors have been inculpated in asthma epidemics, such as in Barcelona, Spain where the unloading of soybeans caused asthma outbreaks [4]. The unloading of soybeans gave rise to a sudden, massive release of soybean dust that reached the urban area under appropriate meteorologic conditions and caused the outbreaks.

Economic factors may influence the prevalence of occupational asthma. Ishizaki and associates demonstrated an association between the numbers of reported cases of allergic symptoms in workers exposed to western red cedar dust and the quantity of western red cedar imported into Japan [109]. Coincidentally with a wider distribution of the wood, cases of western red cedar asthma were reported from all over Japan.

Atopy is stipulated as an important risk factor for occupational asthma, perchance best established for high-molecular-weight (>1,000) compared to low-molecular-weight agents (<1,000) [1, 52, 61]. Why atopy is a host risk factor for sensitization for some low-molecular-weight agents (i.e., platinum salts, ethylenediamine, and dimethyl ethanolamine) but not others (i.e., TDI, western red cedar, trimellitic anhydride, phthalic anhydride, and formaldehyde) is not known [1, 52, 61]. The conflicting data recounting a relationship between atopy and an agent's molecular size with subsequent sensitization to the agent suggest that other factors may play a more important role in allergic sensitization [98].

Cigarette smoking is said to predispose some atopic workers

Fig. 46-2. *Prevalence of clinical diagnoses by questionnaire and abnormal pulmonary function values in isocyanate workers. More abnormalities were noted in employees exposed to more than 20 spills. FEV-1 = forced expiratory volume in 1.0 second; FVC = forced vital capacity; FEF25–75 = forced expiratory flow between 25 and 75 percent of the vital capacity; P = predicted; pred = predicted; SXS = symptoms. (From S. M. Brooks. The evaluation of occupational airway disease in the laboratory and workplace. J. Allergy Clin. Immunol. 70:56, 1982.)*

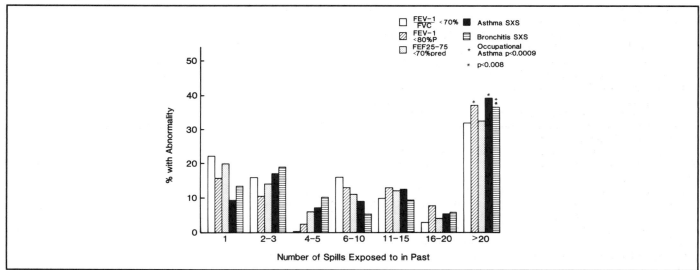

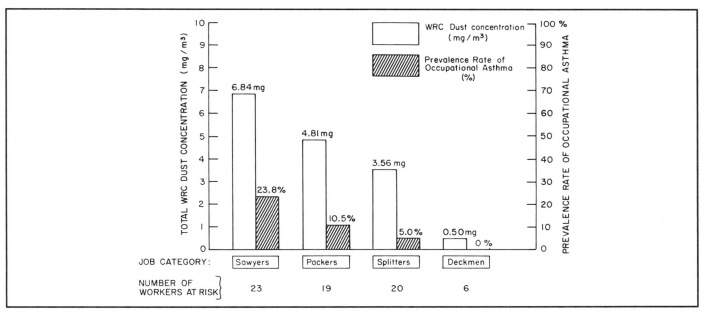

Fig. 46-3. *Prevalence of occupational asthma in western red cedar (WRC) workers according to job category and dust exposure. The diagnosis of occupational asthma was made using clinical and physiologic criteria. A higher prevalence of asthma was noted with higher dust exposure. (From S. M. Brooks, J. J. Edwards, and F. H. Edwards. An epidemiologic study of workers exposed to western red cedar and other wood dusts.* Chest *80[Suppl.]:30, 1981; S. M. Brooks. The evaluation of occupational airway disease in the laboratory and workplace.* J. Allergy Clin. Immunol. *70:56, 1982.)*

to occupational allergic sensitization [7, 196]. A contemplated mechanism to explain the connection between cigarette smoking and allergic sensitization proclaims that the inhalation of cigarette smoke creates an injury to the bronchial epithelium, heightens the bronchial epithelial permeability, and leads to an increased penetration of antigen through the epithelial layer [1].

Workplace airborne irritants may provoke aftermaths similar to cigarette smoking. Hypothetically, occupational exposures to particularly irritating agents (e.g., isocyanates, red cedar dust, trimellitic anhydride) or enzymes (e.g., subtilisin, esperase, protease, papain, amylase) enhance allergic sensitization, at least in part, because of the agent's intrinsic irritant or reactive properties that lead to bronchial mucosal injury and boosted allergen permeability. Industrial operations utilizing irritant agents become doubly dangerous, both from the risk of chronic heavy exposures and from the potential for spills and accidents to occur; the consequences may usher either an allergic or a nonallergic-type asthmatic response. The utilization of irritant gases, such as chlorine and ammonia, in the industrial process of platinum refining may be responsible for inaugurating bronchial epithelial injury. Biagini and associates instanced that platinum salt allergic sensitization in monkeys required concomitant exposure to ozone before allergic sensitization to platinum salts could be invoked [23]. Other animal studies documented that an antecedent exposure to an airborne irritant increases bronchial epithelial permeability and enhances allergic sensitization to an allergen [166, 172].

Nonspecific bronchial hyperresponsiveness may be the aftermath of a self-protective response by a worker to avoid dusty work environments, and promotes self-selection of persons out of such a work force [80]. When observed in a workplace setting, its occurrence is usually attributed to an occupational exposure [1, 28, 52]. Unfortunately, no investigations have prospectively tested airway reactivity before employment and then serially in order to observe which workers are at an increased risk for developing asthma. It is meaningful to discern whether bronchial hyperreactivity is induced or is preexisting because its prevalence

in the general population is more common than previously suspected [8, 41, 174, 203]. To aggrandize the problem, persons with nonspecific bronchial hyperresponsiveness may be completely asymptomatic. A high prevalence was surprisingly found among college athletes reporting minimal or no symptoms [200]. Furthermore, while measurement of bronchial hyperresponsiveness is considered a necessity for diagnosing asthma, there are new insights into its significance and usefulness as a research and clinical tool [105, 168].

An important consideration is whether persons with nonspecific hyperresponsive airways or an atopic state respond more adversely to workplace irritants or pollutants in general than do workers without the condition. It is provocative to hypothesize that there may be this "sensitive" or susceptible subpopulation in the general population [62, 66]. While irritant gases can induce airway inflammation in normal volunteers, a similar exposure in a sensitive population could have more dramatic consequences [16, 112, 151, 162]. A recent report suggested that atopy is an important risk factor for developing obstructive lung disease [113]. Asthmatics, and perhaps atopic persons, are more sensitive to irritant gases, such as sulfur dioxide (SO_2) [126]. Furthermore, the sensitive individual may be analogous to asthmatic subjects with "leaky" airways, in whom epithelial changes are noted on bronchial biopsy specimens, even those persons with the slightest symptoms and who require little or no medication [20, 124, 192].

POSSIBLE MECHANISMS OPERATIVE IN OCCUPATIONAL ASTHMA

Reflex

A number of dusts, gases, fumes, and vapors may cause bronchoconstriction by a direct effect on bronchial irritant receptors. Individuals with preexisting bronchial hyperresponsiveness may develop bronchoconstriction to many and varied airborne irritants at concentrations not affecting "normal" individuals and additionally, will react to the stimuli in a more vigorous manner. Thus, the workplace is an important cause of exacerbations of preexisting asthma. Although they are important to the patient and can be confused for occupational asthma, provocations of symptoms at the workplace by such natural stimuli as exercise, dry air, cold air, stress, and exposure to inert dusts or irritating fumes and gases (i.e., SO_2 or cigarette smoke) are not true examples of this entity.

Alteration in Deposition and Clearance of Particles

The site at which antigen or environmental particles come into contact with responding tissue may be an important determinant of the nature and severity of the asthmatic reaction. Because the number of mast cells is greatest in the terminal bronchioles, deposition of antigen in this area may be more likely to cause an asthmatic reaction than deposition in larger airways. In asthma, the site of deposition of inhaled particles also depends on the degree of airway obstruction present at any time. In the presence of bronchospasm, airway radius decreases and the deposition occurs more by impaction. The net effect is a more central deposition of inhaled material. As bronchial constriction subsides, the particles can reach more peripheral airways. The normal pulmonary defenses may be impaired by environmental and occupational agents indigenous to a workplace, including cigarette smoke, air pollution, chemicals, and dust; this situation may in turn impair particle clearance, possibly leading to a longer persistence of antigen within the lungs. Airway epithelial damage with sloughing of epithelial cells (e.g., Creola bodies) obviously affects mucociliary clearance.

Airway Inflammation

Airway inflammation, discussed in detail in the mechanisms section of this text, seems to play a crucial role in the pathogenesis of nonspecific airway hyperresponsiveness, and leads to many of the other manifestations of asthma. Almost all inflammatory cells in the bronchial wall and lumen have been implicated in the pathogenesis of mucosal inflammation in asthma, but presently, none can be singled out as being the most important [52, 58, 72, 74, 76, 86]. The mast cell's main role appears to be as an initiator of allergen-induced responses. The eosinophil is likely a proinflammatory cell rather than an antiinflammatory cell, and has the capacity to be selectively recruited from the circulation in response to IgE-dependent signals [76]. The eosinophil emits mediators that cause damage to the bronchial epithelium and lead to bronchoconstriction and airway hyperresponsiveness. The role of the other inflammatory cells is not as well defined. The neutrophil's role is better delineated in animal models than in humans. Macrophages have low-affinity receptors for IgE, but whether they act as a proinflammatory cell or have an ability to regulate immunologic responses is not known. Platelets may be important, but their exact role is also not clear. The lymphocyte may play a role as an immunoregulator.

Bronchial Smooth Muscle Hyperresponsiveness

The major control of airway smooth muscle tone is exerted by the parasympathetic nervous system, and the transmitter output from the nerve terminals, which is mainly acetylcholine [126]. The smooth muscle response is modulated not only by acetylcholine, but also by catecholamines, neuropeptides, and autacoids, including histamine and prostaglandins [14, 15, 44]. Inhibitory mechanisms mediated by endogenous prostaglandins in response to acetylcholine release from the nerve terminals of the vagus may also be important [110]. Some possible mechanisms to explain the exaggerated smooth muscle contraction seen in

occupational asthma include a decrease in baseline airway caliber, increased responsiveness of the smooth muscle itself, component(s) of inflammation, an abnormality in the autonomic and/or cholinergic nervous control of the smooth muscle, an increase in the accessibility of the stimuli to target cells, and effects of various peptide neurotransmitters [14, 15].

Adrenergic Influences

The beta-adrenergic receptor is closely associated with adenylate cyclase, an enzyme present in the plasma membrane of many cells that indirectly controls processes such as active secretion, transport, and storage of carbohydrate. Mast cells in the lungs of asthmatic subjects may have lower concentrations of intracellular adenosine $3',5'$-cyclic phosphate (cyclic AMP), which results in the release of the vasoactive mediators that cause the asthmatic reaction. An abnormality in the beta-adrenergic receptor has been noted as an explanation of occupational asthma due to TDI [45], but this hypothesis was negated by others [145, 146]. Vasoactive intestinal peptide (VIP), a potent endogenous bronchoinhibitory peptide, manifests its effects by stimulating cellular adenylate cyclase [15]. Asthma may be related to a lack of protective effect by the muscarinic receptor [6]. Isocyanates have also been implicated for affecting not only receptor proteins, but also enzymes such as acetylcholinesterase [139].

Neuropeptides

In addition to the classic adrenergic and cholinergic mechanisms, neural pathways that are neither adrenergic nor cholinergic (NANC) are receiving great attention [13–15] (see Chap. 18). The NANC nerves affect airway caliber, regulate bronchial vascular resistance and blood flow, influence microvascular leakage, and command mucus secretion. Neuropeptides are stored in nerves and released during mechanical, chemical, or pharmacologic stimulation. The response of this type to stimuli is conceivably important in the pathogenesis of nonallergic occupational asthma following inordinate exposure to irritants. The neuropeptides occur as cotransmitters and interact within the classic adrenergic, cholinergic, and sensory nerves.

VIP, a 28–amino acid peptide, nonadrenergic bronchodilator that is 100 times more potent than isoproterenol, is found in very high concentrations in lung tissue and localizes to efferent nerves, including parasympathetic ganglia. Peptide histidine isoleucine (PHI) and peptide histidine methionine (PHM) may have similar functions, but differ in receptor specificity to different cells. A considerable body of data suggests that VIP has potent antiinflammatory activity in the lung, including inhibiting inflammatory cell function, antagonizing major humoral mediators of inflammation, and attenuating acute edema. It is conceivable that in severe lung airway injury with inflammation (i.e., via allergic or nonallergic pathways), a defect in VIP-inhibiting control of airway smooth muscle can lead to airway hyperresponsiveness. Inflammatory cells (mast cells, neutrophils, eosinophils) release numerous peptidases (e.g., mast cells release tryptase) that rapidly break down VIP. According to Barnes, this may be like "taking the brakes off" cholinergic nerves, resulting in an exaggerated reflex cholinergic bronchoconstriction, and may contribute to the bronchial hyperresponsiveness [15].

Excitatory neuropeptides, including substance P, neurokinin A, and calcitonin gene–related peptide, are characterized by rapid-onset smooth muscle contractile effects (thus, the general designation *tachykinins*). They constitute unmyelinated sensory nerves (C-fibers) and display inflammatory effects. Tachykinins can cause airway smooth muscle contraction, stimulate mucus secretion, increase microvascular permeability and exudation of plasma into the airway lumen, degranulate mast cells, and possibly have chemotactic properties.

Epithelial Damage

Damage to the airway epithelium may represent a critical step in the pathogenesis of occupational asthma (Fig. 46-4). Airway epithelium modulates the bronchoconstrictor effects of many spasmogens, feasibly by releasing a relaxant substance [68, 88]. Once injured, airway epithelium is capable of generating products of the 15-lipoxygenase pathway of arachidonate metabolism, including 8, 15-dihydroxyeicosatetraenoic (diHETE) acids, the chemotactic agents for neutrophils that may augment the airway inflammatory response [156]. Injury to the epithelium may also lead to the production of leukotriene B_4, a potent chemotactic agent that can attract granulocytes, but may also cause smooth muscle contraction and possibly influence airway responsiveness [69, 126].

The damage to the airway epithelium may result in exposure of afferent nerve endings. Stimulation of unmyelinated vagal afferents may introduce axon reflexes and the release of tachykinins; this scenario can prompt bronchoconstriction, increase vascular permeability, and potentiate vagally mediated airway smooth muscle contraction [131]. Bradykinin, for example, may be an inflammatory mediator that can selectively stimulate C-fiber nerve endings and cause release of sensory neuropeptides by an axon reflex [15]. Direct epithelial cell damage due to high-level irritant exposure may produce a "neurogenic inflammation" and subsequent changes similar to allergic occupational asthma. The airway inflammation induced by high-level exposure to irritating inhalants may stimulate tachykinin release, destroy local enzymes that metabolize tachykinins and thereby amplify their effects, or simply expose nerve endings and enhance their triggering [86].

Shedding of epithelium is augmented by eosinophil products, such as cationic major basic protein. Epithelial removal also accentuates the bronchoconstrictor effects of tachykinins, in part because of the lack of metabolism of tachykinins by neutral endopeptidase (NEP) [88, 92, 102, 157]. NEP is bound to the mem-

Fig. 46-4. *Damage to the airway epithelium exposes afferent nerve endings, which can then be stimulated by inflammatory mediators present in the airway lumen. Bradykinin selectively stimulates C-fiber nerve endings and causes the release of sensory neuropeptides by an axon reflex. Excitatory neuropeptides (i.e., substance P [SP]) cause airway smooth muscle contraction, stimulate mucus secretion, increase microvascular permeability and exudation of plasma into the airway lumen, degranulate mast cells, and possibly have chemotactic properties. Epithelial removal accentuates the bronchoconstrictor effects of tachykinins, possibly because of the loss of a relaxant substance. Various cells play a role: The mast cell initiates allergen-induced responses. The eosinophil, recruited from the circulation in response to IgE-dependent signals, emits mediators that cause damage to the bronchial epithelium and lead to bronchoconstriction. Macrophages have low-affinity receptors for IgE, but whether they act as a proinflammatory cell or have an ability to regulate immunologic responses is not known. The lymphocyte may play a role as an immunoregulator. PAF = platelet-activating factor; LTC_4 = leukotriene C_4; ECP = eosinophilic cationic protein; MBP = major basic protein; EDN = eosinophil-derived neurotoxin; IL-2 = interleukin-2; NKA = neurokinin A; VIP = vasoactive intestinal peptide; CGRP = calmodulin gene–related peptide; ACh = acetylcholine; PMN = polymorphonuclear leukocyte.*

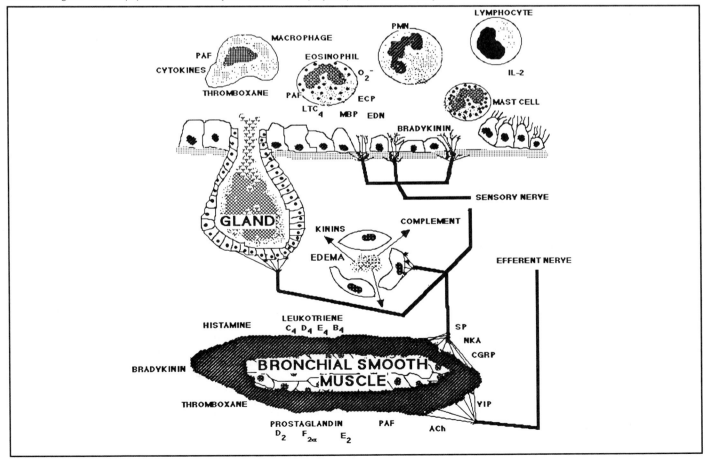

branes of selected airway cells with receptors for tachykinins, which allows the enzyme to cleave tachykinins that come close to the cell-surface receptors [157]. Decreased NEP activity occurs with epithelial removal, leading to an exaggeration of neurogenic inflammation and bronchoconstrictor response. Since substance P also appears to release relaxant factor from airway epithelium, the lack of this factor causes an even more excessive bronchoconstrictor response. An example of the potential importance of the downregulation of NEP by a chemical insult is exemplified by the studies of Sheppard and colleagues [183]. In guinea pigs exposed to TDI, bronchomotor tone responses to inhaled substance P increased and were associated with a decrease in airway tissue NEP activity [183].

Once damage to airway epithelium has occurred, epithelial repair may be delayed by continued exposure to the environmental agent or for other unexplained reasons. Thus, altered epithelial permeability may persist even after termination of exposure, resulting in continued airway hyperreactivity to nonspecific irritants (such as cold air, fumes, odors, and dusts) and asthma symptoms.

Injury to the "tight junctions" between bronchial epithelial cells from potent irritating and toxic substances may facilitate immunologic mechanisms by allowing easier access to the submucosal area of the airways where greater numbers of mast cells are located or by facilitating a formation of hapten-protein conjugates. These structural alterations may become permanent and help to explain how persistent symptoms may be induced by a single high-level exposure or even repetitive lower-level exposures [21].

Microvascular Leakage

Barnes has insinuated that microvascular leakage may be an important factor in the pathogenesis of asthma [14]. The studies of Van De Graaf and others demonstrated an increased plasma exudation into the airways of asthmatic individuals [192]. The leakage occurs at the level of the postcapillary venules, possibly as a result of mediators' effects (i.e., histamine, bradykinin, leukotrienes, platelet-activating factor [PAF]) on vascular endothelium, allowing extravasation to occur. Neuropeptides also greatly enhance microvascular leakage [15]. The microvascular leakage leads to submucosal edema and airway narrowing; it may also contribute to epithelial shedding, and may be important in stimulating mucus secretion and lead to plugging of bronchioles. There can be an effect on mucociliary clearance, and leakage may act as a source of inflammatory mediators, including complement fragments (C3a, C5a, or anaphylatoxins), and kininogen precursor of bradykinin [15].

Pharmacologic Agents

Certain agents in the workplace may directly induce bronchoconstriction. Although these agents evoke a greater response in those with bronchial hyperresponsiveness, all exposed individuals would be expected to demonstrate a response if the exposure is strong enough. Many low-molecular-weight compounds, such as TDI and plicatic acid, may exhibit in vitro pharmacologic actions such as altering receptor proteins; influencing cyclic AMP levels; affecting enzyme systems, such as adenylate cyclase or acetylcholinesterase; inducing nonimmunologic mast cell degranulation; and activating complement. Whether these actions are clinically important is not known [165].

Immunologic Mechanisms

Immunologic mechanisms seem to be operative in the greatest number of cases of occupational asthma [21]. During the latency period, allergens are processed by alveolar macrophages that

Table 46-1. Examples of occupational asthma with specific IgE antibodies

Occupation	Causal agent
Animal handlers	Urine protein, dander
Antibiotic workers	Penicillin, spiramycin
Bakers	Wheat, rye, buckwheat; mites, alpha-amylase, hemicellulase, glucoamylase, papain, soybean
Chemical workers	Sulfonechloramides, azo dyes, ethylenediamine, anthraquinone
Coffee or tea workers	Green coffee, tea dust
Detergent workers	*Bacillus subtilis*, esperase
Entomologists	Locusts, blowfly
Fishery workers	Sea squirts, prawns
Oil extractors, crushers	Castor beans
Pharmaceutical workers	Pepsin, flaviastase, penicillin, cephalosporins, phenylglycine acid chloride, spiramycin
Plastic workers	Phthalic anhydride, trimellitic anhydrides, diisocyanates
Printers	Arabic gum, gum acacia
Processors	Prawns, hoya, egg powder, tobacco leaf
Spice and enzyme workers	Garlic powder, papain, pectinase, trypsin, karaya gum, maiko
Woodworkers	Quillaja bark, red cedar, Douglas fir, African zebrawood, iroko
Insect handlers	Bee moth, cockroach, river flies, locust, meal worm, screw worm
Metal processors	Platinum salts, cobalt, nickel

present antigens to helper T-cells, which in turn stimulate B-cells to produce specific IgE (Table 46-1, Fig. 46-5). Sufficient quantities of antibody are generated to sensitize circulating basophils as well as mast cells [21].

A number of different patterns of response have been recognized in susceptible individuals (Fig. 46-6). An immediate (early) response is characterized by a bronchospastic response peaking in a few minutes and resolving within an hour or 2. This immediate response is readily reversed by bronchodilators, can be prevented by pretreatment with beta-adrenergic agents and disodium cromoglycate but not corticosteroids, and is not followed by an increase in bronchial responsiveness [1]. A late (nonimmediate or delayed) response begins about 1 hour after exposure, peaks in 4 to 6 hours, and may last for 12 to 24 hours after the exposure. The late response, detailed in Chapter 12, is inhibited by pretreatment with corticosteroids or disodium cromoglycate, is more difficult to treat, and is followed by an increase in bronchial responsiveness [22, 55]. A patient may demonstrate an isolated immediate response, an isolated late response, or a dual response. A recurrent late response that has been documented may begin 12 to 24 hours after exposure and is followed by recurrent patterns of recovery and bronchoconstriction for up to 72 hours. This response may be more a reflection of transient increases in bronchial responsiveness than a distinct delayed response [204].

Inhalant high-molecular-weight allergens produce an immediate response in the vast majority of patients. A late response accompanies this response in approximately 50 percent. An isolated late response is unusual. Challenges with low-molecular-weight compounds, by contrast, produce a late response in 90 percent. This is either an isolated response (50%) or a component of the dual response [38, 53, 55, 61].

When specific IgE–antigen reaction takes place on a mast cell, preformed mediators (e.g., histamine, eosinophilic chemotactic factor [ECF-A], neutrophilic chemotactic factor [NCF-A]) are released [52, 54, 55, 58]. Histamine and perhaps metabolites of arachidonic acid are responsible for the bronchospasm. A num-

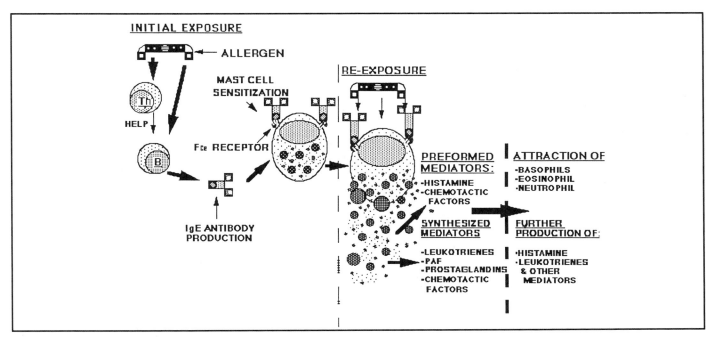

Fig. 46-5. *Mucosal mast cells contain specific IgE receptors on their surface, which can cross-link with antigen and lead to mediator release into the bronchial lumen. The mediators include both preformed (e.g., histamine, various lytic enzymes, and chemotactic peptides such as eosinophil and neutrophil chemotactic [ECF-A and NCF-A] factors) and membrane-derived (i.e., oxidative products of arachidonic acid—cyclooxygenase and lipoxygenase constituents). The late asthmatic response represents a continuation of the early IgE-mediated allergic reaction. The chemotactic factors evolved influence the subsequent inflammatory response noted.*

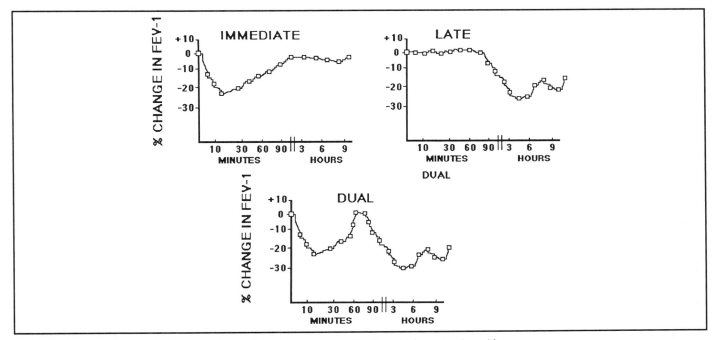

Fig. 46-6. *Patterns of occupational asthmatic reactions that may occur after bronchial provocation with a specific antigen. FEV-1 = forced expiratory volume in 1 second.*

ber of bronchoalveolar lavage (BAL) studies have now documented the release of these mediators during an immediate reaction due to allergen exposure [52, 54, 55, 58]. Inflammatory mediators such as prostaglandin D$_2$ and thromboxane are also released during the immediate reaction [154, 204].

The IgE-antigen interaction is also a stimulus to the production

and release of "newly formed" mediators such as PAF and metabolites of arachidonic acid (e.g., prostaglandins and leukotrienes). The leukotrienes (C$_4$, D$_4$, E$_4$) cause smooth muscle contraction and enhanced mucus production [178]. ECF-A, NCF-A, and leukotriene B$_4$ released from mast cells during the immediate reaction are potent chemotactic factors. Significant increases in eosinophils, eosinophil granule proteins, neutrophils, and lymphocytes during the late-phase reaction have been detected in BAL studies [72, 74, 81, 148]. Recruitment of cells into the airway likely results in airway inflammation.

Increases in nonspecific bronchial responsiveness are generally associated with the late asthmatic response. It appears likely that bronchial hyperresponsiveness is in some way associated with the triggered inflammation. The increase in bronchial hyperresponsiveness due to allergen or sensitizer inhalation may be detected at 3 hours after the exposure and prior to the onset of the late response [78]. The induced increase in bronchial responsiveness lasts for a variable period but usually for several days to weeks. For example, after bronchial challenge tests with TDI, in those subjects demonstrating a late response, increased bronchial responsiveness was still present at 24 hours but returned to baseline in 1 to 4 weeks [141].

Fabbri and colleagues recently found that in subjects with a late asthmatic response induced by TDI, BAL fluid showed an increased number of neutrophils at both 2 hours and 8 hours [81]. Eosinophil counts were increased at 8 hours. The concentration of albumin was increased at the time when leukocytes were increased. This might suggest that the microvascular leak was occurring. No such change occurred in those subjects with an isolated immediate response or in control subjects. To look at the subject of airway inflammation closer, the same investigators pretreated susceptible subjects with corticosteroids prior to challenge. They found that the late response, the increase in bronchial responsiveness, and the migration of neutrophils and eosinophils into the lavage fluid were prevented [26].

HYPOTHETIC MODEL FOR OCCUPATIONAL ASTHMA

The development and progression of occupational asthma embody the culmination of many complex proceedings singularized by constantly evolving and modifying events. The distinction between "asthmatic" and "nonasthmatic" illustrates the extent to which the proceeding has evolved, from the foundational events to the modified complex state. As a part of the evolutionary process, there is sustained divergence and change; some changes are short-lived while others are persisting. The biochemical and physiologic occurrences that precede impact on present and future events. The state at any given time reflects cumulative events of injury and repair, initiation and response, sequence and disarrangement. The lungs play out a systematic biochemical and immunologic stratagem, with "participants" assigned specific roles. The "participators" work in concert but frequently are engaged in discord. Their purpose is to evolve to a counteracting or homeostatic state that redresses previous biochemical and immunologic insults. The outset of occupational asthma melds the various cellular and biochemical phenomena that occur in response to multitudinous signals and stimuli. The enormity and severity of changes reflect the intensity of the signals and stimuli inaugurated. The finality represents the interplaying of reversible and irreversible processes.

At all stages, there is an attempt to maintain homeostasis, balancing cellular and biochemical signals evolving during the asthmatic process. The signals originate from (1) respiratory epithelium, (2) bronchial smooth muscle cells, (3) neural activity, (4) vascular integrity, (5) indigenous leukocyte and monocyte cellular constituents, and (6) endogenous humoral components. Thus, there is fine-tuning and modulation by sensory afferent neural activators (i.e., C-fibers, cough receptors, and rapidly and slowly adapting stretch receptors), adrenergic mechanisms (i.e., alpha- and beta-receptor activity), and NANC nerves and neuropeptides. Other modulators include epithelial smooth muscle in-

hibitory mechanisms (i.e., epithelial-derived relaxant factor), state of microvascular leakage, circulating endogenous hormones (i.e., catecholamines), circulatory mediator (i.e., histamine) influences, and indigenous bronchial mucosal and luminal cells (i.e., macrophage, mast cell, etc.). The airway divergence can be likened to a pendulum, "moving back and forth" in order to maintain a relative constancy of bronchomotor tone and airway cellular balance.

Alteration in the deposition and clearance of allergenic particles may be an important determinant of the nature and severity of the asthmatic reaction. Because the number of mast cells is greatest in the terminal bronchioles, deposition of antigen in this area may be more likely to cause an asthmatic reaction than deposition in larger airways. The normal pulmonary defenses may be impaired by environmental and occupational agents indigenous to a workplace, including cigarette smoke, air pollution, chemicals, and dust; this situation may in turn impair particle clearance, possibly leading to a longer persistence of antigen within the lungs.

Early on, irritant exposures or high-level exposures from spills cause epithelial cell disruption and damage. The attendant outcomes lead to increased respiratory epithelium permeability and enhanced penetration of antigen, possibly into the vicinity of the submucosa where bronchial associated lymphatic tissue (BALT) is located and as a result synthesis of specific IgE and IgG antibodies. Lymphocytes become provoked and begin the immunologic processing that eventually will lead to allergic sensitization (i.e., commencement of IgE and IgG production, cellular immunity, etc.).

Both inhibitory and excitatory neuropeptides influence inflammatory cell function, airway smooth muscle status, mucus secretion, humoral mediators of inflammation, microvascular permeability, and exudation of plasma into the airway lumen. If there is an imbalance, then one or the other of the neural elements predominates. Stimulated release of mast cell mediators, especially secretory peptidases, can modulate the neuropeptide effects. Human mast cell tryptase hydrolyzing VIP results in an exaggerated reflex cholinergic bronchoconstriction and bronchial hyperresponsiveness.

What may be the critical event that launches the whole asthmatic process is injury to bronchial epithelial cells, perhaps from inhaling an allergen, irritant gas, or air pollutant. What exactly transpires is not completely understood, but a damaged epithelium can institute a cascade of biochemical and cellular events, such as generating products of the 15-lipoxygenase pathway of arachidonate metabolism. Mattoli and associates reported that in vitro exposure of bronchial epithelial cells to TDI resulted in a dose-dependent release of 15-HETE that is inhibited by nedocromil [142]. Injury to the epithelium also leads to the production of leukotriene B_4, which not only can attract granulocytes but also may cause smooth muscle contraction, and possibly influence airway responsiveness [69, 126]. Epithelial removal leads to an exaggeration of neurogenic inflammation and the bronchoconstrictor response caused by tachykinins, because of the lack of metabolism of tachykinins by NEP [102, 157]. Substance P may enhance the release of a bronchial smooth muscle relaxant factor from airway epithelium; its lack causes an even more excessive bronchoconstrictor response [92].

Airway inflammation seems crucial in the pathogenesis of occupational asthma. Airway inflammatory products such as bradykinin selectively stimulate C-fiber nerve endings and cause a release of sensory neuropeptides by an axon reflex. Activation of NANC nerves (neurokinin A, substance P, etc.) induces a change in microvascular permeability which leads to submucosal edema and airway narrowing, contributes to epithelial shedding, and stimulates mucus secretion leading to the plugging of bronchioles. Microvascular leakage may act as a source of inflammatory mediators, including complement fragments (C3a, C5a, or anaphylatoxins), and kininogen precursor of bradykinin. Subjects with a late asthmatic response induced by TDI showed BAL fluid changes of an increased concentration of albumin at the time when leukocytes were increased, suggesting that a microvascular leak was occurring [81].

Cellular activation of various inflammatory cells occurs. Alveolar macrophages release increased amounts of O_2^-, thromboxanes, prostaglandins, and PAF. PAF attracts human eosinophils and causes eosinophil infiltration of the airways. As activated eosinophils increase in numbers, the degree and extent of epithelial damage increase. The activated eosinophils manifest enhanced killing properties; intensified toxic oxygen radical production; heightened leukotriene production; and possibly augmentation of other eosinophil functions, such as mounted release of eosinophil cationic protein, peroxidase, or eicosanoids. Mast cells discharge their contents (chemotactic factors and possibly cyclooxygenase and lipoxygenase products). Nervous stimulation can also promote mast cell degranulation, possibly through axon reflexes. Monocytic cellular changes become operative with T-cell activation and the secretion of various cytokines. Secretion of granulocyte chemotactic factors by activated T-lymphocytes and monocytes might be a mechanism whereby granulocytes are attracted to sites of inflammation [63].

Repeated airborne exposures can perpetuate injury of the airways with further shedding of ciliated respiratory epithelium, collagen deposition beneath the epithelial basement membrane, persistent mast cell degranulation, and enhanced infiltration of tissue eosinophils (Fig. 46-7). Frequent and repeated allergen (and possibly irritant) exposures lead to cumulative repercussions, especially when there is a short or absent time period for recovery to occur. What transpires via this evolutionary process is a state where the airways become populated by many and varied activated cells, programmed to react to stimuli in an exaggerated biochemical manner.

The scenario plays out as increasing numbers of activated eosinophils and raised levels of BAL major basic protein (MBP) intensify epithelial damage, airway hyperresponsiveness, and microvascular leakage. Eosinophil release of mediators, including leukotriene C_4, PAF, oxygen radicals, and basic proteins, influences physiologic events. Mast cells continuously release small amounts of presynthesized and synthesized mediators. NANC activity is enhanced with an evolution of axon reflexes, especially as more epithelial cell injury occurs. In a vicious cycle, the presence of eosinophils and other inflammatory cells introduces more widespread and diffuse airway epithelial injury (i.e., macroinjury) and desquamation.

A heavy allergen exposure has serious consequences: Changes become magnified in time and severity and an acute asthmatic attack occurs. The most important significance of a full-blown asthmatic attack is that it causes considerable diffuse injury to the airway: There is massive epithelial damage and denudation, marked vascular and bronchial mucosal permeability, prominent mucus secretion and airway narrowing, and heightened nonspecific airway reactivity.

Nonallergic asthma, such as the RADS, is more of a very precipitous event (Fig. 46-8). The initial massive epithelial damage and disruption is followed by direct activation of NANC pathways (axon reflexes) and institution of neurogenic inflammation. High-level irritant exposure initiates massive epithelial injury. There is nonallergic-related mast cell degranulation and macrophage activation. Chemotactic factors are released and mucosal inflammation ensues. Epithelial cell destruction is substantial. Microvascular leakage introduces more chemotactic factors and further recruitment of inflammatory cells, including eosinophils.

Fig. 46-7. *Repeated low-level encounters to allergens (or irritants?) cause cumulative microinjuries to the airways. A vicious cycle develops: Eosinophil basic protein release produces more diffuse epithelial injury (i.e, macroinjury) and epithelial desquamation. Axon reflexes and neurogenic inflammation are induced. A heavy allergen exposure causes massive epithelial damage and denudation, marked vascular and bronchial mucosal permeability, prominent mucus secretion and airway narrowing, and heightened nonspecific airway reactivity. See Figure 46-4 legend for key to some abbreviations. NEP = neutral endopeptidase; NK = neurokinin; ECF-A = eosinophil chemotactic factor; NCF-A = neutrophil chemotactic factor; BALT = bronchial associated lymphatic tissue; EPI/NE = epinephrine/norepinephrine; EpDRF = epithelial-derived relaxant factor.*

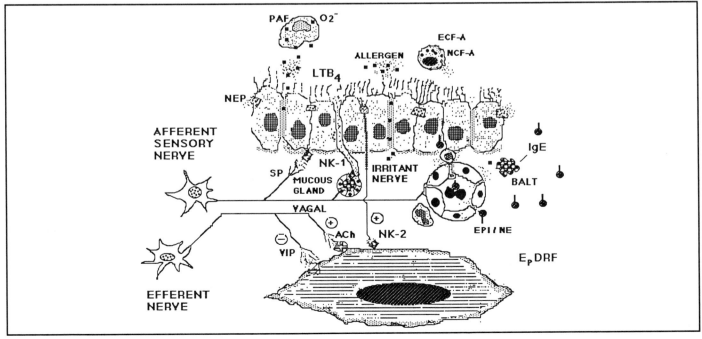

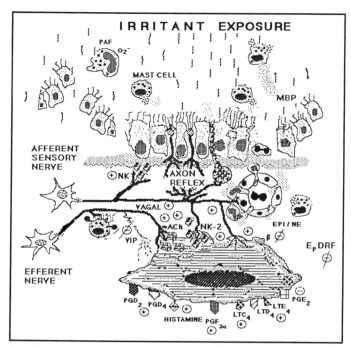

Fig. 46-8. *Mucosal injury occurs from an irritant gas, air pollutant, or allergen, and causes impairment in respiratory epithelium cellular function (i.e., loss of ciliary activity, reduced neutral endopeptidase activity, possibly decreased release of epithelial-derived relaxant factor [EpDRF], etc.). Injury initiates epithelial cell inflammatory mediator release (i.e., leukotriene [LTB]$_4$, 15-lipoxygenase products) and activation of nonadrenergic, noncholinergic nerves (neurokinin [NK], substance P, etc.); the latter invokes changes in microvascular permeability and mucous cell secretion. Stimulated alveolar macrophages release mediators and cell constituents (O_2^-, platelet-activating factor [PAF], etc.) while mast cells release chemotactic factors and possibly cyclooxygenase and lipoxygenase products. Eosinophils are recruited by the release of PAF and other eosinophil chemoattractants. Lymphocytes are primed for specific antibody synthesis (IgE, IgG) and cellular interactions. See Figures 46-4 and 46-7 for key to abbreviations.*

Lung inflammatory cells become activated and answer stimuli with an exaggerated response. The severe airway injury leads to a reduced capacity for recovery. Compensatory upregulation and/or downregulation of receptors and possibly genetic cellular alterations may result.

During recovery, there is resolution of inflammation, epithelial cell repair, neural activity inhibition, and improvement of vascular integrity. The greater the degree and extent of the injury are, the more unlikely it is that complete recovery will occur. There may be a laying down of submucosal collagen and other repair processes may be occurring. Irreversible changes in the airways' mechanical and biochemical status may result. There may be downregulation or upregulation of various receptors in response to persistent stimuli. There may be changes at the gene level with transformation in gene coding.

Bronchial epithelial repair may be delayed by continued exposure to the environmental agent or for other unexplained reasons. Thus, altered epithelial function could persist even after termination of the exposure, resulting in continued airway hyperreactivity to nonspecific irritants and asthma symptoms. Once injured, permanent changes may develop in a nerve ending [179]. Thus, following an airway's injury, sensory nerve damage may initiate an enhancement of the responsiveness of a proportion of C-fiber sensory units, which may translate into an altered release of various neuropeptides or changes in receptor numbers. Once

a major irritant injury occurs, alterations in antigen structure could lead to new antigen determinants and possibly immunologic responsiveness to some modified self-antigen. This scenario could account for the perpetuation of inflammatory aspects of the process and continuation of the hyperreactive state.

The sequela or new state of homeostasis of the foregoing represents the culmination of initiation, evolutionary, and repair processes. Depending on the degree of bronchial injury and the completeness of recovery, the sequela represents the residual of cumulative injuries to the airways. The sequela may be one of complete recovery or may manifest as a chronic persistent asthmatic condition with nonspecific airway hyperresponsiveness.

NONALLERGIC OCCUPATIONAL ASTHMA

Case Examples

A previously healthy, 41-year-old painter and his partner, a 45-year-old man, worked together spray painting a poorly ventilated apartment during the late fall when the weather was cold. The room was sealed and there was poor fresh air recirculation, the windows were covered with a heavy plastic material, duct tape was placed around the edges to ensure a seal, and the main entrance to the apartment was covered to conserve heat. The painters did not wear approved respiratory protective devices, but only paper masks covering their nose and mouth while they spray painted. The paint used was a one-stage vinyl latex primer, reported to be rapid drying and said to contain 25% ammonia, 16.6% aluminum chlorohydrate, and other additives, many documented to be irritants.

Both men spray painted for a total of 12 hours, 4 hours the first day and 8 hours the second. Each individual noted the appearance of an illness beginning at the end of the second day of work, with symptoms consisting of nausea, cough, shortness of breath, paint taste in the mouth, chest tightness, wheezing, and generalized weakness of the limbs. Each subject was subsequently hospitalized for about 2 weeks with provisional diagnoses of "chemical bronchitis." A chest roentgenogram of one subject showed "increased bronchovascular markings" consistent with "chemical pneumonitis." After being discharged from the hospital, both painters consulted private physicians and each was eventually treated with prednisone, oral theophylline, and aerosol adrenergic bronchodilators.

At evaluation 4 months later, there remained persistent symptomatology of wheezing, cough, and exertional dyspnea; one painter also had chest discomfort. Separately, each reported newly developed bronchial irritability symptoms, that is, respiratory manifestations after exposure to many and varied nonspecific stimuli such as cold air, dusts, aerosol sprays, smoke, and fumes. The bronchial irritability symptoms were not acknowledged to be present before the heavy exposure. Each painter denied a past history of asthma, allergies, rhinitis, frequent colds, dyspnea, or any respiratory symptoms. One of the painters admitted to only one short episode of bronchitis 11 years previously, and nothing since. Each subject denied a family history of allergy, asthma, or previous respiratory problems. Each person worked only as a painter in the past, one for 20 years and the other for 25 years. Each stated he never previously spray painted under the environmental conditions of the inciting incident. One subject was a cigarette smoker with a 21 pack/yr history; the other person was essentially a nonsmoker, never consuming more than 20 to 40 cigarettes in his life. A physical examination in one subject disclosed expiratory rhonci. Laboratory findings in the subjects included normal complete blood cell counts with 5 percent eosinophilia in one; normal-appearing chest roentgenograms; and negatives results on radioallergosorbent test (RAST) battery for common airborne allergens. Pulmonary function testing showed mild airway obstruction; the 1-second forced expiratory volume–forced vital capacity ($FEV_{1.0}/FVC$) was 67.7 percent in one man and 70.3 percent in the other; forced expiratory flow in the mid–expiratory phase ($FEF_{25-75\%}$) was 39.8 percent and 31.7 percent of predicted, respectively. Over the next 2 years, the two men were followed with serial clinical evaluations, lung function testing, and methacholine bronchial challenges. The asthma-like symptoms and airway hyperreactivity were noted to persist.

Reactive Airway Dysfunction Syndrome

The entity reactive airway dysfunction syndrome or RADS was first designated in 1985 [30, 31]. Ten individuals developed a persistent asthma-like illness after a single exposure to high levels of an irritant vapor, fume, gas, or smoke. Respiratory symptomatology and continued presence of nonspecific airway hyperresponsiveness were documented in all subjects for about a 3-year-average follow-up period. In 1 person, the persistence of disease was documented to have lasted at least 12 years in duration. Generally, the incriminated exposure was short-lived, often lasting just a few minutes but on occasion may have been as long as 12 hours. There usually was a time interval between the exposure and the development of symptoms; this time period was immediate in 3 but several hours in the other 7 subjects (mean was approximately 9 hours). In almost all instances, the exposure was due to an accident or a situation where there was very poor ventilation and limited air exchange. When tested, all subjects displayed a positive result on a methacholine challenge test. There was no identifiable evidence of preexisting respiratory complaints in any patient studied. Two subjects were found to be atopic but in all others no evidence of allergy was identified. Pulmonary function was normal in 3 of 10 and showed airflow limitation in 7.

Although the incriminating etiologic agents varied in each patient, all were irritants in nature and included uranium hexafluoride gas, floor sealant, spray paint containing significant concentrations of ammonia, heated acid, 35% hydrazine, fumigating fog, metal coating remover, and smoke inhalation. In 2 patients, bronchial biopsied specimens documented bronchial epithelial cell injury and bronchial wall inflammation. There were lymphocytes and plasma cells present but no eosinophilia was observed. Desquamation of respiratory epithelium was seen in one specimen and goblet cell hyperplasia in another. There was no evidence of mucous gland hyperplasia, basement membrane thickening, or smooth muscle hypertrophy.

Other Examples of Irritant-induced Asthma or Reactive Airway Dysfunction Syndrome

Subsequent to the 1985 description of RADS, other examples of RADS were reported. Tarlo and Broder provided a retrospective review of the files of 154 consecutive workers assessed for occupational asthma [189]. Of 59 subjects considered to have occupational asthma, a subset of 10 (and possibly an additional 15) with asthma symptoms for an average of 5 years was characterized by disease initiated by an exposure to high concentrations of an irritant. The clinical criteria for RADS were modified in the study and exposure was not limited to just a single accident or incident at work. It was concluded that irritant-induced occupational asthma is not uncommon in a population referred for an assessment of possible occupational asthma. The prevalence was estimated to be 6 percent for definite irritant-induced asthma and another 10 percent had a possible diagnosis. Boulet implied there was prolonged induction of increased airway hyperresponsiveness after the inhalation of high concentrations of irritants in four "normal" subjects and aggravation of airway hyperresponsiveness in another person with "mild" preexisting asthma [27]. Two of the persons were believed to have developed sensitization after only an intense short-term exposure. Gilbert and Auchincloss reported on a patient with RADS manifested by a restrictive rather than obstructive defect, presumably on the basis of constriction of bronchioles or alveolar ducts [95]. Other examples reported as RADS included three Philadelphia police officers exposed to toxic fumes from a roadside truck accident [170]; a female computer operator exposed to a floor sealant [127]; and workers exposed to TDI [132], possibly acetic acid [171], and possibly SO$_2$ [5]. Moisan described RADS-like illnesses after smoke inhalation in three subjects [150]. Kern reported on 51 of 56 hospital workers exposed to a spill of 100% glacial acetic acid who responded to a self-administered, mailed questionnaire 8 months later [118]. Importantly, information (i.e., patient data base system of health history questionnaire) was available concerning the health status of the exposed persons prior to the spill. The subjects completed methacholine challenges and an industrial hygienist evaluated the extent of the exposure. Eight workers developed an asthma-like illness within 24 hours, with 4 subsequently demonstrating all of the criteria for RADS nearly a year after the accident. The investigator identified a dose-response relationship and concluded that RADS was a valid entity.

Clinical Features

The clinical criteria for confirming a diagnosis of RADS are listed in Table 46-2. A major diagnostic requirement for RADS is the medical history. Malo and coworkers investigated 162 subjects to assess the value of a clinical history (taken by an open medical questionnaire) in predicting the accuracy of the diagnosis of allergic occupational asthma as subsequently confirmed by objective tests [137]. It was estimated that the history alone had a positive predictive value of 63 percent and a negative predictive value of 83 percent. Moreover, there was agreement between the physician's initial assessment and the confirmed diagnosis in only 84 (52%) of the 162 patients. These findings serve to confirm the need for objective testing.

There have been no similar comparisons of the accuracy of the history in predicting documented RADS cases. There is no question that for both RADS and irritant-induced asthma, the history is crucial. In allergic occupational asthma the exact onset of the illness cannot be precisely determined; usually onset is dated to a season, year, or month. RADS, however, can be dated specifically. The patient may even be able to identify the exact time of the day that the illness began. The reason for this clear-cut time discrimination is because RADS is a dramatic event, generally following an accident or unusual precipitous incident. The details become clear in the subject's mind. The exposure is irritant in nature and generally a vapor or gas, but on occasion a high-level dust exposure has been incriminated.

Symptoms of cough, dyspnea, and wheezing suggest asthma as a diagnosis. Characteristically, cough is a predominant symptom and may lead to an incorrect diagnosis of chronic bronchitis or recurrent bouts of acute bronchitis. Some patients have an intractable cough, frequently interrupting an interview with the physician or making spirometric measurements difficult to complete.

The response of symptoms to being away from work may not have the same significance for RADS as it does for allergic occupational asthma. Burge suggested that asking two questions will

Table 46-2. Critieria for reactive airway dysfunction syndrome (RADS)

1. Absence of a preceding asthma-like respiratory disease is documented.
2. Onset occurs after a high-level exposure, usually an accident.
3. Exposure is to a high-level irritant gas, vapor, fume, aerosol, or dust.
4. Onset of symptoms is abrupt and develops within minutes or hours and always by 24 hours.
5. The clinical picture simulates asthma, with unremitting cough, "bronchial irritability" complaints, and wheezing.
6. Pulmonary function testing may show normal findings or reversible airflow limitation.
7. Methacholine (or other agents) challenge is positive in the range noted with asthmatics (i.e., < 8 mg/ml).
8. Other respiratory disorders that simulate asthma are ruled out.

identify the majority of patients with allergic occupational asthma [37]: Are the symptoms improved on days off? Are the symptoms improved during vacation? Persons with RADS (or irritant-induced asthma) may also note improvement away from work because their induced venospecific observing hyperresponsiveness makes them susceptible to many varied low-level irritants and physical factions in their workplace. Symptoms may not improve over a 2-day weekend or occasional day off, but might improve within a period of 2 weeks or so.

An important differentiating chemical designation for RADS and allergic occupational asthma is the temporal relationship between exposure and disease onset. As much knowledge as possible of the incriminated etiologic agent is essential for diagnosis. Allergic occupational asthma does not develop after the initial exposure to the allergen or sensitizer. Sensitization occurs during a latent period. The latent period criteria can be of critical importance in establishing a medical-legal probability of causation [187]. This latent period is variable and may range from weeks to years but usually is several months. Sensitizers such as laboratory animals and the complex salts of platinum produce sensitization within a few months. It has been reported that exposure to isocyanates requires a mean period of 2 years for sensitization to develop; the period is 4 years for colophony and up to 10 years or longer with other agents [38].

The physician considers allergic occupational asthma when a patient has been exposed to a known sensitizing agent [46]. Confusion may occur with a single exposure, which has been reported to cause allergic occupational asthma [152]. A comprehensive set of guidelines for the diagnosis and evaluation of occupational lung disease has been published [22] and concerns of specific bronchoprovocation testing have been elucidated [10, 11, 22].

Consequences of High-level Irritant Exposures

Subjects have been reported to develop persistent respiratory symptoms after a single, high-concentration exposure to an environmental or occupational irritant. Harkonen and coworkers followed seven mine workers involved in a pyrite dust explosion who sustained SO_2-induced lung injury [103]. Four years after the accident, an asthma-like condition characterized by reversible airway obstruction was observed in three persons; four workers showed positive responses to histamine challenges whereas two subjects responded neither to histamine nor to bronchodilators. The authors concluded that nonspecific airway hyperresponsiveness was a frequent sequela of high level SO_2 exposure and could persist for years. In another report, Charan and coworkers described five workers who had accidental high levels of SO_2 exposure, with three survivors developing severe and another showing mild airway obstruction [59]. Flury and colleagues described a 50-year-old man who inhaled substantial quantities of concentrated ammonia vapors, and over the next 5 years serial pulmonary function testing documented the development of an obstructive lung disorder [89]. While methacholine challenges were not performed, the authors indicated that hyperreactive airways were present and likely the direct result of the inhalation injury. Donham and coauthors described an acute toxic exposure to high levels of hydrogen sulfide after agitation of liquid manure [77]. One survivor had respiratory symptoms persisting for over 2 months after the incident. Other reports of persistent obstructive airway disease after high-level irritant exposures include the studies of Murphy and associates on a subject who inhaled vapors liberated from mixing several drain cleaning agents [153] and the studies of Hasan et al. [104], Kennedy et al. [116], Kowitz et al. [205], and Kaufman and Burkons [115] reporting on subjects with chlorine gas exposures. Some individuals exposed to a single heavy exposure of TDI developed respiratory symptoms within 24 hours that persisted for years [132].

Consequences of Low-level Irritant Exposures

Meat wrapper's asthma was the term coined for the three meat wrappers who were treated in an emergency room because of their asthma [33]. Initial epidemiologic investigations recounted a 10 to 57 percent prevalence of respiratory symptomatology among meat wrappers. The etiologic agent was believed to be the emissions from the polyvinyl chloride (PVC) meat wrapping film when it was cut with a hot wire, thus evolving a fine particulate fume of di-2-ethylhexyl adipate combined with an aerosol or vapor of hydrogen chloride [193]. Subsequently, a clinical investigation concluded that it was mainly the emission from thermally activated price labels that was the principal cause of meat wrapper's asthma. The major ingredient of the incriminated price label adhesive is dicyclohexyl phthalate; when heated, it emits irritants, mainly cyclohexyl ether (dicyclohexyl ether) and cyclohexyl benzoate (cyclohexyl ether of benzoic acid) [193]. A potential sensitizer could be phthalic anhydride, a stipulated emission from the heated label [134].

Later investigations failed to demonstrate objective evidence of any major airway disease or chronic respiratory hazard among meat wrappers [33, 193]. For instance, in one study, while lower respiratory complaints were observed in one-third of the meat wrappers, no across shift change in FEV_1 was discerned, even in the most symptomatic workers [33, 193]. When tested in the workplace, phthalic anhydride was not noted in detectable concentrations in the vicinity of the heated price label emissions. Thus, it seems unlikely that this emission is actually present in significant concentrations, that it is present in the air for any reasonable period of time, and that it even remains stable during heating.

Formaldehyde has many applications, including use in the chemical and plastics industries, textile processing, disinfectants, the tanning industry, and the vulcanization process in the rubber industry and as a preservative of anatomic and pathologic material. A major application is in the production of urea formaldehyde foam for mobile home insulation and phenol formaldehyde resin for particle board production. Formaldehyde monomer as well as the degassing of formaldehyde from urea formaldehyde foam insulation has been reported to cause a variety of symptoms, including asthma [62, 70, 91, 122]. Asthma caused by low-level exposure is uncommon; there have been very few cases of formaldehyde-induced asthma documented by bronchial challenge tests, and low levels of exposure will not or rarely result in specific IgE antibody production [122]. Current evidence indicates that occupational asthma from formaldehyde is rare and that most respiratory complaints are the result of the irritative effects of formaldehyde. The occupational study of Nunn and associates found no excess of respiratory symptoms or an accelerated rate of fall of FEV_1 in workers exposed to formaldehyde compared with a group who were not exposed [163]. However, the population studied may have been a "survivor" population, with those workers who developed respiratory symptoms from the previously higher exposure levels leaving employment before the study commenced. There was a suggestion, however, of a possible adverse effect in nonsmokers. The investigation of Krzyzanowski and colleagues concluded that in children there were respiratory effects after prolonged indoor exposure to formaldehyde of less than 0.06 ppm [123]. There was an increased prevalence of physician-diagnosed chronic bronchitis or asthma in children 6 to 15 years old when they were exposed to formaldehyde levels between 0.06 and 0.14 ppm in their homes, with no threshold level identified. The decrement in lung function in adults was smaller than in children, transient, limited to the morning, and seen mainly in smokers exposed to the higher levels. The effects in adults are not clear but the findings in children may be of great concern. It suggests that children are a susceptible subpopulation for adverse health effects from indoor formaldehyde exposure.

The form formaldehyde takes may be important. For example, investigations where formaldehyde is present with respirable dust seem to show adverse effects on pulmonary function [135]. Possibly, gaseous formaldehyde adsorbs to dust particle surfaces and becomes concentrated and allows for longer retention in the lungs. I believe the data are now pretty convincing that prolonged exposure to formaldehyde is rarely associated with immunologically mediated respiratory disease [100].

An occupational airway disorder may occur as a result of exposure to the *dusts of cotton* (i.e., byssinosis), *flax, jute, sisal, or soft hemp*, and may vary clinically from acute dyspnea and chest tightness on 1 or more days of a working week to allegedly a chronic and permanent obstructive airway disease. Tannins constitute a large fraction of the organic material found in both cotton mill dust and cotton bract [176]. They may be leached from inhaled cotton dust and gain access to the pulmonary circulation, causing a cascade of events that might culminate in byssinosis symptoms. Tannins were found to exhibit a dual effect on smooth muscle tone of rabbit pulmonary artery, depending on the degree of initial tone. The contraction effects of tannins appear to be the result of the production and release of thromboxane A_2 from pulmonary endothelial cells. The study by Love and colleagues related airborne dust concentrations and respiratory and allergic symptoms in wool textile workers [129]. The investigators identified endotoxins in a limited series of measurements and hypothesized a possible role in causation of respiratory symptoms [129], as suggested by others.

It has been reported that oxidant-type *air pollution* is likely to cause more respiratory symptoms among allergic patients than nonallergic persons. Bascom and associates addressed this issue utilizing analyses of nasal lavage fluid from asymptomatic allergic rhinitis subjects before and after nasal challenge with antigen (four different doses of antigen) and with and without preexposure to 0.5 ppm of ozone [16]. The study was the first to characterize the upper respiratory response to ozone in asymptomatic allergic subjects and showed that this host factor leads to an enhanced ozone responsiveness. Exposure to ozone alone caused both upper and lower respiratory symptomatology, a mixed inflammatory cell influx in nasal lavage fluid, and an increased albumin concentration in lavage fluid. The ozone exposure caused more pronounced lower respiratory symptoms than upper respiratory symptoms in these asymptomatic allergic rhinitis subjects. Profound inflammatory eosinophilia was produced by ozone exposure but no ozone-induced alteration in nasal antigen challenge sensitivity was observed. This is in contrast to a recent report on asthmatics which documented an increased antigen sensitivity by bronchial inhalation challenges after ozone exposure [151].

Healthy, nonsmoking male volunteers, aged 18 to 35 years, with no history of asthma, allergic rhinitis, or respiratory disease were studied by comparing nasal lavage to BAL [97]. Nasal lavage was found to correlate with the presence of an acute inflammatory response occurring in the lower airways. It was suggested that nasal lavage could be used as a tool to examine other types of irritant pollutants. The nasal neutrophil response, however, did not directly predict the magnitude of the BAL neutrophilic response. Significant attention is placed on ozone, because of the fact that it is the major component of the oxidant-type air pollution, the type of air pollution present in most of this country's larger cities. Devlin and coworkers performed BAL on nonsmoking males randomly exposed to filtered air and either 0.10 ppm or 0.08 ppm of ozone for 6.6 hours with moderate exercise (40 L/min) in order to determine the influence of prolonged exposure of low levels of ozone [73]. A 0.01-ppm concentration resulted in significant increases of neutrophils, protein content, prostaglandin E_2, fibronectin, interleukin-6, and lactate dehydrogenase in BAL fluid, compared to volunteers exposed to filtered air. Additionally, there was reduced alveolar macrophage phagocytosis. Similar changes were observed with the 0.08-ppm level but without a significant increase of protein and fibronectin. There was no observed increase in certain chemoattractants (leukotriene B_4 and complement fragments), which makes one wonder what caused the influx of neutrophils. There was individual variation to the exposure with a considerable range of responses, suggesting a subpopulation that is very sensitive to the low levels of ozone. Ozone exposures (separate 0.00-, 0.08-, 0.10-, and 0.12-ppm exposures) in a climatic chamber for 6.6 hours with inclusions of six 50-minute periods of moderate exercise (total of 5 hours) revealed an approximate twofold increase in nonspecific airway reactivity (as tested by methacholine challenge) [106]. A 12.3 percent decrement in FEV_1 was observed with the 0.12-ppm exposure. Again, a marked variability in response from subject to subject was noted. Frampton and coauthors reported that short-term (3-hour) continuous nitrogen dioxide exposure (1.5 ppm) increased airway reactivity in normal subjects in contrast to brief (15-minute) peaks of nitrogen dioxide at 2.0 ppm, which did not increase reactivity [90]. The question of whether low levels of nitrogen dioxide can alter airway reactivity remains unresolved, perhaps because of the difficulty of comparing studies in which varying levels of exposure were administered under varying conditions to subjects chosen by a variety of screening criteria.

Red-tide toxin, a natural phenomenon caused by the blooms of the unicellular marine algae *Ptychodiscus brevis*, occurs in the Gulf of Mexico, mainly along the west coast of Florida. Red tide has been reported to produce asthma-like symptoms in humans and contraction of in vitro canine airway smooth muscle preparations [173]. Membrane potential and contractility assessments demonstrated that the toxin produced concentration-dependent depolarization and contractions in the canine trachealis smooth muscle preparations, which was inhibited by atropine and the sodium channel blocker tetrodotoxin.

Machining fluids may have irritant properties because of contamination with trace quantities of base metal and there are additives, such as the corrosion inhibitor, antifoam agents, emulsifiers, antioxidants, detergents, viscosity index improver, antiwear agents, extreme pressure agents, and bactericides. Besides the additives, oil-water emulsions provide a good growth media for bacteria and yeast. A study by Kennedy and associates reported an FEV_1 response (5% or greater decrease in FEV_1 across shift change) in 23.6 percent of machinists and only 9.5 percent of the minimally exposed assembly workers [117]. The exact etiologic agent in machining fluids responsible for the FEV_1 changes was not clarified, but microbial contamination with endotoxin from gram-negative bacteria, chemical irritants, and an allergic sensitizer were speculated as potential causes.

REACTIVE AIRWAY INITIATED DYSFUNCTION SYNDROME

It is clear that an irritant can lead to asthma development (i.e., RADS) after a high-level exposure. It appears there are susceptible persons in the general population who respond more adversely to irritant exposures and seem to be at a greater risk for developing asthma from a lower-level irritant gas or vapor exposure [206]. While irritant gas-induced airway inflammation is documented for normal volunteers, a similar exposure in asthmatics and atopic persons seems to produce exaggerated consequences [207]. Furthermore, there is an observed increased antigen sensitivity (as determined by bronchial inhalation challenge) following low-level ozone exposure [208]. Investigations employing low-level ozone exposure document individual variations in responsiveness, suggesting a subpopulation that is very sensitive to the low levels of ozone [209, 210]. Persons with airway hyperresponsiveness are reported to respond more adversely to irritant exposures. Persons with nonspecific bronchial hyperresponsiveness may, however, be completely asymptomatic and this aberration is very common among the young [211]. Furthermore, the prevalence of nonspecific bronchial hyperreactivity in the general population is more common than previously appreciated [212]. Perhaps the increased sensitivity to irritants is due to airway epithelial damage which can be present in asthmatic subjects (and possibly atopic persons) who display minimal symptoms and who require little or no medication [213–215]. Likely, the airways of asthmatics and, possibly some atopics, are "leaky" [216]. Bronchial mucosa-mast cell degranulation and mediator release occurs continuously among atopic asthmatic subjects. Another possibility is that the irritant exposure increases the sensitivity to an allergen and affected subjects respond to lower concentrations of the aeroallergen.

Reactive airways initiated dysfunction syndrome (RAIDS) can be defined as a condition, presumably in persons with an allergic or atopic diathesis, whereby asthma symptoms appear to be initiated by a low- or moderate-level exposure to an irritant substance or material in the workplace or environment, and is characterized clinically by the development of asthma symptoms and physiologically by the finding of an atopic status and the presence of nonspecific airway hyperresponsiveness. The clinical presentation is one of a patient, without preceding respiratory complaints or asthma symptomatology, who develops asthma for the first time after experiencing an irritant exposure lasting a few minutes or hours, or several days or a few weeks. The irritant is generally a gas or vapor, but on occasion, may be in the form of a fume or dust. The exposure levels would not be considered massive, but rather moderate or low-level in nature. Asthma symptoms may develop abruptly or evolve over several days or a few weeks [216]. Initially, upper respiratory symptoms may predominate, including eye, nose, throat and laryngeal symptomatology. Subsequently, the patient develops what seems to be an increased sensitivity to many and varied nonspecific irritants while away from the exposure. This manifestation can be designated as "bronchial irritability"; there is coughing, choking and perhaps wheezing and chest tightness occurring after many and varied nonspecific irritant exposures. When further investigated, the patient is discovered to be atopic or is suspected of having preexisting, but asymptomatic nonspecific airway hyperresponsiveness. In all cases, when tested the methacholine challenge test is positive in the PC_{20} range noted for asthmatic subjects. It is proposed, that the irritant exposure, in these susceptible persons initiated the onset of asthma, perhaps being comparable to a respiratory infection or a large allergen load. The designation *RAIDS* emphasizes the importance of the environmental factors in initiating the onset of asthma. RAIDS is differentiated from classical occupational asthma due to workplace sensitization and RADS due to a massive workplace irritant exposure.

ALLERGIC OCCUPATIONAL ASTHMA

Patients with allergic occupational asthma may have a typical clinical presentation [37]. Several different types of bronchospastic reactions occur in response to workplace exposures [38]. Nonspecific airway hyperresponsiveness may become permanent and symptoms may become persistent after termination of the exposure. Noting a latent period before the development of asthma can be of critical importance in establishing the medical-legal probability of causation [38, 187]. In those individuals with preexisting asthma, or where the exposure is to an irritant, there may be an induction of symptoms at work [61]. This is not generally thought to be occupational asthma.

The initial interview with a patient should include a detailed occupational history. Attention should be paid to potential exposures outside the usual working environment. Asthma may develop as the result of hobbies or a secondary occupation. Exposure may be indirect [47].

Case Example

A 30-year-old spice factory worker without symptoms for the first 5 years of employment noted the gradual onset of cough, which was worse at night [133]. This symptom increased greatly over a period of 1 year and was accompanied by chest tightness, shortness of breath, and wheezing. His symptoms occurred only when garlic powder was being processed in the plant and not at other times; this occurred mainly during the spring and summer periods. His symptoms initiated shortly after exposure to garlic dust in the workplace and persisted throughout the working day, only to improve and disappear by the next morning. He denied allergies, and did not provide a family history of atopy. The subject related that asthma symptoms also developed after ingesting garlic in food.

The subject was a cigarette smoker for 15 years but recently quit. He reported that he was an extremely active person and claimed good health until the development of his respiratory symptoms.

On an initial physical examination, a few scattered wheezes were noted on auscultation of the chest; subsequent examinations were unremarkable.

Laboratory test results were negative except for an elevated total eosinophil count of 1,330/mm³. Skin tests for common airborne allergens were positive for molds, tree pollen, and ragweed. Total IgE antibody was markedly elevated, 4,566 U/ml (normal values <250 U/ml). A prick skin test for garlic extract at 1:10,000 dilution demonstrated a positive response, while an intradermal skin test for garlic extract at 1:10,000 dilution caused dermatographia. Results of the RAST with garlic extract antigen and the methacholine bronchial challenge test were positive.

Specific bronchial inhalation challenges were performed utilizing different concentrations of garlic dust. The dust exposure was simulated by transferring garlic powder from cup to pan near the patient's breathing zone. A personal air sampler located near the mouth measured the dust concentration. Control dust consisted of lactose powder generated alone. Then, two garlic dust exposures were tested by mixing garlic powder concentrations of 1:100 and 1:10 with lactose powder. Tests were performed on separate days. Each exposure lasted for approximately 3 minutes (25 cup transfers) and was followed by serial pulmonary function tests. No response occurred during the control lactose inhalation. A small response was seen with the 1:100 garlic-lactose powder; the personal air sampling measurement was 2.5×10^4 particles per cubic feet (ppcf) of air breathed. With the 1:10 garlic powder concentration of 3.0×10^5 ppcf, a 37 percent fall in FEV_1 was noted. A physical examination at the time of maximal change in FEV_1 revealed generalized wheezing (Fig. 46-9).

Specific Causes

While the number of etiologic agents for allergic occupational asthma is more than 200 and growing, only a few of these agents have been extensively studied and characterized, with many existing only as anecdotal case reports. In some cases, in vitro testing may assist in determining the potential for sensitization [197]. A working knowledge of the more frequent causes and the availability of more extensive lists of agents are available in reviews [21, 28, 32, 52, 53, 61, 165]. Some authors classify responsible agents as (1) microbial products (e.g., *Bacillus subtilis* enzymes in the detergent industry); (2) animal, bird, and arthropod products (e.g., urine protein/dander from small mammals in laboratory settings); (3) plant products (e.g., wheat flour in bakeries); and (4) chemicals (e.g., TDI in the plastics industry). Etiologic agents may also be classified into high-molecular-weight compounds (>1,000). High-molecular-weight compounds are usually proteins, polysaccharides, or peptides of animal, vegetable, bacterial, or insect origin. The prevalence of asthma due

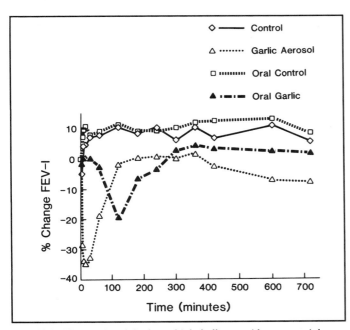

Fig. 46-9. *The results of the bronchial challenge with commercial garlic extract solution. Garlic was aerosolized through a No. 40 DeVilbis nebulizer. A Lowry determination of total protein content was performed on each garlic solution. The maximum fall in 1-second forced expiratory volume (FEV$_{1.0}$) of 35 percent occurred with the highest garlic protein concentration of 1.1 × 10^{-7} gm. The asthmatic reaction could be partially inhibited by cromolyn sodium (not shown). (Reprinted with permission from J. A. Lybarger, et al. Occupational asthma induced by the inhalation and ingestion of garlic. J. Allergy Clin. Immunol. 69:488, 1982.)*

Table 46-3. Substances of animal origin that may cause asthma

Agent	Occupation
Animals	
Laboratory animals (hair, epidermal squamae, mites, pelts, urine and serum protein)	Laboratory animal (rats, mice, guinea pigs, rabbits) handlers
Domestic animals	Farmers, veterinarians, meat processors and inspectors
Animal organ extracts (ACTH, gonadotropic hormone, pituitary peptone powders)	Pharmaceutical workers
Wool	Wool workers
Birds	
Birds (feathers, serum, droppings, egg products)	Bird fanciers, poultry breeders and processors, pluckers, egg processors
Aquatic	
Sea squirt fluid	Oyster and pearl gatherers
Prawns	Prawn processors
Culture oysters (marine organisms)	Oyster shuckers
Crabs	Crab processors
Hoya	Oyster farmers
Pearl shell dust	Pearl shell openers
Marine sponges	Laboratory workers
Amebas and other organisms	Printers using contaminated water
Glue (fish origin)	Bookbinders, postal workers
Animal enzymes	
Hog trypsin, pancreatic extract, flaviastase, amylase, glucose oxidase	Laboratory workers, plastic polymer processors, pharmaceutical workers, fibrocystic children and their parents, enzyme processor workers and messengers, pharmacists
Bacillus subtilis	Detergent enzyme workers
Esperase	Detergent enzyme workers
Human hair	Hairdressers
Insects	
Beatles (*Coleoptera*)	Zoo curators
Grain weevils	Granary workers, dock workers, mill workers
Grain storage mites	Farmers, dock workers
Locusts	Laboratory workers, schoolchildren, and teachers
Mexican bean weevil	Pea and bean sorters
Moths, butterflies	Entomologists
Silkworms (larva, hair, silk glue, sericin)	Silkworm cutters, sericulturists
Stick insects	Field workers, laboratory workers, students
Cockroaches	Laboratory workers, students, field workers
Crickets	Outside workers
Housefly maggots	Anglers
River flies	Outside workers
Sewerworm flies	Outside workers
Sewage flies	Outside workers

to these compounds tends to be relatively high depending on the level of exposure; atopy seems to be a predisposing factor, but not always; and these compounds often result in asthma by inducing immunologic responses characterized by specific IgE antibodies [1]. Positive immediate skin test reactions to extracts are usual and specific IgE may be identified by serologic testing. The pathogenesis of asthma due to high-molecular-weight compounds is no different from that of more common inhalant allergens such as house dust. As a result, occupational asthma due to high-molecular-weight compounds provides a good model for studying extrinsic asthma.

Low-molecular-weight compounds capable of inducing asthma are growing in number. The prevalence of occupational asthma due to low-molecular-weight compounds tends to be lower and atopy generally is not a predisposing factor [1]. These compounds presumably are too small to act as allergens by themselves. They may elicit immunologic responses by acting as a hapten and combining with a protein carrier molecule to form an allergen. The immune response to a hapten-carrier complex can be directed against the hapten, against the carrier, or to a new antigenic determinant [165]. It has been difficult to confirm an IgE-mediated response in many cases of occupational asthma due to low-molecular-weight compounds. Skin testing is usually not helpful and specific IgE antibodies are found in a minority of symptomatic patients. Cellular immunity may be important in this type of asthma [87]. Occupational asthma due to low-molecular-weight compounds may provide a model for studying apparent non–IgE-mediated asthma.

For this chapter, causes of allergic occupational asthma are divided into animal, vegetable, and chemical categories. The causes are shown in Tables 46-3 through 46-5. Examples of allergic causes are presented in the following sections.

Red Cedar

Approximately 4 percent of exposed workers develop asthma [57]. Western red cedar is different from other wood in its unusually high content of water-soluble compounds, including tannin, dyes, pitch, resins, and lignins. Plicatic acid, a major fraction, is a unique component of western red cedar and has not been identified in any other wood. In provocation tests, plicatic acid produced bronchial reactions similar to those produced by a whole extract and is probably the causative agent. BAL studies

Table 46-4. Substances of vegetable origin that may cause asthma

Agent	Occupation
Plants	
Flour, grain dust	Grain elevator workers, bakers, millers, grain workers
Wheat flour	Bakers
Rye flour	Bakers
Buckwheat	Bakers
Wheat gluten derivative	Bakers
Hops	Brewery workers, farmers
Soybean flour and dust	Soybean processors, epidemics
Garlic powder	Spice factory workers
Tamarind seeds	Millers
Tea fluff	Tea makers, sifters, and packers
Green leaf tobacco	Tobacco workers and processors
Green leaf tea	Tea workers
Green and roasted coffee beans	Coffee workers
Castor beans	Farmers, miller, chemists, baggers
Maiko	Japanese food workers, millers
Cottonseed	Bakers, fertilizer workers
Linseed	Oil extractors
Flaxseed	Flax workers
Psyllium	Pharmaceutical workers
Lycopodium clavatum	Dentists
Gum acacia	Printers
Gum tragacanth	Printers, candy and gum workers
Strawberry pollen	Strawberry growers
Potatoes	House wives
Wood	
Western red cedar	Woodworkers, carpenters
African zebrawood	Joiners
Cedar of Lebanon	Shuttle makers
South African boxwood	Pattern makers
Oak	Wood finishers
Mahogany	Wood machinists
Mansonia	Sawmill workers, carpenters, wood finishers
Abiruana	Sawmill workers, carpenters, wood finishers
Cocaballa	Sawmill workers, carpenters, wood finishers
Kejaat	Sawmill workers, carpenters, wood finishers
California redwood	Sawmill workers, carpenters, wood finishers
Ramin	Sawmill workers, carpenters, wood finishers
Quillaja bark	Manufacturers of saponin
Iroko	Sawmill workers
Mulberry	Sawmill workers
Latex	Operating room nurses
Plant enzymes	
Papain	Food technologists
Diastase	Food handlers
Pectinase	Pharmaceutical workers
Bromelain	Pharmaceutical workers
Vegetable gums	
Karaya	Food processors
Arabic	Printers
Acacia	Printers
Tragacanth	Printers
Fungi, molds	
Alternaria and *Aspergillus*	Bakers
Spores of *Cladosporium, Verticillium,* and *Paecilomyces*	Farm workers
Merulius lacrymans	Domestic workers, paprika splitters
Pink rot fungus	Celery pickers
Mushroom molds	Mushroom workers
Molds	Morticians
Fungal amylase	Enzyme processors

Table 46-5. Substances of chemical origin that may cause asthma

Agent	Occupation
Metallic salts	
Platinum	Platinum refiners, chemists
Nickel	Platers, chemical engineers
Aluminum (or fumes)	Chemical workers, potroom workers
Vanadium	Boiler and gas turbine cleaners, mineral ore processors
Cobalt	Refinery and alloy workers, diamond cutters
Stainless steel	Welders
Chromium	Chrome polishers, chemical workers, cement tanning workers
Tungsten carbide	Hard metal grinders
Chemicals	
Akyl cyanoacrylate	Hobbies, home repair
Para-phenylenediamine	Fur dyers, chemical workers
Piperazine	Chemical process workers
Formaldehyde	Nurses, pathologists, laboratory workers
Phenol	Chemical workers, laboratory workers
Chloramine	Brewery workers
Hexachlorophene	Hospital workers
Sulfathiazole	Manufacturers
Sulfonechloramide	Manufacturers
Tannic acid	Sunburn spray users
Orrisroot derivatives	Cosmetic workers, hairdressers
Triethyltetramine	Manufacturing of aircraft filters
Dimethyl ethanolamine	Spray painters
Aminoethanolamine	Aluminum soldering
Ethylenediamine	Rubber and shellac manufacturers, photographers
Pyrethrins	Fumigators
Diisocyanates	Chemical workers, polyurethane foam manufacturing
Phthalic anhydrides	Chemical workers, epoxy resin workers, tool setters, paint manufacturers
Trimellitic anhydride	Manufacturers
Ammonium thioglycate	Beauty operators, cosmetic manufacturers
Aozdicarbaonamide	Rubber workers
Dioazonium salt	Photocopiers
Colophony	Electronic manufacturers
Resin binder systems	Foundry mold makers (MDI, furan-based resins)
Reactive dyes	Dye weighers
Persulfate salts, extract of henna	Hairdressers, chemical workers
Reactive dyes	Textile dyeing
Pharmaceuticals	
Psyllium	Laxative makers, nurses
Amprolium hydrochloride	Poultry feed mixers
Penicillin	Pharmaceutical workers
Pesticides, insecticides	Manufacturers, farmers, fumigators
Tylosin	Pharmaceutical workers
Hydrazine	Pharmaceutical workers
Spiramycin	Pharmaceutical workers
Phenylglycine acid chloride	Pharmaceutical workers
Cephalosporins	Pharmaceutical workers
Methyldopa	Pharmaceutical workers
Salbutamol intermediate	Pharmaceutical workers
Tetracycline	Pharmaceutical workers
Sulfonechloramide	Brewery workers

have documented a release of metabolites of arachidonic acid after inhalation challenges [54, 55, 58].

Clinically, the exposed worker first complains of eye and nose irritation with rhinorrhea and nasal obstruction. After some weeks, a cough develops and is usually worse at the end of the day or at night. Subsequently there may be episodes of nocturnal cough or wheezing. Characteristically, the symptoms, especially those occurring at night, persist for many days or weeks after cessation of the exposure. Symptoms may recur on the first day or evening after return to work, but sometimes they do not reappear for a week or more. Diagnosis may be difficult because some workers have persistent airway obstruction with no change in symptoms over weekends or vacations or even after leaving the industry. Diagnosis is not aided by skin testing, since immediate and delayed skin reactions to cedar extracts have been inconsistent, but specific IgE antibodies to crude cedar extract or plicatic acid–human serum albumin conjugate were found in 40 percent of patients [1, 52, 57]. Inhalation challenge tests seem the best method for confirming the diagnosis.

Colophony
Colophony is a combination of pine tree resins of which the major constituents are abietic, dehydroabietic, and pimaric acid [1, 39, 40, 165]. Asthma among soldering workers in the electronics industry has been associated with exposure to colophony contained in soldering fluxes. Prevalence varies from 4 to 21 percent depending on the exposure. The exact pathogenesis is not certain. Features of the disease suggest an immunologic mechanism but skin tests and in vitro studies have not been able to confirm immunologic sensitization [39, 40].

Acid Anhydrides
Acid anhydride compounds cause IgE-mediated respiratory sensitization in the workplace [21, 165, 195]. The major commercial acid anhydrides include phthalic anhydride, hexahydrophthalic anhydride (HHPA), himic anhydride, tetrachlorophthalic anhydride (TCPA), and trimellitic anhydride. Phthalic anhydride is an essential chemical reagent in the manufacture of a variety of industrial products including plasticizers, epoxy resins, and paints. Epoxy resins show outstanding resistance to heat and chemicals and have wide application in reinforced plastics, adhesives, and encapsulation. The resin is usually prepared from epichlorohydrin and polyhydroxy compound in the presence of a curing agent. The curing involves the use of cross-linking agents known as hardeners. The hardeners include polyamines such as diethylene thiamine, triethyltetramine, and piperazine as well as acid anhydrides (such as phthalic anhydride) and polybasic acids. Although the prevalence of sensitization to phthalic anhydride is unknown, the occurrence of asthma in exposed workers is cited as an important toxic effect. Maccia and coworkers described the case of clinical sensitization in a worker who had symptoms of rhinorrhea, lacrimation, and wheezing after exposure to this chemical [134]. Positive immediate skin test reactions and bronchial challenge results, as well as high serum titers of specific IgE (by RAST) to the phthalic anhydride, corroborated clinical hypersensitivity.

Five workers exposed to epoxy resins had recurrent respiratory symptoms and pulmonary function test abnormalities after exposure to tetrachlorophthalic anhydride [180].

Trimellitic anhydride powder in trimellitic anhydride production was reported to cause acute, IgE-mediated asthma in some workers and symptoms simulating allergic alveolitis in others. In vitro, trimellitic anhydride reacts rapidly with protein to form a trimellitic anhydride–protein complex determined by radioimmunoassay techniques. There have also been reports of extensive and more serious infiltrative pulmonary processes associated with anemia after exposure to trimellitic anhydride fumes,

rather than the dust. The pulmonary syndrome associated with anemia after exposure to trimellitic anhydride fumes, rather than the dust, consists of cough, hemoptysis, dyspnea, pulmonary infiltrates, a restrictive lung defect, hypoxemia, and anemia. The pathogenesis of the disease may be a complex interaction among the chemical toxicity of trimellitic anhydride fumes, the immune reaction against trimellitic anhydride–haptenized proteins by cells of the respiratory tract, and the degree of exposure to trimellitic anhydride fumes of the individual worker.

Diisocyanates
Diisocyanates are widely used in the production of polyurethane foam and have applications in the manufacture of plastics, foam surface coating, elastomers, adhesives, and fibers. The four most common isocyanates are TDI, diphenylmethane diisocyanate, naphthalene diisocyanate, and hexamethylene diisocyanate. HDI and TDI have about the same vapor pressures and are relatively volatile at room temperature, while MDI, with a relatively lower vapor pressure, is not. MDI becomes more volatile and dangerous when it is heated, as with foundry work. Spray painting is a particularly dangerous form of exposure since vapors (HDI, TDI) and particulates (MDI) are airborne and at high levels.

Occupational exposure to TDI, by far the most important commercially and toxicologically, may occur during its production in the vicinity of foam-producing machines, during spraying and molding operations, after accidental leakage or spillage of liquid TDI during bulk or drum handling or drum emptying, after leakage from pumps, during disposal of TDI waste, during welding of polyurethane products, or during the use of polyurethane floor varnish with a TDI activator.

A number of reports detailing various aspects of diisocyanates have been published [2, 5, 10, 11, 25, 26, 27, 34, 45, 47, 50, 75, 81, 84, 87, 99, 114, 128, 132, 139–141, 144–146, 152, 159, 167, 169, 181–183, 185, 198, 199, 201, 204]. Exposure to high concentrations may occur with accidental spillage [32, 34, 114] but low concentrations are usually encountered in industry. Automobile-body spray painting represents an important and high-risk occupation for both asthma and hypersensitivity pneumonias because of the great potential for exposure to high levels of isocyanates, especially HDI. Not infrequently, paint spraying facilities utilize poorly designed control measures. Operations often employ only one or two persons, young and inexperienced, who do not always appreciate the need for proper respiratory protection and protective environmental conditions that are required for this type of work. Workers who get "sick" can be terminated without major repercussions in the smaller companies. There is often a great turnover of employees in this type of work. Thus, affected workers leave the industry, perhaps with respiratory disease. The National Institute for Occupational Safety and Health (NIOSH) estimates that between 50,000 and 100,000 employees in the United States are exposed to isocyanates, and adverse respiratory responses develop in perhaps 5 percent of these [159].

The exact immunologic mechanism in isocyanate asthma is unclear. While there are reports of high levels of IgE antibodies in affected workers [18, 114], these observations have not been confirmed by others [34, 201]. It may be that several immunologic and nonimmunologic mechanisms may be operative [139]. Baur stated that by using HSA-bound (human serum albumin) isocyanates in skin testing, in RAST, and in inhalation challenges, IgE-mediated, diisocyanate-induced disease may be differentiated from nonimmunologic disease [18]. Using these techniques, Baur and associates found that 14 percent of symptomatic workers were immunologically sensitized [19]. Specific bronchial challenge testing, however, may be the only means to document the diagnosis. In a study of 639 factory workers exposed to TDI, the results of RAST measuring specific IgE for p-tolyl isocyanate were positive in less than 5 percent of symptomatic workers [34]. Studies by other investigators reported 15 to 18 percent positive RAST results in affected workers [201]. The presence of serum IgG antibodies has been suggested as being important in the pathogenesis of asthma. An HDI-HSA conjugate followed by specific inhibition after preincubation was considered to support the conclusion that HDI was the cause of asthma in the case of an automobile-body spray painter [182]. Because the significance of IgG antibodies was unclear, the investigators examined serum from 455 isocyanate-exposed persons and 157 unexposed referent subjects. Among the isocyanate-exposed persons, a serum dilution of 20 in the enzyme-linked immunosorbent assay (ELISA) gave positive results for about 10 percent, depending on the job activity group and type of isocyanate studied. For example, "foaming, old equipment" (TDI, MDI) was 33 percent, while "foaming, closed process" (MDI) was 0 percent prevalence. Among 10 patients with isocyanate asthma, 50 percent showed positive tests. When a second criterion for being positive was used (dilution of 100), the prevalence of positive test results was about half, being 5 percent; for patients with asthma it was still 50 percent. While IgG antibodies seem to play only a minor immunopathologic role in isocyanate hypersensitivity pneumonia, they may be important in asthma. This point was emphasized in a study where specific bronchial inhalation challenge to isocyanates was positive in 29 of 65 referred patients [50]. Twenty-one (72%) of 29 with positive bronchial challenges also demonstrated elevated specific IgG levels; 31 percent showed increased specific IgE antibodies. It appears that specific IgG may be a better indicator of isocyanate allergy than IgE antibody determination. Fabbri and associates distinguished the importance of airway inflammation in the pathogenesis of nonspecific airway hyperresponsiveness associated with TDI [81–83]. Fabbri and others also reported a fatal case in a sensitized worker who continued to work [84, 217, 218].

Alkyl Cyanoacrylate
Instant glues containing cyanoacrylate esters are used extensively in home repairs and hobbies. Kopp and coauthors reported on a 32-year-old atopic individual with asthma who used superglue for building remote control model planes [121]. Bronchial provocation to the glue vapors in a manner simulating the home exposure resulted in a late-phase asthmatic response with rhinorrhea and lacrimation. Documented increased airway hyperresponsiveness to methacholine occurred after the bronchial challenge and persisted for several weeks. Complete resolution of asthma symptoms and reversion to a negative methacholine challenge occurred after 6 months of continued avoidance to the glue. There have been additional reports concerning asthma due to this chemical [130, 158].

Aluminum
Potroom workers and aluminum smelters are reported to develop asthma [120, 202]. An irritant response from high-level exposure to potroom fumes is likely the cause of an observed immediate bronchospastic response, while a late-occurring reaction may be immunologically induced. The late response characteristically develops some 4 to 12 hours after exposure and may affect workers during the night while at home. Reports of dual responses have also been noted.

Platinum
Repeated exposure to platinum salts can produce allergic sensitization with both upper and lower respiratory tract symptoms, a syndrome formerly referred to as *platinosis* [7, 29, 196]. The allergic potential of platinum salts is so great that in some studies as many as 60 to 100 percent of exposed persons developed allergy [165]. In most cases sensitization develops within 6 to 7 months, but it may occur as quickly as 10 days or not appear until after 25 years of employment. While asthma has been reported in workers exposed to the halide salts of platinum in the platinum refinery industry, the prevalence of asthma in this industry has been reported to be decreasing in the United Kingdom. The reason given for this reduction in the prevalence of asthma is the policy in England of removing employees from exposure once a positive response on platinum skin tests is identified by surveillance testing.

The asthmatic reaction may be immediate, late, or dual in type and can be reproduced by inhalation challenge tests. Late asthmatic reactions are inhibited by cromolyn sodium. Skin prick tests with low concentrations of chloroplatinates give immediate positive reactions [7]. A RAST has been developed for measuring IgE antibodies to platinum chloride complexes in sensitized workers. Persistence of asthma, elevated levels of IgE, and hyperreactive airways have been demonstrated in workers who have not been exposed for several years [7, 29].

In a recent investigation of platinum workers, cold air challenges were completed in 107 current and 29 terminated employees [7, 29]. Results of cold air challenge testing were positive in 11 percent of the current and 31 percent of the terminated workers; more than one-third of the current workers with positive cold air responses and one-half of the terminated employees with positive cold air responses had positive prick skin reactions to platinum salt. Three individuals with positive cold air challenge and negative skin test responses to platinum were all subsequently found to have positive skin test reactions to platinum when retested 1 year later. Smokers are at increased risk of sensitization to platinum salts [7, 29, 196].

Cobalt
Hard metal is an alloy consisting of tungsten carbide (80–95%) with cobalt (5–20%) as a matrix. Sometimes other metals such as titanium, tantalum, vanadium, nickel, and chromium are added in the carbide form. A number of studies have implicated cobalt as the offending agent in hard metal asthma. The cobalt metal as an alloy causes asthma, which is different from what is found with platinum, nickel, and chromium where asthma and sensitization result from exposure to the metal salt. This implies that cobalt has to be converted to ionized cobalt on the bronchial mucosa to act as a hapten following conjugation with proteins. Sprince and associates surveyed 1,039 tungsten carbide production workers [188]. Roughly 11 percent of workers reported wheezing and there was a 2.1 times greater odds ratio for work-related wheezing in workers exposed to more than 50 $\mu g/m^3$ than in those exposed to less than 50 $\mu g/m^3$. The study of Shirakawa and coworkers also documented specific IgE antibodies in workers [184]. Meyer-Bisch and colleagues investigated 424 workers and 88 control subjects and reported that cough and sputum were common complaints among workers engaged in "soft powder" and presintering workshops, but women in sintering and finishing had more frequent spirometric abnormalities [149].

Ispaghula or Psyllium
The husks and seeds of *Plantago ovata*, also known as ispaghula or psyllium, are hydrophilic and capable of absorbing up to 40 times their own weight in water. Because of this property, they form a mucilaginous material, which is an effective bulk laxative. Inhalation of dusts from pharmaceutical preparations manufactured from husks can cause IgE-mediated allergic respiratory symptoms in workers exposed to this agent, such as nurses, process workers, and home users [12, 43, 48, 96, 143, 160, 175]. In the study of Nelson, 18 percent of the subjects studied reported allergic reactions and 5 percent had dyspnea, wheezing, or hives within 30 minutes of preparing the laxative [160]. There was a reported 3.6 percent prevalence among 130 employees at a pharmaceutical company [12]. Respiratory, nasal, and skin com-

plaints were noted in 48 (52%) of 92 exposed workers in another pharmaceutical company [143]. In this latter study, most of the effects were believed to be irritant in nature, but sensitization occurred in some.

DIAGNOSIS

Overview

A high degree of suspicion must be maintained in the evaluation of any patient of working age who develops asthma or notes a significant deterioration of preexisting symptoms. A necessary first step is to confirm that the patient does indeed have asthma. Although a history of intermittent cough, dyspnea, and wheezing is suggestive, demonstration of reversible airflow limitation must be done for confirmation. A significant improvement in spirometric indices after the inhalation of a bronchodilator would confirm a clinical suspicion of asthma. Substantial improvement of airflow limitation over time or with treatment likewise suggests asthma. Normal spirometry, however, cannot exclude asthma. In this case, a nonspecific bronchoprovocation challenge test may be useful in demonstrating bronchial hyperresponsiveness [61]. A previous diagnosis of asthma does not rule out occupational asthma. A change in the character of the symptoms or the abrupt increase in medication requirement may suggest a new or additional sensitization.

Next, it must be established that symptoms are work related. Although ignoring the workplace as a possible causative source is the more common problem, the physician must avoid leaping to an occupational diagnosis even when the patient has been exposed to a known etiologic agent [46]. On the other hand, the absence or apparent absence of a known allergen or sensitizer in the workplace does not exclude the diagnosis of occupational asthma. An appropriate history may be suggestive, serial measures of pulmonary function may document an appropriate temporal association, and evidence of sensitization to specific workplace compounds may imply exposure. For many purposes, the diagnostic workup may end here. For example, workers who are exposed to a known cause of occupational asthma and in whom a relation between changes in airflow obstruction and airway responsiveness and exposure at work can be established may be assumed to have occupational asthma [46].

Finally, where more diagnostic precision is required or where doubt exists as to the true source of the patient's symptom complex after the initial workup, a specific bronchoprovocation challenge test may be helpful. In many circumstances, it may be the only way to settle the question. Banks and colleagues reported that only approximately 50 percent of patients with symptoms compatible with TDI asthma had a positive response to challenge [10, 11].

The patient with potential occupational asthma should be seen by a physician experienced in the evaluation of such patients before he or she has left work and as early as possible in the disease course, ideally before bronchial hyperresponsiveness has become permanently established [61]. A comprehensive set of guidelines for the diagnosis and evaluation of occupational lung disease was recently published by the American Academy of Allergy and Immunology [22].

History

Malo and coworkers assessed the value of the clinical history taken by an open medical questionnaire in predicting a diagnosis of occupational asthma as confirmed by objective tests in 162 subjects [137]. They found a positive predictive value of 63 percent and a negative predictive value of 83 percent. Moreover,

there was agreement between the physician's initial assessment and the final diagnosis in only 84 (52%) of the 162 patients.

Symptoms often first appear at night or after the work shift has ended, perhaps due to the late response to an exposure encountered at work. Therefore, asking a patient if his or her symptoms are worse at work may miss genuine occupational asthma. Burge suggested asking two questions: Are your symptoms improved on days off? Are your symptoms improved during vacation? The answers will identify the majority of patients with occupational asthma [37]. The latter question may be important in those with more severe disease. Symptoms may not improve over a 2-day weekend or occasional day off but might within a period of 2 weeks or so.

If the workplace exposure is relatively constant, several patterns of asthmatic reactions may be noted [38]. In some circumstances, symptoms and function changes are apparent during each work shift but resolve rapidly, and recovery is complete by the next work shift. A more common presentation may be that of progressive symptoms throughout the work week. Here more severe symptoms and poorer function are noted at the end of the week. At least initially, symptoms may abate with time away from work (e.g., during weekends). However, as the exposure continues, recovery may take longer and may not occur before the new work week begins, resulting in progressive deterioration week by week. At this point, airway hyperresponsiveness may become permanent and symptoms may become persistent. With persistent airway hyperresponsiveness, nonspecific irritants such as exercise, viral infections, cold air, fog, and fumes may elicit symptoms. The workplace becomes one of a number of triggers to symptoms.

Occupational asthma does not develop immediately on exposure to the allergen or sensitizer. Sensitization occurs during a latent period. This period is variable and may range from weeks to years but usually is several months. Potent sensitizers such as laboratory animals and the complex salts of platinum may result in sensitization within a few months. Isocyanates result in sensitization in a mean period of 2 years; colophony, in 4 years; and some agents, up to 10 years [38]. Unless sensitization has been acquired at another job site or through another mechanism, symptoms developing soon after the onset of exposure argue against occupational asthma.

In those individuals with preexisting asthma or where the exposure reaches generally irritant levels, symptoms may occur without a latent period [61]. This is not generally believed to be occupational asthma. Symptoms are related to the general level of irritants in the workplace without specificity. Symptoms are usually absent at night and during time away from work and the irritant exposure. Symptoms do not progress during the work week or over time. Interestingly, a work association may be implied in individuals whose only exertion or environmental exposure occurs during working hours [61]. In contrast to the apparent, but incorrect, workplace-related symptoms of some irritant exposures, nocturnal and weekend symptoms, often prominent in patients with occupational asthma, may lead the physician and patient away from a work association. Irritant-induced worksite bronchospasm may actually appear more work associated.

It is probably obvious but the initial interview with a patient should include a detailed occupational history. Attention should be paid to potential exposures outside the usual working environment. Asthma may develop as the result of hobbies or a secondary occupation. Remember that exposure may be indirect. Carroll and coauthors reported TDI asthma in office workers who inhaled the chemical after it entered the air-conditioning system of their office [47]. The source of the chemical was a neighboring TDI manufacturing factory.

The physical examination may be specific but tends to be very insensitive. The variable nature of asthma and the fact that the worker is away from the worksite when presenting to the physician's office would tend to favor the absence of signs during the examination.

Evidence of Work Relationship

A single measure of pulmonary function is not helpful in diagnosing occupational asthma. Pulmonary function measured on a day away from work may be normal in up to half of those with occupational asthma [37]. Many of the remainder will not demonstrate reversibility. Serial spirometry when the patient has been away from work for a time and repeated when the patient returns to work, if coupled with an appropriate change in symptoms, may help to confirm an association with the work environment [52].

Spirometry before and after a work shift would seem to be a simple method of establishing a work relationship. Burge, however, found that only 22 percent of patients with occupational asthma due to colophony had a significant drop in FEV_1 over a shift, while 11 percent of subjects without occupational asthma had a similar fall in FEV_1 [36]. This method would not identify a late response. This may explain the low incidence of significant falls in the colophony-induced asthmatic group. In keeping with the normal diurnal variation of pulmonary function, spirometric values are the lowest in the early morning and highest in the late afternoon. This diurnal variation is greater in asthmatic patients. Therefore, a true change in function over the usual daytime work shift may be negated or minimized resulting in a false-negative or inconclusive study [37] (Fig. 46-10).

A "stop-resume" work test may provide evidence of work-associated symptoms (Fig. 46-11). Serial measurement of peak expiratory flow rates (PEFRs) by the patient at home and work has been found to be an excellent method [36, 49]. The patient is asked to measure and record PEFR every 2 hours from arising to retiring and to keep a diary of symptoms and medication use. The record should be kept for at least 2 to 3 weeks at work and then for 10 days away from work. Provisions for a paid sick leave during the monitoring period should be arranged [46]. Criteria for interpreting these records have not been firmly established. At present, a graph of the daily maximum, mean, and minimum flow is inspected visually to check for deterioration at work and improvement away from work [38]. A recent study showed that the visual method of assessing the record was as good as a detailed quantitative analysis [52, 53]. These records are subject to the patient's cooperation and honesty, and may therefore prove suspect in an individual with potential secondary gain.

Cote and associates assessed the prolonged recording of PEFR

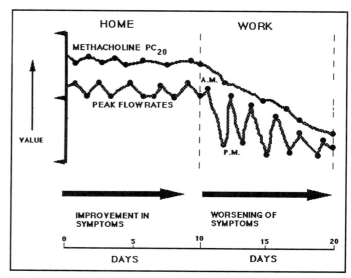

Fig. 46-11. *Objective information provided by noting an increased responsiveness to methacholine with documented falls in PC_{20} suggests that the response is likely allergic in origin and thus, indirectly documenting sensitization. It is an indirect indicator of a late asthmatic attack. Peak expiratory flow rate measurements objectively document the occurrence of reversible airflow limitation and the specific work-relatedness of the airflow limitation.*

in patients with western red cedar asthma, using a specific challenge test as the standard [64]. They found the prolonged PEFR recording to be 86 percent sensitive and 55 percent specific. A positive clinical history was 93 percent sensitive and 45 percent specific. Combining PEFR with a positive clinical history increased the sensitivity to 100 percent; however, specificity decreased to 45 percent.

Serial measurement of nonspecific bronchial responsiveness in conjunction with prolonged recording of PEFR may provide additional evidence of work-relatedness [49]. Significant decreases in airway responsiveness away from work with appropriate changes in PEFR may suggest an occupational association. Cote and coworkers also assessed the value of monitoring changes in bronchial responsiveness [64]. The diagnostic value of changes in bronchial responsiveness alone was found to be relatively low, 62 percent sensitive and 78 percent specific. These investigators concluded that serial measurement of methacholine challenge was not a valuable test in patients suspected of having red cedar asthma [64]. A period of 10 days away from work may not be sufficient time to allow an improvement in responsiveness to take place. The value of including serial measurement of bronchial responsiveness may need to be evaluated for each offending agent.

Nonspecific Bronchial Challenge Testing

The measurement of bronchial responsiveness may be beneficial in the assessment of the patient with occupational asthma. A positive response on a challenge test supports a clinical diagnosis of asthma when baseline pulmonary function is normal. A negative response does not, however, rule out occupational asthma [46]. Bronchial responsiveness may wane when the patient has been away from exposure for a period of time [125], and may never become abnormal in those with immediate asthmatic reactions only. In addition, there are case reports of patients with TDI asthma without bronchial hyperresponsiveness [185]. Guidelines for bronchial provocation in occupational asthma are available [22].

The role of nonspecific bronchial provocation tests in the diag-

Fig. 46-10. *A greater diurnal variation in peak expiratory flow rates at work compared to values made at home may provide confirmatory information for occupational asthma.*

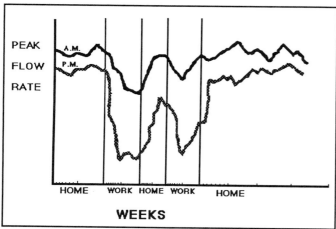

nosis of asthma has been previously discussed, as has the utility of serial measurements of responsiveness in documenting a work association. Additional indications for testing include providing a guide to a safe initial dose of a potential allergen or sensitizer for a specific challenge test and in following the recovery of the patient after cessation of exposure. Cote and coworkers concluded that serial measurement of methacholine challenge was not a valuable test in patients suspected of having red cedar asthma [65].

Skin Tests and Serology

Skin testing with common allergens such as house dust, danders, and grass and tree pollens may be useful in determining the atopic status of the patient. In a few circumstances, especially with high-molecular-weight compounds, appropriate extracts of potential occupational allergens are available for skin testing [42, 101]. For example, skin testing with flour and wheat has a sensitivity of 96 percent and a specificity of 81 percent for baker's asthma [191]. Extracts of animal products, flour, coffee beans, and castor beans have been shown to cause immediate skin test reactions in susceptible individuals [53].

Total serum IgE may be useful in monitoring patients. Increases may indicate exacerbation and decreases, a remission [21, 22]. Specific IgE (occasionally IgG4) antibodies to various occupational allergens, both high molecular weight and low molecular weight when conjugated with protein, may be measured by the RAST and ELISA techniques and may be useful where testing is available. Although serologic testing is highly specific, it is often a less sensitive indicator of sensitization than is skin testing [21, 22]. The RAST has good specificity but cannot be used to exclude a clinical diagnosis when testing results are negative. The ELISA technique is technically easier but appears to be no more sensitive than the RAST. Both skin testing and serologic testing document exposure and sensitization but may not necessarily be associated with symptoms of asthma.

Specific Bronchial Inhalation Challenge

All diagnostic methods discussed thus far may provide evidence of work-associated symptoms and may suggest an etiologic agent. A specific bronchial challenge test is necessary, however, to identify the substance at fault. These studies are time-consuming and carry potential danger. As a result, specific challenge testing is not widely available. Testing should be done by experienced personnel, usually in a hospital setting where the patient may be monitored for a period of time and untoward reactions may be addressed quickly and appropriately (see also Chap. 39).

Specific protocols vary but in general require 3 to 6 days of testing [53, 55]. In one such protocol, on Day 1 the patient is clinically evaluated and a methacholine bronchial provocation test is done. On Day 2, a "mock exposure" is performed. This "placebo day" is important to establish a baseline and defines the extent of the patient's circadian rhythm of function. Day 3 is the first true exposure day. If there is no evidence of decline in lung function on Day 3, the exposure level is increased on Day 4 and Day 5. If no response is detected at the Day 5 exposure, it is concluded that occupational asthma due to the tested substance is not present. In general, the diagnosis can be firmly established in subjects who develop an asthmatic reaction with a greater than 20 percent fall in FEV_1 after exposure to a subirritant level of the offending agent [53, 55].

Testing with occupationally related substances often presents unique problems [53, 55]. Many of the chemicals are irritating, toxic, or too allergenic for testing in the traditional manner. Creative efforts and on-site observations in industry have allowed the development of methods that are safe and simulate the work environment. Where available, testing of aqueous aerosols of allergen extracts may be accomplished in the same manner as testing with histamine or methacholine. First, however, skin testing should be done to identify a safe initial allergen concentration. Bronchial provocation testing of vegetable or chemical dusts may be done by creating a dusty atmosphere from which the subject breathes. Mixing the dust with lactose powder allows a means for diluting the dust. The test substance is placed in a shallow pan. The subject is instructed to transfer the powder from one pan to another for a specified period during which time the subject inhales dust that enters the atmosphere. Vapors or fumes are usually tested in a manner that simulates the work environment. Exposure to low-viscosity liquids can be done by asking the patient to paint the material on a flat surface. Vapors such as TDI may be generated and constantly monitored to give precise levels of exposure and allow successive increases in the exposure up to the threshold limit value. Cloutier and coauthors recently described a new method for conducting specific inhalation challenges with occupational allergens in particulate form [60]. The technical problem of specific inhalation challenge testing is that it is often only performed in a few specialized centers. A modified method may provide wider use of the specific inhalation challenge test and importantly, cost less to develop the necessary equipment and monitoring tools.

Specific bronchial inhalation challenge testing may be indicated in four circumstances: (1) to document a previously unrecognized cause of occupational asthma, (2) to establish a diagnosis where this is in doubt, (3) to determine the precise etiologic agent in a complex working environment, and (4) to confirm the diagnosis for medical-legal purposes [53, 55]. General agreement exists on the first three indications. Whether specific bronchial challenge tests should be performed for medical-legal reasons is controversial.

A specific bronchial inhalation challenge test is considered the "gold standard" when the results are positive. A negative result must be interpreted in context. Several factors must be considered when interpreting the results of a challenge test. A patient who has been away from the exposure for a period of time may lose sensitivity [11]. Therefore, a study should be performed as soon as possible after terminating the exposure. Exposures to a number of chemicals and substances in the workplace are the norm. Challenge testing may show negative results if the wrong substance is being tested or in circumstances where a combination of several substances is required to produce a response. Finally, the method of challenge testing may not provide the correct exposure. Although laboratory exposure may be controlled, it is nevertheless artificial. More studies are needed to define the best method of performing the test to maximize the utility and safety.

PROGNOSIS

A number of studies have now documented the outcome of patients with occupational asthma who have terminated exposure. It appears that symptoms due to occupational asthma may remit when the condition is diagnosed early and the worker is removed from further exposure. More commonly, however, the occupational exposure leads to persistent symptoms and permanent bronchial hyperresponsiveness [52, 56, 65, 67, 152, 165]. Patients continue to have recurrent attacks of asthma that vary in severity from those relieved by occasional inhaled bronchodilator to chronic problems requiring systemic corticosteroid therapy. Persistently symptomatic patients retained their bronchial hyperresponsiveness. In a large follow-up study of 232 patients, 136 patients terminated exposure [56]. Sixty percent had not completely recovered during an average 4-year follow-up. Cote et al. reported the status of 48 patients with western red cedar asthma with continuous exposure for an average of 6.5 years after the diagnosis [65]. None of the patients recovered. Approximately half were stable on medications. Despite treatment, the remaining half deteriorated.

Similar studies in patients with TDI asthma suggest that the majority of patients do not completely recover [136, 138]. Burge followed 45 electronic workers with colophony fume asthma for 1 to 4 years [36]. Of the 20 workers who were available for follow-up and had terminated the exposure, only 2 were free of symptoms. Hudson and associates found that the majority of patients with snow crab asthma failed to recover after cessation of exposure [107].

A favorable outcome was noted with a shorter duration of symptoms before diagnosis, relatively normal pulmonary function, and a lesser degree of bronchial responsiveness [52]. Persistent symptoms after cessation of exposure were associated with a longer duration of symptoms, abnormal pulmonary function, and more marked levels of bronchial responsiveness. These findings suggest that early diagnosis and early cessation of exposure may be important factors influencing prognosis.

Of those individuals who have occupational asthma due to a sensitizing agent and who remain in the same industry or continue exposure for any of a number of reasons, the prognosis is not good. Cote and colleagues reported the status of 48 patients with western red cedar asthma with continuous exposure for an average of 6.5 years after the diagnosis [65]. None of the patients recovered. Approximately half were stable on medications. Despite treatment, the remaining half deteriorated. In patients with TDI asthma, Paggiaro and coworkers found that continued exposure resulted in continuous deterioration [167].

ASSESSMENT OF WORK ENVIRONMENT

Environmental assessment provides important information [190]: (1) Several measurements in the workplace environment may elucidate variability in allergen exposure and its determinants. (2) Environmental monitoring can provide a means for evaluating the effectiveness of interventions aimed at reducing exposures. (3) Environmental measurements provide information on exposure-response relationships. Methods are now available for quantifying airborne allergens using standard analytic industrial hygiene sampling principles and immunoassays [190]. Simply, a known volume of air is sampled using high-volume air samplers. The airborne particles are retained on a filter. Particularly important is a filter medium that permits high flow rates and efficient elution of the allergens in small volumes of buffer. The soluble allergens are extracted from the filter and the amount of retained allergen is assayed by sensitive radioimmunoassay (i.e., RAST or ELISA).

ALLOCATING CAUSE AND EFFECT

The criteria for the diagnosis of occupational asthma includes (1) typical medical and occupational history (i.e., asthma symptoms related to work); (2) specific identification of the offending agent; (3) documentation that the agent can actually cause asthma (i.e., finding similar cases in the literature); (4) presence and/or induction of nonspecific bronchial hyperresponsiveness; (5) documentation of immunologic sensitization, if allergic in nature; (6) documenting work-related changes in pulmonary function testing; and (7) positive response to bronchial inhalation challenges (in hospital or natural, at work) to confirm the diagnosis of an allergic cause. When the subject is no longer working and/or has no possibility of returning to work, then certain pieces of information take on more significance (i.e., Points 1–5). A diagnosis can not be objectively made if the only criterion utilized is a "positive

Table 46-6. Essential features of an occupational history

Chronologically list all full-time jobs beginning with the first. Include a question about part-time jobs and hobbies. If possible, obtain exact dates of employment. For each job:
- Determine what activities the patient performed.
- List all materials used by the patient.
- Identify materials used by workers in the patient's vicinity.
- Ask whether respirators or other protective measures were used.
- Elicit a general evaluation of the workplace ventilation and exhaust.
- Obtain a general estimate of whether exposure was slight, moderate, or intense.
- Figure the duration of exposure to potentially pathogenic materials based on employment dates.
- Calculate the time between the first day of work and the first appearance of symptoms.
- Inquire if any co-workers have similar symptoms.
- Find out if the employers conducted any health monitoring.
- Note whether there is any variation in the severity of symptoms when the patient is away from work evenings, weekends, and vacations.

Source: Adapted from S. M. Brooks. An approach to patients suspected of having occupational pulmonary disease. *Clin. Chest Med.* 2:171, 1981.

history" of work-related symptoms. Table 46-6 summarizes the salient features in obtaining an occupational history.

TREATMENT AND PREVENTION

Accidental high-level exposures such as spills have been reported to have the most serious consequences but provide the greatest opportunity for intervention and development of preventive measures. The planning of procedures to follow in the event of an accident spill is necessary. Engineering controls focusing on proper and effective local exhaust ventilation can reduce worker risks. Other control strategies that may reduce worker exposures include limitation of exposure at the source and installing transmission barriers. Engineering controls require regular maintenance programs and continued evaluation of the industrial process. The use of personal protective devices is generally considered inappropriate, but may be instituted during special situations and generally for only short periods of time. Control options can include the substitution of a sensitizing agent for an agent less likely to cause sensitization. An investigation of the industrial flow schematic may lead to a way of introducing changes in the process that can lower exposure. Various engineering controls methods such as containment, enclosure, or isolation may be an appropriate option. Limiting worker exposure time or job rotation may be possible in some special circumstances. Medical surveillance programs are the keystone for prevention and should identify individuals who are at an increased risk for developing occupational asthma, as well as detect disease at an early stage when intervention options are likely to be successful [9]. An occupational health surveillance program may include preemployment and periodic medical examinations, immunologic monitoring, and periodic spirometric surveys. Informing employees about the potential workplace hazards and proper training for safe work practices are of paramount importance. Tests that measure nonspecific bronchial hyperresponsiveness should not be used as preemployment screening tests to exclude potential individuals at risk. There is no decisive evidence at present that preexisting bronchial hyperresponsiveness represents a risk factor for the development of occupational asthma. It is also inappropriate to exclude atopic persons from employment. Institution of a smoking cessation program is an important option to consider. Specific bronchial provocation studies may be invaluable in certain circumstances, but these studies are indicated (1) for the investigation of a previously unreported sensitizer, (2) for identification of the precise cause where a number of compounds may be at fault, or (3) for medical-legal purposes. Specific bronchial provocation studies should only be carried out by experienced personnel in a hospital setting. A number of modifications of the "stop-resume" work test have been published and can be utilized in suspected cases of occupational asthma. A "stop-resume" work test may provide evidence of work-associated symptoms. Serial measurements of peak expiratory flow rates by the patient at home and work has been found to be an excellent method [36, 49, 64]. Inclusion of testing for nonspecific bronchial responsiveness adds to the specificity of the testing. The demonstration of an increase in responsiveness after returning to work aids in establishing a causal relationship.

For sensitized persons, the best preventive option is complete removal from the work environment because there are reports of fatal consequences of sensitized individuals who continue to work [84, 190]. The early identification of disease, complete cessation of exposure, and complete removal from the work environment may allow the eventual resolution of asthma symptoms and nonspecific airway hyperresponsiveness. On the other hand, a majority of cases persist after exposure is terminated, as a chronic asthmatic condition associated with nonspecific airway hyperresponsiveness. An important observation suggests that the continued exposure of a sensitized individual may lead to a persistent asthmatic condition. A more favorable prognosis is reported to occur with a shorter duration of symptoms before confirming a diagnosis of occupational asthma, maintenance of normal pulmonary function, and the presence of a lesser degree of nonspecific airway hyperresponsiveness at diagnosis [52]. Strategies, such as improving worksite ventilation to reduce exposure or the use of respiratory protective devices, are not medically ethical for an already sensitized individual. When the patient cannot or will not avoid continued exposure, therapy should center on preventing the late asthmatic response. Preventing or minimizing this response may attenuate the induced bronchial responsiveness. As a result, inhaled cromolyn and/or corticosteroids may be beneficial. Inhaled beta agonists, theophylline, and anticholinergic drugs may be useful in alleviating symptoms. Medical therapy to allow a person to better tolerate a workplace exposure is also not generally recommended. However, in situations where the patient cannot or will not avoid continued exposure, the medical-ethical issue arises and can only be resolved on an individual case-by-case basis. An algorithm providing a multidisciplinary approach for determining a pulmonary health hazard is summarized in Fig. 46-12.

Fig. 46-12. *Summary of a multidisciplinary approach for determining a pulmonary health hazard. (Reprinted with permission from S. M. Brooks. An approach to patients suspected of having occupational pulmonary disease.* Clin. Chest Med. *2:171, 1981.)*

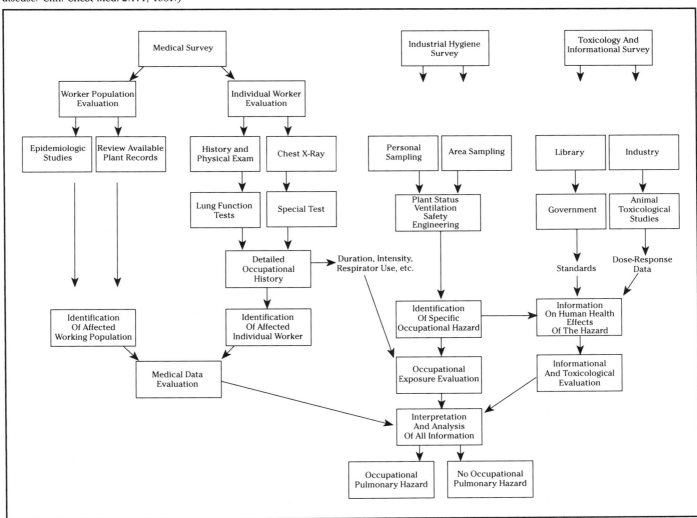

IMPAIRMENT, DISABILITY, AND COMPENSATION

Asthma is becoming a very common occupational disorder. Many, if not most, of those afflicted will be left with persistent asthmatic symptoms. As a result, issues of impairment, disability, and compensation are becoming more and more important.

Impairment refers to the loss of physiologic function or anatomic loss. The American Thoracic Society has defined impairment as "a medical condition resulting from functional abnormality that may be temporary or permanent and that may preclude gainful employment" [3]. Physicians judge impairment. A disability refers to the overall impact of the physiologic loss. Disability awards must therefore take into account not only the degree of impairment but also the job description [71]. A judge, jury, or board determines disability. Compensation is a payment given to a worker who is injured, in this case develops asthma, by the workplace.

Two kinds of legal recourses are available to individuals with a work-related illness, injury, or disease: toxic tort remedies or workers' compensation [164]. The former is adjudicated in a court of law and the recovery is determined by a jury. The plaintiff must show liability based on negligence and that the exposure-induced injury was causally related to the negligence. The latter is a "no-fault" agreement between the company and the worker to the alleged injury and compensation. The case is adjudicated before an administrative law judge and the recovery is based on wages. It must be shown that the disability arose "out of and in the course of employment." The compensation awarded reflects the degree (partial or total) and duration (temporary or permanent) of disability [71].

Chan-Yeung has pointed out that there are no appropriate guidelines for the assessment of impairment or disability in patients with asthma [51]. The American Medical Association (AMA) guidelines for the evaluation of medical impairment are often used by compensation boards or similar agencies [79]. These guidelines primarily incorporate spirometric indices to determine impairment and require the patient to have received optimal treatment. The recommendations seem more appropriate for an individual with a pneumoconiosis and irreversible lung damage. In contrast, persons with asthma show variable airflow obstruction and in fact, if treated, may have "normal" pulmonary function test results at the time of medical evaluation. The important consideration is the presence of nonspecific airway hyperresponsiveness, which can preclude an individual from working in an environment exposing them to irritants, changes in humidity, or cold air. Additionally, exercise-induced bronchospasm may be present and can also limit the ability to engage in certain work activities, especially the type requiring strenuous exertion. A recent working group of the American College of Chest Physicians suggested that the AMA guidelines for the assessment of impairment or disability in subjects with asthma are not adequate [67].

The same working group proposed that the following clinical parameters need consideration when assessing impairment and disability: frequency of asthma symptoms, degree of physical activity limitation, frequency of acute exacerbations, amount of medication required to control disease, duration of asthma state, and perception of severity by the patient. Physiologic measurements must be included, including prebronchodilator and postbronchodilator spirometric measurements and assessment of nonspecific bronchial responsiveness [67].

Malo and associates reported on snow crab workers and discerned that the plateau for symptoms and lung function was reached on average by 1 year and for bronchial hyperresponsiveness by 2 years after cessation of exposure [136]. These data suggest that perhaps an optimum time for evaluating permanent disability in a patient with occupational asthma is preferably 2 years or more after cessation of exposure.

REFERENCES

1. Alberts, W., and Brooks S. Advances in occupational asthma. *Clin. Chest Med.* 13:1, 1992.
2. Allard, C., et al. Occupational asthma due to various agents: Absence of clinical and functional improvement at an interval of four or more years after cessation of exposure. *Chest* 96:1046, 1989.
3. American Thoracic Society. Evaluation of impairment and disability. *Am. Rev. Respir. Dis.* 133:1205, 1986.
4. Anto, J., et al. Community outbreaks of asthma associated with inhalation of soybean dust. *N. Engl. J. Med.* 320:1097, 1989.
5. Axford, A., et al. Accidental exposure to isocyanate fumes on a group of fireman. *Br. J. Ind. Med.* 33:65, 1976.
6. Ayala, L., and Ahmed, T. Is there a loss of a protective muscarinic receptor mechanism in asthma. *Chest* 96:1285, 1989.
7. Baker, D., et al. Cross-sectional study of platinum salts sensitization among precious metals refinery workers. *Am. J. Ind. Med.* 18:653, 1990.
8. Bakke, P., Baste, V., and Gulsvik, A. Bronchial responsiveness in a Norwegian community. *Am. Rev. Respir. Dis.* 143:317, 1991.
9. Balmes, J. Surveillance for occupational asthma. *Occup. Med. State of Arts Rev.* 6:101, 1991.
10. Banks, D., Butcher, B., and Salvaggio, J. Isocyanate induced respiratory disease. *Ann. Allergy* 57:389, 1986.
11. Banks, D., et al. Role of inhalation challenge testing in the diagnosis of isocyanate asthma. *Chest* 95:414, 1989.
12. Bardy, J. D., et al. Occupational asthma and IgE in pharmaceutical company processing psyllium. *Am. Rev. Respir. Dis.* 135:1033, 1987.
13. Barnes, P. Asthma as an axon reflex. *Lancet* 1:242, 1986.
14. Barnes, P. New concepts in the pathogenesis of bronchial hyperresponsiveness and asthma. *J. Allergy Clin. Immunol.* 83:1013, 1989.
15. Barnes, P. Neuropeptides and asthma. *Am. Rev. Respir. Dis.* 143(Suppl.): 28S, 1991.
16. Bascom, R., et al. Effect of ozone inhalation on the response to nasal challenge with antigen of allergic subjects. *Am. Rev. Respir. Dis.* 142: 594, 1990.
17. Bates, D. Workshop summary: Environmental and occupational asthma. *Chest* 98:251S, 1990.
18. Baur, X. New aspects of isocyanate asthma. *Lung* 168(Suppl.):606, 1990.
19. Baur, X., Dewair, M., and Fruhman, G. Detection of immunologically sensitized isocyanate workers by RAST and intracutaneous skin tests. *J. Allergy Clin. Immunol.* 73:610, 1984.
20. Beasley, R., et al. Cellular events in the bronchi in mild asthma and after bronchial provocation. *Am. Rev. Respir. Dis.* 139:806, 1989.
21. Bernstein, D., and Bernstein, I. Occupational Asthma. In E. J. Middleton, C. Reed, and E. Ellis (eds.), *Allergy: Principles and Practice.* St. Louis: C.V. Mosby, 1988. P. 1197.
22. Bernstein, D., and Cohn, J. Guidelines for the diagnosis and evaluation of occupational lung disease: Preface. *J. Allergy Clin. Immunol.* 84:791, 1989.
23. Biagini, R., et al. Ozone enhancement of platinum asthma in a primate model. *Am. Rev. Respir. Dis.* 134:719, 1986.
24. Blanc, P. Occupational asthma in a national disability survey. *Chest* 92: 613, 1987.
25. Borm, P., Bast, A., and Zuiderveld, O. In vitro effects of toluene diisocyanate on beta adrenergic and muscarinic receptor function in lung tissue of the rat. *Br. J. Ind. Med.* 46:56, 1989.
26. Boschetto, P., et al. Prednisone inhibits late asthmatic reactions and airway inflammation induced by toluene diisocyanate in sensitized subjects. *J. Allergy Clin. Immunol.* 80:261, 1987.
27. Boulet, L.-P. Increase in airway responsiveness following acute exposure to respiratory irritants: Reactive airways dysfunction syndrome or occupational asthma? *Chest* 94:476, 1988.
28. Brooks, S. Occupational Asthma. In E. B. Weiss (ed.), *Bronchial Asthma: Mechanisms and Therapeutics.* Boston: Little, Brown, 1985. Pp. 461–493.
29. Brooks, S., et al. Cold air challenge and platinum skin reactivity in platinum refinery workers. *Chest* 1990.
30. Brooks, S. M., Weiss, M. A., and Bernstein, I. L. Reactive airways dysfunction syndrome (RADS): Case reports of persistent airways hyperreactivity after high level irritant exposures. *J. Occup. Med.* 27:29, 1985.
31. Brooks, S., Weiss, M. A., and Bernstein, I. L. Reactive airways dysfunction syndrome: Persistent asthma syndrome after high-level irritant exposure. *Chest* 88:376, 1985.
32. Brooks, S. M. Bronchial Asthma of Occupational Origin. In W. N. Rom (ed.), *Environmental and Occupational Medicine.* Boston: Little, Brown, 1983. Pp. 233–250.

33. Brooks, S. M., and Vandervort, R. Investigation of polyvinyl chloride film thermal decomposition products as an occupational illness of meat wrappers: ii. Clinical studies. *J. Occup. Med.* 19:192, 1977.

34. Brooks, S. M., et al. Epidemiologic Study of Workers Exposed to Isocyanate. In *NIOSH Health Hazard Evaluation Report.* 1980.

35. Brooks, S. M., et al. An epidemiologic study of workers exposed to western red cedar and other wood dusts. *Chest* 80:30, 1981.

36. Burge, P. Occupational asthma in electronic workers caused by colophony fumes: Follow-up of affected workers. *Thoax* 37:348, 1982.

37. Burge, P. Problems in the diagnosis of occupational asthma. *Br. J. Dis. Chest* 81:105, 1987.

38. Burge, P. Diagnosis of occupational asthma. *Clin. Exp. Allergy* 19:649, 1989.

39. Burge, P., et al. Occupational asthma in a factory making flux-colored solder containing colophony. *Thorax* 36:828, 1981.

40. Burge, P. S., et al. Respiratory disease in workers exposed to solder flux fumes containing colophony (pine resin). *Clin. Allergy* 8:1, 1978.

41. Burney, P., et al. Descriptive epidemiology of bronchial reactivity in adult population: Results from a community study. *Thorax* 42:38, 1987.

42. Bush, R., and Kagen, S. Guidelines for the preparation and characterization of high molecular weight allergens used for the diagnosis of occupational lung diseases. *J. Allergy Clin. Immunol.* 84:814, 1989.

43. Busse, W. W., and Schoenwater, W. F. Asthma from psyllium in laxative manufacture. *Ann. Intern. Med.* 83:361, 1975.

44. Butcher, B., Bernstein, I., and Schwartz, H. Guidelines for the clinical evaluation of occupational asthma due to small molecular weight chemicals. *J. Allergy Clin. Immunol.* 84:834, 1989.

45. Butcher, B. T., et al. Toluene diisocyanate (TDI) pulmonary disease: Immunologic and inhalation challenge studies. *J. Allergy Clin. Immunol.* 58:89, 1976.

46. Canadian TS. Occupational asthma: Recommendations for diagnosis, management, and assessment of impairment. *Can. Med. Assoc. J.* 140:1029, 1989.

47. Carrol, K., Secombe, C., and Pepys, J. Asthma due to nonoccupational exposure to toluene diisocyanate. *Clin. Allergy* 6:99, 1976.

48. Cartier, A., Malo, J. L., and Dolovich, J. Occupational asthma in nurses handling psyllium. *Clin. Allergy* 17:1, 1987.

49. Cartier, A., et al. Occupational asthma in snow crab processing workers. *J. Allergy Clin. Immunol.* 74:261, 1984.

50. Cartier, A., et al. Specific serum antibodies against isocyanates: Association with occupational asthma. *J. Allergy Clin. Immunol.* 84:507, 1989.

51. Chan-Yeung, M. Evaluation of impairment/disability in patients with occupational asthma. *Am. Rev. Respir. Dis.* 135:950, 1987.

52. Chan-Yeung, M. Occupational asthma. *Chest* 98:148S, 1990.

53. Chan-Yeung, M. A clinician's approach to determine the diagnosis, prognosis, and therapy of occupational asthma. *Med. Clin. North Am.* 74:811, 1990.

54. Chan-Yeung, M., et al. Histamine, leukotrienes and prostaglandins released in bronchial fluid during plicatic acid-induced bronchoconstriction. *J. Allergy Clin. Immunol.* 84:762, 1989.

55. Chan-Yeung, M., Kinsella, M., and Ostrow, D. Specific bronchoprovocation testing. *Clin. Rev. Allergy* 8:147, 1990.

56. Chan-Yeung, M., MacLean, L., and Paggiaro, P. A follow-up of 232 patients with occupational asthma due to western red cedar (Thuja plicata). *J. Allergy Clin. Immunol.* 80:279, 1987.

57. Chan-Yeung, M., et al. Symptoms, pulmonary function and airway hyperreactivity in western red cedar compared to those in the office workers. *Am. Rev. Respir. Dis.* 130:1038, 1984.

58. Chan-Yeung, M., et al. Evidence for mucosal inflammation in occupational asthma. *Clin. Exp. Allergy* 20:1, 1990.

59. Charan, N., et al. Pulmonary injuries associated with acute sulfur dioxide inhalation. *Am. Rev. Respir. Dis.* 119:555, 1979.

60. Cloutier, Y., et al. New methodology for specific inhalation challenges with occupational agents in powder form. *Eur. Respir. J.* 2:769, 1989.

61. Cockcroft, D. Occupational asthma. *Ann. Allergy* 65:169, 1990.

62. Committee. Formaldehyde and Other Aldehydes. In Board on Toxicology and Environmental Health Hazards, National Academy of Science, 1981.

63. Corrigan, C., and Kay, A. Activated T-lymphocytes in acute and severe asthma: A primary target for both new and conventional asthma therapy. *Immunol. Allergy Pract.* 12:209, 1990.

64. Cote, J., Kennedy, S., and Chan-Yeung, M. Sensitivity and specificity of PC20 and peak expiratory flow rate in cedar asthma. *J. Allergy Clin. Immunol.* 85:592, 1990.

65. Cote, J., Kennedy, S., and Chan-Yeung, M. Outcome of patients with cedar asthma with continuous exposure. *Am. Rev. Respir. Dis.* 141:373, 1990.

66. Cowie, R. Pulmonary dysfunction in gold miners with reactive airways. *Br. J. Ind. Med.* 46:873, 1989.

67. Current State of Knowledge: Epidemiology and Surveillance Working Group. *Chest* 98:240S, 1990.

68. Cuss, F., and Barnes, P. Epithelial mediators. *Am. Rev. Respir. Dis.* 136:32S, 1987.

69. Daniel, E., and O'Byrne, P. Autonomic nerves and airway smooth muscle: Effects of inflammatory mediators on airway nerves and muscle. *Am. Rev. Respir. Dis.* 143:3S, 1991.

70. Day, J. H., Lees, R. E. M., and Clark, R. H. Respiratory effects of formaldehyde and UFFI off-gas following controlled exposure. *J. Allergy Clin. Immunol.* 7(Suppl.):159, 1983.

71. Demeter, S. The many facets of occupational asthma. *Cleve. Clin. Med. J.* 58:137, 1991.

72. DeMonchy, J., et al. Bronchoalveolar eosinophilia during allergen induced late asthmatic reactions. *Am. Rev. Respir. Dis.* 31:373, 1985.

73. Devlin, R., et al. Exposure of humans to ambient levels of ozone for 6.6 hours causes cellular and biochemical changes in the lung. *Am. J. Respir. Mol. Biol.* 4:72, 1991.

74. Diaz, P., et al. Leukocytes and mediators in bronchoalveolar lavage during allergen-induced late-phase asthmatic reactions. *Am. Rev. Respir. Dis.* 139:1383, 1989.

75. Diem, J. E., et al. Five-year longitudinal study of workers employed in a new toluene diisocyanate manufacturing plant. *Am. Rev. Respir. Dis.* 126:420, 1982.

76. Djukanmovic, R., et al. State of the art: Mucosal inflammation in asthma. *Am. Rev. Respir. Dis.* 142:434, 1990.

77. Donham, K., et al. Acute toxic exposure to gases from liquid manure. *J. Occup. Med.* 24:142, 1982.

78. Durham, S., et al. The temporal relationship between increases in airway responsiveness to histamine and late asthmatic responses induced by occupational agents. *J. Allergy Clin. Immunol.* 79:398, 1987.

79. Engleberg, A. (ed.). The Respiratory System: Guides to the Evaluation of Permanent Impairment. Chicago: American Medical Association, 1988.

80. Ernst, P., et al. Relationship of airway responsiveness to duration of work in a dusty environment. *Thorax* 44:116, 1989.

81. Fabbri, L., et al. Bronchoalveolar neutrophilia during late asthmatic reactions induced by toluene diisocyanates. *Am. Rev. Respir. Dis.* 136:36, 1987.

82. Fabbri, L., et al. Prednisone inhibits the late asthmatic reactions and the associated increase in airway hyperresponsiveness induced by toluene-diisocyanate in sensitized subjects. *Am. Rev. Respir. Dis.* 132:1010, 1985.

83. Fabbri, L., et al. Bronchial hyperreactivity: Mechanisms and physiologic evaluation. Airway inflammation during late asthmatic reactions induced by toluene diisocyanate. *Am. Rev. Respir. Dis.* 143:37S, 1991.

84. Fabbri, L. D., et al. Fatal asthma in a subject sensitized to toluene diisocyanate. *Am. Rev. Respir. Dis.* 137:1494, 1988.

85. Figley, K. D. Mayfly (Ephemerida) hypersensitivity. *J. Allergy* 11:376, 1940.

86. Fine, M., and Balmes, J. Airway inflammation and occupational asthma. *Clin. Chest Med.* 9:577, 1988.

87. Finotto, S., et al. Increase in numbers of CD8 positive lymphocytes and eosinophils in peripheral blood of subjects with late asthmatic reactions induced by toluene diisocyanate. *Br. J. Ind. Med.* 48:116, 1991.

88. Flavahan, N., et al. Respiratory epithelium inhibits bronchial smooth muscle tone. *J. Appl. Physiol.* 58:834, 1985.

89. Flury, K., et al. Airway obstruction due to ammonia. *Mayo Clin. Proc.* 58:389, 1983.

90. Frampton, M., et al. Effects of nitrogen dioxide exposure on pulmonary function and airway reactivity in normal humans. *Am. Rev. Respir. Dis.* 143:522, 1991.

91. Frigas, E., Filley, W. V., and Reed, C. E. Asthma induced by dust from urea-formaldehyde foam insulating material. *Chest* 79:706, 1981.

92. Frossard, N., Rhoden, K., and Barnes, P. Influence of epithelium on guinea pig airway in response to tachykinins: Role of endopeptidases and cyclooxygenases. *J. Pharmacol. Exp. Ther.* 248:292, 1989.

93. Gandevia, B. Occupational asthma, part I. *Med. J. Aust.* 2:332, 1970.

94. Gibbons, H. L., Dillie, J. R., and Cowley, R. G. Inhalant allergy to screwworm fly. *Arch. Environ. Health* 10:424, 1965.

95. Gilbert, R., and Auchincloss, J., Jr. Reactive airways dysfunction syndrome presenting as a reversible restrictive defect. *Lung* 167:55, 1989.

96. Goransson, K., and Michaelson, N. G. Ispagula powder. An allergen in the work environment. *Scand. J. Work Environ. Health* 5:257, 1979.

97. Graham, D., and Koren, H. Biomarkers of inflammation in ozone-exposed humans: Comparison of the nasal and bronchoalveolar lavage. *Am. Rev. Respir. Dis.* 142:152, 1990.

98. Grainger, D., et al. The relationship between atopy and nonspecific bronchial responsiveness. *Clin. Exp. Allergy* 20:181, 1990.

99. Grammer, L., et al. Prospective immunologic and clinical study of a population exposed to hexamethylene diisocyanate (HDI). *J. Allergy Clin. Immunol.* 82:627, 1988.

100. Grammer, L., et al. Clinical and immunologic evaluation of 37 workers exposed to gaseous formaldehyde. *J. Allergy Clin. Immunol.* 86:177, 1990.

101. Grammer, L., Patterson, R., and Zeiss, C. Guidelines for the immunologic evaluation of occupational lung disease. *J. Allergy Clin. Immunol.* 84:805, 1989.

102. Grandordy, B., et al. Tachykinin-induced phosphoinositide breakdown in airway smooth muscle and epithelium: Relationship to contraction. *Mol. Pharmacol.* 33:515, 1988.

103. Harkonen, H., et al. Long-term effects from exposure to sulfur dioxide: Lung function four years after a pyrite dust explosion. *Am. Rev. Respir. Dis.* 128:840, 1983.

104. Hasan, F., Gehshan, A., and Fulechan, F. Resolution of pulmonry dysfunction following acute chlorine exposures. *Arch. Environ. Health* 38:76, 1983.

105. Hopp, R., et al. The presence of airway reactivity before the development of asthma. *Am. Rev. Respir. Dis.* 141:2, 1990.

106. Horstman, D., et al. Ozone concentration and pulmonary response relationships for 6.6-hour exposures with five hours of moderate exercise to 0.08, 0.10, and 0.12 ppm. *Am. Rev. Respir. Dis.* 142:1158, 1990.

107. Hudson, P., et al. Follow-up of occupational asthma caused by crab and various agents. *J. Allergy Clin. Immunol.* 76:262, 1985.

108. Industrial Injuries Advisor Council. *Occupational Asthma.* London: Her Majesty's Stationery Office, 1981.

109. Ishizaki, T., et al. Occupational asthma from western red cedar dust (Thujaplicata) in furniture factory workers. *J. Occup. Med.* 15:580, 1973.

110. Ito, Y. Prejunctional control of excitatory neuroeffector transmission by prostaglandins in the airways smooth muscle tissue. *Am. Rev. Respir. Dis.* 143:6S, 1991.

111. Johnson, A., et al. Respiratory abnormalities among workers in an iron and steel foundry in Vancouver. *Br. J. Ind. Med.* 42:94, 1985.

112. Kagamimori, S., et al. The changing prevalence of respiratory symptoms in atopic children in response to air pollution. *Clin. Allergy* 16:299, 1986.

113. Kalliel, J., et al. High frequency of atopic asthma in a pulmonary clinic population. *Chest* 96:1336, 1989.

114. Karol, M. Survey of industrial workers for antibodies to toluene diisocyanate. *J. Occup. Med.* 23:741, 1981.

115. Kaufman, J., and Burkons, D. Clinical, roentgenologic and physiologic effects of acute chlorine exposure. *Arch. Environ. Health* 23:29, 1971.

116. Kennedy, S., et al. Lung health consequences of reported accidental chlorine gas exposure among pulpmill workers. *Am. Rev. Respir. Dis.* 143:74, 1991.

117. Kennedy, S., et al. Acute pulmonary response among automobile workers exposed to aerosols of machining fluids. *Am. J. Ind. Med.* 15:627, 1989.

118. Kern, D. An outbreak of reactive airways dysfunction syndrome following a spill of glacial acetic acid. *Am. Rev. Respir. Dis.* In press.

119. Kobayashi, S. Different Aspects of Occupational Asthma in Japan. In C. Frazier (ed.), *Occupational Asthma.* New York: Van Nostrand Reinhold, 1980. Pp. 229–244.

120. Kongerud, J., and Samuelsen, S. A longitudinal study of respiratory symptoms in aluminum potroom workers. *Am. Rev. Respir. Dis.* 144:10, 1991.

121. Kopp, S., et al. Asthma and rhinitis due to ethylcyanoacrylate instant glue. *Ann. Intern. Med.* 102:613, 1985.

122. Kramps, J., et al. Measurement of specific IgE antibodies in individuals exposed to formaldehyde. *Clin. Exp. Allergy* 19:509, 1989.

123. Krzyzanowski, M., Quackenboss, J., and Lebowitz, M. Chronic respiratory effects of indoor formaldehyde exposure. *Environ. Res.* 52:117, 1990.

124. Laitinen, L., et al. Damage of the airway epithelium and bronchial reactivity in patients with asthma. *Am. Rev. Respir. Dis.* 131:599, 1985.

125. Lam, S., Wong, R., and Chan-Yeung, M. Nonspecific bronchial reactivity in occupational asthma. *J. Allergy Clin. Immunol.* 63:28, 1979.

126. Leff, A. State of the art. Endogenous regulation of bronchomotor tone. *Am. Rev. Respir. Dis.* 137:1198, 1988.

127. Lerman, S., and Kipen, H. Reactive airways dysfunction syndrome. *Am. Fam. Physician* 38:135, 1988.

128. Liss, G., et al. Pulmonary and immunologic evaluation of foundry workers exposed to methylene diphenyldiisocyanate (MDI). *J. Allergy Clin. Immunol.* 82:55, 1988.

129. Love, R., et al. Respiratory and allergic symptoms in wool textile workers I. *Br. J. Ind. Med.* 45:727, 1988.

130. Lozewicz, A., et al. Occupational asthma due to methyl methacrylate and cyanoacrylates. *Thorax* 40:836, 1985.

131. Lundberg, J., Brodin, E., and Saira, A. Effects and distribution of vagal capsaicin-sensitive substance P neurons with special reference to the trachea and lungs. *Acta Physiol. Scand.* 119:243, 1983.

132. Luo, J.-C. J., Nelsen, K., and Fischbein, A. Persistent reactive airway dysfunction after exposure to toluene diisocyanate. *Br. J. Ind. Med.* 47:239, 1988.

133. Lybarger, J., et al. Occupational asthma induced by inhalation and ingestion of garlic. *J. Allergy Clin. Immunol.* 69:448, 1982.

134. Maccia, C. A., et al. In vitro demonstration of specific IgE in phthalic anhydride hypersensitivity. *Am. Rev. Respir. Dis.* 113:701, 1976.

135. Malaka, T., and Kodama, A. Respiratory health effects of plywood workers occupational exposed to formaldehyde. *Arch. Environ. Health* 45:288, 1990.

136. Malo, J., et al. Patterns of improvement in spirometry, bronchial hyperresponsiveness and specific IgE antibody levels after cessation of exposure in occupational asthma caused by snowcrab processing. *Am. Rev. Respir. Dis.* 138:807, 1988.

137. Malo, J., et al. Is the clinical history a satisfactory means of diagnosing occupational asthma? *Am. Rev. Respir. Dis.* 143:528, 1991.

138. Malo, J.-L. Compensation for occupational asthma in Quebec. *Chest* 98(Suppl.):236S, 1990.

139. Mapp, C., et al. Occupational asthma due to isocyanates. *Eur. Respir. J.* 1:273, 1988.

140. Mapp, C., et al. A follow-up study of subjects with occupational asthma due to toluene diisocyanate (TDI). *Am. Rev. Respir. Dis.* 137:1326, 1988.

141. Mapp, C., DiGiacoma, R., and Brosheghini, J. Late, but not early, asthmatic reactions induced by toluene diisocyanate are associated with increased airway responsiveness. *Eur. J. Respir. Dis.* 68:276, 1986.

142. Mattoli, S., et al. Nedocromil sodium prevents the release of 15-hydroxyeicosatetraenoic acid from human bronchial epithelial cells exposed to toluene disiocyanate in vitro. *Int. Arch. Appl. Immunol.* 92:16, 1990.

143. McConnochie, K., Edwards, J., and Fifield, R. Ispaghula sensitization in workers manufacturing a bulk laxative. *Clin. Exp. Allergy* 20:199, 1990.

144. McKay, R., and Brooks, S. Isocyanate measurement (letter to editor). *Am. Ind. Hyg. Assoc.* 44:19, 1983.

145. McKay, R., Brooks, S. M. Effect of toluene diisocyanate on beta adrenergic receptor function: Biochemical and physiologic studies. *Am. Rev. Respir. Dis.* 128:50, 1983.

146. McKay, R., and Brooks, S. M. Hyperreactive airway smooth muscle responsiveness after inhalation of toluene diisocyanate vapors. *Am. Rev. Respir. Dis.* 129:296, 1984.

147. Merchant, J. Priorities for the management of environmental and occupational asthma. *Chest* 98:146S, 1990.

148. Metzger, W., et al. Bronchoalveolar lavage of allergic asthmatic patients following allergen bronchoprovocation. *Chest* 89:477, 1986.

149. Meyer-Bisch, C., et al. Respiratory hazards in hard metal workers: A cross-sectional study. *Br. J. Ind. Med.* 46:302, 1989.

150. Moisan, T. Prolonged asthma after smoke inhalation: A report of three cases and a review of previous reports. *J. Occup. Med.* 33:458, 1991.

151. Molfino, N., et al. Effect of low concentrations of ozone on inhaled allergen responses in asthmatic subjects. *Lancet* 338:199, 1991.

152. Moller, D., et al. Persistent airways disease caused by toluene diisocyanate. *Am. Rev. Respir. Dis.* 134:175, 1986.

153. Murphy, D., et al. Severe airways disease due to the inhalation of fumes from cleaning agents. *Chest* 69:372, 1976.

154. Murray, J., et al. Release of prostaglandin D2 into human airways during acute antigen challenge. *N. Engl. J. Med.* 315:800, 1986.

155. Musk, A., et al. Respiratory symptoms, lung function, and sensitization to flour in a British bakery. *Br. J. Ind. Med.* 46:636, 1989.

156. Nadel, J. Cell to cell communication: Some epithelial metabolic factors affecting airway smooth muscle. *Am. Rev. Respir. Dis.* 138:S22, 1988.

157. Nadel, J., and Borson, B. Modulation of neurogenic inflammation by neutral endopeptidase. *Am. Rev. Respir. Dis.* 143(Suppl.):33S, 1991.

158. Nakazawa, T. Occupational asthma due to alkyl cyanoacrylate. *J. Occup. Med.* 32:709, 1990.

159. National Institute for Occupational Safety and Health. (NIOSH). Criteria for a Recommended Standard: Occupational Exposure to Diisocyanates. In NIOSH. Washington, D.C.: U.S. Department of Health, Education and Welfare, Public Health Service, Centers for Disease Control, 1978.

160. Nelson, W. L. Allergic events among health care workers exposed to psyllium laxatives in the workplace. *J. Occup. Med.* 29:497, 1987.

161. Newman-Taylor, A. Occupational asthma. *Postgrad. Med. J.* 64:505, 1988.

162. Norback, D., Michel, I., and Widstrom, J. Indoor air quality and personal factors related to the sick building syndrome. *Scand. J. Work Environ. Health* 16:121, 1990.

163. Nunn, A., et al. Six year follow up of lung function in men occupationally exposed to formaldehyde. *Br. J. Ind. Med.* 47:747, 1990.

164. Oliver, L. Occupational and environmental asthma: Legal and ethical aspects of patient management. *Chest* 98:220S, 1990.

165. O'Neil, C. Review: Mechanisms of occupational airways diseases induced by exposure to organic and inorganic chemicals. *Am. J. Med. Sci.* 299:265, 1990.

166. Osebold, J., Gershwin, L., and Zee, Y. Studies on the enhancement of allergic lung sensitization by inhalation of ozone and sulfuric acid aerosol. *J. Environ. Pathol. Toxicol. Oncol.* 3:221, 1990.

167. Paggiaro, P., et al. Follow up study of patients with respiratory disease due to toluene diisocyanate (TDI). *Clin. Allergy* 14:463, 1984.

168. Pattemore, P., et al. The interrelationship among bronchial hyperresponsiveness, the diagnosis of asthma, and asthma symptoms. *Am. Rev. Respir. Dis.* 142:1990.

169. Patterson, R., Nugent, K. M., and Eberle, M. E. Immunologic hemorrhagic pneumonia caused by isocyanates. *Am. Rev. Respir. Dis.* 141:226, 1990.

170. Promisloff, R., et al. Reactive airways dysfunction syndrome in three police officers following a roadside chemical spill. *Chest* 98:928, 1990.

171. Rajan, K., and Davies, B. Reversible airways obstruction and interstitial pneumonitis due to acetic acid. *Br. J. Ind. Med.* 46:67, 1989.

172. Reidel, F., et al. Effects of SO_2 exposure on allergic sensitization in the guinea pig. *J. Allergy Clin. Immunol.* 82:527, 1988.

173. Richards, I., et al. Florida red-tide toxins (brevotoxins) produce depolarization of airway smooth muscle. *Toxicon* 28:1105, 1990.

174. Rijcken, B., et al. The relationship of nonspecific bronchial responsiveness to respiratory symptoms in a random population sample. *Am. Rev. Respir. Dis.* 136:62, 1987.

175. Rosenberg, S., et al. Serum IgE antibodies to psyllium in individuals allergic to psyllium and English plantain. *Ann. Allergy* 48:294, 1982.

176. Russell, J., and Rohrbach, M. Tannins induces endothelium-dependent contraction and relaxation of rabbit pulmonary artery. *Am. Rev. Respir. Dis.* 139:498, 1989.

177. Salvaggio, J. Occupational and Environmental Respiratory Disease. In *National Institute of Allergy and Infectious Diseases Task Force Report: Asthma and Other Allergic Diseases.* Washington, D.C.: Department of Health, Education, and Welfare, 1979.

178. Sapienza, S., et al. Role of leukotriene D4 in the early and late pulmonary responses of rats to allergen challenge. *Am. Rev. Respir. Dis.* 142:353, 1990.

179. Sato, J., and Perl, E. Adrenergic excitation of cutaneous pain receptors induced by peripheral nerve injury. *Science* 251:1606, 1991.

180. Schleuter, D. P., et al. Occupational asthma due to tetrachlorophthalic anhydride. *J. Occup. Med.* 20:183, 1978.

181. Seguin, P., et al. Prevalence of occupational asthma in spray painters exposed to several types of isocyanates, including polymethylene polyphenylisocyanate. *J. Occup. Med.* 29:340, 1987.

182. Selden, A., Belin, L., and Wass, U. Isocyanate exposure and hypersensitivity pneumonitis-report of a probable case and prevalence of specific immunoglobulin G antibodies among exposed individuals. *Scand. J. Work Environ. Health* 15:234, 1989.

183. Sheppard, D., et al. Toluene diisocyanate increases airway responsiveness to substance P and decreases airway neutral endopeptidase. *J. Clin. Invest.* 81:1111, 1988.

184. Shirakawa, T., et al. The existence of specific antibodies to cobalt in hard metal asthma. *Clin. Allergy* 18:451, 1988.

185. Smith, A., and Brooks, S. Absence of airway hyperreactivity to methacholine in worker sensitized to toluene diisocyanate (TDI). *J. Occup. Med.* 22:327, 1980.

186. Smith, A., et al. Guidelines for the epidemiologic assessment of occupational asthma. *J. Allergy Clin. Immunol.* 84:794, 1989.

187. Smith, D. Medical-legal definition of occupational asthma. *Chest* 98:1007, 1990.

188. Sprince, N., et al. Cobalt exposure and lung disease in tungsten carbide production. *Am. Rev. Respir. Dis.* 138:1220, 1988.

189. Tarlo, S., and Broder, I. Irritant-induced occupational asthma. *Chest* 96:297, 1989.

190. Task Force on Environment Cancer and Heart and Lung Disease. Workshop on Environmental and Occupational Asthma. *Chest* 98(Suppl.): 145S, 1990.

191. Thiel, H. Baker's Asthma: Epidemiological and Clinical Findings—Needs for Prospective Studies. In J. Kerr and M. A. Glanderston (eds.), *Congress of Allergology and Immunology Proceedings.* Basinstoke: MacMillan, 1983.

192. Van De Graaf, E., et al. Respiratory membrane permeability and bronchial hyperreactivity in patients with stable asthma. Effects of therapy with inhaled steroids. *Am. Rev. Respir. Dis.* 143:362, 1991.

193. Vandervort, R., and Brooks, S. M. Investigation of polyvinyl chloride film thermal decomposition products as an occupational illness of meat wrappers: I. Environmental exposures and toxicology. *J. Occup. Med.* 19:189, 1979.

194. Vedal, S., et al. Symptoms and pulmonary function in western red cedar workers related to duration of employment and dust exposure. *Arch. Environ. Health* 41:179, 1986.

195. Venables, K. Low molecular weight chemicals, hypersensitivity, and direct toxicity: The acid anhydrides. *Br. J. Ind. Med.* 46:222, 1989.

196. Venables, K., et al. Smoking and occupational allergy in workers in a platinum refinery. *Br. Med. J.* 299:939, 1989.

197. Wass, U., and Belin, L. An in vitro method for predicting sensitizing properties of inhaled chemicals. *Scand. J. Work Environ. Health* 16:208, 1990.

198. Wass, U., and Belin, L. Immunologic specificity of isocyanate induced IgE antibodies in serum for 10 sensitized workers. *J. Allergy Clin. Immunol.* 83:126, 1989.

199. Wegman, D. H., et al. A dose-response releationship in TDI workers. *J. Occup. Med.* 16:258, 1974.

200. Weiler, J., et al. Prevalence of bronchial hyperresponsiveness in highly trained athletes. *Chest* 90:23, 1986.

201. Weill, H., et al. Respiratory and Immunologic Evaluation of Isocyanate Exposure in a New Manufacturing Plant. In NIOSH. Washington, D.C.: U.S. Government Printing Office, 1981.

202. Wergeland, E., et al. Respiratory dysfunction after potroom asthma. *Am. J. Ind. Med.* 11:627, 1987.

203. Woolcock, A., et al. Prevalence of bronchial responsiveness and asthma in a rural adult population. *Thorax* 42:361, 1987.

204. Zammit-Tabona, M., et al. Asthma caused by dimethyl methane diisocyanate in foundry workers: Clinical, bronchoprovocation and immunologic studies. *Am. Rev. Respir. Dis.* 128:226, 1983.

205. Kowitz, T. A., et al. Effects of chlorine gas on respiratory function. *Arch. Environ. Health* 14:545, 1967.

206. Committee on Aldehydes, Board on Toxicology and Environmental Health Hazards, Assembly on Life Sciences, National Academy of Sciences. Formaldehyde and Other Aldehydes. Washington, D.C.: National Academy Press, 1981: 204–206.

207. Bascom, R., et al. Effect of ozone inhalation on the response to nasal challenge with antigen of allergic subjects. *Am. Rev. Respir. Dis.* 142: 594, 1990.

208. Molfino, N., et al. Effect of low concentrations of ozone on inhaled allergen responses in asthmatic subjects. *Lancet* 338:199, 1991.

209. Devlin, R., et al. Exposure of humans to ambient levels of ozone for 6.6 hours causes cellular and biochemical changes in the lung. *Am. J. Respir. Mol. Biol.* 4:72, 1991.

210. Horstman, D., et al. Ozone concentration and pulmonary response relationshps for 6.6-hour exposures with five hours of moderate exercise to 0.08, 0.10, and 0.12 ppm. *Am. Rev. Respir. Dis.* 142:1158, 1990.

211. Bakke, P., Baste, V., and Gulsvik, A. Bronchial responsiveness in a Norwegian community. *Am. Rev. Respir. Dis.* 143:317, 1991.

212. Woolcock, A., et al. Prevalence of bronchial responsiveness and asthma in a rural adult popluation. *Thorax* 42:361, 1987.

213. Beasley, R., et al. Cellular events in the bronchi in mild asthma and after bronchial provocation. *Am. Rev. Respir. Dis.* 139:806, 1989.

214. Van De Graaf, E., et al. Respiratory membrane permeability and bronchial hyperreactivity in patients with stable asthma. Effects of therapy with inhaled steroids. *Am. Rev. Respir. Dis.* 143:362, 1991.

215. Laitinen, L., et al. Eosinophilic airway inflammation during exacerbation of asthma and its treatment with inhaled corticosteroid. *Am. Rev. Respir. Dis.* 143:423, 1991.

216. Tarlo, S., and Broder, I. Irritant-induced occupational asthma. *Chest* 96: 297, 1989.

217. Saetta, M., et al. Airway mucosal inflammation in occupational asthma induced by toluene diisocyanate. *Am. Rev. Respir. Dis.* 145:160, 1992.

218. Saetta, M., et al. Effect of cessation of exposure to toluene diisocyanate (TDI) on bronchial mucosa of subjects with TDI-induced asthma. *Am. Rev. Respir. Dis.* 145:169, 1992.

Exercise-Induced Asthma

Ephraim Bar-Yishay
Simon Godfrey

47

Since the publication of the first edition of this text in 1976, the knowledge and understanding of exercise-induced asthma (EIA) have increased to an extraordinary degree. In order to understand the subject and give due credit to the many investigators who have contributed so much, it is useful to follow developments more or less in historic sequence.

Exercise-induced asthma was described as early as the seventeenth century by Sir John Floyer [50], but very little interest was taken in the subject until relatively recently. Herxheimer [62] in 1946 and Jones and his colleagues [66–69] in the early sixties pioneered the scientific investigations. These studies characterized the asthmatic attack provoked by exercise or hyperventilation, and clearly showed EIA to be a normal feature of childhood and young adult asthma. They also related the pattern of EIA to its clinical severity and noted the persistence of EIA in young adults who had "grown out" of childhood asthma. McNeill and coworkers [89] described the diminution of response to further exercise after an initial attack of EIA—the refractory period. These early investigations also clearly established the ability of sympathomimetic agents to prevent EIA, the lesser effects of theophylline and atropine, and the lack of effect from antihistamines and steroids.

By the late 1970s, a new flurry of research began to unravel the importance of the climate of the air being breathed during exercise and the similarities between asthma induced by exercise, isocapnic hyperventilation, and the inhalation of nonisotonic fogs. These issues were introduced by us in the second edition of this book published in 1985, and, even though important work has been undertaken since, the picture today remains far from complete and there is still disagreement on the basic mechanisms of EIA, hyperventilation-induced asthma (HIA), and osmotically induced asthma (OIA).

LUNG FUNCTION CHANGES

The pulmonary response of an asthmatic to exercise, as revealed in the early studies, was quite consistent. This pattern is illustrated in Figure 47-1 [59], which also shows the method for calculating the response. In asthmatics, exercise induces an initial mild bronchodilatation, which is often maintained throughout the exercise period. After stopping exercise, bronchospasm ensues, and lung function reaches its lowest level after 3 to 5 minutes in children and after 5 to 7 minutes in adults. The index most commonly used in quantifying EIA is the percent postexercise fall from the preexercise baseline, often called ΔFEV_1, when the forced expiratory volume in 1 second (FEV_1) is used as the lung function test.

Early studies of EIA used simple measurements, such as peak expiratory flow rate (PEFR) or FEV_1, to document the changes. More recently, lung function has been investigated using whole-body plethysmography to measure lung volumes and airway resistance in addition to the maximum expiratory flow-volume (MEFV) maneuvers. Freedman and associates [52], using static pressure-volume curves as well, found an increased residual volume and reduced elastic recoil pressure during the attack of EIA, suggesting widespread airway closure. A decrease in the elastic recoil would also contribute to the reduction of maximal expiratory flows at low lung volumes. By repeating the MEFV maneuvers using helium-oxygen mixtures, various investigators have shown considerable interpatient variability, with some subjects having predominantly large airways obstruction and others small airways obstruction [19, 86]. Wagner and colleagues [118] recently succeeded in directly measuring the peripheral lung resistance in patients with mild asthma by wedging a retrograde catheter into a subsegmental lobe. They demonstrated a significant increase in peripheral lung resistance in the asthmatic patients as compared to healthy controls, even though the routinely employed lung function parameters (e.g., forced vital capacity, FEV_1, and so on) were comparable. They further noted that bronchodilator therapy did not alleviate this localized condition. Using the forced oscillation technique to measure total respiratory resistance, Mansfield and colleagues [81] found bronchodilatation in their patients during exercise, which persisted throughout the exercise period, irrespective of its length, but this response was less marked in asthmatics than in normals. In a recent study, Rubinstein and colleagues [102], who measured the central airway dimension by an advanced acoustic technique, confirmed Mansfield's finding in that they showed increased dimensions of both extrathoracic and central intrathoracic airways in normal subjects during exercise, but only extrathoracic airway dilatation and main bronchi constriction in asthmatics.

Despite the greater sensitivity of these tests and the freedom from dependence on patient cooperation of some, they have not been convincingly shown to be superior to the simpler indexes such as the ones described in Figure 47-1 [59]. Thus, for example, O'Cain and associates [95] demonstrated that maximal expiratory flow at 30 percent vital capacity has higher sensitivity in detecting small degrees of bronchoconstriction, but Saunders and Rudolf [104] showed the simpler indexes to be adequate, even when lung volume changed.

The effect of exercise on the arterial blood gas values of asthmatics is related to the changes in lung function. During exercise, arterial PO_2 and PCO_2 remain essentially unchanged, but are accompanied by a fall in pH and an accumulation of lactic acid [107]. While some believe these changes to be excessive in asthmatics [107], Silverman and coworkers [109] found no correlation between the pH or lactic acidosis and the severity of EIA. After exercise, and along with the bronchoconstriction, there is moderate arterial hypoxia and occasional hypercapnia [5]. Despite early enthusiasm [62], it has not been possible to show that changes in blood gases or acid-base balance serve as the triggering factors for EIA.

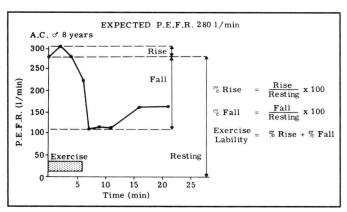

Fig. 47-1. *Typical response to 6 minutes of running by an asthmatic child showing the method of calculating the indexes of bronchial lability. P.E.F.R. = peak expiratory flow rate. (Reprinted with permission from S. Godfrey, et al., Problems of interpreting EIA. J. Allergy Clin. Immunol. 52:199, 1973.)*

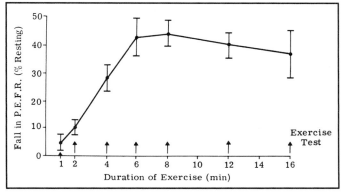

Fig. 47-2. *The effect of the duration of exercise on asthma induced by treadmill running at constant speed and gradient. Each point represents the mean of tests in 10 children who performed each duration of exercise on a different occasion. P.E.F.R. = peak expiratory flow rate. (Reprinted with permission from S. Godfrey, et al., Problems of interpreting EIA. J. Allergy Clin. Immunol. 52:199, 1973.)*

PHYSICAL FACTORS INFLUENCING THE RESPONSE TO EXERCISE

A number of different protocols have been used when performing exercise or hyperventilation challenges, and the way in which the test is performed can influence the result considerably. From 1966 to 1976, there was a great deal of research to define the conditions under which EIA could be demonstrated, the extent to which asthmatics differed from normal subjects, the changes that occurred in lung mechanics and blood gases, and the effect of various therapeutic agents. Silverman and Anderson [108] showed that the severity of EIA increased with increasing work rate and with increasing duration of exercise up to certain plateau values, as illustrated in Figure 47-2 [59]. The maximum response was seen after 6 to 8 minutes of exercise, and patients often experienced reduced asthma after prolonged exercise. They could "run through" their asthma. It has also been known for some time that prior exercise reduces the response to a subsequent challenge [89]. This prior exercise may take the form of brief warming-up periods [105] or a single, more prolonged exercise period [42, 100].

Since the time of Sir John Floyer, it has been known to both asthmatics and their physicians that some types of exercise are more troublesome than others. For this reason, Jones and associates [68] recommended running as the most provocative stimulus. Formal studies conducted under controlled conditions by Fitch and Morton [49] and by Anderson and colleagues [2] showed that running causes more bronchospasm than swimming and that free-range running causes more asthma than cycling. These differences stimulated later investigators to conduct experiments with far-reaching conclusions concerning the mechanism of EIA and other types of provoked asthma.

For a number of years, it has been known that some asthmatics developed bronchospasm if they hyperventilated [30, 62], and even the deep breaths used to perform lung function tests could provoke an attack. HIA resembles EIA in many ways and follows a very similar time course [26] (Fig. 47-3), although there are differences that will be discussed later. Both EIA and HIA have been used in population studies of bronchial reactivity, in attempts to define asthma, in the evaluation of the pathophysiology of asthma, and in the evaluation of drugs used to treat asthma [29, 36, 94, 111, 121]. Both challenges appear to operate through pathways involving a number of steps and are not simply the result of direct action on bronchial smooth muscle, as would appear to be the case with methacholine and histamine challenges. In the following sections, we will consider what is known about the pathophysiology of EIA and HIA, as this is fundamental to the interpretation of results of these challenges.

RELATIONSHIP BETWEEN EIA, HIA, AND OIA

The understanding of the mechanism of EIA has been advanced in recent years in the light of a series of very interesting observations. Weinstein and associates [120], Chen and Horton [32], and Bar-Or and coworkers [15] were the first to note that asthmatic subjects experienced less EIA in a humid climate than in a dry climate. These findings were taken up by Strauss and colleagues [115], who showed that breathing cold and dry air enhances EIA. In a series of studies, they later developed the respiratory heat loss (RHL) hypothesis of EIA, which suggested that airways are cooled when cold and/or dry air is breathed because it must be heated and humidified to meet body conditions before it reaches the alveoli. This requires the evaporation of water and transfer of heat from the airway mucosa. Deal and colleagues [38] then showed that RHL during exercise was reflected by a fall in airway temperature recorded in the esophagus. In later studies, McFadden and coworkers [87, 88] demonstrated airway cooling by direct measurements within the bronchial tree. They went on to show that isocapnic hyperventilation even without exercise can provoke as much asthma as that seen in EIA [39] and that the severity of asthma is related to RHL, however achieved [40]. They concluded that the initial event in EIA was cooling of the airways due to the hyperventilation and that there was no essential difference between EIA and HIA.

There is now, however, some doubt regarding aspects of the RHL hypothesis. Contrary to the findings of Deal and associates [39, 40], later studies have not confirmed a unique relationship between the severity of EIA and the level of minute ventilation or RHL during exercise [7, 31]. For example, we have shown that, at identical levels of RHL, running still caused 39 percent more asthma than did swimming [17]. We also conducted investigations in one subject who consistently developed EIA when breathing warm humid air so that there was no RHL [20], and, in a study by Anderson and coworkers [8], more than half of a group of severe asthmatics developed EIA after exercising while breathing air conditioned to body temperature and humidity. Furthermore, we recently demonstrated [92] that, for the same cooling or water loss, the more intense exercise causes almost twice as much asthma as a lighter challenge (Fig. 47-4). All these findings

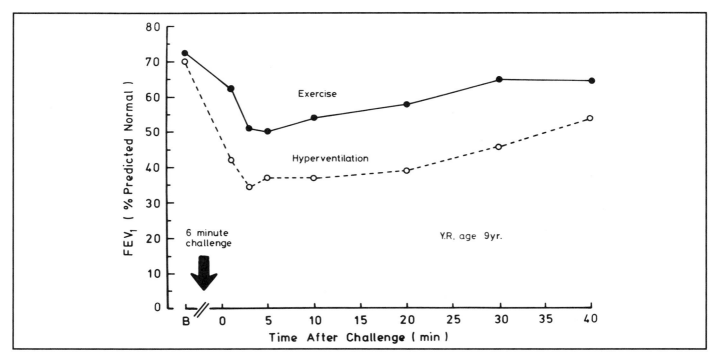

Fig. 47-3. *The response to steady-state exercise and voluntary isocapnic hyperventilation of similar intensity to that occurring during exercise in an asthmatic subject. The pattern of change in lung function is quite similar for the two challenges, although in this instance the change was more marked after hyperventilation.*

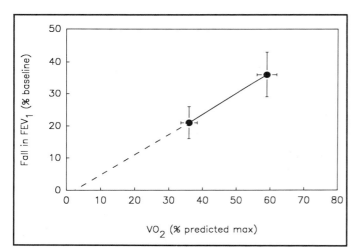

Fig. 47-4. *Severity of exercise-induced asthma in relation to oxygen consumption at two levels of exercise performed with the same amount of heat and water loss from the airways. The results are the mean and standard error for a group of eight children. (Redrawn with permission from N. Noviski, et al., Exercise intensity determines and climatic conditions modify the severity of exercise induced asthma. Am. Rev. Respir. Dis. 136:592, 1987.)*

raise the possibility that the nature of the exercise itself has an independent effect.

Another possible trigger for provoking asthma, which may resemble that of exercise or hyperventilation, is the inhalation of hypotonic or hypertonic salt solutions [106]. When delivered through an ultrasonic nebulizer, quite small quantities of such solutions provoke attacks of asthma in a dose-response fashion. Moreover, there are considerable similarities between OIA and both EIA and HIA; these include the appearance of a refractory period after OIA and protection from OIA by sodium cromogly-

cate administration [4, 18]. Careful inspection of the data relating the severity of induced asthma to the temperature of the air breathed showed that there could be very wide fluctuations of temperature with relatively little difference in the severity of the asthma, provided the water loss was similar [3]. These observations prompted the suggestion that the greater severity of EIA and HIA when breathing cold, dry air is really due to drying of the airways and a resultant increase in the osmolarity of the lining fluid [1]. The more recent observations seem to confirm this suggestion [1, 63]. There has been some argument as to where the evaporation takes place within the airway and whether the volume of fluid available could prevent any significant change in osmolarity [1, 3, 55]. However, Anderson and colleagues [3] have produced compelling evidence to suggest that drying of the mucosa takes place over the most relevant generations of airways.

POSSIBLE MECHANISMS

Since cromolyn sodium (sodium cromoglycate) was shown to inhibit EIA and was thought to act by inhibiting mediator release [35, 110, 115], a simple model was suggested to explain the mechanism of EIA [57], as shown in Figure 47-5. In this model, exercise was believed to have two opposing effects—bronchodilatation due to catecholamine release and bronchoconstriction due to release of stored bronchoconstricting mediators. During exercise these factors were considered to be more or less balanced, with a slight advantage in favor of bronchodilatation. At the end of exercise, the sympathetic discharge rapidly terminates and the unopposed mediators cause bronchospasm. Because mediators require time for resynthesis, the subject who sustains EIA is rendered relatively refractory to further attack. We later showed that this refractory period itself wears off, with a half-life of about 1 hour [42], and so, after about 3 to 4 hours, the subject is fully responsive. While this model accounted for the facts known up to

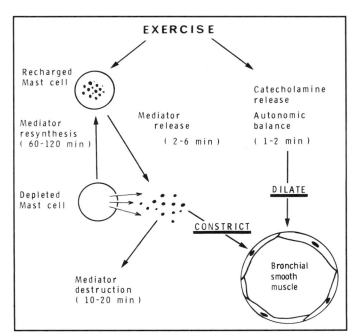

Fig. 47-5. *Hypothetical pathways concerned in exercise-induced asthma. Exercise is envisaged as causing bronchoconstriction by the liberation of stored mediators from mast cells and an opposing bronchodilatation during the exercise period caused by the stimulation of the autonomic nervous system. The net effect on bronchial smooth muscle depends on the balance of these forces and the time factors involved, as discussed in the text. (Reprinted with permission from S. Godfrey, Exercise-induced Asthma. In T. J. H. Clark and S. Godfrey [eds.], Asthma [2nd ed.]. New York: Chapman & Hall, 1983.)*

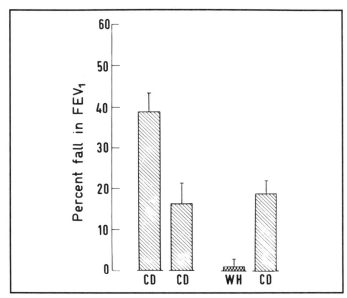

Fig. 47-6. *Postexercise fall in FEV_1 (mean ± S.E.), as a percent of baseline, in subjects who exercised breathing cold dry (CD) air followed 30 minutes later by exercise breathing CD air, and on another occasion exercised first breathing warm humid (WH) air and then CD air after a similar interval. Twelve of 15 subjects were rendered equally refractory by the initial exercise period regardless of the type of air breathed. (Reprinted with permission from I. Ben Dov, et al., Refractory period following exercise-induced asthma unexplained by respiratory heat loss. Am. Rev. Respir. Dis. 125:530, 1982.)*

about 1975, bronchoconstrictor mediators had not been directly identified at that time nor had the stimulus for releasing them.

An alternative mechanism was suggested by Deal and colleagues [41], who found that the blood levels of neither histamine nor neutrophil (leukocyte) chemotactic factor (NCF) change after HIA (see Chap. 10). Their later findings that patients are rendered refractory following exercise but not following hyperventilation [113] led them to suggest further that the refractory period after EIA is related to endogenous catecholamine release persisting in the bloodstream for up to 1 hour after exercise. However, it is well established that, when using the appropriate type of exercise to induce EIA, catecholamine levels return to baseline shortly after the end of exercise [14, 76]. Furthermore, other studies have demonstrated the release of histamine and NCF following EIA and antigen challenge and shown that this release and EIA are suppressed by previous treatment with sodium cromoglycate [9, 12, 77, 78]. The apparent contradiction may be resolved by the findings of Barnes and Brown [12], who showed that, although plasma histamine levels are elevated during exercise in asthmatics, no elevation in histamine levels precedes isocapnic HIA.

The possibility that chemical mediators are involved in the intermediary pathway seems certain in light of further recent findings. Recently, a potent H_1 histamine antagonist, terfenadine, has been shown to markedly reduce the severity of EIA, HIA, and OIA [47, 48, 122]. EIA has also been shown to be reduced by treatment with an inhibitor of leukotriene D_4 [129, 132], and HIA by an inhibitor of 5-lipoxygenase [131]. In animals, HIA is reduced by pretreatment with capsaicin, which reduces the availability of ecosinoids [134]. The eosinophil is now widely believed to be important in the inflammatory process that accompanies asthma [128, 136]. Venge and colleagues [136] showed that levels of serum eosinophil cationic protein (ECP) were higher in those

asthmatics who developed EIA and fell after exercise. Both the level of ECP and the severity of EIA could be reduced by pretreatment with sodium cromoglycate or 4 weeks of taking the inhaled corticosteroid budesonide.

In light of the importance of climatic conditions, we further investigated the refractory period in a study in which subjects performed an initial exercise while breathing either warm humid or cold dry air and then, in both cases, performed a second exercise test while breathing cold dry air [22]. Simply based on the RHL hypothesis, it was expected that the exercise in warm humid air should not induce refractoriness since it would cause neither asthma nor mediator release. This was found in 3 of the 15 subjects tested, but the majority showed quite an unexpected pattern (Fig. 47-6). In these subjects it did not matter whether they breathed cold dry or warm humid air for the first test, as they were rendered equally refractory to the second cold dry test. In other words, exercise per se, not airway cooling and drying or the ensuing bronchoconstriction, was responsible for the refractoriness and presumably for mediator depletion. This observation was recently confirmed by Wilson and coworkers [123] who have extended our finding to show that in asthmatics even a non-EIA–producing exercise using different muscle groups (in their case, arm cranking) induces refractoriness. In contrast, when we carried out a similar test using isocapnic hyperventilation instead of exercise [16], we found temperature (and hence humidity) to be all important, with only hyperventilation in cold dry air rendering our subjects refractory. These findings are in agreement with those of Wilson and associates [124] and, most recently, those of Rosenthal and coworkers [101]. We have further shown that, not only is hyperventilation capable of inducing refractoriness to the following hyperventilation maneuver, but it also renders subjects refractory to exercise and vice versa [24]. Since catecholamine levels do not rise in HIA [14], the fact that refractoriness has been found after both HIA and EIA makes catecholamine release a very unlikely explanation.

A totally new light on the refractoriness issue was shed by recent studies which showed that the prostaglandin inhibitor, indomethacin, could prevent the appearance of refractoriness to EIA and OIA but not to HIA [82, 83, 93]. This suggests that refractoriness, at least to exercise and hyperosmolar challenges, is due to the release of an inhibitory prostaglandin whose effect persists for 30 to 60 minutes or so after the initial challenge, and whose release does not require that the initial challenge cause actual bronchospasm. Further support for this hypothesis can be inferred from the recent findings of O'Byrne and colleagues [64, 80], who showed that inhibitory prostaglandins (i.e., PGE_1) cause bronchodilatation as well as reduced methacholine reactivity.

An alternative hypothesis for the mechanism of the airways obstruction seen with EIA and HIA has been proposed by McFadden and colleagues [55, 56, 85] and Baile and coworkers [11], who attribute the obstruction to reactive hyperemia of the bronchial epithelium. They believe that the airways cool during exercise or hyperventilation and rewarm once the exercise or hyperventilation stops. The rewarming of these cooled airways causes reactive hyperemia and this obstructs the airflow. In support of their idea, they reported greater airways obstruction when the rewarming was increased by breathing warm, humid air at the end of the challenge. However, other investigators have not confirmed that the rate of rewarming affects the degree of obstruction [112]. In any case, this hypothesis seems to be quite untenable, because many asthmatics develop moderate or even marked airways obstruction toward the end of the exercise period while their airways are still cold.

A global model of EIA and HIA is proposed here (Figure 47-7). In this model, exercise results in (1) hyperventilation, (2) a possible direct (intrinsic) effect, (3) increased sympathetic drive, and (4) probable release of an inhibitory prostaglandin. The hyperventilation of exercise, or voluntary isocapnic hyperventilation per se, results in cooling and drying of the airways, which is dependent on the climatic conditions of the inspired air. As a result of the osmotic changes, there is release of mediators from mast cells (or other storage cells) that act on the bronchial smooth muscle and cause bronchospasm. During exercise, the subject is relatively (though not always completely) protected by the increased sympathetic drive. This short-term protection stops as soon as the exercise ends, allowing the bronchospasm to become manifest. There is some suggestion that asthma may appear sooner during hyperventilation, which could be explained by the lack of such fast protection. Another type of protection is built up more slowly through the release of an inhibitory prostaglandin, and this may account for the refractory period after EIA, although not apparently for that following HIA. Finally, the effect of the released mediators depends on the basic level of bronchial reactivity, which, in turn, depends on such factors as the level of allergenic stimulation, recent viral infections, and air pollution (see later discussion).

This model emphasizes the following important points about EIA:

1. EIA is inherently variable because of the many factors that interact to produce the bronchoconstriction.
2. The severity of the response to exercise on any one occasion is largely unpredictable, since not all the variables can be quantified.
3. When using exercise as a challenge in the same subject on different occasions or in different subjects, it is vital to standardize the exercise as well as environmental and allergenic factors as much as possible.

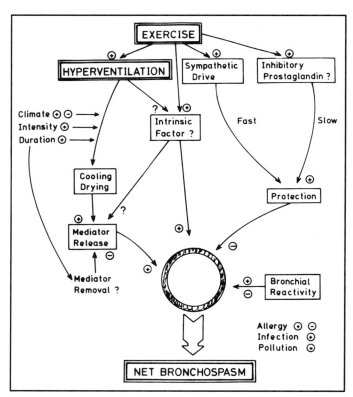

Fig. 47-7. *Updated model of pathways involved in exercise-induced asthma (EIA). Exercise is believed to trigger EIA by increasing ventilation, which, when influenced by climatic conditions, produces cooling and drying of the airways. The total stimulus appears to be influenced by both this drying and the exercise itself. The trigger liberates mediators that act on the airway and cause bronchospasm. The net response of the airway depends on its reactivity, which is influenced by a variety of factors, including the level of allergic stimulation. During exercise, this effect is opposed by increased sympathomimetic drive (short protection), so that in most subjects (but not all) lung function changes little until exercise ceases and the sympathomimetic drive is reduced. In addition, exercise releases protective mediators such as prostaglandins, which cause refractoriness to subsequent exercise (slow protection).*

EIA, BRONCHIAL HYPERREACTIVITY, AND ATOPY

EIA is generally believed to be a manifestation of the increased airway reactivity characteristic of asthma and demonstrable by other means. This hyperreactivity is an order of magnitude greater in asthmatics compared with normal subjects or patients with other lung diseases. Mellis and colleagues [90] studied 50 asthmatic children and compared their responses to exercise and histamine challenge. They found a correlation between the responses to the two challenges, although the incidence of a positive response was greater with histamine (90%) than with exercise (74%). A rather similar conclusion was reached in another study [54], in which 95 percent of the asthmatics responded to a methacholine challenge, 71 percent to ultrasonic fog, and 57 percent to cold air hyperventilation. In our own laboratory, we have found a reasonable correlation between EIA and methacholine sensitivity in children with mild to moderately severe asthma, but a poor correlation in patients with more severe disease who required steroid prophylaxis for management. It is possible that either the disease or its treatment may have different effects on the responsiveness to exercise and methacholine. Increased bronchial reactivity has been noted in subjects other than asthmatics, such as formerly wheezy infants [75], relatives of asthmatic children and wheezy infants [73, 74], and children with cystic fibrosis [79]. However, in all these groups the lability consists of increased bronchodilatation during exercise and a small increase in postexercise bronchoconstriction, which is far less than that seen in asthma.

A number of studies have explored the range of bronchial responsiveness to exercise and the variability of the response in normal subjects and asthmatics [6, 29, 108]. The average rise in peak flow during exercise is about 3 to 4 percent in both normal children and adults, with a maximum postexercise fall of about 9 to 10 percent. Burr and associates [29] studied a group of 812 children, aged 12 years, who were not only healthy themselves but were not related to asthmatic subjects. They found that 92 percent had a postexercise fall in the peak flow rate of less than 10 percent, and 98 percent of them had a fall of less than 15 percent. Backer and colleagues [126] investigated 527 children and found the upper limit of normal for the percentage fall in FEV_1 under controlled conditions to be 12 percent. The consensus from such studies is that a postexercise fall in the PEFR or FEV_1 of greater than 10 percent is suggestive of asthma and, if it is greater than 15 percent, the diagnosis is almost certain [29].

The incidence of EIA in asthmatics and the reproducibility of tests of EIA are greatly influenced by the nature of the exercise test and the conditions under which the exercise is performed. We found a fall in lung function after exercise of greater than 10 percent in 89 percent of the 107 asthmatic children tested. Taking a 15 percent fall in lung function as a cutoff point, Kattan and colleagues [70] detected EIA in 83 to 84 percent of asthmatic children. In the studies of Eggleston and Guerrant [43], using their criteria for optimal test conditions, they found 71 percent of the asthmatics had a positive exercise test but the reproducibility of the challenge was rather poor. Studies in 21 adult asthmatics conducted by Haynes and coworkers [60] showed an incidence of EIA of 82 to 87 percent, using more sensitive tests of lung function. Hence, it seems very likely that EIA will develop in nearly all asthmatics if they exercise vigorously enough under appropriate conditions, but of course many asthmatics, especially adults, never encounter the problem because they engage in little exercise. In addition, the incidence of EIA and the reproducibility of the challenge are most likely affected by basal airway reactivity [33].

Under certain circumstances, an increase in bronchial reactivity can be produced in normal subjects (e.g., by the inhalation of ozone or sulfur dioxide or by viral infection), but this reactivity is small and reverts rapidly to normal [28, 44]. The inhalation of subfreezing air during hyperventilation has also been reported to cause a modest bronchoconstriction in normal subjects [46, 94], but the postchallenge fall in FEV_1 was only about 4 percent—well within the normal response range. The situation with hyperventilation is not so well worked out, but again a postchallenge fall in the FEV_1 of greater than 9 percent makes the diagnosis almost certain when the subject exceeds a ventilation of about 25 times the baseline FEV_1 while breathing cold dry air [121].

A particular problem has been the apparent increased incidence of exercise-induced changes in lung function in subjects with atopic diseases other than asthma, such as hay fever [71]. However, patient classification is all important, and many patients described as having hay fever also wheezed at times. In a careful study in which attention was paid to this point, Deal and colleagues [36] found no overlap between EIA or HIA in hay fever and asthmatic subjects but noted considerable overlap between the hay fever and normal control subjects.

It is well established that nonspecific bronchial reactivity to histamine can be markedly increased for several days or weeks following a specific bronchial provocation challenge with allergen [34]. Equally, removal of individuals from an environment where they are exposed to allergens to which they are sensitive reduces the nonspecific reactivity to histamine [98]. To see if this also applied to exercise, we undertook exercise challenges in asthmatic children on the day before and during the week after a specific allergen bronchial provocation test [91]. We found a clear-cut increase in the response to the same level of exercise, with the fall in FEV_1 almost doubling. This was true whether or not there was both an early and late reaction to the allergen, but, as has been documented before, the histamine responsiveness in our study only increased in those children with both early and late reactions. From these observations it is to be expected that the severity of EIA will vary from time, even for the same severity of stimulus and climatic conditions, depending on the recent exposure of the patient to relevant allergens.

Air pollution, simulated in the laboratory by adding small amounts of sulfur dioxide to the air, has also been shown to considerably enhance EIA [28], further complicating the prediction of the severity of EIA under conditions of natural exposure. To complicate things even further, it was recently shown that nonspecific airway reactivity to either methacholine or histamine challenge is affected by a prior challenge with exercise or isocapnic hyperventilation [53, 64, 114].

EIA closely resembles the immediate response to an allergen inhalation challenge (allergen-induced asthma [AIA]). Both are rapid in onset and pass off relatively quickly, are easily inhibited by pretreatment with sympathomimetic agents and sodium cromoglycate, and are not inhibited by steroids. Some investigators have suggested that EIA may also be characterized in some subjects by a second late-phase fall in lung function a few hours after the challenge [27, 103]. However, others have not confirmed these findings [84, 125] and the issue remains controversial. If EIA and AIA both involve mediator release from the same cells, it would therefore be expected that EIA and AIA should be mutually exclusive, in that the depletion of mediator stored in mast cells caused by EIA may render the subject refractory to AIA. We studied 12 allergic subjects who were first rendered refractory to EIA by repeated exercise and then were exposed to an inhaled antigen [119]. We found two types of response in these subjects; six were refractory to AIA when refractory to EIA and the other six were fully responsive to AIA. There were no obvious clinical or physiologic differences between the groups, and it is possible that in some subjects EIA is due to the release of mediators from sensitized mast cells, while in others the mediators come from different cells. It is also possible that the site of the sensitized mast cells is the determining factor.

DRUGS AND EIA

Because EIA is a safe and simple tool, it has frequently been used as a model for testing the effects of various drugs that are used in the treatment of clinical asthma. The earliest modern investigators determined that EIA could be inhibited by the prior administration of sympathomimetic agents but not by steroids or antihistamines, while the value of theophylline derivatives and atropine was less certain [69, 89]. By 1968, it had been shown that cromolyn sodium also blocked EIA [35]. Since then, relatively little important new information has accrued, except perhaps that relating to the effect of calcium antagonists [13, 96].

The general pattern of action of common agents is shown in Figure 47-8 [58]. Because several of the agents are bronchodilators, the results are expressed on an absolute scale of PEFR and the bronchodilatation following drug administration is shown, along with the subsequent exercise-induced bronchodilatation and the ensuing bronchoconstriction. It can be clearly seen from this figure that the absolute postexercise PEFRs after atropine and theophylline administration were better than those after placebo administration and close to their pre-drug, preexercise values; nevertheless, exercise caused a deterioration in lung func-

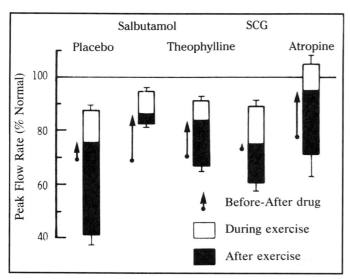

Fig. 47-8. *The effect of drugs on exercise-induced asthma, with values expressed as a percentage of the expected peak flow rate (mean ± SEM PEFR). The arrow indicates the bronchodilatation resulting from the administration of the drug before the exercise test. (N = 15 except for the atropine group in which there were 7 subjects.) SCC = sodium cromoglycate. (Reprinted with permission from S. Godfrey and P. Konig, Inhibition of EIA by different pharmacological pathways. Thorax 31:137, 1976.)*

tion from the post-drug preexercise values. This seems to have given rise to the disputes as to whether theophylline or atropine blocks EIA, with Pollock and colleagues [99] claiming a clear dose-related effect while Bierman and associates [25] were unable to demonstrate such a relationship. Similarly, with atropine Deal and coworkers [37] were unable to show a protective effect on EIA, but others have clearly demonstrated blocking [117]. By contrast, cromolyn sodium did not change the pre-drug lung function (see Fig. 47-8) and clearly inhibited EIA to a considerable degree, while albuterol, although a bronchodilator, so completely abolished any postexercise change that there is no doubt as to its efficacy. In this respect, the relative efficacy of cromolyn sodium was recently found to be related to its total plasma concentration [97], a finding that may explain why some patients are better protected by cromolyn sodium than are others [21, 23]. The position with regard to steroids is currently somewhat confusing. Originally, we and others felt that neither systemic nor inhaled steroids affected EIA [65]. More recently, evidence has accumulated to suggest that the severity of EIA can be diminished by long-term inhaled steroid therapy [61, 135], although this could be due to a more general effect on the resting airway caliber or the prevailing level of bronchial reactivity.

Although sympathomimetic agents are very potent inhibitors of EIA, there is some doubt as to the relative efficacy of oral versus inhaled preparations, even though bronchodilation occurs after administration by either route. Anderson and coworkers [7] found oral salbutamol to be ineffective compared with the inhaled drug, but Francis and associates [51] found both forms to be equally effective.

Recently, there has been interest in the effect of certain other agents on EIA. Enright and colleagues [45] were able to block EIA by the inhalation of a local anesthetic. A promising beneficial effect was obtained with nifedipine, which interferes with the cell-membrane calcium gate mechanism [13, 96]. Of the antihistaminic compounds, the most commonly tested, ketotifen, totally failed to inhibit EIA in carefully controlled studies [72, 116], but a more specific antihistamine drug, terfenadine, has now been shown to block the appearance of EIA [122] and OIA [47, 48] but

not of HIA [122]. Perhaps more exciting has been the finding that the diuretic furosemide can also block both EIA and osmotically induced asthma when given by inhalation [127, 133]. While the mechanism of action of furosemide in preventing EIA is still uncertain, it is tempting to link it to osmotic changes in the airway lining fluid.

Most drug studies that have been performed have shown that these agents have similar effects on EIA and HIA, but two are important because they appear to differentiate between the two types of challenge. Terfenadine can reduce EIA by almost half but has no effect on HIA [122]. A refractory period has been demonstrated after both EIA and HIA, during which it is more difficult to elicit a response to a repeat challenge. It has now been shown that this refractory period following EIA can be eliminated by treatment with indomethacin, but the drug has no effect on the refractory period following HIA [82].

For practical purposes, the most useful way to protect a patient against EIA is to give either a selective beta$_2$ sympathomimetic or cromolyn sodium immediately before exercise by inhalation. In absolute terms, the sympathomimetic is more effective and its duration is longer, but it requires a perfect inhalation technique, which is on the whole easier with the cromolyn sodium spinhaler. The protection falls to about 50 percent of the initial protection in about 4 to 5 hours with salbutamol and in 1.5 to 2 hours with cromolyn sodium. There is no logical reason to use theophylline, either the short- or long-acting form, for the sole purpose of inhibiting EIA.

Although not yet widely available, a new generation of long-acting inhaled beta$_2$ agonists has been developed, and these drugs inhibit EIA for substantially longer than do albuterol or the equivalent beta$_2$ agonists currently in use [130].

REFERENCES

1. Anderson, S. D. Is there a unifying hypothesis for exercise induced asthma. *J. Allergy Clin. Immunol.* 73:660, 1984.
2. Anderson, S. D., Connolly, N., and Godfrey, S. Comparison of bronchoconstriction induced by cycling and running. *Thorax* 26:396, 1971.
3. Anderson, S. D., Daviskas, E., and Smith, C. M. Exercise-induced asthma: a difference in opinion regarding the stimulus. *Allergy Proc.* 10:215, 1989.
4. Anderson, S. D., Schoeffel, R. E., and Finney, M. Evaluation of ultrasonically nebulised solutions for provocation testing in patients with asthma. *Thorax* 38:284, 1983.
5. Anderson, S. D., Silverman, M., and Walker, S. R. Metabolic and ventilatory changes in asthmatic patients during and after exercise. *Thorax* 27:718, 1972.
6. Anderson, S. D., et al. Exercise-induced asthma. *Br. J. Dis. Chest* 69:1, 1975.
7. Anderson, S. D., et al. Inhaled and oral salbutamol in exercise-induced asthma. *Am. Rev. Respir. Dis.* 114:493, 1976.
8. Anderson, S. D., et al. Prevention of severe exercise-induced asthma with hot air. *Lancet* 2:629, 1979.
9. Anderson, S. D., et al. Arterial plasma histamine levels at rest, and during and after exercise in patients with asthma: effects of terbutaline aerosol. *Thorax* 36:259, 1981.
10. Anderson, S. D., et al. Sensitivity to heat and water loss at rest and during exercise in asthmatic patients. *Eur. J. Respir. Dis.* 63:459, 1982.
11. Baile, E. M., et al. Role of tracheal and bronchial circulation in respiratory heat exchange. *J. Appl. Physiol.* 58:217, 1985.
12. Barnes, P. J., and Brown, M. J. Venous plasma histamine in exercise- and hyperventilation-induced asthma in man. *Clin. Sci.* 61:159, 1981.
13. Barnes, P. J., Wilson, N. M., and Brown, M. J. A calcium antagonist, nifedipine, modifies exercise induced asthma. *Thorax* 36:726, 1981.
14. Barnes, P. J., et al. Circulating catecholamines in exercise and hyperventilation induced asthma. *Thorax* 36:435, 1981.
15. Bar-Or, O., Neuman, I., and Dotan, R. Effects of dry and humid climates on exercise-induced asthma in children and adolescents. *J. Allergy Clin. Immunol.* 60:163, 1977.
16. Bhar-Yishay, E., Ben-Dov, I., and Godfrey, S. Refractory period following hyperventilation-induced asthma. *Am. Rev. Respir. Dis.* 127:572, 1983.

17. Bar-Yishay, E., et al. Difference between swimming and running as stimuli for exercise-induced asthma. *Eur. J. Appl. Physiol.* 48:387, 1982.

18. Belcher, N. G., et al. A comparison of the refractory periods induced by hypertonic airway challenge and exercise in bronchial asthma. *Am. Rev. Respir. Dis.* 135:822, 1987.

19. Benatar, S. R., and Konig, P. Maximal expiratory flow and lung volume changes associated with exercise induced asthma in children and the effect of breathing a low-density gas mixture. *Clin. Sci.* 46:317, 1974.

20. Ben-Dov, I., Bar-Yishay, E., and Godfrey, S. Exercise induced asthma without respiratory heat loss. *Thorax* 37:630, 1982.

21. Ben-Dov, I., Bar-Yishay, E., and Godfrey, S. Heterogeneity in the response of asthmatic patients to preexercise treatment with cromolyn sodium. *Am. Rev. Respir. Dis.* 127:113, 1983.

22. Ben-Dov, I., Bar-Yishay, E., and Godfrey, S. Refractory period following exercise induced asthma unexplained by respiratory heat loss. *Am. Rev. Respir. Dis.* 125:530, 1982.

23. Ben-Dov, I., Bar-Yishay, E., and Godfrey, S. Relation between efficacy of sodium cromoglycate and baseline lung function in exercise and hyperventilation induced asthma. *Israel J. Med. Sci.* 20:130, 1984.

24. Ben-Dov, I., et al. Refractory period following induced asthma: comparative contribution of exercise and isocapnic hyperventilation. *Thorax* 38:849, 1983.

25. Bierman, C. W., et al. Acute and chronic theophylline therapy in exercise-induced bronchospasm. *Pediatrics* 60:845, 1977.

26. Blackie, S. P., et al. The time course of bronchoconstriction in asthmatics during and after isocapnic hyperventilation. *Am. Rev. Respir. Dis.* 142:1133, 1990.

27. Boulet, L.-P., et al. Prevalence and characteristics of late asthmatic responses to exercise. *J. Allergy Clin. Immunol.* 80:655, 1987.

28. Boushey, H. A., et al. Bronchial hyperactivity. *Am. Rev. Respir. Dis.* 121:389, 1980.

29. Burr, M. L., Eldridge, B. A., and Borysiewicz, L. K. Peak expiratory flow rates before and after exercise in school children. *Arch. Dis. Child.* 49:923, 1974.

30. Chan Yeung, M. M. W., Vyas, M. N., and Grzybowski, S. Exercise induced asthma. *Am. Rev. Respir. Dis.* 104:915, 1971.

31. Chatham, M., et al. A comparison of histamine, methacholine and exercise airway reactivity in normal and asthmatic subjects. *Am. Rev. Respir. Dis.* 126:235, 1982.

32. Chen, W. Y., and Horton, D. J. Heat and water loss from the airways and exercise-induced asthma. *Respiration* 34:305, 1977.

33. Chung, K. F., et al. Histamine dose-response relationship in normal and asthmatic subjects—the importance of starting airway caliber. *Am. Rev. Respir. Dis.* 126:849, 1982.

34. Cockcroft, D. W., et al. Allergen induced increase in nonallergic bronchial reactivity. *Clin. Allergy* 7:503, 1977.

35. Davies, S. E. The effect of disodium cromoglycate on exercise-induced asthma. *Br. Med. J.* 3:593, 1968.

36. Deal, E. C., et al. Airway responsiveness to cold air and hyperpnea in normal subjects and in those with hay fever and asthma. *Am. Rev. Respir. Dis.* 121:621, 1980.

37. Deal, E. C., et al. Effects of atropine on potentiation of exercise-induced bronchospasm by cold air. *J. Appl. Physiol.* 45:238, 1978.

38. Deal, E. C., et al. Esophageal temperature during exercise in asthmatic and nonasthmatic subjects. *J. Appl. Physiol.* 46:484, 1979.

39. Deal, E. C., et al. Hyperpnea and heat flux: initial reaction sequence in exercise-induced asthma. *J. Appl. Physiol.* 46:476, 1979.

40. Deal, E. C., et al. Role of respiratory heat exchange in production of exercise-induced asthma. *J. Appl. Physiol.* 46:467, 1979.

41. Deal, E. C., et al. Evaluation of role played by mediators of immediate hypersensitivity in exercise-induced asthma. *J. Clin. Invest.* 65:659, 1980.

42. Edmunds, A. T., Tooley, M., and Godfrey, S. The refractory period after exercise induced asthma, its duration and relation to severity of exercise. *Am. Rev. Respir. Dis.* 117:247, 1978.

43. Eggleston, P. A., and Guerrant, J. L. A standardized method of evaluating exercise-induced asthma. *J. Allergy Clin. Immunol.* 58:414, 1976.

44. Empey, D. W., et al. Mechanisms of bronchial hyperreactivity in normal subjects after upper respiratory tract infection. *Am. Rev. Respir. Dis.* 113:131, 1976.

45. Enright, P. L., McNally, J. F., and Souhrada, J. F. Effect of lidocaine on the ventilatory and airway responses to exercise in asthmatics. *Am. Rev. Respir. Dis.* 122:823, 1980.

46. Fanta, C. H., McFadden, E. R., and Ingram, R. H. Effects of cromolyn sodium on the response to respiratory heat loss in normal subjects. *Am. Rev. Respir. Dis.* 123:161, 1981.

47. Finnery, J. P., Wilmot, C., and Holgate, S. T. Inhibition of hypertonic saline-induced bronchoconstriction by terfenadine and flurbiprofen. *Am. Rev. Respir. Dis.* 140:593, 1989.

48. Finney, M. J. B., Anderson, S. D., and Black, J. L. Terfenadine modifies airway narrowing induced by the inhalation of nonisotonic aerosols in subjects with asthma. *Am. Rev. Respir. Dis.* 141:1151, 1990.

49. Fitch, K. D., and Morton, A. R. Specificity of exercise-induced asthma. *Br. Med. J.* 4:577, 1971.

50. Floyer, J. *A Treatise of the Asthma.* London: R. Wilkins & W. Innis, 1698.

51. Francis, P. W. J., Krastins, J. R. B., and Levison, H. Oral and inhaled salbutamol in the prevention of exercise induced bronchospasm. *Pediatrics* 66:103, 1980.

52. Freedman, S., Tattersfield, A. E., and Pride, N. B. Changes in lung mechanics during asthma induced by exercise. *J. Appl. Physiol.* 38:974, 1975.

53. Freedman, S., et al. Abolition of methacholine induced bronchoconstriction by the hyperventilation of exercise or volition. *Thorax* 43:631, 1988.

54. Galdes-Sebaldt, M., McLaughlin, F. J., and Levison, H. Comparison of cold air, ultrasonic mist, and methacholine inhalations as tests of bronchial reactivity in normal and asthmatic children. *J. Pediatr.* 107:526, 1985.

55. Gilbert, I. A., Fouke, J. M., and McFadden, E. R. Heat and water flux in the intrathoracic airways and exercise-induced asthma. *J. Appl. Physiol.* 63:1681, 1987.

56. Gilbert, I. A., Fouke, J. M., and McFadden, E. R. Intra-airway thermodynamics during exercise and hyperventilation in asthmatics. *J. Appl. Physiol.* 64:2167, 1988.

57. Godfrey, S. Exercise-induced Asthma. In T. J. H. Clark and S. Godfrey (eds.), *Asthma.* London: Chapman & Hall, 1983.

58. Godfrey, S., and Konig, P. Inhibition of exercise induced asthma by different pharmacological pathways. *Thorax* 31:137, 1976.

59. Godfrey, S., Silverman, M., and Anderson, S. D. Problems of interpreting exercise induced asthma. *J. Allergy Clin. Immunol.* 52:199, 1973.

60. Haynes, R. L., Ingram, R. H., and McFadden, E. R. An assessment of the pulmonary response to exercise in asthma and an analysis of the factors influencing it. *Am. Rev. Respir. Dis.* 114:739, 1976.

61. Henriksen, J. M. Effect of inhalation of corticosteroids on exercise induced asthma: randomised double blind crossover study of budesonide in asthmatic children. *Br. Med. J.* 291:248, 1985.

62. Herxheimer, H. Hyperventilation asthma. *Lancet* 1:83, 1946.

63. Ingenito, E., et al. Dissociation of temperature-gradient and evaporative heat loss during cold gas hyperventilation in cold-induced asthma. *Am. Rev. Respir. Dis.* 138:540, 1988.

64. Inman, M. D., et al. Methacholine airway responsiveness decreases during exercise in asthmatic subjects. *Am. Rev. Respir. Dis.* 141:1414, 1990.

65. Jaffe, P., et al. Relationship between plasma cortisol and peak expiratory flow rate in exercise induced asthma and the effect of sodium cromoglycate. *Clin. Sci.* 45:533, 1973.

66. Jones, R. H. T., and Jones, R. S. Ventilation capacity in young adults with a history of asthma in childhood. *Br. Med. J.* 2:976, 1966.

67. Jones, R. S. Assessment of respiratory function in the asthmatic child. *Br. Med. J.* 2:972, 1966.

68. Jones, R. S., Buston, M. H., and Wharton, M. J. The effect of exercise on ventilatory function in the child with asthma. *Br. J. Dis. Chest* 56:78, 1962.

69. Jones, R. S., Wharton, M. J., and Buston, M. H. The place of physical exercise and bronchodilator drugs in the assessment of the asthmatic child. *Arch. Dis. Child.* 38:539, 1963.

70. Kattan, M., et al. The response to exercise in normal and asthmatic children. *J. Pediatr.* 92:718, 1978.

71. Kawabori, I., et al. Incidence of exercise-induced asthma in children. *J. Allergy Clin. Immunol.* 58:447, 1976.

72. Kennedy, J. D., et al. Comparison of action of disodium cromoglycate and ketotifen on exercise-induced bronchoconstriction in childhood asthma. *Br. Med. J.* 281:1458, 1980.

73. Konig, P., and Godfrey, S. The prevalence of exercise induced bronchial lability in families of children with asthma. *Arch. Dis. Child.* 48:513, 1973.

74. Konig, P., and Godfrey, S. Exercise-induced bronchial lability and atopic status of families of infants with wheezy bronchitis. *Arch. Dis. Child.* 48:942, 1973.

75. Konig, P., Godfrey, S., and Abrahamov, A. Exercise induced bronchial lability in children with a history of wheezy bronchitis. *Arch. Dis. Child.* 47:578, 1972.

76. Larsson, K., Hjemdahl, P., and Martinsson, A. Sympathoadrenal reactivity in exercise-induced asthma. *Chest* 82:560, 1982.

77. Lee, T. H., et al. Exercise-induced release of histamine and neutrophil chemotactic factor in atopic asthmatics. *J. Allergy Clin. Immunol.* 70:73, 1982.

78. Lee, T. H., et al. Identification and partial characterization of an exercise-induced neutrophil chemotactic factor in bronchial asthma. *J. Clin. Invest.* 69:889, 1982.

79. Levison, H., and Godfrey, S. Pulmonary Aspects of Cystic Fibrosis. In J. A. Mangos and K. C. Talamo (eds.), *Cystic Fibrosis—A Projection into the Future.* New York: Stratton Intercontinental Medical Book Corp., 1976.

80. Manning, P. J., Lane, C. G., and O'Byrne, P. M. The effect of oral prostaglandin E_1 on airway responsiveness in asthmatic subjects. *Pulmon. Pharmacol.* 2:121, 1989.

81. Mansfield, L., et al. Airway response in asthmatic children during and after exercise. *Respiration* 38:135, 1979.

82. Margolski, D. J., Bigby, B. G., and Boushey, H. A. Indomethacin blocks airway tolerance to repetitive exercise but not to eucapnic hyperpnea in asthmatic subjects. *Am. Rev. Respir. Dis.* 137:842, 1988.

83. Mattoli, S., et al. The effect of indomethacin on the refractory period occurring after the inhalation of ultrasonically nebulised distilled water. *J. Allergy Clin. Immunol.* 79:678, 1987.

84. McFadden, E. R. Exercise and asthma. *N. Engl. J. Med.* 317:502, 1987.

85. McFadden, E. R., Lenner, K. A. M., and Strohl, K. P. Postexertional airway rewarming and thermally induced asthma. New insights into pathophysiology and possible pathogenesis. *J. Clin. Invest.* 78:18, 1986.

86. McFadden, E. R., et al. Predominant site of flow limitation and mechanisms of postexertional asthma. *J. Appl. Physiol.* 42:746, 1977.

87. McFadden, E. R., et al. Direct recordings of the temperatures in the tracheobronchial tree in normal man. *J. Clin. Invest.* 62:700, 1982.

88. McFadden, E. R., et al. Thermal mapping of the airways in humans. *J. Appl. Physiol.* 58:564, 1985.

89. McNeill, R. S., et al. Exercise induced asthma. *Q. J. Med.* 35:55, 1966.

90. Mellis, C. M., et al. Comparative study of histamine and exercise challenges in asthmatic children. *Am. Rev. Respir. Dis.* 117:911, 1978.

91. Mussaffi, H., Springer, C., and Godfrey, S. Increased bronchial responsiveness to exercise and histamine after allergen challenge in asthmatic children. *J. Allergy Clin. Immunol.* 77:48, 1986.

92. Noviski, N., et al. Exercise intensity determines and climatic conditions modify the severity of exercise induced asthma. *Am. Rev. Respir. Dis.* 136:592, 1987.

93. O'Byrne, P. M., and Jones, G. M. The effect of indomethacin on exercise-induced bronchoconstriction and refractoriness after exercise. *Am. Rev. Respir. Dis.* 134:69, 1986.

94. O'Byrne, P. M., et al. Asthma induced by cold air and its relation to nonspecific bronchial responsiveness to methacholine. *Am. Rev. Respir. Dis.* 125:281, 1982.

95. O'Cain, C. F., et al. Airway effects of respiratory heat loss in normal subjects. *J. Appl. Physiol.* 49:875, 1980.

96. Patel, K. R. The effect of calcium antagonist nifedipine in exercise-induced asthma. *Clin. Allergy* 11:429, 1981.

97. Patel, K. R., et al. Plasma concentrations of sodium cromoglycate given by nebulisation and metered dose inhalers in patients with exercise induced asthma: relationship to protective effect. *Br. J. Pharmacol.* 22:231, 1986.

98. Platts-Mills, T. A. E., et al. Reduction of bronchial hyperreactivity during prolonged allergen avoidance. *Lancet* 2:675, 1982.

99. Pollock, J., et al. Relationship of serum theophylline concentration to inhibition of exercise-induced bronchospasm and comparison with cromolyn. *Pediatrics* 60:840, 1977.

100. Reiff, D. B., et al. The effect of prolonged submaximal warm-up exercise on exercise-induced asthma. *Am. Rev. Respir. Dis.* 139:479, 1989.

101. Rosenthal, R. R., et al. Analysis of refractory period after exercise and eucapnic voluntary hyperventilation challenge. *Am. Rev. Respir. Dis.* 141:368, 1990.

102. Rubinstein, I., et al. Dichotomous airway response to exercise in asthmatic patients. *Am. Rev. Respir. Dis.* 138:1164, 1988.

103. Rubinstein, I., et al. Immediate and delayed bronchoconstriction after exercise in patients with asthma. *N. Engl. J. Med.* 317:482, 1987.

104. Saunders, D. B., and Rudolf, M. The interpretation of different measurements of airways obstruction in the presence of lung volume changes in bronchial asthma. *Clin. Sci.* 54:313, 1978.

105. Schnall, R. P., and Landau, L. I. The protective effects of short sprints in exercise induced asthma. *Thorax* 35:828, 1980.

106. Schoeffel, R. E., Anderson, S. D., and Altounyan, R. E. Bronchial hyperreactivity in response to inhalation of ultrasonically nebulised solutions of distilled water and saline. *Br. Med. J.* 283:1285, 1981.

107. Seaton, A., et al. Exercise-induced asthma. *Br. Med. J.* 3:556, 1969.

108. Silverman, M., and Anderson, S. D. Standardization of exercise tests in asthmatic children. *Arch. Dis. Child.* 47:882, 1972.

109. Silverman, M., Anderson, S. D., and Walker, S. R. Metabolic changes preceding exercise-induced bronchoconstriction. *Br. Med. J.* 1:207, 1972.

110. Silverman, M., and Andrea, T. Time course of effect of disodium cromoglycate on exercise-induced asthma. *Arch. Dis. Child.* 47:419, 1972.

111. Silverman, M., Konig, P., and Godfrey, S. Use of serial exercise tests to assess the efficacy and duration of action of drugs for asthma. *Thorax* 28:574, 1973.

112. Smith, C. M., et al. Investigation of the effects of heat and water exchange in the recovery period after exercise in children with asthma. *Am. Rev. Respir. Dis.* 140:598, 1989.

113. Stearns, D. R., et al. Reanalysis of the refractory period in exertional asthma. *J. Appl. Physiol.* 50:503, 1981.

114. Stirling, D. R., et al. Characteristics of airway tone during exercise in patients with asthma. *J. Appl. Physiol.* 54:934, 1983.

115. Strauss, R. H., et al. Enhancement of exercise-induced asthma by cold air. *N. Engl. J. Med.* 297:743, 1977.

116. Tanser, A. R., and Elmes, J. A. controlled trial of ketotifen in exercise-induced asthma. *Br. J. Dis. Chest* 74:398, 1980.

117. Tinkelman, D. G., Cauanagh, M. J., and Cooper, D. M. Inhibition of exercise-induced bronchospasm by atropine. *Am. Rev. Respir. Dis.* 114:87, 1976.

118. Wagner, E. M., et al. Peripheral lung resistance in normal and asthmatic subjects. *Am. Rev. Respir. Dis.* 141:584, 1990.

119. Weiler-Ravell, D., and Godfrey, S. Do exercise and antigen induced asthma utilize the same pathways? Antigen provocation in patients rendered refractory to exercise induced asthma. *J. Allergy Clin. Immunol.* 67:391, 1981.

120. Weinstein, R. E., et al. Effects of humidification of exercise-induced asthma (EIA). *J. Allergy Clin. Immunol.* 57:250, 1976.

121. Weiss, S. T., et al. Airway responsiveness in a population sample of adults and children. *Am. Rev. Respir. Dis.* 129:898, 1984.

122. Wiebicke, W., et al. Effect of terfenadine on the response to exercise and cold air in asthma. *Pediatr. Pulmonol.* 4:225, 1988.

123. Wilson, B. A., Bar-Or, O., and Seed, L. G. Effects of humid air breathing during arm or treadmill exercise on exercise-induced bronchoconstriction and refractoriness. *Am. Rev. Respir. Dis.* 142:349, 1990.

124. Wilson, N. M., et al. Hyperventilation-induced asthma: evidence for two mechanisms. *Thorax* 37:657, 1982.

125. Zawadski, D. K., Lenner, K. A., and McFadden, E. R. Re-examination of the late asthmatic response to exercise. *Am. Rev. Respir. Dis.* 137:837, 1988.

126. Backer, V., et al. The distribution of bronchial responsiveness to histamine and exercise in 527 children and adolescents. *J. Allergy Clin. Immunol.* 88:68, 1991.

127. Bianco, S., et al. Prevention of exercise-induced bronchoconstriction by inhaled frusemide. *Lancet* 2:252, 1988.

128. Crimi, E., et al. Airway inflammation and occurrence of delayed bronchoconstriction in exercise-induced asthma. *Am. Rev. Respir. Dis.* 146:507, 1992.

129. Finnerty, J. P., et al. Role of leukotrienes in exercise-induced asthma. Inhibitory effect of ICI 204219, a potent leukotriene D_4-receptor antagonist. *Am. Rev. Respir. Dis.* 145:746, 1992.

130. Henriksen, J. M., Agertoft, L., and Pedersen, S. Protective effect and duration of action of inhaled formoterol and salbutamol on exercise-induced asthma in children. *J. Allergy Clin. Immunol.* 89:1176, 1992.

131. Israel, E., et al. The effects of a 5-lipoxygenase inhibitor on asthma induced by cold, dry air. *N. Engl. J. Med.* 323:1740, 1990.

132. Manning, P. J., et al. Inhibition of exercise-induced bronchoconstriction by MK-571, a potent leukotriene D_4-receptor antagonist. *N. Engl. J. Med.* 323:1736, 1990.

133. Moscato, G., et al. Inhaled furosemide prevents both the bronchoconstriction and the increase in neutrophil chemotactic activity induced by ultrasonic "fog" of distilled water in asthmatics. *Amer. Rev. Respir. Dis.* 143:561, 1991.

134. Ray, D. W., et al. Tachykinins mediate bronchoconstriction elicited by isocapnic hyperpnea in guinea pigs. *J. Appl. Physiol.* 66:1108, 1989.

135. Vathenen, A. S., et al. Effect of inhaled budesonide on bronchial reactivity to histamine, exercise, and eucapnic dry air hyperventilation in patients with asthma. *Thorax* 46:811, 1991.

136. Venge, P., Henriksen, J., and Dahl, R. Eosinophils in exercise-induced asthma. *J. Allergy Clin. Immunol.* 88:699, 1991.

Drug-Induced Asthma

Loren W. Hunt, Jr.
Edward C. Rosenow III

48

A physician caring for patients with asthma may occasionally see those who fail to respond to acceptable therapy, or those whose condition paradoxically becomes worse without an apparent stimulus for increased bronchospasm such as a viral infection or an allergic or irritant exposure. In these instances, the phenomenon of drug-induced asthma should be considered. Although the vast majority of the causes of drug-induced asthma stem from an idiosyncratic pharmacologic reaction to a compound, there are numerous agents that cause asthma via an immunologic or immunoglobulin E (IgE)–related mechanism or via a direct, non-IgE-related release of mediators from mast cells, or by inducing an irritant effect. Table 48-1 lists numerous proposed pathogenetic mechanisms of these reactions and examples thought to be representative of each. Pharmacologic agents can also induce or exacerbate asthma by way of airborne exposure during their manufacture, and a growing list of such agents has been implicated. The numerous agents that have been shown or suspected to cause or aggravate asthma are listed in Table 48-2. This list will undoubtedly grow as additional causes are identified.

ASTHMA CAUSED BY NONSTEROIDAL ANTIINFLAMMATORY AGENTS

Nonsteroidal antiinflammatory agents (NSAIAs) account for a disproportionate 21 percent of all reported adverse drug reactions and make up 5 percent of all reactions associated with outpatient prescriptions [50]. In addition, NSAIAs are by far the most common cause of drug-induced asthma. In a detailed study of 781 asthmatic patients observed over a 2-year period, Iamandescu [75] observed drugs to be a cause of asthma attacks in 10.5 percent of the patients. Of these drug-induced asthmatic reactions, the vast majority, or 64 (77%), were caused by NSAIAs. Aspirin was implicated most commonly among the nonsteroidals, accounting for 42 (51%) of the cases. Aspirin intolerance among asthmatics is usually reported as 4 to 20 percent, depending on whether the diagnosis is based on history alone or on the results of aspirin challenge [141]. In one of the earliest series, reported in 1928, van Leeuwen [177] challenged 100 asthmatic patients with aspirin and this provoked pulmonary reactions in 16. Other authors have reported similar percentages of asthmatics who were unable to tolerate aspirin due to bronchoconstriction [41, 156].

Immediate reactions to the NSAIAs appear to be of two types: (1) urticaria and angioedema, and (2) rhinoconjunctivitis with bronchospasm [154]. The reactions in the former category appear to be either related to aspirin or to a specific NSAIA and may, at least in some cases, be IgE mediated. The reactions in the latter category appear to be distinct in the population of patients affected, the reaction characteristics, and the proposed

mechanism of occurrence [150]. The name *aspirin-induced asthma* has been applied to this distinct-reaction type.

In the majority of patients with aspirin-induced asthma, the first symptoms appear in the third or fourth decade of life and consist of a prominent and intense vasomotor rhinitis with the subsequent development of nasal polyposis. Over 90 percent of the patients have associated sinusitis, with opacification of one or more paranasal sinuses seen on x-ray studies [148]. Familial association is quite rare; Szczeklik [162] identified a familial association in only 2 of 500 aspirin-sensitive asthmatics. Men and women are both affected, and HLA typing reveals no differences in either the frequency of Class I HLA-A, B, or C antigens or of HLA-DR antigens [79]. Mullarkey and associates [114] identified a significant increase in the level of HLA-DQw2 in a group of aspirin-sensitive asthmatics when compared to normals, but the importance of this finding remains unknown. The asthma and aspirin sensitivity usually develop subsequent to the rhinitis, with the asthma running a chronic and protracted course. The asthma is considered by many investigators to be a particularly severe variety; patients have a frequent requirement for corticosteroids and frequent exacerbations during upper respiratory infections [98, 152]. Aspirin-sensitive asthma is not associated with atopy, and skin tests with common aeroallergens are almost always negative [168]. Serum IgE levels are usually normal, and attempts to identify specific anti-aspirin IgE antibodies in association with the asthmatic reactions have failed [150]. Aspirin has no effect on serum IgE levels or peripheral blood eosinophil counts [183]. When acetylsalicylic acid (ASA) challenge causes acute bronchospasm, no acute elevations in the plasma histamine levels, neutrophil chemotactic activity, or complement activity occur relative to baseline levels [146].

Upon ingestion of aspirin, patients with aspirin-induced asthma develop within 1 hour a reaction consisting of wheezing, and flushing of the head and neck, and often have associated rhinorrhea and conjunctival irritation. These reactions may be quite severe, and nausea and vomiting, facial angioedema, and death can occur [171]. The reactions are not prevented by pretreatment with antihistamines, theophylline, or cromolyn sodium [167]. Corticosteroids do not prevent the bronchospasm caused by aspirin challenge [128], but have recently been shown by Nizankowska and colleagues [118] to attenuate the reaction when given preventively for 10 days. Aspirin challenge does not increase methacholine sensitivity [60]. In a review of 92 asthmatic patients who sustained attacks severe enough to warrant intubation and mechanical ventilation, Picado and coworkers [125] found aspirin intolerance to be the precipitating factor in 8 percent. In two of these patients, the life-threatening attack was the first recognized manifestation of aspirin intolerance that the patient had experienced. When oral challenges with aspirin are performed in asthmatics who report a prior reaction to aspirin ingestion, the sensitivity can be confirmed in up to 97 percent

Table 48-1. Pathogenetic mechanisms and clinical patterns of drug-induced asthma

Clinical pattern	IgE	Other antibody	Cyclooxygenase inhibition	Mast cell degranulation	Direct airway irritation	Pharmacologic effect	Noncardiogenic pulmonary edema	Unknown
Immediate	Bromelin Pancreatic extract Papain Penicillin Psyllium Tetracycline?		Aspirin Diclofenac Indomethacin Naprosyn	Steroidal anesthetic Morphine sulfate? Indomethacin? Codeine? Platinum salts Ethylenediamine	Acetate Metabisulfite Marijuana	Beta blockers	Dyazide	Sulfinpyrazone Tartrazine
Delayed		Aldomet? Pancreatic extract Penicillin					Iodides? Imferon	Monosodium glutamate
Prolonged		Carbamazepine				Propranolol Bethanechol		
Anaphylaxis/ anaphylactoid	Cephalosporins						Bleomycin	Podophyllotoxins Zinostatin

[41]. Serial oral challenges performed at the Scripps Clinic showed that an occasional patient can apparently lose aspirin sensitivity over a time frame of 2 or more years [128]. Avoidance of aspirin does not affect the course of the underlying asthma or the number of exacerbations.

There are over 200 drugs that contain aspirin, many of which are over-the-counter preparations. All aspirin-sensitive patients must be made aware of the possible presence of aspirin in medications that they purchase.

The cross-reactivity of aspirin sensitivity and sensitivity to another nonsteroidal antiinflammatory agent, indomethacin, was first reported by Vanselow and Smith [178] in 1967. Reactivity to other NSAIAs was reported the following year by Sampter and Beers [138], who concluded that the pulmonary reaction is probably not immunologic on the basis of prominent structural differences between these compounds. What these compounds had in common was subsequently reported to be the ability to inhibit cyclooxygenase, a key enzyme in arachidonic acid biotransformation [166, 176]. Szczeklik and coworkers, in addition, showed that the potency of these agents in causing bronchospasm is related to their potency as cyclooxygenase inhibitors [166], and that the degree of cross-reactivity to aspirin correlates with the dose of the drug required to inhibit cyclooxygenase in vitro [167]. Drugs that are not cyclooxygenase inhibitors can safely be ingested by these patients, even those that are structurally similar to aspirin, such as salicylamide or sodium salicylate [36]. Table 48-3 includes a list of common antiinflammatory agents that are thought to be safe for use in asthmatics in usual doses.

On rare occasions, however, even some of these "safe" compounds, such as acetaminophen or dextropropoxyphene, have been shown to exacerbate asthma in aspirin-sensitive patients, and tartrazine, sulfinpyrazone, and hydrocortisone have also been reported to cause bronchospasm in rare aspirin-sensitive patients. The mechanism of action of these agents may be weak cyclooxygenase inhibition or an as yet unknown mechanism. It has been found that, if patients who have had reactions to aspirin are challenged with acetaminophen at a dose of 1,000 mg, 28 percent will develop a 20 percent or greater decline in the 1-second forced expiratory volume (FEV_1) [41], but lower doses usually do not produce reactions, as evidenced by Spector and coworkers' [148] study, which showed only 5 percent reacting to a 600-mg dose, and shown by Szczeklik and Gryglewski [165], who were unable to produce a reaction in 11 patients challenged with up to 300 mg of acetaminophen. In challenges performed at the Scripps Clinic, reactivity to a 1,000-mg dose was confirmed in three patients and, in addition, the reactivity failed to recur following aspirin desensitization, suggesting that the mechanism of bronchospasm produced by acetaminophen might stem from

cyclooxygenase inhibition [154]. Stevenson and associates [150, 160] were not able to demonstrate cross-sensitivity between dextropropoxyphene or sodium salicylate, but did observe mild and delayed asthmatic reactions with a challenge dose of 2,000 mg of salsalate.

The cross-reactivity of aspirin with tartrazine (FD & C Yellow No. 5) has not been confirmed in controlled double-blind oral challenge testing [70, 181, 186], despite earlier reports suggesting a prevalence of 8 to 50 percent in aspirin-sensitive asthmatics [142, 148, 149]. Virchow and colleagues [182] studied 156 patients who had confirmed aspirin-induced asthma and found that only four (2.6%) reacted to tartrazine in doses up to 25 mg in a double-blind challenge. Stevenson and associates [159] similarly challenged 150 patients with known ASA sensitivity with 25- and 50-mg doses of tartrazine and found a decline in the FEV_1 values (between 20 and 30%) in only six (4%); however, on subsequent double-blind challenge in five, they could not confirm the sensitivity at the same dose. These studies suggest that tartrazine intolerance is quite rare and probably does not occur on the basis of cross-reactivity with ASA sensitivity.

Hydrocortisone has been reported to occasionally provoke severe bronchoconstriction in patients with aspirin-induced asthma. In 1978, Partridge and Gibson [122] reported on two patients with aspirin-sensitive asthma who experienced severe wheezing upon receiving intravenous hydrocortisone. One patient experienced an apparent anaphylactic reaction and the other developed rapidly increasing bronchospasm necessitating intubation. Hayhurst [72] and Chapman [28] and their colleagues also reported on patients with asthma who sustained severe increased bronchospasm after receiving hydrocortisone intravenously. These authors were able to produce positive immediate skin tests to hydrocortisone in two of the three patients reported. Dajani and associates [37] challenged 11 aspirin-sensitive asthmatics with 100 mg of intravenous hydrocortisone in a single-blind placebo-controlled fashion. They observed chest tightness and wheezing in three patients, and this reaction was reproducible in two of the patients who were later retested in a similar fashion. Skin testing to hydrocortisone showed no reactions in these patients, and the intravenous injection of dexamethasone likewise produced no reaction. Szczeklik and coworkers [170] challenged 32 aspirin-sensitive asthmatics and produced declines in FEV_1 greater than 20 percent in four patients with doses ranging from 50 to 300 mg. These reactions were most prominent at 5 to 15 minutes and cleared spontaneously in 1 hour. There was no response to intravenously administered methylprednisolone, dexamethasone, or betamethasone. The mechanism of these reactions is currently unknown, and these authors caution against the intravenous use of hydrocortisone in the treatment

Table 48-2. Drugs causing or exacerbating asthma

NONSTEROIDAL ANTIINFLAMMATORY AGENTS [154]
Carboxylic acids
  Salicylates
    Acetylsalicylic acid (Aspirin, Easpirin, Zorprin)
  Acetic acid
    Indomethacin (Indocin)
    Indomethacin ophthalmic solution
    Sulindac (Clinoril)
    Tolmetin (Tolectin)
    Zomepirac (Zomax)
    Diclofenac (Voltaren) [167]
    Ketorolac (Toradol) [181]
  Proprionic acids
    Ibuprofen (Motrin, Rufen)
    Naproxen (Naprosyn)
    Naproxen sodium (Anaprox)
    Fenoprofen (Nalfon)
  Fenamates
    Meclofenamate (Meclomen)
    Mefenamic acid (Ponstel)
Enolic acids
  Piroxicam (Feldene)

PYRAZOLONE DRUGS (SULFINPYRAZONE) [164]

ANTIBIOTICS
Nitrofurantoin [134]
Penicillins
Cephalosporins
Tetracycline
Pentamidine aerosol [173]

BETA-ADRENERGIC BLOCKING AGENTS
Systemic
  Antihypertensive therapy
Topical
  Optical treatment for glaucoma
  Transdermal therapy for hypertension
Implicated drugs

Antihypertensive	*Ophthalmic*
Propranolol	Timolol
Nadolol	Betaxolol
Timolol	
Metoprolol	
Atenolol	
Pindolol	
Acebutolol	
Propafenone	

CHOLINERGIC AGONISTS
Methacholine
Carbachol (ophthalmic solution)
Bethanechol (urinary retention) [89]
Echothiophate iodide [59]

CHOLINOMIMETIC ALKALOIDS
Pilocarpine
Muscarine

CORTICOSTEROIDS
IV hydrocortisone
Injectable Kenalog [74]
Inhaled bechlamethasone

DIURETICS
Triamterene/hydrochlorothiazide [55]

MISCELLANEOUS
Imferon [55]
Ipecacuanha [55]
Monosodium glutamate (a drug or food additive) [3]
Pituitary snuff [99]

AGENTS ENCOUNTERED IN PHARMACEUTICAL MANUFACTURING
Antibiotics
  Penicillins
  Cephalosporins
  Spiramycin
  Isoniazid
  Tetracycline [52]
Laxatives
  Psyllium
Opiates
Antihypertensive medications
  Methyl dopa [70]
Cimetidine
Pepsin
Vitamin preparations
  Rose hips
Penicillamine
Enzymes
  Cellulase
  Papain
  Trypsin
  Pepsin
  Diastase [61]
  Pancreatic extract [137]
Phenylglycine acid chloride (added as a side-chain in antibiotic
  synthesis) [82]
Salbutamol intermediate [51]

AGENTS ENCOUNTERED THROUGH OCCUPATIONAL EXPOSURE IN THE
  HOSPITAL OR LABORATORY WORKPLACE
Antibiotics through mixing
Methacholine used during diagnostic testing
Mixing of laxatives
Antibiotics used in laboratory animal feed
Penicillamine
Methyl methacrylate and cyanoacrylate cements
Hexachlorophene (sterilizing agent) [115]

PROPELLANTS OR ADDITIVES TO INHALANT MEDICATIONS
Paradoxical bronchospasm with metered-dose inhalers of beta
  agonists

METABISULFITES USED IN MEDICATIONS AS PRESERVATIVES [153]

AGENTS INDUCING BRONCHOSPASM VIA NON-IgE-RELATED MAST CELL
  DEGRANULATION
Opiates [27]
Radiographic contrast media [20]
Polymyxin
Colistin

MUSCLE RELAXANTS [109]
Suxamethonium
d-Tubocurarine
Alcuronium
Pancuronium
Gallamine

ANESTHETIC AGENTS [29]

AGENTS AGGRAVATING BRONCHOSPASM VIA LOCAL IRRITANT EFFECTS
N-acetylcysteine
Sodium cromoglycate [129]
Aerosolized corticosteroids

DRUG REACTIONS THAT MIMIC ASTHMA
Cough from angiotensin-converting enzyme–inhibiting drugs [64]

DRUGS CAUSING OR EXACERBATING GASTROESOPHOGEAL REFLUX
Theophylline

CHEMOTHERAPEUTIC AGENTS
Bleomycin [187]
Podophyllotoxins [187]
Zinostatin [187]
Methotrexate [80]

Table 48-3. Antiinflammatory drugs that may be safely used by most asthmatics

Sodium salicylate	Chloroquine
Choline salicylate	Paracetamol
Salicylamide	
Dextropropoxyphene	

of acute exacerbations of asthma in aspirin-sensitive asthmatics. We have recently observed a patient who sustained an anaphylactic reaction to injectable Kenalog (triamcinolone acetonide) who, upon skin testing to the components of Kenalog, was found to be allergic to carboxymethylcellulose [74]. It is therefore important, when such reactions to steroid products occur, to fully investigate the reaction with component testing.

The ability to desensitize an aspirin-sensitive asthmatic to aspirin is also an interesting phenomenon. Widal and colleagues [188] in 1922 first reported the ability to block the bronchoconstricting response to aspirin. Stevenson has shown that, with the ingestion of graded doses of aspirin, patients with aspirin sensitivity will lose their ability to respond to aspirin with bronchoconstriction within 24 to 48 hours and will maintain this level of desensitization as long as aspirin is ingested indefinitely in doses of 325 to 650 mg daily. Prolonged desensitization to aspirin may lead to a diminished severity of both the nasal symptoms and the asthma [155, 158]. The degree of aspirin responsiveness in these patients does not correlate with the degree of histamine sensitivity, and neither the histamine [7] nor the methacholine [155] responsiveness change following desensitization. Patients desensitized to aspirin will also maintain desensitization to other cyclooxygenase-inhibiting drugs. If these patients discontinue their maintenance dose of aspirin, they will regain their sensitization within 2 to 7 days [127].

Cyclooxygenase normally converts arachidonic acid into prostaglandins, thromboxane, and prostacyclin. Arachidonic acid is cleaved from membrane phospholipids by phospholipase A_2. A significant shift occurs upon the administration of aspirin, with a shifting of approximately 90 percent of the arachidonic acid metabolism from the cyclooxygenase pathway and prostaglandin (PG) and thromboxane A_2 production to the 5-lipoxygenase pathway and increased leukotriene (LT) production [145]. The 5-lipoxygenase synthesizes LTA_4 from arachidonic acid, which is then metabolized to LTB_4 or LTC_4. LTC_4 is then cleaved to form LTD_4 and LTE_4. LTC_4, LTD_4, and LTE_4 comprise the sulfidopeptide leukotrienes and are potent contractors of bronchial smooth muscle [44]. This shift in the metabolic pathway of arachidonic acid metabolism could result in the loss of bronchoprotective activities afforded by PGE_2, with resultant increased bronchoconstriction, or the shift toward increased production of the leukotrienes could also result in airway obstruction [151, 192]. Both mechanisms may be involved. While these mechanisms have been postulated to explain the phenomenon of aspirin-induced asthma, they do not explain why all patients with asthma do not react in a similar fashion to aspirin ingestion or even why all individuals in general are not aspirin-sensitive with regard to their airways. One must postulate the existence of other factors that might render the aspirin-sensitive asthmatic particularly susceptible to this peculiar type of reaction. These include an increased PGE-dependent bronchodilatory tone, an increased production of the leukotrienes, or an increased sensitivity to the leukotrienes with regard to airway responsiveness.

Arm and associates [7] have recently shown by inhalation challenge that patients with aspirin-sensitive asthma have as much as a 13-fold increased sensitivity to LTE_4 as compared with other asthmatics. Moreover, this increased sensitivity to LTE_4 was not correlated with histamine bronchoprovocation testing, and, after the aspirin-sensitive patients were desensitized to aspirin, their increased sensitivity to LTE_4 was no longer expressed. When nasal washings are examined in aspirin-sensitive patients after aspirin challenge, the levels of histamine and LTC_4 are higher than those seen in non-aspirin-sensitive patients [54]. PGE_2 levels, interestingly, are not lowered [54]. The recent development of various 5-lipoxygenase inhibitors has made possible the ability to further examine the role of leukotrienes and leukotriene sensitivity. A recent trial with a specific leukotriene inhibitor, however, did not attenuate the aspirin-induced asthmatic reaction [118].

Platelets have also been implicated as possible effector cells in asthma and in aspirin-induced asthma [108]. When platelets from aspirin-sensitive asthmatics are incubated with aspirin, there is an increased release of cytotoxic compounds [25]. While this is similar to the release of mediators by platelets when exposed to relevant allergen challenge, a major difference is that only platelet activation induced by aspirin can be inhibited by lipoxygenase inhibitors [140], and that from allergen can be inhibited by anti-FcεRII antibodies [81]. This implies that the platelet activation occurs via a cyclooxygenase inhibiting mechanism in the aspirin-sensitive asthmatics.

In a further characterization of these effects, Ameisen and colleagues [4] have recently demonstrated that peripheral blood platelets from aspirin-sensitive asthmatics respond differently upon exposure to NSAIAs than do platelets recovered from non-aspirin-sensitive asthmatics or from normal controls. The platelets from the aspirin-sensitive patients responded with marked activation, as expressed by high cytotoxic properties, prominent chemiluminescense, and increased cytocidal activity against *Schistosoma mansoni* larvae. These changes were not seen in the platelets from normal controls or those from allergic asthmatics [4]. In the absence of cyclooxygenase-inhibiting drugs, the platelets from aspirin-sensitive asthmatics reacted in a similar fashion to those from controls. The desensitization of four patients to aspirin resulted in failure of their platelets to respond to aspirin activation. These authors were also able to show that the incubation of blood monocytes or basophils failed to produce any detectable increased reactivity. Compounds that are structurally similar to aspirin, such as sodium salicylate or salicylamide, did not produce any platelet activation with this model; in fact, the preincubation of platelets with sodium salicylate successfully prevented platelet activation upon subsequent exposure to aspirin or indomethacin.

This latter observation may be a key indicator of the possible mechanism of aspirin desensitization. Additional studies by these authors using the sera from aspirin-desensitized subjects showed that this sera and sera from controls ingesting aspirin or sodium salicylate daily could block the platelet reactivity of aspirin-sensitive asthmatics to aspirin in vitro [5]. Because the sera from controls ingesting indomethacin do not show this ability to block the platelet response of these patients, and because salicylate, an aspirin metabolite, prevents cyclooxygenase inhibition by aspirin [40], Ameisen and colleagues [5] have suggested that the daily ingestion of ASA may produce enough of the metabolite to act as an inhibitor in preventing this unique reaction.

While these observations are intriguing, a recent report showed no changes in the plasma levels of beta-thromboglobulin, a specific indicator of platelet activation, following inhaled challenges with aspirin-lysine conjugate. Moreover, differences in the platelet chemiluminescense of peripheral blood platelets from aspirin-sensitive patients were not demonstrated [189].

While aspirin does not appear to have a direct effect on the histamine release from peripheral blood basophils [157], Okuda and associates [120] have recently shown that basophils from patients with aspirin-sensitive asthma produce more histamine in response to platelet-activating factor than do those of normals or of patients with asthma who are not aspirin sensitive. Basophilic-rich leukocyte suspensions from aspirin-sensitive patients have also been found to undergo a greater degree of suppression by aspirin of PGE_2 generation compared to the production of LTD_4 generation following anti-IgE challenge. This altered response was thought to be secondary to both a greater inhibition of PGE_2 generation and lack of inhibition of LTD_4 generation [66].

In a recent review, Szczeklik [163] has proposed the hypothesis that aspirin-sensitive asthmatics develop virus-specific cytotoxic T-lymphocytes in response to a chronic viral infection, and these lymphocytes are suppressed by PGE_2 produced by alveolar macrophages. PGE_2 might cause suppression through direct inhibition of the cytotoxic activity of lymphocytes, and this suppression is less effective in interleukin-2–activated lymphocytes. Aspirin ingestion in these patients would thus block PGE_2 production in macrophages and allow unimpeded activation of cytotoxic lymphocytes. While little data support this interesting concept, investigational tools are currently available to test it.

Further investigations involving the mechanism of aspirin-induced asthma will be of great interest, particularly those involving the activation of various effector cells in these patients and those involving specific leukotriene inhibitors. The desensitization of these patients to aspirin, while feasible and effective, is a tool to be used only by physicians and study centers experienced in the methodology, and facilities must be available to monitor these patients closely for emergencies. The practicing physician should caution aspirin-sensitive asthmatics against taking all prescribed and over-the-counter aspirin-containing products and related NSAIAs, as these agents can provoke sudden and severe bronchospasm.

ASTHMA CAUSED BY BETA-ADRENERGIC BLOCKING AGENTS

Beta-blocking agents have become widely used to treat hypertension, angina pectoris, paroxysmal tachycardias, glaucoma, tremor, and, more recently, as prophylaxis for migraine headaches. The more common agents currently used are listed in Table 48-4. The medical histories on asthmatic patients must be taken quite carefully by the physician because many patients may not volunteer the information that they use eyedrops as treatment for glaucoma or use the recently introduced transdermal mepindolol and propranolol patches for the management of hypertensive and cardiac disease [42]. Anecdotally, many allergists and pulmonologists have witnessed an occasional hospitalized patient who responds poorly to treatment for status asthmaticus because he or she continues to receive beta-blocking eyedrops brought into the hospital by the family. Because many of the above-listed indications for beta-blocker usage are for conditions that can occur in younger age groups, it is equally important to remember that concentrations of beta-blocking medications in human breast milk can vary from 3 to 22 percent of the maternal dose for such agents as acebutolol, atenolol, nadolol, or sotalol [11]. These are important considerations for mothers nursing asthmatic infants, particularly since the clearance of these agents is slower in infants less than 6 months of age [12].

Bronchospasm induced by beta-blocking agents can occur after the immediate initiation of these medications or after long-term use lasting several months or years. In some cases, the

Table 48-4. Beta-adrenergic blocking agents

Propranolol	Mepindolol
Nadolol	Acebutolol
Timolol	Sotalol
Metoprolol	Propafenone
Atenolol	Betaxolol
Pindolol	Labetalol

administration of beta blockers has resulted in exacerbations of asthma that have persisted for long periods after withdrawal of the drug [6]. Occasional severe reactions causing death are reported, and, because most of these deaths have occurred in patients with a preexisting history of obstructive airway disease, they are therefore preventable and of major concern [32]. It is of equal concern that the degree of bronchospasm induced in asthmatics or patients with chronic obstructive pulmonary disease is unpredictable on the basis of the severity of their obstruction or chronicity of their disease, or of the sensitivity of the airways to histamine. It is also uncertain which asthmatics will develop severe airway obstruction, even in response to the more cardioselective agents [136, 147].

While the heart contains primarily $beta_1$ receptors and the lung contains primarily $beta_2$ receptors, the beta receptors of each tissue are predominantly, but not exclusively, either one or the other, with as many as 30 percent of the adrenergic receptors in the bronchi of the $beta_1$ type. There are, thus, no true "cardioselective" agents [48, 105]. In addition, the population of beta adrenergic receptors is not static and varies physiologically with age, hormonal concentration, and dietary sodium intake [131]. Various types of disease processes, such as psychiatric, cardiac, or hematologic conditions, can also alter the number of receptors [112]. The administration of beta-receptor antagonists produces upregulation of beta adrenergic receptors [1] and the administration of beta agonists produces downregulation [63].

The dose of the beta-blocking agent also affects the cardioselectivity of the agent, with increasing doses of a cardioselective agent producing by competitive antagonism an increase in the blockade of $beta_2$ receptors [95]. Lennard and associates [93] have also shown that there are different rates of metabolism of various drugs and that the prevalence of individuals who are "poor metabolizers" in populations is often about 10 percent. Hence, the plasma concentrations of beta-blocking agents in poor or slow metabolizers will be significantly increased. Dayer and colleagues [39] showed differences in $beta_1$ blockade between poor and normal metabolizers who were given metoprolol, and Riddell and coworkers [133] demonstrated a decrease in cardioselectivity with metoprolol in the poor metabolizers given the same dosage of beta blocker as the normal metabolizers. Cardioselectivity, thus, is not only difficult to predict based on the specific beta-blocking agent given, but can vary according to the dosage given and the drug-metabolizing characteristics of the particular patient. The response of an asthmatic to a beta blocker can therefore be quite variable and unpredictable, even with the more cardioselective agents.

Ophthalmic beta blockers (eyedrops) are commonly used in the treatment of glaucoma, and impart their effect through lowering intraocular pressure by reducing aqueous secretion [84]. Beta blockers administered as eyedrops pass rapidly into the bloodstream and reach the heart and lungs without being metabolized by the liver. The effect on peripheral organs is determined by the quantity of the beta blocker reaching these organs, the state of the target organ, the type of beta blocker, its fat solubility, and the plasma metabolism [31]. In the airways of susceptible patients, symptoms may occur within a few minutes and attain a maximal response within several hours following administration of the nonselective beta-antagonist timolol.

There are mixed reports as to whether betaxolol, another beta-blocking ophthalmic solution used in the treatment of glaucoma, can induce airway disease. While the original reports [23, 46] stated that there were no adverse effects from betaxolol, two recent reports documented aggravation of obstructive lung disease, especially in asthmatics [71, 186]. Brooks and associates [23] performed a double-blind study in 5 of 29 patients who complained of wheezing or respiratory distress but showed no change in their respiratory function with either betaxolol or placebo. Dunn and colleagues [46] studied 24 asthmatic patients in whom they tested the effects of both timolol and betaxolol. With timolol, the FEV_1 fell a mean of 28 percent. Eight of these patients were then studied with betaxolol and showed no fall in FEV_1. On the other hand, Weinreb and colleagues [186] studied 101 glaucoma patients with obstructive lung disease and found nine patients who developed symptoms and a decline in lung function attributed to betaxolol. Harris and coworkers [71] also found five patients who experienced a worsening in their pulmonary function after starting betaxolol therapy. Further studies should be helpful in clarifying this issue.

The mechanism of beta-blockade–induced bronchoconstriction is not currently resolved. The function of $beta_2$ receptors in the normal lung is uncertain: Stimulation of beta receptors does not result in increased airflow in the normal lung and beta blockade does not usually reduce airflow. Adrenergic stimulation, however, does reduce smooth muscle constriction in an already constricted smooth muscle, thus increasing airflow. Bronchoconstriction can frequently be produced in the asthmatic by allergic or nonspecific stimuli on the basis of bronchial hyperreactivity, and increased sympathetic stimulation may be needed as a protective mechanism. As recently reviewed by Barnes [14], the smooth muscle of human airways lacks sympathetic innervation, and it is likely that the beta receptors there are regulated by endogenous catecholamines. Blockade of the effects of endogenous catecholamines in this system can precipitate or worsen bronchospasm [130].

Animal studies have shown that beta blockers can potentiate the bronchoconstrictive response to both histamine [43] and antigen [126] challenge and these effects are similar to those produced by adrenalectomy; this, again, supports the involvement of endogenous catecholamines [30]. The plasma catecholamine levels, however, are not higher in stable asthmatics than in normals, and no relationship has been found between the plasma catecholamine concentration and the severity of the obstruction to airflow [15]. There may be evidence, however, that the regulation of epinephrine secretion during bronchospasm is abnormal. The rise in the circulating catecholamine levels in normal subjects following exercise is not seen in asthmatics who develop bronchoconstriction secondary to exercise [16]. In addition, various stimuli, such as methacholine challenge [139], antigen challenge [90], propranolol infusion [76], and isocapnic hyperventilation [16], all fail to produce a rise in the circulating catecholamine levels. Ind and coworkers [77], who similarly measured the circulating catecholamine levels in patients admitted to the hospital for the treatment of severe asthma, could not demonstrate an elevation in the plasma epinephrine concentration. Why patients with asthma appear to have poor regulation of their catecholamine response to bronchoconstriction will be an interesting direction for future research.

Beta-adrenergic blockade could thus aggravate this already blunted catecholamine response and increase the degree of bronchoconstriction present. Moreover, beta-adrenergic blockade can prevent the response to exogenous beta agonists given to control bronchospasm. This does not explain, however, the fact that occasional patients without asthma may develop bronchospasm [57], or the observation by Northcote and Ballantyne [119] of progressive loss of lung function over the course of a year in a group of patients without asthma. McNeil and Ingram [103] have also shown that propranolol can occasionally increase airway resistance even in the nonasthmatic patient.

Whether beta blockers can augment a severe Type I allergic response or increase the likelihood of its occurrence is also of particular concern, since many of these reactions can be pulmonary alone or of the systemic anaphylactic form. Numerous reports have described particularly severe forms of anaphylaxis in patients taking beta blockers [58, 68, 78, 116], and the risk may be increased in atopic patients in general and not just isolated to patients with asthma [172]. The release of mediators of immediate hypersensitivity is modulated by neurohumoral mechanisms [92], and beta-adrenergic blockade can augment the release of potent inflammatory mediators from mast cells and leukocytes that can mediate anaphylaxis, vascular permeability, and bronchospasm [10, 106].

ASTHMA INDUCED BY ANTIBIOTICS THROUGH ORAL OR PARENTERAL USE OR BY OCCUPATIONAL EXPOSURE

Several antibiotics, such as the penicillins, cephalosporins, and sulfonamides, have often produced chest and throat tightness, wheezing, or stridor as a result of a systemic allergic reaction (see Table 48-2). Antibiotics such as nitrofurantoin can also cause cough, dyspnea, fever, wheezing, chest x-ray infiltrates, and peripheral blood eosinophilia [134]. While implicating these antibiotics as the cause of these reactions is usually rather straightforward, the ability to detect these agents as a cause of asthma is much more difficult if the patient is developing asthma to them as a result of occupational exposure. Amoxicillin, ampicillin, and penicillin have all been reported to cause asthma through exposure during their manufacture [38, 61, 132]. Atopic patients may be more at risk for such sensitization, and these reactions are thought to be the result of IgE-mediated mechanisms [61]. Coutts and coworkers [34] have also reported the development of asthma from occupational exposure to cephalosporin antibiotics. More rarely, tetracycline has occasionally caused wheezing following oral ingestion or exposure as an aeroallergen during manufacture [104].

Spiramycin, a macrolide antibiotic used by veterinarians as well as being a component of animal feeds, has also caused occupational asthma in as many as 8 percent of the workers who are regularly exposed to it [100]. Although skin testing to spiramycin has yielded equivocal results, both Malo and Cartier [100] and Paggiaro and associates [121] have been able to demonstrate reactions to spiramycin inhalation challenge.

Other pharmacologic agents reported as causing asthma by airborne occupational exposure are isonicotinic acid hydrazide [9], rose hips in the manufacture of over-the-counter vitamin C preparations [87], morphine dust [2], cimetidine, sulfathiazole, sulfonechloramides, amprolium hydrochloride, piperazine [24], and penicillamine [88]. Another reported unusual occupational exposure resulting in asthma has been noted in medical personnel exposed to such agents as methyl methacrylate bone cement [97]. Psyllium, a high-molecular-weight gum widely used as a laxative, can cause occupational asthma through its manufacture and packaging, as well as in hospital and nursing home personnel who are exposed to it while mixing and dispensing it [101].

ASTHMA CAUSED BY EXPOSURE TO ENZYMES

Several enzyme preparations have been reported to cause asthma upon frequent inhalation exposure. Family members of patients with cystic fibrosis have developed asthma as a result of exposure to pancreatic extracts during preparation for use [175]. Other enzymes such as trypsin [190], alpha-amylase [56], papain [19], pepsin [26], and, more recently, cellulase [83] have all caused occupational asthma as the result of airborne exposure during their manufacture. Most affected patients who have been tested either by skin testing or by bronchoprovocation challenge to the enzymes have been positive, suggesting an IgE-mediated cause for the reaction.

ASTHMA AGGRAVATED BY IRRITANT EXPOSURE

One of the hallmarks of the asthmatic response is bronchial hyperreactivity, which is not usually seen in normal individuals. Sodium cromolyn, which is usually well tolerated, has caused harsh coughing and at times wheezing upon inhalation, and this reaction is thought to be mediated by an irritant mechanism [129]. Although Paterson and associates [123] found that skin prick testing of a patient with a bronchospastic reaction documented by inhaled bronchoprovocation challenge was negative, Wass and coworkers [184] recently reported a patient with a prominent reaction, which included wheezing, after using sodium cromolyn and were able to demonstrate a positive skin test response to the drug, in addition to serum-specific IgE antibodies. There are several reported cases of asthma that was paradoxically made worse upon inhalation of a metered-dose of a beta agonist, at times severe enough to cause respiratory arrest. Because many such patients have used beta agonists safely in the past and continue to do so, it is uncertain whether these patients are reacting to a contaminant or whether they might be developing sensitivity to one of the vehicles used as a propellant, the concentration of which might vary [117]. In Nicklas's [117] report of 126 cases, 25 patients developed paradoxical bronchospasm when switching to a new cannister or bottle, suggesting a problem with either an individual metered-dose inhaler or possibly an individual batch of inhalers. There were occasional patients, however, who developed reactions to inhalers that they had formerly used safely. Nebulized isoprenaline has been observed to cause a rebound bronchospasm in some patients. Paterson and coworkers [124] theorized that one of the explanations for this phenomenon is that a metabolite of the drug may be a weak beta blocker. Bisulfites and metabisulfites can also provoke bronchospasm in asthmatics, presumably through release of sulfur dioxide which is then inhaled [153].

COUGH DUE TO ANGIOTENSIN-CONVERTING ENZYME INHIBITORS

It has recently been observed that the angiotensin-converting enzyme (ACE)–inhibiting drugs used for the treatment of hypertension can be associated with the development of harsh coughing, which is often confused with asthma [191]. Reduction of pulmonary airflow is usually not observed in these patients, and the results of methacholine challenges have been negative in most series [22, 174]. Kaufman and associates [85], however, found evidence of bronchial hyperreactivity in eight of nine patients with cough while taking ACE inhibitors as opposed to none of eight patients without cough. It was uncertain if any of these patients had preexistent bronchial hyperresponsiveness, and six of the hyperresponsive patients maintained their bronchial hyperresponsiveness when retested 8 to 24 weeks after cessation of the drug. Hinojosa and coworkers [73] also reported on two patients who developed bronchial hyperresponsiveness simultaneously with cough associated with captopril treatment; the bronchial hyperresponsiveness was not present prior to the symptoms of cough and cleared within 4 weeks following cessation of therapy.

A recent prospective study in a population of hypertensive patients placed on captopril has shown that as many as 30 percent of patients may develop a cough [21], although incidences of 2 to 4 percent are more commonly reported. The cough has been reported as being dry and hacking, often disabling, at times worse at night, and responding poorly to antitussives, bronchodilators, and topical corticosteroids.

Among the ACE inhibitors, the prevalence of cough may be higher with lisinopril and enlapril and less with captopril [33]. The development of cough in association with ACE-inhibiting agents does not appear to have a dose-related effect [33]. Gibson [64] has summarized the results of 209 patients taking enlapril and found that the cough was twice as common among women as among men, and that 10 percent of the patients placed on enlapril had to discontinue its use due to uncontrollable cough. He also found that, in the group of patients who did not discontinue the medication, there was about an equal percentage who continued to cough but to a less severe degree (G. R. Gibson, personal communication, 1991).

The interval from the start of therapy with ACE inhibitors and the onset of cough is variable, and the cough can develop from 1 week to 12 months following the start of therapy and usually clears within 1 to 4 weeks following cessation [94, 161]. The mechanism of the ACE-inhibitor–induced cough remains unclear at the present time. ACE is active in the degradation of substance P and bradykinin, the former a potent neuropeptide which may be involved in lung inflammation [107] and the latter a potent irritant which might result in bronchial irritation [94]. Failure to degrade these potent molecules in the lung could theoretically result in a chronic irritant effect that produces the harsh cough.

In summary, the ACE inhibitors, while exerting a beneficial effect on blood pressure control and cardiac symptoms, can be associated with a bothersome cough in a significant percentage of patients. The mechanism of this cough is currently unclear. Most patients with cough do not have increased bronchial hyperresponsiveness, although bronchial hyperreactivity has been documented in some. Asthmatics do not appear to be at increased risk for the development of cough, and current literature suggests that these agents do not aggravate preexisting asthma and need not be avoided in patients with asthma.

DRUGS CAUSING DIRECT RELEASE OF MAST CELL MEDIATORS

Several drugs are able to cause severe systemic reactions, often associated with wheezing on the basis of a direct, non-IgE-mediated release of mast cell mediators. Iodinated contrast media, polymyxin, various muscle relaxants, morphine, codeine, and pentamidine have all been observed to cause such reactions.

Radiographic contrast media is one of the most common causes of systemic anaphylactic reactions, most of which have associated symptoms of chest tightness and bronchospasm. Although it is not clear if asthmatic patients are at increased risk, patients with a strong history of allergy are about twice as likely to experience a systemic reaction as those without one [144]. It has not been possible to demonstrate an IgE-mediated mechanism behind these reactions, hence the designation of *anaphylactoid reaction*, meaning mast cell degranulation not mediated by the membrane triggering of receptor-bound IgE. Triiodinated contrast agents with a high osmolarity may be much more likely to induce mast cell degranulation than the newer normosmolar agents [13, 20]. Patients who have experienced previous systemic reactions to contrast media agents may have their risk of another reaction reduced significantly if they are pretreated with prednisone, Benadryl (diphenhydramine hydrochloride), and ephedrine [67], or have the procedure performed using a newer normosmolar agent [13].

Recently, several patients have been reported who developed severe bronchospasm following inhalation of cocaine. It is currently unknown whether cocaine-induced asthma is IgE mediated or whether cocaine can similarly cause the direct release of mast cell mediators [135].

Since 1952, anesthetic agents have been known to cause sys-

Table 48-5. Agents used in anesthesia

Anesthetic agents	Muscle relaxants
Propanidid	Succinylcholine
Thiopental	Alcuronium
Propofol	Pancuronium
Etomidate	*d*-Tubocurarine
Methohexital	

temic hypersensitivity reactions, usually including bronchospasm [49] (Table 48-5). The main features of these reactions are hypotension, tachycardia, bronchospasm, laryngeal and facial edema, cyanosis, and gastrointestinal symptoms [17]. Immediate bronchospasm occurs in more than half of the reactions, and delayed reactions after methohexital use have also been seen to occur between 10 and 90 minutes after drug administration [17, 29].

The frequency of reactions depends on the agent given, with reaction rates ranging between 1 of 400 to 1 of 7,000 for alphaxalone, propanidid, and methohexital, and perhaps the frequency is less with thiopental [18, 45, 86, 143]. Previous exposure may be a risk factor for alphaxalone [65], particularly within the first month after use [53].

Prospective studies of the ability of these agents to cause increased plasma histamine release have shown that histamine release commonly occurs following rapid intravenous injection, particularly with thiopental and methohexitol [96]. Similar results can be seen following use of the muscle relaxants [110] (see Table 48-5). Opiate analgesics [109] may cause bronchoconstriction also via an anaphylactoid mechanism.

CHOLINERGIC AGONISTS

Individuals with asthma who work in pulmonary function laboratories can have prominent reactions to inhaled methacholine that is released into the air when patients are undergoing methacholine challenge [62]. Likewise bethanechol, used to treat hypotonic bladder, has also caused dyspnea and wheezing in some patients [89]. Carbachol, an agent used in the treatment of glaucoma, has also caused bronchospasm in rare patients, and echothiophate, a topical anticholinesterase also used for the treatment of glaucoma, has caused severe wheezing [59].

In summary, this chapter illustrates the tremendous spectrum of drugs that can produce airway disease in the individual patient. Many of these medications are over-the-counter nonprescription drugs and therefore patients do not consider them drugs and in turn do not tell the physician that they are using them unless specifically asked. In an asthmatic patient who does not seem to be getting better, it is important for the patient or a family member to bring *all* medications for the clinician to review, including eyedrops, vitamins, cold preparations, and so on. In most situations, just stopping these medications is sufficient for reversing the airway problem or at least bringing about sufficient improvement. In the future, we can anticipate the development of newer medications for the treatment of many different diseases, some of which may have a secondary adverse effect on the airways. The physician must also remember that occasional agents used in the treatment of asthma might themselves cause asthma. Recently, methotrexate has been used successfully to reduce corticosteroid requirements in occasional patients with severe asthma and has gained popularity in the treatment of very severe recalcitrant asthma [113]. Jones and coworkers [80], however, recently reported a patient who developed drug-induced asthma from methotrexate prescribed to treat rheumatoid

arthritis at a dose comparable to that used in the treatment of asthma. Similarly, ethylenediamine, a component of aminophylline, can exacerbate asthma when given intravenously [111]. Finally, the physician must always be vigilant concerning the various pharmacologic agents, which, during their manufacture or distribution, can produce asthma through aerosolized exposure in the workplace.

REFERENCES

1. Aarons, R. D., et al. Elevation of B-adrenergic receptor density in human lymphocytes after propranolol administration. *J. Clin. Invest.* 65:949, 1980.
2. Agius, R. Opiate inhalation and occupational asthma. *Br. Med. J.* 298:323, 1989.
3. Allen, N. D., and Baker, G. J. Chinese restaurant asthma. *N. Engl. J. Med.* 305:1154, 1981.
4. Ameisen, J. C., et al. Aspirin-sensitive asthma: abnormal platelet response to drugs inducing asthma attacks, diagnostic and physiopathological implications. *Int. Arch. Allergy Appl. Immunol.* 78:281, 1985.
5. Ameisen, J. C., et al. Aspirin-sensitive asthma: serum from aspirin desensitized patients inhibits the abnormal platelet response to NSAIDs. *J. Allergy Clin. Immunol.* 77S:182, 1986.
6. Anderson, E. G., et al. Persistent asthma after treatment with beta-blocking drugs. *Br. J. Dis. Chest* 73:407, 1979.
7. Arm, J. P., et al. Airway responsiveness to histamine and leukotriene E4 in subjects with aspirin-induced asthma. *Am. Rev. Respir. Dis.* 140:148, 1989.
8. Asad, S. I., et al. Clinical and biochemical aspects of "aspirin-sensitivity." *NER Allergy Proc.* 7(2):105, 1986.
9. Asai, S., et al. Occupational asthma caused by isonicotinic acid hydrazide (INH) inhalation. *J. Allergy Clin. Immunol.* 80:578, 1987.
10. Assem, E. S. K. Adrenergic mechanisms and immediate-type allergy. *Clin. Allergy* 4:185, 1974.
11. Atkinson, H., and Begg, E. J. Concentrations of beta-blocking drugs in human milk. *J. Pediatr.* 116:156, 1990.
12. Atkinson, H. C., Begg, E. J., and Darlow, B. A. Drugs in human milk: clinical pharmacokinetic considerations. *Clin. Pharmacokinet.* 14:217, 1988.
13. Bagg, M. N. J., Horwitz, T. A., and Bester, L. Comparison of patient responses to high- and low-osmolality contrast agents injected intravenously. *Am. J. Radiol.* 147:185, 1986.
14. Barnes, P. J. Endogenous catecholamines and asthma. *J. Allergy Clin. Immunol.* 77:791, 1986.
15. Barnes, P. J., Ind, P. W., and Brown, J. J. Plasma histamine and catecholamines in stable asthmatic subjects. *Clin. Sci.* 62:661, 1982.
16. Barnes, P. J., et al. Circulating catecholamines in exercise- and hyperventilation-induced asthma. *Thorax* 36:435, 1981.
17. Beamish, D., and Brown, D. T. Delayed adverse responses to i.v. anaesthetics. *Br. J. Anaesth.* 35:279, 1980.
18. Beamish, D., and Brown, D. T. Adverse responses to i.v. anaesthetics. *Br. J. Anaesth.* 53:55, 1981.
19. Beecher, W. Hyperesthetic rhinitis and asthma due to digestive ferments. *IJF* 59:343, 1951.
20. Bettman, M. A. Radiographic contrast agents—a perspective. *N. Engl. J. Med.* 317:891, 1987.
21. Blackie, S. P., et al. Captopril-associated cough is not due to an increase in airways hyperresponsiveness. *Am. Rev. Respir. Dis.* 141(2):A734, 1990.
22. Boulet, L. P., et al. Pulmonary function and airway responsiveness during long term therapy with Captopril. *JAMA* 261:413, 1989.
23. Brooks, A. M., Burden, J. G., and Gillies, W. E. The significance of reactions to betaxolol reported by patients. *Aust. NZ J. Ophthalmol.* 17:353, 1989.
24. Butcher, B. T. Pulmonary reactions to inhaled low-molecular weight chemicals. *Eur. J. Respir. Dis.* 63(S123):13, 1982.
25. Capron, A., et al. New functions for platelets and their pathological implications. *Int. Arch. Allergy Appl. Immunol.* 27:107, 1985.
26. Cartier, A., et al. Occupational asthma due to pepsin. *J. Allergy Clin. Immunol.* 73:574, 1984.
27. Casale, T. B., Bowman, S., and Kaliner, B. A. Mast cell degranulation by opioids. *J. Allergy Clin. Immunol.* 59:420, 1977.
28. Chapman, S. C., Loughnan, B. A., and Somerfield, S. D. Immediate hypersensitivity skin testing in a case of hydrocortisone anaphylaxis: case report. *N. Zealand Med. J.* 90:380, 1979.

29. Clarke, R. S. J., et al. Adverse reactions to intravenous anaesthetics: a survey of 100 reports. *Br. J. Anaesth.* 47:575, 1975.
30. Collier, J. O. J., and James, G. W. O. Humoral factors affecting pulmonary inflation during acute anaphylaxis in the guinea pig in vivo. *Br. J. Pharmacol.* 30:283, 1967.
31. Collignon, P. Cardiovascular and pulmonary effects of beta-blocking agents: implications for their use in ophthalmology. *Surv. Ophthalmol.* 33(suppl):455, 1989.
32. Committee on Safety of Medicines. Fatal bronchospasm associated with beta-blockers. *Curr. Probl.* No. 20, 1987.
33. Coulter, D. M., and Edwards, I. R. Cough associated with captopril and enlapril. *Br. Med. J.* 294:1521, 1987.
34. Coutts, I. I., et al. Asthma in workers manufacturing cephalosporins. *Br. Med. J.* 283:950, 1981.
35. Coutts, I. I., et al. Respiratory symptoms related to work in a factory manufacturing cimetidine tablets. *Br. Med. J.* 288:1418, 1984.
36. Dahl, R. Sodium salicylate and aspirin disease. *J. Allergy* 35:155, 1980.
37. Dajani, B. M., et al. Bronchospasm caused by intravenous hydrocortisone sodium succinate (Solu-Cortef) in aspirin-sensitive asthmatics. *J. Allergy Clin. Immunol.* 68:201, 1981.
38. Davies, R. J., Hendrick, D. J., and Pepys, J. Asthma due to inhaled chemical agents: ampicillin, benzyl penicillin, 6 amino penicillanic acid and related substances. *Clin. Allergy* 30:277, 1974.
39. Dayer, P., et al. Interindividual variation of beta-adrenoceptor blocking drugs, plasma concentration and effect: influence of genetic status on behaviour of atenolol, bopindolol and metoprolol. *Eur. J. Clin. Pharmacol.* 28:149, 1985.
40. Dejana, E., Cerletti, C., and deGaetano, G. Interaction of salicylate and other non-steroidal anti-inflammatory drugs with aspirin on platelet and vascular cyclo-oxygenase activity. *Thromb. Res.* 4(suppl):153, 1983.
41. Delaney, J. C. The diagnosis of aspirin idiosyncrasy by analgesic challenge. *Clin. Allergy* 6:177, 1976.
42. de Mey, C., et al. Transdermal delivery of mepindolol and propranolol in normal man. *Arzneimittelforschung/Drug Res.* 39:1505, 1989.
43. Drazen, J. M. Adrenergic influences on histamine-mediated bronchoconstriction in the guinea pig. *J. Appl. Physiol.* 44:340, 1978.
44. Drazen, J. M., et al. Comparative airway and vascular activities of leukotrienes C-1 and D in vivo and in vitro. *Proc. Natl. Acad. Sci. USA* 77:4354, 1980.
45. Driggs, R. L., and O'Day, R. A. Acute allergic reaction associated with methohexital anesthesia: report of six cases. *J. Oral Surg.* 30:906, 1972.
46. Dunn, T. D. L., et al. The effect of topical ophthalmic instillation of timolol and betaxolol on lung function in asthmatic subjects. *Am. Rev. Respir. Dis.* 133:264, 1986.
47. Dwaselow, A., et al. Rose hips: a new occupational allergen. *J. Allergy Clin. Immunol.* 85:704, 1990.
48. Engel, G. Subclasses of beta-adrenoreceptors: a quantitative estimation of beta-1 and beta-2 adrenoreceptors in guinea pig and human lung. *Postgrad. Med. J.* 57(suppl 1):77, 1981.
49. Evans, F., and Gould, J. Relation between sensitivity to thiopentone, sulphonamides and sunlight. *Br. Med. J.* 1:417, 1952.
50. Faich, G. A. Adverse-drug-reaction monitoring. *N. Engl. J. Med.* 314:1589, 1986.
51. Fawcett, L. W., and Pepys, J. Asthma due to glycyl compound powder: an intermediate in production of salbutamol. *Clin. Allergy* 6:405, 1976.
52. Fawcett, L. W., and Pepys, J. Allergy to a tetracycline preparation. *Clin. Allergy* 6:301, 1976.
53. Fee, J. P. H., et al. Frequency of previous anaesthesia in an anaesthetic population. *Br. J. Anaesth.* 50:917, 1978.
54. Ferreri, N. R., et al. Release of leukotrienes, prostaglandins, and histamine into nasal secretions of aspirin-sensitive asthmatics during reaction to aspirin. *Am. Rev. Respir. Dis.* 137:847, 1988.
55. Fisher, K. H. Drug-induced Asthma Syndromes. In E. B. Weiss, M. S. Segal, and M. Stein (eds.), *Bronchial Asthma: Mechanisms and Therapeutics*, 2nd ed. Boston: Little, Brown, 1985, Pp. 512–521.
56. Flindt, M. L. H. Allergy to alpha-amylase and papain. *Lancet* 1:1407, 1979.
57. Fraley, D. S., et al. Propranolol-related bronchospasm in patients without history of asthma. *S. Med. J.* 73:238, 1980.
58. Frankish, C., McCourtie, D., and Toogood, J. H. Anaphylactic death in a patient on beta blockers. *Clin. Invest. Med.* 8:A42, 1985.
59. Fratto, C. Provocation of bronchospasm by eyedrops. *Ann. Intern. Med.* 88:362, 1978.
60. Frazer, J., et al. Aspirin and methacholine challenges in an ambulatory asthmatic population. *NER Allergy Proc.* 7:38, 1986.
61. Fueko, R. Allergy due to Pharmacologic Dusts. In C. A. Frazier (ed.), *Occupational Asthma*. New York: van Nostrand and Reinhold, 1980, Chap. 14.
62. Fuortes, L. Occupational asthma in a pulmonary functions laboratory (letter). *Ann. Intern. Med.* 111:952, 1989.
63. Galant, S. P., et al. Decreased beta-adrenergic receptors on polymorphonuclear leucocytes after adrenergic therapy. *N. Engl. J. Med.* 299:933, 1978.
64. Gibson, G. R. Enlapril-induced cough. *Arch. Intern. Med.* 149:2701, 1989.
65. Glen, J. B., et al. An animal model for the investigation of adverse responses to i.v. anaesthetic agents and their solvents. *Br. J. Anaesth.* 51: 819, 1979.
66. Goetzl, E. J., et al. Abnormal responses to aspirin of leukocyte oxygenation of arachidonic acid in adults with aspirin intolerance. *J. Allergy Clin. Immunol.* 77:693, 1986.
67. Greenberger, P. A., Patterson, R., and Radin, R. C. Two pretreatment regimens for high-risk patients receiving radiographic contrast media. *J. Allergy Clin. Immunol.* 74:540, 1984.
68. Hannaway, P. J., and Hopper, G. D. K. Severe anaphylaxis and drug-induced beta blockade. *N. Engl. J. Med.* 308:1536, 1983.
69. Harisparsad, D., et al. Oral tartrazine challenge in childhood asthma: effect on bronchial reactivity. *Clin. Allergy* 14:81, 1984.
70. Harries, M. G., et al. Bronchial asthma due to alpha-methyldopa. *Br. Med. J.* 1:1461, 1979.
71. Harris, L. S., Greenstein, S., and Bloom, A. F. Respiratory difficulties with betaxolol. *Am. J. Ophthalmol.* 102:274, 1986.
72. Hayhurst, M., Braude, A., and Benatar, S. R. Anaphylactic-like reaction to hydrocortisone. *S. Afr. Med. J.* 18:259, 1978.
73. Hinojosa, M., et al. Bronchial hyperreactivity and cough induced by angiotensin-converting enzyme-inhibitor therapy. *J. Allergy Clin. Immunol.* 85:818, 1990.
74. Hunt, L. W., and Dunn, W. F. Anaphylaxis following a Kenalog injection: hypersensitivity to carboxymethylcellulose. *J. Allergy Clin. Immunol.* 87(2):A551, 1991.
75. Iamandescu, I. B. NSAIDs-induced asthma: peculiarities related to background and association with other drug or non-drug etiological agents. *Allergol. Immunopathol.* 17(6):285, 1989.
76. Ind, P. W., et al. Propranolol-induced bronchoconstriction in asthma: beta-receptor blockade and mediator release. *Am. Rev. Respir. Dis.* 129: 10, 1984.
77. Ind, P. W., et al. Circulating catecholamines in acute asthma. *Br. Med. J.* 290:267, 1985.
78. Jacobs, R. L., et al. Potentiated anaphylaxis in patients with drug-induced beta-adrenergic blockade. *J. Allergy Clin. Immunol.* 68:125, 1981.
79. Jones, D. H., May, A. G., and Condemi, J. J. HLA-DR typing of aspirin-sensitive asthmatics. *Ann. Allergy* 52:87, 1984.
80. Jones, G., Egils, M., and Karsh, J. Methotrexate-induced asthma. *Am. Rev. Respir. Dis.* 143:179, 1991.
81. Joseph, M., et al. Participation of the IgE receptor in the toxicity of blood platelet against schistosomes. *C. R. Acad. Sci.* (Paris) 298:55, 1984.
82. Kammermeyer, J. K., and Mathews, K. P. Hypersensitivity to phenylglycine acid chloride. *J. Allergy Clin. Immunol.* 52:73, 1973.
83. Kanerva, L., and Tarvainen, K. Occupational skin and respiratory allergy from cellulase and xylanase enzymes. *J. Allergy Clin. Immunol.* 87(2): A246, 1991.
84. Kanski, J. J. Glaucoma. In *Clinical Ophthalmology* (2nd ed.). Stoneham, MA: Butterworth, 1989, P. 197.
85. Kaufman, J., et al. Bronchial hyperreactivity and cough due to angiotensin-converting enzyme inhibitors. *Chest* 95:544, 1989.
86. Kay, B. Brietal Sodium in Children's Surgery. In C. Lehmann (ed.), *Das Ultrakurznarkoticum Methohexital*. Berlin: Springer, 1972, Pp. 149.
87. Kwaselow, A., et al. Rose hips: a new occupational allergen. *J. Allergy Clin. Immunol.* 85:704, 1990.
88. Lagier, F., et al. Occupational asthma in a pharmaceutical worker exposed to penicillamine. *Thorax* 44:157, 1989.
89. Lamid, S., et al. Bethanechol (Urecholin) and bronchoconstriction. *Wis. Med. J.* 81:2, 1981.
90. Larsson, K., Gronneberg, R., and Jhemdahl, P. Bronchodilatation and inhibition of allergen-induced bronchoconstriction by circulating epinephrine in asthmatics subjects. *J. Allergy Clin. Immunol.* 75:586, 1985.
91. Lasser, E. C., et al. Histamine release by contrast media. *Radiology* 100: 683, 1971.
92. Lemanske, R. F., Casale, T. B., and Kaliner, M. The Autonomic Nervous System in Allergic Disease. In A. P. Kaplan (ed.), *Allergy*. New York: Churchill Livingstone, 1985, Pp. 199.

93. Lennard, M. S., et al. Oxidation phenotype: a major determinant of metoprolol metabolism and response. *N. Engl. J. Med.* 307:1558, 1982.

94. Lernhardt, E. B., and Ziegler, M. G. Cough caused by Cilazapril. *Am. J. Med. Sci.* 296:119, 1988.

95. Lertora, J. J. L., et al. Selective beta-1 receptor blockade with oral practolol in man. A dose-related phenomenon. *J. Clin. Invest.* 56:719, 1975.

96. Lorenz, W., and Doenicke, A. Anaphylactoid Reactions and Histamine Release by Intravenous Drugs Used in Surgery and Anaesthesia. In J. Watkins and A. M. Ward (eds.), *Adverse Response to Intravenous Drugs,* London: Academic Press; New York: Grune & Stratton, 1978, P. 83.

97. Lozewicz, S., et al. Occupational asthma due to methyl methacrylate and cyanoacrylates. *Thorax* 40:836, 1985.

98. Lumry, W. R., Curd, J. G., and Stevenson, D. D. Aspirin-sensitive asthma and rhinosinusitis: current concepts and recent advances. *Ear Nose Throat J.* 63:66, 1984.

99. Mahon, W. E., et al. Hypersensitivity to pituitary snuff with miliary shadowing in the lungs. *Thorax* 22:12, 1967.

100. Malo, J. L., and Cartier, A. Occupational asthma in workers of a pharmaceutical company processing spiramycin. *Thorax* 43:371, 1988.

101. Malo, J. L., et al. Prevalence of occupational asthma and immunologic sensitization to psyllium among health personnel in chronic care hospitals. *Am. Rev. Respir. Dis.* 142:1359, 1990.

102. Marcus, A. J., et al. Formation of leukotrienes and other hydroxy acids during platelet-neutrophil interactions in vitro. *Biochem. Biophys. Res. Commun.* 109:130, 1982.

103. McNeil, R. S., and Ingram, R. G. Effect of propranolol on ventilatory function. *Am. J. Cardiol.* 18:473, 1966.

104. Menon, M. P., and Das, A. K. Tetracycline asthma—a case report. *Clin. Allergy* 7:285, 1977.

105. Minneman, K. P., and Molinoff, P. B. Classification and quantitation of beta-adrenergic receptor subtypes. *Biochem. Pharmacol.* 29:1317, 1980.

106. Mjorndal, T. O., et al. Effect of beta-adrenergic stimulation on experimental canine anaphylaxis in vivo. *J. Allergy Clin. Immunol.* 71:62, 1983.

107. Morice, A. J., et al. Angiotensin converting enzyme and the cough reflex. *Lancet* 2:1116, 1987.

108. Morley, J., Page, C. P., and Sanjar, S. Platelets in asthma. *Lancet* 2:726, 1985.

109. Moss, J., and Rosow, C. E. Histamine release by narcotics and muscle relaxants in humans. *Anesthesiology* 59:330, 1983.

110. Moss, J., et al. Histamine release by neuromuscular blocking agents in man. *Klin. Wochenschr.* 60:891, 1982.

111. Motoyoshi, F., et al. Bronchial asthma induced by ethylenediamine in aminophylline injection. *Pediatr. Asthma Allergy Immunol.* 4:295, 1990.

112. Motulsky, H. J., and Insel, P. Adrenergic receptors in man. Direct identification, physiologic regulation, and clinical alterations. *N. Engl. J. Med.* 307:18, 1982.

113. Mullarkey, M. F., et al. Methotrexate in the treatment of corticosteroid-dependent asthma. *N. Engl. J. Med.* 318:603, 1988.

114. Mullarkey, M. F., et al. Association of aspirin-sensitive asthma with HLA-DQw2. *Am. Rev. Respir. Dis.* 133:261, 1986.

115. Nagy, L., and Orosz, M. Occupational asthma due to hexachlorophene. *Thorax* 39:630, 1984.

116. Newman, B. R., and Schultz, L. K. Epinephrine-resistant anaphylaxis in a patient taking propranolol hydrochloride. *Ann. Allergy* 47:35, 1981.

117. Nicklas, R. A. Paradoxical bronchospasm associated with the use of inhaled beta agonists. *J. Allergy Clin. Immunol.* 85:959, 1990.

118. Nizankowska, E., et al. Pharmacological attempts to modulate leukotriene synthesis in aspirin-induced asthma. *Agents Actions* 21:203, 1987.

119. Northcote, R. J., and Ballantyne, D. Influence of intrinsic sympathomimetic activity on respiratory function during chronic B blockade: comparison of propranolol and pindolol. *Br. Med. J.* 293:97, 1986.

120. Okuda, Y., et al. Basophil histamine release by platelet-activating factor in aspirin-sensitive subjects with asthma. *J. Allergy Clin. Immunol.* 86:548, 1990.

121. Paggiaro, P. L., Loi, A. M., and Toma, G. Bronchial asthma and dermatitis due to spiramycin in a chick breeder. *Clin. Allergy* 9:571, 1979.

122. Partridge, M. R., and Gibson, G. J. Adverse bronchial reactions to intravenous hydrocortisone in two aspirin-sensitive asthmatic patients. *Br. Med. J.* 1:1521, 1978.

123. Paterson, I. C., Grant, I. W. B., and Crompton, G. K. Severe bronchoconstriction provoked by sodium cromoglycate. *Br. Med. J.* 2:916, 1976.

124. Paterson, J. W., et al. Isoprenaline resistance and the use of pressurized aerosols in asthma. *Lancet* 2:426, 1968.

125. Picado, C., et al. Aspirin-intolerance as a precipitating factor of life-threatening attacks of asthma requiring mechanical ventilation. *Eur. Respir. J.* 2:127, 1989.

126. Piper, P. J., Collier, J. O. J., and Van, J. R. Release of catecholamines in the guinea pig by substances involved in anaphylaxis. *Nature* 213:838, 1967.

127. Pleskow, W. W., et al. Aspirin desensitization in aspirin-sensitive asthmatic patients: clinical manifestations and characterization of the refractory period. *J. Allergy Clin. Immunol.* 69:11, 1982.

128. Pleskow, W. W., et al. Aspirin-sensitive rhinosinusitis/asthma: spectrum of adverse reactions to aspirin. *J. Allergy Clin. Immunol.* 71:574, 1983.

129. Price, H. V. Asthma attacks precipitated by disodium cromoglycate in boy with alpha-1-antitrypsin deficiency (letter). *Lancet* 2:606, 1982.

130. Prichard, J. Beta-blockers and the patient with bronchial disease. *Ir. Med. J.* 79:303, 1986.

131. Pringle, T. H., and Riddell, J. G. The cardioselectivity of beta adrenoreceptor antagonists. *Pharmacol. Ther.* 45:39, 1990.

132. Reisman, R. E., and Arbesman, C. E. Systemic allergic reactions due to inhalation of penicillin. *JAMA* 203:184, 1968.

133. Riddell, J. G., et al. The dose dependency of the cardioselectivity of metoprolol in man. *Clin. Pharmacol. Ther.* 43:151, 1988.

134. Rosenow, E. C. Drug-induced Hypersensitivity Disease of the Lung. In C. H. Kirkpatrick and H. Y. Reynolds (eds.), *Immunologic and Infectious Reactions of the Lung.* New York: Dekker, 1976.

135. Rubin, R. B., and Neugarten, J. Cocaine-associated asthma. *Am. J. Med.* 88:438, 1990.

136. Ruffin, R. E., et al. Assessment of beta-adrenoreceptor antagonists in asthmatic patients. *Br. J. Clin. Pharmacol.* 13(suppl 2):325S, 1982.

137. Sakula, A. Bronchial asthma due to allergy to pancreatic extract: a hazard in the treatment of cystic fibrosis. *Br. J. Dis. Chest.* 71:295, 1977.

138. Sampter, M., and Beers, R. F. Jr. Intolerance to aspirin. *Ann. Intern. Med.* 68:975, 1968.

139. Sands, M. F., et al. Homeostatic regulation of bronchomotor tone by sympathetic activation during bronchoconstriction in normal and asthmatic humans. *Am. Rev. Respir. Dis.* 132:993, 1985.

140. Sekiya, K., Okuda, H., and Arichi, S. Selective inhibition of platelet lipoxygenase by esculetin. *Biochem. Biophys. Acta* 713:68, 1982.

141. Settipane, G. A. Asthma, aspirin intolerance and nasal polyps. *NER Allergy Proc.* 7:32, 1986.

142. Settipane, G. A., and Pudupakkam, R. K. Aspirin intolerance. III: subtypes, familial occurrence and cross-reactivity with tartrazine. *J. Allergy Clin. Immunol.* 56:215, 1975.

143. Shaw, H. Anaesthetic complications. *NZ Soc. Anaesth. Newsletter* 21:144, 1974.

144. Shehadi, W. H. Contrast media adverse reactions: occurrence, recurrence, and distribution patterns. *Radiology* 143:11, 1982.

145. Sherman, N. A., and Morris, H. G. Aspirin-induced shift in the metabolism of arachidonic acid. *J. Allergy Clin. Immunol.* 71(2):A153, 1983.

146. Simon, R., et al. Plasma mediator studies in aspirin-sensitive asthma. *J. Allergy Clin. Immunol.* 71(2):A146, 1983.

147. Skinner, C., Palmer, K. N. V., and Kerridge, D. F. Comparison of the effects of acebutolol (sectral) and practolol (eraldin) on airways obstruction of asthmatics. *Br. J. Clin. Pharmacol.* 2:417, 1975.

148. Spector, S. L., Wangaard, C. H., and Farr, R. S. Aspirin and concomitant idiosyncrasies in adult asthmatic patients. *J. Allergy Clin. Immunol.* 64:500, 1979.

149. Stenius, B. S. N., and Lemola, M. Hypersensitivity to acetylsalicylic acid (ASA) and tartrazine in patients with asthma. *Clin. Allergy* 6:119, 1976.

150. Stevenson, D. D. Diagnosis, prevention and treatment of adverse reactions to aspirin and nonsteroidal antiinflammatory drugs. *J. Allergy Clin. Immunol.* 74:617, 1984.

151. Stevenson, D. D., and Lewis, R. A. Proposed mechanisms of aspirin sensitivity reactions. *J. Allergy Clin. Immunol.* 80:788, 1987.

152. Stevenson, D. D., and Mathison, D. A. Aspirin sensitivity in asthmatics: when may this drug be safe? *Postgrad. Med.* 78:111, 1985.

153. Stevenson, D. D., and Simon, R. A. Sensitivity to ingested metabisulfites in asthmatic subjects. *J. Allergy Clin. Immunol.* 68:26, 1981.

154. Stevenson, D. D., and Simon, R. A. Aspirin Sensitivity: Respiratory and Cutaneous Manifestations. In E. Middleton, E. C. Reed, and E. F. Ellis (eds.), *Allergy, Principles and Practice.* St. Louis: Mosby, 1989, Pp. 1537–1554.

155. Stevenson, D. D., Simon, R. A., and Mathison, D. A. Aspirin-sensitive asthma: tolerance to aspirin after positive oral aspirin challenges. *J. Allergy Clin. Immunol.* 66:82, 1980.

156. Stevenson, D. D., et al. Provoking factors in bronchial asthma. *Arch. Intern. Med.* 135:777, 1975.

157. Stevenson, D. D., et al. Oral aspirin challenges in asthmatic patients: a study of plasma histamine. *Clin. Allergy* 6:493, 1976.

158. Stevenson, D. D., et al. Aspirin-sensitive rhinosinusitis asthma: a double blind crossover study of treatment with aspirin. *J. Allergy Clin. Immunol.* 73:500, 1984.

159. Stevenson, D. D., et al. Adverse reactions to tartrazine. *J. Allergy Clin. Immunol.* 78:182, 1986.

160. Stevenson, D. D., et al. Salsalate cross-sensitivity in aspirin-sensitive patients with asthma. *J. Allergy Clin. Immunol.* 86:749, 1990.

161. Stoller, J. K., Mehta, A. C., and Vidt, D. G. Captopril-induced cough. *Chest* 93:659, 1988.

162. Szczeklik, A. Analgesics, allergy, and asthma. *Br. J. Clin. Pharmacol.* 303:702, 1980.

163. Szczeklik, A. Aspirin-induced asthma as a viral disease. *Clin. Allergy* 18:15, 1988.

164. Szczeklik, A., Czerniawska-Mysik, G., and Nizankowska, E. Sulfinpyrazone and aspirin-induced asthma (letter). *N. Engl. J. Med.* 303:702, 1980.

165. Szczeklik, A., and Gryglewski, R. J. Asthma and anti-inflammatory drugs: mechanisms and clinical patterns. *Drugs* 25:533, 1983.

166. Szczeklik, A., Gryglewski, R. J., and Czerniawska-Mysik, G. Relationship of inhibition of prostaglandin biosynthesis by analgesis to asthma attacks in aspirin-sensitive patients. *Br. Med. J.* 1:67, 1975.

167. Szczeklik, A., Gryglewski, R. J., and Czerniawska-Mysik, G. Clinical patterns of hypersensitivity to nonsteroidal antiinflammatory drugs and their pathogenesis. *J. Allergy Clin. Immunol.* 60:276, 1977.

168. Szczeklik, A., Nizankowska, E., and Dukes, M. N. G. Drug-Induced Asthma and Bronchospasm. In G. M. Akoun and J. P. White (eds.), *Drug-Induced Disorders.* Amsterdam: Elsevier, Vol. 3, Pp. 189–209.

169. Szczeklik, A., et al. Asthmatic attacks induced in aspirin-sensitive patients by diclofenac and naproxen. *Br. Med. J.* 2:231, 1977.

170. Szczeklik, A., et al. Hydrocortisone and airflow impairment in aspirin-induced asthma. *J. Allergy Clin. Immunol.* 76:530, 1985.

171. Tan, Y., and Collins-Williams, C. Aspirin-induced asthma in children. *Ann. Allergy* 48:1, 1982.

172. Toogood, J. H. Risk of anaphylaxis in patients receiving beta-blocker drugs. *J. Allergy Clin. Immunol.* 81:1, 1988.

173. Toronto Aerosolized Pentamidine Study (TAPS) Group. *Chest* 98:907, 1990.

174. Town, G. I., et al. Angiotensin converting enzyme inhibitors and cough. *NZ Med. J.* 100:161, 1987.

175. Twarog, F. J., et al. Hypersensitivity to pancreatic extracts in parents with cystic fibrosis. *J. Allergy Clin. Immunol.* 59:35, 1977.

176. Vane, J. R. Inhibition of prostaglandin synthesis as a mechanism of action of aspirin-like drugs. *Nature* 231:232, 1971.

177. van Leeuwen, W. S. Pathognomonische Bedeutung der uebe Empfindlichkeit gegen Aspirin bei Asthmatikern. *Munch. Med. Wochenschrift* 37:1588, 1928.

178. Vanselow, N. A., and Smith, J. R. Bronchial asthma induced by indomethacin. *Ann. Intern. Med.* 66:658, 1967.

179. Veale, D., McComb, J. M., and Givson, G. J. Propafenone. *Lancet* 335:979, 1990.

180. Vedanthan, P. K., et al. Aspirin and tartrazine oral challenge: incidence of adverse response in chronic childhood asthma. *J. Allergy Clin. Immunol.* 60:8, 1977.

181. Vicks, S. D., Dean, R. J., and Tenholder, M. F. Ketorolac-induced respiratory failure in an aspirin-sensitive asthmatic. *Immunol. Allergy Proc.* 13:23, 1991.

182. Virchow, C., et al. Intolerance to tartrazine in aspirin-induced asthma: results of a multicenter study. *Respiration* 53:20, 1988.

183. Walters, E., Browne, S., and Settipane, G. A. The effect of aspirin on serum immunoglobulins. *NER Allergy Proc.* 7(2):113, 1986.

184. Wass, U., et al. Assay of specific IgE antibodies to disodium cromoglycate in serum from a patient with an immediate hypersensitivity reaction. *J. Allergy Clin. Immunol.* 81:750, 1988.

185. Weber, R. W., et al. Incidence of bronchoconstriction due to aspirin, azo dyes, non-azo dyes and preservatives in a population of perennial asthmatics. *J. Allergy Clin. Immunol.* 64:32, 1979.

186. Weinreb, R. N., et al. Long-term betaxolol therapy in glaucoma patients with pulmonary disease. *Am. J. Ophthalmol.* 106:162, 1988.

187. Weiss, R. B., and Bruno, S. Hypersensitivity reactions to cancer chemotherapeutic agents. *Ann. Intern. Med.* 94:66, 1981.

188. Widal, M. F., Abrami, P., and Lermoyez, J. Anaphylaxie et idiosyncrasie. *Presse Med.* 30:189, 1922.

189. Williams, R. W., Pawlowicz, A., and Davies, B. H. In vitro tests for the diagnosis of aspirin-sensitive asthma. *J. Allergy Clin. Immunol.* 86:445, 1990.

190. Zweiman, B., et al. Inhalation sensitization to trypsin. *J. Allergy* 39:11, 1966.

191. Rosenow III, E. C. Drug-induced pulmonary disease: an update. *Chest* 102:239, 1992.

192. Kumlin, M., et al. Urinary excretion of leukotriene E_4 and 11-dehydro-thromboxane B_2 in response to bronchial provocations with allergen, aspirin, leukotriene D_4, and histamine in asthmatics. *Am. Rev. Respir. Dis.* 146:96, 1992.

Hypersensitivity Pneumonitis and Allergic Bronchopulmonary Aspergillosis

49

Michael A. Ganz
Paul A. Greenberger
Roy Patterson

HYPERSENSITIVITY PNEUMONITIS

Hypersensitivity pneumonitis, also referred to as *extrinsic allergic alveolitis,* is a term used to describe a group of hypersensitivity lung diseases caused by recurrent exposure and sensitization to inhaled antigens contained in a variety of organic dusts. The resulting pulmonary immunologic response is a diffuse inflammation or pneumonitis of the interstitium, alveoli, and terminal bronchioles. Depending on the intensity and duration of exposure to the etiologic agents, hypersensitivity pneumonitis may present in an acute, subacute, or chronic form. Chronic undiagnosed hypersensitivity pneumonitis can result in pulmonary fibrosis, irreversible lung destruction, and even death.

The number of potential agents capable of causing hypersensitivity pneumonitis will likely continue to expand as the result of increasing recognition, exposures, and understanding of specific antigens. For example, hypersensitivity pneumonitis occurring in association with pulmonary vasculitis and eosinophilia has been recently described in a patient taking a tainted L-tryptophan preparation for insomnia [112]. Many cases of hypersensitivity pneumonitis occur following exposure in an occupational setting [19], which also suggests that preventive measures should be possible.

Etiologic Agents of Hypersensitivity Pneumonitis

A wide variety of agents, such as drugs, chemicals, animal proteins, thermophilic actinomycetes, and fungi can cause hypersensitivity pneumonitis. Some of the most frequently encountered antigens are listed in Table 49-1. Particles that are 4 to 6 μm or smaller can be deposited in the lung and enter the alveoli, causing typical lesions. This is the approximate size of most thermophilic actinomycetes and fungal spores that can cause hypersensitivity pneumonitis [80]. The classic example of hypersensitivity pneumonitis is farmer's lung, caused by long-term exposure to moldy hay. The antigens responsible are thermophilic actinomycetes, a group of organisms classified as bacteria that are also present in contaminated forced-air heating and cooling systems, soil, manure, grain, and vegetable composts (e.g., hay, silage, sugar cane) [4]. These organisms, which include *Micropolyspora faeni, Thermoactinomyces vulgaris, T. viridis, T. candidis,* and *T. sacchari,* may be the most common antigens implicated in hypersensitivity pneumonitis.

Animal proteins, such as avian dust, can be inhaled by pigeon breeders handling dried avian excreta and cause hypersensitivity pneumonitis [83]. Other animal proteins, such as those contained in pituitary snuff and formerly used as treatment by patients with diabetes insipidus, have also been implicated [58]. A recent report describes two women who developed hypersensitivity pneumonitis caused by the inhalation of mollusk-shell dust during the manufacture of nacre buttons [71].

Exposure to industrial chemicals and drugs can result in hypersensitivity pneumonitis, in addition to other pulmonary disorders. Inorganic chemicals, such as trimellitic anhydride and phthalic anhydride, alter the structure of respiratory proteins such as albumin and thereby form new antigens, resulting in sensitization and/or hypersensitivity pneumonitis or asthma. These chemicals are used extensively as curing agents in the plastics industry [21, 59, 103, 124]. Numerous drugs, including amiodarone, gold, methotrexate, nonsteroidal antiinflammatory drugs, penicillamine, trimethoprim and sulfasalazine, have all been implicated as causes of hypersensitivity pneumonitis [46, 60, 104, 126].

Fungi represent a relatively large source of antigens capable of causing hypersensitivity pneumonitis, including *Aspergillus, Alternaria,* and *Penicillium* [80]. Recently, the first reported case of hypersensitivity pneumonitis due to *Aspergillus glaucus* in a mushroom worker was published [122]. Wood dusts contaminated with *Cryptostroma corticale* have been reported to cause hypersensitivity pneumonitis in lumber workers stripping bark from maple logs [17], and hypersensitivity pneumonitis has been encountered in wood trimmers exposed to *Rhizopus, Aspergillus,* or *T. vulgaris* [120], Portuguese workers exposed to cork dust (suberosis) [3], farmers handling wood fuel chips contaminated with *Penicillium* [116], wood pulp workers exposed to moldy wood dust containing *Alternaria* [101], and even from exposure to molds present during the cutting of live trees ("woodman's disease") [16].

In Japan, summer-type hypersensitivity pneumonitis is the most prevalent. The causative agent, *Trichosporon cutaneum,* is extensively distributed in the home environments of the patients, as home construction permits growth of *Trichosporon* underneath floors. Inhalation challenge in these patients has revealed the importance of a specific serotype-related antigen of *T. cutaneum* in the induction of summer-type hypersensitivity pneumonitis [1].

Clinical Characteristics

Despite the wide range of specific organic dusts capable of causing hypersensitivity pneumonitis, the clinical manifestations are basically similar. There are three types of clinical responses (Table 49-2). In the acute form, after a period of asymptomatic exposure, during which sensitization occurs, the inhalation of antigen results in chills, malaise, cough, dyspnea, and temperature ranging from 38.5 to 40.5°C (101–104°F) approximately 4 to 8 hours following exposure. On physical examination, tachycardia, tachypnea, and bibasilar rales may be noted. The patient often appears acutely ill. A peripheral leukocytosis as high as 25,000 cells/mm³ can be observed and infrequently there may be an accompanying eosinophilia. Total serum IgG and IgA levels may be elevated, whereas the IgE level is not, unless the patient is

Supported by U.S.P.H.S. Grant AI11403 and the Ernest S. Bazley Grant.

atopic [75]. The acute form may be mistaken for an infectious process, such as influenza, pneumonitis, or bronchopneumonia, and antibiotics are therefore administered inappropriately. Unless the individual has underlying asthma, bronchospasm and wheezing are not noted [22, 80, 83].

Chest roentgenograms may either be normal or show fine nodular densities and peripheral lung infiltrates (Fig. 49-1). Usually a chest roentgenogram is not available from the time of a previous

Table 49-1. Agents frequently implicated in the etiology of hypersensitivity pneumonitis

Antigen	Disease	Exposure source
ANIMAL PROTEINS		
Bovine and porcine proteins	Pituitary snuff user's lung	Heterologous porcine & bovine pituitary powder
Avian proteins	Bird breeder's lung	Avian excreta
Rodent urinary proteins	Laboratory animal worker's lung	Rodent urine
MOLD		
Graphium sp.	Sequoiosis	Moldy redwood dust
Cryptostroma corticale	Maple bark stripper's disease	Moldy logs
Aspergillus clavatus	Malt worker's lung	Moldy barley
Alternaria	Wood pulp worker's lung	Moldy wood pulp
Penicillium frequentans	Suberosis	Moldy cork dust
Pullularia sp.	Sauna taker's disease	Sauna vapors
Penicillium sp.	Cheese washer's disease	Cheese casings
THERMOPHILIC ACTINOMYCETES		
Micropolyspora faeni	Farmer's lung disease	Moldy hay
Thermoactinomyces vulgaris	Bagassosis	Moldy sugarcane (bagasse)
T. candidis, T. vulgaris	Humidifier lung, air-conditioner lung	Contaminated humidifiers, air-conditioners, & air-ducts
T. vulgaris, T. viridis	Mushroom worker's lung	Moldy compost
OTHER ANTIGENS		
Bacillus subtilis	Detergent worker's disease	Detergent enzymes
Sitophilis granarius	Wheat weevil disease	Contaminated grain
Amoeba	Ventilation pneumonitis	Contaminated water
CHEMICALS		
Phthalic anhydride	Epoxy-resin worker's lung	Epoxy-resin
Toluene diisocyanate	Porcelain refinisher's lung	Paint catalyst
Trimellitic anhydride	Plastic worker's lung	Trimellitic anhydride

acute exposure. A restrictive pattern is typically present on pulmonary function testing, with a decreased forced vital capacity and forced expiratory volume in 1 second (FEV_1). Symptoms generally resolve spontaneously within 12 to 24 hours but may occasionally persist for several days [100].

A second type of clinical response may be observed with prolonged low-level exposure to an antigen. This subacute type occurs in a small number of patients, and these patients develop a more insidious form of hypersensitivity pneumonitis [91]. Symptoms include productive cough, dyspnea, malaise, and weight loss. Restrictive pulmonary function defects occur, although obstruction can sometimes be seen. Chest roentgenograms may be normal or there may be diffuse nodulation and interstitial fibrosis [22, 80]. With long-term avoidance and corticosteroid therapy the signs and symptoms of the disease may resolve. This form of hypersensitivity pneumonitis is often seen among bird breeders and owners, who are subjected to an almost constant exposure to avian proteins in the home.

deGracia and colleagues [15] studied pulmonary function patterns in 22 patients with avian hypersensitivity pneumonitis. At the time of diagnosis, restrictive changes were seen in 72 percent and airway obstruction in 25 percent. Total recovery or significant improvement was observed following termination of exposure in all patients who had been in contact with birds less than 2 years. In contrast, 60 percent of the patients with more than 2 years of contact did not experience complete recovery of lung function. Grammer and coworkers [29], in a study of four children and five adults with chronic avian hypersensitivity pneumonitis, found that the prognosis was very good, provided irreversible damage was not present at the time of diagnosis.

The chronic form of hypersensitivity pneumonitis occurs after recurrent heavy exposure or prolonged low-level exposure. In this form there is progressive development of disabling respiratory symptoms with irreversible physiologic changes. Diffuse infiltrative pulmonary fibrosis predominates, often with dispersed granulomas. A honeycomb pattern is often seen on chest roentgenograms. Reduced diffusing capacity and hypoxemia are frequently present, with a restrictive pattern and reduction of all lung volumes seen on pulmonary function testing. Despite avoidance of exposure and use of corticosteroids, lung function will remain abnormal in these patients due to irreversible damage [8, 22, 41].

Radiographic Findings

Depending on the stage of the disease, radiographic findings will differ. Acute, heavy exposure to antigen causes diffuse air space opacification on x-ray studies. Within a few days, the opacification resolves and is replaced by a fine nodular or reticulonodular pattern, characteristic of the subacute phase. In the chronic stage of hypersensitivity pneumonitis, honeycombing and fibrosis may be seen but are nonspecific. Computed tomography appears to be superior to plain chest radiography in the assessment of the

Table 49-2. Clinical presentations of patients with hypersensitivity pneumonitis

	Acute	Subacute	Chronic
Time course	Hours after exposure	Weeks to months	Months to years
Signs/symptoms	Fever, chills, cough, dyspnea, leukocytosis	Cough, dyspnea, malaise, weight loss	Weight loss, cough, fatigue, progressive shortness of breath
Pulmonary function testing	Restrictive pattern	Restrictive pattern (obstructive on occasion)	Restrictive pattern, hypoxemia, low diffusing capacity
Exposure	Often heavy	Prolonged, low level (common in bird breeders)	Recurrent, heavy exposure or prolonged low level
Prognosis	Good if identification and avoidance instituted promptly	Often good if avoidance measures instituted and no permanent damage at time of diagnosis	Lung function remains abnormal despite avoidance of antigen and use of corticosteroids

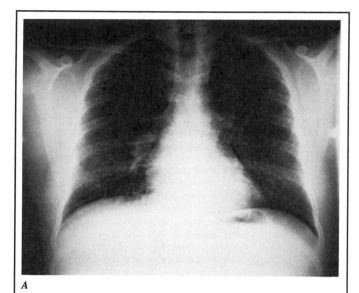

A

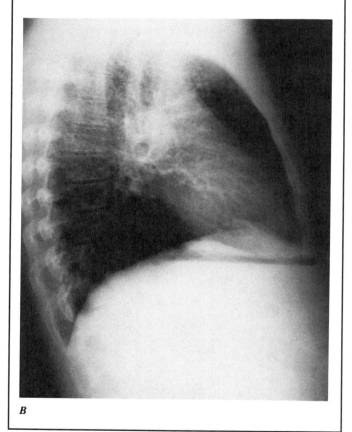

B

Fig. 49-1. *Posteroanterior (A) and lateral (B) chest radiographs of a patient with hypersensitivity pneumonitis due to inhalation of pituitary snuff for the treatment of diabetes insipidus.*

extent of abnormalities present in the subacute and chronic stages. The mid-lung zones are predominantly affected [106].

Pathologic Findings

Lung biopsy specimens from patients with acute hypersensitivity pneumonitis exhibit interstitial pneumonitis with lymphocyte in-

filtration of the alveolar walls, along with plasma cells and foamy macrophages. With progression of disease, there is thickening of the alveoli, obliteration of the alveolar spaces and bronchioles [45, 96] and ultimately large areas of fibrous connective tissue.

Immunology of Hypersensitivity Pneumonitis

Serum precipitating antibodies can be identified in nearly all ill individuals with hypersensitivity pneumonitis, either by gel diffusion or immunoelectrophoresis. These antibodies are not pathognomonic for the disease, however, since they are found in up to 50 percent of exposed but asymptomatic individuals [22]. Serum complement levels are usually within the normal range or are increased, in contrast to the low levels seen in immune complex disease [67].

Peripheral blood lymphocytes and lung lymphocytes obtained from bronchoalveolar lavage fluid from patients with hypersensitivity pneumonitis undergo increased blastogenic activity, with release of lymphokines, such as macrophage migration inhibition factor, when cultured with specific fungal or avian antigens. Lymphocytes from asymptomatic but exposed individuals do not react in this manner. Lavage fluid from patients with hypersensitivity pneumonitis show a marked increase in the number of lymphocytes, especially those of the suppressor T-cell type. This predominance is also observed in asymptomatic individuals [13, 67, 86, 105]. An immunoregulatory defect has been identified in patients with hypersensitivity pneumonitis. Active suppressor T-cell activity has been demonstrated in lavage fluid from asymptomatic but exposed pigeon breeders, whereas symptomatic breeders had depressed suppressor T-cell activity [50].

Pathogenesis of Hypersensitivity Pneumonitis

The pathogenesis of hypersensitivity pneumonitis remains unclear. Early evidence supported a Type III immune complex mechanism (see Chap. 6). The time course of symptoms, the presence of precipitating antibodies against the specific antigen, and the existence of antigen, antibody, and complement in lung biopsy specimens from patients with hypersensitivity pneumonitis all supported this view [76, 102, 119]. However, no vasculitic lesions are usually found and the serum complement level is not depressed. Serum precipitating antibody is present in asymptomatic individuals exposed to specific antigens. In addition, titers of specific antibody in lavage fluid are similar in both ill and asymptomatic individuals [67, 84]. It is currently believed that a Type III mechanism may not play a major role in the pathogenesis. Instead, cellular immunity appears to play a key role in the pathogenesis of hypersensitivity pneumonitis [85, 97]. T-lymphocytes accumulate within the alveolar structures of the lung, particularly CD8$^+$ T-lymphocytes (suppressor T-cells). The interleukin-2 system may play a central role in the mechanisms responsible for lymphocytic alveolitis in hypersensitivity pneumonitis [113]. Other lymphokines, such as macrophage migration inhibition factor, have been detected more consistently in avian-antigen–stimulated peripheral lymphocytes from symptomatic pigeon breeders than from asymptomatic but exposed individuals [11, 20, 40]. The mast cell may also serve an important function in the development of hypersensitivity pneumonitis, based on the findings from animal experiments. When *T. vulgaris* antigen was administered to mice, hypersensitivity pneumonitis–like lesions formed in the lung. Mast cell–deficient mice had less severe lesions. When mast cells were adoptively transferred to the deficient strain, the lung lesions became equally severe [111].

Host factors must be operant, as most exposed individuals remain asymptomatic. As mentioned earlier, immunoregulatory differences between symptomatic and asymptomatic individuals have been demonstrated [50]. A possible pathogenetic sequence may include antigen activation of complement by the alternate pathway. Mediator release, lymphokine generation, and macrophage activation would result in inflammation and development of the typical lesions seen in patients with hypersensitivity pneumonitis. Continued undetected inflammation would result in progressive fibrosis, with consequential clinically irreversible lung damage.

Diagnosis

When a patient presents with a history of intermittent bouts of pneumonitis associated with systemic symptoms and no clear infectious cause or evidence of chronic interstitial lung disease can be identified, a diagnosis of hypersensitivity pneumonitis should be entertained. It is essential to recognize the different clinical patterns that may be seen. A detailed occupational history is of paramount importance, with emphasis on the temporal relationships between symptoms and occupational exposure. At times, obvious accidental exposures will result in high-dose inhalation of agents such as trimellitic anhydride, leading to hypersensitivity pneumonitis or even pulmonary disease anemia–syndrome [125]. Inquiring about hobbies, pets, and heating or filtration systems at home or work is equally important.

Patients may be completely asymptomatic between episodes of hypersensitivity pneumonitis. Pulmonary function testing done several hours before and after work may reveal differences in vital capacity, flow rates, and diffusing capacity. Characteristic acute changes may be diagnostic. At times, an on-site visit to the workplace can be of value; spirometry can be performed there, along with culturing for specific agents and a review of procedures and chemicals present. However, additional expertise, such as that possessed by occupational physicians and hygienists, may be necessary. Workers may be seeking compensation, and some employees may be unaware of the fact that, although a plant facility has documentation of low concentrations of airborne substances, and meets the standards established by O.S.H.A., even lower concentrations can cause disease in a sensitized, exposed patient.

Serum precipitating antibodies can be identified in the vast majority of cases but only confirm exposure, since they are frequently seen in asymptomatic individuals. Immediate skin testing is generally not of diagnostic value. Infrequently, carefully performed bronchial challenges with a suspected antigen in specialized laboratories may be necessary to support a diagnosis. Lung biopsy may help in selected cases of chronic disease of unknown etiology.

The differential diagnosis of hypersensitivity pneumonitis includes other interstitial pulmonary diseases, such as connective tissue disorders, idiopathic pulmonary fibrosis, sarcoidosis, granulomatous disorders, drug reactions, and neoplasms. The sick building syndrome is seen in the case of inadequately ventilated buildings; under these circumstances, the concentrations of formaldehyde or other volatile gases increase and occupants develop irritant respiratory or ocular symptoms. Aside from anxiety, other clinical findings are absent and characteristically the chest roentgenogram is clear [115]. Physicians should have a high level of suspicion when organic dusts are being inhaled, in order to identify new causes of hypersensitivity pneumonitis or even other immunologically mediated diseases. For instance, the development of anaphylaxis and asthma has recently been attributed to the inhalation of deer bone dust [72]. Additionally, in cases of idiopathic pulmonary fibrosis, at times the history and presence of precipitating antibody can help incriminate a cause for end-stage lung disease [36]. Finally, when every reasonable effort has been made to diagnose hypersensitivity pneumonitis and still no antigen is found, the patient may well have idiopathic pulmonary fibrosis, which, in certain cases, may be corticosteroid responsive.

Management

The cornerstone of effective control of hypersensitivity pneumonitis is avoidance of the inciting antigen in all cases. When strict avoidance is not possible, as in certain occupational settings, modifications of the environment, such as filtration and ventilation systems and the wearing of masks, may greatly reduce exposure. For example, the education of farmers has led to an improvement in hay storage techniques, and farmers are now encouraged to use masks when uncapping a silo to remove moldy hay. In acute and subacute forms of hypersensitivity pneumonitis, corticosteroids in doses up to 60 to 80 mg per day are effective after removal of the individual from exposure, and these agents should not be withheld; possible increased recurrence following corticosteroids in farmer's lung is reported [127]. Use of long-term corticosteroids should not be substituted for avoidance measures, and should be used cautiously or not at all in patients who are still exposed to the offending antigen.

ALLERGIC BRONCHOPULMONARY ASPERGILLOSIS

Allergic bronchopulmonary aspergillosis (ABPA) is a lung disease that is increasingly being recognized worldwide. It is characterized by clinical, roentgenographic, serologic, and pathologic evidence of lung involvement attributable to immune-mediated reactions to the common fungus *Aspergillus*. ABPA appears to complicate 1 to 2 percent of all cases of chronic asthma, and the clinical spectrum varies from mild to corticosteroid-dependent asthma to end-stage lung disease with pulmonary fibrosis.

ABPA was originally described by Hinson and coworkers [47] in 1952, when they reported on three patients with severe asthma who exhibited "pyrexial attacks" occurring over the course of months or years. Episodic lobar and segmental collapse were seen on chest radiographs in these patients, who also exhibited peripheral eosinophilia. Mucus plugs were obtained by bronchoscopy, from which *Aspergillus fumigatus* was cultured. Two of the three patients had evidence of bronchiectasis, and all had a history of mold exposure. The first case in North America was reported in 1968 [73].

Aspergillus spores are very common and widely dispersed in nature. The name probably is derived from its resemblance to the brush used for sprinkling holy water (aspergillum) [82]. It is present in large quantities in decaying organic matter, which provides a carbon source; this includes rotting wood chips, fresh-cut grass, compost heaps, potting soil, old hay and grain, and the sewage found in treatment facilities. It is also found in outdoor air. *Aspergillus* is thermotolerant and capable of growing at 15 to 53°C [82]. Hyphae are septate, grow 7 to 10 µg in diameter, and branch at 45-degree angles. Of the *Aspergillus* species that are known to be pathogenic to humans, *A. fumigatus* occurs most frequently.

Aspergillus-related disease is also a significant problem in the agricultural industry in the United States. From 5 to 10 percent of turkey poults succumb to avian aspergillosis yearly, and major outbreaks of respiratory infections can occur in other domesticated fowl such as chickens [98, 121]. In addition, *Aspergillus* infections may cause spontaneous abortions in sheep.

Aspergillus species are quite prevalent in the United States. Solomon and associates [110] were able to detect species of *Aspergillus* during the winter in 47 of 150 homes tested in Michigan, and the inhalation of *A. fumigatus* spores during high seasonal concentrations of mold sporulation has been associated with ABPA exacerbations [81]. There is a recent report of a patient with ABPA resulting from inhalation of *A. fumigatus* originating from a municipal leaf-composting site where collected leaves were stored and composted at a distance of only 250 feet (75 meters) from his residence [54]. Mold spore concentrations in hay and compost have been reported to be extremely elevated [82]. Heat generated during composting is an ideal substrate for a thermotolerant fungus such as *A. fumigatus*. The exact relationship between the proximity to a source of *A. fumigatus* spores and development of ABPA is still not defined.

Diagnosis and Clinical Characteristics

Eight diagnostic criteria for ABPA have been defined. These include: (1) asthma, (2) a history of transient or fixed infiltrates on chest roentgenograms, (3) immediate-type cutaneous reactivity to *Aspergillus*, signifying anti-*Aspergillus* IgE, (4) peripheral blood eosinophilia greater than 1,000 cells/mm³, (5) elevated total serum level of IgE greater than 1,000 ng/ml, (6) demonstration of precipitating antibodies to *A. fumigatus*, (7) elevated serum levels of IgE and IgG antibodies to *A. fumigatus* (IgE-Af and IgG-Af, respectively) compared to sera from *Aspergillus*-sensitive asthmatics in whom ABPA has been excluded [32, 118], and (8) central (proximal) bronchiectasis [94, 99]. Not all of these criteria may be met at the time of initial evaluation (Table 49-3). In some instances, patients with corticosteroid-dependent asthma have been followed for several years before a diagnosis of ABPA became manifest. ABPA has also been diagnosed in patients presenting with seasonal allergic rhinitis and mild asthma [28] and

with lipstick contact dermatitis [89] who had a previous history of pneumonia.

The diagnosis of ABPA is readily apparent if all diagnostic criteria are met [33]. In the absence of central bronchiectasis, however, a diagnosis of ABPA-seropositive (ABPA-S) can be made, as opposed to the more classic presentation of ABPA-CB (central bronchiectasis) [79]. Although patients with ABPA-S may eventually develop central bronchiectasis, preliminary data suggest that ABPA-S represents a less aggressive form of the disease [25]. Alternatively, early diagnosis and appropriate management may prevent lung damage. The only specific diagnostic criteria for ABPA are elevated levels of IgE-Af and IgG-Af compared to control sera [32, 118] and, in the absence of distal bronchiectasis, central bronchiectasis [94, 99]. The other remaining criteria are not specific for ABPA. Approximately 13 to 38 percent of patients with asthma have immediate cutaneous reactivity to *A. fumigatus*, and serum precipitating antibodies to *A. fumigatus* have been noted in 3 percent of nonatopic asthmatics, 25 percent of allergic asthmatics, and approximately 9 percent of all other types of asthma [5, 25, 43, 44]. Furthermore, only 69 to 90 percent of patients with ABPA demonstrate precipitating antibodies to *A. fumigatus* [118]. Other nonspecific findings in ABPA include the isolation of sputum plugs containing *Aspergillus* and immediate and late cutaneous reactivity to *A. fumigatus*.

Associated clinical allergic features seen in patients with ABPA include an increased incidence of allergic rhinitis, allergic conjunctivitis, family history of allergic disease, food allergy, drug allergy, eczema, and urticaria. Virtually all patients in one study demonstrated cutaneous reactivity to molds other than *Aspergillus* [88]. Some patients reported from England have been noted to have a low atopic state, often with the late onset of ABPA [62]. However, this has not been a consistent finding in our patients.

Although unusual at extremes of age, ABPA has been reported in children as young as 14 months [114]. The age at onset can be variable [48, 51, 94]. ABPA may also occur on a familial basis, in patients with cystic fibrosis (see later discussion), in patients with a normal chest roentgenogram [93], and in patients with previously confirmed bronchiectasis.

Staging of ABPA

Five distinct stages of ABPA have been recognized [77]. These include: (I) acute, (II) remission, (III) exacerbation, (IV) corticosteroid-dependent asthma, and (V) end-stage lung disease with pulmonary fibrosis. Although patients may progress through all five stages, they should not be considered as actual phases of the disease (Table 49-4).

Patients in Stage I present with the classic diagnostic signs and symptoms, including asthma, immediate cutaneous reactivity to *A. fumigatus*, serum precipitating antibodies to *A. fumigatus*, ele-

Table 49-3. Diagnostic features of allergic bronchopulmonary aspergillosis

Clinical or laboratory findings	Comments
1. Asthma	Wide range of severity
2. Chest roentgenographic infiltrate(s)	May be absent at initial evaluation
3. Immediate cutaneous reactivity to *Aspergillus* species	Prick or intradermal; essential for diagnosis
4. Elevated total serum IgE level	Useful in following disease activity
5. Precipitating antibodies to *A. fumigatus*	May be seen in some normal individuals
6. Peripheral blood eosinophilia	May be absent if patient has received oral steroids
7. Elevated serum IgE-Af and/or IgG-Af	Essential for diagnosis
8. Central bronchiectasis	Virtually diagnostic for ABPA in absence of distal bronchiectasis; may be absent with ABPA-S

Af = *Aspergillus fumigatus*; ABPA-S = seropositive allergic bronchopulmonary aspergillosis.

Table 49-4. Stages of allergic bronchopulmonary aspergillosis

	Stages				
	I Acute	*II* Remission	*III* Exacerbation	*IV* Corticosteroid-dependent asthma	*V* End-stage lung disease
Chest radiography	Infiltrates; bronchiectasis	Negative	Infiltrates; bronchiectasis	Bronchiectasis	Fibrosis
Total serum IgE	Elevated (at least double from baseline)	Often above normal	Elevated (at least double from baseline)	Normal or above normal	May be low, normal, or elevated
Isotypic antibodies (IgE-Af, IgG-Af)	Elevated (at least double compared to control serum)	Usually elevated; may be normal when remission is long-standing	Elevated	Variable; may be normal	Often normal
Eosinophilia	Present	Absent	Present	Variable	Absent

vated total serum IgE levels, elevated isotypic antibodies (IgE-Af and IgG-Af), peripheral eosinophilia, and pulmonary infiltrates. Central bronchiectasis is present, except in patients with ABPA-S [79]. Treatment with corticosteroids results in resolution of symptoms, clearing of roentgenographic infiltrates, and a decline in the total serum IgE levels and eosinopenia (Fig. 49-2). Following treatment, patients frequently enter Stage II. During this stage, the patient's asthma is easily managed by bronchodilators or inhaled corticosteroids, or both; chest radiographs are clear and the total serum IgE level, although often still elevated, de-

Fig. 49-2. *Posteroanterior (A) and lateral (B) chest radiographs of a patient with acute (Stage I) allergic bronchopulmonary aspergillosis. There are central infiltrates present in both lung fields.*

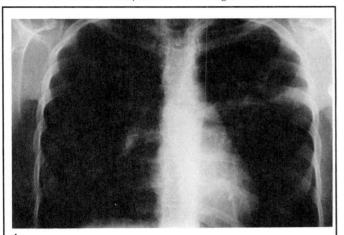

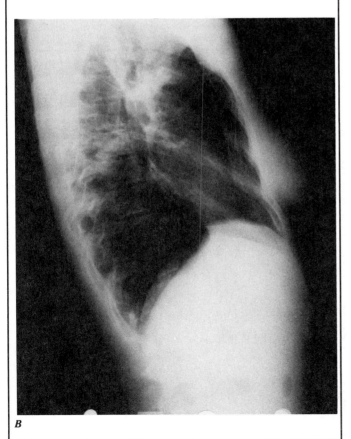

A

B

clines by 35 percent over a 4- to 8-week period. Eosinophilia is absent. Isotypic and precipitating antibodies to *A. fumigatus* may or may not be present. Patients can remain in remission for years, although they are still at risk for recurrences over a prolonged period [38].

When an exacerbation of disease occurs in a patient previously diagnosed with ABPA (Stage III), it is often heralded by an increase in the total serum IgE level [92]. At least a doubling of the IgE level should occur for this finding to be significant. Subclinical exacerbations are common, illustrating the need for serial IgE determinations in order to follow disease activity. Significant IgE elevations require chest roentgenography to determine the presence of pulmonary infiltrates. The treatment of exacerbations is the same as that for acute episodes. Follow-up chest films are necessary after treatment of an exacerbation to document clearing of the infiltrate. Significant elevations in the total serum IgE levels are not always associated with pulmonary infiltrates. Why this occurs is not known, but treatment is not required for an isolated elevated total serum IgE. A persistent elevation of the IgE concentration in the presence of symptoms of increased asthma can indicate an exacerbation of ABPA.

The patient with Stage IV ABPA requires oral corticosteroids to control symptoms of asthma. Patients usually enter this stage when prednisone cannot be tapered further following successful treatment of an exacerbation [79]. Serologic indexes usually remain elevated, and initially the total serum IgE level should be monitored frequently (i.e., monthly) to differentiate a flare-up of the asthma symptoms from an exacerbation associated with a pulmonary infiltrate. One study involving 84 patients with ABPA had the greatest number of patients (45%) in the corticosteroid-dependent asthma stage. While the maintenance prednisone doses in these patients varied between 15 and 30 mg on alternate days, this amount of medication, in addition to inhaled beclomethasone dipropionate, was not sufficient to prevent exacerbations, although symptoms of asthma were controlled [39].

Most patients in Stages I to IV exhibit central bronchiectasis, although some may have only clinical and serologic evidence of disease (ABPA-S). While bronchograms have not been performed in recent years on patients with ABPA, patients with ABPA-S exhibit no bronchiectasis shown by thin-section hilar tomography obtained in the anteroposterior perspective or by thin-section computed tomography. While aggressive treatment with corticosteroids appears to prevent progression to Stage V disease, it is not yet known whether central bronchiectasis can be prevented in this group [77, 79]. By definition, all patients in Stage V have demonstrable bronchiectasis and fixed roentgenographic changes consistent with fibrosis, or fibrosis identified on lung biopsy specimens. Irreversible lung damage is seen on pulmonary function testing, with little or no improvement on corticosteroid therapy. Continued exacerbations with further deterioration of lung function is common, and death can occur from cor pulmonale or respiratory failure. Serologic values are frequently low. In a review of 17 patients with Stage V ABPA, the interval between the onset and diagnosis of disease ranged from 5 months to 35 years [57]. It is likely that failure to diagnose ABPA in patients results in continued lung damage and eventual end-stage disease. Patients who exhibited an FEV_1 of less than 0.8 liter at diagnosis had a uniformly poor prognosis, with death occurring within 7 years [57].

Findings on physical examination also depend on the stage of disease. Acutely ill patients (Stages I and III) may exhibit evidence of consolidation, such as rales, egobronchophony, dullness to percussion, or bronchial breath sounds. Often, however, a patient may have an exacerbation of disease, yet appear well. This can occur in up to 33 percent of the cases of exacerbation [94]. Patients in Stage V frequently exhibit the stigmata of end-stage lung disease (e.g., clubbing, cyanosis, cor pulmonale).

Laboratory Findings

Peripheral eosinophilia greater than 1,000 cells/mm^3 is invariably noted in acute ABPA, unless the patient is being treated with oral corticosteroids [42, 47, 61, 62, 73, 94]. The eosinophil count may be normal if the patient is in remission. Skin testing by prick or by intradermal injection of an *Aspergillus* mix will elicit an immediate cutaneous reaction (i.e., a wheal and flare response). A 1:20 weight-volume (w/v) concentration is used for prick testing and a 1:1,000 w/v concentration for the intradermal test. A late, Arthus-type reaction may infrequently be seen, but is uncommon after a prick test response because so little antigen is absorbed. If immediate skin reactivity is not present, then the diagnosis of ABPA is virtually excluded, assuming that proper technique and a representative extract of *Aspergillus* is used, unless the patient is taking antihistamines or other drugs which might suppress skin test reactivity.

The most important serologic tests are determination of the total serum IgE and isotypic antibody levels (IgE-Af and IgG-Af). The total serum IgE level is generally above 1,000 ng/ml in patients with ABPA. Following treatment, a decline in the total IgE levels helps both to confirm the diagnosis and to document compliance with medication. Even when the patient is in remission, the total serum IgE level may remain elevated in the 2,000 to 4,000 ng/ml range. Documentation of infiltrate clearing and clinical improvement, but not a return of the total IgE level to baseline values, indicates that a disease flare-up has resolved. At times, patients have been overtreated through attempts to return the total IgE to normal values, when instead the goal should be to reduce the total IgE to the plateau level noted during the previous remission of ABPA.

Total serum IgE levels above 20,000 mg/ml are not unusual in acute cases of ABPA and may be useful in distinguishing it from other diseases associated with pulmonary infiltrates and eosinophilia [75]. Most of the elevated serum IgE is nonspecific and not directed against *A. fumigatus* [74]. A persistently elevated total serum IgE level in either a patient in remission or one who has been adequately treated may indicate the presence of an associated disease such as atopic dermatitis or hyper-IgE syndrome, or may simply be the plateau level of IgE for that patient.

The most specific serologic test in ABPA is an elevated IgE and IgG antibody titer specific for *A. fumigatus* (IgE-Af and IgG-Af) [78]. Using an enzyme-linked immunosorbent assay (ELISA), elevated IgE-Af and IgG-Af levels, compared to a population of *Aspergillus*-sensitive asthmatics in whom ABPA has been excluded, can identify patients with ABPA [32, 49]. Raised IgE-Af levels can predict a recurrence of disease in an asymptomatic patient with ABPA [95], and IgA-Af also demonstrates substantially elevated concentrations before and during exacerbations of disease [2]. IgG-Af antibody titers can be an indicator of disease activity in follow-up studies continued over long periods, and may undergo a continuous decline over a 2-year period following an acute episode of ABPA [49]. The disease is associated with a polyclonal antibody response, in which all isotypes are increased [10, 55]. Since several diagnostic features of ABPA, such as elevated levels of total serum IgE and eosinophilia, can vary with disease activity or corticosteroid therapy, elevated IgE-Af and IgG-Af titers may be required to confirm the diagnosis, especially in children [51]. When determining the presence of IgE-Af, IgG-Af, or IgA-Af in sera from children using an ELISA method, it is important to use age-matched control serum or the sensitivity of the assay may be decreased. Adults with asthma but not ABPA have increased serum IgE-Af levels compared to children with asthma [31].

As noted earlier, serum precipitating antibodies using double-gel diffusion techniques are neither sensitive nor specific for ABPA. Absence of precipitating antibody does not exclude the diagnosis. Recovery of *A. fumigatus* from sputum is also not sen-sitive or specific but may be suggestive of ABPA in the appropriate clinical setting [61] (Plate 9).

Radiographic Findings in ABPA

Central (proximal) bronchiectasis, with normal tapering of the distal bronchi and in the absence of cystic fibrosis or congenital ciliary disorders, is virtually pathognomonic for ABPA [23, 63, 66, 99]. Bronchography has been the "gold standard" in determining the presence of bronchiectasis but has largely been supplanted by noninvasive techniques that are nearly as sensitive [37, 66, 68]. Both anteroposterior hilar linear tomography using 1- to 2-mm section widths and high-resolution computed tomography can be used to determine the presence of bronchiectasis in the evaluation of ABPA [23, 69]. Although patients with ABPA-S lack evidence of central bronchiectasis, they should still be considered to have the disease. Pulmonary infiltrates can be identified in this group of patients [25].

Findings on plain chest roentgenograms may be transient or fixed, with a predilection for upper lobe involvement (Fig. 49-3). Proximal bronchiectasis may be evidenced by the existence of either ring or parallel-line shadows. Ring shadows are markings that are 1 to 2 cm in diameter. They represent thick-walled but empty bronchi and are present when the dilated bronchi are viewed *en face*. Seen tangentially, it is referred to as a *parallel-line shadow*. Conventional computed tomography employs an axial view, and therefore can miss some central bronchiectasis, whereas linear hilar anteroposterior tomography views the bronchi longitudinally, which demonstrates parallel-line shadows [23]. Computed tomographic studies have been helpful in identifying bronchiectasis in ABPA [69]. Tramline shadows, which are reversible findings and represent bronchial wall

Fig. 49-3. *Posteroanterior chest radiograph of a patient with allergic bronchopulmonary aspergillosis. There is evidence of mucus-filled bronchi ("gloved finger" shadow).*

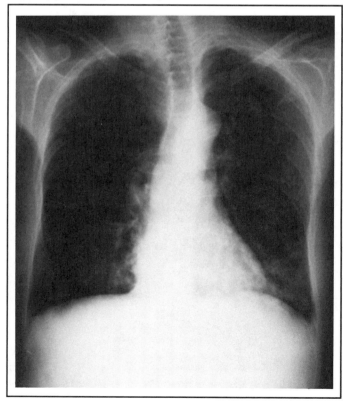

edema, are seen as two parallel lines extending from the hilum and approximate the width of the bronchi at that level. Other findings that are reversible with treatment include distally occluded bronchi ("gloved finger") and dilated bronchi which are impacted with mucus ("toothpaste" shadow) [23, 66, 94]. Spontaneous pneumothorax [87], bullae, and pulmonary fibrosis are seen in end-stage disease [57]. The most common roentgenographic findings in ABPA patients are infiltrates, ring shadows, and parallel-line shadows [66].

Pulmonary Function Tests

Depending on the disease stage, pulmonary function tests may reveal a restrictive, obstructive, mixed, or normal pattern. Patients in remission can have normal lung volumes and flow rates even in the presence of bronchiectasis, provided the asthma is well controlled. During an acute exacerbation, a reduction in lung volumes and diffusing capacity can be demonstrated, consistent with a restrictive pattern. Patients with Stage V disease have reduced lung volumes, a low diffusing capacity, and irreversible airflow obstruction [34, 57]. However, pulmonary function tests are relatively insensitive, and a normal pattern does not exclude a disease exacerbation [70].

Pathologic Findings

Lung biopsy specimens from patients with ABPA are generally nonspecific and the histologic findings may vary even in different areas of the same lung. Dilated, predominantly upper lobe bronchi may contain eosinophils, fungal hyphae, fibrin deposition, Curschmann's spirals, Charcot-Leyden crystals, and thick tenacious mucus, all consistent with bronchial wall inflammation. There is no invasion of the bronchial wall or lung parenchyma by *A. fumigatus*. Mononuclear cell infiltration and granuloma formation can also be seen. Bronchocentric granulomatosis and mucoid impaction of the bronchi are relatively constant findings [7].

Newer histologic techniques have confirmed the largely bronchocentric aspect of ABPA, with demonstration of elastin disruption in the bronchioles. There is no vasculitis or deposition of complement and immunoglobulins in the vessel wall, pointing away from an immune complex mechanism in the pathogenesis of ABPA. Significant amounts of major basic protein, the predominant constituent of eosinophils, have been demonstrated to exist outside eosinophils in scattered foci throughout the tissue as well as in macrophages and interlobular septi. Lymphocytes, plasma cells, monocytes, and numerous eosinophils can also be found [109]. Bronchial wall destruction occurs in areas of inflammation and at sites of parenchymal infiltrates.

Pathogenesis of ABPA

Animal models suggest the need for both IgE and IgG anti-*Aspergillus* antibodies in the pathogenesis of this disease. The passive transfer of serum containing IgE-Af and IgG-Af from a patient with ABPA to rhesus monkeys challenged with *Aspergillus* resulted in pulmonary lesions [27]. IgE-Af and IgG-Af have been shown to be essential for the development of pathologic lesions consistent with ABPA in the primate model [108]. A polyclonal and isotypic antibody host response to fungal antigens has been hypothesized [10]. Proteolytic enzyme release from *Aspergillus* spores could contribute to antigenic exposure. An exaggerated host response, involving cytokine release, lymphocyte sensitization, and complement activation with resultant tissue injury, might then ensue.

There is convincing evidence for the importance of cell-mediated immunity in the pathogenesis of ABPA. Peripheral blood mononuclear cell proliferation, which has been demonstrated to be induced by an extract of *A. fumigatus*, was greater in ABPA

patients than in control subjects [117]. Increased disease activity might be associated with an accumulation of *A. fumigatus*–specific T-lymphocytes in the lung, with a reduced population in the circulation [117]. Peripheral blood basophils from patients with ABPA demonstrate increased in vitro histamine release when stimulated with *Aspergillus* and IgE-Af, as compared to *A. fumigatus*–sensitive asthmatics without ABPA [90]. Studies conducted in patients with cystic fibrosis and ABPA have demonstrated that there are *A. fumigatus* antigen–specific T-cells that proliferate in vitro to *A. fumigatus* and in turn stimulate in vitro B-cell IgE synthesis. B-cells from these patients with cystic fibrosis and ABPA demonstrated previous in vivo activation and spontaneously synthesized IgE [52, 53].

T-cells stimulated with *Aspergillus* antigens secrete cytokines that induce B-cell IgE synthesis in ABPA patients. B-cell IgE hyperactivity has been shown in vivo and in vitro by increased IgE concentrations. Analysis of T-cell regulation and B-cell IgE synthesis appears to distinguish ABPA patients from controls. IgE synthesis in vitro requires antigen recognition, T-cell activation and proliferation, cytokine production such as IL-1, IL-4, and IL-5, and finally B-cell synthesis of IgE. In vitro, interferon gamma downregulates some of the antibody synthesis [52, 53].

Analysis of bronchoalveolar lavage fluid from ABPA patients has shown local (bronchoalveolar lavage compartment) production of IgE-Af and IgA-Af but not IgG-Af, although the IgG-Af was present in lavage fluid. The total IgE level was not elevated in lavage fluid compared with peripheral blood, suggesting that either IgE is not retained in the bronchoalveolar lavage compartment, or is synthesized elsewhere. *A. fumigatus* may serve as a ligand to stimulate isotypic antibody production and total IgE synthesis [35]. It has previously been demonstrated that the *Aspergillus* organisms growing in the respiratory tract are a potent stimulus for nonspecific IgE production [74]. The significance of this is not clear, although total serum IgE measurement is useful clinically in monitoring disease activity.

These studies and the demonstration of mononuclear cell infiltration, granuloma formation, and increased numbers of eosinophils and major basic protein content in biopsy specimens strongly point to cell-mediated immunity as having the major role in the immunopathogenesis of ABPA. A possible scenario begins with spores of *A. fumigatus* becoming trapped in the viscid secretions seen in patients with asthma or cystic fibrosis. The organisms continue to grow and colonize the bronchial tree, shedding antigens that initiate inflammation or may penetrate the lung parenchyma. IgE-Af and *Aspergillus* antigen combine to cause mast cell degranulation. Eosinophils are attracted and then infiltrate the tissue. Major basic protein and other eosinophil products subsequently mediate lung damage. Corticosteroid therapy, which causes eosinopenia, can control inflammation and prevent pulmonary destruction if given early [109]. Corticosteroids decrease bronchial mucus production in that, after treatment, fewer patients have sputum plugs or any sputum at all. Recovery of *A. fumigatus* from sputum can be impossible in such early treated patients. In patients with extensive bronchiectasis, recovery of *A. fumigatus* may be a frequent finding, along with various species of *Pseudomonas* and *Staphylococcus* organisms, among others.

Cystic Fibrosis and ABPA

A well-known association exists between cystic fibrosis and ABPA [9, 65]. The reported incidence of ABPA occurring in patients with cystic fibrosis has varied between 0.6 and 11 percent. This wide range may reflect the fact that underlying lung disease in cystic fibrosis may obscure chest findings considered to be diagnostic for ABPA. The abnormal mucus production and bronchiectasis seen in patients with cystic fibrosis is an ideal medium for the growth and colonization of *Aspergillus*. Many patients with cystic fibrosis have evidence of sensitization to *A. fumigatus* [24, 64], and this has been associated with decreased lung function and possibly lung destruction [18, 123]. A recent study of 137 patients followed over a 3-year period identified eight patients (5.8%) with ABPA [107]. All patients were screened with skin tests, serologic studies, and chest radiographs. A total of 54 new pulmonary infiltrates were identified, of which 11 represented episodes of ABPA. Diagnosis was often confirmed by radiographic and clinical improvement with corticosteroid therapy, where there had been none with conventional antibiotic treatment [107]. ABPA may be underestimated in this population, since exacerbations may be asymptomatic or can occur with normal chest radiographs [93]. Importantly, non-enteric-coated preparations of prednisone or prednisolone should be administered, because enteric-coated corticosteroids may not be adequately absorbed in patients with cystic fibrosis [26].

Differential Diagnosis

Occasional patients with asthma may exhibit proximal bronchiectasis, peripheral eosinophilia, and elevated levels of total serum IgE but lack evidence of sensitization to *A. fumigatus*.

These episodes have been attributed to the effect of other noninvasive fungi such as *Curvularia, Candida, Helminthosporium, Stemphylium, Dreschlera, Aspergillus oryaze,* and *Aspergillus ochraceus* [30, 39, 56]. Allergic bronchopulmonary fungal disease due to fungi other than *Aspergillus* may be a more common occurrence than previously recognized. Researchers in western Australia noted findings of allergic bronchopulmonary disease in 8 patients due to *Bipolaris* and/or *Curvularia* over a 7.5-year period [55a]. Treatment is the same as that for ABPA. Patients strongly suspected of having ABPA or an associated allergic bronchopulmonary fungosis but with negative serologic findings or fungal sputum cultures should be treated as if ABPA were present, and their clinical response observed. Sera can be frozen and tested at a future date.

Pulmonary infiltrates with eosinophilia (PIE syndromes) may be confused with ABPA. These include Löffler's syndrome; localized or persistent parasitic, fungal, or bacterial infections; avian hypersensitivity pneumonitis, such as bird fancier's disease; drug reactions; and chronic eosinophilic pneumonia. Other PIE disorders consist of tropical eosinophilia, allergic granulomatosis with angiitis (Churg-Strauss disease), hypersensitivity vasculitis, and hypereosinophilia syndrome (see Chap. 37). A patient with

Fig. 49-4. *Suggested sequence to confirm or refute diagnosis of allergic bronchopulmonary aspergillosis (ABPA). ABPF = allergic bronchopulmonary fungosis; CB = central bronchiectasis; S = seropositive; AP = anteroposterior; CT = computed tomogram; * = elevated when compared with sera from asthma patients with immediate cutaneous reactivity to* A. fumigatus *in whom ABPA has been excluded.*

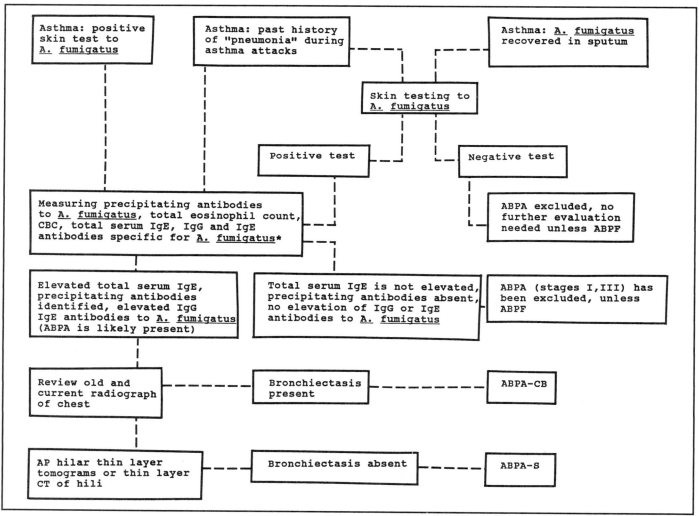

asthma may have peripheral eosinophilia and mucus plugging and may present with an infiltrate on chest radiography. The total serum IgE level may be elevated in eosinophilic pneumonia and eosinophilic vasculitis [12]. Tuberculosis involving the posterior segments of the upper lobes may also simulate ABPA and vice versa. When an infiltrate appears in a patient with asthma, infection, neoplasm, and sarcoidosis should be excluded. An elevated total serum IgE level may be seen in patients with asthma and atopic dermatitis, in the absence of ABPA.

Respiratory diseases associated with *Aspergillus* may also be observed. These include invasive aspergillosis, aspergilloma, hypersensitivity pneumonitis, IgE-mediated *Aspergillus*-sensitive asthma (ABPA excluded), allergic *Aspergillus* sinusitis, and chronic necrotizing pneumonia.

Treatment

Oral corticosteroids are the treatment of choice in acute exacerbations of ABPA. Prednisone (0.5 mg per kilogram of body weight per day) is given as a single morning dose for 2 weeks and then converted to an alternate-day dosing schedule for a total of 3 months of therapy. The drug dose is then tapered and the medication eventually discontinued. Treatment of asthma may require additional medications, such as bronchodilators, inhaled corticosteroids, or cromolyn, and, by definition, prednisone in Stage IV of ABPA. Following a 4- to 6-week period after therapy for acute ABPA has been initiated, clinical improvement should be noted and repeat chest roentgenograms performed to document clearing of the pulmonary infiltrate. A total serum IgE level should also be obtained. An approximate 35 percent decline from the pretreatment value is expected. Total IgE values may remain elevated for a prolonged period once treatment is terminated and the exacerbation has resolved. Repeat measurements should be done monthly for approximately 1 year after treatment; afterwards, the interval between testing can be increased.

Antifungal agents have not been shown to be an effective treatment for ABPA. A recent randomized double-blind, placebo-controlled study demonstrated no efficacy for the nebulized antifungal agent natamycin, either as a steroid-sparing agent or for controlling disease activity in patients with ABPA [14]. When effective anti-*Aspergillus* agents become available and can be taken with minimal risk of toxicity, they may have a role in the care of ABPA patients. It should be remembered that most ABPA patients can be managed with alternate-day prednisone or no prednisone after initial control of the disease is achieved. Prednisone can be tapered and discontinued when remission occurs.

The effective treatment of ABPA depends on early recognition to avoid lung damage (Fig. 49-4). Experience suggests that therapy with oral corticosteroids can prevent progression to end-stage lung disease. The diagnosis of ABPA requires a high index of suspicion. A clue to diagnosis is when a patient with asthma that was previously well controlled becomes unresponsive to the usual medications. In addition, we believe ABPA should be considered and excluded in all patients with chronic asthma. An initial screening test that can be done is to determine immediate cutaneous reactivity to *Aspergillus*. A positive test requires further evaluation, including serologic studies (total IgE, IgG-Af, and IgE-Af) and chest radiography. A negative test excludes ABPA, but not an allergic bronchopulmonary fungosis.

It is hoped that in vitro testing will be improved and be of value in differentiating the patient with asthma, exhibiting anti-*Aspergillus* IgE as demonstrated by immediate-type cutaneous testing and no ABPA, from cases of ABPA. Commercially available in vitro tests can identify anti-*Aspergillus* IgE, compared against sera from nonatopic subjects, but are unable to differentiate levels of anti-*Aspergillus* IgE that distinguish atopic asthma from ABPA. In vitro testing should be helped by the identification of specific molecular-weight bands of *A. fumigatus* that IgE, IgG, or

IgA antibodies are directed against during acute exacerbations of ABPA [6]. Extension of enzyme immunoassays and use of immunoblotting should be of diagnostic value. However, their practical value on a commercial basis remains to be established. Physicians using various laboratories should be aware that false negative serologic tests for ABPA occur, and positive sera from established cases of ABPA should be used as positive controls in any diagnostic laboratory carrying out assays for ABPA.

An increased clinical awareness of ABPA has permitted earlier diagnosis and corticosteroid treatment. Such therapy in new-onset cases seems to prevent emergence of Stage V ABPA. Patients in Stage V disease may still be helped by chest percussion and drainage, antibiotics, prednisone, other antiasthma medications, and oxygen supplementation.

REFERENCES

1. Ando, M., et al. Serotype-related antigen of *Trichosporon cutaneum* in the induction of summer-type hypersensitivity pneumonitis: correlation between serotype of inhalation challenge-positive antigen and that of isolates from patients' homes. *J. Allergy Clin. Immunol.* 85:36, 1990.
2. Apter, A. J., et al. Fluctuation of serum IgA and its subclasses in allergic bronchopulmonary aspergillosis. *J. Allergy Clin. Immunol.* 84:367, 1989.
3. Avila, R., and Villar, T. G. Suberosis respiratory disease in cork workers. *Lancet* 1:620, 1968.
4. Banaszak, E. F., Thiede, W. H., and Fink, J. N. Hypersensitivity pneumonitis due to contamination of an air conditioner. *N. Engl. J. Med.* 283:27, 1970.
5. Bardana, E. J., et al. The general and specific humoral immune response to pulmonary aspergillosis. *Am. Rev. Respir. Dis.* 112:799, 1975.
6. Bernstein, J. A., et al. Immunoblot analysis of sera from patients with allergic bronchopulmonary aspergillosis: correlation with disease activity. *J. Allergy Clin. Immunol.* 86:532, 1990.
7. Bosken, C. H., et al. Pathologic features of allergic bronchopulmonary aspergillosis. *Am. J. Surg. Pathol.* 12:216, 1988.
8. Braun, S. R., et al. Farmer's lung disease: long term clinical and physiologic outcome. *Am. Rev. Respir. Dis.* 119:185, 1979.
9. Brueton, M. J., et al. Allergic bronchopulmonary aspergillosis complicating cystic fibrosis in childhood. *Arch. Dis. Child.* 55:348, 1980.
10. Brummond, W., et al. *Aspergillus fumigatus*–specific antibodies in allergic bronchopulmonary aspergillosis and aspergilloma: evidence for a polyclonal antibody response. *J. Clin. Microbiol.* 25:5, 1987.
11. Calvanico, N. J., et al. Immunoglobulin levels in bronchoalveolar lavage fluid from pigeon breeders. *J. Lab. Clin. Med.* 96:129, 1980.
12. Chandler, M. J., Grammer, L. C., and Patterson, R. Eosinophilic vasculitis with atypical features. *J. Allergy Clin. Immunol.* 77:741, 1986.
13. Cormier, Y., et al. Abnormal bronchoalveolar lavage in asymptomatic dairy farmers: study of lymphocytes. *Am. Rev. Respir. Dis.* 130:1046, 1984.
14. Currie, D. L., et al. Controlled trial of natamycin in the treatment of allergic bronchopulmonary aspergillosis. *Thorax* 45:447, 1990.
15. deGracia, J., et al. Time of exposure as a prognostic factor in avian hypersensitivity pneumonitis. *Respir. Med.* 83:139, 1989.
16. Dykewicz, M. S., et al. Woodman's disease: hypersensitivity pneumonitis from cutting live trees. *J. Allergy Clin. Immunol.* 81:455, 1988.
17. Emanuel, D. A., Wenzel, F. J., and Lawton, B. R. Pneumonitis due to *Cryptostroma corticale* (maple bark disease). *N. Engl. J. Med.* 244:1413, 1966.
18. Feanny, S., et al. Allergic bronchopulmonary aspergillosis in cystic fibrosis: a secretory immune response to a colonizing organism. *Ann. Allergy* 60:221, 1988.
19. Fink, T. N. Hypersensitivity pneumonitis. *J. Allergy Clin. Immunol.* 74:1, 1984.
20. Fink, J. N., Moore, V. L., and Barboriak, J. J. Cell-mediated hypersensitivity in pigeon breeders. *Int. Arch. Allergy Appl. Immunol.* 49:831, 1975.
21. Fink, J. N., and Schlueter, D. P. Bathtub finisher's lung: an unusual response to toluene diisocyanate. *Am. Rev. Respir. Dis.* 118:955, 1978.
22. Fink, J. N., et al. Pigeon breeders' disease: a clinical study of hypersensitivity pneumonitis. *Ann. Intern. Med.* 68:1205, 1968.
23. Fisher, M. R., et al. Use of linear tomography to confirm the diagnosis of allergic bronchopulmonary aspergillosis. *Chest* 87:499, 1985.
24. Forsyth, K. D., et al. IgG antibodies to *Aspergillus fumigatus* in cystic fibrosis: a laboratory correlate of disease activity. *Arch. Dis. Child.* 63:953, 1988.

25. Ganz, M. A., et al. Allergic bronchopulmonary aspergillosis: serologic and clinical correlates in patients with normal chest tomography (abstract). *J. Allergy Clin. Immunol.* 87(No. 1, part 2):140, 1991.

26. Gilbert, J., and Littlewood, J. M. Enteric coated prednisolone in cystic fibrosis. *Lancet* 2:1167, 1986.

27. Golbert, T. M., and Patterson, R. Pulmonary allergic aspergillosis. *Ann. Intern. Med.* 72:395, 1970.

28. Grammer, L. C., Greenberger, P. A., and Patterson, R. Allergic bronchopulmonary aspergillosis in asthmatic patients presenting with allergic rhinitis. *Int. Arch. Allergy Appl. Immunol.* 79:246, 1986.

29. Grammer, L. C., et al. Clinical and serologic follow-up of four children and five adults with bird-fancier's lung. *J. Allergy Clin. Immunol.* 85:655, 1990.

30. Greenberger, P. A. Allergic bronchopulmonary aspergillosis and fungoses. *Clin. Chest Med.* 9:599, 1988.

31. Greenberger, P. A., Liotta, J. L., and Roberts, M. The effects of age on isotypic antibody responses to *Aspergillus fumigatus:* implications regarding *in vitro* measurements. *J. Lab. Clin. Med.* 114:278, 1989.

32. Greenberger, P. A., and Patterson, R. Application of an enzyme-linked immunosorbent assay (ELISA) in diagnosis of allergic bronchopulmonary aspergillosis. *J. Lab. Clin. Med.* 99:288, 1982.

33. Greenberger, P. A., and Patterson, R. Diagnosis and management of allergic bronchopulmonary aspergillosis. *Ann. Allergy* 56:444, 1986.

34. Greenberger, P. A., et al. Late sequelae of allergic bronchopulmonary aspergillosis. *J. Allergy Clin. Immunol.* 66:327, 1980.

35. Greenberger, P. A., et al. Analysis of bronchoalveolar lavage in allergic bronchopulmonary aspergillosis: divergent responses of antigen-specific antibodies and total IgE. *J. Allergy Clin. Immunol.* 82:164, 1988.

36. Greenberger, P. A., et al. End-stage lung and ultimately fatal disease in a bird fancier. *Am. J. Med.* 86:119, 1989.

37. Grenier, P., et al. Bronchiectasis: assessment by thin layer CT. *Radiology* 161:95, 1986.

38. Halwig, J. M., et al. Recurrence of allergic bronchopulmonary aspergillosis after seven years of remission. *J. Allergy Clin. Immunol.* 74:738, 1984.

39. Halwig, M. J., et al. Allergic bronchopulmonary curvulariosis. *Am. Rev. Respir. Dis.* 132:186, 1985.

40. Hansen, P. F., and Penny, R. Pigeon breeder's disease: study of the cell-mediated immune response to pigeon antigens by the lymphocyte culture technique. *Int. Arch. Allergy Appl. Immunol.* 47:498, 1974.

41. Hapke, E. J., et al. Farmer's lung. A clinical, radiographic, functional and serological correlation of acute and chronic stages. *Thorax* 23:451, 1968.

42. Henderson, A. H. Allergic aspergillosis: review of 32 cases. *Thorax* 23:501, 1968.

43. Henderson, A. H., English, M. P., and Vecht, R. J. Pulmonary aspergillosis. A survey of its occurrence in patients with chronic lung disease and a discussion of the significance of diagnosis. *Thorax* 23:513, 1968.

44. Hendrick, D. J., et al. An analysis of skin prick test reaction in 656 asthmatic patients. *Thorax* 30(Suppl.):2, 1975.

45. Hensley, G. T., et al. Lung biopsies of pigeon breeder's disease. *Arch. Pathol.* 87:572, 1969.

46. Higgens, T., and Niklasson, P. M. Hypersensitivity pneumonitis induced by trimethoprim. *Br. Med. J.* 300:1344, 1990.

47. Hinson, K. F. W., Moon, A. J., and Plummer, N. S. Bronchopulmonary aspergillosis: a review and a report of eight new cases. *Thorax* 7:317, 1952.

48. Imbeau, S. A., Cohen, M., and Reed, C. E. Allergic bronchopulmonary aspergillosis in infants. *Am. J. Dis. Child.* 131:1127, 1977.

49. Kauffman, H. F., et al. Immunologic observations in sera of a patient with allergic bronchopulmonary aspergillosis by means of the enzyme-linked immunosorbent assay. *J. Allergy Clin. Immunol.* 74:741, 1984.

50. Keller, R. H., et al. Immunoregulation in hypersensitivity pneumonitis: phenotypic and functional studies of bronchoalveolar lavage lymphocytes. *Am. Rev. Respir. Dis.* 130:776, 1984.

51. Kiefer, T. A., et al. Allergic bronchopulmonary aspergillosis in a young child: diagnostic confirmation by serum IgE and IgG indices. *Ann. Allergy* 56:233, 1986.

52. Knutsen, A. P., and Slavin, R. G. *In vitro* T cell responses in patients with cystic fibrosis and allergic bronchopulmonary aspergillosis. *J. Lab. Clin. Med.* 113:428, 1989.

53. Knutsen, A. P., et al. T and B cell dysregulation of IgE synthesis in cystic fibrosis patients with allergic bronchopulmonary aspergillosis. *Clin. Immunol. Immunopathol.* 55:129, 1990.

54. Kramer, M. N., Kurup, V. P., and Fink, J. N. Allergic bronchopulmonary aspergillosis from a contaminated dump site. *Am. Rev. Respir. Dis.* 140:1086, 1989.

55. Kurup, V. P., et al. Antibody isotype responses in *Aspergillus*-induced disease. *J. Lab. Clin. Med.* 115:290, 1990.

55a. Lake, F. R., et al. Allergic bronchopulmonary fungal disease caused by *Bipolaris* and *Curvularia*. *Aust. N. Z. J. Med.* 21:871, 1991.

56. Lee, T. M., et al. Allergic bronchopulmonary candidiasis: case report and suggested diagnostic criteria. *J. Allergy Clin. Immunol.* 80:816, 1987.

57. Lee, T. M., et al. Stage V (fibrotic) allergic bronchopulmonary aspergillosis. *Arch. Intern. Med.* 147:319, 1987.

58. Mahon, W. E., et al. Hypersensitivity to pituitary snuff with miliary shadowing in the lungs. *Thorax* 22:13, 1967.

59. Malo, J. L., and Zeiss, C. R. Occupational hypersensitivity pneumonitis after exposure to diphenylmethane diisocyanate. *Am. Rev. Respir. Dis.* 125:13, 1985.

60. Martin, W. J. Mechanisms of amiodarone pulmonary toxicity. *Clin. Chest Med.* 11(1):131, 1990.

61. McCarthy, D. S., and Pepys, J. Allergic bronchopulmonary aspergillosis. Clinical immunology: (1) Clinical features. *Clin. Allergy* 1:261, 1971.

62. McCarthy, O. S., and Pepys, J. Allergic bronchopulmonary aspergillosis. Clinical immunology: (2) Skin, nasal and bronchial tests. *Clin. Allergy* 1:415, 1971.

63. McCarthy, D. S., Simon, G., and Hargreave, F. E. The radiological appearances in allergic bronchopulmonary aspergillosis. *Clin. Radiol.* 21:366, 1970.

64. Mearns, M., Longbottom, J., and Batten, J. Precipitating antibodies to *Aspergillus fumigatus* in cystic fibrosis. *Lancet* 1:538, 1987.

65. Mearns, M., Young, W., and Batten, J. Transient pulmonary infiltrations in cystic fibrosis due to allergic aspergillosis. *Thorax* 20:385, 1965.

66. Mintzer, R. A., et al. The spectrum of radiographic findings in allergic bronchopulmonary aspergillosis. *J. Allergy Clin. Immunol.* 127:301, 1978.

67. Moore, U. L., et al. Immunologic events in pigeon breeder's disease. *J. Allergy Clin. Immunol.* 53:319, 1974.

68. Naidich, D. P., et al. Basilar segmental bronchi: thin section CT evaluation. *Radiology* 120:244, 1988.

69. Neeld, D. A., et al. Computerized tomography in the evaluation of allergic bronchopulmonary aspergillosis. *Am. Rev. Respir. Dis.* 142:1200, 1990.

70. Nichols, D., et al. Acute and chronic pulmonary function changes in allergic bronchopulmonary aspergillosis. *Am. J. Med.* 67:631, 1979.

71. Orriols, R., et al. Mollusk shell hypersensitivity pneumonitis. *Ann. Intern. Med.* 113:80, 1990.

72. Patterson, R., Ganz, M. A., and Roberts, M. Anaphylaxis and asthma in a scrimshander due to inhalation of deer bone dust. *Ann. Allergy* 67(suppl.):529, 1991.

73. Patterson, R., and Golbert, T. M. Hypersensitivity disease of the lung. *Univ. Mich. Med. Center J.* 34:8, 1968.

74. Patterson, R., Rosenberg, M., and Roberts, M. Evidence that *Aspergillus fumigatus* growing in the airway of man can be a potent stimulus of specific and nonspecific IgE formation. *Am. J. Med.* 63:257, 1977.

75. Patterson, R., et al. Serum immunoglobulin levels in pulmonary allergic aspergillosis and certain other lung diseases, with special reference to immunoglobulin E. *Am. J. Med.* 54:16, 1973.

76. Patterson, R., et al. IgA and IgG antibody activities of serum and bronchoalveolar lavage fluids from symptomatic and asymptomatic pigeon breeders. *Am. Rev. Respir. Dis.* 120:1113, 1979.

77. Patterson, R., et al. Allergic bronchopulmonary aspergillosis: staging as an aid to management. *Ann. Intern. Med.* 96:286, 1982.

78. Patterson, R., et al. A radioimmunoassay index for allergic bronchopulmonary aspergillosis. *Ann. Intern. Med.* 99:18, 1983.

79. Patterson, R., et al. Allergic bronchopulmonary aspergillosis. Natural history and classification of early disease by serologic and roentgenographic studies. *Arch. Intern. Med.* 146:916, 1988.

80. Pepys, J. Hypersensitivity diseases of the lung due to fungi and organic dusts. *Monogr. Allergy* 4:69, 1969.

81. Radin, R. C., et al. Mold counts and exacerbations of allergic bronchopulmonary aspergillosis. *Clin. Allergy* 13:271, 1983.

82. Raper, K. R., and Fennell, D. I. *The Genus Aspergillus.* Huntington, NY: Robert E. Krieger Publishing Co., 1973.

83. Reed, C. E., Sosman, A. J., and Barbee, R. A. Pigeon breeder's lung. *JAMA* 193:261, 1965.

84. Reyes, C. N., et al. The pulmonary pathology of farmer's lung disease. *Chest* 81:142, 1982.

85. Reynolds, H. Y. Immunologic lung disease. *Chest* 81:745, 1982.

86. Reynolds, H. Y., et al. Analysis of cellular and protein content of bronchoalveolar lavage fluid from patients with idiopathic pulmonary fibrosis and chronic hypersensitivity pneumonitis. *J. Clin. Invest.* 59:165, 1977.

87. Ricketti, A. J., Greenberger, P. A., and Glassroth, J. Spontaneous pneumo-

thorax in allergic bronchopulmonary aspergillosis. *Arch. Intern. Med.* 144:151, 1984.

88. Ricketti, A. J., Greenberger, P. A., and Patterson, R. Immediate-type reactions in patients with allergic bronchopulmonary aspergillosis. *J. Allergy Clin. Immunol.* 71:541, 1983.

89. Ricketti, A. J., Greenberger, P. A., and Patterson, R. Varying presentations of ABPA. *Int. Arch. Allergy Appl. Immunol.* 73:283, 1984.

90. Ricketti, A. J., et al. Hyperactivity of mediator-releasing cells from patients with allergic bronchopulmonary aspergillosis as evidenced by basophil histamine release. *J. Allergy Clin. Immunol.* 72:386, 1983.

91. Riley, D. J., and Saldana, M. Pigeon breeder's lung. Subacute course and the importance of indirect exposure. *Am. Rev. Respir. Dis.* 107:456, 1973.

92. Rosenberg, M., Patterson, R., and Roberts, M. Immunologic responses to therapy in allergic bronchopulmonary aspergillosis: serum IgE values as an indicator and predictor of disease activity. *J. Pediatr.* 91:914, 1977.

93. Rosenberg, M., et al. Allergic bronchopulmonary aspergillosis in three patients with normal chest x-ray films. *Chest* 72:597, 1977.

94. Rosenberg, M., et al. Clinical and immunologic criteria for the diagnosis of allergic bronchopulmonary aspergillosis. *Ann. Intern. Med.* 86:405, 1977.

95. Rosenberg, M., et al. The assessment of immunologic and clinical changes occurring during corticosteroid therapy for allergic bronchopulmonary aspergillosis. *Ann. Intern. Med.* 99:18, 1983.

96. Salvaggio, J. E. Hypersensitivity pneumonitis. *J. Allergy Clin. Immunol.* 74(4):558, 1987.

97. Salvaggio, J. E., and deShazo, R. D. Pathogenesis of hypersensitivity pneumonitis. *Chest* 89:1905, 1986.

98. Savage, A., and Isa, J. M. A note on mycotic pneumonia of chickens. *Sci. Agri.* 13:341, 1933.

99. Scadding, J. G. The bronchi in allergic aspergillosis. *Scand. J. Respir. Dis.* 48:372, 1967.

100. Schleuter, D. P. Response of the lung to inhaled antigens. *Am. J. Med.* 57:476, 1974.

101. Schlueter, D. P., Fink, J. N., and Hensley, G. T. Wood pulp workers' disease: a hypersensitivity pneumonitis caused by *Alternaria*. *Ann. Intern. Med.* 77:907, 1972.

102. Schlueter, D. P., Fink, J. N., and Sosman, A. J. Pulmonary function in pigeon breeder's disease: a hypersensitivity pneumonitis. *Ann. Intern. Med.* 70:457, 1969.

103. Schlueter, D. P., et al. Occupational asthma due to tetrachlorophthalic anhydride. *J. Occup. Med.* 20:183, 1978.

104. Sebostina-Domingo, J. J., et al. Hypersensitivity pneumonitis by sulphasalazine (letter). *Allergy* 44:522, 1989.

105. Semenzato, G., and Trentin, L. Cellular immune responses in the lung of hypersensitivity pneumonitis. *Eur. Respir. J.* 3:357, 1990.

106. Silver, S. F., et al. Hypersensitivity pneumonitis: evaluation with CT. *Radiology* 173:441, 1989.

107. Simmonds, E. J., Littlewood, J. M., and Evans, E. G. U. Cystic fibrosis and allergic bronchopulmonary aspergillosis. *Arch. Dis. Child.* 65:507, 1990.

108. Slavin, R. G., et al. A primate model of allergic bronchopulmonary aspergillosis. *Int. Arch. Allergy Appl. Immunol.* 56:325, 1978.

109. Slavin, R. G., et al. A pathologic study of allergic bronchopulmonary aspergillosis. *J. Allergy Clin. Immunol.* 81:718, 1988.

110. Solomon, W. R., Burge, H. P., and Roise, J. R. Airborne *Aspergillus fumigatus* levels outside and within a large clinical center. *J. Allergy Clin. Immunol.* 62:56, 1978.

111. Takizawa, H., et al. Mast cells are important in the development of hypersensitivity pneumonitis. A study with mast-cell deficient mice. *J. Immunol.* 143(6):1982, 1989.

112. Travis, W. D., et al. Hypersensitivity pneumonitis and pulmonary vasculitis with eosinophilia in a patient taking an L-tryptophan preparation. *Ann. Intern. Med.* 112:301, 1990.

113. Trentin, L., et al. Mechanisms accounting for lymphocytic alveolitis in hypersensitivity pneumonitis. *J. Immunol.* 145(7):2147, 1990.

114. Turner, E. S., Greenberger, P. A., and Sider, L. Complexities of establishing an early diagnosis of allergic bronchopulmonary aspergillosis in children. *Allergy Proc.* 10:63, 1989.

115. Utell, M., and Samet, J. Environmentally mediated disorders of the respiratory tract. *Environ. Med.* 74:291, 1990.

116. Van Asserdelft, A. L. T., Raitio, M., and Turkia, V. Fuel-chip induced hypersensitivity pneumonitis caused by *Penicillium* species. *Chest* 87:394, 1985.

117. Walker, C. A., et al. Lymphocyte sensitization to *Aspergillus fumigatus* in allergic bronchopulmonary aspergillosis. *Clin. Exp. Immunol.* 76:34, 1989.

118. Wang, J. L. F., et al. Serum IgE and IgG antibody activity against *Aspergillus fumigatus* as a diagnostic aid in allergic bronchopulmonary aspergillosis. *Am. Rev. Respir. Dis.* 117:917, 1978.

119. Wenzel, F. J., Emanual, P. A., and Gray, R. L. Immunofluorescent studies in patients with farmer's lung. *J. Allergy Clin. Immunol.* 48:224, 1971.

120. Wimander, K., and Belin, L. Recognition of allergic alveolitis in the trimming department of a Swedish sawmill. *Eur. J. Respir. Dis.* 61(107):163, 1980.

121. Witter, J. F., and Chute, H. L. Aspergillosis in turkeys. *J. Am. Vet. Med. Assoc.* 121:387, 1952.

122. Yoshida, K., et al. Hypersensitivity pneumonitis in a mushroom worker due to *Aspergillus glaucus*. *Arch. Environ. Health* 45(4):245, 1990.

123. Zeaske, R., et al. Immune responses to *Aspergillus* in cystic fibrosis. *J. Allergy Clin. Immunol.* 82:73, 1988.

124. Zeiss, C. R., et al. Trimellitic anhydride-induced airway syndromes: clinical and immunologic studies. *J. Allergy Clin. Immunol.* 60:96, 1977.

125. Zeiss, C. R., et al. A twelve year clinical and immunologic evaluation of workers involved in the manufacture of trimellitic anhydride. *Allergy Proc.* 11(2):71, 1990.

126. Zitnik, R. J., and Cooper, J. A. D. Pulmonary disease due to antirheumatic agents. *Clin. Chest Med.* 11:139, 1990.

127. Kokkarinen, J. I., Tukiainen, H. O., and Terho, E. O. Effect of corticosteroid treatment on the recovery of pulmonary function in farmer's lung. *Am. Rev. Respir. Dis.* 145:3, 1992.

Cough Variant Asthma

Henry Milgrom

Cough is a defense mechanism whose function is to protect against the aspiration of noxious materials into the lungs and to clear the respiratory tract [65]. It is associated with bronchoconstriction and mucus secretion, two processes that enhance its effectiveness [89]. Cough is a reflex whose main afferent pathways, like those of bronchoconstriction, originate in the nerve receptors that lie immediately beneath the respiratory epithelium in the larynx and the tracheobronchial tree, and in extrapulmonary sites: the nose; the paranasal sinuses; the pharynx, ear canals, and ear drums; the pleura; the stomach; the pericardium; and the diaphragm [57]. Nerve impulses that originate in the tracheobronchial tree travel through the vagus nerve, the main afferent pathway for cough [8, 59, 89] (Fig. 50-1). The trigeminal, glossopharyngeal, and phrenic nerves also serve as afferent pathways [57]. Cough is most likely to result from the stimulation of receptors localized in the larynx and proximal airways, while bronchoconstriction can be triggered from the lower airways as well [59]. Cough is an effective clearance mechanism only at high lung volumes [48] because sufficient air velocity to shear mucus from bronchial walls can be achieved only down to the sixth or seventh generation of airway branching [64]. Bronchoconstriction enhances the intensity of the cough reflex [72, 89] and peripherally extends the region of high air velocity and turbulent airflow [59].

It has been shown in animals that physical irritation of the conducting airways [73] or the inhalation of dust [90] or sulfur dioxide [74] stimulates cough and also causes bronchoconstriction. Similar results can be achieved by inhalation challenge or rapid respiratory maneuvers in patients with asthma or chronic bronchitis [85]. Bronchoconstriction, but not the urge to cough, that is induced by these measures can be blocked by pretreatment with intravenous atropine [85]. This is consistent with the view that cholinergic pathways are involved in the efferent limb of reflex bronchoconstriction. In addition, axon reflexes conducted along the branches of sensory end-organs may result in the release of neuropeptides and subsequent smooth muscle contraction, mucus secretion, and epithelial injury [89]. Thus, sensory impulses that trigger or accompany cough may also trigger or enhance bronchospasm [89]. The efferent limb of cough is predominantly autonomic, consisting of recurrent laryngeal, phrenic, and other spinal nerves [57], but it is important to appreciate that the cough reflex is at least partially under voluntary control and may be intensified or suppressed at will [88].

Both cough and bronchoconstriction are provoked by challenge with methacholine or histamine [17]. However, the receptors whose stimulation brings about these reflexes are functionally distinct, and the two reflexes can occur independently [35, 40, 72, 83]. For example, challenge with hyperosmolar solutions causes both cough and bronchoconstriction, but hypoosmolar solutions cause cough alone [35]. Furthermore, induced cough and bronchoconstriction can be distinguished by pretreatment

[41, 83]. When aerosolized water is used as a provoking agent, inhaled lidocaine blocks cough but not bronchoconstriction, while the opposite is true for cromolyn [83]. When inhaled capsaicin is used, cough can be suppressed by opiates administered systemically, while bronchoconstriction is suppressed by opiates administered by inhalation [41]. Moreover, the mechanisms that trigger cough and bronchospasm following exercise or exposure to cold air appear to be different. Cough results from excessive water loss [7], while bronchoconstriction may result from the respiratory loss of heat [24]; cold air-induced bronchoconstriction can be blocked by beta-adrenergic agents, while cough cannot [6]. Thus, cough and bronchospasm are two closely related reflexes that can potentiate one another, but neither depends on the other for its action [29].

Cough is a very common clinical complaint. It is estimated that approximately 12,783,000 office visits in the United States during 1981 were prompted by cough [52], and that as many as 23 percent of nonsmoking adults may have experienced a cough that persisted for a year or longer [5, 91]. The clinical spectrum of chronic cough has changed over the years. Tuberculosis, which had been the leading cause of persistent cough, has been replaced by chronic bronchitis [91]. Current concerns focus on the role of smoking, occupational exposures, and air pollution [91]; clinical conditions such as postnasal drip, asthma, gastroesophageal reflux [56], and viral infection [12, 33, 78]; and iatrogenic factors such as angiotensin-converting enzyme inhibitor therapy [14, 40], all of which are associated with exacerbation of cough, wheezing, and bronchial hyperresponsiveness.

Asthma was defined by the American Thoracic Society in 1962 as [70]

a disease characterized by an increased responsiveness of the trachea and bronchi to various stimuli manifested by a widespread narrowing of the airways that changes in severity either spontaneously or as a result of therapy. Asthma is manifested clinically by episodes of dyspnea, cough and wheezing.

More recently it has been appreciated that asthma is an inflammatory process of the airways that is characterized by the presence of eosinophils and metachromatic cells and the ensuing airway hyperresponsiveness [46] (see Chap. 1). Cough variant asthma may be defined as a presentation of asthma that fulfills all these criteria, in which there is no overt wheezing and cough is the predominant manifestation. It is important to note that there is a poor correlation between the patients' awareness of their symptoms and the degree of airway obstruction which they experience [84]. Thus, pulmonary function abnormalities have been documented in asymptomatic patients [15, 36]. Among the manifestations of asthma, cough may have the distinction of being less subjective than dyspnea or wheezing, and, for this reason, some asthma patients may experience cough alone. The

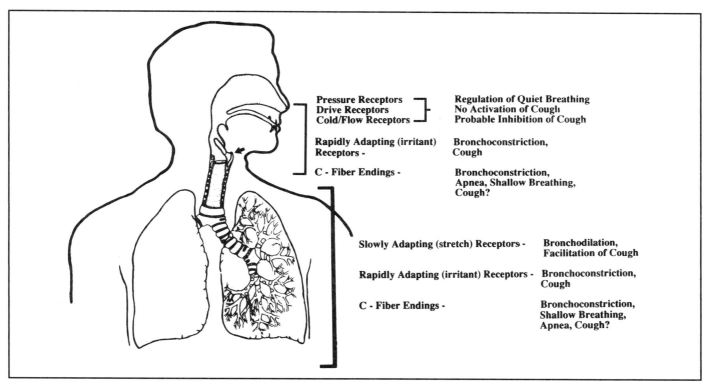

Fig. 50-1. *Vagal afferent nerve receptors involved in the regulation of respiration, cough, and airway tone. (Modified from J.-A. Karlsson, G. Sant-Ambrogio, and J. Widdicombe. Afferent neural pathways in cough and reflex bronchoconstriction. J. Appl. Physiol. 65:1007, 1988.)*

treatment of patients with cough variant asthma is the same as that of all other asthma patients, and it is generally highly effective. Therefore, this diagnosis should be considered in all patients with chronic cough which lasts longer than several weeks.

In 1970, Stanescu and Teculescu [86] reported their observations in a patient whose asthma attacks were initially precipitated by exercise. Subsequent attacks were also caused by cough, either spontaneous or induced, or by respiratory maneuvers requiring high flow rates. The patient was free of symptoms between attacks. His forced expiratory volume in 1 second (FEV_1) was 3.6 liters (92% of predicted), but he had a 19 percent reduction in FEV_1 following exercise, which was prevented by pretreatment with an inhaled beta agonist. His symptoms were eliminated by a week's therapy with oral prednisone. In 1972, Glauser [44] described five patients with paroxysmal nonproductive cough, who did not experience dyspnea or wheezing. Four of the patients had normal findings on examination of the chest, and the fifth manifested localized rhonchi. Three patients had undergone pulmonary function testing, and all showed evidence of airway obstruction with FEV_1 values that, prior to treatment, ranged between 56 and 70 percent of predicted. Treatment with prednisone resulted in the resolution of cough in all five patients.

In 1975, McFadden [69] studied two groups of patients known to have asthma. These patients experienced two to three exacerbations of asthma per year, generally as a result of exposure to a known inciting factor. They required asthma medication intermittently. During the study, they did not experience wheezing, but rather exertional dyspnea or cough. Both groups had airway obstruction that reversed readily after the administration of inhaled isoproterenol. The obstruction in patients with dyspnea as the chief complaint was mainly in the smaller airways, demonstrated by relatively little change in the airway resistance and a marked increase in residual volume. In contrast, patients with cough demonstrated an increase in airway resistance, which

suggested a narrowing located predominantly in the central airways, the site where cough receptors are most abundant [59] (Figs. 50-2 and 50-3).

In 1979, Corrao and colleagues [22] described a group of patients who had chronic cough, but no dyspnea or wheezing. Their baseline spirometry was normal; however, they demonstrated airway hyperresponsiveness following methacholine challenge. All patients experienced improvement after therapy with theophylline or terbutaline, and suffered relapse when the therapy was withdrawn. Two patients later developed overt wheezing. The experience among pediatric patients is similar [19, 45, 62, 75]. Cloutier and Loughlin [19] evaluated 15 children with chronic cough. Ten had normal pulmonary function studies, and minor abnormalities were found in five. Following exercise, all 15 showed exercise-induced bronchospasm. All patients improved after theophylline therapy was instituted. When the theophylline was discontinued, cough recurred in 11 patients. Nine were again studied and found to have recurrence of exercise-induced bronchospasm. Reinstitution of theophylline therapy eliminated cough in these patients. König [62] described 11 children with chronic cough but no wheezing, 10 of whom were old enough to perform an exercise challenge. All showed abnormal results, and all improved when bronchodilator therapy was instituted. Ten patients participated in long-term follow-up, eight of whom suffered attacks of wheezing and dyspnea.

Patients with chronic cough that lasts longer than 4 to 6 weeks require aggressive investigation and treatment [71]. The anatomic approach to the evaluation of chronic cough proposed by Irwin and colleagues [54–56, 77] has been highly successful. It consists of a detailed health history, physical examination, and chest x-ray study. Patients who smoke and those who are exposed to environmental irritants likely to cause coughing do not undergo any additional studies for 4 weeks, while their response to the elimination of the irritants is assessed. If the history, physi-

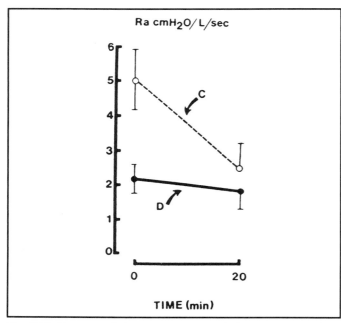

Fig. 50-2. *Response of airway resistance to inhaled isoproterenol. The data points are mean values, and the brackets are 1 standard deviation. The solid line represents the patients with exertional dyspnea (D), and the dotted line, those with cough (C). (Modified from E. R. McFadden. Exertional dyspnea and cough as preludes to acute attacks of bronchial asthma. N. Engl. J. Med. 292:555, 1975.)*

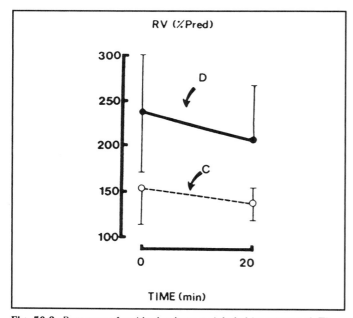

Fig. 50-3. *Response of residual volume to inhaled isoproterenol. The data points are mean values, and the brackets are 1 standard deviation. The solid line represents the patients with exertional dyspnea (D), and the dotted line, those with cough (C). (Modified from E. R. McFadden. Exertional dyspnea and cough as preludes to acute attacks of bronchial asthma. N. Engl. J. Med. 292:555, 1975.)*

cal examination, and chest x-ray findings do not suggest a cause, pulmonary function studies, bronchial challenge, sinus x-ray studies, and allergy evaluation are indicated. Patients whose cause is still uncertain undergo prolonged esophageal pH monitoring because chronic cough may be the sole manifestation of gastroesophageal reflux [58]. Bronchoscopy is of limited value in the evaluation of isolated chronic cough [76], and it is used only in the presence of specific indications. When this approach was instituted in 131 patients, the cause of cough was determined in 99 percent and 24 percent were found to have asthma [56] (Fig. 50-4). It is of note that asthma and conditions commonly associated with it, such as postnasal drip, possibly the result of allergic rhinitis or sinusitis, and gastroesophageal reflux, accounted for 86 percent of the cases of chronic cough. Our own approach is similar; however, we include examination of the vocal cords by fiberoptic rhinolaryngoscopy in the initial evaluation [71]. We have been able to identify a tremor or abnormal adduction of the vocal cords in over 50 percent of the patients (R. P. Wood, et al., unpublished data, 1992). This condition may be analogous to vocal cord dysfunction mimicking or complicating asthma [18] (see Chap. 79). Patients with this condition benefit from breathing exercises [11].

The diagnosis of cough variant asthma can usually be made by documenting a history of episodic cough and reversible airway obstruction. In some patients, especially children, cough may be the only symptom, but the diagnosis of asthma may be confirmed by pulmonary function tests showing reversible airflow obstruction. Some patients may be free of symptoms at the time of their evaluation. In these patients, the history of respiratory disease and physical findings may be difficult to assess, and routine spirometry may not disclose evidence of airway obstruction. In such cases, airway function may be further evaluated by bronchial provocation, usually with methacholine or histamine, to support or exclude the diagnosis of asthma [21, 25, 42, 46]. A definitive diagnosis allows for a more rational use of bronchodilator and steroid therapy [21]. Children with chronic cough benefit from a firm diagnosis because chronic cough is the most common presenting symptom of patients later found to have chronic lung disease [37]. Asthma is the most common diagnosis in these patients [31], but, for reasons that are not clear, many are thought to have chronic bronchitis [87].

The value of bronchial challenge testing, discussed in detail in Chapter 39, is underscored by the fact that the results cannot be predicted accurately. Disagreement between physicians' diagnoses and the results of a methacholine test has been reported in as many as 40 percent of the patients [1], and in epidemiologic studies there has been little correlation between the responses to respiratory questionnaires and airway hyperresponsiveness demonstrated in the pulmonary function laboratory [23, 34, 79]. On the other hand, the results of bronchial challenge studies correlate closely with other indicators of variable airflow obstruction, such as the diurnal variation in peak flow rate [80] and the response of the airways to hyperventilation of cold air or exercise [47], all independent of symptoms [80]. Demonstration of airway hyperresponsiveness is useful to confirm the diagnosis of asthma; however, not all individuals with airway hyperresponsiveness have asthma [68], even when cough is the presenting symptom [13, 20]. Many individuals experience an increase in the reactivity of the airways as a consequence of a viral infection [92]. In one study, nearly 60 percent of the subjects with respiratory symptoms of uncertain etiology showed an abnormal response to histamine challenge [27]. Cockcroft and colleagues [20] reported that airway hyperresponsiveness was present in 47 percent of their patients with cough and no other symptoms, 40 percent with rhinitis and vague chest symptoms, and 22 percent with rhinitis and no chest symptoms at all. Others have shown an increase in the airway responsiveness in patients with rhinitis [30] and those with chronic bronchitis, especially when there is

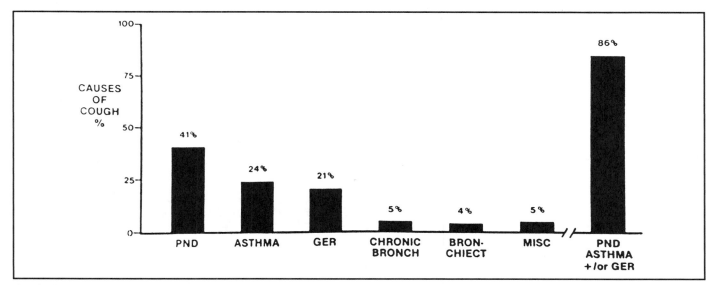

Fig. 50-4. *The causes of chronic cough. The spectrum and frequency of 131 causes of cough were determined in 101 patients. The cause was determined in 99 percent of the patients. The cough was due to a single condition in 73 percent of the patients.* PND = *postnasal drip;* GER = *gastroesophageal reflux;* Bronch = *bronchitis;* Bronchiect = *bronchiectasis;* Misc = *miscellaneous. (Modified from R. S. Irwin, F. J. Curley, and C. L. French. Chronic cough: the spectrum and frequency of causes, key components of the diagnostic evaluation, and outcome of specific therapy. Am. Rev. Respir. Dis. 141:640, 1990.)*

bronchial obstruction [4]. Several studies performed throughout the world have shown that significant numbers of children with airway hyperresponsiveness have no history of asthma [2, 81, 82], although the possibility remains that some of them may develop asthma in the future [53]. In one study, 16 adult patients who presented with chronic cough associated with airway hyperresponsiveness, but no history of wheezing or dyspnea, were evaluated after an interval of 3 to 5 years [13]. All had a good response to bronchodilator therapy. At follow-up, eight no longer experienced cough, did not require bronchodilators, and had a normal response to methacholine challenge. The other eight patients developed typical symptoms of asthma. Thus, a history of cough and presence of airway hyperresponsiveness, although highly suggestive of the diagnosis of cough variant asthma, may not be sufficient to establish this diagnosis. It may be confirmed by the patient's developing unequivocal evidence of reversible airway obstruction later in the clinical course and by his or her response to bronchodilator therapy [13, 21]. A qualification, however, is necessary. Bronchodilators have a beneficial effect on cough that may exceed the degree of bronchodilatation [32, 66], and steroids may have a beneficial effect on cough even in the absence of wheezing or dyspnea, abnormal lung function, or evidence of airway hyperresponsiveness [43].

Bronchial hyperresponsiveness and variable airflow obstruction characteristic of patients with asthma are the result of inflammation [9, 16, 46]. This statement is supported by biopsy [51, 63, 67] and bronchoalveolar lavage [61] studies performed on patients with stable asthma. The eosinophil and eosinophil products play a central role in this process [3, 26, 39], and there is now evidence that it may be initiated by T-lymphocytes [38, 60]. Interestingly, in a recent study of seven children with chronic cough secondary to a lower respiratory tract illness, biopsy specimens obtained from the carina showed evidence of chronic inflammation with a predominance of lymphocytes in all seven. Two patients, both with a reduced FEV_1, had an increased eosinophil count in the respiratory epithelium [49]. These findings are consistent with the hypothesis that the airways of patients with isolated chronic or recurrent cough have undergone morphologic and functional changes comparable to those that occur in

asthma [28]. Furthermore, patients with chronic cough have been reported who show no clinical evidence of asthma or increased airway responsiveness and whose sputum contains eosinophils and metachromatic cells in proportions similar to those of patients with asthma [43]. Thus, inflammatory changes in the airways may result in cough without simultaneously giving rise to hyperresponsiveness.

Studies of the airways of asthmatics show evidence of persistent inflammation [46, 50] (see also Chap. 9). These changes and ensuing airway hyperresponsiveness may be present early in the disease [10] and may precede the development of clinically apparent asthma [53]. Chronic cough may be the first or the sole clinical manifestation of asthma [19, 22, 62]. It may be an important signal of an underlying disease and an indication for evaluation and treatment, based not only on the need for palliative relief but also on an emerging understanding of the inflammatory nature of asthma.

Cough and bronchoconstriction are two important manifestations of asthma. Significantly, both are reflexes that may result from the same stimuli and that share the same afferent pathways. Both may be viewed teleologically as protecting the same structures, and the protective function of cough is enhanced by bronchoconstriction. However, the superimposition is not complete, and areas of dissociation between cough and bronchoconstriction have been identified. In some patients, especially children, cough may be the only symptom of asthma, or it may precede the onset of other symptoms. Spirometry in these patients may reveal unequivocal evidence of airway obstruction and reversibility, or these patients may require bronchial provocation testing to show evidence of airway hyperresponsiveness. Both groups respond to therapy with bronchodilators and corticosteroids. Some aspects of therapy are discussed in Chapter 69.

REFERENCES

1. Adelroth, C., Hargreave, F. E., and Ramsdale, E. H. Do physicians need objective measurements to diagnose asthma? *Am. Rev. Respir. Dis.* 134: 704, 1986.

2. Asher, M. I., et al. International comparison of the prevalence of asthma symptoms and bronchial hyperresponsiveness. *Am. Rev. Respir. Dis.* 138: 524, 1988.

3. Ayars, G. H., et al. Injurious effect of the eosinophil peroxide-hydrogen peroxide-halide system and major basic protein on human nasal epithelium in vitro. *Am. Rev. Respir. Dis.* 140:125, 1989.

4. Bahous, J., et al. Non-allergic bronchial hyperexcitability in chronic bronchitis. *Am. Rev. Respir. Dis.* 129:216, 1984.

5. Banner, A. S. Cough: physiology, evaluation, and treatment. *Lung* 164:79, 1986.

6. Banner, A. S., Chausow, A., and Green, J. The tussive effect of hyperpnea with cold air. *Am. Rev. Respir. Dis.* 131:362, 1985.

7. Banner, A. S., Green, J., and O'Connor, M. Relation of respiratory water loss to coughing after exercise. *N. Engl. J. Med.* 311:833, 1984.

8. Barnes, P. J. Neural control of human airways in health and disease. *Am. Rev. Respir. Dis.* 134:1289, 1986.

9. Barnes, P. J. Allergic inflammatory mediators and bronchial hyperresponsiveness. *Immunol. Allergy Clin. North Am.* 10:241, 1990.

10. Beasley, R., et al. Cellular events in the bronchi in mild asthma and after bronchial provocation. *Am. Rev. Respir. Dis.* 139:806, 1989.

11. Blager, F. B., Gay, M. L., and Wood, R. P. Voice therapy techniques adapted to treatment of habit cough: a pilot study. *J. Commun. Disord.* 21:393, 1988.

12. Braman, S. S., and Corrao, W. M. Cough: differential diagnosis and treatment. *Clin. Chest Med.* 8:177, 1987.

13. Braman, S. S., et al. Cough variant asthma: a 3–5 year followup. *Am. Rev. Respir. Dis.* 125(S):133, 1982.

14. Bucknall, C. E., et al. Bronchial hyperreactivity in patients who cough after receiving angiotensin converting enzyme inhibitors. *Br. Med. J.* 296:86, 1988.

15. Canny, G. J., and Levison, H. Pulmonary function abnormalities during apparent clinical remission in childhood asthma. *J. Allergy Clin. Immunol.* 82:1, 1988.

16. Cartier, A., et al. Allergen-induced increase in bronchial responsiveness to histamine: relationship to the late asthmatic response and change in airway calibre. *J. Allergy Clin. Immunol.* 70:170, 1982.

17. Chausow, A. M., and Banner, A. S. Comparison of the tussive effects of histamine and methacholine in humans. *J. Appl. Physiol.* 55:541, 1983.

18. Christopher, K. L., et al. Vocal cord dysfunction presenting as asthma. *N. Engl. J. Med.* 308:1566, 1983.

19. Cloutier, M. M., and Loughlin, G. M. Chronic cough in children: a manifestation of airway hyperreactivity. *Pediatrics* 67:6, 1981.

20. Cockcroft, D. W., et al. Bronchial reactivity to inhaled histamine: a method and clinical survey. *Clin. Allergy* 7:235, 1977.

21. Corrao, W. M. Methacholine challenge in the evaluation of chronic cough. *Allergy Proc.* 10:313, 1989.

22. Corrao, W. M., Braman, S. S., and Irwin, R. S. Chronic cough as the sole presenting manifestation of bronchial asthma. *N. Engl. J. Med.* 300:633, 1979.

23. Dales, R. E., et al. Prediction of airway reactivity from responses to a standardized respiratory symptom questionnaire. *Am. Rev. Respir. Dis.* 135:817, 1987.

24. Deal, E. C., et al. Role of respiratory heat exchange in production of exercise-induced asthma. *J. Appl. Physiol.* 46:467, 1979.

25. de Benedictis, F. M., Canny, G. J., and Levison, H. Methacholine inhalational challenge in the evaluation of chronic cough in children. *J. Asthma* 23:303, 1986.

26. De Monchy, J. G., et al. Bronchoalveolar eosinophils during allergen-induced late asthmatic reactions. *Am. Rev. Respir. Dis.* 131:373, 1985.

27. Desjardins, A., et al. Non specific bronchial hyperresponsiveness to inhaled histamine and hyperventilation of cold air in individuals with respiratory symptoms of uncertain etiology. *Am. Rev. Respir. Dis.* 137:1020, 1988.

28. Dolovich, J., et al. Early/late response model: implications for control of asthma and chronic cough in children. *Pediatr. Clin. North Am.* 35:969, 1988.

29. Editorial. Cough and wheeze in asthma: are they interdependent? *Lancet* 1:447, 1988.

30. Eggleston, P. A., and Fish, J. E. Upper airway disease and bronchial hyperreactivity. *Clin. Rev. Allergy* 2:429, 1984.

31. Eigen, H., Laughlin, J. J., and Homrighausen, J. Recurrent pneumonia in children and its relationship to bronchial hyperreactivity. *Pediatrics* 70:698, 1982.

32. Ellul-Micallef, R. Effect of terbutaline in chronic "allergic" cough. *Brit. Med. J.* 287:940, 1983.

33. Empey, D. W., et al. Mechanisms of bronchial hyperreactivity in normal subjects after upper respiratory tract infection. *Am. Rev. Respir. Dis.* 113:131, 1976.

34. Enarson, D. A., et al. Predictors of bronchial hyperexcitability in grainhandlers. *Chest* 87:452, 1985.

35. Eschenbacher, W. L., Boushey, H. A., and Sheppard, D. Alteration in osmolarity of inhaled aerosols causes bronchoconstriction and cough, but absence of a permeant anion causes cough alone. *Am. Rev. Respir. Dis.* 129:211, 1984.

36. Ferguson, A. C. Persisting airway obstruction in asymptomatic children with asthma with normal peak expiratory flow rates. *J. Allergy Clin. Immunol.* 82:19, 1988.

37. Fernald, G. W., et al. Chronic lung disease in children referred to a teaching hospital. *Pediatr. Pulmonol.* 2:27, 1986.

38. Frew, A. J., and Kay, A. B. Eosinophils and T-lymphocytes in late-phase allergic reactions. *J. Allergy Clin. Immunol.* 85:533, 1990.

39. Frigas, E., and Gleich, G. J. The eosinophil and the pathophysiology of asthma. *J. Allergy Clin. Immunol.* 77:527, 1986.

40. Fuller, R. W., and Choudry, N. B. Increased cough reflex associated with angiotensin-converting enzyme inhibitor cough. *Br. Med. J.* 295:1025, 1987.

41. Fuller, R. W., et al. Effect of inhaled and systemic opiates on responses to inhaled capsaicin in humans. *J. Appl. Physiol.* 65:1125, 1988.

42. Galvez, R. A., McLaughlin, F. J., and Levison, H. The role of the methacholine challenge in children with chronic cough. *J. Allergy Clin. Immunol.* 79:331, 1987.

43. Gibson, P. G., et al. Chronic cough: eosinophilic bronchitis without asthma. *Lancet* 1:1346, 1989.

44. Glauser, F. L. Variant asthma. *Ann. Allergy* 30:457, 1972.

45. Hannaway, P. J., and Hopper, G. D. K. Cough variant asthma in children. *JAMA* 247:206, 1982.

46. Hargreave, F. E., Gibson, P. G., and Ramsdale, E. H. Airway hyperresponsiveness, airway inflammation, and asthma. *Immunol. Allergy Clin. North Am.* 10:439, 1990.

47. Hargreave, F. E., et al. Inhalation challenge tests and airway responsiveness in man. *Chest* 87(S):202, 1985.

48. Hasani, A., and Pavia, D. Cough as a clearance mechanism. In P. C. Braga and L. Allegra (eds.), *Cough.* New York: Raven Press, 1989, Pp. 39–52.

49. Heino, M., et al. Bronchial epithelial inflammation in children with chronic cough after early lower respiratory tract illness. *Am. Rev. Respir. Dis.* 141:428, 1990.

50. Hogg, J. C. Pathology of Asthma. In P. M. O'Byrne (ed.), *Asthma as an Inflammatory Disease.* New York: Dekker, 1990, Pp. 1–13.

51. Holgate, S. T., et al. Inflammation as the Basis of Asthma. In H. J. Sluiter and R. Vander Lende (eds.), *Bronchitis VI.* Assen: Royal Van Gorcum, 1989. Pp. 163–174.

52. Holinger, L. D. Chronic cough in infants and children. *Laryngoscope* 96:316, 1986.

53. Hopp, R. J., et al. The prevalence of airway reactivity before the development of asthma. *Am. Rev. Respir. Dis.* 141:2, 1990.

54. Irwin, R. S., Corrao, W. M., and Pratter, M. R. Chronic cough in the adult: the spectrum and frequency of causes and successful outcome of specific therapy. *Am. Rev. Respir. Dis.* 123:413, 1981.

55. Irwin, R. S., and Curley, F. J. Is the anatomic, diagnostic work-up of chronic cough not all that it is hacked up to be? *Chest* 95:711, 1989.

56. Irwin, R. S., Curley, F. J., and French, C. L. Chronic cough: the spectrum and frequency of causes, key components of the diagnostic evaluation, and outcome of specific therapy. *Am. Rev. Respir. Dis.* 141:640, 1990.

57. Irwin, R. S., Rosen, M. J., and Braman, S. S. Cough: a comprehensive review. *Arch. Intern. Med.* 137:1186, 1977.

58. Irwin, R. S., et al. Chronic cough as the sole presenting manifestation of gastroesophageal reflux. *Am. Rev. Respir. Dis.* 140:1294, 1989.

59. Karlsson, J.-A., Sant-Ambrogio, G., and Widdicombe, J. Afferent neural pathways in cough and reflex bronchoconstriction. *J. Appl. Physiol.* 65:1007, 1988.

60. Kay, A. B., et al. Cellular Mechanisms. In S. T. Holgate, et al. (eds.), *The Role of Inflammatory Processes in Airway Hyperresponsiveness.* Cambridge, MA: Blackwell Scientific Publications, 1989, Pp. 151–178.

61. Kirby, J. G., et al. Bronchoalveolar cell profiles of asthmatic and non-asthmatic subjects. *Am. Rev. Respir. Dis.* 136:379, 1987.

62. König, P. Hidden asthma in childhood. *Am. J. Dis. Child.* 135:1053, 1981.

63. Laitinen, L. A., et al. Damage of the airway epithelium and bronchial reactivity in patients with asthma. *Am. Rev. Respir. Dis.* 131:599, 1985.

64. Leith, D. E. Cough. *Phys. Ther.* 48:439, 1968.

65. Leith, D. E., et al. Cough. In A. P. Fishman, et al. (eds.), *Handbook of*

Physiology, Section 3: The Respiratory System, Vol. 3, Part 1. Bethesda, MD: American Physiology Society, 1986. Pp. 315–336.

66. Lowry, R., et al. Antitussive properties of inhaled bronchodilators on induced cough. *Chest* 93:1186, 1988.

67. Lozewicz, S., et al. Inflammatory cells in the airways in mild asthma. *Br. Med. J.* 297:1515, 1988.

68. Malo, J.-L., and Tessier, P. Airway Hyperresponsiveness and Asthma. In P. M. O'Byrne (ed.), *Asthma as an Inflammatory Disease*. New York: Dekker, 1990, Pp. 71–102.

69. McFadden, E. R. Exertional dyspnea and cough as preludes to acute attacks of bronchial asthma. *N. Engl. J. Med.* 292:555, 1975.

70. Meneely, G. R., et al. Chronic bronchitis, asthma, and pulmonary emphysema: a statement by the Committee on Diagnostic Standards for Nontuberculous Respiratory Diseases. *Am. Rev. Respir. Dis.* 85:762, 1962.

71. Milgrom, H., et al. Differential diagnosis and management of chronic cough. *Comp. Therapy* 16:46, 1990.

72. Mitsuhashi, M., et al. Hyperresponsiveness of cough receptors in patients with bronchial asthma. *Pediatrics* 75:855, 1985.

73. Nadel, J. A., and Widdicombe, J. G. Reflex effects of upper airway irritation on total lung resistance and blood pressure. *J. Appl. Physiol.* 17:861, 1962.

74. Nadel, J. A., et al. Mechanism of bronchoconstriction during inhalation of sulfur dioxide. *J. Appl. Physiol.* 20:164, 1965.

75. Parks, D. P., et al. Chronic cough in childhood: approach to diagnosis and treatment. *J. Pediatr.* 115:856, 1989.

76. Poe, R. H., et al. Chronic cough: bronchoscopy or pulmonary function testing? *Am. Rev. Respir. Dis.* 126:160, 1982.

77. Poe, R. H., et al. Chronic persistent cough; experience in diagnosis and outcome using an anatomic diagnostic protocol. *Chest* 95:723, 1989.

78. Reisman, J. J., Canny, G. J., and Levison, H. The approach to chronic cough in childhood. *Ann. Allergy* 61:163, 1988.

79. Rijcken, B., et al. The relationship of nonspecific bronchial responsiveness to respiratory symptoms in a random population sample. *Am. Rev. Respir. Dis.* 136:62, 1987.

80. Ryan, G., et al. Bronchial responsiveness to histamine: relationship to diurnal variation of peak flow rate, improvement after bronchodilator and airway calibre. *Thorax* 37:423, 1982.

81. Salome, C. M., et al. Bronchial hyperresponsiveness in two populations of Australian school-children. I. Relation to respiratory symptoms and diagnosed asthma. *Clin. Allergy* 17:271, 1987.

82. Sears, M. R., et al. Prevalence of bronchial reactivity to inhaled methacholine in New Zealand children. *Thorax* 41:283, 1986.

83. Sheppard, D., et al. Mechanism of cough and bronchoconstriction induced by distilled water aerosol. *Am. Rev. Respir. Dis.* 127:691, 1983.

84. Shim, C. S., and Williams, M. H. Evaluation of the severity of asthma: patients versus physicians. *Am. J. Med.* 68:11, 1980.

85. Simonsson, B. G., Jacobs, F. M., and Nadel, J. A. Role of autonomic nervous system and the cough reflex in the increased responsiveness of airways in patients with obstructive airway disease. *J. Clin. Invest.* 46:1812, 1967.

86. Stanescu, D. C., and Teculescu, D. B. Exercise- and cough-induced asthma. *Respiration* 27:377, 1970.

87. Taussig, L. M., Smith, S. M., and Blumenfeld, R. Chronic bronchitis in childhood: what is it? *Pediatrics* 67:1, 1981.

88. Tomori, Z. Protection and Defense Mechanisms of the Respiratory Tract. In J. Korpas and Z. Tomori (eds.), *Cough and Other Respiratory Reflexes* (Progress in Respiration Research, Vol. 12). Basel: S. Karger, 1979, Pp. 1–14.

89. Widdicombe, J. G. Physiology of Cough. In P. C. Braga and L. Allegra (eds.), *Cough*. New York: Raven Press, 1989, Pp. 3–25.

90. Widdicombe, J. G., Kent, D. C., and Nadel, J. A. Mechanism of bronchoconstriction during inhalation of dust. *J. Appl. Physiol.* 17:613, 1962.

91. Wynder, E. L., Lemon, F. R., and Mantel, N. Epidemiology of persistent cough. *Am. Rev. Respir. Dis.* 91:679, 1961.

92. Zoratti, E. M., and Busse, W. W. The role of respiratory infections in airway responsiveness and the pathogenesis of asthma. *Immunol. Allergy Clin. North Am.* 10:449, 1990.

Wheezing

Robert G. Loudon
Raymond L. H. Murphy, Jr.

51

Wheezing is a hallmark of bronchial asthma. Both as a symptom and a sign, it commonly increases and decreases with exacerbations and remission of the disease. Wheezing is often the first clue to the diagnosis of asthma and frequently plays a key role in monitoring the response to therapy. Yet much is unknown about this phenomenon. The relationship between wheezing and other indices of airway obstruction is unclear. Not all asthmatics wheeze and some who do may have less wheezing during exacerbations. Because of recent technological advances, there has been a resurgence of interest in the study of lung sounds, and a considerable body of new information on wheezing now exists. In this chapter, we will discuss the acoustic characteristics, prevalence, mechanism of production, and clinical correlations of wheezing. This evolving knowledge will be discussed in terms of its potential use in diagnosing and monitoring asthma.

The term *wheeze* is used to refer to a high-pitched musical, adventitious sound that is commonly detected by stethoscope. Wheezing, of course, is also often perceived by patients or by persons in their vicinity. This is particularly relevant in the case of young children, where parents may be the key observers. Using this broad definition, wheezing is common. In a population survey, Dodge and Burrows [3] reported that almost 30 percent of those surveyed gave a history of wheezing of some sort. Among 5,422 children in six cities in the United States, persistent wheezing was reported in from 6.6 to 11.6 percent [19]. Knowledge of the precise prevalence of wheezing, however, depends on its definition. When an asthmatic patient perceives himself or herself to be wheezing, confirmation by stethoscope is usual, but wheezing is also commonly heard by chest auscultation when the patient believes the phenomenon to be absent [18]. Another confounding variable in understanding the prevalence of wheezing is observer variability. While this is a considerable problem in auscultation of the lung in general, it is less so with regard to wheezing. Wheezing was found to be correctly identified by respiratory care practitioners more frequently than were any of the other common lung auscultatory findings [20]. Because variability exists in definition and observer perception, more quantifiable descriptions of wheezing have been sought. In this regard, it is useful to review the physical phenomena underlying wheezing.

ACOUSTIC CHARACTERISTICS

Acoustically, wheezing is classified as a "continuous" adventitious sound (Fig. 51-1). The word *continuous* is used to indicate that the duration of the sound is relatively long compared to that of crackles—the brief, explosive "discontinuous" sounds. Crackles have a duration of 25 msec or less, while wheezes have been defined as lasting 250 msec or more [13]. Sounds of intermediate duration (26–249 msec) have been variously called

squeaks, squawks, or *short wheezes.* Wheezes are easily distinguished from crackles and are usually readily distinguished from rhonchi, the other main type of continuous lung sound. Rhonchi have a perceptibly lower pitch than that of wheezes, are more commonly associated with secretions in the airways, and are seen to have a lower dominant frequency on acoustical analysis. Squeaks appear to have dominant frequencies similar to those of wheezes but few examples have been analyzed to date. Squawks have been described as characteristic of [4] alveolitis, but similar sounds can be heard during exacerbations of asthma.

GRAPHIC DISPLAY

Acoustic phenomena are commonly described in the time domain or the frequency domain, or both. In the time domain, the characteristic undulating pattern of a wheeze is readily distinguished from that of normal sounds or crackles, as seen in Figure 51-2.

The relative value of frequency domain analysis can be seen in Figure 51-3. In Figure 51-3A, the sinusoidal time-amplitude plot is seen in the frequency domain to be composed of a single 300-Hz peak, whereas in Figure 3B this signal is composed of combined waves of 150 and 300 Hz.

To allow analysis of the frequency changes over time that occur commonly in wheezing, short intervals of sound (e.g., 100 to 200 msec) are subjected to spectral analysis sequentially and the results displayed serially, as is seen in Figure 51-4.

An alternative method employs color to depict the relative energy content at specific frequencies over time. This method, termed *digital respirosonography,* is illustrated in Plate 10 which contrasts a normal sound (Plate 10A) with that of an asthmatic (Plate 10B).

The choice of method for graphic display will, of course, depend on the clinical application and the equipment available. Of note, analyses such as these can be readily performed at the bedside using a personal computer. The major point is that wheezing can now be documented precisely in terms of its acoustic features. This and recent advances in computer technology have yielded techniques to monitor for the presence and degree of wheezing over long intervals [2]. With this in mind, let us now consider how a wheeze is generated.

MECHANISM OF PRODUCTION

The major mechanism implicated in the production of wheezes is airway narrowing. In experiments on excised lungs, Forgacs [6] observed that wheezes are produced only when the caliber of the airways is narrowed such that the opposite walls touch one another and the linear velocity of the airstream across the nar-

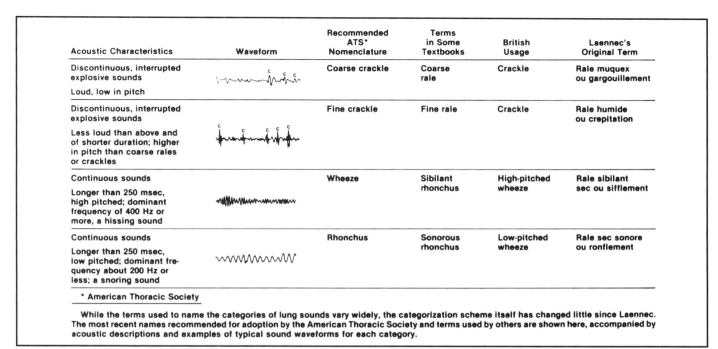

Acoustic Characteristics	Waveform	Recommended ATS* Nomenclature	Terms in Some Textbooks	British Usage	Laennec's Original Term
Discontinuous, interrupted explosive sounds Loud, low in pitch		Coarse crackle	Coarse rale	Crackle	Rale muquex ou gargouillement
Discontinuous, interrupted explosive sounds Less loud than above and of shorter duration; higher in pitch than coarse rales or crackles		Fine crackle	Fine rale	Crackle	Rale humide ou crepitation
Continuous sounds Longer than 250 msec, high pitched; dominant frequency of 400 Hz or more, a hissing sound		Wheeze	Sibilant rhonchus	High-pitched wheeze	Rale sibilant sec ou sifflement
Continuous sounds Longer than 250 msec, low pitched; dominant frequency about 200 Hz or less; a snoring sound		Rhonchus	Sonorous rhonchus	Low-pitched wheeze	Rale sec sonore ou ronflement

* American Thoracic Society

While the terms used to name the categories of lung sounds vary widely, the categorization scheme itself has changed little since Laennec. The most recent names recommended for adoption by the American Thoracic Society and terms used by others are shown here, accompanied by acoustic descriptions and examples of typical sound waveforms for each category.

Fig. 51-1. *Various lung sounds, including their waveform appearance and the nomenclature involved. (Reprinted with permission from R. L. H. Murphy,* A Simplified Introduction to Lung Sounds. *Wellesley Hills, Mass.: Stethophonics.)*

rowed segment reaches a minimal critical velocity. He found that high-pitched musical sounds could be generated by lightly compressing airways of any size. By changing the pressure or the degree of compression of the bronchus, the pitch of the musical note could be varied over more than three octaves. The caliber and thickness of the bronchus chosen for study did not seem to matter. The same range of sounds could be generated from any airway, large or small. He also observed that this pitch is relatively free of gas density. Based on these observations, Forgacs concluded that the pitch of a wheeze reflects the mass, elasticity, and flow velocity through an airway on the point of closure. This pitch does not reflect airway length, as had previously been believed, nor does it reflect airway caliber or the mechanism of closure. Thus it is likely that wheezes occur when air passing through a narrowed airway at high velocity produces a decrease in the gas pressure in the airway at the site of constriction. According to Bernoulli's principle, as the velocity of the gas increases at the constriction, the pressure decreases. If allowed by other forces acting in the airway, collapse will continue progressively until there is substantial resistance and the flow is decreased. Then the internal pressure increases and the lumen enlarges. This alternation of the wall of the airway between almost open and almost closed produces the wheezing noise (Fig. 51-5).

More recently, efforts have been directed toward generating mathematical models to obtain a more fundamental knowledge of wheezing. Grotberg and colleagues [9–11] presented models which assumed that an inviscid and incompressible fluid interacted with a two-dimensional channel possessing flexible walls. Oscillation, presumably of the kind associated with wheezing, could be predicted by these models and related to structural and physiologic models. They stated that for wheeze production both airflow and collapsing walls are required, and that a flutter of airway gas and the airway walls occurs when the airway reaches a critical velocity. Oscillation of the wall rather than of the gas is the dominant mechanism, and the dimensions and physical properties of the gas and walls are such that wheezing, according to their calculations, is most likely to occur in the first five to

seven airway generations. One prediction that arose from these models was that wheezing is always accompanied by flow limitation but that flow limitation is not always accompanied by wheezing. Consonant data have been obtained by Gavriely and associates [8] in physiologic studies of forced expiration carried out in normal subjects, in which the onset of wheezes was associated with a sudden change in transpulmonary pressure. Additional support was obtained by an ingenious series of experiments performed on dried animal lungs [7]. In these experiments, the lung was held at a constant volume by encasement in a plastic carapace with holes drilled in the plastic and the lung surface to provide an isolated lung model in which different flow rates could be produced at a constant lung volume. Wheezing tended to match flow limitation in time of onset. When the lung was frozen to make the airways rigid, the wheeze and the flow limitation were both abolished, only to return when the lung was thawed.

Because of impedance mismatch, higher-frequency sound is poorly transmitted through air-containing fluid. The transmission of wheezing sounds through airways is better than transmission through lung to the surface of the chest wall. This has been demonstrated by the simultaneous recording of sounds with intrabronchial and chest wall microphones. The higher-frequency components heard intrabronchially are attenuated at the chest wall sites [1]. This explains why in many patients wheezing is detected over the trachea but not heard peripherally. This also provides a reason for carefully listening over the trachea in asthmatic patients, as it may be the only site where wheezing can be observed.

While spasm of the bronchial musculature is believed to be the most common cause of wheezing, there are other possible causes, all associated with airway narrowing. These include dynamic airway compression, mucosal edema and thickening, luminal obstruction due to a tumor, foreign body, or mucus plug, and external pressure from a tumor mass. Dynamic compression is believed to be the mechanism responsible for wheezing during a forced expiratory maneuver in normal individuals. It has been

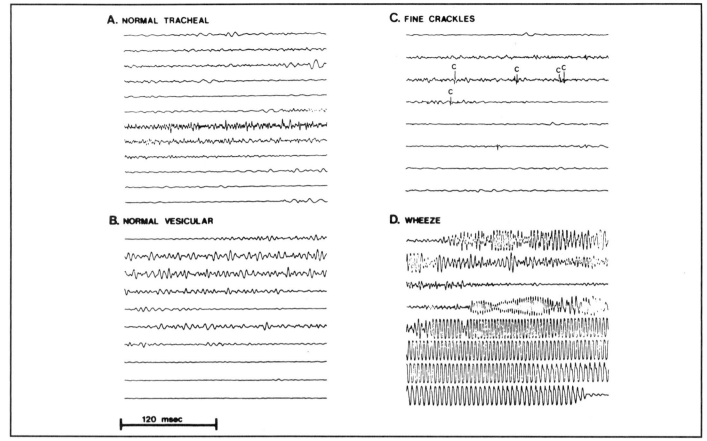

Fig. 51-2. *Time-expanded waveforms of lung sounds. The time-intensity plots in this figure are made from tape recordings of lung sounds stored in a computer memory and then visually displayed on a two-dimensional plot, with amplitude or intensity on the Y axis and time on the X axis. The time axis of the plot is "expanded" or magnified by playing back slowly from the computer memory. A and B illustrate normal tracheal and vesicular sounds. The louder, longer expiratory phase of the tracheal sound is readily recognized, as is the pause between inspiration and expiration. When crackles occur, they produce intermittent ("discontinuous") deflections superimposed on the normal vesicular pattern (C in part C). D shows a "continuous" deflection produced by a wheeze replacing the normal waveform. (Reprinted with permission from R. L. H. Murphy, Auscultation of the lung: past lessons, future possibilities. Thorax 36:99, 1981.)*

suggested that the bronchial hyperresponsiveness occurring in cardiac asthma might result from vasodilation of the bronchial circulation in patients with impaired left ventricular function. Two studies have yielded contradictory evidence, and these were recently reviewed by Fishman [5], who pointed out that further work is necessary before this question can be resolved.

CLINICAL ASSOCIATIONS

Most, but not all, asthmatics wheeze during exacerbations of their illness. The wheezing may be heard over the central airways during expiration in the early stages of the disease, but, as the asthma progresses, wheezing can usually be detected over the entire chest in both phases of respiration. The absence of wheezing in a known asthmatic during an exacerbation is regarded as an ominous sign. It presumably results from mucus plugging or flow rates so low that wheezes are not generated. In our experience, this phenomenon is rare but is important, as it occurs when respiratory failure is imminent.

Wheezing is so commonly associated with bronchial asthma that clinicians have to be reminded of the adage that "all that wheezes is not asthma." Indeed, the rate of wheezing noted in population surveys is often threefold or more higher than the rate of diagnosed asthma [3, 19]. The reason for the high rate of wheezing in such surveys is not clear, but presumably it is most closely related to the prevalence of acute respiratory infection and chronic bronchitis. From the point of view of the clinician, important conditions to be excluded when wheezing is present are generally those, as already noted, that produce airway narrowing. They include upper airway obstruction, cardiac asthma, foreign body or tumor in the airways, and a number of other conditions, including psychogenic stridor and laryngeal dysfunction. Airway obstruction caused by bronchiolitis also tends to be associated with wheezes that are usually brief (see Chap. 37). Chronic bronchitis is commonly associated with wheezing, and usually attributed to the associated airway obstruction.

WHEEZING AND AIRFLOW OBSTRUCTION

The relationship between wheezing and other indices of airflow obstruction is complex. In a study of 83 patients conducted by Marini and colleagues [14], chronic airflow obstruction wheezing scores made during unforced expiratory breathing were independently correlated with the severity of obstruction ($r = 0.42$) and

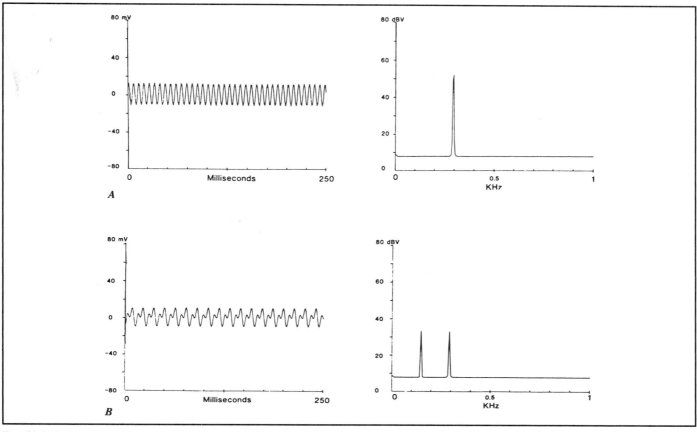

Fig. 51-3. *Continuous adventitious lung sounds. A. Time-amplitude plot and frequency analysis of a 300-Hz sine wave. B. Time-amplitude plot and frequency analysis of a combined sine wave of 160 and 300 Hz. (Reprinted from M. E. Y. Koster, R. P. Baughman, and R. G. Loudon, Continuous adventitious lung sounds. J. Asthma 27:237, 1990. By courtesy of Marcel Dekker, Inc.)*

bronchodilator response (r = 0.46), but these correlations did not permit the consistent prediction of either variable for clinical purposes. The highest wheezing scores, however, were uniformly associated with moderate or severe obstruction. Twenty-nine of 48 patients with wheezing but only 3 of 35 patients without wheezing had a 15 percent or greater improvement in their 1-second forced expiratory volume (FEV_1) after bronchodilator inhalation (p < .001). Eighty of these 83 patients had wheezing on forced expiration, but this bore no relationship to either the degree of obstruction or to the bronchodilator response. An important conclusion was that intense unforced wheezing indicates moderate to severe obstruction; less intense wheezing is associated with a wide range of obstruction.

Shim and Williams [18] examined 93 patients on 320 occasions and noted that the presence of wheezing, either reported by the patients or found on examination, was associated with a significantly lower peak expiratory flow rate (PEFR), but the scatter was great. They noted that biphasic wheezing was associated with a lower PEFR than was expiratory wheezing alone. A high pitch and loudness of wheezing were associated with poorer function. Baughman and coworkers [2] studied 33 outpatient asthmatics who were free of wheeze upon inhalation challenge with histamine or antigen, and noted that about 60 percent of the patients did not exhibit wheezing or dyspnea despite marked obstruction. Both Shim [18] and Baughman [2] and their colleagues concluded that the detection of wheezing by stethoscope was less objective than were pulmonary function studies.

These studies were all based on standard clinical auscultation. Using an objective monitoring device that recorded lung sounds for 30 minutes, Baughman and Loudon [2] noted that the estimated proportion of the breath cycle occupied by wheezing had a good correlation with the FEV_1 (r = 0.893; p < .001). This is important because the correlation was better than any achieved by subjective assessment. This study presents a strong argument for the further development of such noninvasive monitoring devices using automated lung sound analysis.

FUTURE IMPLICATIONS

The acoustic signals arising in the lung that can be detected safely and economically at the surface of the chest are complicated indeed. They vary from breath to breath and from site to site, and not only their production but also their transmission may be affected by changes in the lung. The enormous amount of information provided by lung sounds has been, until recently, impossible to process. New devices and new techniques for recording and analyzing these sounds have been developing quite rapidly in the past two decades, and the relevant information can now be stored, analyzed by signal processing techniques, and graphically displayed for correlation with other clinical indices. Consequently, it is likely that sophisticated tools will soon be available to aid in the diagnosis and monitoring of lung diseases.

Potential applications to aid patients with bronchial asthma include monitoring the duration of action of medications, particularly long-acting medications used to treat nocturnal asthma, and detecting evidence of airway narrowing or mucus plugging in patients unable to undergo pulmonary function testing satis-

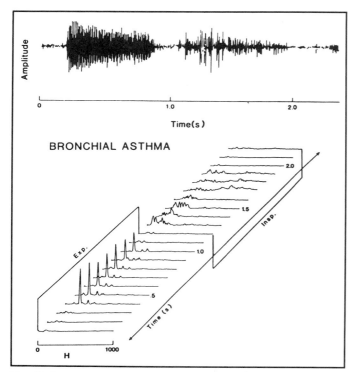

Fig. 51-4. *Time-amplitude plot and frequency analysis of a wheeze recorded in an asthmatic patient. The wheeze is present during a large part of expiration. (Reprinted from M. E. Y. Koster, R. P. Baughman, and R. G. Loudon, Continuous adventitious lung sounds. J. Asthma 27: 237, 1990. By courtesy of Marcel Dekker, Inc.)*

factorily, such as children, the elderly, and patients on mechanical ventilation. In a disease that is by definition variable in its severity and manifestations, and which is influenced by patient activity and by ambient environmental circumstances, it seems likely that monitoring devices will play an important role. Such applications will become more numerous and important as knowledge of the correlation between the acoustic characteristics of wheezing and the pathophysiology of asthma evolves. The technique of histamine challenge in children with asthma analyzed by computerized lung sounds analysis was recently reported [21].

REFERENCES

1. Akasaka, K., et al. Acoustical studies on respiratory sounds in asthmatic patients. *Tohoku J. Exp. Med.* 117:323, 1975.
2. Baughman, R. P., and Loudon, R. G. Lung sound analysis for continuous evaluation of airflow obstruction in asthma. *Chest* 88:364, 1985.
3. Dodge, R. R., and Burrows, B. The prevalence and incidence of asthma and asthma-like symptoms in a general population sample. *Am. Rev. Respir. Dis.* 122:567, 1980.
4. Earis, J. E., et al. The inspiratory "squawk" in extrinsic allergic alveolitis and other pulmonary fibroses. *Thorax* 37:923, 1982.
5. Fishman, A. P. Cardiac asthma—a fresh look at an old wheeze (editorial). *N. Engl. J. Med.* 320(20):1346, 1989.
6. Forgacs, P. Crackles and wheezes. *Lancet* 2:203, 1967.
7. Gavriely, N., and Grotberg, J. B. Flow limitation and wheezes in a constant flow and volume preparation. *J. Appl. Physiol.* 64:17, 1988.
8. Gavriely, N., et al. Forced expiratory wheezes are a manifestation of airway flow limitation. *J. Appl. Physiol.* 62:2398, 1987.
9. Grotberg, J. B., and Davis, S. H. Fluid dynamic flapping of a collapsible channel: sound generation and flow limitation. *J. Biomech.* 13:219, 1980.
10. Grotberg, J. B., and Reiss, E. L. A subsonic flutter anomaly. *J. Sound Vib.* 80:444, 1982.
11. Grotberg, J. B., and Reiss, E. L. Subsonic flapping flutter. *J. Sound Vib.* 92: 349, 1984.
12. Koster, M. E. Y., Baughman, R. P., and Loudon, R. G. Continuous adventitious lung sounds. *J. Asthma* 27(4):237, 1990.
13. Loudon, R., and Murphy, R. L. H. Jr. State of the art: lung sounds. *Am. Rev. Respir. Dis.* 130:663, 1984.
14. Marini, J. J., et al. The significance of wheezing in chronic airflow obstruction. *Am. Rev. Respir. Dis.* 120:1069, 1979.
15. Murphy, R. L. H. Auscultation of the lung: past lessons, future possibilities. *Thorax* 36:99, 1981.
16. Murphy, R. L. H., and Holford, S. Lung sounds. *Basics of RD.* Vol. 4, March 1980.
17. Pasterkamp, H., et al. Digital respirosonography. New images of lung sounds. *Chest* 96:1405, 1989.
18. Shim, O. S., and Williams, H. Relationship of wheezing to the severity of obstruction in asthma. *Arch. Intern. Med.* 143:890, 1983.
19. Speizer, F. E. Asthma and persistent wheeze in the Harvard Six Cities Study. *Chest* 98:191S, 1990.
20. Wilkins, R. L., et al. Lung sound nomenclature survey. *Chest* 98:886, 1990.
21. Beck, R., et al. Histamine challenge in young children using computerized lung sounds analysis. *Chest* 102:759, 1992.

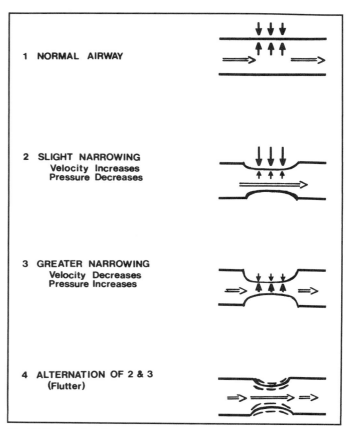

Fig. 51-5. *Postulated wheeze mechanism. The stability of the airway wall depends on a balance between internal air pressure and external forces, and on the mechanical characteristics of the airway itself. When a narrowing of the lumen occurs, the air velocity must increase through the constricted region to maintain a constant mass flow rate. According to the Bernoulli principle, the increased air velocity leads to a decrease in air pressure, thus allowing external forces to further collapse the airway. When the lumen has been reduced so much that the flow decreases, the process begins to reverse itself as the pressure inside the airway begins to increase and reopen the lumen. When conditions are right, the airway wall flutters between nearly occluded and occluded positions and produces wheezing. Short open arrows indicate slower flow; long open arrows indicate faster flow. Large closed arrows indicate higher pressure; small closed arrows indicate lower pressure. (Reprinted with permission from R. L. H. Murphy and S. Holford, Lung sounds. Basics of RD. Vol. 4, March 1980.)*

Sputum

Mauricio J. Dulfano
Sadamu Ishikawa

52

Many of the pathologic changes that characterize bronchial asthma can be recognized, followed, and analyzed upon intelligent observation of the sputum. This material, which is a complex mixture of the secretory activity of a variety of cell types located at different levels within the respiratory tract, is modified by the particular characteristics of a given respiratory disease. Unfortunately, by the time these secretions are expectorated, the sputum has become a heterogeneous mixture from a physicochemical and cytologic point of view, which requires more critical interpretation of the inciting pathologic changes. For example, the topographic site of production, rate of secretion and transport, and adequacy of ventilation may considerably change or age the original secretion. Therefore, there are always significant differences between the secreted mucus and expectorated sputum for clinical examination. These uncertainties create the need for specific technology in the collection, handling, and interpretation of sputum samples according to the specific information desired. For instance, whereas homogenization or concentration methods are perfectly legitimate for purposes of studying the chemistry, cytology, and bacteriology of sputum, they are not appropriate for the study of its rheologic properties; by the same token, even though a 24-hour collection of sputum is acceptable for the study of its chemical properties, it is not the recommended method for evaluating the bacteriology or mycology of a lower respiratory tract acute infection. In any case, a common concern is to obtain a representative sample from the lower respiratory tract and minimize upper passage contamination.

Over the years many different observations have been made on the sputum of asthmatic patients, but only recently have these begun to be sorted into usable patterns. For convenience, this chapter will be considered under five headings: gross appearance, cytology, physical properties, chemical composition, sputum-cilia interaction, and sputum findings in aspiration.

GROSS APPEARANCE

The asthmatic patient usually has great difficulty in expectorating during bronchospastic crises, and the traditional explanation is that the sputum is very scanty, viscid, and composed of mucous plugs. While the difficulty in expectoration is always true, the appearance and volume of the sputum in acute asthma might differ markedly. This was observed by several investigators who noticed in some cases a change in texture and a large volume (bronchorrhea) [49, 75, 81]. Of course these features could not be observed unless patients were followed in a clinical setting where sputum was routinely collected every day. Very frequently asthmatics were literally filling up sputum cups with a cloudy, thin, dirty-looking, opaque expectorate (usually dismissed as "saliva"), which is very tenacious and difficult to raise (Fig. 52-

1). Keal and Reid [50] and Calim [16] describe it as "glairy," and we have called it "slurry" [23]. This material is quite similar to the rhinorrhea of allergic rhinitis, and it can be differentiated from saliva by its histochemical, cellular, and rheologic properties [28]. When freshly expectorated, the material does not adhere to glass and shows few plug aggregates (eosinophilic) floating on a turbid liquid topped by a foam layer. However, when left to stand, the plugs conglomerate and float upwards, giving the sputum a more solid appearance. The functional implications of this type of sputum will be discussed further under the headings Physical Properties and Sputum and Cilia.

EXFOLIATIVE CYTOLOGY AND OTHER PARTICULATES

Observations on the cellular content of respiratory secretions in bronchial asthma go back to the last century, when Bizozzero [7] in 1887 described the Charcot-Leyden crystals in nasal secretions. He called attention to the possible relationship of these crystals to the granules of eosinophils, which were beginning to be recognized at about the same time. Over the years the presence of eosinophils and their association with bronchial asthma have been substantiated. Nevertheless, it took many years until systematic description of the cellular content of sputum in different stages of bronchial asthma (as well as in the differential diagnosis with other bronchopulmonary diseases) started to appear following the earlier work of Bezancon and DeJong [5] and of Von Hoesslin [84]. These efforts were revitalized in 1954, when Papanicolaou [65] described his technique and published the results of exfoliative cytology from different organs. In recent years simplified methods for the study of sputum cytology have been introduced which, along with more quantitative descriptions of cellular events, have greatly enhanced our knowledge of respiratory diseases [19]. The number and relative frequency of different cells that are exudated into the tracheobronchial tree and eventually expectorated as sputum reflect the nature, extent, and severity of various inflammatory or allergic processes taking place in the respiratory tract. Furthermore, the continuous availability of this material allows for repetitive and serial observations of the underlying pathology.

Methodology

Regardless of the method employed, preservation of the cellular structure is essential for interpretation. The best method is to obtain a freshly expectorated sputum sample and immediately examine its cellular content. This method is perfectly adequate if a physician or a trained paraprofessional such as an inhalation therapist or cytologist is present to ascertain that the material obtained is the product of a vigorous deep cough. If that is not

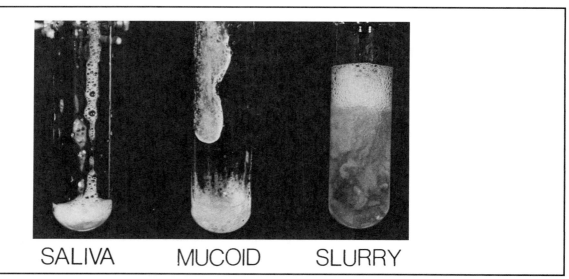

Fig. 52-1. *Saliva and mucoid sputum are both bubbly and transparent, but the latter adheres to the glass wall. The slurry expectorate from acute asthmatics is opaque, nonadherent, and foamy at the top (see text).*

feasible, it is preferable to extend the collection period to include several forced coughs over a period of at least 30 to 60 minutes. Within such periods of time there is no need to add preservatives, and the cell morphology is kept intact within the natural wet environment. If, on the other hand, examination of the sample will be delayed for several hours or more, it is preferable to collect the specimen into a jar containing 70% alcohol/10% buffered formalin, 1:1 volume for 60 minutes, then into 95% ethyl alcohol for 15 minutes, and air dried.

The most critical step in the examination of sputum is the selection of the aliquot. This should start by gross observations of the specimen in a glass container. Usually, one looks for solid particles, plugs, or blood flecks, and basically this is a matter of individual experience. In many cases specimens are sampled by trial and error, and in some laboratories a minimum of two to four selected sputum particles are simultaneously prepared on different slides and the material evenly spread over the entire slide. If the material is to undergo special procedures such as Papanicolaou staining, it is imperative at this step to avoid drying the thin-spread film of sputum because that will quickly alter the morphology of the cells. Thus, as soon as the smear is prepared, the slide is immersed into a fixative mixture of 95% ethyl alcohol and ether, where it is left for at least 1 hour. In this form the sputum can be preserved almost indefinitely, transported, or handled until ready for staining. For differential cell counts, uniformly smeared areas are preferred, and this is carried out best by using an oil immersion objective. Some laboratories are interested not only in the differential counts but also in the quantitative output of each and every cell type [18, 19]. For that purpose it is necessary to obtain 24-hour collections of sputum. This method introduces substantial uncertainty when dealing with a nonhomogenous material such as sputum, because a mistake in the differential count in one single aliquot, when interpreted as representative of 24 hours of output, may magnify a given error into astronomic figures.

Several methods for the observation and identification of the cells in sputum are available. The time-honored examination of unstained specimens is still widely in use. Although the definition of the cells is less precise, it offers the advantage that noncellular structures can simultaneously be seen. This simple technique allows for rapid identification of the general source of the sputum, namely, whether it originates in the lower respiratory tract and/or is highly contaminated by saliva.

An effective unfixed wet preparation is obtained with the addition of aqueous buffered crystal violet [18]. Here an amount of stain equal to the volume of the sputum aliquot is added to the slide and the two gently mixed before the cover slip is replaced on top of the specimen. The presence of the alveolar histiocyte (macrophage) and of ciliated epithelial cells confirms the lower tracheobronchial tree origin of the sputum specimen (Plates 11 and 12). For best results the classic Papanicolaou stain is still the best available method and should be used for final diagnosis [65], particularly in the differentiation of metaplastic or cancer cells. For screening or follow-up, and particularly when one is interested only in a single cell such as the eosinophil in bronchial asthma patients, the Wright's or Hansel stains are very effective yet simple.

Bronchial Epithelial Cells

The cells expectorated by asthmatic patients are derived from two basic sources: (1) the tracheobronchial epithelium shedding bronchial epithelial cells, and (2) the mucosal vascular area and more specifically its reticuloendothelial system (Table 52-1). Shedding of the bronchiolar and bronchial epithelium in chronic bronchial asthma was first described in necropsy specimens by Fraenkel [31] in 1898, and Von Hoesslin referred to them as *epithelialzellballen* [84]. These cells originate in various bronchial epithelial layers from the basal to the columnar mucosa; thus, whereas the nuclei of the epithelial cells remain the same, the cytoplasmic morphology differentiates among them. Typical ciliated bronchial epithelial cells are shown in Plate 12. Bronchial epithelial cells of the nonciliated variety are also often found in sputum; most commonly they belong to the goblet type, an example of which is presented in Plate 13. It must be remembered that bronchial epithelial cells of all varieties are clearly different from the squamous epithelial cell that is characteristic of the upper respiratory tract epithelium (Plate 14). The presence of the latter should alert the observer to the fact that the sputum sample does not originate in the lower respiratory tract. Variation in the number of bronchial epithelial cells in bronchial asthma is of no particular significance. However, bronchial epithelial cells tend occasionally to form large compact clusters, which Naylor termed *Creola bodies* [61] (Plate 15). Studying specimens of 100 asthmatics and 100 nonasthmatic patients, Naylor found these bodies predominantly in asthmatic patients and particularly dur-

Table 52-1. *Sputum cells and particulates in chronic bronchial diseases during clinically stable periods*

Cells	Chronic bronchitis	Chronic bronchial asthma
Curschmann's spirals	Occasionally present	Increased
Charcot-Leyden crystals	Occasionally present	Increased
Creola bodies	Rarely present	Increased [61]
Cell concentration/ml [59]	11.2 ± 4.14*	8.21 ± 2.31*
Bronchial epithelial cells [59]	37.5 ± 3.19*	26.7 ± 19.9*
Polymorphonuclear leukocytes [59]	198 ± 141*	53.4 ± 44.2*
Polymorphonuclear leukocytes with bacteria [59]	18.1 ± 18.7*	4.56 ± 7.64*
Histiocytes [59]	25.4 ± 32.7*	10.3 ± 7.53*
Monocytes [59]	1.77 ± 1.93*	0.23 ± 0.32*
Lymphocytes [59]	1.15 ± 1.14*	0.40 ± 0.71*
Plasma cells [59]	0.32 ± 0.55*	0.01 ± 0.03*
Eosinophils [59]	1.76 ± 2.48*	11.6 ± 10.6*

* Number of cells excreted per day × 10^6.

ing severe asthmatic attacks. Furthermore, it was observed that these cellular aggregates persisted and even increased in patients whose clinical evolution was serious, and they were thus considered of prognostic significance [61].

Creola bodies seem to originate from transudation of edema fluid in the bronchial submucosa, a target area during attacks of bronchial asthma. On occasion these cellular aggregates have been confused with papillary fragments of an adenocarcinoma, and the differential diagnosis can be quite difficult. The most important distinguishing features of the Creola bodies in asthmatic patients are the thoroughly uniform size and shape of the nuclei, the neat peripheral palisading of cells, and the presence of cilia. The latter are particularly important for this differential diagnosis, for according to Naylor and Railey [62], ciliated cells were never found in their cases of adenocarcinoma.

In general, the bronchial epithelial cells that appear in the sputum of chronic stable asthmatic patients are not different in character from those seen in chronic bronchitis. Occasionally, particularly during inflammatory conditions of nonallergic origin, these ciliated bronchial epithelial cells may degenerate in a typical fashion called ciliocytophoria [67] (Plate 16). These particular degenerative forms can be seen in asthmatic or bronchitic patients following a viral infection and tend to disappear with recovery of the patient. In patients with significant eosinophilia, metaplasia of the bronchial epithelium may occur in areas in which the mucosa has been detached and repair is taking place. This can be reflected in the sputum by the presence of metaplastic cells, which sometimes can also be confused with malignant cells [21].

Eosinophils

Although eosinophils (Plate 17) can be observed in many inflammatory responses of the respiratory tract, a marked increase is usually associated with chronic bronchial asthma [30, 54, 68, 86, 95]. In fact, eosinophilic infiltration of the submucosa and thickening of the basement membrane are hallmarks of this disease. However, focal infiltration of eosinophils can also be found in the bronchial mucosa of patients with chronic bronchitis [40]. Therefore, the number of eosinophils in sputum varies considerably, and at times it may be misleadingly low in asthma, particularly at the very beginning of an attack. However, in such cases one will usually find that the sputum contains large quantities of free eosinophilic granules resulting from cell lysis (Plate 18). See Chapter 20 for added details on eosinophil function.

Some investigators have observed characteristic cellular patterns in the sputum of asthmatic patients according to clinical stage. In the acute phase there may be formation of mucous plugs derived from exudation of proteinaceous fluid and eosinophils into the bronchial surface accompanied by increased shedding of the lining epithelium. These elements organize themselves into strips and lamina which, on accumulation into small bronchi, form the core of Curschmann's spirals (see later discussion). If the clinical condition precludes the evacuation of these initial plugs, complex lamina patterns are produced by attrition with conglomeration of degenerative cellular elements and eosinophilic debris. The latter indicates prolonged bronchial obstruction and hence severe asthma [72]. With recovery from asthmatic attacks and renewal of a free flow of sputum, the free eosinophil cell again becomes apparent. Also, it is well known that patients with bronchial asthma treated with corticosteroids reflect the adequacy of treatment by a decrease in the level of eosinophilic cells in the sputum. From all that, it seems evident that eosinophils accompany the attack of asthma, and if at a given time they are not found in large quantities, this probably represents massive lysis or inability to establish adequate mucous drainage; alternatively it may have been caused by steroid administration.

A more difficult question is to define the level or percentage of eosinophils in sputum that is diagnostic of bronchial asthma. In our experience, for patients who are not receiving corticosteroids, a level of eosinophils of 20 percent or more of all cells is usually characteristic of allergic bronchial asthma. However, it must be recognized that some cases of chronic bronchitis may show more than 10 percent of eosinophils in sputum [59].

From a diagnostic point of view, the level of blood eosinophilia is of much less significance. It is well known that blood eosinophils may occasionally be within normal limits in asthmatic patients, regardless of whether it is expressed as a percentage or quantitatively per cubic milliliter of blood; but if blood eosinophilia is present, it is generally a useful index. Attempts to define a correlation between eosinophilia in blood and other secretions or to establish a relation between blood eosinophilia and clinical symptoms have usually not been successful. In a study of 134 children with allergic diseases including bronchial asthma, allergic rhinitis, and atopic dermatitis, simultaneously measured levels of eosinophils in blood and nasal secretions showed significant correlation in only 50 percent of the patients [73]. However, if the blood eosinophilia is very high (more than 10%) in an otherwise asthmatic clinical picture, one should suspect and rule out allergic bronchopulmonary aspergillosis. The cardinal features in that case would be a history of transient pulmonary infiltrates, skin test positive for *Aspergillus* antigen (immediate and delayed), culture of an *Aspergillus* species in sputum, and serum positive precipitins [66] (see Chap. 49). In the typical attack of asthma, the sputum may be scanty and mucoid in appearance or abundant and slurry (as discussed previously). However, it should be remembered that in some cases the expectorate may be yellow or greenish and thick and may look very purulent. Even so, such sputum may contain no pathogenic organisms and may be composed entirely of eosinophils. Clearly, this information is of clinical importance, because in this case administration of antibiotics would be of no value [38]. Thus, the presence of sputum eosinophils indicates an allergic process, perhaps bearing a rough quantitative relationship to the clinical severity, and can also serve as an index of the efficacy of corticosteroids, thereby playing an important role in the diagnosis and treatment of asthma. The significance of eosinophilia in acute asthmatic attacks can also be expressed as an inverse relationship between the number of eosinophils in the sputum and the airflow rates [2]. This relationship does not exist with blood eosinophilia [2].

Charcot-Leyden Crystals

It is commonly assumed today that Charcot-Leyden crystals originate from eosinophils, basophils, or mast cells [3]. They are readily detected in wet, unfixed preparation (Plate 19). These crystals tend to appear in large numbers during acute asthmatic attacks and decrease during clinically stable periods. They may also appear in the sputum of chronic bronchitis and other respiratory conditions but always in association with increased local eosinophilia. Thus, the significance of Charcot-Leyden crystals, clinically and pathogenetically, seems to parallel that of the eosinophilic leukocyte.

Whereas the eosinophilic cell tends to attract the major interest of those studying the cytology of asthmatic sputum, other cellular elements should be considered. In fact, during the clinically stable phase of chronic bronchial asthma the predominant cellular element is the polymorphonuclear leukocyte (neutrophil). Therefore, the predominance of this leukocyte should not necessarily imply infection unless accompanied by a significant proportional decrease in the number of eosinophils and histiocytes as well as a concomitant (e.g., more than 50 bacteria per oil immersion field) increase in the number of bacteria in conjunction with other clinical signs of infection.

Histiocyte

The role of the histiocyte (macrophage) and its origin in pulmonary secretion are still matters of controversy. In general, large numbers of histiocytes in sputum are usually associated with adequate cellular defenses and, therefore, are more common during stable periods of disease or during recuperation from acute insults. Absence or low levels of these scavengers are usually indicators of either the onset of an acute exacerbation of disease and/or the presence of a diminished host defense response. According to Medici and Chodosh [59], an increased bacterial phagocytic activity of histiocytes has also been observed during the resolution of acute infectious episodes in chronic bronchial disease as well as in acute allergic exacerbations in patients with asthma.

Other cells such as lymphocytes and plasma cells have scanty representation in the sputum. In acute bacterial exacerbations of chronic bronchitis and/or bronchial asthma they may appear in increased numbers in the sputum because it is known that they accumulate in the submucosa at such times [40, 71]. As cellular carriers of various immunoglobulins, these cells may have pathogenic significance, but this feature as well as their quantitative distribution in the evolutionary stages of bronchial asthma has not yet been clarified.

Mast Cells

Mast cells are difficult to identify in sputum, although their significance seems to parallel that of the eosinophil. This is reflected in a similar distribution of both cells in tissues exposed to the environmental and immunologic stimuli. Thus, Salvato [71] showed that mast cells were degranulated and decreased in number in the trachea of asthmatic patients, whereas these changes did not occur in chronic bronchitic patients. From this it was inferred that there is a relationship between tissue eosinophilia and degranulation of mast cells. Mast cells and their function are detailed in Chapter 21.

Curschmann's Spirals

First described by Von Leyden in 1872 [85], Curschmann's spirals or coils are associated with the presence of eosinophils and Charcot-Leyden crystals in chronic bronchial asthma. Appearing as twisted spirals of mucinous material around a central thread, the coils are composed of glycoproteins, cells, crystals, and other debris (Plate 20). The origin of these spirals seems to be related to inspissated secretions originating distally in the smaller bronchioles. This is supported by two observations. One, by Gerlach

[33], who many years ago reproduced spiral-like formations by blowing through humidified tubes containing threads of different colors, suggested that the abnormal flow patterns observed in the conducting airways in chronic bronchial disease might be responsible for these formations. A second observation by Dunnill [29] in necropsy material from asthmatic patients indicated that the plugs found in distal airways were mainly composed of Curschmann's spirals along with creola bodies and Charcot-Leyden crystals.

Curschmann's spirals are not uniquely seen in asthmatic patients; they also may be seen in chronic bronchitis, pneumonia, and pulmonary tuberculosis [20, 83]. However, in those cases eosinophils and Charcot-Leyden crystals are not present in the large numbers as seen in bronchial asthma.

PHYSICAL PROPERTIES

Asthmatic sputum during the stable state of the disease appears as a mucoid material (see also Chap. 29). It is mostly colorless, highly translucent, composed of mucinous threads abundantly dispersed with air bubbles adherent to the glass surface, and containing only occasional and small-sized dense plugs. It is shapeless and has a meshlike appearance (see Fig. 52-1). Freshly expectorated sputum is generally nonodorous and has a pH in the range of 6.5 to 8.5. As the number of polymorphonuclear leukocytes increases, the pH tends to be more alkaline and the sputum becomes more purulent [27] (Table 52-2).

The quantity of sputum in asthma, as in other respiratory diseases, bears no direct relationship to the quantity of mucus actually secreted; the latter has never been adequately measured in humans. In the classic allergic asthmatic without superimposed infection, the quantity of sputum may be very small or very large as discussed previously under Gross Appearance. In other cases the beginning of an asthmatic attack is sometimes marked by a distinct decrease in the quantity of sputum, but this may be related to the ability of the patient to raise sputum. To this extent, resumption of a productive cough is one of the best clinical signs to indicate that a lysis in bronchial obstruction is taking place.

The consistency of the asthmatic mucus is that of a gel, and in most cases the solid content is less than 5 percent per unit weight [27]. Actually, *consistency* and *thickness* are not very useful expressions, for they cannot be gauged in precise physical terms, and it is better to express these physical properties in rheologic terms. We have found that variations of viscosity and elasticity of sputum can express quite adequately the difficulties a patient may have in raising the sputum [25].

The rheologic properties of the sputum in asthmatic patients during stable periods are remarkably consistent in that the mate-

Table 52-2. Physical properties of sputum in stable chronic bronchial inflammation

Physical property	Normal	Chronic bronchitis	Bronchial asthma
Quantity (24 hours)	10 ml [79]	24.7 ± 16.3 ml [79]	12.7 ± 8.7 ml [59]
Color	Colorless	Usually yellow or greenish	Colorless
Odor	Nonodorous	Varies according to the kind of infection	Usually nonodorous
pH	7.45–8.15 [52]	6.3–7.9 [60]	5.4–7.6 [60]
Viscosity at 1 sec^{-1}		<400 poises [27]	<400 poises [27]
Elastic recoil at 100 dynes/cm^2		4–8 S$_R$ units [27]	4–8 S$_R$ units [27]

rial shows a high degree of elastic recoil and a comparatively low flow resistance or viscosity [27] (see Table 52-2). This kind of sputum has proved in an animal model in our laboratory under experimental conditions to be best transported by the ciliary escalator (M. J. Dulfano. Unpublished data, 1973). However, during periods of acute exacerbation the rheologic properties of sputum may vary considerably. In some cases the expectoration is very scanty, with a marked increase in viscosity without comparable changes in the elastic recoil [25]. However, in others the expectoration is abundant, semiliquid, and slurry or glairy (as described above), and the glycoprotein bundles that make the matrix of sputum become disorganized and broken (Plate 21A and B). Regardless of this apparent discrepancy, asthmatic patients often exhibit a troublesome but poorly productive cough during the acute attack. Some years ago we examined this slurry sputum and found it to have an exceedingly low viscosity and elastic modulus [23]. Concurrently, this kind of sputum also exhibited a marked decrease in percentage of solids as well as in cell concentrations [23]. With clinical improvement all these changes reversed, the cough decreased, and expectoration became easier. Curiously, it was difficult to reconcile how two opposite kinds of sputa (scanty and "tough" vs. abundant and slurry) could express themselves similarly in a troublesome cough during acute airflow obstruction. A partial explanation was found in our laboratory years ago when we delineated the values of mucus viscoelasticity that would allow for optimal transport of such material by a ciliated mucosa. These values were found to be 1,000 to 3,000 poises and 10 to 25 dynes/cm^2 for the Newtonian viscosity and linear elastic modules, respectively [17]. Thus the surface transport velocity of mucus over a ciliated mucosa significantly decreases when the viscoelastic values deviate widely from the above limits [17]. This proved to be the case with the slurry sputum of acute asthmatics studied by Dulfano where the viscoelastic values were exceedingly low [23]. An additional potential reason for the difficulty in mobilizing the mucus in these patients will be discussed later in the Sputum and Cilia section.

The rheologic properties of the sputum are probably dependent on its molecular structure and particularly on the arrangement of the long and complex glycoprotein fibrils [14, 34, 87, 88]. However, which of these is particularly responsible for the rheologic variations is not yet known; correlations have been attempted with the content of sialic acid [60], the ratio of fucose to sialic acid [50], the degree of hydration, and the quantities of DNA, particularly in purulent sputum [14]. In other studies sputum viscosity is related to the neuraminic acid concentration as well as to the yield of dry macromolecular material. Rheologic findings can also be interpreted in relation to the degree of hydration of the sputum, to an altered synthesis of glycoprotein, or to the addition of a tissue fluid component [50].

Aside from the chemical composition, other factors may well contribute to sputum consistency, including the distributional organization of the water within the sputum, the types of chemical bonding responsible for the gel structure of the secretion, and the alteration of this bonding when the sputum changes from mucoid to purulent. Thus, according to Barton et al. [4], three factors seem to contribute to the abnormal coherence of mucopurulent bronchial secretions: (1) increased disulfide bonding among the structural elements of the bronchial gel, (2) increased covalent crosslinking, and (3) the addition of deoxyribose nucleoprotein fibril material from disintegrated leukocytes. In our own experience significantly higher levels of disulfide bonds are found in purulent as compared to mucoid sputum, and this finding seems to explain best the higher viscosity and elastic modules of purulent sputum [10].

CHEMICAL COMPOSITION

The nonhomogeneous character of sputum and the known difficulties in obtaining a "true," unadulterated secretion preclude a definition of a standard chemical composition of this material. Even when the sputum is mucoid and there is no indication of active infection, its composition may vary widely, depending on the state of hydration, the overall extent of inflammation of the bronchial mucosa, and the uncertain age of the material before its expectoration. As a point of reference, one can use the figures given by Boat and Matthews [8] on the composition of sputum in laryngectomized subjects, which serves in their studies as a prototype for normal (Table 52-3). Some of its features are that the osmolality of respiratory mucus is greater than that of serum, and therefore tracheobronchial secretions are comparably hypertonic. This seems to relate to higher levels of sodium, chloride, potassium, and phosphorus. In asthma water-soluble electrolytes are to some extent bound to soluble macromolecules, with calcium bound in the largest amount. Ultrafiltrable amino acids and oligosaccharide carbohydrates or small glycopeptides are also present. These amino acids are essentially the same as those found in serum, although quantitative differences may appear in their distribution pattern [45]. The amount of inorganic ions in asthmatic sputum has been found to be similar to that from bronchitic patients, but both sodium and chloride are comparably low when compared to laryngectomized patients, particularly if infection is present [12]. The ash content, usually about 1 percent by weight, is apparently decreased in stable asthma and also when the sputum becomes purulent.

Analysis of organic components, which appear in macromolecular form, indicates that approximately 70 percent of the nitrogen is present as protein. Carbohydrate analysis in nonpurulent secretions shows 25 percent hexose, 31 percent hexosamine, 21 percent fucose, and 20 percent sialic acid [11, 31, 57]. Most of

Table 52-3. Chemical composition of sputum in chronic bronchial diseases

| | Blood | Sputum | | |
		Laryngectomy	Asthma	Bronchitis
Sodium	136.00–145.00 mEq/L	165.00 ± 42.00 mEq/L [8]	74.00 mEq/L [41]	116.00 ± 15.00 mEq/L [8]
Potassium	3.50–5.00 mEq/L	13.20 ± 5.40 mEq/L [8]	22.00 mEq/L [41]	18.70 ± 3.20 mEq/L [8]
Chloride	100.00–106.00 mEq/L	162.00 ± 60.00 mEq/L [8]	82.00 mEq/L [41]	97.00 ± 14.00 mEq/L [8]
Calcium	4.50–5.50 mEq/L	6.20 ± 2.00 mEq/L [8]	4.20 mEq/L [41]	—
Proteins	6.00–8.00 gm/100 ml	1.00 ± 0.30 gm/100 ml [8]	Increased [69]	2.04 ± 0.45 gm/100 ml [8]
Carbohydrates	0.08–0.10 gm/100 ml	0.95 ± 0.21 gm/100 ml [8]	—	1.05 ± 0.14 gm/100 ml [8]
Carbohydrates/proteins	$\frac{0.08–0.10}{6.00–8.00}$ gm/100 ml	$\frac{0.95 ± 0.21}{1.00 ± 0.30}$ gm/100 ml [8]	Smaller than	Higher than [8]
Lipids	0.45–0.85 gm/100 ml	0.84 ± 0.27 gm/100 ml [8]	—	1.17 ± 0.43 gm/100 ml [8]
Ash	—	1.13 ± 0.32 gm/100 ml [8]	Decreased [69]	0.88 ± 0.08 gm/100 ml [8]
Osmolarity	285.00–295.00 mOs/L	359.00 ± 56.00 mOs/L [7]	—	—

the carbohydrates are not water soluble and presumably are co-valently bound into mucins, which form the gel of tracheobron-chial secretion. Two-thirds of water-soluble carbohydrates in these secretions are retained after ultrafiltration, suggesting that these carbohydrates are present largely as glycoprotein [8].

Only part of lipids are attached to macromolecules. When the tracheobronchial secretion becomes infected with bacteria, the amount of lipid increases considerably as a result of host cell breakdown [57]. This parallels the observed changes in DNA con-tent, which increases considerably with the appearance of puru-lency. DNA originates in the nuclear material of bronchial and inflammatory cells that have undergone bacterial disintegration, and according to Burgi et al. [15] the increase of DNA in sputum is a reliable indicator of bronchial infection. In one study the sputum from asthmatic patients revealed that the lipid composi-tion consisted mainly of highly saturated triglycerides with large amounts of short chain fatty acids. Phospholipids, mainly leci-thins, were also found [37].

The great variability in the chemical composition of sputum has precluded so far its use as an aid in the differential diagnosis of inflammatory conditions of the bronchial tree. When sputum was analyzed after separation into a sol and gel phase, it was observed that in asthmatic patients the sol phase carries higher concentrations of serum proteins, especially albumin, and a higher protein-carbohydrate ratio than similar sol phases of spu-tum from chronic bronchitic patients [69]. Shimura et al. [75] found that the chemical composition of bronchorrhea sputum in asthmatics showed values intermediate between saliva and mucoid sputum except for a lower pH and histamine concen-tration.

Studies using fluorescein have indicated that the transfer of plasma protein into the bronchial lumen follows its intravenous injection within a few minutes [77]. However, the loss of protein into the sputum of asthmatic patients is usually much less than that observed in bronchitis [9]. Similar observations were made by Honda et al. [42]. Examination of the mucous plugging in the small airways of patients dying from bronchial asthma has disclosed a material of great tenacity [29], which, because of its marked eosinophilic staining properties, has been attributed to the accumulation of serum proteins associated with the inflam-matory response of the allergic reaction [43].

The chemical properties of the mucus secreted by the respira-tory tract are poorly understood. These macromolecules have a high carbohydrate content, comprising 30 to 70 percent of the total weight of various mucin complexes [74]. Certain sugar resi-dues of respiratory mucins appear to be sulfated and are, there-fore, similar to gastrointestinal mucin. The exact carbohydrate composition and arrangement of the sugar residues are not known, nor is it clear whether the heterogeneity of the oligosac-charide chains also occurs in specific mucin molecules. Purifica-tion of mucin components is still very sketchy. Nevertheless, it is known that the sol phase of sputum contains two acidic mucins and two neutral mucins [6]. On the other hand, the gel phase was shown to contain several acidic and at least one neutral mucin [37].

Histologic studies on the mucosa of bronchitic and asthmatic patients disclosed that in chronic bronchitis the mucus was strongly alcian blue positive and thought to consist largely of acid glycoproteins, while in asthma the mucus stained predominantly with the periodic acid–Schiff technique and therefore was pre-sumed to contain many neutral glycoproteins [71].

In the sputum from asthmatic patients, there is considerable increase of a mucin component that contains 12 to 14 percent fucose and is almost devoid of sialic acid. However, an increase in sputum sialomucin has also been reported in patients with bronchial asthma [74]. These contradictions have never been clearly explained. Bukantz and Bern [13] purified mucins exhibit-ing blood group activity from the sputum of patients with asthma.

However, its carbohydrate composition in no way distinguished this mucin from other epithelial mucins. For more detailed stud-ies of tracheobronchial mucins the reader is referred to the re-views of Boat and Matthews [8] and Masson and Heremans [56], recent symposia [93, 94], and to Chapter 29.

Certain proteins found in respiratory tracheobronchial secre-tions fulfill specific functions such as participation in local immu-nologic processes. Among these proteins, lysozyme, lactoferrin, and IgA appear to play a role in the defense of the lungs against microbial invaders [74]. Most important, evidence has accumu-lated that such substances, as well as most other immunoglobu-lins, are actually synthesized and secreted by respiratory tract cells [74]. These chemicals and other proteins found in the mucus from asthmatic patients have been demonstrated by different investigators, particularly during acute attacks. These include IgE [45], histamine [78], slow-reacting substances of anaphylaxis [36], and serotonin [53]. However, their original site of produc-tion and pathways to the lumina of the airways are not entirely clear at this time. Immunoglobulin A is the predominant immuno-globulin in most sputum, and the IgA/IgG ratio has been found to be 10 times higher than in serum, with an average ratio of 0.25 [56]. This ratio seems to be little influenced by the sex or age of the individuals [80]. In patients with acute bronchitis and exten-sive inflammatory response, the content of IgA in sputum has been shown to increase significantly [58]. However, this has not been demonstrated in the sputum of bronchial asthma. In the bronchial mucosa stained with fluorescein antiserum, IgA can be seen in large amounts within the lumina of glandular ducts as well as among cells [56].

The IgG present in sputum is considered to originate mainly from serum by transudation. Therefore, its concentration in spu-tum might be found increased during periods of inflammation, and in some cases of asthma the concentration of IgG may be of the same magnitude as that of IgA [45]. However, not all IgG stems from serum, and there is evidence that there are IgG-pro-ducing cells in the bronchial mucosa that can be detected by immunofluorescence. IgG from this source is referred to as secre-tory IgG [55].

In chronic bronchitis the number of submucosal plasma cells is increased, particularly those containing IgA compared with those with IgG, with no change in those containing IgM [55]. The amount of IgG in sputum is stated to increase with infectious acute asthmatic attacks [22]; however, this was not found in an-other study of asthmatic children [63].

In the sputum of asthmatic patients the immunoglobulin that has received the most attention is IgE, probably because of its known relationship to serum reaginic antibodies responsible for the immediate allergic or Type I response [44]. Normally, the serum concentration of IgE varies from 1 to 80 μg/100 ml and averages from 20 to 30 μg/100 ml. These values have been shown by several investigators to increase tremendously in allergic states [45–47]. In normal bronchial secretions IgE is virtually undetectable, but in sputum from asthmatic patients it has been found to be present in amounts of up to 50 μg/100 ml [56]. Whereas there is no evidence that asthmatic patients have more IgE immunocytes in their bronchial mucosa than normal sub-jects, the IgE/IgG ratios have been found to be higher in the spu-tum than in the serum of allergic patients. Therefore, the exis-tence of secretory IgE in the bronchial mucosa is likely [45]. This is reinforced by reports that IgE can be increased in sputum and not in serum [82]. So far, no structural difference between the IgE found in respiratory secretions and that found in serum has been detected [64].

To some authors [56] the free IgE detected in the sputum may play no pathogenic role, which is reserved for the IgE fraction retained within the bronchial mucosa. This latter fraction be-comes bound to receptor sites in the mast cell, thus initiating the release of reactive substances. This process can be demon-

Table 52-4. Mucus secretagogues in the lower respiratory tract

Mast cell mediators
  Histamine
  Prostaglandins
  Thromboxane A_2
  5- and 15-hydroxyeicosatetraenoic acid
  Leukotrienes C_4 and D_4
  Prostaglandin-generating factor
  Chymase
Neurotransmitters
  Acetylcholine
  α-Adrenergic agonists
  Gastrin-releasing peptide
  Vasoactive intestinal peptide
  Substance P
Inflammatory products
  Eosinophil cationic protein
  Neutrophil elastase
  Macrophage mucus secretagogue

Source: M. A. Kaliner. The clinical significance of mucus in asthma. *J. Respir. Dis.* 12:S18, 1991. Reprinted with permission.

strated by the use of fluorescent antibody or radioautographic methods, using antiserum specific to the heavy chain of IgE (see Chap. 7) [48, 72].

The roles of other biologically active agents present in pulmonary secretions such as kinins, prostaglandins, and cyclic AMP are still to be further defined [70, 82]. In the ferret, platelet-activating factor has been shown to increase mucous secretion directly [91]. A recent review examines the effects of inflammatory mediators on airway mucous secretion [90] (Table 52-4). Among the enzymes present in tracheobronchial secretions, kallikrein seems capable of releasing kinins [36]. Increased antitryptic activity [76] and an increased amount of serotonin [39] have also been described in the sputum of asthmatic patients.

Histamine, which normally can be found in amounts between 10 and 40 μg/gm sputum dry weight, has been reported to be increased in secretions from asthmatic patients, ranging up to 234 μg/gm dry weight [78]. However, these higher values were found not only in asthmatic or allergic individuals but also in people subjected to chronic industrial respiratory irritants.

SPUTUM AND CILIA

Ahmed et al. [1] have pointed out that mucociliary clearance seems to decrease concomitantly with airway conductance during bronchospastic crises in asthmatic patients (see also Chap. 30). This, of course, contributes to stasis and perhaps to dehydration of secretions and expresses itself functionally in a troublesome, ineffective cough. This decrease in clearance can result from a "coupling" defect between cilia and an abnormal mucus, expressed perhaps as the slurry sputum discussed previously under Physical Properties. However, it could also result from some abnormality in the cilia itself of a temporary or permanent nature. Ciliary dyskinetic factors have been described in the blood of asthmatics by Wilson and Fudenberg [89], who remarked on some similarities to the dyskinesia factor present in the serum of cystic fibrosis patients. Similarly, Frigas et al. [32] have found a factor called *major basic protein,* obtained mostly from eosinophils, which may induce ciliotoxic effects.

Studies in our laboratory have shown that ciliary defects may indeed exist in asthmatics. This is expressed as a temporary ciliary inhibition appearing during acute clinical exacerbation of asthma with recovery as the symptoms subside [28]. This ciliary inhibitory factor is present in the sol fraction of sputum but not in serum, and on initial characterization it appears as a sputum protein of low molecular weight [26]. The effects of this cilia inhibitory factor are reproducible in in vitro bioassay test systems, using either frog or human mucosa as substratum [26, 28].

Thus, a common functional pathway can be proposed for the apparently different kinds of sputa seen in the acute stages of many asthmatic patients having bronchospasm and ineffective cough. The expectoration may be either large and slurry or only scanty and thick. These differences may only represent different mucus transit time until expectoration. However, both types of sputum are transported very poorly by the respiratory tract cilia. In the case of slurry sputum, it will contain, in addition, a ciliary inhibitory factor during the acute clinical exacerbation. Chemical isolation of this factor may significantly advance our understanding of the pathogenesis of the asthmatic attack.

SPUTUM FINDINGS IN ASPIRATION

Aspiration of food substances has been recognized increasingly as a cause of acute exacerbations in chronic obstructive pulmonary disease patients [24] (see also Chap. 75). This happens mostly in the debilitated, the elderly, and the edentulous. In most such cases no specific neurologic deficit can be found except a weakness or absence of the gag reflex. The exacerbation of chest symptoms frequently occurs without new chest x-ray findings. The chance of aspiration by faulty deglutition is increased when the traditional liquid and or semiliquid hospital menu is substituted for the regular diet of the patient at home or when the patient's dentures are removed. Finally, if such patients are subjected to endotracheal intubation, with or without the addition of nasogastric tube feeding, aspiration and/or regurgitation is inevitable.

The tendency to aspiration can be easily tested clinically by asking the patient to drink a few sips of water and, after a wait of 20 to 30 seconds, to elicit the appearance of a light throat cough. However, more reliable diagnosis can be made by examination of the sputum or aspirated tracheal secretions. Basically, one would be searching for the presence of food substances that are clearly foreign to the natural respiratory mucus. The most common of such food invaders are starch, fat substances, grains, milk, glucose, and meat fibers. To be reliable, this search must be conducted after the mouth has been properly rinsed and dentures thoroughly cleaned or removed.

Starch

Starch in sputum reacts rapidly with Gram's iodine stain, producing a purple-bluish discoloration. The granules of starch are of various sizes. In potatoes they are round and small and have a rim of cellulose (Plate 22). On consolidation, the granules often take the shape of cotyledons, where the cellulose appears as palisades, circles, and beehives and is always easy to recognize by appropriate and simple microscopic and staining techniques. On direct microscopy, the cellulose fibers are only faintly distinct, since they do not take the iodine stain. However, the reverse is true under polarizing microscopy, where the starch granules' appearance does not change but the cellulose fibers stand out because they are strongly birefringent (Plate 23).

Fatty Substances

Fatty substances are also very ubiquitous and can be detected by their reaction to Sudan IV or Oil red O stains (Plate 24). However, these are useful but nonspecific reactions for fat, and additional techniques may be required for identification of subgroups such as unsaturated fats, triglycerides, glycolipids, phospholipids, and so on [92]. On the other hand, sterols such as cholesterol can be identified readily using a fat stain and polarization. Here,

Table 52-5. Interpretation of sputum findings (see text)

Findings	Clinical significance
General appearance	
Mucoid	"Normal" chronic bronchitis
Purulent	Infective process
Slurry	Allergic process
Particulate components	
Eosinophils >20% or increase in free eosinophil granules	Allergic process
Curschmann's spirals	
Charcot-Leyden crystals	
Mast cells	
Bronchial epithelial cell clusters (creola bodies)	
Polymorphonuclear leukocytes increase >80% with significant decrease of eosinophils and histiocytes	Bacterial infection
Ciliocytophoria	Viral infection
Bronchial casts	Bronchial inspissation
Squamous epithelial cells	Upper respiratory tract sample (discard)

the cholesterol crystals are strongly birefringent and take up the shape of Maltese crosses (Plate 25). When fat substances are found within the macrophage cell, it is an indication that the food has been inside the respiratory tract for at least several hours. It also establishes that such macrophages are viable and capable to act as scavengers.

Meat Fibers

Meat fibers are easy to recognize, particularly those of the striated muscle category. Plate 26 shows such fibers exhibiting dark and light bands as well as very short longitudinal striations.

Milk

Aspirated fluid in intubated patients frequently appears as a cloudy, whitish material, suggesting the presence of milk. A simple procedure to establish this diagnosis is first to try to hydrolize the milk's lactose into glucose and galactose by adding amyloglucosidase to the fluid. After a few minutes, the liberated glucose can be detected readily by the simple glucose-oxidase reaction using Labstix or Dextostix. Glucose is not present as a monomer in our regular diet and thus cannot be expected to be found in aspirated fluid after ingestion of regular food substances, with the possible exception of retention of the food in the mouth allowing for the salivary amylase to break down starch and polysaccharides. However, glucose has become a regular component of many nutrient solutions administered by gastric tube feeding, and the quantity of free glucose can range from 300 to 3,800 mg/ml in reconstituted feeding formulas, such as Osmolite or Sustagen among many. In such cases, it should be easily detectable by Labstix or similar reagents.

A summary of the features of sputum in a variety of airway conditions is shown in Table 52-5.

REFERENCES

1. Ahmed, T., et al. Abnormal mucociliary transport in allergic patients with antigen-induced bronchospasm: Rule of slow-reacting substance of anaphylaxis. *Am. Rev. Respir. Dis.* 124:110, 1981.
2. Alfaro, C., et al. Inverse correlation of expiratory lung volumes and sputum eosinophils in status asthmaticus. *Ann. Allergy* 63:251, 1989.
3. Archer, G. T., and Blackwood, A. Formation of Charcot-Leyden crystals in human eosinophiles and basophils and study of the comparison of isolated crystals. *J. Exp. Med.* 122:173, 1965.
4. Barton, A. D., and Lourenco, R. V. Bronchial secretion and mucociliary clearance. *Arch. Intern. Med.* 131:140, 1973.
5. Bezancon, F., and DeJong, S. I. *Traité de L'Examen des Crachats.* Paris: Masson, 1913.
6. Biserte, R., and Cuvelier, R. Les glycoprotéines des sécrétions bronchiques. *Expos. Annu. Biochim. Med.* 24:85, 1963.
7. Bizzozero, G. *Handbuch der Klinischen Mikroscopie.* Erlangen: Besold, 1887.
8. Boat, T. F., and Matthews, L. W. Chemical Composition of Human Tracheobronchial Secretions. In M. J. Dulfano (ed.), *Sputum: Fundamentals and Clinical Pathology.* Springfield, Ill.: Thomas, 1973.
9. Bonomo, L., and D'Addabbo, A. ^{131}I-albumin turnover and loss of protein into sputum in chronic bronchitis. *Clin. Chim. Acta.* 10:214, 1964.
10. Borentein, O., et al. Disulfide bonds and sputum viscoelasticity. *Biorheology* 15:261, 1978.
11. Brogan, T. D. The carbohydrate complexes of bronchial secretion. *Biochem. J.* 71:125, 1959.
12. Brogan, T. D., et al. Relation between sputum sol phase composition and diagnosis in chronic chest diseases. *Thorax* 26:418, 1971.
13. Bukantz, S. C., and Bern, A. W. Studies with sputum. I. Initial observations on the chemical nature and blood group substance content of asthmatic sputum. *J. Allergy* 29:29, 1958.
14. Burgi, H. Die Viskositat des purulenten und sterilen Sputums bei chronischer Asthmabronchitis. *Medicine Tharacalis* 21:156, 1964.
15. Burgi, H., et al. New objective criteria for inflammation in bronchial secretions. *Br. Med. J.* 2:654, 1968.
16. Calim, A. Bronchorrhea. *Br. Med. J.* 4:274, 1972.
17. Chen, T. M., and Dulfano, M. J. Mucus viscoelasticity and mucociliary transport rate. *J. Lab. Clin. Med.* 91:423, 1978.
18. Chodosh, S. Examination of sputum cells. *N. Engl. J. Med.* 282:854, 1970.
19. Chodosh, S., Zaccheo, C. W., and Segal, M. S. The cytology and histochemistry of sputum cells. I. Preliminary differential counts in chronic bronchitis. *Am. Rev. Respir. Dis.* 85:636, 1961.
20. Clifford, R. *The Sputum: Its Examination and Clinical Significance.* New York: Macmillan, 1932. Pp. 35–36.
21. Cohen, R. C., and Prentice, A. I. D. Metaplastic cells in sputum of patients with pulmonary eosinophilia. *Tubercle* 40:44, 1959.
22. Dennis, E. G., Hornbrook, M. M., and Ishizaka, K. Serum proteins in sputum of patients with asthma. *J. Allergy* 35:464, 1964.
23. Dulfano, M. J. Bronchial mucus—role in acute asthma. *Excerpta Medica Int., Congress Series* 414:285, 1977.
24. Dulfano, M. J. Respiratory Tract Fluid Examination in the Intensive Care Unit. In K. F. MacDonnell et al. (eds.), *Respiratory Intensive Care.* Boston: Little, Brown, 1987.
25. Dulfano, M. J., Adler, K., and Philippoff, W. Sputum viscoelasticity in chronic bronchitis. *Am. Rev. Respir. Dis.* 104:88, 1971.
26. Dulfano, M. J., and Luk, C. K. Sputum and ciliary inhibition in asthma. *Thorax* 37:646, 1982.
27. Dulfano, M. J., and Philippoff, W. Physical Properties. In M. J. Dulfano (ed.), *Sputum: Fundamentals and Clinical Pathology.* Springfield, Ill.: Thomas, 1973.
28. Dulfano, M. J., et al. Ciliary inhibitory effects of asthma patients' sputum. *Clin. Sci.* 63:393, 1982.
29. Dunnill, M. S. The pathology of asthma with special reference to changes in the bronchial mucosa. *J. Clin. Pathol.* 13:27, 1960.
30. Ehrlich, P. *Verhandlung der Physiologischen.* Berlin: Gesellschaft, 1878–79.
31. Fraenkel, A. Z. *Knin. Med.* 35:559, 1898. Cited in Naylor, B. The shedding of the mucosa of the bronchial tree in asthma. *Thorax* 17:69, 1962.
32. Frigas, E., et al. Elevated levels of the eosinophile granule, major basic protein in the sputum of patients with bronchial asthma. *Mayo Clin. Proc.* 56:345, 1981.
33. Gerlach, W. Über die kunstliche Darstellbarkeit Curschmannscher Spiralen. *Dtsch. Arch. Klin. Med.* 50:450, 1892.
34. Gernex-Fieux, C., et al. Etude de l'activite in vitro de dofferents agents reduisans la viscosite de l'expectoration. *Acta Tuberc. Pneumol. Belg.* 3:138, 1964.
35. Harkavy, J. Spasm-producing substance in the sputum of patients with bronchial asthma. *Arch. Intern. Med.* 45:641, 1930.

36. Havez, R., et al. Isolement et caracterisation immonologique de la kallicriene bronchique humaine. *C.R. Acad. Sci.* (*Paris*) 262:309, 1966.

37. Havez, R., et al. Biochemical Exploration of Bronchial Hypersecretions. In H. Peeters (ed.), *Protides of Biological Fluids.* New York: Pergamon, 1968. Pp. 343–360.

38. Helm, W. H., May, J. R., and Livingston, J. L. Long-term oxytetracycline (Terramycin) therapy in chronic respiratory infections. *Lancet* 2:630, 1954.

39. Hepner-Levy, L., Mendes, E., and Ulhoa-Cintra, A. Hydroxytryptamine in the sputum of asthmatic patients. *Acta Allergol.* 16:121, 1961.

40. Hers, J. P. The Pathology of Chronic Relapsing Mucopurulent Bronchitis, With and Without Bronchiectasis. In N. G. M. Orie and H. G. Sluiter (eds.), *Bronchitis.* Assen, Netherlands: Royal Vangorcum, 1961. Pp. 149–158.

41. Hoffman, Von, H., and Ebelt, H. Der Elektrolygehalt des Sputums und des Serums bie Patienten mit Asthma bronchiale und bie Patienten mit chronischer Bronchitis. *Allerg. Asthmaforsch.* 14:227, 1968.

42. Honda, I., et al. Airway mucosal permeability in chronic bronchitics and bronchial asthmatics with hypersecretion. *Am. Rev. Respir. Dis.* 137:866, 1988.

43. Huber, H. L., and Koessler, K. K. The pathology of bronchial asthma. *Arch. Intern. Med.* 30:689, 1922.

44. Ishizaka, T., et al. Pharmacologic inhibition of the antigen-induced release of histamine and slow reacting substance of anaphylaxis (SRS-A) from monkey lung tissue mediated by human IgE. *J. Immunol.* 106:1267, 1971.

45. Ishizaka, K., and Newcomb, R. W. Presence of gamma E in nasal washings and sputum from asthmatic patients. *J. Allergy* 46:197, 1970.

46. Johansson, S. G. O. Raised levels of a new immunoglobulin class (IgND) in asthma. *Lancet* 2:951, 1967.

47. Johansson, S. G. O., et al. Some factors influencing the serum IgE levels in atopic diseases. *Clin. Exp. Immunol.* 6:43, 1970.

48. Kay, A. B., Stechschulte, D. J., and Austen, K. F. An eosinophile leukocyte chemotactic factor of anaphylaxis. *J. Exp. Med.* 133:602, 1971.

49. Keal, E. E. Biochemistry and rheology of sputum in asthma. *Postgrad. Med. J.* 47:171, 1971.

50. Keal, E. E., and Reid, L. Pathological Alterations in Mucus in Asthma Within and Without the Cell. In M. Stein (ed.), *New Direction in Asthma.* Chicago: ACCP, 1975. P. 233.

51. Kohler, H., et al. Der Gehalt des menschlichen Bronchialsekretes an freien Aminosauren. *Z. Erkr. Atmungsorgane* 130:259, 1969.

52. Kwart, H., Moseley, W. W., and Katz, M. The chemical characterization of human tracheobronchial secretions: A possible clue to the origin of fibrocystic mucus. *Ann. N.Y. Acad. Sci.* 106:709, 1963.

53. Levy, L. H., Mendes, E., and Cinta, A. Hydroxytryptamine in sputum of asthmatic patients. *Acta Allergol.* 16:121, 1961.

54. Litt, M. Eosinophiles and antigen-antibody reactions. *Ann. N.Y. Acad. Sci.* 116:964, 1964.

55. Martinex-Tello, F. J., Braun, D. G., and Blanc, W. A. Immunoglobulin production in bronchial mucosa and bronchial lymph nodes, particularly in cystic fibrosis of the pancreas. *J. Immunol.* 101:989, 1968.

56. Masson, P. L., and Heremans, J. F. Sputum Proteins. In M. J. Dulfano (ed.), *Sputum: Fundamentals and Clinical Pathology.* Springfield, Ill.: Thomas, 1973.

57. Matthews, L. W., et al. Studies on pulmonary secretions. I. The overall chemical composition of pulmonary secretions from patients with cystic fibrosis, bronchiectasis, and laryngectomy. *Am. Rev. Respir. Dis.* 88:199, 1963.

58. Medici, T. C., and Burgi, H. The role of immunoglobulin A in endogenous bronchial defense mechanisms in chronic bronchitis. *Am. Rev. Respir. Dis.* 103:784, 1971.

59. Medici, T. C., and Chodosh, S. Nonmalignant Exfoliative Sputum Cytology. In M. J. Dulfano (ed.), *Sputum: Fundamentals and Clinical Pathology.* Springfield, Ill.: Thomas, 1973.

60. Munies, R., Grubb, T. C., and Caliari, R. E. Relationship between sputum viscosity and total sialic acid content. *J. Pharm. Sci.* 57:824, 1963.

61. Naylor, B. The shedding of the mucosa of the bronchial tree in asthma. *Thorax* 17:69, 1962.

62. Naylor, B., and Railey, C. A pitfall in the cytodiagnosis of sputum of asthmatics. *J. Clin. Pathol.* 17:84, 1964.

63. Newcomb, R. W., and DeWald, B. Protein concentrations in sputa from asthmatic children. *J. Lab. Clin. Med.* 73:734, 1969.

64. Newcomb, R. W., and Ishizaka, K. Physiochemical and antigenic studies on human IgE in respiratory fluid. *J. Immunol.* 105:85, 1970.

65. Papanicolaou, G. N. *Atlas of Exfoliative Cytology.* Cambridge, Mass.: Harvard University Press, 1954.

66. Pepys, J., et al. Clinical correlation between long-term (IgE) and short-term (IgG S-TS) anaphylactic antibodies in atopic and non-atopic subjects with respiratory allergic diseases. *Clin. Allergy* 6:645, 1979.

67. Pierce, C. H., and Knox, A. W. Ciliocytophoria in sputum from patients with adenovirus infections. *Proc. Soc. Exp. Bio. Med.* 104:492, 1960.

68. Rich, A. R. Significance of hypersensitivity in infections. *Physiol. Rev.* 21: 70, 1941.

69. Ryley, H. C., and Brogan, T. D. Variation in the composition of sputum in chronic chest diseases. *Br. J. Exp. Pathol.* 49:625, 1969.

70. Said, S. I. The lung as a metabolic organ. *N. Engl. J. Med.* 279:1330, 1968.

71. Salvato, G. Some histological changes in chronic bronchitis and asthma. *Thorax* 23:168, 1968.

72. Sanerkin, N. G., and Evans, D. M. D. The sputum in bronchial asthma: Pathognomonic patterns. *J. Pathol. Bacteriol.* 89:535, 1965.

73. Saracli, T., and Scott, R. B. Comparative study of simultaneous blood and nasal secretion eosinophilia in children with allergic diseases. *J. Asthma Res.* 4:219, 1967.

74. Schultze, H. E., and Heremans, J. F. *Molecular Biology of Human Proteins.* New York: Elsevier, 1966. Vol. 1. Pp. 816–831.

75. Shimura, S., et al. Chemical properties of bronchorrhea sputum in bronchial asthma. *Chest* 94:1211, 1988.

76. Smith, J. M. Interference with tryptic digestion by sputum from asthmatic patients. *Am. Rev. Respir. Dis.* 88:858, 1963.

77. Steinmann, E. P. Die Patho-Physiologic des Bronchialbaumes. *Fortschr. Hals-Mas-Ohren.* 3:40, 1956.

78. Thomas, H. V., and Simmons, E. Histamine content in sputum from allergic and non-allergic individuals. *J. Appl. Physiol.* 26:793, 1969.

79. Toremalm, N. G. The daily amount of tracheobronchial secretions in man: A method for continuous tracheal aspiration in laryngectomized and tracheotomized patients. *Acta Otolaryngol.* (*Stockh.*) [Suppl. 158]: 43, 1960.

80. Turgeon, P., Robert, J., and Turgeon, F. Etude des immunoglobulines sériques et sécrétoires trachéo-bronchiques. *Union Med. Can.* 100:232, 1971.

81. Turief, J., et al. Lesions of the bronchial mucosa in asthma-like disorders: Spasmodic, coriza, laryngotracheitis, and eosinophilic bronchorrhea. *Bull. Mem. Soc. Med. Hosp. Paris* 74:676, 1958.

82. UCLA Conference. Asthma: New ideas about an old disease. *Ann. Intern. Med.* 78:405, 1973.

83. Von Hoesslin, H. *Das Sputum.* Berlin: Springer, 1921.

84. Von Hoesslin, H. *Das Sputum* (2nd ed.). Berlin: Springer, 1926.

85. Von Leyden, E. Zur Kenntnis des bronchial Asthma. *Virchows Arch.* [*Pathol. Anat.*] 54:324, 1872.

86. Walls, R. S., et al. Mechanisms for eosinophilic and neutrophilic leukocytes. *Br. Med. J.* 3:157, 1971.

87. White, J. C., and Elmes, P. C. *Some Rheological Properties of Bronchial Mucus and Mucoprotein: Flow Properties of Blood.* New York: Pergamon, 1960, P. 259.

88. White, J. C., Elmes, P. C., and Walsh, A. Fibrous proteins of pathological bronchial secretions studied by light and microscopy: Deoxyribonucleoprotein and mucoprotein in bronchial secretions. *J. Pathol. Bacteriol.* 67: 105, 1954.

89. Wilson, G. B., and Fudenberg, H. H. Ciliary dyskinesia factors in cystic fibrosis and asthma. *Nature* 266:463, 1977.

90. Widdicombe, J. G., and Webber, S. E. Airway mucus secretion. *News Physiol. Sci.* 5:2, 1990.

91. Wirtz, H., et al. Mechanism of platelet-activating factor (PAF)–induced secretion of mucus from tracheal submucosal glands in the ferret. *Fed. Proc.* 45:418, 1986.

92. Zugibe, F. T. *Diagnostic Histochemistry.* St. Louis: Mosby, 1970. P. 310.

93. Miller, Y. E. Epithelial cell biology and airway disease. *Chest* 101:S3, 1992.

94. Busse, W. W. The role of mucus in asthma management. *J. Respir. Dis.* 12(Suppl.):1991.

95. Pin, I., et al. Changes in the cellular profile of induced sputum after allergen-induced asthmatic responses. *Am. Rev. Respir. Dis.* 145:1265, 1992.

Radiography

Murray L. Janower

53

The increasing incidence, morbidity, and mortality due to asthma are refocusing attention on improved evaluation of patients presenting with an acute attack [3, 15, 17]. A plain chest film remains the major radiologic study, but other anatomic areas of the body may also have to be examined. Modalities such as bronchography, isotopic lung scans, computed tomography, magnetic resonance imaging, and proton emission tomography have limited usefulness in the workup of asthmatic patients.

A physician should only request a radiographic examination if it will be helpful in evaluation and care of the patient. While several studies have documented the low yield of chest films routinely requested on asthmatic patients [1], appropriate indications have come into focus that can exclude other possible diagnoses and exclude complications. In an infant presenting with a first attack of wheezing, possible underlying conditions must be excluded: congenital heart disease, congestive heart failure, vascular ring, mediastinal mass, aspiration pneumonia, and foreign body among others. In an adult with an initial episode of wheezing, chest films are useful to exclude congestive heart failure, tumor, pulmonary embolism, and foreign body. In a patient with a well-established diagnosis, films are usually obtained when the patient has not responded to therapy, is febrile, or is raising purulent sputum. For those asthmatic patients who require hospitalization or whose initial therapy has failed, a number of studies have found that the chest film will reveal positive findings in up to 33 percent of cases [9, 32].

RISK

Essentially no risk is associated with the very small amount of radiation used in obtaining a chest film, even when multiple examinations are required. Assuming that the beam is well collimated, the only tissues radiated are those localized to the thoracic cage (including skin, muscle, bone, and lung); these tissues are extremely radioresistant. Only a small fraction of the more sensitive bone marrow is exposed. Typical marrow doses for a posteroanterior chest film are approximately 5 mrad for an adult and 1 mrad for a child.

To place these doses in perspective, a patient with a lung cancer might receive an entrance dose of 6 million mrad from radiation therapy. All people are exposed to natural background radiation in the environment of approximately 100 mrad/yr; living in a brick rather than a wood house adds about 5 mrad/yr of exposure; living in Colorado instead of Massachusetts, 10 additional mrad; and flying from the East to the West Coast results in additional radiation exposure of 5 mrad from the increased cosmic ray intensity. In an attempt to relate any potential radiation risk to other commonly encountered risks, a relationship has been developed between potential life-shortening (a known effect of large doses of radiation) and known life-shortening due to commonly encountered risks in the environment. These calculations reveal that the risk from one chest film is equivalent to smoking 1.4 cigarettes, eating 40 tablespoons of peanut butter, driving an automobile for 30 miles, or living in Boston for 2 days [33].

TECHNIQUE

Obtaining a chest film of appropriate technical quality is difficult in a child with asthma. A typical child is understandably frightened, crying, and gasping for air simultaneously. Even when the child is calm, the sight of the radiographic equipment is frequently a sufficient stimulus to render the child uncooperative. A further difficulty arises if the child is too young to understand directions to suspend respiration or is unable to do so because of the asthmatic attack. The use of high kilovoltage, with rare-earth screen, and fast film combinations has markedly lowered the exposure times, thus helping to minimize motion artifacts on the resulting film.

While patient cooperation is usually not a problem in adults, adult patients frequently have a marked degree of hyperexpansion of the lungs. An increase in anteroposterior diameter of the chest and the increased amount of air in the lungs frequently mislead the technologist into selecting exposure parameters that result in overpenetration of the chest and overexposure of the lungs. Likewise, if the x-ray machine relies on automatic exposure control, older equipment sometimes will not terminate the exposure in a short enough time to produce a film of optimum density. The resulting overexposed, blackish film hinders evaluation of pulmonary vascularity or detection of minor infiltrates.

RADIOGRAPHIC FINDINGS

Chest Films

A plain film of the chest in an asthmatic patient is usually normal. If positive findings are present, they can be classified into two major categories: (1) Uncomplicated patients may exhibit increased residual air as manifested by changes in the thoracic cage, lung parenchyma, heart, or pulmonary vasculature; and (2) asthma may be complicated by pneumonia, pneumomediastinum, or pneumothorax, among other conditions.

Uncomplicated Patients

As stated previously, in most asthmatic patients the appearance of the chest is normal. The most common abnormality that will be apparent is hyperexpansion of the lungs [13]. The thoracic cage may show an increase in anteroposterior dimension, particularly in children; occasionally, bowing of the sternum (Figs. 53-1 and 53-2), an increase in retrosternal lucency, or bulging of

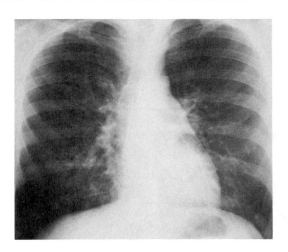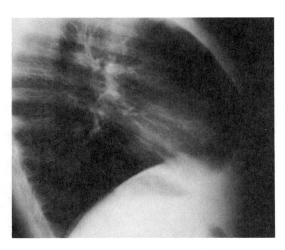

Fig. 53-1. *A 12-year-old asthmatic with marked sternal convexity (pectus carinatum). The anteroposterior diameter of the chest is greater than the transverse diameter. This finding is seen in children with chronic hyperinflation.*

the interspaces may occur. If the patient has been on chronic steroid administration, osteopenia of the vertebral bodies or even compression fractures may be present. The diaphragmatic leaves will appear flat in both anteroposterior and transverse planes (Fig. 53-3), but many normal young adults also can flatten their diaphragmatic leaves by voluntarily taking a deep breath. If fluoroscopy is performed, however, one can see in the asthmatic patient a decreased downward excursion with inspiration and a delayed return to the resting position with expiration; this study is rarely warranted. Similar findings are seen in early to moderate emphysema, and asthma should not be distinguished from emphysema on radiographic signs alone.

Many methods have been proposed for objective radiographic measurements of lung volumes ranging from a combination of measurements of the length, width, and depth of the thoracic cage [28] to methods in which tracings of the boundaries of the thoracic cage are submitted to computer analysis [11]. Although these quantitative measurements may have some validity [24], most observers agree that subjective assessment is almost as meaningful. Regardless of the method used to determine lung hyperinflation, the severity of an attack has little relationship to the apparent lung volumes as seen on the chest film [29].

The image of the lung fields is usually normal. Some observers have noted, however, that the bronchovascular bundles are not sharp and distinct but rather appear to have hazy and indistinct margins; no pathologic correlate explains this change. Related to this peculiar appearance of the lung markings, considerable discussion has been devoted to the possible visualization of thickened bronchial walls [12, 23]. When seen en face, the thickened walls have been described as consisting of thin, radiating white lines likened to tram lines (Fig. 53-4); when seen on end, they have been called ring shadows [7] (Figs. 53-5, 53-6, and 53-7). In an attempt to investigate this finding further, both regular films and plain film laminagraphic studies have been obtained of the hilar bronchi, and measurements have been made of both the wall thickness and the lumen-wall ratio. Some investigators have reported that these measurements are abnormal in asthmatics, with the bronchial walls appearing to be denser and to possess more sharply delineated margins [14]. There are a number of difficulties with these observations. First, the regular film correlates poorly with the laminagraphic examination: In some patients the regular films but not the laminagrams show abnormalities, while in other patients the converse is true. Furthermore, findings in the asthmatic patients considerably overlap findings in the controls, and frequently the asthmatics could not be distinguished from normals on the basis of tomographic measurements of the bronchi. Thin-section, high-resolution computed tomography (CT) is another method for studying bronchial wall thickness, but results with this method are not fully available [18]; the presence of emphysema can be elegantly demonstrated by this technique (Fig. 53-8).

Consideration of the pathologic changes described in the bronchi may help to explain these divergent imaging findings. An accepted standard of bronchial wall pathology is the Reid index, which is expressed as the ratio of the thickness of the bronchial mucous glands to the thickness of the bronchial wall as seen on histologic sections [25]. Even in the comparison of pathologic material from severe chronic bronchitics to that of normals, however, the Reid index is increased by only 18 percent [31]. Thickening of the bronchial walls can certainly occur pathologically in asthma, but the actual increase in depth is measurable in tenths of millimeters. Such gross histologic thickening still represents a microscopic finding with no possibility of seeing it on roentgenographic examination. Not only would such a pathologic finding not result in a change in x-ray density (since x-rays, by the laws of physics, are not capable of demonstrating differences in similar soft-tissue densities), but the walls would appear indistinct from the inflammation and edema rather than sharper. Occasionally reports of this observation recur, however, and this subject will undoubtedly be investigated further.

The size and configuration of the heart are usually unremarkable. True cardiomegaly or cor pulmonale does not occur. More often, the heart is elongated and thin (Fig. 53-9) due to depression of the diaphragmatic leaves. The vascular markings, the main component of which represents the peripheral pulmonary arteries, are usually normal in distribution and caliber. Rarely, the most peripheral markings may appear attenuated, while the more proximal vessels including the main pulmonary arteries may ap-

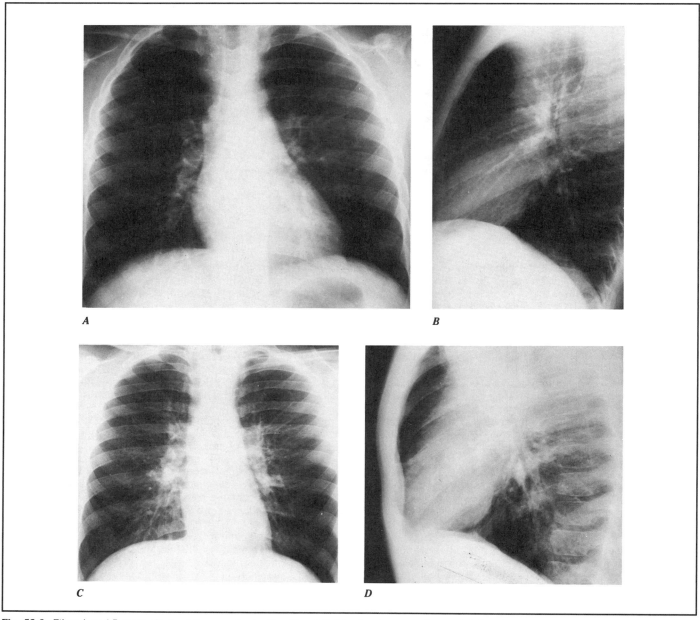

Fig. 53-2. *Films A and B were obtained 1 year prior to films C and D. The development of sternal deformity and increasing anteroposterior diameter of the chest are evident in this patient with asthma. The heart appears smaller on the later study.*

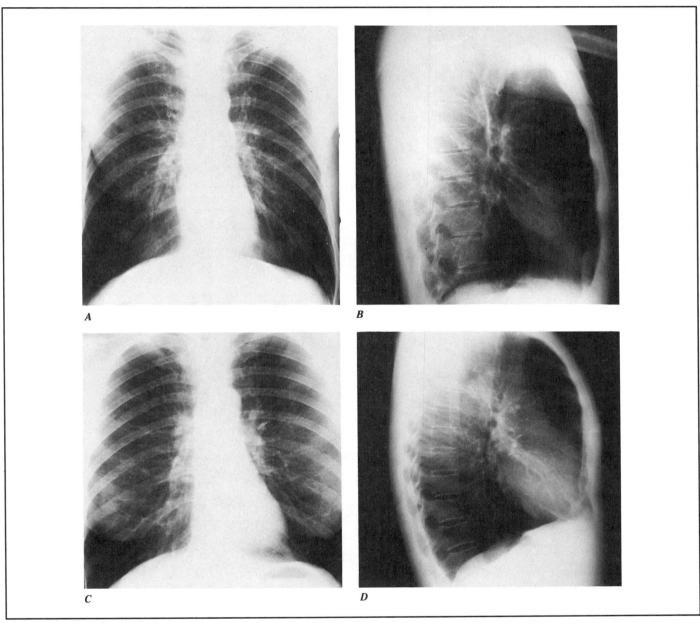

Fig. 53-3. *A 46-year-old male (A, B) and a 47-year-old female (C, D) with lifelong asthma demonstrating hyperaerated lungs, flattened diaphragmatic leaves, and an increase in the retrosternal air space. Both patients are quite thin. Neither has emphysema by standard clinical and laboratory criteria.*

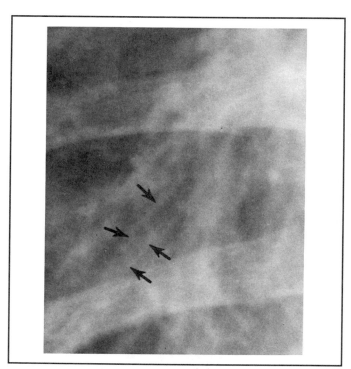

Fig. 53-4. *Tram lines. Detail film, right lower lobe. The parallel white lines (arrows) have been said to represent thickened bronchial walls.*

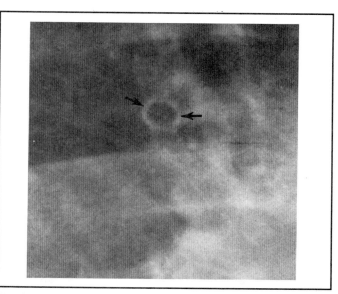

Fig. 53-5. *Ring shadow, right upper lobe bronchus. The wall (arrows) of the bronchus appears minimally thicker than normal.*

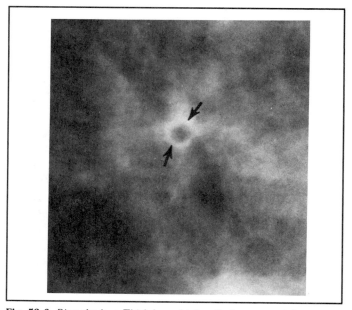

Fig. 53-6. *Ring shadow. Thick bronchial wall of an upper lobe segmental bronchus in a patient with congestive heart failure.*

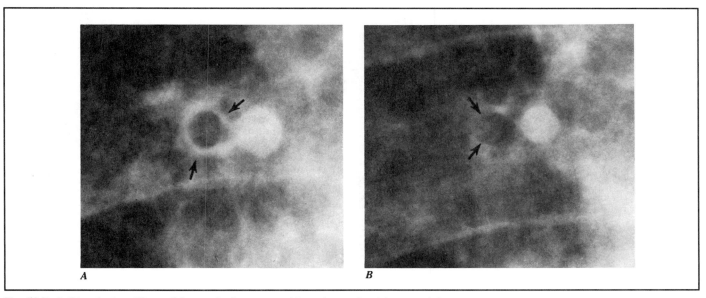

Fig. 53-7. *A. Ring shadow. The wall (arrows) of a segmental bronchus to the right upper lobe appears thickened in this patient in early congestive failure. A dilated artery lies immediately adjacent to the bronchus. B. Following therapy, the bronchial wall is much thinner (arrows).*

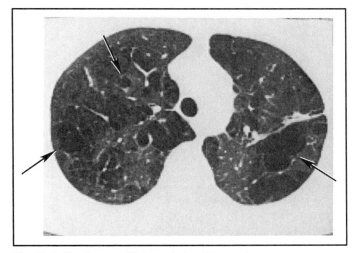

Fig. 53-8. *Emphysema. High-resolution CT scan demonstrates a multitude of irregular lucent spaces (arrows).*

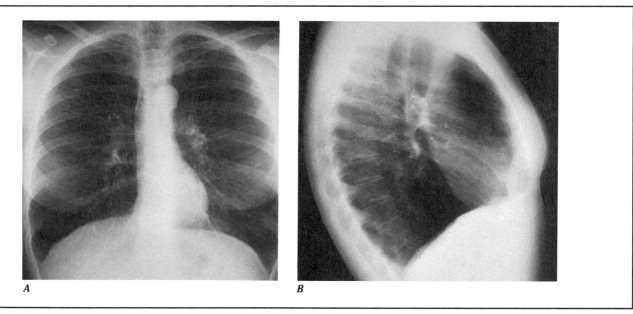

Fig. 53-9. *Small heart. A. The transverse diameter of the heart appears decreased because of the marked hyperexpansion of the lung with depressed diaphragmatic leaves. B. The heart size is normal on lateral projection.*

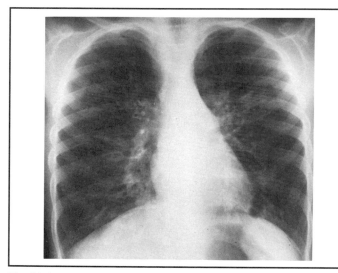

Fig. 53-10. *The peripheral lung fields (outer one-third) are devoid of vascular markings, while the hilar arteries appear slightly prominent. There is an unassociated right lower lobe infiltrate.*

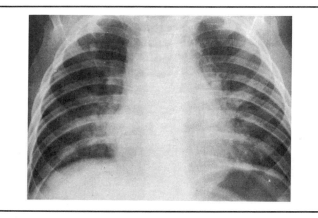

Fig. 53-11. *Diffuse bronchopneumonia.*

pear prominent (Fig. 53-10). These vascular changes do not correlate with the severity of an attack, are reversible, and are probably related to transient pulmonary hypertension.

Complicated Patients

The presence of an abnormality on a chest film cannot be predicted by the clinical status of the patient [10, 34]. Such clinical features as attack severity, respiratory rate, temperature, white blood cell count, arterial blood gases, and the presence or absence of cough and/or sputum production have limited predictive value [6]. Physical examination of the ears, nose, and throat does not aid the prediction. The presence or absence of wheezing and chest retraction is unrelated, but the presence of rales and rhonchi may be more common if a complication is present on the chest film.

Of the possible complications, pneumonia is the most frequent. The offending agent is frequently viral such as respiratory syncytial, adenovirus, rhinovirus, or parainfluenza virus. Common bacteria encountered include *Hemophilus influenzae* and *Streptococcus;* any fungus present almost always is *Aspergillus.* In most cases viral pneumonia cannot be distinguished from bacterial pneumonia by the findings on a chest film. Furthermore, the roentgenographic appearance of infection in asthmatics is identical to that of nonasthmatics. In the earliest stages of infection (infectious bronchitis or bronchiolitis), the hyperaeration and flattened hemidiaphragms will be indistinguishable from those of the patient without an infectious element.

If areas of pneumonic consolidation are present, they vary in size from small to large and occasionally involve an entire lobe. They may be single or multiple and are equally distributed throughout the lung fields. The patches of infiltration are charac-

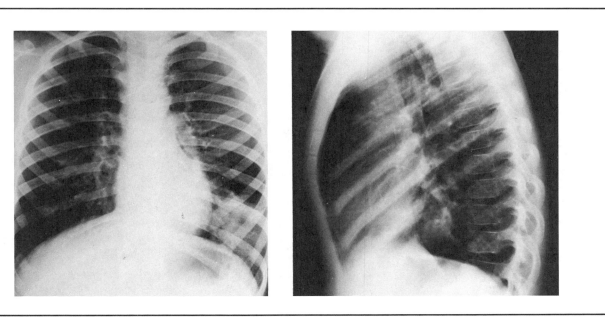

Fig. 53-12. *Bibasilar pneumonia.*

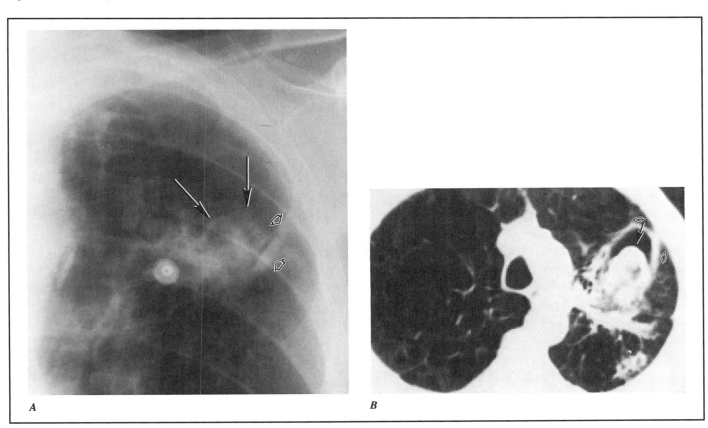

A

B

Fig. 53-13. Aspergillus *fungus ball. A. Plain film. Detail view of the left apex demonstrates an irregular mass (arrows) in a thick-walled cavity (arrowheads). B. The morphology is better demonstrated on the CT scan.*

teristic of air space disease with indistinct borders and frequent air bronchograms (Figs. 53-11 and 53-12). The classically described appearance of viral pneumonia, consisting of increased interstitial markings with enlarged hilar nodes, is most unusual in asthma, as it is in nonasthmatics. Complications such as pleural effusion or empyema are also unusual.

Aspergillosis may take a variety of patterns [8]. (For added radiographs, see Chap. 49.) Again, patches of fungal infiltration may be single or multiple and may range in appearance from amorphous to miliary, nodular, or even round. Cavitation may be seen in up to 20 percent of patients [19] (Fig. 53-13). Aspergillosis is sometimes associated with mucous impaction of bronchi,

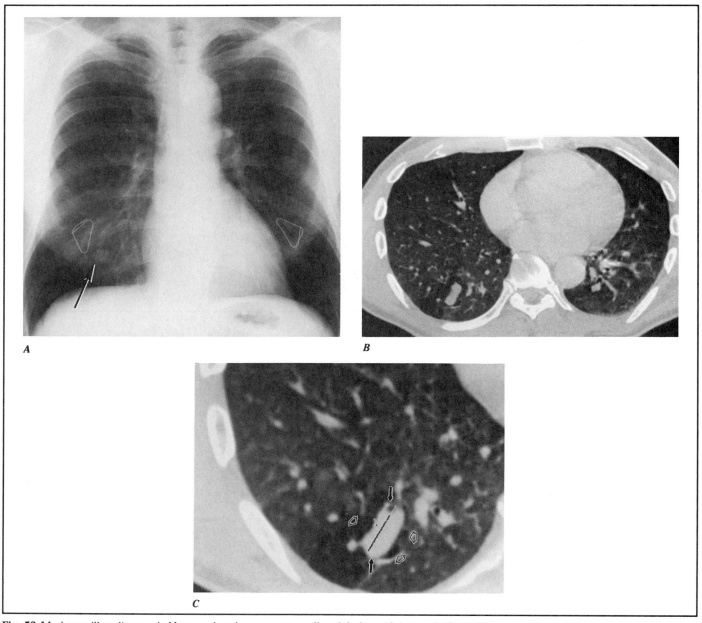

Fig. 53-14. Aspergillus *disease. A. Mucous plug. An apparent small nodule (arrow) is seen in the right lower lung field. (The bilateral dense triangular shadows represent nipple markers.) (B and C. High-resolution CT scan (B) demonstrates a 3 × 2 cm plug (arrows) surrounded by emphysematous air spaces (arrowheads) best seen on the magnification view (C).*

but *Aspergillus* infection is not necessary for production of mucous plugs [2]. If atelectasis occurs, these plugs will be obscured by the atelectatic segments or lobes. Because of collateral air drift, however, the lung distal to the bronchial obstruction may remain aerated, in which event the actual plug may be visible (Fig. 53-14). Their appearance has been likened to that of a cluster of grapes or fingerlike projections (Fig. 53-15). They vary in size from several millimeters to several centimeters, and their longitudinal axes are oriented along the axes of the dilated bronchi. These shadows may be transient, as the patient may expectorate the plugs, or they may be chronic, lasting for years. The usual result of a plug in a bronchus is subsegmental or segmental atelectasis; the radiographic pattern is identical to that of atelectasis from any other cause (Fig. 53-16).

As stated previously, thickened bronchial walls are not visible on films of the chest. If bronchiectasis has resulted from continued bronchial infection with destruction of the bronchial wall, however, the dilated bronchi may sometimes be visible on the chest film either as tubular shadows or saccular patterns sometimes suggesting cavitation. If further investigation is required, high-resolution computed tomography is the procedure of choice [27] (Fig. 53-17). These scans obtained at a slice thickness of 1.5 to 2.0 mm have a sensitivity and specificity approaching that of bronchography. Although bronchography can best reveal the integrity of the bronchi, this hazardous procedure has virtually no role in evaluation of these patients [26]. When bronchography has been performed, marked spasm of the bronchi manifested by decreased caliber and increased peripheral tapering was often

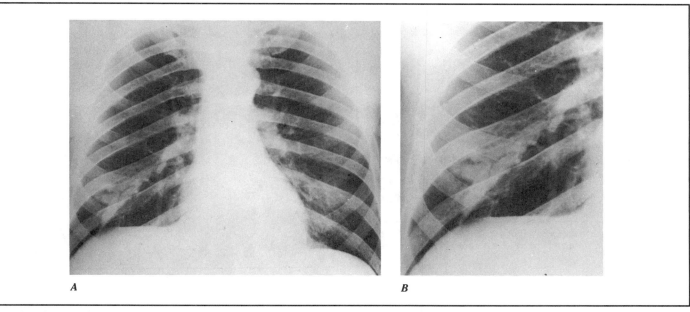

Fig. 53-15. *A. Mucous plugs impacted in right lower lobe bronchi, demonstrating a cluster of tubular shadows likened to a bunch of grapes. B. Close-up of lower lobe.*

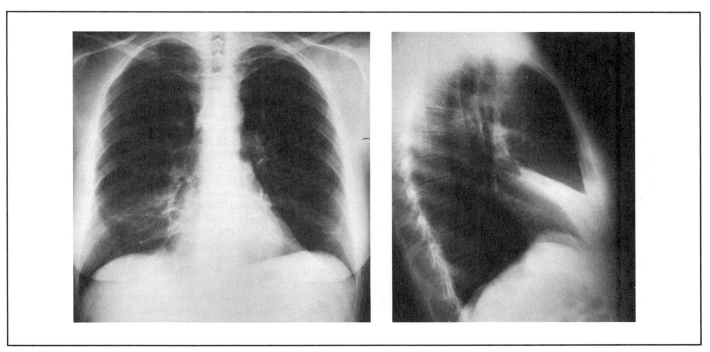

Fig. 53-16. *Atelectasis, right middle lobe.*

demonstrated (Fig. 53-18). Occasionally, signs of bronchitis such as filling of bronchial glands and bronchiolectasis were shown. If bronchiectasis is present its appearance is no different in asthma than in other conditions.

Pneumothoraces are uncommon in asthma, occurring in fewer than 0.5 percent of patients [4]. If present, however, they may compromise a patient with an acute episode and should be radiographically diagnosed. On the other hand, pneumomediastinum

occurs in 5 to 10 percent of asthmatic patients [5, 22]. The presence of a pneumomediastinum is heralded by cough and chest pain during an acute asthmatic attack; occasionally a pneumothorax or pneumomediastinum may occur if the patient has been placed on a ventilator. Subcutaneous emphysema is a common accompanying feature, and on auscultation Hamman's sign is frequently positive. Pneumomediastinum usually follows a benign course, and no therapy is required other than for the bron-

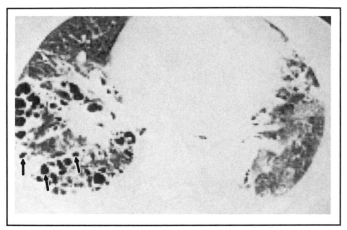

Fig. 53-17. *Bronchiectasis and pneumonia. High-resolution CT scan demonstrates dilated bronchi (arrows) between areas of consolidation.*

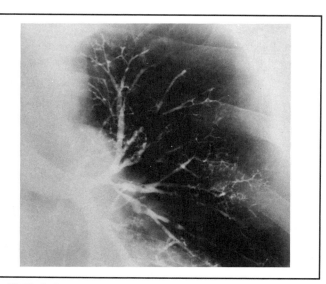

Fig. 53-18. *Left bronchogram in a known asthmatic patient, revealing spasm and irregularity of the bronchi.*

chial constriction that is present. A pneumomediastinum rarely recurs, and it is not accompanied by pneumothoraces. One postulated mechanism involves rupture of peripheral alveolae distal to constricted bronchi with dissection of the air along the pulmonary vascular sheaths into the mediastinum.

On posteroanterior radiographs, a thin band of air on either side of the mediastinum is typical of pneumomediastinum. Sometimes the air adjacent to the heart borders may be confused with pericardial fat (Figs. 53-19 and 53-20). These air streaks can usually be separated from the tracheal air column, and a longitudinal band of gas may also be visible parallel to the wall of the descending aorta. Pneumomediastinum is more easily seen on the lateral projection in which the thin, lucent lines representing the air in the mediastinum are in a retrosternal location or adjacent to the cardiac silhouette or trachea. The thymus gland may be well outlined and uplifted by the gas.

Films of other body areas may occasionally demonstrate findings that are important in patient management. For example, films of the head and neck area may reveal nasal polyps, enlarged adenoids and tonsils, or sinusitis (see Chap. 41). A finding often suggested by an adult patient's history of asthma or nocturnal exacerbations is that of a hiatus hernia with associated reflux; aspiration of gastric contents serves as a stimulus to bronchial spasm (see Chap. 75). The radiology of a tracheal tumor mimicking asthma is shown in Chapter 37. In addition to the previously described bony changes of osteopenia or compression fractures of the dorsal spine caused by steroid administration, osteomyelitis may develop anywhere in the skeleton. Steroid therapy may also lead to the abnormal accumulation of fatty deposits, which appear as mediastinal widening or as increased lucencies in the true bony pelvis.

Ventilation and Perfusion Lung Scans

Isotopic studies occasionally have value in patients with asthma to evaluate for pulmonary embolism or to use as a powerful investigative tool [16, 20, 21]. Ventilatory studies employing xenon 133 or krypton 81m demonstrate abnormal distribution of the single breath inhalation of radioactive gases in almost all cases (Figs. 53-21 and 53-22). The defects are frequently segmental in distribution and can be seen within minutes of the onset of an attack; they are related to bronchial spasm or mucous plugging. Following equilibration, the gas usually assumes a symmetric distribution. If serial films are obtained as the patient breathes room air after equilibration, however, areas of air trap-

ping become manifest by heterogeneous disappearance of the radioactive gas from segments of the lung.

Perfusion scans usually show similar defects: that is, heterogeneous distribution of the radioactive particles (technetium-99m macroaggregated albumin) (see Fig. 53-21). Impairment of perfusion is usually less than that of ventilation (see Fig. 53-22); the areas of lung that are not perfusing generally correspond to the areas of lung that are not ventilating, but some mismatching also occurs. The decreased perfusion appears to be related to hypoxemia secondary to bronchial constriction as well as possibly air trapping and increased intraalveolar and transpulmonary pressure that could interfere with capillary blood flow.

Ventilation-perfusion scanning has been used to study the mechanism of action of aerosol bronchodilators [30]. Specifically, the scans have shown that disturbances of regional ventilation and perfusion do not improve after acute administration of inhaler therapy. Although the peak expiratory flow rate does improve, the ventilation and perfusion defects persist. This indicates that the inhalant is deposited in the more central bronchi, causing dilatation, but does not reach the smaller more peripherally constricted airways. Long-term, more intensive therapy including other agents does result in a marked improvement in the appearance of the scans.

Scanning is of value in occasional patients who present with chest pain and wheezing and the possibility of pulmonary embolism. Assuming a chest film with clear lung fields, the patient with an embolus will show a perfusion defect(s) with a normal ventilation scan. On the other hand, the patient with an asthmatic attack will show multiple perfusion and ventilation defects that are for the most part matched or will show normal perfusion with an abnormal ventilation pattern (Fig. 53-23).

New Radiographic Techniques

A number of new lung imaging techniques are becoming available. High-resolution computed tomography, which is useful in evaluating interstitial fibrosis and the presence and extent of emphysema, has limited use in asthma. Magnetic resonance imaging is now widely available but to date has shown almost no usefulness in the diagnosis of various types of obstructive lung disease. Positron emission tomography is another modality that has yet to show usefulness in the evaluation of the lung.

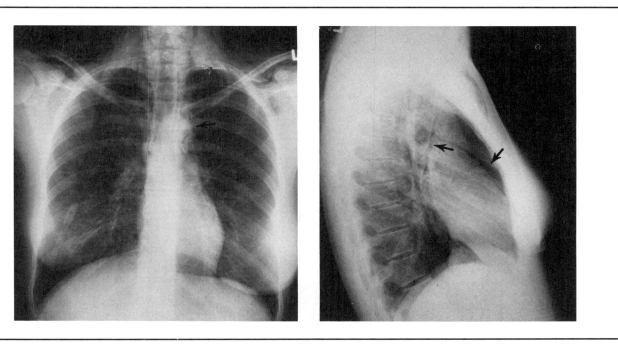

Fig. 53-19. *Pneumomediastinum. Streaks of gas are seen adjacent to the aortic knob (arrows), the mediastinum, and the soft tissues of the neck and axilla on the posteroanterior view; gas is seen in the pretracheal and retrosternal spaces (arrows) on lateral projection.*

Fig. 53-20. *Pneumomediastinum. Air is seen adjacent to the left heart border on the posteroanterior view and anterior to the heart on lateral projection (arrows).*

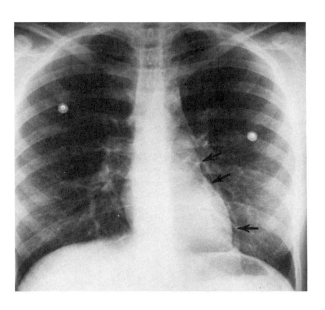
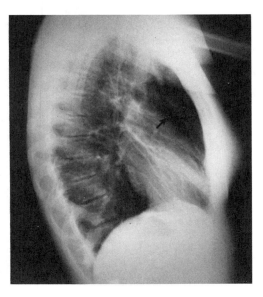

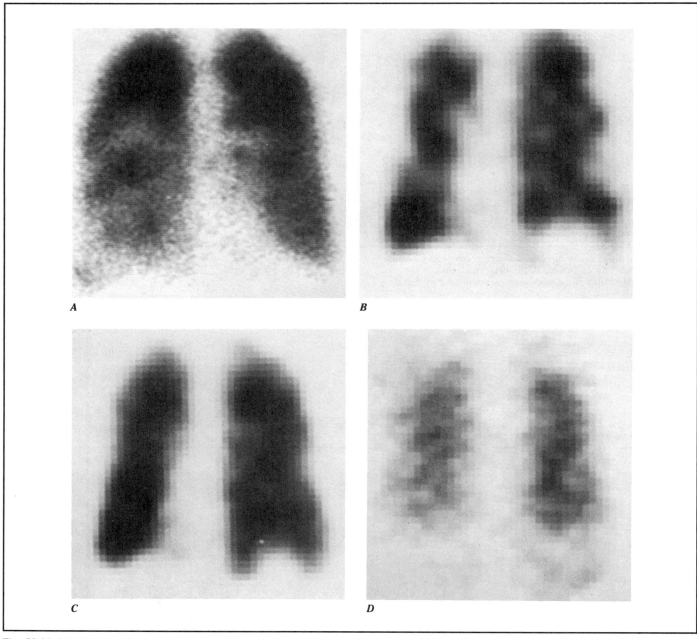

Fig. 53-21. *Ventilation-perfusion scan during an acute asthmatic attack. A. Perfusion: multiple perfusion defects, particularly in the right lung. B. Ventilation: single breath—there are multiple areas of nonventilation. C. Ventilation: equilibrium—most of the lung appears well ventilated. D. Ventilation: delayed washout—diffuse, bilateral air trapping.*

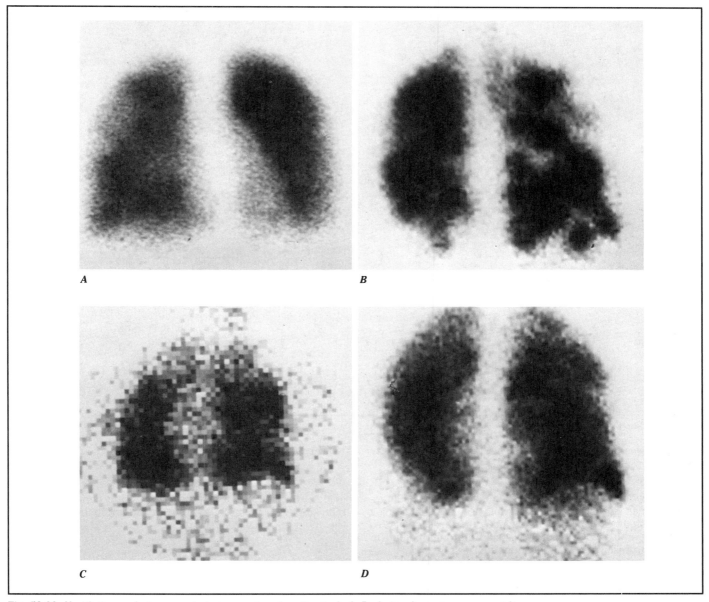

Fig. 53-22. *Ventilation-perfusion scan during an acute asthmatic attack. A. Perfusion: homogenous except for an area in the lateral border of the right upper lobe. B. Ventilation: single breath—multiple areas of nonventilation. C. Ventilation: equilibrium—relatively homogenous opacification of both lung fields. D. Ventilation: delayed washout—diffuse, marked air trapping.*

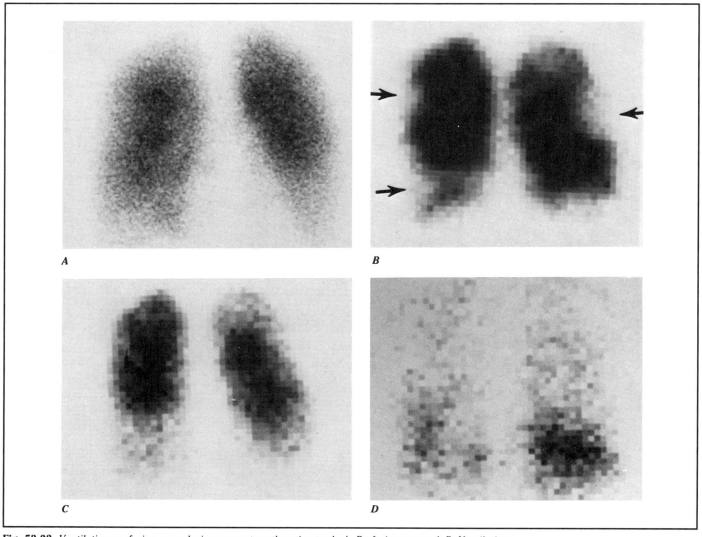

Fig. 53-23. *Ventilation-perfusion scan during an acute asthmatic attack. A. Perfusion: normal. B. Ventilation: single breath—bilateral areas of nonventilation most marked in lateral lungs (arrows). C. Ventilation: equilibrium—most of the lung is ventilated. D. Ventilation: delayed washout—air trapping, most marked at left base.*

In conclusion, the majority of chest films obtained in asthmatics are normal. However, the chest film is useful in evaluating a patient's first attack of asthma to exclude other possible causes of wheezing, and these films are virtually the only method to establish the presence of complications such as pneumonia, atelectasis, pneumomediastinum, and the very rare pneumothorax. A recent prospective study of acute asthma in hospitalized adult patients found, in contrast to the current general consensus, that an admission chest x-ray had a useful role in management decisions. For those patients who failed to respond to emergency room therapy, major radiographic abnormalities were seen in 34 percent of admissions. The authors recommended chest x-ray for all adults admitted to the hospital with acute asthma [31]. The author of a recent study of 135 patients with acute asthma recommended chest films for asthma patients who do not respond rapidly to initial therapy [4a]. High-resolution computed tomography is gaining new respect for evaluation of the integrity of lung parenchyma and bronchi but has yet to assume a definite role in asthmatic patients. Isotopic lung scans have value in identifying the rare patients with pulmonary embolism and asthma. A defined role has yet to emerge for magnetic resonance imaging or positron emission tomography. Used appropriately, various radiographic examinations can be helpful in the evaluation and treatment of asthmatic patients.

REFERENCES

1. Blair, D. N., Coppage, L., and Shaw, C. Medical imaging in asthma. *J. Thorac. Imaging* 1:23, 1986.
2. Braman, S., and Whitcomb, M. Mucoid impaction of the bronchus. *J.A.M.A.* 223:641, 1973.
3. Buist, A. S., and Vollmer, W. M. Reflections on the rise in asthma morbidity and mortality. *J.A.M.A.* 264:1719, 1990.
4. Burk, G. Pneumothorax complicating acute asthma. *S. Afr. Med. J.* 55:508, 1979.
4a. Dalton, A. M. A review of radiological abnormalities in 135 patients presenting with acute asthma. *Arch. Emerg. Med.* 8:36, 1991.
5. Dattwyler, R. J., Goldman, M. A., and Block, K. G. Pneumomediastinum as a complication of asthma in teenage and young adult patients. *J. Allergy Clin. Immunol.* 63:412, 1979.
6. Eggleston, P. A. Radiologic abnormalities in acute asthma in children. *Pediatrics* 54:442, 1974.

7. Fraser, R. G., et al. The roentgenologic diagnosis of chronic bronchitis: A reassessment with emphasis on parahilar bronchi seen end-on. *Radiology* 120:1, 1976.

8. Gefter, W. G., Epstein, D. M., and Miller, W. T. Allergic bronchopulmonary aspergillosis: Less common patterns. *Radiology* 140:307, 1981.

9. Gershel, J. C., et al. The usefulness of chest radiographs in first asthma attacks. *N. Engl. J. Med.* 309:336, 1983.

10. Gillies, J. D., Reed, M. H., and Simons, F. E. R. Radiologic findings in acute childhood asthma. *Can. Assoc. Radiol. J.* 29:28, 1978.

11. Glenn, W. J., and Greene, R. Rapid-computer-aided radiographic calculation of total lung capacity (TLC). *Radiology* 117:269, 1975.

12. Hodson, C. J., and Trickey, S. E. Bronchial wall thickening in asthma. *Clin. Radiol.* 11:183, 1960.

13. Hodson, M. E., Simon, G., and Batten, J. C. Radiology of uncomplicated asthma. *Thorax* 29:296, 1974.

14. Hungerford, G. D., Williams, H. B. L., and Gandevia, B. Bronchial walls in the radiological diagnosis of asthma. *Br. J. Radiol.* 50:783, 1977.

15. McFadden, E. R. Fatal and near fatal asthma. *N. Engl. J. Med.* 324:409, 1991.

16. Mishkin, F., Wagner, H. J., and Tow, D. Regional distribution of pulmonary arterial blood flow in acute asthma. *J.A.M.A.* 203:1019, 1968.

17. Molfino, N. A., et al. Respiratory arrest in near fatal asthma. *N. Engl. J. Med.* 324:285, 1991.

18. Naidich, D. P., et al. Basilar segmental bronchi: Thin-section CT evaluation. *Radiology* 161:95, 1988.

19. Neeld, A. N., et al. Computerized tomography in the evaluation of allergic bronchopulmonary aspergillosis. *Am. Rev. Respir. Dis.* 142:1200, 1990.

20. Novey, H., et al. Early ventilation-perfusion changes in asthma. *J. Allergy* 46:221, 1970.

21. Orphanidori, P., et al. Tomography of regional ventilation and perfusion using krypton 81m in normal subjects and asthmatic patients. *Thorax* 41:542, 1986.

22. Ozonoff, M. Pneumomediastinum associated with asthma and pneumonia in children. *A.J.R.* 95:112, 1965.

23. Petheram, I. S., Kerr, I. H., and Collins, J. V. Value of chest radiographs in severe acute asthma. *Clin. Radiol.* 32:281, 1981.

24. Reich, S. B., Weinshelbaum, A., and Yee, J. Correlation of radiographic measurements and pulmonary function tests in chronic obstructive pulmonary disease. *A.J.R.* 144:695, 1985.

25. Reid, L. Measurement of the bronchial mucus gland layer: A diagnostic yardstick in chronic bronchitis. *Thorax* 15:132, 1960.

26. Robinson, A. E., and Campbell, J. B. Bronchography in childhood asthma. *A.J.R.* 116:559, 1972.

27. Silverman, P. M., and Godwin, J. D. CT/bronchographic correlations in bronchiectasis. *J. Comput. Assist. Tomogr.* 11:52, 1987.

28. Simon, G. The plain radiograph in relation to lung physiology. *Radiol. Clin. North Am.* 11:3, 1973.

29. Simon, G., et al. Radiological abnormalities in children with asthma and their relation to the clinical findings and some respiratory function tests. *Thorax* 28:115, 1973.

30. Sovijarvi, R. A., et al. Effects of acute and long-term bronchodilator treatment on regional lung function in asthma assessed with krypton-81m and technetium-99m labelled macroaggregates. *Thorax* 37:516, 1982.

31. Thurlbeck, W. M., and Angus, G. E. A distribution curve for chronic bronchitis. *Thorax* 19:436, 1964.

32. White, C. S., et al. Acute asthma: Admission chest radiography in hospitalized adult patients. *Chest* 100:14, 1991.

33. Wilson, R. Analyzing the daily risks of life. *Technol. Rev.* 81:40, 1979.

34. Zeiverink, S. E., et al. Emergency room radiography of asthma: An efficacy study. *Radiology* 145:27, 1982.

III Therapy and Patient Management

Staging Therapy to Severity

L. Jack Faling
Gordon L. Snider

54

The pharmacology and rationale for use of the major drugs that are currently available for the management of asthma are each discussed in detail in the various chapters of this book. Also, Chapter 73 deals at length with the management of severe acute asthma or status asthmaticus. Thus, after a brief overview of the pathology and pathogenesis of asthma, in this chapter we will describe a system of grading the severity of asthma. This will be followed by a review of current treatment methods and by presentation of an integrated approach to the management of asthma, with special emphasis on how the various modalities are applied in patients with varying severity of disease.

CLASSIFICATION OF TREATMENT OF DISEASE

The treatment of most human diseases may be divided into two broad categories, specific and symptomatic. Specific treatment is directed at avoiding, preventing, or neutralizing the etiologic effects of the disease. Symptomatic treatment is intended to overcome the anatomic or physiologic effects of the disease without influencing the etiology. For example, avoiding an exposure to animals that are known to produce asthma, such as rats in the case of a laboratory worker, is classified as specific therapy. Bronchodilator therapy is classified as symptomatic therapy.

Asthma is a disease characterized by the development of airflow obstruction in response to stimuli not affecting most persons (see Chap. 1). The airflow obstruction is usually episodic and remits spontaneously or in response to symptomatic treatment. Although the etiology of asthma is discernible in a small proportion of patients (for example, inhalant allergens such as pollens, mold spores, or animal products; ingested allergens in foods and drugs; exposure to occupational chemicals), in most patients the etiology of their asthma is multifactorial or unknown. Consequently, most therapy for this disease is symptomatic. Although much has been learned about the pathogenesis of asthma in the last half century, this information remains incomplete and is still evolving rapidly. As might be expected, changing concepts of pathogenesis have influenced our concepts of symptomatic therapy. A brief review of the anatomy and pathobiology of asthma is in order to provide a rationale for a presentation of tailoring symptomatic therapy to asthma of varying severity.

PATHOGENESIS OF ASTHMA

Pathology of Asthma

Smooth muscle spasm is believed to be an important factor in the etiology of asthma. Although hypertrophy of smooth muscle is observed in persons dying of asthma, bronchial mucous plugs and inflammatory cell reaction are also prominent features and probably outweigh smooth muscle spasm in importance. Degranulated mast cells have been demonstrated in asthma, especially in the bronchial submucosa, but eosinophils are much more numerous; neutrophils, macrophages, and T-lymphocytes are also found. Edema and plasma exudation, expected accompaniments of inflammation, are demonstrable. Goblet cell metaplasia is present in the epithelium, as is thickening of the basement membrane. Focal desquamation of epithelial cells is prominent in both fatal asthma and in bronchial biopsies.

Pathobiology of Asthma

In recent years, inflammation has come to the fore as an important feature even in patients with mild asthma [9, 65] (see Chap. 9). Bronchial hyperresponsiveness has been associated with inflammation in animal studies [23, 93]. Mast cells are likely important in allergic asthma, but their significance in chronic asthma is uncertain. Eosinophils may release basic proteins that are toxic to airway epithelial cells [42] (see Chaps. 20 and 21). Many inflammatory mediators have been implicated in asthma and may contribute to various features of the disease such as bronchoconstriction, congestion, increased vascular permeability, and mucous secretion. Among these are histamine, prostaglandins, leukotrienes, and platelet-activating factor. Cholinergic neural impulses may result in bronchoconstriction and beta-adrenergic impulses in bronchodilation. Recently there has been interest in a third system, the nonadrenergic, noncholinergic nerves whose nerve endings release several neuropeptides that may be important in the asthmatic process [6]. The conclusion to be drawn at this time from these new data is that therapy should be directed against mural inflammation in the airways of asthmatics as well as against the actual components of airway obstruction: bronchospasm, luminal secretory obstruction, and mucosal congestion and edema.

STAGING THE SEVERITY OF ASTHMA

Asthma is a common disease, affecting 4 to 6 percent of persons in the United States and in other industrialized countries (see Chap. 2). The severity of asthma varies widely; the disease is mild in most individuals and attains a severity sufficient to require a hospital admission in less than 5 percent of the asthmatic population. Table 54-1 presents a classification of severity of asthma based primarily on two commonly used tests of airflow limitation, the forced expiratory volume for 1 second (FEV_1) and the peak expiratory flow rate (PEFR) [127].

Mild Asthma

Asthma may be classified as mild when the FEV_1 exceeds 2 liters and the PEFR 200 L/min. Patients with mild asthma may have

Table 54-1. Classification of asthma

Stage	FEV₁ (L)	PEFR (L/min)	Dyspnea and wheezing	Signs		
				Wheezes	Retraction	Hypercapnia
Mild (1)	2.0 +	200 +	±	±	−	−
Moderate (2)	1.0–2.0	80–200	+	+	−	−
Severe (3)	1.0	80	+ +	+ +	+	±

FEV₁ = forced expiratory volume in 1 second; PEFR = peak expiratory flow rate, measured with a Wright peak flowmeter.

Table 54-2. Grading of severe (stage 3) asthma

Grade	FEV₁ (L)	PEFR (L/min)	PaCO₂ (mmHg)	Pulsus paradoxus	Disturbed consciousness
3A	0.75–1.0	60–80	<35	+	−
3B	<0.75	<60	35–45	+ +	±
3C	—*	—*	>45	+ + +	+

FEV₁ = forced expiratory volume in 1 second; PEFR = peak expiratory flow rate, measured with a Wright peak flowmeter.
* Values severely restricted; accurate measurements are not usually possible because of patient's inability to cooperate.

episodic wheezing or occasional mild symptoms such as a feeling of tightness in the chest and increased production of bronchial secretions. They may complain of symptoms only during the night, after exercise, or under some other special circumstances. Patients with mild asthma are often not aware of wheezing and dyspnea; cough, with sputum that is so scanty that it cannot be expectorated but is swallowed, may be the chief complaint (so-called variant asthma; see Chap. 50).

Physical findings in mild asthma are limited to wheezing on auscultation, but in the patient who is symptom-free when studied, all signs may be absent and the FEV₁ and PEFR may be normal. Spirometric tests such as the forced expiratory flow in the middle half of the forced expiratory vital capacity (FEV₂₅₋₇₅%ᵥᶜ), which are relatively independent of effort and represent the geometry of the small poorly supported airways of the lungs, may be abnormal when the FEV₁ and PEFR are normal (see Chap. 26). However, given the episodic nature of the airflow limitation that characterizes asthma, even the more sensitive tests of small airway function may be normal during an asymptomatic period.

Moderate Asthma

In patients with moderate asthma, the FEV₁ falls to between 1 and 2 liters, and the PEFR to between 80 and 200 L/min. Dyspnea and wheezing, although generally episodic, are more frequently manifest. Wheezes and delayed emptying of the chest during forced expiration are uniformly detected on physical examination, but other signs of high-grade airflow limitation are generally absent.

Severe Asthma

In severe asthma, the FEV₁ falls below 1 liter, and the PEFR falls below 80 L/min. Dyspnea and wheezing become prominent and continuous. Most severe asthma occurs in patients with progressive deterioration evolving over days or weeks, or as periods of worsening in those with labile asthma. However, asthma occasionally develops unexpectedly and cataclysmally over a short period of time, giving rise to the need for immediate intubation and ventilatory support or even causing death within a few minutes of onset [109, 141].

Wheezes on chest auscultation are frequent, high-pitched, and widespread; they are often audible during inspiration as well as on exhalation [123] (see Chap. 51). In the most severe asthma, breath sounds are depressed and wheezes disappear as the airflow obstruction becomes so severe that insufficient air is moved to generate appreciable sound. Retraction of intercostal spaces, the use of the accessory muscles of respiration, and diaphoresis are observed. Patients often cannot tolerate recumbency and have difficulty speaking [16]. Pulsus paradoxus becomes evident on physical examination [103]. Disturbances of consciousness may occur [127] (Table 54-2).

Pulsus Paradoxus

In the pulsus paradoxus of asthma, the difference in systolic blood pressure between inspiration and expiration, which is normally limited to no more than 10 mmHg, may increase to as much as 60 mmHg or more [103]. In addition, the electrocardiogram commonly becomes abnormal with P pulmonale and QRS complexes revealing right axis deviation, right bundle block, and occasionally, the findings of right ventricular hypertrophy [44]. These abnormalities all revert to normal with improvement of the asthma. While the precise mechanism of pulsus paradoxus is incompletely understood, high pleural pressure swings during respiration appear to be its major cause. There is an inspiratory fall in left ventricular stroke volume with a simultaneous decline in systolic blood pressure [129]. A reduced cardiac venous return likely contributes to the degree of pulsus, with enhanced ventricular interdependence and increased left ventricular afterload playing additional roles [129]. Inspiratory impairment of right ventricular performance may also be a factor, with high negative intrapleural pressure impeding inward motion of the right ventricular free wall during systole [56]. As pleural pressure falls during expiration, cardiac ejection fraction and systemic blood pressure rapidly return to normal (see Chap. 78).

Severe Acute Asthma (Status Asthmaticus)

The term *status asthmaticus* has been used for generations to designate patients with severe acute asthma not promptly responsive to therapy with epinephrine administered subcutaneously or aminophylline administered intravenously; initial unresponsiveness to inhaled beta-adrenergic bronchodilators is also apparent. Widespread mucus inspissation of airways is characteristic of status asthmaticus and is largely responsible for its refractoriness to conventional bronchodilator therapy and slow recovery of lung function. Airway wall edema and inflammatory cell infiltration may also be contributory; bronchospasm appears to play a less dominant role than it does in acute self-limited asthma.

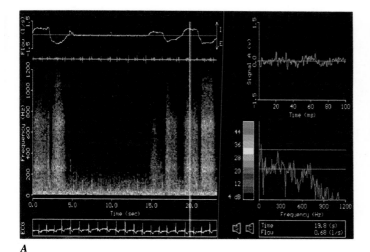

A

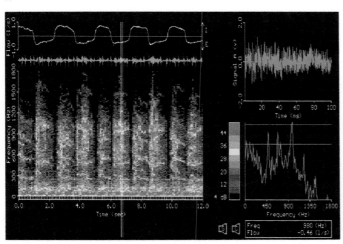

B

Plate 10. *A. Computer screen display of tracheal sounds over 23 seconds, with a respiratory pause over 10 seconds. Calibrated flow is plotted at the top (yellow), and the raw sound signal is displayed below (orange). The respirosonogram shows time on the horizontal and frequencies on the vertical axis. Sound intensity is indicated on a color scale. A simultaneously recorded ECG is plotted at the bottom. The right portion of the monitor screen shows details of a selected 100-msec segment (vertical double bar at 19.8 seconds). The signal waveform is displayed at the top, and the Fourier spectrum of this segment is shown at the bottom. B. Tracheal sounds in a patient with asthma and wheezing after exercise. Polyphonic wheezing is present during both inspiration and expiration. An expiratory segment at 6.7 seconds is shown by its waveform (right top) and by its Fourier spectrum (right bottom). There was no ECG in this patient. (Reprinted with permission from H. Pasterkamp, et al., Digital respirosonography. New images of lung sounds. Chest 96:1405, 1989.)*

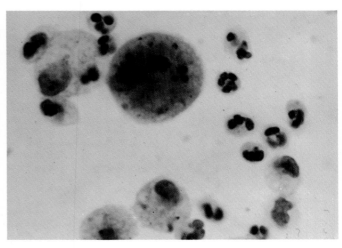

Plate 11. *Macrophages and neutrophils. The former are of various sizes, their cytoplasm is bubbly, and their nucleus is generally eccentric. (Papanicolaou stain, ×1,000.)*

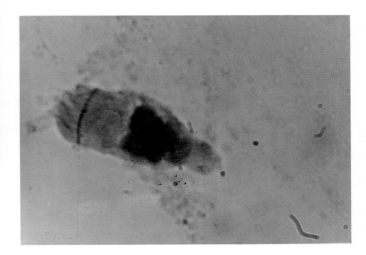

Plate 12. *Bronchial epithelial cell with ciliary tuft at upper left. (Papanicolaou stain, ×1,000.)*

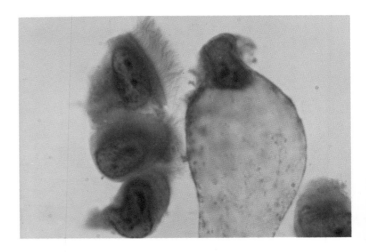

Plate 13. *Goblet cell (right) along with ciliated cell (left). (Methylene blue stain, ×1,000.)*

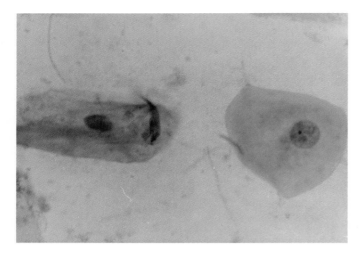

Plate 14. *Sputum specimen from upper respiratory tract showing squamous epithelial cells. (Papanicolaou stain, ×1,000.)*

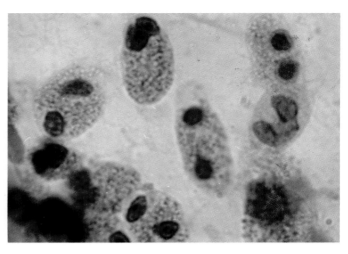

Plate 17. *Eosinophils with prominent and refractile cytoplasmic granulations; nucleus can be bilobed or nonlobed. (Papanicolaou stain, ×1,000.)*

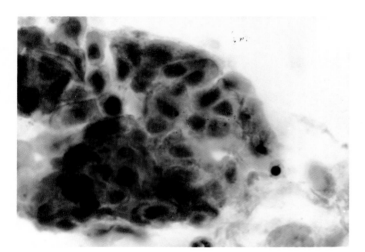

Plate 15. *Creola body formed through accretion of about 300 bronchial epithelial cells. Notice the peripheral palisading and faint cilia. (Papanicolaou stain, ×1,000.)*

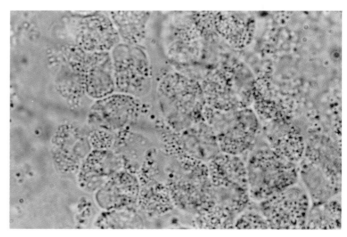

Plate 18. *The whole slide is covered with eosinophilic granules, resulting from disintegration of eosinophils during acute asthmatic attacks. (Papanicolaou stain, ×1,000.)*

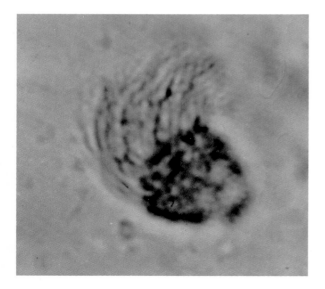

Plate 16. *Degenerated bronchial epithelial cell with complete loss of cytoplasm between nucleus and ciliary tuft (compare with Fig. 52-3). This process is called ciliocytophoria. (Crystal violet stain, unfixed, wet, sputum smear, ×1,000.)*

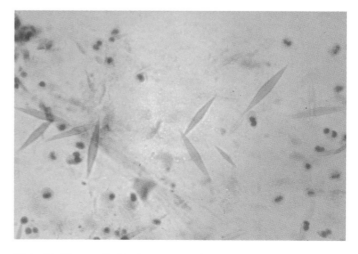

Plate 19. *The needle-like formation of Charcot-Leyden crystals. (Papanicolaou stain, ×1,000.)*

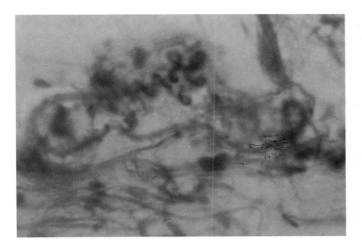

Plate 20. *Curschmann's spirals in their characteristic thread-like appearance. (Papanicolaou stain, ×1,000.)*

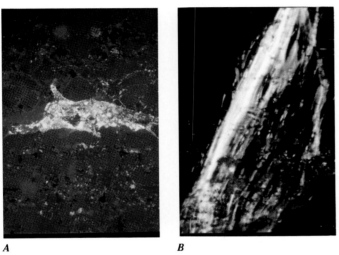

A   B

Plate 21. *Sputum matrix of asthmatic patient during acute clinical exacerbation (A) and after recovery (B). The former shows a marked decrease, fragmentation, and disorganization of the glycoprotein bundles versus the condition after recovery. (Toluidine blue stain, ×1,000.)*

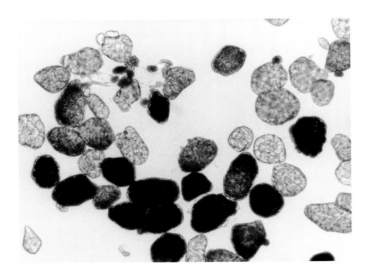

Plate 22. *Potato starch granules encircled by faint cellulose rims. The stain is not taken up uniformly. (Gram's iodine stain, ×400.)*

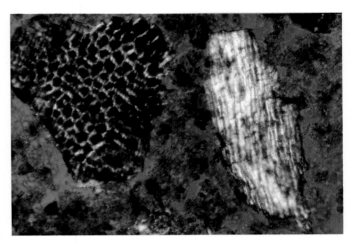

Plate 23. *Cellulose. This material is birefringent and stands out under polarized light. Here, it appears with the shape of palisades (right) and beehive (left). In the latter, the enclosed starch granules do not stand out because they are not birefringent. (Gram's iodine stain, ×1,000.)*

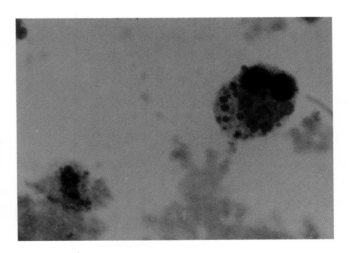

Plate 24. *Histiocyte* (upper right) *filled with ingested fat (red granules and coalesced). Some free fat is also faintly visible in the surrounding area. (Sudan IV stain, ×1,000.)*

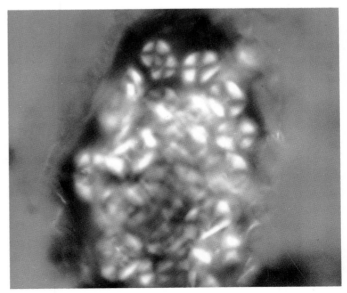

Plate 25. *Cholesterol granules in typical Maltese cross shapes. (Sudan IV stain, polarized light, ×1,000.)*

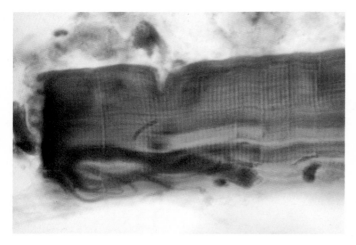

Plate 26. *Meat fiber showing bands and striae. (Papanicolaou stain, ×1,000.)*

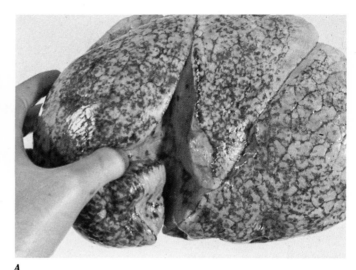

A

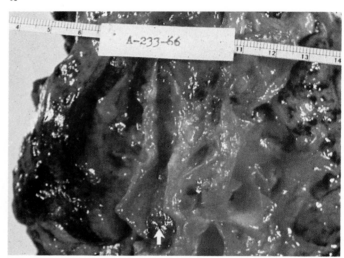

B

Plate 27. *A. Right lung from an autopsy on a patient who died in status asthmaticus. The lungs are stiff and hyperinflated and do not collapse even when squeezed. B. The opened mainstem bronchus and bronchus to the left lower lobe from patient with status asthmaticus. The bronchus is filled with a large mucous plug that is so viscous that the cut end does not retract (arrow). (Reprinted with permission from S. R. Hirsch. The Role of Mucus in Asthma. In M. Stein [ed.], New Directions in Asthma. Park Ridge, Ill.: American College of Chest Physicians, 1975.)*

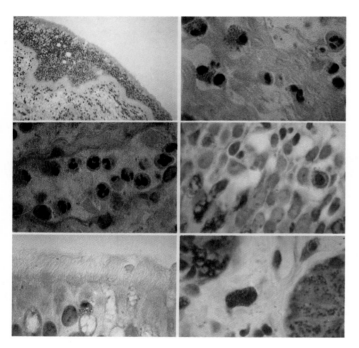

Plate 28. *Relevant features of bronchial biopsy specimens in asthma during clinical remission (light microscopy). Top left. Intact bronchial epithelium with presence of metaplasia and thickened basement membrane. Edema and cell infiltration in the submucosa. (Hematoxylin-eosin stain, original magnification ×100.) Center left. Eosinophils and neutrophils within a vessel in the submucosa. (Hematoxylin-eosin stain, original magnification ×400.) Bottom left. Eosinophil with its granules in the bronchial epithelium. Note the hyperplasia of goblet cells. (Hematoxylin-eosin stain, original magnification ×1,000.) Top right. Inflammatory cells in the submucosa, including eosinophils, neutrophils, and mononucleated cells. (Hematoxylin-eosin stain, original magnification ×400.) Center right. Granulated and partly degranulated mast cell in the bronchial epithelium. Note the presence of epithelial metaplasia and hyperplasia of goblet cells. (Toluidine blue stain, original magnification ×1,000.) Bottom right. Heavily granulated mast cell (center) in close proximity of two mucosal glands and of a vessel. (Toluidine blue stain, original magnification ×1,000.) (Reprinted with permission from Foresi, A., et al. Inflammatory markers in BAL in asthma during remission. Chest 98: 531, 1990.)*

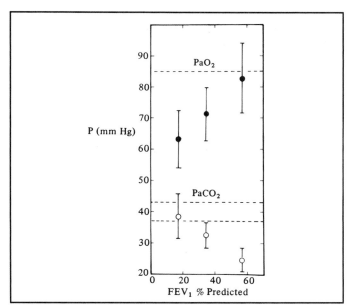

Fig. 54-1. *Arterial PO₂ and PCO₂ (mean ± 1 SD) in 101 asthmatic patients classified into three categories of severity based on the forced expiratory volume for 1 second (FEV₁): mild, greater than 50 percent predicted FEV₁; moderate 25 to 50 percent FEV₁; and severe, less than 25 percent predicted FEV₁. Note the rise in mean PaCO₂ and the fall in mean PaO₂ with increasing severity of disease, but the mean alveolar arterial oxygen difference is similar: 37.7, 39.6, and 40.2 mmHg for the mild, moderate, and severe groups, respectively. (From the data of E. R. McFadden, Jr., and H. A. Lyons. Arterial blood gas tensions in asthma. N. Engl. J. Med. 278:1027, 1968; reprinted with permission from G. L. Snider, Clinical Pulmonary Medicine. Boston: Little, Brown, 1981.)*

Arterial Blood Gases

Arterial blood gas measurements have added an important dimension to ventilatory function tests and lack of responsiveness to bronchodilator agents as a basis for grading severe acute asthma [75, 107, 144] (see Table 54-2). As might be expected with the severe airway narrowing in asthma, there is arterial hypoxemia due to impairment of intrapulmonary distribution of inspired gas. There is a rough correlation between the FEV₁ and the PaO₂—the PaO₂ is increasingly likely to be below 60 mmHg as the FEV₁ falls below 1 liter or 25 percent of predicted value [61, 75]. Although such a correlation has not been found by all investigators [110], arterial blood gas and pH measurement should be a part of evaluation of all severe asthma that is not promptly responsive to bronchodilator drug treatment. A disparity between level of oxygenation and impairment of flow rates has been hypothesized to result from gas exchange abnormalities relating to peripheral airway obstruction, whereas abnormal effort-dependent flow rates are a consequence of large airway narrowing [110]. There tends to be a biphasic relationship between the PaCO₂ and the FEV₁ (Fig. 54-1). The PaCO₂ is generally below 35 mmHg when the FEV₁ is greater than 0.75 liter or 30 percent of the predicted value. In patients with severe acute asthma who have FEV₁ values less than 0.75 liter, the PaCO₂ is increasingly likely to reach or exceed 40 mmHg.

Hypocapnia is the key finding with grade 3A severity asthma. The presence of eucapnia designates grade 3B asthma. However, a eucapnic blood gas value recorded when a patient is first seen must be interpreted in the light of the total clinical presentation; patients with chronic bronchitis complicating their asthma may be eucapnic even in the early stages of exacerbation. The development of normal PaCO₂ values (crossover point) after initially low values should be viewed with concern in asthma of unremit-

ting severity. Hypercapnia (grade 3C asthma) indicates the presence of severe acute respiratory failure [144]. In the hospitalized treated patient in whom hypercapnia persists, vigorous therapeutic measures must continue to be urgently applied, or death may supervene [119, 144]. However, most patients with hypercapnia when first seen respond quickly to pharmacologic therapy and do not require mechanical ventilatory support [12, 82]. In the emergency room setting, the FEV₁ appears to be a better predictor of the outcome of acute asthma than is the extent of arterial blood gas abnormalities [61, 92]. However, as already noted, we still recommend arterial blood gas measurement as a part of the assessment of patients with severe, acute asthma.

SPECIFIC THERAPY

Specific therapy has an important place in the management of mild and moderate asthma in combination with symptomatic therapy; specific treatment has a role in severe asthma only after the disease has been brought under adequate control and a long-term regimen has been established. Provoking factors that can exacerbate asthma, such as sinusitis and eosphageal reflux, require recognition and treatment. Unfortunately, it is often impossible to identify the agents causing a patient's asthma, and hence it is difficult to control the disease by avoiding exposure to the inciting agents. This is often particularly true of household antigens such as mites and molds. Avoidance of exposure to inhalants derived from animals such as dogs, cats, horses, or laboratory rodents may at times result in complete control of asthma. Changing jobs and avoiding exposure to agents in the workplace—for example, the isocyanates (see Chap. 46)—may also result in complete relief of symptoms. So will avoidance of foods containing the preservative sodium metabisulfite in persons allergic to this substance. When complete avoidance to a known allergen is not possible—for example, ragweed or other pollens—a trial of hyposensitization therapy may be undertaken (see Chap. 70). In patients who have drug-induced asthma, such as that due to aspirin, the need for avoidance of aspirin and the coloring agent tartrazine, which is used in some drug formulations and may also induce asthma in aspirin-sensitive individuals, is obvious. The patient must be taught to read the labels of over-the-counter medications and to avoid aspirin even when it is only one of several agents in an analgesic preparation (see Chap. 48). Other nonsteroidal antiinflammatory drugs may also cause severe asthma in aspirin-sensitive persons. Beta-adrenergic antagonist medications should be avoided, including ophthalmic solutions used to treat glaucoma.

All asthmatics should be instructed in the use of a scarf or mask over the nose and mouth when moving about outside in very cold weather. The scarf or mask serves as a heat exchanger, which uses heat from exhalations to warm inspired air. The use of appropriate additional medication before engaging in athletic activity or other exercise, especially if it is outdoors in the winter, should also be taught to all patients (see Chap. 86). All asthmatics should be counseled not to smoke; no asthmatics should add the irritation of tobacco or marihuana smoke to his or her already hyperreactive airways.

SYMPTOMATIC THERAPY

Bronchodilators Versus Antiinflammatory Agents

The management of asthma, especially ambulatory asthma, is undergoing critical reappraisal. What is questioned most is the long-established practice of "step-up" or intensification therapy in which conventional bronchodilators, mainly inhaled and oral beta agonists as well as oral theophylline preparations, are the cornerstone of therapy, with antiinflammatory therapy, such as long-term corticosteroids or cromolyn, added only if control of asthma remains or becomes unsatisfactory. A number of recent observations challenge the validity of this approach. Foremost is the concept that bronchial wall inflammation, not bronchospasm, may be the cardinal event in the pathogenesis of chronic asthma. Both bronchial wall biopsies and bronchoalveolar lavage (BAL) fluid analysis from patients with severe as well as mild stable asthma support this concept (see Chap. 24). Eosinophils appear to play a major role in this process [14], although other cell types such as T-lymphocytes and mast cells are also important [28, 41]. All of these cell types may be present in an activated state [2, 29]. Bronchial epithelial cell shedding, probably as a consequence of mucosal inflammation [57], and epithelial basement membrane thickening are also prominent features noted on bronchial wall biopsies in most asthmatics [41, 57]. Both the delayed or late asthmatic reaction and airway hyperreactivity may relate to airway inflammation and bronchial epithelial disruption [28, 57], and these events can be suppressed by cromolyn sodium inhalation and corticosteroids, while standard bronchodilators fail to accomplish this [7].

A second, recent, albeit preliminary observation is that regularly scheduled inhalation of beta agonists may worsen asthma as compared to as-needed bronchodilator therapy, and such treatment can mildly exacerbate nonspecific bronchial reactivity [120]; tolerance to inhaled methacholine is also reported with long-acting salmeterol [150]. The explanation for this is not presently known but may relate to a "protective" or "masking" effect of beta agonists, allowing greater patient exposure to allergens, irritants, and other injurious environmental agents that can worsen asthma by triggering airway inflammation. One recent mechanism is possible tolerance to nonbronchodilator effects such as mast cell stabilization [149]. It is possible that the escalating use of beta-adrenergic drugs in asthma is one factor promoting a worldwide increase in asthma morbidity and mortality [55, 152]. The number of patients studied is small [120], and more work needs to be done to explore this possibility. We think it currently inappropriate to abandon timed-dose metered-dose inhaler (MDI) beta₂ agonist therapy until extensive confirmation of this initial observation is forthcoming.

Because of the changing concepts of pathogenesis of asthma, there is a trend to introduce antiinflammatory drugs earlier in the course of asthma instead of waiting until the disease becomes more severe. However, it is important to point out that there have been no outcome studies to validate this concept. Further experience is needed to confirm the validity of this proposed therapeutic strategy.

Drugs used to treat asthma are presently classified into two major categories: (1) bronchodilators, which act quickly to relax contracted airway smooth muscle or to reverse one of the other mechanisms of bronchial obstruction such as thick secretions, mucosal congestion, or edema, and (2) antiinflammatory agents, which suppress underlying airway inflammation and inflammatory cell mediator release; the latter must be administered chron-

ically or over a long period of time because they attack underlying mechanisms of asthma but fail to provide immediate bronchodilation. Beta-adrenergic agents, anticholinergic drugs, and theophylline are bronchodilators; corticosteroids, cromolyn sodium, methotrexate, and nedocromil sodium are currently available antiinflammatory agents. The mechanisms of action of drugs used to treat asthma are shown in Table 54-3.

Bronchodilators

Sympathomimetic Amines

Adrenergic agents (see Chap. 55) appear to exert their bronchodilator effect through activation of adenylate cyclase on the exterior surface of the airway smooth muscle membrane via the guanine nucleotide regulatory protein system; adenylate cyclase produces an increase in intracellular cyclic adenosine monophosphate (AMP) concentration, impairing the interaction of myosin and actin to cause smooth muscle contraction [98]. Alpha agonists have their major effects on vascular smooth muscle. Beta-adrenergic agonists give rise to relaxation of bronchial smooth muscle via the beta₂ receptors; cardiac acceleration is produced by binding to beta₁ receptors. Beta-adrenergic agonists also inhibit the release of mediators of asthma such as histamine from airway mast cells as well as the discharge of acetylcholine, a bronchoconstrictor, from postganglionic cholinergic nerve endings in airway walls [108]. They do not inhibit the late asthmatic response or decrease bronchial hyperreactivity [25, 49]. Drugs with mixed properties such as epinephrine and ephedrine produce bronchodilation by their beta₂ properties, but they also produce unwanted side effects such as cardiac acceleration from their beta₁ effects and hypertension from alpha-adrenergic effects. For these reasons, there is no place for ephedrine in the modern treatment of asthma; epinephrine remains useful for subcutaneous administration in severe acute asthma in appropriate patients. There is also no reason to use the older nonselective beta-agonist isoproterenol because of its unwanted beta₁ cardiovascular side effects in addition to its brief duration of action.

A number of drugs with a noncatecholamine ring structure have been developed in recent years that are predominantly beta₂ agonists; that is, they produce effective bronchodilation with relatively little cardiac acceleration. However, it must be remembered that the beta₂ specificity of these newer beta₂ agonists is relative. There is person-to-person variability as well as decreased specificity with higher doses; when these agents are given parenterally, or orally to some patients, there may be quite striking cardiac acceleration (see Chap. 78). Because these drugs are not destroyed in the stomach, they may be given by mouth as well as by aerosol. Furthermore, because they are not destroyed by catechol-o-methyltransferase, as are isoproterenol and isoetharine, they have a much longer duration of action (Table 54-4) [143].

Rapid onset of action, high potency, duration of effect for 4 to 6 hours [3, 121], good patient acceptance, and a wide therapeutic index make the aerosol route, employing a metered-dose inhaler

Table 54-3. Mechanisms of action of drugs used in treatment of asthma

Drug	Block immediate response to allergens	Block delayed response to allergens	Prevent bronchial hyperreactivity	Dilate airway smooth muscle
Beta agonists	+	−	−	+ + +
Anticholinergics	−	−	−	+
Theophylline	+	+	−	+ +
Corticosteroids	− +	+ + +	+ +	− *
Cromolyn	+ +	+ +	+ +	−
Antihistamines	+ + (to histamine)	−	?	+

* Corticosteroids, by preventing and reversing the downregulation of airway β-adrenergic receptors, may prevent the development of tolerance to β-adrenergic agonists, thereby indirectly enhancing bronchial smooth muscle relaxation.
Source: Table derived from data in P. J. Barnes. A new approach to the treatment of asthma. *N. Engl. J. Med.* 321:1517, 1989.

Table 54-4. Sympathomimetic agents

	Recommended dosage per treatment				
	Subcutaneous (ml)	*MDI (mg)*	*Nebulizer[a] (mg)*	*Oral (mg)*	*Duration of action (h)*
Epinephrine (1:1000 solution)	0.1–0.5	0.32–0.9	2.5–22	—	1–2
Isoproterenol	—	0.16–0.39	0.63–3.8	—	1–2
Isoetharine	—	0.68–1.02	1.25–5	—	2–3
Metaproterenol	—	1.3–1.95	10–15	5–20	3–4
Albuterol	—	0.18–0.27	2.5–5	1–4[b]	4–6
Terbutaline	0.25–0.5	0.4–0.6	—	1.25–5	4–6
Bitolterol	—	0.37–1.11	—	—	4–6
Pirbuterol	—	0.40–0.80	—	—	4–6

MDI = metered-dose inhaler.
[a] Dosages vary widely. These are typical treatment doses, usually given at intervals of 3–6 hours.
[b] Long-acting (8- to 12-hour) preparation also available.
Source: L. J. Faling and G. L. Snider. Treatment of chronic obstructive pulmonary disease. *Current Pulmonology* 10:209, 1989. Reprinted with permission.

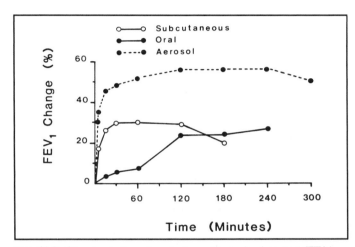

Fig. 54-2. *Changes in forced expiratory volume for 1 second (FEV₁) from baseline value following three different routes of administration of terbutaline. (Redrawn with permission from M. J. Dulfano and O. Glass. The bronchodilator effects of terbutaline: Route of administration and patterns of response.* Ann. Allergy *37:357, 1976.)*

Table 54-5. Steps for appropriate use of metered-dose inhaler (MDI)

1. Remove cap.
2. Shake inhaler.
3. Hold inhaler upright.
4. Tilt head back by 10 to 15 degrees.
5. Position inhaler 2–4 cm in front of open mouth.[a]
6. Begin inhalation and then activate inhaler.
7. Inhale slowly and deeply to total lung capacity.
8. Hold breath for 5–10 seconds.
9. Exhale slowly through nose.[b]
10. Inhale one puff. Wait 3–5 minutes between inhalation of subsequent puffs.

[a] Patients with poor hand to breath coordination should position inhaler between closed lips.
[b] May deliver medication to nose and sinuses with improvement of coexisting rhinitis and sinusitis.
Source: L. J. Faling and G. L. Snider. Treatment of chronic obstructive pulmonary disease. *Current Pulmonology* 10:209, 1989. Reprinted with permission.

(MDI), the ideal method for administering modern beta₂ agonists to manage asthma and prevent exercise-induced bronchospasm (Fig. 54-2). Side effects are fewer than with oral or parenteral beta₂-agonist formulations, presumably because drug action is topical with a lower blood level. The MDI delivery of beta₂ agonist has been shown to be clearly superior in bronchodilator properties to large oral doses of the same beta₂ agonist or to theophylline in stable asthmatics [121, 122]. However, proper technique in the use of an MDI is needed to ensure maximum benefit (Table 54-5) (see Chap. 56). The main side effects are a modest increase in heart rate and mild skeletal muscle tremor in some patients. These usually diminish within a week or two, while tolerance to the bronchodilator effect of MDI-delivered beta₂ agonist is minimal even following extended use [113].

The need to employ MDI extension devices (spacers) routinely to enhance delivery of inhaled beta₂ agonist to the lower respiratory tract is questionable. One well-done study in stable asthmatics documented somewhat greater improvement in FEV₁ following beta₂-agonist delivery by patient-triggered MDI as compared to the inhalation of the beta₂ agonist from a spacer (Fig. 54-3) [32]. As a rule, spacers are only recommended for patients who display poor MDI hand-to-breath coordination after repeated instruction, mainly children under age 5 and elderly patients. Spacers should also be routinely used by patients during severe exacerbations of their asthma when a slow inhalation and a long

end-inspiratory hold—essential steps in the proper use of an MDI—are difficult to perform. Beta₂ agonists administered in this fashion are equally effective to those given by nebulizer treatments, even during the care of asthma in the emergency room or in hospital [115, 136].

The MDI is used on an as-needed basis in patients with only occasional bouts of asthma but is generally prescribed on a fixed schedule in those with frequent asthmatic episodes or with persistent airway obstruction. A combination of a timed-dose and as-needed schedule may be useful—for example, in mild asthma, 3 puffs in the morning and at bedtime and 2 puffs every 4 hours as needed. While it is customary to limit daily dosing to 8 to 12 sprays per day, up to double this amount is generally well tolerated, especially in younger persons, and may be prescribed for patients who require further relief of their airway obstruction; several additional puffs can be taken for breakthrough attacks. However, patients must be cautioned to monitor how frequently they use their MDI, since persistently increased usage generally signals worsening asthma and the requirement to intensify antiinflammatory medications. The patient may be given a peak flow meter for use at home, and the dose of beta₂ agonist (as well as other medications) may be controlled by the fall in peak flow [8, 21] (see Chap. 94).

Metaproterenol, albuterol, terbutaline, bitolterol, and pirbuterol are the noncatecholamine, more selective beta₂ agents available in the United States as MDIs. Patient preference is usually based on acceptance of taste, some variability in side effects, and differences in price. Albuterol has recently become available in the United States as a dry powder, in capsules, which is inhaled from a breath-activated device [76, 135]. Because the powder

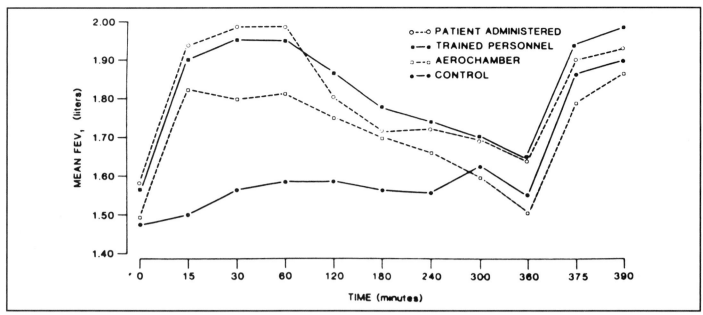

Fig. 54-3. *Change in actual mean forced expiratory volume in 1 second (FEV₁) of 13 stable asthmatic patients over time is shown following inhaled placebo (control) or 200 μg of fenoterol hydrobromide using three different methods of inhalation from a pressurized aerosol metered-dose inhaler (MDI) on each of 4 separate days. At the end of each study (360 minutes), an additional 200 μg of fenoterol by MDI was administered to confirm that patients were capable of a bronchodilator response on the day of study. There was no significant difference in the response to the three methods of active drug administration, but there was a significant difference (p < .05) from the placebo control values. (Reprinted with permission from S. W. Epstein, et al. A comparison of three methods of pressurized aerosol inhaler use. Am. Rev. Respir. Dis. 128:253, 1983.)*

formulation is drawn in by the patient's inspired air stream, successful inhalation does not require good hand-to-breath coordination; also, less pharyngeal impaction of drug occurs. In contrast to conventional MDIs, environmentally harmful fluorocarbons are not generated by this delivery method. Inhaled beta₂ agonists, with a bronchodilating effect lasting for up to 12 hours, are currently undergoing trials [39, 138]. Their release in the United States should improve patient compliance with by-the-clock MDI use and should provide another means for managing nocturnal asthma. Because the long-acting beta₂ agonists take longer to reach peak effect than do the short-acting agents like isoetharine, patients who have used the short-acting catecholamine agents may be reluctant to switch to a longer-acting product because they do not experience the almost immediate relief of symptoms to which they have become accustomed.

Isoetharine, metaproterenol, and albuterol are also available in solution for administration by compressed air-driven or ultrasonic nebulizers. This mode of administration is used for patients who refuse to use an MDI or when it is hoped that dilute bronchodilator aerosol will also lubricate the surface of a bolus of tenacious secretion and make expectoration easier. Such therapy also remains commonplace in hospitalized patients with acute asthma, although it is no more beneficial than beta₂ agonist delivered by an MDI with a spacer attachment [115, 136]. There is no indication for administration of beta₂-agonist solutions by expensive and sometimes hazardous intermittent positive pressure breathing (IPPB) equipment. However, such solutions are beneficial when delivered by ventilator medication nebulizers to intubated patients with status asthmaticus.

Metaproterenol, terbutaline, and albuterol are available in oral preparations but, as already discussed, are less useful than inhaled beta₂ agonists because of the increased frequency of side effects, especially in older persons. An extended oral release preparation of albuterol has activity for as long as 12 hours and is useful in preventing nocturnal asthma [50].

Subcutaneous epinephrine has long been used as effective therapy for managing acute exacerbations of asthma. Terbutaline is also available in a subcutaneous preparation, and the drug has been recommended for management of acute exacerbations of asthma employing one-tenth of its standard oral dose. Although its duration of action is substantially longer than that of epinephrine, terbutaline has decreased beta₂ specificity when administered by the subcutaneous route [125]. Albuterol has been recommended for intravenous use in the management of acute exacerbations of asthma [59, 67] and, unlike intravenous isoproterenol, which has resulted in myocardial ischemia, infarction, and death [64], is said to have relatively few side effects. However, an intravenous preparation of albuterol is not currently available in the United States (see also Chap. 57).

Anticholinergic Agents

There has been a recent renewal of interest in the use of anticholinergic agents as bronchodilators (see Chap. 64). These medications, whose benefit in asthma has been recognized since antiquity, act by competing with acetylcholine for parasympathetic postganglionic receptors on airway smooth muscle cells; bronchodilation is achieved by inhibiting normal cholinergically-mediated bronchomotor tone [47]. This effect is thought to predominate within larger airways. Anticholinergic drugs also block cholinergic nervous system–mediated reflex bronchoconstriction triggered by a wide range of irritants such as inert dusts and cigarette smoke acting on sensory receptors within the upper and lower respiratory tract. Anticholinergic drugs do not inhibit the release of mediators of asthma from mast cells and do not block the late asthmatic response to allergens [52]. They also fail to abolish bronchial hyperreactivity [17]. They are clearly less effective bronchodilators than beta₂ agonists in the treatment of asthma even if inhaled in large doses, and their slower onset of action makes them less useful for the immediate relief of bronchospasm [47].

The only clinically useful route for administering anticholinergic bronchodilators is by aerosol employing either an MDI or nebulized solution. The prototype anticholinergic agent is atropine sulfate, a tertiary ammonium compound, which because it is well absorbed across mucosal surfaces and penetrates the blood-brain barrier causes a wide range of troublesome anticholinergic side effects including tachycardia, mydriasis, ileus, problems with micturition, and mental changes such as confusion and hyperexcitability. While atropine can be administered in doses of up to 0.025 to 0.05 mg/kg using an updraft nebulizer, it is far preferable to employ the atropine derivative ipratropium bromide or another quaternary ammonium compound such as atropine methonitrate. These agents are poorly absorbed across mucosal surfaces and do not cross the blood-brain barrier, thereby freeing them of all serious systemic anticholinergic side effects. Ipratropium is the only anticholinergic agent currently marketed in the United States in an MDI. Glycopyrrolate, another quaternary ammonium compound with long-lasting bronchodilating activity, is the sole agent presently available here as a solution for nebulizer use, although it is not FDA approved for this purpose [139]. Oxitropium bromide, a more potent bronchodilator than ipratropium, is prescribed throughout must of the world and may be released in the United States in the near future.

The MDI delivers approximately 20 μg of ipratropium per puff and can be employed with a spacer. Because its peak bronchodilator action is delayed an hour or longer, significantly later than the peak benefit occurring following inhaled beta$_2$ agonists, ipratropium, like the other anticholinergics, is most effective when administered on a fixed schedule. The standard dose is 2 puffs or 40 μg every 6 hours. Larger doses up to 80 to 120 μg may promote further bronchodilation, but such dosing is controversial and requires further study. Tachyphylaxis does not occur even after long-term use, and side effects are limited to occasional mild xerostomia, short paroxysms of cough, rare paradoxical bronchospasm, and mydriasis with blurred vision if accidentally sprayed into the eyes. Ipratropium does not adversely effect airway mucociliary clearance [140] and unlike beta$_2$ agonists does not worsen hypoxemia or cause tachycardia or skeletal muscle tremor [99].

Occasional asthmatics who respond poorly to beta$_2$ agonists respond well to ipratropium, or a combination of ipratropium with an inhaled or oral beta$_2$ agonist [45] or with theophylline may result in an additive bronchodilator effect. When both ipratropium and a beta$_2$-agonist aerosol are to be used, there may be some advantage to inhaling beta$_2$ agonist about 1 hour following ipratropium; the dilating effect of ipratropium on large airways may promote enhanced penetration of the beta$_2$ agonist to smaller airways where catecholamine bronchodilating activity predominates [18]. Combination therapy with inhaled ipratropium and a beta$_2$ agonist may also be superior to the beta$_2$ agonist alone in the management of a severe exacerbation of asthma [94, 104]. Ipratropium is the preferred treatment in psychogenic asthma and is more effective than a beta$_2$ agonist for bronchospasm induced by beta blockers.

Theophylline

Although theophylline (1,3-dimethylxanthine) has been a mainstay in the management of asthma for more than 60 years, its mechanism of action at the cellular level is uncertain and its current role in therapy of asthma is undergoing reappraisal [66, 112] (see Chap. 58). The bronchodilator action of this drug has long been ascribed to its ability to promote the intracellular accumulation of cyclic AMP through its inhibitory effect on smooth muscle phosphodiesterase, the enzyme responsible for the breakdown of cyclic AMP. However, recent studies indicate that therapeutic concentrations of theophylline (10–20 μg/ml) are well below those required to inhibit phosphodiesterase activity

effectively in human airway smooth muscle [97]. Alternative proposals include stimulation of adrenal catecholamine release, prostaglandin antagonism, inhibition of release of proteolytic enzymes and toxic oxygen metabolites from leukocytes [90], and reduction in cytosolic free calcium concentration, thereby reducing excitation contraction coupling in bronchial smooth muscle [63]. Whatever its mechanism, theophylline can dilate large as well as small airways, and tolerance to its bronchodilator activity does not appear to develop even following long-term use. Unlike beta$_2$ agonists, theophylline inhibits the delayed asthmatic response to inhaled allergens, although certainly less effectively than do corticosteroids and cromolyn sodium [72]. Its ability to improve strength and endurance of diaphragmatic contraction as well as to stimulate respiratory drive is probably a less important pharmacologic action in asthma than in chronic obstructive pulmonary disease (COPD).

Theophylline has fallen into some disfavor, especially as single therapy, because it is a weaker bronchodilator than the beta$_2$ agonists in both stable and acute asthma [122, 126], because it does not diminish bronchial hyperreactivity [31], and because its use is associated with a high frequency of toxicity. While many of its side effects are minor (sleeplessness, nausea, and premature ventricular contractions), others like ventricular arrhythmias and seizures may be fatal. Such severe adverse effects generally develop at serum levels above 30 to 35 mg/L, but some susceptible patients experience them at much lower blood levels. Minor symptoms of theophylline toxicity frequently do not precede arrhythmias or seizures, and such symptoms should not be relied upon as a warning sign or dosing end point [143, 148]. Older patients are especially likely to manifest a narrow therapeutic-toxic index with side effects sometimes occurring at blood levels below 20 mg/L. The toxicity problem is compounded by the substantial variability in theophylline blood level of patients receiving similar daily theophylline doses. This stems from widely varying theophylline clearance rates and serum half-lives due to differing rates of theophylline metabolism by the hepatic microsomal cytochrome P-450 mixed-function oxidase system. In addition to genetically determined rapid and slow metabolizers [80], theophylline clearance decreases with older age and is enhanced or diminished by many factors (Table 54-6). Congestive heart failure, major hepatic dysfunction, and the drugs cimetidine, erythromycin, and ciprofloxacin may so profoundly impair theophylline metabolism by the liver that daily theophylline requirements are reduced by 25 to 50 percent or even more. Severe hypoxemia (PaO$_2$ < 45 mmHg), fever, pneumonia, or viral infections may also retard theophylline metabolism. Diet and time of

Table 54-6. Factors affecting theophylline metabolism

Increase metabolism	Decrease metabolism
Cigarette smoking	Hepatic dysfunction
Marijuana smoking	Congestive heart failure
Phenytoin	Cimetidine
Barbiturates	Erythromycin
Carbamazepine	Troleandomycin
Rifampin	Ciprofloxacin
Hyperthyroidism	Ticlopidine
Cystic fibrosis	Thiabendazole
High protein diet	Oral contraceptives
Children, adolescents	Propranolol
	Severe acute illness
	Viral infections (influenza)
	COPD with severe hypoxemia (PaO$_2$ < 45 mmHg)
	High carbohydrate diet
	Old age

Source: L. J. Faling and G. L. Snider. Treatment of chronic obstructive pulmonary disease. *Current Pulmonology* 10:209, 1989. Reprinted with permission.

dosing can also influence theophylline blood level and rate of drug availability.

The theophylline formulations of choice are the long-acting, slow-release anhydrous theophylline preparations, which are designed to maintain a reasonably stable theophylline blood level when taken on a fixed dosing schedule. Both twice and once a day agents are currently available, although rapid theophylline metabolizers will need to increase dose frequency to avoid excessive fluctuation in theophylline blood concentrations resulting from lower trough levels. Many of the minor but unpleasant caffeine-like side effects of theophylline can be avoided by starting with a reduced dose for up to a week and then gradually increasing to a full dosage. The broad range of the theophylline products presently available in the United States may significantly differ with respect to the completeness, rate, and consistency of their absorption [142]. Physicians should become familiar with and prescribe only one or two of the long-acting formulations.

Given the many factors that impact on theophylline metabolism, measurement of serum theophylline concentration is the only way to make certain that the blood level is in the therapeutic range and the patient is not being threatened by serious theophylline toxicity. Ideally, blood should be drawn when a steady state is achieved after 5 to 6 half-lives of the drug, which is generally 48 to 72 hours after beginning maintenance theophylline therapy. A similarly timed blood level should be done to determine whether a therapeutic intervention has influenced theophylline clearance, whether a particular side effect is related to theophylline, or whether it is safe to increase the dosage of theophylline to enhance therapeutic efficacy.

Despite its many problems, theophylline therapy continues to have a place in asthma management [58]. Once or twice daily dosing with a sustained-release preparation is particularly useful in patients with mild asthma. There is the advantage that patients tend to be more compliant with twice or three times daily oral therapy than with aerosols; this approach is also useful for control of nocturnal asthma. It is important to exclude gastroesophageal reflux as the cause of nocturnal asthma, since theophylline can aggravate this problem by relaxing the lower esophageal sphincter. Theophylline has an additive effect when combined with oral [147] and to a lesser extent with inhaled [122] beta$_2$ agonists. A low dose of oral theophylline taken together with a low dose of an oral beta$_2$ agonist has the efficacy of high-dose single-agent bronchodilator therapy without the serious toxicity of either drug [147]. This approach is warranted in severe asthmatics who fail to control their disease with maximum doses of combined inhaled bronchodilator and inhaled antiinflammatory drugs. This strategy may also be useful in severe chronic, oral corticosteroid-dependent asthma, with theophylline providing some steroid sparing benefit [87].

The value of intravenous aminophylline in the emergency treatment of severe acute asthma is controversial [69] (see Chap. 72). It should not be given as single-agent therapy, but combined aminophylline and subcutaneous beta$_2$-agonist therapy is probably superior to a subcutaneous beta$_2$ agonist given alone [69]. This advantage is lost when aminophylline is used as an adjunct to inhaled beta$_2$ agonists. Similarly, intravenous aminophylline together with systemic corticosteroids appears less effective than beta$_2$ agonists with corticosteroids, but additional studies are needed to clarify this point as well as to address the possible benefit of adding aminophylline to a combination of corticosteroids and beta$_2$ agonists.

A linear relationship between improvement in the FEV$_1$ and the log of the blood theophylline concentration has been demonstrated in asthma [81] (Fig. 54-4). There is much less bronchodilator effect between 15 and 20 μg/ml than between 5 and 10 μg/ml. Put differently, there is only modest further improvement in FEV$_1$ above a serum theophylline level of 10 to 12 μg/ml; there is minimal gain in efficacy but greatly enhanced risk of toxicity as

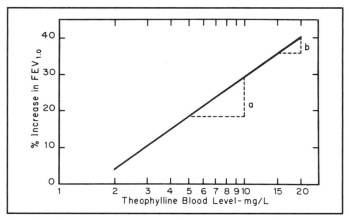

Fig. 54-4. *Dose response relation of increase from baseline value in forced expiratory volume for 1 second (FEV$_1$) in asthmatic subjects, against plasma theophylline concentration, plotted semilogarithmically. Note the much greater change in FEV$_1$ between theophylline blood levels of 5 and 10 mg/L (a) than between levels of 15 and 20 mg/L (b).*

Table 54-7. *Biologic mechanisms of corticosteroids in asthma*

1. Induce formation of lipocortin
2. Through lipocortin, inhibit phospholipase A$_2$ and thereby inhibit eicosanoid release
3. Upregulate beta-adrenergic receptor through increase in beta-adrenergic receptor density
4. Suppress inflammatory airway edema by diminishing microvascular permeability, perhaps through induction of "vasocortin"
5. Inhibit formation and secretion of mucus into airways
6. Inhibit recruitment, proliferation, and activation of various inflammatory cells including mast cells, basophils, eosinophils, lymphocytes, and macrophages
7. Prevent and reduce airway hyperresponsiveness

the maximum tolerable theophylline blood level of 20 μg/ml is approached. That is not to say that some patients, who are mostly younger, may have no toxic effects with blood levels as high as 40 μg/ml.

The oral dose of theophylline that will result in a plasma concentration of 10 μg/ml in ambulatory patients with asthma is in the range of 10 to 15 mg/kg/day. With this dosing, theophylline blood levels are infrequently needed in stable asthma patients. Higher doses will often be needed in patients who are exposed to hepatic enzyme inducers, including those who smoke cigarettes or who require the anticonvulsant medications phenytoin, barbiturates, or carbamazepine.

Antiinflammatory Agents

Corticosteroids

Because of their remarkable ability to suppress inflammation, corticosteroids are acknowledged to play a major role in the management of asthma. They must not be withheld when needed but must be given in such a way as to minimize their toxic side effects. While we do not yet fully understand the mechanisms by which corticosteroids function in asthma, it is clear, as shown in Table 54-7, that these agents interdict the asthma process through multiple effects. Their net benefit is to block the late asthmatic response and to diminish bronchial hyperreactivity [25, 31]. By decreasing the number of airway mast cells, they may reduce the intensity of the early asthmatic reaction. They can minimize beta$_2$ agonist–induced tachyphylaxis by reversing the downregulation of airway beta$_2$-adrenergic receptors [7].

Corticosteroids do not rapidly relieve asthma symptoms; they neither inhibit mast cell mediator release nor do they block the early asthmatic response [116]. Even when given intravenously in severe asthma, corticosteroids take up to 6 hours to begin to relieve airflow obstruction [77]. Accordingly, these drugs must be given on a fixed dose schedule. Because of their safety and efficacy, inhaled corticosteroids are now recognized as first-line drugs in the treatment of asthma. They are considered appropriate therapy in patients with moderate or even mild asthma.

A number of corticosteroids are used systemically for treating asthma. Hydrocortisone, administered only intravenously, has a half-life of 8 to 12 hours. Oral prednisone, prednisolone, and methylprednisone have biologic half-lives of 12 to 36 hours and demonstrate less sodium-retaining potency than hydrocortisone. An intravenous preparation of methylprednisolone is also available. The benefit of parenteral corticosteroids in treating acute asthma in the emergency room setting remains controversial [130]. Most studies demonstrate that such therapy promotes significantly faster recovery than oral corticosteroids alone [35] and reduces the recurrence of asthma for the next 7 to 10 days [20].

Inhaled Corticosteroids

The three MDI-packaged corticosteroids currently available in the United States are beclomethasone dipropionate, triamcinolone acetonide, and flunisolide. All three have potent topical antiinflammatory properties because of their high affinity for glucocorticoid receptors and their high lipid solubility. Budesonide, the most potent of all the aerosolized corticosteroids, is not presently available in this country. These agents manifest low systemic activity and minimal toxicity due to their rapid inactivation by the liver, especially the fraction that undergoes first-pass hepatic metabolism after having been deposited in the mouth during inhalation, swallowed, and absorbed from the gut [22].

In standard low doses, inhaled corticosteroids cause subtle changes in hypothalamic-pituitary-adrenal axis function, which are of questionable importance and cause no clinically significant systemic side effects. With higher doses, endocrine function is adversely affected to a greater but probably still clinically unimportant extent, while systemic side effects remain far less than those with oral corticosteroid therapy. This is true in children as well as in adults [62] (see Chap. 62). Standard doses of inhaled corticosteroids also appear to be safe in pregnant asthmatic women [46].

The beneficial effect of inhaled corticosteroids is dose related. Most childhood asthma can be controlled with beclomethasone doses between 100 and 800 μg/day. One goal of such therapy is to discontinue oral corticosteroids completely or at least to permit reduction of the oral dose to a relatively nontoxic range. This goal, which is especially important in children because of the growth-suppressing effects of corticosteroids, is frequently attainable. In some adult patients, attaining this goal with a beclomethasone MDI requires doses ranging up to 2,000 μg/day, far exceeding the usual dose of 400 μg/day [133]. As a practical matter, such high dosing requires concentrated corticosteroid formulations, which are not currently available in the United States. On occasion, even high doses of inhaled corticosteroids are not sufficient to supplant oral corticosteroid use [106].

Beclomethasone aerosol is effective in a four times daily regimen in mild or moderate asthma, and giving the total dose in a twice daily regimen is often feasible [78]. Four times daily dosing is generally needed in severe disease. A severe relapse of asthma while the patient is on inhaled steroids necessitates the immediate reinstitution of systemic steroid therapy. Inhaled corticosteroids are of benefit in exercise-induced asthma [51], but an inhaled beta₂ agonist or cromolyn is preferred for treating this condition, since both are effective when given as needed, shortly before exercise.

The most common side effects of inhaled steroids are dysphonia (huskiness or hoarseness of the voice), sore throat, and oropharyngeal candidiasis [134]. Dysphonia, the consequence of a steroid myopathy involving muscles controlling the vocal cords, may occur more often in persons who chronically stress their voice. Unlike upper respiratory tract candidiasis, dysphonia does not improve with topical antifungal agents. All these side effects are lessened by mouth rinsing immediately after steroid inhalation and can be totally prevented by using a spacer, which captures the larger nonrespirable particles and minimizes the deposition of corticosteroid in the upper respiratory tract [89]. Less frequent problems with inhaled steroids include the unmasking of allergic conditions previously suppressed by systemic steroid therapy such as allergic rhinitis and allergic bronchopulmonary aspergillosis. The symptoms of systemic steroid withdrawal (arthralgias, myalgias, lethargy, depression and anorexia, or overt hypoadrenalism) may also develop.

Oral Corticosteroids

A short (2- to 4-week) course of an oral corticosteroid, starting at 25 to 30 mg of prednisone or an equivalent dose of another drug such as methylprednisolone, 20 to 24 mg/day, given first in divided doses and then once daily with tapering of the dose as asthma improves, is usually effective in controlling an exacerbation of asthma. Corticosteroids can be taken at the full dose for a few days and stopped abruptly as well as being gradually tapered; there is virtually no risk of serious toxicity with such a course [128].

Daily administration of even low doses of corticosteroids for extended periods is accompanied by a high risk of toxic side effects including osteoporosis, diabetes mellitus, hypertension, increased risk of infection, hypokalemia, and cataracts [1]. The risk of side effects can be minimized by using as low a dose as possible, preferably 10 mg/day or less of prednisone, and by administering the corticosteroid in a single dose in the morning. Giving twice the daily corticosteroid dose on alternate days also decreases toxicity but is not as effective in controlling symptoms. Oral corticosteroids should never be used alone but should supplement inhaled corticosteroids and a bronchodilator regimen.

Cromolyn Sodium

Cromolyn can effectively prevent allergen-induced asthma benefiting both the immediate-onset asthmatic reaction and the delayed-onset reaction, which is associated with pronounced airway inflammatory changes and subsequent bronchial hyperresponsiveness [85]. Though our knowledge of the exact pharmacologic actions of this drug is incomplete, one well-known effect is its inhibition of mast cell mediator release, despite the interaction of IgE and antigen on the mast cell surface [40]. These mediators include both those that are preformed such as histamine and those that are secondary or generated mediators such as leukotrienes.

The new liquid form of cromolyn, prescribed either as an MDI (about 1 mg per puff with most particles 5 μm or less in diameter) or as an ampule containing 20 mg of cromolyn in 2 ml of purified water to be administered by nebulizer, is less irritating than the original dry powder triggered from a gelatin capsule by a specially designed inhaler. Two puffs (2 mg) of cromolyn by MDI is roughly equivalent to 20 mg of the drug administered either as nebulized solution or as inhaled powder. As with other MDIs, delivery of cromolyn to the lungs may be enhanced by a spacer, but the clinical advantage of this is unclear.

Because of its safety with few serious side effects, cromolyn is the antiinflammatory drug of choice in children who have predominantly allergic asthma [7, 85]. Treatment with cromolyn may also help prevent acute asthma attacks in adults whose clinical and laboratory studies indicate that allergic hypersensitivity to some environmental substance is playing a role in triggering their asthma. Cromolyn is of special value when exposure to an allergen cannot be avoided, as in persons whose asthma results from an occupational exposure to laboratory animals. Cromolyn also benefits adults with chronic year-round nonallergic asthma [95], but inhaled corticosteroids remain preferable to cromolyn in adult asthmatics because of their greater efficacy. For seasonal asthma, cromolyn is required just during the seasonal exacerbation. When used on a long-term basis, cromolyn must be administered prophylactically on a fixed dose schedule, initially every 6 hours. A trial period of 4 to 8 weeks is necessary to judge its effectiveness, since it does not benefit all patients. Because cromolyn is expensive, we recommend that its efficacy be documented objectively by improved pulmonary function or by a meaningful reduction in the use of corticosteroids. When patients' symptoms are well controlled, it may be possible to reduce the dose frequency to two or three times daily. Cromolyn is of no benefit in the management of an acute asthma attack but need not be discontinued if a patient has an acute asthma exacerbation while taking this medication.

Cromolyn is also effective in preventing the bronchospasm that follows exercise, cold air inhalation, or exposure to nonimmunologic environmental substances like sulfur dioxide and toluene diisocyanate [85]. If an MDI-delivered beta$_2$ agonist taken prophylactically fails to prevent asthma following these exposures, cromolyn should be taken alone or together with a beta$_2$ agonist employing 2 MDI puffs of the drug 10 to 15 minutes before exposure to these causative factors. If exercise is prolonged or vigorous, additional dosing with a cromolyn MDI can be repeated as needed.

Other Agents

Methotrexate

Methotrexate, a folic acid antagonist with antiinflammatory properties, has been shown by two [84, 124] but not by a third group [33] to have a significant corticosteroid sparing effect in corticosteroid-dependent asthma when used for long periods in a small weekly oral or intramuscular dose of 15 mg. Up to 50 mg/wk of methotrexate has been administered employing drug levels to control dosing [83]. Since severe hypersensitivity-like side effects can occasionally occur with this agent, its use should be limited to severe asthmatics who require high oral corticosteroid dosing (see Chap. 68).

Nedocromil

Nedocromil sodium, a drug not currently available in the United States, is a new inhaled antiinflammatory agent that is more potent than cromolyn sodium, although different in structure. It functions similarly to cromolyn in inhibiting mediator release from mast cells as well as from eosinophils, neutrophils, and macrophages [96]. Like cromolyn, it inhibits both early and late asthmatic responses to inhaled allergens and reduces bronchial hyperreactivity [10]. At present this agent has no apparent advantage over cromolyn (see Chap. 63).

Leukotriene Receptor Antagonists

A number of specific oral leukotriene receptor antagonists are undergoing early trials for managing asthma [24, 53]. While such agents appear to block the protracted bronchospasm induced by leukotrienes, they have been shown so far to have only a modest benefit in treating asthmatic patients [24]. They may also partially prevent exercise and cold air–induced bronchoconstriction [53, 71]. In addition, a blockade of leukotriene production through the use of selective 5-lipoxygenase inhibitors may eventually prove useful in treating asthma [54] (see Chap. 66).

Nonsedating Antihistamines

A number of new nonsedating antihistamines with minimal anticholinergic effects and long duration of activity have been developed; terfenadine and astemizole are the two currently available in the United States. These agents function as specific H$_1$-receptor antagonists and also appear capable of reducing mediator release from mast cells [86]. They have been shown to reduce asthma symptoms and to produce modest bronchodilation in mild atopic asthma [102]. Their greatest benefit is likely to be in patients with atopic, mainly seasonal asthma who also have allergic rhinitis, although further studies are indicated to assess their potential role in managing more severe asthma. Azelastine and ketotifen, oral antihistamines not available in the United States, possess additional antiasthma properties including an ability to attenuate mediator-induced airway smooth muscle contraction [68] and to inhibit the synthesis and release of leukotrienes [60]. However, their overall benefit in treating asthma remains to be documented [132] (see Chap. 65).

Calcium Channel Blockers

Calcium channel blockers like nifedipine and verapamil are weak bronchodilators in patients with chronic stable asthma [118] and provide only modest protection against exercise, cold, histamine, and antigen-induced bronchoconstriction [26, 114]. Their main use in asthma is to treat concomitant systemic hypertension and angina pectoris in preference to beta$_2$ blockers, which often incite bronchospasm in asthmatics (see Chap. 71).

Miscellaneous

A protective effect of inhaled furosemide in allergen-induced early and late asthmatic reactions [11] and bronchodilation promoted by intravenous magnesium sulfate in severe, acute asthma [91] are important preliminary observations, but the exact role of these agents in treating asthma requires further study.

The corticosteroid sparing activity of the macrolide antibiotic troleandomycin for methylprednisolone is well-known and probably due to its inhibitory effect on the hepatic P-450 microsomal enzyme system with delayed methylprednisolone elimination [131]. This effect does not justify its use in asthma unless other efforts to reduce toxic doses of oral corticosteroids have failed (see Chap. 67).

The prescription of oral expectorant agents to thin the often viscid secretions of asthma and improve sputum mobilization remains controversial, with mostly anecdotal evidence of the effectiveness of these agents. Iodinated glycerol in a dose of 60 mg four times daily may be beneficial to asthmatics with excessive mucous secretions [100] and does not cause the many adverse side effects previously noted with oral iodides (see Chap. 69).

Although there is no evidence that overhydration thins bronchial secretions, dehydration clearly gives rise to thickened secretions. Therefore, patients with moderate and severe asthma should be advised to maintain a fluid intake that keeps the urine pale for all except the first voiding following sleep.

Oxygen therapy is important in correcting hypoxemia in severe asthma, especially since bronchodilator agents may cause mild worsening of hypoxemia [43]; low concentrations of oxygen usually suffice. Patients with uncomplicated asthma almost never require long-term oxygen therapy.

STAGING SYMPTOMATIC THERAPY TO SEVERITY OF ASTHMA

Self-Management

Asthma is a recurrent or chronic disease that is highly variable in many patients. It is not possible for the physician to guide the

Table 54-8. Goals in management of asthma

1. Identify and eliminate inciting agents
2. Control symptoms
3. Restore and maintain lung function
4. Prevent long-range loss of lung function
5. Prevent acute attacks of asthma
6. Preserve restful sleep
7. Prevent death from asthma
8. Keep therapy nonintrusive
9. Maintain a normal life-style

patient personally through all the ups and downs of the disease. The key to successful management, especially with severe disease, is educating the patient in self-management, up to the limit of the patient's ability to understand the proposed regimen. The patient should be instructed in how to identify and control trigger mechanisms of asthma, such as allergen exposure, exercise, and inhalation of chilled air. The proper doses of the drugs to be used should be taught. Guidelines should be established on how to adjust therapy on the basis of changing severity of symptoms or changes in lung function as determined with a home peak flowmeter. The patient should also be instructed on when to contact the physician, before or after making a change in therapy, and when to go to the emergency room if the physician cannot be reached. Successful education of the patient in self-management is an ongoing process that may take many months. Evaluation of the effectiveness of education of the patient requires obtaining detailed information on how the patient has dealt with exacerbations since the last visit; the physician then reinforces or adjusts the patient's program. The process is time-consuming but well worth the effort.

Goals and Rationale of Therapy

The goals for managing patients with asthma are set forth in Table 54-8. As already noted, the use of antiinflammatory agents in the treatment of asthma, which has been emphasized in the recent literature, has not yet been shown by outcome studies to be superior to the more conventional management techniques that are based on bronchodilator therapy. Nevertheless, we are convinced on the basis of our clinical experience that antiinflammatory therapy is frequently underutilized. The following sections represent our approach to using this newer information in managing asthma. We take an intermediate position between those who suggest that antiinflammatory agents are to be used only after the most vigorous bronchodilator therapy has failed and those who recommend that inhalations of corticosteroids or cromolyn on a fixed schedule are the keystone of asthma therapy [7, 13, 105, 106]. Table 54-9 summarizes in outline form our approach to asthma, which is given in greater detail in the following pages.

Mild Asthma

The patient with mild asthma, who has only an occasional attack of wheezing and airflow limitation, is most readily managed by the prescription of an MDI containing a long-acting, selective beta$_2$ agonist. The patient should be instructed to activate the MDI early in an inhalation that proceeds slowly from functional residual capacity to total lung capacity. The breath should be held for 5 to 10 seconds at the end of inhalation (see Table 54-5). Two puffs of the aerosol usually suffices to relieve mild asthmatic attacks, but up to 4 additional puffs may be taken, spaced out over 10 to 20 minutes, if adequate relief is not obtained after the initial dose. Similar beta$_2$-agonist aerosol therapy is also often sufficient to control episodic cough in variant asthma.

Table 54-9. Symptomatic management of asthma

MILD ASTHMA
1. Train in use of metered-dose inhaler (MDI).
2. For occasional mild asthma, use beta$_2$-agonist MDI, 2 puffs, followed by 2 puffs once or twice, at 20-minute intervals.
3. For persistent mild asthma, use beta$_2$-agonist MDI, 2–4 puffs on arising and at bedtime, and 1–2 puffs as needed every 4 hours during the day.
4. Beta$_2$-agonist MDI before exercise for exercise-induced asthma.
5. If asthma still not controlled add:
   a. Low-dose corticosteroid MDI in adults or cromolyn inhaler for children *or*
   b. Slowly absorbed theophylline, 200–400 mg bid.

MODERATE ASTHMA
1. Increase beta$_2$-agonist MDI to 4–6 puffs as tolerated on arising and at bedtime and 2 puffs as needed during the day.
2. High-dose steroid MDI; cromolyn is the preferred drug in children.
3. Long-acting oral theophylline, 200–400 mg bid.
4. If symptoms persist, try adding ipratropium MDI.
5. Short course of oral coticosteroid for exacerbation or initial control.

SEVERE ASTHMA
1. Intensified regimen as for moderate asthma, tailored for the patient.
2. Try oral beta$_2$ agonists in younger patients.
3. Educate patient in use of home peak flowmeter.
4. Develop a plan for exacerbations:
   a. PEFR < 300 L/min—double corticosteroid MDI.
   b. PEFR, 80–200 L/min—start oral steroid, e.g., prednisone, 0.5 mg/kg/A.M.; continue until 2 days after full recovery; then taper rapidly.
   c. PEFR < 80 L/min—contact physician.
5. Consider methotrexate for the oral corticosteroid-dependent patient.

The management of mild asthma requires more medication when the patient complains of one or more of the following: Asthma is present for part of each day; asthma is troublesome most nights; asthma of several hours' duration occurs four to six times weekly; or, episodes of asthma are infrequent but protracted, probably representing a late-phase asthmatic reaction. Such patients are advised to take 2 to 4 puffs from a beta$_2$ agonist on arising and at bedtime with additional as-needed aerosol therapy at 4- to 6-hour intervals. A midday beta$_2$-agonist MDI treatment can be regularly scheduled if it seems appropriate. A low dose of a long-acting theophylline preparation every 12 hours or timed-dose corticosteroid MDI or cromolyn inhalations may be added if symptoms persist (400 μg/day). One recent study found that inhaled budesonide was superior to inhaled terbutaline in patients with newly diagnosed mild asthma, suggesting that antiinflammatory inhaled steroids might be considered as primary therapy [151]. Inhaled steroids are more consistently effective in adults; cromolyn is a safer agent in children. Low doses of inhaled corticosteroids (400 μg/day of beclomethasone or its equivalent) are usually sufficient to control mild asthma, but up to twice this dose may occasionally be needed. The choice between oral theophylline and aerosol medication depends on physician and patient preference and side effects from theophylline.

Moderate Asthma

In managing patients with moderate asthma, the frequency and dose of inhaled corticosteroids are increased and given on a fixed schedule. The dose of inhaled corticosteroid may need to be as high as 1,000 to 2,000 μg/day of beclomethasone or an equivalent. A combination of timed-dose and as-needed beta$_2$-agonist MDI treatment is administered; the dose may be increased over that used for mild asthma. A long-acting oral theophylline preparation may be added if the patient continues to experience troublesome asthma on this regimen; an evening dose of a long-acting theophylline is often helpful in preventing nocturnal asthma. Some asthmatics, especially those who also have chronic bronchitis, will improve further when regularly scheduled ipratropium bromide by MDI is added. Cromolyn aerosol remains the preferred drug for antiinflammatory therapy in children.

An exacerbation of asthma occurring while a patient is on full preventive therapy or failure of a newly presenting patient with moderately severe asthma to respond promptly to a regimen of bronchodilators and inhaled steroids is an indication for the administration of a 1- to 2-week course of oral corticosteroids. Prednisone (or equivalent) in a dose of 0.5 mg/kg/A.M. is given until the asthma has been fully controlled for 2 days and is then rapidly tapered.

Purulent sputum in this setting is often the result of a viral infection or nonspecific bronchial inflammation and may even be due to the presence of large numbers of eosinophils in the sputum. Antibiotic therapy is not administered even in the presence of purulent sputum unless the patient is febrile or a sputum Gram's stain shows large numbers of bacteria (see Chap. 44).

In managing a major episode of asthma, even in a patient who was previously relatively symptom-free, it is important to recognize that because of retention of secretions and residual inflammatory changes in small airways, lung function will remain abnormal for some time after all physical signs of asthma have disappeared [74]. Therapy should be continued for an extended period after symptoms have subsided, auscultation has become normal, and lung function has been maximized. Otherwise, airflow obstruction may deteriorate rapidly with an exacerbation of asthma.

Severe Asthma

Severe chronic asthma can be difficult to treat. Many of these patients are never totally free of airflow obstruction even when receiving a wide range of medications. Although such patients constitute only a small percentage of the total asthma population, they make up a relatively large proportion of asthmatics cared for by pulmonary specialists and allergists. These patients need to be seen frequently, with intensive efforts at education in the nature of their disease and involvement in their own management. Treatment plans should be flexible and tailored to the patient's own responses to different medications.

In addition to MDI-delivered beta$_2$ agonists, such patients often receive oral theophylline. Maximal bronchodilatation is obtained with full doses of both agents, albeit at the price of increased toxicity [147]. It is important to monitor blood levels closely if theophylline doses are planned to produce blood levels in the range of 15 to 20 µg/ml. As a rule, younger patients tolerate such aggressive therapy better than older asthmatics, and an oral beta$_2$ agonist may be helpful in this group.

Many of these patients require chronic oral corticosteroid therapy even when they are receiving high doses of inhaled corticosteroids. Inhaled cromolyn sodium may be tried to diminish oral corticosteroid dependence, even though there is no good evidence that corticosteroids and cromolyn have an additive benefit. A low oral dose of methotrexate may contribute a significant corticosteroid sparing effect [83, 84, 124]; close monitoring for hepatic, pulmonary, and bone marrow toxicity is required, especially in patients who are maintained on this therapy for prolonged periods.

Severe Acute Asthma

Management of the acute, severe asthmatic is detailed in Chapter 72; only the salient points will be summarized here.

Site of Treatment

Faced with the problem of managing a patient who is acutely and severely ill with an exacerbation of asthma, usually in the emergency room of a hospital, the physician must decide whether the patient should be admitted to the hospital or whether it is reasonable to treat for a period of time in the emergency room and then send the patient home. A number of clinical features have been identified that indicate the patient who is at increased risk of relapsing shortly after emergency treatment of asthma: a history of severe asthma, especially if the severity was great enough to require previous hospital admission for its treatment [146]; previous need for systemic corticosteroid therapy; failure of usually effective therapy; and increasingly short-lived relief after emergency room therapy [137].

A low FEV$_1$ (less than 0.5 liter) or a low PEFR (less than 16% of predicted) [5] and especially a failure of these indexes to respond to bronchodilator therapy indicate a high probability of relapse after treatment [5, 61]. The physical findings of sternocleidomastoid muscle retraction and pulsus paradoxus have been discussed earlier. Arterial PO$_2$ values of less than 60 mmHg and arterial PCO$_2$ values equal to or greater than 40 mmHg have also been put forward as alarming laboratory values indicating that the patient is at high risk of suffering early relapse or serious consequences of asthma [92, 103].

Ideally, a predictive score utilizing multiple indexes of the asthma severity would allow accurate prediction of the outcome of treatment of acutely ill asthmatics. Unfortunately, the early promise of such an index utilizing seven clinical and laboratory factors selected by multivariate discriminate analysis [37] was not confirmed by two recent prospective studies [19, 111]. Both studies found the ability of the index to predict the outcome of treatment of acute, severe asthma to be little better than that of chance alone, although the index did reflect to some extent the severity of asthma. The index of Fischel and coworkers [37] likely failed because it neglected to take into consideration such variables as duration of emergency room therapy as well as the variability in treatment protocols between hospitals and physicians.

Thus, at present, no predictive method utilizing clinical and physiologic variables can unequivocally predict the outcome of emergency room treatment of asthma or the likelihood of relapse after emergency room discharge. Physicians must consider many factors including the severity of the asthma episode, its duration (the longer the episode the less likely the patient will have prompt and lasting relief), the patient's pattern of asthma in the past, and the response of the patient to emergency room therapy. Hospitalization is advised if there is any doubt as to the course of a patient.

Supportive Care

All patients should receive oxygen as indicated by arterial blood gas analysis. The patient's state of hydration should be assessed and correction of dehydration initiated.

Beta$_2$-Agonist Therapy

Inhaled selective beta$_2$ agonists are the cornerstone of therapy. Emergency room response to these agents does not appear to be impaired by their prior use [113]. They can be effectively delivered by MDI, which should be coupled to a spacer to minimize oropharyngeal impaction of the agent. Alternatively, beta$_2$ agonists may be administered by updraft nebulizer because this device requires less patient cooperation. Serial assessment of physical findings, including improvement in airflow obstruction, pulse rate response, and evidence of cardiac arrhythmias on electrocardiogram may be used to guide dosage. Beta$_2$-agonist aerosols are usually used in standard doses but at increased frequency—for example, 2 to 3 puffs from an albuterol MDI every

20 minutes, or 0.5 ml of 0.5% albuterol solution diluted with 2.5 ml of normal saline in a nebulizer every 1 to 2 hours.

Subcutaneous beta₂ agonists are generally less effective and cause more side effects than inhaled therapy [36] but should be given to severely dyspneic patients who cannot cooperate with inhalation treatment. The preference for inhaled beta₂ agonists also applies to children with acute asthma [88].

Anticholinergic Therapy
In patients who do not promptly respond to beta₂ agonists, an ipratropium bromide MDI should be added to the beta₂ agonists. The treatment is essentially free of toxicity [104].

Intravenous Theophylline
The use of intravenous aminophylline in the treatment of severe, acute asthma remains controversial. Littenberg [69] recently used meta-analysis to assess 13 published controlled trials in which aminophylline therapy alone or together with other bronchodilators was compared to a control non-aminophylline-containing regimen. The 13 reports showed wide differences in their findings; 7 studies found no difference in spirometric results at 1 hour between aminophylline and the control regimen, 3 noted aminophylline therapy to be superior, and 3 found exactly the opposite. After pooling the data, no difference was found between the aminophylline-treated and control groups, although there was a trend toward less improvement in pulmonary function with aminophylline use. Subset analysis showed that aminophylline as single therapy was always inferior to single-agent treatment employing a beta₂ agonist, regardless of the manner in which the beta₂ agonist was administered. Likewise, aminophylline combined with an inhaled beta₂ agonist was no better than an inhaled beta₂ agonist alone. Combination therapy with aminophylline was superior only if subcutaneous epinephrine was the sympathomimetic employed in the combination regimen. Toxicity was also greater in patients receiving aminophylline but appeared to be minor in nature. However, the true incidence of toxic reactions was felt to have been understated.

Littenberg [69] concluded that although aminophylline was clearly inferior to sympathomimetics as single-agent treatment, the available reports failed to provide sufficient evidence to support or refute the usefulness of aminophylline in acute, severe asthma as a component of multimodality therapy. This was because the number of studies was limited, too few patients had been enrolled, pulmonary function change at 1 hour was the only commonly used criterion for improvement with no spirometry at later times, and most studies failed to note the clinical response of their patients.

Thus until the definitive controlled clinical trial with intravenous aminophylline in acute severe asthma is done, it seems reasonable to include intravenous aminophylline in a comprehensive therapeutic regimen for this condition. When patients fail to respond to 1 or 2 hours of inhaled beta₂ agonists and anticholinergic agents, intravenous theophylline should be added. Theophylline dosing in the emergency room should be controlled by initial and serial theophylline blood levels; target blood levels should be 15 to 20 μg/ml in young people and 10 to 12 μg/ml in patients older than 55 years.

Corticosteroids
The institution of corticosteroid therapy is always indicated for severe acute asthma. As discussed earlier, since short courses of corticosteroids are free of side effects and because the benefits are delayed in onset [77], corticosteroid therapy should be started early in the emergency room and continued on discharge; oral corticosteroids are probably as effective as intravenous administration. The benefits of corticosteroids are confirmed in

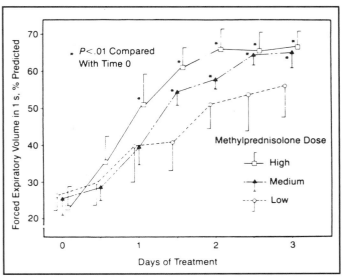

Fig. 54-5. *Responses to intravenous methylprednisolone in status asthmaticus. High dose is 125 mg every 6 hours, medium dose is 40 mg every 6 hours, and low dose is 15 mg every 6 hours. Mean forced expiratory volume in 1 second % predicted (± SEM) is plotted for eight patients in each group. Compared with their initial spirometric values on a half-day basis, the high-dose group significantly improved (p < .01) before the end of the first day, the median-dose group significantly improved (p < .01) early in the second day, and the low-dose group never improved (p > .01). (Reprinted with permission from R. J. Haskell, B. M. Wong, and J. E. Hansen. A double blind randomized clinical trial of methylprednisolone in status asthmaticus. Arch. Intern. Med. 143:1324, 1983. Copyright 1983, American Medical Association.)*

some studies but not in others [35, 70, 130]. Even patients who respond quickly to bronchodilators should be started on oral corticosteroids prior to discharge. Such therapy results in a decreased need for repeat emergency care [20]. Arrangements for follow-up care within 1 to 2 days after discharge from the emergency room are essential.

Hospital Management of Severe Acute Asthma
The management of severe acute asthma in the hospital (status asthmaticus) is presented in detail in Chapter 73; it is discussed briefly here for the sake of completeness. Ideally, all patients with severe acute asthma should be managed in an intensive care unit. The initial investigation and treatment of these patients should proceed in parallel. A complete blood count, serum electrolyte determination, sputum Gram's stain and culture, an electrocardiogram, and arterial blood gas measurements should be obtained. A chest radiograph provides an estimate of the total lung capacity but more importantly may disclose evidence of pneumonia, atelectasis, or pneumothorax (see Chap. 53).

Oxygen by nasal cannula at a flow of 2 to 4 L/min, corticosteroid drugs, and bronchodilator agents should be given. Corticosteroid dose should be in the range of 125 mg of methylprednisolone intravenously every 6 hours for the initial 24 to 48 hours; lower doses can usually be given following this interval [48] (Fig. 54-5). Patients admitted to the hospital with severe asthma are often dehydrated, and as noted earlier, dehydration may give rise to increased viscosity of tracheobronchial secretions. On the other hand, patients with asthma may have the inappropriate secretion of antidiuretic hormone and therefore may be at risk of developing symptomatic hyponatremia [4]. Fluid therapy should be planned to overcome clinically evident dehydration and then to provide enough fluid to meet bodily needs determined by assessment of fluid intake and output every 8 hours.

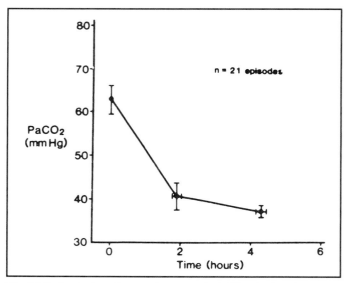

Fig. 54-6. *Resolution of severe hypercapnia in 21 episodes of acute asthma presenting with $PaCO_2 \geq 50$ mmHg not requiring mechanical ventilation. Values are expressed as mean $\pm$ SEM. Five other patients with $PaCO_2 \geq 50$ mmHg required intubation and mechanical ventilation. (Reprinted with permission from R. D. Mountain and S. A. Sahn. Clinical features and outcome in patients with acute asthma presenting with hypercapnia.* Am. Rev. Respir. Dis. *138:535, 1988.)*

The precise role of chest physical therapy, such as vibration, percussion, and postural drainage, is not well defined in severe asthma. The method probably has little to offer the patient with severe high-grade airway obstruction who is producing little secretion. However, as the airway obstruction remits and expectoration begins, these treatments may be of some benefit. Judgment must be exercised so that these techniques do not contribute to fatigue and exhaustion (see Chap. 73).

Many episodes of severe asthma are precipitated by viral infection, but this process has usually subsided by the time the patient comes to medical attention. The integration of sputum data with clinical findings generally permits the judgment to be made as to whether antibiotic therapy should be given for treatment of bacterial infection. Such treatment is not indicated as a routine.

The treatment regimen should be organized into periods with reassessment by means of arterial blood gases and clinical evaluation at 2- to 4-hour intervals. In patients who are acutely ill and not responding rapidly to therapy, the periods of reassessment should occur as often as hourly. Most patients with status asthmaticus who initially manifest hypercapnia can be managed conservatively [82] (Fig. 54-6), but a rising arterial PCO_2, especially in the setting of a full therapeutic regimen, is cause for considering the possibility of endotracheal intubation and mechanical ventilation. This decision should be based on evaluation of the total clinical situation and serial arterial blood gas changes rather than on any single arbitrary level of $PaCO_2$. Fatigue, pending exhaustion, impairment of consciousness, and inability to continue to cooperate all militate in favor of using mechanical ventilation. In contrast to an earlier report [119], recent studies indicate that intubation and mechanical ventilation do not have a high complication rate in patients with asthma [15, 82]. Thus, the decision whether to continue conservative therapy or to proceed to mechanical ventilation should be based on the clinical needs of the patient and not on concerns regarding the risks of mechanical ventilation. Nevertheless, some patients require dangerously high peak ventilator pressure to achieve adequate ventilation; in this group, mechanically controlled hypoventila-

tion can be employed to limit ventilator peak pressures to no greater than 50 to 60 cmH₂O [27, 79]. As-needed intravenous bicarbonate therapy is given to avoid dangerous levels of acidemia. All sedative agents are contraindicated in the management of severe asthma except as part of a mechanical ventilation regimen [34]. Other treatment methods including positive end-expiratory pressure in patients receiving mechanical ventilation [73, 101], intravenous beta₂ agonists [38], bronchoscopy with lavage [30], and general anesthesia with halothane [117] should never be routine therapy for severe asthma; they should be carefully individualized to patients who fail to improve with standard treatment.

As the patient with asthma recovers from a severe attack, a regimen must be developed that can easily be continued after hospital discharge. As with all asthmatics, patients must be educated in the nature of their disease, instructed in the necessity of continuing therapy for a prolonged period after symptoms have subsided, and taught to adjust medication to the severity of their disease.

Patients with very labile asthma should be considered by their physicians as being at risk of dying of their disease. They should be promptly admitted to the hospital if increasing doses of medication, including corticosteroids, have not been successful in controlling symptoms [145]. A vigorous approach is necessary if death is not to occur in this small subset of patients with labile asthma.

Despite the steady accumulation of knowledge on the pathogenesis of asthma over the last decade, no new classes of clinically available drugs have been introduced. Therapy for asthma has evolved during this time mainly by an enhanced understanding of how to use the older, established agents. Antiinflammatory therapy has assumed a primacy it did not have 10 years ago in the management of mild and moderate asthma. The use of inhaled anticholinergics has been added to the use of inhaled beta₂ agonists, and the latter have largely replaced the oral beta₂-agonist preparations. The time-honored use of intravenous aminophylline for the treatment of severe asthma in the emergency room has been questioned. Slowly absorbed, long-acting theophylline has emerged as the oral preparation of choice. Target theophylline blood levels of 10 ± 2 µg/ml have improved the therapeutic index of the drug with little sacrifice of efficacy. But more than ever, asthma represents a challenge to the physician in choosing the correct drug regimen, staging it to the severity of the patient's disease, educating the patient in its use, and successfully relieving suffering and disability.

REFERENCES

1. Adinoff, A. D., and Hollister, J. R. Steroid-induced fractures and bone loss in patients with asthma. *N. Engl. J. Med.* 309:265, 1983.
2. Azzawi, M., et al. Identification of activated T lymphocytes and eosinophils in bronchial biopsies in stable atopic asthma. *Am. Rev. Respir. Dis.* 142:1407, 1990.
3. Backus, B. F., and Snider, G. L. Bronchodilator effects of aerosolized terbutaline: A controlled double blind study. *J.A.M.A.* 238:2277, 1977.
4. Baker, J. W., Yeges, S., and Segar, W. E. Elevated plasma antidiuretic hormone levels in status asthmaticus. *Mayo Clin. Proc.* 51:31, 1976.
5. Banner, A. S., Shah, R. S., and Addington, W. W. Rapid prediction of need for hospitalization in acute asthma. *J.A.M.A.* 235:1337, 1976.
6. Barnes, P. J. Neural control of human airways in health and disease. *Am. Rev. Respir. Dis.* 134:1289, 1986.
7. Barnes, P. J. A new approach to the treatment of asthma. *N. Engl. J. Med.* 321:1517, 1989.
8. Beasley, R., Cushley, M., and Holgate, S. T. A self management plan in the treatment of adult asthma. *Thorax* 44:200, 1989.
9. Beasley, R., et al. Cellular events in the bronchi in mild asthma and after bronchial provocation. *Am. Rev. Respir. Dis.* 139:806, 1989.
10. Bel, E. H., et al. The long-term effects of nedocromil sodium and beclo-

methasone dipropionate on bronchial responsiveness to methacholine in nonatopic asthmatic subjects. *Am. Rev. Respir. Dis.* 141:21, 1990.

11. Bianco, S., et al. Protective effect of inhaled furosemide on allergen-induced early and late asthmatic reactions. *N. Engl. J. Med.* 321:1069, 1989.

12. Bondi, E., and Williams, M. H., Jr. Severe asthma: Course and treatment in hospital. *N.Y. State J. Med.* 77:350, 1977.

13. Bone, R. C. A step care strategy for asthma management. *J. Respir. Dis.* 9(11):104, 1988.

14. Bousquet, J., et al. Eosinophilic inflammation in asthma. *N. Engl. J. Med.* 323:1033, 1990.

15. Braman, S. S., and Kaemmerlen, J. T. Intensive care of status asthmaticus: A 10-year experience. *J.A.M.A.* 264:366, 1990.

16. Brenner, B. E., Abraham, E., and Simon, R. R. Position and diaphoresis in acute asthma. *Am. J. Med.* 74:1005, 1983.

17. Britton, J., et al. Dose related effects of salbutamol and ipratropium bromide on airway calibre and reactivity in subjects with asthma. *Thorax* 43:300, 1988.

18. Bruderman, I., Cohen-Aronovski, R., and Smorzik, J. A comparative study of various combinations of ipratropium bromide and metaproterenol in allergic asthmatic patients. *Chest* 83:208, 1983.

19. Centor, R. M., Yarbrough, B., and Wood, J. P. Inability to predict relapse in acute asthma. *N. Engl. J. Med.* 310:577, 1984.

20. Chapman, K. R., et al. Effect of a short course of prednisone in the prevention of early relapse after the emergency room treatment of acute asthma. *N. Engl. J. Med.* 324:788, 1991.

21. Charlton, I., et al. Evaluation of peak flow and symptoms only self management plans for control of asthma in general practice. *Br. Med. J.* 301:1355, 1990.

22. Check, W. A., and Kaliner, M. A. Pharmacology and pharmacokinetics of topical corticosteroid derivatives used for asthma therapy. *Am. Rev. Respir. Dis.* 141:S44, 1990.

23. Chung, K. F. Role of inflammation in the hyperreactivity of the airways in asthma. *Thorax* 41:657, 1986.

24. Cloud, M. L. A specific LTD$_4$/LTE$_4$-receptor antagonist improves pulmonary function in patients with mild, chronic asthma. *Am. Rev. Respir. Dis.* 140:1336, 1989.

25. Cockcroft, D. W., and Murdoch, K. Y. Comparative effects of inhaled salbutamol, sodium cromoglycate and beclomethasone dipropionate on allergen-induced early asthmatic responses, late asthmatic responses, and increased bronchial responsiveness to histamine. *J. Allergy Clin. Immunol.* 79:734, 1987.

26. Corris, P. A., Nariman, S., and Gibson, G. J. Nifedipine in the prevention of asthma induced by exercise and histamine. *Am. Rev. Respir. Dis.* 128:991, 1983.

27. Darioli, R., and Perret, C. Mechanical controlled hypoventilation in status asthmaticus. *Am. Rev. Respir. Dis.* 129:385, 1984.

28. Diaz, P., et al. Leukocytes and mediators in bronchoalveolar lavage during allergen-induced late-phase asthmatic reactions. *Am. Rev. Respir. Dis.* 139:1383, 1989.

29. Djukanovic, R., et al. Identification of mast cells and eosinophils in the bronchial mucosa of symptomatic atopic asthmatics and healthy control subjects using immunohistochemistry. *Am. Rev. Respir. Dis.* 142:863, 1990.

30. Donaldson, J. C., et al. Acetylcysteine for life-threatening acute bronchial obstruction. *Ann. Intern. Med.* 88:656, 1978.

31. Dutoit, J. J., Salome, C. M., and Woodcock, A. J. Inhaled corticosteroids reduce the severity of bronchial hyperresponsiveness in asthma but oral theophylline does not. *Am. Rev. Respir. Dis.* 136:1174, 1987.

32. Epstein, S. W., et al. A comparison of three means of pressurized aerosol inhaler use. *Am. Rev. Respir. Dis.* 128:253, 1983.

33. Erzurum, S. C., et al. Lack of benefit of methotrexate in severe, steroid-dependent asthma. *Ann. Intern. Med.* 114:353, 1991.

34. Faling, L. J. The Role of Sedatives and Implications of Ventilatory Control in Status Asthmaticus. In E. B. Weiss (ed.), *Status Asthmaticus.* Baltimore: University Park Press, 1978. P. 267.

35. Fanta, C. H., Rossing, T. H., and McFadden, E. R., Jr. Glucocorticoids in acute asthma: A critical controlled trial. *Am. J. Med.* 74:845, 1983.

36. Fanta, C. H., Rossing, T. H., and McFadden, E. R., Jr. Treatment of acute asthma: Is combination therapy with sympathomimetics and methylxanthines indicated? *Am. J. Med.* 80:5, 1986.

37. Fischl, M. A., Pitchenik, A., and Gardner, L. B. An index predicting relapse and need for hospitalization in patients with acute bronchial asthma. *N. Engl. J. Med.* 305:783, 1981.

38. Fitchett, D. H., McNicol, M. W., and Riordan, J. F. Intravenous salbutamol in management of status asthmaticus. *Br. Med. J.* 1:53, 1975.

39. Fitzpatrick, M. F., et al. Salmeterol in nocturnal asthma: A double blind, placebo controlled trial of a long acting inhaled B$_2$ agonist. *Br. Med. J.* 301:1365, 1990.

40. Flint, K. C., et al. Human mast cells recovered from bronchoalveolar lavage: Their morphology, histamine release and effects of sodium cromoglycate. *Clin. Sci.* 68:427, 1985.

41. Foresi, A., et al. Inflammatory markers in bronchoalveolar lavage and in bronchial biopsy in asthma during remission. *Chest* 98:528, 1990.

42. Frigas, E., and Gleich, G. J. The eosinophil and the pathophysiology of asthma. *J. Allergy Clin. Immunol.* 77:527, 1986.

43. Gazioglu, K., et al. Effect of isoproterenol on gas exchange during air and oxygen breathing in patients with asthma. *Am. J. Med.* 50:185, 1971.

44. Gelb, A. F., et al. P pulmonale in status asthmaticus. *J. Allergy Clin. Immunol.* 64:18, 1979.

45. Grandordy, B. M., et al. Cumulative dose-response curves for assessing combined effects of salbutamol and ipratropium bromide in chronic asthma. *Eur. Resp. J.* 1:531, 1988.

46. Greenberger, P. A., and Patterson, R. The management of asthma during pregnancy and lactation. *Clin. Rev. Allergy* 5:317, 1987.

47. Gross, N. J., and Skorodin, M. S. State of the art: anticholinergic, antimuscarinic bronchodilators. *Am. Rev. Respir. Dis.* 129:856, 1984.

48. Haskell, R. J., Wong, B. M., and Hansen, J. E. A double-blind, randomized clinical trial of methylprednisolone in status asthmaticus. *Arch. Intern. Med.* 143:1324, 1983.

49. Hegart, B., Pauwels, R., and Van Der Straeten, M. Inhibitory effect of KWD 2131, terbutaline, and DSCG on the immediate and late allergen-induced bronchoconstriction. *Allergy* 36:115, 1981.

50. Hendeles, L. Asthma therapy: State of the art, 1988. *J. Respir. Dis.* 9(3):82, 1988.

51. Henriksen, J. M. Effect of inhalation of corticosteroids in exercise induced asthma: Randomized double blind crossover study of budesonide in asthmatic children. *Br. Med. J.* 291:248, 1985.

52. Howarth, P. H., et al. Influence of albuterol, cromolyn sodium and ipratropium bromide on the airway and circulating mediator response to allergen bronchial provocation in asthma. *Am. Rev. Respir. Dis.* 132:986, 1985.

53. Israel, E., et al. Effect of a leukotriene antagonist, LY171883, on cold air-induced bronchoconstriction in asthmatics. *Am. Rev. Respir. Dis.* 140:1348, 1989.

54. Israel, E., et al. The effects of 5-lipoxygenase inhibitor on asthma induced by cold, dry air. *N. Engl. J. Med.* 323:1740, 1990.

55. Jackson, R., et al. International trends in asthma mortality: 1970 to 1985. *Chest* 94:914, 1988.

56. Jardin, F., et al. Inspiratory impairment in right ventricular performance during acute asthma. *Chest* 92:789, 1987.

57. Jeffery, P. K., et al. Bronchial biopsies in asthma: An ultrastructural, quantitative analysis and correlation with hyperreactivity. *Am. Rev. Respir. Dis.* 140:1745, 1989.

58. Jenne, J. W. Theophylline is no more obsolete than "two puffs qid" of current beta$_2$ agonists. *Chest* 98:3, 1990.

59. Johnson, A. J., Spiro, S. G., and Pidgeon, J. Intravenous infusion of salbutamol in severe acute asthma. *Br. Med. J.* 1:1013, 1978.

60. Katayakma, S., et al. Effect of azelastine on the release and action of leukotriene C$_4$ and D$_4$. *Int. Arch. Allergy Appl. Immunol.* 83:284, 1987.

61. Kelsen, S. G., et al. Emergency room assessment of treatment of patients with acute asthma. *Am. J. Med.* 64:622, 1978.

62. Kerrebijn, K. F. Use of topical corticosteroids in the treatment of childhood asthma. *Am. Rev. Respir. Dis.* 141:S77, 1990.

63. Kolbeck, R. C., et al. Apparent irrelevance of cyclic nucleotides to the relaxation of tracheal smooth muscle induced by theophylline. *Lung* 156:173, 1979.

64. Kurland, G., Williams, J., and Lewiston, N. J. Fatal myocardial toxicity during continuous infusion intravenous isoproterenol therapy of asthma. *J. Allergy Clin. Immunol.* 63:407, 1979.

65. Laitinen, L. A., et al. Damage of the airway epithelium and bronchial reactivity in patients with asthma. *Am. Rev. Respir. Dis.* 131:599, 1985.

66. Lam, A., and Newhouse, M. T. Management of asthma and chronic airflow limitation: Are methylxanthines obsolete? *Chest* 98:44, 1990.

67. Lawford, P., Jones, P., and Milledge, J. Comparison of intravenous and nebulized salbutamol in initial treatment of severe asthma. *Br. Med. J.* 1:84, 1978.

68. Lee, H. K., and Sperelakis, N. Azelastine inhibits agonist-induced electromechanical activity in canine tracheal muscle. *Chest* 96:665, 1989.

69. Littenberg, B. Aminophylline treatment in severe, acute asthma: A meta-analysis. *J.A.M.A.* 259:1678, 1988.

70. Littenberg, B., and Gluck, E. H. A controlled trial of methylprednisolone in the emergency treatment of acute asthma. *N. Engl. J. Med.* 314:150, 1986.

71. Manning, P. J., et al. Inhibition of exercise-induced bronchoconstriction by MK-571, a potent leukotriene D$_4$-receptor antagonist. *N. Engl. J. Med.* 323:1736, 1990.

72. Mapp, C., et al. Protective effect of antiasthma drugs on late asthmatic reaction and increased airway responsiveness induced by toluene diisocyanate in sensitized subjects. *Am. Rev. Respir. Dis.* 136:1403, 1987.

73. Martin, J. G., Shore, S., and Engel, L. A. Effect of continuous positive airway pressure on respiratory mechanics and pattern of breathing in induced asthma. *Am. Rev. Respir. Dis.* 126:812, 1982.

74. McFadden, E. R., Jr., Kiser, R., and deGroot, W. J. Acute bronchial asthma: Relations between clinical and physiologic manifestations. *N. Engl. J. Med.* 288:221, 1973.

75. McFadden, E. R., Jr., and Lyons, H. A. Arterial-blood gas tension in asthma. *N. Engl. J. Med.* 278:1027, 1968.

76. McFadden, E. R., Jr., and Mills, R. Inhaled albuterol powder for the prevention of exercise-induced bronchospasm. *Immunol. Allergy Practice* 8:29, 1986.

77. McFadden, E. R., Jr., et al. A controlled study of the effects of single doses of hydrocortisone on the resolution of acute attacks of asthma. *Am. J. Med.* 60:52, 1976.

78. Meltzer, E. O., et al. Effect of dosing schedule on efficacy of beclomethasone dipropionate aerosol in chronic asthma. *Am. Rev. Respir. Dis.* 131:732, 1985.

79. Menitove, S. M., and Goldring, R. M. Combined ventilator and bicarbonate strategy in the management of status asthmaticus. *Am. J. Med.* 74:898, 1983.

80. Miller, C. A., Slusher, L. B., and Vesell, E. S. Polymorphism of theophylline metabolism in man. *J. Clin. Invest.* 75:1415, 1985.

81. Mitenko, P. A., and Ogilvie, T. I. Rational intravenous doses of theophylline. *N. Engl. J. Med.* 289:600, 1973.

82. Mountain, R. D., and Sahn, S. A. Clinical features and outcome in patients with acute asthma presenting with hypercapnia. *Am. Rev. Respir. Dis.* 138:535, 1988.

83. Mullarkey, M. F., Lammert, J. K., and Blumenstein, B. A. Long-term methotrexate treatment in corticosteroid-dependent asthma. *Ann. Intern. Med.* 112:577, 1990.

84. Mullarkey, M. F., et al. Methotrexate in the treatment of corticosteroid-dependent asthma: A double-blind crossover study. *N. Engl. J. Med.* 318:603, 1988.

85. Murphy, S. Cromolyn sodium: Basic mechanisms and clinical usage. *Pediatr. Asthma, Allergy Immunol.* 2:237, 1988.

86. Naclerio, R. M., et al. Terfenadine, an H$_1$ antihistamine, inhibits histamine release in vivo in the human. *Am. Rev. Respir. Dis.* 142:167, 1990.

87. Nassif, E. G., et al. The value of maintenance theophylline in steroid dependent asthma. *N. Engl. J. Med.* 304:71, 1981.

88. Nelson, D. R., Sachs, M. I., and O'Connell, E. J. Approaches to acute asthma and status asthmaticus in children. *Mayo Clin. Proc.* 64:1392, 1989.

89. Newhouse, M. T., and Dolovich, M. Aerosol therapy of reversible airflow obstruction. *Chest* 91(Suppl.):58S, 1987.

90. Nielson, C. P., et al. Polymorphonuclear leukocyte inhibition by therapeutic concentrations of theophylline is mediated by cyclic-3',5'-adenosine monophosphate. *Am. Rev. Respir. Dis.* 137:25, 1988.

91. Noppen, M., et al. Bronchodilating effect of intravenous magnesium sulfate in acute severe bronchial asthma. *Chest* 97:373, 1990.

92. Nowak, R. M., et al. Arterial blood gases and pulmonary function testing in acute bronchial asthma: Predicting patient outcomes. *J.A.M.A.* 249:2043, 1983.

93. O'Byrne, P. M., Hargreave, F. E., and Kirby, J. G. Airway inflammation and hyperresponsiveness. *Am. Rev. Respir. Dis.* 136:S35, 1987.

94. O'Driscoll, B. R., et al. Nebulised salbutamol with and without ipratropium bromide in acute airflow obstruction. *Lancet* 1:1418, 1989.

95. Petty, T. L., et al. Cromolyn sodium is effective in adult chronic asthmatics. *Am. Rev. Respir. Dis.* 139:694, 1989.

96. Phillips, G. D., et al. Effect of nedocromil sodium and sodium cromoglycate against bronchoconstriction induced by inhaled adenosine 5'-monophosphate. *Eur. Respir. J.* 2:210, 1989.

97. Polson, J. B., et al. Inhibition of human phosphodiesterase activity by therapeutic levels of theophylline. *Clin. Exp. Pharmacol. Physiol.* 5:535, 1978.

98. Popa, V. Beta-adrenergic drugs. *Clin. Chest Med.* 7:313, 1986.

99. Poppius, H., Salorinne, Y., and Viljanen, A. A. Inhalation of a new anticholinergic drug, SCH 1000, in asthma and chronic bronchitis: Effect on airway resistance, thoracic gas volume, blood gases and exercise-induced asthma. *Bull. Eur. Physiopathol. Respir.* 8:643, 1972.

100. Prenner, B. M. Chronic respiratory disease complicated by mucus: Results of a clinical evaluation of the mucolytic agent iodinated glycerol in a four-week, open trial of adult asthmatics. *Immunol. Allergy Practice* 10:17, 1988.

101. Qvist, J., et al. High-level PEEP in severe asthma. *N. Engl. J. Med.* 307:1347, 1982.

102. Rafferty, P. The European experience with antihistamines in asthma. *Ann. Allergy* 63:389, 1989.

103. Rebuck, A. S., and Read, J. Assessment and management of severe asthma. *Am. J. Med.* 51:788, 1971.

104. Rebuck, A. S., et al. Nebulized anticholinergic and sympathomimetic treatment of asthma and chronic obstructive airways disease in the emergency room. *Am. J. Med.* 82:59, 1987.

105. Reed, C. E. New therapeutic approaches in asthma. *J. Allergy Clin. Immunol.* 77:537, 1986.

106. Reed, C. E. Aerosol glucocorticoid treatment of asthma in adults. *Am. Rev. Respir. Dis.* 141:S82, 1990.

107. Rees, H. A., Miller, J. S., and Donald, K. W. A study of the clinical course and arterial blood gas tension of patients in status asthmaticus. *Q. J. Med.* 37:541, 1968.

108. Rhoden, K. J., Meldrum, L. A., and Barnes, P. J. Inhibition of cholinergic neurotransmission in human airways by beta$_2$-adreno-receptors. *J. Appl. Physiol.* 65:700, 1988.

109. Robin, E. D., and Lewiston, N. Unexpected, unexplained sudden death in young asthmatic subjects. *Chest* 96:790, 1989.

110. Roca, J., et al. Serial relationships between ventilation-perfusion inequality and spirometry in acute severe asthma requiring hospitalization. *Am. Rev. Respir. Dis.* 137:1055, 1988.

111. Rose, C. C., Murphy, J. G., and Schwartz, J. S. Performance of an index predicting the response of patients with acute bronchial asthma to intensive emergency department treatment. *N. Engl. J. Med.* 310:573, 1984.

112. Rossing, T. H. Methylxanthines in 1989. *Ann. Intern. Med.* 110:502, 1989.

113. Rossing, T. H., Fanta, C. H., and McFadden, E. R., Jr. Effect of outpatient treatment of asthma with beta agonists on the response to sympathomimetics in an emergency room. *Am. J. Med.* 75:781, 1983.

114. Russi, E. W., Danta, I., and Ahmed, T. Comparative modification of antigen-induced bronchoconstriction by the calcium antagonists, nifedipine and verapamil. *Chest* 88:74, 1985.

115. Salzman, G. A., et al. Aerosolized metaproterenol in the treatment of asthmatics with severe airflow obstruction: Comparison of two delivery methods. *Chest* 95:1017, 1989.

116. Schleimer, R. P., et al. Effects of dexamethasone on mediator release from human lung fragments and purified human lung mast cells. *J. Clin. Invest.* 71:1830, 1983.

117. Schwartz, S. H. Treatment of status asthmaticus with halothane. *J.A.M.A.* 251:2688, 1984.

118. Schwartzstein, R. S., and Fanta, C. H. Orally administered nifedipine in chronic stable asthma. *Am. Rev. Respir. Dis.* 134:262, 1986.

119. Scoggin, C. H., Sahn, S. A., and Petty, T. L. Status asthmaticus: A nine-year experience. *J.A.M.A.* 238:1158, 1977.

120. Sears, M. R., et al. Regular inhaled beta-agonist treatment in bronchial asthma. *Lancet* 336:1391, 1990.

121. Shim, C., and Williams, M. H., Jr. Bronchial response to oral versus aerosol metaproterenol in asthma. *Ann. Intern. Med.* 93:428, 1980.

122. Shim, C., and Williams, M. H., Jr. Comparison of oral aminophylline and aerosol metaproterenol in asthma. *Am. J. Med.* 71:452, 1981.

123. Shim, C. S., and Williams, M. H., Jr. Relationship of wheezing to the severity of obstruction in asthma. *Arch. Intern. Med.* 143:890, 1983.

124. Shiner, R. J., et al. Randomised, double-blind, placebo-controlled trial of methotrexate in steroid-dependent asthma. *Lancet* 336:137, 1990.

125. Shy, R., Badie, B., and Faciano, J. Comparison of subcutaneous terbutaline with epinephrine in the treatment of asthma in children. *J. Allergy Clin. Immunol.* 59:128, 1977.

126. Siegel, D., et al. Aminophylline increases the toxicity but not the efficacy of an inhaled beta-adrenergic agonist in the treatment of acute exacerbations of asthma. *Am. Rev. Respir. Dis.* 132:283, 1985.

127. Snider, G. L. Staging Therapeutic Schedules to Clinical Severity in Status Asthmaticus. In E. B. Weiss (ed.), *Status Asthmaticus*. Baltimore: University Park Press, 1978. P. 151.

128. Spiegel, R. J., et al. Adrenal suppression after short-term corticosteroid therapy. *Lancet* 1:630, 1979.

129. Squara, P., et al. Decreased paradoxic pulse from increased venous return in severe asthma. *Chest* 97:377, 1990.

130. Stein, L. M., and Cole, R. P. Early administration of corticosteroids in emergency room treatment of acute asthma. *Ann. Intern. Med.* 112:822, 1990.

131. Szefler, S. J., et al. The effect of troleandomycin on methylprednisolone elimination. *J. Allergy Clin. Immunol.* 66:447, 1988.

132. Tinkelman, D. G., et al. Evaluation of the safety and efficacy of multiple doses of azelastine to adult patients with bronchial asthma over time. *Am. Rev. Respir. Dis.* 141:569, 1990.

133. Toogood, J. H., et al. Minimum dose requirements of steroid dependent asthmatic patients for aerosol beclomethasone and oral prednisone. *J. Allergy Clin. Immunol.* 61:355, 1978.

134. Toogood, J. H. Complications of topical steroid therapy for asthma. *Am. Rev. Respir. Dis.* 141:S89, 1990.

135. Tukiainen, H., and Terho, E. O. Comparison of inhaled salbutamol powder and aerosol in asthmatic patients with low peak expiratory flow level. *Eur. J. Clin. Pharmacol.* 27:645, 1985.

136. Turner, J. R., et al. Equivalence of continuous flow nebulizer and metered-dose inhaler with reservoir bag for treatment of acute airflow obstruction. *Chest* 93:476, 1988.

137. Verbeek, P. R., and Chapman, K. R. Asthma: Whom to send home, when to hospitalize. *J. Respir. Dis.* 7(12):15, 1986.

138. Viskum, K. Inhaled salmeterol improves control in moderate to severe asthmatics: A 3 month study. *Eur. Resp. J.* 30:839, 1990.

139. Walker, F. B., et al. Prolonged effect of inhaled glycopyrrolate in asthma. *Chest* 91:49, 1987.

140. Wanner, A. Effect of ipratropium bromide on airway mucociliary function. *Am. J. Med.* 81(Suppl. 5A):23, 1986.

141. Wasserfallen, J.-B., et al. Sudden asphyxic asthma: A distinct entity. *Am. Rev. Respir. Dis.* 142:108, 1990.

142. Weinberger, M., and Hendeles, L. Slow-release theophylline: Rationale and basis for product selection. *N. Engl. J. Med.* 308:760, 1983.

143. Weinberger, M., Hendeles, L., and Ahrens, R. Pharmacologic management of reversible obstructive airway disease. *Med. Clin. North Am.* 65:579, 1980.

144. Weiss, E. B., and Faling, L. J. Clinical significance of $PaCO_2$ during status asthma. *Ann. Allergy* 26:545, 1968.

145. Westerman, D. E., et al. Identification of the high-risk asthmatic patient. *Am. J. Med.* 66:565, 1979.

146. Williams, M. H., Jr. Life-threatening asthma. *Arch. Intern. Med.* 140:1604, 1980.

147. Wolfe, J. D., et al. Bronchodilator effect of terbutaline and aminophylline alone and in combination in asthmatic patients. *N. Engl. J. Med.* 298:363, 1978.

148. Zwillich, C. W., et al. Theophylline-induced seizures in adults. *Ann. Intern. Med.* 82:784, 1975.

149. O'Connor, B. J., Aikman, S. L., and Barnes, P. J. Tolerance to the non-bronchodilator effects of inhaled β_2-agonists in asthma. *N. Engl. J. Med.* 327:1204, 1992.

150. Cheung, D., et al. Long-term effects of a long-acting β_2-adrenoceptor agonist, salmeterol, on airway hyperresponsiveness in patients with mild asthma. *N. Engl. J. Med.* 327:1198, 1992.

151. Haahtela, T., et al. Comparison of a β_2-agonist, terbutaline, with an inhaled corticosteroid, budesonide, in newly detected asthma. *N. Engl. J. Med.* 325:388, 1991.

152. Spitzer, W. O., et al. The use of β-agonists and the risk of death and near death from asthma. *N. Engl. J. Med.* 326:501, 1992.

Beta-Adrenergic Agonists

John W. Jenne
Donald P. Tashkin

55

PHYSIOLOGY AND PHARMACOLOGY

Overview of the Adrenergic Nervous System to the Lungs

The catecholamines norepinephrine and epinephrine are natural compounds that regulate many functions through their action on specific receptor sites. Norepinephrine arises principally from sympathetic nerve endings, while epinephrine comes from the adrenal gland. Adrenergic drugs compete with the natural compounds for these receptors.

Ahlquist [4] in 1948 proposed that adrenergic receptors, stimulating a variety of physiologic responses in various organs, could be classified into two primary types: alpha receptors, responding to agonists in the rank order epinephrine > norepinephrine > isoproterenol; and beta receptors, responding to agonists in the rank order isoproterenol > epinephrine > norepinephrine. Alpha-receptor stimulation causes smooth muscle contraction, while beta-receptor stimulation causes relaxation.

As a result of the physiologic studies conducted by Lands and colleagues [244], beta receptors have been further classified into beta$_1$ and beta$_2$ subtypes. Beta$_1$ receptors display almost equal affinity for epinephrine and norepinephrine, while beta$_2$ receptors are considered more stimulated by epinephrine relative to norepinephrine. Either subtype activates adenylyl cyclase, leading to increased levels of cyclic AMP (cAMP) and activation of cAMP-dependent protein kinases, resulting in the characteristic tissue responses (see Chaps. 14 and 15).

Alpha receptors have also been classified into alpha$_1$ and alpha$_2$ subtypes [180]. Alpha$_1$ stimulation increases the intracellular calcium levels and in many instances phosphoinositol hydrolysis but does not alter the cAMP levels. Alpha$_2$-receptor stimulation inhibits adenylyl cyclase activity and decreases cAMP levels [116].

In humans, bronchial smooth muscle is more densely supplied with cholinergic fibers than is the trachea, but there is no evidence that it receives direct sympathetic innervation, although a very few fibers have been identified [332]. The evidence includes a lack of the dense-core small vesicles of sympathetic varicosities readily seen in other organs [94]. Instead, nerve-mediated relaxation takes place entirely through the nonadrenergic inhibitory system [508], while the adrenergic fibers terminate in bronchial glands and vessels.

The nervous supply to bronchial smooth muscle in humans contrasts with that of other species. In the dog, both cholinergic and sympathetic fibers are supplied, but the nonadrenergic inhibitory system is lacking. In the guinea pig and cat, all three are present [366] (see Chaps. 17 and 18).

In spite of the apparent lack of sympathetic innervation, the smooth muscle membranes of human bronchi contain beta$_2$ receptors that respond to bronchodilators. Circulating epinephrine

(0.2–0.4 nM/L) provides low-level stimulation and may also protect through inhibition of acetylcholine release and mast cell discharge (see later discussion). Spillover of norepinephrine from adjacent structures may also exert some effect.

Fate of Natural Catecholamines

An understanding of beta-adrenergic drug metabolism requires knowledge of the metabolism of natural catecholamines [143]. Norepinephrine released into the junctional cleft activates both alpha and beta receptors. Its action is rapidly terminated by reuptake into the nerve axon (Uptake I), from where it is deaminated by monoamine oxidase (MAO) to dihydroxymandelic acid or taken back into the storage granule. If released by more active nerve impulses in larger quantities, it will also diffuse from the region to be taken up by non-nervous tissue (Uptake II), undergoing methylation at the 3-hydroxyl position by catechol-O-methyltransferase (COMT), forming normetanephrine. It may also diffuse into the circulation and be subjected to MAO and COMT in various tissues and undergo sulfation or glucuronidation in liver and intestinal mucosa. The fate of norepinephrine secreted by the adrenal glands or injected is governed by these extraneuronal metabolic reactions, and its half-life is very short—about 2 minutes. Epinephrine undergoes the same extraneuronal disposition with a similarly short half-life.

Adrenergic Subtype Distribution in Lungs and Heart

Commonly, alpha$_1$ identification is made with [^{3}H]prazosin and alpha$_2$, with [^{3}H]yohimbine. The alpha$_1$ subtype is the classic alpha receptor located on the smooth muscle membranes of most sympathetically innervated tissue and is termed *postsynaptic*; stimulation causes constriction. The alpha$_2$ subtype may, in part, be present in a similar location with a similar function to that of the alpha$_1$ subtype, but it is principally regarded as having a presynaptic location in which it inhibits autonomic ganglia traffic. In human bronchial smooth muscle, there is functional evidence for the existence of alpha receptors, and indeed their activity may be enhanced in asthma and chronic airways disease [230]. However, as discussed by Barnes [25], there are still questions about the specificity of the evidence, and, in any case, their role in asthma seems limited.

Beta-Adrenergic Receptors

Beta-adrenergic subtypes are distinctly different proteins [469]. Mammalian beta$_1$ receptors predominate in the heart and in fat tissue. Beta$_2$ receptors predominate in lung, blood vessels, skeletal muscle, and liver. Both are molecularly distinct from alpha receptors. The consequences of beta$_1$ stimulation are stimulation of the heart and lipolysis, while beta$_2$ compounds cause bronchial and vascular smooth muscle relaxation, skeletal muscle

Table 55-1. Tissue distribution and function of adrenoceptor subtypes

Cell, organ, or process	Receptor type	Response
Lung (human)	Alpha	Bronchoconstriction (weakly); submucosal glands
	Beta$_2$	Bronchodilation; alveolar walls (beta$_2$ > beta$_1$); epithelium (Cl$^-$, H$_2$O transport, EpDRF); submucosal glands (beta$_2$ > beta$_1$); cilia; Clara cell stimulation
Heart	Beta$_1$ > beta$_2$	Increased automaticity, contraction velocity, excitability, and contraction force
Blood vessels	Alpha$_2$	Constriction of arteries and veins
	Beta$_1$	Dilation of coronary vessels
	Beta$_2$	Dilation of most vessels
Mast cells	Alpha	Augmentation of mediator release
	Beta$_2$	Inhibition of mediator release
Glycogenolysis	Alpha (liver)	Stimulation
	Beta$_1$ (heart)	Stimulation
	Beta$_2$ (skeletal)	Stimulation
Insulin release	Beta$_2$	Stimulation
Lipolysis	Beta$_1$	Stimulation
K$^+$ into cells	Beta$_2$	Stimulation
Skeletal muscle	Beta$_2$	Increased force and duration of fast-contracting muscle fibers and decreased force and duration of slow-contracting fibers causing tremor
Noradrenergic nerve terminals	Alpha	Inhibits norepinephrine release
	Beta$_2$	Facilitates norepinephrine release
Cholinergic nerve terminals	Alpha$_2$	Inhibits acetylcholine release
	Beta$_2$	Inhibits acetylcholine release

EpDRF = epithelium-derived relaxant factor.
Source: Adapted from G. M. Lees, A hitch-hiker's guide to the galaxy of adrenoceptors. *Br. J. Med.* 283:173, 1981.

tremor, and stimulation of glycogenolysis. The action of a particular beta agonist is a function not only of the relative affinity for each subtype, but also of the relative preponderance of the subtypes in the tissue. Some selected tissues and their receptor subtypes are listed in Table 55-1.

Airways

Beta-adrenergic receptor subtypes must be identified indirectly by competitive-binding studies using highly selective antagonists such as betaxolol or ICI 89406 for beta$_1$ receptors and ICI 118551 for beta$_2$ receptors [66]. These are used in conjunction with nonselective radioligands such as [^{125}I]iodocyanopindolol for direct radioautography, or with beta agonists for functional discrimination. As found in the airways of several species other than humans, the adrenergic nervous supply to smooth muscle functions through beta$_1$ receptors and can be activated with field stimulation. In humans, however, the muscle subtype is exclusively beta$_2$.

The proportion of beta$_1$ and beta$_2$ subtypes in any species depends on the density of the adrenergic supply for that species, and the level of the bronchial tree. In the densely innervated cat trachea, beta$_1$ receptors predominate. In the guinea pig and dog, tracheal beta$_2$ receptors predominate, particularly more distally. Studies in the guinea pig show an entirely beta$_2$ subtype below the trachea. Relaxation of isolated human bronchial smooth muscle is mediated only by beta$_2$ receptors [146, 509] and, in asthmatics, administration of the beta$_1$-selective agonist prenalterol has no bronchodilator action [264]. Relaxation occurs through the effects of circulating catecholamines and administered beta agonists, which act both directly and indirectly, the latter by inhibiting acetylcholine release at prejunctional beta$_2$ receptors [100, 364] (see later discussion). The epithelium of both guinea pig and human airway has a high density of beta$_2$ receptors, more so than the underlying muscle [66]. These receptors stimulate mucociliary transport by increasing ciliary rate [305] and fluid transport across the membrane. Human submucosal glands are also predominantly beta$_2$, and beta agonists stimulate mucus secretion [345].

Vessels and Parenchyma

Stimulation of the sympathetic nerve trunks in animals reduces flow in the bronchial and tracheal vessels. Vasoconstriction is mediated by alpha adrenergic receptors, and vasodilation by beta receptors [145]. In humans, despite the existence of adrenergic fibers, beta receptors are all the beta$_2$ subtype [66] and stimulation causes an acute fall in pulmonary vascular resistance. Animal studies show that blood flow to the mucosa is enhanced by topically applied beta agonists and reduced by alpha-adrenergic drugs [23]. In guinea pigs, despite increases in flow, beta agonists reduce the leakiness of the subepithelial microvasculature induced by various mediators [338] and may function through the relaxation of elements in the postcapillary venules, thus restoring normal pore size [337].

It is estimated that 90 percent of all beta receptors in the human lung are alveolar in location, and, of these, 30 percent are beta$_1$ in subtype. Their exact location in the alveolar wall (epithelial versus endothelial) has not been identified by histologic means. Mast cell receptors, and those inhibiting the release of histamine and leukotrienes from sensitized lung, are beta$_2$ in subtype. With their potency (pD$_2$) in the nanomolar range, they are likely to respond to tissue levels of beta agonists [64, 509].

Heart

In most animal species, cardiac beta$_2$ adrenergic receptors coexist with beta$_1$ receptors, but are in the minority. However, radioligand studies using highly specific beta$_1$ and beta$_2$ blockers have now shown that human hearts have a higher proportion of beta$_2$ adrenergic receptors than do any other mammals, ranging from 25 to 60 percent of the total [158, 171]. The proportion is highest in the sinoatrial node followed by the atrium and then the ventricle [218]. Right atrial beta$_2$ receptors are believed to be associated with rate rather than force production. As shown by selective antagonists, norepinephrine acts almost exclusively on beta$_1$ receptors, epinephrine equally on beta$_1$ and beta$_2$ receptors, and albuterol exclusively on beta$_2$ receptors [158]. While stimulating either subclass appears to produce the same end result, their population by radioligand binding does not necessarily correlate with their output. Catecholamines are full agonists, completely coupled, and at their maximal effect (E$_{max}$) occupy only a fraction of the total receptor population. Albuterol (also known as salbutamol) acts as a partial agonist. However, it is incompletely coupled, and requires the total population at its E$_{max}$, which is usually lower than the E$_{max}$ from catecholamines. With the current

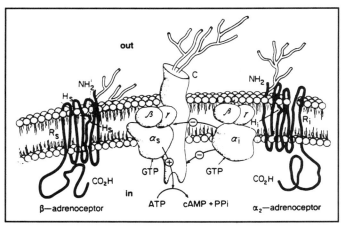

Fig. 55-1. *Receptor control of adenylyl cyclase (C) system. The stimulatory receptor (R_s; beta-adrenergic receptor) and the inhibitory receptor (R_i; alpha$_2$-adrenergic receptor) each possess the classic membrane-receptor structure containing seven transmembrane alpha-helices, and each is coupled to the enzyme through a coupling regulatory protein (G-protein), which is either stimulatory (G_s) or inhibitory (G_i) and consists of three subunits. The complexing of GTP with the alpha$_s$ subunit activates adenylyl cyclase. Its release as GDP (not shown) terminates activation but increases the affinity of the beta-adrenergic receptor for the agonist. The coupling of G_i protein to adenylyl cyclase has not been as well studied. The beta-agonist–binding site (H_s) is estimated to be located about 30 percent within the cell membrane (see text). (Slightly modified from A. Levitzki, Transmembrane signaling to adenylate cyclase in mammalian cells and in* Saccaromyces cervisiae. *Trends Biol. Sci.* 13:298, 1988.*)*

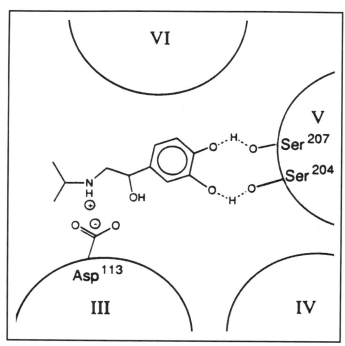

Fig. 55-2. *Model of ligand-binding site of the beta-adrenergic receptor. Isoproterenol is shown in the binding pocket, with postulated interactions with several transmembrane helices, namely at Asp^{113} of helix III, and at Ser^{207} and Ser^{204} of helix V. An interaction with Phe^{289} and Phe^{290} in helix VI is also suspected. (Reprinted with permission from C. D. Strader, I. S. Sigal, and R. A. F. Dixon, Mapping the functional domains of the β-adrenergic receptor.* Am. J. Respir. Cell Mol. Biol. 1:18, 1989.*)*

interest in the use of high doses of beta$_2$-selective agonists given by nebulization and occasionally systemically, their cardiac ramifications are assuming new importance (Chap. 78).

Beta-Adrenergic Receptor Structure and Ligand Binding

The adenylyl cyclase enzyme is depicted in Figure 55-1 in juxtaposition with a stimulatory (beta) and inhibitory (alpha$_2$) adrenergic receptor [256]. The action of these receptors, and a wide variety of hormonal and neurotransmitter receptors, is mediated through a guanine nucleotide–binding regulatory protein (G protein). Receptors acting through G proteins have a primary structure containing seven transmembrane alpha helices. Using site-directed mutagenesis, much work has been done on the beta-adrenergic receptor to identify regions important for ligand binding, G-protein coupling, and the development of agonist-induced subsensitivity [416]. The primary structure of the beta$_2$ receptor consists of 418 amino acids. Figure 55-1 shows the extracellular N-terminal group, the hydrophilic loops, the hydrophobic core in the cell membrane, and the cytoplasmic terminal carboxyl group.

Drug–Receptor Interaction

The pharmacologic action of the drug results from the occupancy of a variable proportion of the receptors to which the drug binds temporarily. Distinction is made between the affinity of the drug for the site and its efficacy. Compounds possessing both affinity and efficacy are termed agonists. Drugs that have affinity but not efficacy are termed antagonists. Weak agonists with sufficient affinity to block other drugs are called partial agonists. These are poorly coupled, but affect all receptors [224]. In contrast, full agonists are well coupled and only a small fraction is required for them to reach their maximum effect. Antagonism between a pure beta agonist such as isoproterenol and a pure antagonist

such as propranolol can be considered to result from competition for two of the three major attachment sites of the receptor. An overdose of one can be counteracted with a sufficient dose of the other. An antagonist such as propranolol binds at its side chain. But the 3- and 4-hydroxyl groups are replaced by an aromatic ring with loss of all activity. A partial antagonist such as pindolol has a point of attachment at the active site but it is not optimal [76].

The ligand-binding domain lies deep within the hydrophobic core. At the pH of the tissues, adrenergic receptor ligands are partly protonated amines at the pH of the tissues, and the binding site contains an acidic counter-ion. Substitution of ASP-113 in the third hydrophobic domain dramatically reduces the affinity of both the agonist and antagonist. The catechol hydroxyl groups of the agonists interact by hydrogen bonding with the side chains of serine residues at positions 204 and 207 in the fifth transmembrane helix, but have no effect on the bonding of beta antagonists lacking the hydroxyl groups. The aromatic ring of agonists undergoes hydrophobic interactions with the PHE-290 in the sixth transmembrane helix. These relationships are shown in Figure 55-2. Work with the fluorochrome agonist carazolol suggests that the agonist site is 30 to 40 percent of the way into the bilayer of the cell membrane [451]. All known beta agonists are phenylethylamine derivatives, and the (−)isomer is two to three orders of magnitude more potent than the (+)isomer.

Radioligand Binding Studies

Binding of an adrenergic agonist to a tissue receptor can be characterized in terms of the maximum number of binding sites and the affinity of the agonist by performing a saturation isotherm with a labeled drug. A Scatchard plot is constructed in which the ratio of bound to free ligand versus the concentration of bound ligand yields a straight line with the slope of $-1/K_D$, and the intercept on the abscissa (B_{max}) gives the total receptor number. Since available radioligands are rather nonspecific in their binding, specific binding must be obtained by substracting the binding determined in the presence of a specifically bound non-labeled drug from the binding in its absence. For beta-adrenergic receptors, propranolol or isoproterenol is used; for alpha receptors, phentolamine is used. A good graphic example of this analysis is the binding of [³H]yohimbine to intact platelets [306]. Phentolamine is used to determine specific binding. Another example is the binding of [¹²⁵I]iodocyanopindolol to beta receptors in human lung section, where specific antagonists are used to establish receptor subtype [407].

From work done on erythrocyte ghosts, it appears that the binding of a catecholamine to the beta receptor also activates two phospholipid methyltransferases, one located on the internal side of the membrane and one on the external surface [179]. Methylation of phosphatidylethanolamine to phosphatidyl-*N*-monomethylethanolamine and thence to phosphatidylcholine increases the fluidity of the local environment and facilitates lateral movement of the beta-adrenergic receptor to interact with the guanylnucleotide coupling factor to stimulate adenylyl cyclase (see subsequent discussion).

G-Protein Coupling to Adenylyl Cyclase

The role of the G protein can be understood with the aid of Figure 55-1 [252]. G proteins consist of three subunits—alpha, beta, and gamma, which couple the receptor to the enzyme, either stimulating or inhibiting it [251]. The GDP–GTP exchange takes place on the alpha fragment, which is anchored to the membrane bilayer by the constant beta and gamma portion. When the beta agonist binds, it causes a conformational change involving residues 223 to 229 to form an amphophilic alpha helix that interacts with the alpha$_S$ subunit [416, 417], with subsequent release of GDP and binding of GTP. The G protein dissociates from the receptor, activating adenylyl cyclase as its GTP is hydrolyzed to GDP. The GDP formed returns to the receptor, greatly enhancing the latter's avidity for new ligand.

The Gi-protein alpha subunit, differing from the Gs alpha subunit, interacts with analogous regions of the alpha$_2$ adrenergic receptor, when its receptor is engaged, resulting in inhibition of adenylyl cyclase (see Fig. 55-1). Other receptors may also be inhibitory, and, in fact, cloned G protein–linked receptors have been shown to couple with various other G proteins, but with varying affinities [104]. At low concentrations of carbocholine, the M$_2$ and M$_4$ receptors inhibit adenylyl cyclase [417].

Receptor Desensitization In Vitro

When a cell or tissue is first exposed to a beta agonist, there is a brisk initial response in the production of cAMP, followed by a decline to nearly the basal level despite the continued presence of drug. The cell becomes "desensitized," "tachyphylactic," or "tolerant" to further stimulation. Desensitization depends on both the concentration of the beta agonist and the time of exposure. All desensitization reactions among cells have in common an acute phase and a chronic phase [251]. With catecholamines, there is generally an uncoupling of the receptor from the catalytic unit of adenylyl cyclase that is expressed as a loss of affinity for the drug, which is rapidly reversed upon drug withdrawal. The chronic phase develops slowly, requires a higher concentration, and is associated with loss of receptors (downregulation). It does not recover quickly. This dissociation between functional desensitization and receptor loss is illustrated in Figure 55-3 from the work of Su and associates [422] with human astrocytoma 1321 Nl cells. There is a rapid reduction of adenylyl cyclase activity, especially in the intact cells, but loss of receptor number is delayed for several hours.

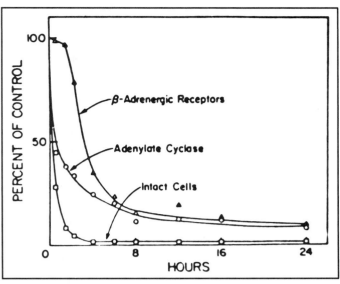

Fig. 55-3. *Time course of decrease in beta-adrenergic receptor density, isoproterenol-stimulated adenylyl cyclase activity, and isoproterenol-stimulated cAMP accumulation during incubation of 1321 Nl cells with 1 μM isoproterenol. (Reprinted with permission from Y. F. Su, et al., Catecholamine-specific desensitization of adenylate cyclase. Evidence for a multistep process. J. Biol. Chem. 255:7410, 1980.)*

Krall and coworkers [236] were able to produce the acute phase of desensitization after exposure of human lymphocytes to only 0.01 n*M* isoproterenol for 60 minutes. There was a nearly complete loss of responsiveness but no loss of number. However, exposure to 1 μ*M* isoproterenol resulted in a 50 percent loss of receptor number. Many workers have shown a loss of lymphocyte responsiveness after long-term treatment with beta agonists. Oral terbutaline therapy in humans produces an associated loss in the numbers of polymorphonucleocytes [382] and lymphocytes [1, 186, 382].

Short-term Desensitization In Vitro

Much progress has been made in understanding the molecular basis of desensitization [169]. Over a time frame of minutes, phosphorylation of the beta receptor takes place by protein kinase A (PKA) and by beta-adrenergic receptor kinase (βARK). PKA is activated by low (nanomole) concentrations of beta agonists, as found with circulating catecholamines or drug therapy. βARK requires high (μ*M*) concentrations, such as exist at sympathetic nerve synapses. Both kinases cause uncoupling of the receptor from the Gs protein by phosphorylating specific sites involved in the coupling. These sites have been deduced by transfecting mutant genes, which code replacements of specific receptor amino acids, into mammalian fibroblasts. As shown in Figure 55-4, PKA phosphorylates amino acids in the third cytoplasmic loop at either low or high beta-agonist concentrations, while βARK involves the terminal 7,000 Daltons of the third cytoplasmic loop and the tail of the receptor. The concerted action of both PKA and βARK results in profound desensitization. βARK is believed to involve a cofactor protein, beta-arrestin, needed in order to bind effectively to the receptor tail. Messenger RNAs (mRNAs) for both βARK and beta-arrestin have been found predominantly in tissues rich in sympathetic innervation. βARK is specific for the beta-adrenergic receptor (homologous desensitization). PKA is not confined to this receptor, but will also act on other receptors linked to adenylyl cyclase (heterologous desensitization).

Simultaneously with uncoupling begins a process of seques-

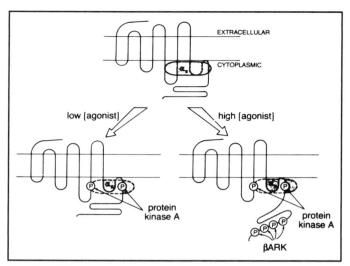

Fig. 55-4. *Model of postulated mechanisms for agonist-induced phosphorylation and desensitization of the beta-adrenergic receptor. At low (nanomolar) agonist concentrations (as with circulating drugs), the cAMP-dependent protein kinase A produced by beta-agonist stimulation phosphorylates one or both of two sites of the receptor adjacent to the $alpha_s$ subunit of the G_s protein, disrupting coupling. At high (micromolar) concentrations of agonist, βARK is also activated, phosphorylating sites on the distal portion of the carboxyl termination of the beta-adrenergic receptor, further disrupting coupling. It has also been postulated that a 48-kDa protein, beta-arrestin, facilitates the phosphorylation process. (Reprinted with permission from R. J. Lefkowitz, W. P. Hausdorff, and M. G. Caron, Role of phosphorylation in desensitization of the β-adrenoceptor. Trends Pharmacol. Sci. 11: 190, 1990.)*

tration of the beta receptor into vesicles and internalization into the cell, effectively removing it from adenylyl cyclase. The internalized receptors are not destroyed, but recycle to the cell surface when the beta agonist is removed.

Long-term Desensitization
Neither PKA or βARK appear to play much of a role in long-termed desensitization. After exposure for several hours, mutant forms of the receptor which lack phosphorylation sites are still desensitized to an extent comparable to the wild type. However, long-term exposure to beta agonists induces a decline in the mRNA encoding for the receptor [155]. This does not appear to be due to a reduction in the production of mRNA, but rather to reduced stability of the RNA. While short-term desensitization could have implications for modifying the airway response to a beta agonist, long-term desensitization could play a role in the subsequent days and weeks of treatment. Such processes may be defined by long-term animal studies. Table 55-2 summarizes these concepts, as published by Lefkowitz and colleagues [251].

Desensitization by Products or the Action of Phospholipase A_2
Evidence is accumulating that one or more products of phospholipase A_2 may be involved in the desensitization process. If, before the desensitization procedure, indomethacin is added to isoproterenol in guinea pig trachea, desensitization is prevented. This seems to be an effect on coupling of the beta receptor with adenylyl cyclase, since there is no effect on the binding of beta agonists to receptors [106, 326]. The direct action of phospholipase on cell membrane lipids may also alter adrenergic receptor function. Guinea pigs challenged after ovalbumin sensitization show enhanced phospholipase activity, and exposure of cell

Table 55-2. *Postulated mechanisms of beta-adrenergic desensitization*

Receptor alteration	Time frame	Mechanism
Uncoupling	Minutes	Phosphorylation by βARK and protein kinase A; action of βARK may involve arrestin-like protein
Sequestration	Minutes	Unknown
Downregulation	Minutes to hours	Increased receptor degradation, possibly as a result of phosphorylation by protein kinase A, and/or by cAMP-independent mechanism; or decreased receptor synthesis by effect of, e.g., protein kinase A at level of mRNA stability

βARK = beta-adrenergic receptor kinase.
Source: R. J. Lefkowitz, W. P. Hausdorff, and M. G. Caron, Role of phosphorylation in desensitization of the β-adrenoceptor. *Trends Pharmacol. Sci.* 11:190, 1990.

membrane to phospholipase A_2 reduces the beta-receptor number and coupling [430]. In vitro studies have shown a good correlation between phospholipase A_2 inhibition and the ability to block isoproterenol-induced desensitization using compounds such as quinacrine and tetracaine, while phospholipase A_2–activating compounds enhance desensitization [277]. In rats administered isoproterenol for several days, loss of beta-receptor number in lung membranes was prevented by the simultaneous administration of quinacrine [448] and, after metaproterenol administration, by corticosteroids [383].

Corticosteroid Reversal at the Receptor Level
As detailed by Davies and Lefkowitz [96], corticosteroids have been shown to increase receptor synthesis, reverse downregulation, and improve coupling, the latter by partially restoring the fraction of receptors in the high-affinity state. Lymphocytes of patients given oral terbutaline become downregulated, but the receptor number may be restored rapidly in vivo over hours with intravenous methylprednisolone [186], oral prednisone, or ketotifen [54]. In neutrophils from volunteers given terbutaline, when hydrocortisone was given prior to collection, or incubated with the cells at the equivalent concentration, it partially restored coupling (affinity) and the generation of cAMP [380]. Improvement of coupling could occur through a change in the receptor membrane milieu (increased fluidity?) by some undefined mechanism, and, certainly, the adverse effects of inflammatory mediators in the asthmatic are reduced.

Mechanisms of Drug Action in Smooth Muscle

The primary modulator of tension in smooth muscle is the level of cytoplasmic calcium. The transition from rest to maximal contraction occurs over a range of about $10^{-7} M$ to $10^{-5} M$ [403]. Like striated muscle, smooth muscle contraction occurs through the conventional sliding-filament mechanism involving actin and myosin. Phosphorylation of myosin filaments by myosin light chain kinase (MLCK) increases its contractile activity and activates its Mg-ATPase. The kinase in turn is activated by its combination with calmodulin, once the latter binds calcium at multiple sites. A mechanism reducing myosin kinase activation is its phosphorylation at sites other than the catalytic site by a cAMP-dependent protein kinase, resulting in a decreased affinity for calmodulin [2].

Much has been learned about the regulation of calcium levels within the cell and the mechanism whereby drugs affect calcium movement [67] (see also Chap. 71). The negative resting potential across the cell membrane of smooth muscle is due to the buildup of ion gradients by active ion pumps. There is an electromechanical force driving calcium in through the cell membrane, with a continuous influx of calcium from its 1.5-mM external concentration (Ca^{++}) to the internal concentration of about $10^{-7}M$ (Ca^{++}). The latter is maintained at this low level by an ATP-dependent calcium extrusion pump. An increase in the low membrane permeability for calcium results in increased influx and activation of the contractile proteins.

Two major mechanisms increase membrane permeability for calcium [39]. One is the opening of slow calcium channels or gates as the membrane potential is reduced, associated with the production of an action potential in some tissues. This is called *electromechanical coupling* and is membrane potential or voltage dependent. The resulting depolarization may spread from cell to cell through gap junctions, particularly abundant in human trachea [94]. A second mechanism is the receptor-operated channel (ROC), in which permeability is increased by union of a receptor with a specific agonist. This is called *pharmacomechanical coupling* and is largely membrane potential independent, with a minor potential-dependent component.

Receptor-Operated Contraction

A framework for discussing receptor-operated contraction and relaxation of smooth muscle is depicted in Figures 55-5 and 55-6. This unfolding story has been a major achievement, and we should understand the broad outlines. As in many other cell processes, two calcium-activated systems are involved. These are the calmodulin-sensitive system, operating through cAMP-dependent PKA, and the protein kinase C (PKC) system [358]. When a contractile agonist combines with its receptor, it stimulates phospholipase C (PLC), a membrane-based phosphodiesterase specific for that agonist, to hydrolyze phosphatidylinositol diphosphate (PIP$_2$) into inositol 1,4,5-triphosphate (IP$_3$) and the lipid-soluble diacylglycerol (DAG). As recently reviewed, IP$_3$ and several related structures (see Fig. 55-6) cause a rapid release of calcium from the endoplasmic reticulum, producing a calcium spike [156]. Calcium also trickles in through the cell membrane as the endoplasmic pool is depleted. The calcium spike loads calcium sites on calmodulin, which then activates MLCK, initiating the rapid-cycling phase of muscle contraction [103, 414] (Chap. 25).

As the spike declines, membrane-bound DAG sensitizes PKC to the lower levels of calcium, which remain; PKC then phosphorylates a variety of cell proteins, and, in this case, various actin-intermediate filament proteins that are involved in the tonic, or "latch-bridge," phase of muscle contraction [330], although myosin light chain phosphorylation continues. PKC can be activated by phorbol esters, and its actions can thus be studied experimentally, including relaxation of its induced contraction by beta agonists [234]. PKC may induce a negative feedback on IP$_3$ formation (Fig. 55-6), as may cAMP.

Relaxation by Beta-Adrenergic Agonists

In smooth muscle preloaded with a fluorescent calcium indicator such as aequorine, the calcium transient produced with a contractile stimulus is rapidly suppressed in the presence of isoproterenol [431] (Fig. 55-7). This could occur through a rise in the cAMP level operating through several mechanisms, such as calcium reuptake into organelles, calcium extrusion from the cell, and cAMP suppression of IP$_3$ formation. cAMP elevation also shifts the equilibrium for MLCK to the inactive (or less active) form, thus allowing phosphorylase to dephosphorylate myosin light chains [321].

A range of agents elevating the cAMP level (i.e., beta agonists,

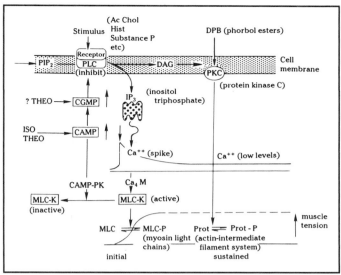

Fig. 55-5. *Two postulated modes of activation of smooth muscle contraction—the calmodulin mode and the protein kinase C (PKC) mode, each activating (phosphorylating) their own set of contractile proteins. Upon receptor stimulation, phosphatidylinositol 4,5-biphosphate (PIP$_2$) is hydrolyzed by phospholipase C (PLC) to the water-soluble myoinositol 1,4,5-triphosphate (IP$_3$), which releases calcium from the sarcoplasmic reticulum to produce a calcium spike. This forms a complex with calmodulin (Ca$_4$ M) to activate myosin light chain kinase (MLC-K), thus catalyzing the phosphorylation of myosin light chains in the initial, rapid-cycling phase of muscle contraction. MLC-K (active) is in equilibrium with MLC-K (inactive), and cyclic AMP (CAMP) generation favors the less active form (through cAMP-dependent protein kinase). cAMP appears to sharply inhibit the action of PLC, and hence the breakdown of PIP$_2$. This is one mechanism of protection against contractile agonists acting at this receptor site. The lipid-soluble diacylglycerol (DAG) sensitizes PKC to low levels of calcium with gradual activation (phosphorylation) of a different set of contractile proteins, the actin-intermediate system, which functions during the sustained phase, along with some contribution from MLC-P. Calcium also continues to trickle in through the cell membrane. The action of cAMP generated by beta agonists (ISO) or theophylline (THEO) in inhibiting PLC is indicated, as well as the possible action of cGMP. (Reprinted with permission from J. W. Jenne and D. P. Tashkin. In S. L. Spector (ed.),* Provocative Challenge Procedures: Background and Methodology. *Mount Kisco, NY: Futura, 1989, P. 461.)*

vasoactive intestinal peptide, forskolin, and phosphodiesterase inhibitors) have been shown to inhibit the inositol phosphate response to histamine [271], and salbutamol produces a potent and rapid inhibition in bovine tracheal smooth muscle [157]. However, this has not been demonstrated with muscarinic agonists in the concentration used, casting some doubt on PLC inhibition as a general mechanism of beta-agonist relaxation [374].

Working with taeniae coli, Bulbring and den Hertog [61] reported that isoproterenol increased $^{45}Ca^{++}$ efflux by about 20 percent, while calcium influx remained the same. They postulated that isoproterenol activates a calcium extrusion pump. Even more striking is a sevenfold increase in calcium efflux from cultured uterine muscle cells on exposure to 1 mM isoproterenol [129].

Using sucrose gap methods in canine tracheal preparations, Ito and Tajima [192] have shown that a concentration of 5×10^{-7} M isoproterenol reduces resting tension, elevates the minimal depolarization required to produce contraction, and suppresses contraction from electrical stimulation. A concentration of 5×10^{-6} M isoproterenol further enhances these effects and increases the resting membrane negative potential. A concentration of 5×10^{-7} M isoproterenol also reduces the amplitude

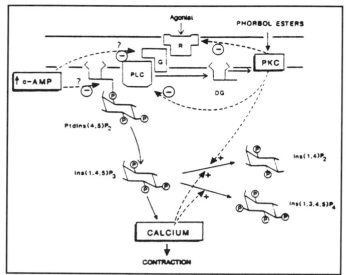

Fig. 55-6. *Action of beta agonist on phospholipase C (PLC) with production of inositol 1,4,5-triphosphate Ins(1,4,5)P₃. Proposed pathways for its formation and metabolism are shown, along with regulation of its concentration by cyclic AMP (c-AMP), protein kinase C (PKC) as activated by diacylglycerol (DG) or phorbol esters, and intracellular calcium (arrows). (Reprinted with permission from J. P. Hall and E. R. Chilvers. Inositol phosphates and airway smooth muscle. Pulmon. Pharmacol. 2:113, 1989.)*

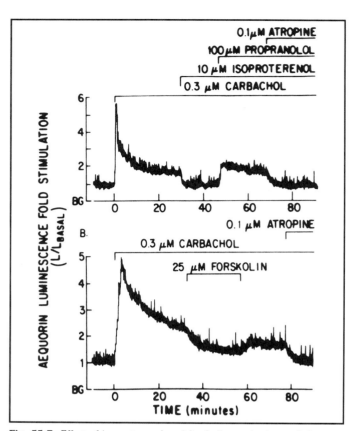

Fig. 55-7. *Effect of isoproterenol and forskolin on the intracellular (Ca⁺⁺) response to carbacholine in bovine trachea. While isoproterenol stimulates adenylyl cyclase through its beta receptor to produce cAMP, forskolin stimulates the enzyme directly. (Reprinted with permission from T. Takuwa, N. Takuwa, and H. Rasmussen. The effect of isoproterenol on intracellular calcium concentration. J. Biol. Chem. 263:762, 1988.)*

of the excitatory junctional potential, with no changes in the membrane potential. The findings of Ito and Tajima [192] indicate an inhibitory action of catecholamines at cholinergic terminals, consistent with early physiologic observations made by Vermeire and Vanhoutte [470] in canine bronchi and with structural correlations made by Jones and colleagues [208] in guinea pig trachea, suggesting prejunctional modulation of acetylcholine release by catecholamines. In canine bronchi, these receptors are of the beta₁ subtype [95], while in human bronchi they are beta₂ [364].

The plasma membrane of airway smooth muscle contains several distinct potassium channels whose activation leads to potassium extrusion, hyperpolarization, and relaxation. Beta agonists stimulate one of these, the calcium-dependent potassium channel whose receptors are densely present on the muscle membrane. Stimulation occurs through both a cAMP-dependent mechanism [238] and, what is even more interesting, a cAMP-independent pathway, the latter through direct stimulation by the alpha fragment of the Gs-protein [237]. The proportion contributed by each mechanism is unknown, but the latest discovery opens the possibility that sensitivity to beta-agonist action occurs even before a rise in the cAMP level. The importance of this channel to beta-agonist action is attested by the fact that in guinea pig trachea its blockage by the specific blocker charybdotoxin causes the dose-response curve for isoproterenol and albuterol to shift 27- and 40-fold to the right, respectively [209]. This has now been shown in human tissues as well [297a].

In summary, there are at least five postulated mechanisms for smooth muscle relaxation by beta-adrenergic agonists in various tissues, all of which may apply to bronchial smooth muscle to some degree. These mechanisms are:

1. Stimulation of cAMP with alteration of myosin kinase by promoting its phosphorylation into a form less avid for calmodulin.
2. cAMP inhibition of PLC with reduction of IP₃ formation.
3. Activation of a calcium extrusion pump.
4. Inhibition of acetylcholine release from cholinergic terminals.

5. Stimulation of the calcium-activated potassium channel.

Factors Modifying the Action of Beta Agonists with Clinical Implications

Functional Antagonism to Smooth Muscle Relaxation

Functional antagonism, which is the antagonism to the action of one agonist by the actions of another through a different receptor, has been well studied in vitro [449] and also been shown to exist in vivo in a canine model [201]. Increasing concentrations of contractile agonists exert a negative feedback on the pD₂ and E$_{max}$ of beta agonists. In vitro antagonism depends on the particular constrictor, however, being much less for histamine or leukotriene LTD₄ than for muscarinic agonists [374]. Even among the latter, there is variability, with much less effect from McN-A-343 than from acetylcholine [461]. Functional antagonism must be important in the response to a beta agonist during an acute attack of asthma, with its high local concentrations of constricting mediators. It is an experimental justification for increasing the dose of beta agonist in more severe attacks.

Studies in bovine trachea and human bronchi have led to the postulate that the differential functional antagonism seen in many tissues is directly related to the degree of inositol phosphate production [461]. Further confirmation of this association comes from studies with human bronchi, where surprisingly little or no difference in functional antagonism exists between hista-

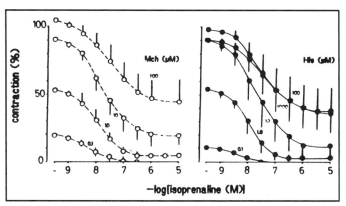

Fig. 55-8. *Relaxation of human bronchial smooth muscle by isoproterenol after contraction by increasing concentrations of methacholine (Mch; left panel) and histamine (His, right panel) at 0.1, 1.0, 10, 100, and 1,000 μM, respectively. Contraction levels are expressed as percentages of the response to 0.1 mM methacholine in each experiment. It is significant that the degree of functional antagonism is relatively similar in human bronchi. (Reprinted with permission from R. G. M. van Amsterdam, et al., Role of phosphoinositide metabolism in human bronchial smooth muscle contraction and in functional antagonism by beta-adrenoceptor agonists. Am. Rev. Respir. Dis. 142:1124, 1990.)*

mine and methacholine (Fig. 55-8), and no difference in inositol phosphate production [462]. Individually, the relationship between functional antagonism and IP_3 production still holds. The locus of negative feedback is not known, but some common process after receptor stimulation must be responsible. Possibilities include negative feedback by PKC [294] (i.e., "cross talk," or perhaps an uncoupling of beta-agonist receptors from adenylyl cyclase at the Gi-protein; see later discussion) [381]. PKC has been shown to directly phosphorylate the $beta_2$ receptor from hamster lung, and can either sensitize or desensitize various beta-agonist–induced adenylyl cyclase systems [43].

Muscarinic Subtypes in the Lung and Interactions with the Adrenergic System

The complexities of the muscarinic system are unfolding, and we should be aware of some interactions. There are five known receptor subtypes. Three concern us in the lung. The M_1 and M_3 subtypes are strongly coupled to phosphoinositol hydrolysis. M_1 receptors facilitate acetylcholine release at parasympathetic ganglia [270], while M_2 receptors inhibit its release at nerve terminals. In many tissues, M_2 receptors inhibit adenylyl cyclase formation by means of pertussis toxin–sensitive G proteins [249], and this has been shown in canine trachea contracted by acetylcholine [207]. M_3 receptors on smooth muscle membranes cause contraction and stimulate mucous glands [370]. $Beta_2$ adrenergic receptors are inhibitory to cholinergic traffic at parasympathetic ganglia, and the severe asthmatic reactions to propranolol could be caused by blocking them [364]. The treatment for these reactions should include atropine. In guinea pigs infected with parainfluenza virus, neuraminidase inactivates the M_2 inhibitory receptor and may lead to airway hyperreactivity [195]. Dysfunction of this receptor must be considered in human asthma (see also Chaps. 16 and 17).

Epithelium Removal

Removal of the epithelium profoundly affects the response to both contractile and relaxing agonists, depending on the species and the airway level examined. The epithelium is believed to produce a relaxing factor (epithelium-derived relaxing factor [EpDRF]) that is stimulated by several bronchoactive agents,

whose nature is still undefined [148]. Relaxation by isoproterenol of fourth-order canine bronchi contracted to 50 percent of maximum (ED_{50}) by acetylcholine is almost completely dependent on the presence of epithelium and to a much greater extent at ED_{80} than at ED_{40} [421]. The clinical relevance of this is not clear, but a denuded bronchus may behave differently. This effect is not present in bronchi constricted by 5-hydroxytryptamine nor relaxed by forskolin. It must depend on activation of epithelial β-adrenergic receptors [421] (Chap. 23).

"Cross-talk:" Desensitization During Acute Anaphylactic Response

In 1982, Meurs and colleagues [293] observed that 24 hours following exposure to antigen, the lymphocytes of allergic subjects had developed a degree of refractoriness to beta-adrenergic stimulation. This involved both homologous and heterologous desensitization. Not only was there a reduction in beta-adrenergic receptor number (downregulation), but also impaired coupling to adenylyl cyclase (loss of affinity). The uncoupling was heterologous; that is, cAMP generation by other agonists stimulating adenylyl cyclase, such as the H_2 action of histamine, was also impaired. Yet, before challenge, the beta-adrenergic response of the lymphocytes from these stable asthmatics was normal. Only in the acute anaphylactic state did it become impaired. Further studies indicated that the impairment was at the Gs-protein, since addition of the GTP analog, Gpp[NH]p, restored sensitivity [295]. Meurs and associates [294] postulated that there was negative feedback (cross-talk) from activation of PKC during the anaphylactic response, since stimulation of lymphocytes by the phorbol ester phorbol 12-myristate 13-acetate (PMA) also produced heterologous desensitization to beta-agonist stimulation [294].

In a similar vein, Nielson [316] showed that, although mediator production of peripheral human granulocytes stimulated by the chemotactic peptide f-Met-Leu-Phe (FMLP) was inhibited initially by isoproterenol, over the next 10 minutes, a refractory state developed that could also be mimicked by the response to PMA. The implication of these results for the responses of inflammatory cells to beta agonists during acute asthmatic attacks is profound. Not only may cellular responses become less sensitive to administered beta agonists, but the protection afforded by endogenous catecholamines is less. Conceivably, similar crosstalk occurs in the smooth muscle of the airway.

Desensitization of Smooth Muscle by Beta-Agonist Exposure and the Effect of Corticosteroids

There is no difficulty in desensitizing bronchial smooth muscle in vitro, provided one uses a sufficient concentration of beta agonist. One recalls that only 0.01 nM isoproterenol for 60 minutes was sufficient to produce the acute phase of desensitization in human lymphocytes [235], and a recent study of lung $beta_2$ receptors and mononuclear leukocytes removed from the lungs of patients briefly exposed to intravenous terbutaline found only the leukocytes to be downregulated [168].

Figure 55-9 shows the shift to the right that occurs when normal human bronchus is exposed to 1 μM isoproterenol for 25 minutes, a concentration tenfold greater than the half-maximal response (EC_{50}) [17]. The results are similar for rat trachea [258]. Pig bronchus is increasingly desensitized upon exposure to 1 and 5 μM isoproterenol [147]. In rats given isoproterenol or terbutaline subcutaneously, the degree of desensitization of the removed trachea is a function of both time and the dose of beta agonist, with progressively decreasing affinity of the drug for the receptor [18]. The desensitization produced is cross-reactive with terbutaline [17, 18]. Thus, the clinical question is whether, over a range of concentrations and time exposures to beta agonists, a significant degree of airway desensitization oc-

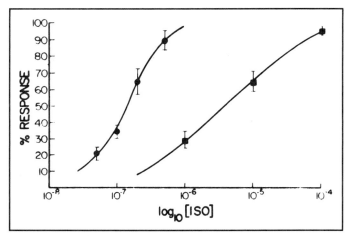

Fig. 55-9. *Log$_{10}$ concentration versus response relationships for isoproterenol (ISO) in control (closed circles) and desensitized (1 × 10^{-6} M, 25 min; closed squares) human bronchial preparations. The means are plotted with the brackets denoting the standard error of the mean. (Reprinted with permission from B. P. Avner and J. W. Jenne, Desensitization of isolated human bronchial smooth muscle to beta receptor agonists.* J. Allergy Clin. Immunol. 68:51, 1981.)

curs and whether it occurs in asthmatics as well as normals. Tissues vary in their susceptibility to desensitization, as do even the airways in asthmatics and normals, the asthmatic seemingly less prone (see later discussion).

Corticosteroids appear to reduce or partially reverse desensitization of smooth muscle as well as leukocytes. Davis and Conolly [99] produced subsensitivity in human bronchi using 4 μM isoproterenol for 60 minutes, and maintained it in the presence of only 1 nM isoproterenol. After drug removal the administration of 0.15 mM hydrocortisone hastened the return of sensitivity over the next 3 hours. Isoproterenol desensitization of pig bronchus was markedly retarded in the presence of 5 μM hydrocortisone, a level reached during treatment of status asthmaticus [147]. In dogs, in which repeated inhalation of isoproterenol had impaired the ability to protect against methacholine constriction, intravenous methylpredisolone appeared to preserve this ability when tested only 75 minutes after steroid administration [413].

Clinically, intravenous methylprednisolone has been shown to restore significant bronchodilator responsiveness within 60 minutes of administration in previously unresponsive asthmatics [113], while intravenous hydrocortisone causes a significant return of bronchial responsiveness to albuterol after only 1 hour (maximum at 3–5 hours) in normal human subjects desensitized by albuterol inhalations over a 4-week period [181] (Chap. 60).

Possible Impaired Response of the Isolated Asthmatic Airway

Some evidence is accumulating that, during fatal attacks of asthma, the smooth muscle response of the airways to beta agonists becomes impaired. Whether asthmatic airways are inherently different from normal airways has been controversial. The airways of asthmatics with mild to moderate disease that were obtained at thoracotomy for lung cancer showed no impairment of response to a beta agonist [486]. Nevertheless, Cerrina and associates [69] found that those bronchi most sensitive to histamine constriction were least sensitive to isoproterenol. Goldie and colleagues [147] examined the airways of asthmatics after a fatal attack and found a four- to fivefold reduction in responses to beta agonists. Tracheal strips with sufficient viability, obtained from seven asthmatics dying from acute attacks, were found by Bai and coworkers [19] to have a four- to fivefold mean reduction

in sensitivity to isoproterenol and theophylline, but increased responses to acetylcholine, histamine, and field stimulation. Detailed study of beta receptors in the airways of a patient dying from asthma showed no reduction in number, but a 10- and 13-fold increase in EC$_{50}$ to isoproterenol and fenoterol, respectively, suggesting a reduction in coupling [407]. While the use of postmortem tissue invites criticism, it is nevertheless provocative to consider that such hyposensitivity is always compared to the findings from postmortem controls. If developing during the attack, postulated mechanisms might include the negative feedback from cross-talk directed toward adenylyl cyclase [295], negative feedback by the surge of arachidonic acid metabolites [326], and residual desensitization from the use of large doses of beta agonist and stress-induced catecholamines. While more studies of postmortem tissue are needed, an alternative approach is to attempt to recreate the in vivo environment of asthmatic tissue to determine its impact on receptors in normal tissue.

Evolution of Beta$_2$-Adrenergic Bronchodilators

The continuing refinement of beta-adrenergic drugs as bronchodilators has consisted of creating compounds with greater beta$_2$ specificity and a prolonged duration of action. The important compounds in evolution are illustrated in Figure 55-10. With the exception of fenoterol, all are available on the U.S. market.

Although isoproterenol has the typically short half-life of catecholamines, more prolonged action was achieved by altering the catechol nucleus, either by changes at the 3-hydroxyl group or by moving the 4-hydroxyl to the 5 position on the ring. These changes eliminate the methylation reaction (COMT) occurring in bronchial tissue at the 3 position and further delay elimination by greatly reducing the rate of sulfate conjugation.

Bitolterol is an inactive "pro-drug," which, aerosolized, undergoes esterase hydrolysis in the bronchial mucosa to become the active drug colterol (N-ter-butylarterenol) [217]. Its action is slightly prolonged over albuterol's. Procaterol (not shown and not available in the United States) is unique because it is several times more potent than isoproterenol with a high degree of beta$_2$ selectivity. It can be given by mouth without gastrointestinal inactivation in a dose of 0.5 to 0.10 mg, or in aerosolized form [511]. Pirbuterol is more recently available in the United States and has approximately the same duration of effect as albuterol and terbutaline.

Formoterol and Salmeterol: New Long-Acting Compounds

The search for compounds with a longer action and greater beta$_2$ selectivity has culminated in two new compounds, formoterol and salmeterol, which promise to revolutionize asthma therapy. Their structure is shown in Figure 55-11. The markedly greater selectivity of these compounds for the trachea over the heart has been demonstrated in several species. However, their most interesting feature is their retention in the tissues and at the receptor site, which allows them to be dosed on a twice daily basis, resulting in much smoother control.

Physiologic Actions of Beta-Adrenergic Agonists

Effects on the Heart

In Vitro Studies. The cardiovascular actions of beta-adrenergic agonists result from direct myocardial effects that increase the rate (chronotropism) and force (inotropism) of contraction and from indirect rate effects that result from baroreceptor reflexes to peripheral dilation. Any increased inotropism is associated with increased myocardial oxygen consumption.

Dose-response curves using guinea pig left and right atrial strips show that, in their effects on contractile force and rate,

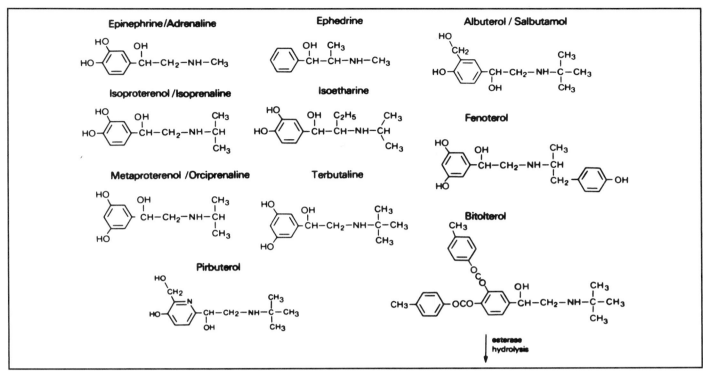

Fig. 55-10. *Beta-adrenergic agonists in use, and their evolution toward more beta₂-selective compounds, with alterations to the N-terminal group of isoproterenol (nonselective) and changes in the catechol ring structure producing more prolonged activity. Only fenoterol is not available in the United States. In some cases, the two names shown represent U.S. and European nomenclature.*

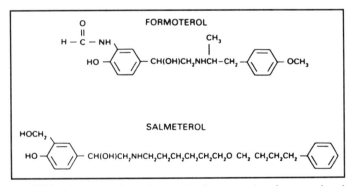

Fig. 55-11. *Structure of new long-acting beta₂ agonists, formoterol and salmeterol, compared to albuterol. Note the addition of lipophilic groupings.*

respectively, isoproterenol and metaproterenol belong to the same family of dose-response curves and are considered full agonists [50]; that is, their curves are parallel and have the same maximal response, although the dose corresponding to ED₅₀, a measure of affinity, differs considerably. This is in contrast to the family of curves containing albuterol and trimetuquinol, which have a shallower slope with a reduced maximal response (Fig. 55-12); these drugs are partial agonists. When similarly compared in human myocardium, the same distinction between isoproterenol and albuterol exists in the effect on contractile force [308]. In the guinea pig atrium, albuterol is 500 to 2,500 times less potent.

Effects on Bronchial Smooth Muscle. Further beta₂ specificity is revealed by in vitro dose-response curves using guinea pig trachea and human bronchial strips obtained from lungs resected for cancer.

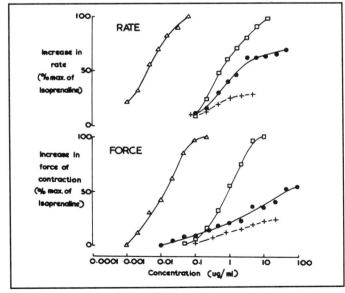

Fig. 55-12. *In vitro dose-response curves showing effects of various beta agonists on contractile force and rate in guinea pig left and right atrium, respectively. Open triangles = isoproterenol; open squares = metaproterenol; closed circles = albuterol; crosses = trimetuquinol. (Reprinted with permission from R. T. Brittain, A comparison of the pharmacology of salbutamol with that of isoprenaline, orciprenaline and trimetuquinol. Postgrad. Med. J. [suppl 47]:11, 1971.)*

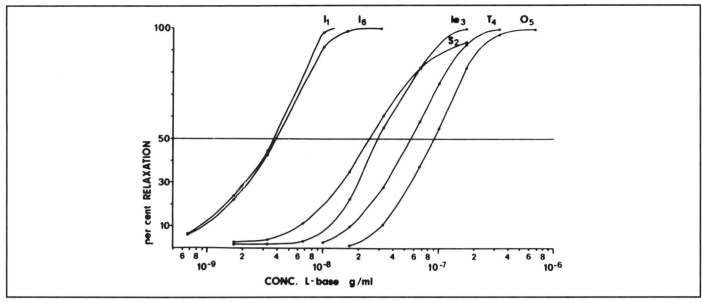

Fig. 55-13. *In vitro dose-response curves showing effects of various beta agonists on smooth muscle relaxation of human bronchial strips precontracted with carbacholine. I_1 and I_6 = isoprenaline given as first and sixth drug, respectively; Ie = isoetharine; S = salbutamol; T = terbutaline; O = orciprenaline. (Reprinted with permission from N. L. V. Svedmyr and G. Thiringer, The effects of salbutamol and isoprenaline on beta receptors in patients with C.O.P.D.* Postgrad. Med. J. *[suppl. 47]:44, 1971.)*

Table 55-3. Bronchodilation activity in human bronchial muscle using carbachol contraction

Drug	ED_{50} (gm/ml)[a]	Ratio[b]
Isoproterenol	0.50×10^{-8}	1
Salbutamol	3.6×10^{-8}	1:7
Terbutaline	5.9×10^{-8}	1:12
Metaproterenol	7.8×10^{-8}	1:16
Isoetharine	3.5×10^{-8}	1:7

[a] ED_{50} (gm/ml) is that concentration giving 50% relaxation (L-base).
[b] The ratio is the concentration required relative to isoproterenol.
Source: N. L. V. Svedmyr and G. Thiringer, The effects of salbutamol and isoprenaline on beta receptors in patients with C.O.P.D. *Postgrad. Med. J.* 47(suppl.):44, 1971. Reprinted with permission.

Based on their findings from human bronchi, Svedmyr and Thiringer [426] constructed the cumulative dose-response curves shown in Figure 55-13. Note that they all fall in the same family of curves. The mean ED_{50} for each drug is tabulated in Table 55-3. These concentrations have the same rank order as the doses required in vivo and are 10 times as great (in the case of terbutaline) as the actual serum concentrations effective during bronchodilator therapy by the systemic route.

Guinea Pig Tissues Used to Determine Beta₂ Selectivity

The comparative properties of beta₂-selective agents are most commonly studied in guinea pig tissues, but the absolute figures may differ between studies and between species. Table 55-4 summarizes the 1982 study of Decker and associates [101], comparing the mean relative affinities (pD_2) of formoterol with those of salbutamol, terbutaline, and isoproterenol. The high affinity of formoterol for trachea provides a 12-fold greater "selectivity ratio" over that of salbutamol. Note, however, that all compounds have rather large "intrinsic activities" (E_{max}) against atria, in contrast to the lower E_{max} for salbutamol shown in Figure 55-12 and Table 55-5, and despite the similarity of the experiments.

Table 55-5 compares the ability of all the major compounds to

Table 55-4. Selectivity of some beta-adrenergic receptor agonists determined in in vitro preparations of guinea pig trachea and atria

	Trachea		Atria		
Drug	pD_2	Intrinsic activity[a]	pD_2	Intrinsic activity[b]	Beta₂-Selectivity[a]
Formoterol	9.29	0.94	6.98	0.94	204
Salbutamol	7.13	0.91	5.90	0.75	17
Terbutaline	6.43	0.83	5.17	0.89	18
Isoprenaline	8.57	1.0	8.62	1.0	0.9

[a] Antilog [pD_2 (trachea) − pD_2 (atria)].
[b] Ratio of maximum response to each compound to the maximum response to isoprenaline.
pD_2 = mean relative affinity.
Source: N. Decker, et al. Effects of N-aralkyl substitution of β-agonists on α and β-adrenoceptor subtypes: pharmacological studies and binding assays. *J. Pharm. Pharmacol.* 34:107, 1982. Reprinted with permission.

Table 55-5. Relative beta-agonist potency at beta₁- and beta₂-adrenergic receptors in guinea pig tissues

Agonist	Guinea pig trachea (beta₂)	Guinea pig left atria (beta₁)	% Isoprenaline maximum (beta₁)
Isoprenaline*	1.0	1.0	100
Orciprenaline	0.05	0.01	89
Salbutamol	0.48	0.0004	14
Clenbuterol	2.0	0.0001	2
Terbutaline	0.08	0.0003	35
Fenoterol	0.9	0.005	100
Procaterol	11.1	0.0001	3
Salmeterol	5.0	0.0001	4
Formoterol	25.0	0.05	100

* Potency of isoprenaline = 1.0.
Data courtesy of M. Johnson, Glaxo Group Research, Ltd., Ware, U.K.

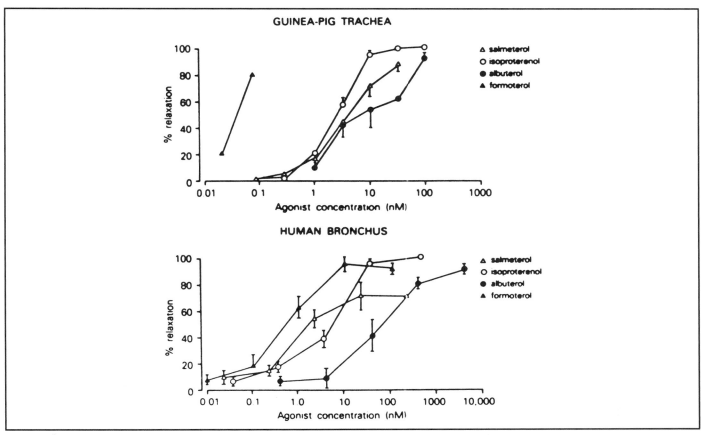

Fig. 55-14. *Action of salmeterol, isoproterenol, albuterol, and formoterol against guinea pig trachea and human bronchus constricted by prostaglandin $F_{2\alpha}$. Note the greater potency of formoterol, particularly in the guinea pig, and the fact that salmeterol is not a full agonist in the human bronchus. (Reprinted with permission from R. A. Coleman, et al., Salmeterol: a potent and long-lasting B_2-adrenoceptor agonist. Am. Rev. Respir Dis. 143:A648, 1991.)*

increase the force of the electrically driven guinea pig left atrium with their ability to relax electrically contracted trachea, all referenced to isoproterenol. These data were provided by Glaxo investigators. Note that fenoterol and formoterol are full agonists (E_{max}) against the heart despite their low potency, and metaproterenol (orciprenaline) nearly so. Such studies provide the needed information to develop beta$_2$-selective compounds.

The "potency" figures given in Table 55-5 are a function of both the EC_{50} and E_{max}, and are the ratio of the concentration of isoproterenol to the concentration of the drug in question producing the same effect. A beta$_2$/beta$_1$ selectivity ratio can be calculated using the formula: potency in trachea/potency in atrium. With the surprisingly low E_{max} and very low potency against atrium, the selectivity ratio for salmeterol becomes enormous at 50,000, compared to 1,200 for salbutamol, 500 for formoterol, and 180 for fenoterol. As mentioned previously, beta$_2$ receptors also exist in guinea pig right atria [170], but are believed to principally act on rate rather than on force.

Guinea Pig Trachea versus Human Bronchi

Figure 55-14 shows the relaxation produced by salmeterol, formoterol, albuterol, and isoproterenol of guinea pig trachea and human bronchi contracted by prostaglandin F_2 (PGF_2) [82]. Note that, in guinea pig trachea, formoterol is far more effective than salmeterol and even isoproterenol, similar to the findings from older studies [101]. The differential is much less in human tissue, but still roughly on the same order.

Table 55-6. Potency and rates of onset and offset of beta-adrenergic receptor agonists in the electrically stimulated guinea pig trachea preparation[a,b]

Agonist	EC_{50}[c] (nM)	Onset time[d] (min)	Offset time[e] (min)
Isoprenaline (N = 4)	29 (13–29)	1–2	1–3
Salbutamol (N = 8)	25 (11–56)	3.2 (2.0–5.4)	11 (8–15)
Clenbuterol (N = 6)	10 (4–25)	5.5 (2.8–10.2)	45 (29–68)
Salmeterol (N = 14)	4 (2–11)	29.0 (24–36)	>420

[a] Guinea pig isolated trachea preparations were electrically field–stimulated under superfusion conditions according to the method of R. A. Coleman and A. T. Nials, The characterization and use of the electrically stimulated, superfused guinea-pig tracheal strip preparation. *Br. J. Pharmacol.* 88:409P, 1986.
[b] 95% confidence limits are shown in parentheses.
[c] The concentration of beta agonist required to inhibit contractile response by 50 percent.
[d] Time required for 50% of the response to an EC_{50} concentration to be achieved.
[e] Time required for 50% recovery from an EC_{50} concentration.
Source: M. Johnson. The pharmacology of salmeterol. *Lung* 168(suppl):115, 1990. Reprinted with permission.

Factors Governing Duration of Action

Interesting studies have been done on the rates of onset and offset of beta agonists in the electrically stimulated superfused guinea pig trachea [20, 205]. As shown in Table 55-6, the EC_{50} for salmeterol, about 4 nM, was less than that for salbutamol, isoproterenol, or clenbuterol, but the mean onset time (50% of

Table 55-7. Various properties against tracheal strip and tracheal tube relaxation as related to lipophilicity

Agonist	Half-life (tracheal strip) (min)	% Max relaxation	Intra pD₂ (potency)	$\dfrac{EC_{50}\ intra}{EC_{50}\ extra}$	Distribution coefficient (octanol/H₂O)	Retention (%)
Salbutamol	0.8	96	5.75	37	0.016	13
Fenoterol	1.1	98	7.20	10.5	0.74	−1
Formoterol	1.7	96	8.51	5.3	2.6	30
Salmefamol	1.6	93	7.46	3.1	2.2	52
Salmeterol	17.6	81	7.97	1.2	63	83

$pD_2 = \log EC_{50}$; EC_{50} = concentration producing 50% relaxation at maximum effect (E_{max}); intra = intraluminal; extra = extraluminal.
Source: A.-B. Jeppsson, et al. Pharmacodynamic and pharmacokinetic aspects of the transport of bronchodilator drugs through the tracheal epithelium of the guinea-pig. *Pulm. Pharmacol.* 2:81, 1989. Reprinted with permission.

effect) was longer (29 versus 3.2 minutes) and the offset time was remarkably prolonged (over 420 versus 11 minutes). This incredible prolongation of activity is the major feature of these new drugs, particularly salmeterol.

More recent studies using the same design include formoterol and show that its time to 50 percent recovery is short, averaging 20 minutes, while salmeterol showed little or no recovery after 7 to 10 hours [82]. When their ability to protect conscious guinea pigs against aerosolized histamine was tested, as judged by the duration of increased respiratory rate, the effects of albuterol lasted less than 1.5 hours and the effects of formoterol were declining at 3.0 hours, but there was little or no loss of salmeterol activity at 6 hours [81]. Thus, a fundamental difference exists in the retention of salmeterol at the receptor site compared to that of formoterol. Formoterol has greater initial affinity, however.

The mechanism for the long retention of the new compounds at the active site in tracheal tissue has been linked to their lipophilicity, although other factors are involved. Current beta₂-selective compounds, such as albuterol, with a duration of action of only 4 hours when given by inhalation, are hydrophilic and easily removed by washing the tissue. The new compounds are lipophilic and difficult to remove. Their intraluminal and extraluminal dynamics have been studied in relation to their lipophilicity using a closed-loop guinea pig trachea [202] (Table 55-7). Although with the conventional tracheal strip salbutamol quickly attained its maximum effect (half-life = 0.8 minute), salmeterol required 17.6 minutes for its half-life onset, despite a much greater final pD₂. When given intraluminally into the tracheal tube, salbutamol required 37 times more drug to achieve the same effect as that when given extraluminally (serosal absorption), as indicated by the ratio of Ec₅₀'s. The more lipophilic compounds had similar EC₅₀'s and were retained at the active site despite vigorous washing. Nevertheless, they were readily displaced by propranolol. Jeppsson and colleagues [202] have concluded that "high lipophilicity and retention in tissues in vitro are factors predictive of a long effect duration after inhalation," but recognize that clenbuterol, a lipophilic compound with only a 4-hour duration, does not fit well into this scheme, so that other factors must be involved.

Most interesting is the fact that, although sotalol rapidly reverses the tissue relaxation by salmeterol, there is a return of the original relaxation when it is washed out (Fig. 55-15). Brittain [51] views the molecule as being anchored by its long nonpolar tail to another portion of the receptor molecule or cell membrane, while its head engages the active site. Sotalol easily competes for the active site, but the head flops back into place when sotalol is removed and relaxation commences anew. Whether formoterol shares this mechanism for its prolonged action is unclear. Both drugs may simply remain in the local lipid environment. Because of this prolonged stimulation of beta₂ receptors, the new compounds must be regarded with some apprehension. Various tissues in the body must undergo the same stimulation when the drugs are given or absorbed systemically. Thus, the

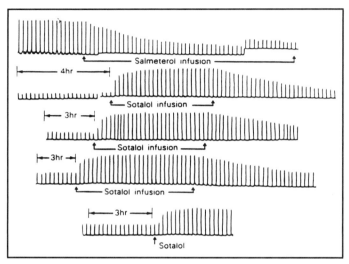

Fig. 55-15. *Transient sotalol reversal of salmeterol-induced relaxant responses in the superfused, electrically stimulated, guinea pig trachea. Note the reassertion of salmeterol inhibition when the sotalol infusion is terminated. The "tail" of salmeterol apparently remains firmly at the active site, although its "head" is temporarily displaced. (Reprinted with permission from M. Johnson, Salmeterol: a novel drug for the treatment of asthma.* Agents Actions *September, 1991. Courtesy of Glaxo, Inc.)*

maximum recommended inhaled dose of salmeterol is 100 μg every 12 hours, since 200 μg causes pulse elevation and plasma potassium concentration reduction.

In Vivo Studies in Humans. Fortified by the in vitro studies, we turn to in vivo comparisons in humans. Here, the effects on heart rate and spirometry are often considered rough measures of relative beta₁ and beta₂ effects, respectively, but the pulse elevation is a hybrid of direct and indirect effects. It underestimates the relative beta₂ specificity. Moreover, beta₂ receptors exist in the sinus node and atrium, which are believed to be involved principally in rate production. Even a beta₃ receptor is now postulated to exist in heart and other tissues [218].

Beta₂ Intravenous Infusion. Svedmyr and Thiringer [426] compared isoproterenol and albuterol infusions in patients with chronic bronchitis. There was a simultaneous increase in pulse and the forced expiratory volume at 1 second (FEV₁) as the dose of isoproterenol was increased, while with albuterol the pulse elevation commenced at a dose ten times higher than that affecting FEV₁. A very similar result was obtained by Paterson and coworkers [333]. By contrast, McEvoy and associates [288] found that the increase in heart rate and FEV₁ with metaproterenol began at the same dose, was similar in manner to that of isoproterenol, and conformed to the findings obtained from in vitro studies.

The very minimal inotropism from albuterol was also evident

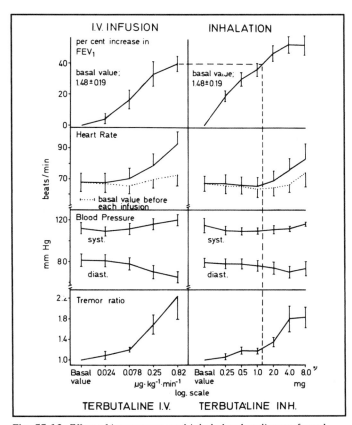

Fig. 55-16. *Effect of intravenous and inhaled terbutaline on forced expiratory volume in 1 second (FEV₁), heart rate, blood pressure, and tremor. (Reprinted with permission from G. Thiringer and N. L. V. Svedmyr, Comparison of infused and inhaled terbutaline in patients with asthma.* Scand. J. Respir. Dis. *57:17, 1976.)*

in the in vivo studies of Gibson and Coltart [141], in which right and left heart catheterization was performed in patients being studied for mitral valve disease. In contrast to isoproterenol, there was little or no effect of albuterol on the systolic ejection rate (a measure of contractile force) when both were infused to equal pulse elevations.

Relative Beta₂ Specificity by the Inhaled Route. The topical application of beta₂ agonists to the airways maximizes bronchial action, while cardiac effects due to absorbed drug are minimized. Figure 55-16 shows the additional freedom from pulse elevation obtained when terbutaline is applied topically by aerosol rather than intravenously. While the dependence of pulse elevation on diastolic pressure drop is apparent in the infusion study, these systemic effects (pulse elevation, diastolic pressure drop, tremor) become a factor only at the highest inhaled doses—doses much higher than normally used clinically (see Chap. 57).

Critical review of the effects of beta-adrenergic drugs on heart rate, whether by the systemic or inhaled route, suggests that normals respond more vigorously than do asthmatic patients [197]. There are at least two possible explanations for this. As shown by Shelhamer and associates [391], atopic asthmatics have a reduced pulse elevation in response to small doses of injected isoproterenol, consistent with a beta defect. Their alpha and cholinergic responsiveness appears to be increased. A second factor is the ongoing tolerance or tachyphylaxis of some tissues to beta agonists stemming from their continued therapeutic use prior to most studies. Impaired cardiac responses were noted by Conolly and coworkers [87] in asthmatics on large doses of inhaled isoproterenol, while Svedmyr and associates [423] re-

ported reduced responses in patients on long-term terbutaline therapy. Relevant to this, the absolute drop in distolic pressure becomes less with the continued oral administration of terbutaline [198].

Antiinflammatory Effects of Beta Agonists
Inhibition of Mediator Release in the Lung. One persistent question is whether bronchodilator inhibition of mediator release from the lung occurs to a significant degree. The modulation of anaphylactic discharge by adrenergic drugs has been framed in terms of their effect on mast cell cAMP [16]. Beta agonists raise the cAMP level and inhibit discharge, while alpha agonists act in the reverse fashion. Tung and Lichtenstein [454] emphasized that the small antigen concentrations encountered by the lung are capable of releasing only a small fraction of the total histamine content of the lung. By analogy with basophil histamine release, inhibition of this smaller amount requires only a tenth of the drug concentration heretofore assumed necessary. Martin and coworkers [283] found that oral terbutaline decreased the release of histamine and neutrophil chemotactic factor into peripheral blood by antigen inhalation, although histamine levels did not correlate with the drop in FEV₁. Borum and Mygind [41] found that a nasal aerosol of fenoterol protected against nasal antigen challenge. One might think that an aerosolized bronchodilator would confer analogous protection to the airway. Indeed, along with bronchodilation, Howarth and colleagues [185] showed that albuterol delivered by metered-dose inhaler (MDI) prevents the rise in plasma histamine and neutrophil chemotactic factor seen after antigen challenge.

There is now renewed interest in this subject because of the current focus on the inflammatory aspects of asthma and the development of the long-acting beta₂ agonists. As discussed by Johnson [205] and outlined in an abstract by Johnson and colleagues [206], the EC₅₀'s for inhibition of mediator release have been determined for isoproterenol, albuterol, formoterol, and salmeterol in a system using passively sensitized human lung fragments (Table 55-8). Figure 55-17 shows the time course of inhibition against repetitive acute challenge. Note, however, that all compounds were used in concentrations about ten times their EC₅₀. The prolonged action of salmeterol, even in comparison with formoterol, is indeed impressive. However, as can be seen, the others are also inhibitory, albeit of shorter duration.

In asthmatics, salmeterol by MDI inhibits both the immediate and late phase response to antigen [455], as does 2.5 mg of albuterol nebulized just before challenge [456a]. In both cases, the authors conclude that the protective effect is present longer than the bronchodilating effect, suggesting that the drug exerts an antiinflammatory action, for example, inhibition of mediator discharge and/or vascular leakage.

"Antipermeability Effects"
In experimental animals beta agonists and xanthines act to prevent the increase in permeability of endothelial capillaries in-

Table 55-8. Inhibition of mediator release from sensitized human lung by beta-adrenergic receptor agonists

Agonist	EC₅₀ (nM) ± SEM (N)		
	Histamine	*LTC₄/D₄*	*PGD₂*
Salmeterol	3.0 ± 1.9 (11)	0.9 ± 0.5 (11)	1.5 ± 0.5 (4)
Isoprenaline	1.1 ± 0.3 (24)	0.4 ± 0.1 (24)	1.4 ± 0.3 (6)
Salbutamol	35.8 ± 14.6 (24)	11.5 ± 2.7 (24)	51.7 ± 32.0 (6)
Formoterol	0.25 (2)	0.03 (2)	NT

EC₅₀ = half-maximal response; LTC₄/D₄ = leukotriene C₄ and D₄; PGD₂ = prostaglandin D₂; NT = not tested.
Source: M. Johnson. The pharmacology of salmeterol. Lung 168(suppl.):115, 1990. Reprinted with permission.

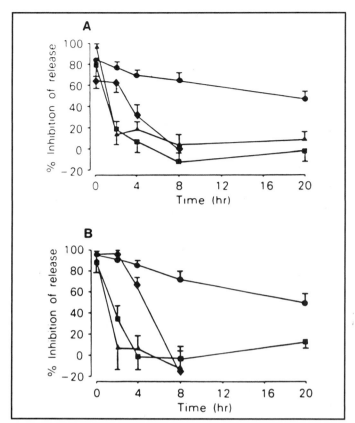

Fig. 55-17. *Duration of equipotent concentrations of beta-adrenergic receptor agonists as inhibitors of mediator release—sensitized human lung fragments when challenged by antigen at intervals. (A) Histamine. (B) Leukotriene C_4 and D_4. Diamonds = formoterol (4 nM); circles = salmeterol (40 nM); triangles = isoproterenol (20 nM); squares = albuterol (200 nM). (Reprinted with permission from M. Johnson, The pharmacology of salmeterol.* Lung *168[suppl] 115, 1990.)*

duced by noxious substances and inflammatory mediators. Terbutaline, given systemically or topically, prevents leakage of plasma into the tracheobronchial lumen [322, 338]. While plasma leakage may be an important defense mechanism initially, if it becomes excessive, it becomes a contributing factor in asthma pathophysiology through the formation of mucosal edema and excessive secretions [337]. An edematous mucosa adversely affects airway dynamics, and probably loosens epithelial tight junctions, causing passage of plasma into the lumen. A sufficient degree of subepithelial hydrostatic pressure may eventually contribute to shedding of the epithelium. The extensive work of the Swedish group in this area has been recently summarized [114].

Exact measurement of beta-agonist action on capillary leak is hampered by the fact that these drugs also decrease hydrostatic pressure and increase flow, with the consequential distortion of measurements of fluid and protein flux which might be attributable to the drug's action on permeability. However, a recent study, in which thrombin was used as the toxic agent on pulmonary capillaries to induce hyperpermeability, was able to demonstrate a direct action of 2 μM isoproterenol in preventing the endothelial cell deformity and actin filament rearrangement which otherwise produced large intercellular pores and increased permeability [297]. This area of pharmacology will benefit greatly from the interest generated by the new long-acting beta$_2$ agonists.

Effects on the Mucociliary System. Using micropipettes to obtain gland secretions from individual ducts, Borson and associates [40] demonstrated cholinergic control of secretion and showed that vagal reflexes stimulated by mechanical contraction of the mucosa stimulate secretion. Alpha- and beta-adrenergic stimulants cause mucous glycoprotein production and secretion, but alpha agonists also stimulate serous cells, increasing the water content of mucus [344]. Beta stimulants increase chloride flux into the lumen of the dog trachea, with presumed passive transfer of water [6]. They also directly or indirectly increase ciliary beat frequency [190]. The net effect of beta agonists is to increase mucociliary clearance [65].

Although beta agonists have been found clinically to relieve cough-variant asthma [191], it is not clear whether this action is related to an effect on mucociliary clearance, on afferent neural pathways mediating cough, or on airway smooth muscle.

Effects on Skeletal Muscle. Skeletal muscle tremor is an unavoidable side effect of beta$_2$ stimulants. Beta$_2$ agonists stimulate receptors on slow motor units and inhibit the fusion of incomplete tetanic contractions, causing reduced tension [325]; in some manner, this enhances tremor. To a lesser extent there may be a cardioballistic "vibration" of the body in synchrony with the heart beat that also contributes to tremor [56], which may also be increased with beta-adrenergic stimulation. There is a fairly close relationship between the initial individual tremor response to oral metaproterenol or terbutaline and the basal tremor [199]. Perception of tremor seems to be related to the relative increase over basal tremor produced by the drug. There is a very large range of normal basal tremor and consequential drug response: this variation appears to reside in the peripheral receptors and their control system. There is still considerable individual variation in discomfort, however, and the most vigorous responders may shake so much that fine movements are impossible. Fortunately, over a 1- or 2-week period of maintenance dosing, the tremor response to a single oral dose subsides markedly (tachyphylaxis) while baseline tremor increases as drug levels accumulate. This contrasts with the bronchodilator response [200]. Thus, elective commencement of these drugs should be initiated at a reduced dose until tolerance develops, although some individuals cannot tolerate even reduced doses.

Metabolic Effects. Metabolic effects include elevation of blood glucose and lactate levels due to stimulation of beta$_2$ receptors in the liver and other tissues, leading to gluconeogenesis and glycogenolysis; an increase in insulin secretion resulting from the stimulation of beta$_2$ receptors in the pancreatic islets (alpha-receptor stimulation inhibits insulin secretion); a decrease in the serum potassium concentration, presumably related to a transcellular shift of potassium due to the action of insulin and to a direct effect of beta-agonist stimulation; and an increase in plasma free fatty acids because of stimulation of beta$_1$ (and alpha) receptors in fat cells [484]. Such effects are usually without clinical significance. The fall in the potassium level has been attributed to stimulation of beta$_2$ receptors stimulating Na$^+$-K$^+$-ATPase at the skeletal muscle membrane [420], although more recent work favors the effect on insulin secretion [385], and is accompanied by a prolongation of the Q-T$_c$ interval. A rise in the plasma cAMP level is readily measured and is a sensitive indicator of drug action on beta$_2$ receptors [463].

Recent studies of the effects of nebulized beta$_2$ agonists on metabolic requirements in the rhesus monkey [313a] and in cystic fibrosis patients [460a] show a surprising increase in oxygen consumption and minute ventilation which could have detrimental effects on energy and ventilatory requirements and might be even counterproductive in selected cases.

Pharmacokinetics of Beta-Adrenergic Drugs

Oral Route

Bronchodilatation occurring after administration of an oral or parenteral drug is closely dependent on serum levels. Beta agonists given orally are incompletely absorbed, and the greater portion is then metabolized by sulfate conjugation, mostly by gut epithelium. Oral terbutaline absorption in five fasting individuals varied from 30 to 61 percent, and, of this only, 25 percent remained unconjugated in urine products [97]. Net bioavailability was thus 10 to 15 percent. The protein binding of terbutaline varies from 14 to 25 percent. A single 5-mg oral dose (terbutaline sulfate) produces a peak level of 6 to 7 ng/ml when taken fasting, and 3 to 4 ng/ml when taken nonfasting, with considerable interindividual variation. On a multiple-dose schedule, the final peak level remains about the same (approximately 3–4 ng/ml), but the trough levels rise as the drug becomes distributed into body compartments, reflected in an increase in basal tremor [319]. With its large mean distribution volume (1.37 L/kg) there is drug accumulation, and, when drug intake is stopped after steady-state is reached, levels decay with a half-life averaging 17 hours [319]! This contrasts with a half-life of only 3 to 4 hours after a single oral or subcutaneous dose [464]. Thus, a maintenance oral dose provides a constant "floor" of beta stimulation, even if a dose is missed. This is a useful alternative to keep in mind for patients who find the inhaled route unsatisfactory.

An oral dose of albuterol is more completely absorbed than is that of terbutaline, and, of this, about 60 percent is conjugated [302]. A single oral dose (4 mg as the base) is rapidly absorbed on a fasting stomach, reaching nearly peak levels at 1 hour [351]. Typically, peak levels are 7 to 9 ng/ml higher than terbutaline's, as are levels on a multiple-dose schedule of 4 mg every 6 hours, averaging about 12 ng/ml [352] (Fig. 55-18). The decay curve after steady-state has a half-life averaging 6.5 hours, longer than the 4.8 to 5.5 hours after a single oral dose [351, 352]. A sustained-release form of albuterol is in common use in the United States, and is particularly valuable in providing good nocturnal levels in brittle asthmatics. An osmotic-delivery, sustained-release form is available outside the United States [260].

It is peculiar that a single oral dose of albuterol is no more effective than a dose of terbutaline [499], although, on a µg/µg basis, albuterol is about twice as potent by inhalation or in vitro, and serum levels twice as high. In patients with chronic obstructive pulmonary disease (COPD), we found the tremor response to a single fasting dose of albuterol (4-mg base) to be only about 37 percent of the response to terbutaline (5-mg sulfate) despite nearly equal bronchodilator responses. The effector compartment distribution kinetics of these drugs may differ.

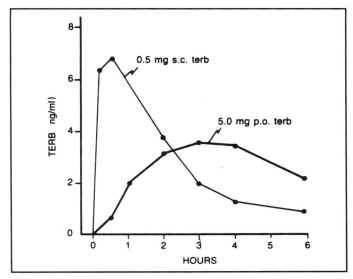

Fig. 55-19. *Comparison of plasma levels and improvement of forced expired volume in 1 second (FEV$_1$) to 5.0 mg of oral terbutaline and 0.5 mg of terbutaline given subcutaneously over time. The oral dose was given under nonfasting conditions. Values are the means in eight asthmatic subjects. Note the close correspondence between FEV$_1$ response and drug levels. (Reprinted with permission from W. Van den Berg, et al., The effects of oral and subcutaneous terbutaline in asthmatic patients. Eur. J. Respir. Dis. 65(suppl 134):181, 1984.)*

Subcutaneous Administration

Subcutaneous administration of terbutaline or epinephrine has an important role, in that it provides almost immediate action and assured delivery. It can supplement the inhaled route and can be used in an emergency. When 0.5 mg of terbutaline is administered subcutaneously, significant levels are present within a few minutes and peak at 20 minutes (Fig. 55-19). As shown by Van den Berg and associates [464], peak levels average about 7.4 ng/ml. Subcutaneous epinephrine has a slightly shorter duration of action. A slow-release form is available as Sus-phrine.

Intravenous Administration

The intravenous route is sometimes employed in patients responding poorly to conventional therapy. With their initial half-life of about 4 to 5 hours, these drugs should first be loaded and then maintained at a much reduced rate. By contrast, isoproterenol, because of its short half-life of only a few minutes, and by analogy to epinephrine, will reach steady-state in about 15 minutes during a constant infusion and effects will cease quickly when the infusion is stopped [124]. As used by Wyatt [506], as of 1987, intravenous terbutaline is loaded at a dose of 1.0 µg/kg/min over 10 minutes, then reduced to 0.1 µg/kg/min, with increases as needed to a maximum of 0.4 µg/kg/min. Intravenous albuterol has been used in children using the same loading dose (1.0 µg/kg/min over 10 minutes) and a maintenance dose of 0.2 µg/kg/min [38]. A constant infusion of 0.133 µg/kg/min of albuterol reaches a plateau at about 20 ng/ml by 5 hours and, when terminated, has a half-life of 6.0 hours [117]. Thus, a loading dose followed by a 0.2 µg/kg/min maintenance dose should produce levels of about 30 ng/ml, or about 2.5 times the levels reached on a 4-mg oral dose every 6 hours.

Intravenous isoproterenol offers great flexibility, and has been used successfully by pediatricians in some centers as a last-ditch effort to avoid intubation. However, it has been as thoroughly studied in animals and found to carry the hazard of myocardial

Fig. 55-18. *Mean plasma concentrations (ng/ml) of albuterol after oral doses of 4 mg (q6h) for five days. Circles and solid line represent the observed and projected plasma levels, respectively. (Reprinted with permission from M. L. Powell, et al., Multiple-dose albuterol kinetics. J. Clin. Pharmacol. 265:643, 1986.)*

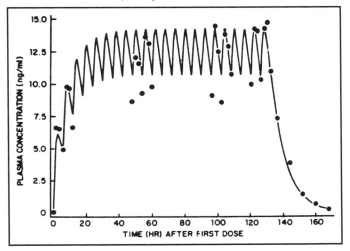

toxicity; toxicity is potentiated by theophylline and possibly corticosteroids [210, 275, 398]. It seems preferable to use beta$_2$-selective agents, again as supported by findings from animal studies (see also Chaps. 57 and 80).

Aerosol

In contrast to systemic administration, bronchodilation after inhaled drug aerosol is a function of drug retained in the airways. The timing of bronchodilation does not coincide with the course of plasma levels. Immediately after aerosolization, there is an effect on airways within seconds, reaching about 80 percent of the peak in 5 minutes. Beta$_2$ agonists reach their peak effect in 30 to 60 minutes, and bronchodilation begins to wane a variable time after this, and is nearly gone at 4 to 5 hours; on the other hand, catecholamine aerosols peak much earlier and last 30 minutes (epinephrine) to 2 hours. Systemic absorption from an MDI begins almost immediately, but drug levels at usual doses are unmeasurable. However, with large doses, indirect measurements are available. Thus, Kung and colleagues [239] delivered 10 puffs of albuterol, at the rate of one puff per minute, and found that plasma insulin levels had peaked and pulse pressure had widened maximally at the first 5-minute measurement. Mouth washing and gargling did not alter the insulin profile, indicating that most drug absorption was taking place in the airways and at the alveolar level. Collier and associates [83] administered 8 puffs (100 μg each) of albuterol from an MDI to asthmatics over 5 minutes and observed a 20 percent rise in pulse rate, which closely correlated with an estimated 36 percent fall in peripheral vascular resistance. Even customary doses of isoproterenol from an MDI will produce a pulse increase that peaks before 5 minutes from the initial wave of absorbed drug from the respiratory tract [225]. This does not occur with usual doses of beta$_2$ agonists.

Another study showed that cAMP generated upon inhaling isoproterenol by MDI peaked at 10 minutes, and the pulse at 5 minutes. Both subsided by 60 minutes [118]. cAMP and pulse elevation produced by fenoterol were substantial at 5 minutes, reached a maximum at 30 minutes, and remained elevated for over 6 hours.

Absorption is also rapid following nebulization, as shown in Fig. 55-20. After 5.0 mg of albuterol, plasma levels had peaked or were nearly peaking at 15 minutes, and then declined with an apparent half-life of 3.0 hours. Levels were higher in patients with cystic fibrosis. After nebulization of 0.15 mg/kg of albuterol, peak levels ranged from 11 to 77 nM/L, averaging 30 nM/L (7.2 ng/ml) [195a]. Older studies show albuterol levels to be about 1.1 ng/ml at 30 minutes after a 3.0-mg nebulization, and after 7.5 mg, about 2.5 ng/ml [476]. Levels of serum terbutaline reached the 2 to 4 ng/ml range 45 minutes after administration of 4.0 mg by nebulizer or MDI [93].

Continuous Nebulization

Some information is available on albuterol plasma levels during continuous nebulization. Children repeatedly nebulized with 0.01 or 0.03 ml/kg (0.05–0.15 mg/kg) of albuterol on an every 20-minute basis for six doses ("low" and "high" dosing) exhibited widely varying levels, ranging from 0.9 to 45 ng/ml, with mean levels of 10 and 19 ng/ml, respectively [386]. Side effects consisted of tremor, headache, vomiting, and increased pulse rate in some patients and correlated poorly with dose.

Deposition and Efficacy of MDI versus Nebulization

A surprisingly difficult problem in respiratory therapy has been to determine the equivalency between beta agonists administered by MDI and by nebulization. How many puffs delivered by MDI are required to equal a standard dose delivered by nebulizer? Generally, nebulized drug is placed in a 3 to 4-ml volume and

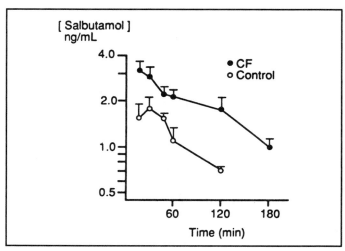

Fig. 55-20. *Mean serum salbutamol concentrations after inhalation by wet nebulizer of 5 mg of salbutamol in patients with cystic fibrosis (CF) and healthy young adults. The dose per kilogram of body weight was comparable for both groups. (Reprinted with permission from N. Vaisman, et al., Pharmacokinetics of inhaled salbutamol in patients with cystic fibrosis versus healthy young adults. J. Pediatr. 111:914, 1987.)*

nebulized "to dryness," the patient inhaling through a mouthpiece or face mask. The efficiency (fraction nebulized) depends on the starting volume, since 0.7 to 1.0 mg is retained in the chamber despite nebulization "to dryness." There is also loss in the apparatus and loss to the atmosphere during the exhalation phase. The rapidity of nebulization depends on the flow rate. Nebulizers differ in their efficiency; this is discussed further in Chapters 32 and 56.

Only those studies that compare a dose-response curve to each modality are valid, since comparing the increase in FEV$_1$ has many pitfalls [435]. In early studies, Newman and associates [312, 313] showed that 8.8 percent of labeled particles delivered by MDI were deposited in the lung, and this was improved to 13 percent using a pear-shaped spacer. Two-thirds of this went to the large airways. The rest of the drug delivered, about 80 percent, impacted on the pharynx and was swallowed. Comparisons with nebulization show nearly equal amounts are delivered to the lung, but very little to the oropharynx. Thus, Zainudin and coworkers [510] compared the distribution of 400 μg of labeled albuterol delivered by MDI–spacer to a dry-powder inhaler (DPI) (Rotahaler) and to a nebulizer with a mouthpiece, nebulizing 4.0 ml to dryness. The MDI delivered 11.2 percent to the lung; DPI, 9.1 percent, and the nebulizer, 9.9 percent. However, despite equal amounts delivered, the mean response in FEV$_1$ was greater for the MDI (35.6%) than for the DPI (25.2%) or nebulizer (25.8%). The reason for this is not apparent, although the large proportion delivered to the gastrointestinal tract by an MDI compared to a nebulizer could have added an absorbed component. A number of studies in which dose-response curves were constructed to establish equivalence are shown in Table 55-9, showing widely varying results. The 1:1 ratio of the Cushley study [93] may owe its high nebulization efficiency to the fact that only the dose leaving the nebulizer was counted, whereas the other authors used the dose placed in the nebulizer.

Using a histamine PC$_{20}$ (provocation concentration producing a 20% fall in FEV$_1$) approach to the end point, Blake and coworkers [36] concluded that 10 puffs administered by MDI was equivalent to a 2.5-mg dose of albuterol delivered by nebulization.

Another way to compare the amounts of beta agonist delivered by MDI versus nebulizer is through their comparative hypokalemic effect, notwithstanding the greater oral deposition, and

Table 55-9. Ratios of equivalent dose (MDI : Neb) in various studies using dose-response curves

Authors	Ratio MDI : Nebulizer	Drug	Spacer?	Nebulizer
Cushley et al., 1983 [93]	1:1	Terbutaline	With and without	Dose leaving nebulizer face mask
Mestitz et al., 1989 [291]	1:2	Terbutaline	No	2.0 ml, face mask
Blake et al., 1992 [36]	1:2.5	Albuterol	Yes	2.0 ml, mouthpiece; PC$_{20}$ end point
Madsen et al., 1982 [272]	1:4	Terbutaline	Yes	2.0 ml, face mask
Weber et al., 1979 [480a]	1:7	Terbutaline	No	1.0 ml, IPPB, Y tube
Harrison et al., 1983 [165]	1:12.5	Albuterol	No	2.0 ml

PC$_{20}$ = provocation concentration producing a 20% fall in FEV$_1$; IPPB = intermittent positive-pressure breathing; MDI = metered-dose inhaler.

Table 55-10. Mean systemic responses to 40 puffs (4,000 μg) of albuterol after 14 days of low and high doses delivered by MDI

2 weeks Premedication	ΔPulse (beats/min)	ΔK$^+$ (mEq/L)	ΔGlucose (M/L)	ΔTremor (% acceleration)
Placebo	+28	−0.92	+1.23	+688
Low dose (800 μg/24 hr)	+24	−0.74	+1.15	+498
High dose (4,000 μg/24 hr)	+15	−0.45	+0.58	+509

MDI = metered-dose inhaler.
Source: B. N. Lipworth et al, Comparison of the effects of prolonged treatment with low and high doses of inhaled terbutaline on beta-adrenoceptor responsiveness in patients with chronic obstructive pulmonary disease. *Am. Rev. Respir. Dis.* 142:338, 1990. Reprinted with permission.

hence gastrointestinal absorption, by MDI. The data available for larger doses suggest that the fall in the potassium level is less per milligram when placed in the nebulization chamber than when delivered by MDI. Thus, 5.0 mg of nebulized albuterol causes a serum potassium drop of 0.4 mEq/L [400], and 10 and 20 mg nebulized to patients on dialysis caused potassium drops of 0.62 and 0.92 mEq/L, respectively [8]. This compares to a fall of 0.46 mEq/L produced by 2,600 μg of albuterol delivered by MDI [501], and the 0.92 mEq/L fall produced by 4,000 μg of albuterol (Table 55-10) [261]. Grossly, on a mg/mg basis, the MDI is several times more efficient.

Comparative Systemic Effects of Inhaled Beta$_2$ Agonists: Is Fenoterol Qualitatively Different?

Fenoterol is a very potent beta$_2$ agonist, 13 times more potent in vitro on human bronchial smooth muscle than albuterol [147]. Moreover, against the beta$_1$ adrenergic receptor, fenoterol is a full agonist, while albuterol and terbutaline are partial agonists [52]. Yet, it is delivered at twice the dose (200 μg/puff) of albuterol. Comparative studies of the systemic effects between beta agonists have been made, stemming from the contention that fenoterol has been associated with an excess number of deaths, compared to albuterol, in recent New Zealand studies [388a] (see later discussion). Wong and colleagues [501] conducted cumulative dose comparisons between 2, 8, and 26 puffs of albuterol, terbutaline, and fenoterol. These produced an acute effect on the serum potassium level and the pulse rate. Twenty-six puffs of albuterol (2,600 μg), terbutaline (6,500 μg), and fenoterol (5,200 μg) produced a fall in the potassium level of 0.46, 0.52, and 0.76 mEq/L and a rise in pulse of 8, 8, and 29 beats/min, respectively. Scheinen and associates [384] studied the systemic effects of 1,200, 1,800, and 2,400 μg administered by MDI to normals. On a weight basis, fenoterol was about twice as potent as albuterol in lowering the potassium or elevating the cAMP levels (Fig. 55-21). The differential effect on pulse was even greater. This same pattern was noted by Crane and associates [90], who compared cardiac responses to 400 and 800 μg of fenoterol, albuterol, and

isoproterenol. At 800 μg, the effect of fenoterol on heart rate and the Q-S$_2$ interval, a measure of inotropic effect, was indistinguishable from the effect of isoproterenol and much greater than the effect of albuterol (Table 55-11). Yet, their effect on lowering diastolic pressure, a beta$_2$ effect, was comparable. Effects were accentuated after a week on theophylline.

As a final caution, while fenoterol is a more potent beta$_2$ agonist than albuterol on a microgram to microgram basis, and in high doses appears superficially to have a proportionately even greater beta$_1$ action and thus less beta$_2$ selectivity, one must still be cautious in claiming this from data obtained in the intact subject, with all its complexities. We now know that the right atrium in man contains a sizeable fraction of beta$_2$ receptors, which also act predominantly on rate [158, 218]. Perhaps a more accurate description of fenoterol's action on the heart is a "beta$_1$-like" effect.

CLINICAL CONSIDERATIONS

Beta-Adrenergic Bronchodilator Compounds

The beta-adrenergic agonists principally used in asthma therapy are listed in Tables 55-12 to 14, along with the manufacturers' current dosage recommendations. These agents will be discussed briefly with regard to their clinical utility.

Epinephrine

Epinephrine was the first synthetic beta-agonist bronchodilator to be used clinically and was introduced in the early 1900s [22]. A potent alpha- and nonselective beta-adrenergic stimulant, epinephrine is still used widely, both by subcutaneous injection for the treatment of severe acute asthma and systemic anaphylaxis and by aerosol inhalation as an over-the counter preparation for the relief of mild asthmatic symptoms.

When administered subcutaneously, epinephrine in aqueous solution has an onset of action within 5 to 15 minutes, a peak effect at 30 to 120 minutes, and a duration of 2 to 3 hours [144, 376, 388]. A longer duration of action (4–8 hours) with a similarly rapid onset may be achieved using an aqueous preparation of epinephrine that is mostly in suspension (Sus-phrine). Side effects of epinephrine stem from stimulation of beta$_1$-, beta$_2$-, and alpha-adrenergic receptors in other tissues and include headache, nervousness, palpitations, tachyarrhythmias, tremor, and systemic hypertension. Parenteral epinephrine should be used cautiously if at all for the treatment of asthma in older patients, especially with known or suspected cardiac disease, as well as in patients with hyperthyroidism. Inadvertent intravenous injection can cause death due to ventricular arrhythmias.

The systemic side effects of epinephrine are reduced but not eliminated when the drug is administered by inhalation. In its aerosol form, epinephrine is administered most commonly using proprietary MDIs (0.16–0.30 mg/puff) and much less often as a wet aerosol of a 1% solution of epinephrine HCl or a 2.25% solu-

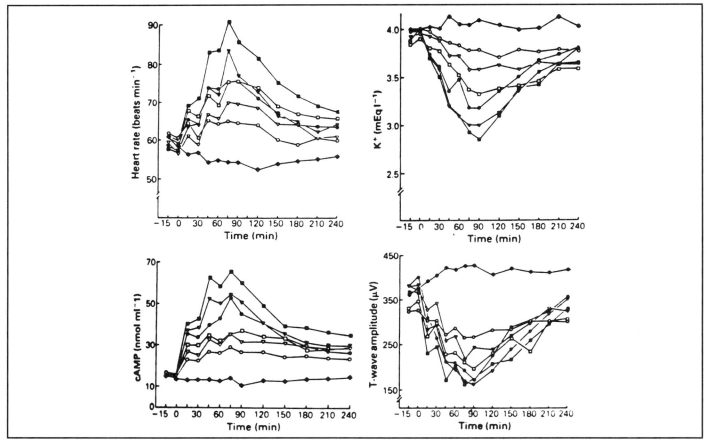

Fig. 55-21. *Effects of large doses of fenoterol and salbutamol delivered by metered dose inhaler on heart rate, K^+, plasma cAMP, and T-wave amplitude in six healthy adults.* Closed diamonds = placebo aerosol; open circles = salbutamol (1,200 μg); open triangles = salbutamol (1,800 μg); open squares = salbutamol (2,400 μg); closed circles = fenoterol (1,200 μg); closed triangles = fenoterol (1,800 μg); closed squares = fenoterol (2,400 μg), all administered over one hour. *(Reprinted with permission from M. Scheinin, Hypokalemic and other non-bronchial effects of inhaled fenoterol and salbutamol: a placebo-controlled dose-response study in healthy volunteers.* Br. J. Clin. Pharmacol. *24:645, 1987.)*

Table 55-11. *Comparative cardiac responses to three beta agonists, 400 and 800 μg, by MDI*

Time (min)	Dose (μg)	Heart rate				Q-S_2 index				Q-T_c interval (msec)			
		Plac	Iso	Fen	Alb	Plac	Iso	Fen	Alb	Plac	Iso	Fen	Alb
15	400	− 2.2	+ 5	+ 4.5	+ 3.4	1.8	− 14.4	− 6.9	− 6.3	− 7	+ 8	+ 8	+ 10
35	800	− 3.3	+ 6.9	+ 16.9	+ 4.1	9.1	− 31	− 30	− 13.2	0	+ 20	+ 30	+ 20

Plac = placebo; Iso = isoprenaline; Fen = fenoterol; Alb = albuterol; MDI = metered-dose inhaler.
Source: J. Crane, C. Burgess, and R. Beasley. Cardiovascular and hypokalemic effects of inhaled salbutamol, fenoterol, and isoprenaline. *Thorax* 44:136, 1989. Reprinted with permission.

tion of racemic (dl-) epinephrine delivered by a compressed air–driven nebulizer. The major disadvantages of aerosolized epinephrine are its relatively short duration of bronchodilation (1–1.5 hours) and transient cardiac and central nervous system side effects resulting from systemic absorption.

Isoproterenol

Isoproterenol, introduced into medicine in the 1940s, gradually replaced epinephrine because of its more potent beta-stimulant properties and its virtual absence of alpha-agonist activity. However, this catecholamine derivative of epinephrine possesses the same major disadvantage of its parent compound, namely, a rela-

tively short duration of action (due to rapid metabolism mainly by COMT and, to a lesser extent, by MAO) [98], undesirable cardiac side effects (due to nonselective stimulation of beta₁ receptors in the myocardium) [333], and lack of effectiveness by the oral route (due to inactivation by sulfate conjugation in the gut). With the more recent introduction of several long-acting beta₂-selective bronchodilators, which are also effective orally, isoproterenol is now used only infrequently. When inhaled from an MDI or a compressed gas-driven nebulizer, the drug produces bronchodilation of rapid onset and short duration (Table 55-12). MDIs of isoproterenol HCl in solution or of crystalline isoproterenol sulfate in suspension generally deliver 0.075 to 0.125 mg per actuation. Wet aerosols consisting of 0.5% to 1% solutions of

Table 55-12. Beta-agonist bronchodilator aerosols (available in United States)

Generic (trade) name	Formulation	Manufacturer's recommended dose[a]	Onset	Peak	Duration[b]	Comments
EPINEPHRINE Medihaler-EPI,[c] Primatene Mist,[c] Bronkaid Mist,[c] AsthmaHaler Mist[c]	MDI, 0.16 mg epinephrine/ puff	1–2 puffs in attack, repeat q3h PRN	1–5 min	<5 min	1–3 hr	Potent bronchodilator; beta$_1$, beta$_2$ actions short-acting (metabolized by COMT); cardiac side effects; discolored solutions of racemic epinephrine should not be used
Various	Nebulizer solution adrenaline, 1% (1:100) Racemic epinephrine, 2.5%	2–6 inhalations, undiluted 4–6 times/day; 0.2–0.4 ml undiluted or diluted in 2–3 ml saline or water q2–6h				
ISOPROTERENOL Isuprel Mistometer Medihaler-Iso Isoprel	MDI, 0.125 mg/puff MDI, 0.125 mg/puff Solutions, 0.5% (1:200) 1.0% (1:100)	1–2 puffs, 4–6 times/day 1–3 puffs, 4–6 times/day 2–15 inhalations, undiluted, q4–6h; 0.2–1.0 ml, diluted in 2–3 ml saline or water, q4–6h 2–7 inhalations, undiluted, q4–6h; 0.1–0.5 ml, diluted in 2–3 ml saline or water, q4–6h	2–5 min	5–30 min	1–3 hr	Potent bronchodilator; short-acting (metabolized by COMT); cardiac side effects; great potential for abuse; V/Q imbalance can produce hypoxemia
ISOETHARINE			5 min	15–60 min	1.5–3 hr	Relatively short-acting (metabolized by COMT); beta$_2$ specific
Bronkometer	MDI, 0.34 mg/puff	1–2 puffs, q4h, more often if necessary				
Bronkosol	Solution, 1%	3–7 inhalations, undiluted, q3–6h; 0.25–1 ml, diluted 1:3 with saline or water, q4h or more often, if needed				
Isoetharine inhalation solution	Unit dose solution: 0.1% (2.5 ml) 0.125% (4 ml) 0.167% (3 ml) 0.2% (2.5 ml) 0.25% (2 ml)	1 unit-dose vial, q4h or more often, if needed				
METAPROTERENOL			2–10 min	30–90 min	1–5 hr (single dose); 1–2.5 hr (repeated doses)	Relatively long-acting (unaffected by COMT); some beta$_2$ specificity; 8% adverse effects
Alupent, Metaprel	MDI, 0.65 mg/puff	2–3 puffs, q3–4h (up to 12 puffs/day)				
Alupent	Solution, 5% (50 mg/ml) Unit dose solution: 0.4% (2.5 ml) 0.6% (2.5 ml)	5–15 inhalations, undiluted, q3–6h; 0.2–0.3 ml, diluted in 2.5 ml saline or water, q4h 1 unit-dose vial, q4h				
ALBUTEROL			<15 min	<60–90 min	3–6 hr	Long-acting (unaffected by COMT or MAO); beta$_2$ specific
Proventil, Ventolin	MDI, 0.09 mg/puff	1–2 puffs, q4–6h; 2 puffs 1.5 min prior to exercise				
Ventolin	Rotocaps, 200 μg, for use with powder inhaler (Rotahaler)	Inhale contents of 1–2 Rotocaps q4–6h or 1 Rotocap 15 min before exercise				
Proventil, Ventolin	Solution. 0.5% (5 mg/ml)	2.5 mg (0.5 ml in 2.5 ml saline), 3–4 times/day				
Proventil	Unit-dose solution, 0.083% (3 ml)	1 unit-dose vial, 3–4 times/ day				
TERBUTALINE Breathaire	MDI, 0.2 mg/puff Nebulized injectable ampule, 1 mg/ml (not FDA approved)	2 puffs, q4–6h (2.5–5.0 mg, followed by 2.5 mg q20 min × 6 doses)[d]	<5–30 min	1–2 hr	3–4 hr	Long-acting, beta$_2$ specific

Table 55-12. *(continued)*

Generic (trade) name	Formulation	Manufacturer's recommended dose[a]	Onset	Peak	Duration[b]	Comments
BITOLTEROL			3–4 min	30–60 min	5–8 hr	Pro-drug hydrolized by esterases to active moiety, colterol. Long-acting, beta₂ specific
Tornalate	MDI, 0.37 mg/puff	2 puffs, q8h (maintenance); 2 puffs, q4–6h, or 3 puffs, q6h PRN				
PIRBUTEROL			<5 min	30–60 min	5 hr	Long-acting, beta₂ specific
Maxair	MDI, 0.2 mg/puff	1–2 puffs, q4–6h (up to maximum of 12 puffs/day)				

MDI = metered-dose inhaler; COMT = catechol-*O*-methyltransferase; V/Q = ventilation/perfusion; MAO = monoamine oxidase.
[a] For adults and children >12 years, unless otherwise specified.
[b] Duration of action generally longer for higher doses and shorter for lower doses.
[c] Preparations available over-the-counter.
[d] Dosage schedule suggested by some authorities (*The Medical Letter on Drugs and Therapeutics: Drugs for Asthma.* (29:11, 1987.)

isoproterenol HCl in doses of 1.25 to 2.5 mg from a compressed gas–driven nebulizer, with or without intermittent positive-pressure breathing (IPPB), have been used to treat patients with severe acute asthma [121, 289, 373a]. In such patients, these doses were found to be effective after refractoriness had developed to home therapy, including MDIs [289], presumably due to the delivery of larger doses of the drug to the lower respiratory tract when inhaled with supervision over several minutes from a nebulizer compared to poorly supervised single inhalations from an MDI.

In the absence of a more suitable drug, isoproterenol has been given *intravenously* for the treatment of life-threatening childhood status asthmaticus with impending respiratory failure [173, 331, 412, 503], with the aim of avoiding the need for intubation and mechanical ventilation. Randomized, controlled studies of the efficacy of intravenous isoproterenol in this setting have been lacking. The rationale for the use of a parenteral beta agonist in severe asthma is that it allows the drug to be delivered via the circulation to sites distal to occlusive plugs, which cannot be penetrated by a bronchodilator aerosol. The rationale for the choice of isoproterenol for intravenous use in this setting is that it permits precise control of the dose, including prompt onset and offset of effect and reversal of undesirable side effects because of the drug's short half-life. In the protocol recommended by Wood and associates [503] for childhood asthma, an intravenous infusion of isoproterenol is initiated with a precalibrated syringe pump at a rate of 0.1 µg/kg/min with continual electrocardiographic monitoring by a physician. The dose is then increased by 0.1 µg/kg/min every 10 to 15 minutes until the heart rate approaches 200 per minute or there is clinical improvement, after which the dose is gradually reduced. In their series of 19 patients, 17 responded favorably within 1.8 to 10.2 hours; one of the two patients representing treatment failures developed ventricular tachycardia that responded promptly to cessation of intravenous isoproterenol. Of 34 children with status asthmaticus treated prospectively according to a similar protocol [331], 27 responded favorably to a mean dose of 0.36 µg/kg/min with an average response time of 1.7 hours; nodal tachycardia that did not require treatment or cessation of intravenous isoproterenol developed in one patient. In a retrospective study of intravenous isoproterenol using a similar protocol in children, most patients also responded favorably, but two of the five failures exhibited cardiotoxocity [412]. In an effort to minimize cardiac toxocity, lower initial and incremental intravenous infusion rates of isoproterenol have also been used successfully, with reversal of impending respiratory failure in children with status asthmaticus [173]. In addition to cardiac dysrhythmias, other cardiac complications of intravenous isoproterenol infusions for the treatment of status asthmaticus in children have included electrocardiographic changes indicating myocardial ischemia [275, 284], fatal focal myocardial

necrosis in an adolescent female [240a], and frequent elevations of the cardiac-specific serum creatine phosphokinase MB isoenzyme (CPK-MB) [275]. The latter observations suggest that this form of therapy frequently may cause subclinical myocardial injury.

In adult patients with severe asthma, Klaustermeyer and associates [229] found that gradually incrementing the dose from 0.0375 to 0.225 µg/kg/min over 2 hours led to progressive bronchodilation with relatively little and nonprogressive tachycardia. They suggested that cautious short-term use of intravenous isoproterenol at these infusion rates might be helpful in treating asthmatics with respiratory failure caused by refractory status asthmaticus to avoid the need for intubation and mechanical ventilation in the lag interval between the initiation of corticosteroid therapy and the expected onset of a significant steroid effect. Asthmatics already on mechanical ventilators who require very high peak inspiratory pressures and who cannot be ventilated effectively or develop hypotension might also benefit. However, extreme caution must be observed if isoproterenol is administered by the intravenous route for treatment of patients with severe acute asthma because of its potentially serious cardiovascular toxocity. All patients receiving intravenous isoproterenol for status asthmaticus should be carefully followed in an intensive care unit with continuous electrocardiographic monitoring and serial determinations of serum CPK-MB levels. Parenteral therapy with a beta₂-selective adrenergic agonist, such as terbutaline administered subcutaneously at suitable intervals or by intravenous infusion (see later discussion), is a safer alternative to intravenous isoproterenol. Albuterol has also been administered intravenously for the treatment of severe acute asthma [38], but is not available in this formulation in the United States (see also Chapters 57 and 80 for added details of intravenous adrenergic usage.)

Ephedrine

Ephedrine, which has been used in herbal form for thousands of years, was introduced into modern medicine in synthetic form in 1923. Because of its effectiveness when given orally and moderate duration of action (3–5 hours), it enjoyed wide popularity, particularly in combination preparations including theophylline, until the advent of the newer, orally effective beta₂-selective adrenergic agents, which are longer-acting and associated with fewer side effects (Table 55-13). Because it causes bronchodilation largely indirectly through release of norepinephrine (itself a weak beta agonist) from storage sites in adrenergic nerve endings [483, 484], ephedrine is a weak bronchodilator and requires doses approximately 2.5 to 10 times those of newer, direct-acting oral sympathomimetic drugs to produce a comparable degree of bronchodilatation. In such large doses, it frequently is associated

Table 55-13. Oral beta-agonist bronchodilators

Generic (trade) name	Formulation	Manufacturer's recommended dose[a]	Onset	Peak	Duration[b]	Comments
EPHEDRINE			Approx 60 min	2–3.5 hr	3–5 hr (non-time-release formulations)	Alpha, beta, beta$_1$, beta$_2$ actions; central nervous system analeptic, usually need sedation, side effects frequent
Various	Capsules 25,[c] 50 mg; elixers/syrups, 4.5, 10,[c] 20 mg/ml	25–50 mg, q3–4h; pediatric age: 2–3 mg/kg daily in 4–6 doses				
Ectasule Minus	Time-release capsules, 15, 30, 60 mg	1 capsule, q12h				
Slo-Fedrin	Capsules, 30, 60 mg	1 capsule, q8–12 h				
METAPROTERENOL			Approx 30 min	2–2.5 hr	4–5 hr	Some beta$_2$ specificity; 17% adverse effects; 10 mg equivalent to 25 mg ephedrine
Alupent, Metaprel	Tablets, 10, 20 mg; Syrup, 10 mg/5 ml	10–20 mg q6–8h, if patient 6–9 yr or under 27 kg; 0.3–2.6 mg/kg per day in divided doses in younger children				
TERBUTALINE			Approx 30 min	2–4 hr	4–7 hr	Beta$_2$ specific, long-acting (unaffected by COMT or MAO); 2.5 mg equivalent to 25 mg of ephedrine; 20–33% rate of tremor (5-mg dose); modest increase in heart rate probably largely baroreceptor-reflex mediated; tachyphylaxis develops to tremorigenic effect
Brethine, Bricanyl	Tablets, 2.5, 5.0 mg	2.5–5 mg, q6–8h; 2.5 mg, 3 times/day, if patient 12–15 yr or if side effects in adult				
ALBUTEROL			Approx 30 min	2–3 hr	4–6 hr (non-extended-release formulations)	Beta$_2$ specific; long-acting (unaffected by COMT or MAO); 2 mg equivalent to 25 mg of ephedrine; similar in efficacy and side effects to equipotent dose of terbutaline
Proventil, Ventolin	Tablets, 2, 4 mg	2–4 mg q6–8h; 2mg 3–4 times/day initially, if patient elderly or unusually sensitive to beta agonists				
Proventil, Ventolin	Syrup, 2 mg/5 ml	2–4 mg (1–2 tsp) 3–4 times/day, adjusted if needed up to a maximum dose of 8 mg 4 times/day. For children 6–14 yr of age, 2 mg (1 tsp) 3–4 times/day, adjusted if needed up to a maximum dose of 24 mg/day in divided doses. For children 2–6 yr of age, 0.1–0.2 mg/day (maximum, 4 mg 3 times/day)				
Proventil Repetabs	Extended release tablets, 4 mg (2 mg released immediately, 2 mg released after several hours)	4–8 mg q12h (maximum, 16 mg bid)				4-mg Repetab bid equivalent to 2-mg regular tablet qid; longer-acting preparation may be useful in treating nocturnal asthma

COMT = catechol-*O*-methyltransferase; V/Q = ventilation/perfusion; MAO = monoamine oxidase.
[a] For adults and children >12 years, unless otherwise specified.
[b] Duration of action generally longer for higher doses and shorter for lower doses.
[c] Preparations available over-the-counter.

with troublesome side effects, including nervousness, anxiety, and insomnia, due to central nervous system stimulation. The nonselective stimulation of beta$_1$, beta$_2$, and alpha receptors in systemic tissues causes other annoying side effects, including hypertension, palpitations, tremor, and symptoms of bladder outlet obstruction (in elderly men). The frequent occurrence of such unwanted systemic effects limits the dose that can be administered for effective bronchodilatation. For all these reasons, ephedrine is generally administered as a fixed-dose combination preparation containing theophylline (usually 130 mg) to enhance its bronchodilator action [285, 440], as well as a sedative or tranquilizer to counteract its stimulant action on the central nervous system. Such combination products are still available as proprie-

tary preparations (but not commonly used) for the intermittent relief of mild asthma.

Isoetharine

Isoetharine, first used in asthma therapy in 1951 [174], is a less potent bronchodilator than isoproterenol but demonstrates some beta$_2$ selectivity, in that it causes relatively less cardiac stimulation for the same degree of bronchodilatation compared to isoproterenol [243]. It also has a slightly longer duration of action (1–3 hours) [254] than isoproterenol and is effective when taken by mouth, although it is not available for oral use in the United States. Aerosol preparations of isoetharine include a metered-dose nebulizer (340 μg per inhalation) and a 0.25% aqueous solution for delivery as a wet aerosol. Its use has largely been superseded by longer-acting beta agonists.

Metaproterenol

This resorcinol derivative of isoproterenol was initially used to treat asthma in 1961. Its major advantages over isoproterenol are its longer duration of action when inhaled in equipotent doses [134, 183] and its effectiveness when given by the oral route. When given intravenously, it does not exhibit any apparent beta$_2$ selectivity [288]. Nevertheless, when inhaled as an aerosol in effective bronchodilator doses, it is associated with mild and relatively infrequent side effects [28, 134, 356, 368], presumably due to the selectivity conferred by the topical route. When given orally in a single dose (20 mg), its bronchodilator effect is noted within 30 minutes and lasts up to 4 to 5 hours [73, 226, 367], although its duration of effectiveness is shorter after multiple dosing. Side effects of tachycardia, palpitations, nervousness, and tremor, although relatively infrequent, can be troublesome. Consequently, a lower oral dose (10 mg) is sometimes preferred. Availability in syrup form (10 mg/5 ml) facilitates pediatric use [71].

Preparations of metaproterenol for aerosol use include an MDI delivering 650 μg per puff and a 5% inhalation solution. Single-dose MDI studies have shown that 1 to 3 puffs produce nearly immediate bronchodilatation of variable duration up to 5 hours, but the duration of effect is shorter (up to only 2.5 hours) after multiple dosing [292]. In single-dose studies of the inhalant solution, increases of FEV$_1$ exceeding 15 percent above baseline are maintained for at least 4 hours following administration of 0.3 ml of 5% metaproterenol (diluted to 2.5 ml), in contrast to only 1 hour following administration of 0.5 ml of isoetharine [368]. Statistically significant bronchodilatation compared to placebo is noted up to 6 hours after administration of 0.3 ml of 5% metaproterenol compared to only up to 1 hour after administration of 0.5 percent isoproterenol [28]. Tachycardia and tremor can occur with moderate frequency from aerosol use via IPPB [368], compared to the virtual absence of side effects from 2 to 3 puffs of the MDI, probably due to the larger dose delivered from the nebulizer.

Terbutaline

Following the studies of Lands and Brown [242] establishing the existence of beta$_1$- and beta$_2$-adrenergic receptors, the pharmaceutical industry increased its efforts to synthesize newer analogs of isoproterenol possessing a greater physiologic ratio of bronchial relaxant (beta$_2$) to cardiac stimulant (beta$_1$) effects. These efforts led to the development of newer agents that, at least in isolated tissue and animal studies, demonstrated particularly marked selectivity for beta-adrenergic receptors in airway smooth muscle over those in myocardium [53, 193, 339]. In addition, the altered structure of these compounds rendered them resistant to the action of COMT and MAO in tissue and to sulfatases in the gut [340], thereby prolonging their biologic activity and allowing them to be administered orally, as well as parenterally and by inhalation.

Terbutaline, the first of these newer compounds to become available in the United States, can be given subcutaneously, orally, and by MDI, but is not yet approved for aerosol solution use. In studies of healthy adult volunteers and patients with stable or acute bronchospastic disease, subcutaneous terbutaline has been found to have little if any therapeutic advantage over epinephrine, either in duration of bronchodilation or in the degree of associated hemodynamic effects [10, 144, 318, 375, 376, 388, 397]. For example, when administered to stable asthmatics as 0.25 mg subcutaneously (the usual dose recommended by the manufacturer), terbutaline produces bronchodilation that is sim-

ilar with respect to onset (within 5 minutes), magnitude, and duration (up to 3 hours) to that produced by 0.25 mg of epinephrine, without any significant differences in heart rate or other side effects [144]. Another study showed similar results, except that terbutaline led to a slightly longer duration of bronchodilatation than did epinephrine (4 hours versus 3 hours) [388]. The apparent discrepancy between these *in vivo* findings in humans and the results of isolated tissue studies indicating a marked dissociation between cardiac and bronchial effects of terbutaline suggests that they are due largely to indirect effects of terbutaline on the heart *in vivo* due to stimulation of beta$_2$ receptors in vascular smooth muscle. The resultant vasodilatation causes both reflex-mediated cardioacceleration and increases in left and right ventricular ejection fractions due to afterload reduction. However, a positive inotropic effect due to direct stimulation of cardiac beta receptors could also contribute to the augmentation in ventricular performance, particularly that of the left heart [46]. Because it is relatively beta$_2$ selective and only a partial agonist for beta$_1$ receptors, parenteral terbutaline may be preferred over epinephrine in the treatment of severe attacks of asthma not responsive to aerosol bronchodilator medication, particularly in the older patient who is at greater risk of serious cardiovascular complications.

Terbutaline has been administered in subcutaneous doses of 0.25 to 0.3 mg as often as every 12 to 15 minutes up to maximum cumulative doses of 4.4 mg in 6 hours and 10 mg in 24 hours to children with status asthmaticus not responding to inhaled beta agonists and intravenous aminophylline [447]. Such frequent subcutaneous doses of terbutaline were not associated with adverse cardiovascular complications. Subcutaneous terbutaline has also been shown to be beneficial when delivered by a continuous infusion (CSIT) using a small portable infusion pump or by 6-hourly injections (QDST) to some patients with severe brittle asthma (diurnal variability in peak expiratory flow rate exceeding 50%) [324]. In the latter series, 13 of 17 patients (76%) with brittle asthma treated with CSIT or QDST in daily doses of 1 to 12 mg of terbutaline (mean, 9–10 mg) for up to 40 months developed sustained improvement in asthma control not previously achieved despite large doses of bronchodilators and corticosteroids given orally and by inhalation. Serious side effects of long-term treatment with subcutaneous terbutaline were few. No patient developed palpitations or hypokalemia, while a few complained of tremor, insomnia, or night cramps, or a combination of these; painful lumps developed at the infusion sites in four patients. In contrast to these results with terbutaline by the subcutaneous route, high-dose oral bronchodilators have been shown to be of only limited benefit in brittle asthmatics [118], perhaps due to variable absorption or a high rate of first-pass metabolism in the liver, resulting in lower blood levels than are obtained with subcutaneous injection.

Intravenous terbutaline, although not approved for use in the United States, has been used in Europe for the treatment of acute severe asthma [471, 491], although little difference in efficacy compared with inhaled terbutaline has been noted. Moreover, for equivalent bronchodilator doses, cardiovascular and tremorigenic side effects are considerably greater when the intravenous route is used [346, 442]. A suggested dosing schedule for the intravenous administration of terbutaline in the treatment of life-threatening asthma consists of a loading dose of 10 μg/kg given over 10 minutes (1 μg/kg/min), followed by a continuous infusion of 0.1 μg/kg/min, with increments of 0.1 μg/kg/min as needed up to a maximum of 0.4 μg/kg/min [221].

In oral form, terbutaline (5 mg) is a more effective bronchodilator than ephedrine (25 mg), with an earlier onset (30 minutes versus 1 hour), greater magnitude (twofold), and longer duration of effect (7 versus 4 hours) [109, 140, 437]. In these oral doses, terbutaline and ephedrine have comparable cardiovascular effects. Compared to oral metaproterenol, terbutaline in single doses causes comparable bronchodilatation but is longer acting [55]. With long-term administration, terbutaline (5 mg) is generally well tolerated without significant attenuation of its bronchodilator effect or production of clinically significant cardiovascular side effects [495]. Tremor is frequently experienced after short-term use of terbutaline (5 mg), reflecting its action on beta$_2$-adrenergic receptors in skeletal muscle [44]. Longer-term use in the same dose is associated with a much lower incidence of annoying tremor [495] due to the preferential development of tachyphylaxis to its tremorigenic (compared to its bronchodilator) effect [200, 245]. In a lower oral dose (2.5 mg), terbutaline has a lower incidence of tremor, yet still causes significant bronchodilatation of relatively long duration, albeit of a lesser magnitude compared to the 5-mg dose [498]. For this reason, the lower dose is sometimes preferred, particularly when initiating oral therapy. A slow-release terbutaline preparation (depot tablets of 5 mg) administered every 12 hours has been shown to provide constant serum levels and to be beneficial in preventing the morning "dip" in FEV$_1$ associated with nocturnal asthma [350]. This formulation is not available in the United States.

In its aerosol form, terbutaline exhibits its greatest bronchoselectivity and least systemic beta$_1$ and beta$_2$ side effects. Metered-dose aerosols of terbutaline (0.5 mg) and metaproterenol (1.5 mg) produce equivalent peak bronchodilatation, but the bronchodilator effect of terbutaline lasts longer (5 versus 3 hours) [128]. Cumulative dose-response studies in clinically stable patients with moderately severe asthma have shown progressive improvement in FEV$_1$ up to a total dose of 1.0 mg when delivered by MDI and 9.0 mg (the maximum dose administered) when given by pressurized nebulizer [480a]. Only negligible cardiovascular side effects and infrequent noncardiac symptoms (headache, tremor, nervousness) were noted at the higher doses. The solution form of terbutaline is not approved for inhalational use in the United States.

Albuterol

Albuterol (also known as salbutamol) is a potent beta$_2$-selective adrenergic bronchodilator, first introduced in 1968. It is now available for oral use as regular and extended-release tablets, as well as a syrup, and for aerosol use as a microcrystalline suspension for inhalation from an MDI, a dry powder for inhalation using a breath-actuated powder aerosol system (e.g., Rotahaler), and a solution for delivery from a jet nebulizer. In regular tablet form, its action is very similar to equipotent doses of terbutaline, with an onset of bronchodilation within 30 minutes, a peak effect at 2 to 4 hours, and a duration of up to 5 hours [253]. In short-term studies, like oral terbutaline, it is associated with generally insignificant cardiovascular side effects [253, 479] but causes tremor in about a third of the patients. The therapeutic effects of the extended-release preparation (4 mg) administered every 12 hours are equivalent to those of the regular 2-mg tablet administered every 6 hours [3]. A syrup formulation of albuterol (2 mg per 5 ml) has been shown to be effective and safe in the treatment of young asthmatic children [355]. Albuterol 2-mg syrup caused greater peak bronchodilatation, a longer duration of action, and less chronotropic effects than did metaproterenol 10-mg syrup in 6- to 9-year-old children with asthma, although both preparations produced similar control of asthma symptoms over 4 weeks of regular drug therapy [500].

Aerosolized albuterol produces a more rapid onset and at least as long-lasting bronchodilatation, with fewer side effects, compared to oral therapy. When given in cumulative doses to maximal tolerance, albuterol produces a greater peak bronchodilatation when inhaled than ingested, because the dose administered by the topical route is less limited by the development of systemic side effects [245]. When administered by MDI, albuterol (200 μg) has a potent bronchodilator action with onset as early

as 1 minute, a peak magnitude at 45 minutes, and a duration as long as 6 hours; at 3 minutes, its bronchodilator effect is approximately 80 percent of peak and at 6 hours, roughly 50 percent of peak [367]. No increase in heart rate and few, if any, side effects are noted with this dose of albuterol aerosol [225, 356, 367, 419]. Dose-response studies of albuterol aerosol administered from an MDI (0.1–2.4 mg) or a dry powder inhaler (Rotahaler) (0.2–4.8 mg) have shown that the bronchodilator potency of these two modes of aerosol delivery is equivalent [424]. Comparisons with metaproterenol have yielded inconsistent results. One group [367] found a consistently greater improvement in FEV$_1$ from 5 to 360 minutes in 21 asthmatics treated with albuterol (200 μg) compared to the improvement seen with metaproterenol (1,500 μg); moreover, albuterol caused a slight decrease in heart rate, whereas metaproterenol produced an immediate, albeit brief, increase in heart rate. In other studies comparing the same doses of aerosolized albuterol and metaproterenol [356, 432], however, no statistically significant differences were found between those two compounds in either their efficacy or toxicity. In general, pressurized aerosols of albuterol and terbutaline in recommended therapeutic doses have yielded comparable results [74, 133, 136, 163].

In solution form, albuterol is commonly administered as a wet aerosol from a power nebulizer for treatment of severe acute asthma in the emergency room or hospital and for domiciliary therapy of chronic asthmatics unable to use MDIs effectively. While the usually recommended dose of albuterol as a wet aerosol is 2.5 mg, significantly greater bronchodilation can be achieved with increasing doses up to 15 mg in stable asthmatics [310], although systemic side effects are also more common as the dose is increased. A number of studies comparing wet and dry aerosols of albuterol (or terbutaline) from power nebulizers and MDIs, respectively, have shown parallel dose-response relationships for the two types of delivery devices and a variable rightward shift of the dose-response curve for the nebulizer compared to that for the MDI [165, 291, 310, 480a]. The magnitude of this rightward shift reflects a variably reduced efficiency of the nebulizer, compared to the MDI, for delivering a bioequivalent dose of the bronchodilator to the lower respiratory tract. The variability in the efficiency ratios of small-volume jet nebulizers to MDIs is wide, ranging from 1:2 to 1:12.5 [257] (see Table 55-9). The reasons for this variable efficiency probably reflect wide variability in the types of nebulizers used, their output characteristics, the manner in which they are operated, and patient inhaling patterns, as well as variability in the technique of MDI use and the employment of MDI-extension devices. It is now clear that what determines the bronchodilator response is not simply the dose added to a nebulizer or the particular aerosol generating device used, but rather the actual dose of the beta agonist that reaches the lower respiratory tract.

Although albuterol is not available for intravenous use in the United States, it has been used abroad by this route, both for experimental purposes [175, 282, 311] and for the treatment of severe asthma [37, 38, 115, 123, 247, 317, 408, 409, 453, 498, 493]. In stable asthmatics, bronchodilator responses to intravenous and inhaled albuterol have been roughly equivalent [175, 311], with cardiovascular, tremorigenic, and metabolic changes noted after intravenous but not aerosol administration. In comparison with equi-bronchodilator doses of intravenous isoproterenol, salbutamol caused longer-lasting bronchodilatation (90 versus 15 minutes following injection) and a 2.5-fold lesser increase in heart rate with similar decreases in diastolic pressure, reflecting its beta$_2$ selectivity [282]. However, the heart rate returned more slowly to baseline after albuterol than after isoproterenol administration. From these findings, albuterol might be considered a safer alternative to isoproterenol for intravenous use in the treatment of severe asthma that is refractory to other measures. However, the longer persistence of the cardioaccelerator effect of albuterol due to slower metabolic inactivation of the drug could be a disadvantage. Several studies have evaluated the efficacy and safety of intravenous albuterol in the management of severe acute asthma. In one study, 500 μg of salbutamol infused at a constant rate over 1 hour produced at least as much bronchodilatation as a similarly timed infusion of 500 mg of aminophylline, with little change in heart rate and fewer side effects than aminophylline [493]. In children with respiratory failure due to status asthmaticus unresponsive to conventional bronchodilator therapy, Bohn and associates [38] administered intravenous albuterol in a loading dose of 0.1 μg/kg/min over 10 minutes, followed by an infusion of 0.2 μg/kg/min that was increased in 0.1 μg/kg steps according to the response up to a maximum rate of 4 μg/kg/min. In 11 of 16 episodes (69%), intravenous albuterol resulted in prompt, sustained reductions in the arterial PCO_2 ($PaCO_2$), with smaller increases in heart rate than previously noted in similar patients treated with intravenous isoproterenol. In adult patients with status asthmaticus, aerosolized albuterol (5 mg) administered via IPPB was less effective than was 200 μg of albuterol injected intravenously over 10 minutes; with gradual recovery, the response to albuterol aerosol was restored [492]. On the other hand, other studies [37, 247] done in patients with severe acute asthma have shown equivalent improvement in lung function with nebulized albuterol (0.5% solution for 3 minutes or 10 mg nebulized continuously over 45 minutes) compared to intravenously infused albuterol (500 μg over 3 minutes or 900 μg over 45 minutes); moreover, the intravenous route was associated with a high incidence of cardiovascular and other systemic side effects not noted with nebulized albuterol. The optimum therapeutic dose of intravenous albuterol has not been established. Doses of 4 μg/kg or 200 to 250 μg injected or infused over 1 to 10 minutes have been used safely in cases of stable and severe asthma [175, 311, 317, 492]. It would seem wise to monitor the electrocardiogram continuously, both during and for at least 20 to 30 minutes following intravenous administration.

Pirbuterol

Pirbuterol, recently released for clinical use in the United States in pressurized aerosol form, is a beta$_2$-selective adrenergic agonist that differs structurally from albuterol only in the substitution of a pyridine for a benzene ring [365]. When administered in equipotent doses, pirbuterol and albuterol show no significant differences in the speed of onset or in the extent or time course of bronchodilatation [34]. Despite apparently greater beta$_2$ specificity in isolated tissue studies [300], the cardiovascular effects of bioequivalent doses of the two drugs when administered orally appear to be comparable [490]. In dose-response studies of pirbuterol administered by MDI in stable asthmatics, 400 μg was found to be the lowest dose producing maximum bronchodilatation without significant changes in blood pressure or heart rate [262].

Bitolterol

Bitolterol mesylate is an inactive pro-drug, 3,4-diester colterol that, after inhalation as an aerosol, undergoes esterase hydrolysis in bronchial tissue to the active drug, colterol (*N*-tert-butyl arterenol) [474]. Available as a solution aerosol in MDI form (350 μg per puff), bitolterol is an effective bronchodilator with a relatively long duration of action (up to 8 hours) and minimal side effects [474]. When compared with two metered doses of albuterol (180 μg) in stable asthmatics, 3 puffs of bitolterol (1,050 μg), the highest recommended dose, produced significantly greater bronchodilatation 4 to 8 hours after inhalation with comparably infrequent side effects [327]. However, a somewhat shorter duration of bronchodilatation after 3 puffs of bitolterol has been noted in other studies [223, 474, 480].

Procaterol

Procaterol, an investigational beta$_2$-adrenergic agent with a unique carbostyrol nucleus, is several times more potent than isoproterenol [429a, 507]. It is also relatively long-acting, causing bronchodilatation for up to 8 hours in an oral dose of 0.10 mg [394] and for up to 7 hours in metered aerosol doses of 10 to 20 μg [415]. When procaterol or albuterol was administered in oral doses of 0.05 mg bid or 2 mg tid, respectively, for 2 weeks, followed by 0.10 mg bid or 4 mg tid, respectively, for 10 weeks, procaterol produced greater short-term improvement in FEV$_1$ than did albuterol initially, as well as after 1 and 2 months, and also comparable control of asthma symptoms [342]. Tolerance was not evident with continued procaterol treatment, in contrast to a diminished duration of response to albuterol during long-term treatment. Tremor was more frequently reported by patients receiving procaterol. In a 12-week study, aerosolized procaterol (10 μg per puff) was compared to albuterol (100 μg per puff), each administered, at least initially, as 2 puffs tid and subsequently, only if needed for more effective asthma control, as 2 puffs qid [286]. A significantly higher percentage of patients receiving procaterol than those receiving albuterol were able to continue dosing on a tid, rather than a qid, schedule, most likely due to the longer duration of action of inhaled procaterol. Tremor and headache are the most common side effects with both oral and aerosol therapy and are dose related.

Fenoterol

Fenoterol, a resorcinol derivative of metaproterenol with relative beta$_2$ specificity in vitro [52, 254], is available outside the United States in both oral and aerosol form. When administered orally in a dose of 5 mg three times daily, it produces improvement in lung function similar to that achieved by the same dose of terbutaline, with a slightly lesser effect on heart rate [72]. Higher doses of fenoterol produce still greater bronchodilatation, but with a higher incidence of cardiovascular side effects and tremor [140]. In a dose of 5 to 10 mg, oral fenoterol may be considered comparable to 4 mg of albuterol and 5 mg of terbutaline [172]. When administered as a pressurized aerosol in single doses of 200 to 400 μg, fenoterol produces long-lasting bronchodilatation (at least 4–5 hours) with a rapid onset (60% of peak within the first few minutes after inhalation), a maximum effect at 60 to 120 minutes, and minimal side effects (mainly tremor) [172]. Higher doses do not improve the response and are accompanied by more frequent side effects.

Most earlier studies did not show any significant differences between fenoterol and albuterol aerosols when given in equivalent doses [172]. However, in higher metered doses, as may be used in the treatment of severe acute asthma, fenoterol exhibits inotropic and chronotropic effects comparable to those produced by isoproterenol [63, 90, 126] and greater than those caused by albuterol or terbutaline [501] administered in bioequivalent doses with respect to bronchodilator efficacy. The hypokalemic effects of fenoterol (see later discussion) are also greater than those of equivalent MDI doses of isoproterenol, albuterol, or terbutaline [90, 384, 501]. It is noteworthy, moreover, that fenoterol MDI is formulated so that each metered dose has approximately twice the bioequivalence of a single dose delivered by other beta-agonist MDIs. The reduced beta$_2$ specificity and greater potency of fenoterol have been proposed as possible contributing factors to the increased asthma mortality in New Zealand occurring during the last decade [91, 335], although this hypothesis has been disputed [60, 323, 410].

Salmeterol

Salmeterol is a new beta$_2$ agonist that is structurally similar to albuterol except for a long lipophilic side chain that is believed to anchor the compound firmly to an exosite in the vicinity of

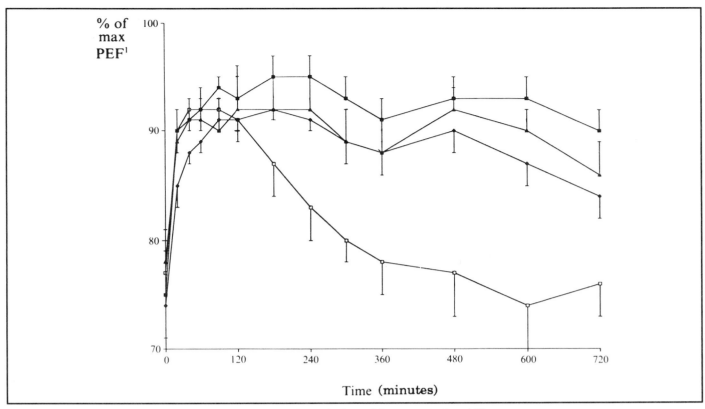

Fig. 55-22. *Peak expiratory flow* (PEF) *after inhalation of 200* μg *of albuterol* (open squares) *and 50* μg (closed diamonds), *100* μg (closed triangles), *and 200* μg (closed squares) *of salmeterol. PEF is expressed as the mean (±1 SEM) percentage of the best-recorded value over four test days. (Reprinted with permission from A. Ullman and N. Svedmyr, Salmeterol, a new long-acting inhaled beta-2 adrenoceptor agonist: comparison with salbutamol in adult asthmatic patients.* Thorax *43:674, 1988.)*

the beta receptor, thereby permitting a much longer duration of action than the parent compound [51]. It is available in Europe and under investigation in the United States. In stable asthmatics, aerosol doses of 50, 100, and 200 μg have been shown to cause a similar peak magnitude of bronchodilatation to that following the administration of albuterol, 200 μg, but a duration of action of at least 12 hours, compared to less than 6 hours for albuterol [460] (Fig. 55-22). The two lower doses of salmeterol caused negligible cardiovascular effects and only a mild tremor comparable to that noted with albuterol, 200 μg, while salmeterol, 200 μg, produced significant, albeit modest, increases in heart rate and more tremor. In a multiple-dose, double-blind crossover study comparing salmeterol, 50 μg bid, and albuterol, 200 μg qid, in 12 asthmatics, most of whom were using inhaled corticosteroids as well, daytime and nocturnal asthma symptoms were less, A.M. and P.M. peak flow rates higher, and use of rescue medication lower during treatment with salmeterol than with albuterol [459].

In placebo-controlled trials, salmeterol given twice daily also reduced nocturnal asthma, as indicated by electroencephalographic evidence of better sleep quality and improvement in overnight and early morning peak flow rates [125]. When inhaled before antigen challenge, salmeterol, 50 μg, abolished not only the early, but also the late-phase, reaction for up to 34 hours, in addition to preventing the increase in nonspecific bronchial hyperreactivity associated with the late-phase reaction [455] (Fig. 55-23). Since salmeterol, 50 μg, inhibited histamine-induced bronchospasm in the same subjects for at least 7.5 to 9.5 hours, but not as long as 32 hours [456], its effect on the hyperresponsiveness associated with the late-phase reaction could not be attributed simply to the prolonged bronchodilatation it produced

and its functional antagonism against mediator agonists. Together with animal studies [205], these results in humans imply that salmeterol may have long-lasting antiinflammatory, as well as bronchodilator, properties. In view of its long duration of bronchodilatation and protection against nonspecific bronchoprovocation, as well as its inhibition of both the early and late phases of antigen-induced bronchospasm and possible antiinflammatory properties, salmeterol appears to be a promising new agent for the maintenance therapy of asthma. This view is supported by comparison studies in which shorter-acting beta agonists administered four times a day demonstrated the superiority of twice-daily administrations of salmeterol in preventing symptoms of asthma and improving lung function [459]. The advantages in terms of improved inhaler compliance are also obvious. On the other hand, salmeterol has a slower rise to peak action than the shorter-acting inhaled beta-agonists, possibly limiting its usefulness as a rescue medication.

Formoterol
Formoterol fumarate, a potent, long-acting, highly selective beta₂ agonist, which is available in Japan in oral form [434], is currently undergoing clinical trials as a metered-dose aerosol. Its pharmacologic properties and therapeutic efficacy have recently been reviewed [122]. Dose-ranging studies of the aerosol formulation have shown 12 μg to provide a greater magnitude and duration of bronchodilatation than 3 and 6 μg. In single-dose comparison studies, formoterol, 12 μg, produced bronchodilatation that was comparable to that produced by albuterol, 200 μg, at 1 hour but was significantly greater than that seen with albuterol use at from

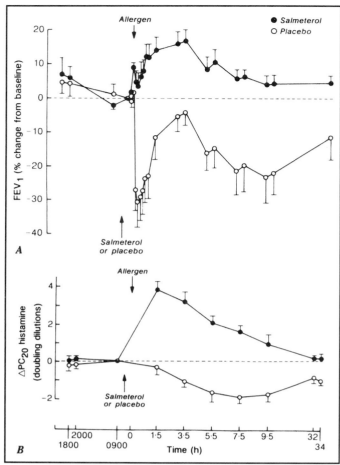

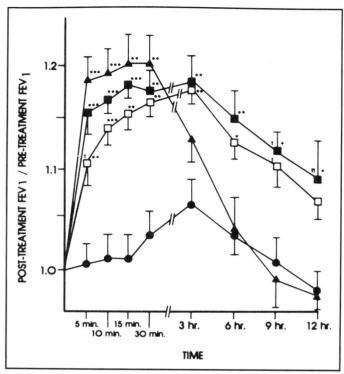

Fig. 55-23. *Effect of inhaled salmeterol, 50 μg (closed circles) or placebo (open circles) on (A) forced expiratory volume in 1 second (FEV₁) response to allergen challenge and (B) histamine responsiveness after allergen challenge, expressed as doubling dilutions of doses of histamine required to provoke a 20 percent decline in FEV₁ from the postdiluent control value. (Reprinted with permission from O. P. Twentyman, et al., Protection against allergen-induced asthma by salmeterol. Lancet 336:1338, 1990. Copyright by The Lancet Ltd., 1990.)*

Fig. 55-24. *Ratio of post- to pretreatment forced expiratory volume at 1 second (FEV₁) following inhalation of placebo (closed circles), salbutamol (closed triangles), and formoterol, 12 μg (open squares) and 24 μg (closed squares), in 16 children with asthma. Values represent means (± 1 SEM). Asterisks denote significant differences from placebo: * = p < .05; ** = p < .01; *** = p < .001. Daggers indicate significant differences between formoterol and salbutamol: † = p < .01; ‡ = p < .01. (Reprinted with permission from P. Arvidsson, et al., Formoterol, a new long-acting bronchodilator for inhalation. Eur. Respir. J. 2:325, 1989.)*

2 to 12 hours; 12 hours after inhalation of formoterol, FEV₁ was still more than 20 percent above baseline [273]. In asthmatic children, doses of 12 and 24 μg of formoterol each led to significant bronchodilatation that lasted for at least 12 hours [30] (Fig. 55-24). Its long duration of action has been attributed to its lipophilicity, which could increase nonspecific binding to the cell membrane in the vicinity of the beta receptor [265]. Although the rise to peak bronchodilatation is slightly slower after inhaled formoterol than albuterol (see Fig. 55-24), formoterol has been used as a rescue, as well as a maintenance, inhaled bronchodilator [15]. Formoterol has also been shown to provide significant protection against methacholine-induced bronchospasm for at least 12 hours, in contrast to a duration of protection by albuterol of only 3 hours [30]. It has also inhibited exercise- and hyperventilation-induced bronchoconstriction for at least 4 hours after inhalation, whereas the duration of protection after albuterol administration was significantly shorter [278, 287]. In 16 asthmatics with chronic stable disease, 15 of whom were using inhaled corticosteroids, a regimen of twice-daily formoterol, 24 μg (two puffs), for four weeks, with additional puffs (12 μg) as needed, led to significantly fewer symptoms of asthma, less disturbed sleep, reduced need for rescue beta₂ agonists, and higher peak

expiratory flow measurements than 1 month of treatment with a shorter-acting beta₂ agonist (albuterol, 400 μg twice daily) plus additional puffs of albuterol (100 mg) when necessary [475].

Formoterol, like salmeterol, is a promising, new long-acting inhaled beta agonist with potential usefulness in the maintenance therapy of asthma, especially nocturnal asthma, using a convenient twice-daily dosing regimen. The basic pharmacology and clinical effects of these new drugs and their potential role in asthma therapy have recently been reviewed [263a]. The therapeutic potential of these long-acting beta₂ agonists in inhibiting allergic inflammation has also been discussed [206a]. Further study of the long-term efficacy and safety of these potent, long-acting inhaled beta₂ agonists is required, however, particularly in view of recent evidence that regular inhalations of a shorter-acting beta agonist (fenoterol) led to poorer control of asthma than did intermittent use only as needed [389] (see later discussion).

Bambuterol

Bambuterol is a lipophilic pro-drug of terbutaline with sustained bronchodilator action due to slow enzymatic conversion to terbutaline in the lung, as well as resistance to metabolic degradation [320]. It is available abroad, but not in the United States. Administered once daily in an oral dose of 20 mg, it has a duration of action of up to 24 hours. When given orally once every evening for 2 weeks, bambuterol provided better bronchodilatation without causing more frequent side effects than did sustained-release terbutaline administered twice daily. Bambuterol has also been shown to be effective in the management of nocturnal asthma not controlled with inhaled beta agonists or inhaled corticosteroids, or both [341].

Routes of Administration

The onset, magnitude, and duration of bronchodilatation of a given dose of beta agonist, the major sites of action within the airways, and the occurrence of extrabronchial side effects are all influenced by the route of drug administration and, for the inhaled route, by the physical characteristics of the aerosol and the technique and sequence of aerosol delivery.

Inhaled Route

The administration of a beta agonist by aerosol has the obvious advantages of rapid onset of bronchodilatation and minimization of cardiac and other unwanted side effects due to the relatively small doses that are delivered topically. Furthermore, the aerosol route yields not only a nearly immediate onset of action but also at least as long-lasting bronchodilatation as that achieved by any other route. The bronchodilator effectiveness of an aerosolized beta agonist is dependent on the dose that is actually delivered to the lower respiratory tract, the sites of deposition of the aerosol within the airways, and a number of host-response characteristics. The delivery of therapeutic aerosols and their deposition in the tracheobronchial tree are influenced by a number of methodologic factors discussed in detail in Chapters 32 and 56. Briefly, these technical considerations include the following: (1) the type of aerosol delivery device, for example: small-volume jet nebulizer (SVJN), ultrasonic nebulizer, MDI with or without an extension device or "spacer," or DPI; (2) the output characteristics of the aerosol delivery device, for example: the number and size of drug-containing particles, particle size distribution, and hygroscopicity of particles; (3) the method of operating the aerosol generating device, for example: for a SVJN, fill volume, driving pressure, continuous versus intermittent nebulization, duration of nebulization, and periodic "tapping" of the nebulizer; for an MDI, shaking and inversion of the canister; for an MDI without a spacer, proper hand–lung coordination; and for a DPI, avoiding high humidity which can cause the powder particles to clump; (4) patient inhaling characteristics: inspiratory flow rate, tidal volume, and end-inspiratory breathhold duration; and (5) the type of airway interface: mouthpiece, mask, endotracheal tube, or tracheostomy tube.

MDIs are currently the most widely used devices for delivering beta-agonist aerosols to the lower airways. However, they require correct technique for optimal effectiveness, including (1) proper coordination between manual actuation of the MDI and inhalation of the aerosol, (2) a slow (0.5–0.75 L/sec), deep inhalation, and (3) a relatively long (≥4 seconds) breath-hold after inhalation [9]. MDIs can be coupled to devices (valved holding chambers or collapsible reservoir bags) that obviate the need for hand–lung coordination and provide audible cues to encourage appropriately slow inhalation of the aerosol. These devices, as well as simple spacers interposed between the mouth and the actuator of the MDI, also decrease particle velocity and deposition in the oropharynx and central airways. Use of these auxiliary devices produces similar, if not better, lower airway deposition of beta-agonist aerosols than that achieved with properly used MDIs alone. They are particularly advantageous for patients who cannot master the proper technique of MDI use. Breath-actuated DPIs are an alternative to spacer devices coupled to MDIs in such patients, although a higher inspiratory flow rate (0.5–2 L/sec) is usually required to generate an effective aerosol from a DPI. An advantage of DPIs is that they do not require a chlorofluorocarbon–propellant system. A number of studies support the equivalent efficacy and greater cost-effectiveness of self-administered MDIs attached to spacer devices compared to jet nebulizers for

delivering beta-agonist aerosols to hospitalized patients with asthma [196, 303], as well as to patients with acute severe asthma [33, 68].

Sites of action of an adrenergic aerosol within the airways are probably closely related to the major sites of deposition. In asthmatics, submicronic beta-agonist aerosols are deposited excessively by inertial inaction at sites of irregular narrowing in central airways, with impaired penetration into the lung periphery [435a]. Consequently, aerosolized beta agonists may be expected to produce dilation preferentially in central airways, particularly when small doses are used [436]. On the other hand, in stable asthmatics, conventional doses of a beta agonist, delivered either by MDI or as a "wet" aerosol, bring about significant improvement in the results of tests of small airways function [74a]. In normal subjects, aerosolized isoproterenol produces a preferential dilatation of peripheral airways [189], whereas atropine causes a relative dilatation of large airways. These findings are consistent with earlier evidence that adrenergic influences predominate in peripheral airways, while the parasympathetic nervous system exerts a constricting influence predominantly in central airways [505].

The response of a patient to a given dose of an inhaled beta agonist depends not only on the dose delivered, but also on a number of host factors [435]. These include: (1) the underlying responsiveness of the airways, which, in turn, is influenced by the degree of inflammation [161] and the thickness of the airway wall [301]; (2) the baseline degree of airflow obstruction; (3) the stability of the obstructive disease (chronic versus acute exacerbation); and (4) the presence and degree of beta-adrenergic tachyphylaxis. For at least three reasons, patients with acute, severe asthma have higher dosage requirements for an aerosolized beta agonist than do those with less severe, stable asthma. First, during acute exacerbations of asthma, the greater degree and extent of airways narrowing due to bronchospasm, inflammatory edema, and mucus secretions impedes delivery of the aerosol to beta-receptor sites in peripheral airways, the major site of increased airways resistance in asthma [473]. Second, constrictor influences are amplified in severe, acute asthma, resulting in greater functional antagonism between the action of beta agonists and that of chemical mediators that are present in higher concentrations [450]. Third, inflammatory mediators may themselves impair beta-receptor function (see earlier discussion).

The *duration* of bronchodilator action of an inhaled beta agonist depends, in part, on the peak magnitude of bronchodilatation and thus on the dose delivered. When adjustments are made to achieve comparable peak effects, the duration of bronchodilatation is determined mainly by (1) the pharmacologic properties of the drug, including its relative resistance to degradation, particularly by COMT, in airway tissue [35] and the affinity with which it binds to beta receptors or sites adjacent to the beta receptor, and (2) host characteristics. Thus, the duration of action of the resorcinol and saligenin derivatives of isoproterenol is considerably longer (4–7 hours) than that of the parent compound (1–2 hours) due to alterations in the phenolic hydroxyl groups which render them resistant to the action of COMT. Moreover, the long duration of action of salmeterol, a derivative of albuterol with a long lipophilic side chain, and formoterol, which is moderately lipophilic, is believed to be due to their lipophilicity, which could increase nonspecific binding to the cell membrane in the vicinity of the beta receptor [45, 265]. Once the dose of a beta agonist achieves saturation levels, a further increase in dose, though not augmenting the magnitude of bronchodilatation, may add to the duration of the effect. Therefore, two different doses of a beta agonist may cause the same peak magnitude of bronchodilatation, but the duration of effect may be shorter following the lower of the two doses.

Host characteristics may also influence the duration of action of an inhaled beta agonist. With increasing severity of asthma, for example, the duration of action of a beta agonist becomes progressively curtailed for reasons similar to those that affect the magnitude of the bronchodilator response. For a given rate of removal of a beta agonist from the beta-adrenergic receptor site, suboptimal bronchodilator doses will occur sooner when higher doses are required to counteract impaired delivery to the lower airways, potent constrictor effects (functional antagonism), and reduced responsiveness (subsensitivity) of the beta receptor. The duration of action of beta agonists is curtailed and more frequent doses are required under these conditions. The duration of action of a beta agonist may also be reduced because of tachyphylaxis, even when the peak magnitude of bronchodilatation is not demonstrably diminished [348].

The bronchodilator effect of an inhaled beta agonist has been shown to last longer than its inhibition of airways responsiveness to various constrictor stimuli, including methacholine [5], histamine [379], and exercise [233]. For example, inhaled metaproterenol produced persistent bronchodilatation for 4 hours, while its protective effect against methacholine-induced bronchoconstriction decreased by 50 percent within 2.25 hours and had disappeared by 4 hours [5] (Fig. 55-25). This dichotomy between

Fig. 55-25. *(A) Activity ratio at serial times after one* (open triangles) *and two* (closed triangles) *puffs of albuterol, two* (open squares) *and four* (closed squares) *puffs of metaproterenol, and placebo aerosol* (closed circles)*. The activity ratio represents the ratio of the provocation concentration producing a 20 percent fall in the forced expiratory volume at 1 second* (FEV_1) *for histamine after drug administration to that before drug administration. (B) The effect of the same drugs in the same doses on* FEV_1*. Note that the maximum bronchodilator effect is sustained for at least 2 hours, whereas the activity ratio is decreasing over the same time period. (Reprinted with permission from R. C. Ahrens, et al., Use of bronchial provocation with histamine to compare the pharmacodynamics of inhaled albuterol and metaproterenol in patients with asthma. J. Allergy Clin. Immunol. 79: 876, 1987.)*

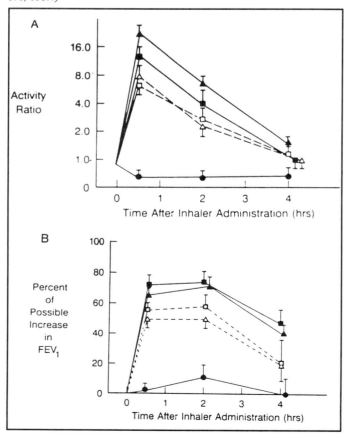

the duration of bronchodilatation and the duration of protection against induced bronchoconstriction following an aerosolized beta agonist has been attributed to differences in the potency of the bronchoconstrictor stimulus in relation to a fixed dose of the beta agonist [5]. Bronchodilation might occur through counteraction of a relatively mild constrictor stimulus responsible for the baseline level of airways obstruction. Conversely, inhibition of induced bronchoconstriction requires a considerably greater beta-agonist action to antagonize a more potent constrictor stimulus that provokes further bronchoconstriction in addition to that which was present initially. The relatively short duration of protection provided by an inhaled beta agonist against bronchoprovocative stimuli has important implications for asthma therapy, particularly since recommendations concerning the dosing frequency for aerosolized beta agonists are usually based on the duration of bronchodilatation they produce and not on the duration of their inhibition of naturally occurring bronchoconstrictor stimuli.

Standard versus Optimal Doses of an Inhaled Beta Agonist. Since the dose requirements for an inhaled beta-adrenergic bronchodilator are influenced by a large number of variables, no standard dose is applicable to all patients under all conditions. The doses and frequency of dosing of beta agonists delivered by an MDI recommended by manufacturers (see Table 55-12) are largely based on studies conducted in trials approved by the Food and Drug Administration (FDA), which consist mostly of clinically stable asthmatics. These dosage regimens often do not suffice for the treatment of severe attacks of asthma for the reasons cited earlier. The maximum recommended doses of the same beta agonists administered in solution form as a wet aerosol are at least ten times higher than those recommended for MDIs (see Table 55-12). The disparity in these dosage recommendations probably reflects the recognition that delivery of beta agonists as a wet aerosol from an SVJN is less efficient than delivery from an MDI. Although most studies demonstrate reduced efficiency of the SVJN in delivering beta agonists to the lower airway, the variability in the efficiency ratios of SVJNs to MDIs is wide, ranging from 1:2 to 1:12.5 [257]. This wide range in relative efficiency is probably due to several factors, including (1) wide variability in the types of SVJNs used, their output characteristics, the manner in which they are operated, and patient inhaling patterns, and (2) variability in the technique of MDI use and the employment of extension devices. Several studies have demonstrated comparable efficacy of the MDI and wet nebulizer when bioequivalent doses are administered. What determines the bronchodilator response to a beta agonist in a given individual is not simply the dose added to the nebulizer or that leaving the actuator of an MDI, but rather the actual dose of the beta agonist that reaches the lower respiratory tract.

"Optimal" dosing regimens vary not only between and within delivery devices, depending on the method of use, but also between patients and even within the same patients, depending on asthma severity. For example, in two small-scale studies [291, 354], asthmatics with moderately severe to severe chronic airflow obstruction were shown to benefit from maintenance doses of aerosolized beta agonists 2½ to 8 times higher than conventional doses, without experiencing significant side effects. In the treatment of acute severe asthma in an emergency room setting, it is well-recognized that inhaled beta agonists must be administered in doses larger than maintenance doses [9, 49, 160]. The inhaled beta agonist may be delivered either by nebulizer powered by 100% oxygen or by MDI with a valved add-on spacer. The use of IPPB for nebulization is not advised because of lack of demonstrably greater effectiveness compared to simple power nebulizers, greater cost and inconvenience, and the potential for causing life-threatening barotrauma [215] (Chap. 83). The recommended adult doses of the beta agonists most commonly administered by power nebulizer are albuterol, 2.5 to 5.0 mg; metaproterenol, 10 to 15 mg; and terbutaline (not FDA approved by this route in the United States), 2 to 5 mg; these doses can be repeated as often as every 20 minutes, if needed. If an MDI with a spacer attachment is used as an alternative to wet nebulization, the following dosing regimen has been recommended: 4 puffs of albuterol (400 μg), metaproterenol (3,000 μg), or terbutaline (1,000 μg) over 2 minutes, followed by one puff every minute until breathlessness abates and forced expiratory flow rates improve or disturbing side effects (e.g., tremor) occur; the initial dose of 4 puffs can be repeated at intervals of 20 to 30 minutes, if needed [160].

In the emergency treatment of children with acute, severe asthma, albuterol has been nebulized in doses of up to 0.15 mg/kg (maximum dose 5.0 mg), followed by as high a dose as 0.05 mg/kg at appropriate intervals, as needed [361, 369, 386]. While common prescribing information recommends a dosage interval of 3 to 4 hours between successive treatments of the longer-acting bronchodilator aerosols (albuterol, terbutaline), the usual practice in the treatment of acute severe asthma is to reduce this interval to 1 or 2 hours, when necessary [220]. In some patients, however, even this interval is too long to prevent worsening asthma in between treatment doses. For example, in acute severe childhood asthma, Robertson and associates [369] found that, after initial treatment with 0.15 mg/kg of albuterol (maximum dose, 5 mg), subsequent nebulization of this same dose at hourly intervals for 2 hours resulted in deterioration before the next scheduled dose and a reduced overall response compared to divided doses of albuterol (0.05 mg/kg; maximum dose, 1.7 mg) delivered every 20 minutes (Fig. 55-26). They attributed the supe-

Fig. 55-26. *Change in the forced expiratory volume at 1 second* (FEV₁) *from baseline at 20-minute intervals in two groups of children with acute severe asthma. Group 1 (closed circles) received salbutamol, 0.15 mg/kg (closed triangles), initially and at hourly intervals; Group 2 (open circles) received salbutamol, 0.15 mg/kg (open triangles), initially and albuterol 0.05 mg/kg every 20 minutes thereafter. Values represent mean changes in FEV₁ from baseline, expressed as the percentage predicted (± 1 SEM). Note that both groups had a similar response to the initial dose of salbutamol. Thereafter, Group 1 continued to improve during the first hour but Group 2 showed deterioration, on the average, prior to the next dose. At 60 minutes, the mean change in FEV₁ was significantly less in group 2 than in group 1 (p < .05). (Reprinted with permission from C. F. Robertson, et al., Response to frequent low doses of nebulized salbutamol in acute asthma. J. Pediatr. 106:672, 1985.)*

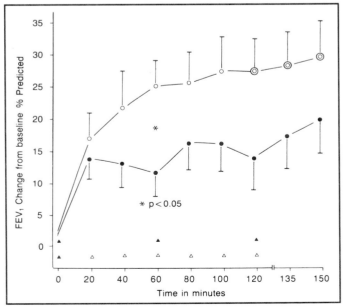

rior results of the more frequent aerosol treatments to the very short duration of bronchodilator response in patients with acute severe asthma and the more effective peripheral penetration of the aerosolized beta agonist when delivered before the airways had been permitted to narrow prior to the next scheduled hourly treatment. In an extension of the latter study, Schuh and coworkers [386] compared albuterol nebulized in high doses (0.15 mg/kg) versus low doses (0.05 mg/kg) administered every 20 minutes for 2 hours in children with acute, severe asthma following initial treatment with a high dose of albuterol. Compared to the low-dose regimen, frequent high doses produced significantly greater improvement in symptoms and forced expired volumes and flow rates and a reduced rate of hospitalization, without causing any greater side effects (tremor, reduced serum potassium levels).

If frequent doses of an aerosolized beta agonist can produce greater improvement in patients with acute severe asthma than less frequently administered doses, even when time-averaged doses are similar, then the continuous nebulization of a beta agonist might prove beneficial in the management of acute severe asthma not responding to intermittent nebulization. In the treatment of 19 children during 27 episodes of acute, severe asthma who were unresponsive to more conservative measures, Moler and colleagues [298] employed continuous nebulization of terbutaline (4 mg/hr in 10 ml) for 3 to 37 hours (mean, 15.4 hours). Asthma symptoms diminished in all patients, elevated PaCO₂ levels declined, and no adverse effects were observed. These authors estimated that the maximum systemically absorbed dose from continuous nebulization of terbutaline (4 mg/hr) in a 15-kg child was 0.58 μg/kg/min, assuming 12 percent delivery to the lung and 1 percent to the mouth and 100 percent absorption from the lung and buccal mucosa; this dose is comparable to the maximum intravenous tocolytic dose used in pregnant women (0.5 μg/kg/min) without causing observable adverse effects to either the mother or fetus.

Side Effects. The side effects of aerosolized beta agonists are due mainly to the pharmacologic effects of the systemically absorbed free compound or to an irritant effect of the aerosolized particles on the airways, or to both causes. Symptoms due to stimulation of beta-adrenergic receptors in extrabronchial tissue (e.g., tremor and palpitations) are minimized by the topical route of administration and are generally absent when even a pharmacologically nonselective beta agonist is administered in conventional doses using an MDI [356]. However, inhaled beta agonists are not without potentially significant toxicity, especially when self-administered in high doses, as is more likely to occur in severe, acute asthma that is refractory to standard doses (see later discussion).

Airway irritation caused by aerosol particles can lead to throat discomfort, cough, or reflex bronchospasm, although the reflex bronchospasm is usually counteracted by the pharmacologic dilator effect of the beta agonist. Infrequent instances of paradoxical bronchospasm following inhalation of isoproterenol aerosols have been noted [219, 362]. Possible mechanisms that might explain these occurrences include stimulation of subepithelial tracheobronchial irritant receptors by inhaled particulate matter leading to vagally mediated bronchospasm, cooling of the airway due to evaporation of the freon propellant from an MDI, or an "allergic" reaction to an additive in the aerosol (e.g., metabisulfite in solution aerosols) [390].

Oral Route

Compared to the topically administered bronchodilator aerosols, oral drugs must be administered in much larger doses to achieve plasma concentrations sufficient to produce a bronchodilator effect. This bronchodilator effect, however, probably extends to a greater range of airways (both peripheral and central) than is generally reached by an aerosol. Although aerosolized bronchodilators can cause dilation of the peripheral airways of asthmatics, as suggested by rapid effects on the density dependence of flow [13, 119], the oral route appears to produce a relatively greater degree of peripheral airways dilatation (reflected by increases in forced vital capacity due to decreases in residual volume) for an equivalent degree of overall bronchodilatation (reflected by increases in FEV_1) [215].

On the other hand, beta agonists provide excellent protection against exercise-induced bronchospasm when administered by the inhaled route, but only negligible protection when taken orally in equivalent bronchodilator doses [12, 232]. Similarly, beta agonists are far more effective against histamine- and methacholine-induced bronchospasm when inhaled than when administered orally [79, 378]. These differences between the protective action of the aerosol and oral forms of a beta agonist could be due to differences in the local concentrations of the drug delivered to different sites in the respiratory tract (e.g., central versus peripheral airways) or to different populations of $beta_2$ receptors—one accessible to the inhaled route and the other to the systemic route [427].

Plasma concentrations of an orally administered beta agonist that are sufficient to cause bronchodilation also produce effects on beta receptors in extrapulmonary tissues, including the heart, systemic blood vessels, skeletal muscle, brain, and bladder, resulting in unwanted side effects (e.g., palpitations, nasal congestion, tremor, insomnia, centrally mediated gastrointestinal symptoms, and aggravation of bladder outlet obstruction). Consequently, less overall bronchodilatation is achieved with cumulative doses of oral drugs than of aerosolized agents before further increases in dose are interdicted by the development of intolerable side effects [245]. On the other hand, additive bronchodilatation may be seen without the addition of systemic side-effects when a beta-adrenergic agonist is administered in aerosol form even after the oral form of the same compound has already begun to produce systemic effects [245].

Long-acting, controlled-release beta agonists have been developed for twice-daily oral dosing. These have potential advantages over immediate-release oral preparations with respect to improvement in patient compliance and therefore better symptom control, as well as more effective prevention of nocturnal asthma and improvement in morning peak flow rates. Albuterol (salbuta-mol) is available abroad in both 4-mg and 8-mg controlled-release tablets containing an osmotic drug delivery system that releases the drug at a constant rate independent of pH and gastrointestinal motility [441]. With multiple dosing, the concentration–time profiles of these formulations at steady-state show little fluctuation in the plasma albuterol levels over a 12-hour dosing interval [260]. The bioavailability is similar to that of immediate-release preparations [428]. Studies comparing long-acting beta agonists with theophylline preparations in stable asthmatic patients have shown comparable efficacy in controlling symptoms, including nocturnal sleep disturbance, and in improving both A.M. and P.M. peak expiratory flow rates, while fewer side effects were reported during treatment with albuterol than with theophylline [176, 472]. A 12-hour sustained-action terbutaline preparation is also available in Europe, but not in the United States.

A repeat-action 4-mg tablet of albuterol with non-osmotically controlled delivery characteristics is available in the United States. This formulation provides rapid release of 2 mg from the tablet coat and delayed release of an additional 2 mg from a barrier-protected core several hours later, thus allowing dosing every 12 hours. At steady-state, the conventional and repeat-action albuterol tablets have comparable bioavailability [353]. Food appears to have a negligible effect on the absorption of albuterol from repeat-action tablets. Moreover, twice-daily administration of this controlled-release preparation has been shown to be as effective in stable asthmatic patients as the standard 2-mg tablet taken four times daily [3].

Subcutaneous and Intravenous Routes

Bronchodilators are given subcutaneously (epinephrine, terbutaline) (Table 55-14) and can be given by slow intravenous injection or infusion (isoproterenol, epinephrine, albuterol, terbutaline) to patients with severe asthma whose response to inhaled drugs is absent, inadequate, or uncertain (see also Chaps. 57 and 80). One rationale for this practice is that, in severe asthma, the parenteral route offers theoretical advantages over the inhaled route by virtue of drug delivery via the systemic circulation to sites in the airway distal to occlusive plugs, and, consequently, inaccessible to the aerosol.

Table 55-14. Beta-agonist bronchodilators for subcutaneous use

Generic (trade) name	Formulation	Manufacturer's recommended dose[a]	Onset	Peak	Duration[b]	Comments
EPINEPHRINE HCL Adrenaline and various others	1:1000 (1 mg/ml) aqueous solution	0.2–0.5 mg (0.01 mg/day in infants and small children) q20 min for 3 doses	5–15 min	0.5–2 hr	2–3 hr	Alpha₁, beta₁, beta₂ action, caution in heart disease, hypertension; arrhythmias may occur; contraindicated in narrow-angle glaucoma, during general anesthesia with halogenated hydrocarbons or cyclopropane, and in organic brain disease
Sus-phrine	1:200 (5 mg/ml) aqueous suspension	0.1–0.3 ml (0.005–0.01 ml/day to maximum of 0.15 ml in infants and small children) q6h or less frequently as needed				
TERBUTALINE Bricanyl, Brethine	1 mg/ml aqueous solution	0.25 mg (0.01 mg/day in infants and small children) repeated in 15–30 min as necessary (maximum dose, 0.5 mg within 4 hr)	5–15 min	0.5–1 hr	1.5–4 hr	Little beta₂ specificity apparent when given parenterally

[a] For adults and children >12 years, unless otherwise specified.
[b] Duration of action generally longer for higher doses and shorter for lower doses.

Despite the theoretical advantage of the parenteral over the inhaled route of administration of beta agonists in acute, severe asthma, most studies have failed to find a significant difference in efficacy between nebulized agents (e.g., isoproterenol, terbutaline, and albuterol) and parenteral therapy (e.g., subcutaneous epinephrine or terbutaline and intravenous albuterol) in either adults [26, 37, 247, 317, 373a, 408, 409, 410, 446, 471, 494] or children [29, 387, 457]. On the other hand, Appel and coworkers [14] found that a significantly greater proportion of patients (18 of 46, or 39%) with severe, acute asthma (peak flow <150 L/min) failed to improve after nebulized metaproterenol (15 mg in 5 ml) than did the proportion (6 of 54, or 11%) not responding to subcutaneous epinephrine (0.3 mg), each agent administered every 30 minutes for 180 minutes ($p < .01$). Moreover, a significantly greater fraction of those who failed to respond to initial therapy with nebulized metaproterenol (13 of 18, or 72%) responded favorably to subsequent treatment with subcutaneous epinephrine, compared with the fraction of those improving with inhaled metaproterenol after a poor response to initial therapy with injected epinephrine (1 of 6, or 17%) ($p < .02$). These findings support the concept that, in some patients with severe, acute asthma, mucous plugs and extensive airway edema impair delivery of nebulized beta agonists to the peripheral airways sufficiently to cause an inadequate therapeutic response that can be circumvented by parenteral therapy. Other possible reasons for a poor response to aerosol therapy include an inefficient aerosol delivery system and inadequate doses of the inhaled drug. As already noted, higher doses of inhaled beta agonists [33, 386] and shorter dosing intervals [220, 369] than are conventionally recommended, including continuous nebulization [298], may enhance the effectiveness of aerosol therapy. Moreover, since side effects tend to occur less frequently with aerosol than with parenteral therapy [14, 26, 29], aerosol treatment should generally be tried first; those patients who fail to respond to inhaled bronchodilator therapy can then be treated with parenteral beta agonists [14, 373a].

The major disadvantage of parenteral therapy is the greater incidence of systemic side effects, particularly those involving the cardiovascular system. Cardiac effects should be less with the use of beta$_2$-selective agents. As already noted, however, equipotent bronchodilator doses of terbutaline and epinephrine given subcutaneously have comparable effects on cardiac output and heart rate [376], although these effects of terbutaline are probably largely indirect consequences of the stimulation of beta$_2$ receptors in vascular smooth muscle [46]. Nonetheless, the resultant increase in heart rate causes an unwanted increase in cardiac work and oxygen requirements. Intravenous salbutamol in bronchodilator doses equivalent to those of isoproterenol produces only 40 to 50 percent of the increase in heart rate noted with isoproterenol, indicating some bronchoselectivity [282]. However, the bronchial-to-cardiac selectivity ratio is only 2 to 2.5:1, which is far less than that noted in studies of isolated tissue. One potential disadvantage of an intravenously infused beta$_2$-selective agent over isoproterenol is the longer duration of action following cessation of the infusion, leading to longer persistence of any unwanted cardiovascular effects.

Interaction of Beta Agonists with Other Drugs

With Theophylline
Theophylline and beta agonists are frequently used in conjunction with one another and given by the same or different routes in both the routine and emergency treatment of asthma. *In vitro* studies demonstrating synergism between these two classes of bronchodilators in the production of leukocyte and smooth muscle cAMP [250a, 330a, 347a], in the relaxation of guinea pig and human tracheobronchial smooth muscle [250a], and in the inhibition of IgE-dependent histamine release from peripheral baso-

phils [257a, 326a] suggest that they might also have additive or synergistic therapeutic effects when used in combination in asthmatic patients. However, the utility of combining these two drugs in asthma therapy depends on the balance of additive therapeutic and toxic effects when administered *in vivo*. While single- and multiple-dose studies of oral ephedrine and theophylline alone and in combination have produced inconsistent results with respect to additive bronchodilatation in asthmatic children [396, 440, 445, 482], the addition of one of the more potent oral beta$_2$-selective agents to theophylline has more consistently produced significant additional bronchodilation [111, 137, 334, 425, 511]. For example, in stable asthmatics, Wolfe and coworkers [497] have shown that the combination of oral terbutaline and aminophylline in either low (2.5 and 200 mg, respectively) or high (5 and 400 mg, respectively) doses produces significantly greater bronchodilation than does either drug when given alone, and that the low-dose combination is equivalent in its bronchodilator effect to that of a high dose of either single agent. Since there are differences in the type and frequency of side effects expected from each of these two classes of drugs, use of both drugs together in relatively low doses could offer therapeutic advantages over a higher dose of either alone in terms of the reduced frequency of side effects. Although such an advantage was not demonstrated in the small number of patients studied either by Wolfe and colleagues [497] or by Eggleston and coworkers [111], using low doses of oral fenoterol with theophylline, the Svedmyrs [425] found that low doses of terbutaline (2.5 mg) and theophylline (280 mg) together produced slightly greater bronchodilation and appreciably *less* tremor than did a high dose of terbutaline alone (5 mg). On the other hand, although combining *high* doses of an oral beta$_2$ agonist and theophylline has the advantage of providing a significant augmentation of bronchodilatation, this is achieved at the cost of a greater frequency of side effects [497]. If an oral beta agonist and an oral theophylline preparation are used together in asthma therapy, it is preferable to administer these agents separately, rather than in a fixed-dose combination, to provide optimal flexibility in adjusting the dose of each agent.

The strategy of using an *inhaled*, rather than an oral, beta agonist in conjunction with oral theophylline has the attractive feature of minimizing additional side effects while offering the possibility of an augmented bronchodilator response [425]. However, Shim and Williams [392] failed to find that the bronchodilator effect of three inhalations of metaproterenol aerosol was significantly enhanced by a single therapeutic dose of aminophylline, possibly because the inhaled beta agonist produced near-maximal bronchodilatation in their patients, or that the aminophylline effect was not present at the start. For long-term use, Smith and colleagues [399] have shown an increased peak expiratory flow rate when aminophylline is added to terbutaline aerosol, particularly in the early morning. On the other hand, in a study of the relative efficacy of maintenance therapy with inhaled albuterol, oral theophylline, and the combination of these two drugs in adolescents with chronic asthma, Joad and associates [204] found that theophylline alone was associated with significantly fewer symptoms, especially at night, compared to albuterol alone, and that the combination regimen was not more effective than was theophylline alone. The poorer results obtained with inhaled albuterol in maintenance therapy, especially for patients with nocturnal asthma, were attributed to its relatively short duration of action, despite greater *acute* bronchodilation and protection against induced bronchospasm. In the same study population, these authors observed no differences between the single- and combination-drug regimens in the frequency of extrapulmonary symptoms (headache, nervousness, tremor, nausea, palpitations, irritability, or impaired ability to concentrate), global perception of side effects, or cardiac arrhythmias [203].

The combined use of beta agonists (particularly in aerosol

form) with oral theophylline in the outpatient management of asthma is widespread. Although less emphasis has been placed on theophylline therapy recently, there is still concern regarding the possibility of augmented cardiotoxicity (ventricular tachyarrhythmias, myocardial necrosis, sudden death) from the coincident administration of these drugs, as suggested by the results of animal studies [127, 210, 315, 487]. Comparable cardiotoxicity from the combined use of these two classes of bronchodilators in humans has not been well documented clinically, possibly due to inadequate study and lack of appropriate cardiac monitoring [314]. In a report describing an increase in the sudden-death rate among young asthmatics in New Zealand [496], at a time when the use of combination theophylline and beta-agonist therapy was increasing, the authors hypothesized that there might be a subgroup of asthmatics who are unduly susceptible to the cardiotoxic effects of this drug combination. Although a number of alternative explanations exist for the recent "epidemic" of asthma mortality in New Zealand, as suggested by these authors [496] as well as others [91, 150, 389, 410], their hypothesis warrants more careful study.

Beta$_2$-selective agonists, even when inhaled, can have significant hemodynamic effects and can increase the blood glucose level and lower the serum potassium concentration (see later discussion). These responses to beta$_2$ stimulation may be augmented by theophylline. For example, studies in patients with stable asthma have shown a potentiation of the positive inotropic effects of nebulized albuterol by the administration of intravenous aminophylline, as indicated by a decrease in total electromechanical systole [62]. However, the enhanced inotropism from combination therapy was judged unlikely to be harmful since it was not associated with any increase in myocardial oxygen consumption. In healthy subjects, maintenance therapy with oral theophylline potentiated the positive inotropic and chronotropic effects of inhaled fenoterol [126]. Theophylline has also been shown to augment the rise in systolic blood pressure caused by subcutaneous or intravenous terbutaline [89, 401] as well as the hypokalemia produced by infused epinephrine [488], albuterol [489], or terbutaline [401]. Although the clinical significance of these findings is unclear, they underscore the importance of monitoring the hemodynamics and serum potassium levels in patients receiving high doses of beta agonists (either by inhalation or parenterally), particularly when administered in combination with theophylline.

Inhaled or injected beta agonists, or both, are frequently used together with either intravenous aminophylline or an oral methylxanthine in the emergency treatment of severe, acute asthma (Chap. 72). In 102 young adults with severe acute asthma, treatment with nebulized isoproterenol (2.5 mg every 20 minutes for 3 doses) alone was no less effective than when intravenous aminophylline or a rapidly acting oral theophylline was administered in combination with the inhaled beta agonist, irrespective of the severity of the initial airflow obstruction; added toxicity of the combination regimens was not observed [120]. A subsequent study from the same group [121] compared single-drug therapy, consisting of either intravenous aminophylline, subcutaneous epinephrine (0.3 mg every 20 minutes for 1 hour), or nebulized isoproterenol (as above), with various combination regimens, including intravenous aminophylline together with either of the above beta agonists or a combination of oral theophylline and inhaled isoproterenol. Theophylline alone yielded the least beneficial response, while the combination of theophylline and a beta agonist was no more efficacious than was inhaled isoproterenol alone (Fig. 55-27). In the subset of patients with more severe airflow obstruction (FEV$_1$ ≤35%), epinephrine as a single agent caused less bronchodilation than did inhaled isoproterenol alone, and the addition of theophylline to epinephrine (but not to inhaled isoproterenol) produced greater bronchodilation than that seen with the parenteral beta agonist alone (see Fig. 55-27),

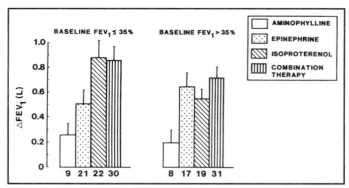

Fig. 55-27. *Change in the forced expiratory volume at 1 second* (FEV$_1$) *from baseline after 1 hour of treatment of acute asthma with intravenous aminophylline, subcutaneous epinephrine, nebulized isoproterenol, or a regimen combining a sympathomimetic and a methylxanthine. Patients with severe airflow obstruction at presentation (FEV$_1$ ≤ 35% of predicted) were analyzed separately from those with less severe baseline obstruction (FEV$_1$ > 35% of predicted). Mean values are denoted by the heights of the bars; arrows represent 1 SEM. Numbers below the bars indicate the number of patients. (Reprinted with permission from C. H. Fanta, T. H. Rossing, and E. R. McFadden Jr., Treatment of acute asthma. Is combination therapy with sympathomimetics and methylxanthines indicated? Am. J. Med. 80:5, 1986.)*

presumably due to submaximal bronchodilation achieved with the latter drug in the more obstructed patients. Aside from nausea, which was more common in patients receiving theophylline, side effects were comparable in all groups. On the other hand, Josephson and coworkers [211] were not only unable to find a significantly greater bronchodilator response to combined therapy with epinephrine and aminophylline compared to epinephrine alone in patients with severe, acute asthma but also noted greater tachycardia and a trend toward more ventricular dysrhythmias, particularly complex ectopy, following combined therapy. In another group of young adults with severe, acute asthma who failed to respond to initial emergency room treatment with nebulized metaproterenol, continued therapy with inhaled metaproterenol (15 mg every hour for 3 hours) along with intravenous placebo was no less efficacious than was treatment with a combination of metaproterenol and intravenous aminophylline, even in patients with the most severe airways obstruction initially (FEV$_1$ 0.8 liter) [394] (Fig. 55-28). Complaints of tremor, nausea, anxiety, and palpitations were significantly more common in the patients receiving theophylline. Overall, the above findings suggest that, in the treatment of severe, acute asthma, theophylline does not add to the efficacy of inhaled beta agonists administered in large, frequent doses or, in general, to the efficacy of parenteral beta agonists, but can increase the toxicity of treatment. Later in the course, however, when the dosing of beta agonists is less intense, theophylline has a role.

With Corticosteroids

Corticosteroids potentiate the effect of adrenergic stimulation in airway smooth muscle [11, 181, 452] and are involved in the regulation of beta-adrenergic receptor density in the lung [130, 279] and other tissues [452]. Beta-agonist drug therapy leads to a reduction in the number (downregulation) of cell-surface beta-adrenergic receptors and the responsiveness to beta-agonist stimulation [85, 138, 304], possibly accounting for the diminished responsiveness (tolerance and subsensitivity) to beta-adrenergic bronchodilator therapy in asthmatics during long-term treatment with these agents [198, 309]. Corticosteroids are capable of restoring responsiveness to adrenergic bronchodilators within

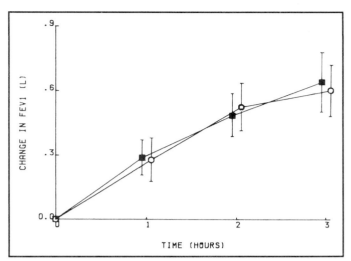

Fig. 55-28. *Change in the forced expiratory volume at 1 second* (FEV$_1$) *in 20 patients with severe acute exacerbations of asthma treated with intravenous aminophylline and inhaled metaproterenol* (open circles) *and in 20 similar patients treated with inhaled metaproterenol alone* (closed squares). *Values represent means ± 1 SEM. Note that the FEV$_1$ improved progressively to a similar extent in both groups. (Reprinted with permission from D. Siegel, et al., Aminophylline increases the toxicity but not the efficacy of an inhaled beta-adrenergic agonist in the treatment of acute exacerbations of asthma. Am. Rev. Respir. Dis. 132:283, 1985.)*

hours in such "tolerant" asthmatics [113, 181], possibly due to upregulation of their beta-adrenergic receptors [186, 436].

With Monoamine Oxidase Inhibitors

MAO inhibitors, used for the treatment of depression, block oxidative deamination of naturally occurring amines, including the catecholamines, following their uptake into storage sites within adrenergic nerve endings. Consequently, caution has been advised in the use of oral beta agonists in patients receiving MAO inhibitors because of the possible potentiation of cardiovascular effects due to inhibition of their metabolic degradation, although COMT plays a much more important role than MAO in the metabolism of circulating catecholamines [483].

With Anticholinergic Bronchodilators

Anticholinergic bronchodilators, ipratropium bromide or atropine in solution, have been used in combination with inhaled beta agonists for the treatment of severe, acute asthma. In this setting, most investigators report an additive bronchodilator effect from ipratropium (0.5–1 mg) and large doses of a beta-agonist solution aerosol (albuterol, 5–10 mg, or fenoterol, 1–1.25 mg) [58, 248, 359, 477]. Furthermore, the effect of the beta agonist appears to be enhanced when ipratropium is administered 60 to 120 minutes prior to the beta agonist [58, 248, 477]. This enhancement may be due to a preferential bronchodilator action of the anticholinergic on the large central airways, thus facilitating delivery of the subsequently administered beta agonist to peripheral sites in the lower respiratory tract where adrenergic influences predominate [189]. On the other hand, one group failed to observe that anticholinergics provided any significant added benefit when inhaled beta agonists were already used in very high, frequent doses for the treatment of acute, severe asthma [216]. However, other investigators have shown that ipratropium, although not improving the overall maximal bronchodilator response to a large dose of nebulized albuterol, may still prolong the duration of the response [178] (Chap. 64).

Adverse Reactions of Beta Agonists

Reduction in PaO$_2$

Beta agonists, while relieving airflow obstruction, usually produce little reduction in the hypoxemia of obstructive airways disease and sometimes even lower the PaO$_2$ further [162, 188, 276, 328, 329, 347, 429]. These decreases in PaO$_2$ are greatest around 5 minutes after the bronchodilator is administered and return toward control values by 30 minutes [222]. Although these falls in PaO$_2$ are generally small, they can sometimes be fairly large [329]. Moreover, not only can beta agonists aggravate the hypoxemia of severe asthma, but hypoxia can also potentiate the myocardial irritability provoked by sympathomimetics in experimental animals [84]. Grant [150] has proposed that uncontrolled hypoxia in asthmatics using large doses of inhaled beta agonists, especially administered via air-driven home nebulizers, for the treatment of severe, acute episodes in an unsupervised domiciliary setting was one factor responsible for the increase in asthma mortality in New Zealand occurring in the late 1970s. As a precautionary measure, therefore, supplemental oxygen should be provided to patients undergoing intensive aerosol or systemic bronchodilator therapy for severe asthma. In such patients, the inspired oxygen concentration can be increased without fear of inducing carbon dioxide retention, since the development of hypercapnia reflects the severity of the airflow obstruction and respiratory muscle fatigue rather than a depressed ventilatory drive.

The mechanism whereby beta agonists can reduce the PaO$_2$ in asthma is thought to involve an increase in pulmonary blood flow to regions where ventilation remains relatively impaired, thereby counteracting the lung's auto regulatory reduction in perfusion to poorly ventilated regions and worsening ventilation–perfusion relationships [328]. The increase in pulmonary blood flow may be secondary to stimulation of beta$_2$ receptors in pulmonary vascular smooth muscle (leading to pulmonary vasodilation) and/or of beta$_1$ receptors in myocardium (leading to increased cardiac output). Since systemic administration of practolol, a beta$_1$-selective adrenergic antagonist, can prevent the fall in arterial PO$_2$ (PaO$_2$) resulting from inhaled isoproterenol [329], the hypoxemic effect of isoproterenol has been attributed to the increase in cardiac output resulting from stimulation of myocardial beta$_1$ receptors. In this regard, it is noteworthy that the aerosol forms of beta$_2$-selective agents, such as albuterol, generally do not have an adverse effect on PaO$_2$ [86, 238a, 263, 377]. However, others have noted small declines in PaO$_2$ on occasion after albuterol aerosol [329], possibly due to its direct pulmonary vasodilator effect or an indirect effect on cardiac output, or to both effects.

Hypokalemia

Reductions in the serum potassium level have been demonstrated following administration of beta agonists by either the parenteral [108, 238a, 255, 311, 371, 385, 386, 393] or the inhaled [90, 154, 261] route. The magnitude of the hypokalemia is greater with the systemic route but is also dependent on both the potency and dose of beta agonists given by inhalation [90, 384]. The precise mechanism of beta-agonist–induced hypokalemia is unclear. However, current evidence suggests that this is a beta$_2$-specific effect [420] which is mediated either directly by beta$_2$-stimulated increases in Na$^+$-K$^+$-ATPase activity [78, 102, 373] or indirectly by pancreatic beta$_2$-receptor stimulation causing increases in the serum insulin concentration [349, 385, 400, 439]; in either case, the increased cellular uptake of potassium is the result, leading to a reduction in the extracellular potassium concentration. In asymptomatic asthmatics, after a therapeutic dose of subcutaneous terbutaline (0.25 mg), the serum potassium level began to decline within 15 minutes, reached a peak decrement (14%) at 30 minutes, and remained depressed for at least 2 hours [240]. A similar time course was noted after subcutaneous, intramuscular, and intravenous albuterol administrations [371]. When cumulative doses (1,200–2,400 μg) of albuterol and fenoterol were given to healthy volunteers by MDI, dose-dependent decreases in the serum potassium level were noted, with mean maximum decreases of 0.67 and 1.13 mEq/L, respectively [384]; significantly greater decrements were observed after fenoterol administration than after equivalent doses of albuterol, consistent with a more potent beta$_2$ effect of the former agent (see Fig. 55-21). Similar findings were reported by Crane and associates [90]. In the latter study, a significant correlation was noted between the magnitude of the hypokalemia and the degree of prolongation of the electrocardiographic Q-T$_c$ interval. The true clinical significance of beta$_2$-agonist–induced hypokalemia is unknown [238a]. However, since hypokalemia can predispose a patient to ventricular dysrhythmias [80, 443], it has been hypothesized that the recent increase in sudden and unexpected deaths due to asthma could be due, in part, to disturbances in cardiac rhythm induced by a combination of stress (associated with an increase in the endogenous catecholamine level) and overuse of inhaled adrenergic agents, leading to hypokalemia [154]. This effect could be enhanced by the concomitant use of diuretics [261] and/or corticosteroids (both of which lead to renal potassium loss), as well as theophylline, which has been shown to cause additional hypokalemia when given in conjunction with a beta agonist [393, 489]. Hypoxemia and acid-base disturbances accompanying severe episodes of asthma could also potentiate the influence of hypokalemia on myocardial irritability. On the other hand, no serious cardiac arrhythmias were observed in 10 patients with near-fatal asthma who were hospitalized in respiratory arrest (or within 20 minutes of its development), despite the fact that all had severe hypercapnia and acidosis and four were hypokalemic, suggesting that asthma mortality is more likely due to severe asphyxia rather than to cardiac arrhythmias [298]. Nevertheless, beta-agonist–induced hypokalemia might still increase the risk of serious cardiac arrhythmias, particularly in older asthmatic patients with coexisting ischemic heart disease who may already have a low serum potassium level due to concomitant diuretic therapy or who may be receiving digitalis, which sensitizes the myocardium to hypokalemia. It is therefore prudent to monitor the serum potassium level in patients receiving large doses of beta agonists for the treatment of severe, acute asthma.

Other Metabolic Effects

Beta$_2$ stimulation can also cause falls in the serum magnesium, calcium, and phosphate levels, possibly due in part to concomitant increases in circulating insulin levels [343, 400]. Despite an increase in the serum insulin concentration due to stimulation of beta$_2$ receptors in the pancreas, blood glucose levels also rise in response to treatment with beta$_2$ agonists, whether administered systemically [240, 343, 371, 385] or by inhalation [311]; the elevation in the blood glucose level is due to beta$_2$-agonist–induced glycogenolysis. After 0.25 mg of terbutaline given subcutaneously, the mean blood glucose level increased transiently from 85 to 103 mg/dl in seven stable adult asthmatics [240]. In 21 asymptomatic asthmatics, 0.3 mg of subcutaneous epinephrine caused a mean maximum rise in the blood glucose concentration of 32 mg/dl. Small, but statistically significant, transient increases in the blood glucose level have also been found after aerosolized albuterol (200 μg) administration [311]. These changes in the blood glucose level after treatment with a beta$_2$ agonist are unlikely to assume clinical significance, except perhaps in diabetic patients in whom intravenous albuterol can rarely cause hyperglycemic ketoacidosis [444]. Although beta$_1$-receptor stimulation is mainly responsible for catecholamine-induced lipolysis, beta$_2$ receptors have some lipolytic activity [357, 402]. Oral albuterol (4 mg), for example, caused a significant increase in the free

fatty acid levels in healthy subjects [439]. Larger increases in the content of nonesterified fatty acids, as well as in ketone body formation, have been found in diabetics given albuterol. There is some evidence that regularly scheduled therapeutic doses of oral terbutaline can raise high-density-lipoprotein–cholesterol concentrations [184].

Myocardial Toxicity

Concern over the potential cardiac toxicity of beta agonists has been rekindled by the puzzling increase in asthma mortality, especially in New Zealand, in the late 1970s and early 1980s. One hypothesis that has been proposed to explain the "epidemic" of fatal asthma in New Zealand is over-reliance on a high-potency, incompletely beta$_2$-selective inhaled beta agonist (fenoterol) possessing cardiac effects similar to those of the nonselective beta agonist isoproterenol [90, 335]. In connection with this epidemic, it has also been hypothesized that the potential cardiac toxicity of inhaled beta agonists, when administered in an unsupervised setting in higher-than-recommended doses for the treatment of severe episodes of asthma, could have been enhanced by uncontrolled hypoxemia [150] (potentially aggravated by the beta agonist), by beta-agonist–induced hypokalemia [90], and by the concomitant administration of oral theophyllines [496].

Beta agonists have well-known effects on the heart, including an increase in the force (inotropic effect) and rate (chronotropic effect) of myocardial contraction and an increase in the rate of conduction of the contractile process through the heart [52]. These effects lead to increases in cardiac output, cardiac work, and myocardial oxygen consumption, the increase in the last variable being disproportionate to the increase in work. Although the beta$_2$-selective adrenergic agonists have quantitatively fewer chronotropic and inotropic effects than do the beta$_1$ stimulants, the cardiac effects of the beta$_2$-selective and nonselective agonists are still qualitatively similar. The hemodynamic effects of the beta$_2$-selective agents have been attributed to the following mechanisms: (1) baroreceptor-mediated increases in sympathetic tone, (2) baroreceptor-mediated withdrawal of parasympathetic activity, (3) stimulation of presynaptic beta$_2$ receptors, thus facilitating the postsynaptic release of norepinephrine, (4) direct stimulation of cardiac beta$_1$ receptors, (5) direct stimulation of cardiac beta$_2$ receptors (see earlier discussion), and (6) arteriolar dilatation, causing a decrease in afterload [418]. The cardiac effects of selective beta$_2$ agonists, most apparent when these agents are given orally or parenterally, can be minimized by aerosol delivery [334]. However, even when administered by MDIs in recommended therapeutic doses, selective beta$_2$ agonists have been shown to retain the potential for hemodynamically significant effects, as indicated by modest, but significant, increases in cardiac output, stroke volume, and the left ventricular mean velocity of circumferential fiber shortening [70].

Catecholamine-induced myocardial necrosis ("contraction-band necrosis") has been observed in animals given large doses of isoproterenol and in humans with pheochromocytoma and other conditions associated with increased sympathetic activity (e.g., severe stress or intracranial catastrophes) [27, 372] (Chap 78). Similar lesions have been found in children dying of acute asthma [107]. These necrotic lesions are distinct in their histologic characteristics and distribution from ischemic infarction due to coronary occlusion. In animals, the range of doses of isoproterenol required to produce these lesions is quite wide, depending on weight, age, and species. Moreover, pretreatment with corticosteroids appears to potentiate the induction of contraction-band necrosis by isoproterenol [153]. Associated arrhythmias have included premature ventricular contractions, ventricular tachycardia, and ventricular fibrillation, which are potentiated by hypoxemia [84]. Proposed mechanisms of myocardial contraction-band necrosis include relative subendocardial ischemia, platelet aggregation, calcium overload, damage to cell membranes produced by elevated levels of free fatty acids, and peroxidation of membrane lipids by catecholamine-derived oxygen free radicals [19a]. Interestingly, although metaproterenol can produce similar lesions, these have not been observed with albuterol, terbutaline, or epinephrine use [274].

These animal studies of catecholamine cardiotoxicity may be relevant to human asthma. For example, 4 of 13 children dying of asthma had myocardial contraction-band necrosis, suggesting that this cardiac lesion may contribute to death in some patients with fatal asthma [107]. Two of these four patients had received isoproterenol parenterally, while data on oral and/or inhaled sympathomimetic treatment for the other two patients are not available. Therefore, the production of this cardiac lesion in asthmatics could be due to catecholamine infusions or to other mechanisms. Myocardial-specific CPK-MB elevations that may be indicative of myocardial injury were found in 15 of 19 patients admitted because of severe childhood asthma and treated with intravenous isoproterenol [275]. These elevations all reverted to normal after intravenous isoproterenol was stopped, despite continuation of intravenous aminophylline and corticosteroids and inhaled beta agonists. Electrocardiographic abnormalities (S-T segment depression or elevation) were noted in six of ten patients with and in two of four without CPK-MB elevation; one of the former patients had associated anginal pain. These findings suggest that intravenous isoproterenol therapy may be associated with frequent, clinically undetected myocardial injury that could be detected by the serial monitoring of serum CPK-MB levels. Although parenteral therapy with beta$_2$-selective stimulants would be expected to cause less cardiotoxicity, systematic studies of the impact of such therapy on serum CPK-MB levels are lacking.

Beta-adrenergic stimulants, especially in combination with theophylline, can cause fatal cardiac arrhythmias in experimental animals [84, 210, 315]. Potentially serious dysrhythmias have also been documented when beta agonists have been administered to humans by the systemic route. For example, disturbing ventricular dysrhythmias have been been induced by isoproterenol when infused intravenously in children with impending respiratory failure due to severe asthma [412, 503]. Moreover, 9 of 41 adults treated for severe, acute asthma with subcutaneous epinephrine (especially those who also received aminophylline) developed dysrhythmias that were attributed to treatment; older patients were more prone to the arrhythmogenic effects of bronchodilator therapy [212]. Since no morbid events were associated with these arrhythmias, their clinical significance may be questionable. Although ventricular arrhythmias have been associated with increased mortality in mainly older patients with acute respiratory failure related to chronic airflow obstruction, the contribution of bronchodilator therapy to this increased mortality is unknown [185a]. Oral terbutaline (5 mg) administration was associated with an increase in ventricular ectopic beats in patients with COPD, although these increases were not impressive [21]. Significant ventricular ectopy (5 or more premature ventricular contractions per minute) was noted in 4 of 15 middle-aged patients with stable asthma after inhalation over a period of 1 to 2 hours of 1,120 to 1,760 μg of fenoterol (7–11 puffs), but not after a comparable dose of albuterol [433]. Higgins and associates [177] performed continuous Holter monitoring in 19 elderly patients with chronic airflow obstruction before and during 24 hours of treatment with albuterol, 5 mg, or terbutaline, 4 mg, four times daily delivered via a compressed-air–driven nebulizer. Four of these patients developed either new or more frequent arrhythmias during nebulized beta-agonist therapy compared to the period prior to initiation of therapy. Although these arrhythmias were not associated with symptoms, the authors concluded that beta agonists delivered with an air-driven nebulizer are not completely safe in elderly patients with severe chronic airflow obstruction.

In contrast to the above findings, most controlled studies in hospitalized or ambulatory patients with asthma fail to document a relationship between clinically significant arrhythmias and treatment with oral or inhaled beta agonists, alone or in combination with theophylline. For example, in 20 patients hospitalized for asthma and treated with repeated doses of inhaled isoproterenol and intravenous aminophylline, 24-hour Holter monitoring failed to reveal the occurrence of potentially dangerous arrhythmias [152]. In young, otherwise healthy asthmatic subjects treated for 1-week periods with either oral terbutaline or sustained-release theophylline, or both agents, 36-hour Holter monitoring did not reveal any significant increase in ventricular ectopy when both agents were combined, although a trend was noted toward an increase in the complexity of the premature beats. In both young and old asthmatics with stable disease treated with maintenance doses of an inhaled beta agonist alone, sustained-release theophylline alone, or the combination, 24-hour electrocardiographic monitoring failed to reveal any cardiotoxic effects from either drug alone or in combination [223]. In clinically stable asthmatic children, hourly doses of inhaled albuterol (180 μg per dose) given over the course of 5 hours failed to induce any arrhythmia [250]. Despite these negative findings, however, one must still be alert to the possibility that beta agonists, particularly when administered in high and frequent inhaled doses or by the parenteral route for the treatment of acute severe asthma, *can*, in individual cases, cause life-threatening arrhythmias [228]. This possibility is of particular concern in the older patient with underlying coronary artery disease. One must also recognize that concomitant hypokalemia, hypoxemia, and acid-base disturbances can predispose to serious rhythm disturbances. Recently, Robin [369a] has raised the possibility that the dose-dependent increase in the Q-T$_c$ interval induced by beta agonists could contribute to sudden death in asthmatics, analogous to the sudden death due to malignant ventricular arrhythmias in nonasthmatic patients with genetically determined or idiopathic acquired prolonged QT interval.

Adverse Effects on Other Organs
Central Nervous System. In conventional doses, the beta agonists are not potent central nervous system stimulants, due largely to the relative inability of these polar compounds to cross the blood-brain barrier. Central nervous system stimulant–like effects of these drugs, including restlessness, apprehension, headache, and tremor, may be secondary, at least partly, to their peripheral cardiovascular, skeletal muscle, and metabolic effects [483].

Skeletal Muscle. Tremor occurs in a dose-dependent manner in response to the acute systemic administration of beta$_2$ bronchodilators [246] and is the most frequently reported side effect from oral beta$_2$ agonists. After multiple dosing with an oral beta agonist, however, the occurrence of tremor declines while its bronchodilator action remains relatively unimpaired ("selective tolerance") [200, 246]. Therefore, tremor can be minimized by initiating therapy with low doses of an oral beta agonist and subsequently (after "selective tolerance" has developed) increasing the dose, if necessary, to achieve greater bronchodilatation. Alternatively, an MDI may be used to minimize tremorigenic and other systemic side effects. Muscle cramps are occasionally experienced during treatment with oral beta$_2$ agents.

Bladder. Stimulation of beta$_2$ receptors in the detrusor muscle of the bladder relaxes the bladder wall, decreasing the driving pressure for micturition, while stimulation of alpha receptors in the vesicle sphincter narrows the bladder outlet. Consequently, bladder outlet obstruction, as in elderly males with prostatism, can be aggravated by any oral sympathomimetic agent, particularly one with both beta- and alpha-stimulant properties (such as ephedrine).

Vascular Smooth Muscle. Due to their vasodilator effect, oral beta$_2$ agonists may reduce diastolic and possibly mean arterial blood pressure, but these reductions are generally very mild and of little clinical significance. In addition, beta$_2$ agonists can occasionally produce or aggravate nasal congestion, particularly in patients with rhinitis. Although congestion of mucosal blood vessels in the tracheobronchial tree is also a theoretically possible outcome of beta-agonist therapy, it is not clear to what extent this occurs or what its clinical significance might be.

Tumorigenicity. Studies in the rat have shown that albuterol, as well as other beta-adrenergic stimulants, causes a dose-related increase in the incidence of benign leiomyomata of the mesovarium in doses 3, 16, and 78 times the maximal human oral dose, but has no effect on fertility [7]. The clinical relevance of these findings to humans is not known. Thus far, studies in mice and hamsters have failed to show evidence of tumorigenicity.

Paradoxical Bronchospasm. Infrequently, beta agonists, especially when inhaled as an aerosol, can paradoxically lead to airway narrowing. Several factors, either alone or in combination, may contribute to this finding. If the apparent bronchospastic reaction is evident only during assessment of the lung function response to a beta-agonist aerosol, it could be due to (1) spirometer-induced bronchospasm related to the deep inhalation preceding a forced exhalation maneuver or (2) dynamic compression, during forced exhalation, of airways made more compliant by bronchial smooth muscle relaxation [42, 266, 411]. If paradoxical bronchospasm is apparent either clinically or during evaluation of the bronchodilator response to therapy, it could be related to (1) reflex bronchospasm due to an irritant effect of the aerosol vehicle, (2) beta-adrenergic tachyphylaxis, uncovering bronchospasm due to one or more of the above factors, or, least likely, (3) a hypersensitivity reaction to the beta agonist itself. Until recently, sulfites were used as preservatives in aqueous solutions of isoproterenol, isoetharine, and metaproterenol for aerosol use. Sulfur dioxide generated by the reaction of sulfites with water and released during nebulization can induce bronchospasm in asthmatics and may have accounted for some paradoxical reactions to bronchodilator aerosols that occurred in the past [231].

Mortality. Although adrenergic agents are of unquestioned value in asthma therapy, misuse of these agents can lead to worsening of asthma and even death. Obviously, however, one can never be certain that drugs are responsible. Sudden death has been reported following epinephrine injections preceded by large and frequent doses of inhaled isoproterenol that had not brought relief [290]. A number of reports describe a relationship between the inhalation of large doses of epinephrine [32, 149] or isoproterenol [151, 266a, 465] and death due to asthma. In nonfatal cases, it has been noted that severe asthma may not remit until inhaled epinephrine [347] or isoproterenol [112, 219, 362, 465] is withdrawn. The most-often-cited examples of the possible relationship between adrenergic drug therapy and mortality in asthma are the startling rise in asthma deaths in several countries, including the United Kingdom, Australia, and New Zealand, among patients aged 5 to 34 years during the early 1960s [132] and the more recent increase in mortality due to asthma in New Zealand in the late 1970s [31, 194]. In investigating the earlier epidemic in the United Kingdom, Speizer and colleagues [405, 406] found that these deaths were most often sudden and unexpected and were closely correlated with the increased use of pressurized adrenergic aerosols. Conolly and associates [87] suggested that these deaths could have been due to the induction of beta-adrenergic tolerance through excessive use of beta-agonist aerosols with consequential loss of protection afforded by endogenous catecholamines against airway constriction. In the late 1960s, following recognition of the potential danger from the overuse of

pressurized adrenergic aerosols and restrictions on their over-the-counter sale, bronchodilator aerosol usage declined; simultaneously, the asthma death rate fell sharply, suggesting that the previously noted relationship between increasing use of beta-adrenergic aerosols and a rising death rate due to asthma might have been a causal one. It is noteworthy, however, that this decline in the asthma death rate occurred concomitantly not only with a more cautious use of adrenergic bronchodilators but also with a greater reliance on corticosteroids for the treatment of asthma resistant to bronchodilator therapy, suggesting that the corticosteroid therapy might also have contributed to the drop in mortality due to asthma.

Because of their cardiotoxicity, the halogenated hydrocarbons (freons), used as propellants for the adrenergic aerosols, have also been incriminated in the epidemic of asthma deaths [77, 438]. It has been found that, if inhaled in large enough doses, sufficient tissue concentrations of these hydrocarbons can be attained to sensitize the canine myocardium to the arrhythmogenic effects of beta agonists [77, 360]. However, conventional doses of MDIs in humans yield blood levels of fluorocarbons corresponding to myocardial concentrations that are far below those required to produce significant toxicity [77, 105]. These data imply little danger of cardiac toxicity from freon propellants when pressurized inhalers are used in recommended doses.

Several hypotheses have been advanced incriminating beta agonists as contributing to the second epidemic of asthma deaths that occurred in New Zealand in the late 1970s and early 1980s. One suggested factor was a change in the country's prescribing practices, in that inhaled beta agonists along with sustained-release theophylline preparations were prescribed in place of inhaled steroids and cromolyn [496], possibly predisposing to fatal cardiac arrhythmias due to the additive cardiac toxicity between theophylline and adrenergic agents [268, 458]. Another proposed factor was an increased use of beta$_2$ agonists delivered by air-driven home nebulizers for the self-treatment of severe episodes of asthma, thus exposing patients to the risk of hypoxic cardiac arrest if large doses of beta agonists were delivered in the face of hypoxemia uncorrected by continuous oxygen therapy [150]. Two case-control studies involving asthma deaths in patients 5 to 45 years of age in New Zealand in 1981 to 1983 [91] and in 1977 to 1981 [335] have led to a particularly contentious hypothesis linking some of the excess asthma mortality to prescribed fenoterol MDI, which was introduced to New Zealand at the outset of the asthma epidemic in 1976. Since fenoterol MDI delivers twice the equivalent bronchodilator dose of albuterol per puff and causes relatively greater cardiac and hypokalemic effects than albuterol [90, 433], it has been speculated that the risk of death due to asthma could be increased by excessive reliance on self-treatment with relatively high doses of this potent, less-selective beta$_2$ agonist [91]. The validity of this hypothesis has been questioned, however, due to problems in the design of the case-control studies and in the analysis of the data [60, 323, 410]. An alternative hypothesis has been proposed, namely that the risks of overuse of any inhaled beta agonist are increased in patients whose overall quality of care and adherence to appropriate therapy, including antiinflammatory agents, is substandard [410]. This hypothesis is consistent with the greater asthma mortality seen among disadvantaged minority groups [485] who have poorer access to high-quality health care and are more likely to rely excessively on self-treatment with beta agonists and to delay seeking appropriate care.

More recently, Spitzer and colleagues [410a] used health insurance data from Saskatchewan, Canada, for a case-control study of fatal or near-fatal asthma. They found an increased risk of death or near death from asthma in association with regular use of inhaled beta$_2$ agonists, especially fenoterol (odds ratio for death from asthma 5.4 per canister), but also including albuterol (odds ratio 2.4 per canister). The authors concluded that these findings could be due to adverse effects of the beta agonists themselves but raised the alternative possibility that increased use of inhaled beta agonists might simply be a marker of more severe disease.

Beta-Adrenergic Tachyphylaxis: A Current Perspective

The use of normal subjects to define questions of tachyphylaxis clearly backfired in the case of airway smooth muscle. While initial studies in normal subjects showed that both airway and metabolic responses were severely blunted after 14 days of exposure to 400 μg of albuterol taken four times daily by MDI and that intravenously administered hydrocortisone restored the airway defect [182], it was later shown by the same group that asthmatic airways showed no decline in responsiveness [167]. The issue became controversial when several studies showed at least some airway subsensitivity development to oral terbutaline [198], albuterol [309], and fenoterol [348], while two studies found a reduction in the duration of the bronchodilatory response curve following inhaled terbutaline or albuterol [363, 481], in the case of albuterol usage requiring between 4 and 8 weeks to become fully manifest. Yet, as critically reviewed by Svedmyr [423b] and Jenne [196a], other studies refuted this. The essential mystery remains: why do asthmatics show little or no development of airway beta-receptor tachyphylaxis compared to normals? They may already be in an altered state.

What about systemic beta$_2$-receptor responses in asthma? When taking oral beta$_2$ agonists, asthmatics clearly develop subsensitivity with regard to a number of beta-receptor–mediated responses. Do inhaled beta agonists reach systemic receptors in sufficient concentration to induce subsensitivity? When asthmatics on long-term low-dose albuterol delivered by MDI were compared to normals, they had about half the response of pulse rate, tremor, blood glucose level, and potassium concentration to a beta-agonist challenge [502]. Since the asthmatics were not tested off the drug, one cannot be certain that these deficiencies were due to tachyphylaxis. It might have been an inherent defect. However, in another study, while low-dose (800 μg daily) albuterol had little effect on systemic responses, 4,000 μg daily caused a significant reduction (see Table 55-10) [261]. Thus, it seems that systemic responses require large doses of beta agonists administered by inhalation in order to develop subsensitivity. Even on 400 μg of albuterol four times daily by MDI, there was no reduction in the beta-receptor number on peripheral lymphocytes [466, 467], although others have shown a trend toward reduction [88].

However, large doses of inhaled fenoterol, a powerful beta$_2$ agonist, used in an asthmatic crisis, or indeed albuterol, could produce some systemic tachyphylaxis, particularly in the inflammatory components in the airways themselves. A hint that this is so follows from the aforementioned study of asthmatics on oral terbutaline [436]. Although developing no subsensitivity in the ability of subcutaneous terbutaline to protect against methacholine challenge, terbutaline's ability to protect against antigen challenge was impaired and, in one patient tested, intravenous methylprednisolone restored the ability. Again, following oral salbutamol therapy, there was no loss of protection afforded by inhaled beta agonists against histamine reactivity [336], but there was against exercise-induced asthma [142]. If, as suggested by Bruynzeel [57], beta receptors that inhibit inflammatory processes are more susceptible to developing tachyphylaxis than those relaxing airway smooth muscle, tachyphylaxis might still become an adverse factor in combating the crisis of an acute attack, and its amelioration by corticosteroids would be crucial. Indeed, there is experimental evidence that antigen challenge itself desensitizes the relaxation response of smooth muscle to epinephrine, and this is reversed by pretreatment with cortico-

steroids or indomethacin [93a]. A growing body of evidence supports the position that inflammatory products adversely affect beta-adrenergic receptor function.

With their use imminent, the question also arises whether the constant beta$_2$ stimulation of salmeterol and formoterol will produce deleterious tachyphylaxis despite their apparent ability to suppress the acute inflammatory response. This remains to be seen. When accompanied by inhaled corticosteroids, they do not lose their bronchodilator efficacy [459]. But, will they lose some efficacy against antigen challenge, especially if not accompanied by a corticosteroid?

Finally, one of the most interesting issues today is the question of hyperreactivity induced by inhaled beta agonists. Several studies have shown a temporary increase in reactivity to histamine upon withdrawal of inhaled beta agonists [227, 235, 467, 468]. The increase is not great, ranging from 0.6 to 1.5 doubling units. Whether this hyperreactivity represents a more subtle index of smooth muscle subsensitivity than can be demonstrated with bronchodilator dose-response curves, or whether it is an independent quality, remains to be seen. Working with an intact guinea pig model, Morley and colleagues [303a] believe that the two are unrelated. Related to this is the recent report by Sears and colleagues [389], which stated that the majority of asthmatics on a constant schedule of inhaled fenoterol, most on inhaled corticosteroids, have increased bronchial hyperreactivity compared to those who use it on an intermittent, as needed, basis. Their morning peak flows and asthma symptoms also worsen. If confirmed, the findings of this study are not necessarily an argument against the use of constant bronchodilation by beta agonists when clearly necessary in the comfortable control of asthma, but probably are an argument for the concomitant use of inhaled corticosteroids, both for their acknowledged antiinflammatory effects and their protection against tachyphylaxis of multiple beta receptors in the airway.

The above experience with airway reactivity, and the New Zealand and Saskatchewan retrospective case-control studies with fenoterol [91, 335, 410a] have unsettled the medical community regarding the potential adverse effects of beta$_2$ agonists on asthma, even with respect to the new, long-acting beta$_2$ agonists. These studies cannot necessarily be extended to preclude the "time-honored" and favorable practices with albuterol and terbutaline, as pointed out in recent, pithy editorials [264a, 309a], provided that antiinflammatory compounds are properly utilized. Nevertheless, we need more information on the mechanisms at work as they may adversely affect the action of these compounds.

Approach to the Treatment of Asthma: Role of Beta-Adrenergic Agonists

Guidelines for the management of asthma, representing the consensus opinions of specialists, including chest physicians, allergists, and pediatricians, have recently been published [48, 49, 160, 307]. The impetus for the establishment of these guidelines was the worldwide increase in morbidity and mortality from asthma, which has been attributed, in part, to underuse of antiinflammatory agents [47, 59, 110] and, by some authorities, to inappropriate use of inhaled beta agonists [91, 389]. Recommendations concerning the use of beta agonists are dependent on both the severity of asthma and whether it is chronically persistent or acutely severe.

Use of Beta Agonists in Acute Severe Asthma

It is uniformly agreed that beta$_2$ agonists should be used at least as required, preferably by inhalation in doses of 1 to 2 puffs from an MDI (or the equivalent dose from a DPI), for relief of acute symptoms of asthma and for prevention of symptoms due to exposure to exercise, allergens, or other stimuli [49, 160, 307]. In patients with infrequent symptoms of asthma and normal or near-normal lung function, this may be the only treatment required. When symptoms are more severe, occur more often, are more persistent, or require more frequent as-needed use of an inhaled beta agonist, and are associated with a greater reduction in forced expiratory flow, regularly scheduled maintenance therapy is required to achieve satisfactory asthma control (i.e., minimal symptoms, normal activity tolerance, and optimum lung function).

Asthma severity and the need for asthma therapy [161, 241] are believed to be linked to the degree of airway inflammation. Therefore, the primary emphasis for *maintenance* treatment of chronic, persistent asthma is now placed on antiinflammatory therapy [24, 160, 504], especially the use of inhaled corticosteroids, supplemented, if necessary, by short courses ("bursts") of oral corticosteroids. In patients with moderate to severe asthma, the usual practice is to continue the use of inhaled beta agonists, not only as needed, but also on a regularly scheduled basis, in conjunction with topical corticosteroids. Beta-agonist aerosols are preferably used prior to the inhalation of the inhaled corticosteroids to enhance penetration of the latter aerosols to the lung periphery. As asthma severity increases, higher doses of inhaled corticosteroids are recommended, and oral bronchodilators (sustained-release theophylline or oral beta agonists, or both), with or without an inhaled anticholinergic, may be added, especially for the relief of nocturnal symptoms. In addition, oral corticosteroids are usually required in relatively short courses for otherwise uncontrolled exacerbations of symptoms. If adequate control cannot be achieved with maximum doses of inhaled corticosteroids, together with 3- to 4-times-daily inhaled beta agonists and around-the-clock oral bronchodilator therapy, as well as periodic "bursts" of oral corticosteroids, maintenance treatment with daily, or preferably alternate-day, oral corticosteroids should be considered.

The results of a recent study raise serious questions concerning the efficacy and safety of regularly scheduled, as opposed to simply as-needed, inhalations of a beta-agonist aerosol [389]. Sixty-four asthmatics with stable disease, most of whom were already receiving maintenance therapy with inhaled corticosteroids, completed a double-blind cross-over trial of regular (four times daily) treatment with inhaled fenoterol plus as-needed treatment with an inhaled beta agonist in comparison with as-needed treatment alone. Each treatment period lasted 24 weeks. The maintenance inhaler contained either fenoterol dispensed as a dry powder (200 μg per dose; two doses per treatment) or a placebo dry powder. The as-needed inhaler consisted of an MDI of either fenoterol (200 μg per puff), albuterol (100 μg per puff), or terbutaline (250 μg per puff). Asthma control was assessed on the basis of nocturnal and daytime symptoms, the need for nocturnal bronchodilator therapy, a change in prednisone requirements, the morning peak expiratory flow, and the degree of methacholine reactivity. Significantly more subjects achieved better control of their asthma during as-needed only bronchodilator inhaler treatment than during regularly scheduled treatment (70% versus 30%, respectively).

It is not clear whether the adverse effects of regular (as opposed to as-needed only) use of an inhaled beta agonist demonstrated in the latter study [389] can be generalized to all inhaled bronchodilators or are specific to fenoterol, which is less beta$_2$ specific than albuterol or terbutaline and is generally dispensed in twice the bioequivalent aerosol dose as that of other inhaled beta agonists. The mechanism, or mechanisms, whereby regular treatment with a beta agonist could lead to deterioration of asthma are unclear but could include the following: (1) a possible adverse effect on mucus [139, 491], (2) protection against the acute (but not the late) phase of antigen-induced asthma, thus predisposing to exposure to greater doses of allergen [389]; and (3) desensitization of beta-adrenergic receptors (on airway

smooth muscle, mast cells, lymphocytes, or other cells) that may play an important homeostatic role in asthma. The small but significant increases in nonspecific airways hyperreactivity noted by several authors several hours after withdrawal of beta-adrenergic therapy [227, 235, 468] would be consistent with tachyphylaxis. However, the latter was considered an unlikely explanation because of the high evening peak expiratory flow rates observed in the patients receiving regular inhaled beta agonists and the lack of the expected protection from inhaled corticosteroids which most of the patients were prescribed. Moreover, others have found a small but significant increase in airways hyperreactivity in asthmatics after inhaling albuterol during one year, without concomitant evidence of tachyphylaxis to the acute bronchodilator effect of the beta agonist [467]. Clearly, additional well-designed studies are required to address the important question of whether regularly scheduled therapy with customary doses of inhaled beta agonists other than fenoterol, especially the longer-acting agents salmeterol and formoterol, leads to better or poorer control of chronic asthma than does as-needed inhaled bronchodilator therapy alone.

Severe exacerbations of asthma are associated with marked airways inflammation, tissue damage, and airflow limitation, accompanied by variable hypoxemia. Although corticosteroids are needed to reverse the inflammatory changes, these changes require hours to days to reverse. Of greater urgency is the need for prompt relief of the symptoms of respiratory distress by reducing airflow obstruction to the maximum extent possible, while simultaneously treating hypoxemia with supplemental oxygen. As discussed earlier, inhaled beta agonists must be administered immediately and in larger and more frequent doses for the treatment of these acute exacerbations than would be the case for maintenance therapy [9, 49, 160], using either an MDI with a valved spacer or a power nebulizer. In most cases, inhaled beta agonists, if administered in sufficiently large and frequent doses, provide relief comparable to that achieved with parenteral beta agonists, with fewer side effects [26, 457, 471]. However, if satisfactory improvement cannot be achieved using the inhaled route, parental beta agonists (subcutaneous epinephrine or terbutaline or intravenous terbutaline or albuterol, if available) may prove effective and obviate the need for intubation and mechanical ventilation. If mechanical ventilation becomes necessary, beta agonists may need to be administered parenterally, since delivery of aerosols from both in-line-solution nebulizers and MDIs (using special adaptors) to intubated, mechanically ventilated patients is far less efficient than delivery to the spontaneously breathing patient [92, 131, 135, 269]. It is important to emphasize that, when beta agonists are given parenterally or in high, frequent doses by inhalation, the patient must be monitored closely for cardiac and other systemic side effects, including hypokalemia.

REFERENCES

1. Aarons, R. D., et al. Decreased beta adrenergic receptor density on human lymphocytes after chronic treatment with agonists. *J. Pharmacol. Exp. Ther.* 224:1, 1983.
2. Adelstein, R. S., et al. Regulation of smooth muscle contractile proteins by calmodulin and cyclic AMP. *Fed. Proc.* 41:2873, 1982.
3. Affrime, M., et al. Therapeutic efficacy of albuterol in asthmatic patients. *Acta Pharmacol. Toxicol.* 59(suppl. 5):228, 1986.
4. Ahlquist, R. P. A study of adrenotropic receptors. *Am. J. Physiol.* 153:586, 1948.
5. Ahrens, R. C., et al. A method for comparing the peak intensity and duration of action of aerosolized bronchodilators using bronchoprovocation with methacholine. *Am. Rev. Respir. Dis.* 129:903, 1984.
6. Al-Bazzaz, F. J., and Cheng, E. Effect of catecholamines on ion transport in dog tracheal epithelium. *J. Appl. Physiol.* 47:397, 1979.
7. Albuterol Product Information. *Physicians' Desk Reference, 1992.* Oradell, N.J.: Medical Economics, 1992. Pp. 583–585.

8. Allon, M., Dunlay, R., and Copkney, C. Nebulized albuterol for acute hyperkalemia in patients on dialysis. *Ann. Intern Med.* 110:426, 1989.
9. American Respiratory Care Foundation (ARCF) and American Association for Respiratory Care (AARC). Consensus statement of the conference on aerosol delivery. *Respi. Care* 36:916, 1991.
10. Amory, D. W., Burnham, S. C., and Cheney, F. W. Jr. Comparison of the cardiopulmonary effects of subcutaneously administered epinephrine and terbutaline in patients with reversible airway obstruction. *Chest* 67:279, 1979.
11. Anderson, R. G. G., and Kovesi, G. The effect of hydrocortisone on tension and cyclic AMP metabolism in tracheal smooth muscle. *Experientia* 30:784, 1974.
12. Anderson, S. D., et al. Inhaled and oral salbutamol in exercise-induced asthma. *Am. Rev. Respir. Dis.* 114:495, 1976.
13. Antic, R., and Macklem, P. T. The influence of clinical factors on site of airway obstruction in asthma. *Am. Rev. Respir. Dis.* 114:851, 1976.
14. Appel, D., Karpel, J. P., and Sherman, M. Epinephrine improves expiratory flow rates in patients with asthma who do not respond to inhaled metaproterenol sulfate. *J. Allergy Clin. Immunol.* 84:90, 1989.
15. Arvidsson, P., et al. Formaterol, a new long-acting bronchodilator for inhalation. *Eur. Respir. J.* 2:325, 1989.
16. Austin, K. F. The chemical mediators of immediate hypersensitivity reactions. In M. Samter, (ed.), *Immunological Disease.* Boston: Little, Brown, 1978. Vol. 1, P. 183.
17. Avner, B. P., and Jenne, J. W. Desensitization of isolated human bronchial smooth muscle to B-receptor agonists. *J. Allergy Clin. Immunol.* 68:51, 1981.
18. Avner, B. P., and Noland, B. In vivo desensitization to beta receptor mediated bronchodilator drugs in the rat: decreased beta receptor affinity. *J. Pharmacol. Exp. Ther.* 207:23, 1978.
19. Bai, T. R. and Prasad, F. W. Abnormalities in airway smooth muscle in fatal asthma. *Am. Rev. Respir. Dis.* 141:552, 1990.
19a. Balazs, T., and Bloom, S. Cardiotoxicity of adrenergic bronchodilator and vasodilating antihypertensive drugs. In E. W. Van Stee (ed.), *Cardiovascular Toxicology.* New York: Raven, 1982, Pp. 199–220.
20. Ball, D. I., et al. Salmeterol, a novel, long-acting β_2-adrenoceptor agonist: Characterization of pharmacological activity in vitro and in vivo. *Br. J. Pharmacol.* 104:665, 1991.
21. Banner, A. S., et al. Arrhythmogenic effects of orally administered bronchodilators. *Arch. Intern. Med.* 139:434, 1979.
22. Barger, G., and Dale, H. H. Chemical structure and sympathomimetic action of amines. *J. Physiol.* (Lond.) 41:19, 1910.
23. Barker, J. A., et al. Tracheal mucosal blood flow responses to autonomic agonists. *J. Appl. Physiol.* 65:829, 1988.
24. Barnes, P. J. The changing face of asthma. *Q. J. Med.* 63(241):359, 1987.
25. Barnes, P. J. Adrenergic regulation of airway fucntion. In M. A. Kaliner and P. J. Barnes (eds.), *The Airways (Vol. 33, Lung Biology in Health and Disease).* New York: Dekker, 1988, P. 57.
26. Baughman, R. P., Ploysongsong, Y., and James, W. A comparative study of aerosolized terbutaline and subcutaneously administered epinephrine in the treatment of acute bronchial asthma. *Ann. Allergy* 53:131, 1984.
27. Beamish, R. W., Singal, P. K., and Dhalla, N. S. Stress and heart disease. In Proceedings of the International Symposium on Stress and Heart Disease, June 26–29, 1984, Winnipeg, Canada. Boston: Martinus-Nijhoff, 1984.
28. Beck, G. J. Controlled clinical trial of a new dosage form of metaproterenol. *Ann. Allergy* 44:19, 1980.
29. Becker, A. B., Nelson, N. A., and Simons, F. E. R. Inhaled salbutamol (albuterol) vs. injected epinephrine in the treatment of acute asthma in children. *J. Pediatr.* 102:465, 1983.
30. Becker, A. B., and Simons, F. E. R. Formaterol, a new long-acting selective β_2-adrenergic receptor agonist: double blind comparison with salbutamol and placebo in children with asthma. *J. Allergy Clin. Immunol.* 84:891, 1989.
31. Benatar, S. Fatal asthma. *N. Engl. J. Med.* 314:423, 1986.
32. Benson, R. L., and Perlman, F. Clinical effects of epinephrine by inhalation. *J. Allergy* 19:120, 1948.
33. Benton, G., et al. Experience with a metered-dose inhaler with a spacer in the pediatric emergency department. *Am. J. Dis. Child.* 143:678, 1989.
34. Beumer, H. M. Pirbuterol aerosol versus salbutamol and placebo aerosols in bronchial asthma. *Drugs Exp. Clin. Res.* 2:77, 1980.
35. Blackwell, E. W., et al. Metabolism of isoprenaline after aerosol and direct intrabronchial administration in man and dog. *Br. J. Pharmacol.* 50:587, 1974.
36. Blake, K., et al. Relative amount of albuterol delivered to lung receptors from a metered dose inhaler and nebulizer solution; bioassay by histamine provocation. *Chest* 101:309, 1992.
37. Bloomfield, P., et al. Comparison of salbutamol given intravenously and by intermittent positive-pressure breathing in life-threatening asthma. *Br. J. Med.* 1:848, 1979.
38. Bohn, D., et al. Intravenous salbutamol in the treatment of status asthmaticus in children. *Crit. Care Med.* 12:892, 1984.
39. Bolton, T. B. Mechanisms of action of transmitters and other substances in smooth muscle. *Physiol. Rev.* 59:606, 1979.
40. Borson, D. B., et al. Adrenergic and cholinergic nerves mediate fluid secretion from tracheal glands of ferrets. *J. Appl. Physiol.* 49:1027, 1980.
41. Borum, P., and Mygind, N. Inhibition of the immediate allergic reaction of the nose by the beta-2 adrenostimulant fenoterol. *J. Allergy Clin. Immunol.* 66:25, 1980.
42. Bouhuys, A., and van de Woestijne, K. P. Mechanical consequences of airway smooth muscle relaxation. *J. Appl. Physiol.* 30:670, 1971.
43. Bouvier, M., et al. Regulation of adrenergic function by phosphorylation. II. Effects of agonist occupancy on phosphorylation of alpha$_1$ and beta$_2$-adrenergic receptors by protein kinase C and the cyclic AMP-dependent protein kinase. *J. Biol. Chem.* 262:3106, 1987.
44. Bowman, W. C., and Knott, M. W. Actions of sympathomimetic amines and their antagonists on skeletal muscle. *Pharmacol. Rev.* 21:27, 1969.
45. Bradshaw, J., et al. The design of salmeterol, a long-acting selective beta$_2$-adrenoceptor agonist. *Br. J. Pharmacol.* 91(suppl):590P, 1987.
46. Brent, B. N., et al. Augmentation of right ventricular performance in chronic obstructive pulmonary disease by terbutaline: a combined radionuclide and hemodynamic study. *Am. J. Cardiol.* 50:313, 1982.
47. British Thoracic Association. Death from asthma in two regions of England. *Br. Med. J.* 285:1251, 1982.
48. British Thoracic Society. Guidelines for management of asthma in adults. I. Chronic persistent asthma. *BMJ* 301:651, 1991.
49. British Thoracic Society. Guidelines for management of asthma in adults. II. Acute severe asthma. *BMJ* 301:797, 1991.
50. Brittain, R. T. A comparison of the pharmacology profile of salbutamol with that of isoproterenol, orciprenaline (metaproterenol) and trimetoquinol. *Postgrad. Med. J.* 47:11, 1971.
51. Brittain, R. T. Approaches to a long-acting, selective beta$_2$-adrenoceptor stimulant. *Lung* 168(suppl):111, 1990.
52. Brittain, R. T., Dean, C. M., and Jack D. Sympathomimetic bronchodilator drugs. *Pharmacol. Ther. Bull.* 2:423, 1976.
53. Brittain, R. T., Jack, D., and Ritchie, A. C. Recent beta-adrenoreceptor stimulants. *Adv. Drug Res.* 5:197, 1970.
54. Brodde, O.-E., et al. Terbutaline-induced desensitization of human lymphocyte B$_2$-adrenoceptors. Accelerated restoration of β-adrenoceptor responsiveness by prednisone and ketotifen. *J. Clin. Invest.* 76:1096, 1985.
55. Brogden, R. N., Speight, T. M., and Avery, G. S. Terbutaline: a preliminary report of its pharmacological properties and therapeutic efficacy in asthma. *Drugs* 6:324, 1973.
56. Brumlik, J. On the nature of normal tremor. *Neurology* 12:159, 1962.
57. Bruynzeel, P. L. B. Changes in the β-adrenergic system due to β-adrenergic therapy: clinical consequences. *Eur. J. Respir. Dis.* 135:62, 1984.
58. Bryant, D. H. Nebulized ipratropium bromide in the treatment of acute asthma. *Chest* 88:24, 1985.
59. Bucknall, C. E., et al. Differences in hospital management. *Lancet* 1:748, 1988.
60. Buist, A. S., et al. Fenoterol and fatal asthma (letter). *Lancet* 334:1071, 1989.
61. Bulbring, E., and den Hertog, A. The action of isoprenaline on the smooth muscle of the guinea pig taenia coli. *J. Physiol.* 304:277, 1980.
62. Burgess, C. D., et al. The hemodynamic effects of aminophylline and salbutamol alone and in combination. *Clin. Pharmacol. Ther.* 40:550, 1986.
63. Burgess, C. D., et al. Lack of evidence for beta-2 receptor selectivity: a study of metaproterenol, fenoterol, isoproterenol, and epinephrine in patients with asthma. *Am. Rev. Respir. Dis.* 143:444, 1991.
64. Butcher, P. R., Cousins, S. A., and Vardey, C. J. Salmeterol: a potent and long-acting inhibitor of the release of inflammatory and spasmogenic mediators from human lung. *Br. J. Pharmacol.* 92:745P, 1987.
65. Camner, P., Strandberg, K., and Philipson, K. Increased mucociliary transport by adrenergic stimulation. *Arch. Environ. Health* 31:79, 1976.
66. Carstairs, J. R., Nimmo, A. J., and Barnes, P. J. Autoradiographic visualization of beta-adrenoceptor subtypes in human lung. *Am. Rev. Respir. Dis.* 132:541, 1985.
67. Casteels, E. Electro and pharmacomechanical coupling in vascular smooth muscle. *Chest* 78(suppl):150, 1980.

68. Cayton, R. M., et al. A comparison of salbutamol given by pressure-packed aerosol or nebulization via IPPB in acute asthma. *Br. J. Dis. Chest* 72:222, 1978.
69. Cerrina, J., et al. Comparison of human bronchial muscle responses to histamine in vivo with histamine and isoproterenol agonists in vitro. *Am. Rev. Respir. Dis.* 134:57, 1986.
70. Chapman, K. R., et al. Hemodynamic effects of an inhaled beta-2 agonist. *Clin. Pharmacol. Ther.* 35:762, 1984.
71. Chervinsky, P. Alupent syrup: results of a six-month trial in asthmatic children. *Ann. Allergy* 34:170, 1975.
72. Chervinsky, P. A. A comparative evaluation of fenoterol and terbutaline in the treatment of asthma. *Ann. Allergy* 40:189, 1978.
73. Chervinsky, P., and Chervinsky, G. Metaproterenol tablets: their duration of effect by comparison with ephedrine. *Cur. Ther. Res.* 17:507, 1975.
74. Choo-Kang, Y. F. J., MacDonald, H. L., and Horne, N. W. A comparison of salbutamol and terbutaline aerosols in bronchial asthma. *Practitioner* 211:801, 1973.
74a. Christensson, P., Arborelius, M. Jr., and Lilja, B. Salbutamol inhalation in chronic asthma bronchiale: dose aerosol vs. jet nebulizer. *Chest* 79:416, 1981.
75. Chung, K. F., Keyes, S. J., and Snashall, P. D. Histamine dose-response relationships in normals and asthmatic subjects. The importance of starting caliber. *Am. Rev. Respir. Dis.* 126:849, 1981.
76. Clark, B. J. Beta-adrenoceptor–blocking agents: are pharmacological differences relevant? *Am. Heart J.* 104:334, 1982.
77. Clark, D. G., and Tinston, D. J. The influence of fluorocarbon propellants on the arrhythmogenic activities of adrenaline and isoprenaline. *Proc. Eur. Soc. Study Drug Toxicity* 13:212, 1972.
78. Clausen, T., and Flatman, J. A. The effect of catecholamines on Na-K transport and membrane potential in rat soleus muscle. *J. Phyiol.* (Lond.) 270:383, 1977.
79. Cockcroft, D. W., et al. Protective effect of drug on histamine-induced asthma. *Thorax* 32:429, 1977.
80. Cole, A. G., Arkin, D., and Soloman R. J. In C. Wood and W. Sommerville (eds.), *International Congress and Symposium Series No. 44.* London: Royal Society of Medicine, 1986, P. 47.
81. Coleman, R. A., Ball, D. I., and Nials, A. T. Potency and duration of action of salmeterol on guinea-pig airways in vitro and in vivo (abstract). *Am. Rev. Respir. Dis.* 143:A468, 1991.
82. Coleman, R. A., Nials, A. T., and Johnson, M. Salmeterol: a potent and long-acting beta₂ adrenoceptor agonist (abstract). *Am. Rev. Respir. Dis.* 143:A648, 1991.
83. Collier, J. G., Dobbs, R. J., and Williams, I. S. Salbutamol aerosol causes a tachycardia due to inhaled rather than swallowed fraction. *Br. J. Clin. Pharmocol.* 9:273, 1981.
84. Collins, J. M., et al. The cardio-toxicity of isoprenaline during hypoxia. *Br. J. Pharmacol.* 36:35, 1969.
85. Conolly, M. E., and Greenacre, J. K. The lymphocyte beta-adrenoceptor in normal subjects and patients with bronchial asthma. The effect of different forms of treatment on receptor function. *J. Clin. Invest.* 58:1307, 1976.
86. Conolly, M. E., et al. A comparison of the cardiorespiratory effects of isoprenaline and salbutamol in patients with bronchial asthma. *Postgrad. Med. J.* 47(suppl):77, 1971.
87. Conolly, M. E., et al. Resistance to beta adrenoceptor stimulants (a possible explanation for the rise in asthma deaths). *Br. J. Pharmacol.* 43:380, 1971.
88. Conolly, M. E., et al. Selective subsensitization of beta-adrenergic receptors in central airways of asthmatics and normal subjects during long-term therapy with inhaled salbutamol. *J. Allergy Clin. Immunol.* 70:423, 1982.
89. Conradson, T. B. Cardiovascular effects of two different xanthines in healthy subjects. Studies at rest, during exercise and in combination with a beta-agonist, terbutaline. *Eur. J. Clin. Pharmacol.* 27:319, 1984.
90. Crane, J., Burgess C., and Beasley, R. Cardiovascular and hypokalemic effects of inhaled salbutamol, fenoterol, and isoprenaline. *Thorax* 44:136, 1989.
91. Crane, J., et al. Prescribed fenoterol and death from asthma in New Zealand, 1981–83: case-control study. *Lancet* 1:917, 1989.
92. Crogan, S. J., and Bishop, M. J. Delivery efficiency of metered dose aerosols given via endotracheal tube. *Anesthesiology* 70:1008, 1989.
93. Cushley, M. J., Lewis, R. A., and Tattersfield, A. E. Comparison of three techniques of inhalation on the airway response to terbutaline. *Thorax* 38:90, 1983.

93a. Daffonchio, L., et al. β-adrenoceptor desensitization induced by antigen challenge in guinea-pig trachea. *Eur. J. Pharmacol.* 178:21, 1990.
94. Daniel, E. E., et al. Ultrastructural studies on the neuromuscular control of human tracheal and bronchial smooth muscle. *Respir. Physiol.* 109, 1986.
95. Danser, A. H. J., et al. Prejunctional β-adrenoceptors inhibit cholinergic transmission in canine bronchi. *J. Appl. Physiol.* 62:785, 1987.
96. Davies, A. O., and Lefkowitz, R. J. In vitro and in vivo desensitization of beta-adrenergic receptors in human neutrophils. Attenuation by corticosteroids. *J. Clin. Invest.* 71:565, 1983.
97. Davies, D. S. The fate of inhaled terbutaline. *Eur. J. Respir. Dis.* 65(suppl 134):141, 1984.
98. Davies, D. S. Metabolism of isoprenaline and other bronchodilator drugs in man and dog. *Bull. Physiopathol. Respir.* 8:679, 1972.
99. Davis, C., and Conolly, M. E. Tachyphylaxis to beta-adrenoceptor agonists in human bronchial smooth muscle. Studies in vitro. *Br. J. Pharmacol.* 10:417, 1980.
100. Davis, C., and Kannan, M. S. Sympathetic innervation of human tracheal and bronchial smooth muscle. *Respir. Physiol.* 68:53, 1987.
101. Decker, N., et al. Effects of N-aralkyl substitution of β-agonists on α- and β-adrenoceptor subtypes: pharmacological studies and binding assays. *J. Pharm. Pharmacol.* 34:107, 1982.
102. De Fronzo, R. A., Bia, M., and Birkhead G. Epinephrine and potassium homeostasis. *Kidney Int.* 20:83, 1981.
103. deLanerolle, P., and Stull, J. T. Myosin phosphorylation during contraction and relaxation of tracheal smooth muscle. *J. Biol. Chem.* 255:9993, 1980.
104. Dohlman, H. G., Caron, M. G., and Lefkowitz, R. J. A family of receptors coupled to guanine nucleotide regulatory proteins. *Biochem. J.* 26:2657, 1987.
105. Dollery, C. T., et al. Arterial blood levels of fluorocarbons in asthmatic patients following use of pressurized aerosol. *Clin. Pharmacol. Ther.* 15:59, 1974.
106. Douglas, J. S., et al. Tachyphylaxis to β-adrenoceptor agonists in guinea pig airway smooth muscle in vivo and in vitro. *Eur. J. Pharmacol.* 42:195, 1977.
107. Drislane, F. W., et al. Myocardial contraction band lesions in patients with fatal asthma: possible neurocardiologic mechanisms. *Am. Rev. Respir. Dis.* 135:498, 1987.
108. D'Silva, J. L. The action of adrenaline on serum potassium. *J. Physiol.* (Lond.) 82:393, 1934.
109. Dulfano, M. J., and Glass, P. Evaluation of a new β₂ adrenergic receptor stimulant, terbutaline, in bronchial asthma. II. Oral comparison with ephedrine. *Curr. Ther. Res.* 15:150, 1973.
110. Eason, J., and Markow, H. L. J. Controlled investigation of deaths from asthma in hospitals in the North East Thames region. *Br. Med. J.* 294:1255, 1987.
111. Eggleston, P. A., Beasley, P. P., and Kindly, R. T. The effects of oral doses of theophylline and fenoterol in exercise-induced asthma. *Chest* 70:399, 1981.
112. Eisenstadt, W. S., and Nicholas, S. S. The adverse effects of adrenergic aerosols in bronchial asthma. *Ann. Allergy* 27:283, 1969.
113. Ellul-Michallef, R., and Fenech, F. F. Effect of intravenous prednisolone in asthmatics with diminished adrenergic responsiveness. *Lancet* 2:1269, 1975.
114. Erjefalt, I., and Persson, C. G. A. Pharmacological control of plasma exudation in the tracheobronchial airways. *Am. Rev. Respir. Dis.* 143:1008, 1991.
115. Evans, W. V., et al. Aminophylline, salbutamol and combined intravenous infusions in acute severe asthma. *Br. J. Dis. Chest* 74:385, 1980.
116. Exton, J. H. Molecular mechanisms involved in alpha-adrenergic responses. *Trends Pharmacol. Sci.* 3:111, 1982.
117. Fairfax, A. J., et al. Slow-release oral salbutamol and aminophylline in nocturnal asthma: relation of overnight changes in lung function and plasma drug levels. *Thorax* 35:526, 1980.
118. Fairfax, A. J., et al. Comparison between the effects of inhaled isoprenaline and fenoterol on plasma cyclic AMP and heart rate in normal subjects. *Br. J. Clin. Pharmacol.* 17:165, 1984.
119. Fairshter, R. D., and Wilson, A. F. Relationship between the site of airflow limitation and localization of the bronchodilator response in asthma. *Am. Rev. Respir. Dis.* 122:27, 1980.
120. Fanta, C. H., Rossing, T. H., and McFadden, E. R. Jr. Emergency room treatment of asthma. Relationship among therapeutic combinations, severity of obstruction and time course of response. *Am. J. Med.* 72:416, 1982.

121. Fanta, C. H., Rossing, T. H., and McFadden, E. R. Jr. Treatment of acute asthma. Is combination theapy with sympathomimetics and methylxanthines indicated? *Am. J. Med.* 80:5, 1986.

122. Faulds, D., Hillingshead, L. M., and Goa, K. L. Formoterol. A review of its pharmacologic properties and therapeutic efficacy in reversible obstructive airways disease. *Drugs* 42:115, 1991.

123. Fitchett, D. H., McNichol, M. W., and Riordan, J. F. Intravenous salbutamol in management of status asthmaticus. *Br. Med. J.* 1:53, 1975.

124. Fitzgerald, G. A., et al. Circulating adrenaline and blood pressure: the metabolic effects and kinetics of infused adrenaline in man. *Eur. J. Clin. Invest.* 10:401, 1980.

125. Fitzpatrick, M. F., et al. Salmeterol in nocturnal asthma: a double-blind, placebo-controlled trial of a long-acting inhaled beta$_2$ agonist. *BMJ* 301:1365, 1990.

126. Flatt, A., et al. The cardiovascular effects of inhaled fenoterol alone and during treatment with oral theophylline. *Chest* 96:1317, 1989.

127. FDA. Interactions between methylxanthines and beta-adrenergic agonists. *FDA Drug Bull.* 11:19, 1981.

128. Formgren, H. Clinical comparison of inhaled terbutaline and orciprenaline in asthmatic patients. *Scand. J. Respir. Dis.* 51:203, 1970.

129. Fortier, M., et al. Beta-adrenergic catecholamine-dependent properties of rat myometrium primary cultures. *Am. J. Physiol.* 245:C84, 1983.

130. Fraser, C. M., and Venter, J. C. The synthesis of beta-adrenergic receptors in cultured human lung cells: induction by glucocorticoids. *Biochem. Biophys. Res. Comm.* 94:390, 1980.

131. Fraser, I., et al. Therapeutic aerosol delivery in ventilator systems (abstract). *Am. Rev. Respir. Dis.* 123(No. 4, Part 2):107, 1981.

132. Fraser, P., and Doll, R. Geographical variations in the epidemic of asthma deaths. *Br. J. Prev. Soc. Med.* 25:34, 1971.

133. Freedman, B. J. Trial of a terbutaline aerosol in the treatment of asthma and a comparison of its effects with those of a salbutamol aerosol. *Br. J. Dis. Chest.* 66:222, 1972.

134. Freedman, B. J., and Hill, G. B. Comparative study of duration of action and cardiovascular effects of bronchodilator aerosol. *Thorax* 26:46, 1971.

135. Fuller, H. D., et al. Pressurized aerosol versus jet aerosol delivery to mechanically ventilated patients. *Am. Rev. Respir. Dis.* 141:440, 1990.

136. Gaddie, J., Legge, J. S., and Palmer, K. N. V. Aerosols of salbutamol, terbutaline, and isoprenaline/phenylephrine in asthma. *Br. J. Dis. Chest* 67:215, 1973.

137. Galant, S. P., et al. The effect of metaproterenol in chronic asthmatic children receiving therapeutic doses of theophylline. *J. Allergy Clin. Immunol.* 61:73, 1978.

138. Galant, S. P., et al. Beta adrenergic receptors of polymorphonuclear particulates in bronchial asthma. *J. Clin. Invest.* 65:577, 1980.

139. Gallagher, J. T., et al. The composition of tracheal mucus and the nervous control of its secretion in the cat. *Proc. R. Soc. Lond [Biol.]* 192:49, 1975.

140. Geumei, A. M., et al. Bronchodilator effect of a new oral beta-adrenoceptor stimulant TH1165a. A comparison with metaproterenol sulfate. *Chest* 70:460, 1976.

141. Gibson, D. G., and Coltart, D. J. Hemodynamic effects of intravenous salbutamol in patients with mitral valve disease: comparison with isoproterenol and atropine. *Medicine* 47:40, 1971.

142. Gibson, G. J., et al. Use of exercise challenge to investigate possible tolerance to beta adrenoceptor stimulation in asthma. *Br. J. Dis. Chest* 72:199, 1978.

143. Gilman, A. G., et al. *The Pharmacological Basis of Therapeutics.* New York: Pergamon Press, 1990, Pp. 102.

144. Glass, P., and Dulfano, M. J. Evaluation of a new β$_2$-adrenergic receptor stimulant, terbutaline, in bronchial asthma. I. Subcutaneous comparison with epinephrine. *Curr. Ther. Res.* 15:141, 1973.

145. Godden, D. J. Reflex and nervous control of the tracheobronchial circulation. *Eur. J. Clin. Pharmacol.* 3(suppl. 12):602s, 1990.

146. Goldie, R. G., et al. Classification of beta-receptors in human isolated bronchus. *Br. J. Pharmacol.* 81:611, 1984.

147. Goldie, R. G., et al. In vitro responsiveness of human asthmatic bronchus to carbachol, histamine, beta-adrenoceptor agonists and theophylline. *Br. J. Pharmacol.* 22:669, 1986.

148. Goldie, R. G., et al. Airway epithelium-derived inhibitory factor. *TIPS* 11:67, 1990.

149. Graeser, J. B. Inhalation therapy of bronchial asthma. *JAMA* 112:1223, 1939.

150. Grant, I. W. B. Asthma in New Zealand. *Br. Med. J.* 286:374, 1983.

151. Greenberg, M. J., and Pines, A. Pressurized aerosols in asthma. (letter). *Br. Med. J.* 1:563, 1967.

152. Grossman, J. The occurrence of arrhythmias in hospitalized asthmatic patients. *J. Allergy Clin. Immunol.* 57:310, 1976.

153. Guideri, G., Barletta, M., and Lehr, D. Extraordinary potentiation of isoproterenol cardiotoxicity by corticoid pretreatment. *Cardiovasc. Res.* 8:775, 1974.

154. Haalboom, J. R. E., Deenstra, M., and Struyvenberg, A. Hypokalemia induced by inhalation of fenoterol. *Lancet* 1:1125, 1985.

155. Hadcock, J. R., Wang, H.-Y., and Malbon, C. C. Agonist-induced destabilization of β-adrenergic receptor mRNA. *J. Biol. Chem.* 264:19928, 1989.

156. Hall, I. P., and Chilvers, E. R. Inositol phosphates and airway smooth muscle. *Pulm. Pharmacol.* 2:113, 1989.

157. Hall, I. P., and Hill, S. J. β-adrenoceptor stimulation inhibits histamine stimulated inositol phospholipid hydrolysis in bovine tracheal smooth muscle. *Br. J. Pharmacol.* 95:1204, 1988.

158. Hall, J. A., Kaumann, A. J., and Brown, M. J. Selective beta$_1$-adrenoceptor blockade enhances positive inotropic rsponses to endogenous catecholamines mediated through beta$_2$-adrenoceptors in human atrial myocardium. *Circ. Res.* 66:1610, 1990.

159. Hargreave, F. E. The drug treatment of asthma: how can it be better applied? *Postgrad. Med. J.* 64(suppl 4):74, 1988.

160. Hargreave, F. E., Dolovich, J., and Newhouse, M. T. The assessment and treatment of asthma: a conference report. *J. Allergy Clin. Immunol.* 85:1098, 1990.

161. Hargreave, F. E., et al. Bronchial responsiveness to histamine and methacholine in asthma. Measurement and clinical significance. *J. Allergy Clin. Immunol.* 68:347, 1981.

162. Harris, L. Comparison of the effect on blood gases, ventilation, and perfusion of ioproterenol-phenylephrine and salbutamol aerosols in chronic bronchitis with asthma. *J. Allergy Clin. Immunol.* 49:63, 1972.

163. Harris, L. Comparison of cardiorespiratory effects of terbutaline and salbutamol aerosols in patients with reversible airways obstruction. *Thorax* 28:59, 1973.

164. Harris, L. H. Effects of isoprenaline plus phenylephrine by pressurized aerosol on blood gases, ventilation and perfusion in chronic obstructive lung disease. *Br. Med. J.* 4:579, 1970.

165. Harrison, B. A., and Pierce, R. J. Comparison of wet and dry aerosol salbutamol. *Aust. NZ J. Med.* 13:29, 1983.

166. Hartnett, B. J. S., and Marlin, G. E. Comparison of terbutaline and salbutamol aerosols. *Aust. NZ J. Med.* 7:13, 1977.

167. Harvey, J. E., and Tattersfield, A. E. Airway response to salbutamol. Effect of regular salbutamol inhalations in normal, atopic and asthmatic subjects. *Thorax* 37:280, 1982.

168. Hauck, R. W., et al. Beta$_2$ adrenoceptors in human lung and peripheral mononuclear leukocytes of untreated and terbutaline-treated patients. *Chest* 98:375, 1990.

169. Hausdorff, W. P., Caron, M. G., and Lefkowitz, R. J. Turning off the signal: desensitization of β-adrenergic receptor function. *FASEB J.* 4:2881, 1990.

170. Hedberg, A., Minneman, K. P., and Molinoff, P. B. Differential distribution of beta$_1$- and beta$_2$-adrenergic receptors in cat and guinea pig heart. *J. Pharmacol. Exp. Ther.* 213:503, 1980.

171. Hedberg, A., et al. Coexistence of beta-1 and beta-2 adrenergic receptors in the human heart: effects of treatment with receptor antagonists or calcium entry blockers. *J. Pharmacol. Exp. Ther.* 234:561, 1985.

172. Heel, R. C., et al. Fenoterol: a review of its pharmacological properties and therapeutic efficacy in asthma. *Drugs* 15:3, 1978.

173. Herman, J. J., Noah, Z. L., and Moody, R. R. Use of intravenous isoproterenol for status asthmaticus in children. *Crit. Care Med.* 11:716, 1983.

174. Herschfus, J. J., et al. A new sympathomimetic amine ("Neosuprel") in the treatment of bronchial asthma. *Ann. Allergy* 9:769, 1951.

175. Hetzel, M. R., and Clark, T. J. H. Comparison of intravenous and aerosol salbutamol. *Br. Med. J.* 2:919, 1976.

176. Higgenbottam, T. W., et al. Controlled release salbutamol tablets versus aminophylline in the control of reversible airways obstruction. *J. Int. Med. Res.* 17:435, 1989.

177. Higgins, R. M., et al. Cardiac arrhythmias caused by nebulized beta-agonist therapy. *Lancet* 2:863, 1987.

178. Higgins, R. M., Stradling, J. R., and Lane, D. J. Should ipratropium bromide be added to beta-agonists in treatment of acute severe asthma? *Chest* 94:718, 1988.

179. Hirata, F. and Axelrod, J. Phospholipid methylation and biological signal transmission. *Science* 209:1082, 1980.

180. Hoffman, B. B., and Lefkowitz, R. J. Alpha adrenergic-receptor subtypes. *N. Engl J. Med.* 302:1390, 1980.

181. Holgate, S. T., Baldwin, C. J., and Tattersfield, A. E. Beta-adrenergic resistance in normal human airways. *Lancet* 2:375, 1977.

182. Holgate, S. T., Baldwin, C. J., and Tattersfield, A. E. Beta-adrenergic resistance in normal human airways. *Lancet* 2:375, 1977.

183. Holmes, T. H. A comparative clinical trial of metaproterenol and isoproterenol as bronchodilator aerosols. *Clin. Pharmacol. Ther.* 9:615, 1968.

184. Hooper, P. L., et al. Terbutaline raises high-density-lipoprotein cholesterol levels. *N. Engl. J. Med.* 305:1455, 1981.

185. Howarth, P. H., et al. Influence of albuterol, cromolyn sodium and ipratropium bromide on the airway circulating mediator response to allergen bronchial provocation in asthma. *Am. Rev. Respir. Dis.* 132:986, 1985.

185a. Hudson, L. D., et al. Arrhythmias associated with acute respiratory failure in patients with chronic airway obstruction. *Chest* 63:661, 1973.

186. Hui, K. K., Conolly, M. E., and Tashkin, D. P. Methylprednisolone reverses the beta agonist–induced decrease in beta receptor number in human lymphocytes. *Clin. Pharmacol. Ther.* 32:566, 1982.

187. Hume, K. M., and Gandevia, B. Forced expiratory volume before and after isoprenaline. *Thorax* 12:276, 1957.

188. Ingram, R. H., Jr., et al. Ventilation-perfusion changes after aerosolized isoproterenol in asthma. *Am. Rev. Respir. Dis.* 101:364, 1970.

189. Ingram, R. J. H. Jr., et al. Relative contributions of large and small airways to flow limitation in normal subjects before and after atropine and isoproterenol. *J. Clin. Invest.* 59:696, 1977.

190. Iravani, J., and Melville, G. N. Mucociliary function of the respiratory tract as influenced by drugs. *Respiration* 34:350, 1974.

191. Irwin, R. S., Corrao, W. M., and Pratter, M. R. Chronic persistent cough in the adult: the spectrum and frequency of causes and successful outcome of specific therapy. *Am. Rev. Respir. Dis.* 123:413, 1981.

192. Ito, Y., and Tajima, K. Dual effect of catecholamines on pre and post junctional membranes in the dog trachea. *Br. J. Pharmacol.* 75:433, 1982.

193. Jack, D. Recent beta-adrenoreceptor stimulants and the nature of beta-adrenoreceptors. *Pharm. J.* 205:237, 1970.

194. Jackson, R. T., et al. Mortality from asthma: a new epidemic in New Zealand. *Br. Med. J.* 285:771, 1982.

195. Jacoby, D. B., and Fryer, A. D. Abnormalities in neural control of smooth muscle in virus-infected airways. *Trends Pharmacol. Sci.* 11(10):393, 1990.

195a. Janson, C. Plasma levels and effects of salbutamol after inhaled or I.V. administration in stable asthma. *Eur. J. Resp. Dis.* 4:544, 1991.

196. Jasper, A. C., et al. Cost-benefit comparison of aerosol bronchodilator delivery methods in hospitalized patients. *Chest* 91:614, 1987.

196a. Jenne, J. W. Whither beta-adrenergic tachyphylaxis? *J. Allergy Clin. Immunol.* 70:413, 1982.

197. Jenne, J. W. Pulmonary Drugs. In R. C. Bone, (ed.), *Critical Care. A Comprehensive Approach.* Park Ridge, IL: American College Chest Physicians, 1984, P. 223.

198. Jenne, J. W., et al. Subsensitivity of beta responses during therapy with a long-acting beta-2 preparation. *J. Allergy Clin. Immunol.* 59:383, 1977.

199. Jenne, J. W., et al. Objective and subjective tremor responses to oral beta-2 agents on first exposure. *Am. Rev. Respir. Dis.* 126:607, 1982.

200. Jenne, J. W., et al. Comparison of tremor responses to orally administered albuterol and terbutaline. *Am. Rev. Respir. Dis.* 134:708, 1986.

201. Jenne, J. W., et al. In vivo functional antagonism between isoproterenol and bronchoconstrictants in the dog. *J. Appl. Physiol.* 63(2):812, 1987.

202. Jeppsson, A.-B., et al. On the predictive value of experiments in vitro in the evaluation of the effect duration of bronchodilator drugs for local administration. *Pulm. Pharmacol.* 2:81, 1989.

203. Joad, J. P., et al. Extrapulmonary effects of maintenance therapy with theophylline and inhaled albuterol in patients with chronic asthma. *J. Allergy Clin. Immunol.* 78:1147, 1986.

204. Joad, J. P., et al. Relative efficacy of maintenance therapy with theophylline, inhaled albuterol, and the combination for chronic asthma. *J. Allergy Clin. Immunol.* 79:78, 1987.

205. Johnson, M. The pharmacology of salmeterol. *Lung* 168(suppl):115, 1990.

206. Johnson, M., Butcher, P. R., and Vardey, C. J. Potency and duration of action of salmeterol as an inhibitor of mediator release from human lung. (abstract) *Am. Rev. Respir. Dis.* 143:655, 1991.

206a. Johnson, M., Vardey, C. J., and Whelan, C. J. The therapeutic potential of long-acting β_2-adrenoceptor agonists in allergic inflammation (editorial). *Clin. Exper. Allergy* 22:177, 1992.

207. Jones, C. A., et al. Muscarinic cholinergic inhibition of adenylate cyclase in airway smooth muscle. *Am. J. Physiol.* 253:C97, 1987.

208. Jones, T. R., Hamilton, J. T., and Lefcoe, N. M. Pharmacological modulation of cholinergic neurotransmission in guinea pig trachea in vitro. *Can. J. Physiol. Pharmacol.* 58:810, 1979.

209. Jones, T. R., et al. Selective inhibition of relaxation of guinea-pig trachea

210. by charybdotoxin, a potent Ca^{++}-activated K^+ channel inhibitor. *J. Pharmacol. Exp. Ther.* 255:697, 1990.

210. Joseph, X., et al. Enhancement of cardiotoxic effects of beta-adrenergic bronchodilators by aminophylline in experimental animals. *Fund. Appl. Toxicol.* 1:443, 1981.

211. Josephson, G. W., et al. The acute treatment of asthma: a comparison of two treatment regimens. *JAMA* 242:639, 1979.

212. Josephson, G. W., et al. Cardiac dysrhythmias during the treatment of acute asthma. A comparison of two treatment regimes by double-blind protocol. *Chest* 78:429, 1980.

213. Juniper, E. F., Frith, P. A., and Hargreave, F. E. Airway responsiveness to histamine and methacholine: relationship to minimum treatment to control symptoms of asthma. *Thorax* 36:575, 1981.

214. Kahn, D. S., Rena, G., and Chappel, C. I. Isoproterenol-induced cardiac necrosis. *Ann. NY Acad. Sci.* 156:285, 1969.

215. Karetsky, M. S. Asthma mortality: an analysis of one year's experience, review of the literature and assessment of current modes of treatment. *Medicine* 54:471, 1975.

216. Karpel, J. P., et al. A comparison of atropine sulfate and metaproterenol sulfate in the emergency treatment of asthma. *Am. Rev. Respir. Dis.* 133: 727, 1986.

217. Kass, I., and Mingo, T. S. Bitolterol mesylate (WIN 32784) aerosol, a new long-acting bronchodilator with reduced chronotropic effect. *Chest* 78: 283, 1980.

218. Kaumann, A. J. Is there a third heart beta-adrenoceptor? *TIPS* 10:316, 1989.

219. Keighly, J. F. Iatrogenic asthma induced by adrenergic aerosols. *Ann. Intern. Med.* 69:985, 1966.

220. Kelly, H. W., et al. Safety of frequent high dose nebulized terbutaline in children with acute severe asthma. *Ann. Allergy* 64(Feb. Part II):229, 1990.

221. Kelly, H. W., Murphy, S., and Jenne, J. W. Appendix V. Intravenous beta agonist for life-threatening asthma. In J. W. Jenne and S. Murphy (eds.), *Drug Therapy for Asthma, Research and Clinical Practice* (Vol. 31, Lung Biology in Health and Disease). New York: Dekker, 1987, P. 1045.

222. Keltz, H., Stone, D. J., and Samortin, T. Nebulization of saline and isoproterenol in chronic bronchitis. *Arch. Intern. Med.* 130:44, 1972.

223. Kemp, J. P., et al. Concomitant bitolterol mesylate aerosol and theophylline for asthma therapy with 24 hr electrocardiographic monitoring. *J. Allergy Clin. Immunol.* 73:32, 1984.

224. Kenakin, T. P., and Ferris, R. M. Effects of in vivo β-adrenoceptor down-regulation on cardiac responses to prenalterol and pirbuterol. *J. Cardiovasc. Res.* 5:90, 1983.

225. Kennedy, M. C. S., and Simpson, W. T. Human pharmacological and clinical studies on salbutamol: a specific β-adrenergic bronchodilator. *Br. J. Dis. Chest* 63:165, 1969.

226. Kerr, A., and Gebbie, T. Comparison of orciprenaline, ephedrine and methoxyphenamine as oral bronchodilators. *NZ Med. J.* 77:320, 1973.

227. Kerrebijn, K. F., van Essen-Zandvleit, E. E. M., and Neijens, H. J. Effects of long-term treatment with inhaled corticosteroids and beta-agonists on the bronchial responsiveness in children with asthma. *J. Allergy Clin. Immunol.* 79:653, 1987.

228. Kinney, E. L., et al. Ventricular tachycardia after terbutaline. *JAMA* 243: 2247, 1978.

229. Klaustermeyer, W. B., Di Bernardo, R. L., and Hale, F. C. Intravenous isoproterenol: rationale for bronchial asthma. *J. Allergy Clin. Immunol.* 55:325, 1975.

230. Kneussl, M. P., and Richardson, J. B. Alpha-adrenergic receptors in human and canine tracheal and bronchial smooth muscle. *J. Appl. Physiol.* 45:307, 1978.

231. Koepke, J. W., Selner, J. C., and Dunhill, A. L. SO_2 derived from bronchodilator solutions. *J. Allergy Clin. Immunol.* 71(suppl.):147, 1983.

232. Konig, P., Eggleston, P. A., and Serby, C. W. Comparison of oral and inhaled metaproterenol for prevention of exercise-induced asthma. *Clin. Allergy* 11:597, 1981.

233. Konig, P., Hordvik, N. L., and Serby, C. W. Fenoterol in exercise-induced asthma. Effect of dose on efficacy and duration of action. *Chest* 84:462, 1984.

234. Kottlikoff, M. I., Murray, R. K., and Reynolds, E. E. Histamine-induced calcium release and phorbol antagonism in cultured airway smooth muscle cells. *Am. J. Physiol.* 253:561, 1987.

235. Kraan, J., et al. Changes in bronchial hyperreactivity induced by 4 weeks of treatment with anti-asthmatic drugs in patients with allergic asthma: a comparison between budesonide and terbutaline. *J. Allergy Clin. Immunol.* 76:628, 1985.

236. Krall, J. F., Connelly, M., and Tuck, M. L. Acute regulation of beta adrener-

gic catecholamine sensitivity in human lymphocytes. *J. Pharmacol. Exp. Ther.* 214:554, 1980.

237. Kume, H., and Kotlikoff, M. I. K_{Ca} in tracheal smooth muscle cells are activated by the subunit of the stimulatory G protein, G_s. *Am. Rev. Respir. Dis.* 145:A204, 1992.

238. Kume, H., et al. Regulation of Ca^{2+}-dependent K^+-channel activity in tracheal myocytes by phosphorylation. *Nature* 341:152, 1989.

238a. Kung, M. Parenteral adrenergic bronchodilation and potassium. *Chest* 89:322, 1986.

239. Kung, M., Croley, S. W., and Phillips, B. A. Systemic cardiovascular and metabolic effects associated with the inhalation of an increased dose of albuterol. Influence of mouth rinsing and gargling. *Chest* 91:382, 1977.

240. Kung, M., White, J. R., and Burki, N. K. The effect of subcutaneously administered terbutaline on serum potassium in asymptomatic adult asthmatics. *Am. Rev. Respir. Dis.* 129:329, 1984.

240a. Kurland, G., Williams, J., and Lewiston, N. Fatal myocardial toxicity during continuous infusion intravenous isoproterenol therapy of asthma. *J. Allergy Clin. Immunol.* 63:407, 1979.

241. Laitinen, L. A., et al. Damage of the airway epithelium and bronchial reactivity in patients with asthma. *Am. Rev. Respir. Dis.* 131:599, 1985.

242. Lands, A. M., and Brown, T. G. Jr. A comparison of the cardiac stimulating and bronchodilator action of selected sympathomimetic amines. *Proc. Soc. Exp. Biol. Med.* 116:331, 1964.

243. Lands, A. M., et al. Comparison of the action of isoproterenol and several related compounds on blood pressure, heart and bronchioles. *Arch. Pharmacol. Ther.* 68:161, 1966.

244. Lands, A. M., et al. Differentiation of receptor systems activated by sympathomimetic amines. *Nature* 214:597, 1967.

245. Larsson, S., and Svedmyr, N. Bronchodilating effect and side effects of beta₂-adrenoceptor stimulants by different modes of administration (tablets, metered aerosol, and combinations thereof). A study with salbutamol in asthmatics. *Am. Rev. Respir. Dis.* 116:861, 1977.

246. Larsson, S., Svedmyr, N., and Thiringer, G. Lack of bronchial beta adrenoceptor resistance in asthmatics during long-term treatment with terbutaline. *J. Allergy Clin. Immunol.* 59:93, 1977.

247. Lawford, P., Jones, B. J., and Milledge, J. S. Comparison of intravenous and nebulized salbutamol in initial treatment of asthma. *Br. Med. J.* 1:84, 1978.

248. Leahy, R. C., Gomm, S. A., and Allen, S. C. Comparison of nebulized salbutamol with nebulized ipratropium bromide in acute asthma. *Br. J. Dis. Chest* 77:159, 1983.

249. Lechleiter, J., Peralta, E., and Clapham, D. Diverse functions of muscarinic acetylcholine receptor subtypes. *Trends Pharmacol. Sci.* [suppl.] (Dec):34, 1989.

250. Lee, H., and Evans, H. E. Lack of cardiac effect from repeated doses of the albuterol aerosol. A margin of safety. *Clin. Pediatr.* 25:349, 1986.

250a. Lefcoe, N. M., Toogood, J. H., and Jones, T. R. In vitro pharmacologic studies of bronchodilator compounds: Interactions and mechanisms. *J. Allergy Clin. Immunol.* 55:94, 1975.

251. Lefkowitz, R. J., Hausdorff, W. P., and Caron, M. G. Role of phosphorylation in desensitization of the β-adrenoceptor. *Trends Pharmacol. Sci.* 11:190, 1990.

252. Lefkowitz, R. J., Kobilka, B. K., and Caron, M. G. The new biology of drug receptors. *Biochem. Pharmacol.* 38:2941, 1989.

253. Legge, J. S., Gaddie, J., and Palmer, K. N. V. Comparison of two oral selective β₂-adrenergic stimulating drugs in bronchial asthma. *Br. Med. J.* 1:637, 1971.

254. Leifer, K., and Wittig, H. The beta-2 sympathomimetic aerosols in the treatment of asthma. *Ann. Allergy* 35:69, 1975.

255. Leitch, A. G., et al. Effect of intravenous infusion of salbutamol on ventilatory response to carbon dioxide and hypoxia on heart rate and plasma potassium in normal men. *Br. Med. J.* 1:365, 1976.

256. Levitzki, A. Transmembrane signaling to adenylate cyclase in mammalian cells and in *Saccaromyces cerevisiae. Trends Biol. Sci.* 13:298, 1988.

257. Lewis, R. A. Inhalation drugs in asthma management: state of the art factors affecting delivery, and clinical response to inhaled drugs. *NER Allergy Proc.* 5(no. 1):23, 1984.

257a. Lichtenstein, L. M., and Margolis, S. Histamine release in vitro: Inhibition by catecholamines and methylxanthines. *Science* 161:902, 1968.

258. Lin, C. S., et al. Mechanism of isoproterenol-induced desensitization of tracheal smooth muscle. *J. Pharmacol. Exp. Ther.* 203:12, 1977.

259. Lipworth, B. J., McDevitt, D. G., and Struthers, A. D. Electrocardiographic changes induced by inhaled salbutamol after treatment with bendrofluazide: effects of replacement therapy with potassium, magnesium and triamterene. *Clin. Sci.* 78:255, 1990.

260. Lipworth, B. J., et al. Single-dose and steady-state phamacokinetics of 4 mg and 8 mg oral salbutamol controlled-release in patients with bronchial asthma. *Eur. J. Clin. Pharmacol.* 37:49, 1989.

261. Lipworth, B. J., et al. Comparison of the effects of prolonged treatment with low and high doses of inhaled terbutaline on beta-adrenoceptor responsiveness in patients with chronic obstructive pulmonary disease. *Am. Rev. Respir. Dis.* 142:338, 1990.

262. Littner, M. R., et al. Acute bronchial and cardiovascular effects of increasing doses of pirbuterol acetate aerosol in asthma. *Ann. Allergy* 48:14, 1982.

263. Littner, M. R., et al. Double-blind comparison of acute effects of inhaled albuterol, isoproterenol or placebo on cardiopulmonary function and gas exchange in asthmatic children. *Ann. Allergy* 50:309, 1983.

263a. Löfdahl, C.-G., and Chung, K. F. Long-acting β₂-adrenoceptor agonists: A new perspective in the treatment of asthma. *Eur. Respir. J.* 4:218, 1991.

264. Löfdahl, C.-G., and Svedmyr, N. Effects of prenalterol in asthmatic patients. *Eur. J. Clin. Pharmacol.* 23:297, 1982.

264a. Löfdahl, C-G, and Svedmyr, N. Beta agonists—friends or foes? *Eur. Resp. J.* 4:1161, 1991.

265. Löfdahl, C.-G., and Svedmyr, N. Formaterol fumarate, a new beta₂-adrenoceptor agonist. Acute studies of selectivity and duration of effect after inhaled and oral administration. *Allergy* 44:264, 1989.

266. Lonky, S. A., and Tisi, G. M. Determining changes in airflow caliber in asthma: the role of submaximal expiratory flow rates. *Chest* 77:741, 1980.

266a. Lowell, F. C., Curry, J. J., and Schiller, I. W. A clnical and experimental study of isuprel in spontaneous and induced asthma. *N. Engl. J. Med.* 140:45, 1949.

267. Lowell, S. A., and Tisi, G. M. Determining changes in airway caliber in asthma: the role of submaximal expiratory flow rates. *Chest* 77:741, 1980.

268. Lubbe, W. F., et al. The role of cyclic adenosine monophosphate in adrenergic effects on ventricular vulnerability to fibrillation in the isolated perfused rat heart. *J. Clin. Invest.* 61:1260, 1978.

269. MacIntyre, N. R., et al. Aerosolized delivery in intubated, mechanically ventilated patients. *Crit. Care Med.* 13:81, 1985.

270. Maclagen, J., and Barnes, P. J. Muscarinic pharmacology of the airways. *Trends Pharmacol. Sci.* [Suppl.]9(12):88, 1989.

271. Madison, J. M., and Brown, J. K. Differential inhibitory effects of forskolin, isoproterenol and dibutyryl cyclic AMP in canine tracheal smooth muscle. *J. Clin. Invest.* 82:1462, 1988.

272. Madsen, E. D., Bundgaard, A., and Hidinger, K. G. Cumulative dose-response study comparing terbutaline pressurized aerosol administered via a pearshaped spacer and terbutaline in a nebulized solution. *Eur. J. Clin. Pharmacol.* 23:27, 1982.

273. Maesen, F. P. V., et al. Bronchodilator effect of inhaled formaterol vs. salbutamol over 12 hours. *Chest* 97:590, 1990.

274. Magnusson, G., and Hansson, E. Myocardial necrosis in the rat. A comparison between isoprenaline, oroprenaline, salbutamol and terbutaline. *Cardiology* 58:174, 1973.

275. Maguire, J. F., Geha, R. S., and Umetsu, D. T. Myocardial specific creatine phosphokinase isoenzyme elevation in children with asthma treated with intravenous isoproterenol. *J. Allergy Clin. Immunol.* 78:631, 1986.

276. Maguire, W. C., and Nair, S. Ventilation and perfusion effects of inhaled alpha and beta agonists in asthma patients. *Chest* 73(suppl):983, 1978.

277. Mallorga, P., et al. Mepacrine blocks beta-adrenergic agonist-induced desensitization in astrocytoma cells. *Proc. Natl. Acad. Sci. USA* 77:1341, 1980.

278. Malo, J.-L., Cartier, A., and Trudeau, C. Formaterol, a new inhaled beta-2 adrenergic agonist has a longer blocking effect than albuterol on hyperventilation-induced bronchoconstriction. *Am. Rev. Respir. Dis.* 142:1147, 1990.

279. Mano, K., Akbarzadeh, A., and Townley, R. G. Effect of hydrocortisone on beta adrenergic receptors in lung membranes. *Life Sci.* 25:1925, 1979.

280. Marlin, G. E., Bush, D. E., and Berend, N. Comparison of ipratropium bromide and fenoterol in asthma and chronic bronchitis. *Br. J. Clin. Pharmacol.* 6:547, 1978.

281. Marlin, G. E., and Turner, P. Intravenous treatment with rimiterol and salbutamol in asthma. *Br. Med. J.* 2:715, 1975.

282. Marlin, G. E., and Turner, P. The relative potencies and β₂-selectivies of intravenous rimiterol, salbutamol and isoprenaline in asthmatic patients. *Int. J. Clin. Pharmacol.* 12:158, 1975.

283. Martin, G. L., et al. The effects of theophylline, terbutaline and prednisone upon antigen-induced bronchospasm and mediator release. *J. Allergy Clin. Immunol.* 66:204, 1980.

284. Matson, J. R., Loughlin, G. M., and Strunk, R. C. Myocardial ischemia

complicating the use of isoproterenol in asthmatic children. *J. Pediatr.* 92:776, 1978.

285. May, C. S., Pickup, M. E., and Paterson, J. W. The acute and chronic bronchodilator effects of ephedrine in asthmatic patients. *Br. J. Clin. Pharmacol.* 2:533, 1975.

286. Mazza, J. A., Tashkin, D. P., and Reed, C. E. An evaluation of procaterol and albuterol (salbutamol) aerosol in the treatment of asthma. *Ann. Allergy* 68:267, 1992.

287. McAlpine, L. G., and Thomas, N. C. Prophylaxis of exercise-induced asthma with inhaled formaterol, a long-acting beta₂-adrenergic agonist. *Respir. Med.* 84:293, 1990.

288. McEvoy, J. D. S., Vall-Spinosa, A., and Paterson, J. W. Assessment of orciprenaline and isoproterenol infusions in asthmatic patients. *Am. Rev. Respir. Dis.* 108:390, 1973.

289. McFadden, E. R., Jr., Kiser, R., and de Groat, W. J. Acute bronchial asthma. Relation between clinical and physiologic manifestations. *N. Engl. J. Med.* 288:221, 1973.

290. McMannis, A. G. Adrenaline and isoprenaline: a warning (letter). *Med. J. Aust.* 2:76, 1964.

291. Mestitz, H., Copland, J. M., and McDonald, C. F. Comparison of outpatient nebulized vs. metered dose inhaler terbutaline in chronic airflow obstruction. *Chest* 96:1237, 1989.

292. Metaproterenol Product Information. *Physicians' Desk Reference, 1992.* Oradell, N.J.: Medical Economics, 1992. Pp. 674–675.

293. Meurs, H., et al. The beta-adrenergic system and allergic bronchial asthma: changes in lymphocyte beta-adrenergic receptor number and adenylate cyclase activity after an allergen-induced attack. *J. Allergy Clin. Immunol.* 70:272, 1982.

294. Meurs, H., et al. Phorbol 12-myristate 13-acetate induces beta adrenergic receptor uncoupling in and non-specific desensitization of adenylate cyclase in human mononuclear lymphocytes. *Biochem. Pharmacol.* 35:4217, 1986.

295. Meurs, H., et al. Regulation of the beta-receptor adenylate cyclase system in lymphocytes of allergic patients with asthma. Possible role for protein kinase C in allergen-induced nonspecific refractoriness of adenylate cyclase. *J. Allergy Clin. Immunol.* 80:326, 1987.

296. Meurs, H., et al. Evidence for a direct relationship between phosphoinositide metabolism and airway smooth muscle contraction induced by muscarinic agonists. *Eur. J. Pharmacol.* 156:271, 1988.

297. Minnear, F. L., et al. Isoproterenol reduces thrombin-induced pulmonary endothelial permeability in vitro. *Am. J. Physiol.* 257:H1623, 1989.

297a. Miura, M., et al. Role of potassium channels in bronchodilator responses in human airways. *Am. Rev. Resp. Dis.* 148:132, 1992.

298. Moler, F. W., Hurwitz, M. E., and Custer, J. R. Improvement in clinical asthma score and PaCO₂ in children with severe asthma treated with continuously nebulized terbutaline. *J. Allergy Clin. Immunol.* 81:1101, 1988.

299. Molfino, N. A., et al. Respiratory arrest in near-fatal asthma. *N. Engl. J. Med.* 324:285, 1991.

300. Moore, P. F., Constantine, J. W., and Barth, W. E. Pirbuterol, a selective beta-2 adrenergic bronchodilator. *J. Pharmacol. Exp. Ther.* 207:410, 1978.

301. Moreno, R. H., Hogg, J. C., and Pare, P. D. Mechanisms of airway narrowing. *Am. Rev. Respir. Dis.* 133:1171, 1986.

302. Morgan, D. J., et al. Pharmacokinetics of intravenous and oral salbutamol and its sulfate conjugate. *Br. J. Clin. Pharmacol.* 22:587, 1986.

303. Morley, T. F., et al. Comparison of beta-adrenergic agents delivered by nebulizer vs. metered dose inhaler with Inspirease in hospitalized asthmatic patients. *Chest* 94:1205, 1988.

303a. Morley, J., Sanjar, S., and Newth, C. Viewpoint: Untoward effects of beta-adrenoceptor agonists in asthma. *Eur. Respir. J.* 3:228, 1990.

304. Morris, H. G. Drug-induced desensitization of beta adrenergic receptors. *J. Allergy Clin. Immunol.* 65:83, 1980.

305. Mossberg, B. Mucociliary transport and its influence by beta adrenoceptor drugs. *Acta Pharmacol. Toxicol.* 44:41, 1979.

306. Motulsky, H. J., and Insell, P. A. Adrenergic receptor in man. Direct identification, physiologic regulation and clinical alterations. *N. Engl. J. Med.* 307:18, 1982.

307. National Heart, Lung and Blood Institute National Asthma Education Program, Expert Panel Report: *Guidelines for the Diagnosis and Management of Asthma.* Bethesda, MD: NHLBI Information Center, 1991.

308. Naylor, W. G. Some observations on the pharmacological effects of salbutamol with particular reference to the cardiovascular system. *Postgrad. Med. J.* 47(suppl):16, 1971.

309. Nelson, H. S., et al. Subsensitivity to the bronchodilator action of albut-

erol produced by chronic administration. *Am. Rev. Respir. Dis.* 116:871, 1977.

309a. Nelson, H. S., Szefler, S. J., and Martin, R. J. Regular inhaled beta-adrenergic agonists in the treatment of bronchial asthma. Beneficial or detrimental? *Am. Rev. Resp. Dis.* 144:249, 1991.

310. Nelson, H. S., et al. The bronchodilator response to inhalation of increasing doses of aerosolized albuterol. *J. Allergy Clin. Immunol.* 72:371, 1983.

311. Neville, A., et al. Metabolic effects of salbutamol: comparison of aerosol and intravenous adminsitration. *Br. Med. J.* 1:413, 1977.

312. Newman, S. P., et al. Deposition of pressurized aerosols in the human respiratory tract. *Thorax* 36:52, 1980.

313. Newman, S. P., et al. Deposition of pressurized aerosol inhaled through extension devices. *Am. Rev. Respir. Dis.* 124:317, 1981.

313a. Newth, C. J. L., et al. The ventilatory and oxygen costs in the anesthetized rhesus monkey of inhaling drugs used in the therapy and diagnosis of asthma. *Am. Rev. Resp. Dis.* 143:766, 1991.

314. Nicklas, R. A., Whitehurst, V. E., and Donohue, R. F. Combined use of beta-adrenergic agonists and methylxanthines (letter). *N. Engl. J. Med.* 307:557, 1982.

315. Nicklas, R. A., et al. Concomitant use of beta-adrenergic agonists and methylxanthines. *J. Allergy Clin. Immunol.* 73:20, 1984.

316. Nielson, C. P. β-adrenergic modulation of the polymorphonuclear leukocyte respiratory burst is dependent upon the mechanism of cell activation. *J. Immunol.* 139:2392, 1987.

317. Nogrady, S. G., Hartley, J. P. R., and Seaton, A. Metabolic effects of intravenous salbutamol in the course of acute severe asthma. *Thorax* 32:559, 1977.

318. Nou, E. A clinical comparison of subcutaneous doses of terbutaline and adrenaline in bronchial asthma. *Scand. J. Respir. Dis.* 52:192, 1971.

319. Nyberg, L. Pharmacokinetic parameters of terbutaline in healthy men. An overview. *Eur. J. Respir. Dis.* 134(suppl. 10):149, 1984.

320. Nyberg, L. Pharmacokinetic properties of bambuterol in solution and tablet—basis for once daily dosage in asthma. *Acta Pharmacol. Toxicol.* 59(suppl 5):229, 1986.

321. Obara, K., and de Lanerolle, P. Isoproterenol attenuates myosin phosphorylation and contraction of tracheal smooth muscle. *J. Appl. Physiol.* 66(5):2017, 1989.

322. O'Donnell, S. R., et al. A histological method for studying the effect of drugs on mediator-induced airway microvascular leakage of rodents. *J. Pharmacol. Methods* 17:205, 1987.

323. O'Donnell, T. V., Rea, H. H., and Holst, P. E. Fenoterol and fatal asthma (letter). *Lancet* 334:1070, 1989.

324. O'Driscoll, B. R. C., et al. Long-term treatment of severe asthma with subcutaneous terbutaline. *Br. J. Dis. Chest* 82:360, 1988.

325. Olsson, O. A. T., et al. Effects of bea-adrenoceptor agonists on airway smooth muscle and slow-contracting skeletal muscle: in vitro and in vivo results compared. *Acta Pharmacol. Toxicol.* 44:272, 1979.

326. Omini, C., et al. Beta-adrenoceptor desensitization in the lung. A phenomenon related to prostanoids. *Prog. Biochem. Pharmacol.* 20:63, 1985.

326a. Orange, R.P., Austin, W. G., and Austen, K. F. Immunologic release of histamine and slow-reactive substance of anaphylaxis from human lung. I. Modulation by agents influencing cellular levels of cyclic 3′,5′-adenosine monophosphate. *J. Exp. Med.* 134(Suppl.):136, 1971.

327. Orgel, H. A., et al. Bitolterol and albuterol metered-dose aerosols: comparison of two long-acting beta-2 adrenergic bronchodilators for treatment of asthma. *J. Allergy Clin. Immunol.* 75:55, 1985.

328. Palmer, K. N. V., et al. Effect of a selective beta-adrenergic blocker in preventing falls in arterial oxygen tension following isoprenaline in asthmatic subjects. *Lancet* 2:1092, 1969.

329. Palmer, K. N. V. Effect of bronchodilator drugs on arterial blood gas tensions in bronchial asthma. *Postgrad. Med. J.* 47(suppl):75, 1971.

330. Park, S., and Rasmussen, H. Carbachol-induced protein phosphorylation changes in bovine tracheal smooth muscle. *J. Biol. Chem.* 261:15734, 1986.

330a. Parker, C. W., and Smith, J. W. Alterations in cyclic adenosine monophosphate metabolism in human bronchial asthma. I. Leukocyte responsiveness to β-adrenergic agents. *J. Clin. Invest.* 52:48, 1973.

331. Parry, W. H., Martorano, F., and Cotton, E. K. Management of life-threatening asthma with intravenous isoproterenol infusions. *Am. J. Dis. Child.* 130:39, 1976.

332. Partanen, M., et al. Catecholamine- and acetylcholinesterase-containing nerves in human lower respiratory tract. *Histochemistry* 76:175, 1982.

333. Paterson, J. W., Courtenay Evans, R. J., and Prime, F. J. Selectivity of bronchodilator action of salbutamol in asthmatic patients. *Br. J. Dis. Chest* 65:21, 1971.

334. Paterson, J. W., Woolcock, A. J., and Shenfield, G. M. Bronchodilator drugs. *Am. Rev. Respir. Dis.* 120:1149, 1979.

335. Pearce, N., et al. Case-control study of prescribed fenoterol and death from asthma in New Zealand, 1977–81. *Thorax* 45:170, 1990.

336. Peel, E. T., and Gibson, G. J. Effects of long-term inhaled salbutamol therapy on the provocation of asthma by histamine. *Am. Rev. Respir. Dis.* 121:973, 1980.

337. Persson, C. G. A. Plasma exudation in tracheobronchial and nasal airways: a mucosal defense mechanism becomes pathogenic in asthma and rhinitis. *Eur. J. Respir. Dis.* 3(suppl. 12):652s, 1990.

338. Persson, C. G. A., Erjefalt, I., and Andersson, P. Leakage of macromolecules from guinea pig tracheobronchial microcirculation. Effects of allergen, leukotrienes, tachykinins and antihistamine drugs. *Acta Physiol. Scand.* 127:95, 1986.

339. Persson, H., and Olsson, T. Some pharmacological properties of terbutaline (INN), 1(3,5-dihydroxyphenyl)-2(t-butylaminol)-ethanol: a new sympathomimetic beta-receptor-stimulating agent. *Acta Med. Scand.* 512(suppl):11, 1970.

340. Persson, K., and Persson, K. The metabolism of terbutaline in vitro by rat and human liver O-methyl-transferase and monoamine oxidases. *Xenobiotica* 2:375, 1972.

341. Petrie, G. R., Choo Kang, J., and Clark, R. A. Bambuterol: efficacy in nocturnal asthma. *Am. Rev. Respir. Dis.* 143:A652, 1991.

342. Petty, T. L., et al. A comparison of oral procaterol and albuterol in reversible airflow obstruction. *Am. Rev. Respir. Dis.* 138:1504, 1988.

343. Phillips, P. J., et al. Metabolic and cardiovascular side effects of the β_2-adrenoceptor agonists salbutamol and rimterol. *Br. J. Clin. Pharmacol.* 9:483, 1980.

344. Phipps, R. J. Adrenergic stimulation of mucus secretion in the human bronchus. *J. Appl. Physiol.* 296:44P, 1979.

345. Phipps, R. J., et al. Sympathetic drugs stimulate the output of secretory glycoprotein from human bronchi in vitro. *Clin. Sci.* 63:23, 1982.

346. Pierce, R. J., et al. Comparison of intravenous and inhaled terbutaline in the treatment of asthma. *Chest* 79:506, 1981.

347. Pierson, R. N. Jr., and Grieco, M. H. Isoproterenol aerosol in normal and asthmatic subjects. *Am. Rev. Respir. Dis.* 100:533, 1969.

347a. Pihlojamaki, K., Kanto, J., and Iisolo, E. Human and animal studies on the interactions between glyphylline and isoprenaline. *J. Asthma Res.* 9: 255, 1972.

348. Plummer, A. L. The development of drug tolerance to beta₂ adrenergic agents. *Chest* 73(suppl):949, 1978.

349. Porte, D. Beta adrenergic stimulation of insulin release in man. *Diabetes* 16:150, 1964.

350. Postma, D. S., et al. Influence of slow-release terbutaline on the circadian variation of catecholamines, histamine, and lung function in nonallergic patients with partly reversible airflow obstruction. *J. Allergy Clin. Immunol.* 77:471, 1986.

351. Powell, M. L., et al. Comparative bioavailability and pharmacokinetics of three formulations of albuterol. *J. Pharmacol. Sci.* 74:217, 1985.

352. Powell, M. L., et al. Multiple dose albuterol kinetics. *J. Clin. Pharmacol.* 26:643, 1986.

353. Powell, M. L., et al. Comparative steady-state bioavailability of conventional and controlled-release formulations of albuterol. *Biopharm. Drug Dispos.* 8:461, 1987.

354. Prior, J. G., Nowell, R. V., and Cochrane, G. M. High-dose inhaled terbutaline in the management of chronic severe asthma: comparison of wet nebulisation and tube-spacer delivery. *Thorax* 37:300, 1982.

355. Rachelefsky, G. S., Katz, R. M., and Siegel, S. C. Albuterol syrup in the treatment of the young asthmatic child. *Ann. Allergy* 47:143, 1981.

356. Racovenanu, C., et al. The bronchodilator effects of orciprenaline and salbutamol—a double-blind study. *Postgrad. Med. J.* 47(suppl):83, 1971.

357. Raptis, J., et al. Effects of cardioselective and non-cardioselective beta-blockade. *Eur. J. Clin. Pharmacol.* 20:17, 1981.

358. Rasmussen, H. The calcium messenger system (the second of two parts). *N. Engl. J. Med.* 314:1164, 1986.

359. Rebuck, A. S., et al. Nebulized anticholinergic and sympathomimetic treatment of asthma and chronic obstructive airways disease in the emergency room. *Am. J. Med.* 82:59, 1987.

360. Reinhardt, C. F., et al. Cardiac arrythmias and aerosol "sniffing." *Arch. Environ. Health* 22:265, 1971.

361. Reisman, J., et al. Frequent administration by inhalation of salbutamol and ipratropium bromide in the initial management of severe acute asthma in children. *J. Allergy Clin. Immunol.* 81:16, 1988.

362. Reisman, R. E. Asthma induced by adrenergic aerosols. *J. Allergy* 46:162, 1970.

363. Repsher, L. H., et al. Assessment of tachyphylaxis following prolonged therapy of asthma with inhaled albuterol aerosol. *Chest* 85:34, 1984.

364. Rhoden, K. J., Meldrum, L. A., and Barnes, P. J. Inhibition of cholinergic neurotransmission in human airways by β-2 adrenoceptors. *J. Appl. Physiol.* 65:700, 1988.

365. Richards, D. M., and Brogden, R. N. Pirbuterol. A preliminary review of its pharmacological properties and therapeutic efficacy in reversible bronchospastic disease. *Drugs* 30:61, 1985.

366. Richardson, J. B., and Ferguson, C. Morphology of the airways. In J. A. Nadel, (ed.), Physiology and Pharmacology of the Airways *(Vol. 15, Lung Biology in Health and Disease)*. New York: Dekker, 1980, P. 1.

367. Riding, W. D., Dinda, P., and Chattergee, S. S. The bronchodilator and cardiac effects of five pressure-packed aerosols in asthma. *Br. J. Dis. Chest* 64:37, 1970.

368. Riker, J. B., and Cocace, L. G. Double-blind comparison of metaproterenol and isoetharine-phenylephrine solutions in intermittent positive pressure breathing in bronchospastic conditions. *Chest* 78:723, 1980.

369. Robertson, C. F., et al. Response to frequent low doses of nebulized salbutamol in acute asthma. *J. Pediatrics* 106:672, 1985.

369a. Robin, E. D., and McCauley, R. Sudden cardiac death in bronchial asthma, and inhaled beta-adrenergic agonists. *Chest* 101:1799, 1992.

370. Roffel, A. F., Elzinga, R. S., and Zaagsma, J. Muscarinic M₃ receptors mediate contraction of human central and peripheral airway smooth muscle. *Pulm. Pharmacol.* 3:47, 1989.

371. Rohr, A. D., et al. Efficacy of parenteral albuterol in the treatment of asthma. Comparison of its metabolic side effects with subcutaneous epinephrine. *Chest* 89:348, 1986.

372. Rona, G. Catecholamine cardiotoxicity. *J. Mol. Cell Cardiol.* 17:291, 1985.

373. Rosa, R. M., et al. Adrenergic regulation of extrarenal potassium disposal. *N. Engl. J. Med.* 302:431, 1980.

373a. Rossing, T. H., et al. Emergency therapy of asthma: Comparison of the acute effects of parenteral and inhaled sympathomimetics and infused aminophylline. *Am. Rev. Respir. Dis.* 122:365, 1980.

374. Russell, J. A. Differential inhibitory effect of isoproterenol on contractions of canine airways. *J. Appl. Physiol.* 57:801, 1984.

375. Sackner, M. A., et al. Bronchodilator effects of terbutaline and epinephrine in obstructive lung disease. *Clin. Pharmacol. Ther.* 16:499, 1974.

376. Sackner, M. A., et al. Hemodynamic effects of epinephrine and terbutaline in normal man. *Chest* 68:616, 1975.

377. Sackner, M. A. Changes in blood oxygen and in cardiac function following beta₂ and other bronchodilator drugs. *Chest* 73(suppl):985, 1978.

378. Salome, C. M., Schoeffel, R. E., and Woolcock, A. J. Effect of aerosol and oral fenoterol on histamine and methacholine challenge in asthmatic subjects. *Thorax* 36:580, 1981.

379. Salome, C. M., et al. Effect of aerosol fenoterol on the severity of bronchial hyperreactivity in patients with asthma. *Thorax* 38:854, 1983.

380. Samuelson, W. M., and Davies, A. O. Hydrocortisone-induced reversal of beta adrenergic receptor uncoupling. *Am. Rev. Respir. Dis.* 130:1023, 1984.

381. Sankary, R. M., et al. Muscarinic cholinergic inhibition of cyclic AMP accumulation in airway smooth muscle. Role of a pertussis toxin–sensitive protein. *Am. Rev. Respir. Dis.* 13:145, 1988.

382. Sano, Y., Watt, G., and Townley, R. G. Decreased mononuclear cell beta-adrenergic receptors in bronchial asthma: parallel studies of lymphocytes and granulocyte desensitization. *J. Allergy Clin. Immunol.* 72:495, 1983.

383. Scarpace, P. J., and Abrass, I. B. Desensitization of adenylate cyclase and down regulation of beta adrenergic receptors after in vivo administration of beta agonist. *J. Pharmacol. Exp. Ther.* 223(suppl. 73):985, 1978.

384. Scheinin, M., et al. Hypokalemia and other non-bronchial effects of inhaled fenoterol and salbutamol. A placebo controlled dose-response study in healthy volunteers. *Br. J. Clin. Pharmacol.* 24:645, 1987.

385. Schnack, C., et al. Effects of somatostatin and oral potassium administration on terbutaline-induced hypokalemia. *Am. Rev. Respir. Dis.* 139:176, 1989.

386. Schuh, S., et al. High- versus low-dose, frequently administered, nebulized albuterol in children with severe, acute asthma. *Pediatrics* 83:513, 1989.

387. Schwartz, A. L., et al. Management of acute asthma in childhood. *Am. J. Dis. Child.* 134:474, 1980.

388. Schwartz, H. J., Trautlein, J. J., and Goldstein, A. R. Acute effects of terbutaline and epinephrine on asthma. *J. Allergy Clin. Immunol.* 58:516, 1976.

388a. Sears, M. R., and Beaglehole, R. Asthma morbidity and mortality: New Zealand. *J. Allergy Clin. Immunol.* 80(Suppl.):383, 1987.

389. Sears, M. R., et al. Regular inhaled beta-agonist treatment in bronchial asthma. *Lancet* 336:1391, 1990.

390. Settipane, G. A. Sulfites in drugs: a new comprehensive list. *NER Allergy Proc.* 7:543, 1986.

391. Shelhamer, J. H., et al. Abnormal adrenergic responsiveness in allergic subjects: analysis of isoproterenol-induced cardiovascular and plasma cyclic adenosine monophosphate responses. *J. Allergy Clin. Immunol.* 66:52, 1980.

392. Shim, C., and Williams, M. H. Comparison of oral aminophylline and aerosol metaproterenol in asthma. *Am. J. Med.* 71:452, 1981.

393. Shires, R., et al. Metabolic studies in acute asthma before and after treatment. *Br. J. Dis. Chest* 73:66, 1979.

394. Siegel, S. C., et al. A placebo-controlled trial of procaterol: a new long-acting oral beta-agonist in bronchial asthma. *J. Allergy Clin. Immunol.* 75:698, 1985.

395. Siegel, D., et al. Aminophylline increases the toxicity but not the efficacy of an inhaled beta-adrenergic agonist in the treatment of acute exacerbations of asthma. *Am. Rev. Respir. Dis.* 132:283, 1984.

396. Sims, J. A., do Pico, G. A., and Reed, C. E. Bronchodilating effect of oral theophylline-ephedrine combination. *J. Allergy Clin. Immunol.* 62:15, 1978.

397. Sly, R. M., Badiei, B., and Faciane, J. Comparison of subcutaneous terbutaline with epinephrine in the treatment of asthma in children. *J. Allergy Clin. Immunol.* 59:128, 1977.

398. Sly, R. M., Jenne, J. W., and Cohn, J. Toxicity of beta-adrenergic drugs. In J. W. Jenne and S. Murphy (eds.), Drug Therapy for Asthma. Research and Clinical Practice *(Vol. 31, Lung Biology in Health and Disease).* New York: Dekker, 1987, P. 953.

399. Smith, J. A., Weber, R. W., and Nelson, H. S. Theophylline and aerosolized terbutaline in the treatment of bronchial asthma. *Chest* 78:816, 1980.

400. Smith, S. R., and Kendall, M. J. Metabolic responses to beta$_2$ stimulants. *J. R. Coll. Physicians London* 18:190, 1984.

401. Smith, S. R., and Kendall, M. J. Potentiation of the adverse effects of intravenous terbutaline by oral theophylline. *Br. J. Clin. Pharmacol.* 21:451, 1986.

402. Smith, U. Adrenergic control of lipid metabolism. *Acta Medica Scand.* 672(suppl):41, 1983.

403. Somlyo, A. P., et al. Calcium and monovalent ions in smooth muscle. *Fed. Proc.* 41:2883, 1982.

404. Spector, S. L., and Gomez, M. G. Dose-response effects of albuterol aerosol compared with isoproterenol and placebo aerosols. *J. Allergy Clin. Immunol.* 59:280, 1977.

405. Speizer, F. E., Doll, R., and Heaf, P. Observations on recent increase in mortality from asthma. *Br. Med. J.* 1:335, 1968.

406. Speizer, F. E., et al. Investigation into use of drugs preceding death from asthma. *Br. Med. J.* 1:339, 1968.

407. Spina, D., et al. Autoradiographic localization of β-adrenoceptors in asthmatic human lung. *Am. Rev. Respir. Dis.* 140:1410, 1989.

408. Spiro, S. G., et al. Effect of intravenous injection in asthma. *Br. J. Clin. Pharmacol.* 2:495, 1975.

409. Spiro, S. G., et al. Intravenous injection of salbutamol in the management of asthma. *Thorax* 30:236, 1975.

410. Spitzer, W. O., and Buist, A. S. Case-control study of prescribed fenoterol and death from asthma in New Zealand, 1977–81 (letter). *Thorax* 45:645, 1990.

410a. Spitzer, W. O., et al. The use of β-agonists and the risk of death and near death from asthma. *N. Engl. J. Med.* 326:501, 1991.

411. Stamm, A. M., Clausen, J. L., and Tisi, G. M. Effects of aerosolized isoproterenol on resting myogenic tone in normals. *J. Appl. Physiol.* 40:525, 1976.

412. Steiner, P., et al. The use of intravenous isoproterenol in the treatment of status asthmaticus. *J. Asthma Res.* 12:215, 1975.

413. Stephen, W. G., et al., Tachyphylaxis to inhaled isoproterenol and the effect of methylprednisolone in dogs. *J. Allergy Clin. Immunol.* 65:105, 1980.

414. Stephens, N. L., et al. Anatomy and physiology of respiratory smooth muscle. In J. W. Jenne and S. Murphy, (eds.), Drug Therapy for Asthma. Research and Clinical Practice *(Vol. 31, Lung Biology in Health and Disease).* New York: Dekker, 1987.

415. Storms, W. W., et al. Procaterol metered-dose inhaler: a multi-clinic study evaluating the efficacy and safety in patients with asthma. *Ann. Allergy* 63:445, 1989.

416. Strader, C. D., Sigal, I. S., and Dixon, R. A. F. Mapping the functional domains of the β-adrenergic receptor. *Am. J. Respir. Cell. Mol. Biol.* 1:81, 1989.

417. Strader, C. D., Sigal, I. S., and Dixon, R. A. F. Structural basis of β-adrenergic receptor function. *FASEB J.* 3:1825, 1989.

418. Strauss, M. H., et al. The role of cardiac beta-1 receptors in the hemodynamic response to a beta-2 agonist. *Clin. Pharmacol. Ther.* 40:108, 1986.

419. Streeton J. A. Salbutamol: a double-blind crossover trial. *Med. J. Aust.* 2:1184, 1970.

420. Struthers, A. D., and Reid, J. L. Adrenaline causes hypokalaemia in man by beta$_2$ adrenoceptor stimulation. *Clin. Endocrinol.* 20:409, 1984.

421. Stuart-Smith, K., and Vanhoutte, P. M. Epithelium, contractile tone, and responses to relaxing beta agonists in canine bronchi. *J. Appl. Physiol.* 69(2):678, 1990.

422. Su, Y. F., Harden, T. K., and Perkens, J. P. Catecholamine-specific desensitization of adenylate cyclase. Evidence for a multistep process. *J. Biol. Chem.* 255:7410, 1980.

423. Svedmyr, N. L. V., Larson, S. A., and Thiringer, G. Development of resistance in beta adrenergic receptors of asthmatic patients. *Chest* 69:479, 1976.

423a. Svedmyr, N. The current place of β$_2$-agonists in the management of asthma. *Lung* (suppl.)105, 1990.

423b. Svedmyr, N. Action of corticosteroids on beta-adrenergic receptors. *Am. Rev. Respir. Dis.* 141(suppl.):S31, 1990.

424. Svedmyr, N., Löfdahl, C.-G., and Svedmyr, K. The effect of powder aerosol compared to pressurized aerosol. *Eur. J. Respir. Dis.* [Suppl.]119:81, 1982.

425. Svedmyr, N., and Svedmyr, K. In vitro and in vivo effects of theophylline and β$_2$-adrenostimulants in combination. *Eur. J. Respir. Dis.* 61(suppl 109):83, 1980.

426. Svedmyr, N. Y., and Thiringer, G. The effects of salbutamol and isoprenaline on β-receptors in patients with COPD. *Postgrad. Med. J.* 47:44, 1971.

427. Sykes, A. P., and Ayres, J. G. Further bronchodilatation from low dose inhaled beta$_2$ agonist in patients receiving infused terbutaline (abstract). *Am. Rev. Respir. Dis.* 143:A646, 1991.

428. Sykes, R. S., Reese, M. E., and Meyer, M. C. Pharmacokinetic properties of a new sustained-release albuterol preparation, Volmax (abstract). *J. Allergy Clin. Immunol.* 79:152, 1987.

429. Tai, E., and Read, J. Response of blood gas tensions to aminophylline and isoprenaline in patients with asthma. *Thorax* 22:543, 1967.

429a. Taira, N. An overview of the pharmacology of procaterol. *J. Respir. Dis.* (January, Suppl.):S22, 1987.

430. Taki, F., et al. The role of phospholipase in reduced beta-adrenergic responsiveness in experimental asthma. *Am. Rev. Respir. Dis.* 133:362, 1986.

431. Takuwa, Y., Takuwa, N., and Rasmussen, H. The effect of isoproterenol on intracellular calcium concentration. *J. Biol. Chem.* 263:762, 1988.

432. Tala, E., Kellomaki, L., and Pylkas, A. Double-blind comparison of isoprenaline, orciprenaline and salbutamol aerosols in patients with asthma. *Postgrad. Med. J.* 47(suppl):61, 1971.

433. Tandom, M. K. Cardiopulmonary effects of fenoterol and salbutamol aerosols. *Chest* 77:129, 1980.

434. Tasaka, K. Formaterol (Atock): a new orally active and selective beta$_2$-receptor stimulant. *Drugs Today* 22:505, 1986.

435. Tashkin, D. P. Measurement and significance of the bronchodilator response. In J. W. Jenne and S. Murphy (eds.), *Drug Therapy for Asthma and Clinical Practice* (Vol. 31, Lung Biology in Health and Disease Series). New York: Dekker, 1987.

435a. Tashkin, D. P., et al. Sites of airway dilation in asthma following inhaled vs. subcutaneous terbutaline: Comparison of physiologic tests with radionuclide lung images. *Am. J. Med.* 68:14, 1980.

436. Tashkin, D. P., et al. Subsensitization of beta-adrenoreceptors in airways and lymphocytes of healthy and asthmatic subjects. *Am. Rev. Respir. Dis.* 125:185, 1982.

437. Tashkin, D. P., et al. Double-blind comparison of acute bronchial and cardiovascular effects of oral terbutaline and ephedrine. *Chest* 68:155, 1975.

438. Taylor, G. J., and Harris, W. S. Cardiac toxicity of aerosol propellants. *JAMA* 214:81, 1970.

439. Taylor, M. W., et al. Metabolic effects of oral salbutamol. *Br. J. Med.* 1:22, 1976.

440. Taylor, W. F., Heimlick, E. M., and Strick, L. Ephedrine and theophylline in asthmatic children: quantitative observations on the combination and ephedrine tachyphylaxis. *Ann. Allergy* 23:437, 1965.

441. Theeuwes, F. Elementary osmotic pump. *J. Pharm. Sci.* 64:1987, 1975.

442. Thiringer, G., and Svedmyr, N. Comparison of infused and inhaled terbutaline in patients with asthma. *Scand. J. Respir. Dis.* 57:17, 1976.

443. Thomas, R., and Hicks, S. Myocardial infarction; ventricular arrhythmias associated with hypokalemia. *Clin. Sci.* 61:32P, 1981.

444. Thomas, D. J. B., et al. Salbutamol-induced diabetic ketoacidosis. *Br. Med. J.* 2:438, 1977.

445. Tinkelman, D. G., and Avner, S. E. Ephedrine therapy in asthmatic children: clinical tolerance and absence of side effects. *JAMA* 137:553, 1977.

446. Tinkelman, D. G., et al. Comparison of nebulized terbutaline (terb) and subcutaneous epinephrine (epi) in the treatment of acute asthma. *Ann. Allergy* 50:398, 1983.

447. Tipton, W. R., and Nelson, H. S. Frequent parenteral terbutaline in the treatment of status asthmaticus in children. *Ann. Allergy* 58:252, 1987.

448. Torda, T., et al., Quinacrine-blocked desensitization of adrenoceptors after immobilization stress or repeated injection of isoproterenol in rats. *J. Pharmacol. Exp. Ther.* 216:334, 1981.

449. Torphy, T. J. Actions of mediators on airway smooth muscle: functional antagonism as a mechanism for bronchodilator drugs. *Agents Actions* 23(suppl):37, 1988.

450. Torphy, T. J., et al. Functional antagonism in canine tracheal smooth muscle: inhibition by methacholine of the mechanical and biochemical response to isoproterenol. *J. Pharmacol. Exp. Ther.* 227:694, 1983.

451. Tota, M. R., et al. Biophysical and genetic analysis of the ligand-binding site of the β-adrenoceptor. *Trends Pharmacol. Sci.* 12:4, 1991.

452. Townley, R. G., et al. The effect of corticosteroids on the beta-adrenergic receptors in bronchial smooth muscle. *J. Allergy* 45:118, 1970.

453. Tribe, A. E., Wong, R. M., and Robinson, J. S. A controlled trial of intravenous salbutamol and aminophylline in acute asthma. *Med. J. Aust.* 2:749, 1976.

454. Tung, R. S., and Lichtenstein, L. M. Cyclic AMP agonist inhibition increases low levels of histamine release from human basophils. *J. Pharmacol. Exp. Ther.* 218:642, 1981.

455. Twentyman, O. P., Finnerty, J. P., and Holgate, S. T. Time course of bronchodilation and functional antagonism of histamine-induced bronchoconstriction after salmeterol. *Thorax* 45:786, 1990.

456. Twentyman, O. P., et al. Protection against allergen-induced asthma by salmeterol. *Lancet* 336:1338, 1990.

456a. Twentyman, O. P., Finnerty, J. P., and Holgate, S. T. Inhibitory effect of nebulized albuterol on the early and late asthmatic reactions and increase in airway responsiveness provoked by inhaled allergen in asthma. *Am. Rev. Resp. Dis.* 144:782, 1991.

457. Uden, D. L., et al. Comparison of nebulized terbutaline and subcutaneous epinephrine in the treatment of acute asthma. *Ann. Emerg. Med.* 14:229, 1985.

458. Ueda, M. D., Loehning, R. W., and Ueyama H. Relationship between sympathetic amines and methylxanthines inducing cardiac arrhythmias. *Anesthesiology* 22:926, 1961.

459. Ullman, A., Hedner, J., and Svedmyr, N. Inhaled salmeterol and salbutamol in asthmatic patients: an evaluation of asthma symptoms and the possible development of tachyphylaxis. *Am. Rev. Respir. Dis.* 142:571, 1990.

460. Ullman, A., and Svedmyr, N. Salmeterol, a new long-acting inhaled beta-2 adrenoceptor agonist: comparison with salbutamol in adult asthmatic patients. *Thorax* 43:674, 1988.

460a. Vaisman, N., Levy, L. D., and Pencharz, P. B. Effect of salbutamol on resting energy expenditure in patients with cystic fibrosis. *J. Pediatr.* 111:137, 1987.

461. van Amsterdam, R. G. M., et al. Role of phosphoinositide metabolism in functional antagonism of airway smooth muscle contraction by beta-adrenoreceptor agonists. *Eur. J. Pharmacol. Molec. Pharmacol. Sect.* 172:175, 1989.

462. van Amsterdam, R. G. M., et al. Role of phosphoinositide metabolism in human bronchial smooth muscle contraction and in functional antagonism by beta-adrenoceptor agonists. *Am. Rev. Respir. Dis.* 142:1124, 1990.

463. Van den Berg, W., et al. Correlation between terbutaline serum levels, cAMP plasma levels and FEV_1 in normals and asthmatics after subcutaneous administration. *Ann. Allergy* 44:233, 1980.

464. Van den Berg, W., et al. The effects of oral and subcutaneous terbutaline in asthmatic patients. *Eur. J. Respir. Dis.* 65(suppl 134):181, 1988.

465. Van Metre, T. E. Adverse effects of inhalation of excessive amounts of nebulized isoproterenol in status asthmaticus. *J. Allergy* 43:101, 1968.

466. Van Schyack, C. P., Visch, M. D., and Van Weel, C. Increased bronchial hyperresponsiveness after inhaling salbutamol during one year is not caused by desensitization to salbutamol. *Am. Rev. Respir. Dis.* 141:A468, 1990.

467. Van Schyack, C. P., et al. Increased bronchial hyperresponsiveness after inhaling salbutamol during one year is not caused by subsensitization to salbutamol. *J. Allergy Clin. Immunol.* 86:793, 1990.

468. Vathenen, A. S., et al. Rebound increase in bronchial responsiveness after treatment with inhaled terbutaline. *Lancet* 1:554, 1988.

469. Venter, J. C., and Fraser, C. M. Beta-adrenergic receptor isolation and characterization with immobilized drugs and monoclonal antibodies. *Fed. Proc.* 42:273, 1983.

470. Vermeire, P. A., and Vanhoutte, P. M. Inhibitory effects of catecholamines in isolated bronchial smooth muscle. *J. Appl. Physiol.* 46:787, 1979.

471. Van Rentergehm, D., et al. Intravenous versus nebulized terbutaline in patients with acute severe asthma: a double-blind randomized study. *Ann. Allergy* 59:313, 1987.

472. Vyse, T., Cochrane, G. M. Controlled release salbutamol tablets versus sustained release theopylline tablets in control of reversible obstructive airways disease. *J. Int. Med. Res.* 17:93, 1989.

473. Wagner, E. M., et al. Peripheral lung resistance in normal and asthmatic subjects. *Am. Rev. Respir. Dis.* 141:584, 1990.

474. Walker, S. B., Kradjan, W. A., and Bierman, C. W. Bitolterol mesylate: a beta-adrenergic agent. Chemistry, pharmacokinetics, pharmacodynamics, adverse effects and clinical efficacy in asthma. *Pharmacotherapy* 5:127, 1985.

475. Wallin, A., et al. Formoterol, a new long-acting beta$_2$ agonist for inhalation twice daily, compared with salbutamol in the treatment of asthma. *Thorax* 45:259, 1990.

476. Walters, E. H., et al. Optimal dose of salbutamol respiratory solution: comparison of three doses with plasma levels. *Thorax* 36:625, 1981.

477. Ward, M. J., et al. Ipratropium bromide in acute asthma. *Br. Med. J.* 282:598, 1981.

478. Warrel, D. A. et al. Comparison of cardiorespiratory effects of isoprenaline and salbutamol in patients with bronchial asthma. *Br. Med. J.* 1:65, 1976.

479. Watson, J. M., and Richens, A. The effects of salbutamol and terbutaline on physiological tremor, bronchial tone and heart rate. *Br. J. Clin. Pharmacol.* 1:223, 1974.

480. Webb, D. R., Mullarky, M. F., and Mingo, T. S. Bitolterol mesylate aerosol in chronic asthma. *J. Allergy Clin. Immunol.* 69:116, 1982.

480a. Weber, R. W., Petty, W. E., and Nelson, H. S. Aerosolized terbutaline in asthmatics. Dosage strength schedule and method of administration. *J. Allergy Clin. Immunol.* 63:116, 1979.

481. Weber, R. W., Smith, K. A., and Nelson, H. S. Aerosolized terbutaline in asthmatics: development of subsensitivity with long-term administration. *J. Allergy Clin. Immunol.* 70:417, 1982.

482. Weinberger, M. M., and Bronsky, E. A. Evaluaton of oral bronchodilator therapy in asthmatic children. *J. Pediatr.* 84:421, 1974.

483. Weiner, N. Norepinephrine, epinephrine and the sympathomimetic amines. In: A. G. Gilman, L. D. Goodman, and A. Gilman (eds), *The Pharmacological Basis of Therapeutics* (6th ed.). New York: Macmillan, 1980, P. 163.

484. Weiner, N. Drugs that inhibit adrenergic nerves and block adrenergic receptors. In A. G. Gilman, L. D. Goodman, and A. Gilman (eds), *The Pharmacological Basis of Therapeutics* (6th ed.). New York: Macmillan, 1980, P. 76.

485. Weiss, K. B., and Wagener, D. K. Changing patterns of asthma mortality. Identifying target populations at high risk. *JAMA* 264, 1683, 1990.

486. Whicker, S. D., Armour, C. L., and Black, J. L. Responsiveness of bronchial smooth muscle from asthmatic patients to relaxant and contractant agents. *Pulm. Pharmacol.* 1:25, 1988.

487. Whitehurst, V. A., et al. Cardiotoxic effects in rats and rabbits treated with terbutaline alone and in combination with aminophylline. *J. Am. Coll. Toxicol.* 2:147, 1983.

488. Whyte, K. F., et al. Methylxanthine and adrenaline-induced hypokalemia—possible contribution to tachyarrhythmias in asthmatic patients. *Clin. Sci.* 66:57P, 1984.

489. Whyte, K. F., et al. Salbutamol induced hypokalemia: the effect of theophylline alone and in combination with adrenaline. *Br. J. Clin. Pharmacol.* 25:571, 1988.

490. Willey, R. F., and Grant, I. W. B. Effects of oral salbutamol and pirbuterol on FEV_1, heart rate and blood pressure in asthmatics. *Br. J. Clin. Pharmacol.* 3:595, 1976.

491. Williams, I. P., et al. Sympathomimetic agonists stimulate mucus secretion into human bronchi. *Thorax* 36:231, 1981.

492. Williams, S., and Seaton, A. Intravenous or inhaled salbutamol in severe acute asthma. *Thorax* 32:555, 1977.

493. Williams, S. J., Parrish, R. W., and Seaton A. Comparison of intravenous aminophylline and salbutamol in severe asthma. *Br. Med. J.* 4:685, 1975.

494. Williams, S. J., Winner, S. J., and Clark, T. J. H. Comparison of inhaled and intravenous terbutaline in acute severe asthma. *Thorax* 36:629, 1981.

495. Wilson, A. F., et al. Cardiopulmonary effects of long-term bronchodilator administration. *J. Allergy Clin. Immunol.* 58:204, 1976.

496. Wilson, J. D., Sutherland, D. C., and Thomas, A. C. Has the change to beta-agonists combined with oral theophylline increased cases of fatal asthma? *Lancet* 1:1235, 1981.

497. Wolfe, B. B., Harden, T. K., and Molinoff, P. B. Beta-adrenergic receptors in rat liver: effects of adrenalectomy. *Proc. Natl. Acad. Sci. USA* 73:1343, 1976.

498. Wolfe, J. D., et al. Bronchodilator effects of terbutaline and aminophylline alone and in combination in asthmatic patients. *N. Engl. J. Med.* 298:363, 1978.

499. Wolfe, J. D., et al. Comparison of the acute cardiopulmonary effects of oral albuterol, metaproterenol, and terbutaline in asthmatics. *JAMA* 253:2068, 1985,

500. Wolfe, J. D., et al. Comparison of albuterol and metaproterenol syrup in the treatment of childhood asthma: a multi-center study. *Pediatrics* 88:312, 1991.

501. Wong, C. S., et al. Bronchodilator, cardiovascular, and hypokalemic effects of fenoterol, salbutamol, and terbutaline in asthma. *Lancet* 336:1396, 1990.

502. Wong, L. B., Miller, I. F., and Yeates, D. B. Stimulation of ciliary beat frequency by autonomic agonists in vivo. *J. Appl. Physiol.* 62:971, 1988.

503. Wood, D. W., et al. Intravenous isoproterenol in the management of respiratory failure in childhood status asthmaticus. *J. Allergy Clin. Immunol* 50:75, 1972.

504. Woolcock, A. J. Therapies to control the airway inflammation of asthma. *Eur. J. Respir. Dis.* 69(suppl 147):166, 1986.

505. Woolcock, A. J., et al. Influence of autonomic nervous system on airway resistance and elastic recoil. *J. Appl. Physiol.* 26:814, 1969.

506. Wyatt, R. Appendix. In J. W. Jenne and S. Murphy (eds.), *Drug Therapy for Asthma. Research and Clinical Practice* (Vol. 31, Lung Biology in Health and Disease). New York: Dekker, 1987, P. 1045.

507. Yagura, T., and Yamamura, Y. A new selective beta-adrenoceptor stimulant (procaterol): its bronchodilator potency and characteristics in asthmatic patients. *Curr. Ther.* 10:45, 1979.

508. Zaagsma, J., et al. Adrenergic control of airway function. *Am. Rev. Respir. Dis.* 136(4):S45, 1987.

509. Zaagsma, J., et al. Comparison of functional beta-adrenoceptor heterogeneity in central and peripheral airway smooth muscle of guinea pig and man. *J. Recept. Res.* 3:89, 1991.

510. Zainudin, B. M. Z., et al. Comparison of bronchodilator responses and deposition patterns of salbutamol inhaled from a pressurized metered dose inhaler, as a dry powder, and as a nebulized solution. *Thorax* 45:569, 1990.

511. Zanetti, C. L., Rotman, H. H., and Dresner, A. J. Efficacy and duration of action of procaterol, a new bronchodilator. *J. Clin. Pharmacol.* 22:250, 1982.

Aerosol Delivery Systems

Archie F. Wilson

56

In recent years, it has been repeatedly suggested that the preferred method of administration of antiasthma drugs is by inhalation [14, 78, 111]. The major advantage that the inhalation route has over the oral or intravenous routes is direct deposition of drug at the site of desired activity and, consequently, use of less drug and the development of fewer side effects [7, 14, 46, 54, 61, 75, 78, 79, 100, 102, 106, 111]. Currently, almost every major type of antiasthma preparation is available in aerosol form; these include beta agonists, anticholinergics, steroids, and other anti-inflammatory preparations; theophylline, which is irritating when inhaled [8, 21, 99], is the only major antiasthma compound not approved for inhalation use.

The therapeutic effectiveness of any inhaled medication is critically dependent on the amount of drug deposited on the walls of specific airways [2, 9, 13, 19, 25, 41, 42, 44, 45, 47, 50, 55, 58, 62, 64, 66–71, 73–75, 78, 80, 84, 87, 89, 94, 111–113]. In turn, where the inhaled medication is deposited is contingent on several technical factors, including the size of the aerosol [9, 31, 58, 78, 112], the hygroscopicity of the drug [24, 39, 40, 82, 83, 90], the particle charge, and the presence of other substances such as diluents [63], surfactants [61], and propellants [37, 60, 61]; additionally, certain patient factors such as the speed of inhalation [26, 65, 66, 68, 80, 85] and the coordination between aerosol release and timing of inhalation [26, 65, 66, 68, 80, 85] play important roles in aerosol deposition.

Where the drug deposits within the respiratory system determines the therapeutic effect: mouth deposition causes little, if any, effect [87, 89]; central deposition tends to cause large-airway dilatation, while more peripheral deposition tends to cause greater small-airway effects [111]; and alveolar deposition is probably rapidly followed by absorption of the soluble aerosol into the circulation and, hence, is often not a desirable site when airway rather than systemic responses are desired [23, 79, 92].

One of the major factors determining both the site of airway deposition and the magnitude of therapeutic effect is particle size [31, 58, 77, 84, 112] (Table 56-1; Fig. 56-1) (see also Chap. 32). The behavior of a particle in an airstream is largely defined by its aerodynamic diameter, which, in turn, is delimited by its diameter, shape, and density [53, 56, 98, 111]. Most therapeutic aerosol particles are round and have a density near unity or slightly larger. The particle diameter of therapeutic aerosols is, however, quite variable over a large range [39, 98, 111] and, in many aerosol-generating systems, may change in the humid conditions of the airways [24, 39, 40, 82, 83, 90]. In general, desirable particle diameters range from about 1 to 7 μm [39, 98, 111]. Particles larger than 10 μm are virtually completely captured by the mouth and oropharynx, while particles less than 1 μm tend to behave like gases and are mostly exhaled [39, 98, 111]. The mass of any therapeutic material is related to particle size by the third power of the radius; an 8-μm-diameter particle has 64 times more mass than a particle of 2-μm diameter. Therefore, large quantities of

inhaled drug may be lost in the tubing and/or mouth and oropharynx.

Aerosol deposition within the thorax is often determined by quantitative assessment of the distribution of aerosol-related radioactivity [44, 49, 68, 70, 80, 89]. Though such measurements may separate gross differences in deposition between the large central airway and peripheral lung (includes small airways and alveoli), such studies cannot clearly separate differences in deposition between medium and large or between medium and small airways or even between small airways and alveoli. Hence, conclusions based on studies of this type must be considered tentative.

In this chapter, aerosol-generation devices and those technical and patient factors that control airway deposition will be discussed.

TYPES OF AEROSOL DELIVERY SYSTEMS

Therapeutic aerosol generation systems, in general, are of two major types: those that create wet particles (*nebulizers* and some *metered-dose inhalers* [MDIs]) and those that deliver preformed aerosol (these include *dry-powder inhalers* [DPIs] and most MDIs). An additional type of device that may be used to potentially improve MDI performance is the *spacer*.

Nebulizers

Nebulizers create liquid droplets from solutions of therapeutic materials. There are two major types of nebulizers: jet and ultrasonic. A typical jet nebulizer consists of a supply of air that by Venturi action draws up liquid through a supply tube; the liquid is broken up into droplets at the end of the feed tube and further shattered against a baffle [29, 50, 57] (Fig. 56-2). Most particles so formed are quite large and collide with the walls of the baffle and the nebulizer, these tend to coalesce into large droplets and are recycled. Some of the smaller particles formed leave the nebulizer constantly. Usually, well over 10 minutes (in some cases, over 30 minutes) is required to complete nebulization. The baffle design is important in determining the size of particles that can escape the nebulizer and become available for patient inhalation; large and multiple baffles produce smaller particles and much longer nebulization times are the result [57]. During the process of nebulization and recycling, solution remaining in the nebulizer becomes progressively more concentrated from evaporation [29, 63]. Consequently, released particles tend to become gradually larger [18, 95]. Because of this evaporation, the nebulizer temperature falls during operation [17, 57]. Additionally, since during operation much of the remaining concentrated solution is, at any moment, on the nebulizer walls, near and at the end of nebulization, jet nebulizers tend to sputter and stop, with a large propor-

Table 56-1. *Mechanisms important in deposition of particles in the lungs*

	Inertia	Sedimentation	Diffusion
Particle size	Large particle diameter, ≥5 μm	Medium particle diameter, 1–6 μm	Smallest particle diameter, ≲1 μm
Anatomic site	Nose, pharynx, larger airways	Smaller airways	Terminal airways, alveolar ducts, alveoli
Aerodynamics	High airflow	Low airflow, breath-hold	Low-to-zero airflow, breath-hold
Geometric factors	Increased bifurcation angles	Horizontal airways, surfaces	Small airspace dimensions, nearby surfaces

Source: J. D. Brain and P. A. Valberg; Deposition of aerosol in the respiratory tract. *Am. Rev. Respir. Dis.* 120:1325, 1979. Reprinted with permission.

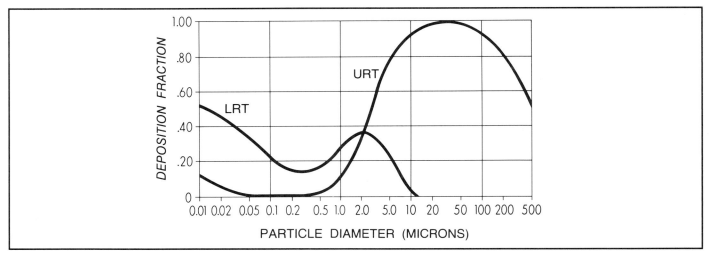

Fig. 56-1. *Particle size and respiratory deposition. The deposition probabilities of particles of different aerodynamic size are indicated for the upper respiratory tract (URT) and the lower respiratory tract (LRT), the demarcation of the two divisions being the epiglottis. These curves can be considered useful for associating the approximate deposition pattern and amount deposited within the human respiratory system during spontaneous respiration through the nose. (Reprinted with permission from P. E. Morrow, Aerosol characterization and deposition. Am. Rev. Respir. Dis. 110:88, 1974.)*

tion (up to 60%) of the mass of the drug adherent to the walls of the device [17, 63].

The amount and diameter of the particles produced by individual jet nebulizers depends on operating conditions as well as design [15–18, 28, 29, 34, 35, 41, 57, 58, 71, 107, 108]. In particular, the fill volume and operating air pressure or flow are important variables [17, 28, 35, 63, 71]. Since the amount of liquid adhering to the walls of all jet nebulizers is about the same when they cease operation, under most conditions, the proportion of the original volume of drug nebulized can be expected to be greater when the fill volume is small. Hence, larger fill volumes, though requiring longer nebulization times, release a higher proportion of contained medication. The driving air pressure (or airflow rate) affects both the amount and size of particles produced [15–18, 28, 35, 57, 71]; high pressure produces a greater number and mass of smaller particles than does lower pressure. It is clear from the above remarks that it is essential for any report about the clinical effects of nebulizers to clearly describe the conditions of use, including the fill volume and driving pressure or airflow rate. Additionally, even though the operating characteristics of individual nebulizers are often not completely understood, it is also important that the type and manufacturer of the nebulizer be reported.

Nebulizers produce particles of greatly varying diameters (heterodisperse). As already noted, larger particles do not reach intrathoracic airways; in the case of nebulizers, the major site of deposition is the tubing connecting the nebulizer with the patient [49]. Similar to MDIs, about 10 percent of the material placed in a nebulizer is deposited within the thorax [49].

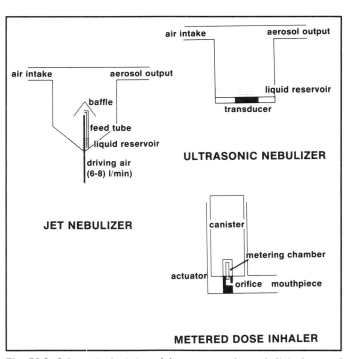

Fig. 56-2. *Schematic depiction of three commonly used clinical aerosol generators.*

When released droplets enter the warmer conditions of human airways, they may theoretically grow or evaporate, depending on the droplet and ambient temperatures as well as on the droplet chemical and osmotic composition [24]. Very little information is available about these potentially important phenomena.

Jet nebulizers may be operated intermittently or continuously. During intermittent operation, air passes through the supply tube only during inspiration. Intermittent operation should be considerably more efficient than continuous operation because nebulization takes place only during that phase of respiration when particles can be inhaled. On the other hand, if there is no nebulization during expiration, gas inspired from the instrumental dead space will not contain particles, and, if the instrumental dead space is large, the amount of aerosol inhaled per breath could be considerably reduced. Intermittent nebulization can be achieved by either occluding a diversion hole in the supply air tube (when the hole is not occluded, air does not traverse the nebulizer chamber) or through positive-pressure (or ventilator)–coordinated nebulization; the latter process is often referred to as *intermittent positive-pressure breathing* (IPPB). Clinically, even in cases of acute asthma, there is little to indicate that IPPB is superior to a continuously operated jet nebulizer [7, 11, 25, 91]. This area requires further investigation, with particular attention to the operating conditions of the nebulizer.

Very-high-frequency (ultrasonic) vibration (see Fig. 56-2) can be used to break liquid up into small particles. The size and number of particles produced by this process depends on the power and speed of oscillation of the energy delivered [29, 111]. The subsequent behavior of particles produced is contingent on principles similar to those discussed earlier for jet nebulizers. In particular, the particles generated exit from the nebulizer only when the volume and speed of intake air are sufficient to carry the aerosol out of the chamber before the baffle or chamber walls are encountered. Similarly, the length and diameter of connecting tubing will affect removal of aerosol by the tubing, in that more particles will exit from the tubing and be available for inhalation if the connecting tubing is short and wide. The output of ultrasonic nebulizers can be quite high; if water is used as a solvent, hypoosmotic damage to the airways can lead to bronchospasm [12].

Metered-Dose Inhalers

MDIs are propellant-driven devices that can form droplets at the orifice where material is released to the atmosphere. Droplets formed consist either of drug dissolved in propellant or solid microparticles suspended in propellant. In either case, a small amount of liquid (in the range of 25–100 μl) is released from a metering chamber when the canister is depressed against the activator (see Fig. 56-2). The most commonly used system releases suspended particles plus a pressurized and liquefied chlorofluorocarbon (CFC) propellant, or propellants, and a surfactant. The less commonly used system releases medication dissolved in alcohol or another cosolvent plus liquefied CFC.

CFC propellants (freons 11, 12, and 114) are simple compounds in which hydrogen atoms of methane and ethane have been replaced by fluorine and chlorine in varying mixtures. These substances have several properties that make them relatively ideal as propellants: they are essentially biologically inert [96, 101]; when pressurized, they become liquid, but when released into the atmosphere, they evaporate rapidly and cause any material that accompanies them to travel at great speed in the direction which the orifice is pointing [37, 61]. The usual pressure within the canister is about 3.5 atmospheres [60, 61]. Canister pressure is important, as can be shown by the effect of canister temperature on aerosol availability; low temperatures (near 0°C) are associated with large particles and reduced aerosol availability; with higher temperatures (around body temperature), particles

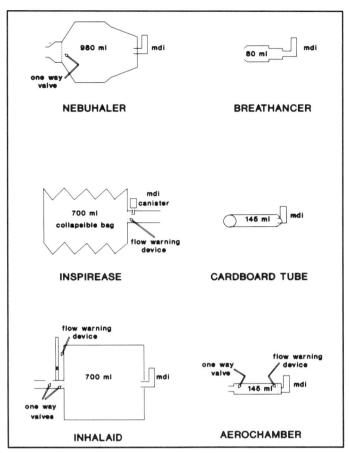

Fig. 56-3. *Schematic depiction of six commonly used metered-dose inhaler spacer devices.*

are smaller and are more respirable [112]. Because these agents have been implicated in the reduction of the Earth's ozone layer [61, 111], their use in refrigeration and other industrial applications will soon disappear in most countries. Though medicinal use of these agents quantitatively accounts for a small fraction of their current total use, it is likely that, even for medicinal use, these materials will also be replaced. Several substitute compounds are being evaluated; potential replacements include pressurized nonchlorinated fluorocarbons and other inert gases.

In the pre-formed delivery type of MDI, surfactants, such as oleic acid, lecithin, and sorbitan trioleate, are added to prevent clumping of the powdered medication [61]. When the canister is pressed into the actuator, a premeasured amount of a mixture of propellant, surfactant, and drug is released. The initial droplet size is quite large—about 30 μm—and the initial particle speed is considerable—about 100 miles per hour [61]. As the propellant evaporates, particle size and speed reduce considerably over a short distance; however, it has been shown that particles may still have considerable momentum 15 cm from the orifice [61]. The final size of the evaporated droplet depends on the number of microparticles present in the original droplet. The output of the MDI is, like nebulizers, heterodisperse with considerable mass in a size range that is not likely to traverse the mouth and oropharynx. Indeed, about 10 to 15 percent of the drug released from an MDI, similar to nebulizer performance, appears in the thorax [49, 113]. The major difference between nebulizer and MDI deposition patterns is where the bulk of the drug deposits; with nebulizer use, about 80 percent of the deposition is in the nebulizer body and connecting tubing; with MDI use, about 80 percent is deposited in the mouth and oropharynx [49].

Particles produced by an MDI are initially enveloped in propellant; as the propellant evaporates from the surface of the particles, the droplets become smaller. Since most antiasthma substances are hygroscopic, the particles may grow considerably as they pass through the humid connections of the airways [39, 40]. What actually happens to inhaled hygroscopic materials in the airways of humans is unknown. To the extent that the particles grow larger, more proximal deposition is likely.

The major disadvantage of an MDI is the necessity to inhale aerosol released in a controlled manner—a significant problem for many patients [36, 43, 93, 111]. It has been shown that it is important to activate an MDI and inhale at the same time; activation of terbutaline MDI either well before or at the end of inhalation was associated with reduced bronchodilatation in asthmatics [65, 86]; our own recent experience with pirbuterol MDI indicates that, though activation at the end of inhalation is relatively ineffective, activation 3 seconds before inhalation is associated with only a slightly less reduction in bronchodilatation, presumably because the aerosol produced by pirbuterol MDI is significantly smaller than that provided by terbutaline MDI. The inspiratory flow rate is another important determinant of MDI effectiveness; a low flow rate of about 0.3 L/sec is associated with less upper airway removal of inhaled aerosol and a better clinical response than a higher flow rate of about 1.5 L/sec [26, 64–66, 68, 111]. Initial lung volume and tidal volume (within limits) have not been clearly shown to be important controlling variables, though the data are somewhat conflicting [26, 64, 65, 85].

Because of the importance and difficulties attendant upon achieving appropriate coordination, breath-activated MDIs have been developed [1, 19]. Though not currently available in the United States, a breath-activated MDI (Autohaler), which is activated at relatively low flow rates (30 L/min), has been introduced in Great Britain. This device will potentially overcome the problem of discoordination but not that of very rapid inspiratory flow rates.

Dry-Powder Inhalers

For a number of years, the only DPI used was the Spinhaler, a device designed for the inhalation of disodium cromoglycate [3, 61, 111]; this device was subsequently supplanted by a much more convenient MDI preparation of disodium cromoglycate. However, interest in the DPI has increased with the realization that some discoordination problems could be eliminated with the use of devices (such as DPIs) that empty only during inspiration. The active medication delivered in the original Spinhaler was greatly diluted with lactose particles, which were included to minimize the clumping of medication particles and adherence of particles to the apparatus [61]. Although a DPI is currently available in the United States which delivers albuterol (Rotahaler) [1], this device has not achieved very much popularity because of its relatively high cost and the relative inconvenience of placing each dose separately into the DPI; a Rotahaler is about equipotent with an MDI [20, 97]. However, there are commercial products available outside the United States that deliver only active medication without an inert filler and require reloading only after many uses (e.g., 200 doses with a Turbuhaler) [1, 30, 36, 81]. Because very small quantities of bronchodilator are effective [77], a potential problem with these new DPIs is that the patient may not be aware when release and inhalation of medication have taken place.

Metered-Dose Inhaler Spacers

Experience with DPIs indicates that discoordination problems can be avoided to a large degree by the use of devices that release aerosol only during inhalation. Another approach to the difficulties associated with discoordination is use of an apparatus that

Table 56-2. Metered-dose inhaler spacers

MDI spacer	Reservoir volume (ml)	Separation of inspired & expired gas	Flow sensor	Available in U.S.
InspirEase	700	No	Yes	Yes
AeroChamber	145	Yes	Yes	Yes
InhalAid	750	Yes	Yes	Yes
Nebuhaler	750	Yes	No	No
Breathancer	80	No	No	Yes
Toilet paper cardboard roll	145	No	No	Yes
Styrofoam cup (infants)	180	No	No	Yes
MDI in bag	980	No	No	Yes

holds aerosol until inhalation takes place. Such reservoirs are usually referred to as *spacers* or *extensions* [48]. Spacers of many designs have been introduced (Fig. 56-3). Spacer reservoir design differs not only in size (volumes vary from 120 to over 1,000 ml) but also in the valving that separates inspired from expired gas and in features such as indicators of inhaled volume and flow rates. Spacers such as the InspirEase [72, 73, 103], InhalAid, Nebuhaler [54, 72], and AeroChamber [27] contain valving that excludes humid exhaled air from the reservoir chamber; such an arrangement tends to minimize the growth of hygroscopic aerosols in a reservoir chamber. InspirEase utilizes a 700-ml collapsible bag, which provides visual evidence of volume inhalation. InspirEase and InhalAid also contain flow-sensing devices that provide feedback and thereby help control the inhalation rate (Table 56-2).

Another potential benefit of spacers is the removal of large particles by sedimentation in the reservoir chamber. Large particles contain a bulk of mass of medication ($V = 4/3\pi r^3$) and deposit primarily in the oral cavity and pharynx. While most medications are inhaled in quantities that have little or no effect except when they deposit on airways, a shift in the deposition of large particles from the oral cavity and pharynx to the reservoir is often not clinically important. However, patients who use medications such as topical steroids, which have potentially deleterious effects on the upper airway mucosa (e.g., thrush and dysphonia), should benefit from the use of spacers [104]. A curious effect noted with a topical steroid inhaled through a spacer is apparently more steroid deposition in the alveoli [104]; that is, morning cortisol levels are lower in patients who use spacers compared to those who do not, suggesting that the spacer, because it promotes increased delivery to the alveoli, causes a greater amount of medication to be absorbed.

Other types of spacers have been developed. Designs include simple tubes (see Fig. 56-3) of varying lengths [32, 52, 59], half cylinders [74], and spherical designs of varying volumes [69]. It is not clear that any design is superior in performance for most patients.

The potential benefits of spacers are many: reduced problems associated with discoordination are noted with most devices; reduced problems associated with too rapid inhalation of aerosol are seen with a few; reduced problems associated with upper airway deposition of medication are found with most. However, the experience has been that, except for a minority of patients who cannot learn how to use MDIs properly [93, 111], spacers are unnecessary [5, 32, 51, 69, 75, 110]. Most patients strongly prefer the convenience of a device that fits easily into a shirt pocket. Even in the case of patients who use inhaled steroids, gargling after inhalation will prevent the complications of thrush and hoarseness, which are, anyway, benign and self-limited.

COMPARISON BETWEEN AEROSOL DELIVERY SYSTEMS

Numerous studies have been conducted that compare the merits of nebulizers, MDIs, DPIs, and MDI spacers. The results of many studies are difficult to interpret because the operating parameters of the studied aerosol delivery systems were not specified. In fact, in most studies in which jet nebulizers were used and in some studies in which MDIs were used, this crucial information was not given. In those studies for which enough information is given to evaluate the procedures used, both the aerosol deposition in the thorax and the clinical response are similar for nebulizers, MDIs, DPIs, and MDI spacers [6, 9a, 22, 30, 32, 33, 34a, 38, 40a, 41a, 51, 54, 55, 76, 97, 105, 109, 113]. Yet, in practice, much more medication is used for the treatment of bronchospasm when nebulizers are used, compared to MDIs and other devices. Obviously, this common practice cannot be supported by the experimental data. The fact that clinical response to these very large doses of nebulized bronchodilator is only slightly greater than that to MDI use illustrates that the typical small doses of bronchodilator utilized with MDIs are very potent and that larger doses of medication, delivered either by nebulizer or MDI, are only minimally more effective because of the log–dose relationship of bronchoactive drugs to spirometric response [77, 102].

REFERENCES

1. Anani, A., Higgins, A. J., and Crompton, G. K. Breath-actuated inhalers: comparison of terbutaline Turbuhaler with salbutamol Rotahaler. *Eur. J. Respir. Dis.* 2:640, 1989.
2. Asmundsson, T., et al. Efficiency of nebulizers for depositing saline in human lung. *Am. Rev. Respir. Dis.* 108:506, 1973.
3. Bell, J. H., Hartley, P. S., and Cox, J. S. Dry powder aerosols. I: A new powder inhalation device. *J. Pharm. Sci.* 60:1559, 1971.
4. Bell, K. A., and Ho, A. T. Growth rate measurements of hygroscopic aerosols under conditions simulating the respiratory tract. *J. Aerosol Sci.* 3:247, 1981.
5. Berry, R. B., et al. Nebulizer vs spacer for bronchodilator delivery in patients hospitalized for acute exacerbations of COPD. *Chest* 96:1241, 1989.
6. Blackhall, M. I., and O'Donnell, S. R. A dose-response study of inhaled terbutaline administered via Nebuhaler or nebulizer to asthmatic children. *Eur. J. Respir. Dis.* 71:96, 1987.
7. Bloomfield, P., et al. Comparison of salbutamol given intravenously and by intermittent positive-pressure breathing in life-threatening asthma. *Br. Med. J.* 1:848, 1979.
8. Bohadana, A. B., et al. The bronchodilator action of theophylline aerosol in subjects with chronic airflow obstruction. *Bull. Eur. Physiopathol. Respir.* 16:13, 1980.
9. Bouchiki, A., et al. Particle size study of nine metered dose inhalers, and their deposition probabilities in the airways. *Eur. J. Respir. Dis.* 1:547, 1988.
9a. Bowton, D. L., Goldsmith, W. M., and Haponik, E. F. Substitution of metered-dose inhalers for hand-held nebulizers. Success and cost savings in a large, acute-care hospital. *Chest* 101:305, 1992.
10. British Thoracic and Tuberculosis Association. A controlled trial of inhaled corticosteroids in patients receiving prednisone tablets for asthma. *Br. J. Dis. Chest* 70:95, 1976.
11. Chang, N., and Levison, H. The effect of a nebulized bronchodilator administered with or without intermittent positive pressure breathing on ventilatory function in children with cystic fibrosis and asthma. *Am. Rev. Respir. Dis.* 106:867, 1972.
12. Cheney, F. W., Jr. and Butler, J. The effects of ultrasonically-produced aerosols on airway resistance in man. *Anesthesiology* 6:1099, 1968.
13. Chung, K. F., Jeyasing, K., and Snashall, P. D. Influence of airway calibre on the intrapulmonary dose and distribution of inhaled aerosol in normal and asthmatic subjects. *Eur. J. Respir. Dis.* 1:890, 1988.
14. Clark, T. J. H. Factors Influencing Route of Administration of Airway Therapy. In P. Sadoul, et al. (eds.), *Small Airways in Health and Disease.* Amsterdam: Excerpta Medica, 1979.
15. Clay, M. M., and Clarke, S. W. Effect of nebulized aerosol size on lung deposition in mild asthma. *Thorax* 42:190, 1987.
16. Clay, M. M., Pavia, D., and Clarke, S. W. Effect of aerosol particle size on bronchodilatation with nebulized terbutaline in asthmatic subjects. *Thorax* 41:364, 1986.
17. Clay, M. M., et al. Assessment of jet nebulizers for lung aerosol therapy. *Lancet* 2:592, 1983.
18. Clay, M. M., et al. Factors influencing the size distribution of aerosols from jet nebulizers. *Thorax* 38:755, 1983.
19. Coady, T. J., Davies, H. J., and Barnes, P. Evaluation of a breath actuated pressurized aerosol. *Clin. Allergy* 6:1, 1976.
20. Crompton, G. K. Clinical use of a dry powder system. *Eur. J. Respir. Dis.* 63(Suppl. 122):96, 1982.
21. Cushley, M. J., and Holgate, S. T. Efficacy of inhaled methylxanthines as bronchodilator in asthma. *Thorax* 38:223, 1983.
22. Cushley, M. J., Lewis, R. A., and Tattersfield, A. E. Comparison of three techniques of inhalation on the airway response to terbutaline. *Thorax* 38:908, 1983.
23. Davies, D. S. Pharmacokinetic studies with inhaled drugs. *Eur. J. Respir. Dis.* 63(Suppl. 119):67, 1982.
24. Davis, S. S., and Bubb, M. D. Physico-chemical studies on aerosol solution for drug delivery. III. The effect of relative humidity on the particle size of inhalation aerosols. *Int. J. Pharmacol.* 7251:303, 1978.
25. Dolovich, M. B., et al. Pulmonary deposition in chronic bronchitis: intermittent positive-pressure breathing versus quiet breathing. *Am. Rev. Respir. Dis.* 115:397, 1977.
26. Dolovich, M. B,. et al. Optimal delivery of aerosols from metered dose inhalers. *Chest* 80(Suppl.):911, 1981.
27. Dolovich, M. B., et al. Clinical evaluation of a simple demand inhalation MDI aerosol delivery system. *Chest* 84:36, 1983.
28. Douglas, J. G., et al. Is the flow rate used to drive a jet nebulizer clinically important? *Br. Med. J.* 290:29, 1985.
29. Ferron, G. H., Kerrebijn, K. F., and Weber, J. Properties of aerosols produced with three nebulizers. *Am. Rev. Respir. Dis.* 114:899, 1976.
30. Fuglsang, G., and Pedersen, S. Comparison of Nebuhaler and nebulizer treatment of acute severe asthma in children. *Eur. J. Respir. Dis.* 69:109, 1986.
31. Godfrey, S., et al. The possible site of action of sodium cromoglycate assessed by exercise challenge. *Clin. Sci. Mol. Med.* 46:265, 1974.
32. Gomm, S. A., et al. Effect of an extension tube on the bronchodilator efficacy of terbutaline delivered from a metered dose inhaler. *Thorax* 35:552, 1980.
33. Gomm, S. A., et al. Dose-response comparison of ipratropium bromide from a metered-dose inhaler and by jet nebulization. *Thorax* 38:297, 1983.
34. Gottschalk, B., Leupold, W., and Woller, P. Deponierung von Aerosolen in den oberen und unteren Atemwegen. *Atemwegs Lungenkrank* 4:378, 1978.
34a. Guidry, G. G., et al. Incorrect use of metered-dose inhalers by medical personnel. *Chest* 101:31, 1992.
35. Hadfield, J. W., Windebank, W. J., and Bateman, J. R. M. Is driving gas flow rate clinically important for nebulizer therapy? *Br. J. Dis. Chest* 80:50, 1986.
36. Hansen, O. R., and Pedersen, S. Optimal inhalation technique with terbutaline Turbuhaler. *Eur. J. Respir. Dis.* 2:637, 1989.
37. Hayton, W. L. Propellant-powered nebulizers. *J. Am. Pharm. Assoc.* 16:201, 1976.
38. Hetzel, M. R., and Clark, T. J. H. Comparison of salbutamol Rotahaler with conventional pressurized aerosol. *Clin. Allergy* 7:563, 1977.
39. Hiller, F. C., et al. Physical properties, hygroscopicity and estimated pulmonary retention of various therapeutic aerosols. *Chest* 77(Suppl.):318, 1980.
40. Hiller, F. C., et al. Effect of low and high humidity on metered-dose bronchodilator solution and powder aerosols. *J. Pharm. Sci.* 69:334, 1980.
40a. Hultquist, C., et al. Effect of inhaled terbutaline sulphate in relation to its deposition in the lungs. *Pulm. Pharmacol.* 5:127, 1992.
41. Johnson, M. A., et al. Delivery of albuterol and ipratropium bromide from two nebulizer systems in chronoic stable asthma: efficacy and pulmonary deposition. *Chest* 96:1, 1989.
41a. Kelly, H. W., and Murphy, S. Beta-adrenergic agonists for acute, severe asthma. *Ann. Pharmacother.* 26:81, 1992.
42. Kim, C. S., Eldridge, M. A., and Sackner, M. A. Oropharyngeal deposition and delivery aspects of metered-dose inhaler aerosols. *Am. Rev. Respir. Dis.* 135:157, 1987.
43. Kim, C. S., Trujillo, D., and Sackner, M. A. Size aspects of metered-dose inhaler aerosols. *Am. Rev. Respir. Dis.* 132:137, 1985.
44. Kohler, D., Fleisher, W., and Matthys, H. New method for easy labeling

of beta-2-agonists in the metered dose inhaler with technetium 99m. *Respiration* 53:65, 1988.

45. Laros, C. D., Van Urk, P., and Rominger, K. L. Absorption, distribution and excretion of the tritium-labelled beta 2 stimulator fenoterol hydrobromide following aerosol administration and instillation into the bronchial tree. *Respiration* 34:131, 1977.

46. Larsson, S., and Svedmyr, N. Bronchodilating effect and side effects of beta 2-adrenoreceptor stimulants by different modes of administration (tablets, metered aerosol, and combinations thereof). *Am. Rev. Respir. Dis.* 116:861, 1977.

47. Laube, B. J., et al. The effect of bronchial obstruction on central airway deposition of a saline aerosol in patients with asthma. *Am. Rev. Respir. Dis.* 133:740, 1986.

48. Lee, H., and Evans, H. E. Evaluation of inhalation aids of metered dose inhalers in asthmatic children. *Chest* 91:366, 1987.

49. Lewis, R. A., and Fleming, J. S. Fractional deposition from a jet nebulizer: how it differs from a metered dose inhaler. *Br. J. Dis. Chest* 79:361, 1985.

50. Lewis, R., et al. Particle sized distribution and deposition from a jet nebulizer: influence of humidity and temperature. *Clin. Sci.* 62:5, 1981.

51. Lewis, R., et al. Is a nebulizer less efficient than a metered dose inhaler and do pear-shaped extension tubes work? *Am. Rev. Respir. Dis.* 125(Pt. 2):94, 1982.

52. Lindgren, S. B., Formgren, H., and Moren, F. Improved aerosol therapy of asthma: effect of actuator tube size on drug availability. *Eur. J. Respir. Dis.* 61:56, 1980.

53. Lourenco, R. V., and Cotromanes, E. Clinical Aerosols. I. Characterization of aerosols and their diagnostic use. *Arch. Intern. Med.* 142:2163, 1982.

54. Madsen, E. B., Bundgaard, A., and Hidinger, K. G. Cumulative dose-response study comparing terbutaline pressurized aerosol administered via a pearshaped spacer and terbutaline in a nebulized solution. *Eur. J. Clin. Pharmacol.* 23:27, 1982.

55. Matthys, H., and Kohler, D. Pulmonary deposition of aerosols by different mechanical devices. *Respiration* 48:269, 1985.

56. Mercer, T. T. Production and characterization of aerosols. *Arch. Intern. Med.* 131:39, 1973.

57. Mercer, T. T., Tillery, M. I., and Chow, H. Y. Operating characteristics of some compressed-air nebulizers. *Am. Ind. Hyg. Assoc. J.* 29:66, 1968.

58. Mitchell, D. M., et al. Effect of particle size of bronchodilator aerosol on lung distribution and pulmonary function in patients with chronic asthma. *Thorax* 42:457, 1987.

59. Moren, F. Drug deposition of pressurized inhalation aerosols. I. Influence of actuator tube design. *Int. J. Pharm.* 1:205, 1978.

60. Moren, F. Drug deposition of pressurized inhalation aerosols. II. Influence of vapor pressure and metered volume. *Int. J. Pharm.* 1:213, 1978.

61. Moren, F. Aerosol Dosage Forms and Formulations. In F. Moren, M. T. Newhouse, and M. B. Dolovich (eds.), *Aerosols in Medicine.* Amsterdam: Elsevier, 1985.

62. Morrow, P. E. Aerosol characterization and deposition. *Am. Rev. Respir. Dis.* 110:88, 1974.

63. Moser, K. M., Butler, E., and Landis, G. A. Fate of radiolabeled isoproterenol aerosol: I. Effect of diluent. *Am. Rev. Respir. Dis.* 96:167, 1967.

64. Newman, S. P., and Pavia, D. Aerosol Deposition in Man. In F. Moren, M. T. Newhouse, and M. B. Dolovich (eds.), *Aerosols in Medicine.* Amsterdam: Elsevier, 1985.

65. Newman, S. P., Pavia, D., and Clarke, S. W. How should a pressurized β-adrenergic bronchodilator be inhaled? *Eur. J. Respir. Dis.* 62:3, 1981.

66. Newman, S. P., Pavia, D., and Clarke, S. W. Improving the bronchial deposition of pressurized aerosols. *Chest* 80(Suppl.):909, 1981.

67. Newman, S. P., Woodman, G., and Clarke, S. W. Deposition of carbenicillin aerosols in cystic fibrosis: effects of nebulizer system and breathing pattern. *Thorax* 43:318, 1988.

68. Newman, S. P., et al. Deposition of pressurized aerosols in the human respiratory tract. *Thorax* 36:52, 1981.

69. Newman, S. P., et al. Deposition of pressurized suspension aerosols inhaled through extension devices. *Am. Rev. Respir. Dis.* 124:317, 1981.

70. Newman, S. P., et al. Effects of various inhalation modes on deposition of radioactive pressurized aerosols. *Eur. J. Respir. Dis.* 63(Suppl. 119):57, 1982.

71. Newman, S. P., et al. Evaluation of jet nebulizers for use with gentamicin solution. *Thorax* 40:671, 1985.

72. Newman, S. P., et al. Enhanced drug delivery from metered dose inhalers with the InspirEase. *Am. Rev. Respir. Dis.* 131:A96, 1985.

73. Newman, S. P., et al. Effect of InspirEase on the deposition of metered-dose aerosol in the human respiratory tract. *Chest* 89:551, 1986.

74. Newman, S. P., et al. Pressurized aerosol deposition in the human lung with and without an "open" spacer device. *Thorax* 44:706, 1989.

75. Noseda, A., and Yernault, J. D. Sympathomimetics in acute severe asthma: inhaled or parenteral, nebulizer or spacer? *Eur. J. Respir. Dis.* 2: 377, 1989.

76. O'Reilly, J. F., et al. Domiciliary comparison of terbutaline treatment by metered dose inhaler with and without conical spacer in severe and moderately severe chronic asthma. *Thorax* 41:766, 1986.

77. Patel, P., Mukai, D., and Wilson, A. F. Dose-response effects of two sizes of monodisperse isoproterenol in mild asthma. *Am. Rev. Respir. Dis.* 141: 357, 1990.

78. Paterson, J. W., Woolcock, D. J., and Shenfield, G. Bronchodilator drugs. *Am. Rev. Respir. Dis.* 129:1149, 1979.

79. Pauwels, R. Pharmacokinetics of inhaled drugs. In F. Moren, M. T. Newhouse, and M. B. Dolovich (eds.), *Aerosols in Medicine.* Amsterdam: Elsevier, 1985, Pp. 219–224.

80. Pavia, D., et al. Effect of lung function and mode of inhalation on penetration of aerosol into the human lung. *Thorax* 32:194, 1977.

81. Persson, G., and Wiren, J. E. The bronchodilator response from inhaled terbutaline is influenced by the mass of small particles: a study on a dry powder inhaler (Turbuhaler). *Eur. J. Respir. Dis.* 2:253, 1989.

82. Porstendorfer, J. Untersuchungen zur Frage des Wachstums von inhalierten Aerosoltielchen im Atemtrakt. *Aerosol Sci.* 2:73, 1971.

83. Porstendorfer, J., Gebhart, J., and Robig, G. Effect of evaporation on the size distribution of nebulized aerosols. *J. Aerosol. Sci.* 8:371, 1977.

84. Rees, P. J., and Clark, T. J. H. The importance of particle size in response to inhaled bronchodilators. *Eur. J. Respir. Dis.* 63(Suppl. 119):73, 1982.

85. Riley, D. J., Weitz, B. W., and Edelman, N. H. The responses of asthmatic subjects to isoproterenol inhaled at different lung volumes. *Am. Rev. Respir. Dis.* 114:509, 1976.

86. Rivlin, J., et al. Effect of administration technique on bronchodilator response to fenoterol in a metered-dose inhaler. *J. Pediatr.* 20:470, 1983.

87. Rodenstein, D., and Stanescu, D. C. Mouth spraying versus inhalation of fenoterol aerosol in healthy subjects and asthmatic patients. *Br. J. Dis. Chest* 76:365, 1982.

88. Roth, M. J., Wilson, A. F., and Novey, H. S. A comparative study of the aerosolized bronchodilators, isoproterenol, metaproterenol and terbutaline in asthma. *Ann. Allergy* 38:16, 1977.

89. Ruffin, R. E., Montgomery, J. M., and Newhouse, M. T. Site of beta-adrenergic receptors in the respiratory tract. *Chest* 74:256, 1978.

90. Scherer, P. W., et al. Growth of hygroscopic aerosols in a model of human airways. *J. Appl. Physiol.* 47:544, 1979.

91. Shenfield, G. M., Evans, M. E., and Paterson, J. W. The effect of a nebulized bronchodilator with and without intermittent positive pressure breathing on the absorption and metabolism of salbutamol. *Br. J. Clin. Pharmacol.* 1:295, 1974.

92. Shenfield, G. W., et al. The fate of nebulized salbutamol (albuterol) administered by intermittent positive pressure respiration to asthmatic patients. *Am. Rev. Respir. Dis.* 108:501, 1973.

93. Shim, C., and Williams, M. H., Jr. The adequacy of inhalation of aerosol from canister nebulizers. *Am. J. Med.* 69:891, 1980.

94. Spiro, S. G., et al. Direct labelling of ipratropium bromide aerosol and its deposition pattern in normal subjects and patients with chronic bronchitis. *Thorax* 39:432, 1984.

95. Sterk, P. J., et al. Physical properties of aerosols produced by several jet- and ultrasonic nebulizers. *Bull. Eur. Physiopathol. Respir.* 20:65, 1984.

96. Stewart, R. D., et al. Physiological response to aerosol propellants. *Environ. Health Perspect.* 26:275, 1978.

97. Svedmyr, N., Lofdahl, C.-G., and Svedmyr, K. The effects of powder aerosol compared to pressurized aerosol. *Eur. J. Respir. Dis.* 63(Suppl. 119): 81, 1982.

98. Swift, D. L. Aerosol characterization and generation. In F. Moren, M. T. Newhouse, and M. B. Dolovich (eds.), *Aerosol in Medicine.* Amsterdam: Elsevier, 1985, Pp. 53–76.

99. Stainforth, N. J., Lewis, R. A., and Tattersfield, A. E. Dosage and delivery of nebulized beta agonist in hospital. *Thorax* 38:751, 1983.

100. Tashkin, D. P., et al. Sites of airway dilatation in asthma following inhaled versus subcutaneous terbutaline. *Am. J. Med.* 68:14, 1980.

101. Thiessen, B., and Pedersen, O. F. Effect of freon inhalation on maximal expiratory flows and heart rhythm after treatment with salbutamol and ipratropium bromide. *Eur. J. Respir. Dis.* 61:156, 1980.

102. Thiringer, G., and Svedmyr, N. Comparison of i.v. administered and inhaled terbutaline with dose-effect curves in patients with chronic obstructive lung disease. *Scand. J. Respir. Dis.* 88(Suppl.):56, 1974.

103. Tobin, M. J., et al. Response to bronchodilator drug administration by a new reservoir aerosol delivery system and a review of other auxiliary delivery systems. *Am. Rev. Respir. Dis.* 126:670, 1982.

104. Toogood, J. H., et al. Use of spacer to facilitate inhaled corticosteroid treatment of asthma. *Am. Rev. Respir. Dis.* 129:723, 1984.

105. Turner, J., et al. Equivalence of continuous flow nebulizer and metered-dose inhalers with reservoir bag for treatment of acute airflow obstruction. *Chest* 93:476, 1988.

106. Walker, S. R., et al. The clinical pharmacology of oral and inhaled salbutamol. *Clin. Pharmacol. Ther.* 13:8651, 1972.

107. Walters, E. H., et al. Optimal dose of salbutamol respiratory solution: comparison of three doses with plasma levels. *Thorax* 36:625, 1981.

108. Weber, B. A., Shenfield, G. M., and Paterson, J. W. A comparison of three different methods of giving nebulized albuterol to asthmatic patients. *Am. Rev. Respir. Dis.* 109:293, 1979.

109. Weber, R. W., Petty, W. W., and Nelson, H. S. Aerosolized terbutaline in asthmatics. Comparison of dosage strength, schedule and method of administration. *J. Allergy Clin. Immunol.* 63:116, 1979.

110. Weeke, E. R. Reported clinical experiences with inhaled terbutaline aerosol via spacer devices. *Eur. J. Respir. Dis.* 63(Suppl. 119):105, 1982.

111. Wilson, A. F. Aerosol Dynamics and Deliver. In J. W. Jenne and S. Murphy (eds.), *Drug Therapy for Asthma: Research and Practice.* New York: Dekker, 1987.

112. Wilson, A. F., Mukai, D. S., and Ahdout, J. J. Effect of canister temperature on performance of metered-dose inhalers. *Am. Rev. Respir. Dis.* 143:1034, 1991.

113. Zainuddin, B. M. Z., et al. Comparison of bronchodilator responses and deposition patterns of salbutamol inhaled from a pressurized metered dose inhaler, as a dry powder, and as a nebulized solution. *Thorax* 45:469, 1990.

Intravenous Sympathomimetic Drugs in Acute Severe Asthma

57

Nils Svedmyr
Claes-Göran A. H. Löfdahl

The efficacy of symptomatic asthma therapy has increased over the past decade partly because of the introduction of relatively long-acting selective beta$_2$-adrenoceptor stimulants, which are effective by several routes of administration. The following basic effects have been suggested to be of clinical importance [62, 66, 78, 83, 84, 89]:

1. Bronchial smooth muscle relaxation
2. Inhibition of mediator release
3. Suppression of permeability edema
4. Stimulation of ion and water secretion into airways in the epithelial cells
5. Increased mucociliary transport
6. Decreased airway reactivity
7. Increased release of epithelial-derived relaxant factor
8. Inhibition of cholinergic neurotransmission

The bronchial smooth muscle relaxation is probably most important. However, the importance of the other effects cannot be ruled out. An inhibition of permeability edema as well as effects on the mucus removal from the airways might also be of importance in an acute situation.

DISTRIBUTION OF BETA$_1$- AND BETA$_2$-ADRENOCEPTORS

The division of beta-adrenoceptors into the beta$_1$ and beta$_2$ subtypes during the 1960s [41, 42] made a separation of cardiac and pulmonary effects of beta-adrenoceptor stimulation possible. At that time, albuterol and terbutaline were registered in Europe as beta$_2$-adrenoceptor stimulating agents with a selective airway effect. A few years later fenoterol was introduced.

Later it was shown in several animal tissues that the beta-adrenoceptor population might be heterogenous. Some species have been found to have beta$_1$-adrenoceptor-mediated bronchial relaxation, such as the guinea pig, in which approximately 25 percent of the relaxation is mediated via beta$_1$-adrenoceptors [37, 105]. In the cat and ferret, tracheal relaxation is mediated mainly via beta$_1$-adrenoceptors [79].

In human bronchial muscle, smooth muscle relaxation is mediated only by beta$_2$-adrenoceptors as shown in vitro [105] and in asthmatic patients using selective beta$_1$ agonists and antagonists [52–54]. Beta-adrenoceptors in skeletal muscle are also important, as the main side effect of the drugs is the skeletal muscle tremor induced by beta-adrenoceptor stimulation. It has been shown that the skeletal muscle receptors are of beta$_2$-adrenoceptor subtype [1, 44, 67, 68]. Attempts have been made to separate the effect of beta$_2$-adrenoceptors in bronchial smooth muscle and skeletal muscle. To date no difference between these receptors has been shown [55].

Circulatory side effects of beta-adrenoceptor stimulation could be due to stimulation of beta-receptors in either peripheral vessels or in the heart. An important reason for tachycardia during beta$_2$-agonist treatment is due to an effect on beta$_2$-adrenoceptors mediating vasodilation in peripheral vessels [2, 3, 71, 90, 93]. In the heart most beta-receptors are of beta$_1$ subtype. However, in the human heart both beta$_1$- and beta$_2$-adrenoceptors have been shown to mediate an increased heart rate. Beta$_2$-adrenoceptors were responsible for 20 percent of the chronotropic effect, whereas beta$_1$-adrenoceptors almost solely mediated inotropic effects [3, 11, 12, 68, 106]. Thus, there is a possibility that the beta$_2$-adrenoceptor agonist induces tachycardia both via a reflex from peripheral vasodilation and from a direct effect of beta$_2$-adrenoceptors in the heart. This direct effect on the heart can only be attenuated by inhalation administration.

Beta-adrenoceptor agonists and various xanthine derivatives have the same maximal relaxant effect on isolated human bronchial muscle in vitro contracted by a moderate dose of carbachol [86]. The potency found clinically is proportional to the relative potency between the drugs in vitro. Unless there is development of substantial tolerance in situ in asthmatic patients for some of these drugs, there is today no reason to believe that the clinical efficacy differs substantially between these two drug classes. Their side effects differ, however, and side effects can make it impossible to achieve this maximal bronchodilating effect in patients with a single drug, especially if they are given systemically. Terbutaline and salbutamol are weak partial agonists on the beta$_1$-adrenoceptor, whereas fenoterol is a full agonist also on the beta$_1$-adrenoceptor [9]. This means that fenoterol, at least at higher doses, has more pronounced beta$_1$-mediated side effects.

PHARMACOKINETICS OF BETA-ADRENOCEPTOR STIMULATING DRUGS

The pharmacokinetic properties of beta-adrenoceptor stimulating drugs vary in several respects (Table 57-1) [61]. The plasma protein binding varies from about 8 percent for salbutamol up to 97 percent for clenbuterol. The plasma half-life varies from less than 5 minutes for isoproterenol and rimiterol to 35 hours for clenbuterol. Terbutaline has a terminal half-life of 17 hours however, with more than 50 percent of the drug disappearing with a half-life of 3 to 4 hours. The oral bioavailability for the drugs varies from 15 to 45 percent. Terbutaline has an oral bioavailability of 15 percent, whereas salbutamol has 45 percent.

SIDE EFFECTS

The importance of side effects of beta-stimulating drugs in asthma treatment is not the same in acute treatment as in mainte-

Table 57-1. Some pharmacokinetic data for oral or intravenous beta-adrenoceptor agonists

	Plasma protein binding (%)	Plasma half-life (hr)	Absorption (%)	Bioavailability (%)
Clenbuterol	97	35	87	?
Fenoterol	55	?	60	?
Isoproterenol	?	0.05	80	25
Rimiterol	?	0.05	47	?
Salbutamol	8	4	75	45
Terbutaline	15	3.5 (>50%), 17	40	15

nance therapy. In maintenance treatment, skeletal muscle tremor is almost always the dose-limiting side effect. Palpitations occur in a few percent of patients [28]. Tachyphylaxis to these side effects occurs after regular treatment for about a week [45]. In the acute treatment, these effects could have some influence on patients, however, with minor importance.

In acute severe asthma, patients often present with tachycardia [35, 36, 91]. Therefore, treatment with a beta-stimulating drug that decreases airway resistance also decreases the respiratory effort needed by the patient. That is the reason why in some studies in acute severe asthma there is a fall of heart rate after treatment even with intravenous beta-stimulating drugs [91].

Beta-stimulators also increase the flux of potassium ions through the cell membrane. Therefore, hypokalemia is seen after intravenous as well as after high doses of inhaled beta-stimulating treatment [14, 36, 51, 63, 80, 97]. It has been argued that this hypokalemia is responsible for serious side effects [17]. This effect is subject to tolerance development under regular treatment, and the most serious consequence of hypokalemia would occur in patients who are not treated with beta-stimulating drugs before their acute asthma attack. It has also been shown that patients on diuretic treatment reach lower levels of serum potassium after combined treatment with beta-stimulating drugs [49]. The most serious consequence of hypokalemia would be an increased risk for cardiac arrhythmias. Minor electrocardiographic (ECG) changes as a T-wave flattening and a slight prolongation of QT time have been described [14, 102]. Supraventricular tachycardias and supraventricular atopic beats are the most common arrhythmias seen. In a few cases, ventricular atopic beats have been described [48, 101]. A 24-hour ECG monitoring showed frequent arrhythmias of various kinds, both supraventricular and ventricular, in patients with acute severe asthma. However, the only arrhythmia that was significantly increased during a 4-hour nebulization period of 20 mg of salbutamol was supraventricular atopic beats. Other arrhythmias were the same during the period after the beta-stimulating drugs as during the rest of the day [48]. Therefore, these authors conclude that high standard doses of beta-agonists given no more than every 6 hours do not seem to be associated with an increased risk of potentially life-threatening arrhythmias. This was in spite of a significant fall of plasma potassium [48]. Intravenous isoproterenol has, however, been reported to give serious cardiac side effects and should no longer be used [57, 64].

Another side effect occurring mainly in acute treatment is the mismatch of ventilation and perfusion with beta-stimulating drugs. Recently, Ballester and coworkers [4] have shown that with intravenous infusion of salbutamol, the ventilation-perfusion mismatch worsened, even if arterial oxygen tension remained unchanged. With inhaled salbutamol there was no mismatch between ventilation and perfusion. Intravenous salbutamol also increased the metabolic rate at the same time as cardiac output increased [4]. Oxygen consumption increased 22 percent after intravenous infusion of 360 μg of salbutamol. Svedmyr [85] showed in 1966 that beta-agonists markedly increased the oxygen consumption, an effect that could be of importance during severe attacks. This further strengthens the recommendation to administer oxygen during an acute attack.

ROUTES OF ADMINISTRATION

Complete dose-response curves in patients with asthma, as well as in vitro studies, show that nonselective and selective beta$_2$-stimulants attain the same maximal bronchodilating effect when given intravenously [90] (Fig. 57-1). The bronchodilator and cardiac stimulant effects of isoprenaline run parallel, suggesting that beta$_1$ and beta$_2$ receptors are equally stimulated. However, with a very high dose of isoprenaline and maximal bronchodilation achieved, the heart frequency continues to increase until it is nearly double at the highest dose; this phenomenon also limits the use of intravenous isoprenaline (non-beta$_2$-selective) in asthma. In the same patients the selective beta$_2$-stimulant (salbutamol) gave the same maximal bronchodilation but was initially not associated with any pulse increase (a sign of selective beta$_2$ effect). The pulse rate did not begin to increase until almost half of the maximum bronchial relaxation had been achieved, and it increased thereafter with increasing salbutamol dose. Yet even with selective beta$_2$-stimulants it is not possible to achieve maximum bronchodilation in severely obstructed patients without a

Fig. 57-1. *Mean dose-response curves ± SEM for isoprenaline and salbutamol for 10 patients with asthma. Each dose was infused during 6 minutes with 30-minute intervals. (Modified from N. Svedmyr and G. Thiringer. The effects of salbutamol and isoprenaline on β-receptors in patients with chronic obstructive lung disease. Postgrad. Med. J. [March Suppl.] 47:44, 1971.)*

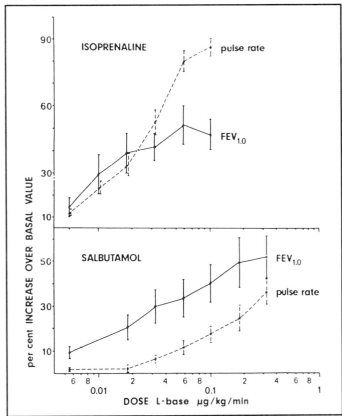

simultaneous increase in pulse rate if the drug is administered systemically, owing to peripheral vasodilation with an ensuing chronotropic effect and to a chronotropic effect with stimulation of the beta$_2$-adrenoceptors in the heart [3, 12]. About the same beta$_2$ selectivity has been established for terbutaline and salbutamol [43, 93], both partial agonists on the beta$_1$-adrenoceptor. Fenoterol is a full agonist on the beta$_1$-adrenoceptor and gives more pronounced side effects [9, 102, 103].

Beta$_2$-adrenoceptor agonists have been compared under controlled conditions with complete dose-response curves in the same patients by inhalation and intravenous routes. Intravenous terbutaline in the upper recommended dose range did not produce maximum relaxation of the bronchial muscle in patients with endogenous asthma (Fig. 57-2), but it did increase the heart rate by 25 beats/min and more than doubled the skeletal muscle tremor [93]. When terbutaline was given by inhalation, the same degree of bronchial relaxation resulted without any effect on heart rate, blood pressure, or tremor, indicating a local effect and increased therapeutic breadth. With higher inhaled terbutaline doses, the maximum bronchodilation was more pronounced than after the highest intravenous dose. The acute margin of safety was notable, the increase of pulse rate after 63 inhalations given cumulatively during 150 minutes of this relatively long-active substance being only 16 beats/min. These side effects are barely noticeable subjectively, implying that very high inhaled doses may be considered in very severe asthma not responding to usual dose therapy. Such high doses can also be inhaled by continuous nebulization.

In a crossover study in 12 asthma patients with acute severe

Fig. 57-2. *Effects of increasing doses of terbutaline by intravenous infusion (during 6 minutes) and dose aerosol on FEV$_1$, heart rate, blood pressure, and skeletal muscle tremor in asthmatics. (Dotted line = heart rate immediately before the next dose.) Means ± SEM from 10 patients. (Modified from G. Thiringer and N. Svedmyr. Comparison of infused and inhaled terbutaline in patients with asthma.* Scand. J. Respir. Dis. *57:17, 1976.)*

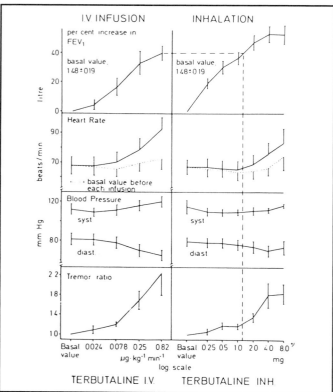

asthma, intravenous salbutamol was compared to the inhaled route [36]. Peak plasma concentration was more than doubled with the intravenous route, and heart rate increased considerably more, with a more pronounced decrease of serum potassium. The bronchodilating effect was, however, less pronounced (Fig. 57-3), again indicating an increased airway selectivity with the inhaled compared to the intravenous route.

In summary, inhalation is the superior route of administration for beta$_2$-stimulants if the patient is able to use the inhaler in a proper way. Better bronchodilation may be obtained with cumulative inhalations with at least 10- to 15-minute intervals than with a single high dose if the inhalations are administered [10, 32].

TOLERANCE

Concern for the development of tolerance to beta$_2$-adrenoceptor stimulants had favoured the use of intravenous theophylline, especially in the United States; however, preference for theophylline is currently challenged because of safety concerns. Many prospective studies in the past few years were conducted to establish whether tolerance of clinical importance to beta-agonists could be demonstrated after conventional doses of regular oral or inhaled beta$_2$-receptor agonists given for periods ranging from 2 weeks to 15 months. Overall the findings suggest that asthmatic patients do not develop tolerance of clinical importance to conventional doses of beta-agonists, in accordance with clinical experience [89].

Also, in emergency room treatment of asthma, inhaled beta-stimulants have recently been shown to be the treatment of choice; in this situation cardiac side effects were much less pronounced than during treatment of mild to moderate chronic asthma [23]. (These studies are discussed later.) This contrasts with the finding in normal subjects where tolerance to the airways' response developed with increasing regular doses of salbutamol [31, 92, 94]. It also contrasts with findings in other tissues in patients with asthma such as skeletal muscle tremor, tachycardia, lymphocyte cyclic adenosine monophosphate (AMP) levels, and metabolic effects as hypokalemia and hyperglycemia, where evidence of tolerance has been frequent after similar doses of beta-agonists [45, 50].

There is, however, often a clinical history of recent overuse of adrenergic bronchodilators, particularly by aerosol, in patients seen in emergency rooms, so in this situation an element of induced beta-adrenergic tolerance cannot necessarily be ruled out. It is, however, easy to overcome this tolerance by increasing the dose of beta$_2$-stimulants. Theoretically, combined treatment with corticosteroids could counteract such a desensitization [88]. It is also important to realize that the duration of bronchodilation is reduced more than the peak effect [70, 96]. Beta$_2$-stimulants should therefore be given in higher doses and with shorter intervals in patients with acute severe asthma than in maintenance therapy.

DRUG COMBINATIONS

Combination with Theophylline

Because beta-stimulants and theophylline have long been thought to act at different sites in the metabolic pathway of cyclic AMP, they have been expected to act synergistically when used together. In clinical practice, beta-stimulants and theophylline have, however, only an additive bronchodilating effect [5, 87].

The role of beta-adrenergic bronchodilators in the emergency treatment of acute asthma has been investigated by McFadden's group [23, 72, 73], who studied the relative effectiveness of var-

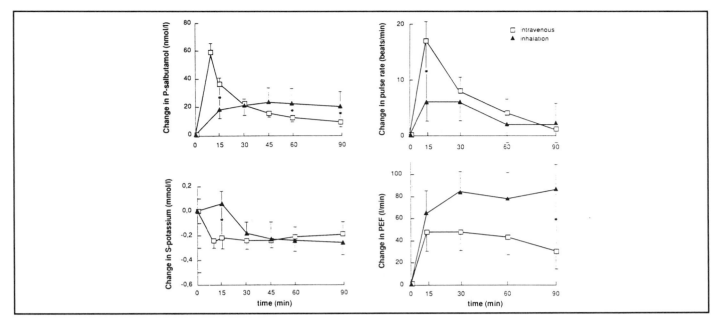

Fig. 57-3. *Plasma concentrations, systemic effects, and ventilatory effects after salbutamol treatment by inhaled route (0.15 mg/kg inhaled during 10–15 minutes from a nebulizer) (open squares) or by intravenous route (5 µg/kg during 10 minutes) (filled triangles). (Modified from C. Jansson. Plasma levels and effects of inhaled and intravenous salbutamol in stable asthma. Pulm. Pharmacol. 4:135, 1991.)*

ious combination regimens (see Chap. 72). In the first of these studies, they showed that a repetitive dose of inhaled isoprenaline (2.5 mg three times with 20-minute intervals) administered by hand-held nebulizer gave much better bronchodilation within 1 hour than intravenous theophylline in conventional therapeutic doses [23]. In the second study, they showed that adrenaline alone (0.3 mg subcutaneously every 20 minutes for three doses) gave less improvement than adrenaline combined with conventional doses of theophylline intravenously or a combination of inhaled isoprenaline (2.5 mg every 20 minutes for three doses) combined with the same dose of theophylline [73]. In the third study, 102 acutely ill patients were randomly assigned to treatment either with inhaled isoprenaline alone (2.5 mg three times with 20-minute intervals) or the same dose of isoprenaline by inhalation combined with intravenous theophylline in conventional doses [72]. The combination of isoprenaline and theophylline was not found to be better than isoprenaline alone. Furthermore, with modern selective, long-acting beta$_2$-adrenoceptor stimulants such as salbutamol and terbutaline, it is possible to achieve even better bronchodilation with fewer cardiovascular side effects than with isoprenaline. Addition of aminophylline only increased the acute toxicity, but not the efficacy of inhaled metaproterenol in acute exacerbations of asthma [77]. These data suggest that the importance of theophylline in the emergency treatment of adults with asthma may have been overemphasized in recent years, leading to underutilization of what is now thought to be possibly the more important component of the treatment, the inhaled adrenergic bronchodilators.

Combination with Corticosteroids

In severe asthma, bronchial muscle constriction is responsible for only part of the airway obstruction. Airway inflammation, manifested as mucosal thickening, edema in the bronchial wall, and mucous plugging, is an important pathogenetic mechanism. While the muscle component may respond to inhaled bronchodilators, the other component could require other types of treatment. Therefore, in the acute treatment, corticosteroids are

needed to act on the inflammatory events in the bronchial mucosa (see Chap. 60).

In maintenance treatment of asthma, it takes at least 1 hour before an effect of corticosteroid treatment can be shown [21], and it takes 6 to 7 hours to achieve the maximum effect of an intravenous corticosteroid as measured by forced expiratory volume in 1 second (FEV$_1$). In acute severe asthma the latency time is longer [15, 20, 24]. It takes at least 6 hours before a significant effect can be shown. That might explain why no effect of corticosteroids has been shown in studies with shorter follow-up time than 6 hours [60]. In clinical trials the steroid effect is often overshadowed by the rapid effect of inhaled beta$_2$-adrenoceptor bronchodilators in high doses. This makes it difficult to show a further significant additional effect of steroids. It should also be questioned whether, for example, acute measurement of FEV$_1$ is an adequate parameter to evaluate corticosteroid effect in acute severe asthma. Several controlled [82] studies show that acute treatment with corticosteroids gives a significantly faster recovery and in some studies also a decreased recurrence rate during the first 10 days, and they also almost completely lack acute side effects [16, 24, 26, 56, 75]. Thus, it is important to introduce corticosteroids early in the treatment of the acute asthma attack to reduce bronchial inflammation and bronchial hyperresponsiveness and improve the distribution of inhaled drugs. Steroids also have the capacity to reverse beta$_2$-adrenoceptor subsensitivity [88]; this subsensitivity is probably without clinical significance.

Combination with Anticholinergic Agents

Several studies have evaluated the effect of anticholinergic treatment, preferentially inhaled ipratropium bromide, in acute asthma and especially the effect when combined with sympathomimetics [39] (see Chap. 64). Due to differences in trial design, it is difficult to evaluate these studies thoroughly. In most studies ipratropium bromide by inhalation adds about a 10 percent increase of ventilatory capacity to standard recommended doses of inhaled beta$_2$ agonists [69]. In most studies the combination seems to have a longer duration of effect [34]. Any influence of this on the long-term clinical outcome has not been shown [81], and it is still not clarified whether the additive effect occurs also with very high doses of inhaled beta$_2$ agonists [39].

INTRAVENOUS BETA AGONISTS IN ACUTE SEVERE ASTHMA—CLINICAL STUDIES

Nonselective Drugs

The first studies with intravenous isoprenaline performed in 1972 and 1973 by Woods and Downes [18, 104] were uncontrolled, emergency room open trials performed in an effort to avoid the use of mechanical ventilation in severely obstructed asthmatics. Similar results were achieved in a study in 1976 [65].

Herman and coworkers [33] reported the result of intravenous treatment with isoproterenol in 37 children in an open uncontrolled study, starting with 0.5 μg/kg body weight/min and increasing the dose at 20-minute intervals. They saw an improvement of PCO$_2$ on a mean dose of 0.2 μg/kg/min seen after a mean time of 0.3 hour. Thus this uncontrolled study showed a positive effect on severely obstructive asthma in children, who initially had a PCO$_2$ of greater than 60 mmHg (8 kPa). The ability of isoprenaline to prevent the need for mechanical ventilation was thus documented. A rebound bronchospasm when decreasing the dose has been described however [65]. Comparative intravenous studies between isoprenaline and salbutamol or other selective beta antagonists have not been performed. However, in asthmatic patients in a stable condition it has been well shown that isoprenaline results in more side effects than salbutamol (see above). Isoprenaline has also been shown to increase theophylline clearance [47].

It has also been described that intravenous isoprenaline causes a small increase in creatine phosphokinase in children with severe status asthmaticus [57]. Other case reports in children showed myocardial ischemia after isoprenaline treatment of acute severe asthma [58, 64] and in one case sudden death due to myocardial damage [40]. These observations indicate a subcellular myocardial injury associated with high doses of isoprenaline treatment given intravenously. This is why a nonselective drug such as isoprenaline preferably should be exchanged for a more selective beta$_2$-adrenoceptor agonist.

Selective Beta$_2$-adrenoceptor Agonists

Salbutamol

The two most commonly used beta$_2$-adrenoceptor agonists at present are salbutamol and terbutaline. There are many more studies published with intravenous salbutamol than with intravenous terbutaline.

Three studies with intravenous salbutamol appeared in 1975. Williams and coworkers [99] compared intravenous salbutamol, 0.5 mg, to intravenous theophylline, 0.5 mg. They showed similar ventilatory effects but an increased incidence of side effects after theophylline treatment. Salbutamol, however, caused a somewhat higher heart rate than theophylline. Another study by May and coworkers [59] showed similar results. Another early study in 1975 with intravenous salbutamol showed improvement of peak expiratory flow (PEF) and increased heart rate but also an unchanged PO$_2$ [27]. Williams and Seaton [98] in an uncontrolled design studied 10 patients with life-threatening asthma using salbutamol both by the inhaled and intravenous route. There was a positive effect of inhalation only in 2 of 10 patients. After 20 minutes intravenous treatment was then given. The study was, however, not designed to compare the effect of the inhaled and intravenous route. Hence conclusions are difficult to draw. Another clinical study in 10 life-threatened asthmatic patients eval-

uated intravenous salbutamol (4 μg/kg) [63]. A positive effect on ventilatory parameters was seen. A decrease of serum potassium and increase of insulin and free fatty acid were also shown. Femi-Pearse and coworkers [25] compared salbutamol and theophylline in a small parallel group design and found similar ventilatory effects and similar effects on heart rate.

Lawford et al. [46] compared salbutamol by nebulization and intravenous routes in a parallel group design involving 16 asthma patients. Two patients were withdrawn from intravenous salbutamol because of side effects. The dose of salbutamol was high—900 μg IV—and the ventilatory effect was increased equally for the intravenous and inhaled route, whereas heart frequency increased by 19 beats/min after intravenous treatment and decreased 10 beats/min after inhaled treatment.

Johnson et al. [38] compared intravenous salbutamol (10 μg/min) to intravenous theophylline (1 mg/min) in 39 patients with acute severe asthma who did not respond to previous treatment with theophylline and salbutamol given by nebulizer. The bronchodilator effect of the intravenous treatment was similar for salbutamol and theophylline, and side effects were also similar.

Bloomfield and coworkers [6] studied inhalation of 10 mg of salbutamol by intermittent positive pressure breathing (IPPB) and compared this to 500 μg of intravenous salbutamol. Inhalation was more effective as judged by reduction in pulsus paradoxus. However, the effect on peak expiratory flow showed no difference between inhaled and intravenous administration. The conclusion from this study could be influenced by the design that compared inhalation followed by intravenous injection after 1 hour with the same treatment given in the opposite order. It is not unlikely that the initial intravenous injection could make the following inhalation more effective, whereas the initial inhalation being less efficacious might not improve the effect of the later intravenous injection. Intravenous administration, however, increased heart rate, while the inhaled drug decreased heart rate frequency.

Evans and coworkers [22] studied 21 patients randomized to either intravenous theophylline, intravenous salbutamol, or a combination of the two. The data revealed a somewhat slower increase of PEF after salbutamol as compared to theophylline and the combination. The changes in heart rate were equal.

Edmunds and Godfrey [19] compared various regimens in children, including salbutamol, theophylline, and other treatments in acute asthma. Intravenous salbutamol was found as effective as inhaled drug in producing bronchodilation. After inhalation, heart rate increased less than after the intravenous route.

Bohn and coworkers [8] performed an open study in 14 children with status asthmaticus needing emergency treatment, whose initial mean PCO$_2$ was 60 mmHg (8 kPa). They were treated with intravenous salbutamol starting with a dose of 1 μg/kg/min during 10 minutes; after that the dose was increased. They found that 69 percent of patients had a decrease in their PCO$_2$ within 4 hours. Compared to historical results in their own department with isoprenaline, they concluded that this treatment is safe. However, they also reported later that they had started to treat patients with inhaled salbutamol.

Greif and coworkers [30] in a crossover, randomized study of 21 acute asthma patients compared aminophylline (6 mg/kg) and salbutamol (4 μg/kg) given IV. Salbutamol showed a better bronchodilating effect with somewhat more pronounced tachycardia.

Cheong and coworkers [13] studied 76 outpatients in a general practice office. The patients were randomly allocated to either intravenous salbutamol (0.5 μg/min) or 5 mg of inhaled salbutamol. Intravenous or inhaled salbutamol was given to patients who did not respond to 5 mg of salbutamol by inhalation initially. In this trial design, intravenous treatment was more effective than inhaled treatment, whereas inhaled treatment did not increase heart rate. However, it is probable that the design of this study, where randomization was performed after first treatment

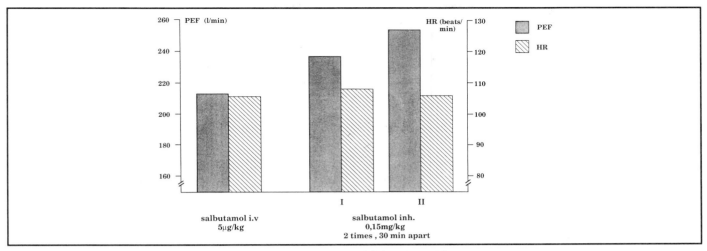

Fig. 57-4. *Mean PEF values and heart rate (HR) in a parallel group study of 176 patients with acute severe asthma treated either with intravenous salbutamol (5 μg/kg) or with inhaled (inh.) salbutamol (0.15 mg/kg), inhaled in two periods 30 minutes apart. The mean basal PEF value before nebulization was 170 ml; the mean basal PEF value before intravenous treatment was 166 ml; and the mean basal HR was 112 and 111, respectively. (Modified and redrawn from Swedish Society of Chest Medicine. High-dose inhaled versus intravenous salbutamol combined with theophylline in severe acute asthma. Eur. Respir. J. 3:163, 1990.)*

with inhaled dose, influenced the results. This study has also been heavily criticized in several letters.

Salmeron et al. [74] compared salbutamol by the inhaled and intravenous routes and found an improved peak flow measurement by the inhaled route as compared to intravenous and a more pronounced decrease of PCO_2 after the inhaled route. No differences concerning side effects were seen in this preliminary report.

A Swedish multicenter study of 176 patients in 1990 compared treatment with two doses of nebulized salbutamol (0.15 mg/kg) given at 30-minute intervals to intravenous salbutamol (0.5 μg/kg [91]. There was a significantly larger increase in PEF after the first inhaled dose compared to intravenous treatment, but there were no differences in side effects between the treatments (Fig. 57-4). After a second inhaled dose, there was a further increase in PEF, but also in systemic side effects. This study confirms that inhalation of beta₂-agonist salbutamol is preferable to systemic treatment in acute severe asthma.

Terbutaline

Terbutaline has about half the potency of salbutamol when given by the intravenous or inhaled route, but it also has a longer half-life. This makes dose-effect comparisons between the two drugs complicated.

Williams and coworkers [100] compared terbutaline by the inhaled and intravenous routes in a randomized, double-blind crossover study. Two doses of 2.5 mg by inhalation followed by two intravenous doses of 250 μg, or vice versa, were given with similar effects on ventilatory parameters. This study confirms that the inhaled route is as effective as the intravenous route despite a very low dose of inhaled drug.

Boe et al. [7] compared two intravenous doses of terbutaline, 4 and 8 μg/kg, given during 5 minutes in a randomized, double-blind parallel group design and a following crossover design. Both in the parallel group design (45 patients) and in the crossover design (19 patients), they did not see a clear-cut dose-response effect on ventilatory parameters, but heart rate and palpitations were more pronounced with the higher dose. It seems that an optimal dose is 4 μg/kg.

Sharma et al. [76] compared intravenous terbutaline, 250 μg, to intravenous theophylline, 250 mg, given during 10 minutes in

a parallel group design in 98 patients. They found better bronchodilation after terbutaline than after theophylline. However, there were more palpitations after terbutaline, whereas nausea and fall of blood pressure only occurred after theophylline treatment.

Van Renterghem and coworkers [95] compared terbutaline by the intravenous and inhaled routes. The inhaled route was quite low, 0.1 mg/kg; the intravenous dose was 6 μg/kg. The doses were repeated after 1 hour. Concerning bronchodilation, inhalation was as good as intravenous treatment. PO_2 was increased after intravenous treatment and was unchanged after inhaled treatment. The pulse rate was significantly higher after intravenous treatment. They used an increasing dose schedule and saw maximum effect on ventilatory parameters when the children received 4.5 μg/kg/hr. Tremor and headache occurred.

Fuglsang and coworkers [29] studied 13 children in a dose-response study, showing that a loading dose of 2 μg/kg and a maintenance dose of 4.5 μg/kg/hr are suitable for treatment of severe bronchoconstriction in children.

For adult asthmatics with acute severe asthma, we would recommend as first treatment high doses of inhaled beta₂ agonists given by continuous nebulization (5–10 mg of salbutamol or 10–20 mg of terbutaline), preferably divided in two inhalation periods within a 10- to 15-minute interval. This can be repeated after 30 minutes, possibly with the addition of inhaled ipratropium bromide. Corticosteroid in high doses should be given early in the treatment. If these measures do not give a satisfactory result, intravenous bronchodilating agents should be considered.

In very severe, life-threatening asthma attacks or in patients with poor compliance to inhalation therapy, intravenous beta₂-stimulating agents could be considered for immediate use. The potential side effects must be weighed against a purported advantage of immediate intravenous drug delivery, thereby permitting time for other therapy to be sufficiently effective to avoid intervention with intubation and mechanical ventilation. Dosages for intravenous treatment in children are given in Chapter 80. Specific guidelines for intravenous terbutaline use are given in Appendix G. Careful monitoring of cardiovascular parameters as well as the basic asthmatic process by means of, for instance, PEF measurements and PO_2 measurements must be followed throughout to ascertain therapeutic/side effect benefit.

REFERENCES

1. Arnold, J. M. O., and McDevitt, D. G. An assessment of physiological finger tremor as an indicator of beta-adrenoceptor function. *Br. J. Clin. Pharmacol.* 16:167, 1983.
2. Arnold, J. M. O., and McDevitt, D. G. Contribution of the vagus to the hemodynamic responses following intravenous doses of isoprenaline. *Br. J. Clin. Pharmacol.* 15:423, 1983.
3. Arnold, J. M. O., and McDevitt, D. G. Heart rate and blood pressure to intravenous boluses of isoprenaline in the presence of propranolol, practolol and atropine. *Br. J. Clin. Pharmacol.* 16:175, 1983.
4. Ballester, E., et al. Ventilation-perfusion mismatching in acute severe asthma: Effects of salbutamol and 100% oxygen. *Thorax* 44:258, 1989.
5. Billing, B., et al. Simultaneous treatment with terbutaline and theophylline. *Eur. J. Respir. Dis. [Suppl.]* 134:211, 1984.
6. Bloomfield, P., et al. Comparison of salbutamol given intravenously and by intermittent positive-pressure breathing in life-threatening asthma. *Br. Med. J.* 1:848, 1979.
7. Boe, J., et al. Acute asthma: Plasma levels and effect of terbutaline i.v. injection. *Eur. J. Respir. Dis.* 67:261, 1985.
8. Bohn, D., et al. Intravenous salbutamol in the treatment of status asthmaticus in children. *Crit. Care Med.* 12:892, 1984.
9. Brittain, R. T., Dean, C. M., and Jack, D. Sympathomimetic Bronchodilator Drugs. In J. Widdicombe (ed.), *Respiratory Pharmacology.* Oxford: Pergamon, 1981. P. 613.
10. Britton, J., and Tattersfield, A. Comparison of cumulative and noncumulative techniques to measure dose-response curves for beta agonists in patients with asthma. *Thorax* 39:597, 1984.
11. Brodde, O.-E., et al. Coexistence of beta-1 and beta-2 adrenoceptors in human right atrium: Direct identification by (±)-125 iodocyanopindolol binding. *Circ. Res.* 53:752, 1983.
12. Brown, J. E., McLeod, A. A., and Shand, S. G. Evidence for cardiac beta-2-adrenoceptors in man. *Clin. Pharmacol. Ther.* 33:424, 1983.
13. Cheong, B., et al. Intravenous beta agonist in severe acute asthma. *Br. Med. J.* 297:448, 1988.
14. Clifton, G. D., et al. Effects of sequential doses of parenteral terbutaline on plasma levels of potassium and related cardiopulmonary responses. *Am. Rev. Respir. Dis.* 141:575, 1990.
15. Collins, J. V., et al. The use of corticosteroids in the treatment of acute bronchial asthma. *Q. J. Med.* 44:259, 1975.
16. Council, M. R. Control trial of effects of cortisone acetate in status asthmaticus. *Lancet* 2:803, 1956.
17. Crane, J. et al. Prescribed fenoterol and death from asthma in New Zealand, 1981–83: Case-control study. *Lancet* 1:917, 1989.
18. Downes, J. J., et al. Intravenous isoproterenol in children with severe hypercapnia due to status asthmaticus: Effects on ventilation, circulation and clinical score. *Crit. Care Med.* 1:63, 1973.
19. Edmunds, A. T., and Godfrey, S. Cardiovascular response during severe acute asthma and its treatment in children. *Thorax* 36:534, 1981.
20. Ellul-Micallef, R., Borthwick, R. C., and McHardy, G. J. R. The effect of oral prednisolone on gas exchange in chronic bronchial asthma. *Br. J. Clin. Pharmacol.* 9:479, 1980.
21. Ellul-Micallef, R., and Fenech, F. F. Effect of intravenous prednisolone in asthmatics with diminished adrenergic responsiveness. *Lancet* 2: 1269, 1975.
22. Evans, W. V., et al. Aminophylline, salbutamol and combined intravenous infusions in acute severe asthma. *Br. J. Dis. Chest* 74:385, 1980.
23. Fanta, C. H., Rossing, T. H., and McFadden, E. J. Emergency room treatment of asthma: Relationships among therapeutic combinations, severity of obstruction and time course of response. *Am. J. Med.* 72:416, 1982.
24. Fanta, C. H., Rossing, T. H., and McFadden, E. R. Glucocorticoids in acute asthma: A critical control trial. *Am. J. Med.* 74:845, 1983.
25. Femi-Pearse, D., et al. Comparison of intravenous aminophylline and salbutamol in severe asthma. *Br. Med. J.* 1:491, 1977.
26. Fiel, S. B., et al. Efficacy of short-term corticosteroid therapy in outpatient treatment of acute bronchial asthma. *Am. J. Med.* 75:259, 1983.
27. Fitchett, D. H., McNicol, M. W., and Riordan, J. F. Intravenous salbutamol in management of status asthmaticus. *Br. Med. J.* 1:53, 1975.
28. Formgren, H. The therapeutic value of oral long-term treatment with terbutaline (Bricanyl) in asthma. *Scand. J. Respir. Dis.* 56:321, 1975.
29. Fuglsang, G., Pedersen, S., and Borgstrom, L. Dose-response relationships of intravenously administered terbutaline in children with asthma. *J. Pediatr.* 114:315, 1989.
30. Greif, J., Markovitz, L., and Topilsky, M. Comparison of intravenous sal-

31. Harvey, J. E., and Tattersfield, A. E. Airway response to salbutamol: Effect of regular salbutamol inhalations in normal atopic and asthmatic subjects. *Thorax* 37:280, 1982.
32. Heimer, D., Shim, C., and Williams, M. H. The effect of sequential inhalations of metaproterenol in asthma. *J. Allergy Clin. Immunol.* 66:75, 1980.
33. Herman, J. J., Noah, Z. L., and Moody, R. R. Use of intravenous isoproterenol for status asthmaticus in children. *Crit. Care Med.* 11:716, 1983.
34. Higgins, R. M., Stradling, J. R., and Lane, D. J. Should ipratropium bromide be added to beta-agonists in treatment of acute severe asthma? *Chest* 94:718, 1988.
35. Janson, C., Herala, M., and Sjogren, I. Nebulization versus injection in ambulatory treatment of acute asthma: A comparative study. *Br. J. Dis. Chest* 82:347, 1988.
36. Jansson, C. Plasma levels and effects of inhaled and intravenous salbutamol in stable asthma. *Pulm. Pharmacol.* 4:135, 1991.
37. Johansson, U., and Waldeck, B. Beta-1-adrenoceptor mediating relaxation of the guinea pig trachea: Experiments with prenalterol, a beta-1-selective adrenoceptor agonist. *J. Pharm. Pharmacol.* 33:353, 1981.
38. Johnson, A. J., et al. Intravenous infusion of salbutamol in severe acute asthma. *Br. Med. J.* 1:1013, 1978.
39. Kelly, H. W., and Murphy, S. Should anticholinergics be used in acute severe asthma? *D.I.C.P. Ann. Pharmacother.* 24:409, 1990.
40. Kurland, G., Williams, J., and Lewiston, N. J. Fatal myocardial toxicity during continuous infusion intravenous isoproterenol therapy of asthma. *J. Allergy Clin. Immunol.* 63:407, 1979.
41. Lands, A. M., Ludena, F. P., and Buzzo, H. J. Differentiation of receptors responsive to isoprenaline. *Life Sci.* 6:2241, 1967.
42. Lands, A. M., et al. Differentiation of receptor systems activated by sympathomimetic amines. *Nature* 214:597, 1967.
43. Larsson, S., and Svedmyr, N. Cumulative dose-response curves for comparison of oral bronchodilating drugs: A study of salbutamol and fenoterol. *Ann. Allergy* 39:362, 1977.
44. Larsson, S., and Svedmyr, N. Tremor caused by sympathomimetics is mediated by beta$_2$-adrenoreceptors. *Scand. J. Respir. Dis.* 58:5, 1977.
45. Larsson, S., Svedmyr, N., and Thiringer, G. Lack of bronchial beta-adrenoceptor resistance in asthmatics during long-term treatment with terbutaline. *J. Allergy Clin. Immunol.* 59:93, 1977.
46. Lawford, P., Jones, B. J. M., and Milledge, J. S. Comparison of intravenous and nebulised salbutamol in initial treatment of severe asthma. *Br. Med. J.* 1:84, 1978.
47. Levy, G., and Koysooko, R. Pharmacokinetic analysis of the effect of theophylline on pulmonary function in asthmatic children. *J. Pediatr.* 86:789, 1975.
48. Lim, R., et al. Cardiac arrhythmias during acute exacerbations of chronic airflow limitation: Effect of fall in plasma potassium concentration induced by nebulised beta 2-agonist therapy. *Postgrad. Med. J.* 65: 449, 1989.
49. Lipworth, B. J., McDevitt, D. G., and Struthers, A. D. Hypokalemic and ECG sequelae of combined beta-agonist/diuretic therapy. *Chest* 98:811, 1990.
50. Lipworth, B. J., Struthers, A. D., and McDevitt, D. G. Tachyphylaxis to systemic but not to airway responses during prolonged therapy with high dose inhaled salbutamol in asthmatics. *Am. Rev. Respir. Dis.* 140: 586, 1989.
51. Lipworth, B. J., et al. The biochemical effects of high-dose inhaled salbutamol in patients with asthma. *Eur. J. Clin. Pharmacol.* 36:357, 1989.
52. Löfdahl, C.-G., Marlin, G. E., and Svedmyr, N. Pafenolol, a highly selective beta1-adrenoceptor-antagonist, in asthmatic patients: Interaction with terbutaline. *Clin. Pharmacol. Ther.* 33:1, 1983.
53. Löfdahl, C.-G., Marlin, G. E., and Svedmyr, N. The effects of pafenolol and metoprolol on ventilatory function and haemodynamics during exercise by asthmatic patients. *Eur. J. Clin. Pharmacol.* 24:289, 1983.
54. Löfdahl, C.-G., and Svedmyr, N. Prenalterol—a selective β$_1$ adrenoceptor agonist—in asthmatics. *Eur. J. Respir. Dis.* 62:111, 1981.
55. Löfdahl, C.-G., et al. Two new beta$_2$-adrenoceptor agonists, D-2343 and QA 25, studied in asthmatic patients. *Allergy* 37:351, 1982.
56. Loren, M. L., et al. Corticosteroids in the treatment of acute exacerbations of asthma. *Ann. Allergy* 45:67, 1980.
57. Maguire, J. F., Geha, R. S., and Umetsu, D. T. Myocardial specific creatine phosphokinase isoenzyme elevation in children with asthma treated with intravenous isoproterenol. *J. Allergy Clin. Immunol.* 78:631, 1986.
58. Matson, J. R., Loughlin, G. M., and Strunk, R. C. Myocardial ischemia

complicating the use of isoproterenol in asthmatic children. *J. Pediatr.* 92:776, 1978.

59. May, C. S., et al. Intravenous infusion of salbutamol in the treatment of asthma. *Br. J. Clin. Pharmacol.* 2:503, 1975.

60. McFadden, E. R., et al. A controlled study of the effects of single doses of hydrocortisone on the resolution of acute attacks of asthma. *Am. J. Med.* 60:52, 1976.

61. Morgan, D. J. Clinical pharmacokinetics of beta-agonists. *Clin. Pharmacokinet.* 18:270, 1990.

62. Nadel, J. A., and Davis, B. Regulation of Na^+ and Cl^- Transport and Mucous Gland Secretion in Airway Epithelium. In R. Porter, J. Rivers, and M. O'Connor (eds.), *Respiratory Tract Mucus.* Amsterdam: Elsevier, 1978. P. 133.

63. Nogrady, S. G., Hartely, J. P. R., and Seaton, A. Metabolic effects of intravenous salbutamol in the course of acute severe asthma. *Thorax* 32:559, 1977.

64. Page, R., et al. Isoproterenol-associated myocardial dysfunction during status asthmaticus. *Ann. Allergy* 57:402, 1986.

65. Parry, W. H., Martorano, F., and Cotton, E. K. Management of life-threatening asthma with intravenous isoproterenol infusions. *Am. J. Dis. Child.* 130:39, 1976.

66. Persson, C. G. A., Ekman, M., and Erjefält, I. Terbutaline preventing permeability effects of histamine in the lung. *Acta Pharmacol. Toxicol.* 42:395, 1978.

67. Perucca, E., Pickles, H., and Richens, A. Effect of atenolol, metoprolol and propranolol on isoproterenol-induced tremor and tachycardia in normal subjects. *Clin. Pharmacol. Ther.* 29:425, 1981.

68. Pringle, T. H., Riddell, J. G., and Shanks, R. G. Characterization of the beta-adrenoceptors which mediate the isoprenaline-induced changes in finger tremor and cardiovascular function in man. *Eur. J. Clin Pharmacol.* 35:507, 1988.

69. Rebuck, A. S., et al. Nebulized anticholinergic and sympathomimetic treatment of asthma and chronic obstructive airways disease in the emergency room. *Am. J. Med.* 82:59, 1987.

70. Repsher, L. H., et al. Assessment of tachyphylaxis following prolonged therapy of asthma with inhaled albuterol aerosol. *Chest* 85:34, 1984.

71. Robinson, B. F., et al. Control of heart rate by the autonomic nervous system. *Circ. Res.* 19:400, 1966.

72. Rossing, T. H., Fanta, C. H., and McFadden, E. J. A controlled trial of the use of single versus combined-drug therapy in the treatment of acute episodes of asthma. *Am. Rev. Respir. Dis.* 123:190, 1981.

73. Rossing, T. H., et al. Emergency therapy of asthma: Comparison of the acute effects of parenteral and inhaled sympathomimetics and infused aminophylline. *Am. Rev. Respir. Dis.* 122:365, 1980.

74. Salmeron, S., et al. Intravenous versus inhaled salbutamol in status asthmaticus: A multicenter double blind study. *Am. Rev. Respir. Dis.* 134:36, 1988.

75. Shapiro, G., et al. Double-blind evaluation of methylprednisolone versus placebo for acute asthma episodes. *Pediatrics* 71:510, 1983.

76. Sharma, T. N., Gupta, P. R., and Gupta, R. B. Intravenous terbutaline and aminophylline in bronchial asthma. *J. Indian Med. Assoc.* 86:92, 1988.

77. Siegel, D., et al. Aminophylline increases the toxicity but not the efficacy of an inhaled beta-adrenergic agonist in the treatment of acute exacerbations of asthma. *Am. Rev. Respir. Dis.* 132:283, 1985.

78. Skoogh, B.-E., and Svedmyr, N. β-2-Adrenoceptor stimulation inhibits ganglionic transmission in ferret trachea. *Pulmonary Pharmacol.* 1:167, 1989.

79. Skoogh, B.-E., et al. Classification of β-adrenoceptors in ferret tracheal smooth muscle by pharmacological responses. *Pulmonary Pharmacol* 1:173, 1989.

80. Spector, S. L. Adverse reactions associated with parenteral beta agonists: Serum potassium changes. *N. Engl. Reg. Allergy Proc.* 8:317, 1987.

81. Storr, J., and Lenney, W. Nebulised iprotropium and salbutamol in asthma. *Arch. Dis. Child.* 61:602, 1986.

82. Storr, J., et al. Early single-dose prednisolone for acute childhood asthma. *Lancet* 1:879, 1987.

83. Stuart-Smith, K., and Vanhoutte, P. M. Airway epithelium modulates the responsiveness of porcine bronchial smooth muscle. *J. Appl. Physiol.* 65:721, 1988.

84. Stuart-Smith, K., and Vanhoutte, P. M. Epithelium, contractile tone, and responses to relaxing agonists in canine bronchi. *J. Appl. Physiol.* 69:678, 1990.

85. Svedmyr, N. Studies on the relationship betwen some metabolic effects of thyroid hormones and catecholamines in animals and man. *Acta Physiol. Scand.* 68:1, 1966.

86. Svedmyr, N. Treatment with beta-adrenostimulants. *Scand. J. Respir. Dis.* 101(suppl.):59, 1977.

87. Svedmyr, K. Beta2-adrenoceptor stimulants and theophylline in asthma therapy. *Eur. J. Respir. Dis.* 116(suppl.):1, 1981.

88. Svedmyr, N. Action of corticosteroids on beta-adrenergic receptors: Clinical aspects. *Am. Rev. Respir. Dis.* 141:S31, 1990.

89. Svedmyr, N., and Löfdahl, C.-G. Physiology and Pharmacodynamics of β-Adrenergic Agonists. In J. Jenne (ed.), *Drug Therapy for Asthma.* New York: Marcel Dekker, 1987. P. 177.

90. Svedmyr, N., and Thiringer, G. The effects of salbutamol and isoprenaline on beta-receptors in patients with chronic obstructive lung disease. *Postgrad. Med. J.* 44, 1971.

91. Swedish Society of Chest Medicine. High-dose inhaled versus intravenous salbutamol combined with theophylline in severe acute asthma. *Eur. Respir. J.* 3:170, 1990.

92. Tashkin, D. P., et al. Subsensitization of beta-adrenoceptors in airways and lymphocytes of healthy and asthmatic subjects. *Am. Rev. Respir. Dis.* 125:185, 1982.

93. Thiringer, G., and Svedmyr, N. Comparison of infused and inhaled terbutaline in patients with asthma. *Scand. J. Respir. Dis.* 57:17, 1976.

94. van den Berg, W., et al. Clinical implications of drug-induced desensitization of the beta receptor after continuous oral use of terbutaline. *J. Allergy Clin. Immunol.* 69:410, 1982.

95. van Renterghem, D., et al. Intravenous versus nebulized terbutaline in patients with acute severe asthma: A double-blind randomized study. *Ann. Allergy* 59:313, 1987.

96. Weber, R. W., Smith, J. A., and Nelson, H. S. Aerosolized terbutaline in asthmatics: Development of subsensitivity with longterm administration. *J. Allergy Clin. Immunol.* 70:417, 1982.

97. Whyte, K. F., et al. The mechanism of salbutamol-induced hypokalaemia. *Br. J. Clin. Pharmacol.* 23:65, 1987.

98. Williams, S., and Seaton, A. Intravenous or inhaled salbutamol in severe acute asthma. *Thorax* 32:555, 1977.

99. Williams, S. J., Parish, R. W., and Seaton, A. Comparison of intravenous aminophylline and salbutamol in severe asthma. *Br. Med. J.* 2:685, 1975.

100. Williams, S. J., Winner, S. J., and Clark, T. J. Comparison of inhaled and intravenous terbutaline in acute severe asthma. *Thorax* 36:629, 1981.

101. Wilson, A. F. Cardiovascular effects: Beta 2 agonists. *J. Asthma* 27:111, 1990.

102. Windom, H. H., et al. The pulmonary and extrapulmonary effects of inhaled beta-agonists in patients with asthma. *Clin. Pharmacol. Ther.* 48:296, 1990.

103. Wong, C. S., et al. Bronchodilator, cardiovascular and hypokalaemic effects of fenoterol, salbutamol and terbutaline in asthma. *Lancet* 336:1396, 1990.

104. Wood, D. W., et al. Intravenous isoproterenol in the management of respiratory failure in childhood status asthmaticus. *J. Allergy Clin. Immunol.* 50:75, 1972.

105. Zaagsma, J., et al. Differentiation of functional adrenoceptors in human and guinea pig airways. *Eur. J. Respir. Dis.* 65:16, 1984.

106. Zerkowski, H.-R., et al. Human muocardial beta-adrenoceptors: demonstration of both beta-1 and beta-2-adrenoceptors mediating contractile responses to beta-agonists on the isolated right atrium. *Naunyn Schmiedebergs Arch. Pharmacol.* 332:142, 1986.

Methylxanthines

Miles M. Weinberger

58

The methylxanthines have been used for various pharmaceutical effects for more than 50 years. Caffeine and theobromine are methylated xanthines found naturally and as additives in various beverages. Theobromine is now rarely used for its pharmacologic properties, although caffeine is still widely used as a self-prescribed central nervous system (CNS) stimulant, and it has also found renewed medical interest as a specific treatment for neonatal apnea [6]. Theophylline is found in small quantities in some dietary substances such as chocolate and has been used in the past as a diuretic, but the most widespread use of this drug has been for bronchodilation. Some of the earliest descriptions of theophylline were following intravenous usage, where it was observed to relieve acute symptoms of asthma not previously responsive to injected epinephrine. More recently, however, the most important use for theophylline has been its role as a major prophylactic agent for controlling the symptoms of chronic asthma. This has occurred as a result of the application of new knowledge related to the pharmacodynamic and pharmacokinetic characteristics of the drug and the availability of rapid, specific serum assays from clinical laboratories. As a result, the efficacy and safety of the drug have increased. In addition, reliably absorbed slow-release formulations have been developed, which provide a highly effective and convenient means of maintaining around-the-clock stabilization of the hyperreactive airways that characterize chronic asthma.

PHARMACEUTICAL CHEMISTRY

Theophylline is a dimethylated xanthine similar in structure to caffeine and theobromine, which are commonly found in coffee, tea, cola beverages, and chocolate (Fig. 58-1). "Salts" of theophylline have been formulated, ostensibly to improve absorption, but the added base in solution only increases solubility by increasing pH with little or no effect on actual absorption. Theophylline can only form a compound with a base (e.g., ethylenediamine) as a result of a tautomeric shift in hydrogen, which occurs at high pH. At physiologic pH, theophylline is a weak base ($PK_a = 8.8$) and incapable of forming a salt with a base. Therefore, so-called salts such as aminophylline and oxtriphylline are merely mixtures of theophylline and base and have no pharmacologic activity other than that attributable to the theophylline [196, 205]. All dosage and labeling of theophylline formulations, therefore, should be in terms of the anhydrous theophylline content. For example, aminophylline injection USP, 25 mg/ml, should more appropriately be labeled "Theophylline Injection, 20 mg/ml."

A number of N-7 substituted methylxanthines have been synthesized (Fig. 58-1). They are stable derivatives and do not dissociate into theophylline in solution and are not converted to theophylline in vivo [189]. They therefore have no more relationship to theophylline than caffeine (which could be identified as 7-methyl theophylline). Of these, only dyphylline is available in the United States. The in vitro dose-response relationship of dyphylline (glyphylline or diprophylline in Europe) suggests a degree of potency only one-tenth that of theophylline [196, 205], and in a clinical study 1,000 mg of dyphylline demonstrated only one-half the bronchodilator effect resulting from a 400-mg dose of theophylline [80]. Smaller doses have been no more effective than placebo [116], and at a peak serum concentration of 15 µg/ml, dyphylline was only slightly more effective than placebo in blocking exercise-induced bronchospasm, whereas theophylline at the same concentration completely inhibited a postexercise decrease in pulmonary function in the same subjects after a standardized exercise stress test [47]. Oral solutions and plain tablets [55] as well as a slow-release product [190] are incompletely absorbed, and elimination is exceedingly rapid with a mean half-life of 2 hours [47, 55, 188]. None of the other methylated xanthines has shown any promise for clinical use in the treatment of asthma.

A possible exception is enprofylline, a new derivative. It is five times more potent than theophylline as a bronchodilator, but produces less CNS stimulation [19, 108, 121]. Unlike theophylline and caffeine, it does not antagonize adenosine [121]; this fact may explain the relative absence of seizures in animal studies. Nausea and headache, however, appear to be common side effects [109], and a 2-hour half-life of elimination may complicate clinical use [19]. It is not clear whether enprofylline will ever see actual clinical usage, but its development has increased our understanding of the structure-function relationship of the methylxanthines. It appears to be the absence of the 1-methyl group on enprofylline that eliminates adenosine receptor inhibition properties with loss of the diuretic effect, cardiac sphincter relaxation, and CNS toxicity (in animal studies) of theophylline. Lengthening of the methyl group on the xanthine nucleus to a propyl group appears to be associated with a greater bronchodilator potency of the enprofylline [156].

PHARMACOLOGY

Theophylline relaxes bronchial smooth muscle [170, 187] but is less potent than the inhaled beta$_2$-agonist sympathomimetic bronchodilators. Theophylline decreases exercise-induced bronchospasm [48, 159] and antigen-induced bronchospasm [125] but not to the same degree as the inhaled beta$_2$ agonists. Theophylline modestly alters nonspecific airway reactivity to histamine or methacholine [90, 99] but again is considerably less potent than the inhaled beta$_2$ agonists [90]. Theophylline also inhibits mast cell degranulation with consequent prevention of the release of mediators that induce bronchospasm and airway inflammation [46, 164], but it is not clear if this is related to its clinical efficacy. Theophylline decreases the secondary increase in airway ob-

Generic name	Structure	Oral bioavailability (%)	Mean adult elimination half-life (hrs)	Estimated potency
Theophylline	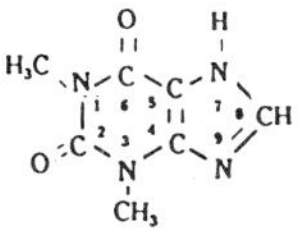 1,3 dimethylxanthine	100	7.7	1
Caffeine	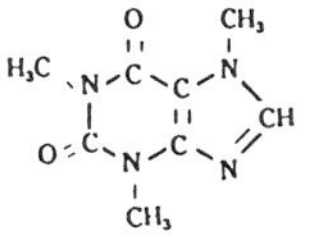 1,3,7 trimethylxanthine	100	6	0.2
Dyphylline	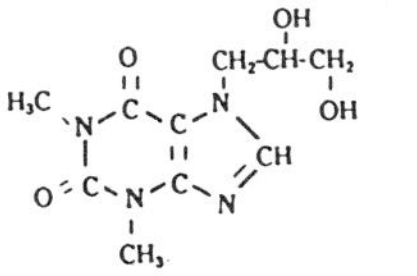 dihydroxypropyl theophylline	88	2.1	0.1
Etophylline	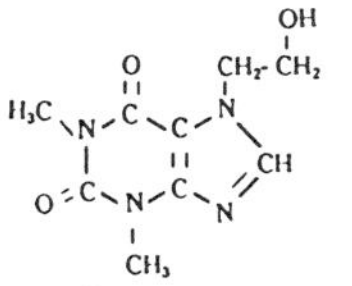 β-hydroxyethyl theophylline	80	4.1	0.14
Proxyphylline	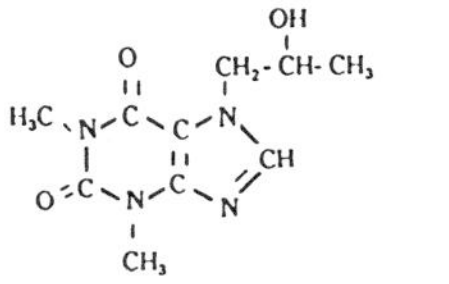 β-hydroxypropyl theophylline	100	6.8	15
Acephylline piperazine	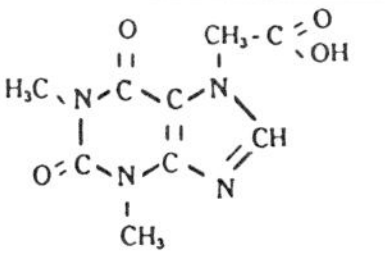 theopylline-7-ylacetic acid	2.5	0.8	0
Bamifylline	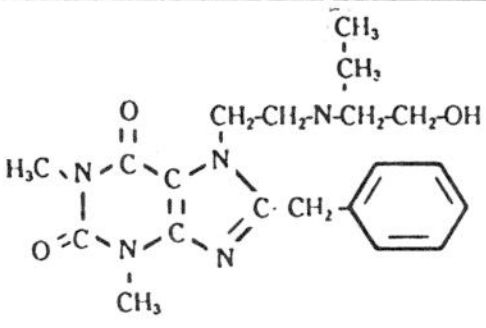 8-Benzyl-7- [2-(N-ethyl-N-2-hydroxyethyamino)ethyl] theophylline	21	20.5	3
Enprofylline	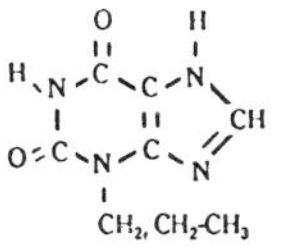 3-propylxanthine	100	2	5

Fig. 58-1. *Comparison of methylxanthines. The various stable derivatives of theophylline are formed by substitution of larger functional groups (R) on the 7-nitrogen of the 1,3-dimethylxanthine structure. Oral bioavailability and half-life data were obtained from an intravenous reference product. In vitro potency was determined from the ability of these compounds to relax human tracheal strips or carbachol-contracted rat tracheas. (Reprinted with permission from L. Hendeles and M. Weinberger. Theophylline: A state-of-the-art review. Pharmacotherapy 3[1]:2, 1983.)*

struction from an allergen challenge, that is, the "late phase" [150–152], and appears also to decrease the consequent increase in nonspecific airway reactivity [31, 77] (Fig. 58-2). Potentially of some relevance to this effect on the inflammatory component of airway obstruction is a report indicating that theophylline inhibits BCG-induced pulmonary inflammatory responses in rats [17].

Other physiologic effects of potential value for respiratory disease include decreased pulmonary arterial resistance [149] and increased diaphragmatic contractility [139]. While these effects have been used as a rationale for theophylline in the treatment of nonreversible chronic obstructive airway disease, the clinical importance of these effects is not established. Central stimulation of respiration from theophylline and the related xanthine, caffeine, is another physiologic effect of theophylline, but this is of clinical importance only for the treatment of recurrent apnea seen in premature infants [4].

As with other methylxanthines such as caffeine, theophylline can potentially induce a transient diuretic effect [203], stimulate the central nervous system [1], produce cerebral vasoconstriction [57], increase gastric acid secretion [45], and inhibit uterine contractions [23]. It also may exert a complex set of actions on the cardiovascular system, including increased biventricular performance both in patients with obstructive pulmonary disease [128] and in normal subjects [147]. A recently described nonpulmonary effect of theophylline is an effect on erythropoietin production that may have clinical usefulness in suppressing erythrocytosis causing polycythemia after renal transplantation [12].

PHARMACODYNAMICS

Efficacy

Theophylline has been repeatedly demonstrated to be effective as monotherapy maintenance medication in the management of chronic asthma. The first studies of this in the early 1970s demonstrated that symptoms were markedly diminished and the need for intervention with measures to treat acute symptoms was virtually eliminated for most patients [230, 231]. Subsequent studies demonstrated fewer asymptomatic days than with cromolyn sodium (disodium cromoglycate) when both were used as monotherapy in patients with severe chronic asthma [61], although efficacy is similar in patients with milder asthma [49, 56, 144]. Comparison with oral beta$_2$ agonists, including metaproterenol [36] and slow-release terbutaline, have shown clinical advantage for theophylline [63, 238]. Although inhaled albuterol is far more potent as a bronchodilator than theophylline, theophylline nonetheless provides more stable clinical effect, which is particularly important for nocturnal symptoms and other times when there will be more than 4 hours between doses of the inhaled agent (Fig. 58-3). Inhaled beta$_2$ agonists are useful as intervention measures for breakthrough symptoms and as a preexercise measure [222] but offer no apparent benefit when added as a routinely scheduled measure [90] and may even cause worsening of asthma [181]. When theophylline is inadequate as monotherapy, it still has substantial additive effect with inhaled or alternate-day oral corticosteroids [22, 140] (Fig. 58-4). In contrast, cromolyn sodium (disodium cromoglycate) has not shown additive effect with either theophylline [61] or inhaled corticosteroids in three placebo-controlled studies [34, 79, 201].

The degree of clinical effect from theophylline described above is most readily apparent when serum concentrations are maintained between 10 and 20 μg/ml [142, 218] (Fig. 58-5). Response of the airways can be demonstrated to parallel changes in serum concentration [113, 159, 170, 187] (Fig. 58-6). Similar to the relationship of serum concentration to bronchodilator activity, effect on stabilizing the responsiveness of the asthmatic airways to exercise can also be demonstrated to relate closely to serum concentration [90] (Fig. 58-7).

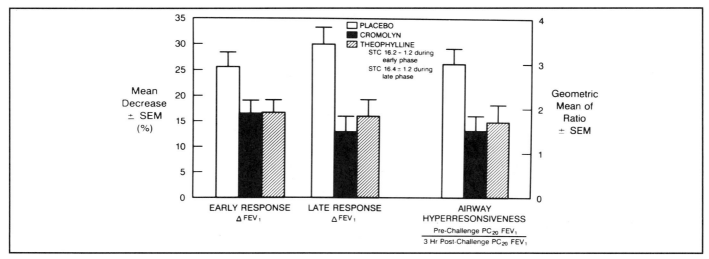

Fig. 58-2. *Comparison of theophylline and cromolyn on the suppression of the early and late phases of antigen-induced airway obstruction and resultant increase in nonspecific airway hyperresponsiveness. FEV_1 = forced-expiratory volume in 1 second; STC = serum theophylline concentration ($\mu g/ml$). (Data from L. Hendeles et al. Theophylline attenuation of allergen induced airway hyperreactivity and late response. J. Allergy Clin. Immunol. 137:A35, 1991.)*

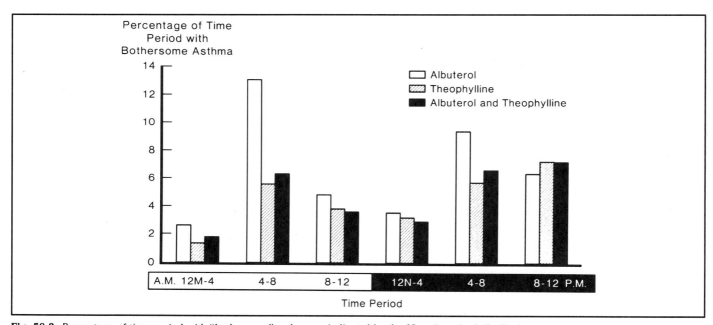

Fig. 58-3. *Percentage of time period with "bothersome" asthma as indicated by the 18 patients in daily diaries during month-long treatment with inhaled albuterol, slow-release theophylline, and the combination. Each day was divided into six time periods of 4 hours each. Differences between the albuterol and the theophylline-containing regimens were greatest from 4:00 to 8:00 A.M. (p = .007 by analysis of variance). (Reprinted with permission from J. Joad et al. Relative efficacy of maintenance therapy with theophylline, and inhaled albuterol, and the combination for the treatment of chronic asthma. J. Allergy Clin. Immunol. 79:78, 1987.)*

In contrast to the continued major role of theophylline as maintenance therapy for chronic asthma, the traditional role of theophylline as an acute intervention measure has been questioned in several clinical trials [3, 14, 166, 177, 184, 202, 239]. In fact a meta-analysis of 13 published studies concluded that theophylline did not contribute significantly to improvement of acute asthma when compared with alternative treatments including beta2 agonists and corticosteroids [117]. Nonetheless, at least one study has supported the use of theophylline as an adjunctive measure in hospitalized adult patients [213], and another controlled study indicated that its use in the emergency room decreased the likelihood of hospitalization [240].

Toxicity

It is the considerable potential for therapeutic benefit from theophylline that continues to justify the use of this 50-year-old medication when so many newer agents have been introduced

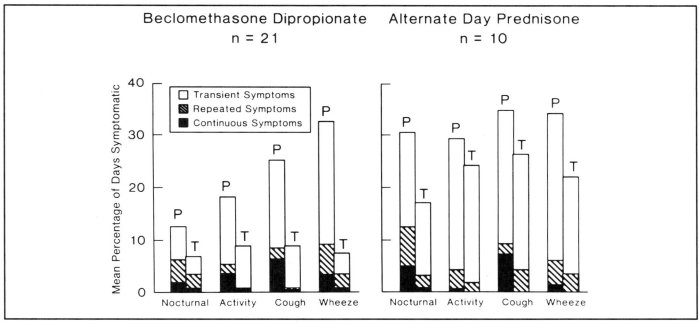

Fig. 58-4. *Mean frequency of symptoms in steroid-dependent asthmatic children during placebo (P) or doses of theophylline (T) previously individualized to achieve a therapeutic serum concentration. The presence of nocturnal symptoms were recorded each morning, and interference with activity, cough, and wheezing were recorded each evening as absent, transient, repeated, or continuous. Inhaled beclomethasone dipropionate was taken by 21 patients (left), while prednisone on alternate mornings was taken by 10 patients (right). These data demonstrate the need to continue therapeutic doses of theophylline in steroid-dependent asthmatics. (Reprinted with permission from E. G. Nassif et al. The value of maintenance theophylline for steroid dependent asthma. N. Engl. J. Med. 304:71, 1981.)*

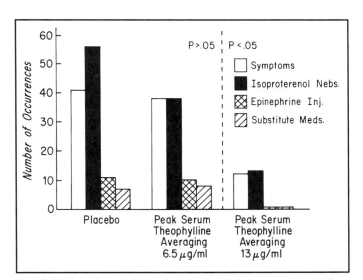

Fig. 58-5. *Frequency and severity of asthmatic symptoms among 12 children with chronic asthma at a residential treatment center. Each patient received, in a double-blind randomized sequence, 1 week's treatment with placebo, an ephedrine-theophylline combination in conventional doses that resulted in peak serum theophylline concentrations averaging 6.5 μg/ml and individualized theophylline doses that resulted in peak serum concentrations averaging 13 μg/ml. Asthmatic symptoms during each 1-week period were promptly treated, when necessary, with inhaled isoproterenol; if symptoms were not rapidly relieved, epinephrine was administered subcutaneously. If the patient was unresponsive to these measures, known drugs were substituted for the double-blind medications. (Reprinted with permission from M. Weinberger, Theophylline for treatment of asthma. J. Pediatr. 92:1, 1978.)*

in the past 20 years. Nonetheless, the prescribing clinician needs to be aware that theophylline has the greatest potential for serious acute toxicity of any medication used for asthma. An extensive review of the world's English language literature of reported cases of theophylline toxicity is recorded elsewhere [68].

Toxicity of theophylline increases in frequency and severity with increasing serum concentrations [73, 83, 246] (Fig. 58-8). Higher serum concentrations appear to be better tolerated from acute overdose than from chronic therapeutic misadventure [148]. Serious toxicity has not been documented at serum concentrations less than 20 μg/ml. Centrally mediated gastrointestinal effects in order of severity include nausea, vomiting, and bloody emesis. Central nervous system stimulatory effects include insomnia, headache, irritability, and seizures. Patients with seizure disorders may experience a lowering of their seizure threshold with uncomplicated seizures similar to those previously experienced by the patient [169]. More serious are the seizures associated with what appears to be a toxic encephalopathy; seizures then are relatively intractable with a protracted course, little response to anticonvulsants, prolonged coma, frequent fatalities, and frequent neurologic residua among survivors [68, 73, 138, 242, 246]. A sinus tachycardia is common as serum concentrations exceed 20 μg/ml. Asymptomatic arrhythmias have been reported at high serum theophylline levels, but more serious cardiac toxicity with ventricular fibrillation has been reported only after rapid infusion through a central venous catheter [24].

Theophylline also has the potential for adverse extrapulmonary effects at serum concentrations well below 20 μg/ml. Like its related xanthine, caffeine, theophylline can cause central nervous system stimulation [1]. Nervousness, insomnia, headache, centrally induced nausea, and even vomiting can occur during initiation of therapy, and the frequency of these symptoms exceed 50 percent if therapeutic serum concentrations are rapidly

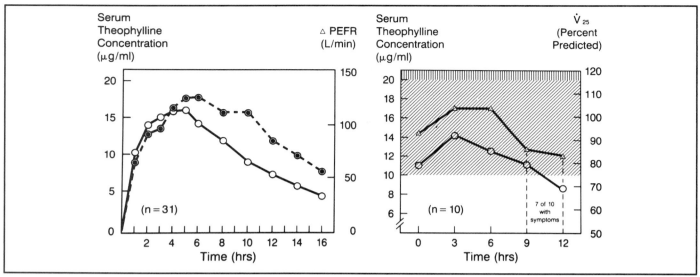

Fig. 58-6. *Relationship between serum theophylline concentration and pulmonary function. Data from the left graph were obtained from 31 adults who received a single 7.5 mg/kg dose of a rapid-release plain tablet. Pulmonary function closely paralleled the rise and fall in serum concentration [170]. Data from the right graph were obtained from 10 children receiving a slow-release theophylline preparation every 12 hours. Symptoms of asthma requiring inhaled albuterol occurred in 7 of the 10 children exclusively during the last 3 hours of the dosing interval when serum concentrations were generally falling below 10 μg/ml; this intervention blunted further fall in pulmonary function [187]. Open circles = serum theophylline concentration; closed circles = ΔPEFR; triangles = percentage of predicted values for the flow rate at $\dot{V}_{25}$.*

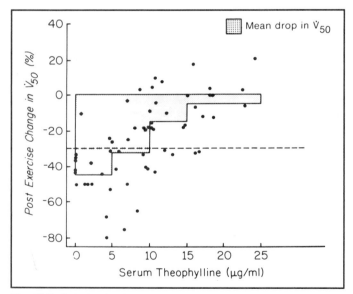

Fig. 58-7. *Relationship between serum theophylline concentration and exercise-induced bronchospasm following a standardized treadmill exercise. The test was performed on 12 children before and at 2, 4, and 6 hours following a 7.5 mg/kg dose of a rapidly absorbed theophylline formulation. The $\dot{V}_{50}$ is the flow rate at 50 percent of vital capacity during a maximal forced expiration. The shaded area represents mean flow-rate changes for the data points in each 5 μg/ml serum concentration interval. The dashed line indicates a 30 percent decrease in pulmonary function conventionally accepted as clinically important. The mean Spearman rank correlation coefficient was 0.75 (p < .01). (Reprinted with permission from J. Pollock et al. Relationship of serum theophylline concentration to inhibition of exercise-induced bronchospasm and comparison with cromolyn. Pediatrics 60:840, 1977. Copyright 1977.)*

attained [71]. However, persistent complaints of side effects are uncommon during chronic therapy, occurring in only 1 or 2 percent of patients when the slow titration process and precautions in the U.S. package inserts are followed, unless serum concentrations exceed 20 μg/ml [133]. Symptoms among those 1 or 2 percent who do not tolerate theophylline include headache, persisting insomnia, or nonspecific central nervous system effects (described in a few patients as "feeling spacy" or "I just don't like the way I feel"). Patients with preexisting migraine may have an increase in the frequency of migraine while taking theophylline (personal observation). In general, however, theophylline has no adverse effects apparent to the patient and specifically is free of effects on daytime cognitive performance and nighttime sleep quality [43a].

Minor neuropsychological and physiologic effects, however, can be measured even during chronic therapy [89]. These are not necessarily adverse effects, however, and include improvement in ability to remember number sequences analogous to the increased alertness associated with caffeine. Other effects include a fine motor tremor that is not clinically apparent for most patients and responses to a structured questionnaire that suggest the possibility of some subtle alterations in mood and subjective feelings of occasional nausea. These effects, however, are small and generally not clinically apparent to the patient when symptom diaries are examined in controlled studies. Small and clinically inapparent mean changes can also be detected in serum and urine calcium (elevated), serum creatinine (elevated), uric acid (elevated), and bicarbonate (lowered). None of these physiologic effects has been demonstrated to be of clinical importance. Concerns about theophylline having an adverse effect on learning and school behavior have been fashionable, but critical examination of evidence available has demonstrated little merit to support this concern [41, 228]. In fact, recent studies have shown no adverse effect on behavior [12a], and performance on standardized achievement tests of asthmatic children in Iowa receiving theophylline was above the national average and identical, on average, with that of nonasthmatic sibling controls [115].

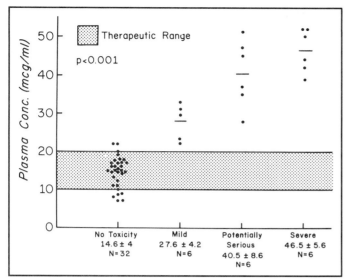

Fig. 58-8. *Relationship of serum concentration and symptoms of toxicity among 50 adults consecutively monitored in the medical intensive care unit of the University of Iowa during constant intravenous infusions of theophylline averaging 0.9 mg/kg/hr as aminophylline. Symptoms of toxicity were recorded by a pulmonary physician before the results of the serum concentration measurement became available. Mild toxicity included nausea, vomiting, headache, nervousness, and insomnia. Moderate toxicity consisted of mild symptoms in conjunction with sinus tachycardia and occasional premature ventricular contractions (PVCs). Patients in the severe category experienced serious arrhythmias such as ventricular tachycardia with runs of PVCs and/or grand mal seizures, which occurred in two patients, one of whom died. Prior symptoms of nausea and vomiting or other minor symptoms of toxicity were absent in half of the patients in the moderate and severe categories. (Reprinted with permission from L. Hendeles et al. Frequent toxicity from IV aminophylline infusions in critically ill patients. Drug Intell. Clin. Pharm. 11:12, 1977.)*

PHARMACOKINETICS

Absorption

Theophylline is rapidly, consistently, and completely absorbed from liquids and plain uncoated tablets [70, 92, 206]. Absorption may be somewhat slowed by concurrent ingestion of food [62, 236] or antacids (aluminum magnesium hydroxide) [7, 183]. In addition to the oral route, theophylline can be given rectally or parenterally. The rate and extent of absorption of theophylline from rectal solutions [126] and experimental polyethylene glycol suppositories [200] approach those of oral solutions, but the usually commercially available rectal suppositories from a cocoa butter base repeatedly have been associated with slow and erratic absorption [15, 171, 200, 203, 216]. Since oral theophylline is reliably absorbed, convenient, and not under the influence of rectal contents or retention time, the only indication for the rectal route is the inability of the patient to take oral medications, such as in the presence of vomiting from causes other than theophylline toxicity or when fasting before surgery.

Since maximum solubility of theophylline in water is about 8 mg/ml at physiologic pH and temperature, intramuscular administration of either the intravenous solution (20 mg/ml) or the intramuscular aminophylline formulation that has been marketed in the past (200 mg/ml) results in precipitation of the drug at the injection site and slow absorption [216]. Moreover, this route is painful and irritating, since these solutions have a pH of about 9.0.

Distribution

Once theophylline enters the systemic circulation, on average 40 percent becomes bound to plasma protein [185], and the remaining amount of free drug distributes throughout the body water. This process is sufficiently rapid that serum concentrations are in equilibrium with tissue concentrations of the drug within 1 hour after an intravenous injection [113]. The apparent volume of distribution (V_d), the space into which theophylline distributes, ranges from 0.3 to 0.7 L/kg (30–70% ideal body weight) and averages about 0.45 L/kg among both children [40, 120] and adults [71, 135]. The mean volume of distribution for premature newborns [5], adults with hepatic cirrhoses [157] or uncorrected acidemia [207], and the elderly [2] is slightly larger, since protein binding is reduced in these patients. In all other circumstances, even when theophylline clearance is altered, the volume of distribution generally remains unaffected. Moreover, the interpatient variability in volume of distribution is much smaller than the interpatient variability in elimination described in the following section.

Theophylline freely crosses the placenta [8, 243] and passes into breast milk [195, 244], although only minor adverse effects have been reported for infants indirectly receiving the drug in this manner. Theophylline crosses the blood-brain barrier more slowly than caffeine. After distribution, however, cerebrospinal fluid concentrations are approximately 90 percent of serum concentrations in premature infants [193] but probably approximate free drug in older patients. Concentrations in saliva average about 60 percent of serum levels [74, 100, 112] and appear to be similar to free drug concentrations in plasma [100, 185]. In vitro measurements of protein binding for theophylline have varied, however, as a result of pH and temperature-dependent effects [185].

Metabolism and Excretion

Theophylline is eliminated from the body by hepatic biotransformation into relatively inactive metabolites, which are excreted in the urine [30]. About 85 to 90 percent of a dose is metabolized [198], probably by cytochrome P-450 [119], the primary component of the mixed-function oxidase system localized in hepatic microsomes. This occurs over multiple parallel pathways by both first-order and capacity-limited kinetic processes [137, 198]. The major metabolite, 1,3-dimethyluric acid, is formed by hydroxylation in the C-8 position, whereas 3-methylxanthine and the intermediate metabolite 1-methylxanthine result from N-demethylation (Fig. 58-9). The intermediate metabolite 1-methylxanthine is rapidly converted by xanthine oxidase to 1-methyluric acid [60]. Since the rate of formation of 1-methylxanthine is slower than its conversion to 1-methyluric acid, highly sensitive assays are able to detect only small amounts of 1-methylxanthine in blood and in urine [198]. About 6 percent of a dose of theophylline is N-methylated to caffeine, which in turn is converted to paraxanthine [197]. Available evidence suggests that N-demethylation and 8-hydroxylation pathways are mediated by two forms of cytochrome P-450, each with a distinctive substrate specificity [16, 58, 59].

Since the hepatic extraction ratio for theophylline is only about 10 percent [146], there is no decrease in oral bioactivity as a result of first-pass metabolism. Renal clearance of theophylline is dependent on urine flow rate [114], but less than 15 percent of a dose is excreted in the urine unchanged beyond the neonatal period (Table 58-1). Therefore, dosage adjustments generally are not required for renal dysfunction except in neonates during the first few months of life. The renal clearance of theophylline metabolites far exceeds the normal glomerular filtration rate, suggesting that tubular secretion plays a role in their elimination [198]. Because the rates of formation of the metabolites are

Table 58-1. Mean percent of total methylxanthines recovered in urine adjusted for differences in molecular weight

Group	Age range	N	Duration of theophylline before urine collection	Theophylline	3-Methylxanthine	1-Methyluric acid	1,3-Dimethyluric acid	Caffeine	Theobromine
Premature [204]	≥2 weeks	10	2 weeks	50.4	1.3	9.3	27.7	9.6	3.8
Neonates [16]	2–31 days	12	2–16 days (mean 5)	44.8	0	13.8	33.6	6.9	—
Young children [16]	1–7 years	6	1–8 days (mean 1.8)	10.1	11.2	32.5	46.1	—	—
Older children [58]	2–12 years	16	Steady state	7.1	16.2	23.5	52.8	0	—
Adults [198]	24–32 years[a]	6	Single IV dose	13.3[b]	15.7	19.8	39.1	0	—

[a] Healthy adult volunteers; smoking history not reported.
[b] Values for this study were calculated as percent of dose administered. Since over 10% of the dose was not recovered, these values are slightly lower than the percentage of total methylxanthine in urine but represent the most accurate method of reporting urinary metabolite excretion patterns.

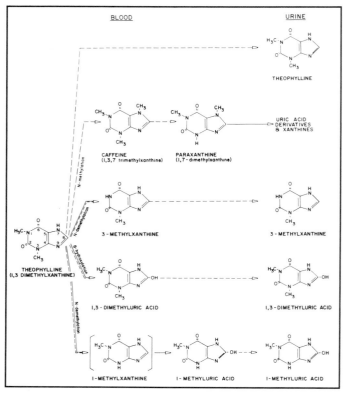

Fig. 58-9. *Hepatic biotransformation of theophylline over multiple parallel pathways by both first-order (broken line) and capacity-limited (combinaton of broken line and unbroken line) processes and urinary excretion of metabolites. The pathway for 7-methylation to caffeine is trivial beyond 1 year of age but is of importance in the neonate, where other pathways are undeveloped and the half-life of caffeine elimination is prolonged.*

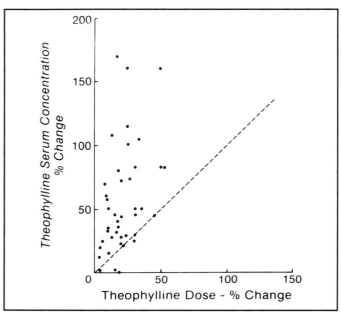

Fig. 58-10. *Relationship between changes in steady-state serum concentration and change in dose among 42 patients who had at least two serum concentration measurements at different doses of the same product (from 200 charts reviewed). In 30 of these children, the percent change in serum concentration was 50 percent greater than the percent change in dose (% change in concentration/% change in dose greater than or equal to 1.5). Thus, dose-dependent kinetics of a sufficient magnitude to be of substantial clinical importance occurred in at least 15 percent of the 200 children examined. (Reprinted with permission from E. Sarrazin et al. Dose-dependent kinetics for theophylline: Observations among ambulatory asthmatic children. J. Pediatr. 97:825, 1980.)*

slower than their rates of excretion, serum levels of metabolite are less than 1 µg/ml when the corresponding theophylline serum concentration is about 10 µg/ml [198]. This explains why 3-methylxanthine, the only active metabolite, has little if any pharmacologic effects. In the neonate about 50 percent of the dose is excreted unmetabolized in the urine, while the remainder undergoes N-methylation to caffeine [11, 20, 21] and C-8 hydroxylation to 1,3-demethyluric acid [16, 204] (Table 58-1).

Early studies suggested that the pharmacokinetics of theophylline could be described by a first-order rate constant—that is, that the rate of metabolism was proportional to the amount remaining because serum concentrations appeared to follow a log-linear decay [40, 135]. However, Tang-Liu et al. [198], using a highly precise and specific assay, demonstrated the unique situation in which the overall clearance appears to be linear but each

metabolic pathway is, in fact, nonlinear. This is a result of the reciprocal nature of the nonlinear process. The renal clearance of unmetabolized theophylline is urine flow rate dependent. At higher serum concentrations (10 µg/ml) after a single dose, theophylline induces a diuresis, and renal clearance of unchanged drug is elevated, but the rate of metabolite formation is relatively slow. At lower concentrations, metabolic clearance is more rapid, but the diuretic effect is decreased, urine flow rate is slower, and the renal clearance of unchanged drug decreases. Thus, the two processes tend to cancel each other. After multiple doses, when tolerance to the diuretic effect has developed, the dose dependency of clearance may be more apparent. Changes in theophylline clearance at different serum concentrations occur in both children [232] and adults [186]. This is clinically relevant in that changes in dosage frequently result in disproportionate changes in serum concentration [87, 178, 232] (Fig. 58-10).

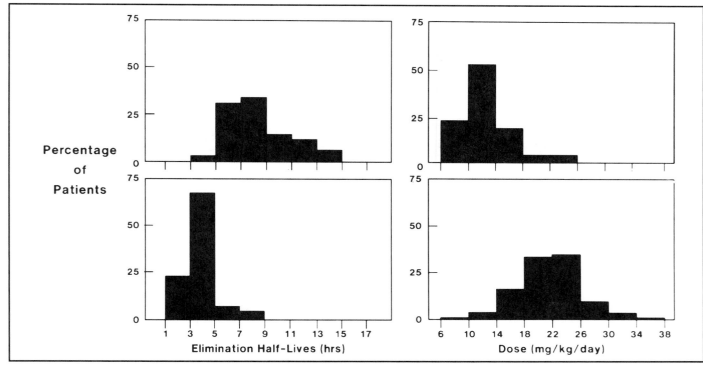

Fig. 58-11. *Distribution of elimination half-lives among 42 young and middle-aged adults* (upper left) *and 40 one- to nine-year-old children* (lower left) *and dosage requirements to attain serum concentrations of 10 to 20 μg/ml among 49 adults, median age 29* (upper right), *and 337 one- to nine-year-old children, median age 6 years* (lower right). *The elimination half-life data are combined from various sources included in Table 58-2 and elsewhere [226] where individual data could be extracted; dosage data are from an ambulatory population of asthmatic patients [133].*

Elimination

In 1972 Jenne et al. [87] first described the relationship between interpatient variation in theophylline elimination rate, dosage requirements, and serum concentration. A fixed dose of oral medication administered continuously to a group of asthmatic adults resulted in a wide range of serum concentrations. When dosage was adjusted to maintain serum concentrations within the 10 to 20 μg/ml range, requirements varied from 320 to 1,600 mg/day. A similar variability in rate of elimination, as determined by total body clearance, was demonstrated for children [54], where the dose required to achieve a therapeutic serum concentration ranged from 16 to 40 mg/kg/day in the age group 1 to 9 years (Fig. 58-11).

Total body clearance, the product of the volume of distribution and the elimination rate constant, most accurately reflects theophylline removal from the body. As a consequence of variability of elimination rate, interpatient variability in clearance is large and appears to be due to differences in the rate of hepatic biotransformation, which changes with age, concurrent illness, smoking, aberrations in diet, and other drugs (Table 58-2). Conflicting reports have been published on the influence of obesity [50, 175], old age [2, 145, 146], and gender [75, 95] on theophylline clearance. Available evidence suggests that there is no clinically important difference in theophylline clearance between obese and normal-weight subjects [175] or between males and females [75]. In contrast, clearance appears to be lower in some elderly patients compared to younger adults as a result of decreased protein binding [2].

Under normal circumstances, clearance [54], serum concentrations [87], and dosage requirements [241] in most patients generally remain acceptably stable over time with little intrapatient variation. Reports of large intrapatient variability in clearance among otherwise healthy children with asthma [110, 215] did not differentiate between variability in the method of clearance determination and actual changes in clearance within those patients.

Theophylline clearance and thus dosage requirements are markedly reduced in neonates [5, 53] and increase during the first year of life [141]. Thereafter, they remain constant for the first 9 years and gradually decline to adult mean values by age 16 [241]. The decrease in theophylline clearance associated with hepatic cirrhoses [123, 157], acute hepatitis [194], cholestasis [194], cardiac decompensation [88, 158, 161], and cor pulmonale [211] can be quite large and of major clinical importance.

Clearance is also reduced during febrile viral respiratory tract infections. Reports have not consistently distinguished the effects of fever versus the effects simply of viral illness [26, 28, 44, 102]. However, experimentally induced fever with etiocholanolone has been shown to reduce the clearance of antipyrine, another drug *N*-demethylated by the cytochrome P-450 system [38], and reduced theophylline clearance in the presence of sustained fever from rubeola [54] and bacterial pneumonia [127] have been reported. Moreover, theophylline clearance was not influenced by induced rhinovirus infection in adult volunteers [10].

There has also been concern and a degree of confusion regarding the potential for influenza immunization to influence theophylline elimination. Kramer and McClain [103] demonstrated that hepatic metabolism of aminopyrine, a sensitive indirect measurement of *N*-demethylation, was reduced in 12 afebrile volunteers 2 to 7 days after immunization with trivalent influenza vaccine, and the effect lasted as long as 21 days in many subjects. They proposed that the vaccine stimulated interferon, which decreased cytochrome P-450 activity as the mechanism for this interaction. Trivalent influenza vaccine has been reported to

Table 58-2. Mean pharmacokinetic parameters of theophylline for various patient populations

Population characteristics	Age, range or mean ± SD (yr)	Number of patients	Total body clearance mean ± SD (ml/kg/min)	Half-life mean ± SD[a] (hr)
Age				
Premature neonates with apnea [5, 53]	3–15 days	6	0.29 ± 0.1	30 ± 6.5
	25–57 days	8	0.64 ± 0.3	20 ± 5.3
Term infants [141]	1–2 days	2	NR	25–26.5
	6–24 weeks	8	NR	14 ± 4
Young children (1–4 years) [120]	2.5 ± 0.9	10	1.7 ± 0.6	3.4 ± 1.1
Older children				
4–12 years [54]	9.4 ± 3.0	17	1.6 ± 0.4	NR
13–15 years [54]	14.0 ± 0.8	6	0.9 ± 0.2	NR
6–17 years [40]	10.7 ± 2.7	30	1.4 ± 0.6	3.7 ± 1.1
Adults: otherwise healthy nonsmoking asthmatics [72]	22–57	16	0.65 ± 0.19	8.2 (6.1–12.8)[b]
Elderly: nonsmokers with normal cardiac, liver, and renal function [2]	70–85	14	0.41 ± 0.1	9.8 ± 4.1
Gender [67]	5–15	49 females	1.08 ± 0.42	NR
		49 males	1.10 ± 0.28	NR
Concurrent illness				
Acute pulmonary edema [158]	71 ± 10	9	0.33 (0.067–2.35)[b]	19 (3.1–82.0)[b]
COPD—elderly, stable nonsmoker >1 year [9]	65.0 ± 1.3	13	0.54 ± 0.05	11.0 ± 0.8
COPD with cor pulmonale [211]	64	8	0.48 ± 0.2	NR
Cystic fibrosis [81]	14–28	10	1.25 ± 0.47	6.0 ± 2.1
Fever associated with acute viral respiratory illness [26]	9–15	6	NR Not measured	During illness: 7.0 ± 3.0 1 month later: 4.1 ± 2.4
Liver disease				
Cirrhosis [123]	56 ± 4	8	0.31 (0.1–0.7)[b]	32 (10–56)[b]
Acute hepatitis [194]	NR	4	0.35 ± 0.05	19.2 ± 1.3
Cholestasis [194]	NR	7	0.65 ± 0.4	14.4 ± 8.7
Smoking history				
Marijuana alone [94]	20–25	7	1.2 ± 0.5	4.3 ± 1.0
Marijuana and cigarettes [94]	19–27	7	1.5 ± 0.4	4.3 ± 1.0
Cigarettes [85]	33	10	Not measured	4.1 ± 1.0
Elderly smokers [33]	67–79	6	0.71 ± 0.2	5.9 ± 0.8
Concurrent drugs				
Allopurinol (high dose, 600 mg/day) [122]	21–30	12	Control: 41.5 ± 6.2 After 28 days: 31.1 ± 5.9	Control: 8.5 ± 1.4 After 28 days: 11.0 ± 1.4
Carbamazepine [176]	11–29	2	—	Control: 3.9–6.5 After 3–4 weeks: 1.6–2.75
Cimetidine [165]	26 ± 2.9	6	Control: 46 ± 11.7 After 1 day: 37.2 ± 10 After 8 days: 31.5 ± 7.1	Control: 7.6 ± 2.1 After 1 day: 10.0 ± 2.4 After 8 days: 11.7 ± 1.6
Erythromycin [163]	23 ± 2.2	8	Control: 0.82 ± 0.17 After 7 days: 0.60 ± 0.11	Control: 6.7 ± 1.9 After 7 days: 8.3 ± 1.8
Influenza trivalent vaccine [131]	25–35	8	Control: 63 ± 23 After 1 day: 47 ± 13	Control: 6.3 ± 1.8 After 1 day: 7.8 ± 1.6
Isoproterenol—IV infusion [65]	4–13	6	Control: 1.6 ± 0.6 During: 1.9 ± 0.7	NR
Oral contraceptives [51]	24.2 ± 2.6	10	Nonusers: 0.85 ± 0.21 Users: 0.62 ± 0.20	Nonusers: 7.8 ± 2.4 Users: 9.6 ± 1.3
Phenobarbital [107]	23–32	4	Control: 0.75 ± 0.35 After 1 month: 1.0 ± 0.5	NR
Phenytoin [124]	19–34	10	Control: 0.72 ± 0.3 After 10 days: 1.3 ± 0.3	Control: 10.1 ± 3.8 After 10 days: 5.2 ± 1.6
Propranolol [29]	27–33	8	Control: 0.82 ± 0.4 After 1 day: 0.49 ± 0.2	Control: 6.8 ± 2.7 After 1 day: 11.1 ± 3.6
Rifampin [173]	NR	6	Control: 104 ± 21[c] After 14 days: 187 ± 43[c]	Control: 7.3 ± 0.9 After 14 days: 5.6 ± 0.9
Troleandomycin (TAO) [229]	39 ± 15	8	Control: 0.70 ± 0.14 After 11 days: 0.34 ± 0.05	NR NR
Ciprofloxacin [67, 180]				
Enoxacin [174]	22–27	4	Control: 117[c] After 5 days: 55, 39, 31 @ 25, 100, 400 mg q12h	Control: 7.8 ± 1.7 After 5 days: 10.5, 13.5, 14.2 @ 25, 100, 400 mg q12h
Aberrant diets				
Low carbohydrate, high protein [96]	22–29	6	Control: 49 ± 4[c] After 2 weeks: 76 ± 5[c]	Control: 8.1 ± 2 After 2 weeks: 5.1 ± 1
High carbohydrate, low protein [42]	7–14	14	Control: 0.98 ± 0.25 After 12 days: 0.8 ± 0.27	—
Charcoal-broiled beef [97]	22–32	8	Control: 70 ± 6[c] After 7 days: 91 ± 9[c]	Control: 6.0 ± 1 After 7 days: 4.7 ± 0.4

NR = not reported; COPD = chronic obstructive pulmonary disease.

[a] While the standard deviation is indicated, the half-lives are not normally distributed—they are somewhat skewed toward higher values.

[b] Median and range. Mean and standard deviations were not meaningful because of large range of values.

[c] Units of clearance are in milliliters per minute.

slow theophylline elimination [168, 214], but in a subsequent study, the interaction could not be demonstrated [43]. Whether the different results of these two studies relate to the type of vaccine used (split versus whole virus) or other factors requires further investigation.

Cigarette smokers [85, 94, 160] and those who use marijuana [94] have clearance that is on average almost twice that in nonsmokers and increases dosage requirements. Similarly, a high-protein, low-carbohydrate diet increases the rate of theophylline elimination about 25 percent, whereas a low-protein, high-carbohydrate meal decreases theophylline clearance about 25 percent compared to a normal diet [42, 96]. Ingestion of charcoal-broiled beef also can increase clearance [97]. The magnitude of these effects, however, is likely to require only modest changes in dose requirements for individuals and then only when radical and persistent alterations in diet occur (e.g., a heavy meat eater becoming a high-carbohydrate vegetarian).

Several drugs affect theophylline metabolism, but the clinical relevance of these interactions is variable. Elimination of theophylline is prolonged in patients receiving propranolol [29]. The more selective beta1 blocker metoprolol does not alter theophylline clearance in nonsmokers but does reduce clearance somewhat less than propranolol in cigarette smokers with high initial clearances [29].

Clearance also is decreased during concurrent administration of macrolide antibiotics erythromycin [104, 129, 163, 167, 245] and troleandomycin [229]. Adverse effects have been observed when these antibiotics have been prescribed concurrently in patients receiving therapeutic doses of theophylline [101, 229]. Erythromycin must be administered for at least 6 days before theophylline clearance is reduced, and the magnitude of the effect is proportional to the steady-state peak erythromycin concentration [163] (Fig. 58-12). Four of the nine controlled studies on this interaction were unable to demonstrate a significant effect of theophylline clearance because the duration of therapy was too short and the erythromycin products used may have been incompletely absorbed [93].

Standard doses of the xanthine-oxidase inhibitor allopurinol block conversion of 1-methylxanthine to 1-methyluric acid without affecting theophylline clearance [60, 212], but larger doses (600 mg/day) as commonly used for tophaceous gout reduce theophylline clearance after 14 days of concurrent therapy [122].

This effect is probably unrelated to the xanthine-oxidase inhibition of allopurinol, since allopurinol also can reduce *N*-demethylase and hydroxylase activity in hepatic microsomes in vitro [210].

The H2 antagonist cimetidine decreases theophylline clearance by an average of 40 percent [82, 165, 172] and has been associated with an approximately twofold increase in serum concentrations when added to a previous therapeutic theophylline regimen [25, 235]. Dosage must therefore be reduced during concurrent administration of these drugs to prevent severe toxicity. The newer H2 antagonist ranitidine does not alter theophylline disposition and is preferable to cimetidine particularly in patients taking theophylline [162].

In contrast, intravenous infusions of isoproterenol for status asthmaticus [65] and anticonvulsant doses of phenobarbital administered for 1 month [107] both increase theophylline clearance, but the magnitude of these effects generally is small and thus not likely to be clinically important unless the serum concentration already is at the low end of the therapeutic range prior to initiation of the second drug.

BIOPHARMACEUTICS

Theophylline has been marketed in a confusing array of formulations. These have included various parenteral preparations and tablets, capsules, solutions, and suspensions for oral use. Oral preparations have also been marketed since at least 1940 as fixed-dose combination products with ephedrine, often also containing a barbiturate or antihistamine; at the time of this writing, some of these are still sold without prescription.

One of the earliest deviations from use of the basic drug was its mixture with ethylenediamine to form a formulation identified as "aminophylline." The high pH of a solution containing the alkaline ethylenediamine improved the solubility of theophylline, which increases sharply at pH 9.0. This had packaging convenience for parenteral preparations; theophylline could then be marketed at concentrations of 20 mg/ml in contrast to 4 mg/ml, the approximate maximum concentration at neutral pH. However, there was no therapeutic advantage, and a parenteral formulation of theophylline without ethylenediamine is now available.

Oral solutions of theophylline were initially hydroalcoholic in the belief that the alcohol was essential for adequate absorption. Subsequently, however, nonalcoholic solutions and at least one suspension were marketed with absorption that matched that of the alcohol-containing formulations. The preferability of avoiding alcohol, particularly for the usual pediatric target population of liquid formulations, has led to the general preference for the newer formulations when a liquid preparation is indicated.

The greater solubility of theophylline with ethylenediamine led to the misguided belief that "aminophylline" and other "salts" would be associated with improved absorption of theophylline in clinical use. Some of the more popular preparations of this sort included, in addition to aminophylline, oxtriphylline (choline theophyllinate), theophylline calcium salicylate, and theophylline glycinate. In point of fact, these formulations offered no therapeutic advantage over unadulterated theophylline. Rectal suppositories were another irrational formulation used because of the misbelief that oral absorption was unreliable. In fact, theophylline has been completely and reliably absorbed from all but enteric-coated tablets and a few poorly formulated slow-release formulations.

Slow-release formulations of theophylline meet a clinical need dictated by the pharmacodynamic and pharmacokinetic characteristics of theophylline, that is, rapid absorption, rapid elimination, and a close relationship between effect and serum concentration. The earliest slow-release formulations were simply enteric-coated tablets designed more to delay dissolution until

Fig. 58-12. *Correlation between peak erythromycin serum concentration and percent change in theophylline total body clearance among eight healthy nonsmoking adult volunteers with a mean ± SD age of 23 ± 2.2 years. Total body clearance was determined from an intravenous dose of theophylline before and on the seventh day of therapy with erythromycin, enteric-coated base, 250 mg QID. (Reprinted with permission from R. A. Prince et al. Effect of erythromycin on theophylline kinetics.* J. Allergy Clin. Immunol. *68:427, 1981.)*

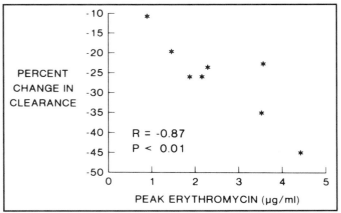

R = -0.87
P < 0.01

the drug was out of the stomach and into the small intestine. Reports as early as 1950 demonstrated erratic and often incomplete absorption from these early preparations. Even as late as 1978, three of the six available slow-release formulations appeared to be incompletely and erratically absorbed [226]. Many (but not all) of the numerous formulations subsequently marketed have had complete absorption, but rate and consistency of absorption have varied considerably [66].

Unfortunately, there has been no standardization in production or requirements by the Food and Drug Administration (FDA) for approval of marketing or claims for dosing interval. Interaction of absorption rate (a product variable), elimination rate (a patient variable), and the dosing interval (a prescribing variable) dictates the resulting fluctuations in serum concentration. Procedures to examine objectively rate and extent of absorption of theophylline from the formulations require determination of the amount and rate of drug absorbed following a dose. This can be determined by calculating the amount of drug in the body represented by a serum concentration and adding to that the amount that was absorbed and already eliminated by the time that serum concentration was measured. When these calculations are performed for multiple sampling following a dose of slow-release theophylline and a reliably and rapidly absorbed reference preparation, an absorption profile can be constructed for the formulation (Fig. 58-13). While a modest lag in the onset of absorption from food is anticipated because of an expected delay in gastric emptying, most formulations show nothing more than consequent slowing of absorption when taken with food in the stomach as compared with an overnight fast. Absorption of some formulations, however, has differed markedly in rate and/or completeness of absorption when taken fasting or following food [76, 98, 105, 134, 153–155, 192, 199, 227] (Fig. 58-14).

The interaction of the rate of absorption of the formulation, the rate of elimination from the patient, and the dosing interval determine the fluctuations in serum concentration and the consequent potential for fluctuations in clinical effect over the selected dosing interval. Considerations of the interaction of these three variables is particularly important to consider, as formulations are marketed for progressively longer dosing intervals. The prescribing clinician should therefore be wary of claims for specified dosing intervals included in advertisements or implied by "uni-" prefixes or "-24" suffixes attached to the brand name [219].

Selection of a slow-release formulation should be limited to products with publicly available data documenting complete absorption after an overnight fast and after a large meal to ensure that these variables will not result in erratic serum concentrations. The data should be presented in a standardized manner as a cumulative fraction absorbed as illustrated in Figure 58-13. From this, estimates of anticipated fluctuations in serum concentration can be determined at defined rates of elimination for specified dosing intervals using standard pharmacokinetic procedures.

Alternatively, a normalized expression of anticipated fluctuation can be calculated from the ratio of the peak to trough or the ratio of the peak-trough difference to the peak or trough. A peak-trough ratio of 2:1 is equivalent to 100 percent fluctuation when the peak-trough difference is expressed as a percent of the trough serum concentration. Fluctuations expressed in this manner can be applied to any target peak serum concentration. Fluctuation in excess of 100 percent (where the peak is twice the trough) can therefore not maintain serum concentrations within the 10 to 20 μg/ml therapeutic range even if the peak is at the upper limit of safe usage, 20 μg/ml. Predicted fluctuations can then be expressed in simple tabular form for different dosing intervals and different elimination half-lives for different formulations under different conditions (Table 58-3). This table illustrates that fluctuations in serum concentrations are influenced by the rate of theophylline absorption from the forumulation, the elimination rate of the patient, and the dosing interval. Thus, differences in forumulation will be less apparent if only fluctuations in serum concentration in adults with average or slower rates of elimination are examined, rather than rates of absorption as illustrated in Figures 58-13 and 58-14.

The predictions in Table 58-3 are based on the assumption of

Fig. 58-13. *Serum concentrations following single doses of a slow-release and reference formulation* (top) *and resulting absorption profile expressed as the cumulative fraction absorbed* (bottom) *calculated by previously described methodology (see text). F_t = fraction absorbed at time* t; *AUC = area under concentration time curve to time* t *or infinity* (∞) *as indicated; C_t = serum theophylline concentration at time* t; β = *elimination rate constant of subject for theophylline.*

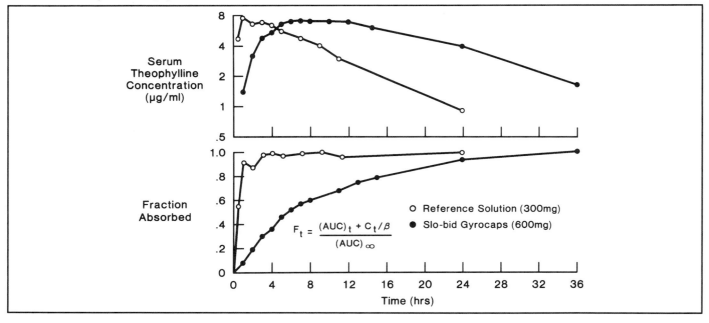

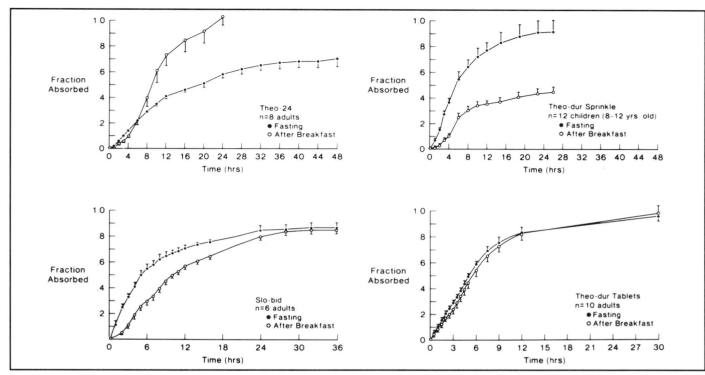

Fig. 58-14. *Paradoxical effects of food on Theo-24* (upper left) *[76] and Theo-Dur Sprinkle* (upper right) *[155].
Major but opposite effects on both the extent and rate of absorption are apparent for these two preparations. In
contrast, no effect on extent and only a modest effect on rate are associated with Slo-Bid Gyrocaps* (lower left)
[227] or Theo-Dur tablets (lower right) *[192].*

Table 58-3. *Predicted fluctuations*[a] *in serum concentration expressed as a percent of trough for selected products based on the rate of
absorption following an overnight fast in adult volunteers and the specified elimination half-life calculated by previously described
methodologies [66, 226, 233]*

Formulation[b]	% Fluctuation during specified dosing interval[c]		Hours < 10 μg/ml during 12-hour dosing interval when peak serum concentration = 15 μg/ml
	8 hours	12 hours	
Plain tablets			
Half-life = 3.7 hr	169	459	8
Half-life = 8.2 hr	61	117	4
Slo-Phyllin Gyrocaps			
Half-life = 3.7 hr	61	225	5
Half-life = 8.2 hr	27	69	2
Slo-bid Gyrocaps			
Half-life = 3.7 hr	24	43	0
Half-life = 8.2 hr	10	18	0
Theo-Dur 200, 300-mg tablets			
Half-life = 3.7 hr	17	38	0
Half-life = 8.2 hr	11	16	0

[a] Actual fluctuations will be somewhat greater than these predicted values, which are based on the same rate of absorption for the evening doses as for the morning fasting
dose from which the rate of absorption is obtained. Both dose-to-dose differences in absorption and the slower absorption following the evening dose will serve to increase
the actual fluctuations. Nonetheless, these idealized values at least provide minimal estimates for the purpose of comparison. Better estimations could be made by including
actual absorption profiles following evening doses if that data were available.
[b] Plain tablets have the most rapid rate of absorption; Slo-Phyllin Gyrocaps are an older slow-release formulation that is considerably more rapidly absorbed than the Slo-
bid Gyrocaps and Theo-Dur tablets. The selected elimination rates of 3.7- and 8.2-hour half-lives represent the means for 1- to 9-year-old children and adults, respectively.
The validity of this methodology has been empirically verified [134, 233].
[c] Note that fluctuations in serum concentration decrease with slower absorption, shorter half-lives, and shorter dosing intervals. Differences in fluctuations of serum
concentration resulting from slow-release formulations will therefore be most apparent at longer dosing intervals in patients with more rapid rates of elimination.

complete absorption, with each dose being absorbed at the rate
measured following a single dose given in the morning after an
overnight fast with no food for 2 hours. Products such as Theo-
Dur Sprinkle [155], Theo-24 [76], and Uniphyl [134] have such
large differences in rate and/or extent of absorption when taken
under differing conditions with regard to meals that this form

of analysis is meaningless for them. All products exhibit some
differences in rate of absorption among doses taken at different
times of the day, with some delay in absorption being common
following an evening dose. However, Theo-Dur Sprinkle is completely absorbed when taken after an overnight fast but is only
about 40 percent absorbed when taken after breakfast [155]. In

contrast, theophylline is paradoxically only about 70 percent absorbed from Theo-24 while fasting, with a marked increase in the rate and extent of absorption when taken after a meal [76]. Absorption of theophylline from Uniphyl increases from about 60 percent fasting to about 80 percent after a meal, although the rate of absorption is little affected [134].

Since the predictions are based on average absorption profiles, dose-to-dose variability of absorption and the potential for lot-to-lot variability of the same formulation can also add variability. The predicted percentage fluctuation in Table 58-3 should be regarded as minimal estimates for the purpose of comparing products. To the extent that real-life conditions do not match those used to calculate the predictions, actual fluctuations will exceed the predicted. *Nonetheless, presentation of data limited only to serum concentrations during multiple dosing in pharmacokinetically uncharacterized patients is of limited interpretability because slow rates of elimination decrease fluctuations in serum concentration as effectively as slow release of theophylline.*

Since patient elimination half-life is generally neither known nor individually determined, dosing interval is initially selected based on population pharmacokinetics. Patients who have above average dose requirements will be expected to have more rapid than average rates of elimination and consequently greater than average fluctuation at the selected dosing interval. If excessive serum concentration is anticipated and the most slowly reliably absorbed formulation is already being used, then a shorter dosing interval should be considered, particularly if a pattern of breakthrough symptoms is apparent.

Because of the lack of standardization and absence of publicly available data providing absorption profiles for many products (fasting and with food), caution should be exercised in substituting one formulation for another. Even certification of bioequivalency by the FDA does not provide assurance because of the lack of appropriate methodology in examining equivalency [220, 227].

CLINICAL USAGE

Therapeutic Decisions

For outpatient use, the bother of theophylline generally no longer provides sufficient additive benefit as an intervention measure for acute symptoms to be worth the bother when a longer-acting inhaled beta$_2$ agonist, such as albuterol, is appropriately and vigorously used. The same argument has been used even for asthma in the emergency room or hospital. There have been several commentaries addressing this issue and even some suggestions that considerations of benefit and risk no longer justify the use of theophylline [39, 86, 106, 130, 143]. Nonetheless, theophylline has been used successfully and safely for over 50 years, and current knowledge regarding its pharmacodynamics and pharmacokinetics, the universal availability of serum theophylline measurements, and newer formulations have provided the ability to further minimize risk and maximize benefit. In reviewing this literature, critically assessing the rationale for continued use of theophylline, and developing appropriate strategies for clinical use, it is helpful to separate acute therapy for intervention of active symptoms, as in the emergency room or hospital, from maintenance therapy used for prevention of symptoms of chronic asthma.

There has been particular controversy regarding the use of theophylline for acute therapy. A meta-analysis of multiple studies in the literature has suggested no benefit [118], but a more recent controlled study suggests that use in the emergency room helps prevent hospitalizations [240], and treatment in hospitalized adults may shorten hospitalization [213]. Although inhaled or parenteral sympathomimetic bronchodilators are the drugs of first choice for treatment of acute symptoms, theophylline may

yet be a useful adjunct in the emergency situation. In fact, the first reports of the clinical response of asthma to theophylline were in patients with poor response to injected epinephrine. However, the development of newer, more beta$_2$ specific sympathomimetic bronchodilators has at least partly supplanted the use of theophylline as an emergency measure for acute asthma. Nonetheless, an inadequate response to a sympathomimetic bronchodilator may still justify a trial of added theophylline.

Dosage for Acute Bronchodilatation

Since acute symptoms of asthma are extremely uncomfortable and potentially life-threatening, rapid attainment of maximal safe effect is desired when the clinical decision to use theophylline is made (Fig. 58-15). Theophylline diffuses into about 0.5 L/kg of body space (with a range of 0.3–0.7 L/kg); each 1 mg/kg of rapidly administered dose will therefore increase the serum concentration by about 2 μg/ml (with a range of 1.4–3.3 μg/ml). An initial infusion of 5 mg/kg will therefore target a serum concentration of 10 μg/ml in patients whose initial serum concentration is zero. Subsequent to attaining levels of 10 to 20 μg/ml with one or more loading doses, a maintenance infusion is given at a dose initially based on mean population pharmacokinetics, again using an initial conservative target serum concentration of 10 μg/ml. Final dosage is guided by measurement of serum concentration [234].

Dosage for Maintenance Therapy of Chronic Asthma

The primary outpatient use of theophylline today is long-term maintenance as prophylaxis for chronic asthma. Slow-release formulations with reliable and complete absorption such as Slo-bid Gyrocaps and Theo-Dur tablets generally maintain acceptably stable blood levels with doses every 12 hours. Initiation of therapy should be with low doses, with final dosage attained after a period of clinical titration as previously described and incorporated into the package inserts of all currently marketed U.S. preparations [225] (Fig. 58-16). Dosage guideline forms specific for the dosage sizes of the most commonly used formulations are available to provide specific printed instructions to patients (Fig. 58-17). Rapid attainment of serum concentrations between 10 and 20 μg/ml are associated with about at least a 50 percent frequency of minor side effects. These include varying degrees of nausea, irritability, and insomnia. In contrast to adverse effects associated with serum concentrations over 20 μg/ml, these adverse effects are generally transient and decrease to about 2 percent with the clinical titration procedure [133]. One to two measurements of serum concentration are generally sufficient to document appropriate dosage. Measurements in ambulatory patients can now be made quickly and simply in an examining room with acceptable clinical accuracy [208], without the need for a laboratory [132]. Once an appropriate maintenance dose is attained, serum concentrations generally remain sufficiently stable so that repeat serum concentrations at 6- to 12-month intervals is generally sufficient in the absence of specific clinical indications for more frequent measurement [133, 134].

Since serum concentrations over 20 μg/ml are associated with a progressive increase in the frequency and severity of theophylline toxicity, a therapeutic range of 10 to 20 μg/ml has been established [221]. While measurable effect sufficient for some patients occurs at lower serum concentration, and toxicity is not apparent universally at higher serum concentrations, this 10 to 20 μg/ml range represents serum concentrations where an optimal likelihood of maximal safe effect can be obtained from theophylline. The dosing interval described in Fig. 58-16 permits that range to be attained with a high degree of safety and acceptance of the medication while efficiently utilizing serum measure-

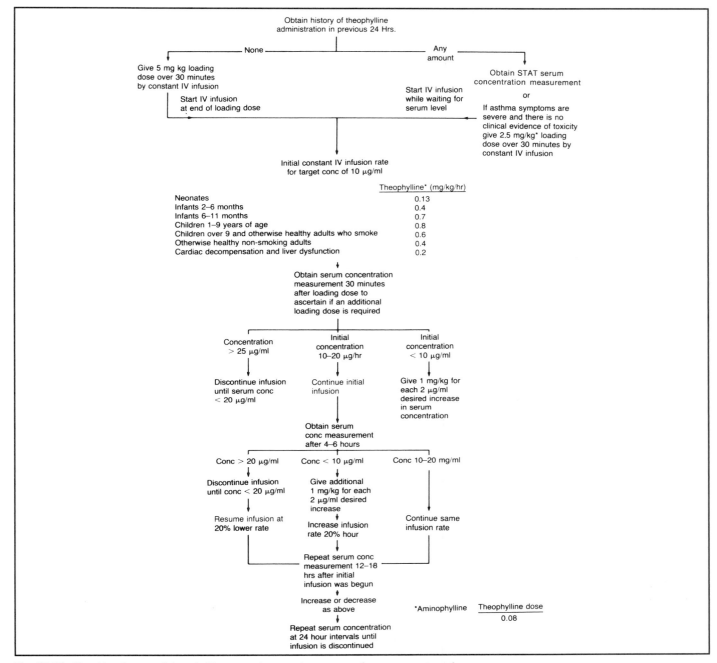

Fig. 58-15. *Algorithm for use of theophylline as an intervention measure for severe acute asthma.*

ments to guide final dosage. Once dosage is established in this manner, it generally remains stable for extended periods [133].

Iatrogenic Causes of Theophylline Toxicity

Although there is the potential for theophylline toxicity from drug interactions or alterations in clearance for other reasons (see Table 58-2), toxicity occurs most commonly from errors in dosage [179, 182]. Fortunately, most cases of toxicity are mild and readily reversible without residual effects. In virtually every case where there has been serious toxicity, such as seizures with neurologic damage, serious errors in dosage occurred, often compounded by other factors such as drug interactions or failing to be alert for early signs of toxicity such as nausea, vomiting, cen-

tral nervous system stimulation, or tachycardia. In the past, errors in intravenous dosage were contributed to, in part, by inappropriately broad recommendations in a prominent journal article [136]. That error was caused by using small numbers of inappropriately selected patients who had rates of elimination that averaged twice that subsequently documented in larger numbers of nonsmoking adult patients (see Table 58-2). Toxicity in infants has been caused by failure to recognize the very slow rates of elimination resulting from immature metabolic pathways under 1 year of age [141]. Poor communication between multiple physicians involved in a patient's care can contribute to risks of toxicity by one physician beginning medications that slow theophylline elimination or discontinuing medications that increase theophylline elimination while neither adjusting or monitoring

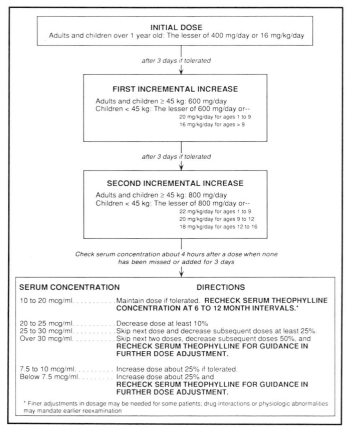

Fig. 58-16. *Dosage schedule for treatment of chronic asthma utilizing slow clinical titration with guidance by measurement of serum concentration. (Corresponding initial daily doses and incremental increases for infants under 1 year are [0.2(age in weeks) + 5]; [0.25(age in weeks) + 6.5]; [0.3(age in weeks) + 8].) It is important that no dose be continued that is not tolerated without overt side effects. When this schedule is followed, adverse effects are minor and apparent in only about 2 percent of patients [133, 134]. (Reproduced with permission from M. Weinberger and L. Hendeles. Slow-release theophylline: Rationale and basis for product selection. N. Engl. J. Med. 308(13):760, 1983.)*

theophylline dosage nor communicating the changes to the physician prescribing the theophylline.

Despite the potential for toxicity and the concerning frequency of dosing errors in some institutions [179], an investigation of extensive clinical use at a large HMO found an exceedingly low frequency of serious toxicity [35]. Among 225,000 theophylline prescriptions for 36,000 patients, only 2 patients (1 child and 1 adult) developed theophylline-induced seizures; it was not indicated whether these were from prescribed doses or ingestions. Thus, iatrogenic theophylline toxicity can be avoided. The following precautions can ensure optimal safe use of theophylline [223]:

1. Always begin with a low dose and titrate slowly; doses should be maintained *only if tolerated.*
2. Always guide final dosage by measurement of serum theophylline concentration.
3. Instruct the patient always to hold a dose of theophylline until a serum concentration can be measured if there is any suggestion of adverse effects, especially persistent headache, nervousness, tachycardia, nausea, or vomiting.
4. Reduce dosage by one-half for fever sustained beyond 24 hours.

5. Reduce maintenance dose by one-third whenever erythromycin or ciprofloxacin is added and by one-half for cimetidine, troleandomycin, and oral contraceptives (a smaller decrease may be adequate for very low estrogen–containing products); recheck theophylline level and readjust the dosage if these are to be maintained; reduce dose by one-half if maintenance therapy with an enzyme inducer such as carbamazepine or phenytoin is discontinued; monitor theophylline levels monthly if cigarette smoking is stopped; consider the possibility of other medications and physiologic abnormalities affecting theophylline elimination, thus altering maintenance dose requirements.
6. Provide adequate instruction (preferably as printed instruction forms) for patient and/or family to understand benefits and risks of theophylline.

METHODS OF MEASURING THEOPHYLLINE IN SERUM

As a result of increased physician demand and improved technology, facilities for measuring theophylline in serum are now readily available. Even if a local clinical laboratory does not provide this service, specimens can be sent to a referral laboratory from most locations. Theophylline remains stable in serum at room temperature for at least 7 days [18], under refrigeration for at least 14 days [18], and when frozen for at least a year [91].

Immunoassay techniques of various types are generally used. They are rapid and specific and can be performed on small volumes. The fluorescence polarization immunoassay (TDx) is particularly popular for large-volume laboratory use because it is more rapid than other conventional methods, the standard curve is stable for at least 2 weeks, thus reducing the reagent expense, and the same equipment can be used for most other drugs that are currently monitored.

Various rapid assays have been developed for use in the doctor's office. Syntex Medical Diagnostics' Acculevel combines the technology of immunoassay with thin-layer chromatography. It requires only a 12 μl drop of whole blood from a finger stick and takes about 15 minutes using a disposable kit. Results are usually accurate within 2 μg/ml [209].

In spite of the intrinsic accuracy and precision of the various available methods under experimental conditions, poor test performance has been a problem in many clinical laboratories in the past because of technician error [18]. Therefore, the accuracy and reproducibility of the laboratory must be determined before its results can be relied on to guide dosage adjustments. Analysis of quality control samples and participation in quality assurance surveys alone do not reflect performance on clinical specimens. Rather, duplicate patient specimens should be sent to a reference laboratory periodically, for comparison to results obtained by the laboratory procedure used for routine sample analysis.

Saliva has been previously recommended to estimate indirectly the concentration of theophylline in serum [112], particularly for children who often vigorously object to venipuncture. While this concept was appealing, subsequent studies demonstrated that the saliva-serum concentration ratio often did not remain constant within the same patient [74]. As a consequence, measurement of salivary levels to estimate serum concentration can lead to errors in dosage adjustment. Since the newer methods require less than 0.05 ml of serum, sufficient blood for analysis can be obtained from a finger or a heel stick.

MANAGEMENT OF THEOPHYLLINE POISONING

Ingestion of an excessive oral dose of theophylline requires discontinuation of the drug and prompt emergency treatment with

Initial Dose: Weight: _42_ kg

    ☒ Adults and children over 25 kg .... 200 mg at _7_ am and _7_ pm
    ☐ Children 20 to 25 kg .... 150 mg at ____ am and ____ pm
    ☐ Children 15 to 20 kg .... 100 mg at ____ am and ____ pm

Increase Dose After 3 Days If Tolerated To:

    ☒ Adults and children over 35 kg .... 300 mg at _7_ am and _7_ pm
    ☐ Children 25 to 35 kg .... 250 mg at ____ am and ____ pm
    ☐ Children 20 to 25 kg .... 200 mg at ____ am and ____ pm
    ☐ Children 15 to 20 kg .... 150 mg at ____ am and ____ pm

Attention: Decrease dose to **Initial Dose** if the increased dose
is not tolerated because of headaches or stomach upset
(nausea, vomiting, diarrhea)

Increase Dose After 3 More Days If Tolerated To:

    ☒ Adults and children over 40 kg .... 400 mg at _7_ am and _7_ pm
    ☐ Children 35 to 40 kg .... 350 mg at ____ am and ____ pm
    ☐ Children 30 to 35 kg .... 300 mg at ____ am and ____ pm
    ☐ Children 20 to 30 kg .... 250 mg at ____ am and ____ pm
    ☐ Children 15 to 20 kg .... 200 mg at ____ am and ____ pm

**CHECK SERUM CONCENTRATION BETWEEN 3 AND 8 HOURS AFTER A DOSE WHEN NONE
HAVE BEEN MISSED OR ADDED FOR AT LEAST 3 DAYS.**

Serum Theophylline Concentration ___ _14_ ___ mcg/ml   Patient: _James Jones_

If serum theophylline is: Directions:

OK—   10 to 20 mcg/ml ....Maintain dose if tolerated. **RECHECK SERUM THEOPHYLLINE
                                           CONCENTRATION AT 6 TO 12 MONTH INTERVALS.***

TOO HIGH—20 to 25 mcg/ml ....Decrease doses by 50 mg.
         25 to 30 mcg/ml ....Skip next dose and decrease subsequent doses by 25% to the
                                           nearest 50 mg.
         Over 30 mcg/ml ....Skip next 2 doses and decrease subsequent doses by 50%. **RECHECK
                                           SERUM THEOPHYLLINE.**

TOO LOW— 7.5 to 10 mcg/ml...............Increase dose by 25% to the nearest 50 mg.****
         5 to 7.5 mcg/ml...............Increase dose by 25% to the nearest 50 mg and **RECHECK SERUM
                                           THEOPHYLLINE FOR GUIDANCE IN FURTHER DOSAGE
                                           ADJUSTMENT.**

*Finer adjustments in dosage may be needed for some patients.
**Dividing the daily dosage into 3 doses administered at 8-hour intervals may be indicated if symptoms occur repeatedly at the end of a dosing interval.

Fig. 58-17. *Dosage guideline form for reliably absorbed slow-release preparations that conservatively follow
the schedule illustrated in Fig. 58-16. Product-specific variations of this form, general information regarding
theophylline, and instructions regarding serum theophylline measurement are available for copying and
provision to patients* [223].

1 gm/kg up to at least 30 gm of activated charcoal [191]. It is
generally not worthwhile to delay administering the activated
charcoal while attempting to induce vomiting. Serum concentrations should be measured frequently and all patients with excessive levels monitored in an intensive care unit. Many patients
survive very high serum theophylline levels unscathed. When
seizures occur, however, death and permanent brain damage are
common sequelae [32, 64, 246]. Charcoal hemoperfusion can rapidly remove theophylline [27, 84] and may be clinically indicated
when the serum concentration is over 60 μg/ml, even in the absence of obvious signs of toxicity [224]. Seizures may thereby be
prevented by promptly reducing the serum concentration to safe
levels. In most cases, however, hemoperfusion has been instituted after the onset of seizures, and the clinical outcome has
not matched the chemical success of the procedure [37]. If risks
of the procedure such as hypotension and thrombocytopenia are
not judged to be excessive and the patient is large enough to gain
vascular access, treatment should be promptly instituted prior
to obvious clinical toxicity. This probably is not warranted when
the serum concentration is less than 40 μg/ml, since the risks of
the procedure probably outweigh the potential benefit. In the
range of 40 to 60 μg/ml the decision must be individualized,
depending on the availability of clinicians experienced with charcoal hemoperfusion and the presence of clinical symptoms such
as nausea, vomiting, headache, tachycardia, irritability, confusion, and so on. If hemoperfusion is not performed, activated
charcoal can be repeated every 2 to 4 hours until the serum level
falls below 20 μg/ml. Even if the theophylline serum level became

excessive as a result of intravenous administration, oral activated
charcoal used in this manner ("gastrointestinal dialysis") shortens the half-life and speeds up removal of the drug [13, 111].
Peritoneal dialysis and other extracorporeal methods of removal
including conventional hemodialysis do not clear theophylline
efficiently and thus are not adequate for the management of
theophylline poisoning [224].

Phenobarbital has been shown to protect laboratory animals
from theophylline-induced seizures [52], but this effect has not
been evaluated clinically. Nonetheless, a 10 to 20 mg/kg intravenous loading dose administered slowly over 30 minutes can be
considered for patients of all ages with serum theophylline levels
greater than 40 μg/ml even if asymptomatic. This would result in
phenobarbital blood level concentration within the therapeutic
range of 15 to 40 μg/ml. When seizures occur, they should be
rapidly terminated with intravenous diazepam or thiopental
while oxygenation and respiratory support are maintained (see
Appendix F, Theophylline Toxicity: A Management Algorithm).

REFERENCES

1. Andersson, K. E., and Persson, C. G. Extrapulmonary effects of theophylline. *Eur. J. Respir. Dis.* [Suppl. 109]61:17, 1980.
2. Antal, E. J., et al. Theophylline pharmacokinetics in advanced age. *Br.
   J. Clin. Pharmacol.* 12:637, 1981.
3. Appel, D., and Shim, C. Comparative effect of epinephrine and aminophylline in the treatment of asthma. *Lung* 159:243, 1981.

4. Aranda, J. V., and Turmen, T. Methylxanthines in apnea of prematurity. *Clin. Perinatol.* 6:87, 1979.

5. Aranda, J. V., et al. Pharmacokinetic aspects of theophylline in premature newborns. *N. Engl. J. Med.* 295:413, 1976.

6. Aranda, J. V., et al. Efficacy of caffeine in treatment of apnea in the low-birth-weight infant. *J. Pediatr.* 90:467, 1977.

7. Arnold, L. A., et al. Effect of antacid on gastrointestinal absorption of theophylline. *Am. J. Hosp. Pharm.* 36:1059, 1976.

8. Arwood, L. L., Dasta, J. F., and Friedman, C. Placental transfer of theophylline: Two case reports. *Pediatrics* 63:844, 1979.

9. Au, W. Y., Dutt, A. K., and Desoyza, N. Theophylline kinetics in chronic obstructive airway disease in the elderly. *Clin. Pharmacol. Ther.* 37:472, 1985.

10. Bachmann, K., et al. Theophylline clearance during and after mild upper respiratory infection. *Ther. Drug Monit.* 9:279, 1987.

11. Bada, H. S., et al. Interconversion of theophylline and caffeine in newborn infants. *J. Pediatr.* 94:993, 1979.

12. Bakris, G. L., et al. Effects of theophylline on erythropoietin production in normal subjects and in patients with erythrocytosis after renal transplantation. *N. Engl. J. Med.* 323:86, 1990.

12a. Bender, B., and Milgrom, H. Theophylline-induced behavior change in children. An objective evaluation of parents' perceptions. *J.A.M.A.* 267(19):2621, 1992.

13. Berg, M. J., et al. Acceleration of the body clearance of phenobarbital by oral activated charcoal. *N. Engl. J. Med.* 307:642, 1982.

14. Beswick, K., Davies, J., and Davey, A. J. A comparison of intravenous aminophylline and salbutamol in the treatment of severe bronchospasm. *Practitioner* 214:561, 1975.

15. Bolme, P., et al. Pharmacokinetics of theophylline in young children with asthma: Comparison of rectal enema and suppositories. *Eur. J. Clin. Pharmacol.* 16:133, 1979.

16. Bonati, M., et al. Theophylline metabolism during the first month of life and development. *Pediatr. Res.* 15:304, 1981.

17. Boner, A. L., et al. Theophylline inhibition of BCG-induced pulmonary inflammatory responses. *Ann. Allergy* 64:530, 1990.

18. Bonham, A., et al. The reliability of serum theophylline determinations from clinical laboratories. *Am. Rev. Respir. Dis.* 122:829, 1980.

19. Borga, O., et al. Enprofylline kinetics in healthy subjects after single doses. *Clin. Pharmacol. Ther.* 34:799, 1983.

20. Bory, C., et al. Metabolism of theophylline to caffeine in premature newborn infants. *J. Pediatr.* 94:988, 1979.

21. Boutroy, M. J., et al. Caffeine, a metabolite of theophylline during the treatment of apnea in the premature infant. *J. Pediatr.* 94:996, 1979.

22. Brenner, M., et al. Need for theophylline in severe steroid-requiring asthmatics. *Clin. Allergy* 18:143, 1988.

23. Buckle, J. W., and Nathanielsz, P. W. Modification of myometrial activity in vivo by administration of cyclic nucleotides and theophylline to the pregnant rat. *J. Endocrinol.* 66:339, 1975.

24. Camarata, S. J., et al. Cardiac arrest in the critically ill: I. A study of predisposing causes in 132 patients. *Circulation* 44:688, 1971.

25. Campbell, M. A., et al. Cimetidine decreases theophylline clearance. *Ann. Intern. Med.* 95:68, 1981.

26. Chang, K. C., et al. Altered theophylline pharmacokinetics during acute respiratory viral illness. *Lancet* 1:1132, 1978.

27. Chang, T. M. S., et al. Albumin-collodion activated charcoal hemoperfusion in the treatment of severe theophylline intoxication in a 3-year-old patient. *Pediatrics* 65:811, 1980.

28. Clark, C. J., and Boyd, G. Theophylline pharmacokinetics during respiratory viral infection. *Lancet* 1:492, 1979.

29. Conrad, K. A., and Nyman, D. W. Effects of metoprolol and propranolol on theophylline elimination. *Clin. Pharmacol. Ther.* 28:463, 1980.

30. Cornish, H. H., and Christman, A. A. A study of the metabolism of theobromine, theophylline and caffeine in man. *J. Biol. Chem.* 228:315, 1957.

31. Crescioli, S., et al. Theophylline inhibits early and late asthmatic reactions induced by allergens in asthmatic subjects. *Ann. Allergy* 66:245, 1991.

32. Culberson, C. G., Langston, J. W., and Herrick, M. Aminophylline encephalopathy: A clinical, electroencephalographic and neuropathological analysis. *Trans. Am. Neurol. Assoc.* 104:224, 1979.

33. Cusack, B., et al. Theophylline kinetics in relation to age: The importance of smoking. *Br. J. Clin. Pharmacol.* 10:109, 1980.

34. Dawood, A. G., Hendry, A. T., and Walker, S. R. The combined use of betamethasone valerate and sodium cromoglycate in the treatment of asthma. *Clin. Allergy* 7:161, 1977.

35. Derby, L. E., et al. Hospital admission for xanthine toxicity. *Pharmacotherapy* 10:112, 1990.

36. Dusdieker, L., et al. Comparison of orally administered metaproterenol and theophylline in the control of chronic asthma. *J. Pediatr.* 101:281, 1982.

37. Ehlers, S. M., Zaske, D. E., and Sawchuck, R. J. Massive theophylline overdose: Rapid elimination by charcoal hemoperfusion. *J.A.M.A.* 240:474, 1978.

38. Elin, R. J., Vesell, E. S., and Wolff, S. M. Effects of etiocholanolone-induced fever on plasma antipyrine half-lives and metabolic clearance. *Clin. Pharmacol. Ther.* 17:447, 1975.

39. Hendeles, L., et al. Safety and efficacy of theophylline in children with asthma. *J. Pediatr.* 120:177, 1992.

40. Ellis, E. F., Koysooko, R., and Levy, G. Pharmacokinetics of theophylline in children with asthma. *Pediatrics* 58:542, 1976.

41. FDA. Theophylline and school performance. *FDA Drug Bull.* 18(3):32, 1988.

42. Feldman, C. H., et al. Effect of dietary protein and carbohydrate on theophylline metabolism in children. *Pediatrics* 66:956, 1980.

43. Fischer, R. G., et al. Influence of trivalent influenza vaccine on serum theophylline levels. *Can. Med. Assoc. J.* 126:1312, 1982.

43a. Fitzpatrick, M. F., et al. Effect of therapeutic theophylline levels on the sleep quality and daytime cognitive performance of normal subjects. *Am. Rev. Respir. Dis.* 145:1355, 1992.

44. Fleetham, J. A., Nakatsu, K., and Munt, P. W. Theophylline pharmacokinetics and respiratory infections. *Lancet* 2:898, 1978.

45. Foster, L. J., Trudeau, W. L., and Goldman, A. L. Bronchodilator effects on gastric acid secretion. *J.A.M.A.* 241:2613, 1979.

46. Fox, C. C. Comparison of human lung and intestinal mast cells. *J. Allergy Clin. Immunol.* 81:89, 1988.

47. Furukawa, C. T., et al. Dyphylline versus theophylline: A double-blind comparative evaluation. *J. Clin. Pharmacol.* 23:414, 1983.

48. Furukawa, C. T., et al. Double blind evaluation of dyphylline, theophylline, and placebo for exercise-induced bronchospasm. *J. Clin. Pharmacol.* 23:414, 1983.

49. Furukawa, C. T., et al. A double-blind study comparing the effectiveness of cromolyn sodium and sustained-release theophylline in childhood asthma. *Pediatrics* 74:453, 1984.

50. Gal, P., et al. Theophylline disposition in obesity. *Clin. Pharmacol. Ther.* 23:438, 1978.

51. Gardner, M. J., et al. Effects of tobacco smoking and oral contraceptive use on theophylline disposition. *Br. J. Clin. Pharmacol.* 16:271, 1983.

52. Gardner, R. A., et al. Unexpected fatality in a child from accidental consumption of antiasthmatic preparation containing ephedrine, theophylline and phenobarbital. *Tex. J. Med.* 46:516, 1950

53. Giacoia, G., et al. Theophylline pharmacokinetics in premature infants with apnea. *J. Pediatr.* 89:829, 1976.

54. Ginchansky, E., and Weinberger, M. Relationship of theophylline clearance to oral dosage in children with chronic asthma. *J. Pediatr.* 91:655, 1977.

55. Gisclon, L. G., Ayres, J. W., and Ewing, G. H. Pharmacokinetics of orally administered dyphylline. *Am. J. Hosp. Pharm.* 36:1179, 1979.

56. Glass, J., et al. Nebulized cromoglycate, theophylline, and placebo in preschool asthmatic children. *Arch. Dis. Child.* 56:648, 1981.

57. Grome, J. J., and Stefanovich, V. Differential effects of methylxanthines on local cerebral blood flow and glucose utilization in conscious rat. *Naunyn Schmiedebergs Arch. Pharmacol.* 333:172, 1986.

58. Grygiel, J. J., and Birkett, D. J. Effect of age on patterns of theophylline metabolism. *Clin. Pharmacol. Ther.* 28:456, 1980.

59. Grygiel, J. J., and Birkett, D. J. Cigarette smoking and theophylline clearance and metabolism. *Clin. Pharmacol. Ther.* 30:491, 1981.

60. Grygiel, J. J., et al. Effects of allopurinol on theophylline metabolism and clearance. *Clin. Pharmacol. Ther.* 26:660, 1979.

61. Hambleton, G., et al. Comparison of cromoglycate (cromolyn) and theophylline in controlling symptoms of chronic asthma. *Lancet* 1:381, 1977.

62. Heimann, G., Murgescu, J., and Bergt, U. Influence of food intake on bioavailability of theophylline in premature infants. *Eur. J. Clin. Pharmacol.* 22:171, 1982.

63. Heins, M., et al. Nocturnal asthma: Slow-release terbutaline versus slow-release theophylline therapy. *Eur. Respir. J.* 1:306, 1988.

64. Helliwell, M., and Berry, D. Theophylline poisoning in adults. *Br. Med. J.* 2:1114, 1979.

65. Hemstreet, M. P., Miles, M. V., and Rutland, R. O. Effects of intravenous

isoproterenol on theophylline kinetics. *J. Allergy Clin. Immunol.* 69:360, 1982.

66. Hendeles, L., Iafrate, R. P., and Weinberger, M. A clinical and pharmacokinetic basis for the selection and use of slow-release theophylline products. *Clin. Pharmacokinet.* 9:95, 1984.

67. Hendeles, L., Vaughan, L., and Weinberger, M. Influence of gender on theophylline dosage requirements in children with chronic asthma. *Drug Intell. Clin. Pharm.* 15:338, 1981.

68. Hendeles, L., and Weinberger, M. Theophylline. In E. Ellis (ed.), *Allergy: Principles and Practice* (2nd ed.). St. Louis: Mosby, 1983. Pp. 535–574.

69. Hendeles, L., and Weinberger, M. Theophylline: A state-of-the-art review. *Pharmacotherapy* 3(1):2, 1983.

70. Hendeles, L., Weinberger, M., and Bighley, L. Absolute bioavailability of oral theophylline. *Am. J. Hosp. Pharm.* 34:525, 1977.

71. Hendeles, L., Weinberger, M., and Bighley, L. Disposition of theophylline after a single intravenous infusion of aminophylline. *Am. Rev. Respir. Dis.* 118:97, 1978.

72. Hendeles, L., Weinberger, M., and Bighley, L. Disposition of theophylline after a single intravenous infusion of aminophylline. *Am. Rev. Respir. Dis.* 118:97, 1978.

73. Hendeles, L., et al. Frequent toxicity from IV aminophylline infusions in critically ill patients. *Drug Intell. Clin. Pharm.* 11:12, 1977.

74. Hendeles, L., et al. Unpredictability of theophylline saliva measurements in chronic obstructive pulmonary disease. *J. Allergy Clin. Immunol.* 60:335, 1977.

75. Hendeles, L., et al. Influence of gender on theophylline dosage requirements in children with chronic asthma. *Drug Intell. Clin. Pharm.* 15:338, 1981.

76. Hendeles, L., et al. Food-induced "dose-dumping" from a once-a-day theophylline product as a cause of theophylline toxicity. *Chest* 87:758, 1985.

77. Hendeles, L., et al. Theophylline attenuation of allergen-induced airway hyperreactivity and late response (Abstract). *J. Allergy Clin. Immunol.* 87:167, 1991.

78. Hendeles, L., et al. Theophylline attenuation of allergen induced airway hyperreactivity and late response. *J. Allergy Clin. Immunol.* 137:A35, 1991.

79. Hiller, E. J., and Milner, A. D. Betamethasone 17 valerate aerosol and disodium cromoglycate in severe childhood asthma. *Br. J. Dis. Chest* 69:103, 1975.

80. Hudson, L. D., Tyler, M. L., and Petty, T. L. Oral aminophylline and dihydroxypropyl theophylline in reversible obstructive airway disease: A single dose, double-blind, crossover comparison. *Curr. Ther. Res.* 15:367, 1973.

81. Isles, A., et al. Theophylline disposition in cystic fibrosis. *Am. Rev. Respir. Dis.* 127:417, 1983.

82. Jackson, J. E., et al. Cimetidine decreases theophylline clearance. *Am. Rev. Respir. Dis.* 123:615, 1981.

83. Jacobs, M. H., Senior, R. M., and Kessler, G. Clinical experience with theophylline: Relationships between dosage, serum concentration and toxicity. *J.A.M.A.* 235:1983, 1976.

84. Jefferys, D. B., et al. Haemoperfusion for theophylline overdose. *Br. Med. J.* 280:1167, 1980.

85. Jenne, J., et al. Decreased theophylline half-life in cigarette smokers. *Life Sci.* 17:195, 1975.

86. Jenne, J. W. Theophylline is no more obsolete than "two puffs qid" of current beta 2 agonists (editorial). *Chest* 98:3, 1990.

87. Jenne, J. W., et al. Pharmacokinetics of theophylline: Application to adjustment of the clinical dose of aminophylline. *Clin. Pharmacol. Ther.* 13:349, 1972.

88. Jenne, J. W., et al. Apparent theophylline half-life fluctuations during treatment of acute left ventricular failure. *Am. J. Hosp. Pharm.* 34:408, 1977.

89. Joad, J., et al. Extrapulmonary effects of maintenance therapy with theophylline and inhaled albuterol in patients with chronic asthma. *J. Allergy Clin. Immunol.* 78:1147, 1986.

90. Joad, J., et al. Relative efficacy of maintenance therapy with theophylline, and inhaled albuterol, and the combination for the treatment of chronic asthma. *J. Allergy Clin. Immunol.* 79:78, 1987.

91. Johnson, C. E., et al. Stability of theophylline in human serum and whole blood. *Am. J. Hosp. Pharm.* 41:2065, 1984.

92. Jonkman, J. H., et al. Disposition and clinical pharmacokinetics of microcrystalline theophylline. *Eur. J. Clin. Pharmacol.* 17:379, 1980.

93. Jonkman, J. H. G., and Hendeles, L. Theophylline-erythromycin interaction (letter). *Chest* 84:309, 1983.

94. Jusko, W. J., et al. Enhanced biotransformation of theophylline in marijuana and tobacco smokers. *Clin. Pharmacol. Ther.* 24:405, 1978.

95. Jusko, W. J., et al. Factors affecting theophylline clearances: Age, tobacco, marijuana, cirrhosis, congestive heart failure, obesity, oral contraceptives, benzodiazepines, barbiturates, and ethanol. *J. Pharm. Sci.* 68:1358, 1979.

96. Kappas, A., et al. Influence of dietary protein and carbohydrate on antipyrine and theophylline metabolism in man. *Clin. Pharmacol. Ther.* 20:643, 1976.

97. Kappas, A., et al. Effect of charcoal-broiled beef on antipyrine and theophylline metabolism. *Clin. Pharmacol. Ther.* 23:445, 1978.

98. Karim, A., et al. Food-induced changes in theophylline absorption from controlled-release formulations: Part I. Substantial increased and decreased absorption with Uniphyl tablets and Theo-Dur Sprinkle. *Clin. Pharmacol. Ther.* 38:77, 1985.

99. Koeter, G. H., et al. Effect of theophylline and enprophylline on bronchial hyperresponsiveness. *Thorax* 44:1022, 1989.

100. Koysooko, R., Ellis, E. F., and Levy, G. Relationship between theophylline concentration in plasma and saliva of man. *Clin. Pharmacol. Ther.* 15:454, 1974.

101. Kozak, P. P., Cummins, L. H., and Gillman, S. A. Administration of erythromycin to patients on theophylline. *J. Allergy Clin. Immunol.* 60:149, 1977.

102. Kraemer, M. J., et al. Altered theophylline clearance during an influenza B outbreak. *Pediatrics* 69:476, 1982.

103. Kramer, P., and McClain, C. J. Depression of aminopyrine metabolism by influenza vaccination. *N. Engl. J. Med.* 305:1262, 1981.

104. LaForce, C. F., Miller, M. F., and Chai, H. Effect of erythromycin on theophylline clearance in asthmatic children. *J. Pediatr.* 99:153, 1981.

105. Lagas, M., and Jonkman, J. H. Greatly enhanced bioavailability of theophylline on postprandial administration of a sustained-release tablet. *Eur. J. Clin. Pharmacol.* 24:761, 1983.

106. Lam, A., and Newhouse, M. T. Management of asthma and chronic airflow limitation: Are methylxanthines obsolete? *Chest* 98:44, 1990.

107. Landay, R. A., Gonzalez, M. A., and Taylor, J. C. Effect of phenobarbital on theophylline disposition. *J. Allergy Clin. Immunol.* 62:27, 1978.

108. Laursen, L. C., et al. Enprofylline-effects of a new bronchodilating xanthine derivative in asthmatic patients. *Allergy* 38:75, 1983.

109. Laursen, L. C., et al. Maximally effective plasma concentrations of enprofylline and theophylline during constant infusion. *Br. J. Clin. Pharmacol.* 18:591, 1984.

110. Leung, P., Kalisker, A., and Bell, T. D. Variation in theophylline clearance rate with time in chronic childhood asthma. *J. Allergy Clin. Immunol.* 59:440, 1977.

111. Levy, G. Gastrointestinal clearance of drugs with activated charcoal. *N. Engl. J. Med.* 307:676, 1982.

112. Levy, G., Ellis, E. F., and Koysooko, R. Indirect plasma-theophylline monitoring in asthmatic children by determination of theophylline concentration in saliva. *Pediatrics* 53:873, 1974.

113. Levy, G., and Koysooko, R. Pharmacokinetic analysis of the effect of theophylline on pulmonary function in asthmatic children. *J. Pediatr.* 86:789, 1975.

114. Levy, G., and Koysooko, R. Renal clearance of theophylline in man. *J. Clin. Pharmacol.* 16:329, 1976.

115. Lindgren, S., et al. Does asthma or treatment with theophylline limit academic performance in children? *N. Engl. J. Med.* 327:926, 1992.

116. Lindholm, B., and Helander, E. The effect on the pulmonary ventilation of different theophylline derivatives compared to adrenaline and isoprenaline. *Acta Allergol.* 21:299, 1966.

117. Littenberg, B. Aminophylline treatment in severe, acute asthma. *J.A.M.A.* 259:1678, 1988.

118. Littenberg, B. Aminophylline treatment in severe, acute asthma: A meta-analysis. *J.A.M.A.* 259:1678, 1988.

119. Lohmann, S. M., and Miech, R. P. Theophylline metabolism by the rat liver microsomal system. *J. Pharmacol. Exp. Ther.* 196:213, 1976.

120. Loughnan, P. M., et al. Pharmacokinetic analysis of the disposition of intravenous theophylline in young children. *J. Pediatr.* 88:874, 1976.

121. Lunell, E., et al. Effect of enprofylline, a xanthine lacking adenosine receptor antagonism, in patients with chronic obstructive lung disease. *Eur. J. Clin. Pharmacol.* 22:395, 1982.

122. Manfredi, R. L., and Vesell, E. S. Inhibition of theophylline metabolism by long term allopurinol administration. *Clin. Pharmacol. Ther.* 29:224, 1981.

123. Mangione, A., et al. Pharmacokinetics of theophylline in hepatic disease. *Chest* 73:616, 1978.

124. Marquis, J., et al. Phenytoin-theophylline interaction. *N. Engl. J. Med.* 307:1189, 1982.

125. Martin, G. L., et al. Effects of theophylline, terbutaline and prednisone on antigen-induced bronchospasm and mediator release. *J. Allergy Clin. Immunol.* 66:204, 1980.

126. Mason, W. D., et al. Bioavailability of theophylline following a rectally administered concentrated aminophylline solution. *J. Allergy Clin. Immunol.* 66:119, 1980.

127. Matthay, R. A., Matthay, M. A., and Weinberger, M. M. Grand mal seizure induced by oral theophylline. *Thorax* 31:470, 1976.

128. Matthay, R. A., et al. Effects of aminophylline upon right and left ventricular performance in chronic obstructive pulmonary disease. *Am. J. Med.* 65:903, 1978.

129. May, D. C., et al. The effects of erythromycin on theophylline elimination in normal males. *J. Clin. Pharmacol.* 22:125, 1982.

130. McFadden, E. R. Methylxanthines in the treatment of asthma: the rise, the fall, and the possible rise again. *Ann. Intern. Med.* 115:323, 1991.

131. Meredith, C. G., et al. Effects of influenza virus vaccine on hepatic drug metabolism. *Clin. Pharmacol. Ther.* 37:396, 1985.

132. Milavetz, G., Vaughan, L., and Weinberger, M. Comparative efficiency of a laboratory and examining room assay for therapeutic drug monitoring of theophylline in ambulatory patients. *Ann. Allergy* 62:453, 1989.

133. Milavetz, G., et al. Evaluation of a scheme for establishing and maintaining dosage of theophylline in ambulatory patients with chronic asthma. *J. Pediatr.* 109:351, 1986.

134. Milavetz, G., et al. Relationship between rate and extent of absorption of oral theophylline from Uniphyl brand of slow-release theophylline and resulting serum concentrations during multiple dosing. *J. Allergy Clin. Immunol.* 80:723, 1987.

135. Mitenko, P. A., and Ogilvie, R. I. Pharmacokinetics of intravenous theophylline. *Clin. Pharmacol. Ther.* 14:509, 1973.

136. Mitenko, P. A., and Ogilvie, R. I. Rational intravenous doses of theophylline. *N. Engl. J. Med.* 289:600, 1973.

137. Monks, T. J., Caldwell, J., and Smith, R. L. Influence of methylxanthine-containing foods on theophylline metabolism and kinetics. *Clin. Pharmacol. Ther.* 26:513, 1979.

138. Mountain, R. D., and Neff, T, A. Oral theophylline intoxication: A serious error of patient and physician understanding. *Arch. Intern. Med.* 144: 724, 1984.

139. Murciano, D., et al. Effects of theophylline on diaphragmatic strength and fatigue in patients with chronic obstructive pulmonary disease. *N. Engl. J. Med.* 311:349, 1984.

140. Nassif, E. G., et al. The value of maintenance theophylline for steroid dependent asthma. *N. Engl. J. Med.* 304:71, 1981.

141. Nassif, E. G., et al. Theophylline disposition in infancy. *J. Pediatr.* 98: 158, 1981.

142. Neijens, J. H., et al. Clinical and bronchodilating efficacy of controlled-release theophylline as a function of its serum concentrations in preschool children. *J. Pediatr.* 107:811, 1985.

143. Newhouse, M. T. Is theophylline obsolete? *Chest* 98:1, 1990.

144. Newth, C. J., Newth, C. V., and Turner, J. A. Comparison of nebulised sodium cromoglycate and oral theophylline in controlling symptoms of chronic asthma in pre-school children: A double-blind study. *Aust. N.Z. J. Med.* 12:232, 1982.

145. Nielsen-Kudsk, F., Magnussen, I., and Jakobsen, P. Pharmacokinetics of theophylline in ten elderly patients. *Acta Pharmacol. Toxicol.* 42:226, 1978.

146. Ogilvie, R. I. Clinical pharmacokinetics of theophylline. *Clin. Pharmacokinet.* 3:267, 1978.

147. Ogilvie, R. I., Fernandez, P. G., and Winsberg, F. Cardiovascular response to increasing theophylline concentrations. *Eur. J. Clin. Pharmacol.* 12:409, 1977.

148. Olson, K. R., et al. Theophylline overdose: Acute single ingestion versus chronic repeated overmedication. *Am. J. Emerg. Med.* 3:386, 1985.

149. Parker, J. O., et al. Hemodynamic effects of aminophylline in chronic obstructive pulmonary disease. *Circulation* 35:365, 1967.

150. Pauwels, R. The effects of theophylline on airway inflammation. *Chest* 92:32S, 1987.

151. Pauwels, R., and Van der Straeten, M. Experimental Asthma and Xanthines. In K. E. Andersson and C. G. A. Persson (eds.), *Anti-Asthma Xanthines and Adenosine.* Amsterdam: Excerpta Media, 1985. Pp. 97–109.

152. Pauwels, R., et al. The effect of theophylline and enprophylline on allergen-induced bronchoconstriction. *J. Allergy Clin. Immunol.* 76:583, 1985.

153. Pedersen, S. Delay in the absorption rate of theophylline from a sus-

154. Pedersen, S., and Moeller-Petersen, J. Influence of food on the absorption rate and bioavailability of a sustained release theophylline preparation. *Allergy* 37:531, 1982.

155. Pedersen, S., and Moeller-Petersen, J. Erratic absorption of a slow-release theophylline sprinkle product. *Pediatrics* 74:534, 1984.

156. Persson, C. G. A., and Kjellin, G. Enprofylline, a principally new antiasthmatic xanthine. *Acta Pharmacol. Toxicol.* 49:313, 1981.

157. Piafsky, K. M., et al. Theophylline disposition in patients with hepatic cirrhosis. *N. Engl. J. Med.* 296:1495, 1977.

158. Piafsky, K. M., et al. Theophylline kinetics in acute pulmonary edema. *Clin. Pharmacol. Ther.* 21:310, 1977.

159. Pollock, J., et al. Relationship of serum theophylline concentration to inhibition of exercise-induced bronchospasm and comparison with cromolyn. *Pediatrics* 60:840, 1977.

160. Powell, J. R., et al. The influence of cigarette smoking and sex on theophylline disposition. *Am. Rev. Respir. Dis.* 116:17, 1977.

161. Powell, J. R., et al. Theophylline disposition in acutely ill hospitalized patients: The effect of smoking, heart failure, severe airway obstruction, and pneumonia. *Am. Rev. Respir. Dis.* 118:229, 1978.

162. Powell, J. R., et al. Inhibition of theophylline clearance by cimetidine but not ranitidine. *Ann. Intern. Med.* 144:484, 1984.

163. Prince, R. A., et al. Effect of erythromycin on theophylline kinetics. *J. Allergy Clin. Immunol.* 68:427, 1981.

164. Proud, D., et al. Pharmacology of upper airways challenge. *Int. Arch. Allergy Appl. Immunol.* 82:493, 1987.

165. Reitberg, D. P., Bernhard, H., and Schentag, J. J. Alteration of theophylline clearance and half-life by cimetidine in normal volunteers. *Ann. Intern. Med.* 95:582, 1981.

166. Femi-Pearse, D., et al. Comparison of intravenous aminophylline and salbutamol in severe asthma. *Br. Med. J.* 1:491, 1977.

167. Renton, K. W., Gray, J. D., and Hung, O. R. Depression of theophylline elimination by erythromycin. *Clin. Pharmacol. Ther.* 30:422, 1981.

168. Renton, K. W., Gray, J. D., and Hall, R. I. Decreased elimination of theophylline after influenza vaccination. *Can. Med. Assoc. J.* 123:288, 1980.

169. Richards, W., Church, J. A., and Brent, D. K. Theophylline associated seizures in children. *Ann. Allergy* 54:276, 1985.

170. Richer, C., et al. Theophylline kinetics and ventilatory flow in bronchial asthma and chronic airflow obstruction: Influence of erythromycin. *Clin. Pharmacol. Ther.* 31:579, 1982.

171. Ridolfo, A. S., and Kohlstaedt, K. G. A simplified method for the rectal instillation of theophylline. *Am. J. Med. Sci.* 237:585, 1959.

172. Roberts, R. K., et al. Cimetidine impairs the elimination of theophylline and antipyrine. *Gastroenterology* 81:19, 1981.

173. Robson, R. A., et al. Theophylline-rifampicin interaction: Non-selective induction of theophylline metabolic pathways. *Br. J. Clin. Pharmacol.* 118:445, 1984.

174. Rogge, M. C., et al. The theophylline-enoxacin interaction: I. Effect of enoxacin dose size on theophylline disposition. *Clin. Pharmacol. Ther.* 44:579, 1988.

175. Rohrbaugh, T. M., et al. The effect of obesity on apparent volume of distribution of theophylline. *Pediatr. Pharmacol.* (New York) 2:75, 1982.

176. Rosenberry, K. R., et al. Reduced theophylline half-life induced by carbamazepine therapy. *J. Pediatr.* 102:472, 1983.

177. Rossing, T. H., et al. Emergency treatment of asthma: Comparison of the acute effects of parenteral and inhaled sympathomimetics and infused aminophylline. *Am. Rev. Respir. Dis.* 122:365, 1980.

178. Sarrazin, E., et al. Dose-dependent kinetics for theophylline: Observations among ambulatory asthmatic children. *J. Pediatr.* 97:825, 1980.

179. Schiff, G. D., et al. Inpatient theophylline toxicity: Preventable factors. *Ann. Intern. Med.* 114:748, 1991.

180. Schwartz, J., et al. Impact of ciprofloxacin on theophylline clearance and steady state concentrations in serum. *Antimicrob. Agents Chemother.* 32:75, 1988.

181. Sears, M. R., et al. Regular inhaled beta agonist treatment in bronchial asthma. *Lancet* 336:1391, 1990.

182. Sessler, C. N. Theophylline toxicity: Clinical features of 116 consecutive cases. *Am. J. Med.* 88:567, 1990.

183. Shargel, L., et al. Effect of antacid on bioavailability of theophylline from rapid and timed-release drug products. *J. Pharm. Sci.* 70:599, 1981.

184. Sharma, T. N., et al. Comparison of intravenous aminophylline, salbutamol and terbutaline in acute asthma. *Indian J. Chest Dis. Allied Sci.* 26: 155, 1984.

tained release theophylline preparation caused by food. *Br. J. Clin. Pharmacol.* 12:904, 1981.

185. Shaw, L. M., Fields, L., and Mayoc, K. R. Factors influencing theophylline serum protein binding. *Clin. Pharmacol. Ther.* 32:490, 1982.

186. Shen, D. D., Fixley, M., and Azarnoff, D. L. Theophylline bioavailability following chronic dosing of an elixir and two solid dosage forms. *J. Pharm. Sci.* 67:916, 1978.

187. Simons, F. E. R., Luciuk, G. H., and Simons, K. J. Sustained-release theophylline for treatment of asthma in preschool children. *Am. J. Dis. Child.* 136:790, 1982.

188. Simons, F. E. R., Simons, K. J., and Bierman, C. W. The pharmacokinetics of dihydroxypropyltheophylline: A basis for rational therapy. *J. Allergy Clin. Immunol.* 56:347, 1975.

189. Simons, K. J., and Simons, F. E. R. Urinary excretion of dyphylline in humans. *J. Pharm. Sci.* 68:1327, 1979.

190. Simons, K. J., Simons, F. E. R., and Bierman, C. W. Bioavailability of a sustained-release dyphylline formulation. *J. Clin. Pharmacol.* 17:237, 1977.

191. Sintek, C., Hendeles, L., and Weinberger, M. Inhibition of theophylline absorption by activated charcoal. *J. Pediatr.* 94:314, 1979.

192. Sips, A. P., et al. Food does not affect bioavailability of theophylline from Theolin Retard. *Eur. J. Clin. Pharmacol.* 26:405, 1987.

193. Somani, S. M., Khanna, N. N., and Bada, H. S. Caffeine and theophylline: Serum/CSF correlation in premature infants. *J. Pediatr.* 96:1091, 1980.

194. Staib, A. H., et al. Pharmacokinetics and metabolism of theophylline in patients with liver disease. *Int. J. Clin. Pharmacol. Ther. Toxicol.* 18: 500, 1980.

195. Stec, G. P., et al. Kinetics of theophylline transfer to breast milk. *Clin. Pharmacol. Ther.* 28:404, 1980.

196. Svedmyr, K., and Svedmyr, N. The role of theophylline in asthma therapy. *Scand. J. Respir. Dis.* [Suppl. 101]:125, 1977.

197. Tang-Liu, D., and Riegelman, S. Metabolism of theophylline to caffeine in adults. *Res. Commun. Chem. Pathol. Pharmacol.* 34:371, 1981.

198. Tang-Liu, D. D. S., Williams, R. L., and Riegelman, S. Non-linear theophylline elimination. *Clin. Pharmacol. Ther.* 31:358, 1982.

199. Thompson, P. J., et al. Slow-release theophylline in patients with airway obstruction with particular reference to the effects of food upon serum levels. *Br. J. Dis. Chest* 77:293, 1983.

200. Tjandramaga, T. B., et al. Comparative systemic availability of rectal and oral preparations of microcrystalline theophylline. *Curr. Med. Res. Opin.* [Suppl. 6]6:142, 1979.

201. Toogood, J. H., Jennings, B., Lefcoe, N. M. A clinical trial of combined cromolyn/beclomethasone treatment for chronic asthma. *J. Allergy Clin. Immunol.* 67:317, 1981.

202. Tribe, A. E., Wong, R. M., and Robinson, J. S. A controlled trial of intravenous salbutamol and aminophylline in acute asthma. *Med. J. Aust.* 2: 749, 1976.

203. Truitt, E. B., McKusick, V. A., and Krantz, J. C. Theophylline blood levels after oral, rectal, and intravenous administration and correlation with diuretic action. *J. Pharmacol. Exp. Ther.* 100:309, 1950.

204. Tserng, K., King, K. C., and Takieddine, F. N. Theophylline metabolism in premature infants. *Clin. Pharmacol. Ther.* 29:594, 1981.

205. Ufkes, J. G., et al. Efficacy of theophylline and its N-7-substituted derivatives in experimentally induced bronchial asthma in the guinea-pig. *Arch. Int. Pharmacodyn. Ther.* 253:301, 1981.

206. Upton, R. A., et al. Evaluation of the absorption from 15 commercial theophylline products indicating deficiencies in currently applied bioavailability criteria. *J. Pharmacokinet. Biopharm.* 8:229, 1980.

207. Vallner, J. J., et al. Effect of pH on the binding of theophylline to serum proteins. *Am. Rev. Respir. Dis.* 120:83, 1979.

208. Vaughan, L., et al. Multicenter evaluation of a disposable visual quantitation device for assaying theophylline from a small capillary blood sample. *Lancet* 1:184, 1986.

209. Vaughan, L. M., et al. Multicenter evaluation of disposable visual measuring device to assay theophylline from capillary blood sample. *Lancet* 1:184, 1986.

210. Vesell, E. S., Passananti, G. T., and Greene, F. E. Impairment of drug metabolism in man by allopurinol and nortriptyline. *N. Engl. J. Med.* 283:1484, 1970.

211. Vicuna, N., et al. Impaired theophylline clearance in patients with cor pulmonale. *Br. J. Clin. Pharmacol.* 7:33, 1979.

212. Vozeh, S., et al. Influence of allopurinol on theophylline disposition in adults. *Clin. Pharmacol. Ther.* 27:194, 1980.

213. Vozeh, S., et al. Theophylline serum concentration and therapeutic effect in severe acute bronchial obstruction: The optimal use of intravenously administered aminophylline. *Am. Rev. Respir. Dis.* 125:181, 1982.

214. Walker, S., Schreiber, L., and Middelkamp, J. N. Serum theophylline levels after influenza vaccination. *Can. Med. Assoc. J.* 125:243, 1981.

215. Walson, P. D., Strunk, R. C., and Taussig, L. M. Intrapatient variability in theophylline kinetics. *J. Pediatr.* 91:321, 1977.

216. Waxler, S. H., and Schack, J. A. Administration of aminophylline (theophylline ethylenediamine). *J.A.M.A.* 143:736, 1950.

217. Weinberger, M. Theophylline for treatment of asthma. *J. Pediatr.* 92:1, 1978.

218. Weinberger, M. The pharmacology and therapeutic use of theophylline. *J. Allergy Clin. Immunol.* 73:525, 1984.

219. Weinberger, M. Clinical and pharmacokinetic concerns of 24-hour dosing with theophylline. *Ann. Allergy* 56:2, 1986.

220. Weinberger, M. Reassurance about generic drugs? (letter). *N. Engl. J. Med.* 317:1412, 1987.

221. Weinberger, M. Treatment of chronic asthma with theophylline. *ISI Atlas Sci: Pharmacology,* 1988, pp. 53–61.

222. Weinberger, M. Development and Implementation of a Treatment Plan. In *Managing Asthma.* Baltimore: Williams & Wilkins, 1989. Pp. 133–139.

223. Weinberger, M. *Managing Asthma.* Baltimore: Williams & Wilkins, 1990. Pp. 275–282.

224. Weinberger, M., and Hendeles, L. Role of dialysis in the management and prevention of theophylline toxicity. *Dev. Pharmacol. Ther.* 1:26, 1980.

225. Weinberger, M., and Hendeles, L. Slow-release theophylline: Rationale and basis for product selection. *N. Engl. J. Med.* 308(13):760, 1983.

226. Weinberger, M., Hendeles, L., and Bighley, L. The relation of product formulation to absorption of oral theophylline. *N. Engl. J. Med.* 299:852, 1978.

227. Weinberger, M., and Milavetz, G. Influence of formulation on oral drug delivery: Considerations for generic substitution and selection of slow-release products. *Iowa Med.* 76:24, 1986.

228. Weinberger, M., et al. Effects of theophylline on learning and behavior: Reason for concern or concern without reason? *J. Pediatr.* 111:471, 1987.

229. Weinberger, M., et al. Inhibition of theophylline clearance by troleandomycin. *J. Allergy Clin. Immunol.* 59:228, 1977.

230. Weinberger, M. M., and Bronsky, E. A. Evaluation of oral bronchodilator therapy in asthmatic children. *J. Pediatr.* 84:421, 1974.

231. Weinberger, M. M., and Bronsky, E. A. Interaction of ephedrine and theophylline. *Clin. Pharmacol. Ther.* 17:585, 1975.

232. Weinberger, M. M., and Ginchansky, E. Dose-dependent kinetics of theophylline disposition in asthmatic children. *J. Pediatr.* 91:820, 1977.

233. Weinberger, M. M., Hendeles, L., and Wong, L. Relationship of formulation and dosing interval to fluctuation of serum theophylline concentration in children with chronic asthma. *J. Pediatr.* 99:145, 1981.

234. Weinberger, M. M., et al. Intravenous aminophylline dosage: Use of serum theophylline measurement for guidance. *J.A.M.A.* 235:2110, 1976.

235. Weinberger, M. M., et al. Decreased theophylline clearance due to cimetidine (letter). *N. Engl. J. Med.* 304:672, 1981.

236. Welling, P. G., et al. Influence of diet and fluid on bioavailability of theophylline. *Clin. Pharmacol. Ther.* 17:475, 1975.

237. Wijnands, W. J., Vree, T. B., and Van Herwaarden, C. L. The influence of quinolone derivatives on theophylline clearance. *Br. J. Clin. Pharmacol.* 22:677, 1986.

238. Wilkens, J. H., et al. Treatment of nocturnal asthma: The role of sustained-release theophylline and oral beta-2-mimetics. *Chronobiol. Int.* 4:387, 1987.

239. Williams, S. J., Parrish, R. W., and Seaton, A. Comparison of intravenous aminophylline and salbutamol in severe asthma. *Br. Med. J.* 4:685, 1975.

240. Wrenn, K., et al. Aminophylline therapy for acute bronchospastic disease in the emergency room. *Ann. Intern. Med.* 115:241, 1991.

241. Wyatt, R., Weinberger, M., and Hendeles, L. Oral theophylline dosage for the management of chronic asthma. *J. Pediatr.* 92:125, 1978.

242. Yarnell, P. R., and Chu, N. S. Focal seizures and aminophylline. *Neurology* 25:819, 1975.

243. Yeh, T. F., and Pildes, R. S. Transplacental aminophylline toxicity in a neonate (letter). *Lancet* 1:910, 1977.

244. Yurchak, A. M., and Jusko, W. J. Theophylline secretion into breast milk. *Pediatrics* 57:518, 1976.

245. Zarowitz, B. J. M., Szefler, S. J., and Lasezkay, G. M. Effect of erythromycin base on theophylline kinetics. *Clin. Pharmacol. Ther.* 29:601, 1981.

246. Zwillich, C. W., et al. Theophylline-induced seizures in adults: Correlation with serum concentrations. *Ann. Intern. Med.* 82:784, 1975.

Standards and Study Design for Asthma Drugs

59

Richard A. Nicklas

Standards for the study of new asthma drugs and study designs required to meet these standards require an enlightened assessment of current issues and trends relating to the clinical use of these drugs. Any current assessment must consider the "asthma paradox"—apparent improvement in therapeutic approaches to asthma management in the face of increasing asthma morbidity and mortality [8, 14, 19, 39, 40, 55, 58]. A number of possibilities have been proposed for such increases [9]. It is generally agreed, however, that reasonable possibilities include prescribing practices of physicians and patient use or misuse of medications prescribed [50].

Recent concern about theophylline has focused on (1) its narrow therapeutic index and the potential for toxicity associated with its use, (2) adverse effects associated with substitution of one product for another [2], (3) modification of pharmacodynamics based on food ingestion, other medications, and underlying disease [28], and (4) potential for alteration in behavior and learning in children [22, 42]. It is not surprising, therefore, that over the past 10 years, associated with availability of inhaled beta agonists, there has been movement away from the use of theophylline as first-line therapy for the treatment of asthma [11, 13, 45]. Such a change was logical based on studies that demonstrated that inhaled beta agonists were more effective in the treatment of acute as well as chronic asthma [20, 27, 53, 61].

At the same time, there has been interest in and concern about the connection, if any, between epidemics of asthma deaths and use of inhaled beta agonists [33, 54]. In this regard, epidemics of asthma deaths have been attributed to overreliance on inhaled beta agonists and underutilization of corticosteroids [7, 46], at a time when there is increasing recognition of the importance of chronic inflammation in the pathogenesis of asthma [10]. This has led to increased awareness of the need for corticosteroids [35, 49] and reexamination of the role of disodium cromoglycate in the treatment of asthma [21, 67].

In addition, recent data suggest that inhaled beta agonists might have a negative therapeutic effect by (1) increasing bronchial hyperreactivity [30, 32, 34a, 62, 63], (2) increasing antigen load to the lower respiratory tract [34, 37], (3) inhibiting heparin release from effector cells [47], and/or (4) producing paradoxical bronchospasm [43]. The potential for diminished therapeutic effect after the regular use of inhaled beta agonists has been recently demonstrated [51]. Although further studies are needed to substantiate these findings, such data have already produced modifications of proposed clinical programs, focusing on use of inhaled corticosteroids and other antiinflammatory agents [21].

Such findings will also have a significant impact on guidelines for the design of future studies with beta-agonist bronchodilators.

Over the same period, consistent with changes in clinical use of asthma medications, two approaches to the development of such medications are evident. One approach has been the modification of already existing classes of drugs—longer-acting forms of theophylline, modifications of devices for the administration of inhaled drugs, and development of "relatively $beta_2$ selective" agonists. Another approach has been the development of new chemical compounds that are designed to prevent or reverse inflammation by inhibition of specific mediators involved in the production of inflammation. This widely divergent group of chemical substances—leukotriene and platelet-activating factor antagonists in particular—may act intracellularly by interfering with mediator production/release or by blocking mediator interaction with receptors on other structures (Fig. 59-1). Of these two approaches, the most successful has been modification of already existing classes of drugs. In the future this approach may lead to (1) longer-acting inhaled beta agonists, (2) theophylline preparations less susceptible to therapeutic modification by food and other factors, (3) continued improvement in devices used to deliver inhaled medications, including modifications to improve compliance in specific subsets of patients, and (4) use of "relatively $beta_2$ selective" agonists by intravenous administration in the treatment of status asthmaticus (Table 59-1).

The development of drugs that are specifically designed to modify the immunopathology of asthma, particularly inflammation, have been less successful. Specific mediator antagonists have been unsuccessful for different reasons, which include (1) tumor development in animals, (2) adverse effects in humans—elevations in liver enzymes, paradoxical bronchospasm from inhaled drugs, or (3) lack of efficacy with repetitive administration. In the case of the latter, this may occur despite the fact that efficacy has been demonstrated in animal models, in vitro, or after single doses prior to challenge with specific mediators and/or allergen. Those evaluating this type of drug must consider the likely specificity of its action. Drugs that effectively prevent a lower respiratory response after inhalation of a specific mediator may have little, if any, effect on patient response to inhaled allergen.

Consideration of therapeutic options, although not recognized formally as a phase of study, is an extremely important prelude to the actual evaluation of new asthma medication. This is a time for enlightened discussion and thought by investigators and sponsors about the type of drugs that are most needed in the patient population for which the drug is intended.

Guidelines [5] will need to consider different approaches related to, and special problems inherent in, the study of different types of drugs. Bronchodilator and nonbronchodilator drugs will require different and, in some cases, unique approaches to their

---

This chapter was written by Dr. Nicklas in his private capacity. No official support or endorsement by the Food and Drug Administration is intended or should be inferred.

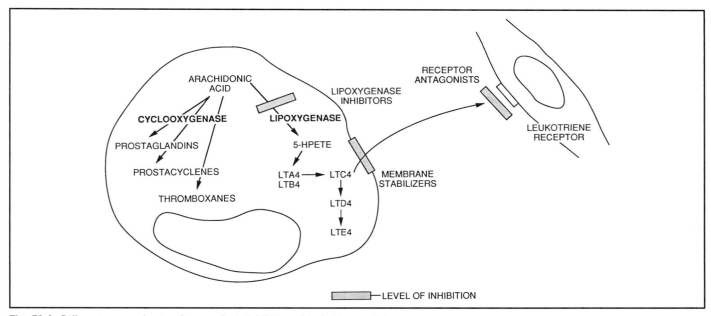

Fig. 59-1. *Different approaches to pharmacologic inhibition of leukotriene activity.*

Table 59-1. *Approaches to development of asthma medications*

Modification of already existing classes of drugs
  Present
    Longer-acting theophylline
    More efficient devices—inhaled drugs
    Relatively selective beta$_2$ agonists
    Inhaled corticosteroids with less systemic effect
    Antihistamines with bronchodilating properties
  Future
    Longer-acting inhaled beta agonists
    Theophylline preparations less susceptible to food, etc.
    Improved devices for delivery of inhaled drugs
    Fixed combination products
    IV use of relatively selective beta$_2$ agonists
Mediator antagonists
  Leukotriene antagonists
  Platelet activating factor antagonists
  Bradykinin antagonists
  Potassium channel activators

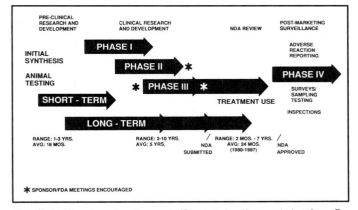

Fig. 59-2. *New drug development. (Reprinted with permission from R. A. Nicklas, The investigative process for new drugs. Ann. Allergy 63: 598, 1989.)*

evaluation within the framework for the evaluation of new drugs as established by the Food and Drug Administration (FDA) [41].

PHASES OF STUDY FOR NEW DRUGS

Following the passage of the Pure Food and Drug Act in 1906, a series of enactments changed the FDA's role in establishing the safety and efficacy of new drugs [69]. In 1938, Congress made it mandatory for the sponsor of "new drugs" to provide the FDA with evidence of safety of such drugs prior to marketing. With the passage of the Kefauver-Harris Amendments to the Food, Drug, and Cosmetic Act in 1962, it became necessary for manufacturers of new drugs to provide substantial evidence of effectiveness as well as safety prior to marketing [6].

The evaluation of investigational medications, including those to be utilized in the treatment of asthma, can appropriately be divided into four periods: a preclinical research and development period, a clinical research and development period, the period of New Drug Application (NDA) review, and postmarketing surveillance period (Fig. 59-2).

After the period of preclinical research and development, the pharmaceutical manufacturer (or occasionally the investigator) who is sponsoring the new drug, will submit an investigational new drug (IND) application for the study of the new drug in humans (Fig. 59-3). There are three phases of study during this clinical research and development period. The initial introduction of the drug into humans, usually in a small number of volunteers (or occasionally the patient population for whom the drug is intended), is considered to be phase 1. The purpose of this phase of study is to determine the dose that is safe for future studies, including the use of dose-ranging studies, and to gather information about the pharmacokinetics of the drug in humans through studies of absorption, distribution, metabolism, and excretion. The primary purpose of phase 1 is to demonstrate that the drug is safe for future study. In addition, however, the effect

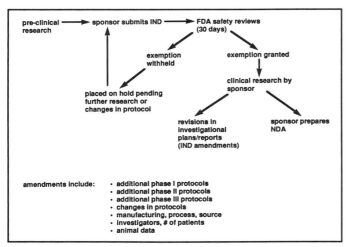

Fig. 59-3. *FDA role in investigational new drug (IND) application process. (Reprinted with permission from R. A. Nicklas, The investigative process for new drugs.* Ann. Allergy *63:598, 1989.)*

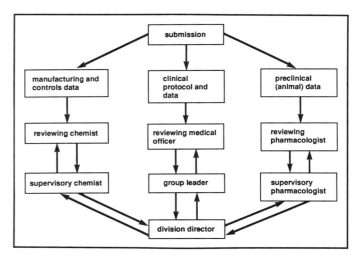

Fig. 59-4. *Interdisciplinary and intradisciplinary interaction within division. (Reprinted with permission from R. A. Nicklas, The investigative process for new drugs.* Ann. Allergy *63:598, 1989.)*

of the drug can be better understood by understanding the pharmacokinetics of the drug.

After phase 1 studies have been completed, the drug is studied in the patient population for whom it is intended, for the purpose of demonstrating the efficacy of the drug. These are considered phase 2 studies and usually involve a relatively small number of patients (50–200) studied over a relatively short period of time. Utilizing double-blind, appropriately controlled protocols, they are, in most cases, designed to show that the drug is efficacious. In the case of medications for the treatment of asthma, these studies are often supplemented by evaluation of the effectiveness of single doses prior to inhalation challenge.

A meeting often takes place at the end of phase 2 between the sponsor and the reviewing division within the Center for Drug Evaluation and Research (CDER) to discuss the sponsor's plans for the study of the drug during phase 3. This phase involves the evaluation of the drug in large numbers of patients for substantially longer periods of time (at least 3 months for bronchodilators and possibly 10–12 months for certain nonbronchodilator asthma drugs). The purpose of phase 3 is to demonstrate the safety of the drug over a longer period of time and continued effectiveness without the development of tolerance in double-blind controlled studies. To provide information that will be useful for setting dosage requirements and for adequately characterizing the drug, close monitoring by the sponsor is necessary during this phase of study.

During the three phases of clinical study, extensive interaction may take place between scientists in the division that is reviewing a new drug and experts outside the division. Intensive interaction always takes place between chemistry, pharmacology, and clinical disciplines within the division (Fig. 59-4). In addition, however, there may be interaction between the reviewing division and other divisions, in particular the Division of Biostatistics and the Division of Biopharmaceutics (Fig. 59-5). Frequent interaction often takes place as well between the reviewers of a drug within a division and the sponsor of that drug. These may include not only planned meetings such as end of phase 2 meetings between the sponsor and the reviewing division, but also unanticipated meetings between the division and the sponsor on issues as they arise.

Guidelines were established for the study of nonbronchodilator asthma drugs in 1984 by the American Academy of Allergy and Immunology, with input from other organizations, including the FDA. In 1978, the FDA developed guidelines for the testing of bronchodilator drugs. These are currently being revised with the

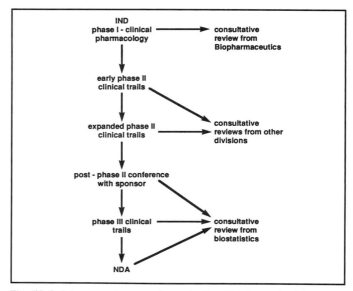

Fig. 59-5. *Interaction between the reviewing division and other divisions. (Reprinted with permission from R. A. Nicklas, The investigative process for new drugs.* Ann. Allergy *63:598, 1989.)*

expert advice of the Pulmonary-Allergy Drugs Advisory Committee to promote state-of-the-art study of this type of drug.

Once the preclinical and clinical research and development periods have been completed, the sponsor will submit data from these studies as well as manufacturing and controls data under an NDA (Fig. 59-6). This submission will contain essential studies that can lead to the approval or nonapproval of the drug. These data will be reviewed not only by the three disciplines within the division, but also by reviewers within the Division of Biostatistics and the Division of Biopharmaceutics and sometimes by microbiologists within the FDA. Furthermore, the data submitted by the sponsor may be reviewed by consultants to the FDA, especially those who sit on Advisory Committees (such as the Pulmonary-Allergy Drugs Advisory Committee, which consults on medications that would be used to treat asthma, among other conditions). Following review of this material, the sponsor will be informed in writing if additional information or analyses are necessary, which can be submitted as an amendment to the NDA.

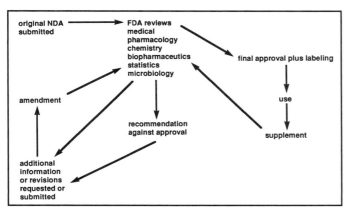

Fig. 59-6. *FDA role in new drug application (NDA) process. (Reprinted with permission from R. A. Nicklas, The investigative process for new drugs. Ann. Allergy 63:598, 1989.)*

Table 59-2. *Study characteristics in evaluation of asthma drugs*

Sample size	Dosage considerations
Age range	Study duration
Patient selection	Inclusion-exclusion criteria
Study blinding	Baseline evaluation
Controls	Efficacy parameters
Parallel versus crossover design	Safety parameters
Center number	

The drug will continue to be evaluated under the fourth recognized period of study for a new drug, postmarketing surveillance, following the approval and marketing of the drug. Adverse effects of the drug that would not have been picked up during previous periods of study because of the infrequency of their occurrence may become apparent during postmarketing surveillance. Therefore, adverse reaction reporting during this period provides additional information on the safety of the drug when analyzed over a longer period of time. Furthermore, additional information may be gathered on patient populations who may not have been adequately studied during premarketing evaluation, such as children and elderly patients.

In summary, there are three phases of clinical study under an investigational new drug application. During phase 1, the initial safety of the drug is demonstrated. By the end of phase 2, the efficacy of the drug will have been determined. Phase 3 is designed to demonstrate the long-term safety and continued efficacy of the drug in studies of longer duration in a large number of patients. Following these phases of study, the drug may be approved for marketing if review of the data generated during these two developmental periods, and subsequently submitted by the sponsor under an NDA, demonstrates the safety and efficacy of the drug. After approval, there will be continuing assessment of the drug through postmarketing surveillance.

The phases of study utilized to demonstrate that a new drug is safe and efficacious are straightforward and clearly defined. The methods that are best used to satisfy these requirements are less clear and more open to interpretation by both sponsors and FDA reviewers. Guidelines for the testing of new drugs are extremely helpful in this regard but will never (and probably never should) take the place of enlightened individual judgement on the part of investigators, sponsors, and FDA reviewers.

Within this general framework, there is great room for flexibility in the design of studies, depending on the type of drug being studied (e.g., bronchodilators or nonbronchodilators), the specific patient population being studied (e.g., pediatric, exercise-induced asthma), and other factors, such as route of administration. It is appropriate, therefore, to look more closely at some of the issues related to appropriate study design for new asthma drugs (Table 59-2).

STUDY DESIGN

Sample Size

While there may be debate over what constitutes an adequate sample size for any phase of study, there is general agreement that the sample size should be large enough to allow for a statistically significant determination on the questions that the study is attempting to answer. This frequently will require input from statisticians prior to initiating the study.

Age Range

Patients over the age of 12 years should in most cases be studied first. Patients between the ages of 6 and 12 years (and certainly younger children) are usually excluded until the safety and efficacy of an asthma drug has been demonstrated in older children and adults and sometimes until preclinical studies have been done to demonstrate the safety of the drug in young animals. Patients less than 6 years of age are generally not studied until efficacy parameters have been adequately defined for 6- to 12-year-old patients and until acute and subacute studies in animals involving the proper route of administration are performed.

Actually, initial clinical studies of asthma medications are usually limited to an evaluation of patients between the ages of 18 and 55 years, approximately. The elderly are sometimes excluded from studies of investigational asthma medications prior to marketing because of the increased potential for cardiovascular effects in this age group, as well as the possibility of drug-drug interaction in a group of patients who are receiving increasingly large numbers of drugs for diseases associated with aging.

Earlier evaluation in children after efficacy has been demonstrated in adults, evaluation of a subset of adolescent asthmatic patients, evaluation of elderly patients, and evaluation of possible differences in response between younger and older patients should be considered in the evaluation of asthma drugs (see Special Considerations).

Patient Selection

The patient population to be studied must be carefully selected on the basis of the study objectives. In some cases, the study population will be reasonably well-defined and homogeneous, such as the study of patients with exercise-induced asthma. In other cases, the study population may represent a heterogeneous accumulation of patients with allergic or nonallergic, mild, moderate, or even steroid-dependent asthma. Studies of patients with perennial asthma may require protocols that are of different length than studies of patients who have strictly seasonal asthma. In addition, the timing of the study must be considered when studying patients who have perennial asthma with seasonal exacerbations.

Patients with severe chronic asthma who may have irreversible lower respiratory changes should obviously not be included in the same study as patients with mild asthma. Controversy still exists, however, over which type of patient is most likely to show improvement after administration of bronchodilators—patients with more severe asthma (FEV_1 40–60% predicted) because there is more room for improvement or patients with milder asthma (FEV_1 60–80% predicted) because they are less likely to have irreversible changes. If the study is designed to evaluate patients with more severe asthma, special consideration must be given to the study design, since these patients will require baseline therapy with bronchodilators and are more likely to require corticosteroid administration during the study. Patients with more severe asthma may best be evaluated, therefore, by recording either their ability to decrease baseline medications while on the study drug or by comparing the use of concomitant medication—number of inhalations of a beta agonist during a 24-hour period, number of steroid bursts required—with the reference control.

If possible, patients should be enrolled only if their asthmatic symptoms are not characterized by wide fluctuations in severity and there is no reason to doubt their compliance. Patients with chronic obstructive pulmonary disease (COPD) should be studied separately.

Study Blinding

Early phase 1 dose-ranging and pharmacokinetic studies may not need to be double-blind, and long-term studies to evaluate safety can be open. Most studies in asthmatic patients, however, especially phase 2 and 3 efficacy studies, must be double-blind, in order to minimize bias when evaluating the efficacy of the drug.

Controls

Phase 2 studies of drugs for the treatment of asthma should include a placebo control, and it is often advisable to include an active-treatment control as well. When nonbronchodilator asthma drugs are being studied, an active-treatment control does not always have to act through the same mechanism as the study drug. For example, an inhaled leukotriene antagonist might be compared with an inhaled corticosteroid, in regard to the long-term efficacy of the study drug. This approach allows the investigator to choose the active-treatment control based on severity of asthma in the patient population to be studied and/or known therapeutic responses in specific subsets of patients. A double-dummy technique should be incorporated into the study design if the patient or physician can visually distinguish one product from the other. A double-dummy technique may be difficult, however, or in some cases impossible, when studying inhaled drugs. In addition, a larger number of inhalations will be required, raising possible concern about the amount of propellant and excipient being delivered to the patient. Therefore, whenever possible, inhaled drugs should be compared to an active-treatment control that utilizes the same delivery system. Innovative approaches to blinding of patients who are comparing two visually different products should be considered.

It is advisable to use controls during each phase of testing for asthma drugs. During phase 1 rising-dose tolerance studies, a placebo control can be utilized, with the placebo randomly placed at different points between rising doses. During phase 2 studies, a placebo or active-treatment control may be appropriate. However, if the response to an active-treatment control is unpredictable, a placebo control should be included. For example, there is such great intrapatient variability in response to inhaled beta agonists (40–60% of patients having a different response to the same product on two separate study days) that a placebo control may be necessary to ensure the validity of the data obtained. During phase 3 studies, both a placebo and active-treatment control should be utilized.

A placebo should be identical to the study drug not only in appearance but also in taste and smell. The composition of the placebo should be identical to the study drug except for the "active" component. Studies of two-component combination products require four arms: (1) study product (drug A + drug B), (2) drug A, (3) drug B, and (4) placebo. For example, the safety and efficacy of a fixed combination of an anticholinergic and a beta-agonist drug must be compared to the same drugs alone, as well as placebo.

Crossover or Parallel Group Study Design

The use of crossover designs has been recommended to decrease the impact of interpatient variability, but substantial intrapatient variability may reduce or obliterate this advantage. Patients may, from one period to the next, have different exposure to the triggers that produce symptoms, increase bronchial inflammation, or increase bronchial hyperreactivity. Because of the substantial potential for intrapatient variability, evaluation of asthma drugs usually does not include crossover studies. In addition, the washout period between treatments must be sufficiently long to prevent any carry-over effect from the first medication administered. Establishment of an adequate washout period is of particular importance in the study of nonbronchodilator asthma drugs because of their prolonged and often variable duration of action. In the evaluation of bronchodilator drugs, an interaction between treatment and period of administration suggestive of a carry-over effect from the active drug has been reported [66]. Therefore, one cannot assume that the treatment effect is the same in both halves of the trial [25] unless there is a sufficiently long washout period between treatments.

Center Number

Independently designed and conducted clinical studies may have distinct advantages during the initial stages of clinical investigation. Multiple independent studies, if well planned, provide opportunities to look at drug response rates and toxicity in a variety of clinical settings, patient populations, and schedules, as well as address specific questions. As a result, valuable information can be obtained about response rates in different subsets of patients, toxicities dependent on age or medical status, and unacceptable adverse reactions. Carefully designed single-center studies by competent investigators should, therefore, be considered in place of multicenter studies in early phases of drug evaluation unless there are strong reasons for not doing so.

The advantages of multicenter studies over multiple independently conducted single-center studies are primarily (1) the accumulation of a sufficient number of patients within a reasonable period of time who can meet the entry criteria for the study and (2) demonstration of the reproducibility of effectiveness and safety by multiple independent investigators utilizing a common protocol under a variety of local conditions. A multicenter study often produces a more representative sampling of the study population than a single-center study in regard to geography, race, socioeconomic status, and life-style.

Dosage Considerations

It is usually possible to determine a safe and effective dose for repetitive-dose studies in patients, based on preclinical data, as well as phase 1 rising-dose tolerance studies in volunteers (or sometimes patients with the clinical condition for which the drug is intended). Such a determination may also require repetitive-dose, rising-dose tolerance studies and should take into account the pharmacokinetics of the drug. The effective dose may also be suggested by the ability of a single dose to inhibit the response to inhalation challenge.

Even then, it may be necessary to study different doses in larger numbers of patients over a longer period of time in randomized, well-controlled double-blind studies to clarify the optimal dose for a particular medication. This may be particularly true for nonbronchodilator asthma drugs, whose effectiveness may not be as readily apparent as that noted after the administration of more rapid-acting bronchodilator drugs.

If the optimal dose is still not apparent when it is otherwise appropriate to initiate phase 3 studies with the drug, protocols for these studies should clearly indicate the specific criteria that will be used for increasing or decreasing the dose, consistent with expected individualization of the dose by practicing physicians.

Study Duration

Traditionally, phase 3 studies of bronchodilator drugs have been of 12 weeks' duration. This has been an empiric determination, based on the need for a study period of sufficient length to demonstrate continuing efficacy, clarify placebo response, determine if tolerance develops, and detect adverse reactions that may not be apparent after shorter periods of drug administration. Because of recent concern about the potential for inhaled beta agonists to produce destabilization of asthma after chronic administration, studies of longer duration may be necessary with this class of drugs in order to evaluate differences in regular or PRN use and/or changes in bronchial hyperresponsiveness. Studies of longer duration than those generally designed for bronchodilator drugs may also be necessary to show effectiveness for drugs that inhibit mediator release or prevent bronchial inflammation. It is clear that a drug may differ in its ability to produce bronchodilation and prevent bronchoconstriction [1, 31]. Studies of different length may, therefore, be necessary to demonstrate one effect or the other.

All studies should have a prestudy baseline period of sufficient duration to (1) determine if patients can be safely entered into the study (see Inclusion-Exclusion Criteria) and (2) identify patients who are likely to be noncompliant.

Following the completion of the study, there should be a follow-up period of sufficient length to determine if there is persistence of abnormal laboratory values or any carry-over effect in terms of efficacy, and ensure that adverse reactions that may have occurred during the study are adequately evaluated. Repeated evaluation of bronchial responsiveness after the completion of the study may provide useful information on the duration of the drug's effect.

Inclusion-Exclusion Criteria

Inclusion-exclusion criteria (Table 59-3) should be defined as specifically as possible prior to initiation of the study and should characterize as clearly as possible the patient population for which the drug is intended. Inclusion and exclusion criteria can be used to effectively eliminate patients with specific medical conditions, patients taking concomitant medication use, or patients whose activities might interfere with interpretation of study results.

Women of Childbearing Potential
Women of childbearing potential should generally be excluded from studies of new drugs until preliminary evidence of the efficacy of the drug has been developed. This allows for an adequate benefit-risk assessment of the use of the drug in this patient population (see Special Considerations).

Children Below the Age of 12 Years
Children who are below the age of 12 years should not generally be studied until the efficacy of the study drug has been demonstrated in patients older than 12 years of age (see Age Range).

Concomitant Disease
Traditionally, patients with clinically significant medical conditions, other than the disease being studied, have been excluded from studies with new drugs for the treatment of asthma to avoid pharmacokinetic/pharmacodynamic alterations that could obscure drug effect and to avoid unexpected adverse events. This

Table 59-3. Generally accepted exclusion criteria in studies of asthma drugs

Women of childbearing potential (until efficacy demonstrated in clinical studies)
Patients less than 12 years of age until efficacy demonstrated in patients older than 12 years
Patients with clinically significant concomitant disease
Patients with clinically significant laboratory values outside the normal reference range
Patients taking concomitant medication that could impact on patient safety or analysis of study results
Patients who have received an investigational drug within 30 days
Heavy smokers
History of alcohol or other drug abuse
History of an upper respiratory infection within 6 weeks
Unavoidable strong allergenic exposure
Patients experiencing an acute exacerbation of asthma
Patients who are grossly overweight or underweight
Patients whose vital signs are outside the normally accepted limits of normal
Patients building up on allergen immunotherapy
Patients with a hypersensitivity to the study drug or any component of the drug product
Patients who have not had a normal chest x-ray within the previous year
Patients who have an abnormal electrocardiogram at baseline
Patients who have been vaccinated with a live attenuated virus within previous 6 weeks
Patients with a history of gastrointestinal surgery or gastrointestinal abnormalities that could interfere with drug absorption (oral tablets, capsules, liquid)

has often excluded patients with clinically significant respiratory (other than asthma), cardiovascular, gastrointestinal, hepatic, renal, endocrine, psychiatric, or neurologic disease. A consequence is that drug-disease interactions are not observed during the development of the drug. There is growing recognition that these exclusions may in the long run be counterproductive and obscure potentially critical information.

Laboratory Values Outside the Normal Reference Range

Protocols for the study of asthma medications will usually include hematology, blood chemistries, and urinalysis as routine assessment of clinical status. Other types of tests may be necessary, however, based on the effect of the study medication (or another drug of the same class) on organ systems or laboratory parameters in preclinical or earlier clinical studies. Since beta agonists, for example, are capable of producing hypokalemia, studies of this class of drugs should ideally include electrolyte determinations (Fig. 59-7).

In most cases, patients with laboratory values outside the normal reference range at baseline are excluded from studies of investigational drugs for the treatment of asthma if they are considered by the investigator to be clinically significant. Clearly, not all laboratory values that are outside the normal reference range are clinically significant or should be the basis for exclusion of patients from the study. Patients can be safely included in studies of asthma drugs with a laboratory value outside the normal reference range if this value is a reflection of the disease being studied, for example a high eosinophil count in a patient with allergic asthma. Patients can also be safely included if the laboratory value when repeated is within the normal reference range (i.e., the initial determination was due to laboratory error). If a laboratory test is repeated and is still outside the normal reference range, it must be determined if the laboratory value is clinically significant, since laboratory values outside the normal

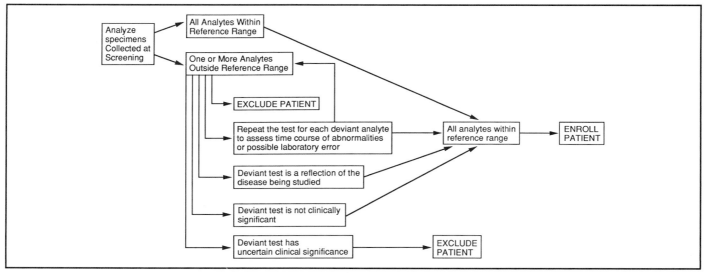

Fig. 59-7. *Approach to evaluation of patients for inclusion in, or exclusion from, studies of asthma drugs.*

reference range can also reflect health (low lipid levels) or the age, activity, or general status of the patient. Increased bilirubin in patients with Gilbert's syndrome and orthostatic proteinuria are examples of laboratory values outside the normal reference range that would not generally exclude patients from studies of asthma drugs.

A specific laboratory value, however, represents only one point in time. Therefore, physicians must often use their knowledge of the patient to interpret the clinical significance of laboratory values that are outside the normal reference range. The investigator should recognize that fasting conditions (low blood sugar), recent exercise (increase in serum glutamic-oxidase transaminase [SGOT]), and periods of rapid growth (increased alkaline phosphatase and phosphorous) can produce variations from normal that are not associated with clinical disease.

Concomitant Medication

The inclusion of patients who are regular users of any prescription or nonprescription drug may increase confusion about study results or decrease patient safety. Medications that are most likely to confound study results or put the asthmatic patient at increased risk are (1) aspirin and other nonsteroidal antiinflammatory drugs [57], (2) beta-adrenergic blocking agents [18], (3) monoamine oxidase inhibitors, (4) tricyclic antidepressants [48], and (5) non-potassium-sparing diuretics [26].

Patients who are receiving asthma medication should be excluded unless they can be stabilized on a consistent regimen for at least 2 weeks prior to initiation of the study. Inclusion or exclusion of patients requiring regular use of corticosteroids may depend on the patient population being studied and the objectives of the study. If patients are included who are receiving continuing therapy with orally inhaled, nasally inhaled, or oral corticosteroids, the daily dose should be carefully noted, and any change in dose should be carefully recorded and analyzed. In studies of non-steroid-dependent patients, it is acceptable to permit a small number of short courses of oral corticosteroids to control symptoms and allow patient continuance in the study, as long as it is specifically indicated prior to the study how these patients will be handled in the analysis of the study results.

If it is necessary to discontinue theophylline prior to inclusion of the patient in the study, the serum theophylline level should be below the therapeutic range and generally less than 3 μg/ml.

Patients who are unable to discontinue use of antihistamines

Table 59-4. *Suggested time period for discontinuing concomitant medications prior to study days*

Medication	Discontinuance time prior to testing
Oral beta agonists	24 hours
Inhaled beta agonists	8 hours
Short-acting theophylline*	24 hours
BID theophylline	48 hours
Once-daily theophylline	72 hours
Inhaled disodium cromoglycate	At least 1 week
Corticosteroids	At least 1 month
Hydroxyzine, terfenadine	96 hours
Astemizole	At least 3 months
Other antihistamines	48 hours

* Caffeine-containing products should not be ingested for 12 hours prior to testing.

should either be excluded from studies or carefully considered in analyses of the study results. Recently approved nonsedating antihistamines can produce bronchodilatation or prevent bronchoconstriction in some patients, making it difficult to determine effectiveness of the study drug [1a, 4a, 48a]. Astemizole is of particular concern, since it can suppress not only dermatologic but also respiratory response to allergen for several months [38]. It is obviously important, therefore, to withhold medications that could confound study results for an appropriate period of time prior to the study. This period is unique for each class of drugs and even for specific drugs within a class. In this regard, Table 59-4 indicates the frequently used periods of abstinence for medications likely to be used by asthmatic patients. Furthermore, patients who have received any investigational drug in the 30 days prior to entering the study should be excluded.

In later phases of drug evaluation, it is desirable to study elderly patients (see Special Considerations). Asthma is not rare in elderly patients. Therefore, substantial use of new drugs for the treatment of asthma can be expected in this patient population, a subset of patients who frequently are receiving medications for hypertension as well as cardiac, renal, or neurologic conditions. Elderly patients may, therefore, be at increased risk from the administration of certain classes of drugs, such as beta-adrenergic agonist bronchodilators. Hypokalemia can be produced by beta agonists, even when given by the inhaled route [17], and augmented by the concomitant administration of theophylline

[65]. This may have special relevance for the elderly asthmatic patient who is receiving diuretics that are not potassium sparing. However, multiple drug regimens in this group of patients is often unavoidable and can provide the opportunity to gather valuable information about drug interactions prior to marketing of the medication.

Patient Habits

Patients who are current smokers or have smoked heavily in the past should be excluded from the study of new drugs for the treatment of asthma. They are more likely to have developed irreversible changes consistent with COPD and are therefore inappropriate for the study of drugs proposed for the treatment of reversible obstructive airway disease.

Patients who have a history of alcohol or other drug abuse should be excluded, since use of these products during the study could (1) interfere with assessment of efficacy, (2) increase the possibility that the patient will not complete the study or in general be noncompliant, or (3) increase the risk for the patient. Urine screening at baseline for drug abuse should include tests for cocaine, opiates, and cannabinoids. Any patient who is not likely to be compliant or who will be a source of confusing data should be excluded.

Other Considerations

Any patient who has had an upper respiratory infection within 6 weeks of entrance into the study should be excluded. Increased bronchial hyperresponsiveness has been demonstrated for up to 6 weeks after an upper respiratory infection [24]. If allergen exposure cannot be stabilized or eliminated as a source of increased symptomatology, it may also influence study results. It has been demonstrated that increased allergen load in the lower respiratory tract may change subsequent patient response to allergen exposure [34]. In fact, any patient who is experiencing an acute exacerbation of asthma or has any acute illness should be excluded, at least until the acute episode and changes associated with it have subsided. Patients who are grossly overweight or underweight should be excluded. Measurement of height and weight is of particular importance when corticosteroid medications are being studied in children and adolescents.

Patients with baseline vital signs outside the normal reference range, often considered to be a blood pressure greater than 140/90 mmHg or less than 90/50 mmHg or a pulse rate greater than 100 beats/min or less than 50 beats/min for adults, should generally be excluded for their safety and for easier interpretation of changes that occur during the study.

Patients who are receiving allergen immunotherapy may be included in studies of new drugs for the treatment of asthma, provided they remain at a constant dose throughout the study.

Patients should not be included unless they have had a normal chest x-ray within the past 6 months or unless the study objectives allow for inclusion of patients with abnormal chest x-rays.

Patients with a history of hypersensitivity to the study drug, to any drug with a similar chemical structure, or to any component of the drug product should be excluded.

Baseline Evaluation

Asthma is a capricious disease, characterized by diverse etiologies and clinical patterns with unpredictable remissions and exacerbations. Therefore, in studies of asthma medications, the characteristics of the patient population must be carefully analyzed to select a patient population that will best answer the questions posed by the study. The relationship of symptoms to aeroallergen exposure should be ascertained and, where appropriate, supported by allergen skin tests.

Baseline pulmonary function testing should be performed and should include at least spirometric measurements of one-second forced expiratory volume (FEV_1), mid-maximal expiratory flow (MMEF), peak expiratory flow rate (PEFR), and forced vital capacity (FVC). To confirm the diagnosis of asthma, and thereby the patient's potential responsiveness to the study drug, reversibility (defined as a 15% improvement in FEV_1) should be demonstrated after the inhalation of a beta-adrenergic agonist bronchodilator. In studies of inhaled bronchodilators, it may be preferable to use a different drug product to demonstrate reversibility than the one that will be evaluated in the study. This will lessen any appearance of bias based on the selection of a patient population that has already responded to the study drug. This is not essential, however, since there may be substantial day-to-day variation in patient response to the same inhaled product.

Patients should have a complete history and physical examination performed at screening, and the forms that will be used to document this evaluation should be included in the protocol submitted by the sponsor.

At screening, a 12-lead electrocardiogram (ECG) should be performed on each patient, and the patient should not be entered into the study unless the ECG is considered normal for the patient population being studied or unless the study objectives allow for inclusion of patients with abnormal ECGs.

Baseline evaluation of patients can be best accomplished if the patient is known to the investigator. It is essential to exclude patients whose ability to comply with the study protocol is questionable. The baseline evaluation period must be of sufficient length that it is possible to reliably assess the patient's symptom pattern and severity.

To ensure a homogeneous patient population, demonstration of bronchial hyperresponsiveness (methacholine challenge) may be necessary in patients with mild asthma. Dependent on the study objectives, other procedures may be necessary to establish a study population that will best answer the questions that the study proposes to answer. Such procedures may include, but are not necessarily limited to, visualization of the sinuses, allergen inhalation challenge, and bronchoalveolar lavage.

When inhaled asthma medications are being evaluated, patients must be carefully instructed in proper inhalation technique and must demonstrate to the investigator their ability to use the product properly.

Efficacy Parameters

Symptom Evaluation

Patient evaluation of symptoms must be performed with a frequency that will ensure that recall of symptoms is adequate for the purposes of the study. If more frequent evaluation of symptoms will lead to more accurate assessment, patients should evaluate symptoms several times during daytime hours. However, most patients do not have the time or motivation to follow such a schedule. It can be argued, moreover, that overall assessment at the end of the day provides more useful information than assessments of shorter duration that may capture only a small isolated segment of the patient's symptoms. It is reasonable for patients to evaluate symptoms twice daily, in the morning upon arising and at night before going to bed. Such an approach can provide meaningful data and better maintain patient compliance. Nighttime symptoms and patterns of sleep should be recorded by the patient when arising in the morning. Quality of sleep, including nighttime awakenings, is an important indicator of the severity of the patient's symptoms and the patient's response to medication.

It is essential, especially in studies of longer duration, that patient compliance with symptom scoring be maintained. Compliance with medication usage has been assessed with reasonable success by pill counting, weighing of canisters (metered-dose inhalers), and specific devices [56]. Unfortunately, no such methods exist for measuring compliance with symptom scoring systems. Careful selection of patients for study becomes, therefore, of great importance in establishing a study group that is most likely to comply with the requirements of the study, including consistent and reliable symptom scoring.

It is difficult to standardize symptom scoring because patients perceive and react to symptoms differently. Inconsistent description of symptoms by patients is a defect inherent in symptom scoring. Prior to the study, therefore, it is essential to establish detailed and clearly understood symptom descriptions, These should be reproducible in the same patient as well as different patients, since intrapatient differences in reporting can be as important to avoid as interpatient differences. Many asthmatic patients are, justifiably, more concerned about nocturnal symptoms. Therefore, the same degree of nocturnal and daytime symptoms may be scored differently by patients. Care in setting up symptom scoring systems should lessen this potential difference in reporting.

Although it is generally felt that patients define their symptoms better than someone else (e.g., investigator, investigator's co-workers, parents), accuracy of symptom reporting can vary tremendously from patient to patient. Generally, children are not good at reporting symptoms because they have poor perception of their symptoms. Therefore, if possible, symptom evaluation in children should not be a primary efficacy parameter. On the other hand, parent evaluation of children may be incomplete, dependent on what the child tells them, and even reflect unfactual and biased reporting and therefore may be less reliable than the child's own evaluation. If the child is reporting to the investigator through an adult, definition of symptoms should maximize the possibility that the adult and the child are describing the same event.

Differences in symptom description by different socioeconomic groups must also be considered when establishing a definition of symptoms.

Although often perceived differently, the four classic symptoms of asthma—cough, wheezing, tightness in the chest, and shortness of breath—generally can be understood and described by patients. On the other hand, symptoms such as fatigue and irritability, although not uncommon in patients with asthma, are more subjective and are less easily quantitated.

Duration of symptoms is an important indicator of symptom severity. Methods for quantitating duration of symptoms depend on patient perception and recall. Therefore, if establishment of symptom duration proves difficult when patients are evaluating symptoms twice daily, consideration should be given to breaking down each 24-hour period into shorter periods. Such periods might include selected periods at work or school. Severity of symptoms can also be assessed by evaluating the patients' ability to function in their environment. Inability to function can be characterized by decreased attendance or productivity at work or school, ability to climb steps, interference with sleep, restriction of activities, or other limitations.

Classifying symptom severity as mild, moderate, or severe is indistinct and should be replaced, if possible, by a less nebulous definition. This should be as analytically reproducible as possible, given differences in patient perception of symptoms and the approach they choose to take in regard to these symptoms. In this regard, "mild" wheezing may motivate one patient to stay home, while another patient with "severe" symptoms may choose to go to work. In an attempt to quantify restrictions on activity, an activity scale can be developed and included in patient analysis. Emergency room and physician office visits may also reflect patient perception of symptoms and the way they choose to handle such symptoms. Hospitalization, intubation, mechanical ventilation, and courses of oral corticosteroids more accurately reflect the severity of the patient's condition but are infrequently noted in most studies of asthma medications. In

studies of longer duration (at least 3 months), quality of life measurements may provide additional information on the severity of the patient's asthma.

Symptom Scoring

The number of categories that should be used for symptom scoring is controversial. Those who feel that too many categories may confuse the patient and lead to a decrease in compliance endorse a maximum of four to five categories recorded twice a day, at least for longer studies where symptom recording may become more of a burden. Others argue quite correctly that too few choices can be as undesirable as too many choices.

Regardless of the number of categories, choices within each category must be defined sharply. This allows as clear a determination as possible between one choice and another.

Clearly, the use of medication to relieve symptoms during the study can have a significant effect on symptom scoring. Most studies provide, at least, for the use of rescue medications to control symptoms and allow patients to continue in the study. Therefore, the patient's symptom diary must clearly document the temporal relationship between medication use and the time of symptom recording. This will make it possible to analyze separately similar symptom scores in patients who have and have not taken concomitant medications. The effect of concomitant medication on symptom scoring is particularly difficult to determine if patients are allowed to take oral corticosteroids during the study (see Concomitant Medications).

Recording of Asthma "Attacks"

The definition of an "attack" of asthma is extremely inconsistent. Therefore, if patients are asked to record asthma attacks during the study, it is essential that an objective measurement, such as pulmonary function, be included in the definition of such an episode. This should ensure that the patient's perception of symptoms correlates with the physiologic response.

In conclusion, symptom scoring, as presently performed, is neither an exact nor an ideal method for evaluating the effectiveness of new medications for the treatment of asthma. This may be due to (1) inaccurate scoring of symptoms, (2) lack of reproducibility, (3) lack of precision in describing symptoms, or (4) lack of correlation with objective measurements. Utilization of a reliable symptom scoring system is essential if this approach is to be considered as anything other than a secondary measure of efficacy.

Bronchoprovocation

Certain classes of asthma drugs can be assessed by their ability to block the respiratory response occurring after inhalation challenge with pharmacologic bronchoconstrictors. Exercise challenge, while relatively easy to perform, is difficult to grade in a dose-response manner. Therefore, it is better suited for demonstrating the ability of a medication to inhibit exercise-induced bronchospasm than for determining an appropriate dose of medication for further study (see Chap. 47). Challenge with pharmacologic bronchoconstrictors, on the other hand, can easily be quantitated but may be less representative of naturally occurring asthma. Such challenge may therefore be most effectively used early in the study of new asthma drugs to establish an effective dose for further study. This should, in most cases, be based on the ability of the drug to inhibit bronchoconstriction produced by pharmacologic challenge appropriate for the class of drug. Thus, platelet-activating factor (PAF) antagonists, anticholinergic bronchodilators, and antihistamines with lower respiratory effects can be evaluated on the basis of their ability to inhibit or modify patient response to PAF, methacholine, or histamine challenge, respectively.

The ability of a medication to inhibit or modify allergen challenge may provide the most clinically relevant information. This may be particularly relevant in the study of antiinflammatory medications, since many asthmatic patients experience late-phase reactions after allergen challenge, reactions felt to reflect airway inflammation and increased bronchial hyperresponsiveness. In addition, challenges with increasing allergen concentrations may help to define the appropriate dose for further study.

In crossover studies or studies utilizing repetitive challenge, there must be an adequate interval between challenges to negate any effect from the previous challenge. With exercise challenge specifically, there may be a refractory period after challenge that could lead to incorrect assessment of the challenge results. Studies using inhalation challenge should be double-blind and placebo-controlled, and the study population must be carefully selected. As a general rule, patients should not be challenged if (1) they have clinically apparent bronchoconstriction, (2) their FEV_1 is 1 liter or less, (3) the baseline FEV_1 is less than 70 percent of predicted normal, or (4) the investigator judges that it is unsafe to perform such a challenge.

Medication that might influence the results of challenge procedures should be discontinued an appropriate time prior to the study procedure (see Table 59-4). Ideally, patients on whom challenge tests are being performed should be nonsmokers. Caffeine-containing foods and beverages should be withheld for at least 12 hours prior to the challenge procedure. Challenge procedures should not be performed in a setting that is likely to influence the test results adversely, that is, a recent viral infection, a recent vaccination, or the presence of airborne irritants or aeroallergens. Ideally, challenge procedures should be done at the same time of day, usually in the early morning.

Challenge solutions should be prepared in buffered isotonic saline, since nonisotonic solutions may produce bronchoconstriction. Methacholine and histamine challenge can also produce irritation of the throat and cough. Therefore, care must be taken to separate adverse effects due to inhaled investigational drugs from adverse effects due to the challenge solution.

Bronchoprovocation should be viewed as desirable but not essential, at the present time. Challenge procedures can provide useful information when performed not only after single doses but after repetitive dosing as well. It should be remembered that steady-state blood or tissue levels may be necessary to maximally block inhalation challenge.

Pulmonary Function Testing

Before measuring pulmonary function, equipment, testing procedures, and interpretation of results must be standardized. Patient effort must be maximized, and appropriate reference standards must be used.

FEV_1 is generally considered the most reproducible spirometric measurement. It incorporates the early effort-dependent portion of the flow-volume curve as well as enough midflow effort-independent determination to maintain its sensitivity. It may not, however, be a sensitive parameter for mild airflow obstruction. FVC, PEFR, and measurement of mid-flows (FEF_{25-75}, MMEF) are other frequently utilized spirometric measurements. In addition, valuable information can be derived from patient measurements of PEFR. Patients trained in the use of peak flowmeters will usually measure PEFR in the morning and evening, but PEFR can be measured at times when the patient notes an increase in symptoms as well. PEFR, however, does not measure small airway function and is very effort dependent.

The best of three acceptable determinations of the above tests should be utilized. Use of a greater number of determinations may produce incorrect readings due to muscle fatigue or effort-induced bronchospasm. Unacceptable variability with poor reproducibility may occur when bronchospasm occurs because of

the FVC maneuver or in patients with significant airway obstruction. Sitting or standing positions are acceptable as long as all testing is done in the same position. Pulmonary function testing usually should be performed at approximately the same time of day, because of diurnal variation. Ideally, studies should be performed in the morning and by the same technician and machinery. The largest FVC and second-largest FVC should not vary by more than 5 percent or 100 cc. The largest FVC and FEV_1 values, even if they come from two different but acceptable determinations, should be utilized.

Bronchodilator response has generally been considered to be a 15, 12, and 25 percent or greater increase over baseline for FEV_1, FVC, and FEF_{25-75}, respectively. With repetitive administration of an asthma medication, baseline pulmonary function may rise throughout the study. For example, the onstudy FEV_1 prior to drug administration 12 weeks after initiation of the study may be significantly higher than the prestudy baseline FEV_1. Analysis of pulmonary function data must take into consideration this response to the medication. This response is commonly seen in studies of asthma drugs and can lead to underestimation of efficacy. Pulmonary function testing should be performed prior to the onset of the study and throughout the study at appropriate time intervals. In repetitive dose studies of 12 weeks' duration, generally used for the evaluation of inhaled beta agonists, measurements are usually made on day 1 and after 30, 60, and 90 days of treatment with the study drug. On each study day, measurements are usually made 5, 15, 30, 60, 90, 120, 180, 240, 300, and 360 minutes after drug administration, although evaluation can be continued for 8 to 12 hours. Measurements should include onset of action, time to peak effect, peak effect, duration of effect, and area under the time-response curve. Onset of action beyond 30 minutes after administration of an inhaled beta agonist should generally be considered unrelated to the study drug. The duration of response should be considered the interval between onset of action and termination of response, often defined as that time point following drug administration when FEV_1 falls below 15 percent above baseline FEV_1 for two consecutive measurements (Fig. 59-8). It is crucial to evaluate not only mean values, but individual patient data as well. Differences in response to two products noted on evaluation of individual patient data may have special relevance for the practicing physician in the management of specific patients.

Fig. 59-8. *Suggested approach to analysis of individual patient response to inhaled bronchodilators.*

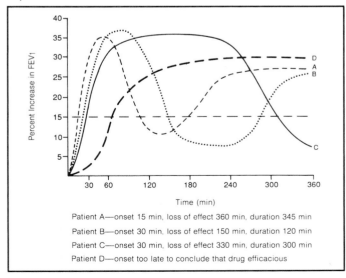

Patient A—onset 15 min, loss of effect 360 min, duration 345 min
Patient B—onset 30 min, loss of effect 150 min, duration 120 min
Patient C—onset 30 min, loss of effect 330 min, duration 300 min
Patient D—onset too late to conclude that drug efficacious

Safety Parameters

Monitoring of Adverse Events

An adverse event can be defined as any expected or unexpected event that occurs during the course of study of an investigational drug, even if related to abuse, overdosage, withdrawal, drug-drug interaction, or failure of the expected pharmacologic effect of the medication under study. Concomitant illness or trauma during the period of investigational drug administration should be considered study drug related until proved otherwise by comparison of the frequency of such events in different treatment groups.

Monitoring adverse events helps to determine (1) the benefit-risk profile of the study drug, (2) the safety of the patient's continued participation in the study, and (3) the appropriate dose or formulation for future studies. In addition, such monitoring provides product information for labeling, which in conjunction with postmarketing surveillance will aid the practicing physician in appropriate clinical use of the drug product.

Separate analyses of total adverse events and those events determined by the investigator to be drug related are necessary to establish that there is no biased assessment of causality. Assessment of causality could conclude that the event is (1) definitely not related to the study drug, (2) probably not related to the study drug, (3) possibly related to the study drug (probability less than 50%), (4) probably related to the study drug (probability greater than 50%), or (5) definitely related to the study drug (positive rechallenge, characteristic clinical or laboratory findings).

To aid in assessment of adverse events, a complete history and physical examination should be performed at least prior to the study and at its conclusion. Under certain conditions, patient evaluation may be required throughout the study.

It is possible to anticipate the development of certain types of adverse events based on knowledge about the class of drugs being studied or the effect of a specific drug in preclinical or previous clinical studies. It is impossible to rule out, however, the appearance in repetitive dose studies of unexpected adverse events that may not have been observed in earlier animal studies or in clinical studies because of (1) study of small numbers of patients for a short duration, (2) utilization of single doses, or (3) subtlety of the adverse experience.

Adverse events should be documented and characterized in regard to (1) date of onset, (2) date of cessation, (3) duration (minutes, hours, days; average duration for intermittent experience; single or continuous experience), (4) severity, (5) clinical significance, and (6) whether information about the event is volunteered or solicited. In addition, it is important to note not just how long after starting the medication the adverse event occurred, but also *how long after drug administration* the adverse event occurred. For example, patients receiving inhaled drugs for treatment of asthma can develop sudden potentially life-threatening bronchospasm. Unless the exact time between drug administration and the adverse event is recorded, it will often be unclear whether asthmatic symptoms are due to the medication or the patient's underlying disease. Severity can be characterized as mild (awareness of event but easily tolerated), moderate (interferes with usual activity), or severe (incapacitating, inability to work or perform usual activity). Changes in severity should be listed as the cessation of an adverse event of a certain severity and the onset of the same event at a different severity.

Clinically significant adverse events include, but are not limited to those (1) related to fatalities, (2) causing discontinuation of the patient from the study, or (3) requiring hospitalization or emergency treatment. The significance of an adverse event may also relate to the organ system involved, whether the event is reversible or irreversible, whether it is disabling, or whether it shortens the patient's life expectancy. Insignificant events are less likely to pose a threat to the patient's health, interfere with the patient's normal life-style, or decrease life expectancy. Significant adverse events warrant further evaluation and follow-up, especially those adverse events that result in patient dropouts or fatalities.

Consideration of Specific Adverse Events

Tremor. Although not life-threatening, tremor is seen frequently in the study of relatively beta2 selective agonists, particularly when administered by the oral route, and can significantly interfere with the patient's ability to function. Tremor is usually obvious to the patient and physician but can also be quantitated, especially when less obvious, by utilization of various devices. Since patients are only able to perceive a twofold or greater change in tremor, there may be a need for objective measurement of this adverse event. At least one study using such objective measurements might be considered in the evaluation of new beta2 selective agonists prior to marketing.

Cardiovascular Events. It is well recognized that beta agonists may, in some patients, produce severe, sometimes life-threatening cardiovascular effects. Even "relatively beta2 selective" agonists have been associated with significant hypokalemia [60], significant changes in blood pressure or pulse rate [54], cardiac arrhythmias [29], ST–T wave changes [16], prolongation of the QT_c interval [15], significant hemodynamic changes [12], and even myocarditis [44].

Methylxanthines can produce a direct cardiac effect through (1) positive inotropic and chronotropic action, (2) arrhythmogenic qualities, or (3) their ability to increase coronary artery flow. Indirectly, theophylline can produce an effect on the heart through its ability to decrease peripheral resistance, pulmonary artery pressure, and cerebral blood flow, as well as elevate or lower blood pressure. Therefore, studies of beta agonists or methylxanthines require careful evaluation of cardiovascular status before, during, and after the study. In many cases, this will require the use of continuous cardiovascular monitoring (see Electrocardiographic Monitoring).

Respiratory Events. Inhaled medications used in the treatment of asthma have the potential to produce paradoxical bronchospasm [43]. Exacerbations of asthma, which can be life-threatening, have been reported after use of inhaled beta agonists [68] (both metered-dose inhalers and solutions for nebulization), corticosteroids [52], ipratropium [3], and disodium cromoglycate [36]. Paradoxical bronchospasm has also been reported after the administration of investigational inhaled mediator antagonists. This type of adverse event must be considered in all studies of asthma medications, especially those that include the administration of inhaled drugs. Product formulations that may be more likely to produce this type of adverse effect should be identified as early as possible to allow sufficient time for reformulation by the sponsor.

Since 50 percent of adverse-reaction reports consistent with paradoxical bronchospasm occur with the first use of a new canister or bottle in patients who have experienced no previous reaction, materials (chemicals) coming in contact with the drug product have been suspected. Such chemicals might leak out of the packaging, produce adverse reactions, interfere with assay procedures, cause hemolysis, or absorb to the study drug.

Laboratory Data

Laboratory tests are an important objective assessment of adverse effect of the study drug on major organ systems and should at least be performed in all patients prior to and at the conclusion of the study. In special situations, laboratory tests may be necessary at selected times during the study as well. They should be drawn in a fasting state, especially if it is possible that the drug has a significant effect on glucose or lipid metabolism. Any laboratory studies that represent a clinically significant deviation from baseline should be repeated as soon as possible and repeated for as long as necessary (even after the study medication is discontinued) to ensure the safety of the patient and the most accurate analysis of the study results. The investigator should not be asked to determine the clinical significance of a laboratory test without knowledge of preclinical and previous clinical data with the study drug.

Different clinical laboratories may be utilized by investigators in multicenter studies. In such cases, attempts should be made to establish reference ranges that have the same standard deviation. It is also important that clinical laboratories not change procedures, standards, or technology after baseline values have been obtained.

Often, newly approved asthma medications will be administered to patients who are already receiving other medications for asthma. In studies of such drugs prior to approval it is important, therefore, to determine if, in regard to laboratory parameters, there is any drug-drug interaction with already available medications. In addition, laboratory tests should be included that can measure activity of concomitant disease while on the study drug. For example, uric acid levels should be followed carefully during the study of asthmatic patients who have gout.

The frequency of laboratory determinations during the study will depend on the type of study, the type of laboratory parameters obtained, and the preclinical and clinical profile of the asthma medication that is being studied. The rapidity with which laboratory values might be expected to change under the influence of the study medication should be considered as well. Laboratory parameters that have been demonstrated in previous studies to be affected by the study medication should be obtained during the study at those times when the peak effect of the drug could be anticipated.

The temporal relationship of the laboratory test to administration of the study drug should be clearly documented in writing, as should the relationship to food ingestion. This may be of particular importance in the study of methylxanthines, where the effect of food on theophylline absorption has obvious clinical relevance.

Electrocardiographic Monitoring

Asthma medications, in particular beta agonists, can have an adverse effect on the cardiovascular system (see Cardiovascular Events). Beta-adrenergic agonists acting through both beta$_1$ and beta$_2$ receptors in the heart and beta$_2$ receptors in the peripheral vasculature can produce clinically significant hemodynamic effects with little, if any, change in blood pressure or heart rate. Based on animal studies, there has also been concern that concomitant administration of beta agonists and methylxanthines could potentiate such cardiac effects [64].

Although 15-second rhythm strips may be helpful in assessing arrhythmogenic potential of the study drug, they are not sufficient to pick up localized ST–T wave changes of myocardial ischemia. On the other hand, 12-lead ECGs of relatively short duration may fail to demonstrate cardiac arrhythmias that could be recognized on continuous ECG (Holter) monitoring.

Continuous ECG monitoring for 24 to 48 hours should therefore be considered at some point after repetitive dosing with any bronchodilator. Whatever type of ECG monitoring is utilized, it should be timed to measure cardiovascular response to the study medication at the time of maximum effect. In addition, 12-lead ECGs should be obtained at times when patients or investigators note any significant cardiovascular symptoms or signs.

Because asthma medication may produce adverse cardiovascular effects and many protocols allow for the use of concomitant asthma medications, ECG monitoring must be done for comparison purposes on all patients in a study, not just those patients who are receiving the study drug. ECG monitoring is particularly important in elderly patients, who are at increased risk of developing cardiovascular complications from administration of asthma drugs. Patients who are experiencing an acute asthmatic attack should also be monitored closely for adverse cardiovascular effects. Such patients may be hypoxic, may be receiving other medications that have the potential to produce or augment adverse cardiovascular effects, and may have electrolyte changes that could predispose them to the development of cardiac arrhythmias.

Vital Signs

Heart rate, respiratory rate, and blood pressure are usually determined prior to the study (at screening and baseline), during the study on evaluation days with repetitive dosing, and at the conclusion of the study. On evaluation days (typically after the first dose of the drug and after 30, 60, and 90 days of drug administration when studying bronchodilators) these measurements are taken at frequent intervals, usually in connection with pulmonary function testing (see Pulmonary Function Testing). The results obtained must be interpreted in relationship to patient age and activity, the severity of the patient's asthma, patient position (sitting, recumbent, standing—especially when studying medications that have the potential to produce orthostatic hypotension), and any other relevant factors. To minimize variability, vital signs should, if possible, be determined by the same person, utilizing the same technique and the same instrument.

Pulmonary Function Testing

Although the frequency of paradoxical bronchospasm after use of inhaled drugs is apparently very low, it has been noted after the administration of inhaled investigational drugs. Lack of improvement in pulmonary function in an asthmatic patient after the administration of an inhaled bronchodilator should be considered paradoxical bronchospasm until proved otherwise.

Decrease in efficacy (tolerance) occurring over time in some patients with the continued administration of beta agonists is a recognized phenomena. The development of tolerance changes the benefit-risk assessment of a drug product. Pulmonary function testing provides an objective base for determining the degree to which tolerance occurs with an investigational drug compared to marketed products of the same class. Accurate assessment of tolerance requires a sufficient washout for other drugs of the same class prior to the onset of the study and adequate washout between treatment regimens in a crossover study. Studies of beta agonists should be of at least 3 months' duration, since loss of efficacy may not be evident in studies of shorter duration. There should be sufficient evaluation points throughout the study to note whether decreased efficacy over time follows a linear pattern.

Serum Levels

Serum levels of new asthma medications are routinely measured during phase 1 rising-dose pharmacokinetic studies. If technology is available and practical, the assessment of new drugs for the treatment of asthma should be based on a correlation between serum levels of the drug and clinical effect. It is important to define the pharmacodynamics of new drugs for the treatment of asthma under variable conditions, such as concomitant administration of other medications or food ingestion.

Special Considerations

Women of Childbearing Potential

Women of childbearing potential are usually not included in phase 1 or 2 studies of investigational asthma medication because of uncertainty about teratogenic effects. This potential produces an unacceptable benefit-risk assessment until the efficacy of the drug has been established. Once the efficacy of a medication has been established, and if there are no teratogenicity concerns based on preclinical studies, women of childbearing potential can be reasonably studied. There is little reason to believe that asthma medications produce a different response in men and women of generally the same age. Therefore, there should be no urgency to study this type of medication in women of childbearing potential until an acceptable benefit-risk ratio has been established.

When women of childbearing potential are studied, pregnancy tests should be performed prior to inclusion in the study. It should be remembered that safe use of an investigational drug in women of childbearing potential does not ensure safe use of the drug in pregnant women. Therefore, women who become pregnant while receiving an investigational drug should be followed through pregnancy and after delivery for a time sufficient to determine if there has been any effect of the medication on the fetus.

Children

The pharmacokinetics of investigational drugs may be different depending on the age and developmental status of the patient. As a result, studies in patients who are less than 12 years of age are generally performed prior to approving the use of a new drug for that patient population. The American Academy of Pediatrics has recognized four stages of development, which need to be considered separately in the evaluation of any new drug [23]: (1) adolescence, (2) childhood (which can be divided into two age ranges: 2–6 years and 6 years to adolescence), (3) infant/toddler (6 weeks to 2 years), and (4) neonatal period (birth to 6 weeks of age). Since asthma rarely occurs in neonates, evaluation of asthma medications in this age group is, under most circumstances, unnecessary.

Adolescence

The complex physiologic and psychologic changes during adolescence and their effect on the efficacy and safety of a drug product need to be considered in the evaluation of asthma drugs. Pharmacokinetics in the adolescent may be modified by endocrine and other biochemical changes. Compliance may also be a problem in this group of patients. Other factors to consider in this subset of patients are (1) the possible abuse of the study drug, (2) the potential for production of psychological and behavioral alterations at an unstable time in the patient's life, (3) the effect on growth (especially with the study of corticosteroids) in puberty, (4) the effect of the study drug on the fetus in the presence of an unknown or hidden early pregnancy, and (5) the potential for asthma to go into natural remission.

Childhood (2 years to adolescence)

The study design must be specialized for pediatric studies. For ethical and medical reasons, investigators or institutional review boards (IRBs) may prefer not to use a placebo control in studies of investigational drugs in children, especially studies of longer duration. If a placebo arm is utilized, baseline medication may be required for control of symptoms. In that case, efficacy determinations may rest on (1) the patient's ability to decrease baseline medication without exacerbation of symptoms or (2) the amount of rescue medication required.

Pharmacokinetic and pharmacodynamic data in adults cannot be predictably extrapolated to children. Therefore, before an investigational drug is administered to large numbers of children, a pediatric dose-ranging pharmacokinetic study should be considered. The effect of the investigational drug on the pharmacoki-

netics of other medications that might be administered concomitantly for the treatment of asthma will also need to be considered.

Pediatric populations need to be assessed differently than adults. For example, patient diaries should include a record of school absences and should be supervised carefully by an informed adult. Particular attention must be paid to regular measurements of height and weight, especially in patients who are receiving investigational corticosteroid preparations.

There has been recent concern about the possible effect of theophylline on school performance in children [22, 42]; however, this has recently been countered [70]. In addition, beta-adrenergic agonists, especially if administered by the oral route, may produce significant tremor, which could interfere with coordination and complicate tasks requiring fine motor movements (see Tremor). Central nervous system adverse effects can include changes in mood, personality, and level of activity, which could interfere with the child's ability to function in school. Therefore, studies of investigational drugs for the treatment of asthma should include an analysis of the child's school performance. This should be done in cooperation with the patient's teacher, utilizing psychological testing appropriate for each patient.

Loss of time from school to fulfill study obligations can be a significant deterrent to study participation or continuation in the study. Therefore, pediatric protocols should be structured to allow as much flexibility as possible and interfere as little as possible with school activities.

Objective measurements will be more difficult to obtain in children who are 2 to 5 years of age. Tests for bronchial hyperresponsiveness, for example, may be difficult or impossible. As a result, studies of this age group cannot generally be built around objective parameters.

It is more difficult to make medications palatable for children than for adults. This factor must be considered in a determination of the appropriate formulation for children. Failure to do so may lead to significantly decreased compliance.

Children may have more difficulty mastering the technique for delivery of aerosolized products. Careful instruction and demonstration of these techniques for both patients and parents are essential to ensure effective delivery of the medication to the younger patient. In general, administration of drug by nebulizer is more reliable in children than administration by metered-dose inhaler, which may be more difficult for the child to coordinate.

Bioavailability and response to drugs administered orally may be influenced by the immaturity of the gastrointestinal tract in infants. Gastric motility comparable to that seen in adults is not achieved until 3 years of age. During this time, gastrointestinal motility is irregular and unpredictable. Certain formulations, such as slow-release products, may be significantly affected by intestinal motility and transit time. Hydrolysis of drug conjugates excreted in the bile may be influenced by the microflora of the infant gastrointestinal tract, which can differ depending on whether the child is breast- or bottle-fed. In addition, gastric emptying is slower during the first months of life. Finally, infants are susceptible to gastroenteritis, which can affect drug absorption.

Prolonged half-lives for some drugs can be expected to occur in infants due to decreased renal clearance. In addition, hepatic clearance of drugs may be increased during early childhood and should be identified for each drug product.

Interpretation of response to investigational drugs must be based on the knowledge that the infant and young child have smaller airway size, deficiency of elastic tissue predisposing to airway closure during tidal ventilation with resultant hypoxemia, inadequate development of alveolar pores, and an increase in the percentage of mucus-secreting glands. Studies of children may be characterized by a less well-defined patient population, since it is more difficult to establish a clear diagnosis of asthma in the infant and young child. In addition, pulmonary function tests are more difficult to perform in the infant and young child, often making it necessary to rely on nonobjective parameters.

Elderly Patients

Changes with older age that are referable to the lower respiratory tract include (1) decreased compliance of the chest wall, (2) doubling of residual volume, (3) reduction of vital capacity, (4) decreased ciliary activity of the bronchial epithelium, (7) increased dead space, and (8) enhanced potential for mechanical and infectious respiratory complications.

The elderly asthmatic patient is at greater risk for the development of adverse cardiovascular effects because of decreased arterial elasticity, decreased coronary blood flow, and the development of atheromatous plaques, which lead to hypertension, coronary artery disease, and cerebrovascular insufficiency. As a result, long-term studies in elderly patients may be associated with increased frequency of naturally occurring adverse cardiovascular events, unrelated to the study drug. On the other hand, beta agonists and methylxanthines have the inherent potential to produce cardiac arrhythmias and other adverse cardiovascular effects (see Cardiovascular Events). Careful monitoring for this type of adverse effect is, therefore, necessary in this age group.

Diseases that occur with greater frequency in the elderly, such as autoimmune conditions, rheumatoid disease, and cancer, could conceivably be triggered by chemical entities in medications. Comparing the frequency of these diseases in patients receiving the study drug to that of control groups is necessary to determine whether there may be a relationship between the administration of the study drug and the development of these conditions.

There may be unintentional failure by elderly patients to comply with study requirements because of decreased cerebrovascular function or increased frequency of diseases associated with memory loss. In addition, elderly patients frequently have decreased finger mobility necessary for repeated use of inhaled asthma medications. The use of device aids for elderly patients so that they can more easily administer inhaled drugs may be helpful.

The effect on the elderly of study medications may be influenced by the 40 to 50 percent decrease in renal function occurring with advanced age. Decrease in renal function may lead to significant increases in blood levels and require modification of dosage.

The increase in medical conditions with increasing age frequently lead to polypharmacy. Prior to inclusion in studies of asthma drugs, elderly patients should be carefully evaluated to reaffirm the need for each medication. The large number of medications taken by elderly patients is more likely to lead to pharmacologic incompatibilities and drug interactions (see Chap. 74).

Studies of Acute Asthma

Special consideration must be given to the study design required to demonstrate the safety and effectiveness of medications for the treatment of patients with acute asthma. Since these patients may have severely compromised respiratory function and increased potential for adverse cardiovascular events, patient entry criteria, monitoring of pulmonary and cardiovascular status, and the general integrity of the study must be scrutinized. In general, unless the investigational drug is specifically proposed for the management of such patients, exclusion should be considered if (1) there is a history of rapid deterioration with previous episodes, (2) the patient can be considered to be fatality prone [59], (3) physical examination demonstrates severe or rapidly progressing bronchial obstruction, (4) the patient has compromised cardiovascular status, (5) $PaCO_2$ is greater than 40 mmHg or pH is less than 7.35, (6) the patient is unable to perform spirometry or peak flow determinations, or (7) the investigator anticipates added risk for any reason from delaying initiation of usual therapy. Studies of acute asthma should include an assessment of the investigational drug's effect on arterial blood gases.

Studies of investigational drugs for the treatment of acute asthma should be designed to permit rapid intervention by the investigator with conventional therapy if the patient's status is deteriorating. Such studies do not necessarily need to be of short duration, since assessment of efficacy may depend on need for intervention—intubation, mechanical ventilation, use of corticosteroids—as well as recurrence or persistence of such exacerbations.

Comparison of the study drug with both an active-treatment and placebo control is desirable. Unless the study design can effectively utilize standard treatment for baseline control of both groups, however, the ethics of utilizing a placebo control can be seriously questioned. Such studies should be double-blind, and parallel groups should be used. Crossover studies under these circumstances are more likely to be associated with sequence effect, and rapidly shifting baselines may offset the advantage of avoiding interpatient variability. Stratification of patients based on pulmonary function (e.g., one group with FEV_1 20–40% predicted and another group with FEV_1 40–60% predicted), concomitant medications, age, and so on are issues that should be determined prior to initiation of the study.

Continuous ECG monitoring should be performed on all patients who are participating in studies with investigational drugs for the treatment of acute asthma. The increased potential for development of cardiac arrhythmias in this setting—hypoxia, other asthma medications, hypokalemia—makes such monitoring essential. Vital signs should be frequently monitored for the same reason.

Careful follow-up of sufficient duration to evaluate the long-term effect of the study drug on the status of patients treated acutely with this medication should be considered.

Generic Issues

There has been recent interest in the most effective method for evaluation of generic forms of inhaled asthma drugs, in particular inhaled beta agonists. The well-established criteria for oral dosage forms based on serum levels cannot be reliably used for inhaled drugs.

It is generally felt that generic preparations should contain the same active ingredient with the same purity as the innovator product. Also the generic product should contain the same excipients, or at least excipients that are generally considered to be safe. The dispersion/release characteristics of the generic preparation should not be significantly different from the reference product. This would imply that the drug is released to the same anatomic portion of the respiratory tract as the marketed drug. In addition, the pharmacologic response to the generic drug should not be significantly different from the innovator product.

The medications currently used to treat asthma will come under close scrutiny in the 1990s. Recent concern about already approved drugs will, logically, have an impact on evaluation of investigational drugs and determination of their approvability for marketing. The medications presently available for the treatment of asthma are, in most cases, more variable in their effect and hence more unpredictable than has previously been appreciated. Assumptions made in the past about pharmacologic intervention may not hold up to careful examination in the future. The benefits and risks of each form of therapy, and the best approach to utilization of that modality will need careful reanalysis. In all likelihood, sponsors of investigational drugs will be encouraged to demonstrate the relationship of their product, if any, to present concerns, just as practicing physicians must be more aware of these concerns and diligent in recognizing and addressing them. As long as asthma morbidity and mortality continue to increase in this country, each drug must be evaluated not only in regard to safety and efficacy but also in regard to its potential impact on these trends. Guidelines for such evaluation are helpful but cannot, and should not, replace enlightened individualized assessment of the most effective methods for achieving this end.

REFERENCES

1. Ahrens, R. C., et al. Use of bronchial provocation with histamine to compare the pharmacodynamics of inhaled albuterol and metaproterenol in patients with asthma. *J. Allergy Clin. Immunol.* 79:876, 1987.
1a. Badier, M., et al. Attenuation of hyperventilation-induced bronchospasm by terfenadine: A new antihistamine. *J. Allergy Clin. Immunol.* 81:437, 1988.
2. Baker, J. R., Jr., et al. Clinical relevance of the substitution of different brands of sustained-release theophylline. *J. Allergy Clin. Immunol.* 81:664, 1988.
3. Beasley, C. R. W., Rafferty, P., and Holgate, S. T. Bronchoconstrictor properties of preservatives in ipratropium bromide (Atrovent) nebulizer solution. *Br. Med. J.* 294:1197, 1987.
4. Becker, A. B., Nelson, N. A., and Simons, F. E. R. Inhaled salbutamol vs. injected epinephrine in the treatment of acute asthma in children. *J. Pediatr.* 465:469, 1983.
4a. Benoit, C., et al. Single-dose effect of astemizole on bronchoconstriction induced by histamine in asthmatic subjects. *Chest* 101:1318, 1992.
5. Bernstein, I. L. (ed.). Report of the American Academy of Allergy and Immunology Task Force on guidelines for clinical investigation of non-bronchodilator antiasthma drugs. *J. Allergy Clin. Immunol.* 78:489, 1986.
6. Botstein, P. Evidence used for approval of new drugs. *Isr. J. Med. Sci.* 22:197, 1986.
7. Bucknall, C. E., et al. Management of asthma in hospital: A prospective audit. *Br. Med. J.* 296:1637, 1988.
8. Buist, A. S. Asthma mortality: Trends and determinants. *Am. Rev. Respir. Dis.* 136:1037, 1987.
9. Buist, A. S. Is asthma mortality increasing? *Chest* 93:449, 1988.
10. Busse, W. W. The role of inflammation in asthma: A new focus. *J. Rev. Respir. Dis.* 10:72, 1989.
11. Canny, G. J., and Levison, H. Management of asthma: A Canadian perspective. *Chest* 90:465, 1986.
12. Chapman, K. R., et al. Hemodynamic effects of an inhaled beta-2 agonist. *Clin. Pharmacol. Ther.* 35:762, 1984.
13. Clark, T. J. H. Asthma therapy in Great Britain. *Chest* 90:67S, 1986.
14. Conway, S. P., and Littlewood, J. M. Admission to hospital with asthma. *Arch. Dis. Child.* 60:636, 1985.
15. Crane, J., Burgess, C., and Beasley, R. Cardiovascular and hypokalemic effects of inhaled salbutamol, fenoterol, and isoprenaline. *Thorax* 44:136, 1989.
16. Crane, J., et al. Hypokalemia and electrocardiographic effects of aminophylline and salbutamol in obstructive airways. *N.Z. Med. J.* 100:309, 1987.
17. Deenstra, M., Haalboom, J. R. E., and Stuyvenberg, A. Decrease of plasma potassium due to inhalation of beta-2 agonists: Absence of an additional effect of intravenous theophylline. *Eur. J. Clin. Invest.* 18:162, 1988.
18. Doshan, H. D., et al. Celiprolol, atenolol, and propranolol: A comparison of pulmonary effects in asthmatic patients. *J. Cardiovasc. Pharmacol.* 8:S105, 1986.
19. Evans, R., et al. National trends in the morbidity and mortality of asthma in the U.S. *Chest* 91:655, 1987.
20. Evans, W. V., et al. Aminophylline, salbutamol and combined intravenous infusion in acute severe asthma. *Br. J. Dis. Chest* 74:385, 1980.
21. Expert Panel Report: National Heart, Lung, and Blood Institute. National Asthma Education Program: Guidelines for the Diagnosis and Management of Asthma. *J. Allergy Clin. Immunol.* 88:453, 1991.
22. Furukawa, C. T., et al. Cognitive and behavioral findings in children taking theophylline. *J. Allergy Clin. Immunol.* 81:83, 1988.
23. *General Guidelines for the Evaluation of Drugs to Be Approved for Use During Pregnancy and for Treatment of Infants and Children: A Report of the Committee on Drugs of the American Academy of Pediatrics to the Food and Drug Administration.* Evanston, IL: American Academy of Pediatrics, 1974. Pp. 1–40.
24. Hall, W. J., Hall, C. B., and Speers, D. M. Respiratory syncytial virus infection in adults. *Ann. Intern. Med.* 88:203, 1978.
25. Hills, M., and Armitage, P. The two period crossover clinical trial. *Br. J. Clin. Pharmacol.* 8:7, 1979.
26. Hollifield, J. W. Electrolyte disarray and cardiovascular disease. *Am. J. Cardiol.* 63:21B, 1989.
27. Josephson, G. W., et al. Emergency treatment of asthma: A comparison of two treatment regimens. *J.A.M.A.* 242:639, 1979.
28. Karim, A., et al. Food-induced changes in theophylline absorption from controlled-release formulations: Substantial increased and decreased absorption with Uniphyl tablets and TheoDur Sprinkle. *Clin. Pharmacol. Ther.* 38:77, 1985.
29. Kinney, E. L., et al. Ventricular tachycardia after terbutaline. *J.A.M.A.* 240:2247, 1978.
30. Kerrebjin, K. F., van Essen-Zandvlict, E. E. M., and Neijens, H. J. Effect of long-term treatment with inhaled corticosteroids and beta agonists on the bronchial responsiveness in children with asthma. *J. Allergy Clin. Immunol.* 79:653, 1987.
31. Konig, P., Hordvik, N. L., and Serby, C. W. Fenoterol in exercise-induced asthma: Effect of dose on efficacy and duration of action. *Chest* 85:462, 1984.
32. Kraan, J., et al. Changes in bronchial hyperreactivity induced by 4 weeks of treatment with antiasthmatic drugs in patients with allergic asthma: A comparison between budesonide and terbutaline. *J. Allergy Clin. Immunol.* 76:628, 1985.
33. Kravis, L. P., and Kolski, G. B. Unexpected death in childhood asthma: A review of 13 deaths in ambulatory patients. *Am. J. Dis. Child.* 139:558, 1985.
34. Lai, C. K. W., Twentyman, O. P., and Holgate, S. T. The effect of an increase in inhaled allergen dose after rimiterol hydrobromide on the occurrence and magnitude of the late asthmatic response and the associated change in nonspecific bronchial responsiveness. *Am. Rev. Respir. Dis.* 140:917, 1989.
34a. Larsson, K., Martinsson, A., and Hjemdahl, P. Influence of β-adrenergic receptor function during terbutaline treatment on allergen sensitivity and bronchodilator response to terbutaline in asthmatic subjects. *Chest* 101:953, 1992.
35. Lewis, L. D., and Cochran, G. M. Systemic steroids in chronic severe asthma. *Br. Med. J.* 292:1289, 1986.
36. Leynadier, F., et al. Death after cromoglycate (letter). *Allergy* 40:540, 1985.
37. Machado, M. L. Early and late allergen-induced bronchial reactions. *Acta Univ. Upsal.,* 1984. P. 504.
38. Malo, J. L., et al. Duration of the effect of astemizole on histamine-inhalation tests. *J. Allergy Clin. Immunol.* 85:729, 1990.
39. Markham, D., et al. Epidemiologic study of deaths from asthma among children in the U.S. 1965–1983. *J. Allergy Clin. Immunol.* 77:161, 1986.
40. Mitchell, E. A. Increasing trends in hospital admission rates for asthma. *Arch. Dis. Child.* 60:376, 1985.
41. Nicklas, R. A. The investigative process for new drugs. *Ann. Allergy* 63:598, 1989.
42. Nicklas, R. A. Theophylline, school performance and the Food and Drug Administration (letter). *Pediatrics* 83:146, 1989.
43. Nicklas, R. A. Paradoxical bronchospasm associated with the use of inhaled beta agonists. *J. Allergy Clin. Immunol.* 85:959, 1990.
44. Nino, A. F., et al. Drug-induced left ventricular failure in patients with pulmonary disease: Endomyocardial biopsy demonstration of catecholamine myocarditis. *Chest* 92:736, 1987.
45. O'Driscoll, B. R. C., and Cochrane, G. M. Emergency use of nebulized bronchodilator drugs in British hospitals. *Thorax* 42:491, 1987.
46. Osman, J., Ormerod, P., and Stableforth, D. Management of acute asthma: A survey of hospital practice and comparison between thoracic and general physicians in Birmingham and Manchester. *Br. J. Dis. Chest* 81:232, 1987.
47. Page, C. P. One explanation of the asthma paradox: Inhibition of natural anti-inflammatory mechanism by B₂ agonists. *Lancet* 337:717, 1991.
48. *Physicians' Desk Reference* (45th ed.). Oradell, NJ: Medical Economics, 1991. P. 587.
48a. Rafferty, P., and Holgate, S. T. Terfenadine (Seldane) is a potent and selective histamine H₁ receptor antagonist in asthmatic subjects. *Am. Rev. Respir. Dis.* 135:181, 1987.
49. Reed, C. E. Basic mechanisms of asthma: Role of inflammation. *Chest* 94:175, 1988.
50. Robin, E. D. Death from bronchial asthma. *Chest* 93:614, 1988.
51. Sears, M. R., et al. Regular inhaled beta agonist treatment in bronchial asthma. *Lancet* 336:1391, 1990.
52. Shim, C., and Williams, M. H., Jr. Cough and wheezing from beclomethasone aerosol. *Chest* 91:207, 1987.
53. Siegel, D., et al. Aminophylline increases the toxicity but not the efficacy

of an inhaled beta adrenergic agonist in the treatment of acute exacerbations of asthma. *Am. Rev. Respir. Dis.* 132:283, 1985.

54. Sinclair, B. L., Clark, D. W., and Sears, M. R. Use of antiasthma drugs in New Zealand. *Thorax* 42:670, 1987.

55. Sly, R. M. Effects of treatment on mortality from asthma. *Ann. Allergy* 56: 207, 1986.

56. Spector, S. L., et al. Compliance of patients with asthma with an experimental aerosol medication: Implications for controlled clinical trials. *J. Allergy Clin. Immunol.* 77:65, 1986.

57. Stevenson, D. D., and Lewis, R. A. Proposed mechanisms of aspirin sensitivity reactions. *J. Allergy Clin. Immunol.* 80:788, 1987.

58. Storr, J., Barrell, E., and Lenney, W. Rising asthma admissions and self referral. *Arch. Dis. Child.* 63:744, 1988.

59. Strunk, R. C. Identification of the fatality-prone subject with asthma. *J. Allergy Clin. Immunol.* 83:477, 1989.

60. Swensen, E. R., and Aitken, S. L. Hypokalemia occurs with inhaled salbutamol (abstract). *Am. Rev. Respir. Dis.* 131:A99, 1985.

61. Vandewalker, M. L., et al. Addition of terbutaline to optimal theophylline therapy: Double-blind crossover study in asthmatic patients. *Chest* 90: 198, 1986.

62. van Schayck, C. P., et al. Increased bronchial hyperresponsiveness after inhaling salbutamol during 1 year is not caused by subsensitization to salbutamol. *J. Allergy Clin. Immunol.* 86:793, 1990.

63. Vathenen, A. S., et al. Rebound increase in bronchial responsiveness after treatment with inhaled terbutaline. *Lancet* 8585:554, 1988.

64. Whitehurst, V. E., et al. The influence of methylxanthines on cardiotoxicity of isoproterenol in rats and minipigs. *Toxicologist* 3:53, 1983.

65. Whyte, K. F., et al. Salbutamol induced hypokalemia: The effect of theophylline alone and in combination with adrenaline. *Br. J. Clin. Pharmacol.* 25:571, 1988.

66. Wilson, N., and Silverman, M. Controlled trial of slow release aminophylline in childhood asthma: Are short-term trials valid? *Br. Med. J.* 284:863, 1982.

67. Woolcock, A. J. Use of corticosteroids in treatment of patients with asthma. *J. Allergy Clin. Immunol.* 84:975, 1989.

68. Yarbrough, J., Mansfield, L. E., and Ting, S. Metered dose inhaler-induced bronchospasm in asthmatic patients. *Ann. Allergy* 55:55, 1985.

69. Ziporyn, T. The Food and Drug Administration: How "those regulations" came to be. *J.A.M.A.* 259:2037, 1985.

70. Lindgren, S., et al. Does asthma or treatment with theophylline limit children's academic performance? *N. Engl. J. Med.* 327:926, 1992.

Corticosteroids

Kian Fan Chung
John Wiggins
John Collins

60

It is now nearly half a century since glucocorticoids were first used in asthma. Toward the end of the 1940s, adrenocorticotrophic hormone (ACTH) and cortisone became available for possible use in several diseases. Immediately following the demonstration of their dramatic action in rheumatoid arthritis, ACTH was given to five asthmatic patients who had obtained only partial relief from aminophylline and adrenaline [19]. They experienced dramatic improvement in asthmatic symptoms within hours or days of ACTH treatment, with gradual return of symptoms following its cessation. Shortly afterward, other groups reported the clinical effectiveness of cortisone in the treatment of asthma [30, 164]. Both intravenous hydrocortisone [29] and oral prednisone [11] were effective in reducing symptoms of patients with chronic asthma, but it soon became clear that prolonged use led to an unacceptable level of systemic side effects, which were also observed when the newer synthetic corticosteroids such as methylprednisolone, dexamethasone, and triamcinolone were introduced.

Attempts at administering glucocorticoids directly to the airways were made during the 1950s, but these generally failed to control asthma despite the fact that enough absorption to cause systemic side effects was observed. The effectiveness of hydrocortisone inhaled as a powder at doses far below those required by systemic administration was reported [26, 70, 98]. On the other hand, hydrocortisone administered by nebulization was shown to be ineffective [26]. It was only in the early 1970s with the development of beclomethasone dipropionate that inhaled corticosteroid therapy became a major therapeutic consideration in the treatment of chronic asthma [28] (see Chap. 61). It has subsequently become clear that the glucocorticoid molecule suitable for inhalation should possess a high affinity for its receptor and should be rapidly inactivated by liver biotransformation [23]. Other topically active glucocorticoids such as triamcinolone acetonide, flunisolide, and budesonide have since been introduced for the treatment of asthma.

MECHANISMS OF ACTION

In the past 20 years, basic understanding of both the mechanisms of action of glucocorticoids and the pathophysiology of asthma has improved. The chronic airway inflammation of asthma is characterized by edema, infiltration with inflammatory cells such as lymphocytes and eosinophils, subepithelial fibrosis, and damage to the epithelium [14, 119]. Several classes of inflammatory mediators including histamine, prostaglandins, leukotrienes, kininogenase, and eosinophil products have been recovered from bronchoalveolar lavage fluid of patients with asthma [36]. The resulting inflammatory processes contribute to airways obstruction and bronchial hyperresponsiveness [35]. Glucocorticoids may act at different levels of these processes in the airways of asthmatic patients, and these actions may underlie their potent beneficial effects in asthma. Studies of inflammatory cell activation in vivo and in vitro illustrate the multiple antiinflammatory actions of glucocorticoids.

The effects of glucocorticoids may be divided into primary and secondary actions, given the complexity of the inflammatory events in asthma. Such a division emphasizes the concept that some cell types are primarily modulated by glucocorticoids, while other cell types may become secondarily involved because mediators that activate them and that are produced by the primary target cells have been regulated by glucocorticoids.

Another important consideration about the pharmacologic actions of glucocorticoids relates to whether these represent an extension of their physiologic effects. Physiologic plasma levels of glucocorticoids exhibit diurnal variation, usually peaking in the morning with frequent, brief surges. Stress, such as that resulting from tissue damage or inflammation, may lead to a surge in plasma glucocorticoid level. These physiologic levels of glucocorticoids may serve to protect the organism from its own activated defense mechanisms, preventing "self-damage" [148]. Thus, endogenous corticosteroids may protect tissues outside a localized area of inflammation or infection against toxic host-defense mechanisms of the body. Endogenous glucocorticoids may be able to induce various acute, as well as prolonged, antiinflammatory activities. In support of this concept, endogenously produced corticosteroids have been shown to inhibit inflammatory responses in the rat [69]. One example of such a stress feedback response is the effect of small doses of interleukin-1 (IL-1), which may be released as a result of immune or infective processes in inducing ACTH and cortisol secretion, which may in turn trigger an antiinflammatory response [17].

Molecular Mechanisms of Action

Glucocorticoids stimulate specific glucocorticoid receptors, which are present in nearly all cell types including those in the airways and lungs. Much progress has been made in our understanding of the subcellular mechanisms by which stimulation of these receptors leads to glucocorticoid activity.

Many of the actions of glucocorticoids can be explained at the molecular levels of gene regulation [88, 121, 149]. Historically, several steps that have led to this finding can be identified. First, the synthesis of labelled steroids with high specific activity has led to the demonstration of high-affinity glucocorticoid receptors on various cell types. Second, the activated receptor has been shown to interact with nuclear DNA and regulate specific genes by binding to specific sequences within the genome. This may result in either increased or decreased transcription of messenger RNAs (mRNAs) of several proteins. Finally, the complementary DNA sequence for the glucocorticoid receptor has been cloned.

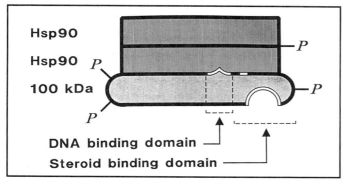

Fig. 60-1. *Proposed model for the nonactivated glucocorticoid receptor. The steroid-binding subunit of the receptor consists of a steroid-binding domain, a DNA-binding domain, and a third domain called "immunogenic." The DNA-binding domain is blocked by the Hsp90 (90 kd heat-shock protein) subunits. On activation of the steroid receptor, Hsp90 subunits are released to expose the DNA-binding domain. Phosphates (P) are indicated. (Reprinted with permission from A. Munck et al. Glucocorticoid receptors and actions. Am. Rev. Respir. Dis. 141:52, 1990.)*

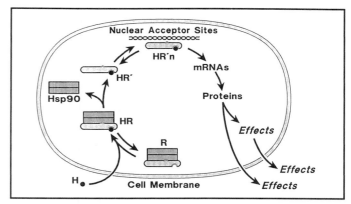

Fig. 60-2. *Genomic mechanism for receptor-mediated action of glucocorticoids. Glucocorticoid hormone H penetrates the cell and binds to nonactivated steroid-receptor complex (R). The resulting activated steroid receptor complex (HR) exposes the DNA-binding site with release of Hsp90 (90 kd heat-shock protein) units. The activated steroid receptor binds to DNA sites in the nucleus (HR'n), resulting in transcription of mRNAs of several proteins, which then mediate the effects of glucocorticoids. (Reprinted with permission from A. Munck et al. Glucocorticoid receptors and actions. Am. Rev. Respir. Dis. 141:52, 1990.)*

Glucocorticoid Receptors

Glucocorticoid receptors are widely distributed in mammalian cells, including those from the lungs as well as the inflammatory cells such as macrophages, lymphocytes, and eosinophils, and are present at an estimated density of several thousand receptors per cell [9]. At physiologic glucocorticoid concentrations, it has been estimated that these receptors are 30 to 40 percent saturated. The precise intracellular site of localization of these receptors has been controversial, although the unactivated receptor is now thought to be present mainly in the cytoplasm, with a little in the nucleus [88]. The binding of a glucocorticoid to its receptor is rapid and reversible, with binding efficacies within the nanomolar range. The human glucocorticoid receptor is a single polypeptide chain of molecular weight ~90,000 containing ~780 amino acids [88]. It has three different recognizable components: a specific steroid-binding site, a DNA-binding site, and another site of unknown function termed the immunogenic domain [76]. In addition, the unactivated steroid hormone receptor contains a heat-shock protein, which dissociates itself from the receptor on activation and exposes the DNA-binding site [101] (Fig. 60-1). It is assumed that the heat-shock protein protects the DNA-binding site of the glucocorticoid receptor.

Glucocorticoid receptor levels are suppressed by glucocorticoid administration in humans in health and disease; conversely, adrenalectomy increases glucocorticoid receptor binding and mRNA in several tissues [109, 172]. The mechanisms for the reduction of glucocorticoid receptor levels probably involve a reduction in the rate of receptor mRNA synthesis and an increase in the rate of degradation of the receptor or of the mRNA by the hormone [152, 171]. Little is known at present about these mechanisms in airway or inflammatory cells found in the lungs of patients with asthma.

Modulation of Gene Transcription

In common with mineralocorticoids, estrogens, and androgens, many of the effects of glucocorticoids are mediated by the transcription and translation of mRNA and synthesis of new proteins (Fig. 60-2). Glucocorticoids penetrate cells by diffusion and are rapidly bound to specific glucocorticoid receptors in the cytoplasm of most mammalian cells. The binding of the corticoid activates the receptor and exposes the binding site of the glucocorticoid-receptor complex to DNA. This complex is rapidly

transported to the nucleus where, with its increased affinity for DNA, it interacts with specific regulatory elements of the DNA of certain genes that encode proteins important in inflammatory responses [153]. Glucocorticoids may also inhibit other genes that regulate the production of cytokines.

Glucocorticoids may therefore increase or decrease the levels of mRNA and the proteins that the mRNA encodes. These proteins are the primary effectors of glucocorticoid action and may be secretory products, enzymes, or regulators of other function including the transcription of other genes. Only a small number of genes that may be expressed, probably 1 to 2 percent, are influenced by glucocorticoids. The response may be dependent on the cell type, its stage of differentiation and development, and perhaps the immediate cellular milieu, such as the presence of inflammatory mediators or other hormones.

Glucocorticoid responses have a relatively slow onset of action because of the time taken for the initiation of RNA transcription and the synthesis of the glucocorticoid-induced protein. In vitro these effects may be undetectable for up to an hour, but other effects such as the increase in stability of the RNA encoding for a particular protein with rapid turnover may have a shorter latent period. The duration of glucocorticoid action may also depend on the turnover time of the induced mRNA and protein. However, some of the observed effects of glucocorticoids may be more rapid, such as inhibition of ACTH release, and cannot be entirely accounted for by transcriptional events and protein synthesis. These immediate effects may involve other pathways such as phosphorylation or processing of newly synthesized protein by activated glucocorticoid receptors [65].

Transcriptional Effects

Glucocorticoids regulate the expression of certain genes that encode proteins that may be important in several aspects of asthma, such as the lipocortins and the beta$_2$-adrenergic receptor. In addition, glucocorticoids may also inhibit the transcription of various cytokines produced by macrophages or lymphocytes. This effect may be mediated by several mechanisms including binding of the activated glucocorticoid receptor to a negative glucocorticoid response element, and interaction of the activated receptor with transcription factors necessary for cytokine synthesis [51a, 177a]. Steroid-induced changes in the levels of these proteins may therefore have secondary influences on several aspects of the inflammatory response in asthma.

Lipocortins

It has been proposed that a major part of the antiinflammatory actions of glucocorticoids is the result of the induction of the synthesis of a group of proteins, the lipocortins [68, 194]. These are now considered to be part of a larger family of calcium- and phospholipid-binding proteins, termed annexins. These proteins have a wide range of different functions such as suppression of inflammation and modulation of cell differentiation and proteins involved in membrane fusion and exocytosis [113]. They inhibit cellular phospholipase A_2, thereby inhibiting the release of arachidonic acid, a precursor of many inflammatory mediators such as prostaglandins and leukotrienes, from membrane phospholipids. One of the first demonstrations of the involvement of lipocortins in glucocorticoid effects was the inhibition of chemotactic activity of neutrophils by glucocorticoids and the marked reduction of the release of arachidonic acid induced by the bacterial peptide f-met-leu-phe (FMLP) [99]. Inhibitors of protein and mRNA synthesis such as cycloheximide and actinomycin D, respectively, could prevent the inhibitory effects of glucocorticoids on arachidonic acid release stimulated by f-met-leu-phe. Glucocorticoids have been shown to inhibit the release of arachidonic acid products shown as prostaglandins and leukotrienes from alveolar macrophages from normal and asthmatic subjects [10]. Human cDNA for lipocortin-1 has been sequenced and cloned [190], and its gene structure has potential glucocorticoid regulatory elements in its promoter region, which suggests that its expression could be under the control of glucocorticoids. Lipocortin-1 has been detected in bronchoalveolar lavage fluid and circulating mononuclear cells obtained from normal volunteers. Lipocortin-1 levels are enhanced by prior administration of oral glucocorticoids [6, 81]. However, one study has failed to show the expression of lipocortin-1 mRNA in human alveolar macrophages by glucocorticoids [27]. Recombinant lipocortin-1 is capable of inhibiting phospholipase A_2 activity in vitro and various inflammatory processes such as the release of thromboxane A_2 and free oxygen radicals or edema formation [38, 136].

The available evidence suggests that lipocortin-1 is synthesized by the action of glucocorticoids and can mimic some of its antiinflammatory actions, probably through an inhibitory action on phospholipase A_2.

Beta₂-Adrenergic Receptor

The effects of glucocorticoids on the airway actions of beta₂-adrenergic agents may partly explain its therapeutic properties in asthma. Glucocorticoids prevent the tachyphylactic bronchodilator response to regular inhalation of beta₂-adrenergic agonist drugs in normal subjects [100] and improve the bronchodilator effect of inhaled isoprenaline in patients with asthma [57] (Fig. 60-3). At the receptor level, in vitro studies on circulating cells such as neutrophils and lymphocytes show that glucocorticoids increase the density of beta-adrenergic receptors after 24 hours of treatment, as a result of an enhancement of beta-receptor synthesis and an increased receptor affinity and coupling to adenyl cyclase [49]. In addition, the reduced beta-receptor density of circulating lymphocytes obtained from both normal and asthmatic subjects treated with beta₂-adrenergic agonists is restored after glucocorticoid treatment [103].

Recent studies in cultured cells have demonstrated that the glucocorticoid-induced increase in beta-adrenergic receptors [72] is due to an enhancement in the transcription rate of mRNA for the beta-receptor (Fig. 60-4) and therefore to an increased synthesis of the beta-receptor [42, 91]. Desensitization of the beta-receptor by treatment with beta-adrenergic agonists results

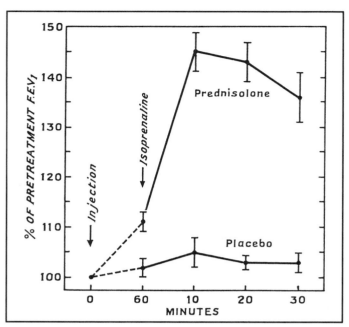

Fig. 60-3. *Effect of intravenous prednisolone phosphate (40 mg) or placebo on airway response to isoprenaline (200 μg) inhaled 1 hour later in eight asthmatic subjects. After prednisolone there was a significant bronchodilator response to isoprenaline, which was also observed 8 hours later. (Reprinted with permission from R. Ellul-Micallef and F. F. Fenech. Effect of intravenous prednisolone in asthmatics with diminished adrenergic responsiveness. Lancet 2:1269, 1975.)*

from a decreased stability of cytoplasmic beta-receptor mRNA [92]. Although this mechanism appears to be unaffected by glucocorticoids, the overall effect of glucocorticoids is to reverse desensitization by an increase in beta-receptor synthesis [92]. Therefore, the beneficial effects of glucocorticoids in asthma may partly result from an increased transcription rate of the beta₂-receptor in the airways.

EFFECT ON INFLAMMATORY CELLS

Many different inflammatory cell types have been implicated in the pathogenesis of asthma, and it is likely that there are complex interactions between these cell types. The precise sequence of cellular inflammatory events is unclear, but interactions between cell types through the release of cytokines or lymphokines from airway macrophages and lymphocytes and other cell types such as mast cells and epithelial cells are likely to occur.

Cytokines form a network of proteins that convey signals for the regulation of cellular proliferation and differentiation [7a]. Increased cytokine gene expression—in particular granulocyte-macrophage colony stimulating factor (GM-CSF), tumor necrosis factor-alpha (TNF-α), IL-1, IL-3, IL-4, IL-5, and IL-6—has been found in the airways of patients with asthma [26a, 26b, 92a].

GM-CSF released from alveolar macrophages obtained from patients with asthma is capable of enhancing leukotriene C_4 generation from human eosinophils [77, 102], which may represent a mechanism by which the activity of circulating eosinophils might be increased in asthma [33]. In addition, IL-5 released from activated T-lymphocytes may also enhance the release of mediators from the eosinophil, and other cytokines such as IL-3 may serve as a growth factor for mast cells and eosinophils [197]. Figure 60-5 summarizes some of the potential interactions between inflammatory cells in asthma and the inhibitory effects of

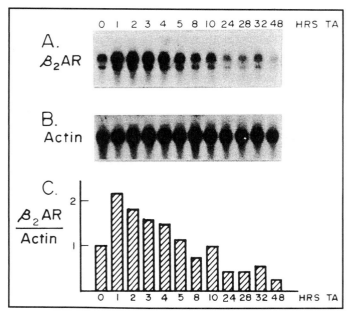

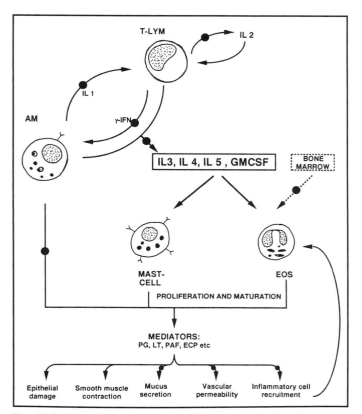

Fig. 60-4. *Effect of glucocorticoid treatment on beta$_2$-adrenergic receptor (β$_2$-AR) and actin mRNA levels in a cultured cell line of hamster smooth muscle cells. Panels A and B show blots of total cellular RNA extracted from these cells and probed with ^{32}P-labelled beta$_2$-adrenergic receptor cDNA (A) or actin cDNA (B). Autoradiographs were quantitated by densitometric scanning (C). Beta$_2$-adrenergic receptor mRNA increases relative to actin mRNA within 1 hour of incubation with triamcinolone acetonide (10^{-7} M). This was paralleled by an increase in beta$_2$-adrenergic receptor number. (Reprinted with permission from S. Collins, M. G. Caron, and K. F. Leftowitz. Beta$_2$-adrenergic receptors in hamster smooth muscle cells are transcriptionally regulated by glucocorticoids. J. Biol. Chem. 263:9067, 1988.)*

Fig. 60-5. *Schematic representation of putative interactions between inflammatory cells, cytokines, and inflammatory mediators to cause many of the features characteristic of asthma. The potential inhibitory effects of glucocorticoids are represented by the closed circles placed on several pathways. Glucocorticoids inhibit the release of IL-1, IL-2, and gamma-interferon (γ-IFN), preventing collaboration between macrophages (AM) and lymphocytes (T-LYM). Release of other interleukins such as IL-3, IL-4, IL-5, and granulocyte-macrophage colony stimulating factor (GMCSF) is also prevented, leading to inhibition of differentiation, proliferation, and activation of mast cells and eosinophils (EOS). In addition, release of inflammatory mediators such as prostaglandins (PG), leukotrienes (LT), platelet-activating factor (PAF), or eosinophil-cationic protein (ECP) may also be prevented by glucocorticoids. Glucocorticoids may therefore be effective at several levels of the inflammatory process in asthmatic airways.*

glucocorticoids on some of these pathways. Glucocorticoids, by inhibiting directly the expression of cytokines in inflammatory cells, prevent cell-to-cell interactions. For example, glucocorticoids inhibit IL-1 beta production from human monocytes by inhibition of both transcriptional and translational steps [111, 123] (see also Chap. 13).

Recent studies have directly examined the antiinflammatory effects of inhaled corticosteroid therapy in bronchial mucosal biopsies obtained from patients with asthma. Inhaled corticosteroid therapy restored epithelial integrity and reduced the number of eosinophils, lymphocytes, mast cells and activated macrophages in bronchial tissues [28a, 52a, 104a, 118a].

Mast Cells

Mast cells are increased in numbers in the airways of patients with asthma, particularly during the pollen season [159], and these more readily release mediators [31, 67], effects that may be dependent on lymphocyte-derived IL-3 and IL-4 [15]. Glucocorticoids do not inhibit the IgE-dependent release of histamine or leukotrienes from cultured human lung mast cells or airway tissue [173, 174]. Conversely, regular treatment with topical corticosteroids reduces the degree of nasal obstruction and the amount of mast cell mediators present after nasal antigen challenge [160]. This effect may result from a reduction in mucosal mast cell numbers through inhibition of IL-3 release from T-lymphocytes [45]. A similar mechanism may underlie the improvement seen in patients with exercise-induced asthma and allergen-induced bronchoconstriction after long-term topical corticosteroid therapy [46, 51]. Finally, glucocorticoids may inhibit IgE-

dependent release of cytokines such as IL-3, and GM-CSF from mast cells [196], thus inhibiting interactions with granulocytes and macrophages (see also Chap. 21).

Eosinophils

Eosinophils have been implicated in the pathogenesis of asthma [53] and may release constituents of their granule contents and lipid-derived mediators such as leukotriene C$_4$ and platelet activating factor [79] (see Chap. 20). IL-3, IL-5, and GM-CSF can increase the survival and function of eosinophils such as the release of leukotriene C$_4$ and cytotoxic activity [179]. Endothelial cells are also able to increase the functional capacity of eosinophils through the release of cytokines, and this effect is inhibited by prior exposure to dexamethasone [120]. Priming of eosinophil survival by several cytokines such as GM-CSF, IL-3, IL-5, and interferon-gamma is inhibited by corticosteroids [119a, 189a]. Therefore, steroids may inhibit the upregulation of eosinophil function. Release of free oxygen radicals and of eosinophil cationic protein from activated human eosinophils is reduced in vitro by glucocorticoids [58, 188]. Studies with bronchoalveolar lavage have shown that topical steroid therapy reduces the influx of eosinophils into the airways following allergen challenge, leading to a reduction in the levels of eosinophilic cationic protein [2]. Steroids may also reduce the capacity for eosinophils to respond to chemotactic signals. Thus, circulating eosinophils from subjects treated with corticosteroids have diminished ability to adhere to nylon fibers with reduced chemotactic activity [5].

Monocytes and Macrophages

Glucocorticoids induce a monocytopenia [168], and part of their antiinflammatory activity may result from inhibition of accumulation of macrophages/monocytes at airway sites of inflammation. Monocytes and macrophages are most sensitive to the effect of glucocorticoids [90]. Glucocorticoids increase the release of lipocortin into bronchoalveolar lavage fluid and from circulating monocytes [6, 81]. The subsequent inhibition of phospholipase A_2 by lipocortin prevents release of arachidonic acid with inhibition of prostaglandin and leukotriene formation [10, 197a]. Release of granule-containing enzymes and of cytokines such as IL-1, tumor necrosis factor, and GM-CSF is markedly reduced by glucocorticoids [111, 155]. Inhibition of IgE-dependent release of lipid mediators such as thromboxane B_2 and leukotriene B_4 alveolar macrophages has also been described [73]. Glucocorticoid-induced inhibition of macrophage activity may be important in reducing interaction of macrophages with other inflammatory cells such as eosinophils and lymphocytes.

Lymphocytes

Lymphocytes may regulate IgE production and mucosal mast cell numbers through the release of IL-3 and IL-4 [161]. T-lymphocytes may also produce GM-CSF and IL-5, which induce eosinophil chemotaxis and activation, and alpha interferon, which activates neutrophils and macrophages. In acute severe asthma, activated T-lymphocytes of the CD4 phenotype can be identified in peripheral blood with increased expression of activation markers such as IL-2R and HLA-DR, accompanied by a raised level of circulating gamma interferon and IL-2 receptor [43] (see Chap. 13). Corticosteroids are very effective in inhibiting proliferation of T-lymphocytes and their production of cytokines [78]. They particularly reduce the release of IL-2, which is a T-cell growth factor, and the expression of IL-2 receptors on T-lymphocytes [166]. In addition, IL-2 production by T-lymphocytes is inhibited through a reduction in the release of IL-1 from macrophages. Hydrocortisone prevents the release of IL-5 from T-cell clones obtained from hypereosinophilic patients [162].

Neutrophils

The role of the neutrophil in asthma is less certain. Neutrophil influx into the nasal mucosa after allergen exposure is inhibited by glucocorticoids [12], but its effects on neutrophil activation in vitro are small or negligible [176]. Production of leukotriene B_4 and release of lysosomal enzymes from activated human neutrophils are not inhibited by glucocorticoids [176]. Adherence of neutrophils to vascular endothelial cells in culture is inhibited to a small extent by glucocorticoids [176], an effect paralleled by a small reduction in the number of the leukocyte adherence receptors, CR3 [156] (see Chap. 9).

Vascular Endothelial Cells

Inhibition of plasma exudation through the endothelial barrier of the bronchial vasculature by glucocorticoids may be a major component of the beneficial effect of glucocorticoids in asthma [20, 37] and lead to a reduction in airway edema. Topically administered glucocorticoids inhibit antigen-induced vascular leakage in the nose of allergic patients [160]. Glucocorticoids may have a direct effect in preventing endothelial cell contraction, which leads to opening up of gap junctions between cells [143], and also inhibit the generation of mediators derived from arachidonic acid metabolism of endothelial cells [126].

EFFECT ON SMOOTH MUSCLE AND MUCOSAL GLANDS

Airway Smooth Muscle

Glucocorticoids have no direct effects on the contractile responses of airway smooth muscle [87]. They potentiate the relaxing effect of beta$_2$ agonists on human airway tissues [50, 75], due to an increase in beta$_2$-adrenergic receptors, and they prevent beta$_2$ receptor downregulation induced by beta$_2$-receptor stimulation [100]. Glucocorticoids may prevent airway smooth muscle contraction indirectly by preventing mediator release from a wide range of inflammatory cells [175] and by reducing the number of mediator-releasing cells, including eosinophils and mast cells in the airways [80]. Hyperplasia of airway smooth muscle has been observed in chronic asthma and may contribute to bronchial hyperresponsiveness. The long-term effect of glucocorticoid treatment on the hyperplasia of airway smooth muscle is not known.

Airway Mucosal Glands

Glucocorticoids reduce baseline mucous glycoprotein production from human and feline airway mucosal glands in vitro [132, 137], an effect probably mediated by the generation of lipocortin [132]. Only small effects were observed on mucus secretion induced by mediators such as histamine from human airways in vitro [137]. However, studies in patients with asthma suggest that steroids reduce the components of sputum such as albumin derived by exudation from serum rather than mucosal gland secretion [110, 145] (see Chap. 29). The beneficial effects of steroid therapy on airway mucosal gland secretion may be indirect through the suppression of both inflammatory cell infiltration and plasma exudation.

BRONCHIAL HYPERRESPONSIVENESS AND LATE-PHASE RESPONSES

Measurements of bronchial hyperresponsiveness (BHR) and of the late-phase response to allergen challenge have been used to gauge the beneficial effects of glucocorticoids in asthma [35, 53] (see Chap. 39). These indices are the best indirect assessment of the potential antiinflammatory effects of glucocorticoids available so far in asthma. More direct evidence for an antiinflammatory effect may be obtained by examination of bronchial biopsies or bronchoalveolar lavage fluid.

Established Bronchial Hyperresponsiveness

Studies using oral glucocorticoids have reported variable results on BHR in asthma, which may in part be explained by the varying doses used. A significant reduction in BHR to methacholine was observed in asthmatic children treated with prednisolone 60 mg/day for 1 week [18]. Oral methylprednisolone also induced a similar improvement in adult asthmatic patients [104] and prevented the increase in bronchial responsiveness observed during the pollen season [181]. By contrast, oral prednisolone at the lower dose of 12.5 mg/day had no effect on BHR over a 3-week period, while inhaled beclomethasone dipropionate (1,200 µg/

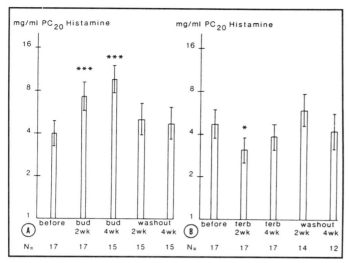

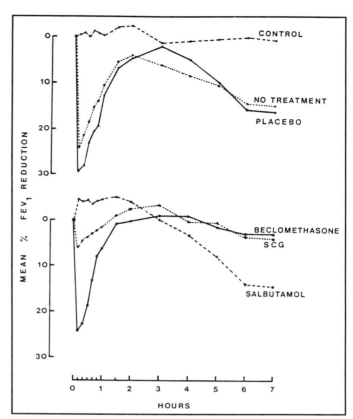

Fig. 60-6. *Effect of treatment with budesonide (*bud*) inhaler (100 μg four times per day,* Ⓐ *) and with terbutaline (*terb*) inhaler (500 μg four times per day,* Ⓑ *) on histamine PC₂₀, the concentration of histamine in mg/ml needed to cause a 20 percent fall in baseline FEV₁ in 17 asthmatic subjects. During the budesonide phase, there was a significant increase in PC₂₀, but during the terbutaline phase a significant decrease in PC₂₀ (* p < .05; *** p < .001). Bars indicate ± SEM; N = number of subjects. (Reprinted with permission from J. Kraan et al. Changes in bronchial hyperreactivity induced by 4 weeks of treatment with antiasthmatic drugs in patients with allergic asthma: A comparison between budesonide and terbutaline. J. Allergy Clin. Immunol. 76:628, 1985.)*

Fig. 60-7. *Time course of mean FEV₁ fall after allergen challenge in atopic asthmatic subjects and the effect of pretreatment with various antiasthmatic medications. The top panel shows the response after control inhalation and after allergen following no treatment and placebo pretreatment. The lower panel shows the effects of pretreatments with inhaled drugs: beclomethasone dipropionate (200 μg), salbutamol (200 μg), and sodium cromoglycate (SCG) (10 mg). Beclomethasone inhibited only the late-phase response, sodium cromoglycate both the early and late responses, and salbutamol only the early response. (Reprinted with permission from D. W. Cockroft and K. Y. Murdoch. Comparative effects of inhaled salbutamol, sodium cromoglycate and BDP on allergen-induced early asthmatic responses, late asthmatic responses and increased bronchial responsiveness to histamine. J. Allergy Clin. Immunol. 79:734, 1987.)*

day) was effective [105], supporting the role for a local action of glucocorticoids in the airways. Significant improvements in BHR to bronchoconstrictor agents such as methacholine or histamine have been observed with inhaled glucocorticoids [54, 112, 116] (Fig. 60-6). In general, most studies have reported a two- to four-fold improvement, although in more severely reactive asthmatics the decrease in BHR can be more substantial [54, 90a]. Increasing the dose of inhaled glucocorticoid does not necessarily result in greater improvements in BHR, which usually remains within the asthmatic range [115]. The component of BHR that is apparently not reversed by glucocorticoid therapy may either represent an inflammatory component of the asthmatic process or permanent structural abnormalities resulting from chronic inflammatory events resistant to glucocorticoid therapy. Persistence of BHR despite inhaled glucocorticoid therapy is associated with presence of subepithelial fibrosis, but with no evidence of inflammatory cell infiltration or of epithelial damage [133]. After a period of treatment of 1 year with inhaled steroids, BHR may disappear in some mild asthmatic patients [108], raising the possibility that treatment for a prolonged period of time at an early stage of the disease may completely reverse BHR. However, after a shorter period of treatment of 6 weeks' duration, the improvement in airway responsiveness was lost within 24 hours [187a].

By contrast, chronic treatment with either beta₂-adrenergic agonists or with theophylline does not improve BHR; indeed, even an increase in BHR has been observed with the beta₂ agonists [54, 112, 116]. These observations in general support the concept that these agents do not posses significant antiinflammatory activity in asthma.

Allergen Challenge

Glucocorticoids in single doses administered prior to allergen challenge prevent the late-phase bronchoconstrictor response

(Fig. 60-7) and the increase in BHR, without affecting the early acute response [39, 59]. Prolonged therapy with either oral prednisolone or inhaled steroids inhibits the early acute response to allergen [46, 51, 138]. This effect of chronic steroid therapy may lead to a reduction in mast cell numbers in the airway mucosa, an effect that has been shown in the nasal mucosa of patients with allergic rhinitis [80, 159] and also in the bronchial mucosa [52a, 104a, 118a]. Chronic inhaled steroid therapy may reduce exercise-induced asthma [46] by a similar mechanism.

OVERALL EFFECTS OF GLUCOCORTICOIDS

Glucocorticoids through action at the genomic level in controlling the transcription of a series of polypeptides or proteins can affect a wide range of responses from diverse cells involved in asthma. The major actions of glucocorticoids are to modulate the composition of the cellular infiltration and the release of mediators such as cytokines, lipid mediators, and enzymes into airway tissues. Interactions between various classes of inflammatory cells are profoundly inhibited (see Fig. 60-5). For example, the reduction in recruitment and activation of the eosinophil in asthma by glucocorticoids results from a concerted effect on T-lymphocytes, endothelial cells, and macrophages, which can produce cytokines and mediators to recruit and activate eosinophils. In addition, there is a major direct inhibitory effect on the release of mediators targeted against various components of the airways such as airway smooth muscle and airway mucosal glands from inflammatory cells already at the airway mucosal site. Therefore, it is clear that glucocorticoids can work at several levels of the inflammatory process. More information will be gathered concerning the effect of inhaled glucocorticoids on the inflammatory process in asthma by examination of airway tissue or cells obtained by bronchoalveolar lavage. Whether all aspects of this process are reversed by glucocorticoids is not known. It is, for example, possible that the process of subepithelial fibrosis is particularly resistant, and it is known that glucocorticoids do not inhibit the release of factors that may be involved in fibrosis [118]. Although further research into the mechanisms of action of glucocorticoids in the airways is necessary, it is also important to examine their extrapulmonary actions such as those on bone or skin. Only then can differences in glucocorticoid mechanism of actions at different sites be identified and the hope for developing glucocorticoids with specific activity in the airways devoid of extrapulmonary side effects be fulfilled.

PHARMACOLOGY

Choice of Oral Glucocorticoid

A number of glucocorticoid preparations are available for the treatment of asthma. Modifications to the basic glucocorticoid molecule (Fig. 60-8) alter both the relative glucocorticoid and mineralocorticoid activities and the plasma and biologic half-lives of the compounds. The choice of an individual preparation depends on the desired biologic half-life (derived from its lymphopenic responses and adrenal suppressive activity) and its antiinflammatory action (Table 60-1).

Betamethasone, dexamethasone, and triamcinolone are inappropriate for use in asthma because their prolonged serum and biologic half-lives result in sustained adrenal suppression and pharmacologic effects, with increased potential for side effects. Prednisolone offers an acceptable balance between a moderately high antiinflammatory potency and a relatively short half-life, which allows recovery of the hypothalamic-pituitary-axis between doses.

Prednisone is inactive until it is reduced at the 11-keto position to form prednisolone in the liver. The former is preferred in some countries because its use theoretically avoids high local concentrations of biologically active glucocorticoid in the upper gastro-

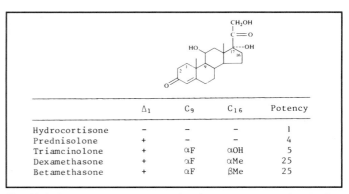

Fig. 60-8. *Basic steroid molecule with relative potencies and radical substitutions of the more common glucocorticoids. (Reprinted with permission from I. F. Skidmore. Anti-inflammatory steroids—the pharmacological and biochemical basis of clinical activity.* Molec. Aspects Med. *4:303, 1981.)*

intestinal tract. However, this consideration appears to be unimportant in clinical practice, and there are disadvantages of prednisone, including impairment of its conversion to prednisolone in liver disease [135], its production of 25 percent lower circulating prednisolone concentration than a comparable dose of prednisolone, and less reliable bioavailability. Other modifications to the glucocorticoid molecule have produced drugs suitable for inhaled use; this is discussed in Chapter 61.

ACTH therapy may be useful in the treatment of childhood asthma, as it may cause less growth disturbance and fewer cushingoid side effects than oral glucocorticoids. However, its disadvantages include the need for parenteral administration, a variable degree and duration of action, prominent androgenic side effects because of generalized adrenal cortical stimulation, and the development of ACTH antibodies following repeat injections.

Pharmacokinetics

Transport and Protein Binding

Glucocorticoids are transported in the circulation in both protein bound and free forms. About 92 percent is protein bound (77% to transcortin and 15% to albumin); the remaining 8 percent is free. Transcortin has a higher binding affinity for cortisol and prednisolone (about 2.5 times stronger) than for other synthetic glucocorticoids such as hydrocortisone [169] and methylprednisolone [184], although its plasma concentration is low. Conversely, albumin has a high plasma concentration but lower affinity for glucocorticoid binding.

Table 60-1. Properties of corticosteroid preparations

Steroid	Antiinflammatory relative potency	Plasma half-life (hr)	Biologic half-life (hr)	Equivalent dose (mg)	Sodium-retaining potency
Short acting					
Hydrocortisone	1	2	12	20.0	2+
Cortisone	0.8	0.5	*	25.0	2+
Intermediate acting					
Prednisone	3.5	1	*	5.0	1+
Prednisolone	4	2–3.5	12–36	5.0	1+
Triamcinolone	5	2–3.5	12–24	4.0	0
Methylprednisolone	5	2–3.5	12–36	4.0	0
Prolonged acting					
Betamethasone ⎱ Dexamethasone ⎰	25–30	5	24–48	0.6–0.75	0

* Prednisone and cortisone must be first converted to prednisolone and hydrocortisone before being active; the half-lives are then compared to the initial compound.

Plasma protein binding of prednisolone is nonlinear because of the high-affinity binding to transcortin [125]. As plasma concentration of prednisolone increases, the limited transcortin binding capacity is saturated and the amount of free drug in the plasma increases. Interestingly, although prednisolone inhibits prednisone binding to transcortin [21], prednisone does not displace prednisolone from plasma protein binding sites [124].

It is generally held that free (unbound) glucocorticoids are the biologically active form and, thus, that patients with hypoalbuminaemia and reduced protein binding will have increased side effects from glucocorticoid therapy. However, many studies have measured only total plasma prednisolone concentrations, and where total, free, and bound concentrations have been estimated, a wide range of free plasma prednisolone concentration has been noted at the same total plasma prednisolone concentration [189]. Studies have shown great within and between subject variability in binding of prednisolone to plasma proteins, possibly caused by changes in endogenous glucocorticoid levels, disease activity, and concomitant drug therapy. The variability in free and bound prednisolone concentrations is the likely explanation for the differing clinical effects in individual patients resulting from uniform prednisolone doses. However, it has also been shown that the development of steroid side effects correlates with slow rates of steroid catabolism, while the therapeutic response does not [114], and the one possible explanation for development of side effects may be failure of adaptation to prednisolone treatment by an increase in the rate of glucocorticoid catabolism.

Bioavailability

The various commercial preparations of both prednisolone [74] and prednisone [71] have similar bioavailability (i.e., the amount of the drug available to the tissues from an individual dose). However, the absorption of prednisolone from enteric-coated tablets, which are formulated to avoid upper gastrointestinal tract side effects, is impaired. Enteric-coated prednisolone tablets are associated with delayed and reduced peak concentrations in comparison with nonenteric-coated preparations. Nevertheless, the bioavailability of the two preparations is similar [157], and there seems to be little hard evidence to support the use of enteric-coated tablets, although some patients prefer them, claiming fewer side effects.

A number of factors may affect the bioavailability of prednisolone. It may be erratic following renal transplantation [97] and ileostomy [4], and it is possible, though unproved, that other small bowel abnormalities can produce poor absorption of enteric-coated prednisolone. The concomitant use of antacids [186] or cimetidine [146] does not affect the absorption of prednisolone. The effect of aging on prednisolone pharmacokinetics was studied by Stuck et al. [183]. It was shown that the interconversion of prednisone to prednisolone and vice versa was independent of age. Elderly subjects appear to have a higher concentration of total and free prednisolone after a given dose than younger subjects because of impaired metabolic clearance. However, despite increased exposure of target tissues to the free drug, there appears to be less suppression of endogenous plasma cortisol concentration following prednisolone than in younger subjects. The bioavailability of glucocorticoids in children is similar to that in adults.

The pharmacokinetics of glucocorticoids may be affected by a number of drugs. Clearance and volume of distribution of both total and unbound prednisolone may be decreased in women taking the oral contraceptive pill, while decreased unbound clearance may occur in patients taking conjugated estrogens [89]. Thus these drugs may expose patients to increased concentrations of unbound prednisolone for an increased time, with the potential for greater pharmacologic and toxic effects. The relationship between ketoconazole and glucocorticoids is un-

Table 60-2. Drug interactions

Drug	Effect with corticosteroids
Phenobarbital	Accelerated cortisol metabolism
Diphenylhydantoin	Accelerated cortisol metabolism
Ethyl biscoumacetate	Anticoagulant effect decreased
Salicylates	Increased renal clearance
Diuretics (except spironolactones)	Increased K^+ loss
Ephedrine	Decreased dexamethasone effect
Rifampin	Decreased corticosteroid effect

clear [198]. Other drugs known to affect the biologic actions of glucocorticoids are shown in Table 60-2.

It has been shown that free prednisolone clearance is increased in obese subjects and that endogenous cortisol (which is higher than normal before exogenous glucocorticoid therapy in obesity) is suppressed at the same rate as in the nonobese and returns to baseline more slowly [144]. This "hyperreactivity" of the adrenal gland in obesity offsets the increased clearance of free prednisolone, and adjustment of prednisolone dose is unnecessary in obese patients.

Differences in prednisolone bioavailability have been noted to be the cause of the "steroid resistance" seen in some asthmatic patients (see Chap. 79). However, in a study of 10 asthmatics whose disease was poorly controlled on oral glucocorticoids, measurements of total plasma clearance, plasma half-life, and volume of distribution were similar to those reported in normal volunteers and other asthmatics [147]. Similar results have been reported recently [5a, 43a]. It seems unlikely, therefore, that steroid resistance is caused by problems with the absorption and elimination of glucocorticoids. Interestingly, prednisolone pharmacokinetics are the same in patients with asthma and those with other steroid-treated disease, such as rheumatoid arthritis [185]; thus variations in the effectiveness of glucocorticoids in different inflammatory diseases do not appear to be caused by pharmacokinetic factors.

Dose-dependent Pharmacokinetics

Prednisolone dose increments do not result in proportionate increases in plasma prednisolone concentrations [140]. In one study, a sixteenfold increase in prednisolone dose from 5 to 80 mg resulted in only a sixfold increase in drug availability to the tissues, measured as area under the plasma concentration-time curve [140]. Thus, to double a clinical effect, a much greater proportionate increase in prednisolone dose would be required. Two other important factors in the pharmacokinetics of prednisolone are that its volume of distribution and systemic clearance both increase with increments of administered dose [140]. It is possible, though unproved, that these two effects act in opposition and serve to eliminate each other. The many variations in prednisolone pharmacokinetics explain why patients do not respond identically to a given dose of prednisolone. It follows that prednisolone therapy should be individually tailored, preferably with monitoring of plasma prednisolone concentrations.

Speed of Action

Glucocorticoid effects on plasma glucose concentration and circulating eosinophil counts occur within minutes of administration. However, changes in airflow in patients with asthma given glucocorticoids occur more slowly. Significant effects on spirometry can be measured about 60 minutes after 40 mg of prednisolone given intravenously, with maximal effects occurring at about 5 hours [40]. Following a similar dose of prednisolone given orally, a significant improvement was detected at 3 hours with a

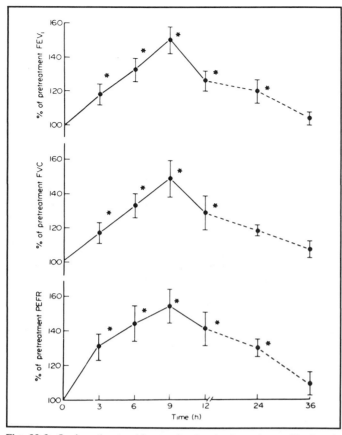

Fig. 60-9. *Oral corticosteroid rate of action in six patients with chronic asthma. Mean (± SEM) FEV_1, FVC, and PEFR values after a single oral dose of 40 mg of prednisolone. Time is after prednisolone administration, expressed as percentages of the immediate pretherapy data. (* = Significant differences at p < .05.) (Reprinted with permission from R. Ellul-Micallef et al. The time-course of response to prednisolone in chronic bronchial asthma. Clin. Sci. 47:105, 1974.)*

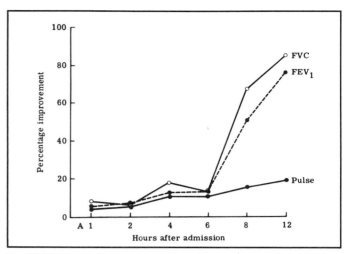

Fig. 60-10. *Percent improvement of cited rates in patients with acute severe asthma after commencing tetracosactrin or intravenous hydrocortisone. (Reprinted with permission from J. V. Collins et al. The use of corticosteroids in the treatment of acute asthma. Q. J. Med. New Series. 44:259, 1975.)*

maximal effect at 9 to 12 hours [56]. Fig. 60-9 illustrates the speed of action of oral prednisolone. Speed of glucocorticoid action may be slower in severe asthma; thus in patients unresponsive to initial beta agonist and theophylline therapy, intravenous hydrocortisone was associated with significant bronchodilation and reduction in pulse rate 6 to 8 hours after the start of glucocorticoid therapy [41] (Fig. 60-10). These differences in speed of action are probably of little clinical relevance, since studies [94, 107] have shown that the administration of glucocorticoids intravenously may offer no advantage over oral therapy in the initial treatment of severe asthma.

Oral Glucocorticoids and the Hypothalamic-Pituitary-Adrenal Axis

Hypothalamic-pituitary-adrenal (HPA) suppression by exogenous glucocorticoid may be reduced by giving the drug in the early morning to coincide with the peak release of ACTH from the pituitary and resultant production of cortisol by the adrenal gland (see Chap. 62). Administration of glucocorticoid later in the day is associated with greater suppression of endogenous cortisol production [60]. Shorter-acting glucocorticoids, such as prednisolone, given in the morning allow recovery of adrenal function before the next dose is given [52]. Conversely, adrenal suppression lasts about 14 hours after a longer-acting glucocorticoid (such as dexamethasone) given in the morning and 24 hours

or more after the same dose given at midnight. A further advantage of giving glucocorticoids as a single daily dose in the morning is the diurnal variation in protein binding, which results in a higher proportion of the drug being non-protein bound, and hence free, than at night [7].

Significant suppression of HPA axis begins when the dose of glucocorticoid is equivalent to daily endogenous glucocorticoid production; for prednisolone this is a dose of about 7.5 to 10.0 mg daily. Higher doses of glucocorticoid result in HPA suppression and adrenal atrophy, the degree of which depends on the time of the day the doses are given [150], the duration of therapy [187], the frequency of doses [63], and the total dosage of glucocorticoid [128]. The minimum duration of glucocorticoid therapy leading to HPA suppression is unknown; minor abnormalities are detectable a few days after starting glucocorticoid therapy, but recovery after short courses is rapid [44]. Significant HPA insufficiency with stress is rarely a problem after 2- to 3-week courses of steroid therapy; depressed basal plasma cortisol levels and decreased response to tetracosactin (synthetic ACTH) return to control levels within 3 days [192]. There is a consistent pattern of recovery after more prolonged HPA suppression (Fig. 60-11). Initially, ACTH levels rise while cortisol levels remain suppressed, and it may take 9 to 12 months for both to return to normal. Where glucocorticoid therapy has yielded levels within the physiologic range (prednisolone dose 7.5–10.0 mg daily) basal plasma cortisol levels usually return to the normal range within 1 month of the end of glucocorticoid therapy [128]. For higher doses and longer durations, insulin stress responses (and presumably clinical stress responses) may still be impaired 1 year after the end of therapy [187].

Attempts to accelerate recovery of HPA suppression using ACTH injections and various combinations for reducing glucocorticoids have proved to be ineffective [8]. The best policy for glucocorticoid withdrawal is slow reduction with tests of adrenal function at regular intervals. These may include measurements of basal plasma cortisol and urinary free cortisol levels and responses to tetracosactrin and insulin stress tests.

With respect to HPA suppression, the optimal scheme for tapering oral glucocorticoids after long-term use is unknown. At higher doses, the rate of reduction can be titrated against asthma control. Once the daily glucocorticoid dose is reduced to levels equivalent to physiologic output, tapering by 1 mg per day per month should allow HPA recovery to occur. If repeated tests

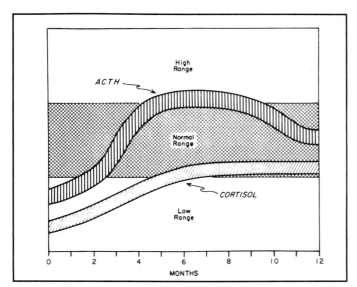

Fig. 60-11. *Hypothalamic-pituitary-adrenal axis recovery patterns following cessation of chronic glucocorticoid administration. (ACTH = adrenocorticotropic hormone.) (Reprinted with permission from R. G. Dluhy et al. Pharmacology and Chemistry of Adrenal Glucocorticoids. In D. L. Azarnoff [ed.], Steroid Therapy. Philadelphia: Saunders, 1975.)*

Table 60-3. Illustration of a program to transfer a patient from 50 mg of prednisone daily to alternate-day therapy* and further reduction after 10 days

Day	Rx mg	Day	Rx mg
1	60	8	10
2	40	9	95
3	70	10	5
4	30	11	85
5	80	12	5
6	20	13	80
7	90	14	5

*This changeover should not be initiated until the patient's symptoms are well controlled.

of adrenal function remain subnormal, further dose reductions should be delayed. Once oral glucocorticoids have been discontinued, adrenal response to ACTH or insulin should be assessed. If this is subnormal, patients should receive adequate replacement doses of glucocorticoid at times of stress, such as acute illness or surgery. It is advisable for the patient to carry a steroid identification card for at least 12 months after the end of long-term oral glucocorticoid therapy [8, 93].

Daily Versus Alternate-Day Therapy

In view of their half-life and duration of pharmacologic action, oral glucocorticoids do not need to be given more often than once daily. Furthermore, HPA suppression can be minimized by giving glucocorticoids as a single early-morning dose to coincide with the natural surge of ACTH production.

The successful use of alternate-day therapy in chronic skin conditions encouraged attempts to use glucocorticoids in this way in asthma. With alternate-day therapy, recovery of HPA function on the nontreatment day is possible [1], and the HPA response to provocation tests may be largely unimpaired [1, 95]. Improvements in both cushingoid features [8] and delayed hypersensitivity responses [134] occur with a change from daily to alternate-day therapy. Further, leukocyte counts, inflammatory responses, and neutrophil half-life, which are impaired on the glucocorticoid day, return to normal on the "off" day [47]. A lowered incidence of infection has been reported with alternate-day therapy [8], partly because of restoration of neutrophil kinetics [47] and the preservation of delayed hypersensitivity responses [62]. Although alternate-day therapy will clearly reduce glucocorticoid complications, its effectiveness in asthma is not well established. Many comparisons of daily and alternate-day therapy [60, 95] have been open to criticism on methodologic grounds, although the satisfactory use of an alternate-day regimen was demonstrated by the study of McAllister [139]. It is not understood why the asthma of some patients, but not others, can be controlled by an alternate-day regimen. Greenberger et al. [85] showed that volume of distribution, half-life, and clearance of prednisolone were the same in patients receiving either daily

or alternate-day regimens, suggesting that differences in pharmacokinetics do not explain requirements for different regimens in similar patients.

When a glucocorticoid is used in an alternate-day regimen, the total dose given should be the sum of the daily doses or somewhat greater. A sample schedule for conversion from a daily to an alternate-day regimen is shown in Table 60-3.

DOSAGE SCHEDULES FOR GLUCOCORTICOIDS IN ASTHMA

Systemic oral glucocorticoids are generally used in the treatment of asthma in two situations: (1) in short courses for exacerbations of asthma that is usually well controlled by inhalers and (2) as maintenance therapy for patients whose disease cannot be stabilized for any reason with inhalers alone. In either situation, the aim is to elevate plasma glucocorticoid levels either by stimulation of endogenous glucocorticoid production (for example, using adrenocorticotrophin or its synthetic analogues) or by provision of exogenous glucocorticoid. There are no firm rules derived from experimental data that determine the choice of dose and route of administration in a given situation.

Exacerbation of Previously Stable Asthma

Acute Severe Asthma (Status Asthmaticus)

Glucocorticoids have been used in the initial treatment of acute severe asthma for many years, and most clinicians would regard this drug as an essential part of its management. The validity of this practice has been addressed by a number of studies. Fanta and colleagues [61] showed that the addition of intravenous hydrocortisone (2 mg/kg loading dose followed by 0.5 mg/kg/hr for 24 hours) was associated with an increased rate of recovery in patients unresponsive to bronchodilators, although benefits were not demonstrated until 12 hours after treatment started. These findings have been supported by the results of other studies in which intravenous methylprednisolone added to bronchodilator therapy resulted in reduced hospital admission rates [96, 127, 177]. Conversely, others have found that early use of intravenous glucocorticoids does not affect hospital admission rates [94, 182], and furthermore, in a study of patients admitted to hospital with severe acute asthma [131], those treated without glucocorticoids had a similar outcome to controls treated conventionally with intravenous hydrocortisone. The author of this report suggested not only that glucocorticoids were of doubtful value in severe acute asthma, but also that the wide use of glucocorticoids in general might have contributed to some asthma deaths. This study was much criticized [84], particularly because the patients not given glucocorticosteroid treatment had a higher rate of mechanical ventilation, which might have been reduced by gluco-corticoid treatment; indeed, many studies have suggested that underuse of glucocorticoids is an important factor associated with asthma deaths [24].

The differences between the studies described are difficult to reconcile, since varying bronchodilator regimens, hospital admission criteria, and follow-up policies were used. Nevertheless, while there is no conclusive proof that systemic glucocorticoids are an essential part of the management of severe acute asthma, most clinicians would consider it unethical to withhold this form of therapy.

It is common practice in severe acute asthma to start treatment with intravenous hydrocortisone. However, provided the patient is able to take tablets, there is good evidence that patients given intravenous glucocorticosteroids fare no better than those given oral glucocorticoids. However, if intravenous glucocorticoids are deemed to be necessary, there is little evidence to dictate which regimen should be used. Recommended intravenous dosages have varied between 100 mg and 1,000 mg in 24 hours [83, 165], although it has been shown that sufficiently high plasma cortisol levels can be achieved using 4 mg/kg body weight given every 4 to 6 hours [41], and this dose has been found to be effective in large numbers of patients [40]. Furthermore, a more recent study comparing 6 and 80 mg/kg/day of hydrocortisone given in four divided doses showed that the extremely high dose conferred no additional benefits [163]. Even doses as low as 50 mg of hydrocortisone intravenously 4 times a day was found to be as effective in resolving acute severe asthma as 200 mg or 500 mg of hydrocortisone 4 times a day [21a].

It is possible that individual patients with severe acute asthma differ in their responsiveness to systemic glucocorticoids. Those who have previously taken glucocorticoids may need higher doses [165], and four different patterns of glucocorticoid requirement were described by Cayton and Howard [32]. However, any enhancement of glucocorticoid clearance in patients who have previously taken the drug does not significantly reduce plasma levels after intravenous hydrocortisone [41] (Fig. 60-12). Further-

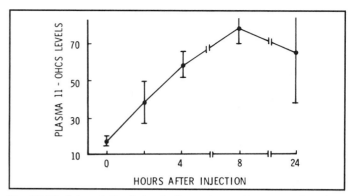

Fig. 60-13. *Adrenal stimulation in five patients with status asthmaticus. Group mean ± 1 S.D. After an initial depot injection of tetracosactrin (1 mg), plasma cortisol levels are depicted. (Reprinted with permission from J. V. Collins et al. The use of corticosteroids in the treatment of acute asthma. Q. J. Med. New Series 44:259, 1975.)*

more, glucocorticoid doses necessary to obtain sustained therapeutic responses are unrelated to either previous corticosteroid doses or HPA status. The use of a loading dose followed by a continuous infusion rather than intermittent injection may allow reduced daily doses of hydrocortisone while maintaining plasma cortisol levels.

Treatment with tetracosactrin, a synthetic ACTH preparation, is an effective alternative to hydrocortisone in the treatment of severe acute asthma [41] (Figs. 60-13 and 60-14). However, this treatment has increased side effects and probably should not be used in preference to hydrocortisone unless the patient is known to have normal adrenal function, has not previously taken glucocorticoids, and is thus free of the possibility of an inadequate adrenal response to stimulation.

Factors that might affect responses to systemic glucocorticoids in acute severe asthma include the mode of onset and duration of the attack [16] and variations in the relative contributions of the pathologic features of asthma and its trigger factors (for example, viral infections may provoke more prolonged and difficult airways obstruction [125]). Patients who have deteriorated rapidly may improve more quickly than those with prolonged attacks, in whom resistant airway narrowing and retention of secretions are more likely to be present and influence treatment response. Studies in both children [158] and adults [169] seem to indicate just such differences in responsiveness.

A recent randomized, double-blind study evaluated the preventative benefit to early asthma relapse after a short course of oral prednisone (40 mg tapered to 0 mg over an 8-day period) given to patients treated in the emergency room for an acute exacerbation of asthma [34]. These patients also received regular antiasthma maintenance therapy during this trial period. A significantly reduced rate of relapse compared to a control group (placebo) was observed. Despite certain study limitations, including the optimal glucocorticoid regimen (dosage and duration) under these conditions, a short course of prednisone may be a useful way to reduce relapse rates after therapy for acute asthma, this beneficial effect being limited to the period of steroid administration and the follow-up of 21 days (Fig. 60-15).

The optimal duration of intravenous glucocorticoid treatment in acute severe asthma is unknown and is probably irrelevant, since it can be replaced by oral glucocorticoids as soon as the patient is able to take treatment by mouth. An initial oral prednisolone dose of 40 to 80 mg daily has been shown to be associated with sustained improvement [25]. There are numerous schedules for tapering oral glucocorticoids in these circumstances. Lederle and colleagues [122] compared a 1-week and a 7-week tapering regimen in a double-blind trial of patients recovering from acute

Fig. 60-12. *Effects of previous corticosteroid treatment on cortisol handling. Plasma half-life of hydrocortisone measured after a single intravenous injection of hydrocortisone, 4 mg/kg body weight in healthy subjects and in patients with severe asthma who had never received previous corticosteroid treatment or had been maintained for at least 6 months with daily doses of prednisolone of 5 to 10 mg (mean 9 mg) or more than 10 mg (mean 16 mg). Results for individuals are shown, and group mean values are shown by bars. The differences for group mean or S.D. between any two groups were not significant at the 10-percent level, and the plasma hydrocortisone levels at any time 6 hours after the injection were also not significantly different between any two groups. (Reprinted with permission from J. V. Collins et al. The use of corticosteroids in the treatment of acute asthma. Q. J. Med. New Series 44:259, 1975.)*

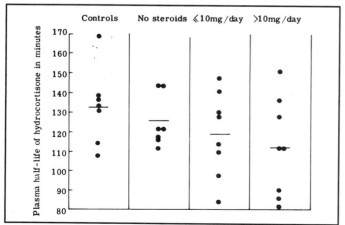

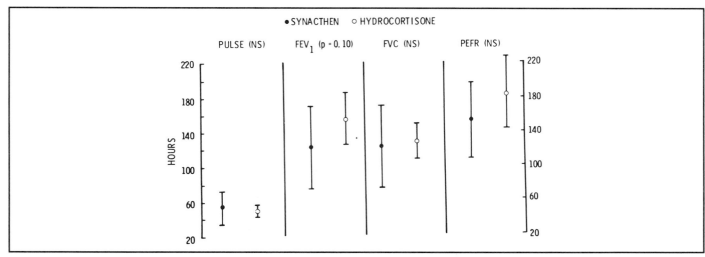

Fig. 60-14. *Comparison of intravenous hydrocortisone (nine patients) and adrenal stimulation with Synacthen (five patients) in status asthmaticus. Time to attain maximum improvement in cited parameters is shown. Group mean ± SEM. (Reprinted with permission from J. V. Collins and D. Jones. Corticosteroid Mechanisms and Therapeutic Schedules. In E. B. Weiss [ed.], Status Asthmaticus. Baltimore: University Park, 1978.)*

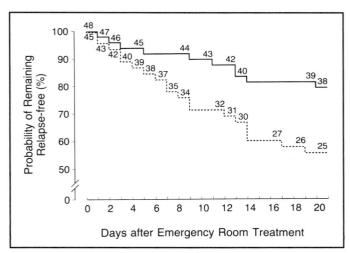

Fig. 60-15. *Kaplan-Meier survival curve showing the probability of remaining relapse-free after emergency room treatment for patients receiving prednisone (solid line) and those receiving placebo (broken line). Values shown are numbers of subjects remaining relapse-free at the beginning of the days on which a relapse occurred. (Reprinted with permission from K. R. Chapman et al. Effect of a short course of prednisone in the prevention of early relapse after the emergency room treatment of acute asthma. N. Engl. J. Med. 324:788, 1991.)*

severe asthma. There was no difference between the two groups with respect to asthma relapse rate, but patients in the prolonged tapering group reported steroid side effects more frequently. The authors' own preference is to continue a high dose until the peak flow has reached the patient's usual best value and then to withdraw glucocorticoids rapidly using peak flow recordings as a guide to response. Aerosol glucocorticoid therapy can be recommenced promptly to facilitate withdrawal of systemic glucocorticoids.

Subacute Asthma

Many exacerbations of asthma do not require in-hospital management, and it is common practice to treat subacute attacks at home with short courses of oral glucocorticoids. The value of

this approach was confirmed by Fiel and colleagues [64] in a study of patients who were treated in an accident and emergency department and then discharged with or without oral methylprednisolone. Patients who received oral glucocorticoids had fewer relapses and less respiratory symptoms than controls given placebo. Short courses of oral glucocorticoids have also been shown to be more effective than single intravenous boluses of methylprednisolone [163], which appeared in this study to offer little advantage over treatment with bronchodilators alone.

The dose response of patients to short courses of oral prednisolone during exacerbations of subacute asthma was studied by Webb [193], who further confirmed the value of oral glucocorticoids in these circumstances and suggested that a minimum daily prednisolone dose of 0.6 mg/kg body weight for a period up to 2 weeks should be used. This recommendation is supported by other studies [32, 56, 191], which suggests that a suitable starting dose of prednisolone for most patients with subacute asthma attacks would be 40 mg daily. There is ample evidence to support the value of administering oral glucocorticoids once daily rather than in divided doses (see Pharmacology).

Although the ideal rate of withdrawal of systemic glucocorticoids in these circumstances is unknown, treatment can be reduced rapidly (providing inhaled glucocorticoids have been continued) using peak flow recordings as a guide. Satisfactory recovery of the HPA axis can be expected when systemic glucocorticoid treatment has not lasted more than 3 weeks [191]. Attempts have been made to identify patients who are most likely to relapse after subacute asthma attacks so that short courses of oral glucocorticoids can be "targeted." However, the liberal use of a short course of oral glucocorticoids seems fully justified in view of current concepts of the inflammatory nature of asthma and the possible links between underuse of glucocorticoids and asthma deaths [24].

Chronic Asthma

Long-term treatment with oral glucocorticoids should be necessary for only a minority of asthmatics because of the development of high-dose glucocorticoid inhalers. Such patients should be maintained on the lowest doses compatible with good asthma control. Frequent attempts to reduce the oral glucocorticoid dose should be made, and reduction rates of 1 mg per month are sometimes helpful. An alternate-day regimen should be adopted where possible.

The natural history of patients requiring long-term oral glucocorticoids was reported by Dykewicz and associates [55]; a review of 40 asthmatics who had taken oral prednisolone for a mean of 6.2 years showed that 10 were able to stop systemic glucocorticoids completely following improvement in their asthma while 3 had increased steroid requirements. This optimistic report may not support the experience of many clinicians who care for a number of asthmatics whose disease control deteriorates markedly when small adjustments are made to the oral glucocorticoid regimen. "Steroid sparing" agents, such as methotrexate and troleandomycin, may also be valuable in selected patients; the use of these drugs is discussed in Chapters 67 and 68.

Some authors believe that intramuscular injection of triamcinolone acetonide allows reduction in prednisolone dose in chronic asthma [141, 193], although the use of this drug is associated with an increased incidence of cutaneous side effects and carries a greater risk of inducing proximal myopathy. Oral or parenteral betamethasone may be used effectively instead of prednisolone in some chronic asthmatics [82].

In a 1991 study the effect of high-dose intramuscular triamcinolone (360 mg over the first 3 days) was compared with oral prednisone (median dose 12.5 mg/day) in chronic, severe life-threatening asthma. High-dose intramuscular triamcinolone was found to be more effective in terms of improved pulmonary function, reduction in emergency room visits and hospitalizations, and reduction in asthma medication requirements. Steroid side effects noted in both treated groups was greater in the triamcinolone group [151]. However, the authors cautioned that further data regarding optimal dosages, preparations, and mode of administration needed to be clarified and such administrations should be utilized only in patients with evidence of reversibility.

COMPLICATIONS OF ORAL GLUCOCORTICOID THERAPY

The potential problems of using long-term oral glucocorticoids in the treatment of asthma are legion and are the same as those encountered in a variety of other diseases (Table 60-4). The overall incidence of glucocorticoid-induced complications in asthma is difficult to assess, since reports vary with respect to the diligence with which complications are sought and the statistical methods and control data used. This is exemplified by the relationship between glucocorticoids and peptic ulceration; in a review of the literature Guss and colleagues [86] noted that many reports were anecdotal and concluded that, contrary to widely held opinion, there is no significant increase in incidence of peptic ulceration in glucocorticoid-treated asthmatics. However, as a general rule, the incidence of complications is proportional to the dose of glucocorticoid used and the patient's age [48]. The relationship to duration of therapy is unclear; some reports have suggested that duration of therapy per se is unimportant [48], while Kwong et al. [117] showed that both ocular and skeletal complications are directly related to total lifetime dosage of corticosteroids.

The general relationship between long-term oral glucocorticoid treatment and osseous complications has been the subject of a number of reviews [13, 130, 178]. The incidence of osteoporosis in Cushing's disease is about 50 percent. However, its incidence in glucocorticoid-treated asthmatics is unknown, although Adinoff [3] found rib or vertebral fractures in 11 percent of 128 patients over 40 years of age who had taken alternate-day glucocorticoids for at least 1 year. It was also shown in this study

Table 60-4. Complications of corticosteroid therapy

Musculoskeletal
  Myopathy
  Osteoporosis—vertebral compression fractures
  Aseptic necrosis of bone
Gastrointestinal
  Peptic ulceration (often gastric)
  Gastric hemorrhage
  Intestinal perforation
  Pancreatitis
Central nervous system
  Psychiatric disorders
  Pseudotumor cerebri
Ophthalmologic
  Glaucoma
  Posterior subcapsular cataracts
Cardiovascular and renal
  Hypertension
  Sodium and water retention—edema
  Hypokalemic alkalosis
Metabolic
  Precipitation of clinical manifestations of genetic diabetes mellitus including ketoacidosis
  Hyperosmolar nonketotic coma
  Hyperlipidemia
  Induction of centripetal obesity
Endocrine
  Growth failure
  Secondary amenorrhea
  Suppression of HPA system
Inhibition of fibroplasia
  Impaired wound healing
  Subcutaneous tissue atrophy
Suppression of the immune response
  Superimposition of a variety of bacterial, fungal, viral, and parasitic infections in steroid-treated patients

that, while bone density was subnormal in glucocorticoid-treated asthmatics, there was no significant correlation with dose or duration of therapy. These results were confirmed by Reid and colleagues [167] in a study that also showed that the reduction in total body calcium in asthmatics treated with oral glucocorticoids (mean daily dose 6.8 mg, mean duration of treatment 12.5 years) was the same as that measured in glucocorticoid-treated patients with rheumatoid arthritis, suggesting that the drug rather than the disease was responsible for demineralization of bone.

The optimal prophylactic and treatment regimens for glucocorticoid-induced bone complications are unknown. Glucocorticoid dose reduction and the use of alternate-day regimens may be helpful, although accelerated bone loss may still occur with low doses, especially in men and postmenopausal women. The study of Reid et al. [167] suggested that the addition of oral calcium supplements was associated with the maintenance of a higher bone mass. However, this was not observed by other studies that suggested that calcitonin injections might be helpful [129]. Other prophylactic possibilities include etidronate, vitamin D and its metabolites, and thiazide diuretics [130]. Hormone replacement therapy should be considered for postmenopausal women receiving long-term glucocorticoids.

Neither the incidence of myopathy in glucocorticoid-treated asthmatics nor the dose at which it is likely to occur are well defined. Bowyer and associates [22] found that 64 percent (16/25) of asthmatics taking more than 40 mg of prednisolone daily had evidence of hip flexor weakness, while muscle weakness was found in only one patient taking less than 30 mg daily, although the duration of treatment was not clear from the paper. Myopathy associated with hydrocortisone therapy also appears to be dose related [178], and the implication of these studies is that an alternative explanation should be considered for myopathy occurring in patients taking relatively low doses of systemic glucocorticoid. Severe generalized myopathy has also been described in patients with asthma who have received high doses of corticosteroids and who have been on mechanical ventilation [178]. It is possible that this acute form of myopathy observed during the treatment of status asthmaticus is the combined effects of corticosteroids and muscle relaxant drugs on the muscle cell [85a].

Complications generally seem to occur less frequently if glucocorticoid doses are maintained below a daily dose of prednisolone of 15 mg (or equivalent), although the clinician should remain vigilant for problems in all asthmatics receiving oral glucocorticoids. The incidence of complications is reduced if alternate-day therapy is adopted. In a review of 85 glucocorticoid-treated asthmatics, whose mean alternate-day prednisolone dosage was 26.2 mg and duration of therapy was 3.2 years, the prevalence of hypertension, peptic ulcer disease, pathologic fracture, and psychosis was not significantly greater than in a control population [66]. A recent review discusses the prevention and treatment of glucocorticoid-induced osteoporosis [199].

Systemic glucocorticoids continue to have an important role in the management of asthma. The pharmacokinetics of this group of drugs are complex and variable, partly explaining interpatient differences in dose responsiveness and susceptibility to side effects.

Oral glucocorticoids are of definite benefit in the management of exacerbations of previously stable asthma and are essential for the long-term management of a minority of patients whose disease cannot be controlled by other means. The complications of systemic glucocorticoid therapy are well-known and potentially serious; they may be minimized by careful clinical practice. There is clearly a need for the development of both better methods of prophylaxis against glucocorticoid-induced side effects and effective alternative antiinflammatory agents for use in asthma. Alternatively, glucocorticoids with specific activity in the airways and devoid of extra-pulmonary side effects should be developed.

REFERENCES

1. Ackerman, G. L., and Nolan, C. M. Adrenocortical responsiveness after alternate-day corticosteroid therapy. *N. Engl. J. Med.* 278:405, 1968.
2. Adelroth, E., et al. Inflammatory cells and eosinophilic activity in asthmatics investigated by bronchoalveolar lavage: The effects of antiasthmatic treatment with budesonide or terbutaline. *Am. Rev. Respir. Dis.* 142:91, 1990.
3. Adinoff, A. D., and Hollister, J. R. Steroid-induced fractures and bone loss in patients with asthma. *N. Engl. J. Med.* 309:265, 1983.
4. Al-Habet, S., et al. Malabsorption of prednisolone from enteric coated tablets after ileostomy. *Br. Med. J.* 281:843, 1980.
5. Altman, L. C., et al. Effect of corticosteroids on eosinophil chemotaxis and adherence. *J. Clin. Invest.* 67:28, 1981.
5a. Alvarez, J., et al. Steroid-resistant asthma: Immunologic and pharmacologic features. *J. Allergy Clin. Immunol.* 89:714, 1992.
6. Ambrose, M. P., and Hunninghake, G. W. Corticosteroids increase lipocortin 1 in alveolar epithelial cells. *Am. J. Respir. Cell Mol. Biol.* 3:349, 1990.
7. Angeli, A., et al. Diurnal variation of prednisolone binding to serum corticosteroid binding globulin in man. *Clin. Pharmacol. Ther.* 23:47, 1978.
7a. Arai, K., et al. Cytokines: Coordinators of immune and inflammatory responses. *Ann. Rev. Biochem.* 59:783, 1990.
8. Axelrod, L. Glucocorticoid therapy. *Medicine* (Baltimore) 55:39, 1976.
9. Ballard, P. L., et al. General presence of glucocorticoid receptors in responsive mammalian tissues. *Endocrinology* 94:998, 1974.
10. Balter, M. S., Eschenbacher, W. L., and Peters-Golden, M. Arachidonic acid metabolism in cultured alveolar macrophages from normal, atopic and asthmatic subjects. *Am. Rev. Respir. Dis.* 138:1134, 1988.
11. Barach, A. L., Bickerman, H. A., and Beck, G. J. Clinical and physiological studies on the use of metacortandracin in respiratory disease: 1. Bronchial asthma. *Dis. Chest* 27:515, 1955.
12. Bascomb, R., et al. Basophil influx occurs after nasal antigen challenge: Effect of topical corticosteroid therapy. *J. Allergy Clin. Immunol.* 81:580, 1988.
13. Baylink, D. J. Glucocorticoid-induced osteoporosis. *N. Engl. J. Med.* 309:306, 1983.
14. Beasley, R., et al. Cellular events in the bronchi in mild asthma and after bronchial provocation. *Am. Rev. Respir. Dis.* 139:806, 1989.
15. Befus, D., et al. Mast cell heterogeneity in man. *Int. Arch. Allergy Appl. Immunol.* 76:232, 1985.
16. Bellamy, D., and Collins, J. V. "Acute" asthma in adults. *Thorax* 34:36, 1979.
17. Besedovsky, H., et al. Immunoregulatory feedback between interleukin-1 and glucocorticoid hormones. *Science* 233:652, 1986.
18. Bhagat, R. G., and Grunstein, M. M. Effect of corticosteroids on bronchial responsiveness to methacholine in asthmatic children. *Am. Rev. Respir. Dis.* 131:902, 1985.
19. Bordley, J. E., et al. Preliminary observations on the effect of adrenocorticotrophic hormone (ACTH) in allergic disease. *Bull. Johns Hopkins Hosp.* 85:396, 1949.
20. Boschetto, P., Rogers, D. F., and Barnes, P. J. Inhibition of airway microvascular leakage by corticosteroids. *Thorax* 44:320, 1989.
21. Boudinot, F. D., and Jusko, W. J. Plasma protein binding interaction of prednisone and prednisolone. *J. Steroid Biochem.* 21:337, 1984.
21a. Bowler, S. D., Mitchell, C. A., and Armstrong, J. G. Corticosteroids in acute severe asthma: Effectiveness of low doses. *Thorax* 47:584, 1992.
22. Bowyer, S. L., LaMothe, M. P., and Hollister, J. R. Steroid myopathy: Incidence and detection in a population with asthma. *J. Allergy Clin. Immunol.* 76:234, 1985.
23. Brattsand, R., and Pipkorn, U. Glucocorticoids: Experimental Approaches. In M. A. Kaliner, P. J. Barnes, and C. G. A. Persson (eds.), *Asthma: Its Pathology and Treatment.* New York: Marcel Dekker, 1990. Pp. 667–709.
24. British Thoracic Society. Deaths from asthma in two regions of England. *Br. Med. J.* 285:1251, 1982.
25. Britton, M. G., et al. High dose corticosteroids in severe acute asthma. *Br. Med. J.* 2:73, 1976.
26. Brocbank, W., and Pengelly, C. D. R. Chronic asthma treated with powder inhalations of hydrocortisone and prednisolone. *Lancet* 1:187, 1958.
26a. Broide, D. H., and Firestein, G. S. Endobronchial allergen challenge: Demonstration of cellular source of granulocyte macrophage colony-stimulating factor by in-situ hybridization. *J. Clin. Invest.* 88:1084, 1991.
26b. Broide, D. H., et al. Cytokines in symptomatic asthmatic airways. *J. Allergy Clin. Immunol.* 89:958, 1992.
27. Bronnegard, M., et al. Human calpactin II (lipocortin 1) messenger ribonucleic acid is not induced by glucocorticoids. *Mol. Endocrinol.* 2:732, 1988.
28. Brown, H. M. The Introduction and Early Development of Inhaled Steroid Treatment. In N. Mygind and T. J. H. Clark (eds.), *Topical Steroid Treatment for Asthma and Rhinitis.* London: Tindall, 1980. Pp. 66–76.
28a. Burke, C., et al. Lung function and immunopathological changes after inhaled corticosteroid therapy in asthma. *Eur. Respir. J.* 5:73, 1992.
29. Burrage, W. S., and Irwin, J. W. Hydrocortisone in the therapy of asthma. *Ann. N. Y. Acad. Sci.* 66:37, 1955.
30. Carryer, H. M., et al. Effects of cortisone on bronchial asthma and hay fever occurring in subjects sensitive to ragweed pollen. *Proc. Mayo Clin.* 25:482, 1950.
31. Casale, T. B., et al. Elevated bronchoalveolar lavage fluid histamine levels in allergic asthmatics are associated with methacholine bronchial hyperresponsiveness. *J. Clin. Invest.* 79:1197, 1987.
32. Cayton, R., and Howard, P. Plasma cortisol and the use of hydrocortisone in treatment of status asthmaticus. *Thorax* 28:567, 1973.
33. Chanez, P., et al. Generation of oxygen free radicals from asthma patients after stimulation with platelet-activating factor and phorbol ester. *Eur. Resp. J.* 3:1002, 1990.
34. Chapman, K. R., et al. Effect of a short course of prednisone in the prevention of early relapse after the emergency room treatment of acute asthma. *N. Engl. J. Med.* 324:788, 1991.
35. Chung, K. F. Role played by inflammation in the hyperreactivity of the airways in asthma. *Thorax* 41:657, 1986.
36. Chung, K. F. Inflammatory Mediators in Asthma. In P. O'Byrne (ed.), *Asthma as an Inflammatory Disease.* New York: Marcel Dekker, 1990. Pp. 159–184.

37. Chung, K. F., et al. The role of increased microvascular permeability and plasma exudation in asthma. *Eur. Respir. J.* 3:329, 1990.

38. Cirino, E., et al. Human recombinant lipocortin 1 has acute local antiinflammatory properties in the rat paw edema test. *Proc. Natl. Acad. Sci. U.S.A.* 86:3428, 1989.

39. Cockroft, D. W., and Murdoch, K. Y. Comparative effects of inhaled salbutamol, sodium cromoglycate and BDP on allergen-induced early asthmatic responses, late asthmatic responses and increased bronchial responsiveness to histamine. *J. Allergy Clin. Immunol.* 79:734, 1987.

40. Collins, J. V., and Jones, D. Corticosteroids in the treatment of severe acute asthma. *Acta Tuberc. Pneumol. Belg.* 68:63, 1977.

41. Collins, J. V., et al. The use of corticosteroids in the treatment of acute asthma. *Q. J. Med.* 44:259, 1975.

42. Collins, S., Caron, M. G., and Lefkowitz, K. F. Beta$_2$-adrenergic receptors in hamster smooth muscle cells are transcriptionally regulated by glucocorticoids. *J. Biol. Chem.* 263:9067, 1988.

43. Corrigan, C. J., and Kay, A. B. CD4 T-lymphocyte activation in acute severe asthma. *Am. Rev. Respir. Dis.* 141:970, 1990.

43a. Corrigan, C. J., et al. Glucocorticoid resistance in chronic asthma: Glucocorticoid pharmacokinetics, glucocorticoid receptor characteristics and inhibition of peripheral blood T-lymphocyte proliferation by glucocorticoids in vitro. *Am. Rev. Respir. Dis.* 144:1016, 1991.

44. Corticosteroids and hypothalamic-pituitary-adrenocortical function. *Br. Med. J.* 1:813, 1980.

45. Culpepper, J. A., and Lee, F. Regulation of IL-3 expression by glucocorticoids in cloned murine T-lymphocytes. *J. Immunol.* 135:3191, 1985.

46. Dahl, R., and Johansson, S.-A. Importance of duration of treatment with inhaled budesonide on the immediate and late bronchial reaction. *Eur. J. Respir. Dis.* 62 (Suppl. 122):167, 1982.

47. Dale, D. C., Fauci, A. S., and Wolff, S. M. Alternate-day prednisone: Leucocyte kinetics and susceptibility to infection. *N. Engl. J. Med.* 291:1154, 1974.

48. David, D. S., Grieco, M. H., and Cushman, P. Adrenal glucocorticoids after 20 years: A review of their clinically relevant consequences. *J. Chronic Dis.* 22:637, 1970.

49. Davies, A. O., and Lefkowitz, R. J. Regulation of beta-adrenergic receptors by steroid hormones. *Ann. Rev. Physiol.* 46:119, 1984.

50. Davies, C., and Conolly, M. E. Tachyphylaxis to β-adrenoceptor agonists in human bronchial smooth muscle. *Br. J. Clin. Pharmacol.* 40:417, 1990.

51. De Baets, F. M., Goeteyn, M., and Kerrebijn, K. F. The effect of two months of treatment with inhaled budesonide on bronchial responsiveness to histamine and house-dust mite antigen in asthmatic children. *Am. Rev. Respir. Dis.* 142:581, 1990.

51a. Diamond, M. I., et al. Transcription factor interactions: Selectors of positive and negative regulation from a single DNA element. *Science* 246:1266, 1990.

52. Di Raimondo, V. C., and Forsham, P. H. Some clinical implications of the spontaneous diurnal variation in adrenal cortical secretory activity. *J. Clin. Endocrinol.* 16:622, 1956.

52a. Djukanovic, R., et al. The effect of an inhaled corticosteroid on airway inflammation and symptoms in asthma. *Am. Rev. Respir. Dis.* 145:669, 1992.

53. Durham, S. R., and Kay, A. B. Eosinophils, bronchial hyperreactivity and late-phase asthmatic reactions. *Clin. Allergy* 15:411, 1985.

54. Du Toit, J. I., Salome, C. M., and Woolcock, A. J. Inhaled corticosteroids reduce the severity of bronchial hyperresponsiveness in asthma, but oral theophylline does not. *Am. Rev. Respir. Dis.* 136:1174, 1987.

55. Dykewicz, M. S., et al. Natural history of asthma in patients requiring long-term systemic corticosteroids. *Arch. Intern. Med.* 146:2369, 1986.

56. Ellul-Michallef, R., Borthwick, R. C., and McHardy, G. J. R. Time course of response to prednisolone in chronic bronchial asthma. *Clin. Sci.* 47:105, 1974.

57. Ellul-Micallef, R., and Fenech, F. F. Effect of intravenous prednisolone in asthmatics with diminished adrenergic responsiveness. *Lancet* 2:1269, 1975.

58. Evans, P. M., Barnes, P. J., and Chung, K. F. Inhibition of human eosinophil superoxide anion production by dexamethasone. *Br. J. Pharmacol.* 100:446P, 1990.

59. Fabbri, L. M., Chiesura-Corona, P., and Dalvecchio, L. Prednisolone inhibits late asthmatic reactions and the associated increase in airway responsiveness induced by toluene diisocyanate in sensitized subjects. *Am. Rev. Respir. Dis.* 132:1010, 1985.

60. Falliers, C. J., et al. Pulmonary and adrenal effects of alternate-day corticosteroid therapy. *J. Allergy Clin. Immunol.* 49:156, 1972.

61. Fanta, C. H., Rossing, T. H., and McFadden, E. J. R. Glucocorticoids in acute asthma: A clinical controlled trial. *Am. J. Med.* 74:845, 1983.

62. Fauci, A. S., and Dale, D. C. Alternate-day prednisone therapy and human lymphocyte subpopulations. *J. Clin. Invest.* 55:22, 1975.

63. Fauci, A. S., Dale, D. C., and Balow, J. E. Glucocorticosteroid therapy: Mechanism of action and clinical considerations. *Ann. Intern. Med.* 84:304, 1976.

64. Fiel, S. B., et al. Efficacy of short-term corticosteroid therapy in outpatient treatment of acute bronchial asthma. *Am. J. Med.* 75:259, 1983.

65. Firestone, G. L., Payvar, F., and Yamamoto, K. R. Glucocorticoid regulation of protein processing and compartmentalization. *Nature* 300:221, 1982.

66. Fitzsimons, R., et al. Prevalence of adverse effects in corticosteroid dependent asthma. *N. Engl. Reg. Allergy Proc.* 9:157, 1988.

67. Flint, K. C., et al. Bronchoalveolar mast cells in extrinsic asthma: Mechanism for the initiation of antigen specific bronchoconstriction. *Br. Med. J.* 291:923, 1985.

68. Flower, R. J. Lipocortin and the mechanism of action of the glucocorticoids. *Br. J. Pharmacol.* 94:987, 1988.

69. Flower, R. J., et al. Comparison of the acute inflammatory response in adrenalectomized and sham-operated rats. *Br. J. Pharmacol.* 87:57, 1986.

70. Foulds, W. S., et al. Hydrocortisone in treatment of allergic conjunctivitis, allergic rhinitis and bronchial asthma. *Lancet* 1:234, 1955.

71. Francisco, G. E., et al. In vitro and in vivo bioequivalence of commercial prednisone tablets. *Biopharm. Drug Dispos.* 5:335, 1984.

72. Fraser, C. M., and Venter, J. C. The synthesis of β-adrenergic receptors in cultured human lung cells: Induction by glucocorticoids. *Biochem. Biophys. Res. Commun.* 94:390, 1980.

73. Fuller, R. W., et al. Dexamethasone inhibits the production of thromboxane B2 and leukotriene B4 by human alveolar macrophages in culture. *Clin. Sci.* 67:653, 1984.

74. Gambertoglio, J. G., Amend, W. J. C., and Benet, L. Z. Pharmacokinetics and bioavailability of prednisone and prednisolone in healthy volunteers and patients: A review. *J. Pharmacokinet. Biopharm.* 8:1, 1980.

75. Geddes, B. A., et al. Interaction of glucocorticoids and bronchodilators on isolated guinea pig trachea and human bronchial smooth muscle. *Am. Rev. Respir. Dis.* 110:420, 1974.

76. Giguere, V., et al. Functional domains of the human glucocorticoid receptor. *Cell* 46:645, 1986.

77. Gilberstein, D. S., et al. Enhancement of human eosinophil cytotoxicity and leukotriene synthesis by biosynthetic (recombinant) pneumocyte-macrophage colony-stimulating factor. *J. Immunol.* 137:3290, 1986.

78. Gillis, S., Crabtree, G. R., and Smith, K. A. Glucocorticoid-induced inhibition of T-cell growth factor production: I. The effect on mitogen-induced lymphocyte proliferation. *J. Immunol.* 123:1624, 1979.

79. Gleich, G. H., and Adolphson, C. R. The eosinophilic leukocyte: Structure and function. *Adv. Immunol.* 39:177, 1986.

80. Gomez, E., et al. Effect of topical corticosteroids on seasonally induced increases in nasal mast cells. *Br. Med. J.* 296:1572, 1988.

81. Goulding, N. J., et al. Antiinflammatory lipocortin 1 production by peripheral blood leucocytes in response to hydrocortisone. *Lancet* 335:1416, 1990.

82. Grandordy, B., et al. Effect of betamethasone on airway obstruction and bronchial response to salbutamol in prednisolone resistant asthma. *Thorax* 42:65, 1987.

83. Grant, I. W. B. Treatment of status asthmaticus. *Lancet* 1:363, 1966.

84. Grant, I. W. B. Are corticosteroids necessary in the treatment of severe acute asthma? *Br. J. Dis. Chest* 76:125, 1982.

85. Greenberger, P. A., et al. Comparison of prednisolone kinetics in patients receiving daily or alternate-day prednisone for asthma. *Clin. Pharmacol. Ther.* 39:163, 1986.

85a. Griffin, D., et al. Acute myopathy during treatment of status asthmaticus with corticosteroids and steroidal muscle relaxants. *Chest* 102:510, 1992.

86. Guss, C., Schneider, A. T., and Chiaramonte, L. T. Perforated gastric ulcer in an asthmatic treated with theophylline and steroids: Case report and literature review. *Ann. Allergy* 56:237, 1986.

87. Gustaffson, B., and Persson, C. G. A. Effect of three weeks' treatment with budesonide on in vitro contractile and relaxant airway effect in the rat. *Thorax* 44:24, 1989.

88. Gustafsson, J., et al. Biochemistry, molecular biology, and physiology of the glucocorticoid receptor. *Endocrine Rev.* 8:185, 1987.

89. Gustavson, L. E., Legler, U. F., and Benet, L. Z. Impairment of predniso-

lone disposition in women taking oral contraceptives or conjugated estrogens. *J. Clin. Endocrinol. Metab.* 62:234, 1986.

90. Guyre, P. M., and Munck, A. Glucocorticoid Actions on Monocytes and Macrophages. In H. N. Clanan and A. R. Oronsky (eds.), *Antiinflammatory Steroids: Basic and Clinical Aspects.* New York: Academic, 1988. Pp. 199–225.

90a.Haahtela, T., et al. Comparison of a β₂-agonist, terbutaline, with an inhaled corticosteroid, budesonide, in newly detected asthma. *N. Engl. J. Med.* 325:388, 1991.

91. Hadcock, J. R., and Malbon, C. C. Regulation of β-adrenergic receptors by "permissive" hormones: Glucocorticoids increase steady-state levels of receptor mRNA. *Proc. Natl. Acad. Sci. U.S.A.* 85:8415, 1988.

92. Hadcock, J. R., Wang, H.-Y., and Malbon, C. C. Agonist-induced destabilization of β-adrenergic receptor mRNA. *J. Biol. Chem.* 264:19928, 1989.

92a.Hamid, Q., et al. Expression of mRNA for interleukin-5 in mucosal bronchial biopsies from asthma. *J. Clin. Invest.* 87:1541, 1991.

93. Harrison, B. D. W., et al. Recovery of hypothalamo-pituitary-adrenal function in asthmatics whose oral steroids have been stopped or reduced. *Clin. Endocrinol.* 17:109, 1982.

94. Harrison, B. D. W., et al. Need for intravenous hydrocortisone in addition to oral prednisolone in patients admitted to hospital with severe asthma without ventilatory failure. *Lancet* i:181, 1986.

95. Harter, J. G., Reddy, W. J., and Thorn, G. W. Studies on an intermittent corticosteroid dosage regimen. *N. Engl. J. Med.* 269:591, 1963.

96. Haskell, R. J., Wong, B. M., and Hansen, J. E. A double-blind, randomised clinical trial of methylprednisolone in status asthmaticus. *Arch. Intern. Med.* 143:1324, 1983.

97. Henderson, R. G., et al. Variation in plasma prednisolone concentrations in renal transplant recipients given enteric coated prednisolone. *Br. Med. J.* 1:1534, 1979.

98. Herxheimer, H., McAllen, M. K., and Williams, C. A. Local treatment of bronchial asthma with hydrocortisone powder. *Br. Med. J.* 2:762, 1958.

99. Hirata, F., et al. A phospholipase A2-inhibitory protein in rabbit neutrophils induced by glucocorticoids. *Proc. Natl. Acad. Sci. U.S.A.* 77:2533, 1980.

100. Holgate, S. T., Baldwin, C. J., and Tattersfield, A. E. Beta adrenergic resistance in normal human airways. *Lancet* 2:375, 1977.

101. Howard, K. J., and Distelhorst, C. W. Evidence for intracellular association of the glucocorticoid receptor with the 90-KDa heat shock protein. *J. Biol. Chem.* 263:3474, 1988.

102. Howell, C. J., et al. Identification of an alveolar macrophage-derived activity in bronchial asthma that enhances leukotriene C4 generation by human eosinophils stimulated by ionophare A23187 as a granulocyte-macrophage colony-stimulating factor. *Am. Rev. Respir. Dis.* 140:1340, 1989.

103. Hui, K. K., Conolly, M. E., and Tashkin, D. P. Reversal of human lymphocyte beta-adrenoceptor desensitization by glucocorticoids. *Clin. Pharmacol. Ther.* 32:566, 1982.

104. Israel, R. H., et al. The protective effect of methylprednisolone on carbachol-induced bronchospasm. *Am. Rev. Respir. Dis.* 130:1019, 1984.

104a.Jeffery, P. K., et al. Effects of treatment on airway inflammation and thickening of basement membrane reticular collagen in asthma: A quantitative light and electron microscopic study. *Am. Rev. Respir. Dis.* 145:1890, 1992.

105. Jenkins, C. R., and Woodcock, A. J. B. Effect of prednisone and beclomethasone dipropionate on airway responsiveness in asthma: A comparative study. *Thorax* 43:378, 1980.

106. Jones, D., et al. The effects of influenza A2 Texas virus infection on pulmonary function in adults with asthma. Proceedings of the 14th Meeting of the International Society of Internal Medicine, Rome, October 1978.

107. Jonsson, S., et al. Comparison of the oral and intravenous routes for treating asthma with methylprednisolone and theophylline. *Chest* 94:723, 1988.

108. Juniper, E. F., et al. Effect of long-term treatment with an inhaled corticosteroid (budesonide) on airway hyperresponsiveness and clinical asthma in nonsteroid-dependent asthma. *Am. Rev. Respir. Dis.* 142:832, 1990.

109. Kalinyak, J. E., et al. Tissue-specific regulation of glucocorticoid receptor-mRNA by dexamethasone. *J. Biol. Chem.* 262:10441, 1987.

110. Keal, E. E. Biochemistry and rheology of sputum in asthma. *Postgrad. Med. J.* 47:171, 1971.

111. Kern, J. A., et al. Dexamethasone inhibition of interleukin 1 beta production by human monocytes: Posttranscriptional mechanisms. *J. Clin. Invest.* 81:237, 1988.

112. Kerrebijn, K. F., Von Essen-Zandvliet, E. E. M., and Neijens, H. J. Effect of long-term treatment with inhaled corticosteroids and beta-agonists on bronchial responsiveness in asthmatic children. *J. Allergy Clin. Immunol.* 79:653, 1987.

113. Klee, C. B. Ca²⁺-dependent phospholipid- (and membrane-) binding proteins. *Biochemistry* 27:6645, 1990.

114. Kozower, M., Veatch, L., and Kaplan, M. M. Decreased clearance of prednisolone: A factor in the development of corticosteroid side effects. *J. Clin. Endocrinol. Metab.* 38:407, 1974.

115. Kraan, J., Koeter, G. H., and Van der Mark, T. W. Dosage and time effects of inhaled budesonide on bronchial hyperreactivity. *Am. Rev. Respir. Dis.* 137:44, 1988.

116. Kraan, J., et al. Changes in bronchial hyperreactivity induced by 4 weeks of treatment with antiasthmatic drugs in patients with allergic asthma: A comparison between budesonide and terbutaline. *J. Allergy Clin. Immunol.* 76:628, 1985.

117. Kwong, F. K., Sue, M. A., and Klaustermeyer, W. B. Corticosteroid complications in respiratory disease. *Ann. Allergy* 58:326, 1987.

118. Lacronique, J. G., et al. Alveolar macrophages in idiopathic pulmonary fibrosis have glucocorticoid receptors, but glucocorticoid therapy does not suppress alveolar macrophage release of fibronectin and alveolar macrophage derived growth factor. *Am. Rev. Respir. Dis.* 130:450, 1984.

118a.Laitinen, L. A., Laitinen, A., and Haahtela, T. A comparative study of the effects of an inhaled corticosteroid, budesonide, and a β₂-agonist, terbutaline, on airway inflammation in newly diagnosed asthma. A randomized, double-blind, parallel-group controlled trial. *J. Allergy Clin. Immunol.* 90:32, 1992.

119. Laitinen, L. A., et al. Damage of the airway epithelium and bronchial reactivity in patients with asthma. *Am. Rev. Respir. Dis.* 131:599, 1985.

119a.Lamas, A. M., Leon, O. G., and Schleimer, R. P. Glucocorticoids inhibit eosinophil responses to granulocyte macrophage colony-stimulating factor. *J. Immunol.* 147:254, 1991.

120. Lamas, A. M., Marcotte, G. V., and Schleimer, R. P. Human endothelial cells prolong eosinophil survival: Regulation by cytokines and glucocorticoids. *J. Immunol.* 142:3978, 1989.

121. Lan, N. C., et al. Mechanisms of glucocorticoid hormone action. *J. Steroid Biochem.* 24:77, 1984.

122. Lederle, F. A., et al. Tapering of corticosteroid therapy following exacerbation of asthma: A randomized, double-blind, placebo controlled trial. *Arch. Intern. Med.* 147:2201, 1987.

123. Lee, S. W., et al. Glucocorticoids selectively inhibit the transcription of the interleukin 1β gene and decrease the stability of interleukin 1β mRNA. *Proc. Natl. Acad. Sci. U.S.A.* 85:1204, 1988.

124. Legler, U. F., and Benet, L. Z. The effect of prednisone and hydrocortisone on the plasma protein binding of prednisolone in man. *Eur. J. Clin. Pharmacol.* 30:51, 1986.

125. Legler, U. F., Frey, F. J., and Benet, L. Z. Prednisolone clearance at steady state in man. *J. Clin. Endocrinol. Metab.* 55:762, 1982.

126. Lewis, G. D., Campbell, W. B., and Johanson, A. R. Inhibition of prostaglandin synthesis by glucocorticoids in human endothelial cells. *Endocrinology* 119:62, 1986.

127. Littenberg, B., and Gluck, E. H. A controlled trial of methylprednisolone in the emergency treatment of acute asthma. *N. Engl. J. Med.* 314:150, 1986.

128. Livanou, T., Ferriman, D., and James, V. H. T. Recovery of hypothalamo-pituitary-adrenal function after corticosteroid therapy. *Lancet* 2:856, 1967.

129. Luengo, M., Picado, C., and Del Rio, L. Treatment of steroid-induced osteopenia with calcitonin in corticosteroid-dependent asthma. *Am. Rev. Respir. Dis.* 142:104, 1990.

130. Lukert, B. P., and Raisz, L. G. Glucocorticoid-induced osteoporosis: Pathogenesis and management. *Ann. Intern. Med.* 112:352, 1990.

131. Luksza, A. Acute severe asthma treated without steroids. *Br. J. Dis. Chest* 76:15, 1982.

132. Lundgren, J. D., et al. Dexamethasone inhibits respiratory glycoconjugate secretion from feline airways in vitro by the induction of lipocortin (lipomodulin) synthesis. *Am. Rev. Respir. Dis.* 137:353, 1988.

133. Lundgren, R., et al. Morphological studies of bronchial mucosal biopsies from asthmatics before and after ten years of treatment with inhaled steroids. *Eur. Respir. J.* 1:883, 1988.

134. MacGregor, R. R., et al. Alternate-day prednisolone therapy: Evaluation of delayed hypersensitivity responses, control of disease and steroid side effects. *N. Engl. J. Med.* 280:1427, 1969.

135. Madsbad, S., et al. Impaired conversion of prednisone to prednisolone in patients with liver cirrhosis. *Gut* 21:52, 1980.

136. Maridonneau-Parini, I., Errasfa, M., and Russo-Marie, F. Inhibition of O_2^--generation by dexamethasone is mimicked by lipocortin 1 in alveolar macrophages. *J. Clin. Invest.* 83:1936, 1989.

137. Marom, Z., et al. The effect of corticosteroids in mucus glycoprotein secretion from human airways in vitro. *Am. Rev. Respir. Dis.* 129:62, 1984.

138. Martin, G. L., et al. Effects of theophylline, terbutaline, and prednisone on antigen-induced bronchospasm and mediator release. *J. Allergy Clin. Immunol.* 66:204, 1990.

139. McAllister, W. A. C. The pharmacokinetics of prednisolone in asthma. M.D. Thesis, University of London, 1984.

140. McAllister, W. A. C., Winfield, C. R., and Collins, J. V. Pharmacokinetics of prednisolone in normal and asthmatic subjects in relation to dose. *Eur. J. Clin. Pharmacol.* 20:141, 1981.

141. McCleod, D. T., et al. Intramuscular triamcinolone acetonide in chronic severe asthma. *Thorax* 840:40, 1985.

142. McFadden, E. R., et al. A controlled study of the effect of single doses of hydrocortisone on the resolution of acute attacks of asthma. *Am. J. Med.* 60:52, 1976.

143. McLeish, K. R., et al. Mechanism by which methylprednisolone inhibits acute immune complex-induced changes in vascular permeability. *Inflammation* 10:321, 1986.

144. Milsap, R. L., Plaisance, K. I., and Jusko, W. J. Prednisolone disposition in obese men. *Clin. Pharmacol. Ther.* 36:824, 1984.

145. Moretti, M., et al. Effects of methylprednisolone on sputum biochemical components in asthmatic bronchitis. *Eur. J. Respir. Dis.* 66:365, 1984.

146. Morrison, P. J., Rogers, H. J., and Bradbrook, I. D. Concurrent administration of cimetidine and enteric coated prednisolone: Effect on plasma levels of prednisolone. *Br. J. Clin. Pharmacol.* 10:87, 1980.

147. Mortimer, O., et al. Bioavailability of prednisolone in asthmatic patients with poor response to steroid treatment. *Eur. J. Respir. Dis.* 71:372, 1987.

148. Munck, A., Guyre, P. M., and Holbrook, N. J. Physiological functions of glucocorticoids in stress and their relation to pharmacological actions. *Endocr. Rev.* 5:24, 1984.

149. Munck, A., et al. Glucocorticoid receptors and actions. *Am. Rev. Respir. Dis.* 141:S2, 1990.

150. Nichols, T. R., Nugent, C. A., and Tyler, F. H. Diurnal variation in suppression of adrenal function by glucocorticoids. *Clin. Endocrinol.* 25:343, 1965.

151. Ogirala, R. G., et al. High-dose intramuscular triamcinolone in severe, chronic, life-threatening asthma. *N. Engl. J. Med.* 324:585, 1991.

152. Okret, S., et al. Down-regulation of glucocorticoid mRNA by glucocorticoid hormones and recognition by the receptor of a specific binding sequence within a receptor cDNA clone. *Proc. Natl. Acad. Sci. U.S.A.* 83:5899, 1986.

153. Payvar, F., et al. Purified glucocorticoid receptors bind selectively in vitro to a cloned DNA fragment whose transcription is regulated by glucocorticoids in vivo. *Proc. Natl. Acad. Sci. U.S.A.* 78:6628, 1981.

154. Pereira, C. A., et al. Sao os corticosteroides necessarios no tratamento da asma aquada nao grave? *Rev. Paul. Med.* 106:28, 1988.

155. Peters-Golden, M., et al. Glucocorticoid inhibition of zymosan-induced arachidonic acid release by rat alveolar macrophages. *Am. Rev. Respir. Dis.* 130:803, 1984.

156. Petroni, K. C., Shen, L., and Guyre, P. M. Modulation of human polymorphonuclear leukocyte IgG Fc receptors and Fc receptor-mediated functions by IFN-gamma and glucocorticoids. *J. Immunol.* 140:3467, 1988.

157. Pickup, M. E., Clinical pharmacokinetics of prednisone and prednisolone. *Clin. Pharmacokinet.* 4:111, 1979.

158. Pierson, W. E., Bierman, C. W., and Kelly, V. C. A. A double-blind trial of corticosteroid therapy in status asthmaticus. *Pediatrics* 54:282, 1974.

159. Pipkorn, U., and Enerback, L. Nasal mucosa mast cells and histamine in hay fever. *Int. Arch. Allergy Appl. Immunol.* 84:123, 1987.

160. Pipkorn, U., et al. Inhibition of mediator release in allergic rhinitis by pretreatment with topical glucocorticoids. *N. Engl. J. Med.* 316:1506, 1987.

161. Platt-Mills, T. A. E. Local production of IgG, IgA and IgE antibodies in grass pollen hay fever. *J. Immunol.* 122:2218, 1979.

162. Raghavachar, A., et al. T-lymphocyte control of human eosinophilic granulopoiesis. *J. Immunol.* 139:3753, 1987.

163. Raimondi, A. C., Figueroa-Casas, J. C., and Roncoroni, A. T. Comparison between high and moderate doses of hydrocortisone in the treatment of status asthmaticus. *Chest* 89:832, 1986.

164. Randolph, T. G., and Rollins, J. P. Effects of cortisone on bronchial asthma. *J. Allergy* 21:288, 1950.

165. Rebuck, A. S., and Read, J. Assessment and management of severe asthma. *Am. J. Med.* 51:788, 1971.

166. Reed, J. C., et al. Effect of cyclosporin A and dexamethasone on interleukin 2 receptor gene and expression. *J. Immunol.* 137:150, 1986.

167. Reid, D. M., et al. Corticosteroids and bone mass in asthma: Comparisons with rheumatoid arthritis and polymyalgia rheumatica. *Br. Med. J.* 293:1463, 1986.

168. Rindhart, J. J., et al. Effects of corticosteroid therapy on human monocyte function. *N. Engl. J. Med.* 292:236, 1975.

169. Rocci, G., et al. Prednisolone binding to albumin and transcortin in the presence of cortisol. *Biochem. Pharmacol.* 31:289, 1982.

170. Rose, J. Q., et al. Prednisolone disposition in steroid dependent asthmatic children. *J. Allergy Clin. Immunol.* 67:188, 1981.

171. Rosewicz, S., et al. Mechanism of glucocorticoid receptor down-regulation by glucocorticoids. *J. Biol. Chem.* 263:2581, 1988.

172. Schlechte, J. A., Ginsberg, B. H., and Sherman, B. M. Regulation of the glucocorticoid receptor in human lymphocytes. *J. Steroid Biochem.* 16:69, 1982.

173. Schleimer, R. P., Schulman, E. S., and MacGlashan, D. W. Effects of dexamethasone on mediator release from human lung fragments and purified human lung mast cells. *J. Clin. Invest.* 71:1830, 1983.

174. Schleimer, R. P., et al. Selective inhibition of arachidonic acid metabolite release from human lung tissue by antiinflammatory steroids. *J. Immunol.* 136:3006, 1986.

175. Schleimer, R. P., et al. Dexamethasone inhibits the antigen-induced contractile activity and release of inflammatory mediators in isolated guinea-pig lung. *Am. Rev. Respir. Dis.* 135:562, 1987.

176. Schleimer, R. P., et al. An assessment of the effect of glucocorticoids on degranulation, chemotaxis, binding to vascular endothelial and formation of leukotriene B4 by purified human neutrophils. *J. Pharmacol. Exp. Ther.* 250:598, 1989.

177. Schneider, S. M., et al. High dose methylprednisolone as initial therapy in patients with acute bronchospasm. *J. Asthma* 25:189, 1988.

177a. Schule, R., et al. Functional antagonism between oncoprotein c-Jun and glucocorticoid receptor. *Cell* 62:1217, 1990.

178. Shee, C. D. Risk factors for hydrocortisone myopathy in acute severe asthma. *Respir. Med.* 84:229, 1990.

179. Silberstein, D. S., Owen, W. F., and Gasson, J. C. Enhancement of human eosinophil cytotoxicity and leukotriene synthesis by biosynthetic recombinant granulocyte-macrophage colony-stimulating factor. *J. Immunol.* 137:3290, 1986.

180. Smith, R. Corticosteroids and osteoporosis. *Thorax* 45:573, 1990.

181. Sotomayor, H., et al. Seasonal increase of carbachol airway responsiveness in patients allergic to grass pollen. *Am. Rev. Respir. Dis.* 130:56, 1984.

182. Stein, L. M., and Cole, R. P. Early administration of corticosteroids in emergency room treatment of acute asthma. *Ann. Intern. Med.* 112:822, 1990.

183. Stuck, A. E., Frey, B. M., and Frey, F. J. Kinetics of prednisolone and endogenous cortisol suppression in the elderly. *Clin. Pharmacol. Ther.* 43:354, 1988.

184. Szefler, S. J., et al. Methylprednisolone versus prednisolone pharmacokinetics in relation to dose in adults. *Eur. J. Clin. Pharmacol.* 30:323, 1986.

185. Taggart, A. T., et al. Prednisolone pharmacokinetics in patients with rheumatoid arthritis, polymyalgia rheumatica and asthma. *Clin. Rheumatol.* 5:327, 1986.

186. Tanner, A. R., et al. Concurrent administration of antacids and prednisone: Effect on serum levels of prednisolone. *Br. J. Clin. Pharmacol.* 7:397, 1979.

187. Treadwell, B. L. J., et al. Pituitary-adrenal function during corticosteroid therapy. *Lancet* 1:355, 1963.

187a. Vathenen, A. S., et al. Time course of change in bronchial reactivity with an inhaled corticosteroid in asthma. *Am. Rev. Respir. Dis.* 143:1317, 1991.

188. Venge, P., and Dahl, R. Are blood eosinophil number and activity important for the development of the late asthmatic reaction after allergen challenge? *Eur. Respir. J.* 2(Suppl. 6):4305, 1989.

189. Wagner, J. G., et al. Plasma protein binding parameters of prednisolone in immune disease patients receiving long term prednisone therapy. *Lab. Clin. Med.* 97:487, 1981.

189a. Wallen, I. L., et al. Glucocorticoids inhibit cytokine-mediated eosinophil survival. *J. Immunol.* 147:3490, 1991.

190. Wallner, B. P., et al. Cloning and expression of human lipocortin, a

phospholipase A2 inhibitor with potential antiinflammatory activity. *Nature* 320:77, 1986.

191. Webb, J., and Clark, T. J. H. Recovery of plasma corticotrophin and cortisol levels after a three-week course of prednisolone. *Thorax* 36:22, 1981.

192. Webb, J., Clark, T. J. H., and Chilvers, C. Time course of response to prednisolone in chronic airflow obstruction. *Thorax* 36:18, 1981.

193. Webb, J. R. Dose response of patients to oral corticosteroid treatment during exacerbations of asthma. *Br. Med. J.* 292:1045, 1986.

194. Whitehouse, B. J. Lipocortins, mediators of the antiinflammatory actions of corticosteroids? *J. Endocrinol.* 123:363, 1989.

195. Willey, C. F., et al. Comparison of oral prednisolone and intramuscular triamcinolone in patients with severe chronic asthma. *Thorax* 39:340, 1984.

196. Wodnar-Filipowicz, A., Heusser, C. H., and Moroni, C. Production of the haemopoietic growth factors GM-CSF and interleukin-3 by mast cells in response to IgE receptor mediated activation. *Nature* 339:150, 1989.

197. Yamaguchi, Y., et al. Highly purified murine interleukin 5 (IL-5) stimulates eosinophil function and prolongs in vitro survival: IL-5 as an eosinophil factor. *J. Exp. Med.* 167:1737, 1988.

197a.Yoss, E. R., et al. Arachidonic acid metabolism in normal human alveolar macrophages: Stimulus specificity for mediator release and phospholipid metabolism, and pharmacologic modulation in vitro and in vivo. *Am. J. Respir. Cell. Mol. Biol.* 2:69, 1990.

198. Zurcher, R. M., Frey, B. M., and Frey, F. J. Impact of ketoconazole on the metabolism of prednisolone. *Clin. Pharmacol. Ther.* 45:366, 1989.

199. Libanati, C. R., and Baylink, D. J. Prevention and treatment of glucocorticoid-induced osteoporosis. *Chest* 102:1426, 1992.

Aerosol Corticosteroids

61

John H. Toogood
Barbara H. Jennings
Jon C. Baskerville
Neville M. Lefcoe

Since their discovery 40 years ago, corticosteroid drugs have played a uniquely valuable role in the treatment of chronic asthma, but it has been difficult to dissociate their beneficial antiasthmatic effects from their undesirable systemic effects because both kinds of response are mediated by the same glucocorticoid receptor [53] (see Chap. 60). Early attempts to achieve a clinically useful separation by administering the drugs by inhalation failed because of too low an antiasthmatic potency (e.g., hydrocortisone, prednisolone) or too high a systemic potency (e.g., dexamethasone) [122, 208]. More recently, a family of corticosteroid drugs has been synthesized whose members share in common the characteristics of enhanced topical antiinflammatory potency and low systemic potency. The former reflects their lipophilic properties coupled with their relatively high affinity for the glucocorticoid receptor. The latter reflects the speed of their biotransformation after systemic absorption, mainly in the liver, to metabolites with little or no glucocorticoid activity.

The members of this family of aerosol corticosteroids (AC) drugs that have proved useful in the treatment of asthma include beclomethasone dipropionate (BDP), betamethasone valerate (BV), budesonide (BUD), triamcinolone acetonide (TA), and flunisolide. BDP, TA, and flunisolide are currently available for clinical use in the United States. BUD, BDP, TA, and flunisolide are available in Canada (Fig. 61-1). Each is effective [109, 143, 211, 219], and there is no convincing evidence that any one is qualitatively superior to another in clinical efficacy per se. However, they differ from one another with respect to the therapeutic index, that is, the ratio of their topical antiinflammatory to their systemic glucocorticoid potencies.

BUD has the most favorable therapeutic index. This confers no practical advantage if conventional low doses are used because none of the AC drugs is discernibly toxic at that dose level. However, it becomes important when the dose is increased above 0.8 mg/day. Direct comparisons of BDP versus BUD at therapeutically equivalent doses show the former has the greater systemic activity [85, 86, 148, 171]. Similar data are not available for TA or flunisolide. These considerations are of practical importance because a substantial number of asthmatic patients require AC doses higher than 0.8 mg/day to control their asthma (Table 61-1).

DRUG DELIVERY

AC drugs are generally administered from a freon-pressurized, metered-dose inhaler (MDI) that emits a measured dose of active

Funding for our clinical studies discussed herein was provided by A. B. Draco (Sweden), Astra Pharmaceuticals (Canada), Fisons Corporation (U.S.A.), the Research Fund of the Medical Associates of Victoria Hospital, Ontario Respiratory Disease Foundation, Schering Corporation (Canada), and Syntex Corporation (U.S.A.).

drug plus the propellants (see Chap. 56). The constituents of the formulations commercially available in the United States, Canada, or Europe are shown in Table 61-2.

The fraction of each dose that reaches the lung, approximately 10 percent or less of the amount actually emitted from the MDI [137], exerts an antiasthmatic effect that is assumed to be proportionate to the topical antiinflammatory potency of the drug as measured by the McKenzie skin blanching test [111, 151]. For BUD, this topical potency is about 1,000 times that of prednisolone. TA and flunisolide have about one-fourth and one-third the topical potency of BUD, respectively [86]. The smallest particles in the inhaled aerosol penetrate to the nonciliated peripheral airways and alveoli, whence they are rapidly absorbed and exert systemic effects that can be measured in terms of changes in blood eosinophil levels or hypothalamic-pituitary-adrenal (HPA) function (see Chap. 62). The systemic glucocorticoid activity of these drugs is weak relative to their topical antiinflammatory potency in the lung, but nevertheless it is three- to sevenfold stronger than that produced by the same amount of prednisolone given by mouth [86].

BIOAVAILABILITY

Systemic glucocorticoid activity may be demonstrated with any AC drug, depending on the dose given and the dosing schedule, the sensitivity and precision of the index chosen to measure the systemic activity, sample size, and how rigorously sources of extraneous variance are controlled [15, 97, 130, 185, 211, 219, 226, 237, 250]. Among the last, patient compliance and the mode of inhalation of the drug may be critically important but are seldom reported in published studies and even more rarely monitored and factored into the analysis. Lack of attention to these factors can reduce the statistical "power" of tests for systemic activity. This in turn may account for many of the published reports that imply a total absence of systemic glucocorticoid activity when AC drugs are used at conventional low-dose levels and for persistence of the erroneous notion that, as a class, they are poorly absorbed from the lung.

LIMITS OF "SAFE" DOSAGE

The "cutoff" generally adopted by most regulatory authorities for the various AC drugs indicates the per diem dose above which a statistically significant degree of reduction in the blood eosinophil count and serum cortisol level at 8:00 A.M. is usually demonstrable in test groups of about 30 human subjects. More sensitive tests of HPA axis function, such as metyrapone responsiveness or measurement of the 24-hour urinary free cortisol output, show unequivocal evidence of systemic activity with doses of AC well

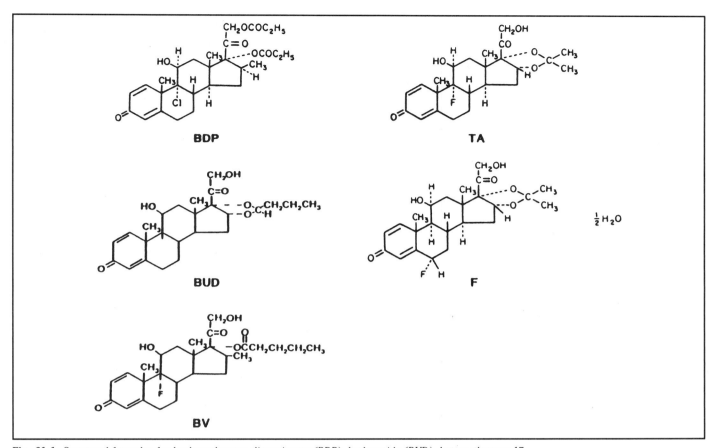

Fig. 61-1. *Structural formulas for beclomethasone dipropionate (BDP), budesonide (BUD), betamethasone 17-valerate (BV), triamcinolone 16,17-acetonide (TA), and flunisolide (F).*

within the approved therapeutic range [15, 97, 130, 132, 226, 237]. However, the clinical importance of these small departures from normal HPA function is problematic.

The systemic activity of any particular dose of AC in different patients and patient groups depends largely on the fraction of the emitted dose that reaches the important absorptive surface in the lung periphery. This fraction is determined by the interaction of numerous factors including variations in normal lung anatomy; the degree of pulmonary functional impairment and the presence or absence of associated chronic bronchitis, each of which reduces peripheral delivery of the inhaled drug [115, 169]; and, in particular, the inspiratory technique used [135]. Also, patients vary widely in their susceptibility to the systemic effects of steroid drugs because of intrinsic or acquired differences in their steroid pharmacokinetics [59, 92]. Children metabolize BUD (and presumably other AC drugs) about 25 percent faster than adults on the average [149, 171]. Finally, because inhaled and oral steroids bind to the same glucocorticoid receptor, they exert additive systemic effects if used together [211, 250].

Since the practicing clinician is chiefly concerned with the needs of individual patients rather than of population groups, it is important to take into consideration these and other factors that can selectively influence the responses of different asthmatic patients to AC drugs. In this way a treatment plan can be formulated that is appropriate to the particular needs and tolerances of each patient. We evaluated some of these factors in a series of studies designed to explore various aspects of the therapeutic performance of AC. Selected data from these studies are discussed in the following pages. A general description of the data-collecting systems and analytic methods used has been published elsewhere [212].

EFFECTIVE DOSAGE

Both the benefits and adverse effects of AC treatment are dose dependent, the relationship being approximately linear on log daily dose (Fig. 61-2). This was first demonstrated with BDP [211] and later with BUD [219]. It applies not only with the indices shown in the Figure 61-2 but also with airway hyperresponsiveness [93]. Patients vary markedly in their responsiveness to AC, as illustrated in Figure 61-1. Some become asymptomatic on 0.2 mg/day of BDP; others need 0.8 mg, and others even more. The dose needed to render half this particular patient group symptom-free (the ED_{50}) was approximately 1.0 mg/day of BDP. Only 25 percent achieved symptom-free status at 0.4 mg/day, the usual recommended starting dose. It was impractical to give enough drug to make the entire group symptom-free. In less severe asthmatics, these response lines would be expected to shift to the left—that is, lower doses would suffice.

Certain patient and disease characteristics have been found to correlate significantly with the degree of responsiveness to inhaled steroid (IS) treatment [204, 210, 216, 225]. However, the usefulness of these variables as predictors of an individual patient's responsiveness in clinical practice is not clearly established. It seems better to rely on a trial of therapy than to restrict the use of the drug according to any particular constellation of patient or disease characteristics. For the purposes of such a trial, dosages higher than the conventional recommended starting dosage of 0.4 mg/day of BDP have been shown to be more efficient because (1) many patients who do not respond to a low dosage do so with a higher dosage [186, 211]; (2) high dosages give more accurately predictable results than low dosages in a trial of limited duration, such as 14 days [210]; (3) a higher dosage

Table 61-1. Distribution of daily doses of budesonide or beclomethasone*

Dosage level	Daily dose (mg)	Number of patients	Percent of total (n = 283)	Cumulative percent (n = 283)	
	0.01	3	1.06	1.06	
	0.05	1	0.35	1.41	
	0.10	1	0.35	1.77	
	0.20	16	5.65	7.42	
	0.25	3	1.06	8.48	
	0.30	12	4.24	12.72	
Low	0.40	40	14.13	26.86	53%
	0.45	3	1.06	27.92	
	0.50	9	3.18	31.10	
	0.60	9	3.18	34.28	
	0.75	3	1.06	35.34	
	0.80	49	17.31	52.65	
	0.90	1	0.35	53.00	
	1.00	32	11.31	64.31	
	1.10	1	0.35	64.66	
	1.20	24	8.48	73.14	
Intermediate	1.50	9	3.18	76.33	41.7%
	1.60	34	12.01	88.34	
	1.75	1	0.35	88.69	
	1.80	3	1.06	89.75	
	2.00	14	4.95	94.70	
	2.40	9	3.18	97.88	
High	3.00	1	0.35	98.23	5.3%
	3.20	5	1.77	100.00	

* AC utilization data from a 1989–1990 audit of 390 adult asthmatic patients receiving ambulatory care from three specialist physicians in a tertiary health care facility [95]. Doses designated above as "low" are generally accepted as free from important adverse systemic effects. Those designated as "high" show systemic activity equivalent to prednisone >15 mg/day (based on bioequivalences of BUD versus prednisone [46]). These designations apply throughout the text.

is required to normalize pulmonary function than simply to control symptoms (Table 61-3) [197, 211]; and (4) normalization of pulmonary function is considered a more efficient goal of long-term asthma treatment than symptomatic treatment alone.

Success of Prednisone Withdrawal

Patients vary not only with respect to their initial responsiveness to AC, as was observed in this study and illustrated in Table 61-1, but also in their minimum dose requirements during long-term therapy [213]. To determine the extent of such variation we titrated the steroid doses down, oral prednisone first and then BDP, to determine the smallest dose each person required to avoid disability and to retain at least half the improvement in $FEF_{25-75\%}$ gained with the initial aggressive treatment [213–215]. The titration schedule used has been described in detail elsewhere [213] and is shown in Table 61-4 in a form adapted for ordinary clinical usage. The minimum maintenance doses (MMD) of BDP and prednisone determined in this way (MMD-B and MMD-P respectively) varied widely, as shown in Figure 61-3. Only four patients could be satisfactorily controlled by the conventional starting dose of 0.4 mg/day or less of BDP; half the group required more than 1.0 mg/day. All patients who previously had been unable to convert to alternate-morning prednisone succeeded in doing so under the aegis of BDP. However, only six were able to stop prednisone and stay off it continuously during the last 6 months of our 18-month follow-up (an 18% success rate). The success rate increases to about 40 percent if one includes the nine others who were able to convert from regular to intermittent prednisone use.

Some other studies report much higher success rates for pred-

nisone withdrawal during AC treatment. The difference relates, at least in part, to the duration of follow-up. This is illustrated by data culled from many trials of BDP, BV, or TA published during a 6-year period. These are presented in Figure 61-4. For each trial the percent of the group completely withdrawn from prednisone during AC treatment is plotted against the duration of the study. It is evident that all the 100 percent successes originate from studies of 4 months' duration or less. The long-term success rate averaged about 30 percent, which is close to our own experience based on an 18-month follow-up. The curve in Figure 61-4 indicates that reliable estimation of patients' minimum requirements for oral and aerosol steroids requires a follow-up of at least 6 months. This is important in clinical practice. In our own study we found we could not reliably discriminate the best responders from the BDP failures until 9 months after steroid weaning commenced [196, 215]. The period of maximum instability of their asthma was between 5 and 8 months [213]. This coincides with the inflexion of the curve shown in Figure 61-4. It is also noteworthy that published reports of asthmatic deaths complicating attempted conversion of chronically prednisone-dependent asthma patients to AC put the time of their occurrence at 4 to 6 months after oral steroid withdrawal [70, 112]. The risks of such morbidity and mortality can and should be minimized by ensuring that every patient keeps an oral steroid on hand and by giving clear instructions about the need to reinstitute the drug or to increase the dose in the event of significant asthma relapse during AC conversion.

The aggregate experience summarized in Figure 61-3 indicates that many asthmatic patients cannot be controlled satisfactorily on conventional low doses of AC alone. Such patients are candidates either for reversion to oral prednisone alone, for combined oral-AC treatment, or for AC treatment at higher than conventional dosage. The relative effectiveness of these alternative steroid regimens is therefore of practical interest.

EFFECTIVENESS OF PREDNISONE VERSUS AC TREATMENT

Current debate about the relative merits of oral versus AC therapy largely revolves around comparisons of the results from unmatched patient groups and dissimilar experimental designs [33, 242]. There are few published studies in which these treatment alternatives have been systematically and prospectively compared over a range of graded doses in the same patients.

Alternate-Morning Prednisone

We used a double-blind, double-dummy, crossover protocol to compare alternate-morning prednisone and AC (BUD) inhaled four times daily via a large volume spacer in 14 steroid-dependent adult asthmatics [220]. These patients had asthma that was stable prior to the study on a combined BDP plus alternate-morning prednisone regimen. Their asthma remained well controlled when they were shifted to BUD alone, and it improved a little as the BUD dose was subsequently increased at 2-week intervals (Fig. 61-5). However, their asthma relapsed when they were given alternate-morning prednisone instead, and this deterioration could not be satisfactorily controlled despite doubling and quadrupling the dose of prednisone (up to 60 mg on alternate days).

In this study, BUD given alone four times daily proved significantly and consistently more effective for asthma control than alternate-morning prednisone given alone, when the two treatments were compared at equivalent levels of systemic activity as reflected by the morning serum cortisol level [220].

The results favor AC over alternate-morning prednisone as the treatment of choice for most patients who require regular steroid therapy for chronic asthma.

Table 61-2. Aerosol corticosteroid (AC) metered-dose inhalers used in the United States, Canada, or Europe

	Dose emitted per puff ($\pm 15\%$)		Recommended adult daily dosage	
AC drug (brand name)	Active drug (mg)	Propellants Stabilizers Cosolvents	Usual dose (mg)	Maximum dose (mg)
Beclomethasone dipropionate (Vanceril, Beclovent, Becotide)	0.05	24 mg freon 11 61 mg freon 12 0.005 mg oleic acid	0.4	1.0
(Becloforte)	0.25	22 mg freon 11 59 mg freon 12 0.025 mg oleic acid	1.0	2.0
Betamethasone 17-valerate (Bextasol)	0.10	85 mg freon 11 61 mg freon 12	0.8	Minimum necessary to control asthma
Budesonide (Pulmicort)	0.05	18 mg freon 11 34 mg freon 12 17 mg freon 114 0.35 mg sorbitan trioleate	0.4	1.0
	0.20	18 mg freon 11 34 mg freon 12 17 mg freon 114 0.35 mg sorbitan trioleate	0.4–0.8	Lowest effective dose
Flunisolide	0.29	17 mg freon 12 35 mg freon 12 17 mg freon 114 0.35 mg sodium trioleate	1.0	2.0
(Aerobid, Bronalide) Triamcinolone acetonide (Azmacort)	0.20	65 mg freon 12 0.65 mg alcohol USP	1.2–1.6	3.2

Note: Some of the dosages shown in the second column are generally adjusted in U.S. literature to allow for estimated losses in the delivery device—to 0.042 mg (beclomethasone) or 0.10 mg (triamcinolone). Logically, similar adjustments ought to be made for each combination of MDI with the different add-on spacer devices now widely used in clinical practice, but this is impractical. Therefore, the daily dosages shown above in the second, fourth, and fifth columns are nominal doses, i.e., as emitted from the valve of the pressurized canister. They may differ from the adjusted doses shown in U.S. literature and the package insert. (Additional dry-powder formulations of AC are listed in Table 61-13.)

Table 61-3. Beclomethasone dose required to attain normal or zero value in 50 percent of treated group (n = 34)*

Response index	ED_{50} BDP (mg/day)
$FEF_{25-75\%}$	>1.6
Oral bronchodilator use	1.6
Attack frequency	1.05
Inhaled bronchodilator use	0.5
Asthma disability score	<0.2

* The required dose of BDP is a function of the goal of treatment.
Source: Adapted from J. H. Toogood et al., A graded dose assessment of the efficacy of beclomethasone dipropionate aerosol for severe chronic asthma. *J. Allergy Clin. Immunol.* 59:298, 1977.

Daily Prednisone

In a separate study [227], we determined the antiasthmatic and systemic potencies of prednisone administered as a single morning dose each day versus BUD inhaled four times daily via a large-volume spacer, over a range of doses extending from low and nontoxic to high and potentially toxic levels.

Either drug appeared equally effective provided a large enough dose was administered. This is illustrated for one representative response index in Figure 61-6. It shows BUD to be 25 times more potent than prednisone. Because estimates of the relative potency of AC drugs versus oral steroid can vary widely depending on which response index is selected for calculating the potencies, we averaged data from four different indices of asthma activity and two indices of systemic steroid activity to derive therapeutic and systemic bioequivalents for BUD versus prednisone. Comparison of these ratios showed that the amount of systemic glucocorticoid activity with BUD was consistently about six times less

Table 61-4. Schedule for converting chronically oral prednisone dependent asthmatic patients to aerosol corticosteroid (AC)

Phase	Approximate duration	Treatment
1	~2 weeks	In severely obstructed patients, precede inhaled steroid with a course of high-dose prednisone, to clear the small airways of mucus. For less severe asthma, skip this step.
2	~2 weeks	Initiate inhaled steroid at high dosage, e.g., >1.0 mg/day of BDP. Convert prednisone rapidly to alternate mornings.
3	~2–4 months	Reduce prednisone at 2-week intervals by 5–10 mg/day. Quit if possible. Continue high-dose inhaled steroid.
4	~2–4 months	If patient cannot stay off prednisone, determine their minimum requirements. High-dose inhaled steroid continues.
5	~6–12 months	Reduce inhaled steroid to lowest dose that maintains optimum control. Minimum prednisone continues if required.

than that of the dose of daily prednisone required to achieve an equivalent level of asthma control in the same patients [227].

Thus, despite its unwanted systemic activity, the use of high-dose BUD appears clinically logical and ethically acceptable as a considered risk in patients with severe asthma in whom the alternative is their continuing dependency on prednisone. These findings may be assumed to apply in principle to the other AC drugs currently used to treat asthma. However, the margin of the therapeutic advantage of the inhaled steroid over prednisone would likely be less if a different AC with lower topical antiinflam-

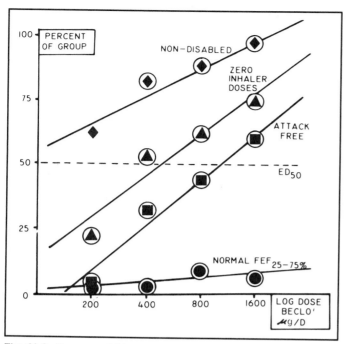

Fig. 61-2. *Response of 34 prednisone-dependent asthmatics to graded doses of BDP. At each encircled point the mean change from the pre-BDP baseline value was significant (p <.05 or better). The effective BDP dose for 50 percent of the group (ED$_{50}$) may be determined by relating the intercepts of the dashed line and each regression line to the abscissa scale. FEF$_{25-75\%}$ = mean forced expiratory flow during the middle half of the forced vital capacity. (Reprinted with permission from J. H. Toogood et al., Tactics for clinical trials of therapy in patients with chronic asthma. J. Asthma 20[Suppl. 1]:51, 1983. Courtesy of Marcel Dekker, Inc.)*

matory potency than BUD were used or if the BUD were administered less frequently than four times a day. Either of these factors may reduce efficacy.

The high therapeutic potency of BUD relative to prednisone accords with other studies that document various antiinflammatory actions of BUD when topically applied to the upper or lower respiratory tract mucosa [3, 7, 8, 16] and also with the fact that the drug's clinical efficacy is fully explainable by these local effects in the airways. The fraction of the AC that is systemically absorbed is therapeutically inactive [229] (Fig. 61-7).

With any of these steroid regimens, oral or inhaled, it is essential that the steroid dose be titrated down to minimum requirements. The frequency distribution of the titrated minimum dosages currently used by adult patients attending our ambulatory care clinic is shown in Table 61-1. Half the patients need more than 1.0 mg/day.

DETERMINANTS OF MINIMUM DOSE REQUIREMENTS OF PREDNISONE AND AC

The airway inflammation that is the primary cause of this disease has been shown to respond to AC therapy [45a, 84a, 94a]. Patients who require relatively high steroid doses to control their asthma show evidence of a greater degree of airway inflammation than do those who do well on lower doses [227]. Furthermore, the factors that determine this variability in dose requirements are the same for inhaled as for oral steroid therapy (Table 61-5); that is, the severity of the ventilatory impairment per se does not selectively limit the therapeutic potential of AC drugs by restricting their access to the lung [227].

Although this commonality of determinants may be seen during short-term AC therapy, it does not hold true during long-term treatment. Factors other than those related to asthma severity per se assume greater importance. This is illustrated in Table 61-6. The data derive from an examination of the reasons for the

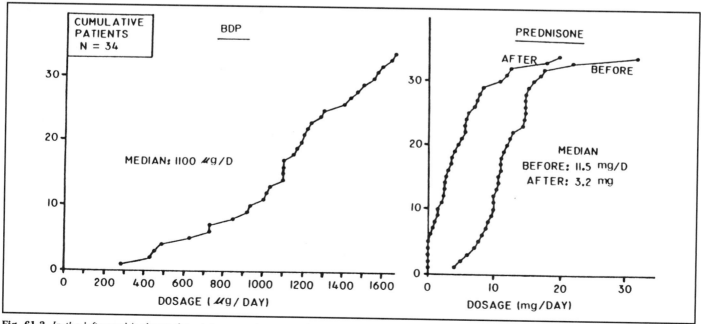

Fig. 61-3. *In the left panel is shown the minimum maintenance dosage of BDP required by 34 patients. Each dot represents one patient's daily usage of BDP averaged over the last 6 months of an 18-month follow-up. Prednisone usage by the same patients is shown in the right panel, before and after weaning to minimum maintenance prednisone dosage. (Reprinted with permission from J. H. Toogood et al., Tactics for clinical trials of therapy in patients with chronic asthma. J. Asthma 20[Suppl. 1]:51, 1983. Courtesy of Marcel Dekker, Inc.)*

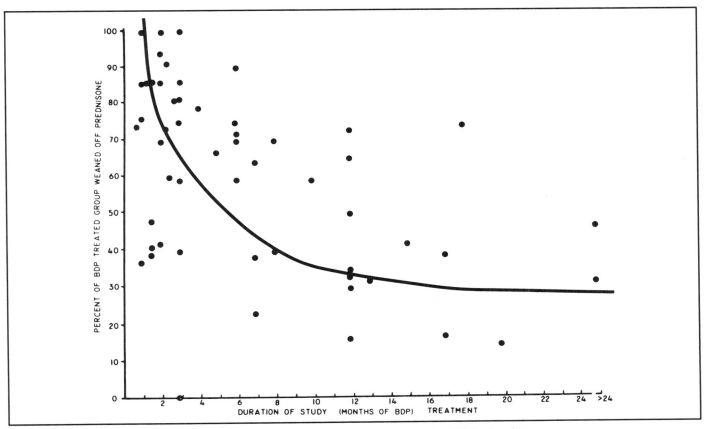

Fig. 61-4. *The success rates for total prednisone withdrawal during different published trials of BDP, plotted in relationship to the duration of each study. (Reprinted with permission from J. H. Toogood et al., Tactics for clinical trials of therapy in patients with chronic asthma.* J. Asthma *20[Suppl. 1]:51, 1983. Courtesy of Marcel Dekker, Inc.)*

Table 61-5. Determinants of occurrence of severe asthma relapses during a crossover comparison of inhaled BUD versus prednisone therapy (n = 34)*

On budesonide	p from X^2	On prednisone	p from X^2
Low FVC	<0.001	Low $FEV_{1.0}$	0.003
High blood eosinophils	0.04	High blood eosinophils	0.001
High blood monocytes	0.001	High blood monocytes	0.009
Predictive accuracy	0.91		0.88

* Strongest correlates among 18 factors analyzed by stepwise logistic regression. These factors characterize the patients who require relatively high doses of steroid to prevent asthma relapses. FVC and $FEV_{1.0}$ could be interchanged without materially altering the predictive power of the equation.
Source: Adapted from J. H. Toogood et al., Bioequivalent doses of budesonide and prednisone in moderate and severe asthma. *J. Allergy Clin. Immunol.* 84:688, 1989.

intersubject variance in the titrated minimum dose requirements for AC and prednisone that is conspicuous in Figure 61-2. Using a modification of the multiple linear regression technique that improves its efficiency in dealing with many explanatory variables, we explored the relationship between these titrated minimum dose requirements and 36 factors selected to represent differences in patient characteristics, disease severity, and past steroid usage and tolerance [205]. Seven factors, listed in Table 61-6, accounted for 69 percent of the observed variability in prednisone requirements (p = <.05), while eight of the variables

accounted for 78 percent of the variability in the same patient's requirements for BDP (p = <.01). Only 2 of the 15 variables that are listed are common to both sets.

Thus, unlike the situation during short-term AC therapy [227], the factors that determine the need for continuing prednisone use during long-term AC therapy are quite dissimilar from those that determine the need for BDP (compare Tables 61-5 and 61-6). This implies that the two drugs play overlapping but distinct therapeutic roles when used for long-term treatment—that they supplement rather than substitute for each other. Coexisting atopy, for example, was associated with a requirement for higher doses of BDP, but it did not increase the need for oral prednisone. Patients with nasal polyps and hyperplastic sinusitis needed more BDP (intranasally) and also more prednisone—both routes of administration needed to control worsening of the upper respiratory tract symptoms caused by the attempted prednisone withdrawal. Patients with associated chronic bronchitis required more prednisone but not more BDP, presumably to minimize mucous plugging and thus ensure continuing access of the inhaled drug to the small airways.

Patient reliability emerged in this analysis as the strongest single correlate of persisting prednisone dependency, more important than age, the pretreatment severity of pulmonary impairment, or the pathogenesis of the asthma (atopic versus nonatopic). The patients who had lower reliability scores needed more prednisone, perhaps because they were as noncompliant about taking BDP as they were about taking their other drugs. Compliance can be assumed to be even more important as a determinant of the success or failure of AC treatment under the

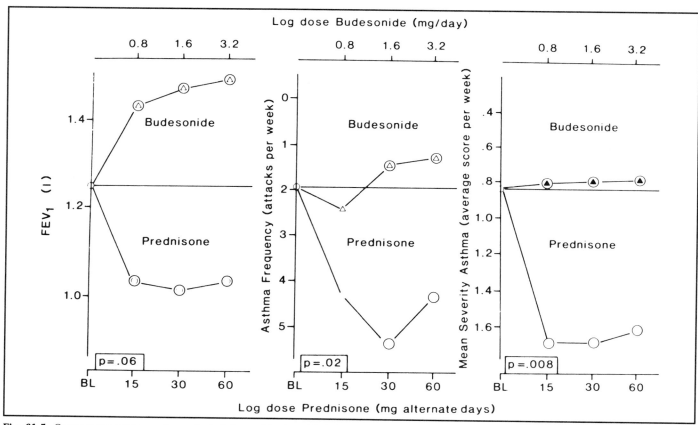

Fig. 61-5. *Group mean responses to graduated doses of budesonide inhaled 4 times daily (Δ) or prednisone given on alternate mornings (○). Encircled symbols identify means that differ statistically significantly from one another according to the t-test. The p values at lower left of the three panels derive from ANCOVA. They quantify the statistical significances of the overall difference between the responses to the two drugs. BL = baseline. (Reprinted with permission from J. H. Toogood et al., Efficacy of Oral vs. Inhaled Glucocorticosteroids. In F. E. Hargreave et al. [eds.],* Glucocorticoids and Mechanisms of Asthma: Clinical and Experimental Aspects. *Amsterdam: Excerpta Medica, 1990. Pp. 87–100.)*

conditions of ordinary clinical practice, since the patients whose data are shown here were preselected to eliminate obvious poor compliers.

RISK VERSUS BENEFIT WITH AEROSOL CORTICOSTEROID TREATMENT

The potential risks of adverse systemic effects are as yet imperfectly defined for the long-term use of intermediate or high doses of AC (see Table 61-1 for the actual doses used to designate low-, intermediate-, and high-dose categories). This issue merits more rigorous study than it has yet received, because currently many patients require and use such doses (see Table 61-1).

However, conventional low doses of AC have been notably free from clinically important systemic adverse effects [21, 35, 144]. This contrasts with the morbidity and mortality known to be associated with theophylline treatment [247] and the less serious adverse effects that limit the usefulness of oral beta-adrenergic bronchodilators [184].

Because of these differences in toxicity, it has been advocated that low-dose AC therapy be viewed as an alternative to oral bronchodilators for the primary treatment of mild asthma [34]. Another consideration supporting its use in such patients is the fact that asthma is primarily an inflammatory process and steroids are the most reliably effective of the known antiinflammatory agents. Logic suggests that preventative intervention with

low-dose AC at an early stage in the course of the disease may be more effective over the long term than allowing the disease to progress until corrective intervention with larger steroid doses is required at a later stage. It has been suggested that such early intervention may prevent progression of asthma to chronic airflow limitation, but this remains speculative at this time.

In patients who have moderately severe asthma but have not previously been dependent on regular oral steroid therapy, it is possible to achieve equivalent (and optimal) levels of asthma control with either alternate-morning prednisone or AC treatment. However, the systemic glucocorticoid activity of the prednisone, as evidenced by weight gain, is greater [132].

Patients who have more severe asthma than has been suboptimally controlled on regular prednisone prior to commencing AC therapy show a favorable overall outcome when given low or intermediate doses of AC regardless of whether they had previously used daily or alternate-morning oral prednisone regimens [195, 213, 224]. Both groups manifest similar degrees of symptom improvement without an accompanying increase in systemic steroid effect, although actual improvement in HPA function may be restricted to those previously dependent on daily prednisone [195]. Furthermore, the adrenocortical function, though improved on AC treatment, may still fall short of normal.

Combined AC-Prednisone Treatment

Largely because of such evidence of persisting suppression of HPA function, it has been suggested that AC therapy confers no

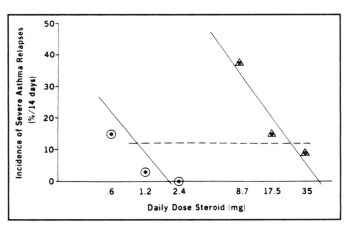

Fig. 61-6. *Incidence of disabling asthma relapses during a double-blind crossover comparison of BUD inhaled four times a day (⊙) versus prednisone (△), single A.M. dose. Every patient took 3 graduated doses of each drug, 2 weeks on each dose level. Doses shown are group means. The individual doses varied depending on the estimated asthma severity of the patient. If a sufficiently large dose is given, either oral or inhaled steroid may effectively control severe chronic asthma. Potency of BUD to prednisone = 25:1. n = 34. (Reprinted with permission from J. H. Toogood, Bronchial Asthma and Glucocorticoids. In R. P. Scheimer, H. N. Claman, and A. Oronsky [eds.], Antiinflammatory Steroid Action: Basic and Clinical Aspects. San Diego: Academic, 1989. Pp. 423–468.)*

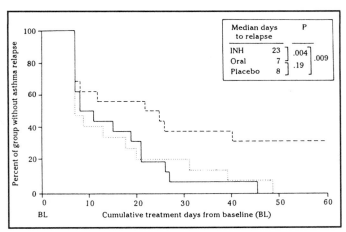

Fig. 61-7. *Interval until asthma relapse (defined as a statistically significant drop in PEFR) after shifting patients whose asthma was well controlled by bronchodilators and high-dose BDP, to either low-dose inhaled BUD (0.4 mg/day), or an oral BUD dose chosen to give 24-hour systemic blood levels 1.5-fold greater than the inhaled BUD, or a placebo. At the dosages compared, the antiasthmatic effect of BUD is fully explainable by its local intrapulmonary activity. --- = inhaled BUD (n = 16); ⋯ = oral BUD (n = 15); — = placebo (n = 16). (Adapted from J. H. Toogood et al., A study of the mechanism of the antiasthmatic action of inhaled budesonide. J. Allergy Clin. Immunol. 85:872, 1990.)*

clinically worthwhile advantage in patients who require higher than usual doses of AC to control severe asthma or in those who must continue to use oral steroid as well [77, 237, 242, 250]. However, in an analysis of long-term therapeutic outcome in a group of AC-treated patients (median dose: 1.1 mg/day of BDP; range: 0.2–1.6), we found the addition of the AC treatment conferred major reductions in asthma symptom frequency and severity, in asthmatic disability, and in iatrogenic hypertension (which implies a corollary increase in life expectancy) [224]. The net

Table 61-6. *Correlates of the variability in minimum dose requirements for prednisone and BDP of 34 patients during long-term therapy*

Variable		Multiple R
Strongest correlation with higher prednisone requirements (MMD-P)		
Low reliability score		0.581
Polyps/sinusitis		0.669
More PM steroid doses (Pre-BDP)		0.718
Higher BDP requirements (MMD-B)		0.757
Associated chronic bronchitis		0.783
More severe hypercortisonism (Pre-BDP)		0.812
Higher prednisone dose (Pre-BDP)		0.833
	R^2:	0.69
	P:	<.05
Strongest correlation with higher BDP requirements (MMD-B)		
Lower pulmonary diffusing capacity		0.549
Allergic rhinitis		0.641
Lower A.M. plasma cortisol		0.745
Higher serum IgE		0.792
Older age		0.826
Polyps/sinusitis		0.845
Shorter duration steroid dependency (Pre-BDP)		0.866
More severe hypercortisonism (Pre-BDP)		0.886
	R^2:	0.78
	P:	<.01

MMD-P and MMD-B = minimum maintenance doses of prednisone and BDP respectively, determined in each patient by 18 months' dose titration.
Note: In this stepwise multiple regression analysis, the strongest correlate emerges at the top, and the combined explanatory power of each set of variables for the interpatient variability in MMD-P and MMD-B is quantified by their respective R^2 (correlation of determination) values.

result therefore appeared clinically worthwhile despite the fact that half the group needed greater than 1.0 mg/day of BDP, that two-thirds needed a combined oral-AC regimen to maintain optimal control of their asthma, and that the prevalence of HPA axis functional suppression in these patients remained unchanged at about 50 percent of the group [224].

These results provide a clinical rationale for using inhaled and oral steroids together whenever it appears clinically necessary. Provided the doses of each drug are titrated to minimum effective levels, the combination regimen can materially improve the level of asthma control without worsening preexisting systemic glucocorticoid effects.

SYSTEMIC ADVERSE EFFECTS

Cortisol Deficiency

The practical importance of the persisting adrenocortical hypofunction that may be found in patients such as those described above should not be exaggerated, since it is known that most steroid-dependent asthmatics, including those with demonstrably subnormal HPA responsiveness to ACTH or insulin-induced hypoglycemia, can safely undergo severe stress such as major surgery, even if preoperative cortisol supplements are purposely withheld [89, 153].*

---

* The latter is not the recommended procedure for ordinary clinical practice. Normal preoperative preparation for patients using inhaled and/or oral steroids should include 100 mg of cortisone acetate orally or intramuscularly at 8-hour intervals during the 24 hours prior to surgery. Intramuscular injection of cortisone is repeated postoperatively every 8 hours until oral usage can be resumed. If emergency surgery is necessary, 4 mg of dexamethasone or 100 mg of hydrocortisone administered intravenously 1 hour preoperatively is preferable, as they are more rapidly effective. If the blood pressure drops, 100 mg of hydrocortisone is given intravenously and repeated as often as needed. See Chapter 82 for added information.

Furthermore, deaths from Addisonian crisis appear remarkably rare in steroid-dependent patients, asthmatic or otherwise [99, 108]. Of greater concern are the potential complications of chronic steroid excess—in particular, growth retardation, cataract formation, and osteoporosis.

Other Effects of Chronic Steroid Excess

Theoretically, there would appear to be no reason why any AC drug, if given to a susceptible person in sufficient dosage, should not cause the aforementioned untoward effects (growth retardation, cataracts, and osteoporosis). Indeed, both BDP and BUD can inhibit growth velocity [246a], occasionally to a clinically important degree [157a, 238a]. However, in practice, conventional doses of AC such as 0.4 to 0.6 mg/day of BDP have been found to exert no discernible growth-inhibiting effect in asthmatic children followed through to adulthood [10]. This accords with and extends the findings in other studies based on shorter periods of surveillance [61, 65, 132]. The minor degrees of growth retardation that have been reported in some low-dose AC-treated children [100] may be explainable by the confounding influence of the transient drop in growth rate that is associated with delayed puberty in many asthmatic children, with or without steroid therapy [11]. Puberty may be delayed in onset in up to 40 percent of children with allergic respiratory disease. The maturational delay and growth retardation relate to pathogenetic correlates such as atopy, rather than to the presence of asthma or its severity [54]. The effects of high doses of AC on growth have not been adequately studied to date.

Published reports of posterior subcapsular ocular cataracts (PSC) occurring in AC-treated patients [91, 168] are very few, but we found a prevalence rate of 27 percent in a group of 48 patients who had received high-dose AC therapy (mean 1.5 mg/day) for an average period of 9.2 years (range 0.01–21 years). The occurrence of PSC in these patients was unrelated to the amount or duration of their inhaled steroid use but correlated significantly with measures of their current and past prednisone usage [48]. Thus, inhaled steroid therapy is more likely to decrease rather than increase the risk of PSC occurrence, by virtue of its capacity to reduce or eliminate the need for prednisone treatment.

The possible effects of AC drugs on calcium, phosphate, vitamin D, and bone metabolism have received little attention until recently. A survey of chronically steroid-dependent adult asthmatics reported a significant reduction in bone mass in patients treated with low-dose BDP or BV [160]. However, the confounding effect of uncontrolled oral steroid usage could not be excluded in these patients [40]. Therefore the attribution of their reduced body calcium levels to the AC therapy remains in doubt. A recent study of BUD inhaled via a spacer found that the short-term administration of conventional or high doses of the drug had no adverse effect on calcium absorption or excretion, or on serum levels of parathyroid hormone or vitamin D, even though the high BUD dose (2.4 mg/day) significantly suppressed endogenous cortisol production and the blood eosinophil count [226].

However, more recent studies show that both BUD and BDP can adversely affect bone turnover and that these effects may be discernible at dose levels sufficiently low that they do not suppress the morning serum cortisol level significantly, that is, 1.2 mg/day of BUD [4, 78, 230]. The clinical significance of these findings is not yet apparent, but it urgently requires study because of the numbers of patients at risk by virtue of their daily dose requirements [204a].

Aside from the effect of different dose levels of AC on bone metabolism, it is also necessary to assess the extent to which different AC drugs and/or different delivery systems may influence the magnitude of these effects. For example, if the drug is administered from an MDI without a spacer, about 10 times more drug would be expected to deposit in the oropharynx, whence it

may be swallowed. The swallowed AC has the potential for acting directly on the small bowel mucosa, as prednisone does, to inhibit calcium and phosphate absorption. The same concern would be expected with the new dry-powder formulations, but there are no relevant data as yet. These issues need to be addressed because of the likelihood that dry-powder devices may eventually replace freon-powered MDI devices in general clinical usage.

Androgen production from the adrenal cortex is inhibited if an AC or oral steroid is administered at a dosage sufficient to suppress the morning serum cortisol level [226]. Because estrogen deficiency is known to be a major risk determinant of osteoporosis in postmenopausal women, and because their residual estrogen supply derives entirely from these androgenic precursors of adrenocortical origin [39], the reduction in androgen output may augment the risk of bone complications in some older female asthmatics if they receive high-dose AC therapy or a combined AC–oral steroid regimen in the absence of an estrogen supplement.

Hyperactivity and behavioral change have been reported in a father and son and acute psychosis in one other child treated with conventional doses of BUD [98, 117]. Florid Cushing's syndrome has been reported in another child who received conventional doses of TA [80], and clinically apparent adrenal suppression in another for whom 0.4 mg/day of BDP had been prescribed [163]. Whether these individuals were slow metabolizers of glucocorticoids or whether they used more than the prescribed quantities of the drug is unknown.

BDP in doses up to 2.0 mg/day has been found to have no adverse effect on the glucose tolerance of young normal subjects or elderly diabetics [51]. The induction or worsening of diabetes has not been reported as a complication of the treatment of asthmatic patients with conventional doses of various AC drugs.

BDP, 1.0 mg/day, has been reported to increase serum cholesterol and insulin levels marginally [94], although these results were not confirmed in a similar study using BDP, 2.0 mg/day [51]. Because these are risk factors for vascular disease, the possibility of augmenting the progress of atherosclerotic major vessel or cardiovascular disease by long-term AC usage is a concern. Currently, the clinical importance (if any) of these reported changes [94] is uncertain.

Reproductive and Cytotoxic Risks

Because of the absence of data from controlled studies in humans, AC drugs have been assigned as a class to the Food and Drug Administration (FDA) Category C with respect to the level of risk they may present to the fetus or infant. This categorization implies that they may be used with due caution in pregnant or nursing women (see also Chap. 81).

Very large doses of AC drugs such as BDP, flunisolide, or BUD have been shown to cross the placental barrier and to be teratogenic and fetotoxic in rabbits and rats. However, the clinical use of normal doses of BDP by pregnant asthmatic patients has not been associated with any discernible increase in the incidence of congenital malformations in the newborn [55, 66]. This accords with similar reports of the safety of oral steroid therapy during pregnancy [231]. Therefore, the well-documented risks of poorly controlled asthma to the fetus and mother [9, 64, 231] coupled with the relative safety of conventional doses of corticosteroid drugs in general, and AC in particular, favor the use of AC in asthmatic patients who have a manifest clinical need [55, 66].

Low levels of some systemically administered glucocorticoids are known to be distributed in human milk [88, 234]. Hence it is conceivable that they might suppress the growth of nursing infants, although this has not, in fact, been documented in human infants [235]. There are no relevant data for the AC drugs currently used to treat asthma.

AC DOSING REGIMENS

Both the efficacy and the therapeutic index of AC treatment may be influenced by varying the dosing regimen.

Dosing Frequency

The ideal dosing frequency is a matter of controversy [198], but there is a reasonable body of objective evidence from controlled studies of BUD or BDP that helps to clarify the issue.

In mild asthmatics, four times daily dosing with BUD has been shown to be more efficient than once daily, that is, the same peak expiratory flow rate (PEFR) response could be achieved with 75 percent less drug per diem if the daily dose was given in divided doses rather than as a single bolus dose [49]. Also once daily treatment proved less effective clinically than 2 doses of BUD or 3 or 4 doses of BDP each day when the same total dose per day was used with each schedule [20, 125].

However, twice daily treatment can be equally as effective as four times daily for periods of several weeks to months, providing the asthma has been well stabilized beforehand [20, 113, 142, 143, 219]. But when asthma is unstable, twice daily dosing is less effective [219]. Furthermore, the difference appears great enough to be clinically important. Figure 61-8 demonstrates that the therapeutically equivalent dose rose from 0.4 mg/day of BUD on four times daily treatment to greater than 3.0 mg/day on twice daily treatment. Thus, halving the dose frequency shifted the therapeutically equivalent dosage from low and nontoxic to high and potentially toxic levels (with a corollary increase in the cost of treatment) [197, 219].

In view of the characteristically variable course of chronic asthma, these findings suggest that it is prudent to maintain four times daily dosing as the standard AC dosing regimen because it is likely to be more efficacious over the long term than less frequent dosing.

This hypothesis was subsequently tested and confirmed in a double-blind, parallel-groups study that compared the effects of 6 months of treatment with BUD given twice daily or four times daily, using the same total dose per day [105]. The patients who received twice daily treatment experienced significantly more acute asthma relapses and three times as many disability days during the 6-month period than the group who received the same treatment in four divided doses (Table 61-7). Furthermore the disparity between the clinical courses of the two treatment groups was continuing to widen at termination of the study. It seems reasonable to assume that this relationship of efficacy to dosing frequency applies to the other antiasthmatic AC drugs, since the available data do not suggest any important pharmacodynamic differences between them.

It has been suggested that reducing the dose frequency of AC may encourage better patient compliance and thus improve the long-term outcome of asthma treatment. This assumption is not based on controlled studies. In fact, the only proven benefit of twice daily dosing of AC is a reduction in the incidence of thrush, as illustrated in Table 61-8 [223].

Our own experience, replicated in three different studies of BUD or BDP during which we measured compliance objectively, has been that the influence of symptom activity on AC usage overrides that of dosing frequency per se, that improved asthma control leads to dose omissions rather than vice versa, and that departures from the prescribed regimen inevitably occur, even in patients selected for high reliability and monitored by frequent clinical follow-up [198, 203]. This is illustrated in Figure 61-9. Inspection of the individual patient data that make up the group means shown in Figure 61-9 revealed that some individuals had used only about 60 percent of the prescribed dose, whereas others had taken as much as 150 percent, depending on differences in the level of asthma control at different times in the study. These extremes of variability in drug use may be assumed to be

Fig. 61-8. *Effect of dosing frequency on the antiasthmatic efficacy of BUD [197]. Each symbol represents the 14-day mean of the lower value of PEFR measured twice each day, plotted against log$_{10}$ puffs/dose for 3 doses of BUD: 0.4 (●), 0.8 (■), and 1.6 (▲) mg/day, given QID or BID to the same patients. n = 34. The difference in potency shown here was entirely attributable to a comparison made in the first half of the study when the asthma was clinically unstable. No difference was discernible when the same comparisons were repeated in the second part of the study when the asthma was stable. Upper line = .05 mg/puff given QID; lower line = 0.2 mg/puff given BID. (Reprinted with permission from J. H. Toogood, Bronchial Asthma and Glucocorticoids. In R. P. Scheimer, H. N. Claman, and A. Oronsky [eds.], Antiinflammatory Steroid Action: Basic and Clinical Aspects. San Diego: Academic, 1989. Pp. 423–468.)*

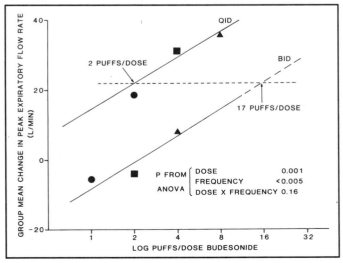

Table 61-7. *Effect of budesonide dosing frequency on incidence of asthma relapse**

	QID dosing	BID dosing
Number	18	18
Rate of relapse	Plateaued after 2 mo	Continued to rise through 6 mo
% of group relapsed within 6 mo	33	72
Disability days/6 mo	147	472 (p = <.001)

* A parallel-groups, double-blind comparative study of 6 months' duration. Both groups received the same dose per day in 2 or 4 divided doses. Therapeutic outcome was more favorable with QID dosing and the difference between the groups increased with time [99].

Table 61-8. *Effect of AC dosing frequency on incidence of thrush**

Budesonide dosing frequency	Nystatin doses/2 weeks (Mean ± SD)	
	Prednisone users (n = 19)	No prednisone (n = 15)
Four times daily	0.965 ± 4.58	0.166 ± 1.58
Twice daily	0.070 ± 0.41	0
p (from paired t)	.05	—
Patients with thrush	5/19	1/15

* Thirty-four asthmatics took the same daily doses of inhaled budesonide twice or four times daily in a balanced crossover comparison.
Source: Adapted from J. H. Toogood et al., Dosing regimen of budesonide and occurrence of oropharyngeal complications. *Eur. J. Respir. Dis.* 65:35, 1984.

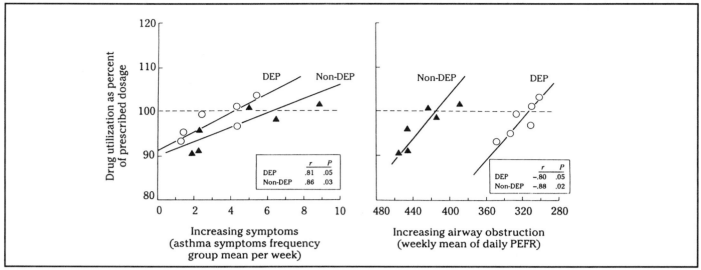

Fig. 61-9. *Shows influence of changes in asthma severity on patient use of an inhaled steroid during a double-blind trial of BUD in 14 prednisone-dependent (○) and 17 nondependent (▲) asthmatic adults [220, 221]. Drug usage was measured objectively from the changes in MDI canister weights at each visit. Group means are shown. r = Pearson correlation coefficient. The p values indicate significant correlations between changes in symptom frequency and peak expiratory flow rate and use of the inhaled steroid; as asthma deteriorated, patients used more than the prescribed dose, and vice versa. (Adapted from J. H. Toogood, High-dose inhaled steroid therapy for asthma.* J. Allergy Clin. Immunol. *83:528, 1989.)*

much wider in ordinary clinical practice than that observed in these supervised clinical trials in patients who had been preselected to exclude those judged likely to be poorly compliant.

Thus it is not necessary to advise patients to reduce the frequency of their AC doses. Most will do that anyway as their symptoms improve [201]. Instead patients ought to be started on four doses per day and then monitored to ensure that an optimum therapeutic response is sustained. If it is not, and lapses in asthma control are associated with reductions in dose frequency, the latter should be corrected.

Dose Scheduling

Giving the entire daily dose of AC in the forenoon might be expected to reduce its systemic activity, as it appears to do with oral prednisone [131]. If this were true, it should permit the upper limits of "safe dosage" of AC to be raised.

We found that morning dosing does indeed conserve a higher 8 A.M. serum cortisol level when intermediate or high doses of AC (BUD) are used [219, 230]. However, there is no parallel sparing of the steroid-induced eosinopenia (Fig. 61-10), and the 24-hour urinary free cortisol output remains the same with either schedule [230]. Thus, it appears unlikely that morning dosing can confer any clinically useful reduction in the risk of adverse systemic effects resulting from AC treatment. Furthermore, morning dosing slightly reduces the efficacy of the drug (Fig. 61-10), and this could be important in some patients with unstable asthma.

EFFICIENT INTRAPULMONARY DELIVERY

The antiasthmatic efficacy of any AC drug depends ultimately on how much gets into the lung. To achieve satisfactory drug delivery in infants or younger children, a solution of BDP and a suspension of BUD have been used by nebulizer, with variable results [28, 62, 110, 116, 132]. In several studies of preschool children with asthma, nebulized BDP proved relatively ineffective [62, 110]. These formulations are not available for clinical use in

the United States. Dry-powder formulations of BDP and BUD (free of additives or propellants) have recently been introduced for clinical use in Europe and Canada. At this time, however, the freon-pressurized MDI remains the delivery system most widely used in the United States and Canada (see also Chap. 56).

Under ideal conditions and in well-trained healthy subjects, about 10 percent of each dose emitted from the MDI enters the lung (Fig. 61-11). This figure is somewhat lower in patients who have obstructive pulmonary impairment (see Table 61-9). About 3 percent of the emitted dose may reach the distal airways [137], while 80 percent deposits in the oropharynx (Fig. 61-11). However, under the less than ideal conditions that prevail in ordinary clinical practice, a number of interacting factors may interfere with AC drug delivery from the MDI. These relate to the delivery device, the inhalation technique, and disease severity (Table 61-10).

Many asthmatic patients who use the MDI coordinate their inspiratory effort poorly [140, 180]. This can significantly reduce the effectiveness of AC treatment. Maximizing the efficiency of intrapulmonary drug delivery requires discharge of the aerosol bolus from the MDI early in the inspiratory effort and a slow inspiration at about 25 L/min, followed by a 10-second breathhold [135]. As shown in Table 61-9, coaching the patient in the correct inhalation technique can materially improve drug delivery, and still further improvement can be achieved by attaching a "spacer" device to the MDI.

Spacers

Spacers of various designs [38, 57, 121, 194] share similar operational principles. They reduce particle velocity and allow more of the propellant to evaporate by increasing the transit distance of the aerosol jet, thus increasing the proportion of small to large particles in the inspired bolus [38]. Only the small particles of inhaled steroid are useful, since the larger ones preferentially deposit in the oropharynx or larger airways, where they may cause oropharyngeal complications or reflex cough.

It has been shown that the oropharyngeal complications of AC

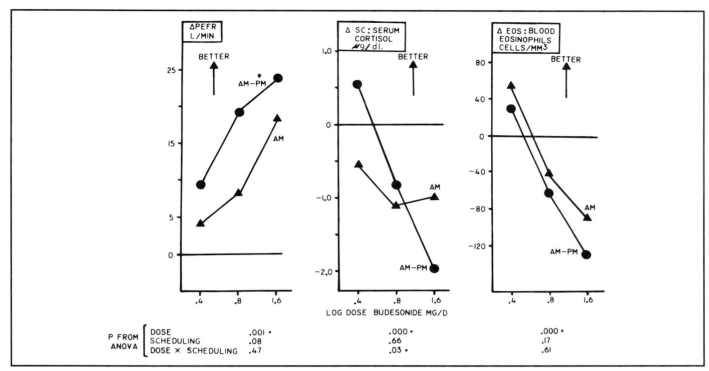

Fig. 61-10. *Effects of* A.M. *versus* A.M./P.M. *dosage schedules on indexes of airflow (Δ PEFR) and systemic glucocorticoid activity (Δ SC, Δ EOS) over a range of BUD dosage. Each point represents the group mean response (2 observations per patient × 34 patients). The p values from ANOVA quantify the significance of the effects of daily dose, scheduling, and dose-scheduling interactions on the three response indexes. Asterisked values are statistically significant (PEFR = peak expiratory flow rate; SC = 0800 hr serum cortisol level; EOS = blood eosinophil count; ANOVA = analysis of variance). (Reprinted with permission from J. H. Toogood et al., Influence of dosing frequency and schedule on the response of chronic asthmatics to the aerosol steroid budesonide.* J. Allergy Clin. Immunol. *70:288, 1982.)*

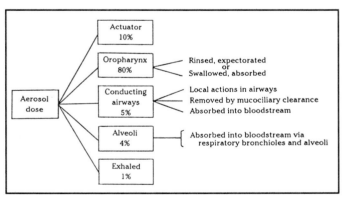

Fig. 61-11. *A typical distribution pattern for a dose of drug inhaled without a spacer from a pressurized MDI. The figures, approximated for simplicity, are derived from direct measurements in vivo, using radiolabelled Teflon particles. (Adapted from S. P. Newman,* Deposition and Effects of Inhalation Aerosols. *Lund, Sweden: A. B. Draco, 1983. P. 97.)*

treatment can be reduced by the use of a spacer [225]. Furthermore, if properly used, the spacer may also double the delivery of the drug to the lung in comparison with what can be achieved with an MDI alone [140, 225] (Fig. 61-12). Efficacy increases commensurately. Large-volume spacers appear potentially more efficient than smaller ones [134] (see Table 61-9). Indeed, if a small spacer is used incorrectly, asthma control may actually deteriorate because of a paradoxic reduction in intrapulmonary drug

delivery consequent to excessive drug losses within the device [222]. Patients often err by expelling more than one puff of drug at a time into the spacer, by allowing more than 2 seconds to elapse before starting to inspire from the spacer, by inspiring too rapidly (faster than 25 L/min), or by failing to breath-hold for 10 seconds at the end of inspiration. Together or separately, these errors can reduce intrapulmonary drug delivery [135, 139].

The presence of one or more of the indications listed in Table 61-11 provide a sufficient basis for prescribing a spacer. Their use ought not to be restricted to patients who obviously use the MDI ineptly because virtually all patients can benefit in terms of a decrease in oropharyngeal complications or augmented delivery of the AC to the lung, or both [225]. Cost-benefit considerations also favor the use of a spacer, even in patients who appear to be doing well on the MDI [225].

Because spacers can increase intrapulmonary drug delivery, and because part of the extra drug is absorbed from the lung in bioactive form, spacers might reasonably be expected to augment the systemic activity of inhaled steroid. In fact they do, as has been shown in adults treated with BUD [225]. However, the magnitude of the effect appears small on the average and clinically unimportant when low or intermediate doses of AC are used [225].

In contrast to the increase in systemic activity that has been seen in adults [225], Prahl and Jensen [156] found that conversion of preschool children from the MDI to a large-volume spacer reduced the systemic glucocorticoid activity of AC (given at high dosage) and that this change was coupled with an improved antiasthmatic response. These contradictory findings (compare [225] versus [156]) might relate to differences between the adult and

Table 61-9. Intrapulmonary deposition of radiolabelled aerosol: MDI versus spacers (% of dose emitted from canister)

	MDI	AC (100 ml)	Tube (110 ml)	Cone (750 ml)	Coaching without spacer	Coaching plus spacer (700 ml)	Spacer's effect on deposition (% relative to MDI)
Normals	10.4[a]	9.85[a]					−5
Bronchitics	8.65[a]	9.02[a]					+5
Asthmatics	7.9[b]		11.5[b]				+46
				13.0[b]			+65
COAD	6.5[c]				11.2[c]		+72
						14.8[c]	+128

MDI = metered-dose inhaler; AC = Aerochamber; COAD = chronic obstructive airways disease.
[a] Data from Dolovich et al. [46].
[b] Data from Newman et al. [138].
[c] Data from Newman et al. [140].

Table 61-10. Factors that diminish intrapulmonary delivery and/or increase oropharyngeal deposition of AC drugs

MDI related
  High-velocity jet
  Short transit distance, valve to airway
  Large particle size (before freons volatilize)
Patient related
  Dose emission uncoordinated with inspiration
  Inspiratory rate greater than 25 L/min
  Failure to breath-hold for 10 seconds after inspiration
Disease related
  Severe obstructive and/or restrictive impairment
  Mucous plugging of small airways due to associated bronchitis or COPD

MDI = metered-dose inhaler; COPD = chronic obstructive pulmonary disease.

pediatric populations studied with respect to the proportion of the active drug distributed to the gut versus the lung while using the MDI. If one postulates inexpert use of the MDI by a child, causing all of the emitted dose to be delivered to the oropharynx and none to the lung, then the swallowed component—of which about 13 percent is bioavailable in the case of BUD [171]—will account for all of the systemic glucocorticoid activity of the AC. The addition of a spacer would be expected to reduce oropharyngeal deposition about tenfold—with a commensurate drop in the amount of drug swallowed and absorbed from the gut. This could more than offset the absolute increase in systemic absorption from the lung resulting from the twofold increase in intrapulmonary delivery achieved with the spacer, and in this way may account for the favorable results some observers have reported [156]. Alternatively, the apparent discrepancies between the effects of spacers in adults versus children might relate to age-dependent anatomic factors such as the ratio of small to large airways at different stages of development or to differences in patient compliance or in inhalation technique. Unfortunately, the inhalation technique used by the children reported by Prahl and Jensen was not described [156].

Inhalation Technique

Simplification of the inhalation procedure has been shown to increase the efficacy of AC treatment [147]. An inhalation technique that involves inhaling the drug from a spacer using several normal inspirations from functional residual capacity has been found to be efficacious in young children [60]. This differs from the slow deep inspiration from residual volume currently advocated for adults [135]. There is a need for comparative studies to determine which inhalation technique confers the most advantageous therapeutic ratio with intermediate and high doses of AC administered by the MDI and whether the optimal technique differs depending on the age of the patient.

Dry-Powder Formulations

The dry-powder formulations of BUD (Turbuhaler) and BDP (Rotahaler or Rotacaps) offer several practical advantages over the MDI, and they appear at least equally as effective [50]. As the devices are breath-activated, they eliminate the problems of coordinating the respiratory effort with release of the AC dose. Patients report they are simpler to use and they reduce the incidence of huskiness or lower airways' irritation from the propellants in the MDI [50]. The multidose Turbuhaler unit offers some advantages over the unit-dose Rotahaler device; it eliminates the need to load each dose manually prior to use, operator errors are reportedly less frequent [41], and the efficiency of intrapulmonary delivery of the active drug is less susceptible to variations in the inspiratory flow rate.

Unlike the MDI, a rapid inspiratory rate is necessary to maximize the efficiency of drug delivery with all the dry-powder devices [67, 146]. The clinical importance of the inspiratory rate is evidenced by the observation that the degree of improvement in airway hyperresponsiveness in response to dry-powder BUD therapy correlates directly with the speed with which the drug is inhaled [50].

Because increasing the rate of inhalation through the Turbuhaler greatly increases the proportion of aerosolized particles of BUD that falls within the "respirable" range (≤ 5 μm) [83], and because these small particles are preferentially distributed to the lung periphery (which is the main site of systemic absorption of the bioactive fraction of the inhaled steroid), one may reasonably anticipate a corollary increase in systemic glucocorticoid activity after switching from the MDI to a dry-powder device. Further, because more than 70 percent of the drug inhaled from the Turbuhaler is deposited in the mouth [141], an increase in candidiasis and thrush might also be expected, especially if the doses are high or given more frequently than twice daily. There are as yet insufficient published data to clarify these uncertainties. They need to be addressed.

Reflex Cough and Bronchospasm

In patients who have chronic airflow limitation along with their asthma, infective exacerbations of mucopurulent bronchitis periodically increase the degree of pulmonary impairment. This shifts the main site of deposition of the inhaled drug toward the more central airways while, at the same time, the accompanying inflammation makes these airways more irritable and hyperresponsive. These changes may persist for weeks after the acute infection. Clinically, they are signalled by the advent of paroxysms of cough or bronchospasm triggered by each AC inhalation in patients who had previously tolerated the drug well. In these circumstances, some may quit the treatment under the mistaken impression they have "become allergic to it" and because they

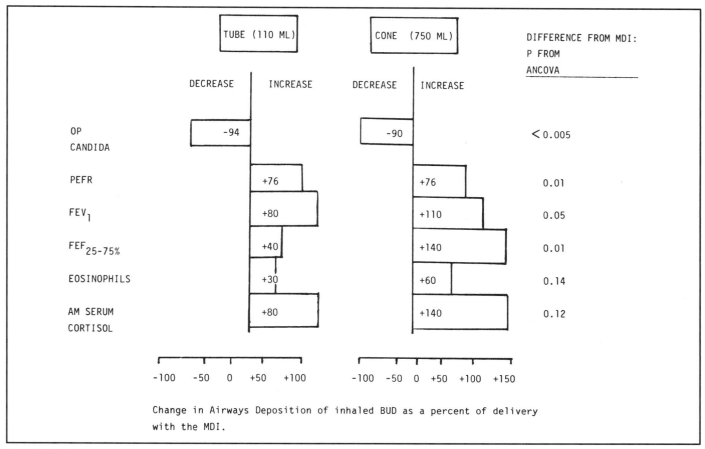

Fig. 61-12. *Effect of two kinds of spacer on deposition of BUD in oropharynx and lung in comparison with the standard MDI (n = 35). The larger the spacer, the greater the augmentation of intrapulmonary delivery of BUD. The reduction in the oropharyngeal deposition of the AC is about the same with either. OP Candida = oropharyngeal colony count; PEFR = peak expiratory flow rate; FEV₁ = forced expiratory volume in one second; FEF = forced expiratory flow; MDI = metered-dose inhaler; ANCOVA = analysis of covariance. (Adapted from J. H. Toogood, Clinical Use of Spacer Systems for Inhaled Glucocorticoid Treatment. In R. Ellul-Micallef, W. K. Lam, and J. H. Toogood [eds.], Advances in the Use of Inhaled Steroids. Hong Kong: Excerpta Medica, Asia Ltd., 1987. Pp. 159–169.)*

Table 61-11. Clinical indications for spacer

Oropharyngeal complications of AC
Suboptimal asthma control
Continuing prednisone dependency, despite AC
Need for > 0.8 mg/day BUD or BDP
Reflex cough or bronchospasm from inhaled drug

perceive a drop in efficacy. The latter is to be expected, since much of each dose is expelled with the reflex cough.

The potential trigger factors for the cough include various constituents of the propellant or the valve assembly, the irritative effect of particulate impaction in the airway, the inspiratory technique, or, rarely, the drug itself [23, 29, 30, 32, 63, 182].

Pretreatment with an inhaled adrenergic [181], slowing the rate of inspiration, or inhaling each dose via a spacer can each improve these symptoms. Switching from BDP to TA may be helpful, partly because of the spacer delivery system supplied with the TA, but also because the switch eliminates the triggering action of the potentially irritating oleic acid constituent that is in the BDP formulation but not in TA [182] (see Table 61-2). However, full resolution of the problem generally requires more aggressive treatment aimed at reversing its primary causes. A burst of prednisone can reduce the airway hyperresponsiveness, accelerate mucociliary clearance of the peripheral airways [12], and improve lung function. The resulting changes in lung dynamics allow deposition of the inhaled aerosol to shift back toward the lung periphery and away from the trachea and carina sites, where deposition of the aerosol bolus triggers the troublesome cough and reflex bronchospasm.

OROPHARYNGEAL COMPLICATIONS

Oropharyngeal candidiasis and dysphonia (huskiness), especially the latter, curtail effective dosage in many AC-treated patients and lead some to abandon the treatment altogether [214]. Both these oropharyngeal complications (like the systemic and antiasthmatic activities of the drugs) are clearly related to the daily dose [211, 214] (see Figs. 61-2 and 61-13). However, their dose dependency is not as consistently discernible as it is with the systemic activities of AC [211, 219, 223, 225]. This implies that factors other than the daily dose per se may act as important codeterminants of these local complications.

Furthermore, the dysphonia and candidiasis may vary independently of one another in the same patients in response to systematic alterations in AC dosage [223]. This implies that they differ in their pathogenesis, and it accords with other evidence

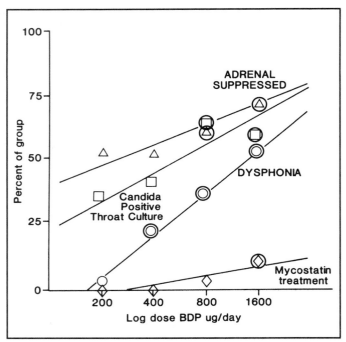

Fig. 61-13. *The occurrence of several adverse responses to beclomethasone dipropionate (BDP) at various dose levels. By comparison with Fig. 61-2, the incidence of these complications can be related to the degree of clinical improvement at any given dosage. Encircled points are statistically significantly different from baseline. (Reprinted with permission from J. H. Toogood et al., A graded dose assessment of the efficacy of beclomethasone dipropionate aerosol for severe chronic asthma.* J. Allergy Clin. Immunol. *59:298, 1977.)*

that shows the pathogenetic correlates of these two problems to be dissimilar [217, 223].

Dysphonia

Dysphonia occurs commonly during AC therapy, whereas laryngeal thrush is extremely rare. The two are not causally related. Therefore nystatin therapy is inappropriate and ineffective for dysphonia. A major causative mechanism for the husky voice is a steroid-induced dyskinesia of the voluntary musculature that controls vocal cord tension [244]. Nonspecific irritation of the larynx due to the propellant freons may also contribute to the huskiness. The problem can be alleviated by anything that reduces deposition of the drug around the larynx, that is, by reducing the daily dose, by slowing the speed with which the AC is inhaled, and/or by inhaling the drug via a spacer designed to selectively remove the larger aerosol particles that ordinarily deposit in the oropharynx and extrathoracic airways when the MDI is used alone [46, 121, 216]. Also a longer postinspiratory breath-hold may help by reducing drug deposition during exhalation [136]. Mouth rinsing immediately after inhaling the drug is recommended to minimize local absorption.

Dysphonia is more common, severe, and persistent in patients whose daily life entails chronic or acute laryngeal stress, such as preachers, teachers, singers, switchboard operators, sports coaches, or employees in a noisy workplace [214]. Compulsive throat clearing commonly aggravates and perpetuates the huskiness. In a few patients, associated hypothyroidism may be a factor [214]. Where one or more of these codeterminants is present, dysphonia may resist all treatment measures, including complete cessation of the AC treatment, until a rigorous voice rest regimen is imposed [214]. Subsequently, the AC treatment can be resumed

at the desired dosage and is usually well tolerated provided laryngeal stress is avoided. Refractory cases may benefit from assessment and treatment by a voice therapist.

Candidiasis and Thrush

Among the pathogenetic determinants of oropharyngeal candidiasis and thrush occurring during AC therapy, the frequency of AC dosing and the concomitant use of prednisone or antibiotics are particularly important [223]. On the other hand, these factors do not relate significantly to dysphonia [217, 223]. The *Candida* overgrowth presumably reflects the inhibitory effect of the drug on the normal host-defense functions of neutrophils, macrophages, and T-lymphocytes at the oral mucosal surface. A 12-hour interval between doses appears sufficient to allow temporary recovery of these functions, as evidenced by the observation that dividing the same daily dose into two rather than four doses prevents the usual dose-dependent increment in the oropharyngeal *Candida* colony count and virtually eliminates thrush (see Table 61-8). This has been shown with BDP and BUD [186, 223], and it probably applies to the other AC drugs as well. Indeed, the advantages that have been claimed for some AC drugs over BDP in terms of a lower incidence of complicating thrush are more likely attributable to differences between their recommended dosing frequencies than to any intrinsic property of the drugs themselves.

Thus, a switch to twice daily dosing while maintaining the same total dose per day may be used to accelerate the clearing of thrush or to prevent its occurrence when the clinical circumstances are such as to increase the likelihood of its occurring, for example, when antibiotics are prescribed for a patient who is already using a high daily dose of AC or combined prednisone-AC therapy [223]. However, reducing the dose frequency to twice daily may result in a clinically important loss of efficacy under some circumstances [219]. Thus, a better alternative in most cases would be a spacer, since the latter can very significantly reduce the amount of oropharyngeal candidiasis even when high doses of AC are administered four times daily [225].

OTHER LOCAL COMPLICATIONS

Esophageal candidiasis is an unusual complication of AC therapy [188] that also reflects the interaction of multiple pathogenetic codeterminants, that is, the topical immunosuppressive activity of the AC in the oropharynx and esophagus plus the effect of systemic steroids if these are used concomitantly, the candidogenic effect of frequent or prolonged broad-spectrum antibiotic therapy, and local damage to the integrity of the lower esophageal mucosa caused by acid reflux resulting from the relaxant effect of theophylline (and/or other drugs such as nitrates or calcium-channel blockers) on the cardiac sphincter. Hiatus hernia, when present, is an added risk factor. Unlike oral candidiasis, which responds well to nystatin, esophageal candidiasis requires ketoconazole or fluconazole therapy. In some patients the problem may prove so intractable as to require AC or theophylline or both to be discontinued.

Several other rare, local complications may occur, even with low doses of AC. These include the painful and protracted atrophic glossitis that may complicate the prolonged and conjoint use of broad-spectrum antibiotics and topical steroid treatment [214] and the severe chronic esophagitis that may result from combined *Candida*–herpes simplex infection [76].

Airway Structure and Function

Long-term AC usage has not been complicated by histologic damage to the epithelium or connective tissues in the airways, as assessed by light and electron microscopy after low-dose [102, 103, 193] or intermediate-dose therapy, that is, 1.6 mg/day of BUD for a year [96]. Indeed, as has been shown with oral steroid treatment [75], AC therapy may encourage bronchial ciliogenesis [102] and the repair of epithelial damage [14].

This contrasts with the atrophy of dermal connective tissue that typically results from chronic application of the same drugs to the skin. The difference presumably reflects the relatively low concentrations of AC per unit surface area in the lung and its much more rapid clearance from the airways than from the skin. Differences in cell sensitivity may also be a factor. In vitro studies of fibroblasts from human lung treated with BUD or BDP found these cells to be approximately 100-fold less sensitive to glucocorticoid effects than skin fibroblasts [173].

BUD and BDP have been found to have no adverse effect on mucociliary clearance [45, 81].

COMPLICATING INFECTIONS

In the immunocompetent patient, the incidence, severity, and duration of viral or bacterial respiratory infections are not increased by AC treatment [56, 192, 214]. There are no reports of "masked" bacterial pneumonia or acute lung abscess complicating the use of AC drugs. Asthmatic patients with a positive tuberculin skin test do not routinely require ancillary treatment with isoniazid if they start regular AC therapy unless there is evidence of active tuberculous disease or recent tuberculin skin test conversion [175–177]. Antituberculous chemotherapy and AC therapy have been used together successfully when active tuberculosis and asthma coexisted [82]. There are no published data to document the safety of AC drugs if they are used in the presence of infection with drug-resistant strains of tubercle bacilli or atypical mycobacteria. In such patients AC must be assumed to carry the same risks of activating the disease as applies with oral steroids.

Pulmonary, bronchial, or systemic fungal infections have not been reported in patients with uncomplicated asthma receiving long-term AC treatment, even with higher than usual doses [214]. However, asthmatic patients who have epithelialized cavities, cysts, or bronchiectatic segments that may harbor a mycetoma might have a measure of increased risk of mycotic superinfection if AC therapy and aggressive prednisone and antibiotic therapy are used conjointly. These factors have been found to correlate significantly with the degree of AC-induced *Candida* overgrowth in the oropharynx [223]. It is not known whether they act similarly to impair local host defenses in lower airways colonized by *Aspergillus fumigatus*. However, we have seen one asthmatic patient with associated chronic obstructive pulmonary disease (COPD) and emphysematous bullae who developed fatal invasive pulmonary aspergillosis after 4 weeks of aggressive treatment with BDP, prednisone, and antibiotics. Also, disseminated aspergillosis has been reported as a complication of the conjoint use of these drugs in a patient with advanced allergic bronchopulmonary aspergillosis [6]. The direct inhibitory effect of *A. fumigatus* spores on normal host defenses in the lung is cautionary [166, 167].

Because of the risks of opportunistic infection, steroids in any form ought to be avoided or used with great caution in the immunocompromised patient.

DURATION OF AC TREATMENT

Like the responses illustrated in Figure 61-2, the effects of AC therapy on bronchial hyperresponsiveness are dose dependent [93]. The effect comprises a prompt response to the AC followed

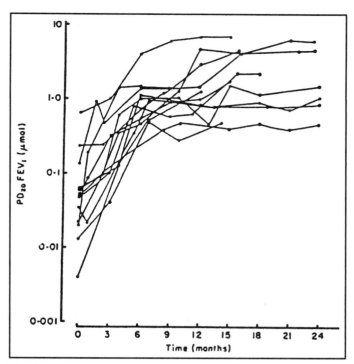

Fig. 61-14. *Changes in airways' hyperresponsiveness of 12 patients during 2 years' treatment with BDP. The response is slowly accumulative. (Data from A. J. Woolcock, K. Yan, and C. M. Salome, Effect of therapy on bronchial hyperresponsiveness in the long-term management of asthma.* Clin. Allergy *18:165, 1988.)*

by a slower accumulative process [236b] measured in terms of weeks, months, or years [87, 90, 93, 200, 211, 248]. The changes in hyperresponsiveness during long-term treatment are well documented in a small group of moderate to severe asthmatics treated with BDP and closely supervised to ensure high compliance with the treatment plan [248]. About 9 months of BDP treatment were required on the average before the improvement in airways' hyperresponsiveness began to plateau, and the improvement was not maximal in some patients until about 15 months (Fig. 61-14). Success was shown to be dependent on the system of patient follow-up care that was used [248].*

In a different group of mild asthmatics treated with low-dose BUD, the impairment in airways' hyperresponsiveness peaked earlier, mainly within 3 months [87]. Nevertheless, some subjects continued to show slowly accumulative improvement even after 1 year. The slow pace of improvement may reflect the time required to dissipate the intramural inflammatory thickening of the airways, which may account for much of the chronic asthmatic patient's exaggerated responsiveness to bronchospastic stimuli [84].

It is doubtful that AC therapy can ever "cure" asthma, in the sense of achieving a remission that can be sustained indefinitely after withdrawal of the drug. We found, in a group of 31 mild asthmatics previously treated with low-dose BDP, that abrupt replacement of the BDP with a therapeutically inert agent under

---

* This approach to asthma therapy is succinctly outlined in the Australian Asthma Management Plan. The plan aims to define the goals of treatment, objectively measure asthma severity by the daily use of a peak expiratory flowmeter, provide the patient with written guidelines for adjusting his or her treatment regimen, and assess each patient's clinical course as frequently as four times per year to ensure that the treatment goals are in fact being met. This regimen provides positive reinforcement via a feedback loop, thus enhancing patient compliance. Interested readers may secure a copy by writing to the Thoracic Society of Australia and New Zealand, 145 Macquire Street, Sydney 2000, Australia.

double-blind conditions resulted in an objectively documented asthma relapse in 50 percent of the group within 10 days and in 100 percent within 48 days [229] (see Fig. 61-7). Fourteen of these patients had received greater than 5 years of regular AC therapy. One had been virtually symptom-free and vigorously active in competitive athletics for 10 years while using BDP or BUD regularly. Other investigators report longer intervals until relapse [18].

Bronchial biopsies of patients treated for 10 years with AC show epithelial healing and significant resolution of the mucosal inflammatory cell infiltration that was present prior to commencing the AC [103]. However, in a few of these patients, some of the metaplastic changes in the respiratory epithelium failed to normalize after 10 years of therapy and the airways' hyperresponsiveness persisted as well [103].

It therefore appears that the need for regular AC therapy must be considered permanent in most asthmatic patients who commence the drug, unless a dominant causative factor can be identified in the home or workplace and removed. In light of this prospect for extended and indefinite usage, and the evidence that cumulative dosage may be the important determinant of such steroid-induced complications as cataract formation [106] and possibly others as well, it is essential that the daily dose of AC be kept as low as is consistent with maintaining good control of the asthma and that ancillary nonsteroidal treatments be used where possible to minimize the AC dose requirements.

ANCILLARY TREATMENT

Concomitant oral bronchodilators, usually slow-release theophylline, should be used where feasible in AC-treated subjects, since they can improve asthma control in patients receiving either inhaled or oral steroid therapy and thus help to keep the steroid doses down [42, 133].

The putative advantages of regular inhaled beta-agonist therapy as a routine supplement to AC treatment require serious reevaluation at this time, in light of recent evidence of the counterproductive results of co-treatment with fenoterol [178]. In this double-blind comparison of routine, four times daily treatment with inhaled fenoterol versus "as needed" usage only, the former regimen was associated with greater airways' hyperresponsiveness, a deeper nocturnal dip in peak expiratory flows, more nocturnal and daytime symptoms, and a more frequent requirement for supplementary prednisone to treat asthma relapses. These adverse effects on therapeutic outcome were not prevented by concomitant AC therapy, given in doses ranging from 0.15 to 3.0 mg/day of BUD or BDP. The notion that preceding each AC treatment with a routine inhalation of a beta agonist can usefully increase the intrapulmonary delivery or efficacy of the inhaled steroid is not supported by any of the studies that have examined the question [104, 123, 225]. This objective can be better accomplished by prescribing a spacer for the AC and training the patient in the principles of efficient inhalation technique [225]. It is our policy to reduce beta-agonist usage as close to zero as possible with the aid of AC therapy. This is an attainable goal in many patients. Currently, 60 percent of the adult asthmatics receiving AC therapy in our clinic use beta agonists only "if needed," and one-half of these need the bronchodilator less frequently than once a month [95].

The addition of cromolyn to an established AC regimen has not been shown to confer any appreciable advantage either in terms of improving asthma control [43, 119] or for facilitating a reduction in the dose of AC in patients whose AC requirements are high enough to perpetuate the HPA suppression caused by their previous prednisone treatment [206]. Similarly, the improvement in asthma symptoms and reduction in AC dosage that

may be attainable by adding ketotifen or nedocromil to an established AC regimen appear marginal at best [79, 101, 170].

Nasal Disease

In our clinic, more than half the patients referred with asthma as their primary problem have some type of upper airway disease as well, and this usually requires treatment [202]. Thus many AC-treated asthmatic patients may be candidates for intranasal topical steroid therapy as well. Despite the theoretic risk of additive systemic effects from the combined use of intranasal and intrapulmonary steroids, the available evidence suggests the magnitude of this risk is negligible under ordinary clinical circumstances. For example, we found the 24-hour urinary free cortisol output was not affected by adding 0.3 mg/day of intranasal flunisolide to an established antiasthmatic regimen averaging 0.52 mg/day of BDP plus 4.3 mg/day of prednisone [218]. These doses were effective for both the rhinitis and asthma. This does not rule out the possibility of additive systemic effects if higher doses are used.

Allergy Management

Atopic allergy is known to be a significant risk factor for the occurrence of asthma both in adults and in children [25, 150, 155, 174], and there is increasingly persuasive evidence that exposure to respirable environmental allergens is one of the most important potentially identifiable and correctable causes of chronic asthma [5, 24, 26, 120, 154, 155, 157, 161, 187, 232, 249]. Therefore an allergy assessment ought to be considered in all asthmatics younger than 50 years of age and also in selected older patients.

In appropriately selected patients, environmental control of allergenic house dust exposure or the elimination of household pets is known to reduce asthma morbidity and drug requirements [126, 127, 152, 238, 239] and to significantly improve airways' hyperresponsiveness [152, 238], provided the control measures are rigorous and sustained for many months [161]. Avoidance of nonallergic trigger factors is similarly important, particularly with respect to environmental tobacco smoke [27, 128, 129]. Tobacco smoke may act not only as a direct respiratory irritant, but possibly as an inducer of atopic sensitization as well [107] (see Chap. 2). Environmental control measures ought therefore to be ancillary to any drug regimen chosen for asthma, and AC therapy cannot adequately substitute for these important avoidance measures.

The relative efficacy of specific immunotherapy for asthma as an adjunct to treatment with AC or other antiasthmatic drugs has not been adequately studied to date. In particular, it is not known whether immunotherapy does (or does not) have any measurable steroid-sparing effect.

ALTERNATIVE TREATMENTS

When a physician has serious concerns about the possible risk of adverse systemic effects accruing after long-term AC usage, cromolyn provides a reasonable alternative, especially in children. Cromolyn has demonstrable inhibitory activity on seasonal exacerbations of allergen-induced airways' hyperresponsiveness and the late asthmatic response [36] (see Chap. 63). It has been shown to be effective for asthma [13, 22, 236], and it is remarkably safe [58, 179, 209]. However, cromolyn is not as effective as AC for the correction of chronic airways' hyperresponsiveness [190]. Where the two drugs have been compared clinically, AC has consistently proved the more effective agent [190, 206]. Similarly the available data for nedocromil and ketotifen show no convincing evidence that either can effectively substitute for AC therapy [44, 79, 170, 191]. Because of the greater efficacy of AC, and because low-dose AC appears to be devoid of clinically important adverse effects, it is inappropriate to rely on cromolyn, nedocromil, or ketotifen as an alternative to AC if they prove incapable of achieving or maintaining optimal asthma control in a particular patient.

AC has been shown to be equally as effective or better than theophylline for chronic asthma and significantly less toxic [158]. It may be more reasonable to view theophylline as an adjunct rather than an alternative to AC because the primary inflammatory process in the airways is not responsive to xanthine therapy [37, 47, 50, 90], whereas it does respond to AC drugs [45a, 84a, 94a]. It is not logical to exclude this important and potentially drug-responsive primary pathogenetic mechanism from the treatment plan.

Similarly, regular inhaled beta-agonist therapy, unlike AC therapy, does not improve the primary airway inflammation [45a, 84a, 94a, 236a], and it is less effective than AC therapy for normalizing pulmonary impairment and symptoms [70a, 94a, 236a].

In "steroid-resistant" asthmatics whose disease requires continued prednisone usage along with AC, methotrexate may be considered. Its capacity to facilitate prednisone weaning has been documented and shown to be specifically drug related [124, 183] (see Chap. 68). However, the magnitude of the reduction in prednisone usage achieved in a recent double-blind multicenter trial appears so small when the change in the parallel group treated with placebo is subtracted, as to be of doubtful value clinically [183]—particularly when offset against the acquired risks of methotrexate toxicity. Some of the latter complications are immediately apparent, while others relate to cumulative dosage [1, 73]. Before committing to methotrexate therapy, due consideration should be given to why the patient continues to be prednisone dependent. Some of the most important reasons are not likely to be changed by methotrexate (see the list of determinants of MMD-P in Table 61-6 and related text). Because of these uncertainties, coupled with the well-documented efficacy of high-dose AC therapy, toxic antimetabolites such as methotrexate ought not to be considered until an adequate trial of high-dose AC has been made. Safety studies have shown that some patients can tolerate high dosages of BUD or BDP for a long time without clinically apparent adverse effects [186, 213, 214, 228]. Similar data for TA and flunisolide are unavailable.

Oral Steroid Preferred

Some advantages and disadvantages of oral versus inhaled steroid therapy are compared in Table 61-12. On the whole, the risk-benefit considerations previously discussed make AC the drug of choice in most cases. However, oral prednisone may be preferred in particular circumstances. This applies to patients in whom adverse socioeconomic circumstances, poor compliance, drug costs, or inept use of the MDI compromises the usefulness of AC treatment. Particular mention needs to be made of the type of unstable high-risk asthmatic patient described by Strunk et al. [189], in whom a recent reduction or withdrawal of prednisone under the aegis of AC treatment (presumably low dose) proved to be one of the harbingers of their death from asthma. Such patients may be assumed to need high doses of AC to achieve adequate control of their asthma. But they cannot be relied on to take the prescribed dose consistently and to continue it indefinitely. As shown in Table 61-6, poor compliance is the major cause of treatment failure during long-term AC treatment, and the consequences of failure in patients such as these are potentially disastrous.

Thus, where severe unstable asthma combines with poor compliance as a prominent behavioral characteristic to create an inordinately high risk of asthmatic death, it is probably safer to rely on prednisone, not on AC alone, to minimize the risk of fatality. The oral prednisone may be given alone or in combination with low- or intermediate-dose AC.

Table 61-12. Some advantages and disadvantages of AC versus oral corticosteroids

Oral	AC
Effective	Effective
Inexpensive	
More convenient, compliance is easy	Compliance too difficult for some
Some subjects are uncontrollable on alternate-morning (low-risk) regimen	Permits conversion of virtually all subjects previously dependent on daily oral steroid to alternate-morning regimen
Essential to control extrapulmonary disease in some subjects	Improved asthma control and/or decreased hypercortisonism in most even if prednisone continued (at reduced dosage)
Abrupt dose increase is usually effective for acute severe asthma	Efficacy of abrupt dose increase for acute asthma exacerbation remains unproved
	At equivalent antiasthmatic dosage, AC consistently shows lower systemic glucocorticoid activity (though not necessarily zero)
Major systemic complications may occur	No major complications observed at conventional low dosage after > 15 years' clinical use

Systemic steroid is also preferred for patients who must continue it for reasons other than asthma. The commonest example of this in ordinary clinical practice is nonatopic perennial hyperplastic rhinosinusitis with recurrent nasal polyposis. However, in the latter patients, low-dose oral prednisone is generally used as a supplement rather than a substitute for AC therapy.

Less common conditions that require continuing systemic steroid therapy include pulmonary infiltration with eosinophilia (PIE syndrome), the various forms of systemic necrotizing vasculitis that may be accompanied by asthma [52], and probably allergic bronchopulmonary aspergillosis (ABPA) (see also Chap. 49).

In patients with ABPA, AC treatment may improve the asthma symptoms without reducing the recurrence rate of the segmental pulmonary consolidations [74, 162, 240]. Oral prednisone, on the other hand, has been shown to prevent these segmental inflammatory lesions [172]. Since it is the destructive effects of the latter, rather than the asthma, that lead to the widespread lung fibrosis characteristic of end-stage ABPA [145], oral steroid therapy should probably remain the mainstay of its long-term management [205].

In patients who have ABPA and require doses of prednisone sufficiently large to carry a risk of significant adverse effects, supplementary bronchodilators ought to be used, and AC may be used, to facilitate reduction of the prednisone dose to less toxic levels. If an AC regimen is adopted, it is advisable that its effectiveness be monitored objectively rather than by symptoms alone. Serial chest radiographs, pulmonary function tests, sputum cultures, total serum IgE, specific IgG *Aspergillus* antibody titers, and blood eosinophil counts provide useful guides to the activity of the disease [145, 164]. Monitoring is advisable because AC treatment has been reported to be associated in some cases with a paradoxic increase in the *Aspergillus* content of the sputum [233]. Also, in at least one patient, disseminated aspergillosis has complicated the use of combined oral and inhaled steroid therapy [6].

The potential for complications such as those mentioned may apply only in those ABPA patients who have advanced disease associated with structural lung defects, such as bronchiectasis. Indeed some experts consider that the use of AC to treat the earlier and milder stages of ABPA may actually prevent the syndrome from evolving into its later stages when bronchiectasis, pulmonary fibrosis, and disabling pulmonary insufficiency dominate the clinical picture.

Acute Asthma: Oral Steroid or AC?

Acute Severe Asthma

The mainstay of treatment for acute severe asthma is prompt aggressive inhaled bronchodilator therapy plus a bolus of 30 to 60 mg of prednisone or 200 mg of hydrocortisone [69, 72]. The steroid is critically important in those patients whose severe airway obstruction is mainly inflammatory rather than bronchospastic in origin, as evidenced by failure of their relatively low airflows to respond within 1 or 2 hours to inhaled bronchodilators [159]. AC is not an appropriate alternative for the systemic steroid because of uncertainties about its efficacy in this potentially dangerous situation. Concurrent AC treatment is therapeutically redundant and may lead to troublesome thrush in some patients because of the candidogenic effects of concomitant administration of high-dose prednisone, antibiotic, and/or AC drugs [76, 188, 223].

After the severe asthma has been optimally controlled and the patient is ready to commence reducing the prednisone dosage, an antiinflammatory drug that is safer for long-term usage should be started. The drug of choice is usually an AC, given at a dose calculated to be sufficient to maintain control of the asthma after the prednisone is withdrawn. Our practice is to convert the prednisone abruptly to alternate-morning usage (while continuing the AC), then titrate toward zero over 2 to 8 weeks. If symptoms recur on the "no prednisone days," the prednisone dose is not reduced further. Instead the patient seeks medical advice.

Exacerbations of Chronic Asthma

A recently published guideline for the management of chronic asthma recommends the daily dose of AC be increased from time to time in response to changes in symptoms and airflow rates and, in particular, that the dose be doubled for about a week at the onset of upper respiratory infection [68]. Another, more detailed set of guidelines for the early treatment of asthma exacerbations recommends that the AC dosage be doubled or quadru-

pled (to 1–2 mg/day) for 1 or 2 days and then followed by a burst of prednisone if the high-dose AC proves ineffective [72]. These recommendations appear essentially empirical, and their efficacy has not been adequately tested by controlled trials. Only one such study has been published to date—a placebo-controlled trial of intermittent high-dose AC (2.25 mg/day of BDP for 5 days), which aimed to control episodic exacerbations of asthma triggered by acute respiratory infection in preschool children. The investigators found a small, statistically significant symptom benefit with the AC, but no reduction in the requirement for hospital admission or the need for a burst of prednisone [246]. Thus the reliability of intermittent high-dose AC therapy for aborting exacerbations of acute asthma remains in doubt.

In older asthmatics, many of whom have associated chronic bronchitis or chronic airflow limitation, it is our practice to rely on a temporary burst of prednisone rather than increasing the AC dose because prednisone is less expensive, predictably effective, and well tolerated by the majority of patients. On the other hand, in patients known to be intolerant of high-dose prednisone, because of acute central nervous system toxicity for example, aggressive treatment with AC may sometimes be effective as a substitute (provided it is started early enough). In these circumstances it is appropriate to maximize the antiasthmatic potency of the drug by increasing the dosing frequency as well as the total dose per day and optimizing intrapulmonary drug delivery by the use of a large-volume spacer. If more than two such interventions with prednisone or high-dose AC are required per year, it probably means the patient's daily dose of AC is too low. It should be increased to provide better protection.

Bronchospasm

It is important to instruct each patient in the correct use of the AC and inhaled bronchodilators and to check them at follow-up to ensure the AC is being used appropriately and not for attempted relief of acute symptoms.

COPD or Asthma?

Although chronic obstructive pulmonary disease (COPD) defined by rigorous criteria does not respond to oral or inhaled steroid

Table 61-13. Patient costs for AC therapy

Generic name	Brand	Dose/puff (mg)	Doses/pkg.	Cost $ per pkg.[a]	Relative antiinflammatory potency[b]	Cost $ per 30 days @ 0.4 mg/day[c]	Cost adjusted for potency[d]
TA	Azmacort	.20	240	15.95	0.27	3.98	1.23
F	Bronalide	.25	100	16.23	0.35	7.79	1.85
BDP	Vanceril	.05	200	11.03	0.64	13.24	1.72
BDP	Beclovent	.05	200	11.32	0.64	13.58	1.77
BDP	Becloforte	.25	200	68.85	0.64	16.52	2.15
BDP	Rotacaps[e]	.20	100	30.49	0.64	18.29	2.38
BDP	Beclodisk[e]	.20	120	36.59	0.64	18.29	2.38
BUD	Pulmicort Turbuhaler[e]	.20	200	65.01	1.0	19.50	1.62
BUD	Pulmicort	.20	100	32.51	1.0	19.51	1.62
BUD	Pulmicort	.05	200	17.25	1.0	20.70	1.72
BDP	Rotacaps[e]	.10	100	22.00	0.64	26.40	3.44
BDP	Beclodisk[e]	.10	100	26.86	0.64	26.86	3.49

[a] Ontario Drug Benefit Formulary prices (Canadian dollars, 1991). Excludes dispensing fee. Approximate U.S. cost/pkg. (U.S. dollars, Northeast U.S.A.):

TA	Azmacort	$39.95
BDP	Vanceril	$32.50
BDP	Beclovent	$31.00

[b] Measured by topical vasoconstrictor assay on human skin.
[c] Items are rank ordered on this column.
[d] In the absence of adequate relative efficacy data for the various AC drugs and formulations, these calculations are based on the topical potencies shown in column b. Other factors may influence relative antiasthmatic potency, e.g., differences in intrapulmonary absorption and metabolism, receptor binding affinities, and the efficiency of intrapulmonary delivery with various delivery devices or AC formulations (see text).
[e] Dry-powder formulations. The others are MDI.

[71], a substantial number of patients who may be categorized as COPD in ordinary clinical practice on the basis of persisting wheeze, breathlessness, and airflow limitation refractory to bronchodilator therapy may benefit materially from high-dose oral or AC treatment [17, 114, 165, 199]. This reflects the preponderance of airway inflammation over bronchospasm as the cause of these patients' airflow limitation. The potential for steroid responsiveness in such patients is not reliably predictable from clinical or pulmonary function criteria, and in particular, it is unrelated to the degree of beta-adrenergic "reversibility" of airflow indices measured by conventional test procedures [17, 207]. Thus a trial of steroid is required. High-dose BDP has been used for this purpose [241], but it is probably more reliable to give a 14-day burst of high-dose prednisone to achieve the initial effect and then convert to an appropriate dose of AC to sustain the improvement in those patients who have responded well.

It is important that therapeutic trials of this type be monitored objectively and not by subjective responses alone. Prednisone therapy, and indeed the very act of participating in a therapeutic trial, can produce statistically significant psychological changes that bias patient-generated indices of dyspnea severity such as the breathlessness score, 12-minute walking distance, or oxygen cost diagram ratings [118]. Failure to appreciate the nonspecific nature of such reports of subjective benefit in the absence of accompanying changes in airflow, forced vital capacity, or the amount of pulmonary hyperinflation [31, 196, 245] may lead to needless and possibly hazardous long-term treatment with steroids, orally or by inhalation, in patients who cannot benefit.

COST AND COST BENEFITS

Cost-benefit data for AC therapy are few and indeterminate. Such as they are, they favor the AC drug. The most detailed evaluation published to date reports a reduction of 50 percent or more in hospitalization rates for asthma after the introduction of BUD treatment and a similar reduction in overall health care costs for inpatient and ambulatory care for asthma [2]. A problem with this and similar cost-benefit assessments is that the beneficial effects of the AC per se cannot be differentiated from those that may result from concomitant improvements in the efficiency of clinical surveillance. (See Chap. 92 for additional discussion.)

Drug costs may be an important consideration for some patients in clinical practice. Table 61-13 compares the AC formulations currently available in Canada in terms of their base cost to the patient.

REFERENCES

1. The ACG Committee on FDA-Related Matters. Methotrexate-induced chronic liver injury: Guidelines for detection and prevention. *J. Gastroenterol.* 88:1337, 1988.
2. Adelroth, E., and Thompson, S. Hogdosinhalationssteroider vid astma—analys av kostnader och vardutnyttjande. *Lakartidninger* 81:4285, 1984.
3. Adelroth, E., et al. Inflammatory cells and eosinophilic activity in asthmatics investigated by bronchoalveolar lavage: The effects of antiasthmatic treatment with budesonide or terbutaline. *Am. Rev. Respir. Dis.* 142:91, 1990.
4. Ali, N. J., Capewell, S., and Ward, M. J. Bone turnover during high dose inhaled corticosteroid therapy. *Thorax* 44(10):900, 1989.
5. Alvareg-Dardet, C. Outbreak of asthma associated with soybean dust. *N. Engl. J. Med.* 321:1127, 1989.
6. Anderson, C. J., Craig, S., and Bardana, E. J., Jr. Allergic bronchopulmonary aspergillosis and bilateral fungal balls terminating in disseminated aspergillosis. *J. Allergy Clin. Immunol.* 65:140, 1980.
7. Andersson, M., Andersson, P., and Pipkorn, U. Topical glucocorticosteroids and allergen-induced increase in nasal reactivity: Relationship between treatment time and inhibitory effect. *J. Allergy Clin. Immunol.* 82:1019, 1988.
8. Andersson, M., Andersson, P., and Pipkorn, U. Allergen-induced specific and non-specific nasal reactions. *Acta. Otolaryngol.* 107:270, 1989.
9. Bahna, S. L., and Bjerkedal, T. The course and outcome of pregnancy in women with bronchial asthma. *Acta Allergol.* (Kbh) 27:397, 1972.
10. Balfour-Lynn, L. Growth in childhood asthma. *Arch. Dis. Child.* 61:1049, 1986.
11. Balfour-Lynn, L. Growth retardation in asthmatic children treated with inhaled beclomethasone dipropionate. *Lancet* 1:475, 1988.
12. Bateman, J. R. M., et al. Tracheobronchial clearance and ventilatory function after medium dose oral corticosteroid therapy in stable asthmatics. *Prog. Respir. Res.* 14:145, 1980.
13. Bernstein, I. L., et al. A controlled study of cromolyn sodium sponsored by the Drug Committee of the American Academy of Allergy. *J. Allergy Clin. Immunol.* 50:235, 1972.
14. Beskow, R., et al. Bronkofiberskopiforbattrad diagnostik och behandling av lungsjukdomar. *Lakartidningen* 72:4731, 1975.
15. Bisgaard, H., et al. Adrenal function in children with bronchial asthma treated with beclomethasone dipropionate or budesonide. *J. Allergy Clin. Immunol.* 81:1088, 1988.
16. Bisgaard, H., et al. Allergen-induced increase of eosinophil cationic protein in nasal lavage fluid: Effect of the glucocorticoid budesonide. *J. Allergy Clin. Immunol.* 85:891, 1990.
17. Blair, G. P., and Light, R. W. Treatment of chronic obstructive pulmonary disease with corticosteroids: Comparison of daily vs. alternate-day therapy. *Chest* 86:524, 1984.
18. Boe, J., et al. Comparison of dose-response effects of inhaled beclomethasone dipropionate and budesonide in the management of asthma. *Allergy* 44:349, 1989.
19. Bone, M. F., et al. Nedocromil sodium in adults with asthma dependent on inhaled corticosteroids: A double blind, placebo controlled study. *Thorax* 44:654, 1989.
20. Boyd, G., Abdallah, S., and Clark, R. Twice or four times daily beclomethasone dipropionate in mild stable asthma? *Clin. Allergy* 15:383, 1985.
21. Brodgen, R. N., et al. Beclomethasone dipropionate: A reappraisal of its pharmacodynamic properties and therapeutic efficacy after a decade of use in asthma and rhinitis. *Drugs* 28:99, 1984.
22. Brompton Hospital. Long-term study of disodium cromoglycate in treatment of severe extrinsic or intrinsic bronchial asthma in adults. *Br. Med. J.* 4:383, 1972.
23. Bryant, D. H., and Pepys, J. Bronchial reactions to aerosol inhalant vehicle. *Br. Med. J.* 1:1319, 1976.
24. Burney, P. G. J., et al. Descriptive epidemiology of bronchial reactivity in an adult population: Results from a community study. *Thorax* 42:38, 1987.
25. Burrows, B., Lebowitz, M., and Barbee, R. A. Respiratory disorders and allergy skin-test reactions. *Ann. Intern. Med.* 84:134, 1976.
26. Burrows, B., et al. Association of asthma with serum IgE levels and skin-test reactivity to allergens. *N. Engl. J. Med.* 320:271, 1989.
27. Canadian Pediatric Society. Secondhand cigarette smoke worsens symptoms in children with asthma. *Can. Med. Assoc. J.* 135:321, 1986.
28. Carlsen, K. H., et al. Nebulised beclomethasone dipropionate in recurrent obstructive episodes after acute bronchiolitis. *Arch. Dis. Child.* 63:1428, 1988.
29. Charpin, D., Beaupre, A., and Orehek, J. Deep-inspiration induced bronchoconstriction: A mechanism for beclomethasone aerosol intolerance. *Eur. J. Respir. Dis.* 64:494, 1986.
30. Charpin, D., and Orehek, J. Reactions to bronchoconstrictor drugs. *Chest* 92:958, 1987.
31. Chrystyn, H., Mulley, B. A., and Peake, M. D. Dose response relation to oral theophylline in severe chronic obstructive airways disease. *Br. Med. J.* 297:1506, 1988.
32. Clark, R. J. Exacerbation of asthma after nebulised beclomethasone dipropionate. *Lancet* 2:574, 1986.
33. Clark, T. J. H. Safety of inhaled corticosteroids. *Eur. J. Respir. Dis.* 63(Suppl. 122):235, 1982.
34. Clark, T. J. H. Inhaled corticosteroid therapy: A substitute for theophylline as well as prednisone? *J. Allergy Clin. Immunol.* 76:330, 1985.
35. Clissold, S. P., and Heel, R. C. Budesonide: A preliminary review of its pharmacodynamic properties and therapeutic efficacy in asthma and rhinitis. *Drugs* 28:485, 1984.
36. Cockcroft, D. W., and Murdock, K. Y. Comparative effects of inhaled salbutamol sodium cromoglycate, and beclomethasone dipropionate on

allergen-induced early asthmatic responses, late asthmatic responses, and increased bronchial responsiveness to histamine. *J. Allergy Clin. Immunol.* 79:734, 1987.

37. Cockcroft, D. W., et al. Theophylline does not inhibit allergen-induced increase in airway responsiveness. *J. Allergy Clin. Immunol.* 83:913, 1989.

38. Corr, D., et al. Design and characteristics of a portable breath actuated particle size selective medical aerosol inhaler. *J. Aero. Sci.* 13:1, 1982.

39. Crilly, R. G., Marshall, D. H., and Nordin, B. E. C. Metabolic effects of corticosteroid therapy in post-menopausal women. *J. Steroid Biochem.* 11:429, 1979.

40. Crompton, G. K. Corticosteroids: In drug therapy for asthma. *Br. Med. J.* 294:123, 1987.

41. Crompton, G. K. The Role of Inhaled β-Agonists and Different Delivery Systems in Asthma. In S. P. Newman, F. Moren, and G. K. Crompton (eds.), *A New Concept in Inhalation Therapy.* Bussum, Netherlands: Medicom Europe, 1987. Pp. 71–76.

42. Dahl, R., and Johansson, S. A. Effect on lung function of budesonide by inhalation, terbutaline s.c. and placebo given simultaneously or as single treatments. *Eur. J. Respir. Dis.* 63(Suppl. 122):132, 1982.

43. Dawood, A. G., Hendry, A. T., and Walker, S. R. The combined use of betamethasone valerate and sodium cromoglycate in the treatment of asthma. *Clin. Allergy* 7:161, 1977.

44. Dawson, K. P., et al. Ketotifen in asthma. *Aust. Paediatr. J.* 25:89, 1989.

45. Dechateau, G. S. M. J. E., Zuidema, J., and Merkus, H. M. The in vitro and in vivo effect of a new non-halogenated corticosteroid—budesonide—aerosol on human ciliary epithelial function. *Allergy* 41:260, 1986.

45a. Djukanovic, R., et al. Effect of an inhaled corticosteroid on airway inflammation and symptoms in asthma. *Am. Rev. Respir. Dis.* 145:669, 1992.

46. Dolovich, M., Ruffin, R., and Newhouse, M. T. Clinical evaluation of a simple demand inhalation device MDI aerosol delivery device. *Chest* 84:36, 1983.

47. Dutoit, J. I., Salome, C. M., and Woolcock, A. J. Inhaled corticosteroids reduce the severity of bronchial hyperresponsiveness in asthma but oral theophylline does not. *Am. Rev. Respir. Dis.* 136:1174, 1987.

48. Toogood, J. H., et al. Risk of posterior subcapsular cataracts (PSC) during oral and inhaled steroid (IS) therapy for asthma. *Clin. Invest. Med.* 15(Suppl. 10):A6, 1992.

49. Ellul-Micallef, R. Acute Dose-response Studies in Bronchial Asthma with Budesonide. In R. Ellul-Micallef, W. K. Lam, and J. H. Toogood (eds.), *Advances in the Use of Inhaled Corticosteroids.* Hong Kong: Excerpta Medica Asia, 1987. Pp. 129–139.

50. Engel, T., et al. Clinical comparison of inhaled budesonide delivered either via pressurized metered dose inhaler or Turbuhaler. *Allergy* 44:220, 1989.

51. Fancourt, G. J., Ebden, P., and McNally, P. The effects of high dose (2000 micrograms/day) inhaled beclomethasone dipropionate (Becloforte) on glucose tolerance in diet controlled elderly diabetic subjects. *Eur. Respir. J.* 1(Suppl. 2):196s, 1988.

52. Fauci, A. S. Vasculitis. *J. Allergy Clin. Immunol.* 72:211, 1983.

53. Feldman, D., Funder, J., and Loose, D. Is the glucocorticoid receptor identical in various target organs? *J. Steroid Biochem.* 9:141, 1978.

54. Ferguson, A. C., Murray, A. B., and Tze, W. J. Short stature and delayed skeletal maturation in children with allergic disease. *J. Allergy Clin. Immunol.* 69:461, 1982.

55. Fitzsimons, R., Greenberger, P. A., and Patterson, R. Outcome of pregnancy in women requiring corticosteroids for severe asthma. *J. Allergy Clin. Immunol.* 78:349, 1986.

56. Frank, A., and Dash, C. H. Inhaled beclomethasone dipropionate in acute infections of the respiratory tract. *Respiration* 48:122, 1985.

57. Freigang, B. Long-term follow-up of infants and children treated with beclomethasone aerosol by a special inhalation device. *Ann. Allergy* 45:13, 1980.

58. Furukawa, C. T., et al. A double blind study comparing the effectiveness of cromolyn sodium and sustained released theophylline in childhood asthma. *Pediatrics* 74:453, 1984.

59. Gambertoglio, J. G., et al. Prednisolone disposition in cushingoid and noncushingoid kidney transplant patients. *J. Clin. Endocrinol. Metab.* 51:561, 1980.

60. Gleeson, J. G. A., and Price, J. F. Controlled trial of budesonide given by the nebuhaler in preschool children with asthma. *Br. Med. J.* 297:163, 1988.

61. Godfrey, S., Balfour-Lynn, L., and Tooley, M. A three to five year follow-

up of the use of the aerosol steroid beclomethasone dipropionate in childhood asthma. *J. Allergy Clin. Immunol.* 62:335, 1978.

62. Godfrey, S., et al. Nebulised budesonide in severe infantile asthma. *Lancet* 2:851, 1987.

63. Godin, J., and Malo, J. L. Acute bronchoconstriction caused by beclovent and not vanceril. *Clin. Allergy* 9:585, 1979.

64. Gordon, M., et al. Fetal morbidity following potentially anoxigenic obstetric conditions: VII. Bronchial asthma. *Am. J. Obstet. Gynecol.* 106:421, 1970.

65. Graff-Lonnevig, V., and Kraepelien, S. Long-term treatment with beclomethasone dipropionate aerosol in asthmatic children with special reference to growth. *Allergy* 34:57, 1979.

66. Greenberger, P. A., and Patterson, R. Beclomethasone dipropionate for severe asthma during pregnancy. *Ann. Intern. Med.* 98:478, 1983.

67. Groth, S., and Dirksen, H. Optimal inhalation procedure for the fenoterol powder inhaler. *Eur. J. Respir. Dis.* 64(Suppl. 130):17, 1983.

68. Guidelines for management of asthma in adults: I. Chronic persistent asthma. Statement by the British Thoracic Society, Research Unit of the Royal College of Physicians of London, King's Fund Centre, National Asthma Campaign. *Br. Med. J.* 390:651, 1990.

69. Guidelines for management of asthma in adults: II. Acute severe asthma. Statement by the British Thoracic Society, Research Unit of the Royal College of Physicians of London, King's Fund Centre, National Asthma Campaign. *Br. Med. J.* 301:797, 1990.

70. Gwynn, C. M., and Smith, J. M. A one year follow up of children and adolescents receiving regular beclomethasone dipropionate. *Clin. Allergy* 4:325, 1974.

70a. Haahtela, T., et al. Comparison of a β₂-agonist, terbutaline, with an inhaled corticosteroid, budesonide, in newly detected asthma. *N. Engl. J. Med.* 325(6):388, 1991.

71. Hall, T. G., et al. The efficacy of inhaled beclomethasone in chronic obstructive airway disease. *Pharmacotherapy* 9:232, 1989.

72. Hargreave, F. E., et al. The assessment and treatment of asthma: A conference report. *J. Allergy Clin. Immunol.* 85(6):1098, 1990.

73. Health and Public Policy Committee, American College of Physicians Position Paper. Methotrexate in rheumatoid arthritis. *Ann. Intern. Med.* 107:418, 1987.

74. Heinig, J. H., et al. High-dose local steroid treatment in bronchopulmonary aspergillosis: A pilot study. *Allergy* 43:24, 1988.

75. Heino, M., et al. Bronchial ciliogenesis and oral steroid treatment in patients with asthma. *Br. J. Dis. Chest* 82:175, 1988.

76. Hemstreet, M. P., Reynolds, D. W., and Meadows, J., Jr. Oesophagitis: A complication of inhaled steroid therapy. *Clin. Allergy* 10:733, 1980.

77. Herxheimer, H. Should corticosteroid aerosols be used in severe chronic asthma? *Thorax* 36:401, 1981.

78. Hodsman, A. B., et al. Differential effects of inhaled budesonide and oral prednisolone on serum osteocalcin. *J. Clin. Endocrinol. Metab.* 72(3):530, 1991.

79. Holgate, S. T. Clinical evaluation of nedocromil sodium in asthma. *Br. J. Clin. Pract.* 41:13, 1987.

80. Hollman, G. A., and Allen, D. B. Overt glucocorticoid excess due to inhaled corticosteroid therapy. *Pediatrics* 81:452, 1988.

81. Holmberg, K., and Pipkorn, V. Influence of topical beclomethasone dipropionate suspension on human nasal mucociliary activity. *Eur. J. Clin. Pharmacol.* 30:625, 1986.

82. Horton, D. J., and Spector, S. L. Clinical pulmonary tuberculosis in an asthmatic patient using a steroid aerosol. *Chest* 71:540, 1977.

83. Jaegfeldt, H., et al. Particle Size Distribution from Different Modifications of Turbuhaler. In S. P. Newman, F. Moren, and G. K. Crompton (eds.), *A New Concept in Inhalation Therapy.* Bussum, Netherlands: Medicom Europe, 1987. Pp. 90–99.

84. James, A. L., Paré, P. D., and Hogg, J. C. The mechanics of airway narrowing in asthma. *Am. Rev. Respir. Dis.* 139:242, 1989.

84a. Jeffrey, P. K., et al. Effects of treatment on airway inflammation and thickening of basement membrane reticular collagen in asthma. *Am. Rev. Respir. Dis.* 145:890, 1992.

85. Jennings, B. H., et al. The assessment of systemic effects of inhaled glucocorticosteroids: A comparison of budesonide and beclomethasone dipropionate in healthy volunteers in assessment of systemic effects of inhaled glucocorticosteroids. Department of Clinical Pharmacology, University of Lund, Sweden, 1990. Pp. VII:1–14.

86. Johansson, S. A., et al. Topical and systemic glucocorticoid potencies of budesonide and beclomethasone dipropionate in man. *Eur. J. Respir. Dis.* 63(Suppl. 122):74, 1982.

87. Juniper, E. F., et al. Effect of long-term treatment with an inhaled corti-

costeroid (budesonide) on airway hyperresponsiveness and clinical asthma in nonsteroid-dependent asthmatics. *Am. Rev. Respir. Dis.* 142: 832, 1990.

88. Katz, F. H., and Burris, R. D. Entry of prednisone into human milk. *N. Engl. J. Med.* 293:1154, 1975.

89. Kehlet, H., and Binder, C. Adrenocortical function and clinical course during and after surgery in unsupplemented glucocorticoid treated patients. *Br. J. Anaesth.* 45:1043, 1973.

90. Kerrebijn, K. F., van Essen-Zandvliet, E. E. M., and Neijens, H. J. Effect of long-term treatment with inhaled corticosteroids and beta-agonists on the bronchial responsiveness in children with asthma. *J. Allergy Clin. Immunol.* 79:653, 1987.

91. Kewley, G. D. Possible association between beclomethasone dipropionate aerosol and cataracts. *Aust. Paediatr. J.* 16:117, 1980.

92. Kozower, M., Veatch, L., and Kaplan, M. M. Decreased clearance of prednisolone, a factor in the development of corticosteroid side effects. *J. Clin. Endocrinol. Metab.* 38:407, 1974.

93. Kraan, J., et al. Dosage and time effects of inhaled budesonide on bronchial hyperreactivity. *Am. Rev. Respir. Dis.* 137:44, 1988.

94. Kruszynska, Y. T., et al. Effect of high dose inhaled beclomethasone dipropionate on carbohydrate and lipid metabolism in normal subjects. *Thorax* 42:881, 1987.

94a. Laitinen, L. A., Laitinen, A., and Haahtela, T. A comparative study of the effects of an inhaled corticosteroid, budesonide, and a β_2-agonist, terbutaline, on airway inflammation in newly diagnosed asthma: A randomized, double-blind, parallel-group controlled trial. *J. Allergy Clin. Immunol.* 90:32, 1992.

95. Laity, A., et al. Profile of ambulatory care for chronic asthma in a tertiary referral clinic. *Clin. Invest. Med.* 14:A6, 1991.

96. Laursen, L. C., et al. Fiberoptic bronchoscopy and bronchial mucosal biopsies in asthmatics undergoing long-term high-dose budesonide aerosol treatment. *Allergy* 43:284, 1988.

97. Law, C. M., et al. Nocturnal adrenal suppression in asthmatic children taking inhaled beclomethasone dipropionate. *Lancet* 1:942, 1986.

98. Lewis, L. D., and Cochrane, G. M. Psychosis in a child inhaling budesonide. *Lancet* 2:634, 1983.

99. Lieberman, P., Patterson, R., and Kunske, R. Complications of long-term steroid therapy for asthma. *J. Allergy Clin. Immunol.* 49:329, 1972.

100. Littlewood, J. M., et al. Growth retardation in asthmatic children treated with inhaled beclomethasone dipropionate. *Lancet* 1:115, 1988.

101. Loftus, B. G., and Price, J. F. Long-term, placebo-controlled trial of ketotifen in the management of preschool children with asthma. *J. Allergy Clin. Immunol.* 79:350, 1987.

102. Lundgren, R. Scanning electron microscope studies of bronchial mucosa before and during treatment with beclomethasone dipropionate inhalation. *Scand. J. Respir. Dis.* 57(Suppl. 101):179, 1977.

103. Lundgren, R., et al. Morphological studies of bronchial mucosal biopsies from asthmatics before and after ten years of treatment with inhaled steroids. *Eur. Respir. J.* 1:883, 1988.

104. Mackay, A. D., and Dyson, A. J. How important is the sequence of administration of inhaled beclomethasone dipropionate and salbutamol in asthma? *Br. J. Dis. Chest.* 75:273, 1981.

105. Malo, J.-L., et al. Four-times-a-day dosing frequency is better than a twice-a-day regimen in subjects requiring a high-dose inhaled steroid, budesonide, to control moderate to severe asthma. *Am. Rev. Respir. Dis.* 140:624, 1989.

106. Manabe, S., Bucala, R., and Cerami, A. Nonenzymatic addition of glucocorticoids to lens proteins in steroid-induced cataracts. *J. Clin. Invest.* 74:1803, 1984.

107. Martinez, F. D., et al. Parental smoking enhances bronchial responsiveness in nine-year-old children. *Am. Rev. Respir. Dis.* 138:518, 1988.

108. Maunsell, K., Pearson, R. S. B., and Livingstone, J. L. Long-term corticosteroid treatment of asthma. *Br. Med. J.* 1:661, 1968.

109. McAllen, M. K., Kochanowski, S. J., and Shaw, K. M. Steroid aerosols in asthma: An assessment of betamethasone valerate and a 12-month study of patients on maintenance treatment. *Br. Med. J.* 1:171, 1974.

110. McCarthy, T. P., and Hultquist, C. Nebulised budesonide in severe childhood asthma. *Lancet* 1:379, 1989.

111. McKenzie, A. W., and Atkinson, R. M. Topical activities of betamethasone esters in man. *Arch. Dermatol.* 89:741, 1964.

112. Mellis, C. M., and Phelan, P. D. Asthma deaths in children—a continuing problem. *Thorax* 32:29, 1977.

113. Meltzer, E. O., Kemp, J. P., and Welch, J. M. Effect of dosing schedule on efficacy of beclomethasone dipropionate aerosols in chronic asthma. *Am. Rev. Respir. Dis.* 131:732, 1985.

114. Mendella, L. A., et al. Steroid response in stable chronic obstructive pulmonary disease. *Ann. Intern. Med.* 96:17, 1982.

115. Messina, M. S., and Smaldone, G. C. Evaluation of quantitative aerosol techniques for use in bronchoprovocation studies. *J. Allergy Clin. Immunol.* 75:252, 1984.

116. Metzger, W. J., Richerson, H. B., and Wasserman, S. I. Generation and partial characterization of eosinophil chemotactic activity and neutrophil chemotactic activity during early and late-phase asthmatic response. *J. Allergy Clin. Immunol.* 78:282, 1986.

117. Meyboom, R. H. B., and de Graff-Breederveld, N. Budesonide and psychic side effects. *Ann. Intern. Med.* 109:683, 1988.

118. Mitchell, D. M., et al. Psychological changes and improvement in chronic airflow limitation after corticosteroid treatment. *Thorax* 39:924, 1984.

119. Mitchell, I., et al. Treatment of childhood asthma with sodium cromoglycate and beclomethasone dipropionate aerosol singly and in combination. *Br. Med. J.* 4:457, 1976.

120. Soliman, M. Y., Rosenstreich, D. L. Natural immunity to dust mites in adults with chronic asthma: I. Mite-specific serum IgG and IgE. *Am. Rev. Respir. Dis.* 134:962, 1986.

121. Moren, F. Drug deposition of pressurized inhalation aerosols I. *Int. J. Pharm.* 1:205, 1978.

122. Morrow Brown, H. The Introduction and Early Development of Inhaled Steroid Treatment. In N. Mygind and T. J. H. Clark (eds.), *Topical Steroid Treatment for Asthma and Rhinitis.* London: Bailliere & Tindall, 1980. Pp. 66–76.

123. Muers, M., and Dawkins, K. Effect of a timed interval between inhalation of beta-agonist and corticosteroid aerosols on the control of chronic asthma. *Thorax* 38:378, 1983.

124. Mullarkey, M. F., et al. Methotrexate in the treatment of corticosteroid-dependent asthma: A double-blind crossover study. *N. Engl. J. Med.* 318:603, 1988.

125. Munch, E. P., et al. Dose frequency in the treatment of asthmatics with inhaled topical steroids. *Eur. J. Respir. Dis.* 67:254, 1985.

126. Murray, A. B., and Ferguson, A. C. Reduction of bronchial hyperreactivity during prolonged allergen avoidance. *Lancet* 2:1212, 1982.

127. Murray, A. B., and Ferguson, A. C. Dust-free bedrooms in the treatment of asthmatic children with house dust or house dust mite allergy: A controlled trial. *Pediatrics* 71:418, 1983.

128. Murray, A. B., and Morrison, B. J. The effect of cigarette smoke from the mother on bronchial responsiveness and severity of symptoms in children with asthma. *J. Allergy Clin. Immunol.* 77:575, 1986.

129. Murray, A. B., and Morrison, B. J. Passive smoking and the seasonal difference of severity of asthma in children. *Chest* 94:701, 1988.

130. Mygind, N., and Hansen, I. Beclomethasone dipropionate aerosol effect on the adrenals in normal persons. *Acta. Allergol.* 28:211, 1973.

131. Myles, A. B., Bacon, P. A., and Daly, R., Jr. Single daily dose corticosteroid treatment. *Ann. Rheum. Dis.* 30:149, 1971.

132. Nassif, E., et al. Extrapulmonary effects of maintenance corticosteroid therapy with alternate-day prednisone and inhaled beclomethasone in children with chronic asthma. *J. Allergy Clin. Immunol.* 80:518, 1987.

133. Nassif, E. G., et al. The value of maintenance theophylline in steroid-dependent asthma. *N. Engl. J. Med.* 304:71, 1981.

134. Newman, S. P. Pressurized aerosols inhaled through extension devices. *J. Aero. Sci.* 14:69, 1983.

135. Newman, S. P., Pavia, D., and Clarke, S. W. How should a pressurized beta-adrenergic bronchodilator be inhaled? *Eur. J. Respir. Dis.* 62:3, 1981.

136. Newman, S. P., Pavia, D., and Garland, N. Effects of various inhalation modes on the deposition of radioactive pressurized aerosols. *Eur. J. Respir. Dis.* 63(Suppl. 119):57, 1982.

137. Newman, S. P., et al. Deposition of pressurized aerosols in the human respiratory tract. *Thorax* 36:52, 1981.

138. Newman, S. P., et al. Deposition of pressurized suspension aerosols inhaled through extension devices. *Am. Rev. Respir. Dis.* 124:317, 1981.

139. Newman, S. P., et al. Improvement of pressurised aerosol deposition with nebuhaler spacer device. *Thorax* 39:935, 1984.

140. Newman, S. P., et al. Effect of Inspir-Ease on the deposition of metered-dose aerosols in the human respiratory tract. *Chest* 89:551, 1986.

141. Newman, S. P., et al. Deposition Patterns in Man from Turbuhaler: A Preliminary Report. In S. P. Newman, F. Moren, and G. K. Crompton (eds.), *A New Concept in Inhalation Therapy.* Bussum, Netherlands: Medicom Europe, 1987. Pp. 104–114.

142. Nyholm, E., Frame, M. H., and Cayton, R. M. Therapeutic advantages of

twice-daily over four-times daily inhalation budesonide in the treatment of chronic asthma. *Eur. J. Respir. Dis.* 65:339, 1984.

143. Orgel, H. A., Meltzer, E. O., and Kemp, J. P. Flunisolide aerosol in treatment of steroid-dependent asthma in children. *Ann. Allergy* 51:21, 1983.

144. Pakes, G. E., et al. Flunisolide: A review of its pharmacological properties and therapeutic efficacy in rhinitis. *Drugs* 19:397, 1980.

145. Patterson, R., et al. Allergic bronchopulmonary aspergillosis: Staging as an aid to management. *Ann. Intern. Med.* 96:286, 1982.

146. Pedersen, S. How to use a rotahaler. *Arch. Dis. Child.* 61:11, 1986.

147. Pedersen, S. Inhaler use in children with asthma. *Dan. Med. Bull.* 34(Suppl. 5):234, 1987.

148. Pedersen, S., and Fuglsang, G. Urine cortisol excretion in children treated with high doses of inhaled corticosteroids: A comparison of budesonide and beclomethasone. *Eur. Respir. J.* 1:433, 1988.

149. Pedersen, S., et al. Pharmacokinetics of budesonide in children with asthma. *Eur. J. Clin. Pharmacol.* 31:579, 1987.

150. Pepys, J., Chan, M., and Hargreave, F. E. Mites and house-dust allergy. *Lancet* 1:1270, 1968.

151. Place, V. A., Velazquez, J. G., and Burdick, K. H. Precise evaluation of topically applied corticosteroid potency. *Arch. Dermatol.* 101:531, 1970.

152. Platts-Mills, T. A. E., et al. Reduction of bronchial hyperreactivity during prolonged allergen avoidance. *Lancet* 2:675, 1982.

153. Plumpton, F. S., Besser, G. M., and Cole, P. V. Corticosteroid treatment and surgery. *Anaesthesia* 24:3, 1969.

154. Pollart, S. M., et al. Epidemiology of emergency room asthma in northern California: Association with IgE antibody to ryegrass pollen. *J. Allergy Clin. Immunol.* 82:224, 1988.

155. Pollart, S. M., et al. Epidemiology of acute asthma: IgE antibodies to common inhalant allergens as a risk factor for emergency room visits. *J. Allergy Clin. Immunol.* 83:875, 1989.

156. Prahl, P., and Jensen, T. Decreased adreno-cortical suppression utilizing the nebuhaler for inhalation of steroid aerosols. *Clin. Allergy* 17:393, 1987.

157. Price, J. A., et al. Measurement of airborne mite antigen in homes of asthmatic children. *Lancet* 336:895, 1990.

157a. Priftis, K., Everard, M. L., and Milner, A. D. Unexpected side-effects of inhaled steroids: A case report. *Eur. J. Pediatr.* 150:449, 1991.

158. Reed, C. E., and American Academy of Allergy and Immunology Study Group. Treatment of mild to moderate asthma: Comparison of aerosol beclomethasone and oral theophylline. *Am. Rev. Respir. Dis.* 143:A625, 1991.

159. Reed, C. E., and Hunt, L. W. The emergency visit and management of asthma (editorial). *Ann. Intern. Med.* 112(11):801, 1990.

160. Reid, D. M., et al. Corticosteroids and bone mass in asthma: Comparisons with rheumatoid arthritis and polymyalgia rheumatica. *Br. Med. J.* 293:1463, 1986.

161. Report of an International Workshop, Bad Kreuznach, Federal Republic of Germany. Dust mite allergens and asthma—a worldwide problem. *J. Allergy Clin. Immunol.* 83:416, 1989.

162. Report to the Research Committee of the British Thoracic Association. Inhaled beclomethasone dipropionate in allergic bronchopulmonary aspergillosis. *Br. J. Dis. Chest* 73:349, 1979.

163. Rhoades, R. B., and Forbes, E. F. Clinically apparent adrenal suppression with beclomethasone (400 μg a day) inhalation. *J. Allergy Clin. Immunol.* 65:218, 1980.

164. Ricketti, A. J., Greenberger, P. A., and Patterson, R. Serum IgE as an important aid in management of allergic bronchopulmonary aspergillosis. *J. Allergy Clin. Immunol.* 74:68, 1984.

165. Robertson, A. S., et al. A double-blind comparison of oral prednisone 40 mg/day with inhaled beclomethasone dipropionate 1500 μg/day in patients with adult onset chronic obstructive airways disease. *Eur. J. Respir. Dis.* 69:565, 1986.

166. Robertson, M. D., et al. Inhibition of phagocyte migration and spreading by spore diffusates of *Aspergillus fumigatus*. *J. Med. Vet. Mycol.* 25:389, 1987.

167. Robertson, M. D., et al. Suppression of host defenses by *Aspergillus fumigatus*. *Thorax* 42:19, 1987.

168. Rooklin, A. R., et al. Posterior subcapsular cataracts in steroid-requiring asthmatic children. *J. Allergy Clin. Immunol.* 63:383, 1979.

169. Ruffin, R. E., et al. Aerosol therapy with Sch 1000: Short-term mucociliary clearance in normal and bronchitic subjects and toxicology in normal subjects. *Chest* 73:501, 1978.

170. Ruffin, R. E., et al. The efficacy of nedocromil sodium (Tilade) in asthma. *Aust. N. Z. J. Med.* 17:557, 1987.

171. Ryrfeldt, A., et al. Pharmacokinetics and metabolism of budesonide, a selective glucocorticoid. *Eur. J. Respir. Dis.* 63(Suppl. 122):86, 1982.

172. Safirstein, B. H., et al. Five-year follow-up of allergic bronchopulmonary aspergillosis. *Am. Rev. Respir. Dis.* 104:450, 1973.

173. Sarnstrand, B., et al. Effect of Glucocorticosteroids on Hyaluronic Acid Synthesis in Vitro in Human Fibroblast-like Cells from Lung and Skin. In J. C. Hogg, R. Eullul-Micallef, and R. Brattsand (eds.), *Glucocorticoids, Inflammation and Bronchial Hyperreactivity*. Amsterdam: Excerpta Medica, 1985, Pp. 157–66.

174. Sarsfield, J. K. Role of house dust mites in childhood asthma. *Arch. Dis. Child.* 49:711, 1974.

175. Schatz, M., and Patterson, R. Asthma, steroid therapy, isoniazid. *Ann. Intern. Med.* 85:538, 1976.

176. Schatz, M., and Patterson, R. Tuberculosis and isoniazid in steroid-treated asthmatic patients. *Ann. Intern. Med.* 85:129, 1976.

177. Schatz, M., et al. The prevalence of tuberculosis and positive tuberculin skin tests in a steroid-treated asthmatic population. *Ann. Intern. Med.* 84:261, 1976.

178. Sears, M. R., et al. Regular inhaled beta-agonist treatment in bronchial asthma. *Lancet* 336:1391, 1990.

179. Settipane, G. A., et al. Adverse reactions to cromolyn. *J.A.M.A.* 241:844, 1979.

180. Shim, C., and Williams, M. H., Jr. The adequacy of inhalation of aerosol from canister nebulizers. *Am. J. Med.* 69:891, 1980.

181. Shim, C. S. Inhalation aids of metered dose inhalers. *Chest* 91:315, 1987.

182. Shim, C. S., and Williams, M. H., Jr. Cough and wheezing from beclomethasone dipropionate aerosol are absent after triamcinolone acetonide. *Ann. Intern. Med.* 106:700, 1987.

183. Shiner, R. J., et al. Randomised, double-blind, placebo-controlled trial of methotrexate in steroid-dependent asthma. *Lancet* 336:137, 1990.

184. Sly, R. M., and Committee on Drugs, The American Academy of Allergy and Immunology. Adverse effects and complications of treatment with beta-adrenergic agonist drugs. *J. Allergy Clin. Immunol.* 75:443, 1985.

185. Smith, M. J., and Hodson, M. E. Effects of long term inhaled high dose beclomethasone dipropionate on adrenal function. *Thorax* 38:676, 1983.

186. Smith, M. J., and Hodson, M. E. High-dose beclomethasone inhaler in the treatment of asthma. *Lancet* 1:265, 1983.

187. Sporik, R., et al. Exposure to house-dust mite allergen (Der p I) and the development of asthma in childhood. *N. Engl. J. Med.* 323:502, 1990.

188. Stein, M. R., Shay, S. S., and Jacobson, K. Monilial esophagitis in asthmatic patients treated with beclomethasone. *J. Allergy Clin. Immunol.* 63:172, 1979.

189. Strunk, R. C., et al. Physiologic and psychological characteristics associated with deaths due to asthma in childhood. *J.A.M.A.* 254:1193, 1985.

190. Svendsen, U. G., et al. A comparison of the effects of sodium cromoglycate and beclomethasone dipropionate on pulmonary function and bronchial hyperreactivity in subjects with asthma. *J. Allergy Clin. Immunol.* 80:68, 1987.

191. Svendsen, U. G., et al. A comparison of the effects of nedocromil sodium and beclomethasone dipropionate on pulmonary function, symptoms, and bronchial responsiveness in patients with asthma. *J. Allergy Clin. Immunol.* 84:224, 1989.

192. Tarlo, S., Broder, I., and Spence, L. A prospective study of respiratory infection in adult asthmatics and their normal spouses. *Clin. Allergy* 9:293, 1979.

193. Thiringer, G., et al. Bronchoscopic biopsies of bronchial mucosa before and after beclomethasone dipropionate therapy. *Scand. J. Respir. Dis.* 57(Suppl. 101):173, 1977.

194. Tobin, M. J., et al. Response to bronchodilator drug administration by a new reservoir aerosol delivery system and a review of other auxiliary delivery systems. *Am. Rev. Respir. Dis.* 126:670, 1982.

195. Toogood, J. H. Steroids in asthma. *Lancet* 2:1185, 1979.

196. Toogood, J. H. How to use steroids in asthma therapy. *J. Respir. Dis.* 3:15, 1982.

197. Toogood, J. H. Concentrated aerosol formulations in asthma. *Lancet* 2:790, 1983.

198. Toogood, J. H. An appraisal of the influence of dose frequency on the antiasthmatic activity of inhaled corticosteroids. *Ann. Allergy* 55:2, 1985.

199. Toogood, J. H. Corticosteroids. In J. W. Jenne and S. Murphy (eds.), *Drug Therapy for Asthma, Research and Clinical Practice*. New York: Marcel Dekker, 1987. Pp. 719–759.

200. Toogood, J. H. Bronchial Asthma and Glucocorticoids. In R. P. Schleimer, H. N. Claman, and A. Oronsky (eds.), *Anti-inflammatory Ste-*

roid Action: Basic and Clinical Aspects. San Diego: Academic, 1989. Pp. 423–468.

201. Toogood, J. H. High-dose inhaled steroid therapy for asthma. *J. Allergy Clin. Immunol.* 83:528, 1989.

202. Toogood, J. H. Some Clinical Aspects of Pharmacotherapy of Rhinitis and Asthma. In N. Mygind, U. Pipkorn, and R. Dahl (eds.), *Rhinitis and Asthma: Similarities and Differences.* Copenhagen: Munksgaard, 1990. Pp. 289–306.

203. Toogood, J. H., and Baskerville, J. Patient compliance during inhaled steroid (IS) therapy. *J. Allergy Clin. Immunol.* 79:144, 1987.

204. Toogood, J. H., Baskerville, J., and Johansson, S.-A. Factors accounting for steroid resistance in chronic asthma. *Chest* 88(1):52S, 1985.

204a. Toogood, J. H., and Hodsman, A. B. Effects of inhaled and oral corticosteroids on bone. *Ann. Allergy* 67(2):87, 1991.

205. Toogood, J. H., Jennings, B., and Baskerville, J. Aerosol Corticosteroids. In E. B. Weiss and M. Segal (eds.), *Bronchial Asthma: Mechanisms and Therapeutics* (2nd ed.). Boston: Little, Brown, 1985. Pp. 698–713.

206. Toogood, J. H., Jennings, B., and Lefcoe, N. M. A clinical trial of combined cromolyn/beclomethasone treatment for chronic asthma. *J. Allergy Clin. Immunol.* 67:317, 1981.

207. Toogood, J. H., Jennings, B. J., and Lefcoe, N. M. Responsiveness of asthmatics to inhaled steroid therapy is unpredictable from tests of bronchodilator "reversibility." *Clin. Invest. Med.* 10(4):B117, 1987.

208. Toogood, J. H., and Lefcoe, N. M. Dexamethasone aerosol for the treatment of "steroid dependent" chronic bronchial asthmatic patients. *J. Allergy* 36:321, 1965.

209. Toogood, J. H., Lefcoe, N. M., and McCourtie, D. R. Multicentre surveillance of longterm safety of sodium cromoglycate. *Allergol. Immunopathol.* 5:448, 1977.

210. Toogood, J. H., et al. Determinants of the response to beclomethasone aerosol at various dosage levels: A multiple regression analysis to identify clinically useful predictors. *J. Allergy Clin. Immunol.* 60:367, 1977.

211. Toogood, J. H., et al. A graded dose assessment of the efficacy of beclomethasone dipropionate aerosol for severe chronic asthma. *J. Allergy Clin. Immunol.* 59:298, 1977.

212. Toogood, J. H., et al. Patient Asthma Monitor (PAM): Interactive Programs for Time-Sequence Analysis of Chronic Obstructive Pulmonary Disease. In D. B. Shires and H. Wolf (eds.), *Medinfo 77.* Amsterdam: North-Holland, 1977. P. 401.

213. Toogood, J. H., et al. Minimum dose requirements of steroid-dependent asthmatic patients for aerosol beclomethasone and oral prednisone. *J. Allergy Clin. Immunol.* 65:355, 1978.

214. Toogood, J. H., et al. Candidiasis and dysphonia complicating beclomethasone treatment of asthma. *J. Allergy Clin. Immunol.* 65:145, 1980.

215. Toogood, J. H., et al. Optimal Dosage in Steroid-Dependent Asthma. In N. Mygind and T. J. H. Clark (eds.), *Topical Steroid Treatment for Asthma and Rhinitis.* London: Bailliere & Tindall, 1980. P. 107.

216. Toogood, J. H., et al. Therapeutic implications of small airways dysfunction in chronic asthma. *Am. Rev. Respir. Dis.* 123:113, 1981.

217. Toogood, J. H., et al. Determinants of oropharyngeal (op) complications during aerosol steroid (as) treatment of chronic asthma. *Am. Rev. Respir. Dis.* 125:120, 1982.

218. Toogood, J. H., et al. Efficacy and safety of concurrent use of intranasal flunisolide and oral beclomethasone aerosols in treatment of asthmatics with rhinitis. *Clin. Allergy* 12:95, 1982.

219. Toogood, J. H., et al. Influence of dosing frequency and schedule on the response of chronic asthmatics to the aerosol steroid, budesonide. *J. Allergy Clin. Immunol.* 70:288, 1982.

220. Toogood, J. H., et al. Bioequivalent doses of inhaled vs. oral steroids for severe asthma. *Chest* 84:349, 1983.

221. Toogood, J. H., et al. Comparison of alternate-morning prednisone vs. inhaled steroid (IS) for asthma. *Ann. R. Coll. Physicians Surg.* 16(4):308, 1983.

222. Toogood, J. H., et al. Proper use of spacers (Sps) to augment the response of asthmatics to inhaled steroids. *Ann. Allergy* 50(5):354, 1983.

223. Toogood, J. H., et al. Dosing regimen of budesonide and occurrence of oropharyngeal complications. *Eur. J. Respir. Dis.* 65:35, 1984.

224. Toogood, J. H., et al. Personal observations on the use of inhaled corticosteroid drugs for chronic asthma. *Eur. J. Respir. Dis.* 65:321, 1984.

225. Toogood, J. H., et al. Use of spacers to facilitate inhaled corticosteroid treatment of asthma. *Am. Rev. Respir. Dis.* 129:723, 1984.

226. Toogood, J. H., et al. Effect of high dose inhaled budesonide on calcium and phosphate metabolism and the risk of osteoporosis. *Am. Rev. Respir. Dis.* 138:57, 1988.

227. Toogood, J. H., et al. Bioequivalent doses of budesonide and prednisone in moderate and severe asthma. *J. Allergy Clin. Immunol.* 84:688, 1989.

228. Toogood, J. H., et al. Safety of long term budesonide (BUD) therapy. *Clin. Invest. Med.* 12(4):B5, 1989.

229. Toogood, J. H., et al. A study of the mechanism of the anti-asthmatic action of inhaled budesonide. *J. Allergy Clin. Immunol.* 85:872, 1990.

230. Toogood, J. H., et al. Effects of dose and dosing schedule of inhaled budesonide on bone turnover. *J. Allergy Clin. Immunol.* 88:572, 1991.

231. Turner, E. S., Greenberger, P. A., and Patterson, R. Management of the pregnant asthmatic patient. *Ann. Intern. Med.* 93:905, 1980.

232. Turner, K. J., et al. Studies on bronchial hyperreactivity, allergic responsiveness, and asthma in rural and urban children of the highlands of Papua New Guinea. *J. Allergy Clin. Immunol.* 77:558, 1986.

233. Turner-Warwick, M., et al. Immunologic lung disease due to aspergillosis. *Chest* 68:346, 1975.

234. United States Pharmacopoeia Dispensing Information. The United States Pharmacopoeial Convention, Inc., Rockville, MD. 1:7, 1983.

235. Update: Drugs in breast milk. *Med. Lett. Drug. Ther.* 21:21, 1979.

236. VanArsdel, P. P., and Paul, G. H. Drug therapy in the management of asthma. *Ann. Intern. Med.* 87:68, 1977.

236a. Van Essen-Zandvliet, E. E., et al. Effects of 22 months of treatment with inhaled corticosteroids and/or beta-2-agonists on lung function, airway responsiveness, and symptoms in children with asthma. *Am. Rev. Respir. Dis.* 146:547, 1992.

236b. Vathenen, A. S., et al. Time course of change in bronchial reactivity with an inhaled corticosteroid in asthma. *Am. Rev. Respir. Dis.* 143:1317, 1991.

237. Vaz, R., et al. Adrenal effects of beclomethasone inhalation therapy in asthmatic children. *J. Pediatr.* 100:660, 1982.

238. Verrall, B., et al. Laminar flow air cleaner bed attachment: A controlled trial. *Ann. Allergy* 61:117, 1988.

238a. Wales, J. K. H., Barnes, N. D., and Swift, P. G. F. Growth retardation in children on steroids for asthma. *Lancet* 338:1535, 1991.

239. Walshaw, M. J., and Evans, C. C. Allergen avoidance in house dust mite sensitive adult asthma. *Q. J. Med.* 58:199, 1986.

240. Wang, J. L. F., et al. The management of allergic bronchopulmonary aspergillosis. *Am. Rev. Respir. Dis.* 120:87, 1979.

241. Wardman, A. G., et al. The use of high dose inhaled beclomethasone dipropionate as a means of assessing steroid responsiveness in obstructive airways disease. *Br. J. Dis. Chest* 82:168, 1988.

242. Weinberger, M. Safety of oral corticosteroids. *Eur. J. Respir. Dis.* 63(Suppl. 122):243, 1982.

243. Welty, C., et al. The relationship of airways responsiveness to cold air, cigarette smoking, and atopy to respiratory symptoms and pulmonary function in adults. *Am. Rev. Respir. Dis.* 130:198, 1984.

244. Williams, A. J., et al. Dysphonia caused by inhaled steroids: Recognition of a characteristic laryngeal abnormality. *Thorax* 38:813, 1983.

245. Williams, I. P., and McGavin, C. R. Corticosteroids in chronic airways obstruction: Can the patient's assessment be ignored? *Br. J. Dis. Chest* 74:142, 1980.

246. Wilson, N. M., and Silverman, M. Treatment of acute, episodic asthma in preschool children using intermittent high dose inhaled steroids at home. *Arch. Dis. Child.* 65:407, 1990.

246a. Wolthers, O. D., and Pedersen, S. Controlled study of linear growth in asthmatic children during treatment with inhaled glucocorticosteroids. *Pediatrics* 89:839, 1992.

247. Woodcock, A. A., Johnson, M. A., and Geddes, D. M. Theophylline prescribing, serum concentrations and toxicity. *Lancet* 2:610, 1983.

248. Woolcock, A. J., Yan, K., and Salome, C. M. Effect of therapy on bronchial hyperresponsiveness in the long-term management of asthma. *Clin. Allergy* 18:165, 1988.

249. Woolcock, A. J., et al. Prevalence of bronchial hyperresponsiveness and asthma in a rural adult population. *Thorax* 42:361, 1987.

250. Wyatt, R., et al. Effects of inhaled beclomethasone dipropionate and alternate-day prednisone on pituitary-adrenal function in children with chronic asthma. *N. Engl. J. Med.* 299:1387, 1978.

Hypothalamic-Pituitary-Adrenal Function in Asthma

62

Roger Ellul-Micallef

The status of the hypothalamic-pituitary-adrenal (HPA) axis in the asthmatic patient has been the subject of interest and research since Kepinov [104] demonstrated increased bronchial sensitivity in an adrenalectomized guinea pig. This was later confirmed by other workers, prominent among whom was Flashman [68]. Wolfram and Zwemer [217] were the first to show conclusively that cortin could protect guinea pigs against anaphylactic shock.

The association of impaired adrenocortical function and bronchial asthma has long been a matter of contention [4]. Ever since it was established that glucocorticoid therapy is frequently of great benefit in the treatment of asthma, it has been tempting to postulate that failure of the adrenal cortex may be an underlying defect in some asthmatic patients. Reports have appeared in the literature of asthma occurring in patients with Addison's disease [85, 91], and, in one of these reports, asthma appeared to be the presenting symptom of adrenal insufficiency [85]. It has also been suggested that occasional cases of chronic asthma may have an autoimmune origin [181]. In a retrospective study reported from the Mayo Clinic [31] concerning 496 patients with hypoadrenalism, only seven (1.4%) showed a definite relationship between the onset of Addison's disease and the development of bronchial asthma. Bronchial asthma is thus only very rarely a presenting feature in patients with Addison's disease. Similarly, signs of impaired adrenocortical function are uncommon in patients admitted to the hospital in status asthmaticus, even in those previously receiving glucocorticoids. Adrenal atrophy has also been an infrequent pathologic finding in patients dying from asthma who had not previously been receiving glucocorticoid treatment [74, 194]. The infrequency of asthma in patients with Addison's disease has made it most unlikely that impaired adrenal function has a close relationship with asthma.

HPA AXIS IN BRONCHIAL ASTHMA

Following Rackemann's [171] initial observation in one asthmatic of low 17-ketosteroid (17-KS) excretion, several papers have been published on the status of pituitary-adrenocortical function in bronchial asthma. Some have reported finding inadequate basal function or an inadequate response to stress [63, 115, 176, 206], while others could find no evidence of impairment of the hypothalamic–pituitary axis [19, 102, 155]. There has also been one report in which increased levels of plasma 17-hydroxycorticosteroids (17-OHCS) were found in children with moderate or severe bronchial asthma [187]. Reviews summarizing the data from earlier reports are found in the papers by Dwyer and coworkers [49] and more recently by Morrish and his colleagues [149].

The apparent discrepancy in the reported findings seems to result from a number of factors. The patient population studied was markedly heterogeneous, and reports often included small patient samples. The type and severity of asthma, the presence or absence of associated complications or other diseases, concomitant drug therapy, and differences in methodology are but a few of the many ways in which the various reports have differed. The nutritional status of the patient may also affect corticosteroid metabolism; thus, even a low-protein, high-carbohydrate diet may result in a decrease in both plasma and urinary corticosteroid levels. Similarly, concomitant endocrine, renal, or liver disease and drugs such as phenobarbital may influence corticosteroid levels [22, 23, 62, 101, 107, 120]. Insufficient data have been provided, making it difficult to know whether some of these factors might have been operative to a significant degree in a number of the patients studied. The majority of these investigations also lacked adequate control groups.

Tests of HPA Axis Status

The wide range of methods used for measuring glucocorticoids and their various metabolites in the endocrinologic assessment of these patients is at least an equally important factor in explaining the contradictory data reported. In addition to plasma cortisol levels and the plasma cortisol response to adrenocorticotropic hormone (ACTH) [19, 49, 109, 149], measurements have included urinary 17-KS, 11-hydroxycorticosteroids (11-OHCS), 17-OHCS, and 17-ketogenic steroids (17-KGS), as well as 11-deoxycorticosteroids. The plasma 17-OHCS [189] and plasma 11-OHCS [25] response to ACTH and the response to metyrapone of 17-KGS and 11-deoxycortisol [7, 149], 17-KS [19], and 17-OHCS [1] have all been used to assess the HPA function in asthmatics. The bioassay procedures used in many of the earlier studies are known to yield rather variable results, especially when comparisons are made between the results from different laboratories. A number of the variables measured may be criticized on the grounds of lack of specificity and sensitivity as well as wide variability. The measurement of 17-OHCS levels used in a number of these studies, in addition to having a low specificity for cortisol (50% and less), is also liable to be interfered with by a number of other substances [87, 138]. On the other hand, while levels of 17-KGS provide a better assessment of glucocorticoid excretion products, they are subject to more variability and interference than 17-OHCS levels. Some workers [19, 63, 171, 214] have based their conclusions on the levels of 17-KS detected, of which less than 10 percent is normally contributed by glucocorticoid metabolism.

The most specific manner of assessing adrenocortical secretion is direct measurement of plasma cortisol levels [88]. At times cortisol has been assayed in serum rather than plasma. This has the advantage of avoiding false high values, which may occur if fibrinogen levels are elevated. A number of methods have been used [98, 133], of which radioimmunoassay appears to be the most sensitive [87, 178]. Fluorometric methods used in the past for measuring cortisol levels are known to systematically overestimate values by 20 to 30 percent, in comparison to those obtained by current radioimmunoassay methods [18, 145].

Single daily measurements of plasma cortisol levels may not provide a true picture of the HPA status. Cortisol secretion is episodic, normally occurring in bursts about ten times a day, and is also subject to circadian variation, with the peak production rate between 4 and 8 A.M. and the nadir between 8 P.M. and midnight [116, 117, 213]; therefore, a single plasma cortisol determination may be misleading. The timing of when the sample is obtained is crucial; preferably it should be taken in the morning before 9 A.M. Serum or plasma cortisol measurements may be affected even by minor stress. In susceptible subjects, the venipuncture or even the apprehension associated with the procedure may be enough to elevate levels.

Measuring the 24-hour excretion of urinary free cortisol integrates the changes in the plasma concentration over an entire day, resulting in a sensitive index of pituitary-adrenal function [17, 30, 185]. Disadvantages of this approach include the problem of making an accurate 24-hour total urine collection. Creatinine determinations may have to be carried out to check the accuracy of collection [87]. Urinary assays may not be widely available and may be technically difficult to perform reliably. Most of the endogenous cortisol is excreted in the urine as metabolites, with only a small fraction existing as free cortisol. A recent study, carried out in normal children and adolescents, has shown that the 17-hydroxysteroid excretion rate, corrected for creatinine values, reflects cortisol adrenal secretion more accurately than does the urinary free cortisol measurement [117]. In asthmatic patients, however, urinary free cortisol levels and the short tetracosactrin test were shown to be specific and equally sensitive as screening tests for HPA suppression, both being much more sensitive than the morning serum cortisol level. In those patients who had a borderline or subnormal HPA function, a close correlation could be shown between the 24-hour urine free cortisol excretion and the maximum serum cortisol level achieved following insulin-induced hypoglycemia [25].

In a further study carried out in patients suffering from rheumatoid arthritis, it was shown that the increase in the plasma cortisol level during surgery was more reliably predicted by the short ACTH test than by the insulin hypoglycemia test. However, the gold standard for testing the integrity and function of the whole HPA axis remains the insulin-induced hypoglycemia stress test [110, 197], which promotes ACTH release, probably through a primary effect on the medial basal hypothalamus [5]. It is, however, unpleasant and time consuming, requires careful clinical supervision, and is not suitable if patients are over 70 years old, have a history of cardiovascular or cerebrovascular disease, or suffer from epilepsy [38].

Other challenge tests use metyrapone [46, 137] or ACTH [218]. Metyrapone activates the feedback loop by blocking the synthesis of cortisol, causing a release of ACTH, and measurements of the cortisol precursor, 11-deoxycortisol in plasma or the cortisol metabolites (17-OHCS) in urine, are then carried out [154]. In studies carried out in both normal volunteers [96] as well as patients with suspected HPA axis dysfunction [94], the single-dose metyrapone test was found to be more sensitive than either the short tetracosactrin (ACTH) or the insulin-induced hypoglycemia test [99].

A new method for diagnosing HPA axis disturbances utilizing corticotropin-releasing factor is little used [86, 126, 216]. The short 30-minute tetracosactrin (ACTH) test remains the one most frequently employed to provide information on adrenal reserve [117, 119]. It is important that this test be carried out exactly 30 minutes after the administration of tetracosactrin, as delay may result in a progressive enhancement of the adrenal response, with failure to detect depression of adrenal function. It carries a small risk of provoking hypersensitivity, which should be kept in mind when testing asthmatics [150].

Although various tests are now available to screen for HPA axis suppression, no single test is established that is clearly the most sensitive, specific, and practical in all cases. Moreover, it has not yet been established which part of the axis is predominantly suppressed by exogenous glucocorticoids, although it has been suggested that suppression may occur at both the hypothalamic-pituitary as well as the adrenal level [92].

The diurnal rhythm of the plasma cortisol level is an extremely sensitive indicator of an intact neuroendocrine function and is the last parameter to revert to normal after glucocorticoid therapy has been stopped. It is technically difficult to measure because of the frequent blood samples required and is therefore not practical for routine use, although it has been described as a more physiologic test of adrenal function than any of the stress tests [200].

Perhaps two of the most interesting investigations evaluating the integrity of the HPA axis in asthmatics not previously treated with glucocorticoids are the study of 16 intrinsic nonatopic asthmatics conducted by Collins and his coworkers [40] and that carried out by Morrish and his colleagues [149] in 25 extrinsic asthmatic patients.

In the first study, all 16 patients showed normal adrenocortical responses to prolonged stimulation with tetracosactrin depot. In a subgroup of six patients, the HPA response to a standard insulin stress test was also normal. The study carried out in the extrinsic group was perhaps even more detailed and included a group of 20 normal, age-matched controls. HPA function was assessed by measuring the plasma levels of ACTH and 11-deoxycortisol after metyrapone stimulation and by measuring plasma cortisol levels following stimulation with cosyntropin: There was no difference shown in any of the measurements between the asthmatic patients and the normal control group (Fig. 62-1). Furthermore, no correlation was detected between the levels of ACTH or of 11-deoxycortisol following metyrapone challenge and the duration or severity of asthma.

These carefully designed studies have failed to show any abnormalities in HPA function in the presence of either intrinsic or extrinsic bronchial asthma. Earlier suggestions of an association between impaired adrenocortical function and asthma have not been confirmed by later more detailed studies employing more sensitive and specific tests. The inverse relationship between the duration of asthma and the response to ACTH [176] has also not been confirmed [40, 149].

Airflow Obstruction and HPA Axis Function

A number of studies carried out in animals have reported that hypoxemia [45, 129, 130, 131], hypercapnia [142, 174], or acidosis [142] could stimulate the HPA axis. This increase in adrenocortical secretion was found to be abolished by hypophysectomy [174], by denervation of the aortic and carotid chemoreceptors [129], and by high doses of dexamethasone [131]. In premature infants with the respiratory distress syndrome [10] and adults with chronic lung disease [209], respiratory failure has been shown to be associated with increased levels of plasma corticosteroids, probably reflecting a response to a stressful situation. Conflicting data have been published showing that adrenocortical function was normal [189, 209] or impaired [114] in patients who were reportedly in a stable phase of their chronic obstructive pulmonary state; in particular, a blunted response to ACTH has been described.

The tests used to detect and monitor HPA function in these studies have in general lacked sensitivity and specificity. More recent evidence seems to point to the fact that airflow limitation of itself does not seem to be associated with impaired adrenocortical function. Cornil and his coworkers [42], in a study of 15

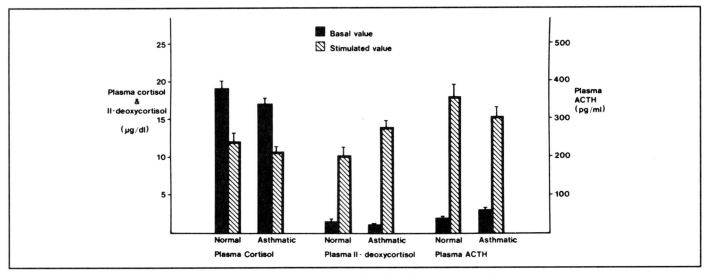

Fig. 62-1. *Results of testing by means of stimulation with metyrapone in asthmatic subjects and normal controls. Bars represent means (± SE). (Reprinted with permission from D. W. Morrish, et al. Hypothalamic-pituitary-adrenal function in extrinsic asthma.* Chest *75:161, 1979.)*

adult patients, most of whom suffered from chronic bronchitis, reported finding markedly elevated plasma cortisol levels when their patients were in acute respiratory failure. This is perhaps not surprising as it is well recognized that stress affects basal plasma cortisol levels. Plasma cortisol levels and the adrenocortical response to ACTH were normal, however, when the patients recovered from acute respiratory failure. These findings were confirmed in a further study of eight patients with stable chronic bronchitis who all had essentially normal cortisol responses to adequate hypoglycemia [183]. Airflow limitation of itself, whether the result of an asthmatic condition or of a bronchitic state, is not associated with impairment of HPA function.

HPA AXIS IN ASTHMATIC PATIENTS ON GLUCOCORTICOID THERAPY

Ever since the first reports by Carryer and his coworkers [32] and Randolph and Rollins [172], glucocorticoids have become firmly established as important therapeutic agents in the management of a condition described by Thomas Willis [215] as "asthma morbus maxime terribilis." Over the past forty years, there has been no lack of controversy [84] as to their usefulness in the treatment of both acute [52, 102a, 144, 184] and chronic [136] bronchial asthma. Objective physiologic data have now confirmed their therapeutic role in asthma [41, 53, 55–57, 59, 60, 64]. It now seems that glucocorticoids generally bring about relief of the asthmatic state by virtue of their general antiinflammatory actions but may also have other effects, such as restoration of beta-adrenergic receptor responsiveness [58].

It is now generally recognized that inflammation is a basic pathologic feature of asthma, arising as the result of the synergized activity of various primary effector cells that, through the release of a whole array of mediators, recruit secondary effector cells responsible for amplifying and perpetating the inflammatory process. The therapeutic success of glucocorticoids in controlling asthma is being increasingly ascribed to their widespread actions on the different components of the inflammatory process. The eosinophils, monocytes, and macrophages are among the most glucocorticoid-sensitive cells involved in the inflammatory process, while the neutrophils and, even more so, the mast cells

are the least sensitive to the action of these drugs. Glucocorticoids are now also known to decrease airway hyperresponsiveness [54].

Suppression of HPA Function in Asthmatics

The suppression of HPA function in asthmatics during prolonged oral [204] and parenteral [141] glucocorticoid therapy and after its withdrawal [143] is well documented, and was recognized within a few years of the introduction of cortisone [75, 180]. The changes it brings about have included a reduction in basal cortisol levels [128, 132], loss of diurnal variation, diminished adrenocortical response to exogenous ACTH [164], decreased response to metyrapone, and blunted to absent responses to insulin-induced hypoglycemia [128]. The onset of suppression is rapid, occurring within minutes or hours, and persists throughout the treatment period. There are, however, conflicting reports regarding the time required for the recovery of normal HPA function after discontinuation of therapy. Adrenal suppression has been reported with daily doses of prednisolone as low as 5 mg [95], and adrenal gland atrophy has been reported in patients who had previously received cortisone for as short a period as 5 days.

Suppression of adrenal function and adrenal atrophy have also been reported to occur within 5 days of a dose of approximately 20 mg of prednisolone per day [13, 110]. This impairment of adrenal function by glucocorticoid therapy may persist for weeks or months [147] and sometimes for as long as 1 year after cessation of treatment [82, 138]. Livanou and his coworkers [122] have shown that, although plasma cortisol levels may reach normal values within a month in the majority of patients, the plasma cortisol response to hypoglycemia may take up to a year to become normal. Other reports, on the other hand, suggest that HPA responses may return to normal within a few days after cessation of treatment [175].

It is perhaps not sufficiently recognized that HPA suppression may also occur with high-dose, short-term glucocorticoid therapy [199, 211]. Streck and Lockwood [199] studied the recovery of the HPA axis in 10 normal subjects following a 5-day course of 25 mg of prednisone given twice daily. Their results suggest that the adrenal component of the HPA stress response was limited for up to 5 days after therapy was concluded. Webb and Clark [211] studied patients with chronic airflow limitation who had been previously treated for a 3-week period with 20 mg of prednisolone given twice daily. They showed that basal plasma cortisol levels were reduced and the response to tetracosactrin was depressed. Basal ACTH levels were also suppressed after such a course and remained so for 4 days. In their study, both the adrenal and the pituitary glands appeared to recover simultaneously, but it is often stated that recovery of the adrenal cortex lags behind that of the pituitary [182]. However, short courses of glucocorticoids (up to 14 days) seem to be associated with hardly any adverse effects of clinical note and only transient HPA axis suppression [220]; on the other hand, if instituted at the appropriate time, they often preempt acute exacerbations of asthma, frequently avoiding the need for hospitalization [28, 66, 90]. This is especially important in children, for whom hospitalization is often a traumatic event. In a study in which the response of the HPA axis to insulin-induced hypoglycemia and synthetic ACTH was tested in a group of chronic asthmatic children, it was concluded that three to four short-term, high-dose systemic glucocorticoid courses of therapy per year did not appear to compromise HPA function [48]. Nonetheless, care must be taken in interpreting such data because individual patients may, at times, exhibit HPA suppression irrespective of the dose used. The recovery of HPA axis responsiveness to stress appears to be slower than the rate of restitution of basal cortisol levels.

Approaches to Glucocorticoid Treatment

During the treatment of chronic asthma, HPA function is said to be better conserved if glucocorticoids are given as a single dose in the morning, mimicking the circadian rhythm, than when the dose is divided throughout the day [151, 157, 188], provided that a rapidly metabolized steroid such as prednisolone is used [135] (Chap. 60). It has been shown in normal subjects that dexamethasone given in the morning caused adrenal suppression lasting for 10 hours, while the same dose given at midnight resulted in a 24-hour suppression of adrenal function [157].

Siegre and Klaiber [188] have reported a much larger decrease in the urinary 17-hydroxyglucocorticoid level when glucocorticoids are taken in the evening than when administered in the morning. There seems to be a diurnal fluctuation in the suppressibility of the pituitary-adrenal axis. Furthermore, the finding of Angeli and coworkers [8] that there is a greater proportion of free, active prednisolone during the day than at night supports the desirability of morning dosing. It has been suggested that there may be two phases of ACTH secretion throughout the day under different control mechanisms. The nocturnal phase appears to be sensitive to physiologic levels of glucocorticoids, while a second phase, responsible for the steady basal activity during the day, responds only to large doses of the hormone [35]. It has long been recognized, both in adults as well as in children, that, if the interval between oral doses is extended to 48 hours, substantially larger amounts of glucocorticoids may be given while the degree of adrenal suppression is reduced [2, 93, 101]. However, even alternate-day treatment has at times been shown to have significant side effects, including HPA axis suppression [148, 179]. Unfortunately, alternate-day treatment not infrequently may fail to adequately control asthmatic symptoms, especially in adults.

Glucocorticoid Aerosol Therapy

In 1951, Gelfland [79] first reported using cortisone as an aerosol suspended in saline. Following this, several attempts were made to introduce glucocorticoid aerosol therapy [9, 16, 21, 44, 67, 69, 162, 191, 205]. These had a markedly limited success, as the doses needed for clinical effectiveness often resulted in signifi-

cant systemic absorption [73, 118, 158]. Siegel and coworkers [187] tested the newly available dexamethasone in asthmatic children and found that, although it improved their asthma, it also significantly suppressed their adrenocortical function; their average ACTH response was reduced by almost half.

The successful introduction of glucocorticoid aerosols with powerful topical activity in the early 1970s has proved to be of unquestionable value in the treatment of the asthmatic condition [24, 36] (Chap. 61). A daily dose of 400 μg of beclomethasone dipropionate was found to be approximately equivalent to 7.5 mg of oral prednisone [20].

Several clinical trials have established the value of glucocorticoid aerosols, either as the only form of glucocorticoid therapy [20, 78] or as a means of reducing the dose of concomitant oral glucocorticoids needed for the control of asthma [20, 72], in an attempt to decrease the incidence of side effects [127]. In conventional doses of 400 μg per day, beclomethasone dipropionate was shown not to interfere with the diurnal variations in plasma cortisol levels [29] and not to suppress HPA function [20, 24, 37, 78, 134]. In non–glucocorticoid-dependent patients, plasma cortisol levels remained within normal limits after 2 years of therapy [190] and the results of stimulation tests with tetracosactrin were also normal [20]. Inhaled glucocorticoids in low doses (200–400 μg/day) are being introduced earlier in the therapeutic regimen of asthma, even in patients with mild asthma, with beneficial effects [124].

It is generally accepted that, at high doses, glucocorticoid aerosols may result in impairment of adrenal function. Gaddie and coworkers [78] reported finding a minor fall in the resting plasma cortisol levels with a dose of 1,600 μg of beclomethasone dipropionate a day, but, at this level, the adrenal response to tetracosactrin stimulation was significantly reduced. In another study, very large doses of beclomethasone dipropionate (2 mg/day) impaired adrenal function in five of seven patients [36]. However, Costello and Clark [43] reported finding no evidence of adrenal suppression in 16 asthmatics treated with 1 mg of beclomethasone dipropionate daily for up to 24 weeks or in a further group of five asthmatics who received 2 mg of beclomethasone dipropionate daily for periods up to 10 weeks. They based their conclusions solely on basal cortisol level measurements and no stimulation tests were carried out.

Recent studies in healthy adult subjects have shown that beclomethasone treatment for 1 week causes suppression of the HPA axis at a dose of 1,600 μg per day, as reflected by a significant reduction in the 24-hour excretion of free cortisol in the urine and in the serum 11-deoxycortisol response to metyrapone [185]. Higher doses of inhaled glucocorticoids are sometimes needed to improve control of the asthmatic state or to reduce the dosage of oral glucocorticoids patients may have been stabilized on. In Europe, high-dose inhalers containing beclomethasone dipropionate and budesonide are also available and are capable of delivering 250 μg per puff and 200 μg per puff, respectively.

Smith and Hodson [192] studied the long-term effects of high-dose beclomethasone dipropionate on adrenal function in 54 asthmatics and reported no significant adrenal suppression in patients taking up to 1,500 μg/day. At this dosage, 91 percent had normal basal plasma cortisol concentrations and normal short tetracosactrin responses, while the 24-hour urinary free cortisol excretion was within the normal range in eight of nine patients tested. However, some evidence of adrenal suppression was found in patients taking 2,000 μg/day, with the basal plasma cortisol level below the normal range in 4 of 11 patients and the 24-hour urinary free cortisol excretion below the normal range in five of 6 patients tested. Similar results have been published by a number of other workers [50, 51, 81], some in patients studied over periods of up to 8 years.

There is often considerable variation between individual patients' HPA response to high-dose inhaled glucocorticoids, and

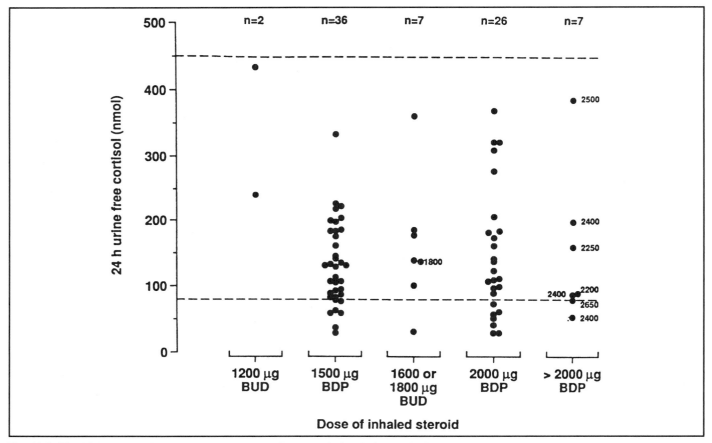

Fig. 62-2. *The 24-hour urine free cortisol excretion in asthmatics inhaling high-dose beclomethasone dipropionate (*BDP*) or budesonide (*BUD*). (Reprinted with permission from P. H. Brown, et al. Hypothalamo-pituitary-adrenal axis suppression in asthmatics inhaling high dose corticosteroids.* Respir. Med. *85:501, 1991.)*

the reasons for this remain largely unknown. In a recent study [26] carried out in 78 adult asthmatics taking long-term, high-dose inhaled glucocorticoids, evidence of HPA axis suppression was found in 16 patients (20%) (Fig. 62-2). Risk factors identified for this suppression included a previous requirement for long-term systemic glucocorticoids and increasing duration of high-dose inhaled therapy. No clear correlation could be identified between the dose and degree of effect on HPA function, whether the dose was corrected for body surface or not. Similarly, no relationship could be shown between suppression and the number of short courses of prednisolone taken in the previous year.

Recent studies of adrenal function in glucocorticoid-dependent asthmatics treated with high-dose inhaled glucocorticoids show there is improvement in HPA axis function when the dose of oral glucocorticoids is reduced. Frequently, patients have been successfully weaned off of oral therapy [3, 111, 198, 201]. The dose of inhaled glucocorticoid required to replace as much of the oral dose of glucocorticoids as possible has to be worked out individually per patient [202]. Occasionally patients experience "withdrawal symptoms" when they are completely weaned off of glucocorticoids [47].

Large-volume spacer devices have been introduced to enable patients with poor inhalation techniques to use metered-dose inhalers properly, and these are especially useful in children and the elderly [61] (Chap. 56). In addition, by reducing upper airway deposition of aerosol, they provide a more selective delivery of an inhaled drug to the lower airway [146, 156, 159]. There were initial suggestions that the use of these spacers increased the potential of adverse side effects [203]. Studies on the use of

spacer devices attached to glucocorticoid metered-dose inhalers have been carried out in healthy subjects [65], asthmatic children [166, 167], and adult asthmatics [27]. In most instances, the use of spacers resulted in a decrease of HPA axis suppression.

Besides the use of spacers, patients should also be advised to rinse out their mouths well after each administration; this simple measure further reduces the amount of orally deposited glucocorticoid available for systemic absorption [182a]. There is considerable interpatient variation in the dose of inhaled glucocorticoid that causes HPA axis suppression whether a spacer is used or not [23a].

It is important to keep in mind that high-dose inhaled glucocorticoids do not constitute the proper treatment for episodes of acute severe asthma; these exacerbations should be treated with systemic glucocorticoids and not by an increase in the dose of inhaled glucocorticoids.

There is still some controversy, especially regarding asthmatic children, as to whether significant suppression of the HPA axis does occur with standard daily doses of inhaled beclomethasone dipropionate. This has followed a report by Wyatt and coworkers [219] stating that, in asthmatic children, early morning serum cortisol levels, urinary free cortisol excretion, and the 11-deoxy-cortisol response to metyrapone were reduced to a similar degree when the effects of 20 to 40 mg of prednisone given on alternate mornings were compared with the effects of 400 to 800 µg per day of inhaled beclomethasone dipropionate given in divided doses. These workers showed that inhaled glucocorticoids have an additive effect on HPA axis suppression when given in conjunction with systemic glucocorticoids. The same group reconfirmed that, in asthmatic children, beclomethasone is absorbed and suppresses HPA function to about the same extent as alternate-day prednisone [152]. Some workers [170] have expressed concern over these results because of the previous use of high-dose oral prednisone in the patients studied without adequate washout intervals to ascertain complete adrenal recovery.

A more recent report from the same group of workers from the University of Iowa cites a decrease in HPA function from the use of inhaled glucocorticoids, similar in magnitude to that detected with alternate-day prednisone on the steroid-free day [153]. Again, oral prednisone was only stopped a month before the start of the study in some of these patients on beclomethasone dipropionate.

These studies are somewhat difficult to interpret, as no individual data points are given. Their findings have been supported by a study conducted by Vaz and colleagues [208]. In a group of 16 asthmatic children, 6 to 15 years old, who had been treated with doses of beclomethasone dipropionate ranging between 300 and 500 μg per day for periods varying from 6 months to 3½ years, baseline cortisol levels were significantly lower than those in a control group of normal children. Following insulin-induced hypoglycemia, the cortisol levels attained were also significantly less in the asthmatic children [208]. This study has been criticized because the control group did not consist of asthmatic patients, the control group was not studied at the same time, more than half the patients studied had previously received some form of systemic glucocorticoid therapy, it cannot be ascertained whether adequate hypoglycemia was achieved, and, furthermore, many of the results obtained may be considered to fall within the normal range [170].

Recent reports of studies in which diurnal cortisol secretion was assessed in asthmatic children inhaling conventional doses of beclomethasone dipropionate have also indicated some suppression of endogenous cortisol secretion [163]. Law and his colleagues [112, 113, 210] sampled plasma every 20 minutes during sleep, starting at midnight and then over a period of 6 hours. They found that nocturnal cortisol secretion decreased as the dose of glucocorticoids increased; there was also a delayed rise from the nocturnal nadir and low early morning levels. Their results have been largely substantiated by a study in which spontaneous cortisol secretion was measured every 30 minutes over a 24-hour period [200] (Fig. 62-3). This study was carried out in 10 children with chronic asthma who inhaled 200 μg of beclomethasone dipropionate at 7 A.M. and 7 P.M. for a 3-month period. Fourteen healthy children served as control subjects. There was a significant reduction in the area under the curve of cortisol in all patients following treatment. This decrease was also reflected in the 24-hour urinary free cortisol measurements. Peak cortisol levels in response to synthetic corticotropin were within normal limits, perhaps indicating that suppression was occurring at the hypothalamic-pituitary level. The maximum induced suppression in cortisol secretion (63%) occurred between 8 P.M. and 2 A.M., after the evening dose, compared with a 29 percent reduction between 8 A.M. and 2 P.M., after the morning dose. Hence, cortisol secretion was not uniformly suppressed during the 24-hour period. In spite of the decrease in cortisol secretion, therapy did not significantly alter the circadian rhythm.

On the other hand, different conclusions have been reached by a number of other workers [15, 77, 80, 103, 105, 106]. Siegel's group [186] found no evidence of suppression of the HPA axis in asthmatic children being given 400 μg of beclomethasone dipropionate per day, as evaluated by diurnal cortisol levels as well as metyrapone and tetracosactrin tests. Similarly, significant reductions in the plasma cortisol levels have rarely been reported after the inhalation of standard doses of other glucocorticoids such as flunisolide [193], triamcinolone acetonide [6a, 14], and budesonide [39].

A newly introduced inhaled glucocorticoid, fluticasone pro-

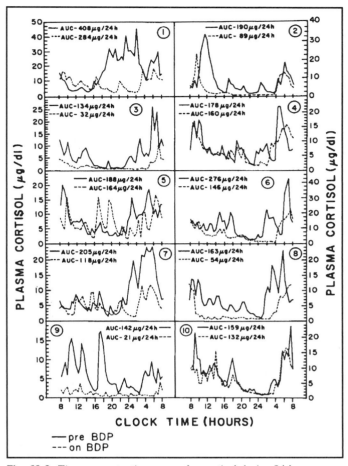

Fig. 62-3. *Time-concentration curves for cortisol during 24-hour period in 10 patients, both before and 3 months after commencement of therapy with inhaled beclomethasone dipropionate* (BDP), *200 μg twice daily.* AUC = *area under curve. (Reprinted with permission from E. Tabachnik and Z. Zadik. Diurnal cortisol secretion during therapy with inhaled beclomethasone dipropionate in children with asthma.* J. Pediatr. *118:294, 1991.)*

pionate, has been said to have no demonstrable effects on the plasma cortisol levels when administered to adult asthmatics [12a, 219a]. It has been claimed that this drug has virtually zero oral bioavailability; budesonide has about 11 percent and flunisolide, about 20 percent [89].

Long-term studies (1 year or longer) in which standard doses of either inhaled beclomethasone dipropionate [70, 76, 140] or budesonide [173, 207] have been used in asthmatic children have also failed to detect significantly impaired adrenal function or to reveal any adverse systemic side effects. In a double-blind, crossover, randomized study from Godfrey's group, comparing the effects of budesonide and beclomethasone dipropionate at equivalent doses of 200 μg twice a day, both drugs were found capable of causing mild adrenal suppression on metyrapone testing [196].

From the many studies performed in children, it appears that daily doses of 400 μg/day or less of inhaled beclomethasone or budesonide do not cause any significant systemic effects; doses of 400 to 800 μg/day may cause some HPA suppression and biochemical effects, while doses greater than 800 μg/day may be clearly associated with impairment of HPA function [17].

Luckily, the vast majority of asthmatic children can be controlled by the administration of 400 μg/day or less of inhaled beclomethasone or budesonide, and changes, if any, are subtle

Table 62-1. Assessment of HPA function

Therapy/assessment	Authors	Test(s) employed
Asthmatics not previously on corticosteroid therapy No impairment of HPA function	Blumenthal et al., 1966 [19]	Plasma cortisol levels Plasma cortisol response to ACTH Urinary 17-ketosteroids and 17-hydroxysteroids
	Dwyer et al., 1967 [49]	Plasma cortisol response to hydrocortisone MCR of cortisol Effect of ACTH on MCR
	Malone et al., 1970 [128]	Plasma 11-OHCS levels Plasma 11-OHCS response to insulin
	Cayton and Howard, 1973 [33]	Plasma cortisol levels Plasma cortisol response to ACTH
	Collins et al., 1975 [41]	Plasma 11-OHCS response to ACTH Plasma 11-OHCS response to insulin
	Wyatt et al., 1978 [219]	Serum cortisol levels; 24-hour urinary free cortisol excretion Serum 11-deoxycortisol response to metyrapone
	Morrish et al., 1979 [149]	Plasma ACTH and plasma 11-deoxycortisol response to metyrapone Plasma cortisol response to cosyntropin
Inadequate basal function	Andersson, 1964 [7]	Urinary 17-KGS
	Abbasy et al., 1967 [1]	Plasma and urinary 17-OHCS
	Weller et al., 1968 [214]	Urinary 17-KS
	Mathé and Knapp, 1971 [132]	Plasma cortisol levels
Inadequate response to stress	Vaccarezza et al., 1961 [206]	Plasma cortisol response to ACTH
	Andersson, 1964 [7]	11-Deoxycortisol response to metyrapone
	Abbasy et al., 1967 [1]	17-OHCS response to metyrapone
	Mathé and Knapp, 1971 [132]	Plasma cortisol response to psychologic stress
Corticosteroid-treated asthmatics: systemic corticosteroid therapy Impaired HPA function	Malone et al., 1970 [128]	Plasma 11-OHCS levels Plasma 11-OHCS response to insulin
	Portner et al., 1972 [164]	Plasma cortisol levels Plasma cortisol response to ACTH
	Cayton and Howard, 1973 [33]	Plasma cortisol levels Plasma cortisol response to ACTH
	Mikhail et al., 1973 [141]	Plasma cortisol levels Plasma cortisol response to insulin Plasma cortisol response to ACTH
	British Thoracic and Tuberculosis Association, 1975 [20]	Plasma cortisol levels Plasma cortisol response to tetracosactrin
	Webb, 1977 [212]	Plasma cortisol levels Plasma cortisol response to metyrapone
Corticosteroid-treated asthmatics: inhaled corticosteroid therapy	Choo-Kang et al., 1972 [36]	Plasma cortisol levels
	Gaddie et al., 1973 [78]	Plasma 11-OHCS levels Plasma 11-OHCS response to tetracosactrin
	Wyatt et al., 1978 [219]	Serum cortisol levels 24-Hour urinary free cortisol excretion
	Vaz et al., 1982 [208]	Plasma cortisol response to insulin Plasma cortisol response to cosyntropin
	Smith and Hodson, 1983 [192] (dose up to 2,000 µg/day)	Plasma cortisol levels; 24-hour urinary free cortisol excretion
	Law et al., 1986 [113]	Nocturnal plasma cortisol levels
	Gordon et al., 1987 [81]	Plasma cortisol levels
	Nassif et al., 1987 [153]	Serum cortisol levels 24-Hour urinary free cortisol excretion Plasma cortisol response to ACTH
	Bisgaard et al., 1988 [17]	24-Hour urinary free cortisol excretion 24-Hour urinary total cortisol metabolite excretion
	Priftis et al., 1990 [169]	Spontaneous cortisol secretion for a 24-hour period
	Tabachnik and Zadik, 1991 [200]	24-Hour urinary free cortisol excretion
Normal HPA function	Costello and Clark, 1974 [43]	Plasma 11-OHCS levels
	Friedman and Frears, 1974 [77]	Plasma cortisol response to insulin Plasma ACTH response to insulin Plasma growth hormone levels Plasma 11-OHCS levels
	Roscoe et al., 1975 [177]	Plasma cortisol response to tetracosactrin Plasma cortisol response to insulin
	British Thoracic and Tuberculosis Association, 1975 [20]	Plasma cortisol levels Plasma cortisol response to tetracosactrin
	Spitzer et al., 1976 [195]	Plasma cortisol levels 24-Hour urinary free cortisol excretion Urinary 17-OHCS levels Plasma cortisol response to insulin

Table 62-1 (continued)

Therapy/assessment	Authors	Test(s) employed
Normal HPA function (*continued*)	Klein et al., 1977 [106]	Plasma cortisol levels Plasma cortisol response to metyrapone Plasma cortisol response to ACTH
	Bhan et al., 1980 [15]	Plasma cortisol levels Plasma cortisol response to tetracosactrin 24-Hour urinary free cortisol excretion
	Smith and Hodson, 1983 [192] (dose up to 1,500 µg/day)	Plasma cortisol levels Plasma cortisol response to tetracosactrin 24-Hour urinary free cortisol excretion
	Goldstein and Konig, 1983 [80]	Plasma cortisol levels 24-Hour urinary free cortisol excretion Plasma cortisol response to tetracosactrin Plasma cortisol response to metyrapone
	Katz et al., 1986 [103]	Plasma cortisol levels Plasma cortisol response to tetracosactrin 24-Hour urinary free cortisol excretion
	Prahl et al., 1987 [168]	Serum cortisol levels 24-Hour urinary free cortisol excretion
	Ribeiro, 1987 [173]	Plasma cortisol levels Plasma cortisol response to tetracosactrin
	Varsano et al., 1990 [207]	Plasma cortisol levels Plasma cortisol response to tetracosactrin
	Freigang and Ashford, 1990 [76]	Plasma cortisol response to tetracosactrin

HPA = hypothalamic-pituitary-adrenal; ACTH = adrenocorticotropic hormone; MCR = metabolic clearance rate; 11-OHCS = 11-hydroxycorticosteroid; 17-KGS = 17-ketogenic steroids; 17-KS = 17-ketosteroid.

and of no clinical significance. Many of the studies have looked at absolute doses used and not attempted to relate them to the body surface area.

In a recent study carried out by Priftis and his colleagues [169], such a relationship between dose and body surface was taken into account. Priftis also measured the total cortisol metabolite excretion during a 24-hour period, as doubts have been raised about the reliability of the 24-hour urinary free cortisol output as an indicator of adrenal insufficiency [97]. They found a dose-dependent suppression of daily cortisol excretion, with cortisol metabolite levels below the normal range when doses of beclomethasone exceeded more than 400 $\mu g/m^2$/day. However, not all their asthmatic children showed a reduction in cortisol production when treated with doses exceeding 400 $\mu g/m^2$/day, even for prolonged periods. Furthermore, no correlation was found between the total cortisol metabolite excretion and the duration of therapy with inhaled glucocorticoids [169].

In an earlier study, Prahl and coworkers [168] reported that a low response to ACTH stimulation in asthmatic children was only detected when doses of beclomethasone were greater than 2,000 $\mu g/1.73m^2$/day. However, it does seem that basal adrenal function is impaired by smaller amounts of the drug than those mentioned in Prahl's study. Children have been found to metabolize budesonide faster than adults, and the drug was undetectable 4 to 8 hours after it was inhaled in a dose of 1 mg [161]. At higher doses (>1,000 μg/day), beclomethasone appears to exert a higher adrenal suppressive effect than does budesonide [160]. Recent studies have shown that the dose of budesonide causing the same plasma cortisol levels may be 70 percent higher than the dose of beclomethasone dipropionate [123, 182a].

Monitoring HPA Function During Aerosol Therapy

As already stated, although the substitution of inhaled glucocorticoids in patients previously receiving oral therapy often helps the HPA axis regain its integrity, a wide individual variation in the time needed for the HPA axis to recover has been reported [177, 195]; in some cases, HPA function had still not returned to normal 6 months or later after the substitution [132]. It is therefore necessary to monitor adrenal function closely in asthmatics, especially children, who are being transferred from systemic to inhaled glucocorticoid therapy.

The importance of long-term surveillance in these patients merits re-stressing. Three children who had been switched to inhaled steroids 5 months previously died suddenly and were found to have atrophic adrenals. One month before death, they had been found to have normal morning plasma cortisol levels and two had had a normal response to ACTH stimulation [139]. The rapid withdrawal of glucocorticoid treatment while inhaled glucocorticoids are being substituted is potentially serious and has proved fatal [34]; some reports have minimized this danger [24, 127].

All this emphasizes a need for caution when substituting inhaled for systemic glucocorticoids and for close surveillance of asthmatics on the higher doses of glucocorticoid aerosols. The clinically relevant issue in patients who have been weaned off of glucocorticoids or switched from systemic to inhaled glucocorticoids is whether the patient is able to respond to a stressful situation. Tests involving insulin-induced hypoglycemia appear to be the most sensitive indices of the ability of the entire HPA axis to respond to stress.

In general, in those cases in which patients cannot be maintained symptom free on inhaled glucocorticoids, attempts to circumvent the problem of HPA suppression by giving the drug on an alternate-day basis or using ACTH have not been completely successful. Control of bronchial asthma, like that of any other chronic condition, often remains a frustrating compromise between attaining maximum relief from symptoms along with the minimum acceptable degree of side effects.

A number of points emerge from the analysis of data obtained from the large number of papers published on the subject. In adults, doses of inhaled steroids up to 1,500 μg/day have not really been associated with significant systemic effects. The corresponding dose in children is 400 μg/day. It is important to realize that, even at these doses, there may be idiosyncratic patients who for some unknown reason show a more pronounced suppression of their HPA axis in response to glucocorticoid therapy. There seems to be little point in performing sophisticated HPA function tests in children up to a dose of about 600 μg/day, and perhaps at this level the most important measurement is that of growth. There are conflicting reports on the growth effects at this dosage; some studies have shown no inhibition [30, 83], while others have shown some growth retardation [12, 121]. Studies using knemometry have detected short-term linear growth in children with mild asthma treated with inhaled glucocorticoids [217a]. Extrapolating such changes in short-term growth velocity to long-term growth in stature is difficult.

Systemic absorption from inhaled glucocorticoids does occur, as the bronchial mucosa offers a very large area for drug absorption. These effects have been shown to have an impact on lipid and carbohydrate metabolism [108] and, perhaps more importantly, on biochemical markers of bone turnover [6, 100, 165].

The demonstration of small changes in cortisol production should not be unconditionally equated with clinically important suppression of HPA axis function. Patients on long-term, high-dose inhaled glucocorticoids should have their HPA axis function checked on a regular basis. Asthmatics being treated with high doses of inhaled glucocorticoids should carry steroid cards with them, just like those for patients on oral therapy. Patients who had previously been on long-term oral glucocorticoids should similarly carry these cards with them until it has been proved that HPA function has recovered completely. The important question to answer is not whether HPA function has returned to its pretreatment status in these patients, assuming pretreatment test values are available, but whether the HPA status can protect the patient from an adrenal crisis during an acute clinical stress after glucocorticoid therapy has been stopped.

To better evaluate the systemic effects of high-dose inhaled glucocorticoids, more long-term studies are needed. It is becoming increasingly obvious that high-dose inhaled glucocorticoids are not entirely free of systemic side effects, but the risk: benefit ratio associated with them seems better than that for systemic glucocorticoids or for undertreated asthma. Table 62-1 summarizes the current status of HPA function in asthma.

REFERENCES

1. Abbasy, A. S., Fahmy, M. S., and Kantoush, M. M. The adrenal cortical glucocorticoid function in asthmatic children. *Acta Paediatr. Scand.* 56: 593, 1967.
2. Ackerman, G. L., and Nolan, C. M. Adrenocortical responsiveness after alternate-day corticosteroid therapy. *N. Engl. J. Med.* 278:405, 1968.
3. Adelroth, E., Rosenhall, L., and Glennow, C. High dose inhaled budesonide in the treatment of severe steroid-dependent asthmatics. A two-year study. *Allergy* 40:58, 1985.
4. Adrenal function and asthma (editorial). *Lancet* 1:853, 1965.
5. Aizawa, T., Yasuda, N., and Greer, M. Hypoglycaemia stimulates ACTH secretion through a direct effect on the basal hypothalamus. *Metabolism* 30:996, 1981.
6. Ali, N. J., Capewell, S., and Ward, M. J. Bone turnover during high dose inhaled corticosteroid treatment. *Thorax* 46:160, 1991.
6a. Altman, L. C., et al. Adrenal function in adult asthmatics during long-term treatment with 800, 1200, and 1600 μg triamcinolone acetonide. *Chest* 101:1250, 1992.
7. Andersson, E. Pituitary function in patients with bronchial asthma measured indirectly by methopyrapone. *Acta Allergol.* (Kbh.) 19:311, 1964.
8. Angeli, A., et al. Diurnal variation of prednisolone binding to serum glucocorticoid binding globulin in man. *Clin. Pharmacol. Ther.* 23:47, 1978.
9. Arbesman, C. E., Bronstein, H. S., and Reisman, R. E. Dexamethasone aerosol therapy for bronchial asthma. *J. Allergy* 34:354, 1963.
10. Baden, M., et al. Plasma glucocorticoids in infants with the respiratory distress syndrome. *Pediatrics* 52:782, 1973.
11. Bakran, I. Jr., et al. The effect of alternate-day prednisone therapy on cortisol secretion rate in corticosteroid-dependent asthmatics. *Int. Clin. Pharmacol. Biopharm.* 15:57, 1977.
12. Balfour-Lynn, L. Growth and childhood asthma. *Arch. Dis. Child.* 61:1049, 1986.
12a. Barnes, N. C., and Payne, S. L. A multi-center, randomized, double-blind, parallel-group study to compare fluticasone propionate 1 mg daily with

beclomethasone dipropionate 2 mg daily in adult patients with severe asthma (abstract). *Am. Rev. Respir. Dis.* 145:743, 1992.
13. Bennett, W. A. Histopathological alteration of adrenal and anterior pituitary glands in patients treated with cortisone. *J. Bone Joint Surg.* 36:867, 1954.
14. Bernstein, I. L., Chervinsky, P., and Felliers, C. J. Efficacy and safety of triamcinolone aerosol in chronic asthma. *Chest* 81:20, 1982.
15. Bhan, G. L., Gwynn, C. M., and Morrison-Smith, J. Growth and adrenal function of children on prolonged beclomethasone dipropionate treatment. *Lancet* 1:96, 1980.
16. Bickerman, H. A., and Itkin, S. E. Aerosol steroid therapy and chronic bronchial asthma. *JAMA* 184:533, 1963.
17. Bisgaard, H., et al. Adrenal function in children with bronchial asthma treated with beclomethasone dipropionate or budesonide. *J. Allergy Clin. Immunol.* 81:1088, 1988.
18. Bjorkheim, I., et al. Accuracy of some routine methods used in clinical chemistry as judged by isotope dilution—mass fragmentography. *Clin. Chem.* 27:733, 1981.
19. Blumenthal, M. N., et al. Adrenal-pituitary function in bronchial asthma. *Arch. Intern. Med.* 117:23, 1966.
20. British Thoracic and Tuberculosis Association. Inhaled glucocorticoids compared with oral prednisolone in patients starting long-term glucocorticoid therapy for asthma. *Lancet* 2:469, 1975.
21. Brockbank, W., and Pengelly, C. D. R. Chronic asthma treated with powder inhalations of hydrocortisone and prednisolone. *Lancet* 2:187, 1956.
22. Brooks, S. M., et al. The effects of ephedrine and theophylline on dexamethasone metabolism in bronchial asthma. *J. Clin. Pharmacol.* 17:308, 1977.
23. Brooks, S. M., et al. Adverse effects of phenobarbital on glucocorticoid metabolism in patients with bronchial asthma. *N. Engl. J. Med.* 286:1125, 1972.
23a. Brown, P. H., Greening, A. P., and Crompton, G. K. High-dose beclomethasone dipropionate (BDP) and hypothalamo-pituitary-adrenal axis function in adults with chronic asthma (abstract). *Am. Rev. Respir. Dis.* 145: 499, 1992.
24. Brown, H. H., Storey, G., and George, W. H. Beclomethasone dipropionate: a new steroid aerosol for the treatment of allergic asthma. *Br. Med. J.* 1:585, 1972.
25. Brown, P. H., et al. Screening for hypothalamic-pituitary-adrenal axis suppression in asthmatics taking high dose inhaled corticosteroids. *Respir. Med.* 85:511, 1991.
26. Brown, P. H., et al. Hypothalamo-pituitary-adrenal axis suppression in asthmatics inhaling high dose corticosteroids. *Respir. Med.* 85:501, 1991.
27. Brown, P. H., et al. Do large volume spacer devices reduce the systemic effects of high dose inhaled corticosteroids? *Thorax* 45:736, 1990.
28. Brunette, M. G., Lands, L., and Thibodeau, L. P. Childhood asthma: prevention of attacks with short-term corticosteroid treatment of upper respiratory tract infection. *Pediatrics* 81:624, 1988.
29. Buisseret, P. D. Effect of beclomethasone dipropionate on the diurnal variations in plasma cortisol levels. *Acta Allergol.* 28:126, 1973.
30. Burch, W. Urine free cortisol determination. A useful tool in the management of chronic hypoadrenal states. *JAMA* 247:2002, 1982.
31. Carryer, H. M., Sherrick, D. W., and Gastineau, C. F. Occurrence of allergic disease in patients with adrenal cortical hypofunction. *JAMA* 172:84, 1960.
32. Carryer, H. M., et al. Effects of cortisone on bronchial asthma and hay-fever occurring in subjects sensitive to ragweed pollen. *Proc. Mayo Clinic* 25:282, 1950.
33. Cayton, R., and Howard, P. Plasma cortisol and the use of hydrocortisone in the treatment of status asthmaticus. *Thorax* 28:567, 1973.
34. Cayton, R. M., and Howard, P. Adrenal failure in bronchial asthma. *Br. Med. J.* 2:547, 1973.
35. Ceresa, F., et al. Once-a-day neurally stimulated and basal ACTH secretion phases in man and their response to corticoid inhibition. *J. Clin. Endocrinol.* 29:1074, 1969.
36. Choo-Kang, Y. F. J., et al. Beclomethasone dipropionate by inhalation in the treatment of airways obstruction. *Br. J. Dis. Chest* 66:101, 1972.
37. Clark, T. J. H. Effect of beclomethasone dipropionate delivered by aerosol in patients with asthma. *Lancet* 1:1361, 1972.
38. Clayton, R. N. Diagnosis of adrenal insufficiency. *Br. Med. J.* 298:271, 1989.
39. Clissold, S. P., and Heel, R. C. Budesonide: a preliminary review of its pharmacodynamic properties and therapeutic efficacy in asthma and rhinitis. *Drugs* 28:485, 1984.

40. Collins, J. V., et al. Hypothalamo-pituitary-adrenal function in intrinsic non-atopic asthma. *Thorax* 30:578, 1975.
41. Collins, J. V., et al. The use of glucocorticoids in the treatment of acute asthma. *Q. J. Med.* 174:259, 1975.
42. Cornil, A., et al. Adrenocortical and somatotrophic secretions in acute and chronic respiratory insufficiency. *Am. Rev. Respir. Dis.* 112:77, 1975.
43. Costello, J. F., and Clark, T. J. H. Response of patients receiving high dose beclomethasone dipropionate. *Thorax* 29:571, 1974.
44. Cotes, P. M., McLean, A., and Sayer, J. B. Absorption of inhaled hydrocortisone. *Lancet* 2:807, 1956.
45. Darrow, D. C., and Sarason, E. L. Some effects of low atmospheric pressure on rats. *J. Clin. Invest.* 23:11, 1944.
46. De Lange, W. E., et al. Plasma 11-deoxycortisol, androstenedione, testosterone and ACTH in comparison with the urinary excretion of tetrahydro-11-deoxycortisol as indices of the pituitary-adrenal response to oral metyrapone. *Acta Endocrinol.* (Copenh.) 93:488, 1980.
47. Dixon, R. B., and Christy, N. P. On the various forms of corticosteroid withdrawal syndrome. *Am. J. Med.* 68:224, 1980.
48. Dolan, L. M., et al. Short-term, high dose, systemic steroids in children with asthma: the effect on the hypothalamic-pituitary-adrenal axis. *J. Allergy Clin. Immunol.* 80:81, 1987.
49. Dwyer, J., Lazarus, L., and Hickie, J. B. A study of cortisol metabolism in patients with chronic asthma. *Aust. Ann. Med.* 16:297, 1967.
50. Ebden, P., and Davies, B. H. High dose corticosteroid inhalers for asthma. *Lancet* 2:576, 1984.
51. Ebden, P., et al. Comparison of two high dose corticosteroid aerosol treatments, beclomethasone dipropionate (1500μg/day) and budesonide (1600μg/day), for chronic asthma. *Thorax* 41:869, 1986.
52. Elbirt, P., et al. Acute asthma: evaluating the role of steroids in preventing relapse (abstract). *Am. Rev. Respir. Dis.* 129:206, 1984.
53. Ellul-Micallef, R. The acute effects of glucocorticoids in bronchial asthma. *Eur. J. Respir. Dis.* 63(suppl. 122):118, 1982.
54. Ellul-Micallef, R. Glucocorticosteroids. The Pharmacological Basis of Their Therapeutic Use in Bronchial Asthma. In P. J. Barnes, I. W. Rodger, and N. C. Thomson (eds.), *Asthma: Basic Mechanisms and Clinical Management.* London: Academic Press, 1988, P. 653.
55. Ellul-Micallef, R., Borthwick, R. C., and McHardy, G. J. R. The time course of response to prednisolone in chronic bronchial asthma. *Clin. Sci.* 47:105, 1974.
56. Ellul-Micallef, R., Borthwick, R. C., and McHardy, G. J. R. The effects of oral prednisolone on gas exchange in chronic bronchial asthma. *Br. J. Clin. Pharmacol.* 9:479, 1980.
57. Ellul-Micallef, R., and Fenech, F. F. Intravenous prednisolone in chronic bronchial asthma. *Thorax* 30:312, 1975.
58. Ellul-Micallef, R., and Fenech, F. F. Effects of intravenous prednisolone in asthmatics with diminished adrenergic responsiveness. *Lancet* 2:1269, 1975.
59. Ellul-Micallef, R., Hansson, E., and Johannson, S. A. Budesonide: a new glucocorticoid in bronchial asthma. *Eur. J. Respir. Dis.* 61:167, 1980.
60. Ellul-Micallef, R., and Johannson, S. A. Acute dose-response studies in bronchial asthma with a new glucocorticoid, budesonide. *Br. J. Clin. Pharmacol.* 15:419, 1983.
61. Ellul-Micallef, R., et al. Use of special inhaler attachment in asthmatic children. *Thorax* 35:620, 1980.
62. Englert, E. R. Jr., et al. Metabolism of free and conjugated 17-hydroxyglucocorticoids in subjects with uremia. *J. Clin. Endocrinol.* 18:36, 1958.
63. Eriksson-Lihr, Z. Function of the suprarenal cortex in allergic diseases. *Acta Paediatr. Scand.* 40(suppl. 83):116, 1951.
64. Fanta, C. H., Rossing, T. H., and McFadden, E. R. Jr. Glucocorticoids in acute asthma: a critical controlled trial. *Am. Rev. Respir. Dis.* 125:94, 1982.
65. Farrer, M., Francis, A. J., and Pearce, S. J. Morning serum control concentrations after 2 mg inhaled beclomethasone dipropionate in normal subjects: effect of a 750 ml spacing device. *Thorax* 45:740, 1990.
66. Fiel, S. B., et al. Efficacy of short-term corticosteroid therapy in outpatient treatment of acute bronchial asthma. *Am. J. Med.* 75:259, 1983.
67. Fisch, B. R., and Grater, W. C. Dexamethasone aerosol in respiratory tract disease. *J. New Drugs* 2:298, 1962.
68. Flashman, D. H. Effect of suprarenalectomy on active anaphylactic shock in white rat. *J. Infect. Dis.* 38:461, 1926.
69. Foulde, W. S., et al. Hydrocortisone in treatment of allergic conjunctivitis, allergic rhinitis and bronchial asthma. *Lancet* 1:234, 1955.
70. Francis, R. S. Long term beclomethasone dipropionate aerosol therapy in juvenile asthma. *Thorax* 31:309, 1976.
71. Francis, R. S. Adrenocortical function during high-dose beclomethasone aerosol therapy. *Clin. Allergy* 14:49, 1984.
72. Franklin, W., and Lowell, F. C. Unapproved drugs in the practice of medicine: beclomethasone—a case in point. *N. Engl. J. Med.* 292:1075, 1975.
73. Franklin, W., et al. Aerosolized steroids in bronchial asthma. *J. Allergy* 3:214, 1958.
74. Fraser, P. M., et al. The circumstances preceding death from asthma in young people in 1968 to 1969. *Br. J. Dis. Chest* 65:71, 1971.
75. Fraser, C. G., Preuss, F. S., and Bigford, W. D. Adrenal atrophy and irreversible shock associated with cortisone therapy. *JAMA* 149:1542, 1952.
76. Freigang, B., and Ashford, D. R. Adrenal cortical function after long-term beclomethasone aerosol therapy in early childhood. *Ann. Allergy* 64:342, 1990.
77. Friedman, M., and Frears, J. Effect of B 17-V inhalation on hypothalamic pituitary-adrenal axis and on growth in asthmatic children. *Arch. Dis. Child.* 49:747, 1974.
78. Gaddie, J., et al. A dose-response study in chronic bronchial asthma. *Lancet* 2:280, 1973.
79. Gelfland, M. L. Administration of cortisone by the aerosol method in the treatment of bronchial asthma. *N. Engl. J. Med.* 245:293, 1951.
80. Goldstein, D., and Konig, P. Effect of inhaled beclomethasone dipropionate on hypothalamopituitary adrenal axis function in children with asthma. *Pediatrics* 72:60, 1983.
81. Gordon, A. C. H., et al. Dose of inhaled budesonide required to produce clinical suppression of plasma cortisol. *Eur. J. Respir. Dis.* 71:10, 1987.
82. Graber, A. L., et al. Natural history of recovery following long-term suppression with corticosteroids. *J. Clin. Endocrinol.* 25:11, 1965.
83. Graff-Lonnevig, V., and Kraepelien, S. Long-term treatment with beclomethasone dipropionate aerosol in asthmatic children with special reference to growth. *Allergy* 34:57, 1979.
84. Grant, I. W. B. Are glucocorticoids necessary in the treatment of severe acute asthma? *Br. J. Dis. Chest* 76:125, 1982.
85. Green, M., and Lim, K. H. Bronchial asthma in Addison's disease. *Lancet* 1:1159, 1971.
86. Grossman, A., et al. New hypothalamic hormone, corticotrophin-releasing factor, specifically stimulates the release of adrenocorticotrophic hormone and cortisol in man. *Lancet* 2:921, 1982.
87. Gwinup, G., and Johnson, B. Clinical testing of the hypothalamic-pituitary adrenocortical system in states of hypo- and hypercortisolism. *Metabolism* 24:777, 1975.
88. Hagg, E., Asplund, K., and Lithner, F. Value of basal plasma cortisol assays in the assessment of pituitary-adrenal insufficiency. *Clin. Endocrinol.* 26:221, 1987.
89. Harding, S. M. The human pharmacology of fluticasone propionate. *Respir. Med.* 84(suppl.):25, 1990.
90. Harris, J. B., et al. Early intervention with short courses of prednisone to prevent progression of asthma in ambulatory patients incompletely responsive to bronchodilators. *J. Pediatr.* 110:627, 1987.
91. Harris, P. W. R., and Collins, J. V. Bronchial asthma in Addison's disease. *Lancet* 1:1248, 1971.
92. Harrison, D. D. W., et al. Recovery of hypothalamo-pituitary-adrenal function in asthmatics whose oral steroids have been stopped or reduced. *Clin. Endocrinol.* 7:109, 1982.
93. Harter, J. A., Redd, W. J., and Thorn, G. W. Studies on an intermittent glucocorticoid dosage regimen. *N. Engl. J. Med.* 269:691, 1963.
94. Hartzband, P. I., et al. Assessment of hypothalamic-pituitary-adrenal axis dysfunction: comparison of ACTH stimulation, insulin-hypoglycaemia and metyrapone. *J. Endocrinol. Invest.* 11:769, 1988.
95. Hicklin, J. A., and Wills, M. R. Plasma "cortisol" response to Synacthen in patients on long-term small-dose prednisone therapy. *Ann. Rheum. Dis.* 27:33, 1968.
96. Holt, P. R., et al. The effect of an inhaled steroid on the hypothalamic-pituitary-adrenal axis—which tests should be used? *Clin. Exp. Allergy* 20:145, 1990.
97. Honour, J. W. The Adrenal Cortex. In C. G. D. Brook (ed.), *Clinical Paediatric Endocrinology.* Oxford: Blackwell, 1989, P. 341.
98. Hsu, T. H., and Bledsoe, T. Measurement of urinary free corticoids by competitive protein-binding radioassay in hypoadrenal states. *J. Clin. Endocrinol. Metab.* 26:1116, 1966.
99. Jasani, M. K., et al. Studies of the rise in plasma 11-hydroxycorticosteroids in corticosteroid treated patients with rheumatoid arthritis during surgery: correlations with the functioning integrity of the hypothalamic-pituitary-adrenal axis. *Q. J. Med.* 37:407, 1968.
100. Jennings, B. H. Assessment of systemic effects of inhaled glucocorticosteroids (Ph.D. Thesis). University of Lund, Sweden, 1990.

101. Jubiz, W., and Meikle, A. W. Alterations of glucocorticosteroid actions by other drugs and disease states. *Drugs* 18:113, 1979.

102. Kass, I., and Appleby, S. The status of the adrenal gland in the asthmatic patient. *Am. J. Med. Sci.* 240:213, 1960.

102a. Kattan, A., Gurwitz, D., and Levison, H. Corticosteroids in status asthmaticus. *J. Pediatr.* 96:S96, 1980.

103. Katz, R. M., et al. Twice daily beclomethasone dipropionate in the treatment of childhood asthma. *J. Asthma* 23:1, 1986.

104. Kepinov, L. Surrénales et anaphylaxie. *Compt. rend. Soc. de Biol.* 87:327, 1922.

105. Kershnar, H., et al. Treatment of chronic childhood asthma with beclomethasone dipropionate aerosol: effect on pituitary-adrenal function after substitution for oral glucocorticoids. *Pediatrics* 62:189, 1978.

106. Klein, R., et al. Treatment of chronic childhood asthma with beclomethasone dipropionate aerosol: a double-blind crossover trial in non-steroid dependent patients. *Pediatrics* 60:7, 1977.

107. Kozower, M., Veatch, L., and Kaplan, M. M. Decreased clearance of prednisone: a factor in development of glucocorticoid side effects. *J. Clin. Endocrinol. Metab.* 38:407, 1974.

108. Kruszynska, Y. T., et al. Effect of high dose inhaled beclomethasone dipropionate on carbohydrate and lipid metabolism in normal subjects. *Thorax* 42:881, 1987.

109. Landon, J., et al. Adrenal response to infused corticotrophin in subjects receiving glucocorticoids. *J. Clin. Endocrinol.* 25:602, 1965.

110. Landon, J., Wynn, V., and James, V. The adrenocortical response to insulin-induced hypoglycaemia. *J. Clin. Endocrinol. Metab.* 27:183, 1963.

111. Laursen, L. C., Taudorf, E., and Weeke, B. High-dose inhaled budesonide in treatment of severe steroid-dependent asthma. *Eur. J. Respir. Dis.* 68:19, 1986.

112. Law, C. M., Preece, M. A., and Warner, J. O. Nocturnal adrenal suppression in children inhaling beclomethasone dipropionate. *Lancet* 1:1321, 1987.

113. Law, C. M., et al. Nocturnal adrenal suppression in asthmatic children taking inhaled beclomethasone dipropionate. *Lancet* 1:942, 1986.

114. Laxenaire, M. C., et al. Fonction cortico-surrénalienne au cours des insuffisances respiratoires chronique. *Ann. Med. Nancy* 8:461, 1969.

115. Lemon, H. M., et al. Endocrine function in bronchial asthma and hay fever. *J. Allergy* 29:384, 1958.

116. Liddle, G. W. Analysis of circadian rhythms in human adrenocortical secretory activity. *Arch. Intern. Med.* 117:739, 1966.

117. Linder, B. L., et al. Cortisol production rate in childhood and adolescence. *J. Pediatr.* 117:892, 1990.

118. Linder, W. R. Adrenal suppression by aerosol steroid inhalation. *Arch. Intern. Med.* 113:665, 1964.

119. Lindholm, J., and Kehlet, H. Re-evaluation of the 30 min ACTH test in assessing the hypothalamic-pituitary-adrenocortical function. *Clin. Endocrinol.* (Oxf.) 26:221, 1987.

120. Lipsett, M. B. Factors influencing the rate of metabolism of steroid hormones in man. *Ann. N.Y. Acad. Sci.* 179:442, 1971.

121. Littlewood, J. M., et al. Growth retardation in asthmatic children treated with inhaled beclomethasone dipropionate. *Lancet* 1:115, 1988.

122. Livanou, T., Ferriman, D., and James, V. Recovery of hypothalamo-pituitary-adrenal function after corticosteroid therapy. *Lancet* 2:856, 1967.

123. Löfdahl, C. G., Mellstrand, T., and Svedmyr, N. Glucocorticoids in asthma. Studies of resistance and systemic effects of glucocorticoids. *Eur. J. Respir. Dis.* 65(suppl. 136):69, 1984.

124. Lorentzson, S., et al. Use of inhaled corticosteroids in patients with mild asthma. *Thorax* 45:733, 1990.

125. Luksza, A. R. Acute severe asthma treated without steroids. *Br. J. Dis. Chest* 76:15, 1982.

126. Lytras, N., et al. Corticotrophin releasing factor: responses in normal subjects and patients with disorders of the hypothalamus and pituitary. *Clin. Endocrinol.* (Oxf.) 20:71, 1984.

127. Maberly, D. J., Gibson, G. J., and Butler, A. G. Recovery of adrenal function after substitution of beclomethasone dipropionate for oral glucocorticoids. *Br. Med. J.* 1:778, 1973.

128. Malone, D. N. S., Grant, I. W. B., and Percy-Robb, I. W. Hypothalamopituitary adrenal function in asthmatic patients receiving long-term glucocorticoid therapy. *Lancet* 2:733, 1970.

129. Marotta, S. F. Roles of aortic and carotid chemoreceptors in activating the hypothalamo-hypophyseal-adrenocortical system during hypoxia. *Proc. Soc. Exp. Biol. Med.* 141:915, 1972.

130. Marotta, S. F. Comparative effects of hypoxia, adrenocorticotropin and methylcholine on adrenocortical secretory rates. *Proc. Soc. Exp. Biol. Med.* 141:923, 1972.

131. Marotta, S. F., Malasanos, L. J., and Boonayathap, U. Inhibition of the adrenocortical response to hypoxia by dexamethasone. *Aerospace Med.* 44:1, 1973.

132. Mathé, A. A., and Knapp, P. H. Emotional and adrenal reactions to stress in bronchial asthma. *Psychosom. Med.* 33:323, 1971.

133. Mattingly, D. A simple fluorimetric method for the estimation of free 11-hydroxycorticoids in human plasma. *J. Clin. Pathol.* 15:374, 1962.

134. McAllen, M. K., Kochanowski, S. J., and Shaw, K. M. Steroid aerosols in asthma: an assessment of betamethasone valerate and 12-month study of patients on maintenance treatment. *Br. Med. J.* 2:171, 1974.

135. McAllister, W. A. C., Mitchell, D. M., and Collins, J. V. Prednisolone pharmacokinetics compared between night and day in asthmatic and normal subjects. *Br. J. Clin. Pharmacol.* 11:303, 1981.

136. Medical Research Council Report. Controlled trial of effects of cortisone acetate in chronic asthma. *Lancet* 2:798, 1956.

137. Meikle, A. W., Jubiz, W., and Hutchings, H. P. A simplified metyrapone test with determination of plasma 11-deoxycortisol. *J. Clin. Endocrinol. Metab.* 29:985, 1969.

138. Melby, J. S. Systemic glucocorticoid therapy: pharmacology and endocrinologic consideration. *Ann. Intern. Med.* 81:505, 1974.

139. Mellis, C. M., and Phelan, P. D. Asthma deaths in children—a continuing problem. *Thorax* 32:39, 1977.

140. Meltzer, E. O., et al. Efficacy of dosing schedule on efficacy of beclomethasone dipropionate aerosol in chronic asthma. *Am. Rev. Respir. Dis.* 131:732, 1985.

141. Mikhail, G. R., Sweet, L. C., and Mellinger, R. C. Parenteral long-acting glucocorticoids: effect on hypothalamic-pituitary-adrenal function. *Allergy* 31:337, 1973.

142. Mittelman, A., et al. Adrenocortical response during corrected and uncorrected hypercapnic acidosis. *Am. J. Physiol.* 188:7, 1957.

143. Miyamoto, T., et al. Adrenal response and side reactions after long-term glucocorticoid therapy in bronchial asthma. *Ann. Allergy* 30:587, 1972.

144. Mok, J., Kattan, M., and Levison, H. Should corticosteroids be used in the treatment of acute severe asthma? A case against the use of corticosteroids in acute severe asthma. *Pharmacotherapy* 5:327, 1985.

145. Moore, A., et al. Cortisol assays: guidelines for the provision of a clinical biochemistry service. *Ann. Clin. Biochem.* 22:435, 1985.

146. Morén, F. Drug deposition of pressurized inhalation aerosols. I. Influence of activator tube design. *Int. J. Pharmacol.* 1:205, 1978.

147. Morris, H. G., and Jorgensen, J. R. Recovery of endogenous pituitary-adrenal function in corticosteroid treated children. *J. Pediatr.* 79:480, 1971.

148. Morris, H. G., Newman, I., and Ellis, E. G. Plasma steroid concentrations during alternate day treatment with prednisone. *J. Allergy Clin. Immunol.* 54:350, 1974.

149. Morrish, D. W., et al. Hypothalamic-pituitary-adrenal function in extrinsic asthma. *Chest* 75:161, 1979.

150. Muller, M., et al. Todlicher Zwischenfall nach intravenoser Injection von synthetischem ACTH. *Dtsch. Med. Wochenschr.* 107:1353, 1982.

151. Myles, A. B., Bacon, B. A., and Daly, J. R. Single daily dose glucocorticoid treatment: effect on adrenal function and therapeutic efficacy in various diseases. *Ann. Rheum. Dis.* 30:149, 1971.

152. Nassif, E., et al. Effects of continuous glucocorticoid therapy for children with chronic asthma. *J. Allergy Clin. Immunol.* 65:219, 1980.

153. Nassif, E., et al. Extrapulmonary effects of maintenance corticosteroid therapy with alternate-day prednisone and inhaled beclomethasone in children with chronic asthma. *J. Allergy Clin. Immunol.* 80:518, 1987.

154. Nelson, J. C., and Tyndall, D. J. A comparison of the adrenal response to hypoglycaemia, metyrapone and ACTH. *Am. J. Med. Sci.* 275:165, 1978.

155. Nelson, J. K., et al. Intemittent therapy with corticotrophin. *Lancet* 2:78, 1966.

156. Newman, S. P., et al. Deposition of pressurized aerosols inhaled through extension devices. *Am. Rev. Respir. Dis.* 124:317, 1981.

157. Nichols, T., Nugent, C. A., and Tyler, F. H. Diurnal variation in suppression of adrenal function by glucocorticoids. *J. Clin. Endocrinol.* 25:343, 1965.

158. Novey, H. S., and Beall, G. Aerosolized steroids and induced Cushing's syndrome. *Arch. Intern. Med.* 115:602, 1965.

159. Padfield, J. M. An evaluation of the use of extension tubes in the treatment of asthma. *Perpect. Ther. N. Eur.* 8:9, 1984.

160. Pedersen, S., and Fuglsang, G. Urine cortisol excretion in children treated with high doses of inhaled corticosteroids: a comparison of budesonide and beclomethasone. *Eur. Respir. J.* 1:433, 1988.

161. Pedersen, S., et al. Pharmacokinetics of budesonide in children with asthma. *Eur. J. Clin. Pharmacol.* 31:579, 1987.

162. Peters, G. A., and Henderson, L. L. Prednisolone aerosol in asthmatic bronchitis: a preliminary report. *Proc. Staff Meet. Mayo Clin.* 33:57, 1958.

163. Phillip, M., et al. Integrated concentration of plasma cortisol levels in asthmatic children treated with long term inhaled steroids (abstract). *Am. Rev. Respir. Dis.* 137:25, 1988.

164. Portner, M. M., et al. Successful initiation of alternate-day prednisone in chronic steroid dependent asthmatic patients. *J. Allergy Clin. Immunol.* 49:16, 1972.

165. Pouw, E. M., et al. Beclomethasone inhalation decreases serum osteocalcin concentrations. *Br. Med. J.* 302:627, 1991.

166. Prahl, P. High-dose steroid aerosol and adrenocortical function in children (abstract). *J. Allergy Clin. Immunol.* 81:317, 1988.

167. Prahl, P., and Jensen, T. Decreased adreno-cortical suppression utilizing the Nebuhaler for inhalation of steroid aerosols. *Clin. Allergy* 17:393, 1987.

168. Prahl, P., Jensen, T., and Bjerregaard-Andersen, H. Adrenocortical function in children on high-dose steroid aerosol therapy. *Allergy* 42:541, 1987.

169. Priftis, K., et al. Adrenal function in asthma. *Arch. Dis. Child.* 65:838, 1990.

170. Rachelefsky, G. S., and Siegel, S. C. Revisited: aerosol corticosteroids in the treatment of childhood asthma. *Pediatrics* 72:130, 1983.

171. Rackemann, F. M. Depletion in asthma. *J. Allergy* 16:136, 1945.

172. Randolph, T. G., and Rollins, J. P. Effect of cortisone on bronchial asthma. *J. Allergy* 21:288, 1950.

173. Ribeiro, L. B. A 12 Month Tolerance Study with Budesonide in Asthmatic Children. In S. Godfrey (ed.), *Glucocorticosteroids in Childhood Asthma.* Amsterdam: Excerpta Medica, 1987, P. 95.

174. Richards, J. B., and Stein, S. M. Effects of CO_2 exposure and respiratory acidosis on adrenal 17-hydroxyglucocorticoids secretion in anesthetized dogs. *Am. J. Physiol.* 188:1, 1957.

175. Robinson, B. H. B., Mattingly, D., and Cope, C. L. Adrenal function after prolonged corticosteroid therapy. *Br. Med. J.* 1:1579, 1962.

176. Robson, A. O., and Kilborn, J. R. Studies of adrenocortical function in continuous asthma. *Thorax* 20:93, 1965.

177. Roscoe, P., Choo-Kang, Y. F. J., and Horne, N. W. Betamethasone valerate in glucocorticoid-dependent asthmatics. *Br. J. Dis. Chest* 69:240, 1975.

178. Ruder, H. S., Guy, R., and Lipsett, M. A radio-immunoassay for cortisol in plasma and urine. *J. Clin. Endocrinol. Metab.* 35:219, 1972.

179. Sadeghi-Nejad, A., and Senior, B. Adrenal function, growth and insulation in patients treated with corticoids on alternate days. *Pediatrics* 43:277, 1969.

180. Salassa, R., Bennet, W., and Keating, F. Post-operative adrenal cortical insufficiency occurrence in patients previously treated with cortisone. *JAMA* 152:1509, 1955.

181. Sanarkin, N. G., and El-Shaboury, A. H. Chronic adrenalitis with bronchial asthma. *Lancet* 2:468, 1965.

182. Seale, J. P., and Compton, M. R. Side effects of corticosteroid agents. *Med. J. Aust.* 144:139, 1986.

182a.Selroos, O., and Halme, M. Effect of a volumatic spacer and mouth rinsing on systemic absorption of inhaled corticosteroids from a metered dose inhaler and dry powder inhaler. *Thorax* 46:891, 1991.

183. Semple, P. d'A., et al. Hypothalamic-pituitary dysfunction in respiratory hypoxia. *Thorax* 36:605, 1981.

184. Shapiro, G. G., et al. Double-blind evaluation of methylprednisolone versus placebo for acute asthma episodes. *Pediatrics* 71:510, 1983.

185. Sherman, B., et al. Further studies of the effects of inhaled glucocorticoids on pituitary-adrenal function in healthy adults. *J. Allergy Clin. Immunol.* 69:208, 1982.

186. Siegel, S. C., Katz, R., and Rachelefsky, G. S. Prednisone and beclomethasone for treatment of asthma. *N. Engl. J. Med.* 300:986, 1979.

187. Siegel, S. C., et al. Plasma 17-hydroxycorticosteroid concentrations in children with bronchial asthma. *J. Allergy* 27:504, 1956.

188. Siegre, E. J., and Klaiber, E. L. Therapeutic utilization of the diurnal variation in pituitary adrenocortical activity. *Calif. Med.* 104:363, 1966.

189. Sjaastad, O. M., et al. Adrenocortical function in chronic pulmonary disease. *N. Engl. J. Med.* 266:801, 1962.

190. Smith, A. P., Booth, M., and Daney, A. J. A controlled trial of beclomethasone dipropionate for asthma. *Br. J. Dis. Chest* 67:208, 1973.

191. Smith, J. M. Hydrocortisone hemisuccinate by inhalation in children with asthma. *Lancet* 2:1248, 1958.

192. Smith, M. J., and Hodson, M. E. Effects of long term inhaled high dose beclomethasone dipropionate on adrenal function. *Thorax* 38:76, 1983.

193. Spangler, D. L., et al. One year trial of aerosolized flunisolide in severe-steroid-dependent asthmatics. *Ann. Allergy* 39:70, 1979.

194. Speizer, F. E., et al. Investigation into use of drugs preceding death from asthma. *Br. Med. J.* 1:339, 1968.

195. Spitzer, S. A., et al. Beclomethasone dipropionate in chronic asthma. *Chest* 70:38, 1976.

196. Springer, C., et al. Comparison of budesonide and beclomethasone dipropionate for treatment of asthma. *Arch. Dis. Child.* 62:815, 1987.

197. Stewart, P. M., et al. A rational approach for assessing the hypothalamo-pituitary-adrenal axis. *Lancet* 1:1208, 1988.

198. Stiksa, G., Nemcek, K., and Glennow, C. Adrenal function in asthmatics treated with high-dose budesonide. *Respiration* 48:91, 1985.

199. Streck, W. F., and Lockwood, D. H. Pituitary adrenal recovery following short-term suppression with glucocorticoids. *Am. J. Med.* 66:910, 1979.

200. Tabachnik, E., and Zadik, Z. Diurnal cortisol secretion during therapy with inhaled beclomethasone dipropionate in children with asthma. *J. Pediatr.* 118:294, 1991.

201. Tarlo, S. M., et al. Six-month double-blind, controlled trial of high dose, concentrated beclomethasone dipropionate in the treatment of severe chronic asthma. *Chest* 93:998, 1988.

202. Toogood, J. H., et al. Minimum dose requirements of steroid-dependent asthmatic patients for aerosol beclomethasone and oral prednisone. *J. Allergy Clin. Immunol.* 61:355, 1978.

203. Toogood, J. H., et al. Use of spacers to facilitate inhaled corticosteroid treatment of asthma. *Am. Rev. Respir. Dis.* 129:723, 1984.

204. Tuft, T., Marks, A. D., and Channick, B. J. Long term glucocorticoid therapy in chronic intractable asthmatic patients. *Ann. Allergy* 29:287, 1971.

205. Uhde, H. Aerosoltherapic mit Prednisolonlosung (Elgene Erfahrungen). *Munchen Med Wochenschr.* 99:891, 1957.

206. Vaccarezza, J. R. The suprarenal function in allergic asthma. *Dis. Chest* 40:121, 1961.

207. Varsano, I., et al. Safety of 1 year of treatment with budesonide in young children with asthma. *J. Allergy Clin. Immunol.* 85:914, 1990.

208. Vaz, R., et al. Adrenal effects of beclomethasone inhalation therapy in asthmatic children. *J. Pediatr.* 100:660, 1982.

209. Voisin, C., et al. La response cortico-surrénalienne au cours des épisodes de décompensation survenant chez l'insuffisance respiratoire chronique. *Lille Med.* 15:1367, 1970.

210. Warner, J. O. The place of Intal in paediatric practice. *Resp. Med.* 83(suppl.):33, 1989.

211. Webb, J., and Clark, T. J. H. Recovery of plasma corticotrophin and cortisol levels after a three-week course of prednisolone. *Thorax* 36:22, 1981.

212. Webb, R. D. Beclomethasone in steroid-dependent asthma. *JAMA* 238:1508, 1977.

213. Weitzman, E. D., et al. Twenty-four hour pattern of the episodic secretion of cortisol in normal subjects. *J. Clin. Endocrinol. Metab.* 33:14, 1971.

214. Weller, H. H., et al. Hormonal pattern in bronchial asthma. *Scand. J. Respir. Dis.* 49:163, 1968.

215. Willis, T. *Pharmaceutice Rationalis.* London: T. Dring, 1679.

216. Wilmsmeyer, W., et al. First-time treatment with steroids in bronchial asthma: comparison of the effects of inhaled beclomethasone and of oral prednisone on airway function, bronchial reactivity and hypothalamic-pituitary-adrenal axis. *Eur. Respir. J.* 3:786, 1990.

217. Wolfram, J., and Zwemer, R. L. Cortin protection against anaphylactic shock in guinea pigs. *J. Exp. Med.* 61:9, 1935.

217a.Wolthers, O. D., and Pedersen, S. Growth of asthmatic children during treatment with budesonide: a double-blind trial. *Br. Med. J.* 303:163, 1991.

218. Wood, J. B., et al. A rapid test of adrenocortical function. *Lancet* 1:243, 1965.

219. Wyatt, R., et al. Effects of inhaled beclomethasone dipropionate and alternate-day prednisone on pituitary-adrenal function in children with chronic asthma. *N. Engl. J. Med.* 299:1387, 1978.

219a.Yernault, J. C. Safety of inhaled fluticasone propionate in adult asthma (abstract). *Eur. Resp. J.* 5(Suppl. 15):325S, 1992.

220. Zora, J. A., et al. Hypothalamic-pituitary-adrenal axis suppression after short-term high dose glucocorticoid therapy in children with asthma. *J. Allergy Clin. Immunol.* 77:9, 1986.

Nonsteroidal Antiallergic Drugs

63

Jonathan A. Bernstein
I. Leonard Bernstein

The concept of mast cell–stabilizing agents began with the discovery of disodium cromoglycate (DSCG), which was subsequently found to be clinically useful in the treatment of asthma and other allergic diatheses. Over the years, experience with DSCG has made it increasingly clear that the stabilization of mast cell membranes only partially accounts for its pharmacologic activity. Therefore, it is overly simplistic to think of DSCG and related compounds as mast cell–stabilizing agents, and most experts now more appropriately refer to these drugs as *antiinflammatory* or *antiallergic* agents.

The clinical success of DSCG resulted in a surge of investigations looking for related compounds with similar but improved pharmacologic and pharmacokinetic properties. Table 63-1 lists some of these agents that have been investigated for their mast cell–stabilizing effects [18, 31, 120, 187]. Interest in the vast majority of these drugs was abandoned as soon as it was determined that their in vitro actions did not predict clinical effectiveness. Table 63-2 compares the in vitro activity of several antiallergic drugs, including DSCG, to their inhibitory effects on allergen-induced bronchoconstriction in patients with asthma. Table 63-3 summarizes the worldwide assessment of these agents gleaned from published therapeutic trials [18].

Several drugs with mast cell–stabilizing effects have been approved for use in Canada, Japan, and Europe, and many of these agents are now undergoing investigation in the United States. It is beyond the scope of this chapter to discuss every investigational drug with mast cell–stabilizing effects. Rather, this chapter will be subdivided into two sections: (1) cromolyn-like agents, and (2) dual-action antihistamines. Although the flavonoids and lodoxamides have not proved to be clinically useful, they remain an invaluable tool for studying the structure–activity relationships of various chromone-like compounds on histamine-releasing cells, and therefore warrant mention in this discussion.

CHROMONE-LIKE COMPOUNDS

Disodium Cromoglycate (FPL 670)

DSCG is a bischromone antiallergic drug that was first discovered in 1965 as a result of pharmacologic investigations of khellin, an antispasmodic agent derived from the Mediterranean plant *Ammi visnaga* (Umbelliferae) [187]. The seeds from these plants were first used centuries ago as smooth muscle relaxants for colic. Further interest in khellin as an antianginal medication grew because of its coronary artery vasodilatory effects. Khellin was observed to also have a bronchodilatory effect, which was useful in treating asthma [65]. The impetus to explore synthetic analogs of khellin arose because its natural alkaloids had undesirable side effects and poor solubility. Researchers focused their attention on the 2-carboxychromone derivatives because they were

soluble compounds and structurally similar to khellin. Many of these related compounds were studied pharmacokinetically before DSCG was recognized to give the best protection against antigen-induced bronchoconstriction [65, 187]. DSCG was subsequently found to be effective in the treatment of many clinically allergic and nonallergic disorders. It has also been used extensively as a research tool for studying the pharmacologic aspects of mast cell heterogeneity in animal and human models [8].

Chemistry
DSCG was synthesized by combining a carboxychromone molecule with an alkylene dioxy chain to form the chemical structure, 1,3-bis-(2-carboxychromone-5-ylosyl)-2-hydroxypropane (Fig. 63-1). DSCG is a lipophobic, polar, and acidic compound (pK_a, 2) with a molecular weight of approximately 500 Daltons. It is 5% water soluble at 20°C and completely insoluble in alcohol. DSCG is slightly soluble in other organic solvents such as dioxane, pyridine, ether, and chloroform. DSCG liquefies at a relative humidity significantly lower than the relative humidity in the lungs [65, 187].

Pharmacokinetics
DSCG has been studied pharmacokinetically after intravenous, oral, inhaled, nasal, and ocular applications [10]. In normal subjects, an intravenous dose of DSCG is rapidly cleared from the plasma. Approximately 50 percent of the drug is excreted unchanged into the urine and the remainder through the biliary system [14]. There are no active metabolites of DSCG. The oral systemic absorption of DSCG ranges between 0.5 to 2 percent in both normal and asthmatic subjects [10, 14, 65].

The amount of DSCG absorbed after inhalation is dependent on the delivery system used and the dose administered [99]. Studies in humans have demonstrated that the highest plasma drug levels are achieved using a spinhaler device, the lowest levels using a pressurized nebulizer, and intermediate levels using a metered-dose inhaler [10]. Peak plasma levels of DSCG after inhalation were also achieved faster using the spinhaler or metered-dose inhaler rather than a nebulizer [10, 223]. Concentrations of DSCG after inhalation were consistently higher in normal subjects compared to those with asthma. This has been attributed to a nonasthmatic's higher inspiratory flow rates and longer breath-holding times [187].

The half-life ($T\frac{1}{2}$) of DSCG ranges between 46 and 99 minutes. Its peak urinary excretion rate occurs 15 to 45 minutes after inhalation, and approximately 45 percent of the total drug dose is excreted in the urine after only 30 minutes [223]. There is no systemic accumulation of DSCG because of its short half-life and low bioavailability [99, 187].

Approximately 7 percent of the total dose of 4 percent intranasal DSCG is absorbed. It is excreted in a manner similar to that

Table 63-1. *Some antiallergic drugs with mast cell–stabilizing effects**

Drug	Administration
Cromolyn-derived	
Proxicromil (FPL 57787)	Oral
Nedocromil sodium	Inhaled
Lodoxamide (U-42585 & U-42718)	Oral
Xanthones	
Doxantrazole (BW 59C)	Oral
AH-7725	Inhaled
RS-7540	Inhaled
Miscellaneous	
BRL-10833	Oral
BRL-2231	Oral
Wy 41195	Oral
Bufrolin	Inhaled
Cinnamoyl anthranilic acid	Inhaled
Cinnarizine	Oral
Azelastine	Oral
Ketotifen (HC 20-511)	Oral
Azatadine	Oral
Oxatomide (KW-4354)	Oral
Tranilast	Oral
Tiaramide	Oral
Zaprinast (M&B-22,948)	Oral
FPL 52694	Oral
FPL 52757	Oral
ICI 74917	Inhaled
Doquilast (Sm 857)	Oral
TBX	Oral
Pemirolast	Oral
Zy 15109 (NAAGA)	Inhaled

* Data from [18, 31, 120, 187].

Table 63-2. *Comparison of the preclinical and clinical activities of antiallergic drugs with disodium cromoglycate*

Compound	Preclinical studies		Clinical studies	
	In vitro[a] human lung	In vivo[b] rat PCA	Prevention of allergen-induced bronchospasm	Asthma therapy
Disodium cromoglycate	1	1	+ + +	+ + +
AH 7725	527	15	±	±
Tixanox	414	112	+ +	±
PRD-92-EA	270	4.5	+ +	±
ICI 74917	205	234	+ +	–
FPL 52757	136	0.12	+	+
FPL 57787	34	0.11	+ +	±
Doxantrazole	92	0.6	+	±

[a] IC_{50} values given in micromolars; IC_{50} = concentration required to inhibit release by 50%.
[b] Intravenous ED_{50} (mg/kg) has been converted to μmol/kg for each analog and compared with the ED_{50} value for disodium cromoglycate; ED_{50} = experimental dose preventing death in animal or inhibiting airway resistance by 50% at a fixed time.
PCA = passive cutaneous anaphylaxis; + = minimal; + + = moderate; + + + = maximal; ± = equivocal.
Source: R. M. Auty, The clinical development of a new agent for the treatment of airway inflammation, nedocromil sodium (Tilade). *Eur. J. Respir. Dis.* 69(suppl. 147):120, 1986. Reprinted with permission.

Table 63-3. *Comparison of antiallergy drugs with disodium cromoglycate in clinical models of asthma and in clinical trials performed in asthmatic patients*

Drug	Route of administration	Effect in challenge tests			Effect in therapeutic trials
		Bronchial antigen (immediate reaction)	Bronchial antigen (delayed reaction)	Exercise	
Disodium cromoglycate	Inhaled	Prevents	Prevents	Prevents	Effective
Doxantrazole	Oral	Inactive	Inactive	Inactive	Poor activity
AH 7725	Oral	Prevents	Inactive	Not known	Poor activity
Nivimedone	Oral	Prevents	Prevents	Not known	Weak activity
FPL 57787	Oral	Prevents	Inactive	Prevents	Weak activity
FPL 52757	Oral	Prevents	Prevents	Not known	Weak activity
ICI 74917	Inhaled	Prevents	Not known	Prevents	Poor activity
Lodoxamide	Oral/inhaled	Prevents	Inactive	Prevents	Poor activity
Oxatomide	Oral	Inactive	Not known	Variable	Poor activity
Ketotifen	Oral	Prevents	Prevents	Variable	Variable activity

Source: R. M. Auty, The clinical development of a new agent for the treatment of airway inflammation, nedocromil sodium (Tilade). *Eur. J. Respir. Dis.* 69(suppl. 147):120, 1986. Reprinted with permission.

of the inhaled form, although some is also lost through the nose and the gastrointestinal tract [10]. In rabbits, less than 0.07 percent of ocularly administered DSCG was absorbed systemically and only 0.01 percent of DSCG entered the aqueous humor. For adequate ocular absorption, DSCG must be applied repeatedly. In human volunteers, the ocular absorption of DSCG was only 0.03 percent and it was excreted unchanged in the bile and urine [10].

Mechanism of Action

After extensive investigation, the mechanism of action of DSCG is still not completely understood. In contrast to the way in which drugs are usually evaluated, DSCG was unique in that much of the early work attempting to define its pharmacologic activity involved human subjects. Altounyan, the drug's first clinical investigator, and himself an asthmatic, volunteered to demonstrate that inhaled DSCG could inhibit the early effects of mast cell–mediator release after antigen inhalation [64]. Extensive in vitro and in vivo work soon followed to investigate the mechanisms of DSCG and its effect on different organ systems using several different cellular and animal models. DSCG had a heterogeneous inhibitory effect in different species and organ systems, which soon became apparent. DSCG was more effective at improving lung function in rhesus monkeys and rats after allergen challenge than it was in guinea pig, calf, and dog animal models [12, 47, 56, 82, 85, 87, 140]. Although DSCG inhibited mast cell–mediated passive cutaneous anaphylaxis in rats, such effects were not observed in mice, guinea pigs, rabbits, monkeys, cows, or human subjects [15, 16, 154, 180, 200, 247, 251]. These

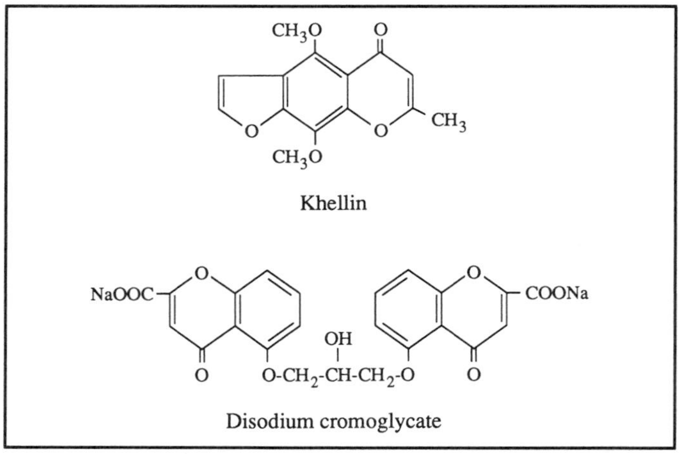

Fig. 63-1. *Structural comparison of khellin and disodium cromoglycate.*

Table 63-4. Species and tissue specificity of disodium cromoglycate

Species	Tissue	Inhibition
Cow	Basophil	−
	Lung	−
	Skin*	−
Dog	Lung	−
Guinea pig	Basophil	−
	Lung	−
	Mesentery	−
	Skin	−
Hamster	Peritoneum	+
Humans	Basophil	−
	Bronchoalveolar lavage	+
	Lung	±
	Skin	−
Monkey	Lung	±
	Skin*	−
Mouse	Peritoneum	−
	Skin*	−
Rabbit	Basophil	−
	Skin*	−
Rat	Intestine	−
	Lung	+
	Peritoneum	+
	Skin	+

* Effect of disodium cromoglycate on cutaneous anaphylactic reactions in vivo.
+ = sensitivity and − = refractoriness to inhibitory action of cromolyn on anaphylactic histamine release from chopped tissue or isolated wells in vitro.
Source: J. D. Foreman and F. L. Pearce, Cromolyn. In E. Middleton, et al. (eds.), *Allergy Principles and Practice.* St. Louis: Mosby, 1988. Reprinted with permission.

experiences emphasized that the use of experimental animal models in assays such as passive cutaneous anaphylaxis could not be used to predict the effect of drugs in humans because mast cell heterogeneity prevents extrapolation of these results from one species to another. Table 63-4 emphasizes this concept of mast cell heterogeneity by summarizing the variable pharmacologic effects of DSCG on different cells and in different species [94].

DSCG was originally proposed to function as a mast cell stabilizer by blocking the entrance of extracellular calcium into the cell. This theory was supported by experiments which demonstrated that DSCG could block antigen-, but not calcium ionophore-A23187–induced histamine release from mast cells [93, 95]. Mazurek and colleagues [25, 165, 167], in an attempt to prove this theory, performed a series of important experiments using rat basophil leukocytes (RBL-2H3) to show that DSCG interacted with a membrane receptor to inhibit histamine release in a cal-

cium-dependent manner. These RBL-2H3 cells were later used to isolate a specific cromolyn receptor (molecular weight, 60,000 Daltons) [164]. This specific membrane receptor, called *cromolyn-binding protein* (CBP), required calcium (Ca^{++}) uptake before immunoglobulin E (IgE)–mediated histamine release could occur. Further evidence for the importance of this receptor was provided by previously unresponsive anti-IgE RBL cell lines that became activated after adding CBP [166]. It was also found that, after the F_c receptor-IgE-CBP complex was inserted into cell membranes unresponsive to anti-IgE or antigen activation, a new conductance gradient formed across the membrane's lipid bilayers. These investigators concluded that one mechanism of DSCG was to block calcium uptake into mast cells or basophils, or both, thereby preventing specific IgE-antigen–induced histamine release [166, 168]. Their conclusions were in contrast to results from other experiments which demonstrated that DSCG could inhibit the release of mast cell mediator "independently" of calcium [152, 191]. Neher [191] used patch-clamp techniques on rat peritoneal mast cell membranes to demonstrate that calcium was neither necessary nor sufficient by itself to cause mediator secretion, regardless of whether an IgE or non-IgE stimulus caused activation. In fact, some investigators failed to find *any* calcium channels in viable mast cell membranes after antigen-IgE stimulation [152]. These discrepancies were partially attributed to the limitations of patch-clamp techniques in detecting calcium channels. As only rat basophilic leukocytes have been shown to contain CBPs but are less sensitive to DSCG inhibition compared to rat mast cells, additional work on other animal mast cell lines is required before the significance of these cromolyn receptors can be explained [94].

Protein phosphorylation has been postulated to play a significant role in DSCG's inhibition of histamine release from mast cells. Several membrane proteins are rapidly phosphorylated after mast cell activation induced by either calcium ionophores or anti-IgE [246]. Interestingly, one of these proteins, with a molecular weight of 78,000 Daltons, became dephosphorylated after Ca^{++}-independent mast cell activation [94, 246]. Artificial phosphorylation of this protein by dibutyryl–cyclic GMP (cGMP) resulted in downregulation of mast cell activation and histamine release [246]. DSCG and structurally related chromone compounds were also shown to induce phosphorylation of this protein [235]. These results suggest an alternate "Ca^{++}-independent" pathway is responsible for inhibiting mast cell histamine release, most likely occurring through activation of cGMP-dependent protein kinase [94, 246].

DSCG has been shown to be effective in attenuating or ablating both the early- and late-phase reactions of allergic diseases by its effect on cells other than mast cells. (See Chapters 8 and 12 for added details.) DSCG inhibited activation of inflammatory cells such as eosinophils and monocytes and end-organ effects of platelet-activating factor (PAF), all of which participate in late-phase reactions [3, 13, 23, 183]. Although DSCG has no direct relaxation effect on smooth muscle, it has been shown to attenuate the smooth muscle contractile responses induced by histamine, serotonin, acetylcholine, bradykinin, and prostaglandin $F_{2\alpha}$, while enhancing smooth muscle relaxation induced by isoproterenol, epinephrine, prostaglandin E and salbutamol [138, 188]. The latter in vitro effects are not clinically significant.

Many of the other proposed, but poorly explained, mechanisms of DSCG were first advanced during clinical drug trials. Although DSCG has been effective in treating asthma induced by exercise, cold, sulfur dioxide, and fog [22, 38, 62, 102, 197, 226–228], investigators have been unable to demonstrate that the release of mast cell mediators is consistently responsible for causing asthma induced by these nonspecific stimuli. It was therefore postulated that the protective effects of DSCG occurred via several neurophysiologic pathways [30]. Its effect on various types of reflex bronchoconstriction are thought to be vagally mediated. DSCG

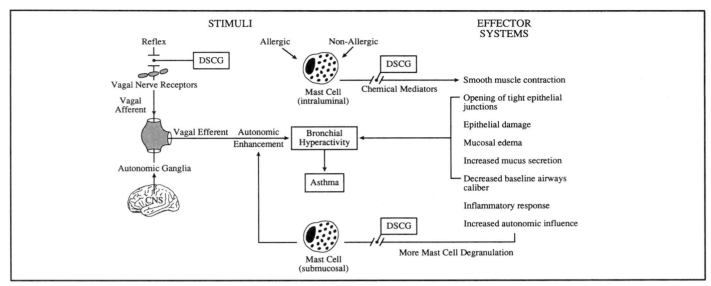

Fig. 63-2. *Sites of action of disodium cromoglycate (DSCG) on the mast cell and the reflex pathways of asthma. (Reprinted with permission from I. L. Bernstein, Cromolyn sodium. Chest 87(suppl.):6S, 1985.)*

Table 63-5. Proposed mechanisms of action of disodium cromoglycate

Stabilizes mast cells
Blocks neutrophilic chemotactic factor-anaphylaxis release
Decreases number of lung inflammatory cells
Inhibits protein kinase C
Inhibits activation of inflammatory cells
Decreases bronchial hyperreactivity
Blocks early and late asthmatic reactions
Decreases airway permeability
Inhibits neuronal reflexes within the lung
Prevents downregulation of $beta_2$ receptors
Inhibits bronchoconstrictor effects of tachykinins
Preserves mucociliary apparatus after bronchial provocation or an
  asthmatic attack

Source: S. Murphy, Cromolyn sodium: basic mechanisms and clinical usage. *Pediatr. Asthma Allergy Immunol.* 2:237, 1988. Reprinted with permission.

was effective in the prophylaxis of asthma induced by sulfur dioxide, metabisulfites, isocyanates, western red cedar, and colophony, all of which have been postulated to occur by reflex bronchoconstriction, thereby supporting a neurophysiologic mechanism [30, 76]. In anesthetized dogs, pretreatment with DSCG was effective in decreasing reflex bronchoconstriction induced by histamine [15]. Studies in dogs have demonstrated that DSCG inhibits reflex bronchoconstriction induced by the stimulation of sensory C fibers with capsaicin, an extract from red pepper that causes release of the neuropeptide substance P from sensory nerves [113]. DSCG inhibited leukotriene D_4–induced bronchoconstriction, which supports a possible vagally mediated mechanism [7]. Figure 63-2 illustrates the sites of action of DSCG on the mast cell and the neuroreflex pathways of asthma, while Table 63-5 summarizes its proposed mechanisms of action [30, 186].

Clinical Efficacy of DSCG

Asthma. Several components of airway inflammation were considered while evaluating the therapeutic potential of DSCG [209] (Fig. 63-3). Early investigations were concerned mainly with DSCG's ability to prevent or decrease bronchial hyperreactivity. Table 63-6 summarizes several of these studies assessing DSCG's effect on bronchial hyperreactivity in response to various specific

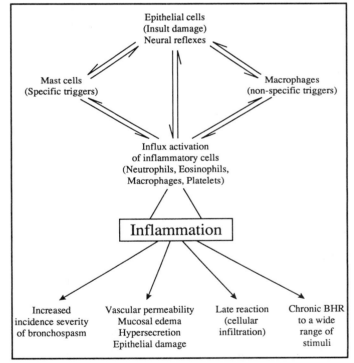

Fig. 63-3. *Factors involved in airway inflammation and bronchial hyperreactivity (BHR). (Reprinted with permission from D. K. Rainey, Nedocromil sodium (Tilade): A review of preclinical studies. Eur. Respir. J. 2:561s, 1989.)*

and nonspecific stimuli [100]. Most of these studies demonstrated significant decreases in bronchial hyperreactivity when DSCG was used on a continuous basis and relapses when the drug was stopped [100]. Results from other studies led to conclusions that DSCG is effective in inhibiting both the early- and late-phase reactions in asthma by its direct stabilizing effect on mast cells and prevention of inflammatory cell influx to the site of action [55, 60, 109, 163, 217]. Bronchoalveolar lavage (BAL) studies (Chap. 24) performed in subjects with exercise-induced asthma

Table 63-6. Review of the studies evaluating the effect of disodium cromoglycate on bronchial hyperreactivity in response to specific and nonspecific stimuli

Investigator	Duration of treatment	Agonist	Decrease in airway responsiveness
Altounyan, 1970	6 wk	Histamine	Yes
Dickson, 1970	1 yr	Histamine	Yes
Ryo, 1971	2 wk	Methacholine	No
Ryo, 1976	2 wk	Antigen	Yes
	2 wk	Histamine	No
	2 wk	Methacholine	No
Cockcroft, 1977	1 wk	Histamine	No
Dickson, 1979	10 yr	Histamine	Yes
Szmidt, 1979	3 wk	Histamine	Yes
Marks, 1981	4 yr	Histamine	Yes
Cole, 1982	6 wk	Histamine	Yes
Bleecker, 1982	4 wk	Antigen	Yes
	4 wk	Methacholine	No
Griffin, 1982	4 wk	Methacholine	No
	4 wk	Cold air	Yes
Griffin, 1983	4 wk	Methacholine	No
Numeroso, 1983	4 wk	Fog	Yes
Lowhagen, 1984(a)	8 wk	Histamine	Yes
Lowhagen, 1984(b)	2 + wk	Histamine	Yes
Stafford, 1984	12 wk	Histamine	Yes
Bierman, 1984	12 wk	Methacholine	Yes
Furukawa, 1984	12 wk	Methacholine	Yes
Orefice, 1984	12 wk	Acetylcholine	Yes
Rocchiccioli, 1984	6 wk	Histamine	Yes
Kraemer, 1985	8 wk	Carbachol	Yes
Lowhagen, 1985	6 wk	Histamine	Yes
Reques, 1985	8 wk	Histamine	No
Laitinen, 1986	4 wk	Histamine	No
Svendsen, 1987	8 wk	Histamine	No
Shapiro, 1988	8 wk	Methacholine	Yes
Petty, 1989	12 wk	Methacholine	Yes

Source: C. T. Furukawa, Anti-asthmatic agents. *Immunol. Allergy Clin. North Am.* 10(3):503, 1990. Reprinted with permission.

have shown that DSCG inhibits neutrophil chemotactic factor and enhances neutrophil and mononuclear cell cytotoxicity [181].

DSCG has been found to be optimally effective in treating children and adults with mild to moderate asthma [33, 84, 99, 122, 146, 171, 176, 184, 205, 240]. It has been effective in treating different types of asthma, including seasonal asthma, chronic perennial allergic asthma, exercise- and cold-induced asthma, cough-variant asthma, animal-induced asthma, and occupational asthma [32]. In children, long-term use of DSCG was shown to be very effective in lowering symptom scores, as evaluated by the subjects, their parents, and their physicians [176, 206]. Active treatment with DSCG has permitted the reduction of other concomitant medications (theophylline, beta$_2$ agonists, and corticosteroids) [84, 101]. In several studies, objective parameters, notably peak expiratory flow rates (PEFRs) and the forced expiratory volume at 1 second (FEV$_1$), also improved in patients treated with DSCG compared to placebo [122, 171, 224]. Double-blinded, placebo-controlled studies performed in adults with chronic asthma have also demonstrated improved symptom scores and pulmonary function measurements [146, 201, 240]. Figure 63-4 illustrates the dramatic improvement in FEV$_1$ from baseline in asthmatics treated over a 12-week period with DSCG compared to the results in controls [201]. As alluded to earlier, most of these studies found that DSCG also reduced bronchial hyperreactivity, with an improvement in FEV$_1$ after bronchial challenge to various stimuli [101, 146, 201, 240] (see Table 63-6). Some studies, however, have failed to detect significant changes in bronchial hyperreactivity or symptom scores after treatment with DSCG. These discrepancies have been attributed to flaws in study design, in-

cluding inadequate length of washout periods during cross-over drug comparison studies, poor patient selection criteria, and small subject groups [36, 144, 148, 234]. Whether these criticisms are valid remains unclear because of the heterogeneous responses patients may exhibit after treatment with DSCG.

DSCG's prophylactic effect in subjects with animal-induced asthma has been well documented [193]. Trials in laboratory workers exposed to animals have shown that DSCG prevents immediate bronchospasm and attenuates the late asthmatic response. In those patients who have casual contact with animals, use of DSCG prior to exposure has been advocated to prevent asthma exacerbations [193].

One of the earliest recognized treatment indications for DSCG is exercise-induced asthma [74]. Studies have conclusively shown that DSCG prevents a decrease in lung function after exercise in a dose-dependent manner, regardless of its mode of delivery [21, 26, 27, 44, 218]. Several investigators have pointed out that pretreatment with DSCG 15 minutes before exercise may result in a heterogeneous therapeutic response because of a variability in the exercise stimulus required to induce asthma [28]. This has been speculated to be the result of differences between mast cell subpopulations distributed throughout the lungs [28]. Asthma induced by nonspecific stimuli such as cold, sulfur dioxide, metabisulfites, and fog has been shown to be attenuated or prevented after pretreatment with DSCG [11, 86, 98, 170, 203, 226]. Several forms of occupational asthma, including baker's asthma, western red cedar asthma, woodworker's asthma, enzyme-induced asthma (papain), and chemically induced asthma (toluene diisocyanate, phthalic anhydride, colophony) have been successfully treated with DSCG [9].

The effectiveness of DSCG has been compared directly to theophylline, beta$_2$ agonists, and inhaled corticosteroids. These studies have revealed that DSCG was comparable to theophylline in reducing symptoms, but with fewer side effects [110, 232]. As expected, beta$_2$ agonists were superior bronchodilators compared to DSCG [114]. Although DSCG has a well-documented steroid-sparing effect, it has not been shown to be more effective than corticosteroids in the treatment of asthma [88].

Allergic Rhinitis. The effects of DSCG on the nasal mucosa have also been studied and found to be effective in the treatment of both seasonal and perennial allergic rhinitis [221]. DSCG attenuates the immediate and late-phase intranasal reaction in a manner similar to that produced by the inhaled form of drug [221]. Several double-blinded, placebo-controlled clinical trials have demonstrated a significant reduction in patients' symptom scores, manifested as a decreased degree of sneezing, rhinorrhea, nasal congestion, and ocular irritation [54, 61, 80, 112]. It has been recommended that intranasal DSCG be initiated prior to the onset of an allergic reaction in order to obtain its maximum therapeutic efficacy [80]. Studies of intranasal biopsy specimens from patients treated with DSCG for allergic rhinitis have shown an increased ratio of normal mast cells to degranulated mast cells, which is consistent with its mast cell–stabilizing effect [103]. The intranasal administration of DSCG has also been studied for the treatment of vasomotor rhinitis and nonallergic rhinitis with eosinophilia syndrome [192]. In contrast to its effectiveness for the treatment of allergic rhinitis, patients with nonallergic nasal diseases have responded poorly to treatment with intranasal DSCG [192, 221].

Allergic Conjunctivitis. Seasonal allergic conjunctivitis is the most common ocular disorder encountered by physicians and is estimated to affect approximately 15 percent of the allergic population [139]. Prior to the introduction of intraocular DSCG, the pharmacologic management of allergic conjunctivitis was restricted to topical and systemic antihistamines, decongestants, and corticosteroids, which were often inadequate [139]. Studies have confirmed that intraocular DSCG is effective in treating ragweed allergic conjunctivitis [108, 248]. Welsh and coworkers

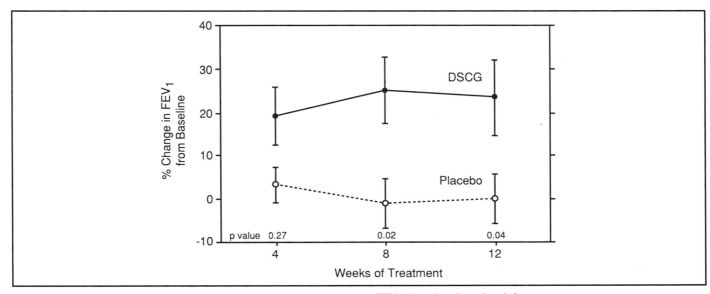

Fig. 63-4. *Mean percentage change in forced expiratory volume at 1 second* (FEV$_1$) *from baseline after 4, 8, and 12 weeks of treatment. DSCG = disodium cromoglycate. (Reprinted with permission from T. L. Petty, et al., Cromolyn sodium is effective in adult chronic asthmatics. Am. Rev. Respir. Dis. 139:694, 1989.)*

[248, 249] attempted to correlate preseason serum IgE antibody levels to the expected degree of response to intraocular and intranasal DSCG used during the ragweed season. Their results were conflicting, in that patients with IgE levels greater than 100 ng/ml had a better intranasal DSCG response whereas those with IgE levels less than 100 ng/ml had a better intraocular DSCG response [248, 249]. The utility of serum IgE levels in predicting nasal and ocular treatment responses is still uncertain.

Vernal keratoconjunctivitis is a chronic, idiopathic, external ocular inflammatory disease, which was also refractory to available treatments prior to the introduction of intraocular DSCG [96]. Several investigations have verified that intraocular DSCG is very effective in the treatment of this disorder [83, 96, 175, 213]. In these studies, the use of DSCG significantly decreased conjunctival hyperemia, superficial punctate keratitis, mucus secretion, and itching [83, 96, 213]. Finally, intraocular DSCG has been very effective in the treatment of giant papillary conjunctivitis, which is a conjunctival inflammatory disorder usually associated with the use of hard or soft contact lenses, ocular prostheses, or postoperative keratoplasty sutures [10, 83, 175]. Prior to the introduction of intraocular DSCG, treatment of this disorder had been frustrating and ineffective [10, 174, 175].

Recently, after its removal from the market, intraocular DSCG became better appreciated by specialists and general practitioners. Patients with these ocular disorders, in particular seasonal allergic conjunctivitis, have not responded as well to alternative topical agents or systemic antihistamines as they have to intraocular DSCG.

Miscellaneous Disorders. DSCG has been used to treat many other disorders, including ulcerative colitis, food allergies, systemic mastocytosis, recurrent aphthous ulcers, interstitial cystitis, and localized seminal fluid hypersensitivity [32, 36a]. The use of DSCG in the treatment of inflammatory bowel disease has been controversial. Some studies have shown that oral DSCG lessened clinical symptoms, which corresponded to decreased inflammation shown by rectal biopsy specimens [159]. Other studies have shown symptomatic improvement without corroborating changes in rectal biopsy specimens [115]. Oral DSCG may also be effective in the treatment of patients with multiple food allergies. Double-blinded, oral food-challenge studies have shown that oral DSCG (Gastrocrom) is effective in preventing allergic reactions

in subjects with documented specific food allergies [32]. Small bowel biopsy specimens in some of these patients have actually shown a decreased eosinophilic inflammatory response when DSCG was administered before the food challenge [32]. Despite these encouraging results in individual patients, oral DSCG has not yet been approved for the treatment of food allergies.

In double-blinded cross-over studies, oral DSCG (Gastrocrom) has been shown to be effective in treating the cutaneous, gastrointestinal, and central nervous system manifestations of systemic mastocytosis [230]. Despite its poor absorption (approximately 1%), oral DSCG reduced symptoms of itching, flushing, diarrhea, abdominal pain, and cognitive dysfunction. However, DSCG had no effect on more objective parameters of this rare mast cell disorder, such as urine histamine levels or peripheral blood eosinophilia [230]. DSCG decreased pain associated with several disorders, including aphthous ulcers and interstitial cystitis, a chronic disabling bladder disorder in women [78, 143, 224]. Cases of successful treatment of localized vaginal seminal plasma hypersensitivity reactions using a topical 4 percent DSCG water-based cream have been reported [36a]. DSCG may have other treatment roles yet to be evaluated.

Dose and Administration
Table 63-7 summarizes the different routes of administration available for DSCG and their recommended dosages [185]. Tachyphylaxis has not been reported to occur with the long-term use of DSCG [148].

Adverse Effects
DSCG is one of the safest medications available on the market. Long-term clinical experience has revealed that side effects are rare (1 in 10,000) [9]. The most common side effects reported by patients include mild irritation of the throat, hoarseness, dry mouth, coughing, chest tightness, and bronchospasm [9]. Less common side effects include nausea, vomiting, facial rash, hives, nasal congestion, and severe urethral burning or dysuria [9]. Rare cases of anaphylaxis occurring after the use of inhaled DSCG have been reported. There have been a few instances of pulmonary infiltrates with eosinophilia and autoimmune disorders developing in patients while using cromolyn sodium. Intraocular DSCG

Table 63-7. Disodium cromoglycate preparations

Product	Concentration	Usage
Intal capsules	20 mg/capsule	1 capsule inhaled 3–4 times a day (used to control asthma)
Ampules	20 mg/2 ml	1 ampule inhaled by nebulization 3–4 times daily (used to control asthma)
Intal metered-dose inhaler	800 mcg/inhalation	2 inhalations 3–4 times daily (used to control asthma)
Nasalcrom	40 mg/ml	2 sprays each nostril 3–4 times daily (allergic rhinitis)
Opticrom	40 mg/ml	2 drops each eye 3–4 times daily (allergic eye disease)

Source: E. C. Morris, Pharmacotherapy of allergic disease. *Primary Care* 14:605, 1987. Reprinted with permission.

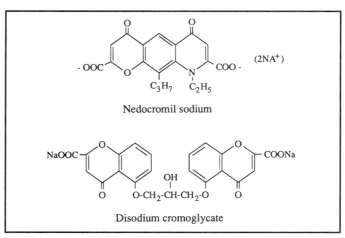

Nedocromil sodium

Disodium cromoglycate

Fig. 63-5. *Structural comparison of nedocromil sodium and disodium cromoglycate.*

Table 63-8. Pharmacokinetics of nedocromil sodium in normal subjects and asthmatics

Parameters	Normal volunteers		Patients (inhalation)
	Oral	Inhalation	
Dose (mg)	70.5	4.0	4.0
C_{max} (μg/L)	5.8	3.3	2.8
t_{max} (min)	54.0	20.0	5–90*
AUC (mg/L·h)	49.1	9.4	5.6
k_a (h^{-1})	0.035	0.34	0.54
$T\frac{1}{2}$ (hr)	21.1	2.3	1.5
Urinary excretion (%)	1.7	5.6	5.0
Bioavailability (%)	3.0	9.2	5.7

* Range.
C_{max} = maximum plasma concentration; t_{max} = time to reach maximum plasma concentrations; AUC = area under plasma concentration–time curve; k_a = terminal rate constant; $T\frac{1}{2}$ = mean terminal half-life.
Source: J. P. Gonzalez and R. N. Brogden, Nedocromil sodium. A preliminary review of its pharmacodynamic and pharmacokinetic properties, and therapeutic efficacy in the treatment of reversible obstructive airways disease. *Drugs* 34:560, 1987. Reprinted with permission.

has been associated with acute chemotic reactions of the conjunctivae [196]. Intranasal DSCG has been well tolerated with negligible side effects [9].

Toxicity studies in animals have confirmed the safety of this drug [24]. One study reported kidney toxicity after using DSCG and this was manifested histologically as blockage of the renal tubules with the precipitated drug. This complication was only elicited after repeated administration of unusually high doses of the drug [24]. Subsequent studies using a conventional therapeutic dose of DSCG could not reproduce this side effect [24].

DSCG has not been found to be carcinogenic after long-term treatment in animal models [9, 24]. DSCG has been considered safe to use during pregnancy, as only 0.08 percent of the drug crosses the placenta after intravenous administration [9]. The incidence of teratogenesis with this drug was less than the risk reported for the normal patient population [9]. Only a negligible amount of DSCG is excreted into breast milk, and therefore it is safe to use while nursing [65].

Cost Effectiveness

Some physicians have hesitated to prescribe DSCG to their patients because of its expense. However, some studies have shown that DSCG was actually more cost effective when the overall total cost of asthma treatment was considered [214]. Thus, asthmatic patients who were better controlled after DSCG treatment required fewer emergency room visits and hospitalizations and missed less days from work each year [214].

Nedocromil Sodium

Nedocromil sodium (NS) is currently available abroad and was recently approved for use in the United States under the trade name Tilade. NS was developed with the intention of finding a drug possessing an improved pharmacologic profile compared to DSCG. It was hoped that NS would prove to be more effective in treating patients unresponsive to DSCG. As we shall see, NS has a therapeutic role in the treatment of asthma but it does not appear to offer dramatic advantages over DSCG, as was initially suggested.

Chemistry

NS is a disodium salt of a pyranoquinoline dicarboxylic acid. It is soluble in water and, to a lesser extent, in alcohol. When solubilized in water, it is stable over several hours at a neutral or slightly acidic pH. NS has a molecular weight of 415 Daltons and has a more rigid configuration than does DSCG (Fig. 63-

5). Structurally, NS and DSCG should be regarded as different compounds, even though they have very similar pharmacologic activities [19, 104, 215].

Pharmacokinetics

NS has been evaluated pharmacokinetically primarily for inhalational delivery. Table 63-8 summarizes the pharmacokinetic parameters of NS after oral administration in normal subjects and inhalational delivery in normal and asthmatic subjects [104]. Inhalation of 4 mg of NS produced a mean maximum plasma concentration (C_{max}) of 3.3 μg/L. NS has a $T\frac{1}{2}$ of 2.3 hours. The rate-limiting factor of the $T\frac{1}{2}$ of NS is its absorption from the lung. NS has a bioavailability of approximately 6 to 9 percent after inhalation, 2.5 percent of which is the result of gastrointestinal absorption. The pharmacokinetic profile for NS after inhalation in normal subjects is essentially the same for asthmatic subjects [104] (see Table 63-8).

After intravenous administration, plasma levels of NS show a biexponential decay. It has a rapid plasma clearance rate of 10.2 ml/min/kg with excretion into the urine and bile. No metabolites of NS have been identified and drug accumulation does not occur with long-term dosing in either normal or asthmatic subjects, making tachyphylaxis less likely [104, 215].

Mechanism of Action

NS has several mechanisms of action similar to DSCG that are incompletely understood [104]. Several different animal models have been used to study the mechanisms of NS. In one of these models, dogs were challenged with inhaled citric acid, a known cough stimulant, which triggers the cough reflex via airway sensory nerves. Pretreatment of these animals with NS eradicated their predicted coughing spasms. The cough reflex was inhibited in cats anesthetized with phenyl diguanide when their C-fiber nerve endings were stimulated. NS was also shown to inhibit bronchial C-fiber nerve endings, which may explain its antitussive effect clinically [104].

Sheep and monkeys sensitized to the parasite *Ascaris suum* have been used to study early- and late-phase asthmatic responses after inhalational challenge with the *Ascaris* antigen [2, 4, 126]. NS and DSCG were equally effective in decreasing the early- and late-phase airway responses, but NS was distinctive in the monkey model because it inhibited the late-phase response when given either before or after the early-phase reaction [2, 4, 126]. Ovalbumin-sensitized guinea pigs have also been used to study the effects of NS on early and late asthmatic reactions. This model was unique in that a triphasic response occurred, which included an early-phase reaction at 2 hours, a late-phase response at 17 hours associated with an influx of neutrophils into the airways, and a late late-phase response at 72 hours associated with an influx of eosinophils. When NS was administered before or after the early-phase reaction, all three of these responses were inhibited, with a corresponding decrease in the numbers of neutrophils and eosinophils in the airways [58]. NS also interfered with passive cutaneous anaphylactic reactions in sensitized guinea pigs, in contrast to DSCG which has no effect in this species [100].

NS has been shown to have direct effects on a variety of cells and their mediators in vitro. NS inhibited neutrophil activation and the subsequent release of cytotoxic mediators [182]. After treatment with NS, parasitized animals succumbed to infestation, presumably because of decreased neutrophil cytotoxic mediators required to kill the parasites [100]. Rabbit neutrophils stimulated by phorbol dibutyrate to release cytotoxic lysosomal enzymes were inhibited by NS but not by DSCG. The inhibitory effect of NS in this model was postulated to occur through its action on protein kinase C, which is specifically activated by phorboldibutyrate [37].

NS has been found to inhibit the PAF-induced chemotaxis of neutrophils and eosinophils to the same degree as experimental PAF antagonists [41]. NS also prevented the release of PAF, leukotriene C_4, and eosinophil cationic proteins from human eosinophils stimulated by either opsonized zymosan or calcium ionophores (i.e., A-23187) [42, 43]. NS had an inhibitory effect on rat and human monocytes and macrophages [100, 132, 236]. In addition, NS interfered with the release of leukotriene B_4 and 5-HETE from passively sensitized BAL macrophages obtained from asthmatic patients [104].

NS effectively inhibited IgE-mediated histamine release from rat peritoneal mast cells, human BAL cells, and enzymatically dispersed lung mast cells [145, 149]. NS inhibited histamine and prostaglandin D_2 release from BAL mast cells obtained from macaque primates [81]. NS also blocked IgE-mediated release of mediators from platelets in rats and humans [132, 236]. Recently, NS has been demonstrated to prevent the in vitro aspirin-induced activation of platelets isolated from aspirin-sensitive asthmatic patients. Although the mechanism for this effect is unknown, it has been proposed that NS binds to a specific platelet receptor or alters platelet metabolism, which prevents platelet activation [162].

Many of these aforementioned in vitro experiments have compared NS's and DSCG's effects on cellular activation and mediator release from eosinophils, neutrophils, monocytes, macrophages, platelets, and mast cells [104]. For example, NS was a more potent inhibitor of histamine release from *Ascaris*-sensitized monkey BAL mast cells than was DSCG [104]. Leung and associates [150] found NS had a greater effect than DSCG in inhibiting anti-IgE–induced histamine release from mast cells isolated by BAL or from enzymatically dispersed lung fragments obtained from nonasthmatic, nonatopic human subjects. The clinical relevance of these in vitro differences between NS and DSCG remains unknown [104].

NS acts on neurophysiologic pathways in a manner similar to that of DSCG. NS was more potent than DSCG in inhibiting coughing symptoms triggered by citric acid challenge. NS was also more effective in inhibiting bronchoconstriction in rats induced by tachykinins such as substance P, neurokinin A, eledoisin, and calcitonin gene–related peptide [72, 100, 131, 198]. Figure 63-6 illustrates the numerous sites of action where NS has been postulated to exert its inhibitory effects [117].

Clinical Efficacy of Nedocromil Sodium

The majority of clinical trials evaluating the efficacy of NS have demonstrated an improvement in patient symptom scores, physician assessment scores, and serial PEFR determinations [215]. Subjects enrolled in these studies varied significantly with respect to the severity of their asthma and known aggravating stimuli. Many of the discrepancies found in early studies evaluating NS have been attributed to poorly selected and controlled patient populations [215]. One of the better designed studies evaluated a highly selected group of patients who were enrolled in the study only if they demonstrated a deterioration in their asthmatic condition, manifested as an overuse of their beta$_2$-agonist inhalers [19]. They found that those subjects who received NS had improved PEFRs and a decreased dependency on their bronchodilator inhalers. Callaghan and associates [46a] have shown that NS allowed reduction or discontinuation of theophylline in adult chronic asthmatics with significant improvement in subjective and objective parameters.

Several studies have attempted to show that NS functions as a corticosteroid-sparing agent and substitutes for DSCG. Lal and associates [141] demonstrated that the majority of patients controlled on inhaled corticosteroids and DSCG could have their medications either stopped or significantly reduced while taking NS. These investigators were able to show subjective improvement in their patients' symptoms, but any changes in more objective parameters, such as PEFR and FEV_1, were less impressive, especially among those subjects who had their inhaled corticosteroid dose reduced or terminated [141]. More recently, a double-blinded, multicenter study conducted by Rebuck and associates [210] demonstrated a modest but significant improvement in symptom scores and PEFRs associated with decreased inhaled bronchodilator use among patients treated with NS compared to placebo [210]. Global analysis of the available controlled clinical investigations reveals that NS is better than placebo and on a par with DSCG.

Clinical trials have confirmed the effectiveness of NS in preventing early- and late-phase asthmatic reactions. Figure 63-7 illustrates the results obtained by Crimi and colleagues [70], who, after administering NS before and after bronchial challenges, found NS was more effective in blocking early- and late-phase reactions if it was administered before the challenge. NS has been shown to reduce bronchial hyperreactivity caused by specific and nonspecific stimuli such as antigens (ragweed), adenosine, sulfur dioxide, metabisulfites, and exercise [71, 77, 125, 189, 202, 225]. Figure 63-8 illustrates the percentage change in FEV_1 improvement in patients with exercise-induced asthma treated with NS compared to placebo [225]. Table 63-9 compares the effects of DSCG and NS on early and late asthmatic responses and bron-

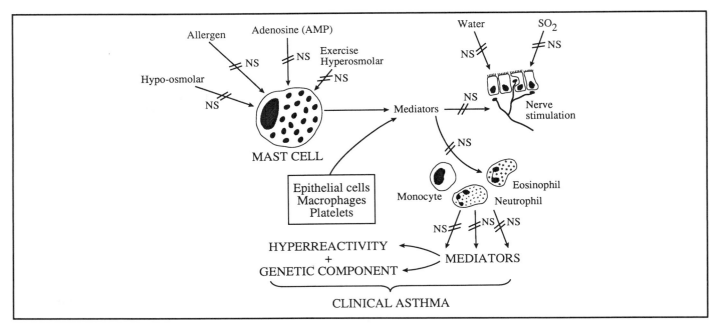

Fig. 63-6. *Inhibitory effects of nedocromil sodium. NS = nedocromil sodium. (Reprinted with permission from S. T. Holgate, Clinical evaluation of nedocromil sodium in asthma. Eur. J. Respir. Dis. 69(suppl. 147):149, 1986.)*

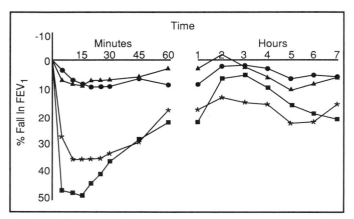

Fig. 63-7. *Changes in the forced expiratory volume at 1 second (FEV₁) in the dual asthmatic response to antigen challenge. Effect of four (prechallenge/postchallenge) treatment combinations; nedocromil sodium/nedocromil sodium (closed circles); nedocromil sodium/ placebo (closed triangles); placebo/nedocromil sodium (closed squares); and placebo/placebo (stars). Numbers in brackets indicate how many patients were excluded from analysis at a specific time point. (Reprinted with permission from E. Crimi, V. Brusasco, and P. Crimi, Effect of nedocromil sodium on the late asthmatic reaction to bronchial antigen challenge. J. Allergy Clin. Immunol. 83:985, 1989.)*

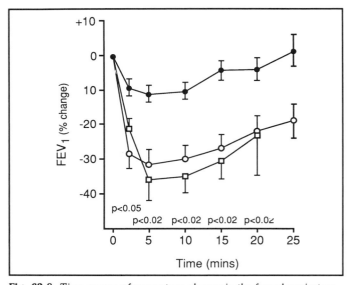

Fig. 63-8. *Time course of percentage change in the forced expiratory volume at 1 second (FEV₁) after exercise in eight asthmatics following preadministration of nedocromil (closed circles), placebo (open circles), or no medication (open squares). (Reprinted with permission from R. J. Shaw and A. B. Kay, Nedocromil, a mucosal and connective tissue mast cell stabilizer, inhibits exercise-induced asthma. Br. J. Dis. Chest 79:385, 1985.)*

chial hyperreactivity to the effects produced by conventional antiasthmatic agents [55].

Limited studies have been performed evaluating the efficacy of NS in asthmatic children. Available information suggests that this medication could serve as a therapeutic adjunct in pediatric asthma, particularly children with exercise-induced bronchospasm [116]. Further clinical trials evaluating the use of NS in children are necessary before any definitive conclusions can be made.

There are also a limited number of studies comparing DSCG with NS. Bronchial provocation studies have shown that NS is more potent in preventing sulfur dioxide–, adenosine–, substance

P–, sodium metabisulfite–, and cold–induced asthma [71, 72, 77, 104, 125, 132a, 202]. Results from these comparative studies have not been consistently reproduced, indicating the need for further investigation [104].

Intranasal Nedocromil Sodium

A few studies have evaluated intranasal NS. Lozewicz and associates [155] obtained nasal biopsy specimens from subjects with seasonal allergic rhinitis before and after treatment with NS. Treatment with intranasal NS demonstrated an improvement in

Table 63-9. *Comparative effects of disodium cromoglycate and nedocromil sodium with other antiasthmatic medications in human asthma*

Drug	EAR	LAR	BHR
Disodium cromoglycate	+	+	+
Nedocromil sodium	+	+	+
Beta stimulants	+	−	−
Theophylline	±	+	±
Corticosteroids	−	+	+

EAR = early asthmatic reaction; LAR = late asthmatic reaction; BHR = bronchial hyperreactivity; + = inhibitory; − = noninhibitory; ± = equivocal.
Source: M. K. Church, Reassessment of mast cell stabilizers in the treatment of respiratory disease. *Ann. Allergy* 62:215, 1989. Reprinted with permission.

patient symptom scores and a decreased need for the use of concomitant antihistamines [155, 216]. Posttreatment biopsy specimens showed a significant decrease in the number of mast cells but not in the number of eosinophils [155]. These investigators postulated that intranasal NS worked by preventing mast cell infiltration into the site of the allergic reaction. Intranasal challenge studies have supported NS's efficacy in the treatment of allergic rhinitis by demonstrating a significant reduction in nasal airway resistance, secretions, and sneezing episodes compared to those findings seen with placebo use [63].

Intraocular Nedocromil Sodium
Two percent NS was used in a multicenter trial conducted to evaluate its potential use for the treatment of seasonal allergic conjunctivitis. The results from this study were promising, as 2% NS was found to be more effective in reducing symptoms and decreasing the need for additional systemic antihistamines than was placebo [147].

Dose and Administration
Inhaled NS is delivered by a metered-dose inhaler (4 mg per inhalation), and the recommended dosage is 4 mg administered two to four times a day and taken on a regular basis [104]. The optimal dosage of intranasal NS is still unknown, but, in clinical studies that have demonstrated clinical efficacy, the dosage used has been one to two intranasal inhalations four times a day [2, 104]. Intraocular NS has been used empirically in studies as a 2% solution with good results, although an actual recommended dose has still not been determined [104, 147].

Adverse Effects
NS appears to be a very safe medication for long-term use in humans. The most significant side effect noted in approximately 5 percent of the patient population has been an unpleasant taste [59, 104]. Other side effects include headaches, nausea, vomiting, and dizziness [59]. Toxicity studies have been performed using NS in several different animal models and have revealed no evidence of fetal malformations or carcinogenicity [59]. Overall, NS has a low order of toxicity with high safety margins, and, although further clinical surveillance is necessary, it appears to be effective in treating asthma, allergic rhinitis, and conjunctivitis.

Lodoxamides
The lodoxamides are a group of very active biologs of DSCG. They were discovered during the performance of passive cutaneous anaphylaxis assays screening for compounds related to DSCG but with more potent pharmacologic profiles [127]. Many of these analogs, such as Wy 41195, were only briefly evaluated before they were abandoned because of the poor correlation between their preclinical screening profile and their clinical activities

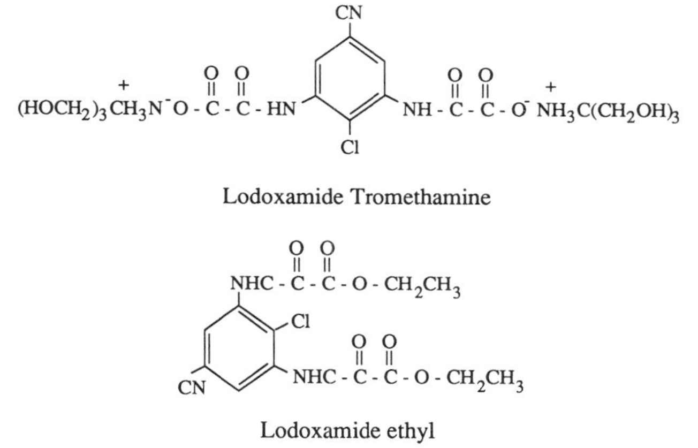

Fig. 63-9. *Chemical structures of the lodoxamides.*

[127]. The lodoxamides were studied more extensively because they initially appeared more promising than their predecessors. Lodoxamide tromethamine (LT or U-42585) and lodoxamide ethyl (LE or U-42718) have both been evaluated and compared to DSCG in preclinical studies [128]. LT has been used more frequently to assess the clinical efficacy of lodoxamides in treating asthma because of its fewer side effects and better solubility. The chemical structures of LT and LE are illustrated in Figure 63-9 [127]. The pharmacokinetics of these compounds have not been evaluated in humans because of their disappointing clinical activity in pilot studies.

Mechanism of Action
The mechanisms of action for the lodoxamides are incompletely understood but are believed to be similar to those of DSCG. They were originally thought to regulate calcium uptake into mast cells by increasing the intracellular cAMP level [127]. Because of the lack of clinical efficacy demonstrated by the lodoxamides, the relevance of this proposed mechanism has not been explored further [127]. Using isolated rat peritoneal mast cells, the lodoxamides have been demonstrated to have differential effects on histamine release [127]. Dose-response studies have shown that, at lower doses, lodoxamide inhibits histamine release by binding to calcium, whereas, at higher doses, lodoxamide forces calcium intracellularly, resulting in increased histamine release [127]. It is unclear which cyclic nucleotides mediate these reactions, but data suggest that LT inhibits cGMP phosphodiesterase while stimulating guanylate cyclase, which results in the intracellular accumulation of cGMP and histamine release. This response was dose dependent, as lower concentrations of LT inhibited histamine release while higher concentrations enhanced histamine release [127].

LT's pharmacologic activity has been evaluated in rat and primate models. Results of single-dose studies comparing the inhibition of histamine release produced by LT and LE to that elicited by DSCG are summarized in Table 63-10 [127]. LT was found to be 2,500 times more potent in rats and 500 times more potent in primates (*Ascaris*-sensitized rhesus monkeys) in inhibiting histamine release compared to DSCG [129, 130]. This effect was more pronounced when the drugs were given simultaneously with the antigen challenge. LT has no significant antibradykinin, antiserotonergic, or anticholinergic end-organ effect [128].

LT and LE have both been evaluated for their effects on allergy skin test reactivity in human subjects [128]. When LT was injected at the skin test site prior to allergen injection, there was a diminished wheal flare reaction not seen with histamine-induced wheal flare reactions [128]. LE had no effect on allergen- or hista-

Table 63-10. Single drug dose (mg/kg) required for 50% inhibition of histamine release

Model	Route of administration	Lodoxamide tromethamine	Lodoxamide ethyl	Disodium cromoglycate
Rat passive cutaneous anaphylaxis	p.o.	1.0	0.1	Inactive
	i.v.	0.001	*	2.5
Rhesus (*Ascaris* sensitized)	p.o.	10.0	1.0	Inactive
	i.v.	0.001	*	0.1
	Intrabronchial	0.01	*	50.0
Isolated purified rat mast cell	—	0.001 μg/ml	*	0.1 μg/ml

* Drug insoluble, cannot be administered by this route.
p.o. = orally; i.v. = intravenously.
Source: H. G. Johnson, New anti-allergy drugs—the lodoxamides. *TIPS* August, 1980, P. 343. Reprinted with permission.

mine-induced skin reactions in humans but inhibited immediate skin test reactions in rodents [97]. These discrepancies have been attributed to intra- and interspecies mast cell heterogeneity [97].

One of the most significant limitations associated with the activity of LT found in rodent and primate animal models was the occurrence of tachyphylaxis. This developed after repeated dosings of the drug, and cross-tachyphylaxis was exhibited with DSCG [127]. This phenomenon has been used as the most plausible explanation for why these and other biologs of DSCG have shown poor clinical activity in treating asthma [127].

Clinical Efficacy

Oral inhaled forms of LT and LE have been evaluated for the treatment of asthma. Preliminary reports suggested that LT and LE were prophylactically effective in treating acute allergen- and exercise-induced bronchospasm [40, 160, 195, 241, 245]. Mann and associates [160], however, evaluated LT in chronic, mildly allergic asthmatics over 4 months and failed to find any significant improvement in symptom scores or pulmonary function readings compared to placebo. A further significance of this study was that a large number of subjects withdrew because of adverse side effects.

Dose and Administration

Johnson [127] performed single dosing studies in humans for LT and found that doses less than or equal to 0.3 mg were generally well tolerated for both inhaled and oral administrations.

Adverse Effects

Most of the side effects associated with LT appear to be cholinergic in origin, manifested as flushing or warmth, headaches, nausea, vomiting, abdominal pain, fatigue, malaise, and dizziness [127, 128].

Other Experimental Uses for Lodoxamide

The lodoxamides, despite their disappointing clinical showing in the treatment of asthma, have been useful experimental agents for studying the pathophysiology of an array of clinical disorders. LT, because of its mast cell–stabilizing and xanthine oxidase–inhibitor properties, has been used to investigate histochemical changes associated with hepatic, pulmonary, cardiac, and spinal cord ischemic injury [20, 75, 90, 91, 136, 156, 220]. Information obtained from these studies has had important ramifications for the improvement of surgical transplantation techniques as well as the management of cardiovascular disease and spinal cord trauma [20, 75].

Flavonoids

The flavonoids are a group of compounds widely distributed in the plant kingdom, having the basic structure 2-phenyl-4-chro-

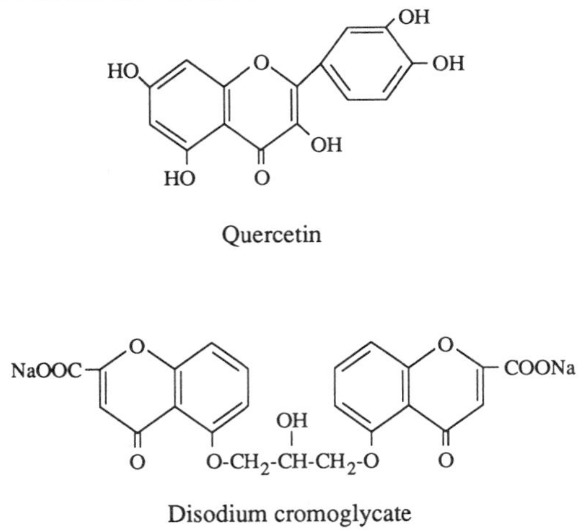

Fig. 63-10. *Structural comparison of quercetin and disodium cromoglycate.*

mone [92]. The most common flavone is quercetin, which naturally exists as quercitrin. Quercitrin is a glycoside of rhamnose and quercetin found in the bark of the North American black oak [92]. Figure 63-10 compares the structures of quercetin and DSCG.

Pharmacologically, the flavonoids have gained notoriety because of their wide spectra of activities. These agents have anticoagulant, antiallergic, antiprostaglandin, and glucose transport inhibitory properties [92, 178]. In addition, they enhance the end-organ effects of vitamin C and epinephrine, while exhibiting anti-inflammatory, antiviral, and mutagenic actions [92]. Many of their proposed activities occur through interference with enzyme systems, some of which include ascorbic acid oxidase, hyaluronidase, catechol-*o*-methyl-transferase, cyclic nucleotide phosphodiesterases, ATPases, prostaglandin synthetase, 5- and 12-lipoxygenases, aldose reductase, histidine decarboxylase, xanthine oxidase, and xanthine dehydrogenase [34, 89, 92, 179].

Because of its structural similarity to DSCG, quercetin has been studied the most extensively of all the flavonoids in order to elucidate the mechanism by which it and similar agents inhibit histamine release from mast cells. Furthermore, these compounds have also been extremely useful in identifying aspects of inter- and intraspecies mast cell heterogeneity [199].

Although the mechanism of action for quercetin on mast cells in unknown, it has been postulated to inhibit the release of histamine by mast cells by increasing the efficiency of calcium ATPase, which is responsible for maintaining low intracellular levels of calcium [89, 92]. Mast cell stabilization results because ATPase prevents the accumulation of high intracellular calcium levels that are ultimately required for mast cell–mediator release

Table 63-11. Effect of flavonoids (at doses of 33 and 100 μM) on antigen-induced histamine secretion from rat mast cells and on Ca⁺⁺-dependent ATPase activity of rabbit skeletal muscle sarcoplasmic reticulum

Table 63-11. *Effect of flavonoids (at doses of 33 and 100 μM) on antigen-induced histamine secretion from rat mast cells and on Ca^{++}-dependent ATPase activity of rabbit skeletal muscle sarcoplasmic reticulum*

Flavonoid	Histamine secretion		Ca^{++}-dependent ATPase activity	
	33 μM	100 μM	33 μM	100 μM
Fisetin	0.31	0.00	0.91	0.57
Kaempferol	0.59	0.24	0.64	0.30
Morin	0.99	0.82	0.95	0.74
Quercetin	0.37	0.00	0.69	0.37
Myricetin	0.42	0.26	0.74	0.37
Rutin	1.00	0.75	0.99	0.91

Source: C. M. S. Fewtrell and B. D. Gomperts, Effect of flavone inhibitors of transport ATPases on histamine secretion from rat mast cells. *Nature* 265:635, 1977. Reprinted with permission.

Table 63-12. *Comparative in vitro effects of disodium cromoglycate and the flavonoid quercetin**

Disodium cromoglycate	Quercetin
1. For maximal inhibitory effect of histamine secretion, DSCG must be added together with the stimulus to the cells.	1. For maximal inhibitory effect of histamine secretion, quercetin can be added before or with the stimulus to the cells.
2. Less effect on rat mast cell–mediator release in the presence of phosphatidyl serine.	2. Equally effective at inhibiting rat mast cell–mediator release in the presence or absence of phosphatidyl serine.
3. Has no effect on calcium ATPase.	3. Inhibits histamine release from mast cells by interfering with calcium–ATPase.
4. Inhibits histamine release from rat peritoneal mast cells.	4. Inhibits histamine release from rat mucosal and peritoneal mast cells.
5. Has no inhibitory effect on histamine secretion from human basophils.	5. Effective inhibitor of histamine secretion from human basophil leukocytes.

* Data from J. C. Foreman, Mast cells and the actions of flavonoids. *J. Allergy Clin. Immunol.* 73:769, 1984.

[89, 92]. Table 63-11 summarizes the effects of various flavones on antigen-induced histamine secretion from rat mast cells and on calcium-dependent ATPase activity [89].

Fewtrell and Gomperts [89] compared the inhibitory effect of quercetin on non-IgE– versus IgE-mediated mast cell histamine release. They found that quercetin was more effective at inhibiting IgE antigen–induced mast cell histamine release. These investigators suggested that quercetin acted to block IgE receptor–activated calcium-transporting mechanisms [92]. At higher concentrations, they found that quercetin could also inhibit calcium ionophore–induced (non-IgE) histamine secretion by interfering with normal oxidative phosphorylation [92].

Quercetin has been shown to affect cells other than mast cells and basophils. Quercetin inhibits oxygen consumption, lysosomal enzyme secretion, and the chemotaxis of neutrophils, possibly by inhibiting phospholipase A_2 and the lipoxygenase enzymes [17, 29, 35, 45, 46]. Quercetin has also been demonstrated to inhibit stimulatory effects directed at cytotoxic T-cells and smooth muscle cells [1, 92].

Fewtrell and Gomperts [89] have compared the features of quercetin with those of DSCG and noted important differences between these two structurally similar compounds. These differences, which are summarized in Table 63-12, emphasize the disparity that often exists between structurally similar compounds

and their mechanisms of action [92]. There have been no clinical trials evaluating the effect of quercetin in the treatment of asthma because of its known toxic side effects.

DUAL-ACTION ANTIHISTAMINES

Over the past thirty years, a great deal of experimental work has been devoted to identifying the pharmacologic properties and mechanisms of H_1 antagonists. The impetus for this work was to understand how these drugs functioned, so that more clinically effective agents could be developed for the treatment of asthma and other allergic disorders.

Lichtenstein and Gillespie [151] observed that H_1 antagonists which were capable of increasing intracellular cAMP levels could also inhibit histamine release from human basophils and monkey lung mast cells. These investigators studied the effects of different classes of antihistamines on human basophils and found that a dose-dependent, bimodal histamine release response occurred. At high concentrations, the antihistamines caused histamine release, whereas, at low concentrations, they inhibited antigen-induced histamine release. Inhibition of histamine release was found to vary among the different classes of H_1 antagonists. For example, the phenothiazine antihistamines were shown to be 10 to 30 times more potent than the other classes of major antihistamines in inhibiting histamine release [151].

The mechanism for the inhibition of histamine release was unexpectedly found to occur through a paradoxical decrease in the intracellular cAMP levels. Church and Gradidge [57] used human lung fragments to evaluate the inhibition of histamine release by H_1 antagonists and structurally related tricyclic antidepressant agents and noted a biphasic effect on histamine release similar to that observed by earlier investigators. There was no correlation between their inhibitory activity on mast cell histamine release and their H_1 receptor antagonist activity, suggesting that the effect of these drugs on mast cells was not mediated through H_1 receptors [57]. Earlier studies evaluating the inhibitory effect of H_1 antagonists, tricyclic antidepressants, neuroleptics, and local anesthetics on histamine release from rat mast cells arrived at similar conclusions [57]. A plausible explanation for this biphasic phenomenon focused on the lipophobic structures of H_1 antagonists. At lower concentrations, H_1 antagonists were rapidly absorbed into cell membranes, where they competitively displaced calcium and prevented adequate calcium uptake into the mast cell and subsequent mediator release. At higher concentrations, the H_1 antagonists dissolved within the cell membrane, which resulted in the cell structure's expansion, disruption, and mediator release [57].

The development of improved laboratory techniques for isolating animal and human mast cells has provided better ways of evaluating the mechanisms of H_1 antagonists. Azatadine, a tricyclic antihistamine in the piperidine class, has been studied for its mast cell–stabilizing effect [238]. In reproducible studies, it has been administered intranasally to allergic individuals and found to decrease the amount of the mast cell–mediator markers (i.e., histamine, kinins, and TAME-esterases) in nasal secretions before and after intranasal challenges [238]. Azatadine administration led to decreased patient symptom scores, which directly corresponded to the decreased levels of several mast cell markers [238]. Daniels and Temple [73] have further shown that the azatadine dose dependently inhibited leukotriene C_4 and D_4 and histamine release from passively sensitized human lung fragments, thereby suggesting a mast cell–stabilizing effect. The new nonsedating H_1 antagonists, which have unique pharmacokinetic and pharmacologic properties, have rekindled the possibility that antihistamines could be used for the treatment of asthma. Large doses of terfenadine (180 mg/day) led to improvement of symptom scores, while allowing for a decrease in bronchodilator use

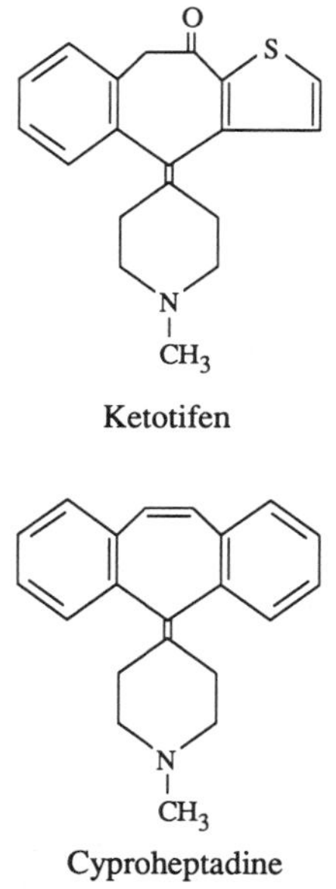

Fig. 63-11. *Structural comparison of ketotifen and cyproheptadine.*

in patients with seasonal allergic asthma [118]. Astemizole and cetirizine have both shown similar promise; however, it is unclear whether the clinical effect of these drugs is simply the result of H₁ antagonism or whether it reflects direct pharmacologic actions on mast cells [118] (see also Chap. 65).

The long-standing warning that H₁ antagonists were contraindicated in the management of asthma has been adequately refuted by many authoritative sources [229].

Although the conventional H₁ antagonists are recognized to have little, if any, clinical benefit in the treatment of asthma, investigation of their mast cell–stabilizing properties led toward the development of dual-action antihistamines [118].

Ketotifen

Ketotifen, or 4-(1-methyl-4-piperidylidene)-4H-benzo[4,5]cyclohepta[1,2-6]thiophen-10(9H)-one hydrogen fumarate, was originally developed for clinical use as an H₁-receptor antagonist. It is a benzocycloheptathiophene compound structurally related to cyproheptadine, an H₁ antagonist with antiserotonergic properties (Fig. 63-11) [242]. During clinical trials evaluating its usefulness as an H₁ antagonist, ketotifen was found coincidentally to be effective as an antiasthmatic agent. This dual-action antihistamine has been available abroad under the trade name Zaditen for several years, but is still awaiting approval for use in the United States.

Pharmacokinetics

Ketotifen is rapidly absorbed after oral dosing and has a peak plasma concentration of approximately 2 to 3 hours [67]. Ketotifen is biphasically eliminated, with mean half-lives of 1.6 and 20.4 hours, respectively [67]. Six metabolites of ketotifen have been isolated and quantitated in human urine, the majority of which consist of the N-glucoronide and 10-hydroxyglucoronide (dihydroketotifen) metabolites [67]. Ketotifen is more rapidly metabolized in children than in adults. Pharmacokinetic studies have revealed similar plasma concentrations and urinary excretion for ketotifen and its main N-glucoronide metabolite in adults and children [68]. Children, regardless of their age or weight, excrete a substantially greater amount of the metabolite, N-desmethyl-

Table 63-13. *Clinical activities of ketotifen*

1. Inhibition of anaphylaxis.
2. Inhibition of bronchial, nasal, and dermal IgE-mediated reactions.
3. Inhibition of mediator release from basophils, neutrophils, and mast cells.
4. Decreased neutrophil activation.
5. H₁ antagonism.
6. Reversal of beta₂-adrenergic tachyphylaxis.
7. Inhibition of calcium uptake in mast cells and smooth muscle.

Source: L. P. Craps, Immunologic and therapeutic aspects of ketotifen. *J. Allergy Clin. Immunol.* 76:389, 1985. Reprinted with permission.

glucoronide, in their urine, indicating a faster rate of drug metabolism compared to adults. Therefore children require higher doses of ketotifen to achieve the same therapeutic effect as in adults [68].

Mechanisms of Action

Ketotifen has a wide spectrum of clinical activity, which is summarized in Table 63-13. Ketotifen has been studied in vitro and clinically in different animal models, including humans, to understand its mechanisms of action. Ketotifen has been shown to inhibit the release of mediators from mast cells and basophils, and its effects on these cells in rats and humans are summarized in Table 63-14. Ketotifen was a more potent and sustained inhibitor of leukotriene release from human lung tissue than it was of histamine release from basophils [67]. Ketotifen has also been shown to inhibit allergen- and estrogen-induced degranulation of circulating blood eosinophils. The latter effect is thought to be important in preventing eosinophil migration into the uterus, the clinical ramifications of which are still not completely understood [231]. The effects of ketotifen on PAF formation and platelet aggregation have also been studied [177]. Ketotifen inhibited adenosine diphosphate–, collagen-, and arachidonic acid–induced platelet aggregation, similar to the effects of DSCG. Ketotifen also inhibited PAF acether–induced platelet secretion in humans [67]. In vitro studies have shown that, at pharmacologic doses, ketotifen induces an insignificant increase in neutrophil adherence and chemotaxis [105, 135]. Ketotifen was shown to inhibit neutrophil chemotactic activity in exercise-induced asthma but not during antigen-induced asthma challenges [67]. More recently, chemoluminescence studies have demonstrated that ketotifen inactivates human alveolar macrophages, but whether this can be equated with its antiasthmatic effect is problematic [133].

Ketotifen acts as a calcium antagonist by directly inhibiting the contraction of smooth muscle fibers in response to various stimuli [69]. Ketotifen has been shown to inhibit calcium uptake in isolated mast cells and smooth muscle cells while inhibiting depolarization-induced contractions of guinea pig taeniae coli [69].

The potent H₁ antagonistic effect of ketotifen occurs through a noncompetitive inhibition of H₁ receptors [69]. The mechanism of its antianaphylactic effect has been shown to be distinct from its H₁ antagonistic mechanism [66]. Sensitized guinea pigs pretreated with ketotifen had a dose-related inhibition of histamine release from lung, heart, and intestinal mast cells. When these cells were pretreated with ketotifen immediately before antigen challenge, no inhibition of mast cell degranulation was observed. However, an attenuation of the acute anaphylactic bronchospasm occurred, which was demonstrated to be the result of ketotifen's H₁ antagonistic effect. It was concluded that ketotifen's antianaphylactic or mast cell–stabilizing capacity occurred over a separate time course than its H₁ antagonistic effect, which could be differentiated by the length of drug treatment prior to challenge [222]. Furthermore, when ketotifen was administered

Table 63-14. Effect of ketotifen on mediator release from isolated mast cells and basophils

Cell type	Challenge	Effect of ketotifen	
		Histamine ($\mu g/ml$)	Leukotrienes ($\mu g/ml$)
Peritoneal rat mast cell	48/80	$IC_{50} = 120$	—
Passively sensitized rat mast cell	Ovalbumin	No effect	—
Basophils of patients with atopy	Rabbit anti-IgE and Ca^{++} ionophore	$IC_{50} = 80$	$IC_{50} = 10$
Basophils of patients with atopy	Grass pollen/house dust	$IC_{50} = 100–500$	—

IC_{50} = concentration required to inhibit mediator release by 50%.
Source: L. P. Craps, Immunologic and therapeutic aspects of ketotifen. *J. Allergy Clin. Immunol.* 76:389, 1985. Reprinted with permission.

Table 63-15. Prevention of bronchospasm in response to various stimuli by ketotifen*

Type of provocation	Degree of prevention of bronchospasm	
	After 1–3 days of treatment	After 3–12 weeks of treatment
Allergen (immediate and delayed reaction)	+ +	+ + +
Histamine	+ +	+ + +
Acetylcholine, carbachol, methacholine	−	+
Sulfur dioxide	+	+ +
Aspirin, benzoic acid	+ +	?
Exercise, cold air, hyperventilation	±	?
Prostaglandin $F_{2\alpha}$	±	?

* Dose 1 mg once or twice daily.
+ + + = marked and consistent; + + = appreciable and consistent; + = moderate and consistent; ± = moderate or inconsistent; − = no preventive effect; ? = not tested.
Source: Data from [67, 69].

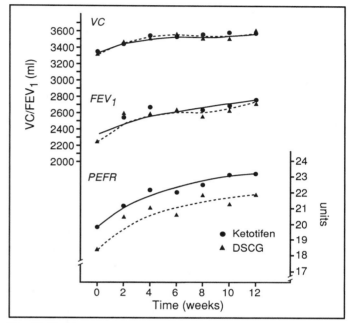

Fig. 63-12. *Changes in respiratory function during treatment with ketotifen or sodium cromoglycate (DSCG). VC = vital capacity; FEV₁ = forced expiratory volume at 1 second; PEFR = peak expiratory flow rate. (Reprinted with permission from L. P. Craps, Ketotifen in the oral prophylaxis of bronchial asthma: a review. Pharmatherapeutica 3: 18, 1981.)*

in combination with another H₁ antagonist, this potentiated an antihistaminic effect in comparison to the negligible antianaphylactic effect observed [66].

Ketotifen has no anticholinergic effect and only weak antiserotonergic activity [67]. Ketotifen is believed to decrease bronchial hyperreactivity by upregulating beta₂-adrenergic receptors, thereby reversing tolerance to beta₂ agonists that may develop in asthmatic patients after long-term use. This effect has been studied in vitro using human peripheral blood lymphocytes possessing beta₂ receptors desensitized by prolonged exposure to isoproterenol [204]. Tolerance to beta₂ agonists in these cells presumably occurs secondary to decreased cAMP accumulation. Studies have demonstrated that ketotifen acts to potentiate isoproterenol-induced cAMP accumulation intracellularly, which supports its role in the reversal of beta₂-agonist tolerance [39, 204]. Because beta₂-agonist tolerance is still considered controversial, the significance of these observations has still not been resolved.

Clinical Utility
Ketotifen has been evaluated extensively for the treatment of asthma. Table 63-15 summarizes some of the results of bronchial provocation studies performed before and after treatment with ketotifen [67]. Ketotifen was found to be most effective at inhibiting allergen- and histamine-induced bronchoconstriction. Its effects on nonspecific stimuli (exercise, cold air, sulfur dioxide) and acetylcholine have been less impressive [57].

Despite the in vitro and human properties of ketotifen, its beneficial role in the treatment of asthma has been inconsistent. Several early multicenter studies demonstrated that ketotifen decreased the frequency and duration of asthmatic attacks while

allowing for decreased use or discontinuation of concomitant medications [206, 237]. Ketotifen had a variable effect in improving objective parameters such as FEV₁ or PEFR [79, 107, 153, 206, 243]. Ketotifen was found to be comparable to DSCG and other dual-action antihistamines (azelastine) in treating chronic asthma [157, 211]. Figure 63-12 shows that the effect of ketotifen on changes in FEV₁, PEFR, and vital capacity is similar to that of DSCG [66]. Studies in children have demonstrated that ketotifen offers no advantages over placebo in decreasing bronchial hyperreactivity, as assessed by pre- and postmethacholine challenges [107]. A more recent double-blinded, controlled, cross-over study performed in children (ages 1 to 3 years) with mild to moderate asthma found that ketotifen had no therapeutic advantages over placebo [243].

Other studies evaluating ketotifen for use in the treatment of exercise-induced and occupational asthma have similarly found this agent to be ineffective [79, 239]. In support of ketotifen's antiasthmatic efficacy were results from two recent large multicenter studies evaluating both children and adults. Investigators found ketotifen to be effective in decreasing patient symptom scores and the use of concomitant medications [173, 206]. Only the Canadian study, which assessed children between the ages of 5 and 17 years, found a significant improvement in FEV₁ from baseline measurements compared to placebo [206]. The steroid-sparing effect of ketotifen has been evaluated in severely corticosteroid-dependent asthmatics. These results found that ketotifen was comparable to DSCG in allowing for a reduction of corticosteroids in these patients [111, 142].

Ketotifen has been evaluated for the treatment of many clinical disorders other than asthma. The pharmacologic properties of ketotifen make it suitable for the treatment of allergic rhinitis, conjunctivitis, and food allergy [67]. Several studies have demonstrated that the drug is effective as an antipruritic, mast cell–stabilizing agent in the treatment of physical urticarias and chronic idiopathic urticaria [121, 169, 233]. It was also effective as an antipruritic agent and in the management of skin eruptions in patients with atopic dermatitis [250]. Ketotifen offered no advantages over existing medications in the treatment of systemic mastocytosis [8, 137].

Ketotifen has been anecdotally used to treat several nonallergic disorders postulated to be caused or aggravated by the release of mast cell mediators. Preliminary data suggest that ketotifen may be effective in the treatment of cluster headaches, idiopathic oligo- or asthenozoospermia, neurofibromatosis, scleroderma, and cheilitis granulomatosa [158, 212, 219, 244].

Dose and Administration

Ketotifen can be given orally, twice a day, which may be advantageous in improving patient compliance. The recommended dose for treating asthma with ketotifen is 1 mg orally twice a day [67].

Adverse Effects

A major disadvantage of ketotifen reported in the majority of clinical studies has been the adverse side effect of drowsiness and fatigue, presumably related to its H₁ antagonist properties. Other commonly reported side effects include lethargy, weight gain, nausea, vomiting, abdominal discomfort, diarrhea, dizziness, nervousness, and rashes, including pityriasis rosea [67, 237].

Azelastine

Azelastine, like ketotifen, can be categorized as a dual-action antihistamine. It is a new oral antiallergic, antiasthmatic agent with potent H₁-antagonistic and mast cell–stabilizing properties [172]. Azelastine has been investigated extensively in animal and human models. Currently, Phase III clinical trials in the United States are in progress to determine whether this agent offers a new therapeutic dimension for the treatment of asthma and other allergic diatheses.

Chemistry

Azelastine is a phthalazinone derivative with the chemical structure of 4-[(p-chlorobenzyl)-2-(hexahydro-1-methyl]-1H-azepin-4-yl)-1-(2H)-phthalazinone hydrochloride [48]. Figure 63-13 compares the structure of azelastine to those of DSCG and NS [172].

Pharmacokinetics

Most of the pharmacokinetic information on azelastine and its major active metabolite, demethyl azelastine, in humans is based on unpublished results. Greater than 95 percent of azelastine is rapidly absorbed after ingestion. Its absorption is unaltered by food, and greater than 80 percent of the drug is protein bound [172]. Both dose- and time-dependent factors influence peak plasma azelastine concentrations in asthmatic subjects [172]. Twice daily dosing has been shown to expedite the time necessary to reach maximal plasma concentrations when compared to single doses (2.3 hours versus 4.2 hours, respectively) [172]. This

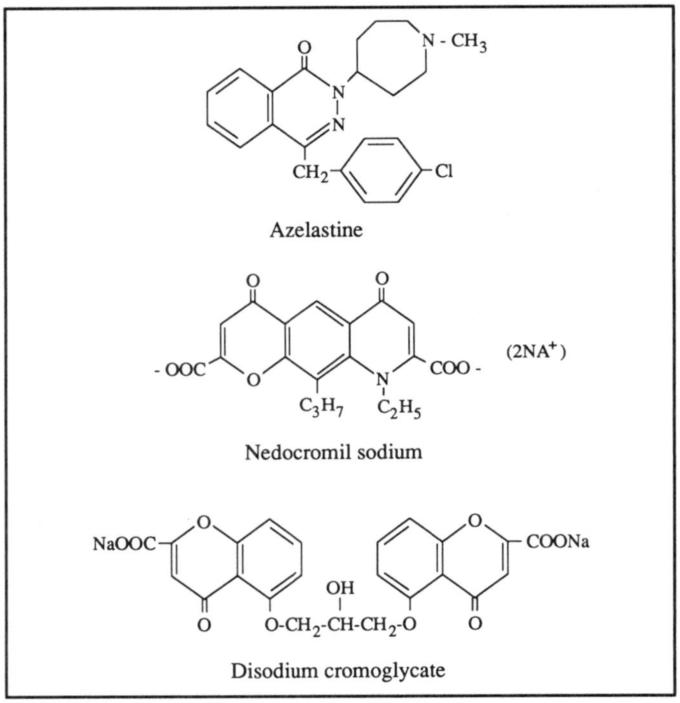

Fig. 63-13. *Structural comparison of azelastine, nedocromil sodium, and disodium cromoglycate.*

is believed to occur because of increased plasma concentrations of the demethylated metabolite, which is quantitatively measured together with its parent compound by the radioimmunoassays employed [172]. Peak plasma concentration levels are achieved faster in children than in adults. The absolute bioavailability of azelastine is greater than 80 percent [172].

Single-dose studies of orally and intravenously administered radioactive azelastine ([¹⁴C]azelastine) have revealed that this drug is primarily distributed within the liver, lung, and kidney. After multiple oral doses of azelastine, its peripheral distribution is changed as higher concentrations of drugs and metabolites are found in the adrenal gland, pancreas, kidney, and spleen. Azelastine does not significantly cross the blood-brain barrier. In animal studies, azelastine has been shown to cross the placenta. Data are not currently available comparing the pharmacokinetic differences among normal, asthmatic, and allergic subjects. Azelastine has not been evaluated in subjects with renal or hepatic dysfunction [172].

The elimination half-life of azelastine in normal subjects is shorter after single dosings (T½ = 25 hours) than that after multiple dosings (T½ = 35.5 hours). This time difference in half-lives after multiple doses has been attributed to the accumulation of the active metabolite, which has a longer elimination half-life (42 hours) [172].

After absorption, azelastine undergoes hydroxylation, demethylation, and oxidation to form zwitterion isomers. The major metabolite, demethyl azelastine, is considered to be responsible for most of the pharmacologic activity. Preliminary [¹⁴C]azelastine elimination studies have revealed that 25 percent of azelastine is excreted in the urine and 50 percent in the feces. It is still unclear whether azelastine undergoes enterohepatic recirculation. In general, results from elimination studies have reported that 75 to 99 percent of a single oral azelastine dose and its metabolites are recovered within 120 to 240 hours. Twenty-five percent of this dose is recovered from the urine and 50 percent from the feces [172].

Mechanisms of Action

The pharmacologic activities of azelastine studied in animals are summarized in Table 63-16 [48]. Studies using radioligand binding assays in animals have demonstrated a high affinity for azelastine to H_1 receptors, with little, if any, affinity binding to beta-adrenergic, acetylcholine, or muscarinic receptors [172]. Azelastine has been demonstrated to inhibit calcium-ionophore–, concanavalin A–, and allergen-induced mast cell and basophil histamine release in rats, rabbits, and guinea pigs [48–50, 172]. The in vitro mast cell stabilization by azelastine has been compared to that of ketotifen and DSCG and was at least 5,000 times more potent than it was for either of these other two agents (Table 63-17) [172].

Chand and associates [51] have suggested that azelastine inhibits histamine release from mast cells by blocking calcium uptake into the mast cells, thereby interfering with a stimulus–excitation coupling process. This hypothesis has not been limited to mast cells, as Nakamura and associates [190] used guinea pig peritoneal macrophages to demonstrate that azelastine, in a dose-dependent manner, inhibited PAF-acether and N-formyl-methionyl-leucyl-phenylalanine–induced intracellular mobilization of Ca^{++}, which resulted in a reduced release of prostaglandin E_2 from these cells. Masuo and associates [162a] used guinea pig ileum smooth muscle cells to demonstrate that azelastine acts as a Ca^{++} antagonist by blocking voltage gated Ca^{++} influx, release, and sensitization.

Azelastine was found to be more potent than conventional antihistamines in inhibiting histamine-induced cutaneous reactions and bronchoconstriction in guinea pigs [52, 172]. In rats, azelastine had a dose-dependent inhibitory effect on the IgE-mediated passive cutaneous anaphylaxis reaction, which was stronger than that of DSCG, ketotifen, or astemizole [53].

Chand and colleagues [52] reported that azelastine was more potent than DSCG and ketotifen in inhibiting the synthesis and

release of leukotrienes. Katayama and coworkers [134] demonstrated that azelastine had a leukotriene antagonistic effect that was more potent than the effect of ketotifen on guinea pig ileum. Azelastine also inhibited calcium ionophore–induced leukotriene release from human polymorphonuclear leukocytes [172]. This leukotriene inhibitory response has been postulated to occur by azelastine's blocking the effects of 5'-lipoxygenase [6, 194].

In vivo studies, for unclear reasons, have been conflicting with regard to the effect of azelastine on bronchial hyperreactivity. Gould and associates [106] were unable to demonstrate significant changes in bronchial hyperreactivity as measured by methacholine challenge in subjects pretreated with azelastine. In contrast, Iwata and colleagues [124] found a significant decrease in airway hyperresponsiveness to methacholine challenge in asthmatic patients treated with azelastine.

Azelastine had a dose-related antagonistic effect on intradermal serotonin-induced passive cutaneous anaphylaxis reactions in rats and a similarly weak effect on serotonin-induced bronchospasm in guinea pigs [53, 172]. Azelastine has been demonstrated to be comparable to ketotifen in inhibiting PAF-induced bronchial reactions in rats and guinea pigs [5]. Azelastine was more effective than ketotifen in inhibiting PAF-induced paw edema reactions in rats [5].

Studies in humans have evaluated the effect of azelastine on skin and airway responsiveness to nonallergic stimuli and these results are summarized in Table 63-18 [207]. The comparative effects of azelastine and ketotifen on the inhibition of histamine-induced bronchoconstriction are similar [172]. Azelastine has more potent bronchodilatory effects than do either DSCG or ketotifen [172]. Azelastine has also been observed to inhibit exercise-induced and distilled water–induced bronchospasm and has been effective in inhibiting allergen-induced bronchoconstriction in atopic asthmatic subjects [172]. Azelastine was also seen to significantly inhibit cutaneous reactivity induced by histamine, codeine, and specific antigens [172].

Preliminary studies examining the effect of azelastine on the early- and late-phase asthmatic reactions have been performed in animal models [172]. These studies showed that azelastine inhibited the early-phase response (1 to 2 hours) by approximately 30 percent and the late-phase response (2 to 8 hours) by 36 to 100 percent [172]. Several investigators have proposed mechanisms for this late-phase response. Busse and coworkers [46] have found that azelastine inhibits neutrophil and eosinophil O_2^- production in a dose-dependent manner, thereby attenuating the late-phase asthmatic reaction. Rafferty and associates [208] suggested that the salutary effect on the late-phase reaction is due to the inhibition of leukocyte activation and mediator release, and their resultant physiologic actions.

Table 63-16. Pharmacologic activities of azelastine

1. Interferes with the synthesis and release of leukotrienes.
2. Inhibits allergic and nonallergic histamine secretion.
3. Inhibits superoxide radical ($\cdot O_2^-$) generation.
4. Inhibits antihistamine-resistant, leukotriene-mediated allergic bronchospasm in guinea pigs.
5. Inhibits IgE-mediated passive cutaneous anaphylaxis in rats.
6. Inhibits aeroallergen-induced bronchospasm in guinea pigs.
7. Antagonizes pharmacologic mediators at their receptor sites, e.g., histamine and leukotrienes.

Source: N. Chand, et al., Inhibition of acute lung anaphylaxis by aerosolized azelastine in guinea pigs sensitized by three different procedures. *Ann. Allergy* 58:344, 1987. Reprinted with permission.

Table 63-17. Mean in vitro concentrations of azelastine, ketotifen, DSCG, and theophylline producing 50% inhibition of histamine release from rat peritoneal mast cells after 0 or 10 minutes' incubation in response to an allergic or nonallergic stimulus

| | IC_{50} ($\mu mol/L$) | | | | | | | |
| | Azelastine | | Ketotifen | | DSCG | | Theophylline | |
Secretory stimulus	0 min	10 min	0 min	10 min	0 min	10 min	0 min	10 min
Allergic stimulus								
Ovalbumin (10 mg/L) + phosphatidyl serine (10 mg/L)	7.62	4.8	—	112	NS	NS	—	2,040
Nonallergic stimulus								
A23187 (0.1 mg/L)	—	5	—	200	NS	NS	NS	NS
Compound 48/40 (0.1 mg/L)	49	42	231	142	223	1,245*	2,769	3,608
Concanavalin A (10 mg/L) + phosphatidyl serine (10 mg/L)	7	2*	62	68	7,526	10,000	217	630*

NS = no significant difference seen over a concentration range of 0.1 to 1,000 $\mu mol/L$; * = $p < .05$ (significant difference between 0 and 10 minutes' incubation time); IC_{50} = concentration required to inhibit mediator release by 50%; DSCG = disodium cromoglycate.
Source: D. McTavish and E. M. Sorkin, Azelastine: a review of its pharmacodynamic and pharmacokinetic properties and therapeutic potential. *Drugs* 38(5):778, 1989. Reprinted with permission.

Table 63-18. The effect of azelastine on airways histamine and methacholine responsiveness and skin wheal response to histamine

		Azelastine (mg)		
	Placebo	4.4	8.8	17.6
PC_{20} histamine (mg/ml)	0.16+ (0.02–1.73)	1.98 (0.13–62)	8.79 (2.24–56)	8.11 (0.92–57)
GM potency ratios to histamine	1	12.8	54.4	50.2
PC_{20} methacholine (mg/ml)	0.16	ND	ND	0.19 (0.01–1.82)
Total wheal area (mm^2)	211 ± 27	146 ± 27	97 ± 19	30 ± 10

ND = not determined; PC_{20} = provocation concentration of agonist producing a 20% decrease in FEV_1 from baseline; + GM = geometric mean (range); mean ± SE (standard error).
Source: P. Rafferty, et al. The *in vivo* potency and selectivity of azelastine as an H_1 histamine–receptor antagonist in human airways and skin. *J. Allergy Clin. Immunol.* 82:1113, 1988. Reprinted with permission.

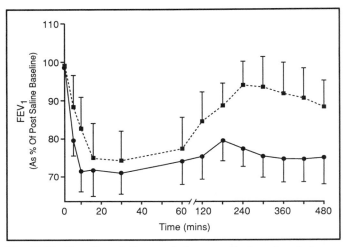

Fig. 63-14. *The effect of allergen challenge on the forced expiratory volume at 1 second (FEV_1) in subjects exhibiting both early and late bronchoconstrictor reactions after treatment with placebo (closed circles) and azelastine, 8.8 mg (closed squares). The bars represent the standard error of the mean for observations in five subjects. (Reprinted with permission from P. Rafferty, et al. The inhibitory actions of azelastine hydrochloride on the early and late bronchoconstrictor responses to inhaled allergen in atopic asthma.* J. Allergy Clin. Immunol. *84:649, 1989.)*

Clinical Efficacy

Azelastine has been evaluated clinically in therapeutic trials for its use in asthma, allergic rhinitis, and atopic dermatitis in children and adults. Many of the early studies were not placebo controlled and the subjects had poorly regulated medical regimens. These studies consistently showed significant symptomatic improvement with the reduction of concomitant medication use. Similar findings were noted in studies evaluating asthmatic children. Some of these studies also reported significant improvement in objective parameters such as the FEV_1 and PEFR [172, 208]. Figure 63-14 illustrates the effect of allergen challenge on FEV_1 in dual asthma responders pretreated with azelastine compared to their response to placebo [208].

One investigational placebo-controlled study evaluating 220 asthmatic subjects found that azelastine use resulted in significant improvement in FEV_1, PEFR, and symptom scores, while the need for bronchodilators decreased [172]. Azelastine has been

Table 63-19. Recommended dose and route of administration of the newer anti-allergic medications

Drug	Route of administration	Adult dose/frequency
Nedocromil sodium	Inhaled	4 mg/inhalation; one puff bid → qid
Lodoxamide tromethamine[a]	Inhaled/oral	0.3 mg in single-dose studies; frequency not determined
Ketotifen[b]	Oral	1 mg bid
Azelastine[b]	Oral	4 mg bid or 8 mg qhs

[a] Not approved for use in humans.
[b] Not available in the United States.

compared to theophylline and ketotifen in preliminary studies. Results have not been overly impressive as far as favoring azelastine over these agents, but further studies are required before more definitive conclusions can be made [172].

Azelastine had a therapeutic effect on seasonal and perennial allergic rhinitis, which was equivalent to chlorpheniramine and terfenadine in reducing the severity of symptom scores (azelastine, 2 mg/day = terfenadine, 120 mg/day = chlorpheniramine, 4 mg four times/day > placebo). One study reported that 4 mg of azelastine a day was more effective in reducing symptoms than was 120 mg of terfenadine per day. Unpublished reports have found that intranasal azelastine is as effective in reducing symptom scores as intranasal corticosteroids [172]. Limited studies comparing azelastine to intranasal DSCG have thus far found these agents to be similar in their therapeutic effect [172].

Limited information regarding the assessment of azelastine as an antipruritic agent in patients with atopic dermatitis and nonspecific eczema is available. Azelastine was more effective in treating the symptoms related to nonspecific eczema than it was in alleviating pruritus associated with atopic dermatitis [172].

Because of its broad spectrum of pharmacologic effects, azelastine holds promise for the treatment of allergic disorders. However, further double-blinded, placebo-controlled clinical trials are needed to assess both the short- and long-term effects of this agent before its precise clinical role can be determined.

Dose and Administration

Azelastine can be administered orally twice daily (4 mg bid) or as a single nighttime dose (8 mg qhs) to effectively treat children (greater than 6 years of age) and adults with asthma [172]. For allergic rhinitis, the recommended dose of azelastine is 1 to 2 mg twice a day and it is not affected by food consumption [172]. Information is unavailable regarding its intranasal use, its use in children less than 6 years of age, or its use in patients with hepatorenal disease. This agent should not be used in pregnant women or nursing mothers [172]. Table 63-19 summarizes the dose and administration route of the newer antiallergic medications. As previously mentioned, only NS is currently slated for use in the United States.

Adverse Effects

Reported side effects from azelastine have varied depending on the dosage, route of administration, and disease processes being treated. Generally, the drug has been rated by physicians and patients as being well tolerated. The most common reported side effects are altered taste perception, drowsiness, and fatigue. Less than 2 percent of all subjects thus far studied have had to be withdrawn from the drug because of adverse side effects [172].

The treatment of asthma has improved over the past thirty years with the introduction of novel drugs possessing a wide spectrum of pharmacologic activities. Many of these agents decrease inflammation, either by interfering with the activity of specific mediators at receptor sites or by direct effects on various cells, including mast cells. Investigation of these multifaceted drugs has facilitated a better understanding of the pathophysiology of asthma. Furthermore, these drugs have acted as models for the development of newer agents such as leukotriene D_4 (MK5-71) and 5′-lipoxygenase (A64077) inhibitors, which have shown potential in the treatment of asthma [123, 161] (Chap. 66). These drugs have sparked renewed interest in the investigation of preexisting agents for different spectra of pharmacologic properties. This is exemplified by recent investigations of albuterol, which, in addition to its bronchodilating capacity, was also found to be a more potent in vivo mast cell stabilizer than DSCG [119].

Although the mast cell–stabilizing agents discussed in this chapter may offer promise as alternative treatment modalities for asthma, none of these drugs as yet possesses substantial advantages over DSCG.

Currently, numerous other oral antiallergic agents are being investigated in preclinical studies. As alluded to earlier, previous experience with evaluating drugs that appeared to be promising by virtue of data obtained from in vitro and animal models was often disappointing in terms of their expected clinical activities. Therefore, it remains to be seen whether newer agents will offer advantages over those currently available.

REFERENCES

1. Abdalla, S., et al. Effects of 3,3′-di-O-methylquercetin on guinea-pig isolated smooth muscle. *J. Pharm. Pharmacol.* 41:138, 1989.
2. Abraham, W. M., Stevenson, J. S., and Sielczak, M. S. Preliminary report on the effect of nedocromil sodium on antigen-induced early and late reactions in allergic sheep. *Eur. J. Respir. Dis.* 69:192, 1986.
3. Abraham, W. M., et al. Cellular markers of inflammation in the airways of allergic sheep with and without allergen-induced late responses. *Am. Rev. Respir. Dis.* 138:1565, 1988.
4. Abraham, W. M., et al. The effect of nedocromil sodium and cromolyn sodium on antigen-induced responses in allergic sheep *in vivo* and *in vitro. Chest* 92:913, 1987.
5. Achterrath-Tuckermann, U., Weischer, C. H., and Szelenyi, I. Azelastine, a new antiallergic/antiasthmatic agent, inhibits PAF-acether–induced platelet aggregation, paw edema and bronchoconstriction. *Pharmacology* 36:265, 1988.
6. Achterrath-Tuckerman, U., et al. Inhibition of cysteinyl-leukotriene production by azelastine and its biological significance. *Agents Actions* 24:217, 1988.
7. Advenier, C., et al. Sodium cromoglycate, verapamil and nicardipine antagonism to leukotriene D_4 bronchoconstriction. *Br. J. Pharmacol.* 78:301, 1983.
8. Alam, R. Role of mast cells and basophils in human diseases. *Insights Allergy* 2:1, 1987.
9. Allansmith, M. R., Petty, T. L., and Schwartz, H. J. Cromolyn sodium: clinical considerations. Excerpta Medica 1987.
10. Allansmith, M. R., et al. Giant papillary conjunctivitis in contact lens wearers. *Am. J. Ophthalmol.* 83:697, 1977.
11. Allegra, L., and Bianco, S. Non-specific broncho-reactivity obtained with ultrasonic aerosol of distilled water. *Eur. J. Respir. Dis.* 61:41, 1980.
12. Anderson, P., and Bergstrand, H. Antigen-induced bronchial anaphylaxis in actively sensitized guinea pigs: effect of long-term treatment with sodium cromoglycate and aminophylline. *Br. J. Pharmacol.* 74:601, 1981.
13. Archer, C. B., et al. Actions of disodium cromoglycate (DSCG) on human skin responses to histamine, codeine and Paf-acether. *Agents Actions* 16:6, 1985.
14. Ashton, J. M., et al. The absorption metabolism and excretion of disodium cromoglycate in nine animal species. *Toxicol. Appl. Pharmacol.* 26:319, 1973.
15. Assem, E. S. K., and Morgan, J. L. Inhibition of allergic reactions in man and other species by cromoglycate. *Int. Arch. Allergy Appl. Immunol.* 38:68, 1970.
16. Assem, E. S. K., and Richter, A. W. Comparison of *in vivo* and *in vitro* inhibition of the anaphylactic mechanism by B-adrenergic stimulants and disodium cromoglycate. *Immunology* 21:729, 1971.
17. Atkins, P. C., Norman, M. E., and Zweiman, B. Antigen-induced neutrophil chemotactic activity in man. *J. Allergy Clin. Immunol.* 62:149, 1978.
18. Auty, R. M. The clinical development of a new agent for the treatment of airway inflammation, nedocromil sodium (Tilade^R). *Eur. J. Respir. Dis.* 69(suppl. 147):120, 1986.
19. Ayres, J. G. Nedocromil sodium: respiratory agent. *Br. J. Clin. Pract.* 41:971, 1987.
20. Ball, T. D., et al. Effects of lodoxamide tromethamine on paraplegia that occurs after infrarenal aortic occlusion in the rabbit. *J. Vasc. Surg.* 5:672, 1987.
21. Bar-Yishay, E., et al. Duration of action of sodium cromoglycate on exercise induced asthma: comparison of 2 formulations. *Arch. Dis. Child.* 58:624, 1983.
22. Bascom, R., and Bleecker, E. G. Bronchoconstriction induced by distilled water. *Am. Rev. Respir. Dis.* 134:248, 1986.
23. Basran, G. S., et al. Cromoglycate inhibits the responses to platelet-activating factor (PAF-acether) in man: an alternative mode of action for DSCG in asthma? *Eur. J. Pharmacol.* 86:143, 1983.
24. Beach, J. E., et al. Cromolyn sodium toxicity studies in primates. *Toxicol. Appl. Pharmacol.* 57:367, 1981.
25. Beaven, M. A., et al. The mechanism of the calcium signal and correlation with histamine release in 2H3 cells. *J. Biol. Chem.* 259:7129, 1984.
26. Ben-Dov, I., Bar-Yishay, E., and Godfrey, S. Relation between efficacy of sodium cromoglycate and baseline lung function in exercise- and hyperventilation-induced asthma. *Isr. J. Med. Sci.* 20:130, 1984.
27. Ben-Dov, I., Bar-Yishay, E., and Godfrey, S. Refractory period after exercise-induced asthma unexplained respiratory heat loss. *Am. Rev. Respir. Dis.* 125:530, 1982.
28. Ben-Dov, I., Bar-Yishay, E., and Godfrey, S. Heterogeneity in the response of asthmatic patients to pre-exercise treatment with cromolyn sodium. *Am. Rev. Respir. Dis.* 127:113, 1983.
29. Bennett, J. P., Gomperts, B. D., and Wollenweber, D. Inhibitory effects of natural flavonoids on secretion from mast cells and neutrophils. *Drug Res.* 31:433, 1981.
30. Bernstein, I. L. Cromolyn sodium. *Chest* 87(suppl.):68S, 1985.
31. Bernstein, I. L. Cromolyn sodium in the treatment of asthma: changing concepts. *J. Allergy Clin. Immunol.* 68:247, 1981.
32. Bernstein, I. L., Johnson, C. L., and Tse, C. S. T. Therapy with cromolyn sodium. *Ann. Intern. Med.* 89:228, 1978.
33. Bernstein, I. L., et al. A controlled study of cromolyn sodium sponsored by the Drug Committee of the American Academy of Allergy. *J. Allergy Clin. Immunol.* 50:235, 1972.
34. Bindoli, A., Valente, M., and Cavallini, L. Inhibitory action of quercetin on xanthine oxidase and xanthine dehydrogenase activity. *Pharmacol. Res. Comm.* 17:831, 1985.
35. Blackburn, W. D. Jr., Heck, L. W., and Wallace, R. W. The bioflavonoid quercetin inhibits neutrophil degranulation, superoxide production, and the phosphorylation of specific neutrophil proteins. *Biochem. Biophys. Res. Comm.* 44:1229, 1987.
36. Blumenthal, M. N., et al. Cromolyn in extrinsic and intrinsic asthma. *J. Allergy Clin. Immunol.* 52:105, 1973.
36a. Bosso, J. V., Aiken, M. J., and Simon, R. A. Successful prevention of local and cutaneous hypersensitivity reactions to seminal fluid with intravaginal cromolyn. *Allergy Proc.* 12:113, 1991.
37. Bradford, P. G., and Rubin, R. P. The differential effects of nedocromil sodium and sodium cromoglycate on the secretory response of rabbit peritoneal neutrophils. *Eur. J. Respir. Dis.* 69(S147):238, 1986.
38. Breslin, F. J., McFadden, E. R. Jr., and Ingram, R. H. Jr. The effects of cromolyn sodium on the airway response to hyperpnea and cold air in asthma. *Am. Rev. Respir. Dis.* 122:11, 1980.
39. Brodde, O. E., et al. Effect of prednisolone and ketotifen on β_2-adrenoceptors in asthmatic patients receiving β_2-bronchodilators. *Eur. J. Clin. Pharmacol.* 34:145, 1988.
40. Brooks, C. D., Maile, M. H., and Wilder, M. A. Attenuation of exercise-induced asthma by inhaled lodoxamide tromethamine (abstract). *J. Allergy Clin. Immunol.* 63:161, 1979.
41. Bruijnzeel, P. L. B., Warringa, R. A. J., and Kok, P. T. M. Inhibition of platelet-activating factor– and zymosan-activated serum–induced chemotaxis of human neutrophils by nedocromil sodium, BN 52021 and sodium cromoglycate. *Br. J. Pharmacol.* 97:1251, 1989.
42. Bruijnzeel, P. L. B., et al. Inhibitory effects of nedocromil sodium on the *in vitro* induced migration and leukotriene formation of human granulocytes. *Drugs* 37(S1):9, 1989.
43. Bruijnzeel, P. L. B., et al. Nedocromil sodium inhibits the A23187- and opsonized zymosan–induced leukotriene formation by human eosinophils but not by human neutrophils. *Br. J. Pharmacol.* 96:631, 1989.
44. Bundgaard, A., Bach-Mortensen, N., and Schmitt, A. The effect of sodium

cromoglycate delivered by spinhaler and by pressurized aerosol on exercise-induced asthma in children. *Clin. Allergy* 12:601, 1982.

45. Busse, W. W., Kopp, D. E., and Middleton, E. Jr. Flavonoid modulation of human neutrophil function. *J. Allergy Clin. Immunol.* 73:801, 1984.

46. Busse, W., Randlev, B., and Sedgwick, J. The effect of azelastine on neutrophil and eosinophil generation of superoxide. *J. Allergy Clin. Immunol.* 83:400, 1989.

46a. Callaghan, B., Teo, N. C., and Clancy, L. Effects of the addition of nedocromil sodium to maintenance bronchodilator therapy in the management of chronic asthma. *Chest* 101:787, 1992.

47. Carney, I. F. IgE mediated anaphylactic bronchoconstriction in the guinea pig and the effect of disodium cromoglycate. *Int. Arch. Allergy Appl. Immunol.* 50:322, 1976.

48. Chand, N., et al. Inhibition of acute lung anaphylaxis by aerosolized azelastine in guinea pigs sensitized by three different procedures. *Ann. Allergy* 58:344, 1987.

49. Chand, N., et al. Inhibition of IgE-mediated allergic histamine release from rat peritoneal mast cells by azelastine and selected antiallergic drugs. *Agents Actions* 16:318, 1985.

50. Chand, N., et al. Changes in aeroallergen-induced pulmonary mechanics in actively sensitized guinea pig inhibition by azelastine. *Ann. Allergy* 64:151, 1990.

51. Chand, N., et al. Inhibition of allergic histamine release by azelastine and selected antiallergic drugs from rabbit leukocytes. *Int. Arch. Allergy Appl. Immunol.* 77:451, 1985.

52. Chand, N., et al. Inhibition of leukotriene (SRS-A)–mediated acute lung anaphylaxis by azelastine in guinea pigs. *Allergy* 41:473, 1986.

53. Chand, N., et al. Inhibition of passive cutaneous anaphylaxis (PCA) by azelastine: dissociation of its antiallergic activities from antihistaminic and antiserotonin properties. *Int. J. Immunopharmacol* 7:833, 1985.

54. Chandra, R. K., Heresi, G., and Woodford, G. Double-blind controlled crossover trial of 4% intranasal sodium cromoglycate solution in patients with seasonal allergic rhinitis. *Ann. Allergy* 49:131, 1982.

55. Church, M. K. Reassessment of mast cell stabilizers in the treatment of respiratory disease. *Ann. Allergy* 62:215, 1989.

56. Church, M. K., Collier, A. O. J. and James, G. W. L. The inhibition by dexamethasone and disodium cromoglycate of anaphylactic bronchoconstriction in the rat. *Br. J. Pharmacol.* 46:56, 1972.

57. Church, M. K., and Gradidge, C. F. Inhibition of histamine release from human lung *in vitro* by antihistamines and related drugs. *Br. J. Pharmacol.* 69:663, 1980.

58. Church, M. K., Hutson, P. A., and Holgate, S. T. Effect of nedocromil sodium on early and late phase responses to allergen challenge in the guinea-pig. *Drugs* 37(S1):101, 1989.

59. Clark, B., et al. Nedocromil sodium preclinical safety evaluation studies: a preliminary report. *Eur. J. Respir. Dis.* 69(S147):248, 1986.

60. Cockcroft, D. W., and Murdock, K. Y. Comparative effects of inhaled salbutamol, sodium cromoglycate, and beclomethasone dipropionate on allergen-induced early asthmatic responses, late asthmatic responses, and increased bronchial responsiveness to histamine. *J. Allergy Clin. Immunol.* 79:734, 1987.

61. Cohan, R. H., et al. Treatment of perennial allergic rhinitis with cromolyn sodium. *J. Allergy Clin. Immunol.* 58:121, 1976.

62. Corkey, C., et al. Comparison of three different preparations of disodium cromoglycate in the prevention of exercise-induced bronchospasm. *Am. Rev. Respir. Dis.* 125:623, 1982.

63. Corrado, O. J., et al. The effect of nedocromil sodium on nasal provocation with allergen. *J. Allergy Clin. Immunol.* 80:218, 1987.

64. Cox, J. S. G. Disodium cromoglycate (FPL 670) ('Intal'): a specific inhibitor of reaginic antibody-antigen mechanisms. *Nature* 216:1328, 1967.

65. Cox, J. S. G., Beach, J. E., and Blair, A. M. J. N. Disodium cromoglycate (Intal). *Adv. Drug Res.* 5:115, 1970.

66. Craps, L. P. Ketotifen in the oral prophylaxis of bronchial asthma: a review. Pharmatherapeutica 3:18, 1981.

67. Craps, L. P. Immunologic and therapeutic aspects of ketotifen. *J. Allergy Clin. Immunol.* 76:389, 1985.

68. Craps, L. P. Prophylaxis of asthma with ketotifen in children and adolescents. A review. *Pharmatherapeutica* 3:314, 1983.

69. Craps, L. P., and Ney, U. M. Ketotifen: current views on its mechanism of action and their therapeutic implications. *Respiration* 45:411, 1984.

70. Crimi, E., Brusasco, V., and Crimi, P. Effect of nedocromil sodium on the late asthmatic reaction to bronchial antigen challenge. *J. Allergy Clin. Immunol.* 83:985, 1989.

71. Crimi, N., et al. Comparative study of the effects of nedocromil sodium

(4 mg) and sodium cromoglycate (10 mg) in adenosine-induced bronchoconstriction in asthmatic subjects. *Clin. Allergy* 18:367, 1988.

72. Crimi, N., et al. Effect of nedocromil on bronchospasm induced by inhalation of substance P in asthmatic subjects. *Clin. Allergy* 18:375, 1988.

73. Daniels, C., and Temple, D. M. The inhibition by azatadine of the immunological release of leukotrienes and histamine from human lung fragments. *Eur. J. Pharmacol.* 123:463, 1986.

74. Davies, S. E. Effect of disodium cromoglycate on exercise-induced asthma. *Br. Med. J.* 3:593, 1968.

75. Dimlich, R. V. W., and Reilly, F. D. Elevated blood glucose after compound 48/80 treatment is not related to hepatic mast cell degranulation in rats (42425). *Proc. Soc. Exp. Biol. Med.* 183:321, 1986.

76. Dixon, M., Jackson, D. M., and Richards, I. M. The effects of sodium cromoglycate on lung irritant receptors and left ventricular cardiac receptors in the anaesthetized dog. *Br. J. Pharmacol.* 67:569, 1979.

77. Dixon, C. M. S., and Ind, P. W. Inhaled sodium metabisulphite induced bronchoconstriction: inhibition by nedocromil sodium and sodium cromoglycate. *Br. J. Clin. Pharmacol.* 30:371, 1990.

78. Doley, A. E., and Walker, D. N. A trial of cromolyn acid in recurrent aphthoris ulceration. *Br. J. Oral Surg.* 12:292, 1975.

79. Dorward, A. J., and Patel, K. R. Inhaled ketotifen in exercise-induced asthma—a negative report. *Eur. J. Respir. Dis.* 67:378, 1985.

80. Dushay, M. E., and Johnson, C. E. Management of allergic rhinitis: focus on intranasal agents. *Pharmacotherapy* 9:338, 1989.

81. Eady, R. P. The pharmacology of nedocromil sodium. *Eur. J. Respir. Dis.* 69(S147):112, 1986.

82. Eady, R. P., et al. The effect of nedocromil sodium and sodium cromoglycate on antigen-induced bronchoconstriction in the ascaris-sensitive monkey. *Br. J. Pharmacol.* 85:323, 1985.

83. Easty, D., Rice, N. S. C., and Jones, B. R. Disodium cromoglycate (Intal) in the treatment of vernal kerato-conjunctivitis. *Trans. Ophthalmol. Soc. U.K.* 91:491, 1971.

84. Edmunds, A. T., et al. Controlled trial of cromoglycate and slow-release aminophylline in perennial childhood asthma. *Br. Med. J.* 281:842, 1980.

85. Eyre, P., Lewis, A. J., and Wells, P. W. Acute systemic anaphylaxis in the calf. *Br. J. Pharmacol.* 47:504, 1973.

86. Fanta, C. H., McFadden, E. R. Jr., and Ingram, R. H. Jr. Effects of cromolyn sodium on the response to respiratory heat loss in normal subjects. *Am. Rev. Respir. Dis.* 123:161, 1981.

87. Farmer, J. B., et al. Mediators of passive lung anaphylaxis in the rat. *Br. J. Pharmacol.* 55:57, 1975.

88. Feldman, B. R., and Davis, W. J. Treatment of asthma with cromolyn and corticosteroids. *Cutis* 17:1103, 1976.

89. Fewtrell, C. M. S., and Gomperts, B. D. Effect of flavone inhibitors of transport ATPases on histamine secretion from rat mast cells. *Nature* 265:635, 1977.

90. Fitzpatrick, J. C., Fisher, H., and Flancbaum, L. Effect of H_1 and H_2 receptor blockers on mobilization of myocardial carnosine to histamine during compound 48/80–induced shock in young rats. *Circ. Shock* 30:145, 1990.

91. Flancbaum, L., Fitzpatrick, J. C., and Fisher, H. Improved survival from compound 48/80–induced lethal stress and inhibition of myocardial histamine and carnosine mobilization by lodoxamide. *Circ. Shock* 27:155, 1989.

92. Foreman, J. C. Mast cells and the actions of flavonoids. *J. Allergy Clin. Immunol.* 73:769, 1984.

93. Foreman, J. C., Hallett, M. B., and Mongar, J. L. Site of action of the antiallergic drugs cromoglycate and doxantrazole. *Br. J. Pharmacol.* 59:473, 1977.

94. Foreman, J. C., and Pearce, F. L. Cromolyn. In E. Middleton, et al. (eds.), *Allergy Principles and Practice,* St. Louis: Mosby, 1988.

95. Foreman, J. C., et al. A possible role for cyclic AMP in the regulation of histamine secretion and the action of cromoglycate. *Biochem. Pharmacol.* 24:538, 1975.

96. Foster, C. S., and Duncan, J. Randomized clinical trial of topically administered cromolyn sodium for vernal keratoconjunctivitis. *Am. J. Ophthalmol.* 90:175, 1980.

97. Frigas, E., and Reed, C. E. Effect of lodoxamide ethyl on allergy skin tests. *J. Allergy Clin. Immunol.* 65:257, 1980.

98. Fuller, R. W., and Collier, J. G. Sodium cromoglycate and atropine block the fall in FEV_1 but not the cough induced by hypotonic mist. *Thorax* 39:766, 1984.

99. Fuller, R. W., and Collier, J. G. The pharmacokinetic assessment of sodium cromoglycate. *J. Pharm. Pharmacol.* 35:289, 1983.

100. Furukawa, C. T. Anti-asthmatic agents. *Immunol. Allergy Clin. North Am.* 10(3):503, 1990.

101. Furukawa, C. T., et al. A double-blind study comparing the effectiveness of cromolyn sodium and sustained-release theophylline in childhood asthma. *Pediatrics* 74:453, 1984.
102. Godden, D., Jamieson, S., and Higenbottam, T. "Fog"-induced broncho-constriction is inhibited by sodium cromoglycate but not lignocaine or ipratropium. *Thorax* 38:226, 1988.
103. Goodman, M. L., and Irwin, J. W. Disodium cromoglycate in anaphylaxis and pollinosis. *Ann. Allergy* 40:177, 1978.
104. Gonzalez, J. P., and Brogden, R. N. Nedocromil sodium. A preliminary review of its pharmacodynamic and pharmacokinetic properties, and therapeutic efficacy in the treatment of reversible obstructive airways disease. *Drugs* 34:560, 1987.
105. Gonzalez, J. A., et al. Action of ketotifen on different functions of neutrophil polymorphonuclear cells. *Allergol. Immunopathol.* 14:215, 1986.
106. Gould, C. A. L., et al. A study of the clinical efficacy of azelastine in patients with extrinsic asthma, and its effect on airway responsiveness. *Br. J. Clin. Pharmacol.* 26:515, 1988.
107. Graff-Lonnevig, V., and Hedlin, G. The effect of ketotifen on bronchial hyperreactivity in childhood asthma. *J. Allergy Clin. Immunol.* 76:59, 1985.
108. Greenbaum, J., et al. Sodium cromoglycate in ragweed-allergic conjunctivitis. *J. Allergy Clin. Immunol.* 59:437, 1977.
109. Gross, N. J. Allergy to laboratory animals: epidemiologic, clinical and physiologic aspects, and a trial of cromolyn in its management. *J. Allergy Clin. Immunol.* 66:158, 1980.
110. Hambleton, G., et al. Comparison of cromoglycate (cromolyn) and theophylline in controlling symptoms of chronic asthma. *Lancet* 1:381, 1977.
111. Hamilos, D. L., and Nealy, T. Adjunctive treatment of severe steroid-dependent asthmatics with ketotifen (Zaditen^R). *Immunol. Allergy Prac.* 12:252/9, 1990.
112. Handelman, N. I., et al. Cromolyn sodium nasal solution in the prophylactic treatment of pollen-induced seasonal allergic rhinitis. *J. Allergy Clin. Immunol.* 59:237, 1977.
113. Harries, M. G. Bronchial irritant receptors and a possible new action for cromolyn sodium. *Ann. Allergy* 46:156, 1981.
114. Hasham, F., Kennedy, J. D., and Jones, R. S. Actions of salbutamol, disodium cromoglycate, and placebo administered as aerosols in acute asthma. *Arch. Dis. Child.* 56:722, 1981.
115. Heatley, R. V., Calcraft, B. J., and Fifield, R. Immunoglobulin E in rectal mucosa of patients with proctitis. *Lancet* 2:1010, 1975.
116. Henriksen, J. M. Effect of nedocromil sodium on exercise-induced bronchoconstriction in children. *Allergy* 43:449, 1988.
117. Holgate, S. T. Clinical evaluation of nedocromil sodium in asthma. *Eur. J. Respir. Dis.* 69(suppl. 147):149, 1986.
118. Holgate, S. T., and Finnerty, J. P. Antihistamines in asthma. *J. Allergy Clin. Immunol.* 83:537, 1989.
119. Howarth, P. H., et al. Influence of albuterol, cromolyn sodium and ipratropium bromide on the airway and circulating mediator responses to allergen bronchial provocation in asthma. *Am. Rev. Respir. Dis.* 132:986, 1985.
120. Hughes, D. T. D. Anti-allergic drugs in the treatment of asthma. *Prog. Respir. Res.* 14:176, 1980.
121. Huston, D. P., et al. Prevention of mast-cell degranulation by ketotifen in patients with physical urticarias. *Ann. Intern. Med.* 104:507, 1986.
122. Hyde, J. S., and Floro, L. D. Pros and cons of cromolyn sodium prophylaxis. *Clin. Pediatr.* 12:525, 1973.
123. Israel, E., et al. The effects of a 5-lipoxygenase inhibitor on asthma induced by cold, dry air. *N. Engl. J. Med.* 323:1740, 1990.
124. Iwata, M., et al. Effect of azelastine, an antiasthmatic drug, on bronchial responsiveness in patients with bronchial asthma. *Chest* 95:1231, 1989.
125. Jackson, D. M., and Eady, R. P. Acute transient SO_2-induced airway hyperreactivity: effects of nedocromil sodium. *J. Appl. Physiol.* 65(3):1119, 1988.
126. Jackson, D. M., and Eady, R. P. Monkeys infected with *Ascaris suum* (a new *in vitro* model of airway disease): protective effect of nedocromil sodium and sodium cromoglycate against bronchial antigen challenge. *Eur. J. Respir. Dis.* 69(S147):202, 1986.
127. Johnson, H. G. New anti-allergy drugs—the lodoxamides. *TIPS* August, 1980. P. 343.
128. Johnson, H. G., and Sheridan, A. Q. The characterization of lodoxamide, a very active inhibitor of mediator release, in animal and human models of asthma. *Agents Actions* 18:301, 1986.
129. Johnson, H. G., VanHout, C. A., and Wright, J. B. Inhibition of allergic reactions by cromoglycate and by a new anti-allergy drug U-42,585E. I. Activity in rats. *Int. Arch. Allergy Appl. Immunol.* 56:416, 1978.
130. Johnson, H. G., VanHout, C. A., and Wright, J. B. Inhibition of allergic reactions by cromoglycate and by a new anti-allergy drug U-42,585E. II. Activity in primates against aerosolized *Ascaris suum* antigen. *Int. Arch. Allergy Appl. Immunol.* 56:481, 1978.
131. Joos, G. F., Pauwels, R. A., and Van Der Straeten, M. E. Effect of nedocromil sodium on the bronchoconstrictor effect of neurokinin A in asthmatics. *Drugs* 37(S1)109, 1989.
132. Joseph, M., et al. Nedocromil sodium inhibition of IgE-mediated activation of human mononuclear phagocytes and platelets from asthmatics. *Drugs* 37(S1)32, 1989.
132a. Juniper, E. F., et al. Airway constriction by isocapnic hyperventilation of cold, dry air: comparison of magnitude and duration of protection by nedocromil sodium and sodium cromoglycate. *Clin. Allergy* 17:523, 1987.
133. Kakuta, Y., et al. Effect of ketotifen on human alveolar macrophages. *J. Allergy Clin. Immunol.* 81:469, 1988.
134. Katayama, S., et al. Effect of azelastine on the release and action of leukotriene C_4 and D_4. *Int. Arch. Allergy Appl. Immunol.* 83:284, 1987.
135. Kato, T., Terui, T., and Tagami, H. Effects of HC 20-511 (ketotifen) on chemoluminescence of human neutrophils. *Inflammation* 9:45, 1985.
136. Keller, A. M., et al. Acute reoxygenation injury in the isolated rat heart: role of resident cardiac mast cells. *Circ. Res.* 63:1044, 1988.
137. Kettelhut, B. V., et al. A double-blind, placebo-controlled, crossover trial of ketotifen versus hydroxyzine in the treatment of pediatric mastocytosis. *J. Allergy Clin. Immunol.* 83:866, 1989.
138. Kitamura, S., Ishihara, Y., and Jakalen, F. Effect of disodium cromoglycate on the action of bronchoactive agents in guinea pig tracheal strips. *Arzneimittelforschung* 34:1002, 1984.
139. Kray, K. T., et al. Cromolyn sodium in seasonal allergic conjunctivitis. *J. Allergy Clin. Immunol.* 76:623, 1985.
140. Krell, R. D., and Chakrin, L. W. An *in vitro* model of canine immediate-type hypersensitivity reactions. *Int. Arch. Allergy Appl. Immunol.* 51:641, 1976.
141. Lal, S., et al. An open assessment study of the acceptability, tolerability and safety of nedocromil sodium in long-term clinical use in patients with perennial asthma. *Eur. J. Respir. Dis.* 69(S147):136, 1986.
142. Lane, D. J. A steroid sparing effect of ketotifen in steroid-dependent asthmatics. *Clin. Allergy* 10:519, 1980.
143. Larson, S. Mast cells in interstitial cystitis. *Br. J. Urol.* 54:283, 1987.
144. Latimer, K. M., et al. Bronchoconstriction stimulated by airway cooling. *Am. Rev. Respir. Dis.* 128:440, 1983.
145. Lebel, B., et al. Spontaneous and non-specific release of histamine and PGD_2 by bronchoalveolar lavage cells from asthmatic and normal subjects: effect of nedocromil sodium. *Clin. Allergy* 18:605, 1988.
146. Lecks, H. I. Appraisals of cromolyn sodium and corticosteroids in the treatment of the asthmatic child. *Clin. Pediatr.* 16:861, 1977.
147. Leino, M., et al. Double-blind group comparative study of 2% nedocromil sodium eye drops with placebo eye drops in the treatment of seasonal allergic conjunctivitis. *Ann. Allergy* 64:398, 1990.
148. Lemire, I., et al. Effect of sodium cromoglycate on histamine inhalation tests. *J. Allergy Clin. Immunol.* 73:234, 1984.
149. Leung, K. B. P., et al. Effects of sodium cromoglycate and nedocromil sodium on histamine secretion from human lung mast cells. *Thorax* 43:756, 1988.
150. Leung, K. B. P., et al. A comparison of nedocromil sodium and sodium cromoglycate on human lung mast cells obtained by bronchoalveolar lavage and by dispersion of lung fragments. *Eur. J. Respir. Dis.* 69(S247):223, 1986.
151. Lichtenstein, L. M., and Gillespie, E. The effect of the H_1 and H_2 antihistamines on "allergic" histamine release and its inhibition by histamine. *J. Pharmacol. Exp. Ther.* 192:441, 1975.
152. Lindau, M., and Fernandez, J. M. IgE-mediated degranulation of mast cells does not require opening of ion channels. *Nature* 319:950, 1986.
153. Lisboa, C., et al. Acute effect of ketotifen on the dose-response curve of histamine and methacholine in asthma. *Br. J. Dis. Chest* 79:235, 1985.
154. Lopez, M., and Bloch, K. J. Effect of disodium cromoglycate on certain passive cutaneous anaphylactic reactions. *J. Immunol.* 103:1428, 1969.
155. Lozewicz, S., et al. Allergen-induced changes in the nasal mucous membrane in seasonal allergic rhinitis: effect of nedocromil sodium. *J. Allergy Clin. Immunol.* 85:125, 1990.
156. Lynch, M. J., et al. Xanthine oxidase inhibition attenuates ischemic-reperfusion lung injury. *J. Surg. Res.* 44:538, 1988.
157. Magnussen, H., The inhibitory effect of azelastine and ketotifen on histamine-induced bronchoconstriction in asthmatic patients. *Chest* 91:855, 1987.
158. Mallet, A. I., et al. The effect of disodium cromoglycate and ketotifen on

the excretion of histamine and N-methylimidazole acetic acid in urine of patients with mastocytosis. *Br. J. Clin. Pharmacol.* 27:88, 1989.

159. Mani, V., Lloyd, G., and Green, F. H. Y. Treatment of ulcerative colitis with oral disodium cromoglycate. A double-blind controlled trial. *Lancet* 2:439, 1979.

160. Mann, J. S., et al. Inhaled lodoxamide tromethamine in the treatment of perennial asthma: a double-blind placebo-controlled study. *J. Allergy Clin. Immunol.* 76:83, 1985.

161. Manning, P. J., et al. Inhibition of exercise-induced bronchoconstriction by MIC-571, a potent leukotriene D$_4$-receptor antagonists. *N. Engl. J. Med.* 323:1736, 1990.

162. Marquette, C. H., et al. The abnormal *in vitro* response to aspirin of platelets from aspirin-sensitive asthmatics is inhibited after inhalation of nedocromil sodium but not of sodium cromoglycate. *Br. J. Clin. Pharmacol.* 29:525, 1990.

162a. Masuo, M., Shimada, T., and Kitazawa, T. Mechanism of inhibitory effects of azelastine on smooth muscle contraction. *J. Pharm. Exp. Ther.* 260:1300, 1992.

163. Mattoli, S., et al. Effects of two doses of cromolyn on allergen-induced late asthmatic response and increased responsiveness. *J. Allergy Clin. Immunol.* 79:747, 1987.

164. Mazurek, N., Baskin, P., and Pecht, I. Isolation of a basophilic membrane protein binding the anti-allergic drug cromolyn. *E.M.B.O. J.* 1:585, 1982.

165. Mazurek, N., Geller-Bernstein, C., and Pecht, I. Affinity of calcium ions to the anti-allergic drug, cromoglycate. *FEBS Lett.* 111:194, 1980.

166. Mazurek, N., et al. Basophil variants with impaired cromoglycate binding do not respond to an immunological degranulation stimulus. *Nature* 303: 528, 1983.

167. Mazurek, N., et al. A binding site on mast cells and basophils for the antiallergic drug cromolyn. *Nature* 286:722, 1980.

168. Mazurek, N., et al. The role of the Fc receptor in calcium channel opening in rat basophilic leukemia cells. *Immunol. Lett.* 12:31, 1986.

169. McClean, S. P., et al. Refractory cholinergic urticaria successfully treated with ketotifen. *J. Allergy Clin. Immunol.* 83:738, 1989.

170. McClellan, M. D., Wanger, J. S., and Cherniack, R. M. Attenuation of the metabisulfite-induced bronchoconstrictive response by pretreatment with cromolyn. *Chest* 97:826, 1990.

171. McLean, W. L., et al. Cromolyn treatment of asthmatic children. *Am. J. Dis. Child.* 125:332, 1973.

172. McTavish, D., and Sorkin, E. M. Azelastine: a review of its pharmacodynamic and pharmacokinetic properties and therapeutic potential. *Drugs* 38(5):778, 1989.

173. Medici, T. C., Radielovic, P., and Morley, J. Ketotifen in the prophylaxis of extrinsic bronchial asthma. *Chest* 96:1252, 1989.

174. Meisler, D. M., Zaret, C. R., and Stock, E. L. Trantas dots and limbal inflammation associated with soft contact lens wear. *Am. J. Ophthal.* 89: 66, 1980.

175. Meisler, D. M., et al. Cromolyn treatment of giant papillary conjunctivitis. *Arch. Ophthalmol.* 100:1608, 1982.

176. Mellon, M. H., Karden, K., and Zeiger, R. S. The effectiveness and safety of nebulizer cromolyn solution in the young childhood asthmatic. *Immunol. Allergy Pract.* 4(5):36/168, 1982.

177. Mesa, M. G., and Valmana, M. de L. A. Effect of ketotifen and disodium cromoglycate on human platelet aggregation. *Allergol. Immunopathol.* 17:33, 1989.

178. Middleton, E. Jr., Drzewiecki, G., and Kirshnanov, D. Quercetin: an inhibitor of antigen-induced human basophil histamine release. *J. Immunol.* 127:546, 1981.

179. Middleton, E. Jr., and Drzewiecki, G. Effects of flavonoids and transitional metal cations on antigen-induced histamine release from human basophils. *Biochem. Pharmacol.* 31:1449, 1982.

180. Mielens, F. E., Ferguson, E. W., and Rosenberg, F. J. Effects of anti-anaphylactic drugs upon passive antibodies in rats. *Int. Arch. Allergy Appl. Immunol.* 47:633, 1974.

181. Moqbel, R., et al. Enhancement of leukocyte cytotoxicity after exercise-induced asthma. *Am. Rev. Respir. Dis.* 133:609, 1986.

182. Moqbel, R., et al. Effects of nedocromil sodium (Tilade^R) on the activation of human eosinophils and neutrophils and the release of histamine from mast cells. *Allergy* 43:268, 1988.

183. Moqbel, R., et al. Enhanced neutrophil and monocytotoxicity after exercise-induced asthma. *Thorax* 40:218, 1985.

184. Moran, F., Bankier, J. D. H., and Boyd, G. Disodium cromoglycate in the treatment of allergic bronchial asthma. *Lancet* 2:137, 1968.

185. Morris, E. C. Pharmacotherapy of allergic disease. *Primary Care* 14:605, 1987.

186. Murphy, S. Cromolyn sodium: basic mechanisms and clinical usage. *Pediatr. Asthma Allergy Immunol.* 2:237, 1988.

187. Murphy, S., and Kelly, H. W. Cromolyn sodium: a review of mechanisms and clinical use in asthma. *Drug Intell. Clin. Pharmacol.* 21:22, 1987.

188. Myers, D. J., Bigby, B. G., and Boushey, H. A. The inhibition of sulfur dioxide–induced bronchoconstriction in asthmatic subjects by cromolyn is dose dependent. *Am. Rev. Respir. Dis.* 133:1150, 1986.

189. Nair, N., Hopp, R. J., and Townley, R. Effect of nedocromil on antigen-induced bronchoconstriction in asthmatic subjects. *Ann. Allergy* 62:329, 1989.

190. Nakamura, T., et al. Effect of azelastine on the intracellular Ca^{2+} mobilization in guinea pig peritoneal macrophages. *Eur. J. Pharmacol.* 148:35, 1988.

191. Neher, E. The influence of intracellular calcium concentration of dialyzed mast cells from rat peritoneum. *J. Physiol.* 395:193, 1988.

192. Nelson, B. L., and Jacobs, R. L. Response of the nonallergic rhinitis with eosinophilia (NARES) syndrome to 4% cromolyn sodium nasal solution. *J. Allergy Clin. Immunol.* 70:125, 1982.

193. Neuman, I., and Lutsky, I. Laboratory animal dander allergy: II. Clinical studies and the potential protective effect of disodium cromoglycate. *Ann. Allergy* 36:23, 1976.

194. Nishihira, J., et al. Effect of azelastine on leukotriene synthesis in murine peritoneal cells and on thromboxane synthesis in human platelets. *Int. Arch. Allergy Appl. Immunol.* 90:285, 1989.

195. Ollier, S., et al. The effect of lodoxamide tromethamine on the immediate asthmatic response to allergen provocation. *Clin. Allergy* 12:587, 1982.

196. Ostler, H. B. Acute chemotic reaction to cromolyn. *Arch. Ophthalmol.* 100:412, 1982.

197. Patel, K. R., Berkin, K. E., and Kerr, J. W. Dose-response study of sodium cromoglycate in exercise-induced asthma. *Thorax* 37:663, 1982.

198. Pauwels, R., Joos, G., and Van Der Straeten, M. Effect of nedocromil sodium on bronchoconstriction induced by adenosine and tachykinins. *Drugs* 37(S1):87, 1989.

199. Pearce, F. L., Befus, A. D., and Bienenstock, J. Mucosal mast cells. *J. Allergy Clin. Immunol.* 73:819, 1984.

200. Perper, R. J., Oronsky, A. L., and Blancuzzi, V. An analysis of the specificity in pharmacological inhibition of the passive cutaneous anaphylaxis reaction in mice and rats. *Int. Arch. Allergy Appl. Immunol.* 193:594, 1975.

201. Petty, T. L., et al. Cromolyn sodium is effective in adult chronic asthmatics. *Am. Rev. Respir. Dis.* 139:694, 1989.

202. Phillips, G. D., et al. Effect of nedocromil sodium and sodium cromoglycate against bronchoconstriction induced by inhaled adenosine 5'-monophosphate. *Eur. Respir. J.* 2:210, 1989.

203. Pichurko, B. M., et al. Influence of cromolyn sodium on airway temperature in normal subjects. *Am. Rev. Respir. Dis.* 130:1002, 1984.

204. Polson, J. B., et al. Effects of ketotifen on the responsiveness of peripheral blood lymphocyte β-adrenergic receptors. *Br. J. Immunopharmacol.* 10: 657, 1988.

205. Prenner, B. M. Safety, efficacy and bronchodilator sparing effects of nebulized cromolyn sodium solution in the treatment of asthma in children. *Ann. Allergy* 49:186, 1982.

206. Rackham, A., et al. A Canadian multicenter study with zaditen (ketotifen) in the treatment of bronchial asthma in children aged 5 to 17 years. *J. Allergy Clin. Immunol.* 84:286, 1989.

207. Rafferty, P., et al. The *in vivo* potency and selectivity of azelastine as an H$_1$ histamine-receptor antagonist in human airways and skin. *J. Allergy Clin. Immunol.* 82:1113, 1988.

208. Rafferty, P., et al. The inhibitory actions of azelastine hydrochloride on the early and late bronchoconstrictor responses to inhaled allergen in atopic asthma. *J. Allergy Clin. Immunol.* 84:649, 1989.

209. Rainey, D. K. Nedocromil sodium (Tilade^R): a review of preclinical studies. *Eur. Respir. J.* 2(6):561s, 1989.

210. Rebuck, A. S., et al. A 3-month evaluation of the efficacy of nedocromil sodium in asthma: a randomized, double-blind, placebo-controlled trial of nedocromil sodium conducted by a Canadian multicenter study group. *J. Allergy Clin. Immunol.* 85:612, 1990.

211. Reques, F. G., et al. Long-term modification on histamine-induced bronchoconstriction by disodium cromoglycate and ketotifen versus placebo. *Allergy* 40:242, 1985.

212. Riccardi, V. M. Mast cell stabilization to decrease neurofibroma growth. *Arch. Dermatol.* 123:1011, 1987.

213. Rice, N. S. C., et al. Vernal kerato-conjunctivitis and its management. *Trans. Ophthalmol. Soc. U.K.* 91:483, 1971.

214. Ross, R. N., et al. Cost-effectiveness of including cromolyn sodium in the

treatment program for asthma: a retrospective, record-based study. *Clin. Ther.* 10:187, 1988.

215. Ruggieri, F., and Patalano, F. Nedocromil sodium: a review of clinical studies. *Eur. Respir. J.* 2:568s, 1989.

216. Ruhno, J., Denburg, J., and Dolovich, J. Intranasal nedocromil sodium in the treatment of ragweed-allergic rhinitis. *J. Allergy Clin. Immunol.* 81: 570, 1988.

217. Ryo, U. Y., Kang, B., and Townley, R. G. Cromolyn therapy in patients with bronchial asthma. *JAMA* 236:927, 1976.

218. Sanguinetti, C. M., et al. Exercise-induced asthma diagnosis and prevention with a metered dose aerosol formulation of sodium cromoglycate. *Respiration* 43:132, 1982.

219. Schill, W.-B., Schneider, J., and Ring, J. The use of ketotifen, a mast cell blocker, for treatment of oligo- and asthenozoospermia. *Andrologia* 18: 570, 1986.

220. Schirmer, W. J., et al. Allopurinol and lodoxamide in complement-induced hepatic ischemia. *J. Surg. Res.* 45:28, 1988.

221. Schwartz, H. J. The effect of cromolyn on nasal disease. *Ear, Nose, Throat J.* 65:449/15, 1986.

222. Sekardi, L., and Friedberg, K. D. Inhibition of immunological histamine release from guinea pig lungs and other organs by mepyramine, ketotifen, and picumast *in vivo*. *Drug Res.* 39:1331, 1989.

223. Shapiro, G. G., and Konig, P. Cromolyn sodium: a review. *Pharmacotherapy* 5:156, 1985.

224. Shapiro, G. G., et al. Double-blind evaluation of nebulized cromolyn, terbutaline, and the combination for childhood asthma. *J. Allergy Clin. Immunol.* 81:449, 1988.

225. Shaw, R. J., and Kay, A. B. Nedocromil, a mucosal and connective tissue mast cell stabilizer, inhibits exercise-induced asthma. *Br. J. Dis. Chest* 79:385, 1985.

226. Sheppard, D., Nadel, J. A., and Boushey, H. A. Inhibition of sulfur dioxide–induced bronchoconstriction by disodium cromoglycate in asthmatic subjects. *Am. Rev. Respir. Dis.* 124:257, 1981.

227. Sheppard, D., et al. Dose dependent inhibition of cold air-induced bronchoconstriction by atropine. *J. Appl. Physiol.* 53:196, 1982.

228. Sheppard, D., et al. Mechanism of cough and bronchoconstriction induced by distilled water aerosol. *Am. Rev. Respir. Dis.* 127:691, 1983.

229. Sly, R. M., et al. Position statement: the use of antihistamine in patients with asthma. *J. Allergy Clin. Immunol.* 82:481, 1988.

230. Soter, N. A., Austen, K. F., and Wasserman, S. I. Oral disodium cromoglycate in the treatment of systemic mastocytosis. *N. Engl. J. Med.* 301:465, 1979.

231. Soto, J., et al. Effect of ketotifen on the distribution and degranulation of uterine eosinophils in estrogen-treated rats. *Agents Actions* 28:198, 1989.

232. Springer, C., et al. Clinical, physiologic, and psychologic comparison of treatment by cromolyn or theophylline in childhood asthma. *J. Allergy Clin. Immunol.* 76:64, 1985.

233. St-Pierre, J. P., Kobric, M., and Rackham, A. Effect of ketotifen treatment on cold-induced urticaria. *Ann. Allergy* 55:840, 1985.

234. Svendsen, U. G., et al. A comparison of the effects of sodium cromoglycate and beclomethasone dipropionate on pulmonary function and bronchial hyperreactivity in subjects with asthma. *J. Allergy Clin. Immunol.* 80:68, 1987.

235. Theoharides, T. C., et al. Antiallergic drug cromolyn may inhibit histamine secretion by regulating phosphorylation of a mast cell protein. *Science* 207:80, 1980.

236. Thorel, T., et al. Inhibition by nedocromil sodium of IgE-mediated activation of human mononuclear phagocytes and platelets in allergy. *Int. Arch. Allergy Appl. Immunol* 85:232, 1988.

237. Tinkelman, D. G., et al. A multicenter trial of the prophylactic effect of ketotifen, theophylline and placebo in atopic asthma. *J. Allergy Clin. Immunol.* 76:487, 1985.

238. Togias, A. G., et al. Demonstration of inhibition of mediator release from human mast cells by azatadine base. *JAMA* 255:225, 1986.

239. Tossin, L., et al. Ketotifen does not inhibit asthmatic reactions induced by toluene diisocyanate in sensitized subjects. *Clin. Exp. Allergy* 19:177, 1989.

240. Turner-Warwick, N., and Batten, J. L. Long-term study of disodium cromoglycate in treatment of severe extrinsic or intrinsic bronchial asthma in adults. *Br. Med. J.* 4:383, 1972.

241. Ungerer, R. G., et al. Effect of inhaled lodoxamide tromethamine in prevention of antigen-induced bronchospasm. *J. Allergy Clin. Immunol.* 68: 471, 1981.

242. v. Wichert, P. Ketotifen, an anti-allergic drug: pharmacological figures and clinical experience. *Prog. Respir. Res.* 14:181, 1980.

243. Volovitz, B., et al. Efficacy and safety of ketotifen in young children with asthma. *J. Allergy Clin. Immunol.* 81:526, 1988.

244. Walker, M., Harley, R., and Leroy, E. C. Ketotifen prevents skin fibrosis in the tight skin mouse. *J. Rheumatol.* 17:57, 1990.

245. Watt, G. D., et al. Protective effect of lodoxamide tromethamine on allergen inhalation challenge. *J. Allergy Clin. Immunol.* 66:286, 1980.

246. Wells, E., and Mann, J. Phosphorylation of a mast cell protein in response to treatment with anti-allergic compounds. *Biochem. Pharmacol.* 32:837, 1983.

247. Wells, P. W., and Eyre, P. The pharmacology of passive cutaneous anaphylaxis in the calf. *Can. J. Physiol. Pharmacol.* 50:255, 1972.

248. Welsh, P. W., et al. Topical ocular administration of cromolyn sodium for treatment in seasonal ragweed conjunctivitis. *J. Allergy Clin. Immunol.* 64:209, 1979.

249. Welsh, P. W., et al. Preseasonal IgE ragweed antibody level as a predictor of response to therapy of ragweed hay fever with intranasal cromolyn sodium solution. *J. Allergy Clin. Immunol.* 60:104, 1977.

250. Yoshida, H., et al. Clinical evaluation of ketotifen syrup on atopic dermatitis: a comparative multicenter double-blind study of ketotifen and clemastine. *Ann. Allergy* 62:507, 1989.

251. Zvaifler, N. J., Bauer, H., and Robinson, J. O. IgE Immunoglobulin in the Rabbit. In K. F. Austen and E. L. Becker (eds.), *Biochemistry of the Acute Allergic Reactions*. Oxford: Oxford University Press, 1971.

Anticholinergic Agents

Nicholas J. Gross

64

The anticholinergic alkaloids such as atropine, which exist in many plants, have been used in herbal remedies for the treatment of respiratory disorders in many traditional medical cultures for many centuries [12]. They were brought to Europe in the early 1800s and rapidly gained enormous popularity as bronchodilators, a position they maintained until well into the present century. When epinephrine was discovered in the 1920s, followed soon by ephedrine, other adrenergic drugs, and then methylxanthines, their use declined. The reasons for their declining popularity at that time included their multiple side effects, together with the fact that they were less effective bronchodilators in asthmatic patients than were the newer agents. Interest in their use has returned with better understanding of the role of cholinergic mechanisms in the control of airway caliber, and the development of synthetic congeners of natural anticholinergic agents that are topically active but much less prone to side effects [20].

RATIONALE FOR THE USE OF ANTICHOLINERGIC BRONCHODILATORS

Anatomy of Airway Autonomic Nerves

In the normal human airways, the bulk of efferent autonomic nerves are branches of the vagus nerve that supply parasympathetic, cholinergic innervation to the airways [27, 44, 45] (Fig. 64-1). Fibers from the vagus nerve enter the lung at the hila and travel along the airways, branching with them and synapsing at peribronchial ganglia that are distributed predominantly among larger airways. Short postganglionic fibers travel from the ganglia to smooth muscle cells, pulmonary arterioles, mucous glands, and possibly ciliated epithelial cells. Acetylcholine released from varicosities and terminals of the postganglionic nerves activates muscarinic receptors on these structures. This results in smooth muscle contraction, liberation of mucus from mucous glands, and, possibly, acceleration of ciliary beating. A low level of cholinergic vagal activity (bronchomotor tone) can be recorded in the normal resting state in experimental animals, but can be considerably augmented in response to stimuli (discussed later) (see also Chap. 17).

Anticholinergic agents compete with acetylcholine at muscarinic receptors. The rationale for their use as bronchodilators, then, is that they inhibit the cholinergic activity responsible for bronchomotor tone and this allows the airways to dilate. They do not inhibit other mechanisms or mediators that may cause airway smooth muscle contraction, nor, indeed, do they affect the numerous other mechanisms of airway obstruction in abnormal states such as asthma.

The small proportion of other efferent autonomic nerves in humans includes branches of the third nervous system, the so-called nonadrenergic, noncholinergic or purinergic system, and branches of the sympathetic system (see Chap. 18). Both of these systems are inhibitory to smooth muscle cells, in that they counteract smooth muscle contraction and have a bronchodilatory effect. However, only those fibers of the third nervous system are believed to end close to smooth muscle cells in humans. Their mediators are believed to be vasoactive intestinal peptide and peptide histidine methionine. There is some evidence that these mediators are released from the same terminals as acetylcholine. This system may be the principal opposition to cholinergic bronchoconstriction. Fibers of the beta-sympathetic system do not end on the smooth muscle cells in humans; instead, they terminate on the peribronchial ganglion cells where they may exert a modulating, inhibitory effect on parasympathetic activity. In addition, there are beta$_2$ receptors on smooth muscle cells through which catecholamines and adrenergic therapy may act.

Vagal Reflexes in Airways

Reflex-mediated bronchoconstriction has been extensively studied in animal models [35, 59]. Two reflex mechanisms have been postulated; a spinal reflex and an axon reflex. In the spinal reflex, a cholinergic bronchomotor activity can be reflexly augmented by a number of stimuli (Fig. 64-2). The territory from which reflex bronchoconstriction can arise is broad and probably includes, in addition to the upper and lower airways, the esophagus and the carotid bodies. Receptors through which the reflex acts include the rapidly adapting irritant receptors and nonmyelinated C fibers, both of which are found in the airway epithelium. The stimuli to which they respond and which result in bronchoconstriction include mechanical irritation, a wide variety of irritant gases, aerosols, and particles of many sorts, and, to some extent, the inhalation of cold dry air and specific mediators such as histamine. Impulses originating from the receptors travel in afferent vagal nerves to the central nervous system (CNS) and back to the lungs in vagal efferents, resulting in bronchoconstriction that occurs in less than 1 second.

A solid body of research derived from elegant physiologic studies, mostly in animals, indicates that bronchoconstriction can be mediated through such vagal reflex mechanisms. However, the extent to which such reflex mechanisms actually contribute to airflow limitation in patients with airways disease is not at all clear. As vagally mediated bronchoconstriction can be entirely ablated by anticholinergic agents and as anticholinergic agents rarely entirely reverse airflow obstruction in any airways disease, one assumes that vagal activity rarely accounts for more than part of the pathophysiology of airflow limitation. This part may be the only reversible component in patients with emphysema, in which airflow obstruction is due mainly to structural damage [21], but it may be a trivial component in diseases such as asthma, in which airflow obstruction is largely due to inflammation. Inflammatory mechanisms can be mitigated by antiinflam-

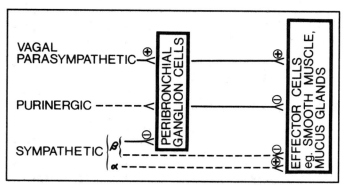

Fig. 64-1. *Diagrammatic representation of efferent autonomic innervation in human airways.* + = *excitatory;* − = *inhibitory;* dashed line = *existence doubtful. (Reprinted with permission from N. J. Gross and M. S. Skorodin, Anticholinergic, antimuscarinic bronchodilators. Am. Rev. Respir. Dis. 129:856, 1984.)*

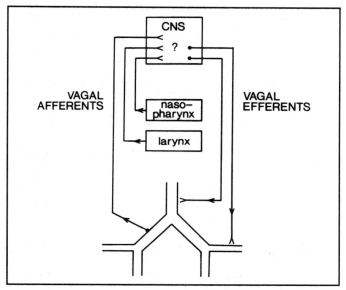

Fig. 64-2. *Diagrammatic representation of vagal reflex pathways from irritant receptors through vagal afferents, central nervous system (CNS), and vagal efferents to effector cells in the airways. (Reprinted with permission from N. J. Gross and M. S. Skorodin, Anticholinergic, antimuscarinic bronchodilators. Am. Rev. Respir. Dis. 129:856, 1984.)*

matory therapy and to some extent by beta-adrenergic agents, but are not amenable to anticholinergic therapy, except to the extent (probably minor) that they are due to cholinergic activity. One might predict from this that anticholinergic agents would be less useful in the treatment of airways inflammation, i.e., asthma, than in the management of chronic bronchitis and emphysema, as is shown later.

A second reflex bronchoconstrictor mechanism is the axon reflex [1]. Activation of airway receptors may release substance P, calcitonin gene-related peptide, and other neurokinins by an antidromic mechanism. The importance of these mechanisms in humans with airways disease is uncertain.

Muscarinic Receptor Subtypes

Muscarinic receptors are a family of polypeptides that have membrane-based ion-channel, phosphoinositol activation, and G-protein activation activities [18]. It has recently become clear that there are numerous muscarinic receptor subtypes, each with

specific properties relating to the above actions. The application of molecular biology has revealed that there are possibly as many as nine muscarinic receptor genes, raising the possibility of this number of unique receptor subtypes, called M_1, M_2, and so on. Three of these are believed to operate in human airways [18]. A detailed discussion of the material is presented in Chapter 16. However, two points are relevant here. One is that airway muscarinic receptors are distributed preferentially in larger airways [2], which corresponds to the distribution of vagal parasympathetic nerves. This implies that the bronchodilator action of anticholinergic agents will also be concentrated on the larger airways.

The second point is that cholinergic activity seems to be inhibited when the M_1 and M_3 receptors (present in peribronchial ganglia and on smooth muscle cells, respectively) are selectively inhibited. Inhibition of the M_2 receptor, which is an autoreceptor, might be expected to augment cholinergic bronchomotor activity. None of the anticholinergic agents that are currently available for clinical use are selective for these subtypes; instead they inhibit all three subtypes. It is possible that inhibitors selective for M_1 and M_3, but not for M_2, for example, have greater bronchodilator potential than all currently available agents. Another approach under consideration is to develop a tertiary ammonium inhibitor that is selective for M_3 receptors and that could be taken by mouth.

ACTION OF ANTICHOLINERGIC AGENTS

Cholinergic Control of Airway Functions

Cholinergic fibers mediate at least three functions in the airways: They promote airway smooth muscle contraction, promote the release of secretions from submucosal glands, and augment the ciliary activity of epithelial cells, although there is some question regarding this last activity [36]. Possibly their most important action is their effect on airway smooth muscle—bronchomotor tone, as discussed earlier—inhibition of which is the principal rationale for administering anticholinergic agents as bronchodilators. They increase airflow even in normal subjects [19]. There is some evidence that basal cholinergic tone is increased in both asthma [48] and chronic obstructive pulmonary disease (COPD) [19], which, if correct, provides additional rationales for using anticholinergic agents in these conditions.

Airway secretion occurring under basal conditions appears not to be inhibitable by anticholinergic agents. However, the augmentation of secretions (such as may occur in asthma) appears to be inhibitable by atropine-like agents [15]. Ciliary activity may follow a similar pattern. The therapeutic role of anticholinergic agents in inhibiting these latter two actions in airways disease, in particular whether it might be beneficial or harmful, is unclear. (See also Chapters 29, 52, and 69.)

Site of Bronchodilatation

When administered systemically, the principal physiologic action of anticholinergic agents tends to be more on central airways as compared to the action of adrenergic bronchodilators [20]. This site conforms to the distribution of both cholinergic nerve terminals and muscarinic receptors in the airways (discussed earlier). Current practice, however, favors the aerosol administration of bronchodilators. When administered by the inhalational route all bronchodilators tend to be preferentially delivered to the larger central airways. Consequently, the site of action of inhaled anticholinergic and alternative bronchodilators is predominantly central. The site of action is not distinguishably different for these different classes of agents.

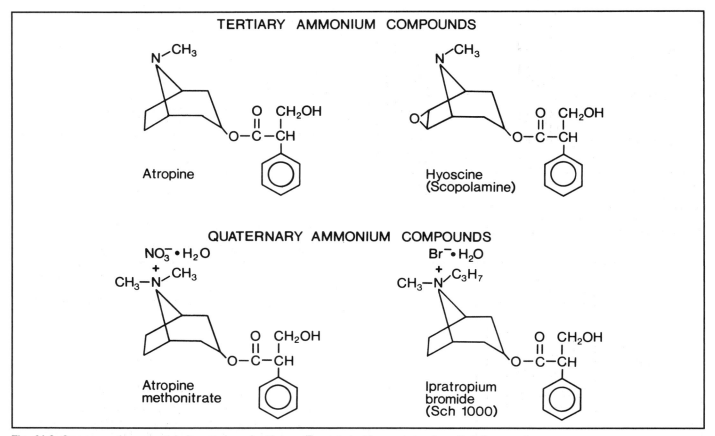

Fig. 64-3. *Structures of some anticholinergic bronchodilators. (Reprinted with permission from N. J. Gross and M. S. Skorodin, Anticholinergic, antimuscarinic bronchodilators. Am. Rev. Respir. Dis. 129:856, 1984.)*

PHARMACOLOGY OF ANTICHOLINERGIC AGENTS

Atropine is the prototype of antimuscarinic agents and is highly selective for muscarinic receptors, although not selective among muscarinic receptor subtypes. Although their chemical structures vary, both agonists and antagonists for muscarinic receptors have an ammonium group and an ester linkage 4.3 to 4.4 Å apart that are essential for binding to the receptor.

Atropine, scopolamine, and all other naturally occurring anticholinergic alkaloids are tertiary ammonium compounds; the nitrogen atom on the tropine ring is 3-valent (Fig. 64-3). The salts of these bases, such as atropine sulfate, are freely water- and lipid-soluble and are well absorbed from mucosal surfaces [23]. Consequently, they are orally active and widely distributed in the body. They counteract parasympathetic, cholinergic activity in almost every system and result in widespread systemic effects. They cross the blood-brain barrier and so also have CNS effects. The dose required for bronchodilatation, 1.0 to 2.5 mg in adults, is sufficient to produce subjective effects in other organs (discussed later). In only slightly higher doses, their effects can be troublesome. Although these effects are rarely dangerous, the therapeutic margin of natural atropine-like agents is thus small.

Pharmaceutical chemists have developed quaternary ammonium anticholinergic agents such as ipratropium bromide in which these side effects are minimal (see Fig. 64-3). In quaternary congeners of atropine, the nitrogen atom in the tropine ring is 5-valent and carries a charge, making the molecule virtually incapable of absorption from mucosal surfaces. Quaternary agents are fully anticholinergic at the site of deposition and will, for example, dilate the pupil if delivered to the eye, or dilate

the bronchi if delivered to the airways. They are not sufficiently absorbed from these sites, however, to produce detectable effects on other organs. They can thus be regarded as topical forms of atropine.

Anticholinergic agents available in the United States include atropine sulfate USP; ipratropium bromide (Atrovent), which has been in use in Europe for about 15 years and in the United States for about 6 years; and glycopyrrolate bromide (Robinul), which has not been approved for respiratory use. Other synthetic quaternary anticholinergic agents include oxitropium bromide (Oxivent), which has recently been made available in some countries in Europe and elsewhere, and atropine methonitrate, both of which are under investigation (Table 64-1).

Atropine and its naturally occurring congeners exist in two optical isomers. Both are present in equal proportions in available preparations but only one of these is pharmacologically active. Synthetic agents such as ipratropium are usually synthesized in the active form. This fact must be taken into account in dose-response studies.

Pharmacokinetics

Atropine sulfate administration by any route results in peak blood levels in 1 hour or less. It has a half-life in the circulation of 3 hours in adults, but longer in children and the elderly [55]. Most of the drug is recovered unchanged in the urine within 24 hours; trace amounts can be found in the feces and in the breast milk of lactating women.

Ipratropium administration by mouth or by inhalation results in very low blood levels, peaking at about 1 to 2 hours, and declining with a half-life of up to 4 hours [9]. Its biologic effect

Table 64-1. *Anticholinergic bronchodilators*

Agent	Trade name	Type	Status	Recommended dose	Duration of action (hr)
METERED-DOSE INHALERS					
Ipratropium bromide	Atrovent	Quaternary	Approved, available	2 puffs (36 μg)	5–6
Oxitropium bromide	Oxivent	Quaternary	Investigational	2 puffs (200 μg)	6–8
Atropine methylnitrate	—	Quaternary	Investigational	?	6–8?
NEBULIZABLE SOLUTIONS					
Atropine sulfate USP	—	Tertiary	Not FDA approved for respiratory use	1–2.5 mg	3–4
Ipratropium bromide	Atrovent	Quaternary	Available (Canada), pending (U.S.)	0.5 mg	4–6
Glycopyrrolate bromide	Robinul	Quaternary	Not FDA approved for respiratory use	1–2.5 mg	6–12

FDA = U.S. Food and Drug Administration.

following inhalation is somewhat longer than that of atropine, probably because it is not removed by absorption. Over 90 percent of the orally administered dose is recovered in the feces; some of the remainder is recovered in the urine as inactive metabolites. It is largely excluded from the CNS. The pharmacokinetics of other synthetic anticholinergic agents are less well known.

Dose Response

The dose response has been extensively reviewed elsewhere [23]. In brief, the optimal dose of nebulized atropine solution has been reported to be 0.025 to 0.04 mg/kg in adults and 0.05 mg/kg in children. The optimal dose of nebulized atropine methonitrate is somewhat less—0.015 to 0.02 mg/kg. The optimal dose of nebulized ipratropium in adults is about 500 μg [24]. The optimal dose of nebulized glycopyrrolate bromide is 0.02 mg/kg. These figures vary according to the severity of airways disease, and the equipment and technique used for nebulization. For metered-dose inhalers (MDIs), the optimal dose of oxitropium bromide has been reported to be 500 μg. The optimal dose of ipratropium delivered by MDI in stable young asthmatics has been variously reported to be in the region of 40 to 80 μg [23]. In stable older patients with COPD the dose response to ipratropium has not been as extensively studied; the optimal dose delivered by MDI may be as much as 160 μg [24]. It seems possible that patients with more severe airways obstruction may need higher doses because of the reduced penetration of particles into the airway tree. In view of the nonabsorbability of the quaternary forms that are now favored for use, little risk is associated with the use of higher than currently recommended doses.

Tolerance and Subsensitivity

Tachyphylaxis to beta-agonist bronchodilators has been reported, although it is not clear whether, if present, it is clinically important. By contrast, tolerance to anticholinergic agents has been repeatedly sought but not found, with one exception [54]. The general lack of tachyphylaxis to anticholinergic agents is in keeping with the concept that agonists may downregulate their receptor, or receptors, but that antagonists have no such effect. Instead, they tend, if anything, to upregulate the receptor [49]. Indeed, one study has shown that patients treated for several weeks with ipratropium developed heightened methacholine responsiveness, suggestive of upregulation [38]. One can conclude from this that tachyphylaxis or tolerance to anticholinergic bronchodilators is unlikely even with long-term administration.

EFFICACY IN ASTHMA

Efficacy Against Specific Stimuli

When given before the application of specific bronchospastic stimuli, anticholinergic agents show varying degrees of protec-

tion (Table 64-2). As would be expected, they protect more or less completely against the bronchospasm induced by cholinergic agonists such as methacholine and carbachol. They provide only partial protection against bronchospasm caused by most other specific stimuli, for example, histamine, prostaglandins, nonspecific dusts and irritant aerosols, exercise, hyperventilation, and the inhalation of cold dry air (reviewed in [20]). In many of the last three instances, adrenergic agents usually provide greater prophylaxis.

There are two interesting and potentially clinically important instances in which anticholinergic agents provide better protection against provocative stimuli—against beta-blocking agents and against psychogenic asthma. Beta-blocking agents can result in catastrophic bronchospasm in asthmatic subjects, presumably because of the inhibition of adrenergic opposition to cholinergic tone. Anticholinergic agents can both prevent beta-blocker–induced bronchospasm and reverse it when it has occurred [10, 25, 26]. Bronchospasm elicited in asthmatic subjects by the suggestion that they were inhaling an agent they believed they were allergic to was prevented by the prior administration of an anticholinergic agent [34, 37]. In another study, subjects whose asthma was considered to be in part due to psychogenic factors were more responsive to ipratropium than were subjects whose asthma was not considered to be psychogenic [42].

Stable Asthma

A very large number of studies have compared the bronchodilator actions of anticholinergic agents with those of adrenergic agents. These provide clinicians with useful information about the comparative actions of these bronchodilators in asthma. Figure 64-4, which shows a comparison typical of most such studies, illustrates many of these points [47]. Anticholinergic agents take longer to reach peak effect, typically 1 to 2 hours, than do adrenergic agents. At their peak effect, they almost invariably result in less bronchodilatation. The quaternary forms may be slightly longer-acting than agents such as salbutamol.

One could criticize most such studies on the grounds that they use recommended doses rather than optimal doses. However, the administration of large cumulative doses of ipratropium to asthmatics was found to result in bronchodilatation that could be considerably augmented by the subsequent administration of an adrenergic agent [53]. Therefore, one must conclude that anticholinergic agents are generally less potent bronchodilators than are adrenergic agents in patients with asthma.

There is among asthmatics substantial variation in responsiveness, however, with some patients responding very little to anticholinergic agents, some responding almost as well to them as to adrenergic agents, and yet others who respond poorly to adrenergic agents but respond better to an anticholinergic agent [6]. Attempts have therefore been made to identify subgroups of asthmatics who are likely to manifest the most responsiveness to anticholinergic agents. Older asthmatics (over 40 years of age)

Table 64-2. *Summary of efficacy of anticholinergic agents against specific bronchospastic stimuli*

Stimulus	Efficacy of anticholinergic agents	Efficacy of adrenergic agents relative to anticholinergic agents
Cholinergic agents	Fully protective	—
Histamine	Partially protective at most	More effective
Various mediators, $PGF_{2\alpha}$, serotonin, bradykinin	Partially protective at most	—
Beta blockade	Effective reversal	Much less effective
Gases, dust, irritants	Variable, usually some protection	—
Antigens	Variable, from none to excellent	More effective
Exercise, hyperventilation, cold air	Moderately effective, possibly more so in large doses	Invariably more effective
Psychogenic factors	Good protection	Probably less effective

$PGF_{2\alpha}$ = prostaglandin $F_{2\alpha}$.
Source: N. J. Gross and M. S. Skorodin, Anticholinergic, antimuscarinic bronchodilators. *Am. Rev. Respir. Dis.* 129:856, 1984. Reprinted with permission.

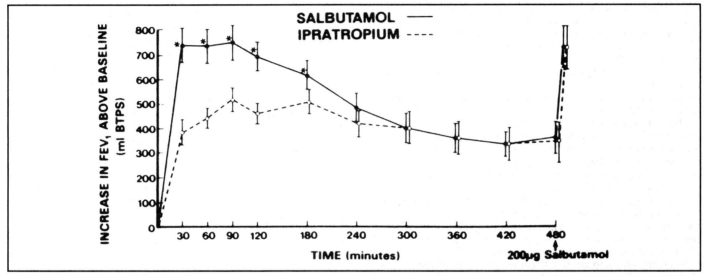

Fig. 64-4. *Increase in the forced expiratory volume at 1 second (FEV$_1$) in 25 patients with asthma after inhalation of 200 μg of salbutamol by metered-dose inhaler (MDI) or 40 μg of ipratropium by MDI on separate days. All patients received an additional dose of salbutamol at 480 minutes. Asterisks denote significant differences (p < .05). (Reprinted with permission from R. E. Ruffin, et al., Combination bronchodilator therapy in asthma. J. Allergy Clin. Immunol. 69:60, 1982.)*

may respond better than younger ones [53], although even children and adolescents aged 10 to 18 years have been shown to benefit [56]. Intrinsic asthmatics and those with a longer duration of asthma may also respond better than extrinsic or younger asthmatics [28], although these too appear to be poor predictors of successful treatment [47]. An individual trial is probably the only reliable way to identify responsiveness [4].

One therefore concludes that the most appropriate role for anticholinergic agents in the therapy of stable asthma is as an adjunct to adrenergic agents. They may provide incremental benefit in those severe asthmatics who are already receiving maximal antiinflammatory and other bronchodilator therapy [61]. A trial use of anticholinergic agents is warranted whenever asthma is poorly controlled because it is hard to predict which patients will respond well to them. They should not be regarded as first-line therapy, except in the event of acute bronchospasm provoked by inadvertent use of a beta-blocking agent or possibly in psychogenic asthma.

Acute, Severe Asthma

As acute, severe asthma is a life-threatening situation, antiinflammatory therapy, that is, corticosteroids, and optimal bronchodi-

latation are required as soon as possible. The optimal bronchodilator therapy in this serious condition has been the subject of many studies, few of them including sufficient numbers of patients to provide valid statistics. In the largest study, Rebuck and coworkers [43] found that 500 μg of nebulized ipratropium resulted in less bronchodilatation than 1.25 mg of nebulized fenoterol during the first 90 minutes of treatment of the acute attack of asthma. However, the combination of both agents was significantly more effective than either was when used alone. Moreover, patients with more severe airways obstruction obtained the greatest benefit from the combination. In contrast, Patrick and colleagues [40] found that 80 μg of ipratropium given by MDI did not augment the bronchodilatation achieved by nebulized albuterol alone. Summers and Tarala [51] were also not able to show that 0.5 mg of nebulized ipratropium solution significantly augmented the bronchodilatation achieved by 5 mg of albuterol alone.

In a similar setting, however, Gilman and coworkers [13] found no difference in the improvement in airflow resulting from 2 mg of nebulized glycopyrrolate as compared to 15 mg of nebulized metaproterenol, though they found fewer side effects in the group that received the anticholinergic agent.

In view of the danger inherent in acute, severe asthma and the safety of agents such as ipratropium and glycopyrrolate, it seems appropriate to recommend that both classes of bronchodilators be given during such attacks, particularly in the early hours of treatment and particularly in patients with more severe airflow obstruction.

CHRONIC BRONCHITIS AND EMPHYSEMA OR COPD

Stable COPD

A very large number of studies have compared the effects of anticholinergic agents with those of other bronchodilators in patients with COPD. In general, patients with COPD do not manifest as much absolute increase in airflow to any agent or combination of agents as do patients with asthma. However, almost all patients with COPD are capable of some bronchodilatation [14]. With very few exceptions, studies in patients with COPD show that the anticholinergic agent provided at least as great and prolonged an increase in airflow as other agents. Most, like the largest such study (Fig. 64-5) [52], show the anticholinergic agent to be a more potent and prolonged bronchodilator than metaproterenol. A similar result was found in a comparison between ipratropium and the most widely used beta$_2$-adrenergic bronchodilator in the United States, namely albuterol [3].

The criticism can again be made that most such studies employed recommended rather than optimal doses of bronchodilators. However, even when large cumulative doses of each agent were given, the anticholinergic agent alone achieved all the available bronchodilatation in these patients [11, 21], as shown in Figure 64-6. As this is clearly not the case in asthmatic patients (discussed earlier), there may thus be a systemic difference between asthmatic and COPD patients with respect to their responsiveness to different bronchodilator agents. The difference between asthmatics and bronchitics is illustrated by a number of studies in which patients with asthma were compared to those with COPD who had similar baseline airflows. All such studies showed results similar to those exemplified in Figure 64-7 [31]. This figure shows that the combination of fenoterol and theophylline resulted in more bronchodilatation than did ipratropium in the asthmatic group, but that ipratropium resulted in more bronchodilatation in the bronchitic group. The reasons for the differ-

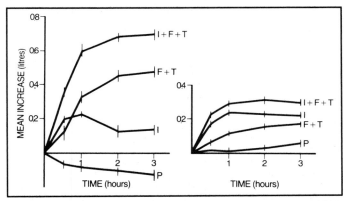

Fig. 64-6. *Responses of 10 patients with emphysema to atropine methonitrate (a) and salbutamol (s) in various sequences. a→s = atropine methonitrate hourly followed by salbutamol at the bold arrow; s→a = same agents in reverse order; a+s = both agents simultaneously; and p = placebo. Pairs of symbols indicate significant difference between values. (Reprinted with permission from N. J. Gross and M. S. Skorodin, Role of parasympathetic system in airway obstruction due to emphysema. N. Engl. J. Med. 311:421, 1984.)*

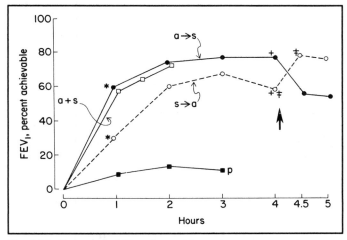

Fig. 64-7. *Increase in the forced expiratory volume at 1 second (FEV$_1$) of 15 patients with asthma (left panel) and 15 patients with chronic bronchitis (right panel). P = placebo; I = ipratropium (40 µg MDI); F+T = fenoterol (5 mg) plus oxtriphylline (400 mg orally). (Reprinted with permission from N. M. Lefcoe, et al., The addition of an aerosol anticholinergic to an oral beta agonist plus theophylline in asthma and bronchitis. Chest 82:300, 1982.)*

Fig. 64-5. *Increase in the forced expiratory volume at 1 second (FEV$_1$) in patients with chronic obstructive pulmonary disease after inhalation of 40 µg of ipratropium by metered-dose inhaler (MDI) (107 patients) or 1.5 µg of metaproterenol by MDI (90 patients). Symbols denote significant differences. (Reprinted with permission from D. P. Tashkin, et al., Comparison of the anticholinergic ipratropium bromide with metaproterenol in chronic obstructive pulmonary disease, a 90 day multicenter study. Am. J. Med. 81(suppl. 5A):81, 1986.)*

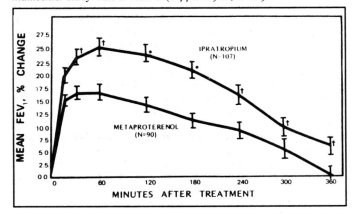

ence between these two groups of patients seem to be due to the fact that the adrenergic combination was much less effective in the bronchitic group, while ipratropium had about the same effect in both groups, and consequently emerged as the more potent agent in the bronchitic patients. This interpretation is consistent with the fact that airflow obstruction in asthma is due to factors related to airway inflammation that are amenable, at least in part, to adrenergic agents but not to anticholinergic agents. These factors are present to a less extent in patients with COPD whose major reversible component is bronchomotor tone, which is best reversed by anticholinergic agents [21]. Whatever the reason, the anticholinergic agents are the most useful bronchodilators in patients with COPD.

One concludes that optimal bronchodilator therapy in COPD might begin with an anticholinergic agent given on a regular maintenance basis because anticholinergic agents produce a greater increase in airflow in these patients than do other bronchodilators. They should be given on a maintenance basis because they take 1 to 2 hours to achieve maximal effect. If additional bronchodilatation is needed in these patients on an as needed or maintenance basis, an adrenergic agent can be used as the adjunct.

Acute Exacerbations of COPD

Recent studies that compared the efficacy of various bronchodilators in acute exacerbations of COPD found no significant differences between adrenergic and anticholinergic agents or their combination [29, 40, 43]. Bronchodilators are clearly indicated in these patients, at least in the initial therapy, so a combination that includes an anticholinergic agent might provide the best therapy in an individual patient, even if its value cannot be statistically validated in larger groups of patients.

Combination with Other Bronchodilators

Combinations of different classes of bronchodilators often provide more improvement in airflow than do single agents, and this effect has been seen in many of the studies cited earlier (for example, see Fig. 64-7). However, this is probably due to the fact that most clinical studies are performed with recommended rather than optimal doses of the bronchodilators, as already noted. Consequently, when two classes of agents are given together, both in the recommended dosage, the effects may simply be additive rather than potentiating. As anticholinergic agents act through a different pathway from that of other bronchodilators, it is not unreasonable to use them in combination with other agents, but the evidence that this is an advantage over using a larger dose of either agent alone is limited to acute asthma (see earlier discussion).

There is no physiologic or pharmacologic contraindication to the combination of anticholinergic agents with other agents used in the treatment of airways diseases. No unfavorable interactions between anticholinergic bronchodilators and other drugs have been reported. When patients are taking both adrenergic and anticholinergic agents by MDI, there is little evidence to suggest that it matters how and in what order they use these agents, though one study suggests that it may be best to administer the anticholinergic agent first [5]. However, a more common practice is to use the adrenergic agent first to obtain an immediate effect, and to follow with the anticholinergic agent. This might improve penetration of the second aerosol into the respiratory tract.

OTHER EFFECTS

Effects on Lung Mechanics, Hemodynamics, and Gas Exchange

Anticholinergic agents, like other bronchodilators, reduce the hyperinflation associated with airflow obstruction [21]. They also improve effort tolerance [32]. The quaternary forms have negligible effects on the hemodynamics [7] and the pulmonary circulation. They also do not carry the risk of increasing hypoxemia, as do adrenergic agents [17], a consideration that might be important in exacerbations of asthma and COPD.

Side Effects

Atropine sulfate results in numerous side effects related to the inhibition of physiologic functions of the parasympathetic system [58]. These effects occur in doses at or only slightly above the bronchodilator dose, and include skin flushing, dryness of the mouth and other mucosae, tachycardia, blurred vision, and mental disturbances. Atropine is contraindicated in patients with glaucoma or prostatic hypertrophy. The principal advantage of quaternary anticholinergic agents is that they are so poorly absorbed from the mucosae that the risk of such effects is insignificant. Even massive, inadvertent overdosage of one such agent resulted in only trivial effects [22]. Ipratropium, the most widely studied quaternary anticholinergic, has been extensively explored for the existence of atropine-like side effects and found to be virtually devoid of them [16]. It can, for example, be given to patients with glaucoma without affecting intraocular tension (provided it is not sprayed directly into the eye). It has not been found to affect urinary flow characteristics in older men, nor has it been found to alter the viscosity and elasticity of respiratory mucus or mucociliary clearance, as does atropine [41, 46, 57, 60].

In terms of normal clinical usage, the only side effect that patients might experience with ipratropium MDI is a brief coughing spell that has been reported to occur in 5 and 10 percent of bronchitic and asthmatic patients, respectively [50, 52]. Rarely, it can result in paradoxical bronchoconstriction. This has been variously attributed to hypotonicity of the nebulized solution, idiosyncrasy to the bromine radical, the benzalkonium preservative, and a selective effect on the M_2 receptor [8, 33, 39]. Unpublished reports suggest that paradoxical bronchoconstriction may also occur with other anticholinergic agents. Although rare, occurring in perhaps 0.3 percent of patients, the possibility of paradoxical bronchoconstriction should be borne in mind, as it would warrant withdrawal of the drug from that patient.

Other than these two effects, very extensive investigation and the worldwide use of ipratropium for over a decade have yielded a remarkably low incidence of untoward reactions during long-term use. Even when taken at four times the currently recommended dosage for 6 months, ipratropium can be well tolerated [30]. Experience with other quaternary anticholinergic agents is less extensive.

CLINICAL APPLICATIONS

The clinical use of anticholinergic bronchodilators is probably best limited to the poorly absorbed quaternary forms, such as ipratropium, oxitropium, atropine methonitrate, and glycopyrrolate, which are best administered by inhalation.

They cannot be regarded as first-line bronchodilators in the treatment of stable asthma, but may have a role as adjuncts to other bronchodilator therapy in this state. They have a more clearly defined role when used in combination with adrenergic agents in the treatment of acute, severe asthma.

The principal role of anticholinergic agents is in the long-term management of stable COPD, where they are probably the most efficacious bronchodilators. Because of their slow onset of action they are best used on a regular maintenance basis, rather than on an as needed basis. The usual dose of ipratropium, the only such agent currently available in the United States, 2 puffs of 20 μg each, is probably suboptimal for many patients with COPD and can safely be doubled or quadrupled [30].

Patients can be advised that these agents act slowly and do not produce any somatic effects other than decreased dyspnea.

REFERENCES

1. Barnes, P. J. Asthma as an axon reflex. *Lancet* 1:242, 1986.
2. Barnes, P. J., Basbaum, C. B., and Nadel, J. A. Autoradiographic localization of autonomic receptors in airway smooth muscle: marked differences between large and small airways. *Am. Rev. Respir. Dis.* 127:758, 1983.
3. Braun, S. R., et al. A comparison of the effect of ipratropium and albuterol in the treatment of chronic obstructive airway disease. *Arch. Intern. Med.* 149:544, 1989.

4. Brown, I. G., et al. Assessment of the clinical usefulness of nebulised ipratropium bromide in patients with chronic airflow limitation. *Thorax* 39:272, 1984.

5. Bruderman, I., Cohen-Aronovski, R., and Smorzik, J. A comparative study of various combinations of ipratropium bromide and metaproterenol in allergic asthmatic patients. *Chest* 83:208, 1983.

6. Burge, P. S., Harries, M. G., and l'Anson, E. Comparison of atropine with ipratropium bromide in patients with reversible airways obstruction unresponsive to salbutamol. *Br. J. Dis. Chest* 74:259, 1980.

7. Chapman, K. R., et al. Hemodynamic effects of inhaled ipratropium bromide alone and in combination with an inhaled beta₂-agonist. *Am. Rev. Respir. Dis.* 132:845, 1985.

8. Connolly, C. K. Adverse reaction to ipratropium bromide. *Br. Med. J.* 285:934, 1982.

9. Deckers, W. The chemistry of new derivatives of tropane alkaloids and the pharmacokinetics of a new quaternary compound. *Postgrad. Med. J.* 51(suppl. 7):76, 1975.

10. De Vries, K. The protective effect of inhaled Sch 1000 MDI on bronchoconstriction induced by serotonin, histamine, acetylcholine and propranolol. *Postgrad. Med. J.* 51(suppl. 7):106, 1975.

11. Easton, P. A., et al. A comparison of the bronchodilating effects of a beta-2 adrenergic agent (albuterol) and an anticholinergic agent (ipratropium bromide), given by aerosol alone or in sequence. *N. Engl. J. Med.* 315:735, 1986.

12. Gandevia, B. Historical review of the use of parasympatholytic agents in the treatment of respiratory disorders. *Postgrad. Med. J.* 51(suppl. 7):13, 1975.

13. Gilman, M. J., et al. Comparison of aerosolized glycopyrrolate and metaproterenol in acute asthma. *Chest* 98:1095, 1990.

14. Gross, N. J. COPD: a disease of reversible airflow obstruction. *Am. Rev. Respir. Dis.* 133:725, 1986.

15. Gross, N. J. Cholinergic Control. In P. J. Barnes, I. W. Rodger, and N. C. Thomson (eds.), *Asthma, Basic Mechanisms and Clinical Management.* London: Academic Press, 1988, Pp. 381–393.

16. Gross, N. J. Ipratropium bromide. *N. Engl. J. Med.* 319:486, 1988.

17. Gross, N. J., and Bankwala, Z. Effects of an anticholinergic bronchodilator on arterial blood gases of hypoxemic patients with COPD. *Am. Rev. Respir. Dis.* 136:1091, 1987.

18. Gross, N. J., and Barnes, P. J. A short tour around the muscarinic receptor. *Am. Rev. Respir. Dis.* 138:765, 1988.

19. Gross, N. J., Co, E., and Skorodin, M. S. Cholinergic bronchomotor tone in COPD: estimates of its amount in comparison to normal. *Chest* 96:984, 1989.

20. Gross, N. J., and Skorodin, M. S. Anticholinergic, antimuscarinic bronchodilators. *Am. Rev. Respir. Dis.* 129:856, 1984.

21. Gross, N. J., and Skorodin, M. S. Role of the parasympathetic system in airway obstruction due to emphysema. *N. Engl. J. Med.* 311:421, 1984.

22. Gross, N. J., and Skorodin, M. S. Massive overdose of atropine methonitrate with only slight untoward effects. *Lancet* 2:386, 1985.

23. Gross, N. J., and Skorodin, M. S. Anticholinergic Agents. In J. W. Jenne and S. Murphy (eds.), *Drug Therapy for Asthma* (Lung Biology in Health and Disease, Vol 31). New York: Dekker, 1987, Pp. 615–668.

24. Gross, N. J., et al. Dose-response to ipratropium nebulized solution in COPD: a 3-center study. *Am. Rev. Respir. Dis.* 139:1188, 1989.

25. Ind, P. W. Anticholinergic blockade of beta-blocker induced bronchoconstriction. *Am. Rev. Respir. Dis.* 139:1390, 1989.

26. Ind, P. W., et al. Anticholinergic blockade of propranolol induced bronchoconstriction. *Thorax* 41:718, 1986.

27. Jeffery, P. K. The Innervation of Bronchial Mucosa. In G. Cumming and G. Bonsignore (eds.), *Cellular Biology of the Lung.* New York, London: Plenum Press, 1981, Pp. 1–25.

28. Jolobe, O. M. P. Asthma versus non-specific reversible airflow obstruction, clinical features and responsiveness to anticholinergic drugs. *Respiration* 45:237, 1984.

29. Karpel, J. P., et al. A comparison of the effects of ipratropium bromide and metaproterenol sulfate in acute exacerbations of COPD. *Chest* 98:835, 1990.

30. Leak, A., and O'Connor, T. High dose ipratropium—is it safe? *Practitioner* 232:9, 1988.

31. Lefcoe, N. M., et al. The addition of an aerosol anticholinergic to an oral beta agonist plus theophylline in asthma and bronchitis. *Chest* 82:300, 1982.

32. Leitch, A. G., et al. The effect of aerosol ipratropium bromide and salbutamol on exercise tolerance in chronic bronchitis. *Thorax* 33:711, 1978.

33. Mann, J. S., Howarth, P. H., and Holgate, S. T. Bronchoconstriction induced by nebulised ipratropium bromide: relation to hypotonicity. *Br. Med. J.* 289:469, 1984.

34. McFadden, E. R., et al. The mechanism of action of suggestion in the induction of acute asthma attacks. *Psychosom. Med.* 31:134, 1969.

35. Nadel, J. A. Autonomic Regulation of Airway Smooth Muscle. In J. A. Nadel (ed.), *Physiology and Pharmacology of the Airways.* New York: Dekker, 1980, Pp. 217–257.

36. Nadel, J. A., Barnes, P. J., and Holtzman, M. J. Autonomic Factors in Hyperreactivity of Airway Smooth Muscle. In P. T. Macklem and J. Mead (eds.), *Handbook of Physiology* Vol. III, Part 2. Bethesda, MD: American Physiological Society, 1986, Pp. 693–702.

37. Neild, J. E., and Cameron, I. R. Bronchoconstriction in response to suggestion: its prevention by an inhaled anticholinergic agent. *Br. Med. J.* 290:674, 1985.

38. Newcomb, R., et al. Rebound hyperresponsiveness to muscarinic stimulation after chronic therapy with an inhaled antimuscarinic agent. *Am. Rev. Respir. Dis.* 132:12, 1985.

39. Patel, K. R., and Tullett, W. M. Bronchoconstriction in response to ipratropium bromide (letter). *Br. Med. J.* 286:1318, 1983.

40. Patrick, D. M., et al. Severe exacerbations of COPD and asthma: incremental benefit of adding ipratropium to usual therapy. *Chest* 98:295, 1990.

41. Pavia, D., et al. Effect of ipratropium bromide on mucociliary clearance and pulmonary function in reversible airways obstruction. *Thorax* 34:501, 1979.

42. Rebuck, A. S., and Marcus, H. I. Sch 1000 in psychogenic asthma. *Scand. J. Respir. Dis.* 103(suppl.):186, 1979.

43. Rebuck, A. S., et al. Nebulized anticholinergic and sympathomimetic treatment of asthma and chronic obstructive airways disease in the emergency room. *Am. J. Med.* 82:59, 1987.

44. Richardson, J. B. Innervation of the lung. *Eur. J. Respir. Dis.* [Suppl] 117:13, 1982.

45. Richardson, J. B., and Ferguson, C. C. Neuromuscular structure and function in the airways. *Fed. Proc.* 38:202, 1979.

46. Ruffin, R. E., et al. Aerosol therapy with Sch 1000: short-term mucociliary clearance in normal and bronchitic subjects and toxicology in normal subjects. *Chest* 73:501, 1978.

47. Ruffin, R. E., et al. Combination bronchodilator therapy in asthma. *J. Allergy Clin. Immunol.* 69:60, 1982.

48. Shah, P. K. D., et al. Clinical dysautonomia in patients with bronchial asthma: study with seven autonomic function tests. *Chest* 98:1408, 1990.

49. Shifrin, G. S., and Klein, W. L. Regulation of acetylcholine receptor concentration in cloned neuroblastoma cells. *J. Neurochem.* 34:993, 1980.

50. Storms, W. W., et al. Use of ipratropium bromide in asthma: results of a multi-clinic study. *Am. J. Med.* 81(suppl. 5A):61, 1986.

51. Summers, Q. A., and Tarala, R. A. Nebulized ipratropium in the treatment of acute asthma. *Chest* 97:425, 1990.

52. Tashkin, D. P., et al. Comparison of the anticholinergic ipratropium bromide with metaproterenol in chronic obstructive pulmonary disease: a 90 day multicenter study. *Am. J. Med.* 81(suppl. 5A):81, 1986.

53. Ullah, M. I., Newman, G. B., and Saunders, K. B. Influence of age on response to ipratropium and salbutamol in asthma. *Thorax* 36:523, 1981.

54. Vaughan, T. R., et al. Development of subsensitivity to atropine methylnitrate: a double-blind, placebo controlled, crossover study. *Am. Rev. Respir. Dis.* 138:771, 1988.

55. Virtanen, R., et al. Pharmacokinetic studies on atropine with special reference to age. *Acta Anaesthesiol. Scand.* 26:297, 1982.

56. Vichyanond, P., et al. Efficacy of atropine methylnitrate alone and in combination with albuterol in children with asthma. *Chest* 98:637, 1990.

57. Wanner, A. Effect of ipratropium bromide on airway mucociliary function. *Am. J. Med.* 81(suppl. 5A):23, 1986.

58. Weiner, N. Atropine, Scopolamine and Related Antimuscarinic Drugs. In A. G. Gilman, L. S. Goodman, and A. Gilman (eds.), *The Pharmacologic Basis of Therapeutics* (6th ed.). New York: Macmillan, 1980, Pp. 120–137.

59. Widdicombe, J. G. The parasympathetic nervous system in airways disease. *Scand. J. Respir. Dis.* [Suppl] 103:38, 1979.

60. Yeates, D. B., et al. Mucociliary tracheal transport rates in man. *J. Appl. Physiol.* 39:487, 1975.

61. Bryant, D. H., and Rogers, P. Effects of ipratropium bromide nebulizer solution with and without preservatives in the treatment of acute and stable asthma. *Chest* 102:742, 1992.

Histamine Antagonists

Richard Wood-Baker
Stephen T. Holgate

65

Histamine was implicated in the pathogenesis of allergic diseases shortly after its structural identification [82] by its ability to mimic features of anaphylaxis in animals following intravenous administration [23]. It was further implicated as a mediator in asthma by the bronchoconstriction it caused in asthmatic subjects, whether administered parenterally [21] or by inhalation [39] (see Chap. 10). This naturally prompted a search for drugs capable of blocking the effects of histamine and this led to the development of the first effective histamine antagonist [31]. A number of similar drugs followed, and findings from studies using these both clinically and experimentally suggested that, in asthma, they were capable of antagonizing the airway effects of histamine [5, 51, 76]. Many of these studies have since been criticized on account of their uncontrolled nature and lack of any objective measurement of respiratory function. Unfortunately, one common feature of the histamine antagonists was the incidence of adverse effects, particularly related to their sedative and anticholinergic actions (Table 65-1). The narrow therapeutic index of the early antihistamines and the introduction of other treatments, notably beta agonists, resulted in their diminished use. Indeed, the theoretical difficulties related to the drying of airway secretions led to their use being positively discouraged [11].

HISTAMINE ANTAGONISTS

Chlorpheniramine and Clemastine

Renewed interest in the role of histamine during the 1970s saw more detailed study of histamine antagonists that was centered on chlorpheniramine and clemastine, both of which were shown to have a bronchodilator effect in resting asthmatic airways [62, 66, 79]. With chlorpheniramine there was a dose effect, which unfortunately occurred at the expense of increased adverse effects. With both drugs, bronchodilatation varied according to the starting airway caliber, and this was suggested to play a role in determining the response to antihistamine treatment. Both drugs antagonized the acute bronchoconstriction caused by inhaled histamine, either by a shift in the dose-response curve [62, 67] or by attenuation of the fall in FEV_1 [38]. Oral or parenteral administration was associated with dose-limiting adverse effects on acetylcholine-induced bronchoconstriction, particularly the anticholinergic activity of chlorpheniramine, which at 10 mg administered intravenously is equivalent to 0.4 mg of atropine administered subcutaneously. These effects appear to be overcome by aerosol administration, inhaled clemastine having no significant effect on methacholine-induced bronchoconstriction in asthmatics [62].

Newer H_1-Receptor Antagonists

Although limited by their adverse effects, the therapeutic efficacy of antagonists to the H_1 receptor in diseases such as seasonal rhinitis led to the search for more potent drugs that were devoid of the limiting adverse effects. Within the last decade, a number of potent and specific H_1-receptor antagonists have been developed, and this has led to a reevaluation of H_1 antihistamines in the treatment of asthma (Fig. 65-1).

Astemizole

Astemizole has no structural relationship to the biogenic amines, particularly histamine, and thus, at doses causing H_1-receptor antagonism, has no anticholinergic or antiserotonergic effects [6, 9]. Although rapidly absorbed orally, there is a delay before the effect on histamine-induced skin wheals [55] or clinical symptoms is seen [41], largely reflecting hepatic uptake followed by release of the parent drug and active metabolites. Once steady-state kinetics have been achieved, astemizole is a potent H_1-receptor antagonist [42] with no evidence of a sedative effect [60], which may be accounted for by its differential (central versus peripheral) H_1-receptor affinity [49]. In the airways of asthmatic subjects, astemizole has not demonstrated a bronchodilator action, possibly as a result of its pharmacodynamic profile, but does antagonize histamine-induced bronchoconstriction. When given at a dose of 10 mg per day for 14 days, astemizole caused a rightward shift in the concentration-response curve, with a geometric mean concentration ratio of 17.4 [40].

Terfenadine

Terfenadine is a piperidine-type antihistamine with effective H_1-receptor antagonism in the absence of significant serotonergic, adrenergic, or cholinergic receptor effects [20]. Following oral administration, it is rapidly absorbed and then extensively metabolized to two main metabolites before excretion [32]. The major metabolite has only one-third the activity of the parent compound at the H_1 receptor [84]. Maximum H_1-receptor antagonism is delayed for several hours after oral dosing, whether evaluated in terms of its inhibition of histamine-induced skin wheals [44, 74] or the improvement of symptoms it brings about [42, 73]. In the asthmatic airways, a single oral dose of terfenadine has a bronchodilator effect and causes a dose-related rightward shift in the concentration-response curve to inhaled histamine [68]. In nine asthmatics a 17 percent improvement in FEV_1 was observed three hours after administration of 120 mg of terfenadine [86]. There is no evidence of a sedative effect nor anticholinergic activity in asthmatic airways [64]. More recent evidence has suggested that terfenadine may possess additional actions of relevance to allergic disease, in particular inhibition of mediator release from inflammatory cells [57, 58].

Cetirizine

Cetirizine has been modified from the antihistamine hydroxyzine by carboxylation of the alcohol side-chain, thereby increasing the H_1-receptor potency while eliminating the unwanted adverse effects, including anticholinergic and antiserotonergic [81]. Carboxylation increases the polarity, thus reducing penetration across the blood-brain barrier, and, together with the receptor selectivity, this accounts for the lack of sedative effects [75]. Cetirizine is rapidly absorbed following oral administration [33] and largely excreted unchanged in the urine [83]. As a conse-

quence, its plasma half-life is highly dependent on renal function [54]. Cetirizine has not been shown to have a bronchodilator action in asthmatic airways but causes a rightward shift in the concentration-response curves to inhaled histamine [13], although quantification of this has not been achieved. In addition to its H_1-receptor antagonism, cetirizine inhibits eosinophil migration in the skin following local allergen challenge [27], and this may provide cetirizine with an additional therapeutic mechanism in asthma.

Loratadine

Loratadine is structurally derived from azatadine and selectively binds to peripheral H_1 receptors [2], with no significant action at alpha-adrenergic or cholinergic receptors [8]. After oral administration, there is rapid absorption followed by extensive metabolism to the major metabolite descarboxyloratadine, which is also pharmacologically active. Most of the drug is excreted in the urine as hydroxydescarboxyloratadine, although renal impairment does not appear to affect its elimination. Although administration of loratadine causes a dose-dependent suppression of the response to intradermal histamine within 2 hours [10, 45, 72], in asthmatic airways there was no bronchodilator activity despite displacing the histamine concentration-response curves rightward [80]. Loratadine had no significant effect on the methacholine concentration-response curves. In vitro investigations indicate that loratadine inhibits the release of a number of mast cell mediators which may be important in allergic disease [48, 78].

Azelastine

Azelastine is a novel phthalazinone derivative, which in vitro has been shown to act as an antagonist at the H_1 and leukotriene

Table 65-1. Pharmacologic profile of nonsedating antihistamines compared with classic antihistamines

	Pharmacologic property		
	Antihistaminic activity	Sedative activity	Anticholinergic activity
Nonsedating			
Terfenadine	+ + +	0	0
Astemizole	+ + +	0	0
Loratadine	+ + +	0/+*	0
Cetirizine	+ + +	0/+*	0
Mequitazine	+ + +	0/+ +*	+/+ +
Classic			
Chlorpheniramine	+ + +	+/+ +*	+/+ +*
Diphenhydramine	+ + +	+ + +	+ +
Promethazine	+ + +	+ + +	+ +
Clemastine	+ + +	+ +	+/+ +
Triprolidine	+ + +	+/+ +	+ +

Source: J. K. Woodward, Pharmacology and toxicology of nonclassical antihistamines. *Cutis* 42(4A):5, 1988. Reprinted with permission.
0 = none; + = slight; + + = moderate; + + + = marked.
* Dose-dependent.

Fig. 65-1. *Chemical structures of some H_1-receptor antagonists. (Reprinted with permission from J. K. Woodward, Pharmacology and toxicology of nonclassical antihistamines. Cutis 42[4A]:5, 1988.)*

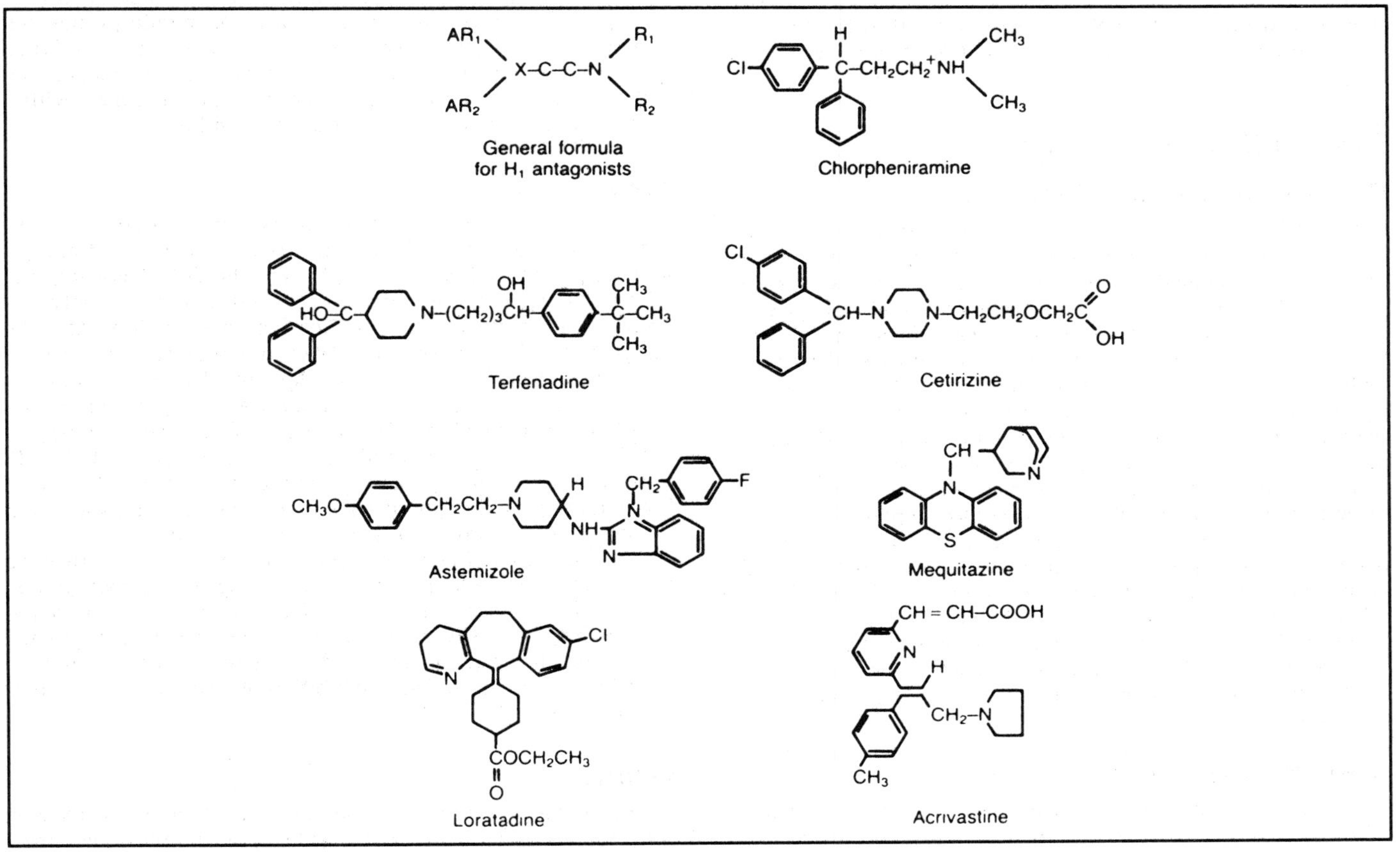

receptors [17]. In animal models it has also been observed to attenuate the response to serotonin and platelet-activating factor in the skin [1, 46, 85]. It is a potent in vitro inhibitor of mast cell degranulation following both immunologic [19] and nonimmunologic [18, 28] stimulation. There is little published data on its pharmacokinetic profile, although significant inhibition of histamine-induced skin wheals occurs within 4 hours of dosing and this may be maintained by regular dosing for up to 6 weeks [36]. Oral doses of azelastine cause bronchodilation [47] lasting up to 6 hours and protect against the bronchoconstrictor action of inhaled histamine [52, 53, 69]. No significant effect was found on methacholine- or leukotriene C_4–induced bronchoconstriction, despite its having significant antileukotriene effects in animal models [3]. (See Chapter 63 for added information.)

TYPES OF ASTHMA

Experimental Asthma

The characteristic variability of clinical asthma and resulting difficulty in assessing new treatments has led to the search for models that may be employed in the laboratory. The principal technique has been the bronchoconstrictor response to allergens occurring immediately (the early asthmatic response) or several hours (the late asthmatic response) following inhalation (Chapter 12). The rise in the plasma histamine [15, 43] and urinary N^τ-methylhistamine [24] concentrations seen following allergen inhalation suggests that mast cell–derived histamine is responsible for at least part of the early bronchoconstrictor response. A contribution by histamine to the late asthmatic response is not as well established [24, 25, 70]. These studies suggest that, although histamine may be responsible for a significant proportion of the early bronchoconstrictor response, it has a less prominent role in the later changes in airway caliber.

As would be expected, predosing with antihistamines has been shown to shift the dose-response curve to inhaled allergen to the right [16, 35, 65, 67], although this effect is less marked when compared to the protection they afford against histamine. In addition, they attenuate the time-course response of the early asthmatic response [12, 22, 56], with greatest inhibition seen during the early part of the bronchoconstrictor response, commensurate with the time-course of histamine release from mast cells.

The effect of H_1 antihistamines on the late asthmatic response has not been as widely studied and the results to date are conflicting. Predosing with triprolidin did not consistently diminish the late bronchoconstrictor response, despite eliciting inhibition of the early response [59]. More recently, loratadine, though causing significant inhibition of the allergen skin wheal response, produced no significant effect on the early or late bronchoconstrictor response [80]. In contrast, azelastine was found to cause significant inhibition of the late asthmatic response when measured as the area under the time-response curve [70]. In both of these studies, the number of subjects exhibiting a consistent late bronchoconstrictor response was small, and, while these findings have to be viewed with caution, azelastine may have additional actions of relevance to the pathogenesis of the late asthmatic response. The effects in LAR were recently reviewed by Townley [87].

Exercise-Induced Asthma

Although the pathogenesis of exercise-induced asthma has not been clearly established, the increase in plasma concentrations of histamine [7] and neutrophil chemotactic factor [50] seen following exercise challenge, together with attenuation of the airway caliber changes produced by salbutamol [4] and sodium cromoglycate [26], suggest mediator release from the mast cell

is a likely mechanism (see Chapter 47). Predosing with antihistamines has usually been shown to attenuate the bronchoconstrictor response to exercise [29, 37, 63], although this has not been a uniform finding [34, 35]. The variable effect of H_1 antagonism on the bronchoconstrictor response to exercise according to the drug used, the dosage, and the route of administration remains unexplained.

Clinical Asthma

The bronchodilator effect of antihistamines has led to the suggestion that there may be a continuous release of small amounts of histamine from mast cells within the asthmatic airways. The resulting low concentrations of histamine may contribute to basal airway tone and, as a result of ablating this, antihistamines cause bronchodilation. One might therefore anticipate antihistamines to cause an increase in airway caliber in addition to an improvement in symptoms. Unfortunately, many of the early studies performed during the 1940s and 1950s lacked any useful measurement of airway caliber [5, 39], relying instead on the reported symptomatology to measure effect. More recently, a small number of studies have appeared that report the effect of newer antihistamines in well-conducted and -controlled studies. To date, these studies have been conducted almost exclusively in mild atopic asthmatics and have shown an encouraging improvement in symptom scores with a concomitant reduction in the use of rescue medication [14, 71, 77], although the effect on airway caliber has been less dramatic. To date, studies in asthmatics with more severe and chronic disease have not been reported. Despite the improvement in symptom scores and airway caliber measurements, studies involving continuous treatment maintained for periods of 2 to 7 weeks have not shown any significant change in airway responsiveness when assessed by methacholine inhalation challenge [30, 36, 71].

The precise role of histamine in the cause of clinical and experimental asthma remains unclear, despite its structural identification at the beginning of this century. In part this has been the result of a lack of potent and specific antagonists devoid of significant adverse effects—that is, until the last decade. The use of these new drugs, together with the measurement of mediators in biologic fluids, has clearly shown that the early bronchoconstrictor response to inhaled allergen results in part from histamine release within the airways. However, the contribution of histamine to the late reaction and the consequence of its pharmacologic antagonism (which is probably of greater relevance to clinical practice) remain unresolved and clearly require further investigation. In a therapeutic setting, H_1-receptor antihistamines clearly bring about subjective and objective improvements in asthmatics with mild atopic disease and are particularly appropriate in those cases where there is coexistent rhinitis. However, their use in patients with more chronic and severe asthma has yet to be assessed, although their bronchodilator action in resting asthmatic airways encourages one to anticipate they may contribute to improved symptom control and airflow measurements in some clinical situations.

SAFETY

The September 1992 FDA Medical Bulletin indicates manufacturers' new boxed warnings for two non-sedating antihistamines. Rare but potentially serious and life-threatening cardiovascular events may be associated with terfenadine (Seldane) and astemizole (Hismanal); these include ECG QT prolongation, torsades de pointes, cardiac arrest, and other ventricular arrhythmias. Patients at risk for the side effects of terfenadine include those receiving concomitant ketoconazole, erythromycin, or troleandomycin; those on dosages above the manufacturer's recommendation; and those with hepatic dysfunction. For astemizole, overdosing appears to be a significant feature. Prodromal syncope or fainting should lead to drug discontinuation and patient evaluation. Patients should be cautioned not to exceed recommended dosages [88] (see Chap. 78).

REFERENCES

1. Acherrath-Tuckermann, U., Weischer, C., and Szelenyi, I. Azelastine, a new antiallergic/antiasthmatic agent, inhibits PAF-acether-induced platelet aggregation, paw edema and bronchoconstriction. *Pharmacology* 36: 265, 1988.
2. Ahn, H.-S., and Barnett, A. Selective displacement of [^{3}H]mepyramine from peripheral vs. central nervous system receptors by loratadine, a non-sedating antihistamine. *Eur. J. Pharmacol.* 127:153, 1986.
3. Albazzaz, M., and Patel, K. Effect of azelastine on bronchoconstriction induced by histamine and leukotriene C_4 in patients with extrinsic asthma. *Thorax* 43:306, 1988.
4. Anderson, S., et al. Inhaled and oral salbutamol in exercise-induced asthma. *Am. Rev. Respir. Dis.* 114:493, 1976.
5. Arbesman, C., Koepf, G., and Lenzer, A. Clinical studies with N'pyridyl N'benzyldi-methylethylenediamine monohydrochloride (pyribenzamine). *J. Allergy* 17:275, 1947.
6. Awouters, F., Niemegeers, C., and Janssen, P. Pharmacology of the specific histamine H1-antagonist astemizole. *Arneimittelforschung* 33:381, 1983.
7. Barnes, P., and Brown, M. Venous plasma histamine in exercise- and hyperventilation-induced asthma in man. *Clin. Sci.* 61:169, 1981.
8. Barnett, A., et al. Evaluation of the CNS properties of SCH 29851, a potential non-sedating antihistamine. *Agents Actions* 14:590, 1984.
9. Bateman, D., Chapman, P., and Rawlings, M. Effects of astemizole on histamine-induced wheal and flare. *Eur. J. Clin. Pharmacol.* 25:547, 1983.
10. Batenhorst, R., et al. Pharmacological evaluation of loratadine (SCH 29851), chlorpheniramine and placebo. *Eur. J. Clin. Pharmacol.* 31:247, 1986.
11. Berkow, R., and Fletcher, A. Antihistamines. In *The Merck Manual* (15th ed.) Rahway, NJ: Merck, Sharpe & Dohme, 1987, P. 2517.
12. Booij-Noord, H., et al. Protection tests on bronchial allergen challenge with disodium cromoglycate and thiazinium. *J. Allergy* 46:1, 1970.
13. Brik, A., et al. Effect of cetirizine, a new histamine H1-antagonist, on airway dynamics and responsiveness to inhaled histamine in mild asthma. *J. Allergy Clin. Immunol.* 80:51, 1987.
14. Bruttmann, G., et al. Protective effect of cetirizine in patients suffering from pollen asthma. *Ann. Allergy* 64:224, 1990.
15. Busse, W., and Swenson, C. The relationship between plasma histamine concentrations and bronchial obstruction to antigen challenge in allergic rhinitis. *J. Allergy Clin. Immunol* 84:658, 1989.
16. Chan, T., Shelton, D., and Eiser, N. Effect of an oral H1-receptor antagonist, terfenadine, on antigen-induced asthma. *Br. J. Dis. Chest* 80:375, 1986.
17. Chand, N., Diamantis, W., and Sofia, R. Antagonism of histamine and leukotrienes by azelastine in isolated guinea pig ileum. *Agents Actions* 19:164, 1986.
18. Chand, N., et al. Inhibition of calcium ionophore (A23187)–stimulated histamine release from rat peritoneal mast cells by azelastine: implications for its model of action. *Eur. J. Pharmacol.* 96:227, 1983.
19. Chand, N., et al. Inhibition of IgE-mediated allergic histamine release from rat peritoneal mast cells by azelastine and selected antiallergic drugs. *Agents Actions* 16:318, 1985.
20. Cheng, H., and Woodward, J. Antihistaminic effect of terfenadine: a new piperidine-type antihistamine. *Drug Dev. Res.* 2:181, 1982.
21. Curry, J. The action of histamine on the respiratory tract in normal and asthmatic subjects. *J. Clin. Invest.* 25:785, 1946.
22. Curzen, N., Rafferty, P., and Holgate, S. Effects of a cyclo-oxygenase inhibitor, flurbiprofen, and an H_1 histamine receptor antagonist, terfenadine, alone and in combination on allergen induced immediate bronchoconstriction in man. *Thorax* 42:946, 1987.
23. Dale, H., and Laidlaw, P. Histamine shock, *J. Physiol.* 52:355, 1919.
24. De Monchy, J., et al. Histamine in late asthmatic reactions following house-dust mite inhalation. *Agents Actions* 16:252, 1985.
25. Durham S., et al. Immunologic studies in allergen-induced late-phase asthmatic reactions. *J. Allergy Clin. Immunol.* 74:49, 1984.
26. Eggleston, P., et al. A double-blind trial of the effect of cromolyn sodium on exercise-induced bronchospasm. *J. Allergy Clin. Immunol.* 50:57, 1972.
27. Fedel, R., et al. Inhibitory effect of cetirizine 2HCl on eosinophil migration in vivo. *Clin. Allergy* 17:373, 1987.
28. Fields, D., et al. Inhibition by azelastine of nonallergic histamine release from rat peritoneal mast cells. *J. Allergy Clin. Immunol.* 73:400, 1984.
29. Finnerty, J., and Holgate, S. Evidence for the roles of histamine and prostaglandins as mediators in exercise-induced asthma: the inhibitory effect of terfenadine and flurbiprofen alone and in combination. *Eur. Respir. J.* 3: 540, 1990.
30. Finnerty, J., Holgate, S., and Rihoux, J.-P. The effect of 2 weeks treatment with cetirizine on bronchial reactivity to methacholine in asthma. *Br. J. Clin. Pharmacol.* 29:79, 1990.
31. Forneau, E., and Bovet, D. Researches sur l'action sympathicolytique d'un nouveau derive du dioxane. *Arch Int. Pharmacodyn. Therap.* 46:178, 1933.
32. Gartiez, D., et al. Pharmacokinetics and biotransformation studies of terfenadine in man. *Drug Res.* 32:1185, 1982.
33. Gengo, F., et al. The relative antihistaminic and psychomotor effects of hydroxyzine and cetirizine. *Clin. Pharmacol. Ther.* 42:265, 1987.
34. Ghosh, S., De Vos, C., and Patel, K. Effect of cetirizine on exercise induced bronchoconstriction in patients with asthma. *Thorax* 45:332, 1990.
35. Gong, H., et al. Effects of oral cetirizine, a selective H_1 antagonist, on allergen- and exercise-induced bronchoconstriction in subjects with asthma. *J. Allergy Clin. Immunol.* 85:632, 1990.
36. Gould, C., et al. A study of the clinical efficacy of azelastine in patients with extrinsic asthma, and its effect on airway responsiveness. *Br. J. Clin. Pharmacol.* 26:515, 1988.
37. Hartley, J., and Nogrady, S. Effect of an inhaled antihistamine on exercise-induced asthma. *Thorax* 35:675, 1980.
38. Hartmann, V., et al. Modulation of histamine-induced bronchoconstriction with inhaled, oral, and intravenous clemastine in normal and asthmatic subjects. *Thorax* 36:737, 1981.
39. Herxheimer, H. Antihistamines in bronchial asthma. *Br. Med. J.* 2:901, 1949.
40. Holgate, S., Emanuel, M., and Howarth, P. Astemizole and other H_1-antihistaminic drug treatment of asthma. *J. Allergy Clin. Immunol.* 76:375, 1985.
41. Howarth, P., Emanuel, M., and Holgate, S. Astemizole, a potent histamine H1-receptor antagonist: effect in allergic rhinoconjunctivitis, on antigen and histamine induced skin wheal and relationship to serum levels. *Br. J. Clin. Pharmacol.* 18:1, 1984.
42. Howarth, P., and Holgate, S. Comparative trial of two non-sedative H1 antihistamines, terfenadine and astemizole, for hay fever. *Thorax* 39:668, 1984.
43. Howarth, P., et al. Influence of albuterol, cromolyn sodium and ipratropium bromide on the airway and circulating mediator responses to allergen bronchial provocation in asthma. *Am. Rev. Respir. Dis.* 132:986, 1985.
44. Huther, K., et al. Inhibitory activity of terfenadine on histamine-induced skin wheals in man. *Eur. J. Clin. Pharmacol.* 12:195, 1977.
45. Kassem, N., et al. Effects of loratadine (SCH 29851) in suppression of histamine-induced skin wheals. *Ann. Allergy* 60:505, 1988.
46. Katayama, S., et al. Antiallergic effect of azelastine hydrochloride on immediate type hypersensitivity reaction in vivo and in vitro. *Drug Res.* 31: 1196, 1981.
47. Kemp, J., Meltzer, E., and Orge, H. A dose-response study of the bronchodilator action of azelastine in asthma. *J. Allergy Clin. Immunol.* 79:893, 1987.
48. Kreutner, W., et al. Antiallergic activity of loratadine, a non-sedating antihistamine. *Allergy* 42:57, 1987.
49. Laduron, P., et al. In vitro and in vivo binding characteristics of a new long-acting histamine H1 antagonist, astemizole. *Mol. Pharmacol.* 21:294, 1982.
50. Lee, T., et al. Exercise-induced release of histamine and neutrophil chemotactic factor in atopic asthmatics. *J. Allergy Clin. Immunol.* 70:73, 1982.
51. Levy, L., and Seabury, J. Spirometric evaluation of benadryl in asthma. *J. Allergy* 18:244, 1947.
52. Magnussen, H. The inhibitory effect of azelastine ar.d ketotifen on histamine-induced bronchoconstriction in asthmatic patients. *Chest* 91:855, 1987.
53. Magnussen, H., et al. Duration of the effect of a single dose of azelastine on histamine-induced bronchoconstriction. *J. Allergy Clin. Immunol.* 83: 467, 1989.
54. Matzke, G., et al. Pharmacokinetics of cetirizine in the elderly and patients with renal insufficiency. *Ann. Allergy* 59:25, 1987.
55. McMillan, J., Simons, K., and Simons, F. Double-blind, cross-over comparison of terfenadine, astemizole, chlorpheniramine and placebo: suppressive effects on histamine-induced wheals and flares. *J. Allergy Clin. Immunol.* 85:255, 1990.
56. Morgan, D., et al. Circulating histamine and neutrophil chemotactic activity during allergen-induced asthma: the effect of inhaled antihistamines and antiallergic compounds. *Clin. Sci.* 69:36, 1985.

57. Nabe, M., et al. Inhibitory effect of terfenadine on mediator release from human blood basophils and eosinophils. *Clin. Exp. Allergy* 19:515, 1989.
58. Naclerio, R., et al. Terfenadine, an H_1 antihistamine inhibits histamine release in vivo in the human. *Am. Rev. Respir. Dis.* 142:167, 1990.
59. Nakazawa, T., et al. Inhibitory effects of various drugs on dual asthmatic responses in wheat flour–sensitive subjects. *J. Allergy Clin. Immunol.* 58:1, 1976.
60. Nicholson, A., and Stone, B. Performance studies with the H_1-histamine receptor antagonists, astemizole and terfenadine. *Br. J. Clin. Pharmacol.* 13:199, 1982.
61. Nogrady, S., and Bevan, C. Inhaled antihistamines—bronchodilatation and effects on histamine- and methacholine-induced bronchoconstriction. *Thorax* 33:700, 1976.
62. Nogrady, S., et al. Bronchodilatation after inhalation of the antihistamine clemastine. *Thorax* 33:479, 1978.
63. Patel, K. Terfenadine in exercise-induced asthma. *Br. Med. J.* 288:1496, 1984.
64. Patel, K. Effect of terfenadine on methacholine-induced bronchoconstriction in asthma. *J. Allergy Clin. Immunol.* 79:355, 1987.
65. Phillips, M., et al. Effect of antihistamines and antiallergic drugs on responses to allergen and histamine provocation tests in asthma. *Thorax* 39:345, 1984.
66. Popa, V. Bronchodilating activity of an H_1-blocker, chlorpheniramine. *J. Allergy Clin. Immunol.* 59:54, 1977.
67. Popa, V. Effect of an H_1-blocker, chlorpheniramine, on inhalation tests with histamine and allergen in allergic asthma. *Chest* 78:442, 1980.
68. Rafferty, P., and Holgate, S. Terfenadine (seldane) is a potent and selective histamine H_1 receptor antagonist in asthmatic airways. *Am. Rev. Respir. Dis.* 135:181, 1987.
69. Rafferty, P., et al. The in vivo potency and selectivity of azelastine as an H_1 histamine-receptor antagonist in human airways and skin. *J. Allergy Clin. Immunol.* 82:1113, 1988.
70. Rafferty, P., et al. The inhibitory actions of azelastine hydrochloride on the early and late bronchoconstrictor responses to inhaled allergen in atopic asthma. *J. Allergy Clin. Immunol.* 84:649, 1989.
71. Rafferty, P., et al. Terfenadine, a potent histamine H_1-receptor antagonist in the treatment of grass pollen sensitive asthma. *Br. J. Clin. Pharmacol.* 30:229, 1990.
72. Roman, I., et al. Suppression of histamine-induced wheal response by loratadine (SCH 29851) over 28 days in man. *Ann. Allergy* 57:253, 1986.
73. Rombaut, N., et al. Therapeutic effect of astemizole and terfenadine in students suffering from seasonal allergic rhinitis: a double-blind comparison. *Drug Dev. Res.* 8:79, 1986.
74. Simons, F., Watson, W., and Simons, K. The pharmacokinetics and pharmacodynamics of terfenadine in children. *J. Allergy Clin. Immunol.* 80:884, 1987.
75. Snyder, S., and Snowman, A. Receptor effects of cetirizine. *Ann. Allergy* 59:4, 1987.
76. Sternberg, L., and Gottesman, J. Clinical observations with thephorin: new antihistaminic drug. *Ann. Allergy* 6:569, 1948.
77. Taytard, A., et al. Treatment of bronchial asthma with terfenadine: a randomised controlled trial. *Br. J. Clin. Pharmacol.* 24:743, 1987.
78. Temple, D., and McCluskey, M. Loratadine, an antihistamine, blocks antigen- and ionophore-induced leukotriene release from human lung in vitro. *Prostaglandins* 35:549, 1988.
79. Thomson, N., and Kerr, J. Effect of inhaled H_1 and H_2 receptor antagonists in normal and asthmatic subjects. *Thorax* 35:428, 1980.
80. Town, G., and Holgate, S. Comparison of the effect of loratadine on the airway and skin responses to histamine, methacholine and allergen in asthmatic subjects. *J. Allergy Clin. Immunol.* 86:806, 1990.
81. Wasserman, S. Histamine and the preclinical pharmacology of cetirizine. *Ann. Allergy* 59:1, 1987.
82. Windaus, A., and Vogt, W. Synthese des Iminazolyethyamins. *Ber. Deutsch Chem. Ges.* 40:369, 1907.
83. Wood, S., et al. The metabolism and pharmacokinetics of ^{14}C-cetirizine in humans. *Ann. Allergy* 59:31, 1987.
84. Woodward, J., and Munro, N. Terfenadine, the first non-sedating antihistamine. *Drug Res.* 32:1154, 1982.
85. Zechel, H.-J., et al. Pharmacological and toxicological properties of azelastine, a novel antiallergic agent. *Drug Res.* 31:1184, 1981.
86. Hopp, R. J., et al. Terfenadine effect on the bronchoconstriction, dermal response, and leukopenia induced by platelet-activating factor. *Chest* 100:994, 1991.
87. Townley, R. G. Antiallergic properties of the second-generation H_1 antihistamines during the early and late reactions to antigen. *J. Allergy Clin. Immunol.* 90:720, 1992.
88. FDA Medical Bulletin 22 (No. 2):2, 1992.

Lipoxygenase, Cyclooxygenase, Alternative Fatty Acids, PAF Inhibitors, Gold, Diuretics, and Alcohol

66

Elliot Israel
Jeffrey M. Drazen

This chapter reviews experimental treatments of asthma. As discussed in previous sections, the currently evolving experimental data support a pathophysiologic paradigm of the asthmatic diathesis in which inflammatory processes, and the mediators of these processes, predispose to airway hyperreactivity or produce actual airway obstruction. Therefore, several novel approaches to therapy have examined the effects of agents that may act by suppressing inflammation and, in the case of newer agents, may act more specifically by interfering with the action or synthesis of putative mediators of inflammation.

This chapter will review the clinical studies concerning the efficacy of agents active on the 5-lipoxygenase pathway, cyclooxygenase pathway, and platelet-activating factor. In addition, it will cover information concerning the utility of alternative fatty acids, diuretics, gold, and alcohol in the treatment of asthma. The data suggesting that agents active on the 5-lipoxygenase pathway, the cyclooxygenase pathway, or platelet-activating factor may contribute to the pathobiology of asthma are discussed in detail elsewhere in this volume. Alternative fatty acids are presumed to act at both the 5-lipoxygenase and the cyclooxygenase pathways, and gold is presumed to have uncharacterized antiinflammatory properties. The putative mechanisms for the action of diuretics and alcohol are not clear. Each section will review the proposed mechanism of action of the agent under consideration and studies of its effect in humans.

AGENTS ACTIVE ON PRODUCTS OF THE 5-LIPOXYGENASE PATHWAY

The sulfidopeptide or cysteinyl leukotrienes (LTC_4, LTD_4, and LTE_4) are molecules derived by the lipoxygenation of arachidonic acid and its subsequent conjugation to glutathione (LTC_4) (Fig. 66-1) (see Chap. 11). Following export of LTC_4 from cells [105] there is sequential removal of glutamic acid (LTD_4) and glycine (LTE_4) from the peptide moiety [160]. In vivo, in the circulation, LTC_4 and LTD_4 are metabolized into the relatively more stable 6-cysteinyl analogue, LTE_4 [111, 140, 142]. In the absence of activated polymorphonuclear leukocytes (PMNs) the major degradation and excretion products of the cysteinyl leukotrienes are native LTE_4, N-acetyl LTE_4, and the products resulting from omega oxidation and beta elimination of LTE_4 [47, 158, 175], namely 16-COOH-LTE_4 and 14-COOH-Δ13-LTE_3. The latter molecules are likely to be bioactive, but this has not been established.

Three lines of evidence have accrued indicating that the cysteinyl leukotrienes may be involved in the asthmatic response and therefore that blockade of their effects or production might be of benefit in asthma:

1. The cells implicated in the pathobiology of asthma are cells capable of the synthesis of the leukotrienes. Although the pathology of severe asthma had been well studied, it was not until recently that biopsy specimens from airways of patients with chronic mild asthma have been examined. These demonstrate mast cells in increased numbers and in various states of activation, eosinophils with granular patterns indicative of activation, T-lymphocytes containing mRNA encoding for the cytokine interleukin-5 (IL-5), as well as loss of epithelial integrity [13, 28, 79, 93, 157]. The mast cells and the eosinophils are capable of producing the leukotrienes de novo. In addition, leukotrienes can be produced when cells capable of donating LTA_4 provide this molecule for effector cells such as vascular endothelial cells or platelets [23, 56, 59, 73, 74, 119]. Therefore the cells implicated in the asthmatic response are a major source of cysteinyl leukotrienes.

2. The physiologic effects of the leukotrienes mimic the physiologic alterations in asthma. The leukotrienes are capable of eliciting physiologic effects at low concentrations. Inhalation of aerosols of leukotrienes by normal subjects results in a decrease in flow rates during a forced exhalation [1, 12, 24–26, 46, 50, 83, 136, 153, 169, 170, 195, 196]. When flow rates low in the vital capacity (determined using partial flow-volume curves) are measured, it has been established that LTC_4 and LTD_4 induce airway narrowing that is prolonged in duration compared to that induced by histamine and that these leukotrienes are over 1,000 times more potent than histamine in normal subjects. In subjects with asthma, LTD_4 is also a potent bronchoconstrictor agonist when the compound is administered by aerosol [1, 46, 72, 136, 153, 169]. LTE_4 is also a potent bronchoactive agonist in normal and asthmatic subjects [3, 46] but is less potent than LTC_4 or LTD_4.

In addition to episodic airway narrowing, asthma is also characterized by increased "irritability" of the airways in response to a variety of distinct stimuli in the environment [125, 135, 165]. Current data suggest that the airway "inflammation" observed in subjects with asthma and airway hyperreactivity are closely linked [11, 78, 120, 136, 143]. Among the mechanisms implicated in the pathobiology of airway hyperresponsiveness is the release of mediators of inflammation; particular importance has been assigned to LTE_4. LTE_4 when incubated with tracheal contractile tissues from guinea pigs induces a state of enhanced airway responsiveness, perhaps through action at a specific LTE_4 receptor subtype [2, 108, 161, 200]. LTE_4 will enhance airway hyperresponsiveness to histamine in subjects with asthma [3].

3. The leukotrienes may be recovered during asthmatic episodes. The cysteinyl leukotrienes have been recovered from human subjects after laboratory challenges that elicit clinical symptoms similar to those that occur in spontaneous asthmatic conditions. For example, leukotrienes have been recovered in the nasal lavage fluid after intranasal challenge with either antigen or cold air [166, 189]. A number of investigative teams have shown

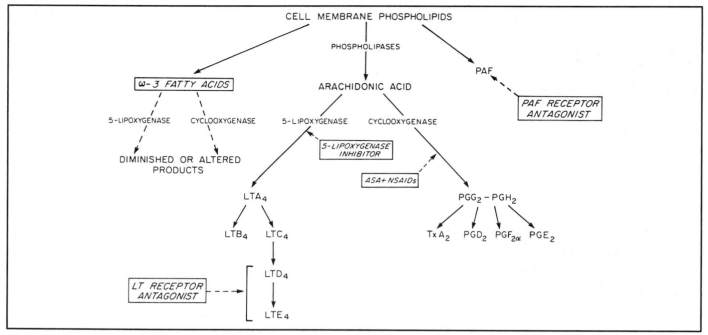

Fig. 66-1. *Modulation of proinflammatory mediators derived from cell membrane phospholipids. Interventions enclosed in solid boxes with dashed arrows indicate inhibition. PAF = platelet-activating factor; ASA = acetylsalicylic acid; NSAIDs = nonsteroidal antiinflammatory drugs; PG = prostaglandin; TxA_2 = thromboxane A_2; LT = leukotriene.*

that leukotrienes can be recovered in significantly greater amounts from bronchoalveolar lavage (BAL) fluid obtained from subjects with symptomatic asthma as compared to subjects with asymptomatic asthma or normal subjects [49, 106, 184, 194, 205].

An important advance has been the development of indices of leukotriene production that rely on measurements made on urine samples [141, 167, 186, 197]. In normal human subjects, after intravenous administration of radiolabeled LTC_4, 5 to 15 percent of the counts are recovered in the urine as intact LTE_4. Not only can exogenous leukotrienes be recovered in the urine, it is now clear that leukotriene recovery can serve as an index of endogenous release of leukotrienes [167, 184, 186]. There is an increase in the recovery of LTE_4 in the urine of subjects with asthma early after antigen challenge; the magnitude of the fall in the forced expiratory volume in 1 second (FEV_1) and the amount of LTE_4 in the urine are well correlated [123]. In spontaneously occurring asthma, there is a clear relationship between LTE_4 production and reversible airway obstruction [50a].

Approaches to modifying the physiologic effects of leukotrienes have recently been aimed in two directions: (1) antagonizing the effects of the cysteinyl leukotrienes at a receptor; and (2) inhibiting the production of the cysteinyl leukotrienes.

It is well established that the cysteinyl leukotrienes exert their effects on airway contractile tissues through action at receptors [172], and in humans only a single leukotriene receptor subtype has been clearly identified [31]. A large number of chemically distinct antagonists have been recognized. However, only a few have been shown to be effective antagonists at the LTD_4 receptor in humans [10, 31, 53, 97, 146, 171], and only a few have been tested in human asthma models, as reported below. Several inhibitors of leukotriene production that work through inhibition of the 5-lipoxygenase enzyme have been examined as well. Only one has been shown to be effective in humans.

Clinical Studies

A number of LTD_4 receptor antagonists have been examined in laboratory-induced asthma. In early studies examining the effi-

cacy of these compounds in the asthmatic response to inhaled antigen, the LTD_4 receptor antagonists L-649,923 and LY-171,883 produced a limited but statistically significant positive effect on the early but not the late asthmatic response [29, 62]. A single oral dose of ICI-204,219, which shifts the dose-response curve to LTD_4 approximately 100-fold "to the right" [171] and thus is almost 30 times more potent than these early compounds, significantly reduced the bronchoconstrictor response resulting from allergen challenge in both the early and the late phase [56a]. The early-phase suppression occurred more "universally" than the late-phase suppression. In addition, this agent suppressed the allergen-induced increase in airway responsiveness to histamine [187]. Preliminary data using MK-571 and SKF-104,353 showed inhibition of both phases of the response to allergen as well [42, 81, 151a]. Not all studies have been positive, however; L-648,051 had no significant protective effect against either the antigen-induced early or the late asthmatic response [14].

Antagonists at the LTD_4 receptor have been shown to be effective in preventing bronchospasm resulting from isocapneic hyperventilation of cold, dry air or due to exercise. Israel and colleagues [89] demonstrated that LY-171,883, an LTD_4 receptor antagonist capable of inducing a three- to fivefold shift in the LTD_4 dose-response curve, had a small but statistically significant effect on the bronchospasm due to cold air inhalation. Manning and colleagues [124] demonstrated a significant amelioration of the asthmatic response resulting from exercise using MK-571. When an area under the curve analysis was used they demonstrated more than a 75 percent inhibition of the exercise response (Fig. 66-2). However, not all of their subjects had a salutary response. More recently, Robuschi and colleagues [156] provided evidence that SKF-104,353, an LTD_4 receptor antagonist, can partially inhibit exercise-induced asthma.

There is only one published study on the effects of an LTD_4 receptor antagonist in subjects with spontaneously occurring asthma [39]. In this study, the antagonist LY-171,883 had a positive effect on lung function as indicated by a small (≈ 0.3 l) but significant improvement in FEV_1. An important finding is that

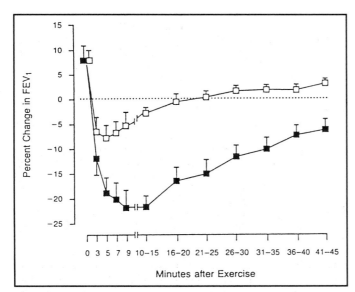

Fig. 66-2. *Mean (± SEM) percent change in FEV$_1$ over time after exercise, after treatment with placebo (■—solid squares) or MK-571 (□—open squares). (Reprinted with permission from P. J. Manning et al. Inhibition of exercise-induced bronchoconstriction by MK-571, a potent leukotriene D4–receptor antagonist. N. Engl. J. Med. 323:1736, 1990.)*

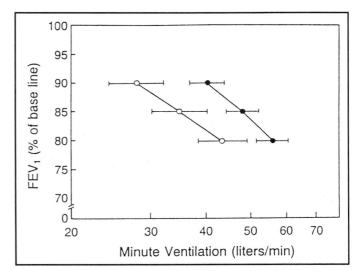

Fig. 66-3. *Composite dose-response curve illustrating the mean (± SEM) percent of baseline FEV$_1$ in relation to ventilation of cold, dry air after treatment with placebo (○) and A-64077 (●). (Reprinted with permission from E. Israel et al. The effects of a 5-lipoxygenase inhibitor on asthma induced by cold, dry air. N. Engl. J. Med. 323:1740, 1990.)*

Table 66-1. Effects of leukotriene D$_4$ receptor antagonists in asthma

| | | | Asthmatic condition | | | | | |
| | | | Laboratory induced | | | Spontaneous | | |
Antagonist	Route	Shift in LTD$_4$ dose-response curve	Allergen	Cold air	Exercise	Bronchodilation	Improved asthma	Comments
LY-171,883	Oral	3–4 fold	+	+	NR	NR	+	Not in development for asthma at this time
MK-571 MK-0679	IV/oral	30–40 fold	+ + +	NR	+ + +	+ +	+ +	Not in development for asthma at this time
SKF-104,353	Inhaled	3–4 fold	+ + +	NR	+	NR	NR	
ICI-204,219	Oral/inhaled	~100 fold	+ + +	NR	NR	+	NR	Inhibits early- and late-phase response to allergen

0–4+ = magnitude of response; NR = not reported.

the subjects with the improved FEV$_1$ had substantially decreased inhaler usage. Interestingly, the effects on FEV$_1$ took approximately 6 weeks to manifest, suggesting that the leukotrienes may affect asthma in part by altering airway responsiveness. This finding is important in that the evaluation of these agents may require months, rather than days to weeks, before the full antiasthmatic effect can be appreciated.

Another strategy to examine antagonists at the LTD$_4$ receptor has been to administer them to subjects with asthma who have withheld their daily asthma medication. In this setting, intravenous MK-571 and ICI-204,219 each resulted in bronchodilation greater than that observed when subjects were given placebo [65, 87]. In contrast a single inhaled dose of SKF-104,353 did not inhibit the response to inhaled prostaglandin D$_2$ (PGD$_2$) or histamine [86]. The effects of antagonists at the LTD$_4$ receptor are summarized in Table 66-1.

In addition to receptor antagonists, another strategy to interfere with the action of leukotrienes in asthma has been to study the effects of inhibitors of the enzyme 5-lipoxygenase on asthmatic responses [64, 90, 122]. In this approach the formation of all 5-lipoxygenase products (as well as lipoxins that derive from initial 5-lipoxygenation) will be prevented. Piriprost (U-60,257) [122] and nafazatrom [64], two first-generation 5-lipoxygenase inhibitors, did not alter the asthmatic response to inhaled antigen or exercise. However, adequate inhibition of 5-lipoxygenase was not demonstrated in these studies. A-64077, a 5-lipoxygenase inhibitor [90] with known in vivo effectiveness, resulted in an amelioration of the asthmatic response to the hyperventilation of cold, dry air indicating the viability of this approach (Fig. 66-3). However, a single dose of A-64077 was only marginally effective against allergen-induced bronchospasm [88], suggesting that mediators other than leukotrienes may be involved in this response or that adequate blockage of production was not achieved.

The use of agents active on the 5-lipoxygenase products in asthma is in its infancy. The initial data are promising. The differing effects seen with agents with different potency suggest that the use of pharmacologic agents of adequate potency is necessary to evaluate adequately the utility of this modality of asthmatic therapy.

CYCLOOXYGENASE INHIBITORS

Prostaglandins are formed from arachidonic acid by the addition of oxygen through action of the enzyme cyclooxygenase. A thorough review of the potential role of prostaglandins in the pathophysiologic mechanisms related to asthma is presented in Chapter 11. Several of the prostaglandins, namely PGD_2, $PGF_{2\alpha}$, and thromboxane A_2, have the capacity to produce constriction of airway smooth muscle [134]. Asthmatics are known to be hyperresponsive to the bronchoconstrictor actions of these compounds [77]; PGD_2 and $PGF_{2\alpha}$ have been shown to increase bronchial responsiveness [63, 80]. Prostaglandins have been detected in the plasma and the airways after inhaled antigen challenge in humans [71, 129]. In addition, PGD_2 and its metabolite $9\alpha,11\beta$-PGF_2 have been detected in the BAL of asthmatics at 10 times the concentration found in rhinitis patients [112].

Nonsteroidal antiinflammatory drugs (NSAIDs) block the action of cyclooxygenase and therefore suppress or prevent the production of prostaglandins; this is their presumed mechanism of action in the treatment of arthritis. By virtue of this action, the NSAIDs, which include aspirin, indomethacin, and ibuprofen among others, should reduce bronchoconstriction resulting from the production of prostaglandins and possibly ameliorate the hyperresponsiveness that might result from the release of these compounds. Despite their availability for centuries, agents inhibiting cyclooxygenase have not been recognized as widely useful in asthma treatment, and only a very small minority of asthmatics appear to benefit from cyclooxygenase inhibition. In fact some asthmatics clearly bronchoconstrict upon the administration of NSAIDs. This may relate to the fact that in addition to the bronchoconstricting prostaglandins mentioned above there is a subset of prostanoids that act to relax bronchial smooth muscle. Nonspecific inhibition of prostanoid synthesis may result in inhibition of the protective effect of these prostaglandins. In addition, recent evidence suggests that in some asthmatics inhibition of cyclooxygenase may result in increased production of potent bronchoconstricting 5-lipoxygenase products [37]. This section will review the data on the utility of cyclooxygenase inhibitors (1) in unselected asthmatics and human asthma models, (2) for desensitization in those asthmatics who bronchoconstrict upon administration of cyclooxygenase inhibitors, and (3) in the small subset of asthmatics who do benefit from cyclooxygenase inhibition.

Clinical Studies

Unselected Asthmatics

Most studies in unselected asthmatics have not demonstrated a beneficial effect of cyclooxygenase blockade. Clinical trials of aspirin and indomethacin have failed to demonstrate a beneficial effect on pulmonary function or clinical symptoms even after 4 weeks of treatment [40, 55, 57, 192].

The effect of cyclooxygenase inhibition in human models of asthma has been variable. Exercise and antigen-induced bronchospasm were not ameliorated by NSAID pretreatment [57, 98, 162, 168]. However, when flurbiprofen, an NSAID with 20 times the potency of indomethacin, was used in atopic asthmatics it inhibited antigen-induced bronchoconstriction by 22 percent, although it did not alter nonspecific airway responsiveness [43]. In another study, indomethacin did ameliorate the fall in FEV_1 after ozone exposure by 75 percent, but it did not prevent the bronchial hyperreactivity that occurred after ozone exposure [204]. It has been suggested that the diverse effects seen in the different challenge models may be related to the fact that some prostanoids such as PGE_2 and PGI_2 can act to relax bronchial smooth muscle or inhibit release of inflammatory mediators. The physiologic effect of cyclooxygenase inhibition may therefore depend on the subsets of prostanoids released by the specific bronchoprovocative stimulus and perhaps on the specific activity of the inhibitor. It is therefore of interest that a selective thromboxane synthetase inhibitor [61] caused a fourfold decrease in acetylcholine reactivity in a group of asthmatics.

Aspirin-Sensitive Asthmatics

It is estimated that up to 10 percent of asthmatics may bronchoconstrict in response to aspirin and NSAIDs (see also Chap. 48). Aspirin desensitization has been used to treat some of these patients. Desensitization is achieved by administering increasing doses of aspirin followed by daily administration of maintenance doses. This approach is derived from the observation that there is a refractory period after aspirin administration [19, 148, 177]. While this approach blunts aspirin sensitivity, the influence of this procedure on underlying asthma symptoms has been variable [36, 113, 114, 117, 130, 132, 177, 178, 182]. Only one of these studies was double-blinded. In this study of 25 aspirin-sensitive individuals [178] there was no change in systemic steroid use, although 16 patients experienced decreases in nasal or asthma symptom scores. A study examining the effect of aspirin desensitization on the PC_{20} FEV_1 showed no change in this measure of nonspecific bronchial reactivity [102]. A recent review of the experience with 107 patients [181] compared those patients who avoided aspirin, those who had been desensitized and stopped desensitization, and those who continued desensitization. In this retrospective report, the patients who underwent desensitization had significantly fewer hospitalizations, emergency room visits, and outpatient visits. In view of the inconsistent results reported with aspirin desensitization and the unblinded and retrospective nature of many of the studies, the use of aspirin desensitization as a treatment modality for general asthma symptoms in aspirin-sensitive asthma remains to be confirmed. It is clearly effective in decreasing NSAID reactions in those sensitive asthmatics who require NSAIDs.

NSAID-Responsive Asthmatics

The existence of a subgroup of asthmatics who bronchoconstrict upon ingestion of NSAIDs suggests that there may be subgroups of asthmatics with differing combinations of mediators responsible for maintaining airway tone, causing bronchoconstriction, and mediating bronchodilation. In addition to those asthmatics "hypersensitive" to aspirin, there is indeed a very small subgroup of patients in whom blockade of cyclooxygenase clearly does produce bronchodilation. Since these cases are rare, only case report data are available [20, 27, 54, 58, 67, 95, 101, 132, 152, 182]. The largest group of such patients was investigated by Szczeklik and Nizankowska [183]. They performed a placebo-controlled, single-blind study on six such patients in which they demonstrated an improvement in pulmonary function tests 1 to 2 hours after aspirin administration. While the patients who bronchodilate with NSAIDs generally appear to be corticosteroid dependent and nonatopic [67], at present the identification of this small minority of patients on clinical or biochemical grounds is not yet possible.

Prostaglandins, depending on the specific moiety, may mediate bronchoconstriction and hyperreactivity or, conversely, bronchodilation and possible bronchoprotective effects. At present only a very few patients can be shown to benefit directly from administration of NSAIDs. These patients remain extremely difficult to identify; paradoxically they also clinically resemble patients who are *hypersensitive* to aspirin. Thus NSAIDs remain an adjunctive modality of treatment for a very select minority of asthmatics. For the vast majority of asthmatics, blockade of cyclooxygenase and inhibition of production of all prostanoids do not produce significant benefits. It is possible that inhibition of the synthesis of specific prostanoid moieties such as thromboxane, or specific receptor antagonism [116] without its attendant stimulation of the products of 5-lipoxygenase, may permit appreciation of bronchoprotective effects in the future.

ALTERNATIVE FATTY ACIDS

As mentioned previously, cyclooxygenase and 5-lipoxygenase products of arachidonic acid have been postulated to play a role in producing the airway narrowing and hyperresponsiveness of asthma. Marine fish oils are rich in eicosapentaenoic acid (EPA) and docosahexaenoic acid (DCHA). Both these fatty acids contain five or more unsaturated carbon-to-carbon bonds as compared to arachidonic acid, which has four such bonds. These particular marine polyunsaturated fatty acids are known as n-3 or omega-3 fatty acids, since the first double bond occurs three carbons removed from the terminal methyl group. In contrast, in arachidonic acid, which is an n-6 fatty acid, the first double bond is six positions removed from the terminal carbon. When included in the diet, EPA and DCHA are incorporated into mammalian tissue phospholipids and may act as alternate substrates for the cyclooxygenase and 5-lipoxygenase enzymes responsible for elaboration of the proinflammatory mediators mentioned above.

When n-3 fatty acids are incorporated into the cell membrane they act to competitively inhibit the conversion of arachidonic acid to prostanoids and leukotrienes. DCHA is poorly metabolized by cyclooxygenase [41]. In addition, some EPA-derived prostaglandin and thromboxane products are less active than those derived from arachidonic acid [131]. EPA metabolites are less effective in causing platelet aggregation and in eliciting chemotaxis of neutrophils [109, 144, 188]. Dietary supplementation with fish oil in humans for 6 weeks has also been shown to decrease the generation of a 5-lipoxygenase product such as LTB_4 by more than 50 percent [109]. EPA also appears to inhibit platelet-activating factor generation from monocyte monolayers [174].

In animals EPA supplementation has been shown to block the progression of autoimmune disease [151]. The effect in animal asthma models has been somewhat variable. While a fish oil diet was shown to enhance the bronchospastic response to intravenous antigen in guinea pigs [110], a study using inhaled antigen showed that such a diet actually produced a significant protective effect [89]. The ability of omega-3 fatty acids to alter both mediator production and inflammatory cellular responses in animal and cell model systems prompted several studies of their effectiveness in modulating human asthmatic responses.

Clinical Studies

Studies in asthmatics using fish oils have generally not shown significant effects on clinical symptoms or reactivity. In a study that examined the effect of 8 weeks of supplementation with high-dose (4 gm/day) or low-dose (0.1 gm/day) EPA supplementation, there was no change in objective pulmonary function or clinical status [99]. A change in neutrophil chemotaxis and LTB_4 generation did occur in the high-dose group despite the lack of clinical efficacy. Of note, of the 12 patients studied, 3 patients were known to be aspirin sensitive. The inclusion of aspirin-sensitive patients may have a direct bearing on outcome, since Picado and colleagues [147] showed that EPA supplementation may actually adversely affect this subset of asthmatics. In a single-blind study of 10 aspirin-sensitive asthmatics treated with placebo followed by a combination of EPA and DCHA for 6 weeks, they found that during the fifth and sixth weeks of therapy, peak expiratory flows fell by approximately 15 percent with a concomitant increase in beta-sympathomimetic use compared to the placebo period.

Arm and colleagues [4] studied the effects of fish oil supplementation in 20 asthmatics for 10 weeks. Twelve subjects received EPA/DCHA and eight received olive oil in a double-blind

manner. Although there was a 50 percent decrease in total LTB production and a decrease in neutrophil chemotaxis, there was no change in spirometry, peak expiratory flow, or histamine responsiveness during the study. However, 11 of the patients who received fish oil were on inhaled steroids, raising the possibility that the response to fish oil may have been eclipsed by the effect of the steroids. In a similar study we investigated asthmatics who were not on inhaled steroids and administered the same dose of EPA/DCHA for 10 weeks in a double-blind manner. We noted no improvement in symptoms, peak expiratory flow rate, histamine responsiveness, or the immediate response to allergen [91]. Of interest, a further study by Arm and colleagues [5] showed that fish oil supplementation blunted the late-phase response to antigen challenge even though it did not produce any clinical response as evidenced by peak flows, medication use, or symptom scores.

In addition to fish oil supplementation, dietary augmentation with oils rich in linolenic acid has been attempted in asthmatics. Linolenic acid can be elongated and desaturated to EPA and can be converted into prostanoids of the 1-series such as PGE_1, which appears to have more bronchodilating effect than PGE_2 [66]. Evening primrose oil, which is high in linolenic acid, was given to 29 asthmatics, 24 of whom were on inhaled steroids and 8 on oral steroids. Despite alterations in the fatty acid composition of cholesterol esters in their plasma, the patients failed to show any significant improvement in their asthma [176]. Other studies with primrose oil, in doses found to produce a beneficial effect in eczema, also failed to demonstrate clinical improvement in asthmatics [51].

Dietary supplementation with alternative fatty acids appears to offer the promise of significant antiinflammatory action via its combined effect on both the cellular and mediator components of inflammation. Alternative fatty acids have been shown to be of potential benefit in rheumatoid arthritis [103, 173] and eczema [201], yet several clinical studies have been unable to demonstrate a beneficial effect in asthmatics. While many of these studies have examined patients already on antiinflammatory agents, even in studies where steroid treatment has been avoided no significant effects have been seen. The apparent lack of efficacy may be due to inhibition of bronchodilator prostanoid production or possibly may be a reflection of the fact that neutrophils may not play a significant role in modulating asthmatic hyperresponsiveness. On the basis of the current studies, alternative fatty acid supplementation does not appear to have a significant role to play in the treatment of asthma.

PLATELET-ACTIVATING FACTOR ANTAGONISTS

The chemical structure of platelet-activating factor (PAF) was elucidated in 1972 from materials released by IgE-stimulated rabbit basophils that caused platelet aggregation [16]. PAF is synthesized from ether-linked phospholipids in cell membrane phospholipids by the action of phospholipase A_2 and PAF synthetase [202]. Multiple cell types implicated in asthma-associated inflammation including neutrophils [118], eosinophils [35], human alveolar macrophages [6], endothelial cells [150], and mast cells [164] have the capacity to produce PAF (see Chap. 22).

PAF has been considered a possible mediator of asthmatic airway narrowing for three reasons. First, although its direct effect on airway smooth muscle varies among species and may be relatively minimal [163], it is a potent inducer of airway microvascular leakage, which can produce luminal obstruction [203]. Second, it has significant eosinophil proinflammatory effects. PAF is the most potent eosinophil chemotactic agent known and activates eosinophils and neutrophils [193]. Third, experiments in humans have suggested that PAF may increase nonspecific bronchial responsiveness. This increase in responsiveness has been observed in normal subjects and not in asthmatics [38, 44, 96, 159]. However, others have not been able to demonstrate such an effect [85, 104], and asthmatics do not appear to be hyperresponsive to PAF when compared to normals [38].

The elucidation of the molecular structure of a receptor for PAF [84] has raised the possibility that the specific antagonism is feasible with potential therapeutic results. On the basis of the in vitro and clinical studies with PAF itself, antagonism of PAF could potentially decrease airway edema, eosinophil-mediated events, and hyperresponsiveness in asthma.

Clinical Studies

The ginkolides, complex organic molecules extracted from the ginko tree, have been used in folk remedies for cough and wheezing and have been shown to be naturally-occurring competitive antagonists of PAF. The discovery of these compounds and synthesis of structural analogues have resulted in the development of several new compounds that antagonize PAF. However, these compounds have only just begun undergoing evaluation in human airways, and as a result, only preliminary reports of small trials in laboratory-induced asthma are available at this time.

WEB-2086, a potent and selective PAF antagonist, has been shown to block PAF-induced contractions [94] in isolated human airways. This compound was also shown to block the potentiating effect of PAF on histamine-induced contractions in this model. Inhaled and oral forms of WEB-2086 were found to be ineffective in blocking allergen-induced bronchoconstriction in asthmatics [60, 198]. Both studies were performed on eight patients with 7 days of pretreatment with WEB-2086. Pretreatment did not modify the early or late response to allergen, nor was there an effect on postallergen methacholine or histamine hyperresponsiveness.

Studies of the effects of additional PAF antagonists in antigen-induced bronchoconstriction have also failed to show an effect. A single dose of MK-287, an agent that can induce a 14- to 34-fold shift in PAF-induced platelet aggregation, given to eight atopic asthmatics failed to affect the early or late response to inhaled house dust [15]. It also failed to alter the allergen-associated hyperresponsiveness to histamine after these challenges.

BN-52063, a mixture of ginkolides that inhibited PAF-induced platelet aggregation, was evaluated in 10 asthmatics [199]. A single dose did not alter the bronchospastic response to isocapnic hyperventilation of cold, dry air, although it did inhibit, by a factor of two, PAF-induced platelet aggregation in the blood. Administration of the compound for 2 days did not change the maximal fall in airway resistance or peak expiratory flow observed in asthmatic subjects after exercise, although there was mild attenuation of the decrease in peak expiratory flow that occurred 20 and 30 minutes after exercise. Of note, there was an increase in the plasma concentration of platelet factor 4 and beta-thromboglobulin postexercise, which was attenuated by BN-52063.

A study of the effect of a single dose of SCH-37370 [48], a combined PAF antagonist-antihistamine, on the bronchoconstriction induced by cold, dry air in 16 asthmatics, produced 16 percent inhibition of reactivity to cold, dry air as judged by a change in the provocative minute ventilation required to produce a 15 percent decrease in FEV_1. There was also a 7.3 percent increase in FEV_1, which persisted even after the challenge. While these results appear promising, similar effects have been reported with antihistamines alone, suggesting that the observed effects may have been due to the antihistaminic properties of this compound.

Although initial studies with PAF suggested that it might produce prolonged bronchial hyperreactivity in normals, these effects have been extremely variable. Preliminary data after short-term administration of the available PAF antagonist have failed to demonstrate significant effects in experimentally-induced

bronchospasm in asthmatics. However, due to PAF's potential role in mediating recruitment of inflammatory cells in the airways, a full evaluation of the potential role of PAF antagonists in asthma will require more prolonged administration of such agents and may require the development of more potent antagonists. The elucidation of the molecular structure of the PAF receptor may make the search for such agents proceed more quickly. This topic is discussed further in Chapter 22.

GOLD

As the focus in asthma therapy shifts to the treatment of underlying inflammation, agents that have been found to be effective in inflammatory diseases such as rheumatoid arthritis have been natural candidates for possible roles in asthma therapy. Chapter 68 discusses methotrexate, a form of therapy useful in rheumatoid arthritis, and its possible utility in the treatment of asthma. Double-blind studies have shown that parenteral gold can be effective in treating rheumatoid arthritis [52], thus raising the possibility that gold salts might offer potential therapeutic benefits in asthma. In vitro, different gold preparations have been shown to decrease histamine release from human basophils [17, 185] and to decrease guinea pig isolated tracheal smooth muscle contractions in response to histamine and LTD_4 [121]. Gold has also been shown to inhibit prostaglandin synthesis [145]. Unfortunately, parenteral gold salt therapy has been associated with a high incidence of side effects (25–50%) including proteinuria, rash, leukopenia, stomatitis, and thrombocytopenia.

Clinical Trials

Gold therapy has been part of conventional chronic asthma therapy in Japan for many years. Most reports of the outcomes of gold therapy have been from uncontrolled studies [139, 179]. Muranaka et al. [127, 128] reported double-blind studies of gold administration. Global physician evaluations improved in 71 percent of the treatment group versus 44 percent of the placebo group. Although less medication was used by the treatment group, obstruction as measured by FEV_1 was unchanged, as was the frequency of acute attacks. Twenty-nine percent of the patients developed side effects, requiring withdrawal in one study, and large numbers of patients dropped out of the therapy group in both studies, making it extremely difficult to evaluate the true efficacy of this treatment regimen.

A partially blinded study in 10 steroid-dependent asthmatics [100] suggested a possible steroid-sparing effect of gold but not without significant toxicity. Five patients showed some improvement in terms of reduced steroid requirement; however, 2 of the 10 patients had to be withdrawn due to proteinuria, and only 2 of the 5 successful medication reductions occurred in the phase where patients and nurses were blinded to study medication. The other three responses occurred during an open trial section of the study.

A recent study by Bernstein et al. [17] looked at the effect of oral gold in an open trial in 20 steroid-dependent asthmatics. In this open trial there was a 34 percent reduction in the mean number of nighttime asthma attacks, and some patients were able to reduce their steroid use. However, the change in steroid use was not significant for the group as a whole. Ten percent of patients were forced to discontinue due to gold side effects in this 5-month trial. Sixty-five percent of patients developed loose stools or diarrhea, which did not require discontinuation of the drug.

Gold is associated with significant morbidity. In view of the incidence and multiplicity of side effects, further controlled clinical trials will be required before we can adopt the use of gold compounds in the treatment of severe asthma. The current data are inadequate to support widespread use of this modality of therapy.

DIURETICS

It has been suggested that dietary salt intake may be a factor in the geographic variation in the prevalence of asthma [32, 33]. Reductions in dietary salt have also been associated with a decrease in histamine responsiveness [34, 92]. In addition, changes in osmolarity and ion composition have been suggested as determinants of the airway response to certain bronchoconstrictor stimuli [76]. Periciliary bronchial lining fluid has also been postulated to play a role in airway narrowing [203]. Recent human experimental data have shown that inhaled diuretics can indeed alter asthmatic responsiveness to physical and antigenic stimulation.

Clinical Studies

In 1988 Bianco and colleagues [21] reported that 28 mg of inhaled furosemide decreased the bronchospastic response to exercise in a group of asthmatics by 35 percent as measured by the fall in FEV_1. They found that this response was dose related and that oral furosemide produced no such effects. They also reported that this effect was only observed when furosemide was inhaled and not when it was administered intravenously. Subsequent work [154] showed that the mean fall in FEV_1 after ultrasonic nebulization of distilled water was also decreased from 26 to 6 percent by prior administration of inhaled furosemide.

The protective effect of inhaled furosemide is not restricted to attenuating the bronchospastic response to physical stimulation. Forty milligrams of inhaled furosemide has been shown to inhibit the early antigen-induced fall in FEV_1 in atopic asthmatics by 69 percent [18] (Fig. 66-4) and by 88 percent [191]. In another report, 28 mg of furosemide inhibited the immediate response to antigen by 73 percent [155].

Of potentially greater interest, inhaled furosemide also blocked the late asthmatic reaction to inhaled antigen by 43 percent [18] (Fig. 66-4). While this effect on the late phase of the reaction to antigen suggested the possibility that the hyperresponsiveness thought to be associated with the late-phase reaction might be blunted as well, these investigators reported no attenuation in methacholine hyperresponsiveness 24 hours after antigen challenge. However, in a subsequent report from this group there was a significant decrease in reactivity to methacholine observed 2 hours after antigen challenge [191].

Furosemide has also been shown to block the bronchospastic response to other "indirect" challenges such as metabisulfite [133], adenosine 5'-monophosphate [149], cold, dry air [75], and acetylsalicylic acid [190]. However, preliminary data suggest that it does not block the bronchospastic response to toluene diisocyanate [126]. It also does not appear to be effective in blocking "direct" bronchial smooth muscle constriction, as evidenced by its minor effects on methacholine-induced bronchoconstriction [75, 133, 149].

It was originally thought that the effects of furosemide may be directly related to its effect on Na^+-K^+ ATPase and subsequent chloride flux. However, bumetanide, a diuretic 40 times more potent than furosemide in its effects on Na^+-K^+ ATPase, has not been shown to prevent bronchoconstriction [137]. Additionally, acetazolamide, a diuretic that acts through inhibition of carbonic anhydrase and has no Na^+-K^+ ATPase effects, produces significant inhibition of cold, dry air–induced bronchoconstriction [138].

Inhaled diuretics appear to inhibit the bronchospastic response to many "indirect" bronchoconstrictors as evidenced by multiple trials in different human asthma models. While the precise mechanism of action is still unclear, the widespread effectiveness suggests that diuretics may play a role in managing asthmatic bronchoconstriction. Potential problems with the diuretics include a possible short duration of action and unwanted diuretic effects at higher doses even when inhaled [138]. The recent report of successful formulation of a metered-dose inhaler of furosemide [22] will permit more rapid evaluation of the true utility of this class of compounds in the management of asthma.

ALCOHOL

Alcohol has been mentioned as a potential treatment for asthma as early as 1550 B.C. in the Ebers papyri [8] in which a combination of honey, wine, and beer was recommended on a daily basis for breathing problems. A mechanism of action has not been established. Although anecdotal reports of the efficacy of alcohol in the treatment of asthma exist throughout the medical literature, controlled trials examining its efficacy have been lacking, and epidemiologic evidence suggests that alcohol actually may be a factor in the development of chronic obstructive lung disease.

Clinical Studies

In an uncontrolled report in 1947 Brown [30] reported that intravenous ethanol was of use in patients with status asthmaticus, resulting in reduced breathlessness and clinical improvement. No objective studies of airway function were reported. Herxheimer and Streseman [82], and subsequently Ayres et al. [7], reported that oral ethanol produced a bronchodilator effect in asthmatics. Although ethanol produced an immediate decrease in specific airway conductance (sG_{AW}), four of five asthmatics had an increase in sG_{AW} 10 to 45 minutes after sipping 40 ml of 60% alcohol [7]. The same group showed, in a single-blind study, that 250 ml of 8% ethanol produced a 33 percent rise in sG_{AW} in asthmatics but not in normals [9]. There was no change in FEV_1, forced vital capacity (FVC), or mid–maximal expiratory flow (MMEF) at this dose of alcohol. A similar amount of 6% ethanol was not effective.

Despite these reports of minor physiologic improvements in isolated aspects of airway function after intravenous or oral ethanol administration, there are numerous reports of bronchoconstriction after ethanol. In particular, inhaled ethanol appears to produce bronchoconstriction [70, 206]. Although this has been

Fig. 66-4. *Mean (± SEM) percent change in FEV_1 after allergen challenge after treatment with placebo (●) and furosemide (○). (Reprinted with permission from S. Bianco et al. Protective effect of inhaled furosemide on allergen-induced early and late asthmatic reactions. N. Engl. J. Med. 321:1069, 1989.)*

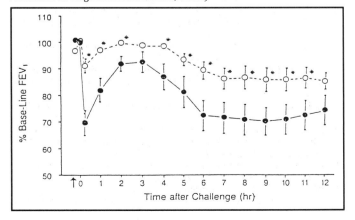

attributed to the nonisotonic nature of the inhaled alcohol, the effect has also been observed when the ethanol was inhaled as an isotonic solution [115]. In addition, certain individuals, possibly more commonly Orientals, may have a sensitivity to alcohol, which results in bronchospasm [69, 70]. This sensitivity may be independent of route of administration and is substantially blocked by antihistamines [69], suggesting that histamine may mediate this response.

In addition to the sensitivity to alcohol in certain subgroups that may not necessarily be asthmatic, it is now well recognized that the other components of certain alcoholic beverages may precipitate airway narrowing in susceptible individuals. It is reported that 10 percent of asthmatics complain of bronchospasm with ingestion of red wine [45]. Study of these patients reveals that some have a particular sensitivity to sulfites, responding with up to a 40 percent decrease in peak expiratory flow after ingestion of wine with added sulfites [45].

While alcohol may cause acute bronchodilation or airway narrowing in subgroups of asthmatics, population studies suggest that alcohol may accelerate the age-related reduction in pulmonary function. A study of a general population in Copenhagen [107] found that alcohol consumption significantly accelerated the loss of FEV_1 and FVC with time, independent of smoking habits. The consumption of greater than 350 gm/week of alcohol was comparable to the effect of smoking 15 gm/day of tobacco. In a study by Garshick and colleagues [68], a significant relationship was demonstrated between cough and phlegm and lifetime alcohol consumption. Alcohol consumption also had a negative effect on FEV_1 over time, although this study suggested that in those patients who both smoked and drank, alcohol may have produced a small protective effect on the deleterious effects of smoking on lung function.

Although some studies suggest a bronchodilating effect of alcohol, these effects are quite small and do not suggest that alcohol would be of additional benefit in the current therapy of asthma. Oral ingestion of alcohol appears to have an initial negative impact on lung function. In addition, a significant number of asthmatics have documented adverse reactions to alcohol or other agents found in certain alcoholic beverages, and epidemiologic data suggest that long-term use of alcohol may have an adverse impact on lung function.

Alternate therapies for asthma are emerging based on our evolving understanding and hypotheses concerning the underlying pathophysiologic mechanisms in asthma. The data in humans presented in this chapter represent the earliest clinical tests of these hypotheses. Initial data with several potent agents affecting the 5-lipoxygenase pathway appear quite promising. Investigations over the next 5 years will be required to define the role of this approach in asthma therapy. Human studies of PAF antagonists appear too preliminary to speculate on the effectiveness of this approach to therapy and will require the development of more potent bioavailable antagonists. It is unclear whether the effectiveness of inhaled diuretics will lead directly to the development of a new therapeutic modality. However, the exploration of the underlying mechanism of the observed bronchoprotective effect in human asthma models may further enhance our understanding of the operative mechanisms in asthma and suggest additional approaches to treatment.

REFERENCES

1. Adelroth, E., et al. Airway responsiveness to leukotrienes C_4 and D_4 and to methacholine in patients with asthma and normal controls. *N. Engl. J. Med.* 315:480, 1986.
2. Aharony, D., Catanese, C. A., and Falcone, R. C. Kinetic and pharmacologic analysis of [3H]leukotriene E_4 binding to receptors on guinea pig lung membranes: Evidence for selective binding to a subset of leukotriene D_4 receptors. *J. Pharmacol. Exp. Ther.* 248:581, 1989.
3. Arm, J. P., Spur, B. W., and Lee, T. H. The effects of inhaled leukotriene E_4 on the airway responsiveness to histamine in subjects with asthma and normal subjects. *J. Allergy Clin. Immunol.* 82:654, 1988.
4. Arm, J. P., et al. Effect of dietary supplementation with fish oil lipids on mild asthma. *Thorax* 43:84, 1988.
5. Arm, J. P., et al. The effects of dietary supplementation with fish oil lipids on the airways response to inhaled allergen in bronchial asthma. *Am. Rev. Respir. Dis.* 139:1395, 1989.
6. Arnoux, B., et al. Antigenic release of PAF-acether and beta-glucuronidase from alveolar macrophages of asthmatics. *Bull. Eur. Physiopathol. Respir.* 23:119, 1987.
7. Ayres, J., Ancic, P., and Clark, T. J. Airways responses to oral ethanol in normal subjects and in patients with asthma. *J. R. Soc. Med.* 75:699, 1982.
8. Ayres, J. G. The history of the use of alcohol in the treatment of respiratory diseases. *Br. J. Dis. Chest* 81:80, 1987.
9. Ayres, J. G., and Clark, T. J. Intravenous ethanol can provide bronchodilatation in asthma. *Clin. Sci.* 64:555, 1983.
10. Barnes, N., Piper, P. J., and Costello, J. The effect of an oral leukotriene antagonist L-649,923 on histamine and leukotriene D_4–induced bronchoconstriction in normal man. *J. Allergy Clin. Immunol.* 79:816, 1987.
11. Barnes, N. C., and Costello, J. F. Airway hyperresponsiveness and inflammation. *Br. Med. Bull.* 43:445, 1987.
12. Barnes, N. C., Piper, P. J., and Costello, J. F. Comparative effects of inhaled leukotriene C_4, leukotriene D_4, and histamine in normal human subjects. *Thorax* 39:500, 1984.
13. Beasley, R., et al. Cellular events in the bronchi in mild asthma and after bronchial provocation. *Am. Rev. Respir. Dis.* 139:806, 1989.
14. Bel, E. H., et al. The effect of an inhaled leukotriene antagonist, L-648,051, on early and late asthmatic reactions and subsequent increase in airway responsiveness in man. *J. Allergy Clin. Immunol.* 85:1067, 1990.
15. Bel, E. H., et al. The effect of a specific oral PAF-antagonist, MK-287, on antigen-induced early and late asthmatic reactions in man (abstract). *Am. Rev. Respir. Dis.* 143:A811, 1991.
16. Benveniste, J., Henson, P. M., and Cochrane, C. G. Leukocyte-dependent histamine release from rabbit platelets: The role of IgE, basophils and a platelet activating factor. *J. Exp. Med.* 136:1356, 1972.
17. Bernstein, D. I., et al. An open study of auranofin in the treatment of steroid-dependent asthma. *J. Allergy Clin. Immunol.* 81:6, 1988.
18. Bianco, S., et al. Protective effect of inhaled furosemide on allergen-induced early and late asthmatic reactions. *N. Engl. J. Med.* 321:1069, 1989.
19. Bianco, S., Robuschi, M., and Petrini, G. Aspirin-induced tolerance in aspirin-asthma detected by a new challenge test. *J. Med. Sci.* 5:129, 1977.
20. Bianco, S., et al. Bronchial response to nonsteroidal anti-inflammatory drugs in asthmatic patients. *Prog. Biochem. Pharmacol.* 20:132, 1985.
21. Bianco, S., et al. Prevention of exercise-induced bronchoconstriction by inhaled frusemide. *Lancet* 2:252, 1988.
22. Bianco, S., et al. Protective effect of furosemide administered by metered aerosol canister on the bronchial obstructive response to ultrasonically nebulized H_2O. *Am. Rev. Respir. Dis.* 143(Suppl.):A548, 1991.
23. Bigby, T. D., and Meslier, N. Transcellular lipoxygenase metabolism between monocytes and platelets. *J. Immunol.* 143:1948, 1989.
24. Bisgaard, H., Groth, S., and Dirksen, H. Leukotriene D_4 induces bronchoconstriction in man. *Allergy* 38:441, 1983.
25. Bisgaard, H., Groth, S., and Madsen, F. Bronchial hyperreactivity to leukotriene D_4 and histamine in exogenous asthma. *Br. Med. J. [Clin. Res.]* 290:1468, 1985.
26. Bisgaard, H., Poulsen, L., and Sondergaard, I. Nebulization and selective deposition of LTD_4 in human lungs. *Allergy* 42:336, 1987.
27. Boszormenyi, N. G., Herjavecz, I., and Hutas, I. Bronchodilators and the preventive effect of aspirin in bronchial asthma. *Orv. Hetil.* 127:627, 1986.
28. Bousquet, J., et al. Eosinophilic inflammation in asthma. *N. Engl. J. Med.* 323:1033, 1990.
29. Britton, J. R., Hanley, S. P., and Tattersfield, A. E. The effect of an oral leukotriene D_4 antagonist L-649,923 on the response to inhaled antigen in asthma. *J. Allergy Clin. Immunol.* 79:811, 1987.
30. Brown, E. A. The use of intravenous ethyl alcohol in the treatment of status asthmaticus. *Ann. Allergy* 5:193, 1947.
31. Buckner, C. K., et al. Pharmacological evidence that human intralobar airways do not contain different receptors that mediate contractions to

leukotriene C_4 and leukotriene D_4. *J. Pharmacol. Exp. Ther.* 237:558, 1986.

32. Burney, P., and Chinn, S. Developing a new questionnaire for measuring the prevalence and distribution of asthma. *Chest* 91:79S, 1987.

33. Burney, P. G., et al. Response to inhaled histamine and 24 hour sodium excretion. *Br. Med. J. [Clin. Res.]* 292:1483, 1986.

34. Burney, P. G., et al: Effect of changing dietary sodium on the airway response to histamine. *Thorax* 44:36, 1989.

35. Capron, M., et al. Role of PAF-Acether in IgE-Dependent Activation of Eosinophils. In P. Braquet (ed.), *New Trends in Lipid Mediators Research: The Role of Platelet-Activating Factor in Immune Disorders.* Basel: Karger, 1988. Pp. 10–17.

36. Chiu, J. T. Improvement in aspirin-sensitive asthmatic subjects after rapid aspirin desensitization and aspirin maintenance (ADAM) treatment. *J. Allergy Clin. Immunol.* 71:560, 1983.

37. Christie, P. E., et al. Urinary leukotriene-E_4 concentrations increase after aspirin challenge in aspirin-sensitive asthmatic subjects. *Am. Rev. Respir. Dis.* 143:1025, 1991.

38. Chung, K. F., and Barnes, P. J. Effects of platelet-activating factor on airway calibre, airway responsiveness and circulating cells in asthmatic subjects. *Thorax* 44:108, 1989.

39. Cloud, M. L., et al. A specific LTD_4/LTE_4-receptor antagonist improves pulmonary function in patients with mild, chronic asthma. *Am. Rev. Respir. Dis.* 140:1336, 1989.

40. Cummings, N. P., Morris, H. G., and Strunk, R. C. Failure of children with asthma to respond to daily aspirin therapy. *J. Allergy Clin. Immunol.* 71:245, 1983.

41. Corey, E. J., Shih, C., and Cashman, J. R. Docosahexaenoic acid is a strong inhibitor of prostaglandin but not leukotriene biosynthesis. *Proc. Natl. Acad. Sci. U.S.A.* 80:3581, 1983.

42. Creticos, P. S., et al. Effects of an inhaled leukotriene antagonist on bronchial challenge with antigen. *J. Allergy Clin. Immunol.* 83:187, 1989.

43. Curzen, N., Rafferty, P., and Holgate, S. T. Effects of a cyclo-oxygenase inhibitor, flurbiprofen, and an H_1 histamine receptor antagonist, terfenadine, alone and in combination on allergen induced immediate bronchoconstriction in man. *Thorax* 42:946, 1987.

44. Cuss, F. M., Dixon, C. M. S., and Barnes, P. J. Effects of inhaled platelet activating factor on pulmonary function and bronchial responsiveness in man. *Lancet* 2:189, 1986.

45. Dahl, R., Henriksen, J. M., and Harving, H. Red wine asthma: A controlled challenge study. *J. Allergy Clin. Immunol.* 78:1126, 1986.

46. Davidson, A. B., et al. Bronchoconstrictor effects of leukotriene E_4 in normal and asthmatic subjects. *Am. Rev. Respir. Dis.* 135:333, 1987.

47. Delorme, D., et al. Synthesis of beta-oxidation products as potential leukotriene metabolites and their detection in bile of anesthetized rat. *Prostaglandins* 36:291, 1988.

48. Dermarkarian, R. M., et al. The effect of SCH-37370, a dual platelet activating factor (PAF) and histamine antagonist, on the bronchoconstriction induced in asthmatics by cold, dry air isocapnic hyperventilation (ISH) (abstract). *Am. Rev. Respir. Dis.* 143:A812, 1991.

49. Diaz, P., et al. Leukocytes and mediators in bronchoalveolar lavage during allergen-induced late-phase asthmatic reactions. *Am. Rev. Respir. Dis.* 139:1383, 1989.

50. Drazen, J. M. Inhalation challenge with sulfidopeptide leukotrienes in human subjects. *Chest* 89:414, 1986.

50a. Drazen, J. M., et al. Recovery of leukotriene-E_4 from the urine of patients with airway obstruction. *Am. Rev. Respir. Dis.* 146:104, 1992.

51. Ebden, P., et al. A study of evening primrose seed oil in atopic asthma. *Prostaglandins Leukotrienes Essent. Fatty Acids* 35:69, 1989.

52. Empire Rheumatism Council. Gold therapy in rheumatoid arthritis: Final report of a multicenter controlled trial. *Ann. Rheum. Dis.* 20:315, 1961.

53. Evans, J. M., et al. L-648,051, a novel cysteinyl-leukotriene antagonist is active by the inhaled route in man. *Br. J. Clin. Pharmacol.* 28:125, 1989.

54. Fairfax, A. J. Inhibition of the late asthmatic response to house dust mite by non-steroidal anti-inflammatory drugs. *Prostaglandins Leukotrienes Med.* 8:239, 1982.

55. Farr, R. S., Spector, S. L., and Wangaard, C. Asthma and nonsteroidal anti-inflammatory drugs (letter). *Ann. Intern. Med.* 89:577, 1978.

56. Feinmark, S. J., and Cannon, P. J. Endothelial cell leukotriene C_4 synthesis results from intercellular transfer of leukotriene A_4 synthesized by polymorphonuclear leukocytes. *J. Biol. Chem.* 261:16466, 1986.

56a. Findlay, S. R., et al. Effect of the oral leukotriene antagonist, ICI 204,219, on antigen-induced bronchoconstriction in subjects with asthma. *J. Allergy Clin. Immunol.* 89:1040, 1992.

57. Fish, J. E., et al. Indomethacin modification of immediate-type immuno-

logic airway responses in allergic asthmatic and non-asthmatic subjects: Evidence for altered arachidonic acid metabolism in asthma. *Am. Rev. Respir. Dis.* 123:609, 1981.

58. Fortuna, M. Aspirin as a bronchodilator. *Plucne Bolesti* 37:221, 1985.

59. Fradin, A., et al. Platelet-activating factor and leukotriene biosynthesis in whole blood: A model for the study of transcellular arachidonate metabolism. *J. Immunol.* 143:3680, 1989.

60. Freitag, A., et al. The effect of treatment with an oral platelet activating factor antagonist (web 2086) on allergen induced asthmatic responses in human subjects. *Am. Rev. Respir. Dis.* 143(Suppl.):A157, 1991.

61. Fujimura, M., et al. Effects of a thromboxane synthetase inhibitor (OKY-046) and a lipoxygenase inhibitor (AA-861) on bronchial responsiveness to acetylcholine in asthmatic subjects. *Thorax* 41:955, 1986.

62. Fuller, R. W., Black, P. N., and Dollery, C. T. Effect of the oral leukotriene D_4 antagonist LY171883 on inhaled and intradermal challenge with antigen and leukotriene D_4 in atopic subjects. *J. Allergy Clin. Immunol.* 83:939, 1989.

63. Fuller, R. W., et al. Prostaglandin D_2 potentiates airway responsiveness to histamine and methacholine. *Am. Rev. Respir. Dis.* 133:252, 1986.

64. Fuller, R. W., et al. Oral nafazatrom in man: Effect on inhaled antigen challenge. *Br. J. Clin. Pharmacol.* 23:677, 1987.

65. Gaddy, J. N., et al. Bronchodilation with a potent and selective leukotriene D_4 (LTD4) antagonist (MK-571) in patients with asthma. *Am. Rev. Respir. Dis.* 146:358, 1992.

66. Gardiner, P. J., and Collier, H. O. Receptors for E and F prostaglandins in airways. *Adv. Prostaglandin Thromboxane Res.* 7:1003, 1980.

67. Garin, P. R., and Frans, A. Aspirin-relieved asthma. *Med. Hypotheses* 32:125, 1990.

68. Garshick, E., et al. Alcohol consumption and chronic obstructive pulmonary disease. *Am. Rev. Respir. Dis.* 140:373, 1989.

69. Geppert, E. F., and Boushey, H. A. An investigation of the mechanism of ethanol-induced bronchoconstriction. *Am. Rev. Respir. Dis.* 118:135, 1978.

70. Gong, H., Jr., Tashkin, D. P., and Calvarese, B. M. Alcohol-induced bronchospasm in an asthmatic patient: Pharmacologic evaluation of the mechanism. *Chest* 80:167, 1981.

71. Green, K., Hedqvist, P., and Svanborg, N. Increased plasma levels of 15-keto-13,14-dihydro-prostaglandin F_{2X} after allergen-provoked asthma in man. *Lancet* 2:1419, 1974.

72. Griffin, M., et al. Effects of leukotriene D on the airways in asthma. *N. Engl. J. Med.* 308:436, 1983.

73. Grimminger, F., Becker, G., and Seeger, W. High yield enzymatic conversion of intravascular leukotriene A4 in blood-free perfused lungs. *J. Immunol.* 141:2431, 1988.

74. Grimminger, F., et al. Potentiation of leukotriene production following sequestration of neutrophils in isolated lungs: Indirect evidence for intercellular leukotriene A_4 transfer. *Blood* 72:1687, 1988.

75. Grubbe, R. E., et al. Effect of inhaled furosemide on the bronchial response to methacholine and cold-air hyperventilation challenges. *J. Allergy Clin. Immunol.* 85:881, 1990.

76. Hahn, A., et al. A reinterpretation of the effect of temperature and water content of the inspired air in exercise-induced asthma. *Am. Rev. Respir. Dis.* 130:575, 1984.

77. Hardy, C. C., et al. The bronchoconstrictor effect of inhaled prostaglandin D_2 in normal and asthmatic men. *N. Engl. J. Med.* 311:209, 1984.

78. Hargreave, F. E., et al. Airway hyperresponsiveness and asthma. *Agents Actions [Suppl.]* 28:205, 1989.

79. Heard, B. E., Nunn, A. J., and Kay, A. B. Mast cells in human lungs. *J. Pathol.* 157:59, 1989.

80. Heaton, R. W., et al. The influence of pretreatment with prostaglandin F_2 alpha on bronchial sensitivity to inhaled histamine and methacholine in normal subjects. *Br. J. Dis. Chest* 78:168, 1984.

81. Hendeles, L., et al. Antigen-induced bronchoconstriction: Attenuation by a specific LTD4 receptor antagonist (abstract). *J. Allergy Clin. Immunol.* 85:197, 1990.

82. Herxheimer, H., and Streseman, E. Ethanol and lung function in bronchial asthma. *Arch. Int. Pharmacodyn. Ther.* 144:310, 1963.

83. Holroyde, M. C., et al. Bronchoconstriction produced in man by leukotrienes C and D. *Lancet* 2:17, 1981.

84. Honda, Z., et al. Cloning by functional expression of platelet-activating factor receptor from guinea-pig lung. *Nature* 349:342, 1991.

85. Hopp, R. J., et al. Effect of PAF-acether inhalation on nonspecific bronchial reactivity and adrenergic responses in normal and asthmatic subjects. *Chest* 98:936, 1990.

86. Hui, K. P., and Barnes, N. C. Effects of a cysteinyl-leukotriene antagonist

in bronchial responsiveness to prostaglandin (PG) D$_2$ and histamine in asthmatics. *Am. Rev. Respir. Dis.* 143:A636, 1991.

87. Hui, K. P., Binks, S., and Barnes, N. C. Effect of a cysteinyl-leukotriene antagonist on resting bronchomotor tone in asthmatics. *Am. Rev. Respir. Dis.* 143(Suppl.):A599, 1991.

88. Hui, K. P., et al. Effect of a 5-lipoxygenase inhibitor on leukotriene generation and airway responses after allergen challenge in asthmatic patients. *Thorax* 46:184, 1991.

89. Israel, E., et al. Fish oil enriched diet modifies the guinea pig pulmonary mechanical responses to inhaled antigen (abstract). *Am. Rev. Respir. Dis.* 131:A277, 1985.

90. Israel, E., et al. The effects of a 5-lipoxygenase inhibitor on asthma induced by cold, dry air. *N. Engl. J. Med.* 323:1740, 1990.

91. Israel, E., et al. Effect of fish oil dietary supplementation in mild asthma. Unpublished.

92. Javaid, A., Cushley, M. J., and Bone, M. F. Effect of dietary salt on bronchial reactivity to histamine in asthma. *Br. Med. J.* 297:454, 1988.

93. Jeffery, P. K., et al. Bronchial biopsies in asthma: An ultrastructural, quantitative study and correlation with hyperreactivity. *Am. Rev. Respir. Dis.* 140:1745, 1989.

94. Johnson, P. R., Armour, C. L., and Black, J. L. The action of platelet activating factor and its antagonism by WEB 2086 on human isolated airways. *Eur. Respir. J.* 3:55, 1990.

95. Joubert, J. R., et al. Non-steroid anti-inflammatory drugs in asthma: Dangerous or useful therapy? *Allergy* 40:202, 1985.

96. Kaye, M. G., and Smith, L. J. Effects of inhaled leukotriene D$_4$ and platelet-activating factor on airway reactivity in normal subject. *Am. Rev. Respir. Dis.* 141:993, 1990.

97. Kips, J. C., et al. MK-571: A potent antagonist of LTD4-induced bronchoconstriction in man. *Am. Rev. Respir. Dis.* 144:617, 1991.

98. Kirby, J. G., et al. Effect of indomethacin on allergen-induced asthmatic responses. *J. Appl. Physiol.* 66:578, 1989.

99. Kirsch, C. M., et al. Effect of eicosapentaenoic acid in asthma. *Clin. Allergy* 18:177, 1988.

100. Klaustermeyer, W. B., Noritake, D. T., and Kwong, F. K. Chrysotherapy in the treatment of corticosteroid-dependent asthma. *J. Allergy Clin. Immunol.* 79:720, 1987.

101. Kordansky, D., et al. Asthma improved by nonsteroidal anti-inflammatory drugs. *Ann. Intern. Med.* 88:508, 1978.

102. Kowalski, M. L., et al. Bronchial hyperreactivity to histamine in aspirin sensitive asthmatics: Relationship to aspirin threshold and effect of aspirin desensitisation. *Thorax* 40:598, 1985.

103. Kremer, J. M., et al. Fish-oil fatty acid supplementation in active rheumatoid arthritis: A double-blinded, controlled, crossover study. *Ann. Intern. Med.* 106:497, 1987.

104. Lai, C. K., et al. Inhaled PAF fails to induce airway hyperresponsiveness to methacholine in normal human subjects. *J. Appl. Physiol.* 68:919, 1990.

105. Lam, B. K., et al. The identification of a distinct export step following the biosynthesis of leukotriene C$_4$ by human eosinophils. *J. Biol. Chem.* 264:12885, 1989.

106. Lam, S., et al. Release of leukotrienes in patients with bronchial asthma. *J. Allergy Clin. Immunol.* 81:711, 1988.

107. Lange, P., et al. Pulmonary function is influenced by heavy alcohol consumption. *Am. Rev. Respir. Dis.* 137:1119, 1988.

108. Lee, T. H., et al. Leukotriene E$_4$–induced airway hyperresponsiveness of guinea pig tracheal smooth muscle to histamine and evidence for three separate sulfidopeptide leukotriene receptors. *Proc. Natl. Acad. Sci. U.S.A.* 81:4922, 1984.

109. Lee, T. H., et al. Effect of dietary enrichment with eicosapentaenoic and docosahexaenoic acids on in vitro neutrophil and monocyte leukotriene generation and neutrophil function. *N. Engl. J. Med.* 312:1217, 1985.

110. Lee, T. H., et al. The effects of a fish-oil-enriched diet on pulmonary mechanics during anaphylaxis. *Am. Rev. Respir. Dis.* 132:1204, 1985.

111. Lewis, R. A., et al. Identification of the C(6)-S-conjugate of leukotriene A with cysteine as a naturally occurring slow reacting substance of anaphylaxis (SRS-A): Importance of the 11-cis-geometry for biological activity. *Biochem. Biophys. Res. Commun.* 96:271, 1980.

112. Liu, M. C., et al. Evidence for elevated levels of histamine, prostaglandin D$_2$, and other bronchoconstricting prostaglandins in the airways of subjects with mild asthma. *Am. Rev. Respir. Dis.* 142:126, 1990.

113. Lockey, R. F. Aspirin-improved ASA triad. *Hosp. Pract.* 13:129, 1978.

114. Lockey, R. F., Rucknagel, D. L., and Vanselow, N. A. Familial occurrence of asthma, nasal polyps and aspirin intolerance. *Ann. Intern. Med.* 78:57, 1973.

115. Lombardi, C., Spedini, C., and Govoni, S. Effect of calcium entry blockade on ethanol-induced changes in bronchomotor tone. *Eur. J. Clin. Pharmacol.* 28:221, 1985.

116. Lumley, P., White, B. P., and Humphrey, P. P. GR32191, a highly potent and specific thromboxane A$_2$ receptor blocking drug on platelets and vascular and airways smooth muscle in vitro. *Br. J. Pharmacol.* 97:783, 1989.

117. Lumry, W. R., et al. Aspirin-sensitive rhinosinusitis: The clinical syndrome and effects of aspirin administration. *J. Allergy Clin. Immunol.* 71:580, 1983.

118. Lynch, J. M., and Henson, P. M. The intracellular retention of newly synthesized platelet-activating factor. *J. Immunol.* 137:2653, 1986.

119. Maclouf, J. A., and Murphy, R. C. Transcellular metabolism of neutrophil-derived leukotriene A$_4$ by human platelets: A potential cellular source of leukotriene C$_4$. *J. Biol. Chem.* 263:174, 1988.

120. Magnussen, H., and Nowak, D. Roles of hyperresponsiveness and airway inflammation in bronchial asthma. *Respiration* 55:65, 1989.

121. Malo, P. E., et al. Inhibition by auranofin of pharmacologic and antigen-induced contractions of the isolated guinea pig trachea. *J. Allergy Clin. Immunol.* 77:371, 1986.

122. Mann, J. S., et al. Effect of inhaled piriprost (U-60, 257) a novel leukotriene inhibitor, on allergen and exercise induced bronchoconstriction in asthma. *Thorax* 41:746, 1986.

123. Manning, P. J., et al. Urinary leukotriene E4 levels during early and late asthmatic responses. *J. Allergy Clin. Immunol.* 86:211, 1990.

124. Manning, P. J., et al. Inhibition of exercise-induced bronchoconstriction by MK-571, a potent leukotriene D$_4$–receptor antagonist. *N. Engl. J. Med.* 323:1736, 1990.

125. McFadden, E. R., Jr. Exercise-induced asthma: Assessment of current etiologic concepts. *Chest* 91:151S, 1987.

126. Moscato, G., et al. Inhaled furosemide does not inhibit the airway response to toluene diisocyanate (tdi). *Am. Rev. Respir. Dis.* 143(Suppl.): A437, 1991.

127. Muranaka, M., Nakajima, K., and Suzuki, S. Bronchial responsiveness to acetylcholine in patients with bronchial asthma after long-term treatment with gold salt. *J. Allergy Clin. Immunol.* 67:350, 1981.

128. Muranaka, M., et al. Gold salt in the treatment of bronchial asthma—a double-blind study. *Ann. Allergy* 40:132, 1978.

129. Murray, J. J., et al. Release of prostaglandin D$_2$ into human airways during acute antigen challenge. *N. Engl. J. Med.* 315:800, 1986.

130. Naeije, N., et al. Effects of chronic aspirin ingestion in aspirin-intolerant asthmatic patients. *Ann. Allergy* 53:262, 1984.

131. Needleman, P., et al. Triene prostaglandins: Prostacyclin and thromboxane biosynthesis and unique biological properties. *Proc. Natl. Acad. Sci. U.S.A.* 76:944, 1979.

132. Nelson, R. P., Stablein, J. J., and Lockey, R. F. Asthma improved by acetylsalicylic acid and other nonsteroidal anti-inflammatory agents. *N. Engl. Reg. Allergy Proc.* 7:117, 1986.

133. Nichol, G. M., et al. Effect of inhaled furosemide on metabisulfite- and methacholine-induced bronchoconstriction and nasal potential difference in asthmatic subjects. *Am. Rev. Respir. Dis.* 142:576, 1990.

134. Oates, J. A., et al. Clinical implications of prostaglandin and thromboxane A$_2$ formation. *N. Engl. J. Med.* 319:689, 1988.

135. O'Byrne, P. M. Allergen-induced airway hyperresponsiveness . *J. Allergy Clin. Immunol.* 81:119, 1988.

136. O'Byrne, P. M. Leukotrienes, airway hyperresponsiveness, and asthma. *Ann. N. Y. Acad. Sci.* 524:282, 1988.

137. O'Connor, B. J., et al. Effect of inhaled furosemide and bumetanide on adenosine 5'-monophosphate– and sodium metabisulfite–induced bronchoconstriction in asthmatic subjects. *Am. Rev. Respir. Dis.* 143:1329, 1991.

138. O'Donnell, W. J., et al. Inhaled acetazolamide attenuates bronchoconstriction induced by cold-air hyperventilation. *Am. Rev. Respir. Dis.* 143(Suppl.):A211, 1991.

139. Okatani, Y. A few clinical statistical observations on the use of Solganal-B-Oleosum in bronchial asthma. *J. Asthma Res.* 17:165, 1980.

140. Orning, L., Bernstrom, K., Hammarstrom, S. Formation of leukotrienes E$_3$, E$_4$ and E$_5$ in rat basophilic leukemia cells. *Eur. J. Biochem.* 120:41, 1981.

141. Orning, L., Kaijser, L., and Hammarstrom, S. In vivo metabolism of leukotriene C$_4$ in man: Urinary excretion of leukotriene E$_4$. *Biochem. Biophys. Res. Commun.* 130:214, 1985.

142. Parker, C. W. et al. Formation of the cysteinyl form of slow reacting substance (leukotriene E4) in human plasma. *Biochem. Biophys. Res. Commun.* 97:1038, 1980.

143. Pauwels, R. The relationship between airway inflammation and bronchial hyperresponsiveness. *Clin. Exp. Allergy* 19:395, 1989.

144. Payan, D. G., et al. Alterations in human leukocyte function induced by ingestion of eicosapentaenoic acid. *J. Clin. Immunol.* 6:402, 1986.

145. Penneys, N. S., et al. Inhibition of prostaglandin synthesis and human epidermal enzymes by aurothiomalate in vitro: Possible actions of gold in pemphigus. *J. Invest. Dermatol.* 63:356, 1974.

146. Phillips, G. D., et al. Dose-related antagonism of leukotriene D$_4$–induced bronchoconstriction by p.o. administration of LY-171883 in nonasthmatic subjects. *J. Pharmacol. Exp. Ther.* 246:732, 1988.

147. Picado, C., et al. Effects of a fish oil enriched diet on aspirin intolerant asthmatic patients: A pilot study. *Thorax* 43:93, 1988.

148. Pleskow, W. W., et al. Aspirin desensitization in aspirin-sensitive asthmatic patients: Clinical manifestations and characterization of the refractory period. *J. Allergy Clin. Immunol.* 69:11, 1982.

149. Polosa, R., Lau, L. C., and Holgate, S. T. Inhibition of adenosine 5′-monophosphate- and methacholine-induced bronchoconstriction in asthma by inhaled frusemide. *Eur. Respir. J.* 3:665, 1990.

150. Prescott, S. M., Zimmerman, G. A., and McIntyre, T. M. Human endothelial cells in culture produce platelet-activating factor (1-alkyl-2-acetyl-sn-glycero-3-phosphocholine) when stimulated with thrombin. *Proc. Natl. Acad. Sci. U.S.A.* 81:3534, 1984.

151. Prickett, J. D., Robinson, D. R., and Steinberg, A. D. Dietary enrichment with the polyunsaturated fatty acid eicosapentaenoic acid prevents proteinuria and prolongs survival in NZB × NZW F1 mice. *J. Clin. Invest.* 68:556, 1981.

151a. Rasmussen, J. B., et al. Leukotriene-D4 receptor blockade inhibits the immediate and late bronchoconstrictor responses to inhaled antigen in patients with asthma. *J. Allergy Clin. Immunol.* 90:193, 1992.

152. Resta, O., et al. Asthma relieved by acetylsalicylic acid and nonsteroid anti-inflammatory drugs. *Respiration* 46:121, 1984.

153. Roberts, J. A., et al. In vitro and in vivo effect of verapamil on human airway responsiveness to leukotriene D$_4$. *Thorax* 41:12, 1986.

154. Robuschi, M., et al. Inhaled frusemide is highly effective in preventing ultrasonically nebulised water bronchoconstriction. *Pulm. Pharmacol.* 1:187, 1989.

155. Robuschi, M., et al. Prevention of antigen-induced early obstructive reaction by inhaled furosemide in (atopic) subjects with asthma and (actively sensitized) guinea pigs. *J. Allergy Clin. Immunol.* 85:10, 1990.

156. Robuschi, M., et al. Prevention of exercise-induced bronchoconstriction by a new leukotriene antagonist (SK&F 104353). *Am. Rev. Respir. Dis.* 145:1285, 1992.

157. Roche, W. R., et al. Subepithelial fibrosis in the bronchi of asthmatics. *Lancet* 1:520, 1989.

158. Rokach, J., et al. Metabolism of peptide leukotrienes in the rat. *Adv. Prostaglandin Thromboxane Leukotriene Res.* 19:102, 1989.

159. Rubin, A. H., Smith, L. J., and Patterson, R. The bronchoconstrictor properties of platelet-activating factor in humans. *Am. Rev. Respir. Dis.* 136:1145, 1987.

160. Samuelsson, B., et al. Leukotrienes and lipoxins: Structures, biosynthesis, and biological effects. *Science* 237:1171, 1987.

161. Saussy, D. L., Jr., et al. Mechanisms of leukotriene E$_4$ partial agonist activity at leukotriene D4 receptors in differentiated U-937 cells. *J. Biol. Chem.* 264:19845, 1989.

162. Schacter, E. N., Kreisman, H., and Bouhuys, A. Prostaglandin-synthesis inhibition and exercise bronchospasm. *Ann. Intern. Med.* 89:287, 1978.

163. Schellenberg, R. R. Airway responses to platelet-activating factor. *Am. Rev. Respir. Dis.* 136:S28, 1987.

164. Schleimer, R. P., et al. Characterization of inflammatory mediator release from purified human lung mast cells. *Am. Rev. Respir. Dis.* 133:614, 1986.

165. Sheppard, D. Airway hyperresponsiveness : Mechanisms in experimental models. *Chest* 96:1165, 1989.

166. Silber, G., et al. In vivo release of inflammatory mediators by hyperosmolar solutions. *Am. Rev. Respir. Dis.* 137:606, 1988.

167. Sladek, K., et al. Allergen-stimulated release of thromboxane A2 and leukotriene E$_4$ in humans: Effect of indomethacin. *Am. Rev. Respir. Dis.* 141:1441, 1990.

168. Smith, A. P. Effect of indomethacin in asthma: Evidence against a role for prostaglandins in its pathogenesis. *Br. J. Clin. Pharmacol.* 2:307, 1975.

169. Smith, L. J., et al. The effect of inhaled leukotriene D$_4$ in humans. *Am. Rev. Respir. Dis.* 131:368, 1985.

170. Smith, L. J., et al. Mechanism of leukotriene D$_4$–induced bronchoconstriction in normal subject. *J. Allergy Clin. Immunol.* 80:340, 1987.

171. Smith, L. J., et al. Inhibition of leukotriene D4–induced bronchoconstriction in normal subjects by the oral LTD4 receptor antagonist ICI 204,219. *Am. Rev. Respir. Dis.* 141:988, 1990.

172. Snyder, D. W., and Krell, R. D. Pharmacological evidence for a distinct leukotriene C$_4$ receptor in guinea-pig trachea. *J. Pharmacol. Exp. Ther.* 231:616, 1984.

173. Sperling, R. I., et al. Effects of dietary supplementation with marine fish oil on leukocyte lipid mediator generation and function in rheumatoid arthritis. *Arthritis Rheum.* 30:988, 1987.

174. Sperling, R. I., et al. The effects of N-3 polyunsaturated fatty acids on the generation of platelet-activating factor-acether by human monocytes. *J. Immunol.* 139:4186, 1987.

175. Stene, D. O., and Murphy, R. C. Metabolism of leukotriene E4 in isolated rat hepatocytes: Identification of beta-oxidation products of sulfidopeptide leukotrienes. *J. Biol. Chem.* 263:2773, 1988.

176. Stenius-Aarniala, B., et al. Evening primrose oil and fish oil are ineffective as supplementary treatment of bronchial asthma. *Ann. Allergy* 62:534, 1989.

177. Stevenson, D. D., Simon, R. A., and Mathison, D. A. Aspirin-sensitive asthma: Tolerance to aspirin after positive oral aspirin challenges. *J. Allergy Clin. Immunol.* 66:82, 1980.

178. Stevenson, D. D., et al. Aspirin-sensitive rhinosinusitis asthma: A double-blind crossover study of treatment with aspirin. *J. Allergy Clin. Immunol.* 73:500, 1984.

179. Sugihara, H. Nonspecific therapy of asthma with gold preparation and insulin. *J. Asthma* 18:51, 1981.

180. Sun, F. F., et al. Identification of a high affinity leukotriene C$_4$–binding protein in rat liver cytosol as glutathione *S*-transferase. *J. Biol. Chem.* 261:8540, 1986.

181. Sweet, J. M., et al. Long-term effects of aspirin desensitization: Treatment for aspirin-sensitive rhinosinusitis-asthma. *J. Allergy Clin. Immunol.* 85:59, 1990.

182. Szczeklik, A., Gryglewski, R. J., and Nizankowska, E. Asthma relieved by aspirin and by other cyclo-oxygenase inhibitors. *Thorax* 33:664, 1978.

183. Szczeklik, A., and Nizankowska, E. Asthma improved by aspirin-like drugs. *Br. J. Dis. Chest* 77:153, 1983.

184. Tagari, P., et al. Measurement of urinary leukotrienes by reversed-phase liquid chromatography and radioimmunoassay. *Clin. Chem.* 35:388, 1989.

185. Takaishi, T., et al. Auranofin, an oral chrysotherapeutic agent, inhibits histamine release from human basophils. *J. Allergy Clin. Immunol.* 74:296, 1984.

186. Taylor, G. W., et al. Urinary leukotriene E4 after antigen challenge and in acute asthma and allergic rhinitis. *Lancet* 1:584, 1989.

187. Taylor, I. K., et al. Effect of cysteinyl-leukotriene receptor antagonist ICI 204.219 on allergen-induced bronchoconstriction and airway hyperreactivity in atopic subjects. *Lancet* 337:690, 1991.

188. Terano, T., Salmon, J. A., and Moncada, S. Biosynthesis and biological activity of leukotriene B$_5$. *Prostaglandins* 27:217, 1984.

189. Togias, A. G., et al. Local generation of sulfidopeptide leukotrienes upon nasal provocation with cold, dry air. *Am. Rev. Respir. Dis.* 133:1133, 1986.

190. Vargas, F. S., et al. Effect of inhaled furosemide on acetylsalicylic acid induced bronchoconstriction in asthmatic subjects. *Am. Rev. Respir. Dis.* 143(Suppl.):A427, 1991.

191. Verdiani, P., et al. Effect of inhaled frusemide on the early response to antigen and subsequent change in airway reactivity in atopic patients. *Thorax* 45:377, 1990.

192. Walters, E. H. Prostaglandins and the control of airways responses to histamine in normal and asthmatic subjects. *Thorax* 38:188, 1983.

193. Wardlaw, A. J., et al. Platelet activating factor: A potent chemotactic and chemokinetic factor for human eosinophils. *J. Clin. Invest.* 78:1701, 1986.

194. Wardlaw, A. J., et al. Leukotrienes, LTC$_4$ and LTB$_4$, in bronchoalveolar lavage in bronchial asthma and other respiratory diseases. *J. Allergy Clin. Immunol.* 84:19, 1989.

195. Weiss, J. W., et al. Bronchoconstrictor effects of leukotriene C in humans. *Science* 216:196, 1982.

196. Weiss, J. W., et al. Airway constriction in normal humans produced by inhalation of leukotriene D: Potency, time course, and effect of aspirin therapy. *J.A.M.A.* 249:2814, 1983.

197. Westcott, J. Y., et al. Measurement of peptidoleukotrienes in biological fluids. *J. Appl. Physiol.* 68:2640, 1990.

198. Wilkens, H., et al. Effects of an inhaled paf-antagonist (web 2086 bs) on allergen-induced early and late asthmatic responses and increased

bronchial responsiveness to methacholine. *Am. Rev. Respir. Dis.* 143(Suppl.):A812, 1991.

199. Wilkens, J. H., et al. Effects of a PAF-antagonist (BN 52063) on broncho-constriction and platelet activation during exercise induced asthma. *Br. J. Clin. Pharmacol.* 29:85, 1990.

200. Winkler, J. D., et al. Leukotriene D_4–induced homologous desensitization in basal and differentiated U-937 cells: Characterization with the partial agonist leukotriene E4 and assessment of receptor reserve. *J. Pharmacol. Exp. Ther.* 247:54, 1988.

201. Wright, S., and Burton, J. L. Oral evening-primrose-seed oil improves atopic eczema. *Lancet* 2:1120, 1982.

202. Wykle, R. L., Malone, B., and Snyder, F. Enzymatic synthesis of 1-alkyl-2-acetyl-sn-glycero-3-phosphocholine, a hypotensive and platelet-aggregating lipid. *J. Biol. Chem.* 255:10256, 1980.

203. Yager, D., et al. Amplification of airway constriction due to liquid filling of airway interstices. *J. Appl. Physiol.* 66:2873, 1989.

204. Ying, R. L., et al. Indomethacin does not inhibit the ozone-induced increase in bronchial responsiveness in human subjects. *Am. Rev. Respir. Dis.* 142:817, 1990.

205. Zehr, B. B., et al. Use of segmental airway lavage to obtain relevant mediators from the lungs of asthmatic and control subjects. *Chest* 95:1059, 1989.

206. Zuskin, E., Bouhuys, A., and Saric, M. Lung function changes by ethanol inhalation. *Clin. Allergy* 11:243, 1981.

Troleandomycin in Corticosteroid Dependency

67

Robert S. Zeiger
Stanley J. Szefler

The corticosteroid-dependent yet resistant asthmatic patient is threatened daily with respiratory catastrophe, constantly posing a major medical challenge. The macrolide antibiotic troleandomycin (TAO), documented nearly 20 years ago as possessing dramatic corticosteroid-sparing activity by research at National Jewish Center, received unfortunately little clinical consideration but now reemerges to the benefit of the corticosteroid-resistant asthmatic. With the recent emphasis on other alternative therapies, such as high-dose inhaled steroids, methotrexate, gold, intravenous gamma globulin, hydroxychloroquine, and dapsone, it is important to review the appropriate use of TAO therapy (see also Chaps. 66 and 68).

STRUCTURE AND PHARMACOLOGY

TAO, the triacetylated derivative of oleandomycin, a product of *Streptomyces antibioticus,* was synthesized initially by Celmer et al. [13] in 1957 for its antimicrobial properties against gram-positive microorganisms. Its parent compound, oleandomycin, consists of two desoxy sugars, L-oleandrose and desosamine, bound in a glycosidic linkage to a lactone nucleus designated as an oleandolide. Drugs possessing such a macrolactone ring have been termed *macrolides.* TAO is synthesized by the sequential acetylation of the three hydroxyl groups (proceeding temporally on desosamine, then L-oleandrose, and lastly oleandolide) present on each of its three chemical moieties [27]. For visual comparison, the chemical structure of TAO, erythromycin, and erythromycin estolate (Ilosone) are noted in Figure 67-1. TAO ($C_{41} H_{67} NO_{15}$), a colorless substance, is relatively stable in aqueous form, even at 37°C. Its sole pharmacologic advantage over oleandomycin rests in improved gastric absorption due to acetylation, which results in higher serum concentrations. However, TAO is deacetylated in vivo, resulting in its antimicrobial activity ultimately deriving from the activity of oleandomycin [27]. Doses of TAO of 22 mg/kg in children repeated every 6 hours result in average peak serum concentrations of oleandomycin in excess of 2.4 μg/ml. TAO is available in capsules (250 mg). For smaller doses, pharmacists can reformulate the capsule to the desired strength. Since it is unavailable for parenteral use (because of poor solubility), oleandomycin phosphate must be used instead [68].

TAO elimination occurs by the biliary and urinary routes. The toxicity of TAO in humans and other animals ($LD_{50} = 100–200$ mg/kg) is quite low. Side effects are predominantly related to the gastrointestinal tract, including nausea, vomiting, diarrhea, esophagitis, and hepatitis [68]. Doses of TAO of 1 gm daily for 2 weeks have caused abnormal liver function tests in 10 to 50 percent of adult patients [63, 78]. SGPT appears to rise more fre-

quently than SGOT with the hepatic toxicity secondary to TAO [71]. Gamma aminotransferase activity may even be an earlier and therefore better discriminator of TAO-induced hepatic toxicity, especially in women taking oral contraceptives [35]. More prolonged use of TAO at 1 gm daily has led to overt clinical illness with hepatocellular and cholestatic hepatic changes in 12 percent of patients [78]. Additionally, prolonged use of TAO at doses of 500 mg or greater daily has led to liver enzyme abnormalities [18]. Characteristically, these liver abnormalities rapidly reverse with discontinuation of TAO [78] (or after rapid tapering of TAO by 50 to 75% or even to alternate-day [personal observation]). Recently Wald et al. [81] reported that successful treatment can begin with TAO at doses of 250 mg/day and then reduced to 250 mg on alternate days. TAO at daily doses of 250 mg or less appears to be very safe and only rarely leads to changes in liver function tests [25, 84].

CLINICAL STUDIES

Following its introduction as an effective antimicrobial agent against gram-positive infections, TAO was naturally studied as a therapeutic agent for infectious asthma. TAO was found to decrease the amount and consistency of sputum and to reduce the necessity for concomitant medications, including corticosteroids, without affecting the bacterial flora of 38 of 44 patients with infectious asthma [42]. Fox [28] noted an excellent or good clinical response in 214 (89%) and a poor response in 26 (11%) of 240 asthmatic or allergic rhinitis patients 2 to 78 years of age with super-imposed mucopurulent secretions treated with TAO for 7 to 21 days (180 patients) and for 1 to 4 months (60 patients). Doses of TAO of 500 mg to 1 gm/day divided were administered throughout the first month and then reduced 25 percent the second and third and 50 percent the fourth month of the therapy. Favorable response was characterized by reduction in sputum, cough, expectoration, rales, wheezing, dyspnea, and symptomatic medication (iodides, bronchodilators, and corticosteroids). No correlation could be discerned between favorable clinical response and the pretreatment bacteria cultured in the secretions prior to TAO.

In a double-blind crossover study in 10 steroid-dependent asthmatics on prednisone or methylprednisolone (MP), Itkin, Menzel, and Townley [41, 54] compared the therapeutic efficacy of 2-week courses of three antibiotics—TAO (250 mg qid), oleandomycin (500 mg qid), and tetracycline (250 mg qid)—and placebo (Table 67-1). Both TAO and its parent compound, oleandomycin, significantly improved clinical (8/10) and spirometric responses (4/10), while tetracycline was no better than placebo. Reductions in steroid doses were not discussed. Two patients who were not on concomitant corticosteroids did not show evidence of either clinical or pulmonary function improvement

Supported in part by Grant FD-R-00278 from the Food and Drug Administration, Program of Orphan Drugs.

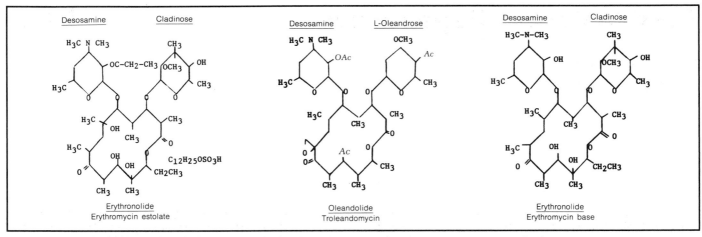

Fig. 67-1. *Chemical structure of macrolide antibiotics.* (Ac = acetyl.)

Table 67-1. *Prospective studies of the clinical and spirometric efficacy of TAO in steroid-dependent asthma*

	Demographic			Study details				Post-TAO response		
Author (yr)	No. of patients	Age x̄ (range)	Atopic component	Initial x̄ MP dose (mg)	Study design	TAO dose (mg)	Duration of TAO	↑ FEV₁	↓ Symptoms	Documented steroid-sparing
Itkin & Menzel (1970) [41]	10	25 (15–53)	9/10	20 D	Double-blind crossover	250 QID	2 wk	Yes (4/10)	Yes (8/10)	N.R.
Spector et al. (1974) [71]	74	N.R. (31–40)	19/74	N.R.	Double-blind crossover	250 QID	2–4 wk	Yes	Yes (N.R.)	63/74 (85%)
Zeiger et al. (1980) [85]	16	43 (13–71)	11/16	29 D	Open	250 QID to 250 QOD	4–18 mo	Yes (13/16)	Yes (16/16)	15/16 (94%)
Eitches et al. (1985) [22]	11	11 (7–13)	8/10	21.5 D	Open	250 mg TID to 250 QOD	12–28 mo	Yes (11/11)	Yes (11/11)	11/11 (100%)
Wald et al. (1986) [81]	15	50 (19–75)	N.R.	38.9 D	Open	250 BID or QD to 250 QOD	3–11 mo	Yes (8/15)	Yes (13/15)	13/15 (87%)

N.R. = not reported; D = daily; MP = methylprednisolone; QID = four times a day; QOD = every other day; TID = 3 times a day; BID = twice a day; QD = once a day.

while on TAO or oleandomycin. The efficacy of TAO could not be correlated with the presence and/or eradication of preexisting infection or with deterioration in liver function. Hydrocortisone metabolism was unchanged by TAO in three normal patients. Increased corticosteroid effects including lymphopenia, eosinopenia, neutrophilia, and more marked cushingoid appearance occurred in those patients benefiting from TAO or oleandomycin. Increased FEV₁ greater than 30 percent was seen within 2 to 5 days of TAO administration and decreased within 2 to 4 days after discontinuation of TAO. These investigators postulated a potentiation of steroid effect by TAO. Although they used both prednisone and MP, it is unclear whether a particular steroid preparation correlated with more favorable results.

The innovative study of Spector and his associates [71] reported in 1974 documented for the first time TAO's steroid-sparing effect and also confirmed its clinical and spirometric efficacy in 74 steroid-dependent asthmatics in a residential center (National Jewish Center) (Table 67-1). Preliminary studies (4 patients) suggested that benefit from TAO was seen more frequently when coadministered with MP than with prednisone as the corticosteroid, dictating use of MP in their study. Response was defined according to corticosteroid reduction as marked in 50/74 (68%) (greater than twofold reduction in alternate-day MP dosage or change from daily to alternate-day dosage that was less than twofold the daily dose), as probable in 13/74 (18%) (reduction in alternate-day steroid dosage 15–50%), and as none in 11/74 (15%). Key clues to responders included the existence of sputum production and possibly a significant non-IgE component to the asthma. Aerosolized bronchodilators were either stopped completely (38%) or decreased by greater than 50 percent (40%) in the marked responders. No relationship was noted between a favorable clinical response and the development of abnormal liver function tests. Methacholine and histamine sensitivity decreased significantly during TAO administration in 11/15 and 5/7 patients, respectively. While on TAO and MP, 92 percent of sputum producers noted either the absence of sputum entirely or a significant decrease in sputum within 3 weeks of combined treatment, but within 1 to 2 weeks after discontinuation of TAO sputum production returned. In 40 of the marked responders, serum morning cortisol levels in 9/15 stayed normal and in 15/25 returned to normal. Increased cushingoid effects were seen in the initial patients studied, in whom MP dosages were not tapered rapidly enough. The metabolic clearance rate for MP was reduced in 6/10 patients while taking TAO, but this reduction was not statistically significant.

The effectiveness of TAO therapy in steroid-dependent yet refractory asthma was restudied by Zeiger et al. [85]. They extended TAO's usefulness for ambulatory patients, developed a clinical strategy that maximized benefit-risk factors, and provided guidelines for long-term use of TAO on an alternate-day regimen. Sixteen severe corticosteroid-dependent asthmatics (14/16 on daily steroids) were treated successfully for 4 to 18 months with the combination of TAO and MP (Table 67-1). Clinical and spirometric improvement was noted within the first weeks (20% increase in FEV_1 in 8/16), with maximal improvement occurring characteristically by 6 weeks (20% increase in FEV_1 in 13/16). The corticosteroid-sparing effect of the TAO and MP combination first noted by Spector et al. [71] was confirmed in this study, as TAO therapy reduced the MP requirement to an average 11 mg every other day from a pre-TAO average MP dosage of 29 mg/day. Moreover, TAO could be reduced to an alternate-day dose of 250 mg in 13/15 patients, while maintaining clinical and spirometric control, though the latter at less than maximal levels. Partial adrenal recovery occurred as documented by morning cortisol levels greater than 5 µg/ml in patients (10/13) in whom MP (4 to 12 mg) could be administered the same alternate day as TAO (250 mg).

Individual differences in the time of partial adrenal recovery were characteristic, probably related in part to dosage, duration, and adrenal effect of prior corticosteroid treatment.

Some of the previous studies cited were performed in adolescents as well as adults. Eitches and colleagues [22] reported their experience with 11 severe steroid-dependent asthmatic children ages 7 to 13 years old. Five subjects required alternate-day steroids, with an average dose of 30 mg of prednisone every other day, and 6 subjects required daily oral steroids, with an average dose of 26.5 mg/day of prednisone. All patients had a cushingoid appearance, 7 were growth retarded, none had obvious cataracts or osteoporosis, but measurements were not detailed on these latter side effects. A protocol similar to that of Zeiger et al. [85] was used.

One year later, MP doses averaged 6 mg every other day for 10 patients, and only 1 patient received daily therapy (4 mg/day). TAO dosages were 250 mg every other day for 9 patients, and 250 mg daily for 2 patients. Patients demonstrated clinical improvement by reduction in their maintenance steroid dose and decrease in hospital and emergency room visits. The FEV_1 increased from a mean baseline value of 54 percent of predicted to 98 percent of predicted. Patients were monitored for changes in ophthalmologic examination, cushingoid facies, and weight gain. Although weight gain and increased cushingoid features were noted initially, they resolved with long-term treatment. No effects on linear growth, bone densitometry, hypertension, or hyperglycemia were mentioned. Four patients received a corticotropin stimulation test at the beginning of the study, and 9 patients were reexamined at the completion of the study. Two of nine patients tested had evidence of adrenal suppression with long-term treatment; however, 3 of 4 patients with adrenal suppression at start of the study had no evidence of adrenal suppression at the end of the study.

A recent advance in the use of TAO is the introduction of a protocol starting with a lower dose of TAO and incorporating a rapid steroid taper. Wald et al. [81] hypothesized that a rapid steroid taper would maintain similar efficacy and reduce the risk for increased steroid side effects. This new TAO protocol provides similar efficacy, with a much lower incidence of the transient increase in acute steroid side effects. With this new approach, 13 of 15 patients tolerated reduction of steroid to an alternate-day dose for the first time in years. Before TAO was begun, the average MP requirement to maintain clinical stability was 38.9 mg/day, and no patient was receiving alternate-day therapy. Within 3 weeks of beginning TAO therapy, 13 of 15 patients tolerated a reduction to alternate-day MP. Mean MP dose at the time of discharge from the National Jewish Center was 25.2 mg on alternate days. Follow-up data were obtained 3 to 11 months after TAO was started. All 13 patients who successfully achieved alternate-day therapy were able to maintain this alternate-day schedule, and furthermore their MP dose was reduced to a mean of 14.8 mg on alternate days.

Studies are in progress to examine the safety and efficacy of this new TAO protocol in children. Ball et al. [3] conducted a 2-week comparison of three treatment regimens including combination of TAO/MP, TAO/prednisone, and MP alone. They reported that patients in all three treatment groups tolerated a 50 percent reduction in their maintenance steroid dose, including those receiving MP alone. Furthermore, patients receiving TAO therapy showed significant improvement in airway hyperresponsiveness, while those receiving MP alone showed no change. Four of five patients on TAO/MP and 2 of 5 patients on TAO/prednisone showed a greater than a twofold concentration improvement in methacholine sensitivity.

DRUG INTERACTIONS

An understanding of the diverse interactions of corticosteroids with other drugs should aid efforts to maintain optimal pharmacologic effects and reduce the toxicity of these agents. Some commonly prescribed drugs that interact with corticosteroids are listed in Tables 67-2 and 67-3. Enhanced beta-adrenergic responsiveness induced by corticosteroids is well established [50]. Less well known, however, is the reversal of corticosteroid-induced impairment of wound healing by vitamin A [39, 73]. Corticosteroids increase acetylsalicylic acid excretion [43], reduce the hypoglycemic effect of oral hypoglycemics, increase the ulcerogenic potential of indomethacin [24], and enhance the potassium-depleting effects of amphotericin and diuretics.

Medications that alter metabolic properties of the microsomal enzyme system influence glucocorticoid elimination (Table 67-3). Concomitant administration of phenobarbital, phenytoin, carbamazepine, and rifampin enhance glucocorticoid elimination via the cytochrome P-450 pathway to form 6-β-hydroxyglucocorticoid [4, 10, 21, 44, 74]. These metabolic enzyme inducers have a greater effect on MP elimination as compared to prednisolone elimination. MP elimination is increased fivefold in the presence of phenobarbital or carbamazepine therapy, while prednisolone elimination is only increased twofold [4].

Medications associated with impaired glucocorticoid elimination include oral contraceptives and ketoconazole. A twofold decrease in prednisolone clearance is observed with oral contraceptives with a dual effect of increased protein binding and impaired metabolism [5]. The increase in protein binding is related to an estrogen-induced increase in corticosteroid binding

Table 67-2. Corticosteroid–drug interaction effect on drug action

Drug	Effect
Beta-adrenergics	Enhance beta-adrenergic responsiveness
Vitamin A	Reverses CS-induced impairment of wound healing
Aspirin	Increased renal ASA excretion by CS
Indomethacin	Increased ulcerogenic potential
Oral hypoglycemics	Reduced hypoglycemic effect by CS
Amphotericin	Enhanced K^+ depletion by CS
Diuretics	Enhanced K^+ depletion by CS

CS = corticosteroids; ASA = acetylsalicylic acid.

Table 67-3. Corticosteroid–drug interaction and effect on corticosteroid metabolism

Corticosteroid	Drug	Effect	Mechanism	References
Cortisol	Beta-adrenergic agonist response	Enhanced beta-agonist affinity	Alteration of beta-receptor	19, 23, 29, 72
	Phenobarbital	Increased elimination	Increased cytochrome P-450 activity	14, 16
	Phenytoin			
	Rifampicin	Decreased steroid effect	Increased elimination	21, 44
Prednisolone	Antacids	Decreased steroid bioavailability	Possible physical adsorption to antacid	81
	Cimetidine	No effect		56, 59, 69
	Ranitidine			
	Ketoconazole	Impaired elimination		87
		No effect		49
	Oral contraceptives	Increased steroid availability	Impaired elimination, increased protein binding	5
	Phenobarbital	Decreased steroid effect	Increased cytochrome P-450 activity	4, 10
	Phenytoin			
	Carbamazepine			
	Rifampicin	Decreased steroid effect	Increased steroid elimination	11, 38
	Troleandomycin	No effect		71, 76
Methylprednisolone (MPn)	Cimetidine	No effect		33
	Diazepam	No effect		74
	Erythromycin	Impaired MPn elimination		45
	Ketoconazole	Impaired MPn elimination		30
	Phenobarbital	Probable diminished steroid effect	Increased cytochrome P-450 activity	4, 74
	Phenytoin			
	Carbamazepine			
	Rifampicin	Decreased steroid effect	Probable increased P-450 activity	11
	Troleandomycin	Enhanced steroid effect	Partially related to impaired MPn elimination	22, 71, 75, 77, 85
Dexamethasone	Cimetidine	No effect		59
	Ephedrine	Enhanced elimination	Possible increased metabolism	9
	Phenobarbital	Increased dexamethasone elimination	Increased cytochrome P-450 activity	10
	Phenytoin			36
	Theophylline	No effect		9

Source: From S. J. Szefler. In R. P. Schleimer, H. N. Claman, and A. Oronsky (Eds.), *Anti-inflammatory Steroid Action.* San Diego: Academic, 1989. Pp. 365–366.

Table 67-4. TAO effect on hepatic microsomal enzyme systems[a]

Microsomal enzyme	TAO action[b]	Effect
Cytochrome P-450	Induction	Forms inactive metabolite complex with reduced Fe in cyto-P-450
Hexobarbital hydroxylase	Inhibition	Prolong sleep
Ethylmorphine *N*-demethylase	Inhibition	Prolong hypnosis
Cholesterol 7α-hydroxylase	Inhibition	↓ Bile acid synthesis
Na⁺-K⁺ ATPase	Stimulation	↑ Bile flow
Theophylline-3-demethylase	Inhibition	↓ Theophylline clearance

[a] Species studied: Rat (all); human (cytochrome P-450).
[b] Requires chronic in vivo administration.

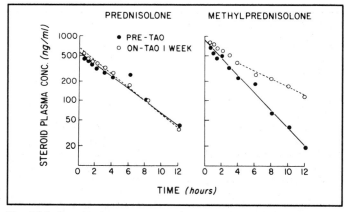

Fig. 67-2. *Steroid plasma concentration versus time plots for patient given Prednisolone (left) and methylprednisolone (right) in 40-mg intravenous doses before and 1 week after initiation of TAO therapy. (Reprinted with permission from S. J. Szefler, et al. Steroid-specific and anticonvulsant interaction aspects of troleandomycin-steroid therapy.* J. Allergy Clin. Immunol. *69:455, 1982.)*

globulin. Although MP elimination is definitely decreased in the presence of ketoconazole [30], there are conflicting reports on the effect of ketoconazole on prednisolone elimination. While one report indicates impaired prednisolone elimination [87], another found no significant change [49]. Cimetidine, a medication usually associated with impaired drug metabolism, has no effect on glucocorticoid pharmacokinetics [33, 56, 59, 69].

TAO appears to induce its own metabolism, forming in rats [61] and humans [62] an inactive metabolite complex with reduced iron in cytochrome-P-450, which inhibits hepatic cytochrome-P-450 drug-metabolizing activity [60]. TAO interacts meaningfully with corticosteroids and other pharmacologic agents. Multiple hepatic microsomal enzyme systems are affected by TAO in vitro, which may inhibit the metabolism of barbiturates [60], morphine [60], and theophylline [48] and inhibit bile acid synthesis [17] or increase bile flow [17] (Table 67-4).

The pharmacologic studies of Szefler and associates [75–77] have helped to elucidate the complex and fascinating interactions of TAO and other macrolide antibiotics with corticosteroids alone and also with concomitant anticonvulsant administration. Measuring plasma concentrations of MP and its metabolites by high-pressure liquid chromatography in 10 severe corticosteroid-dependent asthmatics, Szefler et al. [75] noted that MP elimination in the presence of TAO (14 mg/kg to a maximum 1 gm daily in divided dosage) follows an unusual nonlinear kinetic profile (Fig. 67-2), necessitating the use of a general model-independent pharmacokinetic analysis. Such analyses reveal that,

Table 67-5. *TAO–drug interactions*

Drug	TAO effect on drug clearance	Clinical response	References
Prednisolone	None	None	71, 77
Methylprednisolone (MP)	Inhibition	↑ Steroid effect/toxicity	22, 71, 75, 76, 85
Barbiturate + MP	Reverses ↑ MP elimination ↓ Barbiturate clearance	Restores steroid responses ↑ CNS toxicity	77
Phenytoin + MP	Reverses ↑ MP elimination ↓ Phenytoin clearance	Restores steroid response ↑ Hepatic and CNS toxicity	77
Theophylline (Th)	Inhibition	↑ Th toxicity	83
Carbamazepine	Inhibition	↑ CNS toxicity	55
Ergotamines	Unknown	Ischemic accidents	37
Oral contraceptives	Possible inhibition	Cholestatic jaundice	26
Triazolan	Inhibition	↑ CNS effect	82

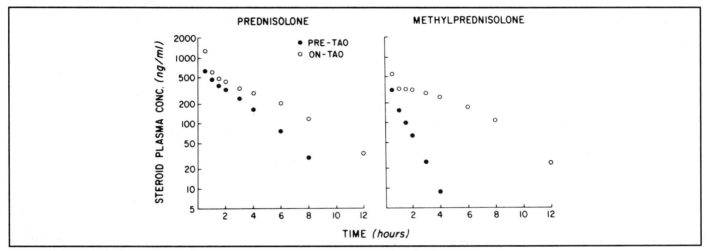

Fig. 67-3. *Steroid plasma concentration versus time plot for patient who received concomitant phenobarbital therapy. Prednisolone* (left) *and methylprednisolone* (right) *were administered in 30-mg intravenous doses before and 1 week after initiation of TAO therapy. (Reprinted with permission from S. J. Szefler et al. Steroid-specific and anticonvulsant interaction aspects of troleandomycin-steroid therapy.* J. Allergy Clin. Immunol. *69: 455, 1982.)*

with respect to TAO/MP drug interaction, clearance and mean residence time are more exact than MP half-life in the evaluation of impaired MP disposition. TAO significantly reduced MP clearance by 66 percent (to 146 ml/min/1.73 m^2). MP half-life increased nearly twofold (from about 2.5 hours to 4.6 hours). MP clearance remained prolonged on even reduced TAO dosage (250 to 500 mg daily) as seen in three patients studied 1 to 5 months on TAO/MP [3], documenting the immediate and continued inhibition of MP clearance by TAO. Further pharmacologic studies on five corticosteroid-dependent asthmatic patients demonstrated that with alternate-day TAO administration (250 mg), MP elimination was impaired on the TAO day to a greater extent than on the non-TAO day. Nevertheless, MP clearance was still impaired on the non-TAO day compared to before TAO was first administered [76]. Therefore, TAO should be coadministered on the same alternate day as MP to maintain the optimal effectiveness of alternate-day TAO/MP treatment.

TAO's effects on corticosteroids are apparently steroid specific since MP but not prednisolone (active metabolite of prednisone) elimination is impaired by TAO (Fig. 67-2) [3]. This steroid specificity in clearance appears to enhance the clinical efficacy that is induced by TAO in combination with MP [3].

On the other hand, the effect that TAO has on MP clearance is not TAO specific, since erythromycin also decreases MP volume of distribution and increases mean residence time and half-life in a nonlinear pattern similar to but to a lesser degree than TAO [45]. Whether erythromycin can induce similar clinical benefit as

TAO in steroid-dependent patients needs to be studied, since the former is potentially less hepatotoxic than TAO.

The interactions of TAO, corticosteroids, and anticonvulsants are extremely complicated (Table 67-5). Hydantoin and barbiturate anticonvulsants increase corticosteroid metabolism, as previously discussed [77], which by reducing corticosteroid availability often reduces corticosteroid effect and/or clinical control [7]. The enhanced MP clearance induced by anticonvulsants can be reversed up to 70 percent by TAO coadministration. This effect of TAO is not steroid specific, as increased prednisolone clearance in the presence of phenobarbital is also reduced by TAO [77] (Fig. 67-3). Anticonvulsant clearance appears inhibited by TAO administration [55], demanding a reduction in anticonvulsant dosage to avoid central nervous system toxicity when TAO is coadministered. Moreover, the risk of liver toxicity, including enzyme abnormalities or frank hepatitis, increases when TAO is administered with hydantoins (and possibly barbiturates) owing to mechanisms yet to be identified but perhaps related to their cohepatic metabolism (personal observation). Though not yet tested, the barbiturates may provide greater safety as the choice anticonvulsant, if effective, for epileptics during TAO/MP treatment, because of its reduced potential for inducing hepatotoxicity compared with the hydantoins [86]. Valproic acid appears to have no effect on glucocorticoid pharmacokinetics (personal observation). Substitution of valproic acid for phenytoin, carbamazepine, and phenobarbital in patients receiving steroid therapy may therefore result in enhanced steroid effect.

Theophylline [83], ergotamine [37], oral contraceptive [26] and triazolam [82] metabolism is inhibited by TAO (Table 67-5), requiring reduction of dosages of these agents to avoid drug toxicity. Low-dose TAO has very little effect on theophylline elimination, and therefore a theophylline dosage adjustment may not be necessary [81]. Isolated clinical anecdotes suggest that corticosteroid-dependent patients who have developed severe liver toxicity from TAO (necessitating discontinuation) may *not* evidence cross-drug toxicity with other macrolides such as erythromycin estolate and therefore not totally lose the clinical benefit derived from macrolides [71]. Studies will need to be performed to determine the correctness of this observation.

PRACTICAL GUIDELINES FOR TROLEANDOMYCIN THERAPY

Candidates for TAO therapy include those steroid-dependent asthmatics (1) whose maintenance asthma regimen requires greater than the equivalent of 10 mg of MP daily; (2) in whom a reversible component exists to spirometry; (3) who have received adequate trials of high-dose conventional antiasthmatic medication (including theophylline, beta-adrenergic agents, anticholinergics, cromolyn, and inhaled corticosteroids); (4) in whom complicating illnesses such as thyroid, cardiac, gastroesophageal reflux, and sinus disease have been adequately treated; and (5) whose psychological problems have or are being approached professionally.

Experience with the treatment of chronic refractory steroid-dependent asthma with TAO has led to the development of a protocol of management (Table 67-6). This protocol serves only as a guide, since therapy must be individualized to be optimal. These guidelines, however, should provide useful clinical strategy for the introduction and long-term use of TAO and MP until more definitive recommendations evolve, in order to maximize benefits and minimize potential side effects. Prudent and rapid reductions in both TAO and MP dosage should prevent or reduce steroid side effects [71, 81, 85].

Steroid- and nonsteroid-related side effects occur frequently during TAO/MP therapy; however, they are usually reversible. Initially, even with new low-dose TAO protocol, some patients experience an increase in steroid-induced cushingoid features, sweating, weight gain, and/or fluid retention. Diets reduced in calories and salt may lessen the latter effects. These steroid effects generally diminish when TAO and MP are tapered to alternate-day dosage. Particular care must be extended to the elderly, as they appear more prone to adverse effects of corticosteroids. The anticipated increased corticosteroid cushingoid side effects that are characteristically induced by TAO may be reduced by reducing initial MP dose by 25 to 50 percent when starting TAO, tapering TAO and MP as rapidly and judiciously as clinically possible (particularly in the elderly), and switching TAO and MP to alternate-day treatment earlier in the tapering course to avoid impending or severe significant existing toxicity, or starting TAO at 250 mg daily [81]. With judicious tapering according to the guidelines in Table 67-6, most patients will tolerate TAO and MP coadministered on the same alternate day [81, 85]. As was mentioned previously, the rapidity of partial adrenal recovery remains individual but usually does not occur until MP (range 4–12 mg QOD) and TAO are administered the same alternate day. Since 4 mg of MP administered with TAO possesses clearance kinetics similar to those of 40 mg of MP when administered without TAO [76], patients unable to be tapered to alternate-day TAO and MP may be at considerable risk for corticosteroid toxicity. These patients probably do not have the benefit-risk ratios suitable for continuation of TAO treatment.

Nonsteroid-related problems, including such gastrointestinal disturbances as nausea, pyrosis, abdominal cramps, and fullness, though common, generally disappear with the reduction of TAO

Table 67-6. TAO/MP protocol for severe, steroid-requiring asthmatics

A. Initiation of therapy
1. Select only severe chronic steroid-requiring asthmatics.
2. Optimize conventional anti-asthmatic therapy (medical, educational, and psychological).
3. Begin measurements of peak expiratory flow twice daily.
4. Carefully assess compliance with present medical regimen.
5. Assess varicella status.
B. MP trial phase
1. Replace prednisone with the corticosteroid equivalent dose of MP.
2. Attempt to decrease the MP dose.
3. Add TAO only if there is:
   a) Absence of liver disease.
   b) Absence of drug allergy to macrolide antibiotics.
   c) There is no response to MP, or MP is still required daily, or frequent steroid bursts are required.
   d) No active or recent exposure to varicella in unimmunized.
C. TAO trial phase
1. Inform and educate the patient (relative to side effects and compliance).
2. Obtain baseline studies, including:
   a) Spirometry (body plethysmography, if possible).
   b) Liver function tests, biochemistry profile, theophylline concentrations, and morning cortisol levels.
   c) Ophthalmology examination for posterior subcapsular cataracts and increased intraocular pressure.
   d) Bone densitometry (as appropriate for age) and bone age.
   e) Obtain baseline blood pressure and weight, and consider photography for comparison of cushingoid features.
   f) Continue peak expiratory flow measurements twice daily.
3. MP reduction:
   a) Empirically reduce theophylline dose by 25% once TAO/MP therapy is begun.
   b) Days 1 and 2—MP in the starting dose (convert baseline prednisone dose to equivalent dose of MP). Days 3–14—Taper the alternate-day MP dose by 20–25% until an alternate-day dose of MP and TAO is obtained (for example, if the starting MP dose is 40 mg, the schedule would be, starting with day 1, 40 mg, 40 mg, 32 mg, 40 mg, 24 mg, 40 mg, 16 mg, 40 mg, 8 mg, 40 mg, 0 mg).
   c) Obtain serum theophylline concentration and liver function tests after 3 days, then weekly for the first month; peak expiratory flow measurements should be obtained twice daily; spirometry should be obtained at 2 weeks and a determination of the patient's response based on peak flow recordings, spirometry, and subjective impressions.
4. TAO dose:
   a) TAO at a dose of 250 mg is given daily along with the MP. There is no reduction in the TAO dose while the patient is on daily corticosteroids.
   b) Once on alternate-day MP, TAO is given only on the same date as the steroid and at a dose of 250 mg every other day.
D. TAO/MP tapering phase
1. Once TAO/MP is administered on an alternate-day schedule, reduce only the MP dose 2–4 mg per dose per week until the dose is less than or equal to 12 mg every other day; then reduce the MP dose by 1–2 mg every other week.
2. If spirometry or peak expiratory flow is decreased by 10–15%, reduce or hold the tapering schedule.
3. Monitor morning cortisol level every month, and if the serum theophylline concentration and liver enzyme tests are normal at the end of the first month, they should be monitored on a monthly basis for at least the next 6 months.
4. Follow growth, blood pressure, bone densitometry, and ophthalmology examination to monitor long-term steroid effects.
5. Consider inhaled corticosteroids and/or nighttime administration of oral beta agonists, such as Proventil Repetabs if a pattern of morning "dipping" is noted and the patient is unable to be tapered further.

Source: Reprinted with permission from B. D. Ball, and S. J. Szefler, Troleandomycin: Present status in the treatment of severe asthmatic children. *Am. J. Asthma Allergy Pediatr.* 2:27, 1988.

and/or theophylline dosage or initiation of pharmacologic therapy (antacids and antiflatulents). To avoid inducing theophylline toxicity during TAO introduction to MP therapy, it is recommended to reduce the theophylline dose empirically by 25 percent, especially if the patient is managed with serum concentrations between 15 and 20 μg/ml. This generally permits maintenance of therapeutic theophylline levels, which must be checked by frequent theophylline blood levels until TAO dosage is stabilized. Hydantoins have recently been shown to enhance theophylline clearance [51], which potentially could be reversed by TAO coadministration, complicating theophylline kinetics even further.

Transient rises in hepatic transaminases occasionally occur during the early phase of TAO introduction, particularly when hydantoins are coadministered. Generally, SGPT appears to be a better indicator of TAO-induced hepatic toxicity than does SGOT. Levels of SGPT greater than 90 units are uncommon during TAO/MP therapy [85], except when potential hepatotoxins (e.g., hydantoins, oral contraceptives) are concurrently administered. Usually gradual reductions in the dosage of TAO as suggested by the guidelines (Table 67-6) are adequate to reduce mildly elevated levels of SGPT. However, more rapid TAO tapering may be necessary when SGPT levels exceed 100 units, as frequently seen in patients on hydantoins (see subsequent discussion). One patient developing prolonged cholestasis following TAO-induced acute hepatitis with treatment consisting of 2 gm/day for 1 week [46]. Jaundice and hypereosinophilia occurred during the treatment period. Jaundice resolved in 3 months but was followed by prolonged anicteric hepatitis. Pruritus resolved within 9 months, and liver enzyme tests normalized in 27 months.

Special consideration must be directed to the steroid-dependent asthmatic on anticonvulsants in whom TAO use is contemplated. Indications and absolute need for anticonvulsants should be reexamined in these patients. If reevaluation indicates that anticonvulsants are unnecessary, they should be tapered slowly and discontinued. As previously discussed, valproic acid could be substituted to avoid the induction of steroid metabolism. When anti-convulsants are essential, their dosages should be empirically reduced 25 to 50 percent to prevent anticonvulsant toxicity during TAO administration. Frequent determination of serum anticonvulsant levels must be performed to ensure adequate seizure control. Similarly, frequent (preferably daily until TAO is reduced to 500 mg daily) liver enzyme determinations should be done to identify quickly any hepatic toxicity, which characteristically occurs during the coadministration of TAO and anticonvulsants. Rapid tapering of TAO to alternate-day dosage may need to be instituted with increasing abnormal hepatic chemistries to avoid frank hepatitis. Alternatively, although not studied yet, TAO could be started at lower doses, or phenobarbital could be substituted in an attempt to avoid liver toxicity from TAO anticonvulsant interactions.

Exacerbations of asthma triggered by TAO/MP tapering, viral illness, and so on do not routinely require large steroid bursts. These relapses generally resolve with small MP increments for a few days (switching to daily MP at same dosage as the maintenance alternate-day dosage or doubling the daily dosage) with or without using daily TAO.

A recent death related to varicella infection occurred during concomitant TAO/MP therapy [47]. It is not clear whether the patient was immunocompromised prior to or as a result of combination TAO/MP or as a result of the varicella infection. Nevertheless, a varicella titer should be obtained before beginning treatment. If negative, the patient should be monitored carefully during times of exposure. Upon exposure, protective antibody, varicella immune globulin, and with any sign of infection, acyclovir should be administered.

MECHANISMS OF TROLEANDOMYCIN ACTION

The mechanism by which TAO exerts a beneficial effect in steroid-dependent asthma remains elusive. Table 67-7 notes certain possible modes of action by which TAO could exert its influence and whether such action appears relevant to asthma.

Although TAO is a macrolide antibiotic with antibacterial properties [40], its effect on asthma appears independent of this action [12, 41, 71]. Aside from macrolide antibiotics (chemically similar to TAO), broad-spectrum antibiotics are ineffective in chronic corticosteroid-dependent asthma. Although TAO has been associated with hepatic dysfunction [20, 63, 78], many patients respond favorably to TAO without evidencing any alteration in liver enzymes, therefore discrediting this mode of action as relevant to improvement in asthma.

In high doses, TAO reduces theophylline clearance [83]; however, it is less likely with lower TAO doses [3, 81]. Possible theophylline toxicity is prevented by reducing existing theophylline dosage by 25 to 50 percent, depending on baseline theophylline blood levels prior to starting TAO. Theophylline levels can be maintained within the therapeutic range of 10 to 20 μg/ml by such manipulation. If therapeutic levels of theophylline do not exist, TAO introduction would tend to increase levels, thereby exerting a beneficial effect. Since therapeutic levels of theophylline were maintained both before and during TAO therapy (by reducing theophylline dosage) in many studies [77, 85], the effect of TAO on theophylline clearance would appear independent and not relevant to its benefit on asthma in these patients.

The interaction of TAO with corticosteroids would appear to be the relevant area for its benefit. It has been demonstrated that histamine lethality in rats could be reduced by the administration of TAO with MP as compared with either agent separately. This benefit was attributed to the elevation of plasma corticosteroid levels seen in those rats being administered the combination of TAO and MP [66].

Selenke et al. [67] demonstrated in animal studies that TAO

Table 67-7. Possible mode of TAO action in corticosteroid-dependent asthma

Mode	Relevant to asthma benefit	Comment
Antibiotic	No	Other broad-spectrum antibiotics ineffective
Hepatic dysfunction	No	Many responders with normal liver function tests
Reduce theophylline clearance	Not usually	Effect independent of improvement; improvement occurs with adequate prior theophyllinization and reduction in theophylline dosage
↑ Adrenal steroid output	No	Required 200 mg/kg TAO (rats)
Reduce steroid clearance	Yes	MP elimination markedly prolonged
Reduce sputum production	Yes	Clue to responder
Enhance steroid inhibition of PHA mitogenesis	?	Indicates TAO/MP interaction at cellular level
Antianaphylactic by itself	No	Required 100 mg/kg/day TAO (guinea pig)
Reduce histamine and methacholine sensitivity	Possible	Correlated with reduction in severity of asthma
Reduce histamine-induced lethality	Possible	Protect against beta-adrenergic blockade (mice)

and MP coadministered in comparison with TAO or MP alone (1) significantly increased liver glycogen deposition in adrenalectomized mice, intact mice, and adrenalectomized rats; (2) protected mice against histamine-induced lethality; (3) increased steroid-induced glucose intolerance in mice; and (4) increased blood corticosteroid levels in rats. TAO's potentiating effect of steroid-induced glycogen deposition occurred also with betamethasone but not hydrocortisone. Interestingly, erythromycin and erythromycin ethylsuccinate, to a lesser degree, in combination with MP also decreased histamine lethality in mice. In these studies lincomycin and tetracycline could not enhance the effects of MP. They concluded from these animal studies (which must be interpreted in light of the recognized corticosteroid sensitivity of rats and mice and relative steroid insensitivity of man) that TAO (and other macrolides) potentiated corticosteroid activity not as antimicrobial agents, adrenocorticotropic hormone-like compounds [31], or quasi-steroids but by functioning as steroid-sparing agents by some yet to be defined mechanism [67].

As discussed previously, corticosteroid metabolic clearance studies in humans have shown marked reductions in MP elimination with the TAO/MP regimen [75], which may contribute in part to TAO's clinical efficacy. TAO and MP interacting together, in contrast to the failure of either drug alone, have been shown to reduce the hypersensitivity both to histamine and methacholine characteristically seen in asthmatics [71]. In contrast, a study of short-term TAO/MP usage in mild asthmatics failed to confirm a change in nonspecific bronchial sensitivity to methacholine [2]. This study incorporated 1 week of treatment with the study medications. In a 2-week treatment course, methacholine bronchial sensitivity improved in four of five patients receiving TAO/MP and two of five patients receiving TAO/prednisone. Since airway hyperresponsiveness appears to be related to inflammation in the airways, this raised the interesting question whether TAO may have some antiinflammatory properties [71]. The finding that TAO increases MP inhibition of mitogen-induced lymphocyte blastogenesis [58] demonstrated for the first time a direct cellular interaction of these drugs, although its relationship to asthma can only be speculative at the moment.

TAO may have other beneficial effects independent of impaired steroid elimination, and concurrently MP may be more effective than oral prednisone. The beneficial effect of MP over prednisone (specifically its active metabolite prednisolone) may be due to better penetration of MP into lung tissue [80]. Recent studies suggest that macrolide antibiotics may have nonantibiotic antiinflammatory properties; for example, erythromycin or TAO may alter neutrophil response to an inflammatory stimulus [34, 57], impair neutrophil response to chemoattractants [33], and inhibit basophil histamine release [53], besides altering T-lymphocyte response to phytohemagglutinin stimulation [58].

The pronounced and rapidly developing cushingoid side effects when TAO and MP are taken together are in contrast to the frequent lack of corticosteroid side effects prior to TAO addition in many patients, even though they were on doses of steroids for periods of time sufficient to produce cushingoid side effects in more responsive asthmatics. The refractoriness of asthma in the partially responsive patients combined with a general failure to develop characteristic corticosteroid side effects at expected doses of traditional steroid therapy suggests that a general end-organ hyporesponsiveness to steroids may exist in these patients, which is reversed in some manner by TAO interaction with corticosteroids.

Steroid requirements in steroid-dependent asthmatics have been shown not to be related to the binding, distribution, or clearance of prednisolone [52, 64, 65]. Speculations as to possible mechanisms for this relative unresponsiveness in steroid-resistant asthmatics include abnormal or diminished steroid receptors, although a recent study failed to demonstrate any TAO effects on corticosteroid receptor number, affinity, or binding properties of skin fibroblasts in vitro [25] (a glucocorticoid receptor–mediator disease has recently been described in humans [15]), defective interaction of corticosteroids with adrenergic or cholinergic receptors, or failure of corticosteroids to stimulate beta-adrenergic receptors, to list just a few. Future studies will define potential mechanisms of action and lead to refined guidelines for the use of TAO.

REFERENCES

1. Alvarez, J., Szefler, S. J., and Gelfand, E. W. Troleandomycin therapy modifies the T-lymphocyte response to glucocorticoids in asthmatics (abstract). *J. Allergy Clin. Immunol.* 85:195, 1990.
2. Andrade, W., et al. Effect of Troleandomycin and methyl prednisolone alone and in combination on bronchial sensitivity to methacholine. *Ann. Allergy* 51:515, 1983.
3. Ball, B. D., et al. Effect of low dose troleandomycin on glucocorticoid pharmacokinetics and airway hyperresponsiveness in severe asthmatic children. *Ann. Allergy* 65:37, 1990.
4. Bartoszek, M., Brenner, A. M., and Szefler, S. J. Prednisolone and methylprednisolone kinetics in children receiving anticonvulsants therapy. *Clin. Pharmacol. Ther.* 42:424, 1987.
5. Boekenoogen, S. J., Szefler, S. J., and Jusko, W. J. Prednisolone disposition and protein binding in oral contraceptive users. *J. Clin. Endocrinol. Metab.* 56:702, 1983.
6. Braude, A. C., and Rebuck, A. S. Prednisone and methylprednisolone disposition in the lung. *Lancet* 2:995, 1983.
7. Brooks, P. M., et al. Effects of enzyme induction on metabolism of prednisolone. *Ann. Rheum. Dis.* 35:339, 1976.
8. Brooks, S. M., Sholiton, L. J., and Altenau, P. The effects of disodium cromoglycate on dexamethasone metabolism. *Am. Rev. Respir. Dis.* 114:1911, 1976.
9. Brooks, S. M., et al. The effects of ephedrine and theophylline on dexamethasone metabolism in bronchial asthma. *J. Clin. Pharmacol.* 17:308, 1977.
10. Brooks, S. M., et al. Adverse effects of phenobarbital on corticosteroid metabolism in patients with bronchial asthma. *N. Engl. J. Med.* 286:1125, 1972.
11. Buffington, G. A., et al. Interaction of rifampin and glucocorticoids: Adverse effect on renal allograft function. *JAMA* 236:1958, 1976.
12. Cabanieu, G. The value and the tolerance of troleandomycin in the long-term treatment of asthma and chronic bronchitis. *Antibiotica* [Quad.] June 1975, P. 110.
13. Celmer, W. D., Els, H., and Murai, K. Oleandomycin Derivatives: Preparation and Characterization. In *Antibiotics Annual, 1957–1958.* New York: Medical Encyclopedia, 1958. P. 476.
14. Choi, Y., et al. Effect of diphenylhydantoin on cortisol kinetics in humans. *J. Pharmacol. Exp. Ther.* 176:27, 1971.
15. Chrousos, G. P., et al. Primary cortisol resistance in man: A glucocorticoid receptor–mediator disease. *J. Clin. Invest.* 69:1261, 1982.
16. Conney, A. H., et al. Induction of liver microsomal cortisol 6β-hydroxylase by diphenylhydantoin or phenobarbital: An explanation for the increased excretion of 6-hydroxycortisol in humans treated with these drugs. *Life Sci.* 4:1091, 1965.
17. Dafniet, M. L., et al. Effects of troleandomycin administration on cholesterol 7-α-hydroxylase activity and bile secretion in rats. *J. Pharmacol. Exp. Ther.* 219:558, 1981.
18. Dasgupta, A., and Marcoux, J. P. Hepatic abnormalities associated with long-term use of troleandomycin in asthma: A case report. *Ann. Allergy* 41:297, 1978.
19. Davies, A. O., and Lefkowitz, R. J.: In vitro desensitization of beta adrenergic receptors in human neutrophils: Attenuation by corticosteroids. *J. Clin. Invest.* 71:565, 1983.
20. Djaczenko, W., Garaci, E., and Damiani, S. Morphometric studies in triacetyloleandomycin-induced ultrastructural modifications of rat hepatocyte mitochondria. *Chemotherapy* 23:167, 1977.
21. Edwards, O. M., et al. Changes in cortisol metabolism following rifampicin therapy. *Lancet* 2:549, 1974.
22. Eitches, R. W., et al. Methylprednisolone and troleandomycin in treatment of steroid-dependent asthmatic children. *Am. J. Dis. Child.* 139:264, 1985.
23. Ellul-Micallef, R., and Fenech, F. F. Effect of intravenous prednisolone in patients with diminished adrenergic responsiveness. *Lancet* 2:1269, 1975.
24. Emmanuel, J. H., and Montgomery, R. D. Gastric ulcer and the anti-arthritic drugs. *Postgrad. Med. J.* 47:227, 1971.
25. Engler, R. J. M., et al. The effects of triacetyloleandomycin and oleandomycin phosphate on the glucocorticoid receptor in cultured skin fibroblasts. *J. Allergy Clin. Immunol.* 75:395, 1985.

26. Fevery, J., et al. Severe intrahepatic cholestasis due to the combined intake of oral contraceptives and triacetyloleandomycin. *Acta Clin. Belg.* 38:242, 1983.

27. Foltz, E. L. Oleandomycin—Its Derivatives and Combinations—in the Treatment of Staphylococcal Infections. In H. Welch and M. Finland (eds.). *Antibiotic Therapy for Staphylococcal Diseases.* New York: Medical Encyclopedia, 1959. P. 39.

28. Fox, J. L. Infectious asthma treated with triacetyloleando-mycin. *Pa. Med. J.* 64:634, 1961.

29. Fraser, C. M., and Venter, J. C. The synthesis of β-adrenergic receptors in cultured lung cells: Induction of glucocorticoids. *Biochem. Biophys.* Res. Commun. 94:390, 1980.

30. Glynn, A. M., et al. Effects of ketoconazole on methylprednisolone pharmacokinetics and cortisol secretion. *Clin. Pharmacol. Ther.* 39:654, 1986.

31. Goncharova, V. J., and Babkova, E. D. Stimulation of adrenal cortex by certain antibiotics of the macrolide group. *Antibiotiki* 8:58, 1963.

32. Green, A. W., et al. Cimetidine-methylprednisolone-theophylline metabolic interaction. *Am. J. Med.* 77:1115, 1984.

33. Greos, L. S., et al. Macrolide antibiotics inhibit neutrophil chemostasis (abstract). *J. Allergy Clin. Immunol.* 85:195, 1990.

34. Greos, L. S., et al. Troleandomycin reduces airways inflammation? (abstract). *Am. Rev. Respir. Dis.* 141:A933, 1990.

35. Haber, I., and Hubens, H. Cholestatic jaundice after triacetyloleandomycin and oral contraceptives: The diagnostic value of gamma-glutamyl transpeptidase. *Acta Gastroenterol. Belg.* 53:475, 1980.

36. Haque, N., et al. Studies on dexamethasone metabolism in man: Effect of diphenylhydantoin. *J. Clin. Endocrinol. Metab.* 34:44, 1972.

37. Hayton, A. C. Precipitation of acute ergotism by triacetyloleandomycin. *N. Z. Med. J.* 69:42, 1969.

38. Hendrickse, W., et al. Rifampicin-induced nonresponsiveness to corticosteroid treatment in nephrotic syndrome. *Br. Med. J.* 1:306, 1979.

39. Hunt, T. K., et al. Effect of vitamin A on reversing the inhibitory effect of cortisone on healing of open wounds in animals and man. *Ann. Surg.* 170: 633, 1969.

40. Isenberg, H., and Karelitz, S. Clinical and Laboratory Evaluation of Triacetyloleandomycin in a Variety of Pyogenic Infections. In H. Welch and F. Marti-Ibanez (eds.), *Antibiotics Annual, 1958–1959.* New York: Interscience, 1959. P. 284.

41. Itkin, I. H., and Menzel, M. L. The use of macrolide antibiotic substances in the treatment of asthma. *J. Allergy* 45:146, 1970.

42. Kaplan, M. A., and Goldin, M. The Use of Triacetyloleandomycin in Chronic Infectious Asthma. In H. Welch and F. Marti-Ibanez (eds.), *Antibiotics Annual, 1958–1959.* New York: Interscience Publishers, 1959. P. 273.

43. Klinenberg, J. R., and Miller, F. Effect of corticosteroids on blood salicylate concentration. *J.A.M.A.* 194:131, 1965.

44. Kyriazopoulou, V., Parparousi, O., and Vagenakis, A. G. Rifampicin-induced adrenal crisis in addisonian patients receiving corticosteroid replacement therapy. *J. Clin. Endocrinol. Metab.* 59:1204, 1984.

45. La Force, C. F., et al. Inhibition of methylprednisolone in the presence of erythromycin therapy. *J. Allergy Clin. Immunol.* 72:34, 1983.

46. Larrey, D., et al. Prolonged cholestasis after troleandomycin-induced acute hepatitis. *J. Hepatol.* 4:327, 1987.

47. Lantner, R., et al. Fatal varicella in a corticosteroid-dependent asthmatic receiving troleandomycin. *Allergy Proc.* 11(2):83, 1990.

48. Lohmann, S. M., and Miech, R. T. Theophylline metabolism by the rat liver microsomal system. *J. Pharmacol. Exp. Ther.* 196:213, 1976.

49. Ludwig, E. A., et al. Ketoconazole effects on prednisolone pharmacokinetics and cortisol suppression. *Drug Intell. Clin. Pharm.* 21:5A, 1987.

50. Marone, G., Lichtenstein, L. M., and Plaut, M. Hydrocortisone and human lymphocytes: Increase in cyclic adenosine 3'5'-monophosphate and potentiation of adenylate cyclase–activating agent. *J. Pharmacol. Exp. Ther.* 215:169, 1980.

51. Marquis, J. F., et al. Phenytoin-theophylline interaction. *N. Engl. J. Med.* 307:1189, 1982.

52. May, C. S., et al. Prednisolone pharmacokinetics in asthmatic patients. *Br. J. Dis. Chest* 74:91, 1980.

53. Mendoza, G. R., Eitches, R. W., and Orner, F. B. Direct effects of oleandomycin on histamine release in human basophils (abstract). *J. Allergy Clin. Immunol.* 71:135, 1983.

54. Menzel, M. K., Itkin, H. L., and Townley, R. G. The effect of TAO upon chronic severe asthma (abstract). *J. Allergy* (Suppl.) p. 55, 1966.

55. Mesdijian, E., et al. Carbamazepine intoxication due to triacetyloleandomycin administration in epileptic patients. *Epilepsia* 21:489, 1980.

56. Morrison, P. J., et al. Concurrent administration of cimetidine and enteric-

coated prednisolone: Effect of plasma levels of prednisolone. *Br. J. Clin. Pharmacol.* 10:87, 1980.

57. Nelson, S., et al. Erythromycin-induced suppression of pulmonary antibacterial defenses in the lung. *Am. Rev. Respir. Dis.* 136:1207, 1987.

58. Ong, K. S., Grieco, N. H., and Rosner, W. Enhancement by oleandomycin of the inhibitory effect of methylprednisolone on phytohemagglutinin-stimulated lymphocytes. *J. Allergy Clin. Immunol.* 62:115, 1978.

59. Peden, N. R., et al. Cortisol and dexamethasone elimination during treatment with cimetidine. *Br. J. Clin. Pharmacol.* 18:101, 1984.

60. Pessayre, D., et al. Hypoactivity of cytochrome P-450 after triacetyloleandomycin administration. *Biochem. Pharmacol.* 30:559, 1981.

61. Pessayre, D., et al. Self-induction by triacetyloleandomycin of its own transformation into a metabolite forming a stable 456-nm-absorbing complex with cytochrome P-450. *Biochem. Pharmacol.* 30:553, 1981.

62. Pessayre, D., et al. Formation of an inactive cytochrome P-450 Fe (II)-metabolite complex after administration of troleandomycin in humans. *Biochem. Pharmacol.* 31:1699, 1982.

63. Robinson, M. M. Hepatic dysfunction associated with triacetyloleandomycin and propionyl erythromycin ester lauryl sulfate. *Am. J. Med. Sci.* 243: 502, 1962.

64. Rose, J. Q., et al. Prednisolone disposition in steroid-dependent asthmatic children. *J. Allergy Clin. Immunol.* 67:188, 1981.

65. Rose, J. W., et al. Prednisolone disposition in steroid-dependent asthmatics. *J. Allergy Clin. Immunol.* 66:366, 1980.

66. Selenke, W., et al. Glucosteroid-sparing effect of certain macrolide antibiotics (abstract). *J. Allergy* 43:156, 1969.

67. Selenke, W. M., Leong, G. W., and Townley, R. G. Nonantibiotic effects of macrolide antibiotics of the oleandomycin-erythromycin group with special reference to their "steroid-sparing" effects. *J. Allergy Clin. Immunol.* 65:454, 1980.

68. Shubin, H., Dumas, K., and Sokmensuer, A. Clinical and Laboratory Studies on a New Derivative of Oleandomycin. In *Antibiotics Annual, 1957–1958.* New York: Medical Encyclopedia, 1958. P. 679.

69. Sirgo, M. A., et al. Effects of cimetidine and ranitidine on the conversation of prednisone to prednisolone. *Clin. Pharmacol. Ther.* 37:534, 1985.

70. Spangler, A. S., et al. Enhancement of the antiinflammatory action of hydrocortisone by estrogen. *J. Clin. Endocrinol. Metab.* 29:650, 1969.

71. Spector, S. L., Katz, F. H., and Farr, R. S. Troleandomycin: Effectiveness in steroid-dependent asthma and bronchitis. *J. Allergy Clin. Immunol.* 54: 367, 1974.

72. Stephen, W. C., et al. Tachyphylaxis to inhaled isoproterenol and the effect of methylprednisolone in dogs. *J. Allergy Clin. Immunol.* 65:105, 1980.

73. Stephens, F. O., et al. Effect of cortisone and vitamin A on wound infection. *Am. J. Surg.* 121:569, 1971.

74. Stjernholm, M. R., and Katz, F. H. Effects of diphenylhydantoin, phenobarbital, and diazepam on the metabolism of methylprednisone and its sodium succinate. *J. Clin. Endocrinol. Metab.* 41:887, 1975.

75. Szefler, S. J., et al. The effect of troleandomycin on methylprednisolone elimination. *J. Allergy Clin. Immunol.* 66:447, 1980.

76. Szefler, S. J., et al. Dose and time-related effect of troleandomycin on methylprednisolone elimination. *Clin. Pharmacol. Ther.* 32:166, 1982.

77. Szefler, S. J., et al. Steroid-specific and anticonvulsant interaction aspects of troleandomycin-steroid therapy. *J. Allergy Clin. Immunol.* 69:455, 1982.

78. Ticktin, H. E., and Zimmerman, H. J. Hepatic dysfunction and jaundice in patients receiving triacetyloleandomycin. *N. Engl. J. Med.* 267:964, 1962.

79. Uribe, M., et al. Decreased bioavailability of prednisone due to antacids in patients with chronic active liver disease and in healthy volunteers. *Gastroenterology* 80:661, 1981.

80. Vichyanond, P., et al. Penetration of corticosteroids in the lung: Evidence for difference between methylprednisolone and prednisolone. *J. Allergy Clin. Immunol.* 84:867, 1989.

81. Wald, J. A., Friedman, B. F., and Farr, R. S. An improved protocol for using troleandomycin (TAO) in the treatment of steroid-requiring asthma. *J. Allergy Clin. Immunol.* 78:36, 1986.

82. Warot, D., et al. Troleandomycin-triazolam interaction in healthy volunteers: Pharmacokinetic and psychometric evaluation. *Eur. J. Clin. Pharmacol.* 32:389, 1987.

83. Weinberger, M., et al. Inhibition of theophylline clearance by troleandomycin. *J. Allergy Clin. Immunol.* 59:228, 1977.

84. Weiner, A. L., and Cohen, W. Hepatic function in acne vulgaris patients treated with triacetyloleandomycin. *J. New Drugs* 2:307, 1962.

85. Zeiger, R. S., et al. Efficacy of troleandomycin in outpatients with severe, corticosteroid-dependent asthma. *J. Allergy Clin. Immunol.* 66:438, 1980.

86. Zimmerman, H. J. *Hepatotoxicity: The Adverse Effects of Drug and Other Chemicals on the Liver.* New York: Appleton-Century-Crofts, 1978. P. 408.

87. Zurcher, R. M., Frey, B. M., and Fret, F. J.: Impact of ketoconazole on the metabolism of prednisolone. *Clin. Pharmacol. Ther.* 45:366, 1989.

Potent Antiinflammatory Agents

Michael F. Mullarkey

The concept that inflammation is a significant pathogenetic event in bronchial asthma is at least 60 years old [1]. In the 1940s, Hench and Kendall used adrenocorticotrophic hormone (ACTH) and adrenal cortical extracts to treat arthritis. Because asthma was believed to be caused by disordered immunity, clinicians considered the possibility that these agents and agents acting like corticosteroids might be useful in the control of asthma. In 1949, Bordley [13] at Johns Hopkins first used cortisone to treat asthma. Between 1944 and 1951, Diaz [18] treated 13 asthmatics with nitrogen mustard. He selected this agent because of "the difficulties of obtaining sufficient amounts of ACTH and cortisone" and because of the then apparent similarity of effects between cortisone and mustards "as regards the phenomena of shock and immunity" [18]. The next year, George Waldbott [60] repeated Diaz's work and treated 21 severe asthmatics with nitrogen mustard. He noted significant improvement in 19 patients, and 5 of the patients remained free of asthma symptoms from 3 to 6 months after treatment. However, toxicity from nitrogen mustard was severe, limiting its use to three courses. Throughout the 1960s and 1970s, clinicians continued to experiment with immunosuppressive agents such as azathioprine in the belief that the suppression of immunity would control inflammation (Table 68-1). With the use of these agents at lower and less frequent doses, the antiinflammatory and immunosuppressive effects were separable. This same dose-dependent property is well appreciated for corticosteroids. At high doses these drugs act rapidly and are immunosuppressive and cytotoxic. When given at lower doses and less frequently, corticosteroids and many of the drugs characterized as immunosuppressive have a slow onset of action and inhibit inflammation with minimal effect on immunity. Rheumatologists and then dermatologists were the first to appreciate and exploit this distinction by controlling drug dose and schedule to capitalize on the use of traditional immunosuppressive drugs to control chronic inflammatory diseases and to avoid the toxicity of prolonged treatment with cortisone.

This chapter will review the very recent perception by physicians that perhaps some of the previous strategies used in the management of chronic inflammation may prove relevant to asthmatic bronchitis.

METHOTREXATE

History

The history of methotrexate shows the evolution of our thought processes regarding the use of low doses of immunosuppressive drugs to control inflammation. In 1947, Sidney Farber [22] in Boston noted that children with acute leukemias produced more myeloblasts when given folic acid. From this observation he concluded that antagonists of folate might prove therapeutically use-

ful. At his urging, the first of a series of antifolates was synthesized by Lederle Laboratories. In 1948 Farber et al. [23] reported that children with leukemias treated with the folate antagonist aminopterin experienced remissions of disease. In 1951, Richard Gubner [25], a cardiologist at Kings County Hospital, used aminopterin to treat seven patients with rheumatoid arthritis. The patients improved significantly. One of the patients also suffered from psoriasis and experienced a remission of her skin lesions when treated with aminopterin. Gubner then treated eight more psoriatics, some with joint involvement, with improvement noted by all of the patients. In this landmark paper, Gubner et al. [25] commented that because of the "unavailability of cortisone and [ACTH], and their untoward effects with protracted administration," they considered another class of agents, which in animal models exerted a similar effect on "experimental disorders characterized by reaction of the mesenchymal tissues. . . ." Aminopterin had previously been shown to be as effective as cortisone in the suppression of adjuvant-induced arthritis.

Throughout the 1950s, high-dose methotrexate, which replaced aminopterin, was utilized in oncology. In 1964, Black and co-workers [10] at the National Institutes of Health (NIH) showed the efficacy of low-dose methotrexate in psoriatic arthritis in a double-blind study. One death from a non-drug-related cause occurred in this study, with the result that this work was not repeated for several years. In 1972, without the benefit of double-blind studies, the Food and Drug Administration (FDA) approved methotrexate for the treatment of psoriasis. Also in that year, Rex Hoffmeister [26] reported on the treatment of 29 refractory rheumatoids with low-dose, once a week methotrexate. Two-thirds of these patients showed significant improvement in their disease. By 1977, Weinstein [66] estimated that 50,000 patients were using low-dose methotrexate. To minimize toxicity, he recommended that the drug be given only once a week in doses of up to 15 mg. Weinstein stressed the toxic role played by alcohol when used with methotrexate as a cause of cirrhosis; thereafter a program of the drug once weekly with the avoidance of alcohol greatly reduced the toxicity of methotrexate without loss of its efficacy. Throughout the 1970s methotrexate was reported to be effective in the treatment of rheumatoid arthritis in uncontrolled studies, but in 1985 four controlled studies, two double-blinded [2, 62], were published showing unequivocally that methotrexate was effective in rheumatoid arthritis.

Mechanism of Action

The mechanisms by which low-dose methotrexate exerts its antiinflammatory effects are unknown. Low-dose methotrexate does not effect T-cell number, B-cell, nonkiller (NK) cell, or macrophage function and does not significantly depress immunoglobulin levels. It does, however, in low doses profoundly depress neutrophil chemotaxis to a wide variety of in vitro and in vivo

Table 68-1. The use of cytotoxic drugs in asthma: 1951–1971

Investigators	Year	Drug(s)	Time	Results (no. responding/ no. treated)
Diaz [18]	1951	Nitrogen Mustard	?	11/13[a]
Waldbott [60]	1952	Nitrogen Mustard	7 wk	19/21[a]
Cohen et al. [16]	1965	Azathioprine	4 mo	1/1[b]
Kaiser and Beall [29]	1966	Azathioprine	3 wk	0/5[a]
Asmundsson et al. [4]	1971	6-Methylprednisolone	12 wk	5/12[a]

[a] Reduction in clinical severity of asthma.
[b] Reduction in corticosteroid use with stability or improvement in severity of asthma.

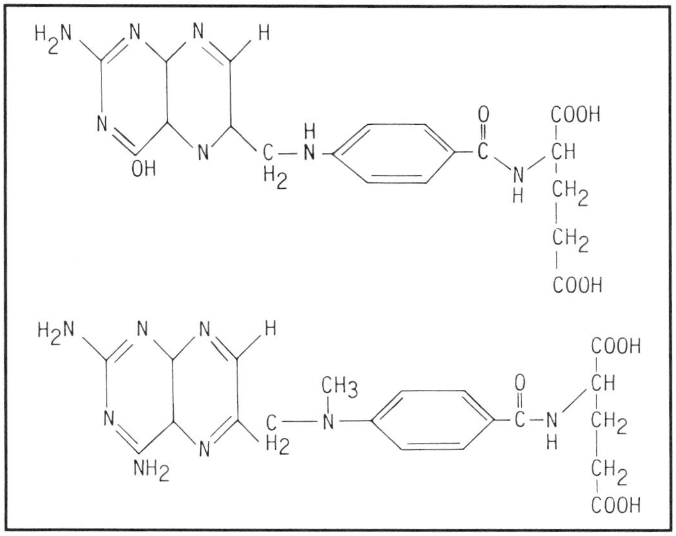

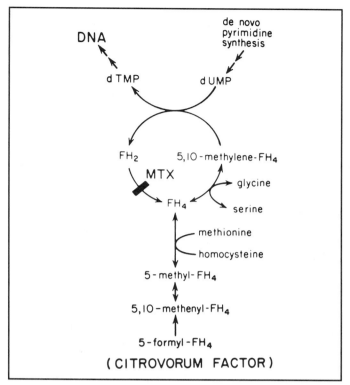

Fig. 68-2. *The folate cycle and the site of action of methotrexate. Also shown is the activation of leucovorin (folinic acid) and its entry point in the cycle bypassing methotrexate (MTX). dTMP = deoxythymidine monophosphate; dUMP = deoxyuridine monophosphate; FH$_2$ = dihydrofolate; FH$_4$ = tetrahydrofolate.*

Fig. 68-1. *Molecular structures of folic acid* (top) *and the folate antagonist methotrexate* (bottom).

Table 68-2. Drugs affecting the renal clearance of methotrexate

Inhibitors of tubular secretion
  Probenecid
  Diuretics
  Nephrotoxins (aminoglycosides, acetaminophen, cyclosporin)
Direct competition for secretion
  Nonsteroidal antiinflammatory drugs
  Aspirin
  Sulfa drugs
  Uric acid
  Penicillin (?)

stimulants in animals and humans [54, 58]. Ternowitz et al. [57] have shown that psoriatics using 15 mg/wk of methotrexate demonstrate a marked inhibition of neutrophil and monocyte chemotaxis. In this study they injected 10 psoriatics and 25 control patients with intradermal C5a. Control subjects and psoriatics tested just before their weekly methotrexate showed equivalent wheal and flare reactions within 4 minutes of injection. This reaction was significantly suppressed when C5a was injected just after methotrexate. In addition, the in vitro chemotactic activity of circulating monocytes and neutrophils to C5a was markedly depressed after methotrexate was taken. More recent studies suggest that methotrexate may block the activity of interleukin-1 (IL-1) but not affect its production [14]. Such an influence by methotrexate on IL-1 would dampen the expression of cell adhesion molecules and the production of other cytokines vital to the generation of inflammation.

Pharmacology

The structures of methotrexate and folic acid are shown in Figure 68-1. Two features of methotrexate's structure determine its efficacy and toxicity. Its homology with folate, an essential dietary factor in the production of tetrafolic acid, enables it to compete for and block the enzyme dihydrofolate reductase (DHR). Its ac-

tions are identical to the antibiotic trimethoprim. Methotrexate's binding to DHR far exceeds that of folate or trimethoprim, and it is therefore able to shut down transfer of one-carbon units in the synthesis of nucleic acids, amino acids, and essential fatty acids (Fig. 68-2).

Methotrexate's primary route of elimination is via the kidney, where it is both filtered and actively secreted [11]. Nearly half of an intravenously administered dose is excreted unchanged in 6 hours, with 90 percent excreted in 24 hours. In low doses, methotrexate's hepatic metabolism and protein binding are insignificant. Methotrexate is a weak organic acid (pK$_a$ 4.8–5.5). This second structural property has great significance in understanding many of methotrexate's potential toxicities. The terminal half-life of methotrexate is thought to be responsible for most of its gastrointestinal and bone marrow toxicity. Therefore drugs that compromise renal function, block tubular secretion, or are themselves weak organic acids will potentiate the toxicity of methotrexate. Examples of such drugs are shown in Table 68-2. Bleyer

[12] has shown that acute toxicity is predictable on the basis of a 24-hour blood level in excess of 1×10^{-7} M.

Toxicity

Drug Interactions
Table 68-2 lists the drug interactions of methotrexate.

Acute Toxicity
In general it is felt that methotrexate toxicity is dose related. Myelosuppression is rare with low-dose methotrexate and usually occurs in the setting of compromised renal function [36, 52]. Nausea, anorexia, diarrhea, and vomiting may occur in 10 percent of patients, while mucositis and dermatitis occur in 6 percent of patients and are usually managed by dose reduction or temporary drug discontinuation [63]. These effects can be reduced or eliminated with daily doses of folic acid of from 1 to 5 mg [38]. Hepatitis is rare and is managed by drug discontinuation with reinstitution after normalization of liver function tests.

Delayed Toxicity
Hepatic fibrosis, occasionally complicated by cirrhosis, was seen when methotrexate was given daily and alcohol use was not controlled. With the use of weekly drug and elimination of alcohol, cirrhosis is unreported below cumulative doses of 4 gm [3, 33, 44, 45]. Hepatic fibrosis is occasionally seen, but whether progression to cirrhosis occurs is unknown. Levels of serum glutamic-oxaloacetic transaminase (SGOT) do not correlate with or predict the development of liver cirrhosis. The cumulative dose of methotrexate at which liver biopsy is recommended is controversial due to the paucity of cases of cirrhosis in patients who do not use alcohol (liver biopsy has been recommended with each cumulative dose of 1,500 mg or every 3 years). It is recommended that a formal consultation with a hepatologist be sought for this decision at a cumulative dose of 1.5 to 2.0 gm and that the liver's synthetic function be checked with the testing of prothrombin time and albumin every 3 to 6 months.

Methotrexate is teratogenic by virtue of its ability to block folate utilization in the fetus. However, it does not damage DNA and therefore is not mutagenic [37]. Patients previously treated with high-dose regimens for cancer have had normal children [47, 48].

Pulmonary fibrosis and interstitial pneumonitis have both been reported to occur with low-dose methotrexate. Unlike other reactions associated with methotrexate, pulmonary toxicity appears to be idiosyncratic and not dose related. While these reactions are rare, it is clear that patients who smoke or have preexisting parenchymal disease are at higher risk [50]. This reaction is treated by drug withdrawal and high-dose corticosteroids. We obtain single-breath carbon monoxide studies (DLCO) on all patients and withhold drug from individuals with DLCO less than 60 percent of predicted. Spirometry is checked with each return visit.

One patient has recently been described by Jones et al. [28] as developing chest tightness and methacholine sensitivity while being treated with low-dose methotrexate for rheumatoid arthritis. While this unusual reaction to methotrexate resolved with subsequent administrations of drug and has not been reported in other patients receiving methotrexate, future explanations of methotrexate's mechanism of action will have to explain such idiosyncratic responses.

Varicella Infection
Patients receiving low-dose methotrexate, just as those receiving troleandomycin (TAO) and prolonged prednisone treatment, are at risk for disseminated varicella [32] (see Chap. 67). Patients at risk should be treated with varicella zoster immune globulin (VZIG) within 96 hours of exposure. Patients with characteristic varicella skin lesions should be treated with oral or intravenous acyclovir and closely followed. Severe abdominal or back pain is a herald of visceral involvement, and these patients should be hospitalized, treated with intravenous acyclovir, and monitored in an intensive care facility.

Negligible Toxicity
Malignancy and mutagenesis are not risk factors in patients treated with methotrexate [5, 7, 53]. Renal dysfunction is not an issue with low-dose methotrexate.

Long-term Studies
Several long-term studies have followed rheumatoids treated with low-dose methotrexate for up to 15 years. These studies show continued efficacy in these patients without serious adverse effects [27, 65]; such long-term data need to be acquired for asthmatics treated with methotrexate.

Methotrexate and Corticosteroid-dependent Asthma

In 1983, this author treated a 63-year-old woman with long-standing psoriasis, psoriatic arthritis, and steroid-dependent bronchial asthma with low-dose methotrexate. As expected, her skin and joint disease improved. Unexpectedly, her asthma showed a marked improvement, and she required no supplemental cortisone for asthma for over a year while taking methotrexate. This led to an open study using low-dose weekly methotrexate in eight corticosteroid-dependent asthmatics. In 1986 we published the observation that seven of eight asthmatics treated with low-dose methotrexate significantly reduced their corticosteroid requirements [40].

To test the validity of the previous observation that methotrexate may be used as a steroid-sparing drug in asthma, as it is used in psoriasis and several rheumatic diseases, we embarked on a double-blind crossover study patterned after the 1985 studies of Weinblatt [62] and Anderson [2] demonstrating the efficacy of methotrexate in rheumatoid arthritis. Twenty-two patients with corticosteroid-dependent asthma treated with maximal bronchodilator therapy, inhaled steroids, and a minimum of 10 mg/day of prednisone were enrolled between February 1986 and March 1987 [41]. Fourteen patients completed the study. The study design was a double-blind crossover of 24 weeks' duration with crossover occurring at 12 weeks. Patients took 15 mg of methotrexate each week in tablet form. Subjects recorded prednisone use and subjective assessments each day. The results of this double-blind crossover study showed a 36.5 percent reduction in the need for prednisone (p = .01), a significant improvement in the patients' subjective assessment of breathing (p = .01) and wheeze (p = .02), and near significant reduction in nocturnal awakenings (p = .08). Pulmonary functions remained stable in spite of significant reductions in prednisone use.

Dyer and colleagues [19] have completed a 28-week double-blind crossover study with oral low-dose methotrexate in 10 corticosteroid-dependent patients. Patients had been steroid dependent for a minimum of 2 years. Investigators attempted to reduce steroid requirements for 3 weeks prior to initiation of the study; those patients able to reduce prednisone continued to taper until steroid requirements were stable. Subjects were then randomized to a 3-month double-blind trial of drug or placebo. Methotrexate was given as 5-mg tablets every 12 hours for three doses each week (the protocol traditionally used in the treatment of psoriasis). At the end of 3 months patients entered a 4-week washout and then were crossed over to drug or placebo for an additional 3 months. The protocol standardized prednisone reduction to 1 to 2 mg/wk until symptoms flared or peak flows declined. At the conclusion of the study patients reduced prednisone use from 11.97 mg/day to 8.37 mg/day (p < .01). No patients were withdrawn because of toxicity.

The largest and longest double-blind placebo-controlled study of the efficacy of low-dose methotrexate in corticosteroid-dependent asthma has been reported by Shiner and associates [51]. Sixty-nine patients referred from 11 centers were seen and evaluated for 4 weeks to ensure steroid dependence. Patients required from 13 to 15 mg/day of prednisolone in addition to over 1,500 mg/day of inhaled budesonide. Stable subjects were enrolled into a double-blind placebo-controlled trial of 15 mg of methotrexate given as a single oral dose once a week. Criteria for steroid reduction were defined before study entry and allowed for 2.5 mg/mo reduction of prednisone if symptoms and spirometry were stable or improved. Drug and placebo were administered for 6 months and then withdrawn, and patients were observed for 10 weeks. Sixty-five patients completed the study. By 12 weeks both placebo and methotrexate patients had reduced prednisone by 16 percent. However, steroid reductions by placebo-treated patients were unstable, and over the remaining 12 weeks placebo-treated patients increased their use of corticosteroids. Methotrexate-treated patients continued to reduce prednisolone and at 24 weeks had reduced prednisone by 50 percent (p < .005). Six of the 38 patients treated with methotrexate discontinued steroids, and 2 additional patients were kept on low-dose steroid because of the discomfort of steroid withdrawal. None of the placebo-treated patients discontinued prednisolone. Ten weeks after discontinuing methotrexate, patients had a return of steroid requirements to enrollment levels.

In 1991 Erzurum et al. [20] reported no benefit from 13 weeks of methotrexate treatment in steroid-dependent asthma. Unlike the three previous studies, patients' steroid requirements were not stabilized before entry. In addition, steroid reduction criteria were not defined. During the 13 weeks of the study, patients taking placebo were able to reduce prednisone by 40 percent. At the end of the study, seven of the nine patients receiving placebo were still reducing prednisone. This rapid and spontaneous reduction of prednisone suggests that the patients in this report may not have been steroid dependent. Clearly they were drawn from a different population of patients than those enrolled in the three previously cited studies. These previous studies indicate that methotrexate treatment does not affect a steroid reduction of more than 30 percent in 13 weeks. Therefore an effect by methotrexate would not be seen in patients able to reduce prednisone by 40 percent in 13 weeks.

We have followed 25 patients with chronic asthma who have been treated with methotrexate for a mean of 22.8 months (range 18–28) and note that 96 percent of patients have reduced corticosteroids by over 50 percent [39]. The mean prednisone dose was reduced from 26.9 mg/day to 6.3 mg/day (p = .0001). Fifteen of the 25 discontinued regular prednisone use, nine patients reduced prednisone use by more than 50 percent, and one patient failed to respond. During treatment with low-dose methotrexate, the forced expiratory volume in 1 second (FEV_1) improved from 1.7 L/sec to 1.9 L/sec (p = .0513), and subjective symptom scores and frequency of nocturnal awakening because of asthma decreased (p < .05). Drug-related toxicity was minimal and consistent with prior experience with the use of low-dose drug. Resistance to methotrexate did not occur. Five patients have discontinued regular prednisone and methotrexate use [31]. This study answers previous concerns regarding the possibility of tachyphylaxis or unusual toxicities unique to asthma when methotrexate is used to treat severe asthma [17].

Clearly asthmatics who have developed corticosteroid side effects despite maximal attempts to reduce cortisone should benefit from a trial of methotrexate. As in the treatment of rheumatologic and dermatologic diseases, methotrexate's risk-benefit profile is preferable to that of long-term prednisone at a dose of 10 mg/day. Methotrexate is neither mutagenic nor oncogenic. It is less efficiently metabolized in patients over 50 years of age [21]. These observations, plus the devastating morbidity of steroid dependence in younger people and methotrexate's success as steroid sparing in juvenile rheumatoid arthritis [46, 61] has made its consideration in younger patients reasonable. Stempel and colleagues [52a] have reported significant steroid-sparing effects after methotrexate therapy in five corticosteroid-dependent children (ages 10 to 16 years), and Guss and Portnoy [25a] reported that four of seven severely steroid-dependent children (ages 3 to 14 years) experienced improvement in pulmonary functions while corticosteroids were reduced or discontinued after low-dose methotrexate treatment.

Appendix H reviews the guidelines we have followed when using low-dose methotrexate in the treatment of corticosteroid-dependent asthma. Careful attention to follow-up and monitoring of patients on this schedule is stressed. Because of the complexity involved in properly evaluating and treating severe asthma, the use of low-dose methotrexate should be restricted to specialists.

GOLD

History

Robert Koch's observation of the inhibition of *Mycobacterium tuberculosis* in vitro led to the successful trial of gold salts in the therapy of rheumatoid arthritis by Forestier in 1929. Dudan in 1932 and Montagna in 1936 reported on the use of gold salts to treat bronchial asthma, while Japanese investigators have reported success with chrysotherapy in asthma therapy since 1959. Unfortunately, these reports have been uncontrolled, and the definition of improvement in these studies has been subjective. Amelioration of asthma may be due to gold's antiinflammatory, immune suppressive, or cytotoxic properties [34].

Clinical Studies

Muranaka et al. [43] reported on 79 patients in a double-blind experience treated with 1.5 gm of gold for 30 weeks. Patients underwent global evaluations on the basis of combined diary and medication scores with clinical evaluation at 19 and 30 weeks. At 19 and 30 weeks about 70 percent of gold-treated patients improved as compared with 45 percent of placebo-treated patients. Unfortunately, symptom scores and medication use were grouped together in assessing response. Patients were not matched with regard to disease severity, duration, and atopic status. The effects of gold on steroid requirements in this study are unclear. Fourteen patients (47%) receiving gold therapy experienced toxicity, with 7 of these discontinuing therapy because of toxicity.

In a second study, published in 1981, Muranaka et al. [42] reported on the clinical course and bronchial reactivity of 24 adult asthmatics treated with injectable gold (aurothiomalate) for 5 to 7 years. Bronchial reactivity was assessed prior to treatment and again 5 to 7 years later with acetylcholine bronchial provocation tests. Two other groups of similar size were treated with conventional therapy alone or with conventional therapy and allergy injections. At the end of the observation period, the patients treated with gold had shown a dramatic decrease in bronchial reactivity, and 5 of 14 patients treated with gold had complete remission of disease, while no remissions were noted in the groups treated with immunotherapy or conventional therapy alone. Again, the patients in this small study were not matched for disease severity, duration, or atopic status.

Klaustermeyer et al. [30] reported in 1987 that 5 of 10 steroid-dependent patients reduced but did not discontinue prednisone after 22 weeks of gold treatment. Toxicity was 60 percent.

In 1988, Bernstein et al. treated 18 patients for 24 weeks in an open study with oral gold (auranofin) [9]. Fifty percent of the patients treated had reduced reactivity to methacholine, and prednisone use was decreased after 24 weeks from 17 mg/day to 11 mg/day. IgE-mediated histamine release was decreased in patients receiving oral gold. Drug-related toxicity was noted in 65 percent of patients. Another study indicates auranofin usefulness in moderately severe asthma [67] (Chap. 66).

Toxicity

Recent data suggest that gold is considerably more toxic than methotrexate [55, 64]. The major toxicities of gold are listed in Table 68-3.

Although parenteral gold salts have proved to be effective in blinded and prospectively controlled studies for the treatment of rheumatoid arthritis, no such body of data currently exists to justify gold's routine use in the treatment of asthma. Convincing long-term and well-controlled trials are required before its use can be considered in other than experimental circumstances. In addition, serious toxic sequelae of gold may limit its clinical use. Careful follow-up of any patient prescribed a gold regimen is mandatory.

ANTIMALARIALS

Tennenbaum and Smith [56] in 1966 first reported efficacy with the use of chloroquine phosphate in the treatment of four steroid-dependent asthmatics. Investigators in France have reported on the efficacy of the antimalarials for the treatment of bronchial asthma in open studies [59].

In 1990 Charous [15] reported on the efficacy of hydroxychloroquine in a pilot study treating 11 severe asthmatics, 7 of whom were corticosteroid dependent. In this study statistically significant reductions in corticosteroid use were demonstrated with concurrent improvement in pulmonary function and reduction in symptom scores. The drug was given in the same dosages employed to treat rheumatoid arthritis and systemic lupus erythematosus.

Table 68-4 outlines the toxicity of hydroxychloroquine. Although the antimalarials are the safest agents discussed in this chapter, their use in asthma should be confined to experimental protocols until confirmation by blinded studies is achieved. Safe

Table 68-3. Gold toxicity

Wide variety of rashes, including exfoliation
Hematologic—usually leukopenia; aplastic anemia ~60% fatal.
Gastrointestinal—hepatic and colitic
Renal—proteinuria 2–10%; nephrotic syndrome rare
Pulmonary fibrosis

Table 68-4. Hydroxychloroquine toxicity

Common
  Abdominal bloating, cramps, nausea
  Headache, irritability, nervousness
  Rash
Rare
  Ocular: decreased vision, double vision, blindness (corneal deposits, retinopathy, defects in accommodation/convergence); preventable by using low dose and regular eye examinations
  Others: decreased cell count, cardiomyopathy, neuropathy, diarrhea, vomiting, convulsions

Table 68-5. Dapsone toxicity

Common—hemolysis with methemoglobinemia in all patients; usually not clinically significant
Rare
  Nausea, vomiting, anorexia
  Peripheral neuropathy, headache, insomnia
  Rashes including exfoliative dermatitis

use of these drugs depends on daily dosage. With the exception of retinopathy, their side effects are reversible. Hydroxychloroquine should be given as 6.0 to 6.5 mg/kg/day based on lean body weight [35]. Patients should have ocular examinations at least twice a year until age 65 and then every 3 months.

DAPSONE

Berlow and colleagues [8] have made the intriguing observation in an open study that dapsone may have significant steroid-sparing properties in bronchial asthma. In their pilot study 10 corticosteroid-dependent asthmatics were treated with 100 mg of dapsone twice a day and followed for up to 13 months. Seven of 10 patients discontinued prednisone, and 2 of the remaining 3 patients reduced steroid requirements by over 50 percent. One patient did not respond. Toxicity in this small study was minimal, with methemoglobinemia and mild anemia occurring in patients and with only 1 patient withdrawn because of drug toxicity. Dapsone, which is used to treat leprosy and some autoimmune diseases, inhibits neutrophil function and chemotaxis. Table 68-5 outlines the toxicity of dapsone.

While the results of a single pilot study appear promising, the use of dapsone in asthma should be restricted to approved experimental protocols. Confirmation of the initial observations by placebo-controlled studies is needed before this agent can be recommended as alternative therapy for bronchial asthma.

CYCLOSPORINE

Cyclosporine is a neutral, lipophilic, cyclic undecapeptide extracted from the fungus *Tolypocladium inflatum*. While the precise mechanism of cyclosporine's immunosuppressive and anti-inflammatory actions is unclear, cyclosporine has been shown to bind to regulatory proteins important in the activation of T-cells and to other regulatory factors important in the generation of cytokines involved in the inflammatory response [13a]. Cyclosporine has been used in open trials in the treatment of corticosteroid-dependent asthma with success [23a, 55a]. A recent double-blind, placebo-controlled, crossover study conducted by Alexander and colleagues [1a] treated 33 corticosteroid-dependent asthmatics with low-dose cyclosporine (5 mg/kg/day) for 12 weeks. Steroid dosage was held constant, and change in pulmonary function during the study period served as the endpoint. Cyclosporine therapy resulted in a mean increase above placebo of 12 percent in morning peak expiratory flow rates and a 17.6 percent increase in forced expiratory flow in 1 second. Dosage of cyclosporine was adjusted by an independent observer on the basis of whole blood trough levels, presence of hypertension, and serum levels of creatinine and potassium. Most adverse events attributable to low-dose cyclosporine, including hypertension, decreased glomerular filtration rate, paresthesias, and multiple biochemical abnormalities, were all mild and reversible upon discontinuation of the drug. Hypertrichosis persisted in some patients for up to 4 months after study completion. This powerful study supports once again the role of inflammation in the pathophysiology of asthma and, in particular, points to the role of activated T-cells and cytokines as probable major factors in the perpetuation of severe disease.

Cyclosporine has been shown to be effective in the treatment of corticosteroid-dependent asthma. Given the toxicity of this drug and the close monitoring required to use this drug, its use should be limited to investigational settings.

COLCHICINE

Colchicine is an antiinflammatory drug useful in the management of acute gout, leukocytoclastic vasculitis, and primary biliary cirrhosis. Its mechanisms of action include inhibition of microtubular assembly, a reported increase in concanavalin A–induced suppressor cells, and effects on cyclic adenosine monophosphate. While it has been widely tried as a therapeutic agent in many chronic inflammatory diseases, its effects in asthma have been disappointing. A recent double-blind study of mild asthmatics demonstrated a modest improvement in symptom scores and frequency of inhaler use [49]. Colchicine had no effect on pulmonary function tests, bronchial provocation, or skin test reactivity. Based on present information there is no reason to recommend this agent for the treatment of bronchial asthma.

Several widely used antiinflammatory drugs with demonstrated steroid-sparing effects in rheumatology and dermatology are now being used or considered for use in the treatment of severe asthma. Given the long history and success of these drugs in treating chronic inflammation, this evaluation seems overdue. At present methotrexate is the only drug shown in double-blind studies to have a major effect, particularly upon corticosteroid use in asthma. Although the response to methotrexate appears high, some patients may take as long as a year to respond, and others may not respond at all. Clearly there is need for the development of additional "steroid-sparing" drugs. Future studies may consider the use of drugs in combination to reduce toxicity and to amplify efficacy, a strategy that has proved useful in both rheumatology and dermatology.

Clinicians must consider the pathology of bronchial asthma [6] and its natural history [24]. As drugs that are safer than corticosteroids become available, they will need to address the question of whether such medications should be reserved for severe disease or used earlier to prevent irreversible damage and disease progression.

REFERENCES

1. Alexander, H. L. Bronchial asthma. In G. M. Piersol and E. I. Bortz (eds.), *The Cyclopedia of Medicine.* Philadelphia: Davis, ii:112, 1933.
1a. Alexander, A. G., Barnes, N. C., and Kay, A. B. Trial of cyclosporin in corticosteroid-dependent asthma. *Lancet* 339:324, 1992.
2. Anderson, P. A., et al. Weekly pulse methotrexate in rheumatoid arthritis: Clinical and immunologic effects in a randomized, double-blind study. *Ann. Intern. Med.* 103:489, 1985.
3. Aponte, J. and Petrelli, M. Histopathologic findings in the liver of rheumatoid arthritis patients treated with long-term bolus methotrexate. *Arthritis Rheum* 31:1457, 1988.
4. Asmundsson, T., et al. Immunosuppressive therapy of asthma. *J. Allergy Clin. Immunol.* 47:136, 1971.
5. Bailin, P. L., et al. Is methotrexate therapy for psoriasis carcinogenic? *J.A.M.A.* 232:359, 1975.
6. Beasley, R., et al. Cellular events in the bronchi in mild asthma and after bronchial provocation. *Am. Rev. Respir. Dis.* 139:806, 1989.
7. Benedict, W. F., et al. Mutagenicity of cancer chemotherapeutic agents in the salmonella/microsome test. *Cancer Res.* 37:2209, 1977.
8. Berlow, B. A., et al. The effect of dapsone in steroid-dependent asthma. *J. Allergy Clin. Immunol.* 87:710, 1991.
9. Bernstein, D. I, et al. An open study of auranofin in the treatment of steroid-dependent asthma. *J. Allergy Clin. Immunol.* 81:6, 1988.

10. Black, R. L., et al. Methotrexate therapy in psoriatic arthritis: Double-blind study of 21 patients. *J.A.M.A.* 189:743, 1964.
11. Bleyer, W. A. The clinical pharmacology of methotrexate: New applications of an old drug. *Cancer* 41:36, 1978.
12. Bleyer, W. A. Clinical pharmacology and therapeutic drug monitoring of methotrexate. *Am. Assoc. Clin. Chem.* 6:1, 1985.
13. Bordley, J. E., et al. Preliminary observations on the effect of adrenocorticotropic hormone (ACTH) in allergic diseases. *Bull. Johns Hopkins Hosp.* 85:396, 1949.
13a. Calderon, E., et al. Is there a role for cyclosporine in asthma? *J. Allergy Clin. Immunol.* 89:629, 1992.
14. Chang, D. M., Baptiste, P., and Schur, P. H. The effect of antirheumatic drugs on interleukin 1 (IL-1) activity and IL-1 and IL-1 inhibitor production by human monocytes. *J. Rheumatol.* 17(9):1148, 1990.
15. Charous, L. B. Open study of hydroxychloroquine in the treatment of severe symptomatic or corticosteroid-dependent asthma. *Ann. Allergy* 65:53, 1990.
16. Cohen, E. P., et al. Clinical and pathological observations in fatal bronchial asthma: Report of a case treated with immunosuppressive drug azathioprine. *Ann. Intern. Med.* 62:103, 1965.
17. Cott, C. R., and Cherniack, R. M. Steroids and "steroid-sparing" agents in asthma. *N. Engl. J. Med.* 318:634, 1988.
18. Diaz, C. J. Treatment of dysreaction diseases with nitrogen mustards. *Ann. Rheum. Dis.* 10:144, 1951.
19. Dyer, P. D., Vaughan, T. R., and Weber, R. W. Methotrexate in the treatment of steroid-dependent asthma. *J. Allergy Clin. Immunol.* 88:208, 1991.
20. Erzurum, S. C., et al. Lack of benefit of methotrexate in severe, steroid-dependent asthma. *Ann. Intern. Med.* 114:353, 1991.
21. Fairris, G. M., et al. Methotrexate dosage in patients over 50 with psoriasis. *Br. Med. J.* 289:801, 1989.
22. Farber, S., et al. Action of pteroylglutamic conjugates on man. *Science* 106:619, 1947.
23. Farber, S., et al. Temporary remissions in acute leukemia in children produced by folic acid antagonist, 4-aminopteroyl-glutamic acid (aminopterin). *N. Engl. J. Med.* 238:787, 1948.
23a. Finnerty, N. A., and Sullivan, T. J. Effect of cyclosporine on corticosteroid-dependent asthma (abstract). *J. Allergy Clin. Immunol.* 87:297, 1991.
24. Finucane, K. E., Greville, H. W., and Brown, P. J. E. Irreversible airflow obstruction: Evolution in asthma. *Med. J. Aust.* 142:602, 1985.
25. Gubner, R., August, S., and Ginsberg, V. Therapeutic suppression of tissue reactivity: II. Effect of aminopterin in rheumatoid arthritis and psoriasis. *Am. J. Med. Sci.* 221:176, 1951.
25a. Guss, S., and Portnoy, J. Methotrexate treatment in severe asthma in children. *Pediatrics* 89:635, 1992.
26. Hoffmeister, R. T. Methotrexate therapy in rheumatoid arthritis (abstract). *Arthritis Rheum.* 15(Suppl.):S114, 1972.
27. Hoffmeister, R. T. Methotrexate therapy in rheumatoid arthritis: 15 years experience. *Am. J. Med.* 75(Suppl. 7A):69, 1983.
28. Jones, G., Mierins, E., and Karsh, J. Methotrexate-induced asthma. *Am. Rev. Respir. Dis.* 143:179, 1991.
29. Kaiser, B. K., Beall, G. N. Azathioprine (Imuran) in chronic asthma. *Ann. Allergy* 24:369, 1966.
30. Klaustermeyer, W. B., Noritake, D. T., and Kwong, F. K. Chrysotherapy in the treatment of corticosteroid-dependent asthma. *J. Allergy Clin. Immunol.* 79:720, 1987.
31. Lammert, J. K., and Mullarkey, M. F. Remission in corticosteroid-dependent bronchial asthma after treatment with methotrexate (MTX) (abstract). *J. Allergy Clin. Immunol.* 85(2):196, 1990.
32. Lammert, J. K., et al. Fatal varicella infection in severe bronchial asthma (submitted).
33. Lanse, S. B., et al. Low incidence of hepatotoxicity associated with long-term, low-dose oral methotrexate in treatment of refractory psoriasis, psoriatic arthritis, and rheumatoid arthritis. *Dig. Dis. Sci.* 30:104, 1985.
34. Lipsky, P. E. Mechanisms of action of slow-acting drugs in rheumatoid arthritis. *Clin. Exp. Rheumatol.* 7(Suppl. 3):S177, 1989.
35. Mackenzie, A. H. Antimalarial drugs for rheumatoid arthritis. *Am. J. Med.* 75(6A):48, 1983.
36. Mackinnon, S. K., Starkebaum, G., and Willkens, R. F. Pancytopenia associated with low dose pulse methotrexate in the treatment of rheumatoid arthritis. *Semin. Arthritis Rheum.* 15:119, 1985.
37. Matheson, D., Brusick, D., and Carrano. Comparison of the relative mutagenic activity for eight antineoplastic drugs in the Ames Salmonella/microsome and TK+/− mouse lymphoma assays. *Drug Chem. Toxicol.* 1:277, 1978.
38. Morgan, S. L., et al. The effect of folic acid supplementation on the toxic-

ity of low-dose methotrexate in patients with rheumatoid arthritis. *Arthritis Rheum.* 33:9, 1990.

39. Mullarkey, M. F., Lammert, J. K., and Blumenstein, B. A. Long-term methotrexate treatment of corticosteroid-dependent asthma. *Ann. Intern. Med.* 112:577, 1990.

40. Mullarkey, M. F., Webb, D. R., and Pardee, N. E. Methotrexate in the treatment of steroid-dependent asthma. *Ann. Allergy* 56:347, 1986.

41. Mullarkey, M. F., et al. Methotrexate in the treatment of corticosteroid-dependent asthma: A double-blind crossover study. *N. Engl. J. Med.* 318:603, 1988.

42. Muranaka, M., Nakajima, K., and Suzuki, S. Bronchial responsiveness to acetylcholine in patients with bronchial asthma after long-term treatment with gold salt. *J. Allergy Clin. Immunol.* 67:350, 1981.

43. Muranaka, M., et al. Gold salt in the treatment of bronchial asthma—a double-blind study. *Ann. Allergy* 40:132, 1978.

44. Rau, R., et al. Liver biopsy findings in patients with rheumatoid arthritis undergoing long-term treatment with methotrexate. *J. Rheumatol.* 16:489, 1989.

45. Reynolds, F. S., and Lee, W. M. Hepatotoxicity after long-term methotrexate therapy. *South. Med. J.* 79:536, 1986.

46. Rose, C. D., et al. Safety and efficacy of methotrexate therapy for juvenile rheumatoid arthritis. *J. Pediatr.* 117:653, 1990.

47. Ross, G. T. Congenital anomalies among children born of mothers receiving chemotherapy for gestational trophoblastic neoplasms. *Cancer* 37:1043, 1976.

48. Rustin, G. J. S., et al. Pregnancy after cytotoxic chemotherapy for gestational trophoblastic tumours. *Br. Med. J.* 288:103, 1984.

49. Schwarz, Y. A., et al. A clinical and immunologic study of colchicine in asthma. *J. Allergy Clin. Immunol.* 85:578, 1990.

50. Searles, G., and Mckendry, R. J. R. Methotrexate pneumonitis in rheumatoid arthritis: Potential risk factors. Four case reports and a review of the literature. *J. Rheumatol.* 14:1164, 1987.

51. Shiner, R. J., et al. Randomised, double-blind, placebo-controlled trial of methotrexate in steroid-dependent asthma. *Lancet* 336:137, 1990.

52. Shupack, J. L., and Webster, G. F. Pancytopenia following low-dose oral methotrexate therapy for psoriasis. *J.A.M.A.* 259:3594, 1988.

52a. Stempel, D. A., Lammert, J., and Mullarkey, M. F. Use of methotrexate in the treatment of steroid-dependent adolescent asthmatics. *Ann. Allergy* 67:346, 1991.

53. Stern, R. S., Zierler, S., and Parrish, J. A. Methotrexate used for psoriasis and the risk of noncutaneous or cutaneous malignancy. *Cancer* 50:869, 1982.

54. Suarez, C. R., et al. Effect of low dose methotrexate on neutrophil chemotaxis induced by leukotriene B$_4$ and complement C5a. *J. Rheumatol.* 14:9, 1987.

55. Suarez-Almazor, M. E., et al. A randomized controlled trial of parenteral methotrexate compared to sodium aurothiomalate (Myochrysine) in the treatment of rheumatoid arthritis. *J. Rheumatol.* 15:753, 1988.

55a. Szczeklik, A., et al. Cyclosporine for steroid-dependent asthma. *Allergy* 46:312, 1991.

56. Tennenbaum, J. I., and Smith, R. E. Antimalarial therapy for resistant asthma. *Ann. Allergy* 24:37, 1966.

57. Ternowitz, T., et al. Methotrexate inhibits the human C5a-induced response in patients with psoriasis. *J. Invest. Dermatol.* 89:192, 1987.

58. Van de Kerkhof, P. C. M., Bauer, F. W., and Maassen-de Grood, R. M. Methotrexate inhibits the leukotriene B$_4$ induced intraepidermal accumulation of polymorphonuclear leukocytes. *Br. J. Derm.* 113:251a, 1985.

59. Voog, R., et al. Asthma therapy with a combination of synthetic antimalarials (83 cases). *Presse Med.* 77:1995, 1969.

60. Waldbott, G. L. Nitrogen mustard in the treatment of bronchial asthma. *Ann. Allergy* 10:428, 1952.

61. Wallace, C. A., et al. Toxicity and serum level of methotrexate in children with juvenile rheumatoid arthritis. *Arthritis Rheum.* 32:677, 1989.

62. Weinblatt, M. E., et al. Efficacy of low-dose methotrexate in rheumatoid arthritis. *N. Engl. J. Med.* 312:818, 1985.

63. Weinblatt, M. E. Toxicity of low-dose methotrexate in rheumatoid arthritis. *J. Rheumatol.* 12(Suppl.):35, 1986.

64. Weinblatt, M. E., Kaplan, H., and Germain, B. F. Low-dose methotrexate compared with auranofin in adult rheumatoid arthritis: A thirty-six-week, double-blind trial. *Arthritis Rheum.* 33:330, 1990.

65. Weinstein, A., et al. Low-dose methotrexate treatment of rheumatoid arthritis: Long-term observations. *Am. J. Med.* 79:331, 1985.

66. Weinstein, G. D. Methotrexate: Drugs five years later. *Ann. Intern. Med.* 86:199, 1977.

67. Nierop, G., et al. Auranofin in the treatment of steroid-dependent asthma: A double-blind study. *Thorax* 47:349, 1992.

Hydration, Humidification, and Mucokinetic Therapy

69

Irwin Ziment

The respiratory tree is lined by a moist membrane that is bathed in mucus whose water content is normally well in excess of 95 percent. Thus water is of considerable importance to the functioning of the respiratory epithelium and the mucociliary escalator, and it is self-evident that fluid balance and airway humidity must have an enormously important role in the treatment of airway disease. The relevance of water as a therapeutic agent in asthma and other obstructive airway disease has been recognized since antiquity. The very earliest treatments offered to patients suffering from coughs and abnormal secretions must have included water in various guises. The water content of the herbal drinks and decoctions that were used was probably of greater therapeutic benefit than the chemical constituents of most of these empiric formulations. Inhalation therapy also had its beginnings in the distant mists of our primitive origins, and steam or scented vapors must have been used along with the burning of incense and other herbal fumes in the inspirational treatment of pulmonary diseases [119].

Most of the current expectorant medications are in fact derived from very old remedies that have enjoyed hallowed reputations in the folk medicine traditions of all major societies. Similarly, many of the still popular spas and thermal bath resorts around the world provide inhalational aromatic vapor therapies, as well as oral and immersional exposure to their products, that have been recommended for hundreds or thousands of years in the treatment of respiratory diseases. A universally respected tradition supports the use of such flavorful hydration remedies as hot teas or tisanes, honey and alcohol, and chicken soup. It is the objective of this chapter to place in perspective these traditional respiratory remedies and their newer derivatives. It is important to realize that many of the newer modalities—such as heated small-particle aerosols—have already accumulated a traditional acceptance equivalent to that of folk remedies in that they are largely devoid of scientifically derived justification.

HYDRATION

There is fairly uniform agreement by authors of current guides to the management of asthma that adequate hydration is of paramount therapeutic importance, although directives are generally presented in very vague terms without any valid evidence offered in support [36, 117]. As a result, it is common for physicians to advise their patients to drink "extra fluids" as part of the daily management of asthma, bronchitis, and other chronic obstructive diseases associated with abnormal respiratory secretions [38, 104]. The need for hydration is emphasized more imperatively for the treatment of status asthmaticus, although cautious authors offer the admonition to avoid the danger of overhydration and the attendant hazard of pulmonary edema [100]. How accurately can the practitioner use water or saline by the oral or intravenous route in the hydration therapy of various degrees of asthma, and is such treatment justified by the published experience?

Unfortunately, assessment of water deficit in any patient is not an accurate science, and both clinical and laboratory findings have to be correlated by the experienced physician who then makes a guess as to the volume by which the patient is depleted [26]. Many sick patients are not only water depleted but also have a deficiency of sodium chloride, and replenishment therapy requires a judicious use of isotonic glucose water and salt solution. If possible, all rehydration should be carried out orally, using water or other beverages or chicken soup, which also offers salt [94], but in patients who are nauseated or vomiting or otherwise unable to drink adequately, intravenous therapy is required. Careful evaluation and management is needed in the acutely ill, dehydrated patient irrespective of any accompanying asthma. The question as to whether the asthmatic patient requires any additional hydration to help loosen respiratory secretions needs to be considered for both the patient with chronic stable asthma and the sick patient with an acute exacerbation of asthma.

Chronic Asthma

There is little evidence to support the need for additional daily fluid intake in patients with chronic stable asthma, although perhaps the majority of clinicians recommend that an increased intake be adhered to [38]. The proffered advice may stipulate that patients drink eight or so glasses of water each day, or more specific instructions may be offered such as to take a cup of hot tea in the morning and follow this with other specific infusions at designated times throughout the day. The use of extra fluid intake is likely to be harmless and may even be beneficial in most patients, although it is not established that a less than normal imbibition of fluid will result in the development of more viscous secretions. However, in a recent study of 12 patients with chronic bronchitis by Shim et al. [95], it was clearly shown that neither a moderate increase in hydration nor a moderate degree of dehydration had any effect on the volume or elasticity of sputum produced or on the respiratory symptoms or spirometry.

Although the state of systemic hydration must be important in chronic asthma, all advice in this regard is based on fallible clinical impressions. One may therefore presume that a "normal" water intake suffices in most asthmatics, and increased intake is justified only if there appears to be increased loss owing to fever, sweating, vomiting, or diarrhea. Perhaps other clinical indices can be used for determining whether the fluid intake is adequate in an asthmatic patient. Thirst is undoubtedly the best and most reliable guide, but in elderly or confused patients the thirst mechanism may be impaired. Objective evidence of the overall adequacy of fluid intake must then be sought. Whether an acute exacerbation of chronic asthma should be regarded as an indication for a further increase in oral fluid intake has not been demonstrated. Perhaps the additional fluid that is usually taken to "wash down" various orally administered bronchodilator or expectorant medications is both appropriate and adequate.

Acute Asthma

Most patients who seek medical help during an exacerbation of asthma are likely to be regarded as being dehydrated to some degree. Hyperventilation or other abnormal respiratory patterns, particularly if associated with breathing through the mouth, may result in a loss of fluid from the airways in excess of the normal daily amount of 200 to 500 ml, but it is difficult to assess the potentially large loss in any individual asthmatic patient. However, Goldberger suggests that a patient with a temperature of 104°F breathing at a rate of 30 to 40 breaths/min may lose as much as 2,500 ml/day from the lungs [41]; even greater amounts could be lost if the patient were to expectorate copiously. The very dyspneic patient may be unable to maintain normal food and fluid intake, and each day of markedly reduced intake may result in a deficit of 1.0 to 1.5 liters. Finally, the overall metabolic cost of severe dyspnea and the associated sweating caused by anxiety or overheating can lead to increased insensible loss of fluid through the skin; this loss may be substantially greater than the normal 300 to 600 ml/day, perhaps amounting to as much as 1.5 liters. As a result of these losses, the patient who has been ill for several days may have a deficit of 2 to 4 liters in moderate asthma. A negative balance exceeding 4 liters could accrue over several days during a severe attack (Table 69-1). Additional losses, such as those resulting from the vomiting that can occur in severe asthma, may need to be taken into account [26, 41, 92].

The total free water deficit can be estimated from a good history, but histories are all too often unreliable. If the patient's stable weight is accurately known, the fluid deficit can be estimated from the loss of weight; however, this information is usually not available. In practice, physicians use a mixture of enlightened guesswork and objective criteria to arrive at a very approximate estimate of the degree of dehydration. Although it is conventional to speak of dehydration, the patient with acute asthma is more correctly diagnosed as being desiccated, since the deficit is mostly free water [97, 98, 106]. *Desiccation* is associated with a loss of interstitial fluid, and this causes considerable thirst. If electrolyte loss has occurred as a result of sweating or vomiting or because of a prolonged reduction in salt intake, the

Table 69-2. Stages of desiccation caused by primary water deficit

Feature	Slight	Moderate	Severe
Percent loss of total body fluid	About 5%	About 10%	About 15%
Actual fluid deficit	1–2 L	2–4 L	>4 L
Typical symptoms			
Thirst	Mild	Severe	Intense
Mental state	Anxious	Confused	Obtunded
Weakness	Slight	Moderate	Profound
Typical findings			
Dry mucous membranes	Slight	Marked	Profound
Skin turgor	Normal	Impaired	Very abnormal
Pulse	Normal	Increased	Rapid
Blood pressure	Normal	Orthostatic hypotension	Hypotension, shock
Laboratory findings			
Urine	Concentrated	Oliguric	Oliguric
Hematocrit	Normal	Normal	Slightly increased
Serum sodium	Normal	Slightly increased	Hypernatremia
Serum osmolality	Slightly increased	Moderately increased	Markedly increased

resulting depletion results in the syndrome of hypovolemia, which is often described as being a sine qua non of true dehydration. Other terms (such as *hypertonic contraction*) are also employed, although in practice the term *dehydration* tends to be used indiscriminately to cover all forms of water and salt depletion. The dehydrated patient who has also lost sodium will manifest depletion of the intravascular volume and will therefore be more likely to demonstrate features of *hypovolemia* (i.e., cardiovascular disturbances including tachycardia, hypotension, and changes in sensorium), but there will be less complaint of thirst, although the tongue may be extremely dry and furrowed. The features of true desiccation are categorized in Table 69-2.

Slight dehydration is suggested by a history of one or two days of moderately severe dyspnea accompanied by reduced oral intake, with the principal limitation being in food intake. Thirst resulting from dehydration is a potent stimulus, and most patients will have drunk some fluid during the course of the attack. These patients usually complain of only moderate thirst, but the oral mucosa will be relatively dry. In such cases, there may be a deficit of 1 to 2 liters, and few physical findings or laboratory abnormalities are likely to be attributable to this small deficit. If the patient requires aminophylline therapy, this will ensure that adequate intravenous fluid is provided, since the drug is generally given in 5% dextrose with water at a rate of about 50 to 100 ml/hr. In general the patient will be able to drink adequately after initial therapy has alleviated the dyspnea, and self-correction of any persisting dehydration will then occur.

Moderate dehydration can result from more severe or more prolonged dyspnea and is particularly likely to develop if there is accompanying vomiting or copious sweating. Patients at greatest risk include the weak or confused and those who have not been able to get help and have therefore failed to maintain their food or fluid intake for 2 or more days. The patient will manifest evidence of extracellular and intracellular fluid deficit, with intense thirst, dry oral and pharyngeal mucosa, cessation of all sweating, and a possible reduction in skin turgor. The latter finding may be completely unreliable in elderly patients, while the dry tongue may be deceiving in any asthmatic patient who has been breath-

Table 69-1. Typical 24-hour water balance during an asthma attack[a]

Water	Normal loss (ml/day)	Possible losses during an attack		
		Mild to moderate asthma (ml/day)	Severe asthma (ml/day)	Severe complicated asthma[b] (ml/day)
Output (O)				
Urine	1,500	1,000	700	400 or less
Lungs	400	700	1,200	2,500
Skin	500	700	1,000	1,500
Stool	100	100	100	100
Total	2,500	2,500	3,000	4,500
Intake (I)[c]	2,500	1,500	1,000	500
Net deficit (O − I)	0	1,000	2,000	4,000

[a] The figures in this table may apply to a typical adult. Considerable additional losses may occur if the asthma is complicated by high fever, marked sweating, and hyperventilation.
[b] Additional losses may occur from vomiting.
[c] Intake is assumed to decrease progressively as attack worsens.

ing through the mouth. The blood pressure may be within the normal range, but an orthostatic response should be demonstrable with a fall in the blood pressure when the patient moves from the recumbent to the erect position. The urine will be decreased to less than 1 L/24 hr, and the specific gravity will usually exceed 1.020. This physiologic conservation of fluid is mediated by antidiuretic hormone. As a consequence of this response, the total fluid deficit is not as great as the patient's dry tongue and respiratory distress may suggest. The serum sodium will be slightly raised, but the hematocrit may not be greatly increased. A further indication of the degree of dehydration could be obtained by measuring the serum osmolality, although this is generally not necessary; however, a value in excess of 290 mOsm/kg would be expected.

The patient with moderate dehydration may not be able to drink sufficient fluid even after initial therapy for the bronchospasm, and intravenous replenishment will usually be deemed appropriate. Half the deficit can readily be replaced in the first 12 hours, with full replenishment being achieved over the next 18 to 24 hours. If the patient has been sweating a great deal, some sodium replacement may be required, and 5% dextrose with 0.5 N saline is advisable (Table 69-3). In general, intravenous fluid replenishment need be given at a rate no greater than 150 ml/hr unless the patient is hypotensive. In small patients and those with cardiac or renal insufficiency, a slower infusion rate (e.g., 100 ml/hr) is advisable, and careful monitoring is required. The urine output should increase, and failure of this to occur is an indication for greater caution in replenishing the intravascular volume.

When restoring fluid volume with intravenous water, care should be taken to avoid causing electrolyte imbalance, and a check of the serum electrolytes should be obtained within 6 to 18 hours. In young children, elderly patients, and those with cardiac, renal, or hepatic insufficiency, there is always a danger of overestimating the fluid deficit with a resulting tendency to overload the patient with intravenous replenishment. Such patients should

be carefully monitored to ensure that the urine output increases appropriately and that signs of congestive heart failure are not precipitated. Restoration of the full fluid deficit should be attained gradually, and this is best achieved by encouraging the patient to drink as dictated by thirst.

Severe dehydration implies a deficit exceeding 10 percent of total body water, and the patient may have signs of a life-threatening illness. Such a condition can develop in a patient who hyperventilates and breathes through the mouth, particularly if there is also increased sweating. However, the daily fluid loss is minimized by the renal retention of water, which causes a pronounced decrease in urine output, so that the eventual daily fluid loss may be only 500 ml greater than normal. If fluid intake is maintained, the patient who has a severe asthma attack lasting 2 to 4 days may develop a total fluid deficit of more than 1 liter, but if fluid intake is markedly decreased the total deficit can approach or exceed 2 L/day. If the asthma is further complicated by high fever or vomiting, the total fluid deficit may exceed 4 to 5 liters in a day, and salt loss will be great. In such cases, severe oliguria, or even anuria, and hypovolemia will be manifested (see Table 69-1).

Thirst is likely to be extreme, although concomitant apathy, confusion, or even obtundation resulting from the dehydration may rob the patient of awareness of this valuable sign. However, the dry, wrinkled or cracked tongue and oral mucosa, and the inelastic skin should point to the severity of the problem. Tachycardia and hypotension with a demonstrable postural fall will be found, and the patient may be unable to tolerate standing. The neck veins, however, are less likely to be reliable in the asthmatic patient who may generate marked negative intrapleural pressure [100], resulting in a spuriously low jugular venous pressure. The hematocrit, serum sodium, and osmolality will be increased while the urine will be reduced in amount and will be highly concentrated. A further complication possible in severely ill asthmatic patients is an inappropriate secretion of antidiuretic hormone leading to hyponatremia, thus making it more difficult to calculate and restore normal fluid balance [6]. Such a situation constitutes a critical emergency. Rapid fluid replenishment will be needed, and pressor support, electrolyte and blood gas control, and other resuscitative measures are likely to be required. Frequent monitoring of vital signs and clinical laboratory data are essential for appropriate management (Table 69-3).

The above discussion relates to the overall problem of dehydration in any patient, irrespective of complicating asthma. It is doubtful whether any additional fluid balance measures are required simply because the patient with asthma is liable to have inspissated secretions. Very few studies have been carried out to demonstrate that dehydration does alter sputum viscosity or mucociliary clearance, and there is no real proof that increased fluid intake has a beneficial effect on respiratory tract secretions [21, 95]. In fact, as Boyd [12] points out in the preface of his book, dehydration such as occurs in persons stranded in a desert does not decrease the output of respiratory tract fluid even after the nose and mouth have become desiccated! Thus, although the need for hydration in the treatment of acute asthma is almost always stressed, it would seem that the asthmatic patient does not require any oral or intravenous replenishment beyond that dictated by the degree of dehydration. Further, it is evident that many milder cases could be treated adequately with oral fluids, but the psychological benefits of intravenous therapy (to both physician and patient) have led to the common practice of using intravenous replenishment even when logic would suggest one need not resort to this route. It is not uncommon to see the hospitalized asthmatic patient receiving the "benefit" of intravenous aminophylline and steroids though he or she is breathing, eating, and drinking without difficulty. Obviously, the intravenous therapy is part of the mystique of management and in no way relates to any special pharmacologic or physiologic de-

Table 69-3. Fluid replenishment[a]

	Degree of Dehydration		
	Mild[b]	*Moderate*[b]	*Severe*
First few hours			
IV fluid	D_5 ½ NS	D_5 ½ NS	D_5 NS
Rate of flow	100–200 ml/hr	100–200 ml/hr	≥200 ml/hr
Next 24 hours			
IV fluid	D_5W or ½ NS	D_5W or ½ NS	D_5 ½ NS
Rate of flow	100–125 ml/hr	125–150 ml/hr	150 ml/hr
Oral fluid intake	Normal intake, e.g., 2–3 L/24 hr	As much as patient desires	As much as patient can tolerate
Monitor			
Serum sodium	Every 24 hr	Every 12–24 hr	Every 12 hr
Urine sodium	Not necessary	Usually not necessary	Every 24 hr for 2 days
Urine volume	Routine monitoring	Routine monitoring	Monitor for oliguria
Pulmonary vascular state	Auscultate	Auscultate	CVP or pulmonary artery catheter

D_5 = 5% dextrose; NS = normal saline; D_5W = 5% dextrose with water; CVP = central venous pressure.

[a] Full replenishment may take 2 to 3 days. Give IV fluids more slowly and with more frequent monitoring in small patients, in the elderly, and in patients with cardiac or renal insufficiency.

[b] In mild to moderate dehydration, intravenous fluid may be required more for administration of aminophylline or a corticosteroid than for reestablishment of fluid balance.

mands imposed by the pulmonary condition. There is undoubtedly a tendency to overdiagnose dehydration in the acutely ill asthmatic patient, since the familiar signs of fluid depletion can be mimicked by the effects of the asthma itself. The dry tongue, flat neck veins, and tachycardia do not necessarily imply intravascular or tissue fluid loss, since these signs may occur in status asthmaticus in a patient who is in perfect fluid balance. The automatic assumption that an asthmatic attack causes dehydration exposes the patient to the risk of iatrogenic pulmonary edema through misguided efforts to restore hydration.

One further comment about hydration can be made. It is a common experience that viscous sputum, such as that expectorated by asthmatic patients, floats or sinks when added to water, and very little absorption of water into the sputum appears to occur. There is evidence that water does not have any gross effect on mucus once it is secreted as sputum, although the state of hydration does have an influence on the secretory mechanism [50]. Thus, oral or intravenous hydration may not have much effect on the structure of sputum already in the airways, but it may result in an increase in the free water separating the mucous sheet from the mucosa, thereby facilitating the mobilization of agglomerations of viscous secretions. Further, water may enter the serous and mucus-secreting cells and thus reduce the viscosity of the mucus that is subsequently secreted. Some authorities believe that in very severe asthma, the dehydrated mucus impacted in the airways can best be dislodged by lavaging it out with large amounts of water or saline selectively instilled into occluded airways through a bronchoscope. Although this form of therapy for status asthmaticus or severe chronic asthma receives occasional glowing reports [69, 96], it is generally felt that any benefits of the procedure are greatly outweighed by the hazards and inconvenience. Thus, lavage will only gain acceptance if further studies demonstrate defensible criteria for its use. (See Chap. 84).

It is common to overestimate the degree of dehydration in asthma and reflexively to order rehydration therapy in any asthmatic patient admitted to the hospital. There is good reason to believe that dehydration may adversely affect the mobility of respiratory secretions, but there is little reason to believe that correction of fluid balance will result in immediate mobilization of the abnormal mucus, and there is no basis for assuming that the asthmatic patient benefits from rehydration more than any other category of patient who has a fluid deficit. In general, adequate fluid is provided by the common routine of giving intravenous aminophylline or corticosteroids in solution at a rate of 100 to 150 ml/hr, and no further efforts to rehydrate most asthmatics are required. The patient with milder asthma will automatically be ensured adequate hydration if allowed to drink freely, while the severely ill patient with hypovolemia requires intravenous hydration for cardiodynamic correction rather than for respiratory purposes. There is clearly a danger in overreacting to the apparent dehydration of the distressed asthmatic, and children and elderly patients are at great risk of being "pushed" into pulmonary edema. It is thus appropriate to suggest that the concept of dehydration should be totally separated from the syndrome of acute asthma, since there is no need for additional fluid replenishment in asthmatic patients beyond that required by any patient with an acute illness that impairs fluid balance.

HUMIDIFICATION

The term *humidity* is often used imprecisely, although it is a quantitative measure of the amount of water vapor in a gas. In clinical practice two major qualifying terms are used. Absolute humidity is the maximal amount of water vapor that a given volume of gas can hold at a given temperature; relative humidity is the ratio of the actual amount to the maximal amount. Room air at a temperature of 21°C has an absolute humidity of 18 mg/L of water; for comfort, a relative humidity approaching 50 percent (9 mg/L) is desirable. When room air is inhaled, it is warmed and fully saturated by the time it reaches the alveoli, where the absolute humidity of 44 mg/L is maintained in a subject at 37°C. Thus, about 35 mg/L of water has to be added to the normal room air as it traverses the respiratory tract. At least half of this is redeposited in the middle and upper respiratory tract during exhalation, but the resulting exhaled air will contain more water vapor than the usual ambient air, thus causing a net daily loss of 200 to 500 ml of water a day.

The nose and pharynx serve as very effective water exchangers, and much of the humidity deficit in inspired air is eliminated by the time the inhaled volume reaches the trachea [27]. The nose can add about 75 percent of the water required to saturate the alveolar air, whereas the mouth can add only about 25 percent of the needed humidity. When the nose is bypassed, as in mouth breathing, the effectiveness of water exchange is decreased since the oral mucosa readily dries out. When both the nose and oropharynx are bypassed in the intubated patient, the inspired air can have a harmful desiccating effect on the tracheobronchial mucosa. Thus, one of the clearest indications for providing added humidity to inspired air is created by endotracheal intubation or tracheostomy. Another indication is the administration of rapid flows of oxygen, since dry gas could quickly desiccate the nose, oropharynx, or tracheobronchial tree. Certain upper or middle respiratory tract conditions including pharyngitis, laryngitis, croup, and tracheitis seem to be helped by humidifying the inspired air. It is far less certain that added water vapor is of value for the treatment of distal airway or alveolar diseases, and the role of humidification in the management of asthma is quite controversial. There is evidence that ciliary activity decreases with lowering of humidity, but the value of humidification has not been clarified in clinical states of mucostasis [4, 53].

Humidity and Asthma

Everyday experience of both patients and their physicians indicates that prevailing weather conditions can affect asthma. Changes in climate are frequently blamed for exacerbations, but there is no universal agreement as to which major characteristics are most blameworthy. Many patients point to smog or fog, while others find fault with rain, wind, or snow. Hot weather is intolerable to some asthmatic patients, whereas cold is more clearly demonstrated asthmogenic stimulus: During the past few years cold air has been shown to act as a potent provocation in patients susceptible to bronchospasm [17, 101] (see Chap. 45).

Humidity remains an enigma, with individual experiences diverging in all directions. Many patients seem to prefer a climate of low humidity, such as that of the desert, and perhaps most asthmatics find that very hot, humid atmospheres are intolerable. Opinions about sea air vary, with some asthmatic patients seeking the seaside for relief and others claiming that the nocturnal mist and dampness get into their chest, exacerbate their asthma, and convert it to bronchitis.

Physicians are often asked by asthmatic patients whether it would be advisable to move to another climate. There is little authoritative information available to use as a basis for making such recommendations, and common sense supplemented by personal experience has to be relied on. Presumably, the best advice is to choose a climate that is neither too hot nor too cold, with limited wind and precipitation, and with a relative humidity of around 30 to 50 percent. However, exacerbations of asthma develop not only outdoors, but also within the relatively controlled living conditions of the patient's home, and often enough during sleep. In fact, the home climate is probably more relevant than the external climate, and of greatest relevance may be the humidity in the patient's bedroom.

Chen and Chai [17] studied eight patients who had nocturnal bronchospasm when breathing air of 17 to 24 percent relative humidity. These subjects experienced less bronchoconstriction when sleeping in a tent containing air warmed to 36° to 37°C with a relative humidity of 100 percent. The authors consider that the benefits are attributable more to the heat than the humidity; the exact benefit of humidification remained undefined, but they suggested that susceptible asthmatic patients should avoid breathing cold air of low humidity. Most asthmatic patients would probably find it unacceptable if not intolerable to sleep in a heated mist tent, but the possible merit of using a simpler humidification device at the bedside deserves further evaluation.

Work by Strauss and coworkers [101] has suggested that breathing cool air of low relative humidity, particularly with exercise or voluntary hyperventilation, provokes bronchospasm. It is postulated that the dry inspired air causes cooling of the respiratory tract as a result of the loss of the latent heat of vaporization that occurs when water from the mucosa evaporates into the dry inspired air. It is thought that cooling of the submucosa causes stimulation of mast cells, which liberate the mediators of bronchospasm. It is of interest that several asthmatic children in Israel were found to have more bronchospasm when exercising in a dry climate than in a humid one and that breathing humidified air could abolish the exercise-induced asthma [7, 40]. The apparent benefit of humidity may explain why asthmatics, who have bronchospasm with exercises such as tennis or running, are often able to swim vigorously without symptoms. However, the topic is further complicated by a report of a boy whose exercise-induced asthma occurred consistently when breathing warm, humidified air [10]. The authors suggest that the protective effect of warm humid air may have been exaggerated in prior reports.

Lilker [58] proposed that asthmatic patients have a basic abnormality of the respiratory mucosa, which makes it more permeable to water molecules. He found that inhalation of distilled water provoked bronchospasm in asthmatic subjects, but not in bronchitic or normal subjects; in contrast, normal saline aerosol did not have an asthmogenic effect. The theory is offered that the asthmatic patient's mucous membrane has an increased osmotic pressure, which draws in solutions of low osmolality (such as water), but not those of higher osmolality (such as normal saline); the transmucosal absorption of water somehow provokes bronchospasm. In support of this concept, Lilker reports that his survey of 93 patients led to the conclusion that by far the most common factor provoking asthma was an increase in humidity or rainy weather. Although his interpretation does not stand up to critical examination, his observation, which is supported by those of others [43], adds further confusion to the role of humidity in asthma. More recently, studies by Aitken et al. [1] have shown that patients with asthma who hyperventilate while breathing heated air at 50°C and 100 percent relative humidity develop bronchospasm, possibly as a result of hypoosmolality. It appears that humidity in excess of water content of 44 mg/L of water is detrimental, and Aitken et al. speculate that a lower level in the inspired air may be optimal for asthmatic subjects.

Humidity and Mucus

Humidity therapy is often provided for patients with respiratory disease to help loosen hyperviscous secretions. This approach is based on precedent, and physicians are led by their patients to believe that this therapy is beneficial. However, there is very little evidence to suggest that humidity therapy has any effect on mucociliary clearance in the human. The subject was reviewed several years ago [39, 107], and it was pointed out that more definitive studies were required to supplement the inconclusive evidence available at that time. In the intervening years, no proof has emerged to support the clinical impression that humidifica-

tion is of therapeutic value in loosening tracheobronchial mucus or in treating asthma [118].

The most relevant observations on the effects of humidity on mucus were reported by Dulfano and coworkers [31, 32], who found that exposure of sputum obtained from subjects with bronchitis to high humidity resulted in an increase in the weight of the material without causing any change in viscosity. In contrast, an aerosol of water caused a greater increase in weight and a decrease in viscosity. In vitro studies by Richards and Marriott [88] led to the opposite conclusion: They found that sputum viscosity does increase as humidity is lowered. At present, there is no good evidence to suggest that humidity therapy is of clinical value in the hospital management of acute asthma in the adequately hydrated patient. Further investigations may clarify the potential benefit of humidity as part of the therapy for asthma that is provoked by such factors as exercise, cold, or sleep (Table 69-4).

Humidification Devices

The simplest humidification devices are showers and kettles or pans of boiling water, and many patients with acute obstructive airway disease believe that exposure to an atmosphere of domestic steam, mist, or vapor leads to symptomatic benefit. Home therapy can be provided by a variety of inexpensive devices including steamers, facial saunas, humidifiers, vaporizers, and misters. The only differences among various products are the relative humidity that they can produce and the temperature of the vapor. Obviously, increasing the temperature results in higher humidity, and if an aerosol is also produced this will ensure 100 percent humidity. Personal preferences rather than scientific criteria determine which device and method of use will be of greatest benefit to the individual patient.

In the hospital setting, more costly and complex devices are used, and a profusion of humidification equipment has been promoted by the very competitive industry that has arisen in the past decade (Table 69-5). The scientific physician will find it virtually impossible to select any particular device, since in spite of the manufacturers' boastful claims there is all too little evidence to suggest that there is any optimal device for the treat-

Table 69-4. Indications for therapeutic humidification

1. To make inspired air comfortable
2. For symptomatic treatment of nasal, sinus, pharyngeal, and laryngotracheal problems
3. To prevent desiccation of mucosa by high-flow gas administration
4. When upper respiratory tract is bypassed, e.g., because of endotracheal tube or tracheotomy
5. Warm humidified air may decrease some forms of bronchospasm, e.g., exercise- or cold-induced, nocturnal
6. Warm humidified air may help improve mucociliary clearance and decrease sputum viscosity in certain patients (however, this has not been substantiated)

Table 69-5. Humidification devices

Device	Value
Shower, steam	Results in over 100% humidity
Facial saunas	Can be effective if heated
Pass-over (blow-by)	Simplest, and of doubtful benefit
Bubbler	Common in hospitals; of little benefit
Underwater jet	Produces moderate humidity
Cascade (diffuser)	Can result in high humidity if heated
Spinning disc	Produces dense mist
Aerosolizers	Can result in 100% humidity
Artificial nose	Can be beneficial after tracheostomy

ment of tracheobronchial disease. The more impressive devices, such as mist tents, were formerly believed to be helpful in loosening mucus in various diseases, such as cystic fibrosis, but their value has been completely discounted during the past two decades [4, 93].

The simplest humidifiers include the pass-over and bubbler devices that can be used with a wide hose and a face mask. They produce such a low output of water vapor that they do not result in any major changes in humidity in the tracheobronchial tree, although the humidified gas may be somewhat more comfortable to the nose and oropharynx than completely dry gas. It has been shown that although these devices are very commonly employed to humidify oxygen given by cannula or mask, they have no detectable advantages at the low flows that are generally used, and they can be justified only for patients requiring gas flows greater than 3 or 4 L/min or an inspired oxygen concentration greater than 30 percent [28, 49].

Dangers of Humidification Therapy

Most humidification devices offer potential for harm to asthmatic patients. Heated devices can add greatly to the humidity of the inspired gas and their use is of possible value, whereas unheated devices are probably of no value. However, heated humidifiers are more dangerous, and their value may be outweighed by their overall potential for severe hazards. If the device overheats, a hot mist that can damage the patient's mucous membrane will result. Of much more serious concern is the humidifier that runs dry, since it will deliver hot gas of zero humidity, which will cause desiccation of the mucosa with thickening of the secretions and impairment of ciliary activity, while the heat itself may cause thermal injury. In all cases a heated humidifier must be carefully monitored to ensure that it is not hazardous and that it is not misused. The humidifier can itself be a source of harm, since those who service them can get scalds or burns or electric shocks. Improper use of an electrically heated device can cause fires and the release of irritating fumes. Fortunately, serious problems of this nature are very rare, but the risk involved contraindicates the use of the more complex devices in a patient's home, unless appropriate use and maintenance can be ensured.

A specific contraindication to the use of heated mist is fever, since a further increase in temperature can result. Many dyspneic patients also complain of a sense of claustrophobia or suffocation when given heated mist therapy, particularly if the mist is dense or if a tight delivery mask is worn. Cold mist may be better tolerated and may even be soothing for a febrile patient. However, cold humidity or mist therapy has relatively little beneficial effect in asthma and may induce or worsen bronchospasm [61].

All humidifiers and aerosolizers can become contaminated with microorganisms. The use of a cold or moderately heated water or saline aerosol can be a potent source of pulmonary infection if the fluid is contaminated with bacteria. Humidifiers are less likely to transmit infection, but they present another risk if they become contaminated with fungi to which the patient is allergic: The resulting "humidifier fever" may be mild or serious and can result in bronchospasm, pulmonary infiltrates, and general malaise [52]. Manufacturers of aerosol delivery units are very conscious of the risk of infection, and many of the available units are sealed and are for individual use only. The ultrasonic nebulizer remains a major risk, and scrupulous care of such devices is mandatory. Humidification units are generally safer, with cascade devices being almost free of the risk of contamination. Inexpensive home humidifiers and vaporizers are unlikely to transmit pulmonary infection but can be responsible for humidifier fever. In this regard, a simple steam kettle is safe and less expensive and requires less upkeep, but the potential for thermal injury must be guarded against.

Although a huge industry has developed a plethora of devices

for providing vapor or mist forms of humidification, there is little reason to believe that the abnormal lower respiratory tract truly benefits from this largesse. The addition of water vapor to the inspired atmosphere is undoubtedly indicated for symptomatic treatment of upper respiratory tract discomfort and for laryngotracheal irritation; it is also mandatory in cases in which intubation results in a loss of the normal humidification provided by the nose. The properties of lower respiratory tract mucus do not change when humidity is added to the inspired air, and abnormal mucociliary clearance is not normalized if the patient is already adequately hydrated. In spite of the common practice of treating acute asthma with added humidification, there is no reason to believe that it is appropriate. Thus, routine thoughtless advocacy of across-the-board humidity therapy is even less justified in asthma than is the automatic assumption that the patient with status asthmaticus must require rehydration.

MUCOKINETIC AGENTS

A large number of pharmacologic agents have been used over the years in the management of mucostasis. Such drugs can be called mucokinetic agents, and the overall process of improving mucociliary clearance and sputum elimination can be referred to as mucokinesis [110]. No classification of mucokinetic agents is entirely satisfactory, but Table 69-6 lists the various categories of the clinically important agents that have been reported to be of clinical value. The topic has been extensively reviewed recently [11, 14, 115, 117, 120, 120a].

It should be recognized that clinical or laboratory investigations into the effectiveness of mucokinetic agents in humans have proved to be extremely difficult to carry out, and there is a dearth of evidence either to support or refute claims that these agents offer major clinical benefits [90, 105]. All of the agents discussed in this section have been shown to have mucokinetic actions in experimental animal models. Much of this work was carried out in Boyd's laboratory in Ontario, Canada, more than 25 years ago. Boyd found that many agents were more effective in the autumn months than at other times, but there is no satisfactory explanation for this discovery [12]. However, if mucokinesis can be affected by such factors as weather, viral infections, and other exogenous and endogenous variables, it is not surprising that the clinical literature is filled with conflict and confusing reports on the mucokinetic responses to the various agents and techniques that are employed. Controversy extends to physical methods for enhancing mucokinesis: Intermittent positive pressure breath-

Table 69-6. Mucokinetic agents

Class of agent	Actions
Airway dilators	
Beta$_2$ agonists	Bronchodilate, stimulate cilia
Alpha agonists	Constrict mucosa, augment secretions
Methylxanthines	Bronchodilate, stimulate cilia
Glucocorticoids	Normalize inflamed mucosa
Antiparasympathomimetics	Bronchodilate, may decrease secretion of mucus
Antibiotics	Normalize infected secretions
Diluents	Add to the water content of secretions
Surfactants	Decrease adhesiveness of mucus
Bronchomucotropics	Stimulate mucous production
Bronchorrheics	Increase osmotic transudation of fluid
Mucolytics	Break down sputum molecules to smaller components
Emetic expectorants	Stimulate gastropulmonary vagal reflex
Mucoregulators	Normalize mucous production

ing, bronchoscopic suctioning, chest percussion or vibration, postural drainage, and even coughing maneuvers all have their critics as well as their supporters [22, 77, 103]. Perhaps in no other area of therapeutics in which the objective is so tangible is there so much doubt regarding the efficacy of the pharmacologic and physical maneuvers that are customarily employed.

Numerous drugs have been reported to have an influence on mucous secretion or quality, but there is relatively little information as to the clinical relevance of their effects. Thus, there are hints that many different classes of agents may be of significance in mucokinesis, for example, anesthetics, sedatives, narcotics, prostaglandins (and antagonists or stimulators of these agents, such as the salicylates), polyamines, peptides, and arachidonic acid derivatives [53, 55, 60, 75, 102]. However, in this chapter no effort will be made to review all these drugs, and only the better-known agents will be described.

Airway Dilators

Drugs that increase the patency of the airways will lead to an improvement in the effectiveness of cough and expectoration [36]. All forms of bronchodilators are capable of enhancing mucociliary clearance and secretion elimination, and therefore appropriate management of asthma with these agents will result in a simultaneous improvement in the patient's ability to cough up sputum. Oral and systemic sympathomimetic bronchodilators (beta$_2$ agonists) and theophylline derivatives (methylxanthines) may be more effective than aerosolized bronchodilators, since the aerosolized drugs fail to reach distal parts of obstructed airways [35, 116]. A further advantage of bronchodilator drugs is that they stimulate the beating of the cilia and result in improved effectiveness of the mucociliary escalator [90, 103, 112].

There is reason to believe that sympathomimetic agonist agents with alpha-adrenergic properties can also enhance mucokinesis [79]. Drugs such as phenylephrine and ephedrine are readily demonstrated to be effective in improving the patency of inflamed nasal passages, and similar mucosal vasoconstriction may occur in the abnormal passages of the lungs of patients with bronchospasm and mucostasis. These agents bring about mucous membrane shrinkage by constricting engorged vessels and reducing edema. A series of studies reported by Nadel and colleagues [9, 56, 71, 72, 79] suggest that alpha-adrenergic agents increase transudation of fluid across the respiratory mucous membrane, thereby causing an increase in the amount of sputum that can then be expectorated; however, this finding does not correspond with clinical experience. These agents, unlike beta-adrenergic stimulators, cause discharge of granules from serous cells in the bronchial mucosa [9], but the full importance of this finding has not been determined.

It is evident that glucocorticoids can also improve mucokinesis, both by reducing inflammation in the airways and by enhancing the effectiveness of beta-adrenergic bronchodilator drugs. It is possible that steroids can directly affect the secretory activities of the bronchial glands: In some patients with abnormal mucus, steroid therapy may restore the respiratory tract secretions to normal. A further suggestion is that glucocorticoids change the permeability of the respiratory mucosa and thereby influence molecular migration into the respiratory tract fluid [50, 89, 109].

Another important class of airway dilators are the antiparasympathomimetics (see Chap. 64). It is known that atropine and ipratropium bromide can cause bronchodilatation in asthma; atropine in large amounts can block normal vagal stimulation of the bronchial glands and cause more viscous secretions. However, when given in relatively small doses by aerosol, they do not cause this antimucokinetic effect [121]. An interesting corollary in airway therapeutics is provided by cholinergic drugs: These can produce discharge of serous cell granules and a marked in-

crease in bronchial gland output, thereby resulting in a considerable mucokinetic effect [9, 13]. Since cholinergic drugs are also liable to induce severe bronchospasm, they are not suitable for therapeutic purposes. Whether mucus-thickening drugs, such as anticholinergics, can be helpful is worth considering. Davis [30] suggests that the mucociliary clearance of watery secretions can be improved by "mucospissic" drugs that thicken the material, thereby allowing more effective coughing. This concept is of great interest, since a known disadvantage of mucolytic agents is their ability to make secretions so watery that they gravitate downwards, causing the patient to "drown" in the material. Perhaps a combination of mucolytic and mucospissic drugs would be of benefit in selected patients [56].

Other agents that have been used in the treatment of bronchospasm have not been shown to have important mucokinetic properties. Cromolyn sodium does not appear to contribute to mucokinesis. Antihistamines, which may be of benefit in the treatment of some forms of asthma, are not of major value in clinical practice, and their antiparasympathomimetic properties may lead to an antimucokinetic effect; however, in clinical practice, such an effect has not been shown [80]. In the future other classes of potential bronchodilators—such as calcium channel–blocking drugs or anti-histaminic mast cell inhibitors such as ketotifen [65]—will need to be examined for their possible effects on mucokinesis.

Antibiotics

For many years it has been recognized that pulmonary infections accompanied by purulent sputum yield to antibiotic therapy and that the abnormal sputum thereby becomes less viscous and decreases in volume. Thus, antibiotic therapy can aid expectoration and can facilitate clearance of sputum from the lungs; in this regard the antibiotic is acting as a mucokinetic agent.

Although the value of antibiotic therapy in chronic bronchitis has been questioned in recent years [3, 73, 91], most practitioners still advise their patients to take a course of an antibiotic whenever their sputum changes for the worse in amount, color, or consistency [113]. In asthma the use of antibiotics is even more controversial, but if the bronchospasm appears to worsen as a consequence of a sinus infection or a severe cold, then infection is generally believed to be involved and an antibiotic is often prescribed. The antibiotic-sensitive organisms that might be pathogenic in "infectious asthma" are poorly defined but are generally believed to be the normal aerobic and anaerobic bacteria that colonize the upper respiratory tract. Agents such as ampicillin, tetracycline, erythromycin, sulfonamide or cotrimoxazole, or a cephalosporin are used in such cases, and the sputum gradually appears to improve along with the other symptoms. It is possible that some agents, such as tetracycline, thicken secretions by a mucospissic effect [30]. However, there is little in the literature to support the use of antibiotics in asthma accompanied by purulent sputum in the absence of other evidence of bacterial infection.

Nebulization of antibiotics was more popular in previous years and was advocated for a variety of pulmonary infections. However, bronchospasm is liable to develop in the asthmatic patient exposed to an aerosolized antibiotic, particularly when a highly allergenic drug such as penicillin is used. There are suggestions that kanamycin sulfate and some sulfonamides have mucolytic properties, but such qualities are certainly not of clinical importance [112].

Diluents

As already explained in the first part of this chapter, water in various forms has long been favored as a mucokinetic. Hydration and humidity have already been discussed, and in this section the use of aerosols will be addressed.

Water does not have any fundamental effect on the biochemical or organic structure of mucus, and if water becomes incorporated into the secretion its only effect is to decrease the concentration of the viscous components. Thus, water serves as a diluent whenever and however it is administered. Oral intake, intravenous therapy, the delivery of humidity, and the use of aerosols all appear to result in similar effects: The mucus may acquire a higher water content with a corresponding lowering of its viscoelasticity. Unfortunately, such theoretic benefits of water administration are not readily demonstrable. Nevertheless, water is frequently prescribed as an aerosol for its supposed mucokinetic effect. Droplets of water have been shown in vitro to be more effective than vaporized water for decreasing the viscosity of sputum specimens [31], but the clinical impression that aerosolized water has beneficial actions in patients with asthma has not been substantiated in controlled in vivo studies [107].

As is the case with humidification therapy, advocates for the therapeutic use of water mist have suggested that denser and warmer aerosols of water are more effective than simpler therapeutic droplet clouds. However, there is no proof to support such allegations, since neither mucociliary clearance nor spirometry findings appear to be noticeably improved by this therapy. Furthermore, numerous studies show that mouth or nasal breathing of a cool aerosol results in only very slight penetration of water particles into the lungs; even with a tracheostomy, only a small proportion of the droplets penetrate into the distal airways [81]. Thus there is surprisingly little proof that mists or aerosols of water benefit patients with hyperviscous secretions or impaired mucociliary clearance [59, 107].

Dense mist therapy is still favored in many hospitals, where it is often administered as an ultrasonic aerosol. The piezoelectric effect that is employed in ultrasonic nebulization results in the production of an extremely dense and stable mist: The vast majority of the particles are uniform in size, with a diameter of 1 to 3 μ. Such devices can nebulize 3 to 6 ml of water per minute and can result in the deposition of relatively large amounts of water in the tracheobronchial tree; indeed, patients receiving prolonged ultrasonic nebulization can become overhydrated. In most patients the deposited fluid can be coughed out, and this expectorated fluid will be accompanied by exfoliated cells and microorganisms from the airways. Because 10 to 40 minutes of ultrasonic aerosol therapy will often result in sputum expectoration in subjects who are otherwise unable to cough up a specimen, the main use of ultrasonic nebulization is to induce the expectoration of sputum for cytologic study and for microbiologic evaluation of possible *Pneumocystis* or mycobacterial infection. The ultrasonic mist of water or saline can be quite irritating, and it is particularly likely to induce coughing in a nonsmoker. Indeed, ultrasonic mist may be as harmful as cigarette smoke, and one wonders what the surgeon-general would feel about the potential outcome on a patient's bronchial mucosa if it should happen to be exposed to 20 ultrasonic aerosol treatments a day given over a period of 20 to 30 years.

Asthmatics are likely to tolerate an ultrasonic aerosol of sterile water poorly, and intense bronchospasm with coughing will develop in many. Indeed, this has been proposed as a test for the presence of asthma [2]. Thus, since the modality is not of proven value and since it is expensive, hazardous, and even self-defeating, ultrasonic nebulization of water should be regarded as being contraindicated in patients with bronchospastic disorders. Whether saline is more desirable than water for this form of therapy is questionable.

For many years propylene glycol was advocated for use in inhalation therapy, although it has lost favor recently. Numerous properties have been ascribed to this agent, but these are not well documented [112]. It has been used as a demulcent or hu-

mectant for its alleged soothing effect, and it is said to stabilize droplets in aerosols; these properties are the outcome of its hygroscopic qualities. It has mild antimicrobial effects, and it has been reported to have mucolytic properties and even mild bronchodilator qualities [112]. However, when added to water it seems to form a relatively inert solution, and it probably has little more than diluent properties. If one elects to use this agent, a 2% solution is probably best, since this is isosmotic and not irritating. Concentrations as high as 20% have been recommended by cytopathologists for use in aerosols (often in combination with hypertonic saline) for inducing sputum; even more concentrated solutions have been advocated by occasional enthusiasts. The agent appears to be well tolerated by asthmatic patients, although it seems to offer no major benefits and therefore is rarely recommended. It should be noted that the propylene glycol may inhibit the growth of pathogenic bacteria on laboratory media, although the specimens of expectorated sputum remain suitable for cytology and for culture of mycobacteria and fungi [112].

Normal saline is often preferred to water for aerosolization; it is less likely to cause airway irritation since the droplets are isosmotic with the tracheobronchial mucosa. Deposited droplets may be incorporated into respiratory secretions, and the diluted mucus may be more readily expectorated. Although normal saline is the most commonly administered aerosol in hospital practice, there is no proof that it improves the function of the mucociliary escalator or that it serves as a mucokinetic [59, 88]. There is some evidence that normal saline has more of a mucolytic effect than does water alone, but this "salt" effect on the viscosity of mucoprotein is a minor one and of little clinical importance [112, 117]. Normal saline may be theoretically preferable to distilled water, but there is little information to suggest that any difference will be noted either objectively or subjectively by the patient other than the taste of the aerosol solution that is deposited in the mouth.

Normal saline is considered to be bland, since it has less effect on the respiratory mucous membrane than either hypotonic or hypertonic solutions. Hypotonic saline is similar to water when given as an aerosol, but theoretically the hypotonic droplets may grow smaller by evaporation whereas water droplets may be more likely to vaporize entirely. The smaller droplets of hypotonic saline are likely to be deposited distally in the tracheobronchial tree, and thus this aerosol may be more effective in causing dilution of mucus in the smaller airways. In practice, this theoretic advantage does not seem to have been recorded. The major clinical indication for hypotonic saline, rather than normal saline, is in cases in which a bland aerosol is required for a patient who is on a salt-restricted diet [114, 118]. Hypotonic saline is available as a half-normal (0.45%) solution, and other concentrations could be made up by adding water to normal saline.

In contrast, hypertonic saline in various concentrations has a more definite effect. The concentrated salt is believed to displace calcium ions from the mucoprotein molecular matrix, and thereby the viscosity of the sputum may be reduced [112]. Furthermore, the hyperosmolar solution will draw fluid out of the respiratory mucosa, further diluting the mucous layer. This osmotic irritant effect can be quite pronounced and may result in bronchorrhea (see Bronchorrheics). The aerosol may also irritate the mucosa and produce coughing, particularly if a dense warm mist or ultrasonic nebulization is administered. The net result of such aerosol therapy could be the induction of a productive cough, and thereby hypertonic saline may be a more effective mucokinetic agent than more dilute solutions [76]. Concentrations of 1.8% to 10%, or even 20%, have been used, and the more concentrated solutions are likely to be more effective; however, frequent use of hypertonic saline aerosols can introduce a major salt load, and congestive cardiac failure or edema may develop in patients who have borderline cardiac compensation or inadequate renal function. Also, repeated topical use of hypertonic saline—or any hyperosmolar solution—is likely to irritate the tracheobronchial mucous membrane.

Other salts have been used in aerosol therapy, but the only important one is sodium bicarbonate, which is usually given as a hypertonic solution [112, 118]. Thus it will have a bronchorrheic effect and a salt effect, thereby resulting in an increased output of mucosal fluid and a mucolytic effect on the mucoprotein molecular network, as well as a surfactant effect (see Surfactants). Salt solutions of various types have been given orally as expectorants, and in previous years solutions of ammonium carbonate, ammonium chloride, antimony potassium tartrate, and potassium or sodium citrate were particularly popular [112, 118], although warm saline solution was regarded by many physicians as being the best of the simple expectorants. None of these hypertonic solutions should be given as an aerosol or as an irrigant solution for more than a few days, since they can eventually cause mucosal irritation.

Surfactants

The adhesiveness of sputum can be reduced in vitro by coating the sample with a wetting agent or a detergent, the action of which is comparable to that of domestic soaps or washing agents. The simplest detergents are alkalis, and sodium hydroxide is an effective agent in vitro; in addition to its ability to decrease the stickiness of mucus, this potent chemical also has marked mucolytic properties. Obviously, sodium hydroxide is not suitable for clinical administration, although sodium bicarbonate is, and it is possible that when the latter is nebulized it is converted in part to sodium carbonate, which then breaks down to liberate sodium hydroxide:

$$2\ NaHCO_3 \xrightarrow{O_2} Na_2CO_3 + H_2O + CO_2 \rightarrow 2\ NaOH + 2\ CO_2$$

In practice hypertonic sodium bicarbonate solutions (1.4–7.5%) seem to be of considerable value for inducing mucokinesis: The solution serves as a surfactant, a mucolytic, a bronchorrheic, and an emetic expectorant [118]. Sodium bicarbonate is also a potentiator of acetylcysteine. Furthermore, it is a useful irrigant for cleansing tracheostomy tubes. In the past, various other surfactants were made available in proprietary products such as Alevaire and Tergemist, and they appeared to be beneficial. These products are no longer marketed, but the readily available hypertonic sodium bicarbonate solutions can be given either by aerosol or by endotracheal instillation, and personal experience has shown that this agent is well tolerated and more effective as a mucokinetic than saline. One problem with sodium bicarbonate is that since it is an alkaline solution it hastens the breakdown of sympathomimetic agents to red or brown adrenochromes; if a bronchodilator is added to the solution, it should be nebulized immediately before major breakdown occurs. Aerosolized or instilled sodium bicarbonate may also irritate the respiratory mucosa if given for more than a few days. The recommended dosage is 2 ml of a 3 to 5 percent solution, which can be given by instillation or nebulization every 4 to 6 hours. A lower concentration (e.g., 1.4%) or a smaller dose (e.g., 0.5 ml) can be given if evidence of irritation of the tracheobronchial mucosa develops.

Bronchomucotropics

The term *bronchomucotropic* was proposed by Boyd [12] for agents that increase the mucus content and the volume of the secreted respiratory tract fluid. Boyd recognized both systemic and inhalant drugs that could be categorized in this class (Table 69-7). However, the term is not generally used, though it is retained here because it does appear to distinguish a specific mechanism.

The traditional aromatic inhalants can be regarded as being bronchomucotropics. These volatile oleoresins are mainly camphenes, pinenes, phenols, terpenes, and *p*-menthane derivatives [12]. Vicks VapoRub, Tiger Balm, eucalyptus, menthol, camphorated oil, Friars' Balsam, and other similar folk remedies are prime examples [115, 119]. Their soothing properties can relieve coughs and appear to be helpful in facilitating expectoration [53, 67]. However, although these agents have an amazingly large following, proof of their effectiveness as mucokinetic agents has not been attained. It would be uncharitable to equate lack of proof with lack of value, and physicians should not shake their patients' faith in such products. Furthermore, one study of patients with colds suggested that inhalation of aromatic vapors (i.e., eucalyptus, menthol, and camphor) had a beneficial effect on the peripheral airway dysfunction that accompanied the coryza [25]. Inhalation of pungent fumes such as those of ammonia (or sal volatile), mustard oil, ground horseradish, and crushed garlic appear to stimulate the respiratory tract and increase mucosal secretion [110]; these agents could also be regarded as bronchomucotropics, although their irritant properties suggest that they should be classified as bronchorrheics (see the following section).

Bronchomucotropics may act by stimulating the bronchial glands to secrete, thereby augmenting the layer bathing the mucosa. Such agents may also have other mucosal or antiasthmatic effects, although these are poorly defined [67]. There is good reason to believe that iodide works by stimulating the bronchial glands, since this ion is clearly taken up by the salivary and nasolacrimal glands, which are then stimulated to activity. It is less clear how inhaled vapors produce effects, but it is presumed that they penetrate the respiratory mucosa and then act on the bronchial glands. Agents with a bronchomucotropic effect that are effective when given by mouth may stimulate the bronchial glands directly after being selectively picked up from the bloodstream, but much of their action is reflex, and therefore these agents are discussed later under the category of expectorants.

Bronchorrheics

Irritants of the respiratory mucosa may result in a marked increase in fluid output, perhaps as a consequence of mast cell mediator release. It is possible that all inhaled fumes or aerosols can cause this effect, and dense or ultrasonic mists of hypertonic agents do appear to have a bronchorrheic action. Thus topical therapy with hypertonic saline, sodium bicarbonate, or aerosol-

Table 69-7. *Bronchomucotropics*

Agent	Administration
Inhalational aromatic volatiles	
Vicks VapoRub	Added to boiling water, rubbed
Tiger Balm	on lips or chest, or fumes
Friars' Balsam	inhaled from fresh product
Other balsams	
Camphorated oil	
Horseradish fumes	
(allyl isothiocyanate)	
Oral (or intravenous) iodide	
SSKI	10–20 drops QID, PO
Potassium iodide	1 gm QID, PO
Hydriodic acid	200 mg QID, PO
Iodinated glycerol	400 mg BID, PO
Sodium iodide	1–3 gm/24 hr, IV

SSKI = saturated solution of potassium iodide.

ized mucolytics such as acetylcysteine can cause osmotic enhancement of mucous secretion [24]. Cigarette smoke is an obvious bronchorrheic, and it is possible that the perceived mucokinesis resulting from aerosols of hypertonic solutions, including saline or concentrated acetylcysteine, is a consequence of their irritant properties rather than any specific mucolytic effect. In former days drugs such as ammonia, mustard oil, and pepper (capsaicin or piperine) were used to stimulate coughing and sneezing, and it is possible that they also have useful mucokinetic effects on the lower airways [117, 118].

In clinical practice it is generally impossible to distinguish a bronchomucotropic or mucolytic effect from the bronchorrheic effect of an aerosol, and bronchorrhea resulting from mucosal irritation probably accounts for much of the increase in expectorated secretions that follows any mucokinetic aerosol administration. Present methods of studying mucociliary clearance do not clearly define the therapeutic site of action of inhaled mucokinetics, and thus expectoration resulting from bronchorrhea produced in the proximal airways may be misinterpreted as the outcome of mucolytic liberation of inspissated secretions.

Mucolytics

Agents that break down the fibrillar molecules of mucoprotein into smaller, less viscous subunits are classified as mucolytics. The most effective agents of this type are derivatives of L-cysteine, an amino acid derived from the acid hydrolysis of the proteins in skin, hair, and feathers. Cysteine itself is poorly tolerated, and the most successful derivative that has been marketed is acetylcysteine, although other cysteine derivatives have also been shown to have mucolytic properties [117].

In common with other mucolytic cysteine derivatives, acetylcysteine has a free thiol (—SH) group; this is an active reducing agent, and it breaks down the disulfide (—S—S—) bridges that bind the glycoproteins and other constituents of mucus, including albumin, lysozyme, and secretory immunoglobulin, thus forming a viscous molecular network. There is some dispute as to whether disulfide bridges occur as part of the innate structure of glycoprotein molecules [68, 105], although there is no doubt that they are important in conferring viscous properties on sputum. Acetylcysteine is extremely effective in vitro, where it can be shown to produce rapid mucolysis in all types of sputum specimens. There is also evidence that it can lyse mucus that is impacted in large airways if given by instillation through an endotracheal tube or a bronchoscope; atelectasis can be treated by instilling 2 to 10 ml of 10% acetylcysteine, while larger amounts can be given during lung lavage [69]. Unfortunately, there is no proof that the drug has mucolytic effects on inspissated secretions when given by aerosol. Most studies fail to demonstrate a major acute clinical benefit after aerosol therapy with acetylcysteine, although patients may claim improved expectoration [8, 86, 90, 112, 117]. As with many mucokinetic agents, investigators suggest the best results are obtained by using daily therapy in chronic bronchitis for several weeks, since measurable improvements do not occur rapidly [5, 18, 20]. There is, thus, reason to regard the drug as being a mucoregulator.

Acetylcysteine is marketed in the United States as Mucomyst and Mucosil; elsewhere it is known by names such as Airbron, Fluimucil, Mucolyticum, and Nac. The solution smells strongly of hydrogen sulfide and burned hair, and its odor may be upsetting to both the clinician and the recipient. The aerosol can be irritating to asthmatic patients and can provoke severe bronchospasm, but this may be prevented by prior or simultaneous administration of an aerosolized bronchodilator. The aerosol may also irritate the throat and cause nausea or gagging, and susceptible patients may vomit. However, other toxicity is rarely caused by the drug, which has been given in large amounts both orally and intravenously in the management of acetaminophen poisoning.

Because of the adverse effects caused by aerosol solution, an odorless crystalline product (Fluimucil), which can be dissolved in water to form a pleasant tasting drink, has been marketed in Europe. Clinical studies in Europe and South America suggest that this oral preparation is very well tolerated when given in a dosage of 100 to 200 mg two to three times a day, and it has been shown to be effective in chronic bronchitis, although acute benefits in asthma have not been clearly demonstrated [37]. Long-term administration of oral acetylcysteine may reduce the frequency of exacerbations of chronic obstructive diseases in patients in whom hyperviscosity of secretions develops periodically [45, 85].

In the United States recommendations for the dosage of acetylcysteine vary, but 2 ml of 10% Mucomyst or Mucosil combined with 2 ml of a diluent (and bronchodilator to prevent bronchospasm) is an average inhalational or nebulizer dose (Table 69-8). Some investigators advocate using 20% acetylcysteine, but the less concentrated solution appears to be effective enough, and it causes fewer side effects. The solution can be aerosolized by a simple nebulizer; some patients tolerate the dense aerosol produced by ultrasonic nebulization. Treatments can be given as often as needed, perhaps four to six times a day, but many patients will not tolerate frequent treatments. Normal saline is the usual diluent, but personal experience suggests that 1.4 to 5.0% sodium bicarbonate results in a more effective mucolytic solution. However, it has been claimed that if sterile water is used as the diluent, less airway irritation is produced. Thus, if a patient has very reactive airways (as in severe asthma) it may be best to use 10% acetylcysteine diluted with an equal volume of sterile water [16]. It is possible that the odorous, irritating solution that is available in the United States will eventually be succeeded by a more benign cysteine derivative; alternatively, oral acetylcysteine granules may be introduced into the United States, or an intramuscular or intravenous form may prove to be worthy of investigation [44, 64].

In recent years, enormous interest has been directed at the potential of acetylcysteine to serve other important uses. The drug is well-known to be a free-radical scavenger [94a], and evidence is emerging that suggests it may be of value in the prevention of damage to the lungs by oxidants in patients with chronic infections or in those exposed to air pollution or cigarette smoke. The drug may also be of value in the early stages of the adult respiratory distress syndrome (ARDS) [55a], and it may prove to have benefits in other organs in addition to the lungs [117]. Recently, evidence has been presented to support the hypothesis that acetylcysteine possesses antiinflammatory properties [57a].

Other cysteine derivatives have been used in Europe, with 2-mercaptoethane sulfonate (Mesna, Mistabron, Mucofluid) being

Table 69-8. Mucolytic agents

Agent	Preparation	Route	Dose
Acetylcysteine	Mucomyst 10%, 20%; Mucosil 10%, 20%	Inhalational	1–2 ml + diluent
	Fluimucil*	PO	200–400 mg
	Other	IV	(Investigational)
Iodide	In Tergemist*	Inhalational	(No longer available)
	SSKI	PO	10–20 drops (1–2 gm)
	Sodium iodide†	IV	50–150 mg/hr
2-Mercaptoethane	Mesna*, Mistabron*	Inhalational	1–2 ml 20% solution

* Not available in the United States for inhalation.
† Not available in the United States.
SSKI = saturated solution of potassium iodide.

the most useful. It is claimed that this agent not only ruptures disulfide bonds of the glycoproteins but also dissociates mucus side-chains by ionization and solubilizes the resulting fragments [112]. Currently, this agent is used as a free-radical scavenger to prevent ifosfamide-induced hemorrhagic cystitis.

Enzymes have been used in the United States as mucolytics, but the old aerosol preparations are no longer available. The value of these agents (e.g., dornase, trypsin, streptokinase) in asthma had never been satisfactorily demonstrated. Recently, a recombinant deoxyribonuclease (rhDNase) has shown promise in reducing purulent sputum viscosity in patients with cystic fibrosis [51a].

Iodide has been shown to be a very effective mucolytic, although this fact is not widely appreciated [63, 64]. Formerly, iodide was actually a favored inhalational drug, being incorporated in the aerosol mucokinetic preparation Tergemist. This is no longer available, although the medication was thought to be useful. In vitro studies have shown that potassium iodide solution can be extremely effective [63], and bedside observations will readily reveal that when saturated solution of potassium iodide (SSKI) is added to sputum it causes almost as much mucolysis as does acetylcysteine. In addition to its direct mucolytic effect on mucoprotein, there is evidence that iodide potentiates the natural proteases usually present in sputum and thereby enhances the proteolytic breakdown of mucoprotein by this secondary action [112]. Iodide has both mucoregulator and expectorant actions, as will be explained later.

Iodide can be given as intravenous sodium iodide (NaI), using a continuous drip of 1 gm in each 1-liter bottle of dextrose water or normal saline, up to a maximum of about 3 gm of NaI a day (Table 69-8). When given in this dosage for several days NaI is well tolerated, and it appears to facilitate expectoration of the hyperviscous secretions that are characteristic of status asthmaticus. Unfortunately, this product is no longer marketed.

In conclusion, it is recognized that although mucolytics are extremely effective in laboratory testing, their value in loosening secretions in asthma is not established, and their delivery by aerosol can induce bronchospasm. The chronic use of these agents in asthmatic bronchitis may lead to subjective improvement with increased ease in expectoration. The mucus-liquefying properties of agents as potent as acetylcysteine may, however, be a problem in patients with airway obstruction and poor cough, since the loosened secretions may gravitate distally in the airways and lead to a worsening in gaseous exchange. Since the aerosolized particles of mucolytic agents tend to be irritating, they can produce cough, bronchorrhea, and bronchospasm, and little of the drug may reach the smaller airways where mucus may be impacted. Further studies are required to determine whether oral or intravenous administration of mucolytic drugs would be effective and whether these routes would be better tolerated and safer than direct delivery into the respiratory tract in asthma.

Expectorants

The generally accepted definition of an expectorant is an agent that is taken by mouth to produce an increased volume of sputum that can be coughed out more easily [111]. Numerous proprietary over-the-counter "cough medicines" contain expectorant agents of different types, and patients who value them feel that they do loosen airway secretions and facilitate expectoration. An enormous number of prescriptions for expectorants are provided by physicians, and considerably more of these medications are purchased without prescription. In spite of this outpouring of faith, there is little evidence to suggest that expectorants result in an outpouring of sputum, and most physicians appear to believe that these agents are placebos.

However, there is one property common to most expectorant

Table 69-9. Oral expectorants

Expectorant	Dosage
Salt solutions	
Sodium chloride	500–1,000 mg
Ammonium salts	500–1,000 mg
Potassium salts	500–1,000 mg
Creosote derivatives	
Guaifenesin	200–600 mg
Guaiacol	500 mg (?)
Terpenes	
Terpin hydrate	125–300 mg (?)
Ipecac syrup	0.25–2 ml
Spices	
Capsaicin (pepper)	10 drops Tabasco sauce
Sinigrin (mustard)	As tolerated
Alliin (garlic)	As tolerated

drugs: In increased dosage they cause nausea and vomiting. Conversely, recognized emetic agents, such as ipecac, have long been classified as expectorants when administered in subemetic doses. Since the lungs are embryologic outgrowths of the foregut, it is not difficult to envisage comparable responses of the airways and stomach to autonomic stimulation. It has therefore been postulated that emetic agents that stimulate gastric receptors evoke a reflex through the vagus nerve whose efferent arc supplies the lungs as well as the foregut [48]. The emetic reflex depends on afferent stimulation activating an emetic center in the reticular formation of the medulla; this causes both vagal and systemic nerve output, which results in antiperistalsis and violent contractions of the diaphragm and abdominal and intercostal muscles, thereby producing vomiting. A lesser stimulation of the gastric afferents may stimulate a "mucokinetic center," which is postulated to exist in the medulla adjacent to the respiratory center [111, 112]. This results in an efferent vagal outflow to the bronchial glands, and these are stimulated to produce airway secretions, thereby enhancing the volume of sputum that can be expectorated (Fig. 69-1). Animal studies have indicated that there is a "gastropulmonary mucokinetic vagal reflex," but the autonomic components may be more complex in the human [12, 71, 108]. Thus it appears that pharyngeal or laryngeal stimulation can evoke a similar mucokinetic response via the ninth cranial nerve [29].

If the above assumptions are correct, any agent that can cause nausea as a result of its irritating effect on the gastric mucosa will have expectorant properties. This implies that nauseants such as salt water, concentrated mustard solution, and other pungent foods or herbs serve as natural expectorants when taken in the diet. Personal experience suggests that people with chronic obstructive lung disease who habitually eat bland foods are more likely to be troubled by retention of mucus than are those whose diet regularly contains pungent spices [111].

A number of the more important expectorant medications will be considered (Table 69-9). Although it is often pointed out that there is no proof that these agents are of clinical benefit [90, 105], such claims are indictments of the unsatisfactory means that have been used for evaluating expectorants. Careful studies have revealed that gastric stimulation by several of these agents does result in enhanced mucous secretion in the tracheobronchial tree [72, 79]. The most effective of the expectorants may also have other actions, including bronchomucotropic, mucolytic, and mucoregulator effects.

Iodide

The oldest of the specific expectorants is probably iodide, and it is available in various formulations [119]. The best known preparation is SSKI, which contains 1,000 mg of potassium iodide per

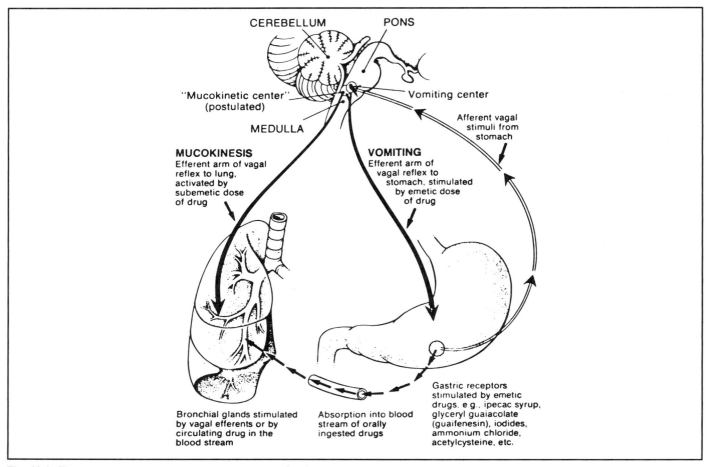

Fig. 69-1. *The gastropulmonary mucokinetic vagal reflex. Orally ingested agents that irritate the stomach can cause reflex emesis. Lesser stimulation evokes a vagal reflex to the bronchial glands, thereby causing them to secrete. Some of these agents will also be absorbed from the bowel, and they can stimulate the bronchial glands directly. (Reprinted with permission from I. Ziment,* Secretions of the Respiratory Tract: Physiology and Pharmacology. *Upper Montclair, N.J.: Projects in Health, 1976.)*

milliliter of solution—although some commercial preparations contain as little as 760 mg/ml. The usual dosage is 10 drops (about 1 ml) of SSKI in a glass of water or beverage three or four times a day, but some patients appear to require two or three times this amount. The additional fluid obtained by means of this prescription can help ensure adequate hydration, as discussed in the early pages of this chapter.

Although there is little proof that SSKI is an effective expectorant, most authorities on asthma recommend that the drug be administered if sputum elimination is a problem. As pointed out earlier, iodide is also a mucolytic and a bronchomucotropic, and there is evidence that it offers other benefits in asthma, including ciliary stimulation and a nonspecific antiasthmatic effect [67, 112]. When given by mouth in large amounts, it can cause gastric irritation, but in smaller doses it can evoke the gastropulmonary mucokinetic vagal reflex without inducing nausea. The iodide is absorbed into the bloodstream where it is picked up by the thyroid and many exocrine glands including the bronchial glands. The bronchial glands are then stimulated to secrete by the direct bronchomucotropic effect, and the iodide that enters the mucoid secretions exerts a mucolytic action. Thus iodide has multiple actions that make it a particularly effective mucokinetic agent with special value in the treatment of asthma.

A major objection of iodotherapy is that it can result in many side effects, but 90 to 95 percent of patients can take the drug without major difficulty. The most common complaint is that iodide leaves an unpleasant taste in the mouth, but this is unacceptable to only a minority of patients. Indeed, if one offers an alternative prescription of 10 to 15 drops of Tabasco sauce in water (which appears to have a mucokinetic action), these patients are likely to look more favorably on the SSKI. Some patients manifest iodine sensitivity by developing an acneiform rash, but more severe rashes or anaphylactoid reactions are exceedingly rare. An enhanced pharmacologic responsiveness to iodide can result in overstimulation of the salivary glands, which may become painful and swollen; this problem is resolved by reducing the dosage. The thyroid gland may be affected by iodide in susceptible individuals: Hyperthyroidism occurs extremely rarely; hypothyroidism may develop in up to 5 percent of patients receiving chronic therapy. It is advisable to limit iodide therapy to courses lasting no more than 4 to 6 weeks, but chronic therapy is often requested by asthmatics who benefit from the drug. It may be appropriate to obtain thyroid tests at 2 months and 4 months, but if abnormalities are not found during this period it is unlikely that hypothyroidism will develop during continued therapy.

Another form of iodide is the organic derivative iodinated glycerol. This has far less toxicity than the inorganic preparations and also has the advantage of proven effectiveness. Since it appears to act as a mucoregulator, it is discussed later under that heading. A related organic iodide, domiodol, which is available in Italy, may have similar properties [14].

Guaifenesin

The most popular expectorant is guaifenesin, which was formerly called glyceryl guaiacolate [118, 119]. Controversy has long raged as to the effectiveness of this drug, and even its theoretic mode of action has been debated. In large amounts the drug is an emetic, and therefore it probably does stimulate the gastropulmonary vagal reflex. Guaifenesin also appears to be picked up by the bronchial glands from the bloodstream, and it exerts a bronchomucotropic effect, stimulating the output of secretions and increasing their water content [19]. Furthermore, it is claimed that the drug is secreted into the mucus, on which it exerts a surfactant effect.

The more prominent manufacturers of this drug recommend that guaifenesin be given to adults in a dosage of 200 mg every 4 hours, up to a maximum of 1,200 mg a day, although Chodosh and Medici [19] recommend that twice this dosage be considered the standard. Hirsch and associates [51] could not detect any major expectorant effect when the drug was given in dosages as high as 1,600 mg a day, and these investigators dispute the claim that larger dosages would be effective. Other studies [54, 57] have failed to provide objective evidence for the effectiveness of this drug in coughs and colds. My impression is that guaifenesin can be helpful in some patients with acute bronchitis, but it is of greater benefit in chronic bronchitics when given for several weeks, as is common with many mucokinetic agents. The drug appears to be less effective in asthma, and it offers negligible benefits in status asthmaticus. The mucokinetic dosage is probably close to the amount likely to produce emesis. In lower dosages the drug is well tolerated, and side effects are rarely encountered. Although this agent is extraordinarily popular, the dosages that are generally employed (e.g., 800 mg/day) are too low, and the medication thus frequently serves as a placebo. It is mostly prescribed as a syrup (e.g., Robitussin), but it is also available in tablets and in numerous combination products. Several side effects of interest, including interference with platelet adhesiveness, have been described, but these properties do not appear to be important clinically.

Ipecac

Over the last several hundred years, ipecac has had a varying reputation as an agent for treating asthma [119], and it has been incorporated in several proprietary cough medicines. There is good evidence from the work of Boyd [12] that the ipecac alkaloids do stimulate sputum production when given in subemetic doses, and this effect appears to be mediated through the gastropulmonary vagal reflex [118].

Although ipecac may be a useful expectorant, especially in children, the drug is used infrequently in current practice. It is of interest, however, that the induction of vomiting by mechanical or pharmacologic stimulation in children with acute asthma may result in simultaneous expectoration of mucous plugs from the airways. Subemetic doses of ipecac may serve to induce "vomiting" of sputum from the lungs without disturbing the stomach. Thus ipecac syrup may be worthy of trial in a dosage of 0.25 to 1 ml three or four times a day in asthmatic children; adults may respond to dosages of up to 2 ml.

Terpin Hydrate

Although turpentine derivatives have long been used as expectorants[119], these agents are poorly tolerated. The most acceptable product is terpin hydrate, which is used to a surprising degree although there is virtually no evidence to suggest it is effective in the usually recommended dose of up to 300 mg every 6 hours [118]. Generally, it is given in much smaller dosages, and it must be concluded that it serves as a placebo. Perhaps larger doses would be more effective, but nausea is likely to be induced.

Thus this agent cannot be recommended, and it is being marketed less commonly.

Other Expectorants

Various salts, herbs, and plant derivatives are used as expectorants, with little evidence as to their effectiveness [86, 119]. Those that are emetics may have a nonspecific reflex mucokinetic action, but their main benefit appears to be a placebo effect. If given in dosages that are close to the amount required to produce vomiting, an expectorant effect may be attained, but such dosages of many of these agents may have additional toxicity, and therefore their therapeutic use cannot be recommended.

Aerosolization of any drug into the lungs tends to result in a major portion of the agent being swallowed. When a mucokinetic drug is given by inhalation, much of the effect may in fact be attributed to gastric deposition with subsequent stimulation of the gastropulmonary mucokinetic reflex. Potentially nauseating drugs, such as the U.S. preparation of acetylcysteine and hypertonic saline, which are given by aerosol, may contribute much of their mucokinetic action through this unintended gastric activation of the vagal reflex.

It is also possible that stimulation of receptors in the pharynx with a potent drug can result in reflex vagal activation of the bronchial glands. For this reason, as was mentioned earlier, it is suggested that Tabasco pepper sauce can be an effective agent when 10 drops are administered in a glass of water. The patient should be encouraged to gargle the solution and then either spit it out or, preferably, swallow it, so as to stimulate both pharyngeal and gastric receptors. Advocates of pungently spiced chicken broth can also attribute its apparent mucokinetic action to its combined effect on pharyngeal and gastric receptors [111, 114].

Mucoregulators

Puchelle and colleagues [82, 83] have identified a group of drugs that alter the biochemical actions of the mucus-secreting glands so as to produce a less viscous output. These mucoregulators are thought to favor the synthesis of sialomucins that contribute a less viscous mucus. Such agents may result in a normalization of the rheologic properties of the secretions, and they may also have an effect on the airways, somehow reducing edema and bronchospasm. Several agents, previously thought of as expectorants or mucolytics, are more correctly categorized as mucoregulators. Thus, the main action of acetylcysteine may be its mucoregulator effect.

Bromhexine

Numerous herbs and plants used in folk remedies have been investigated, and one of the most successful mucokinetic derivatives that has reached the market from this source is bromhexine, which is a very individual molecule, unrelated to prior mucokinetic agents. The drug has been widely used in Europe, where it is mainly known as Bisolvon. It is given principally by mouth in a dosage of 8 to 16 mg three or four times a day, although it has been suggested that intravenous administration may be advantageous [70, 86].

The action of this agent is complex, but it is not a vagus-activating expectorant, nor does it have marked mucolytic effects. It appears to have its major action on the mucus-producing cells, and it results in the release of smaller mucoprotein molecules of lower viscosity. This action is alleged to be brought about by its influence on lysozyme and other cell enzymes [67]. It may also stimulate cilia, and it could possibly have other actions on the airways; indeed, its parent compound was used as an antiasthmatic [112, 119].

Bromhexine has been recommended mainly for the management of chronic bronchitis, but even this indication has been questioned by some investigators who have found little evidence of clinical effectiveness [67, 105]. Overall, it appears that the drug is likely to benefit only a select minority of patients with mucous hypersecretion. The drug has not been adequately studied in asthma, and it is doubtful whether it is of major value in this condition. A derivative of bromhexine, ambroxol (Mucosolvan) appears to have more impressive qualities. This agent has been shown to stimulate surfactant production [115], and it can be of clinical value in bronchitis [34] and asthma [66].

S-Carboxymethylcysteine

For many years *S*-carboxymethylcysteine (SCMC, carbocysteine) has been the subject of a great deal of attention [47]. This agent is a cysteine derivative, but it is a "blocked thiol," lacking the free thiol (—SH) group that makes drugs such as acetylcysteine so potent as mucolytics. It does not appear to be converted to an active thiol, and thus it is not a pro-drug [64]. It has been shown that SCMC has no mucolytic properties, nor does it activate the gastropulmonary reflex. Its effect appears to be at the cellular level in the bronchial glands where it serves as a mucoregulator [33, 82]. It may impair the incorporation of sialic acid residues into glycoprotein. SCMC results in an increased secretion of the less viscous sialomucins with corresponding diminution in production of the more viscous fucomucins. Several careful studies have suggested that daily use of the drug in chronic bronchitis will eventually restore the respiratory tract secretions to a more normal consistency, thereby facilitating sputum elimination [82, 86, 89]. The drug is said to be a possible bronchodilator, and it may reduce mucosal edema. It is also suggested that the drug is a "fluidifier" [33], increasing the volume output of sputum; this could also be described as a bronchomucotropic effect. The postulated effects of SCMC are compared in Table 69-10 with those of the other important mucokinetic agents that have been discussed.

Overall, the clinical value of SCMC remains rather controversial, and it is not clear that it is beneficial in asthma [42]. The drug continues to be studied extensively in Europe, where many practitioners consider it to be one of the mucokinetic agents of choice. In Europe it is known as Mucodyne, and it also has additional trade names such as Actithiol, Bronchipect, Fluifort, Lisomucil, Mucolex, Rhinathiol, Transbronchin, and Visclair-S [86]. It is usually given by mouth in a dosage of 750 to 1000 mg three times a day. Several related drugs have also been used in Europe and elsewhere, for example, carbocysteine-lysine [47], methylcysteine (Acdrile, Acthiol, Actiol, Visclair) [62, 74, 86], ethylcysteine (Daiace, Ethitanin) [86], letosteine [84], and erdosteine [87].

Sobrerol

This agent is relatively popular in Italy. It is obtained by hydration of the epoxide of pinene and thus has a close resemblance to terpin hydrate. It has been variously described as an emetic, an expectorant, a mucolytic, a fluidifier, and a bronchomucotropic, but it could best be described as a mucoregulator [117]. As is the case with other mucoregulators, long-term administration of sobrerol in chronic bronchitis has been reported to result in clinical benefit [15].

Iodinated Glycerol

The most interesting study on a mucokinetic drug in recent years was carried out on a long-established agent marketed in the United States. Iodinated glycerol (Organidin) is an organic iodide, iodopropylidene glycerol, and it had long been utilized as a well-tolerated mucolytic-expectorant. The drug was recently evaluated in 182 patients with chronic bronchitis in 75 different centers and compared in double-blind, randomized fashion with a placebo [78]. The subjects completed 8 weeks on the drug and on placebo, and clinical determinations were made both subjectively and objectively. Iodinated glycerol appeared to produce a significant improvement in pulmonary symptoms and in the ease of expectoration, accompanied by general subjective improvement. Thus, the drug had clinical effects comparable to those reported for other mucoregulators in European studies. No objective measurements of pulmonary function changes or in mucociliary clearance were evaluated. In his report of the study on iodinated glycerol, Petty [78] concluded that the symptomatic parameters of efficacy offered a meaningful index for evaluating mucokinetic therapy in chronic obstructive airway disease. This indeed could serve as a summary of the state of the art of mucokinetic therapeutics.

Garlic

Many of the world's pharmacopoeias list garlic as an expectorant [86, 114], and folk tradition attributes considerable value to this potent herb when used in the treatment of asthma and bronchitis [119]. For these reasons it is worth giving serious consideration to the chemical constituents that are characteristic of garlic. The major component is the nonodoriferous compound, alliin, or *S*-allyl-L-cysteine sulfoxide; when a garlic clove is crushed, the alliin is brought into contact with the intracellular enzyme alliinase, and this converts alliin to garlic's well-known odoriferous flavor, which is diallyl thiosulfinate, also known as allicin. The parent compound, alliin, could be reduced by suitable agents to desoxyalliin, which is *S*-allyl-L-cysteine. This latter molecule bears a remarkable resemblance to *S*-carboxymethylcysteine, and it may be postulated that ingested garlic in the body yields desoxyalliin, which would be expected to have mucoregulator properties (Fig. 69-2). It is worth noting that *S*-carboxymethylcysteine as well as methylcysteine and ethylcysteine are found in various vegetables, such as horseradish, radish, onion, pungent peppers, and mustard—agents that have obvious respiratory mucosal stimulating effects. As Widdicombe [108] points out,

Table 69-10. Actions of major mucokinetic agents

Agent	Mucolytic	Bronchorrheic	Bronchomucotropic	Expectorant emetic	Mucoregulator
Acetylcysteine	+ + +	+ + +	±	+ +	?
Bromhexine	+	−	−	−	+
Guaifenesin	+	−	−	+ +	+ + +
Iodide	+ +	+	+ + +	+ +	+ + *
Saline					
Normal	±	−	−	±	−
Hypertonic	+	+ + +	±	+ + +	−
S-Carboxymethylcysteine	−	−	?	−	+ + +
Sodium bicarbonate	+ +	+ +	±	+ +	−

+ + + = marked effect; + + = moderate effect; + = some effect; ± = equivocal effect; − = no effect; ? = unestablished.
* Organic iodide (iodinated glycerol).

$$CH_2 = CH \cdot CH_2 \cdot SO \cdot CH_2 \cdot CH(NH_2) \cdot COOH$$

(S-allyl-L-cysteine sulfoxide, alliin)

on reduction (perhaps with vitamin C)

$$CH_2 = CH \cdot CH_2 \cdot S \cdot CH_2 \cdot CH(NH_2) \cdot COOH$$

(S-allyl-L-cysteine, desoxyalliin)

Compare this product to the marketed oral mucokinetic drug S-carboxymethylcysteine (Mucodyne):

$$HOOC \cdot CH_2 \cdot S \cdot CH_2 \cdot CH(NH_2) \cdot COOH$$

Fig. 69-2. Alliin, a major constituent of garlic, is converted on reduction to desoxyalliin, which has a marked resemblance to S-carboxymethylcysteine. (Reprinted with permission from I. Ziment [ed]. Practical Pulmonary Disease. New York: Wiley, 1983.)

eating hot curry promotes production of sputum, but this common experience does not appear to have been subjected to laboratory evaluation.

Garlic is not a mucolytic (personal observations), but it could have other mucokinetic properties. It may stimulate the gastropulmonary vagal reflex, and other pungent spices probably do likewise. The volatile components of garlic are obviously excreted by the lung, and they may have local bronchomucotropic and bronchorrheic properties. Since chicken soup is also a well-known mucociliary stimulant [94], it is reasonable to regard a pungent, peppery, garlic-laden chicken broth to be the ideal mucokinetic that is currently available [114], and certainly any other potential expectorant or mucoregulator should be compared to this potent remedy as a standard.

REFERENCES

1. Aitken, M. L., Marini, J. J., and Culver, B. H. Humid air increases airway resistance in asthmatic subjects. *West. J. Med.* 149:289, 1988.
2. Allegra, L., and Bianco, S. Non-specific bronchoreactivity obtained with an ultrasonic aerosol of distilled water. *Eur. J. Resp. Dis.* 61(Suppl. 106): 41, 1980.
3. Anthonisen, N. R., Manfreda, J., and Warren, C. P. W. Antibiotic therapy in exacerbations of chronic obstructive pulmonary disease. *Ann. Intern. Med.* 106:196, 1987.
4. Avery, M. E. Mist Therapy 1973. In J. A. Mangos and R. C. Talamo (eds.), *Fundamental Problems of Cystic Fibrosis and Related Diseases.* Miami: Symposia Specialists, Intercontinental Medical Book, 1973. P. 291.
5. Aylward, M., Maddock, J., and Dewland, P. Clinical evaluation of acetylcysteine in the treatment of patients with chronic obstructive bronchitis: A balanced double-blind trial with placebo control. *Eur. J. Respir. Dis.* [Suppl.] 111:81, 1980.
6. Baker, J. W., Yerger, S., and Segar, W. E. Elevated plasma antidiuretic hormone levels in status asthmaticus. *Mayo Clin. Proc.* 51:31, 1976.
7. Bar-Or, O., Neuman, I., and Dotan, R. Effects of dry and humid climates on exercise-induced asthma in children and pre-adolescents. *J. Allergy Clin. Immunol.* 60:163, 1977.
8. Barton, A. D. Aerosolized detergents and mucolytic agents in the treatment of stable chronic obstructive pulmonary disease. *Am. Rev. Respir. Dis.* 110[Suppl]:104, 1974.
9. Basbaum, C. B., and Finkbeiner, W. E. Mucus-producing Cells of the Airways. In D. Massaro (ed.), *Lung Cell Biology.* New York: Marcel Dekker, 1989. Pp. 37–79.
10. Ben-Dov, I., Bar-Yishay, E., and Godfrey, S. Exercise-induced asthma without respiratory heat loss. *Thorax* 37:630, 1982.
11. Bone, R. C. Managing mucus secretion in patients with asthma or COPD. *J. Respir. Dis.* 11:240, 1990.
12. Boyd, E. M. *Respiratory Tract Fluid.* Springfield, Ill.: Thomas, 1972.
13. Boyd, E. M., and Lapp, M. S. On the expectorant action of parasympathomimetic drugs. *J. Pharmacol. Exp. Ther.* 87:24, 1946.
14. Braga, P. C., and Allegra, L. (eds.). *Drugs in Bronchial Mucology.* New York: Raven, 1989.
15. Castiglioni, C. L., and Gramolini, C. Effect of long-term treatment with sobrerol on the exacerbations of chronic bronchitis. *Respiration* 50:202, 1986.
16. Cato, A. E., Scott, J. A., and Sisson, G. M. The clinical significance of the hypertonicity of acetylcysteine preparations. *Respir. Care* 22:731, 1977.
17. Chen, W. Y., and Chai, H. Airway cooling and nocturnal asthma. *Chest* 81:675, 1982.
18. Chodosh, S. Acetylcysteine in chronic bronchitis. *Eur. J. Respir. Dis.* [Suppl.]111:90, 1980.
19. Chodosh, S., and Medici, T. C. Expectorant effect of glyceryl guaiacolate. *Chest* 64:543, 1973.
20. Chodosh, S., et al. Long-term use of acetylcysteine in chronic bronchitis. *Curr. Ther. Res.* 17:319, 1975.
21. Chopra, S. K., et al. Effects of hydration and physical therapy on tracheal transport velocity. *Am. Rev. Respir. Dis.* 115:1009, 1977.
22. Clarke, S. W. Management of mucus hypersecretion. *Eur. J. Respir. Dis.* 71(Suppl. 153):136, 1987.
23. Clarke, S. W., and Pavia, D. Lung mucus production and mucociliary clearance: Methods of assessment. *Br. J. Clin. Pharmacol.* 9:537, 1980.
24. Clarke, S. W., Thomson, M. L., and Pavia, D. Effect of mucolytic and expectorant drugs on tracheobronchial clearance in chronic bronchitis. *Eur. J. Respir. Dis.* [Suppl.]110:179, 1980.
25. Cohen, B. M., and Dressler, W. E. Acute aromatics inhalation modifies the airways: Effects of the common cold. *Respiration* 43:285, 1982.
26. Condon, R. E., and Nyhus, L. M. (eds.). *Manual of Surgical Therapeutics.* Boston: Little, Brown, 1978. Chap. 9.
27. Cumming, G., and Warwick, W. Water Vapour Handling in the Airways. In J. G. Scadding, G. Cumming, and W. M. Thurlbeck (eds.), *Scientific Foundations of Respiratory Medicine.* London: W. Heinemann, 1981. Chap. 17.
28. Darin, J. The need for rational criteria for the use of unheated bubble humidifiers. *Respir. Care* 27:945, 1982.
29. Davis, B. Mucous Secretion and Ion Transport in Airways. In J. F. Murray and J. A. Nadel (eds.), *Textbook of Respiratory Medicine.* Philadelphia: Saunders, 1988. Pp. 374–388.
30. Davis, S. S. Practical application of viscoelasticity measurements. *Eur. J. Respir. Dis.* [Suppl.]110:141, 1980.
31. Dulfano, M. J., Adler, K., and Wooten, O. Physical properties of sputum: IV. Effects of 100 percent humidity and water mist. *Am. Rev. Respir. Dis.* 107:130, 1973.
32. Dulfano, M. J., and Philippoff, W. Physical Properties. In M. J. Dulfano (ed.), *Sputum: Fundamentals and Clinical Pathology.* Springfield, Ill.: Thomas, 1973. Chap. 6.
33. Edwards, G. F., et al. S-Carboxymethylcysteine in the fluidification of sputum and treatment of chronic airway obstruction. *Chest* 70:506, 1976.
34. Ericsson, C. H., et al. Ambroxol therapy in simple chronic bronchitis: Effects on subjective symptoms and ventilatory function. *Eur. J. Respir. Dis.* 69:248, 1986.
35. Fazio, F., and Lafortuna, C. Effect of inhaled salbutamol on mucociliary clearance in patients with chronic bronchitis. *Chest* 80(Suppl):827, 1981.
36. Foster, W. M., Langenback, E. G., and Bergofsky, E. H. Respiratory drugs influence lung mucociliary clearance in central and peripheral ciliated airways. *Chest* 80(Suppl.):877, 1981.
37. Franceschinis, R., and Lualdi, P. (eds.). Mucolytics and oral acetylcysteine. *Eur. J. Respir. Dis.* [Suppl.] 111:1, 1980.
38. Gershwin, M. E., and Klingelhofer, E. L. *Asthma: Stop Suffering, Start Living.* Reading, MA: Addison Wesley, 1986. P. 127.
39. Gibson, L. E. Use of water vapor in the treatment of lower respiratory disease. *Am. Rev. Respir. Dis.* 110(Suppl.):100, 1974.
40. Godfrey, S. Exercise-induced Asthma. In M. E. Gershwin (ed.), *Bronchial Asthma: Principles of Diagnosis and Treatment.* New York: Grune & Stratton, 1981. Chap. 13.
41. Goldberger, E. *A Primer of Water, Electrolyte and Acid-Base Disturbances* (6th ed.). Philadelphia: Lea & Febiger, 1980.
42. Goodman, R. M., Yergin, B. M., and Sackner, M. A. Effects of S-carboxymethylcysteine on tracheal mucus velocity. *Chest* 74:615, 1978.
43. Graff, T. D. Humidification: Indications and hazards in respiratory therapy. *Anesth. Analg.* 54:444, 1975.
44. Grassi, C., Morandini, G. C., and Frigerio, G. Clinical evaluation of systemic acetylcysteine by different routes of administration. *Curr. Ther. Res.* 15:165, 1973.

45. Grassi, C., et al. Long-term oral acetylcysteine in chronic bronchitis: A double-blind controlled study. *Eur. J. Respir. Dis.* [Suppl.]111:93, 1980.

46. Gross, N. J., et al. Management of acute severe airways obstruction in the asthmatic patient. *American Thoracic Society News*, p. 11, Fall 1978.

47. Guffanti, E. E., Rossetti, S., and Scaccabarozzi, S. Carbocysteine. In P. C. Braga and L. Allegra (eds.), *Drugs in Bronchial Mucology.* New York: Raven, 1989. Pp. 147–170.

48. Gunn, J. A. The action of expectorants. *Br. Med. J.* 2:972, 1927.

49. Hess, D., et al. Subjective effects of dry versus humidified low-flow oxygen on the upper respiratory tract. *Respir. Ther.* 12:71, 1982.

50. Hirsch, S. R. The Role of Mucus in Asthma. In M. Stein (ed.), *New Directions in Asthma.* Park Ridge, IL: American College of Chest Physicians, 1975. Chap. 22.

51. Hirsch, S. R., Viernes, P. F., and Kory, R. C. The expectorant effect of glyceryl guaiacolate in patients with chronic bronchitis. *Chest* 63:9, 1973.

51a. Hubbard, R. C., et al. A preliminary study of aerosolized recombinant human deoxyribonuclease I in the treatment of cystic fibrosis. *N. Engl. J. Med.* 326:812, 1992.

52. Humidifier fever revisited (editorial). *Lancet* 1:1286, 1980.

53. Iravani, J., and Melville, G. N. Mucociliary function in the respiratory tract as influenced by physicochemical factors. *Pharmacol. Ther. B.* 2:471, 1976.

54. Irwin, R. S., and Pratter, M. R. Treatment of cough. *Chest* 82:662, 1982.

55. Jacobs, R., and Kaliner, M. Current Concepts of the Pathophysiology of Allergic Asthma. In R. F. Coburn (ed.), *Airway Smooth Muscle in Health and Disease.* New York: Plenum, 1989. Pp. 277–299.

55a. Jepsen, S., et al. Antioxidant treatment with N-acetylcysteine during adult respiratory distress syndrome: A prospective, randomized, placebo-controlled trial. *Crit. Care Med.* 20:918, 1992.

56. Kaliner, M., et al. Human respiratory mucus. *Am. Rev. Respir. Dis.* 134:612, 1986.

57. Kuhn, J. J., et al. Antitussive effects of guaifenesin in young adults with natural colds. *Chest* 82:713, 1982.

57a. Larson, M. Clinical recognition of N-acetylcysteine in chronic bronchitis. *Eur. Respir. Rev.* 2(7):5, 1992.

58. Lilker, E. S. Asthma is a disease: A new theory of pathogenesis. *Chest* 82:263, 1982.

59. Lourenco, R. V., and Costromanes, E. Clinical aerosols: II. Therapeutic aerosols. *Arch. Intern. Med.* 142:2299, 1982.

60. Lundgren, J. D., and Shelhamer, J. H. Pathogenesis of airway mucus hypersecretion. *J. Allergy Clin. Immunol.* 85:399, 1990.

61. Malik, S. K., and Jenkins, D. E. Alterations in airway dynamics following inhalation of ultrasonic mist. *Chest* 62:660, 1972.

62. Mann, B., Edwards, A., and Laurre, M. Methylcysteine hydrochloride in chronic bronchitis. *Br. J. Dis. Chest* 57:192, 1963.

63. Marriott, C., and Richards, J. H. The effects of storage and of potassium iodide, urea, N-acetylcysteine and triton X-100 on the viscosity of bronchial mucus. *Br. J. Dis. Chest* 68:171, 1974.

64. Martin, R., Litt, M., and Marriott, C. The effect of mucolytic agents on the rheologic and transport properties of canine tracheal mucus. *Am. Rev. Respir. Dis.* 121:495, 1980.

65. Medici, T. C., and Radielovic, P. Effects of drugs on mucus glycoproteins and water in bronchial secretion. *J. Int. Med. Res.* 7:434, 1979.

66. Melillo, G., and Cocco, G. Ambroxol decreases bronchial reactivity. *Eur. J. Respir. Dis.* 69:316, 1986.

67. Melville, G. N., Ismail, S., and Sealy, C. Tracheobronchial function in health and disease: Effect of mucolytic substances. *Respiration* 40:329, 1980.

68. Meyer, F. A., and Silberberg, A. Structure and Function of Mucus. In *Respiratory Tract Mucus* (Ciba Foundation Symposium 54 [New Series]). New York: Elsevier, 1978. P. 203.

69. Millman, M., et al. Repeated bronchoscopy and lavages in a severely ill elderly patient. *Immunol. Allergy Pract.* 12:298, 1990.

70. Mossberg, B., et al. Clearance by voluntary coughing and its relationship to subjective assessment and effect of intravenous bromhexine. *Eur. J. Respir. Dis.* 62:173, 1981.

71. Nadel, J. A. Regulation of fluid and mucous secretion in airways. *J. Allergy Clin. Immunol.* 67:417, 1981.

72. Nadel, J. A. New approaches to regulation of fluid secretion in airways. *Chest* [Suppl.]80:849, 1981.

73. Nicotra, M. B., Rivera, M., and Awe, R. J. Antibiotic therapy of acute exacerbations of chronic bronchitis: A controlled study using tetracycline. *Ann. Intern. Med.* 97:18, 1982.

74. Palmer, K. N. V., Geake, M. R., and Brass, W. Clinical trial of methylcysteine hydrochloride in chronic bronchitis. *Br. Med. J.* 1:280, 1962.

75. Parke, D. V. Pharmacology of mucus. *Br. Med. Bull.* 34:89, 1978.

76. Pavia, D., Thomson, M. L., and Clarke, S. W. Enhanced clearance of secretions from the human lung after the administration of hypertonic saline aerosol. *Am. Rev. Respir. Dis.* 117:199, 1978.

77. Pavia, D., et al. General review of tracheobronchial clearance. *Eur. J. Respir. Dis.* 71(Suppl. 153):123, 1987.

78. Petty, T. L. The national mucolytic study: Results of a randomized, double-blind, placebo-controlled study of iodinated glycerol in chronic obstructive bronchitis. *Chest* 97:75, 1990.

79. Phipps, R. J., Nadel, J. A., and Davis, B. Effects of alpha-adrenergic stimulation on mucus secretion and on ion transport in cat trachea in vitro. *Am. Rev. Respir. Dis.* 121:359, 1980.

80. Popa, V. The classic antihistamines (H₁ blockers) in respiratory medicine. *Clin. Chest Med.* 7:367, 1986.

81. Proctor, D. F., and Swift, D. L. Temperature and Water Vapor Adjustment. In J. D. Brain, D. F. Proctor, and L. M. Reid (eds.), *Respiratory Defence Mechanisms,* Part I. New York: Marcel Dekker, 1977.

82. Puchelle, E., Aug, F., and Polu, J. M. Effect of the mucoregulator S-carboxymethylcysteine in patients with chronic bronchitis. *Eur. J. Clin. Pharmacol.* 14:177, 1978.

83. Puchelle, E., and Sadoul, P. The effect of mucolytic agents on the rheologic and transport properties of canine tracheal mucus. *Am. Rev. Respir. Dis.* 122:808, 1980.

84. Puchelle, E., et al. Drug effects on viscoelasticity of mucus. *Eur. J. Respir. Dis.* [Suppl.]110:195, 1980.

85. Rasmussen, J. B., and Glennow, C. Reduction in days of illness after long-term treatment with *N*-acetylcysteine controlled-release tablets in patients with chronic bronchitis. *Eur. Respir. J.* 1:351, 1988.

86. Reynolds, J. E. F. (ed.). *Martindale: The Extra Pharmacopoeia* (28th ed.). London: Pharmaceutical Press, 1982.

87. Ricevuti, G., et al. Influence of erdosteine, a mucolytic agent, on amoxycillin penetration into sputum in patients with an infective exacerbation of chronic bronchitis. *Thorax* 43:585, 1988.

88. Richards, J. H., and Marriott, C. Effect of relative humidity on the rheologic properties of bronchial mucus. *Am. Rev. Respir. Dis.* 109:484, 1974.

89. Richardson, P. S., and Peatfield, A. C. The control of airway mucus secretion. *Eur. J. Repir. Dis.* 71(Suppl. 153):43, 1987.

90. Richardson, P. S., and Phipps, R. J. The anatomy, physiology, pharmacology and pathology of tracheobronchial mucus secretion and the use of expectorant drugs in human disease. *Pharmacol. Ther. B* 3:441, 1978.

91. Rodnick, J. E., and Gude, J. K. The use of antibiotics in acute bronchitis and acute exacerbations of chronic bronchitis. *West. J. Med.* 149:347, 1988.

92. Rose, B. D. *Clinical Physiology of Acid-Base and Electrolyte Disorders.* New York: McGraw-Hill, 1977.

93. Rosenbluth, M., and Chernick, V. Influence of mist tent therapy on sputum viscosity and water content in cystic fibrosis. *Arch. Dis. Child.* 49:606, 1974.

94. Rosner, F. Hot chicken soup for asthma. *Lancet* 2:1079, 1979.

94a. Sanstrand, B. Is N-acetylcysteine a free radical scavenger *in vivo*? The effect of N-acetylcysteine in oxygen-induced lung injury. *Eur. Respir. Rev.* 2(7):11, 1991.

95. Shim, C., King, M., and Williams, M. H. Lack of effect of hydration on sputum production in chronic bronchitis. *Chest* 92:679, 1987.

96. Shridharani, M., and Maxson, T. R. Pulmonary lavage in a patient in status asthmaticus receiving mechanical ventilation: A case report. *Ann. Allergy* 49:156, 1982.

97. Skillman, J. J. (ed.). *Intensive Care.* Boston: Little, Brown, 1975.

98. Skillman, J. J. Fluid, Electrolyte and Acid-Base Abnormalities. In M. L. Morrison (ed.). *Respiratory Intensive Care Nursing.* Boston: Little, Brown, 1979. Chap. 14.

99. Spector, S. L., Katz, F. H., and Farr, R. S. Troleandomycin: Effectiveness in steroid dependent asthma and bronchitis. *J. Allergy Clin. Immunol.* 54:367, 1974.

100. Stalcup, S. A. and Mellins, R. B. Mechanical forces producing pulmonary edema in acute asthma. *N. Engl. J. Med.* 297:592, 1977.

101. Strauss, R. H., et al. Influence of heat and humidity on the airway obstruction induced by exercise in asthma. *J. Clin. Invest.* 61:433, 1978.

102. Sturgess, J. M. Mucous secretion in the respiratory tract. *Pediatr. Clin. North Am.* 26:481, 1978.

103. Sutton, P. P., et al. Assessment of the forced expiration technique, postural drainage and directed coughing in chest physiotherapy. *Eur. J. Respir. Dis.* 64:62, 1983.

104. Thompson, B. T., et al. Pulmonary Emergencies. In E. W. Wilkins, Jr. (ed.), *Emergency Medicine: Scientific Foundations and Current Practice* (3rd ed.). Baltimore: Williams & Wilkins, 1989. Pp. 143–167.

105. Trembath, P. W. Bronchial Mucus and Mucociliary Transport. In J. G. Scadding, G. Cumming, and W. M. Thurlbeck (eds.), *Scientific Foundations of Respiratory Medicine.* London: W. Heinemann, 1981. Chap. 18.

106. Walker, W. G., and Whelton, A. Water Metabolism. In A. M. Harvey et al. (eds.), *The Principles and Practice of Medicine* (20th ed.). New York: Appleton-Century-Crofts, 1980. Chap. 5.

107. Wanner, A., and Rao, A. Clinical indications for and effects of bland, mucolytic, and antimicrobial aerosols. *Am. Rev. Respir. Dis.* 122 (Suppl.):79, 1980.

108. Widdicombe, J. G. Control of secretion of tracheobronchial mucus. *Br. Med. Bull.* 34:57, 1978.

109. Williams, T. J., and Yarwood, M. Effect of glucocorticosteroids on microvascular permeability. *Am. Rev. Respir. Dis.* 141:S39, 1990.

110. Ziment, I. Mucokinesis: The methodology of moving mucus. *Respir. Ther.*, p. 15, Mar./April 1974.

111. Ziment, I. What to expect from expectorants. *J.A.M.A.* 236:193, 1976.

112. Ziment, I. *Respiratory Pharmacology and Therapeutics.* Philadelphia: Saunders, 1978. Chaps. 2 and 3.

113. Ziment, I. Expectorants in chronic bronchitis. *Respir. Care* 27:1398, 1982.

114. Ziment, I. (ed.). *Practical Pulmonary Disease.* New York: Wiley, 1983. Chaps. 3, 6, and 9.

115. Ziment, I. Mucokinetic Agents. In M. A. Hollinger (ed.), *Current Topics in Pulmonary Pharmacology and Toxicology.* New York: Elsevier Science, 1987. Pp. 122–155.

116. Ziment, I. Theophylline and mucociliary clearance. *Chest* 92(Suppl.): 38S, 1987.

117. Ziment, I. Agents that affect respiratory mucus. *Prob. Respir. Care* 1:15, 1988.

118. Ziment, I. Drugs Modifying the Sol-Layer and the Hydration of Mucus. In P. C. Braga and L. Allegra (eds.), *Drugs in Bronchial Mucology.* New York: Raven, 1989. Pp. 293–322.

119. Ziment, I. Historic Overview of Mucoactive Drugs. In P. C. Braga and L. Allegra (eds.), *Drugs in Bronchial Mucology.* New York: Raven, 1989. Pp. 1–33.

120. Ziment, I. Help for an overtaxed mucociliary system: Managing abnormal mucus. *J. Respir. Dis.* 12:21, 1991.

120a. Ziment, I. Pharmacologic control of mucus secretion. In A. Junod, D. Olivieri, and E. Pozzi (eds.), *Endothelial and Mucus Secreting Cells.* Milan: Masson, 1991. Pp. 269–283.

121. Ziment, I., and Au, J. P. Anticholinergic agents. *Clin. Chest Med.* 7:355, 1986.

Immunotherapy

David F. Graft
Martin D. Valentine

70

Immunotherapy, the administration by subcutaneous injection of graded doses of allergenic extracts, has been part of the therapeutic armamentarium against allergic respiratory disease, including asthma, for over three-fourths of a century. In 1918, Robert Cooke wrote that the asthmatic symptom (of allergy) is controlled (by immunotherapy) far more easily than the nasal manifestation [32], an impression shared by Francis Rackemann [95]. For much of its existence, its use has aroused controversy and the present time is no exception [18, 33, 45, 60, 61a, 63, 64, 69, 86, 120, 124, 126, 127]. It was first used by an English physician, Noon, who showed that immunotherapy produced improvement in patients with hay fever (allergic rhinitis), in whom a stronger concentration of allergen extract was required to elicit conjunctival inflammation after a course of treatment [82]. In relatively short order, the types of extracts and the purported clinical indications for their use expanded markedly, leading to a general mistrust of the technique in the medical community.

Since 1950, about 100 controlled therapeutic trials of allergen immunotherapy have been performed. These, for the most part, have validated that patients with IgE-mediated disease are improved with allergen-specific immunotherapy. The extent of improvement and an analysis of the risks and benefits are discussed later. Several years ago, we reviewed the topic of immunotherapy in the context of allergic respiratory disease, considered the antigens used and the mechanism of its action, and concentrated on its use in the treatment of allergic rhinitis [44]. To consider the role of immunotherapy in the treatment of asthma, one must evaluate the importance of allergy in asthma [76], the mechanism(s) by which allergy might worsen asthma, and the evidence which supports the hypothesis that antiallergic intervention is successful in reducing asthmatic symptoms. The terms *extrinsic* and *intrinsic* asthma were coined by Rackemann and refer to the concept that triggers of wheeze, cough, and chest tightness are either allergic or nonallergic [95]. As we discuss, these situations are neither mutually exclusive nor unrelated inasmuch as there is evidence to suggest that allergic mechanisms can increase nonspecific bronchial reactivity, in turn leading to lowering of the threshold for bronchoconstriction by nonspecific irritants, such as cold air, exercise, or upper respiratory tract infections. We believe allergic asthma to be the result of a several-stage process: First, in the genetically predisposed (atopic) individual, allergen exposure induces the production of allergen-specific IgE, which binds by its Fc portion to the surface of mast cells and basophils. On subsequent exposure, the allergen binds to and cross-links the IgE. A chemical process involving calcium movement culminates in the release of preformed histamine and the synthesis of eicosanoids, potent mediators of bronchospasm; these processes have been detailed in the Mechanisms section.

The importance of allergen-induced inflammation in asthma has recently become more widely appreciated. Alexander found that 52.7 percent of 4,809 bronchial asthma patients had positive skin test responses to pollens, animal danders, or feathers [3]. A higher proportion (84%) of pediatric and adult patients at a London asthma clinic were found to have positive responses on prick skin tests with various aeroallergens [4]. Blair tested 314 patients with a history of wheeze and reversible airway obstruction seen in a large group practice; 66 percent had positive prick test responses to house dust, dust mite, feathers, cat, dog, or horse danders, wool, or five kinds of molds [8]. Chafee and Settipane reported that 76 percent of 1,775 asthmatics seen by a private practice allergist had positive skin test results [27]. Moreover, in the pulmonary clinic at the university hospital in the same city, 42 of 72 consecutive referred adult asthmatics had positive skin test reactivity [59]. Burrows and colleagues studied the relationship of self-reported asthma to serum IgE levels in 2,657 subjects in a stratified random sample in Tucson, Arizona [24]. Geometric means of log IgE values were calculated because IgE values show a lognormal distribution in the general population. Age- and sex-standardized IgE z scores indicated the number of standard deviations by which individual subjects differed from the mean for their age- and sex-specific group. They found that the prevalence of asthma increased as serum IgE increased for all age groups ($p < .0001$). In fact, no asthma was present in the 177 subjects with the lowest IgE levels ($z < -0.46$) for their age and sex. They concluded that asthma is almost always associated with some type of IgE-related reaction and, therefore, has an allergic basis. Furthermore, Sears and colleagues have shown that there is a correlation between airway hyperresponsiveness and serum total IgE level [104a].

There have been many anecdotal reports concerning asthma associated with exposure to animal danders (cats, dogs, horses, or laboratory animals) and other at-home allergens. For example, visiting a house occupied by a cat will cause sneezing, rhinorrhea, and itchy eyes in the cat-allergic individual; if the visitor also has asthma, wheezing and shortness of breath often develop. In the Midwest, ragweed season in August and September can precipitate seasonal asthmatic symptoms.

Another way to assess the role of allergy in asthma is to examine the link between allergic factors and the rate of emergency room visits for asthma, such as in the report from Salvaggio's group, which found epidemic asthma associated with high levels of airborne basidiospores in New Orleans [104]. Reid and associates reported that rises in emergency room and hospital admissions at Travis Air Force Base in northern California for status asthmaticus coincided with rises in rye grass pollen counts (Fig. 70-1) [99]. In a follow-up study during the grass pollen season of 1986, 92 percent of the patients seen for asthma in their emergency room were found to have significant rye grass pollen–specific IgE antibody (Fig. 70-2). This compared to the rate of only 14 percent found in age-matched control patients seen in the emergency room for other reasons or in hospital employees (odds ratio = 69, $p < .001$) [92]. A similar study in Charlottesville,

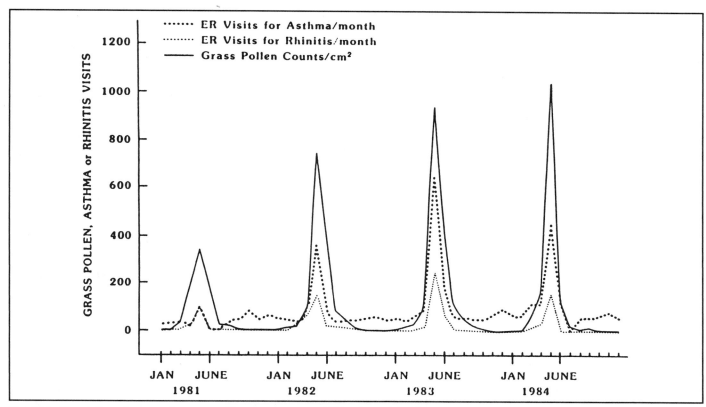

Fig. 70-1. *Correlation of grass pollen count with emergency room (ER) asthma visits. (Reprinted with permission from M. J. Reid, et al. Seasonal asthma in northern California: allergic causes and efficacy of immunotherapy.* J. Allergy Clin. Immunol. *78:590, 1986.)*

Virginia on 102 adults with acute asthma requiring emergency room visits revealed that 70 percent of patients under 50 years old had significant elevations of IgE antibody to one of five common inhalant allergens (dust mite [*Dermatophagoides farinae*], cockroach, cat dander, grass pollen, and ragweed pollen) [93]. Of controls without asthma, only 15 percent had similar levels.

Finally, it has been known for some time that allergic asthma can be simulated in the laboratory. "Bronchoprovocation," in which an allergic asthmatic subject inhales a nebulized extract of the incriminated allergen, results in asthmatic symptoms and measured decreases in 1-second forced expiratory volume (FEV_1) and airway conductance. Initially, the fact that the inhalation of whole pollen grains did not elicit a bronchoconstrictive effect presented an intellectual quandary [128]. Pollen grains at a size of 20 μ in diameter are too large to gain admittance to the bronchi and this seemed to explain why they might not cause symptoms. However, this had to be reconciled with the well-known clinical scenario in which allergic asthmatic patients experience increased symptoms during the pollen season. Agarwal and coworkers at the Mayo Clinic measured airborne antigen E, ragweed allergen, and ragweed pollen grains, and documented that a significant amount of total allergenic activity can be measured in the air as a result of pollen fragments and microaerosol suspensions of specific ragweed antigens, helping to explain the apparent paradox [2]. The Johns Hopkins group showed that bronchoprovocation with fragmented ragweed pollen grains did cause a fall in FEV_1 in the same patients who were unaffected by intact ragweed pollen grains [103].

The reader is referred to a recent national report (NHANES II) sampling approximately 4200 caucasians, age 6-24 years, which reviews the evaluation of specific allergen reactivity associated with asthma and other allergic disorders [132].

How might allergic sensitization result in the chronic asthmatic state? Allergen bronchoprovocation produces an immediate bronchoconstriction that is followed in 4 to 6 hours, in some subjects, by another period of decreased airflow (the late-phase response). A similar process also occurs in the nose with allergic rhinitis. The pathophysiology of the early versus late phases appears quite different. The early phase, initiated by antigen linking with IgE antibodies bound to basophils or mast cells, is due to the effects of mediators, such as histamine, leukotrienes, and prostaglandins, which cause both rapid and slow contractions of airway smooth muscle. It can be abrogated by sympathomimetic bronchodilators or by the prophylactic use of cromolyn sodium. The late-phase reaction, as discussed in Chapter 12, is associated with the development of airway inflammation and increased bronchial reactivity. Chemotactic agents released as a part of the early phase recruit eosinophils and neutrophils into the area. These cells, as well as lymphocytes and platelets, are the source of more mediators, including toxic materials such as major basic protein, platelet-activating factor, and other vasoactive and spasmogenic agents and cytokines, whose presence contributes to a smoldering inflammatory state. The cellular infiltrate is associated with epithelial injury, bronchial edema, mucous gland hyperplasia, and smooth muscle hypertrophy. The late-phase response can be prevented or blunted by using cromolyn or corticosteroid before allergen exposure.

The degree of inflammatory cell infiltrate has been shown to correlate with the amount of bronchial hyperresponsiveness [123]. Fatal asthma is associated with marked inflammatory changes in the submucosa [36], but recent evidence demonstrated that epithelial injury, especially to ciliated cells, is present even in patients with mild asthma [61]. Subepithelial fibrosis has been demonstrated in the bronchi of asthmatics [101]. A recent French report found that the severity of asthma related to the numbers of eosinophils in bronchoalveolar fluid ($p < .001$)

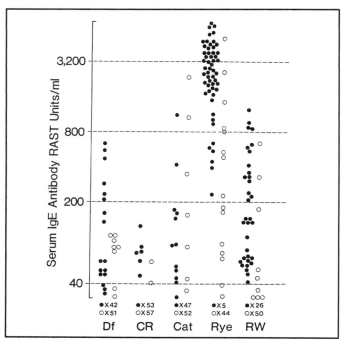

Fig. 70-2. *Elevated titers, as determined by radioallergosorbent testing, to rye grass pollen in emergency room asthmatics. Df = Dermatophagoides farinae; CR = cockroach; RW = ragweed; • = asthma; ○ = no asthma. (Reprinted with permission from S. M. Pollart, et al. Epidemiology of the emergency room asthma in northern California: Association with IgE antibody to rye grass pollen. J. Allergy Clin. Immunol. 82:224, 1988.)*

and in intraepithelial locations ($p < .03$) in bronchial biopsy specimens [17]. The eosinophil is particularly prominent in the allergic inflammatory response, and a role for the eosinophil and eosinophil major basic protein in causing airway epithelial alterations [47] and increased nonspecific airway responsiveness has been suggested by animal experiments [39]. In addition, epithelial damage may result in the loss of an epithelial relaxant factor, which may predispose to bronchoconstriction [118]. Furthermore, exposed epithelial nerves may respond in an exaggerated fashion to nonspecific irritants—bronchial hyperreactivity [6].

More than 40 years ago, Herxheimer argued that the late response provides the best model for studying the asthmatic condition [49] (particularly the late response). More recently, Cockcroft proposed a model in which allergic processes, especially the late-phase portion, lead to the development of bronchial hyperreactivity [28]. Increased bronchial reactivity is the most characteristic feature in asthma [10]. The clinical correlate appears to be an increased response to nonspecific irritants such as cold air, exercise, emotional upsets, upper respiratory tract infections, cigarette smoke, and other air pollutants. In this fashion, allergic factors can set the stage for entirely nonallergic triggers to cause an increase in asthma symptoms. Furthermore, a vicious cycle is set in motion since the same amount of allergen exposure causes more serious symptoms when heightened bronchial reactivity is present [30]. The degree of bronchial reactivity has been correlated to the severity of asthma and to the amount of medication required for symptom control [57]. Bronchial hyperresponsiveness may also predispose an individual to more severe chronic obstructive lung disease of the nonreversible type (chronic bronchitis and emphysema) [40, 85]. Woolcock has asserted that a reduction in reactivity should be the principal goal of asthma therapy [130].

An increase in nonallergic bronchial responsiveness in grass pollen–sensitive asthmatics during natural pollen exposure was

first noted by Altounyan [4]. A decade later, Boulet and associates studied 13 patients with histories of seasonal increases in asthma. Beginning several weeks before and continuing about a month after the ragweed season, symptom diaries, peak expiratory flow rates, and pollen counts were recorded. Repeated methacholine challenges were performed. A decrease in the provocative concentration (PC_{20}) of methacholine required to cause a 20 percent drop in FEV_1 occurred early in the ragweed season (the preseason mean PC_{20} for methacholine was 6.34 mg/ml and the mean lowest PC_{20} for methacholine during the season was 2.63 mg/ml [$p = .004$]) and, most interestingly, did not return to preseason levels for over a month [9]. Studies the following winter showed that the seasonal increase in methacholine responsiveness was limited to the patients who showed a dual (early and late) response to ragweed bronchoprovocation [9]. Sotomayor and coworkers in France studied 10 grass-allergic asthmatics by carrying out carbachol challenges before the season, during the season, and during two study treatments (double-blind, randomized, crossover protocol of oral methylprednisolone, 16 mg/day for 7 days, versus placebo) [108]. They verified that a seasonal increase in bronchial reactivity occurred in pollen-allergic asthmatics and also showed that this increase could be reversed by oral corticosteroid use [108]. Moreover, Eggleston noted a decrease during ragweed season in the amount of exercise required to cause a significant drop in FEV_1 [38].

Cockcroft and associates also showed that allergen bronchoprovocation also leads to increased bronchial hyperreactivity [29]. They measured bronchial reactivity to inhaled histamine and methacholine in 13 asthmatic subjects before and after allergen inhalation in the laboratory. All subjects demonstrated an early asthmatic response; 4 showed definite late-phase responses and an additional 3 had equivocal late responses. The group of 7 subjects who demonstrated elevated nonspecific bronchial reactivity was composed of the 4 patients with definite late responses and 3 of the 5 patients with borderline late responses [29]. The magnitude and duration of the heightened bronchial reactivity were found to correlate with the severity of the late-phase response [26]. It was shown that following allergen challenge, the histamine bronchial hyperresponsiveness increases before the onset of late-phase symptoms [37]. Decreases in exercise tolerance following bronchoprovocation have also been reported [79]. However, not all authors have found a strong association between nonspecific bronchial hyperreactivity and the clinical expression of asthma. Josephs and colleagues reported on several patients in whom exacerbations of asthma occurred in the absence of bronchial hyperreactivity [56]. Much remains to be learned about the interactions of allergy, inflammation, bronchial reactivity, and asthma severity.

A recent 11-year English study evaluated the relation between exposure to mite allergen and the development of allergic sensitization and asthma [109]. All but one of the children with asthma at 11 years old had been exposed at 1 year old to *Der p* allergen levels of more than 10 µg/ml of dust; for this exposure, the relative risk of developing asthma was 4.8-fold higher than if lower levels were present ($p = .05$) [109].

In contrast, there are some promising indications that management of the allergic process by decreasing exposure can lead to a decrease in asthma symptoms. Platts-Mills and coworkers studied the long-term effects of avoiding domestic allergens in nine mite-allergic adult asthmatic subjects by having them live in hospital rooms (very low mite concentrations) for at least 2 months [91]. Symptoms and early morning peak flows improved, and bronchial reactivity decreased. Indeed, five patients had a progressive eightfold or greater increase in the provocative dose (PD_{30}) of histamine required to cause a 30 percent drop in FEV_1, and for the seven patients who could undergo repeated histamine bronchial challenges, the combined p value of the change was less than .001.

Table 70-1. Possible mechanisms of action of immunotherapy

1. Decrease in allergen-specific IgE over time
2. Ablation of expectant postseasonal rise in allergen-specific IgE
3. Increase in allergen-specific IgG-blocking antibodies
4. Increase in allergen-specific IgG and IgA antibodies in nasal secretions
5. Decrease in allergen-induced basophil histamine release in some patients
6. Decrease in antigen-induced proliferation of lymphocyte mediators
7. Generation of antigen-specific suppressor cells

Table 70-2. When to consider immunotherapy for asthma

1. Allergens are demonstrated to be the essential basis for the majority of asthma symptoms.
2. Avoidance measures and medication have not yielded acceptable results.
3. Clinical trials have demonstrated efficacy (pollens, mite, mold? animal danders?).
4. Risks and benefits of immunotherapy with the allergen in question favor its use.

Murray and Ferguson of Vancouver, Canada studied the effects of a dust-free bedroom by supplying zippered vinyl covers for pillows, mattresses, and box springs and made other dust-avoidance suggestions to 10 asthmatic children; no advice was given to a matched group [77]. After 1 month, those with a dust-free bedroom had fewer wheezing days, lower medication use, and better peak flow rates, and bronchial tolerance to histamine was significantly improved [77]. Finally, Walshaw and Evans reported on the benefits of a longer period of allergen avoidance in 50 mite-sensitive adults with asthma. Those who used plastic mattress and pillow covers for 1 year had 100-fold declines in mite levels on the mattresses, and significant improvement in symptom scores, use of medications, peak expiratory flow rates, and histamine PC_{20} [122].

Shampain and colleagues, using neonatally immunized rabbits that produce only IgE antibodies, developed an antigen bronchopulmonary model in which (as in humans) there is an IgE-dependent early and late reaction. The IgG antibody from active or passive immunization ablates the late, but not the early response [105]. Since it has been known for some time that immunotherapy results in an increase in allergen-specific IgG antibodies, this model may provide a mechanism for some of the benefits resulting from immunotherapy. Possible mechanisms of the action of immunotherapy are summarized in Table 70-1.

With this framework in place, one can begin to consider the place of immunotherapy in the treatment of asthma (Table 70-2). What are the goals of this form of treatment? How closely do the results of clinical studies suggest that one can match these expectations? Finally, how do the benefits and risks of immunotherapy compare with alternative methods such as avoidance or treatment with the various classes of pharmacologic agents?

An obvious goal of immunotherapy is to demonstrably reduce that portion of a patient's symptoms of asthma that can be attributed to the allergen in question. An additional, but perhaps more difficult aim is to reduce the patient's comprehensive asthma severity. Obviously, in order to accomplish this, the allergen used in immunotherapy must be the essential basis for the majority of asthma symptoms. As discussed above, an allergen may cause primary symptoms or be the cause of increased bronchial reactivity, which can predispose to secondary symptoms. Alternatively, a combination of allergens may concurrently affect the patient with multiple significant allergic sensitivities. This is the situation that most closely resembles what the allergist deals with in actual practice.

The various allergens present distinct problems. The amount of exposure may be intermittent, seasonal, or nearly constant and findings for one allergen may not be generally applicable to all others. For example, well-standardized extracts (pollens and mites) bear little relationship to molds and dust. Mold extracts are made from both the spores and mycelia; the antigens are more complex than those of plant pollens. House dust has been obtained from vacuum sweepers, mattresses, and so on, and contains a variety of substances including mites, foodstuffs, and human skin scales. One report showed that there was enough cat allergen present in house dust extracts to result in positive results on house dust tests in cat-allergic individuals [21]. See also Chapter 40 for a discussion of this topic.

Immunotherapy trials with house dust (Table 70-3) have yielded mixed results. Part of this can be ascribed to the diverse materials used. In 1949, Bruun studied 189 patients treated with dust extract or placebo for 2 years [23]. Whereas 78 of 95 asthmatic subjects who received dust injections had decreases in severity of symptoms, only 28 of 82 placebo controls improved. The British Tuberculosis Association in 1968 reported the effectiveness of dust versus placebo immunotherapy in 70 patients with asthma [20]. Entry criteria included a history incriminating dust as the cause of paroxysmal wheezing or dyspnea, a positive response to dust on a prick skin test and an absence of seasonal or animal dander–related symptoms. The subjects received 15 weekly injections. Six months of diary records failed to discern a difference between the two groups in wheezing frequency, activity permitted, or medication usage. Expiratory peak flows improved in 18 of 30 patients receiving dust injections and 19 of 35 placebo patients. In a longer study, Aas in 1971 reported improvement in children with asthma receiving either of two extracts as compared to placebo for 3 years [1]. Eighty subjects with a positive skin response and bronchial obstruction following bronchoprovocation with dust extract were enrolled and parents' assessment of asthma severity, number of school days missed, and medication use were recorded. Bronchoprovocation tests were performed at the end of the treatment protocol. The dust group fared better by both the subjective and the objective criteria (although some dissociation of these two variables was found) [1].

Since the mite was identified as the primary cause of house dust sensitivity, most studies have concentrated on the mite (Table 70-4). Two important mites have been identified: the *D. farinae*, which is most prevalent in the United States, and the *Dermatophagoides pteronyssinus*, which dominates in Europe. In 1971 Maunsell and coauthors reported on a 6- to 9-month trial of *Der f* versus dust in asthmatic adults with positive skin responses to both [73]. No injection reactions occurred. When the patient's opinion about his or her asthma condition, the number of attacks, and the daily need for medication were considered, 78 percent of the mite group compared to only 38 percent of the dust group demonstrated improvement. As is a common trend in more recent studies, Formgren and colleagues evaluated allergen-specific bronchial reactivity in a 1-year, double-blind, placebo-controlled study of *Der f* immunotherapy [41]. They found that bronchial allergen sensitivity was lower in the active group. Newton and colleagues found no evidence of clinical improvement but significantly decreased bronchial reactivity to mite [81]. They concluded that an allergic response to mite could be only one of many causes of asthma in those hypersensitive to that allergen. Murray and associates studied the effect of immunotherapy on nonspecific bronchial responsiveness [78]. They reported twofold greater reactivity to histamine in six of seven mite-sensitive asthmatic children following a 1-year treatment course of *Der f* injections [78]. As controls, they used mite-sensitive asthmatics receiving injections of allergens other than mite and eight mite-sensitive children with asthma who did not receive any injections; both of these groups tended to have decreased histamine responses.

Studies with *Der p* in Europe have generally yielded favorable

Table 70-3. Immunotherapy trials with dust extract

Allergen	Author(s)	Year	Length of treatment	Age group	Clinical parameters (no. improved/total) Extract	Placebo	Significant improvement	Decreased bronchial allergen sensitivity	Decreased nonspecific bronchial sensitivity
Dust	Bruun [23]	1949	2 yr	A	74/95	28/82	Yes	—	—
	British Tuberculosis Association [20]	1968	4 mo	A	18/30	19/35	No	—	—
	Aas [1]	1971	3 yr	C	43/51	16/28	Yes	Yes	—

A = adult; C = children.

Table 70-4. House dust mite immunotherapy trials

Allergen	Author(s)	Year	Length of treatment	Age group	Clinical parameters (no. improved/total) Extract	Placebo	Significant improvement	Decreased bronchial allergen sensitivity	Decreased nonspecific bronchial sensitivity
Mite (Der f)	Maunsell et al. [73]	1971	6–9 mo	C, A	14/18	6/16	Yes	—	—
	Newton et al. [81]	1978	1 yr	A	2/7	2/7	No	—	—
	Formgren et al. [41]	1984	1 yr				—	Yes	No
	Murray et al. [78]	1985	1 yr	C	4/7	2/4	No	No	No (↑)
Mite (Der p)	Smith [106]	1971	13 wk	C, A	10/11	3/11	Yes	—	—
	D'Souza [35]	1973	12 wk	C, A	25/40	14/43	Yes	—	—
	Pauli et al. [90]	1984	12 mo	A	3/9	4/9	Yes (limited)	—	—
	Gaddie et al. [43]	1976	13 ½ mo	C, A	—	—	No	—	—
	Marques and Avila [71]	1978	7 ½ mo	C, A	13/16	5/12	Yes	—	—
	Warner et al. [125]	1978	12 mo	C	23/27	12/24	Yes	Yes (late)	—
	British Thoracic Society [19]	1979	12–18 mo	C, A	19/33	9/18	No	—	—
	Bousquet et al. [12]	1985	7 wk	A	—/20*	—/10	—	Yes	—
	Bousquet et al. [14]	1988	1 yr	A, C	Asthma severity score improved from 3.2 to 1.1 in 171 patients	Asthma severity score worsened slightly from 3.0 to 3.2 in 44 patients	Yes	—	—
	Van Bever and Stevens [116]	1989	1 yr	C	13/15	0/8	Yes	Yes(late)	—

A = adult; C = children.
* This study did not examine clinical improvement—it examined changes in bronchial sensitivity to allergen.

results. Particularly interesting was a 1978 report from London by Warner and colleagues in which children receiving tyrosine-absorbed *Der p* or placebo for 1 year were compared in terms of reduction in medication use and bronchoprovocation responses (see Table 70-4) [125]. The strength of the conclusions of the study was increased by a 3-month preinjection assessment period during which all patients were effectively stabilized with mite-avoidance advice, including use of a plastic mattress cover to decrease allergen exposure, and medications were adjusted to achieve maximum benefit with minimum dose. Twenty-three of 27 patients in the mite group compared to 12 of 24 in the placebo group felt they had improved. Continuous attempts were made to reduce drug therapy; 15 of 21 versus only 6 of 21 in the active and placebo group, respectively, were able to completely discontinue medications. On repeat bronchial challenge with mite, the immediate response did not change for either group. However, 10 of 22 mite-treated children lost their late obstructive response while only 1 of 15 controls showed this effect. A series of recent studies from Belgium confirmed this finding [115–117]. Fifteen asthmatic children who demonstrated a late response to inhaled *Der p* were treated with this mite extract for 1 year. The late phase resolved in 5 subjects and as a group, the subjects had less severe late declines in FEV$_1$. They extended their study by taking children who had demonstrated a decline in late-phase

allergen response after a year of mite immunotherapy and randomized them for continued mite or placebo injections. After the second year of immunotherapy, the improvement in late-phase response was maintained but did not improve further. However, in the group who received placebo injections during the second year, a significant worsening of the late-phase response was observed. Nonspecific (methacholine or histamine) bronchial provocation responses were not examined in either study.

Bousquet and colleagues reported that 18 to 36 months of *Der p* immunotherapy led to a decrease in nonspecific (carbachol) sensitivity in mite-sensitive asthmatics [13]. These results differed from those of Murray and associates with *Der f* [78]. The British Thoracic Association compared an 18-month course of *Der p* injections to placebo therapy and obtained mixed results [19]. In asthmatic patients not taking steroids, the treated group did slightly better than controls. In contrast, in steroid-dependent patients, the active treatment group fared slightly worse. Later, in a large French study, Bousquet's group studied 171 mite-treated and 44 placebo-treated asthmatic children and adults [14]. Immunotherapy was initiated with a rush protocol. Using Aas' scoring system, which ranges from 0 to 4 for asthmatic severity, scores for the treated group improved from 3.2 to 1.1, but those for the placebo group showed no significant change from 3.0 to 3.2 ($p < .0001$). Medication scores declined and FEV$_1$ values

Table 70-5. Pollen extract immunotherapy trials

Allergen	Author(s)	Year	Length of treatment	Age group	Clinical parameters (no. improved/total) Extract	Clinical parameters (no. improved/total) Placebo	Significant improvement	Decreased bronchial allergen sensitivity	Decreased nonspecific bronchial sensitivity
Grass pollen	Frankland and Augustin [42]	1954	4 mo	C, A	29/31	8/26	Yes	—	—
	McAllen [74]	1969	3 mo	C, A	17/27	2/8	Yes	—	—
	Hill et al. [51]	1982	6 mo	C	In 1st season, symptom scores increased in both groups; in 2nd season, only placebo scores increased		No	—	—
	Ortolani et al. [88]	1984	10 mo	A	Lower symptom scores in 8 treated vs. 7 placebo patients		Yes	No	—
	Bousquet et al. [11]	1985	4 mo	C, A	23 patients; average symptom/ medication score = 0.9	10 patients; average symptom/ medication score = 2.7	Yes	—	—
	Reid et al. [99]	1986	8 mo	A	9 patients; symptom medication score = 47	9 patients; symptom medication score = 178	Yes	—	—
	Bousquet et al. [16]	1989	4 mo	A	39 patients; average symptom score = 15.1	18 patients; average symptom score = 54.8	Yes	—	—
Ragweed pollen	Bruce et al. [22]	1977	8 mo	A	15 patients; mean physician asthma score = 4.4	17 patients; mean physician asthma score = 4.1	No	No	—
Birch pollen	Rak et al. [97]	1988	4 mo	A	20 patients; average medication score = 2.8	20 patients; average medication score = 18.1	Yes	—	Yes (trend)

A = adult; C = children.

increased in the mite-injected group. The authors also noted that the highest rate of improvement occurred in those under 50 years old and with an FEV_1 greater than 70 percent of the predicted values for age, height, and sex. Additionally, the rate of serious adverse reactions to allergen injections was greater in those with an FEV_1 poorer than 70 percent of predicted [1].

It seems clear from the available evidence that there is little reason to use poorly defined house dust extracts for diagnosis or therapy. One of the reasons this material remains in common use is the high rate of positive skin test responses that occur due to the irritant response to an inappropriately high concentration of dust extract used by some practitioners. Furthermore, variable results can be expected, due to the diversity of source materials and the attendant disparity of the important allergen activities.

Pollen immunotherapy for asthma (Table 70-5) was the subject of a landmark study by Frankland and Augustin in 1954 [42]. Nearly all (29 of 31) of the grass pollen–treated patients improved while only 8 of 26 of the placebo group showed a similar result. In contrast, Hill and colleagues in 1982 reported no significant improvement in grass-allergic asthmatic children following 6 months of immunotherapy initiated with rush protocol 4 months before the grass season [51]. Five other studies demonstrated a positive effect of grass pollen injections. Ortolani and associates found lower symptom scores after only 5 months of grass pollen immunotherapy in eight treated patients when compared to seven who received placebo injections [88]. A study from the Travis Air Force Base in California yielded the graphic demonstration of the synchronous timing of grass pollen counts and emergency room visits for asthma shown earlier (see Fig. 70-1) [99]. The investigators also found that the severity of the grass pollen season, as scored by a combination of symptoms and medication use, was significantly lower (47 versus 178) in the patients receiving grass pollen extract injections (Fig. 70-3). Bousquet and colleagues reported similar results recently [16].

Fewer studies have been conducted with other pollens. The Johns Hopkins group reported negative results in a study with ragweed in 1977 [22]. However, many of the patients failed to show exacerbations of symptoms corresponding to increases in ragweed pollen counts. This finding was attributed to the possibility that many of the autumnal asthma symptoms were actually due to mold sensitivity. The investigators also used lower doses than what is typical for immunotherapy treatment of ragweed allergic rhinitis. A multicenter trial (still in progress) of the use of ragweed immunotherapy for treatment of seasonal asthma in adults has shown that those receiving ragweed had less medication use and better A.M./P.M. peak expiratory flow rates than those in the placebo group (P. S. Norman. Personal communication, 1992.) Finally, a Swedish study found that birch pollen–treated patients had a lower medication score (2.8 versus 18.1) during the spring after 4 months of injections [97]. There was a trend, without statistical significance, for treated patients to have smaller, birch pollen–associated seasonal rises in nonspecific bronchial responsiveness to histamine. Serum levels of eosinophil and neutrophil chemotactic activity and eosinophilic cationic protein were lower in those receiving immunotherapy. It was suggested that this indicated a decreased eosinophilic contribution to airway inflammation [96, 97].

Studies of mold immunotherapy (Table 70-6) in asthma have only appeared recently. Commercial extracts have differed markedly in their composition and allergenic potency [131]. In 1985

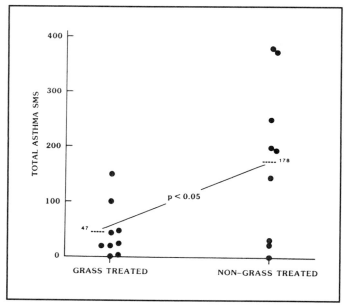

Fig. 70-3. *Total asthma (SMS) for both groups during the study period. SMS = symptom-medication score. (Reprinted with permission from M. J. Reid, et al. Seasonal asthma in northern California: Allergic causes and efficacy of immunotherapy.* J. Allergy Clin. Immunol. 78:590, 1986.)

Reed concluded his review of mold allergy by suggesting that with current information, mold injections and extracts should have a more limited use [98]. However, the situation has improved, at least for two molds, with the recent availability of two standardized extracts for *Cladosporium* and *Alternaria*. Dreborg and colleagues studied the effect of a 10-month course of standardized *Cladosporium herbarum* or placebo in 30 children with asthma [34]. General reactions occurred in 13 of 16 receiving mold therapy. Although symptom scores were similar for both groups, the *Cladosporium*-treated patients used less medication during the 2 weeks of highest mold spore counts. Furthermore, bronchial sensitivity decreased in the active group but not the placebo group. Horst and associates had to screen 6,000 patients to find patients who had no other perennial allergen sensitivity, in order to study the effectiveness of a 1-year, double-blind, placebo-controlled trial of standardized *Alternaria* extract [52]. About 10 of the 24 study patients had asthma. A score averaging symptoms and medications for combined asthma and rhinitis was significantly better in the treated group, although most of the difference appeared to be due to improved rhinitis. Although nasal challenges were improved in the active treatment group, no bronchial challenges were performed. Metzger and coworkers studied six patients treated with *Alternaria* extract and demonstrated a decrease in allergen-induced late-phase response in all subjects [75]. The early phase was reduced significantly in only one patient.

Most allergists recommend dismissal of the animal from the home in the case of dander sensitivity. Nevertheless, several studies have been performed in the last 15 years with animal dander materials (Table 70-7). In 1978, Taylor and coworkers studied 10 patients who had positive results on prick tests and

Table 70-6. Mold extract immunotherapy trials

Allergen	Author(s)	Year	Length of treatment	Age group	Clinical parameters (no. improved/total) Extract	Placebo	Significant improvement	Decreased bronchial allergen sensitivity	Decreased nonspecific bronchial sensitivity
Mold									
Cladosporium	Dreborg et al. [34]	1986	10 mo	C	Median medication scores in 16 extract patients lower than in 11 placebo patients		Yes	Yes	—
Alternaria	Cantani et al. [25]	1988	3 yr	C	31/39	0/40	Yes	—	—
Cladosporium	Malling et al. [70]	1986	5–7 mo	A	5/11	1/11	Yes	—	—
Alternaria	Horst et al. [52]	1990	1 yr	C, A	0.84* in 13 patients	3.55* in 11 patients	Yes	—	—

* Global symptom medication scores.
A = adult; C = children.

Table 70-7. Animal "dander" immunotherapy trials

Allergen	Author(s)	Year	Length of treatment	Age group	Clinical parameters (no. improved/total) Extract	Placebo	Significant improvement	Decreased bronchial allergen sensitivity	Decreased nonspecific bronchial sensitivity
Animal									
Cat	Taylor et al. [112]	1978	4 mo	A	—/5*	—/5	—	Yes	No
	Ohman et al. [87]	1984	4 mo	A	6/9	2/9	Yes	Yes	No
	Van Metre et al. [119]	1988	1 yr	A	11/11	4/11	—	Yes	No
Cat and dog	Sundin et al. [110]	1986	1 yr	C, A	13/22	5/17	Yes	Yes (cat)	Yes (cat)
	Bertelsen et al. [7]	1989	9 mo	C	—/14*	—/13	—	Yes	—
Dog	Valovirta et al. [114]	1986	1 yr	C	8/15	2/12	Yes	Yes	—

A = Adult; C = children.
* This study did not examine clinical improvement—it examined changes in bronchial sensitivity to allergen. Denominator = number of patients.

bronchial challenge to cat pelt extract [112]. The 5 patients who received active treatment for 4 months showed reduced bronchial sensitivity to cat allergen, whereas no improvement was seen in the placebo group. A few years later, the investigators confirmed their work and also demonstrated a parallel clinical correlation in that cat pelt extract treatment resulted in a significant delay in the onset of ocular and pulmonary symptoms on exposure to living cats [87]. A study by Van Metre and colleagues demonstrated similar results [119]. Valovirta and associates in Denmark studied 27 dog-sensitive asthmatic children and found that the active treated group fared better on several hours of natural dog exposure than did the placebo-treated patients [114]. Decreased bronchial sensitivity was also demonstrated.

Several studies have reported combined results of animal dander (cat or dog) injection therapy. A four-part report [48, 65, 67, 110] from Sweden documented the results of a 1-year, double-blind, placebo-controlled trial of cat or dog dander extracts in children and adults with mild to moderate asthma. Patients were matched for age, sex, clinical history, results of bronchial challenge, and IgE specificities in cat- and dog-crossed radioimmuno-electrophoresis. Patients' subjective assessment of the treatment alternatives were as follows: When cat allergen–treated patients were exposed to cat, 9 of 15 had reduced symptoms; for dog allergen–treated patients, 4 of 7 had less symptoms. In the placebo-treated group, only 5 of 17 had decreased symptoms after either cat or dog exposure. The cat allergen–treated patients experienced reduced specific (cat) allergen and histamine bronchial sensitivity, but the dog allergen–treated patients showed no changes. During the second year of the study, both groups received active treatment. Further decreases in cat and histamine bronchial responsiveness occurred in the group that continued on active treatment. In the group transferred to active treatment for the second year, significant decreases in cat and histamine bronchoprovocation thresholds occurred in those receiving cat extract [65]. In 1989, a Danish study used an open controlled protocol to study 27 animal-sensitive asthmatic children [7]. Entry criteria included positive results on skin tests, radioallergosorbent tests, and bronchial provocation tests to dog or cat. Children were excluded if allergy to mite was thought to be more important than dog or cat in causing the symptoms. The investigators found improved specific allergen bronchial tolerance after 9 months of therapy. Rohatgi and coworkers also demonstrated decreased cat- or dog-induced immediate and late asthmatic responses after immunotherapy [102].

In order to simplify and reduce the variables to be considered, most studies have evaluated the clinical or provocation response to a single putative allergen. However, this does not mirror the typical application of immunotherapy in the United States. One of the most intriguing outcomes of immunotherapy as it applies to asthma is a decrease in allergen-specific bronchial reactivity. Most studies that have examined this parameter have shown that immunized individuals could tolerate higher amounts of inhaled allergen before a predetermined decrease in airflow occurred. This improvement was more prominent for the late phase. While this may have some clinical significance, a demonstrated change in nonspecific bronchial reactivity would be more impressive [45, 64]. Although this is the logical outcome of a process that decreases the allergic contribution to airway inflammation and the resultant increase in bronchial responsiveness (as has resulted with strict allergen avoidance), this has not been found in the majority of studies that looked for it. However, since the effects of immunotherapy have been shown to be allergen specific [84], it seems unlikely that immunization to only one allergen in a polysensitized asthmatic patient would necessarily result in decreased nonspecific bronchial sensitivity because exposures to the other culprit allergens would continue to stimulate an inflammatory response.

Although these concepts are modern, the multiple-allergen sensitivity model was examined by Johnstone and coworkers [53–55] in a series of reports over 20 years ago. They concluded a 14-year prospective study in 1968 in which children were immunized to a variety of aeroallergens including pollens, molds, animal danders, and dust that were considered to provoke the perennial allergic asthmatic condition. Patients were randomized to placebo, low-dose, or conventional high-dose treatment regimens and kept diaries recording the number of days of wheezing and missed school days. Of 130 children still in the study by their 16th birthday, 68 percent and 78 percent of the patients receiving low-dose and high-dose treatment, respectively, were free of asthma, compared to only 22 percent of the placebo group. In addition, Tuchinda and Chai demonstrated a reduction in bronchial sensitivity to allergen after 5 to 12 months of immunotherapy with multiple allergens [113]. However, natural history studies have shown that between 30 and 70 percent of children with asthma can expect to be markedly improved or become symptom-free ("outgrowing asthma") by early adulthood [126a].

Another considerable advantage of Johnstone's studies was the length of treatment and observation. Many recent studies evaluated the effectiveness of relatively brief courses of therapy, some as short as 2 months. Although differences may be demonstrated this rapidly, it is possible that prolonged treatment courses induce further advantages. An example is the apparent decreased rate of symptom recrudescence if immunotherapy is continued for 5 years compared to just 2 years. The definitive studies of immunotherapy utilizing well-characterized extracts and modern methods of evaluating clinical responses in pediatric and adult allergic asthma are nearing conclusion (N. F. Adkinson. Personal communication, 1991).

The safety of allergy injections has been the subject of several committee reviews [31, 94, 127]. Untoward reactions following injection therapy are of several types. Local swelling at the injection site occurs in about 20 percent of patients and are a source of discomfort, not danger. Systemic or generalized reactions consist of urticaria, breathing difficulties attributable to laryngeal edema or bronchospasm, and hypovolemic shock which can be life-threatening [133]. They are not uncommon, particularly if a properly high dose (one that can be expected to result in measurable clinical improvement) is employed [62]. In a 6-month prospective French study, systemic reactions occurred in only 0.1 percent of more than 150,000 injections [121]. There were two episodes of anaphylactic shock, but no deaths. However, details of the immunotherapeutic regimen were not disclosed.

Greenberg and coauthors reported on the occurrence rate of injection reactions at four American military treatment centers [46]. Fifty-two systemic reactions (0.3%) resulted from 20,558 injections. Forty-two (7%) of 628 patients experienced systemic reactions. The most interesting finding was that 38 percent of the reactions occurred 35 minutes to 6 hours after the injections. Some studies found pollen [46] or mold extracts to be associated with more severe reactions [58, 89].

Recent attention has focused on fatal allergic reactions to immunotherapy [66, 83, 100]. Lockey and coworkers reported 32 deaths from injections, 8 from skin testing, and 6 others for which the cause was not stated, in the United States from 1945 to 1985 [66]. A portion of the fatalities were attributed to mistakes in dosage. In a 1986 report from the United Kingdom, the Committee on Safety of Medicines noted 26 deaths since 1957, with 5 occurring in the past 18 months [31]. In many of the subjects who died, the injections were given by general practitioners and apparently no facilities or equipment were available for treating general anaphylaxis [60]. In Sweden there has been one death reported in 20 years. Approximately 4 million injections were given during that time [60].

The attention directed at severe injection-induced reactions is particularly germane when considering immunotherapy in the treatment of asthma since asthmatic patients seem to have more severe reactions [15, 66]. In Lockey's report, 53 percent of the fatalities occurred in patients with asthma, suggesting that patients with hyperreactive airways are at particular risk of death should a generalized reaction occur [66]. Bousquet's group studied rush immunotherapy to mite in 125 asthmatic patients and found that 73 percent of subjects with an FEV_1 less than 80 percent of predicted values developed injection-induced wheezing, compared to only 13 percent of those with better pulmonary function results [15].

The role of immunotherapy in the overall treatment plan for asthma requires periodic reassessment [63, 64]. A decrease in exposure to avoidable allergens should be encouraged. A series of studies demonstrated means by which mite exposure can be diminished, and the clinical benefits that accrue [77, 91, 122]. Zippered plastic mattress encasings should be prescribed for every mite-allergic patient. Other allergen-avoidance measures may be ineffective or slow to manifest improvement [80, 129]. Platts-Mills argued that modern homes with wall-to-wall carpeting, central humidifiers, and limited air exchange have encouraged increased mite populations, mite sensitization, and perhaps increased prevalence of (allergic) asthma (T. A. E. Platts-Mills. Personal communication, 1991). Two new products may decrease mite allergen concentrations. Benzyl benzoate (Acarosan) is applied as a moist powder and kills mites. A reduction in allergen content would be expected to follow. Tannic acid solution has been shown to render mite and cat allergen nonallergenic by denaturation. The clinical effectiveness and long-term safety of these products have not been completely established; these measures are discussed further in Chapter 87.

The pharmacologic advances of recent years have resulted in a change in the use of immunotherapy [127]. Sustained-released medications, inhaled sympathomimetics with prolonged durations of action, wider use of cromolyn in pediatric asthma, and most importantly, a growing trend toward the use of inhaled steroids at doses capable of reducing airway inflammation and bronchial hyperresponsiveness [46a] have reduced the need for allergen immunotherapy. The benefits and risks of the various treatment modalities (avoidance, medications, and immunotherapy) need to be examined for each patient. Immunotherapy is a potentially dangerous, tedious treatment. Recurrent visits to the physician's office can be time-consuming, but may allow better "fine-tuning" of the patient's pharmacologic regimen and enhance compliance. What are the dangers of many years of oral theophylline or inhaled steroid use? Does a standard immunotherapy treatment course, for example, 5 years, have an effect into the future on what would have been the natural history of the process? If so, this would affect the cost-benefit comparison for drug versus injection therapy. Refinements in immunotherapy may improve results and decrease risks [5, 68, 72]. It has not been as easy to demonstrate efficacy of immunotherapeutic treatment in asthma as in allergic rhinitis. Nevertheless, well-controlled trials of immunotherapy in mite, pollen, animal dander, and more recently mold allergy have been promising. In practice, allergy injections are generally administered to patients who have significant allergic rhinitis. If a patient also has some degree of asthma, immunotherapy may produce a beneficial response for that problem as well. Whether immunotherapy should be considered for asthma alone depends on the clinical situation, and the parameters governing that decision require further refinement.

In summary, allergy is now generally considered to be important in the pathogenesis of asthma in children and adults. Avoidance measures and medications are frequently recommended. Immunotherapy is commonly employed, although its precise role is still undefined. There is mounting evidence that immunotherapy induces clinical improvement in allergic asthmatics. But most specialists agree that if the improvement gained through immunotherapy can be had through pharmacologic means and manipulation of environmental triggers, then immunotherapy may not be necessary.

REFERENCES

1. Aas, K. Hyposensitization in house dust allergy asthma. *Acta Paediatr. Scand.* 60:264, 1971.
2. Agarwal, M. K., et al. Immunochemical quantitation of airborne short ragweed, *Alternaria*, antigen E, and Alt-1 allergens: A two-year prospective study. *J. Allergy Clin. Immunol.* 72:40, 1983.
3. Alexander, H. L. An evaluation of skin test in allergy. *Ann. Intern. Med.* 5:52, 1931.
4. Altounyan, R. E. C. Changes in Histamine and Atropine Responsiveness as a Guide to Diagnosis and Evaluation of Therapy in Obstructive Airways Disease. In: J. Pepys and A. W. Frankland (eds.), *Disodium Cromoglycate in Allergic Airways Disease.* London: Butterworths, 1970. P. 47.
5. Bacal, E., et al. Polymerized whole ragweed: An improved method of immunotherapy. *J. Allergy Clin. Immunol.* 62:289, 1979.
6. Barnes, P. J. A new approach to the treatment of asthma. *N. Engl. J. Med.* 321:1517, 1989.
7. Bertelsen, A., et al. Immunotherapy with dog and cat extracts in children. *Allergy* 44:330, 1989.
8. Blair, H. The incidence of asthma and hayfever and infantile eczema in an East London group practice of 9145 patients. *Clin. Allergy* 4:389, 1974.
9. Boulet, L., et al. Asthma and increases in nonallergic bronchial responsiveness from seasonal pollen exposure. *J. Allergy Clin. Immunol.* 71:399, 1983.
10. Boushey, H. A., et al. Bronchial hyperreactivity. *Am. Rev. Respir. Dis.* 121:389, 1980.
11. Bousquet, J., et al. Comparison of rush immunotherapy with standardized grass-pollen extract and classical immunotherapy with pyridine extracted alum adjuved extract. *Clin. Allergy* 15:179, 1985.
12. Bousquet, J., et al. Immunotherapy with a standardized *Dermatophagoides pteronyssinus* extract. I. In vivo and in vitro parameters after a short course of treatment. *J. Allergy Clin. Immunol.* 76:734, 1985.
13. Bousquet, J., et al. Nonspecific bronchial hyperreactivity in asthmatic subjects after immunotherapy with a standardized mite extract. *Am. Rev. Respir. Dis.* 135:A135, 1987.
14. Bousquet, J., et al. Specific immunotherapy with a standardized *Dermatophagoides pteronyssinus* extract. II. Prediction of efficacy of immunotherapy. *J. Allergy Clin. Immunol.* 82:971, 1988.
15. Bousquet, J., et al. Immunotherapy with standardized *Dermatophagoides pteronyssinus* extract. III. Systemic reactions during the rush protocol in patients suffering from asthma. *J. Allergy Clin. Immunol.* 83:797, 1989.
16. Bousquet, J., et al. Double-blind, placebo-controlled immunotherapy with mixed grass-pollen allergoids. III. Efficacy and safety of unfractionated and high-molecular-weight preparations in rhinoconjunctivitis and asthma. *J. Allergy Clin. Immunol.* 84:546, 1989.
17. Bousquet, J., et al. Eosinophilic inflammation in asthma. *N. Engl. J. Med.* 323:1033, 1990.
18. Bousquet, J., Hejjaoui, A., and Michel, F. Specific immunotherapy in asthma. *J. Allergy Clin. Immunol.* 86:292, 1990.
19. British Thoracic Association. A trial of house dust mite extract bronchial asthma. *Br. J. Dis. Chest* 73:260, 1979.
20. British Tuberculosis Association. Treatment of house dust mite allergy. *Br. Med. J.* 3:774, 1968.
21. Brown, M., et al. Monoclonal immunoassay for quantitative analysis of Fel d I (Cat-1) in house dust extracts (abstract). *J. Allergy Clin. Immunol.* 79:221, 1987.
22. Bruce, C. A., et al. The role of ragweed pollen in autumnal asthma. *J. Allergy Clin. Immunol.* 52:449, 1977.
23. Bruun, E. Control examination of the specialty of specific desensitization in asthma. *Acta Allergol.* 2:122, 1949.
24. Burrows, B., et al. Association of asthma with serum IgE levels and skin-test reactivity to allergens. *N. Engl. J. Med.* 320:217, 1989.
25. Cantani, A., Businco, E., and Maglio, A. *Alternaria* allergy: A three-year controlled study in children treated with immunotherapy. *Allergol. Immunopathol. (Madr.)* 16:1, 1988.
26. Cartier, A., et al. Allergen-induced increase in bronchial responsiveness

to histamine: Relationship to the late asthmatic response and change in airway caliber. *J. Allergy Clin. Immunol.* 70:170, 1982.

27. Chafee, F. H., and Settipane, G. A. Aspirin intolerance. I. Frequency in an allergic population. *J. Allergy Clin. Immunol.* 53:193, 1973.

28. Cockcroft, D. W. Mechanism of perennial allergic asthma. *Lancet* 2:253, 1983.

29. Cockcroft, D. W., et al. Allergen-induced increase in nonallergic bronchial reactivity. *Clin. Allergy* 7:503, 1977.

30. Cockcroft, D. W., et al. Determinants of allergen-induced asthma: Dose of allergen, circulating IgE antibody concentration, and bronchial responsiveness to inhaled histamine. *Am. Rev. Repir. Dis.* 120:1053, 1979.

31. Committee on Safety of Medicines. Desensitizing vaccines. *Br. Med. J.* 293:948, 1986.

32. Cooke, R. A. Hayfever and asthma: The uses and limitations of desensitization. *NY State J. Med.* 107:577, 1918.

33. Dhillon, M. Current status of mold immunotherapy. *Ann. Allergy* 66:385, 1991.

34. Dreborg, S., et al. A double-blind, multicenter immunotherapy trial in children, using purified and standardized *Cladosporium herbarum* preparation. *Allergy* 41:131, 1986.

35. D'Souza, M. F., et al. Hyposensitization with *Dermatophagoides pteronyssinus* in house dust allergy: A controlled study of clinical and immunological effects. *Clin. Allergy* 3:177, 1973.

36. Dunhill, M. S. The pathology of asthma with special reference to changes in the bronchial mucosa. *J. Clin. Pathol.* 13:27, 1960.

37. Durham, S. R., et al. Increases in airway responsiveness to histamine precede allergen-induced late asthmatic responses. *J. Allergy Clin. Immunol.* 82:764, 1988.

38. Eggleston, P. A. Exercise-induced asthma in children with intrinsic and extrinsic asthma. *Pediatrics* 56(Suppl.):856, 1975.

39. Flavahan, N. A., et al. Human eosinophil major basic protein causes hyperactivity of respiratory smooth muscle. Role of the epithelium. *Am. Rev. Respir. Dis.* 138:685, 1988.

40. Flenley, D. C. Can today's treatment prevent tomorrow's obstruction? *Br. J. Clin. Pract.* 42(Suppl. 59):25, 1988.

41. Formgren, H., et al. Effects of immunotherapy on specific and nonspecific sensitivity of the airways (abstract). *J. Allergy Clin. Immunol.* 73: 140, 1984.

42. Frankland, A. W., and Augustin, R. Prophylaxis of summer hay fever and asthma: A controlled trial comparing crude grass pollen extracts with the isolated main protein component. *Lancet* 1:1055, 1954.

43. Gaddie, J., Skinner, C., and Palmer, K. N. V. Hyposensitization with house dust mite vaccine in bronchial asthma. *Br. Med. J.* 2:561, 1976.

44. Graft, D. F., and Valentine, M. D. Immunotherapy. In A. P. Kaplan (ed.), *Allergy.* New York: Churchill-Livingstone, 1985. P. 679.

45. Grant, I. W. B., Mosbech, H., and Weeke, B. Does immunotherapy have a role in the treatment of asthma? *Clin. Allergy* 16:7, 1986.

46. Greenberg, M. A., et al. Late and immediate systemic-allergic reactions to inhalant allergen immunotherapy. *J. Allergy Clin. Immunol.* 77:865, 1986.

46a. Guidelines for the diagnosis and management of asthma. National Asthma Education Program. Expert Panel Report. U.S. Department of Health and Human Services. August, 1991.

47. Hastie, A. T., et al. The effect of purified human eosinophil major basic protein on mammalian ciliary activity. *Am. Rev. Respir. Dis.* 135:848, 1987.

48. Hedlin, G., et al. Immunotherapy with cat- and dog-dander extracts. II. In vivo and in vitro immunologic effects observed in a 1-year double-blind study. *J. Allergy Clin. Immunol.* 77:488, 1986.

49. Herxheimer, H. The late bronchial reaction in induced asthma. *Int. Arch. Allergy Appl. Immunol.* 3:323, 1952.

50. Herxheimer, H., et al. The evaluation of skin tests in respiratory allergy. *Acta Allergol.* 7:380, 1954.

51. Hill, D. J., et al. Failure of hyposensitization in treatment of children with grass-pollen asthma. *Br. Med. J.* 284:306, 1982.

52. Horst, M., et al. Double-blind, placebo-controlled rush immunotherapy with a standardized *Alternaria* extract. *J. Allergy Clin. Immunol.* 85:460, 1990.

53. Johnstone, D. E. Study of the role of antigen dosage in the treatment of pollinosis and pollen asthma. *Am. J. Dis. Child.* 94:1, 1957.

54. Johnstone, D. E., and Crump, L. Value of hyposensitization therapy for perennial bronchial asthma in children. *Pediatrics* 27:39, 1961.

55. Johnstone, D. E., and Dutton, A. The value of hyposensitization therapy for bronchial asthma in children: A 14-year study. *Pediatrics* 42:793, 1968.

56. Josephs, L. K., et al. Nonspecific bronchial reactivity and its relationship to the clinical expression of asthma: A longitudinal study. *Am. Rev. Respir. Dis.* 140:350, 1989.

57. Juniper, E. F., Frith, P. A., and Hargreave, F. E. Airway responsiveness to histamine and methacholine: Relationship to minimum treatment to control symptoms of asthma. *Thorax* 36:575, 1981.

58. Kaad, P. H., and Ostergaard, P. A. The hazard of mould hyposensitization in children with asthma. *Clin. Allergy* 12:317, 1981.

59. Kalliel, J. N., et al. High frequency of atopic asthma in a pulmonary clinic population. *Chest* 96:1336, 1989.

60. Kay, A. B. Allergen injection immunotherapy (hyposensitization) on trial. *Clin. Exp. Allergy* 19:591, 1989.

61. Laitinen, L. A., et al. Damage of the airway epithelium and bronchial reactivity in patients with asthma. *Am. Rev. Respir. Dis.* 131:599, 1985.

61a. Larsen, G. L. Asthma in children. *N. Engl. J. Med.* 326:1540, 1992.

62. Levine, M. I. Systemic reactions to immunotherapy (abstract). *J. Allergy Clin. Immunol.* 63:209, 1979.

63. Lichtenstein, L. M. An evaluation of the role of immunotherapy in asthma. *Am. Rev. Respir. Dis.* 117:191, 1978.

64. Lichtenstein, L. M., Valentine, M. D., and Norman, P. S. A reevaluation of immunotherapy for asthma. *Am. Rev. Respir. Dis.* 129:657, 1984.

65. Lilja, G., et al. Immunotherapy with cat- and dog-dander extracts. IV. Effects of two years of treatment. *J. Allergy Clin. Immunol.* 83:37, 1989.

66. Lockey, R. F., et al. Fatalities from immunotherapy (IT) and skin testing. *J. Allergy Clin. Immunol.* 79:660, 1987.

67. Lowenstein, H., et al. Immunotherapy with cat- and dog-dander extracts. III. Allergen-specific immunoglobulin responses in a 1-year double-blind placebo study. *J. Allergy Clin. Immunol.* 77:497, 1986.

68. Machiels, J. J. Allergic bronchial asthma due to *Dermatophagoides pteronyssinus* hypersensitivity can be efficiently treated by inoculation of allergen-antibody complexes. *J. Clin. Invest.* 85:1024, 1990.

69. Malling, H. J. Principles of successful immunotherapy. *Clin. Exp. Allergy* 21(Suppl. 1):216, 1991.

70. Malling, H. J., Dreborg, S., and Weeke, B. Diagnosis and immunotherapy of mould allergy. V. Clinical efficacy and side effects of immunotherapy with *Cladosporium herbarum. Allergy* 41:507, 1986.

71. Marques, R. A., and Avila, R. Results of a clinical trial with a *Dermatophagoides pteronyssinus* tyrosine adsorbed vaccine. *Allergol. Immunopathol. (Madr.)* 6:231, 1978.

72. Marsh, D. G., Lichtenstein, L. M., and Campbell, D. H. Studies on "allergoids" prepared from natural occurring allergens. I. Assay of allergenicity and antigenicity of formalinized rye group I component. *Immunology* 18:705, 1970.

73. Maunsell, K., Wraith, D. G., and Hugues, A. M. Hyposensitization in mite asthma. *Lancet* 1:967, 1971.

74. McAllen, M. K. Hyposensitization in grass pollen hay fever. *Acta Allergol.* 24:421, 1969.

75. Metzger, W. J., Donnelly, A., and Richardson, H. B. Modification of late asthmatic responses (LAR) during immunotherapy for alternaria-induced asthma (abstract). *J. Allergy Clin. Immunol.* 71:119, 1983.

76. Moss, R. B. Allergic etiology and immunology of asthma. *Ann. Allergy* 63:566, 1989.

77. Murray, A. B., and Ferguson, A. C. Dust-free bedrooms in the treatment of asthmatic children with house dust or house dust mite allergy: A controlled trial. *Pediatrics* 71:418, 1983.

78. Murray, A. B., Ferguson, A. C., and Morrison, B. J. Non-allergic bronchial hyperreactivity in asthmatic children decreases with age and increases with mite immunotherapy. *Ann. Allergy* 54:541, 1985.

79. Mussaffi, H., Springer, C., and Godfrey, S. Increased bronchial responsiveness to exercise and histamine after allergen challenge in children with asthma. *J. Allergy Clin. Immunol.* 77:48, 1986.

80. Nelson, H. S., et al. Recommendations for the use of residential air-cleaning devices in the treatment of allergic respiratory diseases. *J. Allergy Clin. Immunol.* 82:661, 1988.

81. Newton, D. A. G., Maberly, D. J., and Wilson, R. House dust mite hyposensitization. *Br. J. Dis. Chest* 72:21, 1978.

82. Noon, L. Prophylactic inoculation against hay fever. *Lancet* 1:1572, 1911.

83. Norman, P. S. Fatal misadventures (editorial). *J. Allergy Clin. Immunol.* 79:572, 1987.

84. Norman, P. S., and Lichtenstein, L. M. The clinical and immunologic specificity of immunotherapy. *J. Allergy Clin. Immunol.* 61:370, 1978.

85. O'Conner, G. T., Sparrow, D., and Weiss, S. T. The role of allergy and nonspecific airway hyperresponsiveness in the pathogenesis of chronic obstructive pulmonary disease. *Am. Rev. Respir. Dis.* 140:225, 1989.

86. Ohman, J. L. Allergen immunotherapy in asthma: Evidence for efficacy. *J. Allergy Clin. Immunol.* 84:133, 1989.

87. Ohman, J. L., Findlay, S. R., and Leitermann, K. M. Immunotherapy in cat-induced asthma: Double-blind trial with evaluation of in vivo and in vitro responses. *J. Allergy Clin. Immunol.* 74:230, 1984.

88. Ortolani, C., et al. Grass pollen immunotherapy: A single year double-blind, placebo-controlled study in patients with grass pollen-induced asthma and rhinitis. *J. Allergy Clin. Immunol.* 73:283, 1984.

89. Ostergaard, P. A., Kaad, P. H., and Kristensen, T. A prospective study on the safety of immunotherapy in children with severe asthma. *Allergy* 41:588, 1986.

90. Pauli, G., et al. Clinical and immunological evaluation of tyrosine-absorbed *Dermatophagoides pteronyssinus* extract: A double-blind placebo-controlled trial. *J. Allergy Clin. Immunol.* 74:524, 1984.

91. Platts-Mills, T. A. E., et al. Reduction of bronchial hyperreactivity during prolonged allergen avoidance. *Lancet* 2:675, 1982.

92. Pollart, S. M., et al. Epidemiology of emergency room asthma in northern California: Association with IgE antibody to ryegrass pollen. *J. Allergy Clin. Immunol.* 82:224, 1988.

93. Pollart, S. M., et al. Epidemiology of acute asthma: IgE antibodies to common inhalant allergens as a risk factor for emergency room visits. *J. Allergy Clin. Immunol.* 83:875, 1989.

94. Position Statement. Personnel and equipment to treat systemic reactions caused by immunotherapy with allergic extracts. *J. Allergy Clin. Immunol.* 77:271, 1986.

95. Rackemann, F. M. A clinical study of one hundred and fifty cases of bronchial asthma. *Arch. Intern. Med.* 22:517, 1918.

96. Rak, S., Hakanson, L., and Venge, P. Immunotherapy abrogates the generation of eosinophil and neutrophil chemotactic activity during pollen season. *J. Allergy Clin. Immunol.* 86:706, 1990.

97. Rak, S., Lowhagen, O., and Venge, P. The effect of immunotherapy on bronchial hyperresponsiveness and eosinophil cationic protein in pollen-allergic patients. *J. Allergy Clin. Immunol.* 82:470, 1988.

98. Reed, C. E. What we do and do not know about mold allergy and asthma (editorial). *J. Allergy Clin. Immunol.* 76:773, 1985.

99. Reid, M. J., et al. Seasonal asthma in northern California: Allergic causes and efficacy of immunotherapy. *J. Allergy Clin. Immunol.* 78:590, 1986.

100. Reid, M. J., et al. Fatalities (F) from immunotherapy (IT) and skin testing (ST) (abstract). *J. Allergy Clin. Immunol.* 85:180, 1990.

101. Roche, W. R., et al. Subepithelial fibrosis in the bronchi of asthmatics. *Lancet* 1:520, 1989.

102. Rohatgi, N., Dunn, K., and Chai, H. Cat- or dog-induced immediate and late asthmatic responses before and after immunotherapy. *J. Allergy Clin. Immunol.* 82:389, 1988.

103. Rosenberg, G. L., Rosenthal, R. R., and Norman, P. S. Inhalation challenge with ragweed pollen in ragweed-sensitive asthmatics. *J. Allergy Clin. Immunol.* 71:302, 1983.

104. Salvaggio, J., et al. Relationship between Charity Hospital asthma admission rates, semiquantitative pollen and fungal counts, and total particulate aerometric sampling data. *J. Allergy Clin. Immunol.* 48:96, 1971.

104a. Sears, M. R., et al. Relation between airway responsiveness and serum IgE in children with asthma and apparently normal children. *N. Engl. J. Med.* 325:1067, 1991.

105. Shampain, M. P., et al. An animal model of late pulmonary responses to *Alternaria* challenge. *Am. Rev. Respir. Dis.* 126:493, 1982.

106. Smith, A. P. Hyposensitization with *Dermatophagoides pteronyssinus* antigen: Trial asthma induced by house dust. *Br. Med. J.* 4:204, 1971.

107. Smith, J. M., and Pizzaro, Y. Hyposensitization with extracts of *Dermatophagoides pteronyssinus* and house dust. *Clin. Allergy* 2:281, 1972.

108. Sotomayor, H., et al. Seasonal increase of carbachol airway responsiveness in patients allergic to grass pollen. Reversal by corticosteroids. *Am. Rev. Respir. Dis.* 130:56, 1984.

109. Sporik, R., et al. Exposure to house-dust mite allergen (Der p I) and the development of asthma in childhood: A prospective study. *N. Engl. J. Med.* 323:502, 1990.

110. Sundin, B., et al. Clinical results from a double-blind study on patients with animal dander asthma. *J. Allergy Clin. Immunol.* 77:478, 1986.

111. Taylor, B., Sanders, S. S., and Norman, A. P. A double-blind controlled trial of house dust mite fortified vaccine in childhood asthma. *Clin. Allergy* 4:35, 1974.

112. Taylor, W. W., Ohman, J. L., and Lowell, F. C. Immunotherapy in cat-induced asthma: Double blind trial of bronchial responses to cat allergen and histamine. *J. Allergy Clin. Immunol.* 61:283, 1978.

113. Tuchinda, M., and Chai, H. Effect of immunotherapy in chronic asthmatic children. *Allergy* 51:131, 1973.

114. Valovirta, E., et al. Immunotherapy in allergy to dog: Immunologic and clinical findings of a double-blind study. *Ann. Allergy.* 57:173, 1986.

115. Van Bever, H. P., et al. Modification of the late asthmatic reaction by hyposensitization in asthmatic children to house dust mite. *Allergy* 43:378, 1988.

116. Van Bever, H. P., and Stevens, W. J. Suppression of the late asthmatic reaction by hyposensitization in asthmatic children allergic to house dust mite (*Dermatophagoides pteronyssinus*). *Clin. Exp. Allergy* 19:399, 1989.

117. Van Bever, H. P., and Stevens, W. J. Evolution of the late asthmatic reaction during immunotherapy and after stopping immunotherapy. *J. Allergy Clin. Immunol.* 86:141, 1990.

118. Vanhoutte, P. M. Epithelium-derived relaxing factor(s) and bronchial reactivity. *J. Allergy Clin. Immunol.* 83:855, 1989.

119. Van Metre, T. E., et al. Immunotherapy for cat asthma. *J. Allergy Clin. Immunol.* 82:1055, 1988.

120. Vervloet, D., et al. Immunotherapy in allergic respiratory diseases. *Lung* 120(Suppl.):1013, 1990.

121. Vervloet, D., et al. A prospective national study of immunotherapy. *Clin. Allergy* 10:59, 1980.

122. Walshaw, M. J., and Evans, C. C. Allergen avoidance in house dust mite sensitive adult asthma. *Q. J. Med.* 58:199, 1986.

123. Wardlaw, A. J., et al. Eosinophils and mast cells in bronchoalveolar lavage in subjects with mild asthma: Relationship to bronchial hyperreactivity. *Am. Rev. Respir. Dis.* 137:62, 1988.

124. Warner, J. O. Immunotherapy: Yesterday's Treatment. In C. E. Reed (ed.), *Proceedings of the XII International Congress of Allergology and Clinical Immunology.* St. Louis: CV Mosby, 1986. P. 323.

125. Warner, J. O., et al. Controlled trial of hyposensitization to *Dermatophagoides pteronyssinus* in children with asthma. *Lancet* 2:912, 1978.

126. Weeke, B. The future for immunotherapy. *Clin. Exp. Allergy* 21(Suppl. 1):86, 1991.

126a. Weiss, S. T., and Speizer, F. E. The epidemiology of asthma: risk factors and natural history. In E. B. Weiss, et al. (eds). *Bronchial Asthma* (2nd ed.). Boston: Little, Brown, 1985.

127. WHO/IVIS Working Group Report. Current status of allergen immunotherapy. *Lancet* 1:259, 1989.

128. Wilson, A. F., et al. Deposition of inhaled pollen and pollen extract in human airways. *N. Engl. J. Med.* 288:1056, 1973.

129. Wood, R. A., et al. The effect of cat removal on allergen content in household-dust samples. *J. Allergy Clin. Immunol.* 83:730, 1989.

130. Woolcock, A. J. Therapies to control the airway inflammation of asthma. *Eur. J. Respir. Dis.* 69(Suppl. 147):166, 1986.

131. Yunginger, J. W., Jones, R. T., and Gleich, G. J. Studies on *Alternaria* allergen. II. Measurement of the relative potency of commercial *Alternaria* extracts by the direct RAST inhibition. *J. Allergy Clin. Immunol.* 58:405, 1976.

132. Gergen, P. J., and Turkeltaub, P. C. The association of individual allergen reactivity with respiratory disease in a national sample: Data from the Second National Health and Nutrition Examination Survey, 1976–80 (NHANES II). *J. Allergy Clin. Immunol.* 90:579, 1992.

133. Editorial. Systemic reactions from allergen immunotherapy. *J. Allergy Clin. Immunol.* 90:567, 1992.

Calcium, Calcium Antagonists, and Oxyradicals

71

Wayne H. Anderson
Francis M. Cuss
Earle B. Weiss

CALCIUM AND THE CONTRACTILE PROCESS IN AIRWAY SMOOTH MUSCLE

Smooth muscle contraction, as in all muscle contraction, is initiated when the intracellular calcium $[Ca^{++}]_i$ concentration increases in response to a stimuli. Generally, depending on the smooth muscle type and method of measurement, the basal $[Ca^{++}]_i$ concentration is about 0.1 μM. In "skinned" tracheal smooth muscle, the threshold Ca^{++} concentration for increasing tension was 0.05 μM, with maximum tension occurring at 1.0 μM [292]. Estimates utilizing the fluorescent indicator fura-2 are in good agreement, demonstrating resting calcium levels of 0.165 μM, increasing to 0.5 μM on maximum response to carbachol [306]. Since the extracellular free calcium concentration is approximately 1 to 2 mM, this 10,000-fold gradient demonstrates the ability of smooth muscle to maintain a state of relative Ca^{++} impermeability. Perturbing the processes controlling the low $[Ca^{++}]_i$ concentration leads to contraction.

In striated muscle, Ca^{++} binds to the protein complex tropomyosin, which causes a conformational change allowing for the interaction of actin and myosin and the hydrolysis of adenosine triphosphate (ATP) [91, 92, 294]. The energy released during this hydrolysis is utilized for muscle contraction. In smooth muscle, in addition to a variety of structural differences including the organization of the actin and myosin, a tropomyosin complex has not been identified. Therefore, another mechanism for translating increases in $[Ca^{++}]_i$ to activation of muscle contraction is needed.

It is now established that phosphorylation of the light chain of smooth muscle myosin results in a rapid increase in ATP hydrolysis, a marker of myofibril activation [281], and that this process is reversible by dephosphorylation by phosphatases [228, 265] (Fig. 71-1). The enzyme primarily responsible for phosphorylation of myosin is myosin light-chain kinase, which is dependent on the activation by Ca^{++}-calmodulin [1]. Thus, an increase in $[Ca^{++}]_i$ activates calmodulin, which in turn can bind to and activate myosin light-chain kinase, resulting in the phosphorylation of myosin and energy utilization (ATP hydrolysis) for contraction. Ca^{++} and the phosphorylation of myosin light chains demonstrate a positive cooperativity, such that small increases in $[Ca^{++}]_i$ result in large increases in phosphorylation [306]. Myosin light chains can also be phosphorylated at the same site by a cyclic adenosine monophosphate (AMP)–dependent protein kinase, but the reaction is too slow to be considered physiologically significant [321] (Fig. 71-2).

In canine tracheal smooth muscle contracted with methacholine, a rapid increase in the phosphorylation of myosin can be observed; it precedes the generation of maximum tension and remains constant during maintained tension [76, 77]. The agonist dose-response curve and myosin phosphorylation determined at steady state are superimposable [77, 107]. In the absence of calcium, a transient increase in tension and myosin phosphorylation occurs. Readdition of calcium again results in parallel increases in tension and myosin phosphorylation, demonstrating the calcium dependence of the process [79]. The dependence on steady-state phosphorylation for tension maintenance is not universally accepted [148, 271] and has led to the hypothesis of latch bridges, which maintain force in the presence of declining or dephosphorylated myosin [83].

A second regulatory mechanism in smooth muscle involving Ca^{++}-calmodulin relates to the proposed actin-binding proteins caldesmon and calponin [320]. The inhibitory activity of caldesmon can be reversed by either binding Ca^{++}-calmodulin or by phosphorylation by a Ca^{++}-calmodulin–dependent protein kinase [202]. Both caldesmon and calponin inhibit actin-activated ATPase activity and bind actin and tropomyosin [320] (Fig. 71-3).

Not all phosphorylation of smooth muscle myosin, however, leads to contraction. Protein kinase C, which is activated by a lipid, diacylglycerol (DAG), also has been demonstrated to phosphorylate myosin at a site different from that of myosin light-chain kinase, and results in an inhibition of the ATPase activity [207].

$[Ca^{++}]_i$ can increase the following release from intracellular stores such as the endoplasmic reticulum or intracellular membrane–associated binding sites, or calcium can traverse the membrane down its electrochemical gradient through channels (Fig. 71-4). In airway smooth muscle, two types of channels are proposed to exist: voltage-operated channels (VOCs), which depend on a depolarizing stimuli, and receptor-operated channels (ROCs), which increase calcium flux following ligand-receptor activation.

Voltage-operated Channels

The resting membrane potential of airway smooth muscle is generally in the range of -45 to -60 mV [277]. A range of -20 to -45 mV has been reported for human airway smooth muscle [138, 336]. Some of the variability may depend on the source and viability of the tissue. Depolarizing stimuli to the cell results in an increase in calcium conduction through VOCs. Normally, in response to depolarizing stimuli, airway smooth muscle does not demonstrate action potentials, but depolarizes in a graded fashion, resulting in graded tension development [60, 61]. Two types of calcium channels have been identified in airway smooth muscle: transient (T) and long-lasting (L) [183]. Calcium entering the cell through the L-type channels is sensitive to the class of calcium antagonists exemplified by verapamil and dihydropyridine compounds such as nifedipine. L-channels in the human bronchus seem to be less sensitive to the inhibitory action of these drugs than are other types of smooth muscle [183]. Direct evidence for the existence of L-channels comes from binding studies demonstrating dihydropyridine-binding sites [49, 314]

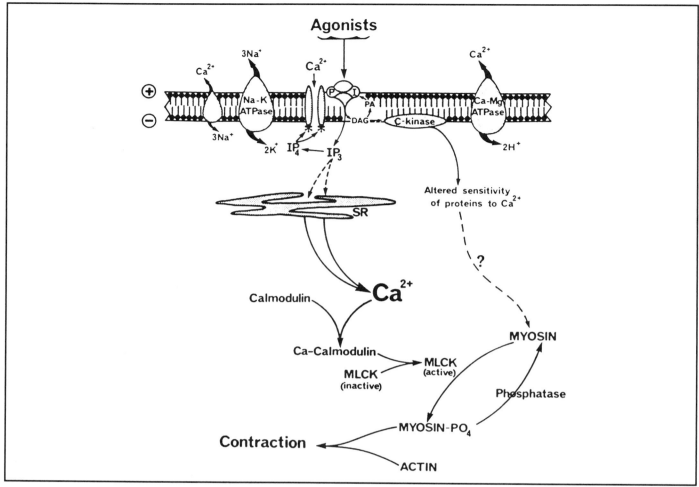

Fig. 71-1. *Summary of the events thought to be involved in excitation-contraction coupling in airway smooth muscle. The initial tension development (phasic response) is determined by the activity of the calmodulin/ myosin light-chain kinase (MLCK) pathway, which is turned on as a consequence of the activator Ca^{++} released from the sarcoplasmic reticulum by inositol-1,4,5-trisphosphate (IP_3). Once generated, IP_3 is metabolized to inositol-1,3,4,5-tetraphosphate (IP_4) as a result of an IP_3 kinase. It has been suggested that IP_4 may be responsible for opening plasmalemmal ion channels, thus permitting a low level of influx of extracellular Ca^{++}. These Ca^{++} may be responsible for maintaining $[Ca^{++}]_i$ slightly above basal levels during maintained tension. The asterisks indicate the points on the inner surface of the membrane at which IP_4 might act. Protein C kinase may be responsible for enhancing the sensitivity of the contractile proteins to Ca^{++}. The C kinase pathway may, therefore, be involved in the maintenance of developed tension (tonic phase of contraction) at a time when $[Ca^{++}]_i$ is low. See text for a fuller description of these events. (Reprinted with permission from I. W. Rodger. Biochemistry of Airway Smooth Muscle Contraction. In P. J. Barnes, I. W. Rodger, and N. C. Thompson (eds.), Asthma: Basic Mechanisms and Clinical Management. New York: Academic Press, 1988. P. 269. Courtesy of Academic Press Inc.)*

and whole-cell patch clamping of human bronchial muscle cells [183]. In guinea pig tracheal smooth muscle, which does exhibit some spontaneous tone, VOCs may be evident in the slow-wave electrical activity that is blocked by calcium antagonists [276]. Human airway smooth muscle appears to be electrically quiescent [227].

Most of the mediators associated with physiologically relevant stimuli (i.e., histamine, acetylcholine, 5-hydroxytryptamine, and leukotrienes) do not induce tension through electromechanical coupling [109], are relatively resistant to the removal of extracellular calcium, and do not generally cause increases in $^{45}Ca^{++}$ influx [251, 252]. While some membrane depolarization may be associated with these agents, generally it is poorly correlated with tension development, or only invokes small changes in membrane potential [109]. Since by definition, VOCs require depolarization as the opening stimulus, it would not be expected

that the calcium antagonists have a major effect on contractions elicited by these agents. In canine tracheal smooth muscle, only responses to low concentrations of acetylcholine were sensitive to verapamil, implying that the strength of the stimulus may be related to different Ca^{++} pools [59]. In guinea pig airway tissue, calcium channel antagonists have been demonstrated to inhibit a portion of the responses to histamine, carbachol, and leukotrienes [50, 328]. While calcium antagonists demonstrated weak antagonist activity toward histamine and acetylcholine, they were more effective in reversing tissue precontracted with these agonists [4, 50]. These data suggest that extracellular calcium influx may be important during the sustained "latch bridge" phase of the response in airway smooth muscle.

Human airway tissue responses to these mediators demonstrate some sensitivity to calcium antagonists [89, 235], and voltage-dependent calcium currents have been demonstrated [183].

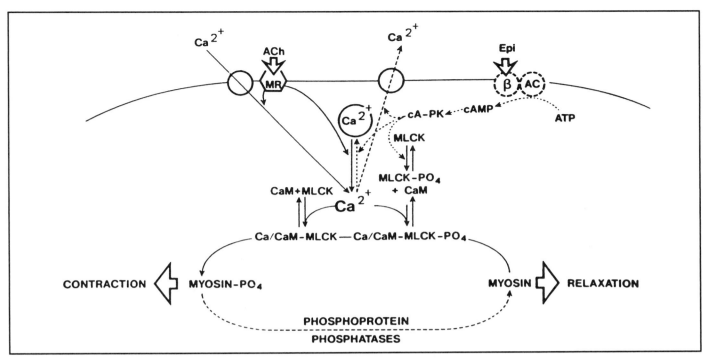

Fig. 71-2. *Cellular events following receptor activation of airway smooth muscle. The solid arrows depict the cellular events associated with contraction; the dotted arrows depict the events involved in relaxation, particularly those associated with an increase in cyclic AMP. The arrows pointing to mechanisms that lead to an increase or a decrease in intracellular calcium following stimulation of either receptor are not designed to specifically identify the underlying mechanisms. Note that the level of myosin phosphorylation is dependent on the balance between myosin light-chain kinase (MLCK) and myosin phosphoprotein phosphatase activity and that a shift in any of the equilibria shown (e.g., by phosphorylation of myosin light-chain kinase) can shift this balance and, hence, the force output of the muscle. ACh = acetylcholine; MR = muscarinic receptor; Epi = epinephrine; β = beta2-adrenergic receptor; AC = adenylate cyclase; cAMP = cyclic AMP; cA-PK = cyclic AMP–dependent protein kinase; MLCK-PO4 = phosphorylated MLCK; CaM = calmodulin; myosin-PO4 = phosphorylated myosin. (Reprinted with permission from P. de Lanerolle. Regulation of Airway Smooth Muscle Responses. In D. Massaro (ed.), Lung Cell Biology. Vol. 41. New York: Marcel Dekker, 1989. P. 178. Courtesy of Marcel Dekker Inc.)*

The greatest inhibitory effects were against histamine, followed by methacholine and then leukotriene D_4, suggesting that human airway smooth muscle may utilize extracellular Ca^{++}, which enters the cells through L-type channels. The concentration of calcium antagonists utilized to affect responses in airway tissue is generally an order of magnitude greater than that required for similar inhibition in vascular tissue, despite the presence of high-affinity binding sites [314]. A comparison of the median inhibitory concentration (IC_{50}) of several calcium antagonists on vascular and tracheal smooth muscle using depolarizing potassium as the stimulus similarly demonstrated a 10- to 20-fold difference in potency in the two tissues [313]. One explanation could be the strong rectifying properties of airway smooth muscle due to potassium channel opening [109, 277]. The resistance to depolarization would maintain the receptor in a low-affinity state, reducing binding of the antagonist to the receptor [26, 260].

T-type voltage-dependent calcium channels have been described by whole-cell voltage clamp experiments in canine airway smooth muscle. T-type calcium currents are induced by depolarization and blocked by Mn^{++} and Cd^{++}, are not sensitive to the dihydropyridine calcium antagonist nifedipine, and demonstrated rapid inactivation [159].

Receptor-operated Channels

ROCs are postulated to open in response to agonist-receptor interactions and by definition are insensitive to the classic L-type calcium antagonists. There is, however, little direct evidence for ROCs in airway smooth muscle. Most agonists can cause contraction in the absence of extracellular Ca^{++} and, as measured by the uptake of $^{45}Ca^{++}$, do not induce calcium influx associated with the induction of tension [3, 237]. Schild plots for the antagonism of calcium in the presence of acetylcholine demonstrated a competitive antagonism for verapamil with a slope of 1 [15, 16]. This indicates the presence of a single affinity site. Since acetylcholine responses are postulated to utilize both VOCs and ROCs for Ca^{++} influx, the Schild plot data could be interpreted that the ROCs and the VOCs are the same site that can be modified by receptor-ligand interactions [252].

Intracellular Calcium

The lack of agonist-mediated calcium influx [3, 237], the relative resistance to the removal of extracellular calcium [60, 154, 235], and the increase in tension elicited by receptor activation in potassium-depolarized tissue [61, 155] collectively suggest that the primary source of receptor-mediated contractile calcium in airway smooth muscle is intracellular.

Many membrane receptor–mediated cellular events are coupled to an effector response by a guanosine triphosphate (GTP)–binding protein (G-protein). G-proteins consist of three subunits that in the unactivated state bind guanosine diphosphate (GDP). Receptor-ligand interactions facilitate the dissociation of GDP and the subsequent binding of GTP. Binding of GTP causes the dissociation of the alpha subunit from the remaining beta-gamma complex. The active alpha subunit interacts with a

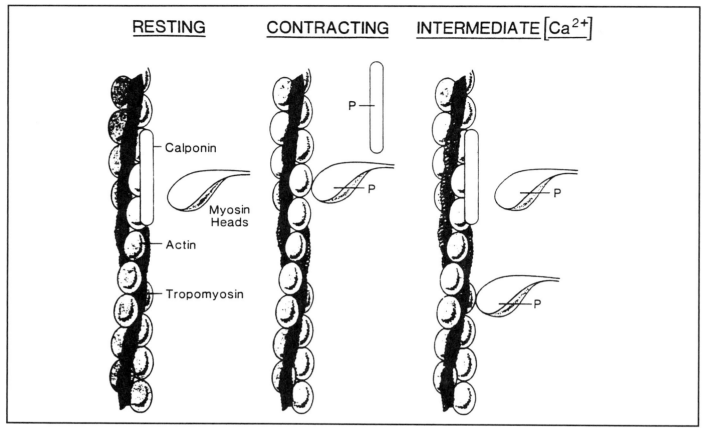

Fig. 71-3. *A model of the postulated physiologic role of calponin in the regulation of smooth muscle actin-myosin interaction. Calponin is shown spanning three actin monomers only because this is the maximum binding stoichiometry determined in vitro; the calponin content in situ is 1 mol per 7 actin monomers. Only the S-1 regions of myosin are included for simplicity. P = phosphorylation. (Reprinted with permission from M. P. Walsh. Calcium-dependent mechanisms of smooth muscle. Biochem. Cell Biol. 69:791, 1991.)*

growing number of effector proteins. Hydrolysis of GTP by a GTPase present on the alpha subunit allows for reassembly of the trimeric inactive complex [111, 298].

Systems that have been identified to be associated with G-protein activation include activation and inhibition of adenylate cyclase [110], phosphodiesterase activation in rod outer segments [105], coupling of muscarinic receptors to potassium channels [37, 231], calcium channels in heart and skeletal muscle T-tubules [38], receptor-coupled phospholipase A_2 activation [13], and coupling of a large number of receptors to phospholipase C and the inositol phosphate second-messenger system [62, 63, 95, 172]. The activation of phospholipase C by receptor-activated G-proteins results in the formation of two intracellular messengers directly involved in $[Ca^{++}]_i$ regulation.

In canine tracheal smooth muscle, cholinergic receptor activation results in a graded fall in membrane phosphatidylinositol and a parallel increase in DAG and phosphatidic acid [24]. In bovine tracheal smooth muscle, a specific loss in phosphatidylinositol-4-phosphate and phosphatidylinositol-4,5-bisphosphate [51, 303], possibly indicates that the phosphorylation of phosphatidylinositol represents a rate-limiting step in the formation of inositol phosphate second messengers [55].

Phospholipase C hydrolysis of the phosphorylated membrane lipid phosphatidylinositol-4,5-bisphosphate results in the release of inositol-1,4,5-trisphosphate (IP_3) (Fig. 71-5). IP_3 can be either phosphorylated to inositol-1,3,4,5-tetraphosphate (IP_4) by a kinase or dephosphorylated by a 5-phosphatase to inositol-1,4-phosphate. Both IP_3 and IP_4 are sequentially dephosphorylated to

inositol, which is recycled into the membrane. Inositol phosphate production is associated with a variety of agonist-induced contractions in airway tissue including cholinergic agonists [191], histamine [122], 5-hydroxytryptamine [167], bradykinin [52], tackykinins, substance P and neurokinins A and B [117], and leukotrienes C_4 and D_4 [115].

IP_3 causes Ca^{++} release from intracellular stores in a variety of smooth muscle, including tracheal smooth muscle [127, 284, 300]. IP_3 binds to a high-affinity stereospecific receptor, most likely on the endoplasmic reticulum. In bovine tracheal smooth muscle, IP_3 has a K_D of 3.8 nM and a B_{max} of 1,003 fmol/mg of protein [53]. Increasing calcium concentrations does not compete with IP_3 binding, as has been demonstrated in neuronal tissue by the calcium-binding protein calmedin [74].

In bovine tracheal smooth muscle, there is a dose-response relationship between receptor occupancy and inositol phosphate accumulation for both histamine and carbachol [114]. There is good agreement between histamine responses and inositol phosphate formation, but with carbachol, a maximum response could be obtained with as little as 20 percent of both inositol phosphate formation and receptor occupancy [114, 116]. It has also been established that the increases in inositol phosphate metabolism precedes contraction [90, 127, 196]. Other metabolites that have been proposed to play a role in calcium mobilization are 1,3,4,5-tetrakisphosphate, the cyclic inositol phosphates, and phosphatidic acid [78, 243].

The hydrolysis of phosphatidylinositol-4,5-phosphate also results in the formation of DAG. Contrary to the water-soluble inosi-

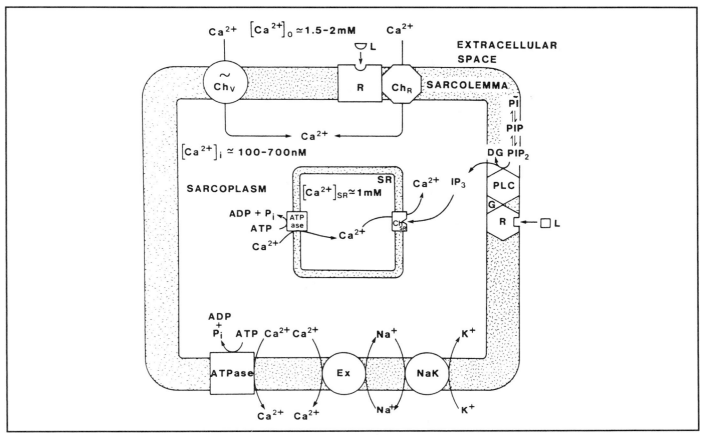

Fig. 71-4. *The principal mechanisms controlling Ca^{++} fluxes across the sarcolemmal and sarcoplasmic reticulum (SR) membranes in smooth muscle. Ch_R = receptor-operated Ca^{++} channel; Ch_{SR} = the SR Ca^{++} release channel–IP_3 receptor; Ch_v = voltage-dependent Ca^{++} channel; DG = 1,2-diacylglycerol; Ex = Na^+/ Ca^{++} exchanger; G = GTP-binding protein; IP_3 = inositol-1,4,5-trisphosphate; L = ligand; NaK = Na^+-K^+- transporting ATPase; PI = phosphatidylinositol; PIP = phosphatidylinositol-4-phosphate; PIP_2 = phosphatidylinositol-4,5-bisphosphate; PLC = phosphoinositide-specific phospholipase C; R = receptor. (Reprinted with permission from M. P. Walsh. Calcium-dependent mechanisms of smooth muscle. Biochem. Cell Biol. 69:773, 1991.)*

tol phosphates that can diffuse through the cell, DAG is hydrophobic and remains associated with the membrane. DAG activates protein kinase C by markedly increasing its affinity for calcium [147, 208]. It has been proposed that one result of protein phosphorylation catalyzed by protein kinase C is the maintenance of smooth muscle tone following activation [102, 242]. Calcium entry induced by calcium ionophores is transient in airway smooth muscle, but when coupled with activators of protein kinase C a response similar to that induced with cholinergic agonists is obtained [213]. However, in cultured airway smooth muscle, increases in $[Ca^{++}]_i$ stimulated with histamine can be abolished by phorbol activators of protein kinase C [160], demonstrating that the role of protein kinase C in airway smooth muscle contraction is not fully understood.

Cyclic AMP and Relaxation

The process of maintaining low levels of $[Ca^{++}]_i$ is autoregulatory, since removing a contractile agonist results in a reversal of the response. There is good evidence in airway smooth muscle that the process of active relaxation in the presence of a contractile agonist can be induced, and that this process is mediated by cyclic AMP [309, 311] (Fig. 71-6).

Cyclic AMP activates a cyclic AMP–dependent protein kinase by binding to the regulatory subunits of the tetrameric protein (two regulatory subunits and two catalytic subunits), causing a conformational change and resulting dissociation of the regulatory subunits [163]. Cyclic AMP–dependent protein kinase exists as two isozymes that can vary in amounts and distribution in different airway smooth muscle [259, 310]. The physiologic significance of the difference of the two isozymes is not known. Two general mechanisms of cyclic AMP/protein kinase effects could result in a reduction in contraction, by mediating a reduction in $[Ca^{++}]_i$ or by altering the sensitivity of the effector contractile system to the Ca^{++} activation process.

Phosphorylation of myosin light-chain kinase reduces its affinity for calcium-calmodulin, thus resulting in a decrease in affinity for myosin light chains. Cyclic AMP–dependent protein kinase can phosphorylate myosin light-chain kinase, resulting in a decrease in phosphorylation of the myosin light chains and a decrease in muscle contraction [76, 78]. Similar results were not, however, observed in bovine tracheal smooth muscle, where no change in the sensitivity of myosin light-chain kinase to Ca^{++}- calmodulin was observed in the presence of the beta agonist isoproterenol [194].

Fura-2 studies on airway smooth muscle demonstrated a reduction in $[Ca^{++}]_i$ to both forskolin-activated adenylate cyclase and beta-receptor stimulation with isoproterenol [98], although a cyclic AMP–dependent, protein kinase–mediated increase in microsomal uptake of Ca^{++} was not observed, as seen in vascular smooth muscle [31, 258]. Alternative mechanisms of cyclic

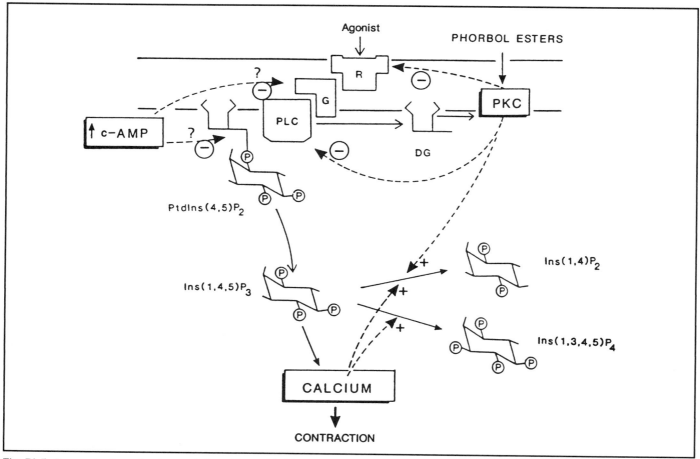

Fig. 71-5. *Proposed scheme for the regulation of inositol-1,4,5-trisphosphate formation and metabolism principally by [Ca^{++}]$_i$, protein kinase C (PKC), and cyclic AMP (cAMP). PLC = phosphoinositide-specific phospholipase C; G = GTP-binding protein; R = receptor; DG = 1,2-diacylglycerol. (Reprinted with permission from E. R. Chilvers and S. R. Nahorski. Phosphoinositide metabolism in airway smooth muscle. Am. Rev. Respir. Dis. 141:S139, 1990.)*

AMP–mediated decreases in [Ca^{++}]$_i$ include activation of a membrane Na-K-ATPase resulting in hyperpolarization [121], inhibition of Ca^{++} influx via VOCs [189], and a reduction in inositol phosphate [122].

For additional information the reader is referred to two recent symposia examining in detail newer basic views on calcium fluxes in cells and recent advances in calmodulin research [44a, 331a].

CALCIUM CHANNEL BLOCKERS IN THE TREATMENT OF ASTHMA

It has been proposed that an anomaly in calcium homeostasis might be an underlying cause of asthma and that any drug that reduced [Ca^{++}]$_i$ concentrations might have therapeutic benefits [193, 329]. Early in their development, it was realized that calcium channel blockers lacked the adverse respiratory effects associated with other antihypertensive drugs [10, 142, 245]. Since they were known to cause vasodilatation by preventing the entry of calcium into vascular smooth muscle, it was logical to assess their effects on bronchial smooth muscle. An increase in [Ca^{++}]$_i$ concentration is the final common pathway of many of the pathologic features of asthma, so it was postulated that in addition to bronchodilatation, calcium channel blockers might have other beneficial effects. Initially studies on models of induced broncho-

spasm showed calcium channel blockers to be very effective [22, 45] and this encouraged further exploration of their effects on other aspects of the asthmatic process. Subsequent studies, however, particularly in clinical asthma, did not confirm the early promise. As new compounds have become available, further studies have been performed in the hope of showing significant therapeutic effects and a more selective action on pulmonary tissue. There have been more than 100 published studies on the effects of calcium channel blockers, but neither formal development programs nor large-scale clinical studies have been performed with this class of drugs in the treatment of asthma.

RATIONALE FOR USE

Calcium ions have a central role in excitation-contraction coupling, stimulus-secretion coupling, and nerve impulse conduction; all are important mechanisms in the pathogenesis of asthma. Thus, it was proposed that there may be an abnormality of calcium homeostasis in asthma that might be amenable to treatment with the broad class of calcium antagonists [193]. The most effective and best known of these are a specific class of heterogeneous compounds called *calcium channel blockers*, which cause vasorelaxation by reducing the entry of calcium ions into the cell through the voltage-sensitive channel in the cell membrane. In vitro studies in smooth muscle showed that calcium channel

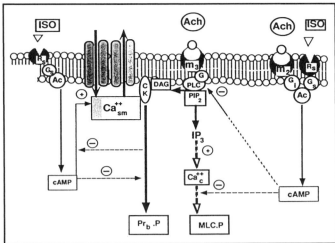

Fig. 71-6. *A schematic model depicting interrelationships between Ca⁺⁺ and cyclic AMP (cAMP) messenger systems in control of airway smooth muscle tone. The plasma membrane (at top) possesses beta-adrenergic receptor (Rₛ) and two types of muscarinic (M) cholinergic receptors: M₂ linked via an inhibitory G-protein (Gᵢ) to adenylate cyclase (AC), and M₃ linked via a G-protein to a phosphoinositol-specific phospholipase C (PLC). When the M₃ receptor is activated by acetylcholine (ACh), there is the production of inositol-1,4,5-trisphosphate (IP₃) and diacylglycerol (DAG). The IP₃ stimulates a release of Ca⁺⁺ from an intracellular Ca⁺⁺ pool, resulting in a transient rise in cytosolic free Ca⁺⁺ concentration (Ca⁺⁺)꜀. This rise in [Ca⁺⁺]꜀ activates myosin light-chain kinase, thereby bringing about a transient increase in the phosphorylation of myosin light chain (MLC.P). This phosphorylation is the key event in initiating muscle contraction. A rise in [Ca⁺⁺]꜀ along with an increase in DAG content of the plasma membrane leads to a translocation of protein kinase C (CK) to the plasma membrane where it exists in a Ca⁺⁺-sensitive form. Activation of M₃ receptor also causes an increase in Ca⁺⁺ influx and hence Ca⁺⁺ cycling, across the plasma membrane, leading to an increase in Ca⁺⁺ concentration in a submembrane domain (Ca⁺⁺ₛₘ). [Ca⁺⁺]ₛₘ regulates CK activity. An increase in CK activity leads directly or indirectly to phosphorylation of a number of proteins (Prᵦ.P), which are involved in sustaining the response. When M₂ receptor is activated, adenylate cyclase activity decreases and cyclic AMP content falls. When a beta-adrenergic agonist such as isoproterenol (ISO) acts, it stimulates adenylate cyclase and causes an increase in cyclic AMP concentration. A rise in cyclic AMP acts at several sites to inhibit events in both branches of the Ca⁺⁺ messenger system: It inhibits ACh-induced hydrolysis of phosphatidylinositol-4,5,-bisphosphate (PIP₂). It acts to inhibit the extent of phosphorylation of both MLC.P and some but not all of the late-phase phosphoproteins (Prᵦ.P). This involves either an inhibition of several kinases and/or an activation of phosphoprotein phosphatase activity. A rise in cyclic AMP also inhibits the ACh-induced increase in Ca⁺⁺ influx by an unknown mechanism. Also, cyclic AMP per se increases Ca⁺⁺ influx, but this effect is markedly inhibited when protein kinase is activated. Hence, a rise in cyclic AMP content in a contracted muscle leads to a decrease in [Ca⁺⁺]ₛₘ in DAG content of membrane and a decrease in state of phosphorylation of both MLC.P and Prᵦ.P. All of these effects appear to participate in relaxing the muscle. (Reprinted with permission from H. Rasmussen, G. Kelley, and J. S. Douglas. Interactions between Ca²⁺ and cAMP messenger system in regulation of airway smooth muscle contraction. Am. J. Physiol. (Lung Cell. Mol. Physiol.) 258:L285, 1990.)*

blockers are most effective at inhibiting K⁺-induced contractions whereas leukotriene-, histamine-, and methacholine-induced contractions are increasingly resistant to the effects of these compounds, presumably because they initiate the release of calcium from alternative sites in the cell [312]. The most obvious action of these drugs would be the attenuation of smooth muscle contraction but there is evidence for modulation of mast cell degranulation [166], sputum clearance [18], and neurotransmission [73].

ASSESSMENT OF CLINICAL UTILITY

The assessment of the therapeutic value of calcium channel blockers is based on their pharmacology, their pharmacokinetics, and their safety and efficacy. The published studies were performed with different compounds, with different trial designs, under different conditions, and with different populations of asthmatic patients, and therefore comparisons have to be made with caution. However, even from such a heterogeneous data base, patterns can be discerned because a large number of studies are available for study.

Clinical Pharmacology

The aim of clinical pharmacology studies is to determine whether a compound shows activity in humans and whether these effects are comparable to those seen in animals. Bronchodilator studies and more complicated inhalational challenge tests have been performed with calcium channel blockers, and are discussed in detail below.

Approximately 100 studies in which pulmonary function was measured after the administration of calcium channel blockers have been performed, but in only a small proportion has statistically significant bronchodilatation been seen either acutely (Table 71-1) or after chronic treatment (Table 71-2). Indeed in three studies, verapamil [100] and diltiazem [131] aerosols and verapamil powder [238] caused significant bronchoconstriction in some patients (see Table 71-1). Bronchodilatation seen after acute administration even in studies showing "positive" responses was clinically insignificant. Overall, none of the calcium channel blockers tested have consistently shown significant bronchodilatation, even when the plasma levels achieved are sufficient to induce vasoactive effects including a fall in blood pressure. While it is a quick and relatively easy test of activity to see if a calcium channel blocker causes bronchodilatation, interpretation of the results can be difficult. For instance, in normal subjects, resting tone is the result of vagal activity, as evidenced by bronchodilatation after the use of anticholinergic drugs [20]. In asthmatic patients, the increased tone may be caused by a release of histamine or leukotrienes, as demonstrated by improvements seen after the administration of specific inhibitors [139, 239]. Although calcium channel blockers have been relatively ineffective in reducing resting tone, nifedipine did attenuate the bronchoconstriction seen after deep inspiration [254]. It is important to note that a lack of acute bronchodilatation does not rule out clinical efficacy; for example, cromolyn has no acute effect on lung function but is efficacious in asthma after longer-term use.

If bronchoconstriction with nonspecific inhalational agents such as histamine and methacholine, which act directly on bronchial smooth muscle, is attenuated, this demonstrates "functional" antagonism of muscle contraction. Protection against exercise-induced bronchospasm may indicate a useful therapeutic effect in those patients with exercise-induced asthma. Bronchial responses that follow the administration of antigen are more complex. The early response is a result of mast cell degranulation, whereas the fall in lung function that occurs in some patients a few hours after antigen administration is associated with an increase in both cellular inflammation and bronchial responsiveness. It has been suggested that therapeutic modification of the late antigen response may be more predictive of an antiinflammatory action and beneficial effects in clinical asthma than other models of induced bronchospasm. Similarly, if a reduction in bronchial responsiveness is observed after prolonged treatment of clinical asthma, it is postulated that this could be a result of a concomitant reduction in bronchial inflammation [257]. This may indicate an important antiasthmatic property of the drug.

Table 71-1. Acute administration

No. of patients[a]	Drug/ formulation	Dose/ frequency	Time before measurement (hr)	Design	Control	FEV_1	FVC	PEFR	Comments	Side effects	Reference
Controlled studies											
10	NIF o	20 mg	2	DX	Alb/PL	b	—	—	3/10 FEV_1 >10%	2/10	263
11	NIF o	10 mg	½	DX	PL	NS	NS	NS	$SGaw^{bd}$	—	217
18	NIF o	20 mg	1½	SX	PL	—	—	d	—	—	142
15	NIF o	10 mg	1½	SX	None	NS	NS	—	From baseline	7/15	198
15	NIF o	20 mg	1½	SX	None	b	b	—	From baseline	7/15	198
15	Ver Neb	20 mg	Immed	SX	PL	NS	b	b	From baseline	8/15	268
8n	Ver Neb	2 mg	½–1½	SX	PL	—	—	—	$SGaw^d$	—	233
10	Ver Neb	1 mg	½–1½	SX	PL	—	—	—	$SGaw^d$	—	233
10	Ver Neb	2 mg	½–1½	SX	PL	—	—	—	$SGaw^d$	—	233
12	PY o	150 mg/ 3 days	1¼	DX	PL	b	b	—	FEF_{25-75} b	5/12	28
Open studies											
5n	NIF o	20 mg	2	Open	None	NS	NS	—	—	—	140
25	NIF o	20 mg	2	Open	None	b	c	—	Decrease PaO_2	1/10	140
15n	NIF sl	20 mg	⅔	Open	None	NS	NS	—	FEF_{25-75} NS	26/60	203
15a	NIF sl	20 mg	⅔	Open	None	b	b	—	FEF_{25-75} NS	26/60	203
15c	NIF sl	20 mg	⅔	Open	None	b	b	—	FEF_{25-75} b	26/60	203
15	NIF sl	20 mg	⅔	Open	None	b	b	—	FEF_{25-75} b	26/60	203
15	NIF sl	20 mg	¾	Open	Amino	—	—	—	Equiv. with amino	8/15	47
Bronchoconstriction											
10	DIL Neb	5–60 mg	⅙	SX	PL	NS			Bronchoconstriction at 60 mg	—	131
9	Ver Neb	5–12.5 mg	⅔	DX	PL	NS			Bronchoconstriction at 12.5 mg	0/9	100
24	Ver Powder	5 mg	½	DX	PL	NS			Bronchoconstriction in 10/24	—	238

NIF = nifedipine; Ver = verapamil; DIL = diltiazem; PY = PY 108-068; Alb = albuterol; Amino = aminophylline; PL = placebo; o = oral; sl = sublingual; Neb = nebulized; D = double-blind; S = single-blind; X = crossover; Immed = immediate; — = not done; NS = not significant; FEV_1 = 1-second forced expiratory volume; FVC = forced vital capacity; PEFR = peak expiratory flow rate; SGaw = specific airway conductance; FEF = forced expiratory flow.
[a] All patients are asthmatic unless indicated otherwise. c = chronic obstructive pulmonary disease; a = angina; n = normal.
[b] $p < .05$.
[c] $p < .02$.
[d] $p < .01$.

Table 71-2. Chronic administration[a]

No. of patients	Drug/ formulation	Dose/ frequency	Duration	Design	Control	PFT	PEFR	Symptoms	Concomitant medication	Side effects	Reference
Controlled studies											
11	NIF o	10 mg tid	4 days	DX	PL	—	b	NS	—	2/11	217
9	NIF o	10 mg qid	2 wk	DX	PL	—	NS	NS	NS	—	106
17	NIF o	20 mg bid	2 wk	SX	PL	b	—	—	—	6/7	142
10	NIF sr	20 mg tid	2 wk	DX	PL	—	NS	NS	—	2/10	279
11	NIF o	10 mg qid	2 wk	DX	PL	—	NS	b	NS	0/11	171
11	NIF o	20 mg tid	3 wk	DX	PL	NS	NS	b	b	5/11	212
14	NIF o	10 mg tid	4 wk	DX	PL	—	NS	NS	NS	7/14	216
21	NIF o	40–120 mg/day	4 wk	DX	—	NS	NS	NS	NS	—	57
12	NIF o	20 mg bid	30 days	DX	PL	NS	—	NS	b	—	293
15	NIF o	10 mg qid	8 wk	DX	PL	—	NS	NS	c (steroids)	4/15	8
12	Ver o	160–240 mg/day	4 wk	DX	Capt	NS	NS	—	—	11/12	247
17	Ver o	160–240 mg/day	4–6 wk	DX	Capt	NS	NS	NS	NS	15/17	246
21	DIL o	240–480 mg/day	4 wk	DX	—	NS	NS	NS	NS	—	57
Open studies											
15c	NIF o	20 mg tid	2 wk	Open	N	N	NS	NS	—	3/15	203
10	NIC o	20 mg tid	3 mo	Open	N	NS	—	—	—	—	108
47	NIF sr	20 mg bid	3–18 mo	Open	N	—	—	—	—	14/47	41
Pediatric study											
22	NIF o	10 mg tid	4 wk	DX	PL	—	—	NS	NS	0/22	275

NIC = nicardipine; sr = slow-release; Capt = captopril; N = none.
[a] See Table 71-1 footnotes for abbreviations not explained here.
[b] $p < .05$.
[c] $p < .02$.

Table 71-3. Exercise-induced and cold air–induced bronchospasm[a]

No. of patients	Drug/ formulation	Dose	Time before challenge (hours)	Design	Significance	Reference
Exercise-induced bronchospasm						
10	NIF o	20 mg	$\frac{3}{4}$	S	b	45
15	NIF o	20 mg	$\frac{1}{2}$	D	b	218
12	NIF o	30 mg	2	D	b	210
11	NIF o	10 mg	$\frac{1}{2}$	D	NS	240
11	NIF o	20 mg	$\frac{1}{2}$	D	b	240
11	NIF o	30 mg	$\frac{1}{2}$	D	b	240
8	NIF sl	20 mg	$\frac{1}{2}$	D	b	22
8	NIF sl	20 mg	$\frac{1}{2}$	D	b	68
8	NIF sl	20 mg	$\frac{1}{2}$	D	b	224
19	NIF sl	20 mg	$\frac{1}{2}$	D	b	269
4	NIF sl	20 mg	1	D	NS	113
8	Ver Neb	3 mg	$\frac{1}{2}$	S	b	221
10	Ver Neb	3 mg	$\frac{1}{2}$	S	b	221
10	Ver Neb	3 mg	$\frac{1}{2}$	D	b	226
10	GAL Neb	3 mg	$\frac{1}{2}$	D	b	226
10	GAL Neb	1 mg	$\frac{1}{2}$	D	NS	184
10	GAL Neb	10 mg	$\frac{1}{2}$	D	b	184
15	GAL Neb	10 mg	$\frac{1}{2}$	D	b	185
10	DIL o	60 mg	4	D	NS	175
10	DIL o	120–180 mg	$1\frac{2}{3}$	D	b	125
15	DIL o	120 mg	$1\frac{1}{2}$	D	NS	184
10	DIL Neb	20–45 mg	$\frac{1}{4}$	D	c	131
10	DIL Neb	10 mg	$\frac{1}{4}$	D	NS	131
9	FEL o	10 mg	10	D	b	225
12	PY o	75 mg	2	D	NS	210
12	PY o	150 mg	2	D	c	210
12	PY o	150 mg	$1\frac{1}{4}$	D	c	28
4	FLO o	25 mg	1	D	NS	113
4	FLO o	50 mg	1	D	NS	113
Pediatric studies						
15	Ver Neb	5 mg/2 ml	$\frac{1}{2}$	D	NS	34
9	Ver Neb	10 mg/4 ml	$\frac{1}{2}$	D	NS	34
7	DIL Neb	5 mg	$\frac{1}{3}$	D	NS	103
7	DIL Neb	10 mg	$\frac{1}{3}$	D	NS	103
13	Ver Neb	5 mg/2 ml	$\frac{1}{2}$	D	d	35
12	Ver Neb	10 mg/2 ml	$\frac{1}{2}$	D	NS	35
Cold air–induced bronchospasm						
8	NIF o	20 mg	$\frac{3}{4}$	D	c	283
8	NIF sl	20 mg	$\frac{1}{2}$	D	b	133
24	Ver Neb	5 mg	$\frac{1}{2}$	D	NS	238
8	Ver IV	Infusion	$\frac{1}{2}$	D	NS	283
10	DIL o	60 mg	4	D	NS	175
Normal subjects						
8	NIF sl	20 mg	$\frac{1}{2}$	D	NS	133

GAL = gallopamil; FEL = felodipine; FLO = floridipine; IV = intravenous.
[a] See Table 71-1 footnotes for abbreviations not explained here.
[b] $p < .01$.
[c] $p < .05$.
[d] $p < .02$.

The first study to test calcium channel blockers in exercise-induced bronchospasm showed that oral nifedipine almost totally blocked the bronchoconstrictive response [45]. Subsequent studies (Table 71-3) using calcium channel blockers by both the oral and inhaled routes showed that while the degree of bronchoconstriction after exercise, compared to that with a placebo, was in general significantly reduced, the proportion of patients with total protection was less than in the earlier studies (Fig. 71-7). When nifedipine was administered after bronchospasm was induced by exercise, it had no effect [181]. Overall pretreatment with verapamil and nifedipine was as effective as pretreatment with cromolyn [68, 225] but less than with beta agonists (see Fig. 71-7). The effects of nifedipine were dose related but with a plateau beyond which larger doses had no greater effect [240]; diltiazem was less effective and showed no dose effect [125, 131,

185]. The protection afforded by diltiazem disappeared relatively quickly and this may explain the negative observations made in some studies [175]. Nifedipine prevents the increase in histamine seen after exercise, suggesting that mediator release inhibition may be as important as smooth muscle effects [22]. In children [34, 35, 103], the effects of neither diltiazem nor verapamil were statistically significantly different from those of placebo, while other comparative drugs were effective in the same studies. Cold air–induced bronchospasm, which is considered to cause bronchoconstriction by a similar mechanism as exercise, has also been studied (see Table 71-3). Nifedipine attenuated the effect of cold air inhalation [133, 283] although verapamil and diltiazem did not [175, 238, 283]. Nifedipine provided no protection in normal subjects.

The effects of calcium channel blockers on bronchoconstric-

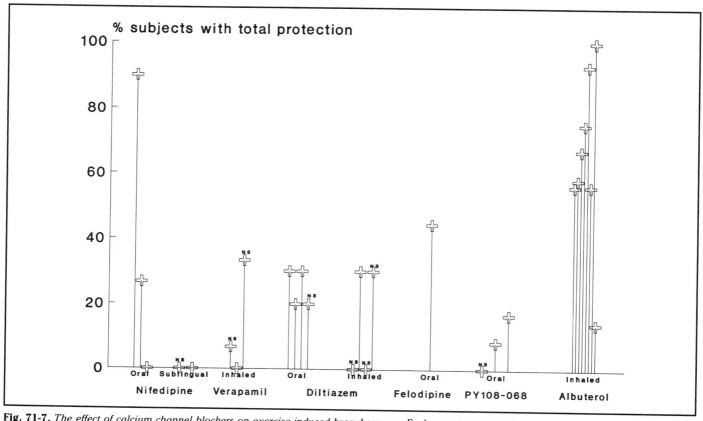

Fig. 71-7. *The effect of calcium channel blockers on exercise-induced bronchospasm. Each cross represents the results of a single published study. The proportion of subjects showing total protection is shown, that is, those subjects whose forced expiratory volume in 1 second (FEV_1) after treatment does not drop below 10 percent of the total fall in FEV_1 after placebo. The group mean is significantly different from the mean with a placebo unless indicated by "NS." The results from published studies conducted with albuterol are included for comparison.*

tion by nonspecific agents are variable but generally positive (Tables 71-4, 71-5, and 71-6). Oral nifedipine appears to offer the greatest degree of protection, although this effect is modest compared to albuterol administered under similar conditions (Figs. 71-8 and 71-9). The effects in normal subjects were also variable; nebulized verapamil was better in normal subjects [6, 233] while oral diltiazem was better in asthmatic subjects [132]. Nebulized verapamil did not significantly shift the provocative dose (PD_{20}) of histamine required to cause a 20 percent drop in forced expiratory volume (FEV_1) in 1 second but did increase the threshold dose needed to cause bronchoconstriction [322], and the administration of nifedipine by aerosol, which would be expected to deliver a greater concentration of the drug to the airways, gave no greater protection than other routes of administration [71]. When the tone was artificially increased with inhaled histamine, nifedipine by aerosol returned pulmonary function to baseline quicker than the control [193]. There was not a dose-related inhibition of methacholine-induced bronchospasm with either oral diltiazem [125] or inhaled gallopamil [185]. In only one [238] out of five studies [126, 132, 220, 248] was any protection noted in normal subjects. In pediatric studies from the same group, nebulized verapamil gave significant protection on one occasion [36] but not on the other [47]. If the degree of effectiveness of these compounds against different bronchoconstricting agents is compared, histamine-induced bronchospasm seems marginally more susceptible to attenuation. However, in one direct comparison [100], nebulized verapamil attenuated methacholine- but not histamine-induced bronchoconstriction. Nebulized verapamil attenuates leukotriene D_4–induced broncho-

constriction in normal [248] but not asthmatic subjects [249]. These data suggest that leukotriene D_4 has a different action in asthmatic subjects, but since verapamil is only able to block bronchoconstriction in normal subjects, this effect is unlikely to be of much value in asthma. Nifedipine has no effect on adenosine-induced bronchoconstriction [69] but is more effective at blocking bronchoconstriction induced by hypotonic saline solution [152] than is nebulized verapamil [153].

Inhalational challenges with various antigens have been performed, although only one study on the effects of calcium channel blockers on the late response has been performed [138a]. Four [5, 67, 134, 256] out of eight controlled studies showed a significant shift in the early response to antigen (Table 71-7), again with nifedipine and gallopamil being more effective than verapamil. The degree of protection was generally modest (Fig. 71-10), although the effects of inhaled gallopamil in one study were considerably superior to those of cromolyn [5]. Overall, these effects presumably reflect blockade both of mediator release and of bronchial smooth muscle contraction. Gallopamil by aerosol had no effect on the late antigen response [138a], and verapamil had no effect on the late response induced by toluene diisocyanate [180].

In summary, therefore, the protective effects of calcium channel blockers against induced bronchoconstriction are modest. In general, the relative potency of individual drugs and their effects in different studies are predictable from in vitro studies. Nifedipine and gallopamil are more effective in these models than the other drugs tested. Therapeutic effects do not appear to be limited by dose since a "plateau" of effect appears to be reached

Table 71-4. Histamine-induced bronchospasm[a]

No. of patients	Drug/ formulation	Dose	Time before challenge (hours)	Design	Significance	Reference
Asthmatic subjects						
8	NIF o	10 mg	2/3	S	NS	308
8	NIF sl	20 mg	1½	D	b	22
15	NIF sl	20 mg	1	D	b	332
10	NIF sl	20 mg	½	D	c	176
10	NIF sl	20 mg	½	D	NS	222
8	NIF sl	20 mg	½	D	c	65
11	NIF sl	20 mg	½	D	c	132
6	NIF Neb	10 mg	¼	D	b	71
10	Ver Neb	3 mg	⅓	D	NS	224
10	Ver Neb	6 mg	⅓	D	NS	224
8	Ver Neb	5 mg	½	D	b	188
10	Ver Neb	3 mg	⅓	D	NS	219
8	Ver Neb	1 mg	1	S	NS	233
8	Ver Neb	2 mg	1	S	NS	233
8	Ver Neb	4 mg	¼	D	c	322
9	Ver Neb	5 mg	2/3	D	NS	100
9	Ver Neb	12.5 mg	2/3	D	NS	100
7	DIL o	60 mg	3/4	D	b	126
Normal subjects						
8	NIF sl	20 mg	½	D	c	132
8	Ver Neb	3 mg	⅓	D	NS	219
7	Ver Neb	1 mg	1	S	NS	233
7	Ver Neb	2 mg	1	S	b	233
8	DIL o	60 mg	3/4	D	NS	126

[a] See Table 71-1 footnotes for explanation of abbreviations.
[b] $p < .05$.
[c] $p < .01$.

before side effects become intolerable. Importantly, gallopamil, a potent drug, administered topically in maximal doses, had no effect in the model most predictive of clinical efficacy, the late antigen response.

Pharmacokinetics and Drug Interactions

Since modest and variable effects are the hallmark of studies with calcium channel blockers, it is important to determine their pharmacokinetics to ensure that a sufficient amount of drug is reaching the site of action. Plasma concentrations were not monitored in the early trials, but more recent studies have shown that there is a threshold below which protective effects are lost as a function of either dose used or time of testing [184, 185]. There is also a plateau beyond which larger doses cause no increase in effect [185, 240]. There is, however, considerable intersubject variability. These studies strongly suggest that higher oral doses are unlikely to offer any further benefits, with the additional risk that vasoactive side effects will become increasingly evident. Theoretically, administration of the compound by the inhaled route may reduce the systemic side effects; however, studies using this method have not shown greater efficacy [71, 185].

Interactions with other antiasthmatic medications have also been studied. Nifedipine was reported to reduce the concentrations of theophylline in one study [279] but not in two others [56, 69]. Diltiazem has no obvious interaction with theophylline [56]. In vitro studies suggested that calcium channel blockers may enhance the effects of beta agonists, and a small additive effect has been shown with nifedipine [70, 168, 301] but not with verapamil [118, 250] in studies in humans. This improvement was minimal and a similar clinical effect would be achieved by increasing the dose of the beta agonist by a small amount.

Clinical Studies

A significant effect on "asthma in the wild" rather than on models of asthma is perhaps the acid test of the efficacy of calcium channel blockers. Thirteen controlled and three open studies have been conducted for periods ranging from 4 days to 3 months in adults (see Table 71-2) and 4 weeks in children [275]. The number of patients in these studies have been very small, ranging from 9 to 21 in controlled studies. Measurements of lung function, patient symptoms, and concomitant medication have been used to assess clinical efficacy, and adverse effects have also been noted. One of the earliest studies showed a significant reduction in the diurnal peak expiratory flow rate after 4 days of nifedipine treatment [217]; however, subsequently the same group found no significant clinical effects after treating patients with nifedipine for 4 weeks [216]. In children, nifedipine had no effect on the diurnal variation in pulmonary function [275]. A large dose of nifedipine given for 3 weeks showed reductions in symptoms and concomitant medication but no changes in lung function [212], while a similar dose given for 2 weeks produced a reduction in symptoms only [171]. Neither verapamil [246, 247], nifedipine [106, 279], nor diltiazem [39] had any significant effect on any clinical parameters in the remaining studies. When nifedipine was given in addition to theophylline, there was a significant reduction in concomitant beta-agonist usage [293] or a reduction in theophylline levels [283] without a change in efficacy. Nifedipine, 10 mg administered 4 times a day for 16 weeks to oral corticosteroid–dependent patients, allowed 12 of the 15 treated patients to significantly reduce their dose of corticosteroids [8], and in a further study the condition of two patients deteriorated after stopping nifedipine treatment [93]. However, these results are not representative of the other clinical studies and should be interpreted with caution. Reductions in blood pressure were noted in most of the studies, especially in those patients with preexisting hypertension. In addition, a variable proportion of patients, ranging from 0 to 95 percent, noted vascular side effects such as flushing, headaches, and peripheral edema.

Overall, the results from the clinical studies showed an inconsistent and small effect in clinical asthma, with a significant num-

Table 71-5. Methacholine-induced bronchospasm[a]

No. of patients	Drug/ formulation	Dose	Time before challenge (hours)	Design	Significance	Reference
13	NIF o	20 mg tid/3 days	$\frac{1}{2}$–$\frac{3}{4}$	D	b	19
8	NIF o	10 mg	$\frac{2}{3}$	S	c	308
12	NIF o	10 mg tid	5 days	D	b	99
8	NIF o	20 mg	1	S	NS	186
8	NIF sl	20 mg	$\frac{1}{6}$	D	NS	39
11	NIF sl	20 mg	$\frac{1}{2}$	D	c	132
8	NIF sl	10 mg	?	?	b	157
7	Ver Neb	3 mg	$\frac{1}{6}$	S	NS	249
8	Ver Neb	2 mg	1	S	NS	233
8	Ver Neb	1 mg	1	S	NS	233
5	Ver Neb	3 mg	$\frac{1}{3}$	D	NS	220
9	Ver Neb	5 mg	$\frac{2}{3}$	D	NS	100
9	Ver Neb	12.5 mg	$\frac{2}{3}$	D	c	100
19	DIL o	120 mg tid	7 days	D	NS	170
8	DIL o	60 mg	$\frac{3}{4}$	D	c	126
12	DIL o	60 mg tid	5 days	D	NS	99
9	DIL o	30–180 mg	$1\frac{2}{3}$	S	NS	125
12	DIL Neb	5–60 mg	$\frac{1}{6}$	S	NS	131
11	GAL Neb	1–20 mg	$\frac{1}{2}$	S	b	185
10	NIC sl	20 mg	Immed	D	NS	25
12	NIS o	10 mg	3	D	b	317
Normal subjects						
8	NIF sl	20 mg	$\frac{1}{2}$	D	NS	132
7	Ver Neb	1 mg	1	S	NS	233
6	Ver Neb	3 mg	$\frac{1}{4}$	S	NS	248
7	Ver Neb	2 mg	1	S	c	233
5	Ver Neb	3 mg	$\frac{1}{3}$	D	NS	220
5	DIL o	60 mg	$\frac{3}{4}$	D	NS	126
Pediatric studies						
15	Ver Neb	5 mg	$\frac{1}{2}$	D	b	36
13	Ver Neb	5 mg/2 ml	$\frac{1}{2}$	D	NS	35
12	Ver Neb	10 mg/2 ml	$\frac{1}{2}$	D	NS	35
Open studies						
9	NIF o	10 mg tid	3 days	Open	b	112
14	NIF sl	20 mg	$\frac{1}{3}$	Open	b	230
9	NIF sl	20 mg	$\frac{3}{4}$	Open	b	199

GAL = gallopamil; NIC = nicardipine; NIS = nisoldipine; ? = not recorded.
[a] See Table 71-1 footnotes for abbreviations not explained here.
[b] $p < .01$.
[c] $p < .05$.

Table 71-6. Bronchospasm induced by other inhalational agents[a]

No. of patients	Drug/ formulation	Dose	Time before challenge (hours)	Type of challenge	Design	Significance	Reference
6	Ver Neb	3 mg	$\frac{1}{4}$	LTD_4	S	NS	249
6n	Ver Neb	3 mg	$\frac{1}{4}$	LTD_4	S	b	248
10	NIF o	20 mg	$\frac{1}{2}$	HS	D	c	152
10	Ver Neb	20 mg	$\frac{1}{2}$	HS	D	NS	153
7	NIF sl	20 mg	?	Ad	D	NS	69
5	NIF sl	20 mg	$\frac{3}{4}$	TDI	D	NS	200
6	Ver sr	120 mg bid	7 days	TDI	D	c (early response) NS (late response)	180

LTD_4 = leukotriene D_4; HS = hypertonic saline; Ad = adenosine; TDI = toluene diisocyanate.
[a] See Table 71-1 footnotes for abbreviations not explained here.
[b] $p < .01$.
[c] $p < .05$.

ber of side effects in many of the studies. The small numbers of patients participating in these studies mean that it is possible that a statistically significant effect could have been missed; however, it remains unlikely that such a result would be clinically significant.

In conclusion, published studies, when reviewed as a group, indicate that presently available calcium channel blockers produce only marginal therapeutic effects in asthma, at the price of systemic vascular effects in some patients. While this precludes a recommendation for their use in asthma, calcium channel

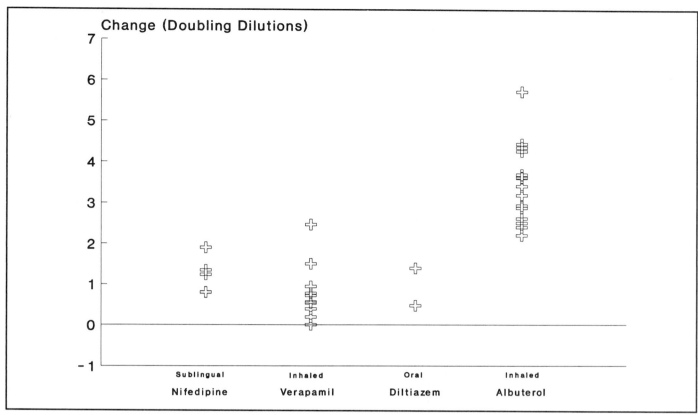

Fig. 71-8. *The effect of calcium channel blockers on histamine-induced bronchospasm. Each cross represents the results of a single published study. The geometric mean change in the dose-effect curve (expressed as the number of doubling dilutions of histamine) is shown following each treatment compared to placebo. The results from published studies conducted with albuterol are included for comparison.*

blockers may offer advantages over other antihypertensive drugs in patients with both hypertension and asthma. Presently available calcium channel blockers have failed to show pulmonary selectivity in clinical trials but this might have been predicted from simple in vitro studies with smooth muscle (Fig. 71-11) [313]. At this stage of our knowledge, it would seem prudent to obtain convincing data showing pulmonary selectivity in vitro before embarking on further studies with calcium channel blockers in humans.

THE ROLE OF CALCIUM IN AIRWAY REACTIVITY

The important action of $[Ca^{++}]_i$ in the muscle excitation-contraction process places it in a potentially critical role for altered airway smooth muscle responses in asthma. The contractile mechanism, indeed even cellular viability, of airway smooth muscle cells is dependent on a critical regulation of free $[Ca^{++}]_i$ concentration. Normally, at rest, airway smooth muscle cell $[Ca^{++}]_i$ concentrations are in the order of 10^{-7} M (about 1/10,000 the concentration $[10^{-3}$ M] of the extracellular fluid); maximal contraction occurs at $[Ca^{++}]_i$ levels of about 10^{-5} M. This calcium concentration differential is achieved by the plasma membrane and by a series of energy-dependent extrusion processes involving sodium-calcium ionic exchange, calcium efflux, and intracellular organelle sequestration. Although contraction in both airway smooth muscle and skeletal muscle is activated by calcium, the mechanisms by which this occurs in smooth muscle are still not definitively established. In airway smooth

muscle, an influx of calcium from the extracellular fluid and a release of calcium from internal pools in stored or bound intracellular sites are likely sources of internal free activator calcium—this in contrast to the reservoir of calcium sequestered in the sarcoplasmic reticulum of skeletal muscle. Calcium fluxing from the extracellular fluid or intracellular sites then diffuses throughout the smooth muscle cells where the smooth muscle fibers are relatively small, conditions sufficient to activate the contractile process. In smooth muscles with a more extensive sarcoplasmic reticulum, a greater rate of contraction results since transmembrane entry is a slower event than is the mobilization of calcium from the sarcoplasmic reticulum. Caveolae, minute cell membrane invaginations in the smooth muscle cell, probably enhance the release of calcium from sarcoplasma tubules following the appropriate stimulus. Additional entry of calcium utilizable for contraction may be via receptor-activated calcium channels in response to hormones or drugs. Overall, an impairment or alteration in any of the critical regulatory processes of calcium balance could result in an increased level of free $[Ca^{++}]_i$ and hence a variety of abnormal responses including those affecting or involving the myocontractile apparatus; abnormal regulation might also include impairment of the myorelaxation process [255].

As discussed, an increase in available or free myoplasmic calcium could contribute to the heightened reactivity of airway smooth muscle to a variety of stimuli, specific or nonspecific, a feature characteristic of the asthmatic airway. A possible abnormality of calcium homeostasis in the pathogenesis of airway smooth muscle reactivity was first reported in 1979 by Weiss and Viswanath [329]. These authors observed an increased sensitivity

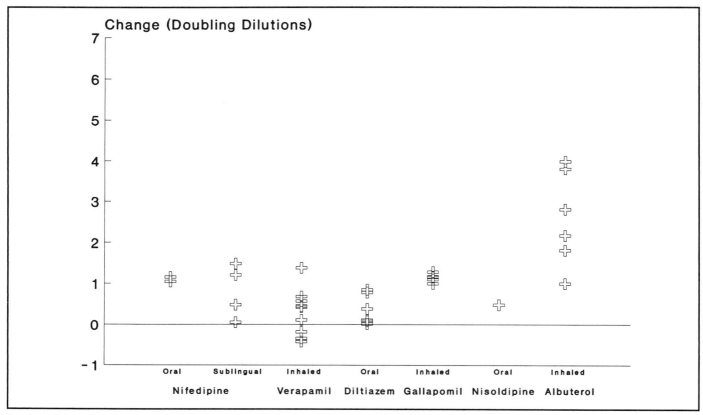

Fig. 71-9. *The effect of calcium channel blockers on methacholine-induced bronchospasm. Each cross represents the results of a single published study. The geometric mean change in the dose-effect curve (expressed as the number of doubling dilutions of methacholine) is shown following each treatment compared to placebo. The results from published studies conducted with albuterol are included for comparison.*

Table 71-7. Antigen-induced bronchospasm[a]

No. of patients	Drug/ formulation	Dose	Time before challenge (hours)	Significance	Reference
Controlled studies					
Early response					
12	NIF o	20 mg	3/4	b	256
8	NIF sl	20 mg	1/2	c	134
7	NIF sl	20 mg	1/2	NS	215
9	NIF sl	20 mg	1/2	c	67
9	Ver Neb	5 mg	2/3	NS	100
9	Ver Neb	12.5 mg	2/3	NS	100
12	Ver o	160 mg	3/4	NS	256
9	GAL Neb	1.05 mg	Immed	b	5
Late response					
6	GAL Neb	20 mg	1/2	NS	138a
Open studies					
23	NIF o	20 mg	1/2	b	158
8	NIF sl	20 mg	1/2	NS	280
8	Ver Neb	2 mg	1/2	NS	280
8	Ver Neb	3 mg	Immed	NS	223
4	Ver Neb	6 mg	Immed	NS	223
10	Ver Neb	20 mg	Immed	d	6
10	Ver o	160 mg	3/4	NS	6
8	Ver o	80 mg tid	1/2	c	192

GAL = gallopamil.
[a] See Table 71-1 footnotes for abbreviations not explained here.
[b] $p < .05$.
[c] $p < .01$.
[d] $p < .02$.

to extracellular calcium following in vitro anaphylaxis in the guinea pig trachealis. The data suggested the following: Normal airway smooth muscle → airway smooth muscle "injury" (e.g., anaphylactic reaction) → acquired calcium homeostatic defect (? increased membrane permeability, altered intracellular binding, etc.) → increased free $[Ca^{++}]_i$ → increased basal muscle tone → nonspecific airway smooth muscle hyperreactivity.

In this scheme the airway smooth muscle becomes altered by some pathophysiologic event(s); its reactivity is not per se the sole consequence of extramyocytic events. The contribution of resting basal muscle tonus to airway reactivity was proposed by Benson [29]. Alterations in excitation-contractile coupling in airway smooth muscle were suggested in a theoretic discussion by Andersson as a basis for bronchial hyperreactivity [11].

While it is emphasized that this concept is currently speculative, several observations have suggested a calcium defect in reactive airway pathogenesis. Dhillon and Rodger [82] observed changes attributable to the utilization or binding of calcium following histamine interaction in calcium-free buffer in the airways of ovalbumin-sensitized guinea pigs. Hedman and Andersson, assaying lungs from sensitized guinea pigs, reported a small but statistically significant difference in ^{45}Ca microsomal binding compared to that in control animals [129]. However, Creese and Bach [66] viewed such hypersensitivity of airway smooth muscle as tested in vitro (and at subphysiologic calcium concentrations) to be caused by an enhanced sensitivity to released or activated leukotrienes and not per se by a defect in calcium homeostasis. It is of interest that the experimental approach of Creese and Bach revealing leukotriene-induced hyperresponsiveness to other bronchoconstrictor agents required low (0.1 mM) extracellular calcium conditions for analysis.

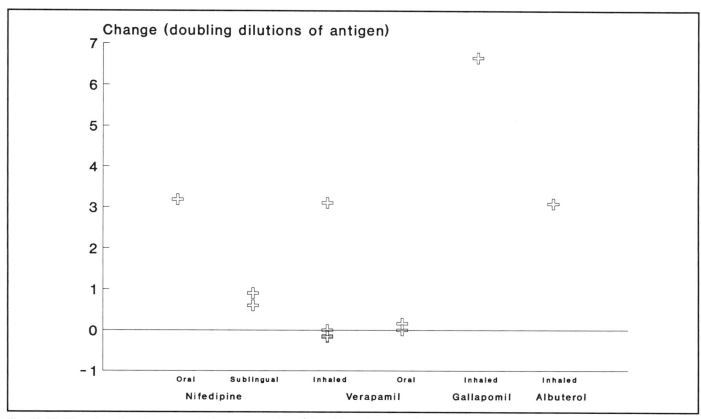

Fig. 71-10. *The effect of calcium channel blockers on antigen-induced bronchospasm. Each cross represents the results of a single published study. The geometric mean change in the dose-effect curve (expressed as the number of doubling dilutions of antigen) is shown following each treatment compared to placebo. The results from published studies conducted with albuterol are included for comparison.*

Fig. 71-11. *Comparison of the activities of calcium antagonists on rat mesenteric arteries and guinea pig trachea.* Dilt = *diltiazem;* Nitr = *nitrendipine;* Nisol = *nisoldipine;* Nimod = *nimodipine. Other compounds are aryl-substituted nifedipine analogs (2NO₂ = nifedipine). (Reprinted with permission from D. S. Triggle. Calcium ions and respiratory smooth muscle function. Br. J. Clin. Pharmacol. 20:2185, 1985.)*

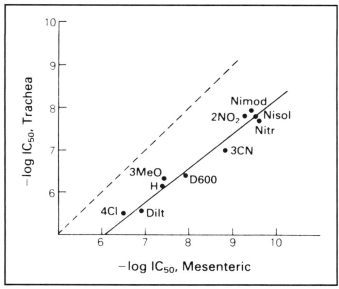

Souhrada and Souhrada [288, 290] reported that sensitization alone alters the electrophysiologic properties of animal airways. Utilizing guinea pig trachealis cells, it was observed that ovalbumin sensitization induced membrane hyperpolarization, an effect demonstrable in vivo and in vitro [285, 289]. While it is possible that agents present in the serum of sensitized animals might produce such changes in membrane potential, these ovalbumin-sensitized trachealis muscles were shown to be hyperresponsive to histamine [286, 287]. It is proposed that an increase in membrane sodium permeability to causative antibodies results in an increase in intracellular sodium; a secondary rise of $[Ca^{++}]_i$ could then explain the above-cited airway smooth muscle response to agonists. In a similar observation, Black and colleagues [33] found that passive sensitization alone with serum derived from *Dermatophagoides farinae* allergen in human bronchial tissue in vitro altered the contractile responses to histamine and concurrently increased the involvement of the calcium voltage-dependent channel (VDC) when exposed to potassium chloride, suggesting an altered calcium mobilization in airway smooth muscle. BAY K8644, a voltage-dependent channel entry agonist, was employed by Raeburn and associates [236] to similarly show an alteration in calcium homeostasis in human bronchial muscle following passive sensitization with antibodies of the house dust mite, *Dermatophagoides pteronyssimus*. A functional difference in the sensitivity to responses mediated by an influx of calcium through VDCs of normal and sensitized bronchial smooth muscles was proposed, with sensitized airways more dependent on calcium entry. The existence of voltage-dependent calcium channels in human bronchial smooth muscles, as determined by the whole-cell patch clamp technique, has been verified by Marthan and colleagues [182]. Small and Foster [278] reviewed the electrophysiologic features of normal and sensitized airway smooth muscle. Stephens and coworkers [295] focused on the role of the mechanical properties of airway smooth muscle in relation to hyperreactivity. In a recent report, an increased shortening capacity of allergic canine tracheal smooth muscle was described. The mechanism for this augmented shortening was speculated to possibly reside in a cytoskeletal protein [295]. The interested reader is directed to Stephens's chapter (Chap. 25) in this textbook for additional information.

Perpina and coworkers [229] investigated the effect of verapamil on contractions of guinea pig lung parenchymal strips to a variety of agonists in unsensitized and sensitized animals. The inhibition of $CaCl_2$-, potassium chloride-, acetylcholine-, and histamine-induced contractions by verapamil in sensitized tissues was considered consistent with an increased calcium influx related to airway hyperreactivity [229]. However, other studies have failed to reveal hyperresponsiveness or only minimal changes employing in vitro models [46, 179, 318, 331].

Animal data in vivo or studies in asthmatic patients analyzing alterations in calcium handling in relation to airway hyperreactivity are limited. Gugger and associates [120] examined ionized plasma calcium concentrations in 12 patients with exercise-induced asthma (EIA) and 20 other asthmatic patients without EIA and compared these with 42 healthy subjects: Plasma ionized calcium concentrations in 12 EIA patients averaged 1.16 ± 0.01 (standard error) mmol/L ($p < .001$) and in 20 asthmatics without EIA, 1.16 ± 0.01 mmol/L ($p < .001$), compared with 1.24 ± 0.01 mmol/L in 42 normal nonexercise controls and 1.20 ± 0.02 mmol/L in 7 normal exercise controls. As shown, there was a small but statistically significant decrease in mean plasma ionized calcium in the asthma subjects, this taking into account changes in inorganic magnesium and phosphorus concentrations, pH, and plasma volumes. However, while a causal relationship between ionized calcium concentrations and bronchial reactivity is possible from these data, as the authors stressed, the relationship is not a simple one and other factors might be involved or operative [120]. Another study utilizing basophils of asthmatic patients revealed the inhibition of calcium ionophore–induced histamine release by nifedipine to be less than observed with normal controls, suggestive of a defective cellular regulation of calcium in asthma [27]. Finally, Downes and Hirshman demonstrated that aerosols of calcium-chelating agents in Basenji dogs increase airway responsiveness to methacholine [88].

At present, the hypothesis of an abnormality in calcium homeostasis contributing to airway smooth muscle hyperresponsiveness in asthma is unresolved. However, there is preliminary information to suggest an increased responsiveness of airway smooth muscle to some defect in calcium control processes following a disturbance in environmental conditions such as in vitro anaphylaxis, chelation, plasma ionized calcium concentrations, or passive sensitization of airway smooth muscle. For a variety of reasons, the limited clinical efficacy of calcium channel inhibitory drugs may have no necessary direct relationship to a fundamental role of calcium disturbance in airway reactivity. Additional studies of this subject are clearly indicated.

OXYRADICALS AND ASTHMA

While oxygen is essential for aerobic life, its activated intermediates are cytotoxic and may be involved in the pathogenesis of a variety of diseases. Oxygen toxic intermediates are free radicals defined as any atom or group of atoms containing one or more unpaired electrons; the term *free* is considered by some as unnecessary. The sequential univalent reduction of molecular oxygen (O_2) yields superoxide anion (O_2^-), hydrogen peroxide (H_2O_2; by definition not a free radical), and the hydroxyl radical ($OH\cdot$):

$$O_2 \xrightarrow{e^-} O_2^- \xrightarrow{e^- + 2H^+} H_2O_2 \xrightarrow{e^- + H^+} OH\cdot \xrightarrow{e^- + H^+} H_2O$$
$$\searrow H_2O$$

Overall,

$$O_2 + 4H^+ + 4e^- \rightarrow 2\ H_2O$$

Superoxide anion radical is very unstable, spontaneously dismutating to yield O_2 and H_2O_2 by the reaction: $2O_2^- + 2H^+ \rightarrow H_2O_2 + O_2$. While superoxide is cytotoxic, its low reactivity suggests that additional biologic effects reside with more reactive, derived metabolites. Superoxide and hydrogen peroxide can yield the more potent and toxic hydroxyl free radical ($OH\cdot$) in the presence of certain hemoproteins (hemoglobin, transferrin), metal chelates, or transition metals in the iron catalyzed Harber-Weiss or O_2^--driven Fenton reaction:

$$O_2^- + Fe^{+++} \rightarrow O_2 + Fe^{++}$$
$$H_2O_2 + Fe^{++} \rightarrow HO\cdot + OH^- + Fe^{+++}$$
$$\text{Net:} \quad O_2^- + H_2O_2 \rightarrow HO\cdot + OH^- + O_2$$

Other reactive oxygen species include singlet oxygen and lipid peroxides. Oxyradicals may also be associated with the metabolism of the arachidonic prostaglandin-thromboxane and lipoxygenase pathways, and superoxide production via cytochrome P_{450} oxygenase metabolism of arachidonate [165, 334]. Chemically or metabolically generated, such radicals exert oxidative stress or biochemical effects in a wide variety of tissues and biologic molecules. For example, free radical effects on proteins result in oxidation of sulfhydryl bound enzymes; on lipids, with peroxidation of membrane fatty acids altering membrane fluidity and permeability; on nuclear DNA, leading to DNA strand modification and even result in cell death (Fig. 71-12).

Biologically active oxyradicals are characterized by a rather brief existence (microseconds), a small radius of toxic activity (30 Å intracellularly), and a low concentration (100 µM–1 nM); hence difficulties may exist in their detection and in clarifying their relationship to disease processes. All mammalian cells possess defense mechanisms to protect against the potentially damaging action of these reactive oxygen species, and a homeostatic balance exists between generation and inactivation processes. The latter antioxidant mechanisms limit or prevent oxidative injury from oxygen reactive products generated during normal metabolic or abnormal pathologic activities. Oxidative damage may ensue where there is either a relative oxidant excess (e.g., hyperoxia, radiation) and/or an insufficient antioxidant capacity. Some of the major protective mechanisms of oxidative stress, whether enzymatic or chemically reactive, include a variety of intracellular and extracellular oxyradical scavengers. Intracellular enzymatic defenses, for example, include catalase ($2\ H_2O_2 \rightarrow 2H_2O + O_2$), superoxide dismutase (SOD) ($2O_2^- + 2H^+ \rightarrow H_2O_2 + O_2$), and glutathione peroxidases ($H_2O_2 + 2GSH \rightarrow 2H_2O + GSSG$, where GSH is reduced glutathione and GSSG is oxidized glutathione). Nonenzymatic antioxidants include vitamin E (cell membrane and extracellular fluids), ascorbic acid (extracellular and intracellular), ceruloplasmin, beta-carotene (membranes of certain tissues), uric acid, and glutathione (-SH compounds). The reader is referred to the text by Halliwell and Gutteridge for a recent detailed review of this subject [123]. The text of Greenwald provides an excellent resource for methodology in oxygen radical research [119]. Doelman and Bast reviewed the subject of oxyradicals in lung diseases [84]; Barnes summarized current information concerning airway inflammation and reactive oxygen species [21].

Sufficient data exist to incriminate reactive oxygen metabolites in some human diseases. In asthma, a significant source of oxy-

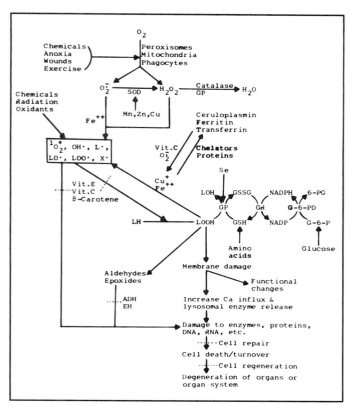

Fig. 71-12. *Possible scheme of free radical–induced lipid peroxidation tissue damage and antioxidant defense. LH = membrane or polyunsaturated lipids; LOOH = lipid hydroperoxides; LOH = hydroxy acid; LOO· = peroxyl radical; L· = alkyl radical; LO· = alkoxy radical; OH· = hydroxyl radical; O$\bar{2}$ = superoxide radical; X· = other free radicals; $'O_2$ = singlet oxygen; H_2O_2 = hydrogen peroxide; SOD = superoxide dismutase; GSH = reduced glutathione; GSSG = oxidized glutathione; GP = GSH peroxidase or phospholipid hydroperoxide GSH peroxidase; GR = GSSG reductase; G-6-PD = glucose 6-phosphate dehydrogenase; 6-PG = 6-phosphogluconate; ADH = aldehyde dehydrogenase/oxidase; EH = epoxide hydrolase; vit. = vitamin; NADPH or NADP = reduced or oxidized nicotinamide adenine dinucleotide phosphate. The dotted lines denote interruption of process or event. (Reprinted with permission from C. K. Chow. Vitamin E and oxidative stress.* Free Radic. Biol. Med. *11:215, 1991.)*

radicals are the resident and migratory cells associated with the inflammatory processes of the airways, including neutrophils, eosinophils, monocytes, mast cells, and alveolar macrophages. The increased activity of the 5-lipoxygenase pathway and the increased complement receptor expression suggest that neutrophils from asthmatics are activated [12, 197]. Not only do activated neutrophils and eosinophils release superoxide anion but also its production and release may be greater in the atopic state [299]. Release of O$\bar{2}$ by activated peritoneal mast cells has also been described [164]. When confronted with an invasive microorganism, polymorphonuclear cells and macrophages become activated and utilize large amounts of oxygen (the "respiratory burst") to generate cytotoxic superoxide anion, which then is converted to other species as H_2O_2, OH·, and singlet oxygen. This conversion is catalyzed at the external cell membrane and in phagocytic vacuoles via bound NADPH-reduced nicotinamide-adenine dinucleotide phosphate. Potent bactericidal hypochlorous acid (HOCl) is subsequently generated from H_2O_2 and various halides by cellular myeloperoxidase. Cellular activation of cytotoxic oxyradicals resulting from viruses or opsonized bacteria as well as immune complexes, immunoglobulins, and chemotactic peptides has been reported to directly damage lung struc-

tures, stimulate histamine release [178], activate the arachidonic acid cascade or platelet-activating factor (PAF) biosynthesis [169], induce smooth muscle contraction [23], and increase vascular permeability or produce secondary bronchoconstricting mediators following lipid peroxidation [80, 81].

Studies utilizing peripheral blood or bronchoalveolar lavage (BAL) cells from asthmatic patients have revealed oxyradical formation and additionally some correlation to airway hyperreactivity. In a 1978 study [135], immune and nonimmune stimulation of human lung mast cells resulted in a parallel release of histamine and superoxide anion. More recently, alveolar macrophages recovered by BAL and assayed by luminol-enhanced chemiluminescence were found to be activated, with the amount of oxyradical release correlating with asthma severity [58, 151]. Calhoun and colleagues reported a greater alveolar macrophage release of superoxide anion from patients with symptomatic asthma contrasted to normal volunteers [43]. Comparing peripheral blood neutrophil O$\bar{2}$ production by N-formyl-methionyl-leucyl-phenylanine (FMLP) with asthma severity, as indexed by methacholine PD_{20}, a significant inverse association was observed [190]. A correlation between the extent of airway hyperresponsiveness and stimulated neutrophil production of H_2O_2 was observed in asthmatic children [75]. In asthmatic adults a similar correlation was observed between neutrophilic superoxide anion release and reduction in expiratory airflow rates; moreover, patients with either an asthma exacerbation or a greater duration of disease exhibited greater changes in FEV_1 reduction and O$\bar{2}$ generation [149] (Fig. 71-13). In another study blood leukocyte O$\bar{2}$ generation was augmented in asthmatic children [205], and was associated with a significant parallel histamine release to the calcium ionophore A23187 and to inhaled histamine bronchoprovocation. Hypodense eosinophils, found in increased numbers in asthma, exhibit augmented inflammatory potential and correlate with airway obstructive severity. Such cells, isolated from the peripheral blood of seven asthmatics, exhibited a small release of O$\bar{2}$ when activated by FMLP or opsonized zymosan; however, eosinophilic heterogeneity was observed dependent on a variety of factors such as cell source and stimulus [264]. Eosinophils from asthmatic subjects appear to be more responsive to PAF release of superoxide anion than are neutrophils, a difference that might contribute to a relationship between PAF and asthma [335]. Furthermore, this eosinophilic release of O$\bar{2}$ is dependent on both transmembrane influx as well as intracellular mobilization of calcium. In patients with chronic obstructive pulmonary disease (COPD), a significant correlation exists between nonspecific airway hyperresponses to aerosol histamine and polymorphonuclear leukocyte O$\bar{2}$ production [234]. In contrast to the above-cited observations, Chilvers and coworkers were unable to demonstrate circulating products of oxygen-derived free radicals in the peripheral blood of patients with acute severe asthma [54]. It should be emphasized that the observations of airway inflammation, enhanced cellular release of oxyradicals, and associated airway obstruction or airway responses to bronchoactive agents in asthmatic patients do not currently provide direct evidence of a causal relationship or explain the mechanism(s) of oxyradical-associated bronchial hyperresponsiveness.

A number of reports on whole-animal studies or in vitro conditions revealed activation and association of oxyradicals with airway responses. For example, H_2O_2 contracts bovine trachealis or canine parenchymal lung strips [296], while in guinea pig tracheal strips, similar contractile responses to H_2O_2 are augmented by removal of the contiguous epithelium [23, 244] (Fig. 71-14); the existence of an epithelial relaxant factor or the removal of antioxidants affecting the H_2O_2 contraction is suggested by the latter finding. In rat lung parenchymal strip models, H_2O_2 causes an initial contractile response followed by a gradual return to resting isometric tension baseline [161]. Concurrently, in rat tracheal

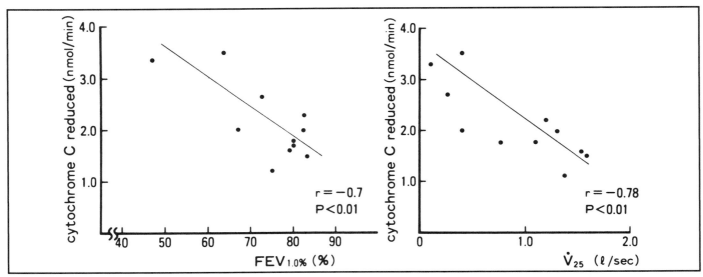

Fig. 71-13. *Correlation between pulmonary function test results and superoxide anion production (ordinate) after stimulation with phorbol myristate acetate. (Reprinted with permission from H. Kanazawa, et al. Role of free radicals in asthmatic patients.* Chest *100:1319, 1991.)*

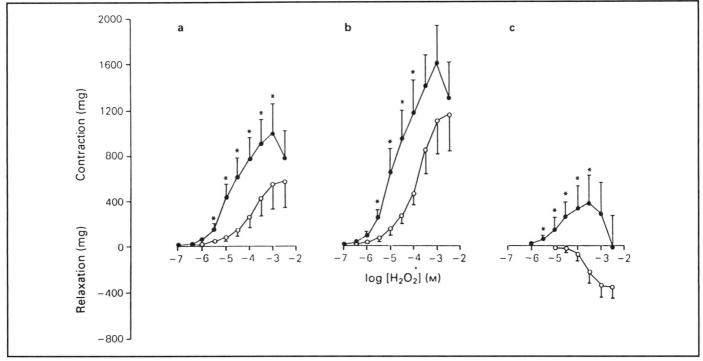

Fig. 71-14. *Effect of hydrogen peroxide (H_2O_2) on guinea pig trachea in the presence (○) and absence (●) of epithelium. a. Mean values of 17 preparations are shown. b. The 10 of 17 preparations, where contraction was observed. c. The 5 of 17 preparations where a relaxation response was observed in the intact preparation. (Reprinted with permission from K. J. Rhoden and P. J. Barnes. Effect of hydrogen peroxide on guinea pig tracheal smooth muscle.* Br. J. Pharmacol. *98:325, 1990.)*

strips, 1 mM H_2O_2 depressed methacholine tension responses by 39 percent (maximal effect) without shifting the PD_2, indicative of an oxidant effect on muscarinic receptors [84]. In other reports cyclooxygenase inhibition by indomethacin of contractile responses induced by low-concentration H_2O_2 in guinea pig trachealis implied activation of bronchoconstricting cyclooxygenase products such as prostaglandin $F_{2\alpha}$ or thromboxane; deepithelialized preparations exposed to H_2O_2 exhibited myore-

laxation ascribed to direct or indirect factors [21, 296]. Since direct in vivo measurement of superoxide anion in tissue can be complex (e.g., electron spin resonance [ESR] spin-trapping), specific enzymes as SOD are often employed to evaluate the presence and effect of O_2^-. For example, a direct bronchoconstrictor action of the xanthine/xanthine oxidase superoxide generation system was shown as an increase in pulmonary resistance in a feline model; this effect was significantly inhibited by pretreatment with SOD or catalase [150]. Finally, while a direct biphasic contraction induced by superoxide radical in guinea pig trachea has been described [206], others have not observed such $O\bar{2}$ contractile responses [21].

Actual concentrations of oxidants at tissue sites that may affect smooth muscle are not precisely known. In the catalytic reduction of xanthine (1 mM) to uric acid by xanthine oxidase (0.01 U/ml), superoxide anion is generated at a rate of ~5 μM/L/min. Human blood neutrophils (10^6 cells) are reported to release ~10^{-5} M H_2O_2 over 2 hours and 14.8 nM $O\bar{2}$ over 5 minutes [190, 307]. In guinea pig trachealis muscle, superoxide anion formation was found to reach a maximum of 15.1 nM over 60 minutes following 10^{-6} M leukotriene D_4 and ~4.85 nM over 30 minutes during in vitro anaphylaxis [324, 326].

Several studies have examined the effect of oxyradicals during immunogenic activation and their relationship to airway reactivity. A direct role for superoxide anion was shown by Weiss where a histamine- and leukotriene D_4–associated trachealis muscle hyperreactivity was induced by superoxide anion; in this model a leftward shift of the median effective concentration (EC_{50}) and an absolute increase in maximal isometric tension were reversed by the $O\bar{2}$ scavenger SOD (Fig. 71-15). The observation proposes a defect in antioxidant protective mechanisms and/or a direct role for $O\bar{2}$ in causing airway hyperreactivity [324]. Generation of $O\bar{2}$ during experimental in vitro immunogenic anaphylaxis has been demonstrated, providing a basis for leukotriene D_4 and $O\bar{2}$ generation, release, and interaction in airway smooth muscle

Fig. 71-15. *Interaction of histamine with leukotriene D_4 (LTD_4) (10^{-7} M) in 2.5 mM (Ca^{++})_E and the effect of pretreatment with superoxide dismutase (SOD): SOD (300 U/ml) inhibited the leukotriene D_4–induced histamine hyperresponse. Both maximal isometric tension and EC_{50} returned to control levels following SOD. (Reprinted with permission from E. B. Weiss. Leukotriene associated toxic oxygen metabolites induce airway hyperreactivity. Chest 89:709, 1986.)*

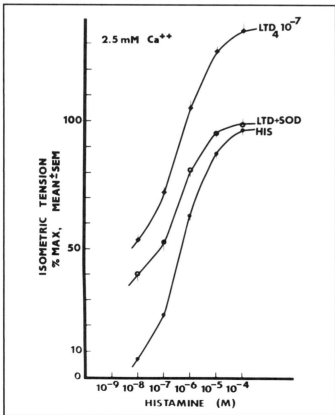

under these conditions [326]. In addition, lipoxygenase product augmentation of histamine responses in human bronchi has been reported [64]. As discussed previously, Katsumata and associates demonstrated direct bronchoconstriction in feline airways in vivo to aerosol xanthine/xanthine oxidase [150]. In this study, concurrent hyperresponsiveness to aerosolized acetylcholine was observed, and this effect was inhibited by vagotomy; under conditions of airway aerosol deposition of a superoxide anion–generating system, these observed bronchoconstrictive and bronchohyperresponsive effects may largely reflect vagally mediated, and not direct myogenic, responses. Airway hyperresponses may be additionally augmented by oxyradical activation of the arachidonic acid cascade, PAF release, and endogenous release of histamine [169, 178]. Other putative mediators or inflammatory cells may be associated with a free radical–asthma process, for example, eosinophil-generated oxyradical epithelial damage by PAF in asthmatics [48], damage to respiratory epithelium from the H_2O_2–halide ion–eosinophil peroxidase system [14], stimulation of PAF biosynthesis by H_2O_2 as demonstrated in bovine endothelial cells [169], H_2O_2 epithelial injury in rat trachea [86], augmented mucus secretion in cultured epithelial cells in the form of high-molecular-weight glycoconjugates in response to superoxide [2], augmented mucus secretion in sheep trachea following ozone exposure [232], and microvascular endothelial disruption injury and increased permeability [81, 144, 304]. In view of the current interest of the potential role of the respiratory epithelium to asthmatic reactivity, some of the above-cited observations appear to implicate interactive effects of the airway structures, beyond the airway smooth muscle itself. Finally, a recent study in ragweed-sensitive patients with allergic rhinitis but without a clinical history of asthma employed BAL and ragweed segmental bronchoprovocation to evaluate superoxide anion production and cellular characteristics following antigen challenge [43a]. The data were consistent with a relatively acellular initial response with activation of alveolar macrophages immediately following ragweed challenge and a delayed (48 hr) appearance of high density alveolar macrophages, which have potentiated superoxide anion release in the late-phase airway response.

Oxygen reactive molecules may react with and may alter cell membrane constituents including beta-adrenoceptor sulfhydryl/disulfide bonds. For example, following exposure to oxyradical-generating systems, beta-adrenergic receptor density in rat lung is decreased, both in vivo and in vitro [161]. In another model the amount of $O\bar{2}$ formed by alveolar macrophages exhibited a high positive correlation with the extent of deterioration of beta-adrenoceptor function in guinea pig trachea [173]. In addition, exposure of rat trachea to H_2O_2 results in a loss of beta-receptor sensitivity to isoproterenol, an effect enhanced by the dietary depletion of antioxidant vitamin E or selenium (reduction of glutathione peroxidase) [84, 85]. In another study, combining isolated tracheal muscle strips and isolated alveolar macrophages, Engels and associates were able to demonstrate hydroxyl radical generation that presumably attenuated tracheal beta-adrenoreceptor function; both catalase and thiouran (hydroxyl scavenger) inhibited this effect [94]. However, Rhodan and coworkers were unable to establish an effect on muscarinic receptors to lipid peroxidation with 4-hydroxy-2,3-transnonenal at concentrations (100 μM) that did reduce beta-adrenoreceptor activity [244]. Doelman and Bast also described a differential sensitivity to oxidative stress preferentially affecting the beta-adrenergic receptor as compared to the muscarinic receptor response [84]. Hence, within the environment of the asthmatic airway, phagocytic/inflammatory cells or free polyunsaturated fatty acids may, via generation of reactive oxygen products, contribute to beta-adrenergic dysfunction presumably by lipid peroxidation or receptor sulfhydryl interaction [162].

Beyond the above-cited factors dealing with the possible interrelationship of oxidative injury in asthma, a small number of observations have involved the role of antioxidants in asthma or asthma models. Two studies reported a reduced selenium concentration in the whole blood of asthmatics [101, 297], trace element selenium being a cofactor for the antioxidant enzyme glutathione peroxidase. The activity of the enzyme glutathione peroxidase, which is cytoprotective of oxyradical injury and involved in arachidonic acid metabolic regulation, is reported to be reduced in whole blood and platelets of asthmatic patients, including those with food and aspirin intolerance [128, 177]. In contrast, Jadot and colleagues observed elevated erythrocytic plasma concentrations of copper-containing and manganese SODs and glutathione peroxidase in all of 29 patients experiencing an asthma exacerbation [141]. Not directly related to asthma, the mucolytic N-acetylcysteine (a glutathione precursor) exhibits some antioxidant properties by its reaction with hypochlorous acid and hydroxyl radicals in dogs exposed to hyperoxic pulmonary stress [319]. A protective action by SOD on free radical–mediated pulmonary vascular permeability is described in a dog model [214]. In the absence of an efficient O_2^- scavenger, the ascorbate system may, as a component of its action, act as a sink for superoxide, and some human and animal studies of experimental asthma cited a beneficial role for ascorbic acid [209, 262]. In addition, infection-associated or infection-induced airway hyperreactivity may also be ameliorated by ascorbate [130]. Alveolar macrophages that release oxidants are also rich in antioxidants [137]; effective scavenging can limit H_2O_2-mediated lung injury [187]. The relationship of a low selenium soil content to a dietary deficiency culpable in an increased relative risk of asthma, as noted in New Zealand, must be currently considered conjectural [101]. While one report observed a decreased alpha-tocopherol activity in asthmatic patients, the effects of vitamin E, which inhibits lipid peroxidation, and beta-carotene, a scavenger, have not been sufficiently evaluated in asthma [9]. Of clinical interest, unrelated to a scavenger role, is the inhibition of superoxide radical generation from guinea pig, rabbit, and human neutrophils by azelastine [42].

Studies examining the effect of oxyradicals on calcium homeostasis in asthma are limited. As discussed, the cytosolic concentration of calcium must be maintained at a low level and within tolerable physiologic limits; concurrently oxyradicals can injure cell membranes and other structures via lipid peroxidation, and overwhelm or injure tightly controlled intracellular regulatory processes [96, 104]. In one paradigm employing a paired experimental sequence, an enhanced (initial rate and maximal reduction) relaxation of resting isometric tension in guinea pig trachealis was observed in muscles previously immunogenically activated and then exposed to ~0 mM extracellular calcium [325]. Inhibition of the late phase of ovalbumin-induced anaphylaxis by FPL 55712 (10 μM) eliminated this enhanced postanaphylactic relaxation following low calcium exposure. Other tracheal muscles, exposed to synthetic leukotriene C_4, exhibited the same enhanced relaxation in a low extracellular calcium environment. Pretreatment with SOD or isocapnic hypoxia (PO_2 10 ± 4 torr) abolished the postanaphylactic and leukotriene C_4–augmented relaxation. Although exposure to low extracellular calcium concentrations may transiently increase cytosolic [Ca^{++}], sequential immersion of control muscles (nonimmune activated) in ~0 mM extracellular calcium did not exhibit any altered effect [302]. It was proposed that an alteration in calcium homeostasis developed following anaphylaxis (or LTD_4 exposure) which affected resting airway isometric muscle tone [325]. Lansing and coworkers [165a] have subsequently demonstrated oxygen-radical induction (employing aerosolized xanthine/xanthine oxidase) of reversible airflow obstruction and hyperresponsiveness to carbachol in a sheep model. An interrelationship between oxyradicals and secondary generation of lipid mediators was proposed to contribute to the free oxygen radical–induced bronchoconstric-

tion and airway hyperreactivity. Hence, while it is reported that oxidants may induce cellular influx and oxidized fatty acids may exhibit calcium ionophore effects, further studies are needed to delineate the relationships between oxidative stress and calcium in cellular injury or in calcium homeostasis in asthma [169, 266].

OTHER CONSIDERATIONS

Sodium and Na^+-K^+-ATPase

A few studies have related the dietary intake of sodium to alterations in bronchial responses to histamine [40, 143]. Other reports indicated a reduced activity of the sodium-potassium–stimulated ATPase in platelet membranes of allergic patients including those with asthma [273]. A circulating Na^+-K^+-ATPase inhibitor responsible for a transport enzyme defect in platelets of allergic patients could affect intracellular cation concentrations [274].

Magnesium

Intravenous magnesium sulfate has been proposed for treatment in patients with severe, intractable asthma (see Chap. 73) [272]. In asthmatic patients, protection against methacholine- or histamine-induced bronchoprovocation by magnesium has been observed [253]. Hypomagnesemia in acute asthma is uncommon and may result from limited gastrointestinal intake or losses (nasogastric suction, diarrhea), use of corticosteroids or diuretics, or other factors. Magnesium, a major intracellular cation, is involved in a variety of processes including neuromuscular activity, phosphorylation reactions, membrane stability, and modulation of ionic calcium transients. While its action may be similar to that of calcium channel antagonists, the observation of a decrease in nerve terminal acetylcholine release suggests that its spasmolytic mechanism may be complex. Extracellular concentrations above 1.2 mM/L inhibit smooth muscle contraction. There is no evidence that magnesium activates the arachidonic acid cascade, but it may enhance prostacyclin release [323].

Potassium

The activity and mechanism of airway smooth muscle potassium channels, which are associated with hyperpolarization and relaxant processes, are presented in detail in Chapter 16 and recently reviewed in [337]. Blockade of K^+ channels could be a contributory mechanism in airway smooth muscle hyperresponsiveness and drugs that open K^+ channels represent a new class of myorelaxants with potential clinical application [7, 124]. Drugs that open potassium channels may cause relaxation by antagonism of intracellular ATP, which functions normally to keep these channels closed [241]. In a recent study, BRL 38227 (lemakalim), the active L-enantiomer of cromakalim, was shown to be an effective relaxant in human bronchi to agonist histamine, neurokinin A, carbachol, resting isometric tone, and contraction provoked by electrical field stimulation [32]. BRL 38227 also protected against morning dipping in asthmatic patients and inhibited histamine-induced bronchoconstriction in healthy volunteers [17, 211]. Interestingly, brain microsomal K^+ channels may be implicated in the regulation of [Ca^{++}]$_i$ and some properties of lemakalim may affect [Ca^{++}]$_i$ [267]. In guinea pig and bovine trachealis muscle, the action of cromakalim in opening K^+ channels was recently reported not to involve the intracellular accumulation of cyclic nucleotides [30]. From studies with human airways Miura and coworkers [197a] recently suggested that charbdotoxin (an inhibitor of smooth muscle large conductance calcium-activated potassium channels)-sensitive potassium channels participate in beta-adrenergic-agonist- and theophylline-induced bronchodilation. Additional studies, both basic and clinical, are warranted to further define the mechanisms and role of K^+ channels and to determine what effect their antagonism has in asthma.

Calmodulin Antagonism

Trifluoperazine, a calmodulin antagonist, exhibits an inhibitory action to a variety of agonists (5-hydroxytryptamine, acetylcholine, histamine, potassium chloride, $CaCl_2$) in sensitized and non-sensitized guinea pig lung strips [261]. Inhibition of calmodulin-calcium binding with subsequent activation of myosin light-chain kinase may afford therapeutic potential.

General Anesthetics

Volatile anesthetics, notably halothane, isoflurane, and enflurane, affect airways by a variety of complex and possibly interrelated mechanisms, including direct smooth muscle relaxation, inhibition of bronchoreactive mediators, and central neural or airway neural reflex blockade (see Chap. 82). The subject was recently reviewed by Hirshman and Bergman [136]. Whatever the fundamental mechanism(s), the clinical use of inhalational anesthetics is generally limited to acute severe asthma when other conventional methods have failed (see Chap. 73). General anesthetics may inhibit oxidative metabolism and calcium mobilization. For example, halothane, enflurane, and isoflurane were shown to inhibit superoxide production by decreased mobilization of $[Ca^{++}]_i$ in human neutrophils stimulated by FMLP [204]. Two recent preliminary reports suggested halothane-mediated relaxant effects in airway smooth muscle to be partially due to a decreased mobilization of $[Ca^{++}]_i$ following cholinergic stimulation; a parallel rise in cytosolic AMP may influence this action [145, 333].

Local Anesthetics

Local anesthetic agents have been administered to asthmatic patients and examined in a variety of experimental conditions. Their action may be multifactorial involving a direct myogenic role, interruption of neural reflexes, and even inhibition of mast cell histamine release, albeit at rather high concentrations [327]. An asthmalytic effect has been observed in some patients but not in others, and aerosol lidocaine is often complicated by bronchospasm in asthmatics [87, 195]. It is suggested that a bronchodilator such as metaproterenol be added to topical lidocaine anesthetic solutions for use in patients with hyperreactive airways [156]. In neural structures, local anesthetics inhibit excitation by decreasing cell membrane permeability to sodium ions, thereby inhibiting cell membrane depolarization. However, in smooth muscle, the spasmolytic action of local anesthetics is not clarified, although some effect on cellular calcium flux or binding has been proposed [44, 97, 338].

REFERENCES

1. Adelstein, R. S., and Klee, C. B. Purification and characterization of smooth muscle myosin light chain kinase. *J. Biol. Chem.* 256:7501, 1981.
2. Adler, K. B., Holden-Stauffer, W. J., and Repine, J. E. Oxygen metabolites stimulate release of high-molecular-weight glycoconjugates by cell and organ cultures of rodent respiratory epithelium via an arachidonic acid-dependent mechanism. *J. Clin. Invest.* 85:75, 1990.
3. Ahmed, F., et al. Some features of the spasmogenic actions of acetylcholine and histamine in guinea-pig isolated trachea. *Br. J. Pharmacol.* 83:227, 1984.
4. Ahmed, F., Foster, R. W., and Small, R. C. Some effects of nifedipine in guinea pig isolated trachealis. *Br. J. Pharmacol.* 84:861. 1985.
5. Ahmed, T., et al. Inhibition of antigen-induced bronchoconstriction by a new calcium antagonist, gallopamil: Comparison with cromolyn sodium. *J. Allergy Clin. Immunol.* 81:852, 1988.
6. Ahmed, T., et al. Comparative effects of oral and inhaled verapamil on antigen-induced bronchoconstriction. *Chest* 88:176, 1985.
7. Akasaka, K., et al. Electromyographic studies of bronchial smooth muscle in bronchial asthma. *Tohoku J. Exp. Med.* 117:55, 1975.
8. al-Waili, N. S. Nifedipine in corticosteroid-dependent asthma: Preliminary study. *Clin. Exp. Pharmacol. Physiol.* 16:715, 1989.
9. Amatuni, V. G., and Safarian, M. D. Metabolite aspects of the differential diagnosis of asthmatic bronchitis and bronchial asthma. *Ter. Arkh.* 58:12, 1986.
10. Anavekar, A. N., et al. A double-blind comparison of verapamil and labetalol in hypertensive patients with co-existing chronic obstructive airways disease. *J. Cardiovasc. Pharmacol.* 3:S374, 1982.
11. Andersson, K. E. Airway hyperreactivity smooth muscle and calcium. *Eur. J. Respir. Dis.* 131(Suppl. 1):49, 1983.
12. Arm, J. P., Walport, J. J., and Loe, T. H. Expression of complement receptors type I (CR1) and type 3 (CR3) on circulating granulocytes in experimentally provoked asthma. *J. Allergy Clin. Immunol.* 83:649, 1989.
13. Axelrod, J., Burch, R. M., and Jelsema, C. L. Receptor mediated activation of phospholipase A_2 via GTP-binding proteins: Arachidonic acid and its metabolites as second messengers. *Trends Neurosci.* 11:117, 1988.
14. Ayars, G. H., et al. Injurious effect of the eosinophil peroxidase-halide system and major basic protein in human nasal epithelium in vitro. *Am. Rev. Respir. Dis.* 140:125, 1989.
15. Baba, K., et al. Effects of verapamil on the contractions of guinea-pig tracheal muscle induced by Ca, Sr and Ba. *Br. J. Pharmacol.* 84:203, 1985.
16. Baba, K., et al. Effects of verapamil on the response of the guinea-pig tracheal muscle to carbachol. *Br. J. Pharmacol.* 88:441, 1986.
17. Baird, A., et al. Cromakalim, a potassium channel activator inhibits histamine induced bronchoconstriction in healthy volunteers. *Br. J. Clin. Pharmacol.* 25:114, 1988.
18. Balfre, K. The effects of calcium and calcium ionophore A23187 on mucin secretion and potential difference in the isolated chicken trachea. *J. Physiol.* 275:80P, 1978.
19. Ballester, E., et al. Effect of nifedipine on arterial hypoxaemia occurring after methacholine challenge in asthma. *Thorax* 41:468, 1986.
20. Barnes, P. J. Neural control of human airways in health and disease. *Am. Rev. Respir. Dis.* 134:1289, 1986.
21. Barnes, P. J. Reactive oxygen species and airway inflammation. *Free Radic. Biol. Med.* 9:235, 1990.
22. Barnes, P. J., et al. A calcium antagonist, nifedipine, modifies exercise-induced asthma. *Thorax* 36:726, 1981.
23. Barnes, P. J., et al. The effect of oxygen derived free radicals on airway smooth muscle responses. *Br. J. Pharmacol.* 90(Suppl.):142, 1987.
24. Baron, C. B., et al. Pharmacomechanical coupling in smooth muscle may involve phosphatidylinositol metabolism. *Proc. Natl. Acad. Sci. USA* 81:6899, 1984.
25. Baronti, A., et al. Effects of acute nicardipine (YC93) on carbachol-induced bronchoconstriction. *Curr. Ther. Res.* 34:142, 1983.
26. Bean, B. P. Nitrendipine block of cardiac calcium channels: High affinity binding to the inactivated state. *Proc. Natl. Acad. Sci. USA* 81:6388, 1984.
27. Bedard, R. M., and Busse, W. W. Inhibition of basophil histamine release by the calcium channel antagonist nifedipine in asthma. *Am. Rev. Respir. Dis.* 129:A9, 1984.
28. Ben-Dov, I., et al. Bronchodilatation and attenuation of exercise-induced bronchospasm by PY 108-068, a new calcium antagonist. *Am. Rev. Respir. Dis.* 133:116, 1986.
29. Benson, M. K. Bronchial hyperreactivity. *Br. J. Dis. Chest* 69:227, 1975.
30. Berry, J. L., et al. Mechanical, biochemical and electrophysiological studies of RP49356 and cromakalim in guinea pig and bovine trachealis muscle. *Pulmonol. Pharmacol.* 4:91, 1991.
31. Bhalla, R. C., et al. Role of cyclic AMP in rat aortic microsomal phosphorylation and calcium uptake. *Am. J. Physiol.* 234:H508, 1978.
32. Black, J. L., et al. The action of a potassium channel activator, BRL 38227 (lemakalim) on human airway smooth muscle. *Am. Rev. Respir. Dis.* 142:1384, 1990.
33. Black, J. L., et al. Sensitization alters contractile responses and calcium influx in human airway smooth muscle. *J. Allergy Clin. Immunol.* 84:440, 1989.
34. Boner, A. L., et al. Comparison of the effects of inhaled calcium antagonist verapamil, sodium cromoglycate and ipratropium bromide on exer-

cise-induced bronchoconstriction in children with asthma. *Eur. J. Pediatr.* 146:408, 1987.

35. Boner, A. L., et al. Effects of different dosages of the calcium antagonist verapamil in exercise- and methacholine-induced bronchospasm in children with chronic asthma. *J. Asthma* 24:81, 1987.

36. Boner, A. L., et al. Nebulised sodium cromoglycate and verapamil in methacholine induced asthma. *Arch. Dis. Child* 62:264, 1987.

37. Breitwieser, G. A., and Szabo, G. Uncoupling of cardiac muscarinic and β-adrenergic receptors from ion channels by a guanine nucleotide analog. *Nature* 317:538, 1985.

38. Brown, A. M., and Birnbaumer, L. Direct G protein gating of ion channels. *Am. J. Physiol. (Heart Circ. Physiol.)* 254:H401, 1988.

39. Burghuber, O. C. et al. Inhibition of acetylcholine-induced bronchoconstriction in asthmatics by nifedipine. *Respiration* 50:265, 1986.

40. Burney, P. G. J., et al. Response to inhaled histamine and 24 hour sodium excretion. *Br. Med. J.* 292:1483, 1986.

41. Bursztyn, M., et al. Long-acting nifedipine in moderate and severe hypertensive patients with serious concomitant diseases. *Am. Heart J.* 110:96, 1985.

42. Busse, W., et al. The effect of azelastine on neutrophil and eosinophil generation of superoxide. *J. Allergy Clin. Immunol.* 81:212, 1988.

43. Calhoun, W. J., et al. Increased superoxide release from alveolar macrophages in symptomatic asthma (abstract). *Am. Rev. Respir. Dis.* 135:A224, 1987.

43a. Calhoun, W. J., et al. Enhanced superoxide production by alveolar macrophages and air-space cells, airway inflammation, and alveolar macrophage density changes after segmental antigen bronchoprovocation in allergic subjects. *Am. Rev. Respir. Dis.* 145:317, 1992.

44. Campbell, A. K. Intracellular Calcium, Its Universal Role as Regulation. Wiley, 1983, P. 32.

44a. Carafoli, E., and Klee, C. New developments in the calmodulin field. *Cell Calcium* 13:353, 1992.

45. Cerrina, J., et al. Inhibition of exercise-induced asthma by a calcium antagonist, nifedipine. *Am. Rev. Respir. Dis.* 123:156, 1981.

46. Cerrina, J., et al. Comparison of human bronchial muscle response to histamine in vivo with histamine and isoproterenol agonists in vitro. *Am. Rev. Respir. Dis.* 134:57, 1986.

47. Chandra, R., et al. Comparative effect of sub-lingual nifedipine and intravenous aminophylline in allergic bronchial asthma. *Indian J. Chest Dis. Allied Sci.* 29:233, 1987.

48. Chanez, P., et al. Increased eosinophil responsiveness to platelet-activating factor in asthma. *Clin. Sci.* 74:5, 1988.

49. Cheng, J. B., Bewtra, A., and Townley, R. G. Identification of calcium antagonist receptor binding sites using (3H)-nitrendipine in bovine tracheal smooth muscle membranes. *Arch. Int. Pharmacodyn. Ther.* 40:267, 1984.

50. Cheng, J. B., and Townley, R. G. Pharmacological characterization of effects of nifedipine on isolated guinea pig and rat tracheal smooth muscle. *Arch. Int. Pharmacodyn. Ther.* 263:228, 1983.

51. Chilvers, E. R., Barnes, P. J., and Nahorski, S. R. Muscarinic receptor stimulated turnover of polyphosphoinositides and inositol phosphates in bovine tracheal smooth muscle. *Br. J. Pharmacol.* 95:778P, 1988.

52. Chilvers, E. R., Barnes, P. J., and Nahorski, S. R. Characterization of agonist-stimulated incorporation of [^{3}H]myo-inositol into phospholipids and [^{3}H]inositol phosphate formation in tracheal smooth muscle. *Biochem. J.* 262:739, 1989.

53. Chilvers, E. R., et al. Characterization of stereospecific binding sites for inositol 1,4,5-triphosphate in airway smooth muscle. *Br. J. Pharmacol.* 99:297, 1990.

54. Chilvers, E. R., et al. Absence of circulating product of oxygen-derived free radicals in acute severe asthma. *Eur. Respir. J.* 2:950, 1989.

55. Chilvers, E. R., and Nahorski, S. R. Phosphoinositide metabolism in airway smooth muscle. *Am. Rev. Respir. Dis.* 141:S137, 1990.

56. Christopher, M. A., et al. Clinical relevance of the interaction of theophylline with diltiazem or nifedipine. *Chest* 95:309, 1989.

57. Christopher, M. A., et al. Efficacy of maintenance therapy with calcium channel blockers for chronic asthma (abstract). *Am. Rev. Respir. Dis.* 137:37, 1988.

58. Cluzel, M., et al. Luminol-dependent chemiluminescence in asthma. *J. Allergy Clin. Immunol.* 80:195, 1987.

59. Coburn, R. F. The airway smooth muscle cell. *Fed. Proc.* 36:2692, 1977.

60. Coburn, R. F. Electromechanical coupling in canine trachealis muscle: Acetylcholine contractions. *Am. J. Physiol.* 236:C177, 1979.

61. Coburn, R. F., and Yamaguchi, T. Membrane potential-dependent and -independent tension in the canine tracheal muscle. *J. Pharmacol. Exp. Ther.* 201:276, 1977.

62. Cockcroft, S. Polyphosphoinositide phosphodisterase: Regulation by a novel guanine nucleotide binding protein, G$_p$. *Trends Biochem. Sci.* 12:75, 1987.

63. Cockcroft, S., and Gomperts, B. D. Role of guanine nucleotide binding protein in the activation of phosphoinositide phosphodiesterase. *Nature* 314:534, 1985.

64. Copas, J. L., Borgeat, P., and Gardiner, P. J. The actions of 5-, 12-, and 15-HETE on tracheobronchial smooth muscle. *Prostaglandins Leukotr. Med.* 8:105, 1982.

65. Corris, P. A., et al. Nifedipine in the prevention of asthma induced by exercise and histamine. *Am. Rev. Respir. Dis.* 128:991, 1983.

66. Creese, B. R., and Bach, M. K. Hyperreactivity of airways smooth muscle produced in vitro by leukotrienes. *Prostaglandins Leukotr. Med.* 11:161, 1983.

67. Crimi, N., et al. Effect of nifedipine on allergen-induced bronchoconstriction. *Allergol. Immunopathol. (Madr.)* 14:263, 1986.

68. Crimi, N., et al. Effect of a calcium antagonist, nifedipine, in exercise-induced asthma. *Respiration* 45:262, 1984.

69. Crimi, N., et al. Effect of sodium cromoglycate and nifedipine on adenosine-induced bronchoconstriction. *Respiration* 53:74, 1988.

70. Cuss, F. M., and Barnes, P. J. Nifedipine prolongs isoprenaline-induced bronchodilatation in normal subjects (abstract). *Clin. Sci.* 67(Suppl. 9):62P, 1984.

71. Cuss, F. M., and Barnes, P. J. The effect of inhaled nifedipine on bronchial reactivity to histamine in man. *J. Allergy Clin. Immunol.* 76:718, 1985.

72. Cuss, F. M., and Barnes, P. J. Inhaled nifedipine and histamine-induced bronchoconstriction (abstract). *Am. Rev. Respir. Dis.* 131(Suppl.):A53, 1985.

73. Cuss, F. M., et al. Effect of nifedipine on autonomic control of airway smooth muscle in vitro. *Am. Rev. Respir. Dis.* 131(Suppl.):A283, 1985.

74. Danoff, S. K., Supattapone, S., and Snyder, S. H. Characterization of a membrane protein from brain mediating the inhibition of inositol(1,4,5) triphosphate receptor binding by calcium. *Biochem. J.* 254:701, 1988.

75. Degenhart, H., et al. Oxygen radicals and their production by leukocytes from children with bronchial hyperresponsiveness. *Clin. Respir. Physiol.* 22:100, 1986.

76. de Lanerolle, P. cAMP, myosin dephosphorylation, and isometric relaxation of airway smooth muscle. *J. Appl. Physiol.* 64:705, 1988.

77. de Lanerolle, P., et al. Myosin phosphorylation, agonist concentration and contraction of tracheal smooth muscle. *Nature* 298:871, 1982.

78. de Lanerolle, P., et al. Increased phosphorylation of myosin light chain kinase after an increase in cyclic AMP in intact smooth muscle. *Science* 223:1415, 1984.

79. de Lanerolle, P., and Stull, J. T. Myosin phosphorylation during contraction and relaxation of tracheal smooth muscle. *J. Biol. Chem.* 255:9993, 1980.

80. Del Maestro, R. F., et al. Oxygen Derived Free Radicals: Their Role in Inflammation. In P. Verge (ed.), *The Inflammatory Process.* Stockholm: A. Lindquist and Wiskell International, 1989. Pp. 113–143.

81. Del Maestro, R. F., Bjork, J., and Arfors, K. E. Increase in microvascular permeability induced by enzymatically generated free radicals. I. In vivo study. *Microvasc. Res.* 22:239, 1981.

82. Dhillon, D. S., and Rodger, I. W. Hyperreactivity of guinea pig isolated airway smooth muscle (abstract). *Br. J. Pharmacol.* 74:180, 1981.

83. Dillon, P. F., et al. Myosin phosphorylation and the cross-bridge cycle in arterial smooth muscle. *Science* 211:495, 1981.

84. Doelman, C. J. A., and Bast, A. Oxygen radicals in lung pathology. *Free Radic. Biol. Med.* 9:381, 1990.

85. Doelman, C. J. A., et al. Vitamin E and selenium regulate the balance between β-adrenergic and muscarinic responses in rat lungs. *FEBS Lett.* 233:427, 1988.

86. Doelman, C. J. A., et al. Mineral dust exposure and free radical-mediated lung damage. *Exp. Lung Res.* 16:41, 1990.

87. Downes, H., and Hirshman, C. A. Lidocaine aerosols do not prevent allergic bronchoconstriction. *Anesth. Analg.* 60:28, 1981.

88. Downes, H., and Hirshman, C. A. Calcium chelators increase airway responsiveness. *J. Appl. Physiol.* 59:92, 1985.

89. Drazen, J. M., Fanta, C. H., and Lacouture, P. G. Effect of nifedipine on constriction of human tracheal strips in vitro. *Br. J. Pharmacol.* 78:687, 1983.

90. Duncan, R. A., et al. Polyphosphoinositide metabolism in canine tracheal smooth muscle (CTSM) in response to a cholinergic stimulus. *Biochem. Pharmacol.* 36:307, 1987.

91. Ebashi, S. Regulation of muscle contraction. *Proc. R. Soc. Lond. [Biol.]* 207:259, 1980.

92. Eisenberg, E., and Hill, T. L. Muscle contraction and free energy transduction in biological systems. *Science* 227:999, 1985.

93. Eliraz, A., et al. Exacerbation of asthmatic symptoms after cessation of nifedipine therapy. *Ann. Allergy* 52:125, 1984.

94. Engels, F., Oosting, R. S., and Nijkamp, F. P. Dual effects of *Haemophilus influenzae* on guinea pig tracheal β-adrenergic receptor: Involvement of oxygen-centered radicals from pulmonary macrophages. *J. Pharmacol. Exp. Ther.* 241:994, 1987.

95. Fain, J. N., Wallace, M. A., and Wojcikiewicz, J. H. Evidence for involvement of guanine nucleotide-binding regulatory proteins in the activation of phospholipases by hormones. *FASEB J.* 2:2569, 1988.

96. Farber, J. L. The role of calcium in cell death. *Life Sci.* 29:1289, 1981.

97. Feinstein, M. B. Inhibition of contraction and calcium excitability in rat uterus by local anesthetics. *J. Pharmacol. Exp. Ther.* 152:516, 1966.

98. Felbel, J., et al. Regulation of cytosolic calcium by cAMP and cGMP in freshly isolated smooth muscle cells from bovine trachea. *J. Biol. Chem.* 263:16764, 1988.

99. Ferrari, M., et al. Differential effects of nifedipine and diltiazem on methacholine-induced bronchospasm in allergic asthma. *Ann. Allergy* 63:196, 1989.

100. Fish, J. E., and Norman, P. S. Effects of the calcium channel blocker, verapamil, on asthmatic airway responses to muscarinic, histaminergic, and allergenic stimuli. *Am. Rev. Respir. Dis.* 133:730, 1986.

101. Flatt, A., et al. Reduced selenium in asthmatic subjects in New Zealand. *Thorax* 45:95, 1990.

102. Forder, J., Scriabine, A., and Rasmussen, H. Plasma membrane calcium flux, protein kinase C activation and smooth muscle contraction. *J. Pharmacol. Exp. Ther.* 232:267, 1985.

103. Foresi, A., et al. Effect of two doses of inhaled diltiazem on exercise-induced asthma. *Respiration* 51:241, 1987.

104. Fuller, B. J., Gower, J. D., and Green, C. J. Free radical damage and organ preservation: Fact or fiction. *Cryobiology* 25:377, 1988.

105. Fung, B. K.-K., Hurley, J. B., and Stryer, L. Flow of information in the light-triggered cyclic nucleotide cascade of vision. *Proc. Natl. Acad. Sci. USA* 78:152, 1981.

106. Garty, M., et al. Effect of nifedipine and theophylline in asthma. *Clin. Pharmacol. Ther.* 40:195, 1986.

107. Gerthoffer, W. T. Calcium dependence of myosin phosphorylation and airway smooth muscle contraction and relaxation. *Am. J. Physiol.* 250:C597, 1986.

108. Gianotti, A., et al. Some effects of prolonged treatment with nicardipine in chronic bronchial asthma. *Curr. Med. Res. Opin.* 10:422, 1987.

109. Giembycz, M. A., and Rodger, I. W. Electrophysiological and other aspects of excitation-contraction coupling in mammalian airway smooth muscle. *Life Sci.* 41:111, 1987.

110. Gilman, A. G. G proteins and dual control of adenylate cyclase. *Cell* 36:577, 1984.

111. Gilman, A. G. G proteins: Transduces of receptor-generated signals. *Annu. Rev. Biochem.* 56:615, 1987.

112. Gonzalez, J. M., et al. Inhibition of airway reactivity by nifedipine in patients with coronary artery disease. *Am. Rev. Respir. Dis.* 127:155, 1983.

113. Gordon, E. H., et al. Comparison of nifedipine with a new calcium channel blocker, flordipine, in exercise-induced asthma. *J. Asthma* 24:261, 1987.

114. Grandordy, B. M., and Barnes, P. J. Phosphoinositide turnover. *Am. Rev. Respir. Dis.* 136(Suppl.):S17, 1987.

115. Grandordy, B. M., et al. Leukotriene C_4 and D_4 induce contraction and formation of inositol phosphates in airways and lung parenchyma. *Am. Rev. Respir. Dis.* 133:A239, 1986.

116. Grandordy, B. M., et al. Phosphatidylinositol response to muscarinic agonist in airway smooth muscle: Relationship to contraction and receptor occupancy. *J. Pharmacol. Exp. Ther.* 238:273, 1986.

117. Grandordy, B. M., et al. Tachykinin-induced phosphoinositide breakdown in airway smooth muscle and epithelium: Relationship to contraction. *Mol. Pharmacol.* 33:515, 1988.

118. Greenspon, L. W., and Levy, S. F. The effect of aerosolized verapamil on the response to isoproterenol in asthmatics. *Am. Rev. Respir. Dis.* 137:722, 1988.

119. Greenwald, R. A. *Handbook of Methods for Oxygen Radical Research.* Boca Raton, Fl.: CRC Press, 1985.

120. Gugger, M., et al. Low plasma concentrations of ionized calcium in patients with asthma. *J. Appl. Physiol.* 64:1354, 1988.

121. Gunst, S. J., and Stropp, J. Q. Effect of Na-K adenosine triphosphatase activity on relaxation of canine tracheal smooth muscle. *J. Appl. Physiol.* 64:635, 1988.

122. Hall, I. P., and Hill, S. J. B$_2$-adrenoceptor stimulation inhibits histamine-stimulated inositol phospholipid hydrolysis in bovine tracheal smooth muscle. *Br. J. Pharmacol.* 95:1204, 1988.

123. Halliwell, B., and Gutteridge, J. M. C. *Free Radicals in Biology and Medicine.* Oxford: Clarendon, 1989.

124. Hamilton, T. C., and Weston, A. H. Cromakalim, nicorandil and pinacidil: Novel drugs which open potassium channels in smooth muscle. *Gen. Pharmacol.* 20:1, 1989.

125. Harman, E., et al. The effect of oral diltiazem on airway reactivity to methacholine and exercise in subjects with mild intermittent asthma. *Am. Rev. Respir. Dis.* 136:1179, 1987.

126. Hartmann, V., and Magnussen, H. Effect of diltiazem on histamine- and carbachol-induced bronchospasm in normal and asthmatic subjects. *Chest* 87:174, 1985.

127. Hashimoto, T., Hirata, M., and Ito, Y. A role for inositol 1,4,5-trisphosphate in the initiation of agonist induced contractions of dog tracheal smooth muscle. *Br. J. Pharmacol.* 86:191, 1985.

128. Hasselmark, L., et al. Lowered platelet gluathione peroxidase activity in patients with intrinsic asthma. *Allergy* 45:523, 1990.

129. Hedman, S. E., and Andersson, R. G. G. Studies on the contracting mechanism induced by slow reacting substance of anaphylaxis (SRS-A) interaction with calcium. *Acta Pharmacol. Toxicol. (Copenh.)* 50:379, 1980.

130. Heffner, J. E., and Repine, J. E. Pulmonary strategies of antioxidant defense. State of the art. *Am. Rev. Respir. Dis.* 140:531, 1989.

131. Hendeles, L., et al. Dose-response of inhaled diltiazem on airway reactivity to methacholine and exercise in subjects with mild asthma. *Clin. Pharmacol. Ther.* 43:387, 1988.

132. Henderson, A. F., and Costello, J. F. The effect of nifedipine on bronchial reactivity to inhaled histamine and methacholine: A comparative study in normal and asthmatic subjects. *Br. J. Dis. Chest* 82:374, 1988.

133. Henderson, A. F., et al. Effect of nifedipine on bronchoconstriction induced by inhalation of cold air. *Thorax* 38:512, 1983.

134. Henderson, A. F., et al. Effects of nifedipine on antigen-induced bronchoconstriction. *Am. Rev. Respir. Dis.* 127:549, 1983.

135. Henderson, W. R., and Kaliner, M. Immunologic and nonimmunologic generation of superoxide from mast cells and basophils. *J. Clin. Invest.* 61:187, 1978.

136. Hirshman, C. A., and Bergman, W. A. Factors influencing intrapulmonary airway calibre during anesthesia. *Br. J. Anaesth.* 65:30, 1990.

137. Hoidal, J. R., et al. Altered oxidative metabolic responses in vitro of alveolar macrophages from asymptomatic cigarette smoke. *Am. Rev. Respir. Dis.* 123:85, 1981.

138. Honda, K., and Tomita, T. Electrical activity in isolated human tracheal muscle. *Jpn. J. Physiol.* 37:333, 1987.

138a. Hoppe, M., et al. The effect of inhaled gallopamil, a potent calcium channel blocker, on the late-phase response in subjects with allergic asthma. *J. Allergy Clin. Immunol.* 89:688, 1992.

139. Hui, K. P., and Barnes, N. C. Lung function improvement in asthma with cysteinyl-leukotriene receptor antagonist. *Lancet* 337:1062, 1991.

140. Ikeda, H., et al. Acute effects of nifedipine on patients with chronic obstructive lung disease. *Arzneimittelforschung* 35:518, 1985.

141. Jadot, G., et al. Antioxidants in asthma. *Bull. Acad. Natl. Med.* 172:693, 1988.

142. Jaiprakash, S. S., et al. Efficacy of nifedipine in the treatment of angina pectoris and chronic airways obstruction. *Postgrad. Med. J.* 56:624, 1980.

143. Javaid, A., Cushley, M. J., and Bone, M. F. Effect of dietary salt on bronchial reactivity to histamine in asthma. *Br. Med. J.* 297:454, 1988.

144. Johnson, K. J., et al. In vivo damage of rat lungs by oxygen metabolites. *J. Clin. Invest.* 67:983, 1981.

145. Jones, K. A., et al. Halothane decreases cytosolic ionized calcium concentration ($[Ca^{2+}]_i$) during acetylcholine-induced contraction of canine trachealis muscle. *Anesthesiology* 75:A639, 1991.

146. Juniper, E. F., et al. Airway responsiveness to histamine and methacholine: Relationship to minimum treatment to control symptoms of asthma. *Thorax* 36:575, 1981.

147. Kaibuchi, K., Takai, Y., and Nishizuka, Y. Cooperative roles of various membrane phospholipids in the activation of calcium activated phospholipid-dependent protein kinase. *J. Biol. Chem.* 256:7146, 1981.

148. Kamm, K. E., and Stull, J. T. Myosin phosphorylation, force, and maximum shortening velocity in neurally stimulated tracheal smooth muscle. *Am. J. Physiol.* 249:C238, 1985.

149. Kanazawa, H ., et al. The role of free radicals in airway obstruction in asthmatic patients. *Chest* 100:1319, 1991.

150. Katsumata, U., et al. Reactive oxygen exposure produces airway hyper-responsiveness. *Am. Rev. Respir. Dis.* 137:285, 1988.

151. Kelly, C. A., et al. Numbers and activity of cells obtained at bronchoalveolar lavage in asthma and their relationship to airway responsiveness. *Thorax* 43:684, 1988.

152. Kivity, S., et al. The combined effect of nifedipine and sodium cromoglycate on the airway response to inhaled hypertonic saline in patients with bronchial asthma. *Eur. Respir. J.* 2:513, 1989.

153. Kivity, S., et al. Combined effect of inhaled verapamil and sodium cromoglycate on the airway response to hypertonic saline. *Ann. Allergy* 64:163, 1990.

154. Kirkpatrick, C. T. Excitation and contraction in bovine tracheal smooth muscle. *J. Physiol (Lond.)* 244:263, 1975.

155. Kirkpatrick, C. T., Jenkinson, H. A., and Cameron, A. R. Interaction between drugs and potassium-rich solutions in producing contraction in bovine tracheal smooth muscle: Studies in normal and calcium depleted tissues. *Clin. Exp. Pharmacol. Physiol.* 2:559, 1975.

156. Kirkpatrick, M. B., Sanders, R. V., and Bass, J. B., Jr. Physiologic effects and serum lidocaine concentrations after inhalation of lidocaine from a compressed gas-powered jet nebulizer. *Am. Rev. Respir. Dis.* 136:1987, 1987.

157. Kneussl, M., et al. Nifedipine protects acetylcholine induced bronchoconstriction: The role of mediator release (abstract). *Am. Rev. Respir. Dis.* 127:108, 1983.

158. Koppermann, G., and Kaukel, G. The influence of nifedipine, a calcium channel blocker, on allergen-induced bronchoconstriction. *Prog. Respir. Res.* 19:271, 1985.

159. Kotlikoff, M. I. Calcium currents in isolated canine airway smooth muscle cells. *Am. J. Physiol.* 254:C793, 1988.

160. Kotlikoff, M. I., Murray, R. K., and Reynolds, E. E. Histamine induced Ca^{2+} release and phorbol antagonism in cultured airway smooth muscle cells. *Am. J. Physiol.* 253:C561, 1987.

161. Kramer, K., et al. A disbalance between β-adrenergic and muscarinic responses caused by hydrogen peroxide in rat airways in vitro. *Biochem. Biophys. Res. Commun.* 145:357, 1987.

162. Kramer, K., et al. Influence of lipid peroxidation on β-adrenoreceptors. *FEBS Lett.* 198:80, 1986.

163. Krebs, E. G., and Beavo, J. A. Phosphorylation-dephosphorylation of enzymes. *Annu. Rev. Biochem.* 48:923, 1979.

164. Kurasawa, M., et al. Superoxide anion formation from activated peritoneal mast cells in vitro measured by MCLA-dependence luminescence. *Immunol. Allergy Pract.* 235:17, 1991.

165. Kuthan, H., and Ullrich, V. Oxidase and oxygen function of the microsomal cytochrome P450 monoxygenase system. *Eur. J. Biochem.* 126:583, 1982.

165a. Lansing, M. W., et al. Lipid mediators contribute to oxygen-radical-induced airway responses in sheep. *Am. Rev. Respir. Dis.* 144:1291, 1991.

166. Lee, V. Y., et al. Verapamil inhibits mediator release from human lung in vitro. *Thorax* 38:386, 1983.

167. Lemoine, H., Pohl, V., and Teng, K. J. Serotonin (5-HT) stimulates phosphatidylinositol (PI) hydrolysis only through the R-state of allosterically regulated 5-HT₂ receptors in calf tracheal smooth muscle. *Naunyn Schmiedebergs Arch. Pharmacol.* 377(Suppl.):R103, 1988.

168. Lever, A. M., et al. Nifedipine enhances the bronchodilator effect of salbutamol. *Thorax* 39:576, 1984.

169. Lewis, M. S., et al. Hydrogen peroxide stimulates the synthesis of platelet-activating factor by endothelium and induces endothelial cell-dependent neutrophil adhesion. *J. Clin. Invest.* 82:2045, 1988.

170. Lichey, J., et al. Effect of diltiazem on methacholine-induced bronchoconstriction in extrinsic asthmatics. *Respiration* 50:44, 1986.

171. Lidji, M., et al. Therapy with nifedipine in asthma: A randomized double-blind crossover trial. *Isr. J. Med. Sci.* 24:1, 1988.

172. Litosch, I., Wallis, C., and Fain, J. N. 5-Hydroxytryptamine stimulated inositol phosphate production in a cell-free system from blowfly salivary glands: Evidence for a role of GTP in coupling receptor activation to phosphoinositide breakdown. *J. Biol. Chem.* 260:5464, 1985.

173. Loesberg, C., Henricks, P. A. J., and Nijkamp, F. P. Inverse relationship between superoxide anion production of guinea pig alveolar macrophages and tracheal β-adrenergic receptor function; influence of dietary polyunsaturated fatty acids. *Int. J. Immunopharmacol.* 11:165, 1989.

174. Lofdahl, C. G., et al. Effects of nifedipine or atenolol on ventilatory capacity and hemodynamics in asthmatic patients: Interaction with terbutaline. *Curr. Ther. Res.* 36:282, 1984.

175. Magnussen, H., et al. Influence of diltiazem on bronchoconstriction induced by cold air breathing during exercise. *Thorax* 39:579, 1984.

176. Malik, S., et al. Effects of sublingual nifedipine on inhaled histamine and methacholine-induced bronchoconstriction in atopic subjects (abstract). *Thorax* 37:230, 1982.

177. Malmgren, R., et al. Lowered glutathione peroxidase activity in asthmatic patients with food and aspirin intolerance. *Allergy* 41:43, 1986.

178. Mannioni, P. F., et al. Free radicals as endogenous histamine releasers. *Agents Actions* 23:129, 1989.

179. Mansour, S., and Daniel, E. E. Responsiveness of isolated tracheal smooth muscle from normal and sensitized guinea pigs. *Can. J. Physiol. Pharmacol.* 65:1942, 1987.

180. Mapp, C., et al. Protective effect of antiasthma drugs on late asthmatic reactions and increased airway responsiveness induced by toluene diisocyanate in sensitized subjects. *Am. Rev. Respir. Dis.* 136:1403, 1987.

181. Marin, J. M., et al. Nifedipine in exercise-induced asthma. *Allergol. Immunopathol. (Madr.)* 14:37, 1986.

182. Marthan, R., et al. Extracellular calcium and human isolated airway muscle: Ionophore A23187 induced contraction. *Respir. Physiol.* 71:157, 1988.

183. Marthan, R., et al. Calcium channel currents in isolated smooth muscle cells from human bronchus. *J. Appl. Physiol.* 66:1706, 1989.

184. Massey, K. L., et al. Duration of protection of calcium channel blockers against exercise-induced bronchospasm: Comparison of oral diltiazem and inhaled gallopamil. *Eur. J. Clin. Pharmacol.* 34:555, 1988.

185. Massey, K. L., et al. Dose response of inhaled gallopamil (D600), a calcium channel blocker, in attenuating airway reactivity to methacholine and exercise. *J. Allergy Clin. Immunol.* 81:912, 1988.

186. Matthews, J. I., et al. Nifedipine does not alter methacholine-induced bronchial reactivity. *Ann. Allergy* 43:462, 1984.

187. McDonald, R. J., Berger, E. M., and Repine, J. M. Alveolar macrophage antioxidants prevent hydrogen peroxide-mediated lung damage. *Am. Rev. Respir. Dis.* 143:1088, 1991.

188. McIntyre, E., et al. Inhaled verapamil in histamine-induced bronchoconstriction. *J. Allergy Clin. Immunol.* 71:375, 1983.

189. Meisheri, K. D., and van Breemen, C. Effects of β-adrenergic stimulation on calcium movements in rabbit aortic smooth muscle: Relationship with cyclic AMP. *J. Physiol.* 331:429, 1982.

190. Meltzer, S., et al. Superoxide generation and its modulation by adenosine in neutrophils of subjects with asthma. *J. Allergy Clin. Immunol.* 83:960, 1989.

191. Meurs, H., et al. Evidence for a direct relationship between phosphoinositide metabolism and airway smooth muscle contraction induced by muscarinic agonists. *Eur. J. Pharmacol.* 156:271, 1988.

192. Miadonna, A., et al. Effect of verapamil on allergen-induced asthma in patients with respiratory allergy. *Ann. Allergy* 51:201, 1983.

193. Middleton, E., Jr. Antiasthmatic drug therapy and calcium ions: Review of pathogenesis and role of calcium. *J. Pharm. Sci.* 69:243, 1980.

194. Miller, J. R., Silver, P. J., and Stull, S. T. The role of myosin light chain kinase phosphorylation in beta-adrenergic relaxation of tracheal smooth muscle. *Mol. Pharmacol.* 24:235, 1983.

195. Miller, W. C., and Awe, R. Effect of nebulized lidocaine on reactive airways. *Am. Rev. Respir. Dis.* 111:739, 1975.

196. Miller-Hance, W. C., et al. Biochemical events associated with activation of smooth muscle contraction. *J. Biol. Chem.* 263:13979, 1988.

197. Mita, H., et al. Increased activity of 5-lipooxygenase in polymorphonuclear leukocytes from asthmatic patients. *Life Sci.* 37:907, 1985.

197a. Miura, M., et al. Role of potassium channels in bronchodilator responses in human airways. *Am. Rev. Respir. Dis.* 146:132, 1992.

198. Molho, M., et al. Nifedipine in asthma. Dose-related effect on resting bronchial tone. *Chest* 91:667, 1987.

199. Moscato, G., et al. Effect of nifedipine on hyperreactive bronchial responses to methacholine. *Ann. Allergy* 56:145, 1986.

200. Moscato, G., et al. Protective effect of nifedipine upon specific bronchial responses to isocyanates. *G. Ital. Med. Lav.* 5:247, 1983.

201. Murray, R. K., et al. Mechanism of phorbol ester inhibition of histamine-induced IP3 formation in cultured airway smooth muscle. *Am. J. Physiol.* 257:L209, 1989.

202. Nagai, P. K., and Walsh, M. P. Inhibition of smooth muscle actin-activated myosin Mg2+ −ATPase activity by caldesmon. *J. Biol. Chem.* 259:13656, 1984.

203. Nair, N., et al. Safety of nifedipine in subjects with bronchial asthma and COPD. *Chest* 86:515, 1984.

204. Nakagawara, M., et al. Inhibition of superoxide production and calcium

mobilization in human neutrophils by halothane, enflurane, and isoflurane. *Anesthesiology* 64:4, 1986.

205. Neyens, H. J., et al. Altered leukocyte response in relation to the basic abnormality in children with asthma and bronchial hyperresponsiveness. *Am. Rev. Respir. Dis.* 130:744, 1984.

206. Nishida, Y., Suzuki, S., and Miyamoto, T. Biphasic contraction of isolated guinea pig tracheal rings by superoxide radical. *Inflammation* 9:333, 1985.

207. Nishikawa, M., Hidaka, H., and Adelstein, R. S. Phosphorylation of smooth muscle heavy meromyosin by calcium activated phospholipid-dependent protein kinase. *J. Biol. Chem.* 258:14069, 1983.

208. Nishizuka, Y. Studies and perspectives of protein kinase C. *Science* 233:305, 1986.

209. Ogilvy, C. S., Dubois, A. B., and Douglas, J. S. Effects of ascorbic acid and indomethacin on the airways of healthy male subjects with and without induced bronchoconstriction. *J. Allergy Clin. Immunol.* 67:363, 1981.

210. Olive, S. R., et al. Comparison of PY 108-068, a new calcium antagonist, with nifedipine in exercise-induced asthma. *Chest* 90:208, 1986.

211. Owen, S., et al. A randomised double blind placebo controlled crossover study of a potassium channel activator in morning dipping (abstract). *Thorax* 44:852, 1989.

212. Ozenne, G., et al. Nifedipine in chronic bronchial asthma: A randomized double-blind crossover trial against placebo. *Eur. J. Respir. Dis.* 67:238, 1985.

213. Park, S., and Rasmussen, H. Activation of tracheal smooth muscle contraction: Synergism between Ca^{2+} and activators of protein kinase C. *Proc. Natl. Acad. Sci. USA* 82:8835, 1985.

214. Parker, J. C., et al. Prevention of free radical-mediated vascular permeability increases in lung using superoxide dismutase. *Chest* 83:52S, 1983.

215. Parrish, R. W., and Davies, B. H. Allergen bronchial challenge and effects of lodoxamide and nifedipine (abstract). *J. Allergy Clin. Immunol.* 71:152, 1983.

216. Patakas, D., et al. Nifedipine treatment of patients with bronchial asthma. *J. Allergy Clin. Immunol.* 79:959, 1987.

217. Patakas, D., et al. Nifedipine in bronchial asthma. *J. Allergy Clin. Immunol.* 72:269, 1983.

218. Patel, K. R. The effect of calcium antagonist, nifedipine, in exercise-induced asthma. *Clin. Allergy* 11:429, 1981.

219. Patel, K. R. Calcium antagonists in exercise-induced asthma. *Br. Med. J.* 282:932, 1981.

220. Patel, K. R. The effect of verapamil on histamine and methacholine-induced bronchoconstriction. *Clin. Allergy* 11:441, 1981.

221. Patel, K. R. Sodium cromoglycate and verapamil alone and in combination in exercise induced asthma. *Br. Med. J.* 286:606, 1983.

222. Patel, K. R., and Al-Shamma, M. R. Effect of nifedipine on histamine reactivity in asthma. *Br. Med. J.* 284:1916, 1982.

223. Patel, K. R., et al. The effect of inhaled verapamil on allergen-induced bronchoconstriction. *Clin. Allergy* 13:119, 1983.

224. Patel, K. R., and Kerr, J. W. Calcium antagonists in experimental asthma. *Clin. Allergy* 12(Suppl.):15, 1982.

225. Patel, K. R., and Peers, E. Felodipine, a new calcium antagonist, modifies exercise-induced asthma. *Am. Rev. Respir. Dis.* 138:54, 1988.

226. Patel, K. R., and Tullett, W. M. Comparison of two calcium antagonists, verapamil and gallopamil (D-600), in exercise-induced asthma. *Eur. J. Respir. Dis.* 67:269, 1985.

227. Paterson, J. W., Woolcock, A. J., and Shenfield, G. M. Bronchodilator drugs. *Am. Rev. Respir. Dis.* 120:1149, 1979.

228. Pato, M. D., and Adelstein, R. S. Dephosphorylation of the 20,000 dalton light chain of myosin by two different phosphatases from smooth muscle. *J. Biol. Chem.* 255:6535, 1980.

229. Perpina, M., et al. Different ability of verapamil to inhibit agonist-induced contraction of lung parenchymal strips from control and sensitized guinea pig. *Respiration* 50:174, 1986.

230. Perpina, M., et al. Nifedipine decreases sensitivity and reactivity to methacholine in mild asthmatics. *Respiration* 51:49, 1987.

231. Pfaffinger, P. J., et al. GTP-binding proteins couple cardiac muscarinic receptors to a K channel. *Nature* 317:536, 1985.

232. Phipps, R. J., et al. The effect of 0.5 ppm ozone on glycoprotein secretion, ion and water fluxes in sheep trachea. *J. Appl. Physiol.* 60:918, 1986.

233. Popa, V. T., et al. The effect of inhaled verapamil on resting bronchial tone and airway contractions induced by histamine and acetylcholine in normal and asthmatic subjects. *Am. Rev. Respir. Dis.* 130:1006, 1984.

234. Postma, D. S., et al. Association between nonspecific bronchial hyperreactivity and superoxide anion production by polymorphonuclear leukocytes in chronic airflow obstruction. *Am. Rev. Respir. Dis.* 137:57, 1988.

235. Raeburn, D., et al. Agonist-induced contractile responses of human bronchial muscle in vitro: Effects of $Ca2+$ removal, $La3+$ and PY108068. *Eur. J. Pharmacol.* 121:251, 1986.

236. Raeburn, D., et al. Concentration-related differences in the effects of the Ca^{2+} agonist BAY K8644 in human bronchus in vitro. *Gen. Pharmacol.* 19:399, 1988.

237. Raeburn, D., and Rodger, I. W. Lack of effect of leukotriene D_4 on calcium-uptake in airway smooth muscle. *Br. J. Pharmacol.* 83:499, 1984.

238. Rafferty, P., et al. Effects of verapamil and sodium cromoglycate on bronchoconstriction induced by isocapnic hyperventilation. *Clin. Allergy* 15:531, 1985.

239. Rafferty, P., and Holgate, S. T. Terfenadine (Seldane) is a potent and selective histamine H1 receptor antagonist in asthmatic airways. *Am. Rev. Respir. Dis.* 135:181, 1987.

240. Rafferty, P., et al. Inhibition of exercise-induced asthma by nifedipine: A dose-response study. *Br. J. Clin. Pharmacol.* 24:479, 1987.

241. Rang, H. P., and Dale, M. M. *Pharmacology* (2nd ed.). London: Churchill-Livingstone, 1991.

242. Rasmussen, H., et al. TPA-induced contraction of isolated rabbit vascular smooth muscle. *Biochem. Biophys. Res. Commun.* 122:776, 1984.

243. Rasmussen, H., Kelley, G., and Douglas, J. S. Interactions between Ca^{2+} and cAMP messenger system in regulation of airway smooth muscle contraction. *J. Physiol.* 258:L279, 1990.

244. Rhoden, K. J., and Barnes, P. J. Effect of hydrogen peroxide in guinea-pig tracheal smooth muscle in vitro: Role of cyclo-oxygenase and airway epithelium. *Br. J. Pharmacol.* 98:325, 1989.

245. Ringqvist, T. Effect of verapamil in obstructive airways disease. *Eur. J. Clin. Pharmacol.* 7:61, 1974.

246. Riska, H., et al. Effects of captopril on blood pressure and respiratory function compared to verapamil in patients with hypertension and asthma. *J. Cardiovasc. Pharmacol.* 15:57, 1990.

247. Riska, H., et al. Comparison of the effects of an angiotensin converting enzyme inhibitor and a calcium channel blocker on blood pressure and respiratory function in patients with hypertension and asthma. *J. Cardiovasc. Pharmacol.* 10(Suppl. 10):S79, 1987.

248. Roberts, J. A., et al. In vitro and in vivo effect of verapamil on human airway responsiveness to leukotriene D_4. *Thorax* 41:12, 1986.

249. Roberts, J. A., et al. Effect of verapamil and sodium cromoglycate on leukotriene D_4 induced bronchoconstriction in patients with asthma. *Thorax* 41:753, 1986.

250. Roberts, J. A., and Thomson, N. C. Effect of verapamil on bronchodilator response to beta receptor agonists in asthma (abstract). *Thorax* 39:171, 1984.

251. Rodger, I. W. Excitation-contraction coupling in airway smooth muscle. *Br. J. Clin. Pharmacol.* 20:255S, 1985.

252. Rodger, I. W. Calcium channels. *Am. Rev. Respir. Dis.* 136:S15, 1987.

253. Rolla, G., et al. Magnesium attenuates methacholine-induced bronchoconstriction in asthmatics. *Magnesium* 6:201, 1987.

254. Rolla, G., et al. Nifedipine inhibits deep-inspiration-induced bronchoconstriction in asthmatics. *Lancet* 1:1305, 1982.

255. Russell, J. A. Tracheal smooth muscle. *Clin. Chest Med.* 7:189, 1986.

256. Russi, E. W., et al. Comparative modification of antigen-induced bronchoconstriction by the calcium antagonists, nifedipine and verapamil. *Chest* 88:74, 1985.

257. Ryan, G., et al. Effect of beclomethasone dipropionate on bronchial responsiveness to histamine in controlled nonsteroid-dependent asthma. *J. Allergy Clin. Immunol.* 75:25, 1985.

258. Sands, H., and Mascali, J. Effects of cAMP and protein kinase on the calcium uptake of various smooth muscle organelles. *Arch. Int. Pharmacodyn. Ther.* 236:180, 1978.

259. Sands, H., Meyer, T. A., and Rickenberg, H. V. Adenosine 3',5'-monophosphate-dependent protein kinase of bovine tracheal smooth muscle. *Biochim. Biophys. Acta* 302:267, 1973.

260. Sanguinetti, M. C., and Kass, R. S. Voltage dependent block of calcium channel current in the calf cardiac Purkinje fiber by dihydropyridine calcium channel antagonists. *Circ. Res.* 55:336, 1984.

261. Sanz, C., et al. Different ability of trifluoperazine to inhibit agonist-induced contraction of lung parenchymal strips from control and sensitized guinea pigs. *J. Pharm. Pharmacol.* 40:120, 1988.

262. Scarpa, M., et al. Superoxide ion as active intermediate in the autoxidation of ascorbate by molecular oxygen. *J. Biol. Chem.* 258:6695, 1983.

263. Schwartzstein, R. S., and Fanta, C. H. Orally administered nifedipine in

chronic stable asthma. Comparison with an orally administered sympathomimetic. *Am. Rev. Respir. Dis.* 134:262, 1986.

264. Sedwick, J. B., Geiger, K. M., and Busse, W. W. Superoxide generation by hypodense eosinophils from patients with asthma. *Am. Rev. Respir. Dis.* 142:120, 1990.

265. Sellers, J. R., Pato, M. D., and Adelstein, R. S. Reversible phosphorylation of smooth muscle myosin, heavy meromyosin and platelet myosin. *J. Biol. Chem.* 256:13137, 1981.

266. Serhan, C., et al. Phosphatidate and oxidized fatty acids are calcium ionophores. *J. Biol. Chem.* 256:2736, 1981.

267. Shah, J., and Pant, H. C. Potassium channel blockers inhibit inositol triphosphate induced calcium release in microsomal fractions isolated from rat brain. *Biochem. J.* 250:617, 1988.

268. Sharma, S. K., and Pande, J. N. Effect of verapamil inhalation on bronchial asthma. *J. Asthma* 27:31, 1990.

269. Sharma, S. K., et al. The effect of nifedipine on exercise-induced asthma. *J. Asthma* 23:15, 1986.

270. Sharma, S. K., et al. Immediate effect of verapamil on pulmonary functions in bronchial asthma. *J. Asthma* 24:179, 1987.

271. Silver, P. J., and Stull, J. T. Regulation of myosin light chain and phosphorylase phosphorylation in tracheal smooth muscle. *J. Biol. Chem.* 257:6145, 1982.

272. Skobelloff, E. M., et al. Intravenous magnesium sulfate for the treatment of acute asthma in the emergency department. *JAMA* 262:1210, 1989.

273. Skoner, D. P., Gentile, D. J., and Evans, R. Decreased activity of the platelet Na$^+$, K$^+$ adenosine triphosphatase enzyme (ATPase) in allergic subjects. *J. Lab. Clin. Med.* 115:535, 1990.

274. Skoner, D. P., Gentile, D., and Evans, R. W. A circulating inhibition of the platelet Na$^+$, K$^+$ adenosine triphosphatase (ATPase) enzyme in allergy. *J. Allergy Clin. Immunol.* 87:476, 1991.

275. Sly, P. D., et al. Does nifedipine affect the diurnal variation of asthma in children? *Pediatr. Pulmonol.* 2:206, 1986.

276. Small, R. C. Electrical slow waves and tone of guinea pig isolated trachealis muscle: Effects of drugs and temperature changes. *Br. J. Pharmacol.* 77:45, 1982.

277. Small, R. C., et al. Airway Smooth Muscle: Electrophysiological Properties and Behavior. In D. K. Agrawal and R. G. Townley (eds.), *Airway Smooth Muscle: Modulation of Receptors and Response.* Boston: CRC Press, 1990. P. 69.

278. Small, R. C., and Foster, R. W. Electrophysiologic behavior of normal and sensitized airway smooth muscle. *Am. Rev. Respir. Dis.* 136:S7, 1987.

279. Smith, S. R., et al. Effect of nifedipine on serum theophylline concentrations and asthma control. *Thorax* 42:794, 1987.

280. So, S. Y., et al. Effect of calcium antagonists on allergen-induced asthma. *Clin. Allergy* 12:595, 1982.

281. Sobieszek, A. Vertebrate Smooth Muscle Myosin. Enzymatic and Structural Properties. In N. L. Stephens (ed.), *The Biochemistry of Smooth Muscle.* Baltimore: University Park Press, 1977. P. 413.

282. Sobue, K., et al. Control of actin-myosin interaction of gizzard smooth muscle by calmodulin and caldesmon-linked flip-flop mechanism. *Biomed. Res.* 3:188, 1982.

283. Solway, J., and Fanta, C. H. Differential inhibition of bronchoconstriction by the calcium channel blockers, verapamil and nifedipine. *Am. Rev. Respir. Dis.* 132:666, 1985.

284. Somlyo, A. V., et al. Inositol trisphosphate-induced calcium release and contraction in vascular smooth muscle. *Proc. Natl. Acad. Sci. USA* 82:5231, 1987.

285. Souhrada, J. F., and Souhrada, M. Significance of the sodium pump for airway smooth muscle. *Eur. J. Respir. Dis.* 64:196, 1983.

286. Souhrada, M., and Souhrada, J. F. Re-assessment of electrophysiological and contractile characteristics of sensitized airway smooth muscle. *Respir. Physiol.* 46:17, 1981.

287. Souhrada, M., Souhrada, J. F. Potentiation of Na$^+$-electrogenic pump of airway smooth muscle by sensitization. *Respir. Physiol.* 47:69, 1982.

288. Souhrada, M., and Souhrada, J. F. Immunologically induced alterations of airway smooth muscle cell membrane. *Science* 225:723, 1984.

289. Souhrada, M., and Souhrada, J. F. Alterations of airway smooth muscle cell membrane by sensitization. *Pediatr. Pulmonol.* 1:207, 1985.

290. Souhrada, M., and Souhrada, J. F. A transient calcium influx into airway smooth muscle cells induced by immunization. *Respir. Physiol.* 67:323, 1987.

291. Souhrada, M., and Souhrada, J. F. Sodium and calcium influx induced by phorbol esters in airway smooth muscle cells. *Am. Rev. Respir. Dis.* 139:927, 1989.

292. Sparrow, M. P., et al. Effect of calmodulin, Ca2+, and cAMP protein kinase on skinned tracheal smooth muscle. *Am. J. Physiol.* 246:C308, 1984.

293. Spedini, C., and Lombardi, C. Long-term treatment with oral nifedipine plus theophylline in the management of chronic bronchial asthma. *Eur. J. Clin. Pharmacol.* 31:105, 1986.

294. Squire, J. Muscle regulation: A decade of the steric blocking model. *Nature* 291:614, 1981.

295. Stephens, N. L., Seow, C. Y., and Kong, S. K. Mechanical properties of sensitized airway smooth muscle: Shortening capacity. *Am. Rev. Respir. Dis.* 143:S13, 1991.

296. Stewart, R. M., et al. Hydrogen peroxide contracts airway smooth muscle: A possible endogenous mechanism. *Respir. Physiol.* 45:333, 1981.

297. Stone, J., et al. Selenium status of patients with asthma. *Clin. Sci.* 77:495, 1989.

298. Stryer, L., and Bourne, H. R. G proteins: A family of signal transducers. *Annu. Rev. Cell Biol.* 2:391, 1986.

299. Styrt, B., Rocklin, R. E., and Klempner, M. S. Characterization of the neutrophil respiratory burst in atopy. *J. Allergy Clin. Immunol.* 81:20, 1988.

300. Suematsu, E., et al. Inositol 1,4,5-trisphosphate releases Ca^{2+} from intracellular store sites in skinned single cells of porcine coronary artery. *Biochem. Biophys. Res. Commun.* 120:481, 1984.

301. Svedmyr, K., et al. Nifedipine—a calcium channel blocker—in asthmatic patients. Interaction with terbutaline. *Allergy* 39:17, 1984.

302. Takemura, H., and Putney, J. W., Jr. Capacitative calcium entry in parotid acinar cells. *Biochem. J.* 258:409, 1989.

303. Takuwa, Y., Takuwa, N., and Rasmussen, H. Carbachol induces a rapid and sustained hydrolysis of phosphotidylinositide in bovine tracheal smooth muscle measurements of the mass of polyphosphoinositides, 1,2-diacylglycerol and phosphatidic acid. *J. Biol. Chem.* 261:14670, 1986.

304. Tate, R. M., et al. Oxygen-radical-mediated permeability edema and vasoconstriction in isolated perfused rabbit lungs. *Am. Rev. Respir. Dis.* 126:802, 1982.

305. Taylor, D. A., Bowman, B. F., and Stull, J. T. Cytoplasmic Ca^{2+} is a primary determinant for myosin phosphorylation in smooth muscle cells. *J. Biol. Chem.* 264:6207, 1989.

306. Taylor, D. A., and Stull, J. T. Calcium dependence of myosin light chain phosphorylation in smooth muscle cells. *J. Biol. Chem.* 263:14456, 1988.

307. Test, S. J., and Weiss, S. J. Quantitative and temporal characteristics of the extracellular H$_2$O$_2$ pool generated by human neutrophils. *J. Biol. Chem.* 259:399, 1984.

308. Tomioka, S., et al. Effect of nifedipine on dose-response curves to acetylcholine and histamine measured during quiet breathing. *Respiration* 50:185, 1986.

309. Torphy, T. J. Biochemical regulation of airway smooth muscle tone: Current knowledge and therapeutic implications. *Rev. Clin. Basic Pharmacol.* 6:61, 1987.

310. Torphy, T. J., et al. Cyclic nucleotide-dependent protein kinase in airway smooth muscle. *J. Biol. Chem.* 257:11609, 1982.

311. Torphy, T. J., and Gerthoeffer, W. T. Biochemical Mechanisms of Smooth Muscle Contraction and Relaxation. In: M. A. Hollinger (ed.), *Current Topics in Pulmonary Pharmacology and Toxicology,* Vol. 1. New York: Elsevier Science, 1986. P. 23.

312. Triggle, D. J. Cellular calcium metabolism: Activation and antagonism. *J. Asthma* 21:375, 1984.

313. Triggle, D. J. Calcium ions and respiratory smooth muscle function. *Br. J. Clin. Pharmacol.* 20:213s, 1985.

314. Triggle, D. J., and Janis, R. A. Nitrendipine: Binding Sites and Mechanism of Action. In A. Scriabine, et al. (eds.), *Nitrendipine.* Baltimore: Urban & Schwarzenberg, 1984. P. 34.

315. Tsuda, T., et al. Bronchodilating effect of inhaled or orally administered calcium channel blocking agents on methacholine-induced bronchoconstriction. *Can. J. Anaesth.* 37:S166, 1990.

316. Twort, C. H. C., and van Breemen, C. Human airway smooth muscle in cell culture: Control on the intracellular calcium store. *Pulmon. Pharmacol.* 2:45, 1989.

317. Verdiani, P., et al. Effect of nisoldipine (BAY k 5552) on methacholine-induced bronchoconstriction in patients with nonspecific bronchial hyperreactivity. *Ann. Allergy* 63:498, 1989.

318. Vincenc, K. S., et al. Comparison of in vivo and in vitro responses to histamine in human airways. *Am. Rev. Respir. Dis.* 128:875, 1983.

319. Wagner, P. D., et al. Protection against pulmonary O₂ toxicity by N-acetylcysteine. *Eur. Respir. J.* 2:116, 1989.

320. Walsh, M. P. Calcium dependent mechanisms of regulation of smooth muscle. *Biochem. Cell Biol.* 69:771, 1991.

321. Walsh, M. P., et al. Is smooth muscle myosin a substrate for cAMP-dependent protein kinase? *FEBS Lett.* 126:107, 1981.

322. Walters, E. H., et al. Effects of calcium channel blockade on histamine induced bronchoconstriction in mild asthma. *Thorax* 39:572, 1984.

323. Watson, K. V., et al. Magnesium sulfate: Rational for its use in pre-eclampsia. *Proc. Natl. Acad. Sci. USA* 83:1075, 1986.

324. Weiss, E. B. Leukotriene-associated toxic oxygen metabolites induce airway hyperreactivity. *Chest* 5:709, 1986.

325. Weiss, E. B. Toxic oxygen products alter calcium homeostasis in an asthma model. *J. Allergy Clin. Immunol.* 75:692, 1985.

326. Weiss, E. B., and Bellino, J. R. Superoxide anion generation during airway anaphylaxis. *Int. Arch. Allergy Appl. Immunol.* 80:211, 1986.

327. Weiss, E. B., Hargraves, W. A., and Viswanath, S. G. The inhibitory action of lidocaine in anaphylaxis. *Am. Rev. Respir. Dis.* 117:859, 1978.

328. Weiss, E. B., Mullick, P. C., and Barbero, L. J. Leukotriene effect in airways smooth muscle: Calcium dependency and verapamil inhibition. *Prostaglandins Leukot. Med.* 12:53, 1983.

329. Weiss, E. B., and Viswanath, S. G. Calcium hypersensitivity in airways smooth muscle: Isometric tension responses following anaphylaxis. *Respiration* 38:266, 1979.

330. Welling, A., et al. Beta-adrenergic receptor stimulates L-type calcium current in adult smooth muscle cells. *Blood Vessels* 28:154, 1991.

331. Whicker, S. D., Armour, C. L., and Black, J. L. Responsiveness of bronchial smooth muscle from asthmatic patients to relaxant and contractile agonists. *Pulmonol. Pharmacol.* 1:25, 1988.

331a. Williams, R. J. P. Calcium fluxes in cells: new views on their significance. *Cell Calcium* 13:273, 1992.

332. Williams, D. O., et al. Effects of nifedipine on bronchomotor tone and histamine reactivity in asthma. *Br. Med. J.* 283:348, 1981.

333. Yamakage, M., and Namiki, A. Effect of halothane on canine tracheal smooth muscle; role of cytosolic Ca^{2+}, cAMP and protein kinase C. *Anesthesiology* 75:A354, 1991.

334. Yamamoto, S. Enzymes in the Arachidonic Acid Cascade. In C. Pace-Ascieak and E. Granstrom (eds.), *Prostaglandins and Related Substances*. Amsterdam: Elsevier Science, 1983. P. 171.

335. Zoratti, E. M., et al. The effect of platelet activating factor on the generation of superoxide anion in human eosinophils and neutrophils. *J. Allergy Clin. Immunol.* 88:749, 1991.

336. Zorychta, E., and Richardson, J. B. Control of smooth muscle in human airways. *Bull. Eur. Physiopathol. Respir.* 16:581, 1980.

337. Small, R. C., et al. Potassium channel activators and bronchial asthma. *Clin. Exp. Allergy* 22:11, 1992.

338. Kai, T., et al. Lidocaine-induced relaxation of airway smooth muscle and intracellular Ca^{2+}. *Anesthesiology* 77:No. 3A, Sept. 1992.

Acute Asthma

Christopher H. Fanta

DEFINITION

A severe attack of acute asthma may develop suddenly or evolve over several days. It represents deterioration from the individual's baseline level of functioning, characterized by worsened airflow obstruction and manifesting usually with dyspnea as the major complaint. Cough, wheezing, and chest tightness commonly accompany the sense of dyspnea, and in some instances may be dominant presenting symptoms. Airflow obstruction of similar severity, if chronic, is not experienced as an "asthmatic attack"; essential features of an attack are a decrease in airway caliber (beyond what the patient experiences as part of normal daily variability in lung function) and the accompanying clinical distress. This chapter refers to such episodes as acute attacks or acute exacerbations of asthma, although it is recognized that some of these events may develop in a subacute manner over a period of days.

EPIDEMIOLOGY

The frequency of acute attacks among an asthmatic population is unknown. It is likely that most asthmatic attacks are self-treated at home by patients themselves; many other episodes are managed in physicians' offices. Treatment in an emergency department is provided for an unknown percentage of episodes. In general, the most severe attacks require emergency department care. However, in urban areas where alternative medical facilities are not readily available to some patients, emergency services may be called on to provide general medical care to asthmatic patients and to treat minor attacks. One can roughly estimate the annual number of emergency department visits for asthma in the United States based on the reported rate of approximately 500,000 annual hospitalizations [77], assuming that hospitalization for asthma generally (90% of the time) occurs only after emergency room treatment has failed to ameliorate an attack completely. In several published series the frequency with which patients who were treated for asthma in an emergency department required hospitalization was approximately 15 to 30 percent [9, 24, 39]. Thus, one can estimate that asthma accounts for as many as 1.5 to 3.0 million emergency department visits each year in the United States. Most of our understanding of acute asthma, including strategies for its management, is derived from clinical studies conducted in emergency departments.

PATHOBIOLOGY

The three major pathobiologic mechanisms of airflow obstruction in acute asthma are airway smooth muscle constriction, airway wall thickening due to inflammation, and luminal mucus plugging. It is likely that these same processes are present in chronic, stable asthma, even mild asthma [13], and differ only in degree during an acute attack. Direct histologic evidence is limited to patients with fatal asthma. Findings from these studies [7, 15] indicate that bronchi and bronchioles are diffusely infiltrated with inflammatory cells, primarily eosinophils. Edema, mucous gland hyperplasia, vascular engorgement, smooth muscle hyperplasia, and subepithelial collagen deposition all contribute to thickening of the airway walls and encroachment on the airway lumina. In most instances, one finds intraluminal accumulation of mucus, sloughed epithelial cells, inflammatory cells, and cellular debris, causing widespread occlusion of airways and clearly contributing to the process of death by asphyxiation. Occasional cases of fatal asthma have been described in which mucus plugging was not prominent; death was attributed to intense bronchoconstriction [62].

Although fatal asthma is considered in greater detail in Chapter 90, it is important to consider the histopathology of severe asthma in the context of this discussion for two reasons. First, because the basic mechanisms of airflow obstruction in fatal asthma differ only in degree from mild stable asthma, it is not surprising that the therapies used to treat asthmatic attacks are generally the same as those used in mild disease, simply administered more intensively. Because of the risk of suffocation, maintenance of adequate gas exchange is a special consideration pertinent to the management of severe asthmatic attacks. Second, one can anticipate that the tempo of response to treatment will differ in asthmatic attacks, depending on the relative contributions to airflow obstruction of inflammation and mucus plugging versus bronchoconstriction. Patients with predominantly airway smooth muscle constriction will be expected to respond rapidly to bronchodilator therapy, whereas patients with predominantly inflamed airway walls and lumina occluded by mucus and cellular material will respond incompletely and possibly not at all to bronchodilators [14]. Even in response to appropriate antiinflammatory therapy, improvement may require a period of many hours to days.

PATHOPHYSIOLOGY

Airflow obstruction is the primary pathophysiologic consequence of these processes in the airways. Patients with asthma who present to an emergency department for treatment of acute exacerbations of their disease vary widely in their degree of airflow obstruction, manifesting a broad spectrum of severities. In one emergency service where lung function was monitored by spirometry, the *average* forced expiratory volume in 1 second (FEV_1) on presentation in an adult population was approximately 1 liter, or 30 to 35 percent of normal [44]. During severe asthmatic attacks, patients may manifest certain physical findings that are useful clinical clues to the severity of the attack. These include pulsus paradoxus [8, 40, 60], use of accessory muscles of respiration (specifically, contraction of sternocleidomastoid muscles) [45, 61], and diaphoresis and refusal to lie supine due to breathlessness [6]. If present, these findings indicate severe obstruction, correlating with an FEV_1 less than approximately 1.5 liter among adult patients. However, as many as half the patients with airflow obstruction of this degree will not manifest these findings [39]. The severity of airflow obstruction is best assessed by direct measurement using spirometry or peak flow determination. Whether pulsus paradoxus, accessory muscle use, and diaphoresis and refusal to lie supine provide additional information regarding disease severity beyond that obtained from direct measurement of airflow obstruction remains unknown.

Other physical findings in severe asthmatic attacks are tachycardia (heart rate > 120 beats/min), tachypnea (respiratory rate > 30 breaths/min), and loud, diffuse wheezing [24]. A "silent chest" due to airflow so severely impaired that wheezes are not generated is well described but infrequently encountered. Also, the parallel respiratory movements of abdomen and chest wall become distorted in severe asthmatic attacks [63]. As airflow obstruction worsens, the anteroposterior expansion of the chest wall is increasingly delayed, lagging behind the outward excursion of the abdomen [29].

Physiologic consequences of severe airflow obstruction include pulmonary hyperinflation and disordered gas exchange. Lung volume measurements made during asthmatic attacks reveal increases in residual volume, functional residual capacity, and often, total lung capacity [80]. Increases in total lung capacity have been confirmed by x-ray planimetry [5] and appear not to be artifacts of the measurement techniques. A proposed mechanism for reversible increases in lung compliance leading to an enlarged total lung capacity relates to stress-relaxation properties of lung elastic tissue. It is hypothesized that prolonged breathing at high lung volumes can modify lung elasticity, causing a shift to the left of the pressure-volume curve [31].

Hyperinflation at functional residual capacity implies that tidal breathing occurs at an increased lung volume during asthmatic attacks. The physiologic advantage to breathing at a larger lung volume is increased elastic recoil of the lungs, with a consequent increase in expiratory airflow. On the other hand, a disadvantageous consequence of an enlarged resting lung volume is that diaphragmatic work during inspiration begins from a shorter resting muscle length, putting the muscle at a mechanical disadvantage. Work of breathing is thereby increased [66], perhaps contributing to the sense of inspiratory dyspnea and chest tightness experienced during asthmatic attacks. Furthermore, electromyographic recordings of diaphragmatic activity during asthmatic attacks have indicated that the diaphragm continues active contraction during exhalation [50], adding to the diaphragmatic workload. At least in some patients, the mechanism of hyperinflation at functional residual capacity appears to be inspiratory muscle contraction during exhalation. In this way the inspiratory muscles perform a braking function, actively preventing complete exhalation to a normal resting lung volume.

The most common derangements in arterial blood gases during asthmatic attacks are hypocapnia and mild-to-moderate hypoxemia: Typical arterial blood gas values are as follows: oxygen tension (PaO_2), 69 mmHg; carbon dioxide tension ($PaCO_2$), 35 mmHg; and pH, 7.44 [47]. When patients present to emergency services for care of asthmatic exacerbations, severe hypoxemia (i.e., PaO_2 < 55 mmHg) is an infrequent initial finding, encountered in only approximately 5 to 10 percent of patients in the absence of pulmonary complications such as lobar collapse, pneumonia, or pneumothorax [39, 47]. Transient falls in PaO_2 may accompany treatment with inhaled beta-adrenergic agonists; medication-induced pulmonary vasodilation with worsened ventilation-perfusion mismatching is the presumed mechanism [34]. Oximetry studies documenting the frequency, duration, and severity of these episodes among adults are lacking, but personal experience suggests that they are generally clinically insignificant.

Alveolar hyperventilation with respiratory alkalosis is the usual response of the ventilatory control center to acute airflow obstruction in asthma. If airflow obstruction becomes increasingly severe, however, alveolar ventilation begins to decrease and the $PaCO_2$ starts to normalize (i.e., increase toward 40 mmHg); wasted ventilation is high and total minute ventilation, though increased above normal, is inadequate to maintain alveolar hyperventilation. A $PaCO_2$ of approximately 40 mmHg in the dyspneic patient with acute asthma is an ominous result, signaling impending ventilatory failure (see Chap. 73). With further worsening of airflow obstruction, total minute ventilation begins to fall and hypercapnia with respiratory acidosis develops. This progressive decline, if unchecked, can ultimately result in apneic respiratory arrest. The contribution of respiratory muscle fatigue to hypercapnic ventilatory failure in acute asthma has not been as well studied as in acute exacerbations of chronic obstructive pulmonary disease, and remains uncertain [56].

There is a significant direct correlation between the FEV_1 and the PaO_2 prior to treatment in acute asthma [39, 43, 47]. However, the correlation is weak so that clinically significant hypoxemia cannot be predicted from the measured airflow obstruction. On the other hand, a clinically useful inverse correlation exists between the FEV_1 and $PaCO_2$. In the absence of sedatives or other respiratory depressants, hypercapnia is rarely observed unless the FEV_1 or peak expiratory flow rate (PEFR) falls to less than 25 percent of predicted [43].

INITIAL ASSESSMENT

Initial assessment of the patient with a severe attack of asthma should be brief, minimizing the delay in instituting treatment. Additional information can be collected later, when the patient is in less respiratory distress. History taking and physical examination are directed at confirming the diagnosis of asthma, assessing its severity, evaluating pertinent comorbid illnesses if present, and excluding potential complications of asthma. In addition, medication use and side effects need to be recorded. However, it should be emphasized that standard blood tests, chest radiographs, and arterial blood gas analyses are not routinely necessary prior to initiating treatment.

A measurement of lung function (spirometry or peak flow determination) prior to treatment can provide information useful later in the course of acute management about the patient's rate of improvement during treatment. In most patients, this testing can be performed without significant stress or worsening of function. It is the best single measure of the severity of the acute attack, and helps to identify patients at risk for hypercapnia, as noted above. In all but the most severely breathless patients, lung function measurement prior to treatment is recommended.

The initial approach is modified for patients in extreme distress with evident or impending respiratory failure. This category includes patients unable to speak because of labored breathing, cyanotic patients, and patients with impaired level of consciousness. In this circumstance, arterial blood gas determinations may provide crucial information and are recommended in parallel with administering bronchodilators and basic life support measures.

Where available, pulse oximetry is a useful and painless means of assessing the adequacy of arterial oxygenation. It does not delay initiation of treatment and can rapidly identify hypoxemic patients, for whom supplemental oxygen is warranted.

TREATMENT

Overview

The primary goal of therapy in acute asthma is the prompt relief of dyspnea and the associated respiratory symptoms while ensuring adequate oxygenation and ventilation. This goal is best achieved by the rapid reversal of airflow obstruction. Therefore, in the absence of severe hypercapnia and/or hypoxemia, treatment is principally directed at improving expiratory airflow. A secondary goal of therapy is an attempt to minimize adverse and unpleasant side effects of treatment. Thus, in evaluating different treatment strategies in the acute care setting, the principal measure of success is the achievement of rapid and large increases in expiratory flow (as measured by FEV_1 or PEFR) while avoiding serious adverse effects from medication.

Repetitive administration of sympathomimetic bronchodilators constitutes the best available means to reverse rapidly the airflow obstruction in acute asthma. These medications have their onset of action within minutes and are potent in effecting relaxation of airway smooth muscle contraction; to the extent that bronchial and bronchiolar smooth muscle constriction is the cause of airflow obstruction, they can achieve effective bronchodilation. Administered repetitively over the first 60 to 90 minutes of therapy in the emergency department, these agents typically bring about a 50 percent or greater increase in FEV_1 in more than half the patients within this same time period [1, 14].

To the extent that airway wall inflammation and intraluminal plugging contribute to a patient's airflow obstruction, systemic corticosteroids provide the most effective therapy. It is generally held that the observable onset of action of corticosteroids is delayed for several (6 or more) hours, and certainly the resolution of inflammation and airway plugging is a gradual process that takes place over hours to days. Thus, while systemic corticosteroids are a crucially important component of therapy in acute, severe asthma and their early administration is favored because of their delayed onset of action, the benefit derived in terms of reduced airflow obstruction may not be observed until after the patient leaves the acute care setting. In general, systemic corticosteroids should be administered early in the course of emergency department care to patients failing to respond promptly to intensive bronchodilator therapy, and they should be administered prior to discharge home to patients at risk for recurrent severe asthmatic symptoms ("relapse").

The management of respiratory failure due to asthma is dealt with in Chapter 73; only brief mention of the topic is made here. Maintenance of adequate gas exchange is of prime importance in the patient with evident or impending respiratory failure. Supplemental oxygen is indicated for documented hypoxemia; the inspired oxygen concentration can be adjusted according to the measured arterial oxygen saturation (by pulse oximetry or arterial blood gas analysis). Often supplemental oxygen is given even in the absence of documented hypoxemia, particularly to patients at risk for complications of severe hypoxia (e.g., patients with known coronary artery or cerebrovascular disease). Empiric oxygen supplementation is best given at low concentrations (e.g., 2 L/min of flow via nasal prongs).

Intubation and mechanically assisted ventilation are indicated for apneic or hypopneic patients and for other patients with worsening hypercapnia despite maximal bronchodilator therapy. This may be instituted in some cases in the emergency department. Even in mechanically ventilated patients, beta-adrenergic agonists can be nebulized in-line using special adaptors fitted to the tubing that connects the ventilator to the patient. In rare instances, effective ventilation cannot be achieved mechanically due to inordinately high airway resistance, and absorption of subcutaneous epinephrine is unreliable due to poor peripheral tissue perfusion. Alternative approaches to this extreme emergency include (1) injection of epinephrine directly into the airways (e.g., 10 ml of epinephrine, 1:10,000 dilution squirted rapidly down the endotracheal tube) or (2) terbutaline administered intravenously (e.g., 0.1–0.4 µg/kg/min by continuous infusion [53] (see Chaps. 55 and 57).

Algorithms summarizing current management strategies in acute asthma have been prepared by the expert panel convened as part of the National Asthma Education Program [50a]. The separate algorithms for adults and children are shown in Figs. 72-1 and 72-2, respectively.

Bronchodilator Therapy

Over the last several years, numerous clinical investigations evaluated the relative efficacy and toxicity of various drugs, both singly and in combinations, in the initial treatment of acute asthmatic attacks. Most of these studies were conducted in emergency departments. In the studies to be cited, the patients were adults, generally less than 50 years old, and free of complicating cardiopulmonary diseases. The measure of drug efficacy was the extent of improvement in FEV_1 or PEFR compared to the value determined prior to treatment, that is, the reduction in expiratory airflow obstruction.

Single-drug Comparisons

A consistent finding throughout all of these studies has been that sympathomimetic drugs—in particular, subcutaneous epinephrine and inhaled beta-adrenergic agonists—are the most effective bronchodilators for acute asthma. Given as a series of three doses spaced every 20 minutes, subcutaneous epinephrine (0.3 mg/dose) and inhaled isoproterenol (2.5 mg/dose) achieved three to four times greater increases in FEV_1 than did intravenous aminophylline in a randomized trial involving 48 asthmatic patients reported from the Peter Bent Brigham Hospital [64] (Fig. 72-3A). In this study, the mean theophylline level measured after 1 hour of treatment in the aminophylline-treated group was in the middle of the recommended therapeutic range (16.2 µg/ml). All patients received only the single bronchodilator agent during the 1-hour study period; no patient was given corticosteroids during this initial hour of treatment. Eight of the 48 patients either failed to show significant improvement or actually deteriorated during this first hour; 7 of these 8 patients had been assigned to the intravenous aminophylline group (Fig. 72-3B). Other investigations confirmed the relatively weak bronchodilator potency of intravenous aminophylline when used alone to treat acute asthma [2, 22, 26, 78].

Sympathomimetic bronchodilators are also more effective than anticholinergic drugs in acute asthma. Karpel and colleagues compared metaproterenol (15 mg) and atropine sulfate (3.2 mg) nebulized twice 30 minutes apart [38]. The inhaled beta-adrenergic agonist caused significantly greater and more rapid bronchodilation than did the anticholinergic agent despite the large doses of the latter [38] (Fig. 72-4). Similar results were obtained comparing single doses of the beta agonist fenoterol (1.25 mg) with the atropine congener ipratropium bromide (0.5 mg), both drugs administered as nebulized solutions [59]. The delayed (20–30 minutes) onset of action of the anticholinergic bronchodilators makes their use as single agents inappropriate for acute asthma.

Several important observations have been made regarding the use of adrenergic agonists in the emergency management of acute asthma. First, the inhalational route of delivery is at least as effective as parenteral administration: Inhaled beta-adrenergic agonists increase lung function as much as subcutaneous epinephrine [1, 64]; in one trial, inhaled epinephrine proved as effective as subcutaneous epinephrine [58]; and in several studies intravenously administered terbutaline proved no more potent

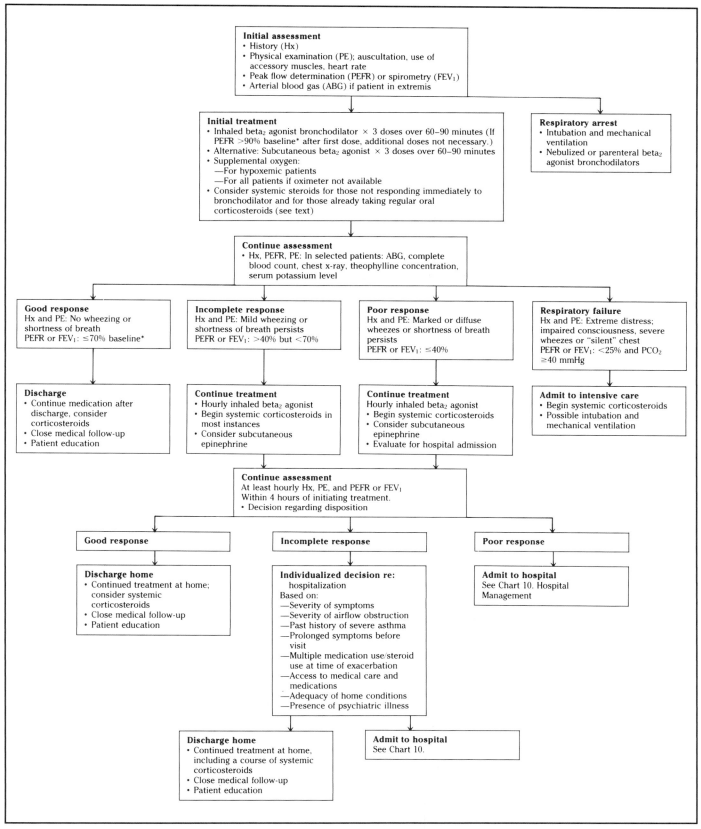

Fig. 72-1. *Acute exacerbations of asthma in adults: emergency department management. Although therapies are often available in a physician's office, most acutely severe exacerbations of asthma require a complete course of therapy in an emergency department. *PEFR % baseline refers to the norm for the individual, established by the clinician. This may be a percentage of standardized norms or a percentage of the patient's personal best. (Reprinted from National Asthma Education Program, Expert Panel Report. Executive Summary: Guidelines for the Diagnosis and Management of Asthma. Publication No. 91-3042A. Bethesda, MD: National Institutes of Health, June 1991. P. 29.)*

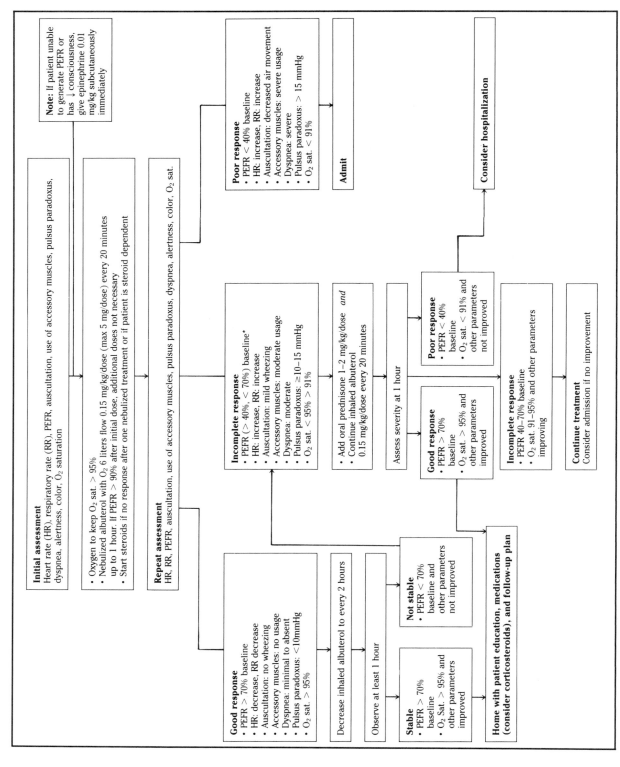

Initial assessment

Heart rate (HR), respiratory rate (RR), PEFR, auscultation, use of accessory muscles, pulsus paradoxus, dyspnea, alertness, color, O₂ saturation

- Oxygen to keep O₂ sat. > 95%
- Nebulized albuterol with O₂ 6 liters flow 0.15 mg/kg/dose (max 5 mg/dose) every 20 minutes up to 1 hour. If PEFR > 90% after initial dose, additional doses not necessary
- Start steroids if no response after one nebulized treatment or if patient is steroid dependent

Note: If patient unable to generate PEFR or has ↓ consciousness, give epinephrine 0.01 mg/kg subcutaneously immediately

Repeat assessment

HR, RR, PEFR, auscultation, use of accessory muscles, pulsus paradoxus, dyspnea, alertness, color, O₂ sat.

Good response
- PEFR > 70% baseline
- HR: decrease, RR decrease
- Auscultation: no wheezing
- Accessory muscles: no usage
- Dyspnea: minimal to absent
- Pulsus paradoxus: <10mmHg
- O₂ sat. > 95%

Incomplete response
- PEFR (> 40%, < 70%) baseline*
- HR: increase, RR: increase
- Auscultation: mild wheezing
- Accessory muscles: moderate usage
- Dyspnea: moderate
- Pulsus paradoxus: ≥10–15 mmHg
- O₂ sat. < 95% > 91%

Poor response
- PEFR < 40% baseline
- HR: increase, RR: increase
- Auscultation: decreased air movement
- Accessory muscles: severe usage
- Dyspnea: severe
- Pulsus paradoxus: > 15 mmHg
- O₂ sat. < 91%

Decrease inhaled albuterol to every 2 hours

- Add oral prednisone 1–2 mg/kg/dose *and*
- Continue inhaled albuterol 0.15 mg/kg/dose every 20 minutes

Admit

Observe at least 1 hour

Assess severity at 1 hour

Stable
- PEFR > 70% baseline
- O₂ Sat. > 95% and other parameters improved

Not stable
- PEFR < 70% baseline and other parameters not improved

Good response
- PEFR > 70% baseline
- O₂ sat. > 95% and other parameters improved

Poor response
- PEFR < 40% baseline
- O₂ sat. < 91% and other parameters not improved

Consider hospitalization

Home with patient education, medications (consider corticosteroids), and follow-up plan

Incomplete response
- PEFR 40–70% baseline
- O₂ sat. 91–95% and other parameters improving

Continue treatment
Consider admission if no improvement

Fig. 72-2. *Acute exacerbations of asthma in children: emergency department management. Although therapies are often available in a physician's office, most acutely severe exacerbations of asthma require a complete course of therapy in an emergency department. *PEFR % baseline refers to the norm for the individual, established by the clinician. This may be a percentage predicted based on standardized norms or the patient's personal best. (Reprinted from National Asthma Education Program, Expert Panel Report. Executive Summary: Guidelines for the Diagnosis and Management of Asthma. Publication No. 91-3042A. Bethesda, MD: National Institutes of Health, June 1991. P. 32).*

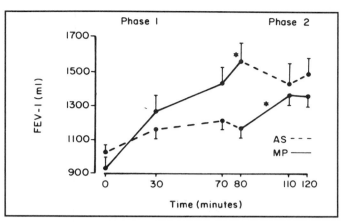

Fig. 72-4. *Cross-over trial comparing the bronchodilator effects of inhaled metaproterenol sulfate (MS) and atropine sulfate (AS). (Reprinted with permission from Karpel, J. P., et al. A comparison of atropine sulfate and metaproterenol sulfate in the emergency treatment of asthma. Am. Rev. Respir. Dis. 133:727, 1986.)*

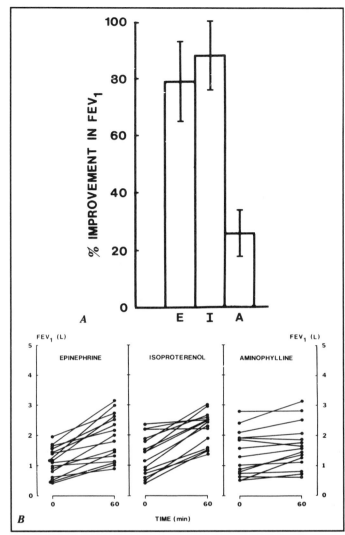

Fig. 72-3*A. Emergency therapy of asthma. Comparison of the bronchodilator responses to epinephrine (E), isoproterenol (I), and aminophylline (A) during the initial hour of emergency department treatment. (Modified from Rossing, T. H., et al. Emergency therapy of asthma: Comparison of the acute effects of parenteral and inhaled sympathomimetics and infused aminophylline. Am. Rev. Respir. Dis. 122:365, 1980.) B. Individual responses to bronchodilator therapy during the initial hour of emergency department treatment. Seven of the eight patients who failed to improve received aminophylline. (Reprinted with permission from Rossing, T. H., et al. Emergency therapy of asthma: Comparison of the acute effects of parenteral and inhaled sympathomimetics and infused aminophylline. Am. Rev. Respir. Dis. 122:365, 1980.)*

than inhaled terbutaline [57, 74, 79]. Concerns regarding the inability to deliver bronchodilator medication by inhalation to severely obstructed patients have proved unfounded. Even when patients with an initial FEV_1 of less than 1 liter or less than 35 percent of predicted are evaluated, the bronchodilator response to inhaled beta agonists is as good as that to subcutaneous epinephrine [20]. Only in the apneic or near-apneic patient would this route of administration need to be modified.

Second, sympathomimetic bronchodilators remain the drugs of choice even among patients using oral or inhaled beta agonists prior to their emergency department visits. Tachyphylaxis or tolerance to the maximal bronchodilator response of sympathomimetic drugs was not detected in a retrospective analysis of 96

emergency room visits for acute asthma [65]; the bronchodilator responses to epinephrine and isoproterenol were identical for patients who had and those who had not used this same class of drugs in the hours and days prior to their arrival at the emergency department [65].

Third, even when given repetitively (every 20–30 minutes for three doses), the inhaled beta agonists and subcutaneous epinephrine are well tolerated hemodynamically: On average, the heart rate increases minimally or not at all, and the blood pressure (systolic and diastolic) tends to fall slightly. Thus, sinus tachycardia is not a contraindication to the use of these agents. Some patients will manifest significant increases in heart rate, but fewer than 5 percent will have increases of 30 beats/min or more [17]. As noted above, most of the reported studies were conducted in young adults free of complicating cardiopulmonary diseases. The safety of these treatment regimens in the elderly or in patients with ischemic heart disease or cardiac arrhythmias has not been established. Unpleasant side effects from beta-agonist bronchodilators are common but generally are not severe: They include tremor, heart pounding, anxiety, and headache.

Two major unanswered questions regarding the use of beta-adrenergic agonists in acute asthma are the optimal method of aerosol delivery and the dose. In all of the studies cited above, the beta-agonist medication was delivered as a "wet aerosol"; that is, a solution of the medication was aerosolized using compressed air or oxygen and a hand-held nebulizer. This technique has the important advantage of allowing the patient to receive the medication during tidal breathing; no special coordination is required. However, the large droplet size and loss of medication out the open end of the exhalation port make the technique relatively inefficient: Only a small fraction of the dose of medication put into the nebulizer container is actually delivered to the patient's airways (see Chap. 56). An alternative approach has been to deliver the same medications from metered-dose medication cannisters, using spacer devices to improve particle delivery to intrathoracic airways. In clinical trials conducted in emergency departments, improvement following as few as three inhalations (spaced 2 minutes apart) from metered-dose inhalers and spacers was identical to that achieved using hand-held nebulizers and standard doses of beta-agonist solutions, despite the 5 to 10-fold smaller doses that are released from the metered-dose cannisters [67, 73]. Advantages of the metered-dose inhalers with spacers include their greater simplicity and reduced cost. A potential disadvantage is the need for supervised administration (without which discoordinated inhalational technique would limit effectiveness). Also, in at least one study of hospitalized asthmatic patients, increases in FEV_1 were significantly smaller with the metered-dose inhaler with the spacer device than with wet aerosols [49].

Optimal use of beta-agonist bronchodilators by metered-dose inhaler in the emergency care of asthma may require larger doses (i.e., a greater number of inhalations), at least among some patients. Dose-response studies in subjects with stable asthma have demonstrated incremental bronchodilation to doses as high as 1,000 to 4,000 µg of albuterol (i.e., 10–40 inhalations from standard preparations) [4, 41]. The dose commonly put into nebulizers when giving three doses every 20 minutes is 7.5 mg (over 1 hour) for albuterol, 7.5 mg for isoetharine, and 45 mg for metaproterenol. Whether larger doses by intermittent or continuous (face mask) nebulization might be more effective with still tolerable side effects is unknown [11]. At present, no evidence is available to favor choice of one selective beta$_2$-adrenergic agonist over another in treating acute exacerbations of asthma [32]. The sympathomimetic drugs and doses commonly used at the present time in the therapy for acute asthma in adults are listed in Table 73-8, and additional information on dosages and dosing schedules can be found in Chap. 55.

Two-drug Combinations

Because different classes of bronchodilators promote smooth muscle relaxation via different intracellular pathways, it is reasonable to consider whether combinations of two or more bronchodilators might be indicated for initial treatment in acute asthma, especially in the most severely obstructed patients. Indeed, when patients are in distress, it is difficult for treating physicians to withhold potentially useful medications, especially if serious adverse effects occur infrequently. Thus, a common practice in emergency departments has been to administer intravenous aminophylline combined with sympathomimetic bronchodilators for severe attacks. However, when subjected to controlled clinical study, this approach has proved unjustified.

The outcomes of several randomized clinical trials demonstrated that when sympathomimetic bronchodilators are administered repetitively over 1 or more hours, the bronchodilator effect is equivalent to two-drug combinations of a sympathomimetic and aminophylline, with fewer side effects [2, 18, 20, 37, 68, 81]. For example, epinephrine administered subcutaneously every 20 minutes for three doses improved expiratory airflow to the same extent with or without concomitant intravenous aminophylline [2, 37]. Likewise, intravenous aminophylline (or oral elixir of theophylline) combined with an inhaled beta agonist is no more effective than multiple doses of the inhaled beta agonist alone, even among a subpopulation of patients with particularly severe airway obstruction (initial $FEV_1 < 1$ liter) [18]. On the other hand, side effects (tremor, anxiety, and palpitations) are more frequent with the two-drug regimens [68]. These observations have been extended to at least 3 hours of emergency department treatment [68]. (Fig. 72-5). A single report suggested a reduced need for hospital admissions among patients in whom intravenous aminophylline is added to nebulized beta agonists and intravenous methylprednisolone during emergency department treatment [81], but this finding could not be explained by corresponding improvements in lung function [81] and is not supported by the results of several previous studies [2, 18, 20, 37, 68].

Current evidence indicates that there is no role for aminophylline in promoting rapid relief of airflow obstruction in the emergency care of acute asthma. For a patient using theophylline or a theophylline-containing medication when he or she develops an acute exacerbation of asthma, it may still be appropriate to measure the serum theophylline concentration and, where appropriate, administer aminophylline or theophylline or adjust the

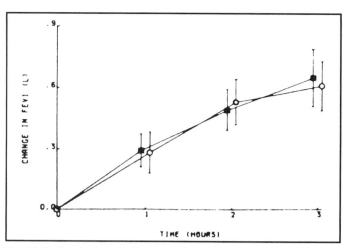

Fig. 72-5. *Comparison of the bronchodilator effect of inhaled metaproterenol (open circles) (administered hourly) versus inhaled metaproterenol plus intravenous aminophylline during three hours of emergency department treatment. (Reprinted with permission from Siegal, D., et al. Aminophylline increases the toxicity but not the efficacy of an inhaled beta-adrenergic agonist in the treatment of acute exacerbations of asthma.* Am. Rev. Respir. Dis. *132:283, 1985.)*

maintenance dose to achieve a therapeutic blood level as part of the subsequent in-hospital or outpatient care. In the acute care setting, however, where beta-agonist bronchodilators are being administered on an intensive, repetitive dosing schedule, no additional bronchodilation will be gained from the use of aminophylline, and no immediate advantage is to be derived from optimizing the serum theophylline concentration.

Concurrent use of two proarrhythmic classes of drugs (sympathomimetics and methylxanthines) has raised concern regarding induction of significant cardiac arrhythmias. Some [36, 79a], not all [16], reports have described an increase in frequency of atrial and ventricular premature beats and tachycardias with the combination of aminophylline and beta-agonist bronchodilators. However, symptomatic arrhythmias are infrequent, and it seems unlikely that bronchodilator-induced cardiac arrhythmias contribute significantly to the incidence of asthmatic deaths [48] (see also Chap. 78). Asphyxia in young and middle-aged patients seems to be a common cause of acute asthma mortality.

Relatively few studies are available regarding the value of combined sympathomimetic and anticholinergic therapy as initial treatment for acute asthma. No studies have specifically addressed whether additive bronchodilation is achieved by administering atropine or atropine derivatives together with repetitive doses of inhaled beta agonists in the first 60 to 90 minutes of treatment. A number of investigators [28, 54, 72, 76] reported the outcome following a single dose of inhaled albuterol with or without nebulized ipratropium in severe asthma (patients treated in the emergency department or newly admitted to the hospital), with variable results at 1 or 2 hours following nebulization. Some researchers found an additive effect from the two-drug combination [54, 76], whereas others did not [28, 72].

In one report describing an advantage to combined therapy, 56 adult patients received either albuterol (10 mg) or albuterol (10 mg) plus ipratropium (0.5 mg) as initial emergency department treatment. The PEFR increased by 31 percent 1 hour after treatment with albuterol alone and 77 percent following therapy with albuterol plus ipratropium; the greatest benefit from the combined therapy was derived by those patients whose initial PEFR was less than 140 L/min [54]. On the other hand, a similarly designed study of 40 asthmatic patients treated on admission to the hospital with albuterol (5 mg) with or without ipratropium

(0.5 mg) found changes in FEV_1 2 hours after treatment to be no different between the two groups [28]. A third study performed in asthmatic children actually noted a negative effect from combined therapy in those who had severe obstruction: Bronchodilation was greater in the group treated with albuterol alone [71].

Although in parts of the world it has become standard practice to treat acute asthma in the emergency department with combined beta-agonist and anticholinergic solutions, in the United States atropine derivatives such as ipratropium bromide and atropine methonitrate are not available as solutions for nebulization. The quaternary ammonium anticholinergic compound glycopyrrolate is available for wet aerosol administration and is an effective bronchodilator in acute asthma [25], but its value in combination with sympathomimetic therapy is unknown. Use of ipratropium bromide by metered-dose inhaler with a spacer device in hospitalized asthmatic patients did not provide additive bronchodilation to conventional therapy [55] and is not likely to have a role in emergency department care. See Chap. 64 for added discussion of ipratropium.

Corticosteroids

There can be little doubt about the crucial role of systemic corticosteroids in relieving acute severe attacks of asthma. A vast body of clinical experience and several controlled clinical trials give strong support to the concept that corticosteroids speed the resolution of severe exacerbations, especially among patients who have failed to improve significantly with bronchodilator therapy alone [19]. Despite this knowledge, some uncertainty still surrounds the use of corticosteroids in the emergency department management of acute asthma. In particular, there is controversy regarding the selection of patients to receive systemic steroids, the timing and route of administration, and the dose. The following discussion reviews some of the pertinent clinical data and offers one approach to the use of steroids in this setting.

In three double-blind, controlled trials, patients presenting to emergency departments with acute asthmatic attacks were randomly assigned to receive corticosteroids or placebo, administered as a single intravenous bolus at the onset of their treatment [42, 46, 70]. All patients also received repeated doses of inhaled beta-agonist bronchodilators. In two of these studies methylprednisolone (125 mg) was the steroid preparation given [42, 70]; in the third, three doses of hydrocortisone were administered to separate patient groups (250, 500, and 1,000 mg) [46]. In all three studies no significant differences in lung function (FEV_1) were observed between the steroid- and placebo-treated groups during the period of emergency care (Fig. 72-6). In one study, in which a trend toward a greater improvement in FEV_1 was found in the steroid-treated group, significantly fewer of the patients who received corticosteroids required hospital admission [42]; however, no difference in admission rate was found in a subsequent investigation of similar design [70].

Two explanations can be offered for this apparent failure of systemic corticosteroids to have an impact on the course of acute asthma in the emergency department. First, some patients improve rapidly with bronchodilators alone; reversal of airway smooth muscle constriction alone corrects the predominant cause of airflow obstruction in these patients. The results reported by McFadden and colleagues [46] support this conclusion: In the patient group treated with hourly inhaled isoproterenol and placebo infusion, after 6 hours the mean FEV_1 reached approximately 80 percent of predicted, leaving little room for improvement with the addition of intravenous hydrocortisone. Second, the onset of action of systemic corticosteroids, although not precisely defined, is generally considered to be delayed for a number of hours after administration. This observed delay is consistent with the pharmacokinetics of corticosteroids (its action requires new protein synthesis) and with its presumed anti-

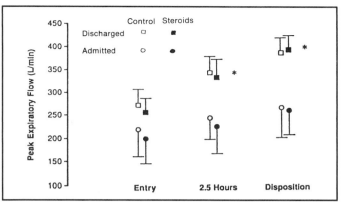

Fig. 72-6. *Trial of systemic corticosteroids (methylprednisolone 125 mg) versus placebo in asthmatic patients treated intensively with bronchodilators in the emergency department. No significant differences were found among patients ultimately hospitalized for their asthma or among patients discharged home. (Reprinted with permission from Stein, L. M., et al. Early administration of corticosteroids in emergency room treatment of acute asthma.* Ann. Intern. Med. *112:832, 1990.)*

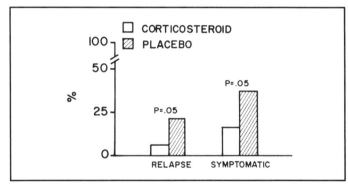

Fig. 72-7. *Reduction in emergency room relapses and in post-discharge respiratory symptoms with a course of oral corticosteroids following emergency department discharge. (Reprinted with permission from Feil, S. B., et al. Efficacy of short-term corticosteroid therapy in outpatient treatment of acute bronchial asthma.* Am. J. Med. *75:259, 1983.)*

inflammatory effects (the resolution of inflammation is a gradual process).

Thus, the major effect of systemic corticosteroids administered in the emergency department is likely to be on the course of the asthmatic attack *after* the patient leaves the emergency care setting, whether the patient is hospitalized or discharged home. Systemic corticosteroids speed the recovery of patients hospitalized for severe asthma [19], and reduce the likelihood of early deterioration and recurrent asthmatic attacks in patients discharged home from the emergency department [10, 21, 30]. This latter benefit is of particular importance to the physician providing emergency care, since he or she is likely to prescribe the treatment regimen for the immediate postdischarge period. Randomized, placebo-controlled trials have documented the benefit of a short course of systemic corticosteroids following emergency department discharge in improving lung function, reducing asthmatic symptoms, and decreasing the incidence of "relapses" (recurrent attacks requiring emergency department care within 7–10 days of initial discharge) [10, 21, 30] (Fig. 72-7). Typical treatment protocols have used 40 to 64 mg of prednisone or methylprednisolone, tapered to zero over 8 days [10, 21]. In one study, a single injection of intramuscular methylprednisolone sodium acetate (40 mg) at the time of discharge also proved effective in reducing asthmatic relapses [30]. The disadvantage of this approach is that once administered, the intramuscular dose cannot be modified according to individual patient needs, a particularly important consideration in the event of an adverse reaction to the medication.

Given the delay in the onset of action of corticosteroids, it is desirable to administer them to severely ill asthmatic patients early in the course of treatment. On the other hand, given their potentially serious adverse effects, it is preferable to avoid their use in patients who improve rapidly to normal or near normal with bronchodilators alone. Indications for the early administration of systemic corticosteroids include the following: patients who develop a severe asthmatic attack despite the use of oral steroids at the time of their deterioration, patients with ventilatory failure, patients with severe obstruction who have no improvement following initial bronchodilator treatment, and patients who after the first 60 to 90 minutes of intensive bronchodilator treatment still have an FEV_1 or PEFR at 40 percent of predicted or less. This last patient group, on average, is unlikely to manifest significant further improvement in airflow obstruction over the ensuing 3 hours of emergency treatment despite continued aggressive use of inhaled and parenteral bronchodilators [18].

A large portion of patients treated for acute asthma will have an intermediate response to the initial bronchodilator treatment, with an FEV_1 or PEFR between 40 and 70 percent of predicted after the first 60 to 90 minutes. Most of these patients will receive continued bronchodilator therapy in the emergency department, and since these patients are less severely ill, the decision regarding their treatment with systemic steroids can be delayed somewhat while their subsequent response is observed. In general, among patients within this broad category, systemic corticosteroids should be given to those with more severe symptoms, worse airflow obstruction, and more gradual response to bronchodilator therapy.

If systemic corticosteroids are given in the emergency department, what dose of which steroid preparation should be given and by what route (oral or intravenous)? No comparative studies are available to help answer these questions. For intravenous administration, methylprednisolone has the slight advantage over hydrocortisone of less mineralocorticoid effect, resulting in less fluid retention and less hypokalemia. A commonly used dose of methylprednisolone is 125 mg by intravenous bolus, although smaller doses (60–80 mg) may be equally effective. The oral route of administration is probably as effective as the intravenous route when identical doses are used [27, 35]. Potential disadvantages to the oral route—namely, delayed effect until absorption is complete, impaired metabolism of prednisone (to prednisolone) in the presence of liver disease, and uncertain absorption in the patient who vomits—are generally not major impediments to oral administration.

REPEAT ASSESSMENT

For some patients in severe respiratory distress, evaluation of their cardiopulmonary status needs to be ongoing while treatment is administered. In all patients, a repeat assessment after the initial 60 to 90 minutes of bronchodilator therapy is warranted. Most patients derive significant relief of their dyspnea from this initial therapy, permitting more detailed history taking and physical examination, as needed. Repeat measurement of lung function with spirometry or peak flow determination should be performed to determine the change in airflow obstruction in response to treatment. It should be noted that two studies have documented a close correlation between FEV_1 and PEFR measurements in the emergency department assessment of acute

asthma [33, 52] and that both techniques require patient coaching and maximal expiratory effort for valid results to be obtained.

Arterial blood gas determination is indicated for patients with persistent severe distress, especially if the FEV_1 or PEFR is less than 25 percent of predicted [43]. The primary purpose of blood gas determination is to assess the adequacy of alveolar ventilation by measuring $PaCO_2$; therefore, pulse oximetry is not an adequate substitute. Patients with a $PaCO_2$ of approximately 40 mmHg or greater after initial intensive bronchodilator therapy should be admitted to the hospital and, in many cases, treated in an intensive care unit.

Although chest radiography is often performed as part of the evaluation of acute asthmatic attacks managed in emergency departments, the yield of diagnostically useful information is low [23, 82] (see Chap. 53). Pulmonary hyperinflation and peribronchial cuffing are common findings, but they have no therapeutic implications. In only approximately 1 to 2 percent of patients will other pertinent abnormalities be found [23, 82]; these findings generally are manifestations of complications of asthma, such as pneumothorax, pneumomediastinum, pulmonary infiltrates (infectious or eosinophilic pneumonias), and atelectasis (from subsegmental to unilateral lung collapse). Chest radiography seems warranted for the following indications: clinical suspicion that one of these complications is present, ventilatory failure ($PaCO_2 \geq 40$ mmHg) or persistent hypoxemia (oxygen saturation < 92% or $PaO_2 < 60$ mmHg), failure to improve despite aggressive therapy in the emergency room, and newly diagnosed asthma. In the majority of patients treated in emergency departments for acute asthmatic attacks, chest radiographs are probably not necessary.

Venous blood studies may be useful to evaluate complicating illnesses, for example, a complete blood cell count with differential if a bacterial infection (e.g., sinusitis or pneumonia) or eosinophilic pneumonia is suspected. Likewise, because of the transient hypokalemia induced by inhaled beta-adrenergic agonists [12], measurement of serum potassium concentration is appropriate if cardiac arrhythmias are observed or if the patient is taking a digitalis preparation. Measurement of serum theophylline concentration in patients taking theophylline-containing preparations at the time of their acute attack is often appropriate, especially if theophylline toxicity is suspected, if the dose has been recently adjusted, or if no measurement has been made in recent months. As suggested by this discussion, it is not necessary to draw venous blood studies on all patients being treated for acute severe asthma.

CONTINUED TREATMENT

Because of persistent symptoms and airflow obstruction, some patients will require continued treatment beyond the initial 60 to 90 minutes. The mainstay of this phase of treatment is continued administration of sympathomimetic agents, preferably inhaled beta$_2$-selective adrenergic agonists. The frequency of administration may need to be adjusted according to the severity of airflow obstruction, the duration of improvement following administration, and the severity of adverse side effects. For the majority of patients, our practice has been to increase the dosing interval to hourly following the initial sequence of treatments (i.e., doses given on presentation and 20, 40, 60, 120, and 180 minutes, etc., thereafter).

The most problematic patients are those who fail to improve significantly with the initial bronchodilator treatments. What medications, other than "more of the same," are available during the subsequent hours as one awaits the beneficial effects of systemically administered corticosteroids? Although no class of bronchodilators is of more proven benefit than the sympathomimetics, several different therapeutic strategies have been tried, some with potential benefit reported. As already discussed, anticholinergic drugs have been shown in some but not all studies to provide additive bronchodilation. Clinical trials conducted among asthmatic patients newly admitted to a hospital presumably include a large fraction of patients who have had an incomplete bronchodilator response to sympathomimetic drugs (with or without aminophylline). In some of these trials, inhaled ipratropium bromide (0.5 mg) provided further bronchodilation when used synchronously or sequentially in combination with inhaled albuterol [75, 76]; in other studies no added benefit was observed [28]. Even in those trials in which a positive effect was found, the incremental bronchodilation beyond that achieved with beta agonists alone was generally small, on the order of 20 percent.

Two studies conducted in emergency departments have specifically addressed the problem of patients who have persistent severe obstruction after initial bronchodilator treatment. In one investigation, patients with an initial PEFR of less than 200 L/min who failed to double their PEFR in response to two doses of nebulized beta agonists were randomly assigned to a 20-minute intravenous infusion of magnesium sulfate (1.2 gm) or placebo [69]. Patients in the placebo group had, on average, stable PEFR during the 20-minute infusion and subsequent 25-minute observation period, while the magnesium-treated group manifested a significant increase in PEFR (by approximately 75 L/min or 33%) during this same interval (Fig. 72-8). It was postulated that magnesium sulfate may relax airway smooth muscle by inhibiting calcium flux into smooth muscle cells through slow calcium channels. The only notable side effect observed was mild fatigue. Additional studies are now needed to confirm this initial observation and to clarify other issues regarding dose, duration of action, and activity when magnesium sulfate is used in combination with other bronchodilators.

In the second investigation, a crossover design was used to compare the bronchodilator effects of subcutaneous epinephrine and inhaled metaproterenol in acute asthma [1]. A sequence of three injections spaced 20 minutes apart was utilized for both agents; 1 hour of observation followed each of the two treatment periods. The study was conducted as a double-blind, randomized protocol with appropriate controls (subcutaneous and inhaled saline solution). For the entire group of patients entered into this trial, no difference could be demonstrated between the two treatments (Fig. 72-9A). However, for those patients who did not significantly improve with the initial sequence of treatments, there was a significant difference during the crossover phase:

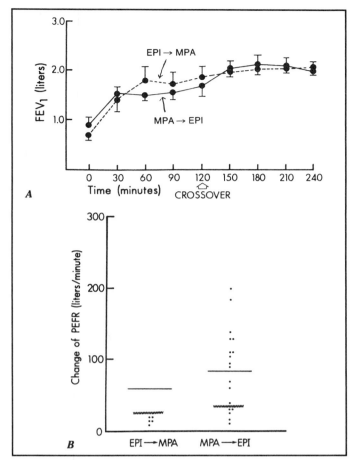

Fig. 72-9A. *Crossover trial comparing subcutaneous epinephrine (epi) and inhaled metaproterenol (meta) in the treatment of acute asthma. (Reprinted with permission from Appel, D., et al. Epinephrine improves expiratory flow rates in patients with asthma who do not respond to inhaled metaproterenol sulfate. J. Allergy Clin. Immunol. 84:90, 1989.)* B. *Among asthmatic patients failing to improve significantly during the first two hours of treatment, the effect of crossover to the alternative bronchodilator. The solid horizontal line indicates the mean value; the zagged horizontal line indicates the threshold for what was considered significant improvement. (Printed with permission from Appel, D., et al. Epinephrine improves expiratory flow rates in patients with asthma who do not respond to inhaled metaproterenol sulfate. J. Allergy Clin. Immunol. 84:90, 1989.)*

Fig. 72-8. *Bronchodilator effect of intravenous magnesium compared to placebo among asthmatic patients with persistent airflow obstruction following treatment with beta-adrenergic agonists. (Reprinted with permission from Skobeloff, E. M., et al. Intravenous magnesium sulfate for the treatment of acute asthma in the emergency department. JAMA 262:1210, 1989. Copyright 1989, American Medical Association.)*

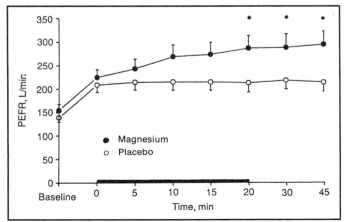

Subcutaneous epinephrine caused bronchodilation among this subpopulation of patients significantly more often than did inhaled metaproterenol (Fig. 72-9B). Expressed in another way, among patients failing to respond to repetitive doses of inhaled beta agonists, subcutaneous epinephrine produced more improvement than would be expected from continued administration of the inhaled beta agonist. Because only 28 patients were available for analysis within this subcategory (i.e., patients who failed to improve significantly with the initial sequence of treatments), it is difficult to draw firm conclusions from this one study.

It should be emphasized that the mainstay of therapy after the initial 60 to 90 minutes in the emergency department remains the frequent administration of sympathomimetic bronchodilators. Slight incremental benefit may be derived from concomitant use of anticholinergic drugs or intravenous magnesium sulfate or from altering the route of adrenergic agonist administration from inhaled to parenteral.

A variety of remedies have been tried for persistent severe

asthma, including intravenous or oral liquid supplementation ("hydration"), mucolytics, antihistamines, and chest physical therapy. None of these ancillary measures has been convincingly shown to be effective in the management of acute asthma, and none is recommended as part of conventional emergency department treatment. Although many patients experience anxiety in response to acute asthma and the stimulatory medicines used to treat it, anxiolytics are contraindicated in this setting because of their respiratory depressant effects.

DECISION REGARDING HOSPITAL ADMISSION

Most hospital admissions for asthma follow intensive treatment of acute asthmatic attacks; patients with an inadequate response to treatment in the emergency department are admitted to the hospital, whether it be to an overnight observation unit, to a general medical or respiratory service, or to an intensive care unit. The assumption underlying this decision to admit is that for the symptomatic patient with persistent airflow obstruction, care that is not reliably available at home can be provided in the hospital. For many years the mainstays of this specialized in-hospital care have been intravenously administered medications, particularly intravenous aminophylline and corticosteroids. However, it has recently become apparent that in most instances, a regimen of oral and inhaled medications is equally effective as a treatment strategy that includes intravenous medicines [35]. Other aspects of in-hospital care should now take a more prominent role in the decision process: ability to provide medication and personal care needs around the clock, clinical observation for the development of respiratory failure, and removal of the patient from potential asthmatic triggers in the home environment.

At either extreme of the spectrum of disease severity, it is easy to decide which patients do or do not require these special, hospital-based services. At the one end, patients who, in response to outpatient or emergency department treatment, have become asymptomatic with normal or near-normal lung function can safely receive their subsequent care on an ambulatory basis. Data extracted from a number of clinical trials indicate that the average FEV_1 or PEFR of patients who are discharged following emergency department care and do not experience recurrent respiratory difficulty over the ensuing 10 to 14 days is approximately 65 to 75 percent of normal [17]. Even among these patients with a good response to emergency treatment, the following precautions should be taken: First, patients should be observed for 30 to 60 minutes following the last bronchodilator treatment, to guard against rapid reversals among patients with highly labile airway function. Second, discharge instructions generally should include an intensification of the medical regimen that the patient was taking at the time of the acute attack. Patients who are sent home to the same environment on the same medications as previously used are vulnerable to recurrent attacks. Third, emergency department discharge provides an excellent opportunity for patient education, including discussion of such topics as medication purpose and use, proper technique for inhalation of medication, avoidance of triggers of asthma, and home monitoring of lung function.

At the other end of the spectrum of disease severity, patients with persistent marked asthmatic symptoms and severe airflow obstruction despite their emergency department treatments require hospital admission. These are patients who unquestionably require frequent treatments and medical observation day and night; they are at risk for developing hypercapnic respiratory failure, necessitating intubation and mechanical ventilation. Such patients are likely to have diffuse wheezes on chest auscultation, dyspnea at rest or on light exertion, and an FEV_1 or PEFR at 40 percent of predicted or less. This suggested value of FEV_1

or PEFR defining "severe" airflow obstruction is somewhat arbitrary, but it finds support in a series of studies that reported the level of lung function at the time of patient disposition from the emergency department. The average value among those patients admitted to the hospital was 35 to 45 percent [17].

A large percentage of the asthmatic patients treated in an emergency department fall in between these extremes of severity. They experience some improvement with treatment but continue to have troublesome symptoms and residual airflow obstruction (FEV_1 or PEFR > 40% but < 70% of normal). Further improvement following discharge will occur in many of these patients, especially if oral corticosteroids are included in their postdischarge treatment regimen. However, others will experience rapid deterioration if discharged home, requiring repeat emergency department care within the next few days because of recurrent severe asthmatic symptoms. Such "relapses" should be considered adverse outcomes of the decision-making process, since these patients will have suffered serious morbidity from their disease and a small but finite risk of death following emergency department discharge.

Current knowledge does not permit reliable identification of those patients within this intermediate category of response who should be hospitalized because of likely deterioration following emergency department discharge. One would predict that characteristics of patients at risk for relapses would include the following: prior history of near-fatal asthma, recent hospitalization or multiple recent emergency department visits for asthma, use of oral corticosteroids at the time of the asthmatic attack, emotional or psychiatric disturbance, serious comorbid illness(es), and inadequate home environment for self-care. Also, an FEV_1 or PEFR at the low end of this intermediate range (i.e., < 55% of predicted) probably indicates a patient at risk. Among patients with emergency department relapses, the average FEV_1 or PEFR at the time of initial discharge from the emergency department was 50 to 55 percent of normal in one collected series of reports (involving patients for whom the postdischarge medical regimen was not specified by experimental protocol) [17].

Among asthmatic patients considered well enough for emergency department discharge, the risk of relapse can be reduced to approximately 6 percent by administration of a course of oral steroids beginning at the time of discharge [10, 21]. One dosing schedule shown to be effective in a placebo-controlled trial [10] is the following: prednisone 40 mg orally at the time of emergency department discharge, 40 mg the following day (single daily dose), and then dose reduction by 5 mg each successive day, resulting in an 8-day tapering schedule. However, the optimal dose, duration, and schedule (single daily dose versus divided doses; tapering doses versus abrupt cessation of a single dose) for such a steroid course are unknown. An "optimal" prescription probably requires tailoring to individual patient needs. Patient-recorded home peak flow monitoring can be useful in this regard, permitting continuation at higher doses for patients whose airflow obstruction is improving slowly and allowing more rapid completion of the course for patients who show prompt improvement but experience adverse side effects. A reliable method to identify the small percentage of patients prone to deterioration despite an outpatient steroid course still awaits development.

It is important to remember that an asthmatic exacerbation has rarely if ever completely resolved at the time a patient is discharged home from the emergency department. Some degree of residual airflow obstruction and airway lability are the rule. Arranging for follow-up medical care within the ensuing week can contribute significantly to favorable outcomes, including fewer emergency department relapses. Likewise, if patient education can be incorporated into emergency department care, the frequency of subsequent emergency department visits can be reduced [42a].

Finally, the practice of detaining asthmatic patients in an emergency department for many hours while awaiting sufficient improvement to permit discharge home should be decried. In most facilities this strategy implies a prolonged period of discomfort for the patient, who is kept on a stretcher or examination table rather than being assigned to a hospital bed. A maximum of 4 hours should suffice to identify patients sufficiently well or sufficiently likely to experience continued improvement that discharge to home is warranted. Similarly, patients who have not improved adequately over 4 hours of intensive emergency department treatment are unlikely to do so during the next 4 hours, and emergency department treatment beyond 8 hours becomes abusive. In fact, in most instances patients definitely requiring hospitalization can be recognized within the first 60 to 90 minutes of intensive emergency department treatment [3, 51, 52]. Hospitalization should be strongly considered following the initial series of bronchodilator treatments if a patient's FEV_1 or PEFR remains at 40 percent of predicted or less [18].

PREVENTION

In many instances severe asthmatic exacerbations represent failures of good preventive care: Opportunities for earlier intervention have been missed. When well, asthmatic persons with normal or near-normal lung function typically have peak flow values in the range of 450 to 650 L/min, but when ill with acute attacks, they may have peak flow rates as low as 100 to 200 L/min or less. Although the deterioration to this latter level of airflow obstruction may be precipitous, occurring over minutes to hours, often it is more gradual, with progressive or stuttering decline over 1 or more days. As the worsening airflow obstruction gradually develops, warning signs often can alert patients and physicians to the evolution of an attack: Persistent cough, nocturnal awakenings due to respiratory symptoms, chest tightness, and exertional dyspnea are common clinical clues. Home monitoring of peak expiratory flow can be useful in this situation, especially if symptoms of an upper respiratory tract illness confound the assessment of asthma severity based on symptoms alone. Both a fall in PEFR that does not respond promptly to a dose of bronchodilators and large diurnal swings in PEFR (characteristically, large decreases in the early morning hours or "morning dipping") are signs of worsening asthma. It is important that patients be educated to recognize these signs and symptoms and to respond appropriately to them.

Home management of the early stages of an acute asthmatic attack is likely to vary from patient to patient and from episode to episode, depending on the particular circumstances of the attack, its severity, the patient's chronic medical regimen for asthma, and experience based on the management of previous attacks. Suggested guidelines for an overall approach should be developed by the patient and physician in collaboration. This "action plan" is then available in advance to the patient and, preferably, to other persons in the home who might also be involved with the patient's care. For example, according to an "action plan" it might be recommended that for a moderate attack the patient increase the frequency of inhaled beta-agonist bronchodilator doses, double the dose of inhaled corticosteroids, and if not better within 24 hours, begin oral corticosteroids (according to a previously specified dosing schedule) and call his or her health care provider.

Probably the single most common omission leading to severe asthmatic attacks is the failure to begin (or increase the chronic dose of) oral corticosteroids during the early phases of a serious attack. Often, when an upper respiratory tract illness is the precipitating event, antibiotics are mistakenly prescribed instead, despite the likelihood that the cause of the infection is viral. A short course of oral corticosteroids instituted at home can often prevent a subsequent, more prolonged course of steroid treatment and obviate the need for emergency department care and, possibly, hospitalization.

REFERENCES

1. Appel, D., Karpel, J. P., and Sherman, M. Epinephrine improves expiratory flow rates in patients with asthma who do not respond to inhaled metaproterenol sulfate. *J. Allergy Clin. Immunol.* 84:90, 1989.
2. Appel, D., and Shim, C. Comparative effect of epinephrine and aminophylline in the treatment of asthma. *Lung* 159:243, 1981.
3. Banner, A. S., Shah, R. S., and Addington, W. W. Rapid prediction of need for hospitalization in acute asthma. *Postgrad. Med. J.* 55:877, 1979.
4. Barnes, P. J., and Pride, N. B. Dose-response curves to inhaled beta-adrenoceptor agonists in normal and asthmatic subjects. *Br. J. Clin. Pharmacol.* 15:677, 1983.
5. Blackie, S. P., et al. Changes in total lung capacity during acute spontaneous asthma. *Am. Rev. Respir. Dis.* 142:79, 1990.
6. Brenner, B. E., Abraham, E., and Simon, R. R. Position and diaphoresis in acute asthma. *Am. J. Med.* 74:1005, 1983.
7. Cardell, B. S., and Pearson, R. S. B. Deaths in asthmatics. *Thorax* 14:341, 1959.
8. Carden, D. L., et al. Vital signs including pulsus paradoxus in the assessment of acute bronchial asthma. *Ann. Emerg. Med.* 12:80, 1983.
9. Centor, R. M., Yarbrough, B., and Wood, J. P. Inability to predict relapse in acute asthma. *N. Engl. J. Med.* 310:577, 1984.
10. Chapman, K. R., et al. Effect of a short course of prednisone in the prevention of early relapse after the emergency room treatment of acute asthma. *N. Engl. J. Med.* 324:788, 1991.
11. Colacone, A., et al. Continuous nebulization of albuterol (salbutamol) in acute asthma. *Chest* 97:693, 1990.
12. Deenstra, M., Haalboom, J. R., and Struyvenberg, A. Decrease of plasma potassium due to inhalation of beta-2-agonists: Absence of an additional effect of intravenous theophylline. *Eur. J. Clin. Invest.* 18:162, 1988.
13. Djukanovic, R., et al. Mucosal inflammation in asthma. *Am. Rev. Respir. Dis.* 142:434, 1990.
14. Drazen, J. M., et al. Recovery of LTE_4 from the urine of patients with acute asthmatic exacerbations. *Am. Rev. Respir. Dis.* 146:104, 1992.
15. Dunnill, M. S. The pathology of asthma with special reference to changes in the bronchial mucosa. *J. Clin. Pathol.* 13:27, 1960.
16. Emerman, C. L., Crafford, W. A., and Vrobel, T. R. Ventricular arrhythmias during treatment for acute asthma. *Ann. Emerg. Med.* 15:699, 1986.
17. Fanta, C. H. Emergency management of asthma. *Clin. Challenge Cardiopulm. Med.* 5:1, 1985.
18. Fanta, C. H., Rossing, T. H., and McFadden, E. R., Jr. Emergency room treatment of asthma: Relationships among therapeutic combinations, severity of obstruction and time course of response. *Am. J. Med.* 72:416, 1982.
19. Fanta, C. H., Rossing, T. H., and McFadden, E. R., Jr. Glucocorticoids in acute asthma: A critical controlled trial. *Am. J. Med.* 74:845, 1983.
20. Fanta, C. H., Rossing, T. H., and McFadden, E. R., Jr. Treatment of acute asthma: Is combination therapy with sympathomimetics and methylxanthines indicated? *Am. J. Med.* 80:5, 1986.
21. Feil, S. B., et al. Efficacy of short-term corticosteroid therapy in outpatient treatment of acute bronchial asthma. *Am. J. Med.* 75:259, 1983.
22. Femi-Pearse, D., et al. Comparison of intravenous aminophylline and salbutamol in severe asthma. *Br. Med. J.* 1(6059):491, 1977.
23. Findley, L. J., and Sahn, S. A. The value of chest roentgenograms in acute asthma in adults. *Chest* 80:535, 1981.
24. Fischl, M. A., Pitchenik, A., and Gardner, L. B. An index predicting relapse and need for hospitalization in patients with acute bronchial asthma. *N. Engl. J. Med.* 305:783, 1981.
25. Gilman, M. J., et al. Comparison of aerosolized glycopyrrolate and metaproterenol in acute asthma. *Chest* 98:1095, 1990.
26. Grief, J., Markovitz, L., and Topilsky, M. Comparison of intravenous salbutamol (albuterol) and aminophylline in the treatment of acute asthmatic attacks. *Ann. Allergy* 55:504, 1985.
27. Harrison, B. D., et al. Need for intravenous hydrocortisone in addition to oral prednisolone in patients admitted to hospital with severe asthma without ventilatory failure. *Lancet* 1(8474):181, 1986.
28. Higgins, R. M., Stradling, J. R., and Lane, D. J. Should ipratropium bromide be added to beta-agonists in treatment of acute severe asthma? *Chest* 94:718, 1988.
29. Hillman, D. R., Prentice, L., and Finucane, K. E. The pattern of breathing in acute severe asthma. *Am. Rev. Respir. Dis.* 133:587, 1986.

30. Hoffman, I. B., and Fiel, S. B. Oral vs repository corticosteroid therapy in acute asthma. *Chest* 93:11, 1988.

31. Holmes, P. W., Campbell, A. H., and Barter, C. E. Acute changes of lung volumes and lung mechanics in asthma and in normal subjects. *Thorax* 33:394, 1978.

32. Hrach, B., and Fanta, C. H. Comparison of beta-agonist bronchodilators in acute asthma. *Clin. Res.* 38:572A, 1990.

33. Hrach, B., and Fanta, C. H. Validity of peak expiratory flow measurements to assess lung function in acute attacks of asthma. *Clin. Res.* 38:274A, 1990.

34. Ingram, R. H., Jr., et al. Ventilation-perfusion changes after aerosolized isoproterenol in asthma. *Am. Rev. Respir. Dis.* 101:364, 1970.

35. Jonsson, S., et al. Comparison of the oral and intravenous routes for treating asthma with methylprednisolone and theophylline. *Chest* 94:723, 1988.

36. Josephson, G. W., et al. Cardiac dysrhythmias during the treatment of acute asthma: A comparison of two treatment regimens by a double blind protocol. *Chest* 78:429, 1980.

37. Josephson, G. W., et al. Emergency treatment of asthma: A comparison of two treatment regimens. *JAMA* 242:639, 1979.

38. Karpel, J. P., et al. A comparison of atropine sulfate and metaproterenol sulfate in the emergency treatment of asthma. *Am. Rev. Respir. Dis.* 133:727, 1986.

39. Kelsen, S. G., et al. Emergency room assessment and treatment of patients with acute asthma: Adequacy of the conventional approach. *Am. J. Med.* 64:622, 1978.

40. Knowles, G. K., and Clark, T. J. H. Pulsus paradoxus as a valuable sign indicating severity of asthma. *Lancet* 2(842):1356, 1973.

41. Lipworth, B. J., Struthers, A. D., and McDevitt, D. G. Tachyphylaxis to systemic but not to airway responses during prolonged therapy with high dose inhaled salbutamol in asthmatics. *Am. Rev. Respir. Dis.* 140:586, 1989.

42. Littenberg, B., and Gluck, E. H. A controlled trial of methylprednisolone in the emergency treatment of acute asthma. *N. Engl. J. Med.* 314:150, 1986.

42a. Maiman, L. A., et al. Education for self-treatment by adult asthmatics. *JAMA* 241:1919, 1979.

43. Martin, T. G., Elenbaas, R. M., and Pingleton, S. H. Use of peak expiratory flow rates to eliminate unnecessary arterial blood gases in acute asthma. *Ann. Emerg. Med.* 11:70, 1982.

44. McFadden, E. R., Jr. Clinical physiologic correlates in asthma. *J. Allergy Clin. Immunol.* 77:1, 1986.

45. McFadden, E. R., Jr., Kiser, R., and deGroot, W. J. Acute bronchial asthma: Relations between clinical and physiologic manifestations. *N. Engl. J. Med.* 288:221, 1973.

46. McFadden, E. R., Jr., et al. A controlled study of the effects of single doses of hydrocortisone on the resolution of acute attacks of asthma. *Am. J. Med.* 60:52, 1976.

47. McFadden, E. R., Jr., and Lyons, H. A. Arterial-blood gas tension in asthma. *N. Engl. J. Med.* 278:1027, 1968.

48. Molfino, N. A., et al. Respiratory arrest in near-fatal asthma. *N. Engl. J. Med.* 324:285, 1991.

49. Morley, T. F., et al. Comparison of beta-adrenergic agents delivered by nebulizer vs metered dose inhaler with InspirEase in hospitalized asthmatic patients. *Chest* 94:1205, 1988.

50. Muller, N., Bryan, A. C., and Zamel, N. Tonic inspiratory muscle activity as a cause of hyperinflation in asthma. *J. Appl. Physiol.* 50:279, 1981.

50a. National Asthma Education Program, Expert Panel Report. *Executive Summary: Guidelines for the Diagnosis and Management of Asthma.* Publication No. 91-3042A. Bethesda, MD: National Institutes of Health, June 1991.

51. Nowak, R. M., et al. Spirometric evaluation of acute bronchial asthma. *JACEP* 8:9, 1979.

52. Nowak, R. M., et al. Comparison of peak expiratory flow and FEV_1 admission criteria for acute bronchial asthma. *Ann. Emerg. Med.* 11:64, 1982.

53. O'Connell, M. B., and Iber, C. Continuous intravenous terbutaline infusions for adult patients with status asthmaticus. *Ann. Allergy* 64(2, part 2):213, 1990.

54. O'Driscoll, B. R., et al. Nebulized salbutamol with and without ipratropium bromide in acute airflow obstruction. *Lancet* 1(8652):1418, 1989.

55. Patrick, D. M., et al. Severe exacerbations of COPD and asthma: Incremental benefit of adding ipratropium to usual therapy. *Chest* 98:295, 1990.

56. Picado, C., et al. Respiratory and skeletal muscle function in steroid-dependent bronchial asthma. *Am. Rev. Respir. Dis.* 141:14, 1990.

57. Pierce, R. J., et al. Comparison of intravenous and inhaled terbutaline in the treatment of asthma. *Chest* 79:506, 1981.

58. Pliss, L. B., and Gallagher, E. J. Aerosol vs injected epinephrine in acute asthma. *Ann. Emerg. Med.* 10:353, 1981.

59. Rebuck, A. S., et al. Nebulized anticholinergic and sympathomimetic treatment of asthma and chronic obstructive airways disease in the emergency room. *Am. J. Med.* 82:59, 1987.

60. Rebuck, A. S., and Pengelly, L. D. Development of pulsus paradoxus in the presence of airways obstruction. *N. Engl. J. Med.* 288:66, 1973.

61. Rebuck, A. S., and Read, J. Assessment and management of severe asthma. *Am. J. Med.* 51:788, 1971.

62. Reid, L. M. The presence or absence of bronchial mucus in fatal asthma. *J. Allergy Clin. Immunol.* 80(3, part 2):415, 1987.

63. Ringel, E. R., et al. Chest wall configurational changes before and during acute obstructive episodes in asthma. *Am. Rev. Respir. Dis.* 128:607, 1983.

64. Rossing, T. H., et al. Emergency therapy of asthma: Comparison of the acute effects of parenteral and inhaled sympathomimetics and infused aminophylline. *Am. Rev. Respir. Dis.* 122:365, 1980.

65. Rossing, T. H., Fanta, C. H., and McFadden, E. R., Jr. Effect of outpatient treatment of asthma with beta agonists on the response to sympathomimetics in an emergency room. *Am. J. Med.* 75:781, 1983.

66. Roussos, C. S., et al. Respiratory muscle fatigue in man at FRC and higher lung volumes. *Physiologist* 19:345, 1976.

67. Salzman, G. A., et al. Aerosolized metaproterenol in the treatment of asthmatics with severe airflow obstruction: Comparison of two delivery methods. *Chest* 95:1017, 1989.

68. Siegal, D., et al. Aminophylline increases the toxicity but not the efficacy of an inhaled beta-adrenergic agonist in the treatment of acute exacerbations of asthma. *Am. Rev. Respir. Dis.* 132:283, 1985.

69. Skobeloff, E. M., et al. Intravenous magnesium sulfate for the treatment of acute asthma in the emergency department. *JAMA* 262:1210, 1989.

70. Stein, L. M., and Cole, R. P. Early administration of corticosteroids in emergency room treatment of acute asthma. *Ann. Intern. Med.* 112:822, 1990.

71. Storr, J., and Lenney, W. Nebulised ipratropium and salbutamol in asthma. *Arch. Dis. Child.* 61:602, 1986.

72. Summers, Q. A., and Tarala, R. A. Nebulized ipratropium in the treatment of acute asthma. *Chest* 97:425, 1990.

73. Turner, J. R., et al. Equivalence of continuous flow nebulizer and metered-dose inhaler with reservoir bag for treatment of acute airflow obstruction. *Chest* 93:476, 1988.

74. Van Renterghem, D., et al. Intravenous versus nebulized terbutaline in patients with acute severe asthma: A double-blind randomized study. *Ann. Allergy* 59:313, 1987.

75. Ward, M. J., et al. Ipratropium bromide in acute asthma. *Br. Med. J.* [*Clin. Res.Ed.*] 282:598, 1981.

76. Ward, M. J., Macfarlane, J. T., and Davies, D. A place for ipratropium bromide in the treatment of severe acute asthma. *Br. J. Dis. Chest* 79:374, 1985.

77. Weiss, K. B. Seasonal trends in US asthma hospitalizations and mortality. *JAMA* 263:2323, 1990.

78. Williams, S. J., Parrish, R. W., and Seaton, A. Comparison of intravenous aminophylline and salbutamol in severe asthma. *Br. Med. J.* 4(5998):685, 1975.

79. Williams, S. J., Winner, S. J., and Clark, T. J. Comparison of inhaled and intravenous terbutaline in acute severe asthma. *Thorax* 36:629, 1981.

79a. Wilson, J. D., Sutherland, D. C., and Thomas, A. C. Has the change to beta-agonists combined with oral theophylline increased cases of fatal asthma? *Lancet* 1(8232):1235, 1981.

80. Woolcock, A. J., and Read, J. Lung volumes in exacerbations of asthma. *Am. J. Med.* 41:259, 1966.

81. Wrenn, K., et al. Aminophylline for acute bronchospastic disease in the emergency room. *Ann. Intern. Med.* 115:241, 1991.

82. Zieverink, S. E., et al. Emergency room radiography of asthma: An efficacy study. *Radiology* 145:27, 1982.

Status Asthmaticus

Nicholas S. Hill
Earle B. Weiss

73

Status asthmaticus is the most critical clinical expression of bronchial asthma because its advanced gas exchange defects are life-threatening. Since status asthmaticus is associated with a 1 to 3 percent mortality rate, a patient with this diagnosis warrants immediate hospitalization with full supportive measures. The clinical state is essentially defined as a severe episode of asthma that is unrelieved by usually effective bronchodilator drugs. This pharmacologic defect is, however, not absolute, for it may be partially overcome in some patients with intravenous isoproterenol or similar adrenergic drugs. This effect of isoproterenol occurs largely (but not exclusively) in children and presumably mainly reflects changes in bronchomotor tone, because these patients are more likely to be suffering from a rapidly reversible bronchial muscle contractile component. This contrasts with the more resistant, slowly resolving patterns associated with airway inflammation and secretional obstruction, in which limited beta-adrenergic drug responses largely occur from the intra-airway mechanical obstruction resulting from glandular secretions, edema, and inflammatory responses. Inasmuch as the majority of affected patients exhibit such secretional airways obstruction, the use of bronchodilator drugs in this context thus becomes a maneuver to identify that such refractory inflammatory, pathomechanical obstruction exists.

While it is well accepted that the term *status asthmaticus* refers to an asthmatic condition possessing two essential features—severe airflow obstruction and little or no improvement in airflow in response to initial bronchodilator therapy [35]—there is no agreement on specific criteria for defining the severity of airflow obstruction or the precise drugs or duration of therapeutic refractoriness necessary to establish the diagnosis. Nevertheless, the general consensus is that the airway obstruction should be life-threatening [5, 57, 163, 263].

A number of other terms have been employed in recent years to describe severe asthma; these include *near fatal asthma* [230], *life-threatening asthma* [350, 384], *acute severe asthma* [6], and *sudden asphyxic asthma* [372], but none satisfactorily replaces *status asthmaticus* because they do not imply refractoriness. Despite the lack of a consensus on an objective definition, acute severe asthma or status asthmaticus can be characterized by a number of clinical and physiologic features (Table 73-1). Persistence of these features, despite adequate acute therapy, would constitute therapeutic refractoriness.

Although there are no specific criteria for defining drug refractoriness in status asthmaticus, general guidelines can be provided. The usual clinical practice is to administer a beta-adrenergic drug by aerosol or by the subcutaneous route, and at times theophylline, to an acutely ill patient with asthma (see Chap. 72) and then to assess the response over the first hour or two of treatment—the temporal course of most beta-agonist agents used in the acute setting. A favorable response is judged according to both subjective clinical features and objective findings—spirometric, peak expiratory flow rate (PEFR), or arterial blood gas measurements; however, spirometric and PEFR testing requires a properly instructed and cooperative patient. Because these findings may vary among patients and as no absolute data exist that define an appropriate therapeutic trial or parameters of response in such patients, no strict criteria can be provided. Nevertheless, in addition to subjective or clinical improvement, as approximate guidelines the forced vital capacity (FVC) should improve to at least 1.5 liters, the first-second forced expiratory volume (FEV_1) by 15 percent or more and at least to 1.0 liter, and the PEFR to at least 100 to 120 liters per minute. Overall, a response in PEFR or FEV_1 of 10 percent or less constitutes a failure of acute therapy; this situation will be clinically obvious. PEFR or FEV_1 values 25 percent or less of the predicted normal identify patients at risk for developing significant hypercapnia or acidosis. A very favorable response to the selected regimen is an improvement in FEV_1 or PEFR of 70 percent or greater than predicted; the response is poor when values remain under 40 percent of the predicted value. In addition, arterial blood gas and pH determinations may be required to validate clinical and spirometric improvement, as some patients may exhibit more subjective or clinical relief than is documented from spirometric or blood gas data; in this context, PaO_2 should be at least 60 mmHg, and $PaCO_2$, 40 to 45 mmHg or less (ambient air) (see further discussion later in this chapter).

Several authors have proposed indices for predicting the need for hospitalization in patients presenting to emergency rooms with severe, acute asthma [13, 97]. Fischl and coworkers [97] concluded that the need for hospitalization could be predicted with 96 percent accuracy if four or more of the following conditions exist before therapy is initiated: (1) pulse rate at least 120/min, (2) respiratory rate at least 30/min, (3) pulsus paradoxus at least 18 mmHg, (4) PEFR 120 L/min or less, (5) moderate to severe dyspnea, (6) accessory muscle use, and (7) wheezing. This grading index could also be applied after initial therapy as an indicator of drug refractoriness. However, two later studies failed to confirm the predictive accuracy of the Fischl index regarding relapse in acute asthma [41, 300], and so the index per se cannot be currently recommended.

The drug schedules proposed in Chapter 72 dealing with the therapy of acute asthma in the adult are recommended for the initial therapeutic strategy. Failure of these approaches usually indicates pharmacologic refractoriness. In the absence of specific criteria for hospitalization, the following constitute general guidelines:

1. Persisting symptoms (dyspnea) and signs (wheezing).
2. PEFR or FEV_1 ($\leq$25–40% predicted) and not improving following acute therapy.
3. Recent repeated emergency room visits; nocturnal difficulties.
4. Arterial blood gas/pH: normal or elevated PCO_2 in a symptomatic patient; acidemic pH; PaO_2 less than 50 to 60 mmHg.

Table 73-1. Indices of acute, severe, or life-threatening refractory asthma

Disturbances of consciousness
Cyanosis (central)
Severe respiratory distress or exhaustion
Recurrent acute episodes over a short period (e.g., 2–7 days)
Increasing bronchodilator requirement with minimal relief
Profuse diaphoresis
Pulsus paradoxus ≥15–18 mmHg
Sternocleidomastoid contraction, intercostal retraction, paradoxical abdominal respiration
Wheezing on inspiration (high pitch) or silent chest
Tachypnea ≥30/min
Tachycardia ≥120 beats/min
Peak expiratory flow rate ≤100–120 L/min, or <25–40% of predicted
Forced vital capacity ≤1–1.5 L, or <25–40% predicted
Forced expiratory volume in 1 second ≤1.0 L, or <25–40% of predicted
PaO_2 ≤60 mmHg (room air)
$PaCO_2$ ≥40–45 mmHg (± acidemia)
Electrocardiographic abnormalities, hypotension
Coexisting pneumonia, pneumothorax, pneumomediastinum

Regardless of the specific criteria applied, once a severe attack of asthma is deemed refractory to therapy and status asthmaticus is diagnosed, three corollaries arise: (1) bronchial asthma is now life-threatening, (2) status asthmaticus is a medical emergency, and monitoring and therapy must be intensified accordingly, and (3) hospitalization is *immediately* required for instituting diagnostic studies, intensive treatment, nursing care, and the elimination of offending agents.

Once initial drug refractoriness to conventional bronchodilators is determined, intravenous corticosteroids should be initiated; 2.0 to 4.0 mg/kg of body weight of hydrocortisone hemisuccinate (or an equivalent preparation) should be given and maintenance doses continued in the hospital (see Chap. 60).

Finally, while a variety of clinical or quantitative methods are available for determining the initial effectiveness of drug therapy (PEFR, spirometry, arterial blood gases, predictive indexes, and so on), no single feature or combination of observations can unequivocally predict the need for hospitalization nor can they supplant the meticulous concerns of the involved physician. In any case of uncertainty as to the patient's course, hospitalization is safer and is strongly recommended.

Considering that the best therapeutic approach would be to avoid the development of status asthmaticus altogether, sections of this chapter will deal with the pathogenesis of status asthmaticus, identification of patients at risk, and strategies that may prevent its development. The goals of management are the restoration of optimal lung function and clinical status, the prevention of mortality, and subsequently the maintenance of stable asthma with prevention of early relapse.

INCITING FACTORS

No unique precipitating factor has been incriminated as the cause of status asthmaticus. The usual incitants are those that may provoke any attack of asthma, including allergen exposure, viral respiratory infection, air pollutants, toxin exposure, cold air, and temperature and humidity changes. In many instances, the initiating event or events, may not be clinically obvious, or many factors may interact to intensify or propagate the process. For most patients, status asthmaticus begins as any other attack of asthma, revealing its true character only as refractoriness to therapy develops. Infectious exacerbations may be more common in patients with intrinsic asthma, whereas allergic insults may be more easily incriminated in those with extrinsic atopy.

Inhalant allergens, because of their sheer incidence, are undoubtedly among the most important incitants. Recently, airborne spores of *Alternaria alternata* have been implicated as a risk factor for respiratory arrest in children and young adults with asthma [250]. Fever, emotional or physical stress, dehydration, and hypermetabolic demands are ancillary factors, but are of therapeutic importance. Occupational hazards also require consideration (see Chap. 46). Asthma has been associated with exposure to isocyanates, enzyme detergents, baking, plastic wrapping, cotton or flax dust, certain wood dusts, and metal compounds such as nickel or platinum salts [312]. Nonasthmatic occupational toxic insults must be distinguished because acute chemical bronchiolitis can mimic status asthmaticus. Of course, cigarette smoking can intensify any insult.

Patients with allergic respiratory diseases exhibit an increased morbidity and mortality during periods of high air pollution with particulates, ozone, oxides of sulfur, carbon monoxide, metals, and photochemicals, as well as during periods of temperature inversion and climate changes. In one serious epidemic in Donora, Pennsylvania, about 90 percent of the asthmatic population was affected, compared with 40 percent of the total population [113]. In addition, hospital emergency room visits in urban areas increase during periods of stagnation; commonly cited examples include such occurrences in New Orleans and Yokohama, Yokohama asthma being a nonspecific effect of air pollutants in susceptible persons [338, 375] (see Chap. 45). In other instances, wind forces from a city dump have been related to similar outbreaks [192]. Even soybean dust has been identified as an asthma epidemic incitant in urban sites [1]. Status asthmaticus and deaths have occurred with such exposure to industrial pollutants, temperature, and atmospheric or geographic changes, and appropriate protective measures should be encouraged.

Respiratory tract infections may precipitate an asthma episode or in some instances develop secondarily. Viral provocations appear to be commonly incriminated, particularly in children, and include respiratory syncytial virus, influenza, parainfluenza, rhinovirus, and adenovirus. Estimates for a viral etiology range from 10 to 40 percent in children requiring hospitalization, with the variability in incidence arising from differences in age, serologic methods, and patient selection [76, 216]. *Mycoplasma pneumoniae* infection, a common cause of community-acquired pneumonia in children and young adults, has been reported to be associated with exacerbations of asthma [20]. The association between viral infections and subsequent airways hyperreactivity is detailed in Chapter 44. *Chlamydia* pneumonia is another causative agent that may be associated with adult-onset asthma [129].

Compared to viruses, bacterial infections are not commonly involved in precipitating asthma attacks but they may be causative in select instances and need to be identified. Bacterial infection in childhood cases of status asthmaticus is perhaps more common in nonatopic children and in those with an immunologic deficiency, while infective bronchitis or sinusitis may be contributory in adults. There may also be an increased risk of infection in corticosteroid-treated patients [63, 223]; this risk may not apply to patients on alternate-day schedules. Whether asthma predisposes a person to subsequent infectious complications is not entirely resolved; in one study, 11 percent of the asthmatic children experienced recurrent bacterial pneumonias [177]. Other data indicate that this is an infrequent problem, possibly because of the brevity of such attacks [209]. In adults, it is becoming clear that the use of routine antimicrobials is not warranted in the management of acute episodes unless specific findings of a bacterial process are present [123] (see Chap. 44).

Certain drugs (nonsteroidal antiinflammatory agents [273] or beta blockers) may precipitate severe asthma attacks, while underuse of necessary medications may amplify the effect of other causative factors (Chap. 48).

MECHANISMS FOR DRUG REFRACTORINESS

A variety of physiochemical and pharmacologic mechanisms have been proposed to explain why patients in status asthmaticus are refractory to therapy (Table 73-2). Several of the pathomechanical findings observed in the lungs of patients who die in status asthmaticus are apparently of sufficient severity to explain refractoriness. Widespread tenacious mucous plugs obstructing the bronchi may physically impede the entry of inhaled drugs, and hence limit the access of aerosolized bronchodilator drugs to the distal or even more central airways; rapid shallow breathing may further reduce aerosol delivery to the peripheral airways. Extensive bronchial wall edema and smooth muscle spasm and hypertrophy may additionally retard the diffusion of drugs from the luminal surface to their site of action. Even with delivery of drug to the sites of action, these pathologic abnormalities are apt to respond slowly. The essential issue, of course, is how and why such critical secretory problems arise in status asthmaticus.

Bronchodilator ineffectiveness could hypothetically result from decreased drug delivery, decreased absorption, increased drug elimination, or alterations in cellular control or homeostatic mechanisms. Evidence has been accruing to suggest that beta-adrenergic receptor hyporesponsiveness to beta agonists is an important mechanism underlying drug refractoriness in patients with severe asthma [118]. Bronchi isolated from subjects who died during asthma attacks are less responsive to beta agonists than are bronchi from subjects without asthma, whereas the responsiveness to theophylline is similar [119]. Other investigators have found a significant negative correlation between beta agonist bronchodilator potency and the severity of asthma [15]. Furthermore, peripheral lymphocytes from atopic asthmatics demonstrate a marked reduction in beta adrenergic receptor function 24 hours after allergen challenge in comparison to lymphocytes from healthy controls, perhaps reflecting impaired coupling between beta adrenergic receptors and adenylate cyclase [222]. These results are compatible with the hypothesis that acute allergic inflammatory responses render beta adrenergic receptors dysfunctional [120]. This hypothesis remains controversial, however, because the apparent receptor hypofunction could also be related to reduced drug access or downregulation brought about by previous beta agonist use. This subject is presented in greater detail in Chapters 14 and 55.

The downregulation of receptors or tachyphylaxis to beta-adrenergic drugs may also be a factor in the refractoriness to therapy [278]. Tachyphylaxis to sympathomimetic drugs such as

Table 73-2. Postulated mechanisms of drug refractoriness

Limited access of aerosolized drugs
   Intense bronchospasm and edema
   Secretional obstruction
   Tachypnea and hypopnea
Beta-adrenergic receptor hyporesponsiveness
   Impaired coupling with adenylate cyclase
   Downregulation of receptors
   Tachyphylaxis
   Metabolic inhibition (isoproterenol)
Inadequate dosages
   Relative to pharmacologic need
   Increased metabolism—clearance
   Drug interactions
Other
   Epithelial damage with inhibition of relaxing factors
   Cholinergic influences
   Corticosteroid "resistance"
   Release of chemoattractant factors and other cytokines
   Epinephrine fastness in acidemia
   Defects in mucociliary function

ephedrine, which acts indirectly through the release of norepinephrine from adrenergic nerve terminals, is well known [42] and results from depletion of norepinephrine stores in the nerve terminals. Other sympathomimetic drugs such as isoproterenol and albuterol act directly on membrane receptors and target cells, causing a different form of tachyphylaxis. Studies done on isolated tissues and in experimental animals have provided evidence that prolonged treatment with such beta-adrenergic agonists decreases the number of functional membrane receptors, thereby reducing the response to a given dose of drug (downregulation) [106, 234]. However, desensitization to beta agonists has not been confirmed by other studies; for example, no reduction has been observed to occur in the number of lymphocytic beta receptors in asthmatics receiving 400 µg of albuterol qid [365].

Clinical studies have shown decreased bronchodilator responsiveness to inhaled albuterol in normal subjects [148] and asthmatic patients [239] and to oral terbutaline in patients with stable asthma or chronic bronchitis [165]. A recent study demonstrated poorer control of asthma in patients using a fenoterol inhaler on a regular rather than an as-needed basis, suggesting that regular therapy impairs bronchodilator responsiveness [317a]. However, not all studies have detected such diminished responsiveness to beta agonists [188], in that the decline in bronchodilator response to beta-adrenergic drugs, when observed, has generally been small, and the clinical relevance of this to status asthmaticus is yet to be clarified. Unquestionably, the first-line therapy for acute, severe asthma remains beta agonists, even though their prior use may have resulted in some hyporesponsiveness. In some instances, corticosteroids may alleviate this problem, since administration restores bronchodilator responsiveness to beta agonists [86, 320].

Among beta agonists, isoproterenol may constitute a special case, as it has been associated with severe refractory asthma and lack of bronchodilator response, with clinical and spirometric improvement occurring after its discontinuation [293, 364]. Therapeutic doses of nebulized isoproterenol have also been reported to induce bronchoconstriction in some patients [174]. Bronchoconstriction following the use of inhaled isoproterenol may result from an irritative effect caused by one or more of the ingredients in the aerosol. A metabolite of isoproterenol, 3-methoxyisoproterenol, is a weak beta-receptor antagonist and may also play a role [266].

The role of alpha-adrenergic pathways in asthma is the subject of continuing study. Although alpha-adrenergic–blocking drugs have been shown to reduce postexercise bronchoconstriction in asthmatics [127, 265], alpha-adrenergic receptors most likely do not play a major role in the regulation of airway tone in either healthy subjects or asthmatic patients [14].

Airway epithelial damage or desquamation may play a role in the refractoriness to therapy in acute, severe asthma. Such damage, aside from causing mechanical obstruction and impairment of the mucociliary apparatus, could impair the secretion of epithelium-derived inhibiting and relaxing factors that may ameliorate bronchospastic responses [99].

Another factor possibly contributing to the refractoriness to therapy is adrenocorticosteroid dependency or resistance. Steroid resistance is characterized by an increased plasma clearance of cortisol, a decreased eosinopenic response to steroids, and poor asthma control despite the use of usually effective corticosteroid doses [314]. Such patients require two to three times the usual steroid doses for control of an asthmatic exacerbation and an immediate increase in dose during any physiologic stress.

Hence, while a variety of factors may contribute to drug refractoriness and these may vary among patients, the precise mechanisms responsible for causing status asthmaticus are currently unresolved. Generally, the presence of widespread, tenacious, and obstructive inflammatory airway secretions and edema appears to be the major problem, but the cause of this is not fully defined. Questions that require answers are: Is it simply a quantitative problem? and How critical is the failure of the mucociliary and clearance activities in this process? Additional biochemical and pharmacologic factors may become additive secondary causes against this background. Diffuse epithelial damage [99] and beta-adrenergic desensitization, either due to beta-adrenergic receptor–adenylate cyclase uncoupling or to drug-induced downregulation, are likely components of the mechanism, or mechanisms, involved. Whether alterations in the sensitivity to or the release of other mediators such as neutrophil chemotactic factors [59], leukotrienes, or platelet-activating factor have a distinctive role in status asthmaticus remains to be established.

Pathology

Our understanding of the pathologic features of status asthmaticus is derived largely from autopsy examinations in fatal cases [38, 84, 150, 151, 221, 383]. The gross and microscopic findings in patients in status asthmaticus have been reviewed by Thurlbeck [354] and Hogg [147] and are discussed in Chapter 28.

At autopsy, the lungs are found to be markedly hyperinflated and do not collapse when removed from the thorax. An almost ubiquitous pathologic finding in patients dying in status asthmaticus presumably reflects a predominant cause of the refractory airways obstruction, namely, the occlusion of airways by thick and extremely tenacious mucous plugs (Plate 27). These may extend diffusely from the upper airways to respiratory bronchioles and coexist with the previously described gross morphologic parenchymal overdistention. In addition to marked compromise of the airways caused by spasm of hypertrophied smooth muscle and epithelial invaginations and evaginations, these inspissated periodic–acid Schiff–positive secretions grossly reduce the effective luminal diameter (Fig. 73-1). These plugs are composed of a mixture of mucus and proteinaceous

Fig. 73-1. *Bronchus from a patient with status asthmaticus. Luminal diameter is reduced by the invagination of the airway, mucous plug in lumen, edema, and muscle hypertrophy and spasm.*

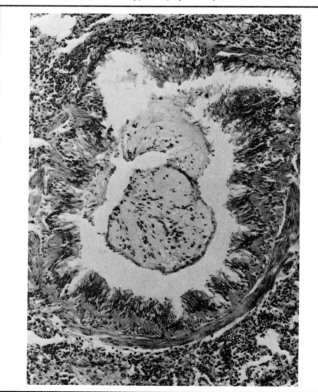

exudate containing large numbers of eosinophils, Charcot-Leyden crystals, and shed airway epithelial cells, either singly or in clumps, which are recognized in expectorated sputum as Creola bodies. Important facets of these secretional phenomena that are yet to be clarified in status asthmaticus include the biochemical changes in such mucus, mucociliary transport, and epithelial mucosal permeability. Additional findings in some patients dying of asthma include occasional patients with "dry" airways and others with areas of atelectasis, subpleural fibrosis, and bronchiectasis [80, 292]. True emphysema with air space enlargement and tissue destruction is seldom seen in cases of fatal asthma [81, 122, 383]. However, interstitial emphysema consisting of disruption and tearing of peribronchial and perivascular connective tissue was recently described in 36 of 53 patients with fatal asthma and was associated with bronchial gland duct ectasia [50].

Typically, the bronchial mucosa shows extensive goblet cell metaplasia and hyperplasia [1a]. Large areas of epithelium are sloughed into the lumen, leaving only the basal layer of the epithelium. Thickening of the basement membrane by deposition of increased amounts of collagen on the nonluminal side of the basal lamina is characteristic of asthma but not pathognomonic, as it is also found in other respiratory diseases [62, 310]. The mucous glands are enlarged and the bronchial wall is heavily infiltrated with eosinophils in patients dying of status asthmaticus. A marked increase in the thickness of bronchial smooth muscle is seen, unlike the situation in chronic bronchitis, and primarily reflects muscle cell hyperplasia rather than hypertrophy [81, 134, 350]. Immunofluorescent staining has identified immunoglobulin E in bronchial epithelial cells, basement membrane, bronchial glands, and intrabronchial mucus in patients with asthma [110]. Recently, inflammation has been described in pulmonary vascular walls adjacent to inflamed bronchi, perhaps contributing to gas exchange abnormalities [307].

Since the classic descriptions of lung pathologic changes in bronchial asthma have been based on the postmortem features of patients dying of acute asthma or status asthmaticus, it has only been inferred that lesser degrees of these characteristic findings occur in milder or nonfatal cases. However, a valuable ultrastructural study of the airways conducted in asthmatic children during clinical remission of their disease, using tissue obtained from lung biopsies performed for other reasons, has been reported [64]. Interestingly, these asymptomatic patients exhibited typical but lesser degrees of mucous plugging, goblet cell hyperplasia, peribronchial smooth muscle hypertrophy, and eosinophilic infiltration. Hence, secretional obstruction seems characteristic of asthma, whether mild or severe, in clinical remission, or in status asthmaticus. Again, this pathomechanical feature not only limits effective aerosol bronchodilator drug dispersion but appears to be the major factor in initial pharmacologic refractoriness.

EPIDEMIOLOGY AND MORTALITY

Asthma affects approximately 3 to 5 percent of the general population [18, 87], but precise statistics on the incidence of status asthmaticus are unavailable. Only a small fraction of asthmatics require hospitalization for the treatment of severe asthma, and the mortality rate for patients who are hospitalized is approximately 1 to 3 percent [25, 82, 171, 316]. In a 20-year follow-up study of 449 patients first seen for asthma before the age of 13, only 2 percent required treatment in-hospital, and only 0.8 percent of the entire group died of asthma [281].

Asthma is a common reason for hospital admission, accounting for 8 percent of the admissions to the medical service and 25 percent of the admissions to the pediatric service of a New York City municipal hospital [172]. When hospitalized for status asthmaticus, children have demonstrated a male predominance [102], and adults a strong female predominance (approximately 2:1) [172, 316, 319].

Although asthma has been recognized for at least a few thousand years [18], during the early 1900s it was commonly believed that acute asthma attacks rarely, if ever, caused death [258]. Several autopsy studies conducted in patients dying from asthma reported during the 1920s through 1950s [150, 151, 383] drew attention to the problem of asthma-related death and described the extensive mucus plugging that characterizes the pathology of asthma. Records of the U.S. National Center for Health Statistics show that the asthma death rate increased from 2.5 per 100,000 population in 1937 to 4.5 in 1951, perhaps related to increased reporting [360]. Subsequently, there was a steady decline in asthma death rates to 0.8 per 100,000 U.S. population in 1978, a period marked by improvements in the pharmacotherapy of asthma, particularly the advent of corticosteroids.

The steady decrease in asthma death rates seen in the United States contrasts with the experience in England, Wales, Australia, Ireland, New Zealand, and Norway, where increases in asthma mortality were observed between 1959 and 1966, affecting all age groups from 5 to 64 years, but especially the 5- to 34-year age group, in which the death rate tripled [18]. The rising death rate paralleled an increase in the use of pressurized aerosols containing isoproterenol, and these were postulated to be responsible for the "epidemic" of asthma-related deaths [158, 335, 336]. This theory has since been disputed by other investigators [107, 287], and as yet there is no satisfactory explanation for the increased mortality occurring during those years. A more recent increase in asthma mortality rates has been reported throughout much of the world, first becoming apparent in New Zealand [126, 162, 236], where between 1975 and 1979 the asthma mortality increased from 1.4 to 4.1 per 100,000 in the 5- to 34-year age group. Initially reports suggested that the use of oral theophylline in combination with high doses of inhaled salbutamol might have contributed to the occurrence of cardiotoxicity and increased rates of sudden death [389]. However, subsequent reports have cast doubt on this association [125, 160, 376]. This subject is further detailed in Chapter 90.

Between 1978 and 1979, asthma mortality increased from 0.8 to 1.2 per 100,000 in the United States, but this may have been related to the implementation in 1979 of the ninth revision of the International Classification of Disease [332]. However, the continued rise in the asthma death rates to 1.6 per 100,000 in 1985 could not be attributed to the reclassification [332]. The increase occurred throughout all age groups and regions of the United States, and occurred in both metropolitan and nonmetropolitan areas. Rates of death were higher among females and blacks, with rates increasing from 1.8 per 100,000 in 1979 to 2.6 per 100,000 in 1984 for black females [332]. Similar increases in asthma death rates have been reported from Australia, England and Wales, Canada, and Denmark. Death rates remain highest in New Zealand, although they have slowly been decreasing since 1980.

RISK FACTORS

The recent alarming increase in the asthma mortality rates in many countries remains unexplained, but has stimulated a number of studies into the risk factors for asthma-related deaths. Based on the findings from these studies, which have been mostly retrospective reviews of death certificates, a profile of the patient at risk for fatal or near-fatal asthma has emerged [30, 51, 141, 199, 286, 306, 317, 340, 346]. Some demographic factors place certain patients at higher risk, namely being in the adolescent or young adult age groups and of non-Caucasian ethnicity [317]. Patients at higher risk usually have a history of severe asthma,

Table 73-3. Risk factors for mortality in asthma

Demographic factors
    Adolescent or young adult
    Non-Caucasion
Historical factors
    Prior life-threatening attacks (prior intubation for asthma)
    Hospitalizations or emergency room visits (3 or more) within the past year
    Emergency room visits or hospitalizations in past month
    Use of 3 or more asthma drugs
    Airway lability (PEFR)
    Corticosteroid use (past/present)
    History of syncope/hypoxic seizures
    Coexisting severe lung disease
Psychosocial factors
    Poor compliance with medications; inability to use devices
    Denial
    Alcoholism
    Continued smoking
    Depression or other major psychiatric illness
    Procrastination in seeking medical care
Physician-related factors
    Failure to diagnose or appreciate severity of attack
    Underutilization of corticosteroids
    Failure to adequately follow up and monitor using objective measures
    Inappropriate use of sedatives or other drugs
    Failure to identify high-risk patient
    Failure to educate patient

PEFR = peak expiratory flow rate.

including prior life-threatening attacks, hospitalization, or emergency room visits within the previous year, and are taking three or more asthma drugs [286]. Airway lability, as determined by marked decreases in the PEFR in the early morning (morning dipping), also identifies patients at risk [142, 381]. Psychosocial factors are also important, including patient denial of the illness or difficulty in recognizing the severity of the disease and poor compliance with medications [224a, 317]. Patients at risk tend to have poor access to medical care and may have difficulties with self-care, emotional disturbances, alcoholism, smoking, depression, or other major psychiatric illnesses [317, 346, 347].

Patients at risk also commonly receive suboptimal care from practitioners, and this includes underutilization of corticosteroids, overreliance on bronchodilator therapy, lack of appreciation by the physician of the severity of the attack, and patient delay in seeking help or physician delay in administering care [332, 340]. These risk factors are summarized in Table 73-3.

Although 86 percent of the patients studied by the British Thoracic Association [30] died outside of the hospital, approximately 50 percent of the deaths in the United States occur in the emergency room or hospital [332]. Factors thought to contribute to in-hospital deaths include underutilization of therapy, especially corticosteroids, lack of frequent physiologic assessments such as spirometry or arterial blood gas analysis [51, 200, 256], and the use of intermittent positive-pressure breathing (IPPB) devices, resulting in pneumothorax [171, 172, 221].

Although patients at higher risk for fatal or near-fatal asthma can be identified, all patients with asthma should be considered at some risk for severe attacks. The British Thoracic Association [30] found that one-third of the patients dying with acute asthma were never previously hospitalized for asthma.

Pre–Status Asthmaticus

A prodromal period of pre–status asthmaticus exists (Table 73-4). This state should be identified because early recognition and intervention may abort the occurrence of overt status asthmat-

Table 73-4. Clues to impending status asthmaticus

History—change in pattern of symptoms
  Wheezing: more severe or frequent, particularly at night
  Worsening dyspnea: progressive exercise limitations, dyspnea at
    rest, orthopnea, or fatigue
  Cough with tenacious sputum: difficult to expectorate or a
    substantial decrease in daily volume; changes in sputum color
    from white to yellow, gray, or green (i.e., purulent)
  Refractoriness to drugs: increasing use with less relief from
    otherwise efficacious drugs; polypharmacy (use of ≥3 drugs)
  Constitutional: personality changes (irritability, confusion), anxiety,
    insomnia
  Large diurnal shifts in PEFR
Examination
  Anxiety, increased respiratory efforts, resting tachypnea
  Expiratory prolongation, onset of inspiratory wheeze
  Respiratory muscle fatigue
Laboratory Data
  Falling flow or volume indexes (FVC, FEV_1, $FEF_{25-75\%}$, PEFR) or
    reduction in FVC with rising FRC
  Limited response to bronchodilator (by spirometry)
  Progressive hypoxemia
  Hypocapnia (<35 mmHg)
  X-ray study: hyperinflation (or pneumonia or atelectasis)
  Eosinophils in blood or sputum: high values or a shift from chronic-
    state levels
  Leukocytosis; purulent sputum

PEFR = peak expiratory flow rate; FVC = forced vital capacity; FEV_1 = forced
expiratory volume in 1 second; $FEF_{25-75\%}$ = mean forced expiratory flow during the
middle half of the FVC; FRC = functional residual capacity.

icus. Perhaps the well-described British epidemic of asthmatic
deaths attributed by some to an unsupervised excessive usage
of concentrated aerosol isoproterenol exemplifies the extreme of
the pre-status problem; here, progressive symptoms presumably
led to more frequent use of a bronchodilator agent rather than
to the seeking of direct medical care.

It is important for the patient and the physician alike to be able
to recognize this period of evolving nonresponsiveness, for it is
easier and safer to abort an impending massive insult than to
treat it once it is maximal. In this regard, patient education and
the enlistment of the patient as a partner in therapy are essential.
Patients should be informed of the purpose of each of their drugs
and should be taught to recognize the features of emerging refractoriness. They should be instructed in the importance of continuing prescribed treatment during asymptomatic periods.

Patients likely to need intermittent oral corticosteroid therapy
may be provided with a reserve supply and instructions on when
and how to take a short course if immediate physician advice is
unavailable. All patients need to know how to obtain prompt
emergency assistance at any time, as delay in reaching medical
assistance can contribute to asthma deaths [30, 199].

At the same time, physicians should not underestimate the
potential for death in patients in status asthmaticus. Since no
single observation or group of observations provides absolute
and reliable prognostic features, all patients must be regarded
as having the potential for a serious episode or even mortality.
Table 73-5 summarizes selected features associated with a poor
prognosis in status asthmaticus.

Physiologic Abnormalities

The physiologic features of status asthmaticus include a spectrum of gas exchange defects associated with airways obstruction. This obstruction is widespread but unevenly distributed
throughout the lungs, and is caused by a variable combination
of factors, including intraluminal secretions, airway wall inflammation and edema, glandular hypertrophy, smooth muscle hy-

*Table 73-5. Features contributing to poor prognosis in status
asthmaticus*

Persisting refractoriness to all bronchodilators and all other
  supportive therapy
Use of inappropriate drugs or inappropriate dosages, or delay in
  initiating therapy
Greater duration of attack
A silent chest reflecting nonmobilization of secretions
Hypercapnia, respiratory ± lactic acidosis
Severe hypoxemia despite full therapy
Cardiac arrhythmias, hypotension
Abuse of sedatives or respiratory depressants
Underlying cardiopulmonary disease

pertrophy and spasm, and expiratory airway compression. Progressive airways obstruction is associated with hyperinflation,
increased work of breathing, and disordered gas exchange, which
in turn are responsible for many of the characteristic symptoms
and signs of status asthmaticus.

Airway Dynamics and Lung Volumes

During an acute asthma attack, the increase in bronchial smooth
muscle tone and other factors tend to close small airways at
higher-than-normal lung volumes. The increased lung volume
raises static transpulmonary pressure and increases outward radial traction on the airways, helping to maintain their patency
[270]. The more severe the asthmatic attack, the greater is the
tendency for airway closure to occur and the higher the lung
volume must be to keep the airways open. Tonic contraction of
inspiratory intercostal and accessory muscles throughout expiration has been shown to contribute to the increase in lung volume in asthma [207]. The diaphragm may also be actively involved in maintaining an increased lung volume, as observed
by Muller and associates [235] during experimental histamine-
induced hyperinflation.

The increased lung volume is manifested clinically and radiographically as hyperinflation of the chest. Functional residual
capacity (FRC) and residual volume (RV) are usually markedly
increased, in some instances by as much as 3 to 5 liters [392].
Total lung capacity (TLC) may be increased or normal [255, 392],
and vital capacity (VC) is usually substantially reduced. For example, Stănescu and Teculescu [342] found a mean VC of 67
percent of predicted (range, 38–99%) during status asthmaticus.
Serial changes in TLC can be used to monitor the course of the
asthmatic attack; even with a constant FEV_1 percent, a fall in
TLC indicates lysis of the obstruction [393]. The increase in RV
accounts for the observed decrease in VC.

The chest hyperinflation may lead to findings that resemble
those of pulmonary emphysema: a chest radiograph showing flat
diaphragms and apparently attenuated pulmonary vasculature
and a physical examination revealing use of accessory musculature (implying a temporary mechanical disadvantage of the diaphragm), low-lying diaphragms, hyperresonance, and a diminished intensity of breath sounds caused by the elevated air-tissue
ratio. However, destructive emphysema is not present, and these
findings are reversible. The chest hyperinflation also results in
positive intrathoracic pressure at the end of expiration, a phenomenon some authors refer to as *intrinsic* or *auto-positive end-
expiratory pressure* (auto-PEEP) [130].

Lung volume measured by the helium dilution method may
underestimate the true lung volume because of impaired ventilation of air spaces distal to severely obstructed airways. The plethysmographic method, on the other hand, measures the entire
thoracic gas volume, whether or not distal air spaces are in free
communication with the airways, but this method may yield spu-

riously increased values of TLC in some patients with severe airways obstruction because of incomplete transmission of alveolar pressure to the mouth [327, 343].

Expiratory airflow obstruction is consistently present. Rebuck and Read [290] found a mean FVC of 1.2 liters and FEV_1 of 0.54 liter among 35 patients hospitalized for the emergency treatment of asthma. A peak expiratory flow of 80 L/min or less has been shown to correlate with deaths in asthma [384]. The possible role of extrathoracic airway obstruction in some asthmatic patients has been investigated by Lisboa and associates [194].

Both large and small (<2 mm in diameter) airways [213] are involved in status asthmaticus. Although the major site of airflow resistance during status asthmaticus may reside in the intermediate or larger airways, small airways resistance also contributes because their large cross-sectional area may also be critically reduced by the presence of intraluminal secretions. These small airway secretions may also contribute to the drug refractoriness, because they impede the distribution of aerosol dilator drugs to peripheral airways. This subject is discussed in additional detail in Chapter 36.

Airflow patterns also contribute to increased airway resistance in advanced asthma. To meet the demands of basal gas exchange as well as those additionally imposed by fever, infection, stress, and the augmented work of the respiratory muscles, total ventilation must be increased. The concurrent increases in airflow through narrowed conduits lead to turbulent flow patterns. Energy losses from the resulting increased gas velocities, eddy currents, and gas vortices must be met by greater changes in alveolar pressure, thus placing greater demands on the respiratory muscles. Resistance to airflow over and through intraairway secretions is estimated to occur with viscid sputum and when secretional thickness exceeds 300 μm [49]. These flow patterns are more extreme in larger airways where turbulence is influenced by gas density. Further, transbronchial pressure gradients are now shifted, so that the peripheral airways are subject to expiratory airflow limitations earlier than they would be in normal subjects. Also, compression of the trachea and large bronchi may complicate the process when active expiration or cough elevates the intrathoracic pressure [72].

Pulmonary Circulation

In acute asthma, blood flow is reduced in poorly ventilated regions of the lung [226]. Ventilation-perfusion lung scans reveal focal areas of reduced perfusion corresponding to areas of abnormal ventilation [388]. The principal mechanism responsible for the redistribution of flow is probably hypoxic vasoconstriction, but an alteration in the intraalveolar pressure and other factors may also play a role. This vasoconstrictive response reduces the degree of hypoxemia that results from perfusion of hypoventilated lung zones. Reversal of this vasoconstriction by certain bronchodilator drugs such as isoproterenol [368, 388] may worsen arterial hypoxemia [131].

Pulmonary vascular resistance is increased by hypoxemia, acidemia, and the effect of increased transmural pressure on pulmonary capillaries at high lung volumes present in acute asthma. Although pulmonary arterial pressure, measured relative to atmospheric pressure, may be normal, the highly negative intrapleural pressure exposes the outer surface of the heart and pulmonary artery to pressures much lower than atmospheric [270, 341]. Hence, transmural pressures across the heart and pulmonary artery are increased and effectively induce a reversible pulmonary hypertension, as the right ventricle must generate more tension during systole. Permutt [270] reported that the average transmural pulmonary arterial pressure approximately doubled in five subjects during severe asthmatic attacks. The hemodynamic effects of the highly negative intrapleural pressure may be responsible for the reversible P pulmonale observed on the

electrocardiogram in severe asthma [109] and have been implicated as a cause of fluid accumulation in the lung in acute asthma [341].

Work of Breathing

The combination of hyperinflation and advanced airways obstruction in severe asthma markedly increases the work of breathing. The elastic work of breathing increases because the slope of the pressure-volume relationship of the thorax falls at high lung volumes [121], and because obstruction of some lung units results in overinflation of nonobstructed units, thereby decreasing dynamic lung compliance. Permutt [270] has pointed out that an increase in the FRC of 2.5 liters with a tidal volume of 500 ml increases the inspiratory work of breathing by 11-fold, even if there is no change in compliance or resistance. However, a reversible increase in compliance has been reported in some patients during acute asthma exacerbations in association with an increased TLC, but the mechanisms involved are unclear [393]. In addition, hyperinflation impairs the efficiency of the diaphragm. As lung volume increases acutely, the muscle fibers of the diaphragm shorten (reducing their force of contraction) and the radius of curvature of the diaphragm increases, thereby decreasing its ability to exert pressure for a given force of its fibers. The increased tidal ventilation at the high lung volume at which the asthmatic patient is forced to breath contributes to the sense of dyspnea during an acute asthmatic attack.

The flow-resistive component of the work of breathing also increases markedly in severe asthma, and expiratory muscle contraction adds further to the work of breathing. Intraluminal secretions impair airflow during inspiration as well as expiration. Clinicians are familiar with complaints of the inability to inspire or of inspiratory wheezing in status asthmaticus, features that can be explained by the inspiratory obstruction as well as by the increase in FRC, which intensifies elastic work. Thus, the inspiratory airways resistance may be almost as high as the expiratory resistance in patients with asthma, in contrast to patients with emphysema whose airflow limitation occurs primarily during expiration [380]. Mean airways resistance values as high as 25 to 56.5 cm H_2O/L/sec (normal, 1.4 to 4.0 cm H_2O/L/sec) have been reported in severe asthma, and the work of breathing has been estimated to be 5 to 25 times that of a normal adult at rest [380].

Breathing patterns may also affect respiratory work. Theoretically, slow deep breaths reduce turbulent airflow and thereby viscous resistance [135]. However, in cases of acute asthma, respiratory frequency is increased by mechanisms that are not yet clearly defined.

As ventilatory demands rise during an attack, oxygen consumption by the respiratory muscles also increases. At increased airway impedances, a given amount of ventilation will consume more oxygen than would occur in normal subjects. As an illustration, if the minute ventilation rises to 60 L/min, the oxygen consumption of the respiratory muscles during an asthma attack may rise to more than 100 to 200 ml/min, in contrast to only 20 ml/min in normal subjects. Besides this inefficiency of the oxygen cost of breathing, the total work may fall below that required to eliminate carbon dioxide, and hypercapnia will ensue. Noelpp and Noelpp-Eschenhagen [243, 244] demonstrated in animals with induced bronchospasm that the work of breathing against elastic resistance increased by 44-fold and the total work of breathing by 12.5-fold. Parallel findings in the context of human asthma for both overall elastic work and expiratory airflow resistances were observed by Attinger and associates [7].

Hence, many factors contribute to the increased work of breathing in asthma: the combined effects of marked increases in the elastic and flow-resistive components of the work of breathing, the decrease in dynamic lung compliance, the reduced efficiency of the respiratory muscles, and the need for active expiratory muscle work all produce a substantial increase in the oxygen requirements of the respiratory muscles, which can lead to respiratory muscle fatigue and eventual hypercapnic ventilatory failure. An increase in the endogenous opioid level during acute methacholine-induced bronchoconstriction may indicate a homeostatic mechanism that operates to minimize inspiratory muscle activity and hence reduce respiratory work and muscle fatigue [17]. The onset of respiratory muscle fatigue, heralded by extreme tachypnea, respiratory muscle incoordination, or paradoxical motion of the abdomen, is a dire development in status asthmaticus, often necessitating intubation and mechanical ventilation.

Gas Exchange

The uneven distribution of inspired gas, owing to marked variations in the time constants of different lung units, leads to gross disturbances in ventilation-perfusion ($\dot{V}/\dot{Q}$) ratios and resulting alterations in arterial blood gas values [351, 388]. The degree of arterial hypoxemia correlates roughly with the severity of airways obstruction and hence the population of low $\dot{V}/\dot{Q}$ units, indicating $\dot{V}A/\dot{Q}$ mismatch as the mechanism of arterial hypoxemia rather than shunt or diffusion limitation. For example, Flenley [100] observed that a PaO_2 of less than 60 mmHg was commonly associated with an FEV_1 of less than 0.5 liter, or less than 30 percent of predicted. In another study of 101 patients, the correlation between the mean FEV_1 and PaO_2 was as follows: mean FEV_1, 59, 35, and 18 percent of predicted; mean PaO_2, 83, 71, and 63 mmHg, respectively [214]. These relationships are further depicted in Figure 73-2A.

In addition, complete airways obstruction may arise from extensive secretions, leading to right-to-left anatomic shunting that may intensify the arterial hypoxemia induced by simple $\dot{V}/\dot{Q}$ mismatch. Shunting, with a $\dot{V}A/\dot{Q}$ ratio of 0, otherwise occurs only when severe airways obstruction develops in patients in status asthmaticus. Valabhji [362] found a mean PaO_2 of 66 mmHg during acute asthma that was attributable mainly to disturbed $\dot{V}/\dot{Q}$ relationships with only a small shunt fraction ($\dot{Q}S/\dot{Q}T$) of 3.7 percent. McFadden and Lyons [214] found an increased $\dot{Q}S/\dot{Q}T$ in only 4 of 30 asthma patients studied during an acute attack; two had hypercapnia and the other two had an FEV_1 less than 15 percent of predicted. Rodriguez-Roisin and coworkers [298] also found an increase in low $\dot{V}/\dot{Q}$ ratio units and no increase in the shunt component among eight ventilator-assisted patients with status asthmaticus.

Compensatory pulmonary vasoconstriction may reduce the impact of the shunt component by diverting blood flow from nonventilated lung zones. In some instances, zones of increased $\dot{V}/\dot{Q}$ ratios occur, resulting in an increase in the physiologic dead space, which can increase respiratory work. Finally, since there is no significant correlation between $\dot{V}A/\dot{Q}$ mismatch and airflow rates, it would seem that gas exchange is largely influenced by the dynamics of the peripheral airways, the effects of which are poorly reflected by usual measurements of airflow.

Diffusion limitations do not appear to contribute significantly to the occurrence of arterial hypoxemia. In fact, although the steady-state carbon monoxide diffusing capacity (D_LCO) has been reported to be reduced in asthma [251], the single-breath D_LCO may be increased, owing to a perfusional redistribution to the lung apices [379]. Arterial hypoxemia may be worsened by the administration of certain drugs such as beta agonists, which act to increase $\dot{V}/\dot{Q}$ inequality by means of an augmented perfusion of underventilated lung units [95, 131]. In severe asthma, including status asthmaticus, dangerous levels of arterial hypoxemia may develop with alarming rapidity, and without hypercapnia. Given the condition of a marginal PaO_2 level (e.g., 60 mmHg), a small critical decrease in airway flow could contribute

to this sudden hypoxemic phenomenon. Finally, at some point in the asthmatic process, overall or net alveolar ventilation may fall and hypoventilation will add its component to arterial hypoxemia.

In a mild asthmatic attack, the primary gas exchange defect is hypoxemia accompanied by hypocapnia, the latter reflecting the increased alveolar ventilation induced by hypoxia, anxiety, and other factors. With progressive airways obstruction, however, effective alveolar ventilation fails, and hypercapnia supervenes (Fig. 73-3). The relationship between FEV_1 and $PaCO_2$ is not linear (see Fig. 73-2B). In a study of acute exacerbations occurring in 101 asthmatics, hypercapnia was present in only 11 patients and was not observed until the FEV_1 fell below 20 percent of its predicted value [214]. Similarly, Nowak and coworkers [247] observed hypercapnia ($PaCO_2 > 42$ mmHg) in 18 of 102 episodes of acute asthma seen in an emergency department; in all hypercapnic patients, the initial FEV_1 was less than 1 liter and less than 25 percent of predicted, and the PEFR was less than 200 L/min. While the incidence of hypercapnia is low, prompt identification of the hypercapnic stage is critical because it is associated with a high mortality rate and because of the potential need for tracheal intubation and mechanical ventilation [261]. Respiratory acidosis develops in only a small number of patients but may be severe when it occurs. Among 101 adults with acute asthma, 7 had respiratory acidosis, 21 had a normal pH, and 73 had respiratory alkalosis [214]; a higher incidence of acidosis may exist in children [78, 330].

A non–anion gap metabolic acidosis caused by renal compensation for hyperventilation is quite common in asthma attacks. Lactic acidosis may be seen in severe asthma [4, 299]; in a series of 12 patients with severe asthma and metabolic acidosis, the plasma lactate concentrations ranged from 2.9 to 9.4 mmol/L [4]. In another series, metabolic acidosis that was thought to be caused by lactate accumulation (average anion gap, 15.8 mEq/L) was found in 28 percent of 229 consecutive episodes of acute asthma [233]. Believed to result from a combination of lactate overproduction by the respiratory muscles and lactate underutilization resulting from hypoperfusion of the liver and skeletal muscles, lactic acidosis reflects severe airways obstruction and possibly impending respiratory failure.

No single pattern of PaO_2, $PaCO_2$, and pH changes is characteristic of status asthmaticus; rather, evolving stages of severity can be arbitrarily categorized (Table 73-6). The use of arterial blood gas and pH profiles, especially with serial observations, is imperative in the management of status asthmaticus, since the severity of the gas exchange and acid-base disturbances cannot be reliably judged on the basis of clinical and spirometric data alone.

Stage I, the mildest stage of gas exchange disturbance, is characterized by hypoxemia with mild hypocapnia and respiratory alkalosis. Here $\dot{V}/\dot{Q}$ disturbances are insufficient to produce ventilatory failure, and respiratory work remains effective in eliminating carbon dioxide. Supplementary oxygen and a sound therapeutic program will often suffice to manage such patients. In Stage II, which reflects a greater severity of airways obstruction, advanced hypoxemia with augmented hyperventilation is observed; these patients are typically rather tachypneic and dyspneic and have frank respiratory distress. When given proper bronchodilator therapy and supportive measures, many of these patients will respond. Disturbingly, other patients in this stage remain refractory to therapy and progress to graver stages of gas exchange impairment in association with pharmacologic refractoriness.

The next phase, Stage III, is a critical point in the evolution of airways obstruction and refractoriness and is a useful index of progressive respiratory impairment, potentially heralding frank ventilatory failure and respiratory acidosis. The salient feature in this stage is the paradoxically "normal" range of values for $PaCO_2$ and pH despite the obvious continued clinical severity of

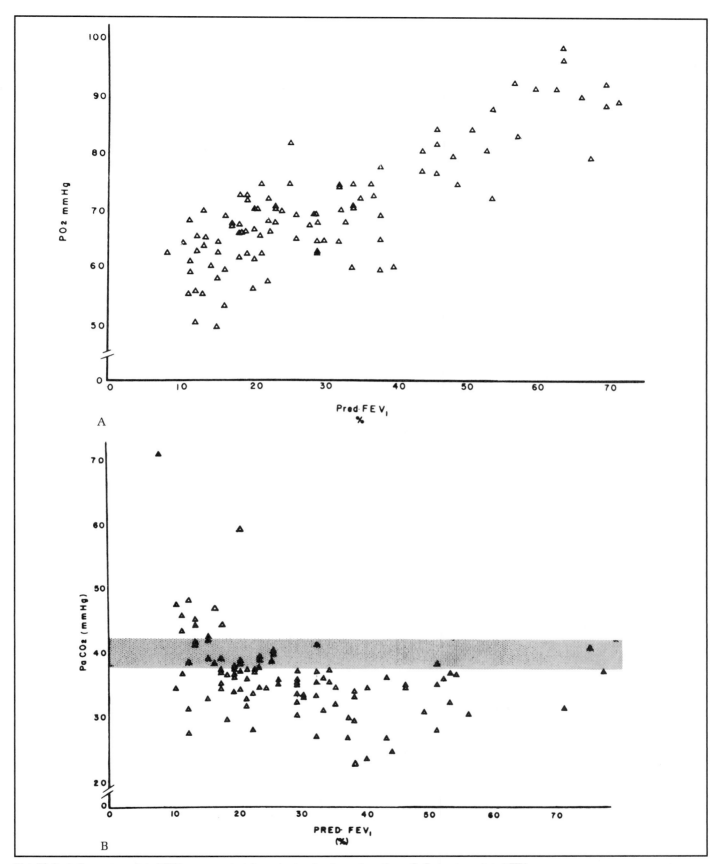

Fig. 73-2. A. Percent predicted FEV₁ versus arterial oxygen tension in acute asthma. B. Percent predicted FEV₁ versus arterial carbon dioxide tension in acute asthma. The normal range of PaCO₂ is shown by the shaded area. (Reprinted with permission from E. R. McFadden, Jr., and H. A. Lyons, Arterial-blood gas tension in asthma. N. Engl. J. Med. 278:1027, 1968.)

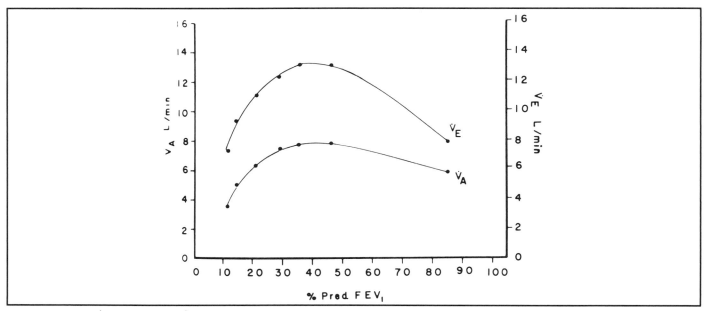

Fig. 73-3. *Minute ($\dot{V}_E$) and alveolar ($\dot{V}_A$) ventilation versus percent predicted FEV_1 in acute asthma. (Reprinted with permission from E. R. McFadden, Jr., and H. A. Lyons, Arterial-blood gas tension in asthma. N. Engl. J. Med. 278:1027, 1968.)*

Table 73-6. Arterial blood gas and pH in asthma[a]

Stage		PaO_2 (mmHg)	$PaCO_2$ (mmHg)	pH	FEV_1 (L)	Dyspnea
I	Mild attack or chronic stable	Normal or mild ↓, 65–80	35–42	7.40	>2.0	+
II	Mild-moderate attack	55–65	<35	>7.45	~1–2	+ +
III	Cross-over	45–55 (or normal[b])	≅40	≅7.40	≤1	+ + +
IV	Severe	<45 (or normal[b])	>45	<7.35	<1	+ + + +

[a] Schema of general range values only.
[b] On therapeutic oxygen.
+ = minimal; + + + + = severe.

the episode. This normalization of $PaCO_2$ and pH reflects progressive failure of effective alveolar ventilation and is, in fact, a state of relative hypoventilation. This is the "cross-over" phase [378] (Fig. 73-4). This phase is stressed to alert physicians to the possible transition from a hyperventilation state seen in Stages I and II to the ensuing phase (Stage IV) of hypoventilation. Since Stage IV, with its overt hypoventilation and respiratory acidosis, is critical in terms of morbidity and mortality and can develop with alarming rapidity from a state of eucapnia, the cross-over phase becomes one of major clinical concern. This stage warrants appropriate clinical and serial blood gas observations as well as the modification and/or intensification, if possible, of all therapeutic modalities. The observations of Mountain and Sahn [232] that essentially no patient with normocapnic, acute, severe asthma progressed to hypercapnia in their series may reflect the beneficial effects of early and appropriate medical therapy, as all their patients were "treated immediately upon presentation by the admitting physician." In this series, patients presenting with hypercapnia on admission presumably evolved through a normocapnic stage without the benefit of timely and appropriate therapeutic intervention.

Patients in Stage IV suffering from advanced hypoxemia, hypercapnia, and respiratory acidosis may well exhibit limited responses to bronchodilator drugs and other supportive measures. While some patients presenting in Stage IV may be successfully managed conservatively, as dictated by the individual clinical circumstances, others will require mechanical ventilatory support if they are exhausted, obtunded, and/or have critical PaO_2, $PaCO_2$, or pH values. Unwarranted causes of hypoventilation, such as sedative use, have no place in managing patients with acute, severe asthma.

CLINICAL CONSIDERATIONS

The onset of status asthmaticus in some patients can be very rapid, and occasionally dramatic, with a terribly oppressive air hunger; in other patients, this evolution may take several days or longer. The salient clinical features include significant dyspnea, wheezing, and cough. These findings follow a variety of incitant causes, as discussed previously, including allergic provocation, infection, nonspecific inhalant-irritant exposure, trigger mechanisms, and drug sensitivity; inappropriate therapy or inappropriate drug schedules will further potentiate the process. The intensity of wheezing is a poor indicator of the actual level of ventilation in severe asthma; extensive peripheral airway plugging may remain undetected until alveolar ventilation is severely limited. Inspiratory wheezing reflects a more advanced obstructive process. A relatively silent chest on auscultation with inability to raise secretions is an ominous finding, suggesting possible widespread inspissation of secretions with bronchial plugging. The significance of wheezing is detailed in Chapter 51.

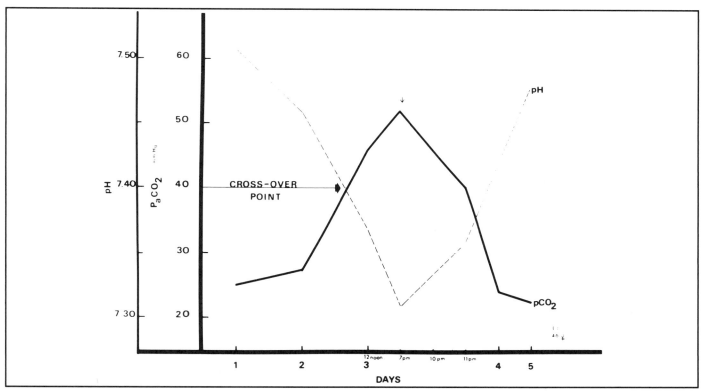

Fig. 73-4. *An example of cross-over Stage III PaCO$_2$ and pH in a 46-year-old woman in status asthmaticus. Note initial hypocapnia and respiratory alkalosis progressing to normal PaCO$_2$-pH relationships as a prelude to frank respiratory acidosis despite full medical therapy. PaO$_2$ on supplemental oxygen at the cross-over point was 80 mmHg. The vertical arrow indicates institution of intubation and ventilatory support. The patient fully recovered. Note the rapid development of acidosis; it can occur in an hour. (Reprinted with permission from E. B. Weiss, and L. J. Faling, Clinical significance of PaCO$_2$ during status asthma: The cross-over point. Ann. Allergy 26:545, 1968.)*

Sputum is rarely copious at the outset, a paucity reflecting its inspissation and adherence to mucosal surfaces. A commonly used clinical guideline suggests that most attacks will not remit until adequate secretion mobilization occurs, although this does not apply to those patients with pure bronchospasm who may respond rapidly to bronchodilator drugs.

Anxiety, tachypnea, tachycardia, monosyllabic speech, diaphoresis, nasal flaring, and accessory muscle use with sternocleidomastoid contraction and intercostal muscle retractions are typical findings in cases of severe asthma. Brenner and colleagues [29] observed that patients who assumed the upright position in bed upon admission generally had more severe asthma attacks, as measured by objective criteria, than did those who assumed a recumbent position; the combination of the upright position and profuse diaphoresis was present in patients with the most severe attacks. Disturbances of consciousness, systemic hypertension, cardiac arrhythmias, and cyanosis are occasionally present. A pulse rate of greater than 130/min may indicate hypoxemia with a PaO$_2$ ranging to less than 40 mmHg, or it may relate to catecholamine response or arise from the use of adrenergic drugs or a combination of factors [291].

The presence of pulsus paradoxus, typically greater than 15 mmHg during severe acute asthma, has been shown to reflect lung hyperinflation, combined with wide fluctuations in intrathoracic pressure that impede pulmonary venous return and decrease left ventricular ejection [339]. It is regarded as a valuable clinical sign, indicating the severity of the obstructive process in asthma [115, 179, 289, 290]. Of 76 patients hospitalized with asthma, Rebuck and Read [290] found a paradox of 10 mmHg or more in 34, all of whom had an FEV$_1$ of 1.25 liters or less. Signifi-

cant paradox was found in all patients with a FEV$_1$ of less than 20 percent of their best FEV$_1$; this often disappeared within hours of starting treatment. In contrast, Shim and Williams [322] observed that pulsus paradoxus was often present with only mild obstruction and often absent in severe obstruction, and they concluded that pulsus paradoxus is an unreliable guide to the severity of obstruction in asthma.

Evaluation of the patient with an acute asthmatic attack requires an assessment of the severity of the attack and of the response to initial therapeutic measures. Unfortunately, symptoms and physical findings correlate poorly with the degree of airflow obstruction, the severity of the gas exchange disturbance, and the responsiveness to initial therapy [176, 212, 290]. The asthmatic patient's self-assessment may be more accurate than the physician's examination in estimating the degree of airways obstruction present [325], but asthmatics vary widely in the degree of functional impairment necessary to elicit symptoms, often tolerating increases of more than 50 percent in RV and airways resistance before experiencing symptoms [304, 305]. In addition, there is considerable variation among physicians in detecting the physical signs of airways obstruction [116]. One study found that the intensity, pitch, and timing of wheezing had a general relationship to the severity of airways obstruction but were not sufficiently reliable to substitute for the measurement of PEFR [326]. Of interest, a recent evaluation compared the diagnostic and therapeutic practice pattern of three Boston teaching hospitals and found considerable variability in the diagnostic evaluation but little variability in the treatment approach to acute asthma [69].

Rebuck and Read [290] found a considerable overlap in FEV$_1$

and VC values among three groups of hospitalized asthmatic patients who were divided on the basis of clinical assessment of severity. McFadden and associates [212] compared the symptoms and physical findings with lung mechanics in patients with acute asthma and found that sternocleidomastoid retraction correlated well with the degree of mechanical impairment, but dyspnea and wheezing did not; when all symptoms and signs had disappeared, marked abnormalities in the FEV_1, FRC, and RV persisted. In another study [176], pulsus paradoxus and sternocleidomastoid contraction were the only physical examination variables that reflected the degree of obstruction present, but even in the presence of severe obstruction ($FEV_1 < 1$ liter), the absence of these signs was the rule.

Clinical circumstances or failure to respond to therapy may suggest other disorders that can mimic acute status asthmaticus; these include acute bronchiolitis (infective, chemical, inhalational), croup, pulmonary embolism (rare), advanced upper airways obstruction (e.g., tumor), angioedema, pulmonary aspiration, and cystic fibrosis (children). A sweat test or quantitative immunoglobulin assay may be indicated if cystic fibrosis or immune deficiency is suspected. Monophonic wheezing arising from a local obstructive process should not be confused with diffuse asthmatic airways wheezing. In the case of a monophonic sound, the intensity of the wheeze clearly diminishes with increasing distance from the site of its generation. Auscultation over the trachea often reveals localized stridor with upper airway obstruction.

The presence of basilar rales, cardiac left ventricular S_3 gallop, or elevated central venous pressure with diffuse wheezing are signs of cardiac failure, although wheezing can at times be the only presenting sign of cardiac decompensation. If severe hypoxemia and hypercapnia supervene, papilledema, neuromuscular abnormalities (asterixis, irritability), confusion, agitation, cardiac arrhythmias, hypotension or shock may ensue and add their respective findings; some patients may present with syncope or be frankly obtunded. These problems require proper clarification.

LABORATORY PROCEDURES

Radiography

The principal value of the chest radiograph is to identify specific coexisting conditions or complications of status asthmaticus, such as pneumonia, pneumothorax, pneumomediastinum [71], atelectasis, or mucoid impaction (see also Chap. 53). Marked hyperinflation is commonly present [96, 272, 288], but, in uncomplicated asthma, the hyperinflation is reversible and the symmetrical pulmonary vascular pattern is preserved, in contrast to the findings in destructive emphysema. Transient opacities may be caused by mucus plugs with or without *Aspergillus* or by foci of pneumonia. Pneumomediastinum, more easily detected on a lateral film [288], is more commonly observed in asthmatic children than in adults [85]. The radiographic identification of pneumomediastinum and pneumothorax, both of which may be undetected by clinical examination, has important therapeutic implications, especially if the use of positive-pressure ventilation is contemplated. The finding of a foreign body or hiatal hernia has obvious clinical implications.

Recent studies conducted in children and adults have suggested that chest radiography is not routinely indicated in the emergency room evaluation of asthma [111, 397]. However, the application of these conclusions to patients with status asthmaticus would be unjustified [112]. Eggleston and colleagues [85] noted infiltrates or pneumomediastinum on admission chest radiographs in 23 percent of 479 children hospitalized with severe asthma. Petheram and coworkers [272] detected clinically unsuspected pulmonary consolidation or collapse on admission radiographs in 9 of 117 adults with acute, severe asthma. A recent prospective study indicated that there were major radiographic abnormalities encountered in 34 percent of the admissions for acute asthma in adults and these findings influenced management decisions [382]. This prompted the authors to recommend chest x-ray studies for all adults admitted to the hospital because of acute asthma. Whenever there is clinical concern that an inciting or complicating process (e.g., pneumonia, pneumothorax, congestive heart failure) might be present, a chest radiograph may be of considerable practical value in determining the approach to management and is recommended.

Electrocardiography

Sinus tachycardia, the most common rhythm disturbance in severe asthma, is influenced both by the pathophysiology of the disease, especially coexistent hypoxemia and acidosis, and by chronotropic drug administration. Elevated plasma levels of norepinephrine found in acute, severe asthma may also be contributory [156].

Other electrocardiographic findings in one series included, in descending order of frequency: right axis deviation, clockwise rotation, right ventricular dominance (R V_1, S V_5 pattern), P pulmonale, ST-T abnormalities, right bundle-branch block, and ventricular ectopic beats [290]. These changes reflect not only the presence of hypoxemia, pH shifts, and pulmonary hypertension but perhaps also mechanical factors, such as impairment of cardiac output and cardiac compression owing to increased intrathoracic pressure. Many of the electrocardiographic changes have been observed to disappear within hours after the initiation of effective asthma therapy [290], but return of the electrocardiogram to normal may be delayed for up to 9 days [329].

P pulmonale (P-wave amplitude ≥ 2.5 mV in leads II, III, or AVF, axis $+ 79 \pm 8$ degrees) was found in 49 percent of patients with a $PaCO_2$ of 45 mmHg or more and arterial blood pH of 7.37 or less during a severe asthma attack and in only 2.5 percent of asthmatics without hypercapnia and acidosis [109]. P pulmonale persisted for 12 to 60 hours after correction of the hypoxemia, hypercapnia, and acidosis and is presumed to result from increased transmural right atrial pressure, which in turn is a reflection of the severity of obstruction in the asthmatic attack [109]. In older patients, the stress of hypoxia during status asthmaticus may provoke cardiac ischemia, multifocal atrial and other serious arrhythmias, or myocardial infarction. (See also Chapter 78.)

Eosinophilia

Eosinophilia may be present in both extrinsic and intrinsic asthma; in adults with intrinsic asthma, the degree of eosinophilia has been reported to correlate with the severity of airway obstruction [149]. The total eosinophil count (TEC), a more accurate index than the percentage of eosinophils in the differential leukocyte count, is less than about 250 cells/mm³ in normal populations and ranges from normal values to 2,000 cells/mm³ or more in allergic asthmatic exacerbations [196]. The TEC may be reduced in acute infections and in patients treated with corticosteroids, epinephrine, isoproterenol, or aminophylline [252]. Corticosteroid-induced eosinopenia (<100 cells/mm³) can be a useful index of steroid efficacy in the treatment of asthmatic airways obstructive processes and assist in evaluating the adequacy of steroid dosage. Steroid-resistant asthmatics with accelerated plasma cortisol clearances tend to have higher TECs and require higher corticosteroid doses to achieve eosinopenia and clinical remission; in one series, the TEC fell 77 percent in steroid-responsive asthmatics but only 36 percent in steroid-resistant patients 4 hours after 40 mg of cortisol had been given intravenously [314].

Sputum eosinophils or Charcot-Leyden crystals have also generally been considered clinically useful in diagnosing allergic asthma. A recent study showed a correlation between sputum eosinophilia and the severity of airflow obstruction [2]. Another careful investigation concluded that (1) blood eosinophilia is not a necessary feature of noninfectious asthmatic exacerbations, (2) the numbers of eosinophils in blood and sputum do reflect the response of such an acute noninfectious exacerbation to corticosteroid therapy, and (3) clinically effective doses of corticosteroids may not necessarily clear eosinophils from the sputum [10]. Finally, in the presence of infection, leukocytosis or immature band shift may occur; dehydration, intercurrent steroid use, or metabolic stress may influence this response.

Chemistry

Electrolyte disturbances may complicate acute, severe asthma. Hypokalemia commonly occurs, and is related to intracellular potassium shifts associated with acute respiratory alkalosis and inhaled or parenteral beta-agonist administration [33]. Hyperkalemia may accompany severe metabolic acidosis. Hypophosphatemia (<0.8 mmol/L) has been reported in 12 of 22 [26] and 11 of 18 [185] patients with acute asthma presenting to an emergency room; severe hypophosphatemia (<0.3 mmol/L) was observed in 3 of the 18 patients in the latter study. Hypophosphatemia is also thought to be related to acid-base shifts and drug administration. It resolves spontaneously as the asthma responds to treatment, and its clinical significance is somewhat unclear. However, severe hypophosphatemia has been implicated as a cause of diaphragm weakness and hence may contribute to respiratory failure or ventilator weaning problems. (See Chapter 91 for further discussion.)

Elevated SGOT, SGPT, and ornithine carbamyltransferase levels during severe asthmatic exacerbations are believed to reflect hypoxic liver injury [52]. Increased activities of lactate dehydrogenase isoenzymes LDH-3, LDH-4, and LDH-5 have been noted in the serum of patients during moderate to severe asthmatic attacks and suggest that both the lung and liver contribute to the increased total LDH activity; neither the total LDH activity nor the isoenzyme pattern correlates with the severity of the attack, however [361]. Serum creatine phosphokinase (CPK) elevations, derived entirely from the skeletal muscle isoenzyme, have been found in asthmatics; levels correlate with the severity of symptoms and of airways obstruction and probably reflect increased respiratory muscle activity [34]. Rhabdomyolysis with acute renal failure was reported in a patient in status asthmaticus; vigorous respiratory muscle contraction, hypoxia, and dehydration were considered responsible [47]. Inhaled or parenteral administration of beta$_2$ agonists induced glycogenolysis that may be responsible for a small and temporary rise in the blood glucose level [33].

High plasma levels of antidiuretic hormone (ADH) may be found in patients with status asthma; the levels decrease toward normal with clinical and spirometric improvement [11]. Factors known to influence ADH secretion that may be operative in status asthmaticus include hypovolemia, decreased left atrial filling pressure, stress, and beta-adrenergic stimulation. Hypotonic fluid therapy in asthmatics with elevated plasma ADH levels can contribute to hyponatremia, water intoxication, and coma. Hyponatremia and an elevated urine-plasma osmolality ratio were noted in 5 of 25 children with acute asthma [143].

Sputum

Sputum examination in status asthmaticus can provide useful clues to the endobronchial pathology and even the inciting events (see also Chap. 52). Initial sputum volumes may be scant, presumably because of widespread inspissation and the entrap-

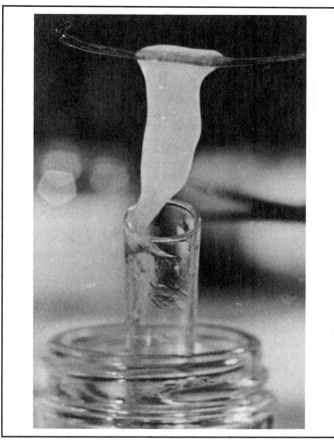

Fig. 73-5. *Mucoid sputum exhibits adhesiveness to the test tube and increased viscosity manifested by the tendency to remain as a bolus. The reader is advised to envision this sputum in the airways. (Reprinted with permission from E. B. Weiss et al., Acute respiratory failure in chronic obstructive pulmonary disease: II. Treatment.* Disease-A-Month, *p. 9, November 1969, H. F. Dowling et al. [eds.]; copyright © 1969 by Mosby–Year Book Medical Publishers, Inc., Chicago.)*

ment of thick tenacious secretions rather than because of hyposecretion. Later in an attack, or with treatment, such sputum becomes thinner and more copious, often containing cylindrical mucus plugs or bronchial casts. On gross examination, the sputum may be mucoid, purulent, or a mixture of both. Mucoid sputum is white, gelatinous, and tenaciously adherent to mucosal surfaces (or sputum containers) (Fig. 73-5), making it difficult to expectorate. Purulent sputum may be tinctured yellow, gray, or green and is often thick and voluminous. Curschmann's spirals are thin, twisted bronchiolar casts composed of mucinous material surrounding a central thread and containing entrapped cells and cellular debris. They may be visible macroscopically or, more often, microscopically and, while not unique to asthma, are frequently present in sputum during or after the asthma attack.

Gram's staining is important for the initial detection and tentative identification of bacteria, pending the results of sputum culture. Golden brown mucus plugs containing mycelia or *Aspergillus* are characteristic of allergic bronchopulmonary aspergillosis which may be seen in adult asthmatics.

Cytologic examination of the sputum simply with an unstained wet preparation can reveal evidence of the damage in the airways mucosa and the response of inflammatory cells; such changes may be useful in establishing the diagnosis and planning therapy (see prior discussion of eosinophils). For example, a predominantly eosinophilic response in sputum may indicate an allergic exacerbation, while a prevalence of polymorphonuclear leukocytes suggests irritative or infectious factors. Individual exfoliated bronchial epithelial cells are easily recognized by their elongated columnar shape, basal nucleus, tapering tail, and ciliated surface. The Creola body, a cluster of such columnar bronchial epithelial cells with intact cilia, implies severe asthma, as intense submucosal edema is presumably required for this cellular dehiscence from the basement membrane. Naylor [237] found Creola bodies in 45 percent of sputum specimens obtained from patients during attacks of asthma and in only 3 percent of specimens from nonasthmatics. The presence of macrophages in sputum is thought to reflect a cellular defense response.

Sputum eosinophilia may be characteristic but not diagnostic of status asthmaticus; occasionally the number of eosinophils is sufficient to give the sputum a purulent appearance. Corticosteroid-treated asthmatics have a lower proportion of sputum eosinophils than do asthmatics not on steroids, and sputum eosinophilia may decrease with steroid therapy [10, 45]. The release of cytoplasmic contents from degenerating eosinophils gives rise to elongated octahedral Charcot-Leyden crystals, which may be found in large numbers in asthmatic sputum. The principal proteinaceous constituent of the eosinophil granule, eosinophil major basic protein (MBP), has been shown to cause exfoliation and cytotoxic damage to human bronchial epithelium [104]. Markedly elevated sputum levels of MBP are found in asthma in contrast to other respiratory diseases; the levels decline with effective treatment and clinical improvement [104] (see also Chaps. 20 and 52).

THERAPY

Once as thorough a clinical and laboratory evaluation of the patient with status asthmaticus as is feasible has been performed and the severity of the gas exchange abnormalities determined, therapy should be instituted without delay. The goal of therapy is to support the patient with whatever measures are necessary while the responsible pathophysiologic processes are reversed.

Most patients respond to conservative but intensive regimens of drug therapy and oxygen, and to measures that aid in the removal of bronchial secretions. Others, particularly those with Stage IV gas exchange abnormalities, may require tracheal intubation and mechanical ventilation.

The severity of the asthma episode on admission does not necessarily reflect the subsequent resolution rate [164]. Delayed recovery may be anticipated under the following conditions: age over 40 years, nonatopic asthma, duration of attack before admission of more than 7 days, poor long-term asthma control, use of maintenance corticosteroids, a PaO_2 of less than 80 mmHg (room air) 48 hours after admission, and failure of PEFR to increase by at least 40 L/min after 6 hours of intensive therapy [19, 164]. During the course of treatment, the adequacy of the patient's response to the therapeutic program should be determined by frequent clinical and laboratory assessments, including arterial blood gases and pH, as indicated. Because status asthmaticus is a life-threatening disease and the clinical deterioration can be precipitous, aggressive management is best conducted in an intensive care unit with continuous cardiopulmonary monitoring and attentive medical and nursing observation around the clock.

Oxygen

The marked gas exchange disturbances resulting from impaired $\dot{V}/\dot{Q}$ relationships, right-to-left intrapulmonary shunting, and alveolar hypoventilation, if present, make hypoxemia a universal finding in severe asthma. The contribution by beta-agonists to hyperoxemia and the mechanism of this effect is detailed in Chapter 55. Extreme hypoxia induces a variety of adverse sequelae,

including pulmonary hypertension and impairment of myocardial, cerebral, and other vital organ functions, and has been implicated in sudden deaths in asthma. *Thus, a PaO_2 sufficient to provide adequate tissue oxygenation must be maintained continuously from the outset in all patients.*

It should be stressed, however, that the PaO_2 does not in itself provide a direct assessment of the adequacy of tissue oxygenation. The blood hemoglobin concentration and its oxygen affinity, cardiac output, and tissue perfusion significantly influence oxygen delivery. The clinical evaluation of individual organs (e.g., brain, heart, kidneys) may afford some indication of the adequacy of their oxygenation, provided consideration is given to other toxic, metabolic, inflammatory, and infectious factors. Elevation of the blood lactate concentration may be utilized as an index of tissue hypoxia, but its value may be limited by its late occurrence.

Despite certain limitations, the mixed venous oxygen tension ($P\bar{v}O_2$) or saturation ($S\bar{v}O_2$) is commonly employed to assess overall tissue oxygenation. Although a very low $S\bar{v}O_2$ probably reflects impaired tissue oxygenation, a normal value does not assure that vital organs are being adequately oxygenated [169]. Hence, a constellation of clinical and laboratory findings, in addition to PaO_2, should be employed to assess the effectiveness of tissue oxygenation in status asthmaticus. Provided that red blood cell mass, oxyhemoglobin affinity (P_{50}), cardiac output, and tissue perfusion are sufficient to meet tissue demands, a PaO_2 of 80 to 100 mmHg provides a margin of safety to protect against the potentially adverse hypoxic effects resulting from suctioning and bronchodilator drugs [108]. In many instances, this level is achieved easily with inspired oxygen concentrations of 30 to 50 percent, delivered by face mask or mechanical ventilator; low-concentration (24% or 28%) face masks are not generally adequate. Since oxygen sources are absolutely dry, supplemental humidification should be provided to minimize bronchial irritation and secretional desiccation. Higher oxygen concentrations are needed in the presence of large right-to-left shunts, as may occur with extensive airways secretions or atelectasis. The proper use of therapeutic oxygen requires longitudinal observations of blood oxygenation status with continuous pulse oximetry and periodic direct arterial analysis as indicated; this need is not supplanted by spirometry or clinical observations.

Oxygen-induced suppression of ventilatory drive is seldom encountered in acute asthma [214, 362], since carbon dioxide retention generally reflects the severity of airflow obstruction and respiratory muscle fatigue (see Chapter 27 for added insight into this discussion). However, caution should be exercised in administering oxygen to patients with mixed disorders who exhibit chronic hypercapnia, coexisting metabolic alkalosis, or inappropriate sedative use. In such cases, low-flow oxygen delivery by nasal cannula or controlled delivery by Venturi mask may alleviate arterial hypoxemia without marked increases in the $PaCO_2$. Inability to provide or maintain adequate oxygenation because of ventilatory suppression is an indication for mechanical ventilation.

Inhalation of low-density mixtures of helium and oxygen has been employed in the treatment of status asthmaticus in an attempt to decrease airflow resistance and thereby increase flow rates and reduce the work of breathing. These advantages, however, depend on the site of obstruction within the airways, which is variable in asthma [73]. Thus, the efficacy and practicability of helium use in status asthmaticus remain to be fully delineated, and use is generally reserved for mechanically ventilated patients who fail to respond to conventional ventilatory modes.

Bronchodilator Agents

Bronchodilator drugs are fundamental in the management of status asthmaticus and should be administered at once. Their primary effect is upon a labile or reversible bronchial smooth muscle contraction, with presumably lesser actions on the inflammatory processes and secretions, which are more fixed and slower to resolve. The relative contribution of these inflammatory and secretory elements varies from case to case, a difference that should be appreciated in evaluating therapeutic effectiveness [167]. Although experimental evidence indicates that both methylxanthines and beta-adrenergics are capable of enhancing mucociliary clearance [101, 348, 369], the clinical significance of this effect is currently unclear. In addition, aminophylline has been shown to improve the contractility of the diaphragm and to render it less susceptible to fatigue, actions that may contribute to its therapeutic efficacy [8].

The evaluation of bronchodilator response in status asthmaticus includes assessments of clinical improvement and changes in spirometry, PEFR, arterial blood gases, and pH. By definition, immediate favorable responses are precluded and drug effectiveness is determined over time by serial observations. *Hence, bronchodilator drugs must be properly prescribed with established effective dosage schedules and the patient observed throughout for both beneficial and adverse effects.*

Theoretical considerations and in vitro studies [190, 349] suggest that methylxanthines and beta agonists may act synergistically on bronchial smooth muscle; however, most clinical studies of such combined therapy have failed to demonstrate synergy either in stable [132, 324, 390] or acute [88, 90, 168, 302] asthma. Indeed, several studies have shown no significant difference in expiratory flow rates between patients who received combined therapy and those treated with a beta-adrenergic agent alone [92, 132, 168, 324, 328]. The latter findings seem to indicate that in many asthmatics the bronchodilating effect of a potent beta-adrenergic agonist is sufficiently great that little additional benefit is derived from the addition of a methylxanthine [92]. However, because these studies focused on the acute therapy of asthma and none was limited to patients with status asthmaticus, the same considerations may not apply to such patients, especially in the presence of severe airway obstruction and refractoriness to beta-agonist therapy. Thus, until carefully controlled studies are available that either confirm or refute the efficacy of the combination of beta agonists and theophyllines in the inpatient management of status asthmaticus, their combined use will continue to be recommended.

Sympathomimetic Drugs

Adrenergic bronchodilator agents are considered to be the primary drugs for both the emergency treatment of acute asthma as well as the subsequent and continuous treatment of status asthmaticus. The obvious goal is to rapidly alleviate airway obstruction and coexistent symptoms as much as feasible; concurrent supplemental oxygen and other supportive means presumably permit time for corticosteroid antiinflammatory actions and endogenous processes to lyse the episode. Rossing and associates [301] demonstrated that, when used as single agents, sympathomimetics raised the FEV_1 by 80 to 90 percent during the first hour of treatment in acute asthma, compared to only 25 percent for aminophylline therapy. A variety of beta-adrenergic drugs and routes of administration are available, and the optimal choice for both the drug and route of administration remains controversial. Although the ease of administration, rapidity of onset, and likelihood of adverse side effects may differ depending on the specific choices made, it is clear that safe, adequate therapy can be achieved using a variety of methods. The choice of a specific treatment depends partly on the characteristics of the patient; for example, parenteral sympathomimetics should be avoided in patients with ischemic cardiac disease. The effective delivery of a proper dose of the selected drug at an appropriate frequency of administration is probably more important than the specific choice of drug.

The subcutaneous route has long been used for the acute administration of beta-adrenergic drugs, although recent studies suggest that this route is usually no more efficacious than the inhaled route and may engender a greater risk of adverse side effects [245]. Subcutaneous delivery has the advantages of ease of administration, rapid onset, and lack of dependence on breathing pattern or patient cooperation. It remains an acceptable route of administration for the emergency treatment of asthma, particularly in children and young adults. Subcutaneous epinephrine (aqueous, 1:1,000) in doses of 0.3 ml (0.1 mg/kg in children) or terbutaline in doses of 0.25 to 0.5 mg may be administered every 20 minutes for three doses unless excessive tachycardia or tremulousness occurs [277]. If there is no response to epinephrine, it should be discontinued. Epinephrine has potent alpha, beta$_1$, and beta$_2$ effects and, in the presence of beta-adrenergic receptor blockade, its alpha-adrenergic effect could theoretically intensify bronchospasm. Although recent studies suggest that it may not be as risky in older patients as previously believed [65], in general, subcutaneous epinephrine should not be employed in the elderly and in patients with hypertension, cardiovascular disease, or marked tachycardia. Terbutaline is generally considered a more selective beta$_2$ agonist than epinephrine, but, when administered subcutaneously, it has similar efficacy and a similar risk of adverse side effects [337]. Pang and associates [262] obtained a good clinical response to subcutaneous terbutaline in 9 of 10 children in status asthmaticus who were refractory to subcutaneous epinephrine and intravenous aminophylline. In another study of subcutaneous adrenergic therapy in acute asthma, 1 mg of terbutaline produced bronchodilation equivalent to that produced by 0.5 mg of epinephrine, but terbutaline, despite its reputed beta$_2$ selectivity, caused a substantially greater increase in heart rate [333].

The aerosolized route for the administration of beta-adrenergic agents has gained popularity in recent years and now must be considered the route of choice in most patients for both the emergency treatment of acute asthma and the sustained treatment of status asthmaticus. This route has the advantage of rapid onset of action with minimal side effects. Aerosolized sympathomimetics are somewhat more difficult to administer than subcutaneous drugs; in patients too young or in too much respiratory distress to cooperate, the subcutaneous route remains the preferred one. In comparison to subcutaneous epinephrine, inhaled isoproterenol has been shown to be as effective, and inhaled terbutaline has been shown to be more effective [92, 355].

Beta-agonist drugs available for aerosolization in the United States are listed in Table 73-7. All have roughly equivalent beta$_2$ selectiveness, but their durations of action differ slightly. Terbutaline sulfate is not available in the United States as an inhalant solution, but the injectable form may be administered undiluted via a nebulizer [279]. Fenoterol, another long-acting beta$_2$-selec-

Table 73-7. Sympathomimetic drugs available in the United States

Drug	Dose interval (hr)	Nebulized dose	MDI dose (μg/puff)
Isoetharine	1–4	5 mg (0.5 cc of 1.0% solution)[a]	340
Metaproterenol	2–6	15 mg (0.3 cc of 5% solution)[a]	650
Albuterol	2–6	2.5 mg (0.5 cc of 0.5% solution)[a]	
Terbutaline	2–6	4 mg (4 cc of 1 mg/ml solution)[b]	90

[a] Dilute into 2–3 cc of normal saline.
[b] Injectable form.

tive agonist, is not available in the United States and has recently been associated with increased asthma death rates in Canada [337a]. During asthma crises, inhaled beta agonists should be administered immediately and, subsequently, at a higher frequency and in larger dosages than is used for maintenance therapy. Following maximal dosing and a positive therapeutic result, the dose schedule is gradually titrated down as the severity of the asthmatic attack subsides.

Recent attention has focused on the optimal route for aerosol administration [245]. Aerosolization may be achieved by compressor-driven nebulizers, metered-dose inhalers (MDIs), or MDIs with spacer devices (see Chap. 56). The MDI with spacer consists of a tube or accordion-like device into which the MDI is discharged. It enhances drug delivery from the MDI by reducing impaction of drug on the tongue and eliminating the need for coordination between MDI discharge and breathing efforts. IPPB devices for the administration of bronchodilator drugs to patients with acute, severe asthma have fallen into disfavor [37, 94, 344]. Fatal pneumothoraces have occurred in asthmatic patients treated with IPPB [170], and a large controlled study found no benefit of IPPB over standard nebulizer treatments in patients with exacerbations of chronic obstructive pulmonary disease (COPD) [159].

Nebulizers have long been considered to be superior to MDIs for the therapy of acute asthma [303, 323], but a number of recent studies suggest that MDIs with spacer devices may be equally efficacious [103, 105, 321, 357]. This is the case despite the fact that doses administered using the MDI and spacer are usually much less than those administered using the nebulizer [103, 321] (Table 73-8). In one recent study, the nebulizer produced a better clinical response than did the MDI with spacer during the first 30 minutes after the initial hospital treatment [231]. However, no significant differences were noted between treatments with the nebulizers versus MDI with spacer for the remainder of the hospitalization. Thus, an acceptable approach to the patient with status asthmaticus is to initiate beta-agonist therapy using a nebulizer and then to switch to an MDI with spacer as soon as the patient's condition stabilizes.

Some groups have recommended rapid sequential administrations of a beta agonist using an MDI with spacer for the treatment of acute, severe asthma [241]. The regimen consists of four initial puffs of a sympathomimetic followed by one puff per minute until subjective or objective benefit is achieved, or until side effects limit continued drug administration. Others have recommended use of continuous nebulization consisting of 4 mg of terbutaline per hour [229] or up to 3 mg every 15 minutes [279] in children. These regimens have not yet been adequately evaluated and cannot currently be recommended for routine use in the treatment of acute asthma.

Administration of adequate doses of inhaled beta agonists (amount and frequency) in most asthmatic patients provides acceptable therapeutic effects comparable to those seen with parenteral dosing but with fewer side effects [359, 366]. However, when an adequate clinical response does not occur using inhaled beta-agonist bronchodilators, then the intravenous route of administration may be beneficial and may even reduce the need for intubation and mechanical ventilation. If subcutaneous dosing has not been attempted in a given patient, it is preferable to attempt this route first (see prior discussion). While the rationale for such parenteral therapy is to deliver bronchoactive drugs by the systemic circulation to distal airway sites affected with high-grade obstruction, this theoretical accessibility advantage has not been fully confirmed in clinical trials. However, Appel and colleagues [3] compared the responses in patients with acute, severe asthma to nebulized metaproterenol versus subcutaneous epinephrine and found that *some* patients exhibit a better response to parenteral (subcutaneous in this study) than to inhaled therapy. This is consistent with the concept that some patients

Table 73-8. Dosages of drugs in acute exacerbations of asthma in adults

INHALED BETA AGONISTS
Albuterol 2.5 mg (0.5 cc of a 0.5% solution, diluted with 2–3 cc of normal saline); or
Metaproterenol 15 mg (0.3 cc of a 5% solution, diluted with 2–3 cc of normal saline); or
Isoetharine 5 mg (0.5 cc of a 1% solution, diluted with 2–3 cc of normal saline); or

SUBCUTANEOUS BETA AGONISTS
Epinephrine 0.3 mg s.q.; or
Terbutaline 0.25 mg s.q.

METHYLXANTHINES
Intravenous
   Aminophylline 0.6 mg/kg/hr by continuous infusion. Lean body weight should be used for these calculations in obese patients. In patients not previously receiving a methylxanthine, a loading dose (6 mg/kg) should be administered. The continuous infusion rate should be adjusted for factors that alter the metabolism of theophylline, including liver disease, congestive heart failure, cigarette smoking, and certain medications (e.g., erythromycin, cimetidine, and ciprofloxacin). The continuous infusion rate should be adjusted according to the serum theophylline level, which should be measured first approximately 6 hours after infusion begins.
Oral
   Daily theophylline dose (mg) = total dose (mg) of aminophylline per 24 hours (times 0.80).
   The dose of theophylline can be given as a sustained-release preparation in two divided doses or as a once-daily preparation.

CORTICOSTEROIDS
Intravenous
   Methylprednisolone 60–80 mg IV bolus every 6–8 hours; or
   Hydrocortisone 2.0 mg/kg IV bolus every 4 hours; or
   Hydrocortisone 2.0 mg/kg IV bolus, then 0.5 mg/kg/hr continuous IV infusion.
Oral
   A typical oral regimen that may be used as a substitute for intravenous corticosteroids might be prednisone or methylprednisolone 60 mg given immediately, then 60–120 mg per day in divided doses, tapered over several days at the discretion of the physician.

With improvement in the patient's condition, corticosteroids are usually tapered to a single daily dose of oral prednisone or methylprednisolone (e.g., 60 mg/day), or divided doses (e.g., 20 mg tid), then gradually further reduced over several days.

If the patient requires a prolonged course of oral corticosteroids, side effects may be minimized by a single AM dose given on alternate days.

Source: National Asthma Education Program, Expert Panel Report. *Executive Summary: Guidelines for the Diagnosis and Management of Asthma.* Publication No. 91-3042A. Bethesda, MD: National Institutes of Health, June 1991. P. 27.

exhibit an inadequate therapeutic response to inhaled drugs because of presumed extensive airway edema and obstructive mucus plugging.

Intravenously administered sympathomimetic drugs are generally reserved for children and young adults who have no history of cardiac disease, who are in respiratory failure, and who have failed to respond satisfactorily (based on clinical and laboratory parameters) to nebulizer treatments. This approach has been used to avert the need for intubation and mechanical ventilation [178], but studies that have directly compared the efficacy of intravenous versus inhaled sympathomimetics have yielded inconsistent results. Intravenous therapy has been shown to be slightly superior [44, 386], equivalent [189], or inferior [23] compared to aerosol therapy. The disparity in results may be partly related to the relative doses of intravenous versus inhaled drugs used in the various studies [245]; inadequate inhaled doses or inefficient aerosol delivery may also be complicating issues. On the other hand, adverse side effects have been reported with intravenous beta-agonist administration, particularly in association with isoproterenol [178]. Tachycardia is common and cardiac ischemia or ventricular tachycardia, or both, have been reported [208]. Combined intravenous aminophylline and terbutaline therapy was associated with severe ventricular arrhythmias (17%) and runs of atrial tachycardia (7%) in a small number of patients with status asthmaticus [184]. These arrhythmias resolved spontaneously and were well tolerated hemodynamically [184]. Oxygen tension declines slightly during intravenous isoproterenol therapy [178], and evidence of cardiotoxicity and fatal arrhythmias with serum CPK elevations have been reported [54, 138, 183, 201]. Thus, although the intravenous route allows for rapid bronchodilation, it may be no more effective than the inhaled route, and it entails a higher risk of adverse side effects [140, 240]. Hence, careful selection of appropriate patients is clearly indicated for such therapy. The reader is referred to Chapter 55 for further discussion of intravenous beta-adrenergic agonists.

If intravenous therapy is to be administered, extreme caution must be exercised. The electrocardiogram should be monitored continuously and an arterial line should be placed for arterial pressure monitoring and frequent arterial blood gas determinations. Drugs available for intravenous use include isoproterenol, starting with a continuous infusion of 0.1 μg/kg/min increased step-wise at 10- to 15-minute intervals in increments of 0.1 μg/kg/min until clinical improvement or excessive tachycardia (>180–200 beats/min) occurs. Beta$_2$-selective agents should induce fewer cardiac effects; yet tachycardia with attendant increases in both cardiac work and oxygen requirement does occur. These agents include albuterol, administered as a bolus dose of 100 to 300 μg intravenously or as 500 to 900 μg over 1 hour [189, 387], and terbutaline, initiated with a dose of 0.25 mg delivered over 5 to 15 minutes and then followed with a continuous infusion of 0.1 to 0.4 μg/kg/min [248]. Intravenous albuterol [61, 98] and terbutaline [248] may be better tolerated than intravenous isoproterenol, but data are limited on the effectiveness of these treatments. This subject is presented in additional detail in Chapters 55, 57, and 80, and, prior to such usage, the reader is strongly urged to review this topic in these chapters for further insight into details of administration and side effects.

Methylxanthines

Methylxanthines are not routinely used as primary drugs in the emergency treatment of acute asthma; they are usually initiated after patients have demonstrated refractoriness to beta agonists. Unfortunately, only a few well-designed studies of methylxanthine therapy in status asthmaticus have been published. Jackson and associates [161] found that symptomatic responses and improvement in pulmonary function test results correlated with serum theophylline concentrations in patients with acute exacerbations of asthma. In a double-blind, placebo-controlled trial of intravenous aminophylline in children hospitalized for status asthmaticus, the aminophylline-treated group had a greater increase in FEV$_1$ and FVC after 1 and 24 hours of treatment than did the control group [276]. Adults treated for acute exacerbations of either asthma or COPD with a high-dose, continuous intravenous aminophylline infusion (mean serum concentration, 19.0 μg/ml) had a greater improvement in FEV$_1$ and FVC and required a shorter duration of aminophylline therapy than did those receiving a low-dose infusion (mean serum concentration, 9.7 μg/ml) [367]; this study concurrently utilized a suboptimal intravenous hydrocortisone dose of 200 mg/day in both patient groups. A recent controlled study suggesting that emergency room use of theophylline may reduce the need for hospitalization for refrac-

tory asthma will require added data to define theophylline use once a patient is hospitalized [394].

Theophylline and aminophylline, the ethylenediamine salt of theophylline that contains 84% anhydrous theophylline by weight, are used for the treatment of status asthmaticus. Theophylline has a potent and sustained bronchodilator action with an average half-life of 3 to 5 hours in normal adults. It also has a number of other potentially beneficial actions in patients with asthma, including improved mucociliary function, central respiratory stimulation, enhancement of cardiovascular function, improved diaphragmatic function, and possible antiinflammatory effects [146]. However, these cited actions are weak and the added benefit of theophylline in patients with status asthmaticus receiving treatment with optimal doses of beta agonists and corticosteroids has not been firmly established.

Nevertheless, intravenous theophylline continues to be recommended for the treatment of status asthmaticus, initiated as a loading infusion of 5 to 6 mg/kg over 30 minutes and followed by a continuous infusion of 0.5 to 0.6 mg/kg/hr in adults [136] (the reader is referred to the flow chart of theophylline dosing in Chapter 58). The continuous infusion rate must be adjusted for smoking status, age, impairment of cardiac or hepatic function, or the presence of drugs that alter theophylline metabolism [136]. Patients already receiving a methylxanthine at the time of their asthma exacerbation should receive a reduced loading dose or should have theophylline administration withheld until a serum level can be obtained. If the theophylline level is in the therapeutic range, the superiority of intravenous theophylline over continued oral therapy has not been demonstrated.

The plasma concentration of theophylline should be maintained in the therapeutic range of 10 to 20 μg/ml, although some bronchodilation is achieved at levels as low as 5 μg/ml [228]. Plasma concentrations exceeding 20 μg/ml are associated with adverse side effects, including anxiety, headache, tremors, anorexia, nausea, vomiting, and diarrhea. Seizures or cardiac arrest may occur at levels exceeding 40 μg/ml [399], and serial monitoring of plasma theophylline concentrations is mandatory. Patients may be switched to oral therapy as soon as their asthma is stabilized. The oral dose is calculated so that it matches the amount of anhydrous theophylline the patient has been receiving by infusion. The oral drug should be administered immediately upon cessation of the intravenous infusion [136]. The reader is referred to Chapter 58 for added details and information regarding aminophylline therapy.

The standard practice of combining beta-agonist and theophylline therapy, often with levels approaching the toxic range, has raised concerns about the increased risk of cardiac arrhythmias contributing to sudden death or morbidity [242, 246, 389]. However, several studies have demonstrated that this combination rarely induces serious arrhythmias in patients with stable asthma [175, 363] or status asthmaticus [184].

Other Bronchodilators

The antimuscarinic agents atropine and ipratropium bromide are effective bronchodilators, with a predominant effect on the central airways [137, 157, 268]. In general, antimuscarinics appear to be most efficacious in patients with chronic bronchitis [28], but they also have efficacy in patients with asthma. In children with stable asthma, bronchodilation was sustained for 5 hours after treatment with nebulized atropine sulfate, 0.1 mg/kg [39] (see also Chap. 64).

Ipratropium bromide, a quaternary ammonium derivative of atropine, became commercially available as an MDI in the United States in 1987. The inhalant solution is not yet available in the United States. Ipratropium bromide is poorly absorbed through the mucosal surfaces and has minimal systemic antimuscarinic effects. The findings of some studies, but not all, suggest that its action is additive to that of beta₂ agonists and theophylline [180, 193]. A 500-μg dose of nebulized ipratropium bromide is as effective a bronchodilator in certain asthmatics as 10 mg of nebulized albuterol [371]. Higgins and associates [145] showed that ipratropium prolonged the action of albuterol, but did not enhance the overall maximal bronchodilator response. The role of antimuscarinics in the therapy of status asthmaticus awaits further evaluation, but their addition to beta agonist and methylxanthine therapy in patients with recalcitrant asthma may enhance benefit with little additional risk of side effects.

Early studies suggested that antihistamines have bronchodilator actions, but their poor efficacy compared with beta agonists and their tendency to produce troublesome sedative and anticholinergic side effects blunted enthusiasm for their use [139]. However, the recent introduction of nonsedating H_1 antagonists such as terfenadine has stimulated new interest in the use of antihistamines for the therapy of asthma. Recent studies suggest that terfenadine is capable of reducing asthma symptoms such as cough and wheeze, but no role has yet been identified for it in the therapy of status asthmaticus [282] (see also Chap. 65).

A number of other bronchodilators have recently received attention as having a possible role in the therapy of acute asthma. Intravenous magnesium sulfate and inhaled furosemide both have acute bronchodilator actions [217, 253], possibly related to effects on calcium handling by the airway smooth muscle cell, but efficacy superior to that of the beta agonists and theophyllines has not been demonstrated. Inhaled anesthetics such as halothane have demonstrable bronchodilator effects [117, 257], but they should be reserved for use as adjuncts during ventilator therapy and will be discussed further under the topic of ventilator management.

Corticosteroids

The appreciation that asthma is primarily an inflammatory disorder characterized by airway hyperresponsiveness underlies the central role corticosteroids play in the treatment of status asthmaticus. The efficacy of corticosteroids in the treatment of status asthmaticus has been established in a number of well-designed, controlled trials [86, 91, 133, 195, 218]. Several studies have questioned the efficacy of corticosteroids in the treatment of status asthmaticus for both adults [56, 124, 197, 215] and children [173], but some of these studies used inadequate steroid doses or had very small study populations. Younger and coworkers [395] demonstrated that, in 49 non-steroid-dependent children hospitalized for status asthmaticus, intravenous methylprednisolone not only resulted in more rapid recovery of airflow rates, but it also led to lowered relapse rates 4 weeks after hospital discharge.

The exact target cells and mechanisms of action of corticosteroids in asthma are uncertain, but it is known that they have wide-ranging effects on a variety of cells and inflammatory mechanisms (see Chap. 60). Membrane stabilization in mast cells, macrophages, and leukocytes, thereby preventing the release of inflammatory mediators [53] and inhibition of phospholipase A_2, and thus preventing the formation of arachidonic acid products including the potent bronchoconstrictors leukotrienes C_4 and D_4, are among their many actions. They also potentiate the bronchodilator response to exogenous catecholamines [320] and restore responsiveness to inhaled beta agonists [86].

Most studies suggest that the response to corticosteroids is not immediate, requiring approximately 6 hours for beneficial effects on airflow to occur [320]. This underscores the need for establishing optimal doses of bronchodilators in the initiation of treatment for status asthmaticus, as well as early administration of corticosteroids. At present, it is recommended that, once bronchodilator refractoriness is established, corticosteroids should be administered immediately.

The risks associated with short courses of corticosteroids are

small; on the other hand, failure to treat with steroids or to employ an adequate dose has been implicated in asthma deaths [30, 51, 200, 256]. Corticosteroid therapy should be initiated without delay in patients currently or recently on maintenance steroids and in patients with a history of similar attacks requiring steroids for lysis. The specific corticosteroid chosen is probably not critical, although most authors have favored methylprednisolone. Studies using hydrocortisone [31, 40] and triamcinolone [249] have also shown benefit. As long as the patient can swallow and has no malabsorption problem, both oral and intravenous steroids are equally effective [285]; however, extremely ill patients will require parenteral dosing. The use of adrenocorticotropic hormone is not recommended because of the uncertainty of adrenocortical responsiveness, although patients with acute asthma not previously treated with corticosteroids respond favorably [55] (see discussion in Chaps. 60 and 62).

The optimal dose of corticosteroids for the treatment of status asthmaticus is unknown, but has received considerable attention and probably depends to a certain extent on individual factors, such as steroid resistance. Haskell and coworkers [133] demonstrated that patients receiving 40 or 125 mg of intravenous methylprednisolone every 6 hours for 3 days had earlier and greater improvements in the FEV_1 than did patients receiving 15 mg every 6 hours. Ratto and associates [285] showed that 80 mg of methylprednisolone given twice daily was as effective as 80 mg given four times daily. Thus, an initial dose of 80 to 125 mg of methylprednisolone or the equivalent given intravenously appears adequate. Thereafter, 50 to 100 mg is given every 8 to 12 hours until definite resolution has begun [353]; adjust regimen as clinically indicated. Alternatively, a regimen of intravenous hydrocortisone hemisuccinate may be employed, beginning with a loading dose of 2 to 4 mg/kg of body weight and continued with doses of 3 mg/kg every 3 hours. In a recent study three different doses of intravenous hydrocortisone in 66 patients with acute severe asthma were compared: low-dose (50 mg qid), medium-dose (200 mg qid), and high-dose (500 mg qid) hydrocortisone for 48 hours, followed by low to high doses of oral prednisone in the respective groups. The low-dose schedule of 200 mg/day was considered effective for resolution; no significant difference in the rate of recovery in lung function was found between the three groups [400]. Total eosinophil counts may be used as an added approximate guide to assess the clinical response and may be especially helpful if steroid resistance is suspected. Effective steroid doses will yield values of 100 cells/mm³ or less within 24 to 36 hours. Monitoring of blood glucose and electrolyte levels and the addition of an antacid regimen are indicated at this time; see Chapter 60 for details on steroid dosages. The dosages of drugs for the treatment of acute exacerbations of asthma in adults recommended by the expert panel report of the National Heart, Lung, and Blood Institute National Asthma Education Program, including corticosteroids, are shown in Table 73-8. Dosing schedules will undoubtedly continue to be evaluated.

When clinical improvement is sustained, steroids may be gradually tapered by the equivalent of 50 mg of methylprednisolone daily over the first 5 to 7 days (about 25% reduction every 2 to 3 days) and then discontinued over the next 10 days to 3 weeks, depending on the patient's clinical course. Any clinical relapse may require a temporary increase in dosage. Patients previously on alternate-day oral schedules are tapered to their previous maintenance level or to an effective inhaled steroid regimen, or both.

Patients who have breakthrough symptoms of their asthma during tapering despite optimal use of inhaled corticosteroids must remain on long-term oral steroid therapy. The importance of adequate corticosteroid treatment in patients with chronic life-threatening asthma has been emphasized [286, 340]. These patients should be discouraged from tapering steroids on their own because of the risk of exacerbation or sudden death.

The complications of brief, high-dose corticosteroid therapy are usually minimal [275], but acute psychotic reactions and fluid and electrolyte disorders related to sodium retention and potassium loss are observed. Furthermore, disuse atrophy or acute myopathy may occur in patients treated with both steroids and neuromuscular blockade [126a, 182], and early physical therapy regimens in patients receiving both agents are encouraged. Complete ophthalmoplegia complicating acute corticosteroid- and pancuronium-associated myopathy was recently reported in a patient with refractory asthma [331]. High-dose corticosteroid use has also been implicated in gastrointestinal ulceration [220], and ulcer prophylaxis should be included in the therapeutic regimen. Nosocomial infection is another serious concern, especially in the mechanically ventilated patient. Fatal disseminated aspergillosis has been reported in such patients [186], and the use of meticulous techniques during tracheal suctioning and ventilator care and good oral hygiene are encouraged.

Antimicrobial Agents

The frequency of bacterial respiratory tract infections as a cause of acute exacerbations of asthma has probably been exaggerated in the past, resulting in an overuse of antimicrobial therapy. However, numerous respiratory tract viruses are associated with exacerbations of asthma, and are implicated in a higher proportion of exacerbations in children than in adults. In three studies conducted in children, a viral or a mycoplasma infection was found in from 32 to 42 percent of the exacerbations of asthma [20, 216, 225]. Among 63 adults hospitalized with severe asthma, 19 percent of the admissions were associated with a viral or mycoplasmal infection [153]. Hudgel and coworkers [152] found that in 19 adult asthmatic patients viral but not bacterial respiratory tract infections were increased during wheezing exacerbations; interestingly, these authors noted that both viral and bacterial infections could occur without inducing an exacerbation of asthma. Viral infection was present in 11 percent of the exacerbations and bacterial infection in 9 percent. Similarly, Clarke [48] found evidence of bacterial or viral infection in only 10.8 percent of asthmatic exacerbations in adults. In another study, transtracheal aspirates obtained from adults with acute asthma did not yield significantly different bacterial or fungal growth from aspirates obtained from controls [21]. The recently described role of *Chlamydia* was discussed earlier in this chapter.

The routine administration of a broad-spectrum antibiotic in 44 children with status asthmaticus who did not have signs of bacterial infection was assessed in a double-blind protocol comparing hetacillin (which is hydrolyzed in vivo to ampicillin) with a placebo [319]. Since the hospital course, length of hospital stay, and complications were similar in the treated and control groups, the authors concluded that there was no obvious advantage to routine antibiotic therapy in such patients. A comparable study in 60 adults hospitalized with acute asthma and treated with either amoxicillin or placebo also disclosed no difference in the rate of improvement in symptoms, length of hospital stay, or pulmonary function at the time of discharge [123].

Thus, the available data do not support the use of antimicrobial agents in patients with status asthmaticus unless there is evidence of bacterial infection. The diagnosis of bacterial lower respiratory tract infection in patients with status asthmaticus may be difficult. Large numbers of eosinophils may impart a purulent appearance to the sputum. While eosinophils cannot be distinguished from neutrophils on a Gram's-stained sputum specimen, a wet mount or Wright stain does permit correct identification. Infiltrates on the chest radiograph may be caused by mucoid impaction and atelectasis rather than pneumonia, and leukocytosis may be present in status asthmaticus without infection. The diagnosis of bacterial infection is supported by the presence of large numbers of neutrophils in the sputum, especially when accompanied by one or two types of bacteria in heavy concentration, and by fever, chills, an increased number of immature neu-

trophils in the peripheral blood, or a compatible chest radiograph. Sinusitis, if present, requires antibiotic treatment. Antimicrobial therapy should be based initially on the pathogens suspected and later modified according to the results of drug susceptibility studies of pathogens isolated from sputum or blood.

Hydration and Sputum Mobilization

In status asthmaticus, hyperpnea, diaphoresis, fever, and reduced fluid intake may contribute to the presence of systemic dehydration. The severity of the fluid deficit may vary considerably and is difficult to assess clinically, since many of the signs of dehydration (e.g., dry mouth, tachycardia, reduced jugular venous pressure) are found during acute asthma in patients who are in normal fluid balance. As in any dehydrated patient, correction of systemic fluid deficits is indicated in order to normalize cardiovascular and cellular function. Although adequate systemic hydration is also thought to have a beneficial effect on respiratory tract secretions, evidence of such an effect is scanty [9, 46]. In mild asthma, adequate hydration may be achieved orally, but, in status asthmaticus, the intravenous route is preferred to ensure sufficient intake. Fluid therapy should be guided by the estimated state of hydration and the initial serum electrolyte concentrations, and modified thereafter as clinically required. Careful observations of fluid intake and output, body weight, and serum and urine sodium concentrations aid in fluid management and the early recognition of fluid retention in susceptible patients (children, the elderly, and those with underlying cardiac disease). Generally, a daily physiologic water intake is sufficient for most patients with status asthmaticus.

Straub and colleagues [345] observed a variable degree of hypovolemia in nine patients during status asthmaticus. Four patients experienced a rise in pulse rate and fall in blood pressure at the time of relief of their airways obstruction. Infusion of 500 to 1,500 ml of plasma led to immediate circulatory improvement. The authors speculated that a combination of hypovolemia and vasodilation in response to hyperventilation may result in circulatory collapse, which in turn may contribute to some of the unexpected deaths in asthmatics. Elevated ADH levels have been found in some patients with status asthmaticus during the acute phase; these levels returned to normal with resolution of the attack [11]. The administration of hypotonic fluids to such patients could result in water intoxication.

Since airway secretions are a major factor in precipitating, intensifying, or perpetuating the acute asthmatic state, the mobilization of secretions is vital. Under normal conditions, inspired air is warmed and saturated with water vapor in the upper respiratory tract and major airways. If this mechanism is impaired or if the upper airway is bypassed by the use of a tracheal tube, it is possible that secretions may desiccate and become thickened and tenacious, and thus more difficult to raise. In addition, mucociliary clearance may be impaired, further favoring secretional stasis. Therapeutic oxygen, if not properly humidified, can contribute to such desiccation; unheated bubble humidifiers produce only 20 percent of the required humidification.

Humidification devices and mist therapy are commonly employed to assist in the mobilization of bronchial secretions. Clinical experience suggests that these measures may be beneficial in selected cases; nevertheless, there is limited evidence to indicate that airways humidification accomplished by currently employed devices has any effect on mucociliary clearance in asthma (see Chap. 69). Studies of the effect of ambient humidity on the viscosity of sputum in vitro have yielded conflicting results [79, 294]. Although aerosols of water or hypertonic saline have been reported to increase the clearance of secretions in patients with chronic bronchitis [260, 267], evidence of their efficacy in asthma is currently inconclusive [370]. Furthermore, the ultrasonic nebulization of distilled water or saline solutions can induce bronchospasm and may not be tolerated by patients during acute asthma attacks [43, 313].

Mucolytic agents, such as acetylcysteine, reduce the viscosity of sputum in vitro. However, the aerosol administration of acetylcysteine in asthmatics induces bronchospasm and worsens hypoxemia [22, 284] and therefore is not recommended. Of limited use, direct intrabronchial instillation of a mixture of 3.0 to 5.0 ml of 10% acetylcysteine with 0.25 ml of 1:200 isoproterenol (or another adrenergic agent) through a tracheal tube or bronchoscope followed by suctioning may be effective in removing life-threatening lobar mucoid impactions [77]. The role of fiberoptic bronchoscopy and bronchial lavage is discussed in Chapter 84.

The efficacy of expectorant drugs, such as iodides and guaifenesin, has not been convincingly demonstrated in asthma (see Chap. 69). Antitussives should be avoided, as their action is contrary to the goal of sputum removal. Once coughing becomes productive, physical measures such as gentle chest percussion and postural drainage can be considered in certain patients, although there is some evidence that these may induce bronchospasm [36] and worsen arterial hypoxemia [154]. Chest physiotherapy, accompanied by supplemental oxygen and preceded by aerosol bronchodilator therapy, should be used only if sputum production is enhanced and bronchospasm is not exacerbated; percussive therapy is generally not indicated in asthma.

Acid-Base and Electrolyte Considerations

The most common acid-base disturbance in status asthmaticus is respiratory alkalosis caused by hyperventilation; it is treated by relief of the underlying asthma. In patients with severe, acute asthma exhibiting hyperventilation of several days' duration, a coexisting non–anion gap metabolic acidosis appears to be common [254]. This base deficit is presumably due to excessive renal bicarbonate excretion as a renal compensatory response during the period of hypocapnia.

The most serious acid-base disturbance in status asthmaticus is respiratory acidosis resulting from progressive hypercapnia; it may be complicated by a metabolic (lactic) acidosis in severe hypoxemic status asthmaticus. Because of the rapidity with which hypercapnic respiratory failure may develop, the compensation provided by renal mechanisms may be inadequate, and severe degrees of acidemia can be seen. The definitive treatment of hypercapnic respiratory failure unresponsive to conservative measures is mechanical ventilation, the indications for which are discussed later.

Metabolic acidosis in acute asthma, aside from hypocapnia-associated renal bicarbonate loss, is due largely to lactic acidosis, which is believed to arise from tissue hypoxia, lactate formation by the respiratory musculature, diminished hepatic removal of lactate, and intracellular alkalosis. Mountain and colleagues [233] recently found that metabolic acidemia may be more common than was previously believed. These authors detected a metabolic acidemia associated with an increased anion gap (mean, 15.8 mEq/L) in 28 percent of 229 episodes of acute asthma; the degree of arterial hypoxemia correlated inversely with the anion gap. The distribution of acid-base disorders in this study is shown in Table 73-9. If the degree of acidemia is severe (pH < 7.15), and especially if there is a delay in instituting mechanical ventilation, 45 to 90 mEq of sodium bicarbonate (in children, 1 mEq/kg) may be infused slowly over 10 to 20 minutes, the required dose titrated to a blood pH of about 7.25. It should be noted, however, that little increase in blood pH will occur unless the carbon dioxide produced from the infused bicarbonate can be eliminated by the lungs [259]. Additionally, a bicarbonate infusion in acute asthma may result in a fall in the PaO_2 level, presumably by increasing the perfusion of underventilated lung regions [224]. Other complications to be avoided include hyperosmolarity, fluid overload, and rebound alkalemia; serum (and urinary) potassium

Table 73-9. Acid-base status at presentation in 229 episodes of acute asthma

Acid-base status	No. (% of episodes)
Normal	28 (12.2)
Respiratory alkalosis	109 (47.6)
Respiratory alkalosis + metabolic acidosis	14 (6.1)
Metabolic acidosis	13 (5.7)
Respiratory acidosis	23 (10.0)
Respiratory acidosis + metabolic acidosis	37 (16.2)
Respiratory alkalosis + metabolic alkalosis	5 (2.2)

Source: R. D. Mountain, et al., Acid-base disturbances in acute asthma. *Chest* 98: 651, 1990.

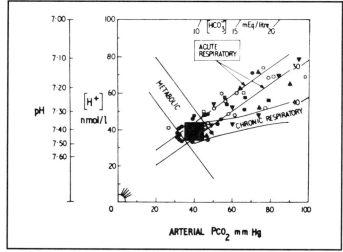

Fig. 73-6. *Acid-base relationships in severe asthma. Closed symbols are from adults, open symbols from children in various series of severe asthma. Ninety-five percent confidence limits of these relationships in pure metabolic acid-base disturbances and in acute and chronic respiratory disturbances are shown. (Reprinted with permission from D. C. Flenley, Blood gas tensions in severe asthma. Proc. R. Soc. Med. 64:1149, 1971.)*

and magnesium levels should be monitored and corrected as needed. The presumed benefits of reducing adverse acidemia may include restoring the responsiveness to adrenergic agents or reducing the morbidity of the acidemia itself. However, a recent report of 14 critically ill patients (none with asthma) described failure to demonstrate improved cardiovascular hemodynamics following the administration of sodium bicarbonate for the treatment of lactic acidosis [58]. The issue of employing sodium bicarbonate in severely acidemic patients seems currently unresolved. Acid-base relationships in severe asthma are depicted in Figure 73-6.

Metabolic alkalosis may result from intravascular volume depletion, from potassium and chloride deficiency owing to vomiting, gastric suction, diuretics, or corticosteroids, or from the administration of bicarbonate. Alkalosis can depress ventilation, decrease cardiac output, induce $\dot{V}$-$\dot{Q}$ mismatching, and lower the seizure threshold, and should be corrected by appropriate replacement of electrolytes and intravascular volume or by alleviation of the primary cause.

Electrolyte abnormalities related to acid-base shifts and drug administration may also complicate status asthmaticus. As discussed previously, hypokalemia and hypophosphatemia are common during acute exacerbations of asthma [26, 185] but they tend to resolve spontaneously with therapy. The clinical significance of these abnormalities is currently unclear, and, unless they are severe (K^+ <3.0 mEq/L, plasma phosphate concentration <0.3 mM/L) treatment may not be necessary. Monitoring the serum potassium level is indicated in any at risk patient, such as the aged, those with ischemic cardiac disease, or those receiving digitalis or diuretics.

Sedatives

Fear, restlessness, and agitation frequently accompany the acute asthma attack and may prompt the physician to administer sedative drugs. Sedated patients, however, experience a false sense of security and this may extend to the physician, while physiologic derangements may continue to worsen without evoking the usual intensity of symptoms. Equally important is the depression of ventilatory drive that various sedatives can induce. In normal subjects, hypoxic and hypercapnic ventilatory responses were depressed by moderate doses of morphine [374], meperidine [181], and diazepam [187, 283]. Other adverse effects of sedative agents are their tendency to suppress cough, thereby impairing the removal of bronchial secretions, and the enhanced metabolism and the consequent reduced effectiveness of corticosteroids when given to patients receiving barbiturates [32].

Sedative use has been identified as a risk factor for respiratory failure with the attendant morbidity of mechanical ventilation in status asthmaticus [204, 316, 350, 381] and has been cited as contributing to asthma deaths [30, 82, 238].

There is no evidence that sedative or tranquilizing drugs reverse the pathophysiologic features of status asthmaticus. In view of their depressant effect on ventilation and their other adverse effects, sedatives should not be used in status asthmaticus except in patients who are receiving mechanical ventilation. The patient's anxiety should be allayed by calm and repeated reassurance offered by the physician and other medical attendants and by prompt, efficient application of therapeutic and supportive measures. Faling [89] has reviewed this subject in detail.

The Airway

Maintenance of a patent airway at all times is essential in the management of status asthmaticus. Patients who are unable to mobilize secretions adequately or who are obtunded, comatose, or in respiratory failure need immediate tracheal intubation. An oral or nasal tracheal tube should be inserted as soon as this need is determined and placed sufficiently early in the course to avoid the complications associated with emergency intubation. Anxious, dyspneic patients are often difficult to intubate and may struggle during the process, with resulting aggravation of the bronchospasm. Hence, intubation should be performed deftly and expeditiously by the most experienced professional available, with care taken to preoxygenate the patient and to avoid the complication of gastric aspiration [309]. We prefer orotracheal intubation using at least a No. 8 endotracheal tube after the patient has been adequately sedated or paralyzed as a way to minimize morbidity.

The use of a low-pressure cuff with the pressure adjusted to allow a minimal leak, proper positioning of the tube, avoidance of undue torsional stresses, a gentle and aseptic suctioning technique, and meticulous nursing care are necessary to minimize the complications of intubation. Atraumatic and careful suctioning techniques can assist in the mobilization of mucus plugs. Complications of the airway are often the most common among series of mechanically ventilated patients [203]. Since tracheal intubation in asthma is seldom necessary for more than a few days, tracheostomy can usually be avoided.

Mechanical Ventilation

Mechanical ventilation is indicated when the patient's ventilatory efforts are insufficient to maintain adequate gas exchange. Con-

currently, appropriate oxygen therapy and suctioning of secretions can be accomplished through the cuffed tracheal tube. Ventilatory failure can be detected by a rise in $PaCO_2$ and can be anticipated by the clinical observation of a marked increase in respiratory effort, a common precursor of fatigue or exhaustion. Since, as we have stressed, $PaCO_2$ is usually reduced during acute asthma, a $PaCO_2$ level at or above the normal range is cause for concern. A steadily rising $PaCO_2$, especially during optimal therapy and when accompanied by incipient or overt respiratory muscle fatigue, is a major indication for mechanical ventilation. Both premature and delayed intubations have their respective hazards. The exact point at which to institute mechanical ventilatory support is determined on the basis of careful longitudinal clinical and gas exchange assessments, observing trends rather than relying on rigid criteria.

From a variety of clinical reports it appears that only a small proportion of patients require mechanical ventilation for status asthmaticus. Approximately 2 to 8 percent of all asthma hospitalizations and from 9 to 16 percent of asthma patients admitted to intensive care units require endotracheal intubation and mechanical ventilatory support [311, 316]. For example, ventilator therapy was instituted in 21 of 811 patients (2.6%) admitted to Colorado General Hospital for status asthmaticus from 1967 to 1975 [316] and in 16 percent of 111 patients admitted with status asthmaticus to a respiratory intensive care unit in Los Angeles from 1968 to 1977 [311]. In both these series, a decline was noted in recent years in the number of asthmatic patients requiring mechanical ventilation. Presumably, early and aggressive therapy reduces the requirement for mechanical ventilation in some patients. Patients with evolving hypercapnia should be admitted to an intensive care unit for aggressive therapy, where facilities for intubation, ventilation, and monitoring are readily available. Supportive intermittent positive-pressure ventilation (IPPV) in asthma patients with severe airflow resistance has its own specific difficulties. Adequate effective alveolar ventilation, in the presence of high and potentially problematic peak inspiratory ventilator pressure with its attendant complications, requires appropriate and careful techniques. Despite many advances in IPPV, the mortality rate in adults in this circumstance can be as high as 10 percent [68].

In the past, it has been emphasized that normocapnia and, in particular, hypercapnia were considered indicators of incipient respiratory failure. However, Mountain and Sahn [232] recently reported in a retrospective analysis that the majority of patients presenting with hypercapnia do not require intubation. They found that only 8.2 percent of 61 patients presenting to an emergency room with hypercapnia required intubation. No patient presenting with normocapnia subsequently required intubation and, among 21 patients with severe hypercapnia ($PaCO_2$, 50–110 mmHg) who did not require mechanical ventilation, the mean time to normalization of $PaCO_2$ was 5.9 hours (Fig. 73-7). Thus, as we have stressed, the value of blood gas measurements in determining the need for mechanical ventilation must be considered in the clinical context. Continuously symptomatic patients with evolving normocapnia or hypercapnia require close observation and maximal therapy.

In an effort to avoid mechanical ventilation and its attendant complications, some authors have advocated the use of continuous positive airway pressure (CPAP) in conjunction with bicarbonate infusion to reduce inspiratory muscle work [202] (see Chap. 91). However, this approach requires further study and should currently be considered investigational.

When frank ventilatory failure occurs despite institution of the intensive therapy described, mechanical ventilatory support must be considered. Clinical features, although suggestive, are not reliable or quantitative indices of effective alveolar ventilation. Measurement of $PaCO_2$ (PaO_2) and pH provide quantitative evidence for ventilatory failure, but these values must be viewed

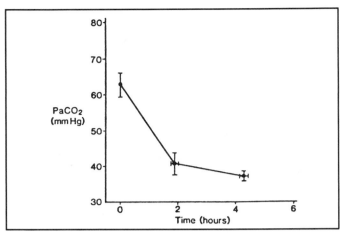

Fig. 73-7. *Resolution of severe hypercapnia in 21 episodes of severe asthma presenting with a PaCO$_2$ exceeding 50 mmHg not requiring mechanical ventilation. Values are expressed as the mean ± SEM. (Reprinted with permission from R. D. Mountain and S. A. Sahn, Clinical features and outcome in patients with acute asthma presenting with hypercapnia. Am. Rev. Respir. Dis. 138:535, 1988.)*

Table 73-10. Guidelines for interventional mechanical ventilation in status asthmaticus (adults)

Clinical
1. Exhaustion, apnea
2. Disturbances of consciousness (obtunded or coma)
3. Extreme tachypnea (>40/min)
4. Overt respiratory muscle fatigue; abdominal paradox
5. Cardiac or hemodynamic instability; hypotension; cardiac arrest

Arterial blood—spirometry
1. Rising PaCO$_2$ greater than 40 to 50 mmHg, with obvious patient distress, despite complete and aggressive therapy. A rise in PaCO$_2$ of 5 to 10 mmHg per hour or more can be a poor prognostic sign when associated with acute respiratory (and lactic) acidosis.
2. Extreme hypercapnia (PaCO$_2$ ≥ 60 mmHg) in the appropriate clinical setting; coexisting acidemia (pH ≤7.20).
3. Refractory hypoxemia despite O$_2$ administration (PaO$_2$ <50 mmHg; FIO$_2$ = 1.0); or O$_2$-induced ventilatory suppression.
4. FEV$_1$ ≤1.0 L (or <25% predicted)
5. PEFR ≤120 L/min (or <25% predicted)

FIO$_2$ = fraction of inspired oxygen; FEV$_1$ = forced expiratory volume in 1 second; PEFR = peak expiratory flow rate.

in the clinical context of the patient. Thus, criteria for intubation and mechanical ventilation (see later discussion) should be best individualized for each patient; hypercapnia or evolving normo-capnia are not necessarily absolute criteria for intubation [35a]. Table 73-10 presents guidelines for ventilatory support in status asthmaticus.

The use of mechanical ventilation in patients in status asthmaticus is not without controversy. Some investigators have reported high mortality rates ranging up to 38 percent [203, 204, 274, 316] associated with high rates of barotrauma, and have discouraged the use of mechanical ventilation except as a last resort [316]. Others have reported very low or no mortality [27, 70, 83, 144, 311] with relatively low morbidity rates. Undoubtedly, some of the differences between these studies are related to differing patient populations. However, those studies reporting low complication rates have generally used low-pressure, controlled mechanical hypoventilation [27, 70, 83]. This ventilator technique eschews use of high peak inspiratory pressures and attendant risks of barotrauma, limiting peak pressure to less than 50 to 55 cmH$_2$O, and allows the PaCO$_2$ to rise, correcting acidemia with bicarbonate infusions, if necessary. Hypercapnia resolves

with the subsequent relief of airflow obstruction. With optimal ventilator technique, patients with acute, severe asthma, including children and pregnant women, can receive mechanical ventilation with relative safety.

If possible, the decision to intubate and initiate mechanical ventilation should neither be a premature one nor delayed to the point where the patient is in respiratory arrest. Only with close clinical observations and serial measurements of gas exchange can the optimal point be selected. Should mechanical ventilation be deemed necessary, we advocate sedating the patient, preferably with a benzodiazepine such as diazepam or lorazepam, or a narcotic, if needed. Some have advocated the use of fentanyl over morphine because of the latter's histamine-releasing properties, although the clinical significance of this effect is minor [24, 396]. Conventional IPPV is instituted with initial ventilator settings employing a volume-preset ventilator to include the assist/control mode, a tidal volume of 8 to 10 ml/kg, a frequency of 12 to 15 cycles/min, and a ventilator inspiratory flow rate of 60 L/min; FIO$_2$ is set to attain a PaO$_2$ of 60 to 80 mmHg (≥95% oxygen saturation).

If the patient encounters difficulty synchronizing with the ventilator and if severe tachypnea or hypercapnia persists, neuromuscular paralysis using pancuronium bromide, vecuronium, or tracrium should be instituted after adequate sedation is achieved [191] (see Chap. 91). Paralyzed patients require close observation in the event of accidental ventilator disconnection.

The goals of mechanical ventilation should include limiting the peak airway pressure (PAP) to less than 50 to 55 cmH$_2$O (preferably ≤40 cmH$_2$O), keeping intrinsic PEEP at less than 15 cmH$_2$O, and normalizing the PaCO$_2$ [130]. Reduction in either the inspiratory flow rate or the tidal volume, or both, may be necessary to limit PAP to under 50 to 55 cmH$_2$O. These goals may be conflicting, particularly if slowing of the ventilator rate is necessary to minimize intrinsic PEEP. If the PaCO$_2$ can be normalized only by increasing PAP or the level of intrinsic PEEP to unacceptable ranges, use of controlled hypoventilation is indicated with acceptance of an elevated PaCO$_2$. Hypercapnia is well tolerated if the pH is maintained at greater than 7.20 to 7.25 by employing a bicarbonate infusion [219]. Generally, this approach is associated with a greater duration of hypercapnia.

Based on evidence suggesting that CPAP reduces the inspiratory work of breathing in patients with induced acute asthma, some investigators have advocated use of PEEP during mechanical ventilation of asthmatics [206, 280]. However, although low levels of PEEP may benefit some patients with severe COPD who have dynamic compression of their airways during expiration, the indications for PEEP in patients with status asthmaticus are unclear [205]. PEEP has been shown to cause excessive increases in lung volumes, airway pressures, and intrathoracic pressures in patients with severe airway obstruction, resulting in hemodynamic compromise [358]. Inasmuch as beneficial effects have not been consistently reported and detrimental effects can ensue, PEEP during ventilatory support cannot currently be recommended in the management of status asthmaticus.

Occasionally, mechanical ventilation may be ineffective despite optimal medical therapy. The progressive rise in PaCO$_2$ necessitates the use of excessively high peak airway pressures. In this situation, a number of additional techniques may be applied. Some investigators advocate the use of inhalational anesthetic agents that have bronchodilator actions [315]. Ether is no longer used, but the halogenated ethers, halothane, enflurane, and isoflurane, have all yielded favorable results in the treatment of severe status asthmaticus unresponsive to standard mechanical ventilation [166, 264]. Isoflurane is currently the preferred anesthetic because it is the least lipid soluble, allowing rapid control of the level of anesthesia, and is less likely to cause arrhythmias or hepatic or renal toxicity [166]. Other anesthetic agents such as ketamine [297] and thiopental [128] have no clear advantages over the inhalational anesthetics, and thiopental may actually extend the period of mechanical ventilation. The use of helium-oxygen mixtures has also been advocated in patients whose condition is recalcitrant to standard mechanical ventilation [114]; peak airway pressures and $PaCO_2$ were abruptly lowered after the initiation of helium-oxygen therapy in seven patients with status asthmaticus [114]. Helium-oxygen is thought to reduce airway resistance by minimizing turbulent airflow, by virtue of helium's lower density. Helium-oxygen mixtures consisting of less than 60% helium are likely to be ineffective because their density approaches that of ambient air [114]. Controlled hypothermia (30°C) has also recently been reported in one patient as a method of minimizing the increase in $PaCO_2$ in status asthmaticus patients failing to respond to conventional mechanical ventilation [33a].

As a last resort, extracorporeal membrane oxygenation has been used successfully in patients with severe asthma unresponsive to mechanical ventilation [211]. There appears to be no role for high-frequency ventilation in cases of expiratory flow limitation because of the dynamic pulmonary hyperinflation it causes [334]. Some have advocated bronchoalveolar lavage as a means of removing airway plugs in patients with severe asthma [377], but one study reported an unacceptably high rate of pulmonary infectious complications associated with this approach [198]. Instillation of *N*-acetylcysteine may produce bronchospasm in asthmatics and should generally be avoided in mechanically ventilated patients (see discussion on sputum hydration in this chapter and Chaps. 69 and 83).

As the airways obstruction is relieved in response to therapy, improvement will be observed as a progressive decrease in the PAP to less than 30 mmH$_2$O and in $PaCO_2$ to the normal range. In most intubated asthma patients, the airway obstruction will resolve substantially within 72 hours. In patients with sudden asphyxic asthma, presumably reflecting a subpopulation of patients with status asthmaticus with ventilatory failure largely due to bronchospasm as the main pathogenetic process, the mean duration of mechanical ventilation was only 33.7 ± 25.3 hours [372]. Therefore, as soon as resolution of the asthmatic process is evident according to clinical and laboratory assessments, weaning from mechanical ventilation can begin. Although a number of ventilatory modes are available for use in weaning, including intermittent mandatory ventilation, pressure-support ventilation, and intermittent use of a T-piece, once the airway obstruction subsides, weaning usually progresses rapidly regardless of the mode chosen. Criteria for the decision to discontinue mechanical ventilation include an alveolar-arterial PO$_2$ difference measured at an FIO$_2$ of 1.0 of less than 300 to 350 mmHg or an adequate PaO$_2$ at an FIO$_2$ of 0.4 or less; a VC of at least 10 to 15 ml/kg of body weight; a normal-range $PaCO_2$ in association with a minute ventilation of less than 10 L/min; and the ability to generate an inspiratory negative pressure of greater than −30 cmH$_2$O [93, 308, 356]. Clinical findings must support these data. Hence, obvious improvement in ausculatory findings, the very important observation of mobilization of secretions, and resolution of contributing factors (e.g., pneumonia, atelectasis, heart failure) should all be apparent.

Difficulty in weaning may be encountered in patients with respiratory muscle weakness resulting from prolonged mechanical ventilation, a deficiency in the total body potassium or phosphate content, or continued use of neuromuscular-blocking drugs [182]. Ventilatory drive may be reduced by the effect of metabolic alkalosis or by the lingering effects of sedatives. Some patients develop a psychologic dependence on the ventilator; in such cases, weaning may be facilitated by the use of intermittent mandatory ventilation or pressure-support ventilation. When mechanical ventilation has been discontinued, the adequacy of ventilation should be assessed during several hours of spontaneous breathing before extubation.

Table 73-11. Complications of assisted ventilation

Complications attributable to intubation and extubation
  Prolonged intubation attempt
  Intubation of right mainstem bronchus
  Premature extubation
  Self-extubation
Complications associated with endotracheal/tracheostomy tubes
  Tube malfunction
  Nasal necrosis
Complications attributable to operation of the ventilator
  Machine failure
  Alarm failure
  Alarm found off
  Inadequate nebulization or humidification
  Overheating of inspired air
Medical complications occurring during assisted ventilation
  Alevolar hypoventilation
  Alveloar hyperventilation
  Massive gastric distention, gastrointestinal bleeding
  Pneumothorax
  Atelectasis
  Pneumonia (nosocomial)
  Hypotension

Source: C. W. Zwillich, et al., Complications of assisted ventilation: a prospective study of 354 consecutive episodes. *Am. J. Med.* 57:161, 1974. Reprinted with permission.

Complications of mechanical ventilation in status asthmaticus include pulmonary barotrauma, impaired cardiac output, and infection, in addition to a variety of ventilator and tracheal tube malfunctions encountered during mechanical ventilation (Table 73-11) [398]. A shorter duration of mechanical ventilation is associated with a decreased rate of complications, including death. The incidence of barotrauma, including pneumothorax, pneumomediastinum, and subcutaneous emphysema, is increased by the high peak inspiratory airway pressures that may be necessary to ventilate patients with severe asthma [271]. Recently, an end-inspiratory lung volume exceeding 1.4 L, measured as the volume expired from peak inspiration to end expiration some 30 to 40 seconds later, was shown to be better than high peak inspiratory airway pressures as a predictor of barotrauma and hypotension in mechanically ventilated patients with acute severe asthma [387a]. Tension pneumothorax may be manifested by a sudden increase in respiratory distress, cyanosis, and absence of breath sounds on chest auscultation. It must be immediately recognized and relieved by the insertion of a large-bore needle or chest tube into the pleural space. In a series of 21 episodes of mechanical ventilation for status asthmaticus, pneumothorax occurred in 33 percent and was associated with decreased survival [316]. In that study, pneumothorax, pneumonia, alveolar hypoventilation, tracheal tube malfunction, and ventilator failure occurred more often during mechanical ventilation in patients with status asthmaticus than in patients receiving mechanical ventilation for other causes. The use of controlled mechanical hypoventilation probably lowers the incidence of barotrauma [70].

The increase in mean intrathoracic pressure resulting from high airway pressures may impair systemic venous return and reduce the cardiac output. The problem may be aggravated by hypovolemia and by the use of drugs that increase venous capacitance, such as morphine and diazepam, and can be minimized by maintaining an adequate intravascular fluid volume and by shortening the inspiratory phase of mechanical ventilation. Cardiac factors and electrocardiographic changes in status asthmaticus are discussed in further detail in Chapter 78.

The incidence of nosocomial respiratory tract infections in intubated and mechanically ventilated patients may be reduced by careful attention to proper technique during airway care and suctioning and by changing ventilator tubing every 48 hours [60].

Table 73-12. Short-term survival in status asthmaticus supported with mechanical ventilation (adults)

Reference	Percent survival
Marchand & van Hasselt, 1966 [204]	79
Misuraca, 1966 [227]	100
Riding & Ambiavagar, 1967 [295]	82
Tabb & Guerrant, 1968 [350]	100
Williams & Crooke, 1968 [385]	89
Iisalo, et al., 1969 [155]	86
Sheehy, et al., 1972 [319]	91
Scoggin, et al., 1977 [316]	62
Westerman, et al., 1979 [381]	90
Santiago & Klaustermeyer, 1980 [311]	100
Picado, et al., 1983 [274]	77
Menitove & Goldring, 1983 [219]	100
Luksza, et al., 1986 [198]	91
Higgins, et al., 1986 [144]	100
Dworkin & Kattan, 1989 [83]	100
Mansel, et al., 1990 [203]	78
Braman & Kaemmerlen, 1990 [27]	100

Prophylactic antimicrobial therapy is not indicated and may, in fact, predispose to infection with resistant bacteria.

Considering the gravity of the attendant pathophysiologic changes, the survival rate in status asthmaticus complicated by ventilatory failure is rather good. An aggregate short-term survival rate of 89 percent was achieved in 17 published series comprising adults treated with mechanical ventilation for status asthmaticus (Table 73-12). The long-term prognosis in one series has been reported by Marquette and associates [205a]. In this analysis, among 121 patients with a near-fatal asthma attack who were followed after discharge from an intensive care unit where they received mechanical ventilation for acute status asthma, the 6-year survival was 77.4 percent; the majority of deaths occurred within the first year following discharge. Cigarette smoking and an age greater than 40 years were identified as risk factors in mortality [205a].

Since only an occasional patient with severe asthma requires intubation and supportive mechanical ventilation, the identification of such high-risk asthma patients could provide clues to preventing this problem. Accordingly, Westerman and coworkers [381] analyzed their retrospective experiences with 39 patients requiring mechanical ventilation for status asthmaticus, and identified the following features as risk factors: patient delay in seeking medical attention, incomplete medical assessment, inadequate preadmission use of corticosteroids, and sedative abuse. Follow-up of the survivors of this study also indicated that clinical patterns characterized by significantly labile asthma or chronic deterioration in airways obstruction were associated with an increased risk of sudden death from asthma. A major point to be emphasized by this and other studies [286, 347] is that patients must be educated by the physician to seek early medical attention for all acute episodes failing to respond to the usual therapy. It is hoped that this will substantially decrease the need for mechanical ventilation with its attendant morbidity.

A summary of the hospital management of acute exacerbations of asthma based on the recent National Heart, Lung, and Blood Institute expert panel report is presented in Figure 73-8.

PREVENTION AND AFTER-CRISIS CARE

Although the cause, or causes, of the recent increase in asthma death rates remain unknown, the ability to identify patients at risk enables the deployment of measures aimed at preventing the development of status asthmaticus. The British Thoracic Association [30] determined that 77 of 90 patients who died of asthma had potentially preventable contributory factors. Of course, not all patients at risk for asthma-related death can be identified prior to the event, and some severe asthma attacks (sudden asphyxic asthma) occur so rapidly that effective therapy cannot be administered. Recently several investigators described sudden death in asthmatics or the precipitous onset of asthma, referred to as *sudden asphyxic asthma* [296, 372]. In a study of 261 consecutive episodes of near-fatal asthma, 13 percent occurred in less than 1 hour [6]. On the other hand, a large majority of severe asthma attacks are slower in onset and preventive therapy is usually feasible.

The general approach to prophylaxis in asthma patients attempts to modify the known risk factors. The first step is to recognize that asthma is present and to identify patients at high risk for severe attacks. These patients require careful evaluation and optimization of their medical regimen. They must be educated regarding the severe nature of their asthma and how to recognize the onset of a severe attack. Instructions to measure and record peak airflow several times daily and to return for regular follow-up visits, at which time objective measures of airflow can be made, are recommended; at this time, educational programs can be reinforced. Patients should be taught to initiate short courses of high-dose oral corticosteroids when signs of significant deterioration occur or when peak flow falls below predetermined levels. If their deteriorating asthmatic state fails to respond to initial therapy, a crisis plan should be in place that includes physician telephone numbers and a means of contacting emergency transport and emergency department personnel [347]. These principles are further detailed in Chapters 90 and 94.

Certainly not all asthma deaths can be prevented with the above-described prophylactic program. As discussed previously, sudden asthma attacks may occur too rapidly to allow treatment, and not all patients will comply with the program outlined. Nevertheless, some reduction in asthma mortality is likely to result, as exemplified by the findings of two recent studies. Mayo and associates [210] randomized 104 adult asthmatics at high risk for severe asthma exacerbations either to an intensive outpatient treatment program or to routine outpatient care. In the intensive program, a vigorous medical regimen and educational program as well as aggressive self-management strategies for asthma exacerbation were provided. The intensive treatment program resulted in a threefold reduction in hospital readmissions and a twofold reduction in hospital day use compared to routine care. A Parisian study [16] examined the effect of improved pre-hospital care on asthma mortality, demonstrating a reduction in death rate from 9 percent to 1.5 percent when delay in physician arrival was shortened from 28.3 to 9.7 minutes.

Another aspect of preventive care is to investigate all possible contributing causes once the acute asthma attack has subsided and to institute a proper program of symptomatic control. The long-term goal is to eliminate offending causes and minimize recurrences. The establishment of an effective relationship between the patient and physician is a critical aspect of management. The knowledge that advice and care are readily available in the event of an emergency provides the patient with a strong measure of reassurance. Prospective case-controlled psychologic and physiologic profiles that attempt to identify the characteristics of fatal asthma (as reported by Strunk and colleagues [346] for children) and status asthmaticus merit continued study for all ages.

Patients may manifest a variety of reactions to the experience of status asthmaticus. As with other life-threatening crises, recollection of the episode may evoke anxiety, even terror. This response may influence the patient's perception of the severity of later asthmatic attacks, thereby influencing medication usage and the frequency of rehospitalization [66, 74, 75]. In contrast, other patients adopt denial as a defense mechanism: by minimizing their symptoms, they may permit a subsequent attack to intensify without seeking appropriate medical attention [74]

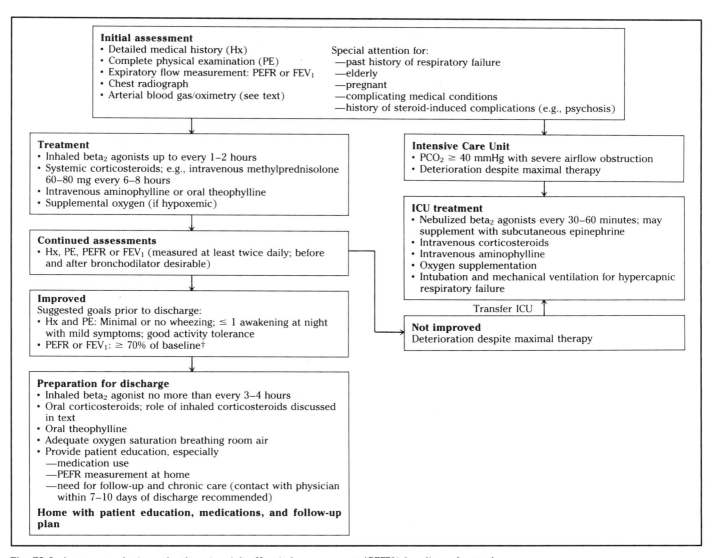

Fig. 73-8. *Acute exacerbations of asthma in adults. Hospital management. †PEFR% baseline refers to the norm for the individual, established by the clinician. This may be percentage predicted based on standardized norms or the patient's personal best percentage. (Reprinted from National Asthma Education Program, Expert Panel Report.* Executive Summary: Guidelines for the Diagnosis and Managment of Asthma. *Publication No. 91-3042A. Bethesda, MD: National Institutes of Health, June 1991. P. 30.)*

(Chap. 85). Both of these responses are maladaptive, and patient education and counseling are required to emphasize that asthma can be well controlled with optimal management and to encourage a realistic perception of the disease. At the same time, there is no place for complacency in the management of these patients, as there is no reliable guide for predicting their course. Throughout management, it is mandatory that careful observations support a rational therapeutic program. For this most critical period in asthma, it is our position that a key factor determining a successful outcome is the commitment by a compassionate, meticulously thoughtful, and knowledgeable physician.

REFERENCES

1. Aceves, M., et al. Identification of soybean dust as an epidemic agent in urban areas by molecular marker and RAST analysis of aerosols. *J. Allergy Clin. Immunol.* 88:124, 1991.

1a. Aikawa, T., et al. Marked goblet cell hyperplasia with mucus accumulation in the airways of patients who died of severe asthma attack. *Chest* 101:916, 1992.

2. Alfaro, C., et al. Inverse correlation of expiratory lung flows and sputum eosinophils in status asthmaticus. *Ann. Allergy* 63:251, 1989.

3. Appel, D., Karpel, J. P., and Sherman, M. Epinephrine improves expiratory flow rates in patients with asthma who do not respond to inhaled metaproterenol sulfate. *J. Allergy Clin. Immunol.* 84:90, 1989.

4. Appel, D., et al. Lactic acidosis in severe asthma. *Am. J. Med.* 75:580, 1983.

5. Apter, A., and Greenberger, P. A. Status asthmaticus. *Allergy Proc.* 11: 168, 1990.

6. Arnold, A. G., Lane, D. J., and Zapata, E. The speed of onset and severity of acute severe asthma. *Br. J. Dis. Chest* 76:157, 1982.

7. Attinger, E. O., Goldstein, M. M., and Segal, M. S. The mechanics of breathing in normal subjects and in patients with cardiopulmonary disease. *Ann. Intern. Med.* 48:1269, 1958.

8. Aubier, M., et al. Aminophylline improves diaphragmatic contractility. *N. Engl. J. Med.* 305:249, 1981.

9. Baetjer, A. M. Effect of ambient temperature and vapor pressure on cilia-mucus clearance rate. *J. Appl. Physiol.* 23:498, 1967.

10. Baigelman, W., et al. Sputum and blood eosinophils during corticosteroid treatment of acute exacerbations of asthma. *Am. J. Med.* 75:929, 1983.

11. Baker, J. W., Yerger, S., and Segar, W. E. Elevated plasma antidiuretic hormone levels in status asthmaticus. *Mayo Clin. Proc.* 51:31, 1976.

12. Ballester, E., et al. Ventilation-perfusion mismatching in acute severe asthma: effects of salbutamol and 100% oxygen. *Thorax* 44:258, 1989.

13. Banner, A. S., Shah, R. S, and Addington, W. W. Rapid prediction of need for hospitalization in acute asthma. *JAMA* 235:1337, 1976.

14. Barnes, P. J. Neural control of human airways in health and disease. *Am. Rev. Respir. Dis.* 134:1289, 1986.

15. Barnes, P. J., and Pride, N. B. Dose-response curves to inhaled B-adrenoceptor agonists in normal and asthmatic subjects. *Br. J. Clin. Pharmacol.* 15:677, 1983.

16. Barriot, P., and Riou, B. Prevention of fatal asthma. *Chest* 92:460, 1987.

17. Bellofiore, S., et al. Endogenous opiates modulate the increase in ventilatory output and dyspnea during severe acute bronchoconstriction. *Am. Rev. Respir. Dis.* 142:812, 1990.

18. Benatar, S. R. Fatal asthma. *N. Engl. J. Med.* 314:423, 1986.

19. Benfield, G. F. A., and Smith, A. P. Predicting rapid and slow response to treatment in acute severe asthma. *Br. J. Dis. Chest* 77:249, 1983.

20. Berkovich, S., Millian, S. J., and Snyder, R. D. The association of viral and mycoplasma infections with recurrence of wheezing in the asthmatic child. *Ann. Allergy* 28:43, 1970.

21. Berman, S. Z., et al. Transtracheal aspiration studies in asthmatic patients in relapse with "infective" asthma and in subjects without respiratory disease. *J. Allergy Clin. Immunol.* 56:206, 1975.

22. Bernstein, I. L., and Ausdenmoore, R. W. Iatrogenic bronchospasm occurring during clinical trials of a new mucolytic agent, acetylcysteine. *Dis. Chest* 46:469, 1964.

23. Bloomfield, P., et al. Comparison of salbutamol given intravenously and by intermittent positive-pressure breathing in life-threatening asthma. *Br. Med. J.* 1:848, 1979.

24. Blumberg, M. Z. Morphine for severe asthma? *N. Engl. J. Med.* 288:50, 1973.

25. Bondi, E., and Williams, M. H., Jr. Severe asthma: course and treatment in hospital. *N.Y. State J. Med.* 77:350, 1977.

26. Brady, A. R., et al. Hypophosphatemia complicating bronchodilator therapy for acute severe asthma. *Arch. Intern. Med.* 149:2367, 1989.

27. Braman, S. S., and Kaemmerlen, J. T. Intensive care of status asthmaticus. A 10 year experience. *JAMA* 264:366, 1990.

28. Braun, S. R., et al. A comparison of the effect of ipratropium and albuterol in the treatment of chronic obstructive airway disease. *Arch. Intern. Med.* 149:544, 1989.

29. Brenner, B. E., Abraham, E., and Simon, R. R. Position and diaphoresis in acute asthma. *Am. J. Med.* 74:1005, 1983.

30. British Thoracic Association. Death from asthma in two regions of England. *Br. Med. J.* 285:5251, 1982.

31. Britton, M. G., et al. High-dose corticosteroids in severe acute asthma. *Br. Med. J.* 2:73, 1976.

32. Brooks, S. M., et al. Adverse effects of phenobarbital on corticosteroid metabolism in patients with bronchial asthma. *N. Engl. J. Med.* 286:1125, 1972.

33. Brown, M. J., Brown, D. C., and Murphy, M. B. Hypokalemia from beta2 receptor stimulation by circulating epinephrine. *N. Engl. J. Med.* 309:1414, 1983.

33a. Browning, D., and Doodram, D. T. Treatment of acute severe asthma assisted by hypothermia. *Anaesthesia* 47:223, 1992.

34. Burki, N. K., and Diamond, L. Serum creatine phosphokinase activity in asthma. *Am. Rev. Respir. Dis.* 116:327, 1977.

35. Busey, H., et al. Statement by committee on therapy. *Am. Rev. Respir. Dis.* 97:735, 1968.

35a. Calhoun, W. J. Management of respiratory failure. *Chest* 101:410S, 1992.

36. Campbell, A. H., O'Connell, J. M., and Wilson, F. The effect of chest physiotherapy upon the FEV-1 in chronic bronchitis. *Med. J. Aust.* 1:33, 1975.

37. Campbell, I. A., et al. Intermittent positive-pressure breathing. *Br. Med. J.* 1:1186, 1978.

38. Cardell, B. S. Pathological findings in deaths from asthma. *Int. Arch. Allergy* 9:189, 1956.

39. Cavanaugh, M. J., and Cooper, D. M. Inhaled atropine sulfate: dose response characteristics. *Am. Rev. Respir. Dis.* 114:517, 1976.

40. Cayton, R. M., and Howard, P. Plasma cortisol and the use of hydrocortisone in the treatment of status asthmaticus. *Thorax* 28:567, 1973.

41. Centor, R. M., Yarbrough, B., and Wood, J. P. Inability to predict relapse in acute asthma. *N. Engl. J. Med.* 310:577, 1984.

42. Chen, K. K., and Meek, W. J. Further studies of the effect of ephedrine on the circulation. *J. Pharmacol. Exp. Ther.* 28:31, 1926.

43. Cheney, F. W., Jr., and Butler, J. The effects of ultrasonically produced aerosols on airway resistance in man. *Anesthesiology* 29:1099, 1968.

44. Cheong, B., et al. A comparison of intravenous with nebulized salbutamol in the treatment of acute severe asthma. *Thorax* 42:731, 1987.

45. Chodosh, S. Sputum: Observations in Status Asthmaticus and Therapeutic Considerations. In E. B. Weiss (ed.), *Status Asthmaticus.* Baltimore: University Park, 1978.

46. Chopra, S. K., et al. Effects of hydration and physical therapy on tracheal transport velocity. *Am. Rev. Respir. Dis.* 115:1009, 1977.

47. Chugh, K. S., Singhal, P. C., and Khatri, G. K. Rhabdomyolysis and renal failure following status asthmaticus. *Chest* 73:879, 1978.

48. Clarke, C. W. Relationship of bacterial and viral infections to exacerbations of asthma. *Thorax* 34:344, 1979.

49. Clarke, S. W., Jones, J. G., and Oliver, B. R. Resistance to two-phase gas-liquid flow in airways. *J. Appl. Physiol.* 29:464, 1970.

50. Cluroe, A., et al. Bronchial gland ectasia in fatal bronchial asthma: association with interstitial emphysema. *J. Clin. Pathol.* 42:1026, 1989.

51. Cochrane, G. M., and Clark, T. J. H. A survey of asthma mortality in patients between ages 35 and 64 in the Greater London hospitals in 1971. *Thorax* 30:300, 1975.

52. Colldahl, H. A study of serum enzymes in patients suffering from periods of respiratory insufficiency, especially asthma and emphysema. *Acta. Med. Scand.* 166:399, 1960.

53. Collins, J. V., and Jones, D. Corticosteroid Mechanisms and Therapeutic Schedules. In E. B. Weiss (ed.), *Staus Asthmaticus.* Baltimore: University Park, 1978.

54. Collins, J. M., et al. The cardiotoxicity of isoprenaline during hypoxia. *Br. J. Pharmacol.* 36:35, 1969.

55. Collins, J. V., et al. The use of corticosteroids in the treatment of acute asthma. *Q. J. Med.* 44:259, 1975.

56. Collins, J. V., et al. Intravenous corticosteroids in treatment of acute bronchial asthma. *Lancet* 2:1047, 1970.

57. Compton, G. K. Severe Acute Asthma. In P. J. Barnes, I. W. Rodger, and N. C. Thomson (eds.), *Asthma, Basic Mechanisms and Clinical Management.* London: Academic Press, 1988.

58. Cooper, D. J., et al. Bicarbonate does not improve hemodynamics in critically ill patients who have lactic acidosis. A prospective, controlled clinical study. *Ann. Intern. Med.* 112:492, 1990.

59. Corrigan, C. J., et al. Cultured peripheral blood mononuclear cells derived from patients with acute severe asthma ("status asthmaticus") spontaneously elaborate a neutrophil chemotactic activity distinct from interleukin-8. *Am. Rev. Respir. Dis.* 143:538, 1991.

60. Craven, D. E., et al. Contamination of mechanical ventilators with tubing changes every 24 or 48 hours. *N. Engl. J. Med.* 306:1505, 1982.

61. Crawford, S. M., and Miles, D. W. Salbutamol and cardiac arrhythmias. *Curr. Med. Res. Opin.* 7:410, 1981.

62. Crepea, S. B., and Harman, J. W. The pathology of bronchial asthma: I. The significance of membrane changes in asthmatic and non-allergic pulmonary disease. *J. Allergy* 26:453, 1955.

63. Cua-Lim, F., and Lim, M. G. Relationship of acute bacterial (suppurative sinusitis) and viral (pneumonitis) infections to status asthmaticus. *J. Asthma Res.* 9:31, 1971.

64. Cutz, E., Levison, H., and Cooper, D. M. Ultrastructure of airways in children with asthma. *Histopathology* 2:407, 1978.

65. Cydulka, R., et al. The use of epinephrine in the treatment of older adult asthmatics. *Ann. Emerg. Med.* 17:322, 1988.

66. Dahlem, N. W., Kinsman, R. A., and Horton, D. J. Panic-fear in asthma: requests for as-needed medications in relation to pulmonary function measurements. *J. Allergy Clin. Immunol.* 60:295, 1977.

67. Dale, D. C., Fauci, A. S., and Wolff, S. M. Alternate-day prednisone: leukocyte kinetics and susceptibility to infections. *N. Engl. J. Med.* 291:1154, 1974.

68. Dales, R. E., and Munt, P. W. Use of mechanical ventilation in adults with severe asthma. *Can. Med. Assoc. J.* 130:391, 1984.

69. Daley, J., et al. Practice patterns in the treatment of acutely ill hospitalized asthmatic patients at three teaching hospitals. *Chest* 100:51, 1991.

70. Darioli, R., and Perret, C. Mechanical controlled hypoventilation in status asthmaticus. *Am. Rev. Respir. Dis.* 129:385, 1984.

71. Dattwyler, R. J., Goldman, M. A., and Bloch, K. J. Pneumomediastinum as a complication of asthma in teenage and young adult patients. *J. Allergy Clin. Immunol.* 63:412, 1979.

72. Dekker, E., and Groen, J. Asthmatic wheezing: compression of the trachea and major bronchi as a cause. *Lancet* 1:1064, 1957.

73. Despas, P. J., Leroux, M., and Macklem, P. T. Site of airway obstruction in asthma as determined by measuring maximal expiratory flow breathing air and a helium-oxygen mixture. *J. Clin. Invest.* 51:3235, 1972.

74. Dirks, J. F., et al. Panic-fear in asthma: rehospitalization following intensive long-term treatment. *Psychosom. Med.* 40:5, 1978.

75. Dirks, J. F., Jones, N. F., and Kinsman, R. A. Panic-fear: a personality dimension related to intractability in asthma. *Psychosom. Med.* 39:120, 1977.

76. Disney, M. E., Matthews, R., and Williams, J. D. The role of infection in the morbidity of asthmatic children admitted to hospital. *Clin. Allergy* 1:399, 1971.

77. Donaldson, J. C., et al. Acetylcysteine for life-threatening acute bronchial obstruction. *Ann. Intern. Med.* 88:656, 1978.

78. Downes, J. J., et al. Arterial blood gas and acid-base disorders in infants and children with status asthmaticus. *Pediatrics* 42:238, 1968.

79. Dulfano, M. J., Adler, K., and Wooten, O. Physical properties of sputum: IV. Effects of 100 percent humidity and water mist. *Am. Rev. Respir. Dis.* 107:130, 1973.

80. Dunnill, M. S. The pathology of asthma, with special reference to changes in the bronchial mucosa. *J. Clin. Pathol.* 13:27, 1960.

81. Dunnill, M. S., Massarella, G. R., and Anderson, J. A. A comparison of the quantitative anatomy of the bronchi in normal subjects, in status asthmaticus, in chronic bronchitis, and in emphysema. *Thorax* 24:176, 1969.

82. Dworetzky, M., and Philson, A. D. Review of asthmatic patients hospitalized in the pavilion service of the New York Hospital from 1948 to 1963, with emphasis on mortality rate. *J. Allergy* 41:181, 1968.

83. Dworkin, G., and Kattan, M. Mechanical ventilation for status asthmaticus in children. *J. Pediatr.* 114:545, 1989.

84. Earle, B. V. Fatal bronchial asthma: a series of 15 cases with review of the literature. *Thorax* 8:195, 1953.

85. Eggleston, P. A., et al. Radiographic abnormalities in acute asthma in children. *Pediatrics* 54:442, 1974.

86. Ellul-Micallef, R., and Fenech, F. F. Effect of intravenous prednisolone in asthmatics with diminished adrenergic responsiveness. *Lancet* 2:1269, 1975.

87. Evans, R., et al. National trends in the morbidity and mortality of asthma in the U.S. *Chest* 91:655, 1987.

88. Evans, W. V., et al. Aminophylline, salbutamol and combined intravenous infusions in acute severe asthma. *Br. J. Dis. Chest* 74:385, 1980.

89. Faling, L. J. The Role of Sedatives and Implications of Ventilatory Control in Status Asthmaticus. In E. B. Weiss (ed.), *Status Asthmaticus.* Baltimore: University Park, 1978.

90. Fanta, C. H., Rossing, T. H., and McFadden, E. R., Jr. Emergency room treatment of asthma: relationships among therapeutic combinations, severity of obstruction and time course of response. *Am. J. Med.* 72:416, 1982.

91. Fanta, C. H., Rossing, T. H., and McFadden, E. R., Jr. Glucocorticoids in acute asthma: a critical controlled trial. *Am. J. Med.* 74:85, 1983.

92. Fanta, C. H., Rossing, T. H., and McFadden, E. R. Treatment of acute asthma. Is combination therapy with sympathomimetics and methylxanthines indicated? *Am. J. Med.* 80:5, 1986.

93. Feeley, T. W., and Hedley-Whyte, J. Weaning from controlled ventilation and supplemental oxygen. *N. Engl. J. Med.* 292:903, 1975.

94. Ferguson, R. J., et al. Nebulized salbutamol in life-threatening asthma: is IPPB necessary? *Br. J. Dis. Chest* 77:255, 1983.

95. Field, G. B. The effects of posture, oxygen, isoproterenol and atropine on ventilation-perfusion relationships in the lung in asthma. *Clin. Sci.* 32:279, 1967.

96. Findley, L. J., and Sahn, S. A. The value of chest roentgenograms in acute asthma in adults. *Chest* 80:535, 1981.

97. Fischl, M. A., Pitchenik, A., and Gardner, L. B. An index predicting relapse and need for hospitalization in patients with acute bronchial asthma. *N. Engl. J. Med.* 305:783, 1981.

98. Fitchett, D. H., McNicol, M. W., and Riordan, J. F. Intravenous salbutamol in management of status asthmaticus. *Br. Med. J.* 1:53, 1975.

99. Flavahan, N. A., et al. Respiratory epithelium inhibits bronchial smooth muscle tone. *J. Appl. Physiol.* 8:834, 1985.

100. Flenley, D. C. Blood gas tensions in severe asthma. *Proc. R. Soc. Med.* 64:1149, 1971.

101. Foster, W. M., Langenback, E. G., and Bergofsky, E. H. Respiratory drugs influence lung mucociliary clearance in central and peripheral ciliated airways. *Chest* 80:877, 1981.

102. Fraser, P. M., et al. The circumstances preceding death from asthma in young people in 1968 to 1969. *Br. J. Dis. Chest* 65:71, 1971.

103. Freelander, M., and van Asperen, P. P. Nebuhaler versus nebulizer treatment of acute severe asthma in children. *Br. Med. J.* 288:1873, 1984.

104. Frigas, E., et al. Elevated levels of the eosinophil granule major basic protein in the sputum of patients with bronchial asthma. *Mayo Clin. Proc.* 56:345, 1981.

105. Fuglsang, G., and Pedersen, S. Comparison of nebuhaler and nebulizer treatment of acute severe asthma in children. *Eur. J. Respir. Dis.* 69:109, 1986.

106. Galant, S. P., et al. Decreased beta-adrenergic receptors on polymorphonuclear leukocytes after adrenergic therapy. *N. Engl. J. Med.* 299:933, 1978.

107. Gandevia, B. Pressurized sympathomimetic aerosols and their lack of relationship to asthma mortality in Australia. *Med. J. Aust.* 1:273, 1973.

108. Gazioglu, K., et al. Effect of isoproterenol on gas exchange during air and oxygen breathing in patients with asthma. *Am. J. Med.* 50:185, 1971.

109. Gelb, A. F., et al. P pulmonale in status asthmaticus. *J. Allergy Clin. Immunol.* 64:18, 1979.

110. Gerber, M. A., Paronetto, F., and Kochwa, S. Immunohistochemical localization of IgE in asthmatic lungs. *Am. J. Pathol.* 62:339, 1971.

111. Gershel, J. C., et al. The usefulness of chest radiographs in first asthma attacks. *N. Engl. J. Med.* 309:336, 1983.

112. Gillies, D. R. N., Conway, S. P., and Littlewood, J. M. Chest x-rays and childhood asthma. *Lancet* 2:1149, 1983.

113. Girsh, L. S. Air Pollutants and Weather and Their Effects on Bronchial Asthma. In C. A. Frazier (ed.), *Annual Review of Allergy 1973.* Flushing, N.Y.: Medical Examination, 1974, Chap. 12, P. 237.

114. Gluck, E. H., Onorato, O. J., and Castriotta, R. Helium-oxygen mixtures in intubated patients with status asthmaticus and respiratory acidosis. *Chest* 98:693, 1990.

115. Gluck, J. C., Busto, R., and Marks, M. B. Pulsus paradoxus in childhood asthma—its prognostic value. *Ann. Allergy* 38:405, 1977.

116. Godfrey, S., et al. Repeatability of physical signs in airways obstruction. *Thorax* 24:4, 1969.

117. Gold, M. I., and Helrich, M. Pulmonary mechanics during general anesthesia: V. Status asthmaticus. *Anesthesiology* 32:422, 1970.

118. Goldie, R. G. Receptors in asthmatic airways. *Am. Rev. Respir. Dis.* 141: S151, 1990.

119. Goldie, R. G., et al. In vitro responsiveness of human asthmatic bronchus to carbachol, histamine, B-adrenoceptor agonists and theophylline. *Br. J. Clin. Pharmacol.* 22:669, 1986.

120. Goldie, R. G., et al. The status of B-adrenoceptor function in asthma. *Pharmacology: Exerpta Medica Congress Series* 750:465, 1987.

121. Goldman, M. D., Grimby, G., and Mead, J. Mechanical work of breathing derived from rib cage and abdominal V-P partitioning. *J. Appl. Physiol.* 41:752, 1976.

122. Gough, J. Post-mortem differences in "asthma" and in chronic bronchitis. *Acta Allergol.* (Kbh.) 16:391, 1961.

123. Graham, V. A. L., et al. Routine antibiotics in hospital management of acute asthma. *Lancet* 1:418, 1982.

124. Grant, I. W. B. Are corticosteroids necessary in the treatment of severe acute asthma? *Br. J. Dis. Chest* 76:125, 1982.

125. Grant, I. W. B. Has the change to beta-agonists combined with oral theophylline increased cases of fatal asthma? *Lancet* 2:36, 1981.

126. Grant, I. W. B. Asthma in New Zealand. *Br. Med. J.* 286:374, 1983.

126a. Griffen, D., et al. Acute myopathy during treatment of status asthmaticus with corticosteroids and steroidal muscle relaxants. *Chest* 102:510, 1992.

127. Gross, G. N., Souhrada, J. F., and Farr, R. S. The long-term treatment of an asthmatic patient using phentolamine. *Chest* 66:397, 1974.

128. Grunberg, G., et al. Facilitation of mechanical ventilation in status asthmaticus with continuous thiopental. *Chest* 99:1216, 1991.

129. Hahn, D. L., Dodge, R. W., and Goulubjatnikov, R. Association of *Chlamydia pneumoniae* (strain twar) infection with wheezing, asthmatic bronchitis, and adult-onset asthma. *JAMA* 226:225, 1991.

130. Hall, J. B., and Wood, L. D. Management of the critically ill asthmatic patient. *Med. Clin. North Am.* 74:779, 1990.

131. Halmagyi, D. F., and Cotes, J. E. Reduction in systemic blood oxygen as a result of procedures affecting the pulmonary circulation in patients with chronic pulmonary diseases. *Clin. Sci.* 18:475, 1959,.

132. Handslip, P. D. J., Dart, A. M., and Davies, B. H. Intravenous salbutamol and aminophylline in asthma: a search for synergy. *Thorax* 36:741, 1981.

133. Haskell, R. J., Wong, B. M., and Hansen, J. E. A double-blind, randomized clinical trial of methylprednisolone in status asthmaticus. *Arch. Intern. Med.* 143:1324, 1983.

134. Heard, B. E., and Houssain, S. Hyperplasia of bronchial muscle in asthma. *J. Pathol.* 110:319, 1973.

135. Hedstrand, U. The optimal frequency of breathing in bronchial asthma. *Scand. J. Respir. Dis.* 52:217, 1971.

136. Hendeles, L., Weinberger, M., and Bighley, L. Disposition of theophylline after a single intravenous infusion of aminophylline. *Am. Rev. Respir. Dis.* 118:97, 1978.

137. Hensley, M. J., et al. Distribution of bronchodilatation in normal subjects: beta agonist versus atropine. *J. Appl. Physiol.* 45:778, 1978.

138. Herman, J. J., Noah, Z. L., and Moody, R. R. Use of intravenous isoproterenol for status asthmaticus in children. *Crit. Care Med.* 11:716, 1983.

139. Herxheimer, H. Antihistamines in bronchial asthma. *Br. Med. J.* 2:901, 1949.

140. Hetzel, M. R., and Clark, T. J. H. Comparison of intravenous and aerosol salbutamol. *Br. Med. J.* 2:919, 1976.

141. Hetzel, M. R., Clark, T. J. H., and Branthwaite, M. A. Asthma: analysis of sudden deaths and ventilatory arrests in hospital. *Br. Med. J.* 1:808, 1977.

142. Hetzel, M. R., Clark, T. J. H., and Houston, K. Physiological patterns in early morning asthma. *Thorax* 32:418, 1977.

143. Higer, R. W., and Holliday, M. A. Acute bronchial asthma and possible inappropriate secretion of antidiuretic hormone. *Pediatr. Res.* 7:428, 1973.

144. Higgins, B., Greening, A., and Crompton, G. Assisted ventilation in severe acute asthma. *Thorax* 41:464, 1986.

145. Higgins, R. M., Stradling, J. R., and Lane, D. J. Should ipratropium bromide be added to beta-agonists in treatment of acute severe asthma? *Chest* 94:718, 1988.

146. Hill, N. S. The use of theophylline in "irreversible" chronic obstructive pulmonary disease. *Arch. Intern. Med.* 148:2579, 1988.

147. Hogg, J. C. Varieties of airway narrowing in severe and fatal asthma. *J. Allergy Clin. Immunol.* 80:417, 1987.

148. Holgate, S. T., Baldwin, C. J., and Tattersfield, A. E. B-adrenergic agonist resistance in normal human airways. *Lancet* 2:375, 1977.

149. Horn, B. R., et al. Total eosinophil counts in the management of bronchial asthma. *N. Engl. J. Med.* 292:1152, 1975.

150. Houston, J. C., DeNevasquez, S., and Trounce, J. R. A clinical and pathological study of fatal cases of status asthmaticus. *Thorax* 8:207, 1953.

151. Huber, H. L., and Koessler, K. K. The pathology of bronchial asthma. *Arch. Intern. Med.* 30:689, 1922.

152. Hudgel, D. W., et al. Viral and bacterial infections in adults with chronic asthma. *Am. Rev. Respir. Dis.* 120:393, 1979.

153. Huhti, E., et al. Association of viral and mycoplasma infections with exacerbations of asthma. *Ann. Allergy* 33:145, 1974.

154. Huseby, J., et al. Oxygenation during chest physiotherapy. *Chest* 70:430, 1976.

155. Iisalo, E. U. M., Iisalo, E. I., and Vapaavuori, M. J. Prolonged artificial ventilation in severe status asthmaticus. *Acta Med. Scand.* 185:51, 1969.

156. Ind, P. W., et al. Circulating catecholamines in acute asthma. *Br. Med. J.* 290:267, 1985.

157. Ingram, R. H., Jr., et al. Relative contributions of large and small airways to flow limitation in normal subjects before and after atropine and isoproterenol. *J. Clin. Invest.* 59:696, 1977.

158. Inman, W. H. W., and Adelstein, A. M. Rise and fall of asthma mortality in England and Wales in relation to use of pressurized aerosols. *Lancet* 2:279, 1969.

159. Intermittent Positive Presure Breathing Trial Group. Intermittent positive pressure breathing in therapy of COPD. *Ann. Intern. Med.* 99:612, 1983.

160. Isles, A. F., and Newth, C. J. L. Combined beta agonists and methylxanthines in asthma. *N. Engl. J. Med.* 309:432, 1983.

161. Jackson, R. H., et al. Clinical evaluation of Elixophyllin with correlation of pulmonary function studies and theophylline serum levels in acute and chronic asthmatic patients. *Dis. Chest* 45:75, 1964.

162. Jackson, R. T., et al. Mortality from asthma: a new epidemic in New Zealand. *Br. Med. J.* 285:771, 1982.

163. Jederlinic, P. J., and Irwin, R. S. Status asthmaticus. *J. Intensive Care Med.* 4:166, 1989.

164. Jenkins, P. F., Benfield, G. F. A., and Smith, A. P. Predicting recovery from acute severe asthma. *Thorax* 36:835, 1981.

165. Jenne, J. W., et al. Subsensitivity of beta responses during therapy with a long-acting beta-2 preparation. *J. Allergy Clin. Immunol.* 59:383, 1977.

166. Johnston, R. G., et al. Isoflurane therapy for status asthmaticus in children and adults. *Chest* 97:698, 1990.

167. Jones, R. S. The physiology and management of childhood asthma. *Postgrad. Med.* 47:181, 1971.

168. Josephson, G. W., et al. Emergency treatment of asthma: a comparison of two treatment regimens. *JAMA* 242:639, 1979.

169. Kandel, G., and Aberman, A. Mixed venous oxygen saturation: its role

170. Karetzky, M. S. Asthma mortality associated with pneumothorax and intermittent positive-pressure breathing. *Lancet* 1:828, 1975.

171. Karetzky, M. S. Asthma mortality: an analysis of one year's experience, review of the literature and assessment of current modes of therapy. *Medicine (Baltimore)* 54:471, 1975.

172. Karetzky, M. S. Asthma in the South Bronx: clinical and epidemiologic characteristics. *J. Allergy Clin. Immunol.* 60:383, 1977.

173. Kattan, M., Gurwitz, D., and Levison, H. Corticosteroids in status asthmaticus. *J. Pediatr.* 96:596, 1980.

174. Keighley, J. F. Iatrogenic asthma associated with adrenergic aerosols. *Ann. Intern. Med.* 65:985, 1966.

175. Kelly, H. W., Menendez, R., and Voyles, W. Lack of significant arrhythmogenicity from chronic theophylline and beta-2 adrenergic combination therapy in asthmatic subjects. *Ann. Allergy* 54:405, 1985.

176. Kelsen, S. G., et al. Emergency room assessment and treatment of patients with acute asthma: adequacy of the conventional approach. *Am. J. Med.* 64:622, 1978.

177. Kjellman, B. Bronchial asthma and recurrent pneumonia in children. Clinical evaluation of 14 children. *Acta Paediatr. Scand.* 56:651, 1967.

178. Klaustermeyer, W. B., DiBernardo, R. L., and Hale, F. C. Intravenous isoproterenol: rationale for bronchial asthma. *J. Allergy Clin. Immunol.* 55:325, 1975.

179. Knowles, G. K., and Clark, T. J. H. Pulsus paradoxus as a valuable sign indicating severity of asthma. *Lancet* 2:1356, 1973.

180. Kreisman, H., et al. Synergism between ipratropium and theophylline in asthma. *Thorax* 36:387, 1981.

181. Kryger, M. H., et al. Effect of meperidine on occlusion pressure responses to hypercapnia and hypoxia with and without external inspiratory resistance. *Am. Rev. Respir. Dis.* 114:333, 1976.

182. Kupfer, Y., et al. Disuse atrophy in a ventilated patient with status asthmaticus receiving neuromuscular blockade. *Crit. Care Med.* 15:795, 1987.

183. Kurland, G., Williams, J., and Lewiston, N. J. Fatal myocardial toxicity during continuous infusion intravenous isoproterenol therapy of asthma. *J. Allergy Clin. Immunol.* 63:407, 1979.

184. Laaban, J. P., et al. Cardiac arrhythmias during the combined use of intravenous aminophylline and terbutaline in status asthmaticus. *Chest* 94:496, 1988.

185. Laaban, J. P., et al. Hypophosphatemia complicating management of acute severe asthma. *Ann. Intern. Med.* 112:68, 1990.

186. Lake, K. B., et al. Fatal disseminated aspergillosis in an asthmatic patient treated with corticosteroids. *Chest* 83:138, 1983.

187. Lakshminarayan, S., et al. Effect of diazepam on ventilatory responses. *Clin. Pharmacol. Ther.* 20:78, 1976.

188. Larsson, S., Svedmyr, N., and Thiringer, G. Lack of bronchial beta adrenoceptor resistance in asthmatics during long-term treatment with terbutaline. *J. Allergy Clin. Immunol.* 59:93, 1977.

189. Lawford, P., Jones, B. J. M., and Milledge, J. S. Comparison of intravenous and nebulized salbutamol in initial treatment of severe asthma. *Br. Med. J.* 1:84, 1978.

190. Lefcoe, N. M., Toogood, J. H., and Jones, T. R. In vitro pharmacologic studies of bronchodilator compounds; interactions and mechanisms. *J. Allergy Clin. Immunol.* 55:94, 1975.

191. Levin, N., and Dillon, J. B. Status asthmaticus and pancuronium bromide. *JAMA* 222:1265, 1972.

192. Lewis, R. Epidemic asthma in New Orleans: A summary of knowledge to date. *J. Louisiana Med. Soc.* 115:300, 1963.

193. Lightbody, I. M., et al. Ipratropium bromide, salbutamol and prednisolone in bronchial asthma and chronic bronchitis. *Br. J. Dis. Chest* 72:181, 1978.

194. Lisboa, C., et al. Is extrathoracic airway obstruction important in asthma? *Am. Rev. Respir. Dis.* 122:115, 1980.

195. Loren, M. L., et al. Corticosteroids in treatment of acute exacerbations of asthma. *Ann. Allergy* 45:67, 1980.

196. Lowell, F. C. Clinical aspects of eosinophilia in atopic disease. *JAMA* 202:875, 1967.

197. Luksza, A. R. Acute severe asthma treated without steroids. *Br. J. Dis. Chest* 76:15, 1982.

198. Luksza, A. R., et al. Acute severe asthma treated by mechanical ventilation: 10 years' experience from a district general hospital. *Thorax* 41:459, 1986.

199. Macdonald, J. B., Seaton, A., and Williams, D. A. Asthma deaths in Cardiff 1963–74: 90 deaths outside hospital. *Br. Med. J.* 1:1493, 1976.

170. (continued) in the assessment of the critically ill patient. *Arch. Intern. Med.* 143:1400, 1983.

200. Macdonald, J. B., et al. Asthma deaths in Cardiff 1963–74: 53 deaths in hospital. *Br. Med. J.* 2:721, 1976.

201. Maguire, J. F., Geha, R. S., and Umetsu, D. T. Myocardial specific creatine phosphokinase isoenzyme elevations in children with asthma treated with intravenous isoproterenol. *J. Allergy Clin. Immunol.* 78:631, 1986.

202. Mansel, J. K., Strogner, S. W., and Norman, J. R. Face-mask CPAP and sodium bicarbonate infusion in acute, severe asthma and metabolic acidosis. *Chest* 96:943, 1989.

203. Mansel, J. K., et al. Mechanical ventilation in patients with acute severe asthma. *Am. J. Med.* 89:42, 1990.

204. Marchand, P., and van Hasselt, H. Last-resort treatment of status asthmaticus. *Lancet* 1:227, 1966.

205. Marini, J. Should PEEP be used in airflow obstruction? (editorial). *Am. Rev. Respir. Dis.* 140:1, 1989.

205a. Marquette, C. H., et al. Long-term prognosis of near-fatal asthma. *Am. Rev. Respir. Dis.* 146:76, 1992.

206. Martin, J. G., Shore, S., and Engel, L. A. Effect of continuous positive airway pressure on respiratory mechanics and pattern of breathing in induced asthma. *Am. Rev. Respir. Dis.* 126:812, 1982.

207. Martin, J., et al. The role of respiratory muscles in the hyperinflation of bronchial asthma. *Am. Rev. Respir. Dis.* 121:441, 1980.

208. Matson, J. R., Loughlin, G. M., and Strunk, R. C. Myocardial ischemia complicating the use of isoproterenol in asthmatic children. *J. Pediatr.* 92:776, 1978.

209. May, J. R. *Chemotherapy of Chronic Bronchitis and Allied Disorders.* London: The English Universities, 1968, P. 83.

210. Mayo, P. H., Richman, J., and Harris, H. W. Results of a program to reduce admissions for adult asthma. *Ann. Intern. Med.* 112:864, 1990.

211. McDonnell, K. F., et al. Extracorporeal membrane oxygenator support in a case of severe status asthmaticus. *Ann. Thorac. Surg.* 31:171, 1981.

212. McFadden, E. R., Jr., Kiser, R., and deGroot, W. J. Acute bronchial asthma: relations between clinical and physiological manifestations. *N. Engl. J. Med.* 288:221, 1973.

213. McFadden, E. R., Jr., and Lyons, H. A. Airway resistance and uneven ventilation in bronchial asthma. *J. Appl. Physiol.* 25:365, 1968.

214. McFadden, E. R., Jr., and Lyons, H. A. Arterial-blood gas tension in asthma. *N. Engl. J. Med.* 278:1027, 1968.

215. McFadden, E. R., Jr., et al. A controlled study of the effects of single doses of hydrocortisone on the resolution of acute attacks of asthma. *Am. J. Med.* 60:52, 1976.

216. McIntosh, K., et al. The association of viral and bacterial respiratory infections with exacerbations of wheezing in young asthmatic children. *J. Pediatr.* 82:578, 1973.

217. McNamara, R. M., et al. Intravenous magnesium sulfate in the management of acute respiratory failure complicating asthma. *Ann. Emerg. Med.* 18:197, 1989.

218. Medical Research Council. Controlled trial of the effects of cortisone acetate in status asthmaticus. *Lancet* 2:803, 1956.

219. Menitove, S. M., and Goldring, R. M. Combined ventilator and bicarbonate strategy in the management of status asthmaticus. *Am. J. Med.* 74:898, 1983.

220. Messer, J., et al. Association of adrenocorticosteroid therapy and peptic-ulcer disease. *N. Engl. J. Med.* 309:21, 1983.

221. Messer, J. W., Peters, G. A., and Bennett, W. A. Causes of death and pathologic findings in 304 cases of bronchial asthma. *Dis. Chest* 38:616, 1960.

222. Meurs, H., et al. The B-adrenergic system and allergic bronchial asthma: changes in lymphocyte B-adrenergic receptor number and adenylate cyclase activity after allergen-induced asthma attack. *J. Allergy Clin. Immunol.* 70:272, 1982.

223. Michel, H., and Zander, M. V. Frequency of bacterial complications in patients treated with corticosteroids for bronchial asthma. *Klin. Wochenschr.* 45:1250, 1967.

224. Milledge, J. S., and Benjamin, S. Arterial desaturation after sodium bicarbonate therapy in bronchial asthma. *Am. Rev. Respir. Dis.* 105:126, 1972.

224a. Miller, T. P., Greenberger, P. A., and Patterson, R. The diagnosis of potentially fatal asthma in hospitalized patients. *Chest* 102:515, 1992.

225. Minor, T. E., et al. Viruses as precipitants of asthmatic attacks in children. *JAMA* 227:292, 1974.

226. Mishkin, F. S., Wagner, H. N., Jr., and Tow, D. E. Regional distribution of pulmonary arterial blood flow in acute asthma. *JAMA* 203:1019, 1968.

227. Misuraca, Le R. Mechanical ventilation in status asthmaticus. *N. Engl. J. Med.* 275:318, 1966.

228. Mitenko, P. A., and Ogilvie, R. I. Rational intravenous doses of theophylline. *N. Engl. J. Med.* 289:600, 1973.

229. Moler, F. W., Hurwitz, M. E., and Caster, J. R. Improvement in clinical asthma score and PaO$_2$ in children with severe asthma treated with continuously nebulized terbutaline. *J. Allergy Clin. Immunol.* 81:1101, 1988.

230. Molfino, N. A., et al. Respiratory arrest in near-fatal asthma. *N. Engl. J. Med.* 324:285, 1991.

231. Morley, T. F., et al. Comparison of beta-adrenergic agents delivered by nebulizer vs. metered dose inhaler with InspirEase in hospitalized asthmatic patients. *Chest* 94:1205, 1988.

232. Mountain, R. D., and Sahn, S. A. Clinical features and outcome in patients with acute asthma presenting with hypercapnia. *Am. Rev. Respir. Dis.* 138:535, 1988.

233. Mountain, R. D., et al. Acid-base disturbances in acute asthma. *Chest* 98:651, 1990.

234. Mukherjee, C., Caron, M. G., and Lefkowitz, R. J. Catecholamine-induced subsensitivity of adenylate cyclase associated with loss of B-adrenergic receptor binding sites. *Proc. Natl. Acad. Sci. USA* 72:1945, 1975.

235. Muller, N., Bryan, A. C., and Zamel, N. Tonic inspiratory muscle activity as a cause of hyperinflation in histamine-induced asthma. *J. Appl. Physiol.* 49:869, 1980.

236. National Health Statistics Center. New Zealand health statistics report—mortality and demographic data, 1959–1979. Wellington, New Zealand.

237. Naylor, B. The shedding of the mucosa of the bronchial tree in asthma. *Thorax* 17:69, 1962.

238. Neder, G. A., Jr., et al. Death in status asthmaticus: role of sedation. *Dis. Chest* 44:263, 1963.

239. Nelson, H. S., et al. Subsensitivity to the bronchodilator action of albuterol produced by chronic administration. *Am. Rev. Respir. Dis.* 116:871, 1977.

240. Neville, A., et al. Metabolic effects of salbutamol; comparison of aerosol and intravenous administration. *Br. Med. J.* 1:413, 1977.

241. Newhouse, M., and Dolovich, M. Aerosol therapy: nebulizer vs. metered dose inhaler. *Chest* 91:799, 1987.

242. Nicklas, R. A., Whitehurst, V. E., and Donohoe, R. F. Combined use of beta-adrenergic agonists and methylxanthines. *N. Engl. J. Med.* 307:557, 1982.

243. Noelpp, B., and Noelpp-Eschenhagen, I. Der experimentelle asthma bronchiale des Meerschweinchens: I. Mitteilung: Methoden zur objektiven Erfasung (Registrierung) des Asth-Maanfallse. *Int. Arch. Allergy Appl. Immunol.* 2:308, 1951.

244. Noelpp, B., and Noelpp-Eschenhagen, I. Der experimentelle asthma bronchiale des Meerschweinchens: II. Mitteilung: Die Rolle bedingter Reflexe in der Pathogenese des Asthma bronchiale. *Int. Arch. Allergy Appl. Immunol.* 2:321, 1951.

245. Noseda, A., and Yernault, J. C. Sympathomimetics in acute severe asthma: inhaled or parenteral, nebulizer or spacer? *Eur. Respir. J.* 2:377, 1989.

246. Novey, H. S. Cardiotoxicity of combined theophylline-beta-adrenergic agonist therapy for asthma. *Immunol. Allergy Pract.* 5:208, 1983.

247. Nowak, R. M., et al. Arterial blood gases and pulmonary function testing in acute bronchial asthma: predicting patient outcomes. *JAMA* 249:2043, 1983.

248. O'Connell, M. B., and Iber, C. Continuous intravenous terbutaline infusions for adult patients with status asthmaticus. *Ann. Allergy* 64:213, 1990.

249. Ogirala, R. G., et al. High-dose intramuscular triamcinolone in severe, chronic, life-threatening asthma. *N. Engl. J. Med.* 324:585, 1991.

250. O'Halloren, M. T., et al. Exposure to an aeroallergen as a possible precipitating factor in respiratory arrest in young patients with asthma. *N. Engl. J. Med.* 324:359, 1991.

251. Ohman, J. L., et al. The diffusing capacity in asthma: effect of airflow obstruction. *Am. Rev. Respir. Dis.* 107:932, 1973.

252. Ohman, J. L., Jr., Lawrence, M., and Lowell, F. C. Effect of propranolol on the responses of cortisol, isoproterenol, and aminophylline. *J. Allergy Clin. Immunol.* 50:151, 1972.

253. Okayane, H., et al. Bronchodilating effect of intravenous magnesium sulfate in bronchial asthma. *JAMA* 257:1076, 1987.

254. Okrent, D., et al. Metabolic acidosis is not due to lactic acidosis in patients with severe acute asthma. *Crit. Care Med.* 15:1098, 1987.

255. Olive, J. T., Jr., and Hyatt, R. E. Maximal expiratory flow and total respiratory resistance during induced bronchoconstriction in asthmatic subjects. *Am. Rev. Respir. Dis.* 106:366, 1972.

256. Ormerod, L. P., and Stableforth, D. E. Asthma mortality in Birmingham 1975–7: 53 deaths. *Br. Med. J.* 280:687, 1980.

257. O'Rourke, P. P., and Crone, R. K. Halothane in status asthmaticus. *Crit. Care Med.* 10:341, 1982.

258. Osler, W. *The Principles and Practice of Medicine* (4th ed). Edinburgh: Pentland, 1901.

259. Ostrea, E. M., Jr., and Odell, G. B. The influence of bicarbonate administration on blood pH in a "closed system": clinical implications. *J. Pediatr.* 80:671, 1972.

260. Palmer, K. N. V. Reduction of sputum viscosity by a water aerosol in chronic bronchitis. *Lancet* 1:91, 1960.

261. Palmer, K. N. V., and Diament, M. L. Hypoxemia in bronchial asthma. *Lancet* 1:318, 1968.

262. Pang, L. M., et al. Terbutaline in the treatment of status asthmaticus. *Chest* 72:469, 1977.

263. Pariente, R. Status Asthmaticus. In F. B. Michel, J. Bousquet, and P. Godard (eds.), *Highlights in Asthmology*. Berlin: Springer-Verlag, 1988.

264. Parness, S. M., et al. Status asthmaticus treated with isoflurane and enflurane. *Anesth. Analg.* 66:193, 1987.

265. Patel, K. R., et al. The effect of thymoxamine and cromolyn sodium on postexercise bronchoconstriction in asthma. *J. Allergy Clin. Immunol.* 57:285, 1976.

266. Paterson, J. W., et al. Isoprenaline resistance and the use of pressurized aerosols in asthma. *Lancet* 2:426, 1968.

267. Pavia, D., Thomson, M. L., and Clarke, S. W. Enhanced clearance of secretions from the human lung after the administration of hypertonic saline aerosol. *Am. Rev. Respir. Dis.* 117:199, 1978.

268. Pavia, D., et al. Effect of ipratropium bromide on mucociliary clearance and pulmonary function in reversible airways obstruction. *Thorax* 34:501, 1979.

269. Pavord, I. D., Wisniewski, A., and Tattersfield, A. E. Inhaled furosemide and exercise-induced asthma. Evidence for a role for inhibitory prostanoids. *Am. Rev. Respir. Dis.* 143:A210, 1991.

270. Permutt, S. Physiologic Changes in the Acute Asthmatic Attack. In K. F. Austen and L. M. Lichtenstein (eds.), *Asthma: Physiology, Immunopharmacology and Treatment*. New York: Academic, 1973.

271. Petersen, G. W., and Baier, H. Incidence of pulmonary barotrauma in a medical ICU. *Crit. Care Med.* 11:67, 1983.

272. Petheram, I. S., Kerr, I. H., and Collins, J. V. Value of chest radiographs in severe acute asthma. *Clin. Radiol.* 32:281, 1981.

273. Picado, C., et al. Aspirin-intolerance as a precipitating factor of life-threatening attacks of asthma requiring mechanical ventilation. *Eur. Respir. J.* 2:127, 1989.

274. Picado, J. M., et al. Mechanical ventilation in severe exacerbations of asthma. *Eur. J. Respir. Dis.* 64:102, 1983.

275. Pierson, W. E., Bierman, C. W., and Kelley, V. C. A double-blind trial of corticosteroid therapy in status asthmaticus. *Pediatrics* 54:282, 1974.

276. Pierson, W. E., et al. Double-blind trial of aminophylline in status asthmaticus. *Pediatrics* 48:642, 1971.

277. Pliss, L. B., and Gallagher, E. J. Aerosol vs. injected epinephrine in acute asthma. *Ann. Emerg. Med.* 10:353, 1981.

278. Plummer, A. L. The development of drug tolerance to beta-2 adrenergic agents. *Chest* 73:949, 1978.

279. Portnoy, J., and Aggarwal, J. Continuous terbutaline nebulization for the treatment of severe exacerbations of asthma in children. *Ann. Allergy* 60:368, 1988.

280. Qvist, J., et al. High-level PEEP in severe asthma. *N. Engl. J. Med.* 307:1347, 1982.

281. Rackemann, F. M., and Edwards, M. C. Asthma in children: a followup study of 688 patients after an interval of twenty years. *N. Engl. J. Med.* 246:815, 1952.

282. Rafferty, P. The European experience with antihistamines in asthma. *Ann. Allergy* 63:389, 1989.

283. Rao, S., et al. Cardiopulmonary effects of diazepam. *Clin. Pharmacol. Ther.* 14:182, 1973.

284. Rao, S., et al. Acute effects of nebulization of N-acetylcysteine in pulmonary mechanics and gas exchange. *Am. Rev. Respir. Dis.* 102:17, 1970.

285. Ratto, D., et al. Are intravenous corticosteroids required in status asthmaticus? *JAMA* 260:527, 1988.

286. Rea, H. H., et al. A case-control study of deaths from asthma. *Thorax* 41:833, 1986.

287. Read, J. The reported increase in mortality from asthma: a clinicofunctional analysis. *Med. J. Aust.* 1:879, 1968.

288. Rebuck, A. S. Radiological aspects of severe asthma. *Australas. Radiol.* 14:264, 1970.

289. Rebuck, A. S., and Pengelly, L. D. Development of pulsus paradoxus in the presence of airway obstruction. *N. Engl. J. Med.* 288:66, 1973.

290. Rebuck, A. S., and Read, J. Assessment and management of severe asthma. *Am. J. Med.* 51:788, 1971.

291. Rees, H. A., Millar, J. S., and Donald, K. W. A study of the clinical course and arterial blood gas tensions of patients in status asthmaticus. *Q. J. Med.* 37:541, 1968.

292. Reid, L. M. The presence or absence of bronchial mucus in fatal asthma. *J. Allergy Clin. Immunol.* 80:415, 1987.

293. Reisman, R. E. Asthma induced by adrenergic aerosols. *J. Allergy* 46:162, 1970.

294. Richards, J. H., and Marriott, C. Effect of relative humidity on the rheologic properties of bronchial mucus. *Am. Rev. Respir. Dis.* 109:484, 1974.

295. Riding, W. D., and Ambiavagar, M. Resuscitation of the moribund asthmatic. *Postgrad. Med. J.* 43:234, 1967.

296. Robin. E. D., and Lewiston, N. Unexpected, unexplained sudden death in young asthmatic subjects. *Chest* 96:790, 1989.

297. Rock, M. J. et al. Use of ketamine in asthmatic children to treat respiratory failure refractory to conventional therapy. *Crit. Care Med.* 14:514, 1986.

298. Rodriguez-Roisin, R., et al. Mechanisms of hypoxemia in patients with status asthmaticus requiring mechanical ventilation. *Am. Rev. Respir. Dis.* 139:732, 1989.

299. Roncoroni, A. J., et al. Metabolic acidosis in status asthmaticus. *Respiration* 33:85, 1976.

300. Rose, C. C., Murphy, J. G., and Schwartz, J. S. Performance of an index predicting the response of patients with acute bronchial asthma to intensive emergency department treatment. *N. Engl. J. Med.* 310:573, 1984.

301. Rossing, T. H., et al. Emergency therapy of asthma: comparison of the acute effects of parenteral and inhaled sympathomimetics and infused aminophylline. *Am. Rev. Respir. Dis.* 122:365, 1980.

302. Rossing, T. H., et al. A controlled trial of the use of single versus combined-drug therapy in the treatment of acute episodes of asthma. *Am. Rev. Respir. Dis.* 123:190, 1981.

303. Rossing, T. H., et al. Effect of outpatient treatment of asthma with beta agonists on the response to sympathomimetics in an emergency room. *Am. J. Med.* 75:781, 1983.

304. Rubinfeld, A. R., and Pain, M. C. F. Perception of asthma. *Lancet* 1:882, 1976.

305. Rubinfeld, A. R., and Pain, M. C. F. Bronchial provocation in the study of sensations associated with disordered breathing. *Clin. Sci.* 52:423, 1977.

306. Ruffin, R. E., Latimer, K. M., and Schembri, D. A. Longitudinal study of near fatal asthma. *Chest* 99:77, 1991.

307. Saetta, M., et al. Quantitative structural analysis of peripheral airways and arteries in sudden fatal asthma. *Am. Rev. Respir. Dis.* 143:138, 1991.

308. Sahn, S. A., and Lakshminaryayan, S. Bedside criteria for discontinuation of mechanical ventilation. *Chest* 63:1002, 1973.

309. Salem, M. R., Mathrubhutham, M., and Bennett, E. J. Difficult intubation. *N. Engl. J. Med.* 295:879, 1976.

310. Salvato, G. Some histological changes in chronic bronchitis and asthma. *Thorax* 23:168, 1968.

311. Santiago, S. M., Jr., and Klaustermeyer, W. B. Mortality in status asthmaticus: a nine-year experience in a respiratory intensive care unit. *J. Asthma Res.* 17:75, 1980.

312. Schlueter, D. P. Response of the lung to inhaled antigens. *Am. J. Med.* 57:476, 1974.

313. Schoeffel, R. E., Anderson, S. D., and Altounyan, R. E. C. Bronchial hyperreactivity in response to inhalation of ultrasonically nebulized solutions of distilled water and saline. *Br. Med. J.* 283:1285, 1981.

314. Schwartz, H. J., Lowell, F. C., and Melby, J. C. Steroid resistance in bronchial asthma. *Ann. Intern. Med.* 69:493, 1968.

315. Schwartz, S. H. Treatment of status asthmaticus with halothane. *JAMA* 251:2688, 1984.

316. Scoggin, C. H., Sahn, S. A., and Petty, T. L. Status asthmaticus: a nine-year experience. *JAMA* 238:1158, 1977.

317. Sears, M. R., and Rea, H. H. Patients at risk for dying of asthma: New Zealand experience. *J. Allergy Clin. Immunol.* 80:477, 1987.

317a. Sears, M. R., et al. Regular inhaled beta-agonist treatment in bronchial asthma. *Lancet* 336:1391, 1990.

318. Shapiro, G. G., et al. A clinical and physiological study of daily versus every-other-day steroids in children with chronic asthma. *J. Allergy Clin. Immunol.* 53:89, 1974.

319. Sheehy, A. F., et al. Treatment of status asthmaticus: a report of 70 episodes. *Arch. Intern. Med.* 130:37, 1972.

320. Shenfield, G. M., et al. Interaction of corticosteroids and catecholamines in the treatment of asthma. *Thorax* 30:430, 1975.

321. Sheppard, D. Equivalence of continuous flow nebulizer and metered-dose inhaler with reservoir bag for treatment of acute airflow obstruction. *Chest* 93:476, 1988.

322. Shim, C., and Williams, M. H., Jr. Pulsus paradoxus in asthma. *Lancet* 1:530, 1978.

323. Shim, C., and Williams, M. H., Jr. The adequacy of inhalation of aerosol from canister nebulizers. *Am. J. Med.* 69:891, 1980.

324. Shim, C., and Williams, M. H., Jr. Comparison of oral aminophylline and aerosol metaproterenol in asthma. *Am. J. Med.* 71:452, 1981.

325. Shim, C. S., and Williams, M. H., Jr. Evaluation of the severity of asthma: patients versus physicians. *Am. J. Med.* 68:11, 1980.

326. Shim, C. S., and Williams, M. H., Jr. Relationship of wheezing to the severity of obstruction in asthma. *Arch. Intern. Med.* 143:890, 1983.

327. Shore, S., Milic-Emili, J., and Martin, J. G. Reassessment of body plethysmographic technique for the measurement of thoracic gas volume in asthmatics. *Am. Rev. Respir. Dis.* 126:515, 1982.

328. Siegel, D., et al. Aminophylline increases the toxicity but not the efficacy of an inhaled beta-adrenergic in the treatment of acute exacerbations of asthma. *Am. Rev. Respir. Dis.* 132:283, 1985.

329. Siegler, D. Reversible electrocardiographic changes in severe acute asthma. *Thorax* 32:328, 1977.

330. Simpson, H., Forfar, J. O., and Grubb, D. J. Arterial blood gas tensions and pH in acute asthma in childhood. *Br. Med. J.* 3:460, 1968.

331. Sitwell, L. D., et al. Complete ophthalmoplegia as a complication of acute corticosteroid and pancuronium-associated myopathy. *Neurology* 41:921, 1991.

332. Sly, M. R. Mortality from asthma, 1979–1984. *J. Allergy Clin. Immunol.* 82:705, 1988.

333. Smith, P. R., et al. A comparative study of subcutaneously administered terbutaline and epinephrine in the treatment of acute bronchial asthma. *Chest* 71:129, 1977.

334. Solway, J., et al. Expiratory flow limitation and dynamic pulmonary hyperinflation during high frequency ventilation. *J. Appl. Physiol.* 60:2071, 1986.

335. Speizer, F. E., Doll, R., and Heaf, P. Observations on recent increase in mortality from asthma. *Br. Med. J.* 1:335, 1968.

336. Speizer, F. E., et al. Investigation into use of drugs preceding death from asthma. *Br. Med. J.* 1:339, 1968.

337. Spiteri, M. A., et al. Subcutaneous adrenaline vs. terbutaline in the treatment of acute severe asthma. *Thorax* 43:19, 1988.

337a. Spitzer, W. O., et al. The use of beta-agonists and the risk of death and near death from asthma. *N. Engl. J. Med.* 326:501, 1992.

338. Spotnitz, M. The significance of Yokohama asthma. *Am. Rev. Respir. Dis.* 92:371, 1965.

339. Squara, P., et al. Decreased paradoxic pulse from increased venous return in severe asthma. *Chest* 97:377, 1990.

340. Stableforth, D. Death from asthma (editorial). *Thorax* 38:801, 1983.

341. Stalcup, S. A., and Mellins, R. B. Mechanical forces producing pulmonary edema in acute asthma. *N. Engl. J. Med.* 297:592, 1977.

342. Stănescu, D. C., and Teculescu, D. B. Pulmonary function in status asthmaticus: effect of therapy. *Thorax* 25:581, 1970.

343. Stănescu, D. C., et al. Failure of body plethysmograhy in bronchial asthma. *J. Appl. Physiol.* 52:939, 1982.

344. Stein, M., and Gelbard, C. The Role of IPPB in Acute Asthma. In E. B. Weiss (ed.), *Status Asthmaticus.* Baltimore: University Park, 1978.

345. Straub, P. W., Buhlmann, A. A., and Rossier, P. H. Hypovolemia in status asthmaticus. *Lancet* 2:923, 1969.

346. Strunk, R. C. Identification of the fatality-prone subject with asthma. *J. Allergy Clin. Immunol.* 83:477, 1989.

347. Strunk, R. C. Death caused by asthma: minimizing the risks. *J. Respir. Dis.* 10:21, 1989.

348. Sutton, P. P., et al. The effect of oral aminophylline on lung mucociliary clearance in man. *Chest* 80:889, 1981.

349. Svedmyr, N. The role of the theophyllines in asthma therapy. *Scand. J. Respir. Dis.* [Suppl.]101:125, 1977.

350. Tabb, W. C., and Guerrant, J. L. Life-threatening asthma. *J. Allergy* 42:249, 1968.

351. Tai, E., and Read, J. Blood-gas tensions in bronchial asthma. *Lancet* 1:644, 1967.

352. Takizawa, T., and Thurlbeck, W. M. Muscle and mucous gland size in the major bronchi of patients with chronic bronchitis, asthma, and asthmatic bronchitis. *Am. Rev. Respir. Dis.* 104:331, 1971.

353. Tanaka, R. M., et al. Intravenous methylprednisolone in adults with status asthmaticus. *Chest* 82:438, 1982.

354. Thurlbeck, W. M. Pathology of Status Asthmaticus. In E. B. Weiss (ed.), *Status Asthmaticus.* Baltimore: University Park, 1978.

355. Tinkelman, D. G., et al. Comparison of nebulized terbutaline and subcutaneous epinephrine in the treatment of acute asthma. *Ann. Allergy* 50:398, 1983.

356. Tobin, M. J. Respiratory muscles in disease. *Clin. Chest Med.* 9:263, 1988.

357. Turner, J. R., et al. Equivalence of continuous flow nebulizer and metered dose inhaler with reservoir bag for treatment of acute airflow obstruction. *Chest* 93:476, 1988.

358. Tuxen, D. V. Detrimental effects of positive end-expiratory pressure during controlled mechanical ventilation of patients with severe airflow obstruction. *Chest* 93:476, 1988.

359. Uden, D. L., et al. Comparison of nebulized terbutaline and subcutaneous epinephrine in the treatment of acute asthma. *Ann. Emerg. Med.* 14:229, 1985.

360. U.S. Dept. Health Education and Welfare. Vital statistucs of the United States: Mortality. Hyattsville, MD: National Center for Health Statistics.

361. Usher, D. J., Shepherd, R. J., and Deegan, T. Serum lactate dehydrogenase isoenzyme activities in patients with asthma. *Thorax* 29:685, 1974.

362. Valabhji, P. Gas exchange in the acute and asymptomatic phases of asthma breathing air and oxygen. *Clin. Sci.* 34:431, 1968.

363. Vandewalker, M. L., et al. Addition of terbutaline to optimal theophylline therapy: double blind crossover study in asthmatic patients. *Chest* 90:198, 1986.

364. Van Metre, T. E., Jr. Adverse effects of inhalation of excessive amounts of nebulized isoproterenol in status asthmaticus. *J. Allergy* 43:101, 1969.

365. Van Schyack, C. P., Visch, M. D., and Van Weel, C. Increased bronchial hyperresponsiveness after inhaling salbutamol during one year is not caused by desensitization to salbutamol. *Am. Rev. Respir. Dis.* 141:A468, 1990.

366. Von Rentergben, D., et al. Intravenous versus nebulized terbutaline in patients with acute severe asthma: a double-blind randomized study. *Ann. Allergy* 59:313, 1987.

367. Vozeh, S., et al. Theophylline serum concentration and therapeutic effect in severe acute bronchial obstruction: the optimal use of intravenously administered aminophylline. *Am. Rev. Respir. Dis.* 125:181, 1982.

368. Wagner, P. D., et al. Ventilation-perfusion inequality in asymptomatic asthma. *Am. Rev. Respir. Dis.* 118:511, 1978.

369. Wanner, A. Clinical aspects of mucociliary transport. *Am. Rev. Respir. Dis.* 116:73, 1977.

370. Wanner, A., and Rao, A. Clinical indications for and effects of bland, mucolytic, and antimicrobial aerosols. *Am. Rev. Respir. Dis.* 122(part 2):79, 1980.

371. Ward, M. J., et al. Ipratropium bromide in acute asthma. *Br. Med. J.* 282:598, 1981.

372. Wasserfallen, J. B., et al. Sudden asphyxic asthma: a distinct entity? *Am. Rev. Respir. Dis.* 142:108, 1990.

373. Webb, A. K., Bilton, R. H., and Hanson, G. Severe bronchial asthma requiring ventilation. A review of 20 cases and advice on management. *Postgrad. Med. J.* 55:161, 1979.

374. Weil, J. V., et al. Diminished ventilatory response to hypoxia and hypercapnia after morphine in normal man. *N. Engl. J. Med.* 292:1103, 1975.

375. Weill, H., et al. Epidemic asthma in New Orleans. *JAMA* 190:811, 1964.

376. Weinberger, M. Asthma deaths and theophylline/beta$_2$-agonist therapy. *Lancet* 2:370, 1981.

377. Weinstein, H. J., Bone, R. C., and Ruth, W. E. Pulmonary lavage in patients treated with mechanical ventilation. *Chest* 72:583, 1977.

378. Weiss, E. B., and Faling, L. J. Clinical significance of PaCO$_2$ during status asthma: the cross-over point. *Ann. Allergy* 26:545, 1968.

379. Weitzman, R. H., and Wilson, A. F. Diffusing capacity and over-all ventilation:perfusion in asthma. *Am. J. Med.* 57:767, 1974.

380. Wells, R. E., Jr. Mechanics of respiration in bronchial asthma. *Am. J. Med.* 26:384, 1959.

381. Westerman, D. E., et al. Identification of the high-risk asthmatic patient: experience with 39 patients undergoing ventilation for status asthmaticus. *Am. J. Med.* 66:565, 1979.

382. White, C. S., et al. Acute asthma: admission chest radiography in hospitalized adult patients. *Chest* 100:14, 1991.

383. Williams, D. A., and Leopold, J. G. Death from bronchial asthma. *Acta Allergol.* (Kbh.) 14:83, 1959.

384. Williams, M. H., Jr. Life-threatening asthma. *Arch. Intern. Med.* 140:1604, 1980.

385. Williams, N. E., and Crooke, J. W. The practical management of severe status asthmaticus. *Lancet* 1:1081, 1968.

386. Williams, S., and Seaton, A. Intravenous or inhaled salbutamol in severe acute asthma? *Thorax* 32:555, 1977.

387. Williams, S. J., Parrish, R. W,. and Seaton, A. Comparison of intravenous aminophylline and salbutamol in severe asthma. *Br. Med. J.* 4:685, 1975.

387a. Williams, T. J., et al. Risk factors for morbidity in mechanically ventilated patients with acute severe asthma. *Am. Rev. Respir. Dis.* 148:607, 1992.

388. Wilson, A. F., et al. The significance of regional pulmonary function changes in bronchial asthma. *Am. J. Med.* 48:416, 1970.

389. Wilson, J. D., Sutherland, D. C., and Thomas, A. C. Has the change to beta-agonists combined with oral theophylline increased cases of fatal asthma? *Lancet* 1:1235, 1981.

390. Wolfe, J. D., et al. Bronchodilator effects of terbutaline and aminophylline alone and in combination in asthmatic patients. *N. Engl. J. Med.* 298:363, 1978.

391. Wood, D. W., et al. Intravenous isoproterenol in the management of respiratory failure in childhood status asthmaticus. *J. Allergy Clin. Immunol.* 50:75, 1972.

392. Woolcock, A. J., and Read, J. Lung volumes in exacerbations of asthma. *Am. J. Med.* 41:259, 1966.

393. Woolcock, A. J., and Read, J. The static elastic properties of the lungs in asthma. *Am. Rev. Respir. Dis.* 98:788, 1968.

394. Wrenn, K., et al. Aminophylline therapy for acute bronchospastic disease in the emergency room. *Ann. Intern. Med.* 115:241, 1991.

395. Younger, R. E., et al. Intravenous methylprednisolone efficacy in status asthmaticus of childhood. *Pediatrics* 80:225, 1987.

396. Zeppa, R., Grossekreutz, D. C., and Sugioka, K. Histamine release into the circulation by meperidin (Demerol). *Proc. Soc. Exp. Biol. Med.* 106:794, 1961.

397. Zieverink, S. E., et al. Emergency room radiography of asthma: an efficacy study. *Radiology* 145:27, 1982.

398. Zwillich, C. W., et al. Complications of assisted ventilation: a prospective study of 354 consecutive episodes. *Am. J. Med.* 57:161, 1974.

399. Zwillich, C. W., et al. Theophylline-induced seizures in adults; Correlation with serum concentrations. *Ann. Intern. Med.* 82:784, 1975.

400. Bowler, S. D., Mitchell, C. A., and Armstrong, J. G. Corticosteroids in acute severe asthma: effectiveness of low doses. *Thorax* 47:584, 1992.

Geriatric Considerations

74

James F. Morris

The specialty of geriatrics has been brought about by the burgeoning of the older segment of the U.S. population. The demographic changes are dramatic, and have been aided by increasing longevity. Medical science can take some credit for this increase in longevity but what has really been accomplished is delay of premature death rather than extension of the projected maximum period of life. This postponement of death will result in a shift toward an older population with an increased incidence of more chronic illnesses. Fries [21] has stated that medicine has passed through the eras of infections, then chronic illnesses, and now is entering the era of senescence. We have increased the maximum age by only one month while increasing the average maximum age to 75 years with a potential for living an average maximum of 85 years. Concurrently there has been a decline in maximum functions such as vital capacity and forced expiratory volume in 1 second (FEV_1), but not in all the homeostatic functions of the body. Thus, it is easier for medicine to improve morbidity but more difficult for it to increase maximum age [9].

It is projected that in thirty years the number of Americans over age 65 will increase from the 30 million recorded in 1990 to 50 million, or 17 percent of the population [28]. Of the elderly, those over age 84 constitute the fastest-growing segment, and this is expected to increase from the 3 million now living to 16 million in the next forty years [15]. The elderly, those age 64 and older, consume a relatively large proportion of the health-care resources of the nation; this is currently one-third. Much of this health care is related to the treatment of diseases of the pulmonary and cardiovascular systems.

In this aging population subject to chronic illnesses, chronic obstructive pulmonary disease (COPD) should increase in prominence, resulting from longer exposure to tobacco smoke and other airborne pollutants as well as to inhaled antigens. This disease group will include asthma, chronic asthmatic bronchitis, and emphysema. When I first proposed the acronym COPD for the Oregon Thoracic Society's manual in 1965, it was intended to include asthma, chronic bronchitis, and emphysema [47]. The definition of asthma at that time emphasized the hyperresponsiveness of the airway smooth muscle and did not appreciate the importance of mucosal inflammation. Currently COPD is the fourth leading cause of death in those over age 65. It is a conservative prediction that the absolute number of patients with COPD, if not the ranking as a cause of death, will increase in the future.

As mentioned earlier, the definitions and separation of asthma and COPD have recently been questioned [20] (Chap. 1). Both have features in common, including potential reversibility of airway obstruction. The diagnostic features, however, are proving to be neither sensitive nor specific.

ASTHMA VERSUS COPD

The confusion between asthma and the other COPD components was delineated by Dodge and associates [18]. In their study of a general population living in Arizona, they found that emphysema developed in older patients whereas asthma developed in a younger age group. This observation was probably an exaggeration explained by the finding that physicians tend to label older men as having emphysema whereas younger men and women in general are more commonly diagnosed as having asthma, despite the disease in both groups exhibiting similar clinical features.

In an editorial, Gross [26] emphasized the responsiveness of COPD patients to bronchodilator therapy and urged the use of bronchodilator drugs in such patients [8]. He questioned the basis for separating the diagnoses of asthma and COPD, especially based on the variability or reversibility of airflow obstruction. In a study conducted by LeDoux and others [37] of patients meeting the American Thoracic Society (ATS) criteria for COPD, the FEV_1 and forced vital capacity response to inhaled anticholinergic and beta-agonist drugs was studied. Unlike other similar studies, no preselection was done based on bronchodilator responsiveness. All 12 patients had significant improvement in airflow after inhaling ipratropium bromide. McWhorter and associates [38] also examined the separation of asthma and COPD, and found the separation was partially successful but imperfect. The prevalence of a diagnosis of asthma was found to be 2.6 percent and was independent of age and cigarette smoking. The prevalence was identical in the two age groups 45 to 54 years and 65 and over. Thus, unlike COPD, the asthma diagnosis did not change with advancing age. Within the asthma group, nonatopic asthma usually began in adult life, in contrast to atopic forms, which usually began before age 8 years.

The issue of bronchial reactivity as a means of distinguishing between asthma and COPD is controversial. Dolovich and colleagues [19] have proposed that the general term *bronchial reactivity* be replaced by *specific responsiveness to methacholine or histamine* because each response is triggered by different bronchial receptors. Obviously, the labels of *asthma* and *COPD* are widely applied without appropriate bronchoprovocation challenge testing and are instead applied based on clinical findings. The other elements of the pathophysiology of asthma, aside from bronchoconstriction, are mucus hypersecretion and airway mucosal inflammation [4]. Both conditions are found as readily in patients with chronic bronchitis and associated pulmonary emphysema as in those with asthma [3a].

In summary, it is difficult to separate the diagnosis of asthma from that of chronic bronchitis and pulmonary emphysema (COPD), especially based on airway responsiveness, and this leads logically to the question, does it matter? Either due to diagnostic bias or the greater likelihood of COPD in association with advancing age, COPD is seen more commonly in the elderly but deserves the same therapeutic approach as that used for asthma.

ASTHMA IN THE ELDERLY

How does asthma present in the elderly and what structural and functional differences are there compared with younger patients?

Table 74-1. Differential diagnosis of causes of airflow obstruction in elderly

1. Asthma
2. Chronic obstructive pulmonary disease
3. Acute nonbacterial bronchitis
4. Endobronchial tumor (bronchogenic carcinoma)
5. Congestive heart failure
6. Gastroesophageal reflux and chronic aspiration

Table 74-2. Age-related decline in respiratory structure and function

ANATOMIC STRUCTURE
1. Atrophy of respiratory muscles (diaphragm, chest wall)
2. Increased anteroposterior chest distance
3. Calcification of costochondral junction
4. Loss of alveolar wall surface area
5. Loss of bronchial muscle fibers
6. Development of panacinar emphysema

PHYSIOLOGIC FUNCTION
1. Decreased vital capacity
2. Increased functional residual capacity
3. Increased closing lung volume
4. Decreased expiratory flows
5. Decreased lung diffusing capacity
6. Increased alveolar-arterial PO_2 gradient
7. Decreased aerobic capacity

Surprisingly, relatively few studies that examine this exist, especially ones that include anatomic investigations. Of those studies addressing the elderly asthmatic, as usual, the distinction between cigarette-induced COPD and asthma, as defined by ATS criteria, is often blurred. If asthmatic airway disease is studied, cigarette smoking should be excluded from the study. The prevalence of asthma in subjects over age 70 is variously reported as 6.5 percent [13], 7.1 percent [17], and 17 percent [10]. These reports all include smokers in their study population. The incidence in the elderly reveals it is uncommon for them to develop asthma. Burrows, Braman and coworkers [10, 13a] studied 25 asthmatic patients over age 70. They separated them into two groups: those with onset of asthma either before or after age 70. A history of allergy occurred in 62 percent of the early-onset group but in none of the late-onset group. Neither onset group had a significant IgE level elevation or immediate skin test hyperreactivity. Of particular interest was the chronic persistent airway obstruction in those with long-standing asthma. Functionally these patients resemble COPD patients. A recent longitudinal study of patients more than 60 years old with asthma who denied a prior history revealed frequent preexisting symptoms; a rapid decline in lung function often occurred around the time of initial diagnosis [66]. Peirson [51] points out the need to recognize the appearance of asthma in the elderly and to differentiate it from other causes of wheezing and airflow obstruction (Table 74-1).

PHYSIOLOGIC ASPECTS OF AGING

The major problem in all of geriatric medicine is determining what are normal bodily changes, both anatomic and functional, versus what are largely due to illness and environmental factors. We know that many unrelated functions deteriorate in a more or less linear fashion with age [9]. Those functions pertaining to the respiratory system can be divided into anatomic and physiologic, as shown in Table 74-2.

It is difficult to generalize regarding the loss of physiologic function concomitant with aging. The diversity may be accounted for by all the factors that influence the erosion of cardiopulmo-

nary fitness, including aging. Admittedly, some elderly men and women function more like middle-aged persons, largely due to life-styles, genetics, and, especially, the newly discovered attention to physical fitness [29, 52].

The basic mechanisms underlying the deterioration of pulmonary function concomitant with aging are unclear. Reasonable explanations include a species-specific intrinsic delay, a sort of biologic clock; an accumulation of prolonged ambient-air pollution consisting of toxic substances; or a lifetime of acute respiratory infections leading to a stepwise decline in pulmonary function. Despite the seemingly linear decline in pulmonary function suggested by linear regression equations, the stepwise decline seems more realistic. This applies both to the airways, where a series of mucosal inflammation and repair events occur, and also to the lung parenchyma, where areas of emphysematous destruction occur without meaningful repair. The insults of cigarette smoking aggravate the aging process and produce more extreme damage.

VENTILATION

A major change that occurs with aging is the alteration of lung parenchyma. The exact structural changes that effectively lead to loss of elastic recoil are uncertain, whether there is a decrease in the number of fibers or, more likely, a change in the relationship of elastic fibers to each other. Notably absent is accompanying inflammatory bronchiolitis, prominent in smokers' centrilobular emphysema, affecting mainly the upper lobes.

Chest wall stiffness or reduced compliance with an enlarged anteroposterior distance results in a small increase in the total lung capacity and a larger increase in functional residual capacity (FRC) and residual volume [33, 36]. Decreased chest wall and diaphragmatic muscle force results in decreased vital capacity and maximum expiratory flows [7, 64] (Fig. 74-1). Most reductions in vital capacity and maximum expiratory flows are expressed as linear decreases when used in predicted regression equations, but, as previously mentioned, it is more likely that greater curvilinearity applies to the elderly. An interesting display, the "lung age," is estimated by spirometry [41]. The age-related linear regression equation calculates the age for which a measured FEV_1 would be normal.

A 15-year longitudinal study of American healthy nonsmokers revealed a mean annual decline in FEV_1 to be 31 ml in men and 26 ml in women [42]. An Australian study of nonsmoking asthmatic men showed an annual FEV_1 decline of 50 ml compared with an annual decrement of 35 ml in normal subjects [48].

The increase in residual volume that occurs with age in nonsmoking men and women is due to premature airway closure. This is worse in dependent lung regions where increased intrathoracic pressure can prematurely collapse noncartilaginous airways. At age 70, slow vital capacity should decrease to 75 percent of the prior maximum value and concurrently a 50 percent increase in residual volume [43]. The deterioration of ventilatory function is accelerated by the inhalation of tobacco smoke with the addition of chronic bronchitis and centrilobular emphysema (COPD).

Distribution of Ventilation

The tethering of elastic parenchymal alveolar wall fibers to the walls of terminal and respiratory bronchioles maintains their luminal patency, especially at lower lung volumes. Aging causes both loss of elastic tissue and elastic recoil. The resulting collapse of unsupported smaller airways results in air trapping. Because of the nonhomogeneity of the airways narrowing, the distribution of inhaled gas is uneven. Measurements of this maldistribution include the single-breath nitrogen washout test and its derivative test, closing volume or capacity [7]. Abnormal test results include an increase in the expired nitrogen slope

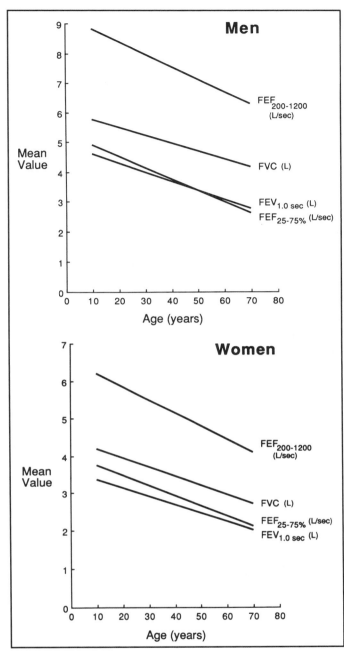

Fig. 74-1. *Decline in ventilatory function with age in men and women.* FEF$_{200-1200}$ = *mean forced expiratory flow between 200 and 1200 ml of FVC; FVC = forced vital capacity; FEV$_{1.0}$ = forced expiratory volume at 1 second; FEF$_{25-75\%}$ = mean forced expiratory flow during the middle half of the FVC.*

and increased closing volume or capacity. Closing capacity may exceed FRC due to premature closure of terminal bronchioles at end-tidal volume. At about age 45, the closing capacity exceeds the supine FRC in healthy individuals. At age 65, the closing capacity may exceed the sitting FRC [16]. This is a rational explanation for the decline in PaO$_2$ with advancing age.

Gas Exchange

The transfer of oxygen and carbon dioxide across the alveolar–capillary membrane is affected by the surface area, qualita-

tive changes in the membrane, and the flows and volumes of inhaled gas and perfused blood. With advancing age, surface area is lost, either because of disease or from the panlobular emphysema secondary to aging. In addition, there is an increasing ventilation perfusion ($\dot{V}/\dot{Q}$) mismatch due primarily to the uneven distribution of ventilation relative to capillary perfusion. As is true for loss in ventilation with increasing age, the decrease is not linear despite the prediction of linear regression equations. Specific factors that are responsible for impairing gas transfer are the changes in the alveolar–capillary membrane, such as thickening which increases resistance to oxygen diffusion, collapse of small airways, and increased $\dot{V}/\dot{Q}$ mismatch. Linear regression equations based on age demonstrate reduced PaO$_2$ and an increased alveolar-arterial oxygen tension gradient P(A-a)O$_2$ [57]. This represents an approximate loss of 0.3 percent of PaO$_2$ per year of adult life. Other age-related factors include a decreasing cardiac output [31]. This plus the decreasing PaO$_2$ reduce oxygen delivery to the tissues. Despite an age-related loss of PCO$_2$ sensitivity, PaCO$_2$ and arterial blood pH are relatively constant throughout the later years [7].

CONTROL OF VENTILATION

The nervous system control of breathing involves peripheral and central chemoreceptors plus central nervous system (CNS) integration. Similar to the attenuation of heart response to exercise, the response to hypoxemia and carbon dioxide retention diminishes with older age [49]. In healthy older men, aged 64 to 73, the ventilatory response to hypoxia is reduced by 51 percent and to carbon dioxide by 41 percent, compared with younger men, aged 22 to 30 [61]. The exact mechanisms responsible for this change are not clear but may include suppression of chemoreceptor sensitivity or impairment of the CNS integrative response. The superimposition of chronic airway obstruction and decreased respiratory muscle strength increases the vulnerability of gas exchange to acute respiratory illnesses.

EXERCISE CAPACITY

The aging process and, in particular, the decline in maximum oxygen consumption is the most challenging universal problem facing physicians. The decrease in aerobic capacity with age, reflected in maximum oxygen consumption ($\dot{V}O_2$max) is well established [3]. Prediction equations for determining $\dot{V}O_2$max are listed in Table 74-3.

Frontera and associates [22] were able to increase $\dot{V}O_2$max in 12 healthy men, aged 60 to 72 years, with the use of strength training but there were no changes in cardiopulmonary function seen in these subjects. Thomas and coworkers [59] increased $\dot{V}O_2$max in healthy, sedentary elderly men using aerobic training. They observed no change in ventilatory threshold for anaerobic metabolism. The components of oxygen delivery as described by Wasserman and colleagues [65] involve pulmonary function, hemoglobin, and cardiac function. At younger ages, exercise ventilation is not the limiting factor in maximum exertion because of the large breathing reserve. Instead, cardiac stroke volume is the major limitation. However, the relative respiratory muscle weakness in the elderly imposes the limitation of exercise ventilation on the lesser degree of reduced cardiac output. The now little used maximum voluntary ventilation (MVV) test is a crude

Table 74-3. Maximum exercise oxygen consumption values

Adult men: $\dot{V}O_2$max, ml/min = (weight, kg + 100 − age, yr) × 21
Adult women: $\dot{V}O_2$ max, ml/min = (weight, kg + 100 − age, yr) × 14

indicator of exercise ventilatory impairment. The FEV_1 has been shown to have a high correlation with the MVV and should be substituted for it [40]. Increasing body weight with age may mask a decrease in the lean or total body muscle mass, and this loss can complicate other causes of decreased exercise capacity. An additional factor in older individuals, especially those with COPD, is the increased potential for protein-calorie malnutrition. This has been shown to lead to decreased respiratory muscle strength [53]. Thus, in the event of an acute exacerbation of asthma or COPD, breathing reserve may be inadequate for maintaining physiologically satisfactory gas exchange.

DEFENSE MECHANISMS

The normal defenses of the lung are listed in Table 74-4. The mucociliary escalator is the major defense mechanism against inhaled particles. Mucociliary transport has been reported to decrease with advanced age but the clinical significance of this is uncertain [50].

The cough reflex is known to diminish with age and may even be absent. The aspiration of microorganisms or food particles occurs more often with advanced age, thus increasing susceptibility to pneumonia. If this is concurrent with impaired mucociliary clearance, the respiratory defenses are seriously compromised.

Serum immunoglobulin levels, especially IgG, are indicators of humoral immunity against bacteria, viruses, *Chlamydia*, and *Mycoplasma*. The serum antibody response to common vaccines such as influenza and pneumococci is especially important in the elderly. Unfortunately, this may be reduced, particularly in the chronically ill elderly patient. Secretory IgA in the respiratory tract appears to be less affected by age.

Cellular immunity is implicated in the host defense against carcinoma as well as mycobacterial and fungal infections. The incidence of lung cancer and tuberculosis is correlated with age as well as with the acknowledged adverse factors of cigarette smoking and malnutrition. Reduced cutaneous, delayed hypersensitivity reactions to antigens such as *Mycobacterium tuberculosis* and systemic and cutaneous fungi are reduced in those over age 60. This impairment appears to be related to reduced helper T-cell and suppressor T-cell activity.

Table 74-4. Lung defense mechanisms

I. Nonspecific
  A. Temperature and humidity
  B. Clearance
    1. Nasopharyngeal—nasal hairs, nonciliated epithelium
    2. Tracheobronchial
      a. Bronchoconstriction
      b. Cough
      c. Mucociliary transport
    3. Alveolar
  C. Secretions
    1. Mucus
    2. Antiproteases
    3. Lysozyme
    4. Complement
    5. Interferon
  D. Cellular
    1. Epithelium
    2. Blood phagocytes
    3. Tissue phagocytes
II. Specific immunologic mechanisms
  A. Humoral antibodies
  B. Cell-mediated immune responses

PHARMACOLOGY AND AGING

The recent introduction of active bronchodilator and antiinflammatory agents has revolutionized the management of reactive airway disease, both asthma and COPD [4]. Much of this improved pharmacologic treatment has derived from newer concepts of the trigger mechanisms responsible for airway hyperresponsiveness as well as awareness of the underlying inflammatory response. Whether or not asthma and COPD should be regarded as essentially similar processes is controversial. Both are characterized by increased bronchial reactivity and chronic inflammation. An intriguing idea relevant to this chapter is the relative influence of the aging process. Could the pharmacologic effects of various airway medications be affected by the age-related deterioration in drug receptors rather than by the difference in causative mechanisms such as heredity, atopy, and cigarette smoking? Does aging affect the response to drugs such as beta agonists and anticholinergics? Answers to these questions could have a major impact on the approach to managing these variations on chronic airway disease at different ages.

Bronchodilators

The two principal types of bronchodilators are beta-agonist and anticholinergic drugs. Both are highly effective as inhaled agents if used properly. Popular usage contends that beta-agonist drugs are the mainstay for relieving, or perhaps preventing, asthmatic bronchoconstriction. An anticholinergic drug, primarily ipratropium bromide (IPR), is useful only when the beta-agonist agent is not fully successful and then is used in combination. The reverse appears to be true in patients with COPD [11].

What does the aging process do to the airway response to bronchodilator therapy? There is no agreement on this important point. Ullah and associates [63] reported that the response to an inhaled beta agonist, salbutamol, declined significantly with age whereas the bronchodilator response to ipratropium bromide did not. In asthmatic patients below age 40, they suggested the drug of choice should be a beta agonist. Because further aging apparently decreases beta-receptor responsiveness, they believed ipratropium bromide to be a relatively superior bronchodilator agent that should be used alone or in combination with an inhaled beta-agonist drug. They speculated that bronchial beta receptors either decrease in number or in function with age. This would be similar to the downregulation of cardiac muscle beta receptors [1]. They further speculated that the published reports of the superiority of beta-agonist drugs in treating asthma and of anticholinergic drugs in treating COPD could be due to the age-related diminution of bronchial beta receptors. In other words, asthma is more prevalent in a younger population and COPD is more prevalent in the older population following many years of cigarette smoking.

In a subsequent report, Barros and Rees [6] confirmed that, in a large group of patients, increased age was associated with a decline in airway response to salbutamol but not to ipratropium bromide. Unfortunately, these authors failed to identify the pulmonary diagnosis. In a review article, Abrams [1] emphasized the diminished cardiac and vascular responsiveness to beta-agonist drugs. He referred to a study by Kendall and colleagues [35] indicating that $beta_2$-mediated responses are unchanged in older individuals and age should not affect bronchodilator response to $beta_2$-selective agonists. This study by Kendall and associates studied the effects of intravenous terbutaline in healthy women. The only pulmonary measurement was the peak flow, which was not significantly different between the younger and older subjects.

A potentially adverse physiologic effect of inhaled bronchodilator drugs was described by Gross and Bankwala [27]. In asthma patients, inhaled beta-agonist drugs were found to worsen gas transfer by increasing $\dot{V}/\dot{Q}$ mismatch. In older patients with COPD, aged 55 to 73, inhaled anticholinergic drugs did not significantly alter gas exchange.

Numerous reports have documented that metered-dose inhalers (MDIs) provide equal or superior bronchodilation compared with nebulized delivery [25]. This is reported for a wide variety of patients, ranging from acute asthmatics [8, 56] to outpatients with stable chronic airway disease [32, 39, 46], to mechanically ventilated patients [23, 24]. Elderly patients may have difficulty using MDIs because of poor hand–lung coordination, brief inspiratory or breathholding durations, or arthritic hands [2]. A better alternative to nebulized aerosols in such patients are spacers or drug reservoirs [44]. Generally, a larger reservoir is preferable, such as one with a volume of 600 to 750 ml, especially when using larger inhaled corticosteroid doses [55, 60]. For maximum inspiratory maneuvers, an audible signal warns of a too rapid inspiratory flow. Another delivery technique is to use four tidal inspiratory breaths per MDI activation [25] (Chap. 56). This requires a spacer that has expiratory valving to ensure persistence of the reservoir aerosol.

Theophylline

Theophylline, formerly a mainstay of bronchodilator therapy, has been overshadowed by safer and more effective medications, especially inhalants [30]. Clearance of theophylline is reduced in elderly patients [45]. This decline with age is reported to be 35 ml/kg/hr. This may result from diseases more common with aging and to a decline in hepatic enzyme activity. Hepatic dysfunction can be caused by primary liver disease, hypoxia, or low blood flow states, as occur in congestive heart failure. Elderly patients are also more likely to take multiple medications, some of which may interact with theophylline (Table 74-5). Drugs of special importance are erythromycin and cimetidine, which decrease theophylline clearance and thus raise blood levels, and phenytoin, which increases theophylline clearance but results in lower levels for both drugs [12]. Toxicity represents a potentially dangerous hazard for the elderly because of variable hepatic metabolism and drug interactions. Even worse, the elderly are less tolerant of serious adverse effects such as cardiac tachyarrhythmia and seizures, both life-threatening. Peculiar to the elderly are toxic manifestations of nervousness, insomnia, and apparent organic brain syndromes, including dementia and psychosis.

Corticosteroids

The role of antiinflammatory drugs in the treatment of all forms of reactive airway disease has achieved preeminence in management [5]. Systemic corticosteroids such has prednisone, when taken on a long-term basis, are especially hazardous in the elderly. The elderly are already more susceptible to associated diseases such as osteoporosis, hypertension, diabetes mellitus, cardiac failure, and peptic ulcer disease, and all of these disorders are potentially worsened by maintenance corticosteroid therapy. At the same time, the possible enhancement of the number and function of bronchial beta receptors and of catecholamine activity are attractive for the older patient. For long-term care, the inhaled corticosteroids are preferable because of low systemic effects, even with the recently recommended higher daily dosage [5, 14, 54, 62].

Sodium cromoglycate has been used primarily for the treatment of allergic asthma but also for nonspecific asthma. Responses have been more favorable in younger patients. A long-term study by Svendsen and associates [58] indicated modest superiority of inhaled corticosteroid over sodium cromoglycate in adult asthmatics over four years. Juniper and coworkers [34] recently reported a one-year study of 29 adult asthmatics receiving inhaled corticosteroids with consequential diminished airway responsiveness and asthma severity. Combining this with inhaled bronchodilators should benefit the elderly patients, particularly in terms of reducing the risks of systemic-medication adverse effects while achieving long-term control of airway obstruction.

Elderly patients with asthma develop important age-related factors that the physician should be aware of in management. Decline in lung function, waning of the immunoregulatory system, the frequent coexistence of other medical disorders affecting oxygen delivery, nutritional status, psychologic and behavioral changes influencing medication compliance, and alterations in drug metabolism and drug interactions are among the prominent considerations. Appropriate attention to these functional and pharmacologic factors is clearly required for the optimal care of elderly patients with asthma.

REFERENCES

1. Abrams, W. B. Cardiovascular drugs in the elderly. *Chest* 98:980, 1990.
2. Allen, S. C., and Prior, A. What determines whether an elderly patient can use a metered dose inhaler correctly? *Br. J. Dis. Chest* 80:45, 1986.
3. Astrand, P., and Rodahl, K. *Textbook of Work Physiology.* New York: McGraw-Hill, 1970, Pp. 171–173.
3a. Bailey, W. C., Richards Jr., J. M., et al. Features of asthma in older adults. *J. Asthma* 29:21, 1992.
4. Barnes, P. J. A new approach to the treatment of asthma. *N. Engl. J. Med.* 321:1517, 1989.
5. Barnes, P. J. Effect of corticosteroids on airway hyperresponsiveness. *Am. Rev. Respir. Dis.* 141:S70, 1990.
6. Barros, M. J., and Rees, P. J. Bronchodilator responses to salbutamol followed by ipratropium bromide in partially reversible airflow obstruction. *Respir. Med.* 84:371, 1990.
7. Bates, D. V. *Respiratory Function in Disease* (3rd ed.). Philadelphia: Saunders, 1989, Pp. 81–86.
8. Berry, R. B., et al. Nebulizer vs spacer for bronchodilator delivery in patients hospitalized for acute exacerbation of COPD. *Chest* 96:1241, 1989.
9. Boss, G. R., and Seegmiller, J. F. Age-related physiologic changes and their clinical significance. *West. J. Med.* 135:434, 1981.
10. Braman, S. S., Kaemerlen, J. T., and Davis, S. M. Asthma in the elderly: a comparision between patients with recently acquired and long-standing disease. *Am. Rev. Respir. Dis.* 143:336, 1991.
11. Braun, S. R., et al. A comparison of the effect of ipratropium and albuterol in the treatment of chronic obstructive airway disease. *Arch. Intern. Med.* 149:544, 1989.
12. Bukowskyk, M., Nakatsu, K., and Munt, P. W. Theophylline reassessed. *Ann. Intern. Med.* 101:63, 1984.

Table 74-5. Antiasthmatic drugs in the elderly

Drug	Adverse effects	Dosage considerations
Beta agonist		
Oral	Tremor, tachycardia	Reduce or discontinue
Inhaled	Uncommon	No changes necessary
Anticholinergic		
Inhaled	Uncommon	No changes necessary
Theophylline		
Oral	Nausea, vomiting, arrhythmias, seizures	Discontinue or maintain serum level 10–20 μg/ml
Corticosteroids		
Oral	Osteoporosis, cataracts, reduces T-cell function, myopathy, aggravates hypertension	Maintenance dose below 20 mg/AM. Avoid or alter dose: cimetidine, erythromycin, phenytoin, rifampin
Inhaled	Oropharyngeal candidiasis	Use a reservoir spacer
Cromolyn		
Inhaled	Uncommon	No changes necessary

13. Burr, M. L., et al. Asthma in the elderly: a review of 11,551 cases. *Br. Med. J.* 1:1041, 1979.

13a. Burrows, B., Barbee, R. A., et al. Characteristics of asthma among elderly adults in a sample of the general population. 100:935, 1991.

14. Check, W. A., and Kaliner, M. A. Pharmacology and pharmacokinetics of topical corticosteroid derivatives used for asthma therapy. *Am. Rev. Respir. Dis.* 141:S44, 1990.

15. Davis Conference. The aging process. *Ann. Inter. Med.* 113:455, 1990.

16. Dhar, S., Shastri, S. R., and Lenoar, R. A. Aging and the respiratory system. *Med. Clin. North Am.* 60:1121, 1976.

17. Dodge, R. R., and Burrows, B. The prevalence and incidence of asthma and asthma-like symptoms in a general population sample. *Am. Rev. Respir. Dis.* 122:567, 1980.

18. Dodge, R., Cline, M. G., and Burrows, B. Comparison of asthma, emphysema, and chronic bronchitis diagnosis in a general population sample. *Am. Rev. Respir. Dis.* 133:981, 1986.

19. Dolovich, J., et al. Asthma terminology: troubles in wordland. *Am. Rev. Respir. Dis.* 134:1102, 1986.

20. Eliason, O. How to define asthma and COPD. *Am. Rev. Respir. Dis.* 136:789, 1987.

21. Fries, J. F. Aging, illness, and health policy: implications of the compression of morbidity. *Perspect. Biol. Med.* 31:407, 1988.

22. Frontera, W. R., et al. Strength training and determinants of VO_2max in older men. *J. Appl. Physiol.* 68:329, 1990.

23. Fuller, H. D., et al. Pressurized aerosol versus jet aerosol delivery to mechanically ventilated patients. *Am. Rev. Respir. Dis.* 141:440, 1990.

24. Gay, P. C., et al. Metered dose inhaler for bronchodilator delivery in intubated, mechanically ventilated patients. *Chest* 99:66, 1991.

25. Gervais, A., and Begin, P. Bronchodilatation with a metered-dose inhaler plus an extension, using tidal breathing vs jet nebulization. *Chest* 92:822, 1987.

26. Gross, N. J. COPD: a disease of reversible air-flow obstruction. *Am. Rev. Respir. Dis.* 133:725, 1986.

27. Gross, N. J., and Bankwala, Z. Effects of an anticholinergic bronchodilator on arterial blood gases of hypoxemic patients with chronic obstructive pulmonary disease: comparison with a beta-adrenergic agent. *Am. Rev. Respir. Dis.* 136:1091, 1987.

28. Guralnik, J. M., and FitzSimmons, S. C. Aging in America: a demographic perspective. *Cardiol. Clin.* 4:175, 1986.

29. Heath, G. W., et al. A physiological comparison of young and older endurance athletes. *J. Appl. Physiol.* 51:634, 1981.

30. Hendeles, L., and Weingerger, M. Theophylline: a "state of the art" review. *Pharmacotherapy* 3:2, 1983.

31. Higginbotham, M. B., et al. Physiologic basis for the age-related decline in aerobic work capacity. *Am. J. Cardiol.* 57:1374, 1986.

32. Jenkins, S. C., et al. Comparison of domiciliary nebulized salbutamol and salbutamol from a metered-dose inhaler in stable chronic airflow limitation. *Chest* 91:804, 1987.

33. Jones, R. L., et al. Effects of age on regional residual volume. *J. Appl. Physiol.* 44:195, 1978.

34. Juniper, E. F., et al. Effect of long-term treatment with an inhaled corticosteroid (budesonide) on airway hyperresponsiveness and clinical asthma in nonsteroid-dependent asthmatics. *Am. Rev. Respir. Dis.* 142:832, 1990.

35. Kendall, M. J., et al. Responsiveness to beta-adrenergic receptor stimulation: the effects of age are cardioselective. *Br. J. Clin. Pharmacol.* 14:821, 1982.

36. Knudson, R. J., et al. Effect of age alone on mechanical properties of the lung. *J. Appl. Physiol.* 43:1054, 1977.

37. LeDoux, E. J., et al. Standard and double dose ipratropium bromide and combined ipratropium bromide and inhaled metaproterenol in COPD. *Chest* 95:1013, 1989.

38. McWhorter, W. P., Polis, M. A., and Kaslow, R. A. Occurrence, predictors, and consequences of adult asthma in NHANESI and follow-up survey. *Am. Rev. Respir. Dis.* 139:721, 1989.

39. Mestitz, H., Copland, J. M., and McDonald, C. F. Comparison of outpatient nebulized vs metered dose inhaler terbutaline in chronic airflow obstruction. *Chest* 96:1237, 1989.

40. Morris, J. F., and Temple, W. P. Reassessment of the maximum voluntary ventilation test. *Am. Rev. Respir. Dis.* 115:143, 1977.

41. Morris, J. F., and Temple, W. P. Spirometric "lung age" estimation for motivating smoking cessation. *Prev. Med.* 14:665, 1985.

42. Morris, J. F., et al. Fifteen-year interval spirometric evaluation of the Oregon predictive equations. *Chest* 93:123, 1988.

43. Murray, J. F., *The Normal Lung* (2nd ed.). Philadelphia: Saunders, 1986, Pp. 339–360.

44. Newhouse, M. T., and Dolovich, M. B. Control of asthma by aerosols. *N. Engl. J. Med.* 315:870, 1986.

45. Nielsen-Kudsk, F., Magnussen, I., and Jakobsen, N. Pharmacokinetics of theophylline in ten elderly patients. *Acta Pharmacol. Toxica* 42:226, 1978.

46. Olivenstein, R., et al. A comparison of responses to albuterol delivered by two aerosol devices. *Chest* 90:392, 1986.

47. Oregon Thoracic Society. *Chronic Obstructive Pulmonary Disease: A Manual for Physicians.* 1965.

48. Peat, J. K., Woolcock, A. J., and Cullen, K. Rate of decline in lung function in subjects with asthma. *Eur. J. Respir. Dis.* 70:171, 1987.

49. Peterson, D. D., et al. Effects of aging on ventilation and occlusion pressure responses to hypoxemia and hypercapnia. *Am. Rev. Respir. Dis.* 124:387, 1981.

50. Phair, J. P., et al. Host defenses in the aged: evaluation of components of the inflammatory and immune responses. *J. Infect. Dis.* 138:67, 1978.

51. Pierson, D. J. Asthma: special challenge in the elderly. *Geriatrics* 37:87, 1982.

52. Pollack, M. L. Effect of age and training on aerobic capacity and body composition of master athletes. *J. Appl. Physiol.* 62:725, 1987.

53. Rochester, D., and Esau, S. Malnutrition and the respiratory system. *Chest* 85:411, 1984.

54. Salmeron, S., et al. High doses of inhaled corticosteroids in unstable chronic asthma. *Am. Rev. Respir. Dis.* 140:167, 1989.

55. Salzman, G. A., and Pyszczynski, D. R. Oropharyngeal candidiasis in patients treated with beclomethasone dipropionate delivered by metered-dose inhaler alone and with Aerochamber. *J. Allergy Clin. Immunol.* 81:424, 1988.

56. Salzman, G. A., et al. Aerosolized metaproterenol in the treatment of asthmatics with severe air flow obstruction. Comparison of two delivery methods. *Chest* 95:1017, 1989.

57. Sorbini, C. A., et al. Arterial oxygen tension in relation to age in healthy subjects. *Respiration* 25:3, 1968.

58. Svendsen, U. G., et al. A comparison of the effects of sodium cromoglyate and beclomethasone dipropionate on pulmonary function and bronchial hyperreactivity in subjects with asthma. *J. Allergy. Clin. Immunol.* 80:68, 1987.

59. Thomas, S. G., et al. Exercise training and "ventilation threshold" in elderly. *J. Appl. Physiol.* 59:1472, 1985.

60. Tobin, M. J., et al. Response to bronchodilator drug administration by a new reservoir delivery system and a review of other auxiliary delivery systems. *Am. Rev. Respir. Dis.* 126:670, 1982.

61. Tockman, M. S. The effects of age on the lung. In *The Merck Manual of Geriatrics.* Rahway, NJ: Merck Sharp & Dohme Research Laboratories, 1990, Pp. 423–459.

62. Toogood, J. H. High-dose inhaled steroid therapy for asthma. *J. Allergy Clin. Immunol.* 83:528, 1989.

63. Ullah, M. I., Newman, G. B., and Saunders, K. B. Influence of age on response to ipratropium bromide and salbutamol in asthma. *Thorax* 36:523, 1981.

64. Wahba, W. M. Influence of aging on lung function—clinical significance of changes from age twenty. *Anesth. Analg.* 62:764, 1983.

65. Wasserman, K., et al. *Principles of Exercise Testing and Interpretation.* Philadelphia: Lea & Febiger, 1986.

66. Burrows, B., et al. Findings before diagnoses of asthma among the elderly in a longitudinal study of a general population sample. *J. Allergy Clin. Immunol.* 88:870, 1991.

Gastroesophageal Reflux and Esophageal Dysfunction

75

Michael K. Farrell

Gastroesophageal reflux, the spontaneous passage of gastric contents from the stomach into the esophagus, occurs frequently. In one survey of presumably normal persons, 10 percent experienced heartburn daily and 50 percent of otherwise healthy adults experienced it intermittently [44]. Reflux is common in infants, due to an immaturity of the lower esophageal sphincter; the vast majority of these infants improve without therapy in the first year of life [8]. Recent studies in normal adults and children have demonstrated that some reflux is "normal," especially in the postprandial period [17, 29].

The patient with gastroesophageal reflux may be asymptomatic or may have symptoms such as chronic cough, hoarseness, nocturnal aspiration, and wheezing. In adults, such diverse pulmonary problems as recurrent bronchitis and pneumonia, asthma, and diffuse interstitial pneumonia have been attributed to reflux [1, 3, 4, 28]. In the pediatric patient, asthma, recurrent pneumonia, apnea, stridor, and episodes of choking and coughing have been attributed to reflux [5, 15, 23, 27, 55]. However, chronic lung disease per se may contribute to gastroesophageal reflux as a consequence of chronic cough, changes in intrathoracic pressure dynamics, and the effect of therapeutic agents on lower esophageal sphincter pressure.

This chapter briefly reviews esophageal physiology, esophageal dysfunction, especially as manifested by esophagitis, and the diagnosis and treatment of gastroesophageal reflux. Potential mechanisms for reflux-associated pulmonary disease will also be reviewed.

ESOPHAGEAL PHYSIOLOGY

In the past, the esophagus was often considered merely a conduit from the pharynx to the stomach. However, recent investigations have demonstrated complex interactions among anatomic factors, local and systemic hormonal factors, and neuronal factors. The esophagus and pulmonary system share similar embryologic origins, the foregut, so it is not surprising that they also share common neurologic pathways.

The esophagus is divided into three distinct portions: the upper sphincter, the body, and the lower sphincter. Striated muscle makes up the upper third and smooth muscle, the lower two-thirds. The upper esophagus has a resting, very high-pressure zone (+ 100 mmHg). The body of the esophagus has a negative pressure identical to the intrathoracic pressure (− 5 mmHg). The distal esophagus contains the lower esophageal sphincter, which is not an actual anatomic sphincter but rather a physiologic high-pressure zone (+ 20 mmHg), the result of the interaction of anatomic, hormonal, and neuronal, primarily vagal, factors. The upper sphincter relaxes following a swallow and the contraction of the superior constrictor muscle of the pharynx initiates peristaltic waves, propelling the swallowed bolus into the esophagus.

A series of sequential contractions, primary peristalsis, follows that propels the bolus down the esophagus. The lower esophageal sphincter then relaxes, allowing the bolus to enter the stomach. The lower esophageal sphincter pressure then returns to normal, forming a barrier against the reflux of gastric contents into the esophagus. The esophagus can vary the strength of the peristaltic contractions as necessary, suggesting an intricate regulatory system.

The esophagus is innervated extrinsically by autonomic nerves originating in the vagus and by branches of the sympathetic nerves; intrinsic innervation is provided by a distinctive myenteric plexus found between muscle layers. The neural control of the esophageal body is chiefly mediated by cholinergic and nonadrenergic, noncholinergic nerves [10].

Recent studies have shown that gastroesophageal reflux occurs in virtually everyone, particularly in the postprandial period [18, 29]. Refluxed acid is promptly cleared from the esophagus, and it is increased saliva production, increased swallowing, and peristalsis that are the major factors responsible for this esophageal clearance [22]. However, the normal reflux barriers are present during sleep and while in the recumbent position. At least three potential mechanisms have been identified that allow reflux: (1) transient inappropriate relaxation of the lower esophageal sphincter, (2) transient increases in intraabdominal pressure, and (3) spontaneous free reflux due to very low resting sphincter tone in the lower esophagus [18, 19]. Most reflux episodes in both normal adults and those with esophagitis are due to inappropriate relaxation of the lower esophageal sphincter. Hence, some amount of reflux must be considered normal, or "physiologic."

ESOPHAGEAL DYSFUNCTION AND PULMONARY DISEASE

The aspiration of gastric contents and subsequent pulmonary disease may occur as a result of primary or secondary esophageal disorders. Asthma, apnea, recurrent pneumonia, and pulmonary fibrosis may result from chronic aspiration. The esophageal disorder may be primary or secondary to neurologic, systemic, or myopathic diseases (Table 75-1). The astute clinician should always suspect esophageal disorders when confronted with unexplained pulmonary disease. Primary esophageal disorders that may be associated with pulmonary disease include achalasia, repaired tracheoesophageal fistulas, and gastroesophageal reflux.

Achalasia is a neurenteric disorder, characterized by the absence of normal peristalsis and failure of the lower esophageal sphincter to relax. A megaesophagus develops as a result and there is frequent overflow aspiration of the esophageal contents [63]. Chronic pulmonary complaints are common in these pa-

Table 75-1. Disease states with esophageal dysfunction

Neurologic	Myopathic	Systemic
Cerebrovascular accidents	Myasthenia gravis	Scleroderma
Multiple sclerosis	Myotonia dystrophica	Diabetes
Amyotrophic lateral sclerosis	Dermatomyositis	Idiopathic intestinal pseudoobstruction
Diphtheria, tetanus	Polymyositis	
Poliomyelitis	Amyloidosis	

tients. Therapy consists of pneumatic dilation of the esophagus or a surgical myotomy (Heller procedure); gastroesophageal reflux may develop after myotomy [43].

Children who have had tracheoesophageal fistulas repaired have a high incidence of pulmonary problems [20, 41]. There is abnormal esophageal peristalsis and an increased incidence of gastroesophageal reflux in such patients, which may contribute to stricture formation. Aspiration is common and results in chronic pulmonary problems, such as apnea and bradycardia episodes and recurrent pneumonia. A surgical antireflux procedure is frequently necessary to eliminate the problem.

The relationship between pulmonary disease and gastroesophageal reflux remains unclear and confusing. The confusion results from the plethora of contradictory reports, often anecdotal in nature, and the paucity of prospective controlled clinical trials. Numerous studies have confirmed the high incidence (45–75%) of reflux in adult and pediatric asthmatic patients [1, 3, 5, 15, 28, 30, 33, 34, 36, 38, 45, 48, 49, 55, 64]. This is independent of bronchodilator use; in addition, approximately 40 percent of adult asthmatic patients have esophagitis [56–58]. What remains unclear is the causal relationship between reflux and asthma. Recent investigations have begun to unravel the connection and place reflux in the proper perspective.

Mendelsohn [40] initially described the severe pulmonary complications that followed aspiration of gastric contents. In 1949, Belcher [4] described 48 patients with esophageal disease and a variety of pulmonary problems, including lung abscesses and bronchiectasis. Iverson and colleagues [28] evaluated 400 adults with esophageal diseases and found that 35 percent had concomitant pulmonary disorders. Mays and associates [38] reported that 44 percent of the patients in their study who suffered from idiopathic pulmonary fibrosis had gastroesophageal reflux, as compared to 5 percent of a control group. Significantly, the esophageal symptoms were often minimal. Using esophageal pH studies, DeMeester and coworkers [17] demonstrated reflux followed by wheezing in eight patients, thus demonstrating for the first time the possibility of a direct causal relationship. An apparent increased incidence of gastroesophageal reflux in children with asthma has been reported [5, 27, 45]. Danus and associates [15] demonstrated reflux in 26 of 43 children with chronic bronchitis; 15 of 20 responded to medical antireflux therapy. Berquist and coworkers [5] evaluated 82 children with recurrent pneumonia or asthma, or both; 40 had gastroesophageal reflux and 32 improved with medical or surgical therapy. However, these studies, although suggesting a possible role for reflux in the pathogenesis of asthma, are flawed. None are prospective, and none adequately address the question: Is the reflux the cause or result of the pulmonary disease? In these early studies, the patients are highly selected and comparable controls groups are lacking. No direct temporal or causal relationships are demonstrated. The documentation of improvement in pulmonary symptoms is subjective and the potential for observer and patient bias is profound. The possibility that the observed reflux might be "physiologic" and incidental was rarely considered.

Varney and Pokorny [65] could find no differences in flow rates and the forced expiratory volume in 1 second (FEV_1) in patients with documented reflux without pulmonary disease as compared to 100 matched controls. In another study, no increase in gastroesophageal reflux or pulmonary changes was noted in asthmatic and control patients studied by prolonged esophageal pH monitoring [27].

Perrin-Fayolle and colleagues [49] described the long-term benefit from the surgical treatment of gastroesophageal reflux in 44 adult patients. Patients were selected on the basis of symptoms but without extensive evaluation. The exact amount of reflux and the presence or absence of esophagitis are unknown. Five years later, 41 percent were deemed "markedly improved" and 66 percent, "improved overall," using an asthma score as the reference criteria. Unfortunately, the study was unblinded and retrospective. However, the authors showed no relationship between obstructive airway disease as well as the duration and severity of the asthma and the response to antireflux therapy. Factors that appeared to predict a favorable outcome were response to medical antireflux therapy, nocturnal asthma attacks, nocturnal tracheitis, and reflux symptoms preceding the onset of asthma symptoms.

Several other recent studies have suggested that, in certain patients, control of gastroesophageal reflux can lessen the asthma. Larrain and coworkers [34] in Chile completed a randomized trial comparing placebo, medical, and surgical therapy. Ninety patients with *intrinsic* asthma were randomized to undergo surgery or to receive cimetidine or placebo. These investigators used a clinical and medication score to assess response after 5 years. Importantly, there were significant responses in all groups, including 40 percent improvement in the placebo group. However, both the medical and surgical groups showed improvement when compared to the placebo group, with the surgical group showing a slight advantage. The factors that predicted success were the onset of reflux symptoms before pulmonary symptoms, nocturnal asthma, laryngeal irritation, and an initial pulmonary response to medical therapy (Fig. 75-1).

Another explanation for the apparent relationship between gastroesophageal reflux and asthma is that the pulmonary disease itself may increase reflux, which in turn may further aggravate the pulmonary dysfunction. Asthmatic patients have been noted to have more and longer reflux episodes during methacholine-induced bronchospasm than controls [42]. Reflux symptoms are also more common in patients with cystic fibrosis than in controls; objective studies have confirmed this observation [54]. Commonly employed medications such as theophylline and beta-adrenergic drugs may decrease lower esophageal sphincter pressure and allow more reflux; this has been documented in the manometry laboratory. However, the exact clinical significance of this remains controversial [6, 7, 26].

Several theories have been proposed to explain pulmonary dysfunction following gastroesophageal reflux. The two most plausible are recurrent microaspiration and bronchospasm mediated via a neuronal reflex arc.

Some evidence for microaspiration in humans exists: several hours after the ingestion of a radioisotope, lung scans have demonstrated isotope in the lung parenchyma. Pellegrini and coworkers [48] evaluated 100 adults with documented reflux. Oral acid regurgitation occurred in 17 patients, but only eight had concurrent symptoms such as cough and wheezing. Microaspiration may perpetuate chronic pulmonary disease. Crausaz and Favez [13] studied adult patients with an FEV_1 of less than 80 percent of the predicted value using scintiscans to demonstrate reflux and subsequent aspiration. There was an increased incidence of reflux (27 of 32 asthmatic patients versus 5 of 13 controls) and aspiration (24 of 32 asthmatic patients versus 5 of 13 controls). Tuchman and associates [61], using adult cats, demonstrated that the intratracheal instillation of minute quantities of acid (0.05 ml of 0.2 N HCl) resulted in a marked increase in total lung

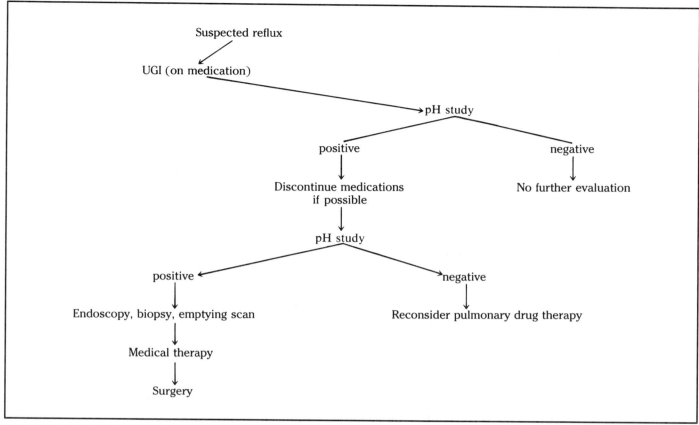

Fig. 75-1. *Evaluation of suspected reflux in the pulmonary patient.* UGI = *upper gastrointestinal series.*

resistance. This increase was much greater following intratracheal as compared to intraesophageal instillation. The increase was pH dependent and was abolished by the prior sectioning of the vagal nerve.

Spaulding and coworkers [59] have postulated that esophageal reflux induces vagally mediated bronchoconstriction in asthmatic adults. They noted that total pulmonary resistance increased following perfusion of the esophagus with acid but not saline. The effect was markedly greater in those asthmatics with distal esophageal sensitivity to acid perfusion, and this is presumed to constitute evidence of esophagitis. Infusion of antacids immediately diminished the increase in pulmonary resistance. In animal studies, the effect was abolished by sectioning the vagal nerves [59]. Andersen and coworkers [2] perfused the esophagus with saline and a dilute acidic solution. The patients in their study were asthmatics with and without esophagitis and patients with esophagitis but no asthma symptoms. Decreases in peak expiratory flow and increases in total airway resistance were observed only in the asthmatic patients with esophagitis. The changes were vagally mediated, since pretreatment with atropine abolished the observed effect. Children with a history of nocturnal asthma and gastroesophageal reflux have responded to acid perfusion of the esophagus with early morning (4:00 A.M.) bronchoconstriction; no response was noted after saline perfusion [16]. This positive response was observed only in those patients with esophagitis, as determined by a positive Bernstein test [16]. These studies suggest that the presence of esophagitis is important; in its absence, no pulmonary response is consistently observed. The proposed mechanism is the exposure of vagal nerves in the inflamed esophageal mucosa.

Mechanical factors may also be important, especially in the young patient. Schey and coworkers [53] demonstrated bradycar-

dia following esophageal distention in infants and neonatal puppies. Herbst and colleagues [23] demonstrated the occurrence of apnea following the infusion of acid into the distal esophagus in premature infants; the presence or absence of esophagitis was not noted.

The reaction to aspirated gastric contents may be significant, since asthmatic patients have hyperactive airways and respond to a wide variety of environmental stimuli. However, skeptics will point out that asthma and gastroesophageal reflux are both common events, so it is not surprising that they may occasionally occur in the same patient; to them, this does not prove a causal relationship.

In spite of the confusion noted above, several very high-risk groups for aspiration and chronic pulmonary disease associated with gastroesophageal reflux can be identified; they include children with repaired tracheoesophageal fistulas and children with severe neurologic impairment.

Following repair of a tracheoesophageal fistula, motility disturbances are universal. In a series of 100 children studied after repair, Dudley and Phelan [20] reported that recurrent bronchitis (more than 3 attacks per year) occurred in 78 percent of children under 3 years of age and 48 percent age 3 and over. Milligan and Levison [41] evaluated 24 children following repair: 23 had abnormal pulmonary function studies in which 18 showed an obstructive pattern and 5, a restrictive pattern. A positive methacholine challenge was documented in 23 of the patients. Medical therapy tends to be unsuccessful; approximately 50 percent of affected patients will eventually require antireflux surgery.

Chronic vomiting is a major problem in severely neurologically impaired children, affecting 10 to 15 percent of institutionalized children. The most common cause of the vomiting in these children is gastroesophageal reflux [66]. Associated problems include poor feeding, poor weight gain with resultant malnutrition, esophagitis with resultant hematemesis and anemia, and eventual stricture formation. These children often have chronic cough, recurrent pneumonia, and wheezing. Conventional medical therapy has not been very successful in these patients; many ultimately require surgery. Morbidity is substantial following surgery, but the quality of life and ease of caring for these children are markedly improved. Morbidity and mortality are equally high in the nonsurgical group, so surgery is frequently the treatment of choice.

DIAGNOSIS

Recent technologic advances have made the precise diagnosis of esophageal dysfunction possible. However, the plethora of available studies reporting varying sensitivity and specificity have created problems for the clinician. The key to diagnosis remains the carefully obtained history and physical examination. The patient with gastroesophageal reflux will frequently complain of dysphagia, effortless regurgitation, and heartburn. Additional symptoms may include nocturnal coughing or choking episodes, awakening with gastric secretions in the pharynx, painful swallowing, chronic hoarseness or voice changes, or a feeling of food sticking in the esophagus. Information on factors that aggravate the symptoms, such as position, specific foods, and medications, should be elicited (Table 75-2). Patients with chronic hoarseness, laryngitis, and nocturnal asthma should be considered to be at particular risk for gastroesophageal reflux–related asthma, as should those whose reflux symptoms preceded the pulmonary complaints [12, 34].

Infants and children with reflux may have unique symptoms; they present with postprandial vomiting that is usually effortless but may be forceful. If the vomiting is severe or caloric intake is subsequently decreased, growth will be affected. Some children, particularly those with neurologic impairment, will exhibit bizarre body positioning (Sandifer's syndrome) or behavior, such as head banging, tooth grinding, and inconsolable crying.

Physical examination will reveal few specific features. Stigmata of chronic lung disease as well as signs of anemia should be noted. The presence of fecal occult blood should raise the suspicion for esophagitis.

A variety of procedures may be helpful in the diagnosis of

Table 75-2. Foods and drugs that affect esophageal sphincter function

Decrease	Increase
Progesterone	Protein meal
Theophylline	Bethanechol
Isoproterenol	Metoclopramide
Anticholinergics	Gastrin
Diazepam	Alkali
Meperidine	Indomethacin
Morphine	Cholinergics
Calcium channel blockers	Histamine
Nicotine	Gastrin
Coffee, caffeine	Motilin
Fat	Beta blockers
Alcohol	Alpha-adrenergic drugs
Chocolate	
Peppermint	
Beta-adrenergic drugs	
Prostaglandins E_2 and A_2	
Dopamine	
Secretin	
Glucagon	

Table 75-3. Diagnostic studies for gastroesophageal reflux

Test	Purpose
Upper gastrointestinal radiography	Assess anatomy and swallowing function
Scintiscan	Amount of reflux and gastric emptying
pH monitoring	Correlate with symptoms risk of esophagitis
Acid perfusion (Bernstein test)	Esophagitis
Endoscopy and esophageal biopsy	Esophagitis

gastroesophageal reflux (Table 75-3). The initial diagnostic study is the upper gastrointestinal series; it can exclude the existence of anatomic abnormalities and may detect esophagitis and peptic ulcer disease. Valuable information regarding swallowing function and the presence of strictures can also be obtained. The presence or absence of a hiatal hernia is of less significance than the reflux of gastric contents. In infants and children, the barium transit should be followed throughout the small intestine to exclude intestinal causes of vomiting, such as malrotation. Because the upper gastrointestinal series is not specific or sensitive for reflux, normal findings do not exclude reflux.

Esophageal motility studies (manometry) have been extensively used in adults to define esophageal motility disturbances. Manometry has been most useful in evaluating motor disturbances such as achalasia and diffuse esophageal spasm and less useful in assessing gastroesophageal reflux because of the overlapping presence of lower esophageal sphincter pressure (LESP) in patients with and without reflux. However, patients with very low LESP (<6 mmHg) are more likely to have esophagitis. Manometry is also useful in assessing patients receiving theophylline products, since they decrease the LESP. A disadvantage of manometry is that it requires expensive equipment and considerable expertise to properly interpret the results. In addition, infants and children require sedation, which affects LESP.

The acid perfusion test (Bernstein test) demonstrates distal esophageal sensitivity to acid and is presumed to identify esophagitis. In adults, the Bernstein test is sensitive and specific, but it has not been extensively evaluated in infants and children [46]. The test does not demonstrate the presence or absence of reflux but rather the consequences of prolonged esophageal exposure to gastric acid. To perform the test, the midesophagus is slowly perfused (100–120 drops per minute) via a nasogastric tube; saline and 0.1 N HCl solutions are alternated. Neither the observer nor the patients should know the order of the solutions. The test is positive when symptoms such as pain appear within 7 to 15 minutes. The patient can then compare the provoked symptoms with the symptoms experienced spontaneously. A negative study does not rule out reflux.

Recently there has been an increasing wave of enthusiasm for monitoring the intraesophageal pH. The major advantages of this technique are that esophageal function can be monitored for longer periods (1–24 hours), and symptoms can be objectively correlated with documented reflux episodes. The effect of position, eating, and physical activity on reflux can be assessed [17, 30, 37]. Esophageal pH monitoring is either done for 1 to 2 hours (Tuttle test, short acid reflux test [SART] or overnight. The SART is usually performed during manometric studies. To perform the test, a dilute acid (300 ml/m² 0.1 N HCl) is instilled into the stomach and the esophageal pH monitored. More than two reflux episodes (pH <4 for 15 seconds or longer) per hour are considered a positive result. Some investigators put the patient through a variety of positions and maneuvers (Valsalva, Mueller, cough), but these may not be physiologic. In addition, a false-positive response may occur following gastric loading since postprandial reflux is common in normal controls.

The overnight pH study is valuable in evaluating the patient with complex symptoms and suspected gastroesophageal reflux. The probe is placed 4 to 5 cm above the lower esophageal sphincter and the pH recorded continuously. Probes with multiple recording sites are available, so it is possible to determine if the reflux extends to the proximal esophagus or to the hypopharynx. Ambulatory systems are available which are scored by computer; these allow the patient to pursue normal activities during the test [37]. The patient's activities and symptoms are recorded throughout the study. The amount and duration of reflux are quantified by a variety of scoring systems, the simplest being the percentage of time during which the esophageal pH is less than 4 [18, 28]. In normal adults and children, the esophageal pH is under 4 less than 5 percent of the time [62]. Esophageal pH monitoring can be combined with other physiologic monitoring for certain complex symptoms (e.g., polysomnography for assessing sleep-related respiratory complaints).

Prolonged pH monitoring has shown that some degree of reflux is normal; this "physiologic" reflux is most likely to occur in the postprandial period. Reflux episodes tend to be more frequent in the awake state, when subjects are upright as opposed to recumbent. These data must be considered, or false positives will occur if pH studies are misinterpreted. False-negative studies can occur if there is achlorhydria or if the probe is placed above a stricture. The most common causes of achlorhydria are the administration of an H_2 antagonist or frequent feedings in infants.

Gastroesophageal reflux can also be evaluated by the scintiscan. In this test, a liquid meal tagged with technetium 99m sulfur colloid is given and the distal esophagus scanned for one hour. More than two episodes of reflux in one hour is considered abnormal. The sensitivity and specificity of this test are good. In addition, this test allows for the assessment of gastric emptying, which is often abnormal in patients with gastroesophageal reflux [25]. An image obtained 12 hours later may demonstrate isotope in the lungs, thus confirming aspiration.

Endoscopy with esophageal biopsy remains the procedure of choice to document esophagitis. Endoscopically normal mucosa may have significant histologic abnormalities, so biopsy specimens should be obtained whenever esophagitis is suspected.

THERAPY

The therapy of gastroesophageal reflux begins with recommendations for simple alterations in life-style. Patients are encouraged to eat three meals a day, not to lie down after eating, and to eat several hours before retiring. The overweight patient is encouraged to lose weight. Smoking, both active and passive, should be prohibited since nicotine causes a marked decrease in the LESP. Foods known to aggravate reflux are eliminated (see Table 75-2); these include fats, alcohol, chocolate, and peppermint [9, 51]. Citrus juices and tomato products may also aggravate reflux symptoms, probably due to osmolarity rather than a direct effect on lower esophageal sphincter function [35]. Medications known to affect LESP are proscribed if possible (see Table 75-2; Fig. 75-1). The head of the bed is elevated 6 inches (15 cm); recent pH studies have shown a decrease in reflux utilizing this therapy. Anticholinergic agents are contraindicated in patients with gastroesophageal reflux; this may be difficult in the asthmatic patient, but alternatives should be sought.

In infants, therapy consists of frequent small feedings, thickened foods, and proper positioning. The infant with reflux should be kept in the prone or upright position as much as possible, since this position decreases reflux episodes. Placing the infant in a conventional car seat only increases reflux.

The major goal in the treatment of gastroesophageal reflux is

to decrease esophageal irritation from refluxed gastric contents. Antacids and H_2 blockers are used to neutralize and decrease gastric acid. Antacids have long been a mainstay in the treatment of reflux disease; they neutralize gastric acid and seem to increase sphincter pressure, thus reducing reflux. Aluminum hydroxide–containing antacids offer the advantage of binding bile acids, thus decreasing this potential source of esophageal irritation. For maximal effectiveness, antacids should be taken 1 hour after meals and before bedtime.

The H_2 antagonists cimetidine, ranitidine, and famotidine decrease gastric acid production but have no effect on esophageal peristalsis or sphincter pressure [21]. Omeprazole, a proton pump inhibitor, markedly suppresses acid production. The H_2 antagonists relieve reflux symptoms and variably promote healing of esophagitis [31]. They provide better symptom relief than do prokinetic agents, which tend to improve pH study parameters but do not reduce symptoms. The H_2 antagonists, especially cimetidine, inhibit hepatic microsomal enzyme activity, leading to delayed clearance of many drugs, including theophylline. Patients should be observed for possible drug toxicity when taking H_2 antagonists along with other drugs. Ranitidine and famotidine have less effect on drug clearance and thus are preferred. Other side effects of the H_2 antagonists include abdominal discomfort, fatigue, and gynecomastia. Absorption of the H_2 blockers may be decreased if taken simultaneously with antacids.

Omperazole is very effective when used for brief periods (6–8 weeks) in the treatment of erosive esophagitis [24, 32]. Experience with longer treatment regimens is slowly accumulating. Current recommendations are that it should be considered when H_2 blockers fail or cannot be tolerated; experience in the pediatric age group is limited.

Sucralfate suspension has been proposed for the treatment of esophagitis, but has not been observed to be more effective than placebo in one study [67]. Sucralfate must be given in an acid environment to be effective and there must be adequate contact time for it to adhere to the esophageal mucosa; hence, it may be more effective in the treatment of severe erosive esophagitis.

Bethanechol is a cholinergic agent that increases lower esophageal sphincter pressure and improves esophageal acid clearance. In several controlled trials, bethanechol was found to reduce symptoms and heal esophagitis in infants and adults (dose in adults, 25 mg qid, and in infants, 9 mg/m^2/day) [50]. Bethanechol may be contraindicated in patients with asthma and should be given carefully because of its cholinergic effect.

Metoclopramide is a dopamine agonist that increases lower esophageal pressure and enhances gastric emptying. McCallum and associates [39] evaluated 31 patients in a double-blind crossover study and demonstrated decreased symptoms and antacid use in the metoclopramide group. Metoclopramide treatment has not been as successful in children [60]. Metoclopramide can cause serious neurologic and psychologic side effects, the most serious being severe extrapyramidal reactions. The very young and very old are at particular risk for this effect. Cisapride is a prokinetic drug that has shown very promising results in trials, but it is not yet available in the United States [14, 52].

Figure 75-1 depicts our present evaluation of the patient with chronic pulmonary disease and suspected reflux. Initial studies are performed while the patient continues taking his or her regular medication. If these studies are negative, no further evaluation is necessary. If the initial studies reveal reflux, medications that could be affecting the lower esophageal sphincter are discontinued and the studies repeated. If the repeat pH study is negative, the patient's medications must be reevaluated. If the pH study remains positive, intensive medical therapy is begun. If medical therapy fails, then antireflux surgery is considered.

Approximately 5 percent of adults and less than 1 percent of children with severe reflux will fail medical therapy and require surgery. Patients at risk for failing medical therapy are the neurologically impaired and those who have had tracheoesophageal fistulas repaired. Recently there has been a proliferation of anti-reflux procedures; the most commonly employed is the Nissen fundoplication. The mortality rate associated with this procedure is 0.2 to 1.5 percent. Complications include failure of the fundoplication, vagal nerve injury, bowel adhesions and subsequent obstruction, and the inability to belch or vomit—"the gas-bloat syndrome"; all these complications have an increased incidence in the neurologically impaired child [47]. A "dumping" syndrome has recently been described to occur after fundoplication; this must be considered in patients with residual abdominal discomfort, bloating, diarrhea, and diaphoresis [11].

Results of surgery are variable. The symptoms directly related to reflux—heartburn and vomiting—are usually well controlled. Postoperative control of pulmonary symptoms ranges from 60 to 90 percent. Predictors of failure to completely control pulmonary symptoms include neurologic dysfunction and swallowing difficulties [30]. No adequately controlled study of medical versus surgical therapy in pulmonary diseases, including asthma, has been performed. The long-range control of reflux in one study was adequate for 5 to 6 years. However, a decrease in LESP and an increase in pH-monitored reflux were noted. The long-term results in infants and children may be better.

REFERENCES

1. Allen, C. J., and Newhouse, M. T. Gastroesophageal reflux and chronic respiratory disease. *Am. Rev. Respir. Dis.* 129:645, 1985.
2. Andersen, L. I., Schmidt, A., and Bundgaard, A. Pulmonary function and acid application in the esophagus. *Chest* 90:358, 1986.
3. Barish, C. F., Wu, W. C., and Castell, D. O. Respiratory complications of gastroesophageal reflux. *Arch. Intern. Med.* 145:1882, 1985.
4. Belcher, J. R. The pulmonary consequences of dysphagia. *Thorax* 4:44, 1949.
5. Berquist, W. E., et al. Gastroesophageal reflux associated with recurrent pneumonia and chronic asthma in children. *Pediatrics* 68:29, 1981.
6. Berquist, W. E., et al. Effects of theophylline on gastroesophageal reflux in normal adults. *J. Allergy Clin. Immunol.* 67:407, 1981.
7. Berquist, W. E., et al. Quantitative gastroesophageal reflux and pulmonary function in asthmatic children and normal adults receiving placebo, theophylline and metaproterenol sulfate therapy. *J. Allergy Clin. Immunol.* 73:253, 1984.
8. Carre, I. J. The natural history of partial thoracic stomach ("hiatus hernia") in children. *Arch. Dis. Child.* 34:344, 1959.
9. Castell, D. O. Diet and the lower esophageal sphincter. *Am. J. Clin. Nutr.* 28:1296, 1975.
10. Castell, D. O., and Johnson, L. F. *Esophageal Function in Health and Disease.* New York: Elsevier, 1983.
11. Caulfield, M. E., et al. Dumping syndrome in children. *J. Pediatr.* 110:212, 1987.
12. Cherry, J., et al. Pharyngeal localization of symptoms of gastroesophageal reflux. *Ann. Otol. Rhinol. Laryngol.* 79:912, 1970.
13. Crausaz, F. M., and Favez, G. Aspiration of solid food particles into lungs of patients with gastroesophageal reflux and chronic bronchial disease. *Chest* 93:376, 1988.
14. Cucchiarra, S., et al. Cisapride for gastroesophageal reflux and peptic esophagitis. *Arch. Dis. Child.* 62:454, 1987.
15. Danus, O., et al. Esophageal reflux—an unrecognized cause of recurrent obstructive bronchitis in children. *J. Pediatr.* 89:220, 1976.
16. Davis, R. S., Larsen, G. L., and Grunstein, M. M. Respiratory response to intraesophageal infusion in asthmatic children during sleep. *J. Allergy Clin. Immunol.* 72:393, 1983.
17. DeMeester, T. R., et al. Technique, implications and clinical use of 24 hour esophageal pH monitoring. *J. Thorac. Cardiovasc. Surg.* 79:656, 1980.
18. Dent, J., et al. Mechanism of gastroesophageal reflux in recumbent asymptomatic human subjects. *J. Clin. Invest.* 65:256, 1980.
19. Dodds, W. J., et al. Mechanisms of gastroesophageal reflux in patients with reflux esophagitis. *N. Engl. J. Med.* 307:1547, 1982.
20. Dudley, N. E., and Phelan, P. D. Respiratory complications of long term survivors of oesophageal atresia. *Arch. Dis. Child.* 51:279, 1976.
21. Feldman, M., and Burton, M. E. Histamine$_2$ receptor antagonists. *N. Engl. J. Med.* 323:1749, 1990.
22. Helm, J. F., Dodds, W. J., and Pelc, L. R. Effect of esophageal emptying and saliva on clearance of acid from the esophagus. *N. Engl. J. Med.* 310: 284, 1984.
23. Herbst, J. J., Minton, S. D., and Book, L. S. Gastroesophageal reflux causing respiratory distress and apnea in newborn infants. *J. Pediatr.* 95:763, 1979.
24. Hetzel, D. J., et al. Healing and relapse of severe peptic esophagitis after treatment with omeprazole. *Gastroenterology* 95:903, 1988.
25. Hillemeier, A. C., et al. Delayed gastric emptying in infants with gastroesophageal reflux. *J. Pediatr.* 98:190, 1981.
26. Hubert, D., et al. Effect of theophylline on gastroesophageal reflux in patients with asthma. *J. Allergy Clin. Immunol.* 81:1168, 1988.
27. Hughes, D. M., et al. Gastroesophageal reflux during sleep in asthmatic patients. *J. Pediatr.* 102:666, 1983.
28. Iverson, L. I. G., May, I. A., and Samson, P. C. Pulmonary complications in benign esophageal disease. *Am. J. Surg.* 126:223, 1973.
29. Jolley, S. G., et al. An assessment of gastroesophageal reflux in children by extended pH monitoring of the distal esophagus. *Surgery* 84:16, 1978.
30. Jolley, S. G., et al. Surgery in children with gastroesophageal reflux and respiratory symptoms. *J. Pediatr.* 96:194, 1980.
31. Klinkenberg-Knol, E. C., et al. Double blind multi-centre comparison of omeprazole and ranitidine in the treatment of reflux esophagitis. *Lancet* 1:349, 1987.
32. Koop, H., and Arnold, R. Long term maintenance treatment of reflux esophagitis with omeprazole. *Dig. Dis. Sci.* 36:552, 1991.
33. Koufman, J., et al. Reflux laryngitis and its sequelae: the diagnostic role of ambulatory 24 hour pH monitoring. *J. Voice* 2:78, 1988.
34. Larrain, A., et al. Medical and surgical treatment of nonallergic asthma associated with gastroesophageal reflux. *Chest* 99:1330, 1991.
35. Lloyd, D. A., and Borda, I. T. Food induced heartburn: effect of osmolality. *Gastroenterology* 80:740, 1981.
36. Martin, M. E., Grunstein, M. M., and Larsen, G. L. The relationship of gastroesophageal reflux to nocturnal wheezing in children with asthma. *Ann. Allergy* 49:318, 1982.
37. Mattox, H. E. Prolonged ambulatory esophageal pH monitoring in the evaluation of gastroesophageal reflux disease. *Am. J. Med.* 89:345, 1990.
38. Mays, E. E., Dubois, J. J., and Hamilton, G. B. Pulmonary fibrosis associated with tracheoesophageal aspiration. *Chest* 69:4, 1976.
39. McCallum, R. W., et al. A controlled trial of metoclopramide in symptomatic gastroesophageal reflux. *N. Engl. J. Med.* 296:354, 1977.
40. Mendelsohn, C. L. The aspiration of stomach contents into the lungs during obstetric anesthesia. *Am. J. Obstet. Gynecol.* 52:191, 1946.
41. Milligan, D. W., and Levison, H. Lung function in children following repair of tracheoesophageal fistula. *J. Pediatr.* 95:24, 1979.
42. Moote, D. W., et al. Increase in gastroesophageal reflux during methacholine induced bronchospasm. *J. Allergy Clin. Immunol.* 78:619, 1986.
43. Murray, G. F., et al. Selective application of fundoplication in achalasia. *Ann. Thorac. Surg.* 37:185, 1984.
44. Nebel, O. T., et al. Symptomatic gastroesophageal reflux incidence and precipitating factors. *Dig. Dis. Sci.* 21:955, 1976.
45. Orenstein, S. R., and Orenstein, D. M. Gastroesophageal reflux and respiratory disease in children. *J. Pediatr.* 112:847, 1988.
46. Orenstein, S. R., et al. Stridor and gastroesophageal reflux: diagnostic use of intraluminal esophageal acid perfusion (Bernstein test). *Pediatr. Pulmonol.* 3:420, 1987.
47. Pearl, R. H., et al. Complications of gastroesophageal anti-reflux surgery in neurologically impaired versus neurologically normal children. *J. Pediatr. Surg.* 25:1169, 1990.
48. Pellegrini, C. A., et al. Gastroesophageal reflux and pulmonary aspiration: incidence, functional abnormality and results of surgical therapy. *Surgery* 56:110, 1979.
49. Perrin-Fayolle, M., et al. Long-term results of surgical treatment for gastroesophageal reflux in asthmatic patients. *Chest* 96:40, 1989.
50. Saco, L. S., et al. Double-blind controlled trial of bethanechol and antacid versus placebo and antacid in the treatment of erosive esophagitis. *Gastroenterology* 82:1369, 1982.
51. Price, S. F., Smithson, K. W., and Castell, D. O. Food sensitivity in reflux esophagitis. *Gastroenterology* 75:240, 1978.
52. Saye, Z., and Forget, P. P. Effect of cisapride on esophageal pH monitoring in children with reflux-associated bronchopulmonary disease. *J. Pediatr. Gastroenterol. Nutr.* 8:327, 1989.
53. Schey, W. L., et al. Esophageal dysmotility in the sudden infant death syndrome. *Radiology* 140:67, 1981.

54. Scott, R. B., O'Loughlin, E. V., and Gall, D. G. Gastroesophageal reflux in patients with cystic fibrosis. *J. Pediatr.* 106:223, 1985.

55. Shapiro, G. G., and Christie, D. L. Gastroesophageal reflux in steroid dependent asthmatic youths. *Pediatrics* 63:201, 1979.

56. Sontag, S., et al. Effect of positions, eating, and bronchodilators on gastroesophageal reflux in asthmatics. *Dig. Dis. Sci.* 35:849, 1990.

57. Sontag, S., et al. Asthmatics have endoscopic esophagitis with or without bronchodilator therapy. *Am. J. Gastroenterol.* 84:A1153, 1989.

58. Sontag, S., et al. Most asthmatics have gastroesophageal reflux with or without bronchodilator therapy. *Gastroenterology* 99:613, 1990.

59. Spaulding, H. S., et al. Further investigation of the association between gastroesophageal reflux and bronchoconstriction. *J. Allergy Clin. Immunol.* 69:516, 1982.

60. Tolia, V., et al. Randomized, prospective, double-blind trial of metoclopramide and placebo for gastroesophageal reflux in infants. *J. Pediatr.* 115:141, 1989.

61. Tuchman, D. N., et al. Comparison of airway responses following tracheal or esophageal acidification in the cat. *Gastroenterology* 87:872, 1984.

62. Vandenplas, Y., and Loeb, H. The interpretation of oesophageal monitoring data. *Eur. J. Pediatr.* 149:598, 1990.

63. Vantrappen, G., et al. Achalasia, diffuse esophageal spasm and related motility disorders. *Gastroenterology* 76:450, 1979.

64. Urschel, H. C., and Paulson, D. L. Gastroesophageal reflux and hiatal hernia. *J. Thorac. Cardiovasc. Surg.* 53:21, 1967.

65. Varney, G. A., and Pokorny, C. Pulmonary function in patients with gastroesophageal reflux. *Chest* 76:678, 1979.

66. Wilkinson, J. D., Dudgeon, D. L., and Sondheimer, J. M. A comparison of medical and surgical treatment of gastroesophageal reflux in severely retarded children. *J. Pediatr.* 99:202, 1981.

67. Williams, R. M., et al. Multi-center trial of sucralfate suspension for the treatment of reflux esophagitis. *Am. J. Med.* 83:61, 1987.

Nocturnal Asthma

Philip W. Ind
Colin T. Dollery
Peter J. Barnes

76

Nocturnal wheezing, first described in the fifth century A.D. [3], remains a common problem, with up to two-thirds of asthma patients waking at night [27, 57, 137, 138].

CLINICAL RELEVANCE

Nocturnal asthma is often an intermittent problem heralding an acute exacerbation of disease. In other patients it may persist for years. Characteristically the patient wakes wheezy or breathless in the early hours of the morning, typically around 4 A.M., but sometimes nocturnal cough [53] may be the only symptom (see also Chap. 50). Surveys confirming a significant excess of deaths and episodes of ventilatory arrest in asthmatics in the early morning [2] underline the clinical importance of nocturnal bronchoconstriction. Sleep disturbance, with or without hypoxemia, probably has a significant morbidity with associated impairment of school or work performance [43]. Treatment remains difficult in many cases, and the precise cause of nocturnal bronchoconstriction remains uncertain. Bronchoalveolar cellular infiltration has recently been reported at night in patients with nocturnal asthma [81], but most evidence favors a relationship with circadian physiologic rhythms.

POSSIBLE MECHANISMS

Many potential pathophysiologic mechanisms of nocturnal asthma have been proposed (Table 76-1).

Allergens

Antigen exposure experimentally can produce nocturnal wheeze on several subsequent nights [96]. Rigorous house-dust mite allergen avoidance has been shown to reduce but not abolish bronchial response to histamine and early-morning wheeze [106]. However, allergen exposure, during the day or at night, is unlikely to be the main explanation as nonatopic asthmatics [24, 27], patients with chronic airflow obstruction [35, 108], and normal individuals [24, 38, 54, 72] all exhibit diurnal variation in airway caliber and responsiveness.

Accumulation of Toxins or Secretions

There is no evidence to support the nocturnal accumulation of hypothetic metabolic toxins [44]. Mucociliary clearance is reduced in asthmatics and in normal subjects in association with sleep rather than posture or a circadian rhythm [101]. Retention of bronchial secretions at night may contribute to early-morning airflow obstruction, but not all such patients produce sputum. Furthermore, the rapid relief of wheeze in most, if not all, patients

by inhaled bronchodilators suggests that smooth muscle contraction is the major mechanism of airway narrowing.

Esophageal Reflux

Esophageal reflux has long been recognized in asthma [99] and may be commoner in nocturnal asthma [80]. However, this may be related to therapy with beta agonists and theophyllines, both of which can reduce tone in the esophageal sphincter [12, 23]. Esophageal acidity may be associated with bronchoconstriction [34, 48, 129] in the absence of microaspiration, possibly as a result of enhanced vagal tone [78]. However, the frequency of "silent" esophageal reflux is probably not increased in asthmatics [104], and reflux is not inevitably associated with bronchoconstriction [12]. Increased histamine responsiveness, in the absence of significant airflow obstruction, was found 90 minutes after drinking dilute hydrochloric acid to mimic acid reflux [146], although the mechanism remains obscure. Issues related to esophageal reflux are discussed more fully in Chap. 75.

Supine Posture

Change to the supine posture commonly causes initially rapid airway narrowing [143], which may also gradually increase [68]. This is not responsible for nocturnal asthma, since bronchoconstriction occurs in patients sleeping seated [24]. Furthermore, daytime bronchoconstriction developing in patients with nocturnal asthma was independent of posture [145]. Posture did not alter histamine responsiveness [143], though pulmonary congestion, which would be anticipated lying supine, may be associated with increased bronchial responsiveness [17].

In shift workers the inversion of peak expiratory flow variation [24, 28] after the first sleep following a change in shift, at a time when other diurnal rhythms, such as body temperature or corticosteroid secretion, usually persist, suggested a contribution of sleep itself to bronchoconstriction. However, sleep deprivation neither prevents nocturnal bronchoconstriction in the majority of patients [18, 56, 119] nor alters morning histamine responsiveness [18].

Marked fluctuations in airway tone have been described in REM sleep in dogs [132]. However, there is still disagreement over whether wheezing is commoner in REM sleep than in other stages [11, 69, 86, 125] or is distributed through various sleep stages according to their relative duration [69]. Most studies rely on airway measurements collected on spontaneous or induced wakening or on indirect evidence of airway narrowing [64, 87, 134]. In one study esophageal and supraglottic pressures were recorded as well as flow at the mouth in asthmatic patients during sleep [11]. Lower respiratory resistance (total lung resistance minus supraglottic resistance) peaks were greatest and longest during stage 3 to 4. The relative rarity of nocturnal asthma in

Table 76-1. *Postulated pathogenetic mechanisms of nocturnal asthma*

Antigen exposure
Accumulation of metabolic toxins
Retention of bronchial secretions
Esophageal reflux and aspiration
Supine posture
Sleep stage or pattern
Sleep apnea
Airway cooling
Interruption of regular therapy
Exaggeration of normal circadian rhythms
Airway inflammation

Table 76-2. *Endogenous circadian rhythms possibly contributing to nocturnal bronchoconstriction*

Physiologic
  Airway caliber
  Bronchial responsiveness
  Sensory mechanisms
  Sympathetic tone
  Parasympathetic tone
  Nonadrenergic noncholinergic nerves
  Receptor responsiveness
  Perception of airflow obstruction
Biochemical
  Circulating catecholamines
  Circulating adrenal corticosteroids
  Opiates
  Drug metabolism
Inflammatory
  Antigen response
  Immunoglobulin E
  Mast cells
  Other inflammatory cells

sleep stages 3 and 4 may relate to a reduced arousal response to increased airflow obstruction [51].

In patients with asthma and sleep apnea, continuous positive airway pressure was effective in reducing nocturnal bronchoconstriction (as well as sleep apnea), suggesting the importance of reflex-induced airway narrowing [20]. It is unclear as to how commonly nocturnal asthma and apneas coexist, but snoring was found to be unusual in nocturnal asthma [86].

Sleep therefore appears to contribute to nocturnal asthma, but more studies that do not involve waking patients or invasive instrumentation are required.

Airway Cooling

There is little information regarding the role of airway cooling in nocturnal asthma. Body temperature falls slightly at night, and breathing warm humidified air at night has been shown to reduce nocturnal bronchoconstriction [21]. Nasal continuous positive airway pressure (CPAP) causes airway cooling but was beneficial rather than detrimental in patients with sleep apnea and nocturnal asthma [20].

Dosing Frequency

Waking patients for regular spacing of medication throughout the 24 hours does not prevent nocturnal wheeze [24], suggesting that interruption of bronchodilator therapy is not of major importance etiologically.

Circadian Rhythms

Chronobiology is the study of biologic rhythms. Many physiologic variables are linked to the light-dark cycle of the solar day. Those that have a periodicity of around 24 hours are called circadian rhythms. They are characterized by amplitude (peak-trough variation), level (baseline around which oscillation occurs), and staging (the precise relationship with other functions, such as sleep-waking activity). Cosinor analysis has generally been applied to the data [52, 94]. Circadian rhythms that could conceivably be involved in nocturnal bronchoconstriction are summarized in Table 76-2.

Circadian Changes in Airway Function

The existence of circadian variation in various measures of airway caliber in normals, as well as asthmatics, has been known for over 30 years [75]. Diurnal rhythms have been described for forced expiratory volume in 1 second (FEV_1) and forced vital capacity (FVC) [50, 75, 82], specific conductance [37, 38, 72], respiratory resistance [76], static lung volumes [72], and dynamic compliance [45], as well as resting ventilation [16], ventilatory response to carbon dioxide [85], and carbon monoxide transfer [22].

Peak expiratory flow (PEF), which is conveniently self-recorded at home, has been the most widely studied index of airway caliber (Fig. 76-1). Peak flow recording in normals showed a statistically significant rhythm in 66 percent of 221 subjects [57]. Mean amplitude by cosinor analysis was 8 percent. In another examination of the normal variation in PEF, the maximum/minimum PEF (%) ratio and the amplitude-to-mean were greater in children aged 6 to 15 years than in adults [111]. Maximum diurnal variation is less than 5 percent for FEV_1 [50, 75, 82] but up to 25 percent for specific conductance [72]. Much larger amplitude rhythms are seen in asthma, but phase has been found to be identical, supporting the hypothesis that nocturnal asthma represents an exaggeration of the normal diurnal variation of airway caliber.

Circadian Rhythm of Bronchial Responsiveness

Bronchial responsiveness to histamine [37, 112, 140] and acetylcholine [117] has long been known to increase markedly at night in asthmatics. Similar degrees of diurnal variation in acetylcholine [117], methacholine [16, 54], and histamine [38] response have been demonstrated in normal subjects. This suggests that increase in bronchial responsiveness at night is unlikely to be simply due to reduction in airway caliber.

A close correlation between the amplitude of diurnal variation of PEF and histamine responsiveness has been demonstrated [15, 123]. The greater the responsiveness, the lower the morning PEF and the greater the bronchodilator response to salbutamol. Similar findings were reported by Martin et al. [79] in patients with nocturnal bronchoconstriction. They found a correlation between overnight change in PEF and methacholine response measured at 4 P.M. and 4 A.M. and bronchodilator response to an inhaled beta$_2$ agonist. Furthermore, they documented markedly increased bronchial response to saline at 4 A.M. with a greater than 20 percent fall in FEV_1 and 8 of 11 patients with the greater nocturnal symptoms and greater overnight fall in PEF. Others have found no correlation between change in airway tone (measured as FEV_1) and circadian variation in bronchial responsiveness [12a, 79, 140]; stability of circadian alterations in lung function including bronchial responsiveness was recently reported [147]. However, this does not invalidate the concept of nocturnal asthma as a manifestation of nonspecific bronchial hyperresponsiveness.

Circadian Change in Inflammatory Responses

Specific bronchial challenge with house dust mite antigen has also been found to produce greater and more long-lasting bron-

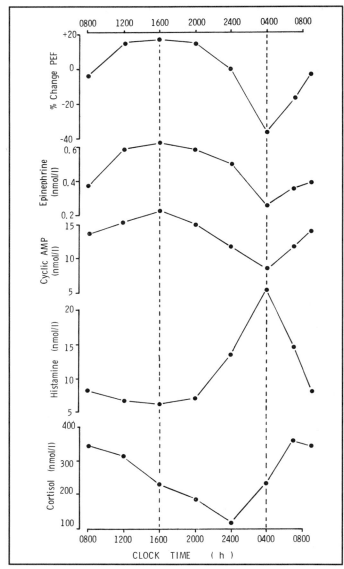

Fig. 76-1. *Mean changes in peak expiratory flow (PEF), venous plasma epinephrine, plasma cyclic adenosine monophosphate (AMP), plasma histamine, and plasma cortisol concentrations over 24 hours in five patients with nocturnal asthma.*

choconstriction at 11 P.M. compared with 3 P.M. [47]. This suggests increased mast cell degranulation or increased response of other inflammatory effector cells.

Upper airways also show circadian rhythms. Nasal symptoms are at a peak in the early hours of the morning in patients with allergic rhinitis [118]. Nasal secretions contain increased concentrations of IgA, IgG, and albumin at night compared with during the day [93].

Cutaneous response to house dust mite antigen is enhanced at night in atopic subjects [116], as is the wheal and flare response to intradermal injections of histamine and the mast cell degranulating compound 48/80 in normal subjects [115]. Antihistamines have been shown to be more effective in antagonizing skin responses at night [114]. Cutaneous response to intradermal tuberculoprotein has also been shown to be significantly reduced at night, suggesting circadian variation of cell-mediated immune responses [29].

Circadian Rhythm of Sensory Mechanisms

Cough threshold to citric acid was significantly higher in the afternoon than in the morning in normal subjects [110]. This may reflect a circadian rhythm of airway sensory receptor mechanisms.

Circadian variation of response to lung inflation has been described [76]. In six asthmatics and six normal subjects challenged with methacholine at 4 A.M. and 4 P.M., similar increased bronchial sensitivity (threshold of response) and bronchial reactivity (slope of response) were found. However the effects of deep inspiration differed. In asthmatics, respiratory resistance increased after deep inspiration, and this effect was greater at 4 A.M. compared to 4 P.M. In normals, resistance decreased to a greater extent at 4 A.M. compared to 4 P.M. The explanation for these findings is unclear, but it may represent differences in cholinergic or nonadrenergic noncholinergic reflexes initiated by sensory receptors.

Circadian Rhythm of Adrenergic Mechanisms

Circadian changes in blood pressure coinciding with changes in plasma norepinephrine [61] suggest an underlying rhythm of sympathetic neural output. Sympathetic tone to pulmonary beta$_2$ adrenoceptors is suggested by the fact that beta-receptor blocking drugs induce bronchoconstriction in asthmatic but not in normal subjects. However, the absence of a functionally significant sympathetic innervation to human bronchial smooth muscle implies modulation of airway caliber by the circulating adrenomedullary hormone epinephrine [62]. Circadian variation in catecholamine excretion was originally described in normal subjects [113, 136] and subsequently in patients with nocturnal asthma [127]. Striking associations of urinary catecholamines and falls in PEF were noted in some but not all patients.

In five patients with nocturnal asthma studied by Barnes et al. [4] plasma epinephrine concentrations were almost three times higher at 4 P.M. compared with values at 4 A.M. Plasma cyclic adenosine monophosphate (AMP) concentrations (reflecting beta-receptor stimulation) varied to the same degree and followed the same pattern. Plasma cortisol concentrations were lowest at 7 A.M. and highest at 12 P.M. There were close correlations of PEF with plasma epinephrine and cyclic AMP and inversely with cortisol, allowing a 4-hour phase shift compatible with the known delayed effects of corticosteroids on the airways. Plasma histamine concentration, thought to reflect mast cell degranulation, inversely mirrored plasma epinephrine. Furthermore, infusion of epinephrine at 0.01 µg/kg/min decreased plasma histamine and increased PEF, suggesting that epinephrine might be "driving" the PEF and plasma histamine rhythms rather than simply being temporally associated [8]. However, the plasma histamine concentrations measured were rather high and may not have accurately reflected pulmonary mast cell activation [63]. In normal subjects, studied as controls, circulating epinephrine concentrations did not differ from those in asthmatic patients and fell similarly at night. Studies measuring urinary catecholamines and histamine have shown similar patterns in patients with chronic airflow obstruction [108] and in children with allergic asthma [140a].

In a similar study Szefler et al. [133] measured plasma concentrations of histamine, cortisol, epinephrine, cyclic AMP, and leukocyte beta-adrenergic receptor density in 7 patients with nocturnal asthma, 10 asthmatics without nocturnal asthma, and 10 normal subjects. A twofold higher plasma histamine concentration was found in all groups at 4 A.M. compared with 4 P.M. Surprisingly, plasma concentrations of cortisol, epinephrine, and cyclic AMP did not differ significantly at the two time points. However, there was a significant 33 percent decrease in mononuclear and polymorphonuclear cell beta-receptor density in nocturnal asthma patients but not in the controls. Beta-adrenergic receptor binding affinity did not change with time in any of the study groups. There was no change in cyclic AMP generation in response to isoproterenol in any of the subject groups.

In a double-blind controlled study in 11 asthmatics, infusion of epinephrine (3.5 ng/kg/min) at 4 A.M. produced no effect on PEF, but subsequent administration of atropine significantly increased PEF, although diurnal variation was not abolished [91]. When atropine was given before epinephrine in 10 asthmatics, the morning dip in PEF was completely corrected and epinephrine had no additional effect. Though these studies can be criticized, alteration of plasma epinephrine within the range of diurnal variation had no effect on PEF in patients with nocturnal asthma. Severe "morning dipping" was observed in a patient with asthma, who had undetectable daytime circulating epinephrine concentrations following adrenalectomy [88]. Systemic beta-receptor blockade with high-dose propranolol did not inhibit the circadian rhythm of airway caliber or of histamine responsiveness [39] in normal subjects.

Circadian Changes in Autonomic Receptors

Significant reductions in lymphocyte beta-receptor density and increased receptor affinity were reported in asthmatic and normal subjects at 8 A.M. compared with 6 P.M. [135]. Similar results were also found in patients with partially reversible airflow obstruction [83]. Increased cyclic AMP generation by leukocytes from normal subjects has been shown at night [100]. However, these findings were not confirmed in a detailed study by Szefler et al. [133]. Circadian rhythms of cholinergic receptors in animal hearts have long been described [130].

Circadian Changes in the Parasympathetic System

The parasympathetic nervous system represents the dominant innervation of human bronchial smooth muscle. A circadian rhythm of parasympathetic outflow is suggested by change in baroreflex response to infused norepinephrine [62]. Cardiac parasympathetic tone is increased at night in humans and animals [10, 25]. Increased vagal tone was implicated in one patient with nocturnal bronchoconstriction who developed bradycardia and increased sinus arrhythmia [127]. The circadian rhythm of parasympathetic tone is reflected in the strong correlation of airway caliber and resting heart rate [38, 70, 89, 108].

In eight nonallergic patients with chronic airflow obstruction, the amplitude of diurnal variation in FEV_1 was 27 ± 2 percent compared with 7 ± 1 percent in controls [108]. Urinary epinephrine excretion was also significantly reduced in patients compared with controls, though there was diurnal variation in both. Electrocardiographic monitoring over 24 hours showed diurnal variation in heart rate and sinus arrhythmia gap (the difference between fast and slow components of sinus arrhythmia during quiet breathing) in both groups. Mean heart rate was lower, and sinus arrhythmia gap (SAG) was significantly higher in patients compared with controls, suggesting increased vagal tone at night in both groups but to a greater extent in patients. Similar results were reported in a group of asthmatic adults [70].

In a single-blind, placebo-controlled study of 10 asthmatics investigated over 2 nights, after a night's acclimatization, vagal blockade with intravenous atropine (30 μg/kg) caused significant bronchodilatation and increase in heart rate and almost completely inhibited overnight fall in PEF [90]. Mean PEF at 4 A.M. after atropine was 390 compared with 260 L/min after placebo (p < .0001). Mean PEF at 4 P.M. after atropine remained significantly higher at 440 L/min (p < .01) so diurnal variation was not abolished. Heart rate at 4 A.M. and 4 P.M. after atropine was the same. Plasma epinephrine concentration and its diurnal variation were unaffected by vagal blockade.

The effect of the anticholinergic ipratropium bromide by nebulizer after increasing doses of atropine intravenously was examined at 4 A.M. and 4 P.M. in seven asthmatics with nocturnal bronchoconstriction in a single-blind and placebo-controlled study [89]. On a separate occasion atropine, 30 μg/kg, was administered intravenously after nebulized ipratropium, 1 mg. Statistically significantly higher (approximately twofold greater) doses of atropine were required for vagal blockade as measured by specific airway conductance (sGaw), PEF, and heart rate response at 4 A.M. compared with 4 P.M. Maximum postatropine effect did not differ at the two time points for sGaw and heart rate, but as previously reported, PEF remained significantly lower at 4 A.M. This suggests either that there is increased efferent parasympathetic discharge to heart and lungs at night or that there are parallel diurnal changes in muscarinic receptor sensitivity in the two tissues. Nebulized ipratropium bromide produced no further bronchodilatation after atropine, but atropine had an additional effect after ipratropium, 1 mg, suggesting that some muscarinic receptors are more accessible from the circulation than by the inhaled route.

In normal subjects parasympathetic blockade by inhaled ipratropium bromide significantly reduced the circadian rhythm of sGaw and inhibited histamine responsiveness but not the circadian rhythm of responsiveness [38]. Changes in parasympathetic tone may be driven by a central clock or be secondary to gastroesophageal reflux, temperature change, or sleep.

Nonadrenergic Noncholinergic Nerves

The nonadrenergic noncholinergic nervous (NANC) system, comprising inhibitory and excitatory components, has been demonstrated in humans as well as animal species [6, 121]. NANC fibers are probably the only significant inhibitory innervation of human airway smooth muscle. Defective bronchodilator vasointestinal peptidergic innervation in asthma could account for nocturnal bronchoconstriction [98]. Sensory neuropeptides including substance P, neurokinins, and calcitonin gene-related peptide may be released from C-fiber endings, and axon reflex mechanisms may be involved [5]. The current state of knowledge is summarized in Chapter 18.

Evidence for a circadian rhythm in NANC nerves has recently been sought by capsaicin response after intravenous atropine and propranolol in normal subjects [77]. Inhibition of NANC function at 6 A.M. compared with 6 P.M. suggested that this may contribute to overnight bronchoconstriction.

Circadian Rhythm of Perception of Breathlessness

In a recent study circadian variation in dyspnea score was found in 40 percent of patients, although 83 percent had significant variation in PEF. There was circadian variation in the relationship between the two with better perception of airflow obstruction during the night when PEF was lowest [103]. Very severe asthmatics have not been studied, and the relationship between airway narrowing and perception of breathlessness is not known for patients at risk of fatal attacks, though there is evidence of poor perception of asthma severity in general in this group of patients.

Airway Inflammation

Airway inflammation is associated with bronchial hyperresponsiveness in experimental animal models, in laboratory asthma, in lavage and biopsy studies of mild asthma, and in asthmatics who die. This evidence is reviewed in Chapter 9. Nocturnal asthma has also been seen as a reflection of bronchial hyperresponsiveness [15, 79, 123].

Direct evidence of airway inflammation at night is provided by a recent bronchoalveolar lavage (BAL) study [81]. BAL was performed at 4 A.M. and 4 P.M., 3 to 6 days apart, in randomized order, in 14 stable atopic asthmatics—7 with nocturnal asthma (>20% reduction in PEF from bedtime to morning wakening) and 7 without (<10% change). There was no difference in BAL return, total cell count, epithelial cell count, or macrophage, lymphocyte, neutrophil, or eosinophil cell count at 4 P.M. in the two groups. At 4 A.M. total white cell, epithelial cell, neutrophil, eosinophil, and lymphocyte counts were increased in the group with nocturnal asthma. BAL total white cells, neutrophils, and eosinophils were increased compared with the 4 P.M. values, although there was no change in peripheral white cells between 4 P.M. and 4 A.M. Overnight fall in PEF correlated with overnight change in percent neutrophils and eosinophils in the whole group of asthmatics, but in the nocturnal asthmatics only the eosinophil percent change correlated with change in PEF. There was no relation to sleep pattern, and the cellular changes were not due to induced bronchoconstriction alone. In this study the observed increase in bronchial responsiveness did not correlate with airway cellularity, unlike previous studies [66, 144]. The mechanism of increase in inflammation at night remains unclear, but subjects with nocturnal asthma appeared to have more severe asthma and ongoing inflammation with greater cell counts at 4 P.M. and lower FEV$_1$ despite increased medication. In two other studies, circadian variation in low-density eosinophils and an enhanced production of oxygen radicals were found to be possible contributors to nocturnal asthma [148, 149].

Other Rhythms Connected with Airway Inflammation

Large circadian variations in total IgE have been described in allergic asthmatics [46], suggesting the possibility that the low plasma levels at night may reflect increased tissue binding and increased mast cell or other inflammatory cell activation. Dahl [31] showed diurnal variation in peripheral blood eosinophil numbers in normals and asthmatics with a maximum at midnight and a nadir at 10 A.M.

Platelet activation has recently been examined in nocturnal asthma. A group of five normals and five asthmatic patients with diurnal variation in PEF greater than 20 percent were studied [92]. A circadian rhythm in B-thromboglobulin (BTG), though not in platelet factor 4 (PF4), was found in all subjects. Platelet activation assessed as the ratio BTG/PF4 correlated inversely with PEF in the asthmatics. Atropine increased early-morning PEF without affecting BTG levels. The significance of these results is unclear.

There are few data regarding circadian variation in inflammatory mediators. Increased plasma histamine concentration or urinary histamine metabolites, as evidence of enhanced mast cell degranulation occurring at night, are somewhat conflicting [4, 108, 133]. No increase in serum neutrophil chemotactic activity was found in patients with or without nocturnal asthma [71]. Circadian variation of arachidonic acid metabolites has been described [74].

The role of airway edema in airway inflammation [105] and its potential consequences [59, 65] have recently been highlighted. Recent experimental evidence that epinephrine [13] and corticosteroids [14] inhibit airway microvascular leakage support the suggestion [7] that reduction in plasma epinephrine and plasma cortisol may predispose to increase in airway edema and bronchoconstriction at night (Fig. 76-2).

Opioids exhibit a diurnal rhythm [36], and there is considerable potential for their involvement as neuromodulatory influences. A nonspecific antagonist revealed no evidence of their involvement in diurnal variation in PEF [1].

Circadian Rhythm and Corticosteroids

The early observation that nocturnal bronchoconstriction coincided with the lowest 4 hourly urinary excretion of 17-hydroxy-

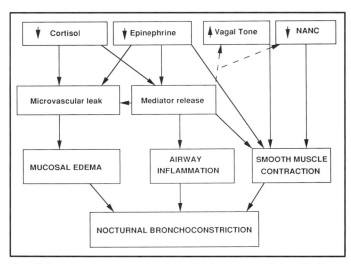

Fig. 76-2. *Inflammatory mechanisms and nocturnal asthma. NANC = nonadrenergic noncholinergic nervous system.*

corticosteroid during the 24 hours led to the suggestion that the rhythm in plasma cortisol might drive the rhythm of airway caliber [128]. Continuous infusion of hydrocortisone to eliminate the overnight fall in plasma hydroxycorticosteroids was unsuccessful however in abolishing nocturnal asthma. Bronchoconstriction recurred in five of the six patients studied, including two out of the three who had complete correction of circadian variation in plasma cortisol. In a recent uncontrolled study, supraphysiologic doses of hydrocortisone sodium succinate (100 mg/h) produced a significant improvement in overnight fall in FEV$_1$ [10a]. In 2 of 11 patients there was complete abolition of nocturnal bronchoconstriction and in 7 others 45 to 87 percent improvement compared with baseline nights, while in the remaining 2 there was no effect. The magnitude of the doses of hydrocortisone required for a benefit may reflect a spectrum of antiinflammatory effects on cell recruitment, activation, mediator production, and the effects of mediators [7]. Extremely low cortisol levels were recorded in a group of patients with nocturnal asthma [71], but this is unlikely to be causal. Neither high-dose steroid therapy [24] nor adrenalectomy prevents the morning dip in PEF [88].

TREATMENT OF NOCTURNAL ASTHMA

The development of nocturnal asthma suggests loss of control and requires increased therapy [119, 139]. A first step is usually to prescribe adequate doses of inhaled steroids [60] or a short course of oral steroids to aim to reduce bronchial inflammation and hyperresponsiveness [73]. However, nocturnal wheezing is commonly resistant to standard asthma therapy, although the bronchoconstriction nearly always responds acutely to inhaled beta$_2$ agonists. Both oral beta$_2$-adrenoceptor agonists and theophyllines would be expected to prevent nocturnal bronchoconstriction by direct actions to relax bronchial smooth muscle and by indirect actions on mast cells and other inflammatory cells. In practice slow-release aminophylline [9] and theophylline preparations [33, 41, 55, 95, 102, 120, 122, 142] appear to be more effective than slow-release oral beta agonists [40, 84, 107, 109, 131, 141], although supraphysiologic plasma concentrations may be achieved. Long-acting oral albuterol may be effective, according to a recent study [150]. Side effects may be minimized and efficacy improved by single doses at nighttime [9, 41, 102, 122], as theophylline pharmacokinetics are altered at night [124] and higher doses are consequently better tolerated. There is also some evidence of circadian rhythms of response to beta agonist and anticholinergic drugs even in normal subjects [45]. Addition of inhaled steroids to oral beta$_2$ agonists results in increased benefit [32]. Cromolyn sodium [58, 67] and nedocromil sodium [49] have not proved very effective in nocturnal asthma.

Inhaled anticholinergic bronchodilators have a longer duration of action than standard beta$_2$ agonists. Inhaled ipratropium bromide [19, 30], oxitropium bromide [26], or intravenous atropine [89, 90] partially inhibit nocturnal bronchoconstriction, though this has not always been found in asthmatic children [126].

High-dose parenteral administration of beta$_2$ agonists is often effective in reducing the morning dip of PEF [97]. Salmeterol, the new long-acting inhaled beta$_2$ agonist, is the first agent that has been shown to improve sleep quality as well as airflow obstruction in nocturnal asthma [42].

Nocturnal asthma is a common, clinically important condition reflecting underlying bronchial hyperresponsiveness. It is probably related to an exaggeration of various normal physiologic circadian rhythms. These include rhythms of airway caliber, bronchial responsiveness, and changes in nerves, the adrenergic system, and vagal parasympathetic tone. The trough in circulating epinephrine and cortisol levels may remove protective antiinflammatory mechanisms, leading to increased bronchial inflammation and inflammatory cell activation producing airway narrowing by increased microvascular leakage, mucosal edema, and smooth muscle constriction. Greater understanding of these mechanisms would have therapeutic implications.

REFERENCES

1. al-Damluji, S., et al. Effect of naloxone on circadian rhythms in lung function. *Thorax* 38:914, 1983.
2. Asthma at night (editorial). *Lancet* 1:220, 1983.
3. Aurelianus Caelius. *De Morbis Acutis et Chronicis.* Amsterdam: Wetsteniand, 1709.
4. Barnes, P., et al. Nocturnal asthma and changes in circulating epinephrine, histamine and cortisol. *N. Engl. J. Med.* 303:263, 1980.
5. Barnes, P. J. Asthma as an axon reflex. *Lancet* 1:242, 1986.
6. Barnes, P. J. Neural control of human airways in health and disease: State of the art. *Am. Rev. Respir. Dis.* 134:1289, 1986.
7. Barnes, P. J. Inflammatory mechanisms and nocturnal asthma. *Am. J. Med.* 85:(suppl. 1B):64, 1988.
8. Barnes, P. J., FitzGerald, G. A., and Dollery, C. T. Circadian variation in adrenergic responses in asthmatic subjects. *Clin. Sci.* 62:349, 1982.
9. Barnes, P. J., et al. Single-dose slow-release aminophylline at night prevents nocturnal asthma. *Lancet* 1:299, 1982.
10. Baust, W., and Bohnert, B. The regulation of heart rate during sleep. *Exp. Brain Res.* 7:169, 1969.
10a. Beam, W. R., Ballard, R. D., and Martin, R. J. Spectrum of corticosteroid sensitivity in nocturnal asthma. *Am. Rev. Respir. Dis.* 145:1082, 1992.
11. Bellia, V., et al. Relationship of nocturnal bronchoconstriction to sleep stages. *Am. Rev. Respir. Dis.* 140:363, 1989.
12. Berquist, W. E., et al. Quantitative gastroesophageal reflux and pulmonary function in asthmatic children and normal adults receiving placebo, theophylline and metaproterenol. *J. Allergy Clin. Immunol.* 73:253, 1984.
12a. Bonnet, R., et al. Circadian rhythm in airway responsiveness and airway tone in patients with mild asthma. *J. Appl. Physiol.* 71:1598, 1991.
13. Boschetto, P., et al. Effect of antiasthma drugs on microvascular leakage in guinea pig airways. *Am. Rev. Respir. Dis.* 139:416, 1989.
14. Boschetto, B., et al. Corticosteroid inhibition of airway microvascular leakage. *Am. Rev. Respir. Dis.* 143:605, 1991.
15. Brand, P. L. P., et al. The relationship of airway hyperresponsiveness to respiratory symptoms and diurnal peak flow in patients with obstructive lung disease. *Am. Rev. Respir. Dis.* 143:916, 1991.
16. Bulow, K. Respiration and wakefulness in man. *Acta Physiol. Scand.* (Suppl. 59):209, 1963.
17. Cabanes, L. R., et al. Bronchial hyperresponsiveness to methacholine in patients with impaired left ventricular function. *N. Engl. J. Med.* 320:1317, 1989.
18. Caterall, J. R., et al. Effect of sleep deprivation on overnight bronchoconstriction in nocturnal asthma. *Thorax* 41:676, 1986.
19. Caterall, J. R., et al. Is nocturnal asthma caused by changes in airway cholinergic activity? *Thorax* 43:720, 1988.
20. Chan, C. S., Woolcock, A. J., and Sullivan, C. E. Nocturnal asthma: Role of snoring and sleep apnoea. *Am. Rev. Respir. Dis.* 137:1502, 1988.
21. Chen, W. Y., and Chai, H. Airway cooling and nocturnal asthma. *Chest* 81:675, 1982.
22. Cinkotai, F. F., and Thomson, M. L. Diurnal variation in pulmonary diffusing capacity for carbon monoxide. *J. Appl. Physiol.* 21:539, 1966.
23. Christensen, J. Effects of drugs on esophageal motility. *Arch. Intern. Med.* 136:532, 1976.
24. Clark, T. J. H., and Hetzel, M. R. Diurnal variation of asthma. *Br. J. Dis. Chest* 71:87, 1977.
25. Clarke, J. M., et al. The rhythm of the normal human heart. *Lancet* 2:508, 1976.
26. Coe, C. I., and Barnes, P. J. Reduction of nocturnal asthma by an inhaled anticholinergic drug. *Chest* 90:485, 1986.
27. Connolly, C. K. Diurnal rhythms in airway obstruction. *Br. J. Dis. Chest* 73:357, 1979.
28. Connolly, C. K. The effect of bronchodilators on diurnal rhythms in airway obstruction. *Br. J. Dis. Chest* 75:197, 1981.
29. Cove-Smith, J. R., et al. Circadian variation in an immune response in man. *Br. J. Med.* 2:253, 1978.
30. Cox, I. D., Hughes, D. T. D., and McDonnell, K. A. Ipratropium bromide in patients with nocturnal asthma. *Postgrad. Med. J.* 60:526, 1984.
31. Dahl, R. Diurnal variation in the number of circulatory eosinophil leukocytes in normal controls and asthmatics. *Acta Allergol.* 32:310, 1977.
32. Dahl, R., Pedersen, B., and Hagglof, B. Nocturnal asthma: Effect of treatment with oral sustained-release terbutaline, inhaled budesonide and the two in combination. *J. Allergy Clin. Immunol.* 79:811, 1989.
33. Davies, D. O., et al. Twice daily slow-release theophylline versus placebo for "morning dipping" in asthma. *Br. J. Clin. Pharmacol.* 17:335, 1984.
34. Davis, R. S., Larsen, G. L., and Grunstein, M. M. Respiratory response to intraoesophageal acid infusion in asthmatic children during sleep. *J. Allergy Clin. Immunol.* 72:393, 1983.
35. Dawkins, K. D., and Muers, M. F. Diurnal variation in airflow obstruction in chronic bronchitis. *Thorax* 36:618, 1981.
36. Dent, R. M. M., et al. Diurnal rhythm of plasma immunoreactive beta endorphin and its relationship to sleep stages and plasma rhythms of cortisol and prolactin. *J. Clin. Endocrinol. Metab.* 52:942, 1981.
37. De Vries, K., et al. Changes during 24 hours in the lung function and histamine hyperreactivity of the bronchial tree in asthmatic and bronchitis patients. *Int. Arch. Allergy* 20:93, 1962.
38. Drehner, D., and Koller, E. A. Circadian rhythms of specific airway conductance and bronchial reactivity to histamine: The effects of parasympathetic blockade. *Eur. Respir. J.* 3:414, 1990.
39. Drehner, D., Passweg, D., and Koller, E. A. Autonomic mechanisms of airway narrowing and increased bronchial reactivity at night. *Experimentia* 44:32, 1988.
40. Fairfax, A. J., MacNabb, W. R., and Davies, H. J. Slow-release oral salbutamol and aminophylline in nocturnal asthma: Relation of overnight changes in lung function and plasma drug levels. *Thorax* 35:526, 1980.
41. Fairshter, R. D., et al. Comparison of clinical effects and pharmacokinetics of once-daily Uniphyl and twice-daily Theo-Dur in asthmatic patients. *Am. J. Med.* 79(Suppl. 6A):48, 1985.
42. Fitzpatrick, M. F., et al. Salmeterol in nocturnal asthma: A double-blind, placebo controlled trial of a long acting inhaled β2 agonist. *Br. Med. J.* 301:1365, 1990.
43. Fitzpatrick, M. F., et al. Sleep quality and daytime cognitive performance in nocturnal asthma. *Thorax* 45:338P, 1990.
44. Francis, A. *The Francis Treatment of Asthma.* London: Heinemann, 1932. Pp. 17–19.
45. Gaultier, C., Reinberg, A., and Girard, F. Etude circadienne de la resistance pulmonaire totale et de la compliance dynamique chez l'enfant sain. *C. R. Acad. Sci.* 280:1253, 1975.
46. Gaultier, C., et al. Circadian rhythm in serum total immunoglobulin E (IgE) in asthmatic children. *Biomed. Pharmacother.* 41:186, 1987.
47. Gervais, P., et al. Twenty-four hour rhythm in the bronchial hyperreactivity to house dust in asthmatics. *J. Allergy Clin. Immunol.* 59:207, 1977.
48. Goodall, R. J. R., et al. Relationship between asthma and gastrooesophageal reflux. *Thorax* 36:116, 1981.
49. Greif, J., et al. A multicenter, double-blind, parallel group comparison of nedocromil sodium in the treatment of bronchial asthma. *Chest* 96:583, 1989.

50. Guberan, E., et al. Circadian variation of FEV₁ in shift workers. *Br. J. Ind. Med.* 26:121, 1969.

51. Gugger, M., et al. Ventilatory and arousal responses to added inspiratory resistance during sleep. *Am. Rev. Respir. Dis.* 140:1301, 1989.

52. Halberg, F., et al. Computer techniques in the study of biological rhythms. *Ann. N.Y. Acad. Sci.* 115:695, 1964.

53. Hannaway, P. J., and Hopper, G. D. K. Cough variant asthma in children. *J.A.M.A.* 247:206, 1982.

54. Heaton, R. W., Gillett, M. K., and Snashall, P. D. Morning-evening changes in airway responsiveness to methacholine in normal and asthmatic subjects: Analysis using partial flow volume curves. *Thorax* 43:727, 1988.

55. Helm, S. G. Diurnal stabilization of asthma with once-daily evening administration of controlled release theophylline: A multi-investigator study. *Allergy Practice* 9:414, 1987.

56. Hetzel, M. R., and Clark, T. J. H. Does sleep cause nocturnal asthma? *Thorax* 34:749, 1979.

57. Hetzel, M. R., and Clark, T. J. H. Comparison of normal and asthmatic circadian rhythms in peak expiratory flow rate. *Thorax* 35:732, 1980.

58. Hetzel, M. R., et al. Is sodium cromoglycate effective in nocturnal asthma? *Thorax* 40:793, 1985.

59. Hogg, J. C., Pare, P. D., and Moreno, R. The effect of submucosal edema on airway resistance. *Am. Rev. Respir. Dis.* 135:S54, 1987.

60. Horn, C. R., Clark, T. J. H., and Cochrane, C. M. Inhaled therapy reduces morning dips in asthma. *Lancet* 1:1143, 1984.

61. Hossmann, V., Fitzgerald, G. A., and Dollery, C. T. Circadian rhythm of baroreflex reactivity and adrenergic vascular response. *Cardiovasc. Res.* 14:125, 1980.

62. Ind, P. W., and Barnes, P. J. Adrenergic Control of Airways in Asthma. In P. J. Barnes, R. I. W. Rodger, and N. C. Thomson (eds.), *Asthma: Basic Mechanisms and Clinical Management.* London: Academy, 1988. Pp. 357–380.

63. Ind, P. W., et al. Measurement of plasma histamine in asthma. *Clin. Allergy* 13:61, 1983.

64. Issa, F. O., and Sullivan, C. E. Respiratory muscle activation and thoracoabdominal motion during acute episodes of asthma during sleep. *Am. Rev. Respir. Dis.* 132:999, 1985.

65. James, A. L., Pare, P. D., and Hogg, J. C. The mechanics of airway narrowing in asthma. *Am. Rev. Respir. Dis.* 139:242, 1989.

66. Jeffery, P. K., et al. Bronchial biopsies in asthma: An ultrastructural, quantitative study and correlation with hyperreactivity. *Am. Rev. Respir. Dis.* 140:1745, 1989.

67. Jenkins, C. J., and Breslin, A. B. X. Long term study of the effect of sodium cromoglycate on non-specific bronchial hyperresponsiveness. *Thorax* 42:664, 1987.

68. Jonsson, E., and Mossberg, B. Impairment of ventilatory function by supine posture in asthma. *Eur. J. Respir. Dis.* 65:496, 1984.

69. Kales, A., et al. Sleep studies in asthmatic adults: Relationship of attacks to sleep stage and time of night. *J. Allergy Clin. Immunol.* 41:164, 1968.

70. Kallenbach, J. M., et al. Heart rate control in asthma: Evidence of parasympathetic overactivity. *Chest* 87:644, 1985.

71. Kallenbach, J. M., et al. Nocturnal events related to "morning dipping" in bronchial asthma. *Chest* 93:751, 1988.

72. Kerr, H. D. Diurnal variation of respiratory function independent of air quality. *Arch. Environ. Health* 26:144, 1973.

73. Kraan, J., et al. Changes in bronchial hyperreactivity induced by 4 weeks treatment with anti-asthmatic drugs in patients with allergic asthma: A comparison between budesonide and terbutaline. *J. Allergy Clin. Immunol.* 76:628, 1985.

74. Kunkel, G., et al. Arachidonic acid metabolites and their circadian rhythm in patients with allergic bronchial asthma. *Chronobiol. Int.* 5:387, 1988.

75. Lewinsohn, H. C., Capel, L. H., and Smart, J. Changes in forced expiratory volumes throughout the day. *Br. Med. J.* 1:462, 1960.

76. Liu, Y.-N., et al. Effect of circadian rhythm on bronchomotor tone after deep inspiration in normal and asthmatic subjects. *Am. Rev. Respir. Dis.* 132:278, 1985.

77. Mackay, T. W., Fitzpatrick, M. F., and Douglas, N. J. Non-adrenergic, non-cholinergic nervous system and overnight airway calibre in asthmatic and normal subjects. *Lancet* 338:1289, 1991.

78. Mansfield, L. E., et al. The role of the vagus nerve in airway narrowing caused by intraesophageal hydrochloric acid provocation and esophageal distension. *Ann. Allergy* 47:431, 1981.

79. Martin, R. J., Cicutto, L. C., and Ballard, R. D. Factors relating to worsening of nocturnal asthma. *Am. Rev. Respir. Dis.* 141:33, 1990.

80. Martin, M. E., Grunstein, M. M., and Larsen, G. L. The relationship of gastroesophageal reflux in children with asthma. *Ann. Allergy* 49:318, 1982.

81. Martin, R. J., et al. Airways inflammation in nocturnal asthma. *Am. Rev. Respir. Dis.* 143:351, 1991.

82. McDermott, M. Diurnal and weekly cyclical changes in lung airways resistance. *J. Physiol.* 186:90P, 1965.

83. Meurs, H., et al. The beta-adrenergic system of non-allergic patients with chronic airflow obstruction and early morning dyspnea. *J. Allergy* 59:417, 1987.

84. Milledge, J. S., and Morris, J. A comparison of slow-release salbutamol with slow release aminophylline in nocturnal asthma. *J. Int. Med. Res.* 7(Suppl. 1):106, 1979.

85. Mills, J. N. Changes in alveolar carbon dioxide tensions by night. *J. Physiol.* 122:66, 1953.

86. Montplaisir, J., Walsh, J., and Malo, J. L. Nocturnal asthma: Features of attacks, sleep and breathing patterns. *Am. Rev. Respir. Dis.* 125:18, 1982.

87. Morgan, A. D., et al. Breathing patterns during sleep in patients with nocturnal asthma. *Thorax* 42:600, 1987.

88. Morice, A., Sever, P., and Ind, P. W. Adrenaline, bronchoconstriction and asthma. *Br. Med. J.* 293:539, 1986.

89. Morrison, J. F. J., and Pearson, S. B. The effect of the circadian rhythm of vagal activity on bronchomotor tone in asthma. *Br. J. Clin. Pharmacol.* 28:545, 1989.

90. Morrison, J. F. J., Pearson, S. B., and Dean, H. G. Parasympathetic nervous system in nocturnal asthma. *Br. Med. J.* 296:1427, 1988.

91. Morrison, J. F. J., et al. Adrenaline and nocturnal asthma. *Br. Med. J.* 301:473, 1990.

92. Morrison, J. F. J., et al. Platelet activation in nocturnal asthma. *Thorax* 46:197, 1991.

93. Mygind, N., and Thomsen, J. Diurnal variation in nasal protein concentration. *Acta Otolaryngol.* 82:219, 1976.

94. Nelson, W., et al. Methods for cosinorrhythmometry. *Chronobiologica* 6:305, 1979.

95. Neuenkirchen, H., et al. Nocturnal asthma and sustained release theophylline. *Eur. J. Respir. Dis.* 66:196, 1985.

96. Newman Taylor, A. J., et al. Recurrent nocturnal asthmatic reactions to bronchial provocation test. *Clin. Allergy* 9:213, 1979.

97. O'Driscoll, B. R. C., et al. Long-term treatment of severe asthma with subcutaneous terbutaline. *Br. J. Dis. Chest* 82:360, 1988.

98. Ollerenshaw, S., et al. Absence of immunoreactive vasointestinal polypeptide in tissue from the lungs of patients with asthma. *N. Engl. J. Med.* 320:1244, 1989.

99. Overholt, R. H., and Astraf, N. M. Oesophageal reflux as trigger in asthma. *N.Y. State J. Med.* 66:3030, 1966.

100. Pauwels, R., and Van der Straeten, M. The leukocytic beta₂-receptor: Effect of circadian rhythm and age in normal people. *Eur. J. Respir. Dis.* 61:26, 1980.

101. Pavia, D. Mucociliary clearance at night: Effect of physical activity, posture, and circadian rhythm. In P. J. Barnes and J. Levy (eds.), *Nocturnal Asthma.* Royal Society of Medicine International Congress and Symposium 1984 series no. 73, pp. 29–38.

102. Pedersen, S. Treatment of nocturnal asthma in children with a single dose of sustained-release theophylline taken after supper. *Clin. Allergy* 15:79, 1985.

103. Peiffer, C., Marsac, J., and Lockhart, A. Chronobiological study of the relationship between dyspnoea and airway obstruction in symptomatic asthmatic subjects. *Clin. Sci.* 77:237, 1989.

104. Perperia, M., et al. The prevalence of asymptomatic gastroesophageal reflux in bronchial asthma and nonasthmatic individuals. *Eur. J. Respir. Dis.* 64:582, 1983.

105. Persson, C. G. A. Role of plasma exudation in asthmatic airways. *Lancet* 2:1126, 1986.

106. Platts-Mills, T. A. E., et al. Reduction of bronchial hyperreactivity during prolonged allergen avoidance. *Lancet* 2:675, 1982.

107. Postma, D. S., et al. The effects of oral slow-release terbutaline on the circadian variation in spirometry and arterial blood gas levels in patients with chronic airflow obstruction. *Chest* 76:628, 1985.

108. Postma, D. S., et al. Influence of parasympathetic and sympathetic nervous system on nocturnal bronchial obstruction. *Clin. Sci.* 69:251, 1985.

109. Postma, D. S., et al. Influence of slow release terbutaline on the circadian variation of catecholamine, histamine and lung function in non-allergic patients with partly reversible airflow obstruction. *J. Allergy Clin. Immunol.* 77:471, 1986.

110. Pounsford, J. C., and Saunders, K. B. Diurnal variation and adaptation

of the cough response to citric acid in normal subjects. *Thorax* 40:657, 1985.

111. Quackenboss, J. J., Lebowitz, M. D., and Krzyzanowski, M. The normal range of diurnal changes in peak expiratory flow rates: Relationship to symptoms and respiratory disease. *Am. Rev. Respir. Dis.* 143:323, 1991.

112. Rachiele, A., et al. Circadian variations of airway response to histamine in asthmatic subjects. *Bull. Eur. Physiopathol. Respir.* 19:465, 1983.

113. Reinberg, A., Chata, J., and Sidi, E. Nocturnal asthma attacks: Their relationship to the circadian adrenal cycle. *J. Allergy* 34:323, 1963.

114. Reinberg, A., and Sidi, E. Circadian changes in the inhibitory effects of an antihistamine drug in man. *J. Invest. Dermatol.* 46:415, 1966.

115. Reinberg, A., Sidi, E., and Ghata, J. Circadian reactivity rhythms of human skin to histamine or allergen and the adrenal cycle. *J. Allergy* 36:273, 1965.

116. Reinberg, A., et al. Circadian reactivity rhythm of human skin to house dust, penicillin and histamine. *J. Allergy* 44:292, 1969.

117. Reinberg, A., et al. Rhythme circadien humain du seuil de la response bronchique a l'acetylcholine. *C. R. Acad. Sci.* 272:1879, 1971.

118. Reinberg, A., et al. Circadian and circannual rhythms of allergic rhinitis: An epidemiological study involving chronobiologic methods. *J. Allergy Clin. Immunol.* 81:51, 1988.

119. Reinhardt, D., et al. Comparison of the effects of theophylline, prednisolone and sleep withdrawal on airway obstruction and urinary cyclic AMP/cyclic GMP excretion of asthmatic children with and without nocturnal asthma. *Int. J. Clin. Pharmacol. Ther. Toxicol.* 8:399, 1980.

120. Rhind, G. B., et al. Sustained release choline theophyllinate in nocturnal asthma. *Br. Med. J.* 291:1605, 1985.

121. Richardson, J., and Beland, J. Non-adrenergic inhibitory nervous system in human airways. *J. Appl. Physiol.* 41:764, 1976.

122. Rivington, R. N., et al. Comparison of morning versus evening dosing with a new once-daily oral theophylline formulation. *Am. J. Med.* 79(Suppl. 6A):67, 1985.

123. Ryan, G., et al. Bronchial responsiveness to histamine: Relationship to diurnal variation of peak flow rate, improvement after bronchodilator and airway calibre. *Thorax* 37:423, 1982.

124. Scott, P. H., et al. Sustained release theophylline for childhood asthma: Evidence for circadian variation of theophylline pharmacokinetics. *J. Pediatr.* 99:476, 1981.

125. Shapiro, C., et al. Do asthmatics suffer bronchoconstriction during rapid eye movement sleep? *Br. Med. J.* 292:1161, 1986.

126. Sly, P. D., Landau, L. I., and Olinski, A. Failure of ipratropium bromide to modify the diurnal variation of asthma in asthmatic children. *Thorax* 42:357, 1987.

127. Soutar, C. A., Carrthers, M, and Pickering, C. A. Nocturnal asthma and urinary adrenaline and noradrenaline excretion. *Thorax* 32:677, 1977.

128. Soutar, C. A., et al. Nocturnal and early morning asthma: Relationship to plasma corticosteroids and response to cortisol infusion. *Thorax* 30:436, 1975.

129. Spaulding, H. S., et al. Further investigation of the association between gastroesophageal reflux and bronchoconstriction. *J. Allergy Clin. Immunol.* 69:516, 1982.

130. Spoor, R. P., and Jackson, D. B. Circadian rhythms: Variation in sensitivity of isolated rat atria to acetylcholine. *Science* 154:782, 1966.

131. Stewart, I. C., et al. Effects of sustained release terbutaline on symptoms and sleep quality in patients with nocturnal asthma. *Thorax* 42:797, 1987.

132. Sullivan, C. E., et al. Regulation of airway smooth muscle tone in sleeping dogs. *Am. Rev. Respir. Dis.* 119:87, 1979.

133. Szefler, S. J., et al. Plasma histamine, epinephrine, cortisol, and leukocyte beta-adrenergic receptors in nocturnal asthma. *Clin. Pharmacol. Ther.* 49:59, 1991.

134. Tabachnik, E., et al. Chest wall mechanics and pattern of breathing during sleep in asthmatic adolescents. *Am. Rev. Respir. Dis.* 124:269, 1981.

135. Titinchi, S., et al. Circadian variation in number and affinity of $beta_2$ adrenoceptors in lymphocytes of asthmatic patients. *Clin. Sci.* 66:323, 1984.

136. Townsend, M. M., and Smith, A. J. Factors influencing the urinary excretion of free catecholamines in man. *Clin. Sci.* 41:253, 1973.

137. Turner-Warwick, M. On observing patterns of airflow obstruction in chronic asthma. *Br. J. Dis. Chest* 71:87, 1977.

138. Turner-Warwick, M. Epidemiology of nocturnal asthma. *Am. J. Med.* 85(1B):6, 1988.

139. Van Aalderan, W. M. C., et al. The effect of reduction of maintenance treatment on circadian variation in peak expiratory flow rate values in asthmatic children. *Acta Pediatr. Scand.* 77:269, 1988.

140. Van Aalderan, W. M. C., et al. Circadian change in bronchial responsiveness and airflow obstruction in asthmatic children. *Thorax* 44:803, 1989.

140a. van Aalderen, W. M. C., et al. Nocturnal airflow obstruction, histamine, and the autonomic central nervous system in children with allergic asthma. *Thorax* 46:366, 1991.

141. Vyse, T., and Cochrane, G. M. Controlled release salbutamol tablets versus sustained release theophylline tablets in the control of reversible obstructive airways disease. *J. Int. Med. Res.* 17:93, 1989.

142. Welsh, P. W., Reed, C. E., and Conrad, E. Timing of once-a-day theophylline dose to match peak blood level with diurnal variation in severity of asthma. *Am. J. Med.* 80:1098, 1986.

143. Wang, Y. T., Coe, C. I., and Pride, N. B. Effect on histamine responsiveness of reducing airway dimensions by altering posture. *Thorax* 45:530, 1990.

144. Wardlaw, A. J., et al. Eosinophils and mast cells in bronchoalveolar lavage in mild asthma: Relationship to bronchial hyperreactivity. *Am. Rev. Respir. Dis.* 137:62, 1988.

145. Whyte, K. F., and Douglas, N. J. Posture and nocturnal asthma. *Thorax* 44:579, 1989.

146. Wilson, N. M., et al. Gastroesophageal reflux and childhood asthma: The acid test. *Thorax* 40:592, 1985.

147. Martin, R. J., Cicutto, L. C., and Ackerson, L. M. Stability of the circadian alteration in lung function in asthma. *J. Allergy Clin. Immunol.* 89:703, 1992.

148. Calhoun, W. J., et al. Characteristics of peripheral blood eosinophils in patients with nocturnal asthma. *Am. Rev. Respir. Dis.* 145:577, 1992.

149. Jarjour, N. N., Busse, W. W., and Calhoun, W. J. Enhanced production of oxygen radicals in nocturnal asthma. *Am. Rev. Respir. Dis.* 146:905, 1992.

150. Storms, W. W., et al. The effect of repeat action albuterol sulfate (Proventil Repetabs) in nocturnal symptoms of asthma. *J. Asthma* 29:209, 1992.

Therapeutic Approaches in the Cardiac-Hypertensive-Diabetic Patient

77

Kenneth R. Chapman
Anthony S. Rebuck

The management of asthma in the presence of coexisting cardiovascular or metabolic disease is a complex task. The nonpulmonary disease may mimic or mask asthma symptoms, making assessment difficult. Medications prescribed for nonpulmonary disease may affect asthma adversely. Antiasthmatic agents also have the potential to produce adverse cardiovascular and metabolic sequelae, although the trend toward topically active inhaled medications helps to minimize such problems. The following review outlines basic pharmacologic and pathophysiologic principles on which sound therapeutic decisions can be based.

CARDIOVASCULAR DISEASE

The forms of cardiovascular disease under discussion comprise the common clinical entities of congestive heart failure, ischemic heart disease, essential hypertension, and supraventricular and ventricular arrhythmias. Our goal is to highlight therapeutic approaches that provide the most effective antiasthmatic therapy least likely to increase myocardial oxygen demand or to provoke significant dysrhythmias.

In asthmatics with coincident impaired left ventricular function, it may be difficult to determine whether episodic dyspnea and wheezing are manifestations of pulmonary or cardiac disease ("cardiac asthma"). Although it has been postulated that "cardiac" asthma may represent underlying occult airway hyperreactivity unmasked by the irritant effects of increased lung water, the lack of methacholine hyperresponsiveness in at least some patients with cardiac asthma argues that this is not the case [75]. When left ventricular dysfunction results in clinical and radiologic manifestations of congestive heart failure, the precise cause of airways' obstruction will be readily apparent, allowing therapy to be directed to improvement of hemodynamic status. However, as has been shown in studies of nonasthmatic patients following myocardial infarction, mild left ventricular impairment in the absence of clinical or radiologic signs of congestive heart failure can result in abnormal tests of small airways' function, ventilation-perfusion mismatch, and an increase in the alveolar-arterial gradient for oxygen [38]. In the asthmatic patient with cardiovascular disease, such changes in respiratory function could result in a misdirected increased effort to treat the pulmonary disease rather than the underlying cause of such deterioration. When confronted by an asthmatic whose respiratory complaints may be in part secondary to cardiac disease, a therapeutic trial may be used to determine where further pharmacologic efforts should be directed. An improvement following more aggressive diuretics or afterload reduction therapy would reasonably suggest that cardiac disease was responsible for the worsening of symptoms. By contrast, improvement following more aggressive bronchodilator therapy would not necessarily rule out left ventricular dysfunction as a cause of respiratory symptoms; adrenergic agonists and methylxanthines have cardiovascular effects that could result in improvement of heart failure. Epinephrine and isoproterenol are inotropic, beta$_2$ selective agents such as terbutaline are vasodilators, and methylxanthines have both inotropic and diuretic properties [64, 86]. A gradual reduction in symptoms with inhaled steroid therapy or sodium cromolyn would suggest more reliably that asthma had been the cause of the symptoms [81].

Cardiovascular Drug Interactions

Drugs used in the treatment of cardiovascular disease may have adverse effects in asthma (Table 77-1). Notable in this respect are the nonselective beta blockers such as propranolol, nadolol, and timolol [89]. While beta blockers have little or no deleterious effect on airway function in healthy nonasthmatic subjects, their use in patients with airway hyperreactivity can have devastating consequences. Such agents should be regarded as absolutely contraindicated for patients with asthma. This caveat applies even to those beta blockers with so-called cardioselectivity (e.g., metoprolol, atenolol) or intrinsic sympathomimetic activity (e.g., pindolol) [32, 52]. The inadvertent use of even small doses of beta-blocking agents can precipitate asthma attacks that are, by definition, resistant to beta-agonist therapy. Should such a clinical scenario of beta blocker–induced bronchospasm occur, relief of symptoms can be achieved only by alternate bronchodilator pathways such as those offered by quaternary anticholinergic compounds, for example, ipratropium bromide [18, 35] (see Chap. 64).

The angiotensin-converting enzyme (ACE) inhibitors used widely in the management of hypertension may cause intractable cough in some patients in the absence of preexisting pulmonary disease [33, 47]. The precise mechanism of ACE inhibitor cough is not clear but is thought to involve increased elaboration of inflammatory mediators such as bradykinin. It appears that asthmatics are no more predisposed to this effect of ACE inhibitor therapy than nonasthmatics [47a]. However, when drug-induced cough complicates reactive or inflammatory airway diseases, much of the therapeutic benefit of standard antiasthmatic drugs is lost. Accordingly, the ACE inhibitors, despite their secure place in the management of hypertension and congestive failure, remain troublesome to physicians in currently managing elderly patients with asthma.

In view of the potential hazard of beta blockers and the nuisance cough induced by ACE inhibitors, the calcium channel blocking agents are those most favored by pulmonary physicians who need to treat hypertension [15, 29]. Diuretics are a low-cost alternative and cause little if any problem for patients with asthma; it has even been suggested that furosemide may decrease bronchial hyperresponsiveness [7, 8]. The sole precautionary note is that diuretics may induce hypokalemia, as may beta agonists [14, 37]. Their use in combination should be under-

Table 77-1. Drugs to avoid or employ with caution in asthmatics with cardiovascular disease

Drug	Problem(s)
Beta-adrenergic blockers	Increase in airways' obstruction
Edrophonium	Increase in airways' obstruction
Aspirin	May increase airways' obstruction
Epinephrine	Increased afterload, arrhythmias
Ephedrine	Vasoconstriction, chronotrophy, tachyphylaxis
Isoproterenol	$Beta_1$ inotrophy, chronotrophy, ?myocardial injury
$Beta_2$ selective agonists	Tachycardia, ? ↑ ectopic beats
Theophylline	Frequent dose adjustment, tachyarrhythmias, hypoxemia
Atropine	Tachycardia, inspissation of bronchial secretions
ACE inhibitors	Cough

Table 77-2. Cardiovascular disorders and asthma therapy

Disorder	Preferred drug(s)	Side effects to minimize
Acute myocardial infarction	Ipratropium bromide	—
	Corticosteroids	
	Aerosol	Oral candidiasis, compliance
	Oral	Sodium retention
	Parenteral	Sodium retention
	Sodium cromolyn	—
Chronic congestive heart failure	β_2-Adrenergic agonists	Chronotropic effect
	Corticosteroids	Fluid retention
	Sodium cromolyn	—
	Ipratropium bromide	—
Essential hypertension	β_2-Adrenergic agonists	Chronotropic effect
	Aerosol corticosteroids	Oral candidiasis, compliance
	Ipratropium bromide	—
	Sodium cromolyn	—

taken with caution, although clinically relevant hypokalemia is rare [16]. In the future, a new class of antihypertensive agent may be particularly helpful in asthmatics; the potassium channel agonists such as cromokalim demonstrate not only useful antihypertensive properties but in both animals and humans have clinically significant bronchodilator properties.

A number of other medications used in the adjunctive therapy of cardiovascular diseases may have minor or major adverse consequences for the asthmatic. Intravenous edrophonium is sometimes used to abort attacks of paroxysmal supraventricular tachycardia; its potent muscarinic properties could provoke attacks of bronchospasm in the predisposed patient. Other arrhythmic drugs such as disopyramide have notable anticholinergic side effects and may produce drying and inspissation of bronchial secretions. Antiplatelet agents such as aspirin may produce airway narrowing in asthmatic subjects, presumably through their effect on prostaglandin metabolism [78, 85]. Some asthmatics, commonly those with nasal polyps, may have bronchospasm following the administration of aspirin (see Chap. 48). Such drug side effects should be sought when asthma appears or becomes worse in a patient with cardiovascular disease.

Some agents used in the treatment of cardiovascular disease may have bronchodilator properties, thus identifying them as preferred agents when a choice can be made from among several alternative drugs. As noted above, calcium channel blockers have been found effective in preventing bronchospasm in both animals and humans and may thus be useful alternatives in the treatment of angina pectoris and systemic hypertension [15, 29, 57]. Although the role of alpha-adrenergic receptors in asthma is not defined clearly, stimulation of alpha receptors could potentially result in bronchoconstriction. Among the alpha-adrenal receptor antagonists, prazosin, administered by the aerosol route, has been found effective in preventing exercise-induced asthma. However, the effect is small and of doubtful clinical significance [5]. Similarly, nitroglycerin has shown inconsistent bronchodilator properties of little clinical worth [48, 53].

Antiasthmatic Therapy

Current concepts in asthma management regard the treatment of asthma to be antiinflammatory therapy and the treatment of symptoms to be inhaled bronchodilators [4, 39, 66]. Indeed, excessive use of bronchodilators is now regarded as a symptom of asthma and an indication that this asthma is uncontrolled and undertreated. So compelling is the concept of first-line antiinflammatory therapy that bronchodilators are now administered more sparingly, usually via inhalation for brief symptomatic relief. Maintenance therapy with bronchodilators, either oral or

Table 77-3. Relative alpha and beta activities of adrenergic bronchodilators

Agent	α	β_2 (airway, vascular smooth muscle)	β_1 (myocardium)
Epinephrine	+ + + +	+ + + +	+ + +
Ephedrine	+ +	+ + + +	+, + +
Isoproterenol	0	+ + + +	+ + + +
Isoetharine	0	+ + + +	+ +
Terbutaline	0	+ + + +	+, + +
Metaproterenol (orciprenaline)	0	+ + + +	+, + +
Salbutamol (albuterol)	0	+ + + +	+, + +
Fenoterol	0	+ + + +	+, + +
Procaterol	0	+ + + +	+, + +
Pirbuterol	0	+ + + +	+, + +

inhaled, is reserved for more troublesome disease [39]. Moreover, some now regard frequent or regular bronchodilator self-administration as more than a mere signpost of unstable asthma but have conjectured that such regular beta agonist use contributes to airway hyperreactivity and asthma instability [74]. A reasonable approach to treating the asthmatic with cardiovascular disease can be derived from the principles summarized in Table 77-2.

Adrenergic Agonists

Subcutaneous epinephrine has been used successfully for several decades in the treatment of acutely ill asthmatics. Although its use is fading, the practice has not altogether disappeared. However, its potent cardiovascular side effects contraindicate its use in asthmatics with significant cardiac or hypertensive disease (Table 77-3). Epinephrine nonselectively stimulates both alpha- and beta-adrenergic receptors, resulting in vasoconstriction, tachycardia, and cardiac inotropy [86]. When used in combination with aminophylline in older, acutely ill asthmatics, epinephrine may induce potentially life-threatening ventricular dysrhythmias [2, 13, 36, 46]. The vasoconstriction produced by this agent has been felt by some to be an advantage by reducing edema of the bronchial mucosa. This potential effect has not, however, been confirmed by physiologic or clinical studies and may not occur to any important degree.

The widespread availability of effective beta$_2$ selective agonists argues strongly against the continued use of epinephrine in any asthmatic [58]. The bronchodilatation of adrenergic agents is achieved by stimulation of the beta$_2$ receptor on bronchial smooth muscle with consequent smooth muscle relaxation and airway dilatation. To minimize all unwanted cardiovascular effects of adrenergic agents, highly selective beta$_2$ agonists have been devised (see Table 77-3). In North America, currently available beta$_2$ agonists comprise albuterol (salbutamol), fenoterol, metaproterenol, pirbuterol, procaterol, and terbutaline. These agents are generally regarded as being almost devoid of cardiovascular effects when given in usual clinical dosages. However, their potential for producing significant hemodynamic changes may be underappreciated. We have found that two metered-dose inhaler puffs of fenoterol (400 μg) produces an average 35 percent increase in cardiac output in normal volunteers [19, 20, 22]. This response is highly variable among individuals, and some may show as much as a doubling in cardiac output to this usual therapeutic dosage. This effect is the result of peripheral vasodilatation with a decrease in afterload and a reflex increase in cardiac output. Such changes are well tolerated by the healthy young asthmatic but may be of concern in the asthmatic with coexisting ischemic heart disease. However, these changes in cardiac output are achieved with relatively little increase in myocardial oxygen consumption and may be relatively benign. In other forms of cardiovascular disease such as congestive failure or hypertension, the peripheral vasodilatation could be regarded as beneficial. Indeed, systemically administered beta$_2$ agonists have been used in the afterload reduction therapy of congestive heart failure [9, 76]. Systemically administered beta$_2$ agonists and corticosteroids have been implicated in the production of pulmonary edema in obstetric patients treated for premature labor [79]. The role of the beta$_2$ agents in this regard is not clear but may reflect beta$_2$ vasodilation, decreased renal blood flow, and oliguria. In the face of incautious fluid administration and with the mineralocorticoid effect of concurrently administered steroids, fluid overload and pulmonary edema could result [27, 31].

Beta$_2$ agonists appear to have relatively little potential for inducing dysrhythmia when administered as single agents. The sinus tachycardia produced by the administration of beta$_2$ drugs is a reflex response to peripheral vasodilatation (see also Chap. 78). Prior et al. [63] found that dysrhythmias were not a problem when they reviewed the case records of 40 patients suffering from deliberate overdosage with oral albuterol. Concern has been expressed for the dysrhythmic potential of beta$_2$ agonists administered in combination with methylxanthines [3]. Animals treated with beta-adrenergic bronchodilators and aminophylline demonstrate infarct-like myocardial lesions, and Wilson et al. [87] postulated such effects might have contributed to the epidemic of asthma deaths in New Zealand [34, 44, 45]. This hypothesis has largely been discounted in favor of more plausible explanations [43, 53a].

Whenever possible, beta$_2$ agonists should be administered by the aerosol route rather than orally or parenterally to minimize systemic and, in particular, cardiac side effects [1, 28, 51, 80]. Comparisons of parenteral versus nebulized sympathomimetics produce bronchodilatation at least equal to that produced via the parenteral route [61]. In exercise-induced asthma, aerosols are more effective than tablets. Although systemic beta$_2$ agonists have been reported to show greater effectiveness than aerosols in small airways, the increased systemic toxicity likely outweighs the putative advantages of this route, particularly in the patient with cardiac disease.

Long-acting beta$_2$ agonists such as formoterol and salmeterol provide useful bronchodilatation to asthmatics for 12 to 16 hours

[49, 84]. Still in the early stages of clinical development, their role in antiasthmatic regimens remains uncertain. Their role in the management of patients with cardiovascular disease remains equally unclear.

Inhaled Corticosteroids

The recommended treatment for asthma of anything more than trivial severity has become the inhalation of antiinflammatory drugs. In mild asthma, the occasional use of inhaled bronchodilator may be sufficient therapy. If the bronchodilator is required more than once or twice daily, a trial of regular cromolyn, nedocromil, or low-dose inhaled steroid is appropriate [12, 30, 39]. If breathlessness or chest tightness with disturbed sleep persists or if the bronchodilator is required more than once or twice daily, high-dose inhaled steroid is indicated. Doses of inhaled beclomethasone or budesonide up to 3,000 to 4,000 μg/day may be used before it is necessary to resort to ingested prednisone (see Chaps. 60 and 61). Such a preventive approach abolishes airway instability, spares the asthmatic patient many unnecessary episodes of wheezing, and reduces the need for inhaled bronchodilators. For asthmatics with cardiac disease, the advantages are obvious. Such patients are less frequently exposed to the cardiovascular sequelae of an acute asthmatic attack, sequelae that include tachycardia, marked fluctuations in systolic blood pressure (pulsus paradoxus), and hypoxemia [21, 65, 77]. They are also spared the need for self-administered bronchodilators and the potential cardiovascular sequelae of those agents.

For most asthmatics, the aggressive use of inhaled steroids obviates the need for oral steroid. Prednisone or equivalent may then be reserved for short-term administration at the time of exacerbation in the ambulatory asthmatic [25]. In severe asthma, the parenteral administration of glucocorticoids may be lifesaving [68]. For the patient with cardiovascular disease, the adverse effects of sodium retention and hypertension are undesirable but unavoidable consequences. When systemic steroid therapy is required, a corticosteroid with high glucocorticoid potency and less mineralocorticoid effect should be selected. For patients with precarious fluid status such as those with congestive failure, systemic blood pressure and fluid status should be monitored carefully with appropriate adjustments made to diuretic and antihypertensive agents.

Anticholinergic Agents

Anticholinergic drugs have been used in the treatment of asthma by Western physicians since smoking of *Datura stramonium* was introduced in Great Britain in the early nineteenth century [56]. The effectiveness of asthma cigarettes containing antimuscarinic alkyloids has been confirmed in this century [83]. Recent advances in the understanding of cholinergic pathways in the control of airway caliber and the development of effective antimuscarinic bronchodilators with minimal systemic toxicity have reawakened interest in this class of bronchodilators [10] (see Chap. 64). The quaternary anticholinergic compounds such as ipratropium bromide are poorly absorbed across biologic membranes so as to produce their bronchodilating effect with minimal systemic absorption and little in the way of side effects [18, 56, 59]. In asthma, these agents are effective bronchodilators when given by inhalation, although they are less potent and less rapid acting than inhaled beta$_2$ agonists [73]. They have useful bronchodilating properties when added to beta$_2$ agonists, methylxanthines, or a regimen of beta$_2$ agonist and methylxanthine in combination [50, 67]. Their efficacy has been demonstrated in the treatment of acute asthma exacerbations as well as in chronic therapy [69]; their effectiveness over long periods of time may prompt their reassessment in light of concerns over asthma instability putatively induced by chronic beta$_2$-agonist therapy.

The available quaternary anticholinergic compounds have

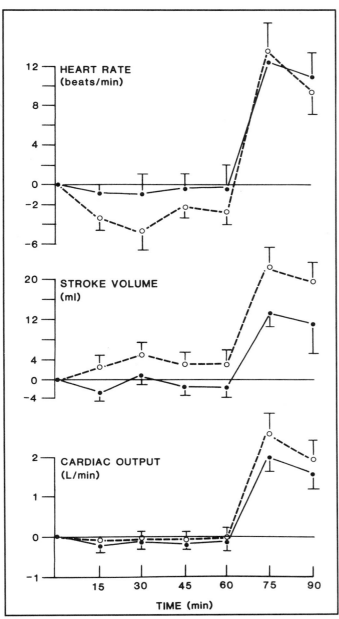

Fig. 77-1. *Hemodynamic effect of inhaled ipratropium bromide. Between time 0 and 60 minutes, 8 puffs of placebo or ipratropium bromide was administered. At time 60 minutes, 2 puffs of fenoterol was administered. The solid line represents placebo plus fenoterol trials; the dashed line represents ipratropium plus fenoterol trials. After ipratropium (0 to 60 minutes), heart rate fell, stroke volume increased, and cardiac output was unchanged. Marked hemodynamic effects after fenoterol were minimally altered by concomitant ipratropium. Bars represent plus or minus 1 standard error. (Reprinted with permission from K. R. Chapman et al. Hemodynamic effects of inhaled ipratropium bromide: Alone and combined with an inhaled beta₂ agonist. Am. Rev. Respir. Dis. 132:845, 1985.)*

minimal cardiovascular impact. Subjects receiving 8 puffs of ipratropium bromide (four times the usual therapeutic dosage in the ambulatory setting) show no significant change in cardiac output when compared to 8 puffs of placebo [20]. In marked contrast to the beta₂ agonists, these agents are essentially devoid of cardiovascular effects (Fig. 77-1). The use of inhaled quaternary anticholinergic compounds would be a reasonable choice for the

older patient with coexisting cardiovascular disease. The agent produces gentle and sustained bronchodilatation without risk of compounding the cardiovascular disease. Inhaled anticholinergics appear to offer greater benefit to older asthmatics than younger asthmatics particularly when compared to adrenergic agents. This is presumably because of downregulation of the adrenergic nervous system, a normal consequence of aging. The cholinergic nervous system shows no such downregulation with aging, and the anticholinergic bronchodilators become, in a relative sense, more potent when contrasted with adrenergic bronchodilators.

Nonsteroidal Antiinflammatories

Following its introduction, sodium cromolyn became widely used as a preventive therapy for asthma of mild severity, particularly in the pediatric population and in those with atopic histories or exercise-induced bronchospasm. It has become clear, however, that sodium cromolyn can play a useful role in patients with asthma of more than mild severity, even in the absence of a clearly defined atopic history [6]. In the elderly, the use of inhaled cromolyn permits a reduction in concomitant therapy with adrenergic drugs and methylxanthines. Given its lack of cardiovascular side effects, cromolyn could be a useful adjunct in the treatment of asthma in patients with myocardial disease. Cromolyn is currently viewed as a prophylactic agent, having no place in the treatment of the acute asthmatic attack. Nedocromil sodium shares properties similar to those of sodium cromolyn [70] (see Chap. 63).

Methylxanthines

Theophylline and its salts are well-known for a narrow therapeutic-toxic ratio and potent cardiovascular and central nervous system side effects [42]. Toxic levels are associated with tachycardia, ventricular dysrhythmias, and cardiac arrest. Even at therapeutic serum levels, theophylline is a potent inotrope and chronotrope, increasing myocardial oxygen demand. Some studies have implicated sympathomimetic and methylxanthine combinations as the cause of arrhythmia in acutely ill asthmatics. Whether true or not, it is difficult to identify any benefit of adding intravenous aminophylline to an effective inhaled bronchodilator regimen in the setting of acute asthma [71, 72].

Theophylline is losing its previous first-line status in the management of asthma. Its present role appears to be as an added bronchodilator in those moderately severe asthmatics who fail to respond to inhaled bronchodilators and regular inhaled antiinflammatory therapy [88]. In this place, it appears to add modest but sustained bronchodilatation over prolonged periods of time [17]. There is no evidence of tachyphylaxis or of induced airway hyperreactivity with its chronic administration. Previously recommended dosing regimens may have been too aggressive; most of the bronchodilator benefit of theophylline is evident at the lower part of the so-called therapeutic range of 10 to 20 mg/L. In clinical practice, "pushing" with theophylline dosage to achieve higher and higher serum levels obeys a law of diminishing returns. This will be particularly true in the elderly patient with coexisting cardiovascular disease. Not only may the diseased myocardium be more susceptible to toxic effects, but the metabolism of theophylline is potentially decreased as a consequence of decreased hepatic blood flow. Thus, any use of theophylline in patients with congestive failure or other cardiac disease must be cautious and resorted to only after less potentially injurious medications have been tried. The mechanism of theophylline's bronchodilatation remains unknown. Previous theories concerning phosphodiastorase inhibition have been discounted; levels of drug required to achieve such inhibition exceed those possible in vivo. Although the biochemical mechanism of theophylline's bronchodilatation remains unknown, more is known about the side effects it induces. It seems likely that adenosine blockade accounts for a number of theophylline's less desirable properties [24]. Adenosine, a naturally occurring autocoid, is thought to be a natural sleep-promoting substance, to be protective against seizures, and to have cardioprotective properties. Thus, by adenosine blockade, theophylline may cause insomnia, seizures (in overdosage), and cardiac arrhythmias. Newer xanthines, which are devoid of adenosine blocking properties, may offer useful clinical bronchodilatation without theophylline's undesirable properties. Agents such as enprofylline have shown promise in early clinical trials [23, 24] (see Chap. 58).

DIABETES MELLITUS

Both asthma and diabetes are common chronic diseases. Curiously, asthma and diabetes coexist less often than would be expected given their prevalence in the general population. This observation dates to the earlier part of this century and has been the subject of sporadic studies since that time [41]. On a trivial level, diabetes complicated by autonomic neuropathy may abolish some of the neural substrate necessary for bronchospasm [11]. This would account for diminished asthma in only a small number of diabetics. A more plausible explanation is that diabetes and asthma are genetically discordant. If so, the genetic study of both diseases could be helpful in understanding the two diatheses.

Antiasthmatic therapy of the diabetic patient must be chosen with two considerations in mind: the adverse metabolic consequences of antiasthmatic drugs, particularly corticosteroids, and the potential complications of coexisting diabetic autonomic neuropathy.

Studies of diabetic autonomic neuropathy have dealt primarily with effects on heart rate, blood pressure regulation, micturation, and (male) sexual function. Information about possible respiratory sequelae of autonomic neuropathy is limited. Neuropathic vagal blockade could result in disease improvement for the diabetic asthmatic given the relative importance of vagal pathways in the control of normal bronchomotor tone. Such an effect has been demonstrated, although its clinical importance is uncertain [40, 60]. However diabetics with autonomic neuropathy are at increased risk of respiratory arrest, particularly following the administration of anesthetics and sedative drugs or when suffering from lower respiratory tract infections [26, 55]. Laboratory studies of diabetics with autonomic neuropathy have demonstrated diminished ventilatory responses to hypoxia. Thus, an asthmatic with coexisting diabetic autonomic neuropathy is at increased risk of respiratory failure. Adrenergic agents and methylxanthines augment ventilatory responsiveness in normal individuals, but their effect in this setting is unknown. Beta₂ agonists must be administered cautiously in patients with autonomic neuropathy, as the vasodilatory effects have the potential to produce significant hypotension. Such a response to subcutaneously administered terbutaline has been described in quadriplegic patients [62]. As a final cautionary note regarding diabetic autonomic neuropathy and asthma, the bladder dysfunction should not be treated with cholinergic agents, as this may precipitate bronchospasm.

The metabolic sequelae of antiasthma drugs are not limited to the corticosteroids. Adrenergic drugs, particularly the beta₂ selective agonists, increase blood glucose [14]. This is most apparent when the drugs are administered orally or parenterally and should be minimal when the aerosol route is used [54]. Nonetheless, the introduction of adrenergic therapy in the diabetic asthmatic should prompt increased attention to blood glucose levels.

When corticosteroid therapy is required in the diabetic patient with asthma, the adverse metabolic consequences of increased blood glucose levels and protein catabolism can be avoided by aggressive treatment with inhaled forms of steroid. In this regard, it is important to note that responsiveness to inhaled steroids is dose related, and dosages up to 3 or 4 mg/day of beclomethasone or budesonide show useful properties. It is difficult to compare the impact of inhaled versus oral steroids with precision, but by one estimate 1,000 μg/day of inhaled budesonide is equivalent to as much as 50 or 60 mg/day of oral prednisone in terms of improved airway control but carries the consequence of only 9 or 10 mg/day of prednisone in terms of metabolic impact [82].

Recommended Asthma Protocol in Diabetes

For diabetic patients with mild asthma, the intermittent, as-needed use of an inhaled bronchodilator would be reasonable initial therapy. Beta₂ agonists are usually tolerated well, but the use of ipratropium bromide or other quaternary anticholinergic would also be a reasonable choice and should have no adverse metabolic consequences. If the inhaled bronchodilator is used more than two or three times daily, a regular inhaled antiinflammatory medication should be added. A useful initial choice would be sodium cromolyn or nedocromil sodium. If adequate airway control is not achieved despite assiduous use for 4 to 8 weeks, inhaled steroid therapy should be undertaken. In the nondiabetic patient, aggressive dosing with inhaled steroids is used before theophylline or other oral bronchodilators are added to the treatment regimen. In the patient with diabetes, theophylline may be resorted to somewhat earlier, given possible metabolic effects of high-dose inhaled steroids. In the severe asthmatic with diabetes, high-dose inhaled steroids are far preferable to oral steroid use. Oral steroids can be resorted to at times of exacerbation and consequent metabolic arrangements dealt with by appropriate titration of insulin or other hypoglycemic agent.

REFERENCES

1. Anderson, S. D., et al. Inhaled and oral salbutamol in exercise induced asthma. *Am. Rev. Respir. Dis.* 114:493, 1976.
2. Banner, A. S., et al. Arrhythmogenic effects of orally administered bronchodilators. *Arch. Intern. Med.* 139:434, 1979.
3. Barclay, J., Smith, W. G. J., and Addis, G. J. Asthma deaths and theophylline/beta₂ agonist therapy. *Lancet* 2:369, 1981.
4. Barnes, P. J. A new approach to the treatment of asthma. *N. Engl. J. Med.* 321:1517, 1989.
5. Barnes, P. J., Willson, N. M., and Vickers, H. Prazosin, an alpha₁-adrenoceptor antagonist, partially inhibits exercise-induced asthma. *J. Allergy Clin. Immunol.* 68:411, 1981.
6. Bernstein, I. L. Cromolyn sodium in the treatment of asthma: Changing concepts. *J. Allergy Clin. Immunol.* 68:247, 1981.
7. Bianco, S., et al. Protective effect of inhaled furosemide on allergen-induced early and late asthmatic reactions. *N. Engl. J. Med.* 321:1069, 1989.
8. Bianco, S., et al. Prevention of exercise-induced bronchoconstriction by inhaled furosemide. *Lancet* 2:252, 1988.
9. Bourdillon, P. D. V., et al. Salbutamol in treatment of heart failure. *Br. Heart J.* 43:206, 1980.
10. Boushey, H. A., et al. Bronchial hyperreactivity. *Am. Rev. Respir. Dis.* 121:389, 1980.
11. Bradley, W. E. (ed.). Aspects of diabetic autonomic neuropathy. *Ann. Intern. Med.* 92:289, 1980.
12. Bulow, B., and Kalen, N. Local and systemic effects of beclomethasone inhalation in steroid-dependent asthmatic patients. *Curr. Ther. Res.* 16:1110, 1974.
13. Camarata, S. J., et al. Cardiac arrest in the critically ill: I. A study of predisposing causes in 132 patients. *Circulation* 44:688, 1971.
14. Carlstrom, S., and Westling, H. Metabolic, circulatory and respiratory effects of a new sympathomimetic β-receptor-stimulating agent, terbutaline, compared with those of orciprenaline. *Acta Med. Scand.* 512:33, 1970.
15. Cerrina, J., et al. Inhibition of exercise-induced asthma by a calcium antagonist, nifedipine. *Am. Rev. Respir. Dis.* 123:156, 1981.

16. Chapman, K. R., and Rebuck, A. S. Bronchodilators, hypokalemia, and fatal asthma. *Lancet* ii(8447):162, 1985.
17. Chapman, K. R. Long-term Efficacy and Tolerability of Theophylline. In R. Pauwels, P. J. Barnes, and N. B. Pride (eds.), *Theophyllin: Symptomatic or Prophylactic Treatment of Asthma and COPD?* London: Medicom, 1989. P. 75.
18. Chapman, K. R. The role of anticholinergic bronchodilators in adult asthma and COPD. *Lung (Suppl.)*:295, 1990.
19. Chapman, K. R., et al. Hemodynamic effects of an inhaled beta$_2$ agonist. *Clin. Pharmacol. Ther.* 35(6):762, 1984.
20. Chapman, K. R., et al. Hemodynamic effects of inhaled ipratropium bromide: Alone and combined with an inhaled beta$_2$ agonist. *Am. Rev. Respir. Dis.* 132:845, 1985.
21. Chapman, K. R., et al. Cardiovascular responses to acute airway obstruction and hypoxia. *Am. Rev. Respir. Dis.* 140:1222, 1989.
22. Chapman, K. R., et al. Effects of atenolol versus diltizem on hemodynamic effects of an inhaled beta$_2$ adrenoreceptor agonist. *Br. J. Clin. Pharmacol.* 27:268, 1989.
23. Chapman, K. R., et al. A placebo-controlled dose-response study of enprofylline in the maintenance therapy of asthma. *Am. Rev. Respir. Dis.* 139:688, 1989.
24. Chapman, K. R., et al. A comparison of enprofylline and theophylline in the maintenance therapy of chronic reversible airways disease. *J. Allergy Clin. Immunol.* 85:514, 1990.
25. Chapman, K. R., et al. Effect of a short course oral prednisone in the prevention of early relapse after the emergency room treatment of acute asthma. *N. Engl. J. Med.* 324:788, 1991.
26. Eagleton, L. E., and Soler, N. G. Hypoventilation in response to hypoxemia in diabetics. *Chest* 80:367, 1981.
27. Elliott, H. R., Abdulla, U., and Hayes, P. J. Pulmonary oedema associated with ritodrine infusion and betamethasone administration in premature labour. *Br. Med. J.* 2:799, 1978.
28. Fairshter, R. D., Novey, H. S., and Wilson, A. F. Site and duration of bronchodilation in asthmatic patients after oral administration of terbutaline. *Chest* 79:50, 1981.
29. Fanta, C. H., et al. Inhibition of bronchoconstriction in the guinea pig by a calcium channel blocker, nifedipine. *Am. Rev. Respir. Dis.* 125:61, 1982.
30. Fein, B. T. Geriatric asthma: Treatment with beclomethasone dipropionate aerosol. *South. Med. J.* 74:1186, 1981.
31. Fogarty, A. J. Cardiac failure in a hypertensive woman receiving salbutamol for premature labour. *Br. Med. J.* 281:226, 1980.
32. Formgren, H. The effect of metoprolol and practolol on lung function and blood pressure in hypertensive asthmatics. *Br. J. Clin. Pharmacol.* 3:1007, 1976.
33. Goldszer, R. C., Lilly, L. S., and Solomon, H. S. Prevalence of cough during angiotensin-converting enzyme inhibitor therapy. *Am. J. Med.* 85:887, 1988.
34. Grant, I. W. B. Has the change to beta-agonists combined with oral theophylline increased cases of fatal asthma? *Lancet* 2:36, 1981.
35. Gross, N. J. SCH 1000: A new anticholinergic bronchodilator. *Am. Rev. Respir. Dis.* 112:823, 1975.
36. Grossman, J. The occurrence of arrhythmias in hospitalized asthmatic patients. *J. Allergy Clin. Immunol.* 57:310, 1976.
37. Haalboom, J. R. E., Deenstra, M., and Struvenberg, A. Hypokalemia induced by inhalation of fenoterol. *Lancet* 1:1125, 1985.
38. Hales, C. A., and Kazemi, H. Small-airways function in myocardial infarction. *N. Engl. J. Med.* 290:761, 1974.
39. Hargreave, F. E., Dolovich, J., and Newhouse, M. T. The assessment and treatment of asthma: A conference report. *J. Allergy Clin. Immunol.* 85:1098, 1990.
40. Heaton, R. W., et al. Diminished bronchial reactivity to cold air in diabetic patients with autonomic neuropathy. *Br. Med. J.* 289:149, 1984.
41. Helander, E. Asthma and diabetes. *Acta Med. Scand.* 162:165, 1958.
42. Hickey, R. F., and Severinghaus, J. W. Regulation of Breathing. Drug Effects. In T. F. Hornbein (ed.), *Regulation of Breathing.* New York: Marcel Dekker, 1981. Vol. 17, Part 2. Chap. 21, P. 1251.
43. Horwitz, R., et al. Clinical complexity and epidemiological uncertainty in case-control research. Fenoterol and asthma management. *Chest* 100:1586, 1991.
44. Interactions between methylxanthines and beta adrenergic agonists. *F.D.A. Drug Bull.* 11:19, 1981.
45. Joseph, X., et al. Enchancement of cardiotoxic effects of β-adrenergic bronchodilators by aminophylline in experimental animals. *Fund. Appl. Toxicol.* 1:443, 1981.
46. Josephson, G. W., et al. Cardiac dysrhythmias during the treatment of acute asthma. *Chest* 78:443, 1981.
47. Kaufman, J., et al. Bronchial hyperreactivity and cough due to angiotensin-converting enzyme inhibitors. *Chest* 95:544, 1989.
47a. Kaufman, J., et al. Angiotensin-converting enzyme inhibitors in patients with bronchial responsiveness and asthma. *Chest* 101:922, 1992.
48. Kennedy, T., et al. Airway response to sublingual nitroglycerin in acute asthma. *J.A.M.A.* 246:145, 1981.
49. Kesten, S., et al. A three month comparison of twice daily inhaled formoterol versus four times daily inhaled salbutamol in the management of stable asthma. *Am. Rev. Respir. Dis.* 144:622, 1991.
50. Kreisman, H., et al. Synergism between ipratropium and theophylline in asthma. *Thorax* 36:387, 1981.
51. Larsson, S., and Svedmyr, N. Bronchodilating effect and side-effects of beta$_2$ adrenoceptor stimulants by different modes of administration (tablets, metered aerosol and combinations thereof): A study with salbutamol in asthmatics. *Am. Rev. Respir. Dis.* 116:861, 1977.
52. Mattson, K., and Popius, H. Controlled study of the bronchoconstriction effect of pindolol administered intravenously or orally to patients with unstable asthma. *Eur. J. Clin. Pharmacol.* 14:87, 1978.
53. Miller, W. C., and Shutz, T. F. Failure of nitroglycerin as a bronchodilator. *Am. Rev. Respir. Dis.* 120:471, 1979.
53a. Molfino, N. A., et al. Respiratory arrest in near-fatal asthma. *N. Engl. J. Med.* 324:285, 1991.
54. Neville, A., et al. Metabolic effects of salbutamol: Comparison of aerosol and intravenous administration. *Br. Med. J.* 1:413, 1977.
55. Page, M. M., and Watkins, P. J. Cardiorespiratory arrest and diabetic autonomic neuropathy. *Lancet* 1:14, 1978.
56. Pakes, G. E., et al. Ipratropium bromide: A review of its pharmacologic properties and therapeutic efficacy in asthma and chronic bronchitis. *Drugs* 20:237, 1980.
57. Patel, K. R. Calcium antagonists in exercise-induced asthma. *Br. Med. J.* 282:932, 1981.
58. Paterson, J. W., Woolcock, A. J., and Shenfield, G. M. Bronchodilator drugs. *Am. Rev. Respir. Dis.* 120:1149, 1979.
59. Pavia, D., et al. Effect of ipratropium bromide on mucociliary clearance and pulmonary function in reversible airways obstruction. *Thorax* 34:501, 1979.
60. Pia Villa, M., et al. Bronchial reactivity in diabetic patients: Relationship to duration of diabetes and degree of glycemic control. *Am. J. Dis. Child.* 142:726, 1988.
61. Pierce, R. J., et al. Comparison of intravenous and inhaled terbutaline in the treatment of asthma. *Chest* 79:506, 1981.
62. Pingleton, S. K., et al. Hypotension associated with terbutaline therapy in acute quadriplegia. *Am. Rev. Respir. Dis.* 126:723, 1982.
63. Prior, J. G., et al. Self-poisoning with oral salbutamol. *Br. Med. J.* 282:1932, 1981.
64. Rall, T. W. Central Nervous System Stimulants: The Xanthines. In A. G. Goodman, L. S. Goodman, and A. Gilman (eds.), *The Pharmacological Basis of Therapeutics* (6th ed.). New York: Macmillan, 1980. P. 592.
65. Rebuck, A. S., and Chapman, K. R. Asthma: Pathophysiology and evaluation of severity. *Can. Med. Assoc. J.* 136:351, 1987.
66. Rebuck, A. S., and Chapman, K. R. Asthma: Trends in pharmacological therapy. *Can. Med. Assoc. J.* 136:483, 1987.
67. Rebuck, A. S., Gent, M., and Chapman, K. R. Anticholinergic and sympathomimetic combination therapy of asthma. *J. Allergy Clin. Immunol.* 71:317, 1983.
68. Rebuck, A. S., and Read, J. Assessment and management of severe asthma. *Am. J. Med.* 51:788, 1971.
69. Rebuck, A. S., et al. Nebulized anticholinergic and sympathomimetic treatment of asthma and chronic obstructive airways disease in the emergency room. *Am. J. Med.* 82:59, 1987.
70. Rebuck, A. S., et al. A three month evaluation of the efficacy of nedocromil sodium in asthma: A randomized, double-blind, placebo-controlled trial of nedocromil sodium conducted by a Canadian multicenter study group. *J. Allergy Clin. Immunol.* 85:612, 1990.
71. Rossing, T. H., Fanta, C. H., and McFadden, E. R., Jr. A controlled trial of the use of single versus combined-drug therapy in the treatment of acute episodes of asthma. *Am. Rev. Respir. Dis.* 123:190, 1981.
72. Rossing, T. H., et al. Emergency therapy of asthma: Comparison of the acute effects of parenteral and inhaled sympathomimetics and infused aminophylline. *Am. Rev. Respir. Dis.* 122:365, 1980.
73. Ruffin, R. E., Fitzgerald, J. D., and Rebuck, A. S. A comparison of the

bronchodilator activity of SCH 1000 and salbutamol. *J. Allergy Clin. Immunol.* 59:136, 1977.

74. Sears, M. R., et al. Regular inhaled beta-agonist treatment in bronchial asthma. *Lancet* 336:1391, 1990.

75. Seibert, A. F., et al. Normal airway responsiveness to methacholine in cardiac asthma. *Am. Rev. Respir. Dis.* 140:1805, 1989.

76. Sharma, B., and Goodwin, J. F. Beneficial effect of salbutamol on cardiac function in severe congestive cardiomyopathy: Effect on systolic and diastolic function of the left ventricle. *Circulation* 58:449, 1978.

77. Silvers, W., Hall, W. D., and Haynes, R. L. Blood pressures in acute asthma. *Chest* 72:412, 1977.

78. Szczeklik, A., Gryglewski, R. J., and Czerniawska-Mysik, G. Clinical patterns of hypersensitivity to nonsteroidal anti-inflammatory drugs and their pathogenesis. *J. Allergy Clin. Immunol.* 60:276, 1977.

79. Tinga, D. J., and Aarnoudse, J. G. Post-partum pulmonary oedema associated with preventive therapy for premature labour. *Lancet* 1:1026, 1979.

80. Tobin, M. J., et al. Response to bronchodilator drug administration by a new reservoir aerosol delivery system and a review of other auxiliary delivery systems. *Am. Rev. Respir. Dis.* 126:670, 1982.

81. Toogood, J. H., et al. A graded dose assessment of the efficacy of beclomethasone dipropionate aerosol for severe chronic asthma. *J. Allergy Clin. Immunol.* 59:298, 1977.

82. Toogood, J. H., et al. Bioequivalent doses of budesonide and prednisone in moderate and severe asthma. *J. Allergy Clin. Immunol.* 84:688, 1989.

83. Trechsel, K., Bachofen, H., and Scherrer, M. Die bronchodilatorische Wirkung der Asthmazigarette. *Schweiz. Med. Wochenschr.* 103:415, 1973.

84. Ullman, A., and Svedmyr, N. Salmeterol, a new long acting inhaled β_2 adrenoceptor agonist: Comparison with salbutamol in adult asthmatic patients. *Thorax* 43:674, 1988.

85. Weber, R. W., et al. Incidence of bronchoconstriction due to aspirin, azo dyes, non-azo dyes, and preservatives in a population of perennial asthmatics. *J. Allergy Clin. Immunol.* 64:32, 1979.

86. Weiner, N. Norepinephrine, Epinephrine and the Sympathomimetic Amines. In A. G. Goodman, L. S. Goodman, and A. Gilman (eds.), *The Pharmacological Basis of Therapeutics* (6th ed.). New York: Macmillan, 1980. P. 138.

87. Wilson, J. D., Sutherland, D. C., and Thomas, A. C. Has the change to beta-agonists combined with oral theophylline increased cases of fatal asthma? *Lancet* 1:1235, 1981.

88. Wolfe, J. D., et al. Bronchodilator effects of terbutaline and aminophylline alone and in combination in asthmatic patients. *N. Engl. J. Med.* 298:363, 1978.

89. Zaid, G., and Beall, G. N. Bronchial response to beta adrenergic blockade. *N. Engl. J. Med.* 275:580, 1966.

Cardiac Interactions, Arrhythmias, and Pathology

78

Curtis N. Sessler
Stephen M. Ayres
Frederick L. Glauser

Asthma and medications used in its treatment can have significant impact on cardiac structure and function. The purpose of this chapter is to critically review (1) the effect of asthma on cardiovascular function, (2) the prevalence, causative factors, and impact of cardiac arrhythmias accompanying asthma and its treatment, and (3) morphologic changes of the heart in fatal asthma.

EFFECTS OF ASTHMA ON THE CARDIOVASCULAR SYSTEM

The effects of respiration on the cardiovascular system have been appreciated for decades [60]. During normal inspiration there is an increase in venous return to the right heart as intrathoracic pressures become more negative [93, 94]. In contrast, maneuvers that increase intrathoracic pressure, such as Valsalva or positive pressure ventilation, may decrease venous return, thus transiently decreasing cardiac output and systemic blood pressure [87]. The Mueller maneuver, a sustained inspiration against a closed glottis, causes an abrupt fall in intrathoracic pressure, which, in addition to increasing venous return, may cause flattening of the cardiac interventricular septum, interfering with ventricular systolic function [10, 40]. During acute asthmatic exacerbation, the interrelationship between ventilation and cardiovascular function becomes much more complex than the events described above and leads to characteristic cardiovascular findings (Table 78-1).

Sinus Tachycardia

Sinus tachycardia is a common finding in patients with acute asthma. Pulse rate typically is 100 beats/min (bpm) or more, and 20 to 25 percent of patients have rates in excess of 120 bpm [44, 75]. Some, but not all, investigators feel tachycardia correlates with the severity of airflow obstruction and is a reliable indicator of a severe asthma attack [30, 103]. Heart rates greater than 130 bpm may reflect a PaO_2 less than 40 mmHg [18]. Tachycardia may be due, at least in part, to the effects of elevated plasma norepinephrine levels found during acute, severe asthma [47]. Other mechanisms may be involved, since histamine-induced bronchoconstriction is accompanied by a modest increase in heart rate despite normal plasma levels of epinephrine and norepinephrine [61]. Sinus tachycardia resolves during appropriate treatment of the acute asthma attack, often despite the use of beta agonists and other positive chronotropes.

Systemic Hypertension and Hypotension

Systolic and diastolic hypertension of modest degree may be seen during severe asthma attacks, particularly in patients with underlying essential hypertension [31]. Normal volunteers made hypoxemic and breathing against expiratory resistive loading mimicking severe asthma develop significant increases in systolic and diastolic blood pressure [14]. The mechanisms probably include the cardiac effects of circulating catecholamines [84]. Systemic hypertension resolves as the asthma attack is brought under control with appropriate treatment, and specific antihypertensive therapy is not required. Rarely, systemic hypotension or frank shock may complicate status asthma, probably from the cumulative effect of multiple factors.

Pulsus Paradox

Pulsus paradox, a fall in inspiratory systolic blood pressure greater than 10 to 15 mmHg, is found during acute asthmatic exacerbation when the forced expiratory volume in 1 second (FEV_1) falls to less than 20 percent of predicted [23, 56, 73, 84, 88, 108]. The absolute amount of paradox, however, is not strictly related to the severity of airway obstruction; for example, a patient with a paradox of 18 mmHg may have worse airway obstruction than a patient with a paradox of 50 mmHg. The degree of arterial hypoxemia may directly influence the amount of paradox [14]. In healthy volunteers expiratory resistive loading (simulating asthmatic airflow obstruction) and hypoxemia (to arterial saturation of 80–90%) each independently causes increases in pulsus paradox over baseline, and the combination (simulating severe acute asthma) produces the greatest increase [14].

The mechanisms of pulsus paradox are complex and controversial [23, 56, 73, 86, 88, 100a, 108, 114, 117] (Table 78-2). The initiating event, lung overinflation secondary to or associated with the severe airway obstruction leads to two deleterious consequences: (1) pulmonary vascular resistance increases as extra-alveolar blood vessels are compressed at these high lung volumes [11, 137] and (2) markedly negative pleural pressures are generated. Peak inspiratory pleural pressures may approach −40 mmHg [115], while mean pleural pressure (peak inspiratory minus peak expiratory pressure) may be in the range of −25 to −30 mmHg.

Negative pleural pressures result in a variety of physiologic consequences including an increase in venous return to the right atrium. This increase in venous return is, in part, offset by the increase in intraabdominal pressure, which compresses the inferior vena cava, narrowing its diameter by up to 50 percent [69, 76]. The negative pleural pressure also increases transmural pressures throughout all heart chambers as well as in the pulmonary arteries [36, 69, 76, 115]. Since the right ventricle and atrium are more compliant and have thinner walls than the left heart chambers, there is right atrial and ventricular enlargement with more blood in these chambers [48]. Additionally, the increased pulmonary vascular resistance is augmented by a "relative pulmonary hypertension," since transmural pressures in the pulmo-

Table 78-1. Cardiovascular manifestations of acute asthma

Cardiac manifestation	Acute exacerbation	Status asthmaticus
Tachycardia	Common (>100 bpm)	Common (>120 bpm)
Systemic hypertension	Sometimes	Sometimes
Systemic hypotension	Absent	Rare
Pulsus paradox (≥15–18 mmHg)	Sometimes	Common
Cor pulmonale	Absent	Rare
Electrocardiographic abnormalities		
P Pulmonale	Rare	Common
Rightward shift of P axis	Rare	Common
Rightward shift of QRS axis	Rare	Sometimes
Nonspecific ST–T changes	Rare	Sometimes

Table 78-2. Mechanisms of pulsus paradox

Marked variability of venous return
Ventricular interdependence
Increased right ventricular afterload with subsequent right ventricular dysfunction
Increased pulmonary vascular resistance ± pulmonary hypertension
Increased left ventricular afterload with subsequent left ventricular dysfunction

nary arteries also increase. These phenomena increase right atrial and ventricular size and cause a leftward septal shift, which encroaches on the left ventricular chamber, that is, so-called ventricular interdependence [10, 40, 78]. The total amount of blood in the left side of the heart is therefore reduced, decreasing cardiac output and leading to a fall in systolic blood pressure, causing pulsus paradox.

Clinical and Electrocardiographic Evidence of Right Heart Dysfunction

The relative increase in pulmonary artery (PA) pressures caused by the negative pleural pressure and the increased pulmonary vascular resistance imposed by lung hyperinflation can lead to right atrial enlargement, resulting in an abnormally vertical P-wave axis and increased P-wave duration and amplitude, "P pulmonale," on the electrocardiogram (ECG) [36, 89, 110]. Gelb et al. [36] studied 129 patients with acute, severe asthmatic attacks. P pulmonale was present in 49 percent of patients with hypercapnia (PaCO$_2$ ≥ 45 mmHg) and acidosis (arterial pH ≤ 7.37), whereas P pulmonale was present in only 2.5 percent of patients without these findings. This phenomenon was transient and disappeared over 12 to 60 hours as gas exchange abnormalities were corrected. P-wave height correlated significantly with PaCO$_2$ and arterial pH, but not PaO$_2$. The authors demonstrated normal PA pressures (relative to atmospheric pressure) in seven patients with P pulmonale; however, peak inspiratory PA transmural pressures (relative to the markedly negative pleural pressures) were increased. The authors hypothesize that the increased right heart transmural pressures result in chamber distention and subsequent P pulmonale. Other ECG abnormalities reported in acute asthma include rightward shift of the QRS axis and nonspecific ST-segment or T-wave abnormalities [36, 110]. In normal volunteers, hypoxemia alone or combined with expiratory resistive loading produces a rightward shift of the QRS and P-wave axes, whereas resistive loading without hypoxemia produced no such ECG changes [14]. Clinical and pathologic evidence of overt cor

pulmonale, although uncommon, is described in patients with severe unrelieved asthma [33, 57].

CARDIAC RHYTHM IN ASTHMA

Cardiac rhythm is variable, depending on a host of factors including the severity of airflow obstruction, the pressure or absence of underlying heart disease (including preexisting arrhythmias, coronary artery disease), age, metabolic derangements such as acidosis or hypoxemia, and medications employed. The impact of various medications depends on the type used, dosage, route of delivery, clinical setting, and the cumulative effect of multiple medications (Table 78-3).

Stable Asthmatics

Prospective continuous ECG recording in otherwise healthy asthmatics not experiencing bronchospasm typically demonstrates normal sinus rhythm and few ventricular or supraventricular premature beats (VPB and SPB, respectively) [16, 43b, 72]. The low prevalence of ventricular arrhythmias in young, otherwise healthy, nonsmoking asthmatics contrasts with data from patients with stable chronic obstructive pulmonary disease (COPD) [107] and likely reflects differences in age or underlying heart disease.

Enhanced parasympathetic nervous activity may lead to accentuated respiratory sinus arrhythmia in asthmatics [51, 123]. Sturani et al. [117] found significantly larger diving reflex-induced drops in heart rate among asthmatics than controls, especially those with intrinsic asthma. There was a strong correlation between the degree of bradycardia and methacholine-induced bronchoconstriction [117]. In children, cholinergic hyperresponsiveness may be a reflection of atopy rather than asthma per se [123].

Bronchodilators and Cardiac Rhythm
Bronchodilators have minimal impact on cardiac rhythm in stable asthmatics (see Table 78-3). Inhaled beta-adrenergic agonists at customary doses produce little or no heart rate change and no significant increase in VPB or SPB number or complexity [49, 65, 68, 72, 128], although higher doses of inhaled albuterol produce a dose-dependent increase in heart rate [68]. Aerosolized beta agonists cause a dose-dependent fall in serum potassium and an increase in QT$_c$ interval on the ECG in stable asthmatics [135a]. The clinical impact of QT$_c$ prolongation is uncertain [137b], although some authors [92a] speculate that sudden death in acute asthma is related. The concomitant use of corticosteroids with inhaled beta agonists does not potentiate any cardiac effects (including effects on QT$_c$), although serum potassium declines are greater than with beta agonists alone [120a]. Standard oral doses of beta-adrenergic agonists terbutaline and albuterol produce mild transient tachycardia or no change in heart rates and are not consistently associated with changes in number or complexity of ventricular or atrial ectopy [43b, 62]. Inhaled ipratropium bromide does not affect heart rate and appears to be free of arrhythmogenic properties [7, 126, 131].

Theophylline causes a dose-dependent increase in heart rate [16, 52, 81] via direct sinus node stimulation (reduced sinoatrial node conduction time and sinus node recovery time) and accelerated intracardiac conduction [26]. This positive chronotropic effect of theophylline has recently been utilized in the treatment of sick sinus syndrome, vasodepressor syncope, and atrial fibrillation with slow ventricular response [1, 1a, 78a]. Adenosine receptor blockage, circulating and locally generated catecholamines, reflex tachycardia from peripheral vasodilatation, and medullary center stimulation probably play a role [125, 129].

Table 78-3. Effects of commonly used bronchodilators on cardiac rhythm in asthma

Agent	Route	Dosage	Population	Clinical setting	Effects on heart rate [refs.]	Effects on rhythm [refs.]
BETA-ADRENERGIC AGONISTS						
Epinephrine	Subcutaneous	0.3–0.5 mg q20min × 3	Adults	Acute asthma	None [22, 27, 28, 50, 113]	SPB ↑ if age >40 [22]
		0.01 mg/kg q20min × 3	Children	Acute asthma	None [124]	
	Nebulized	1% (HCl) 2.25% racemic	Adults	Acute asthma	↓ [19]	
Ephedrine	Oral	25 mg	Adults & children	Stable asthma	↑ [120] or ↓ [25]	
Isoproterenol	Intravenous	0.04–0.23 µg/kg/min	Adults	Status asthma	↑ [55]	VPB, SPB: none [54]
		0.36 µg/kg/min max	Children	Status asthma	↑ ↑ [85, 136]	VPB: rare VT [136]
Isoetharine	Nebulized	2.5 mg q20min × 3	Adults	Acute asthma	None [99]	
Metaproterenol	Nebulized	5 mg	Adults & children	Acute asthma	↓ [138]	
	Nebulized	0.3 ml (15 mg) q20min × 3	Adults	Acute asthma	↓ or none [27, 79]	
		5, 10, 15, 20 mg (dose response)	Children	Acute asthma	None, ↑ with dose >10 mg [106]	
	MDI	1.3 mg (650 µg/act × 2)	Adults	Acute asthma	None [122]	VPB: [43b, 62)
Terbutaline	Intravenous	Load 2 µg/kg, 4.5 µg/kg/hr	Children	Status asthma	↑ [34]	
		4–8 µg/kg injection	Adults	Status asthma	↓ [6]	
	Subcutaneous	0.25–0.5 mg, 1 mg	Adults	Acute asthma	None [113], ↑ with 1-mg dose [112]	
		0.01–0.04 mg/kg	Children	Status asthma	None [84]	
	Oral	15–20 mg/day, divided doses	Adults	Stable asthma	↓ [25], ↑ or none [120]	VPB [43b, 62]
	Nebulized	500 µg	Adults	Acute asthma	None [4]	
		1 mg × 3	Children	Acute asthma	None	
		4 mg/hr continuous	Children	Status asthma	None [77]	
Albuterol	Intravenous	900 µg	Adults	Status asthma	↑ [63]	
	Oral	6–16 mg/day, divided doses	Adults	Stable asthma	None [43b]	SPB: ↑, atrial tachycardia [43b]
		4 mg	Children	Stable asthma	None [128]	
	Nebulized	2.5 mg	Adults	Acute asthma	↓ [19, 43, 64]	
		0.05–0.15 mg/kg q20min × 6	Children	Acute asthma	↑ [102]	
	MDI	200 µg × 4/day, 100–4,000 µg, dose response	Adults	Stable asthma	None [5, 68, 72], ↑ >500 µg [68]	VPB, SPB: same as placebo [72]
		1,080 µg	Children	Stable asthma	None [65]	VPB, SPB: none [65]
Bitolterol mesylate	MDI	350–700 µg × 3/day	Adults	Stable asthma	None [15, 53, 121]	VPB, SPB: none [53]
		350–1,050 µg	Children	Stable asthma	None [105]	
METHYLXANTHINES						
Theophylline	Intravenous	5.6–6.0 mg/kg bolus, then 0.5–0.9 mg/kg/hr	Adults	Stable asthma	None [20], ↑ (dose dependent) [13]	
			Adults	Acute asthma	None [8, 20]	VPB, SPB: no difference vs. epinephrine [28]
					↓ [41, 99, 134]	None [16, 49, 52, 62] VPB: frequent [130], SPB: tachyarrhythmias [130]
	Oral	BID, titrated to STC = 10–20 mg/L	Adults	Stable	None [53]	None VPB, SPB [49, 62]
Enprofylline	Intravenous	1.5 mg/kg bolus, then 0.4 mg/kg/hr	Adults	Acute asthma	↓ [137a]	
ANTIMUSCARINIC						
Ipratropium bromide	Nebulized	500 µg–1 mg	Adults	Acute asthma	None [90], ↓ [64]	
		500 µg	Children	Acute asthma	None [7, 32, 43b]	
	MDI	80 µg × 4/day	Adults	Stable asthma	None [126]	

SPB = supraventricular premature beats; VPB = ventricular premature beats; VT = ventricular tachycardia; MDI = metered-dose inhaler; STC = serum theophylline concentration.

Atrial automaticity is enhanced [67], although SPBs are not increased [16, 49, 52, 62]. Theophylline alone does not appear to increase ventricular ectopy [16, 49, 52, 62].

The combined use of theophylline and beta-adrenergic agonists is common in the outpatient as well as emergency management of asthma. This combination of drugs causes cardiac necrosis and fatal ventricular arrhythmias in experimental animals [35, 55, 133]. Wilson et al. [135] observed an increase in the sudden-death rate of young asthmatics in New Zealand at a time when combined use of these agents was increasing and proposed that episodes of fatal asthma might be related to changes in prescribing habits to more theophylline and beta-adrenergic agonist use. Subsequent correspondence, however, reflected vastly different interpretations of the observations [37, 132]. Although Coleman et al. [16] found that combined therapy with theophylline and a beta-adrenergic agonist in young, otherwise healthy asthmatics does not lead to an increase in the total number of VPBs but increased the degree of complexity, other studies that utilized long-term ECG recording did not demonstrate this combination to be proarrhythmic [52, 53].

Acute Asthma

Sinus tachycardia is common during acute asthma. Clinically significant ventricular ectopy is unusual in otherwise healthy children and young adults, despite treatment with a variety of bronchodilators [22, 28, 50, 75]. Josephson and colleagues [50] prospectively studied patients younger than 50 years of age with no cardiac disease during treatment of acute asthma with epinephrine or aminophylline plus epinephrine. Supraventricular or ventricular arrhythmias were documented in 9 (20%) of 44 episodes, whereas multiform, repetitive, and/or bigeminal ventricular ectopy was limited to 3 (7%) cases, all following epinephrine plus aminophylline. Emerman et al. [28] studied a similar population, who received epinephrine and/or aminophylline, and found ventricular ectopy in 14 (23%) of 60 episodes during the 90-minute ECG recording, although complex ventricular arrhythmias were noted in only 3 (5%). One patient had supraventricular tachycardia (SVT). There was no difference in prevalence of ventricular ectopy among the three treatment groups. In a recent study [130] comparing theophylline and the adenosine nonblocking xanthine enprofylline, arrhythmias were common and of similar frequency in both groups. VPBs were present in 26 (78%) of 33 patients, including nonsustained ventricular tachycardia (VT) in 3 patients, and SVT was noted in 12 (36%) of 33 during 24-hour recordings. These patients were somewhat older (mean age 49 years) than in the previous studies; however, underlying heart disease was rare.

Recently Cydulka et al. [22] studied the effects of subcutaneous epinephrine on cardiac rhythm in acute asthmatics of all ages who had no evidence of acute angina or recent (past 3 years) myocardial infarction. Frequent (> 10/hr) VPBs were noted in 8 (12%) and SPBs in 2 (3%) of the 69 episodes in patients younger than 40 years of age. Two patients had SVT. Frequent VPBs and SPBs were present in 8 (21%) and 6 (16%) of 37 episodes in asthmatics older than 40 years of age. SPBs were statistically more common and VPBs were observed twice as often (although not statistically different) in older versus younger asthmatics. Potentially life-threatening arrhythmias were rare in both age groups. The authors concluded that subcutaneous epinephrine is safe in all acute asthmatics who are free of heart disease, although ECG monitoring should be standard during therapy.

Asthmatics with underlying heart disease may be at increased risk for developing cardiac arrhythmias. In a study of 20 hospitalized asthmatics, 5 had documented heart disease, and 3 of these experienced frequent VPBs, while another developed angina during treatment with intravenous aminophylline and inhaled isoproterenol [38]. After discharge continuous ECG monitoring in these 3 patients demonstrated VPBs but in reduced numbers. Theophylline further increases the exercise-induced rise in the ventricular rate in patients with atrial fibrillation [22a]. Thus theophylline may contribute to difficulties with rate control in acutely ill asthmatics with coexisting atrial fibrillation.

Status Asthmaticus, Acute Severe Asthma, and Respiratory Failure

There is considerable evidence in humans [2, 3, 32] as well as experimental animals [17, 45] that the principal disturbances of respiratory failure, that is, hypoxemia and acidosis, increase the risk of developing cardiac arrhythmias, particularly with concomitant bronchodilator administration. Mechanical ventilation and general anesthesia may place the patient with status asthmaticus at additional risk. In a study of 91 patients with cardiac arrhythmias during respiratory failure (40% had underlying asthma), patients with VPBs had more severe hypoxemia and hypercapnia than patients without ectopy [109]. Although there is a high prevalence of arrhythmias among patients with acute respiratory failure [39, 46], arrhythmias were significantly less common among asthmatics than patients with COPD or pneumonia [39]. It is likely that differences in age or prevalence of coexisting cardiac disease account for some of the difference. In one report, respiratory failure patients with frequent VPBs were of older age than those without ectopy [109].

Several specific therapeutic interventions that are reserved for patients with life-threatening asthma are associated with tachyarrhythmias. Intravenous infusion of beta-adrenergic agonists, including terbutaline, isoproterenol, and albuterol, causes marked sinus tachycardia [34, 54, 63, 85, 136]. Isoproterenol and albuterol infusions have also been associated with cardiac ischemia and/or VT [58, 70, 118, 136]. The combination of intravenous aminophylline and terbutaline was associated with severe ventricular arrhythmias (> 10 VPB/hr, multifocal VPBs, or VT) in 5 (17%) and sustained runs of atrial tachycardia in 2 (7%) of 29 patients with status asthmaticus [59]. All arrhythmias were well tolerated hemodynamically and resolved spontaneously without antiarrhythmic treatment. Use of intravenous epinephrine should be avoided in older patients with status asthmaticus who may have concomitant ischemic heart disease [31a].

In a recent series of acute asthma requiring mechanical ventilation, 7 (22%) of 32 patients had arrhythmias, including supraventricular and ventricular tachyarrhythmias as well as symptomatic bradycardia [71]. These patients had a variety of physiologic derangements and were treated aggressively with bronchodilators. Inhalational general anesthetics are occasionally used in patients with refractory status asthma. Halothane and isoflurane, both potent bronchodilators, are the preferred agents in asthmatics. There are experimental animal data as well as clinical case reports that are suggestive of increased risk of cardiac arrhythmias during halothane administration, particularly in the setting of hypoxemia, hypercapnia, and/or concomitant theophylline or beta-adrenergic agonist therapy [21, 45, 92, 95, 116]. However, several recent series, totaling 34 cases, suggest that halothane may be safely used in status asthma [98, 100]. Cautious administration and ECG monitoring are essential for safe use.

Theophylline Toxicity

Theophylline is widely used in the management of asthma, although there is considerable debate about its role, in large part because of the risk for toxicity. Cardiac arrhythmias constitute one of its most common and important toxic manifestations, which range from sinus tachycardia to ventricular fibrillation

Table 78-4. Cardiac rhythm in theophylline toxicity (STC > 30 mg/L)

	Chronic overmedication		Acute overdose[a]
	Asthma	COPD	
Number of patients	20	60	11
Age (yr)			
Median	38.5	65.5[b]	32
Range	2–76	40–89	1–57
Peak STC (mg/L)			
Median	39.2	38.5	57.2[b]
Range	30.6–57.6	30.3–76.4	34–206
Heart disease	10%	50%[b]	0%
ECG findings			
Normal sinus rhythm	35%	37%	18%
Sinus tachycardia	65%	50%	63%
Supraventricular tachyarrhythmia	0%[c]	23%	27%
Frequent VPBs	20%	35%	18%
Ventricular tachycardia	0%	2%	9%
Ventricular fibrillation	0%	0%	18%

STC = serum theophylline concentration; COPD = chronic obstructive pulmonary disease; ECG = electrocardiogram; VPB = ventricular premature beats.
[a] Eleven acute overdose cases include 10 with asthma and 1 with COPD.
[b] p < .01 versus other groups.
[c] p < .05 versus COPD.
Source: Data derived from Sessler [103] and Sessler and Cohen [104].

(Table 78-4) [83, 103, 104]. Reversible sinus tachycardia is very common [104]. Theophylline enhances atrial automaticity [67] and triggers supraventricular tachyarrhythmias such as multifocal atrial tachycardia (MAT), atrial fibrillation or flutter, and paroxysmal SVT in some toxic patients [5a, 66], particularly in the setting of COPD or acute overdose (see Table 78-4). Supraventricular tachyarrythmias are rare in asthmatics with chronic theophylline overmedication, although they are more common following acute overdose (see Table 78-4).

Frequent VPBs typically are found in toxic older patients and in heart disease [104]. In a recent study in which continuous ECG recording was performed [104], frequent or repetitive VPBs were found in 7 of 16 toxic patients. The VPB number declined significantly during recovery. Although VPBs are often considered to be an indicator of "severe toxicity," only 2 (8%) of the 27 patients with frequent VPBs progressed to sustained VT and received antiarrhythmic therapy (see Table 78-4). Most reported cases of sustained VT occur in patients with COPD and heart disease [104, 111, 119] or following acute theophylline overdose [42, 103]. Ventricular fibrillation typically follows intentional self-poisoning, resulting in peak serum theophylline concentration (STC) greater than 100 mg/L [43a, 83, 103]; this may also occur with rapid central venous infusion [9, 12]. Ventricular fibrillation may occur in young or middle-aged patients who have no known underlying heart disease in these settings. A variety of factors, such as type of ingestion (ingestion of a single excessive dose, i.e., acute overdose, or ingestion of multiple doses, i.e., chronic overmedication [82]), age, and underlying heart disease, influence the risk for developing cardiac arrhythmias [34, 103]. Clinically significant arrhythmias (ventricular or supraventricular tachyarrythmias) are more common in chronic overmedication patients with COPD than with asthma (see Table 78-4), perhaps reflecting documented differences in age or underlying heart disease. Such arrhythmias are also more common in acute overdose patients.

Excessive intravenous doses of the adenosine nonblocking xanthine enprofylline were inadvertently administered to adults with acute asthma in a clinical trial [130]. Four patients with peak serum concentrations of 16 to 42 mg/L (corresponding to theophylline concentrations of 40 to 105 mg/L) had higher heart rates but no more severe ventricular or supraventricular ectopy than patients with lower levels [130].

Cardiac Arrhythmias from Nonsedating Antihistamines

Many asthmatics have concomitant allergic rhinitis. The nonsedating antihistamines, terfenadine and astemizole, are widely used to treat symptoms of this condition, and each have been linked to potentially life-threatening VT and other arrhythmias [99b]. Terfenadine overdose has been associated with ventricular fibrillation, seizures, and death. Ventricular arrhythmias, including torsades de pointes, and death have also occurred rarely in patients taking recommended dosages. Risk factors for serious arrhythmias include liver dysfunction and concurrent therapy with the antifungal ketoconazole or macrolide antibiotics such as erythromycin and troleandomycin. Some experts recommend caution when using terfenadine with any drug that inhibits hepatic metabolism, such as ciprofloxacin, cimetidine, or disulfiram [99b]. In several case reports involving patients using astemizole, VPBs, a prolonged QT interval, atrioventricular block, and symptomatic torsades de pointes have been reported to occur in the setting of elevated serum drug concentration or accidental overdosage [99b]. Recurrent syncope was often the presenting manifestation in more serious cases and should alert the clinician to the possibility of a drug-induced arrhythmia.

CARDIAC PATHOLOGY IN ASTHMA

While the majority of asthma-related deaths are probably related to asphyxia [77a], there is growing concern that cardiac injury may contribute to sudden death [92a, 99a, 101]. The prevalence and spectrum of cardiac pathology remain unclear, however, since most reports consist of single cases or small series [24, 57, 58, 80, 127]. A principle recommendation from a workshop on pathology in asthma [91] was for the establishment of systemic autopsy examination of the heart in all cases of asthmatic death. The pathology should be combined with clinical correlations, particularly as it relates to drug therapy.

Clinical right heart dysfunction occurs in the setting of acute or chronic severe airflow obstruction. Cor pulmonale was the most common cardiac abnormality in one series, being found at autopsy in 5 of 11 children with fatal asthma [57]. Somewhat surprisingly there is also clinical and pathologic evidence of left ventricular ischemia and necrosis in acute, fatal asthma [24, 58, 70, 80, 101, 118, 136].

Morphologic cardiac abnormalities in fatal asthma include focal necrosis, subendocardial myolysis and necrosis, subendocardial mononuclear cellular infiltrate and fibrosis, and myocardial contraction band necrosis (MCBN) [24, 58, 80, 101]. In several cases, multiple small necrotic areas were scattered throughout the ventricular myocardium despite patent coronary arteries [58, 127].

Myocardial contraction band necrosis, a peculiar form of myocardial necrosis, was recently described in 4 of 13 children with fatal asthma [24]. It occurs in a variety of settings including catecholamine infusion, central nervous system stimulation, emotional stress, and transient myocardial ischemia with reperfusion [101]. Grossly left ventricular endocardial surface hemorrhage may be present [101]. Histologically, there is loss of the linear arrangement of myofibrils with areas of dense eosinophilic transverse banding alternating with lighter-staining granular zones of cytoplasm (contraction bands) with sparse neutrophils [101] (Fig. 78-1). There are also mitochondrial deposits of calcium phosphate, which may extend to widespread calcification of entire cells. In contrast to the cellular relaxation that follows typical

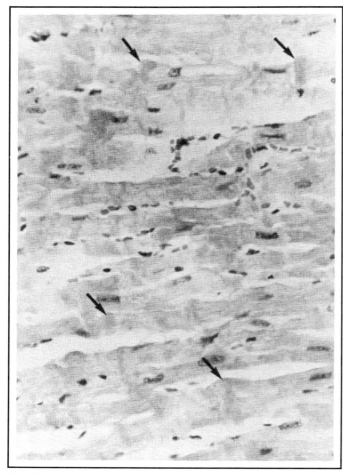

Fig. 78-1. *Histologic findings of myocardial contraction band necrosis in a 13-year-old boy dying of asthma. Contraction bands in necrotic myocytes are indicated by* arrows. *(Hematoxylin-eosin, × 350.) (Reprinted with permission from F. L. Schoen et al., Cardiac pathology in asthma. J. Allergy Clin. Immunol. 70:419, 1987.)*

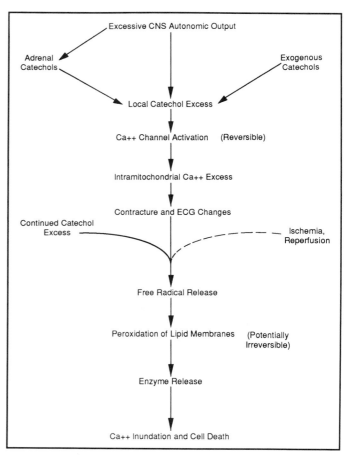

Fig. 78-2. *Proposed mechanisms of pathogenesis of myocardial contraction band necrosis. (Modified from F. W. Drislane et al., Myocardial contraction band lesions in patients with fatal asthma: Possible neurocardiologic mechanisms. Am. Rev. Respir. Dis. 135:498, 1987.)*

ischemic coagulation necrosis, cells undergo tetanic contraction due to intracellular calcium overload [101]. The proposed pathogenesis of MCBN is depicted in Fig. 78-2.

Cardiac pathology in asthma may, in part, be related to drug treatment; however, a cause-and-effect relationship is difficult to establish with certainty. Catecholamines induce myocardial necrosis in a variety of experimental animal models [35, 97], and their use in high doses is associated with clinical and pathologic evidence of ischemia in humans. Cardiac-specific serum creatine kinase MB (CK-MB) isoenzyme was elevated in 15 of 19 children with status asthma during isoproterenol infusion, whereas CK-MB levels were undetectable after drug infusion was discontinued [70]. Other authors have documented reversible ischemic ECG changes during catecholamine administration [74]. Nino et al. [80] reported pathologic features of "catecholamine cardiomyopathy" on endomyocardial biopsy in three asthmatics with left ventricular failure. Morphologic changes produced by high-dose catecholamines include myocardial hypertrophy and myocardial necrosis related to MCBN [96]. Two of four children with MCBN received parenteral catecholamines [24]. These authors [24] emphasize, however, that the other patients did not receive exogenous catecholamines, and other mechanisms as acute stress [29] or neurologic dysfunction (such as seizures in one of their patients) [89] may be important in producing cardiac lesions.

REFERENCES

1. Alboni, P., et al. Clinical effects of oral theophylline in sick sinus syndrome. *Am. Heart J.* 122:1361, 1991.

1a. Alboni, P., et al. Dromotropic effects of oral theophylline in patients with atrial fibrillation and a slow ventricular response. *Eur. Heart J.* 12:630, 1991.

2. Ayres, S. M., and Grace, W. J. Inappropriate ventilation and hypoxemia as causes of cardiac arrhythmias: The control of arrhythmias without antiarrhythmic drugs. *Am. J. Med.* 46:495, 1969.

3. Ayres, S. M., and Mueller, H. Hypoxemia, hypercapnia, and cardiac arrhythmias: The importance of regional abnormalities of vascular distensibility. *Chest* 63:981, 1973.

4. Baughman, R. P., Ploysongsang, Y., and James, W. A comparative study of aerosolized terbutaline and subcutaneously administered epinephrine in the treatment of acute bronchial asthma. *Ann. Allergy* 53:131, 1984.

5. Bellamy, D., and Penketh, A. A cumulative dose comparison between salbutamol and fenoterol metered dose aerosols in asthmatic patients. *Postgrad. Med. J.* 63:459, 1987.

5a. Bitter, G., and Friedman, H. S. The arrhythmogenicity of theophylline. A multivariate analysis of clinical determinants. *Chest* 99:1415, 1991.

6. Boe, J. et al. Acute asthma: Plasma levels and effect of terbutaline i.v. injection. *Eur. J. Respir. Dis.* 67:261, 1985.

7. Boner, A. L., et al. Salbutamol and ipratropium bromide solution in the treatment of bronchospasm in asthmatic children. *Ann. Allergy* 58:54, 1987.

8. Bowler, S. D., et al. Nebulized fenoterol and i.v. aminophylline in acute severe asthma. *Eur. J. Respir. Dis.* 70:280, 1987.

9. Bresnick, E., Woodward, W. K., and Sageman, C. B. Fatal reactions to the intravenous administration of aminophylline. *J.A.M.A.* 136:397, 1948.

10. Brinker, J. A. et al. Leftward septal displacement during right ventricular loading in man. *Circulation* 61:626, 1980.

11. Brower, R. et al. Effect of lung inflation on lung blood volume and pulmonary venous flow. *J. Appl. Physiol.* 58:954, 1985.

12. Camarata, S. J., et al. Cardiac arrest in the critically ill: I. A study of the predisposing causes in 132 patients. *Circulation* 44:688, 1971.

13. Chandler, M. H., et al. Pulmonary function in the elderly: Response to theophylline bronchodilation. *J. Clin. Pharmacol.* 30:330, 1990.

14. Chapman, K. R., et al. Cardiovascular response to acute airway obstruction and hypoxia. *Am. Rev. Respir. Dis.* 140:1222, 1989.

15. Cockcroft, D. W., et al. Comparison of bitolterol mesylate and metaproterenol sulphate. *Curr. Therap. Res.* 30:817, 1981.

16. Coleman, J. J., et al. Cardiac arrhythmias during the combined use of beta-adrenergic agonist drugs and theophylline. *Chest* 90:45, 1986.

17. Collins, J. M., et al. The cardio-toxicity of isoprenaline during hypoxia. *Br. J. Pharmacol.* 36:35, 1969.

18. Cooke, N. J., Cromptom, G. K., and Grant, W. B. Observations on the management of acute bronchial asthma. *Br. J. Dis. Chest* 73:157, 1979.

19. Coupe, M. O., et al. Nebulized adrenaline in acute severe asthma: Comparison with salbutamol. *Eur. J. Respir. Dis.* 71:227, 1987.

20. Crane, J., et al. Hypokalaemic and electrocardiographic effects of aminophylline and salbutamol in obstructive airways disease. *N.Z. Med. J.* 100:309, 1987.

21. Cullen, D. J., and Eger, E. I. The effects of halothane on respiratory and cardiovascular responses to hypoxia in dogs. *Anesthesiology* 33:487, 1970.

22. Cydulka, R., et al. The use of epinephrine in the treatment of older adult asthmatics. *Ann. Emerg. Med.* 17:322, 1988.

22a. Dattilo, G. L., Eiriksson, C. E., and Vestal, R. E. Increased ventricular response rate during exercise in patients with atrial fibrillation treated with theophylline. *Arch. Intern. Med.* 152:797, 1992.

23. Dornhorst, A. C. Pulsus paradoxus. *Intensive Care Med.* 12:387, 1986.

24. Drislane, F. W., et al. Myocardial contraction band lesions in patients with fatal asthma: Possible neurocardiologic mechanisms. *Am. Rev. Respir. Dis.* 135:498, 1987.

25. Dulfano, M., and Glass, P. Evaluation of a new B₂ adrenergic receptor stimulant, terbutaline, in bronchial asthma: II. Oral comparison with ephedrine. *Curr. Therap. Res.* 15:150, 1973.

26. Eiriksson, C. E., Writer, S. L., and Vestal, R. E. Theophylline-induced alterations in cardiac electrophysiology in patients with chronic obstructive pulmonary disease. *Am. Rev. Resp. Dis.* 135:322, 1987.

27. Elenbaas, R. M., et al. Subcutaneous epinephrine vs. nebulized metaproterenol in acute asthma. *Drug Intell. Clin. Pharm.* 19:567, 1985.

28. Emerman, C. L., Crafford, W. A., and Vrobel, T. R. Ventricular arrhythmias during treatment for acute asthma. *Ann. Emerg. Med.* 15:699, 1986.

29. Falconer, B., and Rajs, J., Post-mortem findings of cardiac lesions in epileptics: A preliminary report. *Forensic Sci. Int.* 8:63, 1976.

30. Fischl, M. A. Approach to Acute Asthma in the Emergency Room. In E. B. Weiss, M. S. Segal, and M. Stein (eds.), *Bronchial Asthma: Mechanisms and Therapeutics.* Boston: Little, Brown, 1985. Pp. 802–807.

31. Fischl, M. A., Pitchenik, A. E., and Gardner, L. B. An index predicting relapse and need for hospitalization in patients with acute bronchial asthma. *N. Engl. J. Med.* 305:783, 1981.

31a. Fletcher, D., et al. Cardiac asthma presenting as status asthmaticus: deleterious effect of epinephrine therapy. *Intensive Care Med.* 16:466,1990.

32. Flowers, N. C., and Horan, L. G. Acid-base relationships and the cardiac response to aerosol inhalation. *Chest* 63:74, 1973.

33. Freiberg, D. B., and Colebatch, H. J. Malignant asthma presenting as right heart failure. *Med. J. Aust.* 147:90, 1987.

34. Fuglsang, G., Pedersen, S., and Borgstrom, L. Dose-response relationships of intravenously administered terbutaline in children with asthma. *J. Pediatr.* 114:315, 1989.

35. Gavras, H., et al. Angiotensin and norepinephrine induced myocardial lesions: Experimental and clinical studies in rabbits and man. *Am. Heart J.* 89:321, 1975.

36. Gelb, A. F., et al. P pulmonale in status asthmaticus. *J. Allergy Clin. Immunol.* 64:18, 1979.

37. Grant, I. W. B. Has the change to beta-agonist combined with oral theophylline increased cases of fatal asthma? *Lancet* 2:36, 1981.

38. Grossman, J. The occurrence of arrhythmias in hospitalized asthmatic patients. *J. Allergy Clin. Immunol.* 57:310, 1976.

39. Gulsvik, A., Hansteen, V., and Sivertssen, E. Cardiac arrhythmias in patients with serious pulmonary diseases. *Scand. J. Respir. Dis.* 59:154, 1978.

40. Guzman, P., et al. Transseptal pressure gradient with leftward septal displacement during the Mueller maneuver in man. *Br. Heart J.* 46:657, 1981.

41. Haahtela, T., Venho, K., and Eriksson, G. Comparison of enprofylline and theophylline for intravenous treatment of acute asthma. *Allergy* 41:160, 1986.

42. Hall, K. W., et al. Metabolic abnormalities associated with intentional theophylline overdose. *Ann. Intern. Med.* 101:457, 1984.

43. Harris, L. Comparison of cardiorespiratory effects of terbutaline and salbutamol aerosols in patients with reversible airways obstruction. *Thorax* 28:592, 1973.

43a. Henderson, A., Wright, D. M., and Pond, S. M. Management of theophylline overdose patients in the intensive care unit. *Anaesth. Intensive Care* 20:56, 1992.

43b. al-Hillawi, A. H., Hayward, R., and Johnson, N. M. Incidence of cardiac arrhythmias in patients taking slow release salbutamol and slow release terbutaline for asthma. *Br. Med. J.* 288:367, 1984.

44. Hopewell, P. C., and Miller, R. T. Pathophysiology and management of severe asthma. *Clin. Chest Med.* 5:623, 1984.

45. Horowitz, L. N., et al. Effects of aminophylline on the threshold for initiating ventricular fibrillation during respiratory failure. *Am. J. Cardiol.* 35:376, 1975.

46. Hudson, L. D., et al. Arrhythmias associated with acute respiratory failure in patients with chronic airway obstruction. *Chest* 63:661, 1973.

47. Ind, P. W., et al. Circulating catecholamines in acute asthma. *Br. Med. J. [Clin. Res.]* 290:267, 1985.

48. Jardin, F., et al. Inspiratory impairment in right ventricular performance during acute asthma. *Chest* 92:789, 1987.

49. Joad, J. P., et al. Extrapulmonary effects of maintenance therapy with theophylline and inhaled albuterol in patients with chronic asthma. *J. Allergy Clin. Immunol.* 78:1147, 1986.

50. Josephson, G. W., et al. Cardiac dysrhythmias during the treatment of acute asthma: A comparison of two treatment regimens by a double blind protocol. *Chest* 78:429, 1980.

51. Kallenbach, J. M., et al. Reflex heart rate control in asthma: Evidence of parasympathetic overactivity. *Chest* 87:644, 1985.

52. Kelly, H. W., Menendez, R., and Voyles, W. Lack of significant arrhythmogenicity from chronic theophylline and beta-2-adrenergic combination therapy in asthmatic subjects. *Ann. Allergy* 54:405, 1985.

53. Kemp, J. P., et al. Concomitant bitolterol mesylate aerosol and theophylline for asthma therapy with 24 hr electrocardiographic monitoring. *J. Allergy Clin. Immunol.* 73:32, 1984.

54. Klaustermeyer, W. B., DiBernardo, R. L., and Hale, F. C. Intravenous isoproterenol: Rationale for bronchial asthma. *J. Allergy Clin. Immunol.* 55:325, 1975.

55. Kline, I. K. Myocardial alterations associated with pheochromocytoma. *Am. J. Pathol.* 38:539, 1961.

56. Knowler, G. K., and Clark, T. J. Pulsus paradoxus as a valuable sign indicating severity of asthma. *Lancet* 2:1356, 1973.

57. Kravis, L. P. An analysis of fifteen childhood asthma fatalities. *J. Allergy Clin. Immunol.* 80:467, 1987.

58. Kurland, G., Williams, J., and Lewiston, N. J. Fatal myocardial toxicity during continuous infusion intravenous isoproterenol therapy of asthma. *J. Allergy Clin. Immunol.* 63:407, 1979.

59. Laaban, J. P., et al. Cardiac arrhythmias during the combined use of intravenous aminophylline and terbutaline in status asthmaticus. *Chest* 94:496, 1988.

60. Lanson, H. D., Bloomfield, R. A., and Cournand, A. The influence of the respiration on the circulation in man. *Am. J. Med.* 1:315, 1946.

61. Larsson, K., and Hjemdahl, P. No influence of circulating noradrenaline on bronchial reactivity to histamine in asthmatic patients. *Eur. J. Respir. Dis.* 69:16, 1986.

62. Laursen, L. C., et al. Long-term oral therapy of asthma with terbutaline and theophylline, alone and combined. *Eur. J. Respir. Dis.* 66:82, 1985.

63. Lawford, P., Jones, B. J. M., and Milledge, J. S. Comparison of intravenous and nebulized salbutamol in initial treatment of severe asthma. *Br. Med. J.* 3:84, 1978.

64. Leahy, B. C., Gomm, S. A., and Allen, S. C. Comparison of nebulized salbutamol with nebulized ipratropium bromide in acute asthma. *Br. J. Dis. Chest* 77:159, 1983.

65. Lee, H., and Evans, H. E. Lack of cardiac effect from repeated doses of albuterol aerosol: A margin of safety. *Clin. Pediatr.* (Phila.) 25:349, 1986.

66. Levine, J. L., Michael, J. R., and Guarnieri, T. Multifocal atrial tachycardia: A theophylline induced rhythm. *Lancet* 1:12, 1985.

67. Lin, C., et al. Arrhythmogenic effects of theophylline in human atrial tissue. *Int. J. Cardiol.* 17:289, 1987.

68. Lipworth, B. J., et al. Beta-adrenoceptor responses to high doses of inhaled salbutamol in patients with bronchial asthma. *Br. J. Clin. Pharmacol.* 26:527, 1988.

69. Lloyd, T. C. Effect of inspiration on inferior vena caval blood flow in dogs. *J. Appl. Physiol.* 55:1701, 1983.

70. Maguire, J. F., Geha, R. S., and Umetsu, D. T. Myocardial specific creatine phosphokinase isoenzyme elevation in children with asthma treated with intravenous isoproterenol. *J. Allergy Clin. Immunol.* 78:631, 1986.

71. Mansel, J. K., et al. Mechanical ventilation in patients with acute severe asthma. *Am. J. Med.* 89:42, 1990.

72. Martelli, N. A., Raimondi, A. C., and Lazzari, J. O. Asthma, cardiac arrhythmias, and albuterol aerosol. *Chest* 89:192, 1986.

73. Martin, J., et al. Factors influencing pulsus paradoxus in asthma. *Chest* 80:543, 1981.

74. Matson, J. R., Loughlin, G. M., and Strunk, R. C. Myocardial ischemia complicating the use of isopreterenol in asthmatic children. *J. Pediatr.* 92:776, 1978.

75. McFadden, E. R. Clinical physiologic correlates in asthma. *J. Allergy Clin. Immunol.* 77:1, 1986.

76. Mintz, G. S., et al. Real time inferior vena caval ultrasonography: Normal and abnormal findings and its use in assessing right-heart function. *Circulation* 64:1018, 1981.

77. Moler, F. W., Hurwitz, M. E., and Custer, J. R. Improvement in clinical asthma score and $PaCO_2$ in children with severe asthma treated with continuously nebulized terbutaline. *J. Allergy Clin. Immunol.* 81:1101, 1988.

77a. Molfino, N. A., et al. Respiratory arrest in near-fatal asthma. *N. Engl. J. Med.* 324:285, 1991.

78. Morris, J. et al. Dynamic right ventricular dimension: Relation to chamber volume during cardiac cycle. *J. Thorac. Cardiovasc. Surg.* 91:879, 1986.

78a. Nelson, S. D., et al. The autonomic and hemodynamic effects of oral theophylline in patients with vasodepressor syncope. *Arch. Intern. Med.* 151:2425, 1991.

79. Nelson, S. M., et al. Frequency of inhaled metaproterenol in the treatment of acute asthmatic exacerbation. *Ann. Emerg. Med.* 19:21, 1990.

80. Nino, A. F., et al. Drug-induced left ventricular failure in patients with pulmonary disease: Endomyocardial biopsy demonstration of catecholamine myocarditis. *Chest* 92:732, 1987.

81. Ogilvie, R. I., Fernandez, P. G., and Winsberg, F. Cardiovascular response to increasing theophylline concentrations. *Eur. J. Clin. Pharmacol.* 12:409, 1977.

82. Olson, K. R., et al. Theophylline overdose: Acute single ingestion versus chronic repeated overmedication. *Am. J. Emerg. Med.* 3:386, 1985.

83. Paloucek, F. P., and Rodvold, K. A. Evaluation of theophylline overdoses and toxicities. *Ann. Emerg. Med.* 17:135, 1988.

84. Pang, L. M., et al. Terbutaline in the treatment of status asthmaticus. *Chest* 72:469, 1977.

85. Parry, W. H., Martorano, F., and Cotton, E. K. Management of life-threatening asthma with intravenous isoproterenol infusions. *Am. J. Dis. Child.* 130:39, 1976.

86. Parsons, G. H., and Green, J. F. Mechanisms of pulsus paradoxus in upper airway obstruction. *J. Appl. Physiol.* 45:598, 1978.

87. Payen, D. M., et al. Hemodynamic, gas exchange and hormonal consequences of LBPP during PEEP ventilation. *J. Appl. Physiol.* 62:61, 1987.

88. Rebuck, A. S., and Pengelly, L. D. Development of pulsus paradoxus in the presence of airways obstruction. *N. Engl. J. Med.* 288:66, 1973.

89. Rebuck, A. S., and Read, J. Assessment and management of severe asthma. *Am. J. Med.* 51:788, 1971.

90. Rebuck, A. S., et al. Nebulized anticholinergic and sympathomimetic treatment of asthma and chronic obstructive airways disease in the emergency room. *Am. J. Med.* 82:59, 1987.

91. Reid, L. M. Workshop on pathology: Summary of workshop manuscripts and discussion. *J. Allergy Clin. Immunol.* 80:403, 1987.

92. Richards, W., et al. Cardiac arrest associated with halothane anesthesia in a patient receiving theophylline. *Ann. Allergy* 61:83, 1988.

92a. Robin, E., D., and McCauley, R. Sudden cardiac death in bronchial asthma, and inhaled beta-adrenergic agonists. *Chest* 101:1699, 1992.

93. Robotham, J. L., and Mitzner, W. A. A model of the effects of respiration on left ventricular performance. *J. Appl. Physiol.* 46:411, 1979.

94. Robotham, J. L., et al. Effects of respiration on cardiac performance. *J. Appl. Physiol.* 44:703, 1978.

95. Roizen, M. F., and Stevens, W. C. Multiform ventricular tachycardia due to the interaction of aminophylline and halothane. *Anesth. Analg.* 57:738, 1978.

96. Rona, G. Catecholamine cardiotoxicity. *J. Moll. Cell. Cardiol.* 17:291, 1985.

97. Rona, G., et al. An infarction-like myocardial lesion and other toxic manifestations produced by isoproterenol in the rat. *Arch. Pathol.* 67:443, 1959.

98. Rosseel, P., Lauwers, L. F., and Baute, L. Halothane treatment in life-threatening asthma. *Intensive Care Med.* 11:241, 1985.

99. Rossing, T. H., et al. Emergency therapy of asthma: Comparison of the acute effects of parenteral and inhaled sympathomimetics and infused aminophylline. *Am. Rev. Respir. Dis.* 122:365, 1980.

99a. Ryan, G., et al. Risk factors for death in patients admitted to hospital with asthma: a follow-up study. *Aust. N. Z. J. Med.* 21:681, 1991.

99b. Safety of terfenadine and astemizole. *Med. Lett. Drugs Ther.* 34:9, 1992.

100. Saulnier, F. F., et al. Respiratory and hemodynamic effects of halothane in status asthmaticus. *Intensive Care Med.* 16:104, 1990.

100a. Scharf, S. M. Cardiovascular effects of airways obstruction. *Lung* 169:1, 1991.

101. Schoen, F. J. Cardiac pathology in asthma. *J. Allergy Clin. Immunol.* 70:419, 1987.

102. Schuh, S., et al. High versus low-dose, frequently administered, nebulized albuterol in children with severe, acute asthma. *Pediatrics* 83:513, 1989.

103. Sessler, C. N. Theophylline toxicity: Clinical features of 116 consecutive cases. *Am. J. Med.* 88:567, 1990.

104. Sessler, C. N. and Cohen M. D. Cardiac arrhythmias during theophylline toxicity: A prospective continuous electrocardiographic study. *Chest* 98:672, 1990.

105. Shapiro, G. G., et al. Pediatric dose-response study of bitolterol mesylate aerosol (abstract). Presented at the Sections on Allergy and Immunology Meeting of the American Academy of Pediatrics, Chicago, IL, 1984.

106. Shapiro, G. G., et al. Double-blind, dose-response study of metaproterenol inhalant solution in children with acute asthma. *J. Allergy Clin. Immunol.* 79:378, 1987.

107. Shih, H. T., et al. Frequency and significance of cardiac arrhythmias in chronic obstructive lung disease. *Chest* 94:44, 1988.

108. Shim, C., and Williams, H. Pulsus paradoxus in asthma. *Lancet* 1:530, 1978.

109. Sideris, D. A., et al. Type of cardiac dysrhythmias in respiratory failure. *Am. Heart J.* 89:32, 1975.

110. Siegler, D. Reversible electrocardiographic changes in severe acute asthma. *Thorax* 32:328, 1977.

111. Siemons, L. J., and Parizel, G. Prolonged runs of ventricular tachycardia as a complication of theophylline intoxication: Report of a case. *Acta Cardiol.* 6:457, 1986.

112. Smith, P. R., et al. A comparative study of subcutaneously administered terbutaline and epinephrine in the treatment of acute bronchial asthma. *Chest* 71:129, 1977.

113. Spiteri, M. A., et al. Subcutaneous adrenaline versus terbutaline in the treatment of acute severe asthma. *Thorax* 43:19, 1988.

114. Squara, P., et al. Decreased paradoxic pulse from increased venous return in severe asthma. *Chest* 97:377, 1990.

115. Stalcup, A., and Mellins, R. Mechanical forces producing pulmonary edema in acute asthma. *N. Engl. J. Med.* 297:592, 1977.

116. Stirt, J. A., et al. Arrhythmogenic effects of aminophylline during halothane anesthesia in experimental animals. *Anesth. Analg.* 59:410, 1980.

117. Sturani, C., Sturani, A., and Tosi, I. Parasympathetic activity assessed by diving reflex and by airway response to methacholine in bronchial asthma and rhinitis. *Respiration* 48:321, 1985.

118. Szczeklik, A., Nizankowski, R., and Mruk, J. Myocardial infarction in status asthmaticus. *Lancet* 1:658, 1977.

119. Taniguchi, A., Ohe, T., and Shimorura, K. Theophylline-induced ventricular tachycardia in a patient with chronic lung disease: Sensitivity to verapamil. *Chest* 96:958, 1989.

120. Tashkin, D. P., et al. Double-blind comparison of acute bronchial and cardiovascular effects of oral terbutaline and ephedrine. *Chest* 68:155, 1975.

120a. Taylor, D. R., et al. Interaction between corticosteroid and beta-agonist drugs: Biochemical and cardiovascular effects in normal subjects. *Chest* 102:519, 1992.

121. Tinkelman, D. G., et al. Comparison of aerosols bitolterol mesylate and albuterol (abstract). *J. Allergy Clin. Immunol.* 71:126, 1983.

122. Tobin, M. J., et al. Acute effects of aerosolized metaproterenol on breathing pattern of patients with symptomatic bronchial asthma. *J. Allergy Clin. Immunol.* 76:166, 1985.

123. Tokuyama, K., et al. Beat-to-beat variation of the heart rate in children with allergic asthma. *J. Asthma* 22:285, 1985.

124. Uden, D. L., et al. Comparison of nebulized terbutaline and subcutaneous epinephrine in the treatment of acute asthma. *Ann. Emerg. Med.* 14:229, 1985.

125. Urthaler, F., and Janes, T. N. Both direct and neurally mediated components of the chronotropic actions of aminophylline. *Chest* 70:24, 1976.

126. Vakil, D. V., Ayiomamitis, A., and Nizami, R. M. Use of ipratropium aerosol in the long-term management of asthma. *J. Asthma* 22:165, 1985.

127. van der Bel, J. et al. Fatal nonatherosclerotic myocardial infarction in a young man with allergic bronchial asthma. *Am. J. Forensic Med. Pathol.* 7:344, 1986.

128. Vazquez, C., et al. Oral salbutamol vs. fenoterol in childhood asthma. *Helv. Paediatr. Acta* 42:273, 1987.

129. Vestal, R. E., et al. Effect of intravenous aminophylline on plasma levels of catecholamines and related cardiovascular and metabolic responses in man. *Circulation* 67:162, 1983.

130. Vilsvik, J. S., et al. Comparison between theophylline and an adenosine non-blocking xanthine in acute asthma. *Eur. Respir. J.* 3:27, 1990.

131. Watson, W. T., Becker, A. B., and Simons F. E. Comparison of ipratropium solution, fenoterol solution, and their combination administered by nebulizer and face mask to children with acute asthma. *J. Allergy Clin. Immunol.* 82:1012, 1988.

132. Weinberger, M. Asthma deaths and theophylline/beta$_2$-agonist therapy. *Lancet* 2:370, 1981.

133. Whitehurst, V. E., et al. Cardiotoxic effects in rats and rabbits treated with terbutaline alone and in combination with aminophylline. *J. Am. Coll. Toxicol.* 2:147, 1983.

134. Williams, S. J., Parrish, R. W., and Seaton, A. Comparison of intravenous aminophylline and salbutamol in severe asthma. *Br. Med. J.* 4:685, 1975.

135. Wilson, J. D., Sutherland, D. C., and Thomas, A. C. Has the change to beta-agonists combined with oral theophylline increased cases of fatal asthma? *Lancet* 1:1235, 1981.

135a. Wong, C. S., et al. Bronchodilator, cardiovascular and hypokalemic effects of fenoterol, salbutamol, and terbutaline in asthma. *Lancet* 338:1396, 1990.

136. Wood, D. W., et al. Intravenous isoproterenol in the management of respiratory failure in childhood status asthmaticus. *J. Allergy Clin. Immunol.* 50:75, 1972.

137. Woolcock, A. J., and Read, J. Lung volumes in exacerbations of asthma. *Am. J. Med.* 41:259, 1966.

137a. Youngchaiyud, P., et al. Intravenous enprofylline in the treatment of patients with acute asthma. *J. Int. Med. Res.* 18:473, 1990.

137b. Ziment, I. Infrequent cardiac deaths occur in bronchial asthma. *Chest* 101:1703, 1992.

138. Konig, P., and Hurst, D. J. Nebulized isoetharine and fenoterol in acute attacks of asthma. *Arch. Intern. Med.* 143:1361, 1983.

Chronic Severe Asthma

Harold S. Nelson

Asthma is a disease that varies in severity both from patient to patient and over time in the same patient. Some patients will experience asthma only in conjunction with viral respiratory infections, others only with exercise or with exposure to certain allergens. At the other end of the spectrum are patients with severe asthma. These patients experience virtually daily wheezing and/or dyspnea. Exacerbations are frequent, often severe, and may occur rapidly, resulting in urgent visits to doctors' offices or hospital emergency rooms or in hospitalizations, which may be complicated by respiratory insufficiency and, rarely, the need for intubation. Sudden severe attacks, particularly in children, may result in hypoxic seizures and respiratory arrest. Patients with severe asthma typically will give a history of very poor exercise tolerance with marked limitation of activity. This is not due to exercise-induced bronchoconstriction but rather to preexisting chronic, severe airflow obstruction. They typically experience considerable, almost nightly, sleep interruption due to asthma. Their ability to perform their normal activities at work, at school, or in the home is frequently interrupted.

Patients with severe asthma will typically be receiving a polypharmacy of therapy. This will usually include theophylline, unless they are intolerant of this drug, beta-adrenergic agonists, often by inhalation from metered-dose inhalers and jet nebulizers, and perhaps orally as well, and frequently ipratropium. They will often, of necessity, have been placed on oral corticosteroids either regularly or in the form of short tapering courses, and steroids will frequently be reinstituted as soon as the effects of the preceding course of treatment have been lost, creating a "roller coaster" effect. Both inhaled cromolyn sodium and inhaled steroids will frequently be added, the latter often in relatively low doses. Thus these patients experience not only the frustration caused by the disease itself but in addition a time-consuming and expensive schedule of therapy.

It is the challenge to the physician to completely assess all aspects of the disease in the patient with severe asthma (Table 79-1). First it is important to make certain that the diagnosis is correct. It is exactly among those who appear to have the most severe and refractory asthma that one is most apt to find the patient who has been misdiagnosed as asthmatic and is being treated with inappropriate therapy, accounting for the apparent lack of response. Once it has been established that the patient truly has asthma or reversible obstructive airway disease, it is important, if pulmonary function tests show persistent airway obstruction, to determine to what extent this is reversible. The patient should be assessed for the presence of remediable conditions that may be contributing to the severity of their asthma such as sinusitis and rhinitis, gastroesophageal reflux, allergy, occupational factors, allergic bronchopulmonary aspergillosis, or sleep apnea. The patient should be educated not only regarding the nature of asthma but also regarding the mechanisms of action of the medications with which they are treated. Side effects

of such drugs should also be clarified. The patient's techniques for employing inhaled medications should be assessed. They should be provided with a simple peak flow monitoring device, which may be used to monitor their response to changes in therapy and to allow for a proper therapeutic response to exacerbations of their asthma. They should be placed on an optimal bronchodilator program, and if not already employing inhaled steroids, these should be introduced. If patients have required oral corticosteroids, inhaled corticosteroid dosage should be increased, if possible, to a dose calculated to more than replace their oral steroids. Every attempt should be made to change oral steroids to alternate-day dosing, and then they should be tapered gradually with peak flow and symptom monitoring. If the ultimate dose of corticosteroids required is considered a risk for serious side effects, the use of "steroid-sparing" antiinflammatory agents should be considered. Finally, every patient should be provided with a crisis intervention plan that, based on symptoms and changes in peak flow measurement, provides for escalating medication and, when appropriate, consultation with physicians or emergency care providers.

ASSESSMENT

Establish the Diagnosis of Asthma

Asthma is not a diagnosis of exclusion. Asthma is a chronic inflammatory disease of the airways, characterized by an eosinophilic-lymphocytic submucosal infiltration, epithelial desquamation, and mucous gland hypertrophy and hyperplasia (see Chap. 28). Secondary to this inflammatory process and perhaps also in part on a genetic basis, the airways of patients with asthma are hyperresponsive to bronchoconstrictors such as histamine and methacholine (see Chap. 4). Asthma presents clinically as airway obstruction that is secondary to mucus accumulation, thickening and edema of the bronchial walls, and contraction of the smooth muscle surrounding the airways. All elements of this obstruction are capable of reversal; hence the characteristic feature of asthma is airway narrowing that changes in severity either spontaneously or as a result of therapy [1a]. It is this characteristic reversibility of airflow obstruction that allows a precise diagnosis to be made [40]. Therefore, when patients present with a history of shortness of breath or wheezing, yet have normal pulmonary function tests, it is necessary to establish that at some time they have the airflow obstruction characteristic of asthma. On the other hand, when patients present with airflow obstruction it is mandatory to establish that this is at least partially reversible. While the differential diagnosis of asthma is discussed in Chapter 37, we will consider here only a few of the more frequently encountered problems in differentiation.

In the patient presenting with a history of severe, episodic wheezing dyspnea and no evidence of obstruction on pulmonary function testing, the diagnosis of vocal cord dysfunction must be considered. In some instances vocal cord dysfunction occurs as an apparent conversion reaction in patients who have no evidence of asthma, including negative methacholine challenges [11]. At the time of their attacks these patients have inspiratory stridor, heard best over the larynx. Their expiratory flow-volume loops appear relatively normal, while on inspiration their flow-volume loops will be flattened, as is typical for variable extrathoracic obstruction (Fig. 79-1). If laryngoscopy is performed during an attack, the vocal cords will be seen to be apposed with the only opening a diamond-shaped posterior chink [11]. Often if patients are asymptomatic at the time they are seen, an attack can be brought on by exposure to one of their historical triggers or by performing a methacholine challenge (see Chap. 39). A

Table 79-1. Chronic severe asthma: assessment and treatment

1. Establish the diagnosis of asthma.
2. Establish best achievable pulmonary function.
3. Assess for and treat contributing conditions:
   a. Sinusitis and rhinitis.
   b. Gastroesophageal reflux.
   c. Allergic triggers.
   d. Occupational factors.
   e. Allergic bronchopulmonary aspergillosis.
   f. Obstructive sleep apnea.
4. Educate regarding asthma, medications, and use of devices.
5. Initiate regular home peak flow monitoring.
6. Institute optimal bronchodilator therapy.
7. Begin adequate doses of inhaled corticosteroids. If patient is on oral corticosteroids, attempt to change to alternate day and taper.
8. If ultimate corticosteroid dose is unacceptable, consider alternative antiinflammatory therapy.
9. Provide a crisis intervention plan based on symptoms and objective peak flow values.

more commonly encountered form of vocal cord dysfunction is that complicating true bronchial asthma. Often such patients will be aware of two forms of dyspnea, one associated with tightness in the chest and another associated with a sensation of tightness in the throat, the latter often accompanied by hoarseness or coughing. Again the contribution of lower airway and vocal cord obstruction to the symptoms can often be determined by performing a methacholine challenge, monitoring the response with inspiratory and expiratory flow-volume loops and performing rhinolaryngoscopy upon the appearance of inspiratory loop flattening.

A second common problem in the adult is differentiation of asthma from other forms of chronic airflow obstruction. Although the pathology of chronic obstructive pulmonary disease (COPD) caused by chronic bronchitis and emphysema is quite different from that of asthma, both disorders present with the common complaint of wheezing dyspnea and evidence of expiratory obstruction to airflow on pulmonary function testing. Frequently, despite an impressive history of tobacco use and in the absence of demonstrated reversibility, patients will have been told that they have asthma and they will have been treated as if they had asthma with severe obstruction. A misdiagnosis of asthma is particularly apt to occur in the young patient, with only a moderate smoking history, who presents with emphysema due to alpha₁ antiproteinase deficiency. A careful history will often suggest that patients with COPD do not have asthma. For example, typically they do not have spontaneous episodes of wheezing dyspnea either at night or during the day. Instead, their dyspnea occurs predictably with exercise or after bouts of coughing. The principal clinical differentiation between asthma and COPD is the degree of reversibility [40]. Since these patients often have significantly impaired pulmonary function, an exaggerated estimate of reversibility will be obtained if it is calculated as the percent improvement over baseline [19]. If, instead, the improvement is expressed as a percent of predicted, then 15 percent improvement will reliably identify those patients with the degree of reversibility characteristic of asthma [40].

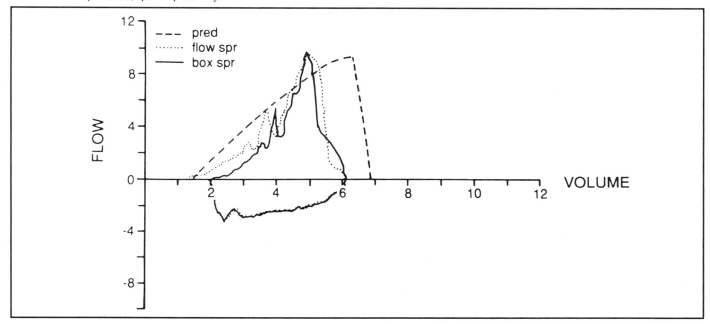

Fig. 79-1. *Flow-volume loop in a patient experiencing vocal cord dysfunction. The flattening of the inspiratory loop with relative preservation of the expiratory loop is characteristic of variable extrathoracic obstruction and is the pattern typically observed during attacks of vocal cord dysfunction. Volume in liters, flow axis in liters/second. Pred = predicted; spr = spirometry.*

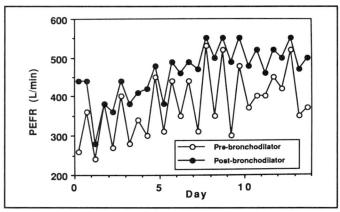

Fig. 79-2. *Response to prednisone, 20 mg bid, in a patient with airflow obstruction not completely reversed by inhaled bronchodilators. Note plateauing of the response after 7 days. PEFR = peak expiratory flow rate.*

Establish Maximum Attainable Reversibility

Patients with chronic severe asthma will usually present with their disease undertreated, as characterized by an unacceptable level of symptoms and evidence of significant airflow obstruction on pulmonary function testing. It is important to bring the asthma under control, to relieve the patient's symptoms, and to establish the degree to which the airflow obstruction is reversible. While it is inappropriate to undertreat patients in the presence of significant residual symptoms of asthma, it is also not good practice to treat with more medication than is required to gain full control of the disease, especially if overtreatment involves the use of medication with a potential for significant side effects.

It has long been appreciated, and now has been carefully established, that airflow obstruction in long-standing asthma may no longer be completely reversible [8]. This is particularly true in those patients who have had long-standing severe asthma [8]. The most effective means of establishing the maximal degree to which airflow obstruction can be reversed is by the administration of oral corticosteroids [63, 67]. For the purpose of inducing full reversibility, prednisone is administered typically in a dose of 20 mg twice daily. Usually the airflow response to this treatment will plateau within 10 to 14 days [67]; however, sometimes the response, although beginning promptly, will take longer to reach its maximal level [63]. Neither the patient's symptoms nor occasional spirometry measured in the clinic or office is adequate to monitor the response to a trial of corticosteroid-induced reversibility. The response should be assessed by twice daily measurement of peak expiratory flow rate by the patient at home. Only with frequent measurements is the inherent variability of asthma overcome so that the plateau of improvement can be appreciated (Fig. 79-2).

Assess and Treat Contributing Factors

A number of associated conditions can contribute to the severity of asthma. There is often disagreement as to the importance of sinusitis [31, 51] or gastroesophageal reflux [16, 56]; however, both have been shown to be capable of contributing to asthma severity and refractoriness and should be sought as indicated and treated if present.

The relation of the upper respiratory tract to asthma is fully discussed in Chapter 41. Here it is sufficient to point out that eosinophilic rhinitis and sinusitis frequently accompany asthma [23]. There are many potential reasons why these conditions, or complicating bacterial sinusitis, could make asthma worse, including loss of the normal conditioning of the air by the nose, irritation of the larynx or lower airway by drainage from the nose of mucoid or purulent secretions initiated by bacteria or mediators [9, 24], or bronchoconstrictive reflexes arising from the nose or sinuses. Double-blind studies have shown that treatment of the upper airway with topical steroids can decrease symptoms of seasonal asthma [68] and blunt bronchial hyperresponsiveness [13]. Both controlled [15] and uncontrolled studies of antibiotic [44] and surgical [32] therapy for chronic sinusitis have also reported significant improvement in refractory asthma, including reduction in corticosteroid requirements. Despite an extensive literature, further controlled studies are needed to establish the relationship of asymptomatic sinus mucous membrane thickening and aggravation of asthma.

Gastroesophageal reflux can potentially contribute to asthma severity by two mechanisms—microaspiration and reflex bronchoconstriction arising from stimulation of afferent receptors in the distal esophagus [39]. As is more fully discussed in Chapter 75, gastroesophageal reflux is very common in both children and adults with asthma. It is also well established that acid stimulation of receptors in the lower esophagus can cause reflex bronchoconstriction. What is less clear is the role of gastroesophageal reflux in patients with chronic, severe asthma. Available data from controlled studies would suggest that it contributes somewhat to nocturnal asthma [18]; however, anecdotal accounts credit it with a major role in chronicity and severity in at least some patients [25].

The role of allergy in asthma is well established and is reviewed in Chapters 34, 42, and 70. Seasonal exacerbations due to pollen and mold exposure are in most parts of the country easily appreciated, as are the symptoms that occur on intermittent contact with animal dander. It is more difficult to assess the contribution of chronic exposure to allergens such as house dust mite, animal dander, cockroaches, and indoor molds to the severity of perennial bronchial asthma. It has been clearly established that elimination of chronic house dust mite exposure can be associated with improvement in symptoms and pulmonary function measurements and reduced bronchial hyperresponsiveness in both children [34] and adults [43]. In the latter study patients who were employing inhaled steroids were able to discontinue their use. Long-term allergen immunotherapy has also been demonstrated to reduce bronchial reactivity not only to the allergen employed in treatment, but also to nonspecific bronchial hyperresponsiveness to histamine [28]. Thus both allergen elimination and specific allergen immunotherapy may have antiinflammatory effects in bronchial asthma, and both should contribute to improvement of chronic severe asthmatics, provided that patients have a significant allergic component to their disease.

It is often difficult to determine the significance of a perennial allergen exposure. There are three lines of evidence, however. The first is to consider the patient's exposures. Does the patient have chronic exposure to animal dander? Does the patient live in an area where levels of humidity allow house dust mites to flourish? Do either geographic area or socioeconomic circumstances suggest the possibility of cockroach infestation in the home? Are there conditions of dampness within the home or is there use of poorly maintained humidifiers, suggesting the possibility of excessive mold spore exposure [53]? The second line of evidence is demonstration of sensitivity to the possible allergens. This is most rapidly, inexpensively, and sensitively accomplished by performing allergen skin testing; however, if these tests are not readily available, similar information can be obtained by in vitro tests [37]. Finally, having established exposure and sensitivity, it is necessary to determine if the patient's asthma symptoms increase at the time of exposure to the allergen. As noted, this is relatively easy with outdoor allergens, since they tend to be present during discrete seasons and in most parts of the country there are periods during which the ambient levels of aeroallergens are low. The importance of an indoor allergen is best established by the response of symptoms to trips away from home, particularly if these are of over a week in duration. Typically symptoms will begin to improve by the end of the week and will be worse for the first 24 hours after returning home. This improvement will only occur if the patient does not have continuing exposure to the allergens while away from home. Continuing exposure is least apt to occur with animal dander but is common with house dust mite allergen unless the trip is to a semi-arid region. Some clues to the importance of indoor allergens can be elicited from the patient's history. Patients with only indoor allergen sensitivity will typically become worse with the onset of cool weather in the fall season, when the doors and windows of the home are closed. Also they will note an exacerbation of symptoms if they are at home during housekeeping chores such as vacuuming and bed making, which tend to resuspend fine-particulate allergens in the air [35].

If there is reasonable evidence to suggest the importance of an indoor allergen, environmental control measures should be instituted. These should be aimed at eliminating the source of allergen if possible and, if complete elimination is not possible, reducing exposure to the allergen, particularly in the bedroom. For further details regarding environmental controls, see Chapter 87.

Recurrent acute episodes of allergic bronchopulmonary aspergillosis or other mycoses can cause exacerbations of chronic asthma, contributing to its severity (see Chap. 49). More importantly, if not recognized and treated, recurrent episodes can lead to bronchiectasis, pulmonary fibrosis, and development of significant irreversible lung damage.

Obstructive sleep apnea is particularly prone to occur in subjects with obesity. A contributing factor may be obstruction of the nasal passages, creating increased negative pressure in the hypopharynx [6]. Nasal obstruction is not uncommon in asthmatics, and patients with chronic severe asthma often develop obesity as a complication of their chronic corticosteroid therapy. Therefore patients with severe corticosteroid-requiring asthma may develop obstructive sleep apnea, which further contributes to their nocturnal awakenings and poor sleep quality. A clue to the development of this problem is pathologic somnolence during the day. It is also worth questioning the patient's spouse regarding the occurrence of snoring and interrupted breathing. If the diagnosis is clinically suggested, a formal sleep study is indicated, since this condition will usually respond to institution of relatively inexpensive therapy with nocturnal nasal continuous positive airway pressure [6].

MANAGEMENT

Educate the Patient Regarding Asthma, Medications, and Devices

It is vital, if patients are to employ their medications and participate in management of their asthma properly, that they receive instruction as to the nature of asthma and asthma triggers, the mode of action and proper use of asthma medication, and how to properly employ any devices that they have been given for either asthma treatment or monitoring. It is particularly important, if reliance is to be placed on medication delivered by metered-dose inhalers that patients be taught their proper use and that they have their technique reassessed at periodic visits. Some individuals, especially the young and the elderly, have difficulty with the necessary coordination between actuation and inhalation from a metered-dose inhaler and will benefit from a spacer device [27]. Use of a spacer will also be helpful to decrease oropharyngeal deposition of inhaled corticosteroids [58] and to allow use of the metered-dose inhaler to treat acute exacerbations of asthma [46] (see Chap. 56).

Initiate Regular Home Peak Flow Monitoring

All patients with chronic, severe bronchial asthma should be provided with a peak flowmeter and be instructed to use it on a daily basis. Peak flow monitoring can provide objective data on airway obstruction to supplement the patient's perception of severity, which may be faulty or insensitive [45]. Measurement of peak flow is not as sensitive as spirometry in detecting minor degrees of airflow obstruction [14] and consistently underestimates the degree of obstruction [65]; nevertheless it does have an overall good correlation with forced expiratory volume in 1 second (FEV_1) [12, 65].

Regular home peak flow monitoring is essential for two purposes. One is to assess the response to corticosteroids, both during the period in which intensive treatment is given to determine maximum reversibility of the patient's obstruction and also during any corticosteroid taper to help detect the minimum dose required to sustain maximum or near maximum lung function. The second major use of home peak flow monitoring is to provide an objective measure of the degree of deterioration in lung function and the response to treatment during exacerbations of asthma. These objective assessments can be used as a component of the patient's crisis intervention plan to determine the intensity of treatment and the requirement for medical assistance.

Place on Optimal Bronchodilator Program

Although the emphasis in asthma therapy is correctly shifting toward antiinflammatory therapy, smooth muscle contraction is a major component of airflow obstruction and often dominates the clinical picture; therefore bronchodilator therapy is required both acutely and chronically. The principal classes of bronchodilators used in asthma are methylxanthines and beta-adrenergic agonists, although anticholinergics can have some benefit [66]. When used for chronic bronchodilator therapy, methylxanthines have been shown to reduce symptoms and the need for supplemental medication in patients receiving both inhaled and oral corticosteroids [36]. Regularly inhaled beta-adrenergic agonists alone have been shown to effect a similar improvement in pulmonary function as the methylxanthines [52], to reduce the occurrence of asthma symptoms [49], and when given to patients already receiving methylxanthines to reduce further the symptoms of asthma and the need for supplemental inhalers [64].

Despite the evidence for efficacy of beta agonists and methylxanthines in chronic asthma, the use of both agents has given rise to concerns [39, 54a]. Use of the methylxanthines, particularly in children, has been questioned on the basis of psychological effects [22] (see Chap. 58) and because of serious side effects usually associated with blood levels above the accepted therapeutic range [62]. Case-control studies from New Zealand have implicated a beta-adrenergic bronchodilator, fenoterol, in an increased risk for death from asthma [41]. However, the methods and conclusions of these studies have been challenged. A crossover comparison of regular versus as-needed use of fenoterol demonstrated that asthma control was worse when the drug was employed on a regular basis [48]. Clearly these concerns will affect what is considered "optimal bronchodilator therapy." It would appear that as-required use of beta-adrenergic bronchodilators is indicated as a first measure. In chronic, severe asthma, limitation of treatment to as-need beta agonists could easily result in an increased requirement for corticosteroids, particularly since the relatively brief bronchodilator action of the beta agonists leaves the patient without coverage during the early-morning hours (see Chap. 76). Bronchodilator therapy during the night is best provided by methylxanthines, perhaps administered as a single dose in the evening or a higher dose in the evening than in the morning (see Chap. 58). Alternatively, a sustained bronchodilator effect through the night can be provided by oral beta agonists, either sustained-release formulations or high doses of rapidly released forms (such as 8–12 mg albuterol at bedtime). The recent concern regarding both beta agonists and methylxanthines may provide an impetus to examine the role of long-acting anticholinergic compounds for chronic asthma therapy [66].

Begin High-dose Inhaled Corticosteroids

Asthma is an inflammatory disease; hence patients with chronic moderate to severe asthma should receive antiinflammatory therapy. Currently the antiinflammatory agents of choice in patients with chronic severe asthma are corticosteroids, which may be administered orally or by inhalation.

It is clear that there is significant absorption and systemic effect from the inhaled corticosteroids when they are administered in doses exceeding those normally employed [57, 59]. Nevertheless, even in high doses, inhaled corticosteroids can be shown to exhibit beneficial ratios of therapeutic to adverse effects compared to oral corticosteroids [57]. Furthermore, inhaled corticosteroids have been shown to exhibit desirable properties, such as reduction in bronchial hyperresponsiveness, not shared by equivalent doses of oral corticosteroids [26]. Therefore inhaled corticosteroids are the preferred chronic antiinflammatory therapy for patients with severe asthma. In patients who are receiving oral corticosteroid therapy, the dose of inhaled steroids should be one calculated potentially to replace their oral therapy. All inhaled corticosteroids are not equal on an actuation for actuation basis [17] (see Chap. 61). In fact they may be close to equivalent on a microgram for microgram basis as discharged from the cannister. High-dose inhaled steroids are best delivered with a spacer to decrease possible oropharyngeal complications and to reduce systemic absorption [7, 20]. There is also evidence, in severe asthma, that the control of asthma symptoms is better, with budesonide at least, if it is delivered in four rather than two daily doses [29].

Once inhaled corticosteroids have been instituted at an appropriate dosage, oral steroids should be rapidly tapered either completely or to alternate-day therapy. Patients will generally tolerate alternate-day corticosteroid therapy if they are given, on the alternate day, a steroid dose three times that previously given on a daily basis. Tapering should then be continued at 2-week intervals with peak flow monitoring until it is apparent that no further reduction is possible. Attempts should then be made to taper the inhaled corticosteroids to the lowest dose sustaining the degree of asthma control [61].

Consider Other "Asthma-sparing" Medications

Asthma pharmacotherapy may be classified according to mechanism of action, as indicated in Table 79-2. Of particular interest are those agents that, with or without bronchodilator properties, have the potential for reducing the inflammatory response that underlies asthma. Some of these compounds, such as inhibitors of platelet activating factor (PAF), neuropeptides, the leukotrienes, and 5-lipoxygenase, thymic hormones, and interferon gamma are currently under investigation but not available for general use. Others such as methotrexate [33, 50], colchicine [47], gold [5, 40a], and cyclosporine [1, 21, 55] have been shown to be effective treatment for asthma in double-blind studies, while gold [5], dapsone [4], hydroxychloroquine [10], cyclosporine [21, 55] and intravenous gamma globulin [30] have shown some promise in open studies (see Chap. 68). Troleandomycin (TAO), alone of these drugs, appears to require concomitant use of oral corticosteroids to be effective [54] (see Chap. 67); hence it should be considered a form of corticosteroid therapy. Cromolyn and nedocromil, although proved to be effective treatment

Table 79-2. Classification of asthma therapy

A. End-organ directed:
  1. Beta-adrenergic agonists
  2. Methylxanthines
  3. Anticholinergics
B. Mediator antagonists and inhibitors:
  1. Histamine
  2. Platelet activating factor (PAF)
  3. Leukotrienes
  4. Bradykinin
  5. Neuropeptides
  6. 5-Lipoxygenase inhibition
C. Antiinflammatory:
  1. Corticosteroids: troleandomycin (TAO)
  2. Methotrexate
  3. Gold
  4. Dapsone
  5. Hydroxychloroquine
  6. Hydroxyurea
  7. Colchicine
D. Immunomodulators:
  1. Intravenous gamma globulin
  2. Thymic hormones
  3. Interferon gamma
  4. Cyclosporine

for mild to moderate asthma [42], have not been demonstrated to have steroid-sparing effects in chronic severe asthma [60].

Most of the aforementioned steroid-sparing agents are either not commercially available or are reviewed elsewhere in this volume and therefore will not be further discussed here. Experience with two, high-dose intravenous gamma globulin and cyclosporin A, is published and the drugs are available. Therefore, their potential usefulness in the treatment of severe asthma should be discussed. Two open studies of cyclosporine, employing an average of 3.5 mg/kg/day for up to 9 months [55] and 5 mg/kg/day for 6 weeks [21], report significant reductions in oral corticosteroid requirements in some [55] or all [21] subjects. A double-blind crossover trial of 5 mg/kg/day for 12 weeks demonstrated both decreased requirement for additional prednisolone and improved pulmonary function. Side effects, including worsening of preexisting hypertension, elevation of serum creatinine, and peripheral neuropathy, were frequent but reversed after cessation of the drug. The improvement in asthma also appeared to be rapidly lost following discontinuation of treatment. Use of high-dose (2 gm/kg/month) intravenous gamma globulin, on the other hand, was not associated with any significant long-term side effects [30]. Eight steroid-requiring pediatric patients received monthly infusions for 6 months. They were able to decrease regular and supplemental steroid use by two-thirds, while experiencing improved symptoms and pulmonary function and decreased immediate skin tests. Again, the improvement waned within 2 to 3 months of discontinuing treatment. The primary disadvantage of high-dose intravenous gamma globulin therapy for severe asthma is the expense. While the preliminary results with cyclosporine and intravenous gamma globulin are encouraging, further controlled studies with cyclosporin A and high-dose intravenous gamma globulin should be conducted before these modalities are widely employed, given the significant side effects with one and the cost of the other.

The patient's corticosteroid dose should be reduced to the minimum that will maintain control of symptoms and pulmonary function near the best attained during intensive oral corticosteroid therapy. The long-term acceptability of this dose should then be determined. In part, this will depend on the presence of corticosteroid side effects from previous therapy, particularly the degree of osteoporosis, as well as the presence of cushingoid habitus, obesity, diabetes, incipient cataracts, and thinning of the

Asthma ━━━━━━━━━━━━━━━━━━━━━━━━━━━━━━━━▶ No! Treat as appropriate for diagnosis.

↓
Yes

1. If not fully reversed with bronchodilators, treat to maximum pulmonary function with oral corticosteroids* 20 mg bid.
2. Assess and treat contributing factors, e.g., rhinosinusitis, GER, allergic triggers, ABPA, sleep apnea.
3. Add inhaled corticosteroids in maximal doses or as estimated to replace oral corticosteroids.
4. Taper oral corticosteroids.

┌──────────────────────────────────▶ If oral steroids replaced, taper inhaled corticosteroids.

↓

1. If ultimate oral corticosteroid dose unacceptable, consider alternative "steroid sparing" medications. First consider drugs proven effective in asthma in double-blind studies:
   a. colchicine
   b. methotrexate
2. If ineffective, consider drugs effective in other inflammatory diseases:
   a. hydroxychloroquine
   b. gold
   c. dapsone
3. If asthma control is inadequate with combination of high dose inhaled and alternate day oral corticosteroids, consider:
   a. trial of TAO-methylprednisolone
   b. trial of high dose intravenous gamma globulin
   c. short course of cyclosporine

Fig. 79-3. *Algorithm for management of the patient with severe asthma. GER = gastroesophageal reflux; ABPA = allergic bronchopulmonary aspergillosis; TAO = troleandomycin; * = prednisone.*

skin. If an alternative antiinflammatory therapy is indicated, its selection should be based on the relative potency and incidence of adverse reactions preferably demonstrated in double-blind, placebo-controlled studies. An algorithm for the management of the patient with severe, chronic asthma is given is Fig. 79-3.

Provide a Crisis Intervention Plan

Asthma is characterized in virtually all patients by periodic exacerbations. If patients are to have optimal control of their asthma, they should be prepared to respond quickly and appropriately to these exacerbations, thereby minimizing interference with their normal activities, need for emergency visits to medical care facilities, and hospitalizations and avoiding the serious complications of asthma, including death.

The crisis intervention plans that have been tested involve maintenance of pulmonary function near maximal and rapid increase in asthma therapy in the face of exacerbations [2, 69]. For implementation of such a plan, it is essential that the patient have available at home and use a device to measure pulmonary function accurately. Although it may be ideal to measure pulmonary function twice daily before and following inhaled bronchodilator, much of the useful information can be obtained by determining peak flows each morning on arising prior to treatment. The peak flow is lowest at about 4 A.M., and in the absence of nocturnal awakening and therapy, this trough is reflected in the reading obtained upon awakening in the morning [3]. Therefore, if patients regularly measure their peak flows each morning on arising, they will likely detect any incipient decline. If the morning peak flow is reduced below the usual range for that time of day, they should employ their bronchodilator and assess the response some 10 to 15 minutes later. If this too falls below the expected range, they should proceed according to their crisis intervention plan (see Table 79-3). A useful strategy for moderate exacerbations of asthma is to temporarily double the dose of inhaled corticosteroids [2]. With more severe exacerbations it is advisable to employ oral corticosteroids. A schedule that works well for most exacerbations is prednisone, 20 mg orally two times

Table 79-3. Crisis intervention plan

PEFR greater than 70 percent potential normal value:
   Continue routine regimen of inhaled beta agonists BID and as needed and inhaled corticosteroids.
PEFR less than 70 percent potential normal value:
   Double dose of inhaled steroids for twice as many days as required to achieve normal baseline.
PEFR less than 50 percent potential normal value:
   Begin oral prednisone 20 mg BID and call physician. Continue BID until sleeping through the night, inhalers providing the usual duration of relief, and PEFR back to baseline.
   Then 20 mg every morning for same number of days.
PEFR less than 30 percent potential normal value:
   Call physician urgently, if not available proceed to emergency room.

PEFR = peak expiratory flow rate.
Source: Modified from R. Beasley, M. Cushley, and S. T. Holgate, A self-management plan in the treatment of adult asthma. *Thorax* 44:200, 1989.

a day until the patient is sleeping through the night, morning peak flows are within the normal range, and inhaled beta agonists are providing relief of the customary duration. At this time prednisone is reduced to 20 mg each morning and continued for the same number of days as the twice daily dose had been administered. Following this, patients return to their previous schedule of antiinflammatory therapy.

There is no one special treatment for patients with severe chronic asthma. What is required is a careful reassessment of patients to be certain that bronchial asthma is indeed the cause of their apparent refractory respiratory symptoms. If asthma is indeed the diagnosis, then patients should be assessed for degree of reversibility so that neither undertreatment nor over treatment occurs. Particular attention should be given to correctable exacerbating factors. Patients should receive education regarding asthma, asthma medications, and devices employed in their treatment program. They should be placed on an optimal regimen of bronchodilators and inhaled corticosteroids, while oral corticosteroids should be tapered with careful peak flow monitoring. If the dose of corticosteroids required to maintain symptoms and pulmonary function within acceptable levels is too great, addition of a steroid-sparing drug should be considered. Finally, all patients should have a written crisis intervention plan, based on alterations in symptoms and peak flow measurements, with graded responses to exacerbations of differing severity. By employing these principles, more optimal control of the chronic severe asthma patient is feasible.

REFERENCES

1. Alexander, A. G., Barnes, N. C., and Kay, A. B. Trial of cyclosporin in corticosteroid-dependent chronic severe asthma. *Lancet* 339:324, 1992.
1a. American Thoracic Society Committee of Diagnostic Standards of Nontuberculous Respiratory Diseases. Chronic bronchitis, asthma and pulmonary emphysema. *Am. Rev. Respir. Dis.* 85:762, 1962.
2. Beasley, R., Cushley, M., and Holgate, S. T. A self-management plan in the treatment of adult asthma. *Thorax* 44:200, 1989.
3. Bellia, V., et al. Validation of morning dip of peak expiratory flow as an indicator of the severity of nocturnal asthma. *Chest* 94:108, 1988.
4. Berlow, B. A., et al. The effect of dapsone in steroid-dependent asthma. *J. Allergy Clin. Immunol.* 87:710, 1991.
5. Bernstein, D. I., et al. An open study of auranofin in the treatment of steroid-dependent asthma. *J. Allergy Clin. Immunol.* 81:6, 1988.
6. Bradley, T. D. Diagnosing and assessing obstructive sleep apnea. *J. Resp. Dis.* 9(3):32, 1988.
7. Brown, P. H., et al. Do large volume spacer devices reduce the systemic effects of high dose inhaled corticosteroids? *Thorax* 45:736, 1990.
8. Brown, P. J., Greville, H. W., and Finucane, K. E. Asthma and irreversible airflow obstruction. *Thorax* 139:131, 1984.
9. Brugman, S. M., et al. Mechanisms for the increase of lower airways hyperresponsiveness induced by experimental sinusitis (abstract). *Am. Rev. Respir. Dis.* 139(2):A107, 1989.
10. Charous, B. L. Open study of hydroxychloroquine in the treatment of severe symptomatic or corticosteroid-dependent asthma. *Ann. Allergy* 65:53, 1990.
11. Christopher, K. L., et al. Vocal cord dysfunction presenting as asthma. *N. Engl. J. Med.* 308:1566, 1983.
12. Connolly, C. K., and Chan, N. S. Relationship between different measurements of respiratory function in asthma. *Respiration* 52:22, 1987.
13. Corren, J., et al. Nasal beclomethasone prevents the seasonal increase in bronchial responsiveness in patients with rhinitis and allergic asthma. *J. Allergy Clin. Immunol.* 90:250, 1992.
14. Cross, D., and Nelson, H. S. The role of the peak flow meter in the diagnosis and management of asthma. *J. Allergy Clin. Immunol.* 87:120, 1991.
15. Cummings, N. P., et al. Effect of treatment of sinusitis on asthma and bronchial reactivity: results of a double-blind study (abstract). *J. Allergy Clin. Immunol.* 73:143, 1984.
16. Davis, R. S., Larsen, G., and Grunstein, M. M. Respiratory response to intraesophageal acid infusion in asthmatic children during sleep. *J. Allergy Clin. Immunol.* 72:393, 1983.
17. Dry, J., et al. A comparison of flunisolide inhaler and beclomethasone dipropionate inhaler in bronchial asthma. *J. Int. Med. Res.* 13:289, 1985.
18. Ekstrom, T., Lindgren, B. R., and Tibbing, L. Effects of ranitidine treatment on patients with asthma and a story of gastroesophageal reflux: a double-blind, cross-over study. *Thorax* 44:19, 1989.
19. Eliasson, O., and DeGraff Jr., A. C. The use of criteria for reversibility and obstruction to define patient groups for bronchodilator trials. Influence of clinical diagnosis, spirometric, and anthropometric variables. *Am. Rev. Respir. Dis.* 132:858, 1985.
20. Farrer, M., Francis, A. J., and Pearce, S. J. Morning serum cortisol concentrations after 2 mg inhaled beclomethasone dipropionate in normal subjects: effect of a 750 ml spacer device. *Thorax* 45:740, 1990.
21. Finnerty, N. A., and Sullivan, T. J. Effect of cyclosporine on corticosteroid-dependent asthma (abstract). *J. Allergy Clin. Immunol.* 87:297, 1991.
22. Furukawa, C. T., et al. Cognitive and behavioral findings in children taking theophylline. *J. Allergy Clin. Immunol.* 81:83, 1988.
23. Harlin, S. L., et al. A clinical and pathologic study of chronic sinusitis: the role of the eosinophil. *J. Allergy Clin. Immunol.* 81:867, 1988.
24. Irwin, R. S., et al. Post nasal drip causes cough and is associated with reversible upper airway obstruction. *Chest* 85:346, 1984.
25. Irwin, R. S., et al. Chronic cough as the sole presenting manifestation of gastroesophageal reflux. *Am. Rev. Respir. Dis.* 140:1294, 1989.

26. Jenkins, C. R., and Woolcock, A. J. Effect of prednisone and beclomethasone dipropionate on airway responsiveness in asthma: a comparative study. *Thorax* 43:378, 1988.
27. Lee, H., and Evans, H. Evaluation of inhalation aids of metered dose inhalers in asthmatic children. *Chest* 91:355, 1987.
28. Lilja, G., et al. Immunotherapy with cat- and dog-dander extracts. IV. Effects of 2 years of treatment. *J. Allergy Clin. Immunol.* 83:37, 1989.
29. Malo, J.-L., et al. Four-times-a-day dosing frequency is better than a twice-a-day regimen in subjects requiring a high-dose inhaled steroid, budesonide, to control moderate to severe asthma. *Am. Rev. Respir. Dis.* 140:624, 1989.
30. Mazer, B. D., and Gelfand, E. W. An open-label study of high-dose intravenous immunoglobulin in severe childhood asthma. *J. Allergy Clin. Immunol.* 87:976, 1991.
31. McFadden Jr., E. R. Nasal-sinus-pulmonary reflexes and bronchial asthma. *J. Allergy Clin. Immunol.* 78:1, 1986.
32. Mings, R., et al. Five-year follow-up of the effects of bilateral intranasal sphenoethmoidectomy in patients with sinusitis and asthma. *Am. J. Rhinol.* 2:13, 1988.
33. Mullarkey, M. F., et al. Methotrexate in the treatment of corticosteroid-dependent asthma: a double-blind crossover study. *N. Engl. J. Med.* 318:603, 1988.
34. Murray, A. B., and Ferguson, A. C. Dust-free bedrooms in the treatment of asthmatic children with house dust or house dust mite allergy—a controlled trial. *Pediatrics* 71:418, 1983.
35. Murray, A. B., Ferguson, A. C., and Morrison, B. J. Diagnosis of house dust mite allergy in asthmatic children: what constitutes a positive history? *J. Allergy Clin. Immunol.* 71:21, 1983.
36. Nassif, E. G., et al. The value of maintenance theophylline in steroid-dependent asthma. *N. Engl. J. Med.* 304:71, 1981.
37. Nelson, H. S. The clinical relevance of IgE. *Ann. Allergy* 49:73, 1982.
38. Nelson, H. S. Is gastroesophageal reflux worsening your patient's asthma? *J. Respir. Dis.* 11:827, 1990.
39. Newhouse, M. T. Is theophylline obsolete? *Chest* 98:1, 1990.
40. Nicklaus, T. M., Burgin Jr., W. W., and Taylor, J. R. Spirometric tests to diagnose suspected asthma. *Am. Rev. Respir. Dis.* 100:153, 1969.
40a. Nierop, G., et al. Auranofin in the treatment of steroid dependent-asthma: a double-blind study. *Thorax* 47:349, 1992.
41. Pearce, N., et al. Case control study of prescribed fenoterol and death from asthma in New Zealand 1977–81. *Thorax* 45:170, 1990.
42. Petty, T. L., et al. Cromolyn sodium is effective in adult chronic asthmatics. *Am. Rev. Respir. Dis.* 139:694, 1989.
43. Platts-Mills, T. A. E., et al. Reduction of bronchial hyperreactivity during prolonged allergen avoidance. *Lancet* 2:675, 1982.
44. Rachelefsky, G. S., Katz, R. M., and Siegel, S. C. Chronic sinus disease associated with reactive airway disease in children. *Pediatr.* 73:526, 1984.
45. Rubinfeld, A. R., and Pain, M. C. F. Perception of asthma. *Lancet* 1:882, 1976.
46. Salzman, G. A., et al. Aerosolized metaproterenol in the treatment of asthmatics with severe airflow obstruction. Comparison of two delivery methods. *Chest* 95:1017, 1989.
47. Schwarz, Y. A., et al. A clinical and immunologic study of colchicine in asthma. *J. Allergy Clin. Immunol.* 85:578, 1990.
48. Sears, M. R., et al. Regular inhaled beta-agonist treatment in bronchial asthma. *Lancet* 2:1391, 1990.
49. Shepherd, G. L., Hetzel, M. R., and Clark, T. J. H. Regular versus symptomatic aerosol bronchodilator treatment of asthma. *Br. J. Dis. Chest* 75:215, 1981.
50. Shiner, R. J., et al. Randomized, double-blind, placebo-controlled trial of methotrexate in steroid-dependent asthma. *Lancet* 336:137, 1990.
51. Slavin, R. G. Relationship of nasal disease and sinusitis to bronchial asthma. *Ann. Allergy* 49:76, 1982.
52. Smith, J. A., Weber, R. W., and Nelson, H. S. Theophylline and aerosolized terbutaline in the treatment of bronchial asthma: double-blind comparison of optimal doses. *Chest* 78:816, 1980.
53. Solomon, W. R. A volumetric study of winter fungus prevalence in the air of midwestern homes. *J. Allergy Clin. Immunol.* 57:46, 1976.
54. Spector, S. L., Katz, F. H., and Farr, R. S. Troleandomycin: Effectiveness in steroid-dependent asthma and bronchitis. *J. Allergy Clin. Immunol.* 54:367, 1974.
54a. Spitzer, W. O. The use of β-agonists and the risk of death and near death from asthma. *N. Engl. J. Med.* 326:501, 1992.
55. Szczeklik, A., et al. Cyclosporine for steroid-dependent asthma. *Allergy* 46:312, 1991.

56. Tan, W. C., et al. Effects of spontaneous and stimulated gastroesophageal reflux on sleeping asthmatics. *Am. Rev. Respir. Dis.* 141:1394, 1990.

57. Toogood, J. H., et al. Budesonide versus prednisone—bioequivalent doses of budesonide and prednisone in moderate and severe asthma. *J. Allergy Clin. Immunol.* 84:688, 1989.

58. Toogood, J. H., et al. Use of spacers to facilitate inhaled corticosteroid treatment of asthma. *Am. Rev. Respir. Dis.* 129:723, 1984.

59. Toogood, J. H., et al. Effect of high-dose inhaled budesonide on calcium and phosphate metabolism and the risk of osteoporosis. *Am. Rev. Respir. Dis.* 138:57, 1988.

60. Toogood, J. H., Jennings, B., and Lefcoe, N. M. A clinical trial of combined cromolyn/beclomethasone treatment for chronic asthma. *J. Allergy Clin. Immunol.* 67:317, 1981.

61. Toogood, J. H., et al. Minimum dose requirements of steroid-dependent asthmatic patients for aerosol beclomethasone and oral prednisone. *J. Allergy Clin. Immunol.* 61:355, 1978.

62. Tsiu, S. J., Self, T. H., and Burns, R. Theophylline toxicity: update. *Ann. Allergy* 64:241, 1990.

63. Turner-Warwick, M. On observing patterns of airflow obstruction in chronic asthma. *Br. J. Dis. Chest* 71:73, 1977.

64. Vandewalker, M. L., et al. Addition of terbutaline to optimal theophylline therapy: double-blind crossover study in asthmatic patients. *Chest* 90:198, 1986.

65. Vaughan, T. R., et al. Comparison of PEFR and FEV_1 in patients with varying degrees of airway obstruction: effect of modest altitude. *Chest* 95:558, 1989.

66. Vichyanond, P., et al. Efficacy of atropine methylnitrate alone and in combination with albuterol in children with asthma. *Chest* 98:637, 1990.

67. Webb, J., Clark, T. J. H., and Chilvers, C. Time course of response to prednisolone in chronic airflow obstruction. *Thorax* 36:18, 1981.

68. Welsh, P. W., et al. Efficacy of beclomethasone nasal solution, flunisolide, and cromolyn in relieving symptoms of ragweed allergy. *Mayo Clin. Proc.* 62:125, 1987.

69. Woolcock, A. J., Yan, Y., and Salome, C. M. Effect of therapy on bronchial hyperresponsiveness in the long-term management of asthma. *Clin. Allergy* 18:165, 1988.

Childhood Asthma

80

Gerard J. Canny
Desmond J. Bohn
John J. Reisman
Henry Levison

Asthma is the leading chronic disease of childhood in industrialized countries. Despite advances in treatment, both mortality [271] and morbidity [157] rates from childhood asthma are increasing (see Chaps. 2 and 90). Although the exact cause of this situation remains unclear, deaths from asthma are usually preventable and result from long-term and short-term deficiencies in management [82]. Similarly, morbidity from asthma is frequently due to underdiagnosis, undertreatment, poor education, and inadequate supervision [43, 111, 144, 240, 293]. By tackling these four problem areas, a significant reduction in the morbidity [48, 240] and, hopefully, mortality [82] rates from asthma could be achieved. The main thrust in this chapter will be to present a practical approach to the diagnosis and management of asthma of varying degrees of severity in children and to focus on features that are unique to childhood asthma.

EPIDEMIOLOGIC ASPECTS

Prevalence

Asthma is common throughout the world, but estimates of its prevalence vary widely. Although this variation may be related to genetic and environmental factors, methodologic differences in data collection (e.g., questionnaires versus interviews versus physician-confirmed diagnosis) and in the definition of asthma are partly responsible [217]. A comprehensive picture of the prevalence of asthma among children in the United States is provided by recently published data from the National Health and Nutrition Examination Survey (NHANES) [91, 222] and the National Health Interview Survey (NHIS) [273] (Table 80-1). It is evident from these surveys that asthma prevalence varies considerably according to the survey design and the questions used to identify asthma. In the United States, the prevalence of asthma among children is higher in males [91, 222, 273], in certain geographic locations (e.g., the South and West) [91], in urban areas [91, 222, 273], and in blacks [91, 222, 273]. In addition, these surveys [91, 222, 273] found that the vast majority of children with asthma develop symptoms in the first few years of life and that the prevalence declines in males during adolescence. The overall prevalence of asthma in the United States is rising, and its severity may also be increasing [91]. Although there is a racial disparity in the prevalence of childhood asthma in the United States [91, 222, 273], this appears to be due largely to the characteristics of a poverty-afflicted environment rather than to genetic differences [222, 273].

The prevalence of asthma in most other countries is similar to that in the United States. For example, in community and school surveys in the United Kingdom [8, 43, 111, 240], the prevalence of wheezing in the preceding year among respondents ranged from 4.9 to 15 percent, a diagnosis of asthma having been made

in up to 9.5 percent of the children surveyed. Estimates of asthma prevalence among Canadian [118], Australian [186, 218], and New Zealand [65] children have also varied considerably, and in New Zealand asthma appears to be particularly severe. Lower prevalence rates of childhood asthma have been reported from Scandinavia, Switzerland, and developing countries [51] (See Chap. 2).

Morbidity and Mortality

Although morbidity is difficult to quantify, it is clear that asthma remains a common cause of school absenteeism [43, 111, 240, 246], restricted activity [240], and visits to both physicians' offices [91] and emergency rooms [37, 178]. In many Western countries, hospitalization rates for childhood asthma have increased dramatically in recent years [157]. During the period 1979 to 1987, asthma hospitalizations among children, aged 0 to 17 years, increased by 4.5 percent per annum in the United States [92] (Fig. 80-1). This increase was most marked in preschool children and among blacks. In Canada, hospital admission rates for asthma have increased by 200 percent between 1971 and 1987 for children under the age of 18 years, the largest increase having occurred in children aged 1 to 4 years [146] (Fig. 80-2). Similarly, hospitalization rates for pediatric asthma have increased in Britain [7, 8], Australia [39], and New Zealand [65]. Although hospital admissions for asthma have increased in recent years, the mean length of stay per hospitalization has decreased [7, 8, 39, 65, 92, 146], and children with acute asthma rarely require admission to critical care units [37, 92]. It is paradoxical that hospital admission rates have risen at a time of increasing availability of effective antiasthmatic medications. Several explanations have been put forward [7, 8, 26, 39, 65, 92, 146], including (1) changes in the international classification of disease (ICD) which occurred in 1979, resulting in the term *asthmatic bronchitis* being coded as asthma, rather than bronchitis; (2) diagnostic transfer, especially from wheezy bronchitis to asthma in young children; (3) an increase in the prevalence and/or severity of asthma; (4) increasing levels of environmental allergens and air pollution; (5) changes in health care access, availability, and utilization; and (6) an increase in the willingness or ability of physicians to diagnose asthma.

Although asthma is an uncommon cause of fatality in children, upward trends in death rates have been reported among children in several Western countries [26, 27, 270]. In the United States, asthma mortality increased by 6.2 percent per annum among children and young adults in the 1980s [26, 270, 271] (Fig. 80-3). Death rates increased faster among children aged 5 to 14 years than among adolescents and young adults and are higher among blacks and in poor urban areas, such as New York City and Cook County, Illinois. The factors that are considered responsible for these rising mortality rates are similar to those put forward to explain the increasing morbidity rates in asthma [26] (see Chap.

Table 80-1. Mean percentages of asthma prevalence among U.S. children by sex and race

		Sex		Race	
Survey and asthma definition	Total	Male	Female	White	Black
National Health and Nutrition Examination Survey II, 1976–1980 (Children 3–17 years)					
Ever diagnosed by physician	7.0	8.3	5.5	6.4	10.1
Currently diagnosed by physician	3.6	4.3	2.9	3.3	5.6
Wheezing[a]	5.3	6.2	4.5	5.0	7.3
Ever diagnosed by physician or wheezing[a]	9.5	11.2	7.8	8.9	13.1
Currently diagnosed by physician or wheezing[a]	6.7	7.8	5.5	6.2	9.4
National Health Interview Survey, 1981 (Children 0–17 years)					
Current asthma[b]	2.8	NA	NA	2.5	4.4

[a] Frequent trouble with wheezing (not counting colds or the flu) during the past 12 months.
[b] Based on parents' reports that their child had asthma at the time of interview, which had been present for longer than 3 months and had not been cured.

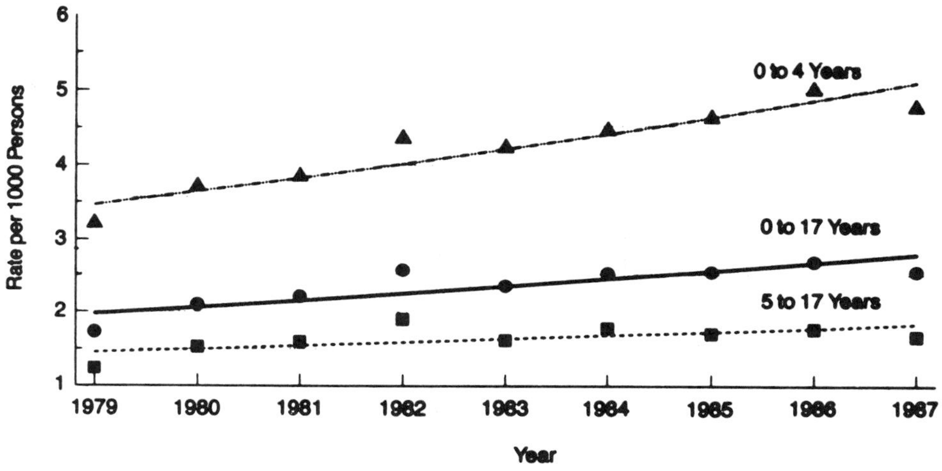

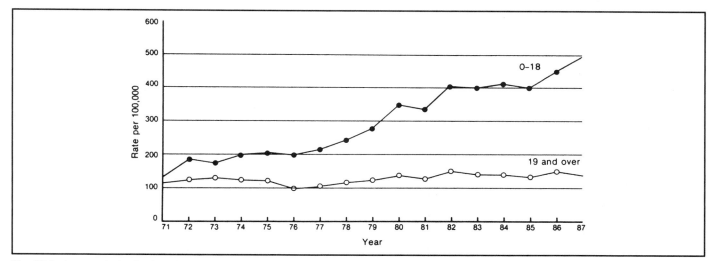

Fig. 80-1. *Asthma hospitalization rates per 1,000 persons for U.S. children and youths aged 0 to 17 years. (Reprinted with permission from P. J. Gergen and K. B. Weiss. Changing patterns of asthma hospitalization among children: 1979 to 1987. J.A.M.A. 264:1688, 1990.)*

Fig. 80-2. *Age-standarized admission rates for asthma, both sexes, Canada 1971 to 1987. (Reprinted with permission from Y. Mao. Canadian Pediatric Asthma: Morbidity, Mortality and Hospitalization Data. In Treatment of Pediatric Asthma: A Canadian Consensus [MEDICINE Publishing Foundation Symposium Series, 29]. Toronto: MES Medical Education Services, 1991.)*

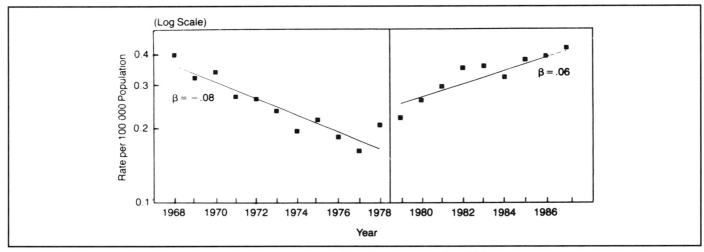

Fig. 80-3. *Asthma mortality rates in the United States, among persons 5 to 34 years from 1968 to 1987. (Reprinted with permission from K. B. Weiss and D. K. Wagener. Changing patterns of asthma mortality: Identifying target populations at risk. J.A.M.A. 264:1683, 1990.)*

90). In addition, it has been suggested that some asthma deaths may be related to therapy, particularly with sympathomimetic agents [195]. Several mechanisms have been postulated to explain this association, including (1) direct cardiotoxic effects of nonselective [195] and selective [187, 241] beta agonists, (2) delivery of beta$_2$ agonists in high dosage without supplementary oxygen by home nebulizers [226], (3) synergistic cardiac toxicity from the concurrent use of beta$_2$ agonists and oral theophylline [278], and (4) paradoxical bronchoconstriction, induced by beta$_2$ agonists [160]. However, the overwhelming evidence from epidemiologic studies is that deaths in asthma are usually due to over-reliance on bronchodilators, resulting in a delay in referral to hospital and treatment with systemic steroids, rather than to a direct toxic effect of beta$_2$ agonists [65, 82, 195].

ETIOLOGIC CONSIDERATIONS

Asthma is a chronic inflammatory disease of the airways characterized by narrowing of the airways that reverses spontaneously or with treatment. Airway obstruction is produced by a combination of airway smooth muscle spasm, edema of the airway mucosa, mucus plugging, and inflammation. The pathologic changes seen at autopsy in children dying from severe acute asthma are similar to those seen in tissue obtained by lung biopsy in children with asthma in remission [61]. These changes are most marked in the peripheral airways and include goblet cell metaplasia, smooth muscle hypertrophy, basement membrane thickening, cellular infiltration, epithelial shedding, and increased collagen deposition beneath the epithelial basement membrane [299]. In patients with mild asthma, however, the bronchial epithelium may be entirely normal [141].

Although the cause of asthma is not completely understood, its major clinical characteristic is an increase in the degree of airway responsiveness to a wide range of stimuli. Up to 90 percent of children with asthma symptoms, for example, demonstrate responsiveness to methacholine [225]. Recent data indicate that bronchial hyperresponsiveness is detectable soon after birth [137], and it has been postulated that the predisposition to wheeze is determined by complex interactions between genetic, atopic, and environmental factors [137, 279].

Genetic Influences

There is much evidence that asthma and other atopic disorders (e.g., eczema, allergic rhinitis) are partially hereditary in nature

(see Chap. 3). Several studies have shown an increased prevalence of asthma among first-degree relatives of index subjects [231–233, 291] and, likewise, that the risk of having an asthmatic child is significantly greater when one or both parents have asthma than when neither parent is affected [43, 64, 108, 117]. Sibbald et al. [233], in a study from a London general practice, showed that 17 percent of parents and 8 percent of the siblings of asthmatic children had asthma, as compared to 4 percent and 3 percent of the respective relatives of control children. Higgins and Keller [108] found that the prevalence of asthma among boys increased from 7.4 percent when neither parent had asthma to 18.3 percent when one or both parent had asthma, and from 4.1 to 11.7 percent for girls. However, other studies have found that the presence of parental atopy/asthma increased the prevalence of asthma in boys but not in girls [64, 117]. A familial component is also thought to exist in the transmission of the bronchial response to methacholine [115, 257]. A recent study has shown that the degree of airway responsiveness to histamine, measured shortly after birth, is increased in the presence of a family history of atopy and asthma [287].

It could be argued that the tendency for asthma to cluster in families is due to the effect of a shared environment rather than to genetic influences. However, twin studies provide more convincing evidence for a genetic component in asthma. A Scandinavian study of 7,000 pairs of twins found that the frequency of concordance for asthma was 19 percent for monozygotic twins, as compared to 5 percent for dizygotic twins [75]. Likewise, Hopp and colleagues [115] found greater concordance for asthma, atopy, and methacholine sensitivity in monozygotic than in dizygotic twins. In a recent twin study from Australia [72], a common genetic influence on asthma and hay fever was reported, although 40 percent of the variation in the liability to these conditions was thought to be environmental in nature.

Atopy

Atopy is defined as a propensity to produce IgE antibodies in response to common environmental antigens and manifests clinically as asthma, allergic rhinitis, and eczema [148]. Family aggregation [64, 232, 233] and twin studies [72, 75, 115] indicate that atopy is at least partly hereditary, and recent data suggest an autosomal dominant pattern of inheritance [52], with the gene locus on chromosome 11 [53]. Transmission of atopy at chromosome 11q is detectable only through the maternal line [297]. The atopic state can be present before the onset of asthma in children and may manifest itself as increased IgE levels in cord blood [59], as well as infantile eczema [117]. Atopy occurs in the majority of patients with asthma [30], and several lines of evidence suggest a causal relationship between these two conditions: (1) atopic patients with asthma have a greater response to methacholine/histamine challenge than their nonatopic counterparts [28, 41, 42]; (2) allergen challenge increases the sensitivity to histamine/methacholine [46]; (3) asthma has been shown to develop in communities newly exposed to certain allergens [71] (e.g., the house dust mite), and airway reactivity decreases when patients are removed from such exposure [191]; (4) the severity and medication requirements of childhood asthma correlate with the number and size of positive skin tests to common environmental allergens [291]; (5) children with eczema and multiple allergen sensitivity appear to be at risk for more persistent asthma [148]; and (6) exposure to high levels of house dust mite antigens during infancy leads to increased bronchial responsiveness in later childhood [242]. The mechanisms linking atopy and asthma have not been elucidated, and the observation that these two conditions can occur independently of one another indicates that allergic factors are not the entire explanation for the development of asthma [279].

The role of food allergens in the pathogenesis of asthma, discussed in detail in Chap. 43, is an even more controversial area. In general, pulmonary reactions to ingested foods are rare [23]. In a recent study of asthmatic children, 5 years of age or less, it was found that 37 of the 109 children studied were allergic to certain foods (e.g., milk, eggs, wheat), as defined by a high serum IgE antibody and a clinical history of a reaction to the food [289]. Although eczema was found to be more common in this subset of patients, as compared to those without food allergies, the severity of asthma did not differ in the two groups. Finally, the question as to whether breast-feeding has a protective effect against the subsequent development of asthma and other atopic conditions remains an unresolved controversy [133, 273, 286].

Respiratory Infections

In children with preexisting asthma, respiratory viruses (e.g., rhinoviruses, respiratory syncytial virus [RSV], influenza and parainfluenza viruses) are the most common precipitating cause of wheezing [31]. Possible mechanisms of virus-induced wheeze include exposure of vagal receptors as a result of epithelial damage, a decreased beta-adrenergic response, and an enhanced release of IgE-mediated histamine from basophils [31]. Respiratory infections, such as bronchiolitis [103, 126, 158, 198, 213, 237], croup [102], and *Chlamydia* pneumonia [272], have also been implicated in the development of airway reactivity and dysfunction. In this regard, the evidence is strongest for RSV-induced bronchiolitis. Moderately severe bronchiolitis in infancy is frequently associated with the development of lung function abnormalities, enhanced airway reactivity, and an increased risk of developing asthma later in childhood [103, 126, 158, 198, 213, 237]. It remains to be clarified whether these infections cause airway reactivity directly or, alternatively, whether an inherited predisposition to airway hyperreactivity or atopy results in more severe infections, which, in turn, are subject to diagnosis at the time or to parental recall in retrospective studies. It has also been suggested that babies who are most likely to wheeze with respiratory infection may have been born with narrower peripheral airways [150]. Based on the epidemiology of asthma and respiratory infections, Burney and colleagues [29] have challenged the theory that there is a direct causal relationship between infection and asthma.

Parental Smoking

In children with asthma, maternal smoking increases the severity of symptoms, adversely affects lung function, and increases airway hyperreactivity [168]. This association is stronger for boys [169] and older children [168, 169] with asthma and is affected by the duration of exposure and the number of cigarettes smoked by the mother each day [168]. On the other hand, the relationship between passive smoking and the acquisition of asthma is less well defined [100, 136, 273]. However, intrauterine exposure to cigarette smoke results in elevated umbilical cord IgE levels [143] and increased airway responsiveness at birth [287] and is a risk factor for the development of atopy [143] and lower respiratory illness in early childhood [255]. Recent data indicate that children who have had atopic dermatitis are more likely to develop asthma if the mother is a smoker than if she is a nonsmoker [170].

Air Pollution

The effect of chemical (e.g., sulfur dioxide, ozone) and particulate pollution on asthma remains controversial. Although a correlation has been noted between the level of ambient pollution and both symptoms and hospitalization rates in children with asthma [40, 194], this is not an invariable finding [264]. Likewise, in view of the low prevalence of asthma in certain highly polluted areas [6], it is unlikely that atmospheric pollution contributes to the development of asthma.

Socioeconomic Factors

The racial discrepancy in the prevalence and morbidity from childhood asthma in the United States appears to be related to social and environmental factors associated with poverty and inner city living [222, 273]. These risk factors for asthma include low family income, low birth weight, young maternal age at the time of the child's birth, crowding in the home, and maternal smoking [222, 273]. Likewise, the difference in the prevalence of asthma between Polynesian children and those of European descent in New Zealand appears to be related to socioeconomic status and home smoking rates [65]. In contrast, no consistent relationship between social status and asthma prevalence has been found in other populations [117, 136].

ESTABLISHING THE DIAGNOSIS OF ASTHMA

The rational treatment of asthma depends on accurate diagnosis and assessment of the severity of asthma in each individual child. Unfortunately, the diagnosis of asthma is hindered by the lack of a pragmatic definition [217] (see Chap. 1). The American Thoracic Society [5] defines asthma as "a disease characterized by increased responsiveness of the trachea and bronchi to various stimuli and manifested by widespread narrowing of the airways that changes in severity either spontaneously or as a result of therapy." Unfortunately, pulmonary function tests are rarely feasible in children under the age of 5 years, and therefore, this definition has limited application in the pediatric population. In addition, some children with asthma have an irreversible component to their disease [35]. We propose that any child, regardless of age, with recurrent (three or more) episodes of wheezing or dyspnea should be considered as having asthma until proved otherwise. The diagnosis of asthma is even more likely if these symptoms are episodic, aggravated by one or more of the factors listed in Table 80-2, and respond to antiasthmatic medications.

Table 80-2. Triggers of asthma

Respiratory infection (viral, mycoplasma)
Exercise
Allergens:
   Inhaled
   Ingested (rare)
Irritants (cigarette smoke, air pollution)
Weather changes
Medications (acetylsalicylic acid)
Chemicals (tartrazine, sulfites, monosodium glutamate)
Emotional stress
Gastroesophageal reflux

The clinician should be aware that about 5 percent of children with asthma present with chronic cough as the sole symptom [206] (see Chap. 50). These children may be diagnosed erroneously as having "bronchitis," and this results in inappropriate treatment [121, 240]. Likewise, some children are misdiagnosed as having persistent/recurrent pneumonia on chest radiographs, when in fact these infiltrates represent atelectasis from mucus plugging of peripheral airways in asthma [76].

A comprehensive history is essential in the initial evaluation of a child with suspected asthma and in planning subsequent therapy. The key points to elicit in the history are listed in Table 80-3. It is also important in the course of the clinical evaluation to identify high-risk patients [173, 251] (Table 80-4) in order to provide them with the special attention they require. Physical examination should focus on overall growth and development and look for clinical evidence of airway obstruction, pulmonary hyperinflation, associated signs of allergy, and drug-related side effects. Finally, the clinical evaluation should be directed at excluding other potential causes of recurrent respiratory symptoms in infants and young children (Table 80-5; see also Chap. 37). Clinical features suggestive of an alternative condition are summarized in Table 80-6, and further investigations may then be necessary (e.g., chest radiograph, sweat testing, barium swallow).

Pulmonary function data can be used to support the diagnosis of asthma. Children from the age of 5 to 6 years onward are

Table 80-3. Asthma history

Nature of symptoms
Pattern of symptoms (severity, frequency, seasonal and diurnal variation)
Precipitating/aggravating factors
Profile of typical acute episode (including emergency room visits, hospitalizations, intensive care unit admissions)
Previous and current drug therapy (response, dosage, delivery, side effects)
Impact of disease on child and family (e.g., exercise tolerance, sleep disturbance, financial difficulties)
Atopic history
School performance and attendance
Psychosocial evaluation of patient/family
Environmental history (including active/passive smoking, housing conditions, pets)
Family history
General medical history of child

Table 80-4. Profile of the high-risk asthmatic

Previous life-threatening episodes, e.g., intensive care unit admission, hypoxic-related seizures
Recent hospitalizations or emergency room visits
Dependency on multiple medications (particularly oral steroids)
Discontinuous medical care
Noncompliance/psychosocial problems (particularly in teenagers)

Source: Data from Newcomb and Akhter [173] and Strunk [251].

Table 80-5. Causes of recurrent wheeze/cough in infants and children

Common	Uncommon	Rare
Asthma	Cystic fibrosis	Tracheomalacia
Recurrent aspiration	Foreign body	Left ventricular failure
	Bronchopulmonary dysplasia	Vascular anomalies
		Mediastinal masses
		Bronchiolitis obliterans
		Immune deficiency states

Table 80-6. Clinical features suggestive of an alternative diagnosis to asthma

History
  Neonatal symptoms/ventilation
  Wheeze associated with feeding/vomiting
  Sudden onset of cough/choking
  Steatorrhea
  Stridor
Physical examination
  Failure to thrive
  Cardiac murmur
  Clubbing
  Unilateral lung signs, focal wheeze
Investigations
  No reversibility of airflow obstruction with bronchodilator
  Focal or persistent chest radiographic findings

usually able to perform simple lung function tests, such as peak flow rate (PFR) and forced expiratory volume in 1 second (FEV_1). If airway obstruction is present at the time of evaluation, the diagnosis of asthma can be confirmed by demonstrating an improvement of at least 15 percent in PFR or FEV_1 after the inhalation of a beta$_2$ agonist from a metered-dose inhaler [209]. In children who have normal lung function at the time of examination and whose history is inconclusive, it may be possible to make a diagnosis of asthma by demonstrating a diurnal variability of 20 percent or more in PFR, measured twice daily at home over a short period of time [106]. In general, however, children have less diurnal lability in lung function than adult asthmatics [120]. A diagnosis of asthma is also supported by demonstrating a decrease of 20 percent or more in PFR/FEV_1 after bronchial challenge with exercise or inhaled methacholine/histamine (see Chap. 39).

Although bronchial provocation tests are useful in the evaluation of asthma, particularly in children with an atypical presentation [66] (e.g., chronic cough), they do have a number of limitations. In the general community, considerable overlap in bronchial responsiveness has been noted between children with asthma and symptom-free children [141, 184]. In addition, bronchial hyperreactivity may occur as a transient phenomenon after upper respiratory infections and in a variety of other pulmonary disorders (e.g., cystic fibrosis) [66]. Although the degree of airway hyperreactivity has been found to correlate with asthma severity and treatment requirements in adult patients [123], this is not invariably the case [122], and we have been unable to reproduce these findings in children with asthma [4]. Finally, the degree of bronchial responsiveness can change over time, depending on exposure to viruses, allergens, and other factors [184].

Lung function and bronchial provocation tests cannot be performed in young children, except in highly specialized laboratories [156]. However, in this age group the diagnosis of asthma can be supported by demonstrating a favorable response to a short trial of an antiasthmatic medication. In this regard, we find it helpful to provide the children's parents with diary cards on which they record the frequency and severity of symptoms; the subsequent response to medications can then be observed (Fig. 80-4).

The majority of asthmatic children over the age of 3 years are atopic [30], and limited skin testing is a reasonable measure to determine sensitivity to environmental antigens. By identifying the offending allergens, the child's parents can then be counseled with respect to appropriate avoidance measures. A skin prick test is preferable to the intradermal technique, which is more likely to produce false-positive reactions [253]. Although negative skin tests exclude clinical allergy with a high degree of reliability, positive results require a confirmatory clinical history [81].

Date this card was started:

1. WHEEZE LAST NIGHT
Good night 0
Slept well but slightly wheezy 1
Woke x 2 3 because of wheeze 2
Bad night, awake most of time 3

2. COUGH LAST NIGHT
None 0
Little 1
Moderately bad 2
Severe 3

3. WHEEZE TODAY
None 0
Little 1
Moderately bad 2
Severe 3

4. NASAL SYMPTOMS
None 0
Mild 1
Moderate 2
Severe 3

5. DAILY READINGS ON PEAK FLOW METER – Morning (M) and Evening (E)
Best of 3 blows

600
500
400
300
200
100

6. MEDICATIONS

Name of medication	Dose Prescribed

Number of doses actually taken during the past 24 hours.

7. COMMENTS Note if you see a Doctor (D) or stay away from school (S) or work (W) because of your chest and anything else important such as an infection (I).

Fig. 80-4. *Asthma daily record card.*

The extracts for skin testing should be selected on the basis of the history. The most important antigens to consider are dust mites (*Dermatophagoides pteronyssinus, D. farinae*), household pets, pollens, and molds. Saline (to exclude dermatographia) and histamine (to exclude recent antihistamine ingestion) controls should also be included. Radioallergosorbent tests (RAST) are an alternative when skin tests are precluded because of skin disease or the risk of anaphylaxis [2]. Finally, bronchial provocation testing with antigens remains essentially a research procedure.

MANAGEMENT

Once the diagnosis of asthma is established, a treatment plan must then be devised that is tailored to meet the needs of the individual child. The management of children with asthma should primarily take place in the community. The long-term goals (Table 80-7) of asthma therapy are to abolish symptoms, maximize lung function, and allow young patients to lead normal lives with minimal interference from their illness. To achieve these objectives, attention must be directed to three fundamental areas: (1) patient education and supervision, (2) environmental control, and (3) drug therapy. In addition, immunotherapy and behavior modification may be indicated for selected children with asthma.

Patient Education and Supervision

Parents of children with asthma frequently have a poor understanding of the disease and its management [261], and this may contribute to the need for hospitalization [50]. Health education programs, emphasizing self-management skills, can reduce morbidity and health care costs and enhance the quality of life for children with asthma [49, 183]. The family members of a child with asthma should have a clear understanding of the nature of asthma, possible aggravating factors, the mechanism of action, mode of administration, and possible side effects of the medications used. They should be provided with written instructions regarding the administration of medications during acute asthma episodes and must be familiar with the signs of deteriorating control, indicating the need for urgent medical attention. As children with asthma approach adolescence, they should be encouraged to assume increasing responsibility for their own care. The control of asthma can be enhanced by having patients measure peak flow rates twice daily at home, thus allowing them to self-adjust therapy (under proper supervision) and make rational decisions about the need for emergency care [60, 295]. We recommend home monitoring of lung function particularly in children with (1) poor asthma control, (2) severe chronic asthma (see Chap. 79), and (3) a history of life-threatening asthma episodes.

Several self-management programs [49] are now available for educating children with asthma and their parents, and a number of educational booklets [36] and videos are also available. Some of this information needs to be transmitted to school personnel to ensure that school attendance and participation in recreational

Table 80-7. Specific goals of asthma therapy

Control symptoms
No emergency room visits/hospitalizations
No school absenteeism
No exercise limitation
No sleep disturbance
Optimal lung function
Limit drug side effects
Normal growth

activities are disrupted as little as possible [110]. Recently, a National Asthma Education Program has been initiated in the United States with the objectives of increasing public awareness of asthma as a serious disease and of facilitating the education of physicians and parents about the management of the condition [183].

For optimal care of the child with asthma, regular follow-up by a consistent health care provider is essential. In this way, the child's progress, response to therapy, compliance, and inhalation technique can be reviewed and lung function monitored. Unfortunately, many children only obtain episodic care for their asthma in the emergency room, and such irregular follow-up has been shown to increase asthma morbidity [37, 281].

Environmental Control

Specific allergic or irritant factors that aggravate the child's asthma should be eliminated or avoided if possible (see Chap. 87). Needless to say, family members should be urged not to smoke while in the house or car with the child. Exposure to wood-burning stoves and kerosene heaters should also be avoided. The observation that 20 percent of teenagers with asthma are cigarette smokers [91] indicates the importance of appropriate counseling in this age group.

Dander from domestic pets, particularly cats [167], is a common trigger of symptoms in children with asthma. If there is clear evidence, based on history and positive skin (or RAST) tests, that the child is sensitive to pets, a trial separation is warranted. Parents should be aware that it may take up to 6 months after the removal of a pet before beneficial results are seen, as animal danders are cleared slowly from the environment [285]. If parents are unwilling to pursue this course of action, they should be encouraged to keep the pet out of the child's bedroom (and outside the house as much as possible) and not to obtain new pets in the future (or replace present ones). Washing the pet regularly [296] and vacuum cleaning with a high-efficiency particulate air (HEPA) filter may also help to reduce the levels of animal allergens in the home [300].

Up to 85 percent of patients with asthma have positive skin tests to house dust mites, the major allergen (Der P 1) being found in mite fecal particles [207]. Mite sensitivity should be suspected if symptoms occur with sweeping, vacuuming, or dusting [166] and can be confirmed by skin (or RAST) testing. Although house mites cannot be totally eradicated, children with asthma do benefit from avoidance measures applied to the bedroom; practical measures are provided in Table 80-8 [165]. If parents are unwilling to institute all of these measures, they should be encouraged at least to cover the child's mattress with a zippered dust-proof cover. House dust mites thrive when the relative humidity is over 50 percent. In humid climates, air conditioning during the summer can keep the relative humidity below this level and significantly decrease the mite concentration in the home. Anti-mite chemicals (e.g., tannic acid, benzylbenzoate) may also help to reduce dust mite concentrations in carpets and upholstered furniture [155]. On the other hand, electrostatic air cleaners appear to be of little help, unless HEPA filters are used [90]. (See also Chaps. 42 and 87.)

Exposure to seasonal pollens and molds can be reduced by closing windows and doors, avoiding the use of window fans, and installing window or central air conditioning [113, 239]. Air conditioning systems are expensive and are probably of limited value in children, who tend to spend much of the day outdoors. Dehumidifiers in damp basements can be helpful, with humidity levels maintained between 25 and 50 percent. However, humidifiers elsewhere in the home are not recommended, as they harbor and aerosolize mold spores and encourage the proliferation of dust mites.

Food allergens rarely trigger asthma symptoms, and exclusion diets are therefore not warranted in the majority of children with

Table 80-8. *How to make a bedroom dust-free*

1. Move all the furniture, carpets, clothes, toys, and books out of the bedroom. The floor surface should be vinyl or hardwood.
2. Seal the hot air vent with tape. Heat the room with an electric baseboard radiator or a hot water heater.
3. Clean the floor, window sills, and shelves with a damp mop or cloth or one that has been treated with oil. Mop the floor once a week.
4. Encase the mattress and box spring in a zippered vinyl cover.
5. Bedding is limited to synthetic fiber or foam chip pillows and to a mattress pad, sheets, cotton thermal blankets or synthetic fiber blankets, and quilts. Launder these every 2–4 weeks (at a temperature of at least 60°C).
6. The room should ideally contain only the specially prepared bed, nonupholstered chairs, and a table. A chest of drawers is permitted but should be cleaned out every few months. Laundered clothes that the child wears from day to day may be kept in these drawers and in the closet.
7. The room should contain no carpets, rugs, mats, stored blankets, books, stuffed toys, pets, or other clutter. One toy, preferably a washable one, and one book may be taken to bed at night. Keep the bedroom door closed, if the child will allow it.

OTHER DUST AVOIDANCE MEASURES
1. Vacuum clean the carpets and furniture in other parts of the house once a week (but not when child is present).
2. Dust and animal danders accumulate in ducts leading from the furnace. Certain companies will clean out these ducts by powerful vacuum suction.

Source: Adapted from A. B. Murray. Avoiding Airborne Allergens in the Home. In *Treatment of Pediatric Asthma: A Canadian Consensus* (MEDICINE Publishing Foundation Symposium Series, 29). Toronto: MES Medical Education Services, 1991.

asthma [23] (see Chap. 43). An occasional child with asthma may be sensitive to aspirin or ingested chemicals, such as tartrazine, sulfites, and monosodium glutamate and will need to be counseled accordingly.

Immunotherapy

Although immunotherapy is widely practiced, its place in the overall management of asthma remains uncertain in view of the variable results of clinical trials [22, 165, 179] (see Chap. 70). For example, in controlled trials of immunotherapy with dust mite extracts in asthma, symptomatic improvement has been shown to occur, but no significant difference in lung function between the mite- and placebo-treated groups has been demonstrated. In addition, the effect of dust mite immunotherapy on airway hyperreactivity is extremely variable [161, 260, 266], and this also applies to immunotherapy with pollen and animal extracts [22, 109, 165, 179]. Bacterial vaccines have no role in the management of asthma, as respiratory infections that induce wheezing in children are rarely bacterial in nature [29, 31].

The authors agree that immunotherapy should be considered only in selected children whose asthma is triggered by one or more specific allergens and is not controlled by environmental measures and optimal pharmacologic therapy [22]. Accurate allergy diagnosis should precede treatment, and this should be based on a careful clinical history and skin (or RAST) testing. Immunotherapy should be used in conjunction with drug therapy and never as the sole form of treatment. Patients should be detained in the physician's office for 30 minutes after each injection to observe for possible adverse reactions [176]. If a child does not show a favorable response after 12 to 18 months, immunotherapy should be discontinued.

Psychological Management

It is generally agreed that psychological factors per se do not play a primary causal role in asthma but can profoundly affect the severity of the condition and the success of treatment [151]. In some children asthma symptoms can be related to emotional stimuli such as excitement, fear, or anger [151]. Psychosocial problems [251] and depression [154] can lead to poor self-management, disregard of symptoms, and interpersonal conflict, factors that have been associated with asthma deaths in children. Theophylline therapy may also lead to psychological and behavioral problems in children with asthma [58]. Finally, some patients can mimic or aggravate asthmatic symptoms by inducing adduction of the vocal cords on inspiration [14].

Effective management of asthma should include close consideration of the psychosocial adjustments of the asthmatic child and his or her family. The primary physician can play a key role in correcting attitude and adjustment problems within a family by providing information concerning the etiologic, therapeutic, and prognostic aspects of asthma [135]. Intervention by a psychiatrist and social worker is indicated for selected children with asthma and can lead to improvement in their clinical status [154]. Behavioral approaches have been used effectively to modify the reaction to situations that provoke episodes of asthma, to deal with manipulative behavior, and to improve compliance with medical regimens. The child's family should be included in such treatment programs, with the objective of bringing about a positive change in family relationships and perceptions. Finally, residential programs with emphasis on family psychotherapy and self-management should be considered for children with severe asthma who fail to respond to outpatient medical and psychosocial care [252, 304].

PHARMACOLOGIC MANAGEMENT

Pharmacotherapy remains the cornerstone of asthma management. Drug therapy of asthma must not only focus on relieving acute asthma episodes but should be used in a preventative fashion, particularly in children with frequent symptoms. For ease of discussion, the drugs currently available for the treatment of asthma can be divided (albeit somewhat artificially) into two main groups, that is, bronchodilators and prophylactic (antiinflammatory) agents. The advantages, disadvantages, and delivery of these medications will be discussed as a background to an overview of their role in the management of asthma of different grades of severity.

Bronchodilators

Beta₂ Agonists

Beta agonists are the most potent bronchodilators available and include albuterol (salbutamol), fenoterol, terbutaline, metaproterenol, bitolterol, and procaterol [32]. The usual doses of beta₂ agonists used at the authors' institution are shown in Table 80-9 (these may differ from manufacturers' recommendations). Depending on the route of administration (and product used), these agents have a duration of action of 4 to 8 hours. Inhaled beta₂ agonists with a more sustained duration of action (up to 12 hours) are undergoing clinical trials (e.g., formoterol, salmeterol) [258].

Beta₂ agonists should be administered by inhalation to ensure a rapid onset of action and to minimize adverse effects. They are the preferred initial treatment for acute exacerbations of asthma and for the prevention of exercise-induced asthma [32]. However, the role of beta₂ agonists in the maintenance treatment of asthma has become extremely controversial, and several considerations account for this. Recent studies have shown that long-term bronchodilator therapy has little effect or may even increase airway reactivity in asthma, unlike antiinflammatory agents, particularly inhaled steroids [131, 263, 305]. In a recent study of adult asthmatics [227], it was found that in two-thirds of the subjects, asthma was better controlled when inhaled beta₂ agonists were used only to control symptoms and not taken regularly four times

Table 80-9. Recommended dosage schedule for bronchodilators*

Bronchodilator	Oral administration	Aerosol administration	
		Formulations	Dose
BETA$_2$ AGONISTS			
Albuterol (salbutamol)	2 mg/5 ml syrup; 2-mg or 4-mg tablets: 0.1–0.15 mg/kg/dose, 3–4 times daily	0.5% solution	0.01–0.03 ml/kg (maximum 1 ml) diluted with 3 ml saline, up to 4 times daily
		Metered aerosol (100 μg/puff)	1–2 puffs, 4 times daily
		Dry powder (200 μg, 400 μg)	200–400 μg, 4 times daily
Fenoterol	2.5-mg tablets: 0.1 mg/kg/dose, 3–4 times daily	0.1% solution	0.01–0.03 ml/kg (maximum 1 ml) diluted with 3 ml saline, up to 4 times daily
		Metered aerosol (200 μg/puff)	1 puff, 4 times daily
Metaproterenol (orciprenaline)	10 mg/5 ml syrup; 20-mg tablets: 0.3–0.5 mg/kg/dose, 3–4 times daily	5% solution	0.01–0.02 ml/kg (maximum 1 ml) diluted with 3 ml saline, up to 4 times daily
		Metered aerosol (750 μg/puff)	1–2 puffs, 4 times daily
Terbutaline	300 μg/ml syrup; 2.5- or 5-mg tablets: 0.075 mg/kg/dose, 3–4 times daily	1% solution	0.03 ml/kg (maximum 1 ml) diluted with 3 ml saline, up to 4 times daily
		Metered aerosol (250 μg/puff)	1 puff, 4 times daily
		Dry powder (500 μg/actuation)	1 dose, 4 times daily
Bitolterol	—	Metered aerosol (370 μg/puff)	1–2 puffs, 4 times daily
Procaterol	—	Metered aerosol (10 μg/puff)	1–2 puffs, 3 times daily
ANTICHOLINERGIC			
Ipratropium bromide	—	Metered aerosol (20 μg/puff)	2 puffs, 4 times daily
		0.025% solution	0.5–1.0 ml, 4 times daily

* Doses given are those used in the authors' unit and may differ from manufacturers' recommendations.

daily in a scheduled fashion. Finally, studies from New Zealand [187] and a very recent Saskatchewan study [241] have found chronic use of beta$_2$ agonists (and possibly theophylline) to be associated with an increased risk of death from asthma; whether this is due to a toxic drug effect or a reflection of severe disease is unclear at this time. In view of the above observations, the general recommendations for the maintenance treatment of asthma are that beta$_2$ agonists should be used as sparingly as possible, usually in combination with a prophylactic antiinflammatory medication and mainly for symptomatic relief [227].

The principal side effects of beta$_2$ agonists are tremor, tachycardia, and hypokalemia [284] and are more common with the oral and systemic routes of administration. Although tolerance (tachyphylaxis) to the bronchodilator effects of beta$_2$ agonists may occur with chronic use, this does not appear to be of major clinical significance and can be reversed by systemic steroids [78]. Recent studies have shown that tolerance to the nonbronchodilator actions [302] of beta agonists and to their protective effect against methacholine challenge [294] can occur when these agents are used regularly.

Anticholinergics

Ipratropium bromide, an atropine derivative, is currently available as a metered aerosol and as a solution for administration by nebulizer (see Table 80-9; see Chap. 64). Although ipratropium has a slower onset of action and provides less maximal bronchodilation than beta$_2$ agonists, it has a more prolonged duration of action (up to 8 hours). In acute asthma, some [15, 205, 267], but not all [202, 248] reports indicate that additional bronchodilation can be achieved when ipratropium is used in combination with a beta$_2$ agonist. Ipratropium has a less clearly defined role in the maintenance treatment of asthma [85, 145]. However, it can be used in combination with a beta$_2$ agonist in children with severe chronic asthma and as an alternative to sympathomimetics or theophylline in children who experience intolerable side effects from these agents. The subset of patients whose asthma is triggered by psychogenic factors appears to respond particularly well to ipratropium [203]. Side effects are very uncommon with ipratropium, although paradoxical bronchoconstriction has been reported, possibly due to the hypotonicity or low pH of the nebulizing solution or to additives such as benzalkonium chloride [201].

Theophyllines

The role of theophylline preparations in the maintenance treatment of asthma has become extremely controversial in recent years [119, 147, 174, 212]. The trend is now toward introducing theophylline later in the therapeutic plan, and several considerations account for this: (1) long-term treatment with theophylline does not appear to reduce airway hyperreactivity in asthma [73] (a recent study has challenged this contention [185]); (2) theophylline preparations result in a high incidence of side effects, particularly in the presence of factors that reduce the metabolism of theophylline (e.g., viruses, erythromycin, liver disease); and (3) theophylline may cause cognitive, behavioral, and learning difficulties in children [58]; a recent study indicates that these side effects are confined largely to children with preexisting attentional and school achievement problems [219]. Lindgren and colleagues [298] found that academic performance was unaffected by theophylline therapy.

Despite these limitations, theophylline remains useful in certain children with asthma, specifically (1) patients with moderate to severe asthma, in whom therapy with beta$_2$ agonists and inhaled steroids is inadequate, (2) children who are unable to use or are noncompliant with inhaled medications, and (3) patients with nocturnal asthma [13]. If theophylline is prescribed, a sustained-release preparation should be chosen, and dosage must be individualized and guided by serum theophylline assays. A suggested dosing regimen for various age groups is shown in Table 80-10 [105]. Adverse side effects at the beginning of therapy can be minimized by commencing the patient on 50 percent of the calculated dose, followed by small increases at 3-day intervals until average doses for age are attained. The final adjustment in theophylline dosage and dosing interval should be based on peak and trough serum theophylline concentrations. After this initial individualization of dosing requirements, subsequent mon-

Table 80-10. Dosage requirements of oral theophylline to maintain serum theophylline concentration within the therapeutic range

Age	Total daily dose (mg/kg)*
Infants 6–52 wk	[0.3 (age in weeks) + 8]
Children 1–9 yr	24
Children 9–12 yr	20
Adolescent 12–16 yr	18
Adults	13 or 900 mg/day (whichever is less)

* Use ideal body weight for age, sex, and height.

itoring of theophylline concentrations at 6- to 12-month intervals is generally adequate. More frequent measurements may be necessary during periods of rapid growth, when control of asthma is suboptimal, or when situations that alter theophylline elimination develop. As a standard precaution, parents should be instructed to reduce the dose of theophylline by 50 percent if their child has a sustained fever and not to administer any other medication without establishing the safety of the combination.

Antiinflammatory Drugs

Cromolyn Sodium

Cromolyn sodium is exclusively a prophylactic agent, as it has no significant bronchodilator action [3]. Although its mechanism of action is unclear, cromolyn inhibits the early and late bronchial responses to allergen challenge and can reduce airway hyperreactivity after several weeks of continuous therapy [45] (see Chap. 63). In some patients, cromolyn has been shown to attenuate bronchoconstriction in response to exercise [54], cold air, and methacholine or histamine [282].

Maintenance therapy with cromolyn sodium should be considered in children with moderately severe asthma [77, 96]. The response to cromolyn therapy in the individual patient is unpredictable, but long-term studies have confirmed its efficacy in 65 percent of children whose asthma is not adequately controlled by bronchodilators [96]. On the other hand, cromolyn appears to be of little value in children who are steroid dependent [84, 112]. For children with predictable seasonal asthma (e.g., grass pollen), best results are obtained if cromolyn is introduced several weeks before anticipated allergen exposure and continued throughout the entire season. In the child with animal-sensitive asthma, cromolyn provides effective prophylaxis if taken 15 to 30 minutes prior to an anticipated encounter with animals. Similarly, exercise-induced asthma can be prevented by taking cromolyn, with or without a beta₂ agonist, 15 to 30 minutes before exercise [54].

Cromolyn is available as a powder (Spinhaler), a solution (for administration by nebulizer), and a metered-dose inhaler. At the onset of treatment it is necessary to administer cromolyn four times daily, but with continued therapy many children can be managed with two to three administrations per day. Table 80-11 provides dosage guidelines for the three formulations of cromolyn available.

Although relatively expensive, a major advantage of cromolyn is a virtual freedom from side effects. Some patients may experience airway irritation after inhaling the dry powder, but this can

Table 80-11. Prescription guidelines for cromolyn therapy

Formulation	Dosage	Administration
Dry-powder capsules	20 mg/capsule	1 capsule, 4 times daily
Solution (1%)	20 mg/2 ml ampule	2 ml, 4 times daily
Metered aerosol*	1 mg/puff	2 puffs, 4 times daily

* A high-dose inhaler (5 mg/puff) is available in some countries.

be alleviated by the prior inhalation of a beta₂ agonist. In view of this irritant property, cromolyn powder should be temporarily withdrawn during acute exacerbations of asthma.

Ketotifen

Ketotifen is an orally active agent with distinct antiallergic and antihistaminic properties [101]. In infants [172], children [200], and adolescents [134] with mild to moderate asthma, ketotifen has been shown to diminish the severity of symptoms, bronchodilator requirements, and the frequency of acute episodes. Its clinical efficacy appears to be equivalent to cromolyn. However, in children with more severe asthma who require multiple medications, the addition of ketotifen is not helpful [139]. A trial is underway in the authors' institution to determine whether ketotifen has a steroid-sparing effect in childhood asthma.

From the studies performed to date, it is clear that a minimum of 6 to 8 weeks is required before the beneficial effects of ketotifen are realized. The recommended dose is 1 mg twice daily in older children, and 0.5 mg twice daily in children less than 3 years of age. The drug appears to be remarkably safe, although weight gain, increased appetite, and sedation are potential problems.

Nedocromil Sodium

Nedocromil is chemically unrelated to cromolyn but has a very similar clinical profile [256]. In adult patients, it has been shown to be effective against antigen challenge and in preventing exercise-induced asthma. It is also effective in the long-term management of asthma (the dosage is 4 mg, four times a day), although no clear advantage over cromolyn has yet emerged [87]. Some studies suggest that nedocromil may allow a reduction in the requirement for oral steroids [21]. Trials in childhood asthma have yet to be performed, and at this time, nedocromil cannot be recommended for young children. Potential side effects include a bitter taste, headache, and nausea. Nedocromil and ketotifen are further detailed in Chap. 63.

Corticosteroids

Inhaled corticosteroids, because of high topical activity but limited systemic absorption, have revolutionized the management of asthma. When administered on a regular basis to children with asthma, inhaled steroids have been shown to control symptoms, improve lung function [132], and cause a gradual reduction in bronchial hyperreactivity [131, 305]. (In adults, this reduction in reactivity may persist for 3 months after inhaled steroids have been discontinued [124].) Inhaled steroid therapy significantly reduces bronchial inflammation and epithelial damage [303], but despite this, airway reactivity rarely returns to the normal range [142]. Inhaled steroids are particularly useful in patients who are dependent on oral steroids in order to eliminate, or at least reduce, the need for systemic steroid therapy [229] (see Chap. 61).

Several inhaled steroid preparations are available (Table 80-12). Although these preparations appear to be equally effective

Table 80-12. Aerosol corticosteroid products

Trade name	Active ingredient	Dose provided
Beclovent	Beclomethasone dipropionate	50 µg/puff 100 µg/rotacap 200 µg/rotacap
Beclodisk	Beclomethasone dipropionate	100 µg/blister 200 µg/blister
Becloforte	Beclomethasone dipropionate	250 µg/puff
Bronalide/AeroBid	Flunisolide	250 µg/puff
Pulmicort	Budesonide	50 µg/puff 200 µg/puff 100, 200, 400 µg/actuation (Turbuhaler)
Azmacort	Triamcinalone	200 µg/puff

clinically, budesonide has the greatest topical activity and may cause less adrenal suppression [132]. Cost, availability, and the delivery system should also influence prescribing decisions. Inhaled steroids are usually delivered by metered-dose inhalers; a spacer device should be attached to increase lung deposition and to prevent the occurrence of oropharyngeal candidiasis [132]. A variety of dry-powder delivery systems are now available, and nebulizing solutions of inhaled steroids are available in some countries.

For children, the generally recommended starting dose of inhaled steroids is 100 μg, four times daily. If a satisfactory clinical response occurs, conversion to a twice daily dosing schedule may eventually be possible in some children, thus improving compliance [132]. Patients with unstable asthma are, however, best advised to adhere to the standard four times daily regimen. Finally, in patients who respond poorly to conventional doses of inhaled corticosteroids, the use of high-dose inhaled steroids (up to 1,600 μg/day) has been shown to improve asthma control and reduce systemic steroid requirements [238], although the risk of adrenal suppression is significantly increased. The introduction of "high-dose" inhalation devices has facilitated the delivery of inhaled steroids in children with severe asthma.

Studies that have examined the effect of inhaled steroids on adrenal function in children are difficult to interpret in view of the discrepancies in steroid dosage, the parameters of adrenal function examined, and the age of the children selected [99, 197, 243, 254]. It is reasonable to conclude that inhaled steroids can cause biochemical derangement in pituitary-adrenal function in some children, and that this effect is dose dependent—a recent study indicates that suppression of adrenal function occurs when the dose exceeds 400 $\mu g/m^2/day$ [197]. Monitoring of adrenal function may be warranted, therefore, in children who require high-dose inhaled steroid therapy. The effect of inhaled steroids on somatic growth is controversial in view of the conflicting results of studies that have examined this question [11, 97, 283, 306]. Recent studies have shown that inhaled steroids may adversely affect bone metabolism [307].

Although oropharyngeal colonization with *Candida* is common in children receiving inhaled steroids, overt infection is rare [230]. The risk of infection can be reduced by rinsing out the mouth with water after each inhalation, by using a spacer device, and by reducing the frequency of inhalations to a twice daily schedule [132]. Dysphonia, caused by an adductor vocal cord paralysis, may occur [277] but responds to temporary withdrawal of corticosteroid therapy. This problem can be avoided by inhaling the drug slowly, preferably through a spacer. Some patients experience airway irritation after inhaling corticosteroids, but this can be prevented by prior inhalation of a beta₂ agonist.

Fortunately, oral steroids are rarely necessary today in the maintenance treatment of pediatric asthma. If this situation does arise, the smallest dose of prednisone/prednisolone compatible with control of symptoms should be given as a single dose, every other morning if possible. Short courses of oral steroids (e.g., prednisone, 1 mg/kg/day for 5–7 days) are extremely effective in treating acute exacerbations of asthma at home and may reduce the need for hospitalization [25, 68, 104]. Although short courses of oral steroids can cause adrenal suppression, rapid recovery in adrenal function occurs [292]. However, children who are treated with more than four short bursts of oral steroids per year may develop more prolonged adrenal suppression [69].

METHODS OF DRUG DELIVERY

Where possible, antiasthmatic medications should be delivered by inhalation [34]. The rationale for using the inhaled route is that medication is deposited directly to the airways, allowing for a rapid onset of drug action, lower dosage requirements, and

fewer systemic side effects as compared to oral therapy. Three inhalation devices are available at the present time for the delivery of aerosolized medications, and each of these will be considered briefly. Delivery devices are also discussed in detail in Chap. 56.

Metered-Dose Inhaler

Cromolyn, ipratropium bromide, and a variety of beta₂ agonists and inhaled steroid preparations can be delivered by inhalers. Metered-dose inhalers (MDIs) are portable, inexpensive, and ideal for children over 7 years of age. However, even with optimal inhalation technique, only 10 percent of the drug released from an MDI reaches the airways; most of the aerosol spray impacts on the oropharynx. In view of this, children must be instructed carefully with respect to the correct use of an inhaler (Table 80-13) and their technique checked at subsequent visits. Unfortunately, inefficient use of MDIs is a common problem in clinical practice and a major cause of treatment failure [32]. Some of the problems encountered include (1) lack of coordination of aerosol actuation with inspiration ("hand-lung" dyscoordination), (2) ceasing to inspire when the aerosol is released into the mouth ("cold freon" effect), (3) rapid inspiration, and (4) inhalation through the nose.

Various extension tubes (spacers) have been designed and marketed to circumvent some of these problems. The use of spacers improves the delivery of aerosols to the lung, best results being obtained with large-volume spacers (≥750 ml) [34]. With valved spacers, tidal breathing can be used, and breath holding is not essential [94]. Spacers are indicated for patients with poor inhaler technique, particularly for young children (3–7 years) who are rarely able to use MDIs effectively. Spacers are advisable when high-dose inhaled steroid therapy is used to reduce the risk of oropharyngeal candidiasis and systemic effects [132]. The addition of a face mask to the spacer may facilitate delivery of aerosolized medications to very young children [177].

Dry-Powder Inhalers

Cromolyn, beta₂ agonists, and inhaled steroids can be delivered by dry-powder inhalers, which are somewhat easier to use than pressurized inhalers and do not contain freons. Recently, dry-powder inhalers with a multidose facility (Diskhaler) and breath-activated inhalers (e.g., Turbuhaler) have become available in some countries. To achieve a maximal effect from dry-powder inhalers, patients must be able to generate high inspiratory flow rates [188]. During acute exacerbations of asthma, when flow rates are reduced, powder inhalers may become less effective.

Nebulizers

Several beta₂ agonists, cromolyn, ipratropium bromide, and, in some countries, corticosteroids can be delivered by nebulizer. Nebulizers are used both in hospital and domiciliary practice with increasing frequency, although this trend is viewed with

Table 80-13. Suggested inhalation technique for metered-dose inhalers

Shake the inhaler and remove the cap.
Hold the inhaler upright and breathe out fully.
Close lips around mouthpiece of inhaler
 or
hold mouthpiece 4 cm in front of open mouth.
Activate inhaler while inspiring slowly and deeply.
Hold breath for 10 seconds (or for as long as possible).
If dose is to be repeated, wait a few minutes.

concern by some clinicians [171]. The main advantage of the nebulizer is that little patient coordination is required and, therefore, can be used to deliver medication to acutely ill or very young children. On the other hand, nebulizers are expensive, not very portable, and an inefficient drug delivery system, although their use in the home may reduce the need for hospitalization [215]. Home nebulizers are of particular benefit in children with severe, chronic asthma, a history of life-threatening asthma episodes, and a demonstrated inability to use MDIs or dry-powder inhalers (e.g, very young children). To ensure the safe use of nebulizers in the home, and to avoid contamination, education of the family is crucial [215]. This topic has been reviewed recently in detail [192] (see Chap. 56). Parents must be reminded that failure on the part of the nebulizer to relieve their child's symptoms is an indication to seek immediate medical help.

PRACTICAL ASPECTS OF DRUG USE IN ASTHMA

The maintenance drug therapy of asthma varies considerably, depending on the frequency and severity of the child's symptoms and the degree of airflow obstruction [290]. Drug therapy should be considered in a stepwise fashion, with the child starting treatment at the level most appropriate for the severity of his or her asthma. Depending on the response to treatment, the intensity of treatment can then be either increased or decreased. The treatment sequence (in whichever direction it is used) is generally applied in the following fashion (Fig. 80-5).

Bronchodilators

About 60 percent of children with asthma have mild and infrequent episodes of coughing and wheezing in the course of the year but otherwise have a normal quality of life (i.e., good exercise tolerance, uninterrupted sleep, regular school attendance) and normal lung function [290]. The intermittent use of a beta$_2$ agonist may suffice in these children. If possible, beta$_2$ agonists should be delivered by inhalation, either by an MDI (with a spacer device if necessary) or a dry-powder inhaler. Treatment can usually be discontinued after 5 to 7 days when symptoms have abated. For young children who are unable to use these inhalation devices, and whose asthma is not severe enough to warrant purchase of a home nebulizer, a liquid formulation of a beta$_2$ agonist, administered orally, may be adequate.

Children with mild asthma may also need to take beta$_2$ agonists (with or without cromolyn) before exposure to stimuli such as exercise, cold air, or allergens (e.g., household pets).

Fig. 80-5. *Drug treatment sequence. *Ketotifen is currently not available in the United States (except on a "compassionate use" basis). TAO = troleandomycin.*

```
        Intermittent bronchodilators (β₂ agonists)
                           ⇅
        Regular prophylactic agent (cromolyn/ketotifen*)
                           ⇅
          Low-dose inhaled steroid ± β₂ agonist
                           ⇅
     Additional bronchodilators (ipratropium/theophylline)
                           ⇅
               High-dose inhaled steroids
                           ⇅
                Maintenance oral steroids
                           ⇅
        ? Steroid-sparing agents (TAO/methotrexate)
```

Regular Antiinflammatory Agents

If the goals of treatment (see Table 80-7) cannot be attained by beta$_2$ agonists alone, continuous prophylactic therapy is indicated. The specific guidelines [32] we use for the introduction of daily prophylactic therapy are listed in Table 80-14. Although the regular administration of a sustained-release theophylline preparation was traditionally used for this purpose, the trend is now toward the introduction of one of the antiinflammatory agents at an earlier stage, that is, cromolyn, ketotifen, or inhaled steroids. In view of the potential for adrenal suppression with inhaled steroids [197, 254], we generally give a trial of a nonsteroidal agent (e.g., cromolyn or ketotifen) initially, at least in children with mild to moderate asthma. Irrespective of which prophylactic agent is chosen, certain rules need to be followed to ensure success with a preventative regimen: (1) Prior to the introduction of a prophylactic medication, the child's asthma should be brought under control (and lung function optimized) by regular treatment with beta$_2$ agonists and a short course of oral steroids, if necessary; (2) the patient/parent must understand the principles of a preventative drug regimen and the importance of compliance and appreciate that several weeks of therapy are required before the full effects of the drug are realized; (3) during this time, a beta$_2$ agonist may need to be used concurrently to maintain asthma control; and (4) while children are maintained on a prophylactic regimen, it is crucial that their parents have access to a beta$_2$ agonist (and appropriate delivery system) to treat acute exacerbations of asthma.

If no therapeutic effect is seen after a 6- to 8-week trial of cromolyn or an 8- to 12-week trial of ketotifen, the child should be switched to low-dose inhaled steroid therapy (400 µg/day). If necessary, this can be combined initially with a beta$_2$ agonist (e.g., albuterol, 200 µg, four times daily). Once symptoms and lung function have improved, the beta$_2$ agonist (and subsequently the inhaled steroid) should be tapered to the lowest dose that maintains adequate control.

Additional Bronchodilators

If control of asthma remains inadequate (as judged by symptoms, lung function, and increased use of beta$_2$ agonists) despite the use of inhaled steroids in standard dosage, the addition of a second bronchodilator may be useful (e.g., ipratropium bromide, 40 µg, three to four times daily, or a sustained-release theophylline product). Alternatively, the regular administration of bronchodilators (beta$_2$ agonists ± ipratropium) in higher doses by home nebulizer may be considered.

High-Dose Inhaled Steroids

Less than 10 percent of the pediatric asthma population suffer from severe, chronic asthma [290], which is characterized by daily symptoms, frequent nocturnal coughing, limitation of exercise tolerance, and persistent airway obstruction. In such children, high-dose inhaled steroid therapy (800–1,000 µg/day)

Table 80-14. Criteria for prophylactic therapy in childhood asthma

Frequent acute episodes (>6/yr) (acute episode = persistent wheeze/cough lasting >24 hr)
Frequent hospital admission (>2–3/yr)
Bronchodilators used routinely twice a day or more
Infrequent but severe asthma episodes (e.g., admission to intensive care unit)
School absenteeism (>3–4 days/month)
Sleep disturbance (1–2 nights/wk)
Persistent airway obstruction (FEV$_1$ < 70%)

should be attempted, preferably administered by a spacer device in three or four divided doses, in conjunction with bronchodilators. If necessary, the dose of inhaled steroids can be increased to a maximum of 1,600 μg/day. All patients with severe asthma should monitor lung function at home, their compliance and inhaler technique should be checked repeatedly, and close attention should be paid to their psychosocial status.

Maintenance Oral Steroids

Maintenance treatment with oral prednisolone/prednisone should be instituted only if adequate control cannot be achieved with maximum doses of inhaled steroid and bronchodilators. If possible, oral steroids should be administered on alternate days, and bronchodilator and high-dose inhaled steroid therapy should be used concurrently. The child's growth and blood pressure need to be monitored, a slit-lamp examination should be performed at 6- to 12-month intervals (to detect early cataract development), and urine samples should be checked regularly for glycosuria. A gradual reduction in steroid dosage should be attempted once the patient is stable.

Steroid-sparing Agents?

In patients with severe asthma who continue to be symptomatic despite the use of oral steroids, a trial of troleandomycin (TAO) has been recommended [265] (see Chap. 67). When used concomitantly with methylprednisolone, this macrolide antibiotic has been shown to improve pulmonary function and symptom control in children with severe asthma and to have a "steroid-sparing" effect. Potential side effects include elevation of hepatic enzymes, a cushingoid appearance, and abdominal pain, which generally resolve when the TAO dose is reduced. As the elimination rate of theophylline is reduced by TAO, serum theophylline concentrations will need to be monitored in patients who are on concomitant theophylline therapy.

Recent studies have shown that the use of low-dose weekly methotrexate in adults with steroid-dependent asthma allows a reduction in steroid dosage without associated clinical deterioration [163]. Pending further investigation, the use of methotrexate in childhood asthma cannot be advocated at the present time. Likewise, gold therapy cannot be recommended at present for the treatment of childhood asthma [18]. (See also Chaps. 66 and 68.)

SPECIFIC PROBLEMS IN PEDIATRIC ASTHMA

Asthma in Infants and Young Children

A variety of physiologic and anatomic factors account for the increased vulnerability of infants and young children to develop airway obstruction and respiratory failure [164]. These include increased peripheral airway resistance, decreased elastic recoil properties of the lung, increased compliance of the rib cage, and decreased collateral ventilation and fatigue-resistant diaphragmatic muscle fibers in infants and young children. It is not surprising, therefore, that the majority of children with asthma develop symptoms in the first few years of life [91, 222, 273] and that hospitalization rates for asthma are particularly high in this age group [92, 146]. Asthma is almost twice as common in boys in early childhood. Although the cause of this is unclear, genetic differences have been suggested [222]. In early life, asthma is typically aggravated by viral respiratory infections, whereas allergic triggers play a relatively unimportant role [8]. A recent study has shown that wheeze in the first 3 years is correlated with abnormal lung function very early in life [150].

Unfortunately, clinicians remain reluctant to apply the term *asthma* in children under 2 years [8], and this frequently leads to inappropriate forms of treatment [293]. Although a variety of conditions may be responsible for recurrent or persistent wheezing in early childhood (see Table 80-5), asthma remains the most common cause. The diagnosis of asthma can be confirmed by demonstrating a favorable response to antiasthmatic medications, as pulmonary function tests are not practical for routine use in this age group [156].

Asthma in early life presents a major therapeutic challenge, largely because of the increased difficulty in administering medications and of the paucity of data concerning the value of many antiasthmatic medications in this age group. In general, inhalation therapy in very young children is only possible with the use of nebulizers, although a spacer device with a face mask may be worth a trial [177]. While the efficacy of beta$_2$ agonists in children less than 18 months of age has been questioned [234], a beneficial clinical response to nebulized albuterol in young children with acute asthma was demonstrated in two recent studies from this institution [16, 17]. For treatment of asthma in early childhood, therefore, we feel that a trial of a nebulized beta$_2$ agonist is warranted (oral beta$_2$ agonists may suffice for the treatment of very mild and infrequent symptoms). If this is not effective, the addition of nebulized ipratropium may be helpful [114]. Children with persistent symptoms should be treated prophylactically with nebulized cromolyn [47, 175] or oral ketotifen [172]. Theophylline therapy may be beneficial in young children, but compliance is poor and side effects are common [140, 175]. If the response to treatment is still inadequate, a trial of nebulized corticosteroids (if available) should be considered, although the efficacy of nebulized steroids in very young children seems quite variable [38, 247, 269]. Preschool children may benefit from inhaled steroids delivered by MDI in conjunction with a spacer and a mask [19, 80, 95]. The appropriate dose of inhaled steroids for young children is unknown; recent data indicate that adrenal suppression does not occur with doses in the range of 200 to 400 μg/day [80, 262]. Finally, in young children with severe, chronic asthma who are still resistant to treatment, the addition of oral steroids, preferably on an alternate-day basis, will be necessary.

Asthma During Adolescence

Although asthma symptoms frequently improve or disappear during adolescence, a deterioration may occur in some patients, and even new cases of asthma may arise in this age group. Specific problems [67] that may need to be addressed in teenagers with asthma include (1) denial of symptoms, (2) noncompliance, (3) psychosocial issues, (4) abuse of MDIs, (5) cigarette smoking, and (6) poor relationship between the patient and the medical team.

Cough-variant Asthma

Children with chronic cough as the sole manifestation of asthma should be given a trial of therapy with bronchodilators, cromolyn, or inhaled steroids [206]. Prevention may be possible by the avoidance of trigger factors. As cough-variant asthma may be related to hyperresponsiveness of cough receptors, antitussive therapy may have a role to play in such children [56] (see Chap. 50).

Exercise-induced Asthma

Exercise-induced asthma (EIA), discussed in Chap. 47, occurs in the majority of patients with asthma and is particularly troublesome in children because of their high level of physical activity [189]. In EIA, the bronchial obstruction reaches its peak 5 to 15 minutes after exertion, whereas a delayed asthmatic response after exercise is uncommon [214]. EIA occurs after strenuous, continuous forms of exercise (e.g., running, skating), whereas team sports and swimming are less likely to provoke symptoms [189]. EIA is more marked with exercise in a cold, dry atmosphere. With adequate prophylaxis, the majority of children with asthma can participate in regular sporting and recreational activities; in fact, physical training programs have been shown to improve exercise tolerance and cardiorespiratory performance in patients with asthma [44, 180] (see Chap. 86).

Warming up before athletic events is helpful. EIA is prevented most effectively by inhalation of a selective beta$_2$ agonist from an MDI or Rotahaler about 5 minutes before exercise [79]. For children who are unable to use these inhalation devices, an appropriate dose of an oral beta$_2$ agonist 2 hours prior to exercise is a useful alternative [83]. Premedication with cromolyn will prevent exercise-induced asthma in about 60 percent of children [54] and, if necessary, can be used in conjunction with a beta$_2$ agonist. Patients who take theophylline for prophylaxis of chronic asthma should be reasonably well protected against EIA, but inhalation of a beta$_2$ agonist may be necessary prior to strenuous exercise. Inhibition of EIA by theophylline occurs predominantly at serum theophylline concentrations greater than 10 mg/L [193].

Nocturnal Asthma

Children with asthma frequently complain of troublesome wheezing and coughing at night and in the early morning ("morning dippers"). The fall in lung function at night reflects an exaggeration of the normal circadian rhythm in airway caliber, that is, a further manifestation of bronchial hyperreactivity in asthma [70]. Treatment of nocturnal symptoms may be difficult. Since bronchial hyperreactivity seems to be the underlying mechanism, the logical first step is to optimize daytime control of asthma with an inhaled bronchodilator and steroid preparation [116]. Control of nocturnal symptoms can be further improved by giving a single dose (10 mg/kg) of a slow-release theophylline preparation at bedtime [13]; the use of an ultra-sustained theophylline preparation may be even more effective in this situation [9]. Long-acting oral beta$_2$ agonists are available in some countries and have been shown to provide effective control of nocturnal symptoms [70]. In the future, long-acting inhaled beta$_2$ agonists (e.g., salmeterol, formoterol) may prove particularly useful in treating nocturnal asthma [259]. Environmental precautions may benefit patients with nocturnal symptoms who exhibit feather or dust mite allergy. Finally, a possible relationship between nocturnal wheezing and gastroesophageal reflux may need to be considered in selected patients [181] (see Chaps. 75 and 76).

"Impossible Asthma"

Some children with asthma continue to have symptoms despite apparently appropriate treatment. Several factors may be responsible for this [12] (Table 80-15). Compliance in particular is very important in the success of treatment. The compliance of an individual patient may be improved through education, by providing consistent medical care, and by maintaining the therapeutic regimen as simple as possible.

Finally, small groups of children with asthma have been described who continue to have peripheral airway obstruction, despite intensive bronchodilator and steroid therapy [1, 35].

ACUTE ASTHMA

Acute asthma is a common, potentially life-threatening medical emergency. At this institution, asthma accounts for 5.6 percent of patient visits to the emergency room [37] and for 11.2 percent of all medical admissions [245]; even higher hospitalization rates for asthma have been reported from other pediatric centers [39, 208]. It should be stressed that severe episodes of asthma can be prevented, or at least ameliorated, by early recognition and intensification of treatment. Unfortunately, deficiencies in both the assessment and treatment of children with acute asthma are common [37] and include (1) failure to measure lung function, (2) underuse of systemic steroids, and (3) inadequate follow-up arrangements on discharge from the emergency room. Acute and severe, refractory problems are also discussed in Chaps. 72 and 73.

Pathophysiology

Regardless of the precipitating factor (see Table 80-2), the central event in acute asthma is widespread airway obstruction that results from bronchial smooth muscle spasm, inflammation, and mucus plugging. Airway obstruction leads to increased airway resistance, reduced flow rates, gas trapping, and pulmonary overdistention. Although pulmonary hyperinflation benefits respiration by helping to maintain patency of the airways, it does so at the expense of a considerable increase in the work of the diaphragm and accessory muscles of respiration.

The changes in airflow resistance are not uniform throughout the bronchial tree; some lung units are overventilated, while others receive inadequate ventilation. This maldistribution of ventilation leads to ventilation-perfusion mismatching and, in turn, arterial hypoxemia. Although significant correlations have been found between the degree of airway obstruction (e.g., FEV_1) and both arterial oxygen tension (PaO_2) [274] and saturation (SaO_2) [130] in children with acute asthma, the scatter among individual values is high.

The changes in arterial carbon dioxide tension ($PaCO_2$) in acute asthma are more complex. As a result of hyperventilation, the majority of patients with acute asthma have a respiratory alkalosis (low $PaCO_2$; alkaline pH) on presentation [274]. However, in the presence of severe airway obstruction ($FEV_1 < 25\%$ predicted), respiratory muscle fatigue and alveolar hypoventilaton ensue, resulting in hypercapnia and respiratory acidosis. Thus, a rising $PaCO_2$, even into the "normal" range, must be regarded as a sign of impending fatigue and respiratory failure in acute asthma. Metabolic acidosis may also occur in severe acute asthma and is primarily due to lactic acidosis, resulting from tissue hypoxia and lactate production by respiratory muscles [162, 274].

Initial Assessment

The intensity of treatment in acute asthma is based on an accurate assessment of the severity of the event. This assessment should not rely alone on history and physical examination but includes simple spirometry, oximetry, and arterial blood gas analysis in selected cases.

History

To avoid delay in management, a relevant, directed history should be obtained. Historical features that should alert the phy-

Table 80-15. Causes of apparent failure of therapy

Incorrect inhaler technique
Inappropriate drug dose or dosing interval
Poor patient compliance
Inadequate trial of preventative agents
Failure to use medications in a systematic fashion
Medical complications, e.g., gastroesophageal reflux, aspirin
  intolerance, allergic bronchopulmonary aspergillosis, sinusitis
Psychosocial factors and vocal cord paralysis
Inappropriate treatment, e.g., antibiotics, antitussives

Table 80-16. Historical features in acute asthma indicating the need for greater caution

Previous episodes of respiratory failure due to asthma
Deterioration despite the use of oral steroids or frequent inhalations of
 bronchodilators at home
Recent hospitalizations or emergency room visits for asthma
Chronic use of oral steroids or high-dose inhaled steroids on presentation
Prolonged duration of symptoms > 24 hours

Table 80-17. Clinical manifestations of severe acute asthma

Tachycardia > 120/min
Tachypnea > 30/min
Dyspnea
Inability to speak
Accessory muscle use
Pulsus paradoxus > 15 mmHg
Life-threatening signs:
 A silent chest on auscultation
 Cyanosis
 Altered consciousness
 Respiratory muscle fatigue (e.g., abdominal paradox)
 Pneumothorax

sician to the possible need for more aggressive therapy are provided in Table 80-16. In addition, it is important to review the family's management of the acute episode prior to the child's presentation to the emergency room. There may be features in their response that will need to be addressed to prevent further episodes of acute asthma in the future.

Physical Examination

A careful, ongoing clinical evaluation is the most important step in determining the severity of acute asthma and the need for hospitalization [129]. Physical signs associated with severe acute asthma in children are shown in Table 80-17 and are reviewed in Chap. 37 also. Of these signs, the degree of accessory muscle use and dyspnea and the level of pulsus paradoxus have been shown to correlate most closely with the severity of airway obstruction, as measured by lung function [130, 204]. As a corollary, significant airway obstruction can exist in the absence of these signs. Wheezing (see Chap. 51) is an unreliable sign in asthma, as, in the presence of severe airway obstruction, airflow is so reduced that wheezing may be absent. Cyanosis, confusion, and fatigue are ominous signs in asthma, and their presence indicates the need for immediate, intensive therapy.

Investigations

In older children, the assessment of acute asthma is incomplete without an objective measurement of the degree of airflow obstruction, using a portable spirometer or a simple peak flow meter [37]. Measurements should be made at baseline and serially to follow the response to treatment; the results should be expressed as a percent of the predicted normal values for height and sex.

Although not all children with acute asthma need arterial blood gas analysis, this procedure is mandatory in patients who are cyanosed, confused, or fatigued, who have severe lung function impairment (e.g., $FEV_1 < 25\%$ predicted), or who are not responding to treatment. Pulse oximetry is a noninvasive method of measuring systemic oxygenation in acute asthma [129, 130] and can be used to determine supplementary oxygen requirements.

Finally, chest radiographs are not routinely necessary in acute

asthma [37] but should be obtained in every episode of severe asthma or if physical findings are suggestive of a complication (e.g., pneumothorax).

Treatment

Children with severe acute asthma require expeditious treatment, close observation, and serial measurements of physical signs and lung function. The goals of treatment in acute asthma are to relieve hypoxemia, reverse airway obstruction by way of bronchodilators and systemic steroids, and prevent early relapse (see Fig. 72-2).

General Measures

In hypoxemic patients, supplementary oxygen should be delivered by face mask. An SaO_2 of 90 percent or greater should be achieved. Nebulized medications should be delivered with oxygen, rather than air, as bronchodilators can aggravate hypoxemia transiently [93].

Some patients presenting with acute asthma are dehydrated and require intravenous fluids to supplement oral intake and to provide access for the administration of medications. Dehydration occurs because of reduced fluid intake, diaphoresis, and hyperventilation. Dehydration should be corrected, but care should be taken to avoid fluid overload, which can predispose to pulmonary edema in the presence of abnormal swings in intrathoracic pressure found in acute asthma [244]. Once the fluid deficit has been corrected, the wisest course is to give maintenance fluid requirements. A conventional hypotonic replacement solution is recommended, and potassium may be necessary, as both sympathomimetics and steroids may cause hypokalemia [33].

Inhaled Bronchodilators

A selective $beta_2$ agonist, administered by the inhaled route, is the most effective initial treatment in acute asthma and has replaced the use of subcutaneous epinephrine in this situation [33]. In children with severe acute asthma, $beta_2$ agonists should be administered by nebulizer. To ensure optimal deposition of drug particles in the lower airways, dilution of the required amount of $beta_2$ agonist with 3 to 4 ml of normal saline is recommended, and the nebulizer should be powered by a continuous flow of oxygen at a rate of 6 L/min [34]. The frequency of administration varies according to the severity of the acute episode and the response to treatment. Two studies from this institution have demonstrated the efficacy and safety of frequent nebulizations of $beta_2$ agonists in severe acute asthma [210, 220]. Based on these studies, our initial approach in severe acute asthma in children is to administer albuterol, 150 μg/kg (maximum 5 mg/dose) every 20 minutes until a clinical response is achieved. Possible side effects include tremor [210, 220], tachycardia [220], and mild hypokalemia [220]. In children with acute asthma who are less severely ill, hourly nebulizations of albuterol may suffice, and in this situation, a larger dose of nebulized albuterol, 300 μg/kg (maximum 10 mg/dose), can be used [221].

Unfortunately, the administration of $beta_2$ agonists by nebulizer in acute asthma is relatively expensive, time-consuming, and dependent on a power source. Some recent studies in children with acute asthma have suggested that $beta_2$ agonists, administered by MDI together with a spacer device, achieve bronchodilation equivalent to that effected by wet aerosol administration [86, 196]. Further studies are needed before this mode of delivery of inhaled $beta_2$ agonists can be recommended, particularly in young, acutely ill children.

In children with moderate to severe asthma, the authors' practice is to administer ipratropium every 4 hours (and hourly if necessary) by nebulizer in combination with albuterol [15, 205]. Based on the dose-response relationship for ipratropium, 125 μg/

dose is recommended in children under the age of 4 years and 250 μg/dose in older children [63]. Unfortunately, ipratropium solution is currently not available in the United States.

Corticosteroids

With one exception [125], beneficial effects have been reported in trials of systemic steroids in children with exacerbations of asthma [25, 68, 104, 249, 288]. It should be realized that any improvement that does occur with the use of corticosteroids in acute asthma may be delayed for several hours. For this reason, corticosteroids should be introduced early, rather than waiting for the child's condition to deteriorate. Systemic steroids are mandatory in children with severe acute asthma and in those who respond poorly to nebulized bronchodilators. The factors listed in Table 80-17 are also indicative of the need for steroid therapy in acute asthma. It should be stressed that systemic steroids represent a supplement to, and not a substitute for, bronchodilator therapy.

The dose of systemic steroids in acute asthma is somewhat arbitrary. Depending on the clinical situation, steroids can be administered either orally (e.g., prednisone, 1–2 mg/kg/day) or intravenously (e.g., hydrocortisone, 4 mg/kg, or methylprednisolone, 1 mg/kg, every 4–6 hours). Although recent data indicate that inhaled steroids may have a role in the treatment of acute asthmatic symptoms at home [280], this form of treatment cannot be recommended for the emergency care of acute asthma at this time (see also Chap. 60).

Theophylline

The value of intravenous theophylline, traditionally a central component of acute asthma management, has been questioned in recent years. Several studies in adults with acute asthma have shown that intravenous aminophylline, when used in combination with frequently administered adrenergic agents, does not effect additional bronchodilation and can lead to an increased incidence of side effects [138]. Unfortunately, only one study [190] (which supports the efficacy of the drug) has evaluated theophylline in acute childhood asthma. It should be pointed out that theophylline, in addition to being a bronchodilator, is a potent respiratory center stimulant and increases respiratory muscle contractility [10], effects that make it potentially useful in severe acute asthma (see Chap. 58).

It is reasonable, therefore, to consider the use of theophylline in hospitalized children with severe acute asthma, particularly if they are not responding satisfactorily to beta$_2$ agonists and steroids. An initial loading dose of aminophylline (6 mg/kg) is administered intravenously over 20 to 30 minutes. For patients who are already on maintenance oral theophylline, a serum theophylline concentration should be determined and the loading dose modified, as appropriate. Following the loading dose, the patient is started on maintenance intravenous aminophylline, which ideally should be given as a continuous infusion rather than by intermittent bolus injections [98]. Suggested maintenance doses of aminophylline are shown in Table 80-18, but the final decision on dosage will depend on the results of serum theophylline assays. A recent study [216] indicates that there may be an advantage in maintaining serum theophylline concentrations close to the upper end of the therapeutic range in acute asthma.

Emergency Room Discharge

After treatment in the emergency room, up to 75 percent of children with acute asthma can be discharged home [37]; the need for hospitalization can be reduced further if a holding room is available, where children can be observed and treated for a more prolonged period of time [276].

Follow-up studies in children recovering from acute exacerba-

Table 80-18. Continuous theophylline^a dosage following an initial loading dose

Patient age/clinical condition	Infusion rate^b (mg/kg/hr)
Infants 2–6 months	0.4
Infants 6–11 months	0.7
Children 1–9 years	1.0
Children 9–12 years	0.8
Children 12–16 years	0.7
>16 years	0.6
Cardiac decompensation, cor pulmonale, and liver dysfunction	0.2

^{a} Aminophylline = theophylline/0.8.
^{b} Use ideal body weight.

tions of asthma indicate that residual pulmonary function and blood gas abnormalities may persist for several weeks [35, 274]. If a decision to discharge the child from the emergency room is taken, it is essential that inhaled bronchodilators be continued at home, administered by an appropriate delivery system. A 5- to 7-day course of oral steroids may also be indicated. Prompt and serial reviews of the child by the primary care physician are mandatory.

Criteria for Hospital Admission

One of the most difficult decisions in the emergency treatment of asthma is whether to admit the child to the hospital. Clearly all critically ill children with asthma should be admitted immediately. Children who continue to have persistent signs and symptoms and residual airflow obstruction (e.g., peak flow rate < 60% predicted) after emergency room treatment should also be hospitalized [129], as should children with complications (e.g., pneumothorax, lobar atelectasis). Greater consideration for admission should be given to children who exhibit any of the features listed in Table 80-16. Finally, recent studies have intimated that children with acute asthma who have SaO$_2$ values of 91 percent or less (in room air) before treatment should be hospitalized [88, 129]. Oxygen saturation measurements in the emergency room also appear to be more predictive of relapse than lung function measurements [88, 89].

In-hospital Management

Virtually all children admitted to hospital with acute asthma will have moderate to severe airway obstruction refractory to initial emergency room treatment [129]. Careful ongoing assessment is therefore essential to determine the response to treatment and detect any deterioration. Lung function measurements, before and after bronchodilators, should be repeated several times each day, and SaO$_2$ should be monitored by oximetry. Serum potassium levels should be checked. Particular attention should be given to children with FEV$_1$ less than 25 percent predicted or PaCO$_2$ 40 mmHg or greater. In-hospital treatment should include hydration, oxygen, regular nebulizations of beta$_2$ agonists and ipratropium, intravenous steroids, and aminophylline (if necessary).

Treatment of Respiratory Failure

Despite optimal therapy, a small number of children with severe acute asthma develop respiratory failure with progressive hypoxia, hypercapnia, and fatigue and require transfer to an intensive care facility. At this institution, approximately 20 children per year are admitted to the intensive care unit with acute asthma [245]. The usual cause of death in asthma is severe asphyxia [159] with acidosis, and correction of these abnormalities is of prime importance. On admission to the intensive care unit (if immediate intubation is not indicated), children are placed in 100% oxygen until arterial blood gas results are available. A nebulized $beta_2$ agonist is administered continuously, a strategy that may obviate the need for intubation [33]; in our unit, nebulized albuterol (150 μg/dose) is used. Nebulized ipratropium can be administered concurrently every hour [205]. An aminophylline infusion is sometimes used, the rate of which is adjusted to maintain theophylline concentrations close to 20 mg/L. Intravenous steroids are administered every 4 to 6 hours. In addition to serial cardiopulmonary measurements, blood gas tensions (from an indwelling arterial catheter) are measured at 15- to 30-minute intervals, as demanded by the child's progress. In the presence of severe acidosis (pH < 7.20), the judicious use of sodium bicarbonate is a useful therapeutic adjunct to restore responsiveness to sympathomimetic agents [153, 162].

In children who fail to respond to the aforementioned measures, a continuous intravenous infusion of a $beta_2$ agonist is warranted and may avert the need for intubation [20, 33]. (See Chaps. 55 and 57 for a detailed discussion of this topic.) In this Canadian unit, intravenous albuterol is used; the infusion is commenced at a rate of 0.5 μg/kg/min and increased by 1 μg/kg every 15 minutes until the patient clinically improves and $PaCO_2$ falls or intubation and ventilation become necessary. The maximum infusion rate of albuterol is 20 μg/kg/min, but patients generally respond to 4 μg/kg/min [20]. The effect of albuterol is followed by cardiovascular and blood gas monitoring, and serum potassium levels should be checked regularly. In the United States, intravenous terbutaline is used as an alternative to albuterol. The recommended dosage schedule for intravenous terbutaline is 10 μg/kg over 10 minutes, followed by 0.2 μg/kg/min.

The patient with severe asthma who requires ventilatory support because of worsening respiratory failure presents one of the most difficult of all ventilator management problems [57]. In the first instance, the physician is frequently presented with a frightened, struggling, and hypoxemic child in whom prompt intubation, without incurring further hypoxemia, is essential. The high airway pressures required to overcome airway resistance, together with the underlying gas trapping, may result in barotrauma, either a pneumomediastinum or a potentially fatal tension pneumothorax. Mortality rates of 0 to 40 percent in adults [62, 107, 224, 268, 275] and 0 to 5 percent in children [55, 57, 74, 235, 236] have been reported in asthmatic patients requiring positive pressure ventilation. For these reasons, the better option is to adopt an aggressive medical approach and only resort to mechanical ventilation where this fails.

Endotracheal Tube Placement

If intubation becomes necessary, this should be done on an elective basis, if possible, prior to the development of cardiorespiratory arrest. The decision to intervene is based on an assessment of the child's clinical condition and response to therapy. Patient exhaustion and somnolence are particularly ominous signs. There is no absolute $PaCO_2$ value above which intubation is mandatory, as some children with very high $PaCO_2$ values respond rapidly to intense medical therapy.

Intubation should be accomplished expeditiously and with the least systemic disturbance to the child. This task should be undertaken by a physician with well-practiced skills in airway management. Somatic sensory input can be blunted by the use of high-dose sedation or an intravenous anesthetic induction agent to render the child unconscious. During intubation in the intensive care setting, we favor the use of intravenous thiopentone or ketamine, combined with a short-acting muscle relaxant (suxamethonium) [57]. Although intravenous thiopentone may cause bronchospasm during induction of anesthesia, it rapidly achieves

loss of consciousness, allowing for prompt intubation. Intravenous ketamine is also widely used for inducing anesthesia during intubation in children with severe asthma [211]. Because of its inherent sympathomimetic properties, it is less likely to produce increased airway resistance in this setting and has the added attraction of not causing a decrease in cardiac output. During intubation, cricoid pressure is applied if there is concern about possible aspiration of gastric contents. An orotracheal tube should be inserted initially to secure the airway before changing to a nasotracheal tube. A tube with an internal diameter 0.5 mm greater than that predicted for age is usually required to allow effective ventilation with a minimal air leak around the tube. Above the age of 9 years, cuffed tubes can be used. After placement of the endotracheal tube, neuromuscular blockade is maintained with a long-acting muscle relaxant (pancuronium bromide) to keep airway pressures at a minimum. The recommended dose of pancuronium during ventilation is 0.1 mg/kg/dose intravenously every 30 minutes as required; if suxamethonium is used at the time of intubation, the initial dose of pancuronium should be decreased by 33 percent.

Ventilation Strategy

To have a successful outcome with positive pressure ventilation in severe asthma, it is important that there is a clear understanding of what one is trying to achieve with ventilatory support. The main objectives are the reversal of hypoxemia, the relief of respiratory muscle work and fatigue, and partial compensation of respiratory acidosis, using the lowest peak airway pressures consistent with these objectives. The objective most definitely is not to achieve a normal $PaCO_2$ during the first few hours of ventilatory support; any attempt to do so may result in increased morbidity due to pulmonary barotrauma. Arterial $PaCO_2$ values in the range of 50 to 60 mmHg are perfectly safe and acceptable as long as they are accompanied by a compensated pH (pH > 7.3) and adequate oxygenation.

A volume-controlled ventilator should be used, set at low ventilatory rates (8–12/min) with an inspiratory time of 1.0 to 1.5 seconds, allowing for an expiratory time of 5 seconds. A tidal volume of 10 to 12 ml/kg should be chosen, with the object of keeping peak airway pressures below 45 cmH_2O. The adequacy of the expiratory time can be gauged by auscultation of the chest or scrutiny of the flow signal from the ventilator. If inspiration commences before the termination of the preceding expiration, gas trapping will occur and carbon dioxide retention will increase.

This ventilatory strategy has been entitled "controlled hypoventilation" by Darioli and Perret [62]. They have reported on the management of 26 adults with severe asthma who required mechanical ventilation on 34 different occasions, where low respiratory frequencies (6–10 cycles/min) and tidal volumes of 8 to 12 ml/kg were used. With these settings, they were able to maintain maximal airway pressures below 50 cmH_2O. There was no mortality in this series, and the mean duration of respiratory support was 2.5 days. Dworkin and Kattan [74] reported a similarly successful outcome with this approach in 10 children who underwent 20 separate episodes of mechanical ventilation. The mean duration of respiratory support was 2 days. We have adopted a similar strategy in the ventilatory management of children with status asthmaticus [57]. In a series of 79 children with severe asthma who required intensive care management, 19 (24%) required ventilatory support (many of these patients had already been intubated at outlying hospitals). The mean $PaCO_2$ was 88 mmHg prior to intubation, which fell to 57 mmHg during the first 3 hours of ventilation. The mean time of ventilation was 42 hours, and all patients survived without long-term sequelae.

Throughout the period of ventilation, all appropriate medical therapy should be continued aggressively. $Beta_2$ agonists can be given by intravenous infusion or nebulized into the inspiratory circuit of the ventilator. Supplementary bicarbonate is given to raise the pH above 7.25 if this cannot be achieved by mechanical ventilation [153, 162]. To keep peak airway pressures at a minimum, muscle paralysis is maintained, and patients are sedated with a continuous narcotic infusion.

The resolution of airway obstruction in a ventilated asthmatic patient will become evident when $PaCO_2$ values fall while the same or lower peak airway pressures are being used. Once the $PaCO_2$ is less than 45 mmHg, peak airway pressures are less than 35 cmH$_2$O, and there is mild or no bronchospasm on auscultation, the muscle paralysis can be stopped. As soon as respiratory muscle function has returned to normal, patients can be placed on spontaneous ventilation. If they maintain a $PaCO_2$ of less than 45 mmHg without assisted ventilation, rapid extubation is advisable.

Although most patients who require ventilatory support can be weaned and extubated within 72 hours, there are occasional patients with severe airway obstruction who have a much more protracted ventilator course, requiring peak airway pressures of up to 60 cmH$_2$O to achieve adequate ventilation. In this situation, there have been anecdotal reports of the successful reversal of bronchospasm with inhaled volatile anaesthetic agents, such as ether and halothane [182, 223], or with high positive end-expiratory pressure [199].

In summary, severe asthma that is associated with respiratory failure of sufficient severity to necessitate the institution of mechanical ventilation is a potentially life-threatening situation, which if not managed appropriately, can result in significant morbidity and mortality. Mechanical ventilation in such circumstances requires the development of a strategy that takes into account the underlying physiology of the disease process rather than applying formulas for ventilation that are based on normal respiratory physiology. It requires an acceptance of the concept that elevated $PaCO_2$ levels are not inherently harmful, but the use of high peak inflation pressures certainly can be. If these concepts are understood, the morbidity and mortality associated with assisted ventilation in severe asthma should be no higher than for any other form of respiratory disease. However, follow-up studies of children who require ventilation for asthma show that they continue to be a high-risk group with ongoing morbidity and mortality [173, 228].

Management During Recovery in Hospital

During the recovery phase of acute asthma, the frequency of inhalation therapy should be reduced gradually, and oral drugs substituted for intravenous medications. The child's inhalation technique should be checked, and reeducation of the family may be indicated. Patients can be allowed home from the hospital once symptoms have cleared and lung function stabilized (e.g., PFR > 75% predicted). Children should be discharged on a course of oral steroids, inhaled bronchodilators, a prophylactic antiinflammatory agent (usually an inhaled steroid), and possibly theophylline. Older children should be supplied with a peak flow-meter on discharge. Early follow-up with the primary care physician is essential. It is hoped that by providing adequate supervision, education, and effective preventative treatment, future episodes of severe acute asthma will be avoided [82].

NATURAL HISTORY OF CHILDHOOD ASTHMA

The most comprehensive information on the natural history of asthma is provided by the Melbourne group, who followed children with asthma prospectively to the age of 28 years [127, 128, 149, 152]. At the age of 21, about 50 percent of the subjects who had mild, infrequent asthma as children had become symptom

Table 80-19. *Factors influencing the outcome of asthma*

Sex	Variable pattern
Age of onset	Unknown
Severity of asthma	Yes
Family history of atopy	Yes
Chronic eczema	Yes
Smoking (active/passive)	Yes
Level of lung function	Probably
Treatment	?

free, whereas this was more the exception than the rule in those who had more severe asthma. Between 21 and 28 years, although some patients improved, others experienced a recurrence of symptoms [127]. It was also found that some adults who had "outgrown" asthma continued to have occult pulmonary function abnormalities and increased airway reactivity; even greater pulmonary function abnormalities were found in symptomatic patients [128]. The factors that may influence the long-term prognosis in childhood asthma are summarized in Table 80-19 [67]. Although some children with asthma may experience some growth retardation around the time of puberty, normal stature is ultimately achieved in the majority of patients [11]. Finally, the relationship between childhood asthma and chronic obstructive lung disease in adult life remains unclear at this time [250].

REFERENCES

1. Akhter, J., Gasper, M. M., and Newcomb, R. W. Persistent peripheral airway obstruction in children with severe asthma. *Ann. Allergy* 63:53, 1989.
2. Allergy Section, Canadian Pediatric Society. Blood tests for allergy in children. *Can. Med. Assoc. J.* 142:1207, 1990.
3. Altounyan, R. E. C. Review of clinical activity and mode of action of sodium cromoglycate. *Clin. Allergy* 10(Suppl.):481, 1980.
4. Amaro-Galvez, R., et al. Grading severity and treatment requirements to control symptoms in asthmatic children and their relationship with airway hyperreactivity to methacholine. *Ann. Allergy* 59:298, 1987.
5. American Thoracic Society. Chronic bronchitis, asthma and pulmonary emphysema. *Am. Rev. Respir. Dis.* 85:762, 1962.
6. Anderson, H. R. Respiratory abnormalities in Papua New Guinea children: The effects of locality and domestic wood smoke pollution. *Int. J. Epidemiol.* 7:63, 1978.
7. Anderson, H. R. Increase in hospital admissions for childhood asthma: Trends in referral, severity, and readmissions from 1970 to 1985 in a health region in the United Kingdom. *Thorax* 44:614, 1989.
8. Anderson, H. R. Is the prevalence of asthma changing? *Arch. Dis. Child.* 64:172, 1989.
9. Arkinstall, W. W. Review of the North American experience with evening administration of Uniphyl tablets, a once-daily theophylline preparation, in the treatment of nocturnal asthma. *Am. J. Med.* 85(Suppl. 18): 60, 1988.
10. Aubier, M., De Troyer, A., and Sampson, M. Aminophylline improves diaphragmatic contractility. *N. Engl. J. Med.* 305:249, 1981.
11. Balfour-Lynn, L. Growth and childhood asthma. *Arch. Dis. Child.* 61: 1049, 1986.
12. Barnes, P. J., and Chung, K. F. Difficult asthma: Cause for concern. *Br. Med. J.* 299:695, 1989.
13. Barnes, P. J., et al. Single-dose slow-release aminophylline at night prevents nocturnal asthma. *Lancet* i:299, 1982.
14. Barnes, S. D., et al. Psychogenic upper airway obstruction presenting as refractory wheezing. *J. Pediatr.* 109:1067, 1986.
15. Beck, R., et al. Combined salbutamol and ipratropium bromide by inhalation in the treatment of severe acute asthma. *J. Pediatr.* 107:605, 1985.
16. Bentur, L., et al. Response of acute asthma to a beta$_2$ agonist in children less than two years of age. *Ann. Allergy* 65:122, 1990.
17. Bentur, L., et al. Controlled trial of nebulized albuterol in children younger than 2 years of age with acute asthma. *Pediatrics* 89:133, 1992.
18. Bernstein, D. I., et al. An open study of auranofin in the treatment of steroid-dependent asthma. *J. Allergy Clin. Immunol.* 81:6, 1988.

19. Bisgaard, H., et al. Inhaled budesonide for treatment of recurrent wheezing in early childhood. *Lancet* 336:649, 1990.

20. Bohn, D. J., et al. Intravenous salbutamol in the treatment of status asthmaticus in children. *Crit. Care Med.* 12:892, 1984.

21. Boulet, L.-P., et al. Tolerance to reduction of oral steroid dosage in severely asthmatic patients receiving nedocromil sodium. *Respir. Med.* 84:317, 1990.

22. Bousquet, J., Hejjaoui, A., and Michel, F.-B. Specific immunotherapy in asthma. *J. Allergy Clin. Immunol.* 86:292, 1990.

23. Bousquet, J., and Michel, F.-B. Food allergy and asthma. *Ann. Allergy* 61(Suppl.):70, 1988.

24. Bronchial inflammation and asthma treatment (editorial). *Lancet* 337:82, 1991.

25. Brunette, M. G., Lands, L., and Thibodeau, L.-P. Childhood asthma: Prevention of attacks with short-term corticosteroid treatment of upper respiratory tract infection. *Pediatrics* 81:624, 1988.

26. Buist, A. S., and Vollmer, W. M. Reflections on the rise in asthma morbidity and mortality. *J.A.M.A.* 264:1719, 1990.

27. Burney, P. Asthma deaths in England and Wales 1931–85: Evidence for a true increase in asthma mortality. *J. Epidemiol. Community Health* 42:316, 1988.

28. Burney, P. G. J., et al. Descriptive epidemiology of bronchial reactivity in an adult population: Results from a community study. *Thorax* 42:38, 1987.

29. Burney, P. G. J., et al. Epidemiology. In S. T. Holgate (ed.), *The Role of Inflammatory Processes in Airway Hyperresponsiveness.* Oxford: Blackwell, 1989. Pp. 222–250.

30. Burrows, B., et al. Association of asthma with serum IgE levels and skin-test reactivity to allergens. *N. Engl. J. Med.* 320:271, 1989.

31. Busse, W. W. Respiratory infections: Their role in airway responsiveness and the pathogenesis of asthma. *J. Allergy Clin. Immunol.* 85:671, 1990.

32. Canny, G. J. The Role of Beta$_2$ Agonists. In *Treatment of Pediatric Asthma: A Canadian Consensus* (MEDICINE Publishing Foundation Symposium Series, 29). Toronto: MES Medical Education Services, 1991. Pp. 41–49.

33. Canny, G. J., Bohn, D., and Levison, H. Sympathomimetics in acute asthma: Inhaled or parenteral? *Am. J. Asthma Allergy Pediatr.* 2(3):165, 1989.

34. Canny, G. J., and Levison, H. Aerosols—therapeutic use and delivery in childhood asthma. *Ann. Allergy* 60:11, 1988.

35. Canny, G. J., and Levison, H. Pulmonary function abnormalities during apparent clinical remission in childhood asthma. *J. Allergy Clin. Immunol.* 82:1, 1988.

36. Canny, G. J., and Levison, H. *Childhood Asthma: A Handbook for Parents* (3rd ed.). Thomson Healthcare Communications, 1991.

37. Canny, G. J., et al. Acute asthma: Observations regarding the management of a pediatric emergency room. *Pediatrics* 83:507, 1989.

38. Carlsen, K. H., et al. Nebulized beclomethasone dipropionate in recurrent obstructive episodes after acute bronchiolitis. *Arch. Dis. Child.* 63:1428, 1988.

39. Carman, P. G., and Landau, L. I. Increased paediatric admissions with asthma in Western Australia: A problem of diagnosis? *Med. J. Aust.* 152:23, 1990.

40. Charpin, D., et al. Respiratory symptoms and air pollution changes in children: The Gardanne Coal-Basin Study. *Arch. Environ. Health* 43:22, 1988.

41. Clifford, R. D., et al. Symptoms, atopy, and bronchial response to methacholine in parents with asthma and their children. *Arch. Dis. Child.* 62:66, 1987.

42. Clifford, R. D., et al. Prevalence of atopy and range of bronchial response to methacholine in 7 and 11 year old schoolchildren. *Arch. Dis. Child.* 64:1126, 1989.

43. Clifford, R. D., et al. Prevalence of respiratory symptoms among 7 and 11 year old schoolchildren and association with asthma. *Arch. Dis. Child.* 64:1118, 1989.

44. Cochrane, L. M., and Clark, C. J. Benefits and problems of a physical training programme for asthmatic patients. *Thorax* 45:345, 1990.

45. Cockcroft, D. W., and Murdock, K. Y. Comparative effects of inhaled salbutamol, sodium cromoglycate, and beclomethasone dipropionate on allergen-induced early asthmatic responses, late asthmatic responses and increased bronchial responsiveness to histamine. *J. Allergy Clin. Immunol.* 79:734, 1987.

46. Cockcroft, D. W., et al. Allergen-induced increase in non-allergic bronchial reactivity. *Clin. Allergy* 7:503, 1977.

47. Cogswell, J. J., and Simpkiss, M. J. Nebulised sodium cromoglycate in recurrently wheezy preschool children. *Arch. Dis. Child.* 60:736, 1985.

48. Colver, A. F. Community campaign against asthma. *Arch. Dis. Child.* 59:449, 1984.

49. Conboy, K. Self-management skills for cooperative care in asthma. *J. Pediatr.* 115:863, 1989.

50. Conway, S. P., and Littlewood, J. M. Admission to hospital with asthma. *Arch. Dis. Child.* 60:636, 1985.

51. Cookson, J. B. Prevalence rates of asthma in developing countries and their comparison with those in Europe and North America. *Chest* 91(Suppl.):97, 1987.

52. Cookson, W. O. C. M., and Hopkin, J. M. Dominant inheritance of atopic immunoglobulin-E responsiveness. *Lancet* 1:86, 1988.

53. Cookson, W. O. C. M., et al. Linkage between immunoglobulin E responses underlying asthma and rhinitis and chromosome 11q. *Lancet* 1:1292, 1989.

54. Corkey, C., et al. Comparison of three different preparations of disodium cromoglycate in the prevention of exercise-induced bronchospasm. *Am. Rev. Respir. Dis.* 125:623, 1982.

55. Cotton, E. K., Parry, W., and Major, M. C. Treatment of status asthmaticus and respiratory failure. *Pediatr. Clin. North Am.* 22:163, 1975.

56. Cough and wheeze in asthma: Are they independent (editorial)? *Lancet* 1:447, 1988.

57. Cox, R., Barker, G. A., and Bohn, D. J. Efficacy, results and complications of mechanical ventilation in children with status asthmaticus. *Pediatr. Pulmonol.*, 11:120, 1991.

58. Creer, T. L., and Gustafson, K. E. Psychological problem associated with drug therapy in childhood asthma. *J. Pediatr.* 115:850, 1989.

59. Croner, S., et al. IgE screening in 1701 newborn infants and the development of atopic disease during infancy. *Arch. Dis. Child.* 57:364, 1982.

60. Cross, D., and Nelson, H. S. The role of the peak flow meter in the diagnosis and management of asthma. *J. Allergy Clin. Immunol.* 87:120, 1991.

61. Cutz, E., Levison, H., and Cooper, D. M. Ultrastructure in airways in children with asthma. *Histopathology* 2:407, 1978.

62. Darioli, R., and Perret, C. Mechanical controlled hypoventilation in status asthmaticus. *Am. Rev. Respir. Dis.* 129:385, 1984.

63. Davis, A., et al. Clinical and laboratory observations: Determination of the dose-response relationship for nebulized ipratropium in asthmatic children. *J. Pediatr.* 105:1002, 1984.

64. Davis, J. B., and Bulpitt, C. J. Atopy and wheeze in children according to parental atopy and family size. *Thorax* 36:185, 1981.

65. Dawson, K. P., and Mitchell, E. A. Asthma in New Zealand children. *J. Asthma* 27:291, 1990.

66. de Benedictis, F. M., Canny, G. J., and Levison, H. Methacholine inhalation challenge in the evaluation of chronic cough in children. *J. Asthma* 23:303, 1986.

67. de Benedictis, F. M., Canny, G. J., and Levison, H. The progressive nature of childhood asthma. *Lung* 168(Suppl.):278, 1990.

68. Deshpande, A., and McKenzie, S. A. Short course of steroids in home treatment of children with acute asthma. *Br. Med. J.* 293:169, 1986.

69. Dolan, L. M., et al. Short-term high-dose systemic steroids in children with asthma: The effect on the hypothalamic-pituitary-adrenal axis. *J. Allergy Clin. Immunol.* 80:81, 1987.

70. Douglas, N. J. Nocturnal asthma. *Q. J. Med.* 264:279, 1989.

71. Dowse, G. K., et al. Prevalence and features of asthma in a sample survey of urban Goroka, Papua New Guinea. *Clin. Allergy* 15:429, 1985.

72. Duffy, D. L., et al. Genetics of asthma and hay fever in Australian twins. *Am. Rev. Respir. Dis.* 142:1351, 1990.

73. Dutoit, J. I., Salone, C. M., and Woolcock, A. J. Inhaled corticosteroids reduce the severity of bronchial hyperresponsiveness in asthma but oral theophylline does not. *Am. Rev. Respir. Dis.* 136:1174, 1987.

74. Dworkin, G., and Kattan, M. Mechanical ventilation for status asthmaticus in children. *J. Pediatr.* 114:545, 1989.

75. Edfors-Lub, M. L. Allergy in 7000 twin pairs. *Acta Allergol.* 26:249, 1971.

76. Eigen, H., Laughlin, J. J., and Homrighausen, J. Recurrent pneumonia in children and its relationship to bronchial hyperreactivity. *Pediatrics* 70:698, 1982.

77. Eigen, H., et al. Evaluation of the addition of cromolyn sodium to bronchodilator maintenance therapy in the long-term management of asthma. *J. Allergy Clin. Immunol.* 80:612, 1987.

78. Ellul-Micallef, R., and Fenech, F. F. Effect of intravenous prednisolone in asthmatics with diminished adrenergic responsiveness. *Lancet* 2:1269, 1975.

79. Exercise and the asthmatic child (editorial). *Pediatrics* 84:392, 1989.

80. Freigang, B. Adrenal cortical function after long-term beclomethasone aerosol therapy in early childhood. *Ann. Allergy* 64:342, 1990.

81. Ferguson, A. C., and Murray, A. B. Predictive value of skin prick tests and radioallergosorbent tests for clinical allergy to dogs and cats. *Can. Med. Assoc. J.* 134:1365, 1986.

82. Fletcher, H. J., Ibrahim, S. A., and Speight, N. Survey of asthma deaths in the Northern region, 1970–85. *Arch. Dis. Child.* 65:163, 1990.

83. Francis, P. W. J., Krastins, I. R. B., and Levison, H. Oral and inhaled salbutamol in the prevention of exercise induced asthma. *Pediatrics* 66:103, 1980.

84. Francis, R. S., and McEnery, G. Disodium cromoglycate compared with beclomethasone dipropionate in juvenile asthma. *Clin. Allergy* 14:537, 1984.

85. Freeman, J., and Landau, L. I. The effects of ipratropium bromide and fenoterol nebulizer solutions in children with asthma. *Clin. Pediatr.* 28:556, 1989.

86. Fuglsang, G., and Pederson, S. Comparison of nebuhaler and nebulizer treatment of acute severe asthma in children. *Eur. J. Respir. Dis.* 69:109, 1986.

87. Geddes, D. M., et al. Nedocromil sodium workshop. *Respir. Med.* 83:265, 1989.

88. Geelhoed, G. C., Landau, L. I., and LeSouef, P. N. Predictive value of oxygen saturation in emergency evaluation of asthmatic children. *Br. Med. J.* 297:395, 1988.

89. Geelhoed, G. C., Landau, L. I., and LeSouef, P. N. Oximetry and peak expiratory flow in assessment of acute childhood asthma. *J. Pediatr.* 117:907, 1990.

90. Georgitis, J. W., and De Mais, J. M. A double-blind study of the effectiveness of a high-efficiency particular air (HEPA) filter in the treatment of allergic rhinitis and asthma. *J. Allergy Clin. Immunol.* 85:1050, 1990.

91. Gergen, P. J., Mullally, D. I., and Evans, R. National survey of prevalence of asthma among children in the United States, 1976–1980. *Pediatrics* 81:1, 1988.

92. Gergen, P. J., and Weiss, K. B. Changing patterns of asthma hospitalization among children: 1979 to 1987. *J.A.M.A.* 264:1688, 1990.

93. Gleeson, J. G. A., Green, S., and Price, J. F. Air or oxygen as driving gas for nebulized salbutamol. *Arch. Dis. Child.* 63:900, 1988.

94. Gleeson, J. G. A., Green, S., and Price, J. F. Nebuhaler technique. *Br. J. Dis. Chest* 82:172, 1988.

95. Gleeson, J. G. A., and Price, J. F. Controlled trial of budesonide given by the Nebuhaler in preschool children with asthma. *Br. Med. J.* 297:163, 1988.

96. Godfrey, S., Balfour-Lynn, L., and Konig, P. The place of cromolyn sodium in the long-term management of childhood asthma based on a 3–5 year follow-up. *J. Pediatr.* 87:465, 1974.

97. Godfrey, S., Balfour-Lynn, L., and Tooley, M. A three- to five-year follow-up of the use of the aerosol steroid, beclomethasone dipropionate, in childhood asthma. *J. Allergy Clin. Immunol.* 62:335, 1978.

98. Goldberg, P., et al. Intravenous aminophylline therapy for asthma: A comparison of two methods of administration in children. *Am. J. Dis. Child.* 134:596, 1980.

99. Goldstein, D., and Konig, P. Effect of inhaled beclomethasone dipropionate on hypothalamo-pituitary-adrenal axis function in children with asthma. *Pediatrics* 72:60, 1983.

100. Gortmaker, S. L., et al. Parental smoking and the risk of childhood asthma. *Am. J. Public Health* 72:574, 1982.

101. Grant, S. M., et al. Ketotifen: A review of its pharmacodynamic and pharmacokinetic properties and therapeutic use in asthma and allergic disorders. *Drugs* 40(3):412, 1990.

102. Gurwitz, D., Corey, M., and Levison, H. Pulmonary function and bronchial reactivity in children after croup. *Am. Rev. Respir. Dis.* 122:95, 1980.

103. Gurwitz, D., Mindorff, C., and Levison, H. Increased incidence of bronchial reactivity in children with a history of bronchiolitis. *J. Pediatr.* 98:551, 1981.

104. Harris, J., et al. Early intervention with short courses of prednisone to prevent progression of asthma in ambulatory patients incompletely responsive to bronchodilators. *J. Pediatr.* 110:627, 1987.

105. Hendeles, L., Weinberger, M., and Wyatt, R. Guide to oral theophylline therapy for the treatment of chronic asthma. *Am. J. Dis. Child.* 132:876, 1978.

106. Hetzel, M. R. The pulmonary clock. *Thorax* 36:481, 1981.

107. Higgins, B., Greening, A. P., and Crompton, G. K. Assisted ventilation in severe asthma. *Thorax* 41:464, 1986.

108. Higgins, M., and Keller, J. Familial occurrence of chronic respiratory disease and familial resemblance in ventilatory capacity. *J. Chronic Dis.* 28:239, 1975.

109. Hill, D. J., et al. Failure of hyposensitisation in treatment of children with grass-pollen asthma. *Br. Med. J.* 284:306, 1982.

110. Hill, R. A., Britton, J. R., and Tattersfield, A. E. Management of asthma in schools. *Arch. Dis. Child.* 62:414, 1987.

111. Hill, R. A., Standen, P. J., and Tattersfield, A. E. Asthma, wheezing and school absence in primary schools. *Arch. Dis. Child.* 64:246, 1989.

112. Hiller, E. J., and Mann, A. D. Betamethasone 17 valerate aerosol and disodium cromoglycate in severe asthma. *Br. J. Dis. Chest* 69:103, 1975.

113. Hirsch, D. J., Hirsch, S. R., and Kalbfleisch, J. H. Effect of central air conditioning and meteorologic factors on indoor spore counts. *J. Allergy Clin. Immunol.* 62:22, 1978.

114. Hodges, I. G. C., et al. Bronchodilator effect of inhaled ipratropium bromide in wheezy children. *Arch. Dis. Child.* 56:729, 1981.

115. Hopp, R. J., et al. Genetic analysis of allergic disease in twins. *J. Allergy Clin. Immunol.* 73:265, 1984.

116. Horn, C. R., Clark, T. J. H., and Cochrane, G. M. Inhaled therapy reduces morning dips in asthma. *Lancet* i:1143, 1984.

117. Horwood, L. J., et al. Social and familial factors in the development of early childhood asthma. *Pediatrics* 75:859, 1985.

118. Infante-Rivard, C., et al. The changing frequency of childhood asthma. *J. Asthma* 24:283, 1987.

119. Jenne, J. W. Theophylline is no more obsolete than "two puffs qid" of current beta₂ agonists. *Chest* 98:3, 1990.

120. Johnston, I. D. A., Anderson, H. R., and Patel, S. Variability of peak flow in wheezy children. *Thorax* 39:583, 1984.

121. Jones, A., and Sykes, A. The effect of symptom presentation on delay in asthma diagnosis in children in a general hospital. *Respir. Med.* 84:139, 1990.

122. Josephs, L. K., et al. Nonspecific bronchial reactivity and its relationship to the clinical expression of asthma. *Am. Rev. Respir. Dis.* 140:350, 1989.

123. Juniper, E. F., Frith, P. A., and Hargreave, F. E. Airway responsiveness to histamine and methacholine and relationship to minimum treatment to control symptoms of asthma. *Thorax* 36:575, 1981.

124. Juniper, E. F., et al. Reduction of budesonide after a year of increased use: A randomized controlled trial to evaluate whether improvements of airway responsiveness and clinical asthma are maintained. *J. Allergy Clin. Immunol.* 87:483, 1991.

125. Kattan, M., Gurwitz, D., and Levison, H. Corticosteroids in status asthmaticus. *J. Pediatr.* 96:596, 1980.

126. Kattan, M., et al. Pulmonary function abnormalities in symptom-free children after bronchiolitis. *Pediatrics* 59:683, 1977.

127. Kelly, W. J. W., et al. Childhood asthma in adult life: A further study at 28 years of age. *Br. Med. J.* 94:1059, 1987.

128. Kelly, W. J. W., et al. Childhood asthma and adult lung function. *Am. Rev. Respir. Dis.* 138:26, 1988.

129. Kerem, E., et al. Predicting the need for hospitalization in children with acute asthma. *Chest* 98:1355, 1990.

130. Kerem, E., et al. Clinical-physiological correlations in acute asthma of childhood. *Pediatrics* 87:481, 1991.

131. Kerrebijn, K. F., van Essen-Zandvlier, E. E. M., and Neijens, H. J. Effect of long term treatment with inhaled corticosteroids and beta-agonists on the bronchial responsiveness in children with asthma. *J. Allergy Clin. Immunol.* 79:653, 1987.

132. Konig, P. Inhaled corticosteroids: Their present and future role in the management of asthma. *J. Allergy Clin. Immunol.* 82:297, 1988.

133. Kramer, M. S. Does breast feeding help protect against atopic disease? Biology, methodology, and a golden jubilee of controversy. *J. Pediatr.* 112:181, 1988.

134. Lamarre, A., et al. Double-blind study comparing ketotifen and DSCG in adolescent asthmatics. *Respiration* 30(Suppl.):16, 1980.

135. Lask, B., and Matthew, D. Childhood asthma: A controlled trial of family psychotherapy. *Arch. Dis. Child.* 54:116, 1979.

136. Leeder, S. R., et al. Influence of family factors on asthma and wheezing during the first five years of life. *Br. J. Prev. Soc. Med.* 30:213, 1976.

137. LeSouef, P. N., et al. Response of normal infants to inhaled histamine. *Am. Rev. Respir. Dis.* 139:62, 1989.

138. Littenberg, B. Aminophylline treatment in severe, acute asthma. *J.A.M.A.* 259:1678, 1988.

139. Loftus, B. G., and Price, J. F. Long-term, placebo-controlled trial of ketotifen in the management of preschool children with asthma. *J. Allergy Clin. Immunol.* 79:350, 1987.

140. Loftus, B. G., and Price, J. P. Treatment of asthma in preschool children with slow release theophylline. *Arch. Dis. Child.* 60:770, 1985.

141. Lozewicz, S., et al. Morphological integrity of the bronchial epithelium in mild asthma. *Thorax* 45:12, 1990.

142. Lundgren, R., et al. Morphological studies of bronchial mucosal biopsies from asthmatics before and after ten years treatment with inhaled steroids. *Eur. Respir. J.* 883, 1988.

143. Magnusson, C. G. Maternal smoking influences cord serum IgE and IgD levels and increases the risk for subsequent infant allergy. *J. Allergy Clin. Immunol.* 78:898, 1986.

144. Management of asthma in the community (editorial). *Lancet* 2:199, 1989.

145. Mann, N. P., and Hiller, E. J. Ipratropium bromide in children with asthma. *Thorax* 37:72, 1982.

146. Mao, Y. Canadian Pediatric Asthma: Morbidity, Mortality and Hospitalization Data. In *Treatment of Pediatric Asthma: A Canadian Consensus* (MEDICINE Publishing Foundation Symposium Series, 29). Toronto: MES Medical Education Services, 1991. Pp. 9–17.

147. Marks, M. B. Theophylline: Primary or tertiary drug? A brief review. *Ann. Allergy* 59:85, 1987.

148. Marsh, D. G., Meyers, D. A., and Bias, B. The epidemiology and genetics of atopic allergy. *N. Engl. J. Med.* 305:1551, 1981.

149. Martin, A. J., et al. The natural history of childhood asthma to adult life. *Br. Med. J.* 280:1397, 1980.

150. Martinez, F. D., et al. Initial airway function is a risk factor for recurrent wheezing respiratory illnesses during the first three years of life. *Am. Rev. Respir. Dis.* 143:312, 1991.

151. Matus, I. Assessing the nature and clinical significance of psychological contributions to childhood asthma. *Am. J. Orthopsychiatry* 51:327, 1981.

152. McNicol, K. N., and Williams, H. B. Spectrum of asthma in children: I. Clinical and physiological components. 4:7, 1973.

153. Menitove, S. M., and Goldring, R. M. Combined ventilator and bicarbonate strategy in the management of status asthmaticus. *Am. J. Med.* 74:898, 1983.

154. Miller, B. D. Depression and asthma: A potentially lethal mixture. *J. Allergy Clin. Immunol.* 80(Suppl.):481, 1987.

155. Miller, J., et al. Effect of tannic acid spray on dust mite antigen levels in carpets. *J. Allergy Clin. Immunol.* 83:262, 1989.

156. Milner, A. D. Lung function testing in infancy. *Arch. Dis. Child.* 65:548, 1990.

157. Mitchell, E. A. International trends in hospital admission rates for asthma. *Arch. Dis. Child.* 60:376, 1985.

158. Mok, J. Y. Q., and Simpson, H. Symptoms, atopy and bronchial reactivity after lower respiratory infection in infancy. *Arch. Dis. Child.* 54:299, 1984.

159. Molfino, N. A., et al. Respiratory arrest in near-fatal asthma. *N. Engl. J. Med.* 324:285, 1991.

160. Morley, J., Sanjar, S., and Newth, C. Viewpoint: Untoward effect of beta-adrenoceptor agonists in asthma. *Eur. Respir. J.* 3:228, 1990.

161. Mosbech, H., et al. Hyposensitization in asthmatics with m PEG modified and unmodified house dust mite extract: II. Effect evaluated by challenge with allergen and histamine. *Allergy* 44:499, 1989.

162. Mountain, R. D., et al. Acid-base disturbances in acute asthma. *Chest* 98:651, 1990.

163. Mullarkey, M. F., et al. Methotrexate in the treatment of corticosteroid-dependent asthma: A double-blind crossover study. *N. Engl. J. Med.* 318:603, 1988.

164. Muller, N. L., and Bryan, A. C. Chest wall mechanics and respiratory muscles in infants. *Pediatr. Clin. North Am.* 26:503, 1979.

165. Murray, A. B. Avoiding Airborne Allergens in the Home. In *Treatment of Pediatric Asthma: A Canadian Consensus* (MEDICINE Publishing Foundation Symposium Series, 29). Toronto: MES Medical Education Services, 1991. Pp. 33–38.

166. Murray, A. B., Ferguson, A. C., and Morrison, A. J. Diagnosis of house dust mite allergy in asthmatic children: What constitutes a positive history? *J. Allergy Clin. Immunol.* 71:21, 1983.

167. Murray, A. B., Ferguson, A. C., and Morrison, B. J. The frequency and severity of cat allergy compared with dog allergy in atopic children. *J. Allergy Clin. Immunol.* 72:145, 1983.

168. Murray, A. B., and Morrison, B. J. The effect of cigarette smoke from the mother on bronchial responsiveness and severity of symptoms in children with asthma. *J. Allergy Clin. Immunol.* 76:575, 1986.

169. Murray, A. B., and Morrison, B. J. Passive smoking by asthmatics: Its greater effect on boys than on girls and on older than on younger children. *Pediatrics* 84:451, 1989.

170. Murray, A. B., and Morrison, B. J. It is children with atopic dermatitis who develop asthma more frequently if the mother smokes. *J. Allergy Clin. Immunol.* 86:732, 1990.

171. The nebulizer epidemic (editorial). *Lancet* 2:789, 1984.

172. Neijens, H. J., and Knol, R. Oral prophylactic therapy in wheezy infants. *Immunol. Allergy Practice* 10:17, 1988.

173. Newcomb, R. W., and Akhter, J. Respiratory failure from asthma: A marker for children with high morbidity and mortality. *Am. J. Dis. Child.* 142:1041, 1988.

174. Newhouse, M. T. Is theophylline obsolete? *Chest* 98:1, 1990.

175. Newth, C. J., Newth, C. V., and Turner, J. A. P. Comparison of nebulized sodium cromoglycate and oral theophylline in controlling symptoms of chronic asthma in preschool children: A double blind study. *Aust. N.Z. Med.* 12:232, 1982.

176. Norman, P. S., and Van Metre, T. E. The safety of allergenic immunotherapy. *J. Allergy Clin. Immunol.* 85:522, 1990.

177. O'Callaghan, C., Milner, A. D., and Swarbrick, A. Spacer device with face mask attachment for giving bronchodilators to infants with asthma. *Br. Med. J.* 298:160, 1989.

178. O'Halloran, S. M., and Heaf, D. P. Recurrent accident and emergency department attendance for acute asthma in children. *Thorax* 44:620, 1989.

179. Ohman, J. L. Allergen immunotherapy in asthma: Evidence for efficacy. *J. Allergy Clin. Immunol.* 84:133, 1989.

180. Orenstein, D. M., et al. Exercise conditioning in children with asthma. *J. Pediatr.* 106:556, 1985.

181. Orenstein, S. R., and Orenstein, D. M. Gastroesophageal reflux and respiratory disease in children. *J. Pediatr.* 112:847, 1988.

182. O'Rourke, P. P., and Crone, R. K. Halothane in status asthmaticus. *Crit. Care Med.* 10:341, 1982.

183. Parker, S. R., Mellins, R. B., and Sogn, D. D. NHLBI Workshop Summary. Asthma education: A national strategy. 140:848, 1989.

184. Pattemore, P. K., et al. The interrelationship among bronchial hyperresponsiveness, the diagnosis of asthma, and asthma symptoms. *Am. Rev. Respir. Dis.* 142:549, 1990.

185. Pauwels, R. A. New aspects of the therapeutic potential of theophylline in asthma. *J. Allergy Clin. Immunol.* 83:548, 1989.

186. Peak, J. K., et al. Asthma and bronchitis in Sydney schoolchildren: I. Prevalence during a six year study. *Am. J. Epidemiol.* 111:721, 1980.

187. Pearce, N., et al. Case-control study of prescribed fenoterol and death from asthma in New Zealand, 1977–81. *Thorax* 45:170, 1990.

188. Pederson, S. How to use a Rotahaler. *Arch. Dis. Child.* 61:11, 1986.

189. Pierson, W. E. Exercise-induced bronchospasm in children and adolescents. *Pediatr. Clin. North Am.* 35:1031, 1988.

190. Pierson, W. E., et al. Double-blind trial of aminophylline in status asthmaticus. *Pediatrics* 48:642, 1971.

191. Platts-Mills, T., et al. Reduction of bronchial hyperreactivity during prolonged allergen avoidance. *Lancet* ii:678, 1982.

192. Plaut, T. F. Using the compressor-driven nebulizer to treat asthma at home. *Am. J. Asthma Allergy Pediatr.* 2:176, 1989.

193. Pollock, J., et al. Relationship of serum theophylline concentration to inhibition of exercise-induced bronchospasm and comparison with cromolyn. *Pediatrics* 60:840, 1977.

194. Pope, C. A. Respiratory disease associated with community air pollution and a steel mill, Utah valley. *Am. J. Public Health* 79:623, 1989.

195. Poynter, D. Fatal asthma: Is treatment incriminated? *J. Allergy Clin. Immunol.* 80(Suppl.):423, 1987.

196. Prendergast, J., et al. Comparative efficacy of terbutaline administered by nebuhaler and by nebulizer in young children with acute asthma. *Med. J. Aust.* 151:406, 1989.

197. Priftis, K., et al. Adrenal function in asthma. *Arch. Dis. Child.* 65:838, 1990.

198. Pullan, C. R., and Hey, E. N. Wheezing, asthma, and pulmonary dysfunction 10 years after infection with respiratory syncytial virus in infancy. *Br. Med. J.* 284:1665, 1982.

199. Qvist, J., Pemberton, M., and Bennike, K.-A. High-level PEEP in severe asthma (letter). *N. Engl. J. Med.* 307:1347, 1982.

200. Rackham, A., et al. A Canadian multicenter study with Zaditen (ketotifen) in the treatment of bronchial asthma in children age 5–17 years. *J. Allergy Clin. Immunol.* 84:286, 1989.

201. Ratterty, P., Beasley, R., and Holgate, S. T. Comparison of the efficacy of preservative free ipratropium bromide and Atrovent nebulizer solution. *Thorax* 43:446, 1988.

202. Rayner, R. J., Cartlidge, P. H. J., and Upton, C. T. Salbutamol and ipratropium in acute asthma. *Arch. Dis. Child.* 62:840, 1987.

203. Rebuck, A. S., and Marcus, H. I. SCH 1000 in psychogenic asthma. *Scand. J. Respir. Dis.* 103(Suppl.):186, 1979.

204. Rebuck, A. S., and Tamarken, J. L. Pulsus paradoxus in asthmatic children. *Can. Med. Assoc. J.* 112:710, 1975.
205. Reisman, J., et al. Frequent administration by inhalation of salbutamol and ipratropium bromide in the initial management of severe acute asthma in children. *J. Allergy Clin. Immunol.* 81:16, 1988.
206. Reisman, J. J., Canny, G. J., and Levison, H. The approach to chronic cough in childhood. *Ann. Allergy* 61:163, 1988.
207. Dust mite allergens and asthma: Report of a second international workshop. *J. Allergy Clin. Immunol.* 89:1046, 1992.
208. Richards, W. Hospitalization of children with status asthmaticus: A review. *Pediatrics* 84:111, 1989.
209. Ries, A. L. Response to Bronchodilators. In J. L. Clausen (ed.), *Pulmonary Function Guidelines and Controversies.* London: Grune & Stratton, 1984. Pp. 215–221.
210. Robertson, C. F., et al. Response to frequent low doses of nebulized salbutamol in acute asthma. *J. Pediatr.* 106:672, 1985.
211. Rock, M. J., et al. Use of ketamine in asthmatic children to treat respiratory failure refractory to conventional therapy. *Crit. Care Med.* 14:514, 1986.
212. Rooklin, A. Theophylline: Is it obsolete for asthma? *J. Pediatr.* 115:841, 1989.
213. Rooney, J. C., and Williams, H. E. The relationship between proved viral bronchitis and subsequent wheezing. *J. Pediatr.* 79:744, 1971.
214. Rubinstein, I., et al. Immediate and delayed bronchoconstriction after exercise in patients with asthma. *N. Engl. J. Med.* 317:482, 1987.
215. Ryan, C. A., Willan, A. R., and Wherrett, B. A. Home nebulizers in childhood asthma: Parenteral perceptions and practices. *Clin. Pediatr.* 27:420, 1988.
216. Sakamoto, Y., Kabe, J., and Horai, Y. Effect of theophylline on improvement of the pulmonary function in the treatment of acute episodes of asthma: The influence of the severity of acute asthma. *Ann. Allergy* 63:21, 1989.
217. Samet, J. M. Epidemiologic approaches for the identification of asthma. *Chest* 91(Suppl.):74, 1987.
218. Schembri, D. A., et al. Bronchial responsiveness in two populations of South Australian rural schoolchildren. *Med. J. Aust.* 152:578, 1990.
219. Schlieper, A., et al. Effect of therapeutic plasma concentrations of theophylline on behavior, cognitive processing, and affect in children with asthma. *J. Pediatr.* 118:449, 1991.
220. Schuh, S., et al. High- versus low-dose, frequently administered, nebulized albuterol in children with severe, acute asthma. *Pediatrics* 83(4):513, 1989.
221. Schuh, S., et al. Nebulized albuterol in acute childhood asthma: Comparison of two doses. *Pediatrics* 86:509, 1990.
222. Schwartz, J., et al. Predictors of asthma and persistent wheeze in a national sample of children in the United States: Association with social class, perinatal events and race. *Am. Rev. Respir. Dis.* 142:555, 1990.
223. Schwartz, S. H. Treatment of status asthmaticus with halothane. *J.A.M.A.* 251:2688, 1984.
224. Scoggin, C. H., Sahn, S. A., and Petty, T. L. Status asthmaticus: A nine-year experience. *J.A.M.A.* 238:1158, 1977.
225. Sears, M. R., Jones, D. T., and Holdaway, M. D. Prevalence of bronchial reactivity to inhaled methacholine in New Zealand children. *Thorax* 41:283, 1986.
226. Sears, M. R., et al. 75 deaths in asthmatics prescribed home nebulizers. *Br. Med. J.* 294:47, 1987.
227. Sears, M. R., et al. Regular inhaled beta-agonist treatment in bronchial asthma. *Lancet* 333:1391, 1990.
228. Seddon, P. C., and Heaf, D. P. Long term outcome of ventilated asthmatics. *Arch. Dis. Child.* 65:1324, 1990.
229. Shapiro, G., et al. Short-term double-blind evaluation of flunisolide aerosol for steroid-dependent asthmatic children and adolescents. *Chest* 80:671, 1981.
230. Shaw, N. J., and Edmunds, A. T. Inhaled beclomethasone and oral candidiasis. *Arch. Dis. Child.* 61:788, 1986.
231. Sibbald, B., Horn, M. E. C., and Gregg, I. A family study of the genetic basis of asthma and wheezy bronchitis. *Arch. Dis. Child.* 55:354, 1980.
232. Sibbald, B., and Turner-Warwick, M. Factors influencing the prevalence of asthma among first degree relatives of extrinsic and intrinsic asthmatics. *Thorax* 34:332, 1979.
233. Sibbald, B., et al. Genetic factors in childhood asthma. *Thorax* 35:671, 1980.
234. Silverman, M. Bronchodilators for wheezy infants? *Arch. Dis. Child.* 59:84, 1984.
235. Simons, F. E. R., Pierson, W. E., and Bierman, C. W. Respiratory failure in childhood status asthmaticus. *Am. J. Dis. Child.* 131:1097, 1977.
236. Simpson, H., et al. Severe ventilatory failure in asthma in children: Experience of thirteen episodes over 6 years. *Arch. Dis. Child.* 53:714, 1978.
237. Sims, D. G., et al. Study of 8-year-old children with a history of respiratory syncytial virus bronchiolitis in infancy. *Br. Med. J.* 1:11, 1978.
238. Smith, M. J., and Hodson, M. E. High-dose beclomethasone inhaler in the treatment of asthma. *Lancet* i:265, 1983.
239. Solomon, W. R., Burge, H. A., and Boise, J. R. Exclusion of particulate allergens by window air conditioners. *J. Allergy Clin. Immunol.* 65:306, 1980.
240. Speight, A. N. P., Lee, D. A., and Hey, E. N. Underdiagnosis and undertreatment of asthma in childhood. *Br. Med. J.* 286:1253, 1983.
241. Spitzer, W. O., et al. The use of β-agonists and the risk of death and near death from asthma. *N. Engl. J. Med.* 326:501, 1992.
242. Sporik, R., et al. Exposure to house-dust mite allergen (Der p 1) and the development of asthma in childhood: A prospective study. *N. Engl. J. Med.* 323:502, 1990.
243. Springer, C., et al. Comparison of budesonide and beclomethasone dipropionate for treatment of asthma. *Arch. Dis. Child.* 62:815, 1987.
244. Stalcup, S. A., and Mellins, R. B. Mechanical forces producing pulmonary edema in acute asthma. *N. Engl. J. Med.* 297:592, 1977.
245. Stein, R., et al. Severe acute asthma in a pediatric intensive care unit: Six years' experience. *Pediatrics* 83:1023, 1989.
246. Storr, J., Barrell, E., and Lenney, W. Asthma in primary schools. *Br. Med. J.* 295:251, 1987.
247. Storr, J., Lenney, C. A., and Lenney, W. Nebulized beclomethasone dipropionate in preschool asthma. *Arch. Dis. Child.* 61:270, 1986.
248. Storr, J., and Lenney, W. Nebulized ipratropium and salbutamol in asthma. *Arch. Dis. Child.* 61:602, 1986.
249. Storr, J., et al. The effect of a single oral dose of prednisolone in acute childhood asthma. *Lancet* 1:879, 1986.
250. Strachan, D. P. Do chesty children become chesty adults? *Arch. Dis. Child.* 65:161, 1990.
251. Strunk, R. C. Workshop on the identification of the fatality-prone patient with asthma: Summary of workshop discussion. *J. Allergy Clin. Immunol.* 80(Suppl.):455, 1987.
252. Strunk, R. L., et al. Outcome of long-term hospitalization for asthma in children. *J. Allergy Clin. Immunol.* 83:17, 1989.
253. Subcommittee of the Allergy Section, Canadian Pediatric Society. Skin testing for allergy in children. *Can. Med. Assoc. J.* 129:828, 1983.
254. Tabachnik, E., and Zadik, Z. Diurnal cortisol secretion during therapy with inhaled beclomethasone dipropionate in children with asthma. *J. Pediatr.* 118:294, 1991.
255. Taylor, B., and Wadsworth, J. Maternal smoking during pregnancy and lower respiratory tract illness in early life. *Arch. Dis. Child.* 62:786, 1987.
256. Thomson, N. C. Nedocromil sodium: An overview. *Respir. Med.* 83:269, 1989.
257. Townley, R. G., et al. Segregation analysis of bronchial response to methacholine inhalation challenge in families with and without asthma. *J. Allergy Clin. Immunol.* 77:101, 1986.
258. Twentyman, O. P., et al. Protection against allergen-induced asthma by salmeterol. *Lancet* 336:1338, 1990.
259. Ullman, A., and Svedmyr, N. Salmeterol: A new long acting inhaled beta$_2$ adrenoceptor agonist: Comparison with salbutamol in adult asthmatic patients. *Thorax* 43:674, 1988.
260. Van Bever, H. P., and Stevens, W. J. Evolution of the late asthmatic reaction during immunotherapy and after stopping immunotherapy. *J. Allergy Clin. Immunol.* 86:141, 1990.
261. Van Asperen, P., et al. Education in childhood asthma: A preliminary study of need and efficacy. *Aust. Pediatr. J.* 22:49, 1986.
262. Varsano, I., et al. Safety of 1 year of treatment with budesonide in young children with asthma. *J. Allergy Clin. Immunol.* 85:914, 1990.
263. Vathenen, A. S., et al. Rebound increase in bronchial responsiveness after treatment with inhaled terbutaline. *Lancet* 1:554, 1988.
264. Vedal, S., et al. Daily air pollution effects on children's respiratory symptoms and peak expiratory flow. *Am. J. Public Health* 77:694, 1987.
265. Wald, J. A., Friedman, B. F., and Farr, R. S. An improved protocol for the use of troleandomycin (TAO) in the treatment of steroid-requiring asthma. *J. Allergy Clin. Immunol.* 78:36, 1986.
266. Warner, J. O., et al. Controlled study of hypo-sensitization to *Dermatophagoides pteronyssinus* in children with asthma. *Lancet* 2:912, 1978.
267. Watson, W. T. A., Becker, A. B., and Simoins, F. E. R. Comparison of ipratropium solution, fenoterol solution and their combination adminis-

tered by nebulizer and face mask to children with acute asthma. *J. Allergy Clin. Immunol.* 82:1012, 1988.

268. Webb, A. K., Bilton, A. H., and Hanson, G. C. Severe bronchial asthma requiring ventilation: A review of 20 cases and advice on management. *Postgrad. Med. J.* 55:161, 1979.

269. Webb, M. S. C., et al. Nebulized beclomethasone dipropionate suspension. *Arch. Dis. Child.* 61:1108, 1986.

270. Weiss, K. B., and Wagener, D. K. Asthma surveillance in the United States: A review of current trends and knowledge gap. *Chest* 98(Suppl.):179, 1990.

271. Weiss, K. B., and Wagener, D. K. Changing patterns of asthma mortality: Identifying target populations at risk. *J.A.M.A.* 264:1683, 1990.

272. Weiss, S. G., Newcomb, R. W., and Beem, M. O. Pulmonary assessment of children after *Chlamydia* pneumonia of infancy. *J. Pediatr.* 108:654, 1986.

273. Weitzman, M., Gortmaker, S., and Sobol, A. Racial, social and environmental risks for childhood asthma. *Am. J. Dis. Child.* 144:1189, 1990.

274. Weng, T. R., et al. Arterial blood gas tensions and acid base balance in symptomatic and asymptomatic asthma in childhood. *Am. Rev. Respir. Dis.* 101:274, 1970.

275. Westerman, D. E., et al. Identification of the high-risk asthmatic patient: Experience with 39 patients undergoing ventilation for status asthmaticus. *Am. J. Med.* 66:565, 1979.

276. Willert, C., et al. Short-term holding room treatment of asthmatic children. *J. Pediatr.* 106:707, 1985.

277. Williams, A. J., et al. Dysphonia caused by inhaled steroids: Recognition of a characteristic laryngeal abnormality. *Thorax* 38:813, 1983.

278. Wilson, J. D., Sutherland, D. C., and Thomas, A. C. Has the change to beta agonist combined with oral theophylline increased cases of fatal asthma? *Lancet* 1:1235, 1981.

279. Wilson, N. M. Wheezy bronchitis revisited. *Arch. Dis. Child.* 64:1194, 1989.

280. Wilson, N. M., and Silverman, M. Treatment of acute, episodic asthma in preschool children using intermittent high dose inhaled steroids at home. *Arch. Dis. Child.* 65:407, 1990.

281. Wissow, L. S., et al. Case management and quality assurance to improve care of inner city children with asthma. *Am. J. Dis. Child.* 142:748, 1988.

282. Woenne, R., Kattan, M., and Levison, H. Sodium cromoglycate-induced changes in the dose-response curve of inhaled methacholine and histamine in bronchial asthma. *Am. Rev. Respir. Dis.* 119:927, 1979.

283. Wolthers, O.D., and Pedersen, S. Growth of asthmatic children during treatment with budesonide: A double blind trial. *Br. Med. J.* 303:163, 1991.

284. Wong, C. S., et al. Bronchodilator, cardiovascular and hypokalaemic effects of fenoterol, salbutamol, and terbutaline in asthma. *Lancet* 336:1396, 1990.

285. Wood, R. A., et al. The effect of cat removal on allergen content in household-dust samples. *J. Allergy Clin. Immunol.* 83:730, 1989.

286. Wright, A. L., et al. Breast feeding and lower respiratory tract illness in the first year of life. *Br. Med. J.* 299:946, 1989.

287. Young, S. The influence of a family history of asthma and parental smoking on airway responsiveness in early infancy. *N. Engl. J. Med.* 324:1168, 1991.

288. Younger, R. E., et al. Intravenous methylprednisolone efficacy in status asthmaticus of childhood. *Pediatrics* 80:225, 1987.

289. Zimmerman, B., Chambers, C., and Forsyth, S. The highly atopic infant and chronic asthma. *J. Allergy Clin. Immunol.* 81:71, 1988.

290. Zimmerman, B., et al. Prevalence of abnormalities found by sinus x-rays in childhood asthma: Lack of relation to severity of asthma. *J. Allergy Clin. Immunol.* 80:268, 1987.

291. Zimmerman, B., et al. The dose relationship of allergy to severity of childhood asthma. *J. Allergy Clin. Immunol.* 81:63, 1988.

292. Zora, J. A., et al. Hypothalamic-pituitary adrenal axis suppression after short-term, high-dose glucocorticoid therapy in children with asthma. *J. Allergy Clin. Immunol.* 77:9, 1986.

293. Canny, G. J. Silent asthma. *Am. J. Asthma Allergy Pediatr.* 5:181, 1992.

294. Cheung, D., et al. Long-term effects of a long-acting β_2-adrenoceptor agonist, salmeterol, on airway hyperresponsiveness in patients with mild asthma. *N. Engl. J. Med.* 327:1198, 1992.

295. Clark, N. M., Evans, D., and Mellins, R. B. Patient use of peak flow monitoring. *Am. Rev. Respir. Dis.* 145:722, 1992.

296. de Blay, F., Chapman, M. D., and Platts-Mills, T. A. E. Airborne cat allergen (Fel d 1) environmental control with the cat in situ. *Am. Rev. Respir. Dis.* 143:1334, 1991.

297. Cookson, W. O., et al. Maternal inheritance of atopic IgE responsiveness on chromosome 11q. *Lancet* 340:381, 1992.

298. Lindgren, S., et al. Does asthma or treatment with theophylline limit children's academic performance? *N. Engl. J. Med.* 327:926, 1992.

299. Lemanske, R. F. Mechanisms of airway inflammation. *Chest* 101(Suppl.): 372, 1992.

300. Luczynska, C. M., et al. Airborne concentrations and particle size distribution of allergen derived from domestic cats (Felis domesticus) *Am. Rev. Respir. Dis.* 141:361, 1990.

301. Martinez, F., et al. Initial airway function is a risk factor for recurrent wheezing respiratory illnesses during the first three years of life. *Am. Rev. Respir. Dis.* 143:312, 1991.

302. O'Connor, B. J., Aikman, S. L., and Barnes, P. J. Tolerance to the nonbronchodilator effects of inhaled β_2-agonists in asthma. *N. Engl. J. Med.* 327:1204, 1992.

303. Djukanovic, R., et al. Effect of inhaled steroid on airway inflammation and symptoms in asthma. *Am. Rev. Respir. Dis.* 145:669, 1992.

304. Weinstein, A. G., et al. Outcome of short-term hospitalization for children with severe asthma. *J. Allergy Clin. Immunol.* 90:66, 1992.

305. Van Essen-Zandvliet, E. E., et al. Effects of 22 months of treatment with inhaled corticosteroids and/or beta₂-agonists on lung function, airway responsiveness, and symptoms in children with asthma. *Am. Rev. Respir. Dis.* 146:547, 1992.

306. Wolthers, O. D., and Pederson, S. Controlled study of linear growth in asthmatic children during treatment with inhaled corticosteroids. *Pediatrics* 89:839, 1992.

307. Packe, G. E., et al. Bone density in asthmatic patients taking high dose inhaled beclomethasone dipropionate and intermittent systemic corticosteroids. *Thorax* 47:414, 1992.

Pregnancy and Menses

81

Sin-Ming J. Chien
Sheldon Mintz

PREGNANCY

Prevention of severe asthma is the most important principle of supervision of the pregnant asthmatic, for the optimal care of both mother and fetus. This principle is highlighted when one realizes that most pregnant females fall within the age group that has seen an increase in mortality in the past two decades. (For a full discussion of this phenomenon, see Chap. 90.)

It is also important to realize that in the young female, both asthma and pregnancy are very common. It is estimated that approximately 1 percent of pregnancies are complicated by asthma and in 1 in 500 pregnancies, the asthma is life-threatening [49, 54, 61, 115, 140]. During pregnancy, asthma is the most common pulmonary condition requiring physician intervention [118]. Thus, it is essential that physicians be aware of the special issues involved in the care of pregnant asthmatic patients in order to ensure both maternal and fetal health.

Many questions need to be addressed about the pregnant asthmatic. How is pulmonary physiology altered during pregnancy? What effect does asthma have on this modified function? Does asthma itself, independent of any effect of drugs used for its treatment, have any deleterious consequences for fetal outcome? Which drugs are safe to use in the pregnant and nursing mother? What is the optimal management of the pregnant asthmatic? This chapter examines each of these topics.

Pulmonary Physiology

Pregnancy is associated with a plethora of mechanical and hormonal changes that affect the static and dynamic functions of the lung; the net effect of these changes, however, is surprisingly mild [3, 4, 44]. On the other hand, ventilatory changes that occur in pregnancy are of greater magnitude. We first review those factors with potential to change pulmonary function and asthma during pregnancy; then we evaluate the *net* effects of these factors on pregnancy and asthma.

Mechanical Changes

During pregnancy, the enlarging uterus itself results in elevation of the diaphragm by a maximum of 4 cm [130]. Furthermore, the transverse diameter of the chest and the subcostal angle gradually increase during pregnancy [138]. There is a reduction in the negative intrathoracic pressures due to a progressive increase in intraabdominal pressures. These changes (Table 81-1) should theoretically lead to a reduction in lung volumes, especially the functional residual capacity (FRC) [3]. (See Pulmonary Function.)

Hormonal Changes

The total range of hormonal changes in pregnancy is beyond the scope of this chapter (for reviews, see [18, 40, 79, 131]). Since the clinical course of asthma during pregnancy is quite variable, varying (or conflicting) hormonal influences are at play and influence either lung function or the asthmatic condition.

Adrenal Corticosteroids. There are clear changes in adrenal corticosteroid metabolism during pregnancy, and these may be important for the asthmatic. Cortisol is the major adrenal glucocorticoid. It is predominantly bound to plasma proteins; only a small fraction of the total plasma cortisol exists in the unbound, biologically active form. During pregnancy, there is an unquestionable increase in total plasma cortisol concentrations [99]. Total cortisol triples, and cortisol bound to cortisol-binding globulin doubles over the course of pregnancy. Although free cortisol remains at a constant 2 percent of the total cortisol level, the resultant free cortisol level is two times higher than that of the nonpregnant female. Thus, there is a true increase in the active form of cortisol during pregnancy.

Why then is there not always an amelioration of asthma during pregnancy? In the first place, this steroid rise is modest, for instance, when compared with that seen in Cushing's disease [25]. Secondly, there may be considerable variability from one patient to the next in corticosteroid levels during pregnancy. This can explain why cushingoid features and striae are occasionally seen during pregnancy. Thirdly, tissue hyporesponsiveness to cortisol may occur, secondary to the high levels of circulating gestational hormones [96]; this would result in decreased biologic activity of the circulating cortisol. Finally, during pregnancy, other hormonal factors that can exacerbate asthma may be present. Thus, the impact of increased free cortisol during pregnancy on asthma must be considered in balance with the other hormonal alterations that occur during pregnancy.

Progesterone and Estrogen. Both progesterone and estrogen are increased throughout the course of pregnancy [66, 144]. The major impact of these hormones is on ventilation, with likely little change in lung mechanics.

The stimulatory effect of progesterone on ventilation has long been well known. Lyons and Antonio in the 1950s showed that intramuscular injection of progesterone into normal subjects resulted in a heightened response in the carbon dioxide stimulation test [82]. Clinical application of this respiratory stimulant effect of progesterone has also met with modest success in patients with sleep apnea [60]. It is thought that the hormone has a direct stimulatory effect on the respiratory center, but how this influence is exerted remains unknown.

The effect of progesterone on airway resistance, however, is much less clear. Progesterone has a dilatory effect on the uterine smooth muscle. It causes membrane hyperpolarization, which results in decreased excitability of the uterine musculature [41]. However, there are no adequate studies of the effect of progesterone on bronchial wall smooth muscle. In a small study, when patients with alveolar hypoventilation associated with obesity were treated with progesterone, decreases in airway resistance

Table 81-1. Effects of the enlarging uterus on pulmonary mechanics

1. Elevation of the diaphragm
   Estimated maximum 4-cm rise in the level of the diaphragm
2. Changes in the thoracic wall configuration
   Increase in the transverse diameter of the chest
   Increase in the subcostal angle
3. Decrease in the negative intrathoracic pressure
   Due to an increase in intraabdominal pressure

Table 81-2. Hormonal influences on pulmonary physiology during pregnancy

Hormone	Changes in pregnancy	Pulmonary effects
Cortisol	↑, Free cortisol doubles	Ameliorates asthma
Progesterone	↑ Up 20 times normal throughout pregnancy	↑ Ventilation; ?? bronchodilatation
Estrogen	↑ Throughout pregnancy	↑ Ventilation
Prostaglandin E_2	↑ Mainly in 3rd trimester and in labor	Bronchodilator, but may have opposite effect in asthmatics
Prostaglandin $F_{2\alpha}$	↑ Throughout pregnancy, especially in labor	Potent bronchoconstrictor
Prostacyclin	↑ Throughout pregnancy	? Prevents bronchoconstriction
Cyclic AMP	↑ In 1st and 3rd trimesters	Possibly bronchodilator
Cyclic GMP	↑ Mainly in 1st trimester	Possibly bronchoconstrictor

and increases in maximum expiratory flow rates were observed; however, the group was likely too small to attain statistical significance [82]. Another study concerning the effect of high-dose birth control pills on flow rates was not able to demonstrate differences by spirometry in control subjects and pill users [17]. This technique may not have had adequate sensitivity to detect small changes in airway function. The latest study on this point details the course of 26 asthmatic patients followed during pregnancy with sequential methacholine challenge tests; there was a great deal of variability, but on the average, airway responsiveness improved. However, there was no strong correlation with the changes in the level of progesterone or estriol [68, 69]. At present, the possibility of a bronchodilating effect of progesterone remains, but is not proved.

There are very few studies concerning the effect of estrogen on pulmonary physiology during pregnancy. Early investigation showed that estrogen may also increase ventilatory drive, an effect that was additive to that of progesterone.

Prostaglandins. Prostaglandins (PG) are a large group of acidic lipids derived from arachidonic acid that share the basic 20-carbon ring and branched structure of prostanoic acids; small variations in double bonds and hydroxyl- or oxy-substitution on this structure lead to widely divergent biologic effects. There are technical difficulties in defining the role of prostaglandins in pregnancy; these difficulties include their short half-lives, their minute quantities, and their rapid metabolism by the lung. Furthermore, prostaglandins may also be produced by fetal or amniotic tissues, with potential release into the maternal circulation [132]. However, current knowledge suggests that PGE_2, $PGF_{2\alpha}$, and prostacyclin may be of significance in pregnant asthmatics.

The serum level of PGE_2 remains unchanged during early pregnancy. However, a small increase in its level is seen during the third trimester and during labor; the hormone is also present in high concentration in amniotic fluid [13]. The role of this prostaglandin on airway dynamics is not clear. In vitro, it usually acts as a bronchodilator, but in one study it caused an increase in airway resistance (interrupter method) in normal pregnant females [123] and variable slight bronchoconstriction in asthmatics [84].

The concentration of $PGF_{2\alpha}$ is increased throughout pregnancy, particularly during labor [23]. It is present in measurable quantities in human venous blood during labor [70]. The metabolites of $PGF_{2\alpha}$ are also increased late in pregnancy. Unlike PGE_2, $PGF_{2\alpha}$ causes constriction of smooth muscles. It has been used in the induction of labor [74]. However, it also is a potent bronchoconstrictor in vivo and in vitro. Asthmatic subjects seem more sensitive to its bronchoconstrictor effects than normal subjects [65]. In fact, the therapeutic infusion of $PGF_{2\alpha}$ to induce labor has resulted in an attack of asthma in at least one pregnant asthmatic woman [35]. Recently, it was demonstrated that another prostaglandin, PGD_2, can also cause a transient increase in airway responsiveness to histamine and methacholine [10]. Its role in pregnancy has yet to be defined.

Prostacyclin is produced by intrauterine tissues and cervix. Its production rate is increased during pregnancy [132]. While the hormone is not clearly a bronchodilator, it can prevent bronchoconstriction in some circumstances [13].

In summary, prostaglandins have antagonistic effects on airway resistance. $PGF_{2\alpha}$ and PGD_2 cause bronchospasm, whereas PGE_2 and prostacyclin have bronchodilatory effects. Pregnancy is associated with increases in the serum levels of these hormones, especially during the third trimester and labor. However, prostaglandins are usually rapidly metabolized by the lung; a single transit will remove 58 percent of $PGF_{2\alpha}$ and 82 percent of PGE_2. This makes it unlikely (but not impossible) that major elevations of these prostaglandins will occur. At present, the role of prostaglandins in the bronchial musculature and airway dynamics during pregnancy remains unclear.

Cyclic Nucleotides. Elevation in the plasma concentration of cyclic adenosine monophosphate (AMP) occurs during the first trimester and the early part of the third trimester [80]. Cyclic guanosine monophosphate (GMP) increases rapidly during the first trimester and then reaches a plateau [72]. It is thought that in general, cyclic AMP is a bronchodilator and cyclic GMP is a bronchoconstrictor [145]. However, as is the case with the prostaglandins, the role of these cyclic nucleotides in pregnant asthmatic patients remains to be clarified.

In summary, the usual hormonal and mechanical changes during pregnancy can have both positive and negative effects on the static and dynamic properties of the lung, and different influences on asthma. These effects are summarized in Table 81-2, and the resultant effects on the lungs are reviewed in the following section.

Pulmonary Function

The consequences of the physiologic changes during pregnancy on pulmonary function have been studied, in somewhat haphazard fashion, since the mid-19th century (see review by Weinberger et al. [138]). Tables 81-3 and 81-4 summarize the current knowledge.

Lung Volumes. Based on results from different reports, the changes in static lung volumes during pregnancy are tabulated in Table 81-3. The largest percentage decreases (about 16% at 36 weeks of gestation [8, 43, 71, 89]) occur in FRC and residual volume (RV). The change in FRC is expected from the alteration of the body contour associated with pregnancy; it occurs gradually throughout the entire gestational period. Expiratory reserve volume (ERV) and RV at term are both decreased, about 8 to 40 percent and 7 to 29 percent less than those of a nonpregnant control subject. On the other hand, both vital capacity (VC) and total lung capacity (TLC) essentially remain constant during late pregnancy.

The increased intraabdominal contents should theoretically just decrease all lung volumes. For example, ascites causes a

Table 81-3. Changes in static lung volumes in normal pregnancy

Study	No. of subjects	Gestation (wk)	Time postpartum (wk)	TLC[a]	VC	RV	FRC
Milne[b] [89]	61	36	?	−4	0	−29	−22
Baldwin et al. [8]	19	26–39	1	−2	0	−7	−11
Alaily and Carrol [4]	38	38–39	<1	−3	+2	−19	−20
Knuttgen and Emerson [71]	13	36+	6	0	+6	−14	−15
Gazioglu et al. [43]	8	36	10	+2	+8	−17	−12
Average				−1	+3	−17	−16

TLC = total lung capacity; VC = vital capacity; RV = residual volume; FRC = functional residual capacity.
[a] All values for pulmonary function tests are expressed as percent change of late pregnancy value from postpartum value.
[b] Calculated from Figure 4 in Milne [89].

Table 81-4. Pulmonary function during pregnancy

1. Static lung volumes (see Table 81-3)
   Functional residual capacity: −16% at 36–38 gestational wk
   Total lung capacity: unchanged (−1%)
   Vital capacity: unchanged (+3%)
2. Spirometry
   Both FEV_1 and FEV_1/FVC: unchanged
3. Diffusion capacity
   Initial ↑ during 1st trimester
   Then ↓ gradually till 3rd trimester
   Returns to prepartum level 2 wk after delivery
4. Ventilation
   Minute ventilation ↑ by up to 48%
5. Arterial blood
   PCO_2: 27–32 mmHg
   PO_2: 106–108 mmHg (1st trimester)
        101–104 mmHg (3rd trimester)
   pH: 7.40–7.45
   Bicarbonate: 18–21 mEq/L
   Alveolar-arterial oxygen gradient: essentially unchanged

FEV_1 = 1-second forced expiratory volume; FVC = forced vital capacity.

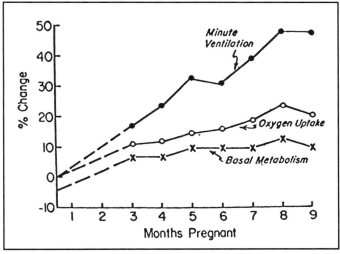

Fig. 81-1. *Temporal relationships of minute ventilation, oxygen uptake, and basal metabolism during the course of pregnancy. (Reprinted with permission from C. M. Prowse and E. A. Gaensler. Respiratory and acid-base changes during pregnancy. Anesthesiology 26:381, 1965.)*

reduction in TLC, VC, FRC, and RV. In fact, in one study, the removal of 12 liters of ascitic fluid resulted in about a 10 percent increase in all four parameters [1]. To counterbalance the augmented intraabdominal pressure and keep a normal VC and TLC, one would need to postulate increased inspiratory muscle function or decreased lung elastic recoil. These factors remain mostly speculative, but one study noted that diaphragmatic excursion was actually increased during pregnancy, which suggests improved net diaphragmatic response [86].

Spirometry. Breathing capacity as measured by spirometry is unchanged during normal pregnancy; the forced expiratory volume in 1 second (FEV_1), the ratio of FEV_1 to FVC, and the forced expiratory flow-volume curve do not alter [2, 3, 8, 91, 107]. This is corroborated by the unchanged maximum voluntary ventilation in pregnant women. These data suggest that physiologic changes during pregnancy have no net effect on the airways. However, two studies of airway resistance, using either the body plethysmographic method or the airway interruption method, have indicated that the airway resistance (Ra) decreases and the conductance (1/Ra) increases in the normal pregnant female near term [44, 107]. One subsequent study, on the other hand, was unable to demonstrate a change in conductance during pregnancy [91]. Thus, the data on large airway function during pregnancy are somewhat conflicting, which is hardly surprising in view of the various hormonal changes associated with pregnancy.

Diffusion Capacity. Studies have shown that pregnancy is associated with changes in the pulmonary diffusion capacity (D_L) [43, 77]. Early studies showed a small, statistically insignificant decrease in diffusion capacity occurring in the third trimester, with a parallel decrease in the membrane component of the diffu-

sion capacity, but capillary blood volume was unchanged [43]. Subsequent studies have demonstrated a drop in diffusion capacity; in the largest series, the drop was about 15 percent, measured by the single-breath test [77]. A longitudinal study showed that there is an initial rise in diffusion capacity during the first trimester, followed by a gradual decline until about 27 weeks. Thereafter, it remains stable and returns to near-normal levels by 2 weeks post partum [90]. A decrease in pulmonary diffusion capacity can be produced by intravenous injection of estrogen (40 mg of conjugated equine urine estrogen), suggesting a possible cause for this decline. In any case, the small change in diffusion capacity is unlikely to be of clinical significance.

Ventilation. It is well known that minute ventilation increases early in pregnancy (in fact, within the first few weeks of conception) and continues to rise throughout gestation (Fig. 81-1). This increase is out of proportion to the metabolic demands of pregnancy and parallels the urinary excretion of the metabolites of progesterone during pregnancy [16, 81, 101]. Prowse and Gaensler showed an increase in minute ventilation of 48 percent above the nonpregnant control; oxygen consumption and basal metabolic rate increased only by 21 percent and 14 percent, respectively [101]. Thus, maternal hyperventilation during pregnancy is likely mediated by the rise in circulating plasma progesterone. Furthermore, the increase in minute ventilation is largely due to an increase in tidal volume of 20 to 40 percent (at term), as respiratory rate remains constant.

The increase in minute ventilation leads to maternal alveolar hyperventilation and a chronic respiratory alkalosis. Normal arterial blood gases of a pregnant female are as follows: oxygen tension (PO_2), about 106 mmHg; carbon dioxide tension (PCO_2), about 27 to 32 mmHg; serum bicarbonate, 18 to 21 mEq/L; and pH, 7.40 to 7.45 [142]. There is a progressive decline in arterial PCO_2 throughout pregnancy. The lowered bicarbonate level indicates metabolic (renal) compensation of the respiratory alkalosis.

Arterial PO_2 ranges from 106 to 108 mmHg during the first trimester, decreasing by 2 to 3 mmHg in the third trimester [138]. There is no significant change in the alveolar-arterial oxygen gradient during pregnancy. The cause for the decline in late pregnancy is unknown; from the data presented earlier, one might postulate that a slight ventilation-perfusion mismatch occurs as a result of earlier airway closure due to the lowered FRC as pregnancy progresses.

In summary, the usual alterations in pulmonary functions during pregnancy include a reduction in FRC and RV, whereas TLC and VC remain unchanged. There is no change in the flow-volume or timed VC curves, but there may be a small reduction in the total pulmonary resistance. Pregnancy is also associated with maternal hyperventilation and respiratory alkalosis, without a significant change in alveolar-arterial oxygen tension.

The Effect of Pregnancy on Asthma

Clinical studies performed since the 1940s confirmed that the clinical course of asthma during pregnancy is extremely variable [133]. Asthma may improve, stabilize, or worsen during the course of pregnancy.

Gluck and Gluck performed a prospective study on 47 pregnant asthmatic subjects [46]. Overall, asthma improved in 13 percent of patients; equal numbers of patients had worsening or no change (43% each). Patients with mild asthma (less than one attack per month) tended to improve during their pregnancy, while those with severe asthma (at least one attack per week) often deteriorated during pregnancy. (It should be noted that in general, their patient population seemed to have relatively mild asthma.) Furthermore, exacerbation of asthma was less common in asthmatics in whom successive levels of IgE decreased during the course of the pregnancy. This important finding has not been corroborated, but their observation that exacerbation of asthma tended to occur during the end of the second trimester was confirmed.

A recent prospective study by Schatz and coworkers [113] found a tendency for asthma to worsen between 29 to 36 weeks of gestation. These authors also noted that in almost all cases, the asthma tended to improve during the last 4 weeks of pregnancy; asthmatic attacks during labor were extremely uncommon. As well, the asthma severity tended to revert to the prepregnant level within the first 3 months post partum.

One study used serial spirometry to follow the course of 27 asthmatics during pregnancy and up to 6 weeks after delivery. When the data were compared with those from 11 nonasthmatic control subjects, no significant effect of pregnancy on asthma was found [122].

Turner and associates [133] reviewed earlier studies reported between 1953 and 1972 on the clinical course of asthma during pregnancy. Eight of the nine studies were retrospective, and assessment of asthmatic severity was subjective (i.e., no spirometry was performed). Of the 1,054 total pregnancies, deterioration occurred in 22 percent; improvement, in 29 percent; and no change, in 49 percent. Two important generalizations were made from reviewing these studies: (1) A patient with severe asthma is likely to have asthma worsen during pregnancy, while those with mild asthma will likely improve. (2) Three of the studies demonstrated that an individual is likely to repeat the same clinical pattern with each pregnancy.

In summary, the course of asthma during pregnancy is quite variable. Women with severe asthma tend to have exacerbations with pregnancy, while those with mild asthma improve. The clinical pattern is likely to repeat with successive pregnancies. Exacerbation tends to occur during the end of the second trimester, with recovery before the end of the third trimester. Severe asthmatic attacks during labor are rare.

It is not known whether the variability of the asthmatic state during pregnancy is due to hormonal or physiologic changes or is a reflection of the natural history of asthma itself. There are problems with most of the studies cited; most were retrospective in nature, and other exacerbating factors of asthma were seldom considered. At present, there are no reported large, controlled, prospective and longitudinal studies of the effect of pregnancy on asthma with modern pulmonary function data.

The Effect of Asthma on Pregnancy

Maternal Aspects
An early study by Bahna and Bjerkedal [7] found a twofold increase in maternal complications (toxemia, postpartum hemorrhage, and hyperemesis gravidarum) in asthmatic females during pregnancy. However, more recent studies have not confirmed this. In one recent study, no maternal deaths occurred during 56 pregnancies in 51 women with severe asthma [36]. Two other studies (one prospective [126], 198 cases; the other retrospective [76], 87 cases) verified the absence of increased maternal complications with asthma, but noted a higher rate of cesarean section and use of epidural analgesia in asthmatic mothers. Other authors have suggested a correlation between gestational hypertension and preeclampsia with poor asthmatic control during pregnancy [112].

Fetal Aspects
Fetal Physiology. Mother and fetus coexist in a host-parasite relationship, with the fetus as the passive partner. Nutrients, oxygen, waste products, and carbon dioxide are exchanged between fetus and mother by concentration and blood flow gradients across the placenta. The chorionic villi provide a large surface area for diffusion. In addition, the blood flow of fetal villous arterial and venous capillaries is in opposite directions, enhancing exchange via countercurrent mechanisms.

Mixing of diffusible substances from maternal arterial and fetal blood occurs in the placenta, which causes the fetal arterial PO_2 to be substantially lower and PCO_2 higher than maternal levels. The approximate value of PO_2 in the umbilical artery is 11 mmHg, with the corresponding PCO_2 at 61 mmHg, while umbilical vein PO_2 and PCO_2 are about 32 and 50 mmHg, respectively (with the mother breathing room air) [54]. The fetus thus exists in a relatively hypoxic environment and there may be very little margin for the fetus to tolerate maternal hypoxia. Wulf and associates demonstrated this elegantly in an experiment using sheep [142]. Maternal PO_2 was reduced from the usual 91 to 65 mmHg by reducing the maternal inspired oxygen content to 15 percent; fetal umbilical vein PO_2 decreased from 32 to 26 mmHg, but a much more substantial decrease in oxygen content occurred because the change was at the steep portion of the fetal oxyhemoglobin dissociation curve.

Maternal hyperventilation and a compensated respiratory alkalosis occur during normal pregnancy, as detailed above. However, during labor or asthmatic attacks, there is often a further decrease in PCO_2. Wulf and associates demonstrated a reduction of PO_2 in fetal scalp vein from 25 to 19 mmHg, when maternal PCO_2 decreased from 22 to 14 mmHg [142]. Two mechanisms were postulated: (1) maternal alkalosis resulting in increased affinity of maternal hemoglobin for oxygen, and decreased oxy-

Table 81-5. Effects of asthma on the outcome of pregnancy[a]

	No. of asthmatic pregnancies	Prematurity	Fetal outcome			
Study			Low birth weight	Congenital malformations	Spontaneous abortions	Mortality (perinatal)
Schaefer and Silverman [109] (1962)[b]	293	—	8.9/6.2	—	11/9.4	—
Gordon et al. [49] (1970)[b]	277	14.4/18	15.2/11.4	—	—	5.9/3.2
Bahna and Berkedel [7] (1972)[b]	381	7.4/5	7.1/3.7	—	—	5.8/3.0
Schatz et al. [114] (1975)[c]	71	14/10	—	2.8/3	1/10	0/2.8
Greenberger and Patterson [53] (1983)[c]	45	7.1/9	—	2.3/3.2	9/11	0/1.6
Fitzsimmons et al. [36] (1986)[c]	56	12.5/9.6	17.2/6.8	0/3	0/11	0/0.7
Stenius-Aarniala et al. [126] (1988)[d]	198	Not ↑	Not ↑	Not ↑	—	1/0.5
Apter et al. [6] (1989)	28	7	0	0	—	0
Lao and Huengsburg [76] (1990)[b]	87	3.4/1.1	10.3/1.1	3/0	—	2/0

[a] Data are presented in the form asthmatics/controls, in percentages.
[b] A concomitant control group was used in the study.
[c] The control value is the percent in the representative general population.
[d] Percent for each category was not available from the original data.

gen delivery, and (2) decreased uterine blood flow caused by maternal alkalosis, as seen in studies performed in sheep. This latter event leads to a drop in fetal pH and arterial PO_2. Thus, poorly compensated maternal respiratory alkalosis can lead to fetal hypoxia [108].

Fetal Outcome. Studies from 1962 to the present are summarized in Table 81-5. Earlier studies suggested a higher incidence of prematurity (<37 weeks of gestation), low birth weight (< 2,500 gm), spontaneous abortion, and perinatal mortality associated with pregnant asthmatics. For instance, Schaefer and Silverman (1962) compared 293 pregnant asthmatics with 30,000 control subjects and reported an increased incidence of low birth weight (8.9% versus 6.2%) and spontaneous abortions (11% versus 9.4%) in asthmatic pregnancies [109]. In 1970, Gordon and coworkers reported on 277 asthmatic pregnancies (30,861 control subjects) [49]. While there was no significant global increase in prematurity and low birth weight as in the former series, there was a twofold increase in perinatal mortality. Fully two-thirds of the mortality occurred in only 16 mothers who had uncontrolled asthma during pregnancy; moreover, the live infants of these mothers had a higher incidence of neurologic abnormality at 1 year old [49]. Bahna and Bjerkedal (1972) similarly found higher perinatal mortality in asthmatic pregnant subjects than in the general population [7]. In these studies, one gets the sense that the asthma was not always well controlled, and that patients with the worst-controlled asthma had worse fetal outcomes.

These studies must be contrasted with subsequent studies which showed that even severe asthma, if well controlled by systemic or inhaled steroids, carried no increased fetal or maternal mortality. As well, no increased incidence of congenital malformations was observed in 171 pregnancies in steroid-dependent asthmatics in three recent studies [36, 53, 114]. The study by Fitzsimmons and colleagues [36] is especially instructive; no neonatal or maternal deaths occurred in 56 pregnancies in 51 women with severe asthma requiring oral prednisone and/or inhaled beclomethasone dipropionate. Among those pregnancies with well-controlled asthma (no emergency therapy with epinephrine), the incidence of prematurity was the same as that in the general population (10% versus 9.6%), but there was a slight increase in low birth weight (12% versus 6.8%). However, among pregnancies requiring emergency therapy for exacerbations, there was a twofold increase in prematurity and fivefold increase in the incidence of low birth weight. These data again imply that improved fetal outcomes can be achieved if maternal asthma exacerbations are prevented during pregnancy. A similar conclusion was reached in a prospective study of 198 asthmatic pregnancies in Finland [126].

Similar results were observed in a recent study by Lao and Huengsburg [76]. Again, there was no increased incidence of prematurity, perinatal mortality, or maternal complications among the 87 asthmatic pregnancies. However, a higher incidence of low-birth-weight babies was observed. It is worthy of note that as in the earlier studies, pregnant asthmatics were more likely to receive epidural analgesia and have cesarean section than were the nonasthmatic control subjects.

The association of asthmatic pregnancy with lower infant birth weight was investigated in the Kaiser-Permanente Asthma-Pregnancy Study. A significant relationship was noted between both decreased birth weight and intrauterine growth retardation, and the decline in maternal pulmonary function during pregnancy [117]. Maternal hypoxia was postulated as the etiologic factor.

In summary, most modern data suggest that asthmatic pregnancies are not associated with an increased risk of prematurity or perinatal mortality if maternal asthma is under proper control during the gestational period. However, infants of asthmatic mothers may have a higher incidence of low birth weight; poor asthmatic control, as expected, leads to poorer fetal outcome.

Drug Safety in Pregnant and Nursing Asthmatics

Any drug used in any pregnancy must be carefully chosen; the potential therapeutic benefit must be weighed against any possible harmful maternal or fetal side effects. As a general rule, most of the drugs ordinarily used for the management of asthma are safe during pregnancy. However, there are some exceptions, and special precautions should be followed in order to avoid prescribing new medications whose effects on the fetus have not yet been fully observed.

The Food and Drug Administration (FDA) has published guidelines for prescribing medications to pregnant women [64, 105]. All drugs are classified into four groups. Class A drugs include those that have undergone proper controlled studies during pregnancy, and have been found to be safe. Among class B drugs are those that have not undergone rigorous studies, but have not thus far been associated with adverse effects in animal or human studies. Many antiasthmatic agents including ipratropium bromide, cromolyn sodium, and terbutaline belong to this group. Drugs that have been associated with adverse effects on fetal health in animals but not (yet) in humans are grouped as class C. Theophylline, prednisone, beclomethasone dipropionate, and metaproterenol fall into this category. Class D drugs are those with demonstrated adverse effects on human fetal health; they should virtually never be prescribed to the pregnant asthmatic. These drugs include inhaled triamcinolone acetonide, tetracy-

Table 81-6. Safety of selected drugs during pregnancy

Drugs	FDA* classification	Safety	Adverse effects/comments
Antibiotics			
Ampicillin/penicillin	—	S	
Cephalosporins	—	U	Not enough data
Chloramphenicol	D	X	Gray syndrome
Erythromycin	B	S	
Trimethoprim-sulfamethoxazole (Septra)	C	X	Hyperbilirubinemia
Tetracycline	D	X	Teeth/bone malformation
Anticholinergics			
Ipratropium bromide	B	S	
Antiinflammatory agents			
Systemic corticosteroids			
Dexamethasone	C	X	Cross into fetal tissue, teratogenic in mice
Hydrocortisone	—	S	
Methylprednisolone	—	S	Cross placenta poorly
Prednisone	C	S	
Prednisolone	C	S	
Inhaled corticosteroids			
Beclomethasone dipropionate	C	S	Beclovent only
Budesonide	—	U	
Flunisolide	C	U	
Triamcinolone	D	X	Teratogenic
Cromoglycates			
Cromolyn sodium	B	S	
Beta agonists			
Albuterol	C	S	May be tocolytic (in high doses)
Ephedrine	—		
Epinephrine	C	U	? Teratogenic
Fenoterol	—	U	
Isoproterenol	C	U	
Metaproterenol	C	U	Teratogenic in mice
Terbutaline	B	S	
Methylxanthines			
Aminophylline	C	S	(May delay labor, transient fetal distress)
Oxtriphylline	C	S	
Theophylline	C	S	
Iodides			
Iodides	D	X	(Fetal goiter)
Iodide-containing expectorants	D	X	

S = safety; X = contraindicated; U = unknown; — = not available.
* According to Food and Drug Administration (FDA) classification: A = drugs proved safe during pregnancy from controlled studies; B = drugs not associated with reported adverse effects in animal/human studies; C = drugs with adverse effects reported in animals, but not human studies; D = drugs with proven adverse effects during human pregnancy.
Source: Data obtained from B. B. Huff (ed.), *Physicians' Desk Reference.* Oradell, NJ: Medical Economics, 1990.

cline, and iodide-containing expectorants. Table 81-6 lists the current FDA recommendations for use in pregnancy of drugs commonly prescribed for asthmatics (see Chap. 59).

Corticosteroids

In the past, there has been some concern over the use of systemic corticosteroids in pregnancy, based mostly on animal studies. Fetal mice and rabbits exposed to systemic corticosteroids often develop congenital malformations (especially cleft palate), but the dosage employed is usually much higher than that recommended for humans [14, 34, 38]. Other concerns include placental insufficiency and neonatal adrenal insufficiency [103, 135]. Earlier studies in humans showed an increased frequency of stillbirth and fetal mortality in fetuses of mothers receiving steroids during pregnancy [136]. As well, two older series (studying patients receiving steroids in early pregnancy for a variety of systemic illnesses) had an incidence of 8.5 and 2.3 percent of cleft palate, which is usually 1.5 percent in the general population (reviewed in [5]). However, more recent clinical studies (which are reviewed below) did not demonstrate on increased risk of congenital malformations, stillbirth, or fetal mortality when the mother used inhaled or systemic corticosteroids during pregnancy [36, 53, 114].

The placental handling and fetal metabolism of specific steroid agents are of importance. Maternal cortisol and corticosterone cross rapidly into fetal tissues, and most of the cortisol is metabolized into an inactive form by fetal enzymes [94]. Dexamethasone and betamethasone cross the placenta in high concentrations [9, 128]. When given to the mother of a premature infant, methylprednisolone does not prevent the respiratory distress syndrome and is therefore thought to cross the placental barrier poorly [15]. Maternal prednisone and prednisolone cross the placenta very poorly; their effect on the fetus is thus likely minimal and may explain the low incidence of adrenal suppression in infants of mothers on prednisone therapy [94]. This suggests that prednisone and methylprednisolone would be the optimal oral and parenteral preparations to treat maternal asthma, with few effects expected on the fetus. As an aside, we note that while pregnant women treated with prednisone have had low urinary estriol secretion, there was none of the expected association with fetal distress or intrauterine growth retardation [93].

Recently, aerosolized corticosteroids have been widely used for the treatment of asthma. Greenberger and Patterson showed that inhaled beclomethasone dipropionate (mean dose, 335 µg/day) was safe during pregnancy, with no increase in perinatal morbidity or congenital malformation observed among 45 pregnancies in 40 women [53]. However, inhaled triamcinolone and flunisolide have been associated with teratogenicity and should be avoided [64, 105].

Beta-adrenergic Agonists

These agents are effective and widely used as bronchodilators, primarily in the inhaled form. We shall examine these agents in terms of their teratogenicity and potential for interference in uterine function.

The Boston Perinatal Collaborative Project (1977) showed that subcutaneous administration of epinephrine during the first trimester of pregnancy was associated with a significant increase in congenital malformations [59, 133]. Although these data are somewhat inconclusive (recall that severe asthma requiring epinephrine results in increased fetal wastage), it seems prudent to avoid epinephrine at least during the early gestational period. (Greenberger suggests that there are not enough data to exclude the use of parenteral epinephrine [52].) Animal studies suggest albuterol and isoproterenol may be teratogenic in mice [87]. However, no teratogenic effects were demonstrated in studies on oral ephedrine in humans [11]. The safety of metaproterenol and terbutaline has not yet been fully established in humans. Data regarding teratogenic effects of other newer beta-adrenergic agents are not available at present.

Sympathomimetic agents have the potential to reduce uteroplacental blood flow. Vasoconstriction in this circulation was demonstrated by intraarterial injection of epinephrine in pregnant monkeys, but was not found after intravenous administration of albuterol or terbutaline in other animal studies [17, 92]. Similar studies on humans have not been done. However, beta agonists are mostly used in the inhaled, low-dose form, and are thus minimally systemically active. Therefore, one would not expect these agents to have a clinically important vasoconstrictive effect on the uteroplacental circulation.

Intravenous beta-adrenergic agonists have also been used as tocolytic agents in premature labor [100, 129]. They inhibit uterine contractility by stimulating the uterine beta receptors, thus increasing intracellular cyclic AMP, which leads to uterine atony. Terbutaline is most frequently used in North America, but albuterol and metaproterenol are occasionally employed. While an interesting syndrome of noncardiogenic pulmonary edema has been associated with the use of these tocolytic agents during the peripartum period, this has not yet been observed in the treatment of asthma. In any case, the potential of these agents to prolong labor is at least a theoretic possibility.

In summary, inhaled beta-adrenergic agents are generally considered safe during pregnancy. The parenteral form of epinephrine may be associated with congenital malformations, and likely should be avoided during early pregnancy. In addition, systemic beta agonists should also be avoided near labor, as they may inhibit or prolong childbirth.

Methylxanthines

Theophylline and aminophylline are the most frequently used methylxanthines. They are discussed in detail in Chapter 58. Although large doses of intravenous aminophylline have been associated with digital malformations in animals [137], no teratogenic effects were observed with the use of theophylline in 117 pregnant women [59] and aminophylline in 76 pregnant females [55].

Maternal theophylline pharmacokinetics change in quantitatively important ways during pregnancy [127]. Higher dosages may be required during the second half of pregnancy due to an increase in the volume of distribution. In the third trimester, there is a 25 to 30 percent reduction in theophylline clearance, and levels may increase [19]. Xanthines have the potential to decrease uterine contractility due to inhibition of phosphodiesterase. On the other hand, one report revealed a *lower* incidence

of perinatal death and respiratory distress syndrome in infants of mothers receiving aminophylline during labor [55].

Theophylline rapidly crosses the placenta, and has the capacity to cause toxic effects on the fetus. Transient tachycardia, jitteriness, and vomiting have been observed in neonates of mothers receiving xanthines near term or during labor, even though the fetal theophylline level was within therapeutic limits [75]. Schatz suggested that theophylline may have a vasoconstrictive effect in certain vascular beds and may be associated with chronic gestational hypertension [111]. This has not been confirmed.

Anticholinergics

Inhaled ipratropium bromide (Atrovent) is sometimes used as a bronchodilator in the treatment of asthma. Ipratropium bromide is poorly absorbed systemically, and atropine-like side effects of dry mouth, visual impairment, and fetal tachycardia are uncommon. Furthermore, no increased risk of congenital malformation has been observed [85], though rigorous studies of its safety are not available.

Disodium Cromoglycate

Cromolyn sodium (Intal) is poorly absorbed after inhalation. About 8 percent of a 20-mg dose of cromolyn is absorbed systemically [28]. It is not known if this substance crosses the placenta, but huge parenteral doses did not show teratogenic effects in mice, rats, and rabbits [110]. In a French study using cromolyn in 296 pregnant females, the incidence of fetal malformation was not increased over that in the general population [141]. There was also no reported incidence of perinatal mortality or prematurity.

Immunotherapy

Allergic immunotherapy is sometimes given to these patients, for example, for allergic rhinitis. A study of 90 pregnant females who received immunotherapy during pregnancy did not demonstrate increased congenital malformations, prematurity, toxemia, or neonatal mortality [88]. The major important side effect seemed to be maternal anaphylactic reactions. Therefore, immunotherapy may be continued in those who have been receiving it prior to pregnancy. However, immunotherapy likely should not be initiated during the gestational period, since severe allergic reactions to the immunotherapy are more common in the first few weeks of hyposensitization.

Others

When taken in large quantities by pregnant women, iodides cross the human placenta and are capable of causing fetal goiter and possibly myxedema. Thus, expectorants containing iodides should be avoided during pregnancy and lactation. Like most drugs, antihistamines should be avoided during early pregnancy. Fetal malformations have been associated with hydroxyzine (Atarax) and possibly diphenhydramine [124]. Similarly, use of decongestants such as phenylpropanolamine and phenylephrine has been associated with congenital malformations and should be avoided [124]. Among antibiotics, tetracycline and estolate-based erythromycin are contraindicated. Sulfonamides should be avoided because they cross the placenta and may lead to kernicterus. Chloramphenicol, if given near birth, may cause the gray syndrome in infants.

This brief review, as well as Table 81-6, is primarily a general guideline. For detailed information concerning possible hazardous effects of specific drugs on maternal and fetal health, the reader is urged to consult FDA guidelines as well as the most recent publications.

Management of Pregnant Asthmatics

In general, the principles involved in the care of pregnant asthmatics are similar to those of nonpregnant patients; the goal is to maintain optimal control and avoid acute exacerbations [22, 52]. From the therapeutic standpoint, pregnancy can be divided into three phases: (1) from conception to term, (2) labor and delivery, and (3) the postpartum period. During each of these phases, there are different areas that require special attention.

Phase 1: Conception to Term

During this period, the goal of therapy is to maintain both maternal and fetal health. This can best be accomplished by keeping maternal asthma under optimal control. There are two important aspects to the management of asthma during this phase: (1) patient education and (2) careful selection of drugs, to minimize the harmful effects of drug therapy on the fetus. This latter is particularly important during the first trimester, when the fetus is particularly susceptible to the teratogenic effects of drugs.

Patient education should start prior to pregnancy; young women of childbearing age should be educated to maintain themselves free of exacerbations that might harm a fetus, even before they are aware that they are pregnant. As well, education is necessary to stress the need for asthmatic control in order to maintain both maternal and fetal health. In patients with labile asthma, home monitoring of peak expiratory flow rates can be very useful in early recognition of exacerbations. It should be emphasized to the patient that the outcome of pregnancy depends on optimal control of the asthma, and physician and mother should work as a team to achieve this goal [97]. One of the major causes of exacerbation of asthma during pregnancy is patient noncompliance [112]. Other aspects of the usual education of the nonpregnant asthmatic should be followed, as well.

The fetus is most sensitive to the teratogenic effects of drugs during the first trimester, especially the first few weeks. It is important for physicians to bear in mind that more than 50 percent of pregnancies are unplanned, and therefore they should prescribe only nonteratogenic drugs to females of the childbearing age. Further, physicians should ask to be notified when a patient is intending to become pregnant, and an effort be made to stabilize the asthma prior to conception. Medication that might have teratogenic effects should be avoided.

Drug treatment of the pregnant asthmatic differs little from that of the nonpregnant asthmatic [10, 21, 27, 52, 118]. For the patient with very mild asthma, one who has only a few attacks a month, these episodes can probably best be treated after onset with the inhalation of a beta-adrenergic bronchodilator. For many asthmatics, this may be all the therapy needed. Excessive use of beta-agonist inhalants should be avoided. Those who require regular use of beta-agonist inhalants should then start on an antiinflammatory inhalant. Inhaled beclomethasone during pregnancy is safe; at present, there are no data on the safety of newer preparations, including budesonide. However, inhaled triamcinolone and flunisolide should be avoided due to their teratogenic effects. Cromolyn can be used as an adjunct to appropriate patients, but should be discontinued if there is no improvement within 4 to 6 weeks.

Theophylline is another commonly used second-line agent after beta agonists. Although it is not associated with congenital malformation, it is transferred rapidly across the placenta and is associated with transient tachycardia and irritability in neonates exposed to the medication. Thus, maternal levels should be monitored carefully especially during the third trimester (when metabolism changes). Patients who have demonstrated a beneficial response to the drug previously may be maintained on it; for most others we believe an inhaled antiinflammatory agent would be a better alternative.

For pregnant asthmatics who continue to have symptoms despite regular use of inhaled beta agonist and corticosteroids, there should be no hesitation about initiating a short course of oral corticosteroids. If steroids are required on a long-term basis, inhaled corticosteroids should be added to reduce the oral dose required. Oral prednisone is usually used: It transfers poorly across the placenta and no teratogenic effects have been proved in humans, while methylprednisolone is the intravenous corticosteroid of choice. Studies have shown that there is no increased risk of congenital malformation and perinatal mortality in steroid-dependent pregnant asthmatics. On the contrary, poorly controlled asthma leads to fetal hypoxia and subsequently prematurity, low birth weight, and increased perinatal mortality.

If a pregnant patient has an acute asthmatic attack, she should be hospitalized if there is evidence of severe decompensation or maternal hypoxia. These patients should be treated aggressively, and oxygen is a cornerstone of therapy. Inhaled beta agonists should usually be administered; if parenteral beta agonists are to be given, terbutaline is preferred over epinephrine, because the latter has been associated with congenital malformations and may decrease uterine blood flow [111]. In addition, intravenous steroids (methylprednisolone) should be started. Patients who previously required theophylline for maintenance therapy may have intravenous aminophylline added after their theophylline level has been measured. It is important to search for precipitating factors (such as infection) and initiate suitable therapy. Patients should have monitoring with oximetry, and an obstetric consultation should be obtained for appropriate fetal monitoring. If the arterial PCO_2 becomes greater than 35 mmHg or arterial pH less than 7.35, the patient should be watched very carefully, and if she worsens, mechanical ventilation may be considered. It is a very rare occurrence for persistent maternal hypoxia or signs of fetal distress to lead to cesarean section if the pregnancy is near term.

Phase 2: Labor and Delivery

As mentioned previously, exacerbation of asthma usually occurs during the second trimester; severe attacks during labor are rare. As always, the key is to have the asthma under control prior to delivery. A few general principles of the management of pregnant asthmatics during labor and delivery are discussed.

In the majority of patients with well-controlled and mild asthma, no specific intervention may be necessary during labor. Therapy with antiasthmatic agents should be continued prior to delivery. The systemic effects of maintenance doses of inhalation beta agonist are minimal and can be used safely. Inhaled (preferably) or nebulized beta agonists can be used to relieve minor symptoms during labor; excessive doses (and the parenteral route) should be avoided because beta agonists can cause uterine relaxation, prolongation of labor, and even possibly uteroplacental insufficiency. Inhalational therapy with anticholinergic agents (Atrovent) and cromolyn can be used safely during labor.

For patients who have been taking systemic adrenal corticosteroids during pregnancy, a stress dose of hydrocortisone (e.g., 100 mg of hydrocortisone sodium succinate intravenously) should be administered on admission to the labor room (or 6 hours before delivery) and every 8 hours after delivery for 24 hours. Hydrocortisone is usually chosen because it crosses the placenta rapidly, and is thus able to provide the required physiologic surge of both maternal and fetal cortisols immediately before delivery [133].

Theophylline attains equal concentration in both maternal and fetal circulations. It can lead to transient distress in neonates exposed to it and decreased uterine contractility. Patients on oral theophylline may be continued with it, provided the level is maintained within the therapeutic range. However, intravenous aminophylline is likely best avoided during labor.

Narcotic analgesics are frequently used to relieve pain and anxiety during labor. Thus, they can reduce maternal hyperventilation, which is harmful. However, adverse effects of narcotics do occur; respiratory suppression and mucus accumulation from inhibition of cough must be watched for. As well, morphine may lead to histamine release and bronchospasm, but this does not occur frequently; morphine should be used judiciously.

Oxytocin increases uterine contractility, and has been frequently used in the induction of labor [48]. It has no effects on bronchial smooth muscle, and can be used safely in pregnant asthmatics. However, $PGF_{2\alpha}$ and PGE_2 (also used to induce labor) can cause severe bronchospasm and must be used cautiously in asthmatics [123].

Local or regional anesthesia has been the technique of choice during delivery in pregnant asthmatics. Spinal, epidural, and caudal techniques have been used successfully [50, 133]. These maneuvers can relieve pain as well as anxiety; this results in lower maternal ventilation and respiratory alkalosis and thus decreases the risk of fetal hypoxia. Furthermore, the trauma of endotracheal intubation is avoided, potent irritant gases are not applied to the lungs, and the patient is awake and able to cough immediately post partum. Furthermore, the risk of aspiration is low. This approach also avoids respiratory depression in the newborn from general anesthesia. Chloroprocaine and bupivacaine are probably the current drugs of choice, since they are better tolerated and more easily eliminated by the fetus [104]. In using spinal and epidural methods, it is essential to avoid respiratory suppression from a high epidural blockade. Supplementary muscle relaxation, if necessary, may be provided with decamethonium [112], which does not cross into the fetus. Vecuronium does not cause the histamine release seen with succinylcholine and tubocurarine, and it has been used in nonpregnant asthmatics [56]. However, its safety in pregnancy is not known at present.

On the other hand, general anesthesia may be necessary under certain conditions, including refusal or inability to tolerate regional anesthesia, status asthmaticus despite maximum therapy and with signs of fetal distress, and difficult breech presentation or complications of pregnancy that require intrauterine manipulation. Premedication or sedatives should be minimal. Narcotic analgesics should be used with caution. Induction should be accomplished with an oxybarbiturate such as methohexital; thiopental, which appears to be deleterious to the asthmatic, should be avoided. Halothane is the inhalational anesthetic agent of choice due to its bronchodilatory effects [62, 106]. Cyclopropane should not be used because it causes bronchoconstriction [47]. Maternal arterial PO_2 should be maintained above normal with supplemental oxygen to avoid fetal hypoxia. This obviates the use of nitrous oxide alone, which does not allow the use of high inspired oxygen tensions. The skill of the anesthesiologist is also an important factor.

Postoperative care will be dictated by the severity of the patient's asthma, and should include vigorous inhalation therapy with bronchodilators and physiotherapy to avoid mucus accumulation. Patients previously taking systemic corticosteroids should be continued with them during the postpartum period and then tapered according to their clinical status.

Phase 3: The Postpartum Period

The asthmatic condition tends to revert to the prepregnant state within 3 months after delivery. One study showed that there is no persistent deterioration of flow rate as a consequence of pregnancy. Patients should be followed frequently at first, and usual adjustments of therapy made, based on symptoms and pulmonary function changes. Once the asthma has been stabilized, routine follow-ups are all that is necessary.

The most frequent question raised by an asthmatic mother is whether she should breast-feed her infant. The advantages of breast-feeding are numerous. Maternal antibodies present in the milk provide immune defense to the infant, and protect infants against infective organisms and allergic antigens [63, 67]. Furthermore, lactation has no effect on the clinical state of maternal asthma [22]. Therefore, physicians should encourage breast-feeding in asthmatics. However, certain medications given to the mother can be transferred to the infant via the breast milk and can cause harmful effects. In general, medications that are considered safe during pregnancy can be administered during lactation. The theophylline level in milk is up to 75 percent of plasma levels [125]. It usually does not have detrimental effects; however, it may cause irritability and jitteriness of infants. One should also be aware of the effects of other medications on the clearance of theophylline, and monitor the levels under appropriate situations. Prednisone crosses poorly into breast milk, and would appear to be safe in moderate doses during breast-feeding. Tetracycline, sulfa drugs, iodides, and chloramphenicol should be avoided. Inhalation of beta agonists and beclomethasone is considered innocuous during breast-feeding. Inhaled cromolyn is poorly absorbed into the maternal circulation, and is probably safe during breast-feeding.

MENSES

Menses is a cyclic endocrinologic phenomenon, with primary manifestations within the female genitourinary tract. The ebb and flow of hormones has its major obvious effect in the "monthly weeping of the uterus," but some case reports and epidemiologic studies have related the menstrual cycle to variations in the severity of asthma. This section reviews the currently available data on the relationships between asthma and the menstrual cycle. We shall see that there is *likely* a premenstrual exacerbation in many women with asthma, most marked in those with more severe asthma. However, the causes for this recurrent phenomenon are far from clear.

Historical Aspects

The association between the menstrual rhythm and exacerbation of asthma in some females has long been observed. Frank, in 1931, was first to describe the phenomenon of worsening asthmatic symptoms prior to menses [37]. His observation was supported subsequently by Claude and Allemany [20] as well as Greene and Dalton [51], who reported, in total, 120 cases of premenstrual exacerbation of asthma. This clinical entity has been termed *premenstrual asthma* [32, 143]. Since then, there have been dramatic case reports correlating recurrent, severe, life-threatening asthmatic attacks within the premenstrual time frame. For instance, Lenoir recently reported three cases of severe premenstrual asthma, documenting the variation of asthmatic symptoms with the onset and cessation of menses [78]. Beynon and coworkers further correlated premenstrual worsening of symptoms with falls in peak expiratory flow rates of up to 400 L/min in three females [12].

Prevalence

Several authors have attempted to quantitate the prevalence of exacerbations of asthma with menses. Rees, in 1963, noted that 27 of 81 female patients out of an "unselected series" of patients from the St. David's Asthma Clinic had premenstrual asthma exacerbations, as noted by symptom scores [102]. This approximately 30 percent prevalence remains constant even in more modern series from different countries. In the United States, in 1986, a survey of 57 consecutive females under 50 years old in a pulmonary practice demonstrated that 19 (33%) of premenopausal females had worsening of asthma premenstrually [31]. Two similar studies in England by Hanley [57] and Gibbs and colleagues [45] revealed a similar percentage (Table 81-7). More

Table 81-7. Studies on premenstrual asthma

		Subjects		Symptoms worsening	Changes in airway function		
Study	Study type	Total	With PMA		PEFR	Spirometry	Methacholine challenge test
Rees [102] (1963)	Retrospective	81	27 (33.3%)	+	—	—	—
Hanley [57] (1981)	Retrospective	102	36 (35%)	+	+	—	—
					(mean ΔPEFR = −40 L/min, based on 8 patients)		
Gibbs et al. [45] (1984)	Retrospective	91	36 (40%)	+	+	—	—
					(mean ΔPEFR = −20 L/min, based on 21 patients)		
Eliasson et al. (1986)	Retrospective	57	19 (33.3%)	+	—	—	—
Pauli et al. [98] (1989)*	Prospective	11		+	+	No change	No change
					(mean ΔPEFR = −15 L/min, based on 11 patients)		

PMA = premenstrual exacerbation of asthma; PEFR = peak expiratory flow rate; — = data not available.
* Total number of subjects in the study was 40, but only 11 were asthmatics and were *not* aware of premenstrual worsening of asthmatic symptoms. Others were nonasthmatic.

importantly, both groups showed that at least in some patients, the worsening symptoms correlated with a slight decline in peak expiratory flow rate. One study suggested the prevalence of premenstrual asthma to be as high as 75 percent; however, the number of subjects was small (n = 27) and the study population might well have been biased toward women with more severe asthma [143]. Thus, in general, it seems likely that as many as one-third of female asthmatics may suffer premenstrual worsening of asthma.

The association of the menstrual cycle with asthmatic attacks is not only limited to the premenstrual period. A small proportion of female asthmatics have exacerbation during menses ("menstrual asthma"), instead of premenstrually: 3 (4%) of 91 females in Rees' study [102] and 2 of 57 asthmatics in Eliasson's study [31].

It should be cautioned that most of the above-mentioned studies were performed retrospectively and predominantly based on (subjective) symptom scores. Only two [32, 57] of the above-mentioned studies attempted to correlate the symptom scores with objective pulmonary function data. This is not just a theoretic concern; Rees, in his study, showed that all females with premenstrual asthma also had some symptoms of the premenstrual syndrome, and this could have had some influence on their perception of symptoms [102].

The best objective data on pulmonary function are found in a unique study from Canada investigating the relationship between airway function and the menstrual cycle in both normal women and asthmatics who were *not* aware of premenstrual exacerbations [98]. No menstrually related changes in peak flows, spirometric parameters, or airway reactivity (on methacholine challenge test) were detected in the normal subjects. The asthmatic women, as a group, had increased symptoms ($p < .001$), and a mild, but significant ($p < .045$) drop in morning peak expiratory flow rates before menses. However, no concomitant change in airway reactivity or spirometric data was observed. The authors made two interesting, but opposing suggestions. Either there really are very mild premenstrual exacerbations in asthma, or airway function is not affected by the menstrual cycle (but other factors that control performance on the peak flow test, e.g., muscle strength, may be influenced by the menstrual cycle). Thus, the association of menstruation with exacerbation of asthma certainly deserves more investigation, and the exact prevalence of premenstrual asthma, in our opinion, is still unknown.

Pathophysiology

What are the potential pathogenic mechanisms relating exacerbations of asthma with the menstrual cycle? Many different fac-

tors including psychological, hormonal, and immunologic processes have been postulated as causative. We start with the hormonal aspects, and examine the changes during a menstrual cycle. The array of hormonal changes that orchestrate the human menstrual cycle is complex, and mostly beyond the scope of this article (see reviews in [33, 119]). However, we summarize the chief events.

During menstruation, estrogen and progesterone levels are low. Production of follicular stimulating hormone (FSH) and luteinizing hormone (LH) by the pituitary starts to rise, and induces follicular growth. The ovarian follicle produces estrogen predominantly, at this time. At about the 10th day after the onset of menstruation, there is a "surge" in secretion of both FSH and LH (and estrogen), and ovulation occurs at the 14th day. Levels of FSH and LH drop thereafter. Estrogen secretion decreases and then increases. Progesterone secretion starts just after ovulation, peaks a week later (concomitant with a secondary peak of estrogen), and then falls to very low levels just at the start of menstruation (Fig. 81-2).

These complex events appear to involve complex regulation by the pituitary gland. Events external to the body can have a role, as well. For instance, close proximity between women in a college dormitory produces a significant degree of synchrony in the onset of menses (reviewed in [119]). As well, it is likely that prostaglandins and prostacyclin as well as catecholamines are involved in menstruation (see below).

The effects of various hormones on airway function have been reviewed in the previous section (see Table 81-2). Recent focus has been on the relationship of progesterone to premenstrual asthma. Progesterone induces uterine smooth muscle relaxation. The fall of progesterone prior to delivery is associated with increased uterine contractility. It has been suggested (with slim evidence) that the hormone may have a similar effect on bronchial smooth muscle, and may be a bronchodilator. During the menstrual cycle, the progesterone level rises after ovulation and falls just prior to menses; this fall has been suggested as a cause of premenstrual exacerbation of asthma. This is supported (in part) by a case report demonstrating that intramuscular injection of progesterone can prevent the premenstrual drop of peak expiratory flow rate in three females with severe premenstrual asthma [12]. However, the doses of progesterone used were high, not physiologic.

More recent investigations into the menstrual cycle have consistently been unable to shed light on the progesterone hypothesis, however. A study by Juniper and colleagues of bronchial hyperreactivity during pregnancy was unable to demonstrate changes in the airways that correlated strongly with progesterone levels [68]. Similarly, two studies failed to correlate changes

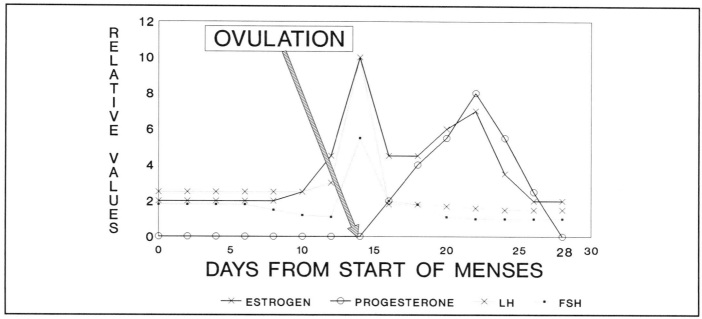

Fig. 81-2. *Hormonal changes during the normal human menstrual cycle. LH = luteinizing hormone; FSH = follicular stimulating hormone. (Redrawn from G. F. Erickson. Follicular Growth and Development. In Speroff, Simpson, and Sciarra (eds.), Gynecology and Obstetrics, Vol. 5. Philadelphia: Lippincott, 1991.)*

in progesterone level during menstrual cycle with pulmonary function tests or airway reactivity in patients with asthma, who had symptomatic changes premenstrually [98, 139]. Furthermore (and most important of all), most premenstrual asthmatic attacks occur 7 to 10 days before menses, which would coincide with the peak instead of the trough in progesterone level.

The other hormone group considered to be potential causative factors of premenstrual asthma are the prostaglandins. $PGF_{2\alpha}$ is a potent bronchoconstrictor and its level varies with different phases of the cycle. Koullapis and Collins reported that the $PGF_{2\alpha}$ metabolite, 13-14-diOH-15-keto-$PGF_{2\alpha}$, has two peaks during the menstrual cycle: the preovulatory and the premenstrual ones [73]. It is postulated that menstrually mediated asthmatic attacks were due to the surge of the $PGF_{2\alpha}$ level. However, Eliasson and associates were unable to document the premenstrual rise in the metabolite level in a subsequent study [30]. Furthermore, the same study showed that the asthmatic reaction to meclofenamate, a potent prostaglandin inhibitor, did not occur during the peak of $PGF_{2\alpha}$ level in the cycle. Thus, the association of $PGF_{2\alpha}$ with premenstrual asthma is, at present, not convincing.

The other factors during the menstrual cycle are many—a review of menstrual diseases mentioned over 100 factors that fluctuate during the menstrual cycle [83]! Rees postulated that important factors may include heightened emotional response during the menstrual period, increased autonomic lability, and increased hydration of bronchial wall [102]. However, the evidence establishing a link between these factors and premenstrual asthma is scanty. We must conclude that the current knowledge concerning causality of premenstrual asthma is quite limited.

Management

The management of females with menstrually related exacerbations of asthma should be no different from that of other asthmatics. Although there are many case reports in the literature of severe premenstrual asthmatic attacks that require assisted ventilation or other heroic therapeutic modalities, conventional antiasthmatic therapy as detailed in the other sections of this book

should be sufficient for the majority of women. Treatment modalities suggested for managing premenstrual asthma include diuretics (see review in [120]), nonsteroidal antiinflammatory agents (meclofenamate) [73], progesterone, and the birth control pill [12, 95]. A recent controlled clinical trial showed that meclofenamate did not prevent premenstrual asthmatic attacks [29]. Although severe premenstrual asthmatic attacks were prevented by intramuscular progesterone injection in three cases reported by Beynon and associates [12], this type of therapy should still be considered as experimental. Similarly, the role of the birth control pill has not been systematically studied, but it appears from some preliminary epidemiologic data that the pill does not influence this syndrome [45, 57]. In summary, there is inadequate knowledge, at present, to justify the use of these modalities in the management of premenstrual asthma. Until more information is available, conventional antiasthmatic therapy should be followed in the management of premenstrual asthma.

In this chapter, an overview of the relationships between pregnancy, menses, and asthma has been presented. Since the last edition of this book, there has been reasonable progress in the understanding of the effects of pregnancy on asthma and vice versa. In the distant past, pregnancy in the asthmatic was considered a high-risk event, associated with significant morbidity and mortality in both fetus and mother. Furthermore, there was concern about the safety of using corticosteroids during early pregnancy. Recent studies have given us the security of knowing that pregnancy in a woman with well-controlled asthma is as safe as that in normal females. Furthermore, corticosteroids can be used safely during pregnancy for controlling asthmatic symptoms, without an increased risk of congenital malformations. Thus, the primary goal in the management of pregnant asthmatics is, in fact, proper control of the asthmatic condition. In the next decade, emphasis in this field will likely focus on the molecular basis of asthma and accumulation of more data on the safety of potent aerosol steroids and other aerosol medications. When the molecular basis of asthma becomes clearer, then the focus in the pregnant asthmatic may (hopefully) shift to the prevention of asthma in the unborn child.

On the other hand, one cannot point to much recent progress in the understanding of the relationship between menses and asthma. An increased prevalence of asthma during the premenstrual period has been suggested; however, large prospective studies correlating worsening of symptoms with objective changes in airway function are needed to firmly establish this. Once this has been better defined, then a whole new area of research in asthma may ensue.

REFERENCES

1. Abelmann, W. H., et al. Effects of abdominal distension by ascites on lung volumes and ventilation. *Arch. Intern. Med.* 93:528, 1954.
2. Agell, D. W., et al. Pulmonary function in pregnancy. I; Serial observation in normal women. *Am. Rev. Tuberc.* 67:568, 1953.
3. Agnostini, E., and Mead, J. Statics of the Respiratory System. In W. O. Fenn and H. Rach (eds.), *Handbook of Physiology: Respiration.* Washington: American Physiological Society, 1964. Pp. 387–410.
4. Alaily, A. B., and Carrol, K. B. Pulmonary ventilation in pregnancy. *Br. J. Obstet. Gynaecol.* 85:518, 1978.
5. Apgar, V. The drug problems in pregnancy. *Clin. Obstet. Gynecol.* 9:623, 1966.
6. Apter, A. J., Greenberger, P. A., and Patterson, R. Outcomes of pregnancy in adolescents with severe asthma. *Arch. Intern. Med.* 149:2571, 1989.
7. Bahna, S. L., and Bjerkedal, T. The course and outcome of pregnancy in women with bronchial asthma. *Acta Allergol.* 27:397, 1972.
8. Baldwin, G. R., et al. New lung functions and pregnancy. *Am. J. Obstet. Gynecol.* 127:235, 1977.
9. Ballard, P. L., Granberg, P., and Ballard, R. A. Glucocorticoid levels in maternal and cord serum after prenatal betamethasone therapy to prevent respiratory distress syndrome. *J. Clin. Invest.* 56:1548, 1975.
10. Barnes, P. J. A new approach to the treatment of asthma. *N. Engl. J. Med.* 321:1517, 1989.
11. Barsky, H. E. Asthma and pregnancy. *Postgrad. Med.* 89:125, 1991.
12. Beynon, H. L. C., Garbett, N. D., and Barnes, P. J. Severe premenstrual exacerbations of asthma: Effects of intramuscular progesterone. *Lancet* 2:370, 1988.
13. Bianco, S., et al. Effects of prostacyclin on aspecifically and specifically induced bronchoconstriction in asthmatic patients. *Eur. J. Respir. Dis. Suppl.* 61:81, 1980.
14. Blackburn, W. R., Kaplan, H. S., and McKay, D. G. Morphological changes in the developing rat placenta after prednisone administration. *Am. J. Obstet. Gynecol.* 92:234, 1965.
15. Block, M. F., Kling, O. R., and Corsby, W. M. Antenatal glucocorticoid therapy for prevention of respiratory distress syndrome in the premature infant. *Am. J. Obstet. Gynecol.* 131:358, 1978.
16. Bonica, J. J. Maternal respiratory changes during pregnancy and parturition. *Clin. Anesthesiol.* 10:1, 1973.
17. Brennan, S. C., McLaughlin, M. K., and Chez, R. A. Effects of prolonged infusion of beta-adrenergic agonist on uterine umbilical blood flow in pregnant sheep. *Am. J. Obstet. Gynecol.* 128:709, 1977.
18. Caldwell, B. V., and Behrman, H. R. Prostaglandins in reproductive processes. *Med. Clin. North Am.* 65:927, 1981.
19. Carter, B. L., Driscoll, C. E., and Smith, G. D. Theophylline clearance during pregnancy. *Obstet. Gynecol.* 68:555, 1986.
20. Claude, F., and Allemany, V. R. Asthma et menstruation. *Presse Med.* 38:755, 1938.
21. Cockcroft, D. W., and Hargreave, F. E. Outpatient management of bronchial asthma. *Med. Clin. North Am.* 74:797, 1990.
22. D'Alonzo, G. E. The pregnant asthmatic patient. *Semin. Perinatol.* 14:119, 1990.
23. Danforth, D. M. *Obstetrics and Gynecology.* New York: Harper & Row, 1977. P. 462.
24. Day, J. H. Paying special attention to the pregnant asthmatic. *Allergy* 3(2):7, 1990.
25. Demey-Ponsart, E., et al. Serum CBG, free and total cortisol and circadian patterns of adrenal function in normal pregnancy. *J. Steroid Biochem.* 16:165, 1982.
26. Derbes, V. J., and Soderman, W. A. Reciprocal influences of bronchial asthma and pregnancy. *Am. J. Med.* 1:376, 1946.
27. DiMarco, A. F. Asthma in the pregnant patient: A review. *Ann. Allergy* 62:527, 1989.
28. Dykes, M. H. M. Evaluation of an antiasthmatic agent, cromolyn sodium. *JAMA* 227:1061, 1974.
29. Eliasson, O., et al. The effect of sodium meclofenamate in premenstrual asthma: A controlled clinical trial. *J. Allergy Clin. Immunol.* 79:909, 1987.
30. Eliasson, O., et al. Serum 13-14-diOH-15-keto-prostaglandin $F_{2\alpha}$ and airway response to meclofenamate and metaproterenol in relation to the menstrual cycle. *J. Asthma* 23:309, 1986.
31. Eliasson, O., Scherzer, H. H., and DeGraff, A. C. Morbidity in asthma in relation to the menstrual cycle. *J. Allergy Clin. Immunol.* 77:87, 1986.
32. Enright, T., et al. Cyclical exacerbation of bronchial asthma. *Ann. Allergy* 58:405, 1987.
33. Erickson, G. F. Follicular Growth and Development. In Speroff, Simpson, and Sciarra (eds.), *Gynecology and Obstetrics*, Vol. 5. Philadelphia: Lippincott, 1991.
34. Fainstat, T. Cortisol induced congenital cleft palate in rabbits. *Endocrinology* 55:502, 1964.
35. Fishburne, J. I., Jr., et al. Bronchospasm complicating prostaglandins $F_{2\alpha}$ for therapeutic abortion. *Obstet. Gynecol.* 39:892, 1972.
36. Fitzsimmons, R., Greenberger, P. A., and Patterson, R. Outcomes of pregnancy in women requiring corticosteroids for severe asthma. *J. Allergy Clin. Immunol.* 78:349, 1986.
37. Frank, R. T. The hormonal causes of premenstrual tension. *Arch. Neurol. Psychiatr.* 26:1053, 1931.
38. Fraser, F. C., Walter, B. E., and Fainstat, T. D. The experimental production of cleft palate with cortisone and other hormones. *J. Cell. Comp. Physiol.* 43:237, 1954.
39. Freedman, S. H., and Anderson, N. E. Spirometry and oral contraceptives. *Am. J. Obstet. Gynecol.* 116:682, 1973.
40. Fuchs, F., and Klopper, A. (eds.), *Endocrinology of Pregnancy.* Hagerstown, Md: Harper & Row, 1977.
41. Garfield, R. E., Kannan, M. S., and Daniell, E. E. Gap-junction formation in the myometrium: Control by estrogen, progesterone and prostaglandins. *Am. J. Physiol.* 238:81, 1980.
42. Garrad, G. S., Littler, W. A., and Redman, C. W. G. Closing volume during normal pregnancy. *Thorax* 33:488, 1978.
43. Gazioglu, K., et al. Pulmonary function during pregnancy in normal woman and in patients with cardiopulmonary disease. *Thorax* 25:445, 1970.
44. Gee, J. B. L., et al. Pulmonary mechanics during pregnancy. *J. Clin. Invest.* 46:945, 1967.
45. Gibbs, C. J., et al. Premenstrual exacerbation of asthma. *Thorax* 39:833, 1984.
46. Gluck, J. C., and Gluck, P. A. The effects of pregnancy on asthma: A prospective study. *Ann. Allergy* 37:164, 1976.
47. Gold, M. I. Anesthesia for the asthmatic patient. *Anesth. Analg.* 49:881, 1970.
48. Goodman, L. S., and Gilman, A. *The Pharmacological Basis of Therapeutics.* New York: Macmillan, 1975. P. 869.
49. Gordon, M., et al. Fetal morbidity following potentially anoxigenic obstetric conditions: VII. Bronchial asthma. *Am. J. Obstet. Gynecol.* 106:421, 1970.
50. Gottschlak, W. General Anesthesia in Obstetrics. In R. M. Wynn (ed.), *Obstetrics and Gynecology Annual.* New York: Appleton-Century-Crofts, 1973.
51. Green, R., and Dalton, K. The premenstrual syndrome. *Br. Med. J.* 1:1007, 1953.
52. Greenberger, P. A. Asthma during pregnancy. *J. Asthma* 27:341, 1990.
53. Greenberger, P. A., and Patterson, R. Beclomethasone dipropionate for severe asthma during pregnancy. *Ann. Intern. Med.* 98:478, 1983.
54. Greenberger, P. A., and Patterson, R. Management of asthma during pregnancy. *N. Engl. J. Med.* 312:897, 1985.
55. Hadjigeorgiou, E., et al. Antepartum aminophylline treatment for prevention of respiratory distress syndrome in premature infants. *Am. J. Obstet. Gynecol.* 135:257, 1979.
56. Hall, J. B., and Wood, L. D. H. Management of the critically ill asthmatic patient. *Med. Clin. North Am.* 74:779, 1990.
57. Hanley, S. P. Asthma variation with menstruation. *Br. J. Dis. Chest* 75:306, 1981.
58. Harman, E. M. Pulmonary problems of pregnancy. *Compr. Ther.* 11:26, 1985.
59. Heinonen, O. P., Slone, D., and Shapiro, S. *Birth Defects and Drugs in Pregnancy.* Littleton, Mass: Publishing Sciences Group, 1977.
60. Hensley, M. J., Saunders, N. A., and Strohl, K. P. Medroxyprogesterone treatment of obstructive sleep apnea. *Sleep* 3:441, 1980.

61. Hernandez, E., Angell, C. S., and Johnson, W. C. Asthma in pregnancy. *Curr. Concepts Obstet. Gynecol.* 55:739, 1980.
62. Hickey, R. F., et al. The effects of halothane and cyclopropane on total pulmonary resistance in dogs. *Anesthesiology* 31:334, 1969.
63. Hide, D. W., and Guyer, B. M. Clinical manifestations of allergy related to breast and cow's milk feeding. *Pediatrics* 76:973, 1985.
64. Huff, B. B. (ed.), *Physicians' Desk Reference.* Oradell, NJ: Medical Economics, 1990.
65. Hyman, A. L., Spannhake, E. W., and Kadowitz, P. J. Prostaglandins and the lung. *Am. Rev. Respir. Dis.* 117:111, 1978.
66. Jaffe, R. B. Endocrine Physiology of Pregnancy. In D. N. Danforth (ed.), *Obstetrics and Gynecology.* Hagerstown, Md: Harper & Row, 1977. Pp. 286–298.
67. Jelliffe, D. B., and Jelliffe, E. F. B. Breast is best: Modern meanings. *N. Engl. J. Med.* 297:912, 1977.
68. Juniper, E. F., et al. Improvement in airways responsiveness and severity during pregnancy. *Am. Rev. Respir. Dis.* 140:924, 1989.
69. Juniper, E. F., et al. Effect of pregnancy on airway responsiveness and asthma severity: Relationship to serum progesterone. *Am. Rev. Respir. Dis.* 143:S78, 1991.
70. Karim, S. M. M. Appearance of prostaglandin $F_{2\alpha}$ in human blood during labour. *Br. Med. J.* 4:618, 1968.
71. Knuttgen, H. G., and Emerson, K. Physiological response to pregnancy at rest and at exercise. *J. Appl. Physiol.* 36:549, 1974.
72. Kopp, L., Paradiz, G., and Tucci, J. R. Urinary excretion of cyclic 3'5' adenosine monophosphate and cyclic 3'5' guanine monophosphate during and after pregnancy. *J. Clin. Endrocrinol. Metab.* 440:590, 1977.
73. Koullapis, E. N., and Collins, L. N. P. The concentration of 13-14-diOH-15-keto-prostaglandin F2-alpha in peripheral venous plasma throughout the normal ovarian and menstrual cycle. *Acta Endocrinol. (Copenh.)* 93:123, 1980.
74. Kreisman, H., Van der Wiel, W., and Mitchell, C. A. Respiratory function during prostaglandin-induced labour. *Am. Rev. Respir. Dis.* 111:564, 1975.
75. Labovitz, E., and Spector, S. Placental theophylline transfer in pregnant asthmatics. *JAMA* 247:786, 1982.
76. Lao, T. T., and Huengsburg, M. Labour and delivery in mothers with asthma. *Eur. J. Obstet. Gynecol. Reprod. Biol.* 35:183, 1990.
77. Lehmann, V. Dyspnea in pregnancy. *J. Perinat Med.* 3:154, 1975.
78. Lenoir, R. J. Severe acute asthma and the menstrual cycle. *Anaesthesia* 42:1287, 1987.
79. Liggins, G. C. Prostaglandins and the onset of labour. *Acta Obstet. Gynecol. Jpn.* 34:1087, 1982.
80. Ling, W. Y., Marsh, J. M., and Lemare, W. J. Adenosine 3'5'-monophosphate in the plasma from human pregnancy. *J. Clin. Endocrinol. Metab.* 44:514, 1977.
81. Lucius, H., et al. Respiratory functions, buffer system and electrolyte concentrations of blood during human pregnancy. *Respir. Physiol.* 9:311, 1970.
82. Lyons, H. A., and Huang, C. T. Therapeutic use of progesterone in alveolar hypoventilation associated with obesity. *Am. J. Med.* 44:881, 1968.
83. Magos, A., and Studd, J. Effects of the menstrual cycle on medical disorders. *Br. J. Hosp. Med.* Feb:68, 1985.
84. Mathe, A. A., et al. Bronchial hyperreactivity to prostaglandin $F_{2\alpha}$ and histamine in patients with asthma. *Br. Med. J.* 1:193, 1973.
85. Mawhinney, H., and Spector, S. L. Optimum management of asthma in pregnancy. *Pract. Ther.* 32:178, 1986.
86. McGinty, A. P. Comparative effects of pregnancy and phrenic nerve interruption on the diaphragm and their relationship to pulmonary tuberculosis. *Am. J. Obstet. Glynecol.* 35:237, 1958.
87. *Med. Lett.* 23:81, 1981.
88. Metzger, W. J., Turner, E., and Patterson, R. The safety of immunotherapy during pregnancy. *J. Allergy Clin. Immunol.* 61:268, 1978.
89. Milne, J. A. The respiratory response to pregnancy. *Postgrad. Med. J.* 55:318, 1979.
90. Milne, J. A., et al. The effect of human pregnancy on the pulmonary transfer factor for carbon monoxide as measured by the single breath method. *Clin. Sci. Mol. Med.* 53:271, 1977.
91. Milne, J. A., et al. Large airways functions during normal pregnancy. *Br. J. Ostet. Gynaecol.* 84:448, 1977.
92. Misenhimer, H. R., et al. Effects of vasoconstrictive drugs on the placental circulation of the rhesus monkey. *Invest. Radiol.* 7:496, 1972.
93. Morrison, J., and Kilpatrick, N. Low urinary estriol excretion in pregnancy associated with oral prednisone therapy. *J. Obstet. Gynaecol. Br. Commonw.* 76:719, 1969.
94. Murphy, B. E., et al. Conversion of maternal cortisol to cortisone during placental transfer to the human fetus. *Am. J. Obstet. Gynecol.* 118:538, 1974.
95. Neinstein, L. S., and Katz, B. Contraceptive use in the chronically ill adolescent female: Part I. *J. Adolesc. Health Care* 7:123, 1986.
96. Nolten, W. E., and Rueckert, P. A. Elevated free cortisol index in pregnancy: Possible regulatory mechanisms. *Am. J. Obstet. Gynecol.* 139:492, 1981.
97. Patterson, R., Greenberger, P. A., and Frederiksen, M. C. Asthma and pregnancy: Responsibility of physicians and patients. *Ann. Allergy* 65:469, 1990.
98. Pauli, B. D., et al. Influence of the menstrual cycle on airway function in asthmatic and normal subjects. *Am. Rev. Respir. Dis.* 140:358, 1989.
99. Peterson, R. E. Cortisol. In F. Fuchs and A. Klopper (eds.), *Endocrinology of Pregnancy.* New York: Harper & Row, 1977. P. 1576.
100. Pisani, R. J., and Rosenow, E. C., III. Pulmonary edema associated with tocolytic therapy. *Ann. Intern. Med.* 110:714, 1989.
101. Prowse, C. M., and Gaensler, E. A. Respiratory and acid-base changes during pregnancy. *Anesthesiology* 26:381, 1965.
102. Rees, L. An aetiological study of premenstrual asthma. *J. Psychosom. Res.* 7:191, 1963.
103. Reinisch, J. M., et al. Prenatal exposure to prednisone in humans and animals retards intrauterine growth. *Science* 202:436, 1978.
104. Reisner, L. S. The Pregnant Patient and Disorders of Pregnancy. In J. Katz, J. Benumof, and L. B. Kadis (eds.), *Anesthesia and Uncommon Diseases.* Philadelphia: Saunders, 1982.
105. Romero, R., and Lockwood, C. The Use of Anti-asthmatic Drugs in Pregnancy. In J. R. Niebyl (ed.), *Drug Use in Pregnancy* (2nd ed.). Philadelphia: Lea & Febiger, 1988. Pp. 67–82.
106. Rosseel, P., Lauwers, L. F., and Baute, L. Halothane treatment in life-threatening asthma. *Intensive Care Med.* 11:241, 1985.
107. Rubin, A., Russon, N., and Goucher, D. The effect of pregnancy upon pulmonary function in normal women. *Am. J. Obstet. Gynecol.* 72:963, 1956.
108. Sachs, B. P., et al. Is maternal alkalosis harmful to the fetus? *Int. J. Gynecol. Obstet.* 25:65, 1987.
109. Schaefer, G., and Silverman, F. Pregnancy complicated by asthma. *Am. J. Obstet. Gynecol.* 82:182, 1961.
110. Schardein, J. L. *Chemically Induced Birth Defects.* New York: Marcel Dekker, 1985. P. 339.
111. Schatz, M. Asthma and pregnancy. *J. Asthma* 27:335, 1990.
112. Schatz, M. Asthma during pregnancy: Control is top priority. *Allergy Observer* 8(3):1, 1991.
113. Schatz, M., et al. The course of asthma during pregnancy, post-partum, and with successive pregnancy: A prospective study. *J. Allergy Clin. Immunol.* 89:509, 1988.
114. Schatz, M., et al. Corticosteroid therapy for the pregnant asthmatic patient. *JAMA* 233:804, 1975.
115. Schatz, M., and Zieger, R. An approach to asthma and rhinitis in pregnancy. *J. Respir. Dis.* 3:89, 1982.
116. Schatz, M., and Zeiger, R. S. Treatment of asthma and allergic rhinitis during pregnancy. *Ann. Allergy* 65:427, 1990.
117. Schatz, M., Zeiger, R. S., and Hoffman, C. P. Intrauterine growth is related to gestational pulmonary function in pregnant asthmatic women. *Chest* 98:389, 1990.
118. Schwartz, D. B. Medical disorders in pregnancy. *Emerg. Med. Clin. North Am.* 5:509, 1987.
119. Schwartz, N. B., and McCormack, C. E. Newer Concepts of Gonadotropin and Steroid Feedback Control Mechanisms. In J. J. Gold and J. B. Josimovich (eds.), *Gynecology and Endocrinology.* Hagerstown, Md: Harper & Row, 1981.
120. Settipane, R. A., and Simon, R. A. Menstrual cycle and asthma. *Ann. Allergy* 63:373, 1989.
121. Shirkey, H. C. Adverse Reactions to Drugs: Their Relation to Growth and Development. In H. C. Shirkey (ed.), *Pediatric Therapy.* St. Louis: Mosby, 1972.
122. Sims, C. D., Chamberlain, C. V. P., and deSwiet, M. Lung function tests in bronchial asthma during and after pregnancy. *Br. J. Obstet. Gynaecol.* 83:434, 1976.
123. Smith, A. P. The effects of intravenous infusion of graded doses of prostaglandins $F_{2\alpha}$ and E_2 on lung resistance in patients undergoing termination of pregnancy. *Clin. Sci.* 44:17, 1973.
124. Stablein, J. J., and Lockey, R. F. Managing asthma during pregnancy. *Compr. Ther.* 10:45, 1984.
125. Stee, G. P., et al. Kinetics of theophylline transfer into breast milk. *Clin. Pharmacol. Ther.* 28:404, 1980.

126. Stenius-Aarnala, B., Piirila, P., and Teramo, K. Asthma and pregnancy: A prospective study of 198 pregnancies. *Thorax* 43:12, 1988.

127. Sutton, P. L., et al. The pharmacokinetics of theophylline in pregnancy. *J. Allergy Clin. Immunol.* 61:174, 1978.

128. Taeusch, H. W., Frigoletto, F., and Kitzmiller, J. Risk of respiratory distress syndrome after prenatal dexamethasone treatment. *Pediatrics* 63:64, 1979.

129. Tepperman, H. M., Beydoun, S. N., and Abdul-Karim, R. W. Drugs affecting myometrial contractility in pregnancy. *Clin. Obstet. Gynecol.* 20:423, 1977.

130. Thomson, K. J., and Cohen, M. E. Studies on the circulation in pregnancy. II: Vital capacity observations in normal pregnant women. *Surg. Gynecol. Obstet.* 66:591, 1938.

131. Tulchinsky, D., and Ryan, K. J. (eds.), *Maternal-fetal Endocrinology.* Philadelphia: Saunders, 1980.

132. Turnbull, A. C., and Anderson, A. B. M. Endocrine control of human parturition. *Acta Obstet. Gynecol. Jpn.* 34:1094, 1982.

133. Turner, E. S., Greenberger, P. A., and Patterson, R. Management of the pregnant asthmatic patient. *Ann. Intern. Med.* 93:905, 1980.

134. Walker, S. R., Richards, A. J., and Paterson, J. W. The absorption, excretion, and metabolism of disodium (^{14}C) cromoglycate in man. *Biochem. J.* 125:27P, 1971.

135. Walsh, S. D., and Clark, F. R. Pregnancy in patients on long term corticosteroid therapy. *Scott. Med. J.* 12:302, 1967.

136. Warrell, B. W., Sheff, M. D., and Taylor, K. Outcomes for the fetus of the mother receiving prednisone during pregnancy. *Lancet* 1:117, 1968.

137. Weinberger, S. E., and Weiss, S. T. Pulmonary Diseases. In *Medical Complications in Pregnancy.*

138. Weinberger, S. E., et al. Pregnancy and the lung. *Am. Rev. Respir. Dis.* 121:559, 1980.

139. Weinmann, G. G., Zacur, H., and Fish, J. E. Absence of changes in airway responsiveness during the menstrual cycle. *J. Allergy Clin. Immunol.* 79:634, 1987.

140. Weinstein, A. M., et al. Asthma and pregnancy. *JAMA* 241:1161, 1979.

141. Wilson, J. Utilisation du cromoglycate de sodium au cours de la grossesse. *Acta Ther. Suppl.* 8:45, 1982.

142. Wulf, K. H., Kunzel, W., and Lehmann, V. Clinical Aspects of Placental Gas Exchange. In Longo and Bartels (eds.), *Respiratory Gas Exchange and Blood Flow in the Placenta.* Bethesda, Md: National Institutes of Health, 1972. Pp. 505–521.

143. Wulfsohn, N. L., and Politzer, W. M. Bronchial asthma during menses and pregnancy. *S. Afr. Med. J.* 38:173, 1981.

144. Yannone, M. E., McCurdy, J. R., and Goldfien, A. Plasma progesterone levels in normal pregnancy, labor, and the puerperium. *Am. J. Obstet. Gynecol.* 101:1058, 1968.

145. Zimert, I. *Respiratory Pharmacology and Therapeutics.* Philadelphia: Saunders, 1978.

Preoperative and Postoperative Considerations

82

Klaus K. Geiger
John Hedley-Whyte

Of 10,000 patients presenting for anesthesia, 3.5 percent suffer from asthma, with no difference between the sexes [35]. Asthmatic patients are more liable to have operative and postoperative complications [47], and the incidence is higher in males than in females. Approximately three-fourths of the complications are pulmonary; 5.6 percent of previously asymptomatic patients developed intraoperative bronchospasm [134]. Cardiac arrest occurred 20 times as frequently in an asthmatic population as in a control nonasthmatic group [24]. No significant correlation seems to exist between the severity of asthma and the complication rate [47]. Individuals with asthma are more prone to have allergies than is the general population [35, 59], and there is evidence that any patient with an allergy is at increased risk of morbidity and mortality from intravenous anesthetics [20, 21, 163–165]. Stein and colleagues [144] found that the frequency of postoperative pulmonary complications in patients with bronchopulmonary disease was 70 percent, as opposed to 3 percent in those with normal preoperative pulmonary function: Careful preoperative and postoperative care can reduce both rate and severity of complications in these patients [112, 134]. Successful management of an asthmatic patient undergoing anesthesia must commence with a thorough preoperative evaluation and proper therapeutic preparation.

IDENTIFICATION OF PATIENTS WITH ASTHMA

Patients may present for anesthesia without a known history of asthma because the symptoms were atypical or because the diagnosis was missed in the past or during the preoperative examination. A history of episodes of shortness of breath at night or during exercise should alert the anesthesiologist to the presence of bronchial asthma. Cholinergic urticaria, a form of physical urticaria precipitated by stimuli that increase core body temperature such as hot showers or physical exercise and episodes of pyrexia, has been associated with alterations in lung function consistent with asthma [138]. Significant falls in forced expiratory volume in 1 second (FEV₁), maximum midexpiratory flow (MMF), and specific conductance and a rise in residual volume have been found in these patients. Chronic persistent cough may be the sole presenting symptom of bronchial asthma [26, 69]. Findings on physical examination, chest roentgenograms, and spirometric tests at baseline may be normal. In this circumstance, only bronchial provocation tests may establish the diagnosis. Patients with a known history of asthma may belong to one of three groups: (1) asymptomatic, (2) asymptomatic with conventional therapy, and (3) symptomatic wheezing despite conventional therapy. Each group requires preoperative evaluation and administration of a proper therapeutic program to support the patient through the perioperative period.

PREOPERATIVE ASSESSMENT

Preoperative assessment of an asthmatic patient starts with a thorough history to identify potentially precipitating factors, seasonal variations, the frequency of attacks, time of the last attack, duration of the present attack, and the dependency on as well as the response to steroids, bronchodilators, and other drugs.

The young adults who had minor wheezes in childhood and who have been wheeze free for at least 3 years generally have normal lung function. However, there is an increasing incidence of abnormal lung function with increasing frequency of wheezing. About 60 percent of the young adults who have ceased wheezing have abnormal bronchial reactivity to inhaled histamine and should probably not be considered to have "grown out" of asthma [88].

The preanesthetic physical examination should consist of determinations of resting blood pressure and pulse rate, pulsus paradoxus, temperature, respiratory rate, accessory muscle use, dyspnea, and wheezing. Gross and microscopic examination of the patient's sputum aids the planning of the preoperative management. A chest roentgenogram should be obtained preoperatively in order to exclude clinically unrecognized pulmonary infiltrates and collapse. An unrecognized pneumothorax or pneumomediastinum can culminate in life-threatening complications during positive pressure ventilation.

The excessive use of bronchodilator therapy or therapeutic failure with bronchodilators increases the difficulties that the asthma patient faces while undergoing anesthesia. Other unfavorable perioperative signs include persistent airway obstruction, arterial hypoxemia, hypercapnia, overinflated lungs, and intercostal retractions. Cyanosis, systemic hypertension, and cardiac arrhythmias are alarming symptoms. Pulsus paradoxus has been proposed as a quantitative clinical index of severe asthma; a paradoxus greater than 10 mmHg indicates an FEV₁ of 1.25 liters or less [114]. Progressive fatigue and exhaustion with mild physical effort also place the patient in a high-risk category.

A disparity often exists between the patient's preoperative subjective assessment of his or her condition and objective assessment of functional performance. Some patients with chronic bronchial asthma do not seem to be aware of obvious airway obstruction. A study [67] on the impact of various behavioral coping styles on the symptomatology of asthmatic patients found that behavioral style and time of testing were more important determinants of the recognition of added resistive loads than was the presence or absence of asthmatic symptoms at the time of testing. Anxious dependent persons are less able to recognize added resistive loads than are adaptive or independent persons. Because of the rapid changes in asthma and the poor correlation between clinical findings and physiologic measurements, pulmonary function tests should be obtained in all asthmatic patients before anesthesia is induced. A clinically asymptomatic patient may still show some airway obstruction on spirometric tests; on the other hand, there may be a sense of irritation and persistent cough with little or no demonstrable airway obstruction. Appropriate therapy may thus reduce perioperative risk.

EVALUATION OF PULMONARY FUNCTION

Preoperative pulmonary testing is essential for two basic categories of patients. First are patients who do not exhibit obvious clinical signs of airway obstruction but do have a history of asthma. Pulmonary function tests in combination with bronchoprovocation tests should help to detect those who may develop complications during and after the period of anesthesia. Second are patients with a known history of asthma for whom pulmonary function tests are helpful (1) to assess the degree and type of airway obstruction, (2) to follow the response to therapeutic maneuvers, (3) to determine the operative and postoperative risk, and (4) to serve as a guide to postoperative care.

There is a good correlation between maximum voluntary ventilation (MVV) and FEV_1. A lack of correlation may reveal respiratory discoordination or fatigue, indicating the inability to sustain respiratory stress, an important factor in preoperative evaluation.

Patients scheduled for major elective surgery may require a more thorough physiologic evaluation. Investigation would include tests such as closing volume, flow-volume curves, frequency dependence of compliance, and body plethysmography. Differential pulmonary function tests are rarely warranted and only if lung resection is planned.

In the evaluation of the patient with asthma, it is equally important to determine the response to bronchodilators. An increase in MMF of 10 to 30 percent following aerosol bronchodilator therapy indicates a mild response; an increase of more than 30 percent is considered a marked response to the drug. In addition, the degree of irreversible abnormality provides a predictive value of the likelihood of complications occurring during recovery from anesthesia. For correct diagnosis and intelligent interpretation of a pulmonary function test, the anesthesiologist has to be familiar with the principle of the test and its limitations. Bronchial reactivity tests with inhaled bronchoconstrictor agents are commonly performed in subjects with asthma [103, 104] (see Chap. 39). An abbreviated methacholine challenge protocol (6–12 minutes) with comparable sensitivity has been described as a screening test for airway reactivity [13]. Unfortunately, these tests are limited in their clinical use because the response is largely determined by the degree of airway obstruction [127]. Use of the FEV_1 as a parameter on bronchial provocation tests can be misleading, since a prior deep inspiration can prevent changes in FEV_1 in some patients with asthma [127]. The usefulness of the maximum expiratory flow-volume curve with air and low-density gas mixtures in following changes in lung function of individual patients must be questioned because within subjects the variability of the $\Delta \dot{V}_{50}$ and $V_{ISO} \dot{V}$ is so great [10, 11, 174]. Body plethysmography may introduce important errors in lung volume measurements in asthmatics. Some of the previously reported acute increases in total lung capacity (TLC) in asthmatic patients may be artifactual [135, 142].

In asymptomatic asthmatic patients, blood gas measurements are often completely normal [161, 172]. On the other hand, patients may demonstrate mild arterial hypoxemia for several weeks despite resolution of their expiratory flow obstruction [156]. A diminished arterial carbon dioxide pressure ($PaCO_2$) is the result of a variety of hyperventilatory stimuli or of a compensatory mechanism to maintain a normal arterial oxygen pressure (PaO_2) and may suggest impaired gas exchange, or an error in performing the arterial puncture. A decrease in PaO_2 and a rise in $PaCO_2$ with exercise suggest limited reserve. Hypoxemia of

varying degrees and a low $PaCO_2$ are sometimes encountered in symptomatic patients, while in status asthmaticus, hypoxemia and hypercapnia with respiratory acidosis may supervene. Hypercapnia is a finding that signals advanced or life-threatening respiratory impairment [168] (see Chap. 73).

There appears to be no close relationship between inequalities in the ratio of alveolar ventilation to perfusion ($\dot{V}_A/\dot{Q}$) and airway obstruction as determined by spirometry [128, 161]. Patients with marked airway obstruction show normal $\dot{V}_A/\dot{Q}$ distribution, while on the other hand, severe $\dot{V}_A/\dot{Q}$ imbalance can be observed in the presence of only mild airway obstruction. It is probably the degree of obstruction of the peripheral airways that determines the extent of impairment of gas exchange.

PREANESTHETIC MANAGEMENT

Asymptomatic Patients

Preoperative therapy of asymptomatic patients should concentrate on the prevention of a new asthma attack, improvement of pulmonary function, and treatment of coexisting disorders. Precipitating factors and offending allergens must be identified and eliminated whenever possible. For example, ethanol has been found to induce asthma in certain individuals [45, 50]. Not only active smoking but also passive smoking may harm the asthmatic. Exposure to sidestream cigarette smoke for 1 hour produces a significant decrease in both FEF_1 and $FEF_{25-75\%}$ (forced expiratory flow, mid–expiratory phase); the impairment in pulmonary function is linear over the 60-minute exposure. Identical conditions cause no measurable effect in nonasthmatic patients [28]. Smoking also interferes with mucociliary transport and alveolar macrophage defense mechanisms, and hence should be stopped at least 1 week before surgery to control bronchoconstriction, sputum production, and cough. Elective surgery should be scheduled with regard to seasonal allergic factors. Since infection is a predisposing factor that can precipitate episodes of bronchial obstruction and mucoid hypersecretion, any active infection should be cleared with the appropriate antibiotics in combination with physical therapy. Hyperreactivity caused by viral infections is present for at least 3 weeks following symptomatic recovery [38]. Sinobronchitic disease and otitis media can trigger an attack and should therefore be treated. In patients with nasal polyps, an aspirin triad that has been described includes aspirin sensitivity, nasal polyps, and asthma; aspirin should be avoided in these patients. Physical exertion and emotional stress have to be avoided, since they can evoke severe bronchospasm. Coexisting medical conditions that may adversely affect the anesthetic and postoperative course, such as anemia, fever, obesity, heart failure, and other pulmonary problems, should be treated.

Symptomatic Patients

No elective surgery should be performed in patients suffering from unstable asthma or an asthmatic attack. Full medical care should be provided and symptoms should be well controlled before anesthesia is delivered. Pharmacologic treatment has to be combined with adequate hydration to promote mobilization and clearance of secretions. A chest x-ray film showing infiltrates, fever, an elevated white blood cell count, and purulent sputum warrants antibiotic therapy. Instruction in breathing exercises, aerosol therapy, and incentive deep breathing modalities is part of successful preoperative management. This instruction helps with the postoperative care by defining the most effective therapy for the patient. Most nonasthmatic children under about 18 months old with wheezing bronchitis do not respond to bronchodilator agents [129]; adequate bronchodilator drugs must be employed in all other asthma patients. The effect of therapy has to be monitored closely by sequential clinical, spirometric, and blood gas measurements; otherwise, frank respiratory failure may develop. A rising $PaCO_2$ to normal values (40–45 mmHg) may signal either an improvement of the pathophysiologic derangement or ventilatory exhaustion as the attack progresses [168]. If a patient does not respond to one kind of therapy, one should always reconsider the underlying pathophysiology of airway obstruction. Clinically, beta-adrenergic resistance is not common [154]; in most instances, there are other causes such as mucus plugging, inflammation, and edema. Beta-adrenergic stimulators do not affect these factors; other agents such as steroids and antibiotics are then indicated. If the acute attack progresses despite full conventional therapy and the patient develops gross respiratory failure as manifested by hypoxemia (PaO_2 < 70 mmHg), hypercapnia ($PaCO_2$ > 50 mmHg), respiratory acidosis, and cardiovascular instability (systemic hypertension or hypotension, arrhythmias), endotracheal intubation and ventilatory support are necessary. Surgery at this point is deferred. When surgery cannot be delayed, a full therapeutic program must be instituted without an extensive preoperative evaluation. Depending on the urgency of the operation, the preoperative workup of the patient should include the measurement of FEV_1 or maximum expiratory flow rate (MEFR) before and after inhalation of a beta-sympathomimetic aerosol to assess the degree of airway obstruction and its reversibility, which is important for postoperative management. If the FEV_1 is reduced to below 40 percent of the total measured vital capacity, one should anticipate possible ventilatory failure and the need for mechanical ventilatory support [168]. An arterial blood gas analysis and appropriate subsequent monitoring guides the postoperative care of the patient. There is enough time before or during the anesthesia period and surgery to obtain a chest roentgenogram and an electrocardiogram (ECG). Blood should always be sampled for determination of hemoglobin, hematocrit, white blood cell count and differential, and electrolyte, blood urea nitrogen (BUN), and blood glucose levels. A sputum examination should be performed. If the patient could not raise any sputum preoperatively, a sample should be aspirated after intubation of the trachea.

Table 82-1 summarizes preoperative risk factors.

EFFECT AND INTERACTION OF THERAPY WITH ANESTHESIA

Aminophylline

Aminophylline is undoubtedly still a widely used bronchodilator agent in the treatment of asthma; however, there is a trend away from its routine use. Its central effects include stimulation of the medullary respiratory center, increase of sensitivity to carbon dioxide [166], decrease in the respiratory threshold for carbon dioxide without altering carbon dioxide sensitivity [34, 46], and an increase of hypoxic ventilatory response [80]. Aminophylline improves the contractility of the diaphragm (fatigued and nonfatigued) and probably also the intercostal and accessory muscles in a dose-related manner [5, 136].

The effect of aminophylline on arterial oxygenation in asthmatic patients is variable [52, 118, 151]. Studies have indicated that large areas of low ventilation persist after bronchodilator use in asthmatic subjects in spite of improvement in airflow rates, and these areas receive a disproportionately high fraction of total pulmonary perfusion [17, 73, 117]. This may be the result of a drug-related loss of pulmonary vasoconstriction to alveolar hypoxia. Aminophylline can produce paradoxical worsening of oxygenation soon after having been given to asthmatics [73, 117]. The effect on the cardiovascular system consists of increases in heart rate, stroke volume, and cardiac output and decreases in venous tone, systemic vascular resistance, and pulmonary capil-

Table 82-1. Preoperative risk factors in asthma

Clinical signs
  Persistent cough
  Sputum production
  Dyspnea
  Reduced exercise tolerance
Physical examination
  Rales and rhonchi
  Wheezing
  Emphysema
  Intercostal retractions, sternocleidomastoid retraction
  Fever
  Tachycardia > 100/min
  Pulsus paradoxus > 30 mmHg of blood pressure
  Cor pulmonale
  Clubbing
  Cyanosis
Radiologic findings
  Air trapping
  Vascular markings
  Enlargement of the heart
  Infiltrates
Laboratory findings
  Leukocytosis with infectious neutrophilic shift to the left
  Eosinophilia
  Sputum: thick, sticky, purulent; possible pathogenic bacteria
Pulmonary function
  FEV_1 < 1.0 liter
  FVC < 1.5 liters
  FEV_1/FVC < 30%
  MEFR < 200 L/min
  MVV < 50% of predicted
  PEFR < 50% of predicted
  Less than 20% improvement in FVC or FEV_1 following
    bronchodilator application
Arterial blood gas analysis
  PaO_2 < 70 mmHg at room air
  $PaCO_2$ < 38 mmHg
  Respiratory alkalosis, metabolic acidemia
Coexisting disorders
  Preexisting pulmonary diseases
  Cardiovascular disease
  Neuromuscular disorders
  Psychogenic disorders
  Infection
  Maxillary sinusitis
  Otitis media
  Kyphoscoliosis
  Limitation of diaphragmatic excursion
  Wasting diseases, malnutrition
  Anemia
  Obesity (> 30% overweight)
  Heavy smoking (> 10 cigarettes/day)
  Older age

FEV_1 = forced expiratory volume in 1 second; FVC = forced vital capacity; MEFR = maximum expiratory flow rate; MVV = maximum voluntary ventilation; PEFR = peak expiratory flow rate.

lary wedge pressure. Preoperative administration of aminophylline followed by halothane anesthesia results in tachycardia and ventricular arrhythmias [7, 123, 147]. The clearance rates of aminophylline are affected by many factors [74, 102]. Patients with pneumonia, heart failure, or liver cirrhosis have lower clearances than do patients with uncomplicated asthma or bronchitis [74, 86, 111]. Heavy smokers have significantly higher theophylline clearance rates than do nonsmokers [72, 74, 111]. Acute fever, obesity, and age decrease the clearance of theophylline [74]. The effects of acidosis and PaO_2 are contradictory [36, 102, 120, 158, 169]. A number of drugs including allopurinol [85], erythromycin [79], cimetidine [71], and phenytoin [87] have been shown to alter the half-life of theophylline. Premature infants have an extremely

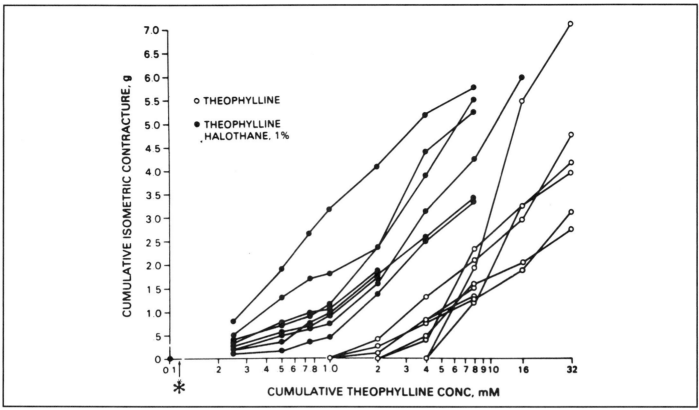

Fig. 82-1. *Cumulative dose-response curve between changes in resting tension (g) and theophylline concentration (mM) (with or without the addition of 1% halothane to the bath), using a logarithmic scale. The asterisk and arrow indicate the upper limit of expected theophylline therapeutic serum concentration, 0.11 mM in humans. Two muscle fascicle responses from each of four patients susceptible to malignant hyperthermia were subjected to each treatment. Theophylline without halothane did not produce a contracture at a concentration of less than 1 mM. From the theophylline dose-response curve, it can be estimated that 1.5 mM would be necessary to initiate a contracture—approximately 10 times the maximal therapeutic level. Extrapolating these results to a clinical setting, sufficient theophylline to induce malignant hyperthermia is not expected to be administered when treating bronchospastic disease. (Reprinted with permission from E. H. Flewellen and T. E. Nelson. Is theophylline, aminophylline, or caffeine (methylxanthines) contraindicated in malignant hyperthermia susceptible patients? Anaesth. Analg. 62:115, 1983.)*

low plasma theophylline clearance rate [4]. Therefore, preoperative monitoring of serum concentration levels is mandatory to avoid intraoperative cardiac complications [146, 147]. Theophylline stimulates the neuromuscular junction [143]. A neuromuscular block by pancuronium has been antagonized by supratherapeutic serum theophylline concentrations [33]. Based on animal studies [81], it has been said that aminophylline is contraindicated in patients susceptible to malignant hyperthermia [149], but a clinical report [42] studying four patients susceptible to malignant hyperthermia does not support this conclusion. The results argue for the cautious administration of aminophylline or theophylline to malignant hyperthermia patients who have a clinical need for these bronchodilators. It is important that serum levels do not exceed the recommended therapeutic range (Fig. 82-1). Such patients, however, should not receive halothane. See also Chapter 58.

Beta Sympathomimetics

Epinephrine and isoproterenol can cause severe arrhythmias (see Chap. 78). This effect is even more pronounced when hypoxemia and acidosis are present. Halothane sensitizes the myocardium to the arrhythmogenic effects of catecholamines and increases the frequency of arrhythmias. Administration of

isoproterenol and epinephrine can lead to worsening of arterial oxygenation despite an improvement in ventilation. The cause is an intrapulmonary redistribution of pulmonary blood flow to areas with low ventilation-perfusion ratios [128, 161]. Terbutaline, a selective beta agonist, decreases systemic arterial pressure and systemic vascular resistance. Severe cardiovascular instability has been observed in patients with acute quadriplegic and autonomic dysfunction [110]. Based on observations in Basenji greyhound dogs that intravenous albuterol (2.5 µg/kg) significantly attenuated the pulmonary response to histamine during halothane anesthesia (beyond the attenuating effect of halothane alone) Tobias and Hirshman concluded that $beta_2$-selective agonists, such as albuterol, are the agents of choice to treat bronchospasm in patients anesthetized with inhalational anesthesia [176].

Steroids and Adrenocortical Function

Preoperatively there is a marked increase in adrenocortical hormone output resulting from fear and anxiety. This response can be abolished by a number of premedication agents such as barbiturates and diazepam. Meperidine lacks this blocking effect when given 1 hour preoperatively in a dose of 2 mg/kg of body weight [107]. No form of general anesthesia can fully suppress the normal pituitary-adrenocortical response to the stressful effect of surgery. Although both spinal and epidural anesthesia will result in considerably less hormonal response than that seen during general anesthesia, there is a small but significant increase in plasma cortisol levels [105, 106]. Muscle relaxants appear not to affect the adrenocortical response.

Steroid treatment causes suppression of the hypothalamic-pituitary-adrenal system [99] (see Chap. 62). The degree of suppression is dependent on the dosages used in steroid therapy and the duration of administration. The use of large doses of topical corticosteroids such as beclomethasone dipropionate can also cause adrenal insufficiency. Supplemental doses of systemic steroids may be required at times of stress. When corticosteroids are administered for a brief period (e.g., 2 weeks), the suppression is transient, and adrenal function will return to normal within 2 weeks after discontinuation of steroid therapy. On the other hand, the administration of any amount of corticosteroid equivalent to or greater than the normal daily output (20 mg of hydrocortisone) for a prolonged period (e.g., >6 months) may result in profound suppression of the hypothalamic-pituitary-adrenal axis. If the dosage and duration of corticosteroid administration are sufficient to suppress endogenous steroid production completely, normal function of the axis may not be restored until 9 to 12 months after discontinuation [51]. Based on these data, it has been recommended to supplement corticosteroids in patients undergoing surgery if they had been taking suppressive doses of steroids at any time within a year of surgery [140]. Various regimens of replacement have been recommended. The regimen of corticosteroid coverage that we apply for patients with proved or suspected hypothalamic-pituitary-adrenal suppression is as follows: 50 to 100 mg of hydrocortisone phosphate or hydrocortisone hemisuccinate as a bolus 30 minutes before the induction of anesthesia, immediately followed by an infusion containing 200 mg of hydrocortisone in normal saline solution at a rate of 10 mg/hr over the next 24 hours. In the following 2 postoperative days the total daily dose is reduced to 150 mg and 100 mg, respectively, given as a continuous infusion over 24 hours. Thereafter, corticosteroids can rapidly be tapered so that at the end of the first postoperative week, steroid therapy can be discontinued or adjusted to the preoperative baseline requirement, provided there are no postoperative stressful complications. The steroid-dependent asthmatic patient should have serial plasma cortisol monitoring so that the dose can be adjusted to maintain plasma cortisol levels at about 100 μg/100 ml [37]. Hydrocortisone is preferred to cortisone acetate. The substance should be given intravenously to ensure adequate steroid levels at a time when they are needed. There is also evidence that the nonsteroid-treated asthmatic patient may likewise be less responsive to adrenocorticotropic hormone (ACTH) stimulation [22, 122]. Under repeated stress, a reduction in adrenocortical reserve is more likely the longer the patient has continuous asthma. Steroid therapy can be responsible for impairment of lung function in obese asthmatic subjects. A decrease in respiratory muscle strength leading to diminished vital capacity and TLC has been demonstrated in some obese asthmatic patients who were on long-term steroid therapy, whereas other asthmatic patients of similar body weight and approximate severity of disease do not show this restrictive pattern when lung volumes were compared [95]. Pharmacologic doses of corticosteroids may interfere with normal wound healing, predispose to infection, and induce catabolic states. Other postoperative problems related to corticosteroid therapy are diabetes mellitus, hypertension, hyperglycemia, hypokalemia, and osteoporosis. A feared complication of steroid therapy presumably is gastrointestinal bleeding; therefore, some patients should prophylactically receive antacid therapy. Cimetidine has been found to aggravate asthma [131, 132, 155].

Table 82-2. Advantages of pulse oximetry

1. Noninvasive
2. Continuous real-time information
3. No calibration
4. No skin heating
5. May be left in place for many hours
6. Rapid response time (5–7 seconds)
7. Minimal saturation error (1–2%) over the range of 60% to 90% saturation
8. Unaffected by skin pigmentation

Source: A. F. Stasic. Monitoring: What Is Helpful and What Is Not. In J. M. Civetta, et al. (eds.), *Critical Care.* Lippincott: Philadelphia, 1988. Reprinted with permission.

Table 82-3. Limitations of pulse oximetry

1. Loss of adequate pulsations
   a. Significant hypothermia
   b. Significant hypotension (i.e., mean arterial pressure less than 50 mmHg)
   c. Infusion of vasoconstrictive drugs (e.g., norepinephrine)
   d. Direct arterial compression
2. Inadequate hemoglobin (e.g., anemia, hemodilution)
3. Intravascular dyes (e.g., indocyanine green, methylene blue, or indigo carmine red)
4. Extraneous movement (e.g., shivering, exercise)
5. Pulsating venous blood (tricuspid regurgitation, cor pulmonale, or hepatic congestion)
6. Dysfunctional hemoglobins (i.e., hemoglobins that are not available for reversible binding to oxygen)
   a. Carboxyhemoglobin (COHb), which results in a *higher* saturation reading, the ratio of which is approximately 1:1. For example, if the pulse oximeter reads 100% and the percentage of COHb is 7%, then the true oxyhemoglobin fraction is 93% (100% − 7%).
   b. Methemoglobinemia (MetHb), which results in a *lower* saturation reading, the ratio of which is approximately 1:1.
7. Fetal hemoglobin (HbF), which results in a lower saturation reading. To obtain the accurate fractional oxyhemoglobin, a correction formula is required.
8. Overestimation of SaO_2 below 65% saturation

Source: A. F. Stasic. Monitoring: What Is Helpful and What Is Not. In J. M. Civetta, et al. (eds.), *Critical Care.* Lippincott: Philadelphia, 1988. Reprinted with permission.

PERIOPERATIVE MONITORING

In symptomatic patients, a central venous line is to be preferred, as it facilitates the management of an asthma attack. Pulse oximetry should be started (Fig. 82-2 and Tables 82-2 and 82-3). High-risk patients should receive a pulmonary artery catheter to guide fluid therapy. An arterial line is very helpful for close monitoring of blood gases and arterial pressure. A temperature probe should be in place in order to control body temperature. ECG monitoring is mandatory for early detection of arrhythmias and ischemic changes. Ventilators equipped with a pressure gauge allow the measurement of the inspiratory pressure. Determination of the expiratory tidal volume with a spirometer enables calculation of the compliance. An increase of the inspiratory pressure may signal the start of, a change in, or a worsening of airway obstruction. Some ventilators allow the continuous registration of airway resistance. A chest drainage set should be on hand in case a pneumothorax develops, a complication more frequent in asthmatic patients [121].

PREANESTHETIC MANAGEMENT

The efforts in preanesthetic management should concentrate on a smooth induction period in order to prevent an acute attack. A prerequisite for achieving this goal is the establishment of a good relationship between the anesthesiologist and the patient.

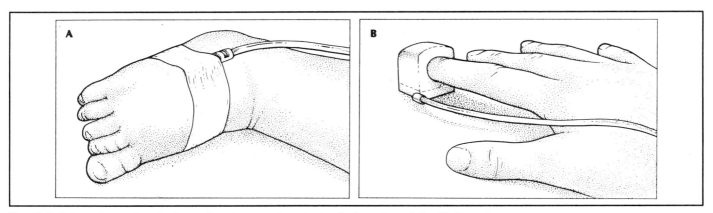

Fig. 82-2. *Pulse oximetry is a simple, noninvasive way of monitoring for hypoxia and should always be employed during anesthesia for asthmatic patients. A variety of pulse oximeters are available, including flexible probes for neonatal and pediatric patients (A) and finger probes for adults and older children (B). (Reprinted with permission from S. Pusker. Painful Procedures. In C. A. Warfield (ed.),* Manual of Pain Management. *Philadelphia: Lippincott, 1991. Pp. 227–230.)*

An open discussion of the problems and the assurance that one understands the worries of the patient help to alleviate anxieties and fears. The patient is concerned not only about anesthesia, the operation, and the result but also about whether the asthma will affect the outcome. Good psychological support will enhance the effect of any type of premedication. A good night's sleep is important; thus, a sedative should be prescribed. The operation should be scheduled for the morning to keep the time of apprehension during the waiting period short. The premedication consisting of a short-acting barbiturate or a sedative such as diazepam should be administered early enough to dampen emotional stress. The route of administration should be carefully considered in children to avoid provoking an acute episode. The use of barbiturates has been criticized on the basis of their metabolic interaction with asthma medications that the patient needs for treatment of his or her disease. The elimination rate of steroids and bronchodilators such as aminophylline has been shown to be enhanced by microsomal enzyme induction [23, 74]. An antihistamine with both sedative and drying properties may be an alternative. Opioids are to be avoided because of their central depressant and other effects [109]. The use of anticholinergic drugs is an advantage due to their bronchodilating properties. A reduction in the resting bronchomotor tone is likely to decrease the bronchoconstrictive response to irritant stimuli such as tracheal intubation. The bronchodilating action of atropine is clinically significant, however, only when large systemic doses (> 1–2 mg) are administered. Such doses effectively block reflex bronchoconstriction caused by airway irritation [133, 137] but produce undesirable side effects including tachycardia and central nervous system symptoms. Glycopyrrolate given in doses commonly used as preanesthetic medication dilates large and small airways to the same extent as atropine, but the effect is more sustained with less cardiac vagal blockade [44]. The use of anticholinergics has been restricted because of concerns that they impair mucus transport by increasing the viscosity of secretions, which in turn causes mucus inspissation and thus increases airway obstruction. Considerable controversy exists with regard to the effect of atropine on total mucociliary clearance by the lung because the effect on both the formation of mucus and the ciliary action is unclear [3, 18, 130]. Nevertheless, systemic hydration should always be ensured before using these drugs [19].

INDUCTION

The induction of anesthesia in an asthmatic patient, particularly an asthmatic child, is a challenge for the anesthesiologist. Well-

sedated children can be induced with an inhalation agent such as halothane, provided the procedure has been carefully explained to the child. If there is any objection to an inhalation technique, administration of an ultrashort-acting barbiturate is an alternative. Thiopental can release histamine and cause coughing and initiate bronchospasm [63, 83], although it has been reported to be useful in facilitating mechanical ventilation in status asthmaticus [177]. Methohexital causes less coughing. Some anesthesiologists recommend alfaxalone (Althesin) or ketamine. Ketamine prevents antigen-induced increases in airway resistance more effectively than does thiopental [61], and directly relaxes airway smooth muscle [84]. The problem with alfaxalone is that certain patients are allergic probably to a preservative component [20, 21]. Ketamine gives rise to problems of altered consciousness postoperatively. When we have given either drug to asthmatic physicians, the majority have complained, preferring methohexital with its slightly increased chance of an asthmatic attack. If the procedure is short and the type of surgery permits, it is best to avoid endotracheal intubation, thus eliminating a cause of reflex bronchoconstriction. Intubation is the most common single factor precipitating an acute asthma attack during surgery [134]. If intubation is necessary, preoxygenation helps to protect against the hypoxemic complications of bronchospasms and cardiac arrhythmias. The hazard of aspiration can be minimized by cricoid pressure applied after the patient is asleep until the intubated trachea is sealed by an inflated tube cuff. The use of succinylcholine for muscle relaxation is not contraindicated.

Since bronchial hyperreactivity to mechanical and inhaled irritants is a characteristic feature of asthma, numerous attempts have been made to attenuate or to abolish the increased bronchomotor response through topical application of local anesthetics [39, 40] as well as through inhalation of ganglionic blocking agents [65] and of anticholinergic substances [14]. Results have been equivocal. If parasympathetic reflexes are an important mechanism, causing airway narrowing, cough, or mucus secretion, these responses are best blocked by halothane, which has, in these respects, less deleterious effects than other general anesthetics [59, 64, 70]. Ketamine also depresses vagal pathways [94] (Fig. 82-3). We believe that a smooth, rapid, and sufficiently deep induction is far more important than the technique and agents used. Capnography should be started prior to induction and pulse oximetry continued.

MAINTENANCE OF ANESTHESIA

All patients undergoing surgery should be monitored at least according to the American Society of Anesthesiologists' guide-

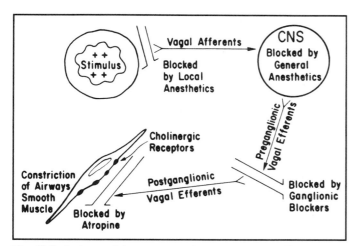

Fig. 82-3. *Pathway of the parasympathetic irritant reflex. This reflex can be interrupted at many different anatomic sites by specific drugs used in anesthesia. CNS = central nervous system. (Reprinted with permission from C. A. Hirshman. Airway reactivity in humans. Anesthesiology 58:171, 1983.)*

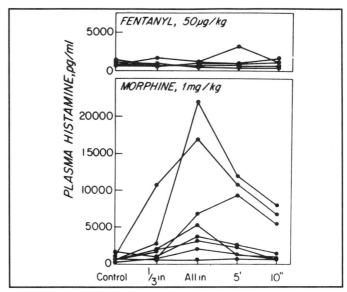

Fig. 82-4. *Effect of morphine and fentanyl on histamine release. Fifteen patients were studied prior to coronary artery bypass surgery. Subjects received an infusion of morphine (1 mg/kg^{-1} intravenously at 100 μg/kg^{-1}/min^{-1} [n = 8]) or fentanyl (50 μg/kg^{-1} intravenously at 5 μg/kg^{-1}/min^{-1} [n = 7]). Patients in the morphine group had an average 750 percent peak increase in plasma histamine levels accompanied by a significant decrease in mean arterial pressure (−27 mmHg) and systemic vascular resistance (−520 dyne/sec/cm^{-5}). The greatest decrease in systemic vascular resistance occurred in those patients with the highest levels of plasma histamine (r = −0.81). Patients in the fentanyl group had no change in plasma histamine level and no decrease in arterial pressure or systemic vascular resistance. (Reprinted with permission from C. E. Rosow, et al. Histamine release during morphine and fentanyl anesthesia. Anesthesiology 56:93, 1982.)*

lines [1, 2]. In addition, continuous anesthesia vapor monitoring is likely to be standard practice [53].

Inhalation agents are preferred for maintenance of general anesthesia. Diethyl ether, cyclopropane, and tribromoethanol have been used in patients with severe bronchial asthma [43, 96, 134]. Newer inhalation anesthetics such as halothane, enflurane, and isoflurane have similar bronchodilating properties and fewer side effects [25, 57, 60, 62, 134, 141]. Halothane has been employed in normocapnic subjects with status asthmaticus [48]. It has been advocated as the best inhalation agent for the surgical patient who has asthma, and we concur.

In contrast to diethyl ether, traditionally utilized in the treatment of status asthmaticus, halothane enables a rapid induction, does not stimulate tracheobronchial secretion, and does not cause laryngeal irritation. Halothane relaxes smooth muscle and suppresses bronchoconstriction evoked by acetylcholine and histamine in guinea pig tracheal smooth muscle isolates [41]. Halothane antagonizes the bronchoconstrictor effect of extrinsic allergen challenge as well as intrinsic vagal and histamine-induced bronchospasm [57, 60]. The mechanism of action is by stimulation of adenyl cyclase activity and to a lesser extent of phosphodiesterase activity, resulting in an increase of intracellular cyclic adenosine monophosphate (AMP) [141, 171], although an effect on cellular calcium has been reported [178]. The known side effects of halothane can give rise to potential complications in an asthmatic. Myocardial depression by halothane may be compounded by hypoxia and hypercarbia. Attenuation or abolition of the hypoxic vascular response in the lung of an asthmatic patient may promote hypoxemia by increasing pulmonary blood flow to areas with low ventilation-perfusion ratios. Monitoring of arterial blood gases and maintenance of normal alveolar ventilation are therefore essential. Caution has to be exercised in asthma patients receiving aminophylline or catecholamines. Aminophylline, epinephrine, and isoproterenol, when used alone or in conjunction with halothane, can cause cardiac arrhythmias. The risk is even greater when hypoxemia and acidosis are present. Scanty human data exist on the effects of aminophylline application during anesthesia. In studies in dogs, aminophylline administration, in a dose yielding serum levels between 10 and 20 mg/L, during induction or maintenance of halothane anesthesia did not produce any arrhythmias [145, 146].

Toxic aminophylline doses are arrhythmogenic when given immediately after halothane anesthesia [146]. Intravenous ami-

nophylline will produce a serum theophylline level of approximately 2 mg/L for every 1 mg/kg given as a loading dose. Arrhythmias have successfully been treated with lidocaine [123]. Halothane anesthesia in patients who have received aminophylline preoperatively may be dangerous and is likely to result in severe and persistent arrhythmias [147]. It has been suggested that one should wait three aminophylline half-lives before administering halothane for elective surgery [123]. An alternate is the use of enflurane, which has been recommended in asthmatic patients [7, 123]. Induction of anesthesia by enflurane following aminophylline does not cause cardiac arrhythmias in dogs [148]. When halothane, aminophylline, and isoproterenol are used together, the incidence of ventricular arrhythmias is higher [152]. There is evidence that heart rate may strongly influence the likelihood of occurrence of cardiac arrhythmias following aminophylline administration [147, 175]; hence, close ECG monitoring is imperative.

The use of narcotics is accompanied by respiratory depression, which persists into the recovery period. In addition, morphine [116] and meperidine [132] release histamine. Fentanyl does not increase serum histamine concentration in therapeutic doses [124] (Fig. 82-4). Histamine release with undesirable release reactions during anesthesia and the value of histamine antagonists have been reviewed by Lorenz and Doenicke [83].

If muscle relaxation is required, pancuronium is superior to *d*-tubocurarine or gallamine. *d*-Tubocurarine produces a dose-related increase in plasma histamine [100]. Pancuronium has no histamine-releasing properties [82]. The simultaneous administration of pancuronium and aminophylline may result in adverse arrhythmogenic effects [9]. Preexisting heart disease may increase this potential. Like pancuronium, clinically effective doses of vecuronium do not release histamine [58]. Similarly, atracurium has only histamine-releasing activity at doses approximately three times those required to produce adequate skeletal muscle relaxation [8]. Curare-like agents can be reversed at the end of surgery with neostigmine, provided a sufficient dose of atropine is given to block its muscarinic effects.

Hyperventilation during anesthesia with depletion of carbon dioxide body stores is dangerous in asthmatic patients whose control of breathing is already compromised by a decreased central carbon dioxide response. Hence, the ventilator has to be adjusted so that normocapnia is maintained. Air trapping, a well-known phenomenon in patients with airflow obstruction, can cause an occult positive end-expiratory pressure (PEEP) in mechanically ventilated patients. The increase of thoracic pressure associated with the "auto-PEEP" phenomenon of alveolar air-trapping can severely affect cardiocirculatory function. Failure to recognize the hemodynamic consequences of auto-PEEP may lead to inappropriate fluid restriction and unnecessary vasopressor therapy. Auto-PEEP should be suspected as exhalatory gas flow continues perceptibly until interrupted at the next inspiratory ventilator cycle. Although not readily apparent during normal ventilator operation, the auto-PEEP effect can be detected and quantified by expiratory port occlusion at the end of the set exhalation period and registering the pressure displayed on the ventilator manometer [108].

Patients with allergic asthma suffer from abnormal autonomic functions, alpha-adrenergic hyperresponsiveness [55], parasympathetic hyperresponsiveness [75], and beta-adrenergic hyporesponsivity [116]. Therefore, agents with autonomic stimulatory effects have to be used judiciously.

Conduction anesthesia for peripheral surgery has been recommended, since it obviates intubation and upper airway stimulation. However, spinal anesthesia for intraperitoneal surgery is associated with a high incidence of adverse reactions in the asthmatic patient [47]. Conduction anesthesia does not entirely protect from bronchospastic complications. Wheezing develops in 1 in 50 asthmatic patients under regional anesthesia [16]. Patients symptomatic at the onset of surgery do not improve with regional anesthesia. This is not surprising in light of the fact that spinal anesthesia blocks the sympathetics (T10–L1) to the adrenal glands with concomitant depression of endogenous catecholamine release, and falling serum catecholamine levels contribute to the development of bronchospasm [6, 27]. In addition, spinal anesthesia blocks the sensory input to the central nervous system from the surgical site and prevents the intraoperative rise in plasma cortisol levels [160].

Table 82-4 summarizes the agents that can be used in the anesthetic management of an asthmatic. No one type of anesthesia is associated with lower rates of postoperative complications. The skill of the anesthesiologist, early recovery from general anesthesia, and good postoperative care greatly reduce the incidence of postoperative complications [53].

BRONCHOSPASM

Bronchospasm is probably the most feared complication in the anesthetic management of an asthmatic patient. In nonventilated patients, labored breathing, intercostal retractions, and minimal

Table 82-4. Anesthetics and asthma

Agent	Recommended	Not recommended	Comment
Premedication			
Barbiturate	(+)		
Diazepam	+		
Antihistamine	+		
Opioid		+	
Atropine	(+)		Promotes mucus inspissation
Glycopyrrolate	+		
Induction			
Thiopental	(+)		Releases histamine; causes coughing
Methohexital	+		
Ketamine	+		
Alfaxalone (Althesin)	(+)		Allergic reaction not uncommon
Maintenance			
Diethyl ether	+		
Cyclopropane	(+)	With catecholamines	
Halothane	(+)	With sympathomimetics	
	(+)	With preoperative aminophylline	
Enflurane	+		
Isoflurane	+		
Morphine		+	
Meperidine		+	
Fentanyl	(+)		
Muscle relaxants			
Succinylcholine	+		
Pancuronium	+		
Alcuronium	+		
Gallamine		+	
d-Tubocurarine		+	
Cholesterinase inhibitor			
Neostigmine	+		Preceded by sufficient dose of atropine to block its muscarinic effect
Local anesthetics			
Amide-type	+		
Ester-type		+	

(+) = not the preferred agent because it may have undesirable effects in asthma patients.

or absent chest excursions indicate bronchoconstriction. On auscultation, inspiratory or expiratory wheezing may be heard. In ventilated patients a progressive rise in inspiratory delivery pressure and a rapidly falling compliance signal airway obstruction. The chest appears inflated, since lung deflation is impeded by the increased airway resistance. Wheezing is not a reliable sign of the severity of bronchoconstriction. Wheezing is a physical phenomenon depending on flow rate. If airflow is minimal because only a little air can be moved as a result of severe obstruction, wheezing may be absent. On the other hand, when airflow is great, turbulence may produce wheezing even though bronchoconstriction is less marked. Because of therapeutic implications, it is important to differentiate an asthma attack from other possible causes of ventilatory impairment such as mechanical obstruction or decreased chest wall compliance, which may arise from light anesthesia without adequate muscle relaxation.

Therapy of intraanesthetic bronchospasm aims at eliminating precipitating factors and modifying bronchomotor tone by an appropriate anesthetic technique and by the administration of bronchodilators. Intraanesthetic bronchospasm frequently develops in lightly anesthetized patients following tracheobronchial instrumentation or surgical stimulation. Such manipulations should be avoided or interrupted and the depth of anesthesia increased. If deepening of anesthesia is not desirable or bronchospasm persists, changing to an anesthetic with more potent bronchodilating properties such as halothane, enflurane, or isoflurane helps. Parasympathomimetic or histamine-releasing substances are to be avoided. When these measures do not relieve bronchospasm, one has to resort to additional therapy. Nebulization of lidocaine (1.0–1.5 mg/kg) can be tried, but is not without problems [93]. It generally relaxes bronchial smooth muscle and blocks respiratory reflexes, but can cause bronchoconstriction [93]. Aerosolized atropine (0.005–0.010 mg/kg) has been shown to be effective in inhibiting bronchoconstriction. The airborne route is preferred because cardiovascular stimulation is less and maximum bronchodilation is achieved [125, 170]. Short-acting sympathomimetics often provide prompt and effective resolution of acute airway obstruction. Selective beta$_2$-adrenergic agonists are preferred to isoproterenol or epinephrine because the former have fewer cardiotoxic side effects. Isoetharine, inhaled dose of 0.5 mg, contained in one to two puffs of the inhaler, and metaproterenol, inhaled dose of 1.0 to 1.5 mg, contained in two or three puffs of the inhaler, are available also as a solution for nebulization; metered albuterol, 0.1 to 0.4 mg, can also be used. The doses may be repeated as long as no adverse side effects occur. There is little information about the relative safety of beta-adrenergic agonists in the presence of halogenated anesthetics.

When bronchospasm does not respond to beta sympathomimetics, aminophylline, 3 mg/kg intravenously over 20 minutes, can be tried. For patients who are not currently receiving aminophylline, 5 mg/kg intravenously over 20 minutes is an appropriate dose. Only 1 mg of aminophylline per kilogram should be given to individuals who have been taking aminophylline medication preoperatively. The combination of sympathomimetics and aminophylline, although according to one study [126] more effective and no more toxic than a sympathomimetic alone, should not be administered in an anesthetic setting because of the dangers of serious arrhythmias that we have already described. In certain instances, correction of metabolic acidemia will enhance the responsiveness to beta-adrenergic agents [98].

In patients in whom bronchodilator therapy has failed, steroids such as methylprednisolone, 4 mg/kg intravenously, may be helpful. However, there is no immediate therapeutic effect, and hours may elapse before improvement can be recorded. Meanwhile, supportive therapy must be provided in order to avoid life-threatening complications. Adequate alveolar ventilation has to be maintained if necessary by means of tracheal intubation, muscle relaxation, and mechanical ventilation. Hypoxemia, hypercapnia, and acidosis cause cardiovascular depression, which can rapidly lead to cardiac arrest. In spontaneously breathing patients, the negative intrathoracic pressure required to overcome the airway obstruction may promote alveolar collapse and fluid accumulation in the lung. Overzealous fluid administration in this situation contributes to the development of pulmonary edema.

POSTOPERATIVE CONSIDERATIONS

The severity of mechanical disturbances caused by surgery is determined primarily by the site of incision. The changes in pulmonary function and hence the incidence of postoperative complications are most severe following upper abdominal and thoracic surgery, less after lower abdominal surgery, and least after surgery on the extremities (Table 82-5). The pain after upper abdominal surgery is a principal factor in reducing vital capacity and effective coughing, but the proximity of the operative site to the diaphragm—responsible for approximately 60 percent of normal ventilation—is of great importance. Prolonged surgery and intraoperative posture of the patient are potentiating factors. Abdominal distention, acute gastric dilatation, and tight restrictive abdominal or chest binders greatly reduce lung volume and thoracopulmonary compliance. The postoperative period is particularly difficult in asthmatic patients who may additionally have abnormalities in ventilation control [68, 91, 115, 153], but careful epidural pain management is not contraindicated [173]. Depression of ventilatory drive is not restricted to symptomatic patients. Persons with a history of severe asthma but normal or nearly normal pulmonary function as measured by spirometry and body plethysmography during remission show a marked decrease in ventilatory response to isocapnic hypoxia and hypercapnia [68] (see Chap. 27). The ventilatory responses to hypoxia and hypercapnia can be deranged separately or together. There appears to be no correlation between the duration of asthma and the ventilatory response. There is evidence that obese asthmatic subjects without primary hypoventilation have a lower ventilatory drive [68]. Asthmatic patients known to have impaired carbon dioxide responses during remission of airway obstruction are more likely to develop hypercapnia during acute episodes than are those who have normal responses when they are asymptomatic. These changes in the control of breathing can be compounded by the effects of anesthesia. Narcotics and volatile anesthetics, even in subanesthetic concentrations, reduce the ventilatory drive to hypercapnia, hypoxemia, and acidosis [76–78, 167]. Thus, in the immediate postoperative period when hypoxemia is likely to develop, the normal response of increased ventilation is not present. Asthmatics are particularly sensitive to narcotics and sedatives. Consequently, they must be administered very carefully; otherwise, frank respiratory failure ensues. Regional techniques for reducing postoperative pain are a better alternative and provide even greater restoration of pulmonary function.

Sympathomimetic agents stimulate the ventilatory response to hypoxemia [12, 54]. There seems to be a direct correlation between adrenocorticosteroid dosage and increased ventilatory hypoxia.

Hypoxemia is almost a constant finding at some time in the postoperative period except after the most minor surgery that does not involve body cavities. Prolonged recovery from anesthesia is nearly always associated with respiratory depression. Incomplete or late return of neuromuscular function encroaches on inspiratory capacity and vital capacity and thereby limits the patient's efforts to overcome increased airway resistance. The

Table 82-5. Effects of surgery and anesthesia on pulmonary function

Lung function	Surgery	Change	Comments	Sequelae
Lung volumes				
Vital capacity	Laparotomy	↓ ~45%[a,b]	Within 1–2 postop. days	Decreased ventilatory reserve
	Upper abdominal	↓ ~55%[a,b]	Within 1–2 postop. days	Decreased ventilatory reserve
	Lower abdominal	↓ ~40%[a,b]	Return to preop. levels over 1–2 wk	Inability of deep breathing (→atelectasis) Ineffective cough (→secretion retention, mucus plugs)
	Nonabdominal Nonthoracic	No change		
Residual volume	Laparotomy	↓ 13%[a,b]		
Functional residual capacity	Laparotomy	↓ 20%[a,b]	Maximal on 4th postop. day	↓ V/Q, ↑ QS/QT (→ ↓ PaO_2)
Expiratory reserve volume	Upper abdominal Lower abdominal	↓ 60%[c] ↓ 25%[c]		If closing volume exceeds ERV→ airway closure
Ventilation pattern				
Respiratory rate	Laparotomy	↑ 26%[a]		↑ V_D/V_T(→ ↑ $PaCO_2$)
Tidal volume	Laparotomy	↓ ~20%[a] Decreased sighing		Airway closure, ↓ compliance (→ ↑ work of breathing → ↑ $\dot{V}O_2$, ↑ $\dot{V}CO_2$)
Gas exchange				
PaO_2		Decrease	Most severe after upper abdominal and thoracic surgery; persists for 5–15 days	Hypoxemia
$PaCO_2$		Compensatory hypocapnia	Increase signals advanced respiratory failure	Hypercapnia Acidosis
Defense mechanism		Cough suppression, mucociliary depression, depressed cellular function (?)	Causative factors: dry and cool anesthesia gases, anticholinergics, narcotics, ↑ FIO_2 Pain	Decreased tracheobronchial clearance
			Artificial airway	Bacterial colonization of upper airway→ pulmonary infection

[a] H. K. Beecher. The measured effect of laparotomy on the respiration. *J. Clin. Invest.* 12:639, 1933.
[b] H. K. Beecher. Effect of laparotomy on lung volume: Demonstration of a new type of collapse. *J. Clin. Invest.* 12:651, 1933.
[c] A. R. Anscombe and R. St. J. Buxton. Effect of abdominal operations on total lung capacity and its subdivisions. *Br. Med. J.* 2:84, 1958.

inability to inspire deeply, to cough effectively, and to clear the airways promotes postoperative atelectasis. Attenuation or abolition of the hypoxic pulmonary vascular response through anesthetics or bronchodilators increases the ventilation-perfusion imbalance in the lung of an asthmatic patient [17, 49, 52, 90, 128]. Hypoxemia can, of course, be prevented by breathing oxygen-enriched gas mixtures. Such therapy should be monitored by pulse oximetry [2] and PaO_2 as indicated.

Tracheal mucociliary transport is impaired in bronchial asthma even in asymptomatic remission [97]. It seems that ciliary beat frequency is not the cause of the dysfunction [92]; other factors such as alteration in the physical characteristics of mucus and periciliary fluid may play a more important role. Cromolyn sodium seems to have the potential of returning impaired mucociliary function toward normal in asymptomatic allergic patients [97]. Beta-adrenergic agents have a stimulatory effect on overall mucociliary transport [92, 159, 162]. Humidification and warming of inspired gases are essential for proper mucociliary function. Lack of humidification depletes the fluid on which the mucus blanket floats and increases the viscosity of mucus itself; secretions are then retained, thereby exaggerating airway obstruction. Incomplete humidification or warming of inspired air, especially in patients with an endotracheal or tracheostomy tube in place, can promote bronchoconstriction [30–32, 101, 150]. The magnitude of the airway obstruction correlates directly with the quantity of the respiratory heat loss and the degree of airway cooling [29, 31]; if heat loss and airway cooling are prevented, bronchial obstruction does not develop. Although most of these findings have been derived from studies examining the role of heat exchange imposed on the airways during physical exertion, they are of clinical relevance in the postoperative care of asthmatic patients. A fall in body temperature of 0.7°C results in an acute asthma attack in most asthmatic patients [16]. When airway mucosa is maintained warm by breathing warm humidified air during body cooling, asthma attacks do not occur [15, 66].

Symptomatic patients will benefit from inhalation of a bronchodilator. It is very useful to know the individual substance to which the patient best responds. Depositing of the aerosol is influenced by the breathing pattern. Total deposition decreases as ventilatory rate increases. Rapid-shallow ventilation results in enhanced large-airway deposition and marked heterogeneity in deposition distribution. Slow-deep breathing produces more uniform deposition throughout the lung, with little aerosol collection in large airways, and the distribution is less homogeneous. Slow-shallow breathing favors deposition in small airways [157]. Hence, slow and deep breaths during inhalation therapy will contribute to a better therapeutic effect.

The patient with a history of asthma needs close supervision during the postoperative period. Many sudden deaths from asthma and many episodes of ventilatory arrest occur during the

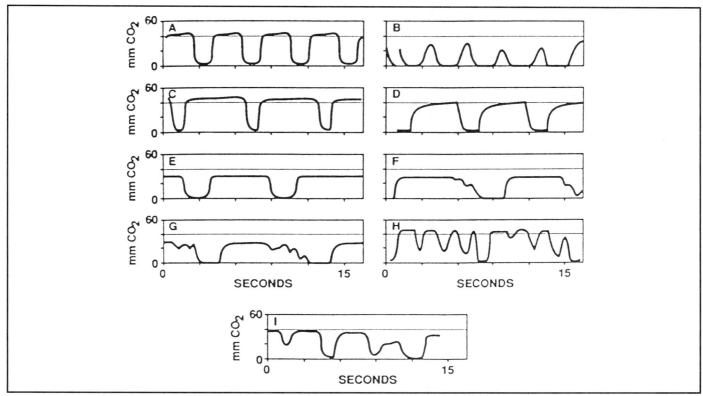

Fig. 82-5. *Capnography waveforms obtained from anesthetized patients using a Perkin-Elmer mass spectrometer. A. Spontaneous respiration in a normal patient. B. Contamination by the flow of fresh gas in a pediatric patient with the sampling port separated from the endotracheal tube by dead space. C. Controlled ventilation in a normal patient. D. Controlled ventilation in a patient with chronic obstructive pulmonary disease. E. Controlled ventilation in a normal patient: low flowmeter flow. The low end-tidal carbon dioxide tension ($P_{ET}CO_2$) could be due to alveolar hyperventilation or to increased alveolar dead space (VD_{ALV}) and resulting increased alveolar-arterial carbon dioxide tension difference ($P(a-A)CO_2$). F. The same patient as in E but with higher flow of fresh gas. At end-expiration, during the period before the ventilator initiates a new inspiration, the sampling catheter draws gas from the circuit, including the fresh gas when the flow is sufficiently high. Note that as in A, a new inspiration usually causes a steep decline from the true end-tidal value to zero. G. Heart beat superimposed on controlled ventilation and, presumably, causing mixing with fresh gas. H. Spontaneous respiration superimposed on controlled ventilation. I. Spontaneous ventilation with varying respiratory pattern. "True" $P_{ET}CO_2$ is 40 mmHg. Spectrometer averages breaths to give a reading of 30 mmHg. (Reprinted with permission from H. B. Fairley. Respiratory Monitoring. In C. D. Blitt (ed.), Monitoring in Anesthesia and Critical Care Medicine (2nd ed.). New York: Churchill-Livingstone, 1990. Pp. 339–372.)*

night and in the early morning [56]. A circadian fall in plasma epinephrine concentration is responsible for acute nocturnal asthma attacks [139]. There is a good correlation between the fall of plasma epinephrine at night and the decrease of peak flow in asthma patients [6]. Plasma cortisol levels do not correlate with the dip in peak flow [119]. Such acute episodes can possibly be prevented by the administration of beta-adrenergic agonists, prescribed appropriately in the immediate postoperative period.

The main indication for mechanical ventilation is deterioration of pulmonary function leading to respiratory muscle exhaustion. Exhaustion is a condition that is easily detected by rising $PaCO_2$ but difficult to quantify clinically. Ascertaining when the moment has come for mechanical ventilatory assistance is a challenging task. An unnecessary intubation with mechanical ventilation does more harm than good. On the other hand, missing the right time may result in cardiac or respiratory arrest with hypoxemic brain damage. It is therefore important to identify those patients who are likely to require ventilatory support. It has been observed that patients with the following changes frequently develop ventilatory failure crisis: FEV_1 of less than 1.0 liter, forced vital capacity (FVC) below 1.5 liters, a ratio of FEV_1 to FVC less than 30 percent, MVV below 50 percent of the predicted value,

tachycardia of greater than 110/min, and a pulsus paradoxus of more than 30 mmHg of arterial blood pressure. These patients should be placed under close supervision and of course monitored with pulse oximetry and capnometry (Figs. 82-5 and 82-6). This will markedly reduce the incidence of unsuspected respiratory arrest (Table 82-6). The use of PEEP expiratory pressure has been considered relatively contraindicated during an asthma attack because of the already existing hyperinflation, the high peak inspiratory pressure, and the potential risk of pneumothorax [49]. On the other hand, it has been shown that in induced asthma, continuous positive airway pressure reduces the load on the inspiratory muscles, thereby improving their efficiency and decreasing the energy cost of their action [89]. The beneficial effect of continuous positive airway pressure on inspiratory muscles critically depends on the magnitude of change in end-expiratory lung volume. PEEP has also successfully been used to combat air trapping during severe bronchospasm [113] (see Chap. 73).

In summary, the perioperative management of asthmatics requires attention to detail, dexterity, careful pulmonary function monitoring, pulse oximetry and capnometry, and a detailed knowledge of the pharmacology of asthma as it relates to anes-

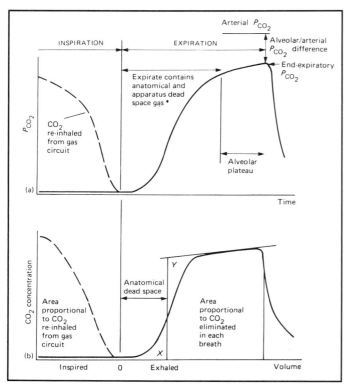

Fig. 82-6. *For capnography, a breathe-through cell may be placed in line with the tracheal tube connector. This adds little to the apparatus dead space and measures carbon dioxide in phase with the measurement of tidal volume. Therefore, carbon dioxide concentrations may be related to volume, allowing derivation of breath-by-breath elimination of carbon dioxide, mean expired carbon dioxide concentration, anatomic dead space, and (in combination with arterial PCO_2) the physiologic dead space. a. The PCO_2 as a function of time as in the normal capnogram. The broken line indicates substantial rebreathing of carbon dioxide in spite of the concentration falling momentarily to zero. b. The additional information that is available when the carbon dioxide concentration is plotted against tidal volumes. (Reprinted with permission from J. A. Bushman, D. T. Mangano, and J. F. Nunn. Monitoring During Anesthesia. In J. F. Nunn, J. E. Utting, and B. R. Brown, Jr. (eds.), General Anesthesia (5th ed.). London: Butterworths, 1989. Pp. 463–492.)*

Table 82-6. Advantages and disadvantages of capnography

Advantages
1. Continuous "devoted" real-time monitor in contrast to "shared" mass spectrometer
2. Noninvasive
3. Detection of air or carbon dioxide embolism
4. Determination of proper endotracheal tube position
5. Life-threatening intraoperative complications (air embolism malignant hyperthermia, endotracheal tube obstruction)

Disadvantages
1. Relatively expensive (up to $6,500 per monitoring station)
2. Prone to mechanical influences (i.e., respiratory cycle time < total transit time)
3. Not useful in neonates and small children because of the high sampling flow rate (about 200–400 ml/min)

Source: A. F. Stasic. Monitoring: What Is Helpful and What Is Not. In J. M. Civetta, et al. (eds.), *Critical Care.* Lippincott: Philadelphia, 1988. Reprinted with permission.

thetics and analgesics. With adequate knowledge and equipment, no asthmatic should be denied indicated surgery, but that surgery may require optimal timing to minimize complications.

REFERENCES

1. American Society of Anesthesiologists. Standards for basic intra-operative monitoring effective January 1, 1991. *Directory of Members* 56:670, 1991.
2. American Society of Anesthesiologists. Standards for postanesthesia care to become effective no later than January 1, 1992. *Directory of Members* 56:672, 1991.
3. Annis, P., Landa, J., and Lichtiger, M. Effect of atropine on velocity of tracheal mucus in anaesthetized patients. *Anesthesiology* 44:74, 1976.
4. Aranda, J. V., et al. Pharmacokinetic aspects of theophylline in premature newborns. *N. Engl. J. Med.* 95:413, 1976.
5. Aubier, M., et al. Aminophylline improves diaphragmatic contractility. *N. Engl. J. Med.* 305:249, 1981.
6. Barnes, P., et al. Nocturnal asthma and changes in circulating epinephrine, histamine and cortisol. *N. Engl. J. Med.* 303:263, 1980.
7. Barton, M. D. Anesthetic problems with aspirin intolerant patients. *Anesth. Analg.* 54:376, 1975.
8. Basta, S. J., et al. Clinical pharmacology of atracurium besylate (BS 23 A): A new nondepolarizing muscle relaxant. *Anesth. Analg.* 61:723, 1982.
9. Belani, K. G., Anderson, W. W., and Buckley, J. J. Adverse drug interaction involving pancuronium and aminophylline. *Anesth. Analg.* 61:473, 1982.
10. Berend, N., et al. The maximum expiratory flow-volume curve with air and low density gas mixture: An analysis of subject and observer variability. *Chest* 80:23, 1981.
11. Berend, N., et al. Small airways disease: Reproducibility of measurements and correlation with lung function. *Chest* 79:263, 1981.
12. Blatteis, C. M., and Lutherer, L. O. Reduction by moderate hypoxia of the calorigenic action of catecholamines in dogs. *J. Appl. Physiol.* 36: 337, 1974.
13. Chatham, M., et al. A screening test for airways reactivity. An abbreviated methacholine inhalation challenge. *Chest* 82:15, 1982.
14. Chen, W. Y., et al. Atropine and exercise-induced bronchoconstriction. *Chest* 79:651, 1981.
15. Chen, W. Y., and Chai, H. Airway cooling and nocturnal asthma. *Chest* 81:675, 1982.
16. Chen, W. Y., and Horton, D. F. Airways obstruction in asthmatics induced by body cooling. *Scand. J. Respir. Dis.* 59:13, 1978.
17. Chick, T. W., Nicholson, D. P., and Johnston, R. L. Effects of isoproterenol on distribution of ventilation and perfusion in asthma. *Am. Rev. Respir. Dis.* 107:869, 1973.
18. Chopra, S. K. Effect of atropine on mucociliary transport velocity in anesthetized dogs. *Am. Rev. Respir. Dis.* 118:367, 1978.
19. Chopra, S. K., et al. Effects of hydration and physical therapy on tracheal transport velocity. *Am. Rev. Respir. Dis.* 115:1009, 1977.
20. Clarke, R. S. J. Hypersensitivity Reactions to Intravenous Anesthetics. In J. W. Dundee (ed.), *Intravenous Anaesthetic Agents.* Current Topics in Anaesthesia Series. London: Arnold, 1979. Pp. 69–76.
21. Clarke, R. S. J., et al. Adverse reaction to intravenous anaesthetics. A survey of 100 reports. *Br. J. Anaesth.* 47:575, 1975.
22. Collins, J. V., et al. Intravenous corticosteroids in treatment of acute bronchial asthma. *Lancet* 2:1047, 1970.
23. Conney, A. H., et al. Induction of liver microsomal cortisol 6-beta-hydroxylase by diphenyl-hydantoin or phenobarbital: An explanation for the increased excretion of 6-hydroxycortisol in humans treated with these drugs. *Life Sci.* 4:1091, 1965.
24. Converse, J. G., and Smotvilla, M. M. Anesthesia and the asthmatic. *Anesth. Analg.* 40:336, 1961.
25. Coon, R. L., and Kampine, J. P. Hypocapnic bronchoconstriction and inhalation anesthetics. *Anesthesiology* 43:635, 1975.
26. Corrao, W. M., Braman, S. S., and Irwin, R. S. Chronic cough as the sole presenting manifestation of bronchial asthma. *N. Engl. J. Med.* 300:633, 1979.
27. Cryer, P. E. Physiology and pathophysiology of the human sympatho-adrenal neuroendocrine system. *N. Engl. J. Med.* 303:436, 1980.
28. Dahms, T. E., Bolin, J. F., and Slabin, R. C. Passive smoking. Effects on bronchial asthma. *Chest* 80:530, 1981.
29. Deal, E. C., Jr., et al. Airway responsiveness to cold air and hyperpnea

in normal subjects and in those with hay fever and asthma. *Am. Rev. Respir. Dis.* 121:621, 1980.

30. Deal, E. C., Jr., et al. Hyperpnea and heat flux: Initial reaction sequence in exercise-induced asthma. *J. Appl. Physiol.* 46:476, 1979.

31. Deal, E. C., Jr., et al. Esophageal temperature during exercise in asthmatic and nonasthmatic subjects. *J. Appl. Physiol.* 46:484, 1979.

32. Deal, E. C., Jr., et al. Role of respiratory heat exchange in production of exercise-induced asthma. *J. Appl. Physiol.* 46:467, 1979.

33. Doll, D. C., and Rosenberg, H. Antagonism of neuromuscular blockage by theophylline. *Anesth. Analg.* 58:139, 1979.

34. Dowell, A. R., et al. Effect of aminophylline on respiratory-center sensitivity in Cheyne-Stokes respiration and in pulmonary emphysema. *N. Engl. J. Med.* 273:1447, 1965.

35. Dundee, J. W., et al. Frequency of atopy and allergy in an anaesthetic patient population. *Br. J. Anaesth.* 50:793, 1978.

36. DuSouich, P., et al. Pulmonary disease and drug kinetics. *Clin. Pharmacokinet.* 3:257, 1978.

37. Dwyer, J., Lazarus, L., and Hickie, J. B. A study of cortisol metabolism in patients with chronic asthma. *Aust. Ann. Med.* 16:297, 1967.

38. Empy, D. W., et al. Mechanisms of bronchial hyperreactivity in normal subjects after upper respiratory tract infections. *Am. Rev. Respir. Dis.* 118:287, 1978.

39. Enright, P. L., McNally, J. F., and Souhrada, J. F. Effect of lidocaine on the ventilatory and airway responses to exercise in asthmatics. *Am. Rev. Respir. Dis.* 122:823, 1980.

40. Fanta, C. H., Ingram, R. H., Jr., and McFadden, E. R., Jr. A reassessment of the effects of oropharyngeal anesthetic in exercise-induced asthma. *Am. Rev. Respir. Dis.* 122:381, 1980.

41. Fletcher, S. W., Flacke, W., and Alper, M. H. The actions of general anesthetic agents on tracheal smooth muscle. *Anesthesiology* 29:517, 1968.

42. Flewellen, E. H., and Nelson, T. E. Is theophylline, aminophylline, or caffeine (methylxanthines) contraindicated in malignant hyperthermia susceptible patients? *Anesth. Analg.* 62:115, 1983.

43. Fuchs, A. M. The interruption of the asthmatic crisis by tribromethanol (Avertin). *J. Allergy* 8:340, 1937.

44. Gall, T. J., and Suratt, P. M. Atropine and glycopyrrolate effects on lung mechanics in normal man. *Anesth. Analg.* 60:85, 1981.

45. Geppert, E. F., and Boushey, H. A. An investigation of ethanol-induced bronchoconstriction. *Am. Rev. Respir. Dis.* 118:135, 1978.

46. Gerhardt, T., McCarthy, J., and Bancalari, E. Effect of aminophylline on respiratory center activity and metabolic rate in premature infants with idiopathic apnea. *Pediatrics* 63:537, 1979.

47. Gold, M. I., and Helrich, M. A study of the complications related to anesthesia in asthmatic patients. *Anesth. Analg.* 42:283, 1963.

48. Gold, M. I., and Helrich, M. Pulmonary mechanics during general anesthesia. V. Status asthmaticus. *Anesthesiology* 32:422, 1970.

49. Gold, M. I., and Ravin, M. B. Anesthesia for the Asthmatic Patient. In M. B. Ravin (ed.), *Problems in Anesthesia: A Case Study Approach.* Boston: Little, Brown, 1981. Pp. 29–36.

50. Gong, H., Jr., Tashkin, D. P., and Calvarese, B. M. Alcohol-induced bronchospasm in an asthmatic patient. Pharmacologic evaluation of the mechanism. *Chest* 80:167, 1981.

51. Graber, A. L., et al. Natural history of pituitary-adrenal recovery following long-term suppression with corticosteroids. *J. Clin. Endocrinol. Metab.* 25:11, 1965.

52. Hales, C. A., and Kazemi, H. Hypoxic vascular response of the lung: Effect of aminophylline and epinephrine. *Am. Rev. Respir. Dis.* 110:126, 1974.

53. Hedley-Whyte, J. (ed.), *Continuous Anesthesia Vapor Monitoring.* Special Technical Publication No. 1090. Philadelphia: American Society for Testing and Materials, 1990.

54. Heistadt, D. D., et al. Effects of adrenergic stimulation on ventilation in man. *J. Clin. Invest.* 51:1469, 1972.

55. Henderson, W. R., et al. Alpha-adrenergic hyperresponsiveness in asthma: Analysis of vascular and pupillary responses. *N. Engl. J. Med.* 300:642, 1979.

56. Hetzel, M. R., Clark, T. J. H., and Branthwaite, M. A. Asthma analysis of sudden deaths and ventilatory arrests in hospital. *Br. Med. J.* 1:808, 1977.

57. Hickey, R. F., et al. The effects of halothane and cyclopropane on total pulmonary resistance in the dog. *Anesthesiology* 31:334, 1969.

58. Hilgenberg, J. D. Comparison of the pharmacology of vecuronium and atracurium with that of other currently available muscle relaxants. *Anesth. Analg.* 62:524, 1983.

59. Hirshman, C. A. Airway reactivity in humans. Anesthetic implications. *Anesthesiology* 58:170, 1983.

60. Hirshman, C. A., and Bergmann, N. A. Halothane and enflurane protect against bronchospasm in an asthma dog model. *Anesth. Analg.* 57:629, 1978.

61. Hirshman, C. A., et al. Ketamine block of antigen-induced bronchospasm in experimental canine asthma. *Br. J. Anaesth.* 51:713, 1979.

62. Hirshman, C. A., et al. Mechanism of action of inhalational anesthesia on airways. *Anesthesiology* 56:107, 1982.

63. Hirshman, C. A., Peters, J., and Cartwright-Lee, J. Leucocyte histamine release to thiopental. *Anesthesiology* 56:64, 1982.

64. Holtzman, M. J., et al. Selective effect of general anesthetics on reflex bronchoconstrictor responses in dogs. *J. Appl. Physiol.* 53:126, 1982.

65. Holtzman, M. J., et al. Effect of ganglionic blockade on bronchial reactivity in atopic subjects. *Am. Rev. Respir. Dis.* 122:17, 1980.

66. Horton, D. J., and Chen, W. Y. Effects of breathing warm humidified air on bronchoconstriction induced by body cooling and by inhalation of methacholine. *Chest* 75:24, 1979.

67. Hudgel, D. W., Cooperson, D. M., and Kinsman, R. A. Recognition of added resistive loads in asthma. The importance of behavioral styles. *Am. Rev. Respir. Dis.* 126:121, 1982.

68. Hudgel, D. W., and Weil, J. V. Depression of hypoxic and hypercapnic ventilatory drives in severe asthma. *Chest* 68:493, 1975.

69. Irvin, R. S., Corrao, W. M., and Pratter, M. R. Chronic persistent cough in the adult: The spectrum and frequency of causes and successful outcome of specific therapy. *Am. Rev. Respir. Dis.* 123:413, 1981.

70. Jackson, D. M., and Richard, I. M. The effects of pentobarbitone and chloralose anesthesia on the vagal component of bronchoconstriction produced by histamine aerosol in the anesthetized dog. *Br. J. Anaesth.* 61:251, 1977.

71. Jackson, J. E., et al. Cimetidine decreases theophylline clearance. *Am. Rev. Respir. Dis.* 123:615, 1981.

72. Jenne, J., et al. Decreased theophylline half-life in cigarette smokers. *Life Sci.* 17:195, 1975.

73. Jezek, V., et al. The effect of aminophylline on the respiration and pulmonary circulation. *Clin. Sci.* 38:549, 1970.

74. Jusko, W. J., et al. Factors affecting theophylline clearances: Age, tobacco, marijuana, cirrhosis, congestive heart failure, obesity, oral contraceptives, benzodiazepines, barbiturates, and ethanol. *J. Pharm. Sci.* 68:1358, 1979.

75. Kaliner, M. The cholinergic nervous system and immediate hypersensitivity. I. Eccrine sweat responses in allergic patients. *J. Allergy Clin. Immunol.* 58:308, 1976.

76. Knill, R. L., Chung, D., and Baskerville, J. Ventilatory responses to acute "Iso-PCO_2" acidosis in awake and anesthetized man. *Clin. Res.* 26:879A, 1978.

77. Knill, R. L., and Gelb, A. W. Ventilatory responses to hypoxia and hypercapnia during halothane sedation and anesthesia in man. *Anesthesiology* 49:244, 1978.

78. Knill, R. L., Manninen, P. H., and Clement, J. L. Ventilation and chemoreflexes during enflurane sedation and anesthesia in man. *Can. Anaesth. Soc. J.* 26:353, 1979.

79. Kozak, P. P., Jr., Cummins, L. H., and Gillman, S. A. Administration of erythromycin to patients with theophylline. *J. Allergy Clin. Immunol.* 60:149, 1977.

80. Lakshminarayan, S., Sahn, S. A., and Weil, J. V. Effect of aminophylline on ventilatory responses in normal man. *Am. Rev. Respir. Dis.* 17:33, 1978.

81. Lefever, G. S., and Rosenberg, H. Aminophylline, halothane and malignant hyperpyrexia in the rabbit. *Fed. Proc.* 39:295, 1980.

82. Levin, N., and Dillon, J. B. Status asthmaticus and pancuronium bromide. *JAMA* 222:1265, 1972.

83. Lorenz, W., and Doenicke, A. H_1 and H_2 blockade: A prophylactic principle in anesthesia and surgery against histamine-release responses of any degree of severity. *N. Engl. Reg. Allergy Proc.* 6:37 and 174, 1985.

84. Lundy, P. M., Gowdey, C. W., and Calhoun, E. H. Tracheal smooth muscle relaxant effect of ketamine. *Br. J. Anaesth.* 46:333, 1974.

85. Manfredia, R. L., and Vesell, E. S. Inhibition of theophylline metabolism by longterm allupurinol administration. *Clin. Pharmacol. Ther.* 29:224, 1981.

86. Mangione, A., et al. Pharmacokinetics of theophylline in hepatic disease. *Chest* 73:616, 1978.

87. Marquis, J. F., et al. Phenytoin-theophylline interaction. *N. Engl. J. Med.* 307:1189, 1982.

88. Martin, A. J., Landau, L. J., and Phelan, P. D. Lung function in young

adults who had asthma in childhood. *Am. Rev. Respir. Dis.* 122:609, 1980.

89. Martin, J. G., Shore, S., and Engel, L. A. Effect of continuous positive airway pressure on respiratory mechanics and pattern of breathing in induced asthma. *Am. Rev. Respir. Dis.* 126:812, 1982.

90. Mather, J. M., Benumof, J. L., and Wahrenbrock, E. A. General anesthetics and regional hypoxic pulmonary vasoconstriction. *Anesthesiology* 46:111, 1977.

91. Matthews, C., and Keyes, T. F. Responses to rebreathing during symptom-free intervals. *Rocky Mt. Med. J.* 63:55, 1966.

92. Maurer, D. R., et al. Role of the ciliary motility in acute allergic mucociliary dysfunction. *J. Appl. Physiol.* 52:1018, 1982.

93. McAlpine, L. G., and Thomson, N. C. Lidocaine-induced bronchoconstriction in asthmatic patients. Relation to histamine airway responsiveness and effect of preservative. *Chest* 96:1012, 1989.

94. McGrath, J. C., MacKenzie, J. E., and Millar, R. A. Effects of ketamine on central sympathetic discharge and the baroreceptor reflex during mechanical ventilation. *Br. J. Anaesth.* 47:1141, 1975.

95. Melzer, E., and Souhrada, J. F. Decrease of respiratory muscle strength and static lung volumes in obese asthmatics. *Am. Rev. Respir. Dis.* 121:17, 1980.

96. Meyer, N. E., and Schotz, S. The relief of severe intractable bronchial asthma with cyclopropane anesthesia. *J. Allergy* 10:239, 1938–39.

97. Mezey, R. J., et al. Mucociliary transport in allergic patients with antigen-induced bronchospasm. *Am. Rev. Respir. Dis.* 118:677, 1979.

98. Mithoefer, J. C., Runser, R. H., and Karetzsky, M. D. The use of sodium bicarbonate in the treatment of acute bronchial asthma. *N. Engl. J. Med.* 272:1200, 1964.

99. Morris, H. G., Neuman, I., and Ellis, E. F. Plasma steroid concentrations during alternate-day treatment with prednisone. *J. Allergy Clin. Immunol.* 54:350, 1974.

100. Moss, J., et al. Role of histamine in the hypotensive action of d-tubocurarine in man. *Anesthesiology* 55:19, 1981.

101. O'Cain, C. F., et al. Airway effects of respiratory heat loss in normal subjects. *J. Appl. Physiol.* 49:875, 1980.

102. Ogilvie, R. I. Clinical pharmacokinetics of theophylline. *Clin. Pharmacokinet.* 3:267, 1978.

103. Orehek, J., and Gayrard, P. Les tests de provocation bronchique non-specifiques dans l'asthma. *Bull. Eur. Physiopathol. Respir.* (*Nancy*) 12:565, 1976.

104. Orehek, J., et al. Influence of the previous deep inspiration on the spirometric measurement of provoked bronchoconstriction in asthma. *Am. Rev. Respir. Dis.* 123:269, 1981.

105. Oyama, T., and Matsuki, A. Plasma levels of cortisol in man during spinal anesthesia and surgery. *Can. Anaesth. Soc. J.* 17:234, 1970.

106. Oyama, T., and Matsuki, A. Plasma cortisol levels during anaesthesia and surgery in man. *Anaesthetist* 20:140, 1971.

107. Oyama, T., et al. Effect of meperidine on adrenocortical function in man. *Can. Anaesth. Soc. J.* 16:282, 1969.

108. Pepe, P. E., and Marini, J. J. Occult positive end-expiratory pressure in mechanically ventilated patients with airflow obstruction. *Am. Rev. Respir. Dis.* 126:166, 1982.

109. Philbin, D. M., et al. The use of H_1 and H_2 histamine antagonists with morphine anesthesia: A double-blind study. *Anesthesiology* 55:292, 1981.

110. Pingleton, S. K., et al. Hypotension associated with terbutaline therapy in acute quadriplegia. *Am. Rev. Respir. Dis.* 126:723, 1982.

111. Powell, J. R., et al. Theophylline disposition in acutely ill hospitalized patients. The effect of smoking, heart failure, severe airway obstruction, and pneumonia. *Am. Rev. Respir. Dis.* 118:229, 1978.

112. Prickman, L. E., and Whitcomb, E. F., Jr. The decreasing hazard of surgical procedures on patients with asthma. *Dis. Chest* 35:30, 1959.

113. Quist, J., et al. High-level Peep in severe asthma. *N. Engl. J. Med.* 307:1347, 1982.

114. Rebuck, A. S., and Read, J. Assessment and management of severe asthma. *Am. J. Med.* 51:788, 1971.

115. Rebuck, A. S., and Read, J. Patterns of ventilatory response to carbon dioxide during recovery from severe asthma. *Clin. Sci.* 41:13, 1971.

116. Reed, C. E. Abnormal autonomic mechanisms in asthma. *J. Allergy Clin. Immunol.* 53:34, 1974.

117. Rees, H. A., et al. Aminophylline in bronchial asthma. *Lancet* 2:1167, 1967.

118. Rees, H. A., Miller, J. S., and Donald, K. W. A study of the clinical course and arterial blood gas tension of patients in status asthmaticus. *Q. J. Med.* 37:541, 1968.

119. Reinberg, A., Ghata, J., and Sidi, E. Nocturnal asthma attacks: Their relationship to the circadian adrenal cycle. *J. Allergy* 34:323, 1963.

120. Resar, R. K., et al. Kinetics of theophylline. *Chest* 76:11, 1979.

121. Rhine, E. J., and Rosales, J. K. Controlled ventilation in the treatment of status asthmaticus in children. *Can. Anaesth. Soc. J.* 17:129, 1970.

122. Robson, A. O., and Kilborn, J. R. Studies of adrenocortical function in continuous asthma. *Thorax* 20:93, 1965.

123. Roizen, M. F., and Stevens, W. C. Multiform ventricular tachycardia due to the interaction of aminophylline and halothane. *Anesth. Analg.* 57:738, 1978.

124. Rosow, C. E., et al. Histamine release during morphine and fentanyl anesthesia. *Anesthesiology* 56:93, 1982.

125. Rossing, T. H., et al. Emergency therapy of asthma: Comparison of the acute effects of parenteral and inhaled sympathomimetics and infused aminophylline. *Am. Rev. Respir. Dis.* 122:365, 1980.

126. Rossing, T. H., Fanta, C. H., and McFadden, E. R., Jr. A controlled trial of the use of single versus combined-drug therapy in the treatment of acute episodes of asthma. *Am. Rev. Respir. Dis.* 123:190, 1981.

127. Rubinfeld, A. R., and Pain, M. D. F. Relationship between bronchial reactivity, airway caliber and severity of asthma. *Am. Rev. Respir. Dis.* 115:381, 1977.

128. Rubinfeld, A. R., Wagner, P. D., and West, J. B. Gas exchanges during acute experimental canine asthma. *Am. Rev. Respir. Dis.* 118:525, 1978.

129. Rutter, N., Milner, H. D., and Hiller, E. J. Effect of bronchodilators on respiratory resistance in infants and young children with bronchiolitis and wheezy bronchitis. *Arch. Dis. Child.* 50:719, 1975.

130. Sadoul, P. Mucociliary function following bronchodilator therapy. *Postgrad. Med. J.* 51(Suppl.):144, 1975.

131. Schachter, E. N., et al. Histamine blocking agents in healthy and asthmatic subjects. *Chest* 82:143, 1982.

132. Schachter, M. The release of histamine by pethidine, atropine, quinine and other drugs. *Br. J. Anaesth.* 7:646, 1952.

133. Sheppard, D., et al. Dose-dependent inhibition of cold air-induced bronchoconstriction by atropine. *J. Appl. Physiol.* 53:169, 1982.

134. Shnider, S. N., and Papper, E. M. Anesthesia for the asthmatic patient. *Anesthesiology* 22:886, 1961.

135. Shore, S., Milic-Emili, J., and Martin, J. G. Reassessment of body plethysmographic technique for the measurement of thoracic gas volume in asthmatics. *Am. Rev. Respir. Dis.* 126:515, 1982.

136. Sigrist, S., et al. The effect of aminophylline on inspiratory muscle contractility. *Am. Rev. Respir. Dis.* 126:46, 1982.

137. Simonsson, B. G., Jacobs, F. M., and Nadel, J. A. Role of autonomic nervous system and the cough reflex in the increased responsiveness of airways in patients with obstructive airway disease. *J. Clin. Invest.* 46:1812, 1967.

138. Soter, N. A., et al. Release of mast-cell mediators and alterations in lung function in patients with cholinergic urticaria. *N. Engl. J. Med.* 302:604, 1980.

139. Soutar, G. A., Carruthers, M., and Pickering, C. A. C. Nocturnal asthma and urinary adrenaline and noradrenaline excretion. *Thorax* 32:677, 1977.

140. Spark, R. F. Hypothalamic-pituitary-adrenal Axis in Surgery. In J. J. Skillman (ed.), *Intensive Care.* Boston: Little, Brown, 1975. Pp. 311–339.

141. Sprague, D. H., Yang, J. C., and Ngai, S. H. Effects of isoflurane and halothane on contractility and the cyclic $3'5'$-adenosine monophosphate system in the rat aorta. *Anesthesiology* 40:162, 1974.

142. Stanescu, D. C., et al. Failure of body plethysmography in bronchial asthma. *J. Appl. Physiol.* 52:939, 1982.

143. Statham, H. E., and Duncan, C. J. Dantrolene and the neuromuscular junction: Evidence for intracellular calcium stores. *Eur. J. Pharmacol.* 39:143, 1976.

144. Stein, M., et al. Pulmonary evaluation of surgical patients. *JAMA* 181:765, 1962.

145. Stirt, J. A., et al. Aminophylline pharmacokinetics and cardiorespiratory effects during halothane anesthesia in experimental animals. *Anesth. Analg.* 59:186, 1980.

146. Stirt, J. A., et al. Arrhythmogenic effects of aminophylline during halothane anesthesia in experimental animals. *Anesth. Analg.* 59:410, 1980.

147. Stirt, J. A., et al. Halothane-induced cardiac arrhythmias following administration of aminophylline in experimental animals. *Anesth. Analg.* 60:517, 1981.

148. Stirt, J. A., et al. Safety of enflurane following administration of aminophylline in experimental animals. *Anesth. Analg.* 60:871, 1981.

149. Stirt, J. A., and Sullivan, S. F. Aminophylline. *Anesth. Analg.* 60:587, 1981.

150. Strauss, R. M., et al. Influence of heat and humidity on the airway obstruction induced by exercise in asthma. *J. Clin. Invest.* 61:433, 1978.

151. Tai, E., and Read, J. Response of blood gas tension to aminophylline and isoprenaline in patients with asthma. *Thorax* 22:543, 1967.

152. Takaori, M., and Loehning, R. W. Ventricular arrhythmias during halothane anesthesia: Effect of isoproterenol, aminophylline and ephedrine. *Can. Anaesth. Soc. J.* 12:275, 1965.

153. Tandon, M. K. Ventilatory response to carbon dioxide in bronchial asthma. *Am. Rev. Respir. Dis.* 99:415, 1969.

154. Tashkin, D. P., et al. Subsensitization of beta-adrenoceptors in airways and lymphocytes of healthy and asthmatic subjects. *Am. Rev. Respir. Dis.* 125:185, 1982.

155. Tashkin, D. P., et al. Effect of orally administered cimetidine on histamine- and antigen-induced bronchospasm in subjects with asthma. *Am. Rev. Respir. Dis.* 125:691, 1982.

156. Valabhaji, P. Gas exchange in the acute and asymptomatic phases of asthma breathing air and oxygen. *Clin. Sci.* 34:431, 1968.

157. Valberg, P. A., et al. Breathing patterns influence aerosol deposition sites in excised dogs' lungs. *J. Appl. Physiol.* 53:824, 1982.

158. Vallner, J. J., et al. Effect of pH on the binding of theophylline to serum proteins. *Am. Rev. Respir. Dis.* 120:83, 1979.

159. Verdugo, P., Johnson, N., and Tam, P. Beta-adrenergic stimulation of respiratory ciliary activity. *J. Appl. Physiol.* 48:868, 1980.

160. Virtue, R. W., Helmreich, M. L., and Gainza, E. The adrenal cortical response to surgery. I. The effect of anesthesia on plasma 17-hydroxycorticosteroid levels. *Surgery* 41:549, 1957.

161. Wagner, P. D., et al. Ventilation-perfusion inequality in asymptomatic asthma. *Am. Rev. Respir. Dis.* 118:521, 1978.

162. Wanner, A. Clinical aspects of mucociliary transport. *Am. Rev. Respir. Dis.* 116:73, 1977.

163. Watkins, J. Anaphylactoid reactions to i.v. substances. *Br. J. Anaesth.* 51:51, 1979.

164. Watkins, J. Adverse Reactions to Intravenous Induction Agents. In J. A. Thornton (ed.), *Adverse Reactions to Anaesthetic Drugs.* Elsevier: North Holland Biomedical, 1980.

165. Watkins, J., Clarke, R. S. J., and Fee, P. H. The relationships between reported atopy or allergy and immunoglobulins: A preliminary study. *Anaesthesia* 36:582, 1981.

166. Wechsler, R. L., Kleiss, L. M., and Kety, S. S. The effect of intravenously administered aminophylline on cerebral circulation and metabolism in man. *J. Clin. Invest.* 29:28, 1950.

167. Weil, J. V., et al. Diminished ventilatory response to hypoxia and hypercapnia after morphine in normal man. *N. Engl. J. Med.* 292:1103, 1975.

168. Weiss, E. B., and Faling, L. J. Clinical significance of $PaCO_2$ during status asthmaticus: The cross-over point. *Ann. Allergy* 26:545, 1968.

169. Westerfield, B. R., Carder, A. J., and Light, R. W. The relationship between arterial blood gases and serum theophylline clearance in critically ill patients. *Am. Rev. Respir. Dis.* 124:17, 1981.

170. Woolcock, A. J. Inhaled drugs in the prevention of asthma. *Am. Rev. Respir. Dis.* 115:191, 1977.

171. Yang, J. C., et al. Effects of halothane on the cycle 3'5'-adenosine monophosphate (cyclic AMP) system in rat uterine muscle. *Anesthesiology* 38:244, 1973.

172. Young, I. H., Corte, P., and Schoeffel, R. E. Pattern and time course of ventilation-perfusion inequality in exercise-induced asthma. *Am. Rev. Respir. Dis.* 125:304, 1982.

173. Younker, D., et al. Bupivacaine-fentanyl epidural analgesia for a parturient in status asthmaticus. *Can. J. Anaesth.* 34:609, 1987.

174. Zeck, R. T., et al. Variability of the volume of isoflow. *Chest* 79:269, 1981.

175. Zink, J., Sasyniuk, B. I., and Dresel, P. E. Halothane-epinephrine-induced cardiac arrhythmias and the role of heart rate. *Anesthesiology* 43:548, 1975.

176. Tobias, J. D., and Hirshman, C. A. Attenuation of histamine-induced airway constriction by albuterol during halothane anesthesia. *Anesthesiology* 72:105, 1990.

177. Grunberg, G., et al. Facilitation of mechanical ventilation in status asthmaticus with continuous thiopental. *Chest* 99:1216, 1991.

178. Jones, K. A., et al. Halothane decreases cytosolic ionized calcium concentration ($[Ca^{2+}]_i$) during acetylcholine-induced contraction of canine trachealis muscle. *Anesthesiology* 75:A639, 1991.

Respiratory Therapy Modalities

83

Steven E. Levy

In a time of increasing cost for the delivery of health care, as reviewed in Chapter 92, it is important to ask the question "Is there a role for respiratory therapy in the treatment of the patient with asthma, and if so, in what setting?" This question is of importance, not just because of the dramatic increase in the cost of respiratory care during the past decade, but also because of the unresolved question as to the proven effectiveness of respiratory therapy modalities [18].

Respiratory therapy has been defined as the therapeutic use of medical gases and administration apparatus, environmental control systems, humidification, aerosols, medication, ventilatory support, bronchopulmonary drainage, pulmonary rehabilitation, cardiopulmonary resuscitation, and airway management [28]. While it is true that most of these respiratory therapy modalities can be used in the treatment of the nonhospitalized patient in the home or the workplace, traditionally they are thought of primarily in the context of their use in the care of the hospitalized patient with an acute respiratory disorder or an acute exacerbation of a chronic respiratory disorder. With the therapy presently available for the patient with bronchial asthma, hospitalization should be required infrequently, and for this reason alone respiratory therapy modalities probably should play a lesser role in the treatment of most asthmatic patients. When hospitalization is necessary, it often represents a medical failure, either on the part of the physician in failing to prescribe adequate therapy or on the part of the patient in failing to understand and adhere to an adequate therapeutic regimen. There will be exceptions to this statement, such as the development of an acute infectious process or an unavoidable exposure to airway irritants or allergies. The patient who requires hospitalization will often be in status asthmaticus, that is, experiencing a life-threatening asthmatic episode that is initially unresponsive to vigorous therapy with epinephrine or comparable beta agonists, aminophylline, aerosolized bronchodilators, and hydration. In such patients the appropriate and expeditious use of respiratory therapy modalities can be life saving [19]. The treatment of status asthmaticus is discussed in Chapter 73 and the emergency room approach to acute asthma is discussed in Chapter 72. A rational and cost-effective respiratory health care system must be a continued component of respiratory therapy modalities. For example, in a recent model for conversion from small volume nebulizer therapy to metered-dose inhaler therapy, substantial annual hours of technician time (5,000 hr) and reduced hospital costs ($43,758) were reported [30].

What then is the role for respiratory therapy modalities in the treatment of the ambulatory patient? The typical ambulatory patient with bronchial asthma will usually do well with beta-adrenergic bronchodilators (nebulized and oral), oral theophylline, adequate intake of water, avoidance of known precipitating factors, the use of antibiotics with the development of a respiratory infection, and the use of corticosteroids (oral and/or nebu-

lized) when the simpler modalities are ineffective [26]. Theoretically, one might, therefore, use any or all of the following treatment modalities: intermittent positive pressure breathing (IPPB) to nebulize a beta-adrenergic bronchodilator; a nebulizer to generate a mist of water or saline solution to loosen secretions; chest percussion, vibration, and postural drainage to facilitate the removal of bronchial secretions; supplemental oxygen to treat hypoxemia; and finally pulmonary rehabilitation. The utility of each modality is considered separately.

INTERMITTENT POSITIVE PRESSURE BREATHING

IPPB was one of the most commonly used respiratory therapy modalities for the treatment of asthma [15]. This is no longer the case. It is now used much less often even though several hypotheses have been advanced regarding the effects of IPPB that might be of value in the patient with bronchial asthma. Metered-dose inhalers (MDIs) and hand-held updraft nebulizers are now the preferred methods of delivering aerosolized bronchodilators in the ambulatory and also the hospitalized patient with asthma. The hypothetical benefits of IPPB include improved aerosol (including bronchodilator drug) delivery, decreased work of breathing, improved ventilation-perfusion relationships with improved oxygenation, bronchodilatation, facilitation of removal of airway secretions, and psychological effect.

Improved Aerosol Delivery

The claim that IPPB can improve aerosol delivery has been made frequently, and previous unproved studies claimed that this form of therapy allows maximum deposition of aerosol in the airways. However, several investigations [6, 7, 20, 25] indicated a similar relief of bronchospasm whether the bronchodilator is delivered by IPPB, an aerosol generator, a freon-activated unit (MDI), or another type of pressurized canister. A study of patients with chronic bronchitis [9] demonstrated no difference in the ratio of aerosol deposition in proximal to peripheral airways when IPPB was compared with spontaneous breathing; furthermore, the total aerosol deposition in the lungs was less following IPPB. However, another study [8] showed an improvement in the relief of bronchospasm when salbutamol was given by IPPB when compared with responses obtained with a pressurized canister. However, the dose given by IPPB was 10 times greater than that by the pressurized canister. In two other studies in patients with severe acute asthma [5, 24], salbutamol inhaled by IPPB produced greater improvement in flow rates than did salbutamol nebulized without IPPB; the improvement was slight and con-

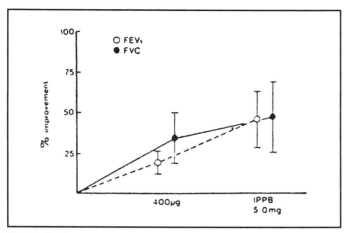

Fig. 83-1. *The percentage improvement in percentage predicted values for 1-second forced expiratory volume (FEV₁) and forced vital capacity (FVC) after the administration of 400 μg of salbutamol from pressure-packed aerosol followed by 5 mg of salbutamol by intermittent positive pressure breathing (IPPB). (Reprinted with permission from R. M. Cayton, et al. A comparison of salbutamol given by pressure-packed aerosol or nebulization via IPPB in acute asthma. Br. J. Dis. Chest 72: 223, 1978.)*

ferred only a marginal advantage to the use of IPPB (Fig. 83-1) [5]. Other studies demonstrated that as many as 80 percent of patients with acute asthma may have problems using an MDI and other devices to deliver a bronchodilator aerosol. IPPB may, therefore, be justified as a means of delivering aerosols when the patient has failed to derive the expected benefit from simpler forms of aerosolization [29].

Decreased Work of Breathing

IPPB may acutely decrease the work of breathing if the patient is relaxed and cooperative. However, in many agitated patients IPPB may actually increase the work of breathing [2]. Furthermore, the question can be raised as to the benefit that can be achieved by improving the work of breathing intermittently for short periods throughout the day. Several studies regarding the effect of continuous positive airway pressure (CPAP) or positive end-expiratory pressure (PEEP) in the treatment of asthma have been published. The effects of CPAP [13] were studied in eight asthmatic patients in whom bronchospasm was induced by the inhalation of an aerosol of histamine. The findings indicated that the load on the inspiratory muscles was reduced, thereby improving their efficiency and decreasing the energy cost of their action. In another study, the use of CPAP was associated with clinical improvement in two patients with severe asthma, suggesting a decrease in the work of breathing [21]. In a randomized crossover study involving 10 stable asthmatics, terbutaline was administered by an MDI connected to a face mask, producing 10 to 15 cm H₂O positive expiratory pressure; an enhanced bronchodilator response was observed with positive expiratory pressure compared to the beta₂ agonist administered alone [11] (Fig. 83-2). However, one study raised a note of caution regarding the use of positive airway pressure. In four patients with asthma requiring mechanical ventilation, PEEP produced improvement in arterial oxygenation, but there were potentially dangerous increases in lung volumes and airway and intrathoracic pressures with circulatory compromise [23]. Thus, the role of CPAP and PEEP in the treatment of asthma remains unclear and requires further study.

Improved Ventilation-perfusion Relationships

Although several earlier studies indicated that IPPB and spontaneous breathing had similar effects on ventilation-perfusion rela-

tionships [10, 22], another study demonstrated that at a given tidal volume, ventilation and perfusion were impaired at the lung bases in normal individuals during IPPB [4]. These studies were done using radioactive-labeled gases administered by IPPB. On the basis of these studies, the authors indicated that spontaneous breathing should be used preferentially to treat atelectasis in supine subjects. Although it was not studied in patients with acute asthma, IPPB apparently disrupts the normal pressure-volume relationship of the lungs [1]. Thus, the normal pattern of ventilation distribution to the lung bases may be altered during IPPB breathing compared with spontaneous breathing.

Bronchodilatation

There is evidence to indicate that IPPB improves bronchospasm at times. The mechanism reflects a passive pulmonary response to an increase in lung volume produced by deep inhalation. However, during spontaneous breathing, similar decreases in airway resistance will occur with increased lung volume. In contrast, significant increases in airway resistance in normal children and asthmatic children have been observed after IPPB [14]. However, one study of positive pressure breathing using positive end-expiratory pressure (PEEP) demonstrated interesting findings that may have significance in regard to IPPB [27]. Bronchoconstriction was induced in five volunteers with a childhood history of asthma, using treadmill exercise. PEEP breathing administered during or after exercise significantly decreased the severity of exercise-induced asthma without any change in end-tidal carbon dioxide tension. It was suggested that the effect during exercise might be related to the reduction of air trapping by PEEP, but that an additional mechanism may be involved since PEEP breathing during work has a lasting effect into recovery.

Facilitation of Removal of Airway Secretions

Despite frequent references to the effectiveness of IPPB in improving mucociliary clearance and the elimination of secretions, there are no reliable data indicating that IPPB positively or negatively affects the physical properties of sputum mucociliary clearance, the effectiveness of cough, or the removal of airway secretions [16]. Any effect of IPPB on mucociliary transport must be distinguished from the effect of concurrent nebulized beta agonists; the issue of significant in vivo effects is still unresolved [12].

Psychological Effect

Many patients who use IPPB find that it provides relief with or without the nebulization of a bronchodilator. In the absence of bronchodilator administration, the subjective improvement could be related to a decreased work of breathing or, possibly, improved ventilation-perfusion relationships or bronchodilatation. Another possible explanation is that there is a psychological effect of IPPB treatment that has yet to be documented because of the ineffectiveness of current techniques of evaluation. Further studies of the overall psychological responses to IPPB therapy in patients with asthma need to be done.

HUMIDIFICATION AND CHEST PHYSIOTHERAPY

Patients with asthma frequently complain of cough with thickened secretions that are difficult to expectorate. Adequate hydration is considered to be a basic need in the treatment of patients with asthma, particularly those with severe asthma, when secretions with mucus plugging can cause life-threatening airway ob-

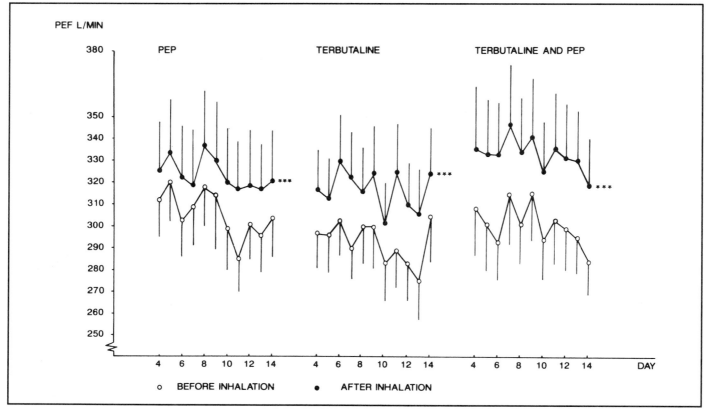

Fig. 83-2. *Peak expiratory flow (PEF) before and after inhalation during the treatment periods (mean and SEM). PEP = positive expiratory pressure. (Reprinted with permission from E. Frischknecht-Christensen, O. Norregaard, and R. Dahl. Treatment of bronchial asthma with terbutaline inhaled by conespacer combined with positive expiratory pressure mask.* Chest *100:317, 1991.)*

struction. Clinical experience suggests that intravenous hydration is effective when the oral intake of fluid is limited. More controversial is the use of bland aerosols in the treatment of mucus production, including patients with asthma; there is no convincing evidence that this form of therapy thins secretions more effectively than oral or intravenous hydration [18]. Moreover, it is important to recognize that in patients with asthma, the administration of aerosols, particularly when generated by ultrasonic nebulizers, may actually induce bronchospasm. Further discussion of this aspect of therapy can be found in Chapter 69.

Chest physiotherapy is another modality often used in the treatment of hospitalized patients with secretions that cannot be expectorated. Chest physiotherapy usually includes postural drainage with chest percussion and vibration. In most patients with stable chronic obstructive pulmonary disease (COPD), the volume of sputum produced after postural drainage and percussion exceeds that produced by cough alone. There is also evidence that physical therapy may improve the clearance of radioactive materials and the velocity of movement of particles from the tracheobronchial tree [18]. Whether similar effects are realized in patients with bronchial asthma is not known. However, since it is the patient with a severe exacerbation of asthma who will usually have a major secretion problem with mucus plugging, and since such patients will usually be hospitalized, it is probable that only in this setting is this therapeutic modality of value.

ADMINISTRATION OF OXYGEN

Since most ambulatory patients with bronchial asthma have adequate arterial oxygenation, supplemental oxygen is rarely

needed. In general, with acute asthma and certainly for status asthmaticus, supplemental oxygen is indicated to provide a physiologic range of oxygen delivery; any potential worsening of ventilation-perfusion relationships during 100% oxygen breathing is offset by the supplemental oxygen enrichment [3]. However, indiscriminate use of high inspired oxygen concentrations in asthma is not warranted. A recent study suggests that use of hyperoxic gas mixtures might contribute to hypercapnia in near-fatal asthma; appropriate oxygen therapy adjusted as indicated by arterial blood gas analysis has been advocated [31, 32].

PULMONARY REHABILITATION AND PHYSICAL TRAINING

Chronic disability is uncommon because of the reversibility of the process, and for this reason pulmonary rehabilitation is probably not indicated in most patients with bronchial asthma. In a recent multidisciplinary pulmonary rehabilitation program involving 24 patients with COPD and 7 patients with asthma, the authors concluded that "the magnitude of change in both physiologic and psychologic parameters was not directly related to lung function, the benefit of rehabilitation can extend to all patients with chronic lung disease, regardless of the severity of preexisting pulmonary disfunction" [17]. Hence, such programs may be of benefit in select patients with asthma. The role of physical training in asthma, including considerations for exercise prescriptions on an individual-based objective criteria of exercise capacity, was recently detailed by Clark [33]. Girodo and colleagues [34] provide a guide to deep diaphragmatic breathing as rehabilitation exercises for asthmatic patients. And a recent editorial stressed the value of regular physical activity for asthmatic children and adults, an important consideration for any rehabilitation program for asthmatics [35].

Although there is a rationale that would justify the use of most respiratory therapy modalities in the treatment of the nonhospitalized ambulatory patient with bronchial asthma, the evidence supporting the use of these modalities is meager. Some patients with bronchial asthma may benefit from the use of one or more of these modalities, but careful consideration should be given to other less costly therapeutic endeavors. At present, the reader will have to draw his or her own conclusions about the value of respiratory treatment for each patient. Further detailed studies are indicated for the use of respiratory therapy modalities in asthma.

REFERENCES

1. Agostini, E., and Miserochi, G. Vertical gradient of transpulmonary pressure with active and artificial lung expansion. *J. Appl. Physiol.* 29:705, 1970.
2. Ayres, S. M., Kozam, R. L., and Lukas, D. S. The effects of intermittent positive pressure breathing on intrathoracic pressure, pulmonary mechanics, and the work of breathing. *Am. Rev. Respir. Dis.* 87:370, 1963.
3. Ballester, E. B. Pulmonary gas exchange in severe chronic asthma; Response to 100% oxygen and salbutamol. *Am. Rev. Respir. Dis.* 141:558, 1990.
4. Bynum, L. J., Wilson, J. E., and Pierce, A. K. Comparison of spontaneous and positive-pressure breathing in supine normal subjects. *J. Appl. Physiol.* 41:341, 1976.
5. Cayton, R. M., et al. A comparison of salbutamol given by pressure-packed aerosol or nebulization via IPPB in acute asthma. *Br. J. Dis. Chest* 72:222, 1978.
6. Chang, N., and Levison, H. The effect of nebulized bronchodilator administered with or without intermittent positive pressure breathing on ventilatory function in children with cystic fibrosis and asthma. *Am. Rev. Respir. Dis.* 106:867, 1972.
7. Chester, E. H., et al. Bronchodilator therapy: Comparison of acute responses to three methods of administration. *Chest* 62:394, 1972.
8. Choo-Kang, K. F. J., and Grant, I. W. B. Comparison of two methods of administering bronchodilator for aerosol to asthmatic patients. *Br. Med. J.* 2:119, 1975.
9. Dolovich, M. D., et al. Pulmonary aerosol deposition in chronic bronchitis: Intermittent positive pressure breathing versus quiet breathing. *Am. Rev. Respir. Dis.* 115:397, 1977.
10. Emmanuel, G. E., Smith, W. M., and Briscoe, W. A. The effect of intermittent positive pressure breathing and voluntary hyperventilation upon the distribution of ventilation and pulmonary blood flow to the lung in chronic obstructive lung disease. *J. Clin. Invest.* 45:1221, 1966.
11. Frischknecht-Christensen, E., Norregaard, O., and Dahl, R. Treatment of bronchial asthma with terbutaline inhaled by conespacer combined with positive expiratory pressure mask. *Chest* 100:317, 1991.
12. Isawa, T., et al. Does a β_2-stimulator really facilitate mucociliary transport in the human lungs in vivo? *Am. Rev. Respir. Dis.* 141:715, 1990.
13. Martin, J. G., Shore, S., and Engel, L. A. Effect of continuous positive airway pressure on respiratory mechanics and pattern of breathing in induced asthma. *Am. Rev. Respir. Dis.* 126:812, 1982.
14. Moore, R. B., Cotton, E. K., and Pinney, M. A. The effect of intermittent positive-pressure breathing on airway resistance in normal and asthmatic children. *J. Allergy Clin. Immunol.* 49:137, 1972.
15. Motley, H. L., Lang, L. P., and Gordon, G. Use of intermittent positive pressure breathing combined with nebulization in pulmonary disease. *Am. J. Med.* 5:853, 1948.
16. Murray, J. F. Review of the state of the art in intermittent positive pressure breathing therapy. *Am. Rev. Respir. Dis.* 110:193, 1974.
17. Niederman, M. S., et al. Benefits of a multidisciplinary pulmonary rehabilitation program, improvements are independent of lung function. *Chest* 99:798, 1991.
18. Pierce, A. K. Conference on the scientific basis of in-hospital respiratory therapy. *Am. Rev. Respir. Dis.* 122:1, 1980.
19. Senior, R. M., Lefrak, S. S., and Korenblat, P. E. Status asthmaticus. *JAMA* 231:1277, 1975.
20. Taylor, W. F., et al. Intermittent positive pressure breathing versus freon mist nebulized isoproterenol in asthmatic children. *Allergy* 38:257, 1966.
21. Tenaillon, A., Salmona, J. P., and Burdin, M. Continuous positive airway pressure in asthma. *Am. Rev. Respir. Dis.* 127:658, 1983.
22. Torres, G., Lyons, H. A., and Emerson, P. The effects of intermittent positive pressure breathing on the intrapulmonary distribution of inspired air. *Am. J. Med.* 29:946, 1960.
23. Tuxen, D. V. Detrimental effects of positive end-expiratory pressure during controlled mechanical ventilator of patients with severe airflow obstruction. *Am. Rev. Respir. Dis.* 140:5, 1989.
24. Webber, B. A., Collins, J. V., and Branthwaite, M. A. Severe acute asthma: A comparison of three months of inhaling salbutamol. *Br. J. Dis. Chest* 76:69, 1982.
25. Weber, R. W., Petty, W. E., and Nelson, H. S. Aerosolized terbutaline in asthmatics. *J. Allergy Clin. Immunol.* 63:116, 1976.
26. Welch, M. H. *Pulmonary Medicine.* Philadelphia: Lippincott, 1977. P. 625.
27. Wilson, B. A., Jackson, P. J., and Evans, J. Effects of positive end-expiratory pressure on exercise induced asthma. *Int. J. Sports Med.* 2:27, 1981.
28. Young, J. A., and Singletary, W. S. History of the Inhalation Therapy-respiratory Care Profession. In G. G. Burton, G. N. Gee, and J. E. Hodgkin (eds.), *Respiratory Care: A Guide to Clinical Practice.* Philadelphia: Lippincott, 1977. P. 11.
29. Ziment, I. Intermittent Positive Pressure Breathing. In G. G. Burton, G. N. Gee, and J. E. Hodgkins (eds.), *Respiratory Care: A Guide to Clinical Practice.* Philadelphia: Lippincott, 1977. P. 555.
30. Tenholder, M. F., Bryson, M. J., and Whitlock, W. L. A model for conversion from small volume nebulizer to metered dose inhaler aerosol therapy. *Chest* 101:634, 1992.
31. Molfino, N. A., et al. Respiratory arrest in near-fatal asthma. *N. Engl. J. Med.* 324:285, 1991.
32. McFadden, E. R. Jr. Fatal and near-fatal asthma. *N. Engl. J. Med.* 324:409, 1991.
33. Clark, C. J. The role of physical training in asthma. *Chest* 101(Suppl.): 293S, 1992.
34. Girodo, M., Ekstrand, K. A., and Metivier, C. J. Deep diaphragmatic breathing: rehabilitation exercises for the asthmatic patient. *Arch. Phys. Med. Rehab.* 73:717, 1992.
35. Schwartzstein, R. M. Asthma: to run or not to run? *Am. Rev. Respir. Dis.* 145:739, 1992.

Fiberoptic Bronchoscopy

Ralph L. Kendall

There are no characteristic endobronchoscopic changes diagnostic of asthma. However, observations from the bronchoscope can help to define the cause of wheezing when it is related to focal airway narrowing or when wheeze is induced by other causes that can mimic asthma. Bronchoscopy was formerly restricted to the use of the rigid instrument until 1968 when Ikeda and coworkers [8] demonstrated the advantages of the flexible bronchofiberscope by which airways could be reached for diagnostic and therapeutic purposes using a procedure that did not require general anesthesia and that could be performed outside the operating room.

The indications for fiberoptic bronchoscopy in patients with wheezing are to diagnose focal airway obstruction caused by an inflammatory process, tumor or foreign body, or any other condition requiring clarification. Flexible bronchoscopy also bypasses narrowed areas to appraise distal airways. While foreign bodies can occasionally be removed via the fiberscope, this procedure is generally best performed with the rigid instrument.

The use of the fiberscope is not without complications, but these occur less frequently than with the rigid bronchoscope [14]. In addition, these complications are usually minor and can generally be averted with adequate local anesthesia. However, Peacock [21] showed that the local application of lidocaine to the major airways caused a significant fall in 1-second forced expiratory volume (FEV_1) and inspiratory and expiratory flow that did not occur with the insertion of the bronchoscope. On occasion, quiescent asthma can be converted to severe iatrogenic bronchospasm. One prospective study by Pereira and associates [22] documented the development of airway obstruction during bronchoscopy, even when the majority of patients were not asthmatic. Epiglottic edema may occur, compounding the existing airway obstruction, when there is undue trauma during the insertion of the instrument. Fiberoptic bronchoscopy produces airway epithelial damage but this is not a mechanism that induces airway hyperresponsiveness [30]. However, even in patients with more severe asthma treated by aerosol corticosteroid, Laursen and coworkers [13] showed that bronchial mucosal biopsies could be performed without precipitating acute symptoms. The pathology of asthma is demonstrated nicely with specimens taken by fiberoptic bronchoscopy (Plate 28).

Bronchoscopy performed while the patient is breathing room air can produce significant hypoxemia, even in patients who are not critically ill. This hypoxemia, occurring when the fiberscope is passed into the trachea, is caused by a variety of mechanisms and is preventable by supplemental oxygen by means of nasal prongs or mask [1]. The inspired oxygen concentration (FIO_2) should be sufficient to maintain an arterial oxygen tension (PaO_2) above 60 mmHg; if this cannot be accomplished, fiberoptic bronchoscopy should not be performed [6]. Concurrently, O_2 saturation should be monitored by continuous oximetry. When the fiberscope is passed through a tracheal tube with a diameter of less than 8.5 mm, there is an unacceptable increase in airway resistance, resulting in airflow rates insufficient for adequate ventilation [25].

Even in the asymptomatic asthmatic patient, bronchoscopy is not without hazard, as there is an increased risk of severe laryngospasm and bronchoconstriction unless a large dose of atropine is used for premedication [29]. The airway narrowing and reduction of forced vital capacity (FVC) and FEV_1 can be counteracted by large doses of intramuscular atropine, 0.8 to 1.0 mg. Prevention of vagally mediated airway obstruction will also reduce secretions and prevent bradycardia during the procedure. Zavala and colleagues [35] showed that atropine administered by aerosol produces excellent bronchodilation and obviates side effects, but this route does not also inhibit the vasovagal response that is abated by parenteral administration. A useful premedication schema includes the administration of an aminophylline as well as atropine: Some advocate giving prednisolone (100-mg intravenous bolus) or an adrenergic agent before the procedure [35]. For example, oral salbutamol (2.5 mg) and nebulized ipratropium bromide (0.5 mg), in addition to local anesthesia to the airways, was suggested by Holgate and colleagues [36] for use in investigative studies. Excessive narcotic premedication that could impair ventilation and gas exchange should be avoided; should this occur, the narcotic effects can be reversed by naloxone. Anesthetic-related deaths can occur before any procedure, and these are not directly related to the bronchoscopic procedure itself. Deaths from fiberoptic bronchoscopy are more frequent in patients with cardiovascular disease and/or chronic obstructive lung disease. Presumably these problems can be minimized or prevented with appropriate electrocardiographic monitoring as well as ear oximetry to monitor and to eliminate hypoxemia [31]. Fatal anesthetic reactions can be prevented by the prudent use of topical lidocaine. Bronchospastic responses to lidocaine may be mediated by prostaglandin $F_{2\alpha}$ as suggested by Weiss and Patwardhan [34]. Atropine prevents bronchoconstriction from lidocaine, which is an important justification for its use as premedication. The low pH of 4% lidocaine in distilled water may increase hyperreactivity, which can be reduced by using a 2% saline solution. While there are many methods for administering local anesthesia, topical spray of the nose and pharynx is an acceptable and easy approach [28]. Prior or concurrent administration of a beta-adrenergic bronchodilator (e.g., metaproterenol) is also recommended to reduce lidocaine-induced bronchospasm in patients with hyperreactive airways [10].

Therapeutic fiberoptic bronchoscopy in asthma patients is primarily utilized to remove critically obstructing, retained secretions and mucus plugs and small bronchi. This has essentially replaced full lung lavage with a catheter, first employed in the treatment of alveolar proteinosis and modified by Kylstra and colleagues [12] for asthma and cystic fibrosis. Ramirez and Kylstra and their respective colleagues used large-volume, gravity filled lavage successfully for patients with refractory asthma who were moderately ill and who were ambulatory but not in status asthmaticus [12, 23]. Rogers and associates [27] demonstrated that large-volume–controlled lavage removed casts in large and small airways, with immediate and long-term clinical improvement in patients requiring ventilatory support who had not responded to optimal bronchodilator therapy and corticosteroids. Volume-controlled lung lavage is a formidable procedure requiring general anesthesia and 100% inspired oxygen, but the bronchial flooding may clear the peripheral airways by removing casts and mucus plugs. Emergency bronchoscopy for acute respiratory distress caused by voluminous secretions in the large airways usually employs the rigid bronchoscope [16].

The flexible bronchofiberscope is primarily utilized when there is accumulation and inspissation of secretions in distal airways not accessible by the rigid instrument. These inaccessible secretions, which may result in respiratory failure requiring mechanical ventilation, can be removed under direct vision. Secretions can be removed during ventilatory support for acute asthma, with the use of an adapter assembly that permits access to distal airways. Supplemental oxygen, FIO_2 1.0, will usually be needed during the procedure to maintain a PaO_2 greater than 60 mmHg, especially if the internal tracheal tube diameter is 8.5 mm or smaller. It has been demonstrated under these conditions that peripheral portions of the tracheobronchial tree can be cleared, improving oxygenation and reducing peak airway pressure [2]. The value of fiberoptic bronchoscopy has also been demonstrated in the management of atelectasis in asthma, where successful aspiration of obstructive mucus plugs results in regional parenchymal expansion and improvement in arterial blood gases [15, 32]. Instillation of 5% N-acetyl-L-cysteine through the fiberscope has been utilized effectively in status asthmaticus with life-threatening bronchial obstruction caused by refractory lobar and peripheral mucus plugging [4]. To avoid added induced bronchospasm, it is recommended that a bronchodilator be concomitantly used. Very careful clinical evaluation is required to determine whether fiberoptic (or rigid) bronchoscopy should be performed and for what advantage in a critically ill asthmatic with advanced secretory obstruction.

Lung lavage with the fiberscope has also been used in asthmatic patients. Large-volume lavage with the fiberscope may enhance peripheral airway secretional clearance, resulting in an improvement FEV_1 and peak flow in asthma [33]. Lavage with smaller volumes (300 ml) of saline solution at room temperature is effective in the removal of alveolar macrophages and proteinaceous material; multiple small-volume lavage can remove mucus plugging in status asthmaticus with a significant increase in oxygenation and lung compliance. Large-volume saline lobar lavage with 1,000 ml through the fiberoptic bronchoscope can also be accomplished with minimal sequelae. Insertion of the bronchoscope and inflation of the lavage tube cuff to occlude the lobar bronchus can produce significant hypoxemia. A fall in PaO_2 by as much as 30 mmHg can occur and also may be seen at the termination of the lavage. This hypoxemia can be reduced but not eliminated by supplemental oxygen and may persist up to 8 hours after the lavage [3]. Ventilation-perfusion abnormalities are also present following lobar lavage, but these return to normal in 24 hours. (The interested reader is referred to the first edition of this book for further information concerning lavage technique [11].)

Pulmonary lavage is presumably used in bronchial asthma despite the paucity both of precise indications and of proved efficacy. Comprehensive prospective controlled trials are indicated to define its role in the management of acute, severe, asthmatic airway obstruction. Interestingly, Millman and associates [17] described the usefulness of bronchoscopy and lavage in a series of patients with chronic bronchial asthma. It is worth reemphasizing that since fiberoptic bronchoscopy may provoke broncho-

spasm in asthmatic patients, the procedure should be performed based on firm indications, and conducted with supplemental oxygen and proper monitoring in addition to adequate bronchodilator therapy and appropriate premedication. In status asthmaticus, intubation and ventilation may be required because of progressive acidemia and refractory hypoxemia. This can be accomplished with continuous intravenous thiopental anesthesia; Grunberg and colleagues [7] showed that gas exchange markedly improved in 1 hour. The concomitant use of bronchial lavage with 5% N-acetyl-L-cysteine, as proposed by Mittman and coauthors [18], could be performed optimally at this time, enhancing the safety of this procedure during severe respiratory distress. The safety and efficacy of bronchoscopy in the critical care unit for retained secretions and mucus plugging have also been demonstrated by Olopade and Drakash [20]. Generally, the use of N-acetyl-L-cysteine in acute asthma should be avoided because of its bronchospastic actions.

Reynolds [26] used bronchoalveolar lavage for investigational purposes in the study on the immunopathogenesis of asthma [19], and Kirby [9] and Rankin [24] and their colleagues demonstrated its safety in patients with mild symptomatic asthma. Djukanovic and coworkers [5] also performed endobronchial biopsies with lavage in patients with more severe asthma without untoward effect, but the authors stressed the need for bronchodilators during the procedure. Bronchoalveolar lavage is discussed in detail in Chapter 24.

In spite of its safety, flexible fiberoptic bronchoscopy should be delayed in most instances until the acute episode has subsided, FEV_1 maximized, and appropriate indications for the examination exist. Table 84-1 provides a summary of guidelines for investigative bronchoscopy in asthma. The safety and use of en-

Table 84-1. *Summary of recommendations and guidelines for investigative bronchoscopy in subjects with asthma and other obstructive airway diseases**

Subjects considered unsuitable	Subjects sensitive to local anesthetics/other medications; individuals exhibiting extreme BHR and severe airflow obstruction; subjects with uncorrected bleeding diathesis (biopsy)
Subjects at high risk from the procedures	Subjects with FEV_1 <60% predicted and/or coexisting cardiopulmonary diseases
Procedural limitations	Instillation of no more than 400 ml fluid; three to six 2-mm biopsies from a combination of the main carina and one or more segmental or subsegmental carinae in a single procedure; brushings limited to two to four areas
Potential hazards	Acute airflow obstruction; laryngospasm; hypoxemia; apnea; bleeding; drug reactions; airway perforation (biopsy); fever; pulmonary infiltrates; infections
Preprocedure evaluation	Complete medical history; physical examination; electrocardiogram; blood pressure; oximetry
Postprocedure monitoring	Gag reflex; pulmonary function; stable clinical status; postdischarge follow-up

BAL = bronchoalveolar lavage; BHR = bronchial hyperresponsiveness; FEV_1 = 1-second forced expiratory volume.
* BAL, bronchial brushing and biopsy, and airway instrumentation can be safely performed in subjects with mild to moderate asthma.
Source: Hurd, S. S. et al. Workshop summary and guidelines—Bronchoscopy. *J. Allergy Clin. Immunol.* 88:808, 1991. Reprinted with permission.

dobronchial biopsy for study purposes in airway inflammation was recently detailed by Holgate and colleagues [36]; for investigational studies, asthma should be clinically stable and mild, and FEV_1 greater than or equal to 70 percent predicted.

REFERENCES

1. Albertini, R. E., Harrell, J. H., II, and Moser, K. M. Management of arterial hypoxemia induced by fiberoptic bronchoscopy. *Chest* 67:134, 1975.
2. Barrett, C. R., Vecchione, J. J., and Bell, A. L. L., Jr. Flexible fiberoptic bronchoscopy for airway management during acute respiratory failure. *Am. Rev. Respir. Dis.* 109:429, 1974.
3. Burns, D. M., et al. Physiological consequences of saline lobar lavage. *Am. Rev. Respir. Dis.* 127:695, 1983.
4. Donaldson, J. C., et al. Acetylcysteine for life-threatening acute bronchial obstruction. *Ann. Intern. Med.* 88:656, 1978.
5. Djukanovic, R., et al. The safety aspects of fiberoptic bronchoscopy, bronchoalveolar lavage, and endobronchial biopsy in asthma. *Am. Rev. Respir. Dis.* 143:722, 1991.
6. Dubrawsky, C., Awe, R. J., and Jenkins, D. E. The effect of bronchofiberscopic examination on oxygenation status. *Chest* 67:137, 1975.
7. Grunberg, G., et al. Facilitation of mechanical ventilation in status asthmaticus with continuous intravenous thiopental. *Chest* 99:1216, 1991.
8. Ikeda, S., Yanai, N., and Ishikawa, S. Flexible bronchofiberscope. *Keio J. Med.* 17:1, 1968.
9. Kirby, J. G., et al. Bronchoalveolar lavage does not alter airway responsiveness in asthmatic subjects. *Am. Rev. Respir. Dis.* 135:554, 1987.
10. Kirkpatrick, M. B., Sanders, R. V., and Bass, J. B., Jr. Physiologic effects and serum lidocaine concentrations after inhalation of lidocaine from a compressed gas-powered jet nebulizer. *Am. Rev. Respir. Dis.* 136:447, 1987.
11. Kovnat, D. Bronchoscopy and Lavage in Asthma. In E. Weiss and M. Segal (eds.), *Bronchial Asthma: Mechanisms and Therapeutics* (1st ed.). Boston: Little, Brown, 1976.
12. Kylstra, J. A., et al. Volume controlled lung lavage in the treatment of asthma, bronchiectasis and mucoviscidosis. *Am. Rev. Respir. Dis.* 103:651, 1971.
13. Laursen, L. C., et al. Fiberoptic bronchoscopy and bronchial mucosal biopsies in asthmatics undergoing long-term high-dose budisonide aerosol treatment. *Allergy* 43:284, 1988.
14. Lukomsky, G. I., Ovchinnikov, A. A., and Bilal, A. Complications of bronchoscopy. Comparison of rigid bronchoscopy under general anesthesia and flexible fiberoptic bronchoscopy under topical anesthesia. *Chest* 79:316, 1981.
15. Mahajan, V. K., Catron, P. W., and Huber, G. L. The value of fiberoptic bronchoscopy in the management of pulmonary collapse. *Chest* 73:817, 1978.
16. Milledge, J. S. Therapeutic fiberoptic bronchoscopy in intensive care. *Br. Med. J.* 2:1427, 1976.
17. Millman, M., et al. Bronchoscopy and lavage for chronic bronchial asthma. *Immunol. Allergy Pract.* 3:10, 1981.
18. Mittman, M., et al. Status asthmaticus use of acetylcysteine during bronchoscopy and lavage to remove mucous plugs. *Ann. Allergy* 50:85, 1983.
19. NHLBI Workshop Summary. Summary and recommendations of a workshop on the investigative use of fiberoptic bronchoscopy and bronchoalveolar lavage in asthmatics. *Am. Rev. Respir. Dis.* 132:180, 1985.
20. Olopade, C. O., and Drakash, U. B. S. *Mayo Clin. Proc.* 64:1255, 1989.
21. Peacock, A. J., Benson-Mitchell, R., and Godfrey, R. Effect of fiberoptic bronchoscopy on pulmonary function. *Thorax* 45:38, 1990.
22. Pereira, W., Jr., Kovnat, D. M., and Snider, G. L. A prospective cooperative study of complications following flexible fiberoptic bronchoscopy. *Chest* 73:813, 1978.
23. Ramirez, J., and Obenour, W. H., Jr. Bronchopulmonary lavage in asthma and chronic bronchitis. Clinical and physiologic observations. *Chest* 59:146, 1971.
24. Rankin, J. A., et al. Bronchoalveolar lavage, its safety in subjects with mild asthma. *Chest* 85:723, 1984.
25. Rauscher, C. R., and Smith, P. F. Therapeutic fiberoptic bronchoscopy. *Ariz. Med.* 31:167, 1974.
26. Reynolds, H. Y. Bronchoalveolar lavage. *Am. Rev. Respir. Dis.* 135:250, 1987.
27. Rogers, R. M., Braunstein, M. S., and Shuman, J. F. Role of bronchopulmonary lavage in the treatment of respiratory failure: A review. *Chest* 62(Suppl., pt 2):95S, 1972.
28. Sackner, M. A. Bronchofiberscopy. *Am. Rev. Respir. Dis.* 111:62, 1975.
29. Sahn, S. A., and Scoggin, C. Fiberoptic bronchoscopy in bronchial asthma: A word of caution. *Chest* 69:39, 1976.
30. Soderberg, M., and Lundgren, R. Flexible fiberoptic bronchoscopy does not alter airway responsiveness. *Respiration* 56:182, 1989.
31. Suratt, P. M., Smiddy, J. F., and Gruber, B. Deaths and complications associated with fiberoptic bronchoscopy. *Chest* 69:747, 1976.
32. Wanner, A., et al. Bronchofiberscopy for atelectasis and lung abscess. *JAMA* 224:1281, 1973.
33. Weinstein, H. J., Bone, R. C., and Ruth, W. E. Pulmonary lavage in patients treated with mechanical ventilation. *Chest* 72:583, 1977.
34. Weiss, E. B., and Patwardhan, A. V. The response to lidocaine in bronchial asthma. *Chest* 72:429, 1977.
35. Zavala, D. C., Godsey, K., and Bedell, G. N. The response to atropine sulphate in patients undergoing fiberoptic bronchoscopy. *Chest* 79:512, 1981.
36. Holgate, S. T., et al. New insights into airway inflammation by endobronchial biopsy. *Am. Rev. Respir. Dis.* 145:S2, 1992.

Psychiatric Aspects

Jonathan Brush
Aleksander A. Mathé

85

For many years, extensive reports have suggested that psychological factors play an important role in the development of bronchial asthma, in precipitating episodes of asthma, and in worsening the course of the illness. Reports from the 1940s [125] found an increased frequency of anxiety and insecurity in asthmatic children, and classic psychoanalytic studies of a small sample of adults during the same period [43, 44] supported the hypothesis that asthma could represent the expression of intense emotion in distorted form—a "suppressed cry for the mother." Alternative formulations [28, 41] were that through learning, particular emotional experiences may have reinforced pulmonary physiologic responses, thus increasing the likelihood of their occurring in the same context.

These early reports have been followed by many investigations, looking at (1) psychoneuroimmunologic pathways and mechanisms, (2) biopsychosocial evidence for connections between asthma and intrapersonal and interpersonal psychological patterns, and (3) evidence for the effectiveness of behavioral or psychological interventions in asthma. This chapter surveys the latter two areas; a separate chapter (Chap. 33) covers the former area. Suffice it to say, however, that accumulated knowledge in the area of psychoneuroimmunology has supported the concept that psychological stress affects the immune system [69] and is associated with increased risk of respiratory infection [20]. Asthma is, in many cases, the result of central nervous system (CNS) interaction with immunologic and endocrinologic processes, with much variation across individuals [108]. Thus, we propose that there is evidence for mechanisms by which psychological influences, along with corresponding events in the CNS extending from there to the peripheral cellular level, play a role in asthma, either in conjunction with allergic processes or independently. Now we turn to evidence that this sequence does in fact occur.

BIOPSYCHOSOCIAL STUDIES

Biopsychosocial evidence for a psychological component in asthma has come from experimental investigations, epidemiologic and sociologic studies, examination of childhood and familial factors, and investigations of the clinical correlates and the clinical course of asthma.

Experimental Investigations

Experimental investigation of psychological factors in asthma dates from 1886 when Sir James MacKenzie [93] described "rose asthma" (acute coryza, congestion, and wheezing) in a young woman disturbed by the sight of a paper rose under glass. Without evidence of reversible obstructive effects in the airways, this remains a suggestive anecdote. Subsequent investigations have been directed increasingly to the effects of stress or learned responses; they have used quantifiable, replicable pulmonary measures. Increasingly more sophisticated psychological assessment has been combined with progressively more precise study of pulmonary function in asthma [46, 50]. Responses to stress present a paradox. Acute attacks of asthma at all ages often occur in a setting of turmoil, characterized by anxiety or anger. Subjective anxiety and elevations in both heart rate and skin temperature have been observed in asthmatic children as compared with normal children [54], providing evidence of sustained activation in parts of the sympathetic nervous system. The following question arises: Why do not these aroused asthmatic patients "cure" themselves [94, 95]?

Induced stress under experimental conditions has thrown some light on this matter. In a general study of pulmonary function, the great sensitivity of a number of respiratory variables to purely emotional arousal stimulated by hypnosis and other techniques has been demonstrated [34, 35]. Longitudinal studies have revealed significant correlations between measures of stress and both airway resistance (Raw) [56] and respiratory movements [57].

In another study [95, 96] two stressors, a disturbing film and a mathematic task carried out under a condition of negative criticism, were allowed to interact, and ascertainment was made of their impact on airway conductance, respiratory and pulse rate, blood pressure, and free fatty acid, plasma cortisol, and urinary catecholamine levels (controlling for dietary and other relevant factors). Subjects had mild asthma, did not require medication, and were matched for age and socioeconomic status with comparison individuals. All subjects responded to the stress condition with expected increases in heart rate, blood pressure, plasma cortisol level, and excretion of urinary norepinephrine. Under stress the asthmatic group responded selectively with a decrease in airway conductance and slowing of respiration, and selectively failed to show a stress-induced elevation in plasma free fatty acid and urinary epinephrine levels. Subjectively both groups reported increases in anxiety and in overall emotion, but the asthmatics reported significantly less provoked anger. A partial replication of this work, confirming the decreased urinary epinephrine excretion, was reported by others [15, 87]. In a population of asthmatic children, the stress of asthmatic attacks also did not increase the excretion of epinephrine in urine [107]. These findings are consistent with the view that an adrenergic defect plays a role in acute asthma [94].

Recent work [77], utilizing a stressful interview as paradigm, demonstrated a drop in mitogenic responsivity after elicitation of, particularly, emotions of anxiety and excitedness, accompanied by elevations of heart rate and blood pressure. While not specifically addressing the issue of asthmatic response to stress, this study provides evidence relevant to the possible pathways by which interpersonal experience may result in increased asthmatic symptoms.

Physiologic considerations are also important in evaluating studies in learning in bronchial asthma. Classic conditioning of asthma was reported [113] by exposing guinea pigs to an allergic stimulus and provoking a dyspneic asthma-like response; later this response was obtained merely by introducing the animals to the same experimental chamber. Conditioning studies must, however, be examined carefully in the light of the demonstration that the preponderant effect observed in attempts at conditioning is hyperventilation, presumably as part of a diffuse stress reaction [130]. By precise measurement of airway resistance, a true asthma-like response was demonstrated, but it was unstable and extinguished rapidly, making extrapolation to the sustained human clinical disorder problematic. In a small number of instances, possible conditioned asthma-like responses were obtained in humans using a classic conditioning paradigm [27, 133] but again chance or suggestive effects could not be excluded. We must conclude that there is little convincing evidence for classic conditioning as a cause of bronchial asthma in the human.

An alternative approach to learning is use of an operant paradigm to bring about visceral learning. Subjects attached to a forced oscillation apparatus [50] yielding second-by-second computer analysis of respiratory resistance were instructed to keep a red light on, which had been programmed to flash when their resistance decreased below a critical level [146]. Two groups with mild asymptomatic asthma (all having elevated baseline airway resistance) showed a "learned" drop in airway resistance. They differed significantly from a control group with comparable mild asthma given purely random reinforcement, who showed no change. The decrease in resistance was modest (about 1.5 cm H_2O/L/sec). Analysis of tidal volumes showed that this was not caused by a shift in lung volume [146]. The same biofeedback paradigm was used to study four asthmatic children and one nonasthmatic child under each of three conditions: biofeedback, isoproterenol, and rest [40]. Biofeedback and isoproterenol produced decreases in airway resistance of equivalent magnitude. Effects on maximum midexpiratory flow (MMEF) and peak expiratory flow rate (PEFR) were variable. Rest had no effect, and none of the experimental treatments influenced the one normal subject. It remains to be seen whether the changes induced in this way can be increased, can be shown to persist over time, and are clinically significant.

Suggestion, which perhaps should be regarded as a variant of learning, capitalizing on acquired associations and implied reinforcement, has also intrigued students of asthma, in the wake of Sir James MacKenzie's experiment. Attacks representing asthma-like responses in the bronchial tree have been reported in subjects exposed to pictorial or verbal suggestions of objects and substances to which they were sensitive [26]. Using direct hypnotic suggestion, asthmatic subjects reported improved breathing, although there were no changes in forced vital capacity (FVC) [149]. In a careful series of experiments, 40 subjects were exposed to aerosolized saline solution; they were told that the vehicle was an allergenic precipitant to which they had been previously found sensitive [92, 99]. Approximately half of the subjects responded with a relatively rapid reduction in airway conductance. This response was reversed when the same saline solution was accompanied by the suggestion that it was a bronchodilator. Atropine blocked the bronchoobstructive effect, implying vagal mediation [91]. Further experiments with suggestion have led to varied results. The effect of suggestion on 1-second forced expiratory volume (FEV_1) was more marked in a group of 10 subjects with intrinsic asthma than in a group of 10 with extrinsic asthma, the latter being defined as those who responded to skin tests, while the former showed no skin reaction to standardized allergic testing [115]. In another study [147] no clear changes from suggestion were obtained in children, possibly because it was difficult to involve them in the experiment and possibly also because measurements were made with the relatively insensitive

Wright peak flowmeter. On the other hand, a significant ameliorative effect of hypnosis on the dose-response curve for the Prausnitz-Küstner–induced allergic skin reaction was reported in four healthy subjects, selected because of their ability to enter a deep hypnotic trance [16].

Subsequently, two carefully controlled experiments were carried out, one with 9 and the other with 22 mildly ill bronchial asthmatics, endeavoring to replicate the previous observations on suggestion [60, 136]. In the first experiment [136], in 6 of 9 patients a clear decrease in specific airway conductance (SGaw) to inhalation of a flavored diluent that had previously been given in combination with methacholine was obtained, partially reversible on exposure to similar suggestion of bronchodilation. Responses to methacholine were greater than to suggestion. Both had maximum effect on Raw and SGaw, which the authors interpreted to indicate the role of the vagus on large airways. The second experiment [60] showed variable responses to pure suggestion, that is, the administration of a vehicle without previous pairing to methacholine; the group effect was statistically significant, although only 6 of 22 subjects had greater than 10 percent reduction in SGaw.

A related approach has consisted of efforts to influence exercise-induced asthma by suggestive means. Exercise asthma elicited by treadmill running not only was inhibited by premedication with salbutamol and disodium cromoglycate, but also was significantly reduced by placebo in 20 of 44 children [48]. The suggestive effect was less than the pharmacologic one and varied among different subject groups, but it seemed to be a promising approach in identifying children whose asthma was sensitive to emotional factors. The efficacy of hypnosis in attenuating exercise-induced asthma was assessed in 10 patients with stable asthma [14]; hypnosis before exercise reduced the drop in FEV_1 from 31.8 percent (on control days) to 15.9 percent, a highly significant effect, nearly as marked as that from pretreatment with cromolyn, which reduced the drop to 7.6 percent. Finally, it was observed that vividly recalled experiences of fear and anger led to decreases in FEV_1 in 60 children [141]. Thus, it is clear that suggestive influences can significantly alter the pathophysiologic responses of some though not all asthmatics. The psychological and biologic characteristics of the subjects affected and the exact conditions and mechanisms, whether involving overall emotional arousal or changes in learned expectancies, are unresolved.

Another set of experiments has taken as a starting point the clinical observation that often when a child was sent away from his or her family, whether to a hospital, school, or camp, the asthma improved, at least initially. The suspicion followed that one might be removing the child from noxious interaction with family members [1, 2]. An obvious question was whether social or allergenic factors were changed. To try to answer that question, children allegedly sensitive to house dust from their homes were hospitalized [86]; exposure in the hospital to large amounts of house dust obtained from each home failed to provoke asthma in 19 of 20 children. A similar experiment involved removing parents from the home and studying respiratory variables and medication demands by a nurse (and parent substitute); 18 of 35 children showed significant improvement in indexes of asthma while their parents were gone [117]. Guided by a specially designed diagnostic interview, the investigators correctly predicted in advance, with one exception, each child's response to this psychosocial manipulation. These experiments all point to differences in reactivity among different asthmatics; they have spurred the effort to find meaningful ways of characterizing subgroups within the disorder.

Epidemiologic Factors and Clinical Groupings

Epidemiologic studies, aside from showing the widespread prevalence of asthma, generally ranging from 2 to 6 percent [118,

148], shed some light on possible etiologic factors. The changing sex distribution, marked by a shift from male predominance among children to a roughly equal ratio among adults, and the elusive phenomenon of "growing out" of asthma [114] suggest that maturational, possibly biologic, and/or familial factors modulate an underlying predisposition. A genetic basis for the predisposition [146] has generally been assumed, based on findings of a family history for allergic disease in 45 to 75 percent of patients [119, 131]. However, in one study [36] of more than 7,000 twin pairs from the Swedish twin registry, a much smaller genetic component was found. Symptom-specific concordance rates in monozygotic (MZ) twins was 19 percent for asthma, 21 percent for hay fever, 15 percent for eczema, and 25 percent for all allergic disorders. Dizygotic (DZ) twins had lower concordance rates than did MZ twins, although they were higher than the general population. Thus, whereas the overall concordance rate was 25 percent for MZ twins, it was 16 percent for DZ twins. More than half of all the MZ pairs with the proper genetic makeup for developing allergy were discordant. This impressive study suggests the need to rethink the relative importance of hereditary versus environmental factors in asthma and other allergic disorders.

Two less well-designed studies of twins yielded conflicting results, one finding a high degree of concordance between MZ twins [55] and the other [19] an extremely low one. Uncertainties regarding the zygosity of the twin pairs and other methodologic shortcomings make their results difficult to interpret.

The search for etiologic specificity in subgroups of asthmatics has prompted a number of clinical epidemiologic surveys. These have yielded uniform but not unequivocal findings. Cases have been seen as exemplifying three major precipitants: allergy (exposure to extrinsic antigens), infection, and emotional distress. Seven such studies [52, 111, 114, 121, 122, 150, 152] have been summarized [146]. There was fair agreement that the major precipitants were distributed roughly as follows: infection in 40 percent and allergy and emotion in roughly 30 percent each. These, however, were retrospective reports and not prospective studies.

Efforts have been made to identify psychological profiles associated with asthma by means of objective personality tests [39, 126, 135]; they have shown lack of consensus, partly owing to the fact that most studies have dealt with a wide spectrum of "allergic" patients. One exception is a study of a relatively homogeneous group of 100 asthmatics receiving antiasthma medication, who were drawn from the public rolls in Finland [143]. The patients were matched for age, sex, and marital status with 100 control subjects not receiving any medication. The Beck Depression Inventory, given to both groups, revealed significantly more pathologic depression in asthmatics than in the normals. A drawing completion test (Wartegg), scored blindly, singled out asthmatics from normals with significant success, especially in males. Asthmatics had lower self-esteem, less ability to make social contacts, and more emotional difficulties, including problems of energy and assertiveness. In a further effort to disentangle the antecedent from the concomitant disturbance, the author searched for and found some suggestive psychosocial precipitants for the 60 percent of his patients whose asthma developed after the age of 21.

An alternative approach has been to focus on the manifest symptoms reported by asthmatic patients [29, 30, 32, 33, 70, 71, 138]. A self-report instrument, the Asthma Symptom Checklist, revealed five groups of symptoms: panic/fear, irritability, hyperventilation/hypercapnia, bronchial obstruction, and fatigue. Most important from the psychiatric point of view was the panic/fear cluster. The investigators found that scores on this scale were closely correlated with a scale empirically derived from the Minnesota Multiphasic Personality Inventory (MMPI), which they believed reflected long-term personality features. Although its face validity is not entirely clear, this long-term MMPI panic/fear scale, used in studies involving several hundred patients, yielded stable

values for given individuals and predicted their behavior during the course of their disease. Patients at the high end of the panic/fear spectrum showed significantly greater use of medications as required, greater likelihood of being discharged from the hospital on steroids, and greater likelihood of being rehospitalized within 6 months. This was not a function of the severity of their illness but appeared to reflect their anxious reaction to it. Interestingly, patients whose scores on the panic/fear scale fell at the low end of the continuum also had excessive hospitalization, reflecting their tendency to deny illness, undermedicate themselves, and be noncompliant. These two contrasting patterns correspond to two major types of management problems, to which we shall return.

The same set of studies examined a further aspect of asthmatic personality, the trait of so-called alexithymia. This term, coined by Sifneos [132] and meaning "no words for mood," was postulated to characterize a wide range of individuals, some of them having psychosomatic disorders, whose feelings emerged through bodily symptoms rather than in words. An original questionnaire [132] to measure this alleged trait and a subsequently derived MMPI [72, 73] appeared to single out at least some asthmatic subjects. However, both the original questionnaire and the derivative MMPI have empirical and statistical weaknesses. The concept of alexithymia does seem to fit some patients, particularly those with severe illness, whose life is absorbed by their symptoms and incapacity and who have great difficulty in recognizing other problems or emotional conflicts. It remains for the future to see how useful the term will be, both in general and in the particular study of asthma.

Recently, efforts have been made to extend this line of research to include children [11]. Fritz and Overholser [45] modified the Asthma Symptom Checklist discussed above, translating items into language suitable for children and sampling independently 162 children, from 6 to 18 years old, and their parents. Factor analyses of both versions of the checklist yielded three interpretable factors: These were labeled general physical symptoms, panic/fear, and hyperventilation/irritability. Parents' factor scores, but not those of their children, were significantly related to medication usage and to hospitalizations. Correlations between children's scores and those of their parents were low, reinforcing the need to gather data from many sources, as in all other assessments of children's disorders.

Family Studies

The structure of families with asthmatic patients has attracted considerable interest. Differences have been postulated in the constellations of families with allergically ill children during periods of eczema (allegedly characterized by more open, dependent gratification) and periods of asthma (allegedly characterized by pressures toward independence along with fears of it) [105]. Early family studies focused principally on mother and child, and utilized samples of already-symptomatic asthmatic children. The early concept of a rejecting mother [104] yielded to that of an engulfing one [1, 2]. One investigation suggested that clinicians working with asthma were only in partial agreement about maternal characteristics, raising the possibility of more than one subgroup of mothers and children [18]. Another investigation postulated an inverse relationship between the allergic potential of a child and psychopathology in the mother, pointing to two subtypes of asthma, one primarily biogenic and the other sociogenic [17]. This view was reinforced by other findings [42]. A further effort was made to divide hospitalized asthmatic children into those who were steroid dependent (primarily biologically ill) and those with rapidly remitting asthma (having a substantial psychogenic component) [118]. A risk in such studies is not only overlooking the complexity of the physiologic processes involved but also at the psychological level overlooking the defense mechanism of denial. Once allergic symptoms have become implicated, individuals or their families may be eager to dismiss psychological factors. Both children and parents might have a powerful need to overemphasize putative biologic factors and to minimize psychosocial conflict. An alternative view was presented in other studies [61, 62] that tested young adult males, some of whom had hay fever and mild asthma, using selected indexes of biologic reactivity along with a battery of projective tests. Allergic subjects perceived their mothers retrospectively as controlling or rejecting or both—their attitudes in this respect differentiated them from a healthy comparison group. It was possible, on the basis of both "allergic potential" alone and "psychological potential" alone, both scored blindly, successfully to select individuals who showed actual manifestations of allergic disease. The hypothesis was additive: that both psychological and biologic factors are widely distributed in the allergic population and that their combined strength determines the severity of the final disorder. Clinical studies [101, 116] support this view of additive etiologic factors rather than single dichotomization into biologic and psychogenic asthma.

More recent studies of family factors in asthma measured both the security of attachment between the asthmatic child and parent [109], and the relationship between early parenting problems and later development of asthma [110]. As predicted by much earlier work [44, 117], severely asthmatic children were significantly more likely to demonstrate insecure attachment than was a control group of healthy children [109], using Ainsworth's strange situation methodology [3]. In a prospective study [110], mothers of children at high genetic risk for asthma (due to the fact that the mothers themselves were asthmatic) were interviewed 3 weeks after the birth of the child. Each parent was coded as to the presence or absence of early difficulty specifically in the parenting role, as well as overall difficulty coping. After 2 years, the children were classified as having either documented asthma, repeated wheezing associated with a respiratory infection, a single incident of wheezing, or no wheezing. Early problems in parenting and coping were predictive of the development of asthma, but the presence of parenting difficulties at 3 weeks was not associated with infectious wheezing. This study supports the hypothesis, put forward earlier, that biologic factors alone do not predict the development of asthma, but interact with psychological factors. Additional data indicate that a difficult infant temperament at 3 weeks *and* elevated MMPI scores in the mothers *and* lower marital satisfaction were *all* independently associated with parenting difficulties, which in turn were associated with the development of asthma. Thus, it appears that infant temperament, parental personality, and quality of the marital relationship were all associated with the parenting difficulty and coping problems which predicted later asthma in this at-risk group. The direction of causality among the psychological factors cannot be inferred given the study's design, but the relationship between parenting difficulty and later asthma was successfully demonstrated.

Relationship difficulties between parents and their asthmatic children aged 7 to 13 years were also found in a study requiring a 5-minute discussion of a mutual problem between parent and child [58]. Mothers of asthmatic children displayed a more critical attitude toward their children than did mothers of healthy controls, a finding that may demonstrate general effects of chronic illness on family functioning, as well as a possible asthma-specific interaction style.

Clinical Case Studies

Conclusions derived from case studies involve intuitive estimates of family constellations and intrapersonal processes. Directly observable behavior may mask hidden contradictory attitudes and feelings. Objective methods to measure such balanced

forces are poorly developed, and we must rely on more complex clinical judgments. These have come chiefly from psychiatric, often psychoanalytically oriented, investigations of small numbers of cases. Some of this work is summarized in what follows, with full recognition of its limitations. It remains to be seen whether future large-scale, methodically more refined research will verify the original clinical judgments. In particular, sampling a broad range of subjects not in psychoanalytic treatment will be necessary in order to test hypotheses generated by case studies.

A promising, but so far exceedingly limited avenue is provided by a few studies in depth of discordant twin pairs. In a pair of MZ male twins discordant for asthma [88], one member had severe asthma from the age of 2, finally requiring placement in a residential center. Treated with psychotherapy, he developed a transient psychotic-like disturbance; the eventual outcome was characterized by marked improvement in both behavior and asthma. His identical twin had an episode of wheezing and was hospitalized briefly in his third year, shortly after the onset of his brother's disease; it never recurred. The authors contended that a more intense attachment to the mother characterized the asthmatic twin's development and may have contributed to his becoming ill. This study again underlines the point that genetic predisposition, while favoring the development of asthma, is not a sufficient determinant. In these twin pairs emotional factors appear to have played a significant role, as they did in the prospective parent-child study mentioned earlier [110].

Psychoanalytically oriented psychotherapy and psychoanalysis in a small number of children disclosed evidence of oscillation between attempts on the part of the asthmatic child to separate from the mother and efforts to achieve intense intimate closeness [65, 66]. Another study reported faulty differentiation between mother and child and a tendency for mothers of asthmatic children, like those of patients with other psychosomatic diseases, to misperceive their children as sick, helpless versions of themselves on whom they could lavish care, thus inadvertently providing powerful and sustained reinforcement of the asthmatic process [137]. A retrospective study [139] of 21 children who died of asthma revealed that more severe psychological problems such as depression, family pathology, and a dysfunctional self-care attitude distinguished those who subsequently died from case control subjects.

Many clinical studies on patients in psychotherapy have found high levels of psychiatric symptomatology in adult patients suffering from asthma [79, 80, 98]. Occasional reports of alternation between asthmatic symptoms and overt psychotic manifestations led to the hypothesis, also entertained for other disorders, that psychosomatic disease and psychosis might be reciprocals of one another. However, subsequent studies indicate that more often, the severe symptoms of personality disturbance are concomitant with disease exacerbations [79]. Other clinical observations have suggested that asthmatics have unusually intense passive and dependent personality trends, reflecting a need to maintain gratification and support from key figures in their lives [75, 79]. These manifestations may be accompanied by intense hostility, appearing only briefly, usually followed by guilty depressive feelings and often by intensification of asthmatic symptoms [10, 78, 81].

Two major hypotheses have sought to describe more specific psychological features. In the first, French and Alexander [44] postulated a particular pattern of emotions relating to a mothering person. This centered around a "suppressed cry," which represented conflict-ridden urges to express anger and at the same time seek dependent protection. The partially inhibited, distorted manifestation of suppressed crying, namely, the asthma attack itself, was seen as a way of uniting the child with a caring mother. An attempt to test this view and closely related hypotheses about other disorders [7] was made by studying 70 patients, 10 in each of six psychosomatic categories. All of them were individuals under 40 years old who had had the onset of their syndromes in adult life. Intensive tape-recorded psychiatric interviews were edited by an internist to delete medical cues. A group of psychoanalyst judges, blind to the medical findings, were able to assign the edited typescripts to correct psychosomatic categories, including asthma, with a highly significant degree of success. As a control, internist judges were asked to perform the same task—their overall success rate was markedly lower than that of the psychoanalysts.

A second psychoanalytic hypothesis [28, 41, 137] suggested that asthma represented specific, unconsciously learned patterns of expression, based on a measure of control gained by the individual over the pulmonary apparatus, so that it communicated in "body language" conflictual fantasies related to both primitive impulses and inhibitory forces. Evidence is scattered from clinical case reports—for instance, a patient whose asthma cleared on recovery of memories of a traumatic scene of strangling witnessed in childhood [90] and cases in which pathologic mother-daughter identification was striking [21, 78, 81]. This hypothesis states that asthma represents a conversion (in the psychological sense) of a conflict into learned, symbolically relevant somatic expressive patterns.

The two hypotheses are actually not so far apart. Primitive fantasies do not exist without strong emotion, and strong emotions do not exist in the absence of fantasied urges toward their expression over bodily pathways. Insofar as French and Alexander talked about use of the vocal respiratory apparatus, they came close themselves to speaking of conversion. Thus, a more comprehensive hypothesis, to which we subscribe, states that in some patients, asthma results when there is simultaneous activation of powerful threatening impulses and efforts to inhibit these, a prior condition being that both these elements have become channelized by biologic and learned predisposition into expression through pulmonary dysfunction. In four psychoanalytically studied patients [75, 78], a dependent relationship with a parental figure coexisted with hidden destructive urges. Arousal of these dangerous impulses was inhibited, and asthma followed.

A controlled retrospective study was carried out of interviews with an asthmatic treated by psychoanalysis [78]. During the course of his treatment he had 25 significant and incapacitating exacerbations. Blinded psychiatric judges, studying edited notes that had been taken routinely before these exacerbations, had significant success in detecting asthmatic occasions from comparison ones (that is, sessions at nearby points in time not followed by asthma). The same data were given to two internists for similar judgments; they searched mainly for residual medical cues, and their results in differentiating the two sets of occasions were only at a chance level.

THERAPEUTIC CONSIDERATIONS

Bronchial asthma is a chronic, sometimes lifelong, at times life-threatening disorder, having multiple etiologic roots and running a fluctuating course. Inevitably, the problem of evaluating therapy is difficult. This consideration applies to all treatment approaches, including medical measures. It has been noted: "In no other common disorder have so many different therapeutic approaches been adopted, and it is suspicious that many of these are credited with improving the condition . . . . Spontaneous improvement and remission are common, often appearing independently of any change in treatment" [12]. One must add that a careful examination of the life circumstances of an individual should be conducted before concluding that changes are purely "spontaneous." As contemporary psychotherapy research has become more rigorous, many studies have examined differing psychological interventions in asthma. Assessment of their effectiveness has varied, from relatively enthusiastic [82] to frankly

pessimistic [5, 124]. Progress has been made in understanding the effect of stress and coping style on asthmatic symptomatology, including the impact of parental dysfunction on children's health status. Demonstrations of specific, clinically significant, interventions have typically focused on small samples or case studies, or on time-limited interventions with the less severely impaired.

At the clinical level there is perhaps the greatest agreement (though also the least precise information) that attention to the behavior of asthmatic patients, particularly their compliance with medical regimes, can help them in coping with their illness. The extremes of patient behavior mentioned earlier [30] can be dealt with so as to minimize the excessive concern and overmedication of patients with hypochondriacal anxiety and to reduce the self-injurious undermedication and noncompliance of those at the denying end of the spectrum. An alternative approach [25] is that "noncompliance" can be adaptive, when patients or their parents are competent in assessing and treating the symptoms of asthma.

More specific efforts at causal intervention have included use of self-management programs, psychotropic drugs, behavioral approaches (relaxation, desensitization, and biofeedback), hypnosis, group psychotherapy, family therapy, residential care, and long-term individual psychotherapy.

Self-Management

At a direct level, asthma self-management programs [51] have been developed, mainly for children, to provide asthmatics and their parents with an understanding of the illness and its treatment. A recent review [74] found that overall, self-management programs increase knowledge, improve compliance and coping strategies, and decrease the number of school absences and the use of emergency medical treatment. Changes in objective physiologic measures are rarely reported, however. The self-management approach has been extended to asthmatic college-age students, in an uncontrolled pilot study [142], which found increased knowledge about asthma, increased control of asthma, increased compliance, and decreased use of the college health service for acute asthma care during the 4 years following an educational workshop.

A nonlinear relationship between knowledge and appropriate asthma self-management was found in a recent study [127] of 91 school-age children with asthma. Specifically, increased knowledge is most helpful to children with lower beginning knowledge levels, and to those with less appropriate beginning behavioral adjustment.

Psychotropic Drugs

Antianxiety medications, even in patients with high panic/fear ratings, have little effect on pulmonary symptoms. Tricyclic antidepressants have been shown to exert a bronchodilatory effect in animals [9] and in some acute human experiments [97]. Their mechanism of action may be pluralistic: The anticholinergic and antihistaminic properties of these compounds are well known; so are their effects as blockers of monoamine uptake. However, early suggestions of their effectiveness in asthma [49, 100, 140] have not been sustained; they seem useful primarily in those patients who show independent signs and symptoms of clinical depression.

Behavioral Approaches

Relaxation

The simplest behavioral approach, relaxation, has been conceptualized and systematized in various ways, varying between the effort to induce relaxation by peripheral muscular maneuvers, as originally proposed by Jacobson [63], and the use of more central psychological state induction [13]. In children, direct suggestions to relax [4–6] have resulted in slight increases in a variety of respiratory measures, relying mostly on PEFR. However, this effect has been "modest and of little clinical significance even in the strongest examples" [6]. Other investigators have reached a similar conclusion about the use of peripheral muscular relaxation [37]. In a potentially significant study [151] transcendental meditation (TM) was used in a 6-month crossover study of 21 patients with stable asthma randomly assigned to either TM or a control condition in which the subjects read about TM. After 3 months, the subjects who practiced TM showed increases in FEV_1 (16%) and PEFR (12%) and, most impressive, a decline in mean Raw (48%). No change was apparent in subjects who received the control (reading) condition first. Independent assessment by physicians indicated greater improvement for both sets of subjects under the TM condition. An additional promising variant of relaxation is found in a single case report of a patient with severe asthma successfully treated by relaxation on cue [145]. Individual differences in hypnotic suggestibility were recently found to relate to improvement in asthmatic symptoms [112] in a study comparing active relaxation with placebo treatment.

Behavior Modification

An approach modeled after classic pavlovian conditioning, behavior modification relies on careful ascertainment of psychosocial triggering stimuli and desensitization of the subject by graduated mental revival of these or by reciprocal inhibition (exposure to other stimuli with a presumed opposite action). This method was successful in one patient with asthma [145] and subsequently used in a controlled study, comparing systematic desensitization with simple suggestion and a relaxation therapy [106]. Twelve subjects, half of them children, participated in a balanced incomplete block design, so that two forms of treatment were given to every patient, and each of the three treatments could be compared across 8 subjects. Significant improvement in PEFR was found in the behavior modification group. This study's strength was that the patients were their own controls. However, a major share of the variance was contributed by 2 subjects who received reciprocal inhibition as their first treatment and improved markedly afterward. It is possible that individual differences in this small group of subjects played the major determining role. Nevertheless, the study represents a promising beginning for systematic controlled investigation of this type of therapeutic approach. A confirmatory study [102] carried out systematic desensitization by reciprocal inhibition in 18 sick children, comparing them with nine control patients who received only routine medical management. Of a large number of variables tested, only FEV_1 showed significant differences between experimental and control subjects after treatment. In the face of comparably reduced steroid medication, the treated patients maintained their pretherapeutic levels of FEV_1, while in control subjects these levels declined. A significant difference was present at follow-up, although the average effect was small and of marginal clinical significance.

Operant Conditioning and Biofeedback

Several observers have remarked on the ready extinction of classic pavlovian conditioning and have suggested that a more clinically applicable model is operant conditioning. In this paradigm the subject actively invokes a response to gain reinforcement, conceivably like a child who "thinks himself into asthma" to avoid school. A substantial reinforcer is biologic feedback, giving information about change of a physiologic parameter in a desired direction. An early study consisted of two phases of training, one a direct reward by verbal praise for production of FEV_1 increases and the other a counterconditioning phase in which bronchocon-

striction was induced and then subjects were reinforced in the same manner for producing positive FEV_1 changes [68]. Children who seemed reactive to psychological stimuli appeared to get long-term benefits—lower medication requirements, fewer emergency room visits, and fewer reported asthma attacks. However, two subsequent studies only partially confirmed these initial findings [23, 67]. Results appeared to be limited to the conditioning sessions, and none of the children showed reductions in asthma symptoms [23]. These somewhat discouraging results do not constitute a fair test of operant conditioning and certainly not of the more restricted form of it, namely biofeedback, since the feedback from routine pulmonary function tests is inevitably delayed. Moreover, the measure used in these studies required a high degree of cooperation, and extraneous motivational factors, not systematically controlled for by these investigators, could have played an unknown role.

More direct feedback is supplied by the forced oscillation method, as already described [40, 144]. In another study [64], forced oscillation before and after a set of five training sessions was used. Fifteen steroid-free subjects with documented chronic asthma were randomly assigned either to feedback contingent on lowering total respiratory resistance (TPR) or to feedback randomly generated by computer. Both groups were required to stay within constant tidal volume limits. At the end of the five trials there was a significant drop in TPR in the experimental group. There were no changes in functional residual capacity (FRC). The authors interpreted their findings as promising evidence for biofeedback-learned decreases in TPR in asthmatic patients. However, their results did not generalize to measurement of airway conductance immediately after the trials, leaving doubt about the duration and clinical relevance of the effect.

A pragmatically simple variation of biofeedback technique has been attained by providing muscular (electromyographic [EMG]) feedback from the facial muscles, especially the frontalis, a maneuver originally designed as an adjuvant to relaxation. It was reported that it led to improved respiratory performance in asthmatic children when compared to relaxation training alone [24], but the evidence was not unequivocal. Additional findings of effectiveness from this form of feedback were provided in studies on children at a summer camp [128, 129]. A total of 44 children were treated with one or another combination of EMG biofeedback and were compared with 44 untreated children. The studies reported that the experimental group showed significantly more improvement on a variety of behavioral and symptomatic measures. Groups were not strictly balanced with respect to pretreatment variables; a more serious defect was the failure to control for nonspecific attentional effects.

To remedy these shortcomings, a rigorous set of studies using the frontalis for feedback employed careful monitoring of EMG tension and observation of the effects of induced relaxation on PEFR in asthmatic children [47, 83, 84]. Controls consisted of both untreated children and children given feedback unrelated to facial tension (using the brachioradialis as the EMG feedback source). A clear-cut increase in PEFR was found in the experimentally treated children. Subsequent studies have extended the approach to adults [85]. Although the effect is clear, the mechanism is less so. The authors argued for a reflex connection between trigeminal and vagal nuclei. An alternative possibility might be that facial muscles are intimately linked to habitual expression of emotion; reducing tension in them might activate habitual emotional effects. The authors were careful to point out that the magnitudes of the laboratory changes they reported are small and their clinical significance unclear. Nevertheless, this work is of interest in pointing to possible specific features that may enhance the applications of relaxation to the treatment of bronchial asthma. A recent behavioral approach [22] taught asthmatic children to understand and discriminate asthmatic symptoms and to manage their symptoms, and at the same time reduced positive reinforcement for symptoms. Children receiving this behavioral intervention reduced their use of medications and improved their school attendance, while maintaining unchanged asthma symptoms.

It is difficult at this time to evaluate the usefulness for asthma of the various behavior therapies. It has been stated that results are "disappointing . . . there is some evidence that meditation and autogenic training bring about improvement . . . [but] neither relaxation nor systematic desensitization yield general beneficial effects" [124]. An alternative view, based on review of 24 behavioral treatment studies, was that "relaxation training and systematic desensitization can produce statistically significant improvement in the respiratory function of asthmatic patients. . . . Such improvement may also be obtainable through operant conditioning techniques . . . (although) the clinical significance and long-term maintenance of the above mentioned improvements are yet to be demonstrated" [82]. More recent studies provide support for the latter, more optimistic view.

Hypnosis

While there is doubt as to the ability of hypnosis to affect the fully established pathophysiologic process of asthma, it is still possible that hypnotherapy may have long-term benefits. In a clinical study, 120 asthmatic patients were treated with brief, rapid-induction hypnosis at weekly intervals [38]. A control group of 115 asthmatics was treated with suggestion to promote body relaxation. By the end of a year, in the hypnotized group, 50 percent were better, 8 percent were worse and 42 percent were unchanged, in contrast to control group figures of 43 percent, 17 percent, and 40 percent, respectively. In another study, ameliorative effects of hypnotherapy to abort acute attacks in 17 children were reported, and some documentation indicated that pulmonary measures as well as long-term courses were favorably affected [8]. A multicenter clinical trial of hypnosis was carried out by the Research Committee of the British Tuberculosis Association [123]. In this study 252 patients with reversible obstructive airway disease were randomly assigned either to deep suggestion under hypnosis once a month, accompanied by autohypnosis daily, or to progressive relaxation and daily breathing exercises. Assessment was by daily diary of wheezing and use of medication as well as FEV measurements. At the end of 1 year, when assessment was carried out by physicians unaware of the therapeutic conditions, the women given hypnosis showed significantly greater improvement on clinical indexes. The most impressive finding was that independent medical assessment showed 59 percent improvement in the total hypnotic group as compared with 43 percent in the control group, a significant between-group difference. Therapists with clinical experience with hypnosis did significantly better than those without it. The study provides strong evidence for the effectiveness of this mode of intervention.

Group Therapy

In a large reported group therapy study [53] involving weekly meetings and an extensive supportive medical and milieu regime, patients were assigned to three groups: (1) symptomatic treatment only, (2) symptomatic treatment plus steroids, or (3) both of the previous treatments plus group therapy. Improvement was found as follows: 17 percent in group 1, 28 percent in group 2, and 73 percent in group 3. The percentages of those "worse or dead" were in the reverse order. The great number of variables involved and the difficulty in knowing initial and final pathophysiologic levels make this interesting endeavor difficult to assess. One study [59] reported results of a behavioral group treatment with asthmatic boys, in which the treated children improved their FEV compared with controls.

Family Therapy

Successful use of family therapy in 7 chronic asthmatic children has also been reported [89]. All were steroid dependent and required frequent additional treatment, including emergency hospital visits: 6 had had prior individual psychological counseling. The parents were described as "overdependent, especially on physicians," and also "overly involved with the patients," becoming "manipulated" by the episodic asthmatic crises. The psychiatrist, working with a pediatrician, treated the family as a whole, giving specific breathing exercises and instruction about emergency treatment, and uncovering disturbed personal relationships. In all 7 patients this program resulted in marked reduction of hospital visits, cessation of positive pressure breathing and of desensitization regimens, and most important, discontinuance of steroids. If such striking results can be replicated in another sample of comparably ill patients, it will establish this form of treatment on an impressive basis.

Long-term Psychoanalytically Oriented Psychotherapy

Long-term psychoanalytic psychotherapy was applied to the original series of 26 adults and children reported by French and Alexander [44]. They described substantial improvement in their series but did not give detailed physiologic or other follow-up data. Others have also applied this approach to severely incapacitated patients [76, 80, 137]. Long-term follow-up studies are lacking, and patients treated in this fashion have had psychiatric diagnoses, as well as asthma. One can argue logically that such a time-consuming approach is indicated if one accepts the evidence of early disturbance in mother-child relationships. Most observers believe that the classic psychoanalytic approach must be modified. Different strategies are possible within a general psychoanalytic framework, such as a nurturant and empathic approach or a confrontative and active attack on the possibly defensive and gratifying "use" of symptoms.

OVERALL EVALUATION OF PSYCHOLOGICAL INTERVENTION

Evaluation of the role of psychological interventions in asthma must be tentative at this time. We have already indicated the highly divergent judgments about the efficacy of behavioral approaches. When other therapies are considered in addition, accurate assessment becomes still more difficult. This problem in the wider field of psychotherapy research was also addressed [134]. A method of meta-analysis was developed to examine data from multiple controlled investigations within a predefined area, transforming studies to commensurable expressions of magnitude of experimental effect as well as defining and measuring features that might mediate the findings and studying their covariation.

As part of an overall survey, this approach was applied to 11 controlled outcome studies on the use of psychotherapy for asthma, in which one group received psychotherapy and a control group received no treatment. The type and duration of psychotherapy, the type of management given to control subjects, the follow-up time, the outcome measures, and the mean age were noted, and an overall statistical estimate of effect size or magnitude of treatment effect was reached. The authors [134] stated: "It is immediately apparent that none of the effect sizes is negative. The odds are overwhelmingly against the possibility, then, that these 11 studies are a sample of a much greater number of studies in which positive findings are outweighed by negative findings."

While measurement methods differed somewhat in different

Table 85-1. Selected psychosocial factors empirically associated with poor outcome or increased risks in bronchial asthma

Sample population	Risk factors	Outcome	Reference
1. Infants with increased genetic loading for bronchial asthma	Early parenting, coping problems determined by prospective interview when child is 3 weeks old	Diagnosis of asthma prior to 2 years more likely ($P < .001$)	108
2. Children 6–18 years old with mild to severe asthma, variety of treatment settings	High panic/fear in child, rated by parent on children's form of Asthma Symptom Checklist	Increased risk of hospitalization (F: 3.04, $P < .05$)	44
3. Children 9–15 years old with asthma	High panic/fear rated by parent on children's form of Battery for Asthma Illness Behavior during psychological interview	Higher intensity of prescribed medication, particularly corticosteroids, independent of spirometric pulmonary tests	11
4. Children 8–18 years old with severe asthma, previously hospitalized	A. Conflict between parents and hospital staff over medical management ($P < .01$) B. Inappropriate asthma self-care ($P < .01$) C. Depressive symptoms ($P < .05$) D. Disregard of perceived asthma symptoms ($P < .06$)	Increased risk of death due to asthma	139
5. Children 11–17 years old with severe asthma who experienced a life-threatening attack of asthma	A. Presence of family dysfunction ($P < .05$) B. History of reaction to reaction or recent loss of important person ($P < .005$) C. Hopelessness and despair in month prior to episode ($P < .05$)	Increased risk of not surviving the respiratory failure	103
6. Adults with asthma, previously hospitalized	Excessive panic/fear or denial of asthmatic symptoms, determined by Asthma Symptom Checklist or MMPI	Increased risk of hospitalization	30, 31
7. Asthmatics aged 10–58 ($\bar{x} = 33$) years, roughly matched for severity	By record review: alcohol problems, personality disorder, depression, recent bereavement, recent unemployment	Greater risk of mortality due to asthma	120

MMPI = Minnesota Multiphasic Personality Inventory.

studies, it was shown by a variety of statistical techniques that handling them as a number of separate studies and even eliminating one outrider study (the least well controlled) did not alter the rather impressive statistical finding. These findings lend support to the view that psychological interventions in this disorder are based on an increasingly solid foundation.

Needless to say, problems still remain. Most experimental investigations of psychotherapy deal with short-term treatments and mildly ill patients. The most serious problems in asthma have to do with chronically incapacitated individuals, frequently having severe illness, including steroid dependence. The psychologic profile of patients with near-fatal asthma may be of some value in management. In a recent study MMPI did not distinguish a group of patients with near-fatal asthma from a group of matched asthmatic controls who never experienced near-fatal asthma. However, individual profiles revealed more frequent personality disturbances with reduced adaptive personality characteristics in the near-fatal asthma group; poor therapy compliance and an increased prevalence of poorly controlled asthma also characterized the near-fatal asthma patients [153]. Psychological features involved in asthmatic therapy compliance was discussed in a recent symposium [154].

What, then, should a psychotherapist advise for an asthmatic patient? Several levels of information are necessary for a full evaluation. At the most surface level, lack of appropriate coping skills specific to asthma would indicate the need for a direct educational approach, whether by the physician or through the use of a teaching package. If signs of a psychiatric syndrome are present, some form of psychotherapeutic and/or pharmacologic intervention is indicated. This may be administered by the primary physician, by a specialist in a mental health discipline, or by both.

Two contrasting cautions are important: The psychotherapist must respect the potential seriousness of the biologic processes in asthma, and must utilize appropriate medical knowledge as part of the total treatment plan. With rare exceptions this means collaboration with a sophisticated medical colleague. However, all therapists and internists should respect the remarkable capacity of psychological conflict to lurk behind a screen of "real" physiologic symptoms, and they must be prepared to adhere to their insights when such conflict is sensed, even though the patient, the family, and even the attending physician may explain it as only an unfortunate by-product of physical suffering.

Time-limited and controlled approaches are valuable for purposes of comparative study, particularly in patients with mild asthma, but for those with severe asthma, the clinician faces complicated problems of long-term management and a long-term relationship with an individual whose somatic and psychic difficulties are significantly intertwined.

In summary, clinical wisdom suggests that emotional factors may indeed play an important part in initiating and sustaining the clinical changes in bronchial asthma. Biologic evidence suggests mechanisms whereby emotional events can influence the pulmonary processes involved in asthma. Acute changes in airway conductance occur in response to psychosocial stimuli in certain subjects. Presumably these are mediated primarily by the parasympathetic nervous system, that is, by vagal influences on the upper airways. More sustained changes in airway conductance, probably involving altered neuroendocrine balance, may be related to specific impairment of epinephrine mobilization, or receptor changes, or the interplay between neuroendocrine mediators (e.g., pituitary hormones, neuropeptides) and immunologic regulation.

There appears to be an interaction between hereditary vulnerability and early environmental factors in many cases of asthma, with evidence now emerging as to the characteristics of the infant-parent relationship that lead to expression of inherited vulnerability.

In some patients with asthma, studied and treated psychoanalytically, fears of separation from caring persons along with fears of aggressive impulses that might precipitate such separation appear to be prominent, though obviously not unique for this disorder.

Classic conditioning has yet to be demonstrated to play a significant role in human asthma, although its participation in triggering attacks cannot be excluded. Possibly more important, preliminary results suggest that operant conditioning can influence airways, although the extent and lasting nature of its influence remain to be determined.

Regardless of the exact nature of mediating mechanisms, there is strong evidence that remission of asthma may be brought about in certain subjects by the interruption of ongoing psychopathogenic interactions, especially with parental figures and perhaps by establishing needed positive relationships. Contrasting patterns of fearful overutilization of medical assistance and denial accompanied by underutilization may be helped by psychologically perceptive management. More specific psychotherapeutic interventions of numerous kinds have been applied in asthma. Antidepressant medications, whose peripheral and CNS actions must be taken into account, seem useful chiefly for patients with concomitant clinical depression. A number of controlled studies have documented benefits from behavioral biofeedback approaches in patients with mild asthma. Positive effects from hypnosis have been demonstrated. One report indicated striking benefits from family therapy for seriously incapacitated children, while another demonstrated the risk of poor management and depression, leading to death, in severely disordered families. Overall these results warrant further investigation; they suggest a need for psychological study and in many cases the use of psychotherapy along with medical management for this complex chronic disorder. Selected psychosocial features empirically associated with a poor outcome or increased risks in asthma are summarized in Table 85-1.

REFERENCES

1. Abramson, H. Evaluation of maternal rejection theory in asthma. *Ann. Allergy* 12:129, 1954.
2. Abramson, H. Group psychotherapy of the parents of intractably asthmatic children. *J. Child. Asthma Res. Institute Hosp.* 1:77, 1961.
3. Ainsworth, M. D. S., et al. *Patterns of Attachment.* Hillsdale, NJ: Lawrence Erlbaum and Associates, 1978.
4. Alexander, A. Systematic relaxation and flow rates in asthmatic children's relationship to emotional precipitants and anxiety. *J. Psychosom. Res.* 16:405, 1972.
5. Alexander, A. Behavioral Medicine in Asthma. In R. Stuart (ed.), *Adherence, Compliance, and Generalization in Behavioral Medicine.* New York: Brunner-Mazel, 1982.
6. Alexander, A., Cropp, G., and Chai, H. The effects of relaxation training on pulmonary mechanics in children with asthma. *J. Appl. Behav. Anal.* 12:27, 1982.
7. Alexander, F., French, T. M., and Pollock, G. *Psychosomatic Specificity,* Vol. I. *Experimental Study and Results.* Chicago: University of Chicago Press, 1968.
8. Aranoff, G., Aranoff, S., and Peck, L. Hypnotherapy in the treatment of bronchial asthma. *Ann. Allergy* 34:356, 1975.
9. Avni, J., and Bruderman, I. The effect of amitriptyline on pulmonary ventilation and the mechanics of breathing. *Pharmacologia* 14:184, 1969.
10. Bacon, C. The role of aggression in the asthmatic attack. *Psychoanal. Q.* 25:309, 1956.
11. Baron, C., et al. Psychomaintenance of childhood asthma: A study of 34 children. *J. Asthma* 23:64, 1986.
12. Bates, D. V., Macklem, P. T., and Christie, R. V. *Respiratory Function in Disease.* Philadelphia: Saunders, 1971.
13. Benson, H. *The Relaxation Response.* New York: Avon, 1975.
14. Ben-Zvi, Z., et al. Hypnosis for exercise induced asthma. *Am. Rev. Respir. Dis.* 125:392, 1982.
15. Bernstein, R. A., et al. Decreased urinary adenosine 3′ 5′ monophosphate (cyclic AMP) in asthmatics. *J. Lab. Clin. Invest.* 80:772, 1972.
16. Black, S. Shifting the dose-response curve of Prausnitz-Küstner reaction by direct suggestion under hypnosis. *Br. Med. J.* 2:324, 1963.
17. Block, J., et al. Interaction between allergic potential and psychopathology in childhood. *Psychosom. Med.* 26:320, 1964.
18. Block, J., et al. Clinicians' conception of the asthmatogenic mother. *Arch. Gen. Psychiatry* 15:610, 1966.
19. Bowen, R. Allergy in identical twins. *J. Allergy Clin. Immunol.* 24:326, 1953.
20. Cohen, S., Tyrell, D. A. J., and Smith, A. P. Psychological stress and susceptibility to the common cold. *N. Engl. J. Med.* 325:606, 1991.
21. Coolidge, J. Asthma in mother and child as a special type of intercommunication. *Am. J. Orthopsychiatry* 26:165, 1956.
22. Dahl, J., Gustafsson, D., and Melin, L. Effects of a behavioral treatment program on children with asthma. *J. Asthma* 27:41, 1990.
23. Danker, P., et al. An unsuccessful attempt to instrumentally condition peak expiratory flow rate in asthmatic children. *J. Psychosom. Res.* 19:209, 1975.
24. Davis, M., Creer, T., and Chai, H. Relaxation training facilitated by biofeedback apparatus as a supplemental treatment in bronchial asthma. *J. Psychosom. Res.* 17:121, 1973.
25. Deaton, A. V., and Olbrisch, M. E. Adaptive Noncompliance: Parents as Experts and Decision Makers in the Treatment of Pediatric Asthma Patients. In M. Wolraich and D. K. Routh (eds.), *Advances in Developmental and Behavioral Pediatrics.* Greenwich, Conn: Jai Press, 1987. Pp. 205–234.
26. Dekker, F., and Groen, J. Reproducible psychogenic attacks of asthma. *J. Psychosom. Res.* 1:58, 1956.
27. Dekker, F., Pelser, H., and Groen, L. Conditioning as a cause of asthmatic attacks. *J. Psychosom. Res.* 2:96, 1957.
28. Deutsch, F. Basic psychoanalytic principles in psychosomatic medicine. *Acta Ther.* 1:102, 1953.
29. Dirks, J., et al. Panic-fear in asthma: Symptomatology as an index of signal anxiety and personality as an index of ego resources. *J. Nerv. Ment. Dis.* 167:615, 1979.
30. Dirks, J., Jones, N., and Kinsman, R. Panic fear: A personality dimension related to intractability in asthma. *Psychosom. Med.* 39:120, 1977.
31. Dirks, J. F., et al. Panic-fear in asthma: Rehospitalization following intensive long-term treatment. *Psychosom. Med.* 40:5, 1978.
32. Dirks, J., Paley, A., and Fross, K. Panic-fear research in asthma and the nuclear conflict theory of asthma: Similarities, differences, and clinical implications. *Br. J. Med. Psychol.* 52:71, 1979.
33. Dirks, J., Schraa, J., and Robinson, S. Patient mislabeling of symptoms: Implications for patient physician communication and medical outcome. *Int. J. Psychiatry Med.* 12:15, 1982.
34. Dudley, D. C., et al. Changes in respiration associated with hypnotically induced emotion, pain and exercise. *Psychosom. Med.* 26:46, 1964.
35. Dudley, D. C., Martin, C. J., and Holmes, T. H. Psychophysiologic studies of pulmonary ventilation. *Psychosom. Med.* 26:645, 1958.
36. Edfors-Lubs, M. Allergy in 7000 twin pairs. *Acta Allergol.* 26:249, 1971.
37. Erskine-Millis, J., and Schonell, M. Relaxation therapy in asthma: A critical review. *Psychosom. Med.* 43:365, 1981.
38. Falliers, C. Treatment of asthma in a residential center—A 15 year study. *J. Allergy* 28:513, 1970.
39. Feingold, B., et al. Psychological studies of allergic women. *Psychosom. Med.* 24:195, 1962.
40. Feldman, C. Effect of biofeedback training on respiratory resistance in children. *Psychosom. Med.* 38:27, 1976.
41. Fenichel, O. Nature and classifications of the so-called psychosomatic phenomena. *Psychoanal. Q.* 14:287, 1945.
42. Freeman, E., et al. Personality variables and allergic skin reactions: A cross validation study. *Psychosom. Med.* 29:312, 1967.
43. French, T. M. Psychogenic factors in asthma. *Am. J. Psychiatry* 98:87, 1939.
44. French, T. M., and Alexander, F. Psychogenic factors in bronchial asthma. *Psychosom. Med. Monogr.* 4:2, 1941.
45. Fritz, G. K., and Overholser, J. C. Patterns of response to childhood asthma. *Psychosom. Med.* 51:347, 1989.

46. Gaensler, E. A., and Lindgren, I. The mechanics of breathing. *Prog. Cardiovasc. Dis.* 1:397, 1959.
47. Glaus, K. D., and Kotses, H. Generalization of conditioned muscle tension: A closer look. *Psychophysiology* 16:563, 1979.
48. Godfrey, S., and Silverman, M. Demonstration of placebo response in asthma by means of exercise testing. *J. Psychosom. Res.* 17:293, 1973.
49. Goldfarb, A., and Venutolo, F. The use of an antidepressant drug in chronically allergic individuals. *Ann. Allergy* 21:667, 1963.
50. Goldman, M. A simplified measurement of respiratory resistance by forced oscillation. *J. Appl. Physiol.* 26:113, 1970.
51. Goldstein, R. A., Green, L. W., and Parker, S. R. Workshop proceedings on self-management of childhood asthma. *J. Allergy Clin. Immunol.* 72:519, 1983.
52. Graham, P. Childhood asthma: A psychosomatic disorder? Some epidemiological considerations. *Br. J. Prev. Soc. Med.* 21:78, 1977.
53. Groen, J. Experience with and results of group therapy with bronchial asthma. *J. Psychosom. Res.* 4:191, 1941.
54. Hahn, W. Autonomic responses of asthmatic children. *Psychosom. Med.* 28:323, 1966.
55. Harvald, B., and Hauge, M. Hereditary Factors Elucidated by Twin Studies. In J. Need, M. Shaw, and W. Shull (ed.), *Genetics and Epidemiology of Chronic Diseases*. Washington, DC: U.S. Dept. of Health, Education, and Welfare, 1965.
56. Heim, E., et al. Airway resistance and emotional state in bronchial asthma. *Psychosom. Med.* 29:450, 1967.
57. Heim, E., et al. Emotion, breathing and speech. *J. Psychosom. Res.* 12:261, 1968.
58. Hermanns, J., et al. Maternal criticism, mother-child interaction, and bronchial asthma. *J. Psychosom. Res.* 33:469, 1989.
59. Hock, R. A., et al. Medicopsychological interventions in male asthmatic children: An evaluation of physiological change. *Psychosom. Med.* 40:210, 1980.
60. Horton, D., et al. Bronchoconstrictive suggestion in asthma: A role for hyperreactivity and emotions. *Am. Rev. Respir. Dis.* 117:1029, 1978.
61. Jacobs, M. A., et al. Interaction of psychologic and biologic predisposing factors in allergic disorders. *Psychosom. Med.* 29:572, 1967.
62. Jacobs, M. A., et al. Incidence of psychosomatic predisposing factors in allergic disorders. *Psychosom. Med.* 28:679, 1966.
63. Jacobson, E. *Progressive Relaxation*. Chicago: University of Chicago Press, 1938.
64. Janson-Bjerklie, S., and Clarke, E. The effects of biofeedback training on bronchial diameter in asthma. *Heart Lung*. 11:20, 1982.
65. Jessner, L. The Psychoanalysis of an Eight-Year-Old Boy with Asthma. In H. I. Schneer (ed.), *The Asthmatic Child: A Psychosomatic Approach to Problems and Treatment*. New York: Harper & Row, 1963.
66. Jessner, L., et al. Emotional impact of nearness and separation for the asthmatic child and his mother. *Psychoanal. Study Child*. 10:353, 1955.
67. Kahn, A. Effectiveness of biofeedback and counter-conditioning in the treatment of asthma. *J. Psychosom. Res.* 21:97, 1977.
68. Kahn, A., Staerk, M., and Bonk, C. Role of counter-conditioning in the treatment of asthma. *J. Psychosom. Res.* 18:89, 1974.
69. Khansari, D. N., Murgo, A. J., and Faith, R. E. Effects of stress on the immune system. *Immunol. Today*. 11:170, 1990.
70. Kinsman, R., et al. Multidimensional analysis of the subjective symptomatology of asthma. *Psychosom. Med.* 35:250, 1973.
71. Kinsman, R., et al. Observations on patterns of symptomatology of acute asthma. *Psychosom. Med.* 36:129, 1974.
72. Kleiger, J., and Jones, N. Characteristics of alexithymic patients in a chronic respiratory illness population. *J. Nerv. Ment. Dis.* 168:465, 1980.
73. Kleiger, J., and Kinsman, R. The development of an MMPI alexithymia scale. *Psychother. Psychosom.* 34:17, 1980.
74. Klingelhofer, E. L., and Gershwin, M. E. Asthma self-management programs: Premises, not promises. *J. Asthma* 25:89, 1988.
75. Knapp, P. Acute bronchial asthma. II: Psychoanalytic observations on fantasy, emotional arousal and partial discharge. *Psychosom. Med.* 22:88, 1960.
76. Knapp, P. The asthmatic and his environment. *J. Nerv. Ment. Dis.* 149:133, 1969.
77. Knapp, P. H., et al. Short term immunological effects of induced emotion. *Psychosom. Med.* 54:133, 1992.
78. Knapp, P., Mushatt, C., and Nemetz, S. The context of reported asthma during psychoanalysis. *Psychosom. Med.* 32:167, 1970.
79. Knapp, P., and Nemetz, S. Personality variations in bronchial asthma: A study of 40 paatients: Notes on the relationship to psychosis and the problem of measuring maturity. *Psychosom. Med.* 19:443, 1957.
80. Knapp, P., and Nemetz, S. Sources of tension in bronchial asthma. *Psychosom. Med.* 19:466, 1957.
81. Knapp, P., and Nemetz, S. Acute bronchial asthma: I. Concomitant depression and excitement and varied antecedent patterns in 406 attacks. *Psychosom. Med.* 32:167, 1960.
82. Knapp, T., and Wells, L. Behavior therapy for asthma: A review. *Behav. Res. Ther.* 16:103, 1978.
83. Kotses, H., et al. Operant reduction in frontalis EMG activity in the treatment of asthma in children. *J. Psychosom. Res.* 20:453, 1976.
84. Kotses, H., et al. Operant muscular reduction and peak expiratory flow rate in asthmatic children. *J. Psychosom. Res.* 22:17, 1978.
85. Kotses, H., and Glaus, K. Application of biofeedback to the treatment of asthma. *Biofeedback Self Regul.* 6:573, 1981.
86. Lamont, J. Psychosomatic study of asthma. *Am. J. Psychol.* 114:890, 1958.
87. Larsson, K. Studies of sympatho-adrenal reactivity and adrenoceptor function in bronchial asthma. *Eur. J. Respir. Dis.* 66(Suppl. 141):1, 1985.
88. Lieberman, M., and Lipton, E. Asthma in Identical Twins. In H. I. Schneer (ed.), *The Asthmatic Child: Psychosomatic Approach to Problems and Treatment*. New York: Harper & Row, 1963.
89. Liebman, R., Minuchin, S., and Baker, L. The use of structural family therapy in the treatment of intractable asthma. *Am. J. Psychiatry* 131:535, 1974.
90. Lofgren, J. B. A case of bronchial asthma with unusual dynamic factors treated by psychotherapy and psychoanalysis. *Int. J. Psychoanal.* 42:414, 1961.
91. Luparello, T., et al. The interaction of psychologic stimuli and pharmacologic agents on airway reactivity in asthmatic subjects. *Psychosom. Med.* 5:512, 1970.
92. Luparello, T., et al. Influence of suggestion on airway reactivity in asthmatic subjects. *Psychosom. Med.* 30:819, 1968.
93. MacKenzie, J. N. The production of "rose asthma" by an artificial rose. *Am. J. Med. Sci.* 91:45, 1886.
94. Mathé, A. A. Decreased circulating epinephrine, possibly secondary to decreased hypothalamic adrenal medullary discharge; a supplementary hypothesis of bronchial asthma pathogenesis. *J. Psychosom. Res.* 15:349, 1971.
95. Mathé, A. A., and Knapp, P. H. Decreased plasma free fatty acids and urinary epinephrine in bronchial asthma. *N. Engl. J. Med.* 281:234, 1969.
96. Mathé, A. A., and Knapp, P. H. Emotional and adrenal reactions to stress in bronchial asthma. *Psychosom. Med.* 33:323, 1971.
97. Mattila, M. J., and Muittari, A. Modification by imipramine of the bronchodilator response to isoprenaline in asthmatic patients. *Ann. Med. Intervae Fenniae* 57:185, 1968.
98. McDermott, N. T., and Cobb, S. A psychiatric survey of 50 cases of bronchial asthma. *Psychosom. Med.* 1:203, 1939.
99. McFadden, E. R., et al. The mechanisms of action of suggestion in the induction of acute asthma attacks. *Psychosom. Med.* 31:134, 1969.
100. Meares, R. A., et al. Amitriptyline and asthma. *Med. J. Aust.* 2:25, 1971.
101. Meijer, A. Conflictual maternal attitudes towards asthmatic children. *Psychother. Psychosom.* 33:105, 1980.
102. Miklich, D. R., et al. The clinical utility of behavior therapy as an adjunctive treatment for asthma. *J. Allergy Clin. Immunol.* 60:285, 1977.
103. Miller, B. D., and Strunk, R. C. Circumstances surrounding the deaths of children due to asthma. *Am. J. Dis. Child.* 143:1294, 1987.
104. Miller, H., and Baruch, D. W. Psychosomatic studies of children with allergic manifestations. I. Maternal rejection: A study of 63 cases. *Psychosom. Med.* 10:245, 1948.
105. Mohr, G., Selesnik, S., and Augenbraun, B. Family Dynamics in Early Childhood Asthma: Some Mental Health Considerations. In H. I. Schneer (ed.), *The Asthmatic Child*. New York: Hoeber, 1963.
106. Moore, N. Behavior therapy in bronchial asthma—A controlled study. *J. Psychosom. Res.* 9:257, 1967.
107. Morris, H., Deroche, G., and Earle, M. Urinary excretion of epinephrine and norepinephrine in asthmatic children. *J. Allergy Clin. Immunol.* 50:138, 1972.
108. Mrazek, D. A. Asthma: Psychiatric Considerations, Evaluation, and Management. In E. Middleton, et al. (eds.), *Allergy: Principles and Practice* (3rd ed.). St. Louis: Mosby, 1988. P. 1176.
109. Mrazek, D. A., Casey, B., and Anderson, I. Insecure attachment in severely asthmatic preschool children: Is it a risk factor? *J. Am. Acad. Child Adolesc. Psychiatry* 26:516, 1987.
110. Mrazek, D. A., et al. Early asthma onset: Consideration of parenting issues. *J. Am. Acad. Child. Adolesc. Psychiatry* 30:277, 1991.

111. Munroe-Ford, R. The causes of childhood asthma. *Med. J. Aust.* 2:128, 1963.
112. Murphy, A. I., Lehrer, P. M., and Karlin, R. Hypnotic susceptibility and its relationship to outcome in the behavioral treatment of asthma. *Psychol. Rep.* 65:691, 1989.
113. Noelpp-Eschenhagen, I., and Noelpp, B. New contributions to experimental asthma. *Prog. Allergy* 4:361, 1954.
114. Pearson, R. S. B. Asthma, allergy and prognosis. *Proc. R. Soc. Med.* 61:467, 1968.
115. Phillipp, R. L., Wilde, G. J. S., and Day, J. H. Suggestion and relaxation in asthmatics. *J. Psychosom. Res.* 16:193, 1972.
116. Pinkerton, P. Correlating physiologic with psychodynamic data in the study and management of childhood asthma. *J. Psychosom. Res.* 11:11, 1967.
117. Purcell, K., et al. The effect on asthma in children of experimental separation from the family. *Psychosom. Med.* 31:144, 1969.
118. Purcell, K., Bernstein, L., and Bukantz, S. A preliminary comparison of rapidly remitting and persistently steroid dependent asthmatic children. *Psychosom. Med.* 23:305, 1961.
119. Ratner, B., and Silberman, E. E. Allergy—Its distribution and the hereditary concept. *Ann. Allergy* 9:1, 1952.
120. Rea, H. A., et al. A case-controlled study of death from asthma. *Thorax* 41:833, 1986.
121. Rees, L. Physical and emotional factors in bronchial asthma. *J. Psychosom. Res.* 1:98, 1956.
122. Rees, L. The importance of psychological, allergic, and infective factors in childhood asthma. *J. Psychosom. Res.* 7:253, 1964.
123. Report to Research Committee of the British Tuberculosis Association. Hypnosis for asthma—A controlled trial. *Br. Med. J.* 4:71, 1968.
124. Richter, R., and Dahme, B. Bronchial asthma in adults: There is little evidence for the effectiveness of behavioral therapy and relaxation. *J. Psychosom. Res.* 26:533, 1982.
125. Rogerson, C. H. Psychological factors in asthma. *Br. Med. J.* 1:406, 1943.
126. Rosenthal, S. V., Aitken, R. C. B., and Zealley, A. K. The Cattell 16PF personality profile of asthmatics. *J. Psychosom. Res.* 17:9, 1973.
127. Rubin, D. H., Bauman, L. J., and Lauby, J. L. The relationship between knowledge and reported behavior in childhood asthma. *J. Dev. Behav. Pediatr.* 10:307, 1989.
128. Scherr, M. S., et al. Effects of biofeedback techniques on chronic asthma in a summer camp environment. *Ann. Allergy* 35:289, 1975.
129. Scherr, M. S., and Crawford, P. L. Three-year evaluation of biofeedback techniques in the treatment of children with chronic asthma in a summer camp environment. *Ann. Allergy* 41:288, 1978.
130. Schiavi, R., Stein, M., and Sethl, B. Respiratory variables in response to a pain-fear stimulus and in experimental asthma. *Psychosom. Med.* 23:485, 1961.
131. Sibbald, B., Horn, M. E. C., and Gregg, I. A family study of the genetic basis of asthma and wheezy bronchitis. *Arch. Dis. Child.* 55:354, 1980.
132. Sifneos, P. The prevalence of "alexithymic" characteristics in psychosomatic patients. *Psychother. Psychosom.* 22:255, 1973.
133. Sloanaker, J., and Luminet, D. Classical conditioning in bronchial asthma. Unpublished doctoral dissertation. Boston: Boston University, 1961.
134. Smith, M. L., Glass, G. V., and Miller, T. S. *The Benefit of Psychotherapy.* Baltimore: Johns Hopkins University Press, 1980.
135. Smith, R. E. A Minnesota Multiphasic Personality Inventory profile of allergy. *Psychosom. Med.* 24:203, 1962.
136. Spector, S., et al. Response of asthmatics to methacholine and suggestion. *Am. Rev. Respir. Dis.* 113:43, 1976.
137. Sperling, M. A Psychoanalytic Study of Bronchial Asthma in Children. In H. I. Schneer (ed.), *The Asthmatic Child.* New York: Harper & Row, 1963.
138. Staudenmeyer, H., Kinsman, R. A., and Jones, N. F. Attitudes toward respiratory illness and hospitalization in asthma: Relationships with personality, symptomatology and treatment responses. *J. Nerv. Ment. Dis.* 166:624, 1978.
139. Strunk, R. C., et al. Physiologic and psychological characteristics associated with deaths due to asthma in childhood. *JAMA* 254:1193, 1985.
140. Sugihara, H., Ishihara, K., and Noguchi, H. Clinical experience with amitriptyline (Tryptanol) in the treatment of bronchial asthma. *Ann. Allergy* 23:422, 1965.
141. Tal, A., and Miklich, D. R. Emotionally induced decreases in pulmonary flow rates in asthmatic children. *Psychosom. Med.* 38:190, 1976.
142. Tehan, N., et al. Impact of asthma self-management education on the health behavior of young adults: A pilot study of the Dartmouth College "Breathe Free" program. *J. Adolesc. Health Care* 10:513, 1989.
143. Teirmaa, O. *Psychosocial Factors in the Onset and Course of Asthma: A Clinical Study on 100 Patients.* Oulu, Finland: University of Oulu Press, 1977.
144. Vachon, L., and Rich, E. S. Visceral learning in asthma. *Psychosom. Med.* 38:122, 1976.
145. Walton, D. Application of Learning Theory to a Case of Bronchial Asthma. In H. Eyesinck (ed.), *Behavior Therapy and the Neuroses.* London: Pergamon, 1960.
146. Weiner, H. *Psychobiology and Human Disease.* New York: Elsevier, 1977.
147. Weiss, J. H., Martin, C., and Riley, J. Effects of suggestion on respiration in asthmatic children. *Psychosom. Med.* 32:409, 1970.
148. Weitzman, M., et al. Maternal smoking and childhood asthma. *Pediatrics* 85:505, 1990.
149. White, D. A., et al. Hypnosis in bronchial asthma. *J. Psychosom. Res.* 5:272, 1958.
150. Williams, D. A., et al. Assessment of the relative importance of the allergic, infective and psychological factors in asthma. *Acta Allergol.* 12:376, 1958.
151. Wilson, A. F., et al. Transcendental meditation and asthma. *Respiration* 32:74, 1975.
152. Wright, G. T. L. Asthma and the emotions. *Med. J. Aust.* 1:961, 1965.
153. Boulet, L.-P., et al. Near-fatal asthma: clinical and physiologic features, perception of bronchoconstriction, and psychologic profile. *J. Allergy Clin. Immunol.* 88:838, 1991.
154. Alt, H. L. Psychiatric aspects of asthma. *Chest* 101:415S, 1992.

Exercise and Sex

Stanley Sabin
Alfred I. Kaplan

86

EXERCISE AND ASTHMA

Bronchoconstriction associated with exercise affects about 12 percent of the population, and is common in asthmatics including those who are atopic without asthma. Exercise-associated bronchospasm in asthmatics [45, 56] has been noted since the beginning of the Common Era [58]. More recently, one study revealed that 80 percent of asthmatics have exercise-related asthma [32]. Despite the awareness and development of increased bronchospasm, properly medicated and physically trained asthmatics can compete at all levels of exertion equal to their nonasthmatic peers [9]. Results of recent Olympic competition support this observation. In the 1984 Los Angeles Olympics [56, 64], forty-one medals were won by athletes with a history of asthma. The 1988 Seoul competition awarded sixteen medals to athletes with a history of bronchospasm [27]. The International Olympic Committee has approved oral theophylline, albuterol, and terbutaline as well as inhaled cromolyn sodium, terbutaline, and albuterol for use by athletes participating in Olympic competition (Table 86-1). Younger asthmatics, males and females equally, are affected more often than are older ones. The symptoms of asthma produced by exercise are not unique but mimic those induced by pollens, infections, and emotion. Eggleston [18] and Phillips [52] found that an asthmatic's response to exercise is unaffected by diurnal variation and that the magnitude of the exercise response is not affected by seasonal allergic sensitivity [17]. Although an unresolved issue, the physician should also be aware that dual and late-phase reactions associated with exercise may contribute to an asthmatic problem, in addition to the obvious acute exercise-induced asthma [69].

All asthmatics have changes in their ventilatory status during and after exercise [47, 56]. This observation suggests that the designation *exercise-induced asthma* (EIA) should be reserved to refer to that small percentage of the population that develops bronchospasm during or after exercise without a previous history of bronchial asthma. These changes in airway caliber that occur in asthmatics during exercise might properly be called *exercise-induced hyperreactivity* [68]. In almost all asthmatics, exercise leads to initial bronchodilation [56] caused by the release of endogenous epinephrine and increased vagal stimulation followed by bronchoconstriction. Exercise lasting longer than 6 minutes results in bronchoconstriction that does not worsen with exercise prolongation (Fig. 86-1). Voy [67] reported that exercise at 85 percent of the maximum oxygen consumption lasting more than 5 minutes is necessary to produce bronchospasm. Several theories have been offered to explain this phenomenon, which is still largely unexplained. Kallenbach [29] postulated a primary hypothalamic abnormality that leads to autonomic imbalance based on his observation of a decreased cortisol response that could not be attributed to the effect of treatment with medications such as beclomethasone. The response to exercise is blunted by nebulized alpha$_1$-adrenergic–receptor blocking agents [6], calcium channel blockers [5], and cromolyn preparations. These observations have suggested a prominent role for mast cells as an etiologic factor in exercise-related bronchospasm [38]. There are reports of increased leukotrienes and neutrophil chemotactic factor in EIA; histamine data are variable [70, 71]. A lesser role has been postulated for a direct relaxant effect on bronchial smooth muscle produced by calcium channel blockers [5]. Crimi and colleagues [72] noted that delayed bronchoconstriction after exercise is not specific to EIA but appears to be associated with airway inflammation.

Previously, physical activities were classified according to how "asthmogenic" they were [7, 23]. Swimming was considered the activity least likely to provoke an attack of bronchospasm, while running, cycling, and "ballgames" were deemed most likely to do so. Current knowledge indicates that such rankings are invalid and erroneous. Asthmatics respond similarly to all types of exercise, as long as significant changes do not occur in the airway temperature [3] and humidity [3], compared with preexercise conditions. If these airway conditions are controlled, then the degree of change in airway caliber and resistance to airflow are proportional to the strenuousness of the activity and the increased ventilation induced by exercise [7, 9, 50, 56]. However, swimming in a pool may be preferred to mountain climbing in air that is often cold and dry.

The appropriate use of inhaled beta-adrenergic drugs and cromolyn preparations prior to exertion and occasionally during exercise allows asthmatics to participate in all activities with confidence and without fear of failing because of their bronchospastic condition [10]. Asthmatics involved in exercise should warm up for prolonged periods prior to engaging in peak exercise [48] and should be informed that nasal breathing, if feasible, can ameliorate exercise-induced hyperreactivity. First described by McNiell in 1966 [45] was the observation that about a half of those patients with exercise-induced asthma are refractory to the asthma for up to four hours. In a more recent study of two women and five men with exercise-induced asthma, Reiff and colleagues [54] found that treadmill running at submaximal levels for a half hour induces a refractory period, during which a given exercise that induces asthma can be performed without the exercise provoking asthma. In this study, after submaximal exercise and a 2-minute rest period, the patients were able to perform maximal exercise for 6 minutes without asthma occurring. Based on these observations, a warm-up period may be a way to prevent or ameliorate the symptoms of EIA [54]. However, with maximal exercise, asthma can still occur in susceptible patients, even though they may be well conditioned; hence, drug therapy is still required to prevent asthma symptoms.

Beta$_2$-adrenergic drugs administered by the inhaled route are the drugs of choice for use before and during exercise, as needed. Cromolyn is effective if taken before exercise. The combination

Table 86-1. Approved and banned antiasthma and antiallergic medications for participants in international athletic events

APPROVED

Beta$_2$ agonists (inhaled or aerosol): albuterol, pibuterol metaproterenol, terbutaline
Theophylline preparations
Cromolyn sodium
Antihistamines
Corticosteroids (inhaled preparations)
Nonnarcotic antitussives or analgesic drugs: dextromethorphan and pholcodine

NOT APPROVED

Beta$_2$ agonists (oral or liquid)
Corticosteroids (oral, intravenous, or intramuscular)
Sympathomimetic amines or stimulants: pseudoephedrine, ephedrine, isoetharine, isoproterenol, phenylephrine, phenylpropanolamine
Narcotic antitussives or analgesic drugs: codeine, dihydrocodeine, oxycodone, hydrocodone

Source: Abstracted from United States Olympic Committee, Division of Sports Medicine, *Drug Education and Doping Control Program: Guide to Banned Medications.* Colorado Springs, CO: U.S. Olympic Committee, 1990, as modified from *J. Respir. Dis.* 12:1110, 1991, with permission.

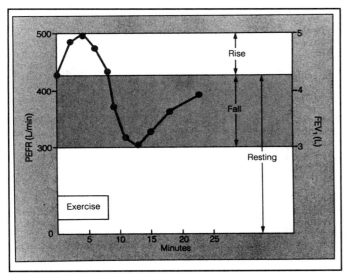

Fig. 86-1. *Lung function changes during and after running in an asthmatic patient who has some airway obstruction while at rest are demonstrated by measurement of peak expiratory flow rate (PEFR) changes. Bronchodilation, which is indicated by an increase in PEFR, occurs initially, but, by the end of the exercise period, PEFR returns to the preexercise level. PEFR continues to decrease after exercise ends and usually reaches its lowest point within the next 5 to 10 minutes. It then begins to normalize, and this period of bronchoconstriction resolves spontaneously within 60 minutes. (Reprinted with permission from M. A. Huftel, et al., Finding and managing asthma in competitive athletes. J. Respir. Dis. 12:1110, 1991; adapted from S. D. Anderson, Exercise induced asthma: current views. Patient Management, October, 1981.)*

of a beta$_2$ agonist with cromolyn is reported to increase the duration of protection [73]. Theophylline preparations have a lesser role in the treatment of exercise-induced asthma. Only a small protective effect is seen with inhaled steroids; ipratropium apparently does not effectively prevent the bronchospasm of EIA; calcium agonists require further study [74]. All acute exacerbations of asthma, whatever the etiology, should be well under control before asthmatics are permitted to indulge in vigorous exercise [48]. The patient with exercise-induced asthma should be advised to take into account other factors, such as the presence of signifi-

cant pollution or cold air, and adjust his or her exercise schedule accordingly; exercise during periods of excessive atmospheric pollutants, such as carbon monoxide and ozone and even aeroallergens, is best tempered. This approach to exercise in asthmatics of all degrees of severity requires the reeducation of healthcare providers and educators [37]. At one time asthmatics were admonished to curtail their physical activities in order to decrease the intensity and frequency of their symptoms. Cochrane [12] noted that the fitness of asthmatics and their cardiorespiratory performance benefit from the use of medically supervised exercise programs. Modern pharmacology, patient education, and training should allow most asthmatics to participate freely in most exercises. Physical fitness achieved through a regular program of appropriate exercise is desirable for most patients with asthma. The role and extent of permissible physical training for asthmatics was recently reviewed by Clark [75]. A sense of physical well-being as well as the psychological benefit of dealing effectively with the asthma process are distinct advantages. Specific advantages of a regular exercise program also include less exercise-induced asthma associated with improved aerobic fitness. A lesser rise in ventilation and heart rate in conditioned asthmatic children has been reported by Orenstein and associates [51]. Regular physical activity and exercise, beside yielding psychological benefits, may decrease the frequency of asthma attacks and school absenteeism [61]. A recent article and editorial stressed the need for education in physical activity for asthmatics; improved communication between physician and patient allows asthma patients to benefit from exercise and improves their quality of life [76, 77].

Specific advice and instructions for preventing exercise-induced bronchospasm are often requested by patients. Schroeckstein [56] has offered the following tips for avoiding exercise-induced asthma:

1. Begin warm-up periods by inhaling the beta$_2$-agonist drug or cromolyn sodium recommended by the physician.
2. Warm up with 10 to 15 minutes of stretching.
3. Work out slowly for 10 to 15 minutes, aiming for a pulse rate below 140 beats/min.
4. If wheezing or shortness of breath develops, inhale the beta agonist again. If cromolyn sodium was the warm-up medication, then use the beta agonist for the first time. When symptoms abate, resume warm-up activity.
5. Following warm-up, go into the full work-out.
6. Follow the work-out with a 10- to 30-minute cool-down period. This may include jogging, stretching, or perhaps weight lifting.

For those patients or physicians desiring more information on sports activities in asthmatics, the following professional organizations may be contacted:

American Academy of Sports Physicians
17113 Gledhill St.
Northbridge, CA   91325

American College of Sports Medicine
Box 1440
Indianapolis, IN   46206-1440

American Physical Therapy Association
1111 N. Fairfax St.
Alexandria, VA   22314

For asthmatic patients interested in more information regarding exercise, the book by Hogshead and Couzens, which is written for patients, is recommended [27].

Recently, concern has been raised about asthmatic scuba divers who may experience barotrauma on ascent (air embolus or pneumothorax) [78]. Banning this activity for such patients has been suggested, and as this issue is currently unresolved, caution is indicated until further objective data are available [79, 80].

SEX AND ASTHMA

Just as asthmatics are able to participate with confidence in physical exercise, so are they capable of engaging in sexual activity. This form of exertion may also precipitate bronchospasm and dyspnea. The treatment of the asthmatic patient should include an understanding of the effects of sexual activity.

Asthma and the various chronic lung diseases have a direct impact on a patient's quality of life. Often there is a loss of self-esteem and the development of anxiety and depression along with dependency. Another facet often overlooked by physicians is sexuality. There are numerous studies on the emotional effects of lung disease [1, 2, 15, 28, 30, 39, 53, 59], but fewer on its effects on sexuality [11, 13, 14, 24, 36, 60, 66]. The report of Masters and Johnson [43] did much to increase the interest in sexuality and its importance to human well-being. With societal attitudes changing, there is now a greater demand by patients seeking information and assistance in sexual dysfunction. Thus, the physician's understanding of not only the physiologic but the psychosocial impact of lung disease on sexual function is very important to the long-term adjustment and well-being of patients with asthma.

As with other diseases, a thorough history often defines the problem. Questions dealing with sexual function must be explored with the asthmatic patient and not avoided. Questions relating to frequency, interest, and satisfaction of sexual activity will often reveal problems [55] that would otherwise go undetected. The effects of a chronic lung disorder on physical sexual expression should be explored, since this may be of greater consequence to the patient than other emotional aspects of the disease [24]. A decrease in sexual frequency seems to be a more common occurrence than other aspects of sexual dysfunction. It is important to question male patients with asthma about problems of impotence, since there are now means of distinguishing psychogenic from organogenic erectile impotence [20]. By determining the patient's erectile capacity, the presence of morning erections, and the status of his libido, one can differentiate organic disease from a psychologic cause [21, 40, 57, 63].

Asthma can affect sexual function, both physically and psychologically. Psychological states can also lead to altered pulmonary physiology, and thus it is important to understand the interaction of these effects. Anger or anxiety can cause a decrease in arterial oxygen tension (PaO_2) by increasing both the work of breathing and skeletal muscle tension. Depression may decrease ventilation. The respiratory distress caused by anxiety or depression can increase the patient's psychological abnormality, and thus produce a vicious cycle. Libido may also greatly diminish with depression, thus exacerbating the sexual difficulty [35]. Other altered psychological states are often present in the asthmatic that also interfere with sexual function [39]: the fears of failure, rejection, guilt, and shame create an environment in which normal sexual relationships cannot exist. The patients also fear the physical difficulties of dyspnea, impotence, and even dying, which further inhibits normal sexual activities.

The physiologic effects of asthma on sexual function are still somewhat controversial. Some believe that only very advanced disease physiologically alters sexual capabilities [13, 66]. Genital intercourse requires the expenditure of 3 to 4 METS—the amount of energy or oxygen consumed per kilogram of body weight per minute [13]. This is equivalent to walking three miles per hour or climbing two flights of stairs. Studies that have used pulmonary function tests to assess this issue have revealed no relationship to sexual function [14, 20]. However, when asthma is in an advanced stage, the combined measurements of the forced expiratory volume in 1 second, the diffusivity of carbon dioxide, PaO_2, and exercise tolerance that define the degree of pulmonary dysfunction do correlate with sexual performance [20]. Chronic hypoxemia can result in neuropsychological abnormalities, and thus the possibility of adversely affected erectile function and libido [22].

A diminished supply of oxygen to the limbic system and other areas of the brain can also result in substantial emotional disturbances that may affect sexual activity. One study revealed 50 percent of such patients had selective brain impairment, particularly in the visual, memory, and perceptive areas [31]. These relationships still require further evaluation. There is little evidence that hormonal function is abnormal or that peripheral vascular disease exists in a higher-than-normal percentage as the etiology of the sexual disturbances in these patients with pulmonary disorders [20]. Likewise, there are no studies showing a difference in the cardiac abnormalities in those patients with sexual dysfunction. It has been reported that sudden death during intercourse is rare [65], and this point should be emphasized to asthmatic patients. There have been reports of both males and females who suffer from exercise-induced asthma who have had episodes of wheezing and dyspnea during sexual intercourse [19, 62]. In the majority of these patients, premedication greatly alleviates the symptoms. The mechanisms involved in the bronchospasm of "sexercise"-induced asthma may be similar to the pathogenesis of exercise-induced asthma, although other etiologic factors have been postulated [19, 62]. The physician should also be aware of the existence of postcoital anaphylaxis, which can include wheezing, that generally occurs 5 minutes after intercourse [49].

Patients with asthma may be prescribed a multitude of therapeutic agents. No correlation has been made between sexual dysfunction or impotence and the four main categories of medication used in the treatment of asthma, namely theophylline, sympathomimetic agents, steroids, and antibiotics [14, 46]. Steroids may, however, decrease fertility and may reduce the number and motility of spermatozoa [42]. Other therapeutic agents that are given to asthmatics who have coexisting disease may interfere with normal sexual function. Digoxin may cause a reduction in libido and the ability to have erections [25]. Antihypertensive drugs have also caused sexual dysfunction, and these include the beta-adrenergic blockers, alpha-adrenergic blockers, and ganglion blockers. Methyldopa and clonidine, which are centrally acting hypotensive drugs, reduce libido and cause failure of erection [8]. Thiazide diuretics can cause erectile difficulty and decreased libido. The antipsychotics, through various pharmacologic actions, can interfere with sexual function, as can the antidepressants [4]. This latter group of drugs, which includes the tricyclics and the monoamine oxidase inhibitors, are often used in patients with chronic asthma and can cause numerous sexual dysfunctions such as decreased libido, delayed ejaculations, decreased erection, and impotence. Alcohol, a potent central nervous system depressant, often causes sexual dysfunction. It is the most common cause of the first episode of secondary impotence [14]; although in the short term it may increase sexual desire, it often simultaneously causes erectile dysfunction. In the long term, alcohol reduces the testosterone level and may decrease libido and increase impotence.

Treatment

For centuries it has been appreciated that a certain configuration of emotional and psychological changes may predispose one to asthmatic attacks. The medical community has come to recognize that asthmatic patients are a heterogeneous group, but possibly possessing a common pathway that can lead to bronchospasm and dyspnea. This symptom complex, when it becomes repetitive, can cause great psychological strain and interfere with normal everyday activities, including sexual relations. The physician should give as much attention to the patient's concerns about sexual function and enjoyment as to the concerns about working capability and other physical performance.

Since a significant cause of sexual dysfunction is psychological, the physician must start the process of treatment by taking a detailed history, including a sexual history. This history taking by itself can be therapeutic, in that it reveals to patients both their concern and knowledge of the problem. Once a problem with deficient sexual performance is revealed, a multidisciplinary approach can be initiated. The patient can be referred for proper counseling if the problem is considered outside the scope of one's expertise or "comfort level." Some suggestions in sexual counseling include:

1. Counsel those patients who appear to be receptive.
2. Counseling sessions should be arranged in private and when interruptions are unlikely.
3. Use a direct approach, selecting easily understood words and few medical terms. Do not be evasive.
4. Include the patient's sexual partner in the session whenever possible. Attempt to reduce the feelings of guilt and anxiety, and increase the sense of self-esteem and security [33, 60].

If the counseling sessions do not lead to an improvement in the patient's sexual function or if performance should worsen, then the patient should be referred to trained psychiatric or psychological personnel. In one study, about 50 percent of the patients indicated a desire to discuss their sexual problems with a physician, and most preferred a physician with expertise in sexual dysfunction [55]. Many different modes of psychiatric and psychological treatments of the asthmatic patient have been claimed to be successful [26, 28], and thus the patient should be encouraged to pursue these therapeutic modalities if necessary. It should be emphasized to the patient that the counseling approach will not alter the underlying respiratory problem and may not greatly alter sexual function, but may provide the patients with better control of their symptoms and improve self-esteem; indirectly this may improve sexual pleasure. One word of caution: one study suggests that certain asthmatics become quite seductive with their physicians [41].

Simultaneously the physician should perform a complete physical examination and laboratory evaluation to exclude other causes of sexual dysfunction; these include diabetes, hypertension, cardiovascular disease including peripheral vascular disease, endocrine disorders, renal insufficiency, and drug or alcohol abuse. It is now possible to monitor nocturnal penile tumescence and to diagnose erectile impotence in the absence of peripheral vascular disease [20]. A thorough review of all medications the patient is taking should be performed and, when feasible, those drugs known to have adverse sexual side effects should be changed or their use discontinued. During this period, the patient should be closely monitored for any improvement in sexual function or worsening of an underlying concomitant disease. Should the patient have no accompanying disease and medication is found not to be a factor, then it may be presumed that the patient's respiratory symptoms are the cause of the sexual difficulties. There are several measures that can be utilized to assist the asthmatic in having a more successful sexual experience (Table 86-2):

1. Sex should be attempted when the patient is well rested, such as after a night's rest. However, this should not occur immediately upon waking up, since some patients may have copious airway secretions.
2. The patient should use an aerosolized bronchodilator and

Table 86-2. Measures to improve sexual experience

1. Well rested
2. Clear secretions
3. Bronchial toilet prior to activity
4. Avoid heavy meals and alcohol
5. Avoid irritating odors
6. Optimal temperature of environment
7. When necessary, use oxygen
8. Assume less dominant positions

other bronchial toilet maneuvers prior to engaging in sexual activity.
3. The consumption of heavy meals or alcohol and sedative use should be avoided prior to sex.
4. The temperature of the room should be adjusted to the comfort level of the patient.
5. Any deodorants, perfumes, or hairsprays which may cause bronchospasm should be avoided.
6. Oxygen may occasionally be required to alleviate dyspnea and shortness of breath.
7. The patient should assume the less dominant position. For the male patient, the partner should assume the superior position, or the lateral position may be preferred. For the female patient, it is important for the male to avoid placing pressure on the patient's chest. Various effective positions have been reported [14, 16].

Sexual activity is a very important component of everyday life. The physician caring for the asthmatic patient must treat this aspect of the disease as aggressively as all other complications that asthmatic patients encounter.

REFERENCES

1. Agarwal, K., and Setha, J. P. A study of psychogenic factors in bronchial asthma. *J. Asthma Res.* 15:191, 1978.
2. Agle, D. P., and Baum, G. L. Psychological aspects of chronic obstructive lung disease. *Med. Clin. North Am.* 61:749, 1977.
3. Anderson, S. D. Sensitivity to heat and water loss at rest during exercise in asthmatic patients. *Eur. J. Respir. Dis.* 63:459, 1982.
4. Baldessarini, R. J. Drugs and the Treatment of Psychiatric Disorders. In L. S. Goodman and A. Gilman (eds.), *The Pharmacological Basis of Therapeutics.* New York: Pergamon Press, 1991.
5. Barnes, P. J. A calcium antagonist, nifedipine, modifies exercise induced asthma. *Thorax* 36:726, 1981.
6. Barnes, P. J., et al. Circulating catecholamines in exercise and hyperventilation induced asthma. *Thorax* 36:435, 1981.
7. Bar-Or, O. Physical conditioning in children with cardiorespiratory disease. *Exerc. Sport Sci. Rev.* 13:305, 1985.
8. Buffum, J. The effects of drugs on sexual function; a review. *J. Psychoactive Drugs* 14(1–2):5, 1982.
9. Bundgaard, A. The importance of ventilation in exercise induced asthma. *Allergy* 36:385, 1981.
10. Bundgaard, A. Exercise and the asthmatic. *Sports Med.* 2:254, 1985.
11. Campbell, M. L. Sexual dysfunction in the COPD patient. *Dimens. Crit. Care Nursing* 6:70, 1987.
12. Cochran, L. J. Benefits and problems of a physical training program for asthmatic patients. *Thorax* 45:345, 1990.
13. Conine, T. A., and Evans, J. H. Sexual adjustment in chronic obstructive pulmonary disease. *Respir. Care* 26:871, 1981.
14. Della Bella, L. Sexuality and the Pulmonary Patient. In J. E. Hodgkin, *Pulmonary Rehabilitation: Guidelines to Success.* Boston: Butterworth, 1984.
15. Dudley, D. L., Wermuth, C., and Hague, W. Psychosocial aspects of care in the chronic obstructive lung disease patient. *Heart Lung* 2:389, 1973.
16. Dudley, D. L., et al. Psychological concomitants to rehabilitation in chronic obstructive pulmonary disease. *Chest* 77:413, 1980.
17. Eggleston, P. A. Exercise induced asthma in children with intrinsic and extrinsic asthma. *Pediatrics* 56(suppl.):856, 1975.

18. Eggleston, P. A., and Guerrant, J. L. A standardized method of evaluating exercise induced asthma. *J. Allergy Clin. Immunol.* 58:414, 1976.
19. Falliers, C. J. Sexercise-induced asthma. *Lancet* 2:1078, 1976.
20. Fletcher, E. C., and Martin, R. J. Sexual dysfunction and erectile impotence in chronic obstructive pulmonary disease. *Chest* 81:413, 1982.
21. Furlow, W. L. Diagnosis and treatment of male erectile failure. *Diabetes Care* 2:18, 1979.
22. Grant, I., et al. Brain dysfunction in COPD. *Chest* 77(Suppl.):308, 1980.
23. Haas, F. Effective aerobic training on forced expiratory air flow in exercising asthmatic humans. *J. Appl. Physiol.* 63:1230, 1987.
24. Hanson, E. I. Effects of chronic lung disease on life in general and on sexuality: perceptions of adult patients. *Heart Lung* 11:435, 1982.
25. Hellerstein, J. K., and Friedman, E. H. Sexual activity and the post coronary patient. *Arch. Intern. Med.* 125:343, 1970.
26. Hindi-Alexander, M. The team approach in asthma. *J. Asthma Res.* 12:79, 1974.
27. Hogshead, N., and Couzens, G. S. *Asthma and Exercise.* New York: H. Holt and Co., 1990, Pp. 46–48.
28. Kahn, A. U. Present status of psychosomatic aspects of asthma. *Psychosomatics* 14:195, 1973.
29. Kallenbach, J. M. The hormonal response to exercise in asthma. *Eur. Respir. J.* 2:171, 1990.
30. Kapotev, C. Emotional factors in chronic asthma. *J. Asthma Res.* 15:5, 1977.
31. Kass, I., Updegraff, K., and Muffly, R. B. Sex in chronic obstructive pulmonary disease. *Med. Aspects Hum. Sexuality* 6:33, 1972.
32. Katz, R. M. Asthma and sports. *Ann. Allergy* 51:153, 1983.
33. Katzin, L. Chronic illness and sexuality. *Am. J. Nurs.* 90:54, 1990.
34. Kivity, S. Dose response like relationship between minute ventilation and exercise induced bronchoconstriction in young asthmatic patients. *Eur. J. Respir. Dis.* 61:342, 1980.
35. Kravitz, H. M. Sexual counseling for the chronic obstructive pulmonary disease patient. *Clin. Challenges Cardiopulm. Med.* 4:1, 1982.
36. Labby, D. H. Sexual concomitants of disease and illness. *Postgrad. Med.* 58:103, 1975.
37. Latinis-Bridges, B. Exercise and sports for children with specific chronic illnesses. *Nurse Pract.* 5:22, 1985.
38. Lee, T. H. The link between exercise respiratory heat exchange and the mast cell in bronchial asthma. *Lancet* 1:520, 1983.
39. Lester, D. M. The Psychological Impact of Chronic Obstructive Pulmonary Disease. In R. F. Johnson (ed.), *Pulmonary Care.* New York: Grune & Stratton, 1973, Pp. 341–345.
40. Levine, S. B. Marital sexual dysfunction: erectile dysfunction. *Ann. Intern. Med.* 85:342, 1976.
41. Luparello, T. J. Asthma and sex. *Med. Aspects Hum. Sexuality* 4:97, 1970.
42. Mancini, R. E., Lavieri, J. C., and Muller, R. Effects of prednisolone upon normal and pathologic human spermatogenesis. *Fertil. Steril.* 17:500, 1966.
43. Masters, W. H., and Johnson, J. E. *Human Sexual Inadequacy.* Boston: Little, Brown, 1970.
44. McCarthy, P. Wheezing or breezing through exercise induced asthma. *Phys. Sports Med.* July 1989, Pp. 125–130.
45. McNeill, R. S., et al. Exercise-induced asthma. *Q. J. Med.* 35:55, 1966.
46. McSweeney, A. M., et al. Chronic obstructive pulmonary disease: socioemotional adjustment and life quality. *Chest* 77(Suppl. 309):2, 1980.
47. Mellis, C. M. Comparative study of histamine and exercise challenges in asthmatic children. *Am. Rev. Respir. Dis.* 117:911, 1978.
48. Mink, B. D. Pulmonary concerns and the exercise prescription. *Clin. Sports Med.* 10(1):111, 1991.
49. Mittman, R. J., et al. Selective desensitization to seminal plasma protein fractions after immunotherapy for post-coital anaphylaxis. *J. Allergy Clin. Immunol.* 86:954, 1990.
50. Noviski, N. Exercise intensity determines and climatic conditions modify the severity of exercise induced asthma. *Am. Rev. Respir. Dis.* 136:592, 1987.
51. Orenstein, D. M., et al. Exercise conditioning in children with asthma. *J. Pediatr.* 106:556, 1985.
52. Phillips, M. J. The effect of sustained release aminophylline on exercise induced asthma. *Br. J. Dis. Chest* 75:181, 1981.
53. Plutchik, R., et al. Emotions, personality and life stresses in asthma. *J. Psychosom. Res.* 22:425, 1978.
54. Reiff, D. B., et al. The effect of prolonged submaximal warm-up exercise on exercise-induced asthma. *Am. Rev. Respir. Dis.* 139:479, 1989.
55. Sadoughi, W., Leshner, M., and Fine, I. A sexual adjustment in chronically ill and physically disabled populations: a pilot study. *Arch. Phys. Med. Rehab.* 311, 1971.
56. Schroeckstein, D. Exercise and asthma: not incompatible. *J. Respir. Dis.* 9:29, 1988.
57. Shrom, E. H., Lief, H. I., and Wein, A. J. Clinical profile of experience with 130 consecutive cases of impotent men. *Urology* 13:511, 1979.
58. Sly, R. M. History of exercise induced asthma. *Med. Sci. Sports Exerc.* 18: 314, 1986.
59. Stein, M., and Luparello, T. J. Psychosomatic aspects of respiratory disorders. *Postgrad. Med.* 47:137, 1970.
60. Straus, S., and Dudley, D. L. Sexual activity for asthmatics—a psychiatric perspective. *Med. Aspects Hum. Sexuality* 63, 1976.
61. Strunk, R., et al. Rehabilitation of a patient with asthma in the outpatient setting. *J. Allergy Clin. Immunol.* 87:601, 1991.
62. Symington, I. S., and Kerr, J. W. Sexercise-induced asthma. *Lancet* 2:693, 1976.
63. Timms, R. J. Sexual dysfunction and chronic obstructive pulmonary disease (editorial). *Chest* 814:398, 1982.
64. Traver, G. Asthma update part II. Treatment. *J. Pediatr. Health Care* 2: 227, 1988.
65. Ueno, M. The so-called coition death. *Jpn. J. Legal Med.* 17:333, 1963.
66. Vemireddi, N. K. Sexual counseling for chronically disabled patients. *Geriatrics* 33:65, 1978.
67. Voy, R. The U.S. Olympic Committee experience with exercise induced bronchospasm 1984. *Med. Sci. Sports Exerc.* 18:238, 1986.
68. Weiler, J. M. Prevalence of bronchial hyperresponsiveness in highly trained athletes. *Chest* 90:23, 1986.
69. Zawadski, D. K., Lenner, K. A., and McFadden, E. R., Jr. Reexamination of the late asthmatic response to exercise. *Am. Rev. Respir. Dis.* 137:837, 1988.
70. Finnerty, J. P., et al. Role of leukotrienes in exercise-induced asthma: inhibitory effect of ICI 204219, a potent leukotriene D_4 receptor antagonist. *Am. Rev. Respir. Dis.* 145:746, 1992.
71. Silvers, W. Exercise-induced allergies: the role of histamine release. *Ann. Allergy* 68:58, 1992.
72. Crimi, E., et al. Airway inflammation and occurrence of delayed bronchoconstriction in exercise-induced asthma. *Am. Rev. Respir. Dis.* 146:507, 1992.
73. Kobayashi, R., and Mellion, M. Exercise-induced asthma, anaphylaxis, and urticaria. *Primary Care* 8:809, 1991.
74. Katz, R., and Pierson, W. Exercise-induced asthma: current perspective. *Adv. Sports Med. Fitness* 1:83, 1988.
75. Clark, C. J. The role of physical training in asthma. *Chest* 101(Suppl.): 293S, 1992.
76. Garfinkel, S. K., et al. Physiologic and nonphysiologic determinants of aerobic fitness in mild to moderate asthma. *Am. Rev. Respir. Dis.* 145: 741, 1992.
77. Schwartzstein, R. M. Asthma: to run or not to run? *Am. Rev. Respir. Dis.* 145:739, 1992.
78. Monaghan, R. The risks of sports diving. *SPUMS J.* 18:53, 1988.
79. U.S. Navy. *Manual of the Medical Department.* Dec. 8:15-58, 15-59, 1987.
80. Hickey, D. D. Outline for medical standards for divers. *Undersea Biomed. Res.* 11:407, 1984.

Air Environmental Controls

Thomas J. Fischer
Michelle B. Lierl

87

The treatment of patients with asthma must be individualized and based on the general principles of avoidance of allergens and irritants, judicious use of pharmacologic therapy, and, if indicated, the administration of immunotherapy (hyposensitization). This individualized approach to the asthmatic patient should be adjusted according to the intensity and severity of the patient's disease, giving consideration to the discomfort, inconvenience, cost, and possible adverse effects of such treatments. Environmental control measures—the avoidance of identifiable or suspected allergens or irritants in the asthmatic's environment—is the most basic and, at times, the most effective method of managing asthma. Asthmatic patients and their families should understand that environmental control measures are essential if the management of asthma and other allergic diseases is to be successful. Drug therapy and immunotherapy are not adequate substitutes for basic avoidance measures.

STANDARD METHODS FOR ENVIRONMENTAL CONTROL

Standard environmental control methods should constitute the initial attempts to reduce allergic and irritant exposure in the home to a minimum without excessive alteration of life-style or the purchase of expensive air-cleaning devices. Molds, house dust mites, animal danders, pollens, and irritating odors can aggravate asthma and other allergic symptoms. Table 87-1 presents basic, standard environmental control measures that should be observed for patients with atopic sensitivities to house dust mite, molds, or various pollens as well as for asthmatic patients whose symptoms are triggered by cigarette smoke, strong odors, or other irritant exposures (see also Tables 42-4 and 42-5). Instruct the patient or family in these measures and regularly review their application, especially if asthmatic symptoms increase without explanation. Excellent video presentations for patient instruction are available through the American Academy of Allergy and Immunology (611 East Wells Street, Milwaukee, WI 53202).

AIR CLEANERS FOR HOME ENVIRONMENTAL CONTROL

In addition to basic environmental control measures, domestic air-cleaning devices, either used by themselves or in conjunction with heating and cooling systems, can help modify the home environment (Table 87-2). There is no ideal heating system for the asthmatic individual. Although hot water, electrical, and other radiant heating systems avoid the blowing of fine particles

Supported in part by the Children's Hospital Research Foundation, Cincinnati, Ohio.

of dust seen with a forced air system, they are unable to filter, humidify, or dehumidify the air unless numerous room units are used. A final decision on heating systems for patients with asthma must be made individually, based on their needs and resources. If duct systems are used, periodic cleaning of the ducts may be necessary, even in a newer home. The vents in the room can be closed (if tolerated) or covered, using aluminum foil [40], Saran wrap [22], or commercially available electrostatic vent guards. Sacca [41] reported potential problems caused by the shedding and dissemination of particles from fiberglass filters and recommended the use of permanent washable metal filters. In addition, patients should exercise caution when placing potentially inflammable materials in contact with metal furnace vents. In addition to filters on furnaces and vents, dust and pollen masks (e.g., 3M Face Mask, Model 9970) may offer some protection during high-level exposure (e.g., housecleaning or yard work). These masks are reasonably priced but have several disadvantages and do not protect against many gases (see Chaps. 42, 45, and 46).

Air Conditioners

The beneficial effect of air conditioning on allergy symptom control has been recognized, and several studies have demonstrated that it can reduce pollen exposure [11, 52, 53]. Because of its reasonable cost, the most common type of air-conditioning device used is the portable refrigeration-type unit. These window units appear to reduce indoor allergen and pollution levels substantially, isolating enclosed rooms from particle-bearing outdoor air. A typical air conditioner (Fig. 87-1) has its basic components divided functionally between two tenuously communicating sections. The indoor division contains a fan that draws room air past cooling coils and returns it in an essentially closed circulation. As the air is cooled, a refrigerant evaporates and is recycled through a condenser (in the outdoor division). This coolant passes through a large surface condenser coil, which is sprayed with water droplets by a second fan to facilitate cooling. The condenser fan has an outdoor intake and thereby exhausts heated air into the free atmosphere. If the door to the room is kept closed, two essentially closed circulations, one indoor directed and the other outdoor directed, are maintained despite a substantial energy exchange. Even with marginally efficient intake filters, window air conditioners produce low particle levels and can effect functional isolation of a room.

Consumer Reports is an excellent source of general information on air conditioning and the ratings of individual air-conditioning units [8]. Because a variety of moist surfaces within these units can support microbial growth, periodic cleaning and the disinfection of intake filters are required. Air-conditioning manufacturers or service companies can provide information on the methods and frequency of cleaning.

Table 87-1. Standard environmental control measures

The patient's bedroom is most important, since a major portion of the day is spent there. Follow these suggestions:
1. The bedroom should contain no stuffed chairs, rugs, or draperies. Linoleum or wood floors, wood or metal furniture, and plastic or washable cotton curtains or Plexiglas window coverings are preferable. If carpets are used, short-pile rugs are preferable to shag rugs. Everything in the room should be washable.
2. Avoid storing blankets, woolens, felt hats, or other dust catchers in bedroom closets. Keep the closet doors closed.
3. If there is a furnace vent in the room, close it (if possible) or cover it with commercially available vent guards. (Exercise caution with inflammable material brought in contact with metal.)
4. Doors and windows in the room must fit tightly. Close windows during major pollen seasons or during pollution alerts.
5. Once or twice a week, clean the room with a damp dust cloth. (The patient should avoid the room during and for 3 to 4 hours after this cleaning.)
6. Use Dacron or foam pillows, and wash pillows and bedding every 1 to 2 weeks with a water temperature greater than 55°C.
7. Vacuum mattresses and springs and completely encase in plastic protectors with a zipper closing.
8. For children, have only wooden, plastic, or nonallergic (not fuzzy) toys.
9. Keep pets out of bedroom.

In the rest of the house, follow these instructions:
1. No smoking should ever be allowed.
2. The patient should not sit on overstuffed furniture or on rugs.
3. Ideally, no pets should be kept indoors, especially in the living quarters.
4. Keep the number of houseplants to a minimum and out of the bedrooms and living room.
5. Do not use room deodorizers, mothballs, or bug sprays (strong odors).
6. Have the furnace cleaned regularly and provide covers for furnace vents if needed.
7. The patient should not be in the house during cleaning.
8. Keep humidifiers and air conditioners clean; replace or, if possible, wash filters according to manufacturer's recommendations.
9. Wearing masks may be helpful during periods of unavoidable allergen exposure.
10. Try to maintain relative humidity between 35 and 50%, and temperatures less than 22°C, especially in the basement.

Table 87-2. Types of domestic air-cleaning devices

Mechanical
    Panel
    Extended surface
    High-efficiency particulate air filter
Electronic
    Negative-ion generator
    Electrostatic precipitator
Hybrid
    Charged media filter
Gas and odor absorbing
    Activated charcoal
    Chemical absorbents
Air conditioning

Source: H. S. Nelson, et al., Recommendations for the use of residential air-cleaning devices in the treatment of allergic respiratory diseases. *J. Allergy Clin. Immunol.* 82:661, 1988. Reprinted with permission.

Central Air-Conditioning Units

A central air-conditioning unit is reasonably efficient in excluding allergens and irritant particles from the home. Hirsch and colleagues [11] concluded that the major mechanism responsible for reducing mold spore counts in centrally air-conditioned homes was that they allowed windows to be kept closed, thus

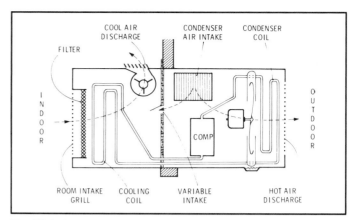

Fig. 87-1. *Operating components of a typical window air conditioner. Note the presence of two continuously communicating compartments and the nominally closed circulations of air that can result. (Reprinted with permission from W. R. Solomon, H. A. Burge, and J. R. Boise, Exclusion of particulate allergens by window air conditioners. J. Allergy Clin. Immunol. 65:305, 1980.)*

excluding particles. The production of a lower relative humidity and filtration were considered less important explanations for low spore counts. The air-conditioned homes in their study had mechanical fiberglass replacement filters, which are only 5 to 10 percent effective in removing particles 2 to 10 µm in diameter, such as smaller mold spores (e.g., *Aspergillus*). No significant differences were found in the percentage distribution of the different genera of molds between air-conditioned and non–air-conditioned homes. Because spore size was apparently not discriminatory in determining the presence of these spores, these filters probably did not decrease spore counts.

Because of the relatively high cost of operating a central air conditioner, however, the system is often used sporadically (only in the hottest weather) or inappropriately (only during the day, while windows are kept open at night for the cooler night air, thus negating the isolation effect). If cost is a major concern for the patient who lives in a climate where bedroom or living room windows can comfortably be kept closed most of the year, a window air-conditioning unit for use on the occasional hot days and nights during the pollen season may be the only device needed. Such an approach would preclude a major investment in a central air-conditioning system.

Because of the progressive increase in the number of vehicles on the road and the miles driven (e.g., 1.43 trillion personal passenger vehicle miles driven in the United States in 1988) [56], particle penetration into the automotive interior assumes added importance in the asthmatic and allergic individual. Driving with the windows closed and air-conditioning operating or driving with the windows closed and vents open decreases the amount of particle concentration compared to that in the outside ambient air [27]. However, alternative sources of bioaerosols within vehicles can result from microbial contamination of air-intake ducts and air-conditioner surfaces [17]. Muilenberg and colleagues [27] quote nonpublished data indicating that the fungus spore output from auto air conditioners usually occurs as an initial 1- to 3-minute "burst," rather than as a sustained emission. Avoiding the car during this cool-down period may be of benefit for allergic or asthmatic patients. Likewise, commercial cleaning services are now available at car service centers and such cleaning can reduce this type of contamination.

Air-Filtration Units

Air-filtration units can reduce airborne particles either by mechanical means (impingement, straining, or diffusion) or by elec-

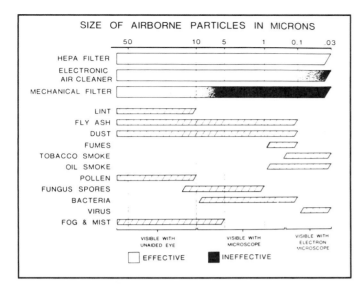

Fig. 87-2. *The effectiveness of various filtering systems in eliminating airborne particles that may precipitate or aggravate allergic diseases.* HEPA = *high-efficiency particulate air. (Reprinted with permission from J. M. Buckley and D. S. Pearlman, Controlling the Environment. In C. W. Bierman and D. S. Pearlman (eds.),* Allergic Diseases of Infancy, Childhood and Adolescence *(1st ed.). Philadelphia: Saunders, 1980.)*

trical attraction. Inertial impaction and gravitational setting are more effective for particles exceeding 1 μm in diameter, but diffusion is particularly effective for particles less than 0.01 μm in diameter. Neither electronic filters nor mechanical devices can effectively remove gases, including odors, though adsorption to activated charcoal or various chemical crystals can partially remove these odors.

Several types of air filters can be placed on central heating and cooling systems: standard filters (e.g., throwaway fiberglass or washable filters), media filters, electronic air cleaners, and "hybrid filters." Each type differs in cleaning efficiency (Fig. 87-2) and cost. Standard filters such as disposable fiberglass filters are available in hardware stores, drugstores, or building supply outlets. The Air Conditioning and Refrigeration Institute (1501 Wilson Boulevard, Arlington, VA 22209) has noted the efficiency of standard filters to be about 3 to 5 percent, according to standard industry comparisons. Media filters are more effective than standard filters but are more expensive, and the filtering material must be replaced at least annually. Efficiency is approximately 25 to 30 percent.

Electronic air cleaners, using two-stage electrostatic precipitators, have the advantages of high efficiency for both large and small particles, low pressure drops, and the ability to collect wet or dry particles; they are also washable. However, their disadvantages include greater initial expense, a requirement for safeguards against high voltage, and the need for frequent cleaning because these filters decrease in efficiency as the plates become loaded with material. Likewise, some units can produce ozone [31], although well-designed and maintained units apparently do not generate ozone in an amount sufficient to be considered a hazard.

Hybrid filters, combining properties of both mechanical and electronic filters, are charged media filters. These filters usually consist of special fibrous material that has been embedded with a permanent electrostatic charge. Air flows through the filter and an electrostatic field is created on the media. Unlike electronic air filters, a voltage source is not required and no ozone, noise, or odor is produced [31].

High-efficiency particulate air (HEPA) filters are a type of me-

chanical filter used in air-cleaning devices but are not regularly placed in central home heating and cooling systems. They were developed during World War II by the Atomic Energy Commission to remove radioactive dust from plant exhaust. These filters are constructed of submicronic glass fibers in a matrix made up of 1- to 4-μm fibers. HEPA filters must meet very stringent standards, including a removal efficiency of 99.97 percent for particles 0.3 μm in diameter, a high efficiency for both large and small particles, and a maximum pressure drop (when clean) of 1 inch (2.5 cm) of water when operated at its rated airflow capacity [32]. This excellent efficiency, along with their modest maintenance requirements (the filter life in the home is usually 2 to 5 years), have made these filters popular in domestic air-cleaning devices. Portable units are available, but central HEPA filter systems are generally not available because of the large blower capacity needed to force air through the HEPA system. A variety of air purifiers using HEPA or electrostatic precipitator filters are available. These units have been extensively studied and rated by *Consumer Reports* [1, 12a].

When electrostatic purifiers and HEPA filters are compared, each shows advantages and disadvantages. HEPA filters collect more material that passes through them, although an electrostatic model can treat more air per minute because of its lower resistance. *Consumer Reports* noted that their testing instruments could not detect levels of ozone at or below 100 parts per billion. However, this same study reported that the Environmental Protection Agency (EPA) has recorded considerably higher ozone levels in homes that use large electrostatic precipitators built into the heating system ducts.

Commonly tested materials for collection by air-cleaning devices have included cigarette smoke, road dust, and pollen, in order to provide a wide spectrum of test particle sizes. One measure of the efficiency of the filtering device is expressed in terms of the "clean air delivery rate," calculated according to the extent that the rate of removal of particles by the cleaning device exceeds that occurring due to natural fallout. This measurement is helpful because it allows for calculations of the number of air exchanges that can be produced for any size room [31] (the usual minimum number of air exchanges noted to have an impact on a moderate contamination problem is one per hour). Additional factors in assessing air-filter machines include noise production, filter access, size and weight, and expense [1, 12a].

While air filtration with HEPA devices or other high-efficiency filtration systems is theoretically helpful for the asthmatic patient, on a practical level, by themselves, they may not greatly alter the asthma or allergic symptoms. Studies attempting to document the benefit of filtration systems have generated conflicting results. In a double-blind study, Kooistra and associates [14] studied the effect of high-efficiency central air cleaners added to central air-conditioning systems on the symptoms of 20 adults with allergic rhinitis sensitive to ragweed or *Alternaria*, or both. Daily medication records and symptom scores were recorded. When the filters were in place, there was a statistically significant decrease in symptoms during the night hours. There was also a trend toward lower symptom scores during daytime and evening hours. These authors concluded that high-efficiency central air cleaners may produce minimal improvement for hay fever patients in comparison with central air conditioning alone. (The filtration device used, the Space Guard Air Cleaner, manufactured by Research Products Corp, Madison, WI, is constructed from glass microfibers formed into a sheet approximately 0.030-inch thick. Particles 6.0 μm and larger are removed with a 99 percent efficiency.)

Several studies have also been performed evaluating the effectiveness of HEPA filters in the control of asthmatic symptoms in children. Zwemer and Karibo [61] studied the night use of an HEPA device in 18 symptomatic asthmatic children. A reduction of allergic symptoms and medications was reported, although statistical methods were not applied in their analysis. Scherr and Peck [45] evaluated HEPA filtration units in a 2-year study conducted at a summer camp for asthmatic children. There was a strong statistical trend ($p < .07$) showing that HEPA filtration units reduced the incidence and severity of nightly asthmatic attacks. Villaveces and coworkers [58] evaluated 13 asthmatic children for 4 weeks in a double-blind cross-over study. Statistically significant improvement in symptom scores during filter use was noted, although peak flows did not significantly improve.

In a recent study, Reisman and associates [37] in a double-blind manner studied the effectiveness of a high-efficiency particulate air filter (Enviracaire) in the treatment of patients with perennial allergic rhinitis and asthma. Thirty-two patients were followed during the fall and winter months. These patients had a positive skin test to house dust or house dust mite extract. The Enviracaire room air cleaner was positioned in the bedroom for 8 weeks; the active filter was used for 4 weeks and a blank placebo filter, for 4 weeks. The active filter produced an average 70 percent reduction in airborne particulate matter that was greater than or equal to 0.3 μm in diameter. The results were also analyzed in terms of the patients' symptoms, medication score, and subjective evaluation. There was no difference in the total symptom/medication scores or individual symptom scores during the placebo and active-filter periods. However, analysis of the last 2 weeks of each filter period (when respiratory infection was absent) demonstrated definite differences in total and individual symptoms, suggesting benefit from use of the active filter. The subjective responses of patients also indicated benefit from the filter. The authors concluded that this type of HEPA filter can reduce allergic respiratory symptoms.

Because the data are incomplete on the merits of high-efficiency filters in the treatment of asthma, the decision to use these devices must be based on the individual asthmatic patient's needs and resources. For asthmatic patients with a high degree of sensitivity to aeroallergens or irritants, those with severe asthma, or those residing in an area of low air quality, the breathing of air (especially at night) from the envelope of clean air provided by these units seems reasonable even if the effects of these devices have not been conclusively demonstrated.

Spurred by the public's concern about the possible harmful effects of polluted air, a large variety of small tabletop or personal air-purifying units have been marketed. Manufacturers of these small units, often priced under $50, may claim that these devices will cleanse the air of large or small particulates, such as dirt, dust, pollen, tobacco smoke, soot, dog and cat dander, lint, hair, mold spores, irritating or undesirable odors, and chemical fumes or gases. A few may claim these devices can even eliminate harmful bacteria or viruses. Such statements, by themselves, do not constitute a therapeutic claim (although that may be implied). If there are medical or health claims on the label (e.g., that it will halt asthma attacks or end allergic reactions), the Food and Drug Administration would regard the air cleaner as a medical device subject to regulation under the Federal Food, Drug and Cosmetic Act. In these cases, the manufacturer or distributor is responsible for assuring that the product will perform the therapeutic function claimed.

As a general rule, the informed patient should remember that, for an efficient filtering system to clear the particulates in a controlled space, sufficient amounts of air must be forced through the system. The careful purchaser realizes that any device powerful and efficient enough to clean a roomful of air is not likely to be inexpensive or contained in a very small unit. A person considering the purchase of an air cleaner to improve breathing conditions should ask its manufacturer for the dioctyl phthalate (DOP) rating of its filters (a test of the efficiency of removing particulate materials), the fan's cubic feet per minute (CFM) displacement rating or power, the filter's CFM capacity, and the space dimensions recommended for use [12] (see Chap. 45).

Humidifiers and Dehumidifiers

The effect of humidity on asthmatic patients is not fully understood, but evidence suggests that both high and low humidity can be detrimental [39]. For optimal results, environmental humidity should be maintained between 35 and 50 percent. The advantages of proper humidification must be weighed against the potential hazards of excessively moist conditions, which can increase mold growth or the propagation of house dust mites. In addition, the aerosol from cool-mist vaporizers, by itself or because of mold contamination [50], has been associated with the precipitation of asthmatic episodes.

There are three general types of humidifiers: reservoir, evaporator, and jet spray [4]. Portable and centrally placed units are available. The appropriate system for a particular house depends on the size, design, and heating system of the house as well as meteorologic conditions in the area. Humidifiers that actively spray water droplets into the air can produce significant aerosol contamination. Evaporative humidifiers can also be contaminated, but do not actively disperse organisms and are less likely to produce adverse health effects unless contamination is severe [5]. Regardless of the type of device used, humidifiers and vaporizers must be cleaned with chlorine bleach before each use [2] to control microbial growth, which can become a source of airborne particles. Subjects who clean contaminated reservoirs especially should be warned that they can be regularly exposed to aerosols of the contaminant organisms and their metabolites.

If excessive humidity is a problem, mechanical dehumidifiers may be necessary. Attempts at energy conservation in homes designed for maximum energy efficiency can produce houses that are especially tight. The relative humidity in these homes can reach levels in excess of 75 percent, even during sub-zero winter weather [5]. However, before a dehumidifier (usually costing $200 to $300) is purchased, several maneuvers can be tried to see if they reduce dampness in the home. Venting fans can reduce humidity caused by cooking or by showers. Clothes dryers should also be vented properly. Wrapping cold-water pipes with insulation will stop them from sweating. In basements with dirt floors or crawl spaces, plastic sheeting placed over the dirt or the installation of insulation with a vapor barrier may help keep out moisture [2]. If these measures do not adequately reduce dampness, a portable dehumidifier may be needed. These units usually remove moisture by passing air over refrigeration coils. Dehumidifiers differ mainly in the amount of water they can remove from the air in a day (usually 40 to 50 pints). As with air conditioners and humidifiers, cleaning of the units is mandatory. *Consumer Reports* is a source of information on individual models [21].

Negative-Ion Generators

Negative-ion generators are controversial because of the medical claims that have been made for them. These devices produce large quantities of electrically charged molecules called *negative ions* that collide with pollutant particles in the air, conveying a negative electrical charge to them. These particles are then drawn through the air to the walls, floors, and other surfaces possessing lower electrical potentials. When tested solely as smoke removers, these units (ranging in cost from $80 to $200) appear effective [35]. However, their role in asthma management, as reviewed by Krueger [16], is less well defined, but initially promising results may warrant further well-controlled studies.

ENVIRONMENTAL CONTROL MEASURES FOR SPECIFIC ALLERGENS OR IRRITANTS

House Dust Mites

House dust is a complex mixture containing fibrous materials of plant and synthetic origin, fungi, bacteria, human epidermis, food remnants, inorganic substances, house dust mites, and, in some homes, animal dander and cockroach and other insect parts (see Chap. 42). During recent years, a major offending allergen in house dust has been identified as the house dust mite of the genus *Dermatophagoides* [13, 34a]. Two major groups of allergens from the genus *Dermatophagoides* have been defined. The Group I allergens (*Der p* I, *Der f* I, and *Der m* I) are heat-labile glycoproteins that are heterogeneous on isoelectric focusing and are excreted in mite feces. The Group II allergens (*Der p* II and *Der f* II) are proteins and are heterogeneous on isoelectric focusing [13].

The presence of mites can be determined by counting them under a microscope after separation from a dust sample, by immunochemical assays (radioallergosorbent test [RAST] inhibition or sandwich radio- or enzyme immunoassay using monoclonal antibodies), or by measuring the guanine level, an excretion product of mites [13]. The measurement of the amount of mites in the home is now possible by sending dust samples to commercial laboratories (ALK Laboratories, Inc., 132 Research Drive, Milford, CT 06460; tel: 1-800-325-7354, and the Johns Hopkins DACI Reference Laboratory, P.O. Box 26037, Baltimore, MD 21224; tel: 1-800-344-3224) or by using a "do-it-yourself" test kit (Acarex; distributed by Fisons Corporation, Bedford, MA). These laboratories can measure other antigens, including those of cat (*Cat fel d* I) and cockroach (cockroach *Bla g* I and *Bla g* II) [10b]. The Acarex test has been shown to correlate with monoclonal antibody tests for dust mites [36, 57] and is relatively simple to use and much less expensive. The use of any method to demonstrate mite presence can lead to patient compliance with mite control measures, as well as alert patients to the presence of mites as possible sensitizing allergens [54].

Optimal growth of *Dermatophagoides* occurs at 25°C and 75 percent relative humidity. Mite density exhibits a seasonal fluctuation, with the highest density occurring in the humid summer months and the lowest in the dryer heating season [3, 30]. Bed and bedroom floor dust often contains the highest concentration of mite allergen [55], although higher mite levels have been observed in heavily used fabric-upholstered furniture and carpeted areas of living and family rooms [3]. Noncarpeted floors have significantly lower mite levels than do carpeted floors despite frequent vacuuming. Although several studies [18, 28, 46] suggest that better-kept houses have fewer mites than those with lower sanitary conditions, other investigations have found no significant positive correlation between mite abundance and the frequency and thoroughness of cleaning and the age of furnishings or dwellings [3]. Although mite numbers and mite allergen levels in dust from carpets or setting in public areas are generally lower than levels in private homes, exceptions have been noted [10a].

With such conflicting data, the use of mite avoidance measures in treating asthmatic patients has also produced variable results. Sarsfield and colleagues [44] studied the response of 14 asthmatic children to the use of mite control measures but did not use a double-blind trial or incorporate cross-over periods into the study. The absolute mite counts were decreased using these measures, and clinical improvement of symptom scores was noted. Burr and associates [7], in a cross-over, controlled trial consisting of 32 adult patients, found no improvement in the daily peak flow readings or drug usage after mite control measures had been employed. The different results of these two studies may relate to different types of patients (adults versus children), different lengths of the trial periods, and beneficial effects too minor to have been detected by the assessment. During an 8-week trial, Mitchell and Elliott [25] used electrostatic precipitators in addition to the usual mite avoidance measures in a study of 10 children with moderate to severe asthma and positive skin test reactions to *D. pteronyssinus*. No significant differences in the mean peak expiratory flow rates between control periods and treatment periods were noted. Criticisms of this study have included

the fact that the electrostatic precipitator may not reduce the number of airborne particles in the actual environment of the mattress and that a 4-week treatment period may be too short to permit accurate assessment.

Although he did not examine the effect on clinical symptoms, Korsgaard [15] evaluated the effect of preventive measures on the concentration of house dust mites in the homes of 23 consecutive patients allergic to house dust mites and the homes of 75 randomly selected control subjects. The high absolute humidity of indoor air was related to a greater concentration of house dust mites. Although the patients' homes were supposedly cleaned more frequently, greater concentrations of house dust mites were found in the dust from bedroom carpeting in the patients' homes than in the homes of control subjects. The author concluded that preventive measures aimed at reducing the concentration of house dust mites should be directed toward lowering the indoor air humidity, and cleaning measures should probably be assigned a lower priority. He also noted that energy conservation measures (e.g., installing insulation) raised the indoor humidity and therefore could increase the frequency or severity of allergic reactions to house dust mites. Evidence for the sensitization of patients with asthma to mite antigens has been reported from many parts of the world. Likewise, these mite antigens can additionally contribute to the occurrence of rhinitis and, perhaps, atopic dermatitis. Two recent controlled studies, in which more extensive cleaning measures were evaluated, have demonstrated the clinical efficacy of cleaning measures in patient homes [29, 59].

Despite the uncertainties of these studies, it appears prudent for anti-mite control measures to be employed for asthmatic patients, especially those with proven dust mite sensitivity. There is now sufficient data to propose that 2 µg of Group I allergens per gram of dust (equivalent to 100 mites per gram or 0.6 mg of guanine per gram) can be regarded as representing a risk for the development of IgE antibody and asthma. Likewise, a higher level of 10 µg of *Der p* I antigen per gram (equivalent to 500 mites per gram of dust) should be regarded as a risk factor for producing acute attacks of asthma in mite-sensitive persons [13, 54].

In the bedroom, where an asthmatic patient can spend 6 to 10 hours a day, mattresses and pillows should be enclosed in plastic zippered covers to isolate mites and prevent rapid re-infestation of bedding. Newer coverings, using vapor-permeable waterproof fabric, are impermeable to house dust mite antigens and may be more comfortable and convenient than plastic covers [33]. These polyurethane-covered encasings reduced mite allergen levels on mattresses up to 98 percent and decreased bronchial hyperreactivity (as measured by provocative aerosol challenges of histamine phosphate) in 24 mite-sensitive asthmatic children [9a]. Washing of the bedding every 1 to 2 weeks, including pillows and mattress pads, is effective if the wash water temperature is 130°F (55°C) or higher. Higher water temperatures may be better but having such hot water in the home can increase the risk of scalding accidents in children. Mosbech and colleagues [26] suggest that house dust mite concentration in bedding can be controlled by the use of electric heating blankets. In their study, such blankets were used during the daytime and washed every 3 months. Mite antigens were reduced by 32 percent in the beds supplied with heating blankets but actually increased by 120 percent in the beds not supplied with heating blankets. Electric heating blankets appear to reduce mites by reducing the relative humidity. Electric blankets must be used in conjunction with current safety concerns about their use.

Another source of mite antigen in the bedroom is the carpet. In addition to serving as an important source of mite allergen, it perhaps provides the source from which bedding is often re-infested. Replacing carpets with hard flooring in the bedroom is often recommended. Alternatively, carpet treatments with a 3 percent tannic acid solution (Allergy Control Solution) has been shown to cause a decrease in mite exposure through protein denaturing of the mite antigen [10, 23]. Benzyl benzoate (Acarosan), also currently available in the United States, can kill mites (and their larvae), and separates and binds allergen-containing waste from carpets for easier removal by vacuum cleaner. These chemicals can be applied to the carpet, either as a powder (Acarosan) or as a fluid (Allergy Control Solution). Neither approach completely solves the problem, as they have proved to be more effective in experimental cultures than they are on carpets and they generally do not have a prolonged effect (that is, greater than 6 months) [10c, 19, 34]. Additional, more definitive studies documenting the beneficial effects of these treatments on the outcome of asthma remain to be performed. Possible adverse effects from these treatments must also be monitored [59a].

In addition to specific measures carried out in the bedroom, the living room and other parts of the house must also be monitored. Weekly vacuum cleaning removes fecal pellets but not live mites. Mite-sensitive patients should not engage in vacuuming, and the area vacuumed should be thoroughly ventilated before such patients return to it. Newer types of vacuum cleaners using filtering systems such as HEPA filters may be of benefit in decreasing the concentrations of airborne particles following vacuuming [20].

Finally, throughout the house, decreasing the absolute humidity below 50 percent (at 22°C) helps control mite growth and decreases the molds upon which mites feed.

Odor Control

Numerous household odors can induce or aggravate asthmatic symptoms. Such odors come from cooking odors, commercial sprays (air fresheners, cleaners), perfumes, soaps, and smoke from fireplaces. Placing lids on cooking containers and using exhaust fans when cooking can reduce odors. Room deodorizers, moth balls, or bug sprays that produce strong odors should be stored away from asthmatic patients and used only when the patient is out of the home. The pine odor of natural Christmas trees and wreaths should be avoided, and plastic Christmas trees and decorations used instead. Natural ornaments also produce mold growth. (See Chapters 42 and 45 for further information on indoor pollution.) Molecules that cause odors and gases cannot be effectively trapped, and their elimination requires far more activated carbon or other absorbent material than many home air-purifier devices currently contain.

Mold Control

Most indoor molds, originating primarily from growth on outdoor vegetation, can readily grow in moist and cool environments in the home. These areas include garbage containers, food storage areas, upholstery, wallpaper, and areas of increased moisture such as damp basements, shower curtains, window moldings, and portable window air-conditioning units [42]. During frost-free periods, emanations of dark-spored forms generally predominate, with indoor levels averaging 25 percent of those in the outside air [51]. Because of size-related undersampling, the yield of open fungal plates often seriously misrepresents actual prevalence levels and occasionally can even exclude recovery of abundant types. If accurate mold counts are to be taken, especially for research experiments (see Chap. 42), volumetric techniques of calculable efficiency should be used in a setting that minimizes contamination from without [5].

Although the complete eradication of molds is impossible, the use of dehumidifying procedures and devices plus fungicides can produce a quantitative reduction in mold concentrations that may benefit the mold-sensitive asthmatic patient. Common sources of mold contamination should be recognized and controlled. These sources include the aerosols from cool-mist vapor-

izers [50] and large numbers of indoor houseplants, which can harbor abundant fungus spores that may become airborne, especially under greenhouse conditions or if the plants are agitated. On the other hand, modest numbers of undisturbed houseplants have been shown to contribute minimally to the prevalence of airborne allergens in homes if the relative humidity is kept low [6]. For the exquisitely mold-sensitive patient (e.g., with allergic bronchopulmonary aspergillosis or hypersensitivity pneumonitis), however, even minimal sources may represent too great an exposure (see Chap. 49).

Excess humidity (relative humidity greater than 60 to 70 percent) enhances mold growth, and the use of dehumidification is helpful. Dehumidification in markedly damp areas plus fungicide use are needed for the sustained reduction of mold growth.

Fungicides can be used by direct application to appropriate surfaces. Phenolated disinfectants (e.g., Lysol) are inexpensive, readily available as sprays or solutions, and effective in controlling mold growth. Other mold disinfectants include halogens (e.g., Clorox) and benzalkonium chloride (e.g., Zephiran Chloride, 1 : 10,000 aqueous solution), a representative of the cationic surface disinfectants [4]. These, of course, should not be inhaled.

Air Pollution Control

The role of air pollution in the production of asthmatic symptoms is detailed in Chapter 45. The immediate control of indoor air pollution should be directed against cigarette smoking. The passive inhalation of smoke can increase symptoms in asthmatic children and can contribute to an increase in the frequency of respiratory infections in normal children. With the increased use of wood-burning stoves to conserve energy, respiratory symptoms can also be aggravated by the increased air pollutant particulates produced by wood fires [2, 43].

Air pollution in urban areas is a continual threat. The results of controlled chamber exposure experiments indicate that air pollutants can adversely affect asthma, although it is not clear to what extent these effects are clinically significant and further research is indicated [38]. Patients in urban areas should be advised to follow their local community guidelines, or similar recommendations, such as those advocated by the Weather and Air Pollution Committee of the American Academy of Allergy and Immunology during air pollution alerts [49] (Table 87-3).

Animal Allergens

Control of animal dander can be problematic because of the emotional attachment to the pet felt by the patient or the family.

Table 87-3. Guidelines for the asthmatic patient during air pollution alerts

1. Avoid unnecessary physical activity.
2. Avoid smoking and smoke-filled rooms.
3. Avoid exposure to dust and other irritants, such as hair sprays, insect sprays, or other sprays; paint; exhaust fumes; smoke from any fire; and other fumes.
4. Avoid exposure to those with colds and respiratory infections.
5. Try to stay indoors in a clean environment. Air conditioning is helpful, if available, as are charcoal filters, electrostatic precipitators, and high-efficiency particulate air filters.
6. If it appears that the air pollution episode is persisting or worsening, it is desirable to leave the polluted area temporarily until the episode subsides.
7. Ask your physician to devise specific instructions to follow. Know what medication to use and when to call your physician. Remember that, in case of an air pollution episode, the physician may be busier than usual and harder to reach. Keep emergency telephone numbers readily available. Know where and when to go to a hospital emergency center.

Source: Adapted from R. G. Slavin, et al., Guidelines for asthmatic patients during air pollution episodes. *J. Allergy Clin. Immunol.* 55:222, 1975.

Table 87-4. Effect of HEPA filter air cleaner on airborne **Fel d** *I in a house with two cats*

Number and type of filter	Height off floor	Airflow (m^3/hr)	Cats present during experiment	Decrease in 3 hr (%)
Living room[a]				
1 HEPA	On floor	300	Yes	70
2 HEPA	On floor	600	Yes	80[b]
1 HEPA	30 cm	600	No	80
2 HEPA	30 cm	1,200	Yes	60
Charcoal	30 cm	1,200	Yes	35
None	On floor	600	Yes	0
Cats' room[c]				
1 HEPA	On floor	300	Yes	30
2 HEPA	On floor	600	No	30
1 HEPA	On floor[d]	600	No	90

[a] Living room: mean background airborne *Fel d* I before experiments, 21.8 ng/m³; mean floor dust, 4 mg/gm *Fel d* I; volume of room, 130 m³.
[b] Mean of two experiments.
[c] Cats' room (containing cat food/litter/bed): mean background airborne *Fel d* I before experiments, 16.5 ng/m³; mean floor dust, 9 mg/gm *Fel d* I; volume of room, 30 m³.
[d] Floor cleaned using aqueous carpet extractor vacuum.
HEPA = high-efficiency particulate air.
Source: C. Luczynska, et al., Airborne concentrations and particle size distribution of allergen derived from domestic cats (*Felis domesticus*). *Am. Rev. Respir. Dis.* 141:361, 1990.

Furthermore, animal allergens, especially cat, can be found in house dust samples even in homes or public places without cats [47], probably originating from cats previously living in the home or brought in by other means. Animal avoidance is the treatment of choice, especially in patients documented to be sensitive to the animal in question. Although easily recommended, complete removal of the antigen (even with the animal gone) is difficult. Wood and coworkers [60] showed that, by 20 to 24 weeks after cat removal, only 8 of 15 study homes had reached levels found in control homes without cats. Cat allergen, unlike dust mite antigen, is widely distributed on wall surfaces, which can provide an important reservoir in the home environment [59b]. More aggressive measures in two homes, including carpet removal, brought about a quicker reduction in the level of cat antigen [60]. Additional materials to speed the removal of cat antigen include the use of room HEPA filters and vacuum cleaners equipped with HEPA filters [20], plus treating carpets with tannic acid to denature cat antigen [47] (Table 87-4).

A recent evaluation of techniques to reduce airborne cat allergens suggests the following procedures: (1) remove the cat from the home or keep it outdoors, (2) polish all floors and use no carpeting, (3) minimize use of upholstered furniture, (4) vacuum clean using an HEPA filter, (5) use air filters in appropriate rooms, and (6) wash the cat weekly [9]. These measures can reduce, but will not totally eliminate, the quantity of *Fel d* I in the ambient home air.

Home Visits by Health Professionals

Home visits by health professionals provide important information on how to improve the home environment, especially for the asthmatic patient with poorly controlled symptoms. Such patients may not recognize an odor or an unusual source of exposure to allergens or irritants. Patients can also be noncompliant. Physicians, social workers, nurses, and allergy technicians can perform these home observations. Analysis of mite, cat, or cockroach exposure can be done, as previously noted. Although mold plates can be exposed for analysis of environmental molds, their limited role must be appreciated. At the conclusion of a home

visit, adequate time should be spent with the asthmatic and his or her family to explain and reinforce the environmental phases of medical management.

Moving to Another Climate

Moving is often unsuccessful in controlling severe asthmatic disease. Furthermore, an impulsive decision to make such a move can produce financial and psychological hardships that can complicate an already difficult situation. Although Skough [48] has demonstrated that patients with chronic upper airway obstruction benefit by moving from a cold, damp climate or an urban environment, experienced asthma specialists [4, 22, 40] advise against making such impulsive moves. If a move is contemplated, a 4- to 6-week trial period is prudent.

REFERENCES

1. Air purifiers. *Consumer Reports* 54(2):88, 1989.
2. ATS Workshop on Environmental Controls and Lung Disease. *Am. Rev. Respir. Dis.* 142:915, 1990.
3. Arlian, L. G., Bernstein, I. L., and Gallagher, J. S. The prevalence of house dust mites, *Dermatophagoides* spp., and associated environmental conditions in homes in Ohio. *J. Allergy Clin. Immunol.* 69:527, 1982.
4. Buckley, J. M., and Pearlman, D. S. Controlling the Environment. In C. W. Bierman and D. S. Pearlman (eds.), *Allergic Diseases of Infancy, Childhood, and Adolescence* (1st ed.). Philadelphia: Saunders, 1980.
5. Burge, H. Bioaerosols: prevalence and health effects in the indoor environment. *J. Allergy Clin. Immunol.* 86:687, 1990.
6. Burge, H. A., Solomon, W. R., and Muilenberg, M. L. Evaluation of indoor plantings as allergen exposure sources. *J. Allergy Clin. Immunol.* 70:101, 1982.
7. Burr, M. L., St. Leger, A. S., and Neale, E. Anti-mite measures in mite-sensitive adult asthma. *Lancet* 1:333, 1976.
8. *Consumer Reports Buying Guide.* Mount Vernon, NY: Consumers Union of the United States, 1990.
9. deBlay, F., Chapman, M. D., and Platts-Mills, T. A. E. Airborne cat allergen (*Fel d* 1): environmental control with the cat *in situ*. *Am. Rev. Respir. Dis.* 143:1334, 1991.
9a. Ehnept, B., et al. Reducing domestic exposure to dust mite allergen reduces bronchial hyperreactivity in sensitive children with asthma. *J. Allergy Clin. Immunol.* 90:135, 1992.
10. Green, W. F. Abolition of allergens by tannic acid. *Lancet* 2:160, 1984.
10a. Green, W. F., et al. House dust mites and mite allergens in public places. *J. Allergy Clin. Immunol.* 89:1196, 1992.
10b. Hamilton, R. G., et al. House dust aeroallergen measures in clinical practice: A guide to allergen-free home and work environments. *Immunol. Allergy Pract.* 14:96, 1992.
10c. Hayden, M. L., et al. Benzyl benzoate moist powder: Investigations of acarical activity in cultures and reduction of dust mite allergen in carpets. *J. Allergy Clin. Immunol.* 89:536, 1992.
11. Hirsch, D. J., Hirsch, S. R., and Kalbfleisch, J. E. Effect of central air conditioning and meteorologic factors on indoor spore counts. *J. Allergy Clin. Immunol.* 62:22, 1978.
12. Hopkins, H. The can's and cant's of air purifiers. *FDA Consumer* October, 1982, Pp. 5–7.
12a. Household Air Cleaners. *Consumer Reports* 57(October 1992):657–662.
13. International Workshop on Dust Mite Allergens and Asthma—A Worldwide Problem, BAD Kreuznach, West Germany, Sept., 1987. *J. Allergy Clin. Immunol.* 83:416, 1989.
14. Kooistra, J. B., Pasch, R., and Reed, C. E. The effects of air cleaners on hay fever symptoms in air conditioned homes. *J. Allergy Clin. Immunol.* 61:315, 1978.
15. Korsgaard, J. Preventive measures in house-dust allergy. *Am. Rev. Respir. Dis.* 125:80, 1982.
16. Krueger, A. P. Air ion as biologic agents: fact or fancy. *Immunol. Allergy Pract.* 6:129, 1982.
17. Kumar, P., Marier, R., and Leech, S. H. Hypersensitivity pneumonitis due to contamination of a car air conditioner. *N. Engl. J. Med.* 305(25):1531, 1981.
18. Lang, J. D., and Mulla, M. S. Abundance of house dust mites, *Dermatopha-*

goides spp., influenced by environmental conditions in homes in Southern California. *Environ. Entomol.* 6:643, 1977.

19. Lau-Schadendorn, S., et al. Short-term effect of solidified benzyl benzoate on mite-allergen concentrations in house dust. *J. Allergy Clin. Immunol.* 87:41, 1991.

20. Luczynska, C., et al. Airborne concentrations and particle size distribution of allergen derived from domestic cats (*Felis domesticus*). *Am. Rev. Respir. Dis.* 141:361, 1990.

21. Machines to Dry Out the Air. *Consumer Reports* 55(7):479, 1990.

22. Mansmann, H. C. Environmental Controls. In E. Middleton, C. E. Reed, and E. F. Ellis (eds.), *Allergy: Principles and Practice.* St. Louis: Mosby, 1975.

23. Miller, J. D., et al. Effect of tannic acid spray on dust mite antigen in carpets. *J. Allergy Clin. Immunol.* 83(1):262, 1989.

24. Miller, J. D., et al. Effect of tannic acid spray on cat allergen levels in carpets (abstract). *J. Allergy Clin. Immunol.* 85(1):226, 1990.

25. Mitchell, E. A., and Elliott, R. B. Controlled trial of an electrostatic precipitator in childhood asthma. *Lancet* 1:559, 1980.

26. Mosbech, H., Korsgaard, J., and Lind, P. Control of house dust mites by electrical heating blankets. *J. Allergy Clin. Immunol.* 81:706, 1988.

27. Muilenberg, M. L., et al. Particle penetration into the automotive interior. *J. Allergy Clin. Immunol.* 87:581, 1991.

28. Mulla, M. S., et al. Some house dust mite control measures and abundance of *Dermatophagoides* mites in Southern California (Acarina: Pyroglyphidae). *J. Med. Entomol.* 12:5, 1975.

29. Murray, A. B., and Ferguson, A. C. Dust-free bedrooms in the treatment of asthmatic children with house dust allergy: a controlled trial. *Pediatrics* 71:418, 1983.

30. Murray, A. B., and Zuk, P. The seasonal variation in a population of house dust mites in a North America city. *J. Allergy Clin. Immunol.* 64:266, 1979.

31. Nelson, H. S., et al. Recommendations for the use of residential air-cleaning devices in the treatment of allergic respiratory diseases. *J. Allergy Clin. Immunol.* 82:661, 1988.

32. Offerman, F. J., et al. Control of respirable particles and radon progeny with portable air cleaners. Berkeley, California: Lawrence Berkeley Laboratory (LBL-16659), February, 1984.

33. Owen, S., et al. Control of house dust mite antigen in bedding. *Lancet* 335:397, 1990.

34. Platts-Mills, T. A. E. Environmental control of house dust mites—new products: what they are and how to use them. Presented at the 47th Annual Meeting of the American College of Allergy and Immunology, San Francisco, California, Nov. 10, 1990.

34a. Platts-Mills, T. A. E., et al. Dust mite allergens and asthma: Report of a second international workshop. *J. Allergy Clin. Immunol.* 89:1046, 1992.

35. Product Testing Department. A test of small air cleaners. *Rodale's New Shelter* July/Aug., 1982, P. 49.

36. Ransom, J. H., Leonard, J., and Wasserstein, R. L. Acarex test correlates with monoclonal antibody test for dust mites. *J. Allergy Clin. Immunol.* 87:886, 1991.

37. Reisman, R. E., et al. A double-blind study of the effectiveness of a high-efficiency particulate air (HEPA) filter in the treatment of patients with perennial allergic rhinitis and asthma. *J. Allergy Clin. Immunol.* 85:1050, 1990.

38. Richards, W. R. Effects of air pollution on asthma. *Ann. Allergy* 65:345, 1990.

39. Rodriguez, G. E., Branch, B. L., and Cotton, E. K. The use of humidity in asthmatic children. *J. Allergy Clin. Immunol.* 56(2):133, 1975.

40. Rosen, F. L., and Green, A. R. An Updated Assessment of the Critical Environmental Factors Involved in the Prevention of Allergic Disease. In C. W. Bierman and K. F. MacDonnell (eds.), *Differential Diagnosis and Treatment of Pediatric Allergy.* Boston: Little, Brown, 1981.

41. Sacca, J. D. Possible hazard with use of fiberglass air filters. *Ann. Allergy.* 34:105, 1975.

42. Salvaggio, J., and Aukrust, L. Mold-induced asthma. *J. Allergy Clin. Immunol.* 68:327, 1981.

43. Samet, J. M., Marbury, M. C., and Spengler, J. D. Health effects and sources of indoor air pollution. *Am. Rev. Respir. Dis.* 136:1486, 1987.

44. Sarsfield, J. K., et al. Mite-sensitive asthma of childhood: trial of avoidance measures. *Arch. Dis. Child.* 49:716, 1974.

45. Scherr, J. S., and Peck, L. W. The effect of high efficiency air filtration system on nighttime asthma attacks. *W. Virginia Med. J.* 73:144, 1977.

46. Sesay, J. R., and Dobson, R. J. Studies on the mite fauna of house dust in Scotland with special reference to that of bedding. *Acarologia* 14:384, 1972.

47. Shamie, S., et al. The consistent presence of cat allergen (Fel d-I) in various types of public places (abstract). *J. Allergy Clin. Immunol.* 85:226, 1990.

48. Skough, B. E. Climate and environmental change in patients with chronic airway obstruction. *Arch. Environ. Health* 31:11, 1976.

49. Slavin, R. G., et al. Guidelines for asthmatic patients during air pollution episodes. *J. Allergy Clin. Immunol.* 55:222, 1975.

50. Solomon, W. R. Fungus aerosols arising from cold mist vaporizers. *J. Allergy Clin. Immunol.* 54:222, 1974.

51. Solomon, W. R. Assessing fungus prevalence in domestic interiors. *J. Allergy Clin. Immunol.* 56:235, 1975.

52. Solomon, W. R., Burge, H. A., and Boise, J. R. Exclusion of particulate allergens by window air conditioners. *J. Allergy Clin. Immunol.* 65:305, 1980.

53. Spiegelman, J., and Friedman, H. The effect of central air filtration and air conditioning on pollen and microbial contamination. *J. Allergy* 42:193, 1968.

54. Sporik, R., et al. Exposure to house-dust mite allergen (Der pI) and the development of asthma in childhood. *N. Engl. J. Med.* 323:502, 1990.

55. Tovey, E. R., et al. The distribution of dust mite allergen in the houses of patients with asthma. *Am. Rev. Respir. Dis.* 124:630, 1981.

56. United States Department of Transportation—Federal Highway Administration. Highway Statistics, 1988. Washington, D.C.: U.S. Government Printing Office, 1990, P. 172.

57. Van der Brempt, X., et al. Comparison of the Acarex test with monoclonal antibodies for the quantification of mite allergens. *J. Allergy Clin. Immunol.* 87:130, 1991.

58. Villaveces, J. W., Rosengren, H., and Evans, J. Use of laminar air flow portable filters in asthmatic children. *Ann. Allergy* 38:400, 1977.

59. Walshaw, M. J., and Evans, C. C. Allergen avoidance in house dust mite–sensitive adult asthma. *Q. J. Med.* 58:199, 1986.

59a. Wolf, S. I. Suffocating odor and asthma after Acarosan-powder carpet treatment. *J. Allergy Clin. Immunol.* 89:637, 1992.

59b. Wood, R. A., Mudd, K. E., and Eggleston, P. A. The distribution of cat and dust mite allergens on wall surfaces. *J. Allergy Clin. Immunol.* 89:126, 1992.

60. Wood, R. A., et al. The effect of cat removal on allergen content in household dust samples. *J. Allergy Clin. Immunol.* 83:730, 1989.

61. Zwemer, R. J., and Karibo, J. Use of laminar control devices as adjunct to standard environmental control measures in symptomatic asthmatic children. *Ann. Allergy* 31:284, 1973.

Inappropriate and Unusual Remedies

88

Irwin Ziment
Myron Stein

HISTORIC BACKGROUND

The reader is referred to the comprehensive presentation by Rosenblatt [60] for an historical perspective on asthma. Rosner [61] has pointed out that earlier physicians may have been relating to a completely different condition when they diagnosed asthma, and it is evident that the disease was not clearly distinguished from bronchitis until the nineteenth century [87]. Many of the historic therapies for asthma were directed at treating the accumulation of phlegm, which was perceived as the fundamental abnormality in most pulmonary disorders. Arguments based on various philosophic concepts of disorders of phlegm led to individualistic justifications for the numerous unproved and often bizarre therapies that were introduced. Thus, there is ample historic precedent for a discussion of inappropriate and unusual therapies of asthma [84].

In the twelfth century, in his "Treatise on Asthma," Maimonides recommended that lettuce, pumpkin, cauliflower, turnip, black beans, peas, garlic, watermelon, peaches, apricots, cucumbers, and sexual intercourse be avoided by the asthmatic. He did endorse as appropriate therapy chicken soup, fresh water fish, fennel, parsley, organum, mint, and radish [61], but it is noteworthy that, although Maimonides showed great holistic and psychological insights, his pharmacologic approaches were rooted in the absurdities of traditional galenic therapy. It is also of considerable interest that most of Maimonides' herbal recommendations were also considered by his contemporaries to be effective as aphrodisiacs [15]. The antiasthma benefits of the medications of today that are based on ancient folk remedies are not always more convincingly demonstrable than are their aphrodisiacal properties.

FOLK REMEDIES

It is interesting to see how many of our current drugs for the treatment of asthma and bronchitis are direct descendants of the traditional folk remedies used in different regions of the world [85] (Table 88-1). Ephedrine is found in Ma Huang, the long-used extract of the Chinese ephedra bush. Atropinic drugs were first used by ancient physicians of India, who burned d'hatura (*Datura stramonium*) to release anticholinergic fumes. Cromolyn is related to khella, an Egyptian antispasmodic agent derived from *Ammi visnaga*. Theophylline comes from tea leaves, and its cousin caffeine, in the form of strong coffee, was one of the most popular asthma drugs of the nineteenth century. Steroids were obtained from such sources as placenta or the urine of pubescent children, or from adrenal gland extracts. Another favorite drug of the nineteenth century was saltpeter (potassium nitrate), which liberated bronchodilator fumes when burned. Many folk remedies are still used today, particularly in Asia, and some may have

the potential for providing more potent derivatives that could offer useful therapy. One enduring folk remedy, marijuana, has been shown to have a definite bronchodilator effect [73], although its irritating smoke may cause bronchitis.

Oriental Folk Remedies

Ancient Chinese drugs remain popular in many oriental communities, and they may appeal to some Westerners. Popular antiasthma agents besides Ma Huang include ginkgo, ardisia, fritillary, kikia root tree, peony, rhododendron, bupleurum (hare's ear), and cinnamon [88]. Many of these are made available in traditional mixtures, with names such as Minor Blue Dragon Combination, or they may be combined in pills such as the Ge Jie Anti-Asthma Pill. The traditional Chinese plant *Ginkgo biloba* is the source of ginkgolides that have been shown to inhibit platelet-activating factor (PAF) [6]; however, its value as an antiasthma drug has not been established in clinical practice, and it is doubtful if it or any of the other popular Chinese plant agents will supplant current drugs.

In India, no traditional Ayurvedic or Unani drug appears to be as effective as d'hatura, although sweetflag, some euphorbias, and *Tylophora asthmatica* (Indian ipecac) may possess antiasthma properties [84, 85, 88]. Numerous additional agents are used throughout Asia, but it appears that none offers uniquely valuable benefits, and thus these agents will fail to be used except in the ethnic societies in which each respective plant derivative has been long established. It is probable that most traditional antiasthma remedies have properties similar to *Tylophora*, in that they have a subemetic action and thus serve as nonspecific expectorants and mucokinetics (see Chap. 69).

Western Folk Remedies

Enormous numbers of antiasthma agents are listed by current writers on herbal medicine. Many of these nostrums first became popular prior to the golden era of Greek medicine, but their persistence in no way relates to their effectiveness. Thus, horehound, hyssop, mullein, and lungwort probably act in similar fashion to ipecac, serving as nonspecific emetic–expectorants [85]. The continuing popularity of coltsfoot (*Tussilago farfara*) as an antitussive and antiasthmatic agent does not appear to be justified clinically, although it has recently been shown that this plant also possesses derivatives with anti-PAF properties [6]. Spices, including onion, garlic, and radish, are of value as mucokinetic agents (Chap. 69); recent studies suggest that some possess antiallergy properties [20]. However, as is the case with most oriental remedies, the hundreds of western plant derivatives for which anecdotal claims are made must be assumed to offer no significant antiasthma effects. Indeed, one should be suspicious of allegedly "potent" unorthodox alternative plant remedies that

Table 88-1. Emergence of major antiasthma drugs

Time	Drug
3000 B.C.–200 A.D.	Ephedrine (China, Greece)
	Atropinic drugs (Middle East, India)
	Chromones (Middle East)
200–1000	Arsenic smoke (introduced in Arabic medicine)
1000–1650	No significant advances
1650 (approx.)	Ipecacuanha (introduced from Brazil into Europe)
1786	Strong coffee (Withering, England)
1802	Stramonium cigarettes (Sims, England)
1840 (approx.)	Iodide (used by Laennec, then Osler, and others)
1840 (approx.)	Potassium nitrate (used in cigarettes in Europe)
1850 (approx.)	Chloroform inhalation (used in Europe)
1900	Adrenaline (recommended, for oral administration by Solis-Cohen, U.S.)
1920	Theophylline (isolated by Kossel in Germany in 1888; used rectally and later intravenously, then orally for asthma)
1924	Ephedrine (introduced by Chen and Schmidt, U.S.)
1940	Isoproterenol (introduced in Germany)
1948	Corticosteroids (introduced in U.S.)
1950	Isoetharine (introduced in U.S.)
1961	Metaproterenol (introduced in Germany)
1967	Fenoterol (introduced in Germany)
1968	Albuterol (introduced in England)
1968	Cromolyn (introduced in England)
1969	Terbutaline (introduced in Sweden)
1972	Beclomethasone (introduced in England)
1974	Ipratropium (introduced in Germany)
1990	Salmeterol (introduced in England)

Table 88-2. Therapy of asthma recommended by Osler in 1895

Few whiffs of chloroform (or in hot whiskey)
Inhalation of amyl nitrate
Injection of morphine/cocaine
Belladonna, henbane, stramonium, lobelia—in solution or as cigarettes
Burning potassium nitrate paper
Potassium iodide solutions
Oxygen

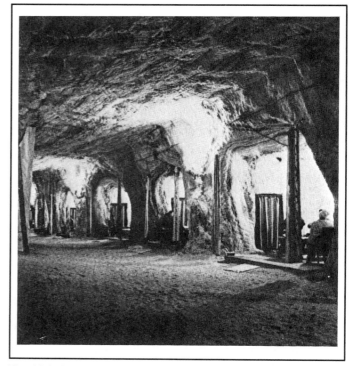

Fig. 88-1. *Salt mine located 200 meters underground in which asthma patients are treated. (Reprinted with permission from C. Holden, Health care in the Soviet Union.* Science *213:1091, 1981. Copyright 1981 by the AAAS.)*

come from other countries, since some simply depend on large amounts of glucocorticosteroids sequestered among the touted herbal components.

HEALTHFUL CLIMATES AND SPAS

In the nineteenth and the earlier part of the twentieth centuries, the therapeutic values of different climates were given serious attention. Thus, the allegedly healthful effects of Saranac Lake helped establish the sanatorium movement for the treatment of tuberculosis in the United States, and places such as Denver and the southwest desert became magnets for asthmatics, as did the European Alps and the French and Italian Riviera.

Many asthmatic patients claim that city air (such as that of smoggy Los Angeles) causes a worsening of their symptoms, and it is a common belief that bracing mountain air or soothing warm beaches offer a salubrious effect. In previous centuries, physicians would advise a sea journey or a sojourn in a balmy winter resort as the perfect treatment for asthma or bronchitis. However, some experts believed the opposite; thus, Henry Salter [62], the most famous writer on asthma in the nineteenth century, recommended smoky city air as being beneficial for some asthmatics! Similarly, many experts, including Osler, Trousseau, and Laennec, advocated the smoking of tobacco products to treat asthma.

The therapeutic approach to asthma recommended by Osler [54] in 1895 is listed in Table 88-2. While the inhalation of smoke from burning powders or cigarettes has been effectively used for many centuries in asthma therapy, this may be associated with harmful accumulations of carbon monoxide, nitrogen oxides, or other irritants. Nevertheless, the possible therapeutic value of anticholinergic smoke from *Datura* cigarettes has been demonstrated [12]. Although certain odors—such as paint, perfumes, and fried foods—are recognized as being aggravating factors in asthma, other olfactory stimulants—such as sea air, menthol, eucalyptus, tar, chloroform, and sniffing the coat of a chihuahua dog—have been reported as being beneficial.

In many countries, a remarkably vibrant health industry exists in certain towns that have long offered spa therapy [19, 87]. Usually these resort areas are endowed with the advantages of good climate, scenic beauty, and pleasurable ambience, while the spas themselves provide mineral baths, medicated vapors, and inhalant aerosols to treat respiratory disorders. Obviously it is difficult to discern the potential benefit of any single component of the healthful package offered by a spa, particularly if the whole therapeutic experience is underwritten by the patient's health insurance policy.

An unusual environmental treatment for asthma is offered in the salt mines of some Eastern European countries (Fig. 88-1). One may assume that cold, dry salt mine air is allergen free and that this will benefit a highly allergic asthmatic patient. However, convincing data indicating the appropriateness or inappropriateness of either salt mine or more conventional spa therapy are lacking in the Western literature. Currently there is no scientific evidence to suggest that any climate or city or geographic area offers particular advantages for patients with asthma, although claims have been made that the absence of the house mite in high mountainous regions may be helpful for allergic patients [13].

It is appropriate to suggest that patients with asthma should not disrupt their lives to seek a new ideal climate or locale, but, if there are compelling reasons to move, a nonpolluted area with few pollens and a relatively constant temperature plus moderate humidity should be selected. However, for obvious reasons, such places are liable to have the disadvantages of being expensive and crowded with victims of chronic pulmonary disease. Initially, patients should reduce their exposure to allergens in their own home, though environmental controls can be carried to extreme measures, thus creating virtually impossible conditions for the patient, the family, and their pets.

DIET

Dietary supplements and, in contrast, elimination diets have often been advocated for the treatment of asthma. Occasionally a true allergy to a food exists and the elimination of such food products, or additives such as sulfites, is important. The addition of vitamins may appear to help patients who invest faith as well as finance in these panaceas; there is some evidence that vitamin C has mild bronchodilator properties [76]. However, many other agents such as fish oil have failed to demonstrate any value [3]. Spices, through their mucus-loosening action, may help [85, 88], and offer a good substitute for salt. A recent theory has been proposed that excess salt in the diet may increase airway hyperresponsiveness in asthma [32], thus providing further reasons for the concerned patient to avoid using too much of this flavoring agent. There is no doubt that coffee may be very helpful in alleviating asthma [7], but alcohol can either provoke or relieve bronchospasm in susceptible patients [4].

OLD DRUGS WITH NEW APPLICATIONS

Several drugs have been periodically described as effective in the treatment of asthma, and usually they fail to attain acceptance; nevertheless, some of these drugs maintain a sub-rosa reputation. Periodically sedatives, cocaine, morphine, and other respiratory depressants are recommended [79]; however, these drugs not only have dangerous side effects, but some may also induce asthma. Antibiotics have been used, both with and without steroids. In particular, troleandomycin (TAO) has been used to reduce steroid dependency; erythromycin may have a similar value. Both agents have recently been reported to be of value in some asthmatics in the absence of steroids [46, 59]. The recognition that *Chlamydia pneumoniae* infection may provoke asthma in adults [29] provides a rationale for using erythromycin or a tetracycline when an "upper respiratory infection" causes bronchospasm. Helium may help relieve severe airway obstruction, and can be useful in life-threatening status asthmaticus [25]. Clonidine taken by inhalation has been reported to relieve asthma [40]. Some representative drugs are listed in Table 88-3, but their possible value is usually based on single unsubstantiated reports [84, 86]. Particular interest in recent years has been accorded to methotrexate, magnesium sulfate, and diuretics, although there is inconclusive data to determine if they will find a meaningful role in asthma therapy.

Methotrexate

Methotrexate was recommended by Mullarkey and coworkers [47, 48], but the initial report was not very convincing. These authors studied 14 patients with asthma who appeared to be dependent on chronic oral steroid therapy [48]. During three

Table 88-3. Unconventional drugs for asthma

Category	Agent
Immunosuppressive agents	Gold (chrysotherapy)
	Methotrexate
	Nitrogen mustard
Nonsteroidal antiinflammatory agents	Aspirin
	Indomethacin
	Levomepromazine
Antimediators	Anti-PAF agents (e.g., ginkgolides, coltsfoot)
	Fish oil
Antispasm agents	Khellin
	Calcium channel blockers
	Magnesium sulfate
	Nitrites
	Dihydroergotoxine
	Phenytoin
Centrally acting agents	Clonidine
	Alcohol
	Marijuana
	Antidepressants
	Sedatives
	General anesthetics
	Ether enemas
Hormones	Progesterone
	Glucagon
	Adrenocorticotropic hormone (ACTH)
	Pituitary extract
Beta₂-adrenergic antagonists	Prazosin
	Methoxamine
Diuretics	Furosemide
	Chlorothiazide
Vitamins	Ascorbic acid
Local anesthetics	Lidocaine
Narcotics	Cocaine
	Morphine
Antibiotics	Triacetyloleandomycin (TAO)
	Erythromycin

PAF = platalet-activating factor.

months of low-dose weekly methotrexate treatment, 13 of the patients were able to reduce their steroid dosage significantly more than was possible when taking placebo. However, the average reduction was 36.5 percent, which is not dramatic enough to make methotrexate a worthwhile agent for most patients who require oral steroids. This result is similar to what may be achieved with TAO, which has a comparable steroid-sparing effect in some patients [67]; however, most experts find that TAO is of limited value in practice, and the same conclusion will probably be applied to methotrexate (Chap. 67).

Magnesium Sulfate

Magnesium sulfate has been repeatedly advocated for the treatment of persistent status asthmaticus, and this drug has recently been resurrected [50]. It is recommended for infusion at the rate of 0.615 mmol/min for 20 minutes. It is believed to have a similar action to that of the calcium channel blockers [45]; however, these latter drugs are of little value in most forms of asthma, although they may be of some benefit in exercise-induced bronchospasm [2]. Thus, it is unlikely that magnesium sulfate will find a significant role in asthma therapy.

Diuretics

Diuretics have long been used to treat cardiac asthma, and occasionally it has been suggested that agents such as chlorothiazide are useful for bronchial asthma [52]. In recent years, great interest has been aroused by the finding that inhaled furosemide can protect against allergen-induced asthmatic reactions and exercise-induced bronchoconstriction, though the exact mechanism remains elusive [9]. It is relevant that inhalation of the diuretic amiloride may improve the quality of mucus in patients with cystic fibrosis, probably by increasing the chloride flux and the amount of water crossing the respiratory epithelium into the luminal mucus [37].

HORMONES

Hormonal extracts from glands have long been used in asthma; early reports suggested that adrenocortical extracts were not beneficial [77] and this did not augur well for corticosteroids, which nevertheless proved to be spectacularly valuable soon after their introduction for the treatment of rheumatoid arthritis. Other adrenocortical and pituitary hormones, including ACTH, have occasionally been recommended for asthma, but have never been generally accepted [83]. Progesterone has gained attention for its value in premenstrual tension, and asthma associated with menstruation may respond to this hormone [8, 22]. Glucagon is another hormone that has been reported to have a bronchodilator action [66]. Epinephrine, which was originally called *adrenaline* to emphasize its origin from the adrenal gland, took many years to become established in the treatment of asthma. Although it has been largely eclipsed by more modern beta-adrenergic aerosols, it maintains an anomalous niche as an over-the-counter aerosol and it appears to be both effective and safe in the management of minor asthma.

IMMUNOTHERAPY

Many allergists believe that highly allergic patients with severe asthma can be helped by injections of standard hyposensitization products of the "guilty" antigens. The exact mechanisms by which immunotherapy works (especially in allergic rhinitis, where it may be very effective) are complex, and include the production of antigen-specific, IgG-blocking antibody, suppression of specific IgE antibody, and decreased mediator release [10]. Extracts of house mites and other insect proteins, animal danders, fungi, and pollens are used most frequently. In Europe, commercial vaccines against bacteria are used in patients with asthma associated with bronchitis. Occasionally other vaccines are still used by unscientific practitioners, including injections with the patient's blood (autohemotherapy), convalescent serum [79], or urine (urotherapy) [53]. More exuberant approaches have included splenic irradiation to remove a potential triggering organ that decreases the immune response [28] and the injection of an extract of thymus called *thymomodulin* to enhance this response [5]. Other forms of unorthodox treatment of allergic asthma include little-known techniques such as enzyme-potentiated transepidermal desensitization (using beta-glucuronidase), treatment of the "dysbiosis" caused by sensitivity to *Candida albicans*, sublingual neutralization, and more bizarre methods that merge into quackery [16]. Plasmapheresis has been used [24], but its value has not been confirmed. Similarly, gold therapy (chrysotherapy) is occasionally recommended [35], but it is still an unestablished modality.

PSYCHOLOGICAL TECHNIQUES

In a significant proportion of patients, asthma can improve when psychological stress is alleviated or when psychoactive therapy is provided that is designed to enable patients to control panic

[27]. Success has been claimed for hypnotherapy [23], verbal desensitization [64], behavior modification [81], and other related lay modalities. Formal psychotherapy is only recommended if indicated for the patient who has a psychological disturbance that is independent of the asthma. Asthmatic patients with depression or anxiety may improve in all respects when given antidepressants [80]. In some patients, reassurance and confidence building will help them feel that they can be in control and thereby reduce the liability for exacerbations of their asthma, or will teach them to keep calm and breathe normally when hyperventilation due to anxiety exacerbates the sense of dyspnea [17].

Transcendental meditation [30], biofeedback training [31], yoga [49, 71], and other techniques can be useful and may be practiced under supervision in rehabilitation programs. Oriental exercises such as tai chi and quigong also have their adherents.

Psychotherapy, breathing exercises, and special techniques may be used inappropriately in the asthmatic. Psychotherapy may add great expense in the hope of providing a cure when simple drug therapy may suffice. On the other hand, failure to consider psychological problems may prolong the intensity and increase the expense of treating the condition. Breathing exercises, which were formerly more popular, may aggravate the asthmatic condition, if used without appropriate drug therapy. Asthma camps and special schools must guarantee expert organization, supervision, and the routine provision of appropriate therapy, if they are to be effective.

SURGICAL AND ANESTHESIOLOGIC APPROACHES

Some patients who wheeze out of proportion to their dyspnea and who fail to show a marked obstructive pattern on pulmonary function testing have vocal cord dysfunction [26] or laryngeal dyskinesia [55]. Such patients were formerly labeled as having "hysterical croup." It is noteworthy that individuals with a nervous cough or habitual throat clearing may have underlying asthma, and their symptoms may abate with bronchodilator therapy. It may help to perform a methacholine challenge test so as to evaluate the underlying tendency to bronchospasm in individuals with variant asthma or unusual coughing or wheezing. Gastroesophageal reflux may provoke bronchospasm, and this possibility needs to be kept in mind [11]. In many cases, it is necessary to exclude an organic abnormality, such as a tumor or foreign body, by means of computerized tomography or endoscopy. In those cases in which aspiration or laryngeal dysfunction may be a cause of asthma, corrective measures, which may include surgery, should be helpful [26, 68].

Specialized oriental techniques occasionally are rediscovered and become fashionable: acupuncture is currently one such favored modality. Although Chinese physicians extol several loci for needling, such as the *fei yu* position adjacent to the third dorsal vertebra [84], controlled studies have failed to demonstrate the benefit of acupuncture [36, 72, 75]. Moxibustion is a variant practice that appears to offer no benefit. Organ vagotonia is a special complex of techniques that has a following in Japan [70]; the nearest equivalent in the West may be bilateral carotid body resection (CBR). This surgical technique has a limited number of adherents, and, although it may help provide a sense of symptomatic benefit [69], the patient who undergoes CBR is liable to experience severe hypoxia that could be fatal. However, as a palliative method in patients with nonresponsive asthma and chronic obstructive pulmonary disease (COPD), bilateral CBR has been described as possibly useful [65, 82].

Other unconventional surgical techniques, such as vagal ablation, have faded into oblivion [21], as have procedures such as irradiation or removal of the spleen or thymus [79]. The excision

Table 88-4. Unconventional therapies for asthma

Category	Therapy
Behavioral	Behavior modification
	Verbal desensitization
	Biofeedback, panic control, hypnosis
	Dancing, tai chi, gentle exercise (e.g., swimming)
	Yoga, chanting, breathing exercises
	Transcendental meditation, relaxation
	Psychotherapy (individual, family, group)
	Chiropractic, homeopathy, ayurveda
	Religion, cults, faith healing
	Speech therapy
Environmental	Mountains, seashore, desert
	Spas, cold washes, baths, aromatic inhalants
	Dust-free rooms, air conditioning, salt mines
	Electrostatic precipitators, filters, ionizers
	Inhalation of carbon dioxide, helium-oxygen
Diet	Elimination (dyes, sulfites, histamine, specific allergens such as nuts and fish)
	Herbs, spices, minerals, megavitamins, pseudovitamins (e.g., pangamic acid)
	Teas, coffee, alcohol
Immunotherapy	Desensitization to blood or urine
	Injections of gamma globulin, convalescent serum
	Urotherapy
	Splenic or tonsil irradiation, plasmapheresis
	Applied kinesiology, radionics
	Anti-*Candida* therapy
	Sublingual neutralization drops
	Vaccines of bacterial lysate (e.g., Broncho-Vaxom)
	Organ vagotonia
Surgical, etc.	Bilateral carotid body resection (glomectomy)
	Vagotomy, injection of atropine into vagus nerve
	Removal of "trigger" organ, e.g., infected teeth or bowel
	Radical sinus, polyp, or nose surgery
	Correction of gastroesophageal reflux
	Cricopharyngeal myotomy
	Glossopharyngealotomy
	Bronchoscopic lavage, instillation of iodized oil
	Acupuncture, moxibustion, shiatsu, massage

of teeth, tonsils, adenoids, hemorrhoids, colon, and other "trigger" organs has undoubtedly benefited the surgeons who advocate such approaches far more than the patients who underwent the procedure. Currently, only nasal polyp and sinus surgery or sinus lavage can be considered as generally accepted surgical approaches in selected patients in whom a sinobronchial relationship appears to explain the presence of asthma [1] (Chap. 41). Therapeutic bronchial lavage is also of value in some asthmatic patients with mucus inspissation in the lower airways [18].

Less radical than surgery are some anesthesiologic approaches. General anesthesia with agents such as halothane [83] or isoflurane [33] has virtually, but not entirely, replaced ether [58]. Local anesthesia of the larynx using xylocaine or its nebulization into the lungs prevents bronchospasm during bronchoscopy, and may be worthy of consideration in other forms of asthma [42, 43]. Nonsteroidal analgesics are rarely thought of as being beneficial in asthma, since aspirin can cause severe bronchospasm. However, occasional reports suggest that these agents can relieve asthma in some patients [38, 51].

Some of the unconventional approaches to asthma therapy are listed in Table 88-4; this complements the drugs listed in Table 88-3.

INAPPROPRIATE USES OF APPROPRIATE THERAPY

Asthma patients sometime make inappropriate use of appropriate therapy. The sudden increase in asthmatic deaths in the United Kingdom in the late 1950s has been attributed to the over-utilization of a readily available form of high-dosage isoproterenol aerosol (see Chap. 2). More recently, the potent, long-acting, relatively nonselective agent fenoterol has been incriminated as a factor in unexpected deaths occurring in asthmatics in New Zealand, and in causing destabilization of asthma in patients living in both New Zealand and Canada [51]. There are also concerns that the regular (as opposed to as-needed) use of beta$_2$ adrenergics by inhalation may destabilize asthma [63, 78]. However, these concerns should not be allowed to offset the many years of experience that have demonstrated the value and safety of these essential drugs. Danger exists from the underuse, overuse, and misuse of both prescription and nonprescription drugs. The reader is referred to the specific chapters on beta-adrenergic aerosols, theophylline, corticosteroids, and so on, to evaluate the benefits gained from the proper use of drug therapy in asthma.

It is well recognized that many patients do not use their metered-dose inhalers (MDIs) properly; sometimes they receive no or poor instruction from their physicians. Patients have failed to remove the cap of the MDI, thus receiving no explicable benefit from their medication, or, of greater concern, some have suffered subsequent aspiration of the inhaler cap. Patients have also inhaled coins or other foreign material stored in an uncapped inhaler. These events have prompted some manufacturers to alter the design of and the instructions for using MDIs. The inappropriate utilization of any beta$_2$-adrenergic drug, theophylline, or corticosteroid is fraught with complications, increased morbidity, and possibly death. Oral beta$_2$-adrenergic agents may require 1 to 2 hours for bronchodilator effects to take place and may not be suitable for rapid relief in an acute attack of asthma. Delays in therapy may result in progression and intractability of the asthmatic episode. Inappropriate therapy with morphine and other sedatives in the asthmatic has already been described. Antihistamines to block H$_1$ receptors may be ineffective in most asthmatic patients. The newer agents may offer benefits [14, 44, 56]; both terfenadine [57] and azelastine [41] have been reported to be useful. Ketotifen is popular in many countries, although its value is controversial and its sedating effect is a major disadvantage [41]. The role of H$_2$ blockers for therapy in asthma is not established, but the blockade of H$_2$ receptors may be dangerous in some asthmatics [74]. Combined preparations of ephedrine, theophylline, and sedatives may produce inadequate levels of theophylline and unwanted effects from ephedrine and sedation. Rapidly released or erratically released and incompletely absorbed preparations of theophylline may be associated with great daily fluctuations in serum levels, ranging from toxic to subtherapeutic; the problem can be exacerbated by "dose-dumping" when some of the sustained-release products are taken with food [34].

Other aspects of inappropriate therapy relate to failure to use blood gas studies, when indicated, to guide therapeutic measures. Staging of the severity of asthma and the application of therapeutic programs based on spirometric changes and blood gas values are described in Chapter 54. Failure to properly assess the asthmatic patient may lead to dangerous complications and death.

INAPPROPRIATE THERAPY RELATED TO INAPPROPRIATE DIAGNOSES

A number of conditions may mimic or complicate asthma (see Chap. 37). The treatment of presumed asthma without appropriate diagnosis may allow morbid progression of the actual underlying condition. Conditions sometimes confused with asthma include pneumothorax, pneumonitis, myocardial infarction, heart failure, collagen vascular diseases, COPD, and organic airways obstruction. There have been descriptions of patients with laryn-

Table 88-5. Inappropriate management of asthma contributing to relapse or complications

Failure to ensure that bronchodilator aerosol is effectively used

Failure to evaluate asthma properly

Failure to stage and treat asthma (e.g., level of care—ambulatory versus hospitalization versus intensive care)

Failure to monitor pulmonary function objectively

Overutilization of adrenergic aerosols in the absence of accompanying treatment with steroids or cromolyn

Failure to utilize theophylline appropriately

Under-, over-, and misutilization of corticosteroids

Reliance on unproven drugs and other forms of therapy

Premature withdrawal of therapy (e.g., therapy based on symptoms or physical examination findings only)

Overcomplication of regimen, resulting in poor compliance

Overtreatment, resulting in excessive dependency on drugs or on prophylactic measures

geal dysfunction who have received intensive therapy for asthma, including corticosteroids, whereas their management should have included speech therapy, psychotherapy, or antidepressants, after appropriate analysis of pulmonary function [55]. Some of the more common errors in patient management are listed in Table 88-5.

GEOGRAPHIC VARIATIONS IN ASTHMA THERAPY

Asthma therapy may vary in different regions, depending on the availability of drugs or specific preparations (e.g., albuterol available in multiple forms—intravenous, subcutaneous, oral, and aerosol—in the United Kingdom versus aerosol and oral only in the United States). However, physicians who treat asthma in other countries indicate that most of the newer beta$_2$-adrenergic agents available to them offer little advantage in terms of onset, peak effect, and duration of action when compared with terbutaline, metaproterenol, or albuterol, although possibly the prolonged action of salmeterol and formoterol may be a valuable advance. Special preparations of herbs or traditional medications continue to be popular in oriental countries and some western ethnic communities; patients who are partial to such therapy may feel that these remedies are more effective than conventional allopathic drugs. Similarly, patients in many countries may prefer homeopathic, chiropractic, osteopathic, naturopathic, and other forms of treatment for milder asthmatic conditions [39].

Over the centuries, numerous forms of therapy for asthmatics have been presented, only to be discarded due to poor or harmful results. The modern era has produced new agents with improved therapeutic effects. Furthermore, older drugs can now be monitored more precisely to maximize benefits and minimize risks (e.g., theophylline). Nevertheless, currently available drug therapies for asthma may be utilized improperly or inappropriately. Some asthmatic patients seek alternative forms of therapy, signaling their dissatisfaction with current remedies. However, alternative and complementary medical systems have recently been thoughtfully reviewed [39], with the conclusion that they have no place in the vast majority of cases of acute, severe asthma, although some patients with persistent asthma could benefit. It is hoped that new approaches to asthma, based on an understanding of the biochemical mechanisms in asthma and described elsewhere in this volume, will bring this condition, at times so difficult to treat, under improved control.

REFERENCES

1. Adinoff, A. D., and Cummings, N. P. Sinusitis and its relationship to asthma. *Am. J. Asthma Allergy Pediatr.* 1:3, 1988.

2. Ahmed, T., D'Brot, J., and Abraham, W. The role of calcium antagonists in bronchial reactivity. *J. Allergy Clin. Immunol.* 81:133, 1988.

3. Arm, J. P., et al. Effect of dietary supplements with fish oil lipids on mild asthma. *Thorax* 43:84, 1988.

4. Ayres, J. G., and Clark, T. J. H. Alcoholic drinks and asthma: a survey. *Br. J. Dis. Chest* 77:370, 1983.

5. Bagnato, A., et al. Long-term treatment with thymomodulin reduces airway hyperresponsiveness to methacholine. *Ann. Allergy* 62:425, 1989.

6. Barnes, P. J., Chung, K. F., and Page, C. P. Platelet-activating factor as a mediator of allergic disease. *J. Allergy Clin. Immunol.* 81:919, 1988.

7. Becker, A. B., et al. The bronchodilator effects and pharmacokinetics of caffeine in asthma. *N. Engl. J. Med.* 310:743, 1984.

8. Beynon, H. L. C., Garbett, N. D., and Barnes, P. J. Severe premenstrual exacerbations of asthma: effect of intramuscular progesterone. *Lancet* 2: 370, 1988.

9. Bianco, S., et al. Protective effect of inhaled furosemide on allergen-induced early and late asthmatic reactions. *N. Engl. J. Med.* 321:1069, 1989.

10. Bush, R. K. Immunotherapy for the treatment of allergic diseases: clinical applications reviewed. *Hosp. Formul.* 23:245, 1989.

11. Castell, D. O. Asthma and gastroesophageal reflux. *Chest* 96:2, 1989.

12. Charpin, D., Orehek, J., and Velardocchio, J. M. Bronchodilator effects of antiasthmatic cigarette smoke (*Datura stramonium*). *Thorax* 34:259, 1979.

13. Charpin, D., et al. Asthma and allergy to house-dust mites in populations living at high altitudes. *Chest* 93:758, 1988.

14. Collins-Williams, C. Antihistamines in asthma. *J. Asthma* 24:55, 1987.

15. Cosman, M. P. A feast for Aesculapius: historical diets for asthma and sexual pleasure. *Annu. Rev. Nutr.* 3:1, 1983.

16. David, T. J. Unorthodox diagnosis and treatment of asthma. *Am. J. Asthma Allergy Pediatr.* 2:71, 1989.

17. Demeter, S. L., and Cordasco, E. M. Hyperventilation syndrome and asthma. *Am. J. Med.* 81:989, 1986.

18. Dietrich, K. A., et al. Therapeutic bronchial lavage in severe asthma. *Ann. Allergy* 63:382, 1989.

19. Dobell, H. *On Winter Cough, Catarrh, Bronchitis, Emphysema, Asthma.* London: J. & A. Churchill, 1875.

20. Dorsch, W., et al. Antiasthmatic effects of onion extracts—detection of benzyl—and other isothiocyanates (mustard oils) as antiasthmatic compounds of plant origin. *Eur. J. Pharmacol.* 107:17, 1984.

21. Dos, S. J., Jacobson, M. J., and Soroff, H. S. The role of surgery in the management of chronic bronchial asthma. In E. B. Weiss and M. S. Segal (eds.), *Bronchial Asthma: Mechanisms and Therapeutics.* Boston: Little, Brown, 1976, P. 1007.

22. Editorial. Asthma, progesterone and pregnancy. *Lancet* 335:204, 1990.

23. Ewer, T. C., and Stewart, D. E. Improvement in bronchial hyper-responsiveness in patients with moderate asthma after treatment with a hypnotic technique: a randomized controlled trial. *Br. Med. J.* 293:1129, 1986.

24. Gartmann, J., Grob, P., and Frey, M. Plasmapheresis in severe asthma. *Lancet* 2:40, 1978.

25. Gluck, E. H., Onorato, D. J., and Castriotta, R. Helium-oxygen mixture in intubated patients with status asthmaticus and respiratory acidosis. *Chest* 98:693, 1990.

26. Goldman, J., and Muers, M. Vocal cord dysfunction and wheezing. *Thorax* 64:401, 1991.

27. Gorman, J. M. Psychobiological aspects of asthma and the consequent research implications. *Chest* 97:514, 1990.

28. Groedel, F. M. Die Roentgenbehandlung des Asthma Bronchiale. In *Roentgenbehandlung Innerer Krankheiten.* Munchen: J. F. Lehman, 1922.

29. Hahn, D. L., Dodge, R. W., and Golubjatnikov, R. Association of *Chlamydia pneumoniae* (strain TWAR) infection with wheezing, asthmatic bronchitis, and adult-onset asthma. *J.A.M.A.* 266:225, 1991.

30. Honsberger, R., and Wilson, A. F. Transcendental meditation in treating asthma. *Resp. Ther.* 3:79, Nov./Dec., 1973.

31. Janson-Bjerklie, S., and Clarke, E. The effects of biofeedback training on bronchial diameter in asthma. *Heart Lung* 11:200, 1982.

32. Javaid, A., Cushley, M. J., and Bone, M. F. Effect of dietary salt on bronchial reactivity to histamine in asthma. *Br. Med. J.* 297:454, 1988.

33. Johnson, R. G., et al. Isoflurane therapy for status asthmaticus in children and adults. *Chest* 97:698, 1990.

34. Jonkman, J. H. G. Food interactions with sustained-release theophylline preparations. A review. *Clin. Pharmacokinet.* 16:162, 1989.

35. Klaustermeyer, W. B., Noritake, D. T., and Wong, F. K. Chrysotherapy in the treatment of corticosteroid-dependent asthma. *J. Allergy Clin. Immunol.* 79:720, 1987.

36. Kleijnen, J., ter Riet, G., and Knipschild, P. Acupuncture and asthma: a review of controlled trials. *Thorax* 46:799, 1991.
37. Knowles, M. R., et al. A pilot study of aerosolized amiloride for the treatment of lung disease in cystic fibrosis. *N. Engl. J. Med.* 332:1189, 1990.
38. Kordansky, D., et al. Asthma improved by non-steroidal anti-inflammatory drugs. *Ann. Intern. Med.* 88:508, 1978.
39. Lane, D. J., and Lane, T. V. Alternative and complementary medicine for asthma. *Thorax* 46:787, 1991.
40. Lundgren, B. R., Ekstrom, T., and Andersson, R. G. G. The effect on inhaled clonidine in patients with asthma. *Am. Rev. Respir. Dis.* 134:266, 1986.
41. Magnussen, H. The inhibitory effect of azelastine and ketotifen on histamine induced bronchoconstriction in asthmatic patients. *Chest* 91:855, 1987.
42. Mathur, U. S., Manchanda, A. K., and Singh, V. Effect of lignocaine aerosol on exercise induced asthma. *Chest* 96(suppl. 2):249S, 1989.
43. McNally, J. F., Jr., et al. The attenuation of exercise-induced bronchoconstriction by oropharyngeal anesthesia. *Am. Rev. Respir. Dis.* 119:247, 1979.
44. Meltzer, E. O. To use or not to use antihistamines in patients with asthma. *Ann. Allergy* 64(Pt. II):183, 1990.
45. Miller, W. F. Consider magnesium sulfate when conventional asthma therapy fails? *J. Crit. Ill.* 6:518, 1991.
46. Miyatake, H., et al. Erythromycin reduces the severity of bronchial hyperresponsiveness in asthma. *Chest* 99:670, 1991.
47. Mullarkey, M. F., Lammert, J. K., and Blumenstein, B. A. Long-term methotrexate treatment in corticosteroid-dependent asthma. *Ann. Intern. Med.* 112:577, 1990.
48. Mullarkey, M. F., et al. Methotrexate in the treatment of corticosteroid-dependent asthma: a double-blind crossover study. *N. Engl. J. Med.* 318:603, 1988.
49. Nagarantha, R., and Nagendra, H. R. Yoga for bronchial asthma: a controlled study. *Br. Med. J.* 291:1077, 1985.
50. Noppen, N., et al. Bronchodilating effect of intravenous magnesium sulfate in acute severe bronchial asthma. *Chest* 97:373, 1990.
51. O'Byrne, P. M., and Jones, G. L. The effect of indomethacin on exercise-induced bronchoconstriction and refractoriness after exercise. *Am. Rev. Respir. Dis.* 134:69, 1986.
52. Odend'hal, S. Chlorothiazide relieves asthmatic wheezing. *Chest* 87:411, 1985.
53. Oriel, G. H. Further observations on the biochemistry of asthma. *Lancet* 2:406, 1933.
54. Osler, W. *The Principles and Practice of Medicine Designed for the Use of Practitioners and Students of Medicine* (2nd ed.). New York: Appleton and Company, 1895.
55. Ramirez, J., Leon, I., and Rivera, L. M. Episodic laryngeal dyskinesia. Clinical and psychiatric characterization. *Chest* 90:716, 1986.
56. Rafferty, P. The European experience with antihistamines in asthma. *Ann. Allergy* 63:389, 1989.
57. Rafferty, P., and Holgate, S. T. Terfenadine (Seldane) is a potent and selective histamine H1 receptor antagonist in asthmatic airways. *Am. Rev. Respir. Dis.* 135:181, 1987.
58. Robertson, C. E., et al. Use of ether in life-threatening acute severe asthma. *Lancet* 1:187, 1985.
59. Rosenberg, S. M., et al. Use of TAO without methylprednisolone in the treatment of severe asthma. *Chest* 100:849, 1991.
60. Rosenblatt, M. B. History of bronchial asthma. In E. B. Weiss and M. S. Segal (eds.), *Bronchial Asthma: Mechanisms and Therapeutics.* Boston: Little, Brown, 1976, P. 5.
61. Rosner, F. Moses Maimonides' treatise on asthma. *Thorax* 36:245, 1981.
62. Salter, H. H. *On Asthma: In Pathology and Treatment.* Philadelphia: Blanchard & Lea, 1864.
63. Sears, M. R., et al. Regular inhaled beta-agonist treatment in bronchial asthma. *Lancet* 336:1391, 1990.
64. Sergeant, H. G., and Yorkston, N. J. Verbal desensitisation in the treatment of bronchial asthma. *Lancet* 2:1321, 1969.
65. Severinghaus, J. W. Carotid body resection for COPD. *Chest* 95:1128, 1989.
66. Sherman, M. S., Lazar, E. J., and Eichaker, P. A bronchodilator action of glucagon. *J. Allergy Clin. Immunol.* 81:908, 1988.
67. Spector, S. L., Katz, F. H., and Farr, R. S. Troleandomycin: effectiveness in steroid-dependent asthma and bronchitis. *J. Allergy Clin. Immunol.* 54:367, 1974.
68. Stein, M., et al. Cricopharyngeal dysfunction in chronic obstructive pulmonary disease. *Chest* 97:347, 1990.
69. Stulbarg, M. S., and Winn, W. R. Bilateral carotid body resection for the relief of dyspnea in severe chronic obstructive pulmonary disease. *Chest* 95:1123, 1989.
70. Takino, M. *Pathogenesis and Therapy of Bronchial Asthma with Special Reference to Organ Vagotonia.* Baltimore: University Park Press, 1976.
71. Tandon, M. K. Adjunct treatment with yoga in chronic severe airways obstruction. *Thorax* 33:514, 1978.
72. Tandon, M. K., and Soh, P. F. T. Comparison of real and placebo acupuncture in histamine-induced asthma. A double-blind crossover study. *Chest* 96:102, 1989.
73. Tashkin, D. P., et al. Effects of smoked marijuana in experimentally induced asthma. *Am. Rev. Respir. Dis.* 12:377, 1975.
74. Tashkin, D. P., et al. Effect of orally administered cimetidine on histamine and antigen-induced bronchospasm in subjects with asthma. *Am. Rev. Respir. Dis.* 125:691, 1982.
75. Tashkin, D. P., et al. A controlled trial of real and simulated acupuncture in the management of chronic asthma. *J. Allergy Clin. Immunol.* 76:855, 1985.
76. Ting, S., Mansfield, L. E., and Yarborough, J. Effects of ascorbic acid on pulmonary functions in mild asthma. *J. Asthma* 20:39, 1983.
77. Unger, L. *Bronchial Asthma.* Springfield, IL: Thomas, 1945.
78. van Schayck, C. P., et al. Bronchodilator treatment in moderate asthma or chronic bronchitis: continuous or on demand? A randomized controlled study. *Br. Med. J.* 303:1426, 1991.
79. Waldbott, G. L. Asthma then and now: are we treating it better? *Ann. Allergy* 43:32, 1979.
80. Yellowlees, P. M., and Kalucy, R. S. Psychobiological aspects of asthma and the consequent research implications. *Chest* 97:628, 1990.
81. Yorkston, N. J., et al. Bronchial asthma: improved lung function after behavior modification. *Psychosomatics* 20:325, 1979.
82. Ziment, I. Carotid body resection—surgical respiratory therapy. *Resp. Ther.* 5:16, Nov./Dec., 1975.
83. Ziment, I. *Respiratory Pharmacology and Therapeutics.* Philadelphia: Saunders, 1978.
84. Ziment, I. Five thousand years of attacking asthma: an overview. *Respir. Care* 31:117, 1986.
85. Ziment, I. Historic overview of mucoactive drugs. In P. C. Braga and L. Allegra (eds.), *Drugs in Bronchial Mucology.* New York: Raven Press, 1989, P. 1.
86. Ziment, I. Bronchial Asthma: Clinical Aspects. In L. Allegra and P. C. Braga (eds.), *Bronchial Mucology and Related Diseases.* New York: Raven Press, 1990, P. 95.
87. Ziment, I. History of the treatment of chronic bronchitis. *Respiration* 58(suppl. 1):37, 1991.
88. Ziment, I. Folk medicines in asthma. *Am. J. Asthma Allergy Pediatr.* 5:155, 1992.

Oral Hyposensitization

Ralph P. Miech

89

A renewed interest in evaluating oral immunotherapy for use in selected patients with various allergic sensitivities is emerging. In the past decade, there were major advances in the understanding of how the immune system might control the initiation, maintenance, and suppression of IgE (reagin) synthesis. Previously, an immunotherapeutic approach to alleviating allergic states was referred to as *desensitization* but this is now known as *hyposensitization*. Hyposensitization has been tried with a variety of classes of allergens, including inhalants, injectants, contactants, and ingestants, which are associated with Type I hypersensitivity.

The classic immunologic theory of hyposensitization states that, if the immune system can be stimulated to produce antigen-specific IgG/IgA antibodies, known as *blocking antibodies*, these blocking antibodies would bind the offending antigen before it could bind to IgE antibodies on the surface of mast cells and thus activate mediator release. Today there are two additional theories concerning mechanisms that may be operative in hyposensitization. Hyposensitization may result in the decreased production of IgE by means of alterations in available lymphokines [4] or a change in the permutation of the idiotypic immune network [5] (see also Chap. 70). For example, in some patients, oral hyposensitization could result in either decreased production of interleukin-4, which potentiates the differentiation of resting B-cells to IgE-producing cells, or in the production of gamma-interferon, which inhibits the action of interleukin-4 on resting B-cells. In other patients, oral hyposensitization may cause a change in the idiotypic immune network profile, so that there is a clonal expansion of antigen-specific suppressor T-cells with a resulting decrease in the production of IgE. A change in the permutation of the idiotypic immune network has been reported for hyposensitization brought about by hypodermic injections if the allergen is administered as an entrapped component of liposomes [1]. Hyposensitization with liposome entrapped allergen resulted in an increase in antigenicity (increased specific IgG) and a decrease in allergic response (decreased specific IgE) to the antigen entrapped within liposomes.

The potential of the oral immunotherapeutic approach is limited to a specific group of asthma patients in which the initiation or exacerbation, or both, of the signs and symptoms of asthma have a positive correlation to the exposure to a specific antigen, i.e., a positive bronchoprovocative challenge and an elevated IgE level. Clinical trials attempting to achieve hyposensitization by the administration of the offending antigen by the oral route were undertaken with the hope of decreasing the incidence and lessening the severity of side effects of hyposensitization stemming from hypodermic injections. Hyposensitization brought about by hypodermic injections of specific allergenic extracts has many disadvantages: the necessity of frequent visits to the physician's office, the frequency of side effects of different degrees of severity, and the risk of a systemic anaphylactic reaction.

Early clinical trials that evaluated oral hyposensitization were unable to demonstrate a statistically significant advantage for this immunotherapy strategy. However, the data did not absolutely rule out the future possibility of its therapeutic effectiveness if appropriate conditions could be identified. These early clinical trials facilitated the performance of further clinical trials of oral hyposensitization. Current clinical trials attempt to utilize appropriate patient selection, purified antigens, quantitation of antigens, proper antigen doses, different vehicles for antigen administration, the use of adjuvants, appropriate antigen administration schedules, and an effective experimental design, i.e., the double-blind placebo-efficacy design. However, there is no agreement as to what should be measured to indicate a beneficial effect for oral hyposensitization—the symptom score, severity score, medication score, provocation tests, skin-prick test, increased IgG levels, decreased IgE levels, or suppression of seasonal increases in IgE levels, or a combination of these.

The incidence and severity of side effects of hyposensitization brought about by hypodermic injections could be markedly decreased if hyposensitization could be achieved by the oral administration of the allergenic extract. In cases of rhinoconjunctivitis and asthma caused by pollen allergies, attempts to use the oral route for the administration of allergenic extracts to achieve hyposensitization has undergone clinical trial [2]. This clinical trial involved the daily oral administration of grass pollen solution until a maximum dose was reached, followed by a maintenance dose administered twice weekly. The investigators concluded that this study did not show a significant advantage for oral hyposensitization over the placebo-treated group. In another clinical trial of oral hyposensitization performed in hay fever patients, a higher-dosage regimen of enterosoluble grass pollen tablets was utilized [8, 9]. In this trial, a double-blind placebo-efficacy experimental design also failed to prove beneficial, as shown by the symptom score, medication score, nasal provocation test, and skin prick test. The authors of this study suggested that clinical improvement "may only be a question of increasing the dose of allergens, adding adjuvants to the allergen powder, or increasing the medication period, or perhaps ensuring delivery of active allergen to a specific, as yet unknown, site in the gastrointestinal tract." A subsequent study with a birch pollen in which high doses of freeze-dried birch pollen extract were administered in enteric-coated gelatin capsules resulted in significantly reduced symptom scores compared with the controls [1a]. Yet, side effects in a few patients and a systemic reaction in one patient were encountered in this clinical trial of oral hyposensitization. In a subsequent report on oral immunotherapy in children with rhinoconjunctivitis due to birch pollen allergy, the treated group had lower symptom scores, significantly decreased skin reactions, increased levels of IgG, and a suppression of the seasonal increase in levels of IgE antibodies against birch pollen [6].

In a report of a clinical trial of oral hyposensitization, large amounts of ragweed antigen E were administered daily via the oral route to selected patients one month before the start of ragweed season [3]. Following this, a small amount of ragweed antigen E was administered orally as a maintenance dose during ragweed season. Treated patients showed a twofold increase in their IgG titer and a significant reduction in clinical symptoms (by 50 to 75%). The nasal and gastrointestinal side effects were similar in both the treated and placebo groups.

Of related interest, topical intranasal immunotherapy for ragweed allergic rhinitis is reported to reduce nasal symptoms during the pollen season; however, its effects on asthma symptoms have not been studied [7].

Currently, oral hyposensitization represents a therapeutic modality for avoiding injection immunotherapy. While the theoretical concept is of fundamental interest, further research and data concerning this approach to asthma therapy are necessary.

REFERENCES

1. Arora, N., and Gangal, S. V. Liposome entrapped allergen on IgE response. *Clin. Exp. Allergy* 22:35, 1992.
1a. Bjorksten, B., et al. Clinical and immunological effects of oral immunotherapy with a standardized birch pollen extract. *Allergy* 41:290, 1986.
2. Cooper, P. J., et al. A controlled trial of oral hyposensitization in pollen asthma and rhinitis in children. *Clin. Allergy* 14:541, 1984.
3. Creticos, P. Oral immunotherapy may yet be a viable alternative. *Allergy Observer* Vol. 8, No. 2, March-April 1991.
4. Ishizaka, K., and Ishizaka, T. Allergy. In W. E. Paul (ed.), *Fundamental Immunology*. New York: Raven Press, 1989.
5. Kearney, J. F. Idiotypic Networks. In W. E. Paul (ed.), *Fundamental Immunology*. New York: Raven Press, 1989.
6. Moller, C., et al. Oral immunotherapy of children with rhinoconjunctivitis due to birch pollen allergy: a double blind study. *Allergy* 41:271, 1986.
7. Nickelsen, J. Local intranasal immunotherapy for ragweed allergy rhinitis. I. Clinical response. *J. Allergy Clin. Immunol.* 68:33, 1981.
8. Taudorf, E., et al. Oral administration of grass pollen to hay fever patients. An efficacy study in oral hyposensitization. *Allergy* 40:321, 1985.
9. Wahn, U., Maasch, H. J., and Geissler, W., Leukocyte histamine release and humoral changes during oral and subcutaneous hyposensitization of grass pollen allergic children. *Helv. Paediatr. Acta* 39:137, 1984.

Fatal Asthma

Joseph N. Gaddy
William W. Busse
Albert L. Sheffer

90

HISTORY

Asthma is a chronic respiratory disease manifested by recurrent bouts of generalized airway obstruction that either resolve following appropriate medical therapy or spontaneously subside. It is not surprising, therefore, that asthma has been portrayed as a nonfatal disorder [186]. Laennec did not consider asthma a cause of death [105], Trousseau stated that, "asthma n'est pas fatale" [asthma is not fatal] [214], and Osler believed that "the asthmatic pants into old age" [142]. Holmes actually considered that there may be some advantage to having asthma and called it "a slight ailment that promotes longevity" [142]. Despite detailed descriptions of the pathologic findings in fatal cases [78], and the noticing of increased asthma deaths in the 1950s [1], the lethal potential of the disease was not fully appreciated until the 1960s' "epidemic," during which marked increases in the rates of death were noted in England and Wales, New Zealand, and Australia [42, 43, 59, 82, 188, 189, 197, 198]. This "epidemic" subsided somewhat in the late 1960s, and the factors that may have contributed to the increased death rates are speculative and have been extensively debated [42, 46, 57, 60, 67, 82, 160, 164, 198, 205]. It is discouraging that, despite changes in medical management and attempts to better educate patients, the overall mortality rate in subjects with severe disease remains at 1 to 2 percent [13, 124, 154, 209].

INCIDENCE

Recent epidemiologic data have revealed a worldwide increase in the asthma mortality (Fig. 90-1). Since the late 1970s, significant increases in deaths have been noted in New Zealand [83, 90,188, 189], England and Wales [23, 24, 164, 189], Australia [189], Canada [23, 189], Sweden [189], Denmark [23, 189], France [15, 23], Hong Kong [196], Germany [23], and the United States [54, 55, 165, 190, 192, 224, 225]. Deaths per 100,000 population increased from 3.4 in 1974 to 6.8 in 1985 in New Zealand, from 3.0 in 1979 to 3.4 in 1984 in England and Wales, from 2.3 in 1978 to 4.2 in 1984 in Australia, from 1.7 in 1979 to 2.0 in 1980 in Canada, from 4.2 in 1975 to 5.6 in 1985 in Sweden, from 1.2 in 1975 to 4.0 in 1985 in Denmark, from 0.32 in 1976 to 0.94 in 1982 in Hong Kong, and from 1.2 in 1979 to 1.6 in 1984 in the United States [54, 55, 165, 190, 192, 224, 225.]

The striking and apparently universal increase in asthma mortality has led investigators to search for factors that may influence the incidence of fatalities.

Age

During the 1980s in the United States, the mortality rates in children and young adults (aged 5 to 34 years) increased by 6.2 ±

1.2 percent per annum, increasing more rapidly among the 5 to 14 year olds than among those aged 15 to 34 years [224]. Age-specific death rates reveal that the most dramatic increase has been in the older age groups, with the rate nearly tripling from 1977 to 1984 in those 85 years or older [165] (Fig. 90-2). However, the largest proportional increase in death rates from 1979 to 1980 occurred in the 10- to 14-year-old age group, with rates increasing from 0.1 to 0.3 per 100,000 [192].

Gender

Asthma death rates in the United States from 1968 to 1984 increased in both sexes, with the rate remaining slightly higher among females than among males [23, 189] (Fig. 90-3).

Race

In 1987, the highest death rate in 5- to 34-year-olds in the United States, was among non-white males, at 13.5 deaths per million population [224]. This rate was nearly five times higher than that among whites of either sex. Overall, the age-adjusted death rates for black subjects are approximately three times the rate for white subjects [165, 191, 224] (Fig. 9-4). Rates for black children aged 15 to 19 years increased from 0.7 per 100,000 population in 1979 to 1.4 in 1986, and black children aged 10 to 14 years had a fourfold increase in death rate (0.3 to 1.2) during the same period [192]. Rates for white children aged 10 to 14 years increased from 0.1 to 0.2 from 1979 to 1986. Thus, by 1986, the rate for subjects 10 to 14 years old was nearly six times higher for black children than for white children. Interestingly, the death rates for American Indians, Japanese, Chinese, and Filipinos living in the United States are lower than the rates for white subjects [189]. A similar racial discrepancy has been noted in New Zealand. From 1981 to 1983, the age-standardized mortality rate for Maoris (indigenous Polynesians) was fivefold higher than that for Caucasian subjects [172]. The prevalence rate of airway hyperresponsiveness and asthma symptoms does not differ significantly between racial groups in Auckland, New Zealand, and therefore cannot account for the differences in fatality rate [72]. Interestingly, however, the utilization of emergency room services for primary care is higher for Maoris than for immigrants and may partially explain the difference in mortality rates [130].

Geographic Location

The rates of death from asthma in subjects between 5 and 34 years of age in the United States have been reported to be higher for blacks in the Northeast and North Central regions, and higher for whites in the West [193]. Additionally, small-area geographic

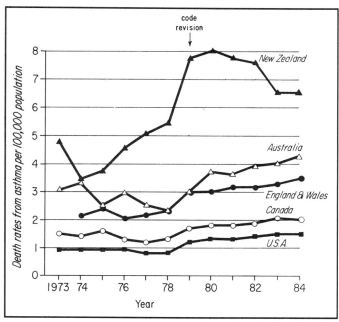

Fig. 90-1. *Asthma death rates per 100,000 population from 1973 to 1984 for the United States (consistently the lowest annual rate) and five other countries. The upward trend since 1977 is accentuated in countries where high-dose isoproterenol preparations were available over-the-counter during that period. (Reprinted with permission from R. M. Sly, Mortality from asthma 1979–84. J. Allergy Clin. Immunol. 82: 705, 1988.)*

analysis revealed that, during the 1980s in patients aged 5 to 34 years, ther were certain areas with persistently high asthma mortality [224, 225]. The four sub-state geopolitical areas (called *state economic areas*) with higher numbers of observed than expected deaths include New York City; Cook County, Illinois; Maricopa County, Arizona; and Fresno, California. The two larger state economic areas (New York City and Cook County) have made a significant contribution to the overall increase in asthma mortality in the United States; these two areas accounted for 21.1 percent of all asthma deaths in 5- to 34-year-olds occurring in 1985 [224]. These results question the role of urban development in contributing to the overall increasing trend in asthma mortality in the United States.

Economic Factors

In the United States, median household incomes have been lower for blacks than for whites, and the black unemployment rates have been higher than those of whites. Interestingly, unemployment rates for blacks have been highest in the North Central region, an area where blacks have a higher asthma death rate than whites [193]. This suggests that economic factors may account for part of the noted racial and regional differences in mortality from asthma. However, there is not a significant difference in the percentage of blacks compared to whites who die from asthma in a hospital [190, 224]. This suggests that lack of hospitalization does not occur because of economic factors and cannot account for the racial or regional differences in asthma mortality rates in the United States.

Although black children with chronic disease are less likely than whites to have health insurance [25], inner-city blacks have been noted to utilize the emergency room more frequently as

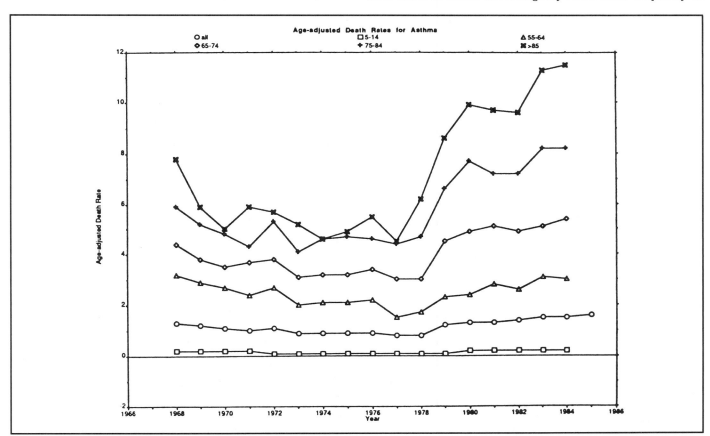

Fig. 90-2. *Relationship of age to asthma deaths. (Reprinted with permission from E. D. Robin, Death from bronchial asthma. Chest 93:64, 1988.)*

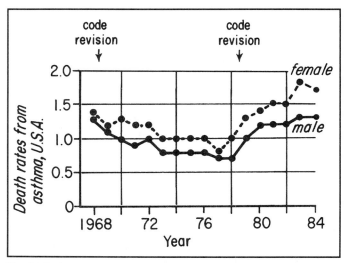

Fig. 90-3. *Asthma death rates per 100,000 general population in the United States by sex and year. (Reprinted with permission from R. M. Sly, Mortality from asthma 1979–84. J. Allergy Clin. Immunol. 82:705, 1988.)*

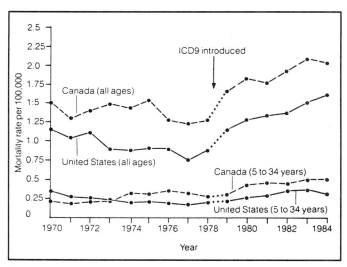

Fig. 90-5. *The effect of the International Classification of Disease revision (ICD9) on asthma mortality. (Reprinted with permission from M. R. Sears, Are deaths from asthma really on the rise? J. Respir. 8:39, 1987.)*

POSSIBLE EXPLANATIONS FOR INCREASING ASTHMA MORTALITY

International Classification of Disease Code Change

The Ninth International Classification of Disease (ICD) revision in 1979 attributes death to asthma if the word *asthma* appears on the death certificate. Previously, if *bronchitis, bronchiolitis,* or *emphysema* was included on the certificate, then death was not attributed to asthma. This revision accounted for most of the 39 percent increase in asthma mortality observed in the United States in 1979, but cannot explain the antecedent increase or the continuing increase in cases of fatal asthma [189]. Interestingly, Denmark and Sweden reported increases in asthma death rates even though they did not revise the ICD code [189, 238]. Furthermore, a code shift from chronic obstructive pulmonary disease (COPD) to asthma could only partially account for the increased asthma mortality rate, as the death rate from COPD has remained stable [189].

It is known that death is inappropriately attributed to asthma in the 15- to 64-year-old age group more than 25 percent of the time [18]. Additionally, asthma deaths are overestimated by as much as 50 percent in subjects older than 55 years [7]. However, it is quite clear that the ICD revision had very little impact on the 5- to 34-year-old age group [176, 204], and that mortality rates in this group have continued to rise (Fig. 90-5).

Asthma Prevalence Change

The prevalence of asthma varies considerably according to the definition used. In the United States, for 3- to 17-year-olds, current asthma, diagnosed by a physician, and/or frequent trouble with wheezing occurring during the previous 12 months occurs in 6.7 percent of youths overall and is significantly higher in black than white children (9.4% versus 6.2%), boys than girls (7.8% versus 5.5%), and urban than rural areas (7.1% versus 5.7%) [64]. Socioeconomic factors such as the poverty index ratio, gross family income, or education of the head of the household are not associated with asthma prevalence in children. However, low income has been shown to be a strong predictor of asthma in adults aged 25 to 74 years, and the higher ratio in blacks appears

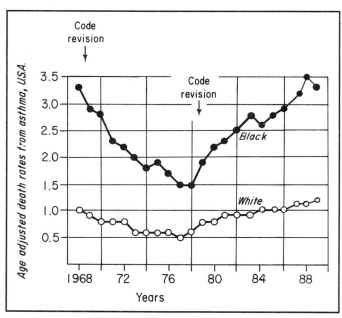

Fig. 90-4. *Age-adjusted rates of death from asthma per 100,000 general population in the United States by race, 1968 to 1986. (Reprinted with permission from R. M. Sly, Mortality from asthma. N. Engl. Reg. Allergy Proc. 7:425, 1986.)*

a primary care source of asthma treatment regardless of their socioeconomic status [115]. The apparent racial differences in emergency room utilization could be due to a different family structure, different social and cultural characteristics, differences in the ease of access to medical care, or more severe disease, but does not appear to be directly related to socioeconomic status. Asthma mortality and socioeconomic status have also been shown to lack correlation in New Zealand [173]. Allergies unique to such economically determined living conditions may be a more significant factor in asthma exacerbation than has been previously recognized.

Table 90-1. Reported prevalence of asthma by sex, race, and age[a]

Survey of age range (yr)	Total	Sex		Race	
		Male	Female	White	Black
6–11					
HES II, 1963–1965	5.3 (0.33)	6.5 (0.52)	4.0 (0.41)	5.2 (0.38)	5.5 (0.65)
NHANES I, 1971–1974	4.8 (0.54)	5.6 (0.84)	3.9 (0.75)	4.7 (0.58)	5.1 (1.2)
NHANES II, 1976–1980	7.6 (0.57)[b]	9.0 (0.82)[b]	6.1 (0.74)[c]	7.2 (0.65)[b]	9.6 (2.0)
12–17					
HES III, 1966–1969	6.0 (0.38)	6.9 (0.62)	5.1 (0.43)	5.8 (0.40)	7.0 (0.67)
NHANES I, 1971–1974	6.0 (0.66)	7.6 (0.91)	4.4 (0.74)	6.3 (0.75)	4.6 (0.94)[d]
NHANES II, 1976–1980	6.5 (0.81)	8.0 (1.2)	4.9 (0.77)	5.9 (0.79)	10.1 (1.8)[b]

HES = Health Examination Survey; NHANES = National Health and Nutrition Examination Survey.
[a] Results are given as mean percentages (±SE).
[b] $p < .01$, NHANES I versus NHANES II.
[c] $p < .05$, NHANES I versus NHANES II.
[d] $p < .05$, HES III versus NHANES I.
Source: P. J. Gergen, D. J. Mullally, and R. Evans, III, National survey of prevalence of asthma among children in the United States, 1976 to 1980. *Pediatrics* 81:1, 1988. Reprinted with permission.

to be explained by their lower income [123]. Interestingly, the reported prevalence of ever having asthma increased by 58 percent (from 4.8 to 7.6%) in 6- to 11-year-old children between the first (1971 to 1974) and second (1976 to 1980) National Health and Nutrition Examination Surveys. For the 12- to 17-year-olds, the asthma prevalence was noted to increase only in black children [64] (Table 90-1).

Asthma prevalence has also been noted to increase in New Zealand (from 7.1% in 1969 to 13.5% in 1982) [128] and in New Guinea (from less than 1% in 1972 to 7.3% in 1988) [234]. However, hospitalization and mortality rates are increasing at a greater pace than prevalence; thus, the increasing prevalence rate alone is not sufficient to explain the increased morbidity and mortality due to asthma.

Changing Asthma Severity

The evidence for a possible increase in asthma severity includes a marked increase in the use of antiasthma medication as well as a marked increase in hospitalization rates. Outpatient prescriptions in the United States from 1972 to 1985 increased by 7 percent for all drug products, and by 200 percent for antiasthma products [14]. However, it is not certain whether the increases are accounted for by increased prescription numbers for a stable number of patients or by increased numbers of subjects taking the same amount of drug. Similarly, there was a striking increase in the sales of antiasthma medication (sympathomimetic aerosols, steroid aerosols, and theophylline) per capita in New Zealand, Australia, and the United Kingdom from 1975 to 1981 [90].

There has been a striking increase in asthma hospitalization rates in the 0- to 14-year age group. From 1969 to 1980, hospitalization rates are reported to have increased tenfold in New Zealand, sixfold in England and Wales, three- to eightfold in Australia, fourfold in Canada, and threefold in the United States [129]. There may have been an increase in the number of admissions per patient, but, at least in New Zealand, the increase was primarily due to an increase in the number of individuals with asthma admitted each year. From 1979 to 1987 in the United States, asthma hospitalizations have increased 4.5 percent per annum in children aged 0 to 17 years [65]. The increase was 2.9 percent per annum in 5- to 17-year-olds, and 5 percent per annum in 0- to 4-year-olds. In addition, the increase in 0- to 4-year-old black children was 1.8 times the increase in whites [65]. Overall, the rates for blacks older than 17 years are 50 percent higher than those for whites, and black children have a rate 150 percent

greater than that of white children [55, 223]. In Maryland, the annual asthma discharge rates are three times higher in blacks than whites aged 1 to 19 years. However, after being adjusted for poverty, rates are only slightly higher in blacks [233]. Interestingly, these increases in hospital admissions for asthma appear to be rising faster than the total hospital admissions [58]. Although the increase in Australia may be largely explained by ICD code changes [29], the increases in Canada [116], England and Wales [4], and New Zealand [131] are not explained by such code changes. The hospitalization rate for asthma from 1979 to 1986 increased by 23 percent in New Zealand [131] and by 55 percent in England and Wales [4]. It is worrisome that asthma hospitalization rates appear to be increasing worldwide. Explanations have included environmental pollution, indoor air pollution, and a change in the perception among physicians of a wheezing illness [65]. However, none of these possibilities seems to adequately explain the increase, and it is possible that a change in the severity of the disease is occurring.

Iatroepidemic

Recently it has been shown that the regular use of inhaled beta[2]-agonist bronchodilators is associated with an increased risk of death or near death from asthma [235]. In addition, it has been demonstrated that approximately 70 percent of stable asthma patients are better controlled when using an inhaled beta agonist on an as-needed rather than regular basis [222]. The adverse effect from regular bronchodilator inhalation was observed to occur in subjects using a bronchodilator as their sole asthma therapy as well as in subjects using inhaled corticosteroids regularly. It has also been shown that the mean airway responsiveness to methacholine increases slightly during the regular use of an inhaled beta agonist. These changes are not likely due to tachyphylaxis brought about by the regular use of a beta agonist, as the morning peak expiratory flow rates were higher in the group of patients treated with an inhaled beta agonist on a regular basis. A possible mechanism for the poorer asthma control seen in patients who routinely use an inhaled beta agonist is that such patients may tolerate a higher initial dose of antigen exposure due to being chronically bronchodilated. It is also possible that regular bronchodilator use results in a blunting of the early asthmatic response without changes in the more significant late asthmatic response. Thus, it has been suggested that the trend toward use of higher doses of long-acting inhaled beta agonists for the treatment of asthma may indeed be an important factor in the worldwide increase in morbidity from this respiratory disease [222].

One possible explanation for deteriorating asthma control during long-term beta-agonist administration is the development of subsensitivity. It has been shown that the peak bronchodilating response as well as the duration of action following beta-agonist inhalation are diminished in asthma subjects following a 12-week period of inhaled terbutaline [159]. However, others have shown that, following regular inhalation of a beta agonist for 13 weeks, there may be a statistically significant decrease in the duration of acute bronchodilatation but that clinically significant tachyphylaxis is quite unusual [216]. Additionally, in a study comparing the effect of routine inhaled beta-agonist therapy versus as-needed beta-agonist treatment, subsensitivity was not noted to be significant [222]. This may be partially explained by the concomitant use of inhaled corticosteroids, which may prevent the development of tachyphylaxis to inhaled beta agonist [41]. It is known that there is a very large variation in the in vitro response to the development of subsensitivity following beta-agonist use [73]. This may explain some of the clinical differences noted in previous studies. Interestingly, normal subjects may be more likely to develop tachyphylaxis to the effects of beta agonists than asthma subjects; however, the changes are not considered to be physiologically significant [99, 212]. Thus, although subsensitization may occur, its clinical significance is unlikely to explain the changes in asthma morbidity and it is not likely to significantly contribute to the overall increasing fatal asthma rate.

Prolonged beta-agonist use in several studies has resulted in no change in response to inhaled histamine [99, 212]. However, others have shown that 4 weeks of regular terbutaline therapy may lead to a temporary increase in bronchial responsiveness to histamine and propranolol [95, 219] as well as to methacholine [62]. In addition, a rebound increase in bronchial responsiveness to histamine has been reported following the abrupt cessation of regular beta-agonist therapy [95]. It is unlikely that the small changes in airway responsiveness following regular beta-agonist usage are causally related to the increase in asthma mortality.

Another potential mechanism through which the use of meter-dose inhalers could contribute to asthma morbidity is via the effects of the freon propellants, the fluorocarbons. These compounds are known to be capable of inducing fatal arrhythmias when inhaled at high concentrations [5]. Potential mechanisms would include a decrease in myocardial contractility, decreased cardiac output, a reflex increase in sympathetic and vagal tone, as well as a potential sensitization of the myocardium to the pro-arrhythmic effect of catecholamines [5, 44]. However, the maximal levels of fluorocarbons noted in humans have been considerably lower than the levels required to sensitize the myocardium in animal models [45, 97].

There are a variety of other adverse effects and potential complications from treatment with beta-adrenergic agonist agents. During an acute asthma episode, the use of beta agonists has been associated with aggravated hypoxia despite a significant decrease in airway obstruction. This is considered to occur through the aggravation of a ventilation-perfusion mismatch secondary to the reversal of compensatory pulmonary vasoconstriction that arises in poorly ventilated lung tissue [81, 228]. However the clinical significance of these changes is believed to be minimal and can be corrected with supplemental oxygen.

The cardiovascular effects of beta-agonist administration in animal models include myocardial necrosis and arrhythmias [37, 70, 152]. These cardiac effects appear to be aggravated by hypoxia [112] as well as by the presence of an increased cardiac workload [232]. The significance of these findings in humans is not entirely clear; however, it is certain that the intravenous administration of beta agonists in adults and children may result in very significant cardiac ischemia [103, 120, 134, 169] (see Chaps. 57 and 78).

Beta$_2$-selective agonists are believed to have less effect on both animal and human myocardium [74]; however, beta$_2$ receptors are known to exist in significant numbers in human cardiac tissue [21, 163]. In addition, there is evidence to suggest that beta$_2$-adrenergic receptors can mediate tachycardia in humans [110], and selective beta$_2$ agonists are known to produce a variety of cardiovascular effects in clinical practice [2, 6, 22, 69, 86, 94, 96, 136, 195, 210, 230]. It could be argued that the administration of an aerosolized beta agonist should not produce significant cardiovascular effects, due to the minute amount of systemic absorption that occurs [9, 32]. However, it is well documented that inhaled beta agonists can produce significant hemodynamic effects, such as an increased cardiac output and stroke volume, without there being a significant change in heart rate or blood pressure [93]. In addition, significant cardiac arrhythmias have been reported to occur following the administration of inhaled beta-agonist drugs [27, 162, 210].

The etiology of the circulatory and arrhythmogenic effects following beta-agonist administration is not entirely clear. These effects may be due to direct stimulation of myocardial beta$_1$ and beta$_2$ receptors, or could be related to the reflex tachycardia that occurs as a compensatory effect, due to vasodilatation which could be related to peripheral beta$_2$ stimulation [135, 168, 227]. Furthermore, hypokalemia is known to occur following systemic or aerosolized beta-agonist administration and could play an important role in the production of the noted cardiovascular effects [3, 40, 102].

Whether the use of a beta agonist results in cardiovascular events that could significantly affect asthma mortality is not entirely clear. During the 1960s' epidemic of fatal asthma, the sales volume of a highly concentrated isoproterenol preparation correlated with the increased asthma mortality in New Zealand, England, and Wales. However, in the Netherlands and Belgium sales of the highly concentrated isoproterenol inhaler did not correlate with fatal asthma. Additionally, Japan had an increased mortality rate at that time but did not market the preparation [205]. Whether the use of highly concentrated beta-agonist inhalers was responsible for the increased mortality noted in the 1960s is not entirely clear and has been extensively debated [42, 46, 57, 60, 67, 82, 160, 164, 197, 198]. It has recently been reported that the use of inhaled fenoterol is associated with an increased risk of death secondary to asthma in patients with severe disease, i.e., those requiring hospitalization within the previous 12 months and requiring oral steroids [145, 179]. However, a causal relationship between asthma death and fenoterol use has been debated, and most large studies reviewing episodes of fatal asthma have not implicated beta-agonist use as a cause of either fatal episodes of asthma or life-threatening arrhythmias, with the exception that beta-agonist overuse may result in a delay in seeking medical care [17, 92, 104, 151, 171, 202, 206, 239].

Theophylline has been used extensively as a bronchodilator for the therapy of asthma [14, 90], and there has been some concern that this agent in some way might be contributing to the noted increase in asthma mortality. There is evidence in animal models that toxic doses of theophylline are capable of producing significant tachycardia, hypotension, and myocardial necrosis [56]. Theophylline is also a positive chronotrope, in that it can produce a dose-dependent increase in heart rate [108, 217, 220], may increase atrial automaticity [106], and accelerate intracardiac conduction [217]. Furthermore, at high concentrations in humans, theophylline has been associated with a variety of supraventricular arrhythmias, including multifocal atrial tachycardia, atrial fibrillation, and paroxysmal supraventricular tachycardia [118, 140, 182, 187]. Additionally, during theophylline toxicity, frequently ventricular premature beats and rarely ventricular tachycardia have been noted [26, 68, 118, 211] (see Chap. 58).

Rapid intravenous infusion and oral overdoses of methylxanthines have also been associated with ventricular fibrillation and cardiac arrest [16, 118, 125, 140, 181]. Despite the known potential cardiovascular effects of theophylline, a recent prospective study has revealed that sustained ventricular or supraventricular tachyarrhythmias that require antiarrhythmic therapy are uncommon during recovery from theophylline toxicity [181]. Furthermore, most prospective studies have revealed that therapeutic doses of theophylline are unlikely to increase the frequency or complexity of ventricular ectopy [36, 38, 52, 86, 87, 91, 144, 171, 185]. Interestingly, patient age appears to be the primary determinant of a life-threatening event such as a seizure or severe arrhythmia in patients with unintentional theophylline intoxication [183], while peak serum theophylline concentrations appear not to predict well which patient with chronic theophylline intoxication will have a life-threatening event. Thus, it would then appear that, although elderly individuals may be at higher risk for a significant cardiovascular event due to theophylline intoxication, reviews of large numbers of asthma deaths have been unable to associate excessive theophylline doses with fatal asthma episodes [175].

The concomitant use of a beta agonist in theophylline preparations has increased dramatically since 1975 [138]. Studies in animal models have also revealed that cardiac lesions and arrhythmias due to beta-agonist administration can be enhanced by concomitant aminophylline usage [85, 229]. Although some investigators have suggested a link between sudden asthma death and the concomitant use of a beta agonist and methylxanthines [231], clinical evidence suggests that the therapeutic levels of theophylline administered with an aerosolized beta agonist do not have a significant cardiotoxic effect [104, 111, 162, 171].

One interesting potential result of the simultaneous use of beta agonists and theophylline is the production of myocardial contraction-band necrosis (MCBN). MCBN is known to occur following severe emotional stress, cardiac reperfusion, intracranial catastrophes, and the administration of large doses of beta agonists, which could be potentiated by aminophylline administration [31, 48, 61, 84, 85, 89, 213]. Some children who have experienced sudden asthma death have been documented to have MCBN [103], which is certainly distinct from the myocardial coagulation necrosis of typical myocardial infarctions. However, the exact relationship between MCBN and sudden asthma death is not entirely clear.

Although there are potential adverse interactions between beta-adrenergic agonists and theophylline, extensive investigations have not implicated theophylline toxicity or beta-agonist–theophylline interactions as a direct cause of death [138, 202]. Long-term bronchodilator use could contribute to a distressed patient's delay in seeking medical attention, thereby increasing the chance of a fatal asthma episode. However, a fatal attack is believed to be more likely to stem from hesitation in prescribing oral corticosteroids than the inappropriate use of theophylline or beta-adrenergic agonists. Thus, the exact role that long-term bronchodilator use has in contributing to the overall increasing asthma mortality is not clear.

Undertreatment

Explanations for asthma deaths which occur in the hospital include an inadequate initial investigation, an inadequate clinical assessment, a delay in instituting appropriate therapy, the inadequate use of corticosteroids, the use of inappropriate sedation, inadequate theophylline monitoring, and failure to institute artificial ventilation at an appropriate time [35, 50, 114, 141]. The most significant factors contributing to hospital asthma deaths are inadequate objective monitoring, including arterial blood gas determination, and an objective measure of airway obstruction, the marked underuse of beta agonists when appropriate, and delayed utilization of systemic steroids [103].

Significant factors that are associated with both outpatient and inhospital asthma deaths include poor patient education, underestimation of the severity of the disease, as well as inadequate assessment and objective monitoring [57, 113, 141, 202]. The gross underuse of beta agonists, the underuse or inappropriate withdrawal of corticosteroids, and the underestimation of the severity of an individual attack by patients, their relatives, and physicians are believed to contribute to the occurrence of fatal asthma episodes [39, 151, 202]. The absence of close follow-up may also be associated with fatal events [236]. These factors result not only in inadequate assessment but also contribute significantly to unnecessary delays in hospital referral as well as inadequate emergency therapy of severe episodes of asthma [151, 175, 177]. Thus, inadequate evaluation and treatment in both the hospital and outpatient management of asthma seem to continue to contribute to the increasing asthma mortality.

The Contribution of Atopy to Fatal Asthma

Sixty percent of the patients who died of asthma and were investigated by the British Thoracic Association in 1979 were atopic, and, interestingly, one-half of these subjects died in May to June or in September to October [19]. Sudden asthma deaths were more frequently noted in the atopic population, as 35 percent of the atopic patients died less than one hour after the beginning of an attack whereas only 15 percent of the nonatopic patients died so acutely [19]. A seasonal variation in the hospitalizations for asthma as well as fatal episodes of asthma has also been noted in the United States [223]. For the 5- to 34-year-old subjects, the peak hospitalization rate occurred from September to November, whereas the peak mortality in the same group occurred between June and August. However, for elderly patients, both the hospitalization rate and mortality rate for asthma tended to peak between December and February [223]. The seasonality of asthma mortality and hospitalization in 15- to 34-year-old subjects has also been demonstrated in Canada [117]. Asthma hospitalization appears to peak in April to May as well as September to October, while mortality tends to peak in October [117]. A seasonal variation in asthma deaths has likewise been reported in Scotland [237]. Interestingly, it has recently been shown that, in children and young adults who reside in the upper Midwest, exposure to *Alternaria* may be a significant risk factor for respiratory arrest [139]. A plausible explanation for the noted seasonal variation in hospitalization and fatal asthma episodes could be that the massive exposure to aeroallergens precipitates severe asthma, resulting in death. However, the contribution of fatal asthma following massive allergen exposure to the general worldwide increase in asthma mortality is not clear.

Although the seasonality of fatal asthma suggests an important role for inhalant allergens in asthma mortality, the indoor environment contains numerous antigens that could also play a role in severe asthma. It is interesting that the ownership of pets is just as likely in families with atopic children as in nonatopic families [75]. Random cross-sectional mattress dust samples obtained from the homes of nonallergic families in the Baltimore area revealed that 77 percent of the samples contained significant amounts of cat dander and 63 percent of the samples contained large quantities of dog dander [109]. In addition, patients sensitive to animal dander are known to experience significant bronchospasm induced by exposure to naturally occurring cat allergen levels [218]. Interestingly, chronic exposure to substantial levels of animal allergen at a young age may influence not only the development of allergy but also significant airway obstruction in children [133]. Therefore, it would appear that, if the indoor animal population were to increase significantly, it could conceivably influence both the prevalence of asthma and its mortality.

Exposure to other relevant indoor allergens such as cockroach antigen could also influence overall asthma morbidity. It has been suggested that an inhalant allergy to cockroach, cat dander, and dust mite is a major risk factor for adults with acute asthma [150]. The combination of exposure to cat and cockroach allergens in addition to sensitization with resultant specific IgE antibody production increases the risk for acute asthma [63]. Cockroach infestation rates are known to vary, depending on geographic location and socioeconomic conditions [63]. Infestation is generally low in suburban populations and increased in crowded urban areas. Additionally, approximately 50 percent of allergic asthma subjects are sensitive to cockroach antigen, as demonstrated by skin testing, and inhalation challenge results in an early asthmatic response in 90 percent of sensitive asthma subjects and a late asthmatic response in 68 percent of such patients [63]. Although cockroach infestation rates for the state economic areas with unusually high asthma mortality rates are not known, it is interesting that conditions favoring high infestation rates also appear to favor higher asthma mortality rates.

The major allergens of house dust mites, *Dermatophagoides pteronyssinus* and *D. farinae,* are known to be significant indoor allergens [109]. It is well documented that exposure to these dust mites may result in prolonged bronchial hyperresponsiveness [34]. It is also known that approximately 65 percent of asthma subjects react to dust mite on skin testing [147], and therefore mite allergy is considered a significant risk factor for asthma. It has also been suggested that exposure to dust mite allergen during early childhood is an important determinant of the subsequent development of asthma, even though it may not be clinically apparent for a number of years [200]. There are a number of additional observations that suggest a very significant role for dust mite allergy in the development and exacerbation of asthma. Mite-allergic patients with acute asthma exacerbations have been shown to be more likely to have high levels of *Der p* I or *Der f* I in their homes [149]. Patients with the new onset of dust mite–sensitive asthma have also been noted to have significantly higher levels of dust mites in their homes than asthma subjects who do not have dust mite–triggered asthma [98]. House dust mite antigen levels have been shown to correlate with increased humidity and tend to be highest in the fall [194]. Interestingly, these higher mite levels appear to occur at a time when the number of fatal asthma episodes in children is also elevated. In school aged children in Japan, *Df*-specific IgE levels are also known to correlate with the incidence of asthma [184]. The marked increase in the prevalence of asthma in Papua New Guinea also appears to be linked to the development of sensitivity to dust mite [47]. Additionally, mite-sensitive children with asthma may outgrow their chronic respiratory symptoms; however, they appear to remain susceptible to airway challenge with mite allergen for years [66]. The association of dust mite allergy and asthma has been strengthened by the demonstration of decreased asthma symptoms and diminished airway responsiveness following prolonged mite antigen avoidance [148]. In addition, sensitization and exposure to dust mite appears to be a risk factor for acute and recurrent asthma [148, 150]. This wealth of information suggests that the development of mite sensitivity followed by prolonged mite antigen exposure may indeed lead to asthma. The exact relationship between dust mite sensitivity and increasing asthma mortality is not clear. However, construction tendencies, including the widespread use of carpeting and less than optimal ventilation, could conceivably promote mite growth and thereby influence asthma morbidity (see Chaps. 42 and 87).

Pollution

Air pollution has long been associated with increased asthma morbidity [11, 20, 80, 170, 201] (Chap. 45). However, the association is not uniform; in Denver, increased asthma symptoms and inhaler use have been found to correlate only with levels of fine nitrates and not with carbon monoxide, sulfur dioxide, or ozone levels, or with temperature and barometric pressure [146]. Recently, pollen or suspended particle numbers have been shown to lack any correlation with emergency room visits or hospitalizations over a 2-year period [12]. It is interesting to note that a cluster of asthma deaths during this time seem to be associated more with patient compliance and inadequate asthma therapy than with air pollution [12]. Whether there is an association between air pollution and the noted increased asthma mortality in certain state economic areas is not clear.

Sudden Asphyxic Asthma

Triggers of acute life-threatening asthma are believed to include emotional upset, thermal inversions, beta-blocker use, as well as aspirin and nonsteroidal antiinflammatory drug use [10]. Interestingly, rare patients have been identified who are either unable to sense the presence of marked airway obstruction [167] or have a markedly decreased hypoxic ventilatory drive [221]. Obviously these subjects, although rare, could be at risk for fatal asthma due to either an absence of symptoms until their respiratory reserve is nearly totally exhausted, or to the absence of a normal hyperventilatory response to bronchial narrowing. There are a number of asthma patients who appear to present with severe hypercapnia and acidosis, which fortunately resolves rapidly [132]. These near-fatal episodes are believed to be triggered by massive allergen exposure or stressful events and are considered to be the result of sudden asphyxia rather than cardiac arrhythmias. This suggests that, in this subset of asthmatics, smooth muscle contraction or sudden mucosal edema formation is the physiologic mechanism associated with a life-threatening event [132]. Although patients may require ventilation for such severe episodes of asthma, the majority of fatalities do not appear to occur as a complication of mechanical ventilation [226]. Whether the percentage of asthma subjects who may be susceptible to sudden asphyxic asthma is changing or is contributing to the overall increased asthma mortality is not clear at this time.

PATHOPHYSIOLOGY

During a severe asthma episode, there is a marked reduction in airflow rates, significant air trapping, a marked ventilation-perfusion mismatch with resulting hypoxia and hypercapnia increased pulmonary vascular resistance, and right ventricular overload [51, 153, 157, 158, 226] (see Chap. 26). If these physiologic changes do not reverse spontaneously or with therapy, death may result.

The typical pathologic findings in cases of fatal asthma include mucus-filled bronchi and bronchioles containing significant numbers of eosinophils and desquamated epithelial cells, distended bronchioles with emphysematous changes, and thickened basement membranes [28, 49, 76] (Chap. 28). Interestingly, however, occasional autopsies do not reveal significant amounts of inflammation, and unsuspected findings that have been noted include the presence of pneumothorax, cor pulmonale, aspiration, bronchopneumonia, and pulmonary edema [100]. These findings occur in a minority of patients, and, in general, the pathologic findings in fatal asthma cases consist of significant airway inflammation and suggest that undertreatment of the inflammatory component of the disease likely contributes significantly to mortality.

IDENTIFICATION OF SIGNIFICANT RISK FACTORS

Reviews of fatal asthma cases have suggested many risk factors, including a poor general understanding of potential disease se-

Table 90-2. Results of the initial case-control study: clusters of variables that distinguished children who died from severity-matched control subjects

Severe disease
  History of hypoxic seizures during asthma attacks
  History of respiratory failure requiring intubation and ventilation
Problems with self-management
  Disregard of perceived asthma symptoms
  Self-care not age appropriate
  Manipulative use of asthma
Poor family-support system
  Difficulties in family cooperation with medical plan
  Parent–child conflict
  Family dysfunction or crisis
Psychological problems in the child
  Psychiatric diagnosis made after referral to a psychiatrist
  Depressive symptoms
  Excessive sensitivity to separation or loss

Source: R. C. Strunk, Identification of the fatality-prone subject with asthma. *J. Allergy Clin. Immunol.* 83:477, 1989. Reprinted with permission.

Table 90-3. Fatal cases compared to patients with a life-threatening episode within the past 3 years

Risk factors present in the 6 months prior to death that were significant included:

1. Respiratory failure requiring intubation
2. Corticosteroid reduction by greater than 50% in the preceding month
3. History of a family disturbance
4. Abnormal reaction to separation or loss
5. Hopelessness or despair
6. Attacks starting during sleep not associated with vomiting
7. Both groups had severe disease, disregarded perceived symptoms, and had similar physician care.

Source: B. O. Miller and R. C. Strunk, Circumstances surrounding the deaths of children due to asthma. *Am. J. Dis. Child.* 143:1294, 1989. Reprinted with permission.

Table 90-4. Results of case-control study: variables that distinguished adults who died from hospitalized severity-matched control subjects.

Life-threatening attack
  Attack in which consciousness was disturbed
  Appreciable hypercapnia was recorded
Psychosocial problems
  Recorded in hospital or general practice records
  Alcoholism
  Personality disorders
  Depression
  Recent bereavement
  Unemployment

Source: H. H. Rea, et al., A case-control study of deaths from asthma. *Thorax* 41: 833, 1986. Reprinted with permission.

verity, inadequate corticosteroid usage, and underuse of beta agonists, as well as the presence of nocturnal bronchoconstriction, infection, sedation, and severe psychopathology [30, 119, 137, 215]. Controlled studies in children have given us considerable insight into which factors may be most important when attempting to identify asthma patients who may be at risk for death [207, 209]. Severe disease, defined by a history of hypoxic seizures or a history of respiratory failure requiring mechanical ventilation, is a significant risk factor. However, these variables do not identify patients at risk of death unless they are associated with one of a variety of psychological variables.

Variables related to psychosocial dysfunction appear to distinguish between subjects who experience fatal asthma and those with severe asthma not resulting in death better than do physiologic variables. Distinguishing psychosocial factors include problems with self-management, a poor family-support system, and psychological problems in the child (Table 90-2). In this controlled study, factors that were not found to be associated with an increased risk of death include inhaler abuse, nocturnal asthma, corticosteroid dependence, adrenal suppression, and emotionally triggered asthma attacks [207]. Recently, fatal asthma cases in children have been compared to patients with a history of a life-threatening episode within the previous 3 years, and significant risk factors present in the 6 months preceding death were identified [127] (Table 90-3). Interestingly, severe disease existed in both groups and the factor that distinguished fatal cases from nonfatal controls was having a history of respiratory failure that required intubation. Surprisingly, both groups appeared to re-

ceive similar medical care and both groups disregarded perceived asthma symptoms. There were, however, a number of psychosocial variables that did distinguish between the fatal and control groups (Table 90-4). The association of psychological factors with fatal asthma raises the question of what neural mechanisms might be involved. For example, there is a known cholinergic predominance in the emotional state of hopelessness and despair [126, 161]. Whether subjects at risk for fatal asthma have significantly different neural tone is not clear at this time (Chap. 85).

One additional interesting physiologic variable has been associated with an increased risk for fatal asthma [100]. It appears that persistent small-airway obstruction has been noted much more frequently in outpatients who eventually experience fatal asthma than in similar subjects who do not die from their disease.

The case-control study of deaths from asthma in New Zealand has contributed significantly to our understanding of risk factors for fatal asthma in adults [155, 156, 166, 174, 175, 177, 178]. Physiologic factors associated with an increased risk of death included the presence of more severe asthma, defined by a history of asthma attacks resulting in decreased consciousness or hypercapnia. Psychosocial problems that distinguished fatal cases from hospitalized controls included alcoholism, personality disorders, depression, recent bereavement, and unemployment. Variables that distinguished fatal cases from community controls included a history of hospitalization or an emergency room visit in the preceding year, the need for three or more antiasthma medications, patient noncompliance, a poor medical care score, and not having had objective airflow measurements performed in the preceding year. Other less strongly associated factors linked to death included a lack of appreciation of asthma severity by the patient, their family, and their physician, overreliance on bronchodilator therapy without adequate steroid treatment, and lack of a crisis plan. It is therefore clear that the presence of severe disease in conjunction with a significant psychosocial problem places adults and children with asthma at risk for fatal episodes. It is also quite clear that undertreatment rather than overtreatment with antiasthma medications likely contributes to asthma mortality.

RECOMMENDATIONS

Management guidelines are essential for fatality-prone asthma patients, as subjects tend to grossly underestimate the potential seriousness of their asthma [53]. Attempts at improving self-management have revealed that educational programs are most likely to benefit those with severe disease [77]. Many programs have shown their utility by decreasing emergency room visits and hospitalization rates in children [33, 107, 122, 203] (Chap. 94). Self-management programs utilizing high-dose inhaled corticoste-

Table 90-5. Recommendations for reducing the risks of asthma deaths

1. Identification of the high-risk patient
   a. Recurrent severe attacks
   b. History of respiratory failure and need for mechanical ventilation
   c. Need for frequent emergency treatment
   d. High-risk age bracket—young children and the elderly
   e. Coexisting cardiovascular disease
   f. Coeisting psychiatric disease, i.e., "sad, mad, or bad"
   g. Long-term corticosteroid requirements
   h. Noncompliance or "mal"-compliance with medications
   i. Evidence of asthma "instability," i.e., increased inhaler use, frequent nocturnal exacerbations
2. Education about asthma and markers of exacerbation
3. Use of peak-flow meters
4. Management of psychosocial problems
5. Home plan of therapy for acute attack
6. Aggressive use of antiinflammatory therapy
7. Eliminate or minimize delays in receiving appropriate medical care
8. Avoid inappropriate medications (i.e., sedatives, adrenergic antagonists, etc.)
9. Be aware of potential drug interactions
10. Provide for close follow-up and continuity of care

roids have also been shown to reduce hospitalization and readmission rates in adults [121]. It therefore seems appropriate to initiate antiinflammatory medication early in the course of asthma therapy [8]. Patients at risk must be identified, and include those with a history of a previous life-threatening asthma episodes and subjects with a history of severe asthma associated with psychosocial problems [208].

Specific recommendations for the management of those patients identified at risk of death should include a written action plan for early treatment of exacerbations. Regular follow-up with objective monitoring of the fatality-prone patient is essential. In addition, psychosocial problems need to be addressed and psychotherapy instituted when indicated to hopefully prevent the fatality-prone subject from dying [71, 127, 207]. Recommendations for reducing the risks for asthma deaths are summarized in Table 90-5.

It is clear that the morbidity and mortality from asthma has increased on a worldwide basis in both children and adults. Unfortunately, the exact etiology of this alarming increase is not clear at the present time. The exact relationship between the disturbing race discrepancy and socioeconomic factors is also not established. The possibility that detrimental effects of anti-asthma medications are somehow contributing significantly to increased asthma mortality is of considerable interest and has generated much debate. However, deleterious effects of medical management could certainly contribute to selected cases of asthma death. Whether asthma severity is increasing is debatable. However, the marked increases in antiasthma medication use and the hospitalization rate suggest that there may indeed be some increase in asthma severity.

Regardless of the etiology of increasing asthma mortality, it seems obvious that we must identify patients at risk and attempt to better inform the public about the potential seriousness of this disease.

REFERENCES

1. Alexander, H. L. A historical account of death from asthma. *J. Allergy* 34:305, 1963.
2. Al-Hillawi, A. H., Hayward, R., and Johnson, N. M. Incidence of cardiac arrhythmias in patients taking slow release salbutamol and slow release terbutaline for asthma. *Br. Med. J.* 288:367, 1984.
3. Allon, M., Dunlay, R., and Copkney, C. Nebulized albuterol for acute hyperkalemia in patients on hemodialysis. *Ann. Intern. Med.* 110:426, 1989.
4. Anderson, H. R., Bailey, P., and West, S. Trends in the hospital care of acute childhood asthma, 1970–8: a regional study. *Br. Med. J.* 281:1191, 1980.
5. Aviado, D. M. Toxicity of aerosol propellants in the respiratory and circulatory systems. IX. Summary of the most toxic: trichlorofluromethane (FC11). *Toxicology* 3:311, 1975.
6. Banner, A. S., et al. Arrhythmogenic effects of orally administered bronchodilators. *Arch. Intern. Med.* 139:434, 1979.
7. Barger, L. W., et al. Further investigation into the recent increase in asthma death rates: a review of 41 asthma deaths in Oregon in 1982. *Ann. Allergy* 60:31, 1988.
8. Barnes, P. J. A new approach to the treatment of asthma. *N. Engl. J. Med.* 321:1517, 1989.
9. Baughman, R. P., Polysongsany, Y., and James, W. A comparative study of aerosolized terbutaline and subcutaneously administered epinephrine in the treatment of acute bronchial asthma. *Ann. Allergy* 53:131, 1984.
10. Benatar, S. R. Fatal asthma. *N. Engl. J. Med.* 314:423, 1986.
11. Bethel, R. A., et al. Interaction of sulfur dioxide and dry cold air in causing bronchoconstriction in asthmatic subjects. *J. Appl. Physiol.* 57:419, 1984.
12. Birkhead, G., et al. Investigation of a cluster of deaths of adolescents from asthma: evidence implicating inadequate treatment and poor patient adherence with medications. *J. Allergy Clin, Immunol.* 84:484, 1989.
13. Blair, H. Natural history of childhood asthma. *Arch. Dis. Child.* 52:613, 1977.
14. Bosco, L. A., et al. Asthma drug therapy trends in the United States, 1972 to 1985. *J. Allergy Clin. Immunol.* 80:398, 1987.
15. Bousquet, J., et al. Asthma mortality in France. *J. Allergy Clin. Immunol.* 80:389, 1987.
16. Bresnick, E., Woodward, W. K., and Sageman, C. B. Fatal reactions to the intravenous administration of aminophylline. *JAMA* 136:397, 1948.
17. British Thoracic Association. Death from asthma in two regions of England. *Br. Med. J.* 285:1251, 1982.
18. British Thoracic Association. Accuracy of death certificates in bronchial asthma. *Thorax* 39:505, 1984.
19. British Thoracic Society. Comparison of atopic and non-atopic patients dying of asthma. *Br. J. Dis. Chest* 81:30, 1987.
20. Brooks, S. M., Weiss, M. A., and Bernstein, I. L. Reactive airways dysfunction syndrome (RADS): persistent asthma syndrome after high level irritant exposures. *Chest* 88:376, 1985.
21. Brown, J. E., McLead, A. A., and Shand, D. G. Evidence for cardiac adrenoreceptors in man. *Clin. Pharmacol. Ther.* 33:424, 1983.
22. Buch, J., and Bundgaard, A. Cardiovascular effects of intramuscular or inhaled terbutaline in asthmatics. *Acta Pharmacol. Toxicol.* 54:183, 1984.
23. Buist, A. S. Asthma mortality: what have we learned? *J. Allergy Clin. Immunol.* 84:275, 1989.
24. Burney, P. Asthma deaths in England and Wales 1931–85; evidence for a true increase in asthma mortality. *J. Epidemiol. Comm. Health* 42:316, 1988.
25. Butler, J. A., et al. Health insurance coverage and physician use among children with disabilities: findings from probability samples in five metropolitan areas. *Pediatrics* 79:89, 1987.
26. Camarata, S. J., et al. Cardiac arrest in the critically ill, I: a study of the predisposing causes in 132 patients. *Circulation* 44:688, 1971.
27. Canepa-Anson, R., Dawson, J. R., and Frankl, W. Beta-2 adrenoceptor agonists—pharmacology, metabolic effects, and arrhythmias. *Eur. Heart J.* 3(suppl. D):129, 1982.
28. Cardell, B. S., and Pearson, R. S. B. Death in asthmatics. *Thorax* 14:341, 1959.
29. Carman, P. G., and Landau, L. I. Increased pediatric admissions with asthma in Western Australia—a problem of diagnosis? *Med. J. Aust.* 152:23, 1990.
30. Carswell, F. Thirty deaths from asthma. *Arch. Dis. Child.* 60:25, 1985.
31. Cebelin, M. S., and Hirsch, C. S. Human stress cardiomyopathy. Myocardial lesions in victims of homicidal assaults without internal injuries. *Hum. Pathol.* 11:123, 1980.
32. Chapman, K. R., et al. Hemodynamic effects of an inhaled beta-2 agonist. *Clin. Pharmacol. Ther.* 35:762, 1984.
33. Clark, N. M., et al. The impact of health education on frequency and

cost of health care use by low income children with asthma. *J. Allergy Clin. Immunol.* 78:108, 1986.
34. Cockcroft, D. W. Mechanisms of perennial allergic asthma. *Lancet* 2:253, 1983.
35. Cochrane, G. M., and Clark, T. J. H. A survey of asthma mortality in patients between the ages of 35 and 64 in the Greater London Hospitals in 1971. *Thorax* 30:300, 1975.
36. Coleman, J. J., et al. Cardiac arrhythmias during the combined use of β-adrenergic agonist drugs and theophylline. *Chest* 90:45, 1986.
37. Collins, J. M., et al. The cardiotoxicity of isoprenaline during hypoxia. *Br. J. Pharmacol.* 36:35, 1969.
38. Conradson, T., et al. Arrhythmogenicity from combined bronchodilator therapy in patients with obstructive lung disease and concomitant ischemic heart disease. *Chest* 91:5, 1987.
39. Conwry, S. P., and Littlewood, J. M. Admissions to hospital with asthma. *Arch. Dis. Child.* 60:636, 1985.
40. Crane, J. et al. Prescribed fenoterol and death from asthma in New Zealand, 1981–83: case-control study. *Lancet* 1:917, 1989.
41. Davis, C., and Conolly, M. E. Tachyphylaxis to beta-adrenoceptors agonists in human bronchial smooth muscle: studies in vitro. *Br. J. Clin. Pharmacol.* 10:417, 1980.
42. Doll, R., and Speizer, F. E. A century of asthma deaths in young people. *Br. Med. J.* 3:245, 1968.
43. Doll, R., et al. Increased deaths from asthma. *Br. Med. J.* 1:756, 1967.
44. Dollery, C. T., et al. Blood concentrations in man of fluorinated hydrocarbons after inhalation of pressurized aerosols. *Lancet* 2:1164, 1970.
45. Dollery, C. T., et al. Arterial blood levels of fluorocarbons in asthmatic patients following use of pressurized aerosols. *Clin. Pharmacol. Ther.* 15:59, 1974.
46. Douglas, E. M., Hillier, T., and Johnson, I. C. Pressurized aerosols in asthma. *Br. Med. J.* 2:53, 1967.
47. Dowse, G. K., et al. The association between *Dermatophagoides* mites and the increasing prevalence of asthma in village communities within the Papua New Guinea highlands. *J. Allergy Clin. Immunol.* 75:75, 1985.
48. Drislane, F. W., et al. Myocardial contraction band lesions in patients with fatal asthma: possible neurocardiologic mechanisms. *Am. Rev. Respir. Dis.* 135:498, 1987.
49. Dunnill, M. S., Massarella, G. R., and Anderson, J. A. A comparison of the quantitative anatomy of the bronchi in normal subjects, in status asthmaticus, in chronic bronchitis, and in emphysema. *Thorax* 24:176, 1969.
50. Eason, J., and Markowe, H. L. J. Controlled investigation of deaths from asthma in hospitals in the North East Thames region. *Br. Med. J.* 294:1255, 1987.
51. Edelson, J. D., and Rebuck, A. S. The clinical assessment of severe asthma. *Arch. Intern. Med.* 145:321, 1985.
52. Eidelman, D. H., et al. Combination of theophylline and salbutamol for arrhythmias in severe COPD. *Chest* 91:808, 1987.
53. Ellis, M. E., and Friend, J. A. R. How well do asthma clinic patients understand their asthma? *Br. J. Dis. Chest* 79:43, 1985.
54. Evans, R., III. Recent observations reflecting increases in mortality from asthma. *J. Allergy Clin. Immunol.* 80:377, 1987.
55. Evans, R., III, et al. National trends in the morbidity and mortality of asthma in the U.S. *Chest* 91(suppl.):65S, 1987.
56. Eriksson, C. E., Writer, S. L., and Vestal, R. E. Theophylline-induced alterations in cardiac electrophysiology in patients with chronic obstructive pulmonary disease. *Am. Rev. Respir. Dis.* 135:322, 1987.
57. Fraser, P. M., et al. The circumstances preceding death from asthma in young people in 1968 to 1969. *Br. J. Dis. Chest* 65:71, 1971.
58. Friday, G. A., and Fireman, P. Morbidity and mortality of asthma. *Pediatr. Clin. North Am.* 35:1149, 1988.
59. Gandevia, B. The changing pattern of mortality from asthma in Australia. *Med. J. Aust.* 1:747, 1968.
60. Gandevia, B. Pressurized sympathomimetic aerosols and their lack of relationship to asthma mortality in Australia. *Med. J. Aust.* 1:273, 1973.
61. Ganote, C. E. Contraction band necrosis and irreversible myocardial injury. *J. Mol. Cell Cardiol.* 15:67, 1983.
62. Garriott, J., and Petty, C. S. Death from inhalant abuse: toxicological and pathological evaluation of 34 cases. *Clin. Toxicol.* 16:305, 1980.
63. Gelber, L., et al. Specific IgE ab and exposure to cat and cockroach allergens as risk factors for acute asthma. *J. Allergy Clin. Immunol.* 87:376a., 1991.
64. Gergen, P. J., Mullally, D. I., and Evans, R., III. National survey of prevalence of asthma among children in the United States, 1976 to 1980. *Pediatrics* 81:1, 1988.
65. Gergen, P. J., and Weiss, K. B. Changing patterns of asthma hospitalization among children: 1979 to 1987. *JAMA* 264:1688, 1990.
66. Gerritsen, J., et al. Change in airway responsiveness to inhaled house dust from childhood to adulthood. *J. Allergy Clin. Immunol.* 85:1083, 1990.
67. Greenberg, M. J., and Pines, A. Pressurized aerosols in asthma. *Br. Med. J.* 1:563, 1967.
68. Hall, K. W., et al. Metabolic abnormalities associated with intentional theophylline overdose. *Ann. Intern. Med.* 101:457, 1984.
69. Hambelton, G., and Shinebourne, E. A. Evaluation of the effects of isoprenaline and salbutamol aerosols on airway obstruction and pulse rates of children with asthma. *Arch. Dis. Child.* 45:766, 1970.
70. Handforth, C. P. Isoproterenol induced myocardial infarction in animals. *Arch. Pathol.* 73:161, 1962.
71. Hargreave, F. E., Dolovich, J., and Newhouse, M. T. The assessment and treatment of asthma: a conference report. *J. Allergy Clin. Immunol.* 85:1098, 1990.
72. Harrison, A. C., et al. Do racial differences in asthma prevalence and severity account for racial differences in asthma admission and mortality rates? *Am. Rev. Respir. Dis.* 133:A176, 1986.
73. Harvey, J. E., and Tattersfield, A. E. Airway response to salbutamol: effect of regular salbutamol inhalations in normal, atopic, and asthmatic subjects. *Thorax* 37:280, 1982.
74. Heitz, A., Schwartz, J., and Velly, J. β-adrenoceptors of the human myocardium: determination of β_1 and β_2 subtypes of radioligand binding. *Br. J. Pharmacol.* 80:711, 1983.
75. Herring, S., et al. The maintenance of pets in allergic families. I. Survey of health beliefs. *Ann. Allergy* 46:24, 1981.
76. Houston, J. C., deNavasquez, S., and Trounce, J. R. A clinical and pathological study of fatal cases of status asthmaticus. *Thorax* 8:207,1953.
77. Howland, J., Bauchner, H., and Adair, R. The impact of pediatric asthma education on morbidity. *Chest* 94:964, 1988.
78. Huber, H. L., and Koessler, K. K. The pathology of bronchial asthma. *Arch. Intern. Med.* 30:689, 1922.
79. Hudgel, D. W., and Weil, J. V. Asthma associated with decreased hypoxic ventilatory drive: a family study. *Ann. Intern. Med.* 80:623, 1974.
80. Imai, M., Yoshida, K., and Kitabatake, M. Mortality from asthma and chronic bronchitis associated with changes in sulfur oxides air pollution. *Arch. Environ. Health* 41:29, 1986.
81. Ingram, R. H., et al. Ventilation-perfusion changes after aerosolized isoproterenol in asthma. *Am. Rev. Respir. Dis.* 101:364, 1970.
82. Inman, W. H. W., and Adelstein, A. M. Rise and fall of asthma mortality in England and Wales in relation to use of pressurized aerosols. *Lancet* 2:279, 1969.
83. Jackson, R. T., et al. Mortality from asthma: a new epidemic in New Zealand. *Br. Med. J.* 285:771, 1982.
84. Jennings, R. B., Reimer, K. A., and Steenberger, C. Myocardial ischemia revisited. The osmolar load, membrane damage, and reperfusion. *J. Mol. Cell Cardiol.* 18:769s, 1986.
85. Joseph, X., et al. Enhancement of cardiotoxic effects of β-adrenergic bronchodilators by aminophylline in experimental animals. *Fund. Appl. Toxicol.* 1:443, 1981.
86. Josephson, G. W., et al. Emergency treatment of asthma: a comparison of two treatment regimens. *JAMA* 242:629, 1979.
87. Josephson, G. W., et al. Cardiac dysrhythmias during the treatment of acute asthma: a comparison of two treatment regimens by a double blind protocol. *Chest* 78:429, 1980.
88. Kang, B. C. Cockroach allergy. *Clin. Rev. Allergy* 8:87, 1990.
89. Karch, S. B., and Billingham, M. E. Myocardial contraction bands revisited. *Hum. Pathol.* 17:9, 1986.
90. Keating, G., et al. Trends in sales of drugs for asthma in New Zealand, Australia, and the United Kingdom, 1975–81. *Br. Med. J.* 289:384, 1984.
91. Kelly, H. W., Menendez, R., and Voyles, W. Lack of significant arrhythmogenicity from chronic theophylline and beta-2-adrenergic combination therapy in asthmatic subjects. *Ann. Allergy* 54:405, 1985.
92. Kelly, H. W., et al. Safety of frequent high dose nebulized terbutaline in children with acute severe asthma. *Ann. Allergy* 64:229, 1990.
93. Kemp, J. P., et al. Concomitant bitolterol mesylate aerosol and theophylline for asthma therapy with 24 hr electrocardiographic monitoring. *J. Allergy Clin. Immunol.* 73:32, 1984.
94. Kendall, M. J., et al. Cardiovascular and metabolic effects of terbutaline. *J. Clin. Hosp. Pharmacol.* 7:31, 1982.
95. Kerrebijn, K. F., van Essen-Zandvliet, E. E. M., and Neijens, H. J. Effect

of long-term treatment with inhaled corticosteroids and beta-agonists on the bronchial responsiveness in children with asthma. *J. Allergy Clin. Immunol.* 79:653, 1987.

96. Kinney, E. L., et al. Ventricular tachycardia after terbutaline. *JAMA* 240: 2247, 1978.

97. Knudson, R. J., and Constantine, H. P. An effect of isoproterenol on ventilation-perfusion in asthmatic versus normal subjects. *J. Appl. Physiol.* 22:402, 1967.

98. Korsgaard, J. Mite asthma and residency: a case-control study on the impact of exposure to house-dust mites in dwellings. *Am. Rev. Respir. Dis.* 128:231, 1983.

99. Kraan, J., et al. Changes in bronchial hyperreactivity induced by 4 weeks of treatment with antiasthmatic drugs in patients with allergic asthma: a comparison between budesonide and terbutaline. *J. Allergy Clin. Immunol.* 76:628, 1985.

100. Kravis, L. P. An analysis of fifteen childhood asthma fatalities. *J. Allergy Clin. Immunol.* 80:467, 1987.

101. Kravis, L. P., and Kolski, G. B. Unexpected death in childhood asthma: a review of 13 deaths in ambulatory patients. *Am. J. Dis. Child.* 13a:558, 1985.

102. Kurg, M., White, J. R., and Burki, N. K. The effect of subcutaneously administered terbutaline on serum potassium in asymptomatic adult asthmatics. *Am. Rev. Respir. Dis.* 129:329, 1984.

103. Kurland, G., Williams, J., and Lewiston, N. J. Fatal myocardial toxicity during continuous infusion of intravenous isoproterenol therapy of asthma. *J. Allergy Clin. Immunol.* 63:407, 1979.

104. Laaban, J. P., et al. Cardiac arrhythmias during the combined use of intravenous aminophylline and terbutaline in status asthmaticus. *Chest* 94:496, 1988.

105. Laennec, R. T. H. Treatise on diseases of the chest and mediate auscultation (translated by John Forbes). London, 1834.

106. Levine, J. L., Michael, J. R., and Guarnier, T. Multifocal arterial tachycardia: a theophylline induced rhythm. *Lancet* 1:12, 1985.

107. Lewis, C. E., et al. A randomized trial of A.C.T. (asthma care training) for kids. *Pediatrics* 74:478, 1984.

108. Lin, C., et al. Arrhythmogenic effects of theophylline in human atrial tissue. *Int. J. Cardiol.* 17:289, 1987.

109. Lind, P., et al. The prevalence of indoor allergens in the Baltimore area: house dust-mite and animal-dander antigens measured by immunochemical techniques. *J. Allergy Clin. Immunol.* 80:541, 1987.

110. Littner, M. R., et al. Double-blind comparison of acute effects of inhaled albuterol, isoproterenol, and placebo or cardiopulmonary function and gas exchange in asthmatic children. *Ann. Allergy* 50:309, 1983.

111. Lloyd, P. R., Covelli, H. D., and Hill, J. C. Dysrhythmic effects of combined theophylline and beta agonist therapy in patients with severe obstructive lung disease. *Chest* 86:282, 1984.

112. Lockett, M. F. Dangerous effects of isoprenaline in myocardial failure. *Lancet* 2:104, 1963.

113. MacDonald, J. B., Seaton, A., and Williams, D. A. Asthma deaths in Cardiff 1963–74: 90 deaths outside hospital. *Br. Med. J.* 1:1493, 1976.

114. MacDonald, J. B., et al. Asthma deaths in Cardiff 1963–74: 53 deaths in hospital. *Br. Med. J.* 1:721, 1976.

115. Mak, H., et al. Prevalence of asthma and health service utilization of asthmatic children in an inner city. *J. Allergy Clin. Immunol.* 70:367, 1982.

116. Mao, Y., et al. Increased rates of illness and death from asthma in Canada. *Can. Med. Assoc. J.* 137:620, 1987.

117. Mao, Y., et al. Seasonality in epidemics of asthma mortality and hospital admission rates, Ontario, 1979–86. *Can. J. Public Health* 81:226, 1990.

118. Marchlinski, F. E., and Miller, J. M. Atrial arrhythmias exacerbated by theophylline: a response to verapamil and evidence for triggered activity in man. *Chest* 88:931, 1985.

119. Mascia, A., et al. Mortality versus improvement in severe chronic asthma: physiologic and psychologic factors. *Ann. Allergy* 62:311, 1989.

120. Matson, J. R., Loughlin, G. M., and Strunk, R. C. Myocardial ischemia complicating the use of isoproterenol in asthmatic children. *J. Pediatr.* 92:776, 1978.

121. Mayo, P. H., Richman, J., and Harris, H. W. Results of a program to reduce admissions for adult asthma. *Ann. Intern. Med.* 112:864, 1990.

122. McNabb, W. L., et al. Self-management education of children with asthma: AIR WISE. *Am. J. Public Health* 75:219, 1985.

123. McWhorter, W. P., Polis, M. A., and Kaslow, R. A. Occurrence, predictors, and consequences of adult asthma in NHANESI and follow-up survey. *Am. Rev. Respir. Dis.* 139:721, 1989.

124. Mellis, C. M., and Phelan, P. D. Asthma deaths in children—a continuing problem. *Thorax* 32:29, 1977.

125. Merrill, G. A. Aminophylline deaths. *JAMA* 123:1115, 1943.

126. Miller, B. O. Depression and asthma: a potentially lethal mixture. *J. Allergy Clin. Immunol.* 80:481, 1987.

127. Miller, B. O., and Strunk, R. C. Circumstances surrounding the deaths of children due to asthma. *Am. J. Dis. Child.* 143:1294, 1989.

128. Mitchell, E. Increasing prevalence of asthma in children. *N. Z. Med. J.* 96:463, 1983.

129. Mitchell, E. A. International trends in hospital admission rates for asthma. *Arch. Dis. Child.* 60:376, 1985.

130. Mitchell, E. A., and Elliott, R. B. Hospital admissions for asthma in children: a prospective study. *N. Z. Med. J.* 94:331, 1981.

131. Mitchell, E. A., et al. Why are hospital admission and mortality rates for childhood asthma higher in New Zealand than in the United Kingdom? *Thorax* 45:176, 1990.

132. Molfino, N. A., et al. Respiratory arrest in near-fatal asthma. *N. Engl. J. Med.* 324:285, 1991.

133. Murray, A. B., Ferguson, A. C., and Morrison, B. J. The frequency and severity of cat allergy vs dog allergy in atopic children. *J. Allergy Clin. Immunol.* 72:145, 1983.

134. Nayler, W. G. Some observations on the pharmacological effects of salbutamol, with particular reference to the cardiovascular system. *Postgrad. Med. J.* 47(suppl.):16, 1971.

135. Neville, A., et al. Metabolic effects of salbutamol: comparison of aerosol and intravenous administration. *Br. Med. J.* 1:413, 1977.

136. Neville, E., et al. Nebulized salbutamol and angina. *Br. Med. J.* 285:796, 1982.

137. Nguyen, M. T., Patterson, K., and Sly, R. M. Causes of death from asthma in children. *Ann. Allergy* 55:448, 1985.

138. Nicklas, R., et al. Concomitant use of beta adrenergic agonists and methylxanthines. *J. Allergy Clin. Immunol.* 73:20, 1984.

139. O'Hollaren, M. T., et al. Exposure to an aeroallergen as a possible precipitating factor in respiratory arrest in young patients with asthma. *N. Engl. J. Med.* 324:359, 1991.

140. Olson, K. R., et al. Theophylline overdose: acute single ingestion versus chronic repeated overmedication. *Am. J. Emerg. Med.* 3:386, 1985.

141. Ormerod, L. P., and Stableforth, D. E. Asthma mortality in Birmingham 1975–7: 53 deaths. *Br. Med. J.* 280:687, 1980.

142. Osler, W. *The Principles and Practice of Medicine.* Edinburgh and London: Young J. Pentland, 1892, P. 498.

143. Paloncek, F. P., and Rodvold, K. A. Evaluation of theophylline overdoses and toxicities. *Ann. Emerg. Med.* 17:135, 1988.

144. Patel, A. K., Skatrud, J. B., and Thomson, J. H. Cardiac arrhythmias due to oral aminophylline in patients with chronic obstructive pulmonary disease. *Chest* 80:661, 1981.

145. Pearce, N., et al. Case-control study of prescribed fenoterol and death from asthma in New Zealand, 1977–81. *Thorax* 45:170, 1990.

146. Perry, G. B., et al. Effects of particulate air pollution on asthmatics. *Am. J. Public Health* 73:50, 1983.

147. Platts-Mills, T. A. E., and Chapman, M. D. Dust mites: immunology, allergic disease, and environmental control. *J. Allergy Clin. Immunol.* 80:755, 1987.

148. Platts-Mills, T. A. E., et al. Reduction of bronchial hyperreactivity during prolonged allergen avoidance. *Lancet* 2:675, 1982.

149. Platts-Mills, T. A. E., et al. Seasonal variation in dust mite and grass-pollen allergens in dust from houses of patients with asthma. *J. Allergy Clin. Immunol.* 79:781, 1987.

150. Platts-Mills, T., et al. Epidemiology of adult asthma in an emergency room (ER). *J. Allergy Clin. Immunol.* 85:237a, 1990.

151. Position Statement, Committee on Drugs, the American Academy of Allergy and Immunology. Adverse effects and complications of treatment with beta-adrenergic agonist drugs. *J. Allergy Clin. Immunol.* 75:443, 1985.

152. Poynter, D., and Spurling, N. W. Some cardiac effects of beta-adrenergic stimulants in animals. *Postgrad. Med. J.* 47(suppl.):21, 1971.

153. Pride, N. B. Physiology of Asthma. In: T. J. H. Clark, and S. Godfrey (eds.), *Asthma* (2nd ed.). London: Chapman and Hall, 1983, P. 12.

154. Rackemann, F. M., and Edwards, M. C. Asthma in children. A follow up study of 688 patients after an interval of 20 years. *N. Engl. J. Med.* 246: 815, 858, 1952.

155. Rea, H. H., et al. A case-control study of deaths from asthma. *Thorax* 41:833, 1986.

156. Rea, H. H., et al. Lessons from the national asthma mortality study: circumstances surrounding death. *N. Z. Med. J.* 100:10, 1987.
157. Rebuck, A. S., and Read, J. Assessment and management of severe asthma. *Am. J. Med.* 51:788, 1971.
158. Rees, H. A., Millar, J. S., and Donald, K. W. A study of the clinical course and arterial blood gas tensions of patients in status asthmaticus. *Q. J. Med.* 37:541, 1968.
159. Repsher, L. H., et al. Assessment of tachyphylaxis following prolonged therapy with inhaled albuterol aerosol. *Chest* 85:34, 1984.
160. Richards, W., and Patrick, J. R. Death from asthma in children. *Am. J. Dis. Child.* 110:4, 1965.
161. Richter, C. P. On the phenomenon of sudden death in animals and man. *Psychosom. Med.* 19:191, 1957.
162. Riding, W. D., Dinda, P., and Chatterjee, S. S. The bronchodilator and cardiac effects of five pressure-packed aerosols in asthma. *Br. J. Dis. Chest* 64:37, 1970.
163. Robberecht, P., et al. The human heart beta-adrenoreceptors. I. Heterogeneity of the binding sites: presence of 50% beta$_1$ and 50% beta$_2$-adrenergic receptors. *Mol. Pharmacol.* 24:169, 1983.
164. Robbins, J. J. Death from asthma. *Br. Med. J.* 2:365, 1968.
165. Robin, E. D. Death from bronchial asthma. *Chest* 93:614, 1988.
166. Rothwell, R. P. G., et al. Lessons from the national mortality study: deaths in hospitals. *N. Z. Med. J.* 100:199, 1987.
167. Rubinfeld, A. R., and Pain, M. C. Perception of asthma. *Lancet* 1:882, 1976.
168. Sackner, M. A., et al. Hemodynamic effects of epinephrine and terbutaline in normal man. *Chest* 68:616, 1975.
169. Santo, M., Sidi, Y., and Pinkhas, Y. Acute myocardial infarction following intravenous salbutamol. *S. Afr. Med. J.* 58:394, 1980.
170. Schrenk, H. H., Heiman, H., and Clayton, G. D. Air pollution in Donora, Pennsylvania: epidemiology of the unusual smog episode of October, 1948. *Public Health Bull.* 1949, P. 306.
171. Sears, M. Fatal asthma: a perspective. *Immunol. Allergy Pract.* 10:25a, 1988.
172. Sears, M. R., and Beaglehole, R. Asthma morbidity and mortality: New Zealand. *J. Allergy Clin. Immunol.* 80:383, 1987.
173. Sears, M. R., O'Donnell, T. V., and Rea, H. H. Asthma mortality and socioeconomic status. *N. Z. Med. J.* 98:765, 1985.
174. Sears, M. R., and Rea, H. H. Patients at risk for dying of asthma. New Zealand experience. *J. Allergy Clin. Immunol.* 80:477, 1987.
175. Sears, M. R., et al. Asthma mortality in New Zealand: a two year national study. *N. Z. Med. J.* 98:271, 1985.
176. Sears, M. R., et al. Accuracy of certification of deaths due to asthma. *Am. J. Epidemio.* 124:1004, 1986.
177. Sears, M. R., et al. Asthma mortality: comparison between New Zealand and England. *Br. Med. J.* 293:1342, 1986.
178. Sears, M. R., et al. Deaths from asthma in New Zealand. *Arch. Dis. Child.* 61:6, 1986.
179. Sears, M. R., et al. 75 deaths in asthmatics prescribed home nebulizers. *Br. Med. J.* 294:477, 1987.
180. Sears, M. R., et al. Regular inhaled beta-agonist treatment in bronchial asthma. *Lancet* 336:1391, 1990.
181. Sessler, C. N., and Cohen, M. D. Cardiac arrhythmias during theophylline toxicity: a prospective continuous electrocardiographic study. *Chest* 98: 672, 1990.
182. Sessler, O. N., Cohen, M., and Garnett, A. R. Cardiac arrhythmias during theophylline toxicity. *Chest* 94(suppl.):8, 1988.
183. Shannon, M., and Lovejoy, F. H. The influence of age vs peak serum concentration on life-threatening events after chronic theophylline intoxication. *Arch. Intern. Med.* 150:2045, 1990.
184. Shibasaki, M., et al. Relation between frequency of asthma and IgE antibody levels against *Dermatophagoides farinae* and total serum IgE levels in school children. *J. Allergy Clin. Immunol.* 82:86, 1988.
185. Shim, C. S., Scher, S. M., and Williams, M. H. Effect of bronchodilator agents on arrhythmia. *NY State J. Med.* 76:1973, 1976.
186. Siegel, S. C. History of asthma deaths from antiquity. *J. Allergy Clin. Immunol.* 80:458, 1987.
187. Siemons, L. J., and Parizel, G. Prolonged runs of ventricular tachycardia as a complication of theophylline intoxication: report of a case. *Acta Cardiol.* 6:457, 1986.
188. Sly, R. M. Increases in deaths from asthma. *Ann. Allergy* 53:20, 1984.
189. Sly, R. M. Mortality from asthma 1979–84. *J. Allergy Clin. Immunol.* 82: 705, 1988.
190. Sly, R. M. Mortality from asthma in children, 1979–84. *Ann. Allergy* 60: 433, 1988.
191. Sly, R. M. Mortality from asthma. *N. Engl. Reg. Allergy Proc.* 7:425, 1986.
192. Sly, R. M. Mortality from asthma. *J. Allergy Clin. Immunol.* 84:421, 1989.
193. Sly, R. M., and O'Donnell, R. Regional distribution of deaths from asthma. *Ann. Allergy* 62:347, 1989.
194. Smith, T. F., et al. Natural exposure and serum antibodies to house dust mite of mite-allergic children with asthma in Atlanta. *J. Allergy Clin. Immunol.* 76:782, 1985.
195. Snider, G. L., and Laguarda, R. Albuterol and isoproterenol aerosols: a controlled study of effect in asthmatic patients. *JAMA* 221:682, 1972.
196. So, S. Y., et al. Rising asthma mortality in young males in Hong Kong, 1976–85. *Respir. Med.* 84:457, 1990.
197. Speizer, F. E., Doll, R., and Heaf, P. Observations on recent increase in mortality from asthma. *Br. Med. J.* 1:335, 1968.
198. Speizer, F. E., et al. An investigation into use of drugs preceding death from asthma. *Br. Med. J.* 1:339, 1968.
199. Sporik, R., Platts-Mills, T. A. E., and Cogswell, J. J. Exposure and sensitization of children admitted to hospital with asthma to house dust mite allergen (Der pI). *J. Allergy Clin. Immunol.* 87:606a, 1991.
200. Sporik, R., et al. Exposure to house-dust mite allergen (Der p I) and the development of asthma in childhood. *N. Engl. J. Med.* 323:502, 1990.
201. Spotnitz, M. The significance of Yokohama asthma. *Am. Rev. Respir. Dis.* 92:371, 1965.
202. Stableforth, D. E. Asthma mortality and physician competence. *J. Allergy Clin. Immunol.* 80:463, 1987.
203. Standenmayer, H., Harris, P. S., and Selner, J. C. Evaluation of a self-help education-exercise program for asthmatic children and their parents: six-month follow-up. *J. Asthma* 74:505, 1981.
204. Stewart, C. J., and Nunn, A. J. Are asthma mortality rates changing? *Br. J. Dis. Chest* 79:229, 1985.
205. Stolley, P. D. Asthma mortality: why the United States was spared an epidemic of deaths due to asthma. *Am. Rev. Respir. Dis.* 105:883, 1972.
206. Strubelt, O., et al. On the pathogenesis of cardiac necrosis induced by theophylline and caffeine. *Acta Pharmacol. Toxicol.* 39:383, 1976.
207. Strunk, R. C. Asthma deaths in childhood: identification of patients at risk and intervention. *J. Allergy Clin. Immunol.* 80:472, 1987.
208. Strunk, R. C. Identification of the fatality-prone subject with asthma. *J. Allergy Clin. Immunol.* 83:477, 1989.
209. Strunk, R. C., et al. Physiologic and psychological characteristics associated with death due to asthma in children. *JAMA* 254:1193, 1985.
210. Tandon, M. K. Cardiopulmonary effects of fenoterol and salbutamol aerosols. *Chest* 77:429, 1980.
211. Taniguchi, A., Ohe, T., and Shimorura, K. Theophylline-induced ventricular tachycardia in a patient with chronic lung disease: sensitivity to verapamil. *Chest* 96:958, 1989.
212. Tashkin, D. P., et al. Subsensitization of beta-adrenoceptors in airways and lymphocytes of healthy and asthmatic subjects. *Am. Rev. Respir. Dis.* 125:185, 1982.
213. Todd, G. L., et al. Experimental catecholamine-induced myocardial necrosis, I. Morphology, quantification and regional distribution of acute contraction band lesions. *J. Mol. Cell Cardiol.* 17:317, 1985.
214. Trousseau, A. Lectures on clinical medicine (translated by Bazire). London, 1867.
215. Turner-Warwick, M. On observing patterns of airflow obstruction in chronic asthma. *Br. J. Dis. Chest* 71:73, 1977.
216. Ullman, A., Hedner, J., and Svedmyr, N. Inhaled salmeterol and salbutamol in asthmatic patients. An evaluation of asthma symptoms and the possible development of tachyphylaxis. *Am. Rev. Respir. Dis.* 142:571, 1990.
217. Urthaler, F., and Janes, T. N. Both direct and neurally mediated components of the chronotropic actions of aminophylline. *Chest* 70:24, 1976.
218. Van Metre, T. E., et al. Dose of cat (*Felis domesticus*) allergen I (Fel d I) that induces asthma. *J. Allergy Clin. Immunol.* 78:62, 1986.
219. Vathenen, A. S., et al. Rebound increase in bronchial responsiveness after treatment with inhaled terbutaline. *Lancet* 1:554, 1988.
220. Vestal, R. E., et al. Effect of intravenous aminophylline on plasma levels of catecholamines and related cardiovascular and metabolic responses in man. *Circulation* 67:162, 1983.
221. Wasserfallen, J.-B., et al. Sudden asphyxic asthma: a distinct entity? *Am. Rev. Respir. Dis.* 142:108, 1990.
222. Weber, R. W., Smith, J. A., and Nelson, H. S. Aerosolized terbutaline in asthmatics: development of subsensitivity with long-term administration. *J. Allergy Clin. Immunol.* 70:417, 1982.

223. Weiss, K. B. Seasonal trends in U.S. asthma hospitalizations and mortality. *JAMA* 263:2323, 1990.

224. Weiss, K. B., and Wagener, D. K. Changing patterns of asthma mortality. Identifying target populations at high risk. *JAMA* 264:1683, 1990.

225. Weiss, K. B., and Wagener, D. K. Geographic variations in asthma mortality: small area analyses of excess mortality, 1981–1985. *Am. J. Epidemiol.* 132(suppl.):107, 1990.

226. Westerman, D. E., et al. Identification of the high-risk asthmatic patient: experience with 39 patients undergoing ventilation for status asthmaticus. *Am. J. Med.* 66:565, 1979.

227. Westling, H. Circulatory effects of β₂ receptor agonists in man. *Acta Pharmacol. Toxicol.* 44(suppl. 2):36, 1979.

228. Wexlar, B. C., Judd, J. T., and Kittinger, G. W. Myocardial necrosis induced by isoproterenol in rats. *Angiology* 19:665, 1968.

229. Whitehurst, V. E., et al. Cardiotoxic effects in rats and rabbits treated with terbutaline alone and in combination with aminophylline. *J. Am. Coll. Toxicol.* 2:147, 1983.

230. Whitsett, T. L., Manion, C. V., and Wilson, M. F. Cardiac, pulmonary, and neuromuscular effects of clenbuterol and terbutaline compared with placebo. *Br. J. Clin. Pharmacol.* 12:195, 1981.

231. Wilson, J. D., Sutherland, D. C., and Thomas, A. C. Has the change to beta-agonists combined with oral theophylline increased cases of fatal asthma? *Lancet* 1:1235, 1981.

232. Winsor, T., et al. Intramyocardial diversion of coronary blood flow: effects of isoproterenol-induced subendocardial ischemia. *Microvasc. Res.* 9:261, 1975.

233. Wissow, L. S., et al. Poverty, race, and hospitalization for childhood asthma. *Am. J. Public Health* 78:777, 1988.

234. Woolcock, A. J., et al. The prevalence of asthma in the South Fore people of Papua New Guinea. A method for field studies of bronchial reactivity. *Eur. J. Respir. Dis.* 64:571, 1983.

235. Spitzer, W. O., et al. The use of β-agonists and the risk of death and near death from asthma. *N. Engl. J. Med.* 326:501, 1992.

236. Molfino, N. A., et al. The fatality-prone asthmatic patient. Follow-up study after near-fatal attacks. *Chest* 101:621, 1992.

237. Mackay, T. W., et al. Factors affecting asthma mortality in Scotland. *Scott. Med. J.* 37:5, 1992.

238. Juel, K., and Pedersen, P. A. Increasing asthma mortality in Denmark 1969–88 not a result of a changed coding practice. *Ann. Allergy* 68:180, 1992.

239. Horwitz, R. I., et al. Clinical complexity and epidemiologic uncertainty in case-control research. Fenoterol and asthma management. *Chest* 100:1586, 1991.

Complications

Guy W. Soo Hoo
Silverio Santiago

91

There are myriad complications associated with asthma. These range from trivial and unusual to universal problems and involve both the pulmonary and extrapulmonary systems. This diversity can be best approached by grouping complications into four broad categories: (1) those related to the pathophysiology of asthma, (2) those associated with the therapy of asthma, (3) other conditions complicated by asthma, (4) and the long-term sequelae of asthma. While there are no complications specific to asthma, awareness of problems compromising asthma and its management is important.

COMPLICATIONS RELATED TO THE PATHOPHYSIOLOGY OF ASTHMA

Reversible bronchoconstriction is the hallmark of asthma. Intense inflammatory responses that contribute to airway caliber narrowing and occlusion [17, 96] (Fig. 91-1) may be coupled with the inhalation of allergens and other irritants that provoke asthma to stimulate cough receptors and induce coughing (Table 91-1. This may be the only manifestation of asthma [54, 95]. Intrathoracic pressures approaching 300 mmHg can be generated during a cough, with a multitude of complications including rectus abdominis muscle rupture, rib fractures, pneumomediastinum, pneumothoraces, and syncope [95, 186] (see also Chap. 50).

Increasing airway obstruction promotes air trapping and hyperinflation; the functional residual capacity may double. Continued inspiratory muscle activity during expiration and expiratory glottic constriction [51, 128, 134] also contribute to lung hyperinflation, which is the most common roentgenographic finding during acute episodes of asthma (about 70%) [63, 72, 173]. Obstruction from mucoid impaction and secondary atelectasis are often associated with allergic bronchopulmonary aspergillosis, but have been reported in asthmatic patients without the disorder [11, 173]. The incidence of segmental and subsegmental atelectasis revealed by chest roentgenograms varies from 3 to 11 percent and appears more frequently in children, possibly related to incomplete development of collateral ventilation. The right lung and particularly the right middle lobe appear most susceptible to mucous plugging and atelectasis [63, 139]. Mucous plugging and atelectasis are usually controlled with respiratory therapy maneuvers, but can occasionally be life-threatening [70, 123], necessitating bronchoscopic removal (Fig. 91-2). Microatelectasis may also contribute to increases in elastic recoil and produce a reversible restrictive defect shown by pulmonary function testing [93].

Continued airways obstruction produces further hyperinflation and increased alveolar pressures that can cause alveolar rupture and dissection of air throughout the thorax. Pneumothoraces and pneumomediastinum are not uncommon complications of asthma; they occur in up to 5 percent of asthmatic patients and can be clinically silent [11, 24, 63, 72, 173] (Fig. 91-3). Prompt recognition of the signs and symptoms associated with barotrauma is important for therapeutic intervention. Less common manifestations of barotrauma include subcutaneous emphysema, encysted pneumothorax, pneumopericardium, and pneumoperitoneum [14, 73, 85, 100, 111, 153]. Barotrauma is generally self-limiting, but some cases require decompression.

Chest wall changes have also been observed during episodes of asthma. A rocking motion of the sternum has been observed during severe obstruction, the result of inward motion of the lower rib cage secondary to diaphragmatic contraction and outward motion of the upper rib cage secondary to accessory muscle contraction [181]. Worsening airflow obstruction also necessitates the generation of large negative intrathoracic pressures to maintain adequate transpulmonary pressures at higher lung volumes. This also translates into an increased left ventricular afterload, which may facilitate the development of pulmonary edema [215]. Adaptation to chronic airflow obstruction may increase inspiratory and expiratory muscle endurance [141].

There appears to be a subset of patients who experience rapidly progressive airways obstruction and asphyxia. Clinically, there appears to be a male predominance, with patients presenting with a severe mixed acidosis, marked hypercapnia, and silent chest examination (no wheezing). A distinguishing characteristic appears to be the paucity of airway secretions or mucous plugs traditionally observed at autopsy in patients who die from asthma. These patients have also been observed to recover more rapidly than a comparison cohort. Inflammation is not the predominant pathophysiologic determinant of this airway obstruction. Instead, bronchospasm appears to be the primary pathogenic mechanism [182, 197, 234]. Exposure to the spores of *Alternaria alternata* has been implicated as a possible precipitant of sudden respiratory arrest in some asthmatics [155]. This underscores the importance of identifying potential etiologic agents or other precipitating factors in order to modify their impact on the susceptible asthmatic patient [140].

There are a number of extrapulmonary complications associated with asthma. Although respiratory alkalosis and acidosis are the predominant acid-base disorders, up to 25 percent of patients may present with a metabolic acidosis secondary to lactic acidosis [4, 9, 148]. The cause of lactic acidosis is multifactorial and includes stimulation of lactate production by respiratory alkalosis and lactate production from both overburdened respiratory muscles and tissue hypoxia. Lactic acidosis is also an indirect marker of the severity of asthma and may portend impending respiratory failure. A non–anion gap metabolic acidosis with normal lactate levels has also been described and has been attributed to renal bicarbonate excretion as a response to respiratory alkalosis during the early stages of asthma [156].

There have been a number of cardiac complications described with asthma. Silent myocardial infarction during episodes of

Table 91-1. Complications related to pathophysiologic changes in asthma

Pathophysiologic event	Complication	Comments
PULMONARY		
1. Airway inflammation and irritation	Cough	Associated complications: rib fracture(s), barotrauma, syncope
2. Airway obstruction	Air trapping and hyperinflation	Present in 70% of chest roentgenograms
3. Mucous production	Mucous plugging and atelectasis	Right lung and right middle lobe most susceptible
4. Increased alveolar pressures	Barotrauma (pneumothorax, pneumomediastinum)	May be clinically silent; may occur in up to 5% of asthma patients
5. Increased intrathoracic pressures and left ventricular afterload	Pulmonary edema	Potential problem
6. Rapidly progressive airways obstruction	Sudden asphyxia	? Etiology of sudden death and respiratory collapse
EXTRAPULMONARY		
1. Tissue hypoxia	Metabolic acidosis	From lactate accumulation
2. Respiratory alkalosis	Metabolic acidosis	Non–anion gap acidosis secondary to renal compensation
3. Hypoxemia, vasospasm	1. Myocardial infarction 2. Myocardial contraction-band necrosis	Dyspnea (may mask myocardial infarction)
4. Chronic hypoxemia	Cor pulmonale, pulmonary hyptertension	
5. Increased insensible fluid losses from diaphoresis, hyperventilation	Hypovolemia	Hypotension
6. Circadian fluctuations in epinephrine and cortisol levels	Sleep disturbances	May need adjustments in medications

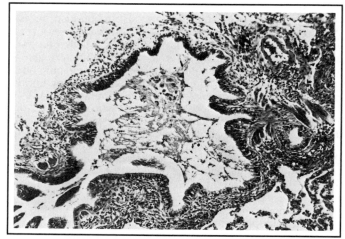

Fig. 91-1. *Bronchiole showing mucus with leukocytes in the lumen as well as edema, with mostly eosinophilic and lymphocytic inflammatory infiltrate in the lamina propria. (H&E, ×100, courtesy of Jerome Wollman.)*

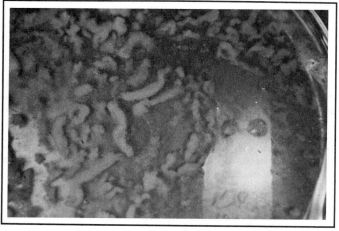

Fig. 91-2. *Mucous plugs obtained after bronchoalveolar lavage of an asthmatic patient using a flexible fiberoptic bronchoscope. (Reprinted with permission from W. B. Klaustermeyer [ed.], Practical Allergy and Immunology. New York: Wiley, 1983. P. 100.)*

asthma is well documented. It is postulated that the dyspnea associated with severe asthma may mask the pain of myocardial ischemia. There are several factors that predispose patients to myocardial damage, including hypoxia, vasospasm related to mediator release, and electrolyte disturbances and dysrhythmias associated with the medications used to treat asthma [44, 98]. Myocardial contraction-band necrosis has also been described in asthmatic patients, which probably reflects the severity of an episode of asthma (see Chap. 78). Although associated with catecholamine use, such necrosis has been found in patients not receiving parenteral catecholamines, thus raising the possibility of damage secondary to alterations in underlying sympathetic activity [60]. An epidemiologic association has also been reported between idiopathic dilated cardiomyopathy and asthma. Asthma precedes cardiac symptoms by several years and is identified as an independent risk factor. This cardiomyopathy may

be the result of long-term exposure to the mediators of asthma, which implies a hypersensitivity mechanism, or alternatively may be the consequence of long-term therapy with beta agonists [55]. Eosinophilic pericarditis has also been reported in association with asthma, but may actually be a manifestation of systemic hypereosinophilia rather than a complication of asthma [101, 229]. Pulmonary hypertension and right ventricular failure are rare in asthma, although they have been reported [42].

Hypovolemia may be a complication of asthma, reflecting increased insensible fluid losses stemming from diaphoresis or hyperventilation with decreased fluid intake in severely dyspneic patients. Clinical assessment of fluid deficits and accurate fluid replenishment are essential, as patients may become hypotensive during therapy [217]. Unexplained hypervolemia has also been reported during asthma exacerbations [110].

A nocturnal deterioration attributed to circadian changes in

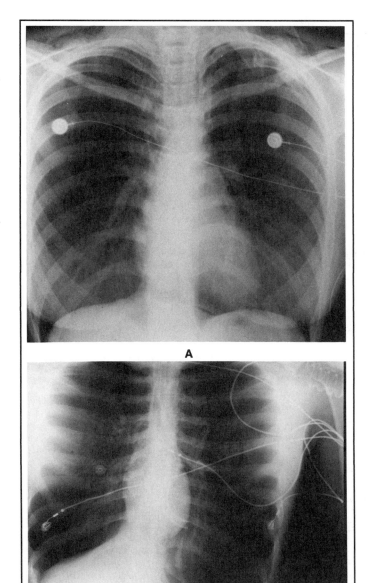

A

B

Fig. 91-3. *Chest roentgenograms taken during two separate episodes of asthma exacerbation. The first roentgenogram (A) demonstrates pneumomediastinum and subcutaneous emphysema. The second roentgenogram (B) demonstrates marked hyperinflation secondary to air trapping. In addition, bilateral pneumothoraces are also present, with the pleural lines visible in the lung apices.*

the circulating cortisol and catecholamine levels may occur in asthma [18]. A reproducible decline in peak expiratory flow rates, increase in bronchial hyperreactivity, and increase in the cellular elements of airway inflammation have been demonstrated [135, 137]. This can produce significant sleep disturbances, including nocturnal cough, difficulty in maintaining sleep, impaired sleep quality, early-morning awakenings, and daytime sleepiness [97, 221]. Recognition of the circadian rhythm of asthma and appropriate pharmacologic measures are important in preventing nocturnal deterioration [136].

Other complications and conditions less commonly associated with asthma include pruritus [34, 58], fatigue [208], vomiting [192], decreased gag reflex [185], subconjunctival hemorrhage [184], prepatellar bursitis [120, 121], clubbing [172], myoclonus [45], and a pseudopolio syndrome [62, 202]. Unusual complications include rectus sheath hematoma [119], spinal epidural emphysema [226], bronchial diverticulitis [50], and clinical dysautonomia [201].

COMPLICATIONS RELATED TO THERAPY

Complications related to the major pharmacologic agents used in asthma are generally well known and appreciated (Table 91-2). They are most often the result of excessive or prolonged use, but may occur with standard-dose therapy. This section will highlight the important and the recently reported complications of therapy. More detailed discussion will be found in respective chapters of this text.

Bronchodilators are the cornerstone of therapy, and complications associated with their use have been well documented [6]. Major toxicities involve the cardiovascular system and electrolyte disturbances. In addition to airway smooth muscle relaxation, beta-adrenergic agents increase cardiac contractility, heart rate, and oxygen consumption. This may produce tachycardia and promotes atrial and ventricular arrhythmias. Although albuterol may produce less cardiac stimulation, it can also produce dysrhythmias, notably atrial fibrillation if there is increased drug delivery, as occurs with the use of spacer devices [32]. Beta-adrenergic agents also dilate the pulmonary vascular bed. This effect alters compensatory ventilation-perfusion relationships and can result in transient arterial hypoxemia [46, 94]. In addition, $beta_2$-receptor stimulation may cause hypokalemia, which can be profound and produce both cardiac dysrhythmias and respiratory arrest [35, 109, 124]. This effect is reported for all beta-agonist agents, but some have greater hypokalemic effects than others [242]. The regular use of inhaled beta-agonist therapy may not be as effective in controlling asthma as intermittent (as-needed) use. In a prospective evaluation comparing regular and intermittent beta-agonist therapy, there was a 40 percent difference in asthma control between the two regimens [198]. Explanations for this included increased reliance on its protective effects, with resultant inadequate steroid therapy, and increased allergen exposure. The association of an increased risk of death or near death from asthma with the regular use of inhaled beta agonists, especially fenoterol, has also been reported [214a]. Beta agonists may also increase mucus production, possibly further worsening asthma [239]. Other complications associated with beta-agonist use include increased airflow obstruction with increasing airway hyperresponsiveness that may be secondary to the effects of other drug constituents or drug tachyphylaxis, or both [6, 230, 231].

Theophylline has been used extensively in the treatment of asthma, but its efficacy is limited by its narrow therapeutic window and systemic toxicity. These drawbacks have currently limited its universal acceptance, and its role remains controversial because of its toxicity profile [39, 115, 125]. In addition to its gastrointestinal effects (nausea, vomiting, gastroesophageal reflux), life-threatening cardiac dysrhythmias and seizures are of particular concern [103, 122, 246]. Theophylline toxicity is not necessarily predictable based on serum levels [2] and may be refractory to standard therapy [23, 25, 78]. Theophylline also stimulates the adrenergic system in the same manner as beta agonists and produces multiple metabolic and electrolyte derangements, including hypokalemia, hypophosphatemia, hypercalcemia, and hyperglycemia [84, 105, 142]. Management of theophylline toxicity includes oral-activated charcoal, with charcoal hemoperfusion reserved for life-threatening toxicity (cardiac dysrhythmias, seizures). Hypermagnesemia has been reported during the treatment of theophylline toxicity consisting of oral-activated charcoal and magnesium-containing cathartics [235].

Table 91-2. Major complications related to drug therapy for asthma

Therapeutic agent	Complication	Comments
1. Beta agonists	a. Atrial and ventricular dysrhythmias	May be potentiated with spacer use
	b. Transient hypoxemia	
	c. Hypokalemia	May predispose to cardiac arrhythmias
	d. Worsening airflow obstruction or hyperresponsiveness	May be exacerbated by regular beta-agonist use
2. Theophylline	Systemic toxicity (cardiac, gastrointestinal, central nervous system)	Narrow therapeutic window; increased risk of toxicity with drugs that decrease theophylline clearance (cimetidine, erthyromycin, etc.; see text for additional agents)
3. Anticholinergic agents	Anticholinergic effects (tachycardia, dry mouth, blurred vision, etc.)	Noted only with nebulized atropine
4. Systemic corticosteroids	a. Musculoskeletal (acute and chronic steroid myopathy, rib and vertebral fractures, bone loss)	Chronic myopathy in up to 50% of patients if daily prednisone dose >40 mg; skeletal complications in about 10% of asthmatic patients
	b. Infectious (increased infection rate)	No increased infection rate if <10 mg of daily prednisone
	c. Gastrointestinal (peptic ulcer disease, bleeding, bowel perforation)	Increased risk with >20 mg of daily prednisone
5. Aerosol corticosteroids	a. Local effects (oral candidiasis, dysphonia)	May be minimized with spacer devices
	b. Cough and wheezing with beclomethasone	Related to propellant preparation
	c. Basal cortisol suppression	With high-dose therapy, but of uncertain clinical significance
6. Cromolyn sodium	Local effects (hoarseness, local irritation, cough, wheezing)	Noted with powder preparation, minimized with metered-dose inhaler
7. Methotrexate	a. Gastrointestinal (nausea, stomatitis, transaminitis)	Controlled with dose reduction
	b. Dermatologic (rash, alopecia)	
	c. Pulmonary (pneumonitis, asthma)	Does not appear to be dose related
8. Gold	a. Gastrointestinal (nausea, dysgeusia)	Controlled by drug cessation
	b. Dermatologic (rash)	
9. Troleandomycin	a. Transaminitis	In up to 50% of patients receiving ≥1 gm daily
	b. Drug interaction (corticosteroids, theophylline)	Increases adverse effects of steroid or theophylline
10. Sedatives	a. Respiratory depression, respiratory failure	? Precipitant of worsening
	b. Potential worsening of bronchospasm	Secondary to histamine release with use of morphine, but may not be of clinical importance

Theophylline interacts with a host of other drugs. Drug toxicity may be accentuated by decreased theophylline clearance in patients treated with erythromycin [179], quinolones [90, 92], isoniazid [91], cimetidine [177], calcium channel blockers [210], propranolol [53], allopurinol [129], oral contraceptives [225], and many other agents [115]. Theophylline clearance is enhanced with phenobarbital [116], phenytoin [131], and intravenous isoproterenol and albuterol [7, 87] use. These interactions may require increasing doses of theophylline in order to maintain therapeutic theophylline levels. Increased theophylline clearance has not been reported with inhaled beta-agonist therapy.

Cognizance of these and other drug interactions is essential to minimize drug toxicity. It has also become evident that dosing errors made by both patients and physicians contribute significantly to the development of toxicity [191, 200]. These include overlapping oral and intravenous medications as well as inappropriate dosing. Dosing without adjustment for drug interactions or without consideration of altered theophylline metabolism due to underlying liver dysfunction or cardiac disease [163, 164] also contributes to the development of theophylline toxicity.

There are also several unusual reactions reported with theophylline use. These include hypersensitivity reactions to the ethylenediamine component of aminophylline solutions [65], theophylline-associated urinary retention [158], and delirium [233]. An association with fibrocystic breast disease has also been reported in asthmatic women [89].

Inhaled anticholinergic agents (atropine and ipratropium bromide) are not as effective as beta agonists when used as sole therapy, but are useful in combination with other bronchodilators [82, 83]. The major toxicity associated with atropine use is related to its systemic absorption and includes tachycardia,

urinary retention, dry mouth, and blurred vision. Ipratropium bromide has almost no systemic absorption, with side effects consisting primarily of dry mouth and dysgeusia. No side effects have been demonstrated with regard to mucus quality or mucociliary function and urinary sphincter tone, as well as in patients with glaucoma. Unlike beta-adrenergic agents, ipratropium bromide does not induce pulmonary vasodilation and arterial hypoxemia [8].

Complications associated with systemic corticosteroid use are well documented [86]. Adverse effects are usually related to the amount taken and the duration of therapy. Although a few weeks of steroid therapy are generally not associated with significant problems, there are reports of an acute steroid myopathy occurring within the first 2 weeks of therapy. This has only been reported in patients requiring mechanical ventilation, and the concomitant use of neuromuscular blocking agents may be an important risk factor. The myopathy, reported for several steroid preparations, affects proximal, distal, and respiratory muscles, and may be associated with myoglobinuria and rhabdomyolysis. Muscle biopsy specimens demonstrate focal and diffuse necrosis without predilection for Type IIB muscle fiber atrophy. Recovery may be prolonged [81a, 165, 241]. This contrasts with chronic steroid-induced myopathy, which primarily involves the proximal skeletal muscles and occasionally respiratory muscles, does not produce myoglobinuria, and exhibits Type IIB muscle fiber atrophy on biopsy specimens. The prevalence of the disorder approaches 50 percent in patients taking doses of prednisone exceeding 40 mg daily [30]. The myopathy usually resolves with discontinuation or reduction in steroid therapy.

Skeletal complications increase in frequency after long-term steroid use [1, 112, 180], with bone densitometry studies revealing trabecular bone loss. About 10 percent of asthmatic patients suffer rib or vertebral fractures, aseptic necrosis of the femoral head, or osteopenia. Rib or vertebral fractures may be a worrisome problem in asthmatic patients because of pain limitations to deep breathing and cough.

Infections are especially worrisome complications of corticosteroid therapy. A recent meta-analysis demonstrated an increased risk of infectious complications in patients taking glucocorticosteroids [218]. Steroid therapy carried an overall relative risk of 1.6 (95% confidence interval, 1.3–1.9), which increased with increasing daily and cumulative doses. The investigators were unable to demonstrate an increased infection rate in patients treated with a daily dose of less than 10 mg or a cumulative total dose of less than 700 mg of prednisone. However, the risk varied with the underlying disease process, with a higher infection risk in patients with underlying neurologic and renal disorders. Of note, patients with underlying pulmonary diseases treated with steroids (daily median dose of 30 mg of prednisone) showed no increased rate or risk of infectious complications. However, opportunistic infections such as disseminated aspergillosis or varicella do occur in patients with asthma whose only risk is corticosteroid administration [114, 209]; a high index of suspicion is key for their proper diagnosis and management.

Corticosteroids have also been implicated as a cause in peptic ulcer disease and gastrointestinal bleeding, although there are data that do not support this [52, 144]. An extensive analysis of this issue led to the conclusion that the risk of peptic ulcer disease and gastrointestinal bleeding increased with daily doses of over 20 mg of prednisone. The risk was also increased, although not significantly, with short-term therapy (less than 30 days) and a cumulative dose greater than 1,000 mg of prednisone. A review of surgical patients suggested that, when treated with steroids, these patients are also at risk for bowel perforation [178]. Although long-term therapy may have increased this risk, a substantial proportion of these patients developed bowel perforation during the perioperative period and within the first 3 weeks of therapy [178]. These observations are irrespective of dose and are applicable although not specific for asthma patients.

Hypersensitivity reactions to corticosteroids are rare. However, reactions ranging from angioedema to diffuse urticaria may occur with topical, oral, or parenteral preparations. The mechanism of hypersensitivity is unknown; such patients who require continued steroid therapy can be managed with desensitization [12, 49].

Although complications are primarily associated with pharmacologic doses of steroids, it is important to adequately treat the inflammatory component of asthma. Underuse of steroids can lead to poorly treated asthma, with an effect as devastating as prolonged corticosteroid use [118, 146].

The high incidence of systemic side effects associated with systemic corticosteroid therapy has prompted the development of alternative therapies. Since their introduction in the early 1970s, inhaled corticosteroids, discussed in detail in Chapter 61, have gained widespread acceptance for the management of asthma. Inhaled steroids allow therapy to be targeted to the airways with minimal systemic absorption. It is not surprising that the systemic side effects from these agents are minimal and dose related. Indications and complications associated with inhaled steroid use have been well chronicled [48, 176, 223].

The most common local side effects of aerosol corticosteroids are oropharyegeal candidiasis and dysphonia. These side effects may become intolerable, prompting discontinuation by some patients, but can be controlled with spacer devices [224]. These spacer devices minimize oropharyegeal deposition and optimize intrapulmonary deposition. Cough and wheezing have also been noted in some patients treated with inhaled beclomethasone dipropionate delivered as a nebulized suspension or with a metered-dose inhaler [47, 205]. Treatment with inhaled triamcin-

olone acetonide resulted in resolution of these symptoms. These side effects have been attributed to either the freon propellant or oleic acid dispersant in the beclomethasone inhaler, which are not part of the triamcinolone acetonide formulation [206]. The offending agent in the nebulized suspension has not been identified.

There has been extensive evaluation of the hypothalamic-pituitary-adrenal axis during inhaled steroid therapy, which has revealed a dose-dependent response. High-dose beclomethasone dipropionate (>2 mg/day) does not appear to suppress basal adrenal cortisol production, but adrenal reserve is not affected [5a, 211]; these effects are of uncertain clinical significance (Chap. 62).

Cromolyn sodium (Chap. 63) acts by preventing mast cell degranulation and thus plays a role in preventing exacerbations of asthma. It is extremely effective in the management of chronic asthma and is well tolerated. Most adverse effects are related to inhalation of the fine powder formulation of the drug (throat irritation, hoarseness, dry mouth, cough, or bronchospasm), but these may be minimized with the use of the cromolyn metered-dose inhaler. These reactions are usually minor and do not necessitate drug cessation [22, 162]. There are few unusual reactions associated with cromolyn sodium use. These include urticaria, angioedema, anaphylaxis, febrile cutaneous eruptions, polymyositis, pericarditis, pulmonary infiltrates with eosinophilia, and pulmonary granulomatosis. These reactions are usually controlled with discontinuation of cromolyn use, but a few patients require corticosteroid treatment for resolution [41, 126, 204].

The high morbidity associated with prolonged steroid administration has spurred investigation of alternative or steroid-sparing agents [175]. Low-dose methotrexate (Chap. 68) has been used in corticosteroid-dependent asthma, with successful reduction in steroid dosage as well as either maintenance or improvement in pulmonary function [149, 150, 207]. This steroid-sparing effect, however, has not been documented by other investigators [66]. Toxicity has been limited to nausea, rash, stomatitis, alopecia, and transaminitis, adverse reactions which are easily managed with adjustments in drug administration. *Pneumocystis carinii* pneumonia was noted in one patient treated with methotrexate and high-dose (60 mg/day) prednisone [66]. No hematologic toxicity, hepatic cirrhosis, or other opportunistic infections have been noted in asthmatic patients. Low-dose methotrexate produces significant morbidity from other diseases when used for extended periods (cumulative doses over 1.5 gm), including cirrhosis requiring liver transplantation [71]. Pulmonary toxicity, including pneumonitis and even asthma, has been reported that does not appear to be dose related [67, 102, 187, 196]. The lower toxicity of methotrexate in asthmatic patients may be a reflection of the younger asthmatic patient population the drug is used in, and deserves continued investigation.

Oral and parenteral gold have also been used as steroid-sparing agents in asthma [20, 108, 151]. With the use of gold, investigators have been able to reduce steroid requirements in asthma patients, with either maintenance or improvement in pulmonary function. Adverse reactions noted with parenteral gold include dysgeusia, minor skin reactions, eosinophilia, and proteinuria [108]. Reported adverse reactions to oral gold are primarily gastrointestinal and mucocutaneous, and necessitated cessation of use in only 5 percent (N = 20) of the patients in one report [20]. In another series, severe eczema necessitated discontinuation of oral gold in 2 (11 percent) of 17 patients [152a]. No significant renal toxicity has been reported. Although promising, the experience with gold has been limited to a small number of patients and awaits further evaluation.

Troleandomycin (TAO) (Chap. 67) is another steroid-sparing agent used in the treatment of asthma. It decreases methylprednisolone metabolism, thereby increasing methylprednisolone's half-life and allowing for a reduction in steroid dosage. Elevated liver function tests are the most common side effect associated with TAO use, affecting up to 50 percent of the subjects receiving daily doses of 1,000 mg. This is probably dose related, since only 7 percent of subjects receiving 250 mg of TAO a day develop elevated liver function tests. Other adverse reactions associated with TAO use include enhancement of steroid-related effects (glucose intolerance, hypertension, and so on). Theophylline toxicity has also been associated with TAO use [237]. These side effects are easily managed by adjustments in the dose of concomitant steroids or theophylline [232, 244].

Antihistamines have had a limited role in the management of asthma because of intolerable sedative and anticholinergic side effects. Severe mucous plugging has been reported with over-the-counter antihistamine use [70]. However, new less-sedating H_1 antihistamine agents appear to be effective and better tolerated, with only minor dysgeusia, dry mouth, and sedation noted as adverse effects [170, 171, 222]. This subject is further detailed in Chapter 65.

Treatment of severe dyspnea and associated agitation during an asthmatic attack with sedatives or anxiolytic agents is potentially deleterious because of their depressive effects on respiratory drive and the cough reflex. They have been implicated by several investigators as the cause of deterioration in the respiratory status, leading to intubation, mechanical ventilation, and death [40, 236, 238]. Morphine and other opiates may stimulate histamine release, which may provoke bronchospasm and emesis and produce dry respiratory secretions. This is of uncertain significance because of the lack of evidence documenting a deleterious effect [27, 203]. However, because of these potential adverse reactions, the use of opiates as well as other sedatives is best avoided in the asthmatic patient. After intubation, benzodiazepines are preferable to opiates if a sedative agent is needed.

Some patients with acute asthma who do not respond to appropriate therapy may eventually require endotracheal intubation and mechanical ventilation. Between 2 and 8 percent of all asthmatic patients admitted to the hospital and between 9 and 15 percent of asthmatic patients admitted to intensive care units require endotracheal intubation and mechanical ventilation [188, 240]. Although extensive criteria for intubation have been published, the decision is best individualized for each patient. Apnea or near apnea, cardiopulmonary arrest, decreased level of consciousness, and an inability to protect the airway are clear indications for endotracheal intubation and mechanical ventilation [56]. Hypercapnia or even normocapnia during an asthmatic attack is associated with severe airflow obstruction and may suggest impending respiratory failure. Hypercapnia, however, is not an absolute criterion for intubation. Several investigators have demonstrated that hypercapnia associated with a moderate to severe respiratory acidosis can often be managed without intubation. Only 10 percent of these hypercapnic patients eventually require intubation and mechanical ventilation. Although associated with a greater severity of illness on presentation, hypercapnia is usually corrected within a day of admission and does not prolong hospitalization [28, 147, 174].

Complications associated with mechanical ventilation are extensive and involve all organ systems [166] (Table 91-3). Asthmatic patients appear to have three times the number of complications as nonasthmatic ventilator patients [195]. Up to a third of asthmatic patients may experience problems with airway management (mainstem bronchus intubation or cuff leaks requiring reintubation and extubation) [127, 130]. Alveolar hypoventilation with worsening hypercapnia and atelectasis has been noted in 30 to 70 percent of mechanically ventilated asthmatic patients. A quarter of the patients may experience significant hypotension after intubation and mechanical ventilation. The delivery of positive intrathoracic pressures during mechanical ventilation in the setting of reduced circulating blood volume decreases venous

Table 91-3. Complications associated with mechanical ventilation

Complication	Comments
1. Airway problems (mainstem bronchus intubation, cuff leaks)	May be related to difficult intubation; may occur in up to one-third of patients
2. Hypotension	Related to decreased circulating volume and delivery of positive intrathoracic pressures
3. Barotrauma	Occurs in up to one-third of asthma patients; increased when airway pressures exceed 55 cm H_2O; requires prompt recognition and decompression
4. Hypophosphatemia	Appearance during correction of respiratory acidosis; occurs in about 10% of asthma patients
5. Pneumonia	May occur three times as often in asthma patients

return and has potentially deleterious consequences. This underscores the importance of adequate hydration in these patients.

Pneumothoraces may occur in up to a third of asthmatic patients requiring mechanical ventilation. This is probably related to the high peak and mean airway pressures necessary to achieve adequate ventilation during bronchospastic episodes. In one series, all episodes of barotrauma occurred when peak airway pressures exceeded 45 cmH_2O, and most occurred when peak airway pressure exceeded 55 cmH_2O. However, there is also evidence suggesting that breathing patterns which promote lung hyperinflation (large tidal volume, short expiratory time) may be equally important in the development of barotrauma and also merit correction [228]. Although life-threatening, barotrauma in asthmatic patients is not a frequent cause of death, accounting for less than 15 percent of deaths of intubated patients in most series; however, this problem should be minimized by appropriate clinical monitoring in such patients.

Other major complications associated with mechanical ventilation include pneumonia, cardiac dysrhythmias, sepsis, and gastrointestinal hemorrhage. These are not unique to asthmatic patients, but appear to occur more frequently in intubated asthmatics.

The majority of asthmatic patients require intubation for less than 72 hours. Most patients have their asthma controlled and are extubated within that time frame. Increasing duration of mechanical ventilation is associated with an increased rate of complications, including death. Other practitioners, however, have reported relatively few complications associated with asthma and mechanical ventilation [88].

Hypophosphatemia may also develop during the management of asthma in both mechanically ventilated patients and non–mechanically ventilated patients after correction of respiratory acidosis. The explanation is multifactorial and includes intracellular shifts of phosphate with reduced urinary phosphate excretion during correction of respiratory acidosis and hypophosphatemia related to bronchodilator therapy [31, 113]. Other mechanisms of hypophosphatemia, including gastrointestinal losses, urinary losses, antacid ingestion, and nutritional causes, are not evident in these patients. Chronic respiratory alkalosis can also produce marked hypophosphatemia; an incidence of about 10 percent in asthma patients has been cited [68]. Hypophosphatemia is implicated as a cause of diaphragmatic weakness contributing to respiratory failure and ventilator weaning difficulties, and thus requires appropriate correction [13, 152].

Complications associated with mechanical ventilation have led to several novel approaches to therapy, but these also have their

Table 91-4. Complications associated with therapy during mechanical ventilation

Therapy	Complication	Comment
1. Controlled hypoventilation	Fluid overload, hypernatremia, hyperosmolarity, metabolic alkalosis	Related to systemic bicarbonate administration
2. Neuromuscular blocking agents (vecuronium)	Prolonged weakness and polyneuropathy	Probably related to cumulative dose and duration of therapy; interaction with steroids (?)
3. Positive end-expiratory pressure	Hyperinflation, hypotension	Relatively small improvement in oxygenation
4. Inhalational anesthetic agents (halothane or enflurane)	Cardiac (myocardial depression, ventricular irritability)	Potentiated in patients receiving beta agonists or theophylline
	Prolonged tetraplegia	Patients who received halothane and enflurane
5. Fiberoptic bronchoscopy	Bronchospasm, hypoxemia noted after bronchoscopy	Average decline in PaO_2 of 20 mmHg; bronchoalveolar lavage associated with increased incidence of pneumonia
6. Acetylcysteine	Bronchospasm	Often administered via bronchoscope

drawbacks (Table 91-4). In order to reduce peak airway pressures and minimize their effects, controlled hypoventilation has been used. That is, severe hypercapnia is accepted, and the acid-base status is normalized with bicarbonate administration. Concomitant management with standard therapy allows the eventual correction of gas exchange abnormalities. Fluid overload, hyperosmolarity, hypernatremia, hypokalemia, and metabolic alkalosis are potential complications of systemic bicarbonate administration [57, 143].

In addition to bicarbonate therapy, controlled hypoventilation may require patient paralysis with neuromuscular blocking agents to facilitate patient-ventilator synchrony, reduce peak airway pressures, and reduce carbon dioxide production and oxygen consumption. This strategy also reduces end-inspiratory lung volume and concomitant dynamic hyperinflation, with further reduction in the incidence of hypotension and barotrauma [241a]. However, there are increasing reports of prolonged weakness and polyneuropathy in asthma patients requiring paralysis, especially in those receiving vecuronium [50a, 59a, 81a, 110a, 130a]. In one report, 7 of 10 of patients infused with vecuronium for more than 6 hours developed evidence of a polyneuropathy [110a]. Higher cumulative doses and longer duration of infusion of vecuronium may predispose to the development of this complication. Creatinine kinase enzymes may not be elevated, and the clinical picture appears to be distinct from steroid-induced myopathy. However, these patients are also treated with high-dose steroids, and it may be impossible to attribute the effect to the vecuronium alone. It is unclear how the interaction of the two agents may predispose to the development of muscle weakness, which may impede liberation from mechanical ventilation. Full recovery eventually occurs, but may take several weeks or months. Minimizing the dose and duration of neuromuscular blockade are important and may reduce the incidence of these complications.

High levels of positive end-expiratory pressure (PEEP) during mechanical ventilation have been used successfully to correct excessive air trapping in patients with severe asthma [169]. How-

ever, a consistent beneficial effect has not been observed [138, 227]. Although arterial oxygenation may improve, concomitant increases in end-inspiratory lung volume and intrathoracic pressures occur at all levels of PEEP including 5 cmH2O, with a significant risk for hypotension at 15 cmH2O [227]. These changes outweigh the small benefits of PEEP and argue against its routine use in patients with severe asthma.

Inhalational anesthetics have also been used successfully in the management of mechanically ventilated patients who are refractory to conventional therapy. Anesthetic use is limited by toxicity (myocardial depression, ventricular irritability), which may be potentiated in patients who are hypoxemic, acidemic, and receiving beta agonists and aminophylline [157, 194]. Enflurane may be less toxic than halothane in this respect, but prolonged tetraplegia has been associated with the administration of both agents [220].

Fiberoptic bronchoscopy and lavage with mucolytic agents have been reported to be of benefit in severe asthma [59, 145]. Although potentially therapeutic, there are complications associated with fiberoptic bronchoscopy. These include laryngospasm, worsening bronchospasm, cardiac dysrhythmias, and hypoxemia. Worsening hypoxemia (average decline in PaO_2 of 20 mmHg) that persists for about 4 hours after bronchoscopy has bee noted in a series of patients undergoing fiberoptic bronchoscopy. This magnitude of hypoxemia may be of greater significance during severe bronchospasm [3, 243]. Acetylcysteine may also precipitate bronchospasm, limiting its use in asthma [21]. Experience with bronchial lavage in acute asthma has been mixed. Although improvement in static compliance was demonstrated in one series, lavage has also been associated with an increased incidence of pneumonia and longer duration of intubation [127]. (See also Chapter 84.)

MEDICAL CONDITIONS COMPLICATED BY ASTHMA

The management of asthma may need to be modified because of the presence of coexistent medical conditions. These conditions usually require appropriate adjustments in medications, but occasionally the disorders may also affect the course of asthma. Optimal management requires the recognition and evaluation of all such conditions.

Gastroesophageal reflux and asthma (Chap. 75) are intricately related [5, 74, 75, 214]. Fifty percent or more of asthmatic subjects may have gastroesophageal reflux, possibly pharmacologically related. Theophylline and beta agonists reduce lower esophageal sphincter tone, thereby increasing acid reflux into the tracheobronchial tree and resulting in chemical tracheobronchitis and vagally mediated bronchoconstriction. Acid can also stimulate midesophageal receptors, resulting in vagally mediated bronchospasm. The elimination of this reflex observed after bilateral vagotomy lends further support to this mechanism. Alternatively, exacerbations of asthma may worsen gastroesophageal reflux. High transdiaphragmatic pressures may facilitate the movement of gastric acid into the esophagus and tracheobronchial tree. Stimulation of asthmatic airways may also cause lower esophageal sphincter relaxation, thus intensifying acid reflux.

In addition to possibly provoking or worsening asthma, gastroesophageal reflux can lead to a host of pulmonary complications. Bronchitis, bronchiectasis, aspiration pneumonia, atelectasis, hemoptysis, and pulmonary fibrosis are potential manifestations of gastroesophageal reflux that may also complicate the management of asthma [16].

Medical or surgical treatment of gastroesophageal reflux may lessen the asthma, although such improvement has been modest [76, 117, 159, 161]. There are also reports that have not documented correlations between intraesophageal acid and bronchoconstriction and an improvement in asthma following treatment of gastroesophageal reflux [64, 219].

The management of asthma in pregnancy has been extensively evaluated [81] (see also Chap. 81). The effect of pregnancy on asthma is individually unpredictable, with about a third of patients experiencing improvement, a third deterioration, and a third no change in their asthma [189]. Some investigators have been able to demonstrate improvement in asthmatic patients, which does not correlate well with the hormonal changes of pregnancy [104]. Clearly, uncontrolled asthma with prolonged periods of hypoxia increase both maternal and fetal morbidity and mortality [77]. Although recent experience has not documented increased fetal mortality, poorly controlled asthma is associated with intrauterine growth retardation [190]. Premature and low-birth-weight infants have also been reported, although this is an inconsistent finding [10]. Status asthmaticus and even respiratory failure requiring mechanical ventilation can be successfully managed in pregnant asthmatics, with good outcomes in both mother and child [193]. The other major issue involves the safety of medications used to control maternal asthma. It appears that all of the commonly used medications can be used safely in pregnant asthmatics [79]. However, beta-agonist therapy (especially terbutaline) may be associated with pulmonary edema [167]. Corticosteroids have been associated with cleft palate in animal studies, but this complication has not been reported with human use. Both systemic and inhaled corticosteroids have been used in pregnant asthmatics with subsequent control of the disease and minimal morbidity [69, 80]. As with nonpregnant patients, close follow-up is essential to minimize complications and optimize disease control.

Exacerbations of asthma may precipitate sickle cell crises in susceptible individuals. The hypoxemia and acidosis associated with severe asthma increase the risk of red blood cell sickling and subsequent crises. Treatment must be directed at both diseases and includes correction of gas exchange abnormalities and exchange transfusions [160].

Adequate control of hypertension in asthmatic patients may be complicated by the interaction of medications used to control both diseases. Sympathomimetic agents may elevate blood pressure, although this not a uniform effect. Epinephrine is the medication most likely to elevate blood pressure, and thus should be avoided in hypertensive patients. The combination of methyldopa and sympathomimetic agents may also exacerbate hypertension [245]. Beta blockers may precipitate cough and bronchospasm and must be avoided in asthmatic patients [37, 168]. Angiotensin-converting enzyme inhibitors may also precipitate cough and bronchospasm in asthmatic patients, but the incidence of cough may be similar to the incidence in the general population (3–15 percent) [104a]. Peripheral adrenergic inhibitors (guanethidine or reserpine) may block the effect of sympathomimetic agents and thus increase susceptibility to bronchospasm as well [199].

The management of patients with psychiatric disturbances and asthma may be complicated by the possibility of steroid-induced psychosis in those patients requiring high-dose or long-term steroids for asthma control [29]. Although there is potential for this complication, it has not been reported by investigators who manage both schizophrenic asthmatics and asthmatics without psychiatric disturbances. Problems that have been noted include medication noncompliance and prednisone phobia (fear of taking adequate doses of prednisone), which have been managed with depot methylprednisolone [213].

LONG-TERM SEQUELAE OF ASTHMA

Recognition of the chronic morbidity in patients with asthma has sparked an interest in the natural history and long-term prognosis of the disease (see Chaps. 2 and 94). Childhood asthma may persist or relapse in adulthood, and may increase the risk for chronic obstructive lung disease. The clinical aphorism that childhood asthma resolves during adolescence may be erroneous. Up to one-fifth of subjects may have disease that persists into adulthood, and over one-quarter experience recurrences after remissions during adolescence. A greater severity of asthma at onset and an atopic history may identify those subjects at risk [26]. The results of a prospective, longitudinal evaluation of asthmatic children and normal controls that extended into adulthood have further clarified these observations. Those subjects whose clinical asthma resolved before puberty continued to demonstrate normal pulmonary function and most had no or mild bronchial reactivity on methacholine provocation testing. However, in those who continued to experience episodes of wheezing into adulthood, the investigators were able to demonstrate a steeper decline in FEV_1/FVC (forced expiratory volume in 1 second/forced vital capacity) and more severe reactivity on methacholine testing. The greatest changes were noted in those with the greatest frequency of wheezing episodes. Sex differences have also been noted, with females experiencing a greater decline in FEV_1 than their male counterparts [237a]. Undertreatment of asthma was noted at all ages, thus underscoring the need for appropriate and adequate therapy. The prevalence of cigarette smoking was the same for all levels and thus could not account for the noted differences [106, 107, 132, 133].

This and other evidence suggests that asthma may be a risk factor in the development of chronic airflow obstruction. Asthma is identified as a factor in the development of chronic bronchitic symptoms in adults, although this relationship does not persist after the stratified analysis of other factors [216]. Persistent airflow obstruction has been noted in a group of patients with chronic asthma after an aggressive course of treatment, suggesting that chronic asthma can produce irreversible airflow obstruction [36]. Pathologic studies of patients with long-standing asthma who die of other causes have demonstrated an increase in the bronchial basement membrane thickness and reduced small airways diameters [212]. These lesions are characteristic of asthma, in contrast to the focal and variable basement membrane thickening noted in patients with chronic obstructive pulmonary disease [99].

Recent immunohistopathologic studies of endobronchial biopsy specimens from patients with mild asthma have demonstrated the presence of subepithelial fibrosis, myofibroblasts, and collagen deposition. In addition, other autopsy studies have demonstrated hypertrophied bronchial smooth muscle involving both large and small airways. These findings provide evidence for structural changes that occur even in mild asthma, and lend support to the possibility that the cumulative effects of these cellular events may lead to chronic irreversible airflow obstruction [19, 33, 61, 183].

However, the relationship between airway hyperreactivity and the development of chronic airflow obstruction remains under investigation. Current evidence for this relationship is only suggestive [38, 154]. While no direct evidence exists to support a causal role for airway hyperresponsiveness in the development of irreversible airflow obstruction, the possibility cannot be excluded.

Growth retardation has also been reported in asthmatic children [43]. In this study, the severity of asthma and the use of systemic steroids had the greatest effects on linear growth. The extent of growth retardation averaged one standard deviation below predicted means. Intermittent steroid use had no effect on growth, while regular daily steroid use produced the greatest growth retardation [43]. However, the subjects in this study were prepubertal, and subsequent investigation has established that delayed puberty is the explanation for the observations of growth retardation [15]. Delayed puberty has been observed in almost one-half of asthmatic children. With the onset of puberty, catch-up growth is seen with ultimate attainment of predicted adult height. Since systemic steroids are detrimental to normal growth, this complication can be minimized with inhaled steroid use or with alternate-day therapy if systemic steroids are absolutely indicated. It should be noted that the stress of delayed puberty may complicate medication compliance and management in the adolescent asthmatic. Concerns over deficits in cognitive function and school performance related to asthma or theophylline use have not been substantiated [124a].

In conclusion, there is a wide spectrum of complications associated with asthma. These include both acute and chronic complications related to the disease as well as complications stemming from therapy and the interaction of asthma with other coexistent conditions. The optimal management of asthma demands the prompt recognition of and attention to complications. This requires constant vigilance and awareness on the part of both the patient and physician. The early recognition of potential problems can minimize the incidence and impact of complications as well as reduce their effect on morbidity and mortality.

REFERENCES

1. Adinoff, A. D., and Hollister, J. R. Steroid-induced fractures and bone loss in patients with asthma. *N. Engl. J. Med.* 309:265, 1983.
2. Aitken, M. L., and Martin, T. Life-threatening theophylline toxicity is not predictable by serum levels. *Chest* 91:10, 1987.
3. Albertini, R. E., et al. Arterial hypoxemia induced by fiberoptic bronchoscopy. *JAMA* 230:1666, 1974.
4. Alberts, W. M., Williams, J. H., and Ramsdell, J. W. Metabolic acidosis as a presenting feature in asthma. *Ann. Allergy* 57:107, 1986.
5. Allen, C. J., and Newhouse, M. T. Gastroesophageal reflux and chronic respiratory disease. *Am. Respir. Rev. Dis.* 129:645, 1984.
5a. Altman, L. C., et al. Adrenal function in adult asthmatics during long-term daily treatment with 800, 1,200, and 1,600 μg triamcinolone acetonide. *Chest* 101:1250, 1992.
6. American Academy of Allergy and Immunology. Adverse effects and complications of treatment with beta-adrenergic agonist drugs. *J. Allergy Clin. Immunol.* 75:443, 1985.
7. Amirav, I., et al. Enhancement of theophylline clearance by intravenous albuterol. *Chest* 94:444, 1988.
8. Anderson, W. M. Hemodynamic and non-bronchial effects of ipratropium bromide. *Am. J. Med.* 81(suppl. 5A):45, 1986.
9. Appel, D., et al. Lactic acidosis in severe asthma. *Am. J. Med.* 75:580, 1983.
10. Apter, A. J., Greenberger, P. A., and Patterson, R. Outcomes of pregnancy in adolescents with severe asthma. *Arch. Intern. Med.* 149:2571, 1989.
11. Anderson, W. M. Mucoid impaction of upper lobe bronchi in the absence of proximal bronchiectasis. *Chest* 98:1023, 1990.
12. Ashford, R. F. U., and Bailey, A. Angioneurotic edema and urticaria following hydrocortisone—a further case. *Postgrad. Med. J.* 56:437, 1980.
13. Aubier, M., et al. Effect of hypophosphatemia on diaphragmatic contractility in patients with acute respiratory failure. *N. Engl. J. Med.* 313:420, 1985.
14. Augelli, N. V., and El-Mallakh, R. S. Pneumopericardium as a complication of acute asthmatic attack. *Ill. Med. J.* 167:311, 1985.
15. Balfour-Lynn, L. Effect of asthma on growth and puberty. *Pediatrician* 14:237, 1987.
16. Barish, C. F., Wu, W. C., and Castell, D. O. Respiratory complications of gastroesophageal reflux. *Arch. Intern. Med.* 145:1882, 1985.
17. Barnes, P. J. A new approach to the treatment of asthma. *N. Engl. J. Med.* 321:1517, 1989.
18. Barnes, P. J., et al. Nocturnal asthma and changes in circulating epinephrine, histamine, and cortisol. *N. Engl. J. Med.* 303:263, 1980.
19. Beasley, R., et al. Cellular events in the bronchi in mild asthma and after bronchial provocation. *Am. Rev. Respir. Dis.* 139:806, 1989.
20. Bernstein, D. I., et al. An open study of Auranofin in the treatment of steroid-dependent asthma. *J. Allergy Clin. Immunol.* 81:6, 1988.
21. Bernstein, I. L., and Ausdenmore, R. W. Iatrogenic bronchospasm occurring during clinical trials of a new mucolytic agent, acetylcysteine. *Dis. Chest* 46:469, 1964.
22. Bernstein, I. L., Johnson, C. K., and Tse, S. D. T. Therapy with cromolyn sodium. *Ann. Intern. Med.* 89:228, 1978.
23. Bertino, J. S., and Walker J. W. Reassessment of theophylline toxicity: serum concentrations, clinical course and treatment. *Arch. Intern. Med.* 147:757, 1987.
24. Berro, E., et al. "Ring around the artery" as a presenting feature in undiagnosed asthma with pneumomediastinum. *South. Med. J.* 83:215, 1990.
25. Biberstein, M. P., Ziegler, M. G., and Ward, D. M. Use of beta-blockade and hemoperfusion for acute theophylline poisoning. *West. J. Med.* 141:485, 1984.
26. Blair, H. Natural history of childhood asthma. *Arch. Dis. Child* 52:613, 1977.
27. Blumberg, M. Z. Morphine for severe asthma? *N. Engl. J. Med.* 288:50, 1973.
28. Bondi, E., and Williams, M. H. Severe asthma: course and treatment in hospital. *NY State J. Med.* 77:350, 1977.
29. Boston Collaborative Drug Surveillance Program. Acute adverse reaction to prednisone in relation to dosage. *Clin. Pharmacol. Ther.* 13:694, 1972.
30. Bowyer, L. S., La Mothe, M. P., and Hollister, J. R. Steroid myopathy; incidence and detection in a population with asthma. *J. Allergy Clin. Immunol.* 76:234, 1985.
31. Brady, H. R., et al. Hypophosphatemia complicating bronchodilator therapy for acute severe asthma. *Arch. Intern. Med.* 149:23, 1989.
32. Breeden, C. C., and Safirstein, B. H. Albuterol and spacer-induced atrial fibrillation. *Chest* 98:762, 1990.
33. Brewster, C. E. P., et al. Myofibroblasts and subepithelial fibrosis in bronchial asthma. *Am. J. Respir. Cell Mol. Biol.* 3:507, 1990.
34. Brown, H. M. Itching and asthma. *Lancet* 2:576, 1984.
35. Brown, M. J., Brown, D. C., and Murphy, M. B. Hypokalemia from beta$_2$-receptor stimulation by circulating epinephrine. *N. Engl. J. Med.* 309:1414, 1983.
36. Brown, P. J., Greville, H. W., and Finucane, K. E. Asthma and irreversible airflow obstruction. *Thorax* 39:131, 1984.
37. Bucca, C., et al. Hyperresponsiveness of the extrathoracic airway in patients with captopril-induced cough. *Chest* 98:1133, 1990.
38. Buist, A. S. Asthma as a risk factor for chronic airways disease. *Chest* 96:314S, 1989.
39. Bukowskyj, M., Nakatsu, K., and Munt, P. W. Theophylline reassessed. *Ann. Intern. Med.* 101:63, 1984.
40. Buranakul, B., et al. Causes of death during acute asthma in children. *Am. J. Dis. Child.* 128:343, 1974.
41. Burger, L. W., Kass, I., and Schenken, J. R. Pulmonary allergic granulomatosis; a possible drug reaction in a patient receiving cromolyn sodium. *Chest* 66:83, 1974.
42. Calverley, P. M. A., et al. Cor pulmonale in asthma. *Br. J. Dis. Chest* 77:303, 1983.
43. Chang, K. C., et al. Linear growth of chronic asthmatic children: the effects of the disease and various forms of steroid therapy. *Clin. Allergy* 12:369, 1982.
44. Chappell, A. G. Painless myocardial infarction in asthma. *Br. J. Dis. Chest* 78:174, 1984.
45. Chee, Y. C., and Poh, S. C. Myoclonus following severe asthma: clonazepam relieves. *Aust. N. Z. J. Med.* 13:285, 1983.
46. Chick, T. W., Nicholson, D. P., and Johnston, R. L. Effects of isoproterenol on distribution of ventilation and perfusion in asthma. *Am. Rev. Respir. Dis.* 107:869, 1973.
47. Clark, R. J. Exacerbation of asthma after nebulised beclomethasone dipropionate. *Lancet* 2:574, 1986.
48. Clark, T. J. H. Inhaled corticosteroid therapy: a substitute for theophylline as well as prednisolone? *J. Allergy Clin. Immunol.* 76:330, 1985.
49. Clee, M. D., et al. Glucocorticoid hypersensitivity in an asthmatic patient: presentation and treatment. *Thorax* 40:477, 1985.
50. Cluroe, A., Beasley, R., and Holloway, L. Bronchial diverticulitis: complication of bronchial asthma. *J. Clin. Pathol.* 41:921, 1988.
50a. Coakley, J. H., et al. Prolonged neurogenic weakness in patients requiring mechanical ventilation for acute airflow limitation. *Chest* 101:1413, 1992.
51. Collett, P. W., Brancatisano, T., and Engel, L. A. Changes in the glottic aperture during bronchial asthma. *Am. Rev. Respir. Dis.* 128:719, 1983.
52. Conn, H. O., and Blitzer, B. L. Non association of adrenocorticosteroid therapy and peptic ulcer. *N. Engl. J. Med.* 294:473, 1976.
53. Conrad, K. A., and Nyman, D. W. Effects of metoprolol and propranolol on theophylline elimination. *Clin. Pharmacol. Ther.* 28:463, 1980.
54. Corrao, W. M., Braman, S. S., and Irwin, R. S. Chronic cough as the sole presenting manifestation of bronchial asthma. *N. Engl. J. Med.* 300:633, 1979.
55. Coughlin, S. S., et al. Idiopathic dilated cardiomyopathy and atopic dis-

ease: epidemiologic evidence for an association with asthma. *Am. Heart J.* 118:768, 1989.

56. Dales, R. E., and Munt, P. W. Use of mechanical ventilation in adults with severe asthma. *Can. Med. Assoc. J.* 130:391, 1984.

57. Darioli, R., and Perret, C. Mechanical controlled hypoventilation in status asthmaticus. *Am. Rev. Respir. Dis.* 129:385, 1984.

58. David, T. J., Wybrew, M., and Hennessen, U. Prodromal itching in childhood asthma. *Lancet* 2:154, 1984.

59. Donaldson, J. C., et al. Acetylcysteine for life threatening acute bronchial obstruction. *Ann. Intern. Med.* 88:656, 1978.

59a. Douglass, J. A., et al. Myopathy in severe asthma. *Am. Rev. Respir. Dis.* 146:517, 1992.

60. Drislane, F. W., et al. Myocardial contraction band lesions in patients with fatal asthma: possible neurocardiologic mechanisms. *Am. Rev. Respir. Dis.* 135:498, 1987.

61. Ebina, M., et al. Hyperreactive site in the airway tree of asthmatic patients revealed by thickening of bronchial muscles. *Am. Rev. Respir. Dis.* 141:1327, 1990.

62. Editorial. Post-asthmatic pseudo-polio in children. *Lancet* 1:860, 1980.

63. Eggleston, P. A., et al. Radiographic abnormalities in acute asthma in children. *Pediatrics* 54:442, 1974.

64. Ekstrom, T., and Tibbling, L. Gastro-oesophageal reflux and triggering of bronchial asthma: a negative report. *Eur. J. Respir. Dis.* 71:177, 1987.

65. Elias, J. A., and Levinson, A. I. Hypersensitivity reactions to ethylenediamine in aminophylline. *Am. Rev. Respir. Dis.* 123:550, 1981.

66. Erzurum, S. C., et al. Lack of benefit of methotrexate in severe, steroid-dependent asthma. *Ann. Intern. Med.* 114:353, 1991.

67. Fertel, D., and Wanner, A. Methotrexate: does it treat or induce asthma? *Am. Rev. Respir. Dis.* 143:1, 1991.

68. Fisher, J., et al. Respiratory illness and hypophosphatemia. *Chest* 83:504, 1983.

69. Fitzsimons, R., Greenberger, P. A., and Patterson, R. Outcome of pregnancy in women requiring corticosteroids for severe asthma. *J. Allergy Clin. Immunol.* 78:349, 1986.

70. Garvin, J. M. Nearly fatal partial obstruction of the upper airway. *Postgrad. Med.* 87(2):81, 1990.

71. Gilbert, S. C., et al. Methotrexate-induced cirrhosis requiring liver transplantation in three patients with psoriasis. *Arch. Intern. Med.* 150:889, 1990.

72. Gillies, J. D., Reed, M. H., and Simons, F. E. R. Radiologic findings in acute childhood asthma. *J. Can. Assoc. Radiol.* 29:28, 1978.

73. Glauser, F. L., and Bartlett, R. H. Pneumoperitoneum in assocation with pneumothorax. *Chest* 66:536, 1974.

74. Goldman, J., and Bennett, J. R. Gastro-oesophageal reflux and respiratory disorders in adults. *Lancet* 2:493, 1988.

75. Goldman, J. M., and Bennett, J. R. Gastro-esophageal reflux and asthma; a common association, but of what clinical importance? *Gut* 31:1, 1990.

76. Goodall, R. J. R., et al. Relationship between asthma and gastro-oesophageal reflux. *Thorax* 36:116, 1981.

77. Gordon, M., et al. Fetal morbidity following potentially anoxigenic obstetric conditions. VII. Bronchial asthma. *Am. J. Obstet. Gynecol.* 106:421, 1970.

78. Greenberg, A., et al. Severe theophylline toxicity: role of conservative measures, antiarrhythmic agents and charcoal hemoperfusion. *Am. J. Med.* 76:854, 1984.

79. Greenberger, P., and Patterson, R. Safety of therapy for allergic symptoms during pregnancy. *Ann. Intern. Med.* 89:234, 1978.

80. Greenberger, P., and Patterson, R. Beclomethasone diproprionate for severe asthma during pregnancy. *Ann. Intern. Med.* 98:478, 1983.

81. Greenberger, P. A., and Patterson, R. Management of asthma during pregnancy. *N. Engl. J. Med.* 312:897, 1985.

81a. Griffin, D., et al. Acute myopathy during treatment of status asthmaticus with corticosteroids and steroidal muscle relaxants. *Chest* 102:510, 1992.

82. Gross, N. J. Ipratropium bromide. *N. Engl. J. Med.* 319:486, 1988.

83. Gross, N. J., and Skorodin, M. S. Anticholinergic, antimuscarinic bronchodilators. *Am. Rev. Respir. Dis.* 129:856, 1984.

84. Hall, K. W., et al. Metabolic abnormalities associated with intentional theophylline overdose. *Ann. Intern. Med.* 101:457, 1984.

85. Harley, E. H. Spontaneous cervical and mediastinal emphysema in asthma. *Arch. Otolaryngol. Head Neck Surg.* 113:1111, 1987.

86. Haynes, R. C. Adrenocorticotropic Hormone; Adrenocortical Steroids and Their Synthetic Analogs; Inhibitors of the Synthesis and Activity of Adrenocortical Hormones. In A. G. Gilman, et al. (eds.), *Goodman and Gilman's The Pharmacological Basis of Therapeutics* (8th ed). New York: Permagon Press, 1990, Pp. 1431–1462.

87. Hemstreet, M. P., Miles, M. V., and Rutland, R. O. Effect of intravenous isoproterenol on theophylline kinetics. *Clin. Pharmacol. Ther.* 69:360, 1982.

88. Higgins, B., Greening, A. P., and Crompton, G. K. Assisted ventilation in severe asthma. *Thorax* 41:464, 1986.

89. Hindi-Alexander, M. C., et al. Theophylline and fibrocystic breast disease. *J. Allergy Clin. Immunol.* 75:709, 1985.

90. Ho, G., Tierney, M. G., and Dales, R. E. Evaluation of the effect of norfloxacin on the pharmacokinetics of theophylline. *Clin. Pharmacol. Ther.* 44:35, 1988.

91. Hoglund, P., Nilsson, L. G., and Paulsen, O. Interaction between isonizid and theophylline. *Eur. J. Respir. Dis.* 70:110, 1987.

92. Holden, R. Probable fatal interaction between ciprofloxacin and theophylline. *Br. Med. J.* 297:1339, 1988.

93. Hudgel, D. W., Cooper, D., and Souhrada, J. Reversible restrictive lung disease simulating asthma. *Ann. Intern. Med.* 85:328, 1976.

94. Ingram, R. H., et al. Ventilation-perfusion changes after aerosolized isoproterenol in asthma. *Am. Rev. Respir. Dis.* 101:364, 1970.

95. Irwin, R. S., Rosen, M. J., and Braman, S. S. Cough: a comprehensive review. *Arch. Intern. Med.* 137:1186, 1977.

96. James, A. L., Pare, P. D., and Hogg, J. C. The mechanics of airway narrowing in asthma. *Am. Rev. Respir. Dis.* 139:242, 1989.

97. Janson, C., et al. Sleep disturbances in patients with asthma. *Respir. Med.* 84:37, 1990.

98. Jazayeri, M. R., Reen, B. M., and Edwards, J. A. Asthma induced myocardial infarction in a patient with normal coronary arteries. *J. Med.* 14:351, 1983.

99. Jeffrey, P. K. Morphology of the airway wall in asthma and in chronic obstructive pulmonary disease. *Am. Respir. Rev. Dis.* 143:1152, 1991.

100. Johnston, S. L., and Oliver, R. M. Cardiac tamponade due to pneumopericardium. *Thorax* 43:482, 1988.

101. Jolobe, O., and Melnick, S. C. Asthma, pulmonary eosinophilia, and eosinophilic pericarditis. *Thorax* 38:690, 1983.

102. Jones, G., Mierins, E., and Karsh, J. Methotrexate-induced asthma. *Am. Rev. Respir. Dis.* 143:179, 1991.

103. Josephson, G. W., et al. Cardiac dysrhythmias during the treatment of acute asthma. *Chest* 78:429, 1980.

104. Juniper, E. F., et al. Improvement in airway responsiveness and asthma severity during pregnancy. *Am. Respir. Rev. Dis.* 140:924, 1989.

104a. Kaufman, J., et al. Angiotensin-converting enzyme inhibitors in patients with bronchial responsiveness and asthma. *Chest* 101:922, 1992.

105. Kearney, T. E., et al. Theophylline toxicity and the beta-adrenergic system. *Ann. Intern. Med.* 102:766, 1985.

106. Kelly, W. J. W., et al. Childhood asthma in adult life: a further study at 28 years of age. *Br. Med. J.* 294:1059, 1987.

107. Kelly, W. J. W., et al. Childhood asthma and adult lung function. *Am. Respir. Rev. Dis.* 138:26, 1988.

108. Klaustermeyer, W. B., Noritake, D. T., and Kwong, F. K. Chrysotherapy in the treatment of corticosteroid-dependent asthma. *J. Allergy Clin. Immunol.* 79:720, 1987.

109. Kolski, G. B., et al. Hypokalemia and respiratory arrest in an infant with status asthmaticus. *J. Pediatr.* 112:304, 1988.

110. Kro, I., and Kuchar, O. Hypervolemia in status asthmaticus. *Lancet* 2:316, 1970.

110a. Kupfer, Y., et al. Prolonged weakness after long-term infusion of vecuronium bromide. *Ann. Intern. Med.* 117:484, 1992.

111. Kusch, M. M., and Orvald, T. O. Mediastinal and subcutaneous emphysema complicating acute bronchial asthma. *Chest* 57:580, 1970.

112. Kwong, F. K., Sue, M. A., and Kaustermeyer, W. B. Corticosteroid complications in respiratory disease. *Ann. Allergy* 58:326, 1987.

113. Laaban, J. P., et al. Hypophosphatemia complicating management of acute severe asthma. *Ann. Intern. Med.* 112:68, 1990.

114. Lake, K. B., et al. Fatal disseminated aspergillosis in an asthmatic patient treated with corticosteroids. *Chest* 83:138, 1983.

115. Lam, A., and Newhouse, M. T. Management of asthma and chronic airflow obstruction: are methylxanthines obsolete? *Chest* 98:44, 1990.

116. Landay, R. A., Gonzalez, M. A., and Taylor, J. C. Effects of phenobarbital on theophylline disposition. *J. Allergy Clin. Immunol.* 62:27, 1978.

117. Larrain, A., et al. Medical and surgical treatment of nonallergic asthma associated with gastroesophageal reflux. *Chest* 99:1330, 1991.

118. Leung, F. W., Santiago, S. M., and Klaustermeyer, W. B. Corticosteroid therapy and death in cases of adult bronchial asthma. *West J. Med.* 138:565, 1983.

119. Lee, T. M., et al. Rectus sheath hematoma complicating an exacerbation of asthma. *J. Allergy Clin. Immunol.* 78:290, 1986.

120. Leung, A. K. Episodic prepatellar bursitis with asthmatic attacks. *J. R. Soc. Med.* 77:806, 1984.
121. Leung, A. K. Prepatellar bursitis associated with asthma. *Br. J. Clin. Pract.* 43:164, 1989.
122. Levine, J. H., Michael, J. R., and Guarnieri, T. Multifocal atrial tachycardia: a toxic effect of theophylline. *Lancet* 1:12, 1985.
123. Lewis, M., et al. Acute respiratory failure in a young asthmatic patient. *Chest* 84:733, 1983.
124. Lim, R., et al. Cardiac arrhythmias during acute exacerbations of chronic airflow limitation: effect of fall in plasma potassium concentration induced by nebulised beta$_2$-agonist therapy. *Postgrad. Med. J.* 65:449, 1989.
124a. Lindgren, S., et al. Does asthma or treatment with theophylline limit children's academic performance? *N. Engl. J. Med.* 327:926, 1992.
125. Littenberg, B. Aminophylline treatment in severe acute asthma—a metaanalysis. *JAMA* 259:1678, 1988.
126. Lobel, H., Machtey, I., and Eldror, M. Y. Pulmonary infiltrates with eosinophilia in an asthmatic patient treated with disodium cromoglycate. *Lancet* 2:1032, 1972.
127. Luksza, A. R., et al. Acute severe asthma treated by mechanical ventilation: 10 years' experience from a distinct general hospital. *Thorax* 41:459, 1986.
128. Macklem, P. T. Hyperinflation. *Am. Rev. Respir. Dis.* 129:1, 1984.
129. Manfredi, R. L., and Vesell, E. S. Inhibition of theophylline metabolism by long-term allopurinol administration. *Clin. Pharmacol. Ther.* 29:224, 1981.
130. Mansel, J. K., et al. Mechanical ventilation patients with acute severe asthma. *Am. J. Med.* 89:42, 1990.
130a. Margolis, B. D., et al. Prolonged reversible quadriparesis in mechanically ventilated patients who received long-term infusions of vercuronium. *Chest* 100:877, 1991.
131. Marquise, J. F., et al. Phenytoin-theophylline interactions. *N. Engl. J. Med.* 307:1189, 1982.
132. Martin, A. J., Landau, L. I., and Phelan, P. D. Lung function in young adults who had asthma in childhood. *Am. Respir. Rev. Dis.* 122:609, 1980.
133. Martin, A. J., et al. The natural history of childhood asthma to adult life. *Br. Med. J.* 1:1397, 1980.
134. Martin, J., et al. The role of respiratory muscles in the hyperinflation of bronchial asthma. *Am. Rev. Respir. Dis.* 121:441, 1980.
135. Martin, R. J., Cicutto, L. C., and Ballard, R. D. Factors related to the nocturnal worsening of asthma. *Am. Rev. Respir. Dis.* 141:33, 1990.
136. Martin, R. J., et al. Circadian variations in theophylline concentrations and the treatment of nocturnal asthma. *Am. Rev. Respir. Dis.* 139:475, 1989.
137. Martin, R. J., et al. Airways inflammation in nocturnal asthma. *Am. Rev. Respir. Dis.* 143:351, 1991.
138. Mathieu, M., et al. Effects of positive end-expiratory pressure in severe acute asthma. *Crit. Care Med.* 15:1164, 1987.
139. Maxwell, G. M. The problem of mucus plugging in children with asthma. *J. Asthma* 22:131, 1985.
140. McFadden, E. R. Fatal and near-fatal asthma. *N. Engl. J. Med.* 324:409, 1991.
141. McKenzie, D. K., and Gandevia, S. C. Strength and endurance of inspiratory, expiratory and limb muscles in asthma. *Am. Rev. Respir. Dis.* 134:999, 1986.
142. McPherson, M. L., et al. Theophylline-induced hypercalcemia. *Ann. Intern. Med.* 105:52, 1986.
143. Menitove, S. M., and Goldring, R. M. Combined ventilator and bicarbonate strategy in the management of status asthmaticus. *Am. J. Med.* 74:898, 1983.
144. Messer, J., et al. Association of adrenocorticosteroid therapy and peptic-ulcer disease. *N. Engl. J. Med.* 309:21, 1983.
145. Millman, M., et al. Status asthmaticus: use of acetylcysteine during bronchoscopy and lavage to remove mucus plugs. *Ann. Allergy* 50:85, 1983.
146. Molfino, N. A., et al. Respiratory arrest in near-fatal asthma. *N. Engl. J. Med.* 324:285, 1991.
147. Mountain, R. D., and Sahn, S. A. Clinical features and outcome in patients with acute asthma presenting with hypercapnia. *Am. Rev. Respir. Dis.* 138:535, 1988.
148. Mountain, R. D., et al. Acid-base disturbances in acute asthma. *Chest* 98:651, 1990.
149. Mullarkey, M. F., Lammert, J. K., and Blumenstein, B. Long-term methotrexate treatment in corticosteroid-dependent asthma. *Ann. Intern. Med.* 112:577, 1990.
150. Mullarkey, M. F., et al. Methotrexate in the treatment of asthma. *N. Engl. J. Med.* 318:603, 1988.
151. Muranaka, M., Nakajima, K., and Suzuki, S. Bronchial responsiveness to acetylcholine in patients with bronchial asthma after long-term treatment with gold salt. *J. Allergy Clin. Immunol.* 67:350, 1981.
152. Newman, J. H., Neff, T. A., and Ziporin, P. Acute respiratory failure associated with hypophosphatemia. *N. Engl. J. Med.* 296:1101, 1977.
152a. Nierop, G., et al. Auranofin in the treatment of steroid-dependent asthma: a double-blind study. *Thorax* 47:349, 1992.
153. Nightingale, R. C., and Flower, C. D. R. Encysted pneumothorax, a complication of asthma. *Br. J. Dis. Chest* 78:98, 1984.
154. O'Connor, G. T., Sparrow, D., and Weiss, S. T. The role of allergy and nonspecific airway hyperresponsiveness in the pathogenesis of chronic obstructive pulmonary disease. *Am. Respir. Rev. Dis.* 140:225, 1989.
155. O'Hollaren, M. T., et al. Exposure to an aeroallergen as a possible precipitating factor in respiratory arrest in young patients with asthma. *N. Engl. J. Med.* 324:359, 1991.
156. Okrent, D. G., et al. Metabolic acidosis not due to lactic acidosis in patients with severe acute asthma. *Crit. Care Med.* 15:1098, 1987.
157. O'Rourke, P. P., and Crone, R. K. Halothane in status asthmaticus. *Crit. Care Med.* 10:341, 1982.
158. Owens, G. R., and Tannebaum, R. Theophylline-induced urinary retention. *Ann. Intern. Med.* 94:212, 1981.
159. Pack, A. I. Acid: a nocturnal bronchoconstrictor? *Am. Respir. Rev. Dis.* 141:1391, 1990.
160. Perin, R. J., et al. Sickle cell disease and bronchial asthma. *Ann. Allergy* 50:320, 1983.
161. Perrin-Fayolle, M., et al. Long-term results of surgical treatment of gastroesophageal reflux in asthmatic patients. *Chest* 96:40, 1989.
162. Petty, T. L., et al. Cromolyn sodium is effective in adult chronic asthmatics. *Am. Rev. Respir. Dis.* 139:694, 1989.
163. Piafsky, K. M. Theophylline kinetics in acute pulmonary edema. *Clin. Pharmacol. Ther.* 21:310, 1977.
164. Piafsky, K. M., et al. Theophylline disposition in patients with hepatic cirrhosis. *N. Engl. J. Med.* 296:1495, 1977.
165. Picado, C., Montserrat, J., and Agusti-Vidal, A. Muscle atrophy in severe exacerbation of asthma requiring mechanical ventilation. *Respiration* 53:201, 1988.
166. Pingleton, S. K. Complications of acute respiratory failure. *Am. Rev. Respir. Dis.* 137:1463, 1988.
167. Pisani, R. J., and Rosenow, E. C. Pulmonary edema associated with tocolytic therapy. *Ann. Intern. Med.* 110:714, 1989.
168. Popa, V. Captopril-related (and -induced?) asthma. *Am. Respir. Rev. Dis.* 136:999, 1987.
169. Qvist, J., et al. High-level PEEP in severe asthma. *N. Engl. J. Med.* 307:1347, 1982.
170. Rafferty, P. Antihistamines in the treatment of clinical asthma. *J. Allergy Clin. Immunol.* 88:647, 1990.
171. Rafferty, P., and Holgate, S. T. Terfenadine (Seldane^R) is a potent and selective histamine H$_1$ receptor antagonist in asthmatic airways. *Am. Rev. Respir. Dis.* 135:181, 1987.
172. Rao, M., et al. Digital clubbing in children with chronic asthma—a clinical experience at Kings County Hospital. *J. Asthma* 18:49, 1981.
173. Rebuck, A. S. Radiological aspects of severe asthma. *Australas. Radiol.* 14:264, 1970.
174. Rebuck, A. S., and Read, J. Assessment and management of severe asthma. *Am. J. Med.* 51:788, 1971.
175. Reed, C. E. New therapeutic approaches in asthma. *J. Allergy Clin. Immunol.* 77:537, 1986.
176. Reed, C. E. Aerosol glucocorticoid treatment of asthma: adults. *Am. Rev. Respir. Dis.* 141:S82, 1990.
177. Reitberg, D. P., Bernhard, H., and Schentag, J. J. Alteration of theophylline clearance and half-life by cimetidine in normal volunteers. *Ann. Intern. Med.* 95:582, 1981.
178. ReMine, S. C., and McIlrath, D. C. Bowel perforation in steroid-treated patients. *Ann. Surg.* 192:581, 1980.
179. Renton, K. W., Gray, J. D., and Hung, O. R. Depression of theophylline elimination by erythromycin. *Clin. Pharmacol. Ther.* 30:422, 1981.
180. Richards, J. M., Santiago, S. M., and Klaustermeyer, W. B. Aseptic necrosis of the femoral head in corticosteroid-treated pulmonary disease. *Arch. Intern. Med.* 140:1473, 1980.
181. Ringle, E. R., et al. Chest wall configurational changes before and during acute obstructive episodes in asthma. *Am. Rev. Respir. Dis.* 128:607, 1983.
182. Robin, E. D., and Lewiston, N. Unexpected, unexplained sudden death in young asthmatic subjects. *Chest* 96:790, 1989.
183. Roche, W. R., et al. Subepithelial fibrosis in the bronchi of asthmatics. *Lancet* 1:520, 1989.
184. Rodriquez-Roisin, R., et al. Subconjunctival hemorrhage: a feature of acute severe asthma. *Postgrad. Med. J.* 61:579, 1985.

185. Ruffin, R., and Rachootin, P. Gag reflex in disease. *Chest* 92:1130, 1987.
186. Sackner, M. A. Cough. In J. F. Murray and J. A. Nadel (eds.), *Textbook of Respiratory Medicine*. Philadelphia: Saunders, 1988, Pp. 397–408.
187. St. Clair, E. W., Rice, J. R., and Snydrman, R. Pneumonitis complicating low-dose methotrexate therapy in rheumatoid arthritis. *Arch. Intern. Med.* 145:2035, 1985.
188. Santiago, S. M., and Klaustermeyer, W. B. Mortality in status asthmaticus: a nine-year experience in a respiratory intensive care unit. *J. Asthma Res.* 17:75, 1980.
189. Schatz, M., et al. The course of asthma during pregnancy, post partum, and with successive pregnancies: a prospective analysis. *J. Allergy Clin. Immunol.* 81:509, 1988.
190. Schatz, M., et al. Intrauterine growth is related to gestational pulmonary function in pregnant asthmatic women. *Chest* 98:389, 1990.
191. Schiff, G. D., et al. Inpatient theophylline toxicity: preventable factors. *Ann. Intern. Med.* 114:748, 1991.
192. Schreier, L., Cutler, R. M., and Saigal, V. Vomiting as a dominant symptom of asthma. *Ann. Allergy* 58:118, 1987.
193. Schreier, L., Cutler, R. M., and Saigal, V. Respiratory failure in asthma during the third trimester: report of two cases. *Am. J. Obstet. Gynecol.* 160:80, 1989.
194. Schwartz, S. H. Treatment of status asthmaticus with halothane. *JAMA* 251:2688, 1984.
195. Scoggin, C. H., Sahn, S. A., and Petty, T. L. Status asthmaticus, a nine-year experience. *JAMA* 238:1158, 1977.
196. Searles, G., and McKendry, R. J. R. Methotrexate pneumonitis in rheumatoid arthritis: potential risk factors. Four case reports and a review of the literature. *J. Rheumatol.* 14:1164, 1987.
197. Sears, N. R., and Dunckley, C. G. Recurrent nocturnal near fatal asthma in a young man. *N. Z. Med. J.* 101:478, 1988.
198. Sears, M. R., et al. Regular inhaled beta-agonist treatment in bronchial asthma. *Lancet* 336:1391, 1990.
199. Segal, M. S. Bronchospasm after reserpine. *N. Engl. J. Med.* 281:1426, 1969.
200. Sessler, C. N. Theophylline toxicity: clinical features of 116 consecutive cases. *Am. J. Med.* 88:567, 1990.
201. Shah, P. K. D., et al. Clinical dysautonomia in patients with bronchial asthma. *Chest* 98:1408, 1990.
202. Shapiro, G. G., et al. Poliomyelitis-like illness after acute asthma. *J. Pediatr.* 94:767, 1979.
203. Sheehy, A. F., et al. Treatment of status asthmaticus. *Arch. Intern. Med.* 130:37, 1972.
204. Sheffer, A. L., Rocklin, R. E., and Goetzl, E. J. Immunologic components of hypersensitivity reactions to cromolyn sodium. *N. Engl. J. Med.* 192:1220, 1975.
205. Shim, C. S., and Williams, M. H. Cough and wheezing after inhalation of beclomethasone dipropionate aerosol in asthma. *Chest* 91:207, 1987.
206. Shim, C. S., and Williams, M. H. Cough and wheezing from beclomethasone dipropionate aerosol are absent after triamcinolone acetonide. *Ann. Intern. Med.* 106:700, 1987.
207. Shiner, R. J., et al. Randomized, double-blind, placebo-controlled trial of methotrexate in steroid-dependent asthma. *Lancet* 336:137, 1990.
208. Shneerson, J. Non-respiratory symptoms of acute asthma. *Thorax* 41:701, 1986.
209. Silk, H. J., et al. Fatal varicella in steroid-dependent asthma. *J. Allergy Clin. Immunol.* 81:47, 1988.
210. Sirmans, S. M., et al. Effect of calcium channel blockers on theophylline deposition. *Clin. Pharmacol. Ther.* 44:29, 1988.
211. Smith, M. J., and Hodson, M. E. Effects of long-term inhaled high dose beclomethasone dipropionate on adrenal function. *Thorax* 38:676, 1983.
212. Sobonya, R. E. Quantitative structural alterations in long-standing allergic asthma. *Am. Respir. Rev. Dis.* 130:289, 1984.
213. Sonin, L., and Patterson, R. Corticosteroid-dependent asthma and schizophrenia. *Arch. Intern. Med.* 144:554, 1984.
214. Spaulding, H. S., et al. Further investigation of the association betweeen gastroesophageal reflux and bronchoconstriction. *J. Allergy. Clin. Immunol.* 69:516, 1982.
214a. Spitzer, W. O., et al. The use of β-agonists and the risk of death and near death from asthma. *N. Engl. J. Med.* 326:501, 1992.
215. Stalcup, S. A., and Mellins, R. B. Mechanical forces producing pulmonary edema in acute asthma. *N. Engl. J. Med.* 297:592, 1977.
216. Strachan, D. P., et al. Asthma as a link between chest illness in childhood and chronic cough and phlegm in young adults. *Br. Med. J.* 296:890, 1988.
217. Straub, P. W., and Buhlmann, A. A. Hypovolemia in status asthmaticus. *Lancet* 2:923, 1969.

218. Stuck, A. E., Minder, C. E., and Frey, F. J. Risk of infectious complications in patients taking glucocorticosteroids. *Rev. Infect. Dis.* 11:954, 1989.
219. Tan, W. C., et al. Effects of spontaneous and simulated gastroesophageal relux on sleeping asthmatics. *Am. Respir. Rev. Dis.* 141:1394, 1990.
220. Tanigaki, T., et al. Transient neuromuscular impairment resulting from prolonged inhalation of halothane and enflurane. *Chest* 98:1012, 1990.
221. Thomson, A. H., Pratt, C., and Simpson, H. Nocturnal cough in asthma. *Arch. Dis. Child.* 62:1001, 1987.
222. Tinkelman, D. G., et al. Evaluation of the safety and efficacy of multiple doses of azelastine to adult patients with bronchial asthma over time. *Am. Rev. Respir. Dis.* 141:569, 1990.
223. Toogood, J. H. Complications of topical steroid therapy for asthma. *Am. Rev. Respir. Dis.* 141:S89, 1990.
224. Toogood, J. H., et al. Use of spaces to facilitate inhaled corticosteroid treatment of asthma. *Am. Rev. Respir. Dis.* 129:723, 1984.
225. Tornatore, K. M., et al. Effect of chronic oral contraceptive steroids on theophylline disposition. *Eur. J. Clin. Pharmacol.* 23:129, 1982.
226. Tsuji, H., et al. CT demonstration of spinal epidural emphysema complicating bronchial asthma and violent coughing. *J. Comput. Assist. Tomogr.* 13:38, 1989.
227. Tuxen, D. V. Detrimental effects of positive end-expiratory pressure during controlled mechanical ventilation of patients with severe airflow obstruction. *Am. Rev. Respir. Dis.* 140:5, 1989.
228. Tuxen, D. V., and Lane, S. The effects of ventilatory pattern on hyperinflation airway pressures and circulation in mechanical ventilation of patients with air-flow obstruction. *Am. Rev. Respir. Dis.* 136:872, 1987.
229. Van Den Bosch, J. M. M., Wagenaar, S. S., and Westermann, C. J. J. Asthma, eosinophilic pleuropneumonia and pericarditis without vasculitis. *Thorax* 41:571, 1986.
230. van Schayck, C. P., et al. Increased bronchial hyperresponsiveness after inhaling salbutamol during one year is not caused by desensitization to salbutamol. *J. Allergy Clin. Immunol.* 86:793, 1990.
231. Vathenen, A. S., et al. Rebound increase in bronchial responsiveness after treatment with inhaled terbutaline. *Lancet* 1:554, 1988.
232. Wald, J. A., Friedman, B. R., and Farr, R. S. An improved protocol for the use of troleandomycin (TAO) in the treatment of steroid-requiring asthma. *J. Allergy Clin. Immunol.* 78:36, 1986.
233. Wasser, W. G., Bronheim, H. E., and Richardson, B. K. Theophylline madness. *Ann. Intern. Med.* 95:191, 1981.
234. Wasserfallen, J. B., et al. Sudden asphyxic asthma: a distinct entity? *Am. Rev. Respir. Dis.* 142:108, 1990.
235. Weber, C. A., and Santiago, R. M. Hypermagnesemia: a potential complication during treatment of theophylline intoxication with oral activated charcoal and magnesium-containing cathartics. *Chest* 95:56, 1989.
236. Webb, A. K., Bilton, A. H., and Hanson, G. C. Severe bronchial asthma requiring ventilation. A review of 20 cases and advice on management. *Postgrad. Med. J.* 55:161, 1979.
237. Weinberger, M., et al. Inhibition of theophylline clearance by troleandomycin. *J. Allergy Clin. Immunol.* 59:228, 1977.
237a. Weiss, S. T., et al. Effects of asthma on pulmonary function in children. A longitudinal population-based study. *Am. Rev. Respir. Dis.* 145:58, 1992.
238. Westerman, D. E., et al. Identification of the high-risk asthmatic patient. *Am. J. Med.* 66:565, 1979.
239. Williams, I. P., et al. Sympathomimetic agonists stimulate mucus secretion into human bronchi. *Thorax* 36:231, 1981.
240. Williams, M. H. Life-threatening asthma. *Arch. Intern. Med.* 140:1604, 1980.
241. Williams, T. J., et al. Acute myopathy in severe acute asthma treated with intravenously administered corticosteroids. *Am. Rev. Respir. Dis.* 137:460, 1988.
241a. Williams, T. J., et al. Risk factors for morbidity in mechanically ventilated patients with acute severe asthma. *Am. Rev. Respir. Dis.* 146:607, 1992.
242. Wong, C. S., et al. Bronchodilator, cardiovascular, and hypokalemic effects of fenoterol, salbutamol, and terbutaline in asthma. *Lancet* 336:1396, 1990.
243. Zavala, D. C. Bronchoscopy, Lung Biopsy and Other Procedures. In J. F. Murray and J. A. Nadel (eds.), *Textbook of Respiratory Medicine*. Philadelphia: Saunders, 1988, Pp. 562–596.
244. Zieger, R. S., et al. Efficacy of troleandomycin in outpatients with severe, corticosteroid-dependent asthma. *J. Allergy Clin. Immunol.* 66:438, 1980.
245. Ziment, I. Management of hypertension in the asthmatic patient. *Chest* 83(suppl.):392, 1983.
246. Zwillich, C. W., et al. Theophylline induced seizures in adults. Correlation with serum concentrations. *Ann. Intern. Med.* 82:784, 1975.

Financial Considerations

Robert N. Ross

92

After adjusting for inflation, total and per capita personal health care expenditures have risen in the United States at annual rates of 5.5 and 4.1 percent since 1950, the proportion of the gross national product devoted to health care has tripled, and by the year 2000 the United States will devote an estimated 15 percent of its total production to health care [1]. There has been a similarly dramatic increase in the number of cost studies in the health care literature over the past few decades (Fig. 92-1); and the rate has been accelerating. One-half of the 39,318 articles published from 1965 through 1990 with "cost" as a key word (as listed in the MEDLINE data base prepared by the U.S. National Library of Medicine) were published since 1984. Publications on the costs of asthma are but a small proportion (0.3%) of the total number of health cost studies; but the number of asthma studies, too, has grown with the intensified interest in medical costs (Fig. 92-2). Of the 115 articles on asthma costs published from 1965 through 1990, 71 of 115 (62%) were published in the years between 1984 and 1990.

The rising cost of health care in the United States has become a major preoccupation of all participants in the health care system. Costs are important to payors because third-party payors assume most of the financial risk for the reimbursement of health care costs. Employers are becoming increasingly concerned because the payors are passing their increased financial exposure on to the employers, who must therefore pay higher premiums. Costs are important to government because government (at all levels) is a major purchaser of both health care and health care coverage; and at the federal level, government is a major payor. The situation is somewhat different for providers and patients. To providers, costs are important if the provider bears some of the financial risk associated with treatment. To patients, costs of care are important only to the extent that personal financial losses due to treatment and incapacitation are greater than reimbursements. Thus what two observers from the Robert Wood Johnson Foundation have called the "national schizophrenia" regarding health care costs: Public opinion surveys show that Americans are deeply concerned about rising health care costs but are unwilling to do anything that might jeopardize their own health care arrangements [2].

Health professionals and policymakers recognize the finiteness of health care resources and are forced to decide on the relative costs and values of goods, services, methods, and outcomes. In an effort to determine whether we are in fact getting good value for money in providing various sorts of health care, the United States Congress asked the Office of Technology Assessment (OTA) in 1978 to explore the applicability of cost-effectiveness and cost-benefit analyses to medical technology. Two years later, OTA published 22 volumes on the subject. The first volume was the main report, *The Implications of Cost-effectiveness Analysis of Medical Technology* [18]. The second report was a review of the cost-effectiveness literature [19]. The succeeding volumes

were presentations of 19 case studies examining the cost and effectiveness of cimetidine, several human immunization programs, and behavioral approaches to the reduction of cardiovascular disease.

The terms *cost-effectiveness* and *cost-benefit* are now widely used; but as Doubilet, Weinstein, and McNeil [9] have noted, they are often used carelessly:

> Examples of its [the term *cost effectiveness*] use abound in the medical literature, in drug and equipment advertisements, and in the hallways and lecture halls of medical institutions. Unfortunately, many who assert that a specified medical practice is cost effective fail to couple that statement with appropriate documentation of associated costs and benefits.

Cost-effective, according to these authors, has been taken variously to mean (1) cost saving with or without regard to effectiveness, (2) effective with or without regard to cost, (3) cost saving with an equal or better health outcome, or (4) having an additional benefit worth the additional cost. When used appropriately, however, cost-effectiveness and cost-benefit studies are conducted to estimate the return on health care investment (whether that return be improved health, reduced utilization of health care resources, enhanced productivity, or improved quality of life).

A cost-effectiveness study measures the cost of a clinical outcome in terms of some other unit, as for instance, dollars per life-year gained or dollars per case of a disease prevented. A cost-benefit study measures the ratio of the cost of a clinical treatment to the saving that results from the benefit. The difficulty with cost-benefit studies, however, is that it is not always clear whose benefit is being considered. The patient, provider, payor, employer, government, and society as a whole may all derive some benefit from the success of a particular treatment, but the benefit may be valued quite differently by these various interests.

Asthma is a perfect candidate for cost-effectiveness and cost-benefit studies. The costs associated with asthma are significant because asthma is a chronic condition, affects large numbers of people, is responsible for a significant decrement in productivity, requires considerable expense for treatment, and has the potential to reduce drastically the quality of life of both the person suffering from asthma and the people associated with the asthmatic. An analysis of the cost-effectiveness or cost-benefit of a treatment of asthma must begin with an accurate estimate of the costs themselves.

ASTHMA COST STUDIES

Several types of costs are associated with asthma. The direct medical costs include the costs of physician office visits, outpa-

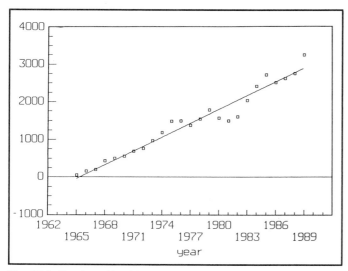

Fig. 92-1. *Number of health cost studies published in the medical literature, 1965–1990.*

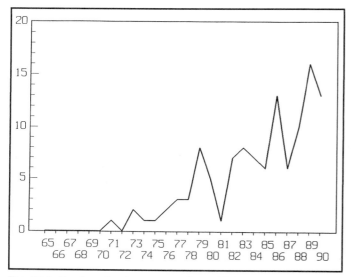

Fig. 92-2. *Number of asthma cost studies published in the medical literature, 1965–1990.*

tient and ancillary care including emergency room visits, medications and procedures, and hospitalizations. Associated with these direct medical costs may be several direct nonmedical costs, such as the cost of transportation, lodging and food, or child care. The indirect costs due to loss of livelihood and loss of life probably far outweigh the direct medical and nonmedical costs. Mortality and decreased productivity or absenteeism during exacerbations of asthma are the major indirect costs. Finally there are the intangible costs attributable to the pain and suffering associated with asthma (that is, reduced quality of life). This last category of costs may be difficult to measure, but it is nevertheless real and must somehow be taken into consideration in any discussion of the costs associated with asthma.

The direct costs of treating asthma may be high. Vance and Taylor [38] reported in 1971 that direct costs of treating severe childhood asthma can require expenditures as high as 31 percent of a family's income, with lower-income families paying a higher proportion of their income. Marion and colleagues [23] studied the direct and indirect costs associated with the management of childhood asthma for the period 1977 to 1980 and found that the average expenditure was $940, or 5.5 percent of the annual family income. Today, at an annual per capita increase in health care costs of 4.1 percent [1], the equivalent expenditure would be more than $1500.

Little has been published on the personal and societal costs of asthma in the United States. Data collection is difficult because only the relative infrequent big-ticket items (e.g., hospitalizations) are well documented. The far more frequent, lower-cost events (e.g., physician office visits, medications) are more difficult to monitor and must be estimated from incomplete data. The indirect costs of asthma (e.g., lost work time, reduced productivity on the job, school absenteeism) and the pain and suffering as a result of asthma are even more difficult to estimate.

It is also difficult to generalize from one set of local findings on asthma costs to the nation as a whole. Costs of care and patients' expectations can differ widely from one region to another. Accepted medical practices can vary widely, too. For example, the relative risk of hospitalization for asthmatic children in Boston, Massachusetts, relative to Rochester, New York, is 3.8 and for New Haven, Connecticut, relative to Rochester 2.3 [31]. The costs of a hospital admission for the treatment of asthma can vary widely both within a hospital and between hospitals. In a recent study of illness severity and costs of admission at teaching and nonteaching hospitals, investigators reported extremely large variances associated with the mean cost of an admission for asthma: $2865 ± 2415 for 248 patients at 6 tertiary teaching hospitals in the Boston area, $2386 ± 2001 for 246 patients at 9 other teaching hospitals, and $2087 ± 1291 for 250 patients at 14 other, nonteaching hospitals [17]. The observed differences in asthma hospitalization rates and costs therefore complicate any effort to generalize local findings to the national level.

Freund and colleagues [12] investigated how the quality, outcomes, and cost of treating asthma vary across three specialty groups (allergists, family physicians, and pediatricians) in the Kansas City area. Patients of allergists took more prescription drugs, rented more medical equipment, and were more likely to receive antiallergy treatment than patients of family physicians or pediatricians. In this regard, the cost of being treated by an allergist was greater than that of being treated by other medical specialists. But patients of physicians other than allergists had two more hospital bed days per year than patients of allergists. The investigators concluded that while costs are higher for patients of allergists, the benefits (e.g., days lost, emergency room visits, hospitalizations) more than offset the additional cost ($62/yr) of treatment by an allergist.

Two published studies give some indication of the costs of asthma. A French evaluation published in 1989 of the medical costs associated with asthma in young adults with no other complicating conditions has shown that the overall costs of asthma are greater than those associated with tuberculosis and at least as great as the costs associated with hypertension or diabetes [34]. The cost of diagnosing asthma in France is estimated to be FF 3250 ($559 at FF 0.1720 to the dollar, May 1991). The costs of monitoring asthma can range from FF 3242 ($558) to FF 14,226 ($2447) depending on severity (Table 92-1). The annual costs of medication for the four levels will also vary with severity, as shown in Table 92-2. Two observations are in order concerning the costs of medication. First, there is a striking difference in cost with increase in severity from mild (level I) to mild-to-moderate (level II) asthma. Second, medical treatment of the most severe cases of asthma (level IV) actually costs less than treatment of the less severe asthma (level III). The costs of hospitalization increase dramatically with increasing severity. The costs of hospitalization are shown in Table 92-3.

Table 92-1. *Estimated annual costs of monitoring asthma by severity of asthma*

Level of severity	Cost of diagnostic services, per year
Level I: 4 exacerbations per year	$558 (FF 3,242)
Level II: approximately 10 exacerbations per year	$2028 (FF 11,791)
Levels III–IV: 2 exacerbations per month with continuous dyspnea	$2447 (FF 14,226)

$ = U.S. dollar; FF = French franc.
Source: Sansonetti et al. Evaluation du cout medical de l'asthme de l'adulte au cours d'une annee de surveillance en milieu hospitalier. *Rev. Mal. Respr.* 6:169, 1989.

Table 92-2. *Estimated annual cost of medical regimen by severity of asthma*

Level	Cost of medication, per year
I	$27 (FF 154)
II	$1001 (FF 5,820)
III	$1198 (FF 6,964)
IV	$889 (FF 5,170)

$ = U.S. dollar; FF = French franc.
Source: Sansonetti et al. Evaluation du cout medical de l'asthme de l'adulte au cours d'une annee de surveillance en milieu hospitalier. *Rev. Mal. Respr.* 6:169, 1989.

Table 92-3. *Estimated annual cost of hospital inpatient care by severity of asthma*

Level	Cost of hospitalization
I	$992 (FF 5,767)
II	$7272 (FF 42,276)
III	$14,753 (FF 85,775)
IV	$20,453 (FF 118,911)

$ = U.S. dollar; FF = French franc.
Source: Sansonetti et al. Evaluation du cout medical de l'asthme de l'adulte au cours d'une annee de surveillance en milieu hospitalier. *Rev. Mal. Respr.* 6:169, 1989.

ESTIMATING THE SOCIETAL COSTS OF ASTHMA IN THE UNITED STATES

Epidemiology

Depending on the definition, there are between 7 and 20 million asthmatics in the United States, of which between 2 and 5 million are children [11]. According to one analysis of data from the National Center for Health Statistics, the prevalence of asthma (defined as ever having been told by a physician) is 10.5 percent, and the prevalence of active asthma within the past 12 months was 7.7 percent [11].

Asthma mortality has been rising (see Chap. 90). During the 1970s, the rate of asthma mortality declined annually by 7.8 percent; but during the 1980s, the mortality rate increased steadily by 6.2 percent annually, increasing fastest among the young (age 5–14), poor, and black [39].

Hospitalization

Not surprisingly, the hospitalization rate has also been rising. Between 1979 and 1987, the hospitalization rate for children 17 years or younger increased annually by 4.5 percent, with the increase largest among the youngest (younger than 4 years), poor, and black [13]. The number of readmissions (as well as new admissions) has been increasing. During the period 1960 to

Table 92-4. *Asthma hospitalization rate in the United States, 1989*

	Total number of hospitalizations	Hospitalization rate/10,000 population	Average length of stay (days)
All patients	475,000	19.3	4.5
Male	204,000	17.1	3.8
Female	271,000	21.3	5.0
By age			
Under 15	168,000	31.2	2.9
15–44	127,000	11.0	4.2
45–64	88,000	19.0	5.2
65 and older	93,000	29.9	7.2

Source: Graves, E. J. 1989 summary: National Hospital Discharge Survey. *Advance Data from Vital and Health Statistics*, no. 199. Hyattsville, MD: National Center for Health Statistics, 1991.

1964, 22 percent of admissions to one hospital had had a previous admission for asthma; during the period 1970 to 1974, that figure rose to 45 percent [26]. A summary of hospitalization statistics for the year 1989 appears in Table 92-4.

In 1987, there were a total of 454,000 hospitalizations for asthma, with an average length of stay of 4.8 days, accounting for 2.2 million hospital inpatient days [28]. The number of hospitalizations in 1989 was 5 percent higher than in 1987, but because of a 6 percent decrease in length of stay, 1989 compared with 1987, there was a net 4 percent decrease in the number of inpatient hospital days.

Emergency Room Visits

In 1980, there were 2.7 million emergency room visits for the treatment of asthma [5]. Estimating from increases in the population from 1980 to the present, we can expect to see more than 3 million emergency room visits for the treatment of acute asthma in the early 1990s. This estimate is conservative because it does not take into account reported increases in the incidence and prevalence of asthma in recent years.

Physician Office Visits

In 1980, there were 5.9 million physician office visits for the treatment of asthma [6]. Looking only at visits to pediatricians classed by diagnosis of asthma, in 1980 there were 3.4 million visits [7]. In 1985, there were 6.5 million office visits [21]. Children aged 11 to 14 years accounted for 297,000 asthma office visits in 1985 [29]. We can expect to see at least 7.2 million office visits in the early 1990s and 9 million visits by the turn of the century. As with estimates for hospitalizations, this figure does not take into account the increasing incidence and prevalence of asthma in the United States.

COSTS OF ASTHMA

The societal cost of asthma is the sum of direct and indirect costs associated with asthma.

The direct medical costs of asthma are physician office visits, emergency room visits, hospitalization, and medications. Table 92-5 shows estimates of major direct costs associated with asthma [32].

Indirect costs associated with asthma are also significant. According to one estimate of the costs of all illnesses, the costs of absenteeism and lost productivity compose 60 percent of the costs of an illness; treatment costs are only 40 percent [22]. Lost time for office visits, emergency room visits, and hospitalizations

Table 92-5. Estimated annual (1991) direct costs associated with the treatment of asthma

Factor	Annual cost ($)
Physician office visits (7.0 million visits × 16.6 minutes per visit × $50/hour)	$94 million
Hospitalization (475,000 hospitalizations × 4.5 days/admission × $1000/day)	$2137 million
Emergency room visits (3 million ER visits × $350/visit)	$1050 million
Medications (6.5 million patients × $550/patient)	$3575 million
Total	$6856 million

Source: Ross, R. N. The costs of managing asthma. *J. Respir. Dis.* (Suppl.):S15, 1989.

(patient's time as well as family time) are major indirect costs of asthma but virtually impossible to evaluate. A further indirect cost is that of patient noncompliance. Patients' failure to take medications as prescribed results in increased costs of physician office visits, emergency room visits, hospitalizations, and a host of other indirect costs.

The largest indirect cost associated with asthma is disability days. An estimated 400,000 persons suffered some limitation of work activity in 1990 because of asthma [32]. The average time out of work was 5.0 days per year [40]. Total disability days due to asthma is thus 400,000 workers × 5.0 days, or 2.0 million lost work days per year. Total indirect costs due to asthma have been estimated to be more than $2 billion [32].

COST-REDUCTION STUDIES

Given the high cost of hospital inpatient care, less intensive alternatives to hospital treatment of asthma are extremely attractive. One French study found that the cost of diagnosis and treatment of severe asthma (42 patients) on an outpatient basis was one-third the cost of hospital inpatient treatment (FF 4,804 versus FF 13,741) [15]. Studies in the United States have shown the clinical effectiveness and cost saving associated with short-term holding room treatment of asthmatic children [30, 41]. For example, Willert and colleagues [41] found that holding room therapy for childhood status asthmaticus is both medically and economically effective, costing $526 ± 226 rather than $1,439 ± 339 for the treatment of hospitalized patients [41]. Two studies have shown that economies can be made possible by introducing short-term holding units for observation and treatment of asthma patients seeking treatment in hospital emergency rooms. In one study of 87 consecutive visits for the treatment of acute asthmatic attacks at Children's Hospital National Medical Center (Washington, D.C.), investigators found that the cost of hospitalization was more than five times the cost of treatment in a holding unit [30]. A second study likewise found that the cost of treating patients for less than a day in a short-term holding room was one-third that of hospitalization [41]. O'Brien found in the study of 434 youngsters treated for recurrent acute asthmatic attacks, 328 of 434 (76%) resolved sufficiently after treatment in the holding room for the patients to go home and 71 of the remaining 106 patients could be released home after additional treatment so that 399 of 434 (92%) patients did not require hospitalization. Four patients did return within a week, however, and did require hospitalization [41]. Willert found that 35 of 52 (67%) children in status asthmaticus could be treated in a holding room and discharged to home and that there was no difference in long-term outcome between children immediately admitted to the hospital and children treated in the holding room [30, 41].

The costs, effectiveness, and benefits of various forms of medical therapy for asthma have been also investigated. A 10-year retrospective study of the costs of asthma therapy in an outpatient clinic at the University of Zurich showed that although the costs of xanthines and antiallergic drugs have come down significantly between the years 1977 and 1987, the overall costs of pharmacotherapy for asthma have remained the same [3]. The best explanation for this paradox is that the treatment of asthma has become increasingly complex and the cheaper drugs are being replaced by more effective, but more expensive medicines. In fact, despite the decreasing cost of xanthines, there is evidence to show that reliance on theophylline is not justified in the emergency room care of most asthmatics on therapeutic or economic grounds [36]. Reliance on theophylline and underuse of proved therapies may actually prolong the hospital stay. Costs associated with theophylline therapy include the drug, serum drug concentration monitoring, and intravenous administration. Published utilization reviews of theophylline assays show that the annual cost of erroneous or inappropriate serum theophylline measurements was $28,860 at one hospital and $77,000 at another [36]. A more recent study by the same investigator has concluded that the inclusion of aminophylline in the inhaled albuterol and oral prednisone treatment of hospitalized adult asthmatics contributes little to their therapy and costs an unnecessary $180 million annually in the United States [37].

Most changes in medical treatment have been cost raising, with the only important cost-saving change in recent years being a significant reduction in the average length of hospital stay [35]. Economical ways of avoiding hospitalization and other extended treatments, of course, are even more cost saving. Consequently, it is very important to note that including medications that directly affect the underlying inflammatory process of asthma are cost saving [10, 33]. Prophylaxis is one of the most cost-effective treatment strategies.

Perhaps the most cost-effective and beneficial intervention in the treatment of asthma is education. Self-management of asthma has emerged as a significant factor in maintaining appropriate care of asthmatic patients and, at the same time, introducing economies into the treatment [27, 42]. Use of the emergency room may resolve acute crises but contribute little to the overall treatment of asthma. A study of 310 low income children from 290 families in New York City showed that health education for the families of the children hospitalized for asthma during the year before the study significantly reduced the number of emergency room visits during the period of the study from 7.4 to 3.5 for the experimental group, but there was no change in visits for the comparison group (8.1 versus 8.2) [4]. Health education can improve adherence to the asthma treatment regimen by 44 percent at an annual cost of $32.03 per patient [43]. It can reduce emergency room utilization and hospitalization, saving $11.22 for every dollar spent on education [4].

A retrospective, record-based study to determine the costs of treating asthma with (27 patients) and without (26 patients) the inclusion of cromolyn sodium in the regular treatment plan showed that the expense of emergency room visits and hospital admissions was significantly reduced in cromolyn sodium-treated patients, $33 versus $624 per year for emergency room costs and $357 versus $1,298 for hospitalization costs [33].

Asthmatic patients were severe enough to have required at least one emergency treatment with epinephrine in the year prior to being referred to the study practice. The only systematic difference between the index group and the comparison group was the inclusion of cromolyn sodium in the treatment program combining bronchodilators, corticosteroids, and other routine asthma medications.

There was a significant reduction in hospitalizations for patients in the cromolyn sodium group: Emergency room visits were reduced by 96 percent for patients treated with cromolyn sodium versus a 3 percent reduction for patients in the comparison group. Mellon and colleagues reported a similar finding of 83

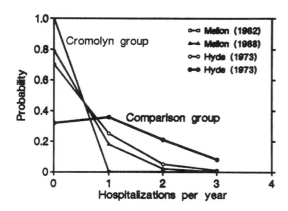

Fig. 92-3. *The probability of zero, one, two, or three hospitalizations per year, cromolyn versus comparison groups.*

percent reduction in emergency room visits during the first 6 months after the introduction of cromolyn sodium [25]. There was a 100 percent reduction in hospitalizations for patients in the cromolyn sodium group versus a 29 percent reduction for the comparison group. The inclusion of cromolyn sodium in the treatment program did not appreciably increase the total number of drugs prescribed over the long term, however. For the period covered by this study, patients in the cromolyn sodium group were prescribed an average of 2.45 ± 0.59 medications per visit period, and patients in the comparison group were prescribed an average of 2.18 ± 0.54 medications per visit period. The aggregate daily cost of all medications prescribed was computed. Daily costs of antiasthma medications did not differ for the two groups of asthma patients. The average daily cost for patients in the cromolyn sodium group was $\$0.93 \pm 0.25$ versus $\$0.84 \pm 0.37$ for the patients in the comparison group. The observed differences between the cromolyn sodium group and the comparison group are so great that further studies (prospective, severity-adjusted studies) will be necessary to test the robustness of the findings. However, as shown in Fig. 92-3, these surprisingly great differences between the cromolyn sodium and comparison groups are not unique. Mellon et al. [24, 25] and Hyde et al. [16] have reported similar findings.

The methodology of cost studies has become popular. But, like all methods, this one easily lends itself to excessive claims and error. The methods were developed by economists, for the most part, and not by physicians. The analyses are accounting systems that must reduce all observable events to some common metric. That metric is usually dollars. But dollars per se cannot reflect the discomfort, disability, and many more subtle, indirect, personal, and societal costs associated with a chronic disease like asthma. The introduction of the QALY—quality adjusted life year—as the common metric for quality of life studies is a gesture toward constructing a general outcome measure that integrates morbidity and mortality into a common unit [20]. But although QALYs make sense in general terms, many problems remain to be resolved at the operational and theoretic level.

The issue raised by all cost studies is that of who the appropriate user of the studies might be. The goal of cost studies is to increase the efficiency of therapy, that is, to provide the maximal incremental health benefit for a fixed amount of resources [8]. Such studies assume as their goal to maximize the net health benefit to the entire target population using fixed resources. They further assume not only that resources are fixed but that programs compete for those fixed resources. Finally, they assume that health benefits accruing as a result of therapy are of equal value to all.

A discussion of these assumptions is beyond the scope of this chapter. But the assumption of competition across programs for finite medical resources deserves special notice. Policymakers who make health resource budgets must decide on the relative value returned on a dollar invested. Clinicians are not faced with such problems in treating individual patients. Thus it must be borne in mind that the ratio of cost to benefit or cost to effectiveness has no absolute value. It is merely a convenient means of rank ordering several competing programs [14]. Physicians and policymakers should not be fooled by the simplicity of the number into thinking that it is an absolute index of therapeutic or fiscal value.

REFERENCES

1. Aaron, H., and Schwartz, W. B. Rationing health care: The choice before us. *Science* 247:418, 1990.
2. Blendon, R. J., and Altman, D. E. Public attitudes about health care costs: A lesson in national schizophrenia. *N. Engl. J. Med.* 311:613, 1984.
3. Bregenzer, T., Mossinger, C., and Medici, T. C. Therapiewandel und Kostenentwicklung des Asthma bronciale: Eine retrospektive Studie uber die letzten 10 Jahre an der Medizinischen Poliklinik des Universitatspitals Zurich. *Pneumologie* 44:960, 1990.
4. Clark, N. M. The impact of health education on frequency and cost of health care use by low income children with asthma. *J. Allergy Clin. Immunol.* 78:108, 1986.
5. Collins, J. G. *Physician Visits, Volume, and Interval Since Last Visit, United States, 1980*, series 10, no. 144. Washington, DC: Public Health Service, 1983.
6. Cypress, B. K. Medication therapy in office visits for selected diagnoses: The National Ambulatory Care Survey, 1980. *Vital and Health Statistics*, series 13, no. 71. Washington, DC: Public Health Service, 1983.
7. Cypress, B. K. Patterns of ambulatory care in pediatrics: The National Ambulatory Medical Care Survey, United States, January 1980–December 1981. National Center for Health Statistics, *Vital and Health Statistics*, series 13, no. 75. DHHS Pub. no. 84-1736. Washington, DC: Public Health Service, 1983.
8. Detsky, A. S., and Naglie, I. G. A clinician's guide to cost-effectiveness analysis. *Ann. Intern. Med.* 113:147, 1990.
9. Doubilet, P., Weinstein, M. C., and McNeil, B. J. Occasional notes: Use and misuse of the term "cost effective" in medicine. *N. Engl. J. Med.* 314:253, 1986.
10. Eigen, H., et al. Evaluation of the addition of cromolyn sodium to bronchodilator maintenance therapy in the long-term management of asthma. *J. Allergy Clin. Immunol.* 80:612, 1987.
11. Evans, R., 3rd, et al. National trends in the morbidity and mortality of asthma in the U.S.: Prevalence, hospitalization and death from asthma over two decades, 1965–1984. *Chest* 91(Suppl. 6):65s, 1987.
12. Freund, D. A., et al. Specialty differences in the treatment of asthma. *J. Allergy Clin. Immunol.* 84:401, 1989.
13. Gergen, P. J., and Weiss, K. B. Changing patterns of asthma hospitalization among children: 1979 to 1987. *J.A.M.A.* 264:1688, 1990.
14. Graves, E. J. 1989 Summary: National hospital discharge survey. *Advance Data from Vital and Health Statistics*, no. 199. Hyattsville, MD: National Center for Health Statistics, 1991.
15. Hirsch, A., et al. Cout-advantages de l'hospitalisation avec hebergement, de l'hopital de jour et de la consultation en pneumologie. A propos de 162 malades. *Rev. Mal. Respir.* 7:331, 1990.
16. Hyde, J. S., Isenberg, P. D., and Floro, L. D. Short- and long-term prophylaxis with cromolyn sodium in chronic asthma. *Chest* 63:875, 1973.
17. Iezzoni, L. I., et al. Illness severity and costs of admissions at teaching and nonteaching hospitals. *J.A.M.A.* 264:1426, 1990.
18. *The Implications of Cost-effectiveness Analysis of Medical Technology.* Washington, DC: U.S. Congress, Office of Technology Assessment, 1980.
19. *The Implications of Cost-effectiveness Analysis of Medical Technology Background Paper #1: Methodological Issues and Literature Review.* Washington, DC: U.S. Congress, Office of Technology Assessment, 1980.
20. Kaplan, R. M., and Ganiats, T. G. QALYs: Their ethical implications. *J.A.M.A.* 264:2502, 1990.
21. Koch, H., and Knapp, D. A. Highlights of drug utilization in office practice: National Ambulatory Medical Care Survey, 1985. *Advance Data from Vital and Health Statistics*, no. 134. DHHS Pub no. 87-1250. Hyattsville, MD: National Center for Health Statistics, 1987.

22. Levy, R. A. How pharmaceuticals cut direct and indirect costs of therapy. *Pharmacy Times* 51:82, 1985.

23. Marion, R. J., Creer, T. L., and Reynolds, R. V. C. Direct and indirect costs associated with the management of childhood asthma. *Ann. Allergy* 54: 31, 1985.

24. Mellon, M. Hospitalizations (H) of asthmatic children (AC) in a health maintenance organization (HMO): A program for reduction. Official abstracts of papers of the XIII International Congress of Allergology and Clinical Immunology (ICACI). *N. Engl. Regional Allergy Proc.* 9:362, 1988.

25. Mellon, M. H., Harden, K., and Zeiger, R. S. The effectiveness and safety of nebulizer cromolyn sodium in the young childhood asthmatic. *Immunol. Allergy Pract.* 4:168, 1982.

26. Mullally, D. I., et al. Increased hospitalizations for asthma among children in the Washington, DC area during 1961–1981. *Ann. Allergy* 53:15, 1984.

27. Mullen, P. D., Mullen, L. R. Implementing asthma self-management education in medical care settings: Issues and strategies. *J. Allergy Clin. Immunol.* 72:611, 1983.

28. National Center for Health Statistics, Hospital Care Statistics Branch. 1987 Summary: National hospital discharge survey. *Advance Data from Vital and Health Statistics*, no. 159 (rev.). DHHS Pub. no. 88-1250. Bethesda, MD: Public Health Service, 1988.

29. Nelson, C. Office visits by adolescents. *Advance Data from Vital and Health Statistics*, no. 196. Hyattsville, MD: National Center for Health Statistics, 1991.

30. O'Brien, S. R., Hein, E. W., and Sly, R. M. Treatment of acute asthmatic attacks in a holding unit of a pediatric emergency room. *Ann. Allergy* 45: 159, 1980.

31. Perrin, J. M., et al. Variations in rates of hospitalization of children in three urban communities. *N. Engl. J. Med.* 320:1183, 1989.

32. Ross, R. N. The costs of managing asthma. *J. Respir. Dis.* (Suppl.):S15, 1989.

33. Ross, R. N., et al. Cost effectiveness of including cromolyn sodium in the treatment program for asthma: A retrospective, record-based study. *Clin. Therap.* 10:188, 1988.

34. Sansonetti, M., et al. Evaluation du cout medical de l'asthme de l'adulte au cours d'une annee de surveillance en milieu hospitalier. *Rev. Mal. Respir.* 6:169, 1989.

35. Scitovsky, A. A. Changes in the costs of treatment of selected illnesses, 1971–1981. *Med. Care* 23:1345, 1985.

36. Self, T. H. et al. Is theophylline use justified in acute exacerbations of asthma? *Pharmacotherapy* 9:260, 1989.

37. Self, T. H., et al. Inhaled albuterol and oral prednisone therapy in hospitalized adult asthmatics: Does aminophylline add any benefit? *Chest* 98: 1317, 1990.

38. Vance, V. J., and Taylor, W. F. The financial cost of chronic childhood asthma. *Ann. Allergy* 29:445, 1971.

39. Weiss, K. B., and Wagener, D. K. Changing pattens of asthma mortality: Identifying target populations at high risk. *J.A.M.A.* 264:1683, 1990.

40. Wilder, C. S. Disability days, United States: 1980. *Vital and Health Statistics*, series, 10, no. 142. Washington, DC: Public Health Service, 1983.

41. Willert, C., et al. Short-term holding room treatment of asthmatic children. *J. Pediatr.* 106:707, 1985.

42. Wilson-Pessano, S. R. An evaluation of approaches to asthma self-management education for adults: The AIR/Kaiser-Permanente study. *Health Ed. Q.* 14:333, 1987.

43. Windsor, R. A., et al. Evaluation of the efficacy and cost effectiveness of health education methods to increase medication adherence among adults with asthma. *Am. J. Public Health* 80:1519, 1990.

Asthma and Alpha₁-Antitrypsin

Charlotte R. Colp
Jack Lieberman

93

The association between alpha₁-antitrypsin (AAT) deficiency and lung disease was first reported by Laurell and Eriksson in 1963 [4]. The type of lung disease involved was primarily emphysema, but an association between AAT abnormalities and asthma has also been suspected since 1969 [3].

AAT is the major constituent of the alpha₁-globulin peak seen by serum protein electrophoresis. The AAT protein is synthesized by the liver, and its relatively low molecular weight of 51 kd allows penetration from blood into the various tissues. Its most important function appears to occur in the lungs, where it constitutes a major defense against proteolytic enzymes, especially the elastase of leukocytes. A consequence of AAT deficiency is destruction of lung parenchyma (emphysema) in the presence of recurrent infection or inflammation. However, AAT abnormalities could also aggravate asthma related to proteases released from mast cells in the course of bronchospasm or to the absence of a normal antiimmunologic effect of AAT [1].

AAT is a polymorphic protein having as many as 75 reported molecular variants distinguishable by isoelectric focusing of serum proteins at an acid pH (4.0–5.0). The variants are named by letters according to their mobility on the isoelectric focused gel: Those moving toward the anode ahead of the normal M type are afforded letters below M, and those moving slower than normal are given letters above M in the alphabet. The protein is inherited as a codominant gene so that the phenotype reflects this inheritance; that is, MM is homozygous normal, ZZ is homozygous, and MZ is heterozygous for the deficient Z gene, which is most prevalent in Northern European populations. The Z gene is the most common cause of AAT deficiency, in that the resultant protein contains an amino acid substitution that blocks completion of molecular synthesis and release of AAT from the liver. The ZZ phenotype causes markedly severe deficiency states (serum AAT < 80 mg/dl), whereas the heterozygous MZ phenotype causes an intermediate deficiency state (serum AAT 80–185 mg/dl), which ordinarily will not lead to emphysema unless the patient has some other cause of increased proteolysis in the lung, such as lifetime cigarette smoking.

The S variant is another slowly moving form of AAT, which leads to only minimal reduction of serum levels of the protein. This variant, which has not been found associated with emphysema unless in combination with the Z in an SZ phenotype, is most prevalent in populations derived from Spain or Portugal. Reports from several countries have indicated increased prevalence of the S and/or Z variants in asthmatic patients as compared to control subjects of the same nationality, while other studies have failed to document such as an association [2] (Table 93-1).

We [2] have noted a markedly increased prevalence of asthma in our clinic patients of Puerto Rican descent in New York City

Table 93-1. Alpha₁-antitrypsin phenotypes in asthmatics and controls

| Population | Group | No. | Phenotype | | | |
			MM (%)	MS (%)	MZ (%)	Other
ADULTS						
Norway	Asthma	39	79.5	15.4	0	SS, FM
	Control	2,830	90	4.4	3	SS, FM
Holland	Asthma	324	86	9	3.4	
	Control	269	90	7	2	
Spain	Asthma	38	66	32	2	
	Atopic dermatitis without asthma	35	73	7	16	SZ 4
Poland	Asthma	240	97	1.25	0.4	
	Control	3,560	96	3	0.29	MV, SS, MF, MI
Cleveland, OH	Asthma	138	94.2	2.9	1.45	
	Control	780	89.6	6	3	SS, SZ
CHILDREN						
French and Spanish	Asthma	110	83	15	2	
	Control	100	88	11	1	
Caribbean, Hispanics in Brooklyn, NY	Asthma	47	89	11		
	Control	56	91	7	2	
Rochester, NY	Asthma	268	91	5	2	SZ, etc.
	Control	930	90	6	2	SZ, etc.
Los Angeles	Asthma	151	85	10.5	1	SZ 1.3
	Control	230	88	9	3	

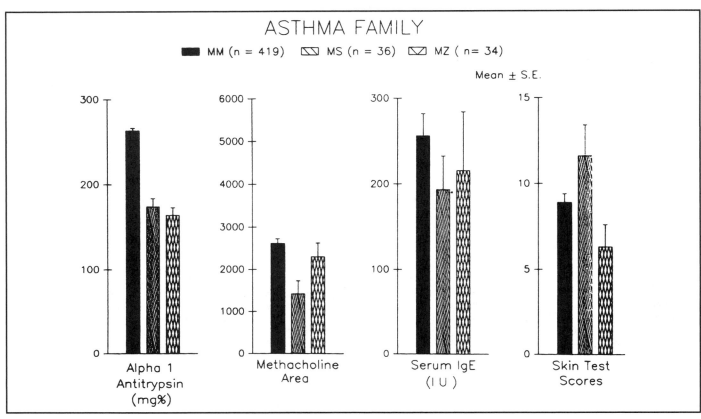

Fig. 93-1. *Mean values (± SE) in homozygous and heterozygous Pi phenotype subjects for α_1-antitrypsin level, methacholine area, serum IgE level, and skin test scores in asthma family members. (Reprinted with permission from R. G. Townley, et al. Association of MS Pi phenotype with airway hyperresponsiveness. Chest 98:594, 1990.)*

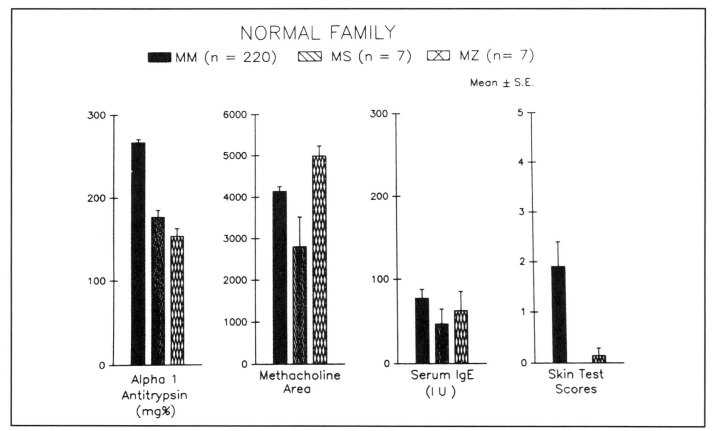

Fig. 93-2. *Mean values (± SE) in homozygous and heterozygous Pi phenotype subjects for α_1-antitrypsin level, methacholine area, serum IgE level, and skin test scores in normal family members. (Reprinted with permission from R. G. Townley, et al. Association of MS Pi phenotype with airway hyperresponsiveness. Chest 98:594, 1990.)*

(60%), as compared to those of non-Hispanic ethnic groups (35%). These Puerto Ricans were also found to have an unusually high prevalence of AAT variants (23%), including both S and Z types, as compared to 10.5% in American whites. While there was no difference in this regard between Puerto Rican asthmatics and control subjects, we found that a significantly larger proportion of individuals with variant phenotypes had a positive family history of asthma: 100 percent versus 68 percent in MM patients in our asthmatics with variant traits.

Also we have noted strikingly reduced smoking histories in those Puerto Ricans with AAT variants, both asthmatics and control subjects (p < .001). Fifteen of 41 MM asthmatics had been heavy smokers, whereas none of 14 with an AAT variant gave a history of having smoked more than 10 packs per year. Among our nonsmoking asthmatics 35 percent were found to have non-MM phenotypes, and a similar proportion has since been found in asthmatic children of Puerto Rican descent.

The propensity for abnormal AAT phenotypes to cause asthma is further substantiated by a recent report from Townley et al. [6] of increased methacholine bronchoreactivity in MS (and to a lesser degree MZ) individuals from both asthmatic and nonasthmatic families (Figs. 93-1 and 93-2). This finding could explain why these individuals are unlikely to smoke. By avoiding tobacco and other respiratory irritants they may be diminishing their risk of having asthma and obstructive pulmonary disease. However, evaluation of the significance of these AAT variant phenotypes is thus made more difficult.

A significant decrease in the functional efficiency of alpha₁-protease inhibitor of the M_1M_1, M_1M_2, and M_2M_2 phenotypes, which may be important in the inflammatory pathogenesis of asthma, was recently reported [7].

Although our asthmatic patients with S and Z trait had normal or near normal serum concentrations of AAT, their propensity to bronchospasm could be increased by an increased liability of variant phenotypes [5], by an inability to increase AAT concentration in the lung to the extent normally achieved in the presence of inflammation, or perhaps by abnormalities of immunologic functions of AAT [1]. With replacement therapy now available for AAT, a therapeutic trial may be considered in the near future in select patients with asthma associated with variant AAT phenotypes.

REFERENCES

1. Arora, P. K., and Miller, H. C. Alpha-1-antitrypsin is an effector of immunological stasis. *Nature* 174:589, 1987.
2. Colp, C., et al. Profile of bronchospastic disease in Puerto Rican patients in New York City: A possible relationship to alpha-antitrypsin variants. *Arch. Intern. Med.* 150:2349, 1990.
3. Fagerhol, M. K., and Hauge, H. E. Serum Pi types in patients with pulmonary diseases. *Acta Allergol.* 24:107, 1969.
4. Laurell, C. B., and Erikson, S. The electrophoretic alpha-globulin pattern in serum alpha-antitrypsin deficiency. *Scand. J. Clin. Lab. Invest.* 15:132, 1963.
5. Lieberman, J. Heat liability of alpha-antitrypsin variants. *Chest* 64:579, 1973.
6. Townley, R. G., et al. Association of MS Pi phenotype with airway hyperresponsiveness. *Chest* 98:594, 1990.
7. Gaillard M. C., et al. Alpha-1-protease inhibitor in bronchial asthma: phenotypes and biochemical characteristics. *Am. Rev. Respir. Dis.* 145:1311, 1992.

Prevention of Asthma: Education and Self-Management Programs

94

Gustave A. Laurenzi

In many respects, bronchial asthma is a model of diseases for which preventive measures can be applied with some degree of success. To minimize the task, however, would be misleading, since the multifactorial aspects, variability, and unpredictability that typify the asthmatic state make a comprehensive program very difficult. Nevertheless, the large body of knowledge relating to basic mechanisms enjoined with clinical experience makes preventive practices an attainable goal (Table 94-1). The strategy for preventive care relates to the nature of the illness: Bronchial asthma is a chronic condition that is characterized by acute exacerbations. Therefore, prevention is dependent on effective maintenance control of the chronic state and the early recognition and treatment of the acute asthmatic attack [23]. For this purpose, individual management goals and therapeutic strategies are necessary [24]. The morbidity and mortality due to bronchial asthma are a complex matter, but in many instances they can be related to the lack of control of chronic asthma activity and the delayed or ineffective treatment of the acute exacerbation [13, 22]. In this sense, prevention takes on a new form and direction and departs from the traditional perception that prevention means avoidance of inciting agents and conditions.

EDUCATION AND SELF-MANAGEMENT

In 1989, the British Thoracic Association reported an analysis of 90 deaths from asthma [3]. The findings revealed startling statistics. The patients were chronic unstable asthmatics who suffered frequent acute attacks. Sixty-one percent of the patients had insufficient medication, and compliance with management was poor in 76 percent. For 71 of the patients the fatal attacks lasted less than 24 hours, and 50 did not receive any medical attention at the time. A panel of reviewers felt that there were potentially preventable factors in 86 percent of the cases, and the underestimation of the severity of attacks was made by 75 percent of the patients and by 69 percent of their doctors. A follow-up report in 1992 identifies the at-risk patient [25]. This unfortunate experience clearly defines the many problems: lack of knowledge, noncompliance, and unavailability of care. These aspects require a change in attitudes and a need for greater educational efforts in the care of asthmatic patients.

The serious impact of asthma on our society prompted a National Institutes of Health workshop in 1988 for the purpose of developing a national strategy to facilitate and promote the dissemination of self-management activities [16]. Emphasis was put on the need for physicians, nurses, therapists, and behavioral scientists to improve their knowledge in the field and combine their expertise in concerted programs of education and care. Community-based programs were singled out as the most effective means to educate patients and coordinate the medical attitudes of the health worker, patient, and the environment. Emphasis was put on education regarding mechanisms, signs and symptoms, individual and combined therapies, early intervention, and contact systems. Continued efforts to translate experience gained from clinical studies into patient care were stressed, and the dissemination of information was felt to be key to this aspect. In all programs, self-management was a central topic of interest, and several studies were cited that established the efficacy of educational intervention in improving asthma care in the home.

Although educational programs may vary in content, emphasis, and degree, they all focus on the patient and family, the home, school and workplace environments, and the patient's activities. Within this context, the education of the professional health worker is paramount, and communication and availability are essential. No program can be successful if, as is the case with many clinic settings, medical help is most available during the usual working day when the patient may need it least and not available at the time of the acute attack. In general, specific information is provided one on one, in group sessions, and by written instructions and published information. Skills regarding peak flowmeter use, medication administration, and the use of spacers are incorporated in a clinic curriculum. Many programs have demonstrated the favorable effect on the overall behavior of the patient and in general found that asthmatics are very interested to learn about their conditions and take an active role in their care [21].

For such broad-sweeping plans to be successful, the complex interrelationships of the disease's effect on the person's daily life, self-image, work and school performance, family, and finances must be taken into account. Clinical trials have demonstrated that educational intervention can improve behavior, compliance, and self-management. Special attention must be given to asthmatic children because of the effect of the illness on the family unit and the psychophysiologic development of the child. In no other medical setting is the patient-parent-doctor relationship more central. Education has led to improved school attendance and performance [8]. As an example, the vital need for young people to keep up with their peers emphasizes the necessity for control of effort asthma in physical education programs. Every effort should be made to understand the special noncompliant attitude of the asthmatic adolescent. Indeed, it is a difficult task to provide instructive programs that instill patient confidence and security without what might be perceived as enforcement strategies that lead to overconcern and confusion. Many of the research studies in self-management have addressed difficult matters such as socioeconomic levels, inner city problems, different ethnic groups, and individual instructions [7]. Rigorous evaluation within these studies requires controlled clinical trials with large numbers of subjects.

Self-management has the advantage of on-site, early treatment of asthma symptoms that might lead to greater distress. The most familiar scenario many authors refer to is to educate the patient to recognize the early onset of an acute exacerbation and admin-

Table 94-1. Principles of asthma prevention

Environmental control
Proper drug prophylaxis and therapy (including immunotherapy)
Crisis plans
Early treatment of acute asthma
Avoidance of known provocations (aspiration, allergens, drugs, cold, exercise, etc (see text)
Worthy of emphasis: no smoking, weight control, adequate nutrition and hydration, control of coexisting diseases, appropriate physical activity programs
Patient education, psychological support
Readily accessible and supportive physician

Table 94-2. Medical treatment of special clinic attenders before and after special clinic enrollment

	Clinic attenders, n = 56	
Medical treatment	Before enrollment	After enrollment
	%	
Daily theophylline	100	82
Oral beta agonist	50	13
Inhaled beta agonist	100	100
Chronic inhaled corticosteroids	20	82
Chronic daily prednisone	25	9
Brief prednisone pulses	0	89
Reservoir device	0	100
Home peak flow meter	0	100

Source: Mayo, P. H., Richman, J., and Harris, J. W. Results of a program to reduce admissions for adult asthma. *Ann. Intern. Med.* 112:864, 1990. Reprinted with permission.

ister a prednisone dose and schedule that will effectively abort its progression. Obviously, the what to do, when, and how in self-management is dependent on education, so that these decisions by patient and family can be made on an informed basis. The ideal is to incorporate self-therapy into the spectrum of treatment modalities so that it complements and expands medical control rather than interferes with it [15]. However, caution is emphasized in some instances in which "home doctors" are created who might delay effective medical aid.

Mayo et al. [14] studied adult asthma patients at a large municipal hospital by a protocol that combined the elements of an outpatient education program with vigorous individualized medical treatment and easy access to the medical system. Patients who previously had multiple hospitalizations were divided into an intensively treated group and a control group that received the usual medical attention. The treatment regimen depended on inhaled beta agonists and corticosteroids and the early use of self-administered prednisone pulses. In general, the use of theophylline and oral beta agonists was abandoned, and daily prednisone needs were markedly diminished by intensive weaning and discontinuation. Spacers and home peak flowmeters were utilized. The study demonstrated that education, access, and carefully monitored therapies markedly improved the control of chronic asthma activity, and prednisone bursts were successful in aborting acute asthmatic attacks. Over a 32-month follow-up period, there was a threefold decrease in hospital admissions, and hospital stays were reduced twofold in the intensively treated ("special clinic group") patients (Tables 94-2 and 94-3). As another example of specific attention to medication regimens, Ross et al. [19] showed that the single addition of cromolyn sodium into therapeutic schedules in the treatment of chronic asthma also significantly reduced office and emergency room

Table 94-3. Readmissions and rehospitalization days for special clinic group and routine clinic group from 1 July 1985 to 28 February 1986

Variable	Special clinic group (n = 47)	Routine clinic group (n = 57)
Hospital admissions	19	70
Hospital admissions per patient	0.4	1.2*
Rehospitalization days	144	384
Rehospitalization days per patient	3.1	6.7†

* $P < 0.004$ compared with special clinic group.
† $P < 0.02$ compared with special clinic group.
Source: Mayo, P. H., Richman, J., and Harris, H. W. Results of a program to reduce admissions for adult asthma. *Ann. Intern. Med.* 112:864, 1990. Reprinted with permission.

visits and hospitalizations with a corresponding decrease in costs.

In another study, Clark instituted an educational program for patients and families in a large population of asthmatic children from a low-income, mixed English and Spanish speaking community [6]. Emphasis was put on self-treatment at home, and a control group was compared with those in the program. The study covered the spectrum of heavy and mild users of the health care system. The education program extended throughout the first year of a 2-year treatment period, and comparisons were made with the 1 year immediately preceding the study. Results showed no changes in the infrequent users, but compared with controls, there was a very significant decrease in emergency room visits and hospitalization among the children whose asthma was severe enough to cause multiple utilizations in the baseline year. Cost analysis found that although the savings did not cover the cost of the entire program, cost decreased significantly in the patients who required more intensive care.

I would like to interject some caution for this approach. In diseases such as asthma, we must be alert to the fact that large-scale study data are not always applicable to the individual patient and the clinical circumstance. The availability of the doctor and other health care providers at the off-times when the patients may need the most attention is clearly required; clinic during the day and emergency room at night might not be the best way. Large programs using multiple people with crossover responsibilities may make the contact system more complex and create confusion. This has happened in psychiatric clinics; the patient often is not sure whom to contact—one person for coping, another for medications, and so on. Obviously, a program associated with self-management requires individualization of responsibilities. After providing medical care in both office and clinic settings, I have always preferred the individual one-on-one relationship, but the complexities of this disease require and have benefitted immensely by the information summarized above. Of course, the physician can and should remain in control and coordinate the outpatient services. No matter the method; it presents a difference, not a distinction, in working toward the goal of effective control. Education and self-management are implicit throughout the rest of this presentation.

CONDITIONS AND INCITING AGENTS

The following conditions and inciting agents are briefly reviewed to stress prevention and self-management (Table 94-4). Avoidance of any incident is primary, but when this is not possible, protection from the effects of an exposure and early and effective treatment are necessary. Education in these areas is fundamental to achieving optimal intervention and proper therapeutic schedules.

Table 94-4. Prevention: control of chronic asthma and acute attack

Knowledge of condition; understanding of goals
Coping styles; compliance, emphasis on childhood and adolescence
Family unit; education, psychological support
Environmental control; home, workplace, weather conditions, pets, allergens, smoking
Immunotherapy
Avoidance of inciting agents; aspirin, other nonsteroidal antiinflammatory agents, beta-adrenergic blockers, angiotensin-converting enzyme inhibitors
Maintenance medications; treatment programs, benefits and side effects of medications, mechanical factors
Recognition of change in asthma pattern; acute attack
Early treatment and contact systems
Special conditions; effort asthma, cough, gastroesophageal reflux
Compliance; awareness of limited or noncompliant patients; drug abuse (i.e., excess use of adrenergic metered-dose inhaler).

Environmental Control

Self-management and education often begin by evaluating the home environment because of the large amount of time spent there. The detailed history is the most important source of information regarding the asthmatic patient's relationship to this environment. Airborne allergens and irritants should be identified to provide a basis for appropriate environmental control. Obviously, a nonallergic, nonirritating atmosphere is impossible, and a constant "nose to the wind" existence is distressful to the patient. However, uncontrolled asthma is a greater misfortune, so that preventive programs of avoidance, elimination, and neutralization of offending agents are necessary. The programs should be ongoing and preferably not descend upon a family unit as an avalanche of change and restriction. Multiple family meetings, explanatory literature, and personal interest are necessary for understanding and cooperation. In instances of acute exposure-reaction experiences, controls may be dramatically successful. The physician should eliminate the important offenders first and then proceed by judgment decisions in a stepwise fashion. Although these measures may not completely satisfy criteria for effectiveness, they are logical, time-tested, and in some situations the only alternative. In practice they are most successful in children but difficult in the adolescent and adult.

The restrictions on the family may be formidable: no smoking in the home, fireplace fires discontinued, plants sequestered, cooking odors vented, and aerosols and sprays forbidden. Incriminated animal pets should be removed or isolated as far as possible from the patient—in any case, always removed from the bedroom. In moldy areas, improved ventilation and dehumidifiers may be necessary, and an occasional fungicide may help. For house dust mites a variety of apparently safe chemicals or insecticides (e.g., pyrethroids, benzyl benzoate) are available for use on rugs; it may be preferable to remove all rugging. Cover mattresses with plastic covers. The last holdout should be the Christmas tree, but if it is a problem, a synthetic variety is advised. In extreme situations, clean zones of the home may be created and the activities of the patient confined to these areas. Foods such as milk, eggs, wheat, chocolate, nuts, malt, shellfish, strawberries, tomatoes, and alcohol may be identified as inciting causes of asthmatic breathing. The outdoor environment is the major source of pollen and pollutants, and climatic and meteorologic conditions are problems for many patients. Highly industrial, humid, cold atmospheres seem to be the worst; however, this is quite variable. The asthmatic seems most vulnerable to season changes, and autumn seems to present the greatest threat; however, individual responses should be identified. Preventive measures should focus on adjustments in medications to prevent attacks during these periods, and pre- or intraseasonal

selective immunotherapy is recommended where applicable. In uncontrollable circumstances a change in geographic location may be suggested. If so, a vacation of 3 to 6 weeks in the prospective area is advised but may not be decisive. This decision should be made on the basis of financial and psychosocial factors as well as health.

The complexities of household allergens are only surpassed by those in the workplace, where exposures to airborne dusts, gases, vapors, and fumes are common. In 1980, the number of substances reported to cause occupational asthma were in excess of 200 [5], and they have increased since then. It is important to understand that the complexities of occupational asthma require an approach that is quite different from that applied to control of the pneumoconioses. Asthma may develop within minutes (acute) or hours (delayed) after exposure, or there may be intervals of weeks, months, or years before it becomes evident. Cooperative efforts among labor, management, and regulatory agencies are necessary, but the responsibility of diagnosis and recommendations for control in relation to health are left to the medical profession. Prevention may begin with the preemployment examination. The detection of thermophilic microorganisms in air-conditioning systems and humidifiers correlated with pulmonary symptoms in office workers represents a situation in which an offending agent can be removed by cleaning or alteration of the system [1]. Air hygiene methodology and personal protection are commonly employed. However, in an established case or one highly suspect, the patient should be given primary consideration, and at this time there seems to be no choice other than complete removal from the exposure. This should lead one to discount selective desensitization in order to keep on the job. Multiple socioeconomic factors may make this impossible, however; so the physician must offer advice for decreasing exposure and prescribe preventive and symptomatic medications. Environmental control factors are detailed in Chapters 42, 45, and 87.

Exercise-Induced Asthma

The demonstration that exercise-induced asthma may be caused by heat loss from airway mucosa as a result of hyperventilation has many preventive implications. The first approach is avoidance of moderate to marked exertion in cold weather. Running produces the most consistent bronchoconstriction, walking and cycling less; swimming is generally best tolerated. Perhaps the high humidity from the water lessens adverse effects, so that swimming may be urged as a substitute for other activities. Warm clothing, masks, scarfs, and nasal breathing are helpful but not sufficient. Asthmatics may have to avoid athletic programs. The observation that exercise-induced asthma is worse in patients in poor control makes readjustment of chronic control and pretreatment of exercise highly desirable so that activity can be continued. Bronchodilators may be used prophylactically. Oral theophylline or adrenergic agents administered 1 to 2 hours before activity may be effective. The indefinite time interval makes inhalation of sympathetic amines preferred. Two inhalations are taken just before or early into the activity and repeated in the postexercise period. The longer-acting albuterol is well adapted for this purpose because asthmatic difficulty usually develops within the exercise period, peaks after cessation, and remains for hours. Sodium cromoglycate is also effective prophylactically, but it is not to be used after effort, since bronchoconstriction will have already occurred. It is taken 15 to 60 minutes before exercise, and the response is dose related [17]. Anticholinergic drugs are not consistently effective, and steroids by any route have no role in the prevention of exercise asthma. See Chapters 47 and 86 for additional details.

Aspirin

Aspirin-induced asthma has emerged as one of the most serious of the many side effects of the drug (see Chap. 48). Its common use and incorporation in many nonprescription and prescription analgesics, antihistamine preparations, and narcotic combinations make the problem a prevalent one. The newer nonsteroidal antiinflammatory agents also cross-react with aspirin and cause asthma in sensitive individuals. Updated lists of drugs with definite or potential harm should be provided and complete avoidance advised. Patients with the triad of rhinosinusitis, nasal polyposis, and asthma are classic, but suspicion should be high in any patient with upper respiratory tract symptoms with or without polyps who develops an asthmatic attack. Unfortunately, the acute attack may result in a protracted siege and set off a more chronic condition that requires steroids. Oral aspirin challenges have been developed, and desensitization techniques are being studied [20]. Food artificially colored with tartrazine dyes (FD&C yellow dye #5) can also cross-react with aspirin; elimination diets are very difficult, but the problem might be partially resolved by prescribing them only in patients with suspected aspirin sensitivity who respond positively to a challenge. Failure of chronic obstructive sinus symptoms may make polypectomy necessary, but it should not be carried out with the expectation that it will alter the aspirin-sensitive condition. The polyps recur, and the relationship of polypectomy to the onset of asthma is not clear.

Beta Blockers

Adrenergic antagonists have the potential to produce bronchoconstriction by beta-receptor blockade. Increased airway resistance, wheezing ventilation, and asthmatic attacks have resulted from their administration; as with other agents, acute and protracted difficulty and onset of chronic asthma have been observed. The widespread therapeutic applications of these agents in medical practice account for the prevalence of side effects; special problems exist in the adult asthmatic with coexisting cardiac disease or hypertension in which beta blockers are indicated. Propranolol is most widely used and has the most potent bronchial effects. Nadolol and trinolol are similar, but the new agents with greater cardioselectivity such as metoprolol and atenolol may offer less threat [10]. Obviously, these agents should be avoided in asthmatic patients, and alternative drugs should be administered when possible to prevent asthma. Tests of airway resistance after a beta-blocker dose are useful, and increased therapy with sympathetic amines may suffice for situations in which the medication is necessary. The ophthalmic medications containing beta-adrenergic receptor blockers for lowering intraocular pressure in open-angle glaucoma are absorbed systematically and may cause bronchospasm. Other opthalmic preparations containing parasympathomimetic drugs (pilocarpine, methacholine) or other agents (indomethacin) may similarly cause bronchospasm and should be avoided or removed if problematic.

Cough

Cough, discussed in Chapter 50, is often the only manifestation of asthma, although it may be caused by acute bronchitis or other conditions. The cough might indicate loss of asthma control and forecast progressive difficulty. The dry, hacking variety may aggravate or provoke further bronchial irritation and posttussive bronchospasm. Sympathetic amines, theophylline, sodium cromoglycate, and steroids may be effective. However, if cough is not controlled by asthma medications, the use of narcotic antitussive therapy is indicated in the asthmatic without respiratory embarrassment. Eosinophilic bronchitis is an asthma variant in which chronic cough is the major symptom [11].

Angiotensin Converting Enzyme Inhibitors

Angiotensin converting enzyme (ACE) inhibitors (captopril, enalapril) are a common cause of protracted irritative cough [4]. Depending on individual sensitivity, the cough may develop within hours of initial administration or after intervals of weeks to months; cough subsides within several days of discontinuation. The cough is more frequent in women; smoking does not seem to be a factor. Less frequently, patients develop asthmatic breathing or exacerbations of preexisting asthma. Both the cough and bronchoconstriction occurs in patients with increased bronchial reactivity. Cough medications, bronchodilators, and sodium cromoglycate may not affect ACE inhibitor–induced cough. With the large choice of antihypertensive agents, it is well advised to avoid ACE inhibitors in patients with bronchial asthma and other bronchial irritation syndromes.

Gastroesophageal Reflux

In patients with increasing nocturnal asthma associated with symptoms of esophageal reflux, peptic esophagitis with or without hiatus hernia should be suspected. This is especially so in elderly patients, but any asthmatic with reflux may be at risk. Dyspepsia and asthma may be markedly improved by a course of cimetidine [12]. Since it is impossible to establish a definite causal relationship between bronchial asthma and gastroesophageal reflux, one should be very cautious in recommending surgical intervention [18]. In most cases, the gastroesophageal reflux precedes the asthma, it is severe and prolonged, and nocturnal tracheitis with cough and bronchospasm are the major symptoms. Response to an antireflux antacid program is not very helpful in making a decision to operate (see Chap. 75).

Chronic Maintenance Control

Adequate maintenance therapy may be accomplished in mild intermittent asthma or in patients with seasonal difficulties by the use of inhaled beta-adrenergic agents. However, if the patient presents weekly to daily difficulties, a specific regimen of inhaled bronchodilators with or without oral methylxanthines is necessary. Medication should be used at specific times during the day; a most important factor is to convince the patients that they should take the medication when they feel well rather than on an as-needed basis. With the emphasis on the inflammatory aspects of asthma, the addition of inhaled corticosteroids and cromoglycate sodium has enhanced chronic control [19]. Among the multiple medications used for asthma, sodium cromoglycate has the singular distinction of being a prophylactic medication by virtue of its pharmacologic action. It can be used prophylactically in both intrinsic and extrinsic asthmatic conditions. Clinician preferences as to patient selection varies. It has been used for allergic asthmatics, allergic patients who are not adequately controlled by a moderate bronchodilator regimen, asthmatics in whom demographic and household irritants play an important role, and exercise-induced asthma. One hopes to reduce the requirement of other medications such as steroids. Cromolyn sodium has no place in the treatment of the acute attack or progressive severe asthma states. Other patients require daily or alternate-day corticosteroids for control. Adjusting therapy to the patient's asthma severity is clearly important and is detailed in Chapter 54.

Adherence to therapy regimens is difficult, especially when they require multiple medications with frequent side effects. Metered-dose inhalers present added problems. Verbal instructions, demonstrations, and observation of the patient during administration are necessary, and the procedure often has to be repeated in follow-up. Specific instructions should be given: Shake the inhaler, breathe out fully, place the mouthpiece in the mouth; keep the mouth open around the instrument; start to breath in; and then depress the canister as one breathes in fully. The breath should be held from 2 to 10 seconds, and then the subject breathes out slowly through pursed lips. A 1- to 10-minute interval is advised between multiple doses. The mouth is kept open to provide a secondary air source that picks up and cyclones the inhalant into the respiratory tract. This process of when to breathe and when to spray may be impossible for children and difficult for the elderly. Hence, spacers in the system, compressor-nebulizer setups, and face masks may be necessary. Patients should be made aware that overuse of inhaled medication may produce severe bronchial irritation. A great advantage may be derived by sessions with a respiratory therapist for instruction in medication use, diaphragmatic breathing, lateral chest expansion, and pursed-lip breathing. The physician must remain alert for the non- or limited complaint patient or those with psychiatric problems as a cause for poorly controlled asthma. Overabuse of drugs is a similar important problem. Resolution of these difficulties will optimize asthma control.

Early Treatment of the Acute Attack

It is important to stress that effective maintenance control of the asthmatic patient is the basis for prevention of the acute attack, and experience shows that poor control before an attack and delay in the initiation of effective treatment predispose to slow recovery and even mortality. Deviations from control highlighted by changes in the asthma pattern forecast the acute episode. Sometimes these are subtle; at other times they are alarmingly rapid and severe. Cough, dyspnea, increasing nocturnal difficulty, increasing medication needs, and medication abuse are danger signals. In such situations, readjustment of medication programs are made to larger doses in combinations given more frequently to effect sustained pharmacologic control. Early treatment is most often successful in preventing progression to severe asthma. The severity of the acute episode is judged by the patient's assessment, which in most cases is fairly accurate; anticipation and recognition of difficulty by patients and family members, early medical contact, and the availability of and trust in the medical sources provided are important factors. The ideal situation is emphasized—a compliant patient who has confidence in an available doctor who has knowledge of the patient's needs. In this regard, the asthmatic's behavior is part of the patient's coping style and compliance. Within this spectrum, there are patients who exaggerate or underestimate degrees of illness and therefore over- or underuse medication and develop inappropriate contact modes. Some aspects of emotional responses are active in most patients and should be taken into account by the physician. The doctor's response depends on previous experience with the patient's acute attacks in terms of onset, rapidity of progression, and the response to therapy in type and amount. Measurements of expiratory flow rate are confirmatory and may forecast progressive difficulty; a patient diary may be of similar benefit. Treatment depends on the maintenance therapy and the acute severity. At the time, inhalant and oral bronchodilators or any other required agent should be increased or added.

Early, short bursts of corticosteroids are very effective in preventing acute asthmatic attacks, emergency room care, and hospitalization. The author has had greatest success with 10 to 15 mg of prednisone, 3 times a day, for 2 days in succession. One should be aware of the frequency of the acute episodes and the length of time of steroid use with each attack. The goal is to produce the desired effect with minimal risk. In reality, steroid side effects are most unusual with short-term high-dose use; they

are related to prolonged administration or abuse. In overall management, the doctor and patient should aim to minimize steroid use. Another factor is the unnecessary employment of overlengthy corticosteroid wean periods. It only prolongs the total time on steroids. At 4-month intervals, I make a "steroid count" on each patient, at which time the number of acute attacks of asthma and total number of days on steroids are recorded. Patients who go through a season of repeated attacks often require a period of weeks on daily prednisone followed by a short wean period, and sometimes an alternate-day program of 10 to 20 mg suffices. Repeated emergency room visits with initial but unsustained response to the usual acute measures are typical. Childhood and adult asthmatics at greatest risk for status asthma are those with long-standing chronic asthma who suffer multiple acute attacks, are steroid dependent, are medication intolerant and resistant, and have poor coping styles. Recurrent bronchitis and continued smoking in adults are additional risk factors.

Acute infectious bronchitis, most often of viral etiology, is a frequent precipitant of the acute attack; *Mycoplasma* is less frequent, and bacterial infection is uncommon. Therefore, antibiotics are of little value in the treatment of acute exacerbations unless there is clinical or laboratory evidence of bacterial disease, and protective antibiotic programs through winter seasons or perennially are not indicated. The chronic asthmatic who suffers recurrent acute episodes should receive influenza and pneumococcal pneumonia immunizations.

In summary, the prevention of asthmatic exacerbations, insofar as realistic, is the primary goal of a therapeutic program. The latter is a multifactorial process involving proper use of the appropriate medications, minimization of drug side effects, environmental control and avoidance of causative incitants, education of patient and family in the asthma process and its treatment, early identification of exacerbations, availability of a personal physician and health care team where indicated, identification of specific complicating disorders, and psychological support. These factors carefully and properly blended and utilized will aid in reducing the morbidity and even the potential mortality of the asthma process. Available educational programs to assist the patient, the family, and the physician are listed in the Appendix.

REFERENCES

1. Banaszak, E. F., Thiede, W. W., II, and Fink, J. N. Hypersensitivity pneumonitis due to contamination of air conditioner. *N. Engl. J. Med.* 283:271, 1970.
2. Bernstein, I. L. Occupational asthma: Coming of age. *Ann. Intern. Med.* 97:125, 1982.
3. British Thoracic Association. Death from asthma in two regions of England. *Br. Med. J.* 285:1251, 1982.
4. Bucknail, C. E., et al. Bronchial hyperreactivity in patients who cough after recurring angiotensin converting enzyme inhibitors. *Br. Med. J.* 296:86, 1988.
5. Chan-Yeung, M. Fate of occupational asthma: A follow-up study of patients with occupational asthma due to Western red cedar (*Thuja plicata*). *Am. Rev. Respir. Dis.* 116:1023, 1977.
6. Clark, N. H. Asthma self management education: Research and duplication for clinical practice. *Chest* 95:1110, 1989.
7. Conboy, K., Self-management skills for cooperative care in asthma. *J. Pediatr.* 115:863, 1989.
8. Evans, D. et al. A school health education program for children with asthma aged 8–11 years. *Health Ed. Q.* 14:267, 1987.
9. Farr, R. S., Spector, S. L., and Wangaord, C. H. Evolution of aspirin and tartrazine idiosyncracy. *J. Allergy Clin. Immunol.* 65:667, 1979.
10. Fishman, W. H. Beta-adrenergic agonists: New drugs and new indications. *N. Engl. J. Med.* 305:500, 1981.
11. Gibson, P. G., et al. Chronic cough: Eosinophilic bronchitis without asthma. *Lancet* 1:1346, 1989.
12. Goodall, R. J. R., et al. Relationship between asthma and gastroesophageal reflux. *Thorax* 36:116, 1981.

13. Laurenzi, G. A. A Clinician's View of Status Asthmaticus, Including Complications and Mortality in Bronchial Asthma. In E. B. Weiss (ed.), *Status Asthmaticus*. Baltimore: University Park Press, 1978. Pp. 363–375.

14. Mayo, P. H., Richman, J., and Harris, H. W. Results of a program to reduce admissions for adult asthma. *Ann. Intern. Med.* 112:864, 1990.

15. Mullen, P. D. Implementing asthma self-management education in medical care settings: Issues and strategies. *J. Allergy Clin. Immunol.* 17:611, 1983.

16. Mellins, R. B. Asthma education, a national strategy (editorial). *Am. Rev. Respir. Dis.* 140:577, 1989.

17. Patel, K. R., Berkin, R. E., and Kerr, J. W. Dose-response study of sodium cromoglycate in exercise-induced asthma. *Thorax* 37:663, 1982.

18. Perrin-Fayolle, M., et al. Long-term results of surgical treatment for gastroesophogeal reflux in asthmatic patients. *Chest* 96:40, 1989.

19. Ross, R. N., et al. Cost-effectiveness of including cromolyn sodium in the treatment program for asthma: A retrospective, record-based study. *Clin. Ther.* 10:188, 1988.

20. Stevenson, D. D., Simon, R. A., and Mathison, D. A. Aspirin sensitive asthma: Tolerance to aspirin after positive oral aspirin challenges. *J. Allergy Clin. Immunol.* 66:82, 1980.

21. Windsor, R. A., et al. Evaluation of the efficacy and cost effectiveness of health education methods to increase medication adherence among adults with asthma. *Am. J. Public Health* 80:1519, 1990.

22. Worth, H. Patient education in asthmatic adults. *Lancet* 168(Suppl.):463, 1990.

23. Baily, W. C., et al. Asthma prevention. *Chest* 102:257S, 1992.

24. Patterson, R. Goals in the management of asthma. *Chest* 101:403S, 1992.

25. British Thoracic Society. The International Clinical Respiratory Group: report of the second meeting. *Chest* 101:1420, 1992.

Current Overview and Unresolved Issues

95

James E. Fish
Stephen P. Peters

A book of this dimension, especially one dealing with a single disease entity, is impressive testimony to the scientific information expansion of our times. The fact that such a book concludes with a chapter that questions the significance of its contents and seeks to define areas of further research is proof, however, that the information on hand is incomplete and that a great deal more important scientific work is yet to come, not to mention another edition of this book.

In this chapter we reflect on the major advances that have shaped our understanding of inflammation as a pathogenetic determinant of asthma and refined our views of the relation between this disorder and abnormal airway responsiveness. How these and other advances in drug development have influenced the treatment of asthma is also considered. The purpose of this exercise is to view the larger picture in an attempt to discern where we are in our understanding of asthma and where there are gaps in our knowledge. We begin with the thesis that the remarkable progress we have made has largely expanded the playing field and extended our range of vision with respect to the possible biologic alterations in asthma. But as the field expands, it also becomes more challenging to predict where the most productive battles will be fought.

Rheumatoid arthritis has been recognized as an inflammatory disorder for decades, yet we grasp almost nothing of its pathogenesis and remain mired at the level of devising improved treatment for symptoms rather than developing definitive therapy. Where, then, does the more recent appreciation of an inflammatory component to asthma place us in terms of truly understanding the causes and possible cures for asthma? What does the term *inflammation* tell us about specific remediable causes of airway obstruction? Do all or even some of the cellular elements that compose evidence of inflammation actually participate in disease pathogenesis, or are they inactive markers of other unrelated events? What is the link between inflammation and abnormal airway responsiveness? And, where are the fruits of the past decade's achievements in terms of improved therapy?

INFLAMMATION

Our view of asthma pathogenesis has rapidly progressed from concepts of aberrant behavior of smooth muscle or receptors that regulate smooth muscle to theories that consider acute and chronic inflammation in the etiologic framework. The term *inflammation* broadly describes an array of cellular and humoral processes that are involved in host defense as well as host injury. Acute and chronic forms of inflammation, by convention, are distinguished on the basis of the primary cell species involved. Whereas polymorphonuclear leukocytes, eosinophils, basophils, and mast cells are generally regarded as components of acute inflammation, other cell types such as lymphocytes, macro-

phages, circulating monocytes, Kupffer cells, and type A synovial lining cells are associated with chronic inflammation. These cellular lines of distinction, however, are becoming obscure as we learn more about the soluble mediators generated by these cells and how they operate to amplify, propagate, and modulate inflammatory reactions via recruitment and activation of different cell types. Recognizing the semantic imprecision in our use of the term *inflammation*, it is worth reviewing briefly the scientific evidence of an inflammatory basis for asthma.

Autopsy studies in asthmatic patients have reported disruption of airway epithelium, mucus gland hyperplasia with mucus plugging of airways, edema, and inflammatory cell infiltration of the submucosa, smooth muscle hypertrophy, and thickening of the basement membrane [11, 18]. In stable asthmatics, bronchoaveolar lavage studies have revealed increased numbers of epithelial cells, mast cells, eosinophils, and lymphocytes, particularly those of the CD8 class [1, 9, 35–37, 70]. Neutrophil numbers have reportedly been increased also, but not significantly [36]. Bronchial biopsies in stable asthmatics have shown increased numbers of eosinophils in the epithelium and submucosa [5, 17]. Two populations of platelets, one with normal survival and one with a shortened life span, have also been found in asthmatics [68]. Together, these studies suggest a potential role for mast cells, eosinophils, and lymphocytes and perhaps even platelets and epithelial cells in the pathogenesis of asthma.

The mere appearance of these cells in tissue specimens or lavage fluid, however, must not be construed as a priori evidence of an active role in the inflammatory process. Cellular recruitment to the lung has been reported to occur without cell activation in some experimental systems [2]. Therefore, it is important to ascertain whether cells are actively participating. One approach has been to document signs of cell "activation," although it should be recognized that there are many facets of cell activation (e.g., locomotion, secretion, surface receptor expression) and little agreement on what they signify in terms of pathogenetic role. Some studies have provided morphologic and histochemical evidence of activation of mast cells, eosinophils, and lymphocytes [5, 17], while others have shown increased chemiluminescence of neutrophils and macrophages obtained from asthmatic airways [35]. There is serologic evidence that platelets are also activated after allergen inhalation challenge [39].

The soluble mediators generated by these cell types are numerous and so, too, are their biologic properties. They include spasmogens (histamine; leukotrienes C_4, D_4, and E_4; thromboxane A_2; and prostaglandin D_2), mucus secretagogues (leukotrienes C_4 and D_4; 5-, 12-, and 15-hydroxyeicosatetraenoic acid), chemotactic factors (leukotriene B_4, eosinophil chemotactic factors, and platelet activating factor), toxic proteins (proteases, hydrolases, major basic protein, and eosinophil derived neurotoxin), reactive oxygen species (superoxide anion, hydrogen peroxide, and hydroxyl radical), and agents that reportedly modify airway reactivity (leukotriene D_4 and platelet activating factor) [2, 68]. This array of mediators is capable of producing all of the major pathophysiologic elements of asthma: (1) smooth muscle constriction, (2) mucus secretion, (3) airway mucosal edema, (4) epithelial destruction, and (5) cellular infiltration. While some, such as histamine and the sulfidopeptide leukotrienes, have long been recognized as important in the causation of reversible airway obstructive processes, others have been described only recently and the full range of their biologic activities is just now being clarified. In addition, macrophage-derived cytokines such as tumor necrosis and interleukin-1 (IL-1) and lymphokines such as those involved in IgE synthesis (IL-4 and IL-6), mast cell maturation (IL-3), and eosinophil maturation (IL-5) are thought to be important, but their role is thus far unproved. Similarly, the role of histamine releasing factors, small-molecular-weight proteins derived from lymphocytes, macrophages, neutrophils, and platelets that trigger histamine release from metachromatic cell in vitro, is unknown but of potential importance [34, 46, 58, 71].

It does not help our understanding of the disease simply to assert that asthma involves elements of acute and chronic inflammation. So too does rheumatoid arthritis, idiopathic interstitial pneumonitis, and a host of other diseases of obscure pathogenesis. The mere appearance of inflammatory cells in a lesion tells us nothing of the role they play in the overall process. Inflammatory cells can exercise any number of different biologic functions that are either directly or indirectly responsible for producing tissue injury. Conversely, inflammatory cells may be recruited to tissues and play a role in the termination of injury and initiation of tissue repair. Circulating inflammatory cells can also migrate to the lung and stand witness to the action without ever participating in it.

Thus, our task now is to advance beyond use of the term *inflammation* as an intellectual shibboleth. We must work to better define the role of individual cell types and the importance of individual mediators. Determining the role of individual mediators should be straightforward as inhibitors of mediator synthesis or receptor binding become available for human use. Clinical trials studying the efficacy of 5-lipoxygenase inhibitors, leukotriene D_4 antagonists, and platelet activating factor antagonists are now underway, and inhibitors of other mediators including various lymphokines and cytokines will soon be available. Because these mediators operate in a complex milieu where several are likely to act synergistically in producing pathologic effects, trials using combinations of inhibitors may be necessary to evaluate their role properly.

Determining the role played by individual cell types will prove to be more challenging, and it will likely require complementary in vivo and in vitro experimentation. One approach in this endeavor entails several interrelated stages of investigation. The first stage involves defining the inflammatory potential of individual cells or the spectrum of inflammatory mediators produced by an individual cell type as well as the control mechanisms regulating mediator release. This work is carried out in vitro and typically requires highly purified cell preparations. Moreover, cells are usually obtained from the circulation. Although much of this work has already been completed, new and important observations continue to emerge, such as the recent discovery that neutrophils synthesize both IL-1 and tumor necrosis factor [45].

In the second stage, the inflammatory potential of individual cell types obtained from the target organ, in this case the lung, is defined. Information regarding differences in behavior of cells obtained from the lung versus the circulation should provide clues as to which mediators are important in altering cell function as well as indication of the role that particular cell type might play in asthma pathogenesis.

In the third stage, hypotheses derived from the above in vitro or ex vivo experiments using cells obtained from the target organ

are confirmed by in vitro experimentation. And finally, in the fourth and fifth stages, selected aspects of cell function are interrupted pharmacologically in clinical studies to provide in vivo confirmation of their role, and then an attempt is made to relate resulting alterations in cell function to modulation of some physiologic process that is characteristic of the disease.

An example should prove illustrative. Segmental lung challenge via bronchoscopy in atopic subjects has recently been employed to model "allergic asthma." In this model, segmental allergen challenge results in recruitment to the lung of a variety of inflammatory cells and in "lung injury" as defined by an influx of albumin to the airways [29, 44, 50]. We have used these techniques with the goal of defining the pathophysiologic role played by specific inflammatory cell types. Using the approaches described above, we can explore the role of the neutrophil.

With regard to the first stage, the inflammatory potential of neutrophils has largely been defined already. These cells show directed movement in response to chemotaxins, they phagocytize particles and release lysosomal hydrolases, and they synthesize toxic oxygen radicals, leukotrienes and other lipid mediators, and cytokines such as IL-1 and tumor necrosis factor [26, 45]. In the second stage of experimentation, neutrophils attracted to the lung by local allergen challenge were characterized and found to display an altered biologic response pattern compared to circulating cells. Specifically, they showed a markedly diminished chemotactic response to leukotriene B_4 (LTB_4), but they demonstrated a normal chemotactic response to the peptide formylmethionyleucylphenylalanine (f-MLP) and a normal oxidative burst in response to phorbol myristate acetate [19, 40].

We can show by in vitro experimentation that incubation of neutrophils with LTB_4 inhibits their subsequent chemotactic response to LTB_4, but it has no effect on their chemotactic response to f-MLP or their oxidative response to phorbol myristate acetate. Thus, from this third stage of experiments we can postulate that LTB_4 is an important chemotaxin in the attraction of neutrophils to the lung after antigen challenge.

In future experiments (stages 4 and 5) it will be necessary to confirm that LTB_4 is important in neutrophil recruitment to the lung in vivo by administering inhibitors of LTB_4 synthesis or binding prior to allergen challenge. If neutrophils are important in this form of lung injury, inhibition of neutrophil influx should also correlate with a decrease in albumin flux into the airways. A similar tactic can be taken to explore the role of different cell types and inflammatory mediators in asthma.

This approach is not without problems, however. First, there is the necessity of having to make assumptions and extrapolations. For example, in the model described above it is assumed that cells retrieved by lavage have similar biologic properties to those in the organ itself. In general, this assumption has proved reasonably accurate for the lung. In addition, it is often possible to confirm lavage findings with small biopsy samples. The availability of small numbers of some cell types for analyses is another problem. This necessitates the use and, in some cases, the development of more sensitive biochemical, histochemical, immunocytochemical, and other analytic techniques. Furthermore, it may be very difficult to obtain a purified population of cells from the target organ. Therefore, techniques that permit analysis of individual cells in a mixed cell population, such as cytochemistry or immunocytochemistry, may prove invaluable. Studies using a number of these principles are in progress, and hopefully they will yield useful and exciting data as we attempt to define inflammation in asthma in more specific terms.

HYPERREACTIVITY

The putative link between inflammation and asthma is abnormal airway responsiveness. Airway inflammation, for reasons yet unknown, is thought to induce a state of hyperresponsiveness that potentiates the degree of airway narrowing provoked by specific agents such as allergens and occupational sensitizers. Abnormal responsiveness is also thought to render the individual more vulnerable to the bronchoconstrictor effects of nonspecific irritants that may operate through neural reflex mechanisms. These hypotheses are based chiefly on evidence from bronchial challenge studies where asthma is conveniently modeled to portray what is considered an abridged pathogenesis and also from longitudinal clinical studies of patients with occupational asthma.

The observation that allergen provocation could produce an early and late airway response and that the latter was followed by an increase in histamine reactivity provided the initial link between airway hyperresponsiveness and late airway reactions [13, 31]. The association between airway reactions and inflammation evolved first from animal studies showing that ozone-induced increases in canine airway responsiveness were associated with neutrophil infiltration of airway mucosa [32] and subsequently from human bronchoalveolar lavage experiments demonstrating that allergen stimulation educed inflammatory changes with both acute and chronic features [29, 44, 50]. Since hyperresponsiveness has been linked to late airway reactions as well as inflammation, late reactions and inflammation have been considered almost synonymous events, as if to imply that critical elements of inflammation in the causation of asthma are the essence of the "late phase."

However appealing these considerations seem, it is important to recognize that they are hypothetic and that there are still many gaps in our understanding of the interrelations between inflammation, airway hyperresponsiveness, and late airway reactions. In fact, the popular view that late airway reactions are linked etiologically to airway hyperresponsiveness has been challenged by the finding that airway responsiveness can increase even before late reactions occur and also by the observation that airway responsiveness can increase after allergen challenge in some patients who do not demonstrate late reactions [12, 20, 69]. It could be argued with compelling logic that late airway reactions and increased airway responsiveness are independent and unrelated consequences of a common initial stimulus, perhaps a critical event in the early airway reaction. For that matter, it could also be argued that allergen bronchial challenge with its early and late phases is not a particularly relevant model of clinical asthma, although in its defense is the importance of early and late reactions in various types of occupational asthma [56]. The usefulness of occupational asthma as a paradigm for the disease in general, however, is uncertain.

Another relevant question is whether increases in airway responsiveness that occur prior to late reactions have the same underlying mechanism as increases that occur 24 hours after allergen challenge. Conceivably, early changes in responsiveness could arise from alterations in airway geometry due to mucosal inflammation, while later increases relate to some other pathology. Certainly, there is reason to believe that hyperresponsiveness can arise from different pathogenetic mechanisms. In fact, the concept of airway hyperresponsiveness evolved not so much on the basis of an understanding of its mechanism, but rather on the basis of an empiric association between asthma and enhanced bronchomotor responsiveness to inhaled smooth muscle agonists. Enhanced responsiveness has also been associated with nonasthmatic chronic obstructive pulmonary disease, interstitial lung disease, congestive heart failure, viral respiratory infections, and irritant exposures [10, 21, 42, 49, 55, 64]. Nevertheless, who would suggest that a single common defect is responsible for enhanced responsiveness in such diverse conditions? Thus, *airway hyperresponsiveness* appears to be as nonspecific a term as *airway inflammation*.

Although we remain largely ignorant of the causes of hyperresponsiveness found in association with any lung disorder, in our search for mechanisms we have learned a great deal about airway physiology and pharmacology. For example, airway smooth muscle in many species, including humans, has been characterized in terms of morphology, contractile properties, and energetics [14, 15, 66, 67]. The importance of cholinergic excitatory and nonadrenergic noncholinergic (NANC) inhibitory control of human airway smooth muscle has also been described [16]. The discovery of muscarinic receptor subtypes in human airway smooth muscle has, at once, extended and complicated our understanding of autonomic influences [7], while the importance of tissue interdependence between airways and lung parenchyma and the interaction between bronchial smooth muscle and other structural elements of the airway wall has gained recognition [33, 47].

These and many other advances have given us a far more sophisticated understanding of human airway function. And yet, for all we have learned, we are still uninformed as to why asthmatic airways are 10- to 1000-fold more responsive than normal airways. It seems likely that further understanding of these mechanisms will rely on experiments using human tissues, in particular asthmatic airways. Animal studies advance our knowledge of biologic systems and facilitate the development of research tools, but it is important to recognize their limitations with regard to extrapolating mechanisms of airway hyperresponsiveness in asthma. The importance of a particular inflammatory cell type or mediator may vary from species to species, not to mention species variation in airway anatomy and autonomic control. For this reason, more work in human tissues, both in vitro and in vivo, will be needed to advance our understanding of the problem. Studies in human smooth muscle to determine whether there are abnormalities with respect to force-length relationships or excitation-contraction coupling mechanisms are vital. Likewise, attempts to assess whether there are differences between asthmatic and normal individuals in terms of the opposing effects that airway wall structures and surrounding parenchyma have on smooth muscle contraction and airway narrowing are important.

Perhaps one of the most important things we have learned from clinical studies is that airway hyperresponsiveness is not the nosologic equivalent of asthma. Studies have shown that airway hyperresponsiveness is not only associated with other disease conditions, but it can also be demonstrated in approximately 10 percent of nonasthmatics individuals who have no history of chest symptoms [22, 28, 48, 60]. Conversely, normal airway responsiveness has also been found in some patients who experience asthma symptoms after workplace exposure to known sensitizers [6, 30, 54]. These findings highlight the limits of tests of airway reactivity in the diagnosis of asthma, and they also raise important questions concerning the natural history of the association between asthma and airway hyperresponsiveness. While hyperresponsiveness may be a consequence of airway inflammation, asthma symptoms may also occur prior to the evolution of hyperresponsiveness. On the other hand, preliminary longitudinal studies [24] have indicated that new incident cases of asthma in laboratory animal workers have occurred most often in patients with abnormal responsiveness at the time of their employment. More extensive prospective longitudinal studies will be necessary to examine this relation between the evolution of asthma symptoms and enhanced responsiveness. Since a sizeable percentage of apparently normal individuals have hyperresponsive airways, such studies will be of special importance in determining whether these individuals are at increased risk for subsequent development of disease. Likewise, follow-up studies of airway responsiveness in children through adolescence and into adulthood may shed light on the role of persistent airway hyperresponsiveness in the natural history of asthma, especially with regard to adolescent remissions and recurrences during adulthood.

TREATMENT

Our greater understanding of pathologic processes in asthma has yet to yield new classes of compounds with proven efficacy, but it has nevertheless influenced treatment rationale and spawned different attitudes toward currently available drugs. For example, the emphasis on inflammation has focused much needed attention on the benefits of prophylactic therapy and the importance of maintaining daily control of the underlying pathophysiology so as to avoid acute exacerbations.

Antiinflammatory drugs have thus been promoted as critical first-line agents to ameliorate inflammatory processes and thereby maintain control of airway reactivity, airway caliber, and symptoms. Corticosteroids and the putative mediator release inhibitor cromolyn fall into the broad category of "antiinflammatory" agents and recently have enjoyed growing popularity in asthma management. It is important to point out, however, that the efficacy of corticosteroids is not a new revelation arising from any enlightened understanding of an inflammatory pathogenesis of asthma. Rather, steroid efficacy has been recognized for several decades and the mechanism of this salutary action is unknown.

In the current wave of enthusiasm for antiinflammatory therapy, the term, inflammation appears to have been taken at generic face value as the potential efficacy of numerous drugs with diverse pharmacodynamic properties is being explored (Table 95-1). Drugs altering folic acid metabolism (methotrexate), lymphocyte function (cyclosporine), and the leukocyte motility (colchicine) are being studied or, in some cases, simply being used without benefit of study [3, 23, 51, 52, 59, 63]. It is not at all clear that any of these immunologic mechanisms are involved directly in the pathogenesis of asthma and, lacking more specific information concerning the role of different mediators and cell types, it is difficult to predict how specific antiinflammatory agents will alter the disease. However, empiricism remains the heart and soul of medicine, and clinical trials with agents such as these are of definite value. Unfortunately, most such trials lack sufficient controls and numbers of subjects to be definitive. Because of the difficulty in measuring outcome with many of these agents, large multicenter clinical trials will be necessary to test the benefits of therapy adequately.

As antiinflammatory agents have been emphasized, so too have the traditional bronchodilator drugs (methylxanthines, beta agonists, and anticholinergics) been deemphasized [76] and, more recently, castigated as having harmful potential. The controversy surrounding the use of methylxanthines centers not only on their low therapeutic index, but also on questions concerning their beneficial effects. Several studies have shown the superiority of both inhaled and injected sympathomimetic agents over theophylline as single therapy for acute asthma episodes [25, 57]. Moreover, a recent study of longer-term effects found that aminophylline offered no significant benefit when added to other standard therapies in hospitalized asthmatics [62].

Given these findings and the well-publicized adverse effects of theophylline, there is likely to be continued emphasis on inhaled corticosteroids as alternative first-line therapeutic agents of choice. While this is probably a sound approach for the majority of young or even middle-aged asthmatics, there are potential problems with inhaled steroid use in children and postmenopausal women that should not be overlooked. Several studies have suggested that conventional doses of inhaled steroids may retard growth in childhood [43, 74]. While it is argued that poorly controlled asthma may by itself retard growth, the significance of this adverse steroid effect merits further documentation, and if proved, alternative means of controlling asthma in this age group should be explored.

As higher-dose formulations of inhaled steroids are made available, we can expect to see diminished use of oral corticosteroids in favor of higher-dose inhaled drug in steroid-dependent or difficult to control patients. As inhaled steroids also gain greater acceptance as first-line therapy, it will be important to discriminate between the use of inhaled steroids as first-line agents versus their role as an alternative to oral steroids in the problem patient. Here the discriminant factor is *dose*, with first-line therapy employing conventional doses and replacement therapy requiring doses exceeding the equivalent of 800 μg of budesonide. The systemic side effects of high-dose inhaled steroids, especially the effects on bone density in postmenopausal women, are not known, but they could prove significant. Since high-dose inhaled steroids may prove no safer than oral steroids in this population, physician and patient education in the proper use of higher-dose formulations will be important.

Recent statements in the lay press have also called attention to the potential dangers of beta-agonist aerosols [72]. These concerns have arisen largely from published studies by Sears et al. [61] and data from a larger study in Canada recently presented to the scientific community [65, 77]. The findings of Sears et al. [61] pertained to a single agent, fenoterol, and suggested that treatment with this agent was associated with more nocturnal symptoms, greater bronchial responsiveness, and poor overall control. The Canadian study examined the effects of different types of beta agonists and found an association between mortality and beta-agonist aerosol use in the asthmatic population. Unfortunately, the latter study did not determine whether beta agonists were the cause of death or whether mortality and beta-agonist use were independently associated with greater disease severity. In any event, the negative attention recently given to bronchodilator drugs combined with the emphasis on antiinflammatory treatment may have some interesting and perhaps untoward consequences. In our attempt to stress the importance of prophylaxis and daily control of asthma with "antiinflammatory" therapy, we might inadvertently deemphasize the importance of achieving airway patency in patients with acute episodes. It is well recognized that asthma deaths are more often a consequence of undertreatment as opposed to overtreatment of the severe episode, and yet the unfavorable publicity given to bronchodilator medications may promote the risk of undertreatment [75]. It is important that we not allow our exuberance over inflammatory mechanisms to cause us to forget that there is more to asthma therapy than prophylaxis and that patients require education in the proper use of "rescue" medications.

Seemingly, we are at a threshold where the remarkable advances we have made in understanding basic pathologic processes will translate to new and more specific forms of therapy. For the near future, however, it is likely that we will see a number of new compounds enter clinical trials with great expectations only to prove disappointing with regard to their salutary effects. On the other hand, these compounds will fulfill another equally important purpose in helping us to define the significance of various mediators and cellular elements that have been implicated in asthma. Several new classes of compounds including

Table 95-1. Antiinflammatory agents in the treatment of asthma

Drug	Reference
Corticosteroids	See Chaps. 60, 61
Cromolyn sodium	See Chap. 63
Gold salts	[8, 38, 53]; see Chaps. 66, 68
Methotrexate	[23, 51, 52, 63]; see Chap. 66
Colchicine	[59]; see Chap. 66
Cyclosporin A	[3, 27]; see Chap. 79
Fish oil	[4]; see Chap. 66
Nonsteroidal antiinflammatory drugs	[41]; see Chap. 63

leukotriene antagonists, platelet activating factor antagonists, lipoxygenase inhibitors, and others are in various stages of clinical trials. As we embark on this period of clinical testing of new drugs, it is important that we ask questions concerning the process of testing therapeutic efficacy itself. For example, when testing antiinflammatory compounds with prophylactic potential, what are the most useful therapeutic end points? Are daily or nocturnal symptoms more important than pulmonary function tests? How useful is concomitant medication usage as an end point variable? What is the optimum or adequate duration of a trial for determining efficacy?

UNRESOLVED ISSUES

Despite recent progress, most of what we really need to know about asthma remains a mystery. Among the many questions yet to be answered, several stand out in terms of their importance to present-day management strategies as well as future progress in solving uncharted aspects of pathogenesis and thence the development of more specific and effective therapy (Table 95-2). In taking the larger view, we believe that the following areas represent the most important areas for investigation over the next decade. A recent state-of-the-art conference summary, "Asthma: What Are the Important Experiments?" [73, 78], is a useful resource for additional perspectives on the issues described herein.

One of the most urgent questions concerns the cause for the recent rise in asthma prevalence, morbidity, and mortality at the same time other chronic lung diseases are in decline [79]. Although untoward drug reactions, environmental factors, and access to medical care have been cited as contributing factors, there are still no satisfactory explanations for these alarming trends. In fact, there is little information at all regarding risk factors for asthma occurrence and severity other than that derived from limited cross-sectional surveys. Family history, allergy, airway hyperresponsiveness, and respiratory viral infections have been identified as risk factors, but the importance of active and passive tobacco smoke exposure, gender, race and socioeconomic issues, and behavioral factors as well is not known. The role of environmental factors as determinants of disease occurrence and severity must also be explored, particularly those factors related to outdoor pollution and allergens in the home environment.

The natural history of asthma is also poorly understood. Is there a relation between asthma and chronic obstructive pulmonary disease (COPD) or a progression from reversible to irreversible pathology with long-standing disease? Longitudinal studies in children as well as adults are key to our understanding how various factors influence disease remission and recurrence.

In light of recent controversy surrounding beta-agonist therapy, it is important that we address questions concerning the long-term consequences of regular beta-agonist use. Controlled longitudinal studies evaluating morbidity, mortality, and quality of life as well as pulmonary function and airway responsiveness are necessary. Likewise, the risks versus benefits of theophylline as regular medication and as rescue therapy for hospitalized asthmatics should be resolved. Multicenter trials involving large numbers of patients will be required to address these issues adequately.

As enthusiasm for antiinflammatory therapy grows, it is imperative that we explore the long-term consequences of such therapy, not only with regard to asthma management but also with regard to other health-related concerns. For example, the long-term effects of inhaled steroids on growth and development in children as well as the effects on bone metabolism in postmenopausal women are uncertain. The effects of these and other classes of antiinflammatory agents on overall immune function must also be explored lest the emerging story of B-cell lymphoproliferative disorders consequent to immunosuppressive therapy in transplant patients be retold in the less tenable context of asthma therapy.

The most important questions concerning our understanding of asthma pathogenesis relate to the link between inflammation, airway hyperresponsiveness, and disease expression. What is the role of specific inflammatory cells, and which of these cells play a primary role in initiating critical inflammatory pathways? The roles of macrophages and T-lymphocytes are of particular importance. Also, which of the many mediators and cytokines are important as signals of cellular responses, and which are primary effectors of end-organ responses such as enhanced vascular permeability, mucus secretion, and smooth muscle contraction? If we can identify those steps in the inflammatory cascade that are key to propagating and sustaining the reaction, we will be far closer to achieving more specific and definitive therapy.

The question concerning whether asthma is causally related to abnormalities of airway smooth muscle or its control is still unresolved. Further investigation using asthmatic airway tissues are necessary to address this issue.

Another important area of investigation concerns the genetic basis of asthma. While genetic determinants of asthma are likely to be quite complicated with multifactorial or polygenic defects, the familial nature of atopy and airway hyperresponsiveness suggest that population and molecular genetic approaches to investigate asthma may bear fruit in terms of defining pathogenesis.

Finally, we believe that future advances will require a more refined view of asthma from a nosologic standpoint. In the past we have tended to regard asthma as a single nosologic entity with unique pathogenesis rather than as a syndrome comprising multiple disorders having common clinical features but their own distinct etiologic mechanisms. It seems likely that progress in the aforementioned clinical, epidemiologic, and basic scientific investigations will shed light on this important question. If there are diverse etiologic pathways leading to the clinical expression of asthma, it is conceivable that different classes of drugs will exhibit varying degrees of efficacy in different groups. Studies attempting to discern these differences are essential if we hope to recognize the benefits of new compounds and achieve a better understanding of asthma.

Table 95-2. Major questions concerning asthma for the 1990s

What is the cause(s) of the recent rise in prevalence, morbidity, and mortality of asthma?

What is the natural history of asthma? Is there a relation between asthma and chronic obstructive pulmonary disease?

What are the long-term consequences of beta agonists when used as regular therapy? What are the risks and benefits of theophylline therapy in hospitalized asthmatics?

What are the long-term consequences of antiinflammatory therapy in asthmatic patients?

What is the link between inflammation, airway hyperresponsiveness, and disease expression?

What are the key inflammatory cells and mediators/cytokines involved in the initiation and propagation of asthmatic airway pathology?

What is the significance of airway hyperresponsiveness in asymptomatic "normal" individuals?

Do abnormalities of airway smooth muscle or its control play a role in asthma pathogenesis or the evolution of airway hyperresponsiveness?

What is the genetic basis of asthma, and what is the link between genetic determinants and environment in the pathogenesis of asthma?

Is asthma a single disease or a syndrome describing multiple disorders with different pathogenetic determinants? How can we better classify asthmatic patients to refine clinical studies regarding pathogenesis and specific therapy?

REFERENCES

1. Adelroth, E., et al. Inflammatory cells and eosinophilic activity in asthmatics investigated by bronchoalveolar lavage: The effects of antiasthmatic treatment with budesonide or terbutaline. *Am. Rev. Respir. Dis.* 142:91, 1990.
2. Albertine, K. H., et al. Morphologic studies during long-term clearance of autologous protein from the air spaces of the sheep lung. *Fed. Proc.* 46: 1422, 1987.
3. Alexander, A., Barnes, N. C., and Kay, A. B. Cyclosporin A (CyA) in chronic severe asthma: A double-blind, placebo-controlled trial. *Am. Rev. Respir. Dis.* 143:A633, 1991.
4. Arm, J. P., et al. Effect of dietary supplementation with fish oil lipids on asthma. *Thorax* 43:84, 1988.
5. Azzawi, M., et al. Identification of activated T lymphocytes and eosinophils in bronchial biopsies in stable atopic asthma. *Am. Rev. Respir. Dis.* 142: 1407, 1990.
6. Banks, D. E., et al. Role of inhalation challenge testing in the diagnosis of isocyanate-induced asthma. *Chest* 95:414, 1989.
7. Barnes, P. J. Muscarinic receptor subtypes: Implications for lung disease. *Thorax* 44:161, 1989.
8. Bernstein, D. I., et al. An open study of auranofin in the treatment of steroid-dependent asthma. *J. Allergy Clin. Immunol.* 81:6, 1988.
9. Bousquet, J., et al. Eosinophilic inflammation in asthma. *N. Engl. J. Med.* 323:1033, 1990.
10. Brooks, S. M., Weiss, M. A., and Bernstein, I. L. Reactive airways dysfunction syndrome (RADS): Persistent asthma syndrome after high level irritant exposures. *Chest* 88:376, 1985.
11. Cardell, B. S., and Pearson, R. S. B Death in asthmatics. *Thorax* 14:341, 1959.
12. Cartier, A., et al. Allergen-induced increase in bronchial responsiveness to histamine: Relationship to the late asthmatic response and change in airway caliber. *J. Allergy Clin. Immunol.* 70:170, 1982.
13. Cockcroft, D. W., et al. Allergen-induced in non-allergic bronchial reactivity. *Clin. Allergy* 7:503, 1977.
14. Daniel, E. E. Control of Airway Smooth Muscle. In M. A. Kaliner and P. J. Barnes (eds.) *The Airways Neural Control in Health and Disease.* New York: Marcel Dekker, 1988. Pp. 485–521.
15. Daniel, E. E., Berezin, I., and O'Byrne, P. M. Structure of Airway Smooth Muscle. In M. A. Kaliner, P. J. Barnes, and C. G. A. Persson (eds.), *Asthma: Its Pathology and Treatment.* New York: Marcel Dekker, 1991. Pp. 189–229.
16. Diamond, L., and Altiere, R. A. Airway Nonadrenergic Noncholinergic Inhibitory Nervous System. In M. A. Kaliner and P. J. Barnes (eds.). *The Airways Neural Control in Health and Disease.* New York, Marcel Dekker, 1988. Pp. 343–394.
17. Djukanovic, R., et al. Quantitation of mast cells and eosinophils in the bronchial mucosa of asymptomatic atopic asthmatics and healthy control subjects using immunocytochemistry. *Am. Rev. Respir. Dis.* 142:863, 1990.
18. Dunnill, M. S. The pathology of asthma, with special reference to changes in bronchial mucosa. *J. Clin. Pathol.* 13:27, 1960.
19. Dupuis, R., et al. Characterization of inflammatory cells recruited to the airways of atopic subjects after local antigen challenge: I. Priming of macrophages but not neutrophils by antigen challenge. *J. Allergy Clin. Immunol.* 87:142, 1991.
20. Durham, S. R., et al. Increases in airway responsiveness to histamine precede allergen-induced late asthmatic responses. *J. Allergy Clin. Immunol.* 82:764, 1988.
21. Empey, D. W., et al. Mechanisms of bronchial hyperreactivity in normal subjects after upper respiratory tract infection. *Am. Rev. Respir. Dis.* 113: 131, 1976.
22. Enarson, D. A., et al. Asthma, asthmalike symptoms, chronic bronchitis, and the degree of bronchial hyperresponsiveness in epidemiologic surveys. *Am. Rev. Respir. Dis.* 136:613, 1987.
23. Erurum, S. C., et al. Lack of benefit of methotrexate in severe, steroid-dependent asthma. *Ann. Intern. Med.* 114:353, 1991.
24. Evans, R., et al. Factors in the risk of asthma in persons exposed to animals in the laboratory. *J. Allergy Clin. Immunol.* 79:A235, 1987.
25. Fanta, C. H., Rossing, T. H., and McFadden, E. R. Treatment of acute asthma: Is combination therapy with sympathomimetics and methylxanthines indicated? *Am. J. Med.* 80:5, 1986.
26. Fantone, J. C., et al. Phagocytic cell-derived inflammatory mediators and lung disease. *Chest* 91:428, 1987.
27. Finnerty, N. A., and Sullivan, T. J. Effect of cyclosporin on corticosteroid dependent asthma. *J. Allergy Clin. Immunol.* 87:297, 1991.
28. Fish, J. E. In Vivo Methods for Study of Allergy: Skin and Mucosal Tests, Techniques and Interpretation—Bronchial Challenge Testing. In E. Middleton, et al. (eds.), *Allergy: Principles and Practice* (3rd ed.). St. Louis: Mosby, 1988. Pp. 447–460.
29. Fish, J. E., Peters, S. P., and Yoss, E. B. Bronchoalveolar Lavage in Asthma: Cellular and Mediator Composition and Macrophage Function Studies. In N. Mygind, U. Pipkorn, and R. Dahl (eds.), *Rhinitis and Asthma.* Sweden: Munksgaard, 1990. Pp. 222–232.
30. Hargreave, F. E., Ramsdale, E. H., and Puglsey, S. O. Occupational asthma without bronchial hyperresponsiveness. *Am. Rev. Respir. Dis.* 130:513, 1984.
31. Herxheimer, H. The late bronchial reaction in induced asthma. *Int. Arch. Allergy* 3:323, 1952.
32. Holtzman, M. J., et al. Importance of airway inflammation for hyperresponsiveness induced by ozone. *Am. Rev. Respir. Dis.* 127:686, 1983.
33. James, A. L., Pare, P. D., and Hogg, J. C. The mechanics of airway narrowing in asthma. *Am. Rev. Respir. Dis.* 139:242, 1989.
34. Kaplan, A. P., et al. A histamine-releasing factor from activated human mononuclear cells. *J. Immunol.* 135:2027, 1985.
35. Kelly, C., et al. Number and activity of inflammatory cells in bronchoalveolar lavage fluid in asthma and their relation to airway responsiveness. *Thorax* 43:684, 1988.
36. Kelly, C. A., et al. Lymphocyte subsets in bronchoalveolar lavage fluid obtained from stable asthmatics, and their correlations with bronchial responsiveness. *Clin. Exp. Allergy* 19:169, 1989.
37. Kirby, J. G., et al. Bronchoalveolar cell profiles of asthmatic and nonasthmatic subjects. *Am. Rev. Respir. Dis.* 136:379, 1987.
38. Klaustermeyer, W. B., Noritake, D. T., and Kwong, F. K. Chrysotherapy in the treatment of corticosteroid-dependent asthma. *J. Allergy Clin. Immunol.* 79:720, 1987.
39. Knauer, K. A., et al. Platelet activation during antigen-induced airway reactions in asthmatic subjects. *N. Engl. J. Med.* 304:1404, 1981.
40. Koh, Y. Y., et al. Characterization of inflammatory cells recruited to the airways of atopic subjects after local antigen challenge: II. Neutrophils recruited to the lung are desensitized to leukotriene B4. *Am. Rev. Respir. Dis.* 143:A38, 1991.
41. Kordansky, D., et al. Asthma improved by nonsteroidal anti-inflammatory drugs. *Ann. Intern. Med.* 88:508, 1978.
42. Little, J. W., et al. Airway hyperreactivity and peripheral airway dysfunction in influenza A infection. *Am. Rev. Respir. Dis.* 118:295, 1978.
43. Littlewood, J. M., et al. Growth retardation in asthmatic children treated with inhaled beclomethasone dipropionate. *Lancet* 1:115, 1988.
44. Liu, M. C., et al. Immediate and late inflammatory responses to ragweed antigen challenge of the peripheral airways in allergic asthmatics. *Am. Rev. Respir. Dis.* 144:51, 1991.
45. Lord, P. C. W., et al. Expression of interleukin-1α and β genes by human blood polymorphonuclear leukocytes. *J. Clin. Invest.* 87:1312, 1991.
46. MacDonald, S. M., et al. Studies of IgE-dependent histamine releasing factors: Heterogeneity of IgE. *J. Immunol.* 139:506, 1987.
47. Macklem, P. T. The clinical relevance of respiratory muscle research. *Am. Rev. Respir. Dis.* 134:812, 1986.
48. Malo, J. L. Reference values of the provocative concentrations of methacholine that cause 6% and 20% changes in forced expiratory volume in one second in a normal population. *Am. Rev. Respir. Dis.* 128:8, 1983.
49. Mellis, C. M., and Levinson H. Bronchial reactivity in cystic fibrosis. *Pediatrics* 61:446, 1978.
50. Metzger, W. J., et al. Local allergen challenge and bronchoalveolar lavage of allergic asthmatic lungs. *Am. Rev. Respir. Dis.* 135:433, 1987.
51. Mullarkey, M. F., Lammert, J. K., and Blumenstein, B. A. Long-term methotrexate treatment in corticosteroid-dependent asthma. *Ann. Intern. Med.* 112:577, 1990.
52. Mullarkey, M. F., et al. Methotrexate in the treatment of corticosteroid-dependent asthma: A double-blind crossover study. *N. Engl. J. Med.* 318: 603, 1988.
53. Muranaka, M., et al. Gold salts in the treatment of bronchial asthma: A double-blind study. *Ann. Allergy* 40:132, 1978.
54. O'Brien, I. M., et al. Toluene di-isocyanate-induced asthma: II. Inhalation challenge tests and bronchial reactivity studies. *Clin. Allergy* 9:7, 1979.
55. Parker, C. D., Bibo, R. E., Reed, C. E. Methacholine aerosol as a test for bronchial asthma. *Arch. Intern. Med.* 115:452, 1965.
56. Pepys, J., and Hutchcroft, B. J. Bronchial provocation tests in etiologic diagnosis and analysis of asthma. *Am. Rev. Respir. Dis.* 112:829, 1975.
57. Rossing, T. H., et al. Emergency therapy of asthma: Comparison of the acute effects of parenteral and inhaled sympathomimetics and infused aminophylline. *Am. Rev. Respir. Dis.* 122:365, 1980.

58. Schulman, E. S., et al. Human lung macrophages induce histamine release from basophils and mast cells. *Am. Rev. Respir. Dis.* 131:230, 1985.

59. Schwartz, Y. A., et al. A clinical and immunologic study of colchicine in asthma. *J. Allergy Clin. Immunol.* 85:578, 1990.

60. Sears, M. R., et al. Prevalence of bronchial reactivity to inhaled methacholine in New Zealand children. *Thorax* 41:283, 1986.

61. Sears, M. R., et al. Regular inhaled beta-agonist treatment in bronchial asthma. *Lancet* 336:1391, 1990.

62. Self, T. H., et al. Inhaled albuterol and oral prednisone therapy in hospitalized adult asthmatics: Does aminophylline add any benefit? *Chest* 98:1317, 1990.

63. Shiner, R. J., et al. Randomized, double-blind, placebo-controlled trial of methotrexate in steroid-dependent asthma. *Lancet* 336:137, 1990.

64. Simonsson, B. G. Clinical and physiological studies on chronic bronchitis: III. Bronchial reactivity to inhaled acetylcholine. *Acta Allergol.* 20:325, 1965.

65. Spitzer, W. O. The relation of use of beta-agonists with asthma deaths and near-deaths. Presented at the First Annual Congress of the European Respiratory Society, Brussels, September 24, 1991.

66. Stephens, N. L. Airway smooth muscle. *Am. Rev. Respir. Dis.* 135:960, 1987.

67. Stephens, N. L., and Jiang, H. Airway smooth muscle mechanics and biochemistry in experimental asthma. *Am. Rev. Respir. Dis.* 143:1182, 1991.

68. Taytard, A., et al. Platelet kinetics in stable atopic asthmatic patients. *Am. Rev. Respir. Dis.* 134:983, 1986.

69. Thorpe, J. E., et al. Bronchial reactivity increases soon after the immediate response in dual-responding asthmatic subjects. *Chest* 91:21, 1987.

70. Wardlaw, A. J., et al. Eosinophils and mast cells in bronchoalveolar lavage in subjects with mild asthma: Relationship to bronchial hyperreactivity. *Am. Rev. Respir. Dis.* 137:62, 1988.

71. White, M. V., and Kaliner, M. A. Neutrophils and mast cells: I. Human neutrophil derived histamine releasing activity. *J. Immunol.* 139:1624, 1987.

72. Winslow, R. Treatment of asthma could change. *Wall Street Journal*, Friday, August 9, 1991.

73. Woolcock, A. J. (ed.). Asthma: What are the important experiments? *Am. Rev. Respir. Dis.* 138:730, 1988.

74. Wothers, O. D., and Pedersen, S. Growth of asthmatic children during treatment with budesonide: A double blind trial. *Br. Med. J.* 303:163, 1991.

75. Ziment, I. Infrequent cardiac deaths occur in bronchial asthma. *Chest* 101:1703, 1992.

76. Haahtela, T., et al. Comparison of a β_2-agonist, terbutaline, with an inhaled corticosteroid, budesonide, in newly detected asthma. *N. Engl. J. Med.* 325:388, 1991.

77. Spitzer, W. O., et al. The use of β-agonists and the risk of death and near death from asthma. *N. Engl. J. Med.* 326:501, 1992.

78. Woolcock, A. J., and Barnes, P. J. Supplement: Asthma: The Important Questions. Part 2. *Am. Rev. Respir. Dis.* 146:1349, 1992.

79. Gergen, P. J., and Weiss, K. B. The increasing problem of asthma in the United States. *Am. Rev. Respir. Dis.* 146:823, 1992.

Appendixes

A. Botanical Regions of the United States and Canada

Region I
North Atlantic: Connecticut, Massachusetts, New Jersey, Pennsylvania, Vermont, Maine, New Hampshire, New York, Rhode Island
Index trees (pollinating season—late winter through spring)
Box elder/maple (*Acer* spp.)
Birch (*Betula* spp.)
Oak (*Quercus* spp.)
Hickory (*Carya ovata*)
Ash (*Fraxinus americana*)
Pine (*Pinus strobus*)
Sycamore (*Platanus occidentalis*)
Cottonwood/poplar (*Populus deltoides*)
Elm (*Ulmus americana*)
Index grasses (pollinating season—spring through early summer)
Redtop (*Agrostis alba*)
Orchard grass (*Dactylis glomerata*)
Fescue (*Festuca elatior*)
Timothy (*Phleum pratense*)
Bluegrass/June grass (*Poa* spp.)
Index weeds (pollinating season—summer through early fall)
Lamb's quarters (*Chenopodium album*)
Ragweed, giant and short (*Ambrosia* spp.)
Cocklebur (*Xanthium strumarium*)
Plantain (*Plantago lanceolata*)
Dock/sorrel (*Rumex* spp.)
Region II
Mid-Atlantic: Delaware, Maryland, Virginia, District of Columbia, North Carolina
Index trees (pollinating season—late winter through spring)
Box elder/maple (*Acer* spp.)
Birch (*Betula nigra*)
Cedar/juniper (*Juniperus virginiana*)
Oak (*Quercus* spp.)
Hickory/pecan (*Carya* spp.)
Walnut (*Juglans nigra*)
Mulberry (*Morus* spp.)
Ash (*Fraxinus americana*)
Cottonwood/poplar (*Populus deltoides*)
Hackberry (*Celtis accidentalis*)
Elm (*Ulmus americana*)
Index grasses (pollinating season—spring through early summer)
Redtop (*Agrostis alba*)
Vernal grass (*Anthoxanthum* spp.)
Bermuda grass (*Cynodon dactylon*)
Orchard grass (*Dactylis glomerata*)
Ryegrass (*Elymus* and *Lolium* spp.)
Timothy (*Phleum pratense*)
Bluegrass/June grass (*Poa* spp.)
Johnson grass (*Sorghum halepense*)
Index weeds (Pollinating season—summer through early fall)
Pigweed (*Amaranthus retroflexus*)
Lamb's-quarters (*Chenopodium album*)

Mexican firebush (*Kochia scoparia*)
Ragweed, giant and short (*Ambrosia* spp.)
Cocklebur (*Xanthium strumarium*)
Plantain (*Plantago lanceolata*)
Dock/sorrel (*Rumex* spp.)
Region III
South Atlantic: Florida (north of Orlando), Georgia, South Carolina
Index trees (pollinating season—late winter through spring)
Box elder/maple (*Acer* spp.)
Birch (*Betula nigra*)
Cedar/juniper (*Juniperus virginiana*)
Oak (*Quercus* spp.)
Hickory/pecan (*Carya* spp.)
Walnut (*Juglans nigra*)
Mesquite (*Prosopis juliflora*)
Mulberry (*Morus* spp.)
Ash (*Fraxinus americana*)
Cottonwood/poplar (*Populus deltoides*)
Hackberry (*Celtis occidentalis*)
Elm (*Ulmus americana*)
Index grasses (pollinating season—spring through early summer)
Redtop (*Agrostis alba*)
Vernal grass (*Anthoxanthum* spp.)
Bermuda grass (*Cynodon dactylon*)
Orchard grass (*Dactylis glomerata*)
Ryegrass (*Elymus* and *Lolium* spp.)
Fescue (*Festuca elatior*)
Timothy (*Phleum pratense*)
Bluegrass/June grass (*Poa* spp.)
Johnson grass (*Sorghum halepense*)
Index weeds (pollinating season—summer through early fall)
Lamb's-quarters (*Chenopodium album*)
Ragweed, giant and short (*Ambrosia* spp.)
Sagebrush (*Artemisia* spp.)
Cocklebur (*Xanthium strumarium*)
Plantain (*Plantago lanceolata*)
Dock/sorrel (*Rumex* spp.)
Region IV
Subtropic Florida: Southern Florida (south of Orlando)
Index trees (pollinating season—winter through spring)
Box elder (*Acer negundo*)
Cedar/juniper (*Juniperus virginiana*)
Oak (*Quercus* spp.)
Pecan (*Carya pecan*)
Privet (*Ligustrum lucidium*)
Palm (*Cocos plumosa*)
Australian pine/beefwood (*Casuarina equisetifolia*)
Sycamore (*Platanus occidentalis*)
Cottonwood/poplar (*Populus deltoides*)
Elm (*Ulmus americana*)
Brazilian peppertree (Florida holly) (*Schinus terebinthifolius*)
Bayberry (wax myrtle) (*Myrica* spp.)
Melaleuca (*Melaleuca* spp.)

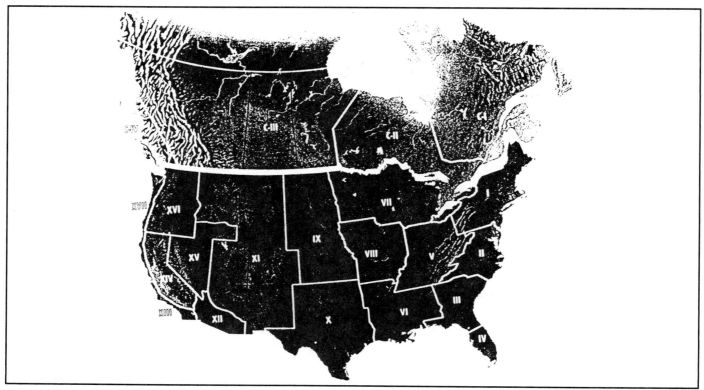

Fig. A-1. *Botanical regions of the United States and Canada. (Courtesy Hollister-Stier.) (Reprinted with permission from R. W. Ausdenmoore, Aeroallergens and Environmental Factors. In G. J. Lawlor, Jr., and T. J. Fischer (eds.),* Manual of Allergy and Immunology: Diagnosis and Therapy. *Boston: Little, Brown, 1981; adapted from* Pollen Guide for Allergy. *Spokane: Hollister-Stier Laboratories, 1978. Copyright Hollister-Stier, 1978.)*

Index grasses (Pollinating season—spring through early summer)
   Redtop (*Agrostis alba*)
   Bermuda grass (*Cynodon dactylon*)
   Salt grass (*Distichlis* spp.)
   Bahia grass (*Paspalpum notatum*)
   Canary grass (*Phalaris minor*)
   Bluegrass/June grass (*Poa* spp.)
   Johnson grass (*Sorghum halepense*)
Index weeds (pollinating season—summer through early fall)
   Pigweed (*Amaranthus spinosus*)
   Lamb's-quarters (*Chenopodium album*)
   Ragweed, giant and short (*Ambrosia* spp.)
   Sagebrush (*Artemisia* spp.)
   Marsh elder/poverty weed (*Iva* spp.)
   Dock/sorrel (*Rumex* spp.)
   Plantain (*Plantago lanceolata*)
Region V
   Greater Ohio valley: Indiana, Ohio, West Virginia, Kentucky, Tennessee
      Index trees (pollinating season—late winter through spring)
         Box elder/maple (*Acer* spp.)
         Birch (*Betula nigra*)
         Oak (*Quercus rubra*)
         Hickory (*Carya ovata*)
         Walnut (*Juglans nigra*)
         Ash (*Fraxinus americana*)
         Sycamore (*Platanus occidentalis*)
         Cottonwood/poplar (*Populus deltoides*)
         Elm (*Ulmus americana*)
      Index grasses (pollinating season—spring through early summer)

Redtop (*Agrostis alba*)
Bermuda grass (*Cynodon dactylon*)
Orchard grass (*Dactylis glomerata*)
Fescue (*Festuca elatior*)
Ryegrass (*Lolium* spp.)
Timothy (*Phleum pratense*)
Bluegrass/June grass (*Poa* spp.)
Johnson grass (*Sorghum halepense*)
Index weeds (pollinating season—summer through early fall)
   Water hemp (*Acnida tamariscina*)
   Pigweed (*Amaranthus retroflexus*)
   Lamb's-quarters (*Chenopodium album*)
   Ragweed, giant and short (*Ambrosia* spp.)
   Sagebrush (*Artemisia* spp.)
   Cocklebur (*Xanthium strumarium*)
   Dock/sorrel (*Rumex* spp.)
   Plantain (*Plantago lanceolata*)
Region VI
   South Central: Alabama, Louisiana, Arkansas, Mississippi
      Index trees (pollinating season—late winter through early spring)
         Box elder/maple (*Acer* spp.)
         Cedar/juniper (*Juniperus virginiana*)
         Oak (*Quercus* spp.)
         Hickory/pecan (*Carya* spp.)
         Walnut (*Juglans nigra*)
         Ash (*Fraxinus americana*)
         Sycamore (*Platanus accidentalis*)
         Cottonwood/poplar (*Populus deltoides*)
         Elm (*Ulmus americana*)
      Index grasses (pollinating season—spring through early summer)

Redtop (*Agrostis alba*)
Bermuda grass (*Cynodon dactylon*)
Orchard grass (*Dactylis glomerata*)
Ryegrass (*Lolium* spp.)
Timothy (*Phleum pratense*)
Bluegrass/June grass (*Poa* spp.)
Johnson grass (*Sorghum halepense*)
Index weeds (pollinating season—summer through early fall)
Pigweed (*Amaranthus retroflexus*)
Lamb's-quarters (*Chenopodium album*)
Ragweed, giant and short (*Ambrosia* spp.)
Sagebrush (*Artemisia* spp.)
Cocklebur (*Xanthium strumarium*)
Dock/sorrel (*Rumex* spp.)
Plantain (*Plantago lanceolata*)

Region VII
Northern Midwest: Michigan, Wisconsin, Minnesota
Index trees (pollinating season—late winter through spring)
Box elder/maple (*Acer* spp.)
Alder (*Alnus incana*)
Birch (*Betula* spp.)
Oak (*Quercus rubra*)
Hickory (*Carya ovata*)
Walnut (*Juglans nigra*)
Ash (*Fraxinus americana*)
Sycamore (*Platanus occidentalis*)
Cottonwood/poplar (*Populus deltoides*)
Elm (*Ulmus americana*)
Index grasses (pollinating season—spring through early summer)
Redtop (*Agrostis alba*)
Bromegrass (*Bromus inermis*)
Orchard grass (*Dactylis glomerata*)
Fescue (*Festuca elatior*)
Ryegrass (*Lolium* spp.)
Canary grass (*Phalaris arundinacea*)
Timothy (*Phleum pratense*)
Bluegrass/June grass (*Poa* spp.)
Index weeds (pollinating season—summer through early fall)
Water hemp (*Acnida tamariscina*)
Lamb's-quarters (*Chenopodium album*)
Russian thistle (*Salsola kali*)
Ragweed, giant and short (*Ambrosia* spp.)
Marsh elder/poverty weed (*Iva* spp.)
Cocklebur (*Xanthium strumarium*)
Dock/sorrel (*Rumex* spp.)
Pigweed (*Amaranthus retroflexus*)
Plantain (*Plantago lanceolata*)

Region VIII
Central Midwest: Illinois, Missouri, Iowa
Index trees (pollinating season—late winter through spring)
Box elder/maple (*Acer* spp.)
Birch (*Betula nigra*)
Oak (*Quercus* spp.)
Hickory (*Carya ovata*)
Walnut (*Juglans nigra*)
Mulberry (*Morus* spp.)
Ash (*Fraxinus americana*)
Sycamore (*Platanus occidentalis*)
Cottonwood/poplar (*Populus deltoides*)
Elm (*Ulmus americana*)
Index grasses (pollinating season—spring through early summer)
Redtop (*Agrostis alba*)
Bermuda grass (*Cynodon dactylon*)
Orchard grass (*Dactylis glomerata*)

Ryegrass (*Lolium* spp.)
Timothy (*Phleum pratense*)
Bluegrass/June grass (*Poa* spp.)
Johnson grass (*Sorghum halepense*)
Corn (*Zea mays*)
Index weeds (pollinating season—summer through early fall)
Pigweed (*Amaranthus retroflexus*)
Lamb's-quarters (*Chenopodium album*)
Mexican firebush (*Kochia scoparia*)
Russian thistle (*Salsola kali*)
Ragweed, giant, short, and western (*Ambrosia* spp.)
Marsh elder/poverty weed (*Iva* spp.)
Plantain (*Plantago lanceolata*)
Dock/sorrel (*Rumex* spp.)
Water hemp (*Acnida tamariscina*)

Region IX
Great Plains: Kansas, North Dakota, Nebraska, South Dakota
Index trees (pollinating season—late winter through spring)
Box elder/maple (*Acer* spp.)
Alder (*Alnus incana*)
Birch (*Betula* spp.)
Hazel (*Corylus americana*)
Oak (*Quercus macrocarpa*)
Hickory (*Carya ovata*)
Walnut (*Juglans nigra*)
Ash (*Fraxinus americana*)
Cottonwood/poplar (*Populus deltoides*)
Elm (*Ulmus americana*)
Index grasses (pollinating season—spring through early summer)
Quack grass/wheat grass (*Agropyron* spp.)
Redtop (*Agrostis alba*)
Brome (*Bromus inermis*)
Orchard grass (*Dactylis glomerata*)
Ryegrass (*Elymus* and *Lolium* spp.)
Fescue (*Festuca elatior*)
Timothy (*Phleum pratense*)
Bluegrass/June grass (*Poa* spp.)
Index weeds (pollinating season—summer through early fall)
Water hemp (*Acnida tamariscina*)
Pigweed (*Amaranthus retroflexus*)
Lamb's-quarters (*Chenopodium album*)
Mexican firebush (*Kochia scoparia*)
Russian thistle (*Salsola kali*)
Ragweed, fall, giant, short, and western (*Ambrosia* spp.)
Sagebrush (*Artemisia* spp.)
Marsh elder/poverty weed (*Iva* spp.)
Cocklebur (*Xanthium strumarium*)
Plantain (*Plantago lanceolata*)
Dock/sorrel (*Rumex* spp.)

Region X
Southwestern Grasslands: Oklahoma, Texas
Index trees (pollinating season—late winter through spring)
Box elder (*Acer negundo*)
Cedar/juniper (*Juniperus virginiana*)
Oak (*Quercus virginiana*)
Mesquite (*Prosopis juliflora*)
Mulberry (*Morus* spp.)
Ash (*Fraxinus americana*)
Cottonwood/poplar (*Populus deltoides*)
Elm (*Ulmus americana*)
Index grasses (pollinating season—spring through early summer)
Quack grass/wheat grass (*Agropyron* spp.)
Redtop (*Agrostis alba*)
Bermuda grass (*Cynodon dactylon*)

Orchard grass (*Dactylis glomerata*)
Fescue (*Festuca elatior*)
Ryegrass (*Lolium* spp.)
Timothy (*Phleum pratense*)
Bluegrass/June grass (*Poa* spp.)
Johnson grass (*Sorghum halepense*)
Index weeds (pollinating season—summer through early fall)
Water hemp (*Acnida tamariscina*)
Careless weed/pigweed (*Amaranthus* spp.)
Saltbush/scale (*Atriplex* spp.)
Lamb's-quarters (*Chenopodium album*)
Mexican firebush (*Kochia scoparia*)
Russian thistle (*Salsola kali*)
Ragweed, false, giant, short, and western (*Ambrosia* spp.)
Sagebrush (*Artemisia* spp.)
Marsh elder/poverty weed (*Iva* spp.)
Cocklebur (*Xanthium strumarium*)
Dock/sorrel (*Rumex* spp.)
Plantain (*Plantago lanceolata*)

Region XI
Rocky Mountain Empire: Arizona (mountainous), Idaho (mountainous), New Mexico, Wyoming, Colorado, Montana, Utah
Index trees (pollinating season—late winter through spring)
Box elder (*Acer negundo*)
Alder (*Alnus incana*)
Birch (*Betula fontinalis*)
Cedar/juniper (*Juniperus scopulorum*)
Oak (*Quercus gambelii*)
Ash (*Fraxinus americana*)
Pine (*Pinus* spp.)
Cottonwood/poplar (*Populus deltoides sargentii*)
Elm (*Ulmus* spp.)
Index grasses (pollinating season—spring through early summer)
Quack grass/wheat grass (*Agropyron* spp.)
Redtop (*Agrostis alba*)
Bromegrass (*Bromus inermis*)
Bermuda grass (*Cynodon dactylon*)
Orchard grass (*Dactylis glomerata*)
Ryegrass (*Elymus* and *Lolium* spp.)
Fescue (*Festuca elatior*)
Timothy (*Phleum pratense*)
Bluegrass/June grass (*Poa* spp.)
Index weeds (pollinating season—summer through early fall)
Water hemp (*Acnida tamariscina*)
Pigweed (*Amaranthus retroflexus*)
Saltbush/scale (*Atriplex* spp.)
Sugar beet (*Beta vulgaris*)
Lamb's-quarters (*Chenopodium album*)
Mexican firebush (*Kochia scoparia*)
Russian thistle (*Salsola kali*)
Ragweed, false, giant, short, and western (*Ambrosia* spp.)
Sagebrush (*Artemisia* spp.)
Marsh elder/poverty weed (*Iva* spp.)
Cocklebur (*Xanthium strumarium*)
Plantain (*Plantago lanceolata*)
Dock/sorrel (*Rumex* spp.)

Region XII
The Arid Southwest: Arizona, Southern California (southeastern desert)
Index trees (pollinating season—winter through spring)
Cypress (*Cupressus arizonica*)
Cedar/juniper (*Juniperus californica*)
Mesquite (*Prosopis juliflora*)
Ash (*Fraxinus velutina*)

Olive (*Olea europaea*)
Cottonwood/poplar (*Populus fremontii*)
Elm (*Ulmus parvifolia*)
Index grasses (pollinating season—spring through early summer)
Bromegrass (*Bromus* spp.)
Bermuda grass (*Cynodon dactylon*)
Salt grass (*Distichlis* spp.)
Ryegrass (*Elymus* and *Iolium* spp.)
Canary grass (*Phalaris minor*)
Bluegrass/June grass (*Poa* spp.)
Index weeds (pollinating season—summer through early fall)
Careless weed (*Amaranthus palmeri*)
Iodine bush (*Allenrolfea occidentalis*)
Saltbush/scale (*Atriplex* spp.)
Lamb's-quarters (*Chenopodium album*)
Russian thistle (*Salsola kali*)
Alkali-blite (*Suaeda* spp.)
Ragweed, false, slender, and western (*Ambrosia* spp.)
Sagebrush (*Artemisia* spp.)
Silver ragweed (*Dicoria canescens*)
Burro brush (*Hymenoclea salsola*)

Region XIII
Southern Coastal California
Index trees (pollinating season—late winter through spring)
Box elder (*Acer negundo*)
Cypress (*Cupressus arizonica*)
Oak (*Quercus agrifolia*)
Walnut (*Juglans* spp.)
Acacia (*Acacia* spp.)
Mulberry (*Morus* spp.)
Eucalyptus (*Eucalyptus* spp.)
Ash (*Fraxinus velutina*)
Olive (*Olea europaea*)
Sycamore (*Platanus racemosa*)
Cottonwood/poplar (*Populus trichocarpa*)
Elm (*Ulmus* spp.)
Index grasses (pollinating season—spring through early summer)
Oats (*Avena* spp.)
Bromegrass (*Bromus* spp.)
Bermuda grass (*Cynodon dactylon*)
Orchard grass (*Dactylis glomerata*)
Salt grass (*Distichlis* spp.)
Ryegrass (*Elymus* and *Lolium* spp.)
Fescue (*Festuca elatior*)
Bluegrass/June grass (*Poa* spp.)
Johnson grass (*Sorghum halepense*)
Index weeds (pollinating season—summer through early fall)
Careless weed/pigweed (*Amaranthus* spp.)
Saltbush/scale (*Atriplex* spp.)
Lamb's-quarters (*Chenopodium album*)
Russian thistle (*Salsola kali*)
Ragweed, false, slender, and western (*Ambrosia* spp.)
Sagebrush (*Artemisia* spp.)
Cocklebur (*Xanthium strumarium*)
Plantain (*Plantago lanceolata*)
Dock/sorrel (*Rumex* spp.)

Region XIV
Central California Valley: Sacramento and San Joaquin Valleys
Index trees (pollinating season—late winter through spring)
Box elder (*Acer negundo*)
Alder (*Alnus rhombifolia*)
Birch (*Betula fontinalis*)
Cypress (*Cupressus arizonica*)
Oak (*Quercus lobata*)

Pecan (*Carya pecan*)
Walnut (*Juglans* spp.)
Ash (*Fraxinus velutina*)
Olive (*Olea europaea*)
Sycamore (*Platanus acerifolia*)
Cottonwood/poplar (*Populus fremontii*)
Elm (*Ulmus* spp.)
Index grasses (pollinating season—spring through early summer)
Redtop (*Agrostis alba*)
Oats (*Avena* spp.)
Bromegrass (*Bromus* spp.)
Bermuda grass (*Cynodon dactylon*)
Orchard grass (*Dactylis glomerata*)
Salt grass (*Distichlis* spp.)
Ryegrass (*Elymus* and *Lolium* spp.)
Fescue (*Festuca elatior*)
Canary grass (*Phalaris minor*)
Timothy (*Phleum pratense*)
Bluegrass/June grass (*Poa* spp.)
Johnson grass (*Sorghum halepense*)
Index weeds (pollinating season—summer through early fall)
Pigweed (*Amaranthus retroflexus*)
Saltbush/scale (*Atriplex* spp.)
Sugar beet (*Beta vulgaris*)
Lamb's-quarters (*Chenopodium album*)
Russian thistle (*Salsola kali*)
Ragweed, false, slender, and western (*Ambrosia* spp.)
Sagebrush (*Artemisia* spp.)
Cocklebur (*Xanthium strumarium*)
Plantain (*Plantago lanceolata*)
Dock/sorrel (*Rumex* spp.)
Region XV
Intermountain West: Idaho (southern), Nevada
Index trees (pollinating season—late winter through spring)
Box elder (*Acer negundo*)
Alder (*Alnus incana*)
Birch (*Betula fontinalis*)
Cedar/juniper (*Juniperus utahensis*)
Ash (*Fraxinus americana*)
Sycamore (*Platanus occidentalis*)
Cottonwood/poplar (*Populus trichocarpa*)
Elm (*Ulmus* spp.)
Index grasses (pollinating season—spring through early summer)
Quack grass/wheat grass (*Agropyron* spp.)
Redtop (*Agrostis alba*)
Bromegrass (*Bromus inermis*)
Bermuda grass (*Cynodon dactylon*)
Orchard grass (*Dactylis glomerata*)
Salt grass (*Distichlis* spp.)
Ryegrass (*Elymus* and *Lolium* spp.)
Fescue (*Festuca elatior*)
Timothy (*Phleum pratense*)
Bluegrass/June grass (*Poa* spp.)
Index weeds (pollinating season—summer through early fall)
Pigweed (*Amaranthus retroflexus*)
Iodine bush (*Allenrolfea occidentalis*)
Saltbush/scale (*Atriplex* spp.)
Lamb's-quarters (*Chenopodium album*)
Mexican firebush (*Kochia scoparia*)
Russian thistle (*Salsola kali*)
Ragweed, false, slender, and western (*Ambrosia* spp.)
Sagebrush (*Artemisia* spp.)
Marsh elder/poverty weed (*Iva* spp.)

Cocklebur (*Xanthium strumarium*)
Plantain (*Plantago lanceolata*)
Dock/sorrel (*Rumex* spp.)
Region XVI
Inland Empire: Oregon (central and eastern), Washington (central and eastern)
Index trees (pollinating season—late winter through spring)
Box elder (*Acer negundo*)
Alder (*Alnus incana*)
Birch (*Betula fontinalis*)
Oak (*Quercus garryana*)
Walnut (*Juglans nigra*)
Pine (*Pinus* spp.)
Cottonwood/poplar (*Populus trichocarpa*)
Willow (*Salix lasiandra*)
Index grasses (pollinating season—spring through early summer)
Quack grass/wheat grass (*Agropyron* spp.)
Redtop (*Agrostis alba*)
Vernal grass (*Anthoxanthum* spp.)
Bromegrass (*Bromus inermis*)
Orchard grass (*Dactylis glomerata*)
Ryegrass (*Elymus* and *Lolium* spp.)
Velvet grass (*Holcus lanatus*)
Timothy (*Phleum pratense*)
Bluegrass/June grass (*Poa* spp.)
Index weeds (pollinating season—summer through early fall)
Pigweed (*Amaranthus retroflexus*)
Saltbush/scale (*Atriplex* spp.)
Lamb's-quarters (*Chenopodium album*)
Mexican firebush (*Kochia scoparia*)
Russian thistle (*Salsola kali*)
Ragweed, false, giant, short, and western (*Ambrosia* spp.)
Sagebrush (*Artemisia* spp.)
Marsh elder/poverty weed (*Iva* spp.)
Plantain (*Plantago lanceolata*)
Dock/sorrel (*Rumex* spp.)
Region XVII
Cascade Pacific Northwest: California (northwestern), Washington (western), Oregon (western)
Index trees (pollinating season—late winter through spring)
Box elder (*Acer negundo*)
Alder (*Alnus rhombifolia*)
Birch (*Betula fontinalis*)
Hazel (*Corylus cornuta*)
Oak (*Quercus garryana*)
Walnut (*Juglans regia*)
Ash (*Fraxinus oregona*)
Cottonwood/poplar (*Populus trichocarpa*)
Willow (*Salix lasiandra*)
Elm (*Ulmus pumila*)
Index grasses (pollinating season—spring through early summer)
Bentgrass (*Agrostis maritima*)
Vernal grass (*Anthoxanthum* spp.)
Oats (*Avena* spp.)
Bromegrass (*Bromus inermis*)
Bermuda grass (*Cynodon dactylon*)
Orchard grass (*Dactylis glomerata*)
Salt grass (*Distichlis* spp.)
Ryegrass (*Elymus* and *Lolium* spp.)
Fescue (*Festuca elatior*)
Velvet grass (*Holcus lanatus*)
Canary grass (*Phalaris arundinacea*)
Timothy (*Phleum pratense*)
Bluegrass/June grass (*Poa* spp.)

Index weeds (pollinating season—summer through early fall)
  Pigweed (*Amaranthus retroflexus*)
  Saltbush/scale (*Atriplex* spp.)
  Lamb's-quarters (*Chenopodium album*)
  Russian thistle (*Salsola kali*)
  Ragweed, false, giant, short, and western (*Ambrosia* spp.)
  Sagebrush (*Artemisia* spp.)
  Cocklebur (*Xanthium strumarium*)
  Plantain (*Plantago lanceolata*)
  Dock/sorrel (*Rumex* spp.)

Region C-I
  Atlantic Provinces and Quebec: Prince Edward Island, New Brunswick, Quebec, Nova Scotia, Newfoundland
    Index trees (pollinating season—late winter through spring)
      Box elder/Manitoba maple (*Acer negundo*)
      Hard maple/sugar maple (*Acer saccharum*)
      Tag alder/speckled alder (*Alnus incana*)
      Paper birch/white birch (*Betula papyrifera*)
      Beech (*Fagus grandifolia*)
      White ash (*Fraxinus americana*)
      Green ash (*Fraxinus pennsylvanica*)
      Butternut (*Juglans cinerea*)
      Sycamore (*Platanus occidentalis*)
      Balsam poplar (*Populus balsamifera*)
      Trembling aspen (*Populus tremuloides*)
      Bur oak (*Quercus macrocarpa*)
      Black willow (*Salix nigra*)
      American elm (*Ulmus americana*)
    Index grasses (pollinating season—spring through early summer)
      Quack grass (couch grass) (*Agropyron repens*)
      Redtop (*Agrostis alba*)
      Bromegrass (*Bromus* spp.)
      Orchard grass (*Dactylis glomerata*)
      Ryegrass (*Elymus* and *Lolium* spp.)
      Timothy (*Phleum pratense*)
      Bluegrass (*Poa* spp.)
    Index weeds (pollinating season—summer through early fall)
      Redroot pigweed (*Amaranthus retroflexus*)
      Ragweed (*Ambrosia* spp.)
      Lamb's-quarters (*Chenopodium album*)
      Plantain (*Plantago lanceolata*)
      Dock/sorrel (*Rumex* spp.)
      Russian thistle (*Salsola kali*)

Region C-II
  Ontario
    Index trees (pollinating season—late winter through spring)
      Box elder/Manitoba maple (*Acer negundo*)
      Hard maple/sugar maple (*Acer saccharum*)
      Tag alder/speckled alder (*Alnus incana*)
      Paper birch/white birch (*Betula papyrifera*)
      Beech (*Fagus grandifolia*)
      White ash (*Fraxinus americana*)
      Green ash (*Fraxinus pennsylvanica*)
      Butternut (*Juglans cinerea*)
      Sycamore (*Platanus occidentalis*)
      Balsam poplar (*Populus balsamifera*)
      Aspen (*Populus tremuloides*)
      Bur oak (*Quercus macrocarpa*)
      Black willow (*Salix nigra*)
      American elm/white elm (*Ulmus americana*)
      Chinese elm/Siberian elm (*Ulmus pumila*)
    Index grasses (pollinating season—spring through early summer)
      Quack grass/couch grass (*Agropyron repens*)
      Redtop (*Agrostis alba*)

Bromegrass (*Bromus* spp.)
Orchard grass (*Dactylis glomerata*)
Ryegrass (*Elymus* and *Lolium* spp.)
Timothy (*Phleum pratense*)
Bluegrass (*Poa* spp.)
Index weeds (pollinating season—summer through early fall)
  Redroot pigweed (*Amaranthus retroflexus*)
  Ragweed (*Ambrosia* spp.)
  Lamb's-quarters (*Chenopodium album*)
  English plantain (*Plantago lanceolata*)
  Dock/sorrel (*Rumex* spp.)
  Russian thistle (*Salsola kali*)

Region C-III
  Prairie Provinces and Eastern British Columbia: Alberta, Manitoba, eastern British Columbia, Saskatchewan
    Index trees (pollinating season—late winter through spring)
      Box elder/Manitoba maple (*Acer negundo*)
      Tag elder/speckled mountain alder (*Alnus incana*)
      Paper birch/white birch (*Betula papyrifera*)
      Green ash (*Fraxinus pennsylvanica*)
      Balsam poplar (*Populus balsamifera*)
      Trembling aspen (*Populus tremuloides*)
      Bur oak (*Quercus macrocarpa*)
      Willow (yellow) (*Salix* spp.)
      Chinese elm/Siberian elm (*Ulmus pumila*)
    Index grasses (pollinating season—spring through early summer)
      Quack grass/couch grass/wheat grass (*Agropyron* spp.)
      Redtop (*Agrostis alba*)
      Common wild oats (*Avena fatua*)
      Bromegrass (*Bromus* sp.)
      Orchard grass (*Dactylis glomerata*)
      Ryegrass (*Elymus* and *Lolium* spp.)
      Timothy (*Phleum pratense*)
      Bluegrass (*Poa* supp.)
    Index weeds (pollinating season—summer through early fall)
      Redroot pigweed (*Amaranthus retroflexus*)
      Ragweed (*Ambrosia* spp.)
      Lamb's-quarters (*Chenopodium album*)
      Sagebrush (*Artemisia* spp.)
      Marsh elder/poverty weed (*Iva* spp.)
      English plantain (*Plantago lanceolata*)
      Dock/sorrel (*Rumex* spp.)
      Russian thistle (*Salsola kali*)

Region C-IV
  Western British Columbia and Vancouver Island
    Index trees (pollinating season—late winter through spring)
      Box elder/Manitoba maple (*Acer negundo*)
      Red alder (*Alnus rubra*)
      Sitka alder (*Alnus sinuata*)
      Paper birch/white birch (*Betula papyrifera*)
      Sycamore (*Platanus occidentalis*)
      Black cottonwood (*Populus trichocarpa*)
      Trembling aspen (*Populus tremuloides*)
      Douglas fir (*Pseudotsuga menziesii*)
      Garry's oak (*Quercus garryana*)
      Yellow willow/Pacific willow (*Salix lasiandra*)
      Chinese elm/Siberian elm (*Ulmus pumila*)
    Index grasses (pollinating season—spring through early summer)
      Quack grass/couch grass (*Agropyron repens*)
      Redtop (*Agrostis alba*)
      Tall oats grass (*Arrhenatherum elatius*)
      Common wild oats (*Avena fatua*)
      Bromegrass (*Bromus* spp.)
      Orchard grass (*Dactylis glomerata*)

Ryegrass (*Elymus* and *Lolium* spp.)
Timothy (*Phleum pratense*)
Bluegrass (*Poa* spp.)
Index weeds (pollinating season—summer through early fall)
Redroot pigweed (*Amaranthus retroflexus*)
Ragweed (*Ambrosia* spp.)
Lamb's-quarters (*Chenopodium album*)
Marsh elder/poverty weed (*Iva* spp.)
English plantain (*Plantago lanceolata*)
Dock/sorrel (*Rumex* spp.)
Russian thistle (*Salsola kali*)
Alaska
Index trees (pollinating season—spring)
Alder (*Alnus incana*)
Aspen (*Populus tremuloides*)
Birch (*Betula papyrifera*)
Cedar (*Thuja plicata*)
Hemlock (*Tsuga hetrophylla*)
Pine (*Pinus contorta*)
Poplar (*Populus balsamifera*)
Spruce (*Picea sitchensis*)
Willow (*Salix* spp.)
Index grasses (pollinating season—late spring and summer)
Bluegrass/June grass (*Poa* spp.)
Bromegrass (*Bromus inermis*)
Canary grass (*Phalaris arundinacea*)
Fescue (*Festuca rubra*)
Orchard grass (*Dactylis glomerata*)
Quack grass/wheat grass (*Agropyron* spp.)
Redtop (*Agrostis alba*)
Ryegrass (*Lolium perenne*)
Timothy (*Phleum pratense*)
Index weeds (pollinating season—summer)
Bulrush (*Scirpus* spp.)
Dock/sorrel (*Rumex* spp.)
Lamb's-quarters (*Chenopodium album*)
Nettle (*Urtica dioica*)

Plantain (*Plantago lanceolata*)
Sagebrush/wormwood (*Artemisia* spp.)
Sedge (*Carex* spp.)
Spearscale (*Atriplex patula*)
Hawaii (all islands) (pollinating season: less defined than in continental regions)
Index trees
Acacia (*Acacia* spp.)
Australian pine/beefwood (*Casuarina equisetifolia*)
Cedar/juniper (*Juniperus* spp.)
Monterey cypress (*Cupressus macrocarpa*)
Date palm (*Phoenix dactylifera*)
Eucalyptus/Gum (*Eucalyptus globulus*)
Mesquite (*Prosopis juliflora*)
Paper mulberry (*Broussonetia papyrifera*)
Olive (*Olea europaea*)
Privet (*Ligustrum* spp.)
Index grasses
Bermuda grass (*Cynodon dactylon*)
Corn (*Zea mays*)
Finger grass (*Chloris* spp.)
Johnson grass (*Sorghum halepense*)
Love grass (*Eragrostis* spp.)
Bluegrass/June grass (*Poa* spp.)
Redtop (*Agrostis alba*)
Sorghum (*Sorghum vulgare*)
Index weeds
Cocklebur (*Xanthium strumarium*)
Plantain (*Plantago lanceolata*)
Kochia (*Kochia scoparia*)
Pigweed (*Amaranthus* spp.)
Ragweed, slender (*Ambrosia* spp.)
Sagebrush (*Artemisia* spp.)
Saltbush/scale (*Atriplex* spp.)

Source: R. W. Ausdenmoore, Aeroallergens and Environmental Factors. In G. J. Lawlor, Jr., and T. J. Fischer (eds.), *Manual of Allergy and Immunology: Diagnosis and Therapy*. Boston: Little, Brown, 1981. Adapted from *Pollen Guide for Allergy*. Spokane: Hollister-Stier Laboratories, 1978. Copyright Hollister-Stier, 1978.

B. Incidence of Individual Molds in the United States[a]

	Northeast U.S.[b]		Southeast U.S.[c]		Central U.S.[d]	
	Indoor	Outdoor	Indoor	Outdoor	Indoor	Outdoor
Hormodendrum	56.7	66.8	66.8	96.5	63.3	81.8
Penicillium	37.0	25.1	31.5	22.8	30.1	27.3
Alternaria	23.4	48.2	18.0	54.3	39.1	72.3
Aspergillus	20.0	7.3	14.7	7.9	16.0	6.3
Pullularia	9.5	19.6	5.4	10.5	4.1	9.1
Geotrichum	11.5	5.5	19.4	8.8	6.1	3.4
Fomes	7.1	16.3	5.8	8.8	5.0	18.2
Epicoccum	6.1	12.6	7.0	20.2	4.1	6.8
Fusarium	5.7	15.1	7.0	21.9	6.4	17.6
Sterile *Mycelia*	5.4	12.3	10.3	12.3	8.1	8.5
Phoma	2.8	12.3	1.4	8.8	3.1	9.7
Rhodotorula	5.3	3.3	4.0		1.7	2.3
Cephalosporium	4.6	9.8	7.2	11.4	3.7	7.4
Stemphylium	4.0	2.5	2.1	3.5	4.0	
Streptomyces	2.4	7.8		8.8	1.2	13.6
Botrytis	3.9	5.0		6.1		
Mucor		7.5	2.8	9.6	1.2	6.3
Poria	3.8	2.8	1.9		2.7	1.7
Trichoderma	2.1	5.0		7.0	2.3	4.0
Helminthosporium	3.6	3.5	5.8	10.5	1.8	4.0
Tetracoccosporium		2.3				
Sporobolomyces	3.1	1.5	1.2		2.0	1.7
Polyporaceae	1.5					1.7
Curvularia			4.9	6.1		
Nigrospora				1.8		
Rhizopus				1.8	2.3	1.7
Spondylocladium						
Verticillium						
Fusidium						
Chaetomium						
Acremonium						
Monosporium						
Unidentified yeast						
Polyporus						
Pleospora						

[a] Expressed as the percent of total exposures when a given fungal genus was recovered.
[b] Delaware, Maryland, Connecticut, Massachusetts, New Jersey, Pennsylvania, New York, Maine, New Hampshire, Rhode Island, and Vermont.
[c] Florida, Georgia, South Carolina, West Virginia, Kentucky, North Carolina, Virginia, Alabama, Arkansas, Louisiana, Tennessee, and Mississippi.
[d] Ohio, Michigan, Wisconsin, Minnesota, Illinois, Missouri, Iowa, and Indiana.
[e] Oklahoma and Texas.
[f] Nevada, New Mexico, Idaho, Colorado, Montana, and Utah.
[g] California.
[h] Oregon and Washington.
Source: R. W. Ausdenmoore. Aeroallergens and Environmental Factors. In G. J. Lawlor, Jr., and T. J. Fischer, *Manual of Allergy and Immunology: Diagnosis and Therapy.* Boston: Little, Brown, 1981. Adapted from *The Role of Molds in Allergy.* Spokane: Hollister-Stier Laboratories, 1977.

Southcentral U.S.[e]		Northwest U.S.[f]		Southwest U.S.[g]		West U.S.[h]	
Indoor	Outdoor	Indoor	Outdoor	Indoor	Outdoor	Indoor	Outdoor
78.6	92.9	62.5	69.6	63.8	93.0	74.5	68.4
25.2	32.1	41.4	40.6	31.9	35.7	35.1	35.9
41.7	85.7	21.1	27.5	42.6	64.3	39.7	47.0
21.3	17.9	15.1	8.7	4.3	7.1	10.1	11.1
1.9		8.0	11.6	6.4	7.1	6.3	12.8
13.6	3.6	6.8	2.9	6.4		2.9	
		2.0	1.4			1.7	5.1
11.7	10.7	2.0	4.3		7.1	16.6	17.1
5.8	46.6	1.2	10.1	4.3	21.4	4.0	11.1
23.3	25.0	4.0	15.9	4.3		7.7	3.4
	7.1	4.8	10.1	6.4	28.6	2.9	8.5
		2.8	7.2	2.1	7.1	2.2	
5.8	21.4	5.2	5.8	4.3	7.1	7.2	4.3
6.8		5.6	11.6	19.1	21.4	10.1	10.3
1.9	17.9	6.8	17.4		35.7	2.9	13.7
		2.4		2.1		4.3	9.4
		3.2	8.7	2.1		3.4	9.4
		1.2	2.9				
		5.2	13.0	2.1			1.7
28.2	25.0	3.6		6.4	14.3	6.3	8.5
		1.2		6.4		1.4	
	32.1	1.6					1.7
4.9	10.7			2.1			
1.9		2.4		6.4	7.1	3.1	5.1
1.9							
	3.6						2.6
	3.6						
			1.4				
				2.1			
				2.1			
					14.3		
						1.2	1.2
							5.1

C. Asthma Education Materials*

PROGRAM MATERIALS FOR TEACHING PATIENTS AND PARENTS—CHILDHOOD ASTHMA

Teaching Manuals or Guides

Living with Asthma—National Heart, Lung, and Blood Institute (NHLBI)
Open Airways (contains materials in Spanish and English)—NHLBI
Air Wise—NHLBI
Air Power—NHLBI
ACT (*Asthma Care Training*)—Asthma and Allergy Foundation of America, Washington, DC

A Kit for Physicians

A Kit for Physicians: Helping Pediatric Patients and Their Parents Manage Asthma—NHLBI
Hispanic *ACT* (*Asthma Care Training*)

PROGRAMS TO ATTEND

Family Asthma Programs—American Lung Association

TEACH YOURSELF AT HOME

For Children with Asthma

Teaching Myself about Asthma, by Guy Parcel, M.D.
Superstuff—Kid's Package, by American Lung Association
Captain Respitore to the Rescue—National Jewish Center for Immunology and Respiratory Medicine
So You Have Asthma Too—Mothers of Asthmatics, Inc.
I'm a Meter Reader—Mothers of Asthmatics, Inc.

For Parents of Children with Asthma

Superstuff—In Control—Parents' Magazine by American Lung Association
Asthma Organizer—Mothers of Asthmatics, Inc.

For Parents and Children

Superstuff—American Lung Association
CALM: Controlling Asthma, Learning to Manage—IOX Associates and Asthma and Allergy Foundation of America
  Prereaders (age 1–7)
  Preadolescents (age 8–12)
  Teenagers (age 13–19)
  Parents
  Attending Physicians
Learn Asthma Control in Seven Days—University of Alabama Hospital

* A major portion of these resources has been reprinted from the National Heart, Lung, and Blood Institute, Bethesda, Maryland (for mailing addresses see Appendix D).

SUPPORT GROUPS

Family Support Group Manual—Asthma and Allergy Foundation of America
Support Group Manual—Mothers of Asthmatics, Inc.
Living with Asthma—NHLBI
Open Airways—NHLBI

BOOKS ON COPING SKILLS AND GENERAL INFORMATION—FOR PARENTS TO READ

Children with Asthma, by Thomas Plaut, M.D. (1987)
Asthma, by Allan Weinstein, M.D. (1987)
The Essential Asthma Handbook, by Francois and Sheila Haas (1987)
Asthma and What You Can Do About It, by Milton Millman, M.D. (1988)
The Asthma Self-Help Book, by Paul J. Hannaway (1989)
A Parent's Guide to Asthma, by Nancy Sander (1989)
The Complete Book of Children's Allergies: A Guide for Parents, by Robert Feldman, M.D.—American Lung Association (1989)
The Best Guide to Allergy, by A. Giannini, M.D., N. Schultz, M.D., and T. Chang, M.D.
Allergy Plants, by M. Jelks, M.D.
Asthma in Schools, by F. Mendoza, M.D., and M. K. Garcia, R.N.
The Asthma Handbook: Guide for Patients and Families, by S. H. Young, M.D., S. Shulman, and M. D. Shulman, Ph.D.

PAMPHLETS ON GENERAL TOPICS

Asthma Facts—American Lung Association
What Happens When a Child Has Asthma—American Lung Association
Asthma: A Matter of Control—American Lung Association of Kansas
Handbook for the Asthmatic—Asthma and Allergy Foundation of America
Asthma: Episodes and Treatment—Public Affairs, Inc.
Your Child and Asthma—National Jewish Center for Immunology and Respiratory Medicine
Understanding Asthma—National Jewish Center for Immunology and Respiratory Medicine
Management of Chronic Respiratory Disease—National Jewish Center for Immunology and Respiratory Medicine
So You Have Asthma Too—Mothers of Asthmatics, Inc.
Living with Asthma—Berlex Laboratories
Asthma—National Institute of Allergy and Infectious Diseases
Respiratory section of *Sources*—Pharmaceutical Manufacturers Association
Check Your Asthma "I.Q."—NHLBI
Tips to Remember—American Academy of Allergy and Immunology (AAAI)
Childhood Asthma: A Handbook for Parents—Hospital for Sick Children, Toronto
Facts About Asthma—NHLBI

PAMPHLETS/ARTICLES FOR COPING

Controlling Asthma—American Lung Association
Asthma Fact and Fiction—National Foundation for Asthma/Tucson Medical Center
Your Asthma Can Be Controlled: Expect Nothing Less—NHLBI

PAMPHLETS ON EXERCISE AND ASTHMA

Exercise and Asthma—Asthma and Allergy Foundation, Washington, DC
Exercise-Induced Asthma—American Allergy Foundation, Menlo Park, CA
Feeling Good with Asthma—Boehringer Ingelheim Pharmaceuticals
Exercise-Induced Asthma and Bronchospasm—AAAI

PAMPHLETS ON SPECIAL TOPICS

Quackery

Quackery and Questionable Treatment in Asthma and Allergy Medicine—Asthma and Allergy Foundation of America

Myths

About Asthma: Facts and Myths—American College of Chest Physicians
Asthma Fact and Fiction—National Foundation for Asthma/Tucson Medical Center

Discovering Asthma

Hidden Asthma . . . and Other Non-Classical Formats—American Allergy Foundation, Menlo Park, CA

Weather

Your Guide to Bad Weather and Chronic and Lung Disease—American College of Chest Physicians

Air Cleaners

Electronic Air Cleaners, and HEPA Filters, Ion Machines, Portable Air Cleaners—American Allergy Foundation, Menlo Park, CA

ASTHMA STATISTICS

Data Fact Sheet: Asthma Statistics—NHLBI

BREATHING EXERCISES

Captain Wonderlung: Breathing Exercises for Asthmatic Children—American Academy of Pediatrics
Management of Chronic Respiratory Disease—National Jewish Center for Immunology and Respiratory Medicine

SCHOOL AND ASTHMA

There Are Solutions for the Student with Asthma—American Lung Association
ASTHMA ALERT for Teachers—American Lung Association

ASTHMA ALERT for School Nurses—American Lung Association
ASTHMA ALERT for Physical Education Teachers—American Lung Association
Tips for Teachers: The Allergic Child—Asthma and Allergy Foundation of America
Asthma and Allergies in the Schools: The Importance of Cooperative Care—Asthma and Allergy Foundation of America
Asthma in the School: Improving Control with the Peak Flow Monitoring—Asthma and Allergy Foundation of America
Open Airways for Schools—American Lung Association
Managing Asthma: A Guide for Schools—NHLBI

ASTHMA DRUGS

From the U.S. Pharmacopoeial Convention, Rockville, Maryland
  Adrenergic Bronchodilators (Oral/Injected)
  Adrenergic Bronchodilators (Inhalation)
  Adrenocorticoids (Oral)
  Adrenocorticoids (Inhaled)
  Cromolyn
  Xanthine Bronchodilators
Sources—Pharmaceutical Manufacturers Association, Washington, DC
. . . About the Allergy and Asthma Drugs You Take—AAAI
Healthfinder: Medications—ODPHP National Health Information Center
"Pharmacologic Therapy of Pediatric Asthma"—American Thoracic Society
What Everyone Needs to Know About Theophylline—Mothers of Asthmatics, Inc.

PEAK FLOW MONITORING

CALM: Controlling Asthma, Learning to Manage—For Prereaders, for Preadolescents, and for Teenagers—IOX Associates and Asthma and Allergy Foundation of America
A User's Guide to Peak Flow Monitoring—Mothers of Asthmatics, Inc.
Peak Performance—Mothers of Asthmatics, Inc.
Asthma in the School: Improving Control with Peak Flow Monitoring—Asthma and Allergy Foundation of America

ALLERGIES IMPORTANT IN ASTHMA

Allergy Plants That Cause Sneezing and Wheezing—AAAI
Dust 'n' Stuff—National Foundation for Asthma/Tucson Medical Center
Allergy in Children—Asthma and Allergy Foundation of America
Drug Allergy—Asthma and Allergy Foundation of America
Food Allergy—Asthma and Allergy Foundation of America
Hay Fever—Asthma and Allergy Foundation of America
Stinging Insect Allergy—Asthma and Allergy Foundation of America
Pollen Allergy—Asthma and Allergy Foundation of America
Sinusitis—Asthma and Allergy Foundation of America
"The Role of Allergy in Asthma"—American Thoracic Society
Allergy Plants—AAAI

MATERIALS FOR ADULTS WITH ASTHMA

Self-Teaching Materials

Learn Asthma Control in Seven Days—University of Alabama Hospital

The Asthma Handbook—American Lung Association
Feeling Good with Asthma—Boehringer Ingelheim Pharmaceuticals

Under Development

Adult *ACT* (*Asthma Care Training*)—Marianne Lewis, M.D., UCLA
Adult *Air Wise/Air Power*—Sandra Wilson-Pisano, M.D., and Gary Arsham, M.D., American Institutes for Research, Palo Alto, CA

FILMS/VIDEOS

Asthma—Family Information Systems
A Regular Kid—American Lung Association
Asthma and Allergies in the School: The Importance of Cooperative Care—Asthma and Allergy Foundation of America
I'm Wonderful and I Have Asthma—AAAI; Pediatric orientation
Jeanette Bolden Story—Asthma and Allergy Foundation of America
Auxiliary Inhalation Devices—Asthma and Allergy Foundation of America
Controlling Allergens in Your Environment—AAAI
So You Have Asthma Too—Mothers of Asthmatics, Inc.
Allergies and Asthma Video—Mothers of Asthmatics, Inc.

SLIDE/AUDIOCASSETTE PACKAGES

An Orientation to Asthma—American Lung Association and American Thoracic Society
Outpatient Management of the Child With Asthma—American Thoracic Society
Pharmacologic Therapy of Pediatric Asthma—American Thoracic Society
The Diagnosis and Treatment of Status Asthmaticus in Children—American Thoracic Society
The Role of Allergy in Asthma—American Thoracic Society

SPECIAL MATERIALS

Scott, the Puppet with Asthma—Kids on the Block Puppets, Columbia, Maryland

SPORTS

Asthma Athletic Scholarship Program—Schering Corporation, Information Services Manager, 2000 Galloping Hill Road, Kenilworth, NJ 07033

INFORMATION LINES

LUNG LINE—800-222-LUNG or 303-355-LUNG—National Jewish Center for Immunology and Respiratory Medicine
Local chapters of American Lung Association
AAAI—information and referral service—800-822-2762 or 800-822-ASMA
American College of Allergy and Immunology—written materials and referral service—1-800-842-7777

RESOURCE LISTS

Asthma Reading and Resource List—NHLBI
Teamwork—Mothers of Asthmatics, Inc.
Asthma Resources Directory: An Essential Resource for Physicians,* edited by Carol Rudoff—Allergy Publications, Menlo Park, CA, 1990 (P.O. Box 640, Menlo Park, CA 94026; very extensive resource)
*Allergy Products Directory**—American Allergy Association (listing of books, foods, cosmetics, services, etc.)

NEWSLETTERS

Asthma and Allergy Advocate—AAAI
The MA Report—Mothers of Asthmatics, Inc.
Allergy Quarterly—Allergy Information Association, 65 Tromley Drive, Islington, Ontario, Canada M9B 5Y7
Allergy Alert—Allergy Foundation of Canada, Box 1904, Saskatoon, Saskatchewan, Canada S7K 3S5
Allergy News—Allergy and Asthma Association of Southern California, 27800 Medical Center Road, Mission Viejo, CA 92691
Asthma Update—quarterly newsletter, 123 Monticello Ave., Annapolis, MD 21401
Rodale's Allergy Relief Newsletter—monthly newsletter from Rodale Press, 33 E. Minor St., Emmas, PA 18049

* Recommended.

D. Professional and Nonprofessional Organizations for Resource Information and Educational Programs*

ALLERGY FOUNDATION OF CANADA
Box 1904
Saskatoon, Saskatchewan
S7K 3S5

ALLERGY INFORMATION ASSOCIATION
65 Tromley Dr., Rm. 10
Islington, Ontario
M9B 5Y7 CANADA
416-244-8585

AMERICAN ACADEMY OF ALLERGY AND IMMUNOLOGY
611 East Wells Street
Milwaukee, WI 53202
414-272-6071

AMERICAN ACADEMY OF PEDIATRICS
141 Northwest Point Blvd.
Box 927
Elk Grove Village, IL 60007
312-569-2025

AMERICAN ALLERGY ASSOCIATION
P.O. Box 7273
Menlo Park, CA 94025-7273
415-322-1663

AMERICAN ASSOCIATION FOR RESPIRATORY CARE
11030 Abales Lane
Dallas, TX 75229-4524
214-243-2272

AMERICAN COLLEGE OF ALLERGY AND IMMUNOLOGY
800 E. Northwest Highway, Suite 1080
Palatine, IL 60067-6516
708-359-2800

AMERICAN COLLEGE OF CHEST PHYSICIANS
911 Busse Highway
Park Ridge, IL 60068
708-359-2800

AMERICAN LUNG ASSOCIATION
1740 Broadway
New York, NY 10019
212-315-8700

AMERICAN THORACIC SOCIETY
1740 Broadway
New York, NY 10019
212-315-8700

ASSOCIATION FOR THE CARE OF ASTHMA
Jefferson Medical College
1025 Walnut St. (ARD)
Philadelphia, PA 19107
215-928-8912

ASTHMA AND ALLERGY FOUNDATION OF AMERICA
1717 Massachusetts Ave. N.W.
Suite 305
Washington, DC 20036
202-265-0265

ASTHMA ASSOCIATION OF CANADA
Box 192
Toronto Dominion Centre
Toronto, CANADA M5K 1H6
416-977-9684

ASTHMA CARE ASSOCIATION OF AMERICA
P.O. Box 568
Spring Valley Road
Ossining, NY 10362
914-762-1941

ASTHMA RESEARCH COUNCIL
12 Pembridge Square
Palace Court
London, W2 4EH ENGLAND

ASTHMATIC CHILDREN'S FOUNDATION
of New York, Inc.
15 Spring Valley Road
P.O. Box 568
Ossining, NY 10562
914-762-2110

CANADIAN LUNG ASSOCIATION
Suite 908
75 Albert Street
Ottawa, Ontario K1P 5E7
613-237-1208

CANADIAN SOCIETY OF ALLERGY AND CLINICAL
IMMUNOLOGY
c/o Montreal General Hospital
Room 7135
1650 Cedar Avenue
Montreal, Quebec H3G 1A4
CANADA

CENTER FOR INTERDISCIPLINARY RESEARCH ON
IMMUNOLOGIC DISEASES
Georgetown University School of Medicine
3900 Reservoir Road N.W.
Washington, DC 20007

HAY FEVER PREVENTION SOCIETY
Rosewall Gardens Ste. 2-G
2300 Sedgwick Ave.
Bronx, NY 10468
212-295-1069

MOTHERS OF ASTHMATICS, INC.
10875 Main Street, Suite 210
Fairfax, VA 22030
703-385-4403

* Resources cited are provided as information only and not as endorsements.

NATIONAL ASTHMA EDUCATION PROGRAM
NHLBI Information Center
Box 30105
Bethesda, MD 20814-0105

NATIONAL CENTER FOR HEALTH EDUCATION
30 E. 29th St. (ARD)
New York, NY 10016-7901
212-769-1886

NATIONAL CENTER FOR HEALTH STATISTICS
Center Building
3700 East West Highway
Hyattsville, MD 20782
301-436-8500

NATIONAL FOUNDATION FOR ASTHMA/TUCSON MEDICAL
  CENTER
P.O. Box 42195
Tucson, AZ 85733

NATIONAL HEART, LUNG, AND BLOOD INSTITUTE
  (NHLBI)
9000 Rockville Pike
Bethesda, MD 20892
301-951-3260

NATIONAL INSTITUTE ON ALLERGY AND INFECTIOUS
  DISEASES (NIAID)
Building 31, Room 7A32
9000 Rockville Pike
Bethesda, MD 20892
301-496-5717; 301-496-4000

NATIONAL JEWISH CENTER FOR IMMUNOLOGY AND
  RESPIRATORY MEDICINE
1400 Jackson Street
Denver, CO 80206
303-388-4461

NEW YORK SUPPORT GROUP FOR PARENTS OF ASTHMATIC
  AND ALLERGIC CHILDREN
201 East 28th Street
New York, NY 10016
212-889-3507

PARENTS OF ASTHMATIC CHILDREN
1 Freeman Avenue
Denville, NJ 07834
201-627-6875

PARENTS OF CHILDREN WITH ASTHMA
9450 Preston Trail East
Ponte Vedra, FL 32082
904-285-1410

E. Summer Camps for Children*

ALASKA
Champ Camp
ALA of Alaska
605 Barrow Street, Suite 2
Anchorage, AK 99501
907-276-5864

ARIZONA
Asthma Day Camp
ALA of Arizona
102 West McDowell Road
Phoenix, AZ 85003
602-258-7505

Camp Not-A-Wheeze
Arizona Asthma Foundation
5410 West Thunderbird Road
Glendale, AZ 85306

ARKANSAS
Asthma Camp
ALA of Arkansas
P.O. Box 3857
Little Rock, AR 72203
501-224-5864

Camp Aldersgate
MedCamps, Inc.
ALA of Arkansas
2000 Aldersgate Road
Little Rock, AR 72205
501-225-1444

CALIFORNIA
Asthma Camp
ALA of Los Angeles County
P.O. Box 36926
Los Angeles, CA 90036-0926
213-935-5864

Breathe Easy Day Camp
ALA of Alameda County
295-27th Street
Oakland, CA 94612
415-893-5474

Camp Concoso
ALA of Contra Costa/Solano
105 Astrid Drive
Pleasant Hill, CA 94523-4399
415-935-0472

Camp Discovery
ALA of Central California
P.O. Box 11187
Fresno, CA 93772-1187
209-266-5864

Camp Sierra
ALA of Central California
P.O. Box 11187
Fresno, CA 93772-1187
209-266-5864

* Modified from M. Holbreith and S. C. Weisberg, Asthma camps: Whom to send, what to look for. *J. Respir. Dis.* 11(4):377, 1990.

Camp Superstuff
ALA of Redwood Empire
P.O. Box 1482
Santa Rosa, CA 95402-1482
707-527-5864

Camp Superstuff
ALA of San Francisco
562 Mission Street, #203
San Francisco, CA 94105
415-543-4410

Camp Superstuff
ALA of Santa Clara-San Benito Counties
1469 Park Avenue
San Jose, CA 95126
408-996-LUNG

Camp Superstuff
ALA of Superior California
2732 Cohasset Road, #A
Chico, CA 95926-0977
916-345-5864

Camp Wheez
ALA of Santa Barbara County
1510 San Andres Street
Santa Barbara, CA 93101-4104
805-963-1426

Club Wheez
ALA of San Mateo County
2250 Palm Avenue
San Mateo, CA 94403-1860
415-349-1111 or 349-1600

Running Springs
AAFA
5410 Wilshire Boulevard, Suite 1005
Los Angeles, CA 90036
213-937-7859

Scamp Camp
ALA of the Inland Counties
371 West 14th Street
San Bernardino, CA 92405
714-884-5864

Scamp Camp
ALA of Orange County
1717 North Broadway
Santa Ana, CA 92706-2675
714-835-5864

Scamp Camp
ALA of San Diego/Imperial Counties
P.O. Box 3879
San Diego, CA 92103
619-297-3901

Scamp Camp
ALA of Ventura County
P.O. Box 1627
Ventura, CA 93002
805-643-2189

Summer Asthma Camp
ALA of Long Beach
1002 Pacific Avenue
Long Beach, CA 90813-3098
213-436-9873

COLORADO
Champ Camp
ALA of Colorado
1600 Race Street
Denver, CO 60206-1198
303-388-4327

CONNECTICUT
Camp Treasure Chest
ALA of Connecticut
45 Ash Street
East Hartford, CT 06108
203-289-5401

DISTRICT OF COLUMBIA
Camp Happy Lungs
ALA of the District of Columbia
475 H Street, N.W.
Washington, D.C. 20001
202-682-5864

FLORIDA
Camp Superstuff
ALA of Dade-Monroe, Inc.
830 Brickell Plaza
Miami, FL 33131-3996
305-377-1771

Sunshine Station
ALA of Florida
P.O. Box 8127
Jacksonville, FL 32239-8127
904-743-2933

GEORGIA
Camp Breathe Easy
ALA of Atlanta
723 Piedmont Avenue, N.E.
Atlanta, GA 30365-0701
404-872-9653

Camp Superstuff
ALA of Georgia
2452 Spring Road
Smyrna, GA 30080
404-434-5864

Superstuff Asthma Day Camp
ALA of Georgia, West Central Branch
2546 Wynnton Road
Columbus, GA 31906
404-323-4700

HAWAII
Hawaii Asthma Camp/Camp Kokokahi
Aloha United Way
99128 Aiea Heights Drive, #107
Aiea, HI 96701

ILLINOIS
Camp Action
Chicago Lung Association
1440 West Washington Boulevard
Chicago, IL 60607-1878
312-243-2000

Camp Ravenwood
AAFA, Greater Chicago Chapter
111 N. Wabash, Suite 909
Chicago, IL 60602
312-346-0745

Camp Superkids
ALA of Illinois
P.O. Box 19239
Springfield, IL 62794-9239
217-528-3441

INDIANA
Camp Superkids
ALA of Indiana
9410 Priority Way West Drive
Indianapolis, IN 46240
317-573-3900

IOWA
Camp Superkids
ALA of Iowa
1025 Ashworth Road, #410
West Des Moines, IA 50265
515-224-0800

KANSAS
Camp Superbreathers
ALA of Kansas
1107 Parklane Office Park, #224
Wichita, KS 67218
316-687-3888

KENTUCKY
Camp Superkids
ALA of Kentucky
P.O. Box 969
Louisville, KY 40201
502-363-2652

MAINE
Camp Opportunity
ALA of Maine
128 Sewall Street
Augusta, ME 04330
207-622-6394

MARYLAND
Camp Superkids
ALA of Maryland
1840 York Road, #K-M
Timonium, MD 21093-2120
301-560-2120

MASSACHUSETTS
Camp Chest Nut
ALA of Massachusetts
803 Summer Street
1st Floor
South Boston, MA 02127-1609
617-269-9720

MICHIGAN
Camp Michi-Mac
ALA of Michigan
403 Seymour Avenue
Lansing, MI 48933-1179
517-484-4541

Camp Sun Deer
ALA of Southeast Michigan
18860 West Ten Mile Road
Southfield, MI 48075
313-559-5100

MINNESOTA
Camp Superkids
ALA of Hennepin County
1829 Portland Avenue
Minneapolis, MN 55404
612-871-7332

Camp Superkids
ALA of Minnesota
480 Concordia Avenue
St. Paul, MN 55103
612--224-4901

MISSOURI
Camp Lakewood
ALA of Missouri
YMCA of the Ozark
1118 Hampton Avenue
St. Louis, MO 63139
314-645-5505

Camp Shawnee
ALA of Western Missouri
Kansas City, MO 64108
816-234-3097

MONTANA
Camp Huff 'n Puff
ALA of Montana
825 Helena Avenue
Christmas Seal Building
Helena, MT 59601
406-442-6556

NEBRASKA
Camp Superkids
ALA of Nebraska
8901 Indian Hills Drive, #107
Omaha, NE 68114
402-393-2222

NEVADA
Camp Superkids
ALA of Nevada, Northern Region
P.O. Box 7056
Reno, NV 89510-7056
702-825-5864

Camp Superkids
ALA of Nevada, Southern Region
P.O. Box 44137
Las Vegas, NV 89116
702-454-2500

NEW HAMPSHIRE
Camp Superkids
ALA of New Hampshire
P.O. Box 1014
Manchester, NH 03105
603-669-2411

NEW JERSEY
Camp Superkids
ALA of Central New Jersey
206 Westfield Avenue
Clark, NJ 07066
201-388-4556

Frost Valley YMCA
ALA of New Jersey
1600 Route 22 East
Union, NJ 07083
201-687-9340

NEW MEXICO
Stephen Lopez Memorial Camp for Asthmatic
   Children
ALA of New Mexico
216 Truman N.E.
Albuquerque, NM 87108
305-265-0732

NEW YORK
Camp Superkids
ALA of Mid-New York
23 South Street
Utica, NY 13501
315-735-9225

Camp Superkids
ALA of Queens
112-25 Queens Boulevard
Forest Hills, NY 11375
718-263-5656

Superkids at Chingachgook
ALA of New York State
8 Mountain View Avenue
Albany, NY 12205
518-459-4197

Wagon Road Camp
Children's Aid Society
Box 47
Chappaqua, NY 10514
914-238-4761

NORTH CAROLINA
Camp Challenge
ALA of North Carolina
P.O. Box 6176
Raleigh, NC 27628
919-782-2888

NORTH DAKOTA
Dakota Super Kids Camp
ALA of North Dakota
P.O. Box 5004
Bismarck, ND 38502
701-223-5613

OHIO
Camp Superkids
ALA of Ohio, South Shore Branch
226 Street-Route 61 East
Norwalk, OH 44857
419-663-LUNG

Camp Superkids/Camp Libbey
ALA of Northwestern Ohio
425 Jefferson Avenue, #902
Toledo, OH 43604-1053
419-255-2378

Camp Superkids/Camp Mowana
ALA of Ohio
2276 Fleming Falls Road
Mansfield, OH 44903
614-279-1700

Camp Superkids XI
ALA of Southwestern Ohio
2330 Victory Parkway
Room 400
Cincinnati, OH 45206
513-751-3650

OKLAHOMA
Camp Breathe Easy
ALA of Oklahoma
P.O. Box 53303
Oklahoma City, OK 73152-3303
405-524-8471

Camp Green Country
ALA of Green Country, Oklahoma
1422 East 71, Suite N
Tulsa, OK 74136
918-747-3441

OREGON
Camp Christmas Seal
ALA of Oregon
P.O. Box 115
Portland, OR 97207
503-224-5145

PENNSYLVANIA
Camp Breathe Easy
ALA of Central Pennsylvania
P.O. Box 1632
Harrisburg, PA 17105-1632
717-234-5991

Camp Huff 'n Puff
ALA of Western Pennsylvania
2851 Bedford Avenue
Pittsburgh, PA 15219
412-621-0400 or 800-553-1990

SOUTH CAROLINA
Camp Puff 'n Stuff
ALA of South Carolina, Coastal Branch
4970A Dorchester Road
Charleston, SC 29418
803-552-2851 or 552-2852

SOUTH DAKOTA
Camp Tepeetonka
South Dakota Lung Association
YMCA
230 South Minnesota
Sioux Falls, SD 57102
605-336-3190

Leif Ericson Day Camp
South Dakota Lung Association
McKennan Hospital
300-21st Street
Sioux Falls, SD 57105
605-339-7677

TEXAS
Jeff A. Green Asthma Camp
ALA of Dallas Area
7616 LBJ Freeway, Suite 100
Dallas, TX 75251
214-239-5864

UTAH
Camp Superkids
ALA of Utah
1930 South 1100 East Street
Salt Lake City, UT 84106
801-484-4456

VIRGINIA
Camp Holiday Trails
P.O. Box 5806
Charlottesville, VA 22905-0806
804-977-3781

Camp Superstuff
ALA of Virginia, Peninsula Region
732 Thimble Shoals Boulevard
Building E, Suite 305B
Newport News, VA 23606
804-886-5864

Camp Superstuff
ALA of Virginia, Southeastern Region
5349 East Princess Anne Road
Norfolk, VA 23502
804-855-3059

WASHINGTON
Camp Breathe Easy
ALA of Washington, Central Region
901 Summitview, #241
Yakima, WA 98902
509-248-4384

Inland Empire Children's Asthma Camp
ALA of Washington, Eastern Region
North 1322 Ash
Spokane, WA 99201
509-325-6516

Summer Asthma Camp
ALA of Washington
King County/NW Field Office
2625 Third Avenue
Seattle, WA 98121
206-441-5100

WISCONSIN
Camp WIKIDAS
ALA of Wisconsin
1330 North 113th Street, #190
Milwaukee, WI 53226-3212
414-258-9100

F. Theophylline Toxicity: A Management Algorithm

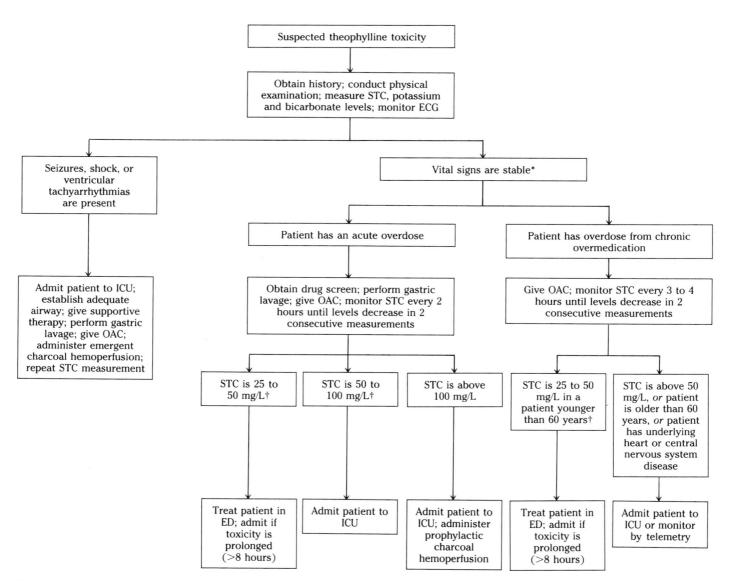

Suspected theophylline toxicity

→

Obtain history; conduct physical examination; measure STC, potassium and bicarbonate levels; monitor ECG

Seizures, shock, or ventricular tachyarrhythmias are present

Admit patient to ICU; establish adequate airway; give supportive therapy; perform gastric lavage; give OAC; administer emergent charcoal hemoperfusion; repeat STC measurement

Vital signs are stable*

Patient has an acute overdose

Obtain drug screen; perform gastric lavage; give OAC; monitor STC every 2 hours until levels decrease in 2 consecutive measurements

STC is 25 to 50 mg/L†

Treat patient in ED; admit if toxicity is prolonged (>8 hours)

STC is 50 to 100 mg/L†

Admit patient to ICU

STC is above 100 mg/L

Admit patient to ICU; administer prophylactic charcoal hemoperfusion

Patient has overdose from chronic overmedication

Give OAC; monitor STC every 3 to 4 hours until levels decrease in 2 consecutive measurements

STC is 25 to 50 mg/L in a patient younger than 60 years†

Treat patient in ED; admit if toxicity is prolonged (>8 hours)

STC is above 50 mg/L, *or patient is older than 60 years, or patient has underlying heart or central nervous system disease*

Admit patient to ICU or monitor by telemetry

STC, serum theophylline concentration; ECG, electrocardiogram; ICU, intensive care unit; OAC, oral activated charcoal; ED, emergency department.
* If seizures, shock, or ventricular tachyarrhythmias develop, transfer patient to the ICU and attempt to perform emergent charcoal hemoperfusion.
† If STC increases to a higher range, follow the algorithm for that range.
Source: Sessler, C. N., and Brady, W. Theophylline toxicity. *J. Crit. Illness* 6:1057, 1991. Reprinted with permission.

G. Guidelines for Intravenous Terbutaline Use in Status Asthmaticus

Donald L. Uden

Terbutaline pharmacokinetics (*Eur. J. Respir. Dis.* 65:195, 1984)
- Oral absorption—25–80%
- Bioavailability—10–15%
- Vd reference compartment—0.5 L/kg
- Vd_{ss}—1.57 ± 0.19 L/kg
- Clearance—3.76 ± 0.86 ml/kg/m
- Half-life
  - Alpha—8–12 minutes
  - Beta—3–4 hours
  - Gamma—17–20 hours

RATIONALE FOR DOSING

Terbutaline has pharmacokinetics similar to aminophylline with respect to a long half-life. Therefore, to achieve therapeutic concentrations rapidly, loading doses must be administered.

TERBUTALINE DOSING GUIDELINES

Loading Guidelines

1. Initiate a continuous infusion at 1 μg/kg/min until the desired outcome is achieved (blood gases, respiratory rate, pulmonary function tests) or unacceptable toxicity occurs (heart rate, serum potassium, serum glucose). (Consult clinical pharmacist on call to determine the most efficient method to deliver the infusion, e.g., syringe pump versus buretrol versus piggyback bag.)
   NOTE: If more than 100 μg/kg (or 100 minutes of infusion) is required and positive therapeutic effects are not obtained, consider an appropriate maintenance infusion and change therapy.

Maintenance Guidelines

2. *If desired therapeutic effect is achieved*, calculate the total dose administered in μg/kg and divide by 200 to determine maintenance infusion rate in μg/kg/min (see nomogram). (For example, 1 μg/kg/min for 60 minutes = total dose of 60 μg/kg divided by 200 = 0.3 μg/kg/min maintenance infusion rate.)
3. *If unacceptable toxicity occurs*, discontinue infusion until toxicity subsides and place patient on a continuous infusion that is 0.05 μg/kg/min less than what would be calculated by the prior equation. (For example, if toxicity occurs at a total load of 70 μg/kg after 70 minutes of 1 μg/kg/min, the maintenance dose would be 70 divided by 200 = 0.35 μg/kg/min; 0.35 μg/kg/min minus 0.05 μg/kg/min = 0.3 μg/kg/min.)

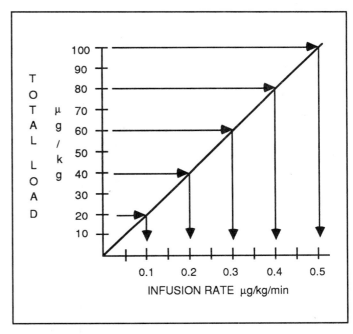

Monitoring Parameters	Desired Therapeutic Outcome
Arterial blood gases	Increased PO_2 and pH, decreased PCO_2
Oxygen saturation	Increased $SO_2 > 90$
Respiratory rate	Decreased respiratory rate
Heart rate	Decreased heart rate secondary to decreased work of respiration

Unacceptable Toxicity	Treatment
Glucose increased	Monitor
Potassium decreased	Add potassium to maintenance fluids
Blood pressure (widening of pulse pressure)	Monitor

H. Guidelines for Methotrexate Use in Severe Bronchial Asthma

Michael F. Mullarkey

Our initial study (see Chap. 68) dealt with the most conventional form of the administration of low-dose methotrexate—that form in which it is administered orally once a week in three divided doses. Since the completion of the study, we are impressed that methotrexate administered parenterally is safer, less expensive, and more effective. We are now treating all patients initially with a single weekly intramuscular injection. Pharmacokinetic studies of oral methotrexate have shown a variation in bioavailability from 25 to 85 percent. The intramuscular administration of this drug ensures a bioavailability that approaches 1.00. Patients receive 7.5 mg IM as their initial dose and then 15 mg IM once a week on the second and all subsequent weekly doses. If a therapeutic response has not been noted after 12 doses, methotrexate should be increased to 25 mg a week. It is known from the oncology literature that a 24-hour blood level of methotrexate in excess of 1×10^{-7} M carries some risk for gastrointestinal and hematologic toxicity. Tablet methotrexate may be used to maintain steroid independence once corticosteroid withdrawal has been accomplished.

The following precautions are suggested in administering methotrexate because of its well-defined toxicities:

1. Cirrhosis with the use of low-dose, pulse methotrexate is essentially rare without the accompanying use of alcohol. Therefore, all patients should abstain from alcohol while using methotrexate.
2. Methotrexate is a weak organic acid and undergoes predominant renal excretion. Agents that prolong its half-life have been responsible for most episodes of hematopoietic suppression with low-dose methotrexate. Avoid the use of diuretics, particularly when used in combination with a nonsteroidal, which decrease glomerular filtration and compete for active secretion at the level of the renal tubule as weak organic acids with methotrexate.
3. Avoid the use of sulfa-containing antibiotics while methotrexate is administered, as there have been several cases of megaloblastic anemia attributed to the concomitant inhibition of folate metabolism by these two agents.
4. Obtain a chest x-ray and DLCO as baseline studies to assess alveolar integrity. Clearly the physician must discontinue the drug in any patient who develops a pneumonia or symptoms suggesting pneumonitis. Do not administer the drug to individuals who lack the pulmonary reserve to sustain an episode of interstitial pneumonitis. Our cutoff point has been to withhold methotrexate in individuals whose DLCOs fall below 60 percent. Routine spirometry assists in determining the effectiveness of the program. Patients responding to low-dose methotrexate should stabilize or improve spirometry as corticosteroids are withdrawn.
5. Obtain a white blood cell count, differential, SGOT, and creatinine the week prior to the first dose, then before the first dose of 15 mg, and then every 3 to 4 weeks thereafter.
6. Methotrexate is teratogenic. All fertile women must understand this potential and practice appropriate birth control. Pregnancy tests are obtained when initiating the drug in fertile women.
7. Patients receiving low-dose methotrexate are at risk for disseminated varicella. Patients at risk should be treated with varicella zoster immune globulin (VZIG) within 96 hours of exposure. Patients with characteristic varicella skin lesions should be treated with oral or intravenous acyclovir and closely followed. Severe abdominal or back pain is a herald of visceral involvement, and these patients should be hospitalized, treated with intravenous acyclovir, and monitored in an intensive care facility.

Stabilization of asthma generally occurs sometime between 6 and 12 weeks, and at that point prednisone is tapered by 5 mg/wk. Patients who have shown no response to methotrexate after 12 weeks of therapy have their dose of methotrexate increased to 25 mg/wk. Twenty-four-hour blood levels are obtained, and precautions as outlined above are followed. After each increase of methotrexate, 24-hour blood levels of methotrexate are measured, and all precautions as outlined above are followed.

I. Technique for Cytologic and Bacteriologic Microscopic Examination of Sputum

Mauricio J. Dulfano

MATERIALS

Fixative—Mix the following in a tightly sealed bottle and store as a stock solution. For daily use, transfer 10 ml to a working bottle.

95% ethyl alcohol—79 ml

Polyethylene glycol, mol wt 1540 (Carbowax)—3 ml

Distilled water—18 ml

3-, 5-, and 10-ml syringes; 18- and 20-gauge needles

Five 15-ml test tubes

Hemocytometer

Isotonic saline solution

Microscope

Crystal violet and Gram's stains

PROCEDURE

1. Spread the sputum sample in a small Petri dish. Divide a solid-looking piece into two aliquots, and place each of them on a slide. Add to the first aliquot an equal amount of buffered crystal violet, and mix thoroughly. Scan to ascertain that the sputum sample originates in the lower respiratory tract. If so, smear the second aliquot for Gram's stain.
2. With a syringe and an 18-gauge needle, aspirate the rest of the sample. If the sample is large, mix well and aspirate 5 ml. Expel air bubbles, and place contents into a test tube and add fixative in an amount equal to twice the volume of the sputum sample. Using a syringe and a 20-gauge needle, mix them in the tube until most of the mucus is broken and the material looks homogeneous. Let stand for 30 minutes in preparation for the differential count. While waiting for the cells to be fixed, aspirate 0.5 ml of the material and mix it in another test tube with 4.5 ml of saline solution for total cell count determination.
3. Pipette several drops of the sputum-fixative solution onto two clean slides; spread and let air-dry completely. Next, immerse only one of the slides in 95% alcohol for 15 minutes, and then rinse again in clean 95% alcohol. The slide is now ready for Papanicolaou staining. The remaining slide, after it has air-dried, preserves its coat of Carbowax and can be stored for any future cytologic or bacteriologic staining.

The homogenization procedure yields a well-distributed and monolayer cell population with total preservation of morphologic characteristics. The differential count is done under oil immersion, counting at least 200 cells. For total cell count, fill the hemocytometer chamber with the saline-sputum mixture (usually a few drops are needed). Count the cells in four of the white cell-counting squares. The total dilution in the chamber mixture is 30 times. (First dilution = 3 times; second dilution, 0.5 ml to 4.5 ml = 10 times; total dilution = $3 \times 10 = 30$ times.) With the above technique, the volume of the four squares in which the cells have been counted = 4×0.1 mm^3 = 0.4 mm^3.

$$\frac{\text{number of cells}}{1 \text{ mm}^3} = \frac{\text{number of cells counted} \times \text{dilution}}{\text{volume of squares}}$$

$$= \frac{\text{number of cells counted in 4 squares} \times 30}{0.4 \text{ mm}^3}$$

Gram's staining is done in the classic way using the fresh sample (see procedure 1); however, a good alternative is to stain the material after it has been fixed and homogenized as described in procedure 3.

The Gram's stain procedure is as follows:

1. Sample (as in procedure 1).
2. Flood smear with crystal violet solution.
3. Let slide stand for 1 minute.
4. Wash with tap water, drain excess water.
5. Flood smear with iodine solution.
6. Let slide stand for 1 minute.
7. Wash with tap water, decolorize with 95% ethyl alcohol or acetone or acetone-alcohol (100 ml of 95% ethyl alcohol plus 100 ml of acetone).
8. Counterstain with safranine, 10 seconds.
9. Wash briefly with tap water.
10. Blot dry. Gram-positive organisms stain blue; gram-negative organisms stain red.

(For various acid-fast staining techniques, see E. H. Lennette, W. J. Hausler, and H. J. Shadomy, *Manual of a Clinical Microbiology* [4th ed.]. Washington, D.C.: American Society of Microbiology, 1985. Pp. 225, 1102.)

J. Medications Available for the Treatment of Asthma, by Class and Generic Name[a]

Steven Kozel
Mauricio J. Dulfano

			ANTICHOLINERGICS		
OTC/RX	Generic name	Proprietary name	Available dosage forms	Suggested dosage—adult	Suggested dosage—pediatric
RX	Atropine sulfate	Dey-Dose atropine sulfate	Solution for inhalation: 0.2% (1 mg/0.5 ml), 0.5% (2.5 mg/0.5 ml)	Nebulizer: 0.025 mg/kg diluted/w 3–5 ml NS q 6–8 hr; max dose = 2.5 mg	Nebulizer: 0.025–0.05 mg/kg diluted in saline q 4–6 hr prn[b]
RX	Ipratropium bromide	Atrovent	MDI: 18 μg/puff	1–2 puffs tid to qid no more often than q 4 hr; max dose = 12 puffs/24 hr; NOTE: initially 4 inh may be required for maximum benefit	Not established
			Solution for inhalation (N/A in US): 0.025% (250 μg/ml)	Nebulizer: 250–500 μg (1–2 ml) of 0.025% diluted with PF NS over 10–15 min q 4–6 hr	< 5 yr: not established; 5–12 yr: 125–250 μg (0.5–1.0 ml) of 0.025% diluted as for adults q 4–6 hr

			ADRENERGIC BRONCHODILATORS		
OTC/RX	Generic name	Proprietary name	Available dosage forms	Suggested dosage—adult	Suggested dosage—pediatric
RX	Albuterol sulfate	Proventil	Tablets: 2, 4 mg	2–4 mg q 6–8 hr; max dose = 32 mg/d	2–6 yr: 100–200 μg/kg/dose q 8 hr, max dose = 4 mg q 8 hr; 6–12 yr: 2 mg q 6–8 hr, max dose = 24 mg/d; > 12 yr: usual adult dose[b]
			Tablets, extended release: 4 mg (Proventil Repetabs)	4–8 mg q 12 hr; max dose = 32 mg/d	< 12 yr: dose not established; > 12 yr: usual adult dose
			Syrup: 2 mg/5 ml	2–4 mg q 6–8 hr; max dose = 32 mg/d	< 2 yr: dose not established; 2–6 yr: 100 μg/kg q 8 hr, max dose = 2 mg q 8 hr; 6–14 yr: 2 mg q 6–8 hr; > 14 yr: usual adult dose
			MDI: 90 μg/puff (as base)	Acute: 2 puffs 1–5 min apart q 4–6 hr; max dose: 16–20 puff/d; prophylaxis: 2 puffs 15 min before exercise	< 12 yr: 1–2 puffs q 6 hr using spacer[b]; > 12 yr: usual adult dose
			Solution for inhalation: 0.083%; 0.5%	2.5 mg (0.083%) (3 ml)/ (0.5%) (0.5 ml) q 6–8 hr via nebulizer/IPPB	Inhalation (0.5%): 0.01–0.05 ml/kg q 4–6 hr; min dose = 0.1 ml, max dose = 1 ml (dilute in 1–2 ml NS)[b]
RX	Albuterol sulfate	Ventolin	Tablets: 2–4 mg	2–4 mg q 6–8 hr; max dose = 32 mg/d	2–6 yr: 100–200 μg/kg/dose q 8 hr, max dose = 4 mg q 8 hr; 6–12 yr: 2 mg q 6–8 hr, max dose = 24 mg/d; > 12 yr: usual adult dose
			Syrup: 2 mg/5 ml	2–4 mg q 6–8 hr; max dose = 32 mg or 4–8 mg q 12 hr	< 2 yr: not established; 2–6 yr: 100 μg/kg q 8 hr, max dose = 4 mg q 8 hr; 6–14 yr: 2 mg q 6–8 hr, max dose = 24 mg/d; > 14 yr: usual adult dose
			MDI: 90 μg/puff (as base)	2–3 puffs 1–5 min apart q 4–6 hr; max dose = 16–30 puffs/d	< 12 yr: not established; > 12 yr: usual adult dose
			Capsules for inhalation: 200 μg/cap (Rotacap)	200–400 μg via "Rotohaler" q 6–8 hr; max dose = 2.4 mg/d	< 12 yr: 1–2 puffs q 6 hr using spacer; > 12 yr: usual adult dose[b]

Medications (continued).

			ADRENERGIC BRONCHODILATORS *(continued)*		
OTC/RX	*Generic name*	*Proprietary name*	*Available dosage forms*	*Suggested dosage—adult*	*Suggested dosage—pediatric*
			Solution for inhalation: 0.5% (5 mg/ml)	2.5 mg (0.5 ml) q 6–8 hr via nebulizer/IPPB	Inhalation (0.5%): 0.01–0.05 ml/kg q 4–6 hr, min dose = 0.1 ml, max dose = 1 ml (dilute in 1–2 ml NS)[b]
RX	Albuterol sulfate (N/A in US)	Ventolin	Injection: 50 μg/ml; 500 μg/ml	IM: 500 μg or 8 μg/kg q 4 hr, max dose = 2 mg/d; IV: 250 μg or 4 μg/kg over 2–5 min, repeat after 15 min if necessary, up to 1 mg/d; IV infusion: 5–20 μg/min	Not established
RX	Bitolterol mesylate	Tornalate	MDI: 370 μg/puff	Acute: 2 puffs 1–3 min apart, MR × 1 prn, then 2 puffs q 4 hr or 3 puffs q 6 hr; prophylaxis: 2 puffs q 8 hr, max dose = 12 puffs/d	< 12 yr: not established; > 12 yr: usual adult dose
RX/OTC	Ephedrine sulfate		Capsules: 25, 50 mg (25-mg capsules OTC)	25–50 mg q 6 hr	3 mg/kg/d in 4–6 divided doses
			Injection: 25 mg/ml, 50 mg/ml	12.5–25 mg SC, IM, slow IV, max dose = 150 mg/24 hr	3 mg/kg/d SC, IV in 4–6 divided doses
OTC	Epinephrine	Bronkaid Mist	MDI: 250 μg/puff	1–2 puffs, 1–2 min apart q 3 hr prn	< 4 yr: individualize; > 4 yr: usual adult dose
OTC	Epinephrine	Primatene Mist	MDI: 200 μg/puff	1–2 puffs 1–2 min apart q 3 hr prn	< 4 yr: individualize; > 4 yr: usual adult dose
OTC	Epinephrine bitartrate	AsthmaHaler Mist	MDI: 300 μg bitartrate equiv to 160 μg base/puff	1–2 puffs, 1 min apart q 3 hr prn	< 4 yr: individualize; > 4 yr: usual adult dose
OTC	Epinephrine bitartrate	Bronitin Mist	MDI: 300 μg bitartrate equiv to 160 μg base/puff	1–2 puffs, 1 min apart q 3 hr prn	< 4 yr: individualize; > 4 yr: usual adult dose
OTC	Epinephrine bitartrate	Medihaler-Epi	MDI: 300 μg as bitartrate equiv to 160 μg base/puff	1–2 puffs 1 min apart q 3 hr prn	< 4 yr: individualize; > 4 yr: usual adult dose
OTC	Epinephrine bitartrate	Primatene Mist suspension	MDI: 300 μg bitartrate equiv to 160 μg base/puff	1–2 puffs 1 min apart q 3 hr prn	< 4 yr: individualize; > 4 yr: usual adult dose
RX/OTC	Epinephrine hydrochloride	Adrenalin chloride	Solution for inhalation 1:100 (1%) (OTC)	8–15 drops in nebulizer, 1–3 inh 1–2 min apart 4–6×/d	< 6 yr: individualize; > 6 yr: usual adult dosage
			Injection 1:1,000 (1 mg/ml) (RX)	0.2–0.5 mg SC q 20 min–4 hr prn	10 μg (0.01 mg)/kg SC to a maximum of 500 μg (0.5 mg) q 15 min × 2 doses, then every 4 hr prn
OTC	Epinephrine hydrochloride, racemic	Vaponefrin	Solution for inhalation: 2% racepinephrine equiv to 1% base	Hand nebulizer: 2–3 inh, repeated in 5 min prn, then q 4–6 hr; nebulization via respirator: 5 ml of 0.1% final concentration for 15 min q 3–4 hr	< 4 yr: individualize; > 4 yr: usual adult dose
OTC	Epinephrine hydrochloride, racemic	AsthmaNefrin	Solution for inhalation: 2.25% racepinephrine HCl equiv to 1.125% base	Hand nebulizer: 2–3 inh, repeated in 5 min prn, then q 4–6 hr; nebulization via respirator: 5 ml of 0.1% final concentration for 15 min q 3–4 hr	< 4 yr: individualize; > 4 yr: usual adult dose
OTC	Epinephrine hydrochloride, racemic	microNefrin	Solution for inhalation: 2.25% racepinephrine equiv to 1.125% base	Hand nebulizer: 2–3 inh, repeated in 5 min prn, then q 4–6 hr; nebulization via respirator: 5 ml of 0.1% final concentration for 15 min q 3–4 hr	< 4 yr: individualize; > 4 yr: usual adult dose

(continued)

Medications (continued).

ADRENERGIC BRONCHODILATORS (continued)

OTC/RX	Generic name	Proprietary name	Available dosage forms	Suggested dosage—adult	Suggested dosage—pediatric
OTC	Epinephrine hydrochloride, racemic	Nephron	Solution for inhalation: 2.25% racepinephrine HCl equiv to 1.25% base	Hand nebulizer: 2–3 inh, repeated in 5 min prn, then q 4–6 hr; nebulization via respirator: 5 ml of 0.1% final concentration for 15 min q 3–4 hr	< 4 yr: individualize; > 4 yr: usual adult dose
RX	Epinephrine hydrochloride, racemic	Racepinephrine	Solution for inhalation: 2.25% racepinephrine HCl equiv to 1.25% base	Hand nebulizer: 2–3 inh, repeated in 5 min prn, then q 4–6 hr; nebulization via respirator: 5 ml of 0.1% final concentration for 15 min q 3–4 hr	< 4 yr: individualize; > 4 yr: usual adult dose
OTC	Epinephrine hydrochloride, racemic	S-2	Solution for inhalation: 2.25% racepinephrine HCl equiv to 1.25% base	Hand nebulizer: 2–3 inh, repeated in 5 min prn, then q 4–6 hr; nebulization via respirator: 5 ml of 0.1% final concentration for 15 min q 3–4 hr	< 4 yr: individualize; > 4 yr: usual adult dose
RX	Epinephrine, long-acting	Sus-Phrine	Injection: 1:200 (5 mg/ml) suspension	0.1 ml (0.5 mg) SC initially, then 0.1 ml (0.5 mg) to 0.3 ml (1.5 mg) q 6 hr	0.005 ml (25 µg)/kg q 6 hr prn; if < 30 kg: do not exceed max dose of 0.15 ml (750 µg)
RX	Ethylnorepinephrine	Bronkephrine	Injection: 2 mg/ml	1–2 mg SC, IM; note: 0.6–1.0 mg may suffice	0.2–1.0 mg SC, IM; varies according to age and wt
	Fenoterol hydrobromide (investigational)	Berotec (Canada); N/A in US	Tablets: 2.5 mg	2.5 mg bid, max dose = 5 mg tid; do not administer more often than q 6 hr	< 12 yr: not established; > 12 yr: usual adult dose
			MDI: 200 µg/puff	1–2 puffs qid; no more often than q 4 hr	< 12 yr: not established; > 12 yr: usual adult dose
			Solution for inhalation: 1 mg/ml	0.5–1 mg via nebulization or IPPB over 10–15 min q 6 hr prn; dilute with 5 ml NS for delivery	< 12 yr: not established; > 12 yr: usual adult dose
RX	Isoetharine hydrochloride	Arm-a-Med Isoetharine HCl	Solution for inhalation: 0.062%, 0.125%, 0.167%, 0.2%, 0.25%	IPPB: 2.5–5 mg q 4 hr; O₂ aerosol: 5 mg over 15–30 min q 4 hr	Not established
RX	Isoetharine hydrochloride	Beta-2	Solution for inhalation: 1%	IPPB: 2.5–10 mg diluted 1:3 with NS q 4 hr; hand nebulizer: 3–7 inh undiluted q 4 hr; O₂ aerosol: 2.5–5 mg diluted 1:3 with NS over 15–30 min q 4 hr	Not established
RX	Isoetharine hydrochloride	Bronkosol	Solution for inhalation: 1%	IPPB: 2.5–10 mg diluted 1:3 in NS q 4 hr; hand nebulizer: 5 mg undiluted delivered in 3–7 inh; O₂ aerosol: 2.5–5 mg diluted 1:3 in NS q 4 hr	Not established
RX	Isoetharine mesylate	Bronkometer	MDI: 340 µg/puff	1 puff repeated in 1–2 min prn, q 4 hr prn	Not established
RX	Isoproterenol hydrochloride/phenylephrine bitartrate	Duo-Medihaler	MDI: 160 µg/puff isoproterenol; 240 µg/puff phenylephrine	Acute: 1–2 puffs; maintenance: 1–2 puffs 4–6 hr; max dose = 2 puffs once or ≯ 6 puffs/hr within 24 hr	Not established
RX	Isoproterenol hydrochloride	Dispos-a-Med Isoproterenol HCl	Solution for inhalation: 0.25% (1:400), 0.5% (1:200)	Bronchodilator: nebulized (0.25%), 6–12 inh repeat q 15 min × 3; max dose = 8 tx/24 hr; acute: 5–15 inh (0.5%) repeat once prn in 5–10 min, then up to 5×/d	Bronchodilator: usual adult dose; acute: 5–15 inh (0.5%) via nebulizer, repeat once prn in 5–10 min; max dose = 5×/d
RX	Isoproterenol hydrochloride	Isuprel, Isuprel Glossets	SL tablets: 10 mg, 15 mg (Glossets)	10–15 mg SL q 6–8 hr; max dose = 60 mg/d	5–10 mg q 8 hr; max dose = 30 mg/d

Medications (continued).

ADRENERGIC BRONCHODILATORS (continued)

OTC/RX	Generic name	Proprietary name	Available dosage forms	Suggested dosage—adult	Suggested dosage—pediatric
			MDI: 131 μg/puff (Isuprel Mistometer)	Acute asthma: 1 puff, may repeat in 1–5 min prn up to q 4–6 hr	Usual adult dose
			Solution for inhalation: 0.5% (1:200), 1.0% (1:100)	Acute bronchial asthma: 5–15 inh (0.5%) or 3–7 inh (1.0%), repeat prn in 5–10 min, then up to 5×/d	Acute bronchial asthma: 5–15 inh (0.5%), repeat prn in 5–10 min, then up to 5×/d
			Injection: 0.2 mg/ml (1:5,000)	Not recommended in USP DI except for bronchospasm during anesthesia (10–20 μg [0.01–0.02 mg]), repeat as needed	(see text)
RX	Isoproterenol sulfate	Medihaler-Iso	MDI: 0.2% (80 μg/puff)	Bronchodilator: 1 puff repeated in 2–5 min prn, up to q 4–6 hr	Usual adult dose
RX	Metaproterenol sulfate	Alupent	Tablets: 10, 20 mg	10 mg q 6–8 hr up to 20 mg q 6–8 hr	6–9 yr or wt < 27 kg: 10 mg q 6–8 hr; > 9 yr or > 27 kg: adult dose
			Syrup: 10 mg/5 ml	10 mg q 6–8 hr up to 20 mg q 6–8 hr	Infants: 400 μg/kg/dose q 8–12 hr; < 2 yr: 400 μg/kg/dose q 6–8 hr; 2–6 yr: 1.0–2.6 mg/kg/d (divided) q 6–8 hr[b]; 6–9 yr or wt < 27 kg: 10 mg q 6–8 hr; > 9 yr or wt > 27 kg: usual adult dose
			MDI: 650 μg/puff	2–3 puffs q 3–4 hr; max dose = 12 puffs/d	< 12 yr: not established
			Solution for inh: 0.4%, 2.5 ml (equiv 0.2 ml, 5%); 0.6%, 2.5 ml (equiv 0.3 ml, 5%)	Nebulizer, hand-held: 5–15 inh q 4 hr	< 12 yr: not established; > 12 yr: usual adult dose
			Solution for inhalation: 5%	Nebulizer, hand-held: 0.2–0.3 ml (5%) diluted/w NS 2.5 ml until nebulized q 4–6 hr; IPPB: 0.2–0.3 ml (5%) diluted/w NS 2.5 ml q 4–6 hr	< 12 yr: (nebulizer) 0.01–0.02 ml/kg (5%) diluted/w 2.5 ml NS q 4–6 hr (min dose = 0.1 ml, max dose = 1.0 ml); > 12 yr: usual adult dose[b]
RX	Metaproterenol sulfate	Arm-a-Med Metaproterenol sulfate	Solution for inh: 0.4%, 2.5 ml (equiv 0.2 ml, 5%); 0.6%, 2.5 ml (equiv 0.3 ml, 5%)	Nebulizer, hand-held: 5–15 inh q 4 hr	< 12 yr: not established; > 12 yr: usual adult dose
RX	Metaproterenol sulfate	Metaprel	Tablets: 10, 20 mg	10 mg q 6–8 hr up to 20 mg q 6–8 hr	6–9 yr or wt up to 27 kg: 10 mg q 6–8 h; > 9 yr or wt ≥ 27 kg: usual adult dose
			Syrup: 10 mg/5 ml	10 mg q 6–8 hr up to 20 mg q 6–8 hr	Infants: 400 μg/kg/dose q 8–12 hr; < 2 yr: 400 μg/kg/dose q 6–8 hr; 2–6 yr: 1.0–2.6 mg/kg/d (divided) q 6–8 hr[b]; 6–9 yr or wt < 27 kg: 10 mg q 6–8 hr; > 9 yr or > 27 kg: usual adult dose
			MDI: 650 μg/puff	2–3 puffs q 3–4 hr; max dose = 12 puffs/d	< 12 yr: not established; > 12 yr: usual adult dose
			Solution for inh: 0.4%, 2.5 ml (equiv 0.2 ml, 5%); 0.6%, 2.5 ml (equiv 0.3 ml, 5%)	Nebulizer, hand-held: 5–15 inh q 4 hr	< 12 yr: not established; > 12 yr: usual adult dose
			Solution for inhalation: 5%	Nebulizer, hand-held: 0.2–0.3 ml (5%) diluted/w NS 2.5 ml until nebulized q 4–6 hr; IPPB: 0.2–0.3 ml (5%) diluted/w NS 2.5 ml q 4–6 hr	< 12 yr: (nebulizer) 0.01–0.02 ml/kg (5%) diluted/w 2.5 ml NS q 4–6 hr (min dose = 0.1 ml, max dose = 1.0 ml)[b]; > 12 yr: usual adult dose

(continued)

Medications (continued).

ADRENERGIC BRONCHODILATORS (continued)

OTC/RX	Generic name	Proprietary name	Available dosage forms	Suggested dosage—adult	Suggested dosage—pediatric
RX	Pirbuterol	Maxair	MDI: 200 μg/puff	1–2 puffs q 4–6 hr; max dose = 12 puffs/d	< 12 yr: not established; > 12 yr: usual adult dose
	Procaterol (N/A in US)	Pro-Air (Canada)	MDI: 10 μg/puff	2 puffs q 8 hr; prophylaxis exercise-induced bronchospasm: 2 puffs 15 min before exercise	< 12 yr: not established; < 12 yr: usual adult dose
RX	Terbutaline sulfate	Brethine	Tablets: 2.5 mg, 5 mg	2.5–5 mg tid q 6 hr intervals; max dose = 15 mg/24 hr	< 12 yr: not established; 12–15 yr: 2.5 mg tid q 6 hr
			MDI: 200 μg/puff	1–2 puffs, 1 min apart q 4–6 hr	< 12 yr: not established; > 12 yr: usual adult dose
			Solution for injection: 1 mg/ml	250 μg SC, repeated in 15–30 min prn; max dose = 500 μg/4 hr; nebulized: 0.01–0.03 ml/kg diluted/w 1–2 ml NS (min dose = 0.1 ml, max dose = 2.5 ml)[b]	< 12 yr: 0.005–0.01 mg/kg/dose SC q 15–20 min × 2 (max = 0.3 mg/dose)[b], nebulized—adult dose[b]; > 12 yr: SC adult dose, nebulized—adult dose[b]
RX	Terbutaline sulfate	Bricanyl	Tablets: 2.5 mg, 5 mg	2.5–5 mg tid at q 6 hr; max dose = 15 mg/24 hr	< 12 yr: not established; 12–15 yr: 2.5 mg tid q 6 hr
			MDI: 200 μg/puff	1–2 puffs, 1 min apart q 4–6 hr	< 12 yr: not established; > 12 yr: usual adult dose
			Solution for injection: 1 mg/ml	250 μg SC, repeated in 15–30 min prn; max dose = 500 μg/4 hr; nebulized: 0.01–0.03 ml/kg diluted/w 1–2 ml NS (min dose = 0.1 ml, max dose = 2.5 ml)[b]	< 12 yr: 0.005–0.01 mg/kg/dose SC q 15–20 min × 2 (max = 0.3 mg/dose)[b], nebulized—adult dose[b]; > 12 yr: SC adult dose, nebulized—adult dose[b]

CORTICOSTEROIDS

OTC/RX	Generic name	Proprietary name	Available dosage forms	Suggested dosage—adult	Suggested dosage—pediatric
RX	Beclomethasone diproprionate	Beclovent	MDI: 42 μg/puff	2 puffs tid–qid; 4 puffs bid; severe asthma 12–16 puffs/day; max dose = 20 puffs/d	< 6 yr: not established; 6–12 yr: 1–2 puffs tid–qid, or 4 puffs bid, max dose = 10 puffs/d
RX	Beclomethasone diproprionate	Beclovent Rotacaps (N/A in US)	Inhalation; (Rotacaps) 100, 200 μg	200 μg tid–qid; maintenance 400 μg/d; max dose = 1 mg/d	100 μg bid–qid; max dose = 1 mg/d
RX	Beclomethasone diproprionate	Vanceril	MDI: 42 μg/puff	2 puffs tid–qid; 4 puffs bid; severe asthma 12–16 puffs/day; max dose = 20 puffs/d	< 6 yr: not established; 6–12 yr: 1–2 puffs tid–qid, or 4 puffs bid, max dose = 10 puffs/d
	Budesonide (investigational)	Pulmicort (Canada)	MDI: 50 μg, 200 μg/puff	Initial: 400–1,600 μg in divided doses bid–qid; maintenance: 200–400 μg bid	< 6 yr: not recommended; 6–12 yr: initial—100–200 μg bid, maintenance—decrease according to response; > 12 yr: usual adult dose
RX	Dexamethasone sodium phosphate	Decadron Phosphate Respihaler	MDI: 100 μg/puff	Initial: 3 puffs tid–qid; maintenance: 2 puffs bid; max dose = 12 puffs/day	6–12 yr: 2 puffs tid–qid; max dose = 8 puffs/d
RX	Flunisolide	Aerobid	MDI: 250 μg/puff	2 puffs bid; max dose = 4 puffs bid	< 4 yr: not established; 4–12 yr: usual adult dose; NOTE: doses > 1 mg/d have not been studied in this age group
RX	Hydrocortisone sodium succinate	A-hydro-Cort	Injection: 100, 250, 500, 1,000 mg	4 mg/kg q 4–6 hr[c]	Status asthmaticus: loading dose 1–2 mg/kg q 6 hr × 24 hr, then 0.5–1.0 mg/kg q 6 hr[b]
RX	Hydrocortisone sodium succinate	Solu-Cortef	Injection: 100, 250, 500, 1,000 mg	4 mg/kg q 4–6 hr[c]	Status asthmaticus: loading dose 1–2 mg/kg q 6 hr × 24 hr, then 0.5–1.0 mg/kg q 6 hr[b]
RX	Methylprednisolone	Medrol	Tablets: 2, 4, 8, 16, 24, 32 mg	4–48 mg/d	Not established

Medications (continued).

			CORTICOSTEROIDS (*continued*)		
OTC/RX	Generic name	Proprietary name	Available dosage forms	Suggested dosage—adult	Suggested dosage—pediatric
RX	Methylprednisolone sodium succinate	A-methaPred	Injection: 40, 125, 500, 1,000 mg	1–2 mg/kg q 4–6 hr[c]	Status asthmaticus: loading dose 2 mg/kg, then 0.5–1.0 mg/kg/dose q 6 hr[b]
RX	Methylprednisolone sodium succinate	Solu-Medrol	Injection: 40, 125, 500, 1,000 mg	1–2 mg/kg q 4–6 hr[c]	Status asthmaticus: loading dose 2 mg/kg, then 0.5–1.0 mg/kg/dose q 6 hr[b]
RX	Prednisolone	Delta-Cortef	Tablets: 5 mg	10–50 mg/d	Acute asthma: 1–2 mg/kg/d in divided doses × 3–5 d[b]
RX	Prednisolone	Prelone	Syrup: 15 mg/ml	10–50 mg/d	Acute asthma: 1–2 mg/kg/d in divided doses × 3–5 d[b]
RX	Prednisone	Deltasone	Tablets: 2.5, 5, 10, 20, 50 mg	10–50 mg/d	Acute asthma: 1–2 mg/kg/d in divided doses × 3–5 d[b]
RX	Prednisone	Liquid Pred	Syrup: 5 mg/ml	10–50 mg/d	Acute asthma: 1–2 mg/kg/d in divided doses × 3–5 d[b]
RX	Prednisone	Meticorten	Tablets: 1 mg	10–50 mg/d	Acute asthma: 1–2 mg/kg/d in divided doses × 3–5 d[b]
RX	Prednisone	Orasone	Tablets: 1, 5, 10, 20, 50 mg	10–50 mg/d	Acute asthma: 1–2 mg/kg/d in divided doses × 3–5 d[b]
RX	Prednisone	Panasol-S	Tablets: 1 mg	10–50 mg/d	Acute asthma: 1–2 mg/kg/d in divided doses × 3–5 d[b]
RX	Prednisone	Prednisone (Roxane)	Oral solution: 5 mg/5 ml	10–50 mg/d	Acute asthma: 1–2 mg/kg/d in divided doses × 3–5 d[b]
RX	Prednisone	Prednisone Intensol concentrate	Oral solution: 5 mg/ml	10–50 mg/d	Acute asthma: 1–2 mg/kg/d in divided doses × 3–5 d[b]
RX	Prednisone	Prednicen-M	Tablets: 5 mg	10–50 mg/d	Acute asthma: 1–2 mg/kg/d in divided doses × 3–5 d[b]
RX	Prednisone	Sterapred/ Sterapred DS	Tablets: 5, 10 mg	10–50 mg/d	Acute asthma: 1–2 mg/kg/d in divided doses × 3–5 d[b]
RX	Triamcinolone acetonide	Azmacort	MDI: 100 μg/puff (delivered)	Initial: 2 puffs tid–qid; severe asthma: 12–16 puffs/d; maintenance: adjust daily dose to bid; max dose = 16 puffs/d	< 6 yr: not established; 6–12 yr: 1–2 puffs tid–qid; max dose = 12 puffs/d

THEOPHYLLINE DOSING GUIDELINES INTRAVENOUS

Comparison of Equivalent Doses and Percent Theophylline Content of Commercially Available Theophylline Salts

Theophylline salt	*Equivalent dose*	*Percentage anhydrous theophylline*
Theophylline (anhydrous)	100 mg	100%
Theophylline monohydrate	110 mg	91%
Aminophylline (anhydrous)	116 mg	86%
Aminophylline dihydrate	127 mg	79%
Oxtriphylline	156 mg	64%
Dyphylline	none	70% by molecular weight ratio (amount equivalent to a given amount of theophylline is unknown)

ALL DOSES EXPRESSED IN TERMS OF THEOPHYLLINE (ANHYDROUS) EQUIVALENTS

	Adult	**Pediatric**
Loading dose:	Not currently receiving a theophylline preparation: 5 mg/kg over 20 min; usually a 0.5-mg/kg (lean body wt) dose will increase the serum theophylline by 1 μg/ml (range: 0.5–1.6 μg/ml)	Loading dose for children up to 16 yr: Same as adult
		Maintenance dose: (acute)
		< 1 yr: dose (mg/kg/hr) = (0.008) (age wks) + 0.21
		1–9 yr: 800 μg/kg/hr
		9–12 yr: 700 μg/kg/hr

(continued)

Medications (continued).

THEOPHYLLINE DOSING GUIDELINES INTRAVENOUS

	Adult	**Pediatric**
	Currently receiving a theophylline preparation and serum theophylline unknown without s/sx of toxicity: 2.5 mg/kg over 20 min	12–16 yr (smokers): 700 µg/kg/hr 12–16 yr (nonsmokers): 500 µg/kg/hr
Maintenance dose: (acute)	Young adult smokers: 700 µg/kg/hr Otherwise healthy nonsmoking adults: 430 µg/kg/hr Older adults and adults with cor pulmonale: 260 µg/kg/hr Adults with CHF or liver failure: 200 µg/kg/hr	

XANTHINE DERIVATIVES, PARENTERAL

RX/OTC	Generic name	Proprietary name	Available dosage forms	Suggested dosage—adult	Suggested dosage—pediatric
RX	Aminophylline	Various	Injection: 250 mg/10 ml	See dosing, theophylline intravenous	See dosing, theophylline intravenous
RX	Dyphylline	Dilor	Injection: 250 mg/ml	See USP DI	Not established
RX	Dyphylline	Lufyllin	Injection: 250 mg/ml	See USP DI	Not established
RX	Theophylline in 5% dextrose	Various	Intravenous, premixed: 4 mg/ml, 3.2 mg/ml, 2 mg/ml, 1.6 mg/ml, 0.8 mg/ml, 0.4 mg/ml	See dosing, theophylline intravenous	See dosing, theophylline intravenous

THEOPHYLLINE DOSING GUIDELINES ORAL IMMEDIATE RELEASE

Comparison of Equivalent Doses and Percent Theophylline Content of Commercially Available Theophylline Salts

Theophylline salt	Equivalent dose	Percentage anhydrous theophylline
Theophylline (anhydrous)	100 mg	100%
Theophylline monohydrate	110 mg	91%
Aminophylline (anhydrous)	116 mg	86%
Aminophylline dihydrate	127 mg	79%
Oxtriphylline	156 mg	64%
Dyphylline	none	70% by molecular weight ratio

ALL DOSES EXPRESSED IN TERMS OF THEOPHYLLINE (ANHYDROUS) EQUIVALENTS

	Adult	**Pediatric**
Loading dose:	Not currently receiving a theophylline preparation: 5–6 mg/kg; usually a 0.5-mg/kg (lean body wt) dose will increase the serum theophylline by 1 µg/ml (range: 0.5–1.6 µg/ml)	Loading dose in children up to 16 yr: Same as adult
	Currently receiving a theophylline preparation and theophylline concentration unknown without s/sx of toxicity; one dose of 2.5 mg/kg	Maintenance dose: (acute) < 6 mos: dose (mg/kg q 8 hr) = (0.07) (age wks) + 1.7 6–12 mos: dose (mg/kg q 6 hr) = (0.05) (age wks) + 1.25 1–9 yr: 5 mg/kg q 6 hr 9–12 yr: 4 mg/kg q 6 hr 12–16 yr: 3 mg/kg q 6 hr
Maintenance dose: (acute)	Young adult smokers: 4 mg/kg q 6 hr Otherwise healthy nonsmoking adults: 3 mg/kg q 8 hr Older adults and adults with cor pulmonale: 2mg/kg q 8 hr* Adults with CHF or liver failure: 2 mg/kg q 12 hr* * Do not exceed 400 mg/d unless serum theophylline monitored at 24-hr intervals	Maintenance dose: (chronic) Initially: 16 mg/kg up to 400 mg/d in 3–4 divided doses at 6–8-hr intervals; increase by 25% q 2–3 d up to the following maximum dosages without monitoring serum theophylline: monitor serum theophylline if doses are exceeded < 1 yr: dose (mg/kg/d) = 0.3 (age wks) + 8.0 1–9 yr: 22 mg/kg/d 9–12 yr: 20 mg/kg/d 12–16 yr: 18 mg/kg/d Adolescent > 16 yr: 13 mg/kg/d or 900 mg/d, whichever is less
Maintenance dose: (chronic)	Initially: 6–8 mg/kg; max dose = 400 mg/d in divided doses tid–qid, at 6–8-hr intervals; increase by 25% q 2–3 d as tolerated; max dose = 13 mg/kg/day or 900 mg/d, whichever is less without checking theophylline; serum theophylline should be monitored if 13 mg/kg/d or 900 mg/d is exceeded	

XANTHINE DERIVATIVES, ORAL IMMEDIATE RELEASE

RX/OTC	Generic name	Proprietary name	Available dosage forms	Suggested dosage—adult	Suggested dosage—pediatric
RX	Aminophylline	Somophyllin	Oral liquid: 105 mg/ml	See dosing, theophylline, oral immediate release	See dosing, theophylline, oral immediate release
RX	Aminophylline	Various	Tablets: 100, 200 mg Oral liquid: 105 mg/5 ml Suppositories: 250, 500 mg	See dosing, theophylline, oral immediate release	See dosing, theophylline, oral immediate release

Medications (continued).

XANTHINE DERIVATIVES, ORAL IMMEDIATE RELEASE *(continued)*

RX/OTC	Generic name	Proprietary name	Available dosage forms	Suggested dosage—adult	Suggested dosage—pediatric
RX	Dyphylline	Dyflex-200/400	Tablets: 200, 400 mg	15 mg/kg q 6 hr or up to qid	Not established
RX	Dyphylline	Neothylline	Tablets: 200, 400 mg	15 mg/kg q 6 hr or up to qid	Not established
RX	Dyphylline	Dilor (* Tablets also available with guaifenesin)	Tablets*: 200, 400 mg Elixir: 160 mg/15 ml	Tablets or elixir: 15 mg/kg q 6 hr or up to qid	Not established
RX	Dyphylline	Lufyllin	Tablets: 200, 400 mg Elixir: 100 mg/15 ml	Tablets or elixir: 15 mg/kg q 6 hr or up to qid	Not established
RX	Oxtriphylline (choline)	Choledyl	Tablets: 100, 200 mg Elixir: 100 mg/5 ml Syrup: 50 mg/5 ml	See dosing, theophylline, oral immediate release	See dosing, theophylline, oral immediate release
RX	Theophylline	Accurbron	Syrup: 150 mg/15 ml	See dosing, theophylline, oral immediate release	See dosing, theophylline, oral immediate release
RX	Theophylline	Aerolate	Oral solution: 150 mg/15 ml	See dosing, theophylline, oral immediate release	See dosing, theophylline, oral immediate release
RX	Theophylline	Aquaphyllin	Syrup: 80 mg/15 ml	See dosing, theophylline, oral immediate release	See dosing, theophylline, oral immediate release
RX	Theophylline	Asmalix	Elixir: 80 mg/15 ml	See dosing, theophylline, oral immediate release	See dosing, theophylline, oral immediate release
RX	Theophylline	Bronkodyl	Capsules: 100, 200 mg	See dosing, theophylline, oral immediate release	See dosing, theophylline, oral immediate release
RX	Theophylline	Elixomin	Elixir: 80 mg/15 ml	See dosing, theophylline, oral immediate release	See dosing, theophylline, oral immediate release
RX	Theophylline	Elixophyllin	Capsules: 100, 200 mg Elixir: 80 mg/15 ml	See dosing, theophylline, oral immediate release	See dosing, theophylline, oral immediate release
RX	Theophylline	Lanophyllin	Elixir: 80 mg/15 ml	See dosing, theophylline, oral immediate release	See dosing, theophylline, oral immediate release
RX	Theophylline	Quibron-T-Dividose	Tablets: 300 mg	See dosing, theophylline, oral immediate release	See dosing, theophylline, oral immediate release
RX	Theophylline	Slo-Phyllin	Tablets: 100, 200 mg Syrup: 80 mg/15 ml	See dosing, theophylline, oral immediate release	See dosing, theophylline, oral immediate release
RX	Theophylline	Theoclear-80	Syrup: 80 mg/15 ml	See dosing, theophylline, oral immediate release	See dosing, theophylline, oral immediate release
RX	Theophylline	Theolair	Tablets: 125, 250 mg Solution: 80 mg/15 ml	See dosing, theophylline, oral immediate release	See dosing, theophylline, oral immediate release
RX	Theophylline	Theostat 80	Syrup: 80 mg/15 ml	See dosing, theophylline, oral immediate release	See dosing, theophylline, oral immediate release

THEOPHYLLINE DOSING GUIDELINES ORAL SUSTAINED RELEASE

Comparison of Equivalent Doses and Percent Theophylline Content of Commercially Available Theophylline Salts

Theophylline salt	Equivalent dose	Percentage theophylline
Theophylline (anhydrous)	100 mg	100%
Theophylline monohydrate	110 mg	91%
Aminophylline (anhydrous)	116 mg	86%
Aminophylline dihydrate	127 mg	79%
Oxtriphylline dihydrate	156 mg	64%

ALL DOSES EXPRESSED IN TERMS OF THEOPHYLLINE (ANHYDROUS) EQUIVALENTS

Adult

Maintenance dose: (chronic) Initially: 4 mg/kg q 8–12 hr or for qd dosage forms 400 mg q 24 hr; increased as tolerated by 2–3 mg/kg/d at 3-d intervals up to 13 mg/kg/d or 900 mg/d, whichever is less without therapeutic monitoring; if these dosage recommendations are exceeded, therapeutic monitoring is recommended

NOTE: The dosage of once-a-day extended release tablets administered in the evening should be limited to no more than 800 mg until more data are available.

Pediatric

Maintenance dose: (chronic) Initially: 4 mg/kg q 8–12 hr or, for once a day dosage forms, 300 mg/d (wt < 30–35 kg) or 400 mg/d (wt > 35 kg) q 24 hr; increase 2–3 mg/kg/d every 3 d up to the following dosages without therapeutic monitoring of serum theophylline; if these dosages are exceeded, therapeutic monitoring is recommended
< 6 yr: not recommended
6–9 yr: 24 mg/kg/d
9–12 yr: 20 mg/kg/d
12–16 yr: 18 mg/kg/d
Adolescent > 16 yr: 13 mg/kg/d or 900 mg/d, whichever is less

NOTE: The dosage of once-a-day extended release tablets administered in the evening should be limited to dosages less than 800 mg until more data are available.
NOTE: Once daily dosing for children < 12 yr has not been established.

(continued)

Medications (continued).

XANTHINE DERIVATIVES, ORAL CAPSULES, SUSTAINED RELEASE

RX/OTC	Generic name	Proprietary name	Available dosage forms	Suggested dosage—adult	Suggested dosage—pediatric
RX	Theophylline	Aerolate, III, JR, SR	Capsules, timed release (8–12 hr): 65, 130, 260 mg	See dosing, theophylline, oral sustained release	See dosing, theophylline, oral sustained release
RX	Theophylline	Elixophyllin SR	Capsules, timed release (8–12 hr): 125, 250 mg	See dosing, theophylline, oral sustained release	See dosing, theophylline, oral sustained release
RX	Theophylline	Slo-bid Gyrocaps	Capsules, timed release (8–12 hr): 50, 75, 100, 125, 200, 300 mg	See dosing, theophylline, oral sustained release	See dosing, theophylline, oral sustained release
RX	Theophylline	Slo-Phyllin Gyrocaps	Capsules, timed release (8–12 hr): 60, 125, 250 mg	See dosing, theophylline, oral sustained release	See dosing, theophylline, oral sustained release
RX	Theophylline	Theo-24	Capsules, timed release (24 hr): 100, 200, 300 mg	See dosing, theophylline, oral sustained release; NOTE: doses > 13 mg/kg or 900 mg once a day should avoid high-fat morning meal or take dose at least 1 hr before eating	See dosing, theophylline, oral sustained release; NOTE: see adult warning
RX	Theophylline	Theo-Dur Sprinkle	Capsules, timed release (12 hr): 50, 75, 125, 200 mg	See dosing, theophylline, oral sustained release; NOTE: capsule may be opened and contents sprinkled on a tsp of soft food; swallow immediately with water/juice and do not subdivide capsule contents	See dosing, theophylline, oral sustained release; see note under suggested dosage, adult
RX	Theophylline	Theobid Duracap	Capsules, timed release (12 hr): 260 mg	See dosing, theophylline, oral sustained release	See dosing, theophylline, oral sustained release
RX	Theophylline	Theobid Jr. Duracap	Capsules, timed release (12 hr): 130 mg	See dosing, theophylline, oral sustained release	See dosing, theophylline, oral sustained release
RX	Theophylline	Theoclear L.A.	Capsules, timed release (12 hr): 130, 260 mg	See dosing, theophylline, oral sustained release	See dosing, theophylline, oral sustained release
RX	Theophylline	Theospan-SR	Capsules, timed release (12 hr): 130, 260 mg	See dosing, theophylline, oral sustained release	See dosing, theophylline, oral sustained release
RX	Theophylline	Theovent	Capsules, timed release (12 hr): 125, 250 mg	See dosing, theophylline, oral sustained release	See dosing, theophylline, oral sustained release

XANTHINE DERIVATIVES, ORAL TABLETS, SUSTAINED RELEASE

RX/OTC	Generic name	Proprietary name	Available dosage forms	Suggested dosage—adult	Suggested dosage—pediatric
RX	Aminophylline	Phyllocontin	Tablets, CR (12 hr): 225 mg	See dosing, theophylline, oral sustained release	See dosing, theophylline, oral sustained release
RX	Oxtriphylline (choline salt)	Choledyl SA	Tablets, sustained action: 400, 600 mg	See dosing, theophylline, oral sustained release	See dosing, theophylline, oral sustained release
RX	Theophylline	Constant-T[e]	Tablets, timed release (8–12 hr): 200, 300 mg	See dosing, theophylline, oral sustained release	See dosing, theophylline, oral sustained release
RX	Theophylline	Quibron-T	Tablets, timed release (8–12 hr) 300 mg	See dosing, theophylline oral sustained release	See dosing, theophylline, oral sustained release
RX	Theophylline	Respbid	Tablets, timed release (8–12 hr): 250, 500 mg	See dosing, theophylline, oral sustained release	See dosing, theophylline, oral sustained release
RX	Theophylline	Sustaire	Tablets, sustained release (8–12 hr): 100, 300 mg	See dosing, theophylline, oral sustained release	See dosing, theophylline, oral sustained release
RX	Theophylline	T-Phyl	Tablets, timed release (8–12 hr): 200 mg	See dosing, theophylline, oral sustained release	See dosing, theophylline, oral sustained release
RX	Theophylline	Theo-Dur	Tablets, timed release (8–24 hr): 100, 200, 300, 450 mg	See dosing, theophylline, oral sustained release	See dosing, theophylline, oral sustained release
RX	Theophylline	Theo-Sav	Tablets, timed release (8–24 hr): 100, 200, 300 mg	See dosing, theophylline, oral sustained release	See dosing, theophylline, oral sustained release
RX	Theophylline	Theochron	Tablets, timed release (12–24 hr): 100, 200, 300 mg	See dosing, theophylline, oral sustained release	See dosing, theophylline, oral sustained release

Medications *(continued)*.

XANTHINE DERIVATIVES, ORAL TABLETS, SUSTAINED RELEASE *(continued)*

RX/OTC	Generic name	Proprietary name	Available dosage forms	Suggested dosage—adult	Suggested dosage—pediatric
RX	Theophylline	Theolair-SR	Tablets, timed release (8–24 hr): 200, 250, 300, 500 mg	See dosing, theophylline, oral sustained release	See dosing, theophylline, oral sustained release
RX	Theophylline	Theophylline SR (various)	Tablets, timed release (12–24 hr): 100, 200, 300 mg	See dosing, theophylline, oral sustained release	See dosing, theophylline, oral sustained release
RX	Theophylline	Uniphyl	Tablets, timed release (24 hr): 400 mg	See dosing, theophylline, oral sustained release	See dosing, theophylline, oral sustained release

MAST CELL STABILIZERS

OTC/RX	Generic name	Proprietary name	Available dosage forms	Suggested dosage—adult	Suggested dosage—pediatric
RX	Cromolyn sodium	Intal	Capsules for inhalation: 20 mg	Bronchial asthma: 20 mg qid; bronchospasm prophylaxis: 20 mg prior to exposure or chronically 20 mg qid; max dose = 160 mg/d	< 2 yr: not established; > 2 yr: usual adult dosage
			MDI: 800 μg/puff	Bronchial asthma: 2 puffs qid; bronchospasm prophylaxis: 2 puffs 10–15 min but not more than 60 min before exposure	≥ 5 yr: usual adult dose
			Solution for inhalation: 20 mg/2 ml ampule	20 mg qid at regular intervals via power nebulizer	< 2 yr: not established; > 2 yr: usual adult dosage
	Ketotifen fumarate (investigational)	Zaditen (Canada)	Tablets: 1 mg; N/A in US	1–2 mg bid; 1 mg bid equivalent to cromolyn powder for inhalation 20 mg qid	< 3 yr: not established; > 3 yr: 1 mg bid with morning and evening meals
			Syrup: 1 mg/5 ml		< 3 yr: not established; > 3 yr: 1 mg bid with morning and evening meals

MISCELLANEOUS

OTC/RX	Generic name	Proprietary name	Available dosage forms	Suggested dosage—adult	Suggested dosage—pediatric
	Azelastine (investigational)	—	N/A in US	4 mg bid (oral)	> 6 yr: 4 mg bid[d]
	Nedocromil (investigational)	Tilade	Inhalation; N/A in US	4 mg/inh; 1 puff bid–qid	< 12 yr: not established

[a] All indicated dosages represent only the averages and, unless otherwise noted, are consistent with the *Physicians' Desk Reference* (PDR), *Drug Information* (12th ed., Rockville, MD: United States Pharmacopeial Convention, 1992) (USP DI 1992), and *Facts and Comparisons* (St. Louis, MO: Facts and Comparisons, 1992). **THE PHYSICIAN MUST INDIVIDUALIZE DOSAGES.** This is particularly important when considering theophylline or its derivatives. **THE PHYSICIAN MUST REFER TO REFERENCE MATERIAL PRIOR TO USE.** Refer to the cited references for additional constituents present in any drug cited in this table.

[b] Taketomo, C. K., Hodding, J. J., and Kraus, D. M. *Pediatric Dosage Handbook, 1992.* Hudson, OH: American Pharmaceutical Association, Lexi-Comp, 1992.

[c] *American Medical Association Drug Evaluations, 1992.* Chicago: American Medical Association, 1992.

[d] McTavish, D., and Sorkin, E. M. Azelastine—a review of its pharmacodynamics and pharmacokinetic properties and therapeutic potential. *Drugs* 38:778, 1989.

[e] No longer being manufactured.

% = percent; < = less than; > = greater than; bid = twice a day; CHF = congestive heart failure; CR = controlled release; d = day; equiv = equivalent; HR = heart rate; hr = hour(s); IM = intramuscular; inh = inhalation(s); IPPB = intermittent positive pressure breathing (device); IV = intravenous; kg = kilogram; max = maximum; μg = microgram; MDI = metered-dose inhaler; mg = milligram; min = minimum; min = minute; ml = milliliter; mos = months; MR = may repeat; N/A = not available; NS = normal saline; OTC = over-the-counter drug; PF = preservative free; prn = as needed, when needed; q = every; qam = each morning; qd = once a day; qid = 4 times a day (in equal intervals); qpm = each evening; RX = prescription drug; s/sx = signs/symptoms; SC = subcutaneous; SL = sublingual; tid = 3 times a day (in equal intervals); tsp = teaspoonful (≅ 5 ml); tx = treatment(s); US = United States; w = with; wks = weeks; wt = weight; x/d = number of times of dosing per day; yr = year(s).

Index

Note: Page numbers in italics indicate figures; page numbers followed by t indicate tables.

A 64077, 120, 891
Acetaminophen, aspirin-induced asthma and, 622
Acetylcholine
    ganglionic and junctional transmission of bronchomotor activity and, *223*, 223–224
    inhalation challenge with, 503
    as neural modulator, 222–223
    vasoactive intestinal peptide cotransmission with, 236–237, *237*
Acetylcysteine, 623t, 926t, 926–927, 964
Achalasia, 1023
Acid anhydrides, occupational asthma and, 601
Acid-base balance
    in severe asthma, 340, *341*
    in status asthmaticus, 1004, *1004*, 1004t
Acquired immunodeficiency syndrome, differential diagnosis of, 465, 476t
Acremonium, 1210–1211
ACTH, synthetic, 810
Actinomycin D, 183
Actinomytes, thermophilic, hypersensitivity pneumonitis and, 633t
Action potential, 166
Acupuncture, 1148
Acute asthma, 972–983
    cardiac rhythm in, 1048
    in childhood. *See* Childhood asthma, acute
    corticosteroids in, 979–980
    definition of, 972
    diagnosis of, 452t, 452–453
    drug combinations in, 978
    drug studies and, 797
    epidemiology of, 972
    hospital admission decisions and, 982–983
    hydration in, 918t, 918–920, 929t
    initial assessment in, 973
    pathobiology of, 972
    pathophysiology of, 972–973
    PEFR in, 982–983
    prevention of, 983, 1192
    repeat assessment of, 980–982
        continued treatment and, 980–982, *981*
    severe. *See* Status asthmaticus
    status asthmaticus. *See* Status asthmaticus
    treatment of, 974–980, *975*, *976*
        bronchodilator therapy in, 974, *977*, 977–979, *978*
        continued, 980–982, *981*
        corticosteroids in, *979*, 979–980
Adenosine, inhalation challenge with, 504

Adenosine
    airway effects of, 253
    bronchoconstriction induced by
        clinical implications of, 255–256
        mechanisms of, 253–255, *254*
    cyclic. *See* Cyclic AMP
    effect on mast cell responses, 255, *255*
Adenosine receptors
    classification of, 199
    muscle relaxation and, 212
Adenylate cyclase
    activation of, 195, *196*
    beta adrenoreceptor coupled to, ternary complex model of, *175*, 175–176
    transcriptional and posttranscriptional controls of regulation by agonists and, 175–176
    cyclic AMP synthesis and, 194
Adenylyl cyclase, G-protein binding to, 194, 703
Adhesion molecules
    in epithelium, 302
    inflammation and, 89
    neural cell, 424
Adhesion receptors, of eosinophils, 259–261, 260t, *261*
Adolescence
    asthma during, 1074
    drug studies and, 795–796
Adrenal function. *See also* Hypothalamic-pituitary-adrenal function
    late asthmatic reactions and, 141
    surgery and, 1102
Adrenal insufficiency, as incitant, 445
Adrenergic agonists, in cardiovascular disease, 1039t, 1039–1040. *See also* Beta-adrenergic agonists; Sympathomimetics
Adrenergic mechanisms, circadian rhythm of, nocturnal asthma and, 1032–1033
Adrenergic nervous system, to lungs, 700
Adrenergic regulation, 165–184
    adrenoceptors and, 171–174, 180–183, 194
        biochemical consequences of adrenergic stimulation and, 173–174, *174*
        downregulation, 175
        experimental asthma and, 393
        G-protein–linked, beta, 172–173
        identification by radioligand technology, 171–172
        pharmacologic classification of, 171
        receptor activation, 193
        reciprocal changes in, 180–183

    responsiveness and mechanisms of regulation of, 174–176, *175*
    in atopic diseases, 176–183
        adrenergically active lymphocytic proteins and, 183–184
        affinity of beta-adrenergic agonists and their receptor sites and, 177–178
        balance of adrenoceptor subtypes and responses and, 179
        blockade of beta receptors by autoantibodies and microbial components and, 177
        "interconversion" controversy and, 179–180
        inverse, reciprocal adrenoceptor activities and, 180–183
        numbers and reactivities of beta receptors and, 178–179
        pattern of mobilization of catecholamines and, 177
    autonomic nervous system and. *See* Autonomic nervous system
Adrenoceptors. *See* Adrenergic regulation; Alpha adrenoceptors; Beta adrenoceptors
Adrenocortical function, anesthesia and, 1102–1103
Adult, infections in, 572–573
Adult respiratory distress syndrome, differential diagnosis of, 465, 476t
Aequorin, 203
Aeroallergens, 545–556, *546*. *See also specific allergens*
    air sampling and, 545–548, 547t, *548*, *549*
    algal, 553
    arthropod, 553, 553t
    bacterial, 555
    epidermal, 552–553. *See also* Epidermal allergens
    fungal, 549–551
        classification of, 551, 552t
        identification of, 550–551
    indoor environmental, 554t, 555t, 556, 580–581. *See also* House dust; House dust mites
    plant, 555–556. *See also* Pollen
    sensitization to, 27
    viral, 553, 555
Aerosol(s), 405–415
    clearance and retention of particles and, 406–407
        mucociliary transport and, 407
        nonciliated regions and, 407
    in occupational asthma, 588

Aerosol(s) (*continued*)
  delivery of, intermittent positive pressure breathing and, 1114, *1115*
  drug. *See also* Aerosol delivery systems; *specific drugs*
    beta-adrenergic agonists, 716, *716*
    generation, delivery, and penetrance of, bronchial provocation tests and, 511
    measuring particle retention and, 414–415
      bronchoalveolar lavage and, 414
      gamma cameras and, 415
      magnetopneumography and, 415
      modeling and, 414
      photometry and, 414
      radioactivity and, 414
      tomography and, 415
    particle deposition and, 409–413, 546, 750t
      anatomy of respiratory tract and, 410, 750
      breathing pattern and, 412
      choice of pathway and, 410
      disease and, 412–413
      hygroscopicity and evaporation and, 411, 412t
      mechanisms of, 405–406, 406t
      particle size and size distribution and, 410–411, 411t, 749
      patterns of, 413, 415
    respiratory effects of, 578–580, *579, 580*
    therapeutic, characterizing and delivering, 408–409, 716
Aerosol delivery systems, 408–409, 749–753, *750, 750t*
  breathing patterns and, 412
  comparison between, 753
  dry-powder inhalers, 752
  freon propellant and morbidity, 1158
  intermittent positive pressure breathing and. *See* Respiratory therapy
  metered dose inhalers, *751,* 751–752. *See also* Metered dose inhalers
  metered-dose inhaler spacers, 752, 752t
  nebulizers, 749–751, *750*
Affinity maturation, 424
Age. *See also* Childhood asthma; *specific age groups*
  drug studies and, 787
  IgE levels and, 28
  mechanical heterogeneity of airway smooth muscle and, 320
  mortality and, 1154, *1155*
  outgrowing asthma and, 528
  prevalence and incidence of asthma related to, 15–16, 16t
Aging. *See* Elderly patients
Airborne irritants, in occupational asthma, 587
Air conditioners, for environmental control, 582, 1137–1138, *1138*
Air-filtration units, for environmental control, 538t, 1138–1140, *1139*
Air pollution, 5, 21
  childhood asthma and, 1065
  environmental control measures for, 1142
  exercise-induced asthma and, 617
  IgE levels and, 28
  indoor, 554t, 580–581, 582t
  occupational asthma and, 597
  outdoor, 577–580, 578t
    respiratory effects of photochemical oxidants and, 580
    respiratory effects of sulfur dioxide and particulate matter and, 578–580, *579, 580*
Air sampling, 545–548, 547t, *548, 549*

Airway. *See also* headings beginning with term Bronchial
  anatomy of autonomic nerves of, anticholinergic agents and, 876, *877*
  beta-adrenergic receptors in, 701
  calcitonin gene-related peptide and, 241–242
  caliber of, antigen challenge in experimental asthma and, *383,* 383–384
  circadian rhythms in function of, nocturnal asthma and, 1031, *1032*
  conducting, functional anatomy of, 352, *353, 354*
  cooling of, nocturnal asthma and, 1031
  disordered anatomy of, functional consequences of, 355
  dynamics of, as risk factor for status asthmaticus, 990–991
  gastrin-releasing peptide and, 245
  inflammation of. *See* Inflammation
  mast cells in, 279
  mucus lining, 356, *357. See also* Mucus
  parasympathetic control of, 217–219
    central-peripheral heterogeneity of cholinergic innervation and, 217
    modulation of neurotransmission and, 217–218
    origins, organization, pathways, and actions and, 217
    parasympathetic ganglia and, 217
    receptor-response coupling mechanisms and, 219, *220*
    receptor types in cholinergic neurotransmission and, 219, 219t
  permeability of, hyperresponsiveness and, 35–36
  reduced caliber of, hyperresponsiveness and, 35
  in status asthmaticus, 1005
  structural changes in asthma, 352, *354,* 354–355
  structure and function of, aerosol corticosteroids and, 832–833
  vagal reflexes in, anticholinergic agents and, 876–877, *877*
  wall of, thickness of, hyperresponsiveness and, 36
Airway dilators, 923
Airway epithelium, 296–307
  barrier function of, 87
  basement membrane, epithelial, 302
  at different levels, structure of, 296
  endothelin and, *306,* 307
  functional anatomy of, 352, *354*
  functions of, 302–306
    absorption permeability across airway mucosa and, 304–305
    epithelium-derived agents and, 87, 302–304, *303,* 304t
    exudation permeability across airway mucosa and, *305,* 305–306
  immunoregulation and, 159
  inflammation of. *See* Inflammation, of airway epithelium
  normal, structure of, 296, *297–299*
  regeneration of, 300–302
    basement membrane and, 302
    effect of treatment on structure and, 302, *303*
    epithelial integrity and cellular adhesion and, 300
    epithelial turnover and, 300, *301*
    extracellular matrix and, 300, 302
  removal, 302–304, 304t

structural changes and bronchial hyperresponsiveness and, 297–300
  asthma and, 297–298, *299–301*
  viral infections and, 298, 300
  tachykinins and, 239, *240*
  water transport, 377
Airway hyperreactivity. *See* Bronchial hyperresponsiveness
Airway obstruction, 449–450
  central, differential diagnosis of, 465–467, *466,* 467t, 476t
  eosinophils and, 266–267
  HPA axis function and, 843–844
  localization of, 336, *337*
  mucociliary dysfunction and, 378–379
  platelet-activating factor and, 290–291
  reduced flow rates and, 335–337, *337*
  reversibility of, 337, 337t
  site of limitation and, bronchoreversibility assessment and, 456–457, *457,* 457t
  wheezing and, 652–653
Airway reactivity. *See* Bronchial hyperresponsiveness; Bronchial reactivity
Airway resistance, 333–334, *335, 336*
  determination of, 9
  variability in, 9
Airway response, late-phase, *157,* 157–158, 159t, *1578*
Airway secretions. *See also* Mucus
  accumulation of, nocturnal asthma and, 1030
  components of, 371, *372*
  inflammation and, 88
  mucociliary apparatus and, 371–372, *372, 373*
  mucociliary transport and, 374–377
  neuropeptide effects on, vasoactive intestinal peptide, 235
  neuropeptide Y and, 245
  regulation of, 371–372
  removal of, intermittent positive pressure breathing and, 1115
  tachykinins and, 239–240
  transport of, 374–377
Airway smooth muscle, 314–330
  abnormalities of, airway hyperresponsiveness and, 38
  in asthma, 320–330
    biochemistry of sensitized muscle and, 323, *323, 324*
    changes in operation of contractile machinery and, 329
    conversion of multiunit muscle to single-unit muscle and, 329
    isometric and isotonic studies of, 321
    leukotrienes and allergic bronchospasm and, 330
    mechanism for increased shortening of sensitized muscle and, 324–325, *324–327*
    nonadrenergic inhibitory system and, 329
    pathophysiology of sensitized muscle and, *321,* 321–323, *322,* 322t
    pharmacology of sensitized muscle and, 325, *328,* 328–329
    pulmonary circulation and, 330
    Schultz-Dale reaction in sensitized canine tracheal muscle and, 321, *321*
  beta-adrenergic agonist actions on, 709–710, *710,* 710t
  calcitonin gene-related peptide and, 241
  contractility of, 318, *318, 319*
  contraction of. *See* Muscle contraction
  corticosteroid effects on, 804

desensitization by beta-agonists exposure, 707–708, *708*
endothelin binding sites in, *306*, 307
force-velocity relationships at loads greater than P$_o$ and, 317, *317*
force-velocity relationships at loads less than P$_o$ and, *315*, 315–316, *316*, 316t
inflammation of, 88
interstitial cells and, 320
length-tension relationships of, 314–315
  hysteresis and, 319
  length-tension curves and, 314–315, *315*
  reduced activation at short lengths and, 315, *315*
maximum force potential and, 318, *318*
mechanical heterogeneity of, 320
  age, temperature, and hormones and, 320
  levels of airway and, 320
  species-engendered differences and, 320
mechanics of cat lung strips and, 320
mechanisms of beta-adrenergic agonist action in, 328, 704–706
  receptor-operated contraction and, 705, *705*, *706*
  relaxation and, 705–706, *706*
neuropeptide effects on, vasoactive intestinal peptide, 235
normally cycling and latch bridges and, *316*, 316–317, *317*
in occupational asthma, 588
parallel elastic component and, 317
physiologic role of, 320
relaxation of, 318–319, *319. See also* Muscle relaxation
sensitized, 321–323, 959–960
  histamine and, 325
  isometric studies of, 321, *321*
  isotonic studies of, 321–323, *322*, 322t
series elastic component and, 317
species-engendered differences in, 320
tachykinins and, 239
tone of. *See* Muscle tone
Albuterol, 687t, 687–688, 723–724
  aerosol, 719t
    pharmacokinetics of, 716, *716*
  continuous nebulization with, pharmacokinetics of, 716
  inhaled, 728, 729, *729*
  intravenous, pharmacokinetics of, 715, 760
  oral, 721t, 730
    pharmacokinetics of, 715, *715*
  in severe acute asthma, 760, *761*
  subcutaneous, 730, 731
Albuterol sulfate, 1224–1225
Alcohol, 895–896
  clinical studies of, 895–896
Algal allergens, 553, 597
Alkyl cyanoacrylate, occupational asthma and, 602
Allergen(s), 50, 441–444, 442t, *443. See also* Aeroallergens; Antigen(s); *specific allergens*
  algal, 553, 597
  animal, 1142
  biochemical studies, 43
  food, sensitization to, 27
  molds, 442
  nocturnal asthma and, 1030
  plant
    botanical regions of the United States and Canada and, 1203–1209
    occupational asthma and, 600t
  for skin testing
    preparation of, 488
    selection of, 486–487

Allergen challenge. *See* Antigen challenge
  exercise-induced asthma and, 617
Allergenic extracts, standardization of, bronchial provocation tests and, 509–510
Allergic asthma, 471
Allergic bronchopulmonary aspergillosis, 635–641
  aerosol steroids and, 835
  cystic fibrosis and, 639–640
  diagnosis and clinical characteristics of, 636, 636t
  differential diagnosis of, 478t, 480, 640–641
  laboratory studies in, 637–638
  pathogenesis of, 639
  pathologic findings in, 639
  pulmonary function tests in, 639
  radiographic findings in, *638*, 638–639
  staging of, 636t, 636–637, *637*
  treatment of, *640*, 641
Allergic bronchopulmonary mycosis, 480
Allergic conjunctivitis, disodium cromoglycate in, 858–859
Allergic pneumonia, 471
Allergic reactions, 51, 56, 545, 834. *See also* Hypersensitivity
  atopic. *See* Atopy
  educational materials on, 1213
  platelet-activating factor as mediator of, 289–290
  platelet activation in, in vivo evidence for, 287
  platelets in, 287
Allergic rhinitis, 537
  disodium cromoglycate in, 858
Alpha-adrenergic blocking agents, bronchial provocation tests and, 511
Alpha-adrenergic system, airway hyperresponsiveness and, 36
Alpha adrenoceptors
  in experimental animal models, 393–394, *394*
  shifting in subtypes and responses of, 179
  smooth muscle, 328
    contraction of, 210
Alpha$_1$-antitrypsin deficiency, 1185, 1185t, *1186*, 1187
Alternaria, 442, *443*, 443, 551, 552t, 986, 1210–1211
  immunotherapy and, 940
Aluminum, occupational asthma and, 602
Alveolar macrophage activation, 148
Alveolitis, allergic, extrinsic. *See* Hypersensitivity pneumonitis
Amantadine hydrochloride, in influenza virus infections, 572, 573
Ambrosia, 549
Aminophylline
  dosage of, 1229, 1230, 1231, 1232
  interaction with anesthesia, 1101–1102, *1102*
Aminophylline dihydrate, 1229, 1230, 1231
Amoxicillin, in sinusitis, 542t
Amoxicillin clavulanate, in sinusitis, 542t
AMP. *See* Adenosine
  cyclic. *See* Cyclic AMP
Ampicillin, in sinusitis, 542t
Analgesics. *See* Aspirin-induced asthma
Anaphylactoid reaction, 627
  acute, desensitization during, 707
Anaphylatoxins, 101
Anesthesia. *See also* Preanesthetic management, Perioperative monitoring
  airway responses and, in experimental animal models, 384
  asthma caused by, 627–628

bronchospasm and, 1106–1107
calcium and, 965
induction of, 1104, *1105*
inhibition of sensory nerve activation by, 244
interaction of therapy with, 1101–1103
  aminophylline and, 1101–1102, *1102*
  beta sympathomimetics and, 1102
  steroids and adrenocortical function and, 1102–1103
maintenance of, 1104–1106, *1105*, 1106t
muscle relaxants, 1105, 1173
ventilator use and, 1006, 1173
Anesthesiologic treatment approaches, 1149
Angina, microvascular, differential diagnosis of, 464, 476t
Angioedema, differential diagnosis of, 468, 476t
Angiotensin-converting enzyme, tachykinin metabolism and, 239
Angiotensin-converting enzyme inhibitors, 1191
  cough due to, 627
Animal dander. *See* Epidermal allergens; *specific animals*
Animal proteins, hypersensitivity pneumonitis and, 632, 633t
Antibiotics. *See also specific drugs*
  asthma caused by, 623t
  asthma induced by, 626
  mucokinetic, 923
  in *Mycoplasma pneumoniae* infections, 572
  in sinusitis, 542, 542t
Anticholinergic agents, 227–228, 688–689, 876–882. *See also specific drugs*
  action of, 877
    cholinergic control of airway functions and, 877
    site of bronchodilation and, 877
  anatomy of airway autonomic nerves and, 876, *877*
  bronchial provocation tests and, 510–511
  in cardiovascular disease, 1040–1041, *1041*
  in childhood asthma, 1070
  cholinergic function and, 227–228
  in chronic obstructive pulmonary disease
    acute exacerbations of, 882
    stable, *881*, 881–882
  clinical applications of, 882
  combination with other bronchodilators, 882
  dosages, 879t
  efficacy in asthma, 879–881
    acute severe, 880–881
    against specific stimuli, 879, 880t
    stable, 879–880, *880*
  interactions with beta agonists, 733
  lung mechanics, hemodynamics, and gas exchange and, 882
  muscarinic receptor subtypes and, 877
  pharmacology of, *878*, 878–879, 879t
    dose response and, 879
    pharmacokinetics and, 878–879
    tolerance and subsensitivity and, 879
  during pregnancy and nursing, 1091
  side effects of, 882
  in status asthmaticus, 695
  vagal reflexes in airways and, 876–877, *877*
Antidiuretic hormone, 997
Antifungal agents, in allergic bronchopulmonary aspergillosis, 641
Antigen(s), 43–47, 50, 545. *See also* Allergen(s); Immune response
  biochemical studies of, 43–44, 44t, *45*, 45t, *46*

Antigen(s) (*continued*)
  compared with other protein antigens, 46–47
  immunologic studies of, 44–46
  inhalation challenge with, 505–506
  modified, as immunotherapeutic reagents, 47
  processed, 54
  purified, from pollens, 549
  recognition of, 50–53, *51*, 51t
    immunoglobulins and, 51–52
    major histocompatibility complex antigens and, 52–53, *53*
    molecular basis for, 51
    T-cell receptors and, 53, *53*
  specificity of IgE biosynthesis and, 63
  storage of, bronchial provocation tests and, 510
Antigen-antibody reactions, 4–5
  dual, 4
Antigen challenge. *See also* Bronchial provocation tests
  airway caliber and, in experimental animal models, 383, 385–386, *386*, *387*
  corticosteroids and, 805, *805*
  eosinophils and, 266–267
  in experimental asthma. *See* Experimental asthma, antigen challenge and
  inflammatory cells and mediators in BAL specimens after, 311–312, 312t
  inhalational, 506–507
Antigen load, 27
Antihistamines. *See also specific drugs*; Histamine antagonists
  dual-action, 865–871
  H₂ antagonists, 1027
  in late asthmatic reactions, 142
  nonsedating, 692
    cardiac arrhythmias from, 1049
Antihypertensive drugs and asthma, 623
Anti-IgE autoantibodies, regulation of IgE synthesis and, 73–77, *75–77*
Antiinflammatory drugs, 690–692, 910–915. *See also specific drugs and drug types*; Aspirin-induced asthma
  bronchodilators versus, 685–686, 686t
  in childhood asthma, 1071–1072, 1073, 1073t
Antimalarials, 914, 914t
Antimicrobials. *See also* Antibiotics
  in status asthmaticus, 1003
Antioxidants, 961–964
Antiparasympathomimetics, mucokinetic effect of, 923
Anxiety. *See* Psychiatric aspects; Psychological factors
Aortic stenosis, definition of, 9
Aquatic substances and asthma, 599t
Arachidonic acid products. *See also* Leukotriene(s)
  control of mucus production and, 367
  immunoregulation and, 149
  late asthmatic reactions and, 141
  leukotriene synthesis and, 112
Aromatic L-amino acid decarboxylase, 167
Arterial blood gases, 450, 685, 973
  gas exchange and, 339t, 339–340, *340*, *341*
  in pulmonary embolism, 461
  in status asthmaticus, 685, *685*, 990–994
Arteriography, in pulmonary embolism, 462–463
Arthropods, 553, 553t
Ascaris lumbricoides, 472
Ascomycetes, 552t
Ascorbic acid
  antioxidant as, 964

blockade of antigen inhalation challenge by, 511
Aspergillosis
  bronchopulmonary, allergic, differential diagnosis of, 478t, 480
  radiographic findings in, 671–672, *671–673*
Aspergillus, 442, *443*, 443, 551, 552t, 1210–1211. *See also* Allergic bronchopulmonary aspergillosis
  reactions induced by, 4
Aspergillus fumigatus, 480, 833
Aspiration, sputum in. *See* Sputum, in aspiration
Aspirin-induced asthma, 124–126, *126*, 449, 621–622, 624t, 624–625, 892
  prevention of, 1191
Aspirin-sensitive asthma
  cyclooxygenase inhibitors in, 892
  differential diagnosis of, 475t
Astemizole, 97, 884
Asthmatic response
  early, correlation of skin test results with clinical history and allergen inhalation test results and, 523–526, 524t
  immediate versus late, bronchial provocation tests and, 507–509, 509t
  late. *See* Late asthmatic reactions
  location of, bronchial provocation tests and, 507
Asymptomatic patients
  diagnosis of, 451
  preanesthetic management of, 1100
Atopic allergens. *See* Antigen(s)
Atopic dermatitis, 183
Atopy, 6, 17–19, *18*, 19t, 56
  adrenergic lymphocyte proteins, 183
  adrenergic regulation in. *See* Adrenergic regulation, in atopic diseases
  in childhood asthma, 1064–1065
  in exercise-induced asthma, 616–617
  familial incidence of, 26, 27t
  fatal asthma and, 1159–1160
  IgE levels and. *See* Immunoglobulin E
  in occupational asthma, 586
  occupational asthma and, 444
  prediction of onset of asthma and, 18–19, 19t
Atropine
  blockade of antigen inhalation challenge by, 510
  in late asthmatic reactions, 142
  mucokinetic effect of, 923
Atropine methonitrate, 879t
  dose response and, 879
Atropine sulfate, 689, 879t, 1224
  pharmacokinetics of, 878
Atrovent. *See* Ipratropium bromide
Atypical asthma, inhalation challenge and, 505
Atypical mast cells, 278
Aureobasidium, 552t
Autoantibodies
  anti-IgE, regulation of IgE synthesis and, 73–77, *75–77*
  beta receptor blockade by, 177
Autodesensitization. *See* Tachyphylaxis
Autonomic nervous system, 165–170. *See also* Adrenergic regulation
  adrenergic transmission and, 166–170
    catecholamine biosynthesis and, 167–168, *168*
    catecholamine degradation and, 170
    catecholamine release and, 169–170
    catecholamine storage and, 168, *169*

neuronal uptake and inactivation of catecholamines and, 170
  information processing in, 166
  sympathetic and parasympathetic divisions of, 165–166
    complementary sympathetic systems and, 165–166
Autonomic receptors, circadian rhythm of, nocturnal asthma and, 1033
Avian hypersensitivity pneumonitis, 553
Axonal conduction, in autonomic nervous system, 166
Axon reflexes, airway hyperresponsiveness and, 37
Azatadine, 865
Azelastine, 868–871, 885–886, 1233
  adverse effects of, 870–871
  chemistry of, 868, *868*
  clinical efficacy of, 870, *870*
  dose and administration of, 870, 870t
  mechanisms of action of, 869, 869t, 870t
  pharmacokinetics of, 868
Azo dyes, asthma caused by, 449

Bacterial allergens, 555
Bacterial infections. *See also* Infections
  IgE levels and, 28
Bakers' asthma, 444
Bambuterol, 726–727
Basement membrane, airway epithelial regeneration and, 302
Basidiomycetes, 552t
Basophils, 280
  in aspirin-induced asthma, 624
  histamine release by, 494–495
  interaction with IgE, 59–60
  passive sensitization of, 494–495
B-cells
  allergens and, 45–46
  immunoregulation and, 150–151
  interaction with IgE, 59
  recognition of foreignness and, 50–51
  T-cell interactions of, 54–55
Beclomethasone, 691
  in sinusitis, 542t
Beclomethasone dipropionate, aerosol, 821t, 1228
  cost of, 836t, 837
  dosing frequency for, 827, *828*
  dry-powder formulations of, 830
  effective dosage of, 819
  HPA axis suppression and, 845, 846, 847, *847*
  minimum maintenance dose of, 820, *822*
Behavior modification, 1126
Bernstein test, 1026
Beta-adrenergic agents
  as bronchodilators. *See* Bronchodilators, beta-adrenergic
  in late asthmatic reactions, 142
Beta-adrenergic agonists, 689, 694, 700–738. *See also* Beta adrenoceptors; *specific drugs*; Sympathomimetics
  adrenergic nervous system to lungs and, 700
    adrenergic subtype distribution in lungs and heart and, 700
    fate of natural catecholamines and, 700
  bronchial provocation tests and, 510
  bronchodilating, evolution of, 708, *709*
  changes in affinity of agonists and their receptor sites and, 177–178
  in childhood asthma, 1069–1070, 1070t
  factors modifying action of, 706–708
    desensitization and, 707–708, *708*, 737
    epithelium removal and, 707

functional antagonism to smooth muscle relaxation and, 706–707, *707*
impaired response of isolated asthmatic airway and, 708
muscarinic subtypes in lung and interactions with adrenergic system, 707
fatality and, 1158
inhaled
  side effects of, 729
  standard versus optimal doses of, 728–729, *729*
interaction with other drugs, 731
mechanisms of action in smooth muscle, 704–706
  contraction and, 705, *705*, *706*
  relaxation and, 705–706, *706*
pharmacokinetics of, 714–717
  aerosols and, 716, *716*
  comparative systemic effects of inhaled beta$_2$ agonists and, 717, 717t, *718*, 718t
  continuous nebulization and, 716
  deposition and efficacy of MDI versus nebulization and, 716–717, 717t
  intravenous administration and, 715–716. *See also* Sympathomimetics
  oral administration and, 714–715, *715*
  subcutaneous administration and, 715, *715*
physiologic actions of, 708–714
  antiinflammatory, 713, 713t, *714*
  antipermeability, 713–714
  on bronchial smooth muscle, 709–710, *710*, 710t
  duration of action and, 711t, 711–712, *712*, 712t
  guinea pig tissues used to determine selectivity and, 710t, 710–711
  on guinea pig trachea versus human bronchi, 711, *711*
  on heart, 708–709, *709*
  inhaled route and, 713, *713*
  intravenous infusion and, 712–713
  in vivo studies in humans, 712
during pregnancy and nursing, 1091
in status asthmaticus, 694–695
tachyphylaxis, 703–704, 704t, 737, 1157–1158
Beta-adrenergic antagonists, bronchial provocation tests and, 510
Beta-adrenergic blocking agents
  airway hyperresponsiveness and, 36
  asthma caused by, 622t, 623t
  asthma induced by, 449, 625t, 625–626, 1039t, 1191
Beta adrenoceptors, 700–704, 701t
  in airways, 701
  blockade and, 176–184, 567
  corticosteroid reversal at receptor level and, 704
  cyclic AMP synthesis and, 192–193, *193*, 194–195, *195*, *196*
  decreases in numbers and reactivities of, 178–179
  desensitization, 703–704, 704t
  distribution of, 756
  drug-receptor interaction and, 702, *702*
  in experimental animal models, 393–394, *394*
  functional responses, 701t
  G-protein coupling to adenylyl cyclase and, 193, 703
  in heart, 701–702
  "interconversion" theory and, 179–180
  kinase (βARK), 703
  muscle relaxation and, 211

in occupational asthma, 588
radioligand binding studies and, 702–703
regulation of, 194
shifting in subtypes and responses of, 179
smooth muscle, 328–329
  desensitization of, 329
structure and ligand binding and, 209, 702, *702*
tissue distribution, 701
transcriptional effects of corticosteroids and, 802, *802*, *803*
in vessels and parenchyma, 701
in vitro desensitization of, *703*, 703–704. *See also* Beta-adrenergic agonists; Tachyphylaxis
  long-term, 704, 704t
  by products or action of phospholipase A$_2$, 704
  short-term, 703–704, *704*
Beta-adrenoceptor stimulators. *See also specific drugs*
  in acute severe asthma, 756–761
    administration routes and, 757, 757–758, *758*
    combination with anticholinergic agents, 759
    combination with corticosteroids, 759
    combination with theophylline, 759
    distribution of beta$_1$ and beta$_2$-adrenoceptors and, 756
    nonselective drugs and, 759–760
    pharmacokinetics of, 756, 757t
    selective drugs and, 760–761, *761*
    side effects of, 729, 733–737, 756–757
    tolerance and, 758–759
Beta-arrestin, atopy and, 183
Beta blocking agents, 1191
Betamethasone, aerosol, 821t
Beta sympathomimetics, interaction with anesthesia, 1102
Betaxolol, asthma caused by, 625–626
Biofeedback, 1126–1127
Birds and asthma, 599
Birth, season of, 27–28
Bitolterol, 687t, 687–688, 724
  aerosol, 720t
Bitolterol mesylate, 1225
Bladder, beta agonists and, 735–736
Blood cell count, 451, 980
Blood chemistry, 451, 957
Blood gas tension, conscious recognition of, 350
Blood vessels, beta-adrenergic receptors in, 701
B-lymphocytes. *See* B-cells
BN-52063, 292, 894
Body rhythms, bronchial provocation tests and, 511
Bombesin, airway effects of, 234, 245
Bone marrow transplantation, 156
Bordetella pertussis, 567
Botanical regions of the United States and Canada, 1203–1209
Botrytis, 1210–1211
Bradykinin, 98–99, 100t
  adenosine-induced bronchoconstriction and, 256
  control of mucus production and, 367
  as inflammatory mediator, 86
  inhalation challenge with, 504
  sensory nerve activation and, 242
Breast feeding, IgE levels and, 27
Breathing
  control of. *See* Ventilatory control
  loaded, conscious recognition of, 350
  work of

decreased, intermittent positive pressure breathing and, 1115, *1116*
as risk factor for status asthmaticus, 991–992
Breathing exercises, educational materials on, 1213
Breathing pattern, particle deposition and, 412
Breathlessness, circadian rhythm of perception of, nocturnal asthma and, 1033
BRL-38227, 964
Bromhexine, 929–930
Bronchi, 296
Bronchial biopsy, inflammation and, 80–81, 298, 834
Bronchial casts, 356, 361
Bronchial challenge testing
  in cough variant asthma, 646
  nonspecific, in occupational asthma, 604–605
  specific, in occupational asthma, 605
Bronchial hyperresponsiveness, 29, 32–39, 81, 936, 1195–1196
  airway permeability and, 35
  airway smooth muscle abnormalities and, 38
  beta$_2$ agonists and, 39
  circadian rhythm and, 1031
  correlating with other factors, inhalation challenge and, 505–506
  corticosteroid effects on, 804–805, *805*, 833
  cough in, 647
  defining, inhalation challenge and, 505
  definition and measurement of, 32–33, *33*
  disodium cromoglycate and, 858
  eosinophils and, 266–267
  in exercise-induced asthma, 616–617
  in experimental asthma. *See* Experimental asthma, airway hyperreactivity in
  genetic factors and, 29
  humoral mediators and, 37t, 37–38
    causing transient bronchoconstriction, 37
    proinflammatory, 37, *38*
  inflammation and, 33–34, *34*
  leukotrienes and, 116–118, *117*, 117t, *118*
  loss of inhibitory mechanisms and, 38–39
    allergen-injection therapy and, 39
    iatrogenic factors and, 39
    inhaled beta$_2$ agonists and, 39
  lymphokines and, 431–432
  neurologic abnormalities and, 36–37
    alpha-adrenergic system and, 36
    beta-adrenergic blockade, 36
    cholinergic overactivity, 36
    local axon reflexes and, 37
    nonadrenergic noncholinergic excitatory nerves and, 36–37
    nonadrenergic noncholinergic inhibitory nervous system and, 36
  in occupational asthma, 587
  physical and structural airway abnormalities and
    airway permeability and, 35–36
    airway wall thickness and, 36
    reduced caliber, 35, *35*
  platelet-activating factor and, 291
  population studies and, 17
  prostanoids and, 122
    pharmacologic modulation of activity of, 124, 125t
  structural changes in airway epithelium and, 297–300
    asthma and, 297–298, *299–301*
    viral infections and, 298, 300

Bronchial hyperresponsiveness (*continued*)
  T-cell(s) and, 429–431, 431t
  T-cells as effector cells of delayed-type
    hypersensitivity in genesis of, 431
Bronchial provocation tests, 489, 501–512
  with acetylcholine, 503
  with adenosine, 504
  aerosol generation, delivery, and
    penetrance and, 511
  with allergens, 506–507
  with carbamylcholine, 503
  circadian and other body rhythms and, 511
  comparison of, 504t, 504–505, 505t
  comparison of skin tests and, 507
  for convincing patients of cause-and-effect
    relationships, 509
  with diluent, 503
  effects of medications on, 510–511
  emotional factors and, 511
  for evaluation of cough, 646
  for evaluation of immunotherapy, 509
  for evaluation of new allergens in
    pulmonary disease, 509
  for evaluation of new treatments that block
    provocative challenges, 509
  with histamine phosphate, 504
  with hypertonic saline, 504
  immediate versus late response and,
    507–509, 509t
  indications for performing, 505–506
  influence of pulmonary function
    measurement, 502, 502t
  interpretation and expression of results of,
    511–512, *512*, 512t
  with leukotrienes, 504
  location of response and, 507
  mediators and mechanisms and, 507
  with methacholine, 503
  in occupational asthma, 604–605
  oral challenge tests, 489
  other disease states and, 511
  patient preparation for, 501, 502t
  pregnancy and, 511
  with prostaglandins, 504
  safety considerations with, 501–502
  with serotonin, 504
  for standardization of allergenic extracts,
    509–510
  storage and standardization of
    pharmacologic bronchoconstrictive
    agents and, 503
  storage of antigens and, 510
  substitutes for skin tests and, 507
Bronchial reactivity, 16–17, 17t, *18*, 936
  calcium and, 957–960
  circadian rhythm of, nocturnal asthma
    and, 1031
  nonspecific, mast cell sensitivity and,
    519–522, *520*, 520t, *521*, 587
  pulmonary function and, 22
Bronchiectasis, in allergic bronchopulmonary
    aspergillosis, 637
Bronchioli, 296
Bronchiolitis
  differential diagnosis of, 469–470, 470t,
    477t
  in infant and young child, 571
Bronchiolitis obliterans, irritant gases
    causing, 471
Bronchitis
  asthmatic, differential diagnosis of, 475t
  chronic
    definition of, 9
    differential diagnosis of, 472, 477t
    eosinophilic, 83

Bronchoalveolar lavage, 309–312
  inflammation and, 80
  inflammatory cells in fluid and, 304,
    309–310, *310*
    after antigen challenge, 311–312, 312t
  inflammatory mediators in fluid and, 80,
    122, 139, 158, 266, 298, 310–311, *311*
    after antigen challenge, 311–312, 312t
    late asthmatic response and, 139, 311
  leukotrienes in fluid and, 118
  measuring particle retention and, 414
Bronchocentric granulomatosis, differential
    diagnosis of, 478t
Bronchoconstriction
  allergic, histamine and, 328
  beta-blockade-induced, 625–626
  in experimental animal models, 384
  leukotriene-induced, mechanisms of, 116
  nocturnal, 342
  stimuli for, 32, *33*
Bronchoconstrictive agents, storage and
    standardization of, 503
Bronchodilation, intermittent positive
    pressure breathing and, 1115
Bronchodilators, 686–690. *See also specific
    drugs and drug types*
  in acute asthma, 974, 977–979
    single-drug combinations and, 974, *977*
    two-drug combinations and, *978*,
      978–979
  anticholinergic. *See* Anticholinergic agents
  antiinflammatory agents versus, 685–686,
    686t
  beta-adrenergic, 717–727. *See also specific
    drugs*
    in asthma treatment, 737–738
    bladder adverse effects of, 735–736
    central nervous system adverse effects
      of, 735
    duration, 727
    evolution of, 708, *709*
    hypokalemia and, 733–734
    inhaled, 727–729, *728*
    interaction with other drugs, 731–733,
      732, *733*
    metabolic effects of, 733–734
    mortality and, 736–737, 1157–1159
    myocardial toxicity of, 734–735,
      1049–1050
    oral, 729–730
    paradoxical bronchospasm and, 736
    reduction in PaO$_2$ and, 733
    selectivity assessment, 709–711
    skeletal muscle adverse effects of, 735
    subcutaneous and intravenous, 730t,
      730–731
    tachyphylaxis and, 703, 707–708, 737
    tumorgenicity of, 736
    vascular smooth muscle adverse effects
      of, 736
  cardiac rhythm and, 1046
  changes after administration to,
    bronchoreversibility assessment and,
    456
  in childhood asthma, 1069–1071, 1073
    acute, 1076–1077
  in chronic severe asthma, 1057–1058
  elderly patients and, 1020–1021
  localization of response to,
    bronchoreversibility assessment and,
    456–457, *457*, 457t
  mode of administration of,
    bronchoreversibility assessment and,
    455–456
  mucokinesis and, 923

reversibility of airflow obstruction and,
    337, 337t
  in stable asthma, cardiac rhythm in, 1046,
    1047t, 1048
  in status asthmaticus, 998–999, 1001–1002
  ventilation-perfusion relationship and, 339
Bronchomotor reflexes, 220
Bronchomucotropics, 925, 925t
Bronchoprovocation, drug studies and,
    792–793
Bronchopulmonary aspergillosis, allergic,
    differential diagnosis of, 478t, 480
Bronchoreversibility, assessment of, 455–457
  criteria for, 337
  density dependence and, 457
  mode of bronchodilator administration
    and, 455–456
  partial expiratory flow-volume maneuvers
    and, *6*, 456
  pulmonary function test selection for, 455
  significance of changes after
    bronchodilator administration and,
    456
  site of airflow limitation and localization of
    bronchodilator response and, *7*,
    456–457, 457t
Bronchorrhea, bronchial mucus in, 361
Bronchorrheics, 925–926
Bronchoscopy, fiberoptic, 1118–1119, 1119t
Bronchospasm, 12
  aerosol corticosteroids and, 830–831
  allergic, leukotrienes and, 330
  anesthesia and, 1106–1107
  exercise, incitants of, 444–445
  induced by viral infection, pathophysiology
    of, *7*, 566–568
  oral versus aerosol steroids and, 836
  paradoxical, beta agonists and, 736
Bronchospastic mediators, 12
Brownian diffusion, 406
Budesonide, aerosol, 821t, 1228
  dosing frequency for, 827
  HPA axis suppression and, 847
Building-related illness, 582, 582t
Byssinosis, 444, 597

Calcitonin gene-related peptide, 241–242
  airway effects of, 241–242
  airway smooth muscle and, 241
  control of mucus production and, 366
  localization of, 241
  vascular effects of, 241, *241*
Calcium
  airway reactivity and, 957–960
  airway smooth muscle contraction and,
    945–950, *946–949*
    cyclic AMP and relaxation and, 203–204,
      949–950, *951*
    inositol-lipid signal and, 182–183, 205
    intracellular calcium and, 947–949, *950*
    receptor-operated channels and, 705,
      947
    voltage-operated channels and, 945–946
  channels, 204–205
  histamine release and, 105
  mast cell secretion and, 277
  mediator release, 105
  mucus and, 366
  oxyradicals and, 964
  plasma ionized, 960
  receptor activation and cellular events
    and, *947*
  reciprocal adrenoceptor activities and,
    182–183, 705
  smooth muscle contraction and, 203–206

electromechanical coupling and, 204–205

pharmacomechanical coupling and, *205*, 205–206

sensitized, 321

smooth muscle relaxation and, 210–211, 705–706

Calcium channel blockers, 692, 950–959. *See also specific drugs*

clinical studies of, 955–957, 959

clinical utility of, 951–957

pharmacokinetics and drug interactions of, 955

pharmacology of, 951, 952t, 953t, 953–955, *954*, 955t, 956t, *957–959*, 958t

rationale for use of, 950–951

Calcium ions, reciprocal adrenoceptor activities and, 182

Caldesmon, 945

Caldwell-Luc procedure, in sinusitis, 542–543

Calmodulin

cellular calcium and, 105, 204, 945

histamine release and, 105

Calmodulin antagonism, 965

Calor, 80

Calponin, 948

Camps, for children, 1217–1219

Candidiasis, aerosol corticosteroids and, 832

Canine allergic inhalant dermatitis, 382

Capnography, 1109

Capsaicin, 238, 242–243, 644

Carbamylcholine, inhalation challenge with, 503

Carbon monoxide, 554, 578

Carbon monoxide diffusing capacity, 340–341, *341*, 341t

S-Carboxymethylcysteine, 930, 930t

Carboxypeptidase, mast cell, 275

Carcinoid syndrome, differential diagnosis of, 469, 477t

Cardiac asthma, 3, 1038

differential diagnosis of, 463–464, 476t

Cardiac pathology, 734, 1049–1050, *1050*

Cardiac rhythm, 735, 1046–1049

in acute asthma, 1048

fatal asthma and, 1158

nonsedating antihistamines and, 1049

in stable asthmatics, 1046, 1049

bronchodilators and, 1046, 1047t, 1049

in status asthmaticus, acute severe asthma, and respiratory failure, 1048

theophylline toxicity and, 1048–1049, 1049t

Cardiovascular disease, 1038–1042, 1168

antiasthmatic therapy in, 1039t, 1039–1042

adrenergic agonists in, 1039t, 1039–1040

anticholinergic agents in, 1040–1041, *1041*

inhaled corticosteroids in, 1040

methylxanthines in, 1041–1042

nonsteroidal antiinflammatories in, 1041

cardiovascular drug interactions and, 1038–1039, 1039t

Cardiovascular system. *See also* Cardiac rhythm; Cardiovascular disease; Electrocardiography; Heart

adverse effects on, drug studies and, 794

anesthesia and, 1105

effects of asthma on, 1045–1046

clinical and electrocardiographic evidence of right heart dysfunction and, 1046

pulsus paradoxus as, 1045–1046, 1046t

sinus tachycardia as, 996, 1045

systemic hypertension and hypotension as, 1038–1039, 1045

Carotid body, ventilation control and, 348, *348*

resection, 1148

Cascade impactors, 409

Case studies, of psychiatric aspects, 1124–1125

Cat dander, 443, 552–553, 1143

Catecholamines

adrenergic transmission and. *See* Autonomic nervous system, adrenergic transmission and

natural, fate of, 700

Catechol-*O*-methyltransferase, in metabolic degradation of catecholamines, 170, 686, 718

Cattle dander, 553

CD3/TCR complex, 53

Cefaclor, in sinusitis, 542t

Cell-surface receptors, 200

Central nervous system, beta agonists and, 735

Cephalosporium, 1210–1211

Cerebral dominance, immune disorders and, 423–424

Cetirizine, 884–885

CFC propellants, 751, 1158

C-fibers, 221, 227, 242

Chaetomium, 1210–1211

Charbtoxin, 244, 964

Charcoal, 778–779

Charcot-Leyden crystals, 354

in sputum, 657–658

Chemical substances, 4–5. *See also specific substances*

challenge with, in experimental animal models, 392–393

hypersensitivity pneumonitis and, 632, 633t

occupational asthma and, 600t

as stimuli to breathing in asthma, *348*, 348–349

Chemotactic factors, in mast cells, 274

Chemotherapeutic agents, asthma caused by, 623t

Chest films, 664–674

in allergic bronchopulmonary aspergillosis, *638*, 638–639

in complicated patients, 670–674, *670–675*

in uncomplicated patients, 664–665, *665–670*, 670

Chest physiotherapy, 695, 1115–1116

Chest tightness, 448

Childbearing, drug studies and, 795–796

Childhood asthma, 1062–1079

acute, 1075–1079

emergency room discharge and, 1077

endotracheal tube placement in, 1078

history in, 1075–1076, 1076t

hospital admission criteria for, 1077

in-hospital management of, 1077

initial assessment in, 1075

investigations in, 1076

management during hospital recovery and, 1079

pathophysiology of, 1075

physical examination in, 1076, 1076t

treatment of, 976t, 1076–1077, 1077t

treatment of respiratory failure in, 1077–1078

ventilation strategy in, 1078–1079

during adolescence, 1074

cough-variant, 646, 1074

epidemiology of, 1062–1064

morbidity and mortality and, 1062, *1063*, 1064, *1064*, *1157*, 1158t

prevalence and, 1062, 1063t

establishing diagnosis of, 1065t, 1065–1066, 1066t, *1067*, 1068

etiology of, 1064–1065

air pollution and, 1065

atopy and, 1064–1065

genetic influences in, 1064

parental smoking and, 1065

respiratory infections and, 1065

socioeconomic factors in, 1065

exercise-induced, 1074–1075

fatal asthma and, 1161, 1161t

growth retardation, 1174

HPA axis in, 846–847

"impossible," 1075, 1075t

in infants and young children, 1074

management of, 1068t, 1068–1072

environmental control in, 1068, 1069t

immunotherapy in, 1068–1069

patient education and supervision in, 1068

pharmacologic, 1069–1072

psychological, 1069

natural history of, 22, 1079, 1079t

nocturnal, 1075

pharmacologic management of, 1069–1074

anticholinergics in, 1070

antiinflammatory drugs in, 1071t, 1071–1073, 1073t

bronchodilators in, 1069–1071, 1070t, 1073

inhaled corticosteroids in, 1073–1074

maintenance oral steroids in, 1074

methods of drug delivery and, 1072t, 1072–1073

steroid-sparing agents in, 1074

Children. *See also* Adolescence; Childhood asthma; Infants

aspiration in, 1024

drug studies and, 796–797

food allergy in, 560–561

infections in, 571–573

summer camps for, 1217–1219

Chlamydia pneumoniae infection, in older children and adults, 573

Chlorella, 553

Chlorpheniramine, 884

Cholecystokinin octapeptide, 246

Cholera toxin, adenylate cyclase activity and, 181, 195, *196*

Cholinergic agonists, 628

asthma caused by, 623t, 628

control of mucus production and, 366

experimental asthma and, *390*, 390–391

inhalation challenge with, in experimental animal models, *390*, 390–391

Cholinergic nervous system, 217

circadian rhythm of, nocturnal asthma and, 1033

contribution to asthma, 225–228

altered ganglionic or postganglionic transmission and, 227

altered output from peripheral receptors and, 226–227

anticholinergic therapy and, 227–228

clinical background of, 225, *225*

increased central output and, 225–226, *226*

control of airways, 217–219

central-peripheral heterogeneity of innervation and, 217

innervation in, 217

mechanisms of receptor-response coupling and, 219, *220*

modulation of neurotransmission and, 217–218

Cholinergic nervous system (*continued*)
  origins, organization, pathways, and
    actions and, 217
  parasympathetic ganglia and, 217
  receptor types in neurotransmission
    and, 219, 219t
  muscle tone and. *See* Muscle tone,
    cholinergic control of
  overactivity of, airway
    hyperresponsiveness and, 36
Cholinomimetic alkaloids, asthma caused by,
    623t
Chromaffin cells, 165–166
Chromogranin, 168
Chromogranin A, 168
Chronic asthma
  control of, 1191
  corticosteroids in, 811–812
  diagnosis of, 452
  exacerbations of, oral versus aerosol
    steroids and, 836
  hydration in, 917–918
Chronic obstructive pulmonary disease, 7t,
    7–8, 12, 1055
  acute exacerbations of, anticholinergic
    agents in, 881–882
  asthma versus, in elderly patients, 1017
  diagnosis of, 452
  oral versus aerosol steroids and, 836–837
  pathology of, versus asthma, 353
  relationship of asthma to, 12, 1174
  stable, anticholinergic agents in, *881*,
    881–882
Churg-Strauss syndrome, differential
    diagnosis of, 474, *474*, 478t, 480, 640
Chymase, mast cell, 275
Chymotrypsin, mast cell secretion and, 277
Cigarette smoking. *See* Smoking
Cigarettes, medicinal, as asthma therapy,
    1040
Cilia. *See also* Mucociliary apparatus
  chemical mediators effect on, 373
  mucociliary transport and, 373–374, *376*
  sputum and, 661
Circadian rhythms
  bronchial provocation tests and, 511
  in mucus production, 357
  nocturnal asthma and. *See* Nocturnal
    asthma
Circulation. *See also* Cardiovascular disease;
    Cardiovascular system; Vasculature
  bronchial, functional anatomy of, 352
  pulmonary, 330
    as risk factor for status asthmaticus, 991
Citric acid, 392
Cladosporium, 442, *443*, 552t
  immunotherapy and, 940
Clara cells, 365
Clemastine, 884
Climate. *See also* Weather
  moving to change, 581, 1143
  in occupational asthma, 586
  therapeutic, 1146
Clinical asthma, histamine antagonists in,
    886
Clinical evaluation, 447–453. *See also*
    Presenting symptoms
  diagnosis and, 451t, 451–452
  laboratory studies in, 450–451, 485–486,
    486t. *See also specific studies*
  physical findings and, 449–450
  presenting symptoms and, 447
  of severity, 452–453
Clinical incitants, 441–445
Clonal expansion, 424
Cluster of differentiation markers, 52

Cobalt, occupational asthma and, 602
Cocaine, asthma caused by, 627
Cocaine toxicity, differential diagnosis of,
    465, 476t
Cockroach allergy, 443
Codfish allergy, 443
Colchicine, 915
Colophony, occupational asthma and, 601
Compensation, occupational asthma and, 608
Complement, 99–101, *100*
  determination of, 494–495
  late asthmatic reactions and, 141
Complement receptors, of eosinophils,
    261–262
Complications, 1167–1175
  long-term sequelae, 1174–1175
  medical conditions complicated by
    asthma, 1173–1174
  related to pathophysiology of asthma,
    1167–1169, *1168*, 1168t, *1169*
  related to therapy, 1007, 1169–1173, 1170t,
    1172t, 1173t
  of ventilation, 1007, 1172t, 1173t
Computed tomography, 674
  in sinusitis, *541*, 542
Conducting airways, functional anatomy of,
    352, *353*, *354*
Congestive heart failure, diagnosis of,
    463–464
Conjunctivitis, allergic, disodium
    cromoglycate in, 858–859
Cor pulmonale, 448
Corticosteroid-dependent asthma,
    methotrexate in, 912–913
Corticosteroids, 690t, 690–691, 800–813. *See
    also specific drugs*
  in acute asthma, 836, *979*, 979–980
    severe, beta-adrenoceptor stimulants
      combined with, 759
  aerosol, 691, 818–837, *819*, 820t, 821t
    airway structure and function and,
      832–833
    alternatives to, 834–837
    ancillary treatment and, 834
    bioavailability of, 818
    in cardiovascular disease, 1040
    in childhood asthma, 1073–1074
    chronic excess effect, 826
    in chronic severe asthma, 836, 1058
    complicating infections with, 833
    COPD and, 836–837
    cortisol deficiency and, 825–826
    cost and cost benefits of, 836t, 837
    dose scheduling for, 828, *829*
    dosing frequency for, *827*, 827t, 827–828,
      828
    drug delivery and, 818, 821t, 828
    dry-powder formulations, 830
    duration of treatment with, *833*, 833–834
    effective dosage of, 819–820, 821t, *822*,
      823
    efficient intrapulmonary delivery and,
      828–831, *829*, 830t, *831*, 831t
    high-dose, 819, 845–846, 850, 1058
    HPA axis function and, 845–847, *846*,
      847, 848t–849t, 849–850
    inhalation technique, 830
    minimum dose requirements for,
      822–824, 823t, 825t
    oral versus, 835
    oropharyngeal complications with, 827t,
      831–832, *832*, 1171
    prednisone versus, 820–822, *824*, *825*
    reproductive and cytotoxic risk of, 826
    risk versus benefit of treatment with,
      824–825
    "safe" dosage for, 818–819

  in allergic bronchopulmonary aspergillosis,
    637, 641
  asthma caused by, 623t
  in asthmatic exacerbations due to viral
    respiratory infection, 573
  beta-adrenergic receptor reversal and, 704
  biologic mechanisms, 690
  bronchial hyperresponsiveness and late-
    phase responses and, 804–805, *805*
  bronchial provocation tests and, 510
  in childhood asthma, 1071t, 1071–1072
    acute, 1077
  in chronic asthma, 811–812
  circadian rhythm in, nocturnal asthma
    and, 1034
  complications of oral glucocorticoid
    therapy and, 812t, 812–813, 1170–1171
  dependency and methotrexate, 912
  desensitization of smooth muscle and,
    707–708, *708*
  dosage schedules for, 809–812
    in chronic asthma, 811–812
    exacerbation of previously stable asthma
      and, 809–811, *810*, *811*
    in subacute asthma, 811
  effect on inflammatory cells, 802–804, *803*
    eosinophils, 803–804
    lymphocytes, 804
    mast cells, 803
    monocytes and macrophages, 804
    neutrophils, 804
    vascular endothelial cells, 804
  effect on smooth muscle and mucosal
    glands, 804
  elderly patients and, 1021
  interactions with beta agonists, 732–733
  interaction with anesthesia, 1102–1103
  in late asthmatic reactions, 142
  mechanisms of action of, 800–802
    glucocorticoid receptors and, 801, *801*
    modulation of gene transcription and,
      801, *801*
    molecular, 800
    transcriptional effects and, 801–802
  oral, 691
  overall effect of, 805–806
  pharmacology of, 806–809
    bioavailability and, 807, 807t
    choice of oral glucocorticoid and, 806,
      806, 806t
    daily versus alternate-day therapy and,
      809, 809t, 820
    dose-dependent pharmacokinetics and,
      807
    hypothalamic-pituitary axis and,
      808–809, *809*
    sparing effect of TAO, 901–908
    speed of action and, 807–808, *808*
    transport and protein binding and,
      806–807
  during pregnancy, 1085
  during pregnancy and nursing, 1090–1091
  resistance and, 835
  in sinusitis, 542t
  in status asthmaticus, 695, 809–811, *810*,
    811, 1002–1003
  in subacute asthma, 811
  withdrawal, 809, 811, 820
Cortisol deficiency, aerosol corticosteroids
    and, 825–826
Cortisol nocturnal patterns, 847
Costs. *See* Economic factors
Cotransmission, nonadrenergic,
    noncholinergic nerves and, 233–234,
    234
  vasoactive intestinal peptide and
    acetylcholine and, 236–237, *237*

Cotton dust, 444
  occupational asthma and, 597
Cottonseed, 556
Cough, 448, 1191
  as manifestation of infectious asthma, 573
  mucociliary dysfunction and, 378
  reflex, aerosol corticosteroids and, 830–831
Cough-variant asthma, 644–647, *645–647*
  in childhood, 1074
Creola bodies, 656–657
Crisis intervention plan, in chronic severe asthma, 1059t, 1059–1060
Cromakalim
  in asthma, 211, 244, 964
  blockade of antigen inhalation challenge by, 511
Cromolyn-binding protein, 855–856
Cromolyn sodium, 691–692, 1233
  adverse effects, 1171
  asthma aggravated by, 627
  bronchial provocation tests and, 510
  in childhood asthma, 1071, 1071t
  in exercise-induced asthma, 618
  in food allergy, 563
  in late asthmatic reactions, *132*, 142
  as MDI, 691
Cross-bridge(s), 203
Cross-bridge cycling, 203
  normally cycling and latch cycling bridges, *316*, 316–317, *317*
Crossover asthma, 340, 685, 995
Crossover study design, for drug studies, 788
Croup, 571–572
  hysterical, 1148
Cryptogenic asthma, 6–7, 8t
Curschmann's spirals, 354
  in sputum, 658
Curvularia, 1210–1211
Cyclic AMP, 173–174, 192–195, *193*
  adrenergic responses and, in experimental animal models, 393
  degradation by cyclic nucleotide phosphodiesterases, 198
  mediator release and, 104–105
  muscle relaxation and, 210–211, 949–950, *951*
  phosphodiesterase activity of, reciprocal adrenoceptor activities and, 181–182
  protein kinases dependent on, 195–198, *197*
  types of, 173–174
  synthesis of, 192–195
    adenylate cyclase and, 194
    beta₂-adrenergic receptor regulation and, 194–195, *195*, *196*
    beta₂-adrenergic receptors and, 192–193, *193*
    guanine nucleotide-binding proteins and, 193, *194*
Cyclic GMP, 199–200, *200*
  degradation by cyclic nucleotide phosphodiesterases, 198
Cyclic nucleotide(s), 192, 197–198. *See also* Cyclic AMP; Cyclic GMP
  during pregnancy, 1086
Cyclic nucleotide phosphodiesterases. *See* Phosphodiesterases, cyclic nucleotide
Cyclooxygenase inhibitors
  following antigen challenge in animal models, 385–386
  aspirin-induced asthma and, 622
  clinical studies of, 892–893
    in aspirin-sensitive asthmatics, 892
    in NSAID-responsive asthmatics, 892–893
    in unselected asthmatics, 892
  prostanoid action and, 123–126

Cyclosporine, 90, 914–915, 1058
Cysteine derivatives, 926t, 926–927
Cystic fibrosis
  allergic bronchopulmonary aspergillosis and, 639–640
  differential diagnosis of, 470–471, 477t
  theophylline and, 772
Cytochalasins, mast cell secretion and, 277
Cytokines, 54t, 429, 430t. *See also*
    Lymphokines; *specific cytokines*
  eosinophil function and, 265
  epithelium-derived, 302
  inflammatory, 431t
  as inflammatory mediators, 86–87, *87*
  in mast cells, 274
  mononuclear cell-derived, *151*, 151–153, 152t
Cytologic sputum examination, technique for, 1223
Cytotoxicity
  of eosinophils, 265
  IgE-dependent, mediators of, 59, 60f
Cytotoxic risks, aerosol corticosteroids and, 826

Dander. *See* Epidermal allergens; *specific animals*
Dapsone, 914, 914t
DCHA. *See* Fish oil, fatty acids derived from
Death. *See* Fatal asthma; Mortality
Defense mechanisms, in elderly patients, 1020, 1020t
Definition of asthma, 3–10, 11–13
  clinical categorization and, 6–8, 7t, 8t
  common features and, 5
  disease concept and, 3–4
  primary, 5–6
  quantitative terms in, 8–9
  severity grading and, 9–10, 10t
Dehumidifiers, for environmental control, 1140
Delayed-type hypersensitivity reaction, T-cells as effector cells of, 431
Delivery, 1092–1093
Delta-PPT, 238
"De novo pathway," 290
Density gradient ultracentrifugation, of bronchial mucus, 359, *359*
Dermatophagoides farinae, 443, 551, *551*, 1160. *See also* House dust mites
Dermatophagoides pteronyssinus, 443, 551–552, 1160. *See also* House dust mites
Dermis, mast cells in, 278
Desensitization. *See also* Immunotherapy; Tachyphylaxis
  to aspirin, 624
  during acute anaphylaxis, 707
Dexamethasone sodium phosphate, 1228
Diabetes mellitus, 1042
  asthma protocol in, 1042
Diacylglycerol, smooth muscle contraction and, 206–207, 948
Diagnosis of allergic bronchopulmonary aspergillosis, 636, 636t
Diagnosis of asthma, 451t, 451–452. *See also specific symptoms and tests*
  in asymptomatic patients, 451
  in children, 1065t, 1065–1066, 1066t, *1067*, 1068
  differential, 459–480, 460t, *461*, *479*
  occupational asthma and. *See*
    Occupational asthma, diagnosis of
  severe asthma and, 1054–1055, *1055*
  in symptomatic patients, 451–452
Diagnosis of esophageal dysfunction, 1026t, 1026–1027

Diagnosis of food allergy, *560*, 560t, 560–561, 561t
Diagnosis of hypersensitivity pneumonitis, 635
Diagnosis of sinusitis. *See* Sinusitis, diagnosis of
Diet(s), 1147, 1149
  aberrant, 772
  elimination, 490, 562
Differential diagnosis of asthma, 452, 459–480, 460t, *461*, 475t–478t, *479*, 480
Diffusing capacity, 340–341, *341*, 341t
  during pregnancy, 1087
5,15-DIHETE, and eosinophils, 262
5,18-DIHETE, and eosinophils, 262
Dihydroalprenolol, 179
Diisocyanates, occupational asthma and, 601–602
Diltiazem, 954–955
Diluents, 923–925
  bronchial provocation tests and, 503
Dipyridamole, adenosine-induced bronchoconstriction and, 254
Disability, in occupational asthma, 608
Disease concept, 3–4
Disease states, bronchial provocation tests and, 511
Disodium cromoglycate (DSCG), 854–860
  adverse effects of, 859–860
  clinical efficacy of, 857–859
    in allergic conjunctivitis, 858–859
    in allergic rhinitis, 858
    in asthma, *857*, 857–858, 858t, *859*
    in other diseases, 859
  chemistry of, 854, *855*
  compared to other antiallergy drugs, 856t
  cost effectiveness of, 860
  dose and administration of, 859, 860t
  mechanism of action of, 855–857, 856t, *857*, 857t
  pharmacokinetics of, 854–855
  during pregnancy and nursing, 1091
  preparations of, 860
Distribution of ventilation, 334–335, *336*
Diuretics, 895
  asthma caused by, 623t
  clinical studies of, 895, *895*
  new applications of, 1147–1148
DNA in secretions, 357
Dog dander, 553
Dolor, 80
Dopamine, 166–167
Downregulation
  adrenoceptors and, 175–176
  IgE biosynthesis and, 62–63
Drive, ventilatory, measurement of, 346–348, *347*
Drug(s). *See also specific drugs and drug types*
  aerosol. *See also* Aerosol delivery systems; *specific drugs and drug types*
    beta-adrenergic agonists, 716, *716*
  educational materials on, 1213
  emergence of, 1146
  hypersensitivity pneumonitis and, 632
  as incitants, 444
  mechanisms of action, 686t
  in occupational asthma, 590
  response to, inhalation challenge and, 506
  therapeutic, 1224–1233
    development of. *See* Drug development
  in exercise-induced asthma, *617*, 617–618
  in late asthmatic reactions, 142–143
  new applications of old drugs, 1147t, 1147–1148

Drug challenges, 490
Drug development, 784–798, *785*, 785t
  phases of study for, 785–787, *785–787*,
    787t
  study design for, 787–798
    acute asthma and, 797
    adolescence and, 796
    age range and, 787
    baseline evaluation and, 791
    center number and, 788
    childhood and, 796–797
    children and, 796
    controls and, 788
    crossover or parallel group, 788
    dosage considerations and, 774, 788–789
    duration and, 789
    efficacy parameters and, 791–793, *793*
    elderly patients and, 797
    generic issues and, 797–798
    inclusion-exclusion criteria and, 789,
      789t
    laboratory values outside normal
      reference range and, 789–791, *790*,
      790t
    patient selection and, 787–788
    safety parameters and, 794–795
    sample size and, 787
    study blinding and, 788
    women of childbearing potential and,
      795–796
Drug-induced asthma, 444, 449, 590, 621–628,
    622t, 623t. *See also* Aspirin-induced
    asthma
  angiotensin-converting enzyme inhibitors
    and, 627
  antibiotics and, 626
  beta-adrenergic blocking agents and, 625t,
    625–626
  cholinergic agonists and, 628
  cough and, 627, 830
  differential diagnosis of, 475t
  enzymes and, 626
  irritants and, 627
  mast cell mediators and, 627–628, 628t
  nonsteroidal antiinflammatory drugs and,
    621–622, 624t, 624–625
Dry-powder formulations, of aerosol
    corticosteroids, 830
Dry-powder inhalers, 409, 752
  breathing pattern and, 412
  in childhood asthma, 1072
Dust
  cotton, 444
  occupational asthma and, 597
  wood, 444
Dyphylline, 1229, 1230, 1231
Dysphonia, inhaled corticosteroids and, 691,
    832
Dyspnea
  in asthma, 447
  conscious sensation of, 350
  exercise and, 444–445
  nocturnal, paroxysmal, 463

Early asthmatic responses, correlation of
    skin test results with clinical history
    and allergen inhalation test results
    and, 523–526, 524t
Economic factors, 1179–1183, *1180*, 1182t
  childhood asthma and, 1065
  cost-reduction studies and, 1182–1183,
    1183
  cost studies and, 1179–1180, 1181t
  emergency room visits and, 1181
  epidemiology and, 1181
  hospitalization and, 1181, 1181t

mortality and, 1155–1156
  in occupational asthma, 586
  physician office visits and, 1181
Educational materials, 1212–1214
Effector cells, 171
Efferent neural activity
  central origin of, 219–220, *221*, 221t
  peripheral inputs to, 220–222, *222*
Eicosanoids, immunoregulation and, 149
Eicosapentaenoic acid, 893
Elderly patients, 1017–1021, 1018t
  asthma versus COPD in, 1017
  defense mechanisms and, 1020, 1020t
  drug studies and, 797
  exercise capacity and, 1019t, 1019–1020
  pharmacology and, 1020–1021
    bronchodilators and, 1020–1021
    corticosteroids and, 1021
    theophylline and, 1021, 1021t
  physiologic aspects of aging and, 1018,
    1018t
  therapy in, 1020–1021
  ventilation and, 1018–1019, *1019*
    control of, 1019
    distribution of, 1018–1019
    gas exchange and, 1019
Electrical forces, particle deposition and, 406
Electrocardiography, 451, 1045–1049
  drug studies and, 795
  in status asthmaticus, 996
Electrolytes
  of mucus, 357–358
  in status asthmaticus, 1004
Electromechanical coupling, 204–205
Elimination diet, 490, 562
Emergency room visits, cost of, 1181
Emotional factors. *See* Psychiatric aspects;
    Psychological factors
Emphysema
  differential diagnosis of, 472, 477t
  hypoventilation in, 349
  parasympathetic activity in, 227
Endobronchial tuberculosis, differential
    diagnosis of, 467–468
Endorphins, 349, 992
Endothelin, *306*, 307
  receptors for, smooth muscle contraction
    and, *209*, 209–210
Endothelium-derived relaxing factor, 199–200
Endotracheal intubation
  in childhood asthma, acute, 1078
  particle deposition and, 410
Endotracheal tuberculosis, differential
    diagnosis of, 476t
Enkephalins, 246
Enprofylline
  in late asthmatic reactions, 142
  adenosine and, 254
Environmental control, 1137–1143, 1190
  air cleaners for home use and, 1137–1140,
    1138t
    air conditioners, 1137–1138, *1138*
    air filtration units, 1138–1140, *1139*,
      1143t
    electrostatic devices, 1139
    negative-ion generators, 1140
  for air pollution, 554t, 555t, 1142, 1142t
  for animal allergens, 1142–1143, 1143t
  in childhood asthma, 1068, 1069t
  home visits by health professionals for,
    1143
  for house dust mites, 1140–1142
  for molds, 1142
  moving to different climate and, 581, 1143
  for odors, 1142
  standard methods for, 1137, 1138t

Environmental factors. *See also* Air pollution;
    Climate; Weather; *specific factors*
  airway inflammation caused by, 17, *18*
  protection from unfavorable air
    environments and, 581–583
    avoidance and, 582
    personal protection and, 582t, 582–583,
      583t
  scientific and clinical evaluation of, 577
  toxins, 471, 477t
Enzyme(s), asthma induced by, 599t, 626
Enzyme allergosorbent test, 493
Enzyme-linked immunoassay, direct
    measurement of antigen-specific
    immunoglobulin E and, 491–492
Enzyme-linked immunosorbent assay,
    489–490
Enzymes, mucolytic, 927
Eosinophil(s), 258–267, 451
  antigen expression in, 262
  asthma and, 265–267
    antigen challenge studies and, 266–267
    in biopsy, 266
  chemotactic activity of
    late asthmatic reactions and, 141
    migration and, 262
  chemotactic factors, 262t
  cord blood and, 259
  corticosteroid effects on, 803–804
  counts of, 495
  cytokines and, 265
  cytotoxicity of, 265
  derived factors, 496
  differentiation of, 258–259
    cytokines in, 258
  heterogeneity of, 259
  hyperresponsiveness and, 266
  as inflammatory cells, 83–84, *84*
  late asthmatic reactions and, 139–140
  Mac-1 expression in, 261–262
  major basic protein in, 258, 264
  mediators secreted by, 262–265, *263*
    eosinophil granule proteins, 264
    granule-stored enzymes, 264
    lipid, 263–264
  migration of, 262, 262t
  morphology of, 258
  PAF and, 262, 263, 291
  parasites and, 258, 265
  production and function of, regulation of,
    156–157
  prolonged tissue survival of, 262
  receptors for, 259–262, *260*
    adhesion, 259–261, 260t, *261*
    complement, 261–262
    immunoglobulin, 261
  secretion and activation of, 265
  sinusitis and asthma and, 536, 536t
  in sputum, 657
  turnover in vivo, 259
Eosinophil cationic protein, 83, 264, 496
  in BAL fluid, 310
Eosinophil chemotactic factor of anaphylaxis
    (ECF-A), 101–102, 262, 274
Eosinophil-derived neurotoxin, 83, 264, 495
Eosinophilia
  airway, platelet-activating factor and,
    291–292
  in allergic bronchopulmonary aspergillosis,
    637–638
  atopy and, 17
  differential diagnosis of idiopathic
    hypereosinophilic syndrome and,
    473–474
  nonallergic rhinitis with eosinophilia
    syndrome and, 537, 538

pulmonary infiltration with, differential
  diagnosis of, 472–473, *473*, 478t
  sputum, 451
  in status asthmaticus, 996–997
  tropical, differential diagnosis of, 473t, 474,
    478t
Eosinophil peroxidase (EPO), 264
Eosinophils, in BAL fluid, 267, 309–310
EPA. *See* Fish oil, fatty acids derived from
Ephedrine, 720–721, 721t
  oral, 721t
Ephedrine sulfate, 1225
Epicoccum, 1210–1211
Epidemiology, 15–21, 16t. *See also specific*
    disorders
  age and sex and, 15–16, 16t
  of airway responsiveness, 16–17, 17t, *18*
  of atopic allergy, 17–19, *18*, 19t
  costs and, 1181
  familial aggregation and, 21
  methodological problems in, 15, 16t
  respiratory infection and, 19
  smoking and, 19–21
    active, 19–20, 20t
    passive, 20–21
  status asthmaticus and, 988
  weather and air pollution and, 21
Epidermal allergens, 443, 552–553. *See also*
    specific animals
  environmental control measures for,
    1142–1143, 1143t
  immunotherapy and, 940t, 940–941
Epinephrine, 687t, 688, 717–718, 1225, 1226
  in acute asthma, 974–981
  aerosol, 719t
  subcutaneous, 730, 730t, 731
    pharmacokinetics of, 715
Epinephrine bitartrate, 1225
Epinephrine hydrochloride, 1225–1226
Epithelial cells, in sputum, 656–657, 657t
Epithelial damage, in occupational asthma,
    589, 589–590
Epithelial mucous glycoprotein, in bronchial
    mucus, *358*, 358–359
Epithelium. *See also* Airway epithelium
  removal of, beta-adrenergic agonists and,
    707
Epithelium-derived relaxant factor, 239
  cholinergic modulation of, 224
  loss of, inflammation and, 87
Erythromycin, in sinusitis, 542t
Esophageal dysfunction, 1023–1028. *See also*
    Gastroesophageal reflux
  diagnosis of, 1026t, 1026–1027
  disease states and, 1024t
  pulmonary disease and, 1023–1026, 1024t,
    1025, 1030, 1173
  thrush, 832
  treatment of, 1027–1028
Esophagus, physiology of, 1023
Estrogen, during pregnancy, 1085–1086
Ethylnorepinephrine, 1226
Evaluation. *See* Clinical evaluation;
    Presenting symptoms
Evaporation, particle deposition and, 411,
    412t
Exercise, 1116, 1132–1133, *1133*, 1133t
  adenosine-induced bronchoconstriction
    and, 256
  breathing, educational materials on, 1213
  capacity for, in elderly patients, 1019t,
    1019–1020
Exercise bronchospasm, incitants of, 444–445
Exercise-induced asthma, 5, 7, 449, 533,
    612–618, 1132
  BAL in, 312

bronchial hyperreactivity and atopy and,
    616–617
  in childhood, 1074–1075
  cromolyn in, 858
  differential diagnosis of, 475t
  drugs and, *617*, 617–618
  histamine antagonists in, 886
  lung function changes in, 612, *613*
  mechanisms of, 614–616, *615, 616*
  physical factors influencing response to
    exercise and, 613, *613, 614*
  prevention of, 1190
  relation to hyperventilation-induced and
    osmotically induced asthma, 613–614,
    614
Expectorants, *8*, 927t, 927–929
Experimental asthma in animals, 382–397
  adrenergic and nonadrenergic responses
    in, 393–394, *394*
  airway hyperreactivity in, 394–397
    genetic factors and, 396–397
    inflammation and, 394–396
    viruses and, 396, *396*
  antigen challenge and, 382–388
    airway caliber changes and, *383*,
      383–384
    immunology and, 382–383
    late-phase reactions and, 386–388
    lung volume changes and, 384
    mediators and, 385–386, *386, 387*
    mucociliary dysfunction and, 386
    ventilation-perfusion abnormalities and,
      384–385, *385*
  histamine antagonists in, 886
  pharmacologic challenge and, 388–392
    cholinergic agonists and, *390*, 390–391
    histamine and, 388–390, *389*
    leukotrienes and, 392
    platelet-activating factor and, 392
    prostaglandins and, 391–392
    serotonin and, 391
  physical and chemical challenges and,
    392–393
  pulmonary mechanics in, 383
Expiratory flow-volume maneuvers, partial,
    bronchoreversibility assessment and,
    456, *456*
Exposure factors, in occupational asthma,
    585–586, *586, 587*
Extracellular matrix, airway epithelial
    regeneration and, 300, 302
Extracorporeal membrane oxygenation, 1007
Extrinsic allergic alveolitis. *See*
    Hypersensitivity pneumonitis
Extrinsic asthma, 8t, 441, 442t
  atopic, 6
  bronchial mucus in, 362t, 362–364, *363*,
    364t
  differential diagnosis of, 475t
  nonatopic, 6

Factitious asthma, differential diagnosis of,
    472, 477t
Family studies, of psychiatric aspects,
    1123–1124
Family therapy, 1127
Fatal asthma, 80, 736–737, 972, 1154–1162,
    1192
  in children, 1062
  history of, 1154
  incidence of, 988, 1154–1156, *1155*
    age and, 1154, *1155*
    economic factors and, 1155–1156
    gender and, 1154, *1156*
    geographic location and, 1154–1155
    race and, 1154, *1156*

increase in, 1156–1160
  allergens and, 1159
  Alternaria alternata and, 986
  asthma prevalence change and,
    1156–1157, 1157t
  atopy and, 1159–1160
  beta agonists and, 736–737, 1157–1158
  disease severity change and, 1157
  iatroepidemic and, 1157–1159
  International Classification of Disease
    code change and, 1156, *1156*
  pollution and, 1160
  season and, 1159
  sudden asphyxic asthma and, 985, 1160,
    1167
  theophylline and, 1158–1159
  undertreatment and, 1159
  pathophysiology of, 1160
  recommendations for prevention of, 1008,
    1161–1162, 1162t
  risk factors for, 1160–1161, 1161t
  subsensitivity in, 1157–1158
Fatty acids, alternative, 893. *See also* Fish oil;
    Tachyphylaxis
  clinical studies of, 893
Fatty substances, in sputum, in aspiration,
    661–662
FcεRII receptor, IgE interactions and, 58–59
FcεRI receptor
  IgE interactions and, 58
  immunoregulation and, 148t, 148–149
Feathers, 443, 553
Felodipine, 954
Fenoterol, 724
  comparative systemic effects of, 717, 717t,
    718, 718t
  in late asthmatic reactions, 142
Fenoterol hydrobromide, 1226
Fenton reaction, 960
Fetus, effect of asthma on, 1088–1089, 1089t
Fiberoptic bronchoscopy, 1118–1119, 1119t
  bronchoalveolar lavage and, 309
Fibrinogen degradation products, in
    pulmonary embolism, 461
Fibrosis, subepithelial, 88
Fish oil. *See also* Fatty acids, alternative
  dietary, 126–129, *127*
  fatty acids derived from
    in bronchial asthma, *128*, 128–129
    in vitro actions and 5-lipoxygenase
      pathway products of, 127
    in vivo incorporation and effects in
      generation of 5-lipoxygenase pathway
      products and leukocyte function, 127
    in vivo incorporation and generation of
      5-lipoxygenase pathway products,
      127–128
Flavonoids, *864*, 864–865, 865t
Flax dust, occupational asthma and, 597
Flow rates, reduced, 335–337, *337*
  localization of airflow obstruction and,
    336, *337*
  reversibility of airflow obstruction and,
    337, 337t
Flow volume curves, 466
Fluid replacement, 919–920
Flunisolide
  aerosol, 821t, 1228
  in sinusitis, 542t
Fluorescent allergosorbent test, 493
Fluticasone propionate, aerosol, HPA axis
    suppression and, 847
Folk remedies, 1145–1146, 1146t
  Oriental, 1145
  Western, 1145–1146
Fomes, 1210–1211

Food allergy, 449, 559–563
  additives and, 560
  allergens and, 27, 443–444. *See also
    specific allergens*
  diagnosis of, *560*, 560t, 560–561, 561t
  food challenge and, 561–562, 562t
  genetic factors, 27
  immunology and sensitization and,
    559–560
  treatment of, 562–563
Food challenge, 561–562, 562t
Food intolerance, 559
Food sensitivity, 559
Food testing, cytotoxic, 496
Foreign bodies, 445
Formaldehyde, 444, 581
  occupational asthma and, 596–597
Formoterol, 708, *709*, 725–726, *726*
Forskolin, 706
FPL 55712, 119, 378
Fungal infections, 28
Fungi
  as aeroallergens, 549–551
    classification of, 551, 552t
    identification of, 550–551
  hypersensitivity pneumonitis and, 632
Fura-2, 203, 949
Furosemide, 692
  inhaled, 895, *895*
  in late asthmatic reactions, 143
Fusarium, 1210–1211
Fusidium, 1210–1211

Galanin, 234, 246
Gallopamil, in late asthmatic reactions,
    142–143, 956
Gamma cameras, measuring particle
    retention and, 415
Gamma globulin infusions, 1058
Ganglionic transmission
  altered, in asthma, 227
  of bronchomotor activity, modulation of,
    222–224, *223*, *224*
Garlic, as mucoregulator, 930–931, *931*, 1145
Gas exchange, 338–340, *339*
  anticholinergic agents and, 882
  arterial blood gases and, 339t, 339–340,
    340, *341*
  in elderly patients, 1019
  status asthmaticus and, 992, *993–995*, 994,
    994t
Gastrin-releasing peptide, 245
  airway effects of, 245
  localization of, 245
Gastroesophageal reflux, 445, 1023, 1191. *See
    also* Esophageal dysfunction
  differential diagnosis of, 468–469, 477t
  nocturnal asthma and, 1030
Gastrointestinal tract
  food allergy and, 560
  mast cells in, 278
Gel phase, constituents of, 361
Gell and Coombs classification, 56t
Gender. *See* Sex
Generator potential, 166
Genetic factors, 21, 26–30, 448
  airway hyperreactivity in experimental
    asthma and, 396–397
  in childhood asthma, 1064
  IgE levels and, 26–29, 27t
  in intrinsic nonatopic asthma, 29–30, *30*
Gene transcription, corticosteroids and, *801*,
    801–802
Geographic location
  asthma therapy and, 995, 1150
  mortality and, 1154–1155
  in occupational asthma, 586

Geotrichum, 1210–1211
Geriatrics. *See* Elderly patients
Ginkgolides, 292, 894, 1145
Glucocorticoid(s). *See also* Corticosteroids
  HPA axis function and, 844–850
    aerosol therapy and, 845–847, *846*, *847*,
      848t–849t, 849–850
    suppression of, 844–845
  mucokinetic effect of, 923
Glucocorticoid receptors, 801, *801*
Glutathione peroxidase, 960, *961*, 964
Glycerol, iodinated
  as expectorant, 928
  as mucoregulator, 930
  in sinusitis, 542t
Glycoconjugates, in bronchial mucus,
    358–359
  epithelial mucous glycoprotein, *358*,
    358–359
  proteoglycans, 359
Glycoproteins, of mucus, 357, 358
  in asthma, 362t, 362–364, *363*, 364t
  epithelial, *358*, 358–359, 365
  normal, 361–362
  in status asthmaticus, 364
Glycopyrrolate, 689
Glycopyrrolate bromide, 879t
  in acute severe asthma, 880
  dose response and, 879
Glycosaminoglycans, of mucus, 358
GMP, cyclic, 199–200, *200*
Gold, 894–895, 913–914
  clinical studies of, 894–895, 913–914
  history of, 913
  toxicity of, 914, 914t, 1171
G-proteins
  beta adrenoreceptors linked to, 172–173
  coupling to adenylyl cyclase, 703
  cyclic AMP synthesis and, guanine
    nucleotide-binding proteins and, 193,
    194
  receptors coupled by, 426, 427t–428t, 702,
    948
Granulocyte-macrophage colony stimulating
    factor
  corticosteroid effects on inflammatory
    cells and, 802–804, *803*
  eosinophil differentiation and, 258
  epithelium-derived, 302–303
  immunoregulation and, 152t, 152–153
  mast cells and, 280
Granulomatosis, bronchocentric, differential
    diagnosis of, 478t
Grasses, pollens from, 549, *550*
Group therapy, 1127
GTPase, 195
Guaifenesin, 929
  in sinusitis, 542t
Guanine nucleotide–binding proteins, cyclic
    AMP synthesis and, 193, *194*
Guanosine monophosphate, cyclic, 199–200,
    200
Guanosine triphosphate–binding proteins,
    histamine release and, 102, 277–278
Guanyl nucleotide regulatory proteins,
    reciprocal adrenoceptor activities and,
    181
Guinea pig, experimental asthma in, 394

Habituation, 425
Health care costs. *See* Economic factors
Heart, 700. *See also* Cardiovascular disease;
    Cardiovascular system
  beta-adrenergic agonist actions on,
    708–709, *709*
  beta-adrenergic receptors in, 701–702

Helium-oxygen mixture, as asthma therapy,
    336, 457, 1007
Helminthosporium, 442, *443*, 552t, 1210–1211
Helminths and eosinophilia, 473
Helodermin, 237–238
Helper/inducer T-cell population, 55
Hematopoietic colony-stimulating factors,
    immunoregulation and, 152t, 152–153
Hemodynamics, anticholinergic agents and,
    882
Hemp dust, occupational asthma and, 597
Heparin, in mast cells, 272–273, 273t
5-HETE, 70
Heterologous desensitization, 176
Hidden asthma, differential diagnosis of, 459,
    475t
Hill's force-velocity relationship, 316
Histamine, 95–97, *96*, 96t
  adenosine-induced bronchoconstriction
    and, 254–255
  airway responsiveness to, 16
  following antigen challenge in animal
    models, 385, *387*
  assays for, 494
  in BAL fluid, 310–311, *311*
  exercise-induced asthma and, 617
  experimental asthma and, 388–390, *389*
  as inflammatory mediator, 85
  inhalation challenge with, 504, 505
    in experimental animal models, 388–390,
      389
  late asthmatic reactions and, 141
  in mast cells, 273–274
  mechanisms of release of, 102–105,
    103–104
    calcium/calmodulin and, 105
    cyclic AMP and, 104–105
    guanosine triphosphate-binding proteins,
      phospholipase C, and inositol
      phosphate pathway and, 102
    phospholipid methylation and turnover
      and, 102–103
  sensitized tracheal smooth muscle and,
    325, 328
    in allergic bronchoconstrictions, 328
    cholinergic component of response and,
      325, 328
    dose-response curves and, 325, *328*
    tachyphylaxis and, 328
  in sputum, 661
  in viral infections, 568
  in vitro antigen-induced leukocyte release
    of, 495–496
    basophil release and, 495–496
    passive sensitization of basophils and,
      496
Histamine antagonists, 884–886
  cardiac arrhythmias from, 1049
  in clinical asthma, 886
  dual action, 865
  in exercise-induced asthma, 886
  in experimental asthma, 886
  pharmacologic properties of, 885t
  safety of, 886, 1049
Histamine equivalent potency, 509
Histamine receptors, smooth muscle
    contraction and, 208
Histamine-releasing factors,
    immunoregulation and, 152t, 153
Histiocytes, in sputum, 658
History, patient
  in acute childhood asthma, 1075–1076,
    1076t
  childhood and, 1066
  correlation between skin test and
    inhalation test results in allergic

asthma. *See* Skin testing, correlation between history and inhalation test results in allergic asthma and
correlation of early asthmatic responses with, 523–526, 524t
in occupational asthma, 603–604
presenting symptoms and, 448–449
provocation tests and, 522–523
negative results and, 523
positive results and, 522–523
severity of asthma and, 13
HLA restriction, 53
HLA system, 52
Hormodendrum, 1210–1211
Hormones, mechanical heterogeneity of airway smooth muscle and, 320
Hormone therapy, 1148
Horse dander, 553
Hospitalization
in acute asthma, 982–983
in children, 1077
cost of, 1181, 1181t
rate in U.S., 1181t
status asthmaticus and, *695*, 695–696, *696*
House dust, *551*, 551–552
as allergen, 443
immunotherapy and, 937–939, 938t
House dust mites, *551*, 551–552, 937, 1160
environmental control measures for, 1140–1142
immunotherapy and, 143, 527t
5-HPETE, 112
H₁-receptor antagonists, 884, *885*
Human leukocyte antigen system, 52–53, *53*
Humidification, 920–922, 1115–1116
dangers of, 922
devices for, 921t, 921–922
mucus and, 921, 921t
Humidifiers, 1140
Humidifying masks, 583
Hydration, 917–920
in acute asthma, 918t, 918–920, 929t
in chronic asthma, 917–918
in status asthmaticus, 1003–1004
Hydrocortisone, 691
aspirin-induced asthma and, 622, 624
in status asthmaticus, 810, *810*
Hydrocortisone sodium succinate, 1228
Hydrogen peroxide, 961–962
Hydroxychloroquine, 914
5-Hydroxytryptamine, 97–98
Hygroscopicity, particle deposition and, 411, *412*
Hymenoptera, 553
Hyohimbine, 703
Hypercapnia
gas exchange and, 339, 973, 992–994
measurement of response to, 346–348, *347*
Hypereosinophilic syndrome, idiopathic, differential diagnosis of, 473–474, 478t
Hyperkalemia, 997
Hypersensitivity, 51, 56. *See also* Allergic reactions
delayed-type, T-cell(s) as effector cells of, 431
type I, 471
Hypersensitivity pneumonitis, 632–635
agents causing, 633t
avian, 553
clinical characteristics of, 632–633, 633t, *634*
diagnosis of, 635
etiologic agents of, 632, 632t
immunology of, 634
management of, 635
pathogenesis of, 634–635

pathologic findings in, 634
radiographic findings in, 633–634
Hypertension, 1038, 1039t, 1045, 1174
Hypertonic saline, mucokinetic effect of, 924–925
Hypervariable regions, 52
Hyperventilation, in experimental animal models, 393
Hyperventilation-induced asthma
mechanisms of, 615–616, *616*
relation to exercise-induced asthma, 613–614, *614*
treatment of, 618
Hypnosis, 1127
Hypokalemia, beta agonists and, 733–734, 757, 997, 1004
Hypophosphatemia, 997, 1004, 1172
Hyposensitization, 63–64
oral, 1152–1153
Hypotension, 1045
Hypothalamic-pituitary-adrenal function, 842–850
airflow obstruction and, 843–844
glucocorticoids and, 808–809, *809*
glucocorticoid therapy and, 844–850
aerosol therapy and, 818, 825, 845–847, *846*, *847*, 848t–849t, 849–850
suppression of HPA function and, 844–845
status in children, 846–849
tests of status of, 842–843, *844*
Hypothyroidism, definition of, 9
Hypoxemia
beta agonists and, 733, 1158
chemical stimuli to breathing and, 348
gas exchange and, 339, 339t, 340, 973, 992–994
measurement of response to, 346–348, *347*
mechanical stimuli to breathing and, 349
nocturnal, 341–342, *341–343*
ventilatory response to, during sleep, 350

Iatrogenic factors, 777, 989t, 1157
ICI 204, 219, 120, 198, 615, 890, 891, 891t
Idiopathic hypereosinophilic syndrome, differential diagnosis of, 473–474, 478t
Immediate asthmatic reactions, bronchial provocation tests and, asthmatic response, 507–509, 509t
Immune complex assays, 495
Immune disorders, cerebral dominance and, 423–424
Immune-neuroendocrine circuitry, 421–432
developmental relationships among cellular and humoral components of, 422–429
cells involved in synthesis, storage, secretion, and release of effector molecules of immunologic reactivities and, 422–423
cerebral dominance and immune disorders and, 423–424
immune regulation molecules and neural cell adhesion molecule and, 424
immune system and nervous system capacity to remember and, 424–426
neural crest interactions in development of immune system and, 423
recognition and communication powers of immune and neuroendocrine systems as shared characteristics and, 426, 427t–428t, 428–429
discovery of, 421–422
future of, 432
lymphocyte as unifying regulatory cell component of, 429–432

bronchial hyperresponsiveness and, 429–432, 431t
bronchial inflammation and, 429, 430t
delayed-type hypersensitivity reaction in genesis of airway hyperreactivity and, 431
emergence and significance of, 432, *433–435*
lymphokines and, 431–432
Immune recognition molecules, neural cell adhesion molecule, 424
Immune response, 50–56. *See also* Antigen(s)
alterations of, 568–569, *570*
clinical applications of, 56
foreignness and, 50
recognition of, 50–53, *51*, 51t
immunoglobulin supergene family and, 53
immunologically related disease and, *55*, 55–56, 56t
lymphokines and, 53–54, 54t
regulation of, 54–55
specific, regulation of, 28–29
supergenes, 53
Immune system. *See also* Immunoregulation
capacity to remember and, 424–426
neural crest interactions in development of, 423
recognition and communication powers of, 426, 427t–428t, 428–429
Immunity, 56
Immunogens. *See* Antigen(s)
Immunoglobulin(s)
antigen recognition and, 51–52
binding factors, 155
Immunoglobulin A, in sputum, 358, 361, 660
Immunoglobulin A receptors, of eosinophils, 261
Immunoglobulin E, 4, 26–29, 57–64, 68–77
in allergic bronchopulmonary aspergillosis, 638
antigen-specific, direct measurement of, 491–492
enzyme-linked immunoassays (ELISA) and, 491–492
fluorescence allergosorbent test (FAST) and, 491
immunoblotting, 492
immunoelectrophoresis, 492
radioallergosorbent test and, 491
atopy and, 17
atopic state and, 26, *27*
biosynthesis of, 60–63, 69–70, 72–73
antigen specificity of, 63
basic pathway of, 60, 61f
helper T-cell types and, 61, 61t
molecules involved in downregulation of, 62–63
molecules involved in upregulation of, 61–62
regulation by anti-IgE autoantibodies, 73–77, *75–77*
regulatory effects of interleukin-4 and interferon and, 70, 72–73, *73*, *74*
T-cell factors in, 69–70
bridging of, biochemical events following, 69, 70t, *70–72*, 71t
cellular interactions of, 58–60
cell types interacting with IgE and, 59–60, *60*
receptors and binding proteins and, 58–59
disodium cromoglycate and, 855
Fc portion of, 148
genetic regulation of, 29
genomic structure of, 57–58
high- and low-affinity receptors for, 68

Immunoglobulin E (*continued*)
hyposensitization and, 63–64
immunopathologic mechanisms in asthma and, 68–69
inflammatory cells and, 69
kinetics of, 57
levels of
determination of, indications for, 491
genetic factors affecting, 28–39
nongenetic factors affecting, 26–28
macrophage receptors for, 148
mast cell sensitivity and, 519, *519*
normal values of, 490
occupational asthma and, 590
peptide structure of, 57, *58*
regulation of synthesis of, 60, 153–156, *154*
dysregulation and, 155–156
upregulation, 61
release mechanisms dependent on, 68
in sputum, 660
total serum, measurement of, 490–491
importance of, 490–491
techniques for, 490
as unique immunoglobulin class, 68
in viral infections, 568
Immunoglobulin E-mediated reactions
mast cells and, 59, 518–522
heterogeneity of, 518
releasability of, 68, 518–519
sensitivity of, *519–521*, 519–522, 520t
in skin and bronchi, 517–522
mast cell heterogeneity and, 518
mast cell releasability and, 518–519
mast cell sensitivity and, 519–522
Immunoglobulin E receptors
of eosinophils, 261
as target for allergy therapy, 69, *73*
Immunoglobulin E response, 73, 74t, 76t
Immunoglobulin G, 4
antigen-specific, subclass determination and, 493–494
Immunoglobulin G receptors, of eosinophils, 261
Immunoglobulin receptors, of eosinophils, 261
Immunoglobulin supergene family, 53
Immunologic mechanisms, in occupational asthma, 590t, 590–592, *591*
Immunoradiometric assay, 490
Immunoregulation, 147–160, *148*
eosinophil production and function and, 156–157
IgE synthesis and, 153–156, *154*
dysregulation and, 155–156
late-phase airway response and, *157*, 157–158, *158*, 159t
lymphocytes and, 150–151, *151*
macrophages and. *See* Macrophage(s)
mononuclear cell-derived cytokines and, *151*, 151–153, 152t
mononuclear cell involvement in cascade of airway inflammation and, 158–160, *159*
mRNA and, 158
Immunotherapy, 5, *36*, 526t, 526–527, *527*, 527t, 934–942, 937t–940t, 1069, 1148, 1152–1153
basic aspects of, 63
evaluation of, bronchial provocation tests and, 509
factors modifying action of beta-adrenergic agonists and, 707–708, *708*
in late asthmatic reactions, 143
mechanisms of, 937t
modified allergens as immunotherapeutic agents and, 47

oral, 1152
during pregnancy and nursing, 1091
safety of, 941
Impairment, in occupational asthma, 608
"Impossible asthma", in childhood, 1075, 1075t
Impulse initiation, in autonomic nervous system, 166
Inappropriate/unusual treatment, 1145–1150, 1149t
diet, 1147
folk remedies, 1145–1146, 1146t
Oriental, 1145
Western, 1145–1146
geographic variations in treatment and, 1150
healthful climates and spas, *1146*, 1146t, 1146–1147
historic background of, 1145
hormones, 1148
immunotherapy, 1148
inappropriate diagnoses and, 1149–1150, 1150t
inappropriate uses of appropriate therapy, 1149
new applications of old drugs, 1147t, 1147–1148
psychological, 1148
surgical and anesthesiologic, 1148–1149, 1149t
Indices of asthma severity, 694, 985
Indomethacin
aspirin-induced asthma and, 622
prostanoid action and, 123, 124, 125t
Indoor environmental pollutants, 554t, 555t, 556, 580–581
Industrial factors
in occupational asthma, 586
toxins, 471, 477t
Inertia, 406
Inertial suction samplers, 547, *549*
Infants
asthma in, 1074
food allergy in, 560–561, 561t
infections in, 571–572
pathogenesis of asthma and, 564–565
sensitization to allergens, 27–28
Infections. *See also* Respiratory infections; *specific infections;* Upper respiratory tract diseases; Viral infections
acute exacerbations of asthma and, 565t, 565–566
aerosol corticosteroids and, 833
in asthmatic patients, clinical approach to, 569, 570t, 571–573
bacterial, IgE levels and, 28
bronchospasm induced by, pathophysiology of, *7*, 566–568
clinical approach to, 569–573
cough as manifestation of infectious asthma and, 573
in epidemiology of asthma, 19
in etiology of asthma, 564–573
fungal, 28
in infant and young child, 571–572
in older children and adults, 572–573
parasitic, IgE levels and, 28
pathogenesis of asthma and, 564–565, 570
of sinuses, 540
in status asthmaticus, 1003
Inflammation, 12, 80–90, *81*, 81t, 1194–1195
adhesion molecules and, 89
of airway epithelium, 87–88
enzymatic degradation of mediators and, 87
loss of barrier and, 87

loss of epithelium-derived relaxant factor and, 87
mediator release and, 88
sensory nerve exposure and, 87–88
airway hyperreactivity in experimental asthma and, 394–396
in dog, 395
in guinea pig, 394
in rabbit, 394–395
in rat, 394
in sheep, 395–396
airway hyperresponsiveness and, 33–34, *34*
of airway smooth muscle, 88
animal models of, 82
bronchial biopsy and, 80–81
bronchoalveolar lavage and, 80
circadian change in, nocturnal asthma and, 1031–1032
effects on target cells, 87–89
eosinophils in, 262
estimation of degree of, 13
fatal asthma and, 80
human models of, 82
IgE-mediated, 50
mononuclear cell involvement in cascade of, 158–160, *159*
mucosal absorption and, 304–305
mucus hypersecretion and, 89
neural effects of, 89
neurogenic, 89, 242–245, 568
modulation of, 243–245, *244*
neuropeptide metabolism and, 243
pattern of innervation and, 243
replacement of neutral endopeptidase and, 245
sensory denervation and, 245
sensory nerve activation and, 242–243, 244–245
sensory nerve depletion and, 243
sensory neuropeptide effects and, 242, *242*, 243
sensory neuropeptide release and, 243–244
nocturnal asthma and, 1033–1034, *1034*
in occupational asthma, 588
plasma extravasation and mucosal edema and, 88–89
effects on airway secretions, 88
generation of plasma-derived mediators and, 88
mucosal edema and, 88–89
subepithelial fibrosis and, 88
symptoms and, 81–82, *82*
therapeutic implications of, 89–90, *90*
new approaches and, 89–90
T-lymphocyte as critical cell of, 429, 430t
vascular responses to, 88
Inflammatory cells. *See also* Eosinophil(s); Macrophage(s); Mast cell(s); Neutrophils; Platelet(s); T-cell(s)
in airway epithelium, 296, *298*, *299*
in bronchoalveolar lavage fluid, 83, 309–310, *310*
after antigen challenge, 311–312, 312t
corticosteroid effects on, 802–804, *804*
IgE and, 69
tachykinins and, 240–241
Inflammatory cytokines, 431t
Inflammatory extravasation, airway mucosa and, 305, *305*
Inflammatory mediators, 12, 84–87, *85*, 85t
bronchial mucus production and, 366–367
in bronchoalveolar lavage fluid, 310–311, *311*
after antigen challenge, 311–312, 312t
cholinergic neurotransmission and, 227

immunoglobulin E as, 50
measurements to, 494
multiple, 87
sinusitis and asthma and, 536t, 536–537
Influenza vaccine, 573
Influenza virus infection
of lower respiratory tract, structural
changes in airway epithelium and
hyperresponsiveness and, 298, 300
in older child and adult, 572–573
Information lines, 1213
Inhalant allergens, sensitization to. *See also*
Aeroallergens; *specific allergens*
Inhalation technique, aerosol corticosteroids
and, 830
Inhalation tests
with concomitant or exclusive bronchial
sensitization causes by non-
IgE–dependent mechanisms, 528–529
negative results and, 523
positive results and, 523
Inhalers
dry-powder. *See* Dry-powder inhalers
metered-dose. *See* Metered-dose inhalers
Inhibitory mechanisms, loss of, airway
hyperresponsiveness and. *See*
Bronchial hyperresponsiveness, loss of
inhibitory mechanisms and
Inorganic ions, in bronchial mucus, 357–358
Inositol-lipid signal pathway, reciprocal
adrenoceptor activities and, 182–183,
705–706, 948–949
Inositol phosphate pathway
histamine release and, 102
muscle contraction and, 205
Insects, 553, 599t
Integrins, leukocyte, 259–261
Interferon, regulation of IgE synthesis and,
62, 70, 72–73, *73, 74*
Interferon alpha, downregulation of IgE
biosynthesis and, 62
Interferon gamma
downregulation of IgE biosynthesis and, 62
immunoregulation and, 152t, 153
Interleukin-1, immunoregulation and, 152t,
153
Interleukin-2, downregulation of IgE
biosynthesis and, 62–63
Interleukin-3, immunoregulation and, 152t,
153
Interleukin-4
immunoregulation and, 152t, 153
regulation of IgE synthesis and, 61–62, 70,
72–73, *73, 74*
Interleukin-5
immunoregulation and, 152t, 153
regulation of IgE synthesis and, 62
Interleukin-6
immunoregulation and, 152t, 153
upregulation of IgE biosynthesis and, 62
Intermittent positive pressure breathing. *See*
Respiratory therapy, intermittent
positive pressure breathing
International Classification of Disease code,
1156, *1156*
Interstitial cells, 320
Intragranular reserve pool, 168
Intrinsic asthma, 6–7, 8t, 441, 442t
bronchial mucus in, 362t, 362–364, *363,*
364t
differential diagnosis of, 475t
nonatopic, genetic factors in, 29–30, *30*
Intubation, endotracheal, in childhood
asthma, acute, 1078
Iodide, 927–928
dosage of, 925t, 926t
mucolytic effect of, 927

Iodinated glycerol
as expectorant, 928
as mucoregulator, 928
in sinusitis, 542t
Ipecac, 929
Ipratropium bromide, 689, 879t
dose response and, 879
mucokinetic effect of, 923
in nocturnal asthma, 1033
pharmacokinetics of, 878–879
Irritant receptors, 221, 227
Isoetharine, 687t, 688, 721–722
aerosol, 719t
Isoetharine hydrochloride, 1226
Isoetharine mesylate, 1226
Isoproterenol, 687t, 718, 719t–720t, 720
aerosol, 719t
pharmacokinetics of, 716
autodesensitization of beta₂-adrenergic
receptors and, 194
bronchodilator response to, 16–17
intravenous, pharmacokinetics of, 715–716,
759
Isoproterenol hydrochloride, 1226
Isoproterenol sulfate, 1227
Ispaghula, occupational asthma and, 602–603

Jet nebulizers, 409, 728
Job type, in occupational asthma, 586
Junction, 166
Junctional transmission
in autonomic nervous system, 166
of bronchomotor activity, modulation of,
222–224, *223, 224*
Jute dust, occupational asthma and, 597

Kallidin, 98
control of mucus production and, 367
Kapok, 555–556
K⁺ channels, muscle relaxation and,
211–212. *See also* Potassium channel
openers
Ketotifen, *866,* 866–868
adverse effects of, 868
in childhood asthma, 1071
clinical utility of, *867,* 867t, 867–868
dose and administration of, 868, 870t
mechanisms of action of, 866t, 866–867,
867t
pharmacokinetics of, 866
Ketotifen fumarate, 1233
Khellin, 855
Kinin(s), 98–99, *99,* 100t
Kininogens, 98
Kulchitzky's cells, 469

L-649, 923, 890
Labor, 1092–1093
Laboratory studies, 450–451, 485–495, 486t.
See also specific tests
Lactic acidosis, 340, 450, 612, 1004, 1167
Laryngeal dysfunction, 1055, 1148
differential diagnosis of, 468, 476t
Laryngotracheobronchitis
in infant and young child, 571–572
irritant gases causing, 471
Latch bridges, *316,* 203, 316–317, *317*
Late asthmatic reactions, 135–143, 528
animal model of, 139
antigen challenge in experimental asthma
and, 386–388
BAL in, 311
bronchial provocation tests and, asthmatic
response, 507–509, 509t
cyclooxygenase inhibitors and, 125

description, frequency, clinical relevance,
and responsible agents and, 135–137,
136, 136t, *137*
eosinophils and, 266
functional aspects and physiologic
consequences of, 137–139, *138, 139,*
139t
historical background of, 135
immune relationships to, 157–158
pathophysiology of, 139–142, *140*
arachidonic acid products and, 141, *142*
circadian pattern in, 138
complement and, 141
eosinophils and, 139–140
histamine and, 141
lymphocytes and, 140
mast cells and, 141
neutrophil and eosinophil chemotactic
activity and, 141
neutrophils and, 140
pathologic changes and, 139
pituitary and adrenal function and, 141
platelet-activating factor and, 141–142
platelets and, 141
viruses and, 137
treatment of, 142–143
antihistamines in, 142
beta₂-adrenergic agents in, 142
corticosteroids in, 142
cromolyn and nedocromil in, 142, *143*
furosemide in, 143
immunotherapy and, 143
theophylline in, 142
Lavage, lung, 1119. *See also* Bronchoalveolar
lavage
Lemakalim, 244, 964
Leukocyte(s). *See also specific leukocytes*
histamine release and, in vitro antigen-
induced, 495–496
Leukocyte integrins, 259–261
Leukocytosis, 451
Leukotriene(s), 70t, 112–120
airway hyperresponsiveness and, 116–118,
117, 117t, *118*
allergic bronchospasm and, 330, 889–890
following antigen challenge in animal
models, 385
aspirin-induced asthma and, 624
B₄, biologic activity of, 114
eosinophilic chemotaxis of, 262
in BAL fluid, 118
biologic activity of, 114
bronchoconstriction induced by,
mechanism of, 116
cellular distribution and transport of, 114
cellular sources of, 112–113
control of mucus production and, 367
experimental asthma and, 392
as inflammatory mediator, 86
inhalation challenge with, 504
in experimental animal models, 392
late asthmatic reactions and, 141, *142*
metabolism of, 113–114
potency of, *115,* 115–116, 116t
receptors for, 114–115, 208
release of, 118–119, *119*
sulfidopeptide, biologic activity of, 114
synthesis of, 112, *113*
treatment and, 119–120
leukotriene antagonists and, 119–120,
692
5-lipoxygenase inhibitors and, 120
Leukotriene receptor(s), smooth muscle
contraction and, 208–209
Leukotriene receptor antagonists, 692

Lidocaine
blockade of antigen inhalation challenge by, 511
effect in asthma, 244, 1965, 1107
Lipid(s), in bronchial mucus, 358, 362
Lipid mediators
of eosinophils, 263–264
macrophage-derived, 149t, 149–150
in mast cells, 274, 274t
Lipid peroxidation, 961
Lipocortins, transcriptional effects of corticosteroids and, 802
5-Lipoxygenase pathway antagonists
agents active on, 889–891, *890*
clinical studies of, 890–891, *891*, 891t
of fish oil-derived fatty acids. *See* Fish oil, fatty acids derived from
mucus and, 367
Load-clamp technique, 318
Local airway challenge, inflammatory cells and mediators in BAL specimens after, 311–312, 312t
Lodoxamides, *863*, 863–864
adverse effects of, 864
clinical efficacy of, 864
dose and administration of, 864, 870t
experimental uses for, 864
mechanism of action of, 863–864, 864t
Löffler's syndrome, differential diagnosis of, 472, 478t, 640
Loratadine, 885
Low-affinity receptor, 50
Lung. *See also* Chronic obstructive pulmonary disease; Respiratory infections; *headings beginning with term* Pulmonary
adrenergic subtype distribution in, 700
aerosols and. *See* Aerosol(s)
function of
in exercise-induced asthma, 612, *613*
during pregnancy, 1086–1088, 1087t
inhibition of mediator release in, by beta-adrenergic agonists, 713, 713t, *714*
mast cells in, 278–279
muscarinic subtypes in, 707
physiology during pregnancy. *See* Pregnancy, pulmonary physiology during
pulmonary rehabilitation and, 1116
Lung compliance, 333, *335*
Lung mechanics, anticholinergic agents and, 882
Lung scans, ventilation and perfusion, 674, *676–678*
Lung sounds, 651
Lung volume(s), 338, *338*
antigen challenge in experimental asthma and, 384
partial expiratory flow-volume maneuvers and, 456, *456*
during pregnancy, 1086–1087
as risk factor for status asthmaticus, 990–991
LY-171, 883, 890–891, 891t
LY 171883, 119, 120
Lymphocyte(s), 150–151, *151*. *See also* B-cells; T-cell(s)
CD markers on, 52
corticosteroid effects on, 804
in hypersensitivity pneumonitis, 634
immune-neuroendocrine circuitry and. *See* Immune-neuroendocrine circuitry, lymphocyte as unifying regulatory cell component of
immunoregulation and, 150–151, *151*
late asthmatic reactions and, 140
subsets, measurement, 495

Lymphocyte proteins and atopy, 183–184
Lymphocyte transformation, 494
Lymphoid organs, 422
Lymphokines, 53–54, 54t. *See also* Cytokines
bronchial hyperresponsiveness and, 431–432
Lyso-PAF, 290
Lysosomal enzymes, in mast cells, 275

Machining fluids, occupational asthma and, 597
Macrophage(s)
corticosteroid effects on, 804
immunoregulation and, 147
as inflammatory cells, 83
lipid mediators derived from, immunoregulation and, 149t, 149–150
platelet-activating factor and, 149
in sputum, 658
T-cell interactions of, 54
Macrophage receptors, for FcεRI, 148t, 148–149
Magnesium, 964
Magnesium sulfate
in acute asthma, 981
new applications of, 1147
Magnetic resonance imaging, 674
Magnetopneumography, measuring particle retention and, 415
Maintenance therapy, chronic, 1191–1192
Major basic protein, 83, 159, 258, 264
in BAL fluid, 309–311
in sputum, 661
Major histocompatibility complex antigens, 52–53, *53*
epithelium and, 304
Management goals, 693, 693t
Marijuana, 772, 1145
Mast cell(s), 271–281, *272*
in asthma, 280–281
atypical, 278
in BAL fluid, 83, 281, 309–310
carboxypeptidase in, 275
chemotactic factors in, 274
d-chymotrypsin, 274
corticosteroid effects on, 803
cytokines in, 274
distribution of, 278–279
genesis of, 279–280
glycosamines of, 273t
granular secretion mechanism, 276
heparin in, 272–273, 273t
heterogeneity of, 278, 518
histamine in, 273–274
immunoglobulin E-mediated reactions and. *See* Immunoglobulin E-mediated reactions, mast cells and
as inflammatory cells, 82–83
interaction with IgE, 59–60
lipid mediators in, 274, 274t
lysosomal enzymes in, 275
mechanism of secretion by, *276*, 276t, 276–278, *277*
mediators, 71t
mucosal, 278
neoplasms and, 280, 280t
proteases in, 274–275
releasability of, 518–519
sensitivity of, 519–522
bronchial nonspecific responsiveness and, 519–522, *520*, 520t, *521*
conditions affecting relationship between skin and bronchial testing results and, 522
serotonin in, 273
specific IgE and, 519, *519*

in sputum, 658
stimuli for secretion, 276t
structure of, 275–276
tryptase in, 275
ultrastructure of, 271–272, *272*
Mast cell chymase, 274–275
Mast cell mediators
drugs causing direct release of, 627–628, 628t
eosinophils and, 267
Mast cell stabilizers, 855
Mastocytosis, systemic, differential diagnosis of, 478t
Meat fibers, in sputum, in aspiration, 662
Meat wrapper's asthma, 596
Mechanical stimuli, to breathing in asthma, 349, *349*
Mechanical ventilation, in status asthmaticus, 1005–1008, *1006*, 1006t–1008t, *1009*
Mediator(s), 50
airway hyperresponsiveness and, 37t, 37–38
proinflammatory mediators, 37, *38*
transient bronchoconstriction and, 37
of allergic reactions, platelet-activating factor as, 289–290
antigen challenge in experimental asthma and, 385–386, *386*, *387*
bronchospastic, 12
clarification of, 507
humoral, 37t, 37–38
causing transient bronchoconstriction, 37
proinflammatory, 37, *38*
of IgE-dependent cytotoxicity, 59, *60*
IgE levels and, 29
inflammatory. *See* Inflammatory mediators
lipid. *See* Lipid mediators
measurement of, 494
release of, cyclic adenosine monophosphate and, 104–105
secreted by eosinophil, 262–265, *263*
eosinophil granule proteins, 264
lipid, 263–264
Mediator cells, 50, 51t
Melittin, 45
Membrane permeabilization, mast cell secretion and, 277–278
Memory, immune and neuronal, 424–426
Menses, 1093–1096
historical aspects of, 1093
management of asthma in, 1095–1096
pathophysiology of asthma exacerbations in, 1094–1095, *1095*
prevalence of asthma exacerbation in, 1093–1094, 1094t
2-Mercaptoethane sulfonate, 926–927
Metabolic acidosis, 340, 1004, 1167
Metabolism
beta-adrenergic agonist effects on, 714
beta-adrenergic bronchodilators and, 733–734
catecholamine degradation and, 170
of leukotrienes, 113–114
of methylxanthines, 769–770, *770*, 770t
of neuropeptides, neurogenic inflammation and, 243
of prostaglandins, 120–121
of tachykinins, 239
of thromboxane, 120–121
Metaproterenol, 687t, 687–688, 722
in acute asthma, 974, 981
aerosol, 719t
inhaled, 728–729
oral, 721t
subcutaneous, 731

Metaproterenol sulfate, 1227
Metered-dose inhalers, 455–456, 686–688, *687*, 687t, *688*, 689, 727, *751*, 751–752, 1000
  in acute asthma, 977
  anticholinergic, 879
  breathing pattern and, 412
  in childhood asthma, 1072, 1072t
  corticosteroid, 818, 821t
  nebulization versus, 716–717, 717t
  spacers and, 752, 752t, 828–830, *831*, 831t
Methacholine
  diagnostic use of, 534
  inhalation challenge with, 503
Methotrexate, 692, 910–913
  in corticosteroid-dependent asthma, 912–913
  history of, 910
  mechanism of action of, 910–911
  new applications of, 1147
  pharmacology of, *911*, 911t, 911–912
  in severe asthma, guidelines for use of, 1222
  toxicity of, 912
  varicella infection and, 912
Methylprednisolone, 691, 1228
Methylprednisolone sodium succinate, 1229
Methylprednisone, 691
Methylxanthines, 764. *See also specific drugs*
  in cardiovascular disease, 1041–1042
  during pregnancy and nursing, 1091
  in status asthmaticus, 1001
Microbial components, beta receptor blockade by, 177
Micropolyspora faeni, 632
Microscopic sputum examination, technique for, 1223
Microvascular angina, differential diagnosis of, 464
Microvascular leakage, in occupational asthma, 590
Mild asthma, 13, 683–684
  treatment of, 693
Milk, in sputum, in aspiration, 662, 662t
MK-571, 119, 120, 292, 890, 891, 891t
MK-0679, 891t
MK-886, 120
Modeling, measuring particle retention and, 414
Moderate asthma, 13, 684
  treatment of, 693–694
Molds, 550, 552t. *See also* Fungi
  as allergens, 442–443, *443*
  environmental control measures for, 1142
  hypersensitivity pneumonitis and, 632, 633t
  immunotherapy and, 939–940, 940t
  incidence in United States, 1210–1211
Monoamine oxidase, in metabolic degradation of catecholamines, 170
Monoamine oxidase inhibitors, interactions with beta agonists, 733
Monocytes, corticosteroid effects on, 804
Monokines, 53
Monosporium, 1210–1211
Morning dippers, 341, 445
Mortality, 23. *See also* Fatal asthma
  beta agonists and, 736–737, 1157–1159
  mucous plug and, 354
  in nocturnal asthma, 342
  pathologic airway changes and, 355
Mucociliary apparatus, 371–379. *See also* Cilia
  beta-adrenergic agonist effects on, 714
  dysfunction of, 372–379
    airflow obstruction and, 378–379

antigen challenge in experimental asthma and, 386
  clearance in asthma, 377t
  cough and, 378
  increased susceptibility to respiratory infection in, 379, *379*, 379t
  interaction, 377
  structure and, 372–373, *374*, *375*
  transport and, 373–378, 407
  mediators and, 377t
  normal function of, 371–372
  secretagogues, 377t
  surgery and, 1108
  transport and, 373–378
    airway secretions and, 374–377
    cilia and, 373–374, *376*
    mucociliary interaction and, 37t, 377–378, *378*
    particle deposition and, 407
Mucoevacuants, in sinusitis, 542t
Mucokinetic agents, 922t, 922–931
Mucolytics, 926t, 926–927. *See specific agents*
Mucor, 552t, 1210–1211
Mucoregulators, 929–931
Mucosa
  edema of, inflammation and, 88–89
  exudation permeability across, *305*, 305–306
Mucosal edema, inflammation and, 88–89
Mucosal glands, corticosteroid effects on, 804
Mucosal mast cells, 278
Mucous casts, 356
Mucous plug, 354
Mucus, 356–367
  cells of origin of, 364–365
  chemical constituents of, 357–359, *358*, 360t
  control of production of, 365t, 365–367, 661
    genes encoding mucin polypeptides and, 367
    inflammatory mediators and, 366–367
    neural, 366
    neuropeptides and, 366
    prostaglandins and, 367
  density gradient ultracentrifugation of, 359, *359*
  genetic encoding of mucin polypeptides, 367
  glycoconjugates, 358
  humidification and, 921, 921t
  hypersecretion of, inflammation and, 89
  immunoglobulins, 358, 361
  importance to clinical problems of asthma, 356
  inorganic ions, 357
  lining airways, 356, *357*
  markers of macromolecular components of, 359–361, 360t
  mucociliary transport and, 375–376
  pH, 357
  physical properties of, 357
  physicochemical studies of, 361–364
    amino acids in, 364
    in extrinsic and intrinsic asthma, 362t, 362–364, *363*, 364t
    normal mucus and, 361–362
    physical properties and, 364
    in status asthmaticus, 364
  sol phase constituents, 361
  volume of secretion and diurnal variation in, 356–357
Multiple allergosorbent test, 492

Muscarinic receptors
  cholinergic neurotransmission and, 219, 219t
  smooth muscle contraction and, 207–208
  subtypes in lung, 707, 877
Muscle contraction, 203–210, *204*
  calcium and. *See* Calcium, airway smooth muscle contraction and
  contractility and, 318, *318*, *319*
  mechanisms of beta-adrenergic agonist action and, 705, *705*, *706*
  receptors mediating, 207–210
    alpha adrenoceptors, 210
    endothelin, *209*, 209–210
    histamine, 208
    leukotriene, 208–209
    muscarinic, 207–208
    prostanoid, 209
    tachykinin, 209
  signal transduction mechanisms for, 203–207
    calcium and, 203–206, *205*
    diacylglycerol-protein kinase C and, 206–207
Muscle relaxants causing asthma, 623t
Muscle relaxation, 210–212, 318–319, *319*
  cyclic AMP and, 949–950, *951*
  functional antagonism of beta-adrenergic agonists to, 706–707, *707*
  intracellular calcium and, 210
  mechanisms of beta-adrenergic agonist action and, 705–706, *706*
  receptors mediating, 211–212
    adenosine, 212
    $beta_2$ adrenoceptors, 211
    K^+ channels, 211–212
    vasoactive intestinal peptide receptors, 212
  signal transduction mechanisms for, 210–211
    cyclic AMP and, 210–211
    cyclic GMP and, 211
Muscle tone, 329
  cholinergic control of, 219–225
    central origin of efferent neural activity and, 219–220, *221*, 221t
    modulation of epithelium-derived relaxant factor and, 224
    modulation of ganglionic and junctional transmission of bronchomotor activity and, 222–224, *223*, *224*
    peripheral inputs to efferent neural activity and, 220–222, *222*
    reasons for, 224–225
  neuropeptide Y and, 245
  prostanoids and, 123–124
Mushrooms, 552t
Mycelia, 1210–1211
Mycoplasma pneumoniae infection, in older child and adult, 572
Myocardial toxicity, of beta agonists, 734–735
Myosin heavy-chain isoenzymes, 323
Myosin light-chain kinase, 197, 203, 210, 704

Nafazatrom, 891
Na^+-K^+-ATPase, 964
Naloxone, mechanical stimuli to breathing and, 349
NARES syndrome, 537, 538
Nasal diseases
  increased lower airway responsiveness in, 534
  treatment of
    aerosol corticosteroids and, 834
    improvement in pulmonary symptoms by, 533–534

Nasal polyps, 538–539
  asthma and, 534, 621
  characteristics of, 538–539
  differential diagnosis of, 475t
  incidence of, 539
  pathogenesis of, 539
  treatment of, 539
Nasal sinus-bronchial reflex, 534–535, 535t
Natural history of asthma, 21t, 21–23
  in adults, 22–23
  in children, 22, 1079, 1079t
Nebulization, metered-dose inhalers versus,
    716–717, 717t
Nebulizers, 749–751, *750*
  in acute asthma, 977
  breathing pattern and, 412
  in childhood asthma, 1072–1073
  jet, 409, 728
  ultrasonic, 409
Nedocromil, 1233
Nedocromil sodium, 692, 860–863
  adenosine-induced bronchoconstriction
    and, 254
  adverse effects of, 863
  chemistry of, 860, *860*
  in childhood asthma, 1071
  clinical efficacy of, 861–862, *862*, 863t
  dose and administration of, 863
  intranasal, 862–863
  intraocular, 863
  in late asthmatic reactions, 142
  mechanism of action of, 861, *862*
  pharmacokinetics of, 860, 860t
Negative-ion generators, for environmental
    control, 583, 1140
Nerves
  in airway epithelium, 296, *297*
  inflammatory effects of, 89
  sensory, neurogenic inflammation and. *See*
    Inflammation, neurogenic
Neural cell adhesion molecule, immune
    recognition molecules and, 424
Neural crest interactions, in development of
    immune system, 423
Neuraminic acid, 359
Neuroeffector junction, 166
Neuroendocrine system, recognition and
    communication powers of, 426,
    427t–428t, 428–429
Neurogenic inflammation. *See* Inflammation,
    neurogenic
Neurokinin A, 238, *238*
Neurokinin B, 238, *238*
Neuropeptide(s). *See also specific*
    neuropeptides
  on airway functions, 233
  bronchial mucus production and, 366
  effects of, 234
  neurogenic inflammation and. *See*
    Inflammation, neurogenic
  in occupational asthma, 588
  opioids and, 243
  in respiratory tract, 233
  role in asthma, 246–247
Neuropeptide receptors, 234
Neuropeptides, sensory, inhibition of effects
    of, 243–244
Neuropeptide Y, 245
  airway tone and, 245
  localization of, 245
  secretions and, 245
  vascular effects of, 245
Neurotransmission
  adrenergic. *See* Adrenergic regulation;
    Autonomic nervous system,
    adrenergic transmission and

cholinergic. *See also* Cholinergic nervous
    system
  receptor types in, 219, 219t
  immune system and nervous system
    memory and, 425
  modulation of, 217–218
    adrenergic modulation of cholinergic
      neurotransmission, 217–218
    cholinergic modulation of cholinergic
      neurotransmission, 218
  neurotransmitters and, 166
    vasoactive intestinal peptide as, 236
    nonadrenergic, noncholinergic nerves and,
      233–234, *234*
    vasoactive intestinal peptide and
      acetylcholine and, 236–237, *237*
    peptidergic, nonadrenergic, noncholinergic
      nerves and, 234
Neutral endopeptidase
  neurogenic inflammation and, 245
  tachykinin metabolism and, 239
Neutrophils
  chemotactic activity of, late asthmatic
    reactions and, 141
  corticosteroid effects on, 804
  as inflammatory cells, 84
  late asthmatic reactions and, 140
Neutrophil chemotactic factor, 274, 499
Newsletters, 1213
Nicotinic receptors, cholinergic
    neurotransmission and, 219
Nifedipine, 692, 952–957
  blockade of antigen inhalation challenge
    by, 511
  in exercise-induced asthma, 618
Nigrospora, 1210–1211
Nitric oxide, 199, 544, 578
  nonadrenergic, noncholinergic nerves and,
    232
Nitrogen dioxide, 554, 578, 581
Nocturnal asthma, 341–342, *341–343*,
    1030–1035
  in childhood, 1075
  clinical relevance of, 1030
  hypoxemia and, 341–342, *341–343*
  incitants of, 445
  mechanisms of, 1030–1034, 1031t
    airway cooling and, 1031
    airway inflammation and, 1033–1034,
      1034
    allergens and, 1030
    circadian change in inflammatory
      responses and, 1031–1032
    circadian changes in airway function
      and, 1031, *1032*
    circadian changes in autonomic
      receptors and, 1033
    circadian changes in parasympathetic
      system and, 1033
    circadian rhythm in corticosteroids and,
      1034
    circadian rhythm of adrenergic
      mechanisms and, 1032–1033
    circadian rhythm of bronchial
      responsiveness and, 1031
    circadian rhythm of perception of
      breathlessness and, 1033
    circadian rhythms and, 1031, 1031t
    dosing frequency and, 1031
    esophageal reflux and, 1030
    nonadrenergic noncholinergic nerves
      and, 1033
    oxyradicals and, 1034
    supine posture and, 1030–1031
    toxin or secretion accumulation and,
      1030

  treatment of, 1034–1035
  ventilatory response to hypoxemia during
    sleep and, 350, 350t
Nonadrenergic noncholinergic nerves,
    232–247, 233t. *See also specific*
    neuropeptides
  cotransmission and, 233–234, *234*
  excitatory, 233, 329
    airway hyperresponsiveness and, 36–37
  inhibitory, 232–233, *233*, 329
    airway hyperresponsiveness and, 36
    nitric oxide and, 232
    purines and, 232
    vasoactive intestinal peptide and,
      232–233
  neuropeptide effects and, 234
  neuropeptide receptors and, 234
  nocturnal asthma and, 1033
  peptidergic neurotransmission and, 234
Nonallergic rhinitis with eosinophilia
    syndrome, 537, 538
Nonspecific responses, 55
Nonsteroidal antiinflammatory drugs
  asthma caused by, 449, 621–622, 623t,
    624t, 624–625
  in cardiovascular disease, 1041
  inhibition of cyclooxygenase by, 892
Normally cycling cross-bridges, *316*, 316–317,
    317
Normal saline, mucokinetic effect of, 924
Nose. *See also* Nasal diseases; Nasal polyps
  filter function failure of, 533
  particle deposition in, 410
NP-gamma, 238
Nucleotides. *See* Cyclic AMP; Cyclic GMP;
    Cyclic nucleotide(s);
    Phosphodiesterases, cyclic nucleotide
Nursing, drug safety and, 1089–1091, 1090t

Obesity, corticosteroid bioavailability and,
    807
Occlusion pressure, 347
Occupational asthma, 585–608. *See also*
    Reactive airway dysfunction
    syndrome; *specific chemicals*
  adrenergic influences and, 588
  airway inflammation and, 588
  allergic, 598–603
    case example of, 598, *599*
    definition of, 585
    specific causes of, 598–599, 599t, 600t,
      601–603
  allocating cause and effect in, 606, 606t
  alteration in deposition and clearance of
    particles and, 588
  animal substances and, 599t
  assessment of work environment and, 606
  bronchial smooth muscle
    hyperresponsiveness and, 588
  definition of, 585
  diagnosis of, 471, 603–605
    evidence of work relationship and, 604,
      604
    nonspecific bronchial challenge testing
      in, 604–605
    skin tests and serology in, 605
    specific bronchial inhalation challenge
      in, 605
  epithelial damage in, *589*, 589–590
  historical features, 606t
  hypothetic model for, 592–594, *593*, *594*
  immunologic mechanisms in, 590t,
    590–592, *591*
  impairment, disability, and compensation
    in, 608
  incitants of, 444

inhalation challenge and, 506
microvascular leakage in, 590
neuropeptides and, 588
nonallergic, 594–597
  case examples of, 594
  clinical features of, 595t, 595–596
  definition of, 585
  high-level irritant exposures and, 596
  low-level irritant exposures and,
    596–597
  occurrence of, 585
  pharmacologic agents and, 590
  predisposing and host factors for, 585–587,
    586, 587
  prognosis of, 605–606
  reflex and, 587–588
  treatment and prevention of, 606–607, *607*
Odors, environmental control measures for,
  1142
Oomycetes, 552t
Operant conditioning, 1126–1127
Ophthalmic drugs causing asthma, 623t, 625
Opioids, inhibition of sensory neuropeptide
  release by, 243
Oral challenge tests, 489
Orrisroot, 556
Orthopnea, in cardiac asthma, 463
Osmotically induced asthma, relation to
  exercise-induced asthma, 613–614, *614*
Oxidant stress, 960
Oxidants, photochemical, respiratory effects
  of, 580
Oxitropium bromide, 879t
  dose response and, 879
Oxtriphylline, 1229, 1230, 1231, 1232
Oxygen, 1116. *See also* Respiratory therapy
  in status asthmaticus, 998
Oxygen therapy, 695, *695*
  ventilatory control and, 349
Oxymetazoline, in sinusitis, 542t
Oxyradicals, 960–964, *961–963*
  in airway reactivity, 963
  as inflammatory mediators, 86
Ozone, 578, 597–598

Papanicolaou stain test, 655–656
Paper immunosorbent test, 490
Parainfluenza virus, 571
Parallel elastic component, 317
Parallel group design, for drug studies, 788
Paranasal sinuses, 539–543. *See also* Sinusitis
  infection of, 540
  nasal sinus-bronchial reflex and, 534–535,
    535t
  structure and function of, 539–540
Parasitic infections
  eosinophils and, 258
  IgE levels and, 28
Parasympathetic nervous system. *See*
  Cholinergic nervous system
Parenchyma, beta-adrenergic receptors in,
  701
Paroxysmal nocturnal dyspnea, 463
Particle(s). *See* Aerosol(s)
Passive transfer reaction, 489
Pathogenesis of allergic bronchopulmonary
  aspergillosis (ABPA), 639
Pathology of asthma, 5, 11–12, 352–355, 353t
  bronchial circulation and, 352
  functional anatomy of conducting airways
    and, 352, *353, 354*
  mechanisms for drug refractoriness of
    status asthmaticus and, 988, *988*
  structural changes and, 352, *354*, 354–355
    functional consequences of, 355

Pathophysiology of asthma
  acute asthma and, 972–973
  childhood asthma and, 1075
  complications related to, 1167–1169, *1168*,
    1168t, *1169*
  exacerbations during menses, 1094–1095,
    1095
  fatal asthma and, 1160
  late asthmatic reactions and. *See* Late
    asthmatic reactions, pathophysiology
    of
  sensitized muscle and, *321*, 321–323, *322*,
    322t
Pathophysiology of bronchospasm, induced
  by viral infection, 566–568, *567*
Patient education, 1133, 1162t, 1188–1189
  in childhood asthma, 1068
  in chronic severe asthma, 1057
Peak expiratory flow rate (PEFR) in clinical
  evaluation, 447, 452, 982–983, 985,
    1031, 1057
Peak flow monitoring, educational materials
  on, 1213
Penicillium, 442, *443*, 550, 551, 552t,
  1210–1211
Peptic ulcer, 1171
Peptide(s). *See also* Neuropeptide(s); *specific
  peptides*
  neurotransmission and, 234
Peptide histidine isoleucine, 237, 588
Peptide histidine methionine, 237, 588
Peptide histidine valine, 237
Perennial nonallergic rhinitis, 537–538
Periciliary fluid, mucociliary transport and,
  376–377
Perioperative monitoring, 1103, 1103t, *1104*
Peripheral sensory fibers, 220
Peroxidase, mast cell, 275
Pertussis toxin, adenylate cyclase activity
  and, 181, 195
PGD_2, 70t, 121–122
PGE_2, 70t, 121–122
$PGF_{2\alpha}$, 70t, 121–122
PGI_2, 70t, 121–122
pH, of bronchial mucus, 358
Phagocytes, airway secretion and, 371
Phagocytic cells, 50
Pharmaceuticals and asthma, 600
Pharmacomechanical coupling, 204, *205*,
  205–206
Phenylephrine, in sinusitis, 542t
Phenylpropanolamine, in sinusitis, 542t
Phenobarbital, 772
Phoma, 1210–1211
Phosphodiesterases, cyclic nucleotide,
  198–199
  reciprocal adrenoceptor activities and,
    181–182
  structural activity relationships of
    inhibitors and, 198
  substrate specificity, kinetic parameters,
    and cellular regulation of enzymatic
    activity and, 198
Phospholipase A_2
  desensitization by, 704
  mast cell secretion and, 277
Phospholipase C, histamine release and, 102,
  948
Phospholipids, methylation and turnover of,
  histamine release and, 102–103
Phosphoprotein phosphatases, 197–198
Photochemical oxidants, respiratory effects
  of, 580
Photochemical smog, 578
Photometry, measuring particle retention
  and, 414

Physical examination
  in acute childhood asthma, 1076, 1076t
  severity of asthma and, 13
Physical findings, 449–450
Physical training, 1116
Physician office visits, cost of, 1181
Physiology of asthma, 11, 333–343. *See also*
  Late asthmatic reactions,
  pathophysiology of; Pathophysiology
  of asthma; *specific tests*
  acid-base balance and. *See* Acid-base
    balance
  acidosis, metabolic and, 340
  acute asthma changes in, 341, 341t,
    972–973
  aging, changes in, 1018–1020
  airflow obstruction
    localized, consequences of, 335
    reversibility of, 337
  airflow resistance and, 333, 337, 457
  blood gas tensions and, 339–340, 339t. *See
    also* Arterial blood gases
  asthma staging and, 684, 992–994
  bronchodilator criteria of reversibility,
    337t, 456–457
  bronchoprovocation criteria, 502
  circadian variations and, 342, 1031
  collateral ventilation and, 325
  compliance and, 333, 335
  diaphragm, 765, 990, 991
  diffusion capacity and, 340
  distribution of ventilation, 334
  elastic recoil in, 338
  equal pressure point, 333
  exercise-induced asthma and, 612
  expiratory flow parameters, 456–457
    density dependency, 456
  flow-volume relationships, 456, *466*, 1055
  forced vital capacity, expiratory volume
    and, 333
  functional residual capacity, 335, 990
  gas exchange and, 338, 992–994
  helium-oxygen. *See* Helium-oxygen mixture
  hypoxemia. *See* Hypoxemia
  hypercapnia. *See* Hypercapnia
  late asthmatic reactions and, 136–137
  lung volumes and, 338, 384, 457, 990–991
  maximum expiratory flow-volume curve in,
    333, 456
  mechanics of breathing in status
    asthmaticus, 991–992
    anticholinergic agents and, 882
  nocturnal changes in, 341–342
  oxygen effects on, 339
  pH and, 339t, 340
  PEFR. *See* Peak expiratory flow rate
    (PEFR), in clinical evaluation
  plethysmography in, 337–338, 990
  pregnancy and, 1086–1088
  preoperative assessment and, 1100
  pulmonary circulation and, 991
  reduced flow rates and, 335
  residual volume and, 335, 990
  scheme functional changes and, 334
  sleep and, 341
  spirometry, 333
    in children, 1076
  status asthmaticus and, 986t, 990–994
  surgical effects upon, 1108
  time constants in, 334
  upper airways and, 336
  ventilatory control, 346–350
  ventilation-perfusion changes and, 338, *339*
  wheeze correlates, 653
  work of breathing, 991, 1155

Physiology of esophagus, 1023
Physiology of lung, during pregnancy. *See* Pregnancy, pulmonary physiology during
Pigeon breeder's disease, 553
Pirbuterol, 687t, 687–688, 724, 1228
   aerosol, 720t
Piriprost, 891
Pituitary adenylate cyclase-activating peptide, 238
Pituitary function. *See also* Hypothalamic-pituitary-adrenal function
   late asthmatic reactions and, 141
Pituitary snuff, 623t
Plantago ovata, 602–603
Plant allergens, 555–556
Planum temporale, 423
Plasma, extravasation of, inflammation and, 88
Platelet(s)
   in aspirin-induced asthma, 624
   functions in human asthma, 289t
   as inflammatory cells, 84
   late asthmatic reactions and, 141
Platelet-activating factor, 289–292
   airway eosinophilia and, 291–292
   airway hyperreactivity and, 291
   airway obstruction and, 290–291
   analogs, 290
   antagonists of, 292, 893–894
      clinical studies of, 894
   chemistry and nomenclature of, 290, *290*
   eosinophil generation and, 263
   eosinophil migration and, 262
   experimental asthma and, 392
   immunoregulation and, 149–150
   increased vascular permeability and, 290
   as inflammatory mediator, 86
   inhalation challenge with, in experimental animal models, 392
   late asthmatic reactions and, 141–142
   as mediator of allergy, 289–290
   as phospholipid mediator, 263–264
   role in asthma, 292
   structure, 290
Platelet activation, 287–289
   allergic reactions and, 287
   in microvasculature, 288
   in vivo evidence for
      in asthma and allergic disease, 287, 288t
      from platelet activation asthmatics, 287–289, 289t
Platelet-derived growth factor, immunoregulation and, 152, 152t
Platelet-derived hyperreactivity factor (PDHF), 291
Platinosis, 602
Platinum, occupational asthma and, 602
Pleospora, 1210–1211
Pleura, mast cells in, 278
Pneumomediastinum, radiographic findings in, 673–674, *675*
Pneumonia
   allergic, 471
   radiographic findings in, *670*, 670–671, *671*
   viral, in infant and young child, 571
Pneumonitis, hypersensitivity. *See* Hypersensitivity pneumonitis
Pollen, 442
   avoidance of, 528
   characteristics and prevalence of, 548–549
   general considerations regarding, 548
   from grasses, 549, *550*
   immunotherapy and, 939, 939t, *940*
   mechanism of production of asthma by, 442
   purified antigens from, 549

seasonal exposure to, 528
   from trees, 442, 548–549
   wind-borne, 442
Pollution. *See also* Air pollution
   fatal asthma and, 1160
Polypeptides, mucin, genes encoding, 367
Polyporaceae, 1210–1211
Polyporus, 1210–1211
Polyp(s), nasal. *See* Nasal polyps
Poria, 1210–1211
Positron emission computed tomography, measuring particle retention and, 415
Postganglionic transmission, altered, in asthma, 227
Postoperative management, 1107–1109, 1108t, *1109*, *1110*, 1110t
Potassium, 757, 964–965
Potassium iodide
   as expectorant, 927–928
   mucolytic effect of, 927
   in sinusitis, 542t
Potentiation, 425
Power stroke, 203
Prausnitz-Küstner reaction, 304, 489
Preanesthetic management, 1100–1101, 1103–1104. *See also* Anesthesia
   in asymptomatic patients, 1100
   in symptomatic patients, 1100–1101, 1101t
Prednisolone, 691, 1229
   bioavailability of, 807
   dose-dependent pharmacokinetics of, 807
   oral, in status asthmaticus, 810
   plasma protein binding of, 807
   speed of action of, 807–808, *808*
Prednisone, 691, 1229
   in allergic bronchopulmonary aspergillosis, 641
   alternate-morning, 820, *824*
   combined with aerosol corticosteroid treatment, 824–825
   daily, 821–822, *825*
   minimum dose requirements of, 822–824, 823t, 825t
   oral, 806
      in status asthmaticus, 810, *811*
   withdrawal of, 820, 821t, *822*, *823*
Pregnancy, 1085–1093, 1174
   bronchial provocation tests and, 511
   drug safety in, 1089–1091, 1090t
   drug schedules in, 1090–1091
   effect of asthma on, 1088–1089
      fetal aspects of, 1088–1089, 1089t
      maternal aspects of, 1088
   effect on asthma, 1088
   management of asthma in, 1092–1093
      during conception to term, 1092
      during labor and delivery, 1092–1093
      postpartum, 1093
   pulmonary physiology during, 1085–1088
      hormonal changes and, 1085–1086
      mechanical changes and, 1085, 1086t
      pulmonary function and, 1086–1088, 1087t
Preoperative assessment, 1099–1100. *See also* Preanesthetic management
   identification of patients with asthma and, 1099
   of pulmonary function, 1100
   of risk factors, 1101t
Presenting symptoms, 447–449
   cor pulmonale as, 448
   cough as, 448
   dyspnea as, 447
   history and, 448–449
   tightness as, 448
   upper airways, 448
   wheezing as, 447–448

Prevention of asthma, 1188–1192, 1189t
   acute asthma and, 983
   conditions and inciting agents and, 1189–1192, 1190t
      angiotensin converting enzyme inhibitors, 1191
      aspirin, 1191
      beta blockers, 1191
      chronic maintenance control and, 1191–1192
      cough, 1191
      early treatment of acute attack and, 1192
      environmental control and, 1190
      exercise-induced asthma and, 1190
      gastroesophageal reflux, 1191
   education and self-management and, 1188–1189, 1189t
   exercise-induced asthma and, 618
   occupational asthma and, 606–607
   status asthmaticus and, 1008–1009
Primary particles, 578
Procaterol, 724, 1228
Professional organizations, 1215–1216
Progesterone, during pregnancy, 1085–1086
Prognosis in long-term asthma, 21
Propranolol, adrenergic responses and, in experimental animal models, 393
Prostaglandin D_2, in BAL fluid, 310
Prostaglandins, 120–124
   airway hyperresponsiveness and, 122
   following antigen challenge in animal models, 385
   biologic activity of, 121
   in biologic fluids, measurements of, 122–123
   biosynthesis and metabolism of, 120–121
   bronchial mucus production and, 367
   experimental asthma and, 391–392
   as inflammatory mediator, 85–86
   inhalation challenge with, 504
      in experimental animal models, 391–392
   late asthmatic reactions and, 141
   metabolites of, 121
   pharmacologic modulation of activity of, 123–124
      airway hyperresponsiveness and, 124, 125t
      airway tone and acute asthmatic responses and, 123–124
      refractory period and, 124
   potency of, 121–122
   during pregnancy, 1086
   receptors for, 121
Prostanoid(s). *See* Prostaglandins; Thromboxane(s)
Prostanoid receptors, smooth muscle contraction and, 209
Proteases, in mast cells, 274–275
Protein(s). *See also specific* proteins
   in bronchial mucus, 358
   of eosinophils, 264
Protein kinase(s), cyclic AMP-dependent, 195–198, *197*
Protein kinase A, 703–704
Protein kinase C
   reciprocal adrenoceptor activities and, 181
   smooth muscle contraction and, 203, 206–207
Proteoglycans, in bronchial mucus, 359
Provocation tests. *See* Bronchial provocation tests
Psychiatric aspects, 1121–1129
   biopsychosocial studies of, 1121–1125
      clinical case studies, 1124–1125
      epidemiologic factors and clinical groupings and, 1122–1123

experimental, 1121–1122
factors associated with poor outcome, 1128t, 1161t
family studies, 1123–1124
fatal asthma profiles, 1128–1161
therapeutic considerations and, 1125–1127
behavior modification and, 1126
evaluation of, 1127–1129, 1128t
family therapy and, 1127
group therapy and, 1127
hypnosis and, 1122, 1127
long-term psychoanalytically oriented psychotherapy and, 1127
operant conditioning and biofeedback and, 1126–1127
pharmacologic, 1125
relaxation and, 1125–1126
self-management and, 1125
Psychogenic factors, 226
Psychological factors, 449. *See also* Psychiatric aspects
bronchial provocation tests and, 511
conscious recognition of asthma and, 350
as incitant, 445
Psychological treatment, 1148
in childhood asthma, 1069
psychotherapeutic, 1127
Psychosomatic illness, differential diagnosis of, 471–472, 477t
Psychotherapy, 1127
Psychotropic drugs, 1125
Psyllium, occupational asthma and, 602–603
Ptychodiscus brevis, 597
Pullularia, 1210–1211
Pulmonary circulation, 330
in status asthmaticus, 991
Pulmonary edema
differential diagnosis of, 452
noncardiogenic. *See* Adult respiratory distress syndrome
Pulmonary embolism, differential diagnosis of, 452, 460–463, *462, 463,* 475t
Pulmonary eosinophilia, tropical, differential diagnosis of, 473–474, 474t
Pulmonary function tests, 450, 793, *793*
airway responsiveness and, 22
in allergic bronchopulmonary aspergillosis, 639
bronchial provocation tests and, 502, 503t
for bronchoreversibility assessment, selection of, 455
in children, 22
drug studies and, 795
in occupational asthma, 604, *604*
Pulmonary infiltration, with eosinophilia, differential diagnosis of, 472–473, *473,* 478t
Pulsus paradoxus, 338, 450, 684, 995, 1045–1046, 1046t
in severe asthma, 684
Purigenic receptors, 199
Purines, nonadrenergic, noncholinergic nerves and, 232
Pyrethrum, 556

Quercitrin, 864–856

Race, mortality and, 1154, *1156*
Radioactivity, measuring particle retention and, 414
Radioallergosorbent test, direct measurement of antigen-specific immunoglobulin E and, 491
Radiographic contrast media, asthma caused by, 627

Radiography, 450–451, 664–678
in acute asthma, 980
in allergic bronchopulmonary aspergillosis, *638,* 638–639, 671
chest films, 664–674
in complicated patients, 670–674, *670–675*
in uncomplicated patients, 664–665, *665–670,* 670
in hypersensitivity pneumonitis, 633
new techniques in, 674, 678
pneumothorax, 673
risk and, 664
in sinusitis, *540,* 540–541, *541*
in status asthmaticus, 996
technique and, 664
ventilation and perfusion lung scans, 674, *676–678*
Radioimmunoassay, 489–490
Radioimmunosorbent test, 489–490
food allergy and, 561
Radioligand technology
adrenoceptor identification by, 172, *173*
binding studies of adrenergic agonists and, 702–703
development of, 171–172
Radon, 554t, 581
Ragweed, 549
Raji cell assay, 49
Rapidly adapting receptors, 221, 226–227
Reactive airway dysfunction syndrome, 595, 597–598
clinical features of, 595t, 595–596
Reactive airways initiated dysfunction syndrome, 598
Receptor(s). *See also specific types of receptors*
adhesion, of eosinophils, 259–261, 260t, *261*
coupled by G-proteins, 426, 427t–428t
irritant, 221, 227
for leukotrienes, 114–115
muscle contraction and. *See* Muscle contraction
muscle relaxation and. *See* Muscle relaxation
rapidly adapting, 221, 226–227
substance P, 238
tachykinin, *238,* 238–239
Receptor-response coupling, parasympathetic airway control and, 219, *220*
Red cedar, occupational asthma and, 599, 601
Red-tide toxin, occupational asthma and, 597
Reflex, in occupational asthma, 587–588
Refractory period, prostanoids and, 124
Rehabilitation. *See* Respiratory therapy
Relaxation therapy, 1125–1126
"Remodeling pathway," 290
Reproductive risks, aerosol corticosteroids and, 826
Resistive loading, response to, 349, *349*
Resource lists, 1213
Respiratory failure
cardiac rhythm in, 1048
in childhood asthma, treatment of, 1077–1078
Respiratory heat loss hypothesis, 613
Respiratory infections, 19, 445. *See also specific infections*
bacterial. *See* Infections
in childhood asthma, 1065
as incitant, 445
increased susceptibility to, mucociliary dysfunction and, 379, *379,* 379t

of upper respiratory tract. *See* Upper respiratory tract diseases
viral. *See* Viral infections
Respiratory syncytial virus, 569–571
Respiratory system, adverse effects on, drug studies and, 794
Respiratory therapy, 1114–1116. *See also* Aerosol delivery systems; Humidification
humidification and chest physiotherapy, 1115–1116
intermittent positive pressure breathing, 751, 1114–1115
bronchodilation and, 1115
decreased work of breathing and, 1115, *1116*
facilitation of removal of airway secretions and, 1115
improved aerosol delivery and, 1114, *1115*
improved ventilation-perfusion relationships and, 1115
psychological effect of, 1115
oxygen administration, 998, 1116
pulmonary rehabilitation, 1116
Resting potential, 166
Rhabdomyolysis, 997, 1170
Rhinitis
allergic, 537
disodium cromoglycate in, 858
chronic, of non–IgE-associated asthma, 538, 538t
nonallergic rhinitis with eosinophilia syndrome and, 537, 538
perennial nonallergic, 537–538
vasoconstrictive, 537–538
vasomotor, 537–538
Rhizopus, 552t, 1210–1211
Rhodotorula, 1210–1211
Right heart dysfunction, 1046
Risk factors, 15, 16t
for fatal asthma, 1160–1161, 1161t
for status asthmaticus. *See* Status asthmaticus, risk factors for
prevention of, 1160–1161, 1192
Rotating arm impactor, 547, *548*
Rubor, 80
Rusts, 552t
Ruthenium red dye, 244, *244*

Salbutamol. *See* Albuterol
Saline, hypertonic, inhalation challenge with, 504
Salmeterol, 708, *709,* 724–725, *725, 726*
Saltatory conduction, 166
Sample size, for drug studies, 787
Sarcoidosis, differential diagnosis of, 464, 476t
SCH-37370, 894
Schistosomes, 265
Schultz-Dale reaction, in sensitized canine tracheal muscle, 320, *321,* 330
Scopolamine, 878
Scuba diving, 1133
Season
avoidance and, 528
of birth, and asthma, 27
infections and, 570t
mortality and, 1159
Secondary particles, 578
Sedatives, in status asthmaticus, 1005
Selectins, 259
Selenium, 964
Self-management, 692–693, 1188–1189
of psychiatric aspects, 1125

Sensory mechanisms, circadian rhythm of, nocturnal asthma and, 1032
Sensory nerves, neurogenic inflammation and. *See* Inflammation, neurogenic
Series elastic component, 317
Serology, in occupational asthma, 605
Serotonin. *See* 5-Hydroxytryptamine
experimental asthma and, 391
inhalation challenge with, 504
in experimental animal models, 391
Severe asthma, 13, 684, 684t, 1054–1060
acute. *See* Status asthmaticus
assessment of, 1054–1057
contributing factors and, 1056–1057
establishing diagnosis of asthma and, 1054–1055, *1055*
establishing maximum attainable reversibility and, 1056, *1056*
in children, 1075
management of, 1057–1060
"asthma-sparing" medications in, 1058t, 1058–1059, *1059*
bronchodilators in, 1057–1058
crisis intervention plan and, 1059t, 1059–1060
inhaled corticosteroids in, 1058
patient education in, 1057
use of methotrexate in, 1222
pulsus paradoxus and, 684
treatment of, 694
guidelines for use of methotrexate in, 1222
Severity of asthma, 9–10, 10t, 12–13
changing, mortality and, 1157
evaluation of, 452t, 452–453
mild asthma, 683–684
moderate asthma, 684
severe asthma, 684, 684t
staging therapy to, 683–696
goals and rationale of therapy and, 693, 693t
in mild asthma, 693
in moderate asthma, 693–694
pathobiology of asthma and, 683
pathogenesis of asthma and, 683
self-management and, 692–693
in severe acute asthma, 694–696
in severe asthma, 694
specific therapy and, 685
symptomatic therapy and, 685–692
status asthmaticus, 684–685
Sex
IgE levels and, 28
mortality and, 1154, *1156*
prevalence and incidence of asthma related to, 15–16, 16t
Sexual activity, 1133–1135
Sexual dysfunction, treatment of, 1134–1135, 1135t
SGOT, 997
SGPT, 997
Sheep wool, 553
Sickle cell anemia, 1174
Signal transduction mechanisms
for muscle contraction. *See* Muscle contraction, signal transduction mechanisms for
for muscle relaxation, 210–211
cyclic AMP and, 210–211
cyclic GMP and, 211
Single-photon emission computed tomography, measuring particle retention and, 415
Sinuses. *See* Paranasal sinuses
Sinusitis
diagnosis of, 540–542

clinical presentation and, 540
computed tomography and, *541*, 542
radiographic appearance and, *540*, 540, *541*
transillumination and, 540–541
ultrasonography and, 541
relationship with asthma, 535t, 535–537, 536t
eosinophils and, 536, 536t
inflammatory mediators and, 536t, 536–537
vagal reflex and, 536, *536*
treatment of, 542t, 542–543
Sinus tachycardia, 1045
Sisal dust, occupational asthma and, 597
Skeletal muscle
beta-adrenergic agonist effects on, 714
beta agonists and, 735
SKF-104, 353, 890, 891, 891t
Skin testing, 486–489
atopy and, 17, *18*
clinical interpretation of, 488
comparison of, 507
with concomitant or exclusive bronchial sensitization causes by non–IgE-dependent mechanisms, 528–529
correlation between history and inhalation test results in allergic asthma and, 517–529
with concomitant or exclusive bronchial sensitization cause by non–IgE-dependent mechanisms, 528–529
early asthmatic responses and, 523–526, 524t
general characteristics of tests and, 522–523
IgE mediated reactions and, 517–522
immunotherapy and, 526t, 526–527, *527*, 527t
late asthmatic reaction and, 528
outgrowing asthma and, 528
seasonal exposure to pollen and avoidance and, 528
correlation of results with clinical history and allergen inhalation test results, 523–526
early asthmatic responses and, 523–526, 524t
in food allergy, 561
grading of results of, 488
negative results and, 523
in occupational asthma, 605
positive results and, 523
preparation of extracts for, 488
procedure for, 486–488
allergen selection and, 486
for epicutaneous test, 487
for intracutaneous test, 487–488
patient preparation and, 486–487
specificity in, 489, 522–523
substitutes for, 507
Sleep
nocturnal asthma and, 226, 341, 1169
ventilatory response to hypoxemia during, 350, 350t
Sleep apnea, 1057
Slowly cycling cross-bridges, *316*, 316–317, *317*
Small airway disease, differential diagnosis of, 472
Smog, 578. *See also* Air pollution
Smoke inhalation, 471
Smoking, 5
active, 19–20, 20t
atopy and, 17–18
IgE levels and, 28

bronchial responsiveness and, 20
childhood asthma and, 1065
occupational asthma and, 586–587
passive, 20–21
theophylline and, 772t, 773
tobacco smoke as incitant and, 445, 581
Smooth muscle, of airway. *See* Airway smooth muscle; Muscle contraction; Muscle relaxation
Smuts, 552t
Sobrerol, 930
Socioeconomic factors. *See also* Economic factors, childhood asthma and, 1065
Sodium, 964, 1147
Sodium bicarbonate
mucokinetic effect of, 925
ventilator therapy and, 1006, 1173
Sodium cromolyn. *See* Cromolyn sodium
Sodium iodide, mucolytic effect of, 927
Sol phase, constituents of, 361
Somatic hypermutation, 425
Somatostatin, 246
Spa(s), *1146*, 1146t, 1146–1147
Spacers
aerosol corticosteroids and, 828–830, *831*, 831t
metered-dose inhalers and, 409, 752, 752t
Specific responses, 55
Spices, as expectorants, 927, 1114
Sphenoethmoidectomy, 536
Spiramycin, asthma induced by, 626
Spirometry, 333–334, *335*, *336*, 450
in occupational asthma, 604
during pregnancy, 1087
severity of asthma and, 13
Spondylocladium, 1210–1211
Sporobolomyces, 1210–1211
Sports, educational materials on, 1213
Sputum, 655–662
analysis of, 451
cytologic and microscopic examination technique and, 1223
exfoliative cytology and particulates and, 655–658
in status asthmaticus, *997*, 997–998
in aspiration, 661–662
fatty substances in, 661–662
meat fibers in, 662
milk in, 662, 662t
starch in, 661
chemical composition of, 659t, 659–661, 661t
cilia and, 661
ciliocytophoria and, 662
exfoliative cytology and particulates in, 655–658
bronchial epithelial cells and, 656–657, 657t
Charcot-Leyden crystals and, 657–658
Creola bodies and, 656–657
Curschmann's spirals and, 658
eosinophils and, 657
histiocytes and, 658
mast cells and, 658
methodology for, 655–656
gross appearance of, 655, *656*
immunoglobulins in, 660
mobilization of, in status asthmaticus, 1003–1004
physical properties of, 658t, 658–659
Stable asthma
anticholinergic agents in, 879–880, *880*
cardiac rhythm in, 1046, 1048
bronchodilators and, 1046, 1047t, 1048
Starch, in sputum, in aspiration, 661

Status asthmaticus, 684–685, 985–1009, 986t.
    See also Childhood asthma
  acid-base abnormalities in, 340, *341*
  anticholinergic agents in, 880–881
  arterial blood gases in, 685, *685*
  beta-adrenergic agonists in, 737–738
  bronchial mucus in, 364
  cardiac rhythm in, 1048
  chemistry in, 997
  clinical considerations in, 994–996
  corticosteroids in, 809–811, *810, 811*
  electrocardiography in, 996
  eosinophilia and, 996–997
  epidemiology and mortality and, 988–989
  guidelines for use of intravenous
      terbutaline in, 1221
  inciting factors for, 986
  mechanisms for drug refractoriness of,
      987t, 987–988
  pathology and, 988, *988*
  prevention and after-crisis care and,
      1008–1009
  radiography in, 996
  risk factors for, 989t, 989–994
    airway dynamics and lung volumes as,
        990–991
    gas exchange and, 992, *993–995*, 994,
        994t
    physiologic abnormalities as, 990
    pre-status asthmaticus and, 989–990,
        990t
    pulmonary circulation and, 991
    work of breathing and, 991–992
  sputum analysis in, *997*, 997–998
  treatment of, 694–696, 998–1008, 1000t,
      1009t
    acid-base and electrolyte considerations
        in, 1004, *1004*, 1004t
    airway and, 1005
    anticholinergics in, 695
    antimicrobial agents in, 1003
    beta-adrenoceptor stimulators in. *See*
        Beta-adrenoceptor stimulators, in
        acute severe asthma
    beta₂-agonists in, 694–695
    bronchodilators in, 998–999, 1001–1002
    complications of, 1007
    corticosteroids in, 695, 1002–1003
    hospital management and, *695*, 695–696,
        696
    hydration and sputum mobilization in,
        1003–1004
    intravenous theophylline in, 695
    ipratropium bromide in, 1001
    mechanical ventilation in, 1005–1008,
        1006, 1006t–1008t, *1009*, 1172
    methylxanthines in, 1001
    oral versus aerosol steroids in, 836
    oxygen in, 998
    sedatives in, 1005
    site of treatment and, 694
    supportive care and, 694
    sympathomimetics in, 999t, 999–1001,
        1000t
Stemphylium, 1210–1211
Steroids. *See* Corticosteroids;
    Glucocorticoid(s)
Stimulus-secretion coupling, 169
Streptomyces, 1210–1211
Subacute asthma, corticosteroids in, 811
Substance P, 238
  airway secretion and, 239–240
  airway smooth muscle and, 239
  control of mucus production and, 366,
      371–372
  effects on inflammatory cells, 240–241

  localization of, 238
  neural effects of, 241
  receptors for, 238
  vascular effects of, 240
Sulfisoxazole, in sinusitis, 542t
Sulfites, 560, 560t
Sulfur dioxide, 578
  respiratory effects of, 578–580, *579, 580*
Sulfur oxide-particulate complex, 578
Summer camps, 1217–1219
Superoxide anion, 960–964
Superoxide dismutase, mast cell, 275, 960
Supine posture, nocturnal asthma and,
    1030–1031
Support groups, 1212
Suppressive factor of allergy, downregulation
    of IgE biosynthesis and, 63
Suppressor/cytotoxic T-cell(s), 55
Surface markers, 52, 52t
Surfactants, 925
Surgery. *See also* Anesthesia; Preanesthetic
    management
  perioperative monitoring and, 1103, 1103t,
      1104
  postoperative management and,
      1107–1109, 1108t, *1109, 1110*, 1110t
  preoperative assessment and. *See also*
      Preanesthetic management
  as treatment approach, 1148–1149
Sweat test, in cystic fibrosis, 471
Sympathomimetics, 686–688, *687*, 687t, *688*
  in exercise-induced asthma, 618
  intravenous, 712, 715, 720, 722, 729,
      756–761, *757, 758*
    in acute severe asthma, 759–761, *761*
    in children, 1078
    combination with anticholinergic agents,
        759
    combination with corticosteroids, 759
    combination with theophylline, 759
    distribution of, 756
    isoproterenol, 759
    pharmacokinetics of, 756, 757t
    salbutamol, 760
    side effects of, 756–757
    terbutaline, 760
    tolerance to, 758–759
  mucokinetic effect of, 923
  routes of administration of, 757
  in status asthmaticus, 999t, 999–1001,
      1000t
Symptomatic patients
  diagnosis of, 451–452
  management of, 693–696
Synapse, 166
Systemic mastocytosis, differential diagnosis
    of, 478t

Tachykinin(s), 238–241
  airway secretion and, 239–240
  airway smooth muscle and, 239
  inflammatory cells and, 240–241
  interactions with epithelium, 239, *240*
  localization of, 238
  metabolism of, 239
  neural effects of, 241
  in occupational asthma, 588
  receptors for, *238*, 238–239
  role in asthma, 246
  vascular effects of, 240
Tachykinin receptors, smooth muscle
    contraction and, 209
Tachyphylaxis
  adenosine-induced bronchoconstriction
      and, 256
  beta-adrenergic, 737

  of beta₂-adrenergic receptors, 194–195, *195*
  to beta-agonists, 703–704, 704t, 737, 879,
      1157–1158
  histamine, 328
Target cells, 50
  effects of inflammation on, 87–89
Tartrazine, aspirin-induced asthma and, 622
Tartrazine challenge, 562
T-cell(s)
  allergens and, 45–46
  B-cell interactions of, 54–55
  bronchial hyperresponsiveness and,
      429–431, 431t
  as critical cell of bronchial inflammation,
      429, 430t
  as effector cells of delayed-type
      hypersensitivity reaction, 431
  helper, IgE biosynthesis and, 61, 61t
  helper/inducer, 55
  IgE synthesis and, 69–70
  immunoregulation and, 147, 150–151, *151*
  as inflammatory cells, 84, *85*
  interaction with IgE, 59
  late asthmatic reactions and, 140
  macrophage interactions with, 54
  recognition of foreignness and, 51
  suppressor/cytotoxic, 55
  surface markers, 150
  T-cell interactions of, 54, *55*
T-cell receptors, 53, *53*
Temperature, mechanical heterogeneity of
    airway smooth muscle and, 320
Temporal course, 10
Terbutaline, 687t, *688*, 722–723
  in acute severe asthma, 760–761
  aerosol, 719t
  inhaled, 729
  intravenous, 761
    guidelines for use of, 1221
  oral, 721t
  subcutaneous, 730, 730t, 731
    pharmacokinetics of, 715, *715*
Terbutaline sulfate, 1228
Terfenadine, 97, 865, 884
  adenosine-induced bronchoconstriction
      and, 254, *254*
  in exercise-induced asthma, 618
Terminal button, 166
Terpin hydrate, 929
Tetracoccosporium, 1210–1211
Tetracosactrin, in status asthmaticus, 810,
    810, 811, 1002
Theophylline, 198–199, *199*, 199t, 689t,
    689–690, *690*, 764–779, 1229, 1230,
    1231, 1232, 1233
  in acute asthma, 978
  in acute severe asthma, beta-
      adrenoreceptor stimulants combined
      with, 759
  adenosine-induced bronchoconstriction
      and, 254
  biopharmaceutics of, 773–776, *774, 775*,
      775t
  bronchial provocation tests and, 510
  chemistry of, 764, *765*
  in childhood asthma, 1070t, 1070–1071
    acute, 1077, 1077t
  clinical usage of, 776–778
    dosage for acute bronchodilation and,
        776, *777*
    dosage for maintenance therapy and,
        776–777, *778*, 779
    therapeutic decisions and, 776
  elderly patients and, 1021, 1021t
  interactions with beta agonists, 731–732,
      732, 733

Theophylline (*continued*)
  intravenous, in status asthmaticus, 695
  in late asthmatic reactions, 142
  measurement in serum, 778
  pharmacodynamics of, 765–768
    efficacy and, 765–766, *766–768*
    toxicity and, 766–768, *769*
  pharmacokinetics of, 769–773
    absorption and, 769
    distribution and, 769
    elimination and, 771, *771*, 772t, 773, *773*
    metabolism and excretion and, 769–770, *770*, 770t
  pharmacology of, 764–765, *766*
  phosphodiesterase and, 198
  structure of, *765*
  toxicity of, 766–768, *769*
    cardiac rhythm and, 1048–1049, 1049t
    fatality and, 1158–1159
    iatrogenic causes of, 777–778
    management algorithm for, 1220
    management of poisoning and, 778–779
Theophylline monohydrate, 1229, 1230, 1231
Thermophilic actinomycetes, 633t
Thromboxane(s)
  airway hyperresponsiveness and, 122
  biologic activity of, 121
  in biologic fluids, measurements of, 123
  biosynthesis and metabolism of, 120–121
  late asthmatic reactions and, 141
  receptors for, 121
  urinary metabolites, 123
Thrush, aerosol corticosteroids and, 832
Thymomodulin, 1148
Time constant, 334–335, *336*
Timolol, 623t
Timothy grass pollen, 549
Tissue-damaging responses, 55–56
Tobacco smoke. *See also* Smoking
  as incitant, 445, 581
Tolerance
  to anticholinergic agents, 879
  to beta-adrenoceptor stimulants, 758–759
Toluene diisocyanate, as allergen, 312, 444, 601. *See also* Acid anhydrides
Tomography, measuring particle retention and, 415
Tort remedies, occupational asthma and, 608
Toxin accumulation, nocturnal asthma and, 1030
Transfer factor. *See* Diffusing capacity
Transforming growth factor-beta, immunoregulation and, 152t, 153
Treatment of asthma, 1197t, 1197–1198. *See also specific modalities and types of asthma*
  drug development for. *See* Drug development
  effect on airway epithelial structure, 302, *303*
  inappropriate. *See* Inappropriate/unusual treatment
  staging to severity. *See* Severity of asthma, staging therapy to
  unresolved issues, 1197–1198
Trees, wind-pollinating, 548–549
Triamcinolone acetonide, 1229
  aerosol, 821t
  in chronic asthma, 812
Trichoderma, 1210–1211
Trimethoprim-sulfamethoxazole regimen, in sinusitis, 542t
Troleandomycin, 692, 901–908
  clinical studies of, 901–903, 902t
  drug interactions of, 903t–905t, 903–905, *904, 905*

mechanisms of action of, 907t, 907–908
  practical guidelines for therapy with, 905–907, 906t
  steroid sparing action of, 902–903
  structure and pharmacology of, 901, *902*
Tropical eosinophilia, differential diagnosis of, 473t, 474, 478t
Tryptase, 82, 275
  assays for, 494
  mast cell, 275
Tuberculosis
  endobrachial, differential diagnosis of, 467–468, 641
  endotracheal, differential diagnosis of, 476t
Tumor, 80
Tumorgenicity, of beta agonists, 736
Tumor necrosis factor-alpha, immunoregulation and, 152t, 153
Twins and atopy, 29

Ultrasonic nebulizers, 409
Ultrasonography, in sinusitis, 541
Unresolved issues, 1194–1198, 1198t
Unusual treatment. *See* Inappropriate/unusual treatment
Upper respiratory tract diseases, 533–543
  causing or associated with asthma, 533–543
    allergic rhinitis and, 537
    chronic rhinitis of non–IgE-associated asthma and, 538, 538t
    filter function failure of nose and, 533
    heat and humidification failure and, 533
    increased lower airway responsiveness during upper respiratory tract infections and, 534
    increased lower airway responsiveness in nasal diseases and, 534
    nasal polyps and, 538–539
    nasal sinus-bronchial reflex and, 534–535, 535t
    nonallergic rhinitis with eosinophilia syndrome and, 538
    relationship of sinusitis and asthma and, 535t, 535–537, *536*, 536t
    sinuses and, 539–540, *540, 541*, 542t
    treatment of nasal symptoms and, 533–534
    vasomotor rhinitis and, 537–538
  infectious, increased lower airway reactivity during, 534
  simulating bronchial asthma, 533, 534t
Upregulation
  heterologous, 176
  immunoglobulin E and, molecules involved in, 61–62
Uptake of catecholamines, 170
Urinary LTE₄, 119, 126, 494, 890
Urticaria pigmentosa, mast cells and, 280

Vagal fibers
  central output and, 225–226, *226*
  cough and, 645
  peripheral output and, 226–227
Vagal reflexes
  in airways, anticholinergic agents and, 876–877, *877*
  in aspiration, 1025
  in cough, 645
  mucokinetic, 928
  sinusitis and asthma and, 536, *536*
Variant asthma, differential diagnosis of, 475t
Varicella infection, methotrexate and, 912
Vascular endothelial cells, corticosteroid effects on, 804

Vascular permeability, platelet-activating factor and, 290
Vascular responses, 88
Vascular smooth muscle, beta agonists and, 736
Vasculature. *See also* Cardiovascular disease; Cardiovascular system
  in airway epithelium, 296, *297*
  effect of neuropeptide Y on, 245
  effects of vasoactive intestinal peptide on, 235–236, *236*
  status asthmaticus and, 991
  tachykinin effects on, 240
Vasoactive intestinal peptide, 234–237
  abnormalities of, 237
  airway secretion and, 235
  airway smooth muscle and, 235
  antiinflammatory actions of, 236
  cholinergic transmission and, 218
  control of mucus production and, 366
  cotransmission with acetylcholine, 236–237, *237*
  as inhibitory nonadrenergic, noncholinergic transmitter, 236
  localization of, 234–235
  neuromodulatory effects of, 236
  nonadrenergic, noncholinergic nerves and, 232–233
  occupational asthma and, 588
  peptides related to, 237–238
  receptors for, 211, 235
    muscle relaxation and, 212
  role in asthma, 246
  vascular effects of, 235–236, *236*
Vasoconstrictive rhinitis, 537–538
Vasodilation, in inflammation, 88
Vasomotor instability, 537–538
Vasomotor rhinitis, 537–538
Vegetable substances, and asthma, 600t
Ventilation
  collateral, 335
  distribution of, 334–335, *336*
  elderly patients and. *See* Elderly patients, ventilation and
  mechanical, in status asthmaticus, 1005–1008, *1006*, 1006t–1008t, *1009*
  during pregnancy, *1087*, 1087–1088
  strategy for, in childhood asthma, acute, 1078–1079
Ventilation-perfusion relationships
  antigen challenge in experimental asthma and, 384–385, *385*
  gas exchange and, 338–339, *339*
  improved, intermittent positive pressure breathing and, 1115
Ventilation-perfusion scans, 674, *676–678*
  in pulmonary embolism, 462, *462*
Ventilatory control, 346–350, *347*
  chemical stimuli to breathing in asthma and, *348*, 348–349
  measurement of ventilatory drives and, 346–348, *347*
  mechanical stimuli to breathing in asthma and, 349, *349*
  recognition of worsening asthma, altered blood gas tension, or loaded breathing and, 350, 350t
Ventilatory drive, measurement of, 346–348, *347*
Verapamil, 692, 952–957
Verticillium, 1210–1211
Viral allergens, 553, 555
Viral infections. *See also* Infections
  acute exacerbations of asthma and, corticosteroids in, 573

airway hyperreactivity in experimental
  asthma and, 396, *396*
  in humans, 570
bronchospasm induced by,
  pathophysiology of, 566–568, *567*
IgE levels and, 28
immune response alterations and, 568–569
in infant and young child, 571
of lower respiratory tract, structural
  changes in airway epithelium and
  bronchial hyperresponsiveness and,
  298, 300
methotrexate and, 912
pneumonia, 571
in older child and adult, 572–573
Viscosity, of sputum, 374

Vital signs, drug studies and, 795
Vitamin E, 964
Volume changes of lungs. *See* Lung
  volume(s)

Warming masks, 583
Water. *See* Humidification; Hydration
Weather, 21, 449, 581. *See also* Climate
WEB-2086, 292, 894
WEB-2170, 292
Weed, 549
Wheezing, 447, 449, 650–654
  acoustic characteristics of, 650, *651*
  airflow obstruction and, 652–653
  clinical associations of, 652
  future implications of, 653–654

graphic display of, 650, *652–654*
  mechanism of production of, 650–652, *654*
Whole-cell patch-clamp method, mast cell
  secretion and, 277
Wood dust, 444
  as allergen, 444
Workers' compensation, occupational asthma
  and, 608

Xanthines. *See* Methylxanthines; *specific
  drugs*
X-ray. *See* Radiography

Yeasts, 1210–1211

Zygomycetes, 552t